西医经典名著集成

菲兹帕里克皮肤病学

FITZPATRICK'S DERMATOLOGY

9TH EDITION

VOLUME 1

Sewon Kang
Masayuki Amagai
Anna L. Bruckner
Alexander H. Enk
David J. Margolis
Amy J. McMichael
Jeffrey S. Orringer

第9版（双语版）

编译委员会主任委员　陈翔　粟娟

上册

McGraw Hill

湖南科学技术出版社

《西医经典名著集成》丛书编译委员会

主 任 委 员 詹启敏

副主任委员（按姓氏笔画排序）

王天有　刘玉村　陈　翔　陈孝平　周宏灏

委　　　员（按姓氏笔画排序）

王晰程　文飞球　付向宁　冯杰雄　刘　钢
李　锋　张小田　张志伟　邱海波　陈明亮
罗小平　赵　爽　施　为　姜玉武　徐崇锐
殷文瑾　郭　莹　曹　杉　彭名菁　粟　娟
舒　焱　雷　霆　燕　翔

秘　　　书 彭文忠

菲兹帕里克皮肤病学
第9版（双语版）
编译委员会

主任委员	陈　翔	中南大学湘雅医院
	粟　娟	中南大学湘雅医院
副主任委员	陈明亮	中南大学湘雅医院
	施　为	中南大学湘雅医院
	赵　爽	中南大学湘雅医院
委　员	（按姓氏拼音排名）	
	黄莹雪	中南大学湘雅医院
	简　丹	中南大学湘雅医院
	李　吉	中南大学湘雅医院
	李　捷	中南大学湘雅医院
	李芳芳	中南大学湘雅医院
	刘芳芬	中南大学湘雅医院
	汪　犇	中南大学湘雅医院
	易　梅	中南大学湘雅医院
	张江林	中南大学湘雅医院
	朱　武	中南大学湘雅医院

图书在版编目（CIP）数据

菲兹帕里克皮肤病学：第9版：双语版：汉、英文. 上册 /[美] 康斯文（Sewon Kang）等主编；陈翔，粟娟等编译.—长沙：湖南科学技术出版社，2020.10
（西医经典名著集成）
ISBN 978-7-5710-0760-7

Ⅰ. ①菲… Ⅱ. ①康… ②陈… ③粟…Ⅲ. ①皮肤病学－汉、英文 Ⅳ. ①R751

中国版本图书馆 CIP 数据核字(2020)第 189071 号

Sewon Kang, Masayuki Amagai, Anna L. Brucker, Alexander H. Enk, David J. Margolis, Amy J. McMichael, Jeffrey S. Orringer
Fitzpatrick's Dermatology, Ninth Edition, 2-Volume Set
ISBN9780071837795
Copyright ©2019 by McGraw-Hill Education.

All Rights reserved. No part of this publication may be reproduced or transmitted in any form or by any means, electronic or mechanical, including without limitation photocopying, recording, taping, or any database, information or retrieval system, without the prior written permission of the publisher.

This authorized Bilingual edition is jointly published by McGraw-Hill Education and Hunan Science & Technology Press. This edition is authorized for sale in the People's Republic of China only, excluding Hong Kong, Macao SAR and Taiwan.

Translation Copyright © 2020 by McGraw-Hill Education and Hunan Science & Technology Press.

版权所有。未经出版人事先书面许可，对本出版物的任何部分不得以任何方式或途径复制或传播，包括但不限于复印、录制、录音，或通过任何数据库、信息或可检索的系统。

本授权双语版由麦格劳-希尔教育出版公司和湖南科学技术出版社合作出版。此版本经授权仅限在中华人民共和国境内（不包括香港特别行政区、澳门特别行政区和台湾省）销售。

翻译版权©2020 由麦格劳-希尔教育出版公司与湖南科学技术出版社所有。

本书封面贴有 McGraw-Hill Education 公司防伪标签，无标签者不得销售。
著作权合同登记号 18-2020-188

西医经典名著集成
FEIZIPALIKE PIFUBINGXUE

菲兹帕里克皮肤病学　第 9 版（双语版）上册

主　　编：	[美]康斯文（Sewon Kang），[日]天谷正之（Masayuki Amagai），[美]安娜 L. 布鲁克纳（Anna L. Brucker），[德]亚历山大 H. 恩（Alexander H. Enk），[美]大卫 J. 马戈利斯（David J. Margolis），[美]艾美 J. 麦克迈克尔（Amy J. McMichael），[美]杰弗里 S. 奥林格（Jeffrey S. Orringer）
编 译 者：	陈翔，粟娟等
责任编辑：	李　忠　杨　颖
出版发行：	湖南科学技术出版社
社　　址：	长沙市湘雅路 276 号
	http://www.hnstp.com
印　　刷：	湖南凌宇纸品有限公司
厂　　址：	长沙市长沙县黄花镇黄花工业园
邮　　编：	410137
版　　次：	2020 年 10 月第 1 版
印　　次：	2020 年 10 月第 1 次印刷
开　　本：	787mm×1092mm　1/16
印　　张：	88.25
字　　数：	4590 千字
书　　号：	ISBN 978-7-5710-0760-7
定　　价：	1050.00 元（上、中、下册）

（版权所有　·　翻印必究）

Fitzpatrick's Dermatology
Ninth Edition

EDITORS

SEWON KANG, MD, MPH

MASAYUKI AMAGAI, MD, PhD

ANNA L. BRUCKNER, MD, MSCS

ALEXANDER H. ENK, MD

DAVID J. MARGOLIS, MD, PhD

AMY J. McMICHAEL, MD

JEFFREY S. ORRINGER, MD

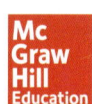

New York   Chicago   San Francisco   Athens   London   Madrid   Mexico City
Milan   New Delhi   Singapore   Sydney   Toronto

SEWON KANG, MD, MPH
Noxell Professor and Chair
Department of Dermatology
Johns Hopkins School of Medicine
Dermatologist-in-Chief
Johns Hopkins Hospital
Baltimore, Maryland

MASAYUKI AMAGAI, MD, PhD
Professor and Chair
Department of Dermatology
Keio University School of Medicine
Tokyo, Japan

ANNA L. BRUCKNER, MD, MSCS
Associate Professor of Dermatology and Pediatrics
University of Colorado School of Medicine
Section Head, Pediatric Dermatology
Children's Hospital Colorado
Aurora, Colorado

ALEXANDER H. ENK, MD
Professor and Chair
Department of Dermatology
University of Heidelberg
Heidelberg, Germany

DAVID J. MARGOLIS, MD, PhD
Professor of Dermatology and Epidemiology
Department of Dermatology
Department of Biostatistics and Epidemiology
University of Pennsylvania Perelman School of Medicine
Philadelphia, Pennsylvania

AMY J. McMICHAEL, MD
Professor and Chair
Department of Dermatology
Wake Forest University School of Medicine
Winston-Salem, North Carolina

JEFFREY S. ORRINGER, MD
Professor and Chief
Division of Cosmetic Dermatology
Department of Dermatology
University of Michigan
Ann Arbor, Michigan

CONTRIBUTORS

Sumaira Z. Aasi, MD
Clinical Professor, Dermatology, Clinical Professor (By Courtesy), Surgery–Plastic and Reconstructive Surgery, Dermatology–North Campus, Stanford University, Redwood City, California [201]

George Agak, PhD
Research Scientist, Dermatology/Medicine, David Geffen School of Medicine at UCLA, Los Angeles, California [78]

Christine S. Ahn, MD
Resident Physician, Wake Forest School of Medicine, Winston Salem, North Carolina [46]

Iris Ahronowitz, MD
Assistant Professor of Clinical Dermatology, Keck School of Medicine, University of Southern California, Los Angeles, California [161]

Murad Alam, MD, MSCI, MBA
Professor of Dermatology, Otolaryngology, and Surgery, Vice-Chair, Department of Dermatology, Chief, Section of Cutaneous and Aesthetic Surgery, Director, Micrographic Surgery and Dermatologic Oncology Fellowship, Northwestern University, Chicago, Illinois [211]

Afsaneh Alavi, MSc, MD, FRCPC
Assistant Professor of Dermatology, Women's College Hospital, University of Toronto, Toronto, Ontario, Canada [149]

Theodore J. Alkousakis, MD
Assistant Clinical Professor, University of Colorado School of Medicine, Medical Director, Adult Dermatology, Aurora, Colorado [140]

Tina S. Alster, MD
Director, Washington Institute of Dermatologic Laser Surgery, Clinical Professor of Dermatology, Georgetown University Medical Center, Washington, DC [209]

Masayuki Amagai, MD, PhD
Professor and Chair, Department of Dermatology, Keio University School of Medicine, Tokyo, Japan [14]

Erin H. Amerson, MD
Associate Professor, University of California, San Francisco, Department of Dermatology, San Francisco, California [1]

Karl E. Anderson, MD, FACP
Departments of Preventive Medicine and Community Health, and Internal Medicine (Division of Gastroenterology and Hepatology), University of Texas Medical Branch, Galveston, Texas [124]

Grant J. Anhalt, MD
Professor of Dermatology and Pathology, Department of Dermatology, Johns Hopkins Hospital, Baltimore, Maryland [53]

Jack L. Arbiser, MD, PhD
Emory University School of Medicine, Department of Dermatology, Atlanta Veterans Affairs Medical Center, Atlanta, Georgia [195]

Roberto Arenas, MD
Mycology Section, Dr. Manuel Gea Gonzalez General Hospital, Mexico City, Mexico [158]

Adam B. Aronson, MD
Resident Physician, Dermatology, University of Iowa Carver College of Medicine, Iowa City, Iowa [128]

Iris K. Aronson, MD
University of Illinois at Chicago, Chicago, Illinois [73]

Arif Aslam, MBChB, MRCP (UK), MRCGP, MRCP (Dermatology)
Consultant Dermatologist and Mohs Surgeon, St Helens and Knowsley Teachings Hospitals NHS Trust, St Helens, United Kingdom [201]

Edwin J. Asturias, MD
The Jules Amer Chair in Community Pediatrics, Children's Hospital Colorado, Associate Professor of Pediatrics and Epidemiology, Division of Pediatric Infectious Diseases, University of Colorado School of Medicine, Center for Global Health, Colorado School of Public Health, Aurora, Colorado [169]

Martine Bagot, MD, PhD
Department of Dermatology, Hôpital Saint-Louis, Paris, France [119, 120]

Fanny Ballieux, MD
Resident, Center for Vascular Anomalies, Division of Plastic Surgery, Cliniques Universitaires St Luc and University of Louvain, Brussels, Belgium [147]

Robert Baran, MD
Honorary Professor, Nail Disease Center, Cannes, France [205]

Raymond L. Barnhill, MD
Professor, Department of Pathology, Institut Curie, and University of Paris Descartes Faculty of Medicine, Paris, France, Department of Pathology, Paris, France [71]

Leslie Baumann, MD
Board Certified Dermatologist, Baumann Cosmetic and Research Institute, Miami, Florida [207]

J. David Beckham, MD
Associate Professor, Director of the Infectious Disease Fellowship Training Program, Division of Adult Infectious Diseases, University of Colorado School of Medicine, Denver, Colorado [169]

Carola Berking, MD
Department of Dermatology, University Hospital Munich, Ludwig-Maximilian University (LMU), Munich, Germany [110]

Christopher Bichakjian, MD
Department of Dermatology, University of Michigan Health System, Ann Arbor, Michigan [202]

Carol M. Black, MD, FRCP
Centre for Rheumatology and Connective Tissue Diseases, UCL Medical School, Royal Free Hospital, London, United Kingdom [63]

Ulrike Blume-Peytavi, MD
Department of Dermatology and Allergy, Charité-Universitätsmedizin, Berlin, Germany [85]

Mark Boguniewicz, MD
Professor, Division of Allergy and Immunology, Department of Pediatrics, National Jewish Health and University of Colorado School of Medicine, Denver, Colorado [22]

Michael Y. Bonner, BA
Emory University School of Medicine, Department of Dermatology, Atlanta, Georgia [195]

Laurence M. Boon, MD, PhD
Coordinator of the Center for vascular Anomalies, Division of Plastic Surgery, Cliniques Universitaires St Luc and Human Molecular Genetics, de Duve Institute, University of Louvain, Brussels, Belgium [147]

Vladimir Botchkarev, MD, PhD, FRSB
Professor and Deputy Director, Centre for Skin Sciences, University of Bradford, United Kingdom, Adjunct Professor, Department of Dermatology, Boston University School of Medicine, Boston, Massachusetts [7]

Francisco G. Bravo, MD
Associate Professor of Dermatology and Pathology, Universidad Peruana Cayetano Heredia, Lima, Peru [158, 171]

Thomas Brenn, MD, PhD
Consultant Dermatopathologist and Honorary Senior Lecturer, Department of Pathology NHS Lothian University Hospitals Trust and the University of Edinburgh, Edinburgh, United Kingdom [122]

Norbert H. Brockmeyer
Walk In Ruhr (WIR) Center for Sexual Health and Medicine, Department of Dermatology, Venerology and Allergology, Ruhr-Universität Bochum, Bochum, Germany [172, 173]

Anna L. Bruckner, MD, MSCS
Associate Professor of Dermatology and Pediatrics, University of Colorado School of Medicine, Section Head, Pediatric Dermatology, Children's Hospital Colorado, Aurora, Colorado [49]

Leena Bruckner-Tuderman, MD, PhD
Professor and Chair of Dermatology, Medical Center-University of Freiburg, Freiburg, Germany [15]

Marie-Charlotte Brüggen, MD, PhD
Department of Dermatology, University Hospital Zurich, Zurich, Switzerland [10]

Jörg Buddenkotte, MD, PhD
Academic Research Scientist, Department of Dermatology and Venereology, Hamad Medical Corporation, Doha, Qatar [79]

Susan Burgin, MD
Assistant Professor, Beth Israel Deaconness Medical Center, Harvard Medical School, Department of Dermatology, Boston, Massachusetts [1]

Craig G. Burkhart, MD
Sylvania, Ohio [178]

Craig N. Burkhart, MD
The University of North Carolina at Chapel Hill, Chapel Hill, North Carolina [178]

Klaus J. Busam, MD
Professor of Pathology and Laboratory Medicine, Weill Medical College of Cornell University, Department of Dermatopathology and Pathology, Memorial Sloan Kettering Cancer Center, New York, New York [115]

Jeffrey Callen, MD
Professor of Medicine (Dermatology), University of Louisville, Chief, Division of Dermatology, Louisville, Kentucky [192]

Avrom Caplan, MD
Department of Dermatology, Hospital of the University of Pennsylvania, Philadelphia, Pennsylvania [184]

Michael A. Cardis, MD
Department of Dermatology, Washington Hospital Center/Georgetown University, Washington, DC [156]

Arival Cardoso de Brito, MD, PhD
Full Professor, Dermatology, Pará Federal University, Belém, Pará, Brazil [159]

Leslie Castelo-Soccio, MD, PhD
Assistant Professor of Pediatrics and Dermatology, The Children's Hospital of Philadelphia and University of Pennsylvania Perlman School of Medicine, Philadelphia, Pennsylvania [89]

Kelly B. Cha, MD, PhD
Department of Dermatology, University of Michigan Health System, Ann Arbor, Michigan [202]

Manasmon Chairatchaneeboon, MD
Clinical Instructor in Dermatology, Department of Dermatology, Faculty of Medicine Siriraj Hospital, Mahidol University, Bangkok, Thailand [134]

Mary Wu Chang, MD
Clinical Professor of Dermatology and Pediatrics, University of Connecticut School of Medicine, Farmington, Connecticut [103, 104]

Joel Charrow, MD
Professor of Pediatrics, Feinberg School of Medicine, Northwestern University, Ann and Robert H. Lurie Children's Hospital of Chicago, Division of Genetics, Birth Defects and Metabolism, Chicago, Illinois [135]

Mei Chen, PhD
Director, USC Laboratories for Investigative Dermatology, The Keck School of Medicine, University of Southern California, Los Angeles, California [56]

Suephy C. Chen, MD, MS
Vice Chair and Associate Professor of Dermatology, Emory University School of Medicine, Atlanta, Georgia [107]

Carol Cheng, MD
Assistant Clinical Professor of Dermatology/Medicine, David Geffen School of Medicine at UCLA, Los Angeles, California [78]

Andy Chern, MD, MPH
Captain, Medical Corps, United States Army, Associate Program Director, Occupational and Environmental Medicine Residency Program, Uniformed Services University of the Health Sciences, F. Edward Hébert School of Medicine, Department of Preventive Medicine and Biostatistics, Bethesda, Maryland [27]

Casey M. Chern, MD
Captain, Medical Corps, United States Army, Dermatology Resident, National Capital Consortium Dermatology Residency Program, Walter Reed National Military Medical Center, Bethesda, Maryland [27]

Anna L. Chien, MD
Assistant Professor, Department of Dermatology, Johns Hopkins School of Medicine, Baltimore, Maryland [106, 185]

Keith A. Choate, MD, PhD
Professor of Dermatology, Genetics and Pathology, Yale University School of Medicine, New Haven, Connecticut [47]

Conroy Chow, MD
Assistant Professor, Department of Dermatology, Loma Linda University, Loma Linda, California [114]

Luisa Christensen, MD
Center for Medical Mycology, University Hospitals Cleveland Medical Center, Case Western Reserve University, Cleveland, Ohio [188]

Sean R. Christensen, MD, PhD
Assistant Professor of Dermatology, Section of Dermatologic Surgery, Yale University School of Medicine, New Haven, Connecticut [204]

Angela M. Christiano, PhD
Department of Dermatology, Department of Genetics and Development, Columbia University, New York, New York [18]

Emily Y. Chu, MD, PhD
Assistant Professor of Dermatology, Hospital of the University of Pennsylvania, Perelman School of Medicine, Philadelphia, Pennsylvania [2]

Jin Ho Chung, MD, PhD
Professor and Chairman, Department of Dermatology, Seoul National University College of Medicine, Seoul, Korea [197]

Matthew Clark, MD
Dermatology Resident, University of Michigan Department of Dermatology, Ann Arbor, Michigan [31]

Roger Clark, DO
Assistant Professor of Medicine, Tufts Medical Center, Brigham and Women's Faulkner Hospital, Boston, Massachusetts [179]

Olivier Cogrel, MD
Dermatologic Surgery and Laser Unit, Dermatology Department, CHU Bordeaux, Hôpital Saint-André, Bordeaux, France [205]

Bernard A. Cohen, MD
Johns Hopkins Hospital Baltimore, Maryland [178]

Jeffrey I. Cohen, MD
Chief, Laboratory of Infectious Diseases, National Institute of Allergy and Infectious Diseases, National Institutes of Health, Bethesda, Maryland [164]

Philip R. Cohen, MD
Professor of Dermatology, University of California San Diego School of Medicine, San Diego, California [36]

Sean C. Condon, MD
Department of Dermatology, Cleveland Clinic, Cleveland, Ohio [186]

Melissa I. Costner, MD
Associate Clinical Professor, Dermatology, UT Southwestern Medical School, North Dallas Dermatology Associates, Dallas, Texas [61]

George Cotsarelis, MD
Milton B. Hartzell Professor and Chair, Department of Dermatology, Perelman School of Medicine University of Pennsylvania, Director, Program on Epithelial Regeneration and Stem Cells, University of Pennsylvania Institute for Regenerative Medicine, Philadelphia, Pennsylvania [7]

Edward W. Cowen, MD
Head, Dermatology Consultation Service, Dermatology Branch, Center for Cancer Research, National Cancer Institute, National Institutes of Health, Bethesda, Maryland [129]

Lauren N. Craddock, MD
Department of Dermatology, University of Wisconsin-Madison, Madison, Wisconsin [160]

Ponciano D. Cruz, Jr., MD
Distinguished Professor, Paul Bergstresser Endowed Chair in Dermatology, Department of Dermatology, The University of Texas, Chief of Dermatology, North Texas Veterans Affairs Medical Center, Dallas, Texas [24]

Jonathan D. Cuda, MD
Assistant Professor of Dermatology, Johns Hopkins School of Medicine, Baltimore, Maryland [108, 115]

Donna A. Culton, MD, PhD
Department of Dermatology, University of North Carolina at Chapel Hill, Chapel Hill, North Carolina [54]

Nika Cyrus, MD
Department of Dermatology, Parkland Health and Hospital System, Dallas, Texas [64]

Adilson da Costa, MD
Emory University School of Medicine, Department of Dermatology, Atlanta, Georgia [195]

Jennifer S. Daly, MD
Clinical Chief, Infectious Diseases and Immunology, Professor of Medicine, Microbiology and Physiological Systems, University of Massachusetts Medical School, Worcester, Massachusetts [182]

Thomas N. Darling, MD, PhD
Professor and Chair of Dermatology, Uniformed Services University of the Health Sciences, Bethesda, Maryland [136]

Mark D. P. Davis, MD
Professor of Dermatology, Mayo Clinic College of Medicine, Department of Dermatology, Rochester, Minnesota [144]

Robert S. Dawe, MBChB, MD(Glasg), FRCP(Edin)
Consultant Dermatologist and Honorary Reader in Dermatology, Department of Dermatology and Photobiology Unit, NHS Tayside and University of Dundee, Dundee, Scotland [95]

Roy H. Decker, MD, PhD
Associate Professor, Vice Chair and Director of Clinical Research, Department of Therapeutic Radiology, Yale School of Medicine, New Haven, Connecticut [200]

Christopher P. Denton, PhD, FRCP
Centre for Rheumatology and Connective Tissue Diseases, UCL Medical School, Royal Free Hospital, London, United Kingdom [63]

Garrett T. Desman, MD
Assistant Professor of Pathology and Dermatology, Icahn School of Medicine at Mount Sinai, New York, New York [71]

Luis A. Diaz, MD
Department of Dermatology, University of North Carolina at Chapel Hill, Chapel Hill, North Carolina [54]

John J. DiGiovanna, MD
Senior Research Physician, DNA Repair Section, Dermatology Branch, Center for Cancer Research, National Cancer Institute, National Institutes of Health, Bethesda, Maryland [130]

Andrzej A. Dlugosz, MD
Poth Professor of Cutaneous Oncology, Departments of Dermatology and Cell and Developmental Biology, University of Michigan Medical School, Ann Arbor, Michigan [19]

Lisa M. Donofrio, MD
Associate Clinical Professor, Department of Dermatology, Yale School of Medicine, Yale University, New Haven, Connecticut [215]

Jeffrey S. Dover, MD, FRCPC
SkinCare Physicians, Chestnut Hill, Massachusetts [208]

Lyn McDivitt Duncan, MD
Professor of Pathology, Harvard Medical School, Chief, Dermatopathology Unit, Department of Pathology, Massachusetts General Hospital, Boston, Massachusetts [109]

Jonathan A. Dyer, MD
Associate Professor of Dermatology and Child Health, Departments of Dermatology and Child Health, University of Missouri, Columbia, Missouri [72]

Lawrence F. Eichenfield, MD
Chief, Pediatric and Adolescent Dermatology, Professor of Dermatology and Pediatrics, Vice Chair, Department of Dermatology, University of California, San Diego School of Medicine, San Diego, California [22]

James T. Elder, MD, PhD
Kirk D. Wuepper Professor of Molecular Genetic Dermatology, Department of Dermatology, University of Michigan, Ann Arbor, Ann Arbor, Michigan [28]

Rosalie Elenitsas, MD
Professor of Dermatology, Director of Dermatopathology, Hospital of the University of Pennsylvania, Perelman School of Medicine, Philadelphia, Pennsylvania [2]

Dana L. Ellis, MD
Clinical Instructor, Department of Dermatology, Yale School of Medicine, Yale University, New Haven, Connecticut [215]

Craig A. Elmets, MD
Professor and Emeritus Chair, Department of Dermatology, University of Alabama at Birmingham, The Birmingham VA Medical Center, Birmingham, Alabama [198]

Joseph C. English III, MD
Professor of Dermatology, University of Pittsburgh, Department of Dermatology, UPMC North Hills Dermatology, Wexford, Pennsylvania [155]

Alexander H. Enk, MD
Professor and Chair, Department of Dermatology, University of Heidelberg, Heidelberg, Germany [116]

Ervin H. Epstein, Jr., MD
Children's Hospital of Oakland Research Institute, UCSF, Oakland, California [111]

Khaled Ezzedine, MD, PhD
Professor, Department of Dermatology, Hôpital Henri Mondor, EA EpiDermE (Epidémiologie en Dermatologie et Evaluation des Thérapeutiques), UPEC-Université Paris-Est Créteil, Créteil, France [76, 171]

Janet A. Fairley, MD
John S. Strauss Professor and Chair, Department of Dermatology, University of Iowa Carver College of Medicine, Iowa City, Iowa [128]

Steven R. Feldman, MD, PhD
Department of Dermatology, Wake Forest University School of Medicine, Winston-Salem, North Carolina [183]

Nicole Fett, MD, MSCE
Associate Professor of Dermatology, Department of Dermatology, Oregon Health and Science University, Portland, Oregon [184]

David Fiorentino, MD, PhD
Professor in the Department of Dermatology and the Department of Immunology and Rheumatology at Stanford University School of Medicine, Redwood City, California [62]

David E. Fisher, MD, PhD
Edward Wigglesworth Professor and Chairman, Department of Dermatology, Harvard Medical School, Director, Melanoma Program MGH Cancer Center, Director, Cutaneous Biology Research Center, Massachusetts General Hospital, Boston, Massachusetts [20]

Joachim W. Fluhr, MD
Oberarzt, Charité-Universitätsmedizin Berlin, Klinik für Dermatologie, Venerologie und Allergologie, Berlin, Germany [96]

John A. Flynn, MD, MBA, MEd
Professor and Associate Dean of Medicine, Johns Hopkins University, Baltimore, Maryland [65]

Ruth K. Foreman, MD, PhD
Instructor of Pathology, Harvard Medical School, Dermatopathology Unit, Department of Pathology, Massachusetts General Hospital, Boston, Massachusetts [109]

Amy K. Forrestel, MD
University of Pennsylvania, Department of Dermatology, Philadelphia, Pennsylvania [133]

Camille Francès, MD
AP-HP, Hôpital Tenon, Université Paris VI, Service de Dermatologie-Allergologie, Paris, France [69]

Nicholas Frank, MD
Dermatology Resident, Vanderbilt University Medical Center, Department of Internal Medicine, Division of Dermatology, Nashville, Tennessee [101]

Esther E. Freeman, MD, PhD
Assistant Professor of Dermatology, Harvard University Medical School, Director, Global Health Dermatology, Massachusetts General Hospital, Department of Dermatology, Boston, Massachusetts [168]

Lars E. French, MD
Professor and Chairman, Department of Dermatology, University of Zurich, Zurich, Switzerland [39]

Sheila Fallon Friedlander, MD
Professor of Dermatology and Pediatrics, University of California, San Diego School of Medicine, Rady Children's Hospital, San Diego, San Diego, California [166]

Adam J. Friedman, MD
Associate Professor of Dermatology, Director of Translational Research, Residency Program Director, Department of Dermatology, George Washington School of Medicine and Health Sciences, Washington, DC [154]

Daniel P. Friedmann, MD
Westlake Dermatology Clinical Research Center, Westlake Dermatology and Cosmetic Surgery, Austin, Texas [212]

Ramsay L. Fuleihan, MD
Professor of Pediatrics, Northwestern University Feinberg School of Medicine, Chicago, Illinois [132]

Abhimanyu Garg, MD
Professor of Internal Medicine, Chief, Division of Nutrition and Metabolic Diseases, Department of Internal Medicine and the Center for Human Nutrition, Distinguished Chair in Human Nutrition Research, Dallas, Texas [74]

Luis Garza, MD, PhD
Associate Professor, Department of Dermatology, Johns Hopkins School of Medicine, Baltimore, Maryland [4]

Mahmoud Ghannoum, PhD, EMBA
Center for Medical Mycology, University Hospitals Cleveland Medical Center, Case Western Reserve University, Cleveland, Ohio [188]

Dee Anna Glaser, MD
Interim Chair and Professor, Director Cosmetic and Laser Surgery, Director of Clinical Research, Department of Dermatology, Saint Louis University School of Medicine, St. Louis, Missouri [81]

Richard G. Glogau, MD
Clinical Professor of Dermatology, University of California, San Francisco, San Francisco, California [216]

Sergij Goerdt, MD
Professor of Dermatology, Chair of Dermatology, Department of Dermatology, Venereology and Allergology, University Medical Center and Medical Faculty Mannheim, University of Heidelberg, Mannheim, Germany [117]

Carolyn Goh, MD
Assistant Clinical Professor of Dermatology/Medicine, David Geffen School of Medicine at UCLA, Los Angeles, California [78]

Chee Leok Goh, MD, MBBS, M. Med (Int. Med), MRCP (UK), FRCP (Edin), Hon FACD, FAMS (Dermatology)
Clinical Professor, National Skin Centre, Singapore [187]

Leonard H. Goldberg, MD
DermSurgery Associates, Houston, Texas [206]

Peter D. Gorevic, MD
Professor of Medicine, Division of Rheumatology, Icahn School of Medicine at Mount Sinai, New York, New York [125]

Eric W. Gou, MD
Department of Internal Medicine, Division of Gastroenterology and Hepatology, University of Texas Medical Branch, Galveston, Texas [124]

Emmy M. Graber, MD, MBA
Dermatologist, The Dermatology Institute of Boston, Boston, Massachusetts [78, 80]

Dorothy Katherine Grange, MD
Professor of Pediatrics, Division of Genetics and Genomic Medicine, Department of Pediatrics, Washington University School of Medicine, St. Louis, Missouri [131]

Clayton B. Green MD, PhD
The Marshfield Clinic, Marshfield, Wisconsin [98]

Justin J. Green, MD
Division of Dermatology, Cooper Medical School of Rowan University, Camden, New Jersey [180]

Roy C. Grekin, MD
Professor of Dermatology, Director, Dermatologic Surgery and Laser Center, University of California, San Francisco, San Francisco, California [114]

Annie Grossberg, MD
Associate Director, Dermatology Residency Program, Assistant Professor, Departments of Dermatology and Pediatrics, Johns Hopkins University, Baltimore, Maryland [102]

Alexandra Gruber-Wackernagel, MD
Medical University of Graz, Research Unit for Photodermatology, Department of Dermatology, Medical University of Graz, Graz, Austria [92]

Johann E. Gudjonsson, MD, PhD
Assistant Professor, Department of Dermatology, Frances and Kenneth Eisenberg Emerging Scholar of the Taubman Medical Research Institute, University of Michigan, Ann Arbor, Michigan [11, 28, 31]

Cheryl J. Gustafson, MD
St. Vincent Carmel Medical Center, Carmel, Indiana [214]

Eva N. Hadaschik, MD
Department of Dermatology, University Hospital Heidelberg, Heidelberg, Germany [112]

Ellen S. Haddock, AB, MBA
University of California, San Diego School of Medicine, La Jolla, California [166]

Alexandra Haden, MD
Assistant Professor of Clinical Dermatology, Department of Dermatology, University of Southern California, Los Angeles, California [143]

Adele Haimovic, MD
SkinCare Physicians, Chestnut Hill, Massachusetts [203]

Russell P. Hall III, MD
J. Lamar Callaway Professor, Department of Dermatology, Duke University Medical Center, Durham, North Carolina [58]

Analisa V. Halpern, MD
Division of Dermatology, Cooper Medical School of Rowan University, Camden, New Jersey [180]

Eckart Haneke, MD, PhD
Clinical Professor (em) of Dermatology, Department of Dermatology, Inselspital, University of Berne, Bern, Switzerland [91]

C. William Hanke, MD, MPH, FACP
St. Vincent Carmel Medical Center, Carmel, Indiana [214]

John E. Harris, MD, PhD
Associate Professor, University of Massachusetts Medical School, Worcester, Massachusetts [76]

Takashi Hashimoto, MD
Professor and Director, Kurume University Institute of Cutaneous Cell Biology, Kurume, Fukuoka, Japan [57]

Jessica C. Hassel, MD
Section Head, DermatoOncology, Department of Dermatology and National Center for Tumor Diseases, University Hospital Heidelberg, Heidelberg, Germany [116]

Roderick J. Hay, DM, FRCP, FRCPath, FMedSci
Professor, Department of Dermatology, Kings College Hospital, Denmark Hill, London, United Kingdom [162]

Masahiro Hayashi, MD, PhD
Associate Professor of Dermatology, Yamagata University Faculty of Medicine, Yamagata, Japan [75]

Kara Heelan, MB BCh, BAO
Dermatology Department, University College London Hospitals, London, United Kingdom [45]

Cara Hennings, MD
University of Tennessee/Erlanger Medical Center, Chattanooga, Tennessee [101]

Markus V. Heppt, MD
Department of Dermatology, University Hospital Munich, Ludwig-Maximilian University, Munich, Germany [110]

Warren R. Heymann, MD
Division of Dermatology, Cooper Medical School of Rowan University, Camden, New Jersey [180]

Michihiro Hide, MD, PhD
Department of Dermatology, Institute of Biomedical and Health Sciences, Hiroshima University, Hiroshima, Japan [41]

Whitney A. High, MD, JD, MEng
Associate Professor of Dermatology and Pathology, University of Colorado School of Medicine, Director of Dermatopathology (Dermatology), Aurora, Colorado [140]

Takaaki Hiragun, MD, PhD
Department of Dermatology, Institute of Biomedical and Health Sciences, Hiroshima University, Hiroshima, Japan [41]

Allen W. Ho, MD, PhD
Resident Physician, Department of Dermatology, Harvard Medical School, Boston, Massachusetts [12]

Melissa B. Hoffman, MD
Resident, Dermatology, Wake Forest School of Medicine, Winston Salem, North Carolina [174]

Jeremy S. Honaker, CNP, PhD
Assistant Professor, Department of Dermatology, Case Western Reserve University, Cleveland, Ohio [190]

Herbert Hönigsmann, MD
Professor of Dermatology, Emeritus Chairman, Department of Dermatology, Medical University of Vienna, Vienna, Austria [38, 199]

Alain Hovnanian, MD, PhD
Professor of Genetics, Department of Genetics, Imagine Institute for Genetic Diseases, Necker Hospital for Sick Children, University Paris Descartes-Sorbonne Paris Cité, Paris, France [50]

Josie Howard, MD
Clinical Faculty, Departments of Psychiatry and Dermatology, University of California, San Francisco, San Francisco, California [100]

Jeffrey T. S. Hsu, MD
Clinical Assistant Professor, Department of Dermatology, University of Illinois College of Medicine at Chicago, Co-Director of Dermatologic, Laser and Cosmetic Surgery, The Dermatology Institute of DuPage Medical Group, Naperville, Illinois [212]

Linden Hu, MD
Professor of Microbiology and Medicine, Tufts University School of Medicine, Boston, Massachusetts [179]

William W. Huang, MD, MPH
Associate Professor of Dermatology, Residency Program Director, Wake Forest School of Medicine, Winston Salem, North Carolina [46]

Raegan Hunt, MD, PhD
Assistant Professor of Dermatology and Pediatrics, Texas Children's Hospital, Baylor College of Medicine, Houston, Texas [103]

Sam T. Hwang, MD, PhD
Department of Dermatology, University of California Davis School of Medicine, Sacramento, California [193]

Omer Ibrahim, MD
SkinCare Physicians, Chestnut Hill, Massachusetts [208]

Alan D. Irvine, MD, DSc
Paediatric Dermatology and National Children's Research Centre, Our Lady's Children's Hospital Crumlin, Dublin, Clinical Medicine, Trinity College, Dublin, Ireland [51]

Carlos M. Isada, MD
Department of Infectious Disease, Cleveland Clinic, Cleveland, Ohio [186]

Heidi T. Jacobe, MD, MSCS
Associate Professor, Department of Dermatology, UT Southwestern Medical Center, Dallas, Texas [64]

Tarannum Jaleel, MD
Instructor, Department of Dermatology, Duke Medical Center, Durham, North Carolina [198]

Camila K. Janniger, MD
Clinical Professor, Dermatology, Rutgers New Jersey Medical School, Englewood, New Jersey [182]

Andrew Johnston, PhD
Department of Dermatology University of Michigan School of Medicine, Ann Arbor, Michigan [193]

Steven R. Jones, MD
Ciccarone Center for the Prevention of Heart Disease, Division of Cardiology, Department of Medicine, Johns Hopkins Hospital, Baltimore Maryland [126]

Natanel Jourabchi, MD
Resident Dermatology Physician, Johns Hopkins School of Medicine, Baltimore, Maryland [37]

Andrea Kalus, MD
Associate Professor, University of Washington School of Medicine, Division of Dermatology, Seattle, Washington [137]

Sewon Kang, MD, MPH
Noxell Professor & Chair, Department of Dermatology, Johns Hopkins School of Medicine, Dermatologist-in-Chief, Johns Hopkins Hospital, Baltimore, Maryland [106, 185]

Varvara Kanti, MD
Department of Dermatology and Allergy, Charité-Universitätsmedizin, Berlin, Germany [85]

Kenneth A. Katz, MD, MSc, MSCE
Department of Dermatology, Kaiser Permanente, San Francisco, California [107]

Stephen I. Katz, MD, PhD
National Institute of Arthritis and Musculoskeletal and Skin Diseases, Bethesda, Maryland [59]

Werner Kempf, MD
Kempf and Pfaltz, Histologische Diagnostik, Department of Dermatology, University Hospital Zurich, Zurich, Switzerland [120]

Michelle L. Kerns, MD
Research Fellow, Department of Dermatology, Johns Hopkins School of Medicine, Baltimore, Maryland [106]

Jay S. Keystone, MD, MSc (CTM), FRCPC
Professor of Medicine, University of Toronto, Tropical Disease Unit, Division of Infectious Diseases, Toronto General Hospital, Toronto, Ontario, Canada [177]

Ellen J. Kim, MD
Sandra J. Lazarus Associate Professor in Dermatology, Department of Dermatology, Perelman School of Medicine at the University of Pennsylvania, Perelman Center for Advanced Medicine, Philadelphia, Pennsylvania [134]

Jenny Kim, MD, PhD
Professor of Dermatology/Medicine/Nutrition, David Geffen School of Medicine at UCLA, Los Angeles, California [78]

Robert S. Kirsner, MD, PhD
Chairman and Harvey Blank Professor, Department of Dermatology and Cutaneous Surgery, Professor, Department of Public Health Sciences, University of Miami Miller School of Medicine, Miami, Florida [149]

Robert Knobler, MD
Associate Professor of Dermatology, Department of Dermatology, Medical University of Vienna, Vienna, Austria [199]

Krzysztof Kobielak, MD, PhD
Group Leader of Laboratory of Stem Cells, Development and Tissue Regeneration, Centre of New Technologies, University of Warsaw, Warsaw, Poland, Principal Investigator, Department of Developmental and Cell Biology, University of California, Irvine, Irvine, California [8]

Heidi H. Kong, MD, MHSc
Investigator, Dermatology Branch, Center for Cancer Research, National Cancer Institute, National Institutes of Health, Dermatology Branch Bethesda, Maryland [16]

John Y. M. Koo, MD
Professor, Psoriasis, Phototherapy, and Skin Treatment Center and Psychodermatology Clinic, Department of Dermatology, University of California San Francisco, San Francisco, California [100]

Neil J. Korman, MD, PhD
Professor, Department of Dermatology, Case Western Reserve University, Cleveland, Ohio [190]

Kenneth H. Kraemer, MD
Chief, DNA Repair Section, Dermatology Branch, Center for Cancer Research, National Cancer Institute, National Institutes of Health, Bethesda, Maryland [130]

Thomas Krieg, MD, FRCP
Department of Dermatology and Venerology, University of Cologne, Cologne, Germany [63]

Daniela Kroshinksy, MD, MPH
Associate Professor, Harvard Medical School, Director of Inpatient Dermatology, Director of Pediatric Dermatology, Massachusetts General Hospital/ MassGeneral Hospital for Children, Boston, Massachusetts [153]

Akiharu Kubo, MD, PhD
Department of Dermatology, Keio University School of Medicine, Tokyo, Japan [14]

Thomas S. Kupper, MD
Thomas B. Fitzpatrick Professor, Department of Dermatology, Brigham and Women's Hospital, Harvard Medical School, Boston, Massachusetts [12]

Anastasia O. Kurta, DO
Dermatology Resident, Department of Dermatology, Saint Louis University School of Medicine, St Louis, Missouri [81]

Drew Kurtzman, MD
Assistant Professor of Medicine (Dermatology), Director, Connective Tissue Disease Clinic, Director, Immunobullous Disease Clinic, The University of Arizona, Tucson, Arizona [145, 192]

Razelle Kurzrock, MD
Professor of Medicine and Chief, Division of Hematology and Oncology; Senior Deputy Center Director, Clinical Science; and Director, Center for Personalized Cancer Therapy and Clinical Trials Office, University of California, San Diego Moores Cancer Center, San Diego, California [36]

Heinz Kutzner, MD
Dermatopathology Friedrichshafen, Friedrichshafen, Germany [121]

Shawn G. Kwatra, MD
Department of Dermatology, Johns Hopkins School of Medicine, Baltimore, Maryland [196]

Avery LaChance, MD, MPH
Dermatology Resident, Harvard Combined Dermatology Residency Training Program, Massachusetts General Hospital, Boston, Massachusetts [153]

Eden Pappo Lake, MD
University of Illinois at Chicago, Chicago, Illinois [73]

Stephan Lautenschlager, MD
Associate Professor University of Zurich, Chairman Outpatient Clinic of Dermatology and Venereology, City Hospital Triemli, Zurich, Switzerland [172, 173]

Gerald S. Lazarus, MD
Professor of Dermatology and Medicine, Johns Hopkins School of Medicine, Baltimore, Maryland [37]

Terry Lechler, PhD
Associate Professor of Dermatology, Duke University Medical Center, Durham, North Carolina [5]

David J. Leffell, MD
David Paige Smith Professor of Dermatology and Professor of Surgery (Otolaryngology and Plastic), Section Chief of Dermatologic Surgery, Yale University School of Medicine, New Haven, Connecticut [204]

Aimee L. Leonard, MD
New England Dermatology and Laser Center, Springfield, Massachusetts [214]

Kieron Leslie, MBBS, DTM&H, FRCP
Professor of Clinical Dermatology, Dermatology Department, University of California, San Francisco, San Francisco, California [161]

Donald Y. M. Leung, MD, PhD
Department of Pediatrics, National Jewish Health, University of Colorado Denver, Denver, Colorado [22]

Benjamin Levi, MD
Director, Burn, Wound and Regenerative Medicine Laboratory, Assistant Professor of Surgery, Ann Arbor, Michigan [99]

Myron J. Levin, MD
Section of Pediatric Infectious Diseases, Department of Pediatrics, University of Colorado School of Medicine, Aurora, Colorado [165]

Matthew Lewis, MD, MPH
Clinical Assistant Professor in the Department of Dermatology at Stanford University School of Medicine, Redwood City, California [62]

Maryam Liaqat, MD
Division of Dermatology, Cooper Medical School of Rowan University, Camden, New Jersey [180]

Henry W. Lim, MD
Emeritus Chair, Department of Dermatology, Henry Ford Hospital, Senior Vice President for Academic Affairs, Henry Ford Health System, Detroit, Michigan [97]

Dan Lipsker, MD, PhD
Professor of Dermatology, Faculté de Medicine, Université de Strasbourg and Clinique Dermatologique, Hôpitaux Universitaires, Strasbourg, France [146]

Adam D. Lipworth, MD
Assistant Professor of Dermatology, Harvard University Medical School, Director, Program for Infectious Diseases of the Skin, Director of Clinical Care Redesign, Dermatology, Brigham and Women's Hospital, Boston, Massachusetts [168]

Robert Listernick, MD
Professor of Pediatrics, Feinberg School of Medicine, Northwestern University, Ann and Robert H. Lurie Children's Hospital of Chicago, Division of General Academic Pediatrics, Chicago, Illinois [135]

Zhi Liu, PhD
Department of Dermatology, University of North Carolina at Chapel Hill, Chapel Hill, North Carolina [54]

Robert Loewe, MD
Associate Professor, Department of Dermatology, Medical University Vienna, Vienna, Austria [9]

Anke S. Lonsdorf, MD
Department of Dermatology, University Hospital Heidelberg, Heidelberg, Germany [112]

Manisha Loss, MD
Department of Dermatology Johns Hopkins School of Medicine, Baltimore, Maryland [196]

Thomas A. Luger, MD
Center of Chronic Pruritus, Department of Dermatology, University of Münster, Münster, Germany [21]

Boris D. Lushniak, MD, MPH
Rear Admiral, United States Public Health Service (Retired), Professor and Chair, Preventive Medicine and Biostatistics, Uniformed Services University of the Health Sciences, F. Edward Hébert School of Medicine, Department of Preventive Medicine and Biostatistics, Bethesda, Maryland [27]

Catherine Maari, MD, FRCPC
Associate Clinical Professor, Division of Dermatology, Montreal University Health Center, University of Montreal, CHU Sainte-Justine, Montreal, Quebec, Canada [70]

Kelly M. MacArthur, MD
Chief Resident, Department of Dermatology, Johns Hopkins University, Baltimore, Maryland [102, 118]

Howard I. Maibach, MD
Department of Dermatology, University of California, San Francisco School of Medicine, San Francisco, California [183]

Aaron R. Mangold, MD
Assistant Professor of Dermatology,
Mayo Clinic, Scottsdale,
Arizona [32, 33]

Matthew D. Mansh, MD
Resident in Dermatology, University
of Minnesota, Minneapolis,
Minnesota [107]

Richard Marchell, MD
Associate Professor of Dermatology
and Dermatologic Surgery,
Residency Program Director,
Medical University of
South Carolina, Charleston,
South Carolina [35]

David J. Margolis, MD, PhD
Professor of Dermatology and
Epidemiology, Department of
Dermatology, Department of
Biostatistics and Epidemiology,
University of Pennsylvania
Perelman School of Medicine,
Philadelphia, Pennsylvania [3, 151]

M. Peter Marinkovich, MD
Attending Physician, VA Palo Alto
Health Care System, Associate
Professor and Director, Blistering
Disease Clinic, Department of
Dermatology, Program in Epithelial
Biology, Stanford University
School of Medicine, Stanford,
California [60]

Seth S. Martin, MD, MHS
Ciccarone Center for the Prevention
of Heart Disease, Division of
Cardiology, Department of
Medicine, Johns Hopkins Hospital,
Baltimore Maryland [126]

Kathryn J. Martires, MD
Clinical Assistant Professor,
Department of Dermatology,
Stanford University School of
Medicine, Palo Alto, California [129]

Erin F. D. Mathes, MD
Associate Professor of Clinical
Dermatology, University of
California, San Francisco,
San Francisco, California [163]

Marcus Maurer, MD
Charité–Universitätsmedizin Berlin,
Department of Dermatology and
Allergy, Berlin, Germany [96]

Aubriana McEvoy
University of Washington, Seattle,
Washington [113]

John A. McGrath, MBBS, PhD
St John's Institute of Dermatology,
King's College London, London,
United Kingdom [18]

Sean McGregor, DO
Resident physician, Wake Forest
University School of Medicine,
Winston-Salem,
North Carolina [175]

Bridget E. McIlwee, DO
Dermatology Resident, Division of
Dermatology University of North
Texas Health Science Center, Fort
Worth, Texas [209]

Amy J. McMichael, MD
Professor and Chair, Department
of Dermatology, Wake Forest
University School of Medicine,
Winston-Salem,
North Carolina [90]

Atul B. Mehta, MA, MB, BChir, MD, FRCP, FRCPath
Professor, University College
London, Royal Free Campus
and Royal Free London NHS
Foundation Trust, London,
United Kingdom [127]

Thomas Mentzel, MD
Consultant Dermatopathologist
and Associated Professor,
Dermatopathologie Bodensee,
Friedrichshafen, Germany [122]

Peter A. Merkel, MD, MPH
Chief, Division of Rheumatology,
Professor of Medicine and
Epidemiology, University of
Pennsylvania, Philadelphia,
Pennsylvania [139]

Robert G. Micheletti, MD
University of Pennsylvania,
Department of Dermatology,
Philadelphia, Pennsylvania [133]

Ashley N. Millard, MD
Marshfield Clinic, Marshfield,
Wisconsin [98]

David Michael Miller, MD, PhD
Clinical Fellow in Medicine,
Division of Hematology/
Oncology, Beth Israel Deaconess
Medical Center, Clinical Associate,
Department of Dermatology,
Massachusetts General Hospital,
Boston, Massachusetts [194]

Jami L. Miller, MD
Department of Internal Medicine,
Division of Dermatology, Vanderbilt
University Medical Center,
Nashville, Tennessee [101]

Lloyd S. Miller, MD, PhD
Associate Professor of Dermatology,
Infectious Diseases and Orthopaedic
Surgery, Johns Hopkins School of
Medicine, Baltimore, Maryland [150]

Leonard M. Milstone, MD
Professor Emeritus of Dermatology,
Yale University School of Medicine,
New Haven, Connecticut [47]

Daniel Mimouni, MD
Associate Professor of Dermatology,
Department of Dermatology,
Beilinson Hospital, Petach Tikva,
Israel, Faculty of Medicine, Tel Aviv
University, Tel Aviv, Israel [53]

Vineet Mishra, MD
Assistant Clinical Professor,
Division of Dermatology and
Cutaneous Surgery, The University
of Texas Health Science Center
at San Antonio, San Antonio,
Texas [212]

Maja Mockenhaupt, MD, PhD
Dokumentationszentrum schwerer
Hautreaktionen (dZh), Department
of Dermatology, Medical Center,
University of Freiburg, Freiburg,
Germany, Dokumentationszentrum
schwerer Hautreaktionen (dZh),
Department of Dermatology,
Medical Center and Medical Faculty,
University of Freiburg, Freiburg,
Germany [43, 44]

Robert L. Modlin, MD, PhD
Klein Professor of Dermatology,
Distinguished Professor of Medicine
and Microbiology, Immunology
and Molecular Genetics, Chief,
Division of Dermatology, Vice
Chair for Cutaneous Medicine
and Dermatology Research,
David Geffen School of Medicine,
UCLA Med-Derm, Los Angeles,
California [11]

Pia Moinzadeh, MD
Department of Dermatology and
Venerology, University of Cologne,
Cologne, Germany [63]

Paul A. Monach, MD, PhD
Division of Rheumatology,
Immunology, and Allergy, Brigham
and Women's Hospital, Chief,
Rheumatology Section, VA Boston
Healthcare System, Boston,
Massachusetts [139]

Gary Monheit, MD
Total Skin and Beauty Dermatology,
Birmingham, Alabama [213]

Robert F. Moore, MD
Resident in Anatomic Pathology, Department of Pathology, Johns Hopkins Hospital, Baltimore, Maryland [115]

Breanne Mordorski, BA
Nanodermatology Research Fellow, Department of Medicine (Division of Dermatology), Albert Einstein College of Medicine, Bronx, New York [154]

Hansgeorg Müller, MD
Dermatopathology Friedrichshafen, Friedrichshafen, Germany [121]

Keisuke Nagao, MD, PhD
Dermatology Branch, National Institutes of Health, Bethesda, Maryland [13]

Mio Nakamura, MD
Clinical Research Fellow, Psoriasis, Phototherapy, and Skin Treatment Center, Department of Dermatology, University of California, San Francisco, San Francisco, California [100]

Zeena Y. Nawas, MD
University of Texas Health Science Center, Houston, Texas [191]

Susan T. Nedorost, MD
Professor, Dermatology and Environmental Health Sciences, Case Western Reserve University, Director, Graduate Medical Education, University Hospitals Cleveland Medical Center, Cleveland, Ohio [25]

Isaac M. Neuhaus, MD
Associate Professor of Dermatology, University of California, San Francisco, San Francisco, California [114]

Sabrina A. Newman, MD
Assistant Professor of Dermatology, Director, Inpatient Dermatology, University of Colorado School of Medicine, Anschutz Medical Campus, Aurora, Colorado [148]

Paul Nghiem, MD, PhD
University of Washington, Seattle, Washington [113]

Quynh-Giao Nguyen, MD
Baylor College of Medicine, Houston, Texas [191]

Matilda W. Nicholas, MD, PhD
Assistant Professor, Department of Dermatology, Duke University Medical Center, Duke University Medical Center, Durham, North Carolina [58]

Elizabeth L. Nieman, MD
Assistant Professor of Dermatology, Division of Dermatology, Department of Medicine, Washington University School of Medicine, St. Louis, Missouri [131]

Scott A. Norton, MD, MPH, MSc
Chief of Dermatology, Children's National Medical Center, Washington, DC [156]

Cathal O'Connor, MD
Paediatric Dermatology, Our Lady's Children's Hospital, National Children's Research Centre, Our Lady's Children's Hospital Crumlin, Dublin [51]

Grainne M. O'Regan, PhD, FRCPI
Paediatric Dermatology, Our Lady's Children's Hospital, National Children's Research Centre, Our Lady's Children's Hospital Crumlin, Dublin [51]

Manabu Ohyama, MD, PhD
Professor and Chairman, Department of Dermatology, Kyorin University School of Medicine, Tokyo, Japan [86]

Ginette A. Okoye, MD
Assistant Professor of Dermatology, Johns Hopkins School of Medicine, Baltimore, Maryland [84]

Ana-Maria Orbai, MD, MHS
Assistant Professor of Medicine, Director Psoriatic Arthritis Program, Johns Hopkins Arthritis Center, Johns Hopkins School of Medicine, Division of Rheumatology, Baltimore, Maryland [65]

Anthony E. Oro, MD, PhD
Department of Dermatology, Stanford University, School of Medicine, Redwood City, California [111]

Jeffrey S. Orringer, MD
Professor and Chief, Division of Cosmetic Dermatology, Department of Dermatology, University of Michigan, Ann Arbor, Michigan [210]

Catherine H. Orteu, MBBS, BSc, MD, FRCP
University College London, Royal Free Campus and Royal Free London NHS Foundation Trust, London, United Kingdom [127]

Stephen M. Ostrowski, MD, PhD
Instructor of Dermatology, Harvard Medical School, Department of Dermatology, Cutaneous Biology Research Center, Massachusetts General Hospital, Boston, Massachusetts [20]

Nina Otberg, MD
Hair Clinic, Skin and Laser Center Potsdam, Potsdam, Germany, Otberg Medical, Hair Transplant Center Berlin–Potsdam, Berlin, Germany [87, 88]

Michael N. Oxman, MD
Division of Infectious Diseases, Department of Medicine, University of California, San Diego and Infectious Diseases Section, Medical Service, Veterans Affairs San Diego Healthcare System, San Diego, California [165]

Vikash S. Oza, MD
Assistant Professor of Dermatology and Pediatrics, The Ronald O. Perelman Department of Dermatology, New York University School of Medicine, New York, New York [163]

Amy S. Paller, MD
Walter J. Hamlin Professor and Chair, Department of Dermatology, Professor of Pediatrics, Northwestern University Feinberg School of Medicine, Chicago, Illinois [132]

Jiun Yit Pan, MBBS, MCI (NUS), GDOM (NUS), DTM&H (Lond), FRCP (Edin)
Dermatologist, National Skin Centre, Singapore [187]

Amit G. Pandya, MD
Department of Dermatology, The University of Texas, Southwestern Medical Center, Dallas, Texas [77]

Deepa Patel, BS
Clinical Research Fellow, The Children's Hospital of Philadelphia, Philadelphia, Pennsylvania [89]

Aimee S. Payne, MD, PhD
Associate Professor of Dermatology, University of Pennsylvania, Philadelphia, Pennsylvania [15, 52]

David R. Pearson, MD
Assistant Professor of Dermatology, University of Minnesota School of Medicine, Minneapolis, Minnesota [151]

David H. Peng, MD, MPH
Chair, Department of Dermatology, University of Southern California, Los Angeles, California [143]

Manuel P. Pereira, MD, PhD
Center of Chronic Pruritus, Department of Dermatology, University of Münster, Münster, Germany [21]

Powell Perng, MD
Johns Hopkins School of Medicine, Department of Dermatology, Baltimore, Maryland [83]

Peter Petzelbauer, MD
Professor of Microvascular Research, Department of Dermatology, Medical University Vienna, Vienna, Austria [9]

Robert G. Phelps, MD
Professor, Departments of Dermatology and Pathology, Icahn School of Medicine at Mount Sinai, New York, New York [125]

Rita O. Pichardo, MD
Associate Professor of Dermatology, Wake Forest University School of Medicine, Winston-Salem, North Carolina [174, 175]

Warren W. Piette, MD
Chair, Division of Dermatology, Department of Medicine, John H Stroger, Jr. Hospital of Cook County, Professor, Department of Dermatology, Rush University Medical Center, Chicago, Illinois [66]

Mark R. Pittelkow, MD
Professor of Dermatology, Mayo Clinic, Chair of Dermatology, Scottsdale, Arizona [32, 33, 67]

Jordan S. Pober, MD, PhD
Bayer Professor of Translational Medicine and Professor of Immunobiology, Pathology and Dermatology, Department of Immunobiology, Yale School of Medicine, New Haven, Connecticut [9]

Brian P. Pollack, MD, PhD
Assistant Professor, Departments of Dermatology and Pathology/Laboratory Medicine, Emory University School of Medicine, The Atlanta VA Medical Center, Atlanta, Georgia [198]

Miriam Keltz Pomeranz, MD
Associate Professor of Dermatology, The Ronald O. Perelman Department of Dermatology, New York University School of Medicine, Chief of Dermatology, NYC Health + Hospitals/Bellevue, New York, New York [105]

Julie Powell, MD, FRCPC
Clinical Professor, Dermatology and Pediatrics, University of Montreal, Director, Pediatric Dermatology, CHU Sainte-Justine, Montreal, Quebec, Canada [70]

Julie S. Prendiville, MB, FRCPC
Clinical Professor in Pediatrics, University of British Columbia, Head, Division of Pediatric Dermatology, BC Children's Hospital, Vancouver, British Columbia, Canada [34]

Katherine Püttgen, MD
Assistant Professor of Dermatology and Pediatrics, Johns Hopkins University, Baltimore, Maryland [118]

Sophia Rangwala, MD
Fellow, Dermatopathology, Johns Hopkins School of Medicine, Baltimore, Maryland [108]

Caroline L. Rao, MD
Assistant Professor, Department of Dermatology, Duke University Medical Center, Duke University Medical Center, Durham, North Carolina [58]

Bobby Y. Reddy, MD
Clinical Fellow, Department of Dermatology, Wellman Center for Photomedicine, Massachusetts General Hospital, Boston, Massachusetts [194]

Michelle Rodrigues, MBBS (Hons), FACD
Chroma Dermatology, Melbourne, Australia, Department of Dermatology, St Vincent's Hospital, Fitzroy, Victoria, Australia [77]

Thomas E. Rohrer, MD
SkinCare Physicians, Chestnut Hill, Massachusetts [203]

Misha Rosenbach, MD
Assistant Professor, Dermatology and Internal Medicine Associate Program Director, Dermatology Residency Director, Inpatient Dermatology Consult Service Director, Cutaneous Sarcoidosis Clinic, Perelman Center for Advanced Medicine, Dermatology Administration, Philadelphia, Pennsylvania [155]

Jean-Claude Roujeau MD, PhD
Emeritus Professor of Dermatology, Université Paris-Est Créteil (UPEC), Créteil, France, Department of Dermatology, Université Paris-Est Créteil, Créteil, France [43, 44]

Anne H. Rowley, MD
Professor of Pediatrics and of Microbiology/Immunology, Feinberg School of Medicine, Northwestern University Attending Physician, Division of Infectious Diseases, Ann and Robert H. Lurie Children's Hospital of Chicago, Chicago, Illinois [142]

Thomas M. Rünger, MD, PhD
Professor of Dermatology, Pathology, and Laboratory Medicine, Department of Dermatology, Boston University School of Medicine, Boston, Massachusetts [17, 130]

Arturo P. Saavedra, MD, PhD
Associate Professor of Dermatology, Harvard University Medical School, Vice-Chairman for Clinical Affairs and Medical Director, Massachusetts General Hospital, Boston, Massachusetts [168]

Mohammed D. Saleem, MD, MPH
Department of Dermatology, Wake Forest University School of Medicine, Winston-Salem, North Carolina [183]

Iman Salem, MD
Center for Medical Mycology, University Hospitals Cleveland Medical Center, Case Western Reserve University, Cleveland, Ohio [188]

Claudio Guedes Salgado, MD, PhD
Associate Professor, Pará Federal University, President of the Brazilian Leprosy Society, Marituba, Pará, Brazil [159]

Ubirajara Imbiriba Salgado, MD
Full Professor, Dermatology, Pará State University, Belém, Pará, Brazil [159]

Liat Samuelov, MD
Senior Physician, Department of Dermatology, Tel-Aviv Sourasky Medical Center, Tel-Aviv, Israel [48]

Khaled S. Sanber, MD, PhD
Baylor College of Medicine, Houston, Texas [191]

Inbal Sander, MD
Assistant Professor of Dermatology and Pathology, Johns Hopkins School of Medicine, Baltimore, Maryland [83]

Julio C. Sartori-Valinotti, MD
Assistant Professor of Medicine and Dermatology, Mayo Clinic College of Medicine, Department of Dermatology, Rochester, Minnesota [144]

Vasanth Sathiyakumar, MD
Ciccarone Center for the Prevention of Heart Disease, Division of Cardiology, Department of Medicine, Johns Hopkins Hospital, Baltimore Maryland [126]

Takashi K. Satoh, MD, PhD, MSc
Postdoctoral Research Fellow, Department of Dermatology University of Zurich, Zurich, Switzerland [39]

Jean-Hilaire Saurat, MD
Professor Emeritus, University of Geneva, Genève, Switzerland [185]

April Schachtel, MD
Dermatology Resident, University of Washington School of Medicine, Division of Dermatology, Seattle, Washington [137]

Knut Schäkel, MD
Professor and Vice Chair of Dermatology, Department of Dermatology, University Hospital, Ruprecht-Karls-University Heidelberg, Heidelberg, Germany [29]

Mark Jordan Scharf, MD
Clinical Professor of Dermatology, University of Massachusetts Medical School, Worcester, Massachusetts [182]

Stefan M. Schieke, MD
Assistant Professor, Department of Dermatology, School of Medicine and Public Health, University of Wisconsin-Madison, Medical Science Center, Madison, Wisconsin [30, 160]

Gabriel Schlager, MD
Department of Dermatology, University Hospital Munich, Ludwig-Maximilian University, Munich, Germany [110]

Kenneth E. Schmader, MD
Duke University Medical Center and Geriatric Research Education and Clinical Center (GRECC), Durham VA Medical Center. Durham, North Carolina [165]

Astrid Schmieder, MD
Senior Consultant, Section Head, Allergology, Psoriasis Competence Center, Department of Dermatology, Venereology and Allergology, University Medical Center and Medical Faculty Mannheim, University of Heidelberg, Mannheim, Germany [117]

Robert A. Schwartz, MD, MPH, DSc (Hon), FRCP Edin, FAAD
Professor and Head, Dermatology, Professor of Medicine, Professor of Pediatrics, Professor of Pathology, Rutgers New Jersey Medical School, Visiting Professor, Rutgers School of Public Affairs and Administration, Honorary Professor, China Medical University, Shenyang, China [181, 182]

Aisha Sethi, MD
Associate Professor of Dermatology, Director Yale Dermatology Global Health Program, Department of Dermatology, Yale University School of Medicine, New Haven, Connecticut [157]

Kara N. Shah, MD, PhD
Kenwood Dermatology, Cincinnati, Ohio [103]

Jerry Shapiro, MD, FRCPC
Hair Clinic, The Ronald. O. Perelman Department of Dermatology, New York University School of Medicine, New York, New York [87, 88]

Neil H. Shear, MD, PhD
Division of Dermatology, Department of Medicine, Sunnybrook Health Sciences Centre, University of Toronto, Division of Dermatology, Department of Medicine, Sunnybrook Health Sciences Centre, Toronto, Ontario, Canada [45]

Jessica M. Sheehan, MD
Derick Dermatology, Northbrook, Illinois [203]

Michael P. Sheehan, MD
Dermatology Physicians, Columbus, Indiana [24]

Hiroshi Shimizu, MD, PhD
Professor and Chairman, Department of Dermatology, Hokkaido University Graduate School of Medicine, Sapporo, Japan [40]

Kanade Shinkai, MD, PhD
Associate Professor, University of California, San Francisco, Department of Dermatology, San Francisco, California [1]

Cathryn Sibbald, BScPhm, MD
Department of Dermatology, Sunnybrook Health Sciences Centre, University of Toronto, Division of Dermatology, Department of Medicine, Sunnybrook Health Sciences Centre, Toronto, Ontario, Canada [45]

Daniel Asz Sigall, MD
Mycology Section, Dr. Manuel Gea Gonzalez General Hospital, Mexico City, Mexico [158]

Jonathan I. Silverberg, MD, PhD, MPH
Assistant Professor of Dermatology, Preventive Medicine and Medical Social Sciences, Northwestern University Feinberg School of Medicine, Director, Northwestern Medicine Multidisciplinary Eczema Center, Director, Patch Testing Clinic, Northwestern Memorial Hospital, Chicago, Illinois [23]

Eric L. Simpson, MD, MCR
Department of Dermatology, Oregon Health and Science University, Portland, Oregon [22]

Noah Smith, MD
Department of Dermatology, University of Michigan Health System, Ann Arbor, Michigan [202]

Clayton J. Sontheimer, MD
Acting Assistant Professor, Pediatric Rheumatology, University of Washington School of Medicine, Seattle Children's Hospital, Seattle, Washington [61]

Richard D. Sontheimer, MD
Professor, Dermatology, University of Utah School of Medicine, Salt Lake City, Utah [61]

Nicholas A. Soter, MD
Professor of Dermatology, New York University School of Medicine, Medical Director, Skin and Cancer Unit, Tisch Hospital, New York, New York [138]

John Stewart Spencer, PhD
Associate Professor, Microbiology, Immunology and Pathology, Colorado State University, Fort Collins, Colorado [159]

Eli Sprecher, MD, PhD
Professor and Chair, Department of Dermatology, Tel Aviv Sourasky Medical Center, Tel-Aviv, Israel and Department of Human Molecular Genetics and Biochemistry, Sackler Faculty of Medicine, Tel Aviv University, Tel Aviv, Israel, Tel Aviv, Israel [48]

Rudolf Stadler, MD, PhD
University Clinic for Dermatology, Johannes Wesling Medical Centre, University of Bochum, Minden, Germany [119, 120]

Sonja Ständer, MD
Center of Chronic Pruritus, Department of Dermatology, University of Münster, Münster, Germany [21]

John R. Stanley, MD
Professor, Department of Dermatology, Perelman School of Medicine, University of Pennsylvania, Philadelphia, Pennsylvania [52]

William G. Stebbins, MD
Vanderbilt University, Nashville, Tennessee [214]

Christopher J. Steen, MD, FAAD
Portland, Maine [181]

Martin Steinhoff, MD, PhD
Chairman, Department of Dermatology and Venereology, Hamad Medical Corporation, Doha, Qatar, Clinical Professor, Weill-Cornell University-Qatar, School of Medicine, and Qatar University, Medical School, Doha, Qatar, Professor, UCD Charles Institute for Translational Dermatology, University College Dublin, Dublin, Ireland [79]

Jane C. Sterling, MB, BChir, MA, FRCP, PhD
Cambridge University Hospitals NHS Foundation Trust, Department of Dermatology, Addenbrooke's Hospital, Cambridge University Hospitals NHS Foundation Trust, Cambridge, United Kingdom [167]

Georg Stingl, MD
Professor and Chair, Division of Immunology, Allergy and Infectious Diseases (DIAID), Department of Dermatology, Medical University of Vienna, Vienna, Austria [10]

Erik J. Stratman, MD
Clinical Professor, Department of Dermatology, University of Wisconsin School of Medicine and Public Health, Marshfield, Wisconsin [98]

Lindsay C. Strowd, MD
Assistant Professor of Dermatology, Wake Forest University School of Medicine, Winston-Salem, North Carolina [175]

Dae Hun Suh, MD, PhD
Professor, Department of Dermatology, Seoul National University College of Medicine, Acne and Rosacea Research Laboratory, Seoul National University Hospital, Seoul, South Korea [26]

Kathryn N. Suh, MD, FRCPC
Associate Professor of Medicine, University of Ottawa, Division of Infectious Diseases The Ottawa Hospital, Ottawa, Ontario, Canada [177]

Tamio Suzuki, MD, PhD
Professor and Chairman of Dermatology, Yamagata University Faculty of Medicine, Yamagata, Japan [75]

Rolf-Markus Szeimies, MD, PhD
Professor of Dermatology, Department of Dermatology and Allergology Klinikum Vest Academic Teaching Hospital Ruhr-University of Bochum, Recklinghausen, Germany [199]

Yoshikazu Takada, PhD
Department of Dermatology, University of California Davis School of Medicine, Sacramento, California [193]

Shunsuke Takahagi, MD, PhD
Department of Dermatology, Institute of Biomedical and Health Sciences, Hiroshima University, Hiroshima, Japan [41]

Junko Takeshita, MD, PhD, MSCE
Assistant Professor of Dermatology and Epidemiology, Department of Dermatology, Department of Biostatistics and Epidemiology, University of Pennsylvania Perelman School of Medicine, Philadelphia, Pennsylvania [3]

Carolina Talhari, MD
Associate Professor of Dermatology, State University of Amazonas, Manaos, Brazil [171]

Jean Y. Tang, MD, PhD
Department of Dermatology, Stanford University, School of Medicine, Redwood City, California [111]

Akiko Tanikawa, MD, PhD
Assistant Professor, Department of Dermatology, Keio University School of Medicine, Tokyo, Japan [68]

Janis M. Taube, MD
Associate Professor of Dermatology, Johns Hopkins School of Medicine, Section Head, Dermatopathology, Baltimore, Maryland [108]

Bailey Tayebi, MD, MBA
Total Skin and Beauty Dermatology, Birmingham, Alabama [213]

Michael D. Tharp, MD
The Clark W. Finnerud, MD Professor and Chair, Department of Dermatology, Rush University Medical Center, Chicago, Illinois [42, 189]

Diane M. Thiboutot, MD
Professor of Dermatology, Associate Dean of Clinical and Translational Research Education, Penn State University College of Medicine, Hershey, Pennsylvania [78, 80]

Thusanth Thuraisingam, MD, PhD
Division of Dermatology, McGill University, Montreal, Quebec, Canada [90]

Kenneth J. Tomecki, MD
Department of Dermatology, Cleveland Clinic, Cleveland, Ohio [186]

Franz Trautinger, MD
Professor of Dermatology and Venereology, Karl Landsteiner University of Health Sciences, Chairman, Department of Dermatology and Venereology, University Hospital of St. Pölten, St. Pölten, Austria [38]

Jeffrey B. Travers, MD, PhD
Chair of Pharmacology and Toxicology, Professor of Dermatology, Boonshoft School of Medicine at Wright State University, Dayton, Ohio [152]

Kenneth Y. Tsai, MD, PhD
Associate Member, Departments of Anatomic Pathology and Tumor Biology, Section Head, Non-Melanoma Skin Cancer and Treatment, Donald A. Adam Melanoma and Skin Cancer Center of Excellence, Moffitt Cancer Center, Tampa, Florida [19]

Hensin Tsao, MD, PhD
Professor of Dermatology, Head, Skin Cancer Genetics Laboratory/ Wellman Center for Photomedicine, Director, Massachusetts General Hospital Melanoma and Pigmented Lesion Center/Department of Dermatology, Director, Massachusetts General Hospital Melanoma Genetics Program/ MGH Cancer Center, Boston, Massachusetts [194]

Susan A. Tuddenham, MD, MPH
Division of Infectious Diseases, Bayview Medical Center, Johns Hopkins University, Baltimore, Maryland [170]

Jake E. Turrentine, MD
Assistant Professor, Division of Dermatology, Department of Medicine, Augusta University, Augusta, Georgia [24]

Stephen K. Tyring, MD, PhD
University of Texas Health Science Center, Houston, Texas [191]

Mark C. Udey, MD, PhD
Dermatology Branch, National Institutes of Health, Bethesda, Maryland [13]

Hideyuki Ujiie, MD, PhD
Assistant Professor, Department of Dermatology, Hokkaido University Graduate School of Medicine, Sapporo, Japan [40]

Robin H. Unger, MD
American Board of Hair Restoration Surgery, International Society of Hair Restoration Surgeons, Assistant Clinical Professor, Dermatology, Mt. Sinai School of Medicine, New York, New York [217]

Walter P. Unger, MD, FRCP (C)
American Board of Dermatology, American Board of Hair Restoration Surgery, International Society of Hair Restoration Surgeons, Clinical Professor, Dermatology, Mt. Sinai School of Medicine, New York, New York [217]

Jochen Utikal, MD
Professor of Dermatology, Section Head Dermato-Oncology, Skin Cancer Unit, German Cancer Research Center (DKFZ), Department of Dermatology, Venereology and Allergology University Medical Center and Medical Faculty Mannheim, University of Heidelberg, Mannheim, Germany [117]

Anders Vahlquist, MD
Professor, Department of Medical Sciences, Dermatology and Venereology, Uppsala University, Uppsala, Sweden [185]

Travis Vandergriff, MD
Assistant Professor of Dermatology and Pathology, Director of Dermatopathology, UT Southwestern Medical Center, Dallas, Texas [93, 94]

Miikka Vikkula, MD, PhD
Head of Laboratory of Human Molecular Genetics, de Duve Institute, University of Louvain, Brussels, Belgium [147]

Ruth Ann Vleugels, MD, MPH
Associate Professor, Harvard Medical School, Director, Autoimmune Skin Diseases Program, Director, Connective Tissue Diseases Clinic, Department of Dermatology, Brigham and Women's Hospital, Boston, Massachusetts [145, 192]

Esther von Stebut, MD
Associate Professor of Dermatology and Infectious Diseases, Department for Dermatology, University Medical Center, Johannes Gutenberg-University, Mainz, Germany [176]

John J. Voorhees, MD, FRPC
Duncan and Ella Poth Distinguished Professor and Chairman, Department of Dermatology, University of Michigan Medical School, Ann Arbor, Michigan [185]

Justin J. Vujevich, MD
Vujevich Dermatology Associates, Pittsburgh, Pennsylvania [206]

Etienne C. E. Wang, BA(Hons), MBBS, MA, MPhil
National Skin Center, Singapore, Department of Dermatology, Columbia University, New York, New York [18]

Stewart Wang, MD, PhD
Professor, Department of Surgery, Chief, Burn Surgery, Division of Plastic Surgery, Department of Surgery, University of Michigan Health Systems, Ann Arbor, Michigan [99]

Roger H. Weenig, MD
Associated Skin Care Specialists, Fridley, Minnesota [67]

Karsten Weller, MD
Department of Dermatology and Allergy, Allergie-Centrum-Charité, Charité-Universitätsmedizin Berlin, Berlin, Germany [96]

Victoria Werth, MD
Professor of Dermatology, Department of Dermatology, University of Pennsylvania School of Medicine, Philadelphia, Pennsylvania [184]

Chikoti M. Wheat, MD
Johns Hopkins School of Medicine, Baltimore, Maryland [178]

Lynn D. Wilson, MD, MPH, FASTRO
Professor, Vice Chairman and Clinical Director, Department of Therapeutic Radiology, Yale School of Medicine, New Haven, Connecticut [200]

Lauren E. Wiznia, MD
The Ronald O. Perelman Department of Dermatology, New York University School of Medicine, New York, New York [105]

Peter Wolf, MD
Professor of Dermatology and Bioimmunotherapy, Vice Chair of the Department of Dermatology, Medical University of Graz, Research Unit for Photodermatology, Department of Dermatology, Medical University of Graz, Graz, Austria [92]

Gary S. Wood, MD
Johnson Professor and Chairman, Department of Dermatology, School of Medicine and Public Health, University of Wisconsin-Madison, Madison, Wisconsin [30]

David T. Woodley, MD
Professor and Emeritus Founding Chair, Department of Dermatology, The Keck School of Medicine, University of Southern California, Los Angeles, California [56]

Sophie M. Worobec, MD
University of Illinois at Chicago, Chicago, Illinois [73]

Albert C. Yan, MD, FAAP, FAAD
Chief, Section of Pediatric Dermatology, Children's Hospital of Philadelphia, Professor, Pediatrics and Dermatology, Perelman School of Medicine at the University of Pennsylvania, Philadelphia, Pennsylvania [123]

Kim B. Yancey, MD
Professor and Chair, Department of Dermatology, University of Texas Southwestern Medical Center, Dallas, Texas [55]

Howa Yeung, MD
Chief Resident in Dermatology, Emory University School of Medicine, Atlanta, Georgia [107]

Andrea L. Zaenglein, MD
Professor of Dermatology and Pediatrics, Penn State College of Medicine, Penn State/ Hershey Medical Center, Hershey, Pennsylvania [78, 80]

Jonathan M. Zenilman, MD
Division of Infectious Diseases, Bayview Medical Center, Johns Hopkins University, Baltimore, Maryland [170]

Christos C. Zouboulis, MD, PhD
Departments of Dermatology, Venereology, Allergology and Immunology, Dessau Medical Center, Brandenburg Medical School Theodor Fontane, Dessau, Germany [6, 82, 141]

PREFACE

A much-treasured legacy of Dr. Thomas B. Fitzpatrick, who served as editor-in-chief for the first four editions of the book, *Fitzpatrick's Dermatology in General Medicine* (DIGM) has always aimed to be a comprehensive source of information for those interested in the clinical and basic science of dermatology. Indeed, from the very first edition of *Fitzpatrick's DIGM*, printed in 1971, this authoritative textbook has been grounded in science. We have continued this tradition in the ninth edition of the book whilst rearranging the discussion to make it more reader friendly and to minimize repetition. With coverage of subject matters expanding beyond General Medicine, we have appropriately modified the book title to *Fitzpatrick's Dermatology*. Important general basic science concepts are extensively covered in dedicated chapters appearing in an early section of the book, allowing subsequent clinical chapters to focus on relevant disease-specific pathophysiology in addition to clinical features, diagnosis, clinical course, and management.

Dermatology is a particularly visual specialty. In the preparation of this edition of the book, we have placed special emphasis on display items (in the form of clinical images, tables, and algorithmic summaries), as we strongly believe that these components are vital for the complete understanding of all readers, but particularly for those in training. What better way to optimize the visual content provided in our chapters than to seek input from trainees themselves? We had trainees review every chapter and provide feedback on additional display items they would find useful.

To further enhance the utility of this gold-standard textbook we have also improved the indexing. A good index is imperative to allow readers, including busy practicing clinicians, to easily and quickly find the particular information about a concept, condition, or therapy that they are interested in at any given time. We hope that you agree the improved indexing allows you to achieve this aim.

No modern textbook is complete without an online presence. The ninth edition is also available in the online format, and we plan to regularly post online updates to the book as new studies and/or guidelines are published. You will also have access to other useful features in the online version of *Fitzpatrick's Dermatology* on *AccessMedicine.com*.

Finally, as a completely new group of editors that is diverse in expertise and international in location of practice, we have endeavored to build on the achievements of previous editorial groups led by Drs. Thomas B. Fitzpatrick, Irwin M. Freedberg, Klaus Wolff, and Lowell A. Goldsmith, whilst providing fresh insight into the content, new thinking regarding the optimal structure of the book, and ultimately helping the book to evolve into the most relevant resource for the modern practicing or trainee dermatologist or skin biologist.

Sewon Kang
Masayuki Amagai
Anna L. Bruckner
Alexander H. Enk
David J. Margolis
Amy J. McMichael
Jeffrey S. Orringer

ACKNOWLEDGMENTS

We thank the many expert authors who wrote chapters for the ninth edition of *Fitzpatrick's Dermatology*. We greatly appreciate the time they dedicated to creating their masterpieces and acknowledge how difficult it must have been to fit the task in with the demands of their dermatology practice, teaching, and research. We are truly grateful. We also appreciate their patience with the editorial team while we reviewed the submissions and then reviewed them again because we wanted to carefully consider all the visual elements included in the book.

With regard to visual elements, we owe much gratitude to Noori Kim and Hester Lim who took the time to carefully read every individual chapter and provide detailed feedback on what additional display items they thought would aid the reader. With more than 200 chapters included in the book, we appreciate the sheer enormity of this task and their dedication to attention to detail.

As a completely new editorial board, we are very grateful for the engagement, advice, and encouragement afforded to us by the previous editor-in-chief Lowell A. Goldsmith. We truly appreciate the time and effort he invested to enable the smooth transition of editorial direction for the new edition of this much-loved book.

A special shout-out to Karen Edmonson, our straight-talking and very patient senior editor at McGraw-Hill Education who kept the whole editorial team motivated and helped to bring our ideas to fruition, and to our editorial project manager Bryony Mearns, who helped to coordinate submission and review of the 217 chapters, keep on top of the status of each chapter, and encourage authors and editors to progress with their book-related tasks. We also appreciate the efforts of Kim Davis and Sonam Arora who expertly coordinated everything from submission of the finalized chapters to the McGraw-Hill team through to print publication.

Finally, we are truly grateful for the understanding and patience of our families. Without their support, this textbook would never have been completed. A book like *Fitzpatrick's Dermatology* demands many evening and weekend hours that would normally be spent with loved ones, and we thank them for allowing us to dedicate many of these hours to *Fitzpatrick's Dermatology*.

Sewon Kang
Masayuki Amagai
Anna L. Bruckner
Alexander H. Enk
David J. Margolis
Amy J. McMichael
Jeffrey S. Orringer

CONTENTS

目 录

Volume 1
上 册

PART 1 FOUNDATIONS OF CLINICAL DERMATOLOGY
第一篇　临床皮肤病学基础

1 Fundamentals of Clinical Dermatology: Morphology and Special Clinical Considerations 1
Erin H. Amerson, Susan Burgin, & Kanade Shinkai
　第一章　临床皮肤病学基本原理：形态学和特殊的临床考虑

2 Pathology of Skin Lesions 19
Rosalie Elenitsas & Emily Y. Chu
　第二章　皮疹的病理学

3 Epidemiology and Public Health in Dermatology 42
Junko Takeshita & David J. Margolis
　第三章　皮肤病流行病学和公共卫生学

PART 2 STRUCTURE AND FUNCTION OF SKIN
第二篇　皮肤的结构和功能

4 Developmental Biology of the Skin 53
Luis Garza
　第四章　皮肤发育生物学

5 Growth and Differentiation of the Epidermis 67
Terry Lechler
　第五章　表皮生长和分化

6 Skin Glands: Sebaceous, Eccrine, and Apocrine Glands 76
Christos C. Zouboulis
　第六章　皮肤腺体：皮脂腺、小汗腺和顶泌汗腺

7 Biology of Hair Follicles 96
George Cotsarelis & Vladimir Botchkarev
　第七章　毛囊生物学

8 Nail 114
Krzysztof Kobielak
　第八章　甲

9 Cutaneous Vasculature 124
Peter Petzelbauer, Robert Loewe, & Jordan S. Pober
　第九章　皮肤血管系统

10 The Immunological Structure of the Skin 139
Georg Stingl & Marie-Charlotte Brüggen
　第十章　皮肤免疫系统

11 Cellular Components of the Cutaneous Immune System 153
Johann E. Gudjonsson & Robert L. Modlin
　第十一章　皮肤免疫系统的细胞成分

12 Soluble Mediators of the Cutaneous Immune System 170
Allen W. Ho & Thomas S. Kupper
　第十二章　皮肤免疫系统的可溶性介质

13 Basic Principles of Immunologic Diseases in Skin (Pathophysiology of Immunologic/Inflammatory Skin Diseases) 204
Keisuke Nagao & Mark C. Udey
　第十三章　皮肤免疫性疾病发生的基本原理(免疫性/炎症性皮肤病的病理生理学)

14 Skin Barrier 219
Akiharu Kubo & Masayuki Amagai
　第十四章　皮肤屏障

15 Epidermal and Dermal Adhesion 246
Leena Bruckner-Tuderman & Aimee S. Payne
　第十五章　表皮和真皮的黏附

16 Microbiome of the Skin 268
Heidi H. Kong
　第十六章　皮肤微生物组学

17　Cutaneous Photobiology ⋯⋯⋯⋯⋯⋯ 280
　　Thomas M. Rünger
　　第十七章　皮肤光生物学

18　Genetics in Relation to the Skin ⋯⋯⋯ 305
　　Etienne C. E. Wang, John A. McGrath,
　　& Angela M. Christiano
　　第十八章　皮肤遗传学

19　Carcinogenesis and Skin ⋯⋯⋯⋯⋯⋯ 328
　　Kenneth Y. Tsai & Andrzej A. Dlugosz
　　第十九章　癌变与皮肤

20　Pigmentation and Melanocyte Biology ⋯⋯ 347
　　Stephen M. Ostrowski & David E. Fisher
　　第二十章　色素沉着和黑素细胞生物学

21　Neurobiology of the Skin ⋯⋯⋯⋯⋯⋯ 371
　　Sonja Ständer, Manuel P. Pereira,
　　& Thomas A. Luger
　　第二十一章　皮肤神经生物学

PART 3　DERMATITIS

第三篇　皮炎

22　Atopic Dermatitis ⋯⋯⋯⋯⋯⋯⋯⋯ 383
　　Eric L. Simpson, Donald Y. M. Leung,
　　Lawrence F. Eichenfield, & Mark Boguniewicz
　　第二十二章　特应性皮炎

23　Nummular Eczema, Lichen Simplex
　　Chronicus, and Prurigo Nodularis ⋯⋯⋯ 406
　　Jonathan I. Silverberg
　　第二十三章　钱币状湿疹、慢性单纯性苔
　　　　　　　　藓和结节性痒疹

24　Allergic Contact Dermatitis ⋯⋯⋯⋯⋯ 416
　　Jake E. Turrentine, Michael P. Sheehan,
　　& Ponciano D. Cruz, Jr.
　　第二十四章　变应性接触性皮炎

25　Irritant Dermatitis ⋯⋯⋯⋯⋯⋯⋯⋯ 436
　　Susan T. Nedorost
　　第二十五章　刺激性皮炎

26　Seborrheic Dermatitis ⋯⋯⋯⋯⋯⋯⋯ 451
　　Dae Hun Suh
　　第二十六章　脂溢性皮炎

27　Occupational Skin Diseases ⋯⋯⋯⋯⋯ 462
　　Andy Chern, Casey M. Chern, & Boris D. Lushniak
　　第二十七章　职业性皮肤疾病

PART 4　PSORIASIFORM DISORDERS

第四篇　银屑病样皮肤疾病

28　Psoriasis ⋯⋯⋯⋯⋯⋯⋯⋯⋯⋯⋯ 483
　　Johann E. Gudjonsson & James T. Elder
　　第二十八章　银屑病

29　Pityriasis Rubra Pilaris ⋯⋯⋯⋯⋯⋯ 525
　　Knut Schäkel
　　第二十九章　毛发红糠疹

30　Parapsoriasis and Pityriasis Lichenoides ⋯ 533
　　Stefan M. Schieke & Gary S. Wood
　　第三十章　副银屑病和苔藓样糠疹

31　Pityriasis Rosea ⋯⋯⋯⋯⋯⋯⋯⋯⋯ 547
　　Matthew Clark & Johann E. Gudjonsson
　　第三十一章　玫瑰糠疹

PART 5　LICHENOID AND GRANULOMATOUS DISORDERS

第五篇　苔藓样皮炎和肉芽肿性皮炎

32　Lichen Planus ⋯⋯⋯⋯⋯⋯⋯⋯⋯⋯ 557
　　Aaron R. Mangold & Mark R. Pittelkow
　　第三十二章　扁平苔藓

33　Lichen Nitidus and Lichen Striatus ⋯⋯⋯ 585
　　Aaron R. Mangold & Mark R. Pittelkow
　　第三十三章　光泽苔藓和线状苔藓

34　Granuloma Annulare ⋯⋯⋯⋯⋯⋯⋯ 595
　　Julie S. Prendiville
　　第三十四章　环状肉芽肿

35　Sarcoidosis ⋯⋯⋯⋯⋯⋯⋯⋯⋯⋯ 603
　　Richard Marchell
　　第三十五章　结节病

PART 6　NEUTROPHILIC, EOSINOPHILIC, AND MAST CELL DISORDERS

第六篇　中性粒细胞、嗜酸性粒细胞、肥大细胞相关性疾病

36　Sweet Syndrome ⋯⋯⋯⋯⋯⋯⋯⋯⋯ 619
　　Philip R. Cohen & Razelle Kurzrock
　　第三十六章　Sweet综合征

37 Pyoderma Gangrenosum · · · · · · · · · · · · · · · · · · 638
  Natanel Jourabchi & Gerald S. Lazarus
  第三十七章　坏疽性脓皮病

38 Subcorneal Pustular Dermatosis
  (Sneddon-Wilkinson Disease) · · · · · · · · · · · · · · 651
  Franz Trautinger & Herbert Hönigsmann
  第三十八章　角层下脓疱病

39 Autoinflammatory Disorders · · · · · · · · · · · · · · · 656
  Takashi K. Satoh & Lars E. French
  第三十九章　自身炎症性疾病

40 Eosinophilic Diseases · 685
  Hideyuki Ujiie & Hiroshi Shimizu
  第四十章　嗜酸性粒细胞疾病

41 Urticaria and Angioedema · · · · · · · · · · · · · · · · · 721
  *Michihiro Hide, Shunsuke Takahagi,
  & Takaaki Hiragun*
  第四十一章　荨麻疹和血管性水肿

42 Mastocytosis · 748
  Michael D. Tharp
  第四十二章　肥大细胞增生症

PART 7　REACTIVE ERYTHEMAS
第七篇　反应性红斑

43 Erythema Multiforme · 763
  Jean-Claude Roujeau & Maja Mockenhaupt
  第四十三章　多形红斑

44 Epidermal Necrolysis (Stevens-Johnson
  Syndrome and Toxic Epidermal Necrolysis) · · · · 774
  Maja Mockenhaupt & Jean-Claude Roujeau
  第四十四章　表皮坏死松解症（Stevens-
  Johnson综合征和中毒性表皮
  坏死松解症）

45 Cutaneous Reactions to Drugs · · · · · · · · · · · · · 791
  Kara Heelan, Cathryn Sibbald, & Neil H. Shear
  第四十五章　药物所致皮肤反应

46 Erythema Annulare Centrifugum and Other
  Figurate Erythemas · 808
  Christine S. Ahn & William W. Huang
  第四十六章　离心性环状红斑和其他形态
  红斑

PART 8　DSORDERS OF CORNIFICATION
第八篇　角化异常性疾病

47 The Ichthyoses · 819
  Keith A. Choate & Leonard M. Milstone
  第四十七章　鱼鳞病

48 Inherited Palmoplantar Keratodermas · · · · · · · 861
  Liat Samuelov & Eli Sprecher
  第四十八章　遗传性掌跖角化病

49 Keratosis Pilaris and Other Follicular
  Keratotic Disorders · 913
  Anna L. Bruckner
  第四十九章　毛周角化病和其他毛囊性
  角化疾病

50 Acantholytic Disorders of the Skin · · · · · · · · · · 924
  Alain Hovnanian
  第五十章　棘层松解性皮肤病

51 Porokeratosis · 949
  *Cathal O'Connor, Grainne M. O'Regan,
  & Alan D. Irvine*
  第五十一章　汗孔角化症

PART 9　VESICULOBULLOUS DISORDERS
第九篇　水疱大疱性疾病

52 Pemphigus · 957
  Aimee S. Payne & John R. Stanley
  第五十二章　天疱疮

53 Paraneoplastic Pemphigus · · · · · · · · · · · · · · · · 983
  Grant J. Anhalt & Daniel Mimouni
  第五十三章　副肿瘤性天疱疮

54 Bullous Pemphigoid · 994
  Donna A. Culton, Zhi Liu, & Luis A. Diaz
  第五十四章　大疱性类天疱疮

55 Mucous Membrane Pemphigoid · · · · · · · · · · 1011
  Kim B. Yancey
  第五十五章　黏膜类天疱疮

56 Epidermolysis Bullosa Acquisita · · · · · · · · · · · 1023
  David T. Woodley & Mei Chen
  第五十六章　获得性大疱性表皮松解症

57 Intercellular Immunoglobulin (Ig)
  A Dermatosis (IgA Pemphigus) · · · · · · · · · · · 1034
  Takashi Hashimoto
  第五十七章　细胞间IgA皮病（IgA天疱
  疮）

58 Linear Immunoglobulin A Dermatosis and
  Chronic Bullous Disease of Childhood · · · · · · 1046
  *Matilda W. Nicholas, Caroline L. Rao,
  & Russell P. Hall III*
  第五十八章　线状IgA皮病和儿童慢性大
  疱性皮病

59 Dermatitis Herpetiformis ⋯⋯⋯⋯⋯⋯⋯⋯ 1057
　　Stephen I. Katz
　　第五十九章　疱疹样皮炎

60 Inherited Epidermolysis Bullosa ⋯⋯⋯⋯ 1067
　　M. Peter Marinkovich
　　第六十章　遗传性大疱性表皮松解症

PART 10　AUTOIMMUNE CONNECTIVE TISSUE AND RHEUMATOLOGIC DISORDERS

第十篇　自身免疫结缔组织病和风湿病

61 Lupus Erythematosus ⋯⋯⋯⋯⋯⋯⋯⋯⋯ 1093
　　Clayton J. Sontheimer, Melissa I. Costner,
　　& Richard D. Sontheimer
　　第六十一章　红斑狼疮

62 Dermatomyositis ⋯⋯⋯⋯⋯⋯⋯⋯⋯⋯⋯ 1118
　　Matthew Lewis & David Fiorentino
　　第六十二章　皮肌炎

63 Systemic Sclerosis ⋯⋯⋯⋯⋯⋯⋯⋯⋯⋯ 1144
　　Pia Moinzadeh, Christopher P. Denton,
　　Carol M. Black, & Thomas Krieg
　　第六十三章　系统性硬皮病

64 Morphea and Lichen Sclerosus ⋯⋯⋯⋯⋯ 1165
　　Nika Cyrus & Heidi T. Jacobe
　　第六十四章　硬斑病和硬化性萎缩性苔藓

65 Psoriatic Arthritis and Reactive Arthritis ⋯⋯ 1187
　　Ana-Maria Orbai & John A. Flynn
　　第六十五章　银屑病性关节炎和反应性关节炎

66 Rheumatoid Arthritis, Juvenile Idiopathic Arthritis, Adult-Onset Still Disease, and Rheumatic Fever ⋯⋯⋯⋯⋯⋯⋯⋯⋯⋯⋯ 1207
　　Warren W. Piette
　　第六十六章　类风湿性关节炎、幼年特发性关节炎、成人Still病和风湿热

67 Scleredema and Scleromyxedema ⋯⋯⋯⋯ 1225
　　Roger H. Weenig & Mark R. Pittelkow
　　第六十七章　硬肿症和硬化性黏液水肿

68 Sjögren Syndrome ⋯⋯⋯⋯⋯⋯⋯⋯⋯⋯ 1232
　　Akiko Tanikawa
　　第六十八章　干燥综合征

69 Relapsing Polychondritis ⋯⋯⋯⋯⋯⋯⋯ 1249
　　Camille Francès
　　第六十九章　复发性多软骨炎

PART 11　DERMAL CONNECTIVE TISSUE DISORDERS

第十一篇　真皮结缔组织异常

70 Anetoderma and Other Atrophic Disorders of the Skin ⋯⋯⋯⋯⋯⋯⋯⋯⋯⋯⋯⋯ 1255
　　Catherine Maari & Julie Powell
　　第七十章　斑状萎缩和其他萎缩性皮病

71 Acquired Perforating Disorders ⋯⋯⋯⋯⋯ 1265
　　Garrett T. Desman & Raymond L. Barnhill
　　第七十一章　获得性穿通性皮病

72 Genetic Disorders Affecting Dermal Connective Tissue ⋯⋯⋯⋯⋯⋯⋯⋯⋯⋯ 1275
　　Jonathan A. Dyer
　　第七十二章　影响真皮结缔组织的遗传性疾病

PART 12　SUBCUTANEOUS TISSUE DISORDERS

第十二篇　皮下脂肪疾病

73 Panniculitis ⋯⋯⋯⋯⋯⋯⋯⋯⋯⋯⋯⋯⋯ 1315
　　Eden Pappo Lake, Sophie M. Worobec,
　　& Iris K. Aronson
　　第七十三章　脂膜炎

74 Lipodystrophy ⋯⋯⋯⋯⋯⋯⋯⋯⋯⋯⋯⋯ 1360
　　Abhimanyu Garg
　　第七十四章　脂肪营养不良

Volume 2
中　册

PART 13　MELANOCYTIC DISORDERS

第十三篇　色素细胞性疾病

75 Albinism and Other Genetic Disorders of Pigmentation ⋯⋯⋯⋯⋯⋯⋯⋯⋯⋯ 1375
　　Masahiro Hayashi & Tamio Suzuki
　　第七十五章　白化病和其他遗传性色素性疾病

76 Vitiligo ⋯⋯⋯⋯⋯⋯⋯⋯⋯⋯⋯⋯⋯⋯⋯ 1397
　　Khaled Ezzedine & John E. Harris
　　第七十六章　白癜风

77 Hypermelanoses ⋯⋯⋯⋯⋯⋯⋯⋯⋯⋯⋯ 1419
　　Michelle Rodrigues & Amit G. Pandya
　　第七十七章　色素沉着过度性疾病

PART 14 ACNEIFORM DISORDERS

第十四篇 痤疮样皮肤病

- **78** Acne Vulgaris 1461
  Carolyn Goh, Carol Cheng, George Agak, Andrea L. Zaenglein, Emmy M. Graber, Diane M. Thiboutot, & Jenny Kim
  第七十八章　寻常痤疮

- **79** Rosacea 1490
  Martin Steinhoff & Jörg Buddenkotte
  第七十九章　玫瑰痤疮

- **80** Acne Variants and Acneiform Eruptions 1520
  Andrea L. Zaenglein, Emmy M. Graber, & Diane M. Thiboutot
  第八十章　痤疮异型和痤疮样疹

PART 15 DISORDERS OF ECCRINE AND APOCRINE SWEAT GLANDS

第十五篇 汗腺疾病

- **81** Hyperhidrosis and Anhidrosis 1531
  Anastasia O. Kurta & Dee Anna Glaser
  第八十一章　多汗症和无汗症

- **82** Bromhidrosis and Chromhidrosis 1543
  Christos C. Zouboulis
  第八十二章　腋臭和色汗

- **83** Fox-Fordyce Disease 1551
  Powell Perng & Inbal Sander
  第八十三章　Fox-Fordyce病

- **84** Hidradenitis Suppurativa 1557
  Ginette A. Okoye
  第八十四章　化脓性汗腺炎

PART 16 DISORDERS OF THE HAIR AND NAILS

第十六篇 毛发和甲疾病

- **85** Androgenetic Alopecia 1575
  Ulrike Blume-Peytavi & Varvara Kanti
  第八十五章　雄激素性脱发

- **86** Telogen Effluvium 1588
  Manabu Ohyama
  第八十六章　休止期脱发

- **87** Alopecia Areata 1599
  Nina Otberg & Jerry Shapiro
  第八十七章　斑秃

- **88** Cicatricial Alopecias 1607
  Nina Otberg & Jerry Shapiro
  第八十八章　瘢痕性脱发

- **89** Hair Shaft Disorders 1621
  Leslie Castelo-Soccio & Deepa Patel
  第八十九章　毛干疾病

- **90** Hirsutism and Hypertrichosis 1640
  Thusanth Thuraisingam & Amy J. McMichael
  第九十章　多毛和多毛症

- **91** Nail Disorders 1655
  Eckart Haneke
  第九十一章　甲疾病

PART 17 DISORDERS DUE TO THE ENVIRONMENT

第十七篇 环境引起的皮肤病

- **92** Polymorphic Light Eruption 1699
  Alexandra Gruber-Wackernagel & Peter Wolf
  第九十二章　多形性日光疹

- **93** Actinic Prurigo 1716
  Travis Vandergriff
  第九十三章　光化性痒疹

- **94** Hydroa Vacciniforme 1723
  Travis Vandergriff
  第九十四章　种痘样水疱病

- **95** Actinic Dermatitis 1728
  Robert S. Dawe
  第九十五章　光化性皮炎

- **96** Solar Urticaria 1740
  Marcus Maurer, Joachim W. Fluhr, & Karsten Weller
  第九十六章　日光性荨麻疹

- **97** Phototoxicity and Photoallergy 1747
  Henry W. Lim
  第九十七章　光毒性与光过敏

- **98** Cold Injuries 1756
  Ashley N. Millard, Clayton B. Green, & Erik J. Stratman
  第九十八章　冻伤

- **99** Burns 1769
  Benjamin Levi & Stewart Wang
  第九十九章　烧伤

PART 18 PSYCHOSOCIAL SKIN DISEASE

第十八篇　心理社会性皮肤病

100 Delusional, Obsessive-Compulsive, and Factitious Skin Diseases · · · · · · · · · · · · · · 1783
Mio Nakamura, Josie Howard, & John Y. M. Koo
第一百章　妄想、强迫症和人为皮肤病

101 Drug Abuse · 1796
Nicholas Frank, Cara Hennings, & Jami L. Miller
第一百零一章　药物滥用

102 Physical Abuse · 1809
Kelly M. MacArthur & Annie Grossberg
第一百零二章　身体虐待

PART 19 SKIN CHANGES ACROSS THE SPAN OF LIFE

第十九篇　皮肤在人一生中的变化

103 Neonatal Dermatology · · · · · · · · · · · · · · · · · 1819
Raegan Hunt, Mary Wu Chang, & Kara N. Shah
第一百零三章　新生儿皮肤病学

104 Pediatric and Adolescent Dermatology · · · · · · 1844
Mary Wu Chang
第一百零四章　儿科和青少年皮肤病学

105 Skin Changes and Diseases in Pregnancy · · · · 1861
Lauren E. Wiznia & Miriam Keltz Pomeranz
第一百零五章　妊娠期的皮肤变化和疾病

106 Skin Aging · 1877
Michelle L. Kerns, Anna L. Chien, & Sewon Kang
第一百零六章　皮肤老化

107 Caring for LGBT Persons in Dermatology · · · · 1892
Howa Yeung, Matthew D. Mansh, Suephy C. Chen, & Kenneth A. Katz
第一百零七章　关于LGBT人群的皮肤病学

PART 20 NEOPLASIA

第二十篇　皮肤肿瘤

108 Benign Epithelial Tumors, Hamartomas, and Hyperplasias · 1901
Jonathan D. Cuda, Sophia Rangwala, & Janis M. Taube
第一百零八章　良性上皮肿瘤、错构瘤和增生性病变

109 Appendage Tumors of the Skin · · · · · · · · · · · 1923
Ruth K. Foreman & Lyn McDivitt Duncan
第一百零九章　皮肤附属器肿瘤

110 Epithelial Precancerous Lesions · · · · · · · · · · · 1961
Markus V. Heppt, Gabriel Schlager, & Carola Berking
第一百一十章　上皮癌前病变

111 Basal Cell Carcinoma and Basal Cell Nevus Syndrome · 1989
Jean Y. Tang, Ervin H. Epstein, Jr., & Anthony E. Oro
第一百一十一章　基底细胞癌和基底细胞痣综合征

112 Squamous Cell Carcinoma and Keratoacanthoma · 2006
Anke S. Lonsdorf & Eva N. Hadaschik
第一百一十二章　鳞状细胞癌和角化棘皮瘤

113 Merkel Cell Carcinoma · · · · · · · · · · · · · · · · · 2026
Aubriana McEvoy & Paul Nghiem
第一百一十三章　梅克尔细胞癌

114 Paget's Disease · 2041
Conroy Chow, Isaac M. Neuhaus, & Roy C. Grekin
第一百一十四章　佩吉特病

115 Melanocytic Nevi · 2052
Jonathan D. Cuda, Robert F. Moore, & Klaus J. Busam
第一百一十五章　黑素细胞痣

116 Melanoma · 2090
Jessica C. Hassel & Alexander H. Enk
第一百一十六章　黑色素瘤

117 Histiocytosis · 2127
Astrid Schmieder, Sergij Goerdt, & Jochen Utikal
第一百一十七章　组织细胞增生症

118 Vascular Tumors · 2152
Kelly M. MacArthur & Katherine Püttgen
第一百一十八章　血管性肿瘤

119 Cutaneous Lymphoma · · · · · · · · · · · · · · · · · 2182
Martine Bagot & Rudolf Stadler
第一百一十九章　皮肤淋巴瘤

120 Cutaneous Pseudolymphoma · · · · · · · · · · · · 2219
Werner Kempf, Rudolf Stadler, & Martine Bagot
第一百二十章　皮肤假性淋巴瘤

121 Neoplasias and Hyperplasias of Muscular and Neural Origin · · · · · · · · · · · · · 2242
Hansgeorg Müller & Heinz Kutzner
第一百二十一章　肌肉和神经源性肿瘤与增生

122 Lipogenic Neoplasms ···················2285
Thomas Mentzel & Thomas Brenn

　　第一百二十二章　　脂肪源性肿瘤

PART 21　METABOLIC, GENETIC, AND SYSTEMIC DISEASES

第二十一篇　代谢性、遗传性和全身性疾病

123 Cutaneous Changes in Nutritional Disease ··························2313
Albert C. Yan

　　第一百二十三章　营养性疾病的皮肤改变

124 The Porphyrias ························2349
Eric W. Gou & Karl E. Anderson

　　第一百二十四章　卟啉病

125 Amyloidosis ···························2374
Peter D. Gorevic & Robert G. Phelps

　　第一百二十五章　淀粉样变性

126 Xanthomas and Lipoprotein Disorders ······2390
Vasanth Sathiyakumar, Steven R. Jones, & Seth S. Martin

　　第一百二十六章　黄色瘤和脂蛋白紊乱

127 Fabry Disease ·························2410
Atul B. Mehta & Catherine H. Orteu

　　第一百二十七章　Fabry病

128 Calcium and Other Mineral Deposition Disorders ···························2426
Janet A. Fairley & Adam B. Aronson

　　第一百二十八章　钙和其他矿物沉积紊乱

129 Graft-Versus-Host Disease ··············2440
Kathryn J. Martires & Edward W. Cowen

　　第一百二十九章　移植物抗宿主病

130 Hereditary Disorders of Genome Instability and DNA Repair ···················2463
John J. DiGiovanna, Thomas M. Rünger, & Kenneth H. Kraemer

　　第一百三十章　基因组不稳定性和DNA修复障碍的遗传性疾病

131 Ectodermal Dysplasias ·················2494
Elizabeth L. Nieman & Dorothy Katherine Grange

　　第一百三十一章　外胚层发育不良

132 Genetic Immunodeficiency Diseases ······2517
Ramsay L. Fuleihan & Amy S. Paller

　　第一百三十二章　遗传性免疫缺陷病

133 Skin Manifestations of Internal Organ Disorders ·····················2549
Amy K. Forrestel & Robert G. Micheletti

　　第一百三十三章　内脏疾病的皮肤表现

134 Cutaneous Paraneoplastic Syndromes ······2566
Manasmon Chairatchaneeboon & Ellen J. Kim

　　第一百三十四章　皮肤副肿瘤综合征

135 The Neurofibromatoses ·················2590
Robert Listernick & Joel Charrow

　　第一百三十五章　神经纤维瘤病

136 Tuberous Sclerosis Complex ·············2606
Thomas N. Darling

　　第一百三十六章　结节性硬化症

137 Diabetes and Other Endocrine Diseases ······2620
April Schachtel & Andrea Kalus

　　第一百三十七章　糖尿病和其他内分泌疾病

Volume 3
下　册

PART 22　VASCULAR DISEASES

第二十二篇　血管性疾病

138 Cutaneous Necrotizing Venulitis ···········2655
Nicholas A. Soter

　　第一百三十八章　皮肤坏死性静脉炎

139 Systemic Necrotizing Arteritis ············2669
Peter A. Merkel & Paul A. Monach

　　第一百三十九章　系统性坏死性动脉炎

140 Erythema Elevatum Diutinum ············2694
Theodore J. Alkousakis & Whitney A. High

　　第一百四十章　持久性隆起性红斑

141 Adamantiades–Behçet Disease ············2701
Christos C. Zouboulis

　　第一百四十一章　白塞病

142 Kawasaki Disease ······················2716
Anne H. Rowley

　　第一百四十二章　川崎病

143 Pigmented Purpuric Dermatoses ··········2728
Alexandra Haden & David H. Peng

　　第一百四十三章　色素性紫癜性皮病

144 Cryoglobulinemia and
Cryofibrinogenemia ·············· 2739
Julio C. Sartori-Valinotti & Mark D. P. Davis

  第一百四十四章　冷球蛋白血症和冷纤维蛋白原血症

145 Raynaud Phenomenon ·············· 2755
Drew Kurtzman & Ruth Ann Vleugels

  第一百四十五章　雷诺现象

146 Malignant Atrophic Papulosis
(Degos Disease) ················ 2774
Dan Lipsker

  第一百四十六章　恶性萎缩性丘疹病

147 Vascular Malformations ·············· 2782
Laurence M. Boon, Fanny Ballieux, & Miikka Vikkula

  第一百四十七章　血管畸形

148 Cutaneous Changes in Arterial, Venous, and Lymphatic Dysfunction ·············· 2817
Sabrina A. Newman

  第一百四十八章　动脉、静脉和淋巴管功能障碍的皮肤表现

149 Wound Healing ·············· 2850
Afsaneh Alavi & Robert S. Kirsner

  第一百四十九章　伤口愈合

PART 23　BACTERIAL DISEASES

第二十三篇　细菌性疾病

150 Superficial Cutaneous Infections and Pyodermas ·············· 2871
Lloyd S. Miller

  第一百五十章　浅部皮肤感染和脓皮病

151 Cellulitis and Erysipelas ·············· 2899
David R. Pearson & David J. Margolis

  第一百五十一章　蜂窝织炎和丹毒

152 Gram-Positive Infections Associated with Toxin Production ·············· 2911
Jeffrey B. Travers

  第一百五十二章　产毒素革兰氏阳性细菌感染

153 Necrotizing Fasciitis, Necrotizing Cellulitis, and Myonecrosis ·············· 2924
Avery LaChance & Daniela Kroshinksy

  第一百五十三章　坏死性筋膜炎、坏死性蜂窝组织炎和肌坏死

154 Gram-Negative Coccal and Bacillary Infections ·············· 2937
Breanne Mordorski & Adam J. Friedman

  第一百五十四章　革兰氏阴性球菌和细菌感染

155 The Skin in Infective Endocarditis, Sepsis, Septic Shock, and Disseminated Intravascular Coagulation ·············· 2971
Joseph C. English III & Misha Rosenbach

  第一百五十五章　感染性心内膜炎、脓毒血症、脓毒性休克和弥散性血管内凝血中的皮肤表现

156 Miscellaneous Bacterial Infections with Cutaneous Manifestations ·············· 2983
Scott A. Norton & Michael A. Cardis

  第一百五十六章　混杂细菌感染引起的皮肤表现

157 Tuberculosis and Infections with Atypical Mycobacteria ·············· 3015
Aisha Sethi

  第一百五十七章　结核和非典型分枝杆菌感染

158 Actinomycosis, Nocardiosis, and Actinomycetoma ·············· 3034
Francisco G. Bravo, Roberto Arenas, & Daniel Asz Sigall

  第一百五十八章　放线菌病、诺卡氏菌病和放线菌瘤

159 Leprosy ·············· 3051
Claudio Guedes Salgado, Arival Cardoso de Brito, Ubirajara Imbiriba Salgado, & John Stewart Spencer

  第一百五十九章　麻风病

PART 24　FUNGAL DISEASES

第二十四篇　真菌性疾病

160 Superficial Fungal Infection ·············· 3085
Lauren N. Craddock & Stefan M. Schieke

  第一百六十章　浅部真菌感染

161 Yeast Infections ·············· 3113
Iris Ahronowitz & Kieron Leslie

  第一百六十一章　酵母菌感染

162 Deep Fungal Infections ·············· 3127
Roderick J. Hay

  第一百六十二章　深部真菌感染

PART 25　VIRAL DISEASES

第二十五篇　病毒性疾病

163 Exanthematous Viral Diseases ·············· 3151

Vikash S. Oza & Erin F. D. Mathes
第一百六十三章　病毒疹性疾病

164 Herpes Simplex······3184
Jeffrey I. Cohen
第一百六十四章　单纯疱疹

165 Varicella and Herpes Zoster······3199
Myron J. Levin, Kenneth E. Schmader, & Michael N. Oxman
第一百六十五章　水痘–带状疱疹

166 Poxvirus Infections······3230
Ellen S. Haddock & Sheila Fallon Friedlander
第一百六十六章　痘病毒感染

167 Human Papillomavirus Infections······3261
Jane C. Sterling
第一百六十七章　人乳头瘤病毒感染

168 Cutaneous Manifestations of HIV and Human T-Lymphotropic Virus······3274
Adam D. Lipworth, Esther E. Freeman, & Arturo P. Saavedra
第一百六十八章　HIV和人类嗜T细胞病毒感染的皮肤表现

169 Mosquito-Borne Viral Diseases······3303
Edwin J. Asturias & J. David Beckham
第一百六十九章　蚊媒病毒性疾病

PART 26　SEXUALLY TRANSMITTED DISEASES

第二十六篇　性传播疾病

170 Syphilis······3315
Susan A. Tuddenham & Jonathan M. Zenilman
第一百七十章　梅毒

171 Endemic (Nonvenereal) Treponematoses······3345
Francisco G. Bravo, Carolina Talhari, & Khaled Ezzedine
第一百七十一章　地方性（非性病性）密螺旋体病

172 Chancroid······3360
Stephan Lautenschlager & Norbert H. Brockmeyer
第一百七十二章　软下疳

173 Lymphogranuloma Venereum······3369
Norbert H. Brockmeyer & Stephan Lautenschlager
第一百七十三章　性病性淋巴肉芽肿

174 Granuloma Inguinale······3380
Melissa B. Hoffman & Rita O. Pichardo
第一百七十四章　腹股沟肉芽肿

175 Gonorrhea, Mycoplasma, and Vaginosis······3387
Lindsay C. Strowd, Sean McGregor, & Rita O. Pichardo
第一百七十五章　淋病、支原体感染和细菌性阴道病

PART 27　INFESTATIONS, BITES, AND STINGS

第二十七篇　虫媒叮咬和感染性疾病

176 Leishmaniasis and Other Protozoan Infections······3405
Esther von Stebut
第一百七十六章　利什曼病和其他原虫感染

177 Helminthic Infections······3434
Kathryn N. Suh & Jay S. Keystone
第一百七十七章　蠕虫感染

178 Scabies, Other Mites, and Pediculosis······3458
Chikoti M. Wheat, Craig N. Burkhart, Craig G. Burkhart, & Bernard A. Cohen
第一百七十八章　疥疮、其他螨类和虱病

179 Lyme Borreliosis······3472
Roger Clark & Linden Hu
第一百七十九章　莱姆病

180 The Rickettsioses, Ehrlichioses, and Anaplasmoses······3492
Maryam Liaqat, Analisa V. Halpern, Justin J. Green, & Warren R. Heymann
第一百八十章　立克次体病、埃氏立克次体病和无浆体病

181 Arthropod Bites and Stings······3511
Robert A. Schwartz & Christopher J. Steen
第一百八十一章　节肢动物咬伤和蜇伤

182 Bites and Stings of Terrestrial and Aquatic Life······3526
Camila K. Janniger, Robert A. Schwartz, Jennifer S. Daly, & Mark Jordan Scharf
第一百八十二章　陆生和水生生物的叮咬和蜇伤

PART 28　TOPICAL AND SYSTEMIC TREATMENTS

第二十八篇　外用和系统药物治疗

183 Principles of Topical Therapy······3553
Mohammed D. Saleem, Howard I. Maibach, & Steven R. Feldman
第一百八十三章　外用药物的治疗原则

184 Glucocorticoids ⋯⋯⋯⋯⋯⋯⋯⋯⋯⋯⋯ 3573
Avrom Caplan, Nicole Fett, & Victoria Werth
第一百八十四章　糖皮质激素

185 Retinoids ⋯⋯⋯⋯⋯⋯⋯⋯⋯⋯⋯⋯⋯⋯ 3587
Anna L. Chien, Anders Vahlquist,
Jean-Hilaire Saurat, John J. Voorhees, & Sewon Kang
第一百八十五章　维甲酸类药物

186 Systemic and Topical Antibiotics ⋯⋯⋯⋯ 3600
Sean C. Condon, Carlos M. Isada,
& Kenneth J. Tomecki
第一百八十六章　系统使用和外用抗生素

187 Dapsone ⋯⋯⋯⋯⋯⋯⋯⋯⋯⋯⋯⋯⋯⋯ 3617
Chee Leok Goh & Jiun Yit Pan
第一百八十七章　氨苯砜

188 Antifungals ⋯⋯⋯⋯⋯⋯⋯⋯⋯⋯⋯⋯⋯ 3631
Mahmoud Ghannoum, Iman Salem,
& Luisa Christensen
第一百八十八章　抗真菌药

189 Antihistamines ⋯⋯⋯⋯⋯⋯⋯⋯⋯⋯⋯ 3647
Michael D. Tharp
第一百八十九章　抗组胺药

190 Cytotoxic and Antimetabolic Agents ⋯⋯ 3659
Jeremy S. Honaker & Neil J. Korman
第一百九十章　细胞毒性和抗代谢药

191 Antiviral Drugs ⋯⋯⋯⋯⋯⋯⋯⋯⋯⋯⋯ 3690
Zeena Y. Nawas, Quynh-Giao Nguyen,
Khaled S. Sanber, & Stephen K. Tyring
第一百九十一章　抗病毒药

192 Immunosuppressive and
Immunomodulatory Drugs ⋯⋯⋯⋯⋯⋯ 3715
Drew Kurtzman, Ruth Ann Vleugels, & Jeffrey Callen
第一百九十二章　免疫抑制药和免疫调节药

193 Immunobiologics: Targeted Therapy Against Cytokines, Cytokine Receptors, and Growth Factors in Dermatology ⋯⋯⋯⋯⋯ 3730
Andrew Johnston, Yoshikazu Takada, & Sam T. Hwang
第一百九十三章　免疫生物制剂：皮肤病学中针对细胞因子、细胞因子受体和生长因子的靶向治疗

194 Molecular Targeted Therapies ⋯⋯⋯⋯⋯ 3758
David Michael Miller, Bobby Y. Reddy, & Hensin Tsao
第一百九十四章　分子靶向治疗

195 Antiangiogenic Agents ⋯⋯⋯⋯⋯⋯⋯⋯ 3790
Adilson da Costa, Michael Y. Bonner,
& Jack L. Arbiser
第一百九十五章　抗血管生成抑制药

196 Other Topical Medications ⋯⋯⋯⋯⋯⋯ 3810
Shawn G. Kwatra & Manisha Loss
第一百九十六章　其他外用药

197 Photoprotection ⋯⋯⋯⋯⋯⋯⋯⋯⋯⋯⋯ 3824
Jin Ho Chung
第一百九十七章　光保护剂

PART 29　PHYSICAL TREATMENTS

第二十九篇　物理治疗

198 Phototherapy ⋯⋯⋯⋯⋯⋯⋯⋯⋯⋯⋯⋯ 3837
Tarannum Jaleel, Brian P. Pollack, & Craig A. Elmets
第一百九十八章　光疗

199 Photochemotherapy and Photodynamic
Therapy ⋯⋯⋯⋯⋯⋯⋯⋯⋯⋯⋯⋯⋯⋯ 3867
Herbert Hönigsmann, Rolf-Markus Szeimies,
& Robert Knobler
第一百九十九章　光化学疗法和光动力疗法

200 Radiotherapy ⋯⋯⋯⋯⋯⋯⋯⋯⋯⋯⋯⋯ 3891
Roy H. Decker & Lynn D. Wilson
第二百章　放疗

PART 30　DERMATOLOGIC SURGERY

第三十篇　皮肤外科

201 Cutaneous Surgical Anatomy ⋯⋯⋯⋯⋯ 3903
Arif Aslam & Sumaira Z. Aasi
第二百零一章　皮肤外科解剖学

202 Perioperative Considerations in
Dermatologic Surgery ⋯⋯⋯⋯⋯⋯⋯⋯ 3913
Noah Smith, Kelly B. Cha, & Christopher Bichakjian
第二百零二章　皮肤科手术的围手术期注意事项

203 Excisional Surgery and Repair,
Flaps, and Grafts ⋯⋯⋯⋯⋯⋯⋯⋯⋯⋯ 3934
Adele Haimovic, Jessica M. Sheehan,
& Thomas E. Rohrer
第二百零三章　肿物切除术和修复、皮瓣和皮片移植

204 Mohs Micrographic Surgery ⋯⋯⋯⋯⋯⋯ 3970
Sean R. Christensen & David J. Leffell
第二百零四章　莫氏显微外科

205 Nail Surgery ⋯⋯⋯⋯⋯⋯⋯⋯⋯⋯⋯⋯ 3984
Robert Baran & Olivier Cogrel
第二百零五章　甲部手术

206 Cryosurgery and Electrosurgery ⋯⋯⋯⋯ 4002

Justin J. Vujevich & Leonard H. Goldberg

第二百零六章　冷冻疗法和电疗法

PART 31　COSMETIC DERMATOLOGY

第三十一篇　美容皮肤学

207 Cosmeceuticals and Skin Care in Dermatology ·················· 4015
Leslie Baumann

第二百零七章　化妆品和皮肤护理

208 Fundamentals of Laser and Light-Based Treatments ·················· 4033
Omer Ibrahim & Jeffrey S. Dover

第二百零八章　激光原理和光学治疗

209 Laser Skin Resurfacing: Cosmetic and Medical Applications ················ 4048
Bridget E. McIlwee & Tina S. Alster

第二百零九章　激光皮肤表皮重建：美容和医疗应用

210 Nonablative Laser and Light-Based Therapy: Cosmetic and Medical Indications ·········· 4061
Jeffrey S. Orringer

第二百一十章　非剥脱激光和以光为基础的治疗：美容和医学适应证

211 Noninvasive Body Contouring ············ 4073
Murad Alam

第二百一十一章　无创塑形

212 Treatment of Varicose Veins and Telangiectatic Lower-Extremity Vessels ······ 4088
Daniel P. Friedmann, Vineet Mishra, & Jeffrey T. S. Hsu

第二百一十二章　下肢静脉曲张和毛细血管扩张的治疗

213 Chemical Peels and Dermabrasion ·········· 4113
Gary Monheit & Bailey Tayebi

第二百一十三章　化学剥脱术和磨削术

214 Liposuction Using Tumescent Local Anesthesia ························ 4125
C. William Hanke, Cheryl J. Gustafson, William G. Stebbins, & Aimee L. Leonard

第二百一十四章　局部麻醉下的肿胀吸脂术

215 Soft-Tissue Augmentation ················ 4130
Lisa M. Donofrio & Dana L. Ellis

第二百一十五章　软组织填充术

216 Botulinum Toxin ···················· 4142
Richard G. Glogau

第二百一十六章　肉毒杆菌毒素

217 Hair Transplantation ·················· 4153
Robin H. Unger & Walter P. Unger

第二百一十七章　毛发移植

Foundations of Clinical Dermatology

PART 1

第一篇 临床皮肤病学基础

Chapter 1 :: Fundamentals of Clinical Dermatology: Morphology and Special Clinical Considerations
:: Erin H. Amerson, Susan Burgin, & Kanade Shinkai

第一章
临床皮肤病学基本原理：形态学和特殊的临床考虑

中文导读

皮肤病具有独特的形态学和分布特点，皮肤的形态和反应模式提示疾病的病理生理学特点，有助于鉴别诊断。详细询问病史，运用皮肤病学专业术语，全面（包括毛发和甲）的皮肤黏膜检查，对诊断非常重要。

本章从以下几个方面全面阐述了临床皮肤病学基本原理。

1. 皮肤病诊断的艺术和科学 本部分作者讲到了识别皮肤病的原发皮疹与反应模式，对诊断与治疗皮肤病是至关重要的。运用皮肤病专业术语，获得患者详细的病史与整体健康状态，准确识别皮疹形态，是皮肤病诊断的艺术。

2. 接触病人

（1）病史询问：询问病史非常重要，而且要与患者的主观症状结合起来。对于已经诊断的病例，要验证诊断是否正确，并评估治疗和监测病情进展与并发症，提出修改治疗意见。表1-1概述了采集病史的方法。

（2）体格检查：完整的皮肤检查包括对整个皮肤表面的检查，不要忽略以下区域，如头皮、眼睑、鼻、口腔、耳朵、生殖器、臀部、肛门、会阴和指趾间。全面评估可以提高诊断率，降低漏诊率。体格检查指南详见表1-2。

3. 皮肤病的形态学 本部分详细介绍了各种原发皮损和继发皮损的形态、颜色、分布、是否曝光部位、皮脂溢出部位、局部性、泛发性、对称性等。具体见表1-4、表1-5。另外表1-6概述了一些临床症状和体征与某些特殊皮肤病或系统性疾病的关系。

4．皮疹的反应模式 当没有明显的形态特征、构型或分布时，反应模式是特别有用的工具，确定反应模式可以帮助制订指南（表1-7~表1-15）和初始治疗。确定反应模式的第一步是识别原发皮损，要注意某些皮肤病不只是一种反应模式。

5．结论 形态学是皮肤病学的重中之重，可以获得正确的诊断并加深了解皮肤病临床与病理的关系。仔细评估皮肤和全身状况，是皮肤病诊断学中至关重要的。

〔陈明亮〕

AT-A-GLANCE

- Skin diseases have characteristic morphology and distribution.
- Morphologic characteristics and reaction patterns of the skin suggest disease pathophysiology, helping focus the differential diagnosis.
- The history is indispensable in elucidating complex diagnoses.
- Knowledge and appropriate use of dermatologic terminology is essential.
- The comprehensive mucocutaneous examination, including hair and nails, should always be performed.

THE ART AND SCIENCE OF DERMATOLOGIC DIAGNOSIS

The diagnosis and treatment of cutaneous diseases requires the physician's ability to recognize the primary lesions and reaction patterns of the skin, and to put these visual clues into context with the patient's history and overall health. In this chapter, we discuss a fundamental approach to the patient presenting with a skin problem. We introduce the technical vocabulary of dermatologic description, also known as morphology. Accurately identifying morphology is an essential step in generating a differential diagnosis. Use of standard dermatologic terminology is also critical for effective clinical documentation, research, and communication with other health care providers.

The process of examining and describing skin lesions requires perception of subtle details: appreciation of a specific hue of erythema, a shape or distribution, or the presence of characteristic findings on nails or mucous membranes often hold the key to the correct diagnosis. Repeated patient encounters help to train the eye to recognize such patterns. With time and experience, the physician can associate clinical skin findings with histopathologic features, enabling a rich understanding of the pathophysiology of skin disease, as well as clinical-pathologic correlation.

APPROACH TO THE PATIENT

HISTORY

Dermatology is a visual specialty, and some skin conditions may be diagnosed at a glance. History may be crucial in complex cases, such as the patient with rash and fever, or the patient with generalized pruritus. There is therapeutic value in receiving a patient's narrative thread, as they feel heard, and they may reveal information relevant to treatment choice or invite opportunities for education and reassurance. In practice, many dermatologists take a brief history, perform a physical examination, then undertake more detailed questioning based on the differential diagnosis that the examination suggests.

In taking a history from a patient presenting with a new skin complaint, the physician's primary goal is to establish a diagnosis, with a secondary goal of evaluating the patient as a candidate for therapy. In patients whose diagnosis is already established, the physician's goals are to reevaluate the original diagnosis, monitor disease progress and complications, and modify treatment accordingly.

Table 1-1 presents an approach to obtaining the history in a patient presenting with a skin problem. The physician may choose to customize the history depending on whether the chief complaint is a growth or an eruption, a nail or hair disorder, or another condition, and whether it is a new problem or a followup visit for an ongoing condition.

TABLE 1-1
History Taking in Dermatologic Diagnosis

Chief Complaint and History of the Present Illness
- **Duration:** When the condition was first noted and dates of recurrences or remissions
- **Timing:** Constant, intermittent, worst at night, worst in winter
- **Evolution:** How the condition has changed or progressed over time
- **Location:** Where lesions were first noted, and how they have spread, if applicable
- **Symptoms:** Pruritus, pain, bleeding, nonhealing, change of preexisting skin lesions, associated with fever or other systemic signs
- **Severity:** Ask patient to rate severity of pain or pruritus on a 10-point scale to follow severity over time
- **Ameliorating and Exacerbating Factors:** Sun exposure, heat, cold, trauma, exposures (such as chemicals, medications, cosmetics, perfumes, plants, or metals), relation to menses or pregnancy
- Preceding illness, new medications, new topical products, or exposures
- Therapies tried, including nonprescription or home remedies, and response to therapy
- Prior similar problems, prior diagnosis, results of biopsies or other studies performed

Medical History
- A history of all chronic illnesses, particularly those that may manifest in the skin, (diabetes, renal and hepatic disease, infection with HIV or other viruses, polycystic ovarian syndrome, lupus, thyroid disease) and those that are associated with skin disease (asthma, allergies)
- History of surgical procedures, including organ transplantation
- *Immunosuppression:* iatrogenic, infectious, or inherited
- Pregnancies
- Psychiatric disease
- History of blistering sunburns, exposure to arsenic or ionizing radiation
- **Medication History:** A detailed history, including prescriptions, nonprescription medications, vitamins, dietary supplements, herbal remedies, with particular attention to those medications started recently
- **Allergies:** To medications, foods, environmental antigens, and contactants
- **Social History:** Occupation, hobbies and leisure activities, alcohol and tobacco use, illicit drug use, sexual history (including high-risk activities for sexually transmitted diseases), diet, bathing habits, pets, living conditions (eg, alone, with family, homeless, in an institution), history of travel or residence in endemic areas for infectious diseases, cultural or religious practices
- **Family History:** Of skin disease, atopy (atopic dermatitis, asthma, hay fever) or skin cancer
- **Review of Systems:** May be focused or comprehensive depending on the diagnosis (asking about specific symptoms that may accompany a dermatologic condition, such as joint symptoms in psoriasis; asking a comprehensive ROS in the setting of cutaneous signs of systemic disease such as palpable purpura)

PHYSICAL EXAMINATION

SCOPE OF THE COMPLETE CUTANEOUS EXAMINATION

The complete cutaneous examination includes inspection of the entire skin surface, including often-overlooked areas such as the scalp, eyelids, ears, genitals, buttocks, perineum, and interdigital spaces; the hair; the nails; and the mucous membranes of the eyes, nose, mouth, genitals, and anus. Patients presenting with a highly focused complaint, such as a single wart or acne, may not require a comprehensive skin examination in routine clinical practice. There are many advantages to performing a complete cutaneous examination, including identification of potentially harmful lesions, such as skin cancers, providing reassurance for benign skin findings, locating additional diagnostic clues (Wickham's striae on the buccal mucosa in lichen planus, for instance), opportunities for patient education (eg, lentigines are a sign of sun damage and suggest the need for improved sun protection), and an opportunity to convey the physician's concern about the patient's skin health through a thorough examination. A thorough evaluation increases the possibility of making a diagnosis at the bedside and mitigates the risk of overlooking another diagnosis. A guide to performing the physical examination of the patient presenting with a skin problem is presented in Table 1-2.

IDEAL CONDITIONS FOR THE COMPLETE SKIN EXAMINATION

A complete skin examination is most effective when performed under ideal conditions. Excellent lighting, preferably bright, natural light, is paramount; without good lighting, subtle but important details may be missed. The patient should be fully undressed, and gowned with additional draping, if desired.

TABLE 1-2
Physical Examination in Dermatologic Diagnosis

General Impression of the Patient
- Well or ill
- Obese, cachectic, or normal weight
- **Skin Color:** Degree of pigmentation, pallor (anemia), jaundice
- **Skin Temperature:** Warm, cool, or clammy
- **Skin Surface Characteristics:** Xerosis (dryness), seborrhea (excessive oil), turgor, hyper- or hypohidrosis (excessive or decreased sweating), and texture
- **Degree of Photoaging:** Lentigines, actinic purpura, rhytides

Morphology
- Define the primary lesion
- Describe their color, texture
- Describe any secondary changes
- Describe their shape and configuration
- Describe the Distribution of Lesions: Localized (isolated), grouped, regional, generalized, universal, symmetrical, sun-exposed, flexural, extensor extremities, acral, intertriginous, dermatomal, follicular

Aspects of General Physical Examination That May Be Helpful
- Vital signs
- Abdominal examination for hepatosplenomegaly
- Pulses
- Lymph node examination (especially in cases of suspected infection and malignancy)

Underwear, socks, shoes, makeup, and eyeglasses should be removed. The examining table should be at a comfortable height, with a head that reclines, an extendable footrest, and gynecologic stirrups. The examining room should be at a comfortable temperature for the lightly dressed patient. It should contain a sink for hand washing and disinfecting hand foam, as patients are reassured by seeing their physician wash hands before the examination. If the patient and physician are of opposite genders, having a chaperone in the room may be required.

RECOMMENDED TOOLS FOR THE COMPLETE SKIN EXAMINATION

Although the physician's eyes and hands are the only essential tools for examination of the skin, the following are often useful and highly recommended:

- A magnifying tool such as a loupe, magnifying glass, and/or dermatoscope.
- A bright focused light such as a flashlight or penlight.
- Glass slides for diascopy and viral direct fluorescent antibody (DFA) testing, fungal scrapings and touch preparations, Tzanck smears, scabies prep.
- Alcohol pads to remove scale or surface oil.
- Gauze pads or tissues with water for removing makeup.
- Gloves: when any contagious condition is suspected, when contact with body fluids is possible, when examining mucous membranes and genital areas, and when performing any procedure.
- A ruler for measuring lesions.
- No. 15 and No. 11 scalpel blades for scraping and incising lesions, respectively.
- Diagnostic solutions: potassium hydroxide solution, oil, Tzanck smear, bacterial, viral, and fungal culture media.
- A camera for photographic documentation.
- A Wood lamp (365 nm) for highlighting subtle pigmentary changes.

TECHNIQUE OF THE DERMATOLOGIC PHYSICAL EXAMINATION

Consistency in a comprehensive mucocutaneous examination is essential to ensure that no areas are overlooked. One approach to the complete skin examination is presented here. First, observe the patient at a distance for general impressions (eg, asymmetry due to a stroke, cachexia, jaundice). Next, examine the patient in a systematic way, usually from head to toe, uncovering one area at a time to preserve patient modesty. Move the patient and the illumination as needed for the best view of each body area. Sometimes side lighting best reveals depth and details of skin lesion borders. Palpate lesions to determine whether they are soft, firm, tender, or fluid-filled. A magnifier worn on the head leaves both hands free for palpation of lesions. Certain lesions, especially pigmented lesions, are best examined with a dermatoscope to identify characteristic concerning features. Mucosal sites should be carefully examined with additional illumination with a penlight or flashlight. During the examination, patients may be reassured by the physician's reporting of benign lesions as they are encountered.

Special examination techniques for hair and nail disorders are discussed in Chaps. 85 through 91.

After completing the examination, it is important to document the skin findings, including the type of lesions and their locations, either descriptively or on a body map. Specific documentation using photography and triangulation based on anatomic landmarks is particularly important for lesions suspicious for skin malignancy undergoing biopsy, so that the exact location may be found and definitively treated at a later date.

INTRODUCTION TO MORPHOLOGY

Joseph Jakob von Plenck's (1738–1807) and Robert Willan's (1757–1812) work in defining basic morphologic terminology laid the foundation for the description and comparison of fundamental lesions, thereby facilitating characterization and recognition of skin disease.

The eminent dermatology professors Wolff and Johnson have asserted: to read words, one must recognize letters; to read the skin, one must recognize the basic lesions. The "letters," or elemental building blocks of morphology, are the primary lesion and secondary (epidermal) change. The skilled clinician uses macroscopic characteristics noted on examination to understand where and what types of microscopic pathologic changes are present, achieving clinical–pathologic correlation. For example, flat-topped or planar papules and plaques tend to be processes affecting the epidermis and superficial dermis, while dome-shaped or nodular lesions often exhibit deeper infiltration into the dermis or subcutis. Scaling or crusting indicates that the epidermis is affected, while a smooth, intact surface on a palpable lesion reflects a purely dermal or subcutaneous process.

The combination of primary morphology and secondary change (or absence of secondary change) determine a diagnostic category, also known as the "reaction pattern." For example, when the primary lesion is a circumscribed papule or plaque with scale, it likely falls into the "papulosquamous" reaction pattern, which suggests a specific set of diagnostic possibilities. Once the reaction pattern has been determined, a differential diagnosis comes into focus. This differential diagnosis may be further honed by other lesional characteristics, including shape or color, and the arrangement of lesions in relationship to one another (configuration)

TABLE 1-3
Primary Morphology

PRIMARY LESION	SIZE	TOPOGRAPHY	CONTENTS
Macule	<1 cm	Flat	N/A (color change only)
Patch	≥1 cm	Flat	N/A (color change only)
Papule	<1 cm	Raised/Depressed	Solid
Plaque	≥1 cm	Raised/Depressed	Solid
Nodule	≥1 cm	Raised	Solid or fluid
Vesicle	<1 cm	Raised	Fluid (serum, blood, lymph)
Bulla	≥1 cm	Raised	Fluid (serum, blood, lymph)
Pustule	<1 cm	Raised	Fluid (pus)
Erosion	Any	Depressed	N/A
Ulceration	Any	Depressed	N/A

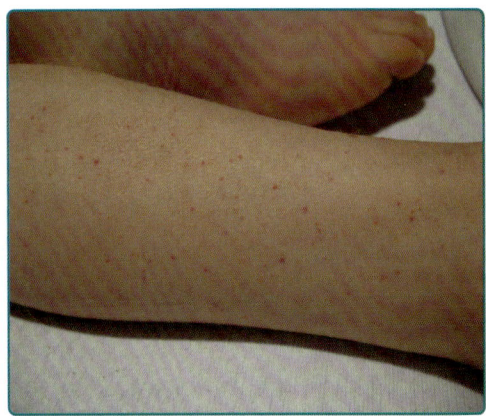

Figure 1-1 Macule, petechiae.

and on the body (distribution).

It is important for the dermatologist in training to be aware that variation and ambiguity in definitions of morphologic terms exist among the dermatology community. For example, in dermatology textbooks, a papule has been described as no greater than 1 cm in size, no less than 0.5 cm, or ranging from the size of a pinhead to that of a split pea. In this chapter, the authors have selected definitions that reduce the subjectivity inherent in some morphologic frameworks.

PRIMARY MORPHOLOGY

The primary morphology describes 3 lesional characteristics: size, topography, and the character of contents (Table 1-3). The primary morphology should be the "noun" which all other "adjectives" (such as color, shape, size, texture) describe. A macule or patch is not palpable (a color change only) and raised or depressed lesions that are palpable are papules or plaques. Erosions and ulcerations may be primary or secondary.

FLAT (NONPALPABLE) PRIMARY LESIONS

Macule: A macule is flat, even with the surface level of surrounding skin or mucous membranes, and perceptible only as an area of color different from the surrounding skin or mucous membrane. Macules are less than 1 cm in size (Fig. 1-1).

Patch: A patch, like a macule, is a flat area of skin or mucous membranes with a different color from its surrounding. Patches are 1 cm or larger in size (Fig. 1-2).

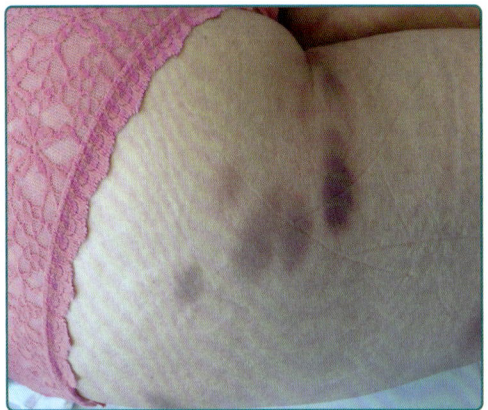

Figure 1-2 Patch, fixed drug eruption.

RAISED (PALPABLE) PRIMARY LESIONS

Papule: A papule is an elevated or depressed lesion less than 1 cm in size, which may be solid or cystic. Among other characteristics, papules may be further described by their topography. Some examples include papules that are sessile, pedunculated, dome-shaped,

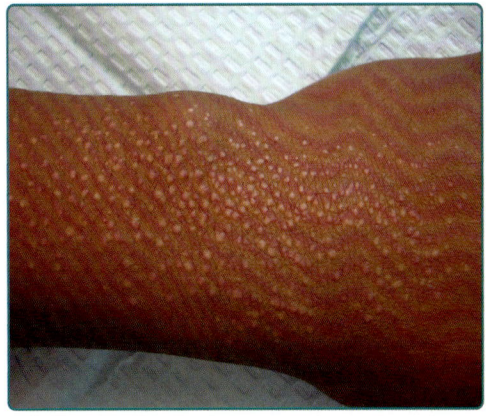

Figure 1-3 Papule, lichen nitidus.

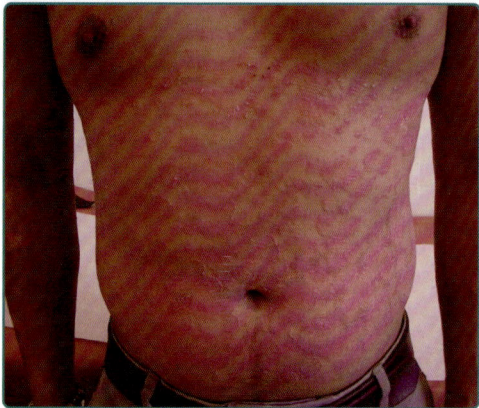

Figure 1-4 Plaque, psoriasis.

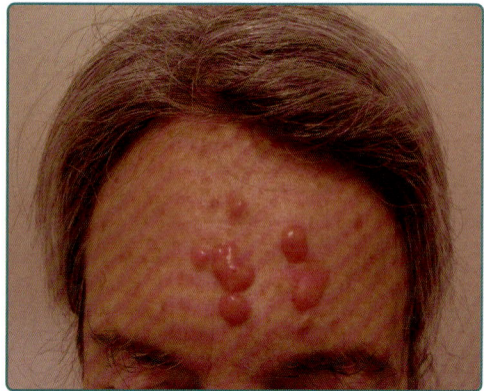

Figure 1-5 Nodule, lymphoma cutis.

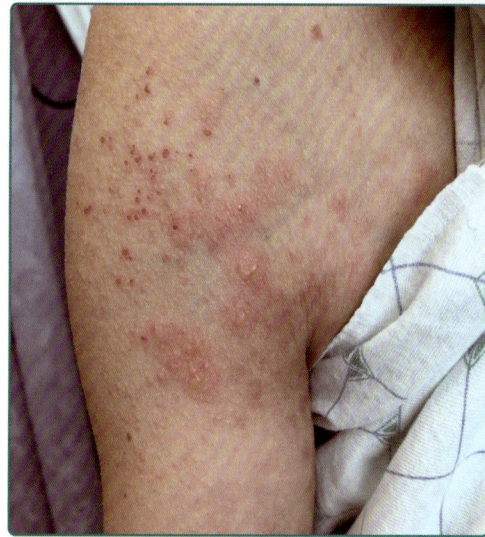

Figure 1-6 Vesicle, bullous lupus erythematosus. Note brown incipient crusts marking the sites of earlier blisters now ruptured.

flat-topped, filiform, mammillated, acuminate (conical), or umbilicated (Fig. 1-3).

Plaque: A plaque is a solid plateau-like elevation or depression that has a diameter of 1 cm or larger (Fig. 1-4).

Nodule: A nodule is a palpable lesion greater than 1 cm with a domed, spherical or ovoid shape. They may be solid or cystic. Depending on the anatomic component(s) primarily involved, nodules are of 5 main types: (1) epidermal, (2) epidermal–dermal, (3) dermal, (4) dermal–subdermal, and (5) subcutaneous. Texture is an important additional feature of nodules: firm, soft, boggy, fluctuant, etc. Similarly, different surfaces of nodules, such as smooth, keratotic, ulcerated, or fungating, also help direct diagnostic considerations (Fig. 1-5). *Tumor*, also sometimes included under the heading of nodule, may be used to describe a more irregularly shaped mass, benign or malignant.

FLUID-FILLED PRIMARY LESIONS

Vesicle and Bulla: A vesicle is a fluid-filled papule smaller than 1 cm (Fig. 1-6), whereas a bulla (blister) measures 1 cm or larger (Fig. 1-7). By definition, the wall is thin and translucent enough to visualize the contents, which may be clear, serous, or hemorrhagic. Vesicles and bullae arise from cleavage at various levels of the epidermis (intraepidermal) or the dermal–epidermal interface (subepidermal), sometimes extending into the dermis. The tenseness or flaccidity of the vesicle or bulla may help determine the depth of the split. However, reliable differentiation requires histopathologic examination of the blister edge.

Pustule: A pustule is a circumscribed, raised papule in the epidermis or infundibulum containing visible pus. The purulent exudate, composed of leukocytes with or without cellular debris, may contain organisms or may be sterile. The exudate may be white, yellow, or greenish-yellow in color. Pustules may vary in size and, in certain situations, may coalesce to form "lakes" of pus. When associated with hair follicles, pustules may appear conical and contain a hair in the center (Fig. 1-8).

SECONDARY CHANGE (EPIDERMAL OR SURFACE CHANGE)

Scale is a macroscopic finding indicating a change in the epidermis, usually the stratum corneum. Scale may have many different descriptive characteristics, for instance, soft, rough, gritty, bran-like, or micaceous (Table 1-4).

Crust describes dried fluid on the skin's surface due to serum, blood, pus, or a combination. When crust is round or oval, it points to the former presence of a vesicle, bulla or pustule (as seen in Fig. 1-6). Linear or

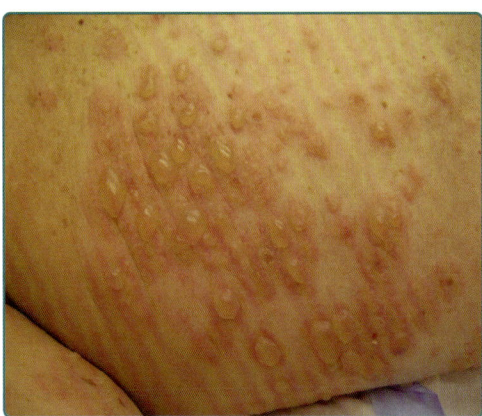

Figure 1-7 Vesicles and bullae, linear IgA disease.

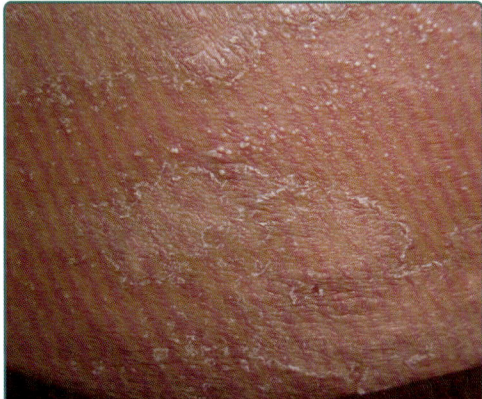

Figure 1-8 Pustule, pustular psoriasis.

angulated crusts are indicative of excoriations. Other specialized types of crust include eschar, which is dry, adherent, and dark red-purple, brown, or black in color and signals skin necrosis (Fig. 1-11), or fibrin, which is a soft, yellow crust on the surface of some ulcers.

Lichenification is a thickening and accentuation of the skin lines that results from repeated rubbing or scratching of the skin. It is found primarily in chronic eczematous processes or neurogenic processes (Fig. 1-12).

Atrophy of the epidermis results in a shiny quality with "cigarette-paper" wrinkling. Atrophy of the dermis results in a depressed lesion.

A *fissure* is a linear loss of continuity of the skin's surface or mucosa that results from excessive tension or decreased elasticity of the involved tissue. Fissures frequently occur on the palms and soles where the thick stratum corneum is least expandable.

OTHER LESIONAL CHARACTERISTICS

In addition to primary morphology, other features of lesions can be important in narrowing a differential diagnosis; sometimes, these other characteristics are the most important determinants of the differential. For instance, the most notable feature of a rash or lesion might be its shape or distribution, which points the clinician to a specific list of possible diagnoses.

TABLE 1-4 Types of Scale

TYPE OF SCALE	DESCRIPTION
Craquelé/xerotic	Desquamation giving the appearance of dried, cracked skin. Combination of hyperkeratosis and fissuring, which appears like the cracked bed of a dry river.
Cutaneous horn	Conical projection of compact stratum corneum.
Exfoliative/desquamative	Scales split off from the epidermis in finer scales or in sheets.
Follicular	Scales appear as keratotic plugs, spines, or filaments.
Gritty	Densely adherent scale with a sandpaper texture.
Ichthyosiform	Scales are regular, polygonal plates arranged in parallel rows or diamond patterns (fish-like, tessellated, Fig. 1-9).
Keratotic/hyperkeratotic	Scales appear as thick, compact, adherent layers of stratum corneum.
Lamellar	Scales are thin large plates or shields attached in the middle and looser around the edges.
Pityriasiform	Scale is small and branny.
Psoriasiform (micaceous and ostraceous)	Scale is silvery and brittle and forms thin plates in several loose sheets, like mica (micaceous scale). Large scales may accumulate in heaps, giving the appearance of an oyster shell (ostraceous scale, Fig. 1-10).
Seborrheic	Scales are thick, waxy or greasy, yellow-to-brown, flakes.
Shellac-like	Scale is shiny with a sheet-like desquamating edge, like peeling paint.
Wickham striae	Scale appears as a lacy white pattern overlying violaceous flat-topped papules.

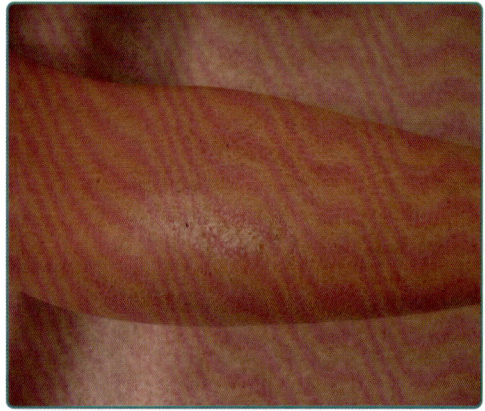

Figure 1-9 Ichthyosiform scale, ichthyosis vulgaris.

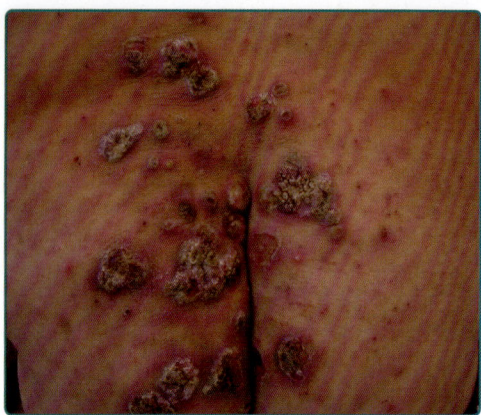

Figure 1-10 Ostraceous scale, psoriasis.

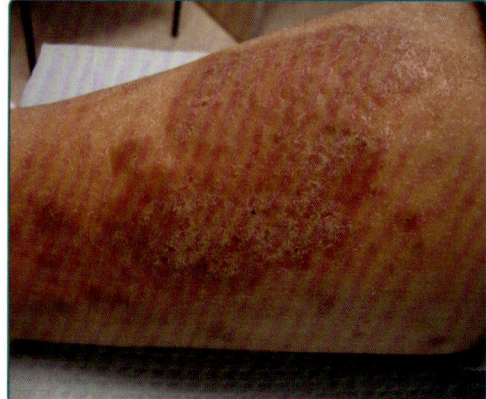

Figure 1-12 Lichenification, lichen simplex chronicus.

COLOR

Perhaps the most important additional feature of a lesion other than primary morphology is color. The experienced dermatologist will notice subtle variations in hue and saturation of a particular color, and can ascribe meaning to these variations. The most common types of color on the skin are variations in brown (hyperpigmentation) and red (erythema), which will be discussed in depth below. Other colors and their histopathologic correlations are described in Table 1-5.

Brown: Brown color is most often representative of melanin, either within melanocytes or outside of melanocytes. Less frequently, a brown hue also may be caused by deposition of other pigments, cells, or materials in the dermis (such as deposition of hemosiderin, amyloid, or mucin; certain types of inflammation, including inflammation that is granulomatous, histiocytic, plasmacytic, or mixed). Mast cells induce melanin production in the overlying epidermis, often leading to brown color overlying the focus of mast cells in the dermis. Melanin in the epidermis, whether contained within or outside of melanocytes, appears tan to muddy brown; when it is very concentrated, as in some nevi or melanomas or heavily pigmented seborrheic keratoses, it may appear brown-black. Melanin in the dermis, either within melanocytes or extracellular, may appear brown, gray, or blue. This gray-blue color results from the "Tyndall effect," named for the 19th-century physicist John Tyndall, who described the preferential transmission of longer wavelengths (blue photospectrum) when particles are suspended in a medium (in this case, melanin or other brown pigment suspended in the dermis). Differentiation between epidermal and dermal melanin also can be aided by a Wood lamp, which accentuates epidermal but not dermal melanin.

Oxidized keratin, (within an infundibular cyst, for instance) and foreign pigmentation (such as tattoos) can also exhibit the Tyndall effect when located in the dermis.

When the epidermis is inflamed or damaged, melanin often drops to into the dermis. Therefore, many subacute, chronic, or recently resolved epidermal inflammatory diseases or injuries have a brown or gray-brown tone. The more constitutive pigment in an individual's skin, the more prominent these changes will be.

Red: Also known as "erythema," red can have infinite hues. Pale red, pink, or purple may result from inflammation leading to hyperemia (subtle vascular dilation). More saturated red to purple can indicate intense hyperemia or vascular congestion (also called rubor, as seen in erysipelas); even more saturated red to purple hue can result from the either malformed or ectopic blood vessels (Fig. 1-13) or extravasated erythrocytes (petechiae or purpura, see "vascular reaction pattern" below). Variations in the hue of erythema are vast and provide subtle clues to the type of inflammation present. True red is often associated with neutrophilic inflammation (as seen in cellulitis or Sweet syndrome); red-purple (violaceous erythema, Fig. 1-14) with lymphocytic inflammation (lymphoma cutis, connective tissue disease, interface reactions such as lichen planus). Granulomatous inflammation may appear red-brown (sarcoidosis, marked by the classis "apple jelly" color seen in Fig. 1-15, or a juvenile xanthogranuloma) to orange or yellow (Fig. 1-16, necrobiosis lipoidica). One

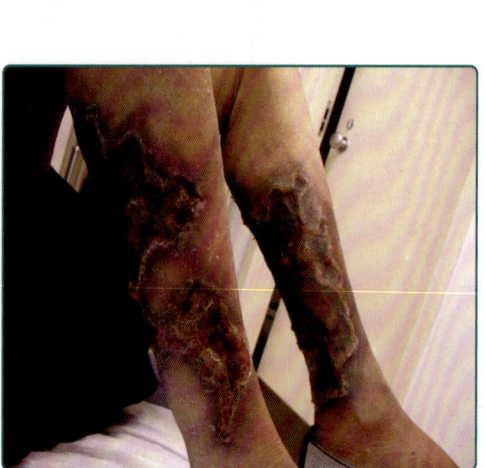

Figure 1-11 Eschar overlying stellate purpura, calciphylaxis.

TABLE 1-5
Implications of Color Changes in Altered Skin

COLOR	PATHOLOGY	DIAGNOSTIC EXAMPLES
White	Reduced or absent melanin synthesis	Tinea versicolor, vitiligo
	Keratin	Milium
	Calcium deposit	Calcinosis cutis
	Scar	Atrophie blanche
Black	Dense melanin	Melanoma
	Intraepidermal hemorrhage	Talon noir
	Necrosis	Cutaneous anthrax
	Oxidized keratin (brown to black)	Open comedone
Brown	Melanin	Melanocytic nevus, melasma
Red-brown	Hemosiderin ("cayenne pepper")	Pigmented purpuric dermatosis
	Granulomatous inflammation ("apple jelly")	Sarcoidosis (Fig. 1-15)
	Histiocytic inflammation	Langerhans cell histiocytosis
	Mixed inflammation	Granuloma faciale
	Plasmacytic inflammation ("copper"- or "ham"-colored)	Secondary syphilis
	Mast cell inflammation	Urticaria pigmentosa
	Mucin deposition	Pretibial myxedema
	Amyloid deposition	Lichen amyloidosis
	Infiltration with smooth muscle	Cutaneous leiomyoma
	Subacute or chronic epidermal inflammation	Subacute lupus erythematosus
Red	Vascular dilation or congestion	Erysipelas
	Neutrophilic inflammation	Sweet syndrome
	Vascular neoplasm	Cherry angioma
Pink or salmon	Acute inflammation with dilation of superficial dermal vessels	Eczema, drug eruptions, urticaria, pityriasis rubra pilaris, psoriasis
Orange	Granulomatous inflammation with histiocytes having abundant cytoplasm	Juvenile xanthogranuloma
Yellow	Pus	Folliculitis
	Lipid	Xanthelasma
	Histiocytic inflammation	Necrobiosis lipoidica (Fig. 1-16)
	Elastolysis	Pseudoxanthoma elasticum
	Sebaceous glands	Sebaceous hyperplasia
	Bilirubin	Jaundice
Green	Deep hemosiderin	Ecchymosis
	Pyocyanin pigment	Pseudomonas infection
	Myeloperoxidase	Chloroma
	Tissue eosinophilia	Wells syndrome
Blue/gray	Deep dermal melanin	Blue nevus
	Deep deposition of other pigment	Argyria, tattoo
Violet to lilac	Acute lymphocytic inflammation with dilation of deep dermal blood vessels	Borders of evolving morphea, dermatomyositis, lichen planus
Plum	Vascular neoplasm	Kaposi sarcoma
	Dense lymphocytic inflammation	Lymphoma cutis
	Malignant neoplasm	Nodular amelanotic melanoma
	Hemorrhage	Ecchymosis

major caveat is that the true hue of erythema is easiest to visualize in acute conditions affecting fair skin. Subacute or chronic conditions, particularly with epidermal involvement, will have epidermal alteration causing epidermal pigment drop-out into the dermis, making lesions appear more brown or gray. Hemorrhage can also alter the hue, making lesions appear more purple.

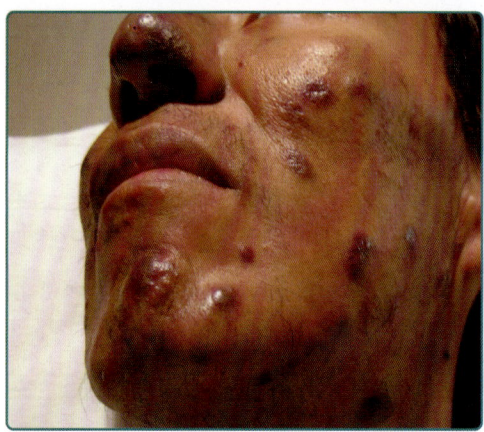

Figure 1-13 Purple papules, Kaposi sarcoma.

SHAPE AND CONFIGURATION OF LESIONS

"Shape" describes an individual macule, patch, papule, or plaque; "configuration" refers to shapes made from the arrangement of individual primary lesions in relation to one another. For example, *annular* or *linear* may be the shape of a single plaque, or a configuration of discrete papules. *Demarcation* refers to the edge of an individual lesion and whether it is sharply defined from or blends into the surrounding skin.

Annular: Ring-shaped; implies that the edge of the lesion has a color and/or texture change that is more prominent on the leading edge than the center (as seen in granuloma annulare, tinea corporis, erythema annulare centrifugum) (Fig. 1-17).

Round/Nummular/Discoid: Coin-shaped; solid circle or oval; usually with uniform morphology from the edges to the center (nummular eczema, plaque-type psoriasis, discoid lupus) (Fig. 1-18).

Arcuate: Arc-shaped; often a result of incomplete formation of an annular lesion (urticaria, subacute cutaneous lupus erythematosus).

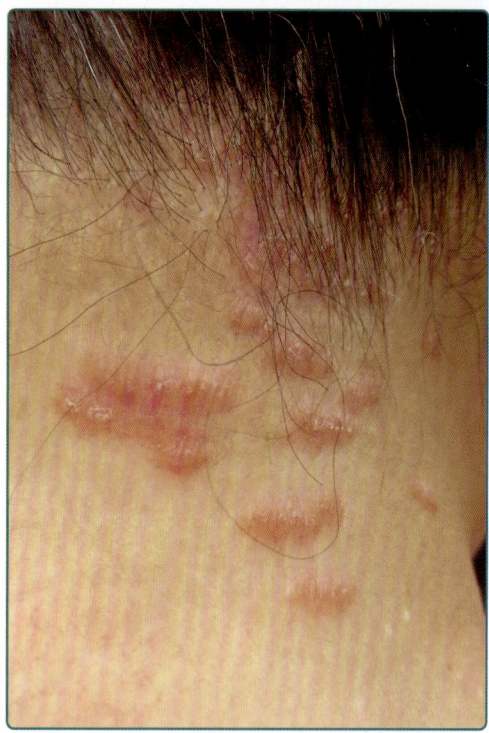

Figure 1-15 Apple-jelly sign, sarcoidosis.

Linear: Resembling a straight line; often implies an external contactant or Koebner phenomenon has occurred in response to scratching; may apply to a single lesion (such as a scabies burrow, poison ivy dermatitis, or bleomycin pigmentation) or to the arrangement of multiple lesions (as seen in lichen nitidus or lichen planus).

Geographic: A shape similar to a land mass; edges are reminiscent of a coastline

Reticular or Retiform: Net-like or lacy in appearance, with somewhat regularly spaced rings or crossing lines with sparing of intervening skin (as seen in livedo reticularis, cutis marmorata) (Fig. 1-19).

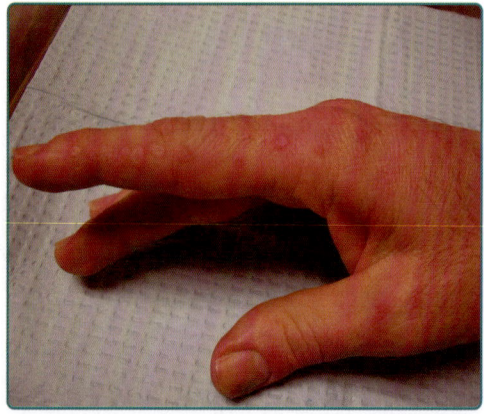

Figure 1-14 Violaceous Gottron papules, dermatomyositis.

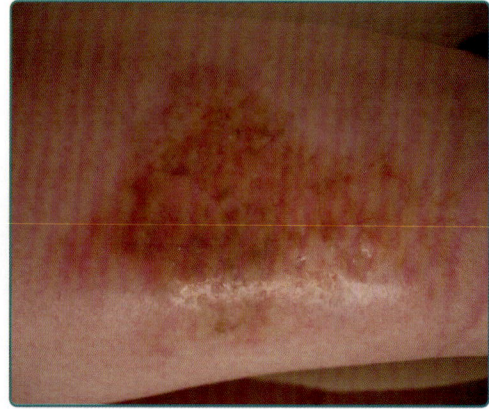

Figure 1-16 Yellow, necrobiosis lipoidica diabeticorum.

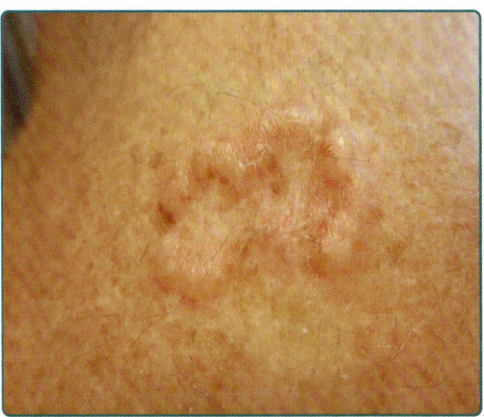

Figure 1-17 Annular lesion, granuloma annulare.

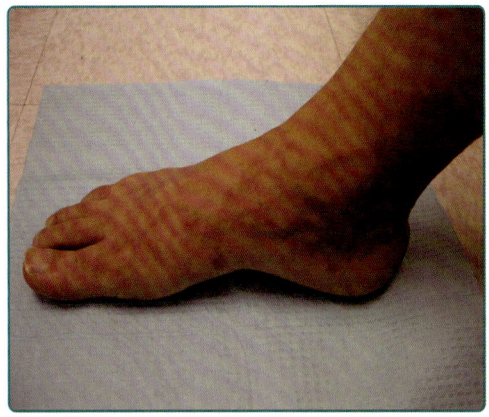

Figure 1-19 Reticular eruption, livedo racemosa.

Stellate: Having multiple angulated edges, resembling a star (Fig. 1-11).

Serpiginous: Serpentine or snake-like (cutaneous larva migrans, for instance, in which the larva migrates this way and that through the skin in a wandering pattern) (Fig. 1-20).

Targetoid: Target-like, with a center darker than the periphery. *Typical targets* (eg, erythema multiforme) have 3 zones: a dark red-purple or dusky center, encircled by a paler pink zone, followed by a rim of darker erythema. *Atypical targets* have just 2 zones, a dark or dusky center with a paler pink rim. Note that both have a center darker in comparison to the outer zone; if the center is paler than the outer zone, it should be termed "annular" (Fig. 1-21).

Whorled: Like marble cake, with 2 distinct colors interspersed in a wavy pattern; usually seen in mosaic disorders in which cells of differing genotypes are interspersed (as seen in incontinentia pigmenti, hypomelanosis of Ito, linear and whorled nevoid hypermelanosis).

Grouped/Herpetiform: Lesions clustered together (a classic example is herpes simplex virus reactivation noted as grouped vesicles on an erythematous base; also seen with certain arthropod bites).

Scattered: Sparse lesions that are irregularly distributed.

Polycyclic: Formed from coalescing circles, rings, or incomplete rings (as seen in urticaria, subacute cutaneous lupus erythematosus) (Fig. 1-22).

DISTRIBUTIONS OF MULTIPLE LESIONS

Dermatomal/Zosteriform: Unilateral and lying in the distribution of a single spinal afferent nerve root; the classic example is herpes zoster (Chap. 165).

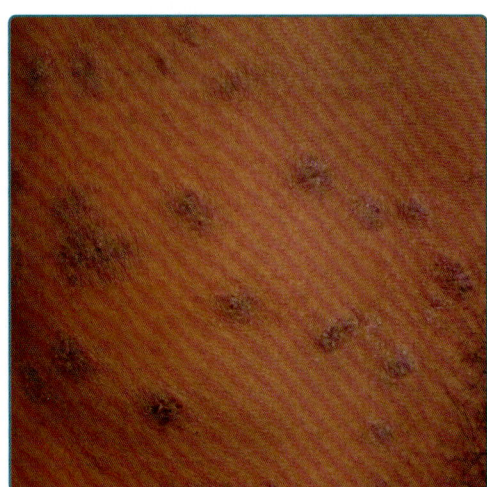

Figure 1-18 Nummular lesion, nummular dermatitis.

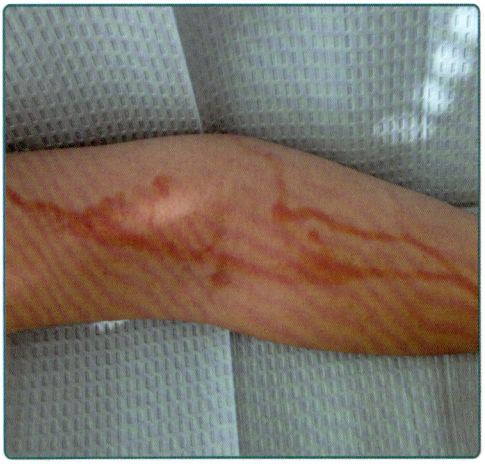

Figure 1-20 Serpiginous erythema, jellyfish sting.

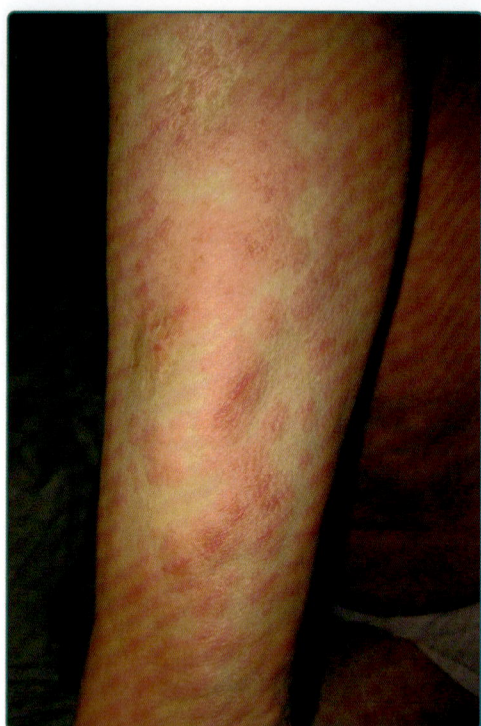

Figure 1-21 Atypical targetoid lesions, Stevens-Johnson syndrome due to medication.

Blaschkoid: Following lines of skin cell migration during embryogenesis; generally longitudinally oriented on the limbs and circumferential on the trunk, but curvilinear rather than perfectly linear; described by Alfred Blaschko and implies a mosaic disorder (such as incontinentia pigmenti, inflammatory linear verrucous epidermal nevus).

Lymphangitic and Sporotrichoid: Lying along the distribution of a lymph vessel; implies an infectious agent that is spreading centrally from an acral site. Lymphangitic lesions are usually a red streak along a limb due to a staphylococcal or streptococcal cellulitis. When individual papules or nodules lie along the distribution of a lymphatic network, this pattern is termed "sporotrichoid" and suggests a particular infectious differential.

Sun Exposed/Photodistributed: Occurring in areas usually not covered by clothing, namely the face, dorsal hands, and a triangular area corresponding to the opening of a V-neck shirt on the upper chest (examples include photodermatitis, subacute cutaneous lupus erythematosus, polymorphous light eruption, squamous cell carcinoma). *Photo-accentuated* means the sun-exposed skin has a more dense distribution of lesions compared to non-sun-exposed skin.

Sun Protected: Occurring in areas usually covered by one or more layers of clothing; usually a dermatosis that is improved by sun exposure (such as parapsoriasis, mycosis fungoides).

Acral: Occurring in distal locations, such as on the hands, feet, wrists, ankles, ears, or penis.

Truncal: Occurring on the trunk or central body.

Extensor: Occurring over the dorsal extremities, overlying the extensor muscles, knees, or elbows (psoriasis is a classic example).

Flexor: Overlying the flexor muscles of the extremities, the antecubital and popliteal fossae (childhood atopic dermatitis, for instance).

Intertriginous: Occurring in the skin folds, where 2 skin surfaces are in contact, namely the axillae, inguinal folds, inner thighs, inframammary skin, and under an abdominal pannus; often related to moisture and heat generated in these areas.

Seborrheic: Favoring the hair-bearing locations of the skin, including scalp, eyebrows, beard, central chest, axillae, genitals. Also often favors the nasolabial and postauricular creases.

Follicular: Papules centered around hair follicles.

Localized: Confined to a single body location.

Generalized: Widespread. A generalized eruption consisting of inflammatory (red) lesions is called an *exanthem* (rash). A macular exanthem consists of macules, a papular exanthem of papules, a vesicular exanthem of vesicles, etc.

Bilateral Symmetric: Occurring with mirror-image symmetry on both sides of the body.

Universal: Involving the entire cutaneous surface (as in erythroderma, alopecia universalis).

Table 1-6 describes some clinically relevant maneuvers that point to particular cutaneous or systemic diseases.

REACTION PATTERNS

Certain combinations of primary and secondary morphologies point the clinician to a subset of diseases.

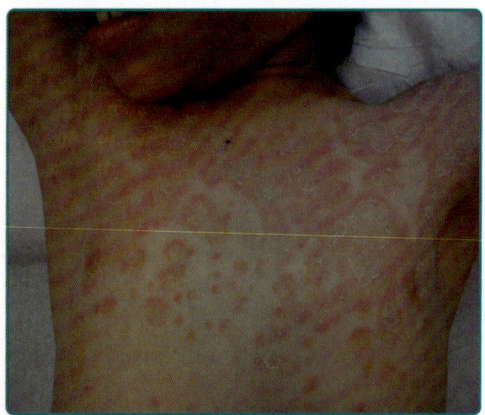

Figure 1-22 Polycyclic eruption, pityriasis rosea.

TABLE 1-6
A Selection of Cutaneous Diagnostic Signs[a]

CUTANEOUS SIGN	DESCRIPTION	SIGNIFICANCE
Apple-jelly sign	A yellowish hue is produced from pressure on the lesion with a glass slide	Noted in granulomatous processes (Fig. 1-15)
Asboe–Hansen sign	Lateral extension of a blister with downward pressure	Noted in blistering disorders in which the pathology is above the basement membrane zone
Auspitz sign	Pinpoint bleeding at the tops of ruptured capillaries with forcible removal of outer scales from a psoriatic plaque	Not entirely sensitive or specific for psoriasis
Buttonhole sign	A flesh-colored, soft papule feels as though it can be pushed through a "buttonhole" into the skin	Noted in a neurofibroma
Carpet tack sign	Horny plugs at the undersurface of scale removed from a lesion	Noted in lesions of chronic cutaneous lupus
Darier sign	Urticarial wheal produced in a lesion after it is firmly rubbed with a finger or the rounded end of a pen; the wheal, which is strictly confined to the borders of the lesion, may not appear for several minutes	Noted in urticaria pigmentosa and rarely with cutaneous lymphoma or histiocytosis
Dermatographism	Firmly stroking unaffected skin produces a wheal along the shape of the stroke within seconds to minutes	Symptomatic dermatographism represents a physical urticaria
Pseudo-Darier sign	Transient induration of a lesion or piloerection after rubbing	Noted in congenital smooth muscle hamartoma
Fitzpatrick (dimple) sign	Dimpling of the skin with lateral compression of the lesion with the thumb and index finger produces dimpling as a result of tethering of the epidermis to the dermal lesion	Characteristic of dermatofibroma
Nikolsky sign	Lateral pressure on unblistered skin with resulting shearing of the epidermis	Noted in blistering disorders in which the pathology is above the basement membrane zone; relevant entities include pemphigus vulgaris and toxic epidermal necrolysis

[a]Others are discussed in the chapters on diseases in which the signs occur.

Groups of diagnoses that share similar morphologic characteristics are termed "reaction patterns," suggesting a particular list of differential diagnosis. Reaction patterns are an especially useful tool when no characteristic shape, configuration, or distribution is apparent. Determining the reaction pattern can also help guide workup (Tables 1-7 through 1-15) and initial treatment.

The first step to determining the reaction pattern is identifying the primary lesion. In generalized eruptions, or when mixed morphologies are present, it is useful to go to the edge of a larger lesion or group of lesions to determine the primary morphology. It is important to note that some diseases with variable morphologies may fall into more than one reaction pattern.

TABLE 1-7
Papulosquamous Reaction Pattern—Common Examples

Psoriasis
Lichen planus
Pityriasis rosea
Pityriasis rubra pilaris
Pityriasis lichenoides chronica
Syphilis (secondary)
Mycosis fungoides (MF)/parapsoriasis
Drug (lichenoid, pityriasis rosea-like)
Subacute and discoid lupus, dermatomyositis
Tinea corporis
Tinea versicolor
Seborrheic dermatitis
Nutritional deficiency
Lichenoid id reaction
Porokeratosis
Superficial basal cell carcinoma
Squamous cell carcinoma in situ

Toolbox
History
Distribution
Examine scalp, nails, mucous membranes
KOH preparation, fungal culture
Rapid plasma reagin (RPR)
Biopsy for routine histology

REACTION PATTERNS WITH SURFACE CHANGE

PAPULOSQUAMOUS

In papulosquamous eruptions, the primary lesion is a relatively thin or flat-topped papule or plaque with scale. Crust or lichenification is usually not present.

ECZEMATOUS

Eczematous eruptions consist of thin erythematous papules and plaques with epidermal change. On the surface of an acute eczematous process, there is enough epidermal spongiosis (edema between keratinocytes) to cause the formation of serous crusting, microvesicles, or sometimes frank bullae. When microvesicles collapse, they form characteristic tiny round crusts often admixed with scale and subtle or overt fissuring. When subacute to chronic, the surface is often dry, scaly, fissured, and/or lichenified from rubbing or scratching. Compared with papulosquamous eruptions, eczematous primary lesions are typically ill demarcated, and individual lesions vary widely in their size and spacing. Because most eczematous eruptions share a common histology, the distribution and history are key in differentiating among them (Table 1-8).

Histopathologically, these processes involve the epidermis and superficial to mid-dermis. Individual papules or plaques are typically well demarcated, and there is often normal skin visible between each discrete papule or plaque (Table 1-7).

TABLE 1-8
Eczematous Reaction Pattern—Common Examples

Same or Similar Histology
- Atopic
- Irritant contact
- Allergic contact
- Nummular
- Dyshidrosis Dishidrotic
- Xerotic/asteatotic
- Stasis
- Photoallergic drug eruption
- Actinic dermatitis/actinic prurigo
- Id or "autoeczematization"
- Eczematous drug eruption
- Seborrheic dermatitis
- Lichen simplex chronicus

Mimickers-Scraping, Biopsy May Be Helpful
- Scabies
- Tinea
- Some blistering disorders (bullous pemphigoid, dermatitis herpetiformis)
- Mycosis fungoides
- Nutritional deficiency
- Polymorphous light eruption

Toolbox
- History
- Distribution
- Examine scalp, nails, mucous membranes
- Patch testing
- Scraping (scabies, KOH)
- Biopsy for routine histology, direct immunofluorescence (DIF)
- Bacterial culture, HSV culture (if superinfection suspected)

VESICULOBULLOUS

Sometimes vesicles and bullae are quite obvious; other times, when all the blisters have ruptured, the clinician must recognize their "footprints"—clues to their recent presence. Because blisters are filled with fluid, when they collapse, they often leave behind round, oval, arcuate, or geographic erosions or crusts. When small ruptured vesicles are grouped together, as in herpes simplex, they form crust with "scalloped" edges. Other subtle clues include erosions with "mauserung" desquamation, a rumpled rim of epidermis hanging from the erosion's edge, or milia, which can result from healing of deeper blisters (Table 1-9).

TABLE 1-9
Vesiculobullous Reaction Pattern—Common Examples

Pustules
- Psoriasis
- Acute generalized exanthematous pustulosis (AGEP)
- Sneddon–Wilkinson/IgA pemphigus
- Candida
- Herpes Simplex Virus (HSV) or Varicella Zoster Virus (VZV) infections
- Follicular pustules (acne/rosacea, bacterial folliculitis; Majocchi granuloma, pityrosporum folliculitis, eosinophilic folliculitis)
- Impetigo
- Miliaria pustulosa

Vesicles/Bullae
- Acute eczematous process
- Allergic contact dermatitis
- Bullous arthropod
- HSV/VZV
- Coxsackie
- Bullous tinea
- Autoimmune blistering diseases
- Porphyria cutanea tarda, pseudoporphyria
- Polymorphous light eruption
- Inherited blistering diseases
- Impetigo
- Miliaria crystallina
- Bullous diabeticorum

Vesicles/Pustules as Secondary Processes
- Infection (cellulitis, necrotizing fasciitis, deep fungal, atypical mycobacteria, leishmaniasis, scabies, nocardiosis)
- Edema
- Chemical/thermal/Ultraviolet burn
- Necrosis
- Fixed drug eruption, erythema multiforme, Stevens–Johnson syndrome, Toxic epidermal necrolysis
- Neutrophilic dermatoses (leukocytoclastic vasculitis, Sweet syndrome, pyoderma gangrenosum)
- Halogenodermas

Toolbox
- History
- Distribution
- Examine scalp, nails, mucous membranes
- KOH and/or fungal culture—blister roof, pustule
- Bacterial culture—blister fluid, pustule
- DFA, Viral culture—blister base
- Biopsy for routine histology, DIF, tissue culture (bacterial, mycobacterial, fungal)

TABLE 1-10
Dermal "Plus" Reaction Pattern—Common Examples

Infections
Mycobacteria: TB and atypical mycobacteria
Fungal: kerion, subcutaneous mycoses, deep fungal mycoses, mycetomas
Parasites: leishmaniasis, Chagas, nodular scabies
Bacteria: bartonella, botryomycosis, blastomycosis-like pyoderma, anthrax, gonococcus, syphilitic gumma
Viral: molluscum, disseminated VZV, verrucous HSV, poxviruses
Neoplasias: Kaposi sarcoma, SCC, BCC, Merkel cell carcinoma, amelanotic melanoma, metastases, etc.
Inflammatory: Neutrophilic (Sweet syndrome, pyoderma gangrenosum, halogenodermas), lymphoma (tumor-stage CTCL, B-cell lymphomas), sarcoidosis, polyarteritis nodosa, palisaded neutrophilic and interstitial granulomatous dermatitis

Toolbox
History
Distribution
Examine scalp, nails, mucous membranes, lymph nodes
Culture surface (viral, bacterial, fungal)
Biopsy for routine histology
Biopsy for culture (bacterial, fungal, mycobacterial)

TABLE 1-11
Macular Reaction Pattern—Common Examples

Pink
Vascular anomaly or neoplasm (such as nevus simplex)
Exanthems (drug, viral)
Macular granuloma annulare, interstitial granulomatous drug eruption
Tinea versicolor (can induce scale)

Red
Red to red-purple
Vascular anomaly or neoplasm (such as telangiectasia, port-wine stain)
Petechiae (due to trauma, thrombocytopenia, Rocky Mountain spotted fever, Parvovirus, scurvy)
Ecchymosis
Red to red-brown
Pigmented purpura
Telangiectasia macularis eruptive perstans (TMEP)
Erythema ab igne
Fixed drug eruption

Brown
Melasma
Lentigo
Junctional melanocytic nevus
Melanoma
Some birthmarks (Café au lait macule, nevus spilus)
Postinflammatory pigmentation
Tinea versicolor
Patch-stage KS
Flat warts
Diabetic dermopathy

White
Vitiligo
Contact leukoderma
Inherited (piebaldism, ash-leaf macule, nevus anemicus)
Postinflammatory pigmentation
Pityriasis alba
Hypopigmented MF
Tuberculoid leprosy
Guttate hypomelanosis
Flat warts
Progressive macular hypomelanosis
Bier spots

Gray/Blue
Blue nevus
Nevus of Ota
Mongolian spot
Lichen planus pigmentosa and related disorders
Drug effect (minocycline, amiodarone, hydroxychloroquine)
Deposition (ochronosis, silver)
Tattoo

Toolbox
History
Shape
Distribution
Examine mucous membranes
Wood lamp
KOH (for tinea versicolor)
Biopsy for routine histology

Some diseases with prominent surface change defy categorization into papulosquamous, eczematous, or vesiculobullous reaction patterns. The astute clinician can recognize an eruption as difficult to characterize and is aware this actually suggests a differential diagnosis in itself. Some examples include scabies, acantholytic diseases (Grover, Darier disease), some drug eruptions, some "id" reactions, and some paraneoplastic conditions.

DERMAL "PLUS"

These are dermally infiltrated papules, nodules or plaques with surface change: hyperkeratotic scale, crust, vesicles, pustules, erosion, or ulceration (Table 1-10).

REACTION PATTERNS WITHOUT SURFACE CHANGE

In the absence of surface change, the epidermis and its melanin are unaltered, often allowing color and topography to be the defining characteristics. Shape, configuration, and distribution are also helpful.

MACULAR

Macules can derive their color changes from changes in the epidermis or dermis (Table 1-11).

TABLE 1-12
Dermal Reaction Pattern—Common Examples

Inflammatory
Neutrophils (Sweet syndrome, pyoderma gangrenosum, neutrophilic eccrine hidradenitis)
Lymphocytes (tumid lupus, cutaneous lymphoid hyperplasia, morphea, lichen sclerosus)
Histiocytes (xanthomas, xanthogranulomas, granuloma annulare, sarcoidosis, Rosai-Dorfman, Multicentric Reticulohistiocytosis, palisaded neutrophilic, and interstitial granulomatous dermatitis)
Mixed (erythema elevatum diutinum, granuloma faciale)
Mastocytoma
Plasmacytoma
Well syndrome
Angiolymphoid hyperplasia with eosinophilia

Infectious
Cellulitis, Erysipelas, bartonella (Bacillary angiomatosis, cat scratch)
Mycobacteria (TB, leprosy, atypical mycobacteria)
Subcutaneous and deep fungal infection

Neoplastic
Kaposi sarcoma (plaque, tumor-stage)
Lymphomas (CTCL, B-cell)
Leukemia cutis
Adnexal neoplasms
Vascular neoplasms
BCC, SCC, nevus, melanoma, spindle cell neoplasms, Merkel cell
Cutaneous metastases
Keloid, hypertrophic scar
Dermatofibroma, Dermatofibrosarcoma protuberans

Depositional
Colloid milium
Amyloid
Mucin
Gout
Calcium

Toolbox
History
Distribution
Examine lymph nodes, mucous membranes
Biopsy for routine histology, tissue culture

TABLE 1-13
Subcutaneous Reaction Pattern

Inflammatory
Erythema nodosum
Lupus and other connective tissue-related panniculitis
Subcutaneous Sweet syndrome, GA, sarcoidosis (Darier-Roussy)

Infectious
Erythema induratum
Nocardia, actinomyces

Physical
Traumatic
Cold

Other
Lipodermatosclerosis
Enzyme-mediated (pancreatic, alpha-1 antitrypsin)
Steroid and other drug injections
Subcutaneous fat necrosis of the newborn
Panniculitis-like CTCL

Toolbox
History
Distribution
Biopsy for routine histology, tissue culture

DERMAL

A dermal reaction pattern is a papule or plaque without surface change where the infiltrative process is in the dermis (Table 1-12).

SUBCUTANEOUS

Subcutaneous reaction pattern is a deeper papule or plaque, usually without surface change, though occasionally they may ulcerate and crust. The infiltrative or inflammatory process is in the subcutis (Table 1-13).

PURPURIC

Purpura are red or purple macules, patches, papules, or plaques that result from bleeding into the skin. Because blood has extravasated, they do not blanch when pressure is applied. They may range in color from true red to red-purple or magenta to red-brown ("cayenne pepper"). Purpuric macules are sometimes called "petechiae"; purpuric patches are sometimes called "ecchymoses." Ecchymosis may also overlie a plaque or nodule from dermal or subdermal hemorrhage, known as hematoma, and may appear yellow-green when a few days old. Purpuric papules, or "palpable purpura," typically represent inflammation of small vessels associated with hemorrhage, as in leukocytoclastic vasculitis, a coagulopathy affecting small vessels, as in cryoglobulinemia, or very small emboli. Purpuric plaques represent ischemia, embolism, infarction, intravascular infection, or inflammation of small-medium or medium vessels, that may lead to necrosis of the overlying epidermis. These can manifest as pink papules (usually medium vessels) or stellate dark purple plaques (Fig. 1-23), and may be accompanied by pink, red, or purple net-like ("retiform") hyperemia ("livedo"). If the overlying epidermis becomes necrotic, bullae, ulcer, and/or eschar may form at the surface (Table 1-14).

ERYTHEMAS

Erythemas are blanching red-pink macules, patches, papules, or plaques, or a combination, usually without surface change. This reaction pattern may be subdivided into *morbilliform erythemas*, *figurate erythemas*, *urticarial erythemas*, and *targetoid erythemas* (Table 1-15).

TABLE 1-14
Purpuric Reaction Pattern—Common Examples

Vasculitis
Small vessel
Hypersensitivity vasculitis (to drug or infection)
Henoch–Schoenlein purpura (IgA vasculitis)
ANCA+
Connective-tissue disease associated
Medium vessel
Polyarteritis nodosa
Churg–Strauss
Levamisole hypersensitivity
Macular arteritis

Infectious
Meningococcemia
Purpura fulminans
Ecthyma gangrenosum
Hyperinfection strongyloidiasis
Aspergillus, mucor, and other vasculotropic fungi

Embolic
Cholesterol emboli
Septic emboli (endocarditis and others)

Vasculopathy
Calciphylaxis
Cryoglobulin, cryofibrinogen
Antiphospholipid antibody syndrome, livedoid vasculopathy, livedo racemosa
Coumadin/heparin necrosis
Levamisole hypersensitivity
Other hypercoagulable states

Other
Vascular or intravascular neoplasms (Kaposi sarcoma, angiosarcoma, intravascular lymphoma)
Cutis marmorata
Petechiae (trauma, thrombocytopenia, Rocky Mountain spotted fever, Parvovirus, scurvy)
Ecchymoses

Toolbox
History
Distribution
Other lab workup depending on morphology and history
Biopsy for routine histology
Biopsy for DIF
Biopsy for tissue culture

TABLE 1-15
Erythemas

Exanthems
Viral
Bacterial (toxic shock syndrome, scarlet fever, meningococcus, mycoplasma)
Drug (morbilliform eruption, drug-induced hypersensitivity syndrome)
Graft-vs-host disease
Kawasaki disease
Miliaria rubra

Figurate
Erythema annulare centrifugum
Deep gyrate erythemas
Erythema migrans
Erythema marginatum

Urticaria/Urticaria
Urticaria
Neutrophilic urticaria
Papular urticaria
Urticarial vasculitis
Dermal hypersensitivity reaction
Polymorphous eruption of pregnancy
Urticarial bullous pemphigoid
Acute hemorrhagic edema of childhood

Targetoid
Erythema multiforme
Mycoplasma-induced rash and mucositis
Fixed drug eruption
Urticarial vasculitis
Paraneoplastic pemphigus
Rowell-type lupus

Toolbox
History
Distribution
Examine mucous membranes
Biopsy for routine histology, DIF
Viral studies
Other lab workup depending on morphology and history

- *Morbilliform erythemas* are exanthems that are typically consist of diffuse symmetric blanching pink, red, or magenta macules and papules.
- *Figurate erythemas* are annular, arcuate, or polycyclic blanching pink to red plaques. They generally do not have surface change, with the exception of erythema annulare centrifugum, which exhibits prototypical "trailing scale."
- *Urticarial erythemas* are pink, blanching macules, papules, or plaques, often exhibiting a characteristic "wheal and flare" appearance, with blanching of the skin surrounding the primary lesion (Fig. 1-24).
- *Targetoid erythemas* have at least 2 zones of color, with a darker center compared to the periphery. The center often has a "dusky," or gray-violet, hue, owing to epidermal necrosis, or vesiculates as the necrotic epidermis detaches.

CONCLUSION

In the age of digital photography, the basic art and science of morphology remains paramount in dermatology to achieve accurate diagnosis and a deeper understanding of clinical–pathologic correlation. As Siemens (1891–1969) wrote, "he who studies skin diseases and fails to study the lesion first will never learn dermatology." Careful evaluation of the skin and systematic identification of primary morphology, secondary changes, and reaction pattern

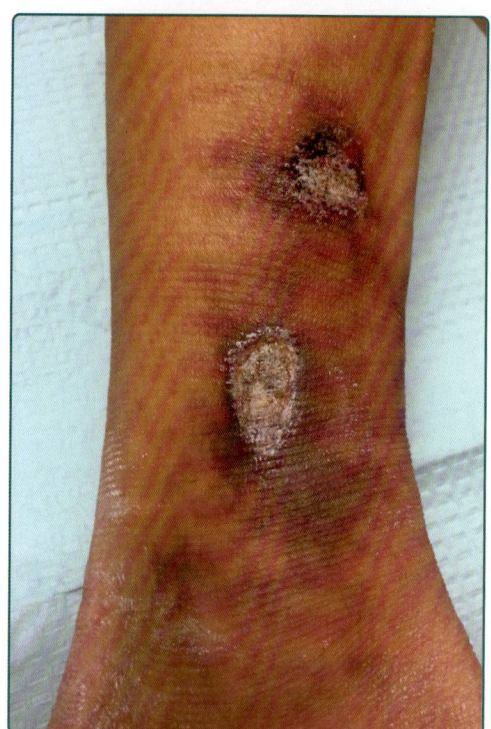

Figure 1-23 Retiform purpura with ulceration and eschar, cutaneous polyarteritis nodosa.

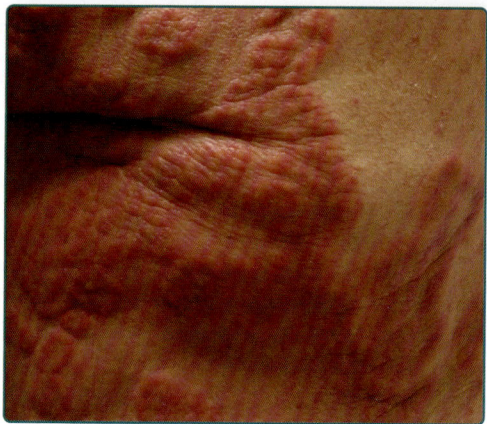

Figure 1-24 Urticarial phase, bullous pemphigoid.

is essential to the art and science of dermatologic diagnosis.

ACKNOWLEDGMENTS

The authors are truly grateful for the opportunity to build upon the work of Amit Garg, Nikki A. Levin, and Jeffrey D. Bernhard, authors of a previous version of this chapter. The authors thank Lindy P. Fox and Ilona J. Frieden for sharing materials and insights that informed this work.

SUGGESTED READINGS

Burgin S. *A Guidebook to Dermatologic Diagnosis.* New York, NY: McGraw-Hill. In press.

duVivier A. *Atlas of Clinical Dermatology*, 4th ed. Philadelphia, PA: Saunders; 2012.

Ghatan HEY. *Dermatological Differential Diagnosis and Pearls*, 2nd ed. Boca Raton, FL: CRC Press; 2002.

Schneiderman P, Grossman ME. *A Clinician's Guide to Dermatologic Differential Diagnosis.* Boca Raton, FL: CRC Press; 2006.

White GM, Cox NH. *Diseases of the Skin: A Color Atlas and Text*, 2nd ed. Maryland Heights, MO: Mosby; 2005.

Wolff K, Johnson R, Saavedra A, et al. *Fitzpatrick's Color Atlas and Synopsis of Clinical Dermatology*, 8th ed. New York, NY: McGraw-Hill; 2017.

Chapter 2 :: Pathology of Skin Lesions
:: Rosalie Elenitsas & Emily Y. Chu

第二章
皮疹的病理学

中文导读

不同皮肤组织解剖上相互连接且相互作用，这就是皮肤的反应单元。浅表反应单元包括表皮、真表皮交界区和真皮乳头，第二反应单元是含深部血管丛的网状真皮，第三反应单元是具有间隔和小叶成分的皮下组织，第四反应单元是毛囊和腺体，嵌入在第三个反应单元中。

皮肤组织的遗传异质性和相互作用，导致多种临床和病理反应模式。本章作者从以下几个方面介绍。

1. 皮肤病理学导论　作者介绍了皮肤活检在皮肤病诊断中至关重要。皮肤活检过程复杂，涉及20个步骤。其中重点介绍了活检方法、活检部位、组织保存和送检、组织病理学评估。

2. 皮肤的炎症反应　本部分介绍了3种皮肤反应单元及其特点。

3. 皮肤肿瘤性疾病　讨论了如何评估皮肤肿瘤良恶性、肿瘤细胞起源和特征，介绍了表皮来源肿瘤、真皮来源肿瘤、不同来源良恶性肿瘤的病理特点和鉴别要点。

〔陈明亮〕

AT-A-GLANCE

- Different tissue compartments interconnect anatomically and interact functionally. These are the reactive units of the skin.
- The superficial reaction unit comprises the epidermis, the junctional zone, and the papillary body with its vascular system.
- The reticular dermis with the deeper dermal vascular plexus is the second reactive unit.
- The third reactive unit is the subcutaneous tissue with its septal and lobular compartments.
- Hair follicles and glands are a fourth reactive unit embedded into these three units.
- Pathologic processes may involve these reactive units alone or several of them together in a concerted fashion.
- The heterogeneity and interaction of these individual cutaneous compartments explains why a few basic pathologic reactions lead to a multiplicity of clinical and pathologic reaction patterns.

INTRODUCTION TO SKIN PATHOLOGY

Skin biopsies play an important role in the care of patients with dermatologic disorders. Adequate knowledge of dermatopathology is crucial not only for interpreting the pathology report from the laboratory, but also for deciding how and where to perform the biopsy. The process of a skin biopsy is more complex than meets the eye, as it has been estimated that there are approximately 20 "handoff" steps in this process.[1] Errors can occur at any one of these steps, and accurate communication at all points is important in minimizing medical mishaps.[1,2]

CHOOSING THE TYPE OF BIOPSY

Before performing a biopsy one must review the clinical differential diagnosis, which will assist in deciding whether a shave, punch, or excisional specimen is best (Table 2-1). One must also consider the anatomical location of the biopsy, and how it will affect the cosmetic result. Shave biopsies are best for cases where most of the pathology is in the epidermis or superficial dermis. Examples include nonmelanoma skin cancer (basal cell carcinoma, squamous cell carcinoma), seborrheic keratosis, actinic keratosis, verruca vulgaris, and some melanocytic nevi. For most inflammatory dermatoses, a punch biopsy produces the best results. Excisional biopsies are used for complete removal of a cutaneous neoplasm as well as in cases of panniculitis or fasciitis where substantial deep tissue is needed. Curettage should be restricted to lesions with a known diagnosis, such as a seborrheic keratosis, verruca, or basal cell carcinoma, where histopathologic examination is less important, and mostly performed for confirmation. Curettage results in fragmented and distorted tissue making evaluation by the pathologist extremely difficult.

CHOOSING THE SITE TO BIOPSY

Although a biopsy of a cutaneous neoplasm is obvious, inflammatory dermatoses can be more challenging. Choosing the site to biopsy can be just as important as the biopsy itself. It is best to choose lesions that have not been treated, excoriated, or secondarily infected. In general, it is better to choose fully evolved lesions rather than a brand-new lesion. The exception is blistering disorders, when a new blister is ideal. In this scenario, it is important to include the edge of the blister as well as the surrounding skin that has not yet blistered. When assessing vasculitis and connective tissue disease, the age of the lesion is critical as often very early or old lesions may lack diagnostic findings. Elston[3] has eloquently reviewed important issues in biopsies of specific skin diseases. For patients with unusual or persistent dermatoses, or if cutaneous T-cell lymphoma is suspected, more than one biopsy can be beneficial. When a biopsy is performed for alopecia, two 4-mm punch biopsies are optimal: one for horizontal sections and one for vertical sections. Alternative methods, such as the HoVert technique and Tyler technique, allow for horizontal and vertical sections from one punch biopsy.[4,5]

SUBMISSION OF THE BIOPSY

All routine skin biopsies are submitted in 10% neutral buffered formalin. At the time of the biopsy, one must ensure that there is adequate formalin in the bottle (approximately 10 times the volume of the specimen), and also confirm that the specimen is actually in the bottle and submerged in the fluid. A double check to confirm that the skin tissue is not stuck to the punch, the shave tool, or the bottle cap can help prevent a medical mishap. In cold weather, 95% ethyl alcohol (10% of the formalin volume) must be added to the formalin to prevent freezing of the tissue and subsequent freeze artifacts, which can lead to misdiagnosis.

Direct immunofluorescence may be of benefit in some disease processes, such as autoimmune blistering diseases, discoid lupus erythematosus, and vasculitis. In this case, a separate piece of skin is submitted in Michel medium (a solution containing ammonium sulfate, *N*-ethyl maleimide, and magnesium sulfate in citrate buffer), with specific instructions to the

TABLE 2-1
Choosing the Type of Biopsy

SUSPECTED DIAGNOSIS	BIOPSY TYPE
Actinic keratosis	Shave
Seborrheic keratosis	Shave
Verruca	Shave
BCC, SCC	Shave most common; punch/excision
Blistering disease	Punch or deep shave edge of blister
Contact dermatitis	Punch
Connective tissue disease	Punch
Mycosis fungoides	Punch
Vasculitis	Punch
Granulomatous process	Punch
Atypical nevi	Deep shave, punch, or excision
Panniculitis	Punch (minimum 6 mm) or ellipse

BCC, basal cell carcinoma; SCC, squamous cell carcinoma.

laboratory that immunofluorescence is requested. If your laboratory is in the same building or within walking distance, the specimen can be transported on saline-soaked gauze in a sterile cup. This latter option should only be used if immediate delivery to the laboratory is possible because tissue that is not fixed in formalin or put into a holding medium such as Michel medium will begin to autolyze.

If possible, skin biopsies should be submitted to a dermatopathology laboratory. Dermatopathology laboratories are advantageous because the histotechnologists have the experience of proper embedding of small pieces of skin. Maloriented skin sections are extremely challenging to interpret even for experienced pathologists. Choosing a dermatopathology laboratory also ensures that the specimen will be interpreted by a dermatopathologist. All biopsies must be submitted with clinical information. Minimal information includes: age, sex of patient, anatomical location of the biopsy, clinical description and/or clinical diagnosis. With electronic medical records, often this can be printed directly onto the pathology form. Submitting a clinical photograph may assist in clinical pathologic correlation of both neoplastic and inflammatory disorders. Pathology reports are not always "black and white" with only one diagnosis. For inflammatory disorders, a descriptive diagnosis may result from the pathology laboratory, and the dermatologist must correlate those findings with the dermatologist's differential diagnosis. In all cases, one must always correlate the pathology findings with the clinical presentation. If the results do not make sense, one should consider either additional sampling or a discussion with the pathologist.

ASSESSMENT OF HISTOPATHOLOGY

Commonly used immunohistochemical and histochemical stains are shown in Tables 2-2 and 2-3, respectively. The skin is composed of different tissue compartments that interconnect anatomically and interact functionally. Conversely, epidermis, dermis, and subcutaneous tissue are heterogeneous in nature and an analysis of pathologic processes involving the skin, and this heterogeneity, explains how a few basic reactions lead to a multiplicity of reaction patterns within this tissue.

INFLAMMATORY REACTIONS IN THE SKIN

Pathophysiologically, the skin can be subdivided into 3 reactive units that extend beyond anatomic boundaries (Fig. 2-1); they overlap and can be divided into different subunits that respond to pathologic stimuli according to their inherent reaction capacities in a coordinated pattern: (a) superficial reactive unit, (b) reticular dermis, and (c) subcutaneous fat. Hair follicles and glands are a separate reactive unit that are predominantly in the reticular dermis.

SUPERFICIAL REACTIVE UNIT

The superficial reactive unit is composed of epidermis, the junction zone, the subjacent loose, delicate connective tissue of the papillary dermis and its capillary network, and the superficial vascular plexus (see Fig. 2-1).

EPIDERMIS

Keratinocytes represent the bulk of the epidermis. The epidermis, an ectodermal epithelium, also harbors a number of other cell populations such as melanocytes, Langerhans cells, and Merkel cells. The basal cells of the epidermis undergo proliferation cycles that provide for the renewal of the epidermis and, as they move toward the surface of the skin, undergo a differentiation process that results in surface keratinization. Thus, the epidermis is a dynamic tissue in which cells are constantly nonsynchronized replication and

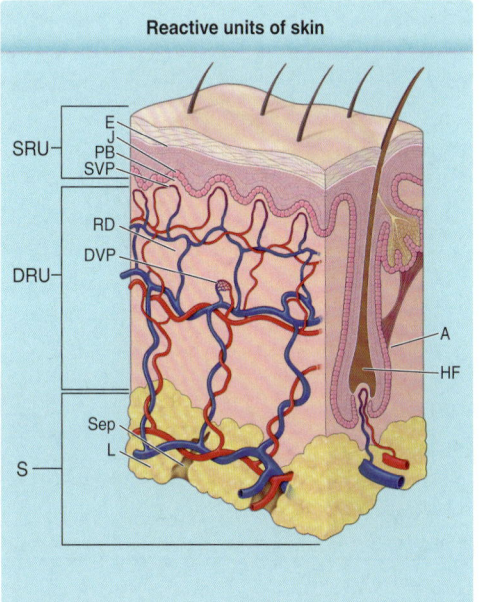

Figure 2-1 Reactive units of skin. The superficial reactive unit (*SRU*) comprises the epidermis (*E*), the junction zone (*J*), and the papillary body (*PB*, or papillary dermis) with the superficial microvascular plexus. The dermal reactive unit (*DRU*) consists of the reticular dermis (*RD*) and the deep dermal microvascular plexus (*DVP*). The subcutaneous reactive unit (*S*) consists of lobules (*L*) and septae (*Sep*). A fourth unit is the appendages (*A*; hair and sebaceous glands are the only appendages shown). *HF,* hair follicle.

TABLE 2-2
Commonly Used Immunohistochemical Stains

IMMUNOHISTOCHEMICAL STAIN	ASSOCIATED CONDITION(S)
Epithelial Markers	
P63	Cutaneous spindle cell squamous carcinoma
CAM5.2	Paget disease, extramammary Paget disease
CK7	Paget disease, extramammary Paget disease
CK20	Merkel cell carcinoma
Epithelial membrane antigen (EMA)	Squamous cell carcinoma
Carcinoembryonic antigen (CEA)	Sweat gland neoplasms, Paget disease, extramammary Paget disease
Mesenchymal Markers	
Desmin	Skeletal and smooth muscle tumors (leiomyoma)
Smooth muscle actin (SMA)	Glomus tumor, leiomyosarcoma
CD34	Dermatofibrosarcoma protuberans, trichoepitheliomas
Factor XIIIa	Dermatofibroma
CD31	Vascular tumors
D2-40 (podoplanin)	Lymphatic endothelial marker
GLUT1	Infantile hemangiomas
Vimentin	Sarcomas
Neuroectodermal Markers	
S100	Desmoplastic melanoma, Langerhans cell histiocytosis, granular cell tumor
HMB-45	Desmoplastic melanoma, blue nevus
Melan-A, Mart-1	Desmoplastic melanoma
Hematopoietic Markers	
CD45Ra (LCA)	Hematolymphoid proliferations
CD20	B-cell lymphomas
CD10 (CALLA)	Atypical fibroxanthomas, clear-cell hidradenoma, sebaceous tumors
CD79a	Plasma cell, B-cell marker
CD138 (syndecan-1)	Plasma cell marker
CD3	T-cell lymphomas
CD4	T-helper lymphocytic marker
CD5	Mantle cell lymphoma, chronic lymphocytic leukemia
CD7	Most commonly lost antigen in T-cell lymphoma
CD8	T-cell cytotoxic/suppressor marker
CD30	Anaplastic large cell lymphoma, lymphomatoid papulosis, chronic arthropod bites (scabies, tick)
CD1a	Langerhans cell histiocytosis
Langerin CD207	Langerhans cells
BCL2	B-cell lymphoproliferative disorders
Infectious Diseases	
HHV8	Kaposi sarcoma

HHV8, human herpesvirus 8.
Data from Elston DM, Ferringer T. *Dermatopathology*, 2nd ed. Philadelphia: Saunders, 2013.

differentiation; this precisely coordinated physiologic balance between progressive keratinization as cells approach the epidermal surface to eventually undergo programed cell death and be sloughed, and their continuous replenishment by dividing basal cells, is in contrast to the relatively static minority populations of Langerhans cells, melanocytes, and Merkel cells.

Disturbances of Epidermal Cell Kinetics:

Enhanced cell proliferation accompanied by an enlargement of the germinative cell pool and increased mitotic rates lead to an increase of the epidermal cell

TABLE 2-3
Commonly Used Histochemical Stains

HISTOCHEMICAL STAIN	FEATURE VISUALIZED
Verhoeff-Van Gieson stain	Elastic fibers (black)
Toluidine blue	Mucin (blue)
	Mast cell granules (metachromatic)
Masson's trichrome	Collagen (blue-green)
	Smooth muscle (red)
Leder stain	Mast cell cytoplasm (red)
Periodic acid–Schiff	Glycogen (red)
	Fungi (red)
Alcian blue	Acid mucopolysaccharides, such as mucin (blue)
Colloidal iron	Acid mucopolysaccharides (blue)
Mucicarmine	Mucopolysaccharides (pink/red)
Congo red	Amyloid (red, but apple green birefringence with polarized light)
Thioflavin T	Amyloid (yellow/yellow-green)
Crystal violet	Amyloid (red-purple metachromatically)
Prussian blue (Perls stain)	Iron (deep blue)
Fontana-Masson	Melanin (black)
Von Kossa	Calcium (black)
Alizarin red	Calcium (orange-red)
Oil red O	Lipids (red)
Sudan black	Lipids (black)
Gomori methenamine silver	Fungus (gray-black)
Ziehl-Neelsen; Fite acid-fast stain	Mycobacteria (red)
Auramine-rhodamine	Mycobacteria (red-yellow)
Warthin-starry	Spirochetes (black)
Giemsa	Myeloid cells (blue)
	Mast cells (blue)
	Leishmania, Histoplasma

Data from Elston DM, Ferringer T. *Dermatopathology*, 2nd ed. Philadelphia: Saunders, 2013.

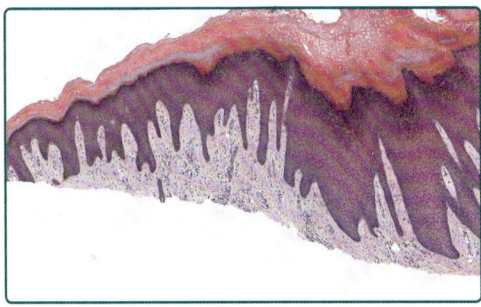

Figure 2-2 Acanthosis. The epidermis on the right side of this photomicrograph is thicker than normal because of a proliferation of keratinocytes.

pattern, one sees retained nuclei in the stratum corneum. Parakeratosis can be the result of incomplete differentiation (eg, squamous cell carcinoma), or the result of reduced transit time, which does not permit epidermal cells to complete the entire differentiation process (eg, psoriasis).

Dyskeratosis represents altered, often premature or abnormal, keratinization, of individual keratinocytes, but it also refers to the morphologic presentation of apoptosis of keratinocytes. Dyskeratotic cells have an eosinophilic cytoplasm and a pyknotic nucleus and are packed with keratin filaments arranged in perinuclear aggregates. It is important to remember that although both premature or abnormal keratinization and apoptosis may produce an end-product referred to as "dyskeratosis," the early events and mechanisms responsible are different. Whereas cells early in the process of abnormal keratinization often have increased eosinophilic keratin aggregates within their cytoplasm with viable-appearing nuclei, apoptotic cells during early evolutionary stages have shrunken, pyknotic, and sometimes fragmented nuclei in the setting of normal-appearing cytoplasm.

In some diseases, dyskeratosis is the expression of a genetically programed disturbance of keratinization as is the case in Darier disease. Dyskeratosis may occur

population and thus to a thickening of the epidermis (*acanthosis*, Fig. 2-2). In contrast to acanthosis is epidermal *atrophy* (thinning of epidermis, Fig. 2-3). Although there are many causes of atrophy, one primary etiology is a decrease in epidermal proliferative capacity, as may be seen with physiological aging or after the prolonged use of potent topical or systemic steroids. With atrophy, the epidermal rete ridges are initially lost, followed by progressive thinning of the epidermal layer.

Disturbances of Epidermal Cell Differentiation: A simple example of disturbed epidermal differentiation is *parakeratosis*, in which faulty and accelerated cornification leads to retention of pyknotic nuclei of epidermal cells at the epidermal surface. Instead of the normal anucleate "basket-weave"

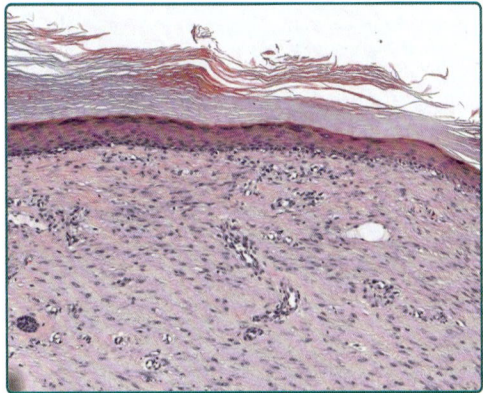

Figure 2-3 Atrophy. The epidermis is thin and there is flattening of the rete ridge architecture.

in actinic keratosis and squamous cell carcinoma. Dyskeratosis may also be caused by direct physical and chemical injuries. In the sunburn reaction, eosinophilic apoptotic cells—so-called sunburn cells—are found within the epidermis within the first 24 hours after irradiation with ultraviolet B (UVB); similar cells may occur after high-dose systemic cytotoxic treatment. Individual cell death within the epidermis is a regular phenomenon in graft-versus-host disease and in erythema multiforme.

Disturbances of Epidermal Cohesion:

Epidermal cohesion is the result of intercellular attachment devices (desmosomes) and the related intercellular molecular interactions. Desmosomes dissociate and reform at new sites of intercellular contact as cells migrate through the epidermis and keratinocytes mature toward the epidermal surface. The most common result of disturbed epidermal cohesion is the intraepidermal vesicle, a small cavity filled with fluid. Table 2-4 shows a classification of blistering diseases.

Three basic morphologic patterns of intraepidermal vesicle formation are classically recognized. *Spongiosis* is an example of the *secondary* loss of cohesion between epidermal cells caused by the influx of tissue fluid into the epidermis. Serous exudate may extend from the dermis into the intercellular compartment of the epidermis; as it expands, epidermal cells remain in contact with each other only at the sites of desmosomes, acquiring a stellate appearance and giving the epidermis a sponge-like morphology (spongiosis). As the intercellular edema increases, increased white space is noted between keratinocytes (Fig. 2-4), individual cells rupture and lyse, and microcavities (spongiotic vesicles) result. Confluence of such microcavities leads to larger blisters. Leukocytes then migrate into the epidermis with spongiotic edema, which is best illustrated in acute

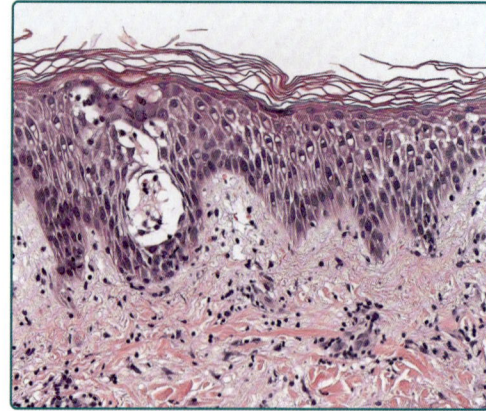

Figure 2-4 Spongiosis. Accumulation of fluid in the epidermis is manifested by white space between the keratinocytes.

allergic contact dermatitis. The accumulation of polymorphonuclear leukocytes within the epidermis eventually leads to the formation of a pustule.

Acantholysis is a *primary* loss of cohesion of epidermal cells. This is initially characterized by a widening and separation of the interdesmosomal regions of the cell membranes of keratinocytes, followed by splitting and a disappearance of desmosomes. The cells are intact but are no longer attached; they revert to their smallest possible surface and round up (Fig. 2-5). Intercellular gaps result, and the influx of fluid from the dermis leads to a cavity, which may form in a suprabasal, midepidermal, or even subcorneal location. Acantholysis occurs in a number of different pathologic processes that do not have a common etiology and pathogenesis. In the pemphigus group, acantholysis results from the interaction of autoantibodies and antigenic determinants on the keratinocyte membranes and related desmosomal adhesive proteins, and in the staphylococcal scalded-skin syndrome,

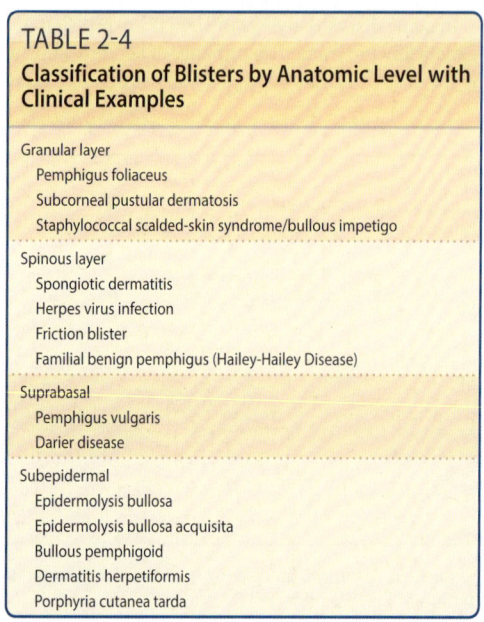

TABLE 2-4
Classification of Blisters by Anatomic Level with Clinical Examples

Granular layer
  Pemphigus foliaceus
  Subcorneal pustular dermatosis
  Staphylococcal scalded-skin syndrome/bullous impetigo

Spinous layer
  Spongiotic dermatitis
  Herpes virus infection
  Friction blister
  Familial benign pemphigus (Hailey-Hailey Disease)

Suprabasal
  Pemphigus vulgaris
  Darier disease

Subepidermal
  Epidermolysis bullosa
  Epidermolysis bullosa acquisita
  Bullous pemphigoid
  Dermatitis herpetiformis
  Porphyria cutanea tarda

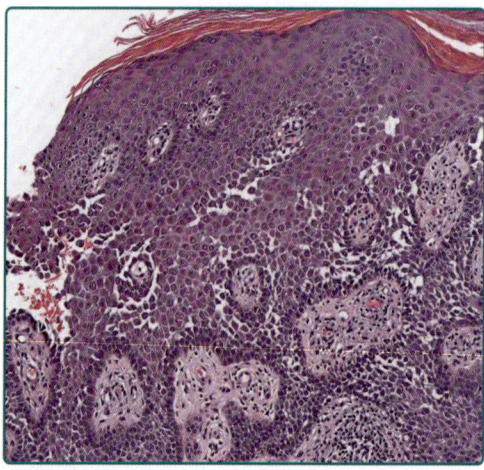

Figure 2-5 Acantholysis. Epidermal keratinocytes separate from each other and take on a rounded, rather than elongate, appearance.

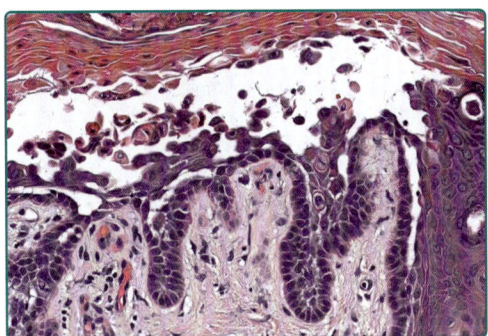

Figure 2-6 Acantholysis and dyskeratosis. This combination of features can be seen in Darier disease, warty dyskeratoma, and Grover disease.

it is caused by a staphylococcal exotoxin. In familial benign pemphigus, it results from the combination of a genetically determined defect of the keratinocyte cell membrane and exogenous factors. A similar phenomenon, albeit more confined to the suprabasal epidermis, occurs in Darier disease, where it is combined with dyskeratosis in the upper epidermal layers (Fig. 2-6) and a compensatory proliferation of basal cells. When acantholysis results from viral infection, it is usually combined with other cellular phenomena such as ballooning, giant cells, and nuclear moulding.

Indeed, a loss of epidermal cohesion can also result from a primary dissolution of cells (ie, cytolysis). In the epidermolytic forms of epidermolysis bullosa, genetically defective and thus structurally compromised basal cells rupture as a result of trauma so that the cleft forms through the basal cell layer. Cytolytic phenomena in the stratum granulosum are characteristic for epidermolytic hyperkeratosis, bullous congenital ichthyosiform erythroderma, ichthyosis hystrix, and some forms of hereditary palmoplantar keratoderma.

DERMAL–EPIDERMAL JUNCTION

Epidermis and dermis are structurally interlocked by means of the epidermal rete ridges and the corresponding dermal papillae, and foot-like submicroscopic cytoplasmic microprocesses of basal cells that extend into corresponding indentations of the dermis. Dermal–epidermal attachment is enforced by hemidesmosomes that anchor basal cells onto the basal lamina; this, in turn, is attached to the dermis by means of anchoring filaments and microfibrils. These structural relationships correlate with complex molecular interactions that serve to bind the epidermis, basement membrane, and superficial dermis in a manner that promotes resistance to potentially life-threatening epidermal detachment. The basal lamina is not a rigid or impermeable structure because leukocytes, Langerhans cells, or other migratory cells pass through it without causing a permanent breach in the junction. After being destroyed by pathologic processes, the basal lamina is reconstituted; this represents an important phenomenon in wound healing and other reparative processes. Functionally, the basal lamina is part of a unit that, by light microscopy, appears as the periodic acid–Schiff–positive "basement membrane" and, in fact, represents the entire junction zone. This consists of the lamina lucida, spanned by microfilaments, and subjacent anchoring fibrils, small collagen fibers, and extracellular matrix. The junction zone is a functional complex that is primarily affected in a number of pathologic processes.

Disturbances of Dermal–Epidermal Cohesion: The destruction of the junction zone or its components usually manifests as disturbance of dermal–epidermal cohesion and leads to blister formation. In these processes, the entire epidermis forms the roof of the blister, and the floor of the blister is composed of dermis without epidermal keratinocytes. In bullous pemphigoid (Fig. 2-7), cleft formation runs through the lamina lucida of the basal membrane and is caused by autoantibodies directed against specific antigens on the cytomembrane of basal cells (*junctional blistering*). Junctional blistering also occurs in the junctional forms of epidermolysis bullosa, but here it is due to the hereditary

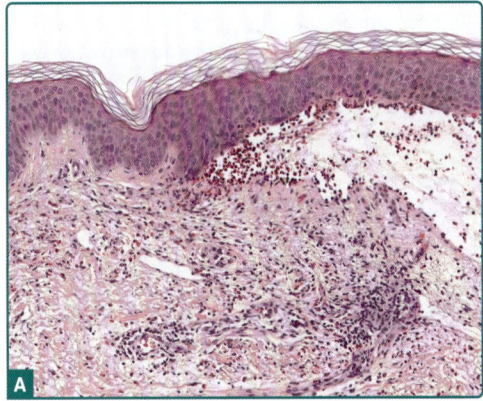

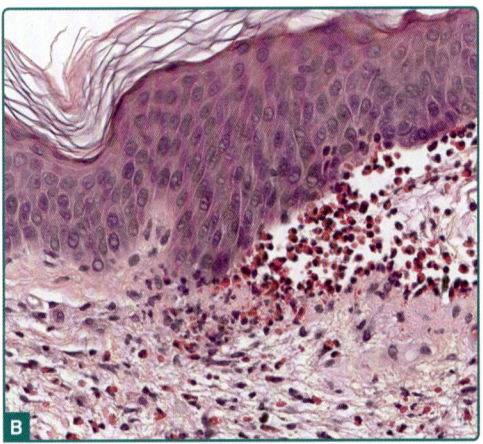

Figure 2-7 Bullous pemphigoid. **A,** There is subepidermal blister formation associated with an eosinophil-rich infiltrate. **B,** At the edge of the blister, eosinophils align at the dermal–epidermal junction.

impairment or absence of molecules important for dermal–epidermal cohesion.

In *dermolytic blistering*, the target of the pathologic process is below the basal lamina. These blisters look similar on hematoxylin and eosin (H&E) staining with the roof composed of intact epidermis. Reduced anchoring filaments and increased collagenase production result in dermolytic dermal–epidermal separation in recessive epidermolysis bullosa. Circulating autoantibodies directed against type VII collagen in anchoring fibrils are the cause of dermolytic blistering in acquired epidermolysis bullosa. Other disorders that result in dermolytic blistering include dermatitis herpetiformis, and porphyria cutanea tarda.

PATHOLOGIC REACTIONS OF THE ENTIRE SUPERFICIAL REACTIVE UNIT

Most pathologic reactions of the superficial skin involve the epidermis and the papillary dermis with the superficial microvascular plexus. This is a highly reactive tissue compartment consisting of capillaries, pre- and postcapillary vessels, mast cells, fibroblasts, macrophages, dendritic cells, and peripatetic lymphocytes, all embedded in a loose connective tissue and extracellular matrix. The prominence of involvement of one of the components over the others may lead to the development of different clinical pictures. A few examples of reaction patterns are detailed below.

Spongiotic Dermatitis: In spongiotic dermatitis such as nummular, contact, and atopic dermatitis, there is an inflammatory reaction of the papillary dermis and superficial microvascular plexus and spongiosis of the epidermis. Lymphocytes infiltrate the epidermis early in the process and aggregate around Langerhans cells, and this is followed by spongiotic vesiculation (Fig. 2-8). Parakeratosis develops as a consequence of epidermal injury and proliferative responses, and the inflammation results in acanthosis and hyperkeratosis in chronic lesions.

Psoriasis: The initial pathologic events in psoriasis appear to be the perivascular accumulation of lymphocytes within the papillary dermis and focal migration of leukocytes (often neutrophils, although T cells are also integral to pathogenesis) into the epidermis. Acanthosis caused by increased epidermal proliferation, elongation of rete ridges sometimes accompanied by an undulant epidermal surface (papillomatosis), and edema of the elongated dermal papillae together with vasodilatation of the capillary loops develop almost simultaneously (see Fig. 2-9). The disturbed differentiation of the epidermal cells results in parakeratosis, and small aggregates of neutrophils infiltrating the upper epidermis (spongiform pustules), in the parakeratotic stratum corneum (Munro microabscesses). Therefore, the composite picture characteristic of psoriasis results from a combined pathology of the papillary dermis with participation of superficial venules, the epidermis, and circulating cells. Psoriasis is an instructive example of the limited specificity of histopathologic reaction patterns within the skin because psoriasiform histologic features occur in a number of diseases unrelated to psoriasis.

Interface and Lichenoid Dermatitis: In both interface and lichenoid processes, lymphocytes are present along the dermal–epidermal junction associated with vacuolar alteration of basal layer keratinocytes. In an interface reaction, the infiltrate is sparse, and in lichenoid reactions, the infiltrate is dense and band-like at the dermal–epidermal junction. Subsequently there is dyskeratosis of keratinocytes, hyperkeratosis, and, occasionally, hypergranulosis (lichen planus, Fig. 2-10). Depending on the disease state, the epidermis may be thickened (lichen planus) or atrophic (lupus erythematosus).

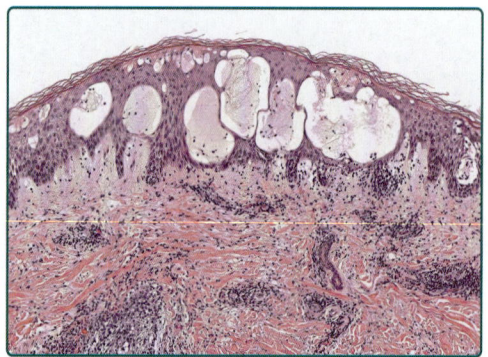

Figure 2-8 Spongiotic dermatitis. Accumulation of fluid in the epidermis leads to formation of an intraepidermal microvesicle.

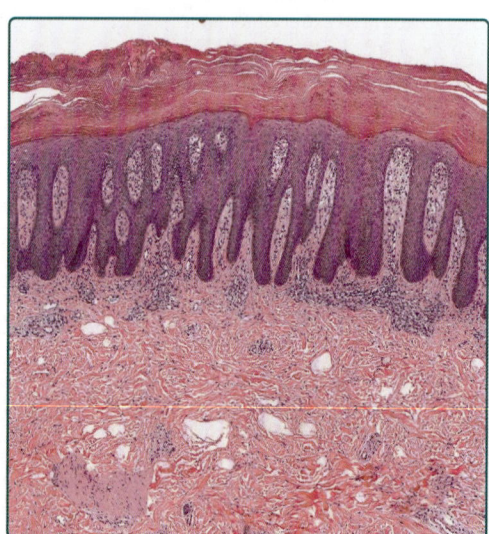

Figure 2-9 Psoriasis. There is uniform thickening of the epidermis with elongate rete ridges and a diminished granular layer.

In addition to lupus erythematosus and lichen planus, interface/lichenoid changes can be seen in dermatomyositis, erythema multiforme, secondary syphilis, fixed drug reaction, graft-versus-host disease, and lichenoid drug reactions. Differentiating these entities depends on the cellular makeup of the infiltrate (lymphocytes, eosinophils, plasma cells) and, importantly, the clinical presentation.

Subepidermal Blistering Processes: In subepidermal blistering processes, the roof of the blister is composed of full-thickness intact epidermis, and the floor of the blister is dermis without attached keratinocytes. In evaluating this group of diseases, one studies the edge of the blister and the character of the inflammatory cells. For example, in bullous pemphigoid, eosinophils align at the dermal–epidermal junction, at the edge of the blister (see Fig. 2-7). If neutrophils are seen in this area, the differential diagnosis includes dermatitis herpetiformis, linear immunoglobulin A disease, bullous lupus erythematosus, and inflammatory epidermolysis bullosa acquisita. Subepidermal blistering with little to no inflammatory cells generally indicates porphyria cutanea tarda, epidermolysis bullosa acquisita, or the cell-poor variant of pemphigoid. Direct and indirect immunofluorescence testing and/or enzyme-linked immunosorbent assay (ELISA) testing for antibodies to BP180/BP230 are often helpful in distinguishing entities in the subepidermal blister disease group.

RETICULAR DERMIS

The reticular layer of the dermis represents a second reactive unit and is composed of coarse connective tissue and the deeper dermal vascular plexus (see Fig. 2-1). The dermis represents a strong fibroelastic tissue with a network of collagen and elastic fibers embedded in an extracellular matrix with a high water-binding capacity. In contrast to the tightly interwoven fibrous components of this reticular layer of the dermis, the papillary dermis is composed of finer elastic fibers and collagen bundles that follow the structures they surround.

PATTERN EVALUATION

The dermis contains a superficial and deep vascular network. In the upper dermis, the superficial plexus supplies individual vascular districts consisting of several dermal papillae. Superficial and deep networks are connected so intimately that the entire dermal vascular system represents a single three-dimensional network. In dermal-based processes, the epidermis is relatively normal in appearance. In evaluation of pathological states, one can classify these processes into perivascular (*angiocentric*: around blood vessels), *periadnexal* (around hair follicles and/or eccrine glands), and *nodular* or diffuse inflammatory patterns. Additionally, there may be alterations of the dermal connective tissue (collagen, elastin) or deposition of material in the dermis.

***Angiocentric* Pattern (Fig. 2-11):** In the superficial microvascular system, two reaction patterns occur: (a) acute inflammatory processes in which the epidermis and junctional zone are often involved together with the vascular system, and (b) more chronic processes that often remain confined to the perivascular compartment. In this context, it should be noted that the cytologic composition of the infiltrate is important: neutrophils, eosinophils, lymphocytes, mast cells. For example, an infiltrate composed mostly of neutrophils associated with fibrin and hemorrhage is typical of small vessel or leukocytoclastic vasculitis that presents clinically as palpable purpura. In contrast, perivascular lymphocytes with hemorrhage is typical of Schamberg's pigmented purpuric dermatosis.

***Periadnexal* Pattern (Fig. 2-12):** Follicular units (hair follicle with sebaceous gland), eccrine ducts/glands, and apocrine glands constitute the skin adnexal structures. Inflammatory processes concentrated predominantly around hair follicles raise a differential diagnosis of folliculitis, acneiform processes, and infectious folliculitis by bacteria, fungus, or

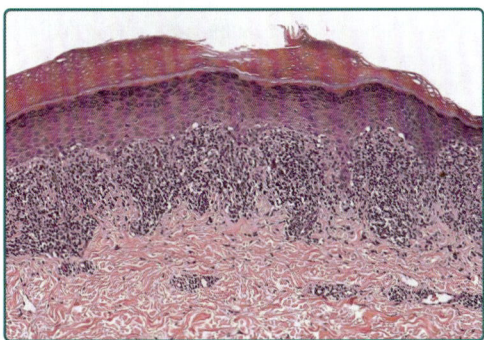

Figure 2-10 Lichen planus. An acanthotic epidermis with a band-like lymphocytic infiltrate that approximates the dermal–epidermal junction.

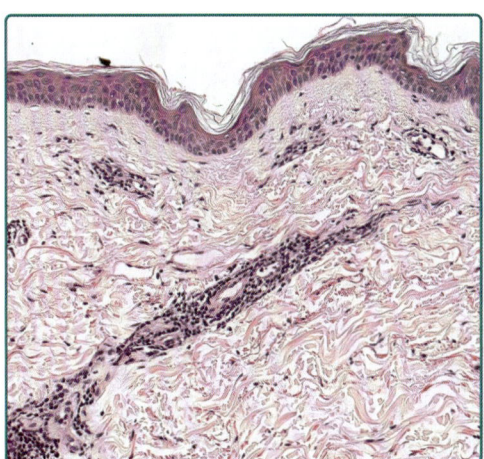

Figure 2-11 Angiocentric pattern. Inflammatory cells are seen primarily around small vessels in the dermis.

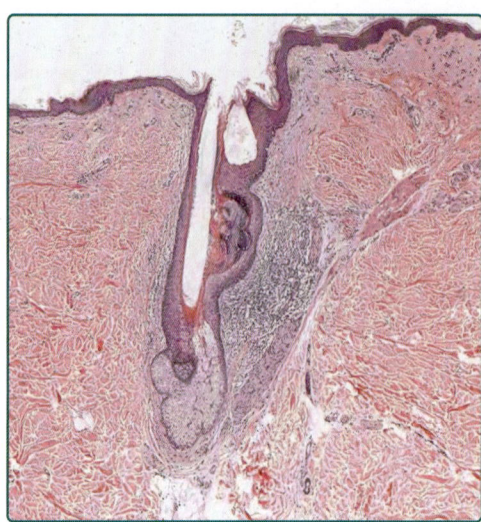

Figure 2-12 Perifollicular pattern. In this example of folliculitis, inflammatory cells surround a follicle.

herpesvirus. Perieccrine inflammation is not specific, but it is often a clue that leads to a diagnosis of lupus erythematosus, neutrophilic eccrine hidradenitis, perniosis, or syringotropic mycosis fungoides. Evaluation of the character of the infiltrate is important in the pattern.

Nodular or Diffuse Pattern (Fig. 2-13): In this pattern of inflammation, the collections of dermal cells form larger aggregates than what is seen in the angiocentric pattern. Similar to other patterns, one must evaluate the cellular make-up of the infiltrate. Nodular collections of lymphocytes raise a differential diagnosis of cutaneous B-cell lymphoma, cutaneous lymphoid hyperplasia (pseudolymphoma), and angiolymphoid hyperplasia. In these cases, immunohistochemical staining for various T-cell and B-cell antigens is helpful in establishing the diagnosis. If neutrophils predominate in a nodular infiltrate, one considers Sweet syndrome, pyoderma gangrenosum, follicular rupture, or abscess formation associated with infection.

COMPOSITION OF THE INFILTRATE

Once a pattern is established at low magnification, one can proceed to evaluation of the specific composition of the infiltrate. Evaluation includes determining both the predominant and less prominent cell types: lymphocytes, histiocytes (with or without granulomas), neutrophils, eosinophils, plasma cells, or mast cells.

Lymphocytes: Lymphocytes have small round/oval nuclei and very little cytoplasm. Although lymphocytic infiltrates occur in the majority of inflammatory dermatoses, there are a number of pathologic processes in which lymphocytes predominate, and thus determine the histologic picture. Lymphocytic

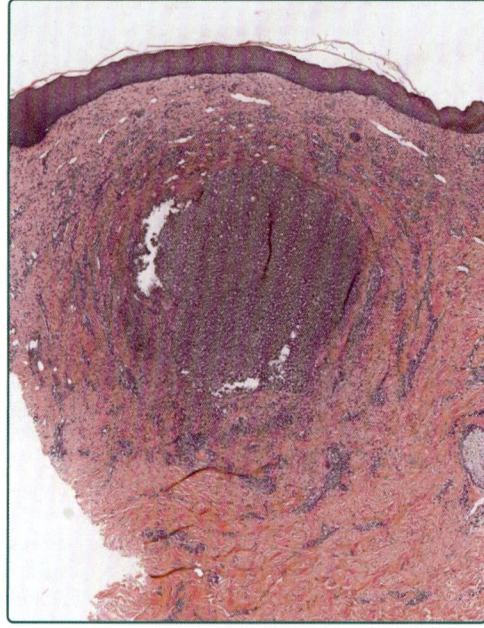

Figure 2-13 Nodular pattern. Dense aggregates of inflammatory cells are present in the dermis.

infiltrates are formed in inflammatory or proliferative conditions, and in proliferative conditions, may represent a benign or malignant process.

Among the many possible reaction patterns characterized by lymphocytic infiltrates, several typical patterns can be distinguished.

- Lymphocytic cuffing of venules without involvement of the papillary dermis and the epidermis may occur in figurate erythemas, viral exanthema, and in drug eruptions. The infiltrates of chronic lymphocytic leukemia show a similar distribution pattern but are usually more pronounced.
- Perivascular lymphocytic infiltrates with a mucinous infiltration of the nonperivascular connective tissue is often a clue to a differential diagnosis of lupus erythematosus or dermatomyositis.
- Nodular lymphocytic infiltrates, often mimicking lymph node tissue, are typical of lymphocytoma cutis or cutaneous lymphoid hyperplasia. Atypical lymphocytic infiltrates involving both the superficial and deeper dermis, and cytologically characterized by pronounced pleomorphism of the cellular infiltrate, are characteristic of lymphomatoid papulosis, one of the spectrum of CD30+ lymphoproliferative disorders. This condition exemplifies the problems that arise when the histopathology of a lesion is used alone to determine whether a process is benign or malignant. Without knowledge of the clinical features and the course of disease, a definitive diagnosis is extremely difficult.

Neutrophils and Eosinophils: Eosinophils are recognized by their characteristic bilobed nucleus and eosinophilic granular cytoplasm (Fig. 2-14). The

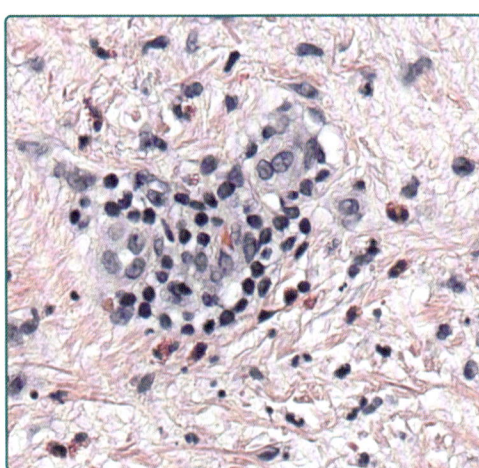

Figure 2-14 Eosinophils. The nuclei are bilobed and the cytoplasm is bright pink and granular. The lymphocytes have small dark nuclei and scant cytoplasm.

presence of many eosinophils in a dermal infiltrate can be helpful in diagnosing an allergic reaction (insect bite, medication reaction, scabies), but also in the differential diagnosis of Wells syndrome (eosinophilic cellulitis), angiolymphoid hyperplasia with eosinophilia, and the prodromal stage of pemphigoid. Neutrophils have multilobed nuclei and a less-eosinophilic cytoplasm than eosinophils. Neutrophil-rich infiltrates often imply an infectious etiology especially if neutrophils aggregate in the dermis forming an abscess. In contrast, there are many noninfectious neutrophilic processes in the skin, such as Sweet syndrome, pyoderma gangrenosum, urticaria, and vasculitis.

Granulomatous Reactions: Skin is an ideal tissue for granuloma formation in which histiocytes play a key role. The proliferation and focal aggregation of histiocytic cells are termed a *granuloma*. When such cells are closely clustered they resemble epithelial tissue, hence the designation *epithelioid cells*. Granulomas usually lead to destruction of preexisting tissue, particularly elastic fibers, and in such instances result in atrophy, fibrosis, or scarring. Tissue damage or destruction manifests either as necrobiosis or fibrinoid or caseous necrosis, or it may result from liquefaction and abscess formation or from replacement of preexisting tissue by fibrohistiocytic infiltrate and fibrosis.

Sarcoidal granulomas are typically characterized by nodules of epithelioid histiocytic cells, occasional Langerhans giant cells, and only a small number of lymphocytes. In addition to sarcoidosis, silica, zirconium, and beryllium granulomas, and a number of foreign-body granulomas may have such histopathologic features (Fig. 2-15).

Granulomatous reactions of the skin comprise a large spectrum of histopathologic features. Palisading granulomas surround hypocellular areas of the connective tissue with histiocytes in radial alignment (Fig. 2-16). Granuloma annulare, necrobiosis lipoidica,

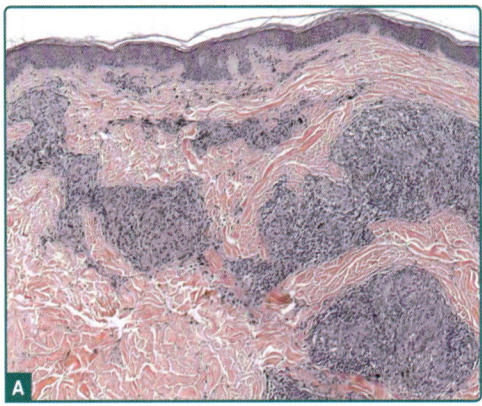

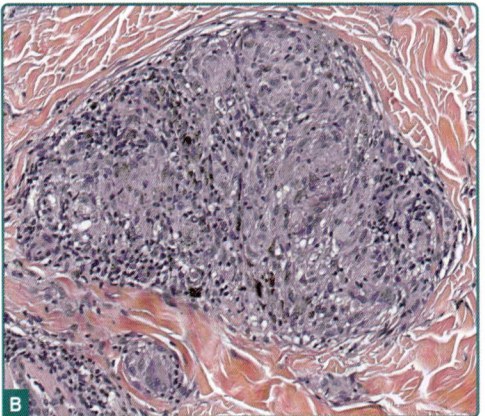

Figure 2-15 Granuloma. **A,** This foreign-body granuloma shows an aggregate of lymphocytes, histiocytes, and multinucleated giant cells forming a nodule. **B,** Higher magnification of epithelioid histiocytes and foreign material (black pigment).

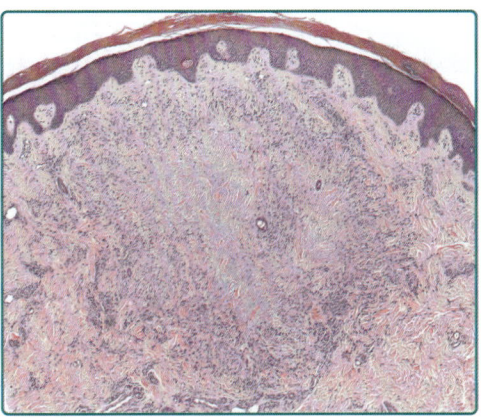

Figure 2-16 Granuloma annulare. In granuloma annulare, histiocytes and giant cells surround a zone of hypocellular collagen that shows few to no nuclei.

and rheumatoid nodules belong to this group. These reactions may have significance as signs of systemic disease.[6] Rheumatoid nodules can be associated with rheumatoid arthritis, and interstitial granulomatous dermatitis can be associated with arthritis and immune-mediated disorders.

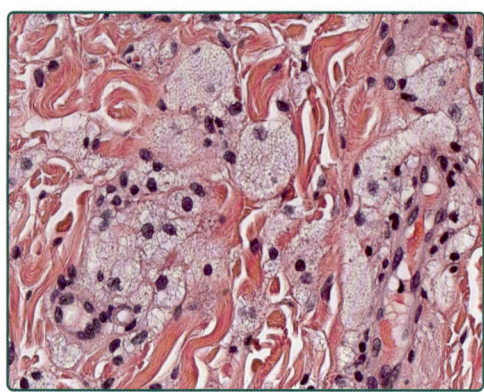

Figure 2-17 Xanthoma cells. The cytoplasm is enlarged and shows a vacuolated (bubbly) appearance.

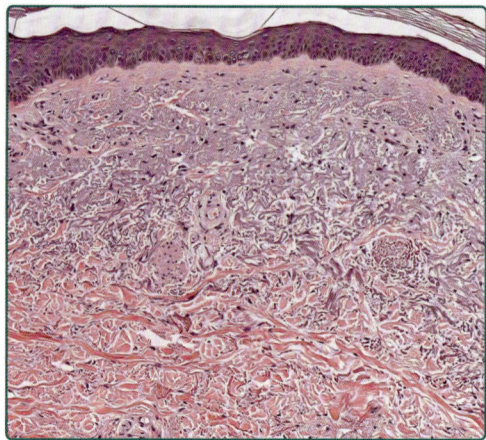

Figure 2-18 Actinic (solar) elastosis. The superficial dermis show many gray-colored elastotic fibers from chronic sun damage. In the lower portion of the photomicrograph, the collagen shows the normal pink color.

Infectious granulomas with a sarcoidal appearance may occur in tuberculosis, syphilis, leishmaniasis, leprosy, and atypical mycobacterial or fungal infections. Necrosis can also develop within the granuloma proper, as is the case for fibrinoid necrosis in sarcoidosis, caseation in tuberculosis, or the necrosis developing in mycotic granulomas. Many of the infectious granulomas are associated with epidermal hyperplasia, often exhibiting intraepidermal abscesses. In the dermis, there is a mixture of cells, including histiocytes, epithelioid cells, eosinophils, neutrophils, and lymphocytes.

A specific form of granulomatous reaction results when the cellular infiltrate consists almost exclusively of the key granuloma cell, the *histiocyte*. One property of this cell is its capacity to store phagocytosed material. In xanthomatous reaction patterns, histiocytes take up, store fat, and are thus transformed into foam cells (Fig. 2-17). These cells are characteristic of various types of xanthomatous processes including tuberous and eruptive xanthomas as well as xanthelasma.

FIBROUS DERMIS AND EXTRACELLULAR MATRIX

Sclerosing processes of the skin involve mainly the connective tissue of the dermis. The hallmark of scleroderma and morphea is the homogenization, thickening, and dense packing of the collagen bundles, and a narrowing of the interfascicular clefts within the reticular dermis. There is also a perivascular infiltrate of lymphocytes and plasma cells. Sclerodermoid changes may be found in the toxic oil syndrome and L-tryptophan disease, eosinophilic fasciitis, and mixed connective tissue disease.

Faulty synthesis or crosslinking of collagen results in a number of well-defined diseases or syndromes but leads to relatively few characteristic histopathologic changes. In the different types of the Ehlers-Danlos syndrome, the faulty collagen cannot be recognized histopathologically, and only the relative increase of elastic tissue may indicate that something abnormal has occurred in the dermis. The fragmentation and curled and clumped appearance of elastic fibers are diagnostic in pseudoxanthoma elasticum. On the other hand, in actinic elastosis, a consequence of chronic sun damage, all components of the superficial connective tissue are involved. Except for a narrow grenz zone below the epidermis, the papillary dermis, and the superficial layers of the reticular dermis are filled with clumped and curled fibers that progressively become homogenized and basophilic (Fig. 2-18). They are stained by dyes that have an affinity for elastic tissue and thus histochemically behave similar to elastic fibers.

Alterations in elastic tissue generally cannot be visualized on routine H&E staining except for actinic elastosis, and the use of special stains is necessary. Verhoeff-van Gieson staining is often used to highlight presence, absence, or alteration of elastic fibers in the dermis.

Endogenous and exogenous materials can also alter the dermis. Examples of endogenous materials include the accumulation of mucinous ground substance as one can see in pretibial myxedema, or deposits of proteinaceous amyloid as nodular aggregates in the dermis or surrounding vessels and adnexal structures (systemic amyloidosis). Materials that are not produced by the body can be introduced into the dermis accidentally or in cosmetic procedures (tattoos: Fig. 2-19, filler agents).

SUBCUTANEOUS FAT

The third reactive unit, the subcutaneous tissue, is composed of lobules of adipocytes and the intervening bands of fibrous connective tissue called septa.[7]

Inflammation of subcutaneous fat reflects either an inflammatory process of the fat lobules (lobular panniculitis) or a process arising in the septum (septal

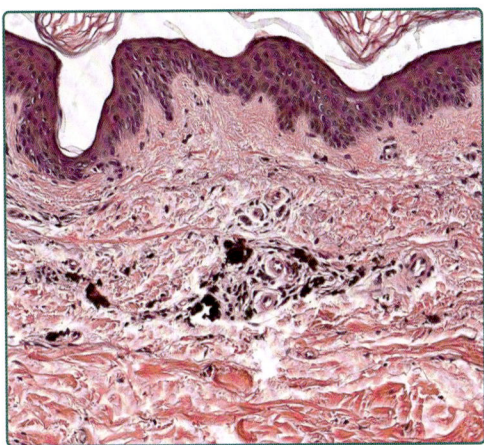

Figure 2-19 Tattoo. Foreign substances can be deposited in the dermis. Tattoo pigment is seen here as course clumps of black pigment in the superficial dermis.

panniculitis).[8,9] There may or may not be associated vasculitis. Destruction of fat, be it of a traumatic or inflammatory nature, leads to the release of fatty acids that by themselves are strong inflammatory stimuli, attracting neutrophils and scavenger histiocytes and macrophages; phagocytosis of destroyed fat usually results in lipogranuloma formation.

Septal panniculitis that follows inflammatory changes of the trabecular vessels is usually accompanied by edema, infiltration of inflammatory cells, and a histiocytic reaction. This is the classic appearance in erythema nodosum (Fig. 2-20). Recurring septal inflammation may lead to a broadening of the interlobular septa, fibrosis, and the accumulation of histiocytes and giant cells.

Lobular panniculitis refers to an inflammatory process predominantly in the subcutaneous lobules with less involvement of the septa. The lipid material derived from damaged adipocytes contains free and esterified cholesterol, neutral fats, soaps, and free fatty acids, which, in turn, exert an inflammatory stimulus. Histiocytic cells migrate into the inflamed fat, and phagocytosis leads to foam cell formation.

Exogenous factors may affect the subcutaneous tissue. Traumatic panniculitis leads to necrosis of fat lobules and a reactive inflammatory and granulomatous tissue response. After the injection of oils or silicone, large cystic cavities may be formed. Oily substances may remain within the adipose tissue for long periods without causing a significant tissue reaction; oil cysts evolve that are surrounded by multiple layers of residual connective tissue, so that the tissue acquires a "Swiss cheese" appearance.

Panniculitis also occurs as a result of infectious agents (bacteria, mycobacteria, and fungal organisms) in which neutrophil-rich inflammation and/or granulomatous inflammation is characteristic.

NEOPLASTIC DISORDERS OF THE SKIN

This section discusses how to approach the evaluation of skin neoplasms based on the cell type(s) of origin, as well as features to consider in determining benignancy versus malignancy. Select neoplasms of the skin are also reviewed in greater detail, although this chapter is intended to provide only a general overview of the many skin tumors that exist.

ASSESSMENT OF SKIN TUMORS

CELL TYPES IN THE SKIN

The normal epidermis is composed of 4 cell types: keratinocytes, melanocytes, Langerhans cells, and

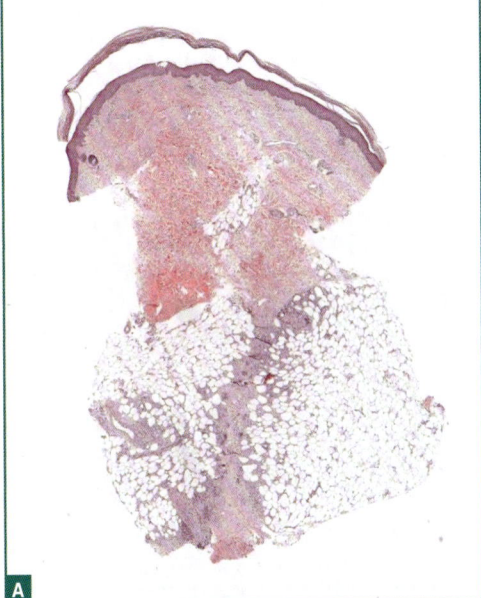

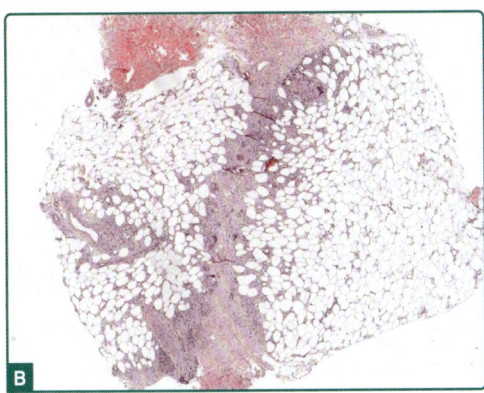

Figure 2-20 **A** and **B**, Erythema nodosum. The subcutaneous septa are thickened by fibrosis and inflammation.

Merkel cells. The cellular components of the normal dermis includes fibroblasts, endothelial cells lining vascular channels, smooth muscle cells, and nerve fibers. These cells types are reviewed in detail in Chap. 5.

FACTORS IN DETERMINING BENIGNANCY VERSUS MALIGNANCY OF TUMORS

The factors commonly used to assess skin tumors are (a) symmetry, (b) pattern of infiltration, (c) cytology, and (d) mitotic activity. Although specific criteria may apply for certain tumor types, benign tumors generally demonstrate reasonably good symmetry if a vertical line is drawn through the center of the tumor. Benign lesions are more likely to be well-circumscribed, whereas those with malignant potential often have a more infiltrative pattern into the surrounding tissue. Tumors that are benign tend to have cells with smaller, bland-appearing, and uniform nuclei compared to those that are malignant; in the malignant category, larger nuclei, nuclear pleomorphism, and sometimes prominent nucleoli are observed. Finally, mitotic figures can be observed in benign lesions, but are more frequently seen in malignant tumors. Atypical mitotic figures (those that are asymmetric and/or multipolar) are also more likely to appear in the setting of a malignant tumor.

TUMORS OF EPIDERMAL ORIGIN

KERATINOCYTIC TUMORS

Verruca Vulgaris: Verrucae vulgaris demonstrate marked hyperkeratosis, papillomatosis, and acanthosis (Fig. 2-21A). Verrucae vulgaris prominently feature koilocytes, cells which have structural changes secondary to human papillomavirus (HPV) infection. Koilocytes are identified by small round nuclei, perinuclear halos, and clumping of keratohyaline granules (Fig. 2-21B). They tend to be localized in the upper stratum spinosum and stratum granulosum in newer warts, and may be absent in more mature verrucae. Parakeratosis may be seen in the stratum corneum, most often localized to the areas directly overlying koilocytes. The epidermal rete within verrucae are elongated, and the rete at the periphery of the lesions often are oriented toward the center of the warts.

Verruca Plana: Histologically, verrucae plana show hyperkeratosis and epidermal acanthosis, but lack the papillomatosis seen in verrucae vulgaris. Koilocytes are observed in the granular layer of the epidermis.

Condyloma Acuminatum: Condyloma acuminata display slight hyperkeratosis and prominent acanthosis (Fig. 2-22A). While papillomatosis is a common feature, the surface of condyloma acuminata show rounded crests (so-called knuckling) as compared to verrucae vulgaris, which demonstrate elongated, pointed spires. Compared to other types of viral warts, koilocytes are not as prominently observed in condyloma acuminata (Fig. 2-22B). HPV immunostaining may be employed to help assess for viral change within condyloma acuminata, although in our experience immunostaining is commonly negative when koilocytes are not readily observed on H&E-stained sections.

Seborrheic Keratosis: Seborrheic keratoses show marked hyperkeratosis, papillomatosis, and acanthosis on histology (Fig. 2-23). In some cases, thin strands of anastomosing epithelium are seen within seborrheic keratoses, resulting in a reticulated pattern. Pseudo horn cysts and horn cysts are frequently observed in the acanthotic epidermis. There is often keratinocyte pigmentation. The keratinocytes within seborrheic keratoses are usually small and bland in appearance, although when lesions are irritated or inflamed the nuclei may become enlarged. Squamous eddies, which are composed of whorls of squamous

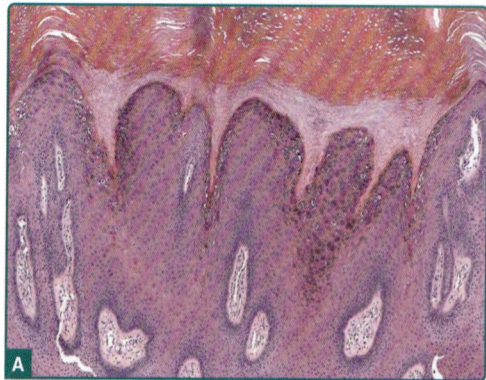
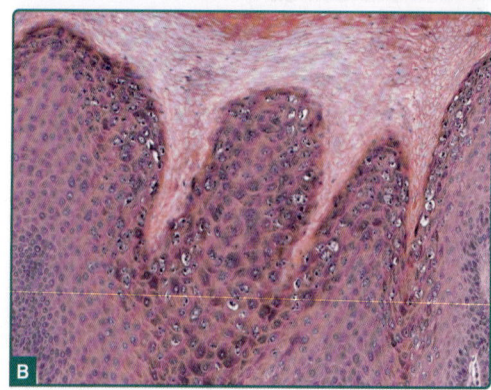

Figure 2-21 **A,** Verruca vulgaris showing hyperkeratosis, acanthosis and papillomatosis of the epidermis. **B,** Koilocytes seen in a verruca, showing clumping of keratohyaline granules and perinuclear halos.

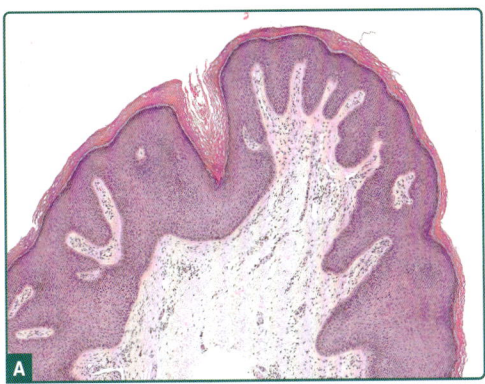

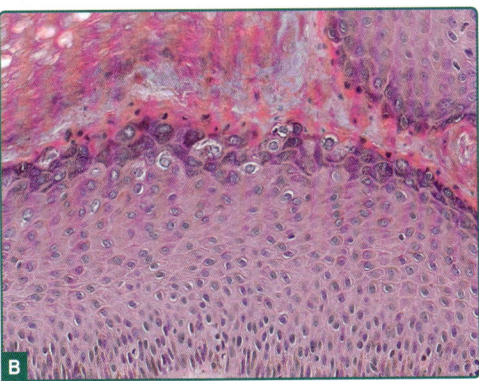

Figure 2-22 **A,** Condyloma acuminatum demonstrating hyperkeratosis and acanthosis. In contrast to verruca vulgaris, there are rounded, rather than pointed, epidermal crests. **B,** Koilocytes in condyloma acuminatum, which are frequently less prominent than those seen in verruca vulgaris.

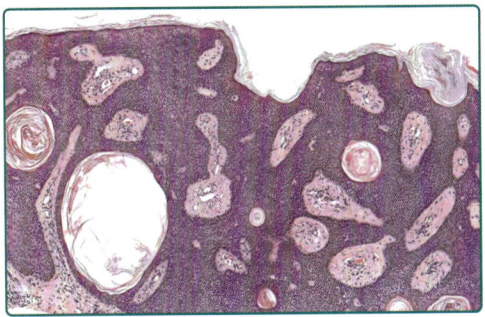

Figure 2-23 Seborrheic keratosis with hyperkeratosis, acanthosis, and multiple pseudo horn cysts.

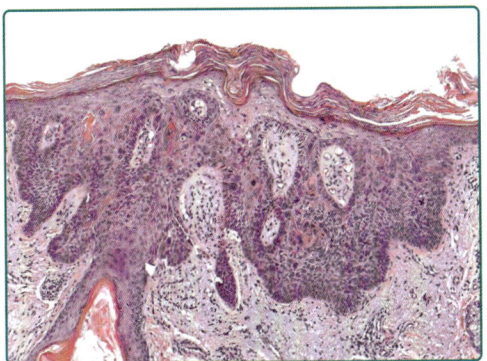

Figure 2-24 Squamous cell carcinoma in situ demonstrating full-thickness keratinocyte atypia within the epidermis. Enlarged, hyperchromatic keratinocyte nuclei are easily seen.

epithelial cells, are more frequently observed in inflamed or irritated seborrheic keratoses.

Inverted follicular keratoses are considered variants of seborrheic keratoses. Inverted follicular keratoses have an endophytic architecture compared to other types of seborrheic keratoses. Squamous eddies are a prominent feature in this variant.

Squamous Cell Carcinoma: When squamous cell carcinoma (SCC) is restricted only to the epidermis, it is referred to as SCC in situ. Such lesions show full-thickness atypia of the epidermis with keratinocytes that have enlarged nuclei, nuclear pleomorphism, and increased mitotic activity (Fig. 2-24). Apoptotic or dyskeratotic keratinocytes are also commonly observed in SCC in situ. There is typically parakeratosis in the stratum corneum, with underlying loss of the granular layer. By definition, SCC in situ does not invade the underlying dermis, but may show extension of the atypical keratinocytes along adnexal structures including hair follicles and eccrine ducts. The term "Bowen disease" is often used interchangeably with "SCC in situ," although in our practice "Bowen disease" is reserved for SCC in situ of sun-protected anatomic sites such as the anogenital region.

Invasive SCC shows acanthosis of the epidermis, composed of atypical keratinocytes, as well as lobules of keratinocytes that have broken away from the epidermis and are embedded within the dermis (Fig. 2-25). The keratinocytes may be enlarged and glassy in appearance, with associated horn pearls composed of parakeratin. This type of pattern is seen frequently in well to moderately differentiated SCCs. More poorly differentiated tumors lack significant keratinization and often have an infiltrative pattern within the dermis. Solar elastosis is frequently observed in invasive SCCs.

Keratoacanthoma: Keratoacanthomas are very similar in appearance to well-differentiated SCCs, both clinically and histologically. However, unlike SCCs, they involute spontaneously within several months to a year after they arise. Multiple keratoacanthomas may arise spontaneously, in the context of genetic syndromes such as in Muir-Torre syndrome, or as a side effect of taking certain medications, notably the BRAF (v-raf murine sarcoma viral oncogene homolog B) inhibitors sorafenib, vemurafenib, and dabrafenib.[10,11]

Microscopically, mature keratoacanthomas show a cup-shaped epithelial proliferation, exhibiting prominent acanthosis consisting of glassy keratinocytes. There is usually a central keratin-filled crater, and the epidermis extends medially over the crater to form a

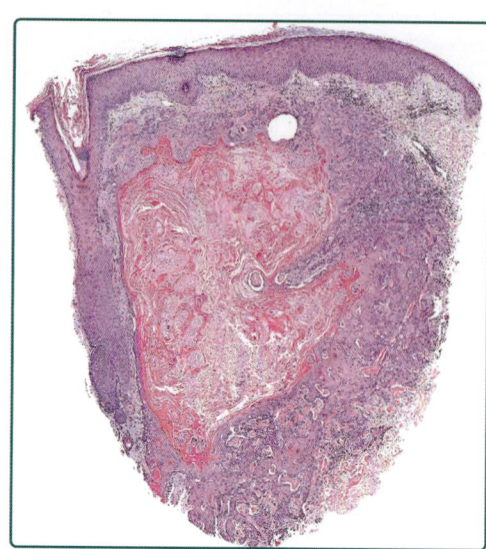

Figure 2-25 Invasive squamous cell carcinoma characterized by a nodule of atypical keratinocytes in the dermis with prominent keratinization consisting of parakeratin.

"lip." The epithelial proliferation invaginates into the underlying dermis, which often displays solar elastosis. A characteristic finding of keratoacanthomas is the presence of neutrophilic microabscesses within the atypical epithelium. A lymphocyte-rich inflammatory infiltrate is frequently observed in the surrounding dermis.

Involuting keratoacanthomas show atypia of the epidermis as described above, associated with a lymphocytic infiltrate at the base of the lesion and often the presence of dyskeratotic keratinocytes. This is accompanied by fibrosis of the surrounding stroma, which eventually forms a scar.

Basal Cell Carcinoma: Histopathologically, basal cell carcinomas (BCCs) are comprised of lobules of purple or basophilic cells, which most closely resemble the cells found in the basal layer of the epidermis. The lobules display palisading of columnar cells at the periphery (Fig. 2-26A). Within the lobules, mitotic figures and apoptotic cells (often referred to as single-cell necrosis) are observed (Fig. 2-26B). The basaloid lobules typically demonstrate connection to the epidermis, and may also be seen arising from hair follicles. In superficial BCC, the basaloid lobules are small and arise from the epidermis, without deeper involvement. In the nodular type of BCC, larger basaloid lobules with deeper dermal involvement are observed. The stroma surrounding the basaloid lobules is distinctive as it is fibromyxoid in appearance, composed of fibroblasts set within a loose mucinous matrix. Stromal retraction, or spaces between the basaloid lobules and the surrounding fibromucinous connective tissue, is commonly seen.

The infiltrative type of BCC is made up of smaller, elongated islands of basaloid cells, as compared to the tumor lobules seen in nodular BCC, and may invade deeply into the dermis. Morpheaform BCC display similarly small, elongated islands, but in association with thickened collagen bundles. These latter two histologic types, along with the micronodular type of BCC, which is composed of small tumor lobules in the dermis, represent the types of BCC at highest risk for aggressive behavior and local recurrence following surgery or other destructive treatment methods.

ADNEXAL TUMORS

This category of tumors includes those with differentiation toward various epidermal appendages including hair follicles, sweat glands (eccrine and apocrine), and sebaceous glands. Selected entities within these categories are discussed below.

Trichoepithelioma: Trichoepitheliomas demonstrate lobules of basaloid cells in embedded in the dermis, which have a cribriform or lace-like appearance (Fig. 2-27). Horn cysts are often present within the basaloid lobules. The stroma surrounding the basaloid lobules shows an increased number of

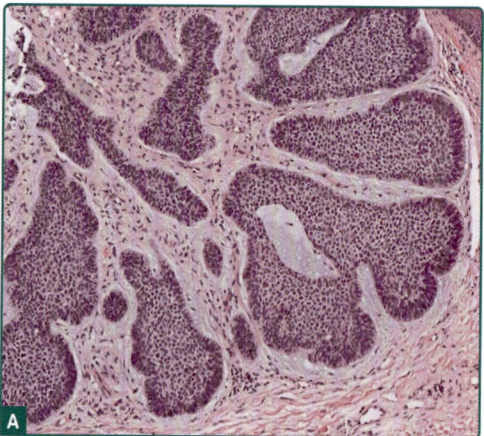

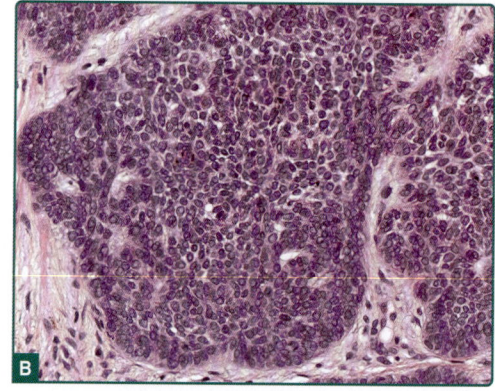

Figure 2-26 **A,** Basal cell carcinoma with lobules of purple basaloid cells exhibiting peripheral palisading in the dermis, set within a fibromyxoid stroma. **B,** Single-cell necrosis within a basaloid lobule.

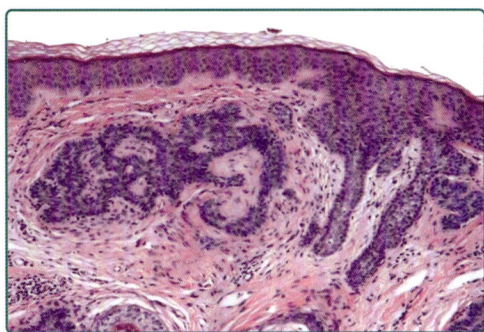

Figure 2-27 Trichoepithelioma showing cribriform basaloid lobules with a dense fibrous stroma. Papillary mesenchymal bodies are observed.

fibroblasts, and lacks the mucinous ground substance typically observed in the stroma of BCCs. Papillary mesenchymal bodies are a characteristic feature of trichoepitheliomas. They form invaginations into the basaloid tumor lobules, showing many fibroblasts and strongly resembling the papillae of normal hair follicles.

A variant of a trichoepithelioma is the desmoplastic trichoepithelioma, which classically occurs on the face of young adult women. In contrast to conventional trichoepitheliomas, desmoplastic trichoepitheliomas show elongated thin islands of basaloid cells set within a fibrotic (desmoplastic) stroma. Horn cysts are commonly seen, indicating follicular differentiation of these benign tumors. In addition, areas of calcification are frequently present.

Trichoblastoma: Trichoblastomas are benign follicular tumors, and are thought to be growths of follicular germinative cells. Trichoblastomas may be mistaken microscopically for BCCs, since they show lobules of basaloid epithelium situated in the dermis and demonstrate peripheral palisading. Unlike BCC, however, epidermal connections are not commonly observed in trichoblastomas. Another distinguishing feature compared to BCC is the stroma surrounding the basaloid islands, which is richer in fibroblasts and compacted, lacking mucinous ground substance. The stroma of trichoblastomas and trichoepitheliomas are therefore virtually identical in appearance. One variant of a trichoblastoma is the so-called trichoblastic fibroma, which shows similar epithelial and mesenchymal elements as trichoblastomas, but the basaloid islands in trichoblastic fibromas are smaller and the surrounding stroma is a more prominent feature.

Syringoma: These benign neoplasms demonstrate eccrine differentiation, and are specifically composed of collections of small eccrine ducts set with a fibrous stroma. These epithelial islands are often described as having a "tadpole-like" appearance. The individual ducts show central lumina that are lined by 2 rows of bland epithelial cells. Occasionally, the epithelial cells have a clear cell morphology, which is the result of glycogen accumulation.

Sebaceous Tumors: Sebaceous tumors may be solitary or present in multiples, particularly in the context of Muir-Torre syndrome.[12] Sebaceous tumors may be classified according to the proportion of cells within the neoplasm that exhibit sebaceous (versus basaloid) differentiation, as well as the amount of cytologic atypia observed. Given this framework, sebaceous tumors are grouped into one of the following categories: sebaceous adenoma, sebaceous epithelioma, or sebaceous carcinoma.

Sebaceous adenomas are benign tumors, which are composed of both cells with sebaceous differentiation and basaloid cells. The sebaceous cells predominate over the basaloid cells, so that most of the tumor is sebaceous in appearance. The cells are arranged in lobules and the tumor is well-circumscribed overall, lacking infiltrative growth patterns. Mitotic activity may be seen within the basaloid component of sebaceous adenomas.

In contrast to sebaceous adenomas, sebaceous epitheliomas are composed of more than 50% basaloid cells, with a smaller population of cells demonstrating sebaceous differentiation. Like sebaceous adenomas, the basaloid compartment of the tumor may exhibit mitotic activity, and infiltrative growth is not observed. However, there may be some increased nuclear atypia compared to sebaceous adenomas.

Sebaceous carcinomas are malignant neoplasms, displaying prominent cytologic atypia in both sebaceous cell and basaloid cell types, with enlarged and pleomorphic nuclei. The tumor cells are frequently arranged in irregularly shaped lobules, and often show infiltration into the surrounding stroma. Mitoses are easily identified within the lesional cells.

MELANOCYTIC LESIONS

Common Nevi: Melanocytic nevi may involve the epidermis only, the dermis only, or both the epidermis and dermis, and accordingly are classified as being junctional, intradermal, or compound. Many nevi evolve over time, progressing from junctional to compound to primarily intradermal nevi. Common nevi are composed of nests of nevic cells, which involve in the tips of the epidermal rete in junctional and compound nevi, and the dermis in intradermal and compound nevi. Within the dermal compartment, the nevus cells show maturation, a term that refers to the distribution of larger nests of melanocytes in the superficial dermis and smaller nests, and/or single nevic cells at the base of the lesion. In common nevi, the melanocytes are typically round, with varying amounts of cytoplasm (Fig. 2-28), although nevic cells that are neurotized (resembling neural cells) are also frequently encountered.

Dysplastic Nevi: Under the microscope, dysplastic nevi exhibit architectural disorder and random (as opposed to uniform) cytologic atypia. Some of the architectural features used to render a diagnosis of a dysplastic nevus include the presence of a shoulder, bridging of melanocytic nests between adjacent epidermal rete, lamellar fibroplasia, pagetoid spread, and lentiginous growth of melanocytes along the dermal epidermal junction (Fig. 2-29). The "shoulder" refers to the junctional component of a nevus that extends at least 3 rete pegs beyond a central area of dermal nevus cells. Melanocytic bridging is a phenomenon in which nests of nevic cells from adjacent rete appear to grow toward each other and fuse. Lamellar fibroplasia is commonly observed in dysplastic nevi, and indicates fibrosis in the papillary dermis that runs in parallel to areas of bridging in the epidermis. Pagetoid spread is seen to some degree in dysplastic nevi, although not as extensively in melanomas, and denotes upward spread of melanocytes in the epidermis away from the basilar epidermis. Finally, dysplastic nevi may exhibit increased growth of single melanocytes (as opposed to merely nested growth) along the dermal–epidermal junction, a finding that is described as a lentiginous growth pattern.

Cytologic atypia is frequently observed within dysplastic nevi, and may be graded as mild, moderate, or severe. In contrast to melanomas, the cytologic atypia of dysplastic nevi is typically isolated to a subset of melanocytes (random atypia), rather than affecting nearly all the lesional melanocytes.

Spitz Nevi: Spitz nevi are melanocytic nevi that are composed of spindled and/or epithelioid melanocytes. Because of some of their architectural and cytologic features, there can be difficulty in distinguishing these lesions from melanoma. Spitz nevi typically occur in children and young adults, although are sometimes also seen in older adults.

Spitz nevi may be compound, junctional, or intradermal. Compound lesions are most frequently observed, and demonstrate a proliferation of large nested spindled and/or epithelioid melanocytes, sometimes pigmented, along the dermal–epidermal junction, with similar nests in the underlying dermis. The epidermis is usually hyperplastic. There is often clefting around the nests of melanocytes in the epidermis (Fig. 2-30). Pagetoid spread may be seen, predominantly in the center of the lesion. Kamino bodies are a characteristic feature of Spitz nevi. These are acellular, globular

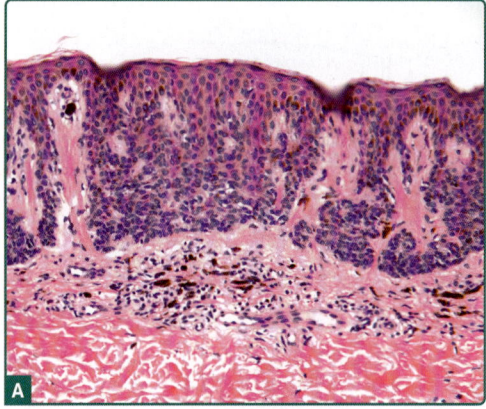
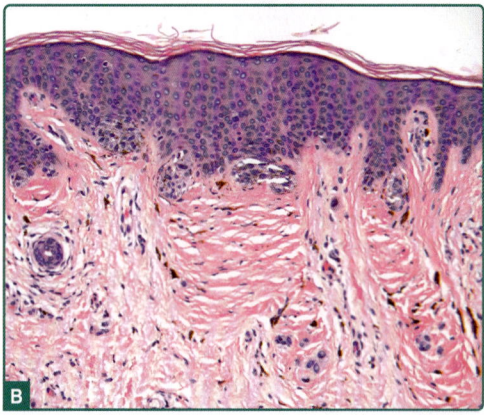

Figure 2-29 **A,** Dysplastic nevus displaying bridging of nests of melanocytes between adjacent epidermal rete pegs. **B,** Lamellar fibroplasia, a common finding in dysplastic nevi.

eosinophilic inclusions in the epidermis, which are thought to be derived from basement membrane material. Conventional Spitz nevi show symmetry and sharp lateral circumscription. The dermal nevus cells exhibit maturation, a term that indicates the tendency of nevus cells at the base of Spitz nevi to be smaller than those in the more superficial dermis. Although dermal mitoses may be observed in Spitz nevi, the mitotic rate does not usually exceed 2 per mm^2.

Melanoma: Malignant melanomas may arise from preexisting nevi, or occur de novo. These tumors may be restricted to the epidermis only, in which case they are referred to as *melanoma in situ*. Invasive malignant melanoma usually involves the epidermis and the underlying dermis, although in a small number of cases, primary dermal melanomas are observed. Melanomas are classified as having a radial growth phase and/or vertical growth phase. Melanomas that have only a radial growth phase are those that are restricted to the epidermis, or the epidermis and the superficial dermis, in the absence of expansile tumor masses in the dermis. Vertical growth phase melanomas have dermal tumor masses that are larger than nests of melanocytes seen in the epidermis and/or have dermal mitoses.

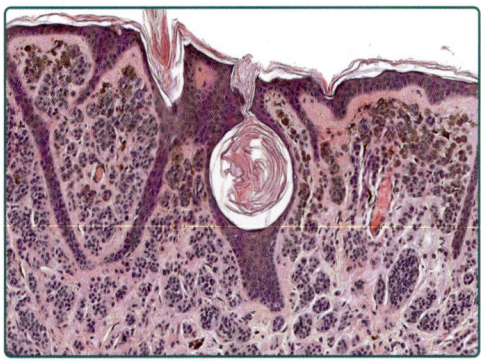

Figure 2-28 Dermal nevus. Nests of nevic cells, some showing melanin pigmentation, are present within the dermis.

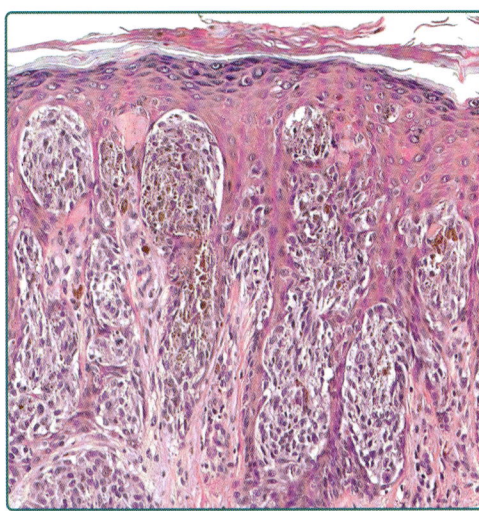

Figure 2-30 Spitz nevus with vertically oriented nests of epithelioid and spindled melanocytes. Kamino bodies are also seen.

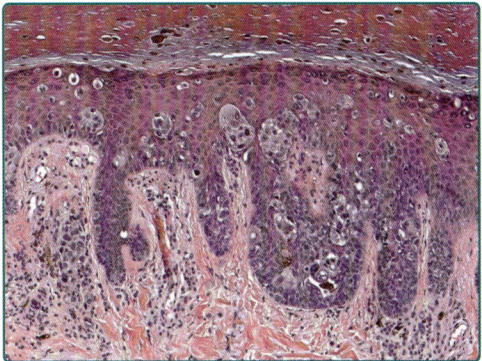

Figure 2-31 Malignant melanoma characterized by highly crowded growth of atypical melanocytes along the dermal–epidermal junction and extensive pagetoid spread. Atypical melanocytes are also present in the dermis.

While radial growth phase melanomas may be classified into several histologic types (superficial spreading, lentigo maligna, acral lentiginous, and mucosal lentiginous), a disorganized growth pattern with cytologic atypia is common to all of them (Fig. 2-31). Intraepidermal melanomas are commonly found to have confluent or near confluent growth of nested and single melanocytes along the dermal–epidermal junction. Lesions are often markedly asymmetrical. The lesional cells classically harbor uniform severe cytologic atypia. Pagetoid spread is commonly observed, to a greater extent than seen in dysplastic nevi. Solar elastosis is also frequently present, particularly in the superficial spreading and lentigo maligna types.

Superficial spreading melanomas usually display more nested growth of melanocytes compared to lentigo maligna types, and also show more extensive pagetoid spread up to the granular layer. The epidermis is thickened in superficial spreading melanoma and often atrophic in lentigo maligna melanoma. There is usually a greater degree of sun damage in the lentigo maligna type of melanoma. Acral lentiginous and mucosal lentiginous melanomas, similar to lentigo maligna melanomas, show a predominance of single melanocytes over nested growth along the dermal–epidermal junction. Pagetoid spread is seen but may not be extensive. By virtue of the sites of acral lentiginous and mucosal lentiginous melanomas, solar elastosis is minimal.

Vertical growth phase melanomas are divided into those that have a radial growth phase and those that do not. Nodular melanomas are melanomas that have only a vertical growth phase. Whereas nodular melanomas harbor an intraepidermal component, the in situ melanoma does not extend significantly beyond the lateral borders of the dermal portion of the melanoma. The vertical growth phase component of melanomas that also have a radial growth phase may be conventional, or less commonly, desmoplastic or spindle cell in morphology. Conventional vertical growth phase melanomas demonstrate dermal cells that are similar in morphology to the overlying radial growth phase. Uniform cytologic atypia and mitoses are often found. Melanocytes in the dermis do not exhibit maturation as compared to intradermal nevi.

Desmoplastic vertical growth phase melanomas are commonly found in association with lentigo maligna or mucosal lentiginous radial growth phases. Desmoplastic melanomas feature elongated, spindled nuclei set within a fibrotic stroma rich in thickened collagen bundles. Nuclear atypia may be subtle. One helpful clue to the diagnosis of desmoplastic melanoma is the presence of nodular lymphocytic aggregates in the dermis. Of note, desmoplastic melanomas have a distinct immunohistochemical staining profile compared to conventional melanomas; they are typically MART-1 negative and positive for S-100 and SOX10 stains.

TUMORS OF DERMAL ORIGIN

Many tumors of dermal origin are derived from one of several cell types, including fibroblasts, endothelial cells, neural cells, and smooth muscle cells. These tumors may exhibit a spindle cell morphology, and certain morphologic clues are helpful in distinguishing the cell type of origin, and thus rendering an accurate diagnosis. For instance, smooth muscle cells have cigar-shaped nuclei with rounded, blunt ends that are accompanied by a perinuclear halo. Neural cells have wavy S-shaped nuclei with tapered ends. Cells that exhibit fibroblastic differentiation have elongated nuclei with tapered ends.

FIBROHISTIOCYTIC TUMORS

Dermatofibroma: Dermatofibromas exhibit fibroblastic differentiation, and are often classified as "fibrohistiocytic" because they may also display histiocytic

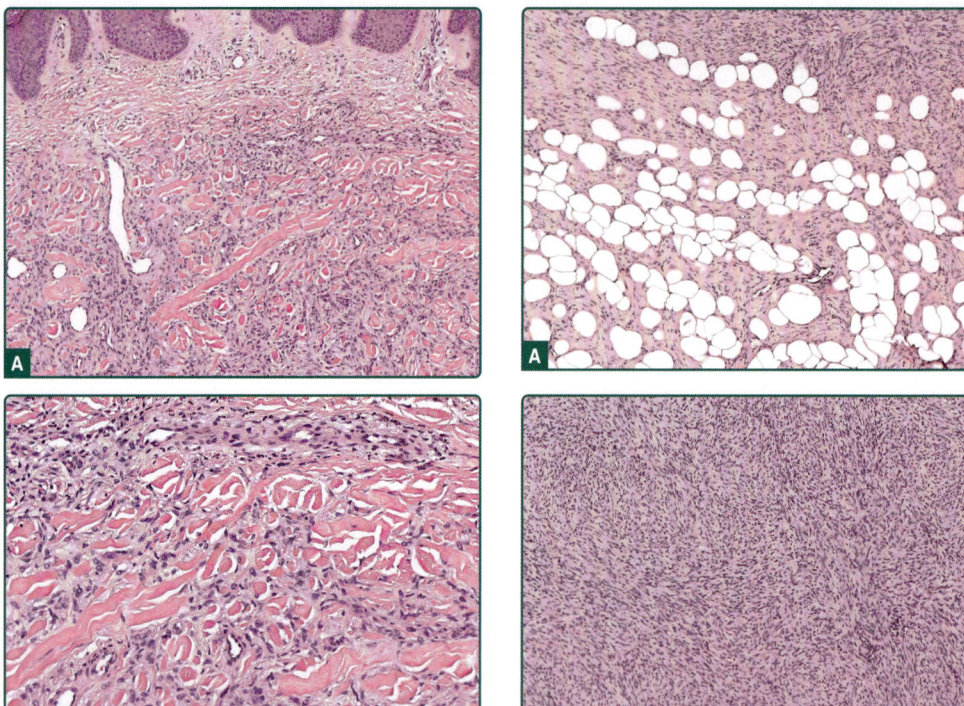

Figure 2-32 **A,** Dermatofibroma, demonstrating a proliferation of bland-appearing spindled cells in the dermis with associated collagen wrapping. **B,** Higher power view of collagen wrapping.

Figure 2-33 **A,** Dermatofibrosarcoma protuberans with elongated spindled cells intercalating between adipose cells in the subcutaneous fat, also known as "honeycombing." **B,** Storiform pattern of spindled cells in the dermis.

differentiation in the form of foamy and/or giant cells. Dermatofibromas are benign lesions, which tend to have a hyperplastic epidermis and hyperpigmented, flattened rete, which are described as "dirty feet." Follicular induction is also commonly observed in the epidermis, which may closely resemble superficial BCCs. In the reticular dermis, bland-appearing spindled cells with tapered ends are observed (Fig. 2-32A), sometimes in association with round cells with foamy cytoplasm and/or giant cells. The degree of cellularity in dermatofibromas vary, as some lesions are relatively paucicellular while others are more densely cellular. "Collagen wrapping" is frequently seen, particularly at the periphery of dermatofibromas, in which spindle cells encircle collagen bundles (Fig. 2-32B). Immunohistochemical stains may be helpful in the diagnosis of dermatofibromas, as the fibrohistiocytic cells are positive for Factor XIIIa stains and negative for CD34 stains.

Dermatofibrosarcoma Protuberans: Dermatofibrosarcoma protuberans is a malignant neoplasm that is typically locally aggressive without a high incidence of metastasis. These tumors are characterized by a proliferation of bland-appearing spindle cells in the reticular dermis and subcutaneous fat. The cells intercalate between adipocytes in the subcutaneous fat, resulting in a "honeycomb" appearance (Fig. 2-33A). A storiform or whorled pattern of the cells is commonly observed in the dermal compartment (Fig. 2-33B). There is often very little cytologic atypia. The lesional cells are positive for CD34 immunohistochemical stains but negative for Factor XIIIa stains, allowing differentiation from cellular dermatofibromas.

Atypical Fibroxanthoma: In contrast to dermatofibrosarcoma protuberans, atypical fibroxanthomas (AFXs) demonstrate marked cytologic atypia of spindled and epithelioid cells in the dermis. The lesional cells harbor markedly enlarged nuclei, nuclear pleomorphism, and mitotic figures are easily identified. Despite this prominent cytologic atypia, AFXs are readily treated with local excision and only very rarely metastasize. A panel of immunohistochemical stains including CD34, pan-cytokeratin, p63, S-100, and CD10 may be helpful in distinguishing AFX from other spindle cell tumors, including dermatofibrosarcoma protuberans, spindle-cell SCC, and spindle-cell/desmoplastic melanoma. Although CD10 is frequently positive in AFX, it is not a specific marker as it has also been reported to be positive in some carcinomas and melanomas. A biopsy of the surface of an undifferentiated pleomorphic sarcoma, a lesion with potential for metastatic disease, is indistinguishable from AFX.

TUMORS OF VASCULAR ORIGIN

PYOGENIC GRANULOMA

Also known by the name *lobular capillary hemangioma*, pyogenic granuloma is a benign vascular lesion. Pyogenic granulomas are exophytic clinically, and the polypoid architecture under the microscope reflects this. Typically, there is an epidermal collarette around the dermal vascular proliferation (Fig. 2-34A). In the dermis are clusters of small capillaries lined by bland endothelial cells (Fig. 2-34B). The lobules of capillaries are set within a loose stroma containing fibroblasts.

ANGIOSARCOMA

Angiosarcomas are malignant vascular tumors. In relatively well-differentiated lesions, irregular vascular channels are seen in the dermis, which are lined by atypical endothelial cells (Fig. 2-35). The endothelial cells have variably enlarged nuclei and nuclear pleomorphism. The lesional cells are highlighted by endothelial cell markers, including CD31 and

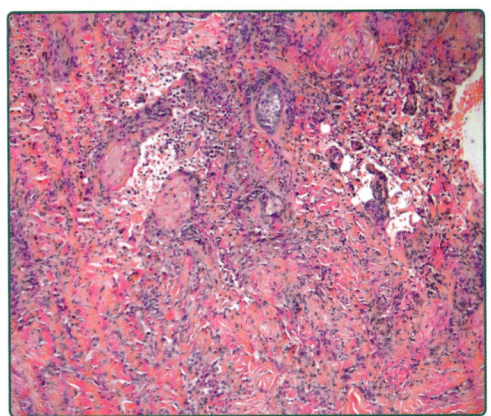

Figure 2-35 Angiosarcoma with a proliferation of atypical endothelial cells in the dermis and associated irregular vascular spaces.

CD34. Poorly differentiated angiosarcomas may display increased cellularity, increased nuclear atypia, and increased number of mitoses compared to well-differentiated lesions.

TUMORS OF NEURAL ORIGIN

NEUROFIBROMA

Neurofibromas are benign lesions that may occur sporadically or in the context of neurofibromatosis. They are dermal tumors that consist of small, bland neural cells with wavy, S-shaped nuclei, set within a light pink stroma (Fig. 2-36). The stroma may be myxoid. Neurofibromas tend to be well circumscribed within the dermis. Mast cells are commonly observed within neurofibromas.

SCHWANNOMAS

Also known as neurilemomas, schwannomas are as their name suggests, benign proliferations of Schwann

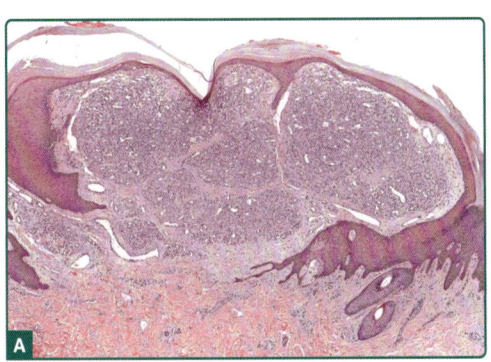

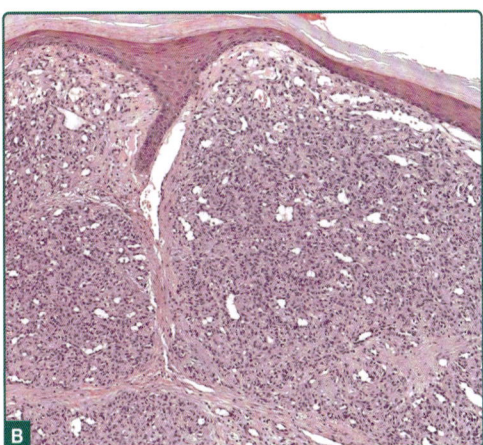

Figure 2-34 **A,** Pyogenic granuloma characterized by an epidermal collarette and clusters of capillaries in the dermis. **B,** Higher power view of lobules of capillaries in the dermis.

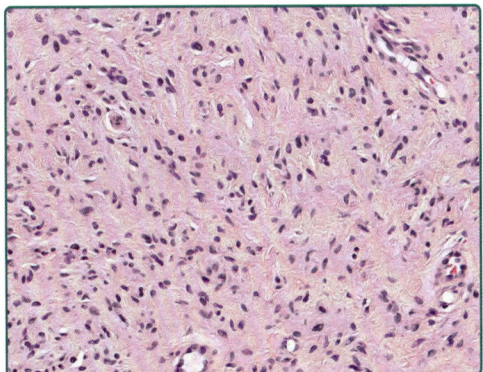

Figure 2-36 Neurofibroma showing spindled cells with wavy nuclei and characteristic pink stroma.

cells. They are well-circumscribed but nonencapsulated lesions in the dermis, and are easily recognizable because there are two distinct patterns of tissue seen within them, namely Antoni A and Antoni B areas. Antoni A areas are more cellular, with areas of palisading of nuclei in parallel to one another around a relatively an acellular extracellular matrix, also referred to as *Verocay bodies*. Antoni B areas demonstrate spindled cells within a looser and often myxoid extracellular matrix.

TUMORS OF SMOOTH MUSCLE ORIGIN

LEIOMYOMA

The leiomyoma is a benign smooth muscle neoplasm, and in the skin is derived from either pilar muscle (piloleiomyoma) or from vascular smooth muscle (angioleiomyoma). In the former, there is a proliferation of smooth muscle bundles in the reticular dermis (Fig. 2-37A). The cells are pink in color and elongated, with cigar-shaped nuclei that have tapered ends (Fig. 2-37B). While mitoses are sometimes observed, the mitotic rate is generally very low. The typical angioleiomyoma appears as a well-circumscribed nodule in the deep reticular dermis and subcutaneous fat (Fig. 2-37C). A central vascular lumina may be seen, in addition to smaller vascular channels amid bundles of smooth muscle.

LEIOMYOSARCOMA

Similar to their benign counterparts, leiomyosarcomas may be derived from pilar muscle or vascular smooth muscle. These malignant tumors may display atypical, enlarged nuclei, increased cellularity, frequent mitoses, and/or infiltrative growth patterns (Fig. 2-38).

ACKNOWLEDGMENTS

The authors wish to acknowledge the previous authors, Drs. Martin C. Mihm, Abdul-Ghani Kibbi, George F. Murphy, and Klaus Wolff for their contributions to this chapter.

REFERENCES

1. Watson AJ, Redbord K, Taylor JS, et al. Medical error in dermatology practice: development of a classification system to drive priority setting in patient safety efforts. *J Am Acad Dermatol*. 2013;68:729-737.
2. Stratman EJ, Elston DM, Miller SJ. Skin biopsy: Identifying and overcoming errors in the skin biopsy pathway. *J Am Acad Dermatol*. 2016;74(1):19-25.

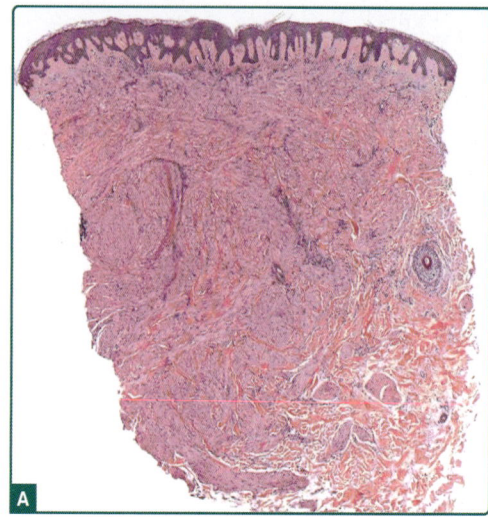
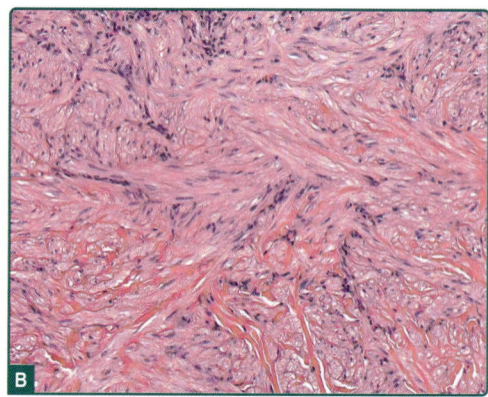
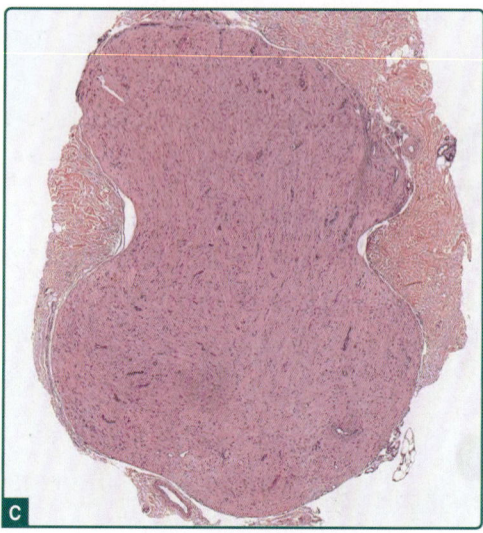

Figure 2-37 **A,** Pilar leiomyoma exhibiting fascicles of spindled cells in the reticular dermis. **B,** Higher power view of pilar leiomyoma. The spindled cells have cigar-shaped nuclei with blunt ends. **C,** Angioleiomyoma, showing characteristic deeply seated well-circumscribed nodules in the deep reticular dermis.

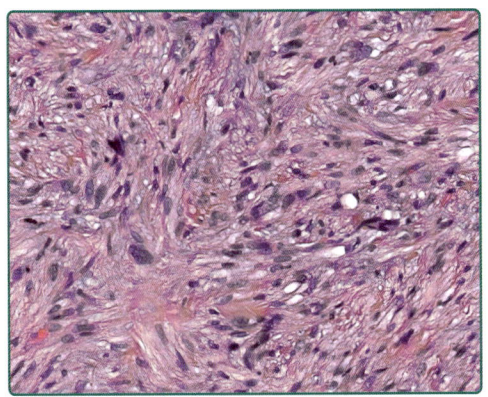

Figure 2-38 Leiomyosarcoma. The spindle cells show scattered enlarged atypical nuclei.

3. Elston, DM, Stratman EJ, Miller SJ. Biopsy issues in specific diseases. *J Am Acad Dermatol*. 2016;74:1-16.
4. Nguyen JV, Hudacek K, Whitten JA, et al. The HoVert technique: a novel method for the sectioning of alopecia biopsies. *J Cutan Pathol*. 2011;38(5): 401-406.
5. Elston D. The "Tyler technique" for alopecia biopsies. *J Cutan Pathol*. 2012;39(2):306.
6. Magro CM, Crowson AN, Regauer S. Granuloma annulare and necrobiosis lipoidica tissue reactions as a manifestation of systemic disease. *Hum Pathol*. 27:50, 1996.
7. Requena L. Normal subcutaneous fat, necrosis of adipocytes and classification of the panniculitides. *Semin Cutan Med Surg*. 2007;26(2):66-70.
8. Requena L, Yus ES. Panniculitis. Part I. Mostly septal panniculitis. *J Am Acad Dermatol*. 2001;45(2): 163-183.
9. Requena L, Sánchez Yus E. Panniculitis. Part II. Mostly lobular panniculitis. *J Am Acad Dermatol*. 2001;45(3): 325-361; quiz 362-364.
10. Chu EY, Wanat KA, Miller CJ, et al. Diverse cutaneous side effects associated with BRAF inhibitor therapy: a clinicopathologic study. *J Am Acad Dermatol*. 2012;67(6): 1265-1272.
11. Kong HH, Cowen EW, Azad NS, et al. Keratoacanthomas associated with sorafenib therapy. *J Am Acad Dermatol*. 2007;56(1):171-172.
12. John AM, Schwartz RA. Muir-Torre syndrome (MTS): an update and approach to diagnosis and management. *J Am Acad Dermatol*. 2016;74(3):558-566.

Chapter 3 :: Epidemiology and Public Health in Dermatology
:: Junko Takeshita & David J. Margolis

第三章
皮肤病流行病学和公共卫生学

中文导读

流行病学研究是对人群中疾病的发病率、流行率、分布、病因和疾病自然史的研究，它不仅有助于了解疾病的自然史和治疗方法，而且有助于了解疾病的公共卫生政策。流行病学研究可以是分析性的，也可以是描述性的。

1. 基本概念　本节介绍了临床试验、卫生服务研究、以患者为导向的研究、疾病自然史、疾病负担、干预、风险因素、偏倚、混淆、效应、有效性、比较有效性、队列等基本概念。

2. 研究设计　本节介绍了大多数研究的两个基本类型为分析性和描述性，包括实验研究、观察性研究、Meta分析、描述性研究、质量报告和评估证据等。

3. 流行病学方法　本节介绍了流行病学的多种方法，包括描述性的、分析性的和患者报告的结果。

4. 结论　流行病学是增进我们对人群中疾病理解的基础。流行病学中以病人为导向的健康服务研究，对促进人们了解人群中和个体中皮肤病发生水平，是必不可少的。了解流行病学及其研究方法和措施的基本知识，能够帮助临床医生解读原始文献和实践循证医学。

〔陈明亮〕

AT-A-GLANCE

- Epidemiology is the study of disease in a population.
- Epidemiologic studies may be analytic (including meta-analyses, clinical trials, and cohort and case-control studies) or descriptive.
- Most epidemiologic studies measure association; causality is difficult to establish with nonexperimental studies.
- Bias and confounding are important limitations to be aware of, especially in observational studies.

INTRODUCTION

Epidemiology is the study of disease in the population, and it includes the incidence, prevalence, distribution, cause, and natural history of disease. The study of epidemiology is concerned with the health of populations and helps to inform not only the natural history and treatment of disease but also the public health policy of a disease. Epidemiologic studies are often used to help guide evidence-based practice. Most epidemiologic studies are observational, which means that epidemiologists, in their quest to understand a disease, observe a population and how it is affected by a disease without intervening on the population. On the other hand, in experimental studies, a clinical trialist will determine how an intervention affects an individual's health by actively exposing individuals in a population to an exposure, such as a drug, of interest.

Understanding a disease includes not only identifying the cellular, genetic, and molecular causes and consequences of the illness but also assessing how the disease affects patients and the population in which they reside. Epidemiology is the basic science underpinning this exploration, and epidemiologic techniques are the foundation for nearly all clinical research. Comprehensive clinical training requires knowledge of both the basic science underlying the pathophysiology of disease as well as the epidemiology and natural history of disease. Because the techniques of an epidemiologist are often the basic science of evidence-based medicine, as a practitioner of dermatology, a good foundation in epidemiologic cutaneous science is as important as understanding the molecular basis of skin disease.

BASIC CONCEPTS

DEFINITIONS

The following are basic terms often used to describe epidemiologic studies.

Clinical trials are interventional studies that include randomized controlled trials (RCTs). These studies are considered experimental studies in that the investigator has a direct influence on the subjects in the study via an intervention and evaluates the effect of the intervention. The experimental environment is tightly controlled, allowing an investigator to determine the efficacy an intervention (ie, the effect of an intervention in an ideal setting). Although these studies provide the highest level of proof of an effect by minimizing bias (ie, internal validity), randomized clinical studies many not generalize well to all members of a population (ie, external validity).

Health services research evaluates how an individual receives health care and interacts with the health care system. These studies can include evaluations of access to care, interactions between health care providers and patients, and a patient's perception of his or her illness. Epidemiologic techniques, including clinical trials as well as techniques more common to economics, anthropology, sociology, and psychology, are often used in health services research studies.

Patient-oriented research has been defined in many different ways. At present, it most commonly refers to studies of how patients interact with their health care and disease. Outcomes of these studies are often directed by or informed by individuals with an illness of interest.

The **natural history of disease** is the course of the disease from its onset until its, or the patient's, end or resolution, the latter of which may be study outcomes of interest. It includes not just interactions with health care providers but the course of the disease within the patient's experience as well.

The **burden of disease** is a measure of how an individual is affected by an illness. Burden can include measures of how an illness changes an individual's life including economic and social costs. Burden can also be measured at the population level. For example, the prevalence of a disease can be a measure of the burden of that disease in the population.

An **outcome** is the observation of primary interest. Outcomes could include death; the onset, resolution, or change in the status of an illness; and quality of life, among others. Outcomes often have clinical relevance and should be defined before a study commences.

In many situations, the strongest association between a risk factor or intervention and an outcome is a **causal association**. In experimental studies such as a randomized clinical trial, causation is easier to establish because of the careful design of the study. When an intervention is thought to directly cause an outcome of interest, this suggests a causal association between the two. Causality can only be established with properly designed studies in which there is a clear temporal relationship between the intervention and measured outcome; the outcome is explicitly defined; the study is without noticeable bias; there is an underlying biologically plausible explanation for the relationship between the intervention and the outcome; and the measured effect between the intervention and outcome is reproducible, strong, and statistically significant. Establishing a causal association in observational studies is more difficult because of the potential for bias in these studies. Simply identifying a statistically significant association between a risk factor and an outcome is not necessarily sufficient to suggest causation. Many have opined about how to determine causation in an observational study. Sir Bradford Hill's criteria for observational studies are often cited as necessary to demonstrate causation;[1] however, not all agree. These criteria are based on the notions that a risk factor needs to occur before the outcome, the risk factor is not part of another factor's causal pathway, prior knowledge of the risk factor provides evidence that it could cause the outcome, there is a strong and dose-dependent association between the risk factor and outcome, and the association is reproducible. Although the criteria that are used to determine if an association noted in an observational study is causal are often attributed to Sir Bradford Hill, that was not his purpose when he proposed these criteria. His purpose was to begin a discussion on what might be noted in an observational study that could be used to determine causation.

An **intervention** is the application of a substance or an action to subjects in an experimental study.

A **risk factor** is an attribute that increases the likelihood of developing a disease or other outcome of interest. A risk factor could be environmental, genetic, ancestral, economic, or medication related, among others. Risk factors are important to measure, particularly in observational studies.

An **association** occurs when an attribute or other factor is found to be related to an outcome of interest. The magnitude of an association is often measured by an effect estimate, and the likelihood that the association is real is often documented by statistical significance.

Bias is a systematic error that causes the results of a study to deviate from the truth. In epidemiologic studies, bias is defined in several ways. For the purpose of this discussion, we will categorize bias into two broad categories, **selection bias** and **information bias**. **Selection bias** is a systematic error in a study caused by how subjects are selected or not selected for a study. This also applies to the selection process for an intervention or exposure to a risk factor. For example, in a cohort study evaluating whether a topical therapy used to treat psoriasis is more effective than a systemic therapy, selection bias would occur if those selected for treatment with a topical steroid had less severe disease than those selected for the systemic therapy. In a case-control study, selection bias can occur if the source population from which the cases are drawn is different from the control source population. For example, in a hypothetical case-control study evaluating the association between nonsteroidal antiinflammatory drug (NSAID) use and colon cancer, comparing cases of colon cancer drawn from patients admitted to the hospital with control participants drawn from patients with arthritis admitted to the hospital may result in a falsely low effect estimate because the control participants likely have had a high exposure to NSAIDs. **Information bias** is bias that occurs because of reporting. For example, in a case-control study evaluating the association between cigarettes and lung cancer, because of previous reports and package warnings about cigarettes, it is likely that those with cancer are more likely to recall and report a history of cigarette use than those without lung cancer. In a cohort study evaluating the risk of cancer among patients with psoriasis, information bias could be introduced if the method of information gathering (ie, psoriasis subjects answer survey questions while waiting patiently for phototherapy) elicits more detailed responses about cancer risk factors, such as cigarette use, in the psoriasis patient cohort than in the cohort of patients without psoriasis (ie, subjects without psoriasis answer survey questions while completing an office visit after a wart treatment). The ultimate problem with bias is that it cannot be measured, and as a result, it is difficult to determine the net effect of the bias on the study results.

Confounding occurs when two risk factors or exposures are associated with each other and the outcome of interest. This association often distorts the estimated effect of either risk factor on the outcome. For example, in a cohort study of the risk of malignancy in those with psoriasis, it might be important to understand the impact of cigarette use and alcohol use. This can be problematic because smoking and alcohol use has been reported to be more prevalent among patients with psoriasis than those without psoriasis, and people who smoke and drink more alcohol are more likely to develop a malignancy. When evaluating the association of any of these variables on cancer risk, it is important to assess whether the estimate is "confounded" by the other risk factors.

Efficacy is the measure of an effect in an ideal setting. Ideal settings tend to maximize the internal validity (minimize potential errors or confounding) of the study's results. For example, randomized clinical trials use precise definitions of a disease and how to use an intervention, randomization (the selection of an intervention or treatment is not based on the investigators preference but based on a pre-specified numerical formula), blinding (investigators collecting data from study participants are not aware of treatment assignment), and other specifications that ensure internal validity. These design elements maximize the likelihood that the results of the study will be unbiased. Studies that minimize bias are thought to be **internally valid**, which means that if the study was repeated using the same study design and the same study cohort, the same results would be found. Because a random sample from the population at large is not usually selected for a randomized clinical trial, these studies may not generalize to the full population. In addition, the inclusion and exclusion criteria for randomized clinical trials (eg, how a patient is determined to be eligible for enrollment) tend to be very selective and may not correspond to how a disease is defined by most health care workers. Studies that measure efficacy are called **explanatory studies**.

Effectiveness is how well an intervention works in the real world. As noted earlier, in clinical settings, the definition of a disease may lose precision, patients may not take their medications, and providers may not properly prescribe medications. Effectiveness measures allow for this loss of precision. These studies tend to be more generalizable in that they are representative of the "real" world and not the idealized world of a clinical trial. Studies that represent results that are reproducible in many other study settings are thought to be **externally valid** or generalizable.

Comparative effectiveness refers to studies that compare two or more treatments that are generally accepted to be effective. These studies use real-world treatment settings, thus allowing for imprecisions that occur in daily care. These studies are often called **pragmatic studies** in that they lack the regulatory oversight that is required by federal agencies when treatments receive initial approval, thereby allowing the study design to be more consistent with routine patient–physician interactions.

A **cohort** is a group of people. In observational studies, a cohort is often defined based on disease status or having a risk factor of interest.

STUDY DESIGNS

An understanding of epidemiologic study designs is essential to properly addressing clinical questions and interpreting published literature. Many different types of epidemiologic study designs exist, the most common of which will be reviewed here. Most studies can be divided into two basic categories: analytic and descriptive (Fig. 3-1).

ANALYTIC STUDIES

Analytic studies examine the association between an exposure and outcome. Two main types of analytic studies are experimental and observational studies.

EXPERIMENTAL STUDIES

Experimental studies are those in which subjects receive an active intervention (ie, drug or other treatment). Clinical trials are the most commonly used and recognized of the experimental studies. Clinical trials are often classified based on guidance from federal agencies such as the Food and Drug Administration (FDA). This nomenclature was created to help establish an orderly and reproducible process allowing for the evaluation of novel interventions that require federal approval before human experimentation can begin and establish a foundation for the justification for the approval of a new treatment. The FDA algorithm includes the following:

1. *Phase I studies* are the first studies performed in humans and are often designed with the notion that they are human pharmacology studies. The goal of phase I studies is to evaluate a drug's dose range, safety, tolerability, pharmacokinetics, and pharmacodynamics.
2. *Phase II studies* are also called initial efficacy studies and are conducted to initially determine the effect of an intervention on patients with the disease of interest. These studies are also conducted to obtain additional information required to properly design phase III trials.
3. *Phase III studies*, also called comparative efficacy studies, are designed to assess the efficacy of an intervention compared with that of a "control" treatment (either active treatment or placebo). Sometimes called pivotal studies, phase III studies provide the data necessary for regulatory agencies such as the FDA to decide whether or not to approve a drug. Randomization and blinding are important aspects of phase III studies that ensure their internal validity and reduce bias. These studies are often considered the best design to evaluate a new treatment.
4. *Phase IV studies*, or postmarketing studies, are usually conducted after a treatment obtains FDA approval for marketing. They may also be called effectiveness studies because of their focus on how well the approved drug works in the general population and how safe the drug is in a larger population and over a longer period of time. Sometimes phase IV studies assess the effectiveness of the intervention for uses other than the approved indication.

Given the limitations of explanatory trials, such as poor external validity or generalizability, relatively short study periods, and focus on how interventions work in the ideal setting, an increasing emphasis has been placed on studying interventions' effects in the real-world setting. As such, **pragmatic trials** have gained popularity in recent years.[2] Pragmatic trials, also known as large simple studies or Peto studies,

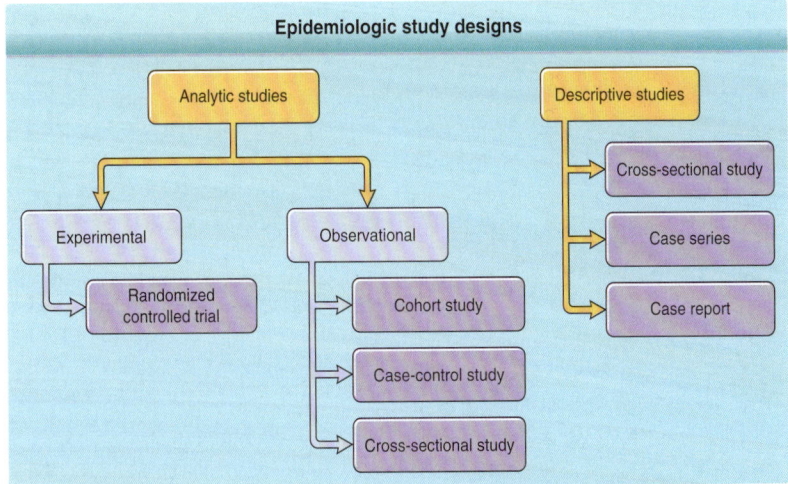

Figure 3-1 Epidemiologic study designs.

are effectiveness studies that focus on understanding how an intervention works in the routine clinical setting. As opposed to explanatory trials, the goal of pragmatic trials is to maximize the generalizability of the results to many practice settings and minimize the scientific (with respect to internal validity), regulatory, and administrative burden common to explanatory trials. Examples of pragmatic RCTs in dermatology include a Dutch study of home versus outpatient ultraviolet B phototherapy for psoriasis (PLUTO)[3] and a UK study of prophylactic antibiotics for prevention of cellulitis (PATCH II).[4] Differences between explanatory and pragmatic trials are summarized in Table 3-1. In reality, however, few trials can be defined as purely explanatory or pragmatic and instead display a mix of explanatory and pragmatic trial characteristics. As such, tools have been developed to help classify trials as explanatory or pragmatic, including the tool by Gartlehner and coworkers[5] and the PRECIS (pragmatic-explanatory continuum indicator summary) tool by Thorpe and coworkers[6] Additionally, guidelines for quality reporting of pragmatic trials have been developed as an extension of the Consolidated Standards of Reported Trials (CONSORT) statement for RCTs.[7]

OBSERVATIONAL STUDIES

Observational studies are those in which subjects are observed and exposures and outcomes are measured in routine care without any effort to intervene or otherwise influence any measured factors. The most common types of observational studies include cohort studies, case-control studies, and cross-sectional studies.

A **cohort study**, sometimes called a prospective study, follows a cohort (group of patients) over time and monitors the effect of a risk factor or exposure on the development of an outcome. For example, in an effort to answer the question of whether or not treatment of acne with isotretinoin increases the risk of developing inflammatory bowel disease (IBD), a cohort study could be designed. Individuals with acne and no prior history of IBD who are treated with isotretinoin (the exposed group) could be followed and compared with individuals who have not been treated with isotretinoin (the unexposed group) to determine if there is a difference between the two groups in risk of developing IBD. Alhusayen and coworkers performed such a study.[8] Advantages of cohort studies include the ability to evaluate for multiple outcomes in a single study and calculate incidence rates. On the other hand, cohort studies tend to be large and time consuming and are subject to bias. It is also important to recognize that many cohort studies are conducted using medical records or administrative databases, which allows for use of data that have already been collected. Thus, the data collection is retrospective. Nevertheless, the direction of observation for cohort studies using these data remains prospective in that a study start date is determined and study subjects are observed prospectively from that date for development of the outcome of interest. An example is Barbieri and coworkers' study of duration of tetracycline treatment and use of topical retinoids for treatment of acne.[9]

A **case-control study** is sometimes also called a retrospective study. These studies sample a group with a disease of interest (cases) and another that does not have the disease (controls). The study subjects are then interrogated or preceding data are examined to determine the prevalence of a risk factor. For example, Palmer and coworkers used a case-control study to identify loss-of-function variants of filaggrin that are associated with atopic dermatitis.[10] This example highlights the advantage of being able to evaluate multiple potential risk factors for a single outcome in case-control studies. An effect estimate, typically an odds ratio, is calculated based on the prevalence of exposure in the two groups. Case-control studies are often smaller than cohort studies, are particularly useful for studying rare outcomes, take much less time (subjects are not followed for the outcome to occur), and are particularly subject to selection and recall biases.

META-ANALYSIS

A **meta-analysis** is a quantitative study of studies. It is a systematic review that attempts to combine the results of multiple studies in order to create a pooled effect estimate of an outcome of interest. Meta-analyses may summarize experimental or observational studies. Because of inherent variability due to study designs, many who conduct meta-analyses favor combining only randomized clinical trials as a way to minimize bias. The outcome of interest for a meta-analysis is

TABLE 3-1
Differences between Efficacy and Effectiveness Research

EFFICACY HOW WELL DOES THE INTERVENTION WORK IN THE IDEAL SETTING?	EFFECTIVENESS HOW WELL DOES THE INTERVENTION WORK IN THE REAL WORLD?
Stringent patient selection criteria to optimize safety	Heterogeneous patient population more susceptible to adverse events
Highly motivated patients with strict adherence to research protocol	Variations in patient motivation and ability to adhere to prescribed regimen
Highly trained investigators with expertise in the study drug	Variation in experience and knowledge of the drug by prescriber
Clinical response determined at arbitrary "short-term" time points	Clinical response determined in routine clinical visits
Maximize internal validity	Maximize external validity

not always the primary outcome of the original studies that are included. By combing multiple studies, the "meta" estimates are often more precise than the individual estimates in the original studies. However, meta-analyses need to be carefully designed and interpreted because combination of results can lead to biased estimates. As a result, the analyst needs to carefully evaluate study designs, including the reproducibility and consistency between studies of the outcome of interest, as well as the heterogeneity among studies before creating the meta-estimate and providing an interpretation of results. An example meta-analysis evaluated the efficacy of oral antibiotics and oral contraceptives for the treatment of acne vulgaris.[11] Recent meta-analytic techniques called network of evidence or mixed treatment comparison have been developed to enable comparisons between treatments that were never directly compared in individual studies.

DESCRIPTIVE STUDIES

Descriptive studies are designed to report the distribution of disease or other health outcomes in a population. Descriptive studies may include **case reports** and **case series** that provide a detailed profile of single or multiple patients observed in the clinical setting. Cross-sectional studies may also be descriptive, for example, in the instance of measuring the prevalence of a particular disease or other outcome in a population.

QUALITY REPORTING AND ASSESSING EVIDENCE LEVELS

Standardized recommendations for quality reporting and levels of evidence rating scales can aid in the interpretation of epidemiologic studies and clinical recommendations or guidelines, respectively.

QUALITY REPORTING

Transparency and standardized reporting of clinical and epidemiologic studies are necessary to ensure reproducibility and allow for critical assessment and proper interpretation of study methods and results. Recommendations for quality reporting have been created with the purpose to improve study reporting. Quality reporting tools and checklists exist for systematic reviews, meta-analyses, and experimental and observational studies. Some examples include AMSTAR (A Measurement Tool to Assess Systematic Reviews),[12,13] PRISMA (Preferred Reporting Items for Systematic Reviews and Meta-Analyses),[14] and QUOROM (Quality of Reporting of Meta-Analyses) for systematic reviews or meta-analyses;[15] CONSORT (Consolidated Standards of Reporting Trials) for clinical trials;[16] and STROBE (Strengthening the Reporting of Observational Studies in Epidemiology) for observational studies,[17] among others.

LEVELS OF EVIDENCE

The ability to assess and classify evidence levels for clinical recommendations is essential for the practice of evidence-based medicine. More than 100 grading scales exist to aid in assessing levels of evidence and are used by variety of publications.[18] A few of the more commonly used scales include the SORT (Strength-of-Recommendation Taxonomy),[19] GRADE (Grading of Recommendations, Assessment, Development and Evaluation),[20] and Oxford Centre for Evidence-Based Medicine (OCEBM)[21,22] scales. The SORT scale has been adopted as the preferred grading scale by several family medicine and primary care journals, including *American Family Physician*, *Journal of the American Board of Family Practice*, and *Journal of Family Practice*, among others. The GRADE scale is the Cochrane group's recommended scale for grading quality of evidence and strength of recommendations. The OCEBM scale allows for grading of evidence for diagnostic tests, prognostic markers, and harm that many other scales do not.

MEASURES IN EPIDEMIOLOGY

Various types of measures exist in epidemiology, including descriptive, analytic, and patient-reported outcome measures. These measures are necessary for describing a population, assessing associations, and understanding the patient perspective, respectively.

DESCRIPTIVE MEASURES

Descriptive measures are used in descriptive studies and characterize an outcome of interest in a population. **Prevalence** is the frequency of a disease or other outcome of interest over a given period of time. It is measured as the number of individuals with a disease divided by the number of individuals sampled over a specified time period. Measuring prevalence is especially important and relevant for chronic diseases. Prevalence can be measured as point prevalence (ie, does an individual have the disease today), yearly prevalence (ie, does an individual have a disease during a 12-month period), lifetime prevalence, or any other given time period of interest.

Incidence is the frequency of new cases of a disease or other outcome among those who are at risk of the disease or outcome of interest within a specified period of time. The "at-risk population" refers to those who have the potential to develop the disease or other outcome of interest. For example, men would not be included in the at-risk population for a study of ovarian cancer. Generally, a new case occurs only once, and after an individual develops the disease or other outcome, he or she is removed from the population at risk. In a given time frame, incidence is measured by dividing the number of individuals who developed a disease by the number of individuals in the at-risk population.

The **duration** of a disease is how long it affects an individual. Some diseases are acute and only last for a short period of time (eg, cellulitis), and otherwise are chronic and last for a lifetime (eg, psoriasis). The magnitude of the prevalence and incidence of a disease can differ greatly because of long duration of a disease. For example, the prevalence of psoriasis in adults in the U.S. population is estimated at 2 to 4 per 100 (2% to 4%),[23,24] but the incidence is less than 1 per 1000 per person-year (0.1%).[25,26]

TABLE 3-2
Effect Estimates: An Example of Mortality Risk among Patients with Severe Psoriasis[27]

	NO PSORIASIS (N = 15,075)	SEVERE PSORIASIS (N = 3951)
Incidence rate of mortality per 1000 person-years (95% CI)	12.0 (11.3-12.8)	21.3 (19.0-23.9)
Overall hazard ratio (95% CI)	Reference	1.5 (1.3-1.7)
Overall attributable risk: number of deaths per 1000 patient-years	Reference	6.0

CI; confidence interval.

MEASURES OF ASSOCIATION

Many epidemiologic studies attempt to measure the impact of a risk factor on an outcome of interest. An effect estimate is a measure of this effect. A typical effect estimate is the **risk ratio** or **relative risk**, also called a **hazard ratio** in time-to-event analyses. This is a ratio of how an outcome is measured in those with a disease versus those without a disease (ie, the ratio of the incidence of the outcome in the persons exposed versus the incidence of the outcome in the group not exposed). For example, Gelfand and coworkers found the incidence of death in those with severe psoriasis is 21.3 per thousand person-years versus 12.0 per thousand person-years in those without psoriasis.[27] The overall risk ratio is 1.5, which means that those with psoriasis have a 50% increased risk of death. **Attributable risk** or **risk difference** is a variation on this measure. It is the absolute risk in the exposed persons minus the absolute risk in the nonexposed persons. Using the example above, the overall attributable risk is 6 per thousand person-years, which means that in a cohort of 1000 patients with psoriasis, 6 deaths occurred that can be associated with having psoriasis compared with not having psoriasis (Table 3-2).

Many studies use the **odds ratio** as an effect estimate. An odds ratio is the ratio of the odds that a case is exposed compared with the odds that a control is exposed. Classically, odds ratios have been associated with case-control studies. However, now odds ratios are often measured because they are easily calculated in a commonly used statistical analysis called logistic regression. When measuring risk, odds ratios and relative risks are equivalent measurements when the outcome is rare (prevalence of less than 5%), but the odds ratio overestimates the relative risk when the outcome is common. In most settings, reports of odds ratios or risk ratios are "adjusted" because study subjects rarely experience a single exposure, and thus confounding by other exposures or risk factors is of concern. Adjustment can be done by statistical manipulation and can control for confounding factors. Considering psoriasis again, those with psoriasis might be older or more likely to have cardiovascular disease than the control population. To properly estimate the risk ratio or odds ratio, it would be appropriate to remove (or adjust for) the effect of age or cardiovascular disease from the measure of the risk of death. It is important to remember that these effect estimates are measures of association and not necessarily indicative of causality; other criteria need to be met to establish causal relationships.

TEST CHARACTERISTICS

In studies of diagnostic test performance, **sensitivity** and **specificity** are important test characteristics that should be reported (Fig. 3-2). The **sensitivity** of a test is the proportion of truly diseased individuals (ie, true positives and false negatives) who are defined as having the disease by a test (ie, true positives). It is also called the true positive rate. The **specificity** of a test is the proportion of individuals who truly do not have the disease (ie, false positives and true negatives) who are defined by the test as not having the disease (ie, true negatives). It is also called the true negative rate. In clinical situations, health care providers tend to care more about the **positive** or **negative predictive value** of a test as they answer the more clinically relevant questions of how likely a patient is to have or not have a disease given a positive or negative test, respectively. The **positive predictive value** is the proportion of individuals who have a positive test that truly have the disease, and the **negative predictive value** is the proportion of individuals who have a negative test who truly do not have the disease. Whereas the sensitivity and specificity of a diagnostic test are fixed characteristics, the positive and negative predictive values of a test may vary depending on the prevalence of the

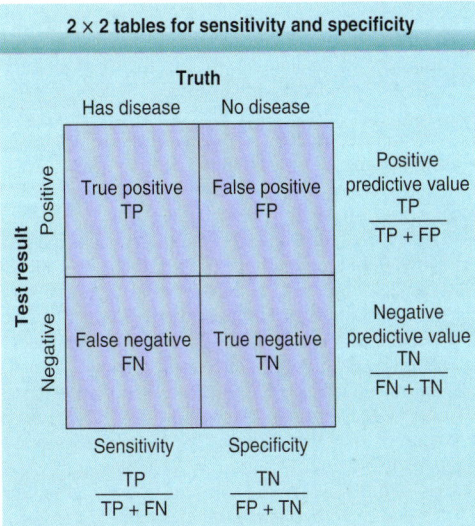

Figure 3-2 2 × 2 tables for sensitivity and specificity.

disease in the population being tested. Depending on how these parameters are determined, the estimates can be influenced by disease definition and certainty of diagnosis; the prevalence, incidence, or frequency of the disease within the studied cohort; and the diagnostic criteria used to assure that the patient has the disease of interest.

PATIENT-REPORTED OUTCOME MEASURES

Our current health care and research environment places increasing importance on incorporation and consideration of the patient experience of disease and health care. As such, **patient-reported outcome measures** (PROMs), tools that assess the experience of disease and health care directly from the patient's self-report, have become a major focus of research and clinical care. PROMs vary in their focus of assessment from generic measures of overall health or quality of life (QoL) to skin-, disease-, and symptom-specific measures (Table 3-3). On a national level, the National Institutes of Health initiated the Patient-Reported Outcomes Measurement Information System (PROMIS),[28] which is a publicly available system of validated generic measures of patient-reported health status for physical, mental, and social well-being across multiple medical conditions. PROMs are particularly important in the field of dermatology in which many of the conditions that are evaluated and treated do not directly impact hard health outcomes, such as mortality, but do significantly affect patients' QoL. Several PROMs are specific to dermatology, including the skin-related QoL instruments Dermatology Life Quality Index,[29] Skindex-29,[30] and Skindex-16[31] as well as several condition-specific (eg, Patient-Oriented Eczema Measure[32]) and symptom-specific (eg, Itchy-Quant[33]) tools.

CONCLUSIONS

Epidemiology forms the basis for advancing our understanding of disease among populations. Epidemiologic, patient-oriented, and health services research is essential for furthering our knowledge of dermatologic diseases at both a population and individual level. A basic understanding of epidemiology and its study methods and measures enables the clinician to interpret primary literature and practice evidence-based medicine.

REFERENCES

1. Hill AB. The environment and disease: association or causation? *Proc R Soc Med*. 1965;58:295-300.

TABLE 3-3
Examples of Instruments Used to Measure Patient Reports

DOMAIN	TYPICAL INSTRUMENT(S)	COMMENT
Overall quality of life	Medical Outcomes Study Short-Form instruments (SF-36)[34] and (SF-12)[35]	36 or 12 items; commonly used in clinical research; interpretable scores
Skin-related quality of life	Dermatology Life Quality Index[36] Skindex-29,[37] Skindex-16[31]	10 items; most commonly used; focuses on functioning 29 or 16 items; focuses on emotional effects, symptoms, and functioning
Disease-specific severity	Patient-Oriented Eczema Measure (POEM),[32] Self-Administered Psoriasis Area and Severity Index (SAPASI)[38]	Correlate well with clinician measures
Symptoms: pruritus	Itch Severity Scale,[39] Pruritus-Specific Quality-of-Life Instrument,[40] ItchyQuant[33]	Demonstrate promising measurement properties
Patient satisfaction	Consumer Assessment of Healthcare Providers and Systems (CAHPS) survey[41]	Correlates with adherence, quality of life, and quality of care
Patient preferences	Utilities,[42] Willingness to Pay[43]	Correlations among different measures of preferences can be weak

2. Patsopoulos NA. A pragmatic view on pragmatic trials. *Dialogues Clin Neurosci.* 2011;13(2):217-224.
3. Koek MB, Buskens E, van Weelden H, et al. Home versus outpatient ultraviolet B phototherapy for mild to severe psoriasis: pragmatic multicentre randomised controlled non-inferiority trial (PLUTO study). *BMJ.* 2009;338:b1542.
4. Thomas K, Crook A, Foster K, et al. Prophylactic antibiotics for the prevention of cellulitis (erysipelas) of the leg: results of the UK Dermatology Clinical Trials Network's PATCH II trial. *Br J Dermatol.* 2012;166(1):169-178.
5. Gartlehner G, Hansen RA, Nissman D, et al. A simple and valid tool distinguished efficacy from effectiveness studies. *J Clin Epidemiol.* 2006;59(10):1040-1048.
6. Thorpe KE, Zwarenstein M, Oxman AD, et al. A pragmatic-explanatory continuum indicator summary (PRECIS): a tool to help trial designers. *J Clin Epidemiol.* 2009;62(5):464-475.
7. Zwarenstein M, Treweek S, Gagnier JJ, et al. Improving the reporting of pragmatic trials: an extension of the CONSORT statement. *BMJ.* 2008;337:a2390.
8. Alhusayen RO, Juurlink DN, Mamdani MM et al. Isotretinoin use and the risk of inflammatory bowel disease: a population-based cohort study. *J Invest Dermatol.* 2013;133(4):907-912.
9. Barbieri JS, Hoffstad O, Margolis DJ. Duration of oral tetracycline-class antibiotic therapy and use of topical retinoids for the treatment of acne among general practitioners (GP): a retrospective cohort study. *J Am Acad Dermatol.* 2016;75(6):1142-1150 e1141.
10. Palmer CN, Irvine AD, Terron-Kwiatkowski A, et al. Common loss-of-function variants of the epidermal barrier protein filaggrin are a major predisposing factor for atopic dermatitis. *Nat Genet.* 2006;38(4):441-446.
11. Koo EB, Petersen TD, Kimball AB. Meta-analysis comparing efficacy of antibiotics versus oral contraceptives in acne vulgaris. *J Am Acad Dermatol.* 2014;71(3):450-459.
12. Shea BJ, Grimshaw JM, Wells GA, et al. Development of AMSTAR: a measurement tool to assess the methodological quality of systematic reviews. *BMC Med Res Methods.* 2007;7:10.
13. Shea BJ, Hamel C, Wells GA, et al. AMSTAR is a reliable and valid measurement tool to assess the methodological quality of systematic reviews. *J Clin Epidemiol.* 2009;62(10):1013-1020.
14. Liberati A, Altman DG, Tetzlaff J, et al. The PRISMA statement for reporting systematic reviews and meta-analyses of studies that evaluate healthcare interventions: explanation and elaboration. *BMJ.* 2009;339:b2700.
15. Moher D, Cook DJ, Eastwood S, et al. Improving the quality of reports of meta-analyses of randomised controlled trials: the QUOROM statement. Quality of Reporting of Meta-analyses. *Lancet.* 1999;354(9193):1896-1900.
16. Schulz KF, Altman DG, Moher D, et al. CONSORT 2010 statement: updated guidelines for reporting parallel group randomised trials. *BMJ.* 2010;340:c332.
17. von Elm E, Altman DG, Egger M, et al. The Strengthening the Reporting of Observational Studies in Epidemiology (STROBE) statement: guidelines for reporting observational studies. *Lancet.* 2007;370(9596):1453-1457.
18. Systems to rate the strength of scientific evidence. Evidence report/technology assessment: number 47. AHRQ publication no. 02-E015. Rockville (MD): Agency for Healthcare Research and Quality; 2002.
19. Ebell MH, Siwek J, Weiss BD, et al. Strength of recommendation taxonomy (SORT): a patient-centered approach to grading evidence in the medical literature. *Am Fam Physician.* 2004;69(3):548-556.
20. Guyatt GH, Oxman AD, Vist GE, et al. GRADE: an emerging consensus on rating quality of evidence and strength of recommendations. *BMJ.* 2008;336(7650):924-926.
21. Howick J, Chalmers I, Glasziou P, et al. The 2011 Oxford CEBM Levels of Evidence (Introductory Document). http://www.cebm.net/index.aspx?o=5653.
22. Howick J, Chalmers I, Glasziou P, et al. Explanation of the 2011 Oxford Centre for Evidence-Based Medicine (OCEBM) Levels of Evidence (Background Document). http://www.cebm.net/index.aspx?o=5653.
23. Kurd SK, Gelfand JM. The prevalence of previously diagnosed and undiagnosed psoriasis in US adults: results from NHANES 2003-2004. *J Am Acad Dermatol.* 2009;60(2):218-224.
24. Rachakonda TD, Schupp CW, Armstrong AW. Psoriasis prevalence among adults in the United States. *J Am Acad Dermatol.* 2014;70(3):512-516.
25. Bell LM, Sedlack R, Beard CM, et al. Incidence of psoriasis in Rochester, Minn, 1980-1983. *Arch Dermatol.* 1991;127(8):1184-1187.
26. Icen M, Crowson CS, McEvoy MT, et al. Trends in incidence of adult-onset psoriasis over three decades: a population-based study. *J Am Acad Dermatol.* 2009;60(3):394-401.
27. Gelfand JM, Troxel AB, Lewis JD, et al. The risk of mortality in patients with psoriasis: results from a population-based study. *Arch Dermatol.* 2007;143(12):1493-1499.
28. Cella D, Yount S, Rothrock N, et al. The Patient-Reported Outcomes Measurement Information System (PROMIS): progress of an NIH Roadmap cooperative group during its first two years. *Med Care.* 2007;45(5 suppl 1):S3-S11.
29. Basra MK, Fenech R, Gatt RM, et al. The Dermatology Life Quality Index 1994-2007: a comprehensive review of validation data and clinical results. *Br J Dermatol.* 2008;159(5):997-1035.
30. Chren MM, Lasek RJ, Quinn LM, et al. Skindex, a quality-of-life measure for patients with skin disease: reliability, validity, and responsiveness. *J Invest Dermatol.* 1996;107(5):707-713.
31. Chren MM, Lasek RJ, Sahay AP, et al. Measurement properties of Skindex-16: a brief quality-of-life measure for patients with skin diseases. *J Cutan Med Surg.* 2001;5(2):105-110.
32. Charman CR, Venn AJ, Williams HC. The patient-oriented eczema measure: development and initial validation of a new tool for measuring atopic eczema severity from the patients' perspective. *Arch Dermatol.* 2004;140(12):1513-1519.
33. Haydek CG, Love E, Mollanazar NK, et al. Validation and Banding of the ItchyQuant: A Self-Report Itch Severity Scale. *J Invest Dermatol.* 2017;137(1):57-61.
34. Ware J. *SF-36 Health Survey Manual and Interpretation Guide.* Boston: The Health Institute, New England Medical Center; 1993.
35. Ware J Jr, Kosinski M, Keller SD. A 12-Item Short-Form Health Survey: construction of scales and preliminary tests of reliability and validity. *Med Care.* 1996;34(3):220-233.
36. Finlay AY, Khan GK. Dermatology life quality index (DLQI)—a simple practical measure for routine clinical use. *Clin Exper Dermatol.* 1994;19:210-216.

37. Chren MM et al. Improved discriminative and evaluative capability of a refined version of Skindex, a quality-of-life instrument for patients with skin diseases. *Arch Dermatol*. 1997;133(11):1433-1440.
38. Fleischer AB et al. Patient measurement of psoriasis disease severity with a structured instrument. *J Invest Dermatol*. 1994;102:967-969.
39. Majeski CJ et al. Itch Severity Scale: a self-report instrument for the measurement of pruritus severity. *Br J Dermatol*. 2007;156(4):667-673.
40. Desai NS et al. A pilot quality-of-life instrument for pruritus. *J Am Acad Dermatol*. 2008;59(2):234-244.
41. Adult Specialty Care Questionnaire 1.0: Agency for Health Care Research and Quality (AHRQ); 2010. http://www.cahps.ahrq.gov/content/products/CG/PROD_CG_CG40Products.asp?p=1021&s=213.
42. Chen SC et al. A catalog of dermatology utilities: a measure of the burden of skin diseases. *J Investig Dermatol Symp Proc*. 2004;9(2):160-168.
43. Delfino M Jr, Holt EW, Taylor CR, et al. Willingness-to-pay stated preferences for 8 health-related quality-of-life domains in psoriasis: a pilot study. *J Am Acad Dermatol*. 2008;59(3):439-447.

PART 2

Structure and Function of Skin

第二篇　皮肤的结构和功能

Chapter 4 :: Developmental Biology of the Skin
:: Luis Garza

第四章
皮肤发育生物学

中文导读

本章共分为13节：①皮肤的细胞类型；②皮肤的结构；③胚胎发育概论；④神经嵴与体节发育；⑤表皮分化；⑥间充质/成纤维细胞与脂肪发育；⑦黑素细胞分化；⑧皮肤神经的发育；⑨附属器发育；⑩脉管系统；⑪皮肤中的造血细胞；⑫嵌合体；⑬结论。全面讨论了皮肤的发育，介绍了皮肤的结构，并讲述了有皮肤表现的遗传性疾病中，皮肤的正常发育是如何被扰乱的。

第一节介绍了皮肤发育过程中的细胞类型及其作用，以及发育过程中的重要中枢发育信号通路，包括Wnt配体、β-catenin、P63、Shh配体、EDAR外营养不良蛋白A受体等。

第二节介绍了皮肤分为表皮层、真皮层及皮下组织。表皮层主要细胞为角质形成细胞，角蛋白丰富；真皮层主要细胞是成纤维细胞，产生胶原蛋白；皮下组织脂肪细胞含量丰富，同时与真皮层共享血管、神经等成分。

第三节介绍了皮肤发育开始于胚胎形成的2周内，原肠胚是皮肤发育与其他器官发育分离的第一个阶段，原肠胚形成的外胚层最终形成表皮、黑素细胞及神经系统。中胚层发育为成纤维细胞、血管、肌肉和骨骼。

第四节介绍了神经嵴的发育有助于黑素细胞和成纤维细胞等结构的形成，在皮肤发育中很重要；体节是真皮成纤维细胞的前体细胞。

第五节介绍了表皮是在羊膜的液体环境中发育的，经历了周皮形成、中间层形成，以及完全成熟三个阶段。若在发育过程中出现基因突变导致皮肤屏障缺陷，则出现鱼鳞病等综合征。

第六节介绍了真皮是由胚胎中胚层形

成,主要细胞是成纤维细胞,具有很强的异质性,表现为身体不同部位的成纤维细胞起源不一样,皮肤特定部位的成纤维细胞功能也不一样。同时介绍了脂肪细胞是由真皮成纤维细胞祖细胞发育而来的,具有多样性,不仅拥有能量平衡作用,同时在免疫监测等方面起作用。

第七节介绍了黑素细胞来源于神经嵴,前体是SOX10阳性的祖细胞,当分化为黑素细胞时,关键的表达转录因子为MITF,DCT和KIT蛋白。若丢失MITF和KIT表达,则转变为黑素母细胞-成体黑素细胞干细胞,位于毛囊球干细胞域,为头发提供色素。黑素细胞发育异常与蓝痣及斑驳病发生等相关。

第八节介绍了皮肤的感觉神经元分布广泛,从三叉神经或背根神经节发育,可以根据感觉、位置以及髓鞘化程度来进行分类。默克尔细胞是一种特殊的调节哺乳动物触觉的感受器,从基底层角质形成细胞发育而来,可以形成恶性肿瘤。

第九节介绍了附属器的发育中关于毛发的胚胎发育研究,新的观念认为由β-连环蛋白信号在角质形成细胞和成纤维细胞中同时启动发育。其次为皮脂腺的发育在胎儿第13至14周由SOX9+LRIG1+毛囊干细胞在球茎期发育而成。其他附属器结构了解不多,汗腺和指甲的发育依赖EDAR通路,而大汗腺相关研究极少。

第十节介绍了血管的发育是由血管母细胞而来,通过Ihh、FGF2、BMPs和VEGF等信号介导从中胚层向内皮细胞系分化,随后形成有内腔的管。淋巴管发育是由成熟的表达PROX1的静脉内皮细胞,在外侧中胚层的VEGF-C表达区域萌发并迁移以建立淋巴管。脉管系统异常可引起如Sturge-Weber综合征等疾病。

第十一节介绍了皮肤中的造血细胞主要包括淋巴细胞和髓样细胞,其中朗格汉斯细胞由胚胎的卵黄囊产生。而其他免疫细胞定居皮肤并不只是从血液和淋巴结循环而来,而是有一套专门的皮肤特异性记忆T细胞库,它可能与驻留在淋巴结中的中央记忆T细胞共享一个共同的幼稚T细胞前体。造血细胞发育不良会引起高IgE综合征等皮肤综合征。

第十二节介绍了与皮肤病相关的一个重要的发育因素是嵌合体,即胚胎在发育过程中获得了新的突变。

第十三节介绍了Shinya Yamanaka因首次明确了将皮肤成纤维细胞转化为诱导多能干细胞的基因混合物而被授予2012年诺贝尔医学奖。对于皮肤发育的认识是最终采用细胞疗法作为全新治疗领域的第一步。

〔粟 娟〕

AT-A-GLANCE

- The skin is divided into 3 layers:
  - *Epidermis:* Forms the barrier to outside world and is the locus of immune surveillance and activation to prevent and combat infections.
  - *Dermis:* Provides the main structural substance (collagen) of skin. Forms a main interface to vasculature and nervous system in the skin, and intimately interfaces with epidermis to coordinate skin function.
  - *Hypodermis:* The area beneath the collagen-rich dermis that is characterized by subcutaneous adipose tissue with a role in energy balance, as well as recently defined roles in epidermis crosstalk and immune surveillance.
- Skin development, as for other organs, occurs in the stepwise progression from more pluripotent to increasingly differentiated cells with specialized function.

How does your entire body form from a single cell? The process of development is perhaps one of the most complicated events in biology, yet occurs with startling fidelity. This chapter discusses how the skin develops as a means to introduce the reader to the structures of the skin; to create a framework to understand normal skin function; and to learn how its normal development is disrupted in a variety of inherited genetic diseases that manifest with skin symptoms.

As science and medicine increasingly converge, knowledge of normal skin development is increasingly important. For example, knowing the normal function of skin structure allows the clinician greater insight into the clinical phenotype during its disruption in the context of skin disease. This is most clearly the case for inherited skin disorders. Also, with the advent of personalized medicine and personal genome sequencing, clinicians will be responsible for interpreting how different inherited polymorphisms will affect patients. Although the field is challenged with making assumptions that findings in mice hold true for humans, the careful study of skin development is not simply an academic exercise, but a method for enhancing patient care.

TYPES OF SKIN CELLS

CELLS OF THE SKIN FORMED DURING DEVELOPMENT

- *Keratinocytes* are the central cells of the epidermis and form the intermediate filament keratins that, among other roles, provide structural resiliency to cells.
- *Fibroblasts* are the central cells of the dermis that, among other roles, secrete collagen, which provides the substance for the dermis.
- *Appendages* are organized structures of keratinocytes and fibroblasts that act together to make hair follicles, eccrine sweat glands, apocrine glands, and the nail unit.
- *Melanocytes* are cells that reside predominantly in the epidermis and synthesize melanin whose primary function is to absorb and block the sun's damaging ultraviolet light.
- *Langerhans cells* are immune cells that reside predominantly in the epidermis, and internalize and present potentially harmful antigens encountered in the environment to initiate an immune response.
- *Sensory neurons* monitor touch, pressure, temperature, and hair follicle movement.
- *Arterioles* and *venules* connect to the cardiovascular system.
- *Lymph vessels* return interstitial fluid to the circulatory system.
- *Merkel cells* live in the epidermis and sense touch.
- *Immune cells* develop elsewhere, but are important components of the skin and include T cells, B cells, dendritic cells, macrophages, neutrophils, and mast cells.

CENTRAL DEVELOPMENTAL SIGNALING PATHWAYS

- *Wnt ligands* are extracellular secreted proteins that likely have important posttranslational modifications such as palmitoylation and activate the frizzled receptors to eventually stabilize β-catenin, causing its nuclear translocation from cytoplasmic-associated or cytoskeletal-associated structures. β-Catenin controls epithelial differentiation, stem cell function, appendage function.
- *p63* is a transcription factor with multiple isoforms that is perhaps the central regulator of epithelial identity. Without p63, epidermis fails to stratify or fully form, which leads to failure of appendage formation.
- *Shh ligands* are extracellular secreted proteins that bind the smoothened receptor and eventually activate the *Gli* family of transcription factors. Shh is very important to hair follicle formation and function.
- *EDAR* (ectodysplasin A receptor) is a receptor for the EDA (ectodysplasin A) ligand and part of the tumor necrosis factor (TNF) receptor family. It is critically important for the development of appendages.
- The ligands Delta or Jagged bind the receptor *Notch* which initiates transcription and epidermal differentiation.
- *BMP* (bone morphogenic protein) ligands are a family of ligands that bind BMP receptors and, among other functions, regulate hair follicle cycling and growth.
- *HOX* (homeobox) transcription factor family is important in large-scale body patterning.

STRUCTURES OF THE SKIN

The structures of the skin are defined by how they support skin function, and the process of development is the acquisition of this final functional unit (Fig. 4-1). For example, because the foremost function of skin is as a barrier to prevent outside materials from entering the body, the *epidermis*, or outer layer of the skin, develops an intricate layered arrangement with the most mature surface layer being the most resistant for ingress of foreign material. Other important functions include resisting trauma, protecting from ultraviolet light, repelling infections, sensing the environment, thermoregulation, and energy metabolism. These different systems within the skin develop at different rates, and are discussed in more depth below.

As mentioned, the outermost layer of the skin is the epidermis. The cell that composes the majority

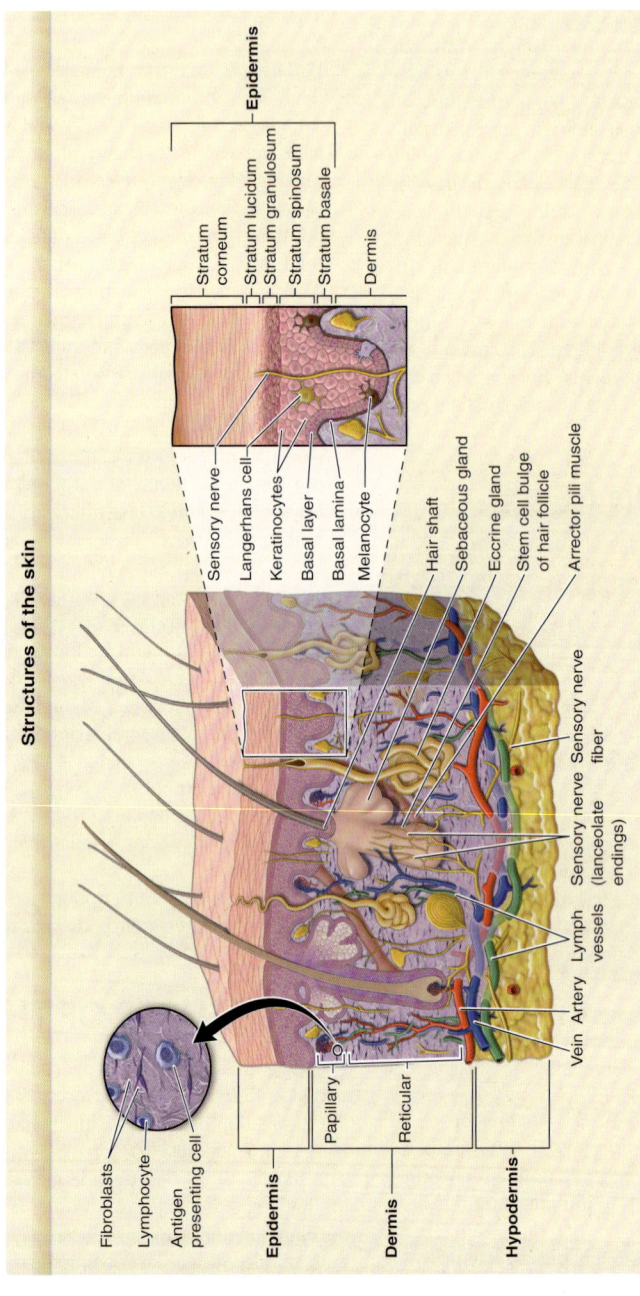

Figure 4-1 Structures of the skin. In this schematic, the general architecture of skin is depicted and makes clear the complexity required during development for formation of all elements.

TABLE 4-1
Summary of Important Developmental Stages of Skin Development

TRIMESTER	ESTIMATED GESTATIONAL AGE IN WEEKS (APPROXIMATE)	EPIDERMAL DEVELOPMENT	DERMAL DEVELOPMENT	APPENDAGEAL DEVELOPMENT
First Transition from embryo to fetus:	2	Gastrulation begins and ectoderm is formed; single-layer germinativum		
	3	Periderm forms		
	8	Intermediate layer forms		Dental placodes forming
	8	Melanocytes present	Distinct boundary between epidermis and dermis	
	9			Nail placodes form
	10	Langerhans cells present		Hair follicle placodes form
	12	Merkel cells present	Dermal–epidermal junction and basement membrane matures	Sweat gland placodes form on volar sites
Second	13		Papillary distinct from reticular dermis	
	24	Periderm sloughs	Elastic fibers visible	
Third	27			
	40	Birth		

Data from Bolognia JL, Jorizzo JL, Rapini RP, eds. *Dermatology*. New York: Mosby Elsevier; 2003.

of the epidermis is the *keratinocyte*, so named because the structural protein keratin is abundant in that cell. Keratinocytes are stacked in layers of increasingly more mature states until they are effectively ghosts of cells that serve only as a barrier and have little to no energy consumption. In aggregate, the epidermal layers are thicker in areas of the palms and soles, which are subjected to more pressure, and thinner in areas without such pressure, such as the eyelids. Each layer is defined by different keratins, and keratins also differ by body site. In fact, the same general arrangement of keratinocytes that mature from normal epidermis toward dead cells in the epidermis also is how teeth and hair are formed. Although in the general epidermis the dead keratinocytes are regularly released to allow for the next layer to mature and replace it, in hair and teeth those cells are retained to form the final "keratinized" structure. It is important to emphasize that many cells besides keratinocytes reside in the epidermis, including nerve cells that pierce the basal lamina, a vital scaffolding structure that separates the epidermis from the dermis, the next most internal layer of skin.

While keratins are the protein most abundant in the epidermis, collagens are the most abundant protein in the dermis. Leather used in clothing is effectively dermis and represents well the strength that collagens afford to the skin. As discussed in section "Mesenchyme/Fibroblast and Adipose Development", there are also a wide variety of unique collagens with different functions. The primary cell of the dermis is the fibroblast, which produces collagens but has a large repertoire of other functions. Within the general area of the dermis are also structures such as the invaginated epithelium of the hair follicle or the sweat gland. These invaginated areas of epithelium often become a hub for the other components of the dermis: blood vessels, lymphatic vessels, nerves, and a host of cells of hematopoietic origin.

The final layer is the *hypodermis* or the subcutaneous tissue, which transitions to the fascial layers. Although there is a greater abundance of adipocytes and much less collagen, many of the other components of the dermis are shared with the hypodermis, but, for example, with vessels and nerves of higher caliber.

GENERAL SUMMARY OF EMBRYONIC DEVELOPMENT

Human development occurs through 40 weeks of gestation, and is commonly subdivided into trimesters (Table 4-1). The week of development is typically counted beginning from the last menstrual period. The developing human is called a fetus at around 8 weeks after arms and legs have developed and show motion. This occurs during the first trimester, from weeks 0 to 12 of estimated gestational age, when organogenesis has mostly completed. The second trimester occurs from weeks 12 to 26 and is marked by continuous development, for example, the appearance of downy hair in the infant. The third trimester runs from weeks 26 to 40 and is when most development completes, including the formation of the vernix caseosa from the skin whose function is thought to lubricate for the passage through the birth canal. Interestingly, skin function is not complete even at birth as final full-barrier formation occurs afterward.

The most complicated steps of development occur at the earliest times when the skin begins to form within the first 2 weeks of development. Several canonical structures characterize early development: *morula*, *blastula*, *gastrula*, and then *somatogenesis*, and *organogenesis*. After fertilization, the initial unstructured multiplication of cells leads to the formulation of a morula. The morula divides to form a more complicated structure called a blastula, which has 2 main parts. The first is the trophoblast, which is destined to become the parts of the placenta of fetal (as opposed to maternal) origin, namely the chorion, amnion, allantois. The second is the inner cell mass (ICM), which is destined to become the actual embryo. As the ICM differentiates into 3 germ layers it becomes the gastrula, which is the first stage where skin development separates from the development of other organs.

The 3 germ layers that form during gastrulation include the *ectoderm*, the *mesoderm*, and the *endoderm*. The ectoderm forms eventually the epidermis and melanocytes, but also the nervous system. The mesoderm forms fibroblasts, blood vessels, muscles, and bone. The endoderm does not contribute to skin development. There are some exceptions to these generalities, such as some fibroblast subpopulations that actually originate from the ectoderm, as they are thought to be derived from the neural crest.

NEURAL CREST AND SOMITE DEVELOPMENT

Neural crest development is important in the skin as it contributes to structures such as melanocytes and fibroblasts, and is therefore also involved in some clinical diseases where neural crest does not mature correctly.

Neural crest development initiates during the third week of fetal life when the ectoderm forms the neural plate within it. The ectoderm is the outermost layer of the ICM and sits upon the mesoderm. A plate of cells within the ectoderm differentiates into the future central nervous system. However, at the junction between the neural plate and the ectoderm, a distinct group of cells, known as the neural crest form. During gastrulation, the neural plate forms a valley in the ectoderm, and as it does, the edges of the valley actually rise up; this raised area is the boundary between the ectoderm and the neural plate and is termed the *neural crest*, as the crest of a hill. Eventually the valley becomes so deep and narrow that top parts of the ectoderm fuse and the neural plate detaches to become the neural tube. The neural crest cells, however, are not retained in either the ectoderm or the neural tube, but instead remain free in the mesoderm. Interestingly, there are some differences in terms of when the neural tube closes and when the neural crest cells migrate away, probably as a clue to their function. In the head, the neural crest migrate even before neural tube closure, and contribute to dermal fibroblasts in the face and anterior scalp. In the trunk, it is the last event. Neural crest cells are thought to specifically secrete the Wnt1 ligand, an important signaling molecule that activates the transcription factor and cytoskeletal protein, β-catenin.

Neural crest cells continue to migrate after neural tube morphogenesis. After detaching from the ectoderm or the neural tube, neural crests migrate either dorsally or ventrally. Persistent neural crest cells that do not complete migrations and differentiate into melanocytes are hypothesized to contribute to common blue nevi.

By the third week of human development, the mesoderm condenses into regular-spaced cuboidal segments termed *somites*, which are lateral to the neural tube. Although they mostly contribute to the axial skeleton and muscles, early somite fibroblasts are also precursors for dermal fibroblasts. Many of these fibroblasts—especially from body locations such as the back—originate from the dorsolateral portions of the somite, which is also called the *dermatomyotome*. Many diseases are associated with defects in neural crest migration, some of which affect melanocytes (see section "Melanocyte and Differentiation"). Non–melanocyte-related diseases of neural crest migration include DiGeorge syndrome where 22q11.2 deletion results in defects in cardiac, craniofacial, and endocrine organs, among others.[1]

EPIDERMIS DIFFERENTIATION

The final epidermis is a strong barrier consisting of a carefully stratified sequential layer of keratinocytes, so named because of their abundant synthesis of keratins, which are intermediate filaments with broad roles in regulating cell function even outside of their central role of providing structural support.[2] The final mature layers of the epithelium are very well defined with characteristic keratins expressed at each stage, typically with unique pairs of both a type I keratin and a type II keratin. The lack of development of some these keratins through mutations causes some blistering epidermolysis bullosa diseases, and is just one example of a family of proteins necessary for epidermal function. Understanding epithelial development (Fig. 4-2) will guide understanding of these diseases.

The development of the epidermis is unique in that it is destined to function at the air interface, but develops in the liquid environment of the amnion, and thus undergoes some unique stages that are never repeated in life. These stages are named after the layers that form such that the first is periderm formation, followed by intermediate layer formation, and, finally, full maturation.

Epidermal development begins soon after gastrulation. Although it is mostly complete in the first trimester, it is not fully complete until after birth. Skin forming begins when the ectoderm converts to a single layer known as the *germinativum*—a cuboidal, mitotically

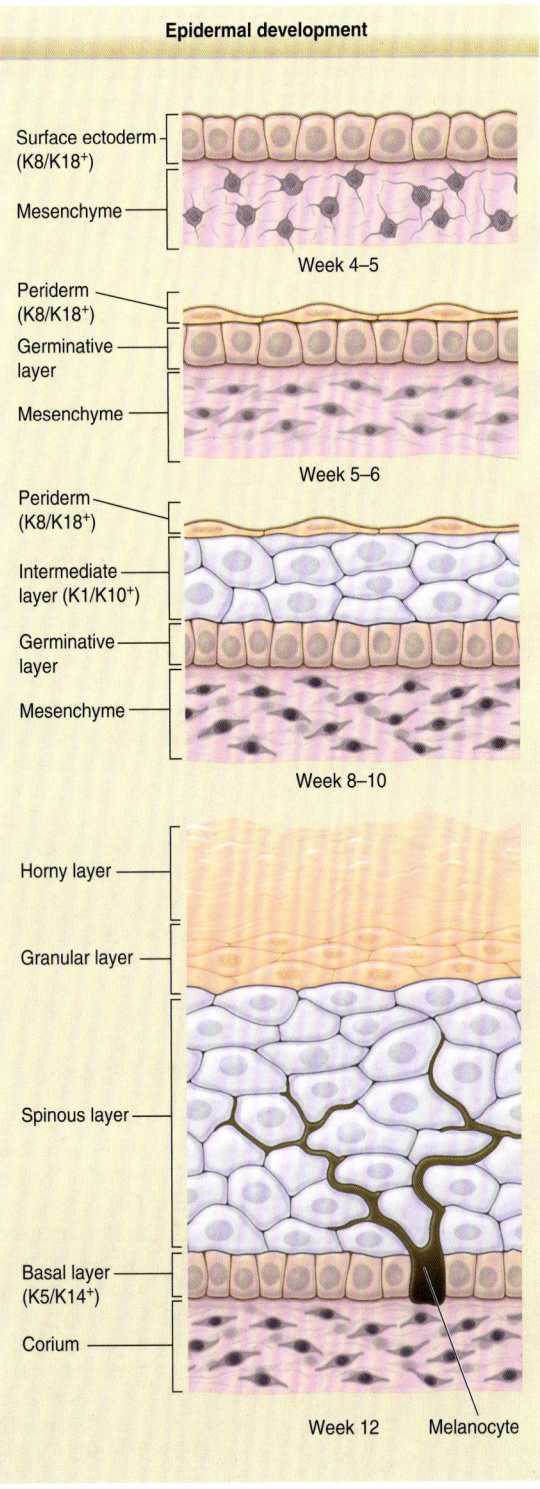

Figure 4-2 Epidermis development. Shown are the intermediate stages of skin development and acquisition of postnatal keratin expression.

active and undifferentiated layer. It expresses the gene *p63*, which is vital for epidermal differentiation and also corrupted in the EEC syndrome. Coincident with p63 expression is conversion from the more primitive cytokeratins KRT8 and KRT18 to the more mature basal layer keratins KRT5 and KRT14.[3] At 15 days the periderm layer forms above it, which appears as flattened cells with tight junctions and polarized cytoskeletal adhesions. The periderm initially expresses the cytokeratin KRT17 and then cytokeratin KRT6. Genes that control periderm formation include *SFN*, *IRF6*, and *IKKα*, likely partially through the nuclear factor kappa B (NF-κB) pathway. Hypothesized functions for the periderm include transport of and/or protection from material from the amnion, regulation of the dermis, and contribution to epithelial maturation. Recent evidence suggests it is also a protective layer that prevents pathologic adhesions to adjacent epithelium, so that lack of periderm formation leads to the human cocoon syndrome.[4]

At around 60 days of gestation, the intermediate layer is formed between the periderm on the outside and the germinativum layer. The intermediate layer probably forms through asymmetric cell divisions in basal layer keratinocytes,[5] much as is thought to occur for suprabasal layer formation in adults. In this case, 1 daughter cell continues to function as a stem cell in the basal layer, while its asymmetric sibling cell moves upward to begin differentiation. Following the formation of these 3 layers of embryonic skin, stratification of the epidermis begins coincident with the conversion to a fetus. Barrier formation is patterned, at least in mice, initiating at the dorsum and head. From there, it moves posteriorly and toward dorsal and ventral midlines. Characteristics of low transepidermal water loss and full exclusion of dyes as tests of mature epidermis are not reached until after birth.

Defects in the establishment of the skin barrier in humans are related to the clinical ichthyosis syndromes, also called defects in cornification. A wide variety of genes are important in the establishment of the skin barrier, and disruption of any of them can, in varying degrees, cause disease. Perhaps the most common is ichthyosis vulgaris with defects in the filaggrin protein, which is present in keratohyalin granules in the upper epidermis, from which the term *granular* layer derives. But others include defects in keratins of the suprabasal layer (KRT1 and KRT10), or in enzymes that crosslink proteins to make an impermeable layer (transglutaminases), or in lipid-metabolizing enzymes whose products are important for cornification (ALOX).[6]

MESENCHYME/FIBROBLAST AND ADIPOSE DEVELOPMENT

The dermis is formed from the mesodermal layer of the embryo; consequently, it is referred to as mesenchyme. Important structures, such as blood vessels and nerves, are discussed in sections "Development of the Cutaneous Nerves and Vasculature". Besides these, the primary cell type that supports the dermis is the fibroblast, which—despite a monomorphic appearance on histology—is likely a very heterogenous population. Although fibroblasts are most appreciated for their ability to abundantly secrete collagens and other extracellular matrix molecules, they are very critical even to epithelial cell function in many contexts, often depending on their location in the body and their subtype within that area of skin.[7]

The first type of fibroblast heterogeneity is the diversity of distinct lineages found at distinct body locations such as those at the distal fingertips compared to the proximal arm. Whereas fibroblasts from the ventral body are thought to derive from lateral plate mesoderm, fibroblasts from the head are thought to develop more from neural crest precursors, and those, for example, of back skin are more likely to develop from somites (and more specifically dermatomyotomes). This heterogeneity of fibroblast origin might partially explain the different features of skin in these areas, such as the high density of hair follicles in the head compared to the abdomen (see next paragraph). Even within a body part such as the limb, fibroblasts have distinct developmental origins whose signature is retained even in adulthood.[8] In particular, fibroblasts are programmed with a specific combination of *HOX* genes, which, even after culturing of fibroblasts, are retained to specify, for example, proximal to distal location with functional consequences such as the thick hairless skin on the palms and soles. This is consistent with the vital role of HOX in specifying body patterning, where mutations can lead to large-scale changes, such as legs appearing where antennae should be in Antennapedia *Drosophila* mutants.

Although the evidence is somewhat mixed, the mesenchymal cells are considered to be regulators of keratinocyte function.[9] In tissue-swapping studies where positionally mismatched epidermis and dermis layers are juxtaposed (eg, palmo-plantar dermis with haired epidermis), fibroblasts can "reprogram" keratinocyte function in some cases. Although contamination remains a theoretical concern,[10-14] this is one example suggesting that fibroblasts are not merely important for synthesis of extracellular proteins, but actually help dictate epidermal identity and function.

There is also heterogeneity of fibroblasts within a given location of skin. A common fibroblast progenitor (in mice characterized by the markers PDGFRa, Dlk1, and Irig1) gives rise to two general linages of fibroblasts, one destined for the upper dermis and one for the lower dermis. The upper dermal fibroblast progenitor (PDGFRa+, Blimp1+, Dlk–, Irig1+) become dermal papillae (a ball of fibroblasts that control hair keratinocytes), arrector pili muscle (muscle attached to hair that causes goosebumps), and the fibroblast of the upper dermis termed *papillary fibroblasts*. These fibroblasts are unique in their greater density and biased synthesis of collagens such as collagen III over collagen I. Interestingly, more detail is emerging on how these precursors differentiate and localize, such as the role of nephronectin as a maturation signal in the hair follicle stem cell compartment to induce arrector pili muscle differentiation.[15] The lower dermal fibroblast progenitor (PDGFRa+, Blimp1–, Dlk1+) give rise to not only adipocytes but to the reticular fibroblasts (lower density and biased collagen I over collagen III production). These reticular fibroblasts also differentiate to myofibroblasts during wounding, which promotes wound closure and likely also scarring. A separate group has defined another population of fibroblasts that promotes scarring in wounds and is classified by high engrailed (eng1) expression during development.[16] Although more work is needed to define the intersections of these populations and what differentially controls them, the startling heterogeneity of fibroblasts is quite clear.

One interesting developmental feature of fibroblasts is that they maintain their mesodermal capacity to transdifferentiate, for example, into bone and fat in culture, especially those from the dermal papillae, or fibroblasts surrounding the hair follicle in the hair sheath. These are classic defining features of mesenchymal stem cells derived from the bone marrow, but mesenchymal stem cells are thought to be distinct from most resident dermal fibroblasts, and not a normal component of the dermis, and do not contribute to dermis formation.[7,17] Similarly, pericytes, which are fibroblasts closely associating with blood vessels, also likely do not contribute to dermis formation.

Adipose cells have long been appreciated to have important roles in energy balance. Recently, however, a wider role has been appreciated, such as in immune surveillance[18] and coordinating hair cycling.[19] Adipocytes develop from lower dermal fibroblast progenitors. Similar to the diversity of fibroblasts, there also is an important diversity of adipocytes. Perhaps the central distinction is between white adipose cells, which function to store energy as lipid, and brown adipose, which function to burn energy through the uncoupling of oxidative phosphorylation to generate heat. In humans, brown adipose cells are thought to be located in the subcutaneous tissue at the paracervical/interscapular and supraclavicular areas.[20] Even though peroxisome-proliferator-activated receptor γ (PPARγ) is an important transcription factor for both white and brown adipose development, Prdm16 appears to be uniquely important for brown adipose development.[21] How brown adipocytes might modulate skin function in health and disease is an important area of future study.

Hallmark clinical syndromes of defects in mesenchymal development include focal dermal hypoplasia or Goltz syndrome caused by mutations in the *PORC* gene, which is important for Wnt molecule secretion. In Goltz syndrome, dermal atrophy manifests as fat herniations appearing as soft yellow to red nodules appearing in Blaschko lines and ulcers at sites of absent skin, among other symptoms. Analogous clinical syndromes for adipose tissue include the lipodystrophy syndromes such as Berardinelli-Seip where a lack of adipose development occurs from defects in the lipid synthesizing *AGPAT2* gene.[22]

MELANOCYTE DIFFERENTIATION

The dynamics of melanocyte development are clues to multiple human pigmentation inherited diseases, and perhaps even melanoma. For example, multiple hypotheses exist to explain the treatment-resistance and metastatic potential of melanomas such as their intrinsic ability to resist oxidative damage. Another posits that their considerable migration during development might be recapitulated in metastatic potential. Indeed, the great distances melanoblasts migrate beg the question on how the behavior might be different among less versus more migratory populations once the melanoblasts reach their destination. Melanocytes can be detected by the eighth week estimated gestational age (EGA)[23] in human epidermis.

Melanocytes derive from the neural crest as described in section "Neural Crest and Somite Development" migrating from the closing neural tube. Their precursor is a *SOX10*-positive progenitor, which also can differentiate into glial cells in addition to melanocytes. When differentiating into melanocytes, they begin to express the critical transcription factor MITF (microphthalmia-associated transcription factor), and also DCT and KIT proteins. These precursor cells actually can lose expression of MITF and KIT to revert to a melanoblast—the adult melanocyte stem cells—that live in the hair follicle bulge stem cell compartment. These melanoblasts differentiate through asymmetric divisions to mature melanocytes (expressing TYR [Tyrosinase]) that populate the hair follicle to give pigment to hair.[24] In addition to populating hair follicles, melanoblasts are thought to home to sweat glands where they might contribute to acral melanomas. These melanocyte stem cells supply interfollicular melanocytes as well, most dramatically during ultraviolet light therapy for patients with vitiligo.

There are a number of clinical correlates to the development of melanocytes. Melanocytes are present in the dermis more in development and less in adults. However, dermal melanocytes are thought to persist after birth in several locations, including the dorsa of the hands and feet, the sacrum/buttocks, and the scalp. These areas are clinically important because they are also common sites for blue nevi. Another example of defective melanocyte development is piebaldism where disrupted melanocyte migration secondary to defects in, for example, c-kit growth factor signaling lead to areas of albinism.

DEVELOPMENT OF THE CUTANEOUS NERVES

The skin has an extensive array of sensory neurons which during development requires careful orchestration for correct placement. Multiple types of sensory nerves can be divided based on their sensation (touch

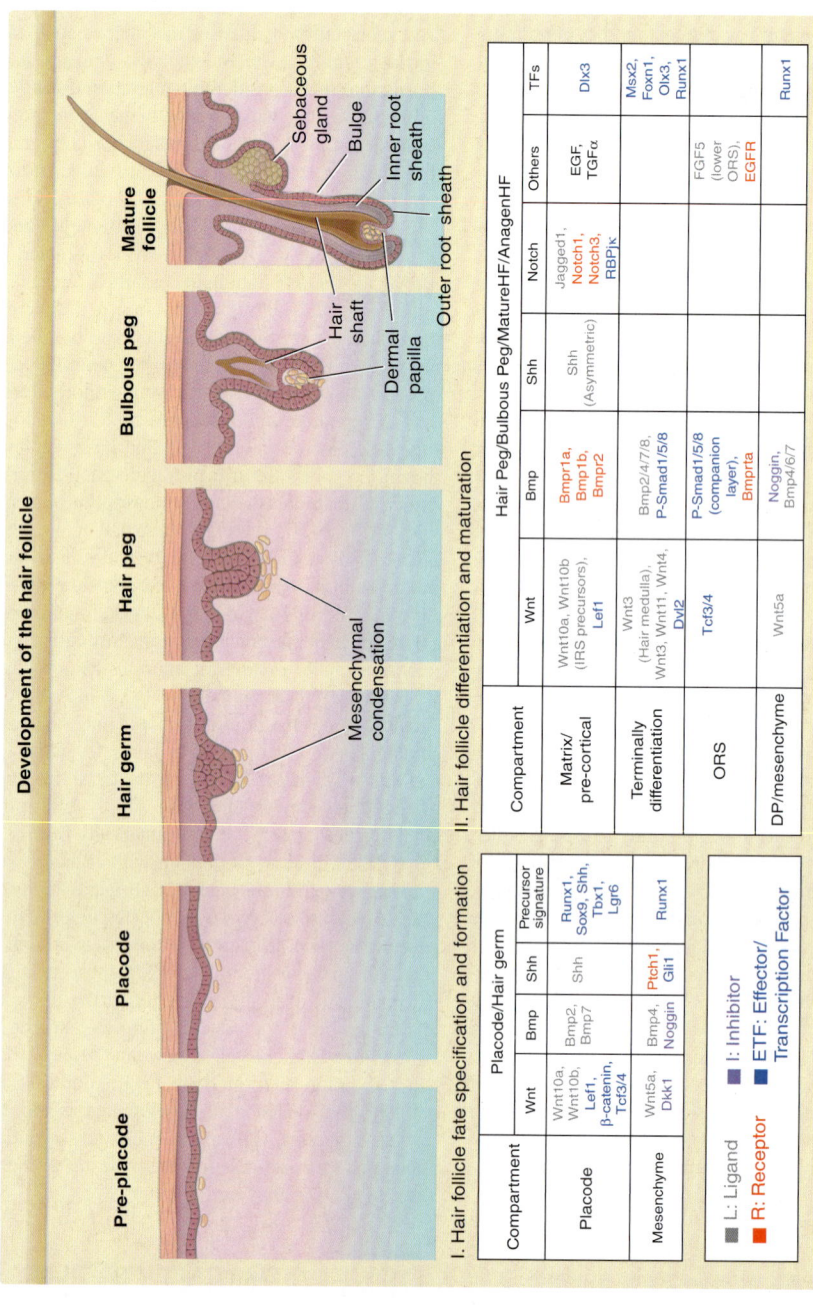

Figure 4-3 Hair follicle development. Shown are the stages of hair follicle during development, with a focus on the overlapping signaling pathways between initial hair follicle morphogenesis and postnatal hair cycling. (Adapted from Lee J, Tumbar T. Hairy tale of signaling in hair follicle development and cycling. *Semin Cell Dev Biol.* 2012;23(8):906-916, with permission. Copyright © Elsevier.)

versus temperature), their location (deeper dermal Pacini pressure sensor versus hair-based touch pressure), and, most commonly, the degree of myelination (Aβ, Aδ, or C fibers).[25]

In the skin, sensory neurons develop from the trigeminal (head) or dorsal root ganglia (elsewhere). The sensory nerves of the skin begin development following motor neurons.[26] However, rather than terminating in muscles as do motor neurons, somatosensory nerves of the skin continue toward the tissue periphery. The cues for this divergence likely originate from keratinocytes, and current suggestions for the identity of these cues include heparin sulfate proteoglycans and the leukocyte-antigen–related family receptors on neurons. How they are regulated differentially in more densely innervated areas such as volar sites is an exciting question that has not been firmly resolved.

Merkel cells, which are the cause of a very malignant cutaneous neoplasm, act to tune mammalian touch receptors.[27] They develop from basal-layer keratinocytes, as proven with their absence in mice where the gene *Atoh1* is deleted in the KRT14+ keratinocytes.[28] Consistent with their function, Merkel cells are found as early as 12 weeks EGA with particular high density at volar sites, appendages, and nerves.[29] Another example of the development of epithelial sensors from keratinocytes are the taste buds of the tongue, which, consistent with a shared ectodermal heritage, are evidence of the developmental plasticity between keratinocytes and neuronal-like cells.[30]

ADNEXAL DEVELOPMENT

Adnexal structures refer to all the skin appendages, or specialized arrangements of keratinocytes for unique functional purposes such as hair, nail, or sweat production. These appendages actually have similarities in development to actual limb appendages, as seen in mice where deletions in β-catenin or p63 lead to embryos with limb deformations as well as skin appendage formation.

The best studied of these appendages is the hair follicle. The exciting analogy to development of the hair follicle is that even in the adult, the hair goes through repeating cycles of apoptosis followed by regeneration, which partially recapitulates development. During normal hair cycling, however, the bulge stem cell compartment is maintained, unlike during development where it is formed de novo. Nevertheless, it has been rediscovered that—at least in mice—adults may fully recapitulate the organogenesis of hair follicles, with even the reformation of the stem cell compartment.[31]

How does embryogenesis of a hair occur (Fig. 4-3)? One consensus is that the earliest step in hair development is initiated by the activity of β-catenin in keratinocytes rather than fibroblasts, but this opinion has shifted and it is now thought that initiation of development by β-catenin activity in keratinocytes and fibroblasts might be effectively simultaneous. These epidermal and dermal signals determine how the regular spacing of hair follicles is generated. Mathematical models of reaction–diffusion involving both activators and inhibitors can effectively generate regular repeating nodes of activity, which, given the similarity to hair follicle regular arrangement, suggests that this occurs in vivo.[32] Signals involved in patterning are thought to include Wnt, but also BMP and FGF (fibroblast growth factor) signaling, among others. In this complete process, signals emanate at first broadly, and then become more localized and patterned to reflect the final tissue architecture. The broad outline of hair development shares similarities with the development of both teeth and mammary glands, among other structures.

The earliest morphologic changes are the formation of a hair placode in the epidermis, where the keratinocytes become thinner, columnar, and tightly packed. This occurs around 75 days EGA, and is accompanied by accumulations of congregated or condensed fibroblasts beneath the epidermis. The following stage is the hair germ phase (80 days EGA; sometimes referred to as hair bud), which is the more pronounced downward movement of epithelium forming a clear nubbin, followed by continued downward epithelial invasion through the peg stage (100 days EGA). During the peg stage, the epithelium begins to wrap around and encompass the associated inductive fibroblast population, which is now called the dermal papillae. Some authors include a final bulbous peg stage, by the end of which the sebaceous glands are formed. At the end of hair follicle development, the follicle is capable of creating a keratinized shaft, lanugo hair. Lanugo hair refers to the first wave of hair production and emerges around 130 days EGA. Interestingly, not all hairs develop simultaneously, and most lanugo hair is shed before birth.

The hair follicle stem cell compartment, termed *the bulge*, is so named because during development this area (located roughly between the arrector pili muscle and the sebaceous gland in the area termed *the isthmus*) is rounded out as a bulge in the otherwise straighter edge of the hair follicle.[33] In recent years, novel, distinct, stem cell populations of the hair follicle are being defined, some even outside of the bulge region, with many marked by the specific members of the LGR family of Wnt coreceptors.[34]

As mentioned above, an array of signals helps define the patterning of hair follicle development. Similarly, an orchestra of signals coordinate the final steps of morphogenesis. The activity of β-catenin is perhaps the most important for appendage development. Mice with activated versions of β-catenin in keratinocytes, for example, form supernumerary hair follicles. Downstream genes that are activated and necessary for morphogenesis include the ectodysplasin ligand (EDA) and receptor (EDAR) functions. For example, human mutations in EDAR cause syndromes where individuals are born with fewer hair follicles and sweat glands. Other genes important for hair development include the *Shh*, *BMP*, and *FGF* pathways.[35] Interestingly, different structures within the hair respond to these signals differently. For example, sebaceous gland differentiation is dependent on low activity of the β-catenin pathway, but also c-Myc, the androgen receptor, and p53, among others.[36]

Sebaceous glands develop during the bulbous peg phase from SOX9+ LRIG1+ hair follicle keratinocyte stem cells during 13th to 14th weeks of fetal life. Interestingly, while sebaceous glands have a dip in activity during childhood, they are more active during embryogenesis (in the production of the vernix caseosa) and puberty.[36] Classic sebaceous glands are always associated with hair follicles and do not exist alone, but variations of the sebaceous gland labeled as orphan sebaceous glands include the meibomian gland of the eye, the Fordyce spots of the mouth, the Tyson glands of the prepuce, and the Montgomery glands of the female areola.

Despite increased attention, less is known regarding the developmental dynamics of other appendage structures, such as the orphan sebaceous glands. Many overlaps exist, such as the primacy of epithelial–mesenchymal interactions and the involvement of the β-catenin and EDAR pathways. For example, sweat gland and nail development require EDAR, as evidenced even in small natural variants of EDAR (V370A), which confer changes in humans such as thick hair, incisor tooth shoveling, and increased eccrine sweat gland density.[37] Other similarities are that just as lanugo hair is an initial wave of keratinization, nails also have a preliminary nail that is complete and then shed in utero during the second trimester. Nail development also requires HOX programming (see HOX discussion in section "Mesenchyme/Fibroblast and Adipose Development") as is evident by patients with nail-patella with mutations in the HOX gene *LMX1b*.[21] Sweat glands in the volar skin develop around 12 to 13 weeks EGA, and the rest of the body at 20 weeks, following the same pattern of placode formation as a hair follicle.

Besides hair, nails, and sweat glands, the final appendage of the skin is the apocrine gland found in the hormonally responsive areas of the axillae and genitals. As apocrine glands are absent from most, if not all, regions of the mouse, little research has defined their developmental biology. Also, besides the above appendageal organs, there are other specialized keratinized structures, such as dermatoglyphs, the technical term for ridges responsible for characteristic fingerprints. Volar dermatoglyphics development begins around week 7 EGA when protuberances in palms and soles, called *volar pads*, appear.[38] The substance of volar pads are accumulations of grouped fibroblasts. As the volar pads involute, epidermal ridges appear as a result of local hyperproliferation of the basal layer of epidermis. There are several rounds of epidermal ridge development and also much more to learn about this process.

VASCULATURE

The vasculature are an essential development step for the continued growth and viability of the skin. The stem cells that contribute to the development of vessels are called *angioblasts*, and develop from mesoderm differentiating toward the endothelial lineage through signals such as Indian hedgehog (Ihh), FGF2, BMPs, and vascular endothelial growth factor (VEGF).[39] The angioblasts begin as scattered cells in the mesoderm, but then coalesce and form tubes with lumens as they complete their differentiation toward endothelial cells. Following this, they arborize and sprout to extend themselves[39] to mature in reactions involving TGF-β and platelet-derived growth factor (PDGF). Angiopoietin-1 is required for the recruitment of associated cells such as pericytes.

Current models posit that cutaneous vasculature develops following cues from previously established skin peripheral sensory neurons.[40] For example, in mutants where nerve branching is misrouted, arteries follow these spurious patterns, likely through the activity of the provascular growth hormone, VEGF. This still begs the question of how veins and arteries generate a parallel alignment. This alignment is important to minimize heat loss, such that arteries warm returning venous blood along the vascular plexus. While the EphrinB2 released by arteries as a ligand for EphB4 receptor on veins is important to maintain the arteriovenous (A-V) plexus,[41] how arteries and veins are juxtaposed has only recently been elucidated. In one current model, the signaling agent Apelin is produced from arterial endothelial cells, and stimulates chemotaxis and expression of APJ, a G-protein–coupled receptor, on venous endothelial cells to promote A-V alignment.[42]

Explanations regarding the differential density of vasculature according to skin site—such as the higher density of vessels in the scalp versus the back dermis—are likely related to local cues such as from Netrins, VEGF, Slit, and Semaphorins. Contributing to this will be differences in nerve development, but also in appendageal development such as hair follicles. Given that appendageal formation often precedes full sensory neuronal development, the further elucidation of secreted factors by hair follicles or sweat glands, for example, that guide the development of nerves and vasculature is an important future area of investigation.

Lymphatic development occurs through the maturation of established venous endothelial cells that express PROX1. These cells bud and migrate off to establish lymph vessels, first in regions of VEGF-C expression in the lateral mesoderm.

There exists also a large variety of clinical syndromes with aberrant development of the vasculature. One hallmark disease is the Sturge-Weber syndrome where defects in the gene *GNAQ* cause prominent port-wine stains on the face, as well as intracranial vascular anomalies leading to seizures and mental retardation, among other symptoms, and which is more concerning than the port-wine stains.

HEMATOPOIETIC CELLS IN THE SKIN

Hematopoietic cells of the skin are of numerous types, with novel subsets often being defined, but which generally include lymphocytes and myeloid cells. Their development is varied, and, of course, the earliest development of blood cells occurs outside of the skin.[43] The yolk sac of the developing embryo is the first to contribute blood cells by supplying the nucleated red cells which supply oxygen to the developing embryo. The yolk sac also generates some important myeloid lineages, such as the skin-specific antigen presenting cells known as the Langerhans cell. Langerhans cells are detectable by 10 weeks of gestation.[44] The second wave of development of hematopoietic cells occurs in the dorsal aorta, with later contributions from the liver. Here, the hematopoietic stem cells are generated that eventually can give rise to all blood cell lineages, as well as reconstitute an entire bone marrow.

Besides Langerhans cells, how do other immune cells take residence in the skin? Recent work highlights that not all T cells simply cycle through the epidermis from the blood and lymph nodes, but that a dedicated repertoire of resident tissue memory T cells are important to maintain immunity. Resident central memory T cells, which reside in lymph nodes, likely share a common naïve T-cell precursor for these skin-specific T cells, but are developed in adults and not in embryos.[45]

Defective hematopoietic cell development can cause hallmark syndromes in the skin, including hyperimmunoglobulin E (hyper-IgE) syndrome or Job syndrome where signal transducer and activator of transcription 3 (STAT3) mutations—a vital signaling molecule in lymphocytes—leads to impaired T-helper cell 17 (TH17) development and, instead, to excessive T-helper cell 2 (TH2) profile of eosinophilia and hyper-IgE characterized by chronic eczema and recurrent skin *Staphylococcus aureus* infections.

MOSAICISM

An important developmental correlate to skin diseases is mosaicism, where an embryo acquires a novel mutation in the process of development.[48] This results in the birth of a child where a subset of cells–the daughter cell lineage from the first cell to acquire the mutation– are mutated at that DNA, while the remaining cells are comparatively healthy. The geographic pattern of disease on the individual is then a direct window on the patterns of development and expansion from the original cell. The distinct morphologies in mosaicism are varied and important, but the most classic is commonly referred to as Blaschko's lines that consists of either linear expansions, or curving patterns of the growing mutant clone that are affected by the new mutation.[48]

CONCLUSIONS

The 2012 Nobel Prize in Medicine was awarded to Shinya Yamanaka for the first defined cocktail of genes that would convert a skin fibroblast into a totipotent embryonic stem cell capable of making any tissue, the induced pluripotent stem cell (IPSC). This has ushered in a new race to understand the exact cues necessary to engineer every cell in the body. In this way, patient-specific stem cells could be generated with simultaneous correction of genetic lesions before reimplantation into affected areas. Alternatively, unique genetic models could be made for research tools. For skin biologists, the careful understanding of skin development is a first step toward eventually harnessing the power of cellular therapy as an entirely new therapeutic domain. Although the field of developmental skin biology has been very productive, there still remain large gaps in our knowledge that are relevant to this and other avenues to improving human health.

REFERENCES

1. Menendez L, Kulik MJ, Page AT, et al. Directed differentiation of human pluripotent cells to neural crest stem cells. *Nat Protoc*. 2013;8(1):203-212.
2. Pan X, Hobbs RP, Coulombe PA. The expanding significance of keratin intermediate filaments in normal and diseased epithelia. *Curr Opin Cell Biol*. 2013;25(1):47-56.
3. Sumigray KD, Lechler T. Cell adhesion in epidermal development and barrier formation. *Curr Top Dev Biol*. 2015;112:383-414.
4. Richardson RJ, Hammond NL, Coulombe PA, et al. Periderm prevents pathological epithelial adhesions during embryogenesis. *J Clin Invest*. 2014;124(9):3891-3900.
5. Lechler T, Fuchs E. Asymmetric cell divisions promote stratification and differentiation of mammalian skin. *Nature*. 2005;437(7056):275-280.
6. Williams ML, Elias PM. Genetically transmitted, generalized disorders of cornification. The ichthyoses. *Dermatol Clin*. 1987;5(1):155-178.
7. Driskell RR, Watt FM. Understanding fibroblast heterogeneity in the skin. *Trends Cell Biol*. 2015;25(2):92-99.
8. Chang HY, Chi JT, Dudoit S, et al. Diversity, topographic differentiation, and positional memory in human fibroblasts. *Proc Natl Acad Sci U S A*. 2002;99(20):12877-12882.
9. Pearton DJ, Yang Y, Dhouailly D. Transdifferentiation of corneal epithelium into epidermis occurs by means of a multistep process triggered by dermal developmental signals. *Proc Natl Acad Sci U S A*. 2005;102(10):3714-3719.
10. Billingham RE, Silvers WK. Studies on the conservation of epidermal specificities of skin and certain mucosas in adult mammals. *J Exp Med*. 1967;125(3):429-446.
11. Doran TI, Vidrich A, Sun TT. Intrinsic and extrinsic regulation of the differentiation of skin, corneal and esophageal epithelial cells. *Cell*. 1980;22(1 Pt 1):17-25.
12. Mackenzie IC, Hill MW. Connective tissue influences on patterns of epithelial architecture and keratinization in skin and oral mucosa of the adult mouse. *Cell Tissue Res*. 1984;235(3):551-559.
13. Boukamp P, Breitkreutz D, Stark HJ, et al. Mesenchyme-mediated and endogenous regulation of growth and differentiation of human skin keratinocytes derived from different body sites. *Differentiation*. 1990;44(2):150-161.
14. Konstantinova NV, Lemak NA, Duong DM, et al. Artificial skin equivalent differentiation depends on fibroblast donor site: use of eyelid fibroblasts. *Plast Reconstr*

Surg. 1998;101(2):385-391.
15. Fujiwara H, Ferreira M, Donati G, et al. The basement membrane of hair follicle stem cells is a muscle cell niche. *Cell*. 2011;144(4):577-589.
16. Rinkevich Y, Walmsley GG, Hu MS, et al. Skin fibrosis. Identification and isolation of a dermal lineage with intrinsic fibrogenic potential. *Science*. 2015; 348(6232):aaa2151.
17. Higashiyama R, Nakao S, Shibusawa Y, et al. Differential contribution of dermal resident and bone marrow-derived cells to collagen production during wound healing and fibrogenesis in mice. *J Invest Dermatol*. 2011;131(2):529-536.
18. Zhang LJ, Guerrero-Juarez CF, Hata T, et al. Innate immunity. Dermal adipocytes protect against invasive *Staphylococcus aureus* skin infection. *Science*. 2015;347(6217):67-71.
19. Festa E, Fretz J, Berry R, et al. Adipocyte lineage cells contribute to the skin stem cell niche to drive hair cycling. *Cell*. 2011;146(5):761-771.
20. Virtanen KA, Lidell ME, Orava J, et al. Functional brown adipose tissue in healthy adults. *N Engl J Med*. 2009;360(15):1518-1525.
21. Harms M, Seale P. Brown and beige fat: development, function and therapeutic potential. *Nat Med*. 2013;19(10):1252-1263.
22. Nolis T. Exploring the pathophysiology behind the more common genetic and acquired lipodystrophies. *J Hum Genet*. 2014;59(1):16-23.
23. Holbrook KA, Underwood RA, Vogel AM, et al. The appearance, density and distribution of melanocytes in human embryonic and fetal skin revealed by the anti-melanoma monoclonal antibody, HMB-45. *Anat Embryol (Berl)*. 1989;180(5):443-455.
24. Mort RL, Jackson IJ, Patton EE. The melanocyte lineage in development and disease. *Development*. 2015;142(7):1387.
25. Lumpkin EA, Caterina MJ. Mechanisms of sensory transduction in the skin. *Nature*. 2007;445(7130):858-865.
26. Wang F, Julien DP, Sagasti A. Journey to the skin: somatosensory peripheral axon guidance and morphogenesis. *Cell Adh Migr*. 2013;7(4):388-394.
27. Maksimovic S, Nakatani M, Baba Y, et al. Epidermal Merkel cells are mechanosensory cells that tune mammalian touch receptors. *Nature*. 2014;509(7502):617-621.
28. Morrison KM, Miesegaes GR, Lumpkin EA, et al. Mammalian Merkel cells are descended from the epidermal lineage. *Dev Biol*. 2009;336(1):76-83.
29. Moll I, Moll R, Franke WW. Formation of epidermal and dermal Merkel cells during human fetal skin development. *J Invest Dermatol*. 1986;87(6):779-787.
30. Castillo D, Seidel K, Salcedo E, et al. Induction of ectopic taste buds by SHH reveals the competency and plasticity of adult lingual epithelium. *Development*. 2014;141(15):2993-3002.
31. Ito M, Yang Z, Andl T, et al. Wnt-dependent de novo hair follicle regeneration in adult mouse skin after wounding. *Nature*. 2007;447(7142):316-320.
32. Sick S, Reinker S, Timmer J, et al. WNT and DKK determine hair follicle spacing through a reaction-diffusion mechanism. *Science*. 2006;314(5804):1447-1450.
33. Cotsarelis G, Sun TT, Lavker RM. Label-retaining cells reside in the bulge area of pilosebaceous unit: implications for follicular stem cells, hair cycle, and skin carcinogenesis. *Cell*. 1990;61(7):1329-1337.
34. Barker N, Tan S, Clevers H. Lgr proteins in epithelial stem cell biology. *Development*. 2013;140(12): 2484-2494.
35. Biggs LC, Mikkola ML. Early inductive events in ectodermal appendage morphogenesis. *Semin Cell Dev Biol*. 2014;25-26:11-21.
36. Niemann C, Horsley V. Development and homeostasis of the sebaceous gland. *Semin Cell Dev Biol*. 2012;23(8):928-936.
37. Kamberov YG, Wang S, Tan J, et al. Modeling recent human evolution in mice by expression of a selected EDAR variant. *Cell*. 2013;152(4):691-702.
38. Babler WJ. Embryologic development of epidermal ridges and their configurations. *Birth Defects Orig Artic Ser*. 1991;27(2):95-112.
39. Bautch VL, Caron KM. Blood and lymphatic vessel formation. *Cold Spring Harb Perspect Biol*. 2015; 7(3):a008268.
40. Mukouyama YS, Shin D, Britsch S, et al. Sensory nerves determine the pattern of arterial differentiation and blood vessel branching in the skin. *Cell*. 2002;109(6):693-705.
41. Pasquale EB. Eph receptor signalling casts a wide net on cell behaviour. *Nat Rev Mol Cell Biol*. 2005;6(6):462-475.
42. Kidoya H, Naito H, Muramatsu F, et al. APJ regulates parallel alignment of arteries and veins in the skin. *Dev Cell*. 2015;33(3):247-259.
43. Golub R, Cumano A. Embryonic hematopoiesis. *Blood Cells Mol Dis*. 2013;51(4):226-231.
44. Fujita M, Furukawa F, Horiguchi Y, et al. Regional development of Langerhans cells and formation of Birbeck granules in human embryonic and fetal skin. *J Invest Dermatol*. 1991;97(1):65-72.
45. Gaide O, Emerson RO, Jiang X, et al. Common clonal origin of central and resident memory T cells following skin immunization. *Nat Med*. 2015;21(6):647-653.
46. Lee J, Tumbar T. Hairy tale of signaling in hair follicle development and cycling. *Semin Cell Dev Biol*. 2012;23(8):906-916.
47. Bolognia JL. *Dermatology*. New York, NY: Mosby; 2003.
48. Happle R. The categories of cutaneous mosaicism: A proposed classification. *Am J Med Genet A*. 2016 Feb;170A(2):452-459. doi: 10.1002/ajmg.a.37439. Epub 2015 Oct 22.

Chapter 5 :: Growth and Differentiation of the Epidermis
:: Terry Lechler

第五章
表皮生长和分化

中文导读

本章共分为5节：①概述；②表皮的生长；③表皮的分化；④表皮分化调控；⑤结论。全面阐述了干细胞在毛囊间上皮中的作用、基底细胞的增殖调控以及表皮屏障的形成。

第一节概述了表皮既有重要的屏障功能，同时又能快速更替。为完成这些不同的功能，表皮具有高度调节的增殖/分化程序。位于表皮基底层的祖细胞具有很强的增殖和自我更新能力，而分化细胞主要是产生屏障。

第二节介绍了表皮中存在干细胞，其中毛囊间上皮干细胞表达β1整合素、LRIG1和CD46等基因，能在完整的皮肤中形成团簇。其干细胞龛可能分布在整个基底层，或上皮嵴的顶部或底部。若出现表皮异常增殖，则会发生癌症和银屑病等疾病，提出了揭示调控表皮增殖的潜在机制对于治疗选择具有重要作用。

第三节介绍了表皮各层细胞的分化，基底细胞的最主要标记蛋白为角蛋白5和14，棘细胞以角蛋白1和10表达为特征，颗粒细胞的特点是含有透明角质颗粒，提供水合和紫外线防护功能，也能防止液体流失。颗粒细胞死亡后形成表皮末端分化产物角化包膜，主要为兜甲蛋白，协作形成皮肤屏障。

第四节介绍了表皮的分化包括转录因子、角蛋白和其他结构蛋白质的表达以及超微结构分析，其调控涉及了信号通路、转录控制、表观遗传因子和转录后调控。

第五节总结了表皮的增殖和分化是受到高度调控的，平衡失调则引起包括皮肤癌、银屑病和鱼鳞病等病理改变。对于增殖和分化的生理和病理调控的认识有望指导疾病更好的治疗，同时提及了基底层干细胞/祖细胞已经在临床上用来治疗烧伤和遗传性皮肤病。

〔粟 娟〕

AT-A-GLANCE

- Epidermal homeostasis and wound healing are driven by proliferation of stem/progenitor cells in the basal layer.
- Epidermal differentiation is a tightly regulated process that is controlled by the interplay between transcription factors, chromatin modifiers, and posttranscriptional regulators.
- Terminal differentiation results in 2 barriers, tight junctions and the cornified envelopes, which protect us from the external environment.

INTRODUCTION

The epidermis must maintain a largely impenetrable barrier to the outside world over the course of a lifetime. Simultaneously, it rapidly turns over, replacing itself every 2 weeks, and retains the ability to heal wounds. To accomplish these divergent roles, the epidermis has a highly regulated proliferation/differentiation program. Progenitor cells within the basal layer of the epidermis have a very high capacity for proliferation and self-renewal, whereas the major role for differentiated cells is generation of a barrier. In this chapter, we will discuss the current understanding of the roles of stem cells in interfollicular epidermis, how proliferation is controlled in basal cells, and how multiple pathways and structures collaborate to generate an epidermal barrier. Of note, some of these findings are drawn from studies in mouse skin, which is architecturally distinct from human epidermis. However, in many cases, there are studies of cultured human cells or human disease correlates that substantiate some of the findings in mice.

EPIDERMAL GROWTH

EPIDERMAL STEM CELLS

Stem cells are progenitor cells that can both renew themselves and give rise to differentiated progeny over an extended time period. The ability of the epidermis to continually regenerate itself and to heal wounds indicates that it must contain stem cells. Further, the pioneering work of Howard Green and colleagues allowed for the growth of these epidermal stem cells in culture, which was a great boon to understanding many aspects of epidermal stem cell biology. In addition, their work allowed for the clinical use of cultured epidermal stem cells in treating burn wounds, an early example of the utility of adult stem cells in regenerative therapy.[1] Here, we will describe some current aspects of the state of knowledge of stem cells within interfollicular epidermis. Of note, however, is that this has lagged behind our understanding of stem cells of the hair follicle (discussed in Chap. 7).

When cells are cultured from the human epidermis under standard conditions, they are heterogeneous in their self-renewing ability. Some undergo only a few rounds of division and may reflect transit-amplifying cells, a highly proliferative but short-lived cell population. The cells that self-renew robustly are putative stem cells. Consistent with this difference in activity, isolated basal cells express varying levels of a number of genes, including β1 integrin, LRIG1, and CD46.[2-4] Cells with high expression of these genes have higher self-renewing capacity in vitro and tend to form clusters in intact skin. This data are consistent with the presence of a distinct stem cell pool within the basal layer. Single-cell sequencing approaches have further demonstrated that there is likely to be heterogeneity even in this enriched pool of stem cells.[4] Although it is difficult to determine the functional roles and consequences of this heterogeneity in human skin in situ, these types of studies are possible in the mouse. However, there has been continued debate about the hierarchical makeup of progenitors within the mouse epidermis. Although some studies suggest that the basal layer is composed of a single unipotent population, others have provided evidence for at least 2 types of progenitor cells that differ in proliferation dynamics and marker expression.[5-9] It is expected that in the next few years, a much clearer picture of the regulation and functions of these distinct cell types will emerge.

EPIDERMAL STEM CELL NICHE

The tissue microenvironment in which stem cells normally exist is called their niche. Niches are continually being more thoroughly defined and include factors such as direct cell-cell and cell-matrix communication, soluble secreted factors (including inflammatory, nervous, and other tissue resident cells), and local tissue mechanical properties. The niche for stem cells in the human interfollicular epidermis is not clear. Various studies have suggested that they are located dispersed throughout the basal layer, or at either the tops or bottoms of rete ridges. Part of this may reflect regional differences in skin architecture as well as the early stages of our ability to mark and track these specific cell types. Regardless of their position, the progenitor cells in the basal layer largely produce differentiated progeny that form in columns directly above them.[10] Although progenitor cells can be lost or can expand laterally (to a limited degree) in a stochastic manner, they give rise to differentiated cells that move through the layers without significant lateral movement.[5,7,11]

EPIDERMAL PROLIFERATION

The epidermis requires continuous proliferation for both homeostatic turnover and wound healing. However, inappropriate proliferation occurs in many pathologic conditions, including cancer and psoriasis. Uncovering the underlying mechanisms regulating proliferation is therefore expected to reveal pathologic mechanisms and treatment options. It is thus important to understand the hierarchy/types of progenitor cells to determine whether there are specific kinds of cells that are amplified or hyperproliferative in response to different stimuli, whether cells are inhibited from differentiating and what molecular pathways are driving the overproliferation.

This is a complex area as many diverse external cues (chemical and mechanical) as well as genetic mutations can impact proliferation. These include endothelial signals, inflammatory signals, and extracellular matrix rigidity to name a few. Many of the major developmental signaling pathways including Wnt, Notch, Yap, and Hedgehog regulate epidermal proliferation in both physiologic and pathogenic states. Major downstream targets include the Ras-MAPK pathway and the PI3K/AKT/PTEN, which regulate growth and entry into and passage through the cell cycle.[12]

EPIDERMAL DIFFERENTIATION

BASAL CELLS

Basal progenitor cells are characterized by their mitotic activity, which is necessary for normal epidermal turnover and wound healing. These cells are most often marked by the expression of keratins 5 and 14 (Fig. 5-1). Keratins are members of the intermediate filament family of proteins and are obligate heterodimers that assemble to form polymers in the cell.[13] This large family of proteins shows tissue and cell type–specific expression (Table 5-1). In the epidermis, the keratin filaments stabilize both cell-cell adhesions called desmosomes and cell-substratum adhesions called hemidesmosomes. Both of these provide mechanical anchoring roles, and mutations in hemidesmosomal, desmosomal, and keratin genes result in various forms of epidermolysis bullosa (discussed in detail in Chap. 60; see Table 5-2). In addition to hemidesmosomes, basal keratinocytes are attached to the underlying substratum by focal adhesions, which bind to filamentous actin in the cell and play many roles, including promoting survival and proliferation of keratinocytes.[14] All keratinocytes, including basal keratinocytes, have cell-cell adhesions

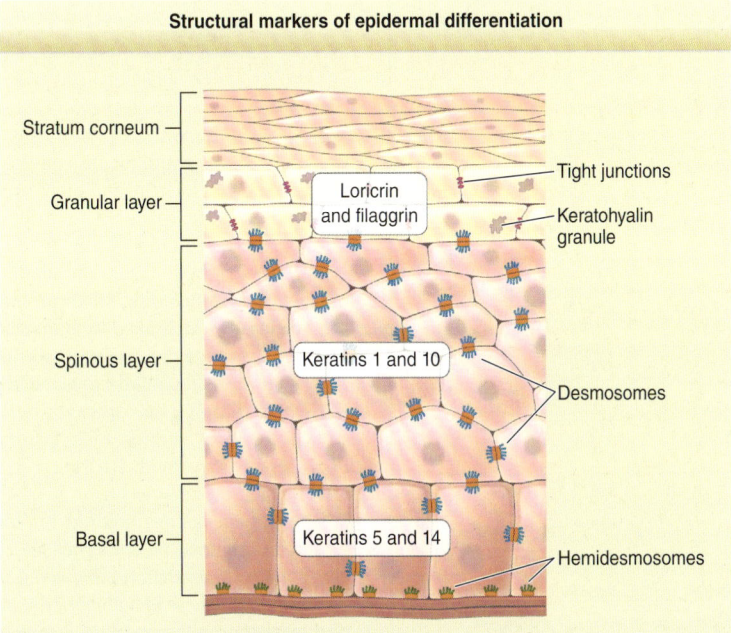

Figure 5-1 Structural markers of epidermal differentiation. Basal cells are defined by basement membrane attachment, the presence of hemidesmosomes, and the expression of keratins 5 and 14. Keratin 1 and 10, in contrast, mark all differentiated cell layers, whereas loricrin and filaggrin are expressed in upper spinous and granular cells. All cells contain desmosomes, though the makeup of desmosomes changes, with desmoglein 3 (Dsg3) and plakophilin 2 (Pkp2) being highly expressed in basal cells whereas Dsg1 and Pkp1 are highly expressed in differentiated epidermis. Tight junctions and keratohyalin granules mark the granular cells.

called adherens junctions, which are actin-based structures. Adherens junctions' components have diverse functions from regulating cellular architecture to growth control and inflammation.[15]

Basal keratinocytes give rise to spinous cells during epidermal homeostasis. The production of cells in the suprabasal cell layers is driven by mitotic spindle reorientation and asymmetric cell divisions during embryonic development.[16,17] However, in the adult mouse skin, delamination of basal cells from the underlying basement membrane and their subsequent migration upward appears to predominate.[7] The relative contributions of cell division orientation and delamination is not yet clear in the human epidermis. However, the pathways that control the commitment to differentiation are established in some detail. Here we will first describe characteristics of differentiated cell types followed by the intricate pathways that control differentiation.

SPINOUS CELLS

Basal to spinous differentiation is a highly regulated transition. Cells switch from a mitotic, keratin 5/14–expressing type to a postmitotic state characterized by the expression of keratins 1 and 10. There is an upregulation of desmosomes in these cells that gives them a spiny appearance in histologic sections. The composition of desmosomes also changes on differentiation. Although basal cells are high in the desmosomal cadherin, Dsg3, the levels of this protein decrease through differentiation whereas Dsg1 is upregulated.[18] Consistent with this, disruption of Dsg3-based junctions (as occurs in pemphigus vulgaris) results in disruption of cell-cell adhesion between basal cells and between the basal cells and the first layer of spinous cells. Perturbation of Dsg1 (which occurs in pemphigus foliaceus) results in blistering in more superficial layers of the epidermis.

GRANULAR CELLS

The identifying feature of these cells is keratohyalin granules. These granules are composed of keratins, profilaggrin and loricrin, and other proteins that make up the bulk of the cornified envelopes. Filaggrin and loricrin are also commonly used markers for these cell layers. Upon secretion, keratins and loricrin as well as other proteins, including small proline-rich proteins, become highly crosslinked by transglutaminase to the plasma membrane to generate cornified envelopes. Profilaggrin is eventually metabolized into amino acids and pyrrolidone carboxylic acid and urocanic acid (sometimes referred to as natural moisturizing factor [NMF]) to provide hydration and UV protective functions.

Many of the genes required for formation of the terminal differentiated epidermis are contained in the epidermal differentiation complex, a region on chromosome 1q21. These include loricrin, involucrin, small proline-rich proteins, and late cornified envelope proteins to name a few. The transcriptional regulation of this complex is under tight control and is one of the major targets of the differentiation cascade.

It is also in the granular cells that one barrier to loss of fluids occurs. Tight junctions are cell-cell adhesions that restrict the flow of fluids and ions and act as a bar-

TABLE 5-1
Keratin Family Members and Their Sites of Expression[a]

TYPE I KERATINS		TYPE II KERATINS	
NAME	MAIN SITE(S) OF EXPRESSION	NAME	MAIN SITE(S) OF EXPRESSION
K9	Epidermis (suprabasal)	K1	Epidermis (suprabasal)
K10	Epidermis (suprabasal)	K2	Epidermis (suprabasal)
K12	Cornea	K3	Cornea (suprabasal)
K13	Oral mucosa	K4	Oral mucosa (suprabasal)
K14	Complex epithelia	K5	Complex epithelia (basal layer)
K15	Complex epithelia	K6a	Epithelial appendages
K16	Epithelial appendages	K6b	Epithelial appendages
K17	Epithelial appendages	K6c	Skin (needs confirm)
K18	Simple epithelia	K7	Simple epithelia
K19	Broad distribution	K8	Simple epithelia
K20	Gut epithelium		
K23	Pancreas (needs confirm)		
K24	unknown		
K25-K28	Inner root sheath (hair follicles)	K71-K74	Inner root sheath (hair follicles)
		K75	Companion layer (hair follicles)
		K76	Oral mucosa
		K77	Sweat gland ducts
		K78	Tongue
		K79	Skin
		K80	Tongue
K31-K38	Hair shaft (hair follicles)	K81-K86	Hair shaft (hair follicles)
K39	Hair shaft (hair follicles)		
K40	Hair shaft (hair follicles)		

[a]This list was originally generated by Pierre Coulombe, John Stanley, and Tung-Tien Sun and published in the previous edition of this book.

TABLE 5-2
Keratin-Based, Inherited Skin Bullous Disease Affecting Primarily the Epidermis[a]

DISEASE	RELEVANT OMIM CATALOG NUMBER(S)[a]	TARGET GENES	AFFECTED CELL TYPE	COMMENTS
Epidermolysis bullosa simplex	131800 (Koebner subtype) 131800 (Weber-Cockayne) 131760 (Dowling-Meara)	K5 or K14	Basal keratinocyte	K, WC, and DM correspond to different degrees of severity; the position/nature of the mutation in K5 or K14 is a key determinant. Rare mutations in the same genes result in recessive inheritance (OMIM #60100)
Epidermolysis bullosa simplex with mottled pigmentation	131960	K5	Basal keratinocyte	A single dominant allele, K5P28L, has been found in multiple pedigrees. Typified by hyperpigmentation of healed skin blisters
Epidermolysis bullosa simplex with limb girdle muscular dystrophy	226670 (also,131950)	Plectin	Basal keratinocyte	Plectin is a cytolinker protein attaching IFs to adhesive complexes and F-actin/microtubules in keratinocytes and myocytes
Dowling-Degos disease	179850	K5 (null)	Basal keratinocyte	Inherited recessively; features multiple aberrations in skin pigmentation
Epidermolytic hyperkeratosis	113800	K1 or K10	Spinous keratinocyte	Same as bullous congenital ichthyosiform erythroderma. As for EBS, there is wide variation in severity of clinical presentation, correlating with the position and nature of the mutation affecting either K1 or K10
Ichthyosis hystrix (Curth-Macklin)	146490; 146600	K1 or K10	Spinous keratinocyte	Characteristic ridges or spikes present at the skin surface. Ultrastructurally, presence of large bundles of densely packed IFs around nucleus
Ichthyosis bullosa of Siemens palmoplantar keratodermas:	146800	K2e	Granular keratinocyte	Affects primarily flexural areas; blistering confined to the upper suprabasal layers; can be confused with mild EHK/BCIE Confined to the epidermis of palms and soles
▪ Epidermolytic	144200	K9	Spinous keratinocyte	Reflects the unique distribution of this large type I keratin
▪ Nonepidermolytic	139350 (diffuse) 600962 (focal)	K1 or K16	Spinous Keratinocyte	This is one of the rare conditions for which the Pathogenesis is not indicative of cell fragility; may reflect a nonmechanical role for keratins
▪ Striate	607654	DP, Dsg1, or K1	Spinous keratinocyte	Desmoplakin (DP) and desmoglein 1 (Dsg1) are structural components of desmosomes, to which keratin IFs are attached in epidermis

[a]Note: See the Intermediate Filament Database (www.interfil.org) and Online Mendelian Inheritance in Man (www.ncbi.nlm.nih.gov/omim/) websites for further information.

rier to membrane diffusion. These structures form specifically in the granular layer, thus allowing diffusion in the intercellular spaces of live cells within the lower layers of the epidermis. At the core of tight junctions are claudins and genetic disruption of claudin 1 results in lethal barrier defects in mice and neonatal ichthyosis in humans.[19,20] The mechanisms underlying the specific formation of tight junctions in granular cells are not currently known.

The last function of granular cells is to die. The resulting cornified envelopes are not living cells, and thus nuclear and cytoplasmic contents must be eliminated. This is thought to be a modified form of programmed cell death.

STRATUM CORNEUM

Cornified envelopes are the products of terminal differentiation in the epidermis. They are acellular and anuclear structures. The core consists of keratins surrounded by highly crosslinked networks of proteins, especially loricrin. Specialized lipids surround these, rich is ceramides that are also crosslinked. The crosslinking is largely contributed by transglutaminases. Transglutaminase expression begins in the spinous layer, but it is inactive there. Both increased calcium and cofactors are thought to specifically activate transglutaminase in the upper granular layer. The crosslinking of proteins and the presence of specialized lipids result in mechanical stability and relative impermeability of the epidermis. While the stratum corneum forms an outside-in barrier, the tight junctions form an inside-out barrier and thus collaborate to form an effective barrier to the external environment.

REGULATION OF EPIDERMAL DIFFERENTIATION

As discussed above, a number of criteria are used to describe differentiation in epidermis. These include, but are not limited to, proliferation rate, expression of transcription factors, keratins and other structural proteins, and ultrastructural analyses. The structural changes that accompany differentiation are highly regulated by a cascade of pathways, including signaling pathways, transcriptional control, epigenetic factors, and posttranscriptional regulation. Though complex, we present some of the major players below that highlight the roles of these various pathways in generating the differentiated structures that are necessary for epidermal barrier formation.

TRANSCRIPTIONAL REGULATORS

p63 controls epidermal specification, but it also plays an important role in maintaining basal cell fate/proliferation and induction of differentiation.[21] Direct targets of p63 include both structural proteins and other transcription factors that regulate differentiation. One of these transcription factors, ZNF750, is in turn required for expression of another transcription factor Klf4, which plays a major role in expression of granular genes.[22] Klf4 upregulates the expression of a number of lipid-modifying enzymes and structural proteins important for cornified envelope production.[23,24] p63 also acts by controlling the epigenetic status of the genome, discussed below.

Notch signaling is a commitment factor for transition of basal cells to spinous cells.[25-27] It is absent in basal cells and activated in spinous cells. Inhibiting Notch signaling prevents many aspects of spinous cell fate, whereas activating it in basal cells is sufficient for some aspects of spinous differentiation. Although some direct targets of Notch are known, such as Hes1, a direct pathway to spinous gene expression is unclear. In some contexts, Notch collaborates with transcription factors of the AP-2 gene family to function. For example, Notch induces the expression of a transcription factor, C/EBP, in spinous cells that binds along with AP-2 factors to the promoter of keratin 10, regulating its expression.[28,29]

Transcription factors of the Grainyhead-like (GRHL) are also key promoters of epidermal differentiation. Most prominently, GRHL3 is required for efficient barrier formation, in part through regulating the expression of transglutaminase-1.[30]

Some major regulators of epidermal differentiation are highlighted in Fig. 5-2, which shows their general expression profiles and sites of action.

EPIGENETIC REGULATORS

Epigenetic regulators control the organization and/or accessibility of chromatin for transcriptional regulation. In the epidermis, differentiation is driven by coincident expression of transcription factors and chromatin states.[31]

DNA METHYLATION

Methylated DNA is usually associated with a repressive transcriptional environment. In the epidermis, this is important for suppressing expression of differentiation genes in the basal layer. Loss of the methyltransferase DNMT1 results in loss of progenitor function and premature expression of differentiation-associated genes.[32]

HISTONE MODIFICATIONS

Chromosomal DNA is organized by histones that are subject to regulatory posttranslational modifications, including methylation and acetylation, that regulate transcription factor occupancy. A specific methylation (lysine 27 of Histone H3) of many epidermal differentiation genes, including those from the epidermal differentiation complex, represses their expression in basal cells, whereas loss of methylation promotes differentiation.[33] Methylation also inhibits other cells' fates, such as keratinocytes giving rise to mechanosensory Merkel cells.[34] Regulated histone acetylation is also essential for epidermal differentiation. In part this is due to binding of histone deacetylases to the same gene promoters that p63 represses, highlighting the central role of the p63 axis in epidermal homeostasis.[35]

CHROMATIN REMODELERS

This final category of epigenetic regulators is also important for proper differentiation. The SWI/SNF complex is active in differentiated cells of the epidermis, and mutations in these genes result in differentiation and barrier defects.[36] In contrast, when they are activated in basal cells, premature differentiation occurs.[37] In part, the activity of the SWI/SNF complex acts through expression of KLF4, one of the key terminal differentiation-inducing transcription factors. The physical localization of the EDC complex is also con-

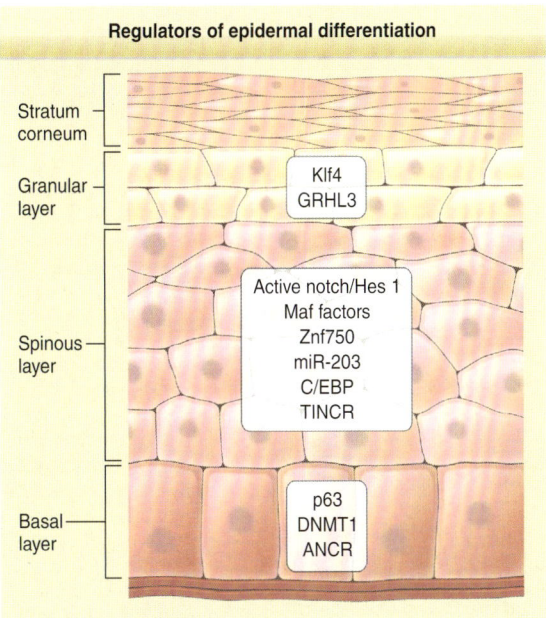

Figure 5-2 Regulators of epidermal differentiation. Transcription factors and epigenetic regulators of epidermal proliferation and differentiation are indicated. The position of the labels corresponds to the area of the epidermis where the factor is first expressed. Although direct interactions and regulations are known between some of these factors, this is both complex and incompletely understood. The text provides additional insight into cross-regulation and structural target genes.

trolled by chromatin remodeling factors such as Satb and Brg1, thus exposing another layer of regulation of expression of terminal differentiation genes.[38]

POSTTRANSCRIPTIONAL REGULATION

Once transcripts are generated, there is additional control over mRNA stability and translation. This level of regulation is also key to an ordered differentiation program in the epidermis.

miRNA: miRNAs are short noncoding RNAs that generally function to modulate the levels/translation of a number of target mRNAs. One important example in the epidermis is mIR-203, which is expressed in spinous cells where it represses p63 expression, among other targets, thus ensuring proper differentiation.[39]

lncRNA: A second class of regulatory RNAs is the long noncoding (lncRNAs). In the epidermis, the 2 best characterized are ANCR and TINCR, which work to promote basal cell fate and differentiated cell fate, respectively. ANCR acts, in part, by recruiting histone methyltransferase to certain promoters. TINCR, in contrast, is upregulated in differentiated cells, where it stabilized the differentiation promoting mRNAs such as Klf4 and Grhl3.[40]

Transcript Regulation: In addition to the above pathways, recent work has highlighted roles for regulated translation/degradation of mRNAs. For example, GRHL3 is expressed at low levels in basal cells because of its mRNA being unstable. Loss of the machinery that promotes GRHL3 degradation caused increased GRHL3 expression and premature differentiation.[41] Similarly, a separate subset of mRNAs of proliferation-promoting genes is positively regulated at the translational level to maintain high levels in basal cells.[42]

CONCLUSIONS

As the epidermis needs to provide an essential barrier to the outside world and to continuously renew itself, the decisions of proliferation and differentiation are highly regulated. Pathologies resulting from dysregulation of this balance, including skin cancers, psoriasis, and ichthyosis, to name a few, are many. Further understanding of the physiologic and pathologic control of proliferation and differentiation decisions is expected to lead to better treatments. In addition, the incredible regenerative capacity of stem/progenitor cells within the basal layer has already been clinically harnessed to treat burns and genetic skin conditions.

REFERENCES

1. De Luca M, Pellegrini G, Green H. Regeneration of squamous epithelia from stem cells of cultured grafts. *Regen Men.* 2006;1:45-57.
2. Jensen KB, Watt FM. Single-cell expression profiling of human epidermal stem and transit-amplifying cells: Lrig1 is a regulator of stem cell quiescence. *Proc Natl Acad Sci U S A.* 2006;103:11958-11963.
3. Jones PH, Watt FM. Separation of human epidermal stem cells from transit amplifying cells on the basis of differences in integrin function and expression. *Cell.* 1993;73:713-724.
4. Tan DW, Jensen KB, Trotter MW, et al. Single-cell gene expression profiling reveals functional heterogeneity of undifferentiated human epidermal cells. Development (Cambridge, England). 2013;140:1433-1444.
5. Clayton E, Doupé DP, Klein AM, et al. A single type of progenitor cell maintains normal epidermis. *Nature.* 2007;446:185-189.
6. Gomez C, Chua W, Miremadi A, et al. The interfollicular epidermis of adult mouse tail comprises two distinct cell lineages that are differentially regulated by Wnt, Edaradd, and Lrig1. *Stem Cell Reports.* 2013;1:19-27.
7. Rompolas P, Mesa KR, Kawaguchi K, et al. Spatiotemporal coordination of stem cell commitment during epidermal homeostasis. *Science.* 2016;352:1471-1474.
8. Sada A, Jacob F, Leung E, et al. Defining the cellular lineage hierarchy in the interfollicular epidermis of adult skin. *Nat Cell Biol.* 2016;18:619-631.
9. Sanchez-Danes A, Hannezo E, Larsimont JC, et al. Defining the clonal dynamics leading to mouse skin tumour initiation. *Nature.* 2016;536:298-303.
10. Ghazizadeh S, Taichman LB. Organization of stem cells and their progeny in human epidermis. *J Invest Dermatol.* 2005;124:367-372.
11. Mascre G, Dekoninck S, Drogat B, et al. Distinct contribution of stem and progenitor cells to epidermal maintenance. *Nature.* 2012;489:257-262.
12. Lopez-Pajares V, Yan K, Zarnegar BJ, et al. Genetic pathways in disorders of epidermal differentiation. *Trends Genet.* 2013;29:31-40.
13. Pan X, Hobbs RP, Coulombe PA. The expanding significance of keratin intermediate filaments in normal and diseased epithelia. *Curr Opin Cell Biol.* 2013;25:47-56.
14. Watt FM, Fujiwara H. Cell-extracellular matrix interactions in normal and diseased skin. *Cold Spring Harb Perspect Biol.* 2011;3(4). pii:a005124.
15. Sumigray KD, Lechler T. Cell adhesion in epidermal development and barrier formation. *Curr Top Dev Biol.* 2015;112:383-414.
16. Lechler T, Fuchs E. Asymmetric cell divisions promote stratification and differentiation of mammalian skin. *Nature.* 2005;437:275-280.
17. Williams SE, Beronja S, Pasolli HA, et al. Asymmetric cell divisions promote Notch-dependent epidermal differentiation. *Nature.* 2011;470:353-358.
18. Simpson CL, Patel DM, Green KJ. Deconstructing the skin: cytoarchitectural determinants of epidermal morphogenesis. *Nat Rev Mol Cell Biol.* 2011;12:565-580.
19. Furuse M, Hata M, Furuse K, et al. Claudin-based tight junctions are crucial for the mammalian epidermal barrier: a lesson from claudin-1-deficient mice. *J Cell Biol.* 2002;156:1099-1111.
20. Hadj-Rabia S, Baala L, Vabres P, et al. Claudin-1 gene mutations in neonatal sclerosing cholangitis associated with ichthyosis: a tight junction disease. *Gastroenterology.* 2004;127:1386-139.
21. Koster MI. p63 in skin development and ectodermal dysplasias. *J Invest Dermatol.* 2010;130:2352-2358.
22. Sen GL, Boxer LD, Webster DE, et al. ZNF750 is a p63 target gene that induces KLF4 to drive terminal epidermal differentiation. *Dev Cell.* 2012;22:669-677.
23. Patel S, Xi ZF, Seo EY, et al. Klf4 and corticosteroids activate an overlapping set of transcriptional targets to accelerate in utero epidermal barrier acquisition. *Proc Natl Acad Sci U S A.* 2006;103:18668-18673.
24. Segre JA, Bauer C, Fuchs E. Klf4 is a transcription factor required for establishing the barrier function of the skin. *Nat Genet.* 1999;22:356-360.
25. Blanpain C, Lowry WE, Pasolli HA, et al. Canonical notch signaling functions as a commitment switch in the epidermal lineage. *Genes Dev.* 2006;20:3022-3035.
26. Moriyama M, Durham AD, Moriyama H, et al. Multiple roles of Notch signaling in the regulation of epidermal development. *Dev Cell.* 2008;14:594-604.
27. Rangarajan A, Talora C, Okuyama R, et al. Notch signaling is a direct determinant of keratinocyte growth arrest and entry into differentiation. *EMBO J.* 2001;20:3427-3436.
28. Lopez RG, Garcia-Silva S, Moore SJ, et al. C/EBPalpha and beta couple interfollicular keratinocyte proliferation arrest to commitment and terminal differentiation. *Nat Cell Biol.* 2009;11:1181-1190.
29. Wang X, Pasolli HA, Williams T, et al. AP-2 factors act in concert with Notch to orchestrate terminal differentiation in skin epidermis. *J Cell Biol.* 2008;183:37-48.
30. Ting SB, Caddy J, Hislop N, et al. A homolog of Drosophila grainy head is essential for epidermal integrity in mice. *Science.* 2005;308:411-413.
31. Perdigoto CN, Valdes VJ, Bardot ES, et al. Epigenetic regulation of epidermal differentiation. *Cold Spring Harb Perspect Med.* 2014;4(2). pii:a015263.
32. Sen GL, Reuter JA, Webster DE, et al. DNMT1 maintains progenitor function in self-renewing somatic tissue. *Nature.* 2010;463:563-567.
33. Ezhkova E, Pasolli HA, Parker JS, et al. Ezh2 orchestrates gene expression for the stepwise differentiation of tissue-specific stem cells. *Cell.* 2009;136:1122-1135.
34. Bardot ES, Valdes VJ, Zhang J, et al. Polycomb subunits Ezh1 and Ezh2 regulate the Merkel cell differentiation program in skin stem cells. *EMBO J.* 2013;32:1990-2000.
35. LeBoeuf M, Terrell A, Trivedi S, et al. Hdac1 and Hdac2 act redundantly to control p63 and p53 functions in epidermal progenitor cells. *Dev Cell.* 2010;19:807-818.
36. Indra AK, Dupé V, Bornert JM, et al. Temporally controlled targeted somatic mutagenesis in embryonic surface ectoderm and fetal epidermal keratinocytes unveils two distinct developmental functions of BRG1 in limb morphogenesis and skin barrier formation. Development (Cambridge, England). 2005; 132:4533-4544.
37. Bao X, Tang J, Lopez-Pajares V, et al. ACTL6a enforces the epidermal progenitor state by suppressing SWI/SNF-dependent induction of KLF4. *Cell Stem Cell.* 2013;12:193-203.
38. Mardaryev AN, Gdula MR, Yarker JL, et al. p63 and Brg1 control developmentally regulated higher-order chromatin remodelling at the epidermal differentiation complex locus in epidermal progenitor cells. Development (Cambridge, England). 2014;141:101-111.

39. Yi R, Poy MN, Stoffel M, et al. A skin microRNA promotes differentiation by repressing "stemness." *Nature*. 2008;452:225-229.
40. Lopez-Pajares V, Qu K, Zhang J, et al. A LncRNA-MAF:MAFB transcription factor network regulates epidermal differentiation. *Dev Cell*. 2015;32:693-706.
41. Mistry DS, Chen Y, Sen GL. Progenitor function in self-renewing human epidermis is maintained by the exosome. *Cell Stem Cell*. 2012;11:127-135.
42. Wang Y, Arribas-Layton M, Chen Y, et al. DDX6 orchestrates mammalian progenitor function through the mRNA degradation and translation pathways. *Mol Cell*. 2015;60:118-130.

Chapter 6 :: Skin Glands: Sebaceous, Eccrine, and Apocrine Glands
:: Christos C. Zouboulis

第六章
皮肤腺体：皮脂腺、小汗腺和顶泌汗腺

中文导读

本章共分为3节：①概述；②皮脂腺；③汗腺。全面介绍了皮脂腺、小汗腺和顶泌汗腺的解剖、胚胎发生、生理功能及其调节因素等。

第一节总体概述了皮肤腺体由分泌室、腺体或螺旋和排泄部分组成，腺细胞起源于上皮细胞。腺体分泌有分泌细胞破裂的全分泌以及分泌细胞排泄两种方式，产物排入毛囊管或直接排出到皮肤表面。

第二节皮脂腺，介绍了其解剖特点、分布、胚胎发生，介绍了皮脂的分泌、成分及功能，以及皮脂产生的调节因素。重点提到了即使在同一个体或同一解剖区域，皮脂腺的大小差异也很大；皮脂腺的生理功能是通过全分泌形式分泌脂质，脂质为非极性(中性)脂类的混合物，具有抗菌和保持皮肤柔软光滑作用，同时参与了先天免疫过程；皮脂腺受多种因素调节，主要为雄激素和维甲酸。

第三节汗腺，详细介绍了小汗腺和顶泌汗腺。关于小汗腺介绍了其发育，解剖与功能，出汗的神经调控，出汗率的药物控制，汗液的成分及汗液分泌的机制，以及汗腺导管具有重吸收机制等，重点讲述了小汗腺出汗的神经调控机制主要为下丘脑中央机制产生热汗，而汗液分泌机制主要为ACh诱导的胞内$Ca2^+$介导途径。因大量汗液的产生，汗腺导管进化到具有重吸收NaCl功能，可最大限度地减少电解质损失。关于顶泌汗腺，介绍了其分泌的最新方式为分泌型，由肾上腺素能激动剂控制，可能具有性引诱剂、区域标记和警告信号的作用，但目前功能已退化。

〔栗 娟〕

INTRODUCTION

The human skin has several types of exocrine glands (Latin, *glandulae cutis*), which release their biochemical products onto the skin surface. All skin glands consist by a secretory compartment, the gland or coil (tubulus), and an excretory part, the duct (ductus). Skin gland cells are of epithelial origin, but their secretory compartments are located at different depths in the dermis.

Three major types of skin glands are recognized according to their product, the excretory function, and the location, where the excretory ducts release their products (diseases of these glands are listed in

Table 6-1). Regarding their product, skin glands are classified into glands secreting sebum (sebaceous glands) and sweat (sweat glands). Concerning their secretory function, skin glands are classified into holocrine glands, whose fully differentiated secretory cells burst and release both the cytoplasmic content and the cell membranes into their ducts, and merocrine glands, which excrete their product via exocytosis from secretory cells. Regarding the location where their ducts release their product, the ducts of sebaceous glands, in most cases, and apocrine sweat glands excrete their products into the hair follicle canal, and the eccrine sweat glands excrete directly onto the skin surface. Sebaceous glands are holocrine glands, and sweat glands (both eccrine and apocrine ones) are merocrine glands.

SEBACEOUS GLANDS

AT-A-GLANCE

- Sebaceous glands are multilobular structures that consist of acini connected to a common excretory duct and are usually associated with a hair follicle.
- Sebaceous glands vary considerably in size, even in the same individual and in the same anatomic area.
- The sebaceous glands excrete lipids by disintegration of entire cells, a process known as holocrine secretion.
- Human sebum, as it leaves the sebaceous gland, contains squalene, cholesterol, cholesterol esters, wax esters, and triglycerides.
- Sebaceous glands are regulated by several molecules, among them androgens and retinoids.

TABLE 6-1
Diseases of the Major Skin Glands

Diseases of the Sebaceous Glands
Increased activity/volume
Acne vulgaris
Rosacea
(Hyper)seborrhea
Periorificial dermatitis
Hair follicle naevus
Congenital sebaceous gland hyperplasia
Senile sebaceous gland hyperplasia
Sebaceoma (sebaceous gland epithelioma)
Sebaceous carcinoma
Muir-Torre Syndrome
Decreased activity/volume
Senile xerosis cutis
Psoriasis
Lichen planopilaris
Pseudopelade Brocq
Hidradenitis suppurativa
Linear morphea
Chlor- /dioxin-induced acne
Chemotherapy-induced diffuse alopecia
Zouboulis syndrome

Diseases of the Eccrine Glands
Increased activity
Hyperhidrosis (primary and secondary)
Eccrine carcinoma
Decreased activity
Hypohidrosis/Anhidrosis
Abnormal activity/Obstruction of the eccrine duct
Neutrophilic eccrine hidradenitis
Coma bullae
Erythema multiforme
Cystic fibrosis
Miliaria (crystallina, rubra, and profunda)
Syringosquamous metaplasia

Diseases of the Apocrine Glands
Abnormal activity
Bromhidrosis
Chromhidrosis
Fox-Fordyce disease (apocrine miliaria)
Hidradenitis suppurativa (initially considered as a disease of the apocrine glands; currently as a disease of the terminal hair follicles)

ANATOMY OF THE SEBACEOUS GLANDS

HISTOLOGY

Human sebaceous glands are multilobular structures of epithelial origin that consist of acini connected to a common excretory duct, the sebaceous duct (ductus seboglandularis) (Fig. 6-1). Sebaceous glands are composed of sebocytes, which are lipid-producing uniquely differentiated epithelial cells.[1,2] On the other hand, the sebaceous duct is lined by undifferentiated keratinocytes and is usually associated with a hair follicle which is composed of stratified squamous epithelium. The periphery of the sebaceous gland is a basal cell layer composed of small, cuboidal, nucleated, highly mitotic sebocytes.[1,3] Cells progress toward the middle of the gland and accumulate lipid droplets (LDs) as they transform into terminally differentiated cells, full of lipids.[3] The latter lack all other cellular organelles, burst, and die, excreting their entire contents to the duct in a holocrine manner (Fig. 6-2). Surrounding the glands are connective tissue capsules composed of collagen fibers that provide physical support.[4]

LOCATION

Sebaceous glands are associated with hair follicles all over the body. A sebaceous gland associated with a hair follicle is termed a *pilosebaceous unit* (see Fig. 6-1). The glands may also be found in certain nonhairy sites, including the eyelids (Meibomian glands, tarsal glands), the nipples (Montgomery glands, areolar glands), around the genitals (Tyson glands), and the

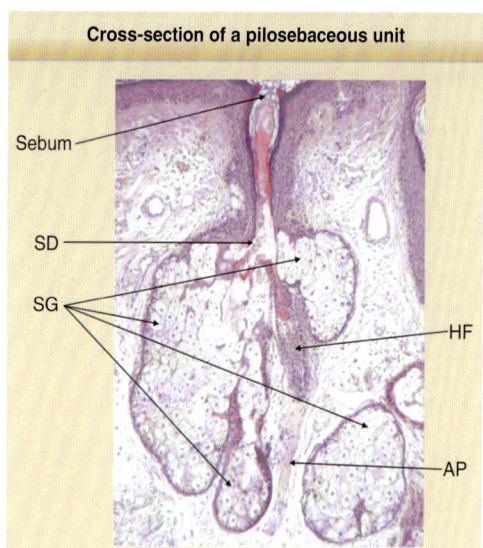

Figure 6-1 Cross-section of a pilosebaceous unit: a multiacinar sebaceous gkland associated with a hair follicle (HF). AP, arrector pili muscle (×20); SD, sebaceous duct, Sebum, sebum and keratin. (Modified with permission from: Zouboulis CC, Tsatsou F. Anatomy of the sebaceous gland. In: Zouboulis CC, Katsambas AD, Kligman AM, eds. *Pathogenesis and Treatment of Acne and Rosacea.* Berlin: Springer; 2014:27-31. Copyright © 2014.)

mucosa (lips, gums and inner cheeks, and genitals; Fordyce spots).[1] Fordyce spots open and release their content directly to the epithelial surface. The latter are visible to the unaided eye because of their large size (up to 2 to 3 mm) and the transparency of the oral epithelium (Fig. 6-3). Only the palms and soles, which have no hair follicles, are totally devoid of sebaceous glands. In addition, the dorsal surfaces of the hand and foot have sparse sebaceous glands.[5] Sebaceous glands vary considerably in size, even within the same individual and within the same anatomic area. On the external body surface, most glands are only a fraction of a millimeter in size. The largest glands and greatest density of glands are located on the nose (1600 glands/cm^2) followed by the face and scalp (up to 400 to 900 glands/cm^2).[4] The hairs associated with these large glands are often tiny, and the total structure is more specifically termed *sebaceous follicles*, being a pilosebaceous unit variant, the other two being the terminal hair follicle and the vellus hair follicle.

EMBRYOGENESIS AND MORPHOGENESIS

The development of the sebaceous glands is closely related to the differentiation of hair follicles and

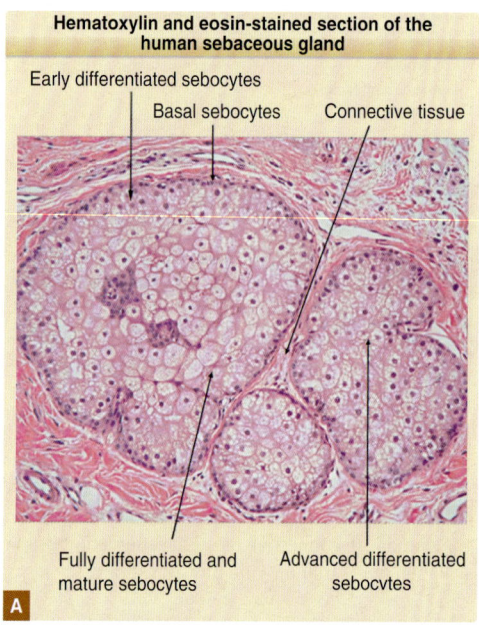
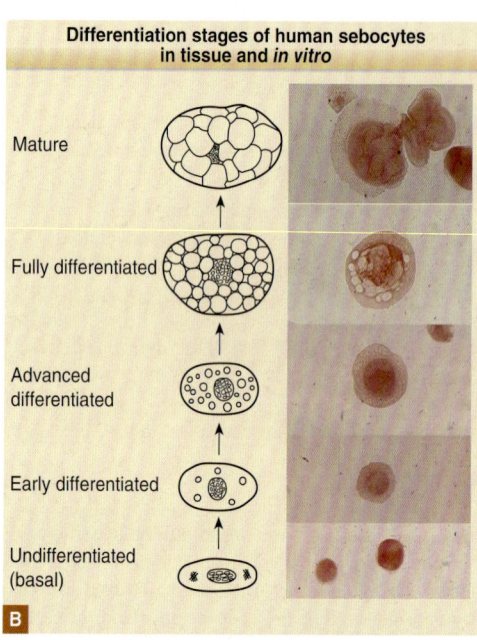

Figure 6-2 **A,** Hematoxylin and eosin–stained section of the human sebaceous gland showing the different stages of sebocyte differentiation. Cells progress toward the middle of the gland, lose their nuclei, and organelles, and accumulate lipid droplets. **B,** Differentiation stages of human sebocytes in tissue *(left)*[19] and in vitro *(right)*[3] according to Tosti[17] and McEwan Jenkinson and coworkers.[18] Undifferentiated sebocytes are small cells with a high nucleocytoplasmic ratio. Early differentiated sebocytes are larger cells with a decreased nucleocyloplasmic ratio compared with the undifferentiated sebocytes and a few lipid droplets arranged in the perinuclear area. Advanced differentiated sebocytes are cells with further increases in size and decreases of the nucleocytoplasmic ratio. Multiple cytoplasmic lipid droplets are distributed inside the cytoplasm. Fully differentiated sebocytes are cells with abundant, partially large, cytoplasmic lipid droplets. Mature sebocytes are disorganized large cell with denatured nuclei; the lack of cytoplasmic lipids is caused by lysis of the cell blood cell membrane.

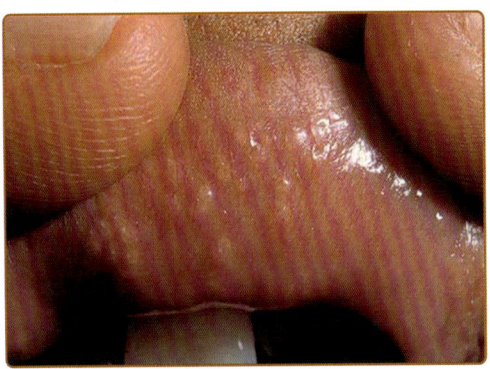

Figure 6-3 Fordyce spots at the upper lip mucosa.

epidermis.[6-8] At the 10th to 12th weeks of fetal life, a stratum intermedium becomes apparent, and at about the same time, developing hair germs are quite distinct. In the following weeks, the follicles extend downward into the dermis, and the rudiments of the sebaceous glands appear on the posterior surfaces of the hair pegs. By 13 to 16 weeks, the glands are clearly distinguishable, arising in a cephalocaudal sequence from bulges (epithelial placodes) of the hair follicles. The latter contain the epidermal stem cells that generate multiple cell lineages, including epidermal and follicular keratinocytes, as well as sebaceous glands. As daughter cells migrate from the bulge region, changes in the expression patterns of numerous transcription factors determine their final cell lineage. Despite continuous differentiation of its cells, the sebaceous gland can be regenerated by the reservoir of stem cells in the hair follicle bulge. However, retroviral lineage marking has provided strong evidence that the sebaceous gland might arise and be maintained independently of the hair follicle bulge.[9]

Wnt or wingless (Wnt) and Sonic hedgehog (Shh) signaling pathways are intricately involved in embryonic patterning and cell fate decisions. Cells destined to become sebocytes have increased Shh and Myc signaling and decreased Wnt signaling (Fig. 6-4A).[10,11] In human SZ95 sebocyte and transgenic mouse models, whereas intact Wnt signaling promotes hair follicle differentiation, inhibition of Wnt signaling by preventing the Lef1–β-catenin interaction leads to sebocyte differentiation.[11,12] Loss of function and gain of function in both models demonstrated that blocking Shh signaling inhibited normal sebocyte differentiation, and constitutively activating Shh signaling increased the number and size of human sebocytes and mouse sebaceous glands in skin.

Several important molecular aspects of sebaceous gland development have been identified, mostly with the aid of genetically modified cell lines. The earliest known signal necessary for sebaceous gland development is SOX9, which is in fact essential for the specification of early hair follicle stem cells and therefore for the morphogenesis of both structures (Fig. 6-5).[9] Further studies indicate that later in embryonic development, a subpopulation of these stem cells expressing PRDM1 (formerly known as BLIMP1) is established near the entrance of the sebaceous gland. PRDM1

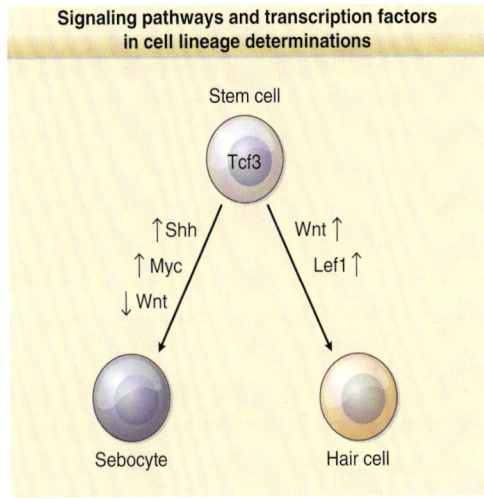

Figure 6-4 Simplified signaling pathways and transcription factors that are involved in cell lineage determinations.[9-11] As daughter cells migrate from the bulge region, changes in the expression patterns of numerous transcription factors determine their final cell lineage. Additional pathways and transcription factors play a significant role in determining each cell lineage. Lef1, lymphoid enhancer binding factor 1; Myc, myelocytomatosis oncogene; Shh, Sonic hedgehog; Tcf3, transcription factor 3; Wnt, wingless (wg)/int.

(BLIMP-1) acts as a marker of terminal epithelial cell differentiation.[13,14] Loss of PRDM1 (BLIMP-1) results in increased gene expression of c-myc, an essential player in sebaceous gland homeostasis.[15] Overexpression of c-myc in transgenic mice results in enlarged and more numerous sebaceous gland at the expense of the hair follicle lineage. Moreover, skin-specific deletion of c-myc negatively affects sebaceous gland development. In skin, c-myc and β-catenin exert opposing effects on sebocyte differentiation (see Fig. 6-4). Antagonizing Wnt–β-catenin signaling constitutes an important prerequisite for normal sebaceous differentiation in postnatal skin tissue. Stem cells expressing LRIG1, which has been suggested to be multipotent stem cells giving rise to epidermal lineages, can act under homeostatic conditions as sebocyte progenitor cells.[16]

Sebaceous gland cells at first contain glycogen. This lingers at the periphery of the gland but is quickly lost at the center, where lipid drops are visible at 17 weeks.[13,14] The future common excretory duct, around which the acini of the sebaceous gland attach, begins as a solid cord. The cells composing the cord are filled with sebum, and eventually they lose their integrity, rupture, and form a channel that establishes the first pilosebaceous canal, the duct, through which sebum flows into the follicular canal and subsequently to the skin surface. New acini result from buds on the peripheral sebaceous duct wall. The cell organization of the neonatal sebaceous acini consists of undifferentiated (basal), differentiating (early, advanced and fully differentiated), and mature sebaceous gland cells (see Fig. 6-2).[3,17-19] Undifferentiated

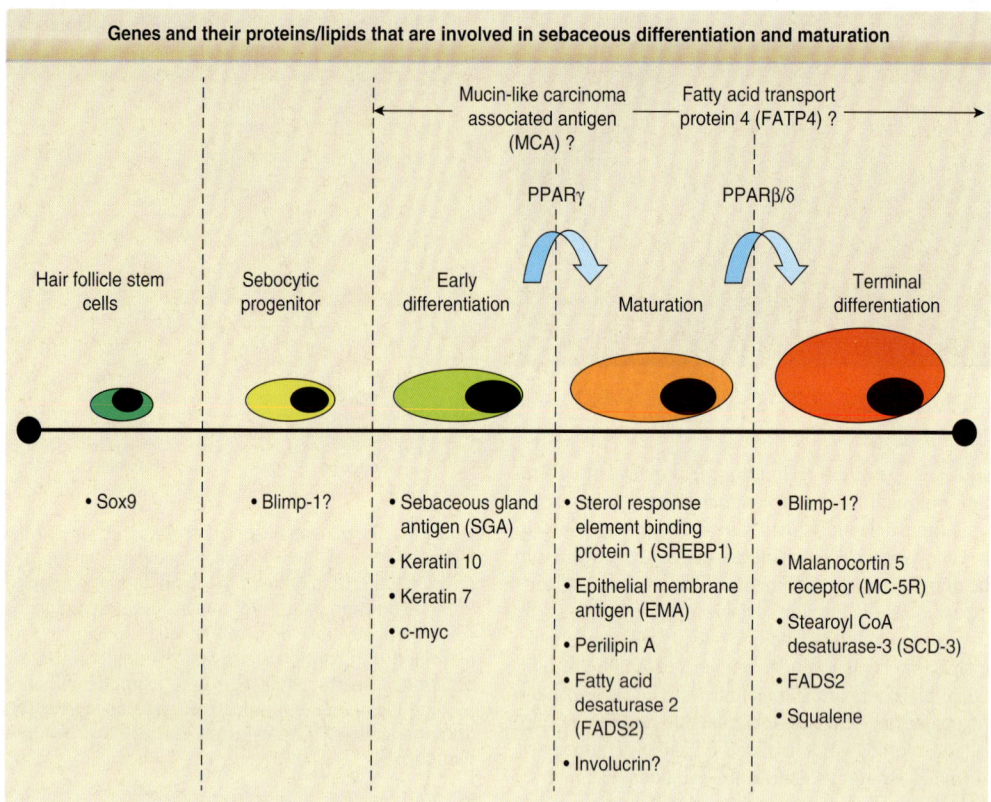

Figure 6-5 Genes and their proteins/lipids reported to be involved in sebaceous differentiation and maturation.[9] PPAR, peroxisome-proliferator-activated receptor.

cells arranged in a single layer facing the basal lamina, comparable to the epidermal basal layer; they represent the germinative cells of the gland, flattened or cuboidal in shape, showing round and densely basophilic nuclei.[20] These bear characteristics of stem cells because they give rise to a continual flux of proliferating and differentiating cells. The basal cells of the peripheral zone form about 40% of the gland. Growing toward the center of the gland lobules, the basal cells gradually differentiate into an early differentiated cell type, an advanced differentiated cell type, a fully differentiated cell type, and the mature sebocyte.[3,21] The maturation zone also represents about 40% of the sebaceous gland.

PHYSIOLOGY OF THE SEBACEOUS GLAND

HOLOCRINE SECRETION

The sebaceous glands exude lipids by disintegration of entire cells, a process known as *holocrine secretion*. Holocrine secretion by sebaceous gland cells does not occur mechanically via increased cell volume, as considered previously, but rather from a multistep, cell-specific lysosomal DNase2-mediated mode of programmed cell death, which differs from apoptosis, necroptosis, and cornification.[22]

As sebaceous gland cells are displaced into the center of the gland, they begin to produce lipids, which accumulate in droplets. With approaching the sebaceous duct, they disintegrate and release their content. Only neutral lipids reach the skin surface. Proteins, nucleic acids, and the membrane phospholipids are digested and are apparently recycled during the disintegration of the cells.[2] Sebaceous gland secretion can be enhanced with increased rates of induced terminal sebocyte differentiation.

LIPID COMPOSITION OF SEBUM

Sebum production is a continuous event. The exact mechanisms underlying its regulation are not fully defined. *Complexity* and *uniqueness* are the two terms that best characterize sebaceous lipids. Δ6 desaturation, wax ester synthesis, and squalene accumulation are examples that manifest sebaceous lipid biology.[22-24] Genetic knockout animal models of lipid synthesis demonstrate dramatic changes in skin physiology and pathology, resulting from impairment of sebaceous lipid pathways.[25] Human sebum, as it leaves the sebaceous gland, contains a mixture of nonpolar (neutral) lipids, mainly triglycerides, wax esters, squalene, and smaller amounts of cholesterol and cholesterol esters (Fig. 6-6). During passage of sebum through the hair canal, bacterial enzymes hydrolyze some of the triglycerides, so that the lipid mixture reaching the skin surface contains free fatty acids and small proportions of mono- and diglycerides, in addition to the original components. Triglycerides, diglycerides, and free fatty acids form 40% to 60% of total skin surface lipids followed by wax esters (25% to 30%), squalene (12% to 15%), cholesterol esters (3% to 6%), and cholesterol (1.5% to 2.5%).[26,27] The wax esters and squalene distinguish sebum from the lipids of human internal organs, which contain no wax esters and little squalene. However, human sebaceous glands appear to be unable to transform squalene to sterols, such as cholesterol. The patterns of unsaturation of the fatty acids in the triglycerides, wax esters, and cholesterol esters also distinguish human sebum from the lipids of other organs. The "normal" mammalian pathway of desaturation involves inserting a double bond between the 9th and 10th carbons of stearic acid (18:0) to form oleic acid (18:1Δ9). However, in human sebaceous glands, the predominant pattern is the insertion of a Δ6 double bond into palmitic acid (16:0). The resulting sapienic acid (16:1Δ6) (see Fig. 6-6) is the major fatty acid of adult human sebum. Elongation of the chain by two carbons and insertion of another double bond gives sebaleic acid (18:2Δ5,8), a fatty acid thought to be unique to human sebum.[22-24]

Sebaceous fatty acids and alcohols are also distinguished by chain branching. Methyl branches can occur on the penultimate carbon of a fatty acid chain (iso branching), on the third from the last (antepenultimate) carbon (anteiso branching), or on any even-numbered carbon (internal branching). Examples of these unusual unsaturated and branched-chain moieties are included in the lipid structures in Fig. 6-6.

FUNCTION OF SEBUM

Sebum in humans was initially considered to solely cause acne.[28,29] Subsequently, it has been suggested that sebum reduces water loss from the skin's surface and functions to keep skin soft and smooth, although evidence for these claims in humans is minimal; however, as demonstrated in the sebaceous gland–deficient (Asebia) mouse model, glycerol derived from triglyceride hydrolysis in sebum is critical for maintaining stratum corneum hydration.[30] Sebum has later been shown to have mild antibacterial action, protecting the skin from infection by bacteria and fungi because it contains antiinflammatory lipids and immunoglobulin A, which is secreted from most exocrine glands.[31-33] Vitamin E delivery to the upper layers of the skin protects the skin and its surface lipids from oxidation. Thus, sebum flow to the surface of the skin may provide the transit mechanism necessary for vitamin E to function.[34] The current concept is that sebum is involved in the multimodal activities of the sebaceous glands (Table 6-2).

INNATE IMMUNITY

Antimicrobial peptides, including cathelicidin, psoriasin, β-defensin 1, and β-defensin 2, are expressed within the sebaceous gland. Functional cathelicidin peptides have direct antimicrobial activity against *Propionibacterium acnes* but also initiate cytokine production and inflammation in the host organism.[35,36] In addition, free fatty acids in human sebum are bactericidal against gram-positive organisms as a result of its ability to increase β-defensin 2 expression.[31,36] Innate immune Toll-like receptors 2 and 4 (TLR2, TLR4) as well as CD1d and CD14 molecules are also expressed in sebaceous glands and immortalized human sebocytes.[37] With the expression of innate immune receptors and antibacterial peptides, the sebaceous gland may play an important role in pathogen recognition and protection of the skin surface.[38-41]

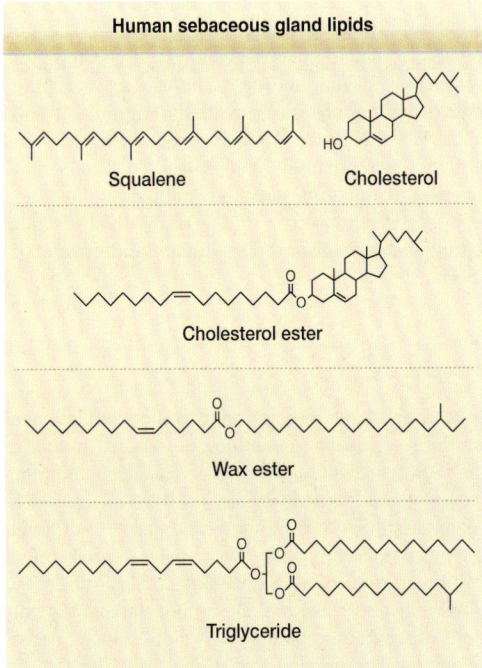

Figure 6-6 Human sebaceous gland lipids. The structures of the cholesterol ester, wax ester, and triglyceride are representative of the many species that are present. Two sebaceous-type unsaturated fatty acid moieties are shown: sapienic acid (16:1Δ6) (in the wax ester structure) and sebaleic acid (18:2Δ5,8) (in the triglyceride structure). Anteiso branching is shown in the alcohol moiety of the wax ester, and iso branching is shown in the triglyceride.

FACTORS REGULATING SEBACEOUS GLAND SIZE AND SEBUM PRODUCTION

Sebocytes preserve characteristics of stem-like cells despite their programming for terminal differentiation because they present a remarkable potential of

TABLE 6-2
Sebaceous Gland Functions
Embryology, Development, and Differentiation
■ Expression of terminal differentiation-triggering transcription factors, including CCAAT and enhancer binding proteins and peroxisome-proliferator-activated receptors
■ Partial responsibility for the three-dimensional organization of skin surface lipids and the integrity of the skin barrier
■ Influence on follicular differentiation
■ Highly complex acetylcholine receptor expression pattern
■ Preservation of characteristics of stem-like cells despite their terminal cell differentiation program
Synthetic Activity
■ Production of vernix caseosa
■ Production of sebum
■ Histamine-1 receptor expression and inhibition of squalene synthesis by antihistamines
Protection
■ Natural photoprotective activity against ultraviolet B irradiation
■ Thermoregulatory and repelling properties
■ Possible involvement in wound healing
Transportation
■ Delivery of antioxidants from and to the skin surface
■ Sebum as vehicle of fragrance
Inflammation and Immunity
■ Direct pro- and antiinflammatory properties
■ Production of proinflammatory and of antiinflammatory lipids
■ Toll-like receptor 2–induced upregulation of lipogenesis
■ Lipid-induced innate antimicrobial activity
■ Presence of antimicrobial protective immunoglobulin A and cytokine and chemokine mRNA in normal sebaceous glands
■ Synthesis of antibacterial peptides and proinflammatory cytokines and chemokines in the presence of bacteria with some of the peptides being bacteriotoxic
■ Expression of ectopeptidases
■ Contribution to skin inflammation by promoting the differentiation of Th17 lymphocytes
■ Response to lipid-mediated redox stress
■ Influence of macrophage polarization and activation via sebaceous lipids
Endocrine Properties
■ Regulation of the independent endocrine function of the skin
■ Expression of all steroidogenic enzymes
■ Regulation of local androgen synthesis
■ Substantial involvement in the hormonally induced skin aging process
■ Modification of lipid synthesis by combined androgens and peroxisome-proliferator-activated receptor ligands, estrogens and the insulin-like growth factor 1–insulin-like growth factor 1 complex
■ Expression of vitamin D receptor and vitamin D–metabolizing enzymes
■ Expression of retinoid-metabolizing cytochrome P450 enzymes
■ Selective control of the action of hormones and xenobiotics on the skin
■ Exhibition and affection by a regulatory neuropeptide program

bipotential differentiation.[42,43] The sebaceous gland might be maintained by unipotent stem cells that are replenished by multipotent stem cells in the hair follicle bulge.[13] However, it is an emerging view that there might be at least three distinct niches for skin stem cells: the follicle bulge, the base of the sebaceous gland, and the basal layer of the epidermis.[44]

The average transit time of sebaceous gland cells from formation to discharge, has been calculated as 7.4 days in the human gland, with 4 to 7 days in undifferentiated and 14 to 25 in differentiated lipid-producing cells.[1] Within any one glandular unit, the acini vary in differentiation and maturity. The synthesis and discharge of the lipids contained in the sebaceous cells require more than 1 week. The size of sebaceous glands increases with age. The mean size rises from $0.2 \text{ mm}^2 \pm 0.5 \text{ mm}^2$ to $0.4 \text{ mm}^2 \pm 2.1 \text{ mm}^2$. The sebaceous cells of prepubertal and hypogonadal boys and men are qualitatively similar to those of normal adults, even though the glands are smaller.[45] In general, whereas the number of sebaceous glands remains approximately the same throughout life, their size tends to change with age.[46] The turnover of the sebaceous glands in older adults is slowed down compared with young adults.

A variety of experimental models are used to study the factors involved in sebaceous gland regulation, including cell culture of isolated human sebaceous glands, primary sebocytes, immortalized sebocyte cell lines, and three-dimensional models, as well as mouse and hamster animal models.[47-50] Results from these investigations clearly indicate that sebaceous glands are multifactional (see Table 6-2),[51,52] regulated, among others, by ligands of sebaceous gland cell receptors (Table 6-3), such as androgen and estrogen receptors, peroxisome-proliferator-activated receptors (PPAR) and liver-X receptor (LXR), neuropeptide receptors, retinoid, and vitamin D receptors.[53-56] The ligand–receptor complexes activate pathways involving lipogenesis but also cell proliferation, differentiation, hormone metabolism, and cytokine and chemokine release.[57]

ANDROGENS

Sebaceous glands require androgenic stimulation to produce significant quantities of sebum. Individuals with a genetic deficiency of androgen receptors (complete androgen insensitivity) have no detectable sebum secretion and do not develop acne.[58] Although the most powerful androgens are testosterone and its end-organ reduction product, 5α-dihydrotestosterone (DHT), levels of testosterone do not parallel the patterns of sebaceous gland activity. For example, testosterone levels are many fold higher in males than in females, with no overlap between the sexes. However, the average rates of sebum secretion are only slightly higher in males than in females, with considerable overlap between the sexes. Also, sebum secretion starts to increase in children during adrenarche, a developmental event that precedes puberty by about 2 years.

TABLE 6-3
Hormone Receptors Expressed in Human Sebaceous Gland Cells

RECEPTORS	NATURAL LIGANDS	EFFECT ON CULTURED SEBOCYTES
Peptide Hormone and Neurotransmitter Receptors		
Serpentine (Seven-Transmembrane Domain) Receptors		
■ Corticotropin-releasing hormone (CRH) receptors 1 and 2 (CRH-R1 > CRH-R2)	CRH, urocortin	↓ Proliferation, ↑ Δ^{5-4} 3β-hydroxysteroid dehydrogenase (CRH), ↑ lipid synthesis (CRH), ↑ IL-6 and IL-8 release (CRH)
■ Melanocortin-1 and 5 receptors (MC-1R and MC-5R)	α-Melanocyte-stimulating hormone (α-MSH)	↓ IL-1–induced IL-8 synthesis (MC-5R), differentiation marker (MC-1R)
■ μ-Opiate receptors (OPRs)	β-Endorphin	↓ EGF-induced proliferation, ↑ lipid synthesis
■ VPAC receptors	Vasoactive intestinal polypeptide (VIP), receptors for neuropeptide Y and calcitonin gene-related peptide (CGRP)	Neuropeptide Y stimulates IL-6 and IL-8 release
■ Cannabinoid receptors CR1 and CR2	Cannabinoid	
■ Histamine receptor 1	Histamine	Regulation of squalene synthesis
Single-Transmembrane Domain Receptors with Intrinsic Tyrosine Kinase Activity		
■ Insulin-like growth factor (IGF) I receptor	IGF-I, insulin	↑ Lipogenesis
Single-Transmembrane Domain Receptors without Intrinsic Tyrosine Kinase Activity		
■ Growth hormone (GH) receptor	GH	↑ Differentiation, ↑ DHT effect on lipogenesis
Nuclear Receptors		
Steroid Receptors		
■ Androgen receptor	Testosterone, 5α-dihydrotestosterone (DHT)	↑ Proliferation (with PPAR ligands ↑ lipogenesis)
■ Progesterone receptor	Progesterone	?
Thyroid Receptors		
■ Estrogen receptors (ER-α- and -β)	17β-Estradiol	↑ Polar lipid production
■ Retinoic acid receptors (RAR-α and -γ)	*All-trans* retinoic acid (atRA)	↓ Proliferation
■ Retinoid X receptors (RXR-α, > PXR-β, -γ)	9-*cis* RA	Regulate lipogenesis (?)
■ Vitamin D receptor	Vitamin D_3	Regulates cell proliferation, cell cycle, lipid content, and IL-6 and IL-8 secretion
■ Peroxisome proliferator-activated receptors (PPARα, PPARγ > PPARβ)	Linoleic acid (RRARβ/Δ), leukotrien-B4 (LTB4)	↑ Lipogenesis, ↑ prostaglandin E2 release, ↑ IL-6 release, ↑ COX2 synthesis
■ Liver X receptors (LXRα and -β)	22(R)-Hydroxycholesterol	↓ Proliferation, ↑ lipogenesis, ↓ COX2 and inducible NOS

COX, cyclooxygenase; DHT, 5α-dihydrotestosterone; EGF, epidermal growth factor; IGF, insulin-like growth factor; IL, interleukin; NO, nitric oxide synthase; VPAC, vasoactive intestinal peptide receptor.

The weak adrenal androgen, dehydroepiandrosterone sulfate (DHEAS), is probably a significant regulator of sebaceous gland activity through its conversion to testosterone and DHT in the sebaceous gland.[59] Levels of DHEAS are high in newborns, very low in 2- to 4-year-old children, and start to rise when sebum secretion starts to increase. In adulthood, DHEAS levels show considerable individual variation but are only slightly higher in men than in women on the average. There is a decline in DHEAS levels in both sexes starting in early adulthood and continuing throughout life; this decline parallels the decline of sebum secretion. DHEAS is present in the blood in high concentration. The enzymes required to convert DHEAS to more potent androgens are present in sebaceous glands.[60] These include 3β-hydroxysteroid dehydrogenase, 17β-hydroxysteroid dehydrogenase, and 5α-reductase. Each of these enzymes exists in two or more isoforms that exhibit tissue-specific differences in their expression. The predominant isozymes in the sebaceous gland include the type 1 3β-hydroxysteroid dehydrogenase, the type 2 17β-hydroxysteroid dehydrogenase, and the type 1 5α-reductase.[61,62]

RETINOIDS

Isotretinoin (13-*cis*-retinoic acid, 13-*cis*-RA) is the most potent pharmacologic inhibitor of sebum secretion. Significant reductions in sebum production can be observed as early as 2 weeks after use.[63,64] Histologically, sebaceous glands are markedly reduced in size, and individual sebocytes appear undifferentiated lacking the characteristic cytoplasmic accumulation of sebaceous lipids.[3,65]

Isotretinoin does not interact with any of the known retinoid receptors. It may serve as a prodrug for the synthesis of all-*trans*-retinoic acid, which interacts with retinoid receptors expressed in sebaceous gland cells (retinoic acid receptors [RARs; isotypes α and γ] and retinoid X receptors [RXRs; isotypes α, β, γ]).[66] However, it has greater sebosuppressive action than do all-*trans*- or 9-*cis*-retinoic acid.[67] 13-*cis*-RA exerts pluripotent effects on human sebaceous gland cells and their lipogenesis.[63] Inhibition of androgen synthesis, cell cycle arrest, and apoptosis by 13-*cis*-RA may explain the reduction of sebaceous gland size after treatment.

PEROXISOME-PROLIFERATOR-ACTIVATED RECEPTORS

PPARs are members of the nuclear hormone receptor family and act as transcriptional regulators of a variety of genes, including those involved in lipid metabolism in adipose tissue, liver, and skin. PPARs are similar to retinoid receptors in many ways. Each of these receptors forms heterodimers with retinoid X receptors to regulate the transcription of genes involved in a variety of processes, including lipid metabolism and cellular proliferation and differentiation. PPARα, δ, and γ receptor subtypes have been detected in basal sebaceous gland cells.[54] PPARγ is also detected within differentiated cells. Pharmacologic PPAR-γ modulation regulates sebogenesis and inflammation in SZ95 human sebaceous gland cells.[68] In patients receiving fibrates (PPAR-α ligands) for hyperlipidemia or thiazolidinediones (PPAR-γ ligands) for diabetes, sebum secretion rates are increased.[69]

PPAR-γ–RXR-α and LXR–RXRα promoter interactions are of crucial importance for the regulation of key genes of lipid metabolism. Although various fatty acids, eicosanoids, and prostanoids activate PPARs, oxysterols and intermediate products of the cholesterol biosynthetic pathway activate LXRs. PPAR-α agonists and PPAR-γ antagonists may reduce sebaceous lipid synthesis and as such may be useful in the treatment of acne. On the other hand, whereas PPAR-γ agonists may be beneficial in aging skin, PPAR-δ agonists may be involved in sebaceous tumorigenesis.

LXR

LXRs, which are members of the NHR family, play a critical role in cholesterol homeostasis and lipid metabolism.[70] Treatment of SZ95 sebaceous gland cells with the LXR ligands TO901317 or 22(R)-hydroxycholesterol enhanced accumulation of LDs in the cells, which could be explained through induction of the expression of the LXRα receptor and known LXR targets, such as fatty acid synthase and sterol regulatory element–binding protein-1 (SREBP-1).[54,71]

FOXO1

FoxO1 is expressed in most lipid-metabolizing cells, including the prostate, liver, fat tissue, and skin.[72] Human sebaceous gland cells also express FoxO1. Acne and increased sebaceous lipogenesis are associated with a relative nuclear deficiency of FoxO1 caused by increased growth hormone–insulin–insulin-like growth factor 1 or fibroblast growth factor 2 signaling.

STRUCTURAL PROTEINS

During sebogenesis, lipids are stored in LDs. LDs are limited by a membrane containing phospholipids and numerous proteins and enzymes. The most relevant membrane proteins are the perilipin (PLIN) family, which possesses structural and regulatory properties. In particular, PLIN2, the major form expressed during the differentiation process, regulates the gland size in vivo and regulates sebaceous lipid accumulation.[73] Experimental downmodulation of the PLIN2 expression significantly modifies the composition of neutral lipids with a significant decrease in the unsaturated fatty acid component caused by a marked decrease in the expression of specific lipogenic enzymes. On the other hand, PLIN3 has currently been shown to modulate specific lipogenic pathways in human sebaceous gland cells.[74] Another structural protein, angiopoietin-like 4, is strongly induced during human sebocyte differentiation and regulates sebaceous lipogenesis.[75]

CONCLUSION

The regulation of sebaceous glands and human sebum production is complex. Advances are being made in this area, which may lead to alternative therapies for the reduction of sebum and improvements in acne.

SWEAT GLANDS

AT-A-GLANCE

- A human has 2 to 4 million sweat glands (200 to 400/cm² of skin surface).
- Up to 10 L/day of sweat is produced by acclimatized individuals.
- In humans, sweat glands are generally classified into apocrine and eccrine types.
- Hypothalamic temperature is the strongest stimulus for sweating.
- Acetylcholine is the major stimulus of eccrine sweat glands secreted by sympathetic nerves.
- Adrenergic stimulation controls apocrine gland secretion.
- Botulinum toxin inhibits sweating by preventing acetylcholine release.
- Oxidative metabolism of glucose is a major source of eccrine gland adenosine triphosphate.
- Ductal reabsorption conserves NaCl.
- Bacteria are necessary for apocrine odor.
- Odiferous precursors secretion is controlled by the MRP8 encoded by ABCC11.

Eccrine gland sweat allows the body to control its internal temperature in response to thermal stress. Apocrine gland function is more obscure but likely includes pheromone production. Although the eccrine and apocrine secretory portions of sweat glands are clearly morphologically distinctive, their ducts are histologically indistinguishable if the duct orifice cannot be detected. Immunohistological distinction can be performed by the stage-specific embryonic antigen-4 (SSEA-4), which is a marker of ductal cells of eccrine but not of apocrine sweat glands.[76]

ECCRINE SWEAT GLANDS

DEVELOPMENT OF THE ECCRINE SWEAT GLANDS

A human has approximately 2 to 4 million sweat glands (200 to 400/cm² of skin surface).[77] Sweat glands are found over nearly the entire body surface and are especially dense on the palms, soles, forehead, and upper limbs.[78] However, they are absent at the margins of the lips, the eardrums, and the nailbeds of fingers and toenails. Anlagen of eccrine sweat glands first appear in 3.5-month-old fetuses on the palms and soles (see Chap. 4), then develop in the axillary skin in the fifth fetal month, and finally develop over the entire body by the sixth fetal month.[78] The anlagen of the eccrine sweat gland, which develops from the epidermal ridge, is double layered and develops a lumen between the layers between the fourth and eighth fetal months. By the eighth fetal month, eccrine secretory cells resemble those of an adult; by the ninth fetal month, myoepithelial cells form around the secretory coil and the excretory duct.

ANATOMY AND FUNCTION OF THE ECCRINE SWEAT GLANDS

Two distinct segments, the secretory coil (tubulus) and the duct, form the eccrine sweat gland. The secretory coil secretes a sterile, dilute electrolyte solution with primary components of bicarbonate, potassium, sodium chloride (NaCl), and other minor components such as glucose, pyruvate, lactate, cytokines, immunoglobulins, antimicrobial peptides (eg, dermcidin,[79] β-defensin,[80] cathelicidines[81]). Relative to the plasma and extracellular fluid, the concentration of Na$^+$ ions is much lower in sweat (~40 mM versus ~150 mM in plasma and extracellular fluid). The eccrine excretion has a high concentration of Na$^+$ ions. However, Na$^+$ ions are partially reabsorbed via the epithelial sodium channels (ENaC) that are located on the apical membrane of the eccrine gland duct cells.[82] This reuptake of Na$^+$ ions reduces the loss of Na$^+$ during the process of perspiration.

Secretory Coil: The secretory coil contains three distinct cell types: (1) clear (secretory), (2) dark (mucoid), and (3) myoepithelial.[83] The clear and dark cells occur in approximately equal numbers but differ in their distribution. Although the dark cells border the apical (luminal) surfaces, the clear cells rest either directly on the basement membrane or on the on the myoepithelial cells. The clear cells directly access the lumen by forming intercellular canaliculi (Fig. 6-7). Spindle-shaped contractile myoepithelial cells lie on the basement membrane and abut the clear cells. An adult secretory coil is approximately 2- to 5-mm long and approximately 30 to 50 μm in diameter. Heat accumulation results in larger sweat glands and ducts, and their dimensions in turn correlate with enhanced sweat output.[84] Clear cells contain abundant mitochondria and an autofluorescent body, called the lipofuscin granule, in the cytoplasm. The clear cell plasma membrane forms many villi. The clear cell secretes water and electrolytes. Dark cells have a smooth cell surface and contain abundant dark cell granules.[83] The function of dark cells is unknown. Myoepithelial cells contain actin filaments and are contractile,[85,86] producing pulsatile sweat.

Duct: The duct of the eccrine sweat gland consists of an outer ring of peripheral or basal cells and an inner ring of luminal or cuticular cells. It seems that the proximal (coiled) duct is functionally more active than the distal straight portion in pumping Na$^+$ for ductal Na$^+$ reabsorption because Na$^+$, K$^+$-adenosine triphosphatase (ATPase) activity and the number of mitochondria are higher in the proximal portion (Fig. 6-8).[83,85,87,88] In contrast, the luminal ductal cells have fewer mitochondria, much less Na$^+$, K$^+$-ATPase

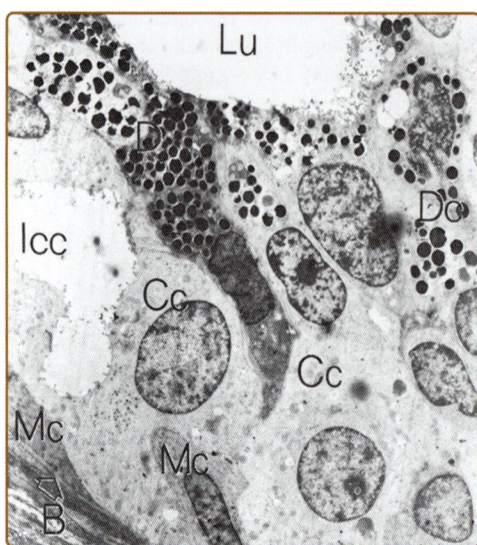

Figure 6-7 Electron micrograph of the secretory coil of a human eccrine sweat gland. B with *arrow*, basal lamina; CC, clear cell; DC, dark cell; ICC, intercellular canaliculi; Lu, lumen; MC, myoepithelial cell.

temperature effect is speculated to be due to increased release of periglandular neurotransmitters.

The sweating in menopausal "hot flashes" reinforces the concept of a central hypothalamic mechanism for thermal sweating but also shows that the response of individuals to the same changes in core temperature can vary. Although hormonal factors influence sweating during menopause, excessive sweating does not correlate simply with hormonal levels. Instead, menopausal hot flashes seem to be caused by a hypersensitive brain response (particularly the hypothalamus but perhaps the insula, anterior cingulate, amygdala, and primary somatosensory cortex as well). In asymptomatic menopausal women and premenopausal women, the core temperature can change up to 0.4°C (33°F) without eliciting a response. In symptomatic

activity, and a dense layer of tonofilaments near the luminal membrane, which is often referred to as the *cuticular border*. The cuticular border provides structural resilience to the ductal lumen, which may dilate whenever ductal flow of sweat is blocked. The entire structural organization of the duct is well designed for the most efficient Na^+ absorptive function. The luminal membrane serves as the absorptive surface by accommodating both Na^+ and Cl^- channels, and the basal ductal cells serve in Na^+ pumping by providing maximally expanded Na^+ pump sites and efficient energy metabolism. The lumen and the duct contain β-defensin, an antimicrobial, cysteine-rich, low-molecular-weight peptide.[80,81] In the epidermis, the duct spirals tightly upon itself.

NEURAL CONTROL OF ECCRINE SWEATING

The preoptic hypothalamic area plays an essential role in regulating body temperature: whereas local heating of the preoptic hypothalamic tissue activates generalized sweating, vasodilatation, and rapid breathing, local cooling of the preoptic area causes generalized vasoconstriction and shivering. Whereas the elevation of hypothalamic temperature associated with an increase in body temperature provides the strongest stimulus for thermoregulatory sweating responses, cutaneous temperature exerts a weaker influence on the rate of sweating.[84,89] On a degree-to-degree basis, an increase in internal temperature is about nine times more efficient than an increase in mean skin temperature in stimulating the sweat center. The local

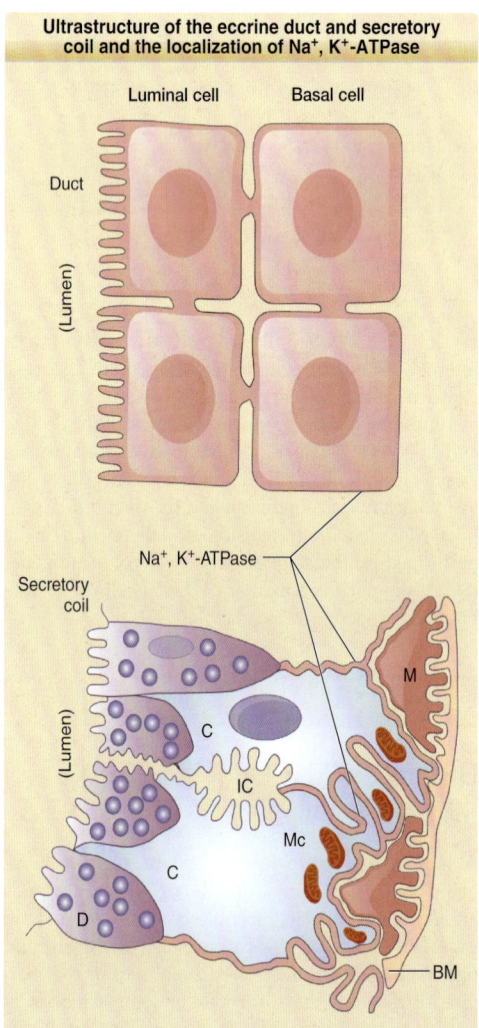

Figure 6-8 The ultrastructure of the eccrine duct and secretory coil and the localization of Na^+, K^+-adenosine triphosphatase (ATPase). The thick lines indicate the localization of Na^+, K^+-ATPase. BM, basement membrane; C, clear cell; D, dark cells; IC, intercellular canaliculi; M, myoepithelial cell; Mc, mitochondria.

postmenopausal women, changes as small as 0.1°C (32°F) trigger peripheral vasodilation and sweating. Why the brain is hypersensitive to small changes in core temperature is poorly understood, but increased levels of brain norepinephrine appear to influence the response to small changes in core temperature through their action on α_2-adrenergic receptors in the brain; higher levels of the norepinephrine metabolite 3-methoxy-4-hydroxyphenylglycol have also been found in symptomatic menopausal women compared with asymptomatic women. Decreased norepinephrine release is postulated as the mechanism by which clonidine relieves hot flashes in symptomatic women. Decreased core temperature may be the reason that women with decreased body mass index tend to have fewer symptoms even though their estrogen levels probably are lower than those in women with increased body mass index. Levels of estrogen, luteinizing hormone, and β-endorphins also were originally thought to influence hot flashes, but later studies have suggested no association.[90]

Innervation: Efferent nerve fibers originating from the hypothalamic preoptic sweat center descend through the ipsilateral brainstem and medulla and synapse in the intermediolateral cell columns of the spinal cord without crossing (although sympathetic vasomotor fibers may partially cross).[91] The myelinated axons rising from the intermediolateral horn of the spinal cord (preganglionic fibers) pass out in the anterior roots to reach (through white ramus communicans) the sympathetic chain and synapse. Unmyelinated postganglionic sympathetic class C fibers arising from sympathetic ganglia join the major peripheral nerves and end around the sweat gland. The supply to the skin of the upper limb is commonly from T2 to T8. The face and the eyelids are supplied by T1 to T4, so that resection of T2 for the treatment of palmar hyperhidrosis is likely to cause Horner syndrome. The trunk is supplied by T4 to T12 and the lower limbs by T10 to L2. Unlike the sensory innervation, a significant overlap of innervation occurs in the sympathetic dermatome because a single preganglionic fiber can synapse with several postganglionic fibers.

The major neurotransmitter released from the periglandular nerve endings is acetylcholine (Ach), an exception to the general rule of sympathetic innervation, in which noradrenaline is the peripheral neurotransmitter.[92] In addition to ACh, adenosine triphosphate (ATP), catecholamine, vasoactive intestinal peptide, atrial natriuretic peptide, calcitonin gene-related peptide, and galanin have been localized in the periglandular nerves. The significance of these peptides or neurotransmitters in relation to sweat gland function is not fully understood.

Botulinum toxin interferes with ACh release. Its heavy chain binds the neurotoxin selectively to the cholinergic terminal, and the light chain acts within the cells to prevent ACh release. Type A toxin cleaves sensory nerve action potential-25, a 25-kDa synaptosomal-associated protein; the type B light chain cleaves vesicle-associated membrane protein (also called *synaptobrevin*). Botulinum toxins are used for symptomatic relief of hyperhidrosis.[93] A more detailed description can be found in Chaps. 81 and 216.

Denervation: In humans, the sweating response to intradermal injection of nicotine or ACh disappears within a few weeks after denervation of the *postganglionic* fibers,[93,94] and the sweating response to heat ceases immediately after resection of the nerves. In contrast, after denervation of *preganglionic* fibers (caused by spinal cord injuries or neuropathies), pharmacologic responsiveness of the sweat glands is maintained from several months to 2 years, even though their thermally induced sweating is no longer present.[95]

EMOTIONAL SWEATING

Sweating induced by emotional stress (emotional sweating) can occur over the whole skin surface in some individuals, but it is usually confined to the palms, soles, axillae, and forehead. Emotional sweating on the palms and soles ceases during sleep, but thermal sweating occurs even during sleep if the body temperature rises. Because both types of sweating can be inhibited by atropine, emotional sweating is cholinergically medicated.

PHARMACOLOGY OF THE ECCRINE SWEAT GLAND AND SWEATING RATE

Sweat glands respond to cholinergic agents, α- and β-adrenergic stimulants, and other periglandular neurotransmitters, such as vasoactive intestinal peptide and ATP. Periglandular ACh is the major stimulant of sweat secretion, and its periglandular concentration determines the sweat rate in humans.[96] When dissociated clear cells are stimulated in vitro by cholinergic agents, they lose K^+ and Cl^-, increase intracellular Ca^{2+}, and shrink, mimicking actions seen in vivo. Striking individual differences exist in the degree of sweating in response to a given thermal or physical stress. In general, males perspire more profusely than females.[97] The sweat rate in a given area of the skin is determined by the number of active glands and the average sweat rate per gland. The maximal sweat rate per gland varies from 2 to 20 nL/min^2. Sweat rate increases during acclimatization, but the morphologic and pharmacologic bases of the individual and regional differences in sweating rate during acclimatization are still poorly understood (Fig. 6-9). In thermally induced sweating, the sweat rate can be mathematically related to the body and skin temperatures in a given subject only in the low sweat rate range. Cholinergic stimulation yields a 5 to 10 times higher sweating rate than does β-adrenergic stimulation. α-Adrenergic stimulation (by phenylephrine) is no more potent than isoproterenol (ISO) (a β-adrenergic agonist) in humans in vivo.[98] Whereas cholinergic sweating begins immediately on intradermal injection, β-adrenergic sweating requires a latent period of from 1 to 2 minutes, which suggests that the intracellular mechanism of sweat induction

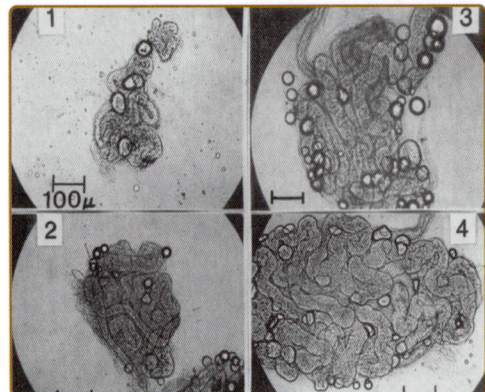

Figure 6-9 Individual variation in the size of the sweat gland in four male adults, aged 22 to 28 years. Sweat glands were isolated from skin biopsy specimens obtained from the upper back behind the axilla. Whereas subject 1 is a sedentary man who does not exercise regularly, subject 4 is a well-acclimatized athletic individual.

may be different for methacholine and for ISO. Because the sweat rate in response to adrenergic agents is rather low, it may be reasonable to surmise that adrenergic stimulation in periglandular nerves may be involved in the regulation of sweat gland function but not in the induction of sweat secretion. One consequence of dual cholinergic and adrenergic innervation is to maximize tissue accumulation of cyclic adenosine monophosphate (cAMP), which may be instrumental in stimulating the synthesis of sweat and glandular hypertrophy of the sweat gland. The possibility that periglandular catecholamine is directly involved in emotional sweating or sweating associated with pheochromocytoma[99] may be ruled out because these sweating responses can be blocked by anticholinergic agents.

PHARMACOLOGY AND FUNCTION OF ECCRINE MYOEPITHELIUM

The periodicity of sweat secretion in vivo is caused by the periodicity of central nerve impulse discharges, which occur synchronously with vasomotor tonus waves. Myoepithelial contraction occurs with cholinergic stimulation, but neither α- nor β-adrenergic agents induce tubular contraction.[100] Although the myoepithelium may contribute to sweat production via pulsatile contractions, it also seems to provide structural support for the secretory epithelium, especially under conditions in which stagnation of sweat flow (caused by ductal blockade) results in an increase in luminal hydrostatic pressure.[86]

ENERGY METABOLISM

Sweat secretion is mediated by the energy (ie, ATP)-dependent active transport of ions, so a continuous supply of metabolic energy is mandatory for sustained sweat secretion. Endogenous glycogen stored in the clear cells can sustain sweat secretion for less than 10 minutes; thus, the sweat gland must depend almost exclusively on exogenous substrates for its energy metabolism. Mannose, lactate, and pyruvate are used nearly as readily as glucose; other hexoses, fatty acids, ketone bodies, intermediates of the tricarboxylic acid cycle, and amino acids are either very poorly used or not used as substrates. The physiologic significance of lactate or pyruvate utilization by the sweat gland is not yet clear. However, because the plasma level of glucose (5.5 mM) is much higher than that of lactate (1 to 2 mM) or pyruvate (<1 mM), glucose may play a major role in sweat secretion. Oxidative metabolism of glucose is favored as the major route of ATP formation for secretory activity.[100]

COMPOSITION OF HUMAN ECCRINE SWEAT

Inorganic Ions: Sweat is formed in two steps: (1) secretion of a primary fluid containing nearly isotonic NaCl concentrations by the secretory coil and (2) reabsorption of NaCl from the primary fluid by the duct. Although a number of factors affect ductal NaCl absorption, the sweat rate (and thus the transit time of sweat) has the most important influence

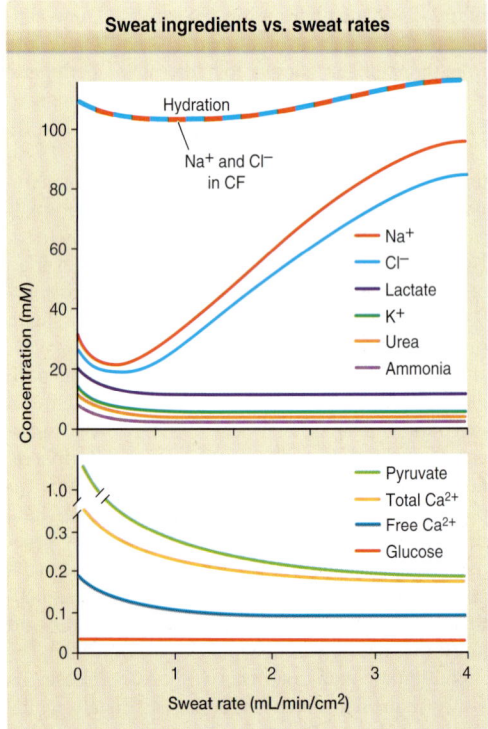

Figure 6-10 Relationship between the concentration of sweat ingredients and the sweat rate in thermally induced human sweat in normal individuals and in persons with cystic fibrosis (CF).

on final NaCl concentration. Sweat NaCl concentration increases with increasing sweat rate to plateau at around 100 mM (Fig. 6-10). Potassium (K^+) concentration in sweat is relatively constant. It ranges from 5 to 10 mM, which is slightly higher than plasma K^+ concentration. HCO_3^- concentration in the primary sweat fluid is approximately 10 mM, but that of final sweat is less than 1 mM, which indicates that HCO_3^- is reabsorbed by the duct, presumably accompanied by ductal acidification.[101] Sweat NaCl concentration is increased in individuals with cystic fibrosis.[102] Aquagenic wrinkling of the palms (whitened, wrinkling, and papillation of the palms after brief water exposure) is seen more frequently in carriers and patients with cystic fibrosis (see Chap. 81).

Lactate: The concentration of lactate in sweat usually depends on the sweat rate. At low sweat rates, lactate concentration is as high as 30 to 40 mM, but it rapidly drops to a plateau at around 10 to 15 mM as the sweat rate increases. Whereas acclimatization is known to lower sweat lactate concentrations, arterial occlusion rapidly raises sweat NaCl and lactate concentrations and reduces the sweat rate.[100] Sweat lactate is probably produced by glycolysis of glucose by the secretory cells.[103]

Urea: Urea in sweat is derived mostly from serum urea.[104] Sweat urea content is usually expressed as a sweat–plasma ratio (S/P urea). S/P urea is high (2 to 4) at a low sweat rate range but approaches a plateau at 1.2 to 1.5 as the sweat rate increases.

Ammonia and Amino Acids: The ammonia concentration in sweat is 0.5 to 8 mM,[105] which is 20 to 50 times higher than the plasma ammonia level. The concentration of sweat ammonia is inversely related to the sweat rate and sweat pH. Free amino acids are present in human sweat,[106] although it is not clear what proportion of measured amino acids derive from epidermal contamination.

Proteins Including Proteases: The concentration of sweat protein in the least contaminated, thermally induced sweat is approximately 20 mg/dL, with the major portion being low-molecular-weight proteins (ie, molecular weight <10,000). Because sweat samples collected by simple scraping (and even those collected with a plastic bag) can be massively contaminated with plasma or epidermal proteins, previous reports on the presence of α- and γ-globulins, transferrin, ceruloplasmin, orosomucoid, albumin,[106,107] and immunoglobulin E must be carefully reexamined. The sweat samples collected over an oil barrier placed on the skin (the least-contaminated sweat) contain no or trace of γ-globulin and a very small amount of albumin. Yokozeki and coworkers[108] also reported the presence of cysteine proteinases and their endogenous inhibitors in sweat and the sweat gland. Dermcidin is an antimicrobial peptide produced and secreted in sweat.[79] Other organic compounds reported to be present in sweat include histamine,[109] prostaglandin,[110] and vitamin K–like substances.[111] Sweat also contains traces of pyruvate and glucose. Sweat glucose increases concurrently with a rise in plasma glucose level. Some orally ingested drugs, including griseofulvin,[112] ketoconazole,[113] amphetamines,[114] and various chemotherapeutic agents,[115] are secreted in sweat.

MECHANISMS OF SWEAT SECRETION

Several distinct sequential processes lead to eccrine gland sweat production[116]: (1) stimulation of the eccrine sweat gland by ACh via increased intracellular Ca^{2+}; (2) Ca^{2+}-stimulated loss of cellular K^+, Cl^-, and H_2O, which leads to eccrine gland cell shrinkage; and (3)

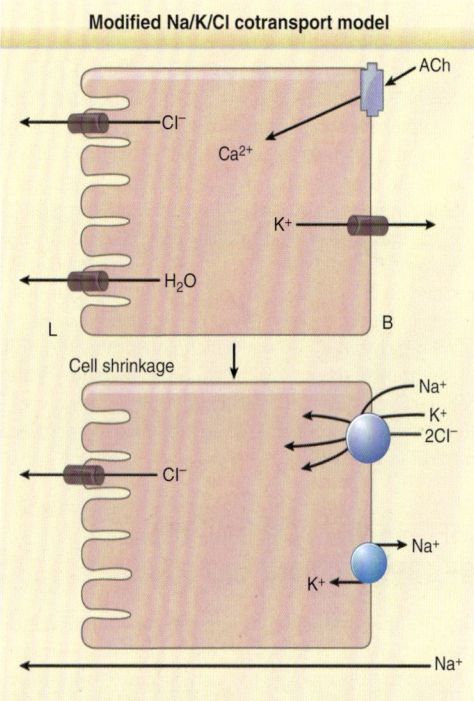

Figure 6-11 Modified Na/K/2Cl cotransport model for the ionic mechanism of cholinergic eccrine sweat secretion. Periglandular neurotransmitters, such as acetylcholine (ACh), bind to receptors on the basolateral membrane, which leads to increased intracellular Ca^{2+}; this in turn activates K^+ and Cl^- channels, mediating K^+, Cl^-, and H_2O efflux from the cell. The resulting cell shrinkage activates the basolateral $Na^+/K^+/2Cl^-$ antiporter, which leads to Na^+, K^+, and Cl^- influx. The Na^+ and K^+ fluxes are recycled across the basolateral membrane by the Na^+, K^+-adenosine triphosphatase. In contrast, Cl^- fluxes flow unopposed into the lumen, causing an electrical gradient that drives Na^+ exit from the tissue into the lumen via a paracellular pathway. Net fluxes: H_2O, Cl^-, and Na^+ (isotonic) flow into the lumen. pH of the secreted fluid is neutral. Paracellular Na^+ fluxes across the cell junction are indicated with an *arrow* at the bottom of the figure. B, basolateral membrane; L, luminal or apical membrane.

volume-activated transcellular plus paracellular fluxes of Na^+, Cl^-, and H_2O, which leads to net flux of largely isotonic NaCl solution into the glandular lumen. These processes are illustrated in Fig. 6-11.

Sweating initially is stimulated when ACh is released from periglandular cholinergic nerve endings in response to thermal or emotional stimuli. ACh binds to cholinergic receptors on the clear cell plasma membrane, stimulating intracellular Ca^{2+} release and influx, and increasing cytosolic Ca^{2+} concentrations. Increased intracellular Ca^{2+}, in turn, opens Ca^{2+}-sensitive Cl^- and K^+ channels in the clear cell basolateral membrane, which allows Cl^- and K^+ to escape. Because H_2O follows K^+ and Cl^-, to maintain cell iso-osmolarity, the cell shrinks.[116,117]

This decrease in cell volume sets off a second cascade of cell signaling events. First, decreased cell volume stimulates the NKCC1[118] class of Na/K/2Cl cotransporters, which carry Na^+, K^+, and $2Cl^-$ into the cell in an electrically neutral fashion (ie, two cations and two anions cancel out net charges). The resulting increase in cytosolic Na^+ activates the Na^+, K^+-ATPase, located in the basolateral membrane, which recycles Na^+ and K^+ across the basolateral membrane. The net movement of the negatively charged Cl^- ion across the apical membrane into the lumen in turn drives the positively charged Na^+ ion into the lumen as well, along a paracellular pathway. Therefore, the final product of glandular secretion is the net movement of Na^+, Cl^-, and H_2O into the glandular lumen to form the isotonic NaCl precursor of sweat.

ACh-induced sweating, which constitutes the bulk of sweat production, appears to be mediated by intracellular Ca^{2+}, as detailed earlier. In contrast, adrenergic-induced sweating appears to be mediated by increased intracellular cAMP.[119]

MECHANISM OF DUCTAL REABSORPTION

Because the production of large sweat volumes could lead to dangerous losses of NaCl, the sweat duct has evolved to reabsorb NaCl, which minimizes electrolyte loss, even at high sweat volumes (Fig. 6-12).

Ductal Na^+ reabsorption is accomplished through the coordinated activities of intracellular enzymes and plasma membrane ion channels, pumps, and exchangers. These mechanisms not only reabsorb electrolytes but also acidify the sweat, which results in a final sweat product that is hypotonic and acidic. Na^+ reenters the duct cells through the apical membrane via amiloride-sensitive[120] epithelial Na^+ channels (ENaC)[5] and is transported across the basolateral membrane by ouabain-sensitive[88] Na^+, K^+-ATPase pumps. Cl^- transport appears to be both transcellular and paracellular, with the cystic fibrosis transmembrane regulator (CFTR) Cl^- channels playing an important role in transcellular fluxes.[118] In cystic fibrosis, CFTR Cl^- channels are mutated, and eccrine duct Cl^- reabsorption is defective but not completely abolished.[27] Na^+ is increased in the duct and the sweat at the skin surface.[121] Unlike in the lung, CFTR mutations do not lead to increased ENaC-mediated Na^+ influx, which suggests that the CFTR–ENaC interactions seen in other tissues differ from that in the eccrine duct. Sweat acidification appears to be mediated via the enzyme carbonic anhydrase, the HCO_3^-/Cl and Na^+/H^+ exchangers, and the V-type H^+ ATPase. The intracellular enzyme carbonic anhydrase catalyzes HCO_3^- and H^+ production. Whereas intracellular HCO_3^- is cleared via the HCO_3^-/Cl antiporter, H^+ is pumped into the luminal sweat by the V-type H^+ ATPase.[122] The Na^+/H^+ antiporter NHE1 (Na^+/H^+ exchanger isoform 1),[123,124] found in the basolateral membrane, is important in intracellular pH regulation.

The transfer of sweat to the skin surface without leakage is important for the homeostatic regulation of skin and is impaired in atopic dermatitis; lesional skin presents a decreased claudin-3 expression in sweat glands, which is accompanied by sweat leakage.[122]

Several drugs are known to modify ductal NaCl reabsorption. When aldosterone is injected systemically or locally, the Na/K ratio in sweat begins to decrease within 6 hours, reaching a nadir at 24 hours and returning to the preinjection level in 48 to 72 hours.[121] Na^+ deprivation stimulates both renin and aldosterone secretion, but high thermal stress per se (a single 1-hour exposure of humans to a temperature of 40°C [104°F]) is a potent stimulator of renin and aldosterone secretion in either the presence or absence of sodium deprivation. In an in vitro sweat gland preparation, neither acetazolamide (a carbonic anhydrase inhibitor) nor antidiuretic hormone changed ductal or secretory function. However, more potent carbonic anhydrase inhibitors, such as topiramate,[125] have been reported to induce oligohidrosis.

APOCRINE SWEAT GLANDS

Apocrine sweat glands are found in humans, largely confined to the regions of the axillae, the perineum, and the areolae of the breast.[126] Differentiated apocrine sweat glands are present at the external auditory canal (ceruminous glands). Apocrine sweat glands do not become functional until just before puberty; thus, it is assumed that their development is associated with the hormonal changes at puberty, although the exact hormones have not been identified.

ANATOMY

Apocrine glands are coiled and localized in the subcutaneous fat near the dermis. The gland consists of a single layer of cuboidal or columnar cells. These secretory cells rest on a layer of myoepithelial cells.[127] The duct is composed of a double layer of cuboidal cells and empties into hair follicle infundibulum. Sweat and sebum are mixed in the hair follicle and arrive mixed at the epidermal surface. The apocrine sweat is cloudy, viscous, initially odorless, and at a pH of 6 to 7.5.

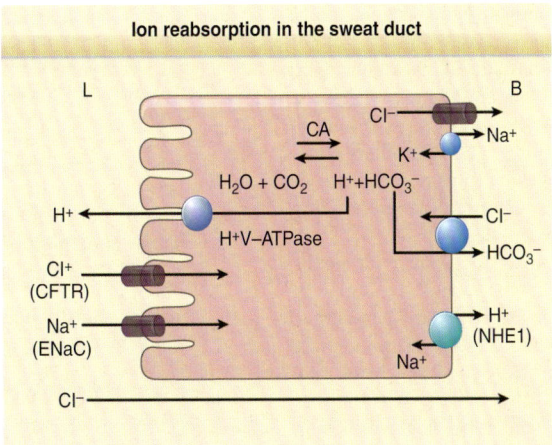

Figure 6-12 Illustration of ion reabsorption in the sweat duct. Na⁺ enters the apical (luminal) membrane through epithelial Na⁺ channels (ENaC) and is transported across the basolateral membrane by Na⁺, K⁺-adenosine triphosphatase (ATPase). Cl⁻ enters the cell through the cystic fibrosis transmembrane regulator Cl⁻ channel (CFTR) and is transported across the lumen via a paracellular pathway. H⁺ generated by the enzyme carbonic anhydrase (CA) is pumped into the lumen by a V-type H⁺ ATPase (H⁺ V-ATPase). Intracellular pH homeostasis is maintained by parallel HCO_3^-/H^+ and Na⁺/H⁺ (NHE1) exchangers. The activity of these enzymes, transporters, and channels results in H⁺ secretion and Na⁺ and Cl⁻ reabsorption, which produces a final sweat that is hypotonic and acidic. Paracellular Cl⁻ fluxes across the cell junction are indicated with an *arrow* at the bottom of the figure. B, basolateral membrane; L, luminal or apical membrane.

The sweat of apocrine sweat glands only attains its characteristic odor upon being degraded by bacteria, which releases volatile odor molecules. More bacteria (especially corynebacteria) leads to stronger odor. The presence of axillary hair also makes the odor even more pungent because secretions, debris, keratin, and bacteria accumulate on the hair.

Like the eccrine gland, the myoepithelium fulfills dual functions in both providing structural support and pumping out preformed sweat.

β-Adrenergic receptors and purinergic receptors have been identified on apocrine glands.[94] However, nerve fibers and muscarinic receptors have not been identified, suggesting that any cholinergic stimulation acts humorally.[128]

FUNCTIONS

A number of functions have been attributed to the apocrine glands, including roles as odoriferous sexual attractants, territorial markers, and warning signals. These glands play a role in increasing frictional resistance and tactile sensibility as well as in increasing evaporative heat loss in some species. The production of pheromones by the apocrine glands of many species is well established.[129]

Because the apocrine glands of humans do not begin to function until puberty and are odor producing, it is attractive to speculate that they have some sexual function, which may now be vestigial. There are high levels of 15-lipoxygenase-2 in the secretory cells of the apocrine gland. Its product, 15-hydroxyeicosatetraenoic, a ligand for the nuclear receptor PPARγ, may function as a signaling molecule and in secretion or differentiation.[128]

COMPOSITION OF SECRETION

When it is first secreted, the apocrine sweat of humans is milky, viscid, and without odor. Apocrine sweat contains three types of precursors: fatty acids, sulfanyl alkanols, and odiferous steroids, which are converted by bacteria on axillary skin, particularly corynebacterium striatum, into odiferous substances. Secretion of amino acid and steroid precursors is controlled by an ATP-dependent efflux pump multidrug resistance protein 8 (MRP8), encoded by the gene *ABCC11*, which is expressed in apocrine sweat glands. Axillary odor is significantly reduced in Asian populations that carry a single nucleotide polymorphism in this gene, which also affects earwax characteristics.[130]

MODE OF SECRETION

Despite previous reports for apocrine (decapitation), holocrine, and merocrine types of secretion in apocrine glands, current data indicate that the secretion of apocrine glands is merocrine. Cannulation of the duct of the human apocrine sweat gland has shown that secretion is pulsatile, and it is assumed that contractions of the myoepithelial cells surrounding the secretory cells are responsible for these pulsations.[131]

CONTROL OF SECRETION

The apocrine sweat glands of humans respond to emotive stimuli only after puberty. They can be stimulated by either epinephrine or norepinephrine given locally or systemically. Studies have shown that the apocrine glands are controlled mainly by adrenergic agonists,[132] although some cholinergic control also has been reported.[128,133] This is in contrast to the eccrine glands, which are under cholinergic control.

Although an intact nerve supply is a functional requirement of apocrine sweating, the demonstration of nerve endings or varicosities in close proximity to the glands has been difficult.[128,133] Local capillary circulation likely assists in conveying transmitter substance to the sweat gland cells, a form of neurohumoral transmission.

As would be expected, drugs that affect adrenergic systems also have an effect on apocrine sweat glands. Adrenergic neuron-blocking agents inhibit sweating, as do drugs that deplete the stores of transmitter substance in adrenergic neurons. Drugs that block specific adrenergic receptors also inhibit sweating, but the types of receptors that must be blocked differ in various species. The type of receptor that mediates the response of the apocrine glands of humans has not been elucidated.

REFERENCES

1. Zouboulis CC, Fimmel S, Ortmann J, et al. Sebaceous glands. In: Hoath SB, Maibach HI, eds. *Neonatal Skin—Structure and Function*, 2nd ed. New York: Marcel Dekker; 2003:59-88.
2. Pappas A. Sebum and sebaceous lipids. In: Zouboulis CC, Katsambas AD, Kligman AM, eds. *Pathogenesis and Treatment of Acne and Rosacea*. Berlin: Springer; 2014:33-41.
3. Zouboulis CC, Krieter A, Gollnick H, et al. Progressive differentiation of human sebocytes in vitro is characterized by increased cell size and altered antigenic expression and is regulated by culture duration and retinoids. *Exp Dermatol*. 1994;3:151-160.
4. Downie MMT, Guy R, Kealey T. Advances in sebaceous gland research: potential new approaches to acne management. *Int J Cosmet Sci*. 2004;26:291-311.
5. Benfenati A, Brillanti F. Sulla distribuzione delle ghiandole sebacee nella cute del corpo umino. *Arch Ital Dermatol*. 1939;15:33-42.
6. Montagna W. An introduction to sebaceous glands. *J Invest Dermatol*. 1974;62:120-123.
7. Thody AJ, Shuster S. Control and function of sebaceous glands. *Physiol Rev*. 1989;69:383-416.
8. Deplewski D, Rosenfield RL. Role of hormones in pilosebaceous unit development. *Endocrine Rev*. 2000;21:363-392.
9. Zouboulis CC, Nikolakis G, Dessinioti C. Molecular aspects of sebaceous differentiation. In: Zouboulis CC, Katsambas AD, Kligman AM, eds. *Pathogenesis and Treatment of Acne and Rosacea*. Berlin: Springer; 2014:19-26.
10. Merrill B, Gat U, DasGupta R, et al. Tcf3 and Lef1 regulate lineage differentiation of multipotent stem cells in skin. *Genes Dev*. 2001;15:1688-1705.
11. Niemann C, Unden AB, Lyle S, et al. Indian hedgehog and β-catenin signaling: role in the sebaceous lineage of normal and neoplastic mammalian epidermis. *Proc Natl Acad Sci U S A*. 2003;100(suppl 1):11873-11880.
12. Allen M, Grachtchouk M, Sheng H, et al. Hedgehog signaling regulates sebaceous gland development. *Am J Pathol*. 2003;163:2173-2178.
13. Lo Celso C, Berta MA, Braun KM, et al. Characterization of bipotent epidermal progenitors derived from human sebaceous gland: contrasting roles of c-myc and β-catenin. *Stem Cells*. 2008;26:1241-1252.
14. Magnúsdóttir E, Kalachikov S, Mizukoshi K, et al. Epidermal terminal differentiation depends on B lymphocyte-induced maturation protein-1. *Proc Natl Acad Sci U S A*. 2007;104:14988–14993.
15. Horsley V, Elder HY, Montgomery I, et al. Blimp1 defines a progenitor population that governs cellular input to the sebaceous gland. *Cell*. 2006;126:597-609.
16. Niemann C, Horsley V. Development and homeostasis of the sebaceous gland. *Semin Cell Dev Biol*. 2012;23:928-936.
17. Tosti A. A comparison of the histodynamics of sebaceous glands and epidermis in man: a microanatomic and morphometric study. *J Invest Dermatol*. 1974;62:147-152.
18. Jenkinson DM, Elder HY, Montgomery I, et al. Comparative studies of the ultrastructure of the sebaceous gland. *Tissue Cell*. 1985;17:683-698.
19. Kurokawa I, Mayer-da-Silva A, Gollnick H, et al. Monoclonal antibody labeling for cytokeratins and filaggrin in the human pilosebaceous unit of normal, seborrhoeic and acne skin. *J Invest Dermatol*. 1988;91:566-571.
20. Zouboulis CC, Tsatsou F. Anatomy of the sebaceous gland. In: Zouboulis CC, Katsambas AD, Kligman AM, eds. *Pathogenesis and Treatment of Acne and Rosacea*. Berlin: Springer; 2014:27-31.
21. Xia L, Zouboulis C, Detmar M, et al. Isolation of human sebaceous glands and cultivation of sebaceous gland-derived cells as an in vitro model. *J Invest Dermatol*. 1989;93:315-321.
22. Fischer H, Fumicz J, Rossiter H, et al. Holocrine secretion of sebum is a unique DNase2-dependent mode of programmed cell death. *J Invest Dermatol*. 2017;137:587-594.
23. Nicolaides N. Skin lipids: their biochemical uniqueness. *Science*. 1974;186:19-26.
24. Picardo M, Ottaviani M, Camera E, et al. Sebaceous gland lipids. *Dermatoendocrinol*. 2009;1:68-71.
25. Georgel P, Crozat K, Lauth X, et al. A TLR2-responsive lipid effector pathway protects mammals against Gram-positive bacterial skin infections. *Infect Immun*. 2005;73:4512-4521.
26. Camera E, Ludovici M, Galante M, et al. Comprehensive analysis of the major lipid classes in sebum by rapid resolution high-performance liquid chromatography and electrospray mass spectrometry. *J Lipid Res*. 2010;51:3377-3388.
27. Nikkari T. Comparative chemistry of sebum. *J Invest Dermatol*. 1974;62:257-267.
28. Kligman AM. The uses of sebum? In. Montagna W, Ellis RA, Silver AF, eds. *Advances in Biology of Skin. Vol IV. The Sebaceous Glands*. Oxford: Pergamon Press; 1963:110-112.
29. Cunliffe WJ, Shuster S. Pathogenesis of acne. *Lancet*. 1969;1(7597):685-687.
30. Flurh JW, Mao-Qiang M, Brown BE, et al. Glycerol regulates stratum corneum hydration in sebaceous gland deficient (Asebia) mice. *J Invest Dermatol*. 2003;120:728-737.
31. Zouboulis CC, Jourdan E, Picardo M. Acne is an inflammatory disease and alterations of sebum composition initiate acne lesions. *J Eur Acad Dermatol Venereol*. 2014;28:527-532.

32. Wille JJ, Kydonieus A. Palmitoleic acid isomer (C16:1d6) is the active antimicrobial fatty acid in human skin sebum. *Skin Pharmacol Appl Skin Physiol*. 2003;16:176-187.
33. Gebhart W, Metze D, Jurecka W. Identification of secretory immunoglobulin A in human sebaceous and sweat glands. *J Invest Dermatol*. 1989;92:648.
34. Thiele JJ, Weber SU, Packer L. Sebaceous gland secretion is a major physiologic route of vitamin E delivery to skin. *J Invest Dermatol*. 1999;113:1006-1010.
35. Lee DY, Yamasaki K, Rudsil J, et al. Sebocytes express functional cathelicidin antimicrobial peptides and can act to kill propionibacterium acnes. *J Invest Dermatol*. 2008;128:1863-1866.
36. Lai Y, Gallo RL. AMPed up immunity: how antimicrobial peptides have multiple roles in immune defense. *Trends Immunol*. 2009;30:131-141.
37. Nakatsuji T, Kao MC, Zhang L, et al. Sebum free fatty acids enhance the innate immune defense of human sebocytes by upregulating beta-defensin-2 expression. *J Invest Dermatol*. 2010;130:985-984.
38. Oeff MK, Seltmann H, Hiroi N, et al. Differential regulation of Toll-like receptor and CD14 pathways by retinoids and corticosteroids in human sebocytes. *Dermatology*. 2006;213:266.
39. Lovászi M, Mattii M, Eyerich K, et al. Sebum lipids influence macrophage polarization and activation. *Br J Dermatol*. 2017;177:1671-1682.
40. Mattii M, Lovászi M, Garzorz N, et al. Sebocytes contribute to skin inflammation by promoting the differentiation of Th17 cells. *Br J Dermatol*. 2018;178(3):722-730.
41. Lovászi M, Szegedi A, Zouboulis CC, et al. Sebaceous immunobiology is orchestrated by sebum lipids. *Dermatoendocrinol*. 2018;10:e1375636.
42. Zouboulis CC, Baron JM, Böhm M, et al. Frontiers in sebaceous gland biology and pathology. *Exp Dermatol*. 2008;17:542-551.
43. Zouboulis CC, Adjaye J, Akamatsu H, et al. Human skin stem cells and the ageing process. *Exp Gerontol*. 2008;43:986-997.
44. Fuchs E. Skin stem cells: rising to the surface. *J Cell Biol*. 2008;180:273-284.
45. Serri F, Huber WM. The development of sebaceous glands in man. In: Montagna W, Ellis RA, Silver AF, eds. *Advances in Biology of Skin. Vol. IV. Sebaceous Glands*. Oxford: Pergamon; 1963:1-18.
46. Fenske NA, Lober CW. Structural and functional changes of normal aging skin. *J Am Acad Dermatol*. 1986;15:571-585.
47. Zouboulis CC, Dessinioti C. Experimental models of the sebaceous gland. In: Zouboulis CC, Katsambas AD, Kligman AM, eds. *Pathogenesis and Treatment of Acne and Rosacea*. Berlin: Springer; 2014:43-49.
48. Zouboulis CC, Xia L, Akamatsu H, et al. The human sebocyte culture model provides new insights into development and management of seborrhoea and acne. *Dermatology*. 1998;196:21-31.
49. Zouboulis CC, Schagen S, Alestas T. The sebocyte culture—a model to study the pathophysiology of the sebaceous gland in sebostasis, seborrhoea and acne. *Arch Dermatol Res*. 2008;300:397-413.
50. Schneider M, Zouboulis CC. Primary sebocytes and sebaceous gland cell lines for studying sebaceous lipogenesis and sebaceous gland diseases. *Exp Dermatol*. 2018;27(5):484-488.
51. Nikolakis G, Stratakis CA, Kanaki T, et al. Skin steroidogenesis in health and disease. *Rev Endocr Metab Disord*. 2016;17:247-258.
52. Zouboulis CC, Picardo M, Ju Q, et al. Beyond acne: current aspects of sebaceous gland biology and function. *Rev Endocr Metab Disord*. 2017;17:319-334.
53. Hong I, Lee MH, Na TY, et al. LXRα enhances lipid synthesis in SZ95 sebocytes. *J Invest Dermatol*. 2008;128:1266-1272.
54. Schmuth M, Watson RE, Deplewski D, et al. Nuclear hormone receptors in human skin. *Horm Metab Res*. 2007;39:96-105.
55. Zouboulis CC. Sebaceous cells in monolayer culture. *In Vitro Cell Dev Biol*. 1992;28A:699.
56. Zouboulis CC. Sebaceous gland in human skin—the fantastic future of a skin appendage. *J Invest Dermatol*. 2003;120:xiv-xv.
57. Alestas T, Ganceviciene R, Fimmel S, et al. Enzymes involved in the biosynthesis of leukotriene B4 and prostaglandin E2 are active in sebaceous glands. *J Mol Med*. 2006;84:75-87.
58. Imperato-McGinley J, Gautier T, Cai LQ, et al. The androgen control of sebum production. Studies of subjects with dihydrotestosterone deficiency and complete androgen insensitivity. *J Clin Endocrinol Metab*. 1993;76:524-528.
59. Chen W, Tsai SJ, Sheu HM, et al. Testosterone synthesized in cultured human SZ95 sebocytes mainly derives from dehydroepiandrosterone. *Exp Dermatol*. 2010;19:470-472.
60. Chen W, Thiboutot D, Zouboulis CC. Cutaneous androgen metabolism: basic research and clinical perspectives. *J Invest Dermatol*. 2002;119:992-1007.
61. Fritsch M, Orfanos CE, Zouboulis CC. Sebocytes are the key regulators of androgen homeostasis in human skin. *J Invest Dermatol*. 2001;116:793-800.
62. Azmahani A, Nakamura Y, Felizola SJ, et al. Steroidogenic enzymes, their related transcription factors and nuclear receptors in human sebaceous glands under normal and pathological conditions. *J Steroid Biochem Mol Biol*. 2014;144B:268-279.
63. Zouboulis CC. Isotretinoin revisited—pluripotent effects on human sebaceous gland cells. *J Invest Dermatol*. 2006;126:2154-2156.
64. Ganceviciene R, Zouboulis CC. Isotretinoin for acne vulgaris: state-of-the-art treatment for acne vulgaris. *J Dtsch Dermatol Ges*. 2010;8(suppl 1):S47-S59.
65. Zouboulis CC, Korge B, Akamatsu H, et al. Effects of 13-*cis*-retinoic acid, all-*trans*-retinoic acid and acitretin on the proliferation, lipid synthesis and keratin expression of cultured human sebocytes in vitro. *J Invest Dermatol*. 1991;96:792-797.
66. Tsukada M, Schröder M, Roos TC, et al. 13-*cis* Retinoic acid exerts its specific activity on human sebocytes through selective intracellular isomerization to all-*trans* retinoic acid and binding to retinoid acid receptors. *J Invest Dermatol*. 2000;115:321-327.
67. Hommel L, Geiger JM, Harms M, et al. Sebum excretion rate in subjects treated with oral all-*trans*-retinoic acid. *Dermatology*. 1996;193:127-130.
68. Mastrofrancesco A, Ottaviani M, Cardinali G, et al. Pharmacological PPARγ modulation regulates sebogenesis and inflammation in SZ95 human sebocytes. *Biochem Pharmacol*. 2017;138:96-106.
69. Trivedi NR, Cong Z, Nelson AM, et al. Peroxisome proliferator-activated receptors increase human sebum production. *J Invest Dermatol*. 2006;126:2002-2009.
70. Zouboulis CC. Sebaceous gland receptors. *Dermatoendocrinol*. 2009;1:77-80.

71. Russell LE, Harrison WJ, Bahta AW, et al. Characterization of liver X receptor expression and function in human skin and the pilosebaceous unit. *Exp Dermatol*. 2007;16:844-852.
72. Gross DN, van den Heuvel AP, Birnbaum MJ. The role of FoxO in the regulation of metabolism. *Oncogene*. 2008;27:2320-2336.
73. Dahlhoff M, Camera E, Picardo M, et al. PLIN2, the major perilipin regulated during sebocyte differentiation, controls sebaceous lipid accumulation in vitro and sebaceous gland size in vivo. *Biochim Biophys Acta Gen Subjects*. 2013;1830:4642-4649.
74. Camera E, Dahlhoff M, Ludovici M, et al. Perilipin 3 modulates specific lipogenic pathways in SZ95 sebocytes. *Exp Dermatol*. 2014;23:759-761.
75. Dahlhoff M, Camera E, Picardo M, et al. Angiopoietin-like 4, a protein strongly induced during sebocyte differentiation, regulates sebaceous lipogenesis but is dispensable for sebaceous gland function in vivo. *J Dermatol Sci*. 2014;75:148-150.
76. Borowczyk-Michalowska J, Zimolag E, Konieczny P, et al. Stage-specific embryonic antigen-4 (SSEA-4) as a distinguishing marker between eccrine and apocrine origin of ducts of sweat glands. *J Invest Dermatol*. 2017;137(11):2437-2440.
77. Szabo G. The number of eccrine sweat glands in human skin. In: Montagna W, Ellis R, Silver A, eds. *Advances in Biology of Skin*. New York: Pergamon; 1962:1.
78. Sato K, Dobson RL. Regional and individual variations in the function of the human eccrine sweat gland. *J Invest Dermatol*. 1970;54(6):443-449.
79. Schittek B, Hipfel R, Sauer B, et al. Dermcidin: a novel human antibiotic peptide secreted by sweat glands. *Nat Immunol*. 2001;2(12):1133-1137.
80. Ali RS, Falconer A, Ikram M, et al. Expression of the peptide antibiotics human beta defensin-1 and human beta defensin-2 in normal human skin. *J Invest Dermatol*. 2001;117(1):106-111.
81. Murakami M, Lopez-Garcia B, Braff M, et al. Postsecretory processing generates multiple cathelicidins for enhanced topical antimicrobial defense. *J Immunol*. 2004;172(5):3070-3077.
82. Hanukoglu I, Boggula VR, Vaknine H, et al. Expression of epithelial sodium channel (ENaC) and CFTR in the human epidermis and epidermal appendages. *Histochem Cell Biol*. 2017;147(1):733-748.
83. Ellis R. Eccrine sweat glands: electron microscopy, cytochemistry and anatomy. In: Jadassohn J, ed. *Handbuch der Haut und Geschlechtskrankheiten*. Berlin: Springer-Verlag; 1967:223.
84. Sato F, Owen M, Matthes R, et al. Functional and morphological changes in the eccrine sweat gland with heat acclimation. *J Appl Physiol*. 1990;69(1):232-236.
85. Saga K, Sato K. Ultrastructural localization of ouabain-sensitive, K-dependent p-nitrophenyl phosphatase activity in monkey eccrine sweat gland. *J Histochem Cytochem*. 1988;36(8):1023-1030.
86. Sato K, Nishiyama A, Kobayashi M. Mechanical properties and functions of the myoepithelium in the eccrine sweat gland. *Am J Physiol*. 1979;237(3):C177-C184.
87. Hashimoto K, Gross BG, Lever WF. The ultrastructure of the skin of human embryos. I. The intraepidermal eccrine sweat duct. *J Invest Dermatol*. 1965;45(3):139-151.
88. Sato K, Dobson RL, Mali JW. Enzymatic basis for the active transport of sodium in the eccrine sweat gland. Localization and characterization of Na-K-adenosine triphosphatase. *J Invest Dermatol*. 1971;57(1):10-16.
89. Nadel ER, Bullard RW, Stolwijk JA. Importance of skin temperature in the regulation of sweating. *J Appl Physiol*. 1971;31(1):80-87.
90. Freedman RR. Hot flashes: behavioral treatments, mechanisms, and relation to sleep. *Am J Med*. 2005;118(suppl 12B):124-130.
91. Johnson R, Spalding J. *Disorders of the Autonomic Nervous System*. Philadelphia: FA Davis; 1974.
92. Hu Y, Converse C, Lyons MC, et al. Neural control of sweat secretion: a review. *Br J Dermatol*. 2018;178(6):1246-1256.
93. Kreyden OP, Scheidegger EP. Anatomy of the sweat glands, pharmacology of botulinum toxin, and distinctive syndromes associated with hyperhidrosis. *Clin Dermatol*. 2004;22(1):40-44.
94. Coon J, Rothman S. The sweat response to drugs with nicotine-like action. *J Pharmacol Exp Ther*. 1941;23:1.
95. Faden AI, Chan P, Mendoza E. Progressive isolated segmental anhidrosis. *Arch Neurol*. 1982;39(3):172-175.
96. Suzuki Y, Ohtsuyama M, Samman G, et al. Ionic basis of methacholine-induced shrinkage of dissociated eccrine clear cells. *J Membr Biol*. 1991;123(1):33-41.
97. Buceta JM, Bradshaw CM, Szabadi E. Hyperresponsiveness of eccrine sweat glands to carbachol in anxiety neurosis: comparison of male and female patients. *Br J Clin Pharmacol*. 1985;19(6):817-822.
98. Sato K, Sato F. Defective beta adrenergic response of cystic fibrosis sweat glands in vivo and in vitro. *J Clin Invest*. 1984;73(6):1763-1771.
99. Prout BJ, Wardell WM. Sweating and peripheral blood flow in patients with phaeochromocytoma. *Clin Sci*. 1969;36(1):109-117.
100. Sato K. The physiology, pharmacology, and biochemistry of the eccrine sweat gland. *Rev Physiol Biochem Pharmacol*. 1977;79:51-131.
101. Sato K, Sato F. Na^+, K^+, H^+, Cl^-, and Ca^{2+} concentrations in cystic fibrosis eccrine sweat in vivo and in vitro. *J Lab Clin Med*. 1990;115(4):504-511.
102. Pagaduan JV, Ali M, Dowlin M, et al. Revisiting sweat chloride test results based on recent guidelines for diagnosis of cystic fibrosis. *Pract Lab Med*. 2018;10(1):34-37.
103. Sato K, Dobson RL. Glucose metabolism of the isolated eccrine sweat gland. II. The relation between glucose metabolism and sodium transport. *J Clin Invest*. 1973;52(9):2166-2174.
104. Brusilow SW, Gordes EH. The permeability of the sweat gland to nonelectrolytes. *Am J Dis Child*. 1966;112(4):328-333.
105. Brusilow SW, Gordes EH. Ammonia secretion in sweat. *Am J Physiol*. 1968;214(3):513-517.
106. Page CO Jr, Remington JS. Immunologic studies in normal human sweat. *J Lab Clin Med*. 1967;69(4):634-650.
107. Jirka M, Blanicky P. Micro-isoelectric focusing of proteins in pilocarpine-induced sweat. *Clin Chim Acta*. 1971;31(2):329-332.
108. Yokozeki H, Hibino T, Takemura T, et al. Cysteine proteinase inhibitor in eccrine sweat is derived from sweat gland. *Am J Physiol*. 1991;260(2 Pt 2):R314-R320.
109. Garden JW. Plasma and sweat histamine concentrations after heat exposure and physical exercise. *J Appl Physiol*. 1966;21(2):631-635.
110. Forstrom L, Goldyne ME, Winkelmann RK. Prostaglandin activity in human eccrine sweat. *Prostaglandins*. 1974;7(6):459-464.
111. Seutter E, Sutorius AH. The vitamin K derivatives of some skin-mucins. 3. A route of oxygen transfer. *Int J Vitam Nutr Res*. 1971;41(4):529-536.

112. Shah VP, Epstein WL, Riegelman S. Role of sweat in accumulation of orally administered griseofulvin in skin. *J Clin Invest*. 1974;53(6):1673-1678.
113. Harris R, Jones HE, Artis WM. Orally administered ketoconazole: route of delivery to the human stratum corneum. *Antimicrob Agents Chemother*. 1983;24(6):876-882.
114. Vree TB, Muskens AT, van Rossum JM. Excretion of amphetamines in human sweat. *Arch Int Pharmacodyn Ther*. 1972;199(2):311-317.
115. Bolognia JL, Cooper DL, Glusac EJ. Toxic erythema of chemotherapy: a useful clinical term. *J Am Acad Dermatol*. 2008;59(3):524-529.
116. Sato K. The physiology and pharmacology of the eccrine sweat gland. In: Goldsmith L, ed. *Biochemistry and Physiology of the Skin*. Oxford: Oxford University Press; 1983:596.
117. Takemura T, Sato F, Saga K, et al. Intracellular ion concentrations and cell volume during cholinergic stimulation of eccrine secretory coil cells. *J Membr Biol*. 1991;119(3):211-219.
118. Reddy MM, Quinton PM. Cytosolic potassium controls CFTR deactivation in human sweat duct. *Am J Physiol Cell Physiol*. 2006;291(1):C122-C129.
119. Sato K, Sato F. Cyclic AMP accumulation in the beta adrenergic mechanism of eccrine sweat secretion. *Pflugers Arch*. 1981;390(1):49-53.
120. Garty H, Palmer LG. Epithelial sodium channels: function, structure, and regulation. *Physiol Rev*. 1997;77(2):359-396.
121. Granger D, Marsolais M, Burry J, et al. Na^+/H^+ exchangers in the human eccrine sweat duct. *Am J Physiol Cell Physiol*. 2003;285(5):C1047-C1058.
122. Yamaga K, Murota H, Tamura A, et al. Claudin-3 loss causes leakage of sweat from the sweat gland to contribute to the pathogenesis of atopic dermatitis. *J Invest Dermatol*. 2018;138(6):1279-1287.
123. Granger D, Marsolais M, Burry J, et al. V-type H^+-ATPase in the human eccrine sweat duct: immunolocalization and functional demonstration. *Am J Physiol Cell Physiol*. 2002;282(6):C1454-C1460.
124. Nejsum LN, Praetorius J, Nielsen S. NKCC1 and NHE1 are abundantly expressed in the basolateral plasma membrane of secretory coil cells in rat, mouse, and human sweat glands. *Am J Physiol Cell Physiol*. 2005;289(2):C333-C340.
125. de Carolis P, Magnifico F, Pierangeli G, et al. Transient hypohidrosis induced by topiramate. *Epilepsia*. 2003;44(7):974-976.
126. Shappell SB, Keeney DS, Zhang J, et al. 15-Lipoxygenase-2 expression in benign and neoplastic sebaceous glands and other cutaneous adnexa. *J Invest Dermatol*. 2001;117(1):36-43.
127. Charles A. An electron microscopic study of the human axillary apocrine gland. *J Anat*. 1959;93(2):226-232.
128. Lindsay SL, Holmes S, Corbett AD, et al. Innervation and receptor profiles of the human apocrine (epitrichial) sweat gland: routes for intervention in bromhidrosis. *Br J Dermatol*. 2008;159(3):653-660.
129. Mykytowycz R. The behavioural role of the mammalian skin glands. *Naturwissenschaften*. 1972;59(4):133-139.
130. Martin A, Saathoff M, Kuhn F, et al. A functional ABCC11 allele is essential in the biochemical formation of human axillary odor. *J Invest Dermatol*. 2010;130(2):529-540.
131. Sato K. Pharmacological responsiveness of the myoepithelium of the isolated human axillary apocrine sweat gland. *Br J Dermatol*. 1980;103(3):235-243.
132. Wu JM, Mamelak AJ, Nussbaum R, et al. Botulinum toxin a in the treatment of chromhidrosis. *Dermatol Surg*. 2005;31(8 Pt 1):963-965.
133. Robertshaw D. Apocrine sweat glands. In: Goldsmith L, ed. *Physiology, Biochemistry and Molecular Biology of the Skin*. Oxford: Oxford University Press; 1991:763.

Chapter 7 :: Biology of Hair Follicles
:: George Cotsarelis & Vladimir Botchkarev

第七章
毛囊生物学

中文导读

本章共分为6节：①毛发的演变/进化和功能；②毛发胚胎学；③毛发解剖学；④毛囊周期；⑤毛发色素形成；⑥结论。本章详细地阐述了毛囊的发育生物学等功能。

第一节介绍了毛发的功能除了常规的隔离和保护作用外，随着社会的发展，其对社会交往的影响更受关注。

第二节介绍了毛囊发育分为八个阶段，重点介绍了第一阶段初级毛胚，提到Wnt/β连环蛋白途径、Eda、FGF、Bmp等调节毛囊发育的重点信号通路分子。

第三节介绍了毛发解剖学，不仅从宏观层面阐述了不同个体，以及同一个体在不同时期的头发类型和头发的弯曲度的差异，而且从显微层面介绍了毛发从外到内主要包括结缔组织鞘、外根鞘、内根鞘、角质层、发干皮质和发干髓质，每一部分都以不同的毛囊特有角蛋白表达为特征。

第四节介绍了毛囊周期分为生长期、退行期、休止期，毛囊干细胞被认为是毛囊周期性再生的控制因素。近来米尔纳等提出了毛囊的第四个周期概念"外生期"，即脱发到再生的阶段，认为这是一个主动过程。

第五节毛发色素形成，介绍了这是黑素合成和运输相互紧密协作的结果。毛发中存在毛囊黑素细胞干细胞，受TGF-β和Notch信号通路的调控，不断补充毛囊中产色素的黑素细胞，维持毛发色素。

第六节总结了毛囊是上皮和间质之间复杂的信号相互作用的结果，许多分子在毛囊形成中起到了作用。

〔粟　娟〕

AT-A-GLANCE

- The primary purpose of hair in humans is to influence social interactions.
- Hair follicle development depends on interactions between epithelial and mesenchymal cells. The genes important for this interaction are slowly being elucidated.
- Genes important for hair follicle development also play a role in hair follicle cycling.
- The hair follicle bulge possesses stem cells important for the continual regeneration of the follicle during cycling.
- Hair pigmentation depends on melanocyte stem cells and differentiated cells in the follicle. Many genes important for melanocyte behavior and hair pigmentation have been defined.

EVOLUTION AND FUNCTION OF HAIR

Hair is found only in mammals, in which during the course of evolution, its primary roles were to serve as insulation and protection from the elements. In contemporary humans, however, hair's main purpose revolves around its profound role in social interactions. Loss of hair (alopecia) and excessive hair growth in unwanted areas (hirsutism and hypertrichosis) can lead to significant psychological and emotional distress that supports a multibillion-dollar effort to reverse these conditions.

Much progress has been made in understanding hair growth, and as a result, new treatments for alopecia are on the horizon.[1,2] These advances resulted from the interest of developmental biologists and other investigators in the hair follicle as a model for a wide range of biological processes. As each hair follicle cyclically regenerates, it recapitulates its initial development. Many growth factors and receptors important during hair follicle development also regulate hair follicle cycling.[3,4] The hair follicle possesses keratinocyte and melanocyte stem cells, nerves, and vasculature that are important in healthy and diseased skin.[5-7] To appreciate this emerging information and to properly assess a patient with hair loss or excess hair (see Chaps. 85-90), an understanding of the anatomy and development of the hair follicle is essential.

EMBRYOLOGY

Morphologically, hair follicle development has been divided into eight consecutive stages, several of which are illustrated in Fig. 7-1. Each stage is characterized by unique expression patterns for growth factors and their receptors, growth factor antagonists, adhesion molecules, and intracellular signal transduction components.[8-10] Promising advances in understanding the molecular mechanisms behind hair follicle development arose through the discovery that mammalian counterparts (homologs) of genes important for normal *Drosophila* (fruit fly) development also affect hair follicle development. *Decapentaplegic (Dpp/BMP), engrailed (en), Homeobox (hox), hedgehog/patched (hh/ptc), notch, wingless/armadillo (wg/wnt/catenin),* and *branchless (Fgf)* genes are all critical for hair follicle and vertebrate development in general (reviewed in [8-10]). These genes were all first discovered in *Drosophila*; thus, most of the names assigned to them describe the peculiar appearance (phenotype) of the flies carrying mutations in these genes.[11]

Follicle formation begins on the head and then moves downward to the remainder of the body in utero. The first hairs formed are lanugo hairs, which are nonpigmented, soft, and fine. Lanugo hair is typically shed between the 32nd and 36th weeks of gestation, although approximately one third of newborns still retain their lanugo hair for up to several weeks after birth.

Patterning genes, called homeobox genes, which are precisely organized in the genome so that they are expressed in strict temporal sequences and spatial patterns during development, likely are responsible for the nonrandom and symmetrical distribution of hair follicles over the body.[11,12] In adult mice, homeobox gene expression reappears in hair follicles and serves to maintain normal hair shaft production.[13] *Engrailed*, a type of homeobox gene, is responsible for dorsal-ventral patterning, and mice lacking *engrailed* develop hair follicles on their footpads.[14]

Although hair follicles and hairs all share the same basic anatomy, their growth, size, shape, pigmentation and other characteristics differ widely based on body location and variation among individuals. Many of these characteristics are established during development but are then profoundly altered by hormonal influences later in life. We are beginning to understand the genes controlling hair length, curl, and distribution because of elegant genetic studies on dogs. These studies reveal that fibroblast growth factor-5 (FGF-5), Keratin 71, and R-spondin 2 influence length, curl, and distribution, respectively.[15] In humans, thicker hair found in Asians is associated with increased activity of Edar.[16]

The size of many types of follicles changes drastically several times throughout life. For example, lanugo hair follicles, which produce hair shafts several centimeters long, convert to vellus follicles that produce small hairs that protrude only slightly from the skin surface. Later in life, vellus follicles on the male beard enlarge into terminal follicles that generate thick, long hairs. On the scalp of genetically predisposed individuals, terminal follicles miniaturize and form effete, microscopic hairs.

EPITHELIAL PLACODE OR PRIMARY HAIR GERM

In the human fetus, hair follicles develop from small collections of cells, called epithelial placodes, which corresponds to stage 1 of hair follicle development and first appear around 10 weeks of gestation (see Fig. 7-1). The epithelial placode then expands to form the "primary hair germ" whose progeny eventually generate the entire epithelial portion of the hair follicle.[17]

The hair follicle placode is formed through the centripetal migration of the basal epidermal cells and their compaction.[18] The cells of the hair placode and germ express placental cadherin and become oriented vertically, losing their desmosomes, hemidesmosomes, and epithelial cadherin, which decreases their adhesion to their neighbors.[19-21] Dermal cells beneath the hair follicle placode form a condensation, which later develops into the dermal papilla.[22] Signaling between the epithelial and mesenchymal cells during placode formation involves several signaling pathways (Wnt, Eda, Fgf, Bmp) operating via multiple feedback mechanisms[23] (see Fig. 7-1). Extensive signaling between epithelial and mesenchymal cells results in the appearance of

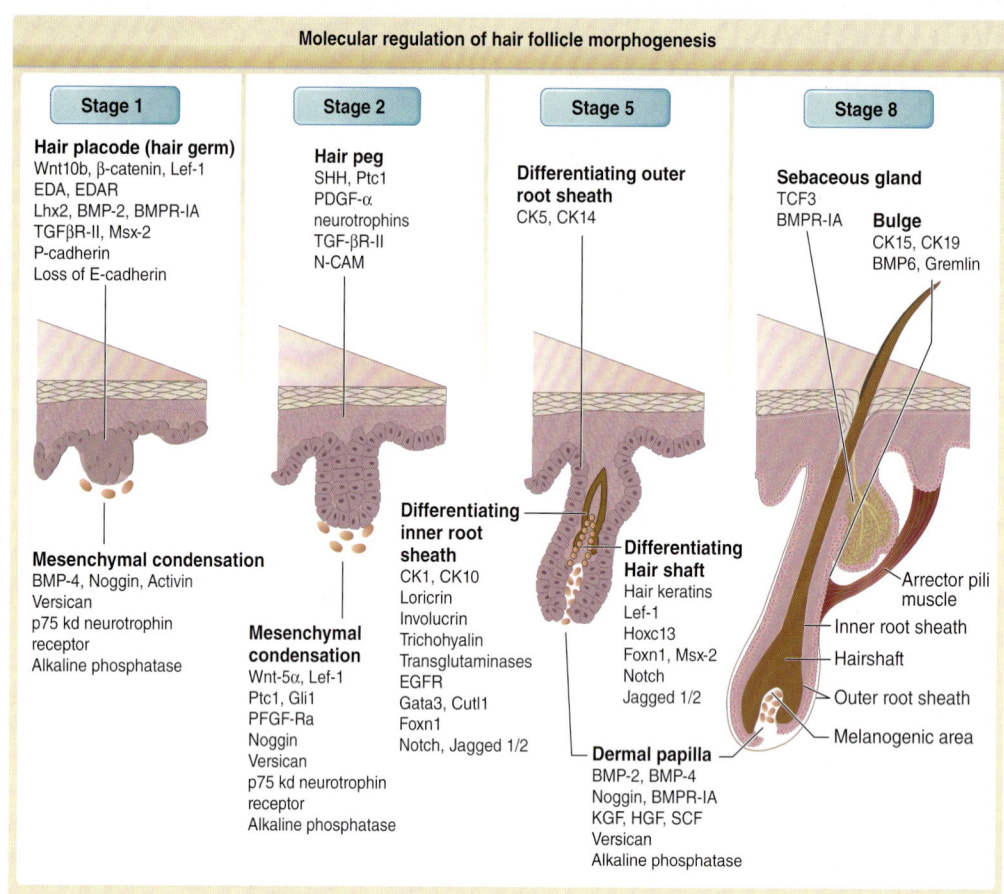

Figure 7-1 Molecular regulation of hair follicle morphogenesis. The schematic shows the expression of different growth factors, their receptors, adhesion, and cell matrix molecules; transcriptional regulators in hair follicle epithelium; and mesenchyme during distinct stages of hair follicle development. BMP, bone morphogenetic protein; BMPR-IA, bone morphogenetic protein receptor, type IA; CK, keratin 5; Cutl1, cut-like 1; E-cadherin, epithelial cadherin; EDA, ectodysplasin; EDAR, ectodysplasin receptor; EGFR, epidermal growth factor receptor; Foxn1, forkhead box N1; Gata3, GATA binding protein 3; Gli1, glioma-associated oncogene homolog 1; HGF, hepatocyte growth factor; Hoxc13, homeobox C13; KGF, keratinocyte growth factor; Lef-1, lymphoid enhancer factor 1; Lhx2, LIM homeobox 2; N-CAM, neural cell adhesion molecule; P-cadherin, placental cadherin; PDGF-α, platelet-derived growth factor α polypeptide; PFGF-Rα, platelet-derived growth factor receptor α; Ptc1, patched1; SCF, stem cell factor; Shh, sonic hedgehog; TCF3, transcription factor 3; TGF-βR-II, transforming growth factor-β receptor 2.

distinct sets of lineage-specific transcription factors (Lhx2, Sox9, Msx2, Foxi3) in the epithelial progenitor cells that promote differentiation toward a hair follicle fate. In turn, the dermal condensate beneath the hair placode expresses the extracellular matrix proteoglycan versican, p75 kD neurotrophin receptor, as well as the transcription factors Tbx18 and Sox2 (reviewed in [24-26]). These factors allow for maturation of the dermal condensate into the dermal papilla. The dermal papilla drives the growth of the fully formed follicle. These reciprocal signals pass through the intervening basement membrane, which undergoes alterations in its morphology and chemical composition that may alter its ability to sequester growth factors and binding proteins, thus possibly modulating the epithelial–mesenchymal interactions.

Many of these regulatory molecules important for the formation of the hair follicle have been defined, but how they interact to generate hair follicles in an otherwise homogeneous epithelium has yet to be determined. In one model, the spacing and size of placodes are regulated by a dermal signal, which varies in character in different body regions. The dermal signal occurs uniformly within each body region and triggers the activation of promoters and repressors of follicle fate in the epithelium that then compete with one another, resulting in the establishment of a regular array of follicles.[9,27-29] Differences in the levels of promoter and repressor activation could account for regional differences in the size and spacing of follicles. Consistent with this model, several positive and negative regulators of hair follicle fate are initially expressed uniformly in the epidermis and subsequently become localized to placodes.

One of the earliest molecular pathways that positively regulate hair follicle initiation is the WNT/β-catenin pathway. β-catenin is the downstream mediator of WNT signaling. WNT proteins bind to receptors on the cell membrane and, through a series of signals, inhibit the degradation of cytoplasmic β-catenin. β-Catenin then translocates to the nucleus, forming a complex with the LEF/TCF family of transcription factors and resulting in expression of downstream genes.[9] Activation of the β-catenin pathway appears necessary for establishing epithelial competence, a state in which the epithelial tissue has the potential to form a hair follicle. Normally, the β-catenin pathway is inactive in the adult epidermis, but by artificially activating β-catenin in epidermal basal cells of adult transgenic mice, hair follicles develop de novo.[30] This remarkable finding could eventually have therapeutic implications, although constant activation of this pathway in the hair follicle also results in pilomatricomas and trichofolliculomas, two types of relatively rare cutaneous tumors.[30,31] Whereas dermal Wnt/β-catenin signaling is also important for the survival and specification of the mesenchymal condensate cells, loss of dermal β-catenin results in arrest of hair follicle development.[32]

Ectodysplasin (*EDA*), a molecule related to tumor necrosis factor (TNF), and its receptor (*EDAR*) also are part of another major pathway that stimulate early follicle development in both mouse and human.[27,33] *EDA* gene mutations cause X-linked anhidrotic ectodermal dysplasia, a syndrome associated with decreased numbers of hair follicles, and defects of the teeth and sweat glands (see Chap. 131).[34] The *EDAR* gene is mutated in autosomal recessive and dominant hypohidrotic ectodermal dysplasias, causing identical phenotypes to those resulting from *EDA* mutations. The mouse *Edar* gene is expressed ubiquitously in the epithelium before placode formation and then becomes restricted to placodes, but the *Eda* gene is ubiquitously expressed even after placode formation.[27] Mice with mutations in these genes have the same phenotype as humans with similar mutations, and mice overexpressing Eda in the epidermis show formation of "fused" follicles because of the loss of proper spacing between neighboring hair placodes.[27,35,36] Variations in the *EDAR* gene causing higher EDAR activity are associated with thicker hair.[16]

In contrast to EDA and EDAR, which promote hair follicle development, members of the bone morphogenetic protein (BMP) family inhibit follicle formation. Whereas *Bmp2* is expressed diffusely in the ectoderm but then localizes to the early placode and underlying mesenchyme, *Bmp4* is expressed in the early dermal condensate.[37,38] BMP signaling inhibits placode formation, and neutralization of BMP activity by its antagonist Noggin promotes placode fate, at least in part via positive regulation of Lef-1 expression.[37,39-41] Mice lacking Noggin have fewer hair follicles than normal and delayed follicular development.[41] The Notch pathway also appears to play a role in determining the follicular pattern. The Notch ligand delta-1 is normally expressed in the mesenchyme underlying the placode,[42-44] and when misexpressed in a small part of the epithelium, it promotes and accelerates placode formation while suppressing placode formation in surrounding cells.[42,45]

Another secreted protein present in the follicular placode that plays a major role in epithelial-mesenchymal signaling is Sonic hedgehog (SHH).[46,47] Skin from mice lacking Shh have extremely effete hair follicles with poorly developed dermal papillae.[48-50] Patched1 (PTC1), the receptor for SHH, is expressed in the germ cells and the underlying dermal papilla, suggesting that SHH may have both autocrine and paracrine inductive properties necessary for hair germ and dermal papilla formation.[51] Patched is the gene deficient in basal cell nevus syndrome.[52]

THE BULBOUS PEG OR HAIR BUD

In the next stage of development, the bulbous peg or hair bud (or stage 2 of hair follicle development; see Fig. 7-1) is formed by elongation of the hair germ into a cord of epithelial cells. The mesenchymal cells at the sides of the peg will develop into the connective tissue sheath of the hair follicle, and those at the tip of the peg will develop into the dermal papilla. Proliferation of the epithelial cells and lateral expansion of the follicular placode are regulated by Shh, which also promotes morphogenesis of the dermal papilla expressing the corresponding receptors.[48,49] The deepest portion of the follicle peg forms a bulbous structure surrounding the dermal papilla and goes on to form the matrix of the hair follicle, which gives rise to the hair shaft and inner root sheath. The outer root sheath forms two bulges on the side of the hair follicle farthest from the epidermis. The superficial bulge develops into the sebaceous gland. The deeper bulge serves as the future site of epithelial stem cells that generate the new lower follicle during hair follicle cycling. The arrector pili muscle usually attaches to the bulge area, and contraction of the muscle erects the hair shaft leading to "goose bumps." In the axillae, anogenital region, areolae, periumbilical region, eyelids, and external ear canals, a third bulge develops superficial to the sebaceous gland bud and gives rise to the apocrine gland.

MATURE HAIR FOLLICLE

As the hair follicle bulb appears during the bulbous peg stage, at least eight different cell layers constituting all of the components of the mature hair follicle form. Understanding which genes determine these specific cell lineages within the follicle is an important question. The inner root sheath cells express hair follicle-specific keratins Krt25-28/Krt81-86, epidermal keratins Krt1/10, components of the cornified cell envelope (loricrin, involucrin, trichohyalin, transglutaminases, and so on).[53] Differentiation of the inner root sheath is regulated by the epidermal growth factor receptor signaling and its ligand transforming growth factor (TGF-α), as well as by the enzymes involved in the TGF-α ectodomain shedding (TNF-α–converting enzyme and lysophosphatidic acid–producing enzyme

PA-PLA1$_\alpha$), which prevent premature keratinization in the inner root sheath cells, leading to the formation of curly hair.[54-56] Also, BMP and Notch signaling pathways, as well as Cutl1, Dlx3, Gata-3, and Msx-2 transcription factors, are involved in the control of inner root sheath differentiation (reviewed in [57,58]).

The central lumen where the hair shaft will emerge is formed by necrosis and cornification of epithelial cells in the infundibulum. As the hair shaft is produced, several signaling pathways are involved in the control of its differentiation. Hair shaft–specific differentiation is characterized by expression of hair-specific keratins (Krt31-37, Krt81-86) and keratin-associated proteins in hair progenitor cells.[53] Wnt, Bmp, Edar, FGF, Hedgehog, IGF, and Notch signaling pathways, as well as a number of transcription factors, including Dlx3, Foxn1, Hoxc13, Krox20, and Msx2 (reviewed in [57,58]) regulate this hair shaft differentiation program. Some transcription factors, such as Foxn1, Lef1, and Hoxc13, directly regulate transcription of the hair keratin or keratin-associated protein genes.[57,58] WHN[59-61] is mutated in nude mice and rarely in humans with hair, nail, and immune defects.[62,63] Comprehensive RNAseq profiling data of the distinct cell populations in mature murine hair follicles described by Rezza and colleagues[64] reveal signaling interaction networks implicated in epithelial–mesenchymal interactions and provide a comprehensive platform linked to an interactive online database to identify and further explore the crosstalk between stem cells and their progeny in regulating hair follicle growth.

This process of hair follicle formation is repeated in several waves, with the formation of secondary follicles alongside the initial follicle. In human scalp skin, the follicles are primarily clustered into groups of three and possess an oblique orientation with a similar angle to their neighbors.

ANATOMY

HAIR TYPES

After formation of the lanugo hair that is characteristic of the prenatal period, there are two major types of hair classified according to size (Table 7-1). Terminal hairs are typically greater than 60 μm in diameter, possess a central medulla, and can grow to well over 100 cm in length. The duration of the growing stage (anagen) determines the length of the hair. The hair bulb of terminal hairs in anagen is located in the subcutaneous fat. In contrast, vellus hairs are typically less than 30 μm in diameter, do not possess a medulla, and are less than 2 cm in length. The hair bulb of vellus hairs in anagen is located in the reticular dermis. Terminal hairs are found on the scalp, eyebrows, and eyelashes at birth. Vellus hairs are found elsewhere, and, at puberty, vellus hair follicles in the genitalia, axillae, trunk, and beard area in men transform into terminal hair follicles under the influence of sex hormones. Terminal hair follicles in the scalp convert to vellus-like or miniaturized hair follicles during androgenetic alopecia (see Chap. 85).[1,65]

The curvature of the hair varies greatly among different individuals and races and ranges from straight to tightly curled. Curved hair shafts arise from curved hair follicles. The shape of the inner root sheath is thought to determine the shape of the hair. Curled hair in cross section is more elliptical or flattened in comparison with straight hair, which is rounder. Several genes influencing hair shape have been identified. Mutations in the epidermal growth factor receptor (EGFR) pathway and in insulinlike growth factor binding protein 5 result in curly hair in mice.[28,66]

MICROSCOPIC ANATOMY

The upper follicle consists of the infundibulum and the isthmus, and the lower follicle consists of the suprabulbar and the bulbar areas (Fig. 7-2).[67,68] The upper follicle is permanent, but the lower follicle regenerates with each hair follicle cycle. The major compartments of the hair from outermost to innermost include the connective tissue sheath, the outer root sheath, the inner root sheath, the cuticle, the hair shaft cortex, and the hair shaft medulla, each characterized by distinct expression of the hair follicle–specific keratins (Table 7-2).[69,70]

OUTER ROOT SHEATH

The outer root sheath is continuous with the epidermis (see Fig. 7-2) at the infundibulum and continues down to the bulb. The cells of the outer root sheath change considerably throughout the follicle. The outer root sheath in the infundibulum resembles epidermis and forms a granular layer during its keratinization. In the isthmus, the outer root sheath cells keratinize in a trichilemmal fashion, lacking a granular layer. Trichilemmal keratinization occurs where the inner root sheath begins to slough. Desmoglein expression markedly changes here as well, and trichilemmal or pilar cysts retain these characteristics.[71] Keratinocytes in the outer root sheath form the bulge at the base of the isthmus (see section "Hair Follicle Stem Cells"). These cells generally possess a higher nuclear-to-cytoplasmic ratio than other areas of the follicle. Moving downward, the outer root sheath cells become much larger and contain abundant glycogen in the suprabulbar follicle. In the bulb, the outer root sheath consists of

TABLE 7-1
Hair Types and Characteristics

TYPE OF HAIR	ANAGEN DURATION	SIZE (DIAMETER, LENGTH)
Lanugo	1-3 months	40 μm, 1-2 cm
Vellus	1-2 weeks	<30 μm, <2 cm
Terminal	>1 year	>60 μm, 10≥100 cm
Miniaturized	<1 week	<30 μm, <2 cm

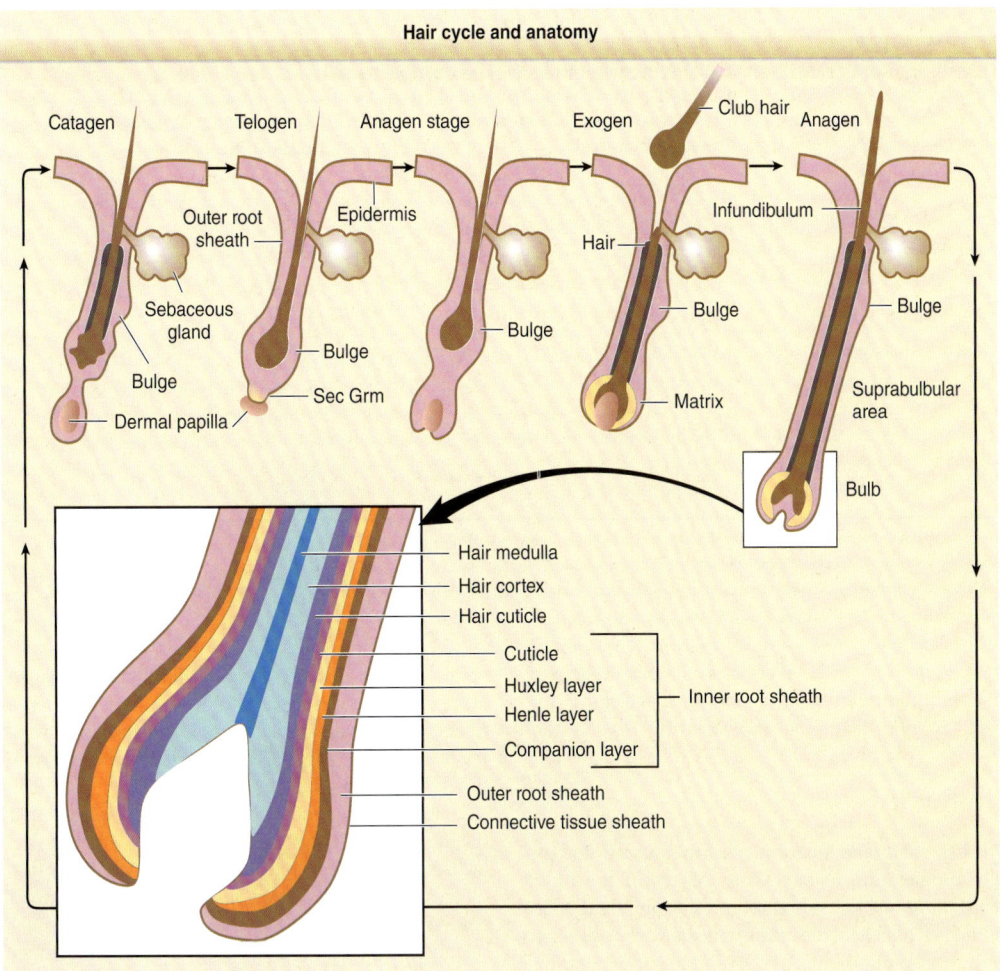

Figure 7-2 Hair cycle and anatomy. The hair follicle cycle consists of stages of rest (telogen), hair growth (anagen), follicle regression (catagen), and hair shedding (exogen). The entire lower epithelial structure is formed during anagen and regresses during catagen. The transient portion of the follicle consists of matrix cells in the bulb that generate seven different cell lineages, three in the hair shaft and four in the inner root sheath. Sec Grm, secondary germ.

only a single, flattened cell layer that can be traced to the base of the follicle.

INNER ROOT SHEATH

The inner root sheath extends from the base of the bulb to the isthmus and contains four parts from outermost to innermost: the companion layer, Henle layer, Huxley layer, and inner root sheath cuticle. The companion layer (see Fig. 7-2) has been referred to as the innermost layer of the outer root sheath, but recent evidence indicates that it is more like inner root sheath than outer root sheath.[67,72] The companion layer attaches to the Henle layer and moves upward with the rest of the inner root sheath; thus, it provides a slippage plane between the outer root sheath, which is stationary, and the inner root sheath.[72] The companion layer is prominent in some follicles (eg, the beard) compared with others. The cells of the companion layer are flat compared to the cuboidal outer root sheath cells and express a type II cytokeratin, K6hf.[72] The Henle layer is one cell layer thick and is the first to develop keratohyalin granules and the first to keratinize. The Huxley layer is two to four cell layers thick and keratinizes above the Henle layer at the region known as *Adamson fringe*. Some cells within the Huxley layer protrude through the Henle layer and attach directly to the companion layer. These cells are called *Fluegelzellen* or *wing cells*.[73] The cells of the inner root sheath cuticle partially overlap, forming a "shingled roof" appearance, and they intertwine precisely with the cuticle cells of the hair shaft. This association between the two cuticles anchors the hair shaft tightly to the follicle. The inner root sheath, composed of hard keratins and associated proteins (see Table 7-2), is thought to dictate hair shape by funneling the hair shaft cells as they are produced. The

TABLE 7-2
Expression of Keratin Genes in Distinct Hair Follicle (HF) Compartments

HF COMPARTMENTS	TYPE I KERATINS, NEW NOMENCLATURE (OLD NOMENCLATURE)	TYPE II KERATINS, NEW NOMENCLATURE (OLD NOMENCLATURE)
Outer root sheath	K14 (K14), K15 (K15), K16 (K16), K17 (K17), K19 (K19)	K5 (K5)
Inner root sheath, companion layer	K16 (K16), K17 (K17)	K75 (K6hf), K6 (K6)
Hair matrix or precortex	K35 (Ha5)	K85 (Hb5)
Inner root sheath, Henle layer	K25 (K25irs1), K27 (K25irs3), K28 (K25irs4)	K71 (K6irs1)
Inner root sheath, Huxley layer	K25 (K25irs1), K27 (K25irs3), K28 (K25irs4)	K71 (K6irs1), K74 (K6irs4)
Inner root sheath, cuticle	K25 (K25irs1), K26 (K25irs2), K27 (K25irs3), K28 (K25irs4)	K71 (K6irs1), K72 (K6irs2), K73 (K6irs3)
Hair, cuticle	K32 (Ha2), K35 (Ha5)	K82 (Hb2), K85 (Hb5)
Hair, mid- and upper cortex	K31 (Ha1), K33a (Ha3-I), K33b (Ha3-II), K34 (Ha4), K35 (Ha5), K36 (Ha6), K37 (Ha7), K38 (Ha8)	K81 (Hb1),[a] K83 (Hb3), K85 (Hb5), K86 (Hb6)[a]
Hair, medulla	K16 (K16), K17 (K17), K25 (K25irs1), K27 (K25irs3), K28 (K25irs4), K33 (Ha3), K34 (Ha4), K37 (Ha7)	K5 (K5), K6 (K6), K75 (K6hf), K81 (Hb1)[a]

[a]Autosomal dominant mutations of K81 and K86 lead to monilethrix (alopecia caused by increased hair fragility).
Data from Langbein L, Rogers MA, Praetzel-Wunder S, et al. K25 (k25irs1), K26 (k25irs2), k27 (k25irs3), and k28 (k25irs4) represent the type I inner root sheath keratins of the human hair follicle. *J Invest Dermatol*. 2006;126:2377; and Langbein L, Schweizer J. Keratins of the human hair follicle. *Int Rev Cytol*. 2005;243:1.

transcription factor GATA-3 is critical for inner root sheath differentiation and lineage. Mice lacking this gene fail to form an inner root sheath.[74]

HAIR SHAFT

The hair shaft (and inner root sheath) arises from rapidly proliferating matrix keratinocytes in the bulb, which have one of the highest rates of proliferation in the body. The cells of the future hair shaft are positioned at the apex of the dermal papilla and form the medulla, cortex, and hair shaft cuticle (see Fig. 7-2). Immediately above the matrix cells, hair shaft cells begin to express specific hair shaft keratins in the prekeratogenous zone. The differentiation of hair shaft cells in this zone is dependent on the Lef-1 transcription factor. Lef-1 binding sites are present in most hair keratin genes. BMP receptor type 1a is also critical for matrix cell differentiation into the hair shaft because loss of this receptor prevents hair shaft differentiation.[67,75,76]

The hair shaft cuticle covers the hair, and its integrity and properties greatly impact the appearance of the hair. When the hair exits the scalp, the cuticle endures weathering, and it is often completely lost at the distal ends of long hairs. Inside the cuticle, the cortex comprises the bulk of the shaft and contains melanin. The cortex is arranged in large cable-like structures called *macrofibrils*. These, in turn, possess microfibrils that are composed of intermediate filaments. The medulla sits at the center of larger hairs, and specific keratins expressed in this layer of cells (see Table 7-2) are under the control of androgens.[68]

DERMAL PAPILLA

The dermal papilla (see Fig. 7-1) is a core of mesenchymally derived tissue enveloped by the matrix epithelium. It is comprised of fibroblasts, collagen bundles, a mucopolysaccharide-rich stroma, nerve fibers, and a single capillary loop. It is continuous with the perifollicular sheath (dermal sheath) of connective tissue that envelops the lower follicle.

Tissue recombination experiments have shown that the dermal papilla has powerful inductive properties, including the ability to induce hair follicle formation when transplanted below non–hair-bearing footpad epidermis.[77,78] This shows that the tissue patterning established during the fetal period can be altered under appropriate conditions. In human follicles, the volume of the dermal papilla correlates with the number of matrix cells and the resulting size of the hair shaft.[79] In mice, the sizes of the hair bulb and hair diameter strongly depend of the proliferative activity of the matrix keratinocytes.[80]

Many soluble growth factors that appear to act in a paracrine manner on the overlying epithelial matrix cells originate from the dermal papilla. Specifically, keratinocyte growth factor (KGF) is produced by the anagen dermal papilla, and its receptor, FGF receptor 2 (FGFR2), is found predominantly in the matrix keratinocytes. Injections of KGF into nude mice produce striking hair growth at the site of injection,[81] suggesting that KGF is perhaps necessary for hair growth and cycling. However, surprisingly, KGF knockout mice develop morphologically normal hair follicles that produce "rough" or "greasy" hair; thus, KGF's effects on hair follicle morphogenesis and cycling appear dispensable or replaceable by other growth factors with redundant functions.[82]

HAIR FOLLICLE INNERVATION

Myelinated sensory nerve fibers run parallel to hair follicles, surrounding them and forming a network (reviewed in [83]). Smaller nerve fibers form an outer circular layer, which is concentrated around the bulge of terminal follicles and the bulb of vellus follicles. Several different types of nerve endings, including free nerve endings, lanceolate nerve endings, Merkel cells, and pilo-Ruffini corpuscles are found associated with hair follicles.[84] Each nerve ending detects different forces and stimuli. Free nerve endings transmit pain, lanceolate nerve endings detect acceleration, Merkel cells sense pressure, and pilo-Ruffini structures detect tension. Perifollicular nerves contain neuromediators and neuropeptides, such as substance P and calcitonin gene-related peptide, that influence follicular keratinocytes and alter hair follicle cycling.[41,85-88] In addition to neuropeptides, nerve fibers innervating hair follicles produce Shh that signals to a population of cells in the bulge marked by the Hedgehog response gene *Gli1*.[89] The progeny of Shh-responding perineural bulge cells incorporate into healing skin wounds where, notably, they can change their lineage into epidermal stem cells. The perineural niche (including Shh) is dispensable for the follicle's contribution to wound healing but is necessary to maintain bulge cells capable of becoming epidermal stem cells.[89]

In turn, hair follicle keratinocytes produce neurotrophic factors that influence perifollicular nerves and stimulate their remodeling in a hair cycle–dependent manner.[88,90] Merkel cells, which are considered neuroendocrine cells, also produce neurotrophic factors, cytokines, or other regulatory molecules. Because Merkel cells are concentrated in the bulge area, some have postulated that these secreted factors may influence the cycling of the hair follicle.[91]

PERIFOLLICULAR SHEATH

The perifollicular sheath envelops the epithelial components of the hair follicle and consists of an inner basement membrane called the *hyaline* or *vitreous (glassy) membrane* and an outer connective tissue sheath. The basement membrane of the follicle is continuous with the interfollicular basement membrane. It is most prominent around the outer root sheath at the bulb in anagen hairs. During catagen, the basement membrane thickens and then disintegrates.

Surrounding the basement membrane is a connective tissue sheath composed primarily of type III collagen. Around the upper follicle, there is a thin connective tissue sheath continuous with the surrounding papillary dermis and arranged longitudinally. Around the lower follicle, the connective tissue sheath is more prominent, with an inner layer of collagen fibers that encircles the follicle surrounded by a layer of longitudinally arranged collagen fibers.

When transplanted under the skin, this perifollicular connective tissue has the remarkable ability to form a new dermal papilla and induce new hair follicle formation.[92] Even when the connective tissue sheath is transplanted to another individual, these follicles survive without evidence of immunologic rejection.

HAIR FOLLICLE CYCLE

Each individual hair follicle perpetually traverses through three stages: (1) growth (anagen), (2) involution (catagen), and (3) rest (telogen).[6] The length of anagen determines the final length of the hair and thus varies according to body site; catagen and telogen duration vary to a lesser extent depending on site. Scalp hair has the longest anagen of 2 years to more than 8 years. Anagen duration in young males at other sites is shorter: legs, 5 to 7 months; arms, 1.5 to 3.0 months; eyelashes, 1 to 6 months; and fingers, 1 to 3 months. In contrast to most mammals, including mice and newborn humans, in adult humans, the hairs of the scalp grow asynchronously. Approximately 90% to 93% of scalp follicles are in anagen, and the rest are primarily in telogen.[65] Applying these figures to the 100,000 to 150,000 hairs on the scalp indicates that approximately 10,000 scalp hairs are in telogen at any given time. However, because an adult loses only 50 to 100 hairs per day, this indicates that telogen is a heterogenous state. The follicles that are shedding their hair shafts are thus in "exogen," which comprises approximately 1% of the telogen hair follicles (see Fig. 7-2 and later discussion). Hair on the scalp grows at a rate of 0.37 to 0.44 mm/day or approximately 1 cm/month.

HAIR FOLLICLE STEM CELLS

Because the lower portion of the follicle cyclically regenerates, hair follicle stem cells were thought to govern this growth. Historically, hair follicle stem cells were assumed to reside exclusively in the "secondary germ" (see Fig. 7-2), which is located at the base of the telogen hair follicle. It was thought that the secondary germ moved downward to the hair bulb during anagen and provided new cells for production of the hair. At the end of anagen, the secondary germ was thought to move upward with the dermal papilla during catagen to come to rest at the base of the telogen follicle. This scenario of stem cell movement during follicle cycling was brought into question when a population of long-lived presumptive stem cells was identified in an area of the follicle surrounding the telogen club hair.[93] Subsequently, it was shown that the secondary germ is a transient structure that forms at the end of catagen from cells in the lower bulge.[94] The concept that hair follicle stem cells are permanently located in the bulge has now been confirmed using lineage analysis, which showed that the bulge cells give rise to all epithelial layers of the hair follicle.[5,95,96] In line with this, ablation of bulge cells results in destruction of the follicle.[97] These findings support the notion that loss of hair follicle stem cells in the bulge leads to permanent or cicatricial types of alopecia (see Chap. 88).

Progress has been made in defining subsets of cells within the hair follicle that serve as different stem and progenitor populations. Markers that have been shown through genetic lineage analysis to contribute

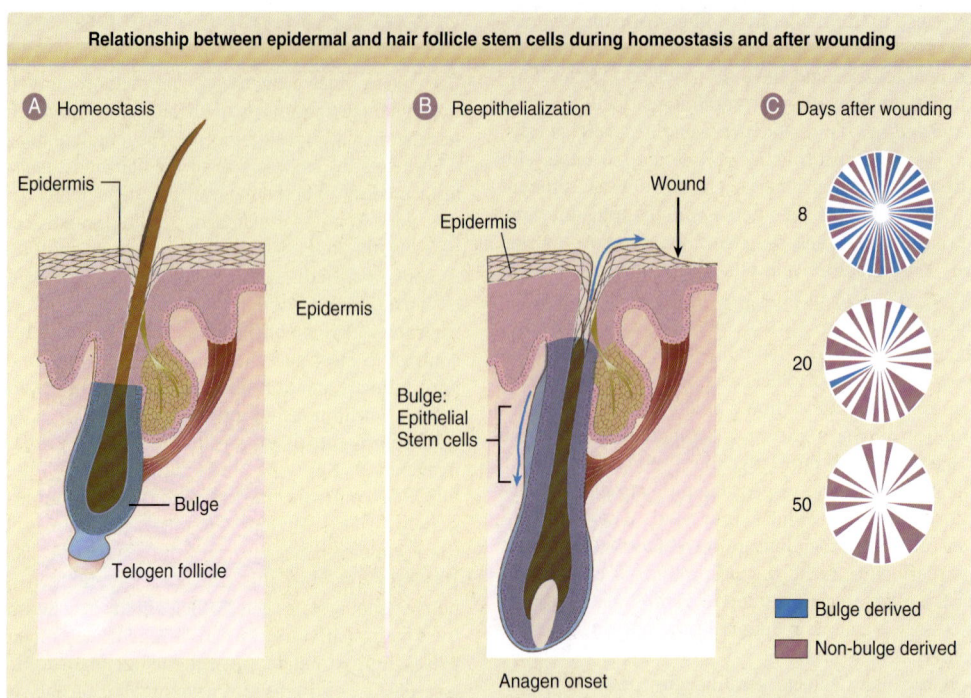

Figure 7-3 Relationship between epidermal and hair follicle stem cells during homeostasis and after wounding. **A,** During normal conditions, epidermal renewal is dependent on cell proliferation within the epidermis. Epithelial stem cells in the hair follicle bulge do not contribute to epidermal renewal. **B,** After full-thickness wounding, bulge cells contribute cells to the epidermis for immediate wound closure (*blue upward arrow*). Bulge cells also are required for hair follicle cycling (*blue downward arrow*) **C,** Over time, bulge-derived cells diminish, and non–bulge-derived cells (from the interfollicular epidermis and infundibulum) appear to predominate in the reepithelialized wound.

to the perpetual cycling of the hair follicle include cytokeratin 15 and Lgr5.[97,98] Lgr5, although sometimes touted as an exclusive marker of secondary germ cells, also marks bulge cells. Lgr6, a gene related to Lgr5, is expressed in an area above the bulge in the upper isthmus. The cells marked by Lgr6 migrate to the epidermis during homeostasis and after wounding.[99] In addition to these markers, several others demonstrate the heterogeneity of the hair follicle epithelium.[100]

Are bulge cells the "ultimate" stem cells within the skin epithelium? For example, do they generate epidermis and sebaceous glands during homeostasis and after wounding? To answer these questions, lineage analysis and transgenic techniques were again used. As illustrated in Fig. 7-3, bulge cells do not normally move to the epidermis, but after full-thickness excision of the skin, bulge cell progeny migrate into the wound during reepithelialization.[5,97] These cells comprise approximately 30% of the cells in the regenerated epidermis. The role of bulge cells in sebaceous gland maintenance is still not clear but is under investigation.

ANAGEN

The formation of a new lower follicle and hair at anagen onset recapitulates folliculogenesis in the fetus. Anagen can be divided into seven stages: (1) stage I—growth of the dermal papilla and onset of mitotic activity in the germlike overlying epithelium; (2) stage II—bulb matrix cells envelop the dermal papilla and begin differentiation, and the evolving bulb begins descent along the fibrous streamer; (3) stage III—bulb matrix cells show differentiation into all follicular components; (4) stage IV—matrix melanocytes reactivate; (5) stage V—hair shaft emerges and dislodges telogen hair; (6) stage VI—new hair shaft emerges from skin surface; and (7) stage VII—stable growth.[101]

During proliferation and migration of keratinocytes into the dermis to reform the new lower follicle, enzymes such as proteases and collagenases appear at the leading edge of the downgrowth, and growth factors and their receptors are upregulated similar to an epithelial wound.[6] Pathways of keratinocyte differentiation that are seen in the epidermis during wound healing, such as expression of keratin 6, are activated. Mice lacking Stat3, a regulator of cell migration in the cutaneous epithelium, show defects in wound healing and a failure of hair follicles to enter anagen,[102] thus further illustrating the similarity between wound healing and the early events of anagen. Remarkably, the dermal papilla in the midst of this degradative milieu survives and moves downward. Neurocutaneous and vascular networks are remodelled.[90,103] Melanocytes proliferate and repopulate the new hair bulb.[104] Finally, a burst of endothelial proliferation and angiogenesis in the dermal papilla marks the time point when the lower follicle is completely restored and is actively producing the new hair shaft.[105]

CATAGEN

The onset of catagen is marked by cessation of the mitotic activity of the matrix cells and by well-coordinated apoptosis in the cyclic portion of the hair follicle.[6,7] Pigment production by melanocytes ceases before matrix cell proliferation stops, thus leading to a nonpigmented proximal end in the telogen club hair (see Fig. 7-2). Melanin is often found in the surrounding dermis and papilla, where it is engulfed by macrophages. The perifollicular sheath collapses, and the vitreous or glassy membrane thickens. The lower follicle retracts upward with the dermal papilla. The perifollicular sheath forms a fibrous streamer composed of fibroblasts, small blood vessels, and collagen.[1] Eventually, the dermal papilla becomes situated immediately below the bulge at the lower portion of the isthmus.

During catagen, the largest follicles, on the scalp, for example, shorten their length from 2- to 5-mm-long structures whose deepest portion, the bulb, extends down into the subcutaneous fat to truncated 0.25- to 0.5-mm follicles in telogen. As the basement membrane around the lower follicle thickens, the dermal papilla, protected from the surrounding apoptosis and destruction (perhaps because it expresses Bcl-2, an antiapoptotic factor[6]), condenses and begins to move upward to come to rest below the bulge during telogen. The migration of the dermal papilla from the subcutaneous fat to the dermis during catagen is necessary for continued follicle cycling. This is illustrated by the syndrome of atrichia with papules.[106,107] These patients have mutations in either their hairless gene or in their vitamin D receptor gene, in which case they also have rickets. Mice with similar mutations have the hairless phenotype. We know from these mice that folliculogenesis is normal; however, when the follicles enter catagen for the first time, the lower portion of the follicle does not involute and contract properly, and the dermal papilla remains stranded in the subcutaneous fat.[93] Although bulge cells are still present, no new anagen follicles ever form, presumably because the stem cells cannot interact with the dermal papilla.[93]

The study of mouse mutants has also resulted in several key findings that have increased our understanding of the molecular events at catagen onset. Specifically, Hebert and coworkers[108] discovered that mice lacking the *Fgf5* gene have hair that is 50% longer than their wild-type littermates and that mutations in this gene are responsible for the angora phenotype that was described more than 30 years ago. Although these findings were rather unexpected, careful evaluation of *Fgf5* expression throughout the normal hair cycle demonstrated that its expression was upregulated in the outer root sheath and hair matrix cells just before the onset of catagen, suggesting that *Fgf5* may trigger catagen onset.

Interestingly, the follicle still eventually entered catagen, even in the absence of FGF-5, suggesting redundancy in the FGF-5 pathway or an intrinsic finite proliferative capability of the matrix cells.[93] Further studies also demonstrated that other FGF family members and their receptors are expressed during anagen and probably also play a role in the hair follicle cycle.[109] The hair phenotype of FGF-5–deficient mice is substantially reversed by ectopic expression of the antiapoptotic gene $bcl\text{-}xL_x$ in the outer root sheath, suggesting that regulation of cell survival in the outer root sheath may play a role in control of the hair growth cycle.[110]

Although it has been known for many years that exogenous EGF administered to sheep results in catagen induction,[111] only through more recent transgenic and knockout studies in mice has the importance of the EGFR system in hair cycle regulation been realized.[66,112] For example, knockout mice lacking TGF-α, the major ligand for EGFR, have abnormal hair follicle development and manifest the waved hair phenotype.[55,113] When EGFR is functionally downregulated in the basal layer of the epidermis and hair follicle using a dominant negative transgenic strategy, the resulting hair is not only waved but also longer than normal.[66] Transition of the hair follicles from anagen to catagen is delayed in these mice. Hair follicles in mouse skin that completely lack EGFR also do not progress from anagen to telogen.[112] Thus, EGFR and its ligand are required for normal hair follicle development and cycling. Given the complexity of the EGFR family, which includes four receptors (ErbB1–4) and at least six ligands, future studies are needed to clarify the role of individual family members in hair follicle cycling.

In addition to FGF-5 and EGF, neurotrophins and TGF-β1 induce premature catagen. Neurotrophin-3 and brain-derived neurotrophic factor transgenic mice show premature catagen development, and brain-derived neurotrophic factor overexpression leads to the shortening of hair length by 15%, most likely via stimulation of proapoptotic signaling through p75 kDa neurotrophin receptor.[114,115] TGF-β1 induces premature catagen in isolated human hair follicles and in mouse skin in vivo, and TGF-β1 knockout mice display delay in catagen onset.[116-118]

TELOGEN AND EXOGEN

When catagen is complete and a club hair is formed (see Fig. 7-2), the hair follicle prepares the hair for expulsion from the scalp. About 1% of telogen hairs are shed each day. Milner and colleagues[119] have proposed distinguishing hair shedding as a separate phase called *exogen*. Exogen is a highly controlled and timed event in mammals that shed on a seasonal basis. That exogen is an active stage is supported by Headington's description of one type of telogen effluvium he termed *immediate telogen release*.[120] This type of hair loss can be seen soon after starting medications, such as minoxidil, or in response to rapid fluctuations in light–dark cycles. It consists of an increase in shedding of club hairs within weeks of the precipitating event (too soon to be caused by follicles prematurely entering telogen from anagen), suggesting that club hairs that are normally retained in the follicle can be actively shed. The heterogeneity of telogen is further supported by the work of Guarrera and Rebora,[121] who followed individual hairs in situ using macrophotographs for more than 2 years and showed that several months could transpire between hair shedding and regrowth. This "lag period" is normally not present or is very short but often lasts several months in patients with androgenetic alopecia.

HAIR PIGMENTATION

Hair becomes pigmented as a result of a tightly coordinated program of melanin synthesis and transport from the hair bulb melanocytes to differentiating hair shaft keratinocytes.[122-124] This process is strictly coupled to anagen and ceases during catagen and telogen. Numerous signaling molecules, structural proteins, enzymes, cofactors, and transcriptional regulators control hair pigmentation (Figs. 7-4 and 7-5).[122,124,125]

HAIR MELANOCYTE DEVELOPMENT

Melanoblasts can be identified in the epidermis of human embryos at 50 days of estimated gestational age before the onset of hair follicle morphogenesis.[126-128] These melanocytes originate in the neural crest and migrate first to the dermis and then epidermis.[129] New data reveal that melanocytes in the skin arise from two sources: from neural crest cells migrating in the dorsolateral pathway and from Schwann cell progenitors located in cutaneous nerves.[130] Commitment of neural crest cells to the melanocyte lineage is regulated by Pax3 and microphthalmia transcription factors (Mitf), which stimulate the expression of dopachrome tautomerase (or tyrosinase-related protein 2[131]), an enzyme involved in melanin biosynthesis that also functions as an early melanoblast marker.[128] Subsequent steps of melanoblast development (migration into the dermis and epidermis) are controlled by signaling mechanisms activated through endothelin receptor type B (Ednrb) and c-kit receptor, which are mutated in humans with Hirschsprung disease and piebaldism, respectively, resulting in formation of unpigmented hairs.[129]

After entering the placode of the developing hair follicle, melanoblasts proliferate and become produce pigment synchronously with the onset of hair fiber formation.[132] Experimental and genetic data suggest that migration of melanoblasts into the hair follicle and their differentiation to pigment producing melanocytes depends on stem cell factor (SCF)/c-kit signaling. SCF is a ligand that binds to its receptor (c-kit). Pharmacologic blockade of c-kit during embryogenesis, as well as genetic ablation of SCF or c-kit in corresponding mouse mutants results in unpigmented hairs.[133-135]

HAIR FOLLICLE MELANOCYTE STEM CELLS AND PIGMENT-PRODUCING MELANOCYTES

Melanocyte stem cells located in the hair follicle bulge generate progeny that repopulate the melanocytes in the new hair bulb formed at the onset of anagen.[104,136] Melanocyte stem cells express Trp2, Bcl-2, Pax3, and other melanogenic enzymes (tyrosinase, tyrosinase-related protein 1[131]) and signaling molecules (c-kit, Ednrb, Sox10, Mitf, and Lef1)[137] are expressed at low levels. Melanocyte stem cells can be first detected in the bulge area during late stages of hair follicle morphogenesis and similar to epithelial stem cells they are quiescent.[136-138] TGF-β signaling plays an important role in controlling melanocyte stem cells entering into a noncycling (dormant) state during hair follicle morphogenesis.[139]

Maintenance of melanocyte stem cells during hair follicle cycling is controlled by TGF-β and Notch signaling pathways. Notch signaling plays a crucial role in the survival of melanocyte stem cells and immature melanoblasts by preventing apoptosis.[140] Cross-talk between the TGF-β pathway and Bcl2 is also important for maintenance of melanocyte stem cells: Bcl2 plays a key role in maintenance of melanocyte stem cells, and Bcl2 knockout mice show progressive hair graying because of the depletion of melanocyte stem cells.[137-139,141,142] However, Bcl2 deficiency may be compensated by overexpression of SCF, which rescues loss of melanocyte stem cells in the hair follicle bulge of Bcl2 knockout mice.[137]

Melanocytes producing pigment are located in the hair bulb above the dermal papilla.[104,124] These cells synthesize and transport melanin to hair shaft keratinocytes and express a full set of enzymes and other proteins involved in melanin biosynthesis including tyrosinase, Trp1, Trp2 (in mice), and pMel17 (in humans).[104,137] Keratinocytes, as pigment recipient cells, produce Foxn1 and its target Fgf2 to identify themselves as the targets for pigment transfer.[143]

HAIR CYCLE–DEPENDENT CHANGES IN MELANOCYTES

Hair follicle melanocytes undergo substantial remodeling during hair follicle cycling.[104,124] In telogen, hair follicle melanocytes are found in the bulge, secondary hair germ, and connective tissue.[104] In humans, melanocytes in the telogen hair follicle do not express Trp1- and tyrosinase, do not proliferate, and can be visualized by expression of pMel17. Some of these cells also express c-kit receptor, and others remain c-kit-negative and represent melanocyte stem cells

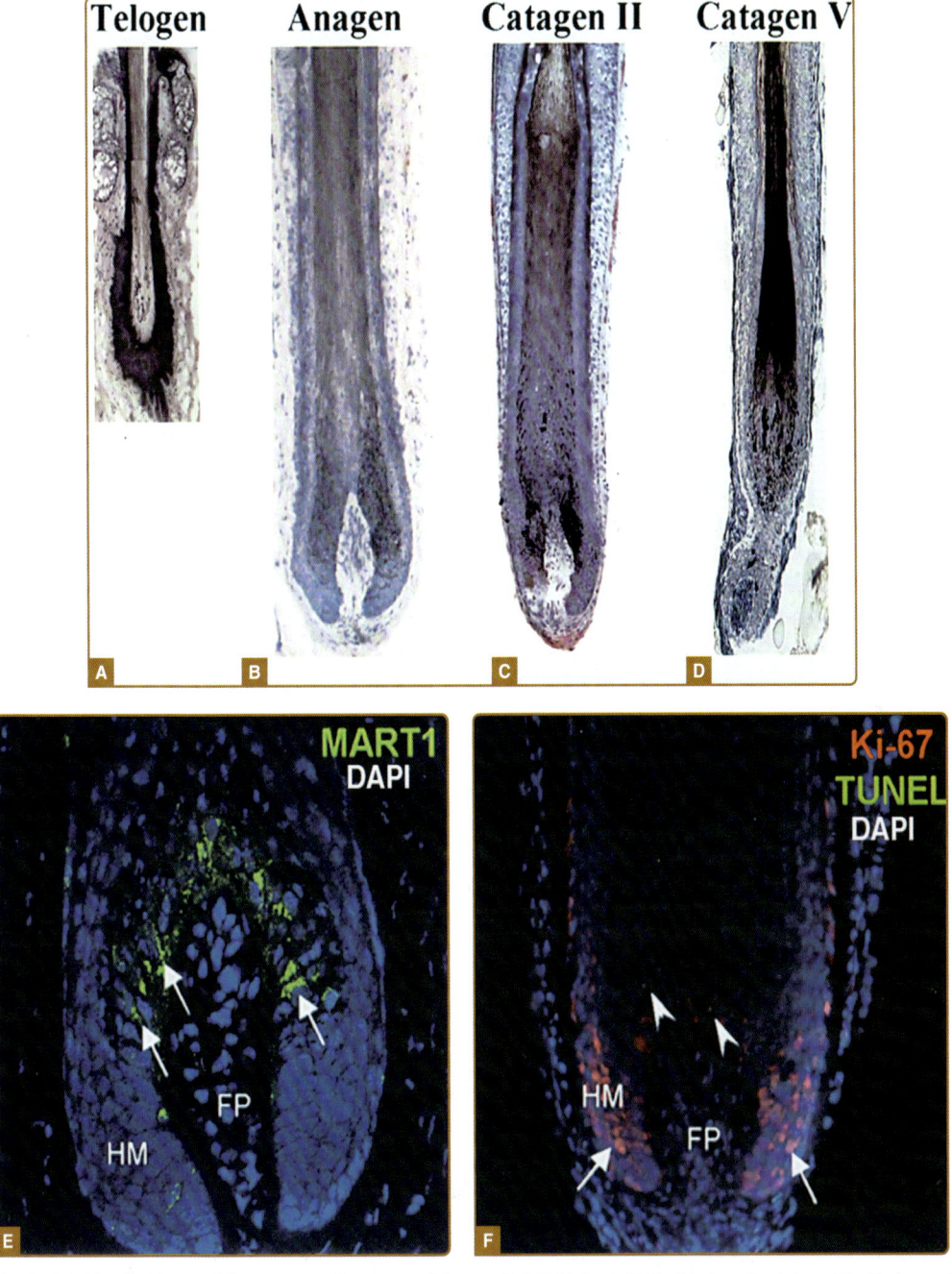

Figure 7-4 Morphology and fluorescent microscopy of human hair follicle at distinct hair cycle stages. Morphology of human hair follicle during telogen (**A**), late anagen (**B**), and early and late catagen (**C, D**). **E,** Immunofluorescent visualization of the melanocytes (*arrows*) in the hair bulb of late anagen hair follicle with antimelanoma-associated antigen recognized by T cells antibody. **F,** Immunofluorescent detection of proliferative marker Ki-67 (*arrows*) and apoptotic TUNEL+ cells (*arrowheads*) in early catagen hair follicle. FP, follicular papilla; HM, hair matrix.

(MCSCs).[104,136,137] Wnt activation in MCSCs drives their differentiation into pigment-producing melanocytes.[144] TGF-β signaling is activated in melanocyte stem cells when they reenter the quiescent noncycling state during the hair cycle, and this process requires Bcl2 for cell survival.[139] After wounding or ultraviolet type B irradiation, McSCs in the hair follicle are capable of exiting the stem cell niche and migrate to the epidermis followed by their differentiation into functional epidermal melanocytes in a melanocortin 1 receptor (Mc1r)–dependent manner.[145,146]

During early anagen, resting melanocytes proliferate, differentiate, and migrate within the hair follicle synchronously with regeneration of the hair follicle

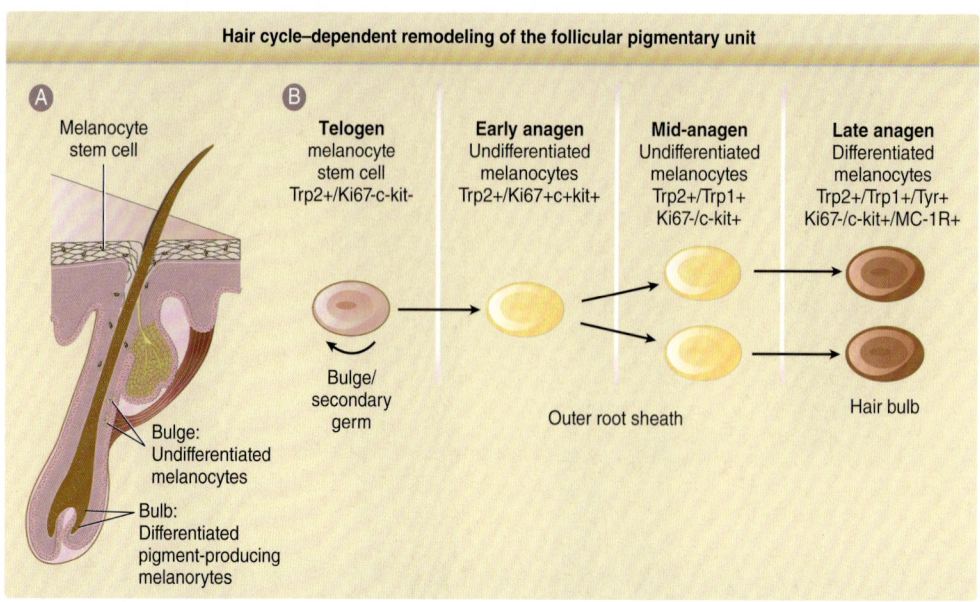

Figure 7-5 Hair cycle–dependent remodeling of the follicular pigmentary unit. **A,** Schematic illustrating localization of distinct subpopulations of melanocytes in anagen hair follicle. **B,** Dynamics of the follicular melanocytes during anagen. Expression of melanogenic markers and growth factor receptors indicated is based on the data obtained from murine hair follicles. Note that human follicular melanocytes do not express tyrosinase-related protein 2 (Trp2). c-kit, c-kit oncogene. (Data from Botchkareva NV, Khlgatian M, Longley BJ, et al. SCF/c-kit signaling is required for cyclic regeneration of the hair pigmentation unit. *FASEB J.* 2001;15:645-658.)

bulb. Hair follicle melanocytes are maximally proliferative during early and midanagen, and their transition to melanogenic competence is accompanied by the appearance of Trp1 and tyrosinase protein.[104] However, this process is stringently controlled, and Notch signaling is necessary to prevent differentiation of melanoblasts into pigment-producing melanocytes before they reach the hair bulb, as well as for their proper positioning in the hair matrix.[147]

Similar to embryonic and early postnatal development, SCF/c-kit signaling plays a critical role in repopulation of the bulb with pigment-producing melanocytes. Whereas c-kit is expressed on proliferating, differentiating and melanocytes producing pigment, overexpression of SCF in the epidermis of transgenic mice significantly increases the number of hair follicle melanocytes and their proliferative activity.[104] Similarly, administration of the ACK45 antibody blocking c-kit signaling dramatically reduces melanocyte number in anagen hair follicles, resulting in hair depigmentation.[104] However, in the next hair cycle, the previously treated animals grow fully pigmented hairs with the normal number and distribution of melanocytes, suggesting that melanocyte stem cells are not dependent on SCF/c-kit.[104]

During catagen, melanogenic activity in the follicular melanocytes abruptly ceases. Immunohistochemical and electron microscopic data suggest that some pigment-producing melanocytes located above the follicular papilla undergo apoptosis, and others drop into the dermal papilla of the follicle.[148,149]

MOLECULAR CONTROL OF HAIR COLOR

Follicular melanocytes synthesize pigment via a cascade of enzymatic conversions of phenylalanine or tyrosine into brown-black eumelanin or yellow pheomelanin that requires melanogenic enzymes (tyrosinase, tyrosinase-related proteins 1/2, -glutamyltranspeptidase, peroxidase) and essential co-factors, such as 6-tetrahydrobiopterin.[122,148] The balance between black and yellow pigment synthesis (eumelanin and pheomelanin, respectively) is regulated by signaling through the melanocortin type 1 receptor (MC-1R) that has long been implicated in the controlling hair color.[150,151]

After binding to MC-1R, α-melanocyte stimulating hormone (α-MSH) stimulates adenylyl cyclase, resulting in elevation of intracellular cyclic adenosine monophosphate (cAMP) levels. This leads to increase of transcriptional activity of MITF that stimulates synthesis of enzymes (tyrosinase, Trp1/2) involved in eumelanin formation.[152,153] Pheomelanin synthesis in the hair follicle melanocytes of mice occurs when MC-1R signaling is inhibited by Agouti signal protein (ASP) that competes with α-MSH in binding to MC-1R.[151,152] In mice, ASP expression is positively regulated by BMP signaling, and transgenic mice overexpressing the BMP antagonist Noggin show hair darkening.[149] Although ASP is expressed in human skin, its role in human pigmentation remains unclear.[153]

Recent data also demonstrate the existence of a proopiomelanocortin (POMC)–MC-1R pathway in human hair follicles: MC-1R is expressed by hair follicle melanocytes, and its ligands α-MSH and adrenocorticotrophic hormone (ACTH) are able to promote melanocyte proliferation, dendricity, and pigment production.[154] Another POMC-derived peptide, β-endorphin, that interacts with the μ-opiate receptor expressed by hair follicle melanocytes has a similar effect.[154] However, signaling through the μ-opiate receptor may regulate hair pigmentation via modulating the activity of protein kinase C (PKC)-β, a known positive regulator of pigment production.[155]

Follicular melanocytes are sensitive to aging, which results in their premature loss and hair greying.[156] In contrast to normally pigmented hair follicles, fewer melanocytes are found in the bulb of a grey hair; however, these melanocytes still express tyrosinase and synthesize then transfer melanin to keratinocytes.[157] In addition, a population of inactive melanocytes (melanoblasts including stem cells) in the outer root sheath is markedly reduced in follicles producing grey hairs compared with ones producing pigmented hairs.[157] The fact that melanocyte stem cells are damaged in hair follicles producing grey hairs was confirmed in mice by applying ionizing radiation, which triggered premature differentiation of melanocyte stem cells in the follicular bulge into mature, pigment-producing melanocytes followed by their depletion and irreversible hair graying.[158] Deficiency of ATM-kinase, a central transducer of the DNA-damage response, sensitizes MSCs to ectopic differentiation, demonstrating its role in protecting melanocyte stem cells from their premature differentiation.[158]

CONCLUSION

A hair follicle is formed as the result of a complex interplay of signals between epithelium and mesenchyme. Many molecular pathways important in development also play roles in hair follicle formation. The product of this process is a miniature organ with distinctive vertical and concentric architecture. Both epithelial stem cells and melanocyte stem cells in the follicle are important for the constant regeneration of the follicle.

REFERENCES

1. Nieves A, Garza LA. Does prostaglandin D2 hold the cure to male pattern baldness? *Experimental Dermatology* 2014;23(4):224-227.
2. Guo H, Gao WV, Endo H & McElwee KJ. Experimental and early investigational drugs for androgenetic alopecia. *Expert Opinion on Investigational Drugs*. 2017; 26:8,917-932. doi: 10.1080/13543784.2017.1353598.
3. Fuchs E. Scratching the surface of skin development. *Nature*. 2007;445:834-842.
4. Schneider MR, Schmidt-Ullrich R, Paus R. The hair follicle as a dynamic miniorgan. *Curr Biol*. 2009;19: R132-R142.
5. Cotsarelis G. Epithelial stem cells: a folliculocentric view. *J Invest Dermatol*. 2006;126:1459-1468.
6. Stenn KS, Paus R. Controls of hair follicle cycling. *Physiol Rev*. 2001;81:449-494.
7. Botchkarev VA, Yaar M, Peters EM, et al. Neurotrophins in skin biology and pathology. *J Investig Dermatol Symp Proc*. 2006;126:1719-1727.
8. Botchkarev VA. Neurotrophins and their role in pathogenesis of alopecia areata. *J Investig Dermatol Symp Proc*. 2003;8:195-198.
9. Millar S. Molecular mechanisms regulating hair follicle development. *J Invest Dermatol*. 2002;118:216-225.
10. Schmidt-Ullrich R, Paus, R. Molecular principles of hair follicle induction and morphogenesis. *Bioessays*. 2005;27:247-261.
11. Krumlauf R. Hox genes in vertebrate development. *Cell*. 1994;7:191-201.
12. Chuong CM, Oliver G, Ting SA, et al. Gradients of homeoproteins in developing feather buds. *Development*. 1990;110:1021-1030.
13. Godwin AR, Capecchi MR. Hoxc13 mutant mice lack external hair. *Genes Dev*. 1998;12:11-20.
14. Loomis CA, Harris E, Michaud J, et al. The mouse Engrailed-1 gene and ventral limb patterning. *Nature*. 1996;382:360-363.
15. Cadieu E, Neff MW, Quignon P, et al. Coat variation in the domestic dog is governed by variants in three genes. *Science*. 2009;326:150-153.
16. Mou C, Thomason HA, Willan PM, et al. Enhanced ectodysplasin-A receptor (EDAR) signaling alters multiple fiber characteristics to produce the East Asian hair form. *Hum Mutat*. 2008;29:1405-1411.
17. Levy V, Lindon C, Harfe BD, et al. Distinct stem cell populations regenerate the follicle and interfollicular epidermis. *Dev Cell*. 2005;9:855-861.
18. Ahtiainen L, Lefebvre S, Lindfors PH, et al. Directional cell migration, but not proliferation, drives hair placode morphogenesis. *Dev Cell*. 2014;28:588-602.
19. Jamora C, DasGupta R, Kocieniewski P, et al. Links between signal transduction, transcription and adhesion in epithelial bud development. *Nature*. 2003;422: 317-322.
20. Nanba D, Hieda Y, Nakanishi Y. Remodeling of desmosomal and hemidesmosomal adhesion systems during early morphogenesis of mouse pelage hair follicles. *J Invest Dermatol*. 2000;114:171-177.
21. Rhee H, Polak L, Fuchs E. Lhx2 maintains stem cell character in hair follicles. *Science*. 2006;312:1946-1999.
22. Hardy MH. The secret life of the hair follicle. *Trends Genet*. 1992;8:55-60.
23. Sennett R, Rendl M. Mesenchymal-epithelial interactions during hair follicle morphogenesis and cycling. *Semin Cell Dev Biol*. 2012;23:917-927.
24. Botchkarev VA, Paus R. Molecular biology of hair morphogenesis: development and cycling. *J Exp Zool B Mol Dev Evol*. 2003;298:164-180.
25. Driskell RR, Clavel C, Rendl M, et al. Hair follicle dermal papilla cells at a glance. *J Cell Sci*. 2011;124:1179-1182.
26. Sennett R, Wang Z, Rezza A, et al. An integrated transcriptome atlas of embryonic hair follicle progenitors, their niche, and the developing skin. *Dev Cell*. 2015;34:577-591.
27. Bazzi H, Getz A, Mahoney MG, et al. Desmoglein 4 is expressed in highly differentiated keratinocytes and trichocytes in human epidermis and hair follicle. *Differentiation*. 2006;74:129-140.
28. Sick S, Reinker S, Timmer J, et al. WNT and DKK determine hair follicle spacing through a reaction-diffusion mechanism. *Science*. 2006;314:1447-1450.
29. Stark J, Andl T, Millar SE. Hairy math: insights into hair-follicle spacing and orientation. *Cell*. 2007;128:17-20.

30. Gat U, DasGupta R, Degenstein L, et al. De Novo hair follicle morphogenesis and hair tumors in mice expressing a truncated beta-catenin in skin. *Cell*. 1998;95:605-614.
31. Chan EF, Gat U, McNiff JM, et al. A common human skin tumour is caused by activating mutations in beta- catenin. *Nat Genet*. 1999;21:410-413.
32. Tsai SY, Sennett R, Rezza A, et al. Wnt/beta-catenin signaling in dermal condensates is required for hair follicle formation. *Dev Biol*. 2014;385:179-188.
33. Mikkola ML, Thesleff I. Ectodysplasin signaling in development. *Cytokine Growth Factor Rev*. 2003; 14:211-224.
34. Kere J, Srivastava AK, Montonen O, et al. X-linked anhidrotic (hypohidrotic) ectodermal dysplasia is caused by mutation in a novel transmembrane protein [see comments]. *Nat Genet*. 1996;13:409-416.
35. Mustonen T, Ilmonen M, Pummila M, et al. Ectodysplasin A1 promotes placodal cell fate during early morphogenesis of ectodermal appendages. *Development*. 2004;131:4907-4919.
36. Zhang M, Brancaccio A, Weiner L, et al. Ectodysplasin regulates pattern formation in the mammalian hair coat. *Genesis*. 2003;37:30-37.
37. Noramly S, Morgan BA. BMPs mediate lateral inhibition at successive stages in feather tract development. *Development*. 1998;125:3775-3787.
38. Jung HS, Francis-West PH, Widelitz RB, et al. Local inhibitory action of BMPs and their relationships with activators in feather formation: implications for periodic patterning. *Dev Biol*. 1998;196:11-23.
39. Jiang TX, Jung HS, Widelitz RB, et al. Self-organization of periodic patterns by dissociated feather mesenchymal cells and the regulation of size, number and spacing of primordia. *Development*. 1999;126: 4997-5009.
40. Patel K, Makarenkova H, Jung HS. The role of long range, local and direct signalling molecules during chick feather bud development involving the BMPs, follistatin and the Eph receptor tyrosine kinase Eph-A4. *Mech Dev*. 1999;86:51-62.
41. Botchkarev VA, Botchkareva NV, Roth W, et al. Noggin is a mesenchymally derived stimulator of hair-follicle induction. *Nat Cell Biol*. 1999;1:158-164.
42. Viallet JP, Prin F, Olivera-Martinez I, et al. Chick Delta-1 gene expression and the formation of the feather primordia. *Mech Dev*. 1998;72:159-168.
43. Crowe R, Henrique D, Ish-Horowicz D, et al. A new role for Notch and Delta in cell fate decisions: patterning the feather array. *Development*. 1998;125:767-775.
44. Powell BC, Passmore EA, Nesci A, et al. The Notch signalling pathway in hair growth. *Mech Dev*. 1998;78: 189-192.
45. Crowe R, Niswander L. Disruption of scale development by Delta-1 misexpression. *Dev Biol*. 1998;195:70-74.
46. Iseki S, Araga A, Ohuchi H, et al. Sonic hedgehog is expressed in epithelial cells during development of whisker, hair, and tooth. *Biochem Biophys Res Commun*. 1996;218:688-693.
47. Bitgood MJ, McMahon AP. Hedgehog and Bmp genes are coexpressed at many diverse sites of cell-cell interaction in the mouse embryo. *Dev Biol*. 1995;172:126-138.
48. St-Jacques B, Dassule HR, Karavanova I, et al. Sonic hedgehog signaling is essential for hair development. *Curr Biol*. 1998;8:1058-1068.
49. Chiang C, Swan RZ, Grachtchouk M, et al. Essential role for Sonic hedgehog during hair follicle morphogenesis. *Dev Biol*. 1999;205:1-9.
50. Karlsson L, Bondjers C, Betsholtz C. Roles for PDGF-A and sonic hedgehog in development of mesenchymal components of the hair follicle. *Development*. 1999;126:2611-2621.
51. Platt KA, Michaud J, Joyner AL. Expression of the mouse Gli and Ptc genes is adjacent to embryonic sources of hedgehog signals suggesting a conservation of pathways between flies and mice. *Mech Dev*. 1997;62:121-135.
52. Oro AE, Higgins KM, Hu Z, et al. Basal cell carcinomas in mice overexpressing sonic hedgehog. *Science*. 1997;276:817-821.
53. Schweizer J, Langbein L, Rogers MA, et al. Hair follicle-specific keratins and their diseases. *Exp Cell Res*. 2007;313, 2010-2020.
54. Luetteke NC, Phillips HK, Qiu TH, et al. The mouse waved-2 phenotype results from a point mutation in the EGF receptor tyrosine kinase. *Genes Dev*. 1994;8:399-413.
55. Luetteke NC, Qiu TH, Peiffer RL, et al. TGF alpha deficiency results in hair follicle and eye abnormalities in targeted and waved-1 mice. *Cell*. 1993;73:, 263-278.
56. Inoue A, Arima N, Ishiguro J, et al. LPA-producing enzyme PA-PLA(1)alpha regulates hair follicle development by modulating EGFR signalling. *EMBO J*. 2011;30:4248-4260.
57. Schneider MR, Schmidt-Ullrich R, Paus R. The hair follicle as a dynamic miniorgan. *Curr Biol*. 2009;19:R132-142.
58. Lee J, Tumbar T. Hairy tale of signaling in hair follicle development and cycling. *Semin Cell Dev Biol*. 2012;23:906-916.
59. Nehls M, Pfeifer D, Schorpp M, et al. New member of the winged-helix protein family disrupted in mouse and rat nude mutations. *Nature*. 1994;372:103-107.
60. Segre JA, Nemhauser JL, Taylor BA, et al. Positional cloning of the nude locus: genetic, physical, and transcription maps of the region and mutations in the mouse and rat. *Genomics*. 1995;28:549-559.
61. Brissette JL, Li J, Kamimura J, et al. The product of the mouse nude locus, Whn, regulates the balance between epithelial cell growth and differentiation. *Genes Dev*. 1996;10:2212-2221.
62. Meier N, Dear TN, Boehm T. Whn and mHa3 are components of the genetic hierarchy controlling hair follicle differentiation. *Mech Dev*. 1999;89:215-221.
63. Frank J, Pignata C, Panteleyev AA, et al. Exposing the human nude phenotype [letter]. *Nature*. 1999; 398:473-474.
64. Rezza A, Wang Z, Sennett R, et al. Signaling networks among stem cell precursors, transit-amplifying progenitors, and their niche in developing hair follicles. *Cell Rep*. 2016;14:3001-3018.
65. Linch CA, Whiting DA, Holland MM. Human hair histogenesis for the mitochondrial DNA forensic scientist. *J Forensic Sci*. 2001;46:844-853.
66. Murillas R, Larcher F, Conti CJ, et al. Expression of a dominant negative mutant of epidermal growth factor receptor in the epidermis of transgenic mice elicits striking alterations in hair follicle development and skin structure. *Embo J*. 1995;14:5216-5223.
67. Yuhki M, Yamada M, Kawano M, et al. BMPR1A signaling is necessary for hair follicle cycling and hair shaft

differentiation in mice. *Development (Cambridge, England)*. 2004;131:1825-1833.
68. Jave-Suarez LF, Winter H, Langbein L, et al. HOXC13 is involved in the regulation of human hair keratin gene expression. *J Biol Chem*. 2002;277:3718-3726.
69. Langbein L, Schweizer J. Keratins of the human hair follicle. *Int Rev Cytol*. 2005;243:1-78.
70. Langbein L, Rogers MA, Praetzel-Wunder S, et al. K25 (K25irs1), K26 (K25irs2), K27 (K25irs3), and K28 (K25irs4) represent the type I inner root sheath keratins of the human hair follicle. *J Invest Dermatol*. 2006;126:2377-2386.
71. Wu H, Stanley JR, Cotsarelis G. Desmoglein isotype expression in the hair follicle and its cysts correlates with type of keratinization and degree of differentiation. *J Invest Dermatol*. 2003;120:1052-1057.
72. Botchkareva NV, Ahluwalia G, Shander D. Apoptosis in the hair follicle. *J Invest Dermatol*. 2006;126:258-264.
73. Langbein L, Rogers MA, Praetzel S, et al. A novel epithelial keratin, hK6irs1, is expressed differentially in all layers of the inner root sheath, including specialized huxley cells (Flugelzellen) of the human hair follicle. *J Invest Dermatol*. 2002;118:789-799.
74. Kaufman CK, Zhou P, Pasolli HA, et al. GATA-3: an unexpected regulator of cell lineage determination in skin. *Genes Dev*. 2003;17:2108-2122.
75. Andl T, Ahn K, Kairo A, et al. Epithelial Bmpr1a regulates differentiation and proliferation in postnatal hair follicles and is essential for tooth development. *Development*. 2004;131:2257-2268.
76. Kobielak K, Pasolli HA, Alonso L, et al. Defining BMP functions in the hair follicle by conditional ablation of BMP receptor IA. *J Cell Biol*. 2003;163:609-623.
77. Jahoda CA, Horne KA, Oliver RF. Induction of hair growth by implantation of cultured dermal papilla cells. *Nature*. 1984;311:560-562.
78. Reynolds AJ, Jahoda CA. Cultured dermal papilla cells induce follicle formation and hair growth by transdifferentiation of an adult epidermis. *Development*. 1992;115:587-593.
79. Elliott K, Stephenson TJ, Messenger AG. Differences in hair follicle dermal papilla volume and cell number: implications for the control of hair follicle size and androgen responses. *J Invest Dermatol*. 1999;113:873-877.
80. Sharov AA, Sharova TY, Mardaryev AN, et al. BMP signaling controls hair follicle size and modulates the expression of cell cycle-associated genes. *Proc Natl Acad Sci U S A*. 2006;103:18166-18171.
81. Danilenko DM, Ring BD, Yanagihara D, et al. Keratinocyte growth factor is an important endogenous mediator of hair follicle growth, development, and differentiation. Normalization of the nu/nu follicular differentiation defect and amelioration of chemotherapy-induced alopecia. *Am J Pathol*. 1995;147:145-154.
82. Guo L, Degenstein L, Fuchs E. Keratinocyte growth factor is required for hair development but not for wound healing. *Genes Dev*. 1996;10:165-175.
83. Paus R, Peters EM, Eichmuller S, et al. Neural mechanisms of hair growth control. [Review]. *J Investig Dermatol Symp Proc*. 1997;2:61-68.
84. Halata Z. Sensory innervation of the hairy skin (light- and electronmicroscopic study. *J Invest Dermatol*. 1993;101:75S-81S.
85. Paus R, Heinzelmann T, Schultz KD, et al. Hair-growth induction by substance-p. *Lab Invest*. 1994;0071:134-140.
86. Hordinsky M, Ericson M, Snow D, et al. Peribulbar innervation and substance P expression following nonpermanent injury to the human scalp hair follicle. *J Investig Dermatol Symp Proc*. 1999;4:316-319.
87. Hordinsky MK, Ericson ME. Relationship between follicular nerve supply and alopecia. *Dermatol Clin*. 1996;14:651-660.
88. Peters EM, Botchkarev VA, Botchkareva NV, et al. Hair-cycle-associated remodeling of the peptidergic innervation of murine skin, and hair growth modulation by neuropeptides. *J Invest Dermatol*. 2001;116:236-245.
89. Brownell I, Guevara E, Bai CB, et al. Nerve-derived sonic hedgehog defines a niche for hair follicle stem cells capable of becoming epidermal stem cells. *Cell Stem Cell*. 2011;8:552-565.
90. Botchkarev VA, Eichmüller S, Johansson O, et al. Hair cycle-dependent plasticity of skin and hair follicle innervation in normal murine skin. *J Comp Neurol*. 1997;386:379-395.
91. Narisawa Y, Hashimoto K, Nakamura Y, et al. A high concentration of Merkel cells in the bulge prior to the attachment of the arrector pili muscle and the formation of the perifollicular nerve plexus in human fetal skin. *Arch Dermatol Res*. 1993;285:261-268.
92. Reynolds AJ, Lawrence C, Cserhalmi-Friedman PB, et al. Trans-gender induction of hair follicles. *Nature*. 1999;402, 33-34.
93. Cotsarelis G, Sun TT, Lavker RM. Label-retaining cells reside in the bulge area of pilosebaceous unit: implications for follicular stem cells, hair cycle, and skin carcinogenesis. *Cell*. 1990;61:1329-1337.
94. Ando H, Watabe H, Valencia JC, et al. Fatty acids regulate pigmentation via proteasomal degradation of tyrosinase: a new aspect of ubiquitin-proteasome function. *J Biol Chem*. 2004;279:15427-15433.
95. Morris RJ, Liu Y, Marles L, et al. Capturing and profiling adult hair follicle stem cells. *Nat Biotechnol*. 2004;22:411-417.
96. Oshima H, Rochat A, Kedzia C, et al. Morphogenesis and renewal of hair follicles from adult multipotent stem cells. *Cell*. 2001;104:233-245.
97. Ito M, Liu Y, Yang Z, et al. Stem cells in the hair follicle bulge contribute to wound repair but not to homeostasis of the epidermis. *Nat Med*. 2005;11:1351-1354.
98. Jaks V, Barker N, Kasper M, et al. Lgr5 marks cycling, yet long-lived, hair follicle stem cells. *Nat Genet*. 2008; 40:1291-1299.
99. Snippert HJ, Haegebarth A, Kasper M, et al. Lgr6 marks stem cells in the hair follicle that generate all cell lineages of the skin. *Science*. 2010;327, 1385-1389.
100. Jaks V, Kasper M, Toftgard R. The hair follicle-a stem cell zoo. *Exp Cell Res*. 2010;316:1422-1428.
101. Müller-Röver S, Handjiski B, van der Veen C, et al. A comprehensive guide for the accurate classification of murine hair follicles in distinct hair cycle stages. *J Invest Dermatol*. 2001;117:3-15.
102. Sano S, Tarutani M, Yamaguchi Y, et al. Keratinocyte-specific ablation of stat3 exhibits impaired skin remodeling, but does not affect skin morphogenesis. *EMBO J*. 1999;18:4657-4668.
103. Mecklenburg L, Tobin DJ, Müller-Röver S, et al. Active hair growth (anagen) is associated with angiogenesis. *J Invest Dermatol*. 2000;114:909-916.
104. Botchkareva NV, Khlgatian M, Longley BJ, et al. SCF/c-kit signaling is required for cyclic regeneration of the hair pigmentation unit. *FASEB J*. 2001;15:645-658.

105. Pierard GE, de la Brassinne M. Modulation of dermal cell activity during hair growth in the rat. *J Cutan Pathol*. 1975;2:35-41.
106. Ahmad W, Faiyaz ul Haque M, Brancolini V, et al. Alopecia universalis associated with a mutation in the human hairless gene. *Science*. 1998;279:720-724.
107. Miller J, Djabali K, Chen T, et al. Atrichia caused by mutations in the vitamin D receptor gene is a phenocopy of generalized atrichia caused by mutations in the hairless gene. *J Invest Dermatol*. 2001;117:612-617.
108. Hebert JM, Rosenquist T, Gotz J, et al. FGF5 as a regulator of the hair growth cycle: evidence from targeted and spontaneous mutations. *Cell*. 1994; 78:1017-1025.
109. Rosenquist TA, Martin GR. Fibroblast growth factor signalling in the hair growth cycle: expression of the fibroblast growth factor receptor and ligand genes in the murine hair follicle. *Dev Dyn*. 1996;205:379-386.
110. Pena JC, Kelekar A, Fuchs EV, et al. Manipulation of outer root sheath cell survival perturbs the hair-growth cycle. *Embo J*. 1999;18:3596-3603.
111. Hollis DE, Chapman RE. Apoptosis in wool follicles during mouse epidermal growth factor (mEGF)-induced catagen regression. *J Invest Dermatol*. 1987;88: 455-458.
112. Hansen LA, Alexander N, Hogan ME, et al. Genetically null mice reveal a central role for epidermal growth factor receptor in the differentiation of the hair follicle and normal hair development. *Am J Pathol*. 1997;150 1959-1975.
113. Mann GB, Fowler KJ, Gabriel A, et al. Mice with a null mutation of the TGF alpha gene have abnormal skin architecture, wavy hair, and curly whiskers and often develop corneal inflammation. *Cell*. 1993;73:249-261.
114. Botchkarev VA, Botchkarev NV, Albers KM, et al. Neurotrophin-3 involvement in the regulation of hair follicle morphogenesis. *J Invest Dermatol*. 1998; 111:279-285.
115. Botchkarev VA, Botchkareva NV, Albers KM, et al. A role for p75 neurotrophin receptor in the control of apoptosis-driven hair follicle regression. *FASEB J*. 2000;14:1931-1942.
116. Foitzik K, Lindner G, Mueller-Roever S, et al. Control of murine hair follicle regression (catagen) by TGF-beta1 in vivo. *FASEB J*. 2000;14:752-760.
117. Philpott MP, Sanders D, Westgate GE, et al. Human hair growth in vitro: a model for study of hair follicle biology. *J Dermatol Sci*. 1994;7(suppl):S55-S72.
118. Blair HJ, Uwechue IC, Barsh GS, et al. An integrated genetic and man-mouse comparative map of the DXHXS674-Pdha1 region of the mouse X chromosome. *Genomics*. 1998;48:128-131.
119. Milner Y, Sudnik J, Filippi M, et al. Exogen, shedding phase of the hair growth cycle: characterization of a mouse model. *J Invest Dermatol*. 2002;119:639-644.
120. Headington JT. Telogen effluvium. New concepts and review. *Arch Dermatol*. 1993;129:356-363.
121. Guarrera M, Rebora A. Anagen hairs may fail to replace telogen hairs in early androgenic female alopecia. *Dermatology*. 1996;192:28-31.
122. Slominski A, Tobin DJ, Shibahara S, et al. Melanin pigmentation in mammalian skin and its hormonal regulation. *Physiol Rev*. 2004;84:1155-1228.
123. Magerl M, Tobin DJ, Müller-Röver S, et al. Patterns of proliferation and apoptosis during murine hair follicle morphogenesis. *J Invest Dermatol*. 2001;116:947-955.
124. Tobin DJ, Slominski A, Botchkarev V, et al. The fate of hair follicle melanocytes during the hair growth cycle. *J Invest Dermatol*. 1999;4:323-332.
125. Slominski A, Wortsman J, Plonka PM, et al. Hair follicle pigmentation. *J Invest Dermatol*. 2005;124:13-21.
126. Holbrook KA, Underwood RA, Vogel AM, et al. The appearance, density and distribution of melanocytes in human embryonic and fetal skin revealed by the anti-melanoma monoclonal antibody, HMB-45. *Anat Embryol (Berlin)*. 1989;80:443-455.
127. Jordan S, Beermann F. Nomenclature for identified pigmentation genes in the mouse. *Pigment Cell Res*. 2000; 13:70-71.
128. Yoshida H, Kunisada T, Kusakabe M, et al. Distinct stages of melanocyte differentiation revealed by anlaysis of nonuniform pigmentation patterns. *Development*. 1996; 122:1207-1214.
129. Boissy RE, Nordlund JJ. Molecular basis of congenital hypopigmentary disorders in humans: a review. *Pigment Cell Res*. 1997;10:12-24.
130. Adameyko I, Lallemend F, Aquino JB, et al. Schwann cell precursors from nerve innervation are a cellular origin of melanocytes in skin. *Cell*. 2009;139:366-379.
131. Bertolotto C, Buscà R, Abbe P, et al. Different cis-acting elements are involved in the regulation of TRP1 and TRP2 promoter activities by cyclic AMP: pivotal role of M boxes (GTCATGTGCT) and of microphthalmia. *Mol Cell Biol*. 1998;18:694-702.
132. Botchkareva NV, Botchkarev VA, Gilchrest BA. Fate of melanocytes during development of the hair follicle pigmentary unit. *J Investig Dermatol Symp Proc*. 2003;8:76-79.
133. Kunisada T, Yoshida H, Yamazaki H, et al. Transgene expression of steel factor in the basal layer of epidermis promotes survival, proliferation, differentiation and migration of melanocyte precursors. *Development*. 1998;125:2915-2923.
134. Kunisada T, Lu SZ, Yoshida H, et al. Murine cutaneous mastocytosis and epidermal melanocytosis induced by keratinocyte expression of transgenic stem cell factor. *J Exp Med*. 1998;187:1565-1573.
135. Zsebo KM, Williams DA, Geissler EN, et al. Stem cell factor is encoded at the Sl locus of the mouse and is the ligand for the c-kit tyrosine kinase receptor. *Cell*. 1990;63:213-224.
136. McGill GG, Horstmann M, Widlund HR, et al. Bcl2 regulation by the melanocyte master regulator Mitf modulates lineage survival and melanoma cell viability. *Cell*. 2002;109:707-718.
137. Mak SS, Moriyama M, Nishioka E, et al. Indispensable role of Bcl2 in the development of the melanocyte stem cell. *Dev Biol*. 2006;291:144-153.
138. Nishimura EK, Granter SR, Fisher DE. Mechanisms of hair graying: incomplete melanocyte stem cell maintenance in the niche. *Science*. 2005;307:720-724.
139. Nishimura EK, Suzuki M, Igras V, et al. Key roles for transforming growth factor beta in melanocyte stem cell maintenance. *Cell Stem Cell* 2010;6:130-140.
140. Moriyama M, Osawa M, Mak SS, et al. Notch signaling via Hes1 transcription factor maintains survival of melanoblasts and melanocyte stem cells. *J Cell Biol*. 2006;173:333-339.
141. Veis DJ, Sorenson CM, Shutter JR, et al. Bcl-2-deficient mice demonstrate fulminant lymphoid apoptosis, polycystic kidneys, and hypopigmented hair. *Cell*. 1993;75, 229-240.
142. Yamamura K, Kamada S, Ito S, et al. Accelerated disappearance of melanocytes in bcl-2-deficient mice. *Cancer Res*. 1996;56:3546-3550.
143. Weiner L, Han R, Scicchitano BM, et al. Dedicated epithelial recipient cells determine pigmentation patterns. *Cell*. 2007;130:932-942.

144. Rabbani P, Takeo M, Chou W, et al. Coordinated activation of Wnt in epithelial and melanocyte stem cells initiates pigmented hair regeneration. *Cell*. 2011;145:941-955.
145. Chou WC, Takeo M, Rabbani P, et al. Direct migration of follicular melanocyte stem cells to the epidermis after wounding or UVB irradiation is dependent on Mc1r signaling. *Nat Med*. 2013;19:924-929.
146. Takeo M, Lee W, Rabbani P, et al. EdnrB governs regenerative response of melanocyte stem cells by crosstalk with Wnt signaling. *Cell Rep*. 2016;15:1291-1302.
147. Aubin-Houzelstein G, Djian-Zaouche J, Bernex F, et al. Melanoblasts' proper location and timed differentiation depend on Notch/RBP-J signaling in postnatal hair follicles. *J Invest Dermatol*. 2008;128:2686-2695.
148. Schallreuter KU, Beazley WD, Hibberts NA, et al. Pterins in human hair follicle cells and in the synchronized murine hair cycle. *J Invest Dermatol*. 1998;111:545-550.
149. Sharov A, Tobin DJ, Sharova TY, et al. Changes in different melanocyte populations during hair follicle involution (catagen). *J Invest Dermatol*. 2005;125:1259-1267.
150. Abdel-Malek Z, Suzuki I, Tada A, et al. The melanocortin-1 receptor and human pigmentation. *Ann N Y Acad Sci*. 1999;885:117-133.
151. Barsh GS. What controls variation in human skin color? *PLoS Biol*. 2003;1:E27.
152. Abdel-Malek ZA. Melanocortin receptors: their functions and regulation by physiological agonists and antagonists. *Cell Mol Life Sci*. 2001;58:434-441.
153. Adan RA, Hillebrand JJ, De Rijke C, et al. Melanocortin system and eating disorders. *Ann N Y Acad Sci*. 2003;994:267-274.
154. Kauser S, Thody AJ, Schallreuter KU, et al. A fully-functional POMC/MC-1R system regulates the differentiation of human scalp hair follicle melanocytes. *Endocrinology*. 2005;146(2):532-43.
155. Cable J, Jackson IJ, Steel KP. Light (Blt), a mutation that causes melanocyte death, affects stria vascularis function in the mouse inner ear. *Pigment Cell Res*. 1993;6:215-225.
156. Tobin DJ. Human hair pigmentation—biological aspects. *Int J Cosmet Sci*. 2008;30:233-257.
157. Commo S, Gaillard O, Thibaut S, Bernard BA. Absence of TRP-2 in melanogenic melanocytes of human hair. *Pigment Cell Res*. 2004;17:488-497.
158. Inomata K, Aoto T, Binh NT, et al. Genotoxic stress abrogates renewal of melanocyte stem cells by triggering their differentiation. *Cell*. 2009;137:1088-1099.
159. Wood JM, Decker H, Hartmann H, et al. Senile hair graying: H2O2-mediated oxidative stress affects human hair color by blunting methionine sulfoxide repair. *FASEB J*. 2009;23:2065-2075.

Chapter 8 :: Nail
:: Krzysztof Kobielak

第八章
甲

中文导读

本章共分为6节：①概述；②甲结构(解剖学)和功能；③甲的生长和分化；④甲干细胞池；⑤甲上皮在指再生中的作用；⑥结论。

第一节概述了甲生物学的新发现及其生长规律以及甲分化的机理，尤其是甲的干细胞群及甲的再生能力。

第二节甲结构(解剖学)和功能，介绍了甲始于远端指骨表面的甲上皮，包含甲近端皱襞、侧甲皱襞、甲基质、甲板、甲床。甲板具有保护作用及维持手指精细操作功能，甲皱襞能保护甲免受毒素和异物的侵害。

第三节甲的生长和分化，介绍了目前普遍支持甲是仅由甲基质产生的假说。

第四节甲干细胞池，目前研究表明甲器官中有两种皮肤干细胞池，分别是双功能甲近端皱襞干细胞池和快速循环甲干细胞池。

第五节甲上皮在指再生中的作用，介绍了人的指尖受伤后可完全再生，这与位于甲近端基质中的神经干细胞及其分化密切相关。甲上皮的Wnt/β-连环蛋白信号是指再生、甲形成和分化关键机制，若通路发生突变，可出现遗传性无甲症等疾病。

第六节总结了甲器官中的干细胞群体及其相互关系的发现，以及干细胞和干细胞微环境之间的相互作用，有助于揭开干细胞生物学的新概念，具有极大的转化潜力，为截肢者开发新的疗法。

〔粟 娟〕

AT-A-GLANCE

The nail appendage is composed of several layers that organize the nail organ:

- The eponychium creates a border between skin epidermis and nail organ at the dorsal limit of the nail proximal fold (NPF), forming a protective seal.
- The NPF forms after skin epidermis bends inward ventrally at the eponychium's border and becomes the nail epidermis, creating the NPF, which localizes slow-cycling bifunctional nail proximal fold stem cells (NPFSCs). NPFSCs actively deliver progeny to the perinail epidermis and nail matrix along with differentiated nail plate upon nail regeneration.
- The matrix, a ventral continuation of the proximal fold after it bends dorsally and distally, is composed of actively proliferating cells called onychocytes. In the proximal nail matrix, fast-proliferating nail stem cells are located. Their differentiation is coupled directly with the ability to orchestrate digit regeneration.
- Nail matrix differentiates, forming the keratogenous zone, which finally deposit cells into the overlying nail plate.
- Hyponychium is the most distal part of the nail epithelium located peripherally to the nail bed, and beneath the nail plate at the junction between the free edge and the skin epidermis of the fingertip, it forms a seal that protects the nail bed.

INTRODUCTION

The nail organ is one of the skin appendages located on the distal phalanx of each finger and toe in human body. Interestingly, nails exhibit continuous growth under physiological conditions and can fully regenerate upon removal. This chapter covers new discoveries of nail appendage biology, its growth regulation, and the mechanism of nail differentiation. Scientists have been intensely searching for stem cells in various organs in hopes of understanding and taking advantage of their regenerative abilities. Indeed, the skin is a complex organ containing a number of different "mini-organs," skin appendages that are maintained by independent stem cell populations.

For the past several years, there have been active investigations and discussion about whether the nail organ alone possess stem cells that can regenerate the whole nail appendage or if other cells appear to contribute to nail regeneration. This chapter presents new discoveries about the coexistence of two independent populations of skin stem cells localized in the nail organ, with quite opposite cell cycle dynamics, namely a slow-cycling population of bifunctional nail proximal fold stem cells (NPFSCs) and fast-cycling nail stem cells (NSCs). In addition, their reciprocal dependence and interactions during nail organ regeneration have been discussed. Thus, nails contain a gradient of slow- to fast-cycling cells, with slow-cycling NPFCs and then more active cells in the intermediate zone (IZ) that separate them from highly proliferative stem cells in the nail proximal matrix.

We also present a new function of nail organ, specifically newly discovered NSCs in the nail proximal matrix and their adjacent progenitors in the nail distal matrix that contribute actively to nail differentiation and their surprising critical role in orchestrating digit regeneration in mammals. Moreover, stem cell isolation from nail organs and their gene expression profiling revealed their molecular characteristics, in which bone morphogenetic protein (BMP) and wingless-type MMTV integration site family (Wnt) signaling pathways were identified to be an essential in nail fate differentiation as well as in digit regeneration. Thus, current research has begun to unveil that also other skin appendages, including nails, possess their own stem cells with regenerative capacities. However, more studies are needed for further characterization of these stem cells in the nail organ that may shed some light on putative stem cell regenerative potential in human nails in the future. Therefore, because of its extraordinary regenerative potential, further studies of mechanisms regulating stem cell populations in nails and their interaction with mesenchymal cells may lead to new routes to treat various nail disorders, including amputations in humans.

NAIL ORGAN STRUCTURE (ANATOMY) AND FUNCTION

Nails belong to one of the skin appendages and are located on the distal phalanx of each finger and toe in the human body (Fig. 8-1). The nail appendage begins as an extension of the distal phalanx skin epidermis at the border called the eponychium (Fig. 8-2). At that point, the skin epidermis bends inward ventrally and becomes the nail epidermis, forming the nail proximal fold (NPF) (see Fig. 8-2). Interestingly, normal epidermal differentiation ceases just after the proximal fold folds inward at the eponychium border; thus, nail layers continuing beyond this point do not form the granular layer typically observed in normal skin epidermis. As a ventral continuation of the proximal fold after it bends dorsally and distally is the nail matrix composed of actively proliferating nail cells called onychocytes (see Figs. 8-2 and 8-3).[1] Above the matrix lies the keratogenous zone (KZ) where matrix cells differentiate, flatten out, die, and deposit into the overlying nail plate (see Figs. 8-2 and 8-3). The nail plate is a hard structure that serves as a protective covering by preventing trauma to the tips of toes and fingers; it is also used as a tool to pick up small objects, which is important for fine manipulations and subtle finger functions. Through the nail plate, the whitish crescent-shaped base is called the lunula ("small moon"), the visible part of the matrix (see Fig. 8-1). The lunula can best be seen in the thumb and may not be visible in the little finger.

Within the nail organ, the nail plate contains a hard keratinized structure composed of flattened and anucleated cells called corneocytes overlying the distal phalange (see Figs. 8-1 and 8-2). Corneocytes are formed during nail differentiation from nail cells, onychocytes. The nail plate exerts counterpressure at the fingertips for protection and enhances sensitivity. Distal to the nail matrix is the nail bed, composed of a basal layer and one or two layers of suprabasal postmitotic keratinocytes, contributing a few horn cells to

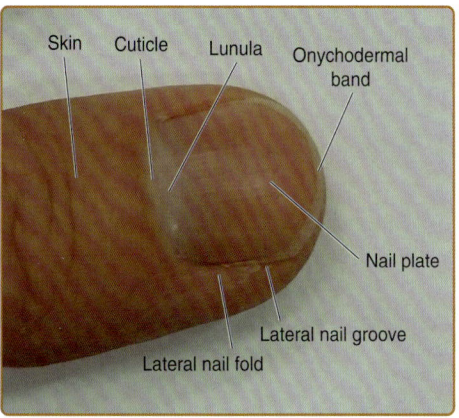

Figure 8-1 Picture of a human fingertip with the nail organ. Visible structure include the skin, cuticle, nail plate with the proximally located lunula, and the distally located onychodermal band. On the side, the nail plate is separated by the lateral nail groove and lateral nail fold.

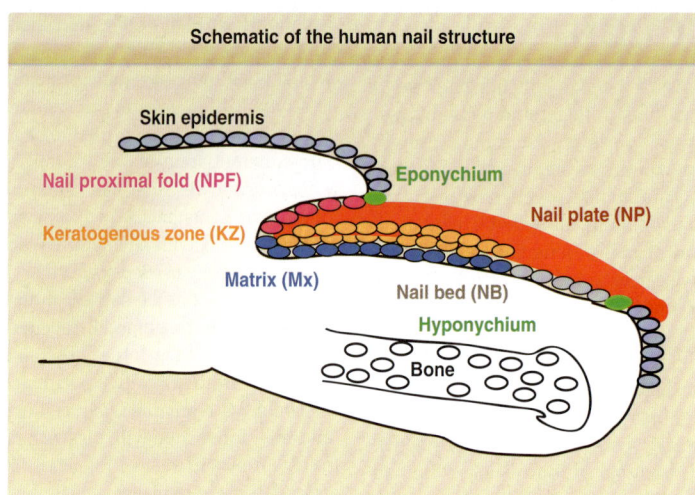

Figure 8-2 Schematic of the human nail structure (longitudinal section through the middle of nail). Different nail layers and structures with color include the nail proximal fold (*pink*), matrix (*blue*), keratogenous zone (*orange*), nail bed (*light grey*), nail plate (*red*), and flanking from both sides by eponychium and hyponychium (*green*), which separates the nail structure from the skin epidermis (*dark grey*).

the undersurface of the distal nail plate (see Fig. 8-2).[2] The nail plate is attached to the finger by interdigiting with the underlying nail bed (see Fig. 8-2). The nail cuticle extends from the edge of the proximal fold onto the nail plate, sealing the proximal end of the nail and protecting it from toxins and foreign substances (see Fig. 8-1). Laterally, the nail plate is surrounded by lateral nail grooves and lateral nail folds (see Fig. 8-1). Similarly, at the distal end border of the nail unit, the hyponychium seals the nail plate to the nail bed under the onychodermal band to prevent infection (see Figs. 8-1 and 8-2).

Comparing human nails with those of other mammals (eg, mouse nail in this example), it is apparent that the shape is very different, likely owing to differences in evolution and function. The human nail is flatter (see Figs. 8-1 and 8-3); a mammal's claw is a near conical structure with greater curvature. This shape is influenced by the underlying distal phalanx and the distribution of the matrix.[1,3]

NAIL GROWTH AND DIFFERENTIATION

So far, it is believed that the matrix is largely responsible for nail plate production. However, previously, it was unclear whether the matrix is the sole source of nail differentiation or if other parts of the nail unit, such as the nail bed, also contribute to the nail plate. In the past, Lewis observed that the nail plate is composed of three different layers and proposed that they arise from three different parts of the nail unit. It was theorized that the superficial layer of the dorsal nail originates from the proximal nail fold, the intermediate nail arises from the matrix, and the deep ventral nail is produced by the nail bed.[4]

About a decade later, Zaias and Alvarez used radioactive tritiated glycine to mark and follow nail cells in squirrel monkeys, demonstrating that the uptake in the label moves from the matrix into the nail plate over time.[5] Only small amounts of radioactive tritiated glycine were incorporated in the nail bed and were therefore dismissed as a source of nail production because of its inactivity. Taken together, the nail matrix was proposed to be solely responsible for nail plate formation.[5] Similar studies were also conducted on human volunteers using both tritiated thymidine (^{3}H-thymidine) and glycine in which matrix cells were proposed to migrate into the nail bed in addi-

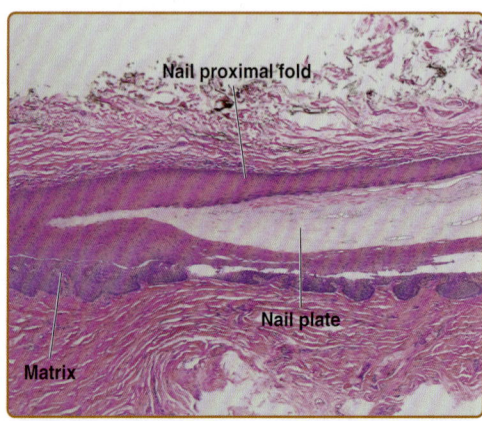

Figure 8-3 The nail apparatus. Histologic appearance of the elements that make up the nail unit (hematoxylin and eosin staining of longitudinal section through the middle of nail; original magnification ×20). Nail histologic layers are the nail proximal fold, matrix, and nail plate. (Used with permission from Dr. Sébastien de Feraudy, MD, PhD, Associate Professor & Director of Dermatopathology, UC Irvine Dermatopathology Laboratory, Irvine, CA.)

tion to the nail plate.[6] The hypothesis that the nail is produced only by the matrix was further supported by Berker and Angus, who demonstrated that the matrix cells were highly proliferative compared with the relatively inactive nail bed.[7] In other studies, it has been proposed that although the matrix produces the bulk of the nail plate, the nail bed also contributes to the nail plate based on nail thickness and mass.[8,9] It is argued that the contribution of the nail bed to the ventral nail plate allows distal movement of the nail plate as it grows. Thus, in conclusion, there appear to be a general consensus that the nail plate is produced by matrix cells.

TWO POOLS OF STEM CELLS EXIST IN NAIL ORGAN (HOMEOSTASIS AND REGENERATION)

Whether the matrix cells are the only source of progenitor cells required for nail production or if the other layers including NPF also contribute to portion of the nail during the lifetime, meeting the criteria of being stem cells per se is evaluated in this section.

Adult stem cells found in various organs throughout the body are responsible for maintaining the normal turnover of organs as well as tissue repair in the event of an injury.[10] These are made possible by its ability to self-renew and differentiate into the different specialized cell types in its respective organs.[10] Because stem cells are required for tissue homeostasis and regeneration throughout life, they must have long-term self-renewal capacity. Moreover, it has been proposed that stem cells divide infrequently to avoid incorporation of mutations associated with cell division. In each organ, stem cells reside in specialized microenvironments called niches, which helps maintain quiescence or regulate proliferation and differentiation, which are important for tissue homeostasis and repair.[10-13]

Upon activation, these stem cells divide and leave the niche to form more differentiated transit-amplifying (TA) progenitor cells. In contrast to the relatively quiescent stem cells, TA cells rapidly proliferate and differentiate into cells needed for regeneration or repair.[10] Adult stem cells are theoretically present in all regenerative tissues, but their localization and characterization are often difficult because little is known about these organs. Therefore, scientists have used the slow-cycling property to label and identify putative stem cells in various organs. In early pulse-chase studies, animals were injected with ^{3}H-thymidine, which gets incorporated into the newly synthesized DNA of dividing cells. After efficient labeling, the animal undergoes a period of chase when dividing cells dilute out the ^{3}H-thymidine label and slow-cycling cells retain this radioactive label. This method allowed for the identification of slow-cycling label-retaining cells (LRCs).

In 1990, Cotsarelis and coworkers identified a unique population of slow-cycling LRCs in the bulge region of the hair follicle using ^{3}H-thymidine pulse chase experiments. They demonstrated that these bulge LRCs can be stimulated to proliferate upon treatment with a tumor promoter (12-O-tetradecanoylphorbol-13-acetate [TPA]) and went on to hypothesize that these LRCs are stem cells of the hair follicle.[14] Before identifying LRCs in the hair follicle bulge, Cotsarelis and coworkers also reported on LRCs in the cornea limbus using similar pulse chase experiments.[15] These limbal LRCs were also preferentially activated in response to injury and can also be stimulated by TPA. These data support the theory that stem cells persist throughout the lifetime of an animal to contribute to the tissue during regeneration and wound repair.

Using radioactive labeling, however, researchers were unable to probe for colocalization of potential markers through immunological histology. Soon after, scientists began to use a new synthetic thymidine analog, bromodeoxyuridine (BrdU).[16] In contrast to ^{3}H-thymidine, BrdU is not radioactive. In addition, antibodies against BrdU allow for immunohistochemistry to probe for markers that colocalize with BrdU-marked LRCs.[17] Pulse-chase studies with BrdU have been widely used to identify LRCs in numerous tissues.

More recently, a new method for identifying LRCs using transgenic mice with tetracycline-induced histone 2B-green fluorescent protein (H2B-GFP) has been described.[18] With this system, a specific or ubiquitous promoter can be used to drive inducible H2B-GFP expression in the tissues of interest. One advantage of this system is that it can more efficiently label the cells before chase, but the BrdU method can only label cells that are actively dividing in the synthesis phase during pulse. Moreover, this H2B-GFP transgenic label-retaining system allows for the isolation of live LRCs for further characterization and analysis. For the first time, this method allowed the isolation of live hair follicle label-retaining stem cells for gene expression profiling to determine the molecular characteristics of these stem cells independent of any other markers such as keratin 15 (K15) or CD34.[18] Over the years, this method allowed understanding of how hair follicles and their stem cells are regulated.

SLOW-CYCLING BIFUNCTIONAL NAIL PROXIMAL FOLD STEM CELLS IN THE NAIL ORGAN

Subsequently, in addition to the hair follicle in many skin appendages, such as the cornea and sweat glands, slow-cycling stem cell characteristics were demonstrated[14,15,19-21]; however, little was known about other skin appendages such as nails.

Therefore, recent studies tried to address whether such a quiescent stem cell population also exists in continuously growing nails. First notice of existence of LRCs in the nail after BrdU pulse-chase experiments suggested the presence of LRCs in the basal layer of the nail matrix adjacent to the nail bed in the mouse nail; however, further characterization has not been performed.[22] In contrast to this localization, using immunohistochemical staining, Sellheyer and coworkers showed that the ventral proximal fold in human nails expresses hair follicle stem cell (hfSC) markers (eg, K15; keratin 19 [K19]; and pleckstrin homology-like domain, family A, member 1 protein [PHLDA1]) during embryogenesis and contains very few Ki67+ cells (a nuclear protein associated with cell proliferation), making them more quiescent similar to hfSCs, suggesting that the proximal fold may represent the human NSC niche.[23]

These discrepancies have been addressed in recent studies using H2B-GFP LRCs system in transgenic mice for the in vivo detection of quiescent, slow-cycling skin cells.[24] This method allows identifying a previously unreported population of nail LRCs within the basal layer of the NPF (Fig. 8-4).[24] Interestingly, in mice, the nail exists as a three-dimensional near-conical structure; therefore, LRCs are organized in a ringlike configuration.[24] Nail LRCs express the hfSC marker K15, and in vivo lineage tracing experiments show that K15-labeled cells, originating in the NPF, contribute to both the nail structure (see Fig. 8-4, *black arrow #2*, long term) and more predominantly to the perinail epidermis (see Fig. 8-4, *green arrow #1*), thus possessing a bifunctional stem cell characteristic. Upon nail regeneration, these K15-derived NPFSCs actively deliver progeny to the nail matrix and differentiate into the nail plate (see Fig. 8-4, *black arrow #2*). Similarly, in vivo engraftment experiments demonstrate that the nail LRCs can actively participate in functional nail regeneration. Transcriptional profiling of isolated nail LRCs revealed a requirement for BMP signaling in proper nail formation and differentiation (Fig. 8-5). Thus, BMP signaling guides NPFSCs toward nail differentiation, and without this pathway, matrix cells proliferate less, and a KZ is not observed above the matrix region (see Fig. 8-5).[24] Also, proper nail plate differentiation is compromised, and without BMP signaling, the nail adopts an epidermal fate in vivo (see Fig. 8-5). It manifests the extension of the skin epidermis granular layer throughout the nail with typical epidermal markers such as keratin 1 (K1) and loricrin expression observed in the nail plate (see Fig. 8-5). In contrast, typical differentiation nail plate marker AE13 (keratin expressed in both the hair cortex and nail plate) was undetectable (see Fig. 8-5).[24] Interestingly, a similar role of BMP signaling was observed in proper hair follicle differentiation.[25] This observation was also consistent, and the phenotype was even more severe than a phenotype of the *Msx2* and *Foxn1* double mutant; both genes previously have been showed as downstream targets of BMP signaling regulating normal nail differentiation.[26] It was also similar to *Foxn1* and *Hoxc13* single mutants, with aberrant extension of the epidermal stratum granulosum within the nail structure (see Fig. 8-5).[2,27] In addition, the role of BMP signaling is also required for maintenance

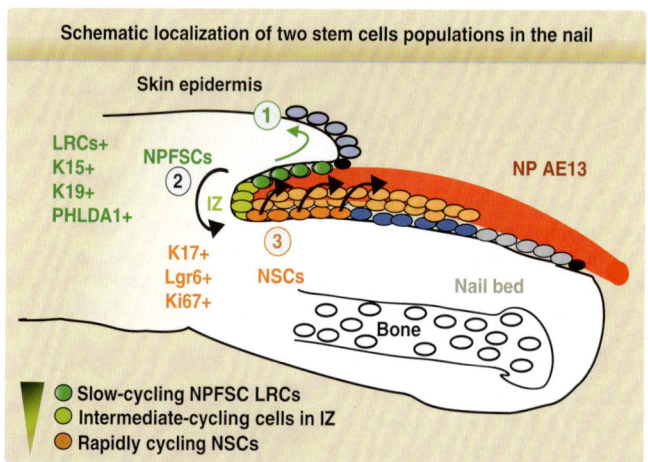

Figure 8-4 Schematic localization of two stem cells populations in the nail. Localization of nail proximal fold stem cells (NPFSCs) with slow-cycling label-retaining characteristic (LRCs) in the nail proximal fold and fast-proliferating nail stem cells (NSCs) in the proximal matrix. NPFSCs express keratin 15 (K15); keratin 19 (K19); and pleckstrin homology-like domain, family A, member 1 protein (PHLDA1). K15-marked NPFSCs contribute predominantly to the perinail epidermis (*1, green arrow*) but also to the nail matrix and nail differentiation (*2, black arrow*) during nail homeostasis. NSCs, when marked by Lgr6, participate in nail matrix structure and nail plate (NP) differentiation (*3, black arrows*). AE13, keratin that is expressed in the hair cortex and nail plate; IZ, intermediate zone; Ki67, a nuclear protein associated with cell proliferation; Lgr6, leucine-rich repeat containing G protein–coupled receptor 6.

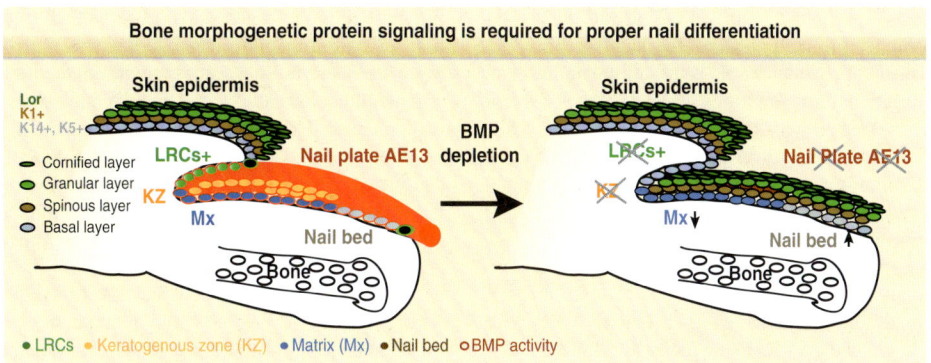

Figure 8-5 Bone morphogenetic protein (BMP) signaling is required for proper nail differentiation. Active BMP signaling is found in nail proximal fold and the nail matrix (indicated by *circles with red encasements*). BMP depletion in nails demonstrates the absence of the keratogenous zone (KZ, *orange circles*), hyperplasia of the nail bed (*grey circles*), and loss of label-retaining cells (LRCs), and an ectopic granular layer extends over the whole nail plate (layer of skin epidermis marked by *green circles*). Keratin 1 (K1) and Loricrin (Lor) epidermal markers are ectopically expressed in the absence of BMP signaling. Positive K1 staining is found in the proximal fold and ventral nail of control mice. Ectopic K1 expression (layer of skin epidermis marked by *brown circles*) is observed instead of expression of the nail plate marker AE13 (*red color*). Loricrin expression is found in the proximal fold until eponychium and is absent in the dorsal nail plate of control mice. Ectopic loricrin expression (layer of skin epidermis marked by *dark green circles*) is observed instead of expression of the nail plate marker AE13 (*red color*). The amount of proliferating cells in Mx (marked by *blue circles*) appears to be decreased, and AE13, a marker of the nail plate differentiation, is compromised without BMP signaling. Thus, the ectopic expression of epidermal markers demonstrates that BMP signaling may be required for the nail fate, and without it, the nail structure acquires an epidermal-like phenotype.

of the LRC characteristic of NPFSCs (see Fig. 8-5), as previously observed in hfSCs.[28] Taken together, a novel population of bifunctional stem cells within the NPF region displays plastic homeostatic dynamics capable of responding to injury and suggests a common, coordinated mechanism of protective barrier formation that could occur between the nail and adjacent epidermis.[24]

RAPIDLY CYCLING UNIPOTENT NAIL STEM CELLS IN THE NAIL ORGAN

The nail matrix is a morphological continuation of the NPF cells that attach to each other through the IZ wrapping around the proximal end of the nail plate (see Fig. 8-4). Thus, proliferating matrix progenitor cells are found in the near vicinity of the NPF region and differentiate into cells of the KZ to form the external nail plate.

In terms of the cell proliferation dynamic, a clear distinction was observed between slow-cycling nail LRCs in the NPF and the actively dividing matrix cells after only 1 week of chase.[24] At that time point, Ki67 immunolabeling primarily is localized to proliferating matrix cells and a minority of weakly H2B-GFP+ cells immediately adjacent to Ki67 negative strongly H2B-GFP+ proximal fold (PF) LRCs, indicating increased proliferation within the matrix in comparison with the adjacent PF region (see Fig. 8-4).

Thus, the area between both regions—the proliferating matrix and the quiescent PF IZ—has been described as containing weakly H2B-GFP+ and Ki67+ cells, which arise from H2B-GFP label dilution after cell division. The IZ gradually decreases in size with increasing periods of chase, being minimal just after a 2-week chase to completely disappearing after a 4-week chase. This indicates the existence of a gradient in cell division expanding from relatively quiescent slow-cycling LRCs in the NPF (through the IZ of more active cells) to rapidly dividing matrix cells (see Fig. 8-4).[24]

Thus, it was demonstrated that the nail matrix contains rapidly dividing progenitor cells responsible for nail differentiation. However, whether matrix cells alone possess stem cell characteristics and can generate the whole nail appendage was investigated and is addressed further later in this chapter.

To locate stem cells in nails, Takeo and coworkers used a transgenic mouse lineage tracing system. Under control of keratin 14 (K14) promoter-driven Cre recombinase–mutated estrogen receptor (Cre-ER) (K14–Cre-ER), they marked keratinocytes in the basal layer of the skin epidermis and the nail epidermis by activating LacZ expression.[29] In that system, LacZ expression was driven by the Rosa26 promoter, and its activation followed Cre-mediated removal of the floxed stop cassette. Thus, it allowed labeling genetically a small subset of K14 nail basal epidermal cells, including nail matrix cells and bed cells, using a single injection of tamoxifen and then assessing participation of LacZ-labeled cells in nail regeneration over an extended period of time. Over 5 months, the number of LacZ+ descendants of the labeled K14 nail epithelial cells extended linearly and distally, persisting as streaks that emerged only from the proximal matrix but not from the distal matrix. Proximal matrix cells possessed characteristics of undifferentiated epidermal cells expressing keratin 17 (K17) in addition to K14 with highly proliferative Ki67 marker (see Fig. 8-4). The isolated proximal matrix cells had the highest colony-forming ability in vitro, a general characteristic of epithelial stem cells. Thus, prolonged labeling results along with in vitro culture data demonstrated that the rapidly dividing proximal matrix contains self-renewing cells, meeting the criteria to be per se NSCs that sustain nail growth (see Fig. 8-4).[29]

Interestingly, a gene expression analysis between proximal matrix versus distal matrix revealed that proximal matrix cells were enriched with NSCs with downregulated Wnt signaling pathway.[29] Indeed, analyses using two different Wnt reporter mice confirmed that although the Wnt signal started from the distal part of the K17-positive NSC region and persisted into the distal matrix of K17-negative distal matrix, both signals were absent in the proximal end of the nail matrix. Consistently, Wnt signaling pathway components such as Tcf1 (also known as hepatocyte nuclear factor 1a), a nuclear mediator of Wnt signaling, and Wls (Wntless homologue) were not expressed in the proximal end of NSCs, but several keratins that contained a TCF1 and LEF1 consensus binding site were upregulated in the distal matrix, thus suggesting direct involvement of Wnt signaling in nail differentiation. This was verified by deletion of Wnt signaling activation in the nail epithelium by removing β-catenin (an essential mediator of Wnt signaling) in adult epithelium revealed by the lack of AE13, a marker for keratinized nail cells. Interestingly, without β-catenin or Wntless, the entire nail epithelium showed characteristics of the NSC region with K17-positive and highly proliferating Ki67-positive cells, thus confirming the essential role of Wnt signaling in nail differentiation.

Moreover, in a recent study, scientists identified a cell population expressing a mediator of Wnt signaling, Lgr6 (leucine-rich repeat containing G protein–coupled receptor 6), as key stem cells marker for the nail, which was localized within the nail proximal matrix, thus being consistent and confirming previous discoveries by Takeo and coworkers.[30] Indeed, Lgr6 is a molecular marker specific to the NSCs, giving rise to the nail plate and contributing to the growth of nail over time (see Fig. 8-4). Thus, these data confirmed that canonical Wnt signaling (which results in β-catenin localization to the nucleus of the nail matrix) broadly correlates with the expression of Lgr6-expressing nail matrix cells.

ROLE OF NAIL EPITHELIUM IN DIGIT REGENERATION

The tips of the digits of humans, similar to those of some mammals, including mice, are capable of complete regeneration after injury like those of amphibians.[31,32] Interestingly, this capacity is limited to the area associated with the nail, and previous studies showed that nail transplantation after amputation at the middle phalanx can induce ectopic digit bone differentiation.[31-33] Thus, this observation suggests that the nail epithelium has a special function, creating a permissive regenerative environment for digit regeneration. Recently, some cellular and molecular components of the digit regeneration process have been discovered by Takeo and associates.[29] Indeed, the process is orchestrated and depends on the presence of the overlaying nail organ and its reciprocal interaction with underlying blastema. It has been shown that nail epithelium, particularly NSCs located in the proximal nail matrix and their differentiation, is coupled directly with ability to orchestrate digit regeneration. On a molecular level in the mouse model, Wnt/β-catenin signaling from nail epithelium has been shown to be necessary for digit regeneration. The current proposed model is that NSCs in the proximal matrix give rise to distal matrix cells with Wnt activation (through Wntless), and, simultaneously, NSCs and distal matrix cells differentiate into the nail plate (Fig. 8-6). After distal amputation at the level of the distal matrix expressing Wntless (but NSCs in proximal matrix remain intact), the wound site is covered by regenerating nail epithelial cells, which in turn activate Wnt signaling (Wntless) to differentiate into distal matrix cells and the nail plate (see Fig. 8-6). The Wnt pathway activation promotes blastema innervations through semaphorin 5a (Sema5a, an axon-guidance molecule), which is upregulated in control nail epithelium 3 weeks after amputation. Conversely, innervations are necessary for fibroblast growth factor 2 (FGF2) expression in the regenerating nail epithelium (see Fig. 8-6). Then FGF2 promotes proliferation of either Runx2-positive progenitors or Sp7 osteoblasts, ultimately leading to coupled digit regeneration (see Fig. 8-6). Interestingly, receptor for FGF2 ligand FGFR1 is expressed in mesenchymal blastema (a Runx2 progenitor); thus, the ERK pathway could be recruited to activate and maintain their proliferation (see Fig. 8-6).

Thus, nail differentiation is regulated by a WNT-dependent mechanism that is linked to digit regeneration. Indeed, Wnt deletion (in β-catenin conditional knockout [KO] mice) results in a lack of nail differentiation that manifests by absence of TopGal expression in the nail matrix (a gene reporter for WNT pathway) and AE13 expression (a marker for keratinized nail plate cells), and bone regeneration is blocked. Moreover, Runx2 progenitor cells, mesenchymal cells, and Sp7 osteoblasts underneath the nail matrix epithelium in β-catenin conditional KO mice were not stimulated to proliferate or produce BMP4. Moreover, Wnt-dependent innervation can promote digit regeneration because Sema5a is downregulated in the nail epithelium 3 weeks after amputation in β-catenin conditional KO mice. These data are in agreement that denervation (nerves removed surgically before amputation) suppresses blastema growth similar to that observed in conditional KO mice without FGF2 expression in the nail epithelium after denervation.[34,35] Interestingly, although after proximal amputation of nail matrix cells, stabilization of β-catenin induces TCF1 expression and regeneration of the distal matrix and formation of well-innervated blastema cells, β-catenin

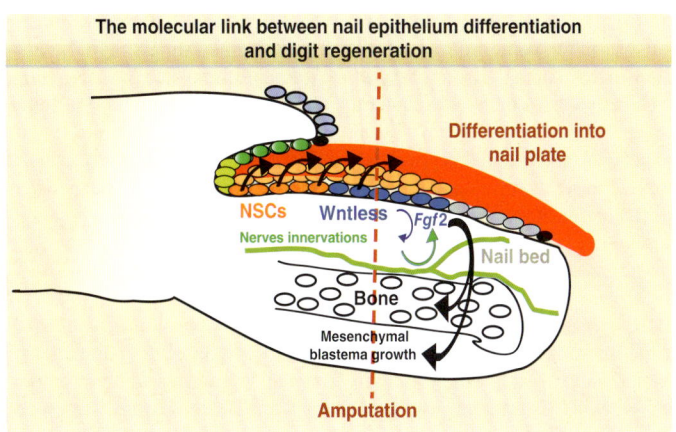

Figure 8-6 The molecular link between nail epithelium differentiation and digit regeneration. Nail stem cells (NSCs) in the proximal matrix (*dark orange circles*) give rise to distal matrix cells (*blue circles*) with Wnt activation (Wntless) under homeostatic conditions. Both proximal and distal matrix cells differentiate into the nail plate (*red color*). After distal-level amputation (*red dotted line*), the nail epithelial cells begin to regenerate the wound site along with activation Wnt signaling to differentiate into distal matrix cells and the nail plate. This Wntless activation in nail epithelium is required to promote (*blue arrow*) blastema innervations (*green*), which is necessary (*green arrow*) for Fgf2 expression in the regenerating nail epithelium (*blue circles*). Subsequently, fibroblast growth factor 2 (FGF2) promotes (*black arrow*) proliferation of Runx2-positive mesenchymal cells, ultimately leading to digit regeneration. (Adapted from Takeo M, Chou WC, Sun Q, et al. Wnt activation in nail epithelium couples nail growth to digit regeneration. *Nature*. 2013;499(7457):228-232.)

stabilization in the nail epithelium does not promote digit regeneration after amputation proximal to the NSC niche. Therefore, the remaining proximal matrix epidermis is not able to respond to β-catenin stabilization, and digit regeneration cannot be restored, which is in contrast to distal matrix function.

This results are consistent with inhibition of proper digit-tip regeneration after ablation of Lgr6, an important agonist of the Wnt pathway that marks NSCs and gives rise to the nail plate.[30] In addition, Lgr6 expression is not only limited to the nail matrix but is more broadly expressed within a subset of cells in the digit tip, namely, in the bone osteoblasts and eccrine sweat glands. Therefore, Lgr6-expressing cells not only mark NSC epithelium but also contribute to the blastema, which suggest not only direct but also a potential indirect role for Lgr6-expressing cells during digit-tip regeneration.[30] Indeed, this role has been confirmed by analysis of Lgr6-deficient mice, which have both a nail and bone regeneration defect, but it remains unclear whether the Lgr6-positive osteoblasts contribute to this phenotype. Thus, the role of these cells in normal skeletal homeostasis and digit regeneration remains to be determined in the future.

Collectively, the dual function of Wnt signaling in the NSC lineage that directs nail formation and differentiation and digit regeneration appears to be a key mechanism that coordinates the regeneration of epithelial and mesenchymal tissues in mammalian digit-tip regeneration (see Fig. 8-6). Indeed, interestingly, some nail disorders in humans that may affect only nails include inherited anonychia and isolated congenital nail dysplasia. Affected families with inherited anonychia have severe hypoplasia of the nails in which mutations in R-spondin 4 (Rspo4), which is implicated in the Wnt signaling pathway, were identified, suggesting an important role of Rspo4 in nail development.[36]

CONCLUSIONS

Stem cells have long term self-renewal potential and are capable of differentiating into a variety of different cell types. This persistence and multipotency are crucial for the maintenance of tissue during homeostasis and repair. Because of its extraordinary regenerative potential, understanding its maintenance and regulation will prove its usefulness in tissue regeneration and treatment of various disorders.

Current discoveries unveiled the model in which stem cells in nail organs exist in two different activation mode—slow-cycling and actively proliferating ones—to fulfill the demands of continuously growing nails.[24,29] These data demonstrated that the nail organ contains a gradient of slow- to fast-cycling stem cells, with slow-cycling NPFSCs in the proximal fold, more active cells in the IZ, and finally rapidly proliferative NCSs in the nail proximal matrix regions.

Collectively, this model supports the current view about adult stem cell dynamics and potency in several organs and tissues during homeostasis and regeneration. For example, the label-retaining, NPFSCs, and rapidly proliferative NCSs present a dynamic hierarchy similar to that described in hfSCs in which some hfSCs participate in the new hair cycle and other hfSCs of the upper outer root sheath (ORS) of growing follicles reestablish the new bulge with quiescent hfSCs.[37] During this bulge activation, a gradient of slow- to fast-cycling cells is observed within the ORS extending from the bulge region toward the matrix, respectively.

Why does the nail organ possess two populations of stem cells? One answer might come from observation of similar system of two stem cell populations with different cell cycling dynamics in the intestine. In the intestine, slow-cycling LRCs stem cells have been identified in the +4 position of intestinal crypts that expressed Bmi1.[38,39] In contrast, fast-cycling stem cells were also found at the bottom of the crypts expressing Lgr5,[40] and both stem cell populations are capable of differentiating into all intestinal lineages.[39] Interestingly, recently, in the absence of rapidly proliferating Lgr5+ stem cells, Bmi1 stem cells can maintain the normal turnover of the intestines while repopulating the Lgr5+ stem cell population.[41] This suggests that Bmi1+ cells, localized where LRCs are found, act as a reserve stem cell population. Thus, a similar backup system between two populations of stem cells in nails, namely NPFSCs and NSCs, might exist to protect overall nail organ maintenance. Thus, it will be interesting to further address this in the future. Overall, this suggest that NSCs in the proximal matrix[29] integrate the adjacent neighboring proximal fold as a location of bifunctional NPFSCs.[24] Collectively, these examples underscore an inherent plasticity of the adult stem cell populations within nail epithelia, and slow-cycling NPFSCs in these highly proliferative tissues might represent a backup system for NSCs during times of stress, injury, or depletion of the stem cell population.

All these exciting discoveries about stem cell populations in the nail organ and their mutual relationships as well as reciprocal interactions between stem cells and stem cell niches help unravel new concepts in stem cell biology and have great translational potential that could considerably impact regenerative medicine. Indeed, in mouse digit-tip regeneration, it has been demonstrated that although nail epithelium with its stem cells is critical to orchestrate this process, crosstalk with other germ-layer and lineage-restricted stem/progenitor cells is essential to successfully complete this regeneration.[42] Thus, in the future, this research might potentially restore anatomical and functional structures by orchestrating full-digit regeneration, including bone, innervations, and vasculature with skin and skin appendages along with nail, therefore benefiting individuals with digit amputations.

These results have established a direct relationship between NSC differentiation and digit regeneration and suggest that NSCs may have therapeutic potential to contribute toward the development of novel treatments for amputees. This is a very important problem because many people are affected by accidental amputation of fingers or toes worldwide. Recent nail and digit regeneration data have begun to pave the way toward unveiling the underlying mechanisms required to expose this regenerative potential. Therefore, new discoveries in nail biology will very likely enhance our understanding of the fundamental mechanisms required to orchestrate digit regeneration with the potential to unlock the broad regenerative potential to reconstitute the whole limb beyond digit regeneration.

Although more studies are needed for further characterization of these stem cell population in the nail organ, these data may shed some light on putative stem cells markers for human nails in the future. Indeed, interestingly, initial observation in human of the ventral proximal fold was proposed to be the NSCs in the developing embryonic human nail based on the expression of bulge stem cell markers, K15, K19, and PHLDA1 with quiescent characteristics that might represent NPFSCs in the mouse model.[23] In contrast, the human nail matrix contains highly proliferative cells marked by Ki67, similar to the mouse nail matrix, which might be similar as NSCs highly proliferating stem cells in the proximal matrix in mice.[23] Thus, further identification, characterization, and isolation of those two distinct populations of stem cells in nail organ in humans at the ventral proximal fold and nail matrix might provide crucial understanding of nail organ biology at the molecular level, which can potentially provide insight into designing translational therapies for regrowing greater portions of the limbs and other nonregenerative tissues in the future. Therefore, defining the regenerative potential of these NSCs and NPFSCs and the molecular mechanisms by which they are regulated in vivo (with the intent that novel therapies) may emerge toward the successful nail organ regeneration and wound healing, including treatment of amputee patients.

ACKNOWLEDGMENTS

I express my apologies to colleagues whose work could not be included in this chapter. I thank Dr. Sébastien de Feraudy, MD, PhD, associate professor and director of dermatopathology, UC Irvine Dermatopathology Laboratory (Irvine, CA), for providing the figure with hematoxylin and eosin staining of a human nail after biopsy. I thank Dr. Agnieszka Kobielak for critical reading of this manuscript and members of Dr. Krzysztof Kobielak laboratories for helpful discussions. KK is supported by the National Science Centre (NCN) Opus Grant 2015/19/B/NZ3/02948 and the National Institute of Arthritis and Musculoskeletal and Skin Diseases of the National Institutes of Health Grant R01-AR061552.

REFERENCES

1. de Berker DAR, Baran R. Science of the nail apparatus. In: Baran R, de Berker DAR, Holzberg M, Thomas L, eds. *Baran & Dawber's Diseases of the Nails and their Management*, 4th ed. Oxford, UK: Wiley-Blackwell; 2012:1-50.
2. Mecklenburg L, Paus R, Halata Z, et al. FOXN1 is critical for onycholemmal terminal differentiation in nude (Foxn1) mice. *J Invest Dermatol*. 2004;123(6):1001-1011.
3. Dawber RPR, de Berker DAR, Baran R. Science of the nail apparatus. In: Baran R, Dawber RPR, de Berker DAT, et al, eds. *Baran and Dawber's Diseases of the Nails and Their Management*, 3rd ed. Oxford, UK: Blackwell Science Ltd; 2001:1-47.
4. Lewis BL. Microscopic studies of fetal and mature nail and surrounding soft tissue. *AMA Arch Derm Syphilol*. 1954;70(6):733-747.
5. Zaias N, Alvarez J. The formation of the primate nail plate. An autoradiographic study in squirrel monkey. *J Invest Dermatol*. 1968;51(2):120-136.

6. Norton LA. Incorporation of thymidine-methyl-H3 and glycine-2-H3 in the nail matrix and bed of humans. *J Invest Dermatol*. 1971;56(1):61-68.
7. de Berker D, Angus B. Proliferative compartments in the normal nail unit. *Br J Dermatol*. 1996;135(4) 555-559.
8. Johnson M, Comaish JS, Shuster S. Nail is produced by the normal nail bed: a controversy resolved. *Br J Dermatol*. 1991;125(1):27-29.
9. Johnson M, Shuster S. Continuous formation of nail along the bed. *Br J Dermatol*. 1993;128(3):277-280.
10. Fuchs E, Tumbar T, Guasch G. Socializing with the neighbors: stem cells and their niche. *Cell*. 2004;116(6): 769-778.
11. Spradling A, Drummond-Barbosa D, Kai T. Stem cells find their niche. *Nature*. 2001;414(6859):98-104.
12. Lin H. The stem-cell niche theory: lessons from flies. *Nat Rev Genet*. 2002;3(12):931-940.
13. Watt FM, Hogan BL. Out of Eden: stem cells and their niches. *Science*. 2000;287(5457):1427-1430.
14. Cotsarelis G, Sun TT, Lavker RM. Label-retaining cells reside in the bulge area of pilosebaceous unit: implications for follicular stem cells, hair cycle, and skin carcinogenesis. *Cell*. 1990;61(7):1329-1337.
15. Cotsarelis G, Cheng SZ, Dong G, et al. Existence of slow-cycling limbal epithelial basal cells that can be preferentially stimulated to proliferate: implications on epithelial stem cells. *Cell*. 1989;57(2):201-209.
16. Albers KM, Setzer RW, Taichman LB. Heterogeneity in the replicating population of cultured human epidermal keratinocytes. *Differentiation*. 1986;31(2):134-140.
17. Bickenbach JR, Chism E. Selection and extended growth of murine epidermal stem cells in culture. *Exp Cell Res*. 1998;244(1):184-195.
18. Tumbar T, Guasch G, Greco V, et al. Defining the epithelial stem cell niche in skin. *Science*. 2004;303 (5656):359-363.
19. Leung Y, Kandyba E, Chen YB, et al. Label retaining cells (LRCs) with myoepithelial characteristic from the proximal acinar region define stem cells in the sweat gland. *PLoS One*. 2013;8(9):e74174.
20. Lu CP, Polak L, Rocha AS, et al. Identification of stem cell populations in sweat glands and ducts reveals roles in homeostasis and wound repair. *Cell*. 2012; 150(1):136-150.
21. Nakamura M, Tokura Y. The localization of label-retaining cells in eccrine glands. *J Invest Dermatol*. 2009;129(8):2077-2078.
22. Nakamura M, Ishikawa O. The localization of label-retaining cells in mouse nails. *J Invest Dermatol*. 2008; 128(3):728-730.
23. Sellheyer K, Nelson P. The ventral proximal nail fold: stem cell niche of the nail and equivalent to the follicular bulge—a study on developing human skin. *J Cutan Pathol*. 2012;39(9):835-843.
24. Leung Y, Kandyba E, Chen YB, et al. Bifunctional ectodermal stem cells around the nail display dual fate homeostasis and adaptive wounding response toward nail regeneration. *Proc Natl Acad Sci U S A*. 2014;111(42):15114-15119.
25. Kobielak K, Pasolli HA, Alonso L, et al. Defining BMP functions in the hair follicle by conditional ablation of BMP receptor IA. *J Cell Biol*. 2003;163(3):609-623.
26. Cai J, Ma L. Msx2 and Foxn1 regulate nail homeostasis. *Genesis*. 2011;49(6):449-459.
27. Godwin AR, Capecchi MR. Hoxc13 mutant mice lack external hair. *Genes Dev*. 1998;12(1):11-20.
28. Kobielak K, Stokes N, de la Cruz J, et al. Loss of a quiescent niche but not follicle stem cells in the absence of bone morphogenetic protein signaling. *Proc Natl Acad Sci U S A*. 2007;104(24):10063-10068.
29. Takeo M, Chou WC, Sun Q, et al. Wnt activation in nail epithelium couples nail growth to digit regeneration. *Nature*. 2013;499(7457):228-232.
30. Lehoczky JA, Tabin CJ. Lgr6 marks nail stem cells and is required for digit tip regeneration. *Proc Natl Acad Sci U S A*. 2015;112(43):13249-13254.
31. Borgens RB. Mice regrow the tips of their foretoes. *Science*. 1982.217(4561):747-750.
32. Mohammad KS, Day FA, Neufeld DA. Bone growth is induced by nail transplantation in amputated proximal phalanges. *Calcif Tissue Int*. 1999;65(5):408-410.
33. Zhao W, Neufeld DA. Bone regrowth in young mice stimulated by nail organ. *J Exp Zool*. 1995;271(2): 155-159.
34. Mohammad KS, Neufeld DA. Denervation retards but does not prevent toetip regeneration. *Wound Repair Regen*. 2000;8(4):277-281.
35. Brockes JP. The nerve dependence of amphibian limb regeneration. *J Exp Biol*. 1987;132:79-91.
36. Blaydon DC, Ishii Y, O'Toole EA, et al. The gene encoding R-spondin 4 (RSPO4), a secreted protein implicated in Wnt signaling, is mutated in inherited anonychia. *Nat Genet*. 2006;38(11):1245-1247.
37. Hsu YC, Pasolli HA, Fuchs E. Dynamics between stem cells, niche, and progeny in the hair follicle. *Cell*. 2011.144(1):92-105.
38. Potten CS, Owen G, Booth D. Intestinal stem cells protect their genome by selective segregation of template DNA strands. *J Cell Sci*. 2002;115(Pt 11):2381-2388.
39. Sangiorgi E, Capecchi MR. Bmi1 is expressed in vivo in intestinal stem cells. *Nat Genet*. 2008;40(7):915-920.
40. Barker N, van Es JH, Kuipers J, et al. Identification of stem cells in small intestine and colon by marker gene Lgr5. *Nature*. 2007;449(7165):1003-1007.
41. Tian H, Biehs B, Warming S, et al. A reserve stem cell population in small intestine renders Lgr5-positive cells dispensable. *Nature*. 2011;478(7368):255-259.
42. Rinkevich Y, Lindau P, Ueno H, et al. Germ-layer and lineage-restricted stem/progenitors regenerate the mouse digit tip. *Nature*. 2011;476(7361):409-413.

Chapter 9 :: Cutaneous Vasculature
:: Peter Petzelbauer, Robert Loewe, & Jordan S. Pober

第九章 皮肤血管系统

中文导读

本章共分为7节：①皮肤血管系统的结构和组织；②正常皮肤血管的特点和功能；③急性炎症的真皮血管改变；④慢性炎症的真皮血管改变；⑤特定疾病的真皮血管改变；⑥创伤愈合和癌症中的皮肤血管系统；⑦结论。

第一节皮肤血管系统的结构和组织，介绍了浅血管丛和深血管丛相互连接组成的皮肤血管网络。浅血管丛由成对的小动脉和小静脉组成，深血管丛走行于真皮网状层与皮下组织交界处。其中重点讲述了毛细血管后小静脉周围各种常驻的白细胞群体与内皮细胞和前体细胞一起，形成了毛细血管后小静脉的"管周渗出单元"，为附属器炎症相关的白细胞或网状真皮内炎症的入口。

第二节正常皮肤血管的特点和功能，介绍了皮肤血管具有止血、对液体和溶质的"渗透选择性"、调节局部血流灌注、皮肤体温调节、免疫监测等功能。

第三节急性炎症的真皮血管改变，介绍了皮肤血管系统的不同部分以不同方式促成急性炎症，主要观点仍是集中在血管内皮细胞发生的变化。小动脉内皮细胞释放的血管舒张分子的平衡发生变化，局部出现高灌注，表现为皮温升高及发红。静脉的内皮细胞粘附破坏，血浆蛋白外渗出现肿胀，有助于组织修复。

第四节慢性炎症的真皮血管改变，介绍了微血管内皮细胞中E-选择蛋白的持续表达可能为慢性炎症的皮肤特异性特征。

第五节特定疾病的真皮血管改变，介绍了急慢性皮肤炎症中血管内皮细胞表达表面分子不一样。急性皮肤炎症中，内皮细胞高水平表达E-选择素和P-选择素，中等水平表达VCAM-1和ICAM-1，炎性浸润主要由CLA和CD45RO阳性的记忆T细胞组成，而在一些慢性炎症皮损中，内皮细胞表达中等数量的E-选择素和大量的VCAM-1。同时介绍了银屑病血管改变中的"接吻现象"和"喷射乳头"。

第六节创伤愈合和癌症中的皮肤血管系统，介绍了在组织损伤或肿瘤生长的情况下会形成新的血管，在成人中，新血管是通过已有的血管萌发而来。特别介绍了伤口愈合过程中有局部萌发的传统血管生成和干细胞来源的血管生成两种途径；缺氧的皮肤肿瘤，通过套叠式血管生成、血管生成模拟、血管选择等模式增加血液供应，可能也在肿瘤转移中发挥作用。

第七节总结了皮肤血管系统位置不一，功能不一。不同的血管节段可单独或联合对各种刺激做出反应，进而影响皮肤病。

〔栗　娟〕

AT-A-GLANCE

- The cutaneous vasculature is divided into a superficial, a deep, and a subcutaneous vascular plexus. The superficial vascular plexus is formed by parallel pairs of arterioles and venules connected via capillary loops that extend into the dermal papillae. These segments may individually or conjointly respond to exogenous or endogenous stimuli, thereby influencing skin disease expression.
- Skin microvessels are formed from an endothelial cell lining that is supported by mural cells that are pericytes in most of the microvasculature but smooth muscle cells in the larger arterioles and venules and resident perivascular leukocytes, including T cells, macrophages, mast cells, and dendritic cells.
- Skin microvessels, like other microvessels, perform three important constitutive functions: regulating fluidity of the blood, forming a barrier that separates and controls transfer of molecules and cells between circulating blood and tissue, and regulating local blood flow.
- Control of blood flow through skin microvessels have a special and critical role in thermoregulation not performed by other segments of the vasculature.
- Skin microvascular cell morphology and gene expression and function are altered by acute or chronic inflammatory skin diseases and in cancers. These processes may involve formation of new blood vessels (angiogenesis) or remodeling of preexisting vessels.
- Skin-specific microvascular responses may be influenced by keratinocyte-derived and other environmental-derived factors.

INTRODUCTION

The blood vascular system is a continuous series of hollow tubes that are lined by a one-cell-thick layer of epithelium-like mesenchymal cells, the endothelium, and are supported by various mural cells, typically pericytes (PCs) in microvessels and smooth muscle cells (SMCs) in larger caliber vessels. All vascular endothelial cells (ECs) share common features and functions and hence may be collectively described as one cell type. However, ECs from one segment of the vascular system may differ in significant ways from the ECs at other anatomic sites. Blood vessel ECs also differ from lymphatic ECs, which are not discussed in this chapter. Mural cells have distinct embryologic origins throughout the blood vasculature, but little is known about their variation with anatomic location. Consequently, these cells will be discussed as if they were homogeneous, but such descriptions should be regarded with caution.

STRUCTURE AND ORGANIZATION OF THE SKIN VASCULATURE

Approximately 3 decades ago, Irwin Braverman[1] described the organization of the vascular network of human skin. The human dermal vasculature consists of two interconnected systems, a superficial and a deep vascular plexus (DVP) with additional vascular networks surrounding sweat glands and hair follicles (Fig. 9-1).

The superficial vascular plexus (SVP) is composed of paired arterioles and venules that form an interconnected network of vessels coursing on a plane parallel to and just beneath the epidermal surface. Capillaries arise from the arterioles, extend upward within the papillary dermis at sites between the epidermal rete ridges, and then loop back down to the venules, forming arcade-like structures. Whereas the basement membrane of the arterioles appears homogeneous by electron microscopy, that of the venules is multilayered. In normal skin, most of the capillary loop is invested with a basement membrane that resembles that of the arteriole, acquiring a venule-like investiture only at the level of the deepest rete just proximal to the anastomosis with the venule of the SVP. There are no ultrastructural differences between capillary loops at different sites of the skin. The arterioles and venules of the SVP are connected by short, straight vessels to the arterioles and venules of a deeper planar network of anatomizing vessels, called the DVP (see Fig. 9-1). The plane of the DVP is parallel to that of the SVP and courses above the boundary between the reticular dermis and the underlying subcutis. The arterioles of the DVP are fed through penetrating vessels from the subcutis. The

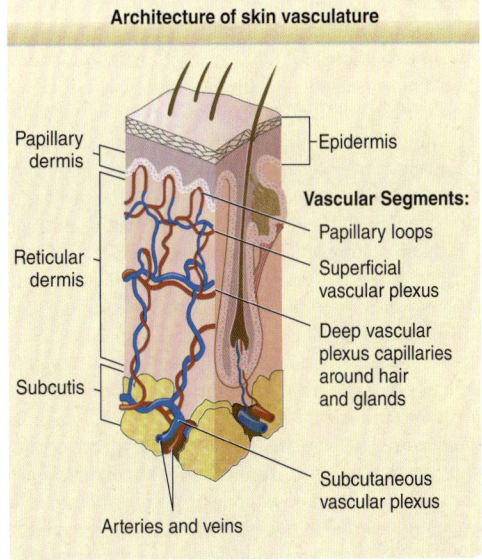

Figure 9-1 Schematic diagram of the architecture of the skin vasculature.

venules of DVP are drained by valve-containing veins that return to the subcutaneous fat. Capillary networks connecting the arterioles and venules of the DVP provide nourishment for the adnexal structures within the reticular dermis. The venules of the DVP serve as portals of entry for leukocytes associated with inflammation of the adnexa or for inflammation within the reticular dermis itself.

The walls of dermal arterioles are made of three layers: an intima composed of ECs, a media consisting of SMCs, and an adventitia containing some connective tissue-type cells. In the terminal arterioles, SMCs may be replaced by PCs that reside within the basement membrane of the ECs instead of in a distinct medial compartment. The walls of veins and venules have a similar structure, but compared with the corresponding arteries and arterioles, vessels of the venous circulation have a larger lumen and a thinner muscular wall and contain valves positioned at sites where the small vessels connect to larger ones. The walls of dermal capillaries and postcapillary venules consist of a monolayer of fenestrated ECs sitting on a simple basement membrane (Fig. 9-2). Capillaries are typically lined by a single file of highly curved ECs that enclose the lumen and are tightly connected to the adjacent ECs on either end, forming a tube with a lumen that is typically less than 10 µm in diameter.

Postcapillary venules are of a somewhat larger caliber, are circumferentially lined by more than one EC, have looser connections between neighboring ECs, and have a multilayered basement membrane. The fenestrae of dermal capillary ECs are formed primarily by a protein called plasmalemmal vesicle protein (PV)-1 that was previously designated as Pathologische Anatomie Leiden-endothelial (PAL-E) antigen and used as a marker of microvascular ECs. PCs that reside within the basement membrane of dermal microvessels provide structural integrity to the walls of both capillaries and postcapillary venules and contribute to basement membrane synthesis, and when it occurs, remodeling. ECs outnumber PCs in skin microvessels, and each PC contacts multiple ECs and form adherens junctions. Postcapillary venules of the SVP are also associated with various resident populations of leukocytic cells, including T cells, macrophages, dendritic cells, and mast cells. These cells, along with ECs and PCs, form the "perivascular extravasation unit"[2] of the postcapillary venules, the segment of the vasculature through which circulating leukocytes can be recruited into the dermis. These perivascular resident leukocyte populations were identified more than 20 years ago and for the most part have not been reclassified as newer understandings of leukocyte lineages and developmental programs have been elucidated. For example, it is now appreciated that memory T cells can take up long-term residence in tissues, acquiring characteristics and functions distinct from those of circulating T-cell populations.[3] The populations of perivascular T cells in noninflamed skin have not yet been categorized in comparison with circulating T cells or epidermal resident T cells with this new information in mind. Dendritic cells are now known to be quite heterogeneous with distinct developmental programs; each dendritic cell type serves different immunologic functions. Again, the types of perivascular dendritic cells have not been defined by these new criteria. Mast cells are also heterogeneous in terms of their granule contents and biosynthetic profiles, and it is unclear what human dermal perivascular mast cells may synthesize. Resident tissue macrophages are now known to originate either from more primitive embryonic origins, such as yolk sac or fetal liver, or from bone marrow–derived monocytes, and these populations also have distinct properties.[4] Finally, dermal dendrocytes, also known as veil cells, form a resident population that envelop microvessels of the SVP, associate with T cells and mast cells, and express coagulation factor XIIIa and stabilin 1 in addition to other macrophage-like markers. There has been much debate as to whether these cells are bone marrow or mesenchyme derived, and with the new appreciation of resident macrophage heterogeneity, they may in fact be neither. In general, it is proposed that all such perivascular leukocyte cell types serve as sentinels for infection or injury, but it is possible that some of these populations also have constitutive vascular functions.

Veins of the dermis form three kinds of anastomosing connections; large anastomoses of main trunks of the ascending veins, small anastomoses in the ascending sections of the small veins, and very small anastomoses from the small ascending veins reaching the papillary dermis. This anastomosing network of dermal veins is organized in polygons of various sizes, which is thought to play a role it outcomes of skin flap surgery.

PROPERTIES OF AND FUNCTIONS OF NORMAL SKIN VASCUALTURE[5]

See Table 9-1.

HEMOSTASIS

Blood is a fluid that is poised to become a gel at sites where vessel integrity is disrupted, beneficially forming a clot to limit extravasation but typically avoiding formation of a thrombus within the vessel lumen that could occlude the vessel and limit perfusion. Vascular ECs are the principal cell responsible for maintaining blood fluidity, and they may be altered when needed to actively promote clot formation. Blood plasma contains the proteins of the coagulation system that produce fibrin gels as well as platelets that can form a primary hemostatic plug. The EC lining prevents intravascular activation both of the coagulation system and of platelets yet keeps both systems poised to respond to injury. The key inhibitors of

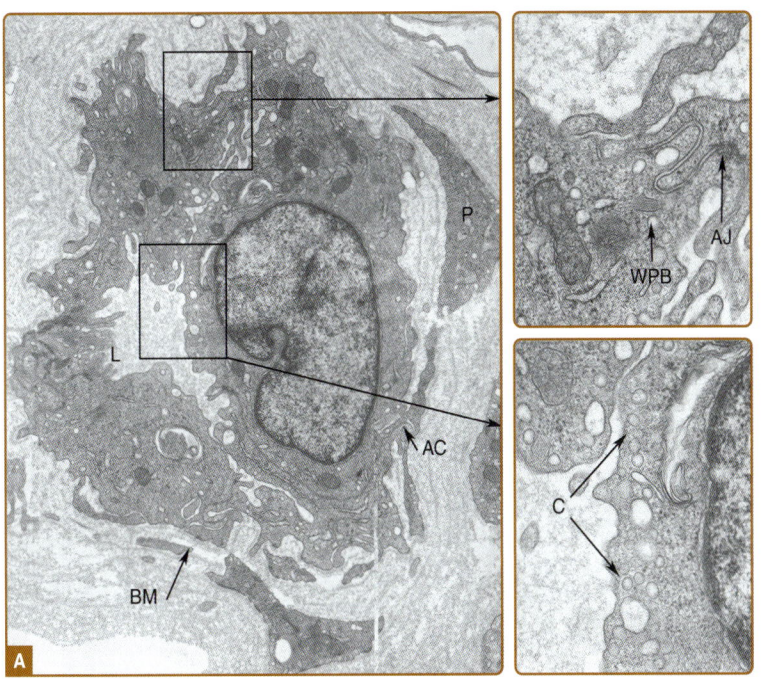

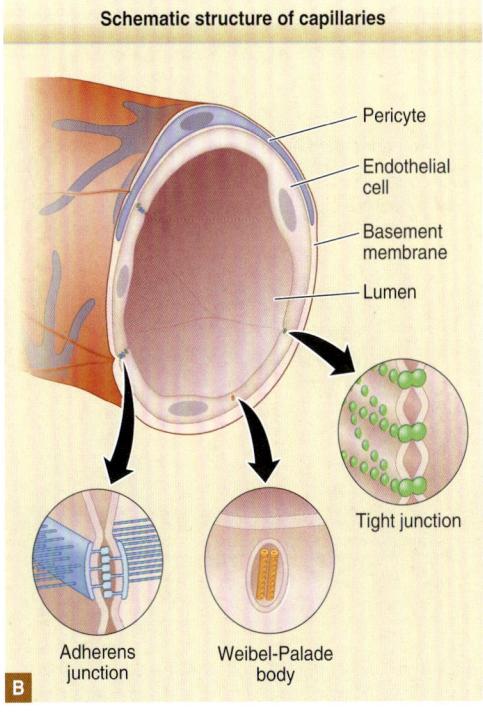

Figure 9-2 **A,** Ultrastructure of a postcapillary venule. AC, area of contact between endothelial cell and pericyte; AJ, adherens junction; BM, basement membrane; C, caveolae; L, lumen; P, pericyte; WPB, Weibel-Palade body. **B,** A schematic diagram of **A**.

coagulation basally expressed by ECs are tissue factor pathway inhibitor (which prevents the dramatic increases of the enzymatic activity of factor VIIa on factors IX and X that is catalyzed by tissue factor), thrombomodulin (which redirects thrombin from cleaving and thereby converting fibrinogen to fibrin to target and activate protein C instead), and anticoagulant heparan sulfates (which activate antithrombin III to function as an inhibitor of thrombin and factor Xa). ECs also basally limit platelet activation

TABLE 9-1
Properties and Functions of Normal Skin Vasculature
1. Hemostasis
2. Permselectivity
3. Perfusion
4. Thermoregulation
5. Immune surveillance

by (1) producing nitric oxide and prostacyclin (also called prostaglandin I_2), which inhibits platelet activation by elevating intracellular cyclic guanosine monophosphate and cyclic adenosine monophosphate, respectively), (2) expressing ectoenzymes that degrade platelet-activating adenosine triphosphate and adenosine diphosphate to inert adenosine monophosphate, (3) minimizing the activation of thrombin (which activates platelets by cleaving protease activated receptor 1), and (4) masking basement membrane and interstitial collagens (which can be recognized by platelet surface proteins and serve as alternative activators of platelets) (Fig. 9-3).

PERMSELECTIVITY

Dermal ECs form a barrier that permits limited passage of fluid and solutes, allowing the blood to nourish the tissues while displaying "permselectivity" for macromolecules (Fig. 9-4). ECs also basally present a virtually impenetrable barrier for blood cells (except at specialized sites of high permeability and leukocyte trafficking). In general, arterioles and capillaries are less permeable to macromolecules because ECs lining these vessels are connected to each other by tight junctions containing claudins (mostly claudin 5), junctional adhesion molecules (mostly JAM-A), and occludin (although occludin appears dispensable based on gene disruption in mice). Tight junctions prevent paracellular passage of macromolecules, limiting their crossing of the capillary EC lining to fenestrae or to vesicular transport, thereby enabling control of which molecules may pass (permselectivity). PCs may influence the barrier by stabilizing EC–EC contacts but are too sparse in skin microvessels to form a continuous surface that can directly block macromolecular transit. The capillaries, although narrower in diameter than other microvessels, have a cumulative surface area that vastly exceeds other parts of the microvasculature so that most transit takes place

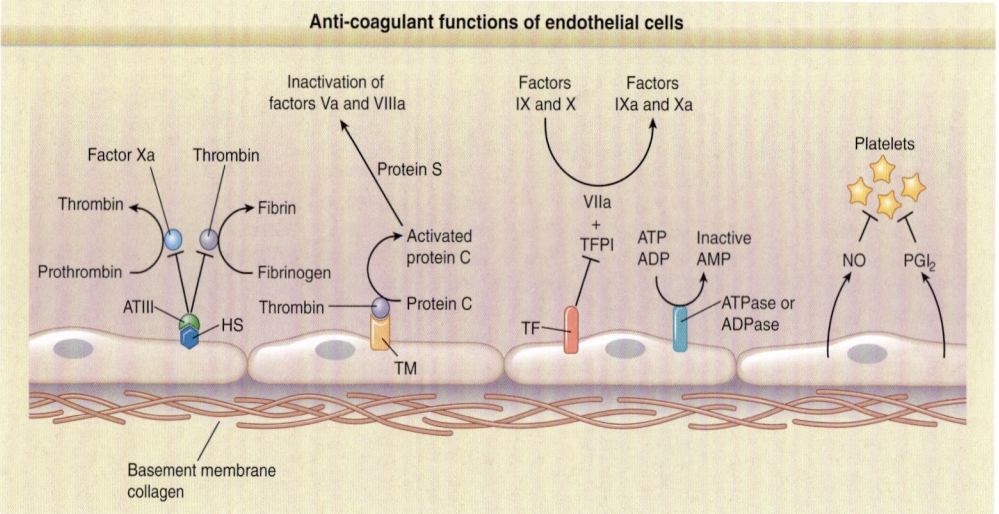

Figure 9-3 Anticoagulant and thrombotic functions of endothelial cells. To prevent coagulation, endothelial cells (1) express anticoagulant heparan sulfates (HS) that can bind and activate antithrombin III (ATIII), which then blocks the enzymatic activity of factor Xa, which converts prothrombin to thrombin, and of thrombin, which converts fibrinogen to fibrin; (2) express thrombomodulin (TM), which binds thrombin and changes it from a procoagulant enzyme that cleaves fibrinogen to fibrin into an anticoagulant enzyme that activates protein C that, in combination with protein S, then cleaves and inactivates factors V and VIII (which serve as cofactors for factors Xa and IXa, respectively); and (3) express tissue factor pathway inhibitor, which prevents tissue factor from accelerating the catalytic activity of factor VIIa, which cleaves and activates factors IX and X to factors IXa and Xa, respectively. To prevent platelet activation, endothelial cells (1) express ectoenzymes that convert extracellular adenosine triphosphate (ATP) and adenosine diphosphate (ADP), which are activators of platelets, to adenosine monophosphate (AMP), which cannot activate platelets; (2) synthesize and release inhibitors of platelet activation such as nitric oxide (NO) and prostacyclin (PGI_2); and (3) prevent platelets from coming in contact with basement membrane collagen, another activator of platelet activity. These functions are mutually reinforcing as thrombin is an activator of platelets and activated platelets provide lipid surfaces that bind coagulation factors to promote the clotting cascade.

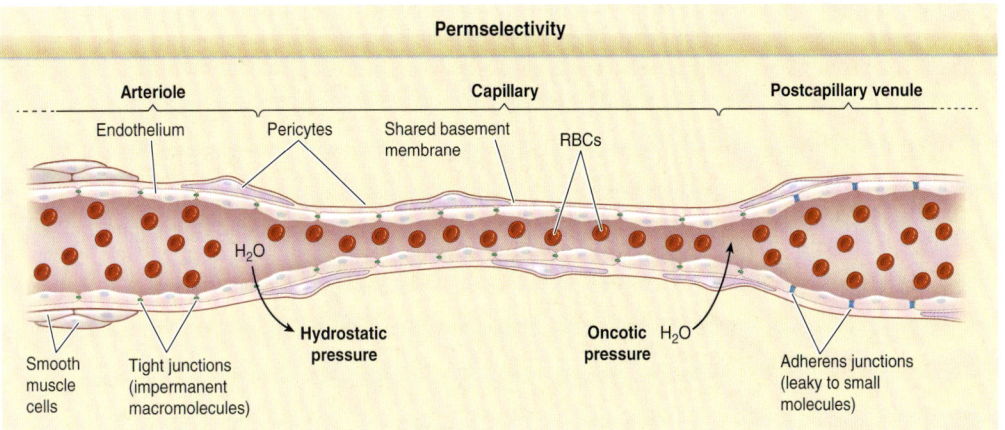

Figure 9-4 Endothelial cells establish permselective barriers. Permselectivity refers to the ability of the endothelial lining of the microvasculature to permit passage of water and solutes but not that of macromolecules. Tight junctions (TJs), which are expressed in the arterioles and capillaries, allow passage of water and solutes but prevent the passage of macromolecules and cells. Some small molecules, but not others, can pass based on size and charge. Hydrostatic pressure in the arteriolar end of the capillary forces water and solutes across the TJs and the retained macromolecules draw back water and small molecules at the venular end of the capillary through oncotic pressure. The postcapillary venules lack TJs, and their adherens junctions are dynamically regulated to allow some macromolecules to enter the tissue in the context of inflammation. RBC, red blood cell.

across this portion of the SVP. By allowing fluid and solutes to cross the EC lining by the paracellular route while preventing macromolecules to do so, dermal capillaries of the SVP allow hydrostatic pressure gradients near the arteriolar side of the capillary loop to drive fluid and solutes into the tissue and then draw them back into the bloodstream on the venular side of the capillary loop through oncotic gradients formed by the proteins retained within the vessel lumen. ECs of the postcapillary venules form few, if any, tight junctions and are instead held together primarily by adherens junctions, which are largely formed by VE-cadherin and associated catenins. (Skin arteriolar and capillary ECs also form adherence junctions, but these seem dispensable once tight junctions form.) Venules are somewhat leaky to macromolecules under basal conditions, but macromolecular escape into the tissue is limited by the relatively small (in comparison with capillary) surface area of the venular EC lining. The net result of these structural features is that dermal vascular ECs regulate rather than prevent molecular exchange between blood and tissues.

PERFUSION

ECs regulate local blood flow primarily by acting on SMCs surrounding arterioles (Fig. 9-5). These are oriented almost parallel to the vessel's circumferential or radial axis. ECs control SMC tone, which regulates the size of the vessel lumen and the resistance of the vessel to dilation. Vascular resistance along with blood pressure determines blood flow. PCs, which are also contractile, function largely to provide structural integrity to the terminal arterioles, capillaries, and postcapillary venules but may also contribute some to vascular resistance. Under normal circumstances, ECs synthesize both vasodilators, such as nitric oxide and prostacyclin, that reduce SMC tone and vasoconstrictors, such as endothelin, that increase tone. EC also express angiotensin-converting enzyme, which can generate a vasoconstrictor, angiotensin II, from angiotensin I, a circulating inert precursor. The balance between vasodilators and vasoconstrictors may be regulated by neural or hormonal signals. Importantly, inhibiting nitric oxide synthase-3 (also known as endothelial NOS) in ECs will cause vasoconstriction and increased resistance, suggesting that vasodilation is normally dominant. Recent evidence suggests that resident perivascular memory T cells specific for certain oxidized lipid adducts, can induce vasoconstriction through elaboration of cytokines such as tumor necrosis factor (TNF)-α and interleukin (IL)-17A, although it is not known if this occurs in skin.[6]

THERMOREGULATION

The skin is the source of thermal information and is an executive organ for thermal homeostasis. Temperature is sensed through primary somatosensory afferent nerves; skin blood flow is modified through sympathetic vasodilation or vasoconstriction. To conserve heat, cutaneous vessels constrict; for convective heat transfer from the core to the periphery, cutaneous vessels dilate, and blood flow increases. The skin blood flow is normally 250 to 300 mL/min but can vary

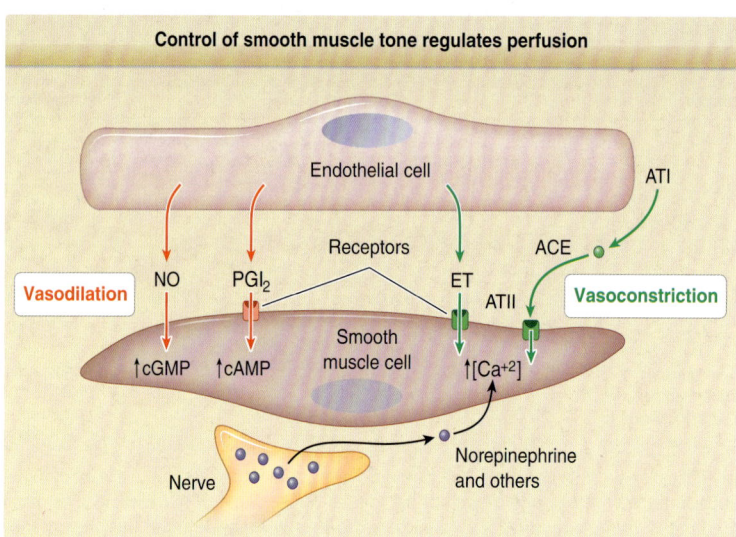

Figure 9-5 Control of perfusion by regulating smooth muscle cell tone. The active resistance of blood vessels can be modulated by altering the contractile tone mural vascular smooth muscle cells in muscular arteries and arterioles. Endothelial cells can produce vasodilators such as nitric oxide (NO) and prostacyclin (PGI_2). NO directly activates soluble guanylate cyclase to elevate cyclic guanosine monophosphate (cGMP) levels, and PGI_2 interacts with a membrane G–protein coupled receptor that activated adenylate cyclase to increase cycle adenosine monophosphate (cAMP). Both reduce the degree of actomyosin contraction. Endothelial cells can also produce vasocontrictors such as endothelin (ET) or, via the ectoenzyme angiotensin-converting enzyme (ACE), convert inactive angiotensin I (ATI) to vasoactive angiotensin II (ATII). Both ET and ATII signal through G protein–coupled receptors to increase the level of cytosolic free calcium ion, increasing the degree of actomyosin contraction. Nerves may release neurotransmitters that also bind to G protein–coupled receptors to increase cytosolic free calcium and actomyosin contraction. Increased actomyosin contraction shortens the length of the smooth muscle cells, which are arranged radially, thereby reducing the vessel lumen diameter and increasing resistance to flow.

from nearly zero in cold to as much as 6 to 8 L/min, which then covers approximately 60% of the cardiac output.[7] Nonglabrous skin is subject to reflex thermoregulation by the sympathetic nervous system. The noradrenergic vasoconstrictor system is tonically active and is activated by cold exposure. Initial vasodilation to body heating is achieved by reflex removal of active vasoconstrictor tone. With further heating, the parasympathetic cholinergic nerves release predominantly acetylcholine, causing active vasodilation. Concomitantly, autonomic and sensory nerve fibers release neurotransmitters, such as substance P, calcitonin gene-related peptide, vasoactive intestinal peptide, and pituitary adenylate cyclase activating polypeptide, which directly or indirectly induce vasodilatation. Local factors such as venous congestions and increased transmural pressure also modulate skin blood flow. Glabrous skin contributes to thermoregulation through shunts from the arterial directly into the venous beds, thereby bypassing capillary loops, the thermosensitivity of the hand being significantly greater than that of soles (Table 9-2).

Dysregulation in the skin thermoregulation is seen in postmenopausal hot flushes related to changed estrogen levels. Estrogen has vasodilator function as demonstrated in estrogen receptor knockout mice. Estrogen replacement relieves hot flashes and reduces resting body temperature in these individuals.

Individuals with Type 1 diabetes have greater skin blood flow relative to healthy control participants, potentially related to moderate vasodilation induced by a hyperinsulinemia and an impaired thermoregulatory response of skin vessels. The underlying mechanisms related to impaired heat responses remain largely unresolved. The absence of C-peptide produced in β cells or reduced nitric oxide bioavailability because of diminished NOS activity may play a role.

TABLE 9-2
Thermoregulation in Nonglabrous and Glabrous Skin

Nonglabrous Skin
  -Ambient temperature
Basal activity of noradrenalic system
  -Cold: vasoconstriction
Activation of noradrenalic system
  -Heat: vasodilation
Shutdown of noradrenalic system
  -Further heating
Parasympathetic cholinergic nerves
- Acetylcholine

Autonomic and sensory nerve fibers
- Substance P
- Calcitonin gene-related peptide
- Vasoactive intestinal peptide
- Pituitary adenylate cyclase activating polypeptide

Glabrous Skin
Additional thermoregulatory capacity through opening arteriovenous shunts or closing arteriovenous shunt

A pathological thermoregulatory reflex is seen in Raynaud disease; patients have an exaggerated vasospastic response to cold or emotion, resulting in ischemia of the digits. Vasospastic attacks in Raynaud disease are restricted to cutaneous arteries supplying skin sites with a rich density of arteriovenous anastomosis, a situation at glabrous sites. These sites are normally targeted by sympathetic adrenergic vasoconstrictive activity in response to cold. Patients with Raynaud disease have increased sympathetic vasoconstrictive activity, which results in increased blood flow through arteriovenous anastomosis. Of note, bosentan, antagonizing endothelin A and endothelin B receptors, which has promising clinical effects in scleroderma, does not influence vasospasm in Raynaud disease.

Patients with erythromelalgia have burning pain and vasodilation with erythema of the extremities. It is caused by mutations affecting the encoding *SCN9A* gene that leads to channelopathies. Although the primary cause of the abnormal vascular reaction is unknown, most patients have abnormal quantitative sudomotor axon reflex tests (measuring resting skin temperature, resting sweat output, and stimulated sweat output), some have abnormal adrenergic function, and others an abnormal cardiovagal function. Erythromelalgia most severely affects the palms and soles. It is therefore thought that arteriole–venule shunts are abnormally innervated or show an abnormal response. As pointed out earlier, these arteriole–venule shunts are mainly found in glabrous skin.

IMMUNE SURVEILLANCE

In addition of being a physical barrier, the skin has features of an immunologic barrier. Among resident cells housing in the skin are semiprofessional antigen-presenting cells such as keratinocytes, ECs, and macrophages and professional antigen-presenting cells such as Langerhans cells and dermal dendritic cells. In addition, the skin is populated by T cells. The majority of these cutaneous T cells are resident, largely within the epidermis, but as noted earlier, there also appear to be T cells resident in the perivascular compartment of the venules.

In addition to resident populations, there are circulating T cells with a predilection for homing to skin. More than 30 years ago, the term *skin-associated lymphoid tissues* was created (subsequently renamed the *skin immune system*), which postulated the existence of subsets of T lymphocytes displaying special affinity for the skin and that the acquisition of this affinity by T cells is determined signals received from resident cutaneous cells. After an immune response within the skin, a subset of memory T cells develops that can exit from the skin via the lymphatics to enter draining lymph nodes. These T cells may then reenter the skin upon rechallenge by the same anitigen,[8] and they may retain a preference for skin sites. The first skin-associated protein expressed on a population of memory T lymphocytes was described and termed *cutaneous lymphocyte antigen* (CLA).[9] CLA is a carbohydrate moiety on the surface of T cells closely related to sialylated Lewis X, which has homology to the core structure of P-selectin glycoprotein-1. CLA was shown to bind to E-selectin expressed on activated endothelium, but the latter is ubiquitously expressed on activated endothelium (albeit perhaps more transiently than in skin), suggesting that this is not the only mechanism regulating skin-specific leukocyte homing. A potential candidate providing additional specificity is the chemokine TARC (also called cutaneous T cell-attracting chemokine or CCL17) (Fig. 9-6), which is produced by cutaneous venules, induced in inflamed skin and absent on intestinal vessels.[10] Its receptor, CCR4, is expressed on the CLA-positive memory T cells. The interaction of TARC and CCR4 triggers E-selectin–mediated adhesion of CLA positive T cells. However, skin infiltration in CCR4-/- mice is not impaired, indicating that further regulatory pathways exist. Another candidate for skin-specific recruitment of CLA[hi+] T cells is the chemokine CTACK (also called thymus and activation-regulated chemokine or CCL27). CTACK is constitutively expressed by basal keratinocytes and is detectable on ECs and fibroblasts of the papillary dermis.[11] It is thought that CTACK is mainly expressed and secreted by keratinocytes in the epidermis and captured and presented by dermal cells through glycosaminoglycans or through its receptor, CCR10 (see Fig. 9-6). CCR10 is expressed on T cells and is critical for their migration into the noninflamed skin. Knockout of CCR10 changes the balance of resident regulatory T cells (Tregs) and CD4+ effector T cells in the skin and causes overreactive inflammation after topical application of ovalbumin in a sensitized mouse. Using neutralizing anti-CTACK antibodies, the homing of CD4/CLA/CCR10-positive T cells is blocked.[11]

Circulating dendritic cells may also use CLA–E-selectin interactions to extravasation into the skin.

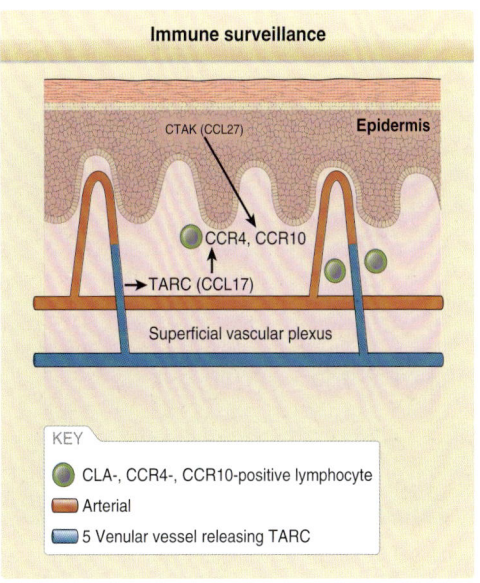

Figure 9-6 Immune surveillance.

A subset of B cells also may express CLA and exhibit enhanced binding to E-selectin, potentially enabling cutaneous migration. Indeed, although very rare, B cells are present in normal human skin.[12] These cells display a clonally restricted pattern, indicating recognition of a restricted antigenic repertoire—most likely against skin-associated antigens—alluding to the possibility of a skin-resident memory B-cell population. They have been shown to recirculate from the skin to regional lymph nodes by using CCR6–CCL20 interactions.

The blood also contains a population of circulating T cells, characterized as effector memory T cells that function to seek out the presence of microbial antigens to which a prior immune response had been made. These, like other T cells, detect antigen using a clonally distributed repertoire of receptors that were selected to detect microbial peptides bound to class I major histocompatibility complex (MHC) molecules (human leukocyte antigen [HLA]-A, -B, or -C of CD8+ T cells) or bound to class II MHC molecules (HLA-DR, -DP, or -DQ) but not peptides derived from self-proteins. Dermal microvascular ECs express high levels of MHC molecules of both classes under basal (noninflamed conditions) and can efficiently form peptide–MHC molecule complexes. These cells also express surface proteins, such as LFA-3, 4-1BB ligand, Ox40-ligand, and ICOS-ligand, that can provide antigen-independent enhancing signals ("costimulation") required for circulating memory T-cell activation. Recognition of antigen on the luminal surface of ECs in an infected tissue not only activates these cells but also triggers their diapedesis across the EC lining into the skin. The cell biology of this process is unique in that T-cell recognition of antigen on the EC surface causes cells to round up, rather than spread, and cross between ECs by extending a cytoplasmic protrusion containing the microtubule organizing center and cytoplasmic granules rather than these structures following the cell body and nucleus in a trailing uropod. This antigen presenting function of ECs may be redundant with presentation of antigen by perivascular dendritic cells or macrophages that also display peptide–MHC molecule complexes on extensions that protrude into the vascular lumen. Both types of signals may supplement the initiation of immunity by resident or recirculating T cells located within the perivascular unit.

DERMAL VASCULAR ALTERATIONS OF ACUTE INFLAMMATION[13]

Different segments of the microvasculature contribute in different ways to acute inflammation. Historically, much of the focus has been on changes that occur in the EC lining. Local sites of inflammation are perfused at a higher level, primarily because of a shift in the balance of vasodilatory molecules released by the EC of the arterioles and, to a lesser extent, the capillaries. The principal mediator for this change is an increase in the synthesis of prostacyclin, likely resulting from a cytokine-induced increase in the expression of cyclooxygenase (COX)-2 (also known as prostaglandin H synthase 2), which is more active than constitutively expressed COX-1. The resultant increase in blood flow results in local warming ("calor") and increased redness ("rubor") of the inflamed site. Venular EC disrupt their intracellular adherens junctions (Fig. 9-7), allowing the extravasation of large plasma proteins such as fibronectin and fibrinogen, the latter being converted to fibrin within the extravascular space, producing swelling ("tumor"). These proteins form a provisional matrix in the tissue that will allow extravasating leukocytes to attach and migrate and will serve for ultimate tissue repair. Other changes are in the display of surface molecules by the venular ECs that can serve to capture circulating leukocytes. Selectins expressed by EC cause tethering and rolling of leukocytes. Chemokines, especially IL-8 (CXCL8) for neutrophils and monocyte chemoattractant protein 1 (MCP-1, also known as CCL2), for monocytes cause spreading and firm attachment

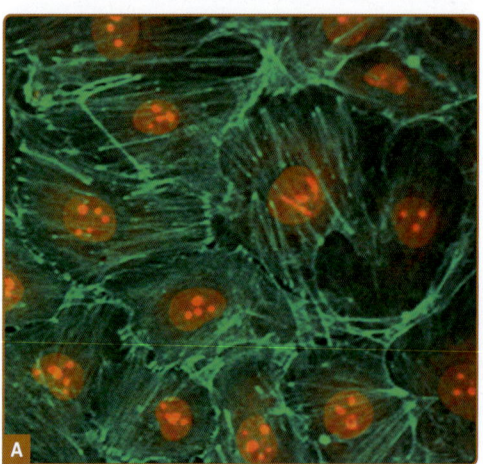
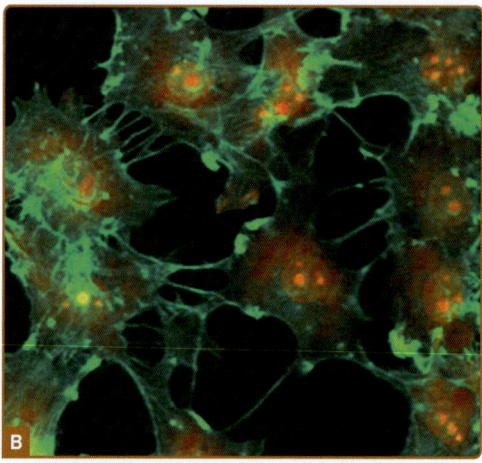

Figure 9-7 Cultured venular endothelial cells forming a continuous monolayer (**A**), thrombin-treated endothelial cells with disrupted intercellular junctions mimicking a leaky vessel (**B**). The phalloidin-staining of the actin skeleton is in *green*, and nuclei are in *red*; 1000× magnification.

of leukocytes. Leukocyte crawling on the EC surfaces toward the extracellular junctions is mediated primarily by ICAM (intercellular adhesion molecule)-1. For mononuclear leukocytes, vascular cellular adhesion molecule (VCAM)-1 may aid in capture, rolling, and crawling. Chemokines may be made by the ECs or may be produced by sentinel cells of the perivascular unit and become displayed by attaching noncovalently to heparin sulfates on the EC luminal surface. These changes in ECs have been referred to as endothelial activation. Certain autacoids or enzymes such as thrombin may induce transient, protein synthesis–independent changes such as P-selectin translocation from intracellular storage granules (known as Weibel-Palade bodies) to the cell surface or synthesis of chemotactic lipids, such as platelet activating factor. Such changes are sometimes referred to as Type I activation, but the transient nature of such changes typically results in short-term effects, such as a wheal and flare reaction, rather than leukocyte recruitment. The latter is more dependent on new gene transcription and protein synthesis induced by inflammatory cytokines such as TNF-α, IL-1α, or IL-1β. Cytokine activation of EC can also promote coagulation by down-regulating thrombomodulin synthesis while inducing expression of tissue factor. Coagulation may be propagated by EC release of plasma membrane–derived microparticles containing tissue factor.

When leukocytes reach the intracellular junctions of postcapillary venular ECs, they engage additional proteins that contribute to extravasation. Several of these, such as platelet endothelial cell adhesion molecule (PECAM)-1, poliovirus receptor, and CD99, are stored in invaginations of the lateral border plasma membrane (known as the lateral border recycling compartment) that are brought to the cell surface to engage receptors expressed on the leukocyte. (Sometimes these molecules can line short-lived transcellular channels located near but not at the actual intercellular junction, allowing leukocytes to pass through rather than between ECs. It is not known if this distinction has any physiological significance.) After the leukocyte has passed through the EC layer, it engages basement membrane proteins and PCs that express elevated levels of ICAM-1 and chemokines in response to the same cytokines that activate ECs. The interaction with PCs may extend for 30 minutes or more as PCs contract to open gaps in the basement membrane and guide extravasating leukocytes to these areas. When outside the basement membrane, extravasated leukocytes continue to interact with PCs and perhaps with other cells of the perivascular unit, migrating along adventitial surface of the vessel.

TNF-α and IL-1 induce proinflammatory changes in ECs that typically do not distinguish among different leukocyte types. However, the kinetics of induction of different adhesion molecules varies. Whereas E-selectin is made within the first 2 hours and correlates with the onset neutrophil recruitment, VCAM-1 is synthesized later (ie, in about 6 to 12 hours) and correlates with the onset of mononuclear leukocyte recruitment (Fig. 9-8). Polarizing cytokines, such as interferon (IFN)-γ or IL-4 and IL-13, favor the production of chemokines that preferentially activate T cells and effector cells mostly associated with T_H1 or T_H2-type adaptive immunity, respectively. IL-17 has little effect on ECs but instead acts on PCs to induce factors that prolong neutrophil survival (granulocyte-macrophage colony-stimulating factor and granulocyte-colony stimulating factor), favoring prolongation of neutrophilic inflammation characteristic of T_H17-type inflammation.[14]

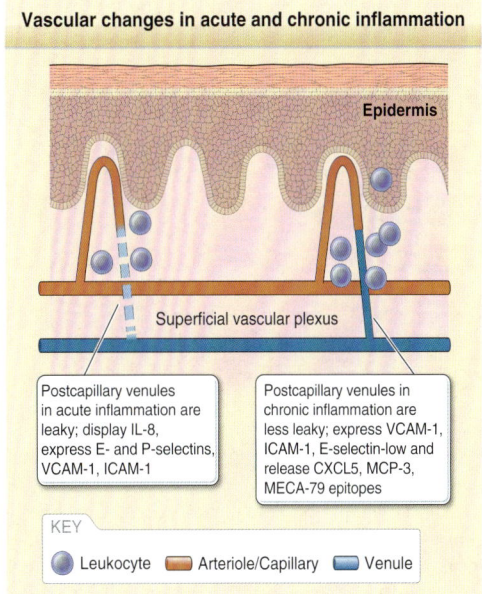

Figure 9-8 Vascular changes in acute and chronic inflammation. ICAM, intercellular adhesion molecule; IL, interleukin; MCP-3, monocyte chemoattractant protein 3; VCAM, vascular cellular adhesion molecule.

DERMAL VASCULAR ALTERATIONS OF CHRONIC INFLAMMATION

Continuous activation of ECs is possible and results in distinct changes compared with the acute activation. Transgenic mice overexpressing TNF in an endothelium-specific manner display an inflammatory skin phenotype with epidermal hyperproliferation and fibrosis. In culture, whereas chronic TNF-stimulated EC display a continuous and high ICAM-1 and VCAM-1 expression, E-selectin is absent and cannot be reinduced by additional TNF stimulation (ie, ECs are desensitized in regard to E-selectin expression). Interestingly, these chronic TNF-stimulated cells continuously overexpress CXCL5 and MCP-3.[15] Cultured skin ECs show sustained and higher expression of E-selectin and slower internalization and degradation of E-selectin protein compared with umbilical vein endothelium, but this may be a general property of microvascular ECs.[16] Nevertheless, sustained expression of E-selectin, although not unique to skin, is generally described as a skin-specific feature of chronic inflammation (see Fig. 9-8).

DERMAL VASCULAR CHANGES IN SPECIFIC DISEASES

ACUTE VERSUS CHRONIC SKIN INFLAMMATION: GENERAL CONSIDERATIONS

In acute dermatitis, ECs express high levels of E- and P-selectin and moderate amounts of VCAM-1 and ICAM-1. The inflammatory infiltrate consists mainly of CLA and CD45RO-positive memory T cells. In chronic skin lesions, such as psoriasis, chronic lupus erythematosus, and mycosis fungoides, ECs express moderate amounts of E-selectin and high amounts of VCAM-1. They may also undergo morphologic changes and acquire a phenotype reminiscent of high endothelial venules. This type of EC has a cuboidal appearance, different from the flat morphology of ECs lining the other vessels. High endothelial venules express sialyted, fucosylated, and sulfated carbohydrate moieties corresponding to peripheral node addressins, which are recognized by antibody MECA-79. These addressins are constitutively expressed on high endothelial venules of lymph nodes; they bind to L-selectin expressed on leukocytes and control recirculation of T cells through lymph nodes. These sialyted, fucosylated, and sulfated carbohydrate moieties may also be expressed in chronic skin lesions such as cutaneous T-cell lymphoma.[17] Also in cutaneous melanoma, blood vessels express MECA-79 moieties, and the amount of MECA-79-reactive vessels correlates with the amount of tumor infiltrating lymphocytes and with histologic signs of tumor regression.[18] In squamous cell carcinoma, numbers of MECA-79–positive vessels were found to correlate with survival.

PSORIASIS

As mentioned previously, leukocytes primarily exit the blood stream through postcapillary venules. The capillary loops within the papillary tips of the dermis have an arteriolar phenotype; hence, leukocytes can exit the bloodstream through the SVP below but not within the tips of the papillae. The situation is different in psoriasis. In this disease, the capillary loops elongate and change morphology. Whereas normal capillaries at the turnaround point sit on an arteriolar basement membrane, psoriatic capillary loops at the turnaround point touch the epidermis, a phenomenon called "kissing," and remodel the basement membrane to resemble that of the postcapillary venule. ECs within the loop proliferate, producing both elongation and an increase in diameter. (The proliferation of the ECs is sometimes misinterpreted as angiogenesis, but no new vessels are actually formed.) Furthermore, the ECs of the remodeled psoriatic loop express adhesion molecules normally associated with cytokine-activated venular ECs, supporting tethering, rolling, and extravasation of leukocytes.[19] Lymphocytes and neutrophils can now exit the vessel lumen within the tips of the papillae and migrate into the epidermis. This histologic picture of lymphocytes and neutrophils extravasation within the tips of the papillae has been termed "squirting papillae" and is a typical feature of psoriasis and contrasts findings in chronic eczema, in which leukocytes extravasate across post-capillary venules of the SVP (Fig. 9-9).

LICHEN RUBER PLANUS

Another chronic skin disease, lichen ruber planus, has an enlarged blood microcirculatory bed within the papillary dermis compared with healthy skin. Specifically, oral lichen planus has tortuous capillaries with enlarged capillary loop diameter. Intralesional bevacizumab, anti-VEGF antibody, injections induced lesion resolution without relapse during a 3-month follow-up in a small series of patients. In this setting, vascular endothelial growth factor (VEGF) not only induces angiogenesis but is also proinflammatory by inducing endothelial adhesion molecule expression which may explain effects of the anti-VEGF antibody.

SKIN VASCULATURE IN WOUND HEALING AND CANCER

ANGIOGENESIS AND VASCULOGENESIS

In healthy adults, blood vessels are stable structures with a very slow turnover of ECs. In settings of chronic inflammation, tissue injury, or tumor growth, new vessels may be formed, and existing vessels may undergo remodeling. Much of the process of vessel formation has been learned by studying the formation of the vascular system during embryogenesis. In embryos, ECs arise from angioblasts, which migrate to peripheral tissues and form primitive blood vessels (vasculogenesis). Subsequently, new blood vessels arise from preexisting ones (angiogenesis) (Fig. 9-10). Mesenchymal cells are then recruited into the vessel wall, where they subsequently differentiate into SMCs and PCs, a process called vascular remodeling. In adults, new blood vessels develop through angiogenesis (sprouting from preexisting blood vessels); it has been proposed that circulating endothelial progenitor cells, mesoangioblasts, and multipotent adult progenitor cells contrib-

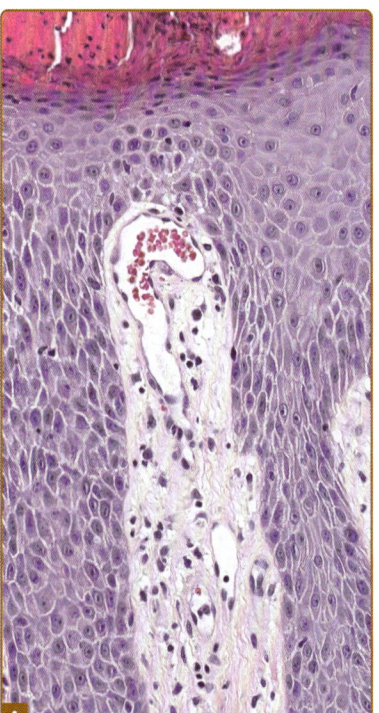 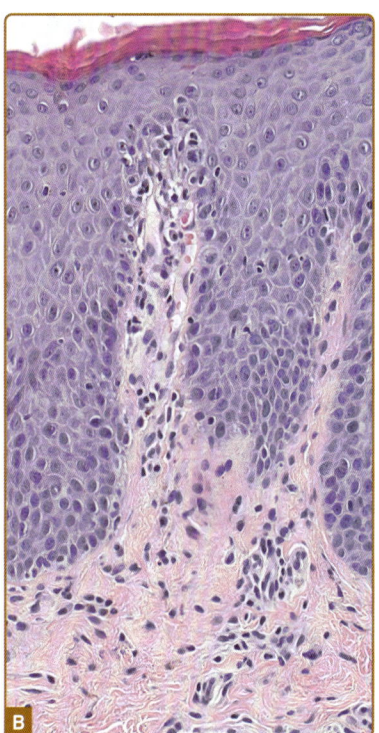

Figure 9-9 **A,** Vascular changes in psoriasis; the capillary loops within the tips of the papillae dilate, elongate, and at the turnaround point touch the epidermis, a phenomenon called "kissing." **B,** Leukocytes exit the vessel lumen within the tips of the papillae ("squirting papillae"); 20× magnification.

ute to new vessel formation (adult vasculogenesis). Several investigators have proposed that these progenitors arise in the bone marrow, just as angioblasts arise in the embryonic blood island. However, it is unclear that bone marrow–derived cells give rise to stable ECs, and many such observations have now been reinterpreted to imply a role for monocytes that express EC markers, promote angiogenesis, and then disappear as the new vessels become stable. Stem cells and endothelial progenitor cells have been identified in vessel walls as resident cells. Such cells are thought to reside in a niche, awaiting appropriate stimuli such as vessel injury to take part in the repair of damaged and the formation of new blood vessels. Among such vascular wall progenitor cells are CD34+/CD31- cells that differentiate into ECs. Other resident vascular wall progenitor cells are SMC progenitors and mesenchymal stromal cells that may arise from PCs.

Signals inducing new vessel formation in the skin follow the principal mechanisms given in all organs. Molecules of the VEGF family—VEGF A through E—most prominently act on ECs. Fibroblast growth factor (FGF) 1 and 2 are also potent EC mitogens but also act on SMCs, PCs, and fibroblasts. In adults, FGF-1 and FGF-2 are stored in the cytoplasms of a variety of cells and are released when cells are injured, acting

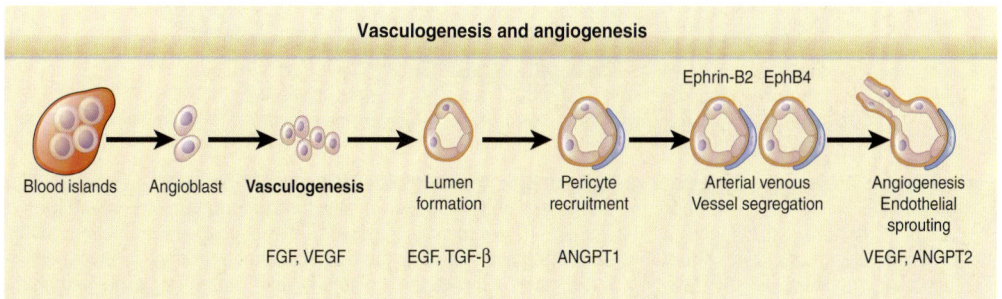

Figure 9-10 Vasculogenesis and angiogenesis. ANGPT, angiopoietin; FGF, fibroblast growth factor; TGF-β, transforming growth factor-β; VEGF, vascular endothelial growth factor.

as "wound hormones" to stimulate local angiogenesis and connective tissue growth. Other polypeptide factors have also been found to act on ECs in vivo and in vitro, including epidermal growth factor (EGF), heparin-binding EGF–like growth factor, and hepatocyte growth factor (HGF) or scatter factor (SF). For vascular remodeling and stabilization, tyrosine kinase receptor 1 (Tie) and 2 are required. Tie-2 mediates the dialogue between mesenchymal cells and the endothelium of the immature blood vessel through binding to angiopoietins (Fig. 9-11). The eph family of receptor tyrosine kinases and their corresponding ephrin ligands are membrane bound and appear to mediate bidirectional cell-to-cell signaling. During vascular development, ephrin-B2 marks the ECs of early arterial vessels, and ephrin-B4 marks the ECs of early veins. Platelet-derived growth factor (PDGF) and transforming growth factor (TGF)-β are secreted by ECs and promote migration of mesenchymal cells, matrix biosynthesis, and differentiation. Matrix glycoproteins such as fibronectin and laminin and receptors for matrix glycoproteins such as β_1 and β_3 integrins are also believed to play a role in vasculogenesis and angiogenesis. This seems intuitive because neither ECs nor mesenchymal cells can survive unless they interact with matrix proteins via integrin receptors.

WOUND HEALING

Full-thickness wounds heal in interconnected and overlapping stages involving coagulation, inflammation, proliferation, and remodeling. Immediately after wounding, disrupted blood vessels contract to stop bleeding. The activation of the coagulation cascade leads to platelet clot and subsequently to fibrin clot formation. At this stage, wounded vessels function as guiding structures for circulating inflammatory cells. Complement activation and the release of CXC chemokines by platelets and keratinocytes results in the recruitment of circulating neutrophils. Surrounding capillaries become leaky, resulting in further plasma and cell accumulation within wounds. The vascular leakiness gradually decreases but persists for the next 3 to 7 days. The formation of a capillary network occurs by capillary tip extension from a parent vessel, maturation of capillary tips into capillary sprouts, anastomosis, and further branching. After this rapid formation of blood vessels during the inflammatory and proliferative stages of healing, the vascular system is remodeled, regressed, or both. The angiogenic response is mainly driven by VEGF, FGF-2, PDGF, and members of the TGF-β family (Fig. 9-12). Macrophages are the major sources of VEGF during an early healing

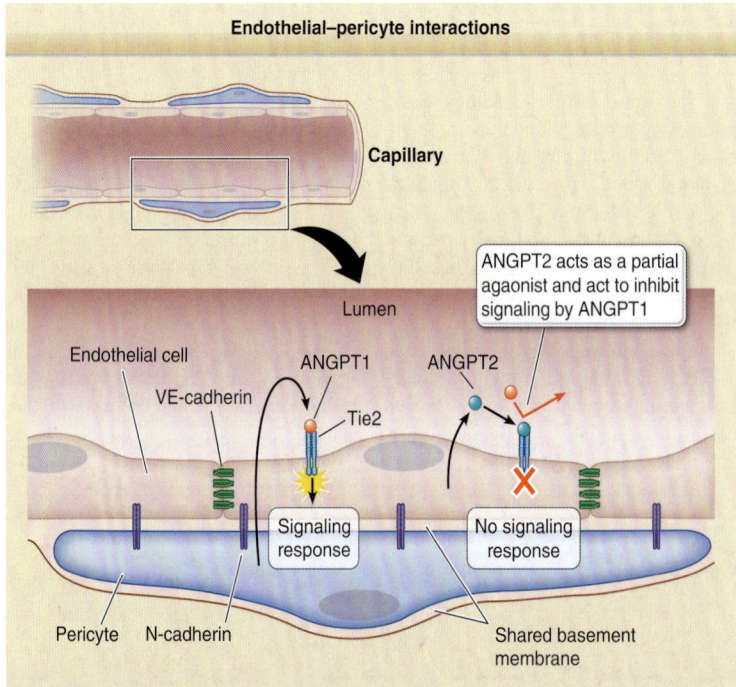

Figure 9-11 Endothelial cell (EC)–pericyte interactions. Pericytes are localized to within the basement membrane of the EC lining of microvessels and contribute to its synthesis and maintenance, and the composition and organization of the basement membrane may modify EC functions. Pericytes directly contact ECs, forming adherens junctions involving N-cadherin linkages. Pericytes also stabilize ECs by paracrine signals; the best understood of which involves pericyte secretion of angiopoietin 1 (ANGPT1), which binds to and activates the receptor tyrosine kinase Tie2 expressed on the endothelium. ANGPT1 binding prevents EC-derived ANGPT2 from binding to the same receptor. ANGPT2 acts as a partial agonist, and when its levels increase, it prevents ANGPT1-mediated signaling, leading to disruption of endothelial cell junctions associated with capillary leak, angiogenesis, or both.

stage; at later stages, most VEGF-expressing cells are found within the neoepithelium.[20] Under conditions of injury, hypoxia, or inflammation, keratinocytes produce and release a wide range of angiogenic factors, including members of the FGF or TGF protein family, PDGF, or VEGF. Concomitantly, VEGFR-2 is upregulated on ECs, which augments endothelial responses to VEGF. FGF-2 is derived from infiltrating macrophages but also from ECs themselves. Antibodies against FGF-2 inhibit wound angiogenesis nearly completely.

Stem cells from the skin stem cell niches and endogenous stem cells outside the niche support wound healing. These include hair follicle bulge and dermal sheath stem cells surrounding hair follicles, epidermal stem cells, and bone marrow–derived mesenchymal stem cells. Despite all preclinical wound-healing studies, translation of stem cell–based strategies in the clinical settings has had only limited success.[21] The quantitative contribution of stem cell–derived angiogenesis compared with conventional angiogenesis through local sprouting is unknown.

TUMOR ANGIOGENESIS

Skin tumors, like any other solid tumor, acquire their blood supply from the neighboring blood capillaries. Rapid tumor growth without adequate blood supply induces hypoxia. Hypoxia is augmented because of the leaky and disorganized tumor vasculature, resulting in acute fluxes in oxygen tension and in diffusion-limited regions within the tumor. Both the tumor and the stroma compartments respond to hypoxia by expressing the hypoxia-inducible factor (HIF) family of transcription factors.[22] Hypoxia stimulates tumor cells and macrophages to secrete TGF-β, PDGF, CXCL2, and endothelin, which activate fibroblasts. In fibroblasts, hypoxia stimulates extracellular matrix remodeling and the release of angiogenetic factors. Hypoxia directly effects vascular barrier function by decreasing the association between PCs and ECs. Tumors themselves may produce VEGF, FGF-2, EGF, and HGF or SF (see Fig. 9-12). Additionally, tumors may augment blood supply by intussusceptive angiogenesis (splitting of an existing blood vessel in two), vasculogenic mimicry (the formation of fluid-conducting channels by tumor cells), vessel co-option (tumor cells migrate along the preexisting vessels), and vasculogenesis.[23] Vascular mimicry appears to play a specific role in metastatic melanoma (not in primary lesions) because patients with this type of vascular channel formation have a worse 5-year survival rate.[24] Another interesting phenomenon observed in the tumor associated vasculature is endothelial-to-mesenchymal transition, which generates cancer-associated myofibroblasts that stimulate inflammation and fibrosis and augment vascular dysfunction and as a result increase hypoxia. TGF-β is one of the driving factors of endothelial-to-mesenchymal transition.[25]

CONCLUSIONS

The skin vascular system is unique in several respects. It is organized into functionally distinct vascular

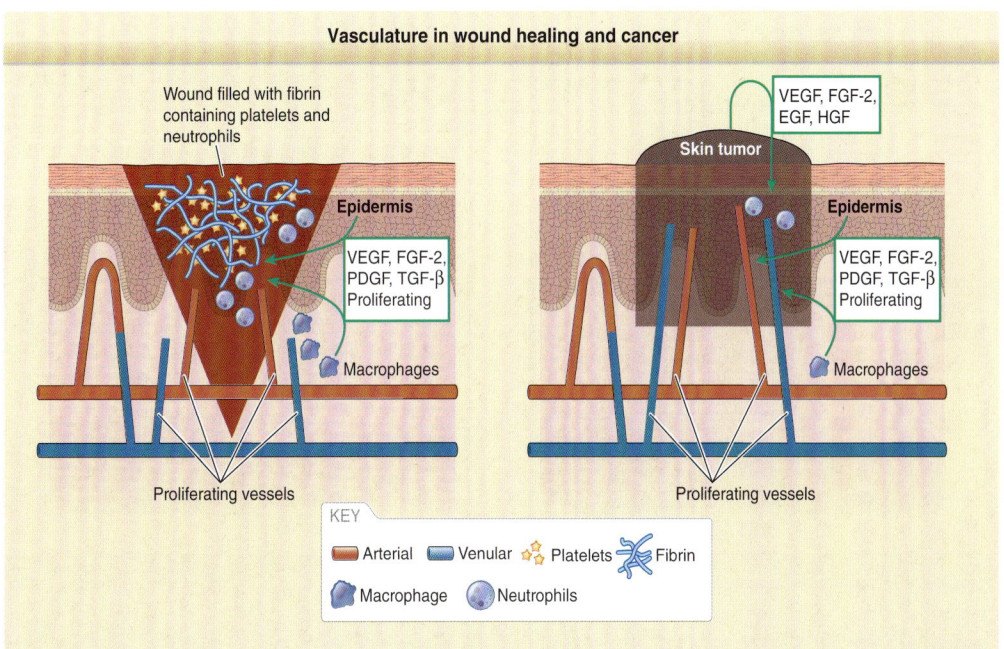

Figure 9-12 Vasculature in wound healing and cancer. EGF, endothelial growth factor; FGF, fibroblasst growth factor; HGF, hepatocyte growth factor; PDGF, platelet-derived growth factor; TGF-β, transforming growth factor-β; VEGF, vascular endothelial growth factor.

segments: the loops within the tips of the papillae, the SVP, and the DVP. These segments may individually or conjointly respond to exogenous or endogenous stimuli, thereby influencing skin disease expression. Because of their proximity to the epidermis, ECs of the SVP may directly respond to keratinocyte-derived factors such as cutaneous T cell–attracting chemokine or VEGF, which results in an altered vascular architecture, phenotype, and function. Moreover, skin EC may be directly exposed to environmental antigens. In this context, the constitutive expression of HLA class II molecules by postcapillary venules implies that ECs play a role in antigen presentation, which may increase the likelihood that the antigen is recognized in a timely manner to efficiently recruit memory T cells to sites of danger.

REFERENCES

1. Braverman IM. Ultrastructure and organization of the cutaneous microvasculature in normal and pathologic states. *J Invest Dermatol*. 1989;9(suppl)3:2S-9S.
2. Weninger W, Biro M, Jain R. Leukocyte migration in the interstitial space of non-lymphoid organs. *Nat Rev Immunol*. 2014;14:232-246.
3. Fan X, Rudensky AY. Hallmarks of tissue-resident lymphocytes. *Cell*. 2016;164:1198-1211.
4. Ginhoux F, Guilliams M. Tissue-resident macrophage ontogeny and homeostasis. *Immunity* 2016;44: 439-449.
5. Pober JS, Sessa WC. Inflammation and the blood microvascular system. *Cold Spring Harb Perspect Biol*. 2015;7:a016345.
6. Wu J, Saleh MA, Kirabo A, et al. Immune activation caused by vascular oxidation promotes fibrosis and hypertension. *J Clin Invest*. 2016;126:1607.
7. Charkoudian N. Skin blood flow in adult human thermoregulation: how it works, when it does not, and why. *Mayo Clin Proc*. 2003;78:603-612.
8. Bromley SK, Yan S, Tomura M, et al. Recirculating memory T cells are a unique subset of CD4+ T cells with a distinct phenotype and migratory pattern. *J Immunol*. 2013;190:970-976.
9. Berg EL, Yoshino T, Rott LS, et al. The cutaneous lymphocyte antigen is a skin lymphocyte homing receptor for the vascular lectin endothelial cell-leukocyte adhesion molecule 1. *J Exp Med*. 1991;174:1461-1466.
10. Reiss Y, Proudfoot AE, Power CA, et al. CC chemokine receptor (CCR)4 and the CCR10 ligand cutaneous T cell-attracting che.mokine (CTACK) in lymphocyte trafficking to inflamed skin. *J Exp Med*. 2001;194:1541-1547.
11. Homey B, Alenius H, Muller A, et al. CCL27-CCR10 interactions regulate T cell-mediated skin inflammation. *Nat Med*. 2002;8:157-165.
12. Nihal M, Mikkola D, Wood GS. Detection of clonally restricted immunoglobulin heavy chain gene rearrangements in normal and lesional skin: analysis of the B cell component of the skin-associated lymphoid tissue and implications for the molecular diagnosis of cutaneous B cell lymphomas. *J Mol Diagn*. 2000;2:5-10.
13. Muller WA. Localized signals that regulate transendothelial migration. *Curr Opin Immunol*. 2016;38:24-29.
14. Lui R, Lauridsen H, Amezquita R, et al. Interleukin-17 promotes neutrophil-mediated immunity by activating microvascular pericytes and not endothelium. *J Immunol*. 2016;197(6):2400-2408.
15. Rajashekhar G, Grow M, Willuweit A, et al. Divergent and convergent effects on gene expression and function in acute versus chronic endothelial activation. *Physiol Genomics*. 2007;31:104-113.
16. Kluger MS, Johnson DR, Pober JS. Mechanism of sustained E-selectin expression in cultured human dermal microvascular endothelial cells. *J Immunol*. 1997;158: 887-896.
17. Lechleitner S, Kunstfeld R, Messeritsch-Fanta C, et al. Peripheral lymph node addressins are expressed on skin endothelial cells. *J Invest Dermatol*. 1999;113:410-414.
18. Martinet L, Le GS, Filleron T, et al. High endothelial venules (HEVs) in human melanoma lesions: major gateways for tumor-infiltrating lymphocytes. *Oncoimmunology*. 2012;1:829-839.
19. Petzelbauer P, Pober JS, Keh A, et al. Inducibility and expression of microvascular endothelial adhesion molecules in lesional, perilesional, and uninvolved skin of psoriatic patients. *J Invest Dermatol*. 1994;103:300-305.
20. Minutti CM, Knipper JA, Allen JE, et al. Tissue-specific contribution of macrophages to wound healing. *Semin Cell Dev Biol*. 2017;61:3-11.
21. Cerqueira MT, Pirraco RP, Marques AP. Stem cells in skin wound healing: are we there yet? *Adv Wound Care (New Rochelle)*. 2016;5:164-175.
22. LaGory EL, Giaccia AJ. The ever-*expanding* role of HIF in tumour and stromal biology. *Nat Cell Biol*. 2016;18: 356-365.
23. Krishna PS, Nagare RP, Sneha VS, et al. Tumour angiogenesis—origin of blood vessels. *Int J Cancer*. 2016;139:729-735.
24. Cao Z, Bao M, Miele L, et al. Stem cells in skin wound healing: are we there yet? Tumour vasculogenic mimicry is associated with poor prognosis of human cancer patients: a systemic review and meta-analysis. *Eur J Cancer*. 2013;49:3914-3923.
25. Xiao L, Kim DJ, Davis CL, et al. Tumor endothelial cells with distinct patterns of TGFbeta-driven endothelial-to-mesenchymal transition. *Cancer Res*. 2015;75:1244-1254.

Chapter 10 :: The Immunological Structure of the Skin
:: Georg Stingl & Marie-Charlotte Brüggen

第十章 皮肤免疫系统

中文导读

本章共分为4节：①背景；②皮肤免疫系统：细胞和分子成分；③动态平衡下的皮肤免疫系统；④病理条件下的皮肤免疫系统。本章系统地介绍了皮肤先天性和适应性免疫系统的基本结构要素，提出了在生理和病理条件下免疫功能的概念。

第一节背景，介绍了皮肤免疫发现的历程。目前对于皮肤免疫学的起源有两种说法，一是儿科医生Clemens von Pirquet和Béla Schick描述的血清病皮疹可能是皮肤免疫的第一个证明；二是更多的皮肤科医生则认为Beutner和Jordon发现的天疱疮和大疱性类天疱疮患者可出现自身抗体为皮肤免疫的开端。

第二节皮肤免疫系统：细胞和分子成分，介绍了皮肤免疫系统有先天和后天两个组成部分，分别有不同的细胞和分子成分。参与先天免疫的白细胞和非白细胞都配备了模式识别受体，能够快速感知危险信号。在天然免疫系统中，中性粒细胞是大多数皮肤损伤后的第一反应细胞，此外，还有嗜酸性粒细胞、先天性淋巴细胞、巨噬细胞以及具有先天免疫功能的树突状细胞。皮肤适应性免疫系统的反应细胞是激发和表达获得性免疫所必需的细胞，主要为树突状抗原提呈细胞和T淋巴细胞。

第三节动态平衡下的皮肤免疫系统，介绍了维持细胞和组织的动态平衡需要防止对无害物质的过度反应，以及亚临床水平的宿主防御反应。这种"隐藏的"宿主防御反应在先天和适应性水平都起作用，举例阐述了宿主防御反应过程：寄生于表皮的共生菌诱导依赖于不同类型树突状细胞之间相互作用的免疫反应，这种相互作用导致Tc17细胞的产生，这些CD8+T细胞产生和释放的IL-17与角质形成细胞上的IL-17受体结合，并触发能够防止真正病原体过度生长的介质产生。

第四节病理条件下的皮肤免疫系统，介绍了皮肤接收到危险信号或其他致病或促病因子的传递，会对其细胞和分子调节产生宿主防御反应，其通常的临床表现是组织炎症。同时描述了银屑病Koebner反应中侵入皮肤或在皮肤中放大的第一个过路细胞通常是具有天然免疫反应的细胞。而在大多数情况下，炎症性皮肤病的特点是T淋巴细胞的浸润。同时也介绍了皮肤癌中的免疫与肿瘤患者的预后及免疫治疗等密切相关。目前根据所涉及的T细胞亚群可分类为Th1型、Th2/Th22型、Th1/Th17型、Th17型、Th9型、细胞毒性T型等不同类型的炎症。最后提到了针对炎症的转化研究是未来临床研究的趋势。

〔栗 娟〕

AT-A-GLANCE

- Skin is a "Grenzorgan" equipped with the capacity to mount and execute immune responses.
- The cutaneous immune system disposes of an innate and adaptive arm to exert these functions.
- Molecular constituents of the cutaneous immune system include pattern recognition receptors and effector molecules.
- Tissue homeostasis requires the prevention of exaggerated responses to innocuous substances and the occurrence of host-defense reactions at a subclinical level, ie, in the absence of inflammation.
- Under pathological conditions, danger signals or other disease-eliciting/-promoting factors in the skin elicit a coordinated (host defense) reaction of its cellular and molecular elements.

The skin is a border organ ("Grenzorgan") separating the host's structural constituents from the environment and, at the same time, allowing the communication between the inside and the outside world. This dual role of the skin is commonly referred to as "skin barrier function." Its major task is to secure and maintain tissue homeostasis and, thus, to preserve host integrity. In case of a major danger signal such as the overwhelming assault of pathogenic microorganisms, it must allow for the rapid generation and mobilization of effective host defense reactions leading to the neutralization of the pathogen. To fulfill these obligations, the skin contains a variety of structural, cellular, and molecular elements, which confer physical, chemical, and immunological protection. The immunological barrier consists of the different constituents of both the innate and active immune response, which, dependent on the situation, are either productive and—at the expense of tissue destruction—protective or nonproductive and downregulating, thus preventing overreaction to an otherwise innocuous substance. This chapter describes the basic structural elements of the cutaneous innate and adaptive immune system and, based on this information, develops a concept of its functionality under physiologic and pathologic conditions.

BACKGROUND

In 1905, the pediatricians Clemens von Pirquet and Béla Schick published their monography named "Die Serumkrankheit" ("serum sickness") and meticulously described the clinical symptoms of children that had received sera of horses previously vaccinated with *Corynebacterium diphtheriae* (Fig. 10-1).[1] This serum treatment was quite successful in mitigating or even abrogating the diphtherial infection, but, as a complication, the children later developed a transitory disease attack consisting of fever, arthritis, nephritis, encephalitis, and, very notably, a skin rash. Because the intensity of the symptoms directly correlated with the amount of serum administered, Pirquet and Schick correctly speculated that serum sickness is an undesired (immunological?) host reaction against animal proteins. The validity of this assumption was not confirmed until the 1950s when investigators at the Scripps Research Institute showed that rabbits immunized with foreign proteins would develop a clinical disease complex similar to that of serum-injected children and, microscopically and serologically, characterized by the occurrence of immune complexes.[2,3] It is very likely that the skin rash in serum sickness was the first demonstration of the skin being a target of immune responses. Despite this, most dermatologists would date the actual beginning of modern immunodermatology to Beutner and Jordon's critical observations that patients with pemphigus and bullous pemphigoid exhibit pathogenic autoantibodies against desmosomal and basement membrane–associated antigens, respectively.[4,5] In this context, it is interesting that with very few exceptions, the skin, although a preferential target in several antibody-mediated diseases, is essentially devoid of B lymphocytes.

Edward Jenner's successful smallpox vaccination showed for the first time that host defense responses can also originate in the skin.[6] In this heroic experiment performed on his gardener's son, Jenner introduced, by scraping, material obtained from an infectious cowpox pustule (of a dairymaid) into the skin. Upon reinoculation with material from a fresh smallpox lesion a few weeks later, the boy was protected from the disease. Almost 100 years later, Coley's seminal observation that an ulcerated sarcoma of the breast regressed upon streptococcal superinfection implied that the (skin's) immune/defense system can also be mobilized in the combat of cancer.[7] In fact, Besredka and Gross showed in 1935 that mice that had been repeatedly immunized with homogenates of tissue sarcomas via the skin were protected against a later challenge with the wild-type cancer, whereas mice that had been vaccinated via other routes (ie, intramuscularly or intravenously) would succumb to the disease.[8] The authors speculated about the existence of a unique immunologic milieu in the skin that would preferably promote the generation of (cancer) protective immune responses. It was not until the late 1960s that we would learn more about the mechanistic details of the skin's peculiar role in the elicitation of an immune response. Based on Landsteiner's discovery[9] that allergic contact dermatitis is a lymphocyte-mediated reaction that usually begins and invariably ends in the skin, Macher and Chase, in a series of legendary experiments, came to the conclusion that in hapten-specific immune responses an antigenic depot is formed in the skin that needs to leave this organ for a successful hapten-specific sensitization to occur.[10] The finding of Frey and Wenk that patent lymphatics are a prerequisite for a successful skin-induced sensitization implied that this event would take place in the skin-draining

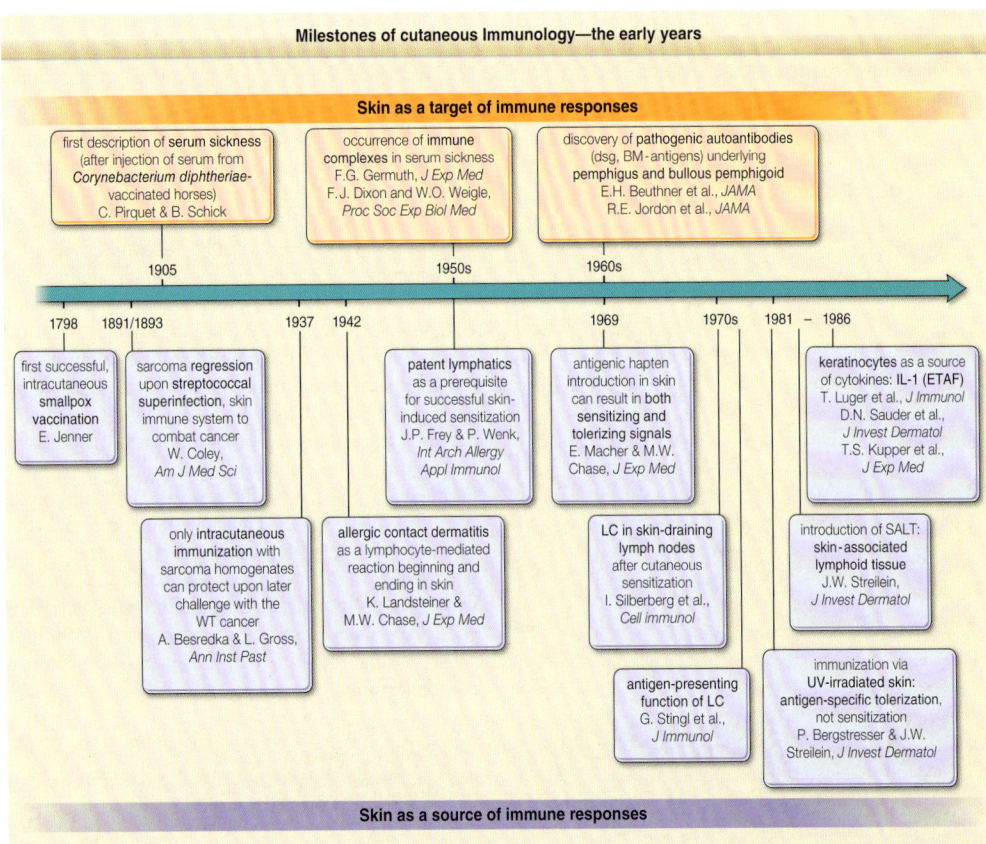

Figure 10-1 Milestones of cutaneous immunology—the early years. Major discoveries unraveling the role of the skin as a targer (upper part) and source (lower part) of immune responses.

lymph nodes.[11] Interestingly enough, Macher and Chase reported also that early removal of the cutaneous antigenic depot would result in antigen-specific unresponsiveness rather than in a null even.[12] This demonstrated clearly that introduction of an antigenic hapten in the skin can evoke not only sensitizing but also tolerizing signals. The medical relevance of this finding became obvious when it was shown that the attempt of immunization via ultraviolet (UV)-irradiated skin results in antigen-specific tolerization rather than sensitization.[13,14] Based on the original ultrastructural observation by Silberberg and Baer of the presence of Langerhans cells (LCs) in skin-draining lymph nodes after cutaneous sensitization with dinitrochlorobenzene (DNCB)[15] and the first demonstration of the antigen-presenting function of LCs,[16] the concept emerged that LCs and, later, other dendritic cells of the skin play a crucial role in capturing haptens and other exogenous antigens to induce activation of naïve T cells in skin-draining lymph nodes. Wayne Streilein coined the term *skin-associated lymphoid tissues* for this cutaneous immune circuit[17] and postulated that soluble mediators, for example, proinflammatory cytokines, produced by both leukocytes and resident skin cells such as keratinocytes,[18-20] would modulate antigen-presenting cell (APC) function and, thus, influence the outcome of the cutaneous immune response. As is shown in this review and in other chapters of this book, the skin represents an immunologic orchestra capable of generating quantitatively and qualitatively different functional voices. The enormous progress in drug discovery and development during the past decade now allows us to selectively and precisely tune the individual instruments of this network.

THE SKIN IMMUNE SYSTEM: CELLULAR AND MOLECULAR CONSTITUENTS

The skin is an organ equipped with the capacity to mount and execute immune responses. The cells and molecules needed for this exercise are summarized under the term *skin immune system*.[21] The skin immune system has an innate and an adaptive component (Table 10-1). The innate component is characterized by (a) its rapid onset, (b) its capacity to discriminate

TABLE 10-1
Cellular Constituents of the Cutaneous Immune System

CELL "FAMILY"	MEMBERS
A) Innate Immune System of the Skin	
Resident cells (nonleukocytic)	Keratinocytes
	Fibroblasts
	Sebocytes
	Endothelial cells
	Nerve cells
Granulocytes	Neutrophils (polymorphonuclear neutrophils [PMNs])
	Eosinophils
	Basophils
Macrophages	
Mast cells	
Innate lymphoid cells (ILCs)	Cytotoxic ILCs: natural killer (NK) cells
	Helper ILC: ILC1
	ILC2
	ILC3
Dendritic cells (DC)	Inflammatory DC[a]
	Plasmacytoid dendritic cell[a]
B) Adaptive Immune System of the Skin	
Dendritic cells	Langerhans cells
	CD141+ DC
	Dermal DC
	Inflammatory DC[a]
	pDC[a]
T lymphocytes (αβ) (details: see Fig. 10-4)	Naïve T cells
	Memory T cells

[a]As a consequence of their molecular and structural equipment, plasmacytoid DCs and inflammatory DCs can fulfill both innate and adaptive immune functions.

between danger and nondanger only, instead of distinguishing between individual antigenic specificities, and (c) its lack of memory. Adaptive immunity, by contrast, needs 10 to 14 days to develop, but it is characterized by an exquisite peptide specificity brought by the enormous polymorphism of human leukocyte antigens on APCs and a set of rearranged antigen receptors on B cells and T cells. Another distinguishing feature of the adaptive response is to react in an enhanced fashion to a repeated antigenic challenge (memory).[22]

Cells of the cutaneous innate response consist of both leukocytes (Table 10-1A, Fig. 10-2A) and nonleukocytes such as keratinocytes and fibroblasts. Leukocytes belonging to the innate immune system include granulocytes, mononuclear phagocytes, mast cells, innate lymphoid cells (ILCs), and two particular types of dendritic cells (DCs), namely plasmacytoid DC (pDC) and inflammatory DC. Within normal human skin (NHS), all these innate leukocytes are present in only small (mononuclear phagocytes, mast cells) or even negligible numbers (the rest).

MOLECULAR CONSTITUENTS: RECEPTORS AND EFFECTORS

To do their job, both leukocytes and nonleukocytes involved in innate immunity are equipped with pattern recognition receptors (PRRs). PRR constitute a large family of either surface-bound and/or cytoplasmic receptors (eg, toll-like receptors, TLR) that are capable of rapidly sensing danger signals such as microbes and their constituents, haptens, and UV radiation (Table 10-3 lists the members of TLR familiy).[23,24] As a consequence, innate immunocytes either expand in situ or are recruited from the circulation (see Fig. 10-2B) and begin to elaborate mediators destined to neutralize and/or eliminate the pathogen (Table 10-2). These include the production of proinflammatory cytokines, chemokines, lytic molecules, proteases, complement components, and arachidonic acid metabolites, as well as a group of antimicrobial peptides (AMPs). AMPs[25] are produced in a constitutive or induced fashion and can eliminate pathogenic bacteria, viruses, fungi, and parasites, and, in addition, subserve other biologic functions such as chemotaxis or wound repair promotion.

CELLULAR CONSTITUENTS

INNATE IMMUNE SYSTEM

Granulocytes, Mast Cells: Among the leukocytes of the innate immune system, neutrophils usually act as the so-called first responders after most forms of skin injury. As an example, microbial assault results in the production/release of different types of chemotactic factors, such as chemokines, leukotrienes, and complement components. This allows neutrophils to abundantly enter the skin from the peripheral blood and migrate toward the site of injury. The main effector function of neutrophils is to eliminate microbes, either by phagocytosis (ingestion and killing) or by using their neutrophil extracellular traps,[26] which enable them to kill extracellular pathogens. Eosinophils are much less efficient phagocytes than polymorphonuclear neutrophils. However, by releasing preformed cationic proteins (eg, eosinophilic cationic proteins) that are toxic to several parasites, eosinophils provide efficient protection against the parasites. Basophils contain histamine-filled granules and are a rich source of cytokines such as interleukin (IL)-4 and IL-13. In this regard, basophils resemble mast cells and, similar to mast cells, play an important role in allergic tissue inflammation. Mast cells exhibit membrane-bound and cytoplasmic granules, which contain preformed mediators (eg, histamine, serotonin) and molecules synthesized upon activation (eg, tumor necrosis factor [TNF], IL-3, IL-4, IL-13), respectively. Important activation mechanisms of mast cells resulting in the release and production of molecular mediators are the

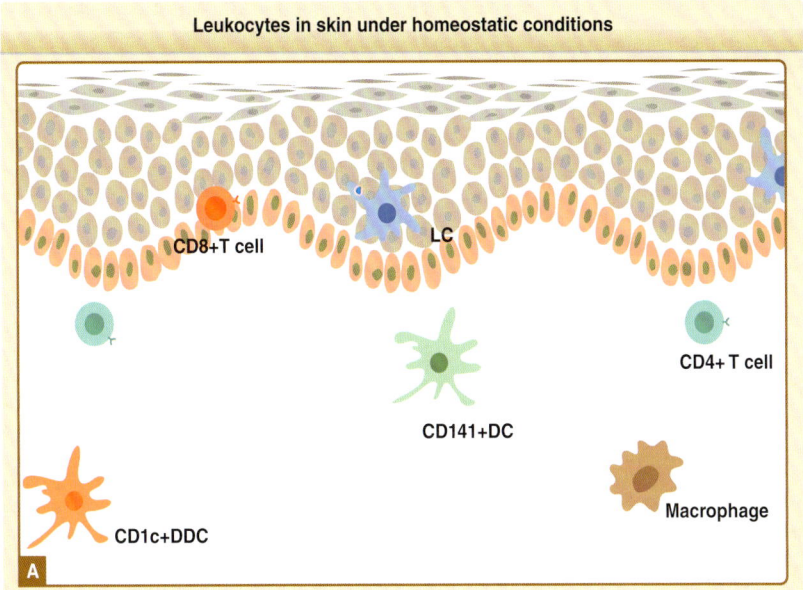

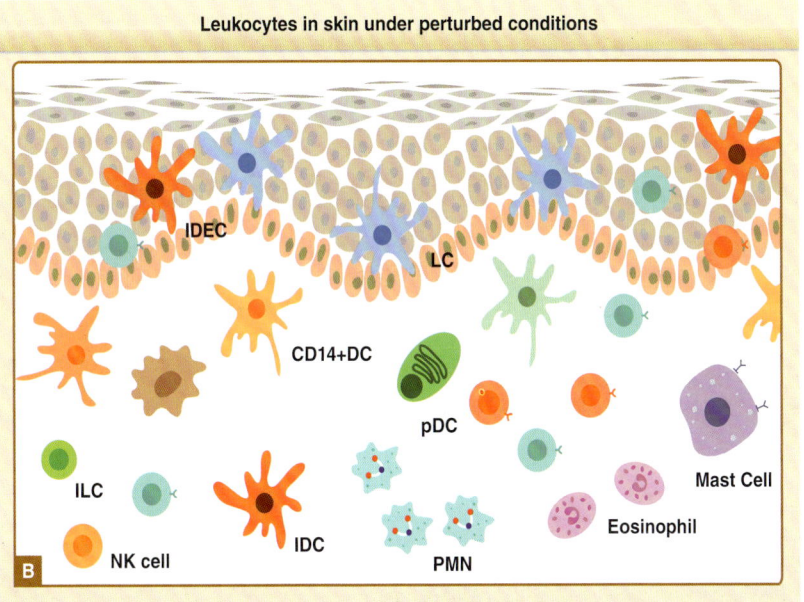

Figure 10-2 Leukocyte populations in human skin under homeostatic and inflammatory conditions. **A,** Leukocytes in skin under homeostatic conditions. Normal human skin harbors a resident T-cell population (CD4+ and CD8+) as well as various dendritic cell (DC) subsets (Langerhans cells [LC] in the epidermis; CD141+ and CD1c+ DC in the dermis). Only a few innate leukocytes are found in normal human skin, notably macrophages. **B,** Leukocytes in skin under perturbed conditions (inflammation). Under inflammatory conditions, a plethora of cells belonging to either the innate (macrophages, granulocytes, plasmacytoid dendritic cell [pDC], inflammatory DC [IDC], mast cells, innate lymphoid cell [ILC]) or adaptive immune system (CD4+ and CD8+ T cells) infiltrate the skin. IDEC, inflammatory dendritic epidermal cells; NK, natural killer; PMN, polymorphonuclear neutrophil.

interaction of complement cleavage products C3a and C5a with their respective receptors, as well as Fc-mediated binding of immunoglobulin E. In the situation of Fc-mediated binding of immunoglobulin E, immunoglobulin E crosslinking by the respective antigen results in type I hypersensitivity reactions.

Innate Lymphocytes: Much attention has focused on a family of non-T non-B lymphoid cells that includes not only cytotoxic (natural killer [NK] cells) but also so-called helper ILCs. Among the best known roles of NK cells are the recognition and killing of virally infected and neoplastic cells and the

TABLE 10-2
Overview of Effector Substances of the Innate Immune System in Skin

FAMILY OF MOLECULES	EXAMPLES
Cytokines	- Tumor necrosis factor (TNF), interleukin (IL)-1β, IL-6, IL-8, IL-12 - IL-10, transforming growth factor (TGF)-β
Chemokines	- CXCL1, CXCL8, CCL3, CCL5, CCL20
Antimicrobial peptides (AMPs)	- Human cathelicidin LL-37 - Human beta-defensins hBD-2, hBD-3 - Psoriasin S100A - Dermcidin - Ribonuclease (RNAse) 7 - Lysozyme
Complement components	- C3a, C5a, C3b
Arachidonic acid metabolites	- PGE4, LKTs, etc.
Reactive oxygen species (ROS)	
Lytic molecules	- Granulysin, perforin, tumor necrosis factor–related apoptosis-inducing ligand (TRAIL), granzyme B
Proteases	- Matric metalloproteases (MMPs) - Serine proteases (eg, kallikreins)
Pattern recognition receptors (PRRs)	- Toll-like receptors (TLRs) - Nucleotide-binding oligomerization domain (NOD)-like receptors (NLR) - Retinoic acid inducible gene I (Rig1)-like receptors (RLRs) - C-type lectin receptors (CLRs)

secretion of interferon (IFN)-γ, a main immunoregulatory cytokine. As opposed to CD8+ T cells, which use the recognition of major histocompatibility complex (MHC) I antigen complexes to induce killing, MHC I is recognized by inhibitory receptors on NK cells and results in the inhibition of lytic responses. On the other hand, contact with cells exhibiting altered MHC I (eg, virus-infected cells) or ligands of activating NK cell receptors at their surface induces a cytotoxic killing cascade. Helper ILCs can be subdivided into 3 subsets (ILC1, ILC2, ILC3) according to their transcription factor and cytokine profiles, which show striking similarities with T helper (Th) cell subsets. Thus both ILC1s and Th1 cells are TBET (a Th1 pathway transcription factor)-positive and produce IFN-γ; ILC2s are differentiating under the influence of GATA3 (a Th2 pathway transcription factor) and are secreting IL-5 and IL-13; and ILC3s and Th17/Th22 cells abundantly express RORC/AHR, respectively, and are a rich source of IL-17 and IL-22.[27] The exact role of helper ILCs in skin remains to be elucidated.

Macrophages: Next to polymorphonuclear neutrophils, macrophages and mononuclear phagocytes are heavily involved in the elimination of invading microbes. They accomplish this by phagocytosis and the subsequent killing of the pathogen by reactive oxygen species. Thereafter, they switch their functional program to clean up the stage and promote tissue regeneration and repair. However, we wouldn't do justice to the macrophages by simply labeling them as phagocytes given that they also exert an APC function and, by doing so, play a great role in shaping cutaneous immune responses.[28]

Dendritic Cells with Innate Immune Functions: As to DC subsets with proper innate immune functions, pDCs play a major role in antiviral defense by the massive production of type I interferons (IFN-α, IFN-β) upon activation of TLR7 and TLR9 (Table 10-3). In this context, it is noteworthy that the artificial TLR7 ligand imiquimod provides a strong activation signal for pDC, resulting not only in IFN-α production, but also in the expression of lytic molecules such as tumor necrosis factor–related apoptosis-inducing ligand.[29] This mechanism is probably responsible for the therapeutic efficacy of topical imiquimod in patients with genital warts, actinic keratosis, and basal cell carcinomas.[30] Inflammatory DCs include various subsets (eg, tipDC [TNF-α/inducible nitric oxide synthase–producing DC], inflammatory dendritic epidermal cells)[31] and exert proinflammatory functions such as the production of TNF and inducible nitric oxide synthase[32] and the priming of Th cell responses.[33-35]

ADAPTIVE IMMUNE SYSTEM

Cells of the cutaneous adaptive response are the ones needed for the elicitation and expression of adaptive immunity. These are dendritic APC and T lymphocytes (see Table 10-1B and Fig. 10-2A).

TABLE 10-3
Toll-Like Receptors and Ligands

TOLL-LIKE RECEPTOR (TLR)	LIGAND	
TLR1	Triacylated lipoproteins (TLR 2/1)	Gram-negative bacteria, mycobacteria
TLR2	Diacylated lipoproteins (TLR 2/6)	Gram-positive bacteria (*Propionibacterium acnes*)
TLR3	Virus-derived double-stranded RNA (dsRNA)	Viruses (dsRNA)
TLR4	Lipopolysaccharide (LPS)	Gram-negative bacteria
TLR5	Flagellin	Flagellated bacteria
TLR6	Lipopeptides	Mycobacteria
TLR7	Virus-derived single-stranded RNA (ssRNA)	Viruses (ssRNA)
TLR8	Virus-derived ssRNA	Viruses (ssRNA)
TLR9	Unmethylated DNA sequences (bacterial DNA)	Bacteria

TABLE 10-4
Main Characteristics of DC Populations in Human Skin

	LC	DDC	CD141+ DC	PDC	IDEC
Precursor	Self-maintaining? Monocytic?	Myeloid	Myeloid	Plasmacytoid	Monocytic
Markers	Langerin, CD1a, CD11c (low), CD11b, E-cadherin, DEC-205, CD39	CD1c (BDCA-1), CD1a, CD1b, CD11c, CD11b, CD33, CD172, DEC-205, CLEC6A, CLEC7A, CD206 (mannose receptor)	CD141 (BDCA-3), CD11c, DEC-205, CLEC9A	CD303 (BDCA-2), CD304 (BDCA-4), CD45RA, CD123 (IL-3R), DEC-205	CD1a, CD1c, CD11c, CD11b, CD206, CD209
Fc receptors	FcεRI, FcγRII	–	–	FcαR, FcγRIIa, FcεRI	FcεRI
TLR	TLR1, TLR2, TLR6	TLR1–8	TLR1–3, TLR6, TLR8	TLR1, TLR6, TLR7, TLR9	–
Main function	Initiation/regulation of T-cell responses	Stimulation of naïve T cells	Cross presentation	Antiviral immune response	Induction Th17-response
Cytokine production	TNF-α, IL-6, IL-8, IL-10, IL-12	TNF-α, IL-8, IL-10, IL-12, IL-23	TNF-α, (CXCL10), IFN-γ	Type-1 interferons (IFN-α)	IL-1β, TNF-α, IL-6, IL-23

All the cells listed above lack the expression of so-called lineage markers (CD3, CD14, CD19, CD20, CD56, glycophorin A) but express CD45 as well as human leukocyte antigen-D related (HLA-DR).

DC, dendritic cell; DDC, dermal dendritic cell; IFN, interferon; IL, interleukin; LC, Langerhans cell; Th, T-helper cell; TLR, toll-like receptor; TNF, tumor necrosis factor.

Dendritic Cells: As outlined in Chapter 11 in greater detail, normal (unperturbed) human skin contains 3 distinct populations of antigen-presenting DCs: epidermal LCs, dermal DCs (DDCs), and CD141+ DC. They are all derived from bone marrow precursors, although for LCs there still remains some debate; Table 10-4 lists the major phenotypic features and functions of skin DC. LCs[36] express CD1a, a formalin-resistant, sulfhydryl-dependent adenosine triphosphatase/CD39, as well as surface receptors for the uptake of native and complexed antigens such as DEC-205, the FcγRII/CD32 and FcεR1. Most notably, LCs contain endocytic organelles called Birbeck granules (Fig. 10-3B),[37] whose major constituent is the C-type lectin langerin/CD207.[38] CD207 enables LCs, together with CD1a, to present nonpeptide antigens (eg, *Mycobacterium leprae*) to T cells.[39,40] MHC I and II antigens (Fig. 10-3A) are mostly located within the cytoplasm of resident LCs.[41,42] DDC are MHC II-positive, express CD1c rather than CD1a, display the mannose receptor as well as DC-SIGN (dendritic cell–specific intercellular adhesion molecule-3-grabbing nonintegrin) for antigen uptake, but are devoid of Birbeck granules/Langerin (as opposed to the situation in humans, a subpopulation of murine DDC is Langerin-positive).[43-45] Another DC subset, namely CD141 (also known as BDCA-3 or thrombomodulin)-expressing DC, was initially identified in the peripheral blood, but has been found to also constitute a very small cell population in the human dermis.[46] CD141+ DCs are characterized by the expression of CD11c and DEC-205, as well as the receptors CLEC9A, TLR3, and TLR7, which enable them to take up extracellular necrotic cells and viral nucleic acids. Functionally, the 3 different types of "resident" skin DCs exhibit the characteristic features of bone marrow–derived DCs: migration (from the skin to the draining lymph nodes during primary immune responses) and induction of helper or cytotoxic antigen-specific immune responses in naïve resting T cells.[31] In the case of CD141+ DCs, the T-cell response is usually cytotoxic in nature and directed against antigenic moieties expressed by and taken up from surrounding symbionts and then channeled in the MHC class I presentation pathway. This phenomenon is termed *cross presentation*.[47] Some evidence exists that LCs also can take up antigens from surrounding keratinocytes and present the relevant peptides to CD8+ T cells in the context of MHC I.[48] Similar to DCs from other tissues, skin DCs exhibit an antigen uptake and, at the same time, immunoinhibitory mode when located in situ.[49] Resident LCs, for instance, extend their dendrites through and beyond the tight junctions formed between keratinocytes of the stratum corneum.[50] On the other hand, LCs carry only small amounts of costimulatory molecules on their surface and produce just negligible amounts of immunostimulatory cytokines such as IL-1β, IL-6, IL-12, and IL-23. In other words, LCs display phenotypic features that favor and facilitate the activation of regulatory T cells (Tregs). In fact, when they are kept in a resting state, as by glucocorticosteroids, they preferentially promote the expansion of Treg.[51]

Upon the receipt of danger signals, LCs,[52] and probably also DDCs,[44] mature into very potent immunostimulators for both CD4+ and CD8+ naïve, as well primed, T cells. The in vivo significance of these in vitro findings is evidenced by the occurrence of similar maturation events on DC[53,54] migrating from the skin to the draining lymph nodes under danger conditions.

T Lymphocytes: In most of the older textbooks of dermatology and immunology, the skin was often referred to as "nonlymphoid tissue." If such a term refers

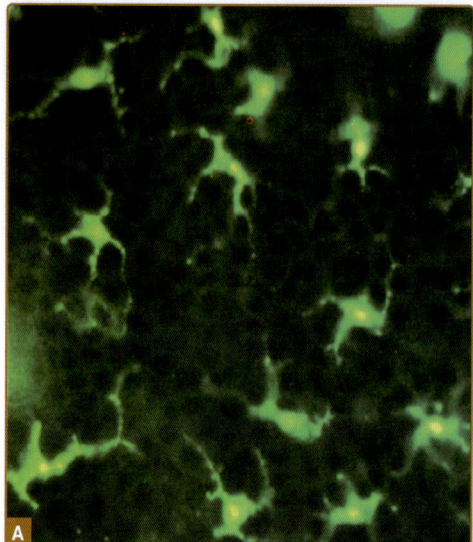
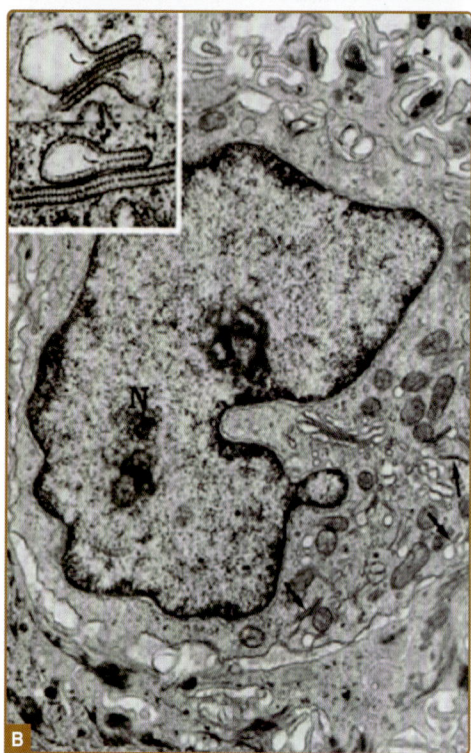

Figure 10-3 Langerhans cells (LCs). **A,** LCs in a sheet preparation of murine epidermis as revealed by anti–major histocompatibility complex class II (fluorescein isothiocyanate [FITC]) immunostaining. **B,** Electron micrograph of a LC in human epidermis. Arrows denote Birbeck granules. N, nucleus. (From Stingl G. New aspects of Langerhans cell functions. *Int J Dermatol*. 1980;19:189, with permission.) *Inset:* High-power electron micrograph of Birbeck granules. The curved arrows indicate the zipper-like fusion of the fuzzy coats of the vesicular portion of the granule. The delimiting membrane envelops 2 sheets of particles attached to it and a central lamella composed of 2 linear arrays of particles. (Copyright © 1967 Wolff. Originally published in Wolff K. The fine structure of the LC granule. *J Cell Biol*. 1967;35:468-473.)

to those tissues in which primary immune responses, that is, lymphocyte sensitization, are not or only very rarely taking place, the skin may well deserve such a designation. This, however, doesn't mean that the skin is devoid of lymphocytes. Just the opposite is true. Notwithstanding the existence of small numbers of ILCs and NK cells (see "Innate Lymphocytes" section), T lymphocytes[55] are by far the largest, and probably the most important, lymphocyte population within NHS (see Figs. 10-2A and 10-4). In fact, its size exceeds that of the T-cell population in the peripheral blood.[56] Most skin T cells are localized in the dermis and only 10% in the epidermis. T cells can be subdivided according to different criteria such as (a) antigenic experience, (b) the type of T-cell receptors (α/β vs. γ/δ), (c) type of accessory molecules expressed (CD4 vs CD8), and (d) functional differentiation (type of transcription factor; helper vs cytotoxic; cytokine secretion pattern). According to these distinguishing features, T cells of NHS, unlike skin T cells of rodents, express predominantly α/β T-cell receptors.[55] Whereas dermal T cells are mainly CD4+, epidermal T cells preferentially display the CD8+ phenotype. In their vast majority, T cells in skin express the memory (CD45RO+) rather than the naïve (CD45RA+) phenotype. According to the existing nomenclature, memory T cells are generally subdivided into central (Tcm) and effector memory (Tem) cells (Fig. 10-5).[57] Tcm cells exhibit the CCR7+/CD62L+ phenotype and are mainly found in secondary lymphoid organs such as lymph nodes and spleen. They are only sparsely scattered within NHS, but present in slightly larger numbers in chronic inflammatory (eg, eczema, psoriasis) and neoplastic (eg, cutaneous T-cell lymphoma) skin diseases.[58,59] Tem cells can be subdivided into recirculating memory T cells and tissue-resident memory T (Trm) cells. Recirculating Tem cells (CD62L-/CCR7+) constantly recirculate between nonlymphoid tissues and lymphatic organs. In contrast, Trm cells permanently reside in the skin, and, thus, can provide an extremely rapid onsite protection upon exposure to previously encountered antigens, that is, before other Tem cells are recruited from the circulation. All Trm cells are characterized by the expression of CD69 and some of them (mostly CD8+ Trm cells) by the αE integrin CD103.[57] They may have a very long life span and may thus not only be of crucial importance for the skin's immunosurveillance function, but also for the reactivation of inflammatory skin diseases (see "The Skin Immune System under Pathologic Conditions" section).

THE SKIN IMMUNE SYSTEM UNDER HOMEOSTATIC CONDITIONS

Maintenance of cellular and tissue homeostasis requires (a) the prevention of exaggerated responses to innocuous substances (eg, human dander, plant pollen, nutrients) and (b) the occurrence of host-defense reactions at

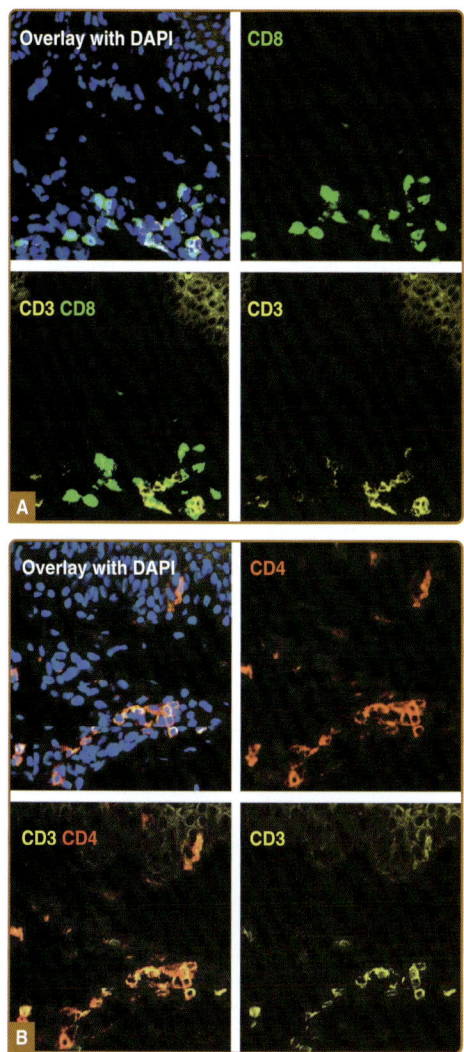

Figure 10-4 T cells in normal human skin. **A,** CD8 stained with fluorescein isothiocyanate (FITC; green); CD3 stained with APC; DAPI nuclear staining. The epidermis is located on the upper side of the images. **B,** Double immunofluorescence staining of CD4+ T cells in normal human skin (NHS): CD4 stained with tetramethylrhodamine isothiocyanate (TRITC; red); CD3 stained with allophycocyanin (APC; yellow); DAPI (4,6-diamidino-2-phenylindole) nuclear staining.

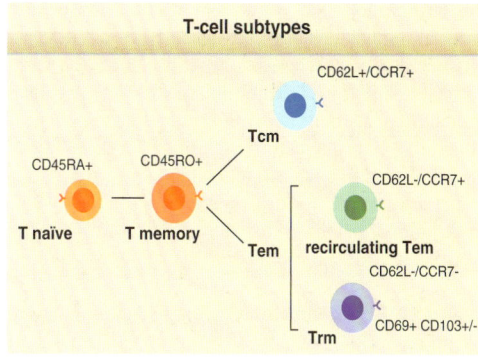

Figure 10-5 T-cell subtypes. Scheme of the different T-cell subsets as defined by their naïve/memory state. Tcm, central memory T cell; Tem, effector memory T cell; Trm, tissue-resident memory T cell.

a subclinical level, that is, in the absence of inflammation. Concerning host-defense reactions at a subclinical level, we must assume that the overgrowth of pathogenic microorganisms in normal skin is prevented by constitutively produced mediators such as proteins with antimicrobial properties (eg, ribonucleotidases 1, 4, 5, and 7), different proteases,[60] and certain AMPs. The S100 calcium-binding protein A7 (S100A7), also known as Psoriasin, is an AMP with a baseline production by keratinocytes. Its antimicrobial effect is mainly directed against *Escherichia coli*.[61] Evidence exists that "hidden" host defense reactions are not only operative at both the innate and the adaptive levels. Commensals (eg, *Staphylococcus epidermidis*) colonizing the epidermis are capable of inducing an immune response that is dependent on the interplay between different types of DC, which interplay ultimately results in the generation of Tc17 cells. The IL-17 produced and released by these CD8+ T cells binds to IL-17 receptors on keratinocytes and triggers the production of mediators capable of preventing the overgrowth of true pathogens such as *Staphylococcus aureus*.[62]

Contrary to the original belief that antigen presentation by DCs invariably results in sensitization, it is now clear that this is luckily (!) not the case. Otherwise, every harmless environmental substance would evoke a massive tissue response. This implies that professional APCs must exist that in the absence of danger signals induce negative (ie, downregulating or tolerizing) signals. In this context, the role of LCs has been heavily debated over the years. In the older literature, LCs were generally regarded as the principal sensitizing cells in skin-derived immune responses. This theory was mainly based on the demonstration, by electron microscopy, of Birbeck granule–containing LCs in the draining lymph nodes of hapten-sensitized guinea pigs[15] and on the observation that hapten application to animal (mouse, hamster) skin with normal LC numbers would result in sensitization, whereas exposure of LC-deficient skin to the very same hapten would lead to tolerization.[14] Later, however, it became clear that LCs are dispensable for the occurrence of protective immune responses against certain microorganisms causing skin infections (eg, herpes simplex virus).[63]

The finding of migrating LCs not only under danger conditions,[64,65] but also under noninflammatory homeostatic conditions, was of crucial importance for our understanding of LC in vivo functions. In fact, LCs carrying melanosomes and/or apoptotic bodies have been detected in lymph vessels of normal skin.[66] In line with this was the demonstration of immature LCs in lymph nodes draining chronically inflamed skin.[67] Consequently, we must assume that antigen-bearing LCs and DCs are constantly trafficking between skin and lymph nodes. That the functional outcome of this event is often that of antigen-specific unresponsiveness can be deduced from the observation that most individuals without any clinical sign of nickel (Ni) allergy have circulating, Ni-specific Tregs, whereas only those suffering from contact allergy to Ni exhibit Ni-specific CD8+ cells.[68] In a similar fashion, LCs can cross-present keratinocyte-derived antigens to lymph node T cells without any clinical sign of sensitization.[69]

The important question remains whether all DC populations of the skin, dependent only on the composition of the milieu in which they reside, can evoke either sensitizing or tolerizing responses, or, alternatively, whether one given DC type is more prone to induce one or the other. An important role of the cytokine milieu DCs act in is suggested by data showing that thymic stromal lymphopoietin strongly influences DCs and LCs to skew T-cell responses toward a Th2 direction.[70,71] On the other hand, evidence exists that mice whose LC population had been depleted by genetic manipulation would develop stronger T-cell reactions to haptens or microbial antigens than would wild-type animals.[72] These findings led to the hypothesis that LCs are intrinsically destined to generate downregulating or tolerizing T-cell responses. The validity of either concept has yet to be proven.

THE SKIN IMMUNE SYSTEM UNDER PATHOLOGIC CONDITIONS

Upon the receipt of danger signals (eg, microbial invasion, exposure to irritants, sensitizing haptens and/or drugs, UV radiation, trauma, heat, cold) or the delivery of other, often ill-defined, disease-eliciting or disease-promoting factors, the skin reacts with a coordinated (host defense) reaction of its cellular and molecular elements. A major component of this tissue response is immunologic in nature. Its magnitude and quality depend on the type of danger signal involved but its usual clinical manifestation is tissue inflammation (see Fig. 10-2B). As exemplified by and probably best investigated in the kinetics of the Koebner reaction in psoriasis, the first passenger cells invading the skin or amplifying in skin are usually cells of the innate response, that is, granulocytes, monocytes, NK cells, ILCs, and pDCs. pDCs are usually detected on the (active) margins of the individual lesions.[73] ILCs of psoriatic lesions belong in their majority to the ILC3 subset and are often located in close proximity to lesional T cells.[74,75] In certain inflammatory skin diseases, infiltrating cells belong almost exclusively to the innate immune system. Examples include pustular psoriasis, pyoderma gangrenosum, acute generalized exanthematous pustulosis, Job syndrome, acne inversa, rosacea, and autoinflammatory syndromes (neutrophils), as well as eosinophilic fasciitis, eosinophilic cellulitis, and hypereosinophilic syndrome (eosinophils). It is not entirely clear whether some of these reactions have an adaptive component or not. In acne and rosacea,[76,77] for example, T cells of the Th17 lineage have been identified in lesional skin, and in the case of acne have been shown to recognize *Propionibacterium acnes*-derived peptides.[77]

In their majority, inflammatory skin diseases are characterized by a prominent, often predominating, lymphocytic infiltrate consisting mostly of T lymphocytes. B cells, interestingly enough, tend to avoid the skin, with few notable exceptions such as cutaneous *Leishmania* infection.[78,79] Now that it is possible to functionally characterize T-cell subsets in situ or freshly isolated from tissue on the basis of cytokines and transcription factors expressed,[74,80,81] many inflammatory skin diseases can now be classified according to the T-cell subset(s) involved (Table 10-5). Psoriasis, for example, is the prototype of a Th17-driven disease, whereas atopic dermatitis has a strong Th2/Th22 signature.[81] Some evidence indicates that lichen planus lesions are characterized by a Th1 pattern.[82] Allergic contact dermatitis had initially been considered as a Th1-/cytotoxic T-cell–mediated disease,[83,84] but newer evidence speaks for an important role of IL-17–producing T cells in its pathogenesis.[85-87] UV obviously favors the expansion of Treg.[88] Certain illnesses, such as graft-versus-host disease, exhibit different molecular patterns in different stages and subtypes of the disease.[89] It is not clear whether similar differences exist between the various forms (acute, subacute, and chronic) of cutaneous lupus erythematosus. Some data speak for an important role of the type I IFN–Th1 axis and for a dysregulation of Treg.[90,91] The role of Th17 cells, if any, is controversially debated.[92,93] It is not unreasonable to assume that a molecular map of most (inflammatory) skin diseases will be available in the not too distant future. This will probably result in the molecular, and thus functional, subclassification of skin diseases, which on purely morphologic grounds are considered homogeneous. In psoriasis, this may be true for the small group of patients who do not or only poorly respond to the novel TNF or IL-17A antagonists. As mentioned earlier in this section, the recurrence of an inflammatory skin disease is not only caused by the

TABLE 10-5
Examples of T-Cell–Driven Skin Diseases

T-CELL PATTERN	SKIN DISEASES
Th1	Lichen planus
	Allergic contact dermatitis
	Tuberculoid leprosy
	Cutaneous leishmaniasis
Th2/Th22	Atopic dermatitis
	Acute graft-versus-host disease (GVHD)
	Lepromatous leprosy
	Diffuse leishmaniasis
Th9	To be determined (tumors?)
Th1/Th17	Chronic lichenoid GVHD
Th17	Acne vulgaris
	Psoriasis
Cytotoxic T cells	Allergic contact dermatitis
	Toxic epidermal necrolysis (?)

influx of pathogenic leukocytes from the blood, but can also be caused by the activation of T memory cells in the skin, notably Trm. It is not entirely clear which types of APC are involved in this process. These must not necessarily be the APCs (ie, LCs and DDCs) residing in normal skin. In fact, the population of tipDCs[94] and 6-sulfo poly-*N*-acetyllactosamine DCs (slan-DCs)[95] are probably the major IL-23–producing cells in psoriatic lesions that are responsible for the differentiation of T-helper cells in Th17 cells and for their survival. In contrast, inflammatory-type DCs of myeloid origin are apparently needed for the expansion of Th2 cells in atopic dermatitis.[96] Biologic drugs now exist that allow us to interfere with the pathologic tissue response not only at the lymphocyte, but also at the APC level. In fact, the anti–IL-23p19 antibodies guselkumab, tildrakizumab, and risankizumab show excellent efficacy in the treatment of plaque psoriasis.[97-99]

A discussion of the skin immune system under pathologic conditions is incomplete without mentioning the immune contexture in human skin cancers. As already discussed earlier (see "Background"), ample evidence exists that mobilization of cells and molecules of the immune system can often result in the successful elimination of cancer cells that manifests clinically as tumor regression. This phenomenon is not infrequently seen in skin cancers such as melanoma and actinic keratoses. The cancer-destructive capacity of immune cells becomes weaker and weaker the longer the (primary) tumor persists. In other words: the cancer avoids immune destruction by slowly shifting the tumor microenvironment from a tumoricidal into a tumor-promoting mode.[100-102] All types of immune cells can be found within or around the tumor. These infiltrates are heterogeneous between different types of cancer and can be very diverse from patient to patient. It appears that the presence of high numbers of intratumoral and peritumoral granulocytes, pDCs, myeloid-derived suppressor cells, and so-called M2 macrophages, producing IL-4, IL-10, IL-13, and transforming growth factor (TGF)-β, heralds a bad prognosis, whereas large numbers of CD3+ T cells, CD8+ cytotoxic T lymphocytes, and CD45RO+ memory T cells of both the CD4 and the CD8 type are associated with a longer disease-free survival.[102] Attention is now focused on the role of IL-9–producing T cells, so-called Th9 cells, in cancer immunity.[103] In mice, they possess potent anticancer properties, especially against melanoma.[104] Studies in human (skin) cancers are urgently needed to determine the anticancer potential of Th9 cells and, thus, their possible relevance for cancer immunotherapy.

POST SCRIPTUM

In a remarkable speech delivered at the Annual Meeting of the Society of Clinical Investigation in 1981, the late immunologist Dr. William Paul predicted a golden era of clinical investigation.[105] He thought that the introduction of certain technologies (production of monoclonal antibodies and the cloning of cells and genes) would result in true accomplishment. Today, we can safely state that his prophecy was true. Technology-driven, ground-breaking discoveries at the bench are today being translated into true benefit for our patients. That dermatology is at the forefront of this development is encouraging and at the same time a challenge.

REFERENCES

1. Pirquet CP, Schick B. *Die Serumkrankheit*. Leipzig, Germany: Deuticke; 1905.
2. Germuth FG Jr. A comparative histologic and immunologic study in rabbits of induced hypersensitivity of the serum sickness type. *J Exp Med*. 1953;97(2):257-282.
3. Weigle WO, Dixon FJ. Relationship of circulating antigen-antibody complexes, antigen elimination, and complement fixation in serum sickness. *Proc Soc Exp Biol Med*. 1958;99(1):226-231.
4. Beutner EH, Lever WF, Witebsky E, et al. Autoantibodies in pemphigus vulgaris response to an intercellular substance of epidermis. *JAMA*. 1965;192: 682-688.
5. Jordon RE, Beutner EH, Witebsky E, et al. Basement zone antibodies in bullous pemphigoid. *JAMA*. 1967; 200(9):751-756.
6. Jenner E. *An Inquiry into the Causes and Effects of the Variolae Vaccinae, a Disease Discovered in Some of the Western Countries of England, Particularly Gloucestershire, and Known by the Name of "The Cow Pox."* London, UK: Sampson Low; 1798.
7. Coley WB. The treatment of malignant tumors by repeated inoculations of erysipelas: with a report of ten original cases. *Am J Med Sci*. 1893;105(5): 487-511.
8. Besredka A, Gross L. De l'immunisation contre le sarcome de la souris par la voie intracutanée. *Ann Inst Pasteur (Paris)*. 1935;(55):491-500.
9. Landsteiner K, Chase MW. Studies on the sensitization of animals with simple chemical compounds: VI. Experiments on the sensitization of guinea pigs to poison ivy. *J Exp Med*. 1939;69(6):767-784.
10. Macher E, Chase MW. Studies on the sensitization of animals with simple chemical compounds. XI. The fate of labeled picryl chloride and dinitrochlorobenzene after sensitizing injections. *J Exp Med*. 1969;129(1): 81-102.
11. Frey JR, Wenk P. Experimental studies on the pathogenesis of contact eczema in the guinea-pig. *Int Arch Allergy Appl Immunol*. 1957;11(1-2):81-100.
12. Macher E, Chase MW. Studies on the sensitization of animals with simple chemical compounds. XII. The influence of excision of allergenic depots on onset of delayed hypersensitivity and tolerance. *J Exp Med*. 1969;129(1):103-121.
13. Kripke ML. Antigenicity of murine skin tumors induced by ultraviolet light. *J Natl Cancer Inst*. 1974;53(5): 1333-1336.
14. Streilein JW, Bergstresser PR. Langerhans cell function dictates induction of contact hypersensitivity or unresponsiveness to DNFB in Syrian hamsters. *J Invest Dermatol*. 1981;77(3):272-277.
15. Silberberg-Sinakin I, Thorbecke GJ, Baer RL, et al. Antigen-bearing Langerhans cells in skin, dermal lymphatics and in lymph nodes. *Cell Immunol*. 1976;25(2):137-151.
16. Stingl G, Katz SI, Clement L, et al. Immunologic functions of Ia-bearing epidermal Langerhans cells. *J Immunol*. 1978;121(5):2005-2013.

17. Streilein JW. Skin-associated lymphoid tissues (SALT): origins and functions. *J Invest Dermatol*. 1983;80(suppl):12s-16s.
18. Luger TA, Stadler BM, Katz SI, et al. Epidermal cell (keratinocyte)-derived thymocyte-activating factor (ETAF). *J Immunol*. 1981;127(4):1493-1498.
19. Kupper TS, Ballard DW, Chua AO, et al. Human keratinocytes contain mRNA indistinguishable from monocyte interleukin 1 alpha and beta mRNA. Keratinocyte epidermal cell-derived thymocyte-activating factor is identical to interleukin 1. *J Exp Med*. 1986;164(6):2095-2100.
20. Sauder DN, Carter CS, Katz SI, et al. Epidermal cell production of thymocyte activating factor (ETAF). *J Invest Dermatol*. 1982;79(1):34-39.
21. Bos JD, Kapsenberg ML. The skin immune system Its cellular constituents and their interactions. *Immunol Today*. 1986;7(7-8):235-240.
22. Abbas A, Lichtman AH, Pillai S. *Cellular and Molecular Immunology*. 8th ed. Philadelphia, PA: Elsevier Saunders; 2014:544.
23. De Nardo D. Toll-like receptors: activation, signalling and transcriptional modulation. *Cytokine*. 2015;74(2):181-189.
24. Kumagai Y, Akira S. Identification and functions of pattern-recognition receptors. *J Allergy Clin Immunol*. 2010;125(5):985-992.
25. Takahashi T, Gallo RL. The critical and multifunctional roles of antimicrobial peptides in dermatology. *Dermatol Clin*. 2017;35(1):39-50.
26. Hoffmann JH, Enk AH. Neutrophil extracellular traps in dermatology: caught in the NET. *J Dermatol Sci*. 2016;84(1):3-10.
27. Klose CS, Artis D. Innate lymphoid cells as regulators of immunity, inflammation and tissue homeostasis. *Nat Immunol*. 2016;17(7):765-774.
28. Okabe Y, Medzhitov R. Tissue biology perspective on macrophages. *Nat Immunol*. 2016;17(1):9-17.
29. Stary G, Bangert C, Tauber M, et al. Tumoricidal activity of TLR7/8-activated inflammatory dendritic cells. *J Exp Med*. 2007;204(6):1441-1451.
30. Wagstaff AJ, Perry CM. Topical imiquimod: a review of its use in the management of anogenital warts, actinic keratoses, basal cell carcinoma and other skin lesions. *Drugs*. 2007;67(15):2187-2210.
31. Haniffa M, Gunawan M, Jardine L. Human skin dendritic cells in health and disease. *J Dermatol Sci*. 2015;77(2):85-92.
32. Serbina NV, Salazar-Mather TP, Biron CA, et al. TNF/iNOS-producing dendritic cells mediate innate immune defense against bacterial infection. *Immunity*. 2003;19(1):59-70.
33. Nakano H, Lin KL, Yanagita M, et al. Blood-derived inflammatory dendritic cells in lymph nodes stimulate acute T helper type 1 immune responses. *Nat Immunol*. 2009;10(4):394-402.
34. Hammad H, Lin KL, Yanagita M, et al. Inflammatory dendritic cells—not basophils—are necessary and sufficient for induction of Th2 immunity to inhaled house dust mite allergen. *J Exp Med*. 2010;207(10):2097-2111.
35. Segura E, Touzot M, Bohineust A, et al. Human inflammatory dendritic cells induce Th17 cell differentiation. *Immunity*. 2013;38(2):336-348.
36. Romani N, Brunner PM, Stingl G. Changing views of the role of Langerhans cells. *J Invest Dermatol*. 2012;132(3, pt 2):872-881.
37. Birbeck MS, Breathnach AS, Everall JD. An electron microscope study of basal melanocytes and high-level clear cells (Langerhans cells) in vitiligo. *J Invest Dermatol*. 1961;37(1):51-64.
38. Valladeau J, Ravel O, Dezutter-Dambuyant C, et al. Langerin, a novel C-type lectin specific to Langerhans cells, is an endocytic receptor that induces the formation of Birbeck granules. *Immunity*. 2000;12(1):71-81.
39. Hunger RE, Sieling PA, Ochoa MT, et al. Langerhans cells utilize CD1a and langerin to efficiently present nonpeptide antigens to T cells. *J Clin Invest*. 2004;113(5):701-708.
40. Pena-Cruz V, Ito S, Dascher CC, et al. Epidermal Langerhans cells efficiently mediate CD1a-dependent presentation of microbial lipid antigens to T cells. *J Invest Dermatol*. 2003;121(3):517-521.
41. Vermeer BJ, Mommaas AM, Wijsman MC, et al. Ultrastructural localization of HLA-DR and HLA-DQ molecules in Langerhans cells and B cells: an immunoelectronmicroscopic study. *Reg Immunol*. 1988;1(2):85-91.
42. De Panfilis G, Manara GC, Ferrari C, et al. Simultaneous colloidal gold immunoelectronmicroscopy labeling of CD1a, HLA-DR, and CD4 surface antigens of human epidermal Langerhans cells. *J Invest Dermatol*. 1988;91(6):547-552.
43. Cerio R, Griffiths CE, Cooper KD, et al. Characterization of factor XIIIa positive dermal dendritic cells in normal and inflamed skin. *Br J Dermatol*. 1989;121(4):421-431.
44. Lenz A, Heine M, Schuler G, et al. Human and murine dermis contain dendritic cells. Isolation by means of a novel method and phenotypical and functional characterization. *J Clin Invest*. 1993;92(6):2587-2596.
45. Nestle FO, Zheng XG, Thompson CB, et al. Characterization of dermal dendritic cells obtained from normal human skin reveals phenotypic and functionally distinctive subsets. *J Immunol*. 1993;151(11):6535-6545.
46. Haniffa M, Shin A, Bigley V, et al. Human tissues contain CD141hi cross-presenting dendritic cells with functional homology to mouse CD103+ nonlymphoid dendritic cells. *Immunity*. 2012;37(1):60-73.
47. Bevan MJ. Cross-priming for a secondary cytotoxic response to minor H antigens with H-2 congenic cells which do not cross-react in the cytotoxic assay. *J Exp Med*. 1976;143(5):1283-1288.
48. Stoitzner P, Tripp CH, Eberhart A, et al. Langerhans cells cross-present antigen derived from skin. *Proc Natl Acad Sci U S A*. 2006;103(20):7783-7788.
49. Jonuleit H, Schmitt E, Schuler G, et al. Induction of interleukin 10-producing, nonproliferating CD4(+) T cells with regulatory properties by repetitive stimulation with allogeneic immature human dendritic cells. *J Exp Med*. 2000;192(9):1213-1222.
50. Kubo A, Nagao K, Yokouchi M, et al. External antigen uptake by Langerhans cells with reorganization of epidermal tight junction barriers. *J Exp Med*. 2009;206(13):2937-2946.
51. Stary G, Klein I, Bauer W, et al. Glucocorticosteroids modify Langerhans cells to produce TGF-beta and expand regulatory T cells. *J Immunol*. 2011;186(1):103-112.
52. Schuler G, Steinman RM. Murine epidermal Langerhans cells mature into potent immunostimulatory dendritic cells in vitro. *J Exp Med*. 1985;161(3):526-546.

53. Romani N, Lenz A, Glassel H, et al. Cultured human Langerhans cells resemble lymphoid dendritic cells in phenotype and function. *J Invest Dermatol*. 1989;93(5):600-609.
54. van de Ven R, van den Hout MF, Lindenberg JJ, et al. Characterization of four conventional dendritic cell subsets in human skin-draining lymph nodes in relation to T-cell activation. *Blood*. 2011;118(9):2502-2510.
55. Foster CA, Yokozeki H, Rappersberger K, et al. Human epidermal T cells predominantly belong to the lineage expressing alpha/beta T cell receptor. *J Exp Med*. 1990;171(4):997-1013.
56. Clark RA, Chong BF, Mirchandani N, et al. A novel method for the isolation of skin resident T cells from normal and diseased human skin. *J Invest Dermatol*. 2006;126(5):1059-1070.
57. Watanabe R, Gehad A, Yang C, et al. Human skin is protected by four functionally and phenotypically discrete populations of resident and recirculating memory T cells. *Sci Transl Med*. 2015;7(279):279ra39.
58. Gelb AB, Smoller BR, Warnke RA, Picker LJ. Lymphocytes infiltrating primary cutaneous neoplasms selectively express the cutaneous lymphocyte-associated antigen (CLA). *Am J Pathol*. 1993;142(5):1556-1564.
59. Akdis M, Akdis CA, Weigl L, et al. Skin-homing, CLA+ memory T cells are activated in atopic dermatitis and regulate IgE by an IL-13-dominated cytokine pattern: IgG4 counter-regulation by CLA- memory T cells. *J Immunol*. 1997;159(9):4611-4619.
60. Iwase T, Uehara Y, Shinji H, et al. *Staphylococcus epidermidis* Esp inhibits *Staphylococcus aureus* biofilm formation and nasal colonization. *Nature*. 2010;465(7296):346-349.
61. Gläser R, Meyer-Hoffert U, Harder J, et al. The antimicrobial protein Psoriasin (S100A7) is upregulated in atopic dermatitis and after experimental skin barrier disruption. *J Invest Dermatol*. 2009;129(3):641-649.
62. Naik S, Bouladoux N, Linehan JL, et al. Commensal-dendritic-cell interaction specifies a unique protective skin immune signature. *Nature*. 2015;520(7545):104-108.
63. Allan RS, Smith CM, Belz GT, et al. Epidermal viral immunity induced by CD8alpha+ dendritic cells but not by Langerhans cells. *Science*. 2003;301(5641):1925-1928.
64. Cumberbatch M, Illingworth I, Kimber I. Antigen-bearing dendritic cells in the draining lymph nodes of contact sensitized mice: cluster formation with lymphocytes. *Immunology*. 1991;74(1):139-145.
65. Larsen CP, Steinman RM, Witmer-Pack M, et al. Migration and maturation of Langerhans cells in skin transplants and explants. *J Exp Med*. 1990;172(5):1483-1493.
66. Stoitzner P, Pfaller K, Stössel H, et al. A close-up view of migrating Langerhans cells in the skin. *J Invest Dermatol*. 2002;118(1):117-125.
67. Geissmann F, Dieu-Nosjean MC, Dezutter C, et al. Accumulation of immature Langerhans cells in human lymph nodes draining chronically inflamed skin. *J Exp Med*. 2002;196(4):417-430.
68. Cavani A, Nasorri F, Ottaviani C, et al. Human CD25+ regulatory T cells maintain immune tolerance to nickel in healthy, nonallergic individuals. *J Immunol*. 2003;171(11):5760-5768.
69. Holcmann M, Stoitzner P, Drobits B, et al. Skin inflammation is not sufficient to break tolerance induced against a novel antigen. *J Immunol*. 2009;183(2):1133-1143.
70. Soumelis V, Reche PA, Kanzler H, et al. Human epithelial cells trigger dendritic cell mediated allergic inflammation by producing TSLP. *Nat Immunol*. 2002. 3(7):673-680.
71. Ito T, Wang YH, Duramad O, et al. TSLP-activated dendritic cells induce an inflammatory T helper type 2 cell response through OX40 ligand. *J Exp Med*. 2005;202(9):1213-1223.
72. Kaplan DH, Jenison MC, Saeland S, et al. Epidermal Langerhans cell-deficient mice develop enhanced contact hypersensitivity. *Immunity*. 2005;23(6):611-620.
73. Nestle FO, Conrad C, Tun-Kyi A, et al. Plasmacytoid pre-dendritic cells initiate psoriasis through interferon-alpha production. *J Exp Med*. 2005;202(1):135-143.
74. Brüeggen MC, Bauer WM, Reininger B, et al. In situ mapping of innate lymphoid cells in human skin: evidence for remarkable differences between normal and inflamed skin. *J Invest Dermatol*. 2016;136:2396-2405.
75. Villanova F, Flutter B, Tosi I, et al. Characterization of innate lymphoid cells in human skin and blood demonstrates increase of NKp44+ ILC3 in psoriasis. *J Invest Dermatol*. 2014;134(4):984-991.
76. Buhl T, Sulk M, Nowak P, et al. Molecular and morphological characterization of inflammatory infiltrate in rosacea reveals activation of Th1/Th17 pathways. *J Invest Dermatol*. 2015;135(9):2198-2208.
77. Kistowska M, Meier B, Proust T, et al. Propionibacterium acnes promotes Th17 and Th17/Th1 responses in acne patients. *J Invest Dermatol*. 2015;135(1):110-118.
78. Palma GI, Saravia NG. In situ characterization of the human host response to *Leishmania panamensis*. *Am J Dermatopathol*. 1997;19(6):585-590.
79. Egbuniwe IU, Karagiannis SN, Nestle FO, et al. Revisiting the role of B cells in skin immune surveillance. *Trends Immunol*. 2015;36(2):102-111.
80. Newell EW, Sigal N, Bendall SC, et al. Cytometry by time-of-flight shows combinatorial cytokine expression and virus-specific cell niches within a continuum of CD8+ T cell phenotypes. *Immunity*. 2012;36(1):142-152.
81. Nograles KE, Zaba LC, Shemer A, et al. IL-22-producing "T22" T cells account for upregulated IL-22 in atopic dermatitis despite reduced IL-17-producing TH17 T cells. *J Allergy Clin Immunol*. 2009;123(6):1244-1252 e2.
82. Terlou A, Santegoets LA, van der Meijden WI, et al. An autoimmune phenotype in vulvar lichen sclerosus and lichen planus: a Th1 response and high levels of microRNA-155. *J Invest Dermatol*. 2012;132 (3, pt 1):658-666.
83. Kehren J, Desvignes C, Krasteva M, et al. Cytotoxicity is mandatory for CD8(+) T cell-mediated contact hypersensitivity. *J Exp Med*. 1999;189(5):779-786.
84. Xu H, Dilulio NA, Fairchild RL. T cell populations primed by hapten sensitization in contact sensitivity are distinguished by polarized patterns of cytokine production: interferon gamma-producing (Tc1) effector CD8+ T cells and interleukin (II) 4/II-10-producing (Th2) negative regulatory CD4+ T cells. *J Exp Med*. 1996;183(3):1001-1012.
85. He D, Wu L, Kim HK, et al. CD8+ IL-17-producing T cells are important in effector functions for the elicitation

of contact hypersensitivity responses. *J Immunol*. 2006;177(10):6852-6858.
86. He D, Wu L, Kim HK, et al. IL-17 and IFN-gamma mediate the elicitation of contact hypersensitivity responses by different mechanisms and both are required for optimal responses. *J Immunol*. 2009;183(2):1463-1470.
87. Kish DD, Li X, Fairchild RL. CD8 T cells producing IL-17 and IFN-gamma initiate the innate immune response required for responses to antigen skin challenge. *J Immunol*. 2009;182(10):5949-5959.
88. Schwarz A, Beissert S, Grosse-Heitmeyer K, et al. Evidence for functional relevance of CTLA-4 in ultraviolet-radiation-induced tolerance. *J Immunol*. 2000;165(4):1824-1831.
89. Brueggen MC, Klein I, Greinix H, et al. Diverse T-cell responses characterize the different manifestations of cutaneous graft-versus-host disease. *Blood*. 2014;123(2):290-299.
90. Wenzel J, Wörenkämper E, Freutel S, et al. Enhanced type I interferon signalling promotes Th1-biased inflammation in cutaneous lupus erythematosus. *J Pathol*. 2005;205(4):435-442.
91. Freutel S, Gaffal E, Zahn S, et al. Enhanced CCR5+/CCR3+ T helper cell ratio in patients with active cutaneous lupus erythematosus. *Lupus*. 2011;20(12):1300-1304.
92. Jabbari A, Suárez-Fariñas M, Fuentes-Duculan J, et al. Dominant Th1 and minimal Th17 skewing in discoid lupus revealed by transcriptomic comparison with psoriasis. *J Invest Dermatol*. 2014;134(1):87-95.
93. Stannard JN, Kahlenberg JM. Cutaneous lupus erythematosus: updates on pathogenesis and associations with systemic lupus. *Curr Opin Rheumatol*. 2016;28(5):453-459.
94. Lowes MA, Chamian F, Abello MV, et al. Increase in TNF-alpha and inducible nitric oxide synthase-expressing dendritic cells in psoriasis and reduction with efalizumab (anti-CD11a). *Proc Natl Acad Sci U S A*. 2005;102(52):19057-19062.
95. Brunner PM, Koszik F, Reininger B, et al. Infliximab induces downregulation of the IL-12/IL-23 axis in 6-sulfo-LacNac (slan)+ dendritic cells and macrophages. *J Allergy Clin Immunol*. 2013;132(5):1184-1193e8.
96. Wollenberg A, Kraft S, Hanau D, et al. Immunomorphological and ultrastructural characterization of Langerhans cells and a novel, inflammatory dendritic epidermal cell (IDEC) population in lesional skin of atopic eczema. *J Invest Dermatol*. 1996;106(3):446-453.
97. Kopp T, Riedl E, Bangert C, et al. Clinical improvement in psoriasis with specific targeting of interleukin-23. *Nature*. 2015;521(7551):222-226.
98. Blauvelt A, Papp KA, Griffiths CE, et al. Efficacy and safety of guselkumab, an anti-interleukin-23 monoclonal antibody, compared with adalimumab for the continuous treatment of patients with moderate to severe psoriasis: Results from the phase III, double-blinded, placebo- and active comparator-controlled VOYAGE 1 trial. *J Am Acad Dermatol*. 2017;76(3):405-417.
99. Gordon KB, Duffin KC, Bissonnette R, et al. A phase 2 trial of guselkumab versus adalimumab for plaque psoriasis. *N Engl J Med*. 2015;373(2):136-144.
100. Schreiber RD, Old LJ, Smyth MJ. Cancer immunoediting: integrating immunity's roles in cancer suppression and promotion. *Science*. 2011;331(6024):1565-1570.
101. Hanahan D, Weinberg RA. Hallmarks of cancer: the next generation. *Cell*. 2011;144(5):646-674.
102. Fridman WH, Pagès F, Sautès-Fridman C, et al. The immune contexture in human tumours: impact on clinical outcome. *Nat Rev Cancer*. 2012;12(4):298-306.
103. Rivera Vargas T, Humblin E, Végran F, et al. TH9 cells in anti-tumor immunity. *Semin Immunopathol*. 2017;39(1):39-46.
104. Purwar R, Schlapbach C, Xiao S, et al. Robust tumor immunity to melanoma mediated by interleukin-9-producing T cells. *Nat Med*. 2012;18(8):1248-1253.
105. Paul WE. Clinical investigation—on the threshold of a golden era? Presidential address. *J Clin Invest*. 1981;68(3):823-826.

Chapter 11 :: Cellular Components of the Cutaneous Immune System
:: Johann E. Gudjonsson & Robert L. Modlin

第十一章
皮肤免疫系统的细胞成分

中文导读

本章共分为3节：①概述；②先天免疫系统和获得性免疫系统；③免疫系统的细胞成分。详细地介绍了皮肤免疫系统的各种细胞成分及其功能和相互作用。

第一节概述，介绍了皮肤除了是人体最大的器官之外，还是内外环境之间的保护性屏障。皮肤细胞免疫网络的进化，确保了对病原体的充分反应，以及促进体内平衡和控制过度炎症反应的机制。皮肤免疫系统的细胞成分涉及多种细胞类型、免疫细胞亚型，通常涉及角质形成细胞、内皮细胞和成纤维细胞等实质细胞的参与。这些细胞之间的相互作用是高度复杂的，每种细胞类型在免疫反应中往往既有特殊性又有其他作用。

第二节先天免疫系统和获得性免疫系统，介绍了皮肤先天免疫系统的主要功能是提供快速的第一道防线来抵御微生物病原体，同时促进了适应性免疫系统的激活，决定了针对入侵病原体的适应性免疫反应的类型。两个系统协同作用保护宿主，但如果异常激活会导致各种炎症和疾病。

第三节免疫系统的细胞成分，详细介绍了T细胞、B细胞、非常规的先天T细胞和先天淋巴细胞、自然杀伤细胞、树突状细胞、巨噬细胞、肥大细胞、粒细胞等。

〔粟 娟〕

AT-A-GLANCE

- Human immune system consists broadly of innate vs adaptive immune responses.
- Innate immune system has multiple different cellular subsets that have in common rapid response to infection and injury but are restricted in their ability to recognize and respond to all pathogens, instead relying on germline encoded pattern recognition receptors and danger signals.
- Adaptive immune system is a slower but more adaptive arm of the immune system that can respond to near limitless range of pathogens.
- Recently identified immune cells, such as innate lymphoid cells and unconventional T cells, span the spectrum between the innate and the adaptive immune system.

INTRODUCTION

Apart from being one of the largest organs in the human body, the skin acts as a protective barrier between the internal and external environments. Although the epidermis acts as a physical and physiologic barrier to the entry of commensals and pathogens, the near constant exposure to an array of both benign and harmful microorganisms and other stressors in the skin has promoted the evolution of a complex cellular immune network, involving both the innate and adaptive parts of the immune system. This ensures adequate responses against pathogens as well as mechanisms to promote homeostasis and control excessive inflammatory response. This network in the skin has been named the skin immune system and consists of a large number of specialized skin-resident immune cells as well as circulating lymphocytes constantly recirculating between the skin, skin-draining lymph nodes, and the peripheral circulation.[1] The cellular constituents of the skin immune system involve multiple cell types, subtypes of immune cells, and often involve participation of parenchymal cells including keratinocytes, endothelial cells and fibroblasts (Fig. 11-1). The interactions between these are highly complex, with each cell type often having both specific and redundant roles in immune responses.

INNATE AND ADAPTIVE IMMUNE SYSTEM

The skin immune system includes components of both the innate and adaptive immune components (Fig. 11-2). The innate immune system recognizes specific motifs, such as proteins, lipids, nucleotides, and other metabolites, associated with broad classes of pathogens, and with the receptors for these encoded in germline DNA. In contrast, the adaptive immune system is based on the generation of near limitless antigen receptor or antibody diversity through somatic recombination, which in turn provides the foundation for immunologic memory through differentiation, expansion, and persistence of long-lived antigen-specific lymphocytes.[2] This expansion and persistence of antigen-specific lymphocytes in turn allow a more rapid and robust response in the event of subsequent immunologic challenge. In recent years, this distinction has been somewhat challenged as it has become clear that many immune cells have properties of both the innate and adaptive immune systems, and that the innate immune system can adapt to repeated challenges. Such innate immune memory response has been termed "trained immunity" and provides protection against reinfection in a T- and B-cell–independent manner.[3]

Whereas T and B cells are the primary cells of the adaptive immune system, dendritic cells and macrophages with their prominent expression of pattern-associated receptors are the key players of the innate immune system, in terms of either directly dealing with microbial infection and/or instructing the adaptive immune response. Other cell types that participate in innate immune responses include mast cells, neutrophils, and resident tissue cells such as keratinocytes, endothelial cells and fibroblasts. Several cell types have dual characteristics of the innate and adaptive immune system, including innate lymphoid cells (ILCs), and innate-like T cells, as discussed in greater detail later in this chapter.

The primary function of the innate immune system is to provide a rapid first line of defense against microbial pathogens to contain them, while the much slower but more powerful adaptive part of the immune system is being activated. The activation of the innate immune system promotes activation of the adaptive immune system and dictates what type of adaptive immune response is mounted against the invading pathogen. Therefore, these 2 systems act in synergy to defend the host, but abnormal activation of these systems can frequently lead to various inflammatory conditions and diseases (Fig. 11-3).

CELLULAR COMPONENTS OF THE IMMUNE SYSTEM

T CELLS

T cells are derived from multipotent hematopoietic stem cells in the bone marrow. Progenitor T cells migrate through the blood to the thymus, where they mature. This is the reason for the naming of these cells, where the "T" in *T cells* stands for "thymus-dependent." The majority of human T cells rearrange their alpha and beta chains on the T-cell receptor in the thymus and are termed αβ T cells, whereas a small minority of T cells in the thymus have γδ T-cell receptors. The γδ receptors have limited diversity and are considered to be part of the innate immune system. These two, αβ and γδ, are the key lineages of T cells.

T cells that have completed their primary development in the thymus, and have not yet encountered their specific antigen, are known as naïve T cells and circulate through the bloodstream to secondary lymphoid organs including lymph nodes and the spleen. Once a naïve T cell meets its specific antigen, presented to it as a peptide MHC complex on the surface of an antigen-presenting cell in secondary lymphoid organs, it is able to develop into an effector T cell and a longer-lived central memory T cells. In contrast to naïve T cells, effector T cells are able to mount a response to antigens. T cells can be either CD4+ or CD8+. Naive CD8+ T cells recognize peptide antigens in the binding pocket of MHC class I molecules such as HLA-A, HLA-B, or HLA-C, and differentiate into cytotoxic effector T cells, which recognize and kill infected cells. Some αβ CD8+ T cells with limited TCR diversity are able to respond to lipid antigens by MHC class I–like antigen-presenting molecules, including the CD1 family of proteins. CD8+ effector T cells are often defined by the major cytokine that they produce, including

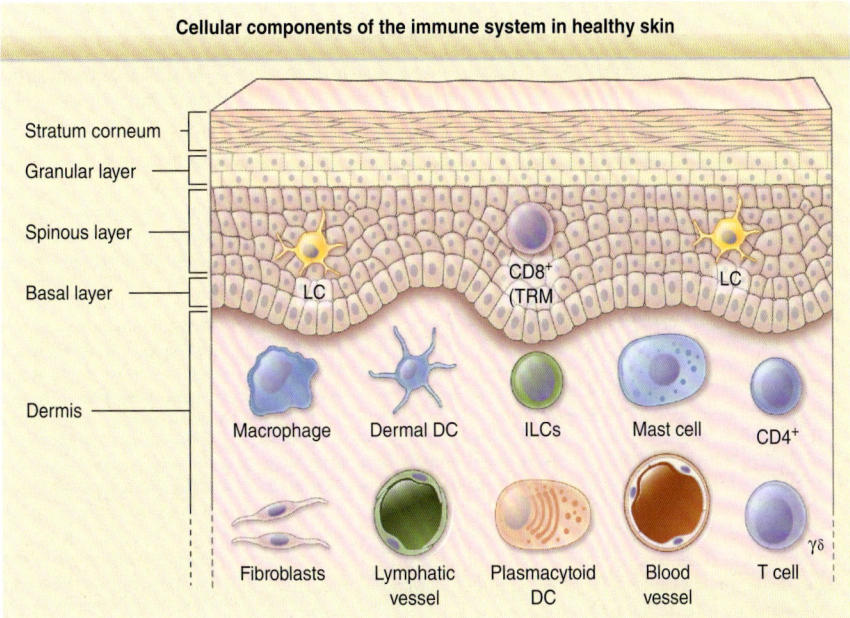

Figure 11-1 Components of the cellular immune system in healthy skin. Multiple different immune cell populations are present in healthy skin. Langerhans cells and resident memory T cells, primarily CD8+, reside in the epidermal layer, whereas CD4+ and γδ T cells are found in the upper dermis. Innate lymphoid cells (ILCs) are found in proximity to the dermal-epidermal junction, whereas mast cells are often in proximity to dermal blood vessels. Dermal dendritic cells and macrophages are found in the dermis. Other cells may contribute to immune responses in skin such as fibroblasts, lymphatic blood vessels, nerves (not shown), and melanocytes (not shown).

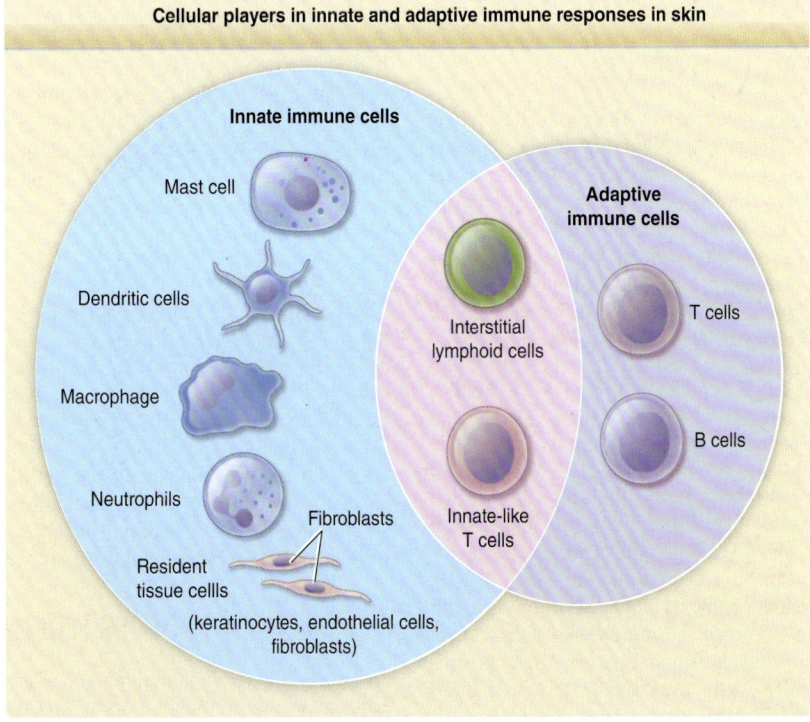

Figure 11-2 Innate and adaptive cells. Interstitial lymphoid cells and innate-like T cells have both innate and adaptive immune functions.

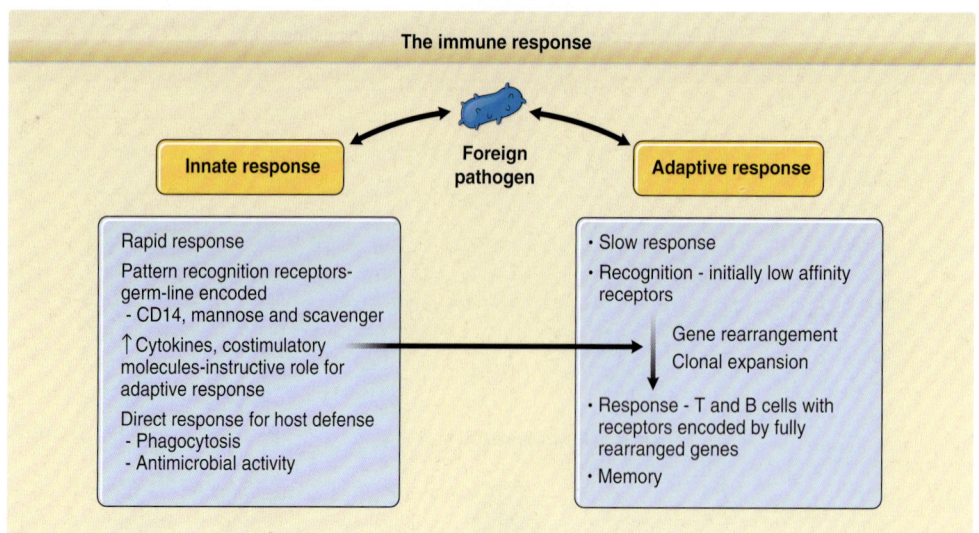

Figure 11-3 The immune system of higher vertebrates uses both innate and adaptive immune responses. These immune responses differ in the way they recognize foreign antigens and the speed with which they respond, yet they complement each other in eradicating foreign pathogens.

IFN-γ, IL-4, and IL-17, as T-cytotoxic (T_C)1, T_C2, and T_C17s, respectively. Naïve CD4+ T cells recognize peptide antigens in the binding pocket of MHC class II molecules such as HLA-DR, HLA-DQ, and HLA-DP on antigen-presenting cells and differentiate into effector subsets that have broader and different immunologic functions. This includes the main CD4+ T-cell subsets, T helper 1 (T_H1), T_H2, T_H17, and T follicular-helper (T_{FH}), and T regulatory cells (Tregs) (Fig. 11-4).

T HELPER 1 (T_H1) CELLS

T_H1 cells are characterized by the production of the cytokines IL-2, IFN-γ, and TNF-α. T_H1 cells are the main mediators of cell-mediated immunity. These cells are characterized by the expression of the T-box transcription factor T-bet, which induces both transcriptional activation of the IFN-γ gene locus and responsiveness to the T_H1-polarizing cytokine IL-12. T_H1 cells, primarily by the release of IFN-γ, activate macrophages to kill or inhibit the growth of pathogens and trigger cytotoxic T-cell responses.

T HELPER 2 (T_H2) CELLS

T_H2 cells are characterized by the production of the cytokines IL-4, IL-5, and IL-13. The zinc-finger transcription factor GATA-3 is critical for inducing the T_H2 program in these cells. In contrast to T_H1 cells, T_H2 cells facilitate humoral (antibody) responses and inhibit some cell-mediated immune responses. There is significant crossregulation between those 2 arms of the immune system. Thus, the T_H1 cytokine IFN-γ downregulates T_H2 responses, and conversely, IL-4 downregulates both Th1 responses and macrophage function.

T HELPER 9 (T_H9) CELLS

IL-9 is produced by a population of T cells, which is distinguished from other T-cell lineages such as T_H1, T_H2, and T_H17 cells. These T_H9 cells coproduce TNF-α, but unlike mouse T_H9 cells, do not produce IL-10. T_H9 cells are found primarily among the skin homing (cutaneous leukocyte antigen [CLA] positive) T-cell population and are present in healthy human skin. IL-9 promotes upregulation of other proinflammatory cytokines including IFN-γ, IL-13, and IL-17, suggesting that T_H9 activation can initiate inflammatory reactions and amplify activation and cytokine production of other T_H subsets.[4]

T HELPER 17 (T_H17) CELLS

T_H17 cells are characterized by the production of the cytokines IL-17A, IL-17F, IL-21, IL-22, and recently IL-26.[5] They depend on IL-23 for their survival and expansion,[6] and are regulated by the transcription factor RORγt. T_H17 cells are involved in antigen responses against extracellular pathogens including both bacteria and fungi. These cells have been implicated as key players in the pathogenesis of psoriasis.

T REGULATORY CELLS (TREGS)

Tregs play a key role in maintaining tolerance to self-antigens in the periphery. Loss of Tregs, as happens in IPEX (immune dysregulation, polyendocrinopathy, enteropathy, and X-linked) syndrome, results in

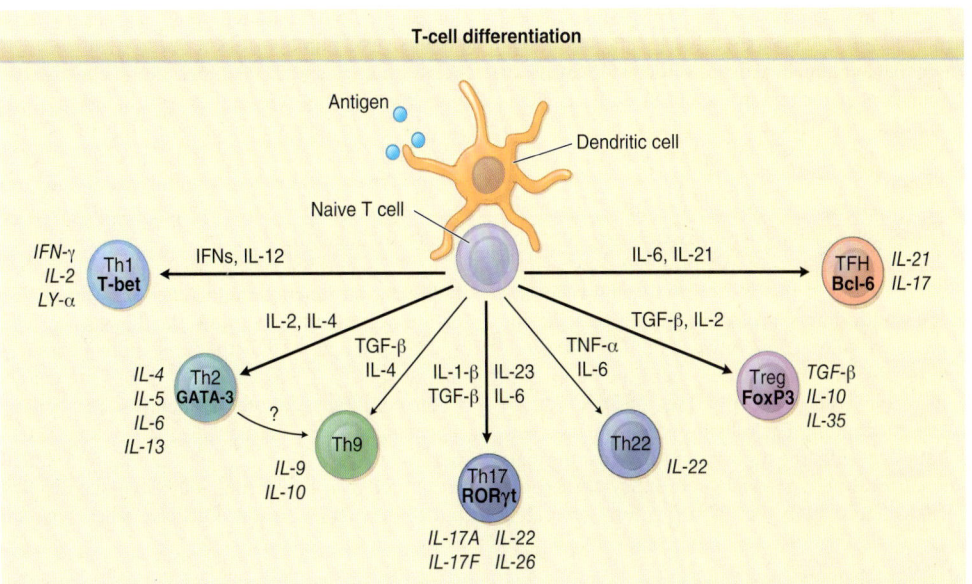

Figure 11-4 Schematic view of events governing and occurring in T-cell differentiation. Depending on the type and activation status of the antigen-presenting dendritic cells (DCs) and on the type and amounts of cytokines secreted by these and/or other cells, naïve T cells will expand and differentiate into various subsets, that is, T_H1, T_H2, T_H9, T_H17, T_H22, Treg, and T_{FH}. They exhibit different types of transcription factors and secrete different types of cytokines.

multiorgan autoimmune disease. Tregs function by suppressing the activation, cytokine production, and proliferation of other T cells.[7] They are characterized by expression of the transcription factor FOXP3, the genetic cause of IPEX syndrome. About 5% to 10% of the T cells resident in normal human skin are FOXP3+ T regs.[8] Other populations of Tregs have been reported in humans, including IL-10 producing FOXP3-negative cells, and have been implicated in systemic lupus erythematosus.

T FOLLICULAR HELPER CELLS (T_{FH})

T_{FH} represent a distinct subset of CD4+ T cells primarily found in B-cell areas of lymph nodes, spleen, and Payer patches. T_{FH} trigger the formation and maintenance of germinal centers in lymph nodes and spleen through the expression of CD40 ligand (CD40L) and the secretion of IL-21 and IL-4. These cells play a crucial role in orchestrating selection and survival of B cells that go on to differentiate into either antibody-producing plasma cells or memory B cells.

SKIN HOMING

To gain entry into the skin, T cells need to express the right surface molecules and receptors. This includes the cutaneous lymphocyte antigen (CLA),[9] and expression of specific chemokine receptors including CCR4 and CCR10.[10] CLA is an inducible carbohydrate modification of P-selecting glycoprotein ligand-1 (PSGL-1), a known surface glycoprotein that is expressed constitutively on all human peripheral-blood T cells. This modification enables it to bind E-selectin, which is highly expressed on skin endothelial cells.[9] CCR4 binds to the chemokines CCL17 and CCL22, whereas CCR10 binds to the chemokine CCL27. CCR4 is present on essentially all skin-homing cells, whereas CCR10 is only present on a subset of skin-homing T cells.[10] This specific and highly controlled trafficking of T cells to the skin explains the greater than 100-fold enrichment of antigen-reactive T cells at the site of cutaneous inflammation compared with blood.

TISSUE RESIDENT (T_{RM}), EFFECTOR (T_{EM}), AND CENTRAL MEMORY (T_{CM}) T CELLS

Healthy human skin contains about twice as many T cells as are present in the entire blood volume, or about 20 billion. Of skin-tropic (CLA+) memory T cells, 98% are located in human skin under non-inflamed conditions and only 2% are present in the circulation.[11] These findings radically changed the long-held assumption that memory T cells continuously recirculate between peripheral organs via the blood and secondary lymphoid structures and are rapidly recruited to the site of infection when needed. Instead, a substantial number of T cells are static and reside in the skin, where they can provide rapid defense against invading pathogens. This also explains observations made from the xenotransplant model of human skin inflammation. In these studies, healthy-appearing skin of patients with psoriasis was grafted onto immunodeficient mice. After few weeks, the uninvolved skin spontaneously developed psoriasis, whereas no changes were seen for skin from nonpsoriatic healthy controls. These elegant studies demonstrated that T cells that reside in noninflamed human skin are sufficient to create an inflammatory pathology in the absence of recirculating lymphocytes.[12] These observations and others led to the naming of these T cells as "resident memory T cells," or T_{RM}.

T_{RM} cells are nonrecirculating memory T cells that are found in epithelial barrier tissues, including the GI tract, lung, skin, and reproductive tract.[13] The physiologic role of this is to provide these epithelial sites with highly protective T cells specific for the pathogens most commonly encountered through these tissues, and at the sites where they are readily available when needed[13] (Fig. 11-5). Evidence for this function of T_{RM} cells derives from vaccination studies with the live vaccinia virus through skin scarification, in which keratinocytes become infected. Vaccination via scarification generated long-term T cell–mediated immunity—characterized by increased number of skin resident memory CD8+ cells—that was 100,000 times more effective than subcutaneous, intradermal, and intramuscular vaccination in protecting against reinfection of the skin.[14] Although illustrative of the function of T_{RM} cells, this study also questions the value of traditional routes of vaccination, particularly against pathogens that primarily infect the skin.[14]

T_{RM} cells have been suggested to exist as 2 phenotypically and functionally distinct populations. Both of these populations express the T_{RM} marker CD69 and are distinguished by the expression of the surface marker CD103. CD69+CD103+ T_{RM} cells are enriched in the epidermis, are predominantly CD8+, and have a tendency for increased effector cytokine production, whereas CD103− T_{RM} cells are more frequently encountered in the dermis and have slightly lower but still potent effector functions when compared

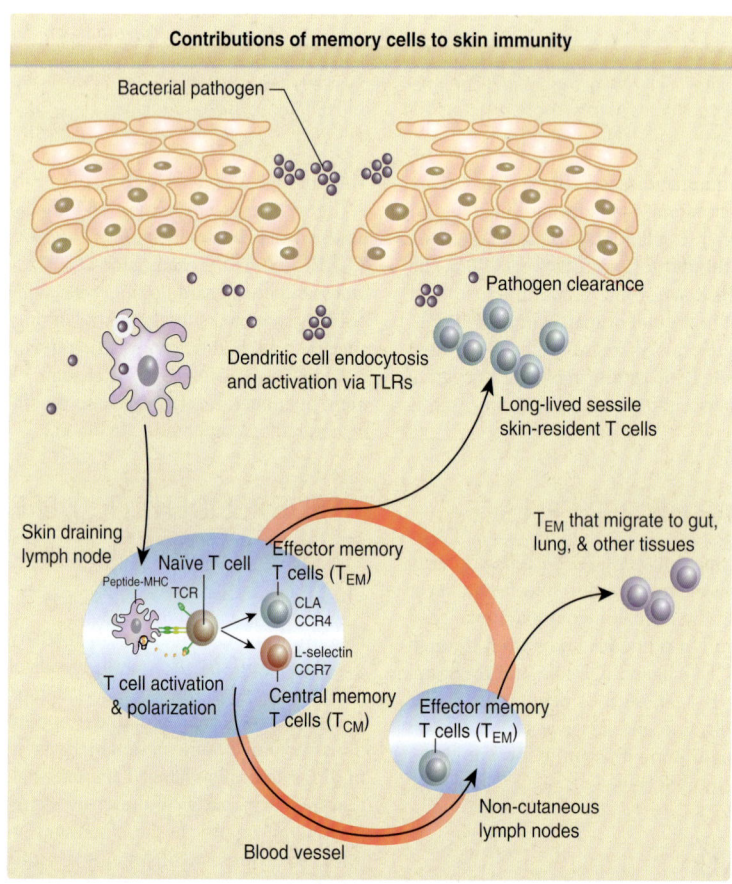

Figure 11-5 Contributions of T effector memory, central memory, and resident memory cells to skin immunity. After exposure to bacterial pathogens, resident dendritic cells in the skin become activated (ie, through activation of toll-like receptors (TLR)) and migrate to skin-draining lymph nodes. Naïve T cells recognizing bacterial peptide antigens on the surface of dendritic cells differentiate and polarize into skin homing effector memory T cells (T_{EM}) and central memory T cells (T_{CM}). Skin homing T_{EM} enter all areas of the skin but in highest number at the site of pathogen exposure. These cells will contribute to pathogen clearance, and some will become long-lived tissue-resident memory T cells (T_{RM}). T cells are also released from the skin draining lymph nodes and migrate to secondary lymphoid tissue including noncutaneous lymph nodes, giving rise to new populations of T_{EM} that home to other nonskin peripheral tissues such as the gut and lungs. (Adapted from Clark RA. J Invest Dermatol. 2010;130(2):362-370, with permission. Copyright © The Society for Investigative Dermatology.)

with recirculating T cells.[15] In contrast, CD103+ T_{RM} cells have more limited proliferative capacity compared with CD103- T_{RM} cells. CD103 expression was enhanced by keratinocyte contact and is TGF-β dependent,[15] and through its binding to E-cadherin in the epidermis is responsible for retaining these cells within the epidermis.

Human skin also contains populations of recirculating memory T cells. These cells coexpress both the skin homing receptor CLA and CCR4 and the central memory markers CCR7/L-selectin (CD62L). Based on variable expression of L-selectin, these cells have been named migratory memory T cells (T_{MM}) (L-selectin negative) in contrast to central memory T cells (T_{CM}, L-selectin+).[15] T_{CM} have higher sensitivity to antigenic stimulation and are less dependent on costimulation compared to naïve T cells. Following TCR triggering, T_{CM} produce mainly IL-2, but after proliferation they differentiate into effector T cells (T_{EM}), which are characterized by rapid effector function and are capable of producing large amounts of effector cytokines including IFN-γ, IL-4, and IL-17, as well as perforin in the case of CD8+ T_{EM}.

Importantly, the biology of these T-cell subsets can help explain many of the clinical characteristics of various skin diseases. As T_{RM} do not migrate or recirculate, inflammatory lesions caused by these cells tend to be sharply demarcated, with abrupt cut-off from normal skin, a classic feature of skin lesions in diseases such as psoriasis. It also explains why lesions tend to persist long-term in a particular location, and often recur in the same location on discontinuation of effective therapy. Furthermore, as these cells are already on-site, they can respond to repeated antigen challenges extremely rapidly, often within hours of exposure—such as that seen in fixed drug eruptions. Finally, the biology of the T_{RM} cells can also help explain differences between types of cutaneous lymphomas, such as mycosis fungoides and Sezary syndrome, with the former being mediated by T_{RM} cells and the latter by circulating central memory T cells (T_{CM}).[15] Finally, as T_{RM} cells have a tendency to progressively accumulate in tissues with repeated antigen exposure, T_{RM}-mediated inflammatory diseases tend to worsen over time, with an increasingly rapid onset of inflammation and increasing severity of inflammation with each exposure.[13]

B CELLS

B cells form the humoral arm of the immune system, which is characterized by antibody production. Antibodies produced by B cells have various functions, they can bind to and neutralize pathogens by preventing their ability to enter and infect cells, and similarly they may bind and neutralize bacterial toxins. Antibodies also facilitate the uptake of pathogens by phagocytes in a process called opsonization that facilitates binding to the cell surface Fc receptor. Lastly antibodies bound to pathogens can activate proteins of the classical pathway of the complement system. As evident from the description above, the humoral immune response mainly protects extracellular spaces, blocks infection of all cells but permits uptake by phagocytes with the capacity to destroy the pathogen. B cells emigrate from the bone marrow, following which cells migrate to secondary lymphoid organs such as the spleen, peripheral lymph nodes, and gut-associated lymphoid tissue (Payer patches and mesenteric lymph nodes). B-cell activation usually requires help from T_{FH} cells. Activated B cells differentiate into either memory B cells or antibody-secreting plasma cells. Cytokines made by T_{FH} cells direct the choice of the antibody isotype in human: that is, IL-4 promotes immunoglobulin G1, G4, and E responses; IFN-γ induces immunoglobulin G3; whereas TGF-β induces immunoglobulin A responses. They also have antibody-independent roles, acting as antigen-presenting cells, and producing cytokines with potent effects on both localized and systemic immunity.

B cells are infrequently found in normal skin under homeostatic conditions and the role of B cells in cutaneous immunity remains poorly defined. For the limited number of B cells found in skin, it is unclear if they represent a specific skin-resident population or whether they are derived from circulation populations of B cells. Of note, B cells have been observed in chronic inflammatory skin conditions such as cutaneous leishmaniasis, diffuse cutaneous sclerosis, cutaneous lupus, and atopic dermatitis, and plasma cells can similarly be found under certain inflammatory conditions such as syphilis and leprosy. IL-10-producing B cells have been found to have an anti-inflammatory effect, and have therefore been named B-regulatory cells or Bregs, but so far these findings have only been demonstrated in murine models of skin inflammation. The presence of these cells have recently been described in human skin.

UNCONVENTIONAL AND INNATE-LIKE T CELLS AND INNATE LYMPHOID CELLS (ILCs)

In recent years, a number of other nonrecirculating lymphocyte populations have been characterized. These lymphocyte populations are residents of nonlymphoid tissue and organs and include invariant natural killer T (iNKT) cells, mucosal-associated invariant T (MAIT) cells, γδ T cells, and intestinal intraepithelial lymphocytes (IELs), as well as the emerging family of ILCs. These tissue-resident lymphocytes span the continuum between the innate and adaptive immune system and share a number of features pertaining to their tissue-resident functions.[2] It is thought that these cell populations act as sensors of perturbed tissue integrity such as from infection or injury and help recruit additional immune cells from blood as well as amplifying local inflammatory responses through their effect on parenchymal cells.[2]

INNATE LYMPHOID CELLS

ILCs are defined by 3 main features: the absence of recombinant activating gene (RAG)–dependent rearranged antigen receptors; a lack of myeloid and dendritic cell phenotypical markers (negative lineage markers), and their lymphoid morphology.[16] ILCs uniformly express the IL-7 receptor alpha chain CD127 and require IL-7 for their development.[17] Keratinocytes express and secrete IL-7 and are an important source of IL-7. ILCs have striking similarities to T cells regarding their transcription factor expression and cytokine profiles. Mirroring T helper polarization of conventional CD4+ T cells, ILCs can be similarly subdivided into group 1 (ILC1), 2 (ILC2), and 3 (ILC3) based on cytokine patterns.[18] ILC1s, similar to T_H1 cells, generate IFN-γ and TNF-α, have no cytotoxic molecules, and are dependent on the transcription factor T-bet. ILC2 express and produce T_H2 cytokines, including IL-4, IL-5, and IL-13, and have a high expression of the GATA-3 transcription factor. Lastly, ILC3s constitute a group of cells expressing variable levels of the transcription factors RORγt, aryl-hydrocarbon receptor (AHR), and T-bet, and release variable amounts of IFN-γ, IL-22, and IL-17[19] (Fig. 11-6).

ILCs are mainly clustered beneath the dermal-epidermal junction and exhibit a close spatial relationship to T lymphocytes.[19] This localization, and the existence of different ILC populations, suggests that these cells may have evolved to respond rapidly to pathogenic signals and to facilitate adaptive immune responses.[20] ILC respond quickly to epithelial cell–derived mediators, and respond almost exclusively by producing cytokines. This innate response is important in activating other innate immune responses in the skin, as well as initiating and orchestrating involvement of the adaptive immune system.[21,22] The outcome of this activation, depending on the ILC subset involved, and their interplay with other cell populations, is complex and may result in either amplification of the inflammatory response or its downregulation. How ILCs are regulated in the skin, the array of effector mechanisms they employ, and their potential role in maintaining skin barrier homeostasis is still incompletely understood.[20]

UNCONVENTIONAL AND INNATE-LIKE T CELLS

Unconventional or innate-like T cells express T-cell receptors of limited diversity, which recognize antigens in the context of nonclassical MHC-like molecules, or independent of MHC-related presenting molecules altogether. Lymphocytes belonging to this group include iNKT cells, MAIT cells, and γδ T cells[2]

(Fig. 11-7). In addition, T cells and NKT cells have been shown to recognize nonpeptide antigens in the context of CD1 molecules.

The human cluster of differentiation 1 (CD1) gene family consists of a small number of genes that are structurally related to the MHC class I genes; however, unlike MHC class I molecules, CD1 proteins are nonpolymorphic. The CD1a, b, and c molecules are more closely homologous to one another than to CD1d,[23] and are absent in mice. In skin, CD1a and c isoforms are present on the surface of Langerhans cells, whereas, CD1a, b, and c are expressed on dermal dendritic cells.[24] CD1 molecules present a universe of lipid-based antigens to T cells and the process involves endosomal acidification, which facilitates high-affinity interaction of CD1 molecules with their cognate antigens.[25]

Autoreactive as well as CD1a-restricted T-cell responses against lepromatous leprosy and tuberculosis antigens have been reported, with the demonstration that CD1a can present a large variety of antigens including host-derived sulfatides, "headless antigens,"[26] pollen phospholipids, and mycobacterium-derived dideoxymycobactin. CD1a-autoreactive T cells home to skin, recognizing CD1a loaded with skin-derived lipids,[26] including lipids processed into free fatty acids, which allows direct interaction between the T-cell receptor and CD1a.

Langerhans cells are epidermal dendritic cells that mediate innate immune responses in skin, with phagocytic[27] and antimicrobial function, as well as a key role in antigen presentation to T cells. Langerhans cells are characterized by their high expression of CD1a and unique expression of langerin (CD207). Langerin is required for Birbeck granule formation, endosomal structures unique to Langerhans cells.[27] Langerin and CD1a colocalize in those endosomal structures, and CD1a is targeted to these endosomes through a Rab22-dependent pathway. Upon antigen capture, Langerhans cells mature and migrate to regional lymph nodes, where they activate T cells, which then return to the skin.

CD1-restricted T cells have a role in and contribute to host defense against microbial pathogens. Thus, group I CD1-restricted T cells secrete Th1 cytokines; are cytolytic against infected targets, as in case of mycobacterial infections; and trigger antimicrobial activity.[24] These antimicrobial T cells express perforin, granzyme B, and the antimicrobial protein granulysin in intracellular granules.[24] Granzyme B cooperates with granulysin in killing intracellular bacteria. The expression of granulysin, as has been shown in leprosy, correlates with containment of infection, and is approximately 6-fold more frequent in tuberculous leprosy than lepromatous leprosy skin lesions.[24] Furthermore, the ability of these T cells to release IFN-γ potentially leads to induction of the vitamin D–dependent antimicrobial response.[28]

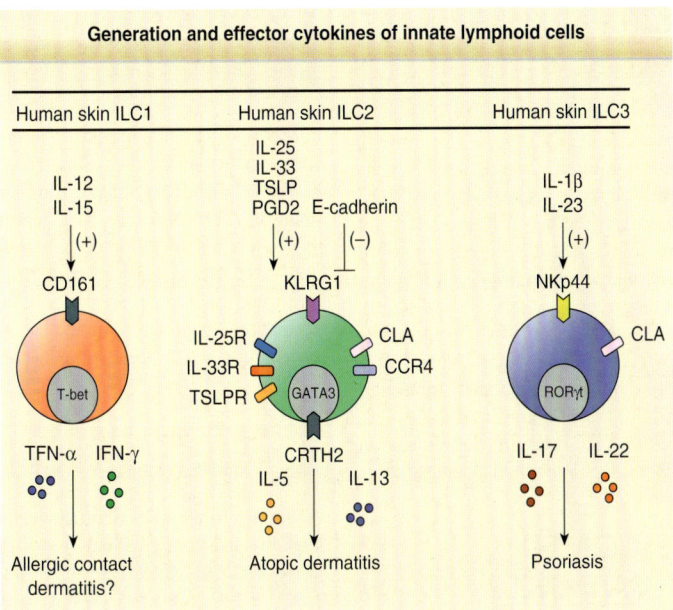

Figure 11-6 Generation and effector cytokines of innate lymphoid cells. Three populations of ILCs are found in human skin (ILC1-3). ILC1 express the surface molecule CD161 and are thought to be activated by IL-12 and IL-15. The primary cytokines produced by ILC1s are TNF-α and IFN-γ. ILC1 are implicated in the pathogenesis of allergic contact dermatitis. ILC2 are activated by the Th2 cytokines IL-25 and IL-33, TSLP, and prostaglandin PGD2. ILC2 express the receptor KLRG1 and CRTH2, CCR4, and receptors for IL-25 (IL-25R), IL-33 (IL-33R), and TSLP (TSLPR). The main effector cytokines from ILC2 include LI-5 and IL-13, and these cells have been implicated in the pathogenesis of atopic dermatitis. ILC3 are activated by IL-1 and IL-23, express the receptor NKp44, and produce IL-17 and IL-22. They are implicated in the pathogenesis of psoriasis. Each ILC subset is characterized by expression of TF factors in similar manner as Th subsets. Thus, similar to T_H1 cells, ILC1 express T-bet; ILC2 similar to T_H2 cells express GATA3 and ILC3 express RORγt similar to T_H17 cells. (Adapted from Kim BS. *J Invest Dermatol*. 2015;135(3):673-678, with permission. Copyright © The Society for Investigative Dermatology.)

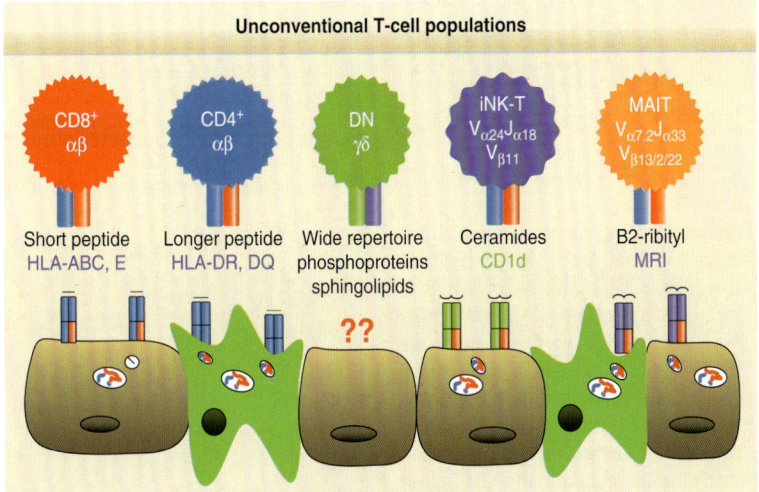

Figure 11-7 Unconventional T-cell populations. Unconventional T cells respond more quickly compared with their conventional counterparts (CD8 and CD4 αβ T cells). These cells are characterized by their limited TCR rearrangement. However, they expand the repertoire of antigens recognized by T cells. Thus, invariant natural killer (iNK) T cells are able to respond to lipid antigens presented by CD1d. Other T-cell subsets including γδ and αβ T cells are also able to recognize lipid antigens bound by members of the CD1 family of proteins (not shown). γδ T cells are able to recognize a diverse array of structures including phosphoantigens and sphingolipids apparently independent of major histocompatibility complex (MHC)-antigen presentation. Mucosal-associated invariant T (MAIT) cells recognize antigens presented in the context of an MHC-like molecule, MR1, on the surface of antigen-presenting cells or epithelia. MAIT cells respond to antigens derived from the structures of vitamins B_2 and B_9 containing a ribityl carbohydrate group. (Adapted from Johnston A, Gudjonsson JE. *J Invest Dermatol*. 2014;134(12):2864-2866, Fig. 1, with permission. Copyright © The Society for Investigative Dermatology.)

INVARIANT NATURAL KILLER CELLS (iNKT CELLS)

iNKT cells are a subset of T cells that express an invariant T-cell receptor α-chain (Vα24-Jα18 in human), paired with a TCRβ of limited diversity. iNKT cells recognize glycolipid antigens presented by the MHC class I–like molecule CD1d, and can be activated by potent bacterial ligands such as cell wall sphingolipids. They can also sense changes in host lipid metabolism through recognition of less potent, transiently expressed, rare, or unstable endogenous lipids.[2] Five major distinct iNKT cell subsets express and mirror T helper cell subsets in cytokine production, including iNKT1, iNKT2, and iNKT17, analogous to the T_H1, T_H2, and T_H17, respectively. iNKT cells are dependent on the transcriptional factor PLZF for their development.

MUCOSAL-ASSOCIATED INVARIANT T (MAIT) CELLS

MAIT cells are a special subset of T cells that express a semi-variant T cell receptor combining a unique TCRα chain (Vα7.2-Jα33 in humans) with a restricted set of TCRβ chains. These cells are evolutionarily conserved and have a capacity for rapid effector function. MAIT cells are activated by bacterial riboflavin biosynthesis intermediates that are presented by the MHC class I–like molecule MR1. As mammals do not synthesize riboflavin, but instead rely on certain bacteria and yeast, MAIT cells provide a means to control certain commensal bacteria and assess and control for either overgrowth or infection by these organisms. Consistent with this scenario, only microbes with a functional biosynthetic pathway for riboflavin synthesis are able to activate MAIT cells. Distinct subsets of MAIT cells can produce IFN-γ and IL-17.[2]

γδ T-CELLS

γδ T cells are characterized by the expression of the γδ T cell receptor, and in contrast to the strict MHC restriction of αβ T-cells, several modes of antigen-recognition by γδ T cells have been described. Thus, different subsets of γδ T cells have been shown to recognize lipid-based antigens presented on the CD1 family of molecules, MHC class I–like molecules such as MICA, and even soluble ligands. As discussed here above, the CD1 gene family consists of a small number of genes that are structurally related to the MHC class I genes. However, unlike MHC class I molecules, CD1 proteins are nonpolymorphic, CD1a and c are present on the surface of Langerhans cells, whereas CD1a, b, c, and d are expressed on dermal dendritic cells. γδ T cells have an ability to self-renew in tissues independently of circulating precursors. While representing the majority of lymphocytes in mouse skin, γδ T cells only represent a small fraction (1% to 2%) of resident T cells in human skin.

NATURAL KILLER (NK) CELLS

Natural killer cells appear as large granular lymphocytes. In humans, these cells are characterized by being CD16+ CD56+ CD94+ CD161+ but negative for the T-cell markers CD3. NK cells have a role in surveying the body, looking for altered cells, either transformed or infected with viruses or parasites. The cells harboring these pathogens are killed directly via perforin/granzyme/granulysin or Fas/Fas-ligand dependent mechanisms or indirectly via the secretion of cytokines.

DENDRITIC CELLS

The main function of dendritic cells is to process antigen material and present it on the cell surface and activate T cells. Dendritic cells were first described in the late 19th century by Paul Langerhans. However, the term "dendritic cells" was first used in 1973 by Ralph Steinman and Zanvil Cohn, but Steinman was later awarded the Nobel Prize for his discovery of the central role of dendritic cells in adaptive immune response.[29]

MYELOID DENDRITIC CELLS

Dendritic cells (DCs) are a heterogenous population of cells in the immune system. Dendritic cells arise primarily from myeloid progenitors within the bone marrow, and migrate via the blood to tissues throughout

TABLE 11-1
Dendritic Cell (DC) Subsets Found in Skin[a]

CONVENTIONAL DCs	PLASMACYTOID DC	LANGERHANS CELLS
CD141+ myeloid DCs: CD141+ (BDCA-3) CLEC9A+, CD11b−	CD123+, CD303+ (BDCA-2), CD304+, TLR7, TLR9	Langerin+++, CD1a++, E-cadherin++, Birbeck granules
CD1c+ myeloid DCs: TLR3+, FLT3+, CD11c^{low} CD11c^{hi}, CD11b+, CD1c+ (BDCA-1), CD1a+		
Monocyte-derived DCs: CD14+ CD11b+, CX3CR1+, CD209+		

[a]Three major populations of dendritic cells (apart from inflammatory dendritic cells) are found in skin. These include CD141+ and CD1c+ myeloid dendritic cells and monocyte-derived DCs that are characterized by expression of CD14. Plasmacytoid dendritic cells are characterized by expression of CD123 (interleukin-3 receptor α-chain) and CD303 (BDCA-2), express TLR7 and TLR9, and are major producers of type I interferons. Langerhans cells are characterized by CD1a and langerin expression.

the body, or directly to secondary lymphoid organs. There are 3 cutaneous dendritic cell populations in healthy skin: epidermal Langerhans cells, resident dermal conventional dendritic cells, and plasmacytoid dendritic cells[30] (Table 11-1). Conventional (previously called myeloid) dendritic cells are abundant at barrier tissue sites where they are in close contact with surface epithelia. During inflammation there is an additional population of myeloid dermal "inflammatory" dendritic cells.[30] Under normal homeostatic conditions, when there is no infection or tissue injury, dendritic cells are in an immature state, and in that state they efficiently take up antigens but have low levels of costimulatory molecules and not equipped to stimulate naïve T cells.

Dendritic cells are active in ingesting antigens by phagocytosis using both complement receptors and Fc receptors. Antigens taken up through these mechanisms are processed and presented in the binding pocket of MHC class II molecules for recognition by CD4+ T cells. When antigen directly enters the cytosol of dendritic cells, it is processed in the proteasome, transported into the endoplasmic reticulum, and presented on the cell surface within the binding pocket of MHC class I molecules for activation of naïve CD8+ T cells. Dendritic cells are also effective at cross-presentation. Cross-presentation permits the presentation of exogenous antigens, which are normally presented by MHC class II molecules, to be presented by MHC class I molecules. Cross-presentation pathways are important for immune defenses against many viruses and in elimination of autoreactive CD8+ T cells.

Dermal dendritic cells are also a major source of cytokines in inflammatory conditions such as psoriasis. The inflammatory dendritic cells in psoriasis produce TNF-α and have inducible nitric oxide synthetase (iNOS) and have been termed "Tip-DCs." Pathogenicity of these cells in psoriasis is suggested by the rapid downregulation of Tip-DCs products TNF-α, IL-20, and IL-23 during treatment with effective therapies.[31] Tip-DCs can also stimulate the differentiation and activation of Th17 cells. The potential role of these DCs as sources of inflammatory mediators is in contrast to the classic role of DCs as antigen-presenting cells.[30]

PLASMACYTOID DENDRITIC CELLS

Plasmacytoid dendritic cells are a unique population of resident cutaneous dendritic cells, initially described by their morphology, which is similar to plasma cells.[32] Plasmacytoid dendritic cells are thought to act as sentinels in early defences against viral infection, particularly given their expression of Toll-like-receptors 7 and 9 (TLR7 and TLR9), and intracellular nucleic acid sensor such as RIG-1, that functions as a pattern recognition receptor for certain single stranded RNA viruses. In contrast to conventional dendritic cells, plasmacytoid dendritic cells express fewer MHC class II and co-stimulatory molecules on their surface, and the process antigens less efficiently. Given the focus of this dendritic cell subsets towards viral pathogens,

their ability to produce large amounts of type 1 interferons during infections is not surprising—this has been estimated to about 10,000-fold more than any other cell type.[33] Viral RNA- and DNA-containing repeated CG nucleotides (CpG) binding to TLR7 and TLR9 are the main inducers of this type 1 interferon response. Plasmacytoid dendritic cells have been implicated in the pathogenesis of psoriasis, appearing to have a critical role in triggering the onset of psoriatic lesions, through binding of the antimicrobial peptide cathelicidin (LL37) to self-DNA and subsequent activation of TLR9.[34]

LANGERHANS CELLS

Langerhans cells are a specialized subset of dendritic cells that reside in the epidermal layer of the skin. These cells were initially described by Paul Langerhans in 1868, who described the presence of nonpigmentary dendritic cells in the epidermis and thought them to be a part of the nervous system. These cells remained an enigma for more than a century until the recognition that Langerhans cells are leukocytes derived from the bone marrow.[35] Langerhans cells account for 2% to 4% of cells in the epidermis[36] and are arranged in a dense network in between epidermal keratinocytes.[35] Langerhans cells are characterized by a unique cytoplasmic organelle, the electron-dense Birbeck granules, which have a unique "tennis-racket" shape. Langerhans cells are characterized by high expression of CD1a.[37] Langerhans cells also express CD207, also known as langerin, which is localized in the Birbeck granules and is a C-type lectin receptor, and may shuttle antigens to a nonclassical antigen-processing pathway, leading to cross-presentation of antigens on MHC class I molecules.[27] Langerhans cells require the cytokines IL-34 and TGF-β, both derived from keratinocytes, for their development and epidermal residence.[38] The role of Langerhans cells is not yet fully clear. They can cross-prime and activate CD8+ T cells' responses in an IL-15-dependent manner,[39] as well as contribute to expansion of Tregs, suggesting a role of Langerhans cells in tissue homeostasis.[40]

MACROPHAGES

Macrophages are an essential component of innate immunity and play a central role in inflammation. Macrophages reside in tissue and function as immune sentinels, where they are uniquely equipped to sense and respond to tissue invasion by infectious microorganisms and tissue injury through various scavenger, pattern recognition, and phagocytic receptors.[41] In most healthy tissues, macrophages are maintained with minimal contribution of circulating monocytes. In contrast, during injury or infection a large influx of monocytes enter injured tissues and differentiate into macrophage-like and DC-like cells.

Macrophages have been divided into 2 main populations; M1 and M2 macrophages (Table 11-2). M1

TABLE 11-2
Molecules Involved in the Polarization of M1 and M2 Macrophages

	M1	M2
iNOS production	↑	—
Surface expression	MHC class II, CD40, CD68, CD80, CD86, CD25 (IL-2Rα), CD127 (IL-7Rα)[a]	MHC class II, CD206, CD209 (DC-SIGN), CD302, Dectin-1[a]
Response to stimulus	IFN-γ, LPS, GM-CSF	IL-4, IL-13, M-CSF, helminths
Arginase 1	—	↑
Cytokine production	IL-1β, IL-6, IL-12, IL-15, IL-18, IL-23, TNF	IL-10, TGF-β
Transcription factors	IRF5	STAT6, IRF4
NFκB participation	p65	p50

[a]CD40, CD80, and CD86 are costimulatory molecules on antigen-presenting cells. CD25 and CD127 are receptors for the cytokines IL-2 and IL-7 respectively. CD206 (mannose receptor) is a pattern recognition receptor, belonging to the C-type lectin superfamily. CD302 is another C-type lectin receptor involved in cell adhesion, migration, and phagocytosis. Dectin-1 is another C-type lectin that functions as a pattern recognition receptor for a variety of glucans from fungi and plants.
Data from Chavez-Galan L et al. *Front Immunol.* 2015;6:263.

macrophages, or classically activated macrophages, are activated primarily by IFN-γ, and produce pro-inflammatory cytokines such as IL-1β, TNF-α, IL-12, and IL-18. They have a high expression of MHC class II molecules, and express CD68 and the costimulatory molecules CD80 and CD86. These macrophages have the ability to phagocytize large numbers of pathogens and kill intracellular bacteria. Interestingly, for efficient intracellular killing macrophages, vitamin D is required for the adaptive immune responses to overcome the ability of intracellular pathogens to avoid this killing.[28] M2 macrophages, or alternatively activated macrophages, are activated primarily by stimuli such as IL-4, IL-10, TGF-β, and IL-13. M2 macrophages are thought to play a central role in response to parasites, tissue remodeling, and allergic diseases, and may have a role in resolution of skin inflammation.[41]

MAST CELLS

Mast cells are usually most abundant at epithelial sites, such as the skin and mucosal tissue, where they are ideally situated to act as a first line of defense against external pathogens and other environmental insults.[42] Mast cells are derived from pluripotent bone marrow precursors. After egression from the bone marrow, mast cell progenitors circulate in the blood before they enter various tissues and develop into mature mast cells. Key factors influencing the maturation of mast cells, including stem cell factor (SCF, also known as KIT ligand), which binds to the c-kit receptor (CD117), and interleukin-3 (IL-3).

Mast cells are long-lived cells that can survive in tissues for months to years and have retained the ability to proliferate in response to appropriate signals.[43] Mast cells are heterogeneous and differ in some of their properties from submucosal or connective tissue mast cells, but both can be involved in allergic reactions.

Mast cells express the receptor for immunoglobulin E (FCεRI) constitutively on their surface, and the best-known cause of mast cell activation is when antigens crosslink immunoglobulin E bound to these receptors. A relatively low level of allergen is sufficient to trigger degranulation of mast cells. Mast cells can also bind immunoglobulin G antibodies through FcγRII receptors. Mast cells can also act as sentinels of infection and are equipped with pattern recognition receptors, including various TLRs, which are activated in response to conserved pathogen-associated molecular patterns. The responses elicited to pathogens depend on the stimulus. Thus, when TLR4 is activated by lipopolysaccharide on mast cells, it leads to cytokine production in the absence of degranulation. In contrast TLR2 activation by peptidoglycans induces both degranulation and cytokine production.[43] Other factors that can induce mast cell activation besides the ones mentioned above, including complement activation (C3a and C5a), neuropeptides (substance P) and certain toxins (venom-derived, and certain bacteria-derived peptides).[42]

Mast cells have a high content of electron-dense lysosome-like secretory granules that occupy a major proportion of the cytoplasm of mature mast cells, leading to the initial nomenclature of these cells "mastung," which means "well fed" or "fattened." These granules are filled with a plethora of preformed compounds. Histamine is probably the most well known, but other amines, such as serotonin, are also found in mast cell granules. Mast cell granules include various cytokines such as TNF-α, vascular endothelial growth factor (VEGF), various proteases, antimicrobial proteins such as cathelicidins, and chemokines. Mast cells can also produce a large number of cytokine following activation, including TNF-α, IL-3, IL-4, IL-5, and IL-6,[43] as well as lipid mediators such as leukotrienes, prostaglandins, and platelet-activating factor—these factors, when released, contribute to increased vascular permeability and edema at the site of infection or insult—the so-called wheal and flare response that occurs within minutes. As a result of these preformed mediators, which are rapidly released upon activation (in a process called degranulation), mast cells are specialized for first-line surveillance function, and regulation of the subsequent innate and adaptive immune response that follows. Thus, mast cell–derived TNF can induce upregulation of adhesions molecules on local vascular endothelium including E-selectin (which binds CLA on T cells) as well as other adhesion molecules, promoting the influx of T cells and dendritic cells. Chemokines such as CCL20 will add to this influx of inflammatory cells. Furthermore, mast cell products can directly modulate dendritic cell activation and antigen presentation by promoting antigen uptake and cross-presentation, and upregulation of costimulatory molecules required for T-cell activation. Overall, given the presence of cytokines such as IL-4, these responses are more directed toward T_H2 responses.[43] The cutaneous reactions most commonly attributed directly to mast cell activation include urticaria and anaphylaxis.

GRANULOCYTES

Basophils, neutrophils, and eosinophils are classified as granulocytes, which are characterized by the presence of lobulated nuclei and secretory granules in the cytoplasm (Table 11-3).

NEUTROPHILS

Neutrophils are the most abundant leukocytes in the blood accounting for about 35% to 70% of the peripheral blood leukocytes. Neutrophils are short-lived, with a life span somewhere between 5 and 90 hours. Generation of neutrophils is controlled by granulocyte colony-stimulating factor (G-CSF), and can reach up to 2×10^{11} cells per day. They are the hallmark cell of acute inflammation secondary to their high mobility and are usually recruited to sites of injury within minutes. They are powerful effector cells that destroy infectious threats through several different processes, including phagocytosis, degranulation, reactive oxygen species (ROS), and neutrophil extracellular traps. Neutrophils lead the first wave of host defense against infection or tissue damage.[44] Neutrophils must therefore sense, prioritize, and integrate chemotactic cues to migrate toward sites of infection or tissue damage. Neutrophils express more than 30 different receptors, including G protein–coupled, Fc, adhesion, cytokine, and pattern recognition receptors.

Once in the tissue, neutrophils contribute to the recruitment, activation, and programming of antigen-presenting cells. Neutrophils release chemokines and proinflammatory mediators that attract monocytes and dendritic cells, and influence whether macrophages differentiate to a pro- or anti-inflammatory state.[45] On a per-cell basis, neutrophils make fewer molecules of a given cytokine than macrophages or

TABLE 11-3
Secretory Granules

	MAST CELLS	EOSINOPHILS	BASOPHILS	NEUTROPHILS
Amines	Histamine		Histamine	
	Serotonin			
	Dopamine			
Cytokines	TNF	TNF	IL-4, 13	TNF
	IL-4, 5, 6, 15	IL-3, 4, 5, 6, 10, 12, 13		IL-1
	bFGF	VEGF		
	VEGF	TGF-β		
	TGF-β	NGF		
	NGF	TGF-α		
	SCF	GM-CSF		
Enzymes	Cathepsin B, C, L, D, E	Acid phosphatase	Neutral protease	Elastase
	Tryptase	Collagenase (MMP1)	Cathepsin G	Myeloperoxidase
	Chymase	Arylsulfatase B	Carboxypeptidase A	Collagenase (MMP1)
	Carboxypeptidase 3	Histaminase		Proteinase 3
	Cathepsin G	Phospholipase D		Cathepsin B, D, G
	MMP9	Catalase		Phospholipase A2
	ADAMTS5			Lysozyme
	Arylsulfatase A			
	Hexosaminidase			
Lipid mediators	Leukotrienes C4, B4, D4, E4	Leukotrienes C4, D4, E4	Leukotrienes C4	
	Platelet-activating factor	Thromboxane B2		
	Prostaglandin D2	Prostaglandin E1, E2		
		Platelet-activating factor		
Other	Heparanase	Major basic protein	Major basic protein	Alpha-defensins
	Cathelicidin (LL37)	Eosinophil cationic protein		
	Renin			

lymphocytes, but neutrophils often outnumber other leukocytes at inflammatory sites by several orders of magnitude and can therefore by important sources of proinflammatory cytokines such as TNF-α.[45] Neutrophil recruitment can be amplified exponentially in a phase termed "neutrophil swarming." This process is driven by signals from early recruited cells including neutrophils and macrophages to recruit more neutrophils both directly and indirectly through further activation of tissue and tissue resident cells.

Several different processes are critical for neutrophils to assert their destructive capabilities (Fig. 11-8). These include degranulation of preformed proinflammatory mediators, ability to mount a respiratory burst, and neutrophilic extracellular traps.

Neutrophils have several different types of granules. The first granules to be discharged on activation are peroxidase-negative. These include proteins such as lactoferrin, lipocalin, and cathelicidin (LL37) along with several metalloproteinases, which function by degrading laminin, collagen, proteoglycans, and fibronectin and therefore have an important role in facilitating neutrophil recruitment and tissue breakdown.[45] The next granules to be emptied, usually occurring as the concentration of chemoattractants increases, are peroxidase-positive, and contain the antimicrobial proteins alpha-defensins and serprocidins; serine proteases cathepsin G, neutrophil elastase, and proteinase 3; and myeloperoxidase (MPO), the iron-containing enzyme that colors pus green. Myeloperoxidase produces hypochlorous acid (HOCl) from hydrogen peroxide (H_2O_2) and chloride anion (Cl^-).[45] The serine proteases released by neutrophils have been shown to cleave the IL-36 family cytokines (IL-36α, IL-36β, and IL-36γ) into their more active forms, increasing their biologic activity approximately 500-fold.[46] Interestingly, neutrophil elastase has been shown to cleave the IL-36 receptor antagonist into its highly active antagonistic form.[47] IL-36-mediated responses have been shown to be a driver of neutrophil infiltration in pustular psoriasis, and these studies show that neutrophils may both promote inflammation and help control it.

Neutrophils use respiratory burst to degrade bacteria and particles that have been ingested via their phagocytic receptors. Respiratory burst is the rapid release of reactive oxygen species (ROS) driven by the NADPH oxidase. The NADPH oxidase reaction results in a transient increase in oxygen consumption by the cells, and leads to generation of superoxide anions within the lumen of the phagolysosomes. This is converted by the enzyme superoxide dismutase (SOD) into hydrogen peroxide (H_2O_2). Further chemical and enzymatic reactions produce a range of toxic ROS including hydroxyl radial (*OH), hypochlorite (OCl^-), and hypobromite (OBr^-).

In addition to killing microbes in the phagolysosomes, neutrophils use another mechanism of destruction that is directed at extracellular pathogens. During activation, some neutrophils undergo a unique form of cell death in which the nuclear chromatin is released into the extracellular space and forms a matrix known as neutrophil extracellular traps, or NETs. NETs

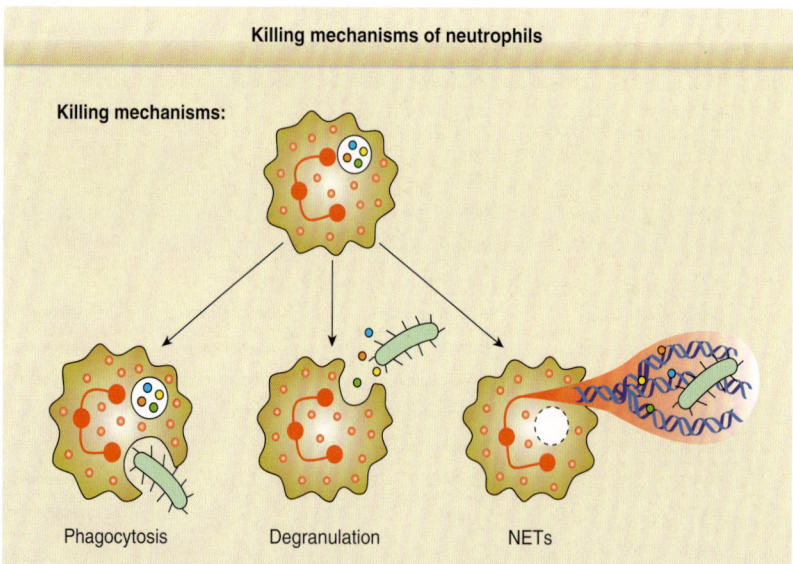

Figure 11-8 Killing mechanisms of neutrophils. Neutrophils can eliminate pathogens by multiple means, both intra- and extracellular. Neutrophils are able to ingest bacterial and other pathogens through phagocytosis and subsequently kill the pathogens using NADPH dependent mechanisms through release of reactive oxygen species or antibacterial proteins (lactoferrin, lysozymes, cathepsins, or defensins). Neutrophils have multiple cytoplasmic granules that they can release into their surroundings. Neutrophils can also eliminate extracellular microorganisms by releasing neutrophil extracellular traps (NETs). These NETs are composed of DNA to which neutrophil derived antimicrobial proteins and enzymes (myeloperoxidase, elastase) are attached to. NETs immobilize pathogens, preventing them from spreading and facilitate subsequent phagocytosis. They can also directly kill pathogens by means of proteases and antimicrobial proteins. (Adapted by permission from Springer Nature: Kolaczkowska E. *Nat Rev Immunol*. 2013;13(3):159-175; Fig. 1. Copyright © 2013.)

facilitate capturing of microorganisms, which may then be more efficiently phagocytosed by other neutrophils or macrophages.[44] NET formation requires the generation of ROS, and patients with chronic granulomatous disease, apart from having defective respiratory burst, also have reduced NET formation

Neutrophil activation can lead to substantial tissue damage, as is evident from disorders such as pyoderma gangrenosum. Therefore, it is crucial to prevent tissue damage by promoting resolution of inflammation through the removal of neutrophils from the site of injury. This clearance of neutrophils can occur through necrosis and subsequent phagocytosis by macrophages, or apoptosis. Recent studies have showed that neutrophils can also leave sites of inflammation in a process termed neutrophil reverse migration.[48]

EOSINOPHILS

Eosinophils were first described by Paul Ehrlich in 1879, who noted their capacity to be stained by acidophilic dyes. Eosin is one of these acidic dyes that bind to and form salts with basic, or eosinophilic, compounds like proteins containing amino acid residues such as arginine and lysine, staining them dark red, leading to the name eosinophils for these cells. Eosinophils are derived from pluripotent progenitors in the bone marrow and released into the peripheral blood in a mature state.

Eosinophils are readily recruited into tissues in response to appropriate stimuli such as interleukin-5 (IL-5) and the eotaxin chemokines CCL11 (eotaxin-1), CCL13, and CCL26 (eotaxin-3). Eosinophils account for somewhere between 0 and 5% of peripheral blood leukocytes. These cells can be readily distinguished from neutrophils by the virtue of their bilobed nuclei and large specific granules. The granules in eosinophils contain 4 major proteins; eosinophilic peroxidase, major basic protein, and the ribonucleases eosinophilic cationic protein and the eosinophil-derived neurotoxin. The granules also store numerous cytokines, enzymes and growth factors.[49] Eosinophils are characterized by expression of the interleukin-5-receptor subunit alpha (IL-5Rα) and the CC-chemokine receptor 3 (CCR3), which binds CCL11, CCL13, and CCL26. The cytokines IL-5 has a profound role in all aspects of eosinophil development, and can by produced by both T-cells and mast cells. The epithelial cell–derived cytokines thymic stromal lymphopoietin (TSLP), a common cytokine in atopic dermatitis, IL-25 (IL-17E), and IL-33 all promote eosinophilia by inducing IL-5 production.[49]

When eosinophils are in tissues, they are usually found in proximity to mast cells, with which they communicate extensively. The crosstalk that occurs between eosinophils and mast cells is thought to involve both physical and various soluble mediators, leading to modulation of allergic inflammation.

BASOPHILS

Basophils account for less than 1% of peripheral blood leukocytes and are the least common type of granulocyte. Since the discovery of basophils by Paul Ehrlich at the end of the 19th century, the role of this small population of cells in the blood has remained an enigma.[50] Basophils were for a long time thought to be a redundant variant of mast cells in the blood, but this does not seem to be the case as basophils differ from mast cells in many important ways. In contrast to mast cells, which mature in tissues, basophils complete their maturation in the bone marrow before they enter the peripheral blood. Basophils are short-lived, having a life span of several days in contrast to weeks to years for mast cells. Finally, basophils do not retain the ability to proliferate unlike mast cells.[50] Basophils are defined by the presence of basophilic granules in the cytoplasm, by the surface expression of the high-affinity Fc receptor for immunoglobulin E (FceRI) and by the release of chemical mediators such as histamine, after stimulation.[50] Basophils are an important source of Th2-type cytokines, and basophils secrete large quantities of IL-4, suggesting that basophils may be involved in mediating allergic diseases and immunity against parasites, and can under such conditions be recruited to peripheral tissues, although in small numbers.

KERATINOCYTES

Keratinocytes are the most abundant cell type in skin and form the epidermis. The epidermis forms a physical barrier between the "inside" and "outside," and prevents invasion of pathogens, entry of chemicals, and loss of water and other soluble mediators through the skin. In addition, the low pH of the skin inhibits growth of bacteria, and creates optimal condition for the function and activity of skin derived antimicrobial proteins, which include human beta defensin-2 (hBD2), RNAse7, dermcidin, and cathelicidin (LL37). Keratinocytes play an active role in inflammatory responses and express multiple different Toll-like receptors including TLR1, -2, -3, -4, -5, and -10. Keratinocytes are also an important source of cytokines, either constitutively or upon induction. These cytokines include IL-1, IL-6, IL-7, IL-15, IL-20, TNF-α, TSLP, TGF-β1, IL-36, and a broad range of chemoattractants such as the S100A family of proteins, and chemokines including CXCL1, CXCL2, IL-8 (CXCL8), CCL4, CCL5, CCL17, CCL22, CXCL9, CXCL10, CCL20, which attract various inflammatory cell types, such as neutrophils (CXCL1, CXCL2, CXCL8), macrophages and dendritic cells (CCL4), Th1 cells (CXCL9, CXCL10), Th2 cells (CCL17, CCL22), and Th17 cells (CCL20). This production of antimicrobial peptides, cytokines, and chemokines by keratinocytes has multiple consequences for the migration of various subsets of inflammatory cells, influence proliferation and differentiation processes of infiltrating leukocytes, and finally affect the production of other cytokines in skin, justifying the term "cytokinocyte", which is sometimes used for keratinocytes.

REFERENCES

1. Egbuniwe IU, Karagiannis SN, Nestle FO, et al. Revisiting the role of B cells in skin immune surveillance. *Trends Immunol.* 2015;36:102-111.
2. Fan X, Rudensky AY. Hallmarks of tissue-resident lymphocytes. *Cell.* 2016;164:1198-1211.
3. Netea MG, Joosten LA, Latz E, et al. Trained immunity: a program of innate immune memory in health and disease. *Science.* 2016;352(6284):aaf1098.
4. Schlapbach C, Gehad A, Yang C, et al. Human TH9 cells are skin-tropic and have autocrine and paracrine pro-inflammatory capacity. *Sci Transl Med.* 2014;6(219):219-218.
5. Meller S, Di Domizio J, Voo KS, et al. T(H)17 cells promote microbial killing and innate immune sensing of DNA via interleukin 26. *Nat Immunol.* 2015;16(9):970-979.
6. Harrington LE, Hatton RD, Mangan PR, et al. Interleukin 17-producing CD4+ effector T cells develop via a lineage distinct from the T helper type 1 and 2 lineages. *Nat Immunol.* 2005;6(11):1123-1132.
7. Sakaguchi S, Sakaguchi N. Regulatory T cells in immunologic self-tolerance and autoimmune disease. *Int Rev Immunol.* 2005;24:211-226.
8. Clark RA, Huang SJ, Murphy GF, et al. Human squamous cell carcinomas evade the immune response by down-regulation of vascular E-selectin and recruitment of regulatory T cells. *J Exp Med.* 2008;205(10):2221-2234.
9. Fuhlbrigge RC, Kieffer JD, Armerding D, et al. Cutaneous lymphocyte antigen is a specialized form of PSGL-1 expressed on skin-homing T cells. *Nature.* 1997;389:978-981.
10. Soler D, Humphreys TL, Spinola SM, et al. CCR4 versus CCR10 in human cutaneous TH lymphocyte trafficking. *Blood.* 2003;101:1677-1682.
11. Clark RA, Chong B, Mirchandani N, et al. The vast majority of CLA+ T cells are resident in normal skin. *J Immunol.* 2006;176(7):4431-4439.
12. Boyman O, Hefti HP, Conrad C, et al. Spontaneous development of psoriasis in a new animal model shows an essential role for resident T cells and tumor necrosis factor-alpha. *J Exp Med.* 2004;199(5):731-736.
13. Clark RA. Resident memory T cells in human health and disease. *Sci Transl Med.* 2015;7:269rv261.
14. Liu L, Zhong Q, Tian T, et al. Epidermal injury and infection during poxvirus immunization is crucial for the generation of highly protective T cell-mediated immunity. *Nat Med.* 2010;16(2):224-227.
15. Watanabe R, Gehad A, Yang C, et al. Human skin is protected by four functionally and phenotypically discrete populations of resident and recirculating memory T cells. *Sci Transl Med.* 2015;7(279):279ra239.
16. Spits H, Artis D, Colonna M, et al. Innate lymphoid cells—a proposal for uniform nomenclature. *Nat Rev Immunol.* 2013;13(2):145-149.
17. Kang J, Coles M. IL-7: the global builder of the innate lymphoid network and beyond, one niche at a time. *Semin Immunol.* 2012;24:190-197.
18. De Obaldia ME, Bhandoola A. Transcriptional regulation of innate and adaptive lymphocyte lineages. *Annu Rev Immunol.* 2015;33:607-642.
19. Bruggen MC, Bauer WM, Reininger B, et al. In situ mapping of innate lymphoid cells in human skin: evidence for remarkable differences between normal and inflamed skin. *J Invest Dermatol.* 2016;136(12):2396-2405.
20. Kim BS. Innate lymphoid cells in the skin. *J Invest Dermatol.* 2015;135:673-678.
21. Eberl G, Colonna M, Di Santo JP, et al. Innate lymphoid cells. Innate lymphoid cells: a new paradigm in immunology. *Science.* 2015;348:aaa6566.
22. Sonnenberg GF, Artis D. Innate lymphoid cells in the initiation, regulation and resolution of inflammation. *Nat Med.* 2015;21:698-708.
23. Calabi F, Bradbury A. The CD1 system. *Tissue Antigens.* 1991;37:1-9.
24. Ochoa MT, Loncaric A, Krutzik SR, et al. "Dermal dendritic cells" comprise two distinct populations: CD1+ dendritic cells and CD209+ macrophages. *J Invest Dermatol.* 2008;128:2225-2231.
25. Niazi K, Chiu M, Mendoza R, et al. The A' and F' pockets of human CD1b are both required for optimal presentation of lipid antigens to T cells. *J Immunol.* 2001;166(4):2562-2570.
26. de Jong A, Cheng TY, Huang S, et al. CD1a-autoreactive T cells recognize natural skin oils that function as headless antigens. *Nat Immunol.* 2014;15(2):177-185.
27. Valladeau J, Ravel O, Dezutter-Dambuyant C, et al. Langerin, a novel C-type lectin specific to Langerhans cells, is an endocytic receptor that induces the formation of Birbeck granules. *Immunity.* 2000;12(1):71-81.
28. Fabri M, Stenger S, Shin DM, et al. Vitamin D is required for IFN-gamma-mediated antimicrobial activity of human macrophages. *Sci Transl Med.* 2011;3(104):104ra102.
29. Banchereau J, Steinman RM. Dendritic cells and the control of immunity. *Nature.* 31998;92:245-252.
30. Zaba LC, Krueger JG, Lowes MA. Resident and "inflammatory" dendritic cells in human skin. *J Invest Dermatol.* 2009;129:302-308.
31. Zaba LC, Cardinale I, Gilleaudeau P, et al. Amelioration of epidermal hyperplasia by TNF inhibition is associated with reduced Th17 responses. *J Exp Med.* 2007;204(13):3183-3194.
32. Corcoran L, Ferrero I, Vremec D, et al. The lymphoid past of mouse plasmacytoid cells and thymic dendritic cells. *J Immunol.* 2003;170(10):4926-4932.
33. Ito T, Amakawa R, Inaba M, et al. Plasmacytoid dendritic cells regulate Th cell responses through OX40 ligand and type I IFNs. *J Immunol.* 2004;172(7):4253-4259.
34. Lande R, Gregorio J, Facchinetti V, et al. Plasmacytoid dendritic cells sense self-DNA coupled with antimicrobial peptide. *Nature.* 2007;449(7162):564-569.
35. Merad M, Ginhoux F, Collin M. Origin, homeostasis and function of Langerhans cells and other langerin-expressing dendritic cells. *Nat Rev Immunol.* 2008;8:935-947.
36. Valladeau J, Saeland S. Cutaneous dendritic cells. *Semin Immunol.* 2005;17:273-283.
37. Fithian E, Kung P, Goldstein G, et al. Reactivity of Langerhans cells with hybridoma antibody. *Proc Natl Acad Sci U S A.* 1981;78(4):2541-2544.
38. Wang Y, Szretter KJ, Vermi W, et al. IL-34 is a tissue-restricted ligand of CSF1R required for the development of Langerhans cells and microglia. *Nat Immunol.* 2012;13(8):753-760.
39. Klechevsky E, Morita R, Liu M, et al. Functional specializations of human epidermal Langerhans cells and CD14+ dermal dendritic cells. *Immunity.* 2008;29(3):497-510.
40. Seneschal J, Clark RA, Gehad A, et al. Human epidermal Langerhans cells maintain immune homeostasis

in skin by activating skin resident regulatory T cells. *Immunity.* 2012;36:873-884.
41. Lavin Y, Mortha A, Rahman A, et al. Regulation of macrophage development and function in peripheral tissues. *Nat Rev Immunol.* 2015;15:731-744.
42. Wernersson S, Pejler G. Mast cell secretory granules: armed for battle. *Nat Rev Immunol.* 2014;14:478-494.
43. Abraham SN, St John AL. Mast cell-orchestrated immunity to pathogens. *Nat Rev Immunol.* 2010;10:440-452.
44. de Oliveira S, Rosowski EE, Huttenlocher A. Neutrophil migration in infection and wound repair: going forward in reverse. *Nat Rev Immunol.* 2016;16:378-391.
45. Nathan C. Neutrophils and immunity: challenges and opportunities. *Nat Rev Immunol.* 2006;6:173-182.
46. Henry CM, Sullivan GP, Clancy DM, et al. Neutrophil-derived proteases escalate inflammation through activation of IL-36 family cytokines. *Cell Rep.* 2016;14(4):708-722.
47. Macleod T, Doble R, McGonagle D, et al. Neutrophil Elastase-mediated proteolysis activates the anti-inflammatory cytokine IL-36 Receptor antagonist. *Sci Rep.* 2016;6:24880.
48. Nourshargh S, Renshaw SA, Imhof BA. Reverse migration of neutrophils: where, when, how, and why? *Trends Immunol.* 2016;37:273-286.
49. Rosenberg HF, Foster PS. Reply to eosinophil cytolysis and release of cell-free granules. *Nat Rev Immunol.* 2013;13:902.
50. Karasuyama H, Mukai K, Tsujimura Y, et al. Newly discovered roles for basophils: a neglected minority gains new respect. *Nat Rev Immunol.* 2009;9:9-13.

Chapter 12 :: Soluble Mediators of the Cutaneous Immune System
:: Allen W. Ho & Thomas S. Kupper

第十二章
皮肤免疫系统的可溶性介质

中文导读

本章共分为6节：①可溶性介质的概念；②细胞因子生物学；③基于细胞因子生物学的治疗意义；④趋化因子：白细胞动员中心的次级细胞因子；⑤趋化因子在疾病中的作用；⑥可溶性介质网络：治疗意义和应用。本章重点介绍两个主要的有助于调定有效免疫反应的可溶性介质：细胞因子和趋化因子。

第一节可溶性介质的概念，介绍了可溶性介质在细胞与组织需要进行通信交流时发挥的作用。细胞因子是一种可溶性的多肽介质，在造血系统细胞与体内其他细胞之间的信号交流中起着关键作用。趋化因子是一个小细胞因子超家族，是细胞运输的重要介质。

第二节细胞因子生物学，首先介绍了细胞因子命名的变化，新发现的细胞因子都是根据用于分离和鉴定活性分子的生物学分析来命名的。接下来介绍了细胞因子在T细胞亚群分类中的价值。除了功能分类外，同时介绍了基于细胞因子的三维结构进行的分类。此外，本节内容重点介绍了细胞因子以特异性和高亲和力与应答细胞表面上的受体结合，然后借助信号转导机制来完成其功能。

第三节基于细胞因子生物学的治疗意义，介绍了细胞因子和细胞因子拮抗剂正在用于临床治疗，并且正在进行药物研发。基于细胞因子的疗法将会提供一种更有针对性的方法来破坏潜在的疾病过程。同时介绍了一些临床应用成功的例子，最常见的是应用于银屑病治疗的细胞因子拮抗药，TNF-α阻断药物、IL-12/IL-23拮抗药，针对IL-17A的人类单克隆抗体。

第四节趋化因子：白细胞动员中心的次级细胞因子。本节内容首先概述了趋化因子的两个主要特殊功能：①通过组织中的趋化梯度引导Leu-2核细胞，将效应器细胞带到需要的地方；②能够通过整合素增加白细胞与内皮细胞表面配体的结合，促进白细胞在组织中的牢固黏附和外渗。在皮肤发育、免疫、炎症和癌症中起着重要作用。

第五节趋化因子在疾病中的作用，介绍了趋化因子在特应性皮炎、银屑病、皮肤癌、传染病等多种皮肤疾病中的作用。

第六节可溶性介质网络：治疗意义和应用，介绍了细胞因子和趋化因子的不平衡会导致慢性疾病。细胞因子和趋化因子目前正被用于临床治疗，这可能是未来临床的核心。

〔粟 娟〕

AT-A-GLANCE

- Cytokines are polypeptide mediators that function in communication between hematopoietic cells and other cell types.
- Cytokines often have multiple biologic activities (pleiotropism) and overlapping biologic effects (redundancy).
- Chemokines and their receptors are vital mediators of cellular trafficking.
- Chemokines are synthesized constitutively in some cells and can be induced in many other cell types.
- Cytokine and chemokine-based therapeutics now in use include recombinant cytokines, inhibitory monoclonal antibodies, fusion proteins composed of cytokine receptors and immunoglobulin chains, topical immunomodulators such as imiquimod, prevention of T-cell arrest on activated endothelium or blocking infection of T cells by human immunodeficiency virus 1 using CC chemokine receptor 5 analogs, and cytokine fusion toxins.

THE CONCEPT OF SOLUBLE MEDIATORS

When cells and tissues in complex organisms need to communicate over distances greater than one cell diameter, soluble factors must be used. A subset of these factors is most important when produced or released transiently under emergent conditions (Table 12-1). When faced with an infection- or injury-related challenge, the host must orchestrate a complex and carefully choreographed series of steps. It must mobilize certain circulating white blood cells precisely to the relevant injured area (but not elsewhere) and guide other leukocytes involved in host defense, particularly T and B cells, to specialized lymphatic tissue remote from the infectious lesion but sufficiently close to contain antigens from the relevant pathogen. After a limited period of time in this setting (ie, lymph node [LN]), antibodies produced by B cells and effector-memory T cells, can be released into the circulation and localize at the site of infection. Soluble factors produced by resident tissue cells at the site of injury, by leukocytes and platelets that are recruited to the site of injury, and by memory T cells ultimately recruited to the area, all coordinate an evolving and effective response to a challenge to host defense. Most important, the level of this response must be appropriate to the challenge, and the duration of the response must be transient, that is, long enough to decisively eliminate the pathogen but short enough to minimize damage to healthy host tissues. This chapter focuses on two major categories of soluble mediators that help regulate an effective immune response: cytokines and chemokines.

Cytokines are soluble polypeptide mediators that play pivotal roles in communication between cells of the hematopoietic system and other cells in the body.[1] Cytokines influence many aspects of leukocyte function, including differentiation, growth, activation, and migration. Although many cytokines are substantially upregulated in response to injury to allow a rapid and potent host response, cytokines also play important roles in the development of the immune system and in homeostatic control of the immune system under basal conditions. The growth and differentiation effects of cytokines are not limited to leukocytes, but we will not discuss soluble factors that principally mediate cell growth and differentiation of cells other than leukocytes in this chapter. The participation of cytokines in many aspects of immune and inflammatory responses has prompted the examination of a variety of cytokines or cytokine antagonists (primarily antibodies and fusion proteins) as agents for pharmacologic manipulation of immune-mediated diseases. Therapeutic targeting of cytokines has proven valuable in treating dermatologic disorders. Indeed, a detailed appreciation of cytokine biology sheds light onto a host of cutaneous diseases that result from immune dysfunction.

Chemokines are a large superfamily of small cytokines that are accepted as vital mediators of cellular trafficking. Since the discovery of the first *chemo*attractant *cytokine* or chemokine in 1977, 50 additional new chemokines and 17 chemokine receptors have been discovered. Initially associated only with recruitment of leukocyte subsets to inflammatory sites,[2] it has become clear that chemokines play roles in angiogenesis, neural development, cancer metastasis, hematopoiesis, and infectious diseases. This chapter includes a review of chemokine function in inflammatory conditions but touches on the role of these molecules in other settings as well.

CYTOKINE BIOLOGY

General features of cytokines are their pleiotropism and redundancy. Before the advent of a systematic nomenclature for cytokines, most newly identified cytokines were named according to the biologic assay that was being used to isolate and characterize the active molecule (eg, T-cell growth factor for the molecule that was later renamed *interleukin 2*, or IL-2). Very often, independent groups studying quite disparate bioactivities isolated the same molecule that revealed the pleiotropic effects of these cytokines. For example, before being termed *interleukin 1* (IL-1), this cytokine had been variously known as *endogenous pyrogen*, *lymphocyte-activating factor*, and *leukocytic endogenous mediator*. Many cytokines have a wide range of activities, causing multiple effects in responsive cells and a different set of effects in each type of cell capable of responding. The redundancy of cytokines typically means that in any single bioassay (eg, induction of T-cell proliferation), multiple cytokines display activity. In addition, the absence of a single cytokine (eg, in mice with targeted mutations in a cytokine gene) can often be largely or even completely compensated for by other cytokines with overlapping biologic effects.

CLASSIFICATIONS OF CYTOKINES

The first cytokines described had distinct and easily recognizable biological activities, exemplified by IL-1, IL-2, and the interferons (IFNs). The term *cytokine* was first coined by Cohen in 1975 to describe several such activities released into the supernatant of an epithelial cell line.[3] Before this, such activities had been thought to be the exclusive domain of lymphocytes (lymphokines) and monocytes (monokines) and were considered a function of the immune system. Keratinocyte cytokines were first discovered in 1981,[4] and the list of cytokines produced by this epithelial cell rivals nearly any other cell type in the body.[5,6] The number of molecules that can be legitimately termed cytokines continues to expand and has brought under the cytokine rubric molecules with a broad range of distinct biological activities. The progress in genomic approaches has led to identification of novel cytokine genes based on homologies to known cytokine genes. Making sense of this plethora of mediators is more of a challenge than ever, and strategies to simplify the analysis of the cytokine universe are sorely needed.

TABLE 12-1
Primary Soluble Mediators Constitutively Expressed by Human Keratinocytes

MEDIATOR	UPREGULATING STIMULI
Cytokines	
IL-1α	IL-1α, TNF-α, LPS, UVB, IFN-γ
IL-1α	IL-1α, TNF-α, LPS, UVB
IL-1RA	IL-1α, TNF-α, LPS, UVB, IFN-γ
IL-6	IL-1α, IFN-γ, IL-17, LPS
IL-18	TNF-α, UVB, LPS, dsRNA
TGF-α	TNF-α, IFN-γ
TGF-β	UVB, LPS, RA
Chemokines	
CXCL8	TNF-α, IL-1α, IFN-γ, IL-17, UVB, dsRNA, flagellin
CCL17	IFN-γ, TNF-α
CCL20	TNF-α, IL-1α, IL-1β, IFN-γ, IL-17, CD40L, dsRNA
CCL27	TNF-α, IL-1β, dsRNA

dsRNA, double-stranded RNA; IFN, interferon; IL, interleukin; LPS, lipopolysaccharide; TNF, tumor necrosis factor; UVB, ultraviolet B; RA, retinoic acid.

T-CELL SUBSETS DISTINGUISHED BY PATTERN OF CYTOKINE PRODUCTION

Another valuable concept that has withstood the test of time is the assignment of many T cell–derived cytokines into groups based on the specific helper T-cell subsets that produce them (Fig. 12-1). The original two helper T-cell subsets were termed *Th1* and *Th2*.[7] Commitment to one of these two patterns of cytokine secretion also occurs with CD8 cytotoxic T cells and γ/δ T cells. Dominance of type 1 or type 2 cytokines in a T-cell immune response has profound consequences for the outcome of immune responses to certain pathogens and extrinsic proteins capable of serving as allergens. More than 2 decades after the original description of the Th1 and Th2 subsets, strong evidence has emerged that there are other functionally significant patterns of cytokine secretion by T cells. Most prominent among these newer T-cell lineages are *Th17 cells* and *regulatory T cells* (or *Treg cells* for short). The Th17 subset is distinguished by production of a high level of IL-17, but many Th17 cells also secrete IL-21 and IL-22. Th17 cells promote inflammation, and there is consistent evidence from human autoimmune diseases and mouse models of these diseases that IL-17-producing cells are critical effectors in autoimmune disease.[8] A subset of T cells known as Treg cells has emerged as a crucial subset involved in the maintenance of peripheral self-tolerance.[9] Two of the most distinctive features of Treg cells are their expression of the FoxP3 transcription factor and production of transforming growth factor-β (TGF-β), a cytokine that appears to be required for Treg cells to limit the excess activity of the proinflammatory T-cell subsets.[10] IL-10 is also a significant contributor to the suppressive activity of Treg cells, particularly at some mucosal interfaces.[11] Additional proposed helper T-cell subsets are follicular helper T (Tfh) cells that specialize in providing B cell help in germinal centers, Th9 cells distinguished by high levels of IL-9 production that function in antiparasite and antimelanoma immunity,[12] and Th22 cells associated with skin inflammation that produce IL-22 but not other Th17-associated cytokines. Not only does each of these T-cell subsets exhibit distinctive patterns of cytokine production, but cytokines are also key factors in influencing the differentiation of naïve T cells into these subsets. IL-12 is the key Th1-promoting factor; IL-4 is required for Th2 differentiation; and IL-6, IL-23, and TGF-β are involved in promoting Th17 development.

STRUCTURAL CLASSIFICATION OF CYTOKINES

Not all useful classifications of cytokines are based solely on analysis of cytokine function. Structural biologists, aided by improved methods of generating homogenous preparations of proteins and establishment of new analytical methods (eg, solution magnetic resonance spectroscopy) that complement the classical

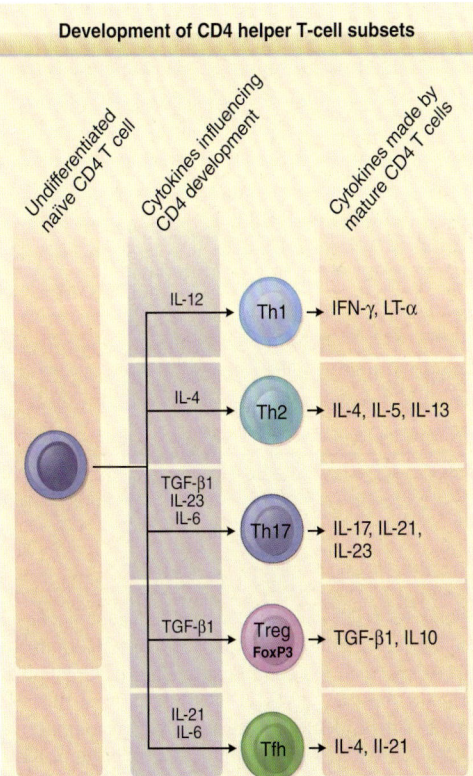

Figure 12-1 Cytokines control the development of specific CD4 helper T-cell subsets. The cytokine milieu at the time of activation of naïve undifferentiated CD4 T cells has a profound influence on the ultimate pattern of cytokine secretion adopted by fully differentiated T cells. Subsets of effector CD4 T cells with defined patterns of cytokine secretion include T helper 1 (Th1), Th2, Th17, and T follicular helper (Tfh) cells. Regulatory CD4 T cells (Treg cells) express the FoxP3 transcription factor, and their effects are mediated in part by their production of transforming growth factor-β1 (TGF-β1) and/or interleukin 10 (IL-10). IFN, interferon; LT, lymphotoxin. (Adapted from Swain SL, McKinstry KK, Strutt TM. Expanding roles for CD4+ T cells in immunity to viruses *Nat Rev Immunol.* 2012;12:136-148.)

x-ray crystallography technique, have determined the three-dimensional structure of many cytokines. These efforts have led to the identification of groups of cytokines that fold to generate similar three-dimensional structures and bind to groups of cytokine receptors that also share similar structural features. For example, most of the cytokine ligands that bind to receptors of the hematopoietin cytokine receptor family are members of the four-helix bundle group of proteins. Four-helix bundle proteins have a shared tertiary architecture consisting of four antiparallel α-helical stretches separated by short connecting loops. The normal existence of some cytokines as oligomers rather than monomers was discovered in part as the result of structural investigations. For example, IFN-γ is a four-helix bundle cytokine that exists naturally as a noncovalent dimer. The bivalency of the dimer enables this ligand to bind and oligomerize two IFN-γ receptor complexes, thereby facilitating signal transduction. TNF-α and TNF-β are both trimers that are composed almost exclusively of β-sheets folded into a "jelly roll" structural motif. Ligand-induced trimerization of receptors in the TNF receptor family is involved in the initiation of signaling.

SIGNAL TRANSDUCTION PATHWAYS SHARED BY CYTOKINES

To accomplish their effects, cytokines must first bind with specificity and high affinity to receptors on the cell surfaces of responding cells. Many aspects of the pleiotropism and redundancy manifested by cytokines can be understood through an appreciation of shared mechanisms of signal transduction mediated by cell surface receptors for cytokines. In the early years of cytokine biology, the emphasis of most investigative work was the purification and eventual cloning of new cytokines and a description of their functional capabilities, both in vitro and in vivo. Most of the cytokine receptors have now been cloned, and many of the signaling cascades initiated by cytokines have been described in great detail. The vast majority of cytokine receptors can be classified into a relatively small number of families and superfamilies (Table 12-2), the members of which function in an approximately similar fashion. Table 12-3 lists the cytokines of particular relevance for cutaneous biology, including the major sources, responsive cells, features of interest, and clinical relevance of each cytokine. Most cytokines send signals to cells through pathways that are very similar to those used by other cytokines binding to the same class of receptors. Individual cytokines often use several downstream pathways of signal transduction, which accounts in part for the pleiotropic effects of these molecules. Nevertheless, we propose here that a few major signaling pathways account for most effects attributable to cytokines. Of particularly central importance are the nuclear factor κB (NF-κB) pathway and the Janus kinase (JAK)/signal transducer and activator of transcription (STAT) pathway, described in the following sections.

NUCLEAR FACTOR κB, INHIBITOR OF κB, AND PRIMARY CYTOKINES

A major mechanism contributing to the extensive overlap between the biologic activities of the primary cytokines IL-1 and TNF is the shared use of the NF-κB signal transduction pathway. IL-1 and TNF use completely distinct cell surface receptor and proximal signaling pathways, but these pathways converge at the activation of the NF-κB transcription factor. NF-κB is of central importance in immune and inflammatory processes because a large number of genes that elicit

TABLE 12-2
Major Families of Cytokine Receptors

RECEPTOR FAMILY	EXAMPLE	MAJOR SIGNAL TRANSDUCTION PATHWAY(S) LEADING TO BIOLOGIC EFFECTS
IL-1 receptor family	IL-1R, type 1	NF-B activation via TRAF6
TNF receptor family	TNFR1	NF-B activation involving TRAF2 and TRAF5 Apoptosis induction via "death domain" proteins
Hematopoietin receptor family (class I receptors)	IL-2R	Activation of JAK/STAT pathway
IFN/IL-10 receptor family (class II receptors)	IFN-R	Activation of JAK/STAT pathway
Immunoglobulin superfamily	M-CSF R	Activation of intrinsic tyrosine kinase
TGF-receptor family	TGF-R, types I and II	Activation of intrinsic serine/threonine kinase coupled to Smad proteins
Chemokine receptor family	CCR5	Seven transmembrane receptors coupled to G proteins
IL-17 receptor family	IL-17R	NF-B activation via Act1 and TRAF

CCR, CC chemokine receptor; IFN, interferon; IL, interleukin; JAK, Janus kinase; M-CSF, macrophage colony stimulating factor; NF-B, nuclear factor B; STAT, signal transducer and activator of transcription; TGF, transforming growth factor; TNF, tumor necrosis factor; TRAF, tumor necrosis factor receptor-associated factor.

or propagate inflammation have NF-κB recognition sites in their promoters.[13] NF-κB–regulated genes encode cytokines, chemokines, adhesion molecules, nitric oxide synthase, cyclooxygenase, and phospholipase A2.

In unstimulated cells, NF-κB heterodimers formed from p65 and p50 subunits are inactive because they are sequestered in the cytoplasm as a result of tight binding to inhibitor proteins in the IκB family (Fig. 12-2). Signal transduction pathways that activate the NF-κB system do so through the activation of an IκB kinase (IKK) complex consisting of two kinase subunits (IKKα and IKKβ) and a regulatory subunit (IKKγ). The IKK complex phosphorylates IκBα and IκBβ on specific serine residues, yielding a target for recognition by an E3 ubiquitin ligase complex. The resulting polyubiquitination marks this IκB for rapid degradation by the 26S proteasome complex in the cytoplasm. After IκB has been degraded, the free NF-κB (which contains a nuclear localization signal) is able to pass into the nucleus and induce expression of NF-κB–sensitive genes. The presence of κB recognition sites in cytokine promoters is very common. Among the genes regulated by NF-κB are *IL-1β* and *TNF-α*. This endows *IL-1β* and *TNF-α* with the capacity to establish a positive regulatory loop that favors persistent inflammation. Cytokines besides IL-1 and TNF that activate the NF-κB pathway as part of their signal transduction mechanisms include IL-17 and IL-18.

Proinflammatory cytokines are not the only stimuli that can activate the NF-κB pathway. Bacterial products (eg, lipopolysaccharide, or LPS), oxidants, activators of protein kinase C (eg, phorbol esters), viruses, and ultraviolet (UV) radiation are other stimuli that can stimulate NF-κB activity. TLR4 is a cell surface receptor for the complex of LPS, LPS-binding protein, and CD14. The cytoplasmic domain of TLR4 is similar to that of the IL-1 receptor type 1 (IL-1R1) and other IL-1R family members and is known as the *TIR* domain (for Toll/IL-1 receptor).[14] When ligand is bound to a TIR domain-containing receptor, one or more adapter proteins that also contain TIR domains are recruited to the complex. Myeloid differentiation primary response 88 (MyD88) was the first of these adapters to be identified; the other known adapters are TIRAP (TIR domain-containing adapter protein), TRIF (TIR domain-containing adapter inducing IFN-β), and TRAM (TRIF-related adapter molecule). Engagement of the adapter, in turn, activates one or more of the IL-1R-associated kinases (IRAK1 to IRAK4) that then signal through TRAF6, a member of the TRAF (TNF receptor–associated factor) family, and TAK1 (TGF-β–activated kinase) to activate the IKK complex.[15]

JAK/STAT PATHWAY

A major breakthrough in the analysis of cytokine-mediated signal transduction was the identification of a common cell surface to nucleus pathway used by the majority of cytokines. This JAK/STAT pathway was first elucidated through careful analysis of signaling initiated by IFN receptors (Fig. 12-3) but was subsequently shown to play a role in signaling by all cytokines that bind to members of the hematopoietin receptor family.[16] The JAK/STAT pathway operates through the sequential action of a family of four nonreceptor tyrosine kinases (the JAKs or *J*anus family *k*inases) and a series of latent cytosolic transcription factors known as *STATs* (*s*ignal *t*ransducers and *a*ctivators of *t*ranscription). The cytoplasmic portions of many cytokine receptor chains are noncovalently associated with one of the four JAKs (JAK1, JAK2, JAK3, and tyrosine kinase 2 [Tyk2]).

The activity of JAK kinases is upregulated after stimulation of a cytokine receptor. Ligand binding to the cytokine receptors leads to the association of two or more distinct cytokine receptor subunits and brings the associated JAK kinases into close proximity with each other. This promotes cross-phosphorylation or autophosphorylation reactions that in turn fully acti-

TABLE 12-3
Cytokines of Particular Relevance for Cutaneous Biology

CYTOKINE	MAJOR SOURCES	RESPONSIVE CELLS	FEATURES OF INTEREST	CLINICAL RELEVANCE
IL-1	Epithelial cells	Infiltrating leukocytes	Active form stored in keratinocytes	IL-1Ra used to treat rheumatoid arthritis
IL-1	Myeloid cells	Infiltrating leukocytes	Caspase 1 cleavage required for activation	IL-1Ra used to treat rheumatoid arthritis
IL-2	Activated T cells	Activated T cells, Treg cells	Autocrine factor for activated T cells	IL-2 fusion toxin targets CTCL
IL-4	Activated Th2 cells, NKT cells	Lymphocytes, endothelial cells, keratinocytes	Causes B-cell class switching and Th2 differentiation	—
IL-5	Activated Th2 cells, mast cells	B cells, eosinophils	Regulates eosinophil response to parasites	Anti–IL-5 depletes eosinophils
IL-6	Activated myeloid cells, fibroblasts, endothelial cells	B cells, myeloid cells, hepatocytes	Triggers acute-phase response, promotes immunoglobulin synthesis	Anti–IL-6R used to treat rheumatoid arthritis
IL-10	T cells, NK cells	Myeloid and lymphoid cells	Inhibits innate and acquired immune responses	—
IL-12	Activated APCs	Th1 cells	Promotes TH1 differentiation, shares p40 subunit with IL-23	Anti-p40 inhibits Crohn disease and psoriasis
IL-13	Activated Th2 cells, nuocytes	Monocytes, keratinocytes, endothelial cells	Mediates tissue responses to parasites	—
IL-17	Activated Th17 cells	Multiple cell types	Mediates autoimmune diseases	Potential drug target in autoimmune disease
IL-22	Activated Th17 cells and Th22 cells	Keratinocytes	Induces cytokines and antimicrobial peptides	Contributes to psoriasis
IL-23	Activated dendritic cells	Memory T cells, Th17 cells	Directs Th17 differentiation, mediates autoimmune disease	Anti-p40 inhibits Crohn disease and psoriasis
IL-25	Activated Th2 cells, mast cells	Th17 cells	Promotes Th2 differentiation, inhibits Th17 cells	—
IL-26	Th17 cells, natural killer cells, macrophages	Epithelial cells and microorganisms	Promotes inflammation and has intrinsic anti-microbial properties	—
IL-27	Activated APCs	Th1 cells	Promotes Th1 differentiation	—
IL-31	Th2 cells, mast cells, macrophages, dendritic cells	Macrophages, epithelial cells, eosinophils	Promotes inflammation and pruritus	Potential drug target in atopic dermatitis
IL-35	Treg cells	Th17 cells and Treg cells	Inhibits Th17 cells and expands Treg cells	—
TNF-α	Activated myeloid, lymphoid, and epithelial cells	Infiltrating leukocytes	Mediates inflammation	Anti–TNF-effective in psoriasis
IFN-α and IFN-β	Plasmacytoid dendritic cells	Most cell types	Major part of innate antiviral response	Elicited by topical imiquimod application
IFN-γ	Activated Th1 cells, CD8 T cells, NK cells, dendritic cells	Macrophages, dendritic cells, naïve T cells	Macrophage activation, specific isotype switching	IFN used to treat chronic granulomatous disease
TSLP	Epithelial cells including keratinocytes	Dendritic cells, B cells, Th2 cells	Promotes Th2 differentiation	Involved in atopic diseases

APC, antigen-presenting cell; CTCL, cutaneous T-cell lymphoma; IFN, interferon; IL, interleukin; NKT, natural killer T cell; Th, T helper; TNF, tumor necrosis factor; Treg, T regulatory; TSLP, thymic stromal lymphopoietin.

vate the kinases. Tyrosines in the cytoplasmic tail of the cytokine receptor as well as tyrosines on other associated and newly recruited proteins are also phosphorylated. A subset of the newly phosphorylated tyrosines can then serve as docking points for attachment of additional signaling proteins bearing Src homology 2 (SH2) domains. Cytoplasmic STATs possess SH2 domains and are recruited to the phosphorylated cytokine receptors via this interaction. Homodimeric or heterodimeric STAT proteins are phosphorylated by the JAK kinases and subsequently translocate to the nucleus. In the nucleus, they bind recognition sequences in DNA and stimulate transcription of specific genes, often in cooperation with other transcription factors. The same STAT molecules can be involved in signaling by multiple different cytokines. The specificity of the response in these instances may depend on the formation of complexes involving STATs and other

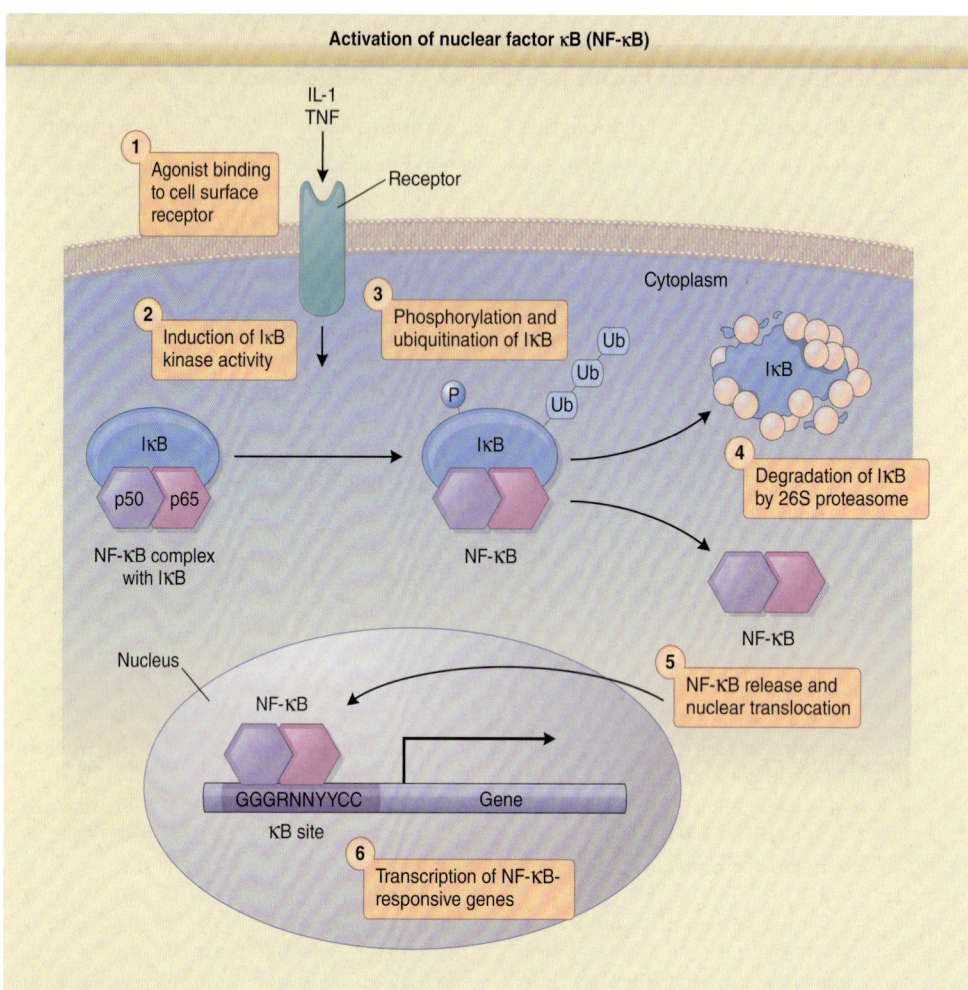

Figure 12-2 Activation of nuclear factor κB (NF-κB)–regulated genes after signaling by receptors for primary cytokines or by Toll-like receptors (TLRs) engaged by microbial products. Under resting conditions, NF-κB (a heterodimer of p50 and p65 subunits) is tightly bound to an inhibitor called IκB that sequesters NF-κB in the cytoplasm. Engagement of one of the TLRs or the signal transducing receptors for interleukin-1 (IL-1) or tumor necrosis factor (TNF) family members leads to induction of IκB kinase activity that phosphorylates IκB on critical serine residues. Phosphorylated IκB becomes a substrate for ubiquitination, which triggers degradation of IκB by the 26S proteasome. Loss of IκB results in release of NF-κB, which permits it to move to the nucleus and activate transcription of genes whose promoters contain κB recognition sites. Ub, ubiquitin.

transcription factors that then selectively act on a specific set of genes.

Therapeutic targeting of the JAK/STAT pathway has been met with recent enthusiasm in the treatment of cutaneous autoimmune and autoinflammatory disorders. Tofacitinib is a small molecule inhibitor that targets JAK1, JAK3, and, to a lesser extent, JAK2. It has been found to be effective in the treatment of psoriasis and psoriatic arthritis, being noninferior to the anti-TNF biologic, etanercept.[17] Recent reports have also indicated efficacy in the treatment of alopecia areata.[18] Furthermore, the JAK1 and JAK2 inhibitor ruxolitinib has been beneficial in the treatment of dermatomyositis,[19] with similar efficacy of tofacitinib being reported.[20] Clinical trials are currently being undertaken to evaluate the clinical efficacy of JAK inhibition in the treatment of patients with stimulator of interferon genes (STING)-associated vasculopathy with onset in infancy, an autoinflammatory disorder that targets the skin, blood vessels, and lungs. Indeed, further work must be done to fully exploit targeting the JAK/STAT pathway for maximal clinical benefit.

INTERLEUKIN-1 FAMILY OF CYTOKINES

The IL-1 family is a group of cytokines that induces a complex network of proinflammatory cytokines and regulates and initiates inflammatory responses via expression of integrins on leukocytes and endothelial cells. The IL-1 family includes a number of cytokines; however,

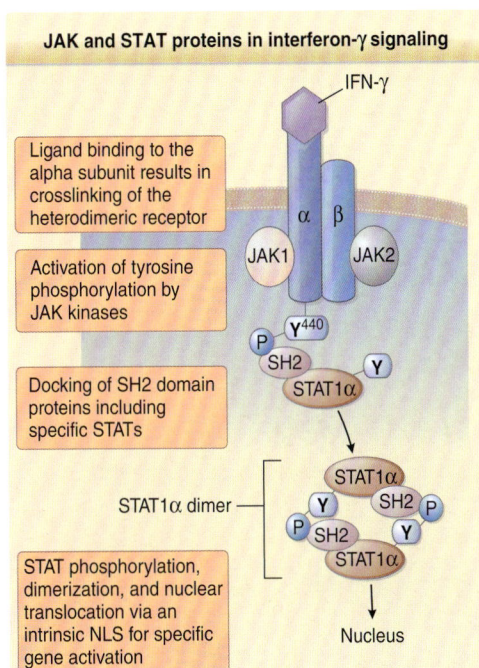

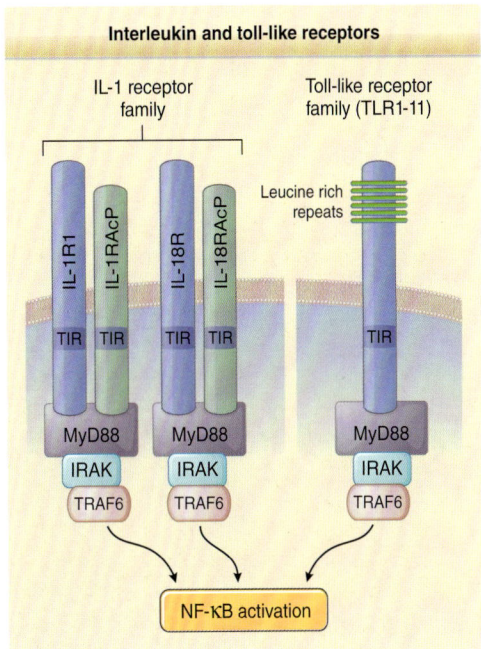

Figure 12-3 Participation of JAK (Janus kinase) and STAT (signal transducer and activator of transcription) proteins in interferon-γ (IFN-γ) signaling. Binding of human IFN-γ (a dimer) to the alpha subunit of the receptor complex results in the crosslinking of the alpha and beta subunits. The nonreceptor protein tyrosine kinases JAK1 and JAK2 are activated and phosphorylate critical tyrosine residues in the receptor such as the tyrosine at position 440 of the α chain (Y^{440}). STAT1α molecules are recruited to the IFN-γ receptor based on the affinity of their Src homology 2 (SH2) domains for the phosphopeptide sequence around Y^{440}. Receptor-associated STAT1α molecules then dimerize through reciprocal SH2-phosphotyrosine interactions. The resulting STAT1α dimers translocate to the nucleus via the nuclear localization signal (NLS) and stimulate transcription of IFN-γ–regulated genes.

Figure 12-4 The interleukin 1 receptor (IL-1R) family and Toll-like receptors (TLRs) use a common intracellular signaling pathway. Receptors for cytokines in the IL-1 family (typified by the IL-1 and IL-18 receptors) share a common signaling domain with the TLRs (TLR1 to TLR11) called the *Toll/IL-1 receptor (TIR)* domain. The TIR domain receptors interact with TIR domain-containing adapter proteins such as MyD88 that couple ligand binding to activation of IL-1R-associated kinase (IRAK) and ultimately activation of nuclear factor κB (NF-κB). IL-1RAcP, IL-1R accessory protein; TRAF, tumor necrosis factor receptor-associated factor.

the archetypal members, interleukins 1α and 1β along with IL-18, will be discussed further here (Fig. 12-4).

IL-1 is the prototype of a cytokine that has been discovered many times in many different biologic assays. Distinct genes encode the α and β forms of human IL-1, with only 26% homology between these proteins at the amino acid level. Both IL-1s are translated as 31-kDa molecules that lack a signal peptide, and both reside in the cytoplasm. This form of IL-1α is biologically active, but 31-kDa *IL-1β* must be activated by cleavage by caspase 1 (initially termed *interleukin-1β-converting enzyme*) in a multiprotein cytoplasmic complex called the *inflammasome* (Fig. 12-5) to generate an active molecule.[21]

In general, whereas IL-1β appears to be the dominant form of IL-1 produced by monocytes, macrophages, Langerhans cells (LCs), and dendritic cells (DCs), IL-1α predominates in epithelial cells, including keratinocytes. This is likely to relate to the fact that epithelial IL-1α is stored in the cytoplasm of cells that comprise an interface with the external environment. Such cells, when injured, release biologically active 31-kDa IL-1α and, by doing so, can initiate inflammation.[22] However, if uninjured, these cells will differentiate and ultimately release their IL-1 contents into the environment. Leukocytes, including dendritic and LCs, carry their cargo of IL-1, and its unregulated release could cause significant tissue damage. Thus, biologically active IL-1β release from cells is controlled at several levels: IL-1β gene transcription, *caspase 1* gene transcription, and availability of the adapter proteins that interact with caspase 1 in the inflammasome to allow the generation of mature activated IL-1β. IL-1β stimulates the egress of LCs from the epidermis during the initiation of contact hypersensitivity, a pivotal event that leads to accumulation of LCs in skin-draining LNs. Studies of mice deficient in *IL-1α* and *IL-1β* genes suggest that both molecules are important in contact hypersensitivity but that IL-1α is more critical.

Active forms of IL-1 bind to the IL-1R1 or type 1 IL-1 receptor.[14] This is the sole signal-transducing receptor for IL-1, and its cytoplasmic domain has little homology with other cytokine receptors, showing greatest homology with the *Toll* gene product identified in *Drosophila*. A second cell surface protein, the IL-1R accessory protein, or IL-1RAcP, must associate with

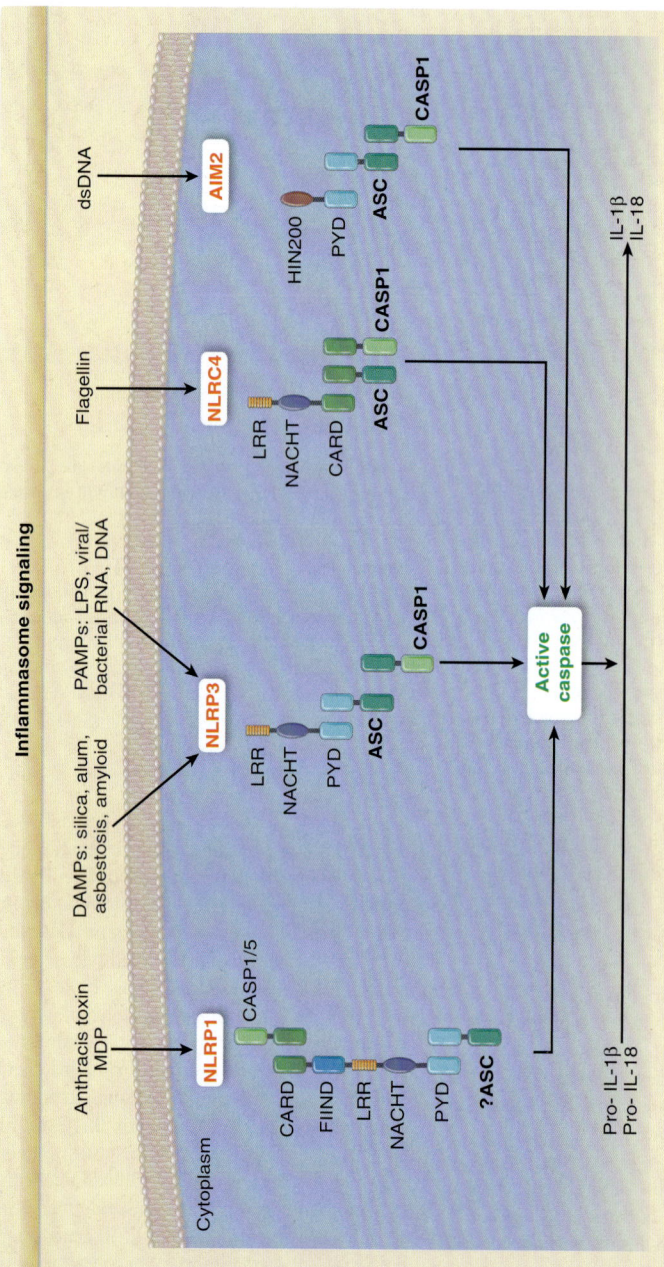

Figure 12-5 Inflammasomes are multimeric protein complexes that assemble in the cytosol after sensing various stimuli. Although there are fundamental differences between inflammasomes depending on stimuli, canonical inflammasomes oligomerize upon activation, leading to the recruitment of the adapter ASC (apoptosis-associated speck-like protein containing a caspase activation and recruitment domain), which serves as a scaffold to recruit the inactive pro-caspase-1. Oligomerization of pro-caspase-1 proteins induces their autoproteolytic cleavage into active caspase-1. Active caspase-1 is a cysteine-dependent protease that cleaves the precursor cytokines pro–IL-1β and pro–IL-18, generating the biologically active cytokines IL-1β and IL-18, respectively. AIM2, absent in melanoma 2; CARD, caspase activation and recruitment domain; DAMP, danger-associated molecular pattern; HIN200, hematopoietic interferon-inducible nuclear antigens with 200 amino acid repeats; LRR, leucine-rich repeat; MDP, muramyl dipeptide; NACHT, NAIP (neuronal apoptosis inhibitor protein), C2TA (MHC class 2 transcription activator), HET-E (heterokaryon incompatibility) and TP1 (telomerase-associated protein 1); PAMP, pathogen-associated molecular pattern; PYD, pyrin domain. (Adapted from Guo H, Callaway JB, Ting JP. Inflammasomes: mechanism of action, role in disease, and therapeutics. *Nat Med*. 2015;21(7):677-687.)

IL-1R1 for signaling to occur. When IL-1 engages the IL-1R1–IL-1RAcP complex, recruitment of the MyD88 adapter occurs followed by interactions with one or more of the IRAKs. These kinases in turn associate with TRAF6. Stepwise activation and recruitment of additional signaling molecules culminate in the induction of IKK activity. The net result is the activation of a series of NF-κB–regulated genes.

A molecule known as the *IL-1 receptor antagonist*, or IL-1ra, can bind to IL-1R1 but does not induce signaling through the receptor. This IL-1ra exists in three alternatively spliced forms, and an isoform produced in monocytes is the only ligand for the IL-1R1 that both contains a signal peptide and is secreted from cells. Two other isoforms of IL-1ra, both lacking signal peptides, are contained within epithelial cells. The function of IL-1ra seems to be as a pure antagonist of IL-1 ligand binding to IL-1R1, and binding of IL-1ra to IL-1R1 does not induce the mobilization of IL-1RAcP. Consequently, although both IL-1α/β and IL-1ra bind with equivalent affinities to IL-1R1, the association of IL-1R1 with IL-1RAcP increases the affinity for IL-1α/β manyfold while not affecting the affinity for IL-1ra. This is consistent with the observation that a vast molar excess of IL-1ra is required to fully antagonize the effects of IL-1. The biologic role of IL-1ra is likely to be in the quenching of IL-1–mediated inflammatory responses, and mice deficient in IL-1ra show exaggerated and persistent inflammatory responses.

A second means of antagonizing IL-1 activity occurs via expression of a second receptor for IL-1, IL-1R2. This receptor has a short cytoplasmic domain and serves to bind IL-1α/β efficiently but not IL-1ra. This 68-kDa receptor can be cleaved from the cell surface by an unknown protease and released as a stable, soluble 45-kDa molecule that retains avid IL-1–binding function. By binding the functional ligands for IL-1R1, IL-1R2 serves to inhibit IL-1–mediated responses. It is likely that IL-1R2 also inhibits IL-1 activity by associating with IL-1RAcP at the cell surface and removing and sequestering it from the pool available to associate with IL-1R1. Thus, whereas soluble IL-1R2 binds to free IL-1, cell surface IL-1R2 sequesters IL-1RAcP. Expression of IL-1R2 can be upregulated by a number of stimuli, including corticosteroids and IL-4. However, IL-1R2 can also be induced by inflammatory cytokines, including IFN-γ and IL-1, probably as a compensatory signal designed to limit the scale and duration of the inflammatory response. Production of IL-1R2 serves to make the producing cell and surrounding cells resistant to IL-1-mediated activation. Interestingly, some of the most efficient IL-1–producing cells are also the best producers of the IL-1R2.

IL-18 was first identified based on its capacity to induce IFN-γ. One name initially proposed for this cytokine was IL-1γ because of its homology with IL-1α and IL-1β. Like IL-1β, it is translated as an inactive precursor molecule of 23 kDa and is cleaved to an active 18-kDa species by caspase 1. It is produced by multiple cell types in skin, including keratinocytes, LCs, and monocytes. IL-18 induces proliferation, cytotoxicity, and cytokine production by Th1 and natural killer (NK) cells, mostly synergistically with IL-12. The IL-18 receptor bears striking similarity to the IL-1 receptor.[14] The binding chain (IL-18R) is an IL-1R1 homolog, originally cloned as IL-1Rrp1. IL-18R alone is a low-affinity receptor that must recruit IL-18RAcP (a homolog of IL-1RAcP). As for IL-1, both chains of the IL-18 receptor are required for signal transduction. Although there is no IL-18 homolog of IL-1ra, a molecule known as *IL-18-binding protein* binds to soluble mature IL-18 and prevents it from binding to the IL-18R complex. More recently, it has become clear that there is a family of receptors homologous to the IL-1R1 and IL-18R molecules,[14] which have a TIR motif in common. All of these share analogous signaling pathways initiated by the MyD88 adapter molecule.

When IL-1 produced by epidermis was originally identified, it was noted that both intact epidermis and stratum corneum contained significant IL-1 activity, which led to the concept that epidermis was a shield of sequestered IL-1 surrounding the host, waiting to be released on injury. More recently, it was observed that high levels of the IL-1ra coexist within keratinocytes; however, repeated experiments show that in virtually all cases, the amount of IL-1 present is sufficient to overcome any potential for inhibition mediated by IL-1ra. Studies have now shown that mechanical stress to keratinocytes permits the release of large amounts of IL-1 in the absence of cell death. Release of IL-1 induces expression of endothelial adhesion molecules, including E-selectin, intercellular adhesion molecule-1 (ICAM-1), and vascular cell adhesion molecule-1 (VCAM-1), as well as chemotactic and activating chemokines. This attracts not only monocytes and granulocytes but also a specific subpopulation of memory T cells that bear cutaneous lymphocyte antigen on their cell surfaces. Memory T cells positive for cutaneous lymphocyte antigen are abundant in inflamed skin, comprising the majority of T cells present. Therefore, any injury to the skin, no matter how trivial, releases IL-1 and attracts this population of memory T cells. If they encounter their antigen in this microenvironment, their activation and subsequent cytokine production will amplify the inflammatory response. This has been proposed as the basis of the clinical observation of inflammation in response to trauma, known as the *Koebner reaction*.

Several biologics that act by inhibiting IL-1 function have been developed for clinical use, including recombinant IL-1Ra (anakinra), an antibody to IL-1β (canakinumab), and an IgG Fc fusion protein that includes the ligand binding domains of the type I IL-1R and IL-1RAcP (rilonacept, also known as IL-1 Trap). All of these agents are efficacious in countering the IL-1–induced inflammation associated with a group of rare autoinflammatory diseases called the cryopyrin-associated periodic syndromes. Anakinra was initially US Food and Drug Administration (FDA) approved as a therapy for adult rheumatoid arthritis. IL-1 inhibition is also being tested as a therapy for gout, an inflammatory arthritis triggered by uric acid–mediated activation of inflammasomes that generate IL-1β.

TUMOR NECROSIS FACTOR

TNF-α is the prototype for a family of signaling molecules that mediate their biologic effects through a family of related receptor molecules. TNF-α was initially cloned on the basis of its ability to mediate two interesting biologic effects: (1) hemorrhagic necrosis of malignant tumors and (2) inflammation-associated cachexia. Although TNF-α exerts many of its biologically important effects as a soluble mediator, newly synthesized TNF-α exists as a transmembrane protein on the cell surface. A specific metalloproteinase known as *TNF-α-converting enzyme (TACE)* is responsible for most TNF-α release by T cells and myeloid cells. The closest cousin of TNF-α is TNF-β, also known as *lymphotoxin α (LT-α)*. Other related molecules in the TNF family include lymphotoxin β (LT-β) that combines with LT-α to form the LT-α1β2 heterotrimer, Fas ligand (FasL), TNF-related apoptosis-inducing ligand (TRAIL), receptor activator of NF-κB ligand (RANKL), and CD40 ligand (CD154). Although some of these other TNF family members have not been traditionally regarded as cytokines, their structures (all are type II membrane proteins with an intracellular *N*-terminus and an extracellular *C*-terminus) and signaling mechanisms are closely related to those of TNF. The soluble forms of TNF-α, LT-α, and FasL are homotrimers, and the predominant form of LT-β is the membrane-bound LT-α1β2 heterotrimer. Trimerization of TNF receptor family members by their trimeric ligands appears to be required for initiation of signaling and expression of biologic activity.

The initial characterization of TNF receptors led to the discovery of two receptor proteins capable of binding TNF-α with high affinity. The p55 receptor for TNF (TNFR1) is responsible for most biologic activities of TNF, but the p75 TNF receptor (TNFR2) is also capable of transducing signals (unlike IL-1R2, which acts solely as a biologic sink for IL-1). TNFR1 and TNFR2 have substantial stretches of close homology and are both present on most types of cells. Nevertheless, there are some notable differences between the two TNFRs.

Unlike cytokine receptors from several of the other large families, TNF signaling does not involve the JAK/STAT pathway. TNF-α evokes two types of responses in cells: (1) proinflammatory effects, and (2) induction of apoptotic cell death (Fig. 12-6). The proinflammatory effects of TNF-α, which include upregulation of adhesion molecule expression and induction of secondary cytokines and chemokines, stem in large part from activation of NF-κB and can be transduced through both TNFR1 and TNFR2. Induction of apoptosis by signaling through TNFR1 depends on a region known as a *death domain* that is absent in TNFR2, as well as interactions with additional proteins with death domains within the TNFR1 signaling complex. Signaling initiated by ligand binding to TNFR1, Fas, or other death domain–containing receptors in the TNF family eventually leads to activation of caspase 8 or 10 and the nuclear changes and DNA fragmentation characteristic of apoptosis.

At least two TNFR family members (TNFR1 and the LT-β receptor) also contribute to the normal anatomic development of the lymphoid system. Mice deficient in TNF-α lack germinal centers and follicular DCs. *TNFR1* mutant mice show the same abnormalities plus an absence of Peyer patches. Mice with null mutations in *LT-α* or *LT-β* have further abnormalities in lymphoid organogenesis and fail to develop peripheral LNs.

TNF-α is an important mediator of cutaneous inflammation, and its expression is induced in the course of almost all inflammatory responses in skin. Normal human keratinocytes and keratinocyte cell lines produce substantial amounts of TNF-α after stimulation with LPS or UV light. Cutaneous inflammation stimulated by irritants and contact sensitizers is associated with strong induction of TNF-α production by

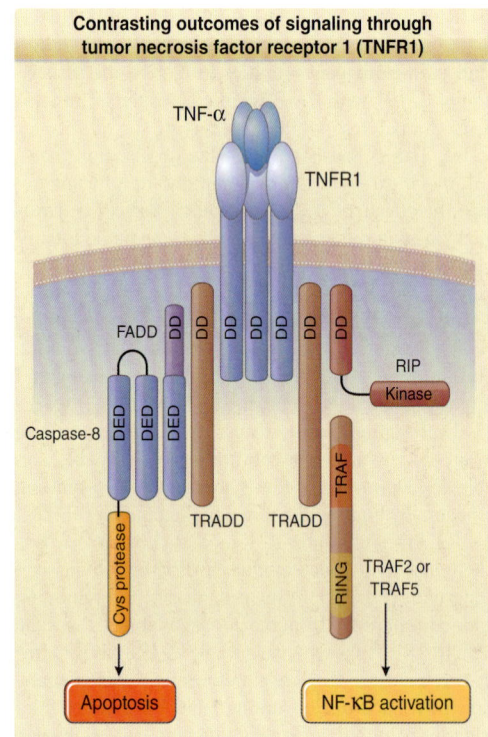

Figure 12-6 Two contrasting outcomes of signaling through tumor necrosis factor receptor 1 (TNFR1). Engagement of TNFR1 by trimeric tumor necrosis factor-α (TNF-α) can trigger apoptosis and/or nuclear factor κB (NF-κB) activation. Both processes involve the adapter protein TNFR-associated death domain (TRADD), which associates with TNFR1 via interactions between "death domains" (DD) on both proteins. For NF-κB activation, TNFR-associated factor 2 (TRAF2) and receptor-interacting protein (RIP) are required. Induction of apoptosis occurs when the death domain-containing protein Fas-associated death domain protein (FADD) associates with TRADD. FADD also contains a "death effector domain" (DED) that interacts with caspase 8 to initiate the apoptotic process. Cys, cysteine. (Adapted from Brenner D, Blaser H, Mak TW. Regulation of tumour necrosis factor signaling: live or let die. *Nat Rev Immunol.* 2015;15:362-374.)

keratinocytes. Exposure to TNF-α promotes LC migration to draining LNs, allowing for sensitization of naïve T cells. One molecular mechanism that may contribute to TNF-α–induced migration of LCs toward LNs is reduced expression of the E-cadherin adhesion molecule after exposure to TNF-α. Induction of CC chemokine receptor 7 (CCR7) on both epidermal and dermal antigen-presenting cells (APCs) correlates with movement into the draining lymphatics. The predominant TNFR expressed by keratinocytes is TNFR1. Autocrine signaling loops involving keratinocyte-derived TNF-α and TNFR1 lead to keratinocyte production of a variety of TNF-inducible secondary cytokines.

The central role of TNF-α in inflammatory diseases, including rheumatoid arthritis and psoriasis, has become evident from clinical studies. Clinical drugs that target the TNF pathway include the humanized anti–TNF-α antibody infliximab, the fully human anti–TNF-α antibody adalimumab, and the soluble TNF receptor etanercept. Drugs in this class are FDA approved for the treatment of several autoimmune and inflammatory diseases, including Crohn disease and rheumatoid arthritis. These three anti-TNF drugs are also FDA approved for the treatment of psoriasis and psoriatic arthritis. This class of drugs also has the potential to be valuable in the treatment of other inflammatory dermatoses. Paradoxically, they are not effective against all autoimmune diseases—multiple sclerosis appears to worsen slightly after treatment with these agents. The TNF antagonists are powerful immunomodulating drugs, and appropriate caution is required in their use. Cases of cutaneous T-cell lymphoma initially thought to represent psoriasis have rapidly progressed to fulminant disease after treatment with TNF antagonists. TNF antagonists can also allow the escape of latent mycobacterial infections from immune control, with a potentially lethal outcome for the patient.

IL-17 FAMILY OF CYTOKINES

IL-17 (also known as IL-17A) was the first described member of a family of related cytokines that now includes IL-17B through F. IL-17A and IL-17F have similar proinflammatory activities, bind to the same heterodimeric receptor composed of the IL-17RA and IL-17RC receptor chains, and act to promote recruitment of neutrophils and induce production of antimicrobial peptides. These IL-17 species normally function in immune defense against pathogenic species of extracellular bacteria and fungi. Mutations in *STAT3* associated with the hyper-IgE syndrome block the development of Th17 cells, an important cellular source of IL-17, and lead to recurrent skin infections with *Staphylococcus aureus* and *Candida albicans*.[23,24] Less is currently known about the actions of IL-17B, C, and D. IL-17E, also known as IL-25, is a product of Th2 cells and mast cells that signals through IL-17RB. A total of five receptor chains for IL-17 family cytokines have been identified, but how each of these individual receptor chains associates to form receptors for all the members of the IL-17 family remains to be elucidated. These IL-17 receptor chains are homologous to each other but display very limited regions of homology to the other major families of cytokine receptors. Recent expansion of interest in Th17 cells and the entire IL-17 family is closely linked to observations that the immunopathology of autoimmune disease in human patients and mouse models is often associated with an inappropriate expansion of Th17 cells. These findings have generated intense interest in targeting the IL-17 signaling axis in the treatment of a number of cutaneous disorders. Indeed, anti–IL-17 biologic therapies have proven tremendously successful in treating patients with psoriasis. Two human monoclonal antibodies against IL-17A, secukinumab and ixekizumab, are currently approved for use in moderate to severe chronic plaque psoriasis with a number of other therapies in clinical trials. Thus, the cytokines produced by Th17 cells and the receptors that transduce these signals may turn out to be useful targets for therapies designed to dampen autoimmunity (Fig. 12-7).

LIGANDS OF THE CLASS I (HEMATOPOIETIN RECEPTOR) FAMILY OF CYTOKINE RECEPTORS

The hematopoietin receptor family (also known as the *class I cytokine receptor family*) is the largest of the cytokine receptor families and comprises a number of structurally related type I membrane-bound glycoproteins. The cytoplasmic domains of these receptors associate with nonreceptor tyrosine kinase molecules, including the JAK kinases and Src family kinases. After ligand binding and receptor oligomerization, these associated nonreceptor tyrosine kinases phosphorylate intracellular substrates, which leads to signal transduction. Most of the multiple-chain receptors in the hematopoietin receptor family consist of a cytokine-specific α chain subunit paired with one or more shared receptor subunits. Five shared receptor subunits have been described to date: (1) the common γ chain (γ_c); (2) the common β chain shared between the IL-2 and IL-15 receptors; (3) a distinct common β chain shared between the granulocyte-macrophage colony-stimulating factor (GM-CSF), IL-3, and IL-5 receptors; (4) the IL-12Rβ2 chain shared by the IL-12 and IL-23 receptors; and (5) the glycoprotein 130 (gp130) molecule, which participates in signaling by IL-6 and related cytokines.

CYTOKINES WITH RECEPTORS THAT INCLUDE THE γ_c CHAIN

The receptor complexes using the γ_c chain are the IL-2, IL-4, IL-7, IL-9, IL-13, IL-15, and IL-21 receptors. Two of these receptors, IL-2R and IL-15R, also use the IL-2Rβ$_c$ chain. The γ_c chain is physically associated with JAK3, and activation of JAK3 is critical to most signaling initiated through this subset of cytokine receptors.[25]

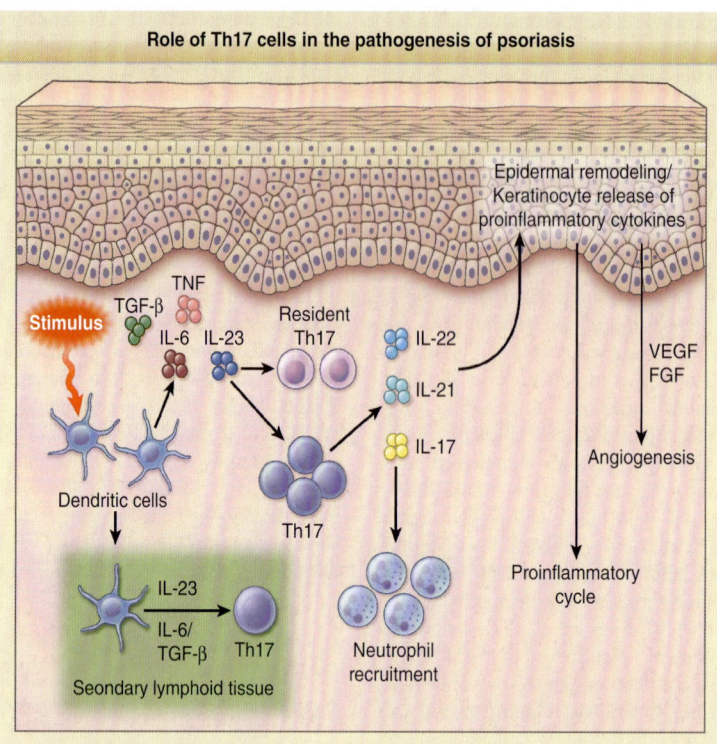

Figure 12-7 The Th17 soluble mediator axis plays a central role in the pathogenesis of psoriasis. After a stimulus such as trauma or infection in a genetically predisposed person, resident dendritic cells produce proinflammatory cytokines both at the site of injury and in the secondary lymphoid tissue, resulting in the generation of pathogenic Th17 cells. Th17 cells produce cytokines such as interleukin (IL)-17, IL-21, and IL-22. Cytokines such as IL-22 and tumor necrosis factor-α (TNF-α) induce keratinocyte hyperplasia. The cytokine milieu generated by Th17 cells also results in neutrophil recruitment and induce keratinocyte to release proangiogenic mediators and other inflammatory cytokines, leading to an inflammatory cycle of disease. FGF, fibroblast growth factor; TGF, transforming growth factor; VEGF, vascular endothelial growth factor.

Interleukin-2 and Interleukin-15: IL-2 and IL-15 can each activate NK cells and stimulate proliferation of activated T cells. IL-2 is a product of activated T cells, and IL-2R is largely restricted to lymphoid cells. The *IL-15* gene is expressed by nonlymphoid tissues, and its transcription is induced by UVB radiation in keratinocytes and fibroblasts and by LPS in monocytes and DCs. Multiple isoforms of IL-15Rα are found in various hematopoietic and nonhematopoietic cells. The IL-2R and IL-15R complexes of lymphocytes incorporate up to three receptor chains, but most other cytokine receptor complexes have two. The affinities of IL-2R and IL-15R for their respective ligands can be regulated, and to some extent, IL-2 and IL-15 compete with each other. The highest affinity receptor complexes for each ligand ($\sim 10^{-11}$ M) consist of the IL-2Rβ$_c$ and γ$_c$ chains, as well as their respective α chains (IL-2Rα, also known as CD25, and IL-15Rα). γ$_c$ and IL-2Rβ$_c$ without the α chains form a functional lower affinity receptor for either ligand (10^{-8} to 10^{-10} M). Although both ligands transmit signals through the γ$_c$ chain, these signals elicit overlapping but distinct responses in various cells. Activation of naïve CD4 T cells by T-cell receptor and costimulatory molecules induces expression of IL-2, IL-2Rα, and IL-2Rβ$_c$, which leads to vigorous proliferation. Prolonged stimulation of T-cell receptor and IL-2R leads to expression of FasL and activation-induced cell death. Although IL-2 signaling facilitates the death of CD4 T cells in response to sustained exposure to antigen, IL-15 inhibits IL-2–mediated activation-induced cell death as it stimulates growth. Similarly, whereas IL-15 promotes proliferation of memory CD8 T cells, IL-2 inhibits it. IL-15 is also involved in the homeostatic survival of memory CD8 T cells, NK cells, and NK T cells. These contrasting biologic roles are illustrated by mice deficient in IL-2 or IL-2Rα that develop autoimmune disorders and mice deficient in IL-15 or IL-15Rα, which have lymphopenia and immune deficiencies. Thus, whereas IL-15 appears to have an important role in promoting effector functions of antigen-specific T cells, IL-2 is involved in reining in autoreactive T cells.[26]

Interleukin-4 and Interleukin-13: IL-4 and IL-13 are products of activated Th2 cells that share limited structural homology (~30%) and overlapping but distinct biologic activities. A specific receptor for IL-4, which does not bind IL-13, is found on T cells and NK cells. It consists of IL-4Rα (CD124) and γ$_c$ and transmits signals via JAK1 and JAK3. A second receptor complex that can bind either IL-4 or IL-13 is found on keratinocytes, endothelial cells, and other nonhematopoietic cells. It consists of IL-13Rα1 and IL-4Rα and transmits signals via JAK1 and JAK2. These receptors are expressed at low levels in resting cells, and their expression is increased by various activating signals. Curiously, whereas exposure of monocytes to IL-4 or IL-13 suppresses expression of IL-4Rα and IL-13Rα1, the opposite effect is observed in keratinocytes. Both signal transduction pathways appear to converge with the activation of STAT6, which is both necessary and sufficient to drive Th2 differentiation. IL-13Rα2 is a cell surface receptor homologous to IL-13Rα1 that specifically binds to IL-13 but is not known to transmit any signals.[25]

The biologic effects of engagement of the IL-4 receptor vary depending on the specific cell type but most pertain to its principal role as a growth and differentiation factor for Th2 cells. Exposure of naïve T cells to IL-4 stimulates them to proliferate and differentiate into Th2 cells, which produce more IL-4, which in turn leads to autocrine stimulation that prolongs Th2 responses. Thus, the expression of IL-4 early in the immune response can initiate a cascade of Th2 cell development that results in a predominately Th2 response. The genes encoding IL-4 and IL-13 are located in a cluster with IL-5 that undergoes structural changes during Th2 differentiation that are associated with increased expression. Although naïve T cells can make low levels of IL-4 when activated, IL-4 is also produced by activated NK T cells. Mast cells and basophils also release preformed IL-4 from secretory granules in response to FcεRI-mediated signals. A prominent activity of IL-4 is the stimulation of class switching of the immunoglobulin genes of B cells. Nuocytes and natural helper cells are recently identified populations of innate immune effector cells that provide an early source of IL-13 during helminth infection. As critical factors in Th2 differentiation and effector function, IL-4 and IL-13 are mediators of atopic immunity. Indeed, therapeutic targeting of IL-4 has proven beneficial in the treatment of atopic dermatitis.[27] In addition to controlling the behavior of effector cells, they also act directly on resident tissue cells, such as in inflammatory airway reactions.[28]

Interleukin-9 and Interleukin-21: IL-9 is a product of activated Th2 cells exposed to TGF-β that acts as an autocrine growth factor as well as a mediator of inflammation.[29] It is also produced by mast cells in response to IL-10 or stem cell factor. It stimulates proliferation of T and B cells and promotes expression of immunoglobulin E by B cells. It also exerts proinflammatory effects on mast cells and eosinophils. IL-9–deficient mice exhibit deficiencies in mast cell and goblet cell differentiation. IL-9 can be grouped with IL-4 and IL-13 as cytokines that function as effectors of allergic inflammatory processes and may play an important role in asthma and allergic disorders. However, recent evidence has emerged implicating the important role that IL-9 plays in mediate antimelanoma activity.[12,30] IL-21 is also a product made by the Th2, Th17, and Tfh lineages that signals through a receptor composed of a specific α chain (IL-21R) homologous to the IL-4R α chain and γ_c.[31] Absence of an intact IL-21 receptor is associated with impaired Th2 responses.[32]

Interleukin-7 and Thymic Stromal Lymphopoietin: Mutations abrogating the function of IL-7, IL-7Rα (CD127), γ_c, or JAK3 in mice or humans cause profound immunodeficiency as a result of T- and NK-cell depletion.[25] This is principally due to the indispensable role of IL-7 in promoting the expansion of lymphocytes and regulating the rearrangement of their antigen receptor genes. IL-7 is a potent mitogen and survival factor for immature lymphocytes in the bone marrow and thymus. The second function of IL-7 is as a modifier of effector cell functions in the reactive phase of certain immune responses. IL-7 transmits activating signals to mature T cells and certain activated B cells. Like IL-2, IL-7 has been shown to stimulate proliferation of cytolytic T cells and lymphokine-activated killer cells in vitro and to enhance their activities in vivo. IL-7 is a particularly significant cytokine for lymphocytes in the skin and other epithelial tissues. It is expressed by keratinocytes in a regulated fashion, and this expression is thought to be part of a reciprocal signaling dialog between dendritic epidermal T cells and keratinocytes in murine skin. Keratinocytes release IL-7 in response to IFN-γ, and dendritic epidermal T cells secrete IFN-γ in response to IL-7.

An IL-7–related cytokine using one chain of the IL-7 receptor as part of its receptor is thymic stromal lymphopoietin (TSLP). TSLP was originally identified as a novel cytokine produced by a thymic stromal cell line that could act as a growth factor for B- and T-lineage cells. The TSLP receptor consists of the IL-7Rα and a second receptor chain (TSLPR) homologous to but distinct from the γ_c chain. TSLP has attracted interest because of its ability to prime DCs to become stronger stimulators of Th2 cells. This activity may permit TSLP to foster the development of some types of allergic diseases.[33,34]

CYTOKINES WITH RECEPTORS USING THE INTERLEUKIN-3 RECEPTOR β CHAIN

The receptors for IL-3, IL-5, and GM-CSF consist of unique cytokine-specific α chains paired with a common β chain known as *IL-3Rβ* or β_c (CD131). Each of these factors acts on subsets of early hematopoietic cells.[35] IL-3, which was previously known as *multilineage colony-stimulating factor*, is principally a product of CD4+ T cells and causes proliferation, differentiation, and colony formation of various myeloid cells from bone marrow. IL-5 is a product of Th2 CD4+ cells and activated mast cells that conveys signals to B cells and eosinophils. IL-5 has a costimulatory effect on B cells in that it enhances their proliferation and immunoglobulin expression when they encounter their cognate antigen. In conjunction with an eosinophil-attracting chemokine known as *CC chemokine ligand 11* or *eotaxin*, IL-5 plays a central role in the accumulation of eosinophils that accompanies parasitic infections and some cutaneous inflammatory processes. IL-5 appears to be required to generate a pool of eosinophil precursors in bone marrow that can be rapidly mobilized to the blood, but eotaxin's role is focused on recruitment of these eosinophils from blood into specific tissue sites. GM-CSF is a growth factor for myeloid progenitors produced by activated T cells, phagocytes, keratinocytes, fibroblasts, and vascular endothelial cells. In addition to its role in early hematopoiesis, GM-CSF has potent effects on macrophages and DCs. In vitro culture of fresh LCs in the presence of GM-CSF promotes their transformation into mature DCs with maximal immunostimulatory potential for naïve T cells. The effects of GM-CSF on DCs probably account for the dramatic ability of GM-CSF to evoke therapeutic antitumor immunity when tumor cells are engineered to express it.[36,37]

INTERLEUKIN-6 AND OTHER CYTOKINES WITH RECEPTORS USING GLYCOPROTEIN 130

Receptors for a group of cytokines, including IL-6, IL-11, IL-27, leukemia inhibitory factor, oncostatin M, ciliary neurotrophic factor, and cardiotrophin-1, interact with a hematopoietin receptor family member, gp130, which does not appear to interact with any ligand by itself. The gp130 molecule is recruited into signaling complexes with other receptor chains when they engage their cognate ligands resulting in signal transduction.

IL-6 is the most thoroughly characterized of the cytokines that use gp130 for signaling and serves as a paradigm for discussion of the biologic effects of this family of cytokines. IL-6 is yet another example of a highly pleiotropic cytokine with multiple effects. A series of different names (including *IFN-β_2, B-cell stimulatory factor 2, plasmacytoma growth factor, cytotoxic T cell differentiation factor,* and *hepatocyte-stimulating factor*) were used for IL-6 before it was recognized that a single molecular species accounts for all of these activities. IL-6 acts on a wide variety of cells of hematopoietic origin. IL-6 stimulates immunoglobulin secretion by B cells and has mitogenic effects on B lineage cells and plasmacytomas. IL-6 also promotes maturation of megakaryocytes and differentiation of myeloid cells. Not only does it participate in hematopoietic development and reactive immune responses, but IL-6 is also a central mediator of the systemic acute-phase response. Increases in circulating IL-6 levels stimulate hepatocytes to synthesize and release acute-phase proteins.

There are two distinct signal transduction pathways triggered by IL-6. The first of these is mediated by the gp130 molecule when it dimerizes upon engagement by the complex of IL-6 and IL-6Rα. Homodimerization of gp130 and its associated JAK kinases (JAK1, JAK2, Tyk2) leads to activation of STAT3. A second pathway of gp130 signal transduction involves Ras and the mitogen-activated protein kinase cascade and results in phosphorylation and activation of a transcription factor originally designated *nuclear factor of IL-6*.

IL-6 is an important cytokine for skin and is subject to dysregulation in several human diseases, including some with skin manifestations. IL-6 is produced in a regulated fashion by keratinocytes, fibroblasts, and vascular endothelial cells as well as by leukocytes infiltrating the skin. IL-6 can stimulate the proliferation of human keratinocytes under some conditions. Psoriasis is one of several inflammatory skin diseases in which elevated expression of IL-6 has been described. Human herpesvirus 8 (HHV8) produces a viral homolog of IL-6 that may be involved in the pathogenesis of HHV8-associated diseases, including Kaposi sarcoma and body cavity–based lymphomas.

The other cytokines using gp130 as a signal transducer have diverse bioactivities. IL-11 inhibits production of inflammatory cytokines and has shown some therapeutic activity in patients with psoriasis. Exogenous IL-11 also stimulates platelet production and has been used to treat thrombocytopenia occurring after chemotherapy.

The IL-6 family member IL-31 has been recognized as an important mediator of cutaneous allergic diseases and atopic dermatitis, possibly through itch stimulation.[38] Major sources for IL-31 production are activated CD4+ T lymphocytes, in particular Th2 cells, mast cells, macrophages, and DCs. In contrast to all other IL-6 family members, IL-31 does not use gp130 as a receptor subunit. Rather, its cognate receptor complex is composed of the OSMRβ subunit and the IL-31RA subunit, which bears 28% sequence homology to gp130.[39] Serum IL-31 levels have been directly correlated with disease severity in atopic dermatitis, and animal models have demonstrated the role of IL-31 in the complex pathogenesis of itch symptoms in atopic dermatitis. Moreover, IL-31 acts directly to inhibit keratinocyte differentiation and filaggrin expression, thereby impairing skin barrier function in atopic dermatitis. Encouragingly, early trials of monoclonal antibodies targeting IL-31 in patients with atopic dermatitis have been efficacious in decreasing pruritus and sleeplessness. Further work on IL-31 may provide novel therapeutics for the treatment of atopic dermatitis and itch.

INTERLEUKIN-12, INTERLEUKIN 23, INTERLEUKIN-27, AND INTERLEUKIN-35: PIVOTAL CYTOKINES REGULATING T HELPER 1 AND T HELPER 17 RESPONSES

The IL-12 cytokine family includes IL-12, IL-23, IL-27, and IL-35. IL-12 is different from most other cytokines in that its active form is a heterodimer of two proteins, p35 and p40. IL-12 is principally a product of APCs such as DCs, monocytes, macrophages, and certain

B cells in response to bacterial components, GM-CSF, and IFN-γ. Whereas activated keratinocytes are an additional source of IL-12 in skin. Human keratinocytes constitutively make the p35 subunit, expression of the p40 subunit can be induced by stimuli including contact allergens, phorbol esters, and UV radiation.

IL-12 is a critical immunoregulatory cytokine that is central to the initiation and maintenance of Th1 responses. Th1 responses that are dependent on IL-12 provide protective immunity to intracellular bacterial pathogens. IL-12 also has stimulatory effects on NK cells, promoting their proliferation, cytotoxic function, and the production of cytokines, including IFN-γ. IL-12 has been shown to be active in stimulating protective antitumor immunity in a number of animal models.[40]

Two chains that are part of the cell surface receptor for IL-12 have been cloned. Both are homologous to other β chains in the hematopoietin receptor family and are designated β1 and β2. The β1 chain is associated with Tyk2 and the β2 chain interacts directly with JAK2. The signaling component of the IL-12R is the β2 chain. The β2 chain is expressed in Th1 but not Th2 cells and appears to be critical for commitment of T cells to production of type 1 cytokines. IL-12 signaling induces the phosphorylation of STAT1, STAT3, and STAT4, but STAT4 is essential for induction of a Th1 response.

IL-23 is a heterodimeric cytokine in the IL-12 family that consists of the p40 chain of IL-12 in association with a distinct p19 chain. IL-23 has overlapping activities with IL-12 but also induces proliferation of memory T cells. Interest in IL-23 has been sparked by the observation that IL-23 promotes the differentiation of T cells producing IL-17 (Th17 subset). The IL-23 receptor consists of two chains: (1) the IL-12Rβ1 chain that forms part of the IL-12 receptor and (2) a specific IL-23 receptor.[41]

The third member of the IL-12 family to be discovered was IL-27. IL-27 is also a heterodimer and consists of a subunit called *p28* that is homologous to IL-12 p35 and a second subunit known as *EBI3* that is homologous to IL-12 p40. IL-27 plays a role in the early induction of the Th1 response. The IL-27 receptor consists of a receptor called *WSX-1* that associates with the shared signal-transducing molecule gp130.[41,42]

The newest member of the IL-12 family is IL-35. The IL-35 heterodimer is composed of the p35 chain of IL-12 associated with the IL-27β chain EBI3. In contrast to the other IL-12 family cytokines, IL-35 is selectively made by Treg cells, promotes the growth of Treg cells, and suppresses the activity of Th17 cells.[43]

The IL-12 family of cytokines has emerged as a promising new target for anticytokine pharmacotherapy. The approach that has been developed the furthest to date is targeting both IL-12 and IL-23 with monoclonal antibodies directed against the p40 subunit that is part of both cytokines. Ustekinumab is an antihuman p40 monoclonal antibody that has shown therapeutic activity against psoriasis comparable to that of TNF inhibitors and has received FDA approval for the treatment of psoriasis.[44] The development of anti-p40 therapies is several years behind anti-TNF-α drugs, but development of additional anti-p40 biologics for clinical use is anticipated. Novel therapies targeting p19, which would specifically block IL-23, are also in development for clinical use in psoriasis.

LIGANDS OF THE CLASS II FAMILY OF CYTOKINE RECEPTORS

A second major class of cytokine receptors with common features includes two types of receptors for IFNs, IL-10R, and the receptors for additional IL-10-related cytokines, including IL-19, IL-20, IL-22, IL-24, and IL-26.

Interferons: Prototypes of Cytokines Signaling through a JAK/STAT Pathway:

IFNs were one of the first families of cytokines to be characterized in detail. The IFNs were initially subdivided into three classes: (1) IFN-α (the leukocyte IFNs), (2) IFN-β (fibroblast IFN), and (3) IFN-γ (immune IFN). The α and β IFNs are collectively called *type I IFNs*, and all of these molecules signal through the same two-chain receptor (the IFN-αβ receptor).[45] The second IFN receptor is a distinct two-chain receptor specific for IFN-γ. Both of these IFN receptors are present on many cell types within skin as well as in other tissues. Each of the chains comprising the two IFN receptors is associated with one of the JAK kinases (Tyk2 and JAK1 for the IFN-αβR, and JAK1 and JAK2 for the IFN-γR). Only in the presence of both chains and two functional JAK kinases will effective signal transduction occur after IFN binding. A new class of IFNs known as *IFN-λ* or *type III IFNs* has now been identified that has a low degree of homology with both type I IFNs and IL-10.[46] The current members of this class are IL-28A, IL-28B, and IL-29. Although the effects of these cytokines are similar to those of the type I IFNs, they are less potent. These type III IFNs use a shared receptor that consists of the β chain of the IL-10 receptor associated with an IL-28 receptor α chain.

Viruses, double-stranded RNA, and bacterial products are among the stimuli that elicit release of the type I IFNs from cells. Plasmacytoid DCs have emerged as a particularly potent cellular source of type I IFNs. Many of the effects of the type I IFNs directly or indirectly increase host resistance to the spread of viral infection. Additional effects mediated through IFN-αβR are increased expression of major histocompatibility complex (MHC) class I molecules and stimulation of NK cell activity. Not only does it have well-known antiviral effects, but IFN-α also can modulate T-cell responses by favoring the development of a Th1 type of T-cell response. Finally, the type I IFNs also inhibit the proliferation of a variety of cell types, which provides a rationale for their use in the treatment of some types of cancer. Forms of IFN-α enjoy considerable use clinically for indications ranging from hairy cell leukemia, various cutaneous malignancies, and papillomavirus infections. Some of the same conditions that respond to therapy with type I IFNs also respond to topical immunomodulatory agents such as imiquimod. This synthetic imidazoquinoline drug is an agonist for the TLR7 receptor, whose natural ligand is single-stranded RNA. Imiquimod stimulation of cells expressing TLR7 elicits local release of large amounts of type I IFNs from plasmacytoid DCs, which can trigger clinically useful antiviral and tumor inhibitory effects against genital warts, superficial basal cell carcinoma, and actinic keratoses. Resiquimod is a related synthetic compound that activates both TLR7 and TLR8, eliciting a slightly different spectrum of cytokines.[47]

Production of IFN-γ is restricted to NK cells, CD8 T cells, and Th1 CD4 T cells. Th1 cells produce IFN-γ after engagement of the T-cell receptor, and IL-12 can provide a strong costimulatory signal for T-cell IFN-γ production. NK cells produce IFN-γ in response to cytokines released by macrophages, including TNF-γ, IL-12, and IL-18. IFN-γ has antiviral activity, but it is a less potent mediator than the type I IFNs for induction of these effects. The major physiologic role of IFN-γ is its capacity to modulate immune responses. IFN-γ induces synthesis of multiple proteins that play essential roles in antigen presentation to T cells, including MHC class I and class II glycoproteins, invariant chain, the Lmp2 and Lmp7 components of the proteasome, and the TAP1 and TAP2 intracellular peptide transporters. These changes increase the efficiency of antigen presentation to CD4 and CD8 T cells. IFN-γ is also required for activation of macrophages to their full antimicrobial potential, enabling them to eliminate microorganisms capable of intracellular growth. Similar to type I IFNs, IFN-γ also has strong antiproliferative effects on some cell types. Finally, IFN-γ is also an inducer of selected chemokines (CXC chemokine ligands 9 to 11) and an inducer of endothelial cell adhesion molecules (eg, ICAM-1 and VCAM-1). Because of the breadth of IFN-γ's activities, it comes the closest of the T-cell cytokines to behaving as a primary cytokine.

Interleukin-10: An "Antiinflammatory" Cytokine: IL-10 is one of several cytokines that primarily exert regulatory rather than stimulatory effects on immune responses. IL-10 was first identified as a cytokine produced by Th2 T cells that inhibited cytokine production after activation of T cells by antigen and APCs. IL-10 exerts its action through a cell surface receptor found on macrophages, DCs, neutrophils, B cells, T cells, and NK cells. The ligand-binding chain of the receptor is homologous to the receptors for IFN-α/β and IFN-γ, and signaling events mediated through the IL-10 receptor use a JAK/STAT pathway. IL-10 binding to its receptor activates the JAK1 and Tyk2 kinases and leads to the activation of STAT1 and STAT3. The effects of IL-10 on APCs such as monocytes, macrophages, and DCs include inhibition of expression of class II MHC and costimulatory molecules (eg, B7–1, B7–2) and decreased production of T cell-stimulating cytokines (eg, IL-1, IL-6, and IL-12). At least four viral genomes harbor viral homologs of IL-10 that transmit similar signals by binding to the IL-10R.[48]

A major source of IL-10 within skin is epidermal keratinocytes. Keratinocyte IL-10 production is upregulated after activation; one of the best-characterized activating stimuli for keratinocytes is UV irradiation. UV radiation–induced keratinocyte IL-10 production leads to local and systemic effects on immunity. Some of the well-documented immunosuppressive effects that occur after UV light exposure are the result of the liberation of keratinocyte-derived IL-10 into the systemic circulation. IL-10 also likely plays a dampening role in other types of cutaneous immune and inflammatory responses because the absence of IL-10 predisposes mice to exaggerated irritant and contact sensitivity responses.

Novel Interleukin-10–Related Cytokines: Interleukins 19, 20, 22, 24, and 26: A series of cytokines related to IL-10 have been identified and shown to engage a number of receptor complexes with shared chains.[49] IL-19, IL-20, IL-24, and IL-26 transmit signals via a complex consisting of IL-20Rα and IL-20Rβ. IL-22 signals through a receptor consisting of IL-22R and IL-10Rβ. The receptors for these IL-20 family cytokines are preferentially expressed on epithelial cells including keratinocytes. Increased expression of these cytokines and their receptors is associated with psoriasis. The IL-20 family cytokines have profound effects on the proliferation and differentiation of human keratinocytes in culture.[50] Transgenic mice overexpressing IL-20, IL-22, or IL-24 develop epidermal hyperplasia and abnormal keratinocyte differentiation.[51] All of these findings point to a significant role for these cytokines in the epidermal changes associated with cutaneous inflammation. T cells producing IL-22 that elaborate a distinct set of cytokines from Th1, Th2, and Th17 cells have been isolated from the epidermis of patients with psoriasis and other inflammatory skin disorders. The IL-22 produced by these T cells promotes keratinocyte proliferation and epidermal acanthosis.[52,53] IL-26 is produced by T cells, in particular Th17 cells, NK cells, and macrophages, and has been demonstrated to play an important role in mediating proinflammatory signals in inflammatory bowel disease and rheumatoid arthritis. However, a novel functional characteristic of IL-26 has also been established. IL-26 has structural properties uniquely reminiscent of antimicrobial peptides (AMPs). Analogous to canonical AMPs, the cationic and amphipathic nature of IL-26 allows it to kill select gram-negative bacteria, including *Pseudomonas aeruginosa*, *Klebsiella pneumoniae*, and *Escherichia coli*, as well as gram-positive *S. aureus* at effector concentrations similar to traditional AMPs. Therefore, a more nuanced role for these cytokines is emerging.

TRANSFORMING GROWTH FACTOR-β FAMILY AND ITS RECEPTORS

TGF-β1 was first isolated as a secreted product of virally transformed tumor cells capable of inducing normal cells in vitro to show phenotypic characteristics associated with transformation. More than 30 additional members of the TGF-β family of cytokines have now been identified. They can be grouped into several families: the prototypic TGF-βs (TGF-β1 to TGF-β3), the bone morphogenetic proteins, the growth and differentiation factors, and the activins. The TGF name for this family of molecules is somewhat of a misnomer because TGF-β has antiproliferative rather than proliferative effects on most cell types. Many of the TGF-β family members play an important role in development, influencing the differentiation of uncommitted cells into specific lineages. TGF-β family members are made as precursor proteins that are biologically inactive until a large prodomain is cleaved. Monomers of the mature domain of TGF-β family members are disulfide linked to form dimers that strongly resist denaturation.

Participation of at least two cell surface receptors (type I and type II) with serine/threonine kinase activity is required for biologic effects of TGF-β.[54] Ligand binding by the type II receptor (the true ligand-binding receptor) is associated with the formation of complexes of type I and type II receptors. This allows the type II receptor to phosphorylate and activate the type I receptor, a "transducer" molecule that is responsible for downstream signal transduction. Downstream signal transmission from the membrane-bound receptors in the TGF-β receptor family to the nucleus is primarily mediated by a family of cytoplasmic Smad proteins that translocate to the nucleus and regulate transcription of target genes.

TGF-β has a profound influence on several types of immune and inflammatory processes. An immunoregulatory role for TGF-β1 was identified in part through analysis of TGF-β1 knockout mice that develop a wasting disease at 20 days of age associated with a mixed inflammatory cell infiltrate involving many internal organs. This phenotype is now appreciated to be a result in part of the compromised development of regulatory T cells when TGF-β1 is not available. Development of cells in the DC lineage is also perturbed in the TGF-β1–deficient mice, as evidenced by an absence of epidermal LCs and specific subpopulations of LN DCs. TGF-β–treated fibroblasts display enhanced production of collagen and other extracellular matrix molecules. In addition, TGF-β inhibits the production of metalloproteinases by fibroblasts and stimulates the production of inhibitors of the same metalloproteinases (tissue inhibitors of metalloproteinase, or TIMPs). TGF-β may contribute to the immunopathology of scleroderma through its profibrogenic effects.[55]

THERAPEUTIC IMPLICATIONS BASED ON CYTOKINE BIOLOGY

Cytokines and cytokine antagonists are being used therapeutically by clinicians, and development of additional agents continues, with a few specific examples described in the previous sections. Cytokine-based therapeutics may offer a more targeted approach to disrupting the underlying disease process; however, their immunosuppressive properties may increase the risk of infections and malignancy. Examples of successful therapeutic targeting of cytokines in a number of cutaneous disorders will be discussed.

TNF-α blockade has proven to be efficacious in the treatment of plaque psoriasis. Patients with active skin disease have elevated levels of TNF-α in both blood and lesional skin. More recently, the efficacy of TNF-α inhibitors in treating psoriasis has been attributed to their inhibition of Th17 cells.[56] The TNF-α antagonists approved to treat psoriasis include infliximab and adalimumab (anti–TNF-α monoclonal antibodies) and etanercept (a human TNF receptor 2 Fc fusion protein). All three agents bind to both soluble and transmembrane forms of TNF-α, interrupting TNF-α–mediated inflammatory pathways. Despite their utility clinically, these agents should be monitored closely when prescribed to patients given the risk of serious infections (eg, tuberculosis) and the potential for increased risk of malignancies or major adverse cardiovascular events.

Ustekinumab, an approved treatment for moderate to severe plaque psoriasis, is a fully human IgG1κ monoclonal antibody with high affinity and specificity for the common p40 subunit shared by IL-12 and IL-23. Increased levels of IL-23 and Th17 cytokines have been detected in human psoriatic skin, and IL-23 has been shown to induce psoriasis-like skin inflammation in mice.[57] Ustekinumab has been successful in the treatment of moderate to severe plaque psoriasis, with superior efficacy over etanercept demonstrated in the ACCEPT trial.[44] Ustekinumab has also been shown to achieve sustained clinical responses with a favorable safety profile for up to 4 years of treatment in the PHOENIX 1 and 2 trials.[58] Evidence is accumulating to suggest that IL-23 and its resulting Th17 pathway play a more important role in psoriasis than IL-12. Indeed, selective inhibition of the IL-23-specific p19 subunit improves psoriasis. Currently, there are multiple antibody-based therapeutics targeting p19 in phase III development for the treatment of psoriasis with encouraging results. Neutralization of IL-23 results in decreased numbers of skin infiltrating T cells, DCs, and neutrophils, while epidermal LCs remain unaffected.[59] Further investigation is required to fully define the role of IL-23 in the pathogenesis of psoriasis; however, the clinical results of selective IL-23 inhibition have been, thus far, promising.

IL-17 is a key cytokine in the pathogenesis of psoriasis at the keratinocyte level.[60] As such, there is heightened interest in exploiting the IL-17 cytokine axis in the treatment of psoriasis. Secukinumab and ixekizumab are human monoclonal antibodies that target IL-17A and are approved for the treatment of moderate to severe plaque psoriasis. In two phase III clinical trials, ERASURE and FIXTURE, secukinumab was proven to be efficacious in the treatment of plaque psoriasis, with superior efficacy over etanercept demonstrated in the FIXTURE trial.[61] Two phase 3 trials, UNCOVER-2 and

UNCOVER-3, showed that ixekizumab was superior to placebo and etanercept in the treatment of moderate to severe plaque psoriasis.[62] Brodalumab is a human IgG2 monoclonal antibody that binds to and blocks the IL-17 receptor and is currently undergoing the approval process for the treatment of psoriasis.

Apremilast is a novel small molecule inhibitor of phosphodiesterase 4 (PD-4) that has been recently approved for the treatment of moderate to severe plaque psoriasis and psoriatic arthritis. PD-4 is expressed predominantly in immune cells, including DCs, neutrophils, and monocytes but also in keratinocytes. Normally, PD-4 causes degradation of the secondary messenger cyclic AMP, leading to increased production of proinflammatory soluble mediators such as TNF-α, IL- 2, -12 and -23, and chemokine ligands 9 (CXCL9) and 10 (CXCL10).[63] Therefore, PD-4 inhibition by apremilast results in the reduction of proinflammatory cytokine and chemokine production. Indeed, the phase III trials, ESTEEM 1 and ESTEEM 2 demonstrated favorable efficacy and safety of apremilast compared with placebo in patients with moderate to severe plaque psoriasis.[64] Further investigation of the safety profile with long-term use is needed.

Tofacitinib, a novel oral JAK inhibitor, disrupts cytokine signaling through inhibition of JAK1 and JAK3, leading to altered lymphocyte function. There is excitement in developing tofacitinib as a viable therapeutic option for psoriasis, alopecia areata, and dermatomyositis because cytokine signaling through the JAK-STAT pathway is a major component in cutaneous inflammatory disorders. A recent phase II clinical trial demonstrated clinical improvement in psoriasis patients treated with tofacitinib compared with placebo.[65] Serendipitously, a patient with concurrent psoriasis and alopecia areata treated with tofacitinib for his psoriasis noted improvement in his alopecia as well.[66] Subsequently, a larger cohort of 90 patients with alopecia areata who were treated with tofacitinib was published, with 77% of patients achieving clinical improvement.[67] Furthermore, tofacitinib and ruxolitinib, a JAK1 and JAK2 inhibitor, respectively, have been beneficial in the treatment of dermatomyositis.[19,20] Further investigations with rigorous trials is warranted to fully evaluate the efficacy of tofacitinib in the treatment of inflammatory skin disorders.

Dupilumab is a monoclonal antibody in development for the treatment of adult patients with inadequately controlled moderate to severe atopic dermatitis. It is directed against the α-subunit of the IL-4 receptor, and through this effect blocks IL-4 and IL-13, the drivers of Th2-mediated inflammation responsible for the hallmark symptoms of atopic dermatitis. In two randomized, placebo-controlled, phase 3 trials, SOLO 1 and SOLO 2, dupilumab improved the signs and symptoms of atopic dermatitis in adult patients, including pruritus, anxiety, depression, and quality of life, compared with placebo.[27] Studies are ongoing to access the efficacy and safety of dupilumab in the pediatric population and for the treatment of asthma.

Therapeutic blockade of the IL-22–IL-22R axis has the potential to be a viable area of development in the treatment of atopic dermatitis and psoriasis. In animal models of psoriasis, IL-22 deficiency and blockade resulted in reduction of disease burden.[68] However, the initial clinical trials evaluating antihuman IL-22 antibodies have been disappointing. Therefore, the effect of inhibiting the IL-22–IL-22R pathway in psoriasis remains to be determined. In atopic dermatitis, IL-22–producing T cells appear to play a significant role in mediating disease.[69] As such, there are ongoing efforts to develop IL-22 inhibitors in the treatment of atopic dermatitis.

With certain notable exceptions, systemic cytokine therapy has been disappointing and is often accompanied by substantial morbidity. As an example, high-dose intravenous recombinant IL-2 for patients with metastatic melanoma results in low response rates (~6%) and significant morbidity occurring because of drug toxicity. Moreover, the use of high-dose IFN-α2b as adjuvant therapy for high-risk surgically resected melanoma (stage IIB or III) produced sustained improvement in relapse-free survival; however, the therapy also results in significant morbidity. More recently, however, low-dose IL-2 has proven to be beneficial in the treatment of chronic graft-versus-host disease.[70] Although current cytokine-based therapies are limited, a better understanding of cytokine biology will lead to the development and enhancement of clinical efficacious therapies.

There is increasing evidence to support the use of cytokines and cytokine antagonists for the treatment of a range of dermatologic disorders. However, this will require an understanding of the fundamental biology governing inflammatory responses at cutaneous tissues. Further investigation is needed to establish the efficacy and safety of the biological therapies currently available and to support the development of new treatments options.

CHEMOKINES: SECONDARY CYTOKINES CENTRAL TO LEUKOCYTE MOBILIZATION

Although cytokines help coordinate the different cellular mediators of an inflammatory response, chemokines, a large superfamily of small cytokines, have two major specialized functions. First, they guide leukocytes via chemotactic gradients in tissue. Typically, this is to bring an effector cell to where its activities are required. Second, a subset of chemokines has the capacity to increase the binding of leukocytes via their integrins to ligands at the endothelial cell surface, which facilitates firm adhesion and extravasation of leukocytes in tissue. Therefore, an appreciation of chemokine biology is critical because it plays an important role in skin development, immunity, inflammation, and cancer.

An overview of the structure of chemokines and chemokine receptors will be provided that will detail the molecular signaling pathways initiated by the binding of a chemokine to its cognate receptor. Expression patterns of chemokine receptors will be highlighted because of the many types of immune cells that potentially can be recruited to skin under inflammatory conditions. Individual chemokine receptors will be highlighted in regard to biologic function, including facilitation of migration of effector T cells into the skin and the egress of APCs out of the skin. Finally, the roles of chemokines and their receptors in several cutaneous diseases—atopic dermatitis, psoriasis, cancer, and infectious disease—provide a better idea of the diversity of chemokine function in skin.

STRUCTURE OF CHEMOKINES

Chemokines are grouped into four subfamilies based on the spacing of amino acids between the first two cysteines. The CXC chemokines (also called α-chemokines) show a C–X–C motif with one nonconserved amino acid between the two cysteines. The other major subfamily of chemokines lacks the additional amino acid and is termed the CC subfamily (or β-chemokines). The two remaining subfamilies contain only one member each: the C subfamily is represented by lymphotactin, and fractalkine is the only member of the CXXXC (or CX3C) subfamily. Chemokines can also be assigned to one of two broad and, perhaps, overlapping functional groups. One group (eg, regulated upon activation, normal T cell expressed and secreted [RANTES], macrophage inflammatory protein (MIP)-1α/β liver and activation-regulated chemokine [LARC]) mediates the attraction and recruitment of immune cells to sites of active inflammation, but others (eg, secondary lymphoid-tissue chemokine (SLC) and stromal-derived factor-1 [SDF-1]) appear to play a role in constitutive or homeostatic migration pathways.[71]

The complexity and redundancy in the nomenclature of chemokines has led to the proposal for a systematic nomenclature for chemokines based on the type of chemokine (C, CXC, CX3C, or CC) and a number based on the order of discovery as proposed by Zlotnik and Yoshie.[71] For example, SDF-1, a CXC chemokine, has the systematic name CXCL12. Because both nomenclatures are still in wide use, the original names (abbreviated in most cases) as well as systematic names will be used interchangeably. Table 12-4 provides a list of chemokine receptors of interest in skin that are discussed as well as the major chemokine ligands that bind to them.

Chemokines are highly conserved and have similar secondary and tertiary structure. Based on crystallography studies, a disordered amino terminus followed by three conserved antiparallel β-pleated sheets is a common structural feature of chemokines. Fractalkine is unique in that the chemokine domain sits atop a mucin-like stalk tethered to the plasma membrane via a transmembrane domain and short cytoplasmic tail.[72] Although CXC and CC chemokines form multimeric structures under conditions required for structural studies, these associations may be relevant only when chemokines associate with cell-surface components such as glycosaminoglycans (GAGs) or proteoglycans. Because most chemokines have a net positive charge, these proteins tend to bind to negatively charged carbohydrates present on GAGs. Indeed, the ability of positively charged chemokines to bind to GAGs is thought to enable chemokines to preferentially associate with the luminal surface of blood vessels despite the presence of shear forces from the blood that would otherwise wash away the chemokines.

CHEMOKINE RECEPTORS AND SIGNAL TRANSDUCTION

Chemokine receptors are seven transmembrane spanning membrane proteins that couple to intracellular heterotrimeric G-proteins containing α, β, and γ subunits.[71] They represent a part of a large family of G protein–coupled receptors (GPCR), including rhodopsin, that have critical biologic functions. Leukocytes express several Gα protein subtypes—s, i, and q—and the β and γ subunits each have 5 and 11 known subtypes, respectively. This complexity in the formation of the heterotrimeric G protein may account for specificity in the action of certain chemokine receptors. Normally G proteins are inactive when guanosine diphosphate (GDP) is bound, but they are activated when the GDP is exchanged for guanosine triphosphate (GTP) (Fig. 12-8). After binding to a ligand, chemokine receptors rapidly associate with G-proteins, which in turn increases the exchange of GTP for GDP. Pertussis toxin is a commonly used inhibitor of GPCR that irreversibly ADP-ribosylates Gα subunits of the α_i class and subsequently prevents most chemokine receptor–mediated signaling.

Activation of G proteins leads to the dissociation of the G_α and $G_{\beta\gamma}$ subunits (see Fig. 12-6). The G_α subunit has been observed to activate protein tyrosine kinases and mitogen-activated protein kinase, leading to cytoskeletal changes and gene transcription. The G_α subunit retains GTP, which is slowly hydrolyzed by the GTPase activity of this subunit. This GTPase activity is both positively and negatively regulated by GTPase-activating proteins (also known as regulator of G-protein signaling [RGS] proteins). The $G_{\beta\gamma}$ dimer initiates critical signaling events in regard to chemotaxis and cell adhesion. It activates phospholipase C (PLC),[73] leading to formation of diacylglycerol (DAG) and inositol triphosphate (Ins[1,4,5]P$_3$). Ins(1,4,5)P$_3$ stimulates Ca^{2+} entry into the cytosol, which along with DAG, activates protein kinase C isoforms. Whereas the $G_{\beta\gamma}$ subunits have been shown to be critical for chemotaxis, the G_α subunit has no known role

TABLE 12-4
Chemokine Receptors in Skin Biology

CHEMOKINE RECEPTOR	CHEMOKINE LIGAND	EXPRESSION PATTERN	COMMENTS
CCR1	MIP-1 (CCL3), RANTES (CCL5), MCP-3 (CCL7)	T, Mo, DC, NK, B	Migration of DCs and monocytes; strongly upregulated in T cells by IL-2
CCR2	MCP-1 (CCL2), -3, -4 (CCL13)	T, Mo	Migration of T cells to inflamed sites; replenish LC precursors in epidermis; involved in skin fibrosis via MCP-1
CCR3	Eotaxin (CCL11) > RANTES, MCP-2 (CCL8), 3,4	Eo, Ba, Th2, K	Migration of Th2 cells and "allergic" immune cells
CCR4	TARC (CCL17), MDC (CCL22)	T (benign and malignant)	Expression in Th2 > Th1 cells; highly expressed on CLA+ memory T cells; TARC expression by keratinocytes may be important in atopic dermatitis; may guide trafficking of malignant as well as benign inflammatory T cells
CCR5	RANTES, MIP-1, (CCL3,4)	T, Mo, DC	Marker for Th1 cells; migration to acutely inflamed sites; may be involved in transmigration of T cells through endothelium; major HIV-1 fusion coreceptor
CCR6	LARC (CCL20)	T, DC, B	Expressed by memory, not naïve, T cells; possibly involved in arrest of memory T cells to activated endothelium and recruitment of T cells to epidermis in psoriasis
CCR7	SLC (CCL21), ELC (CCL 19)	T, DC, B, melanoma cells	Critical for migration of naïve T cells and "central memory" T cells to secondary lymphoid organs; required for mature DCs to enter lymphatics and localize to lymph nodes; facilitates nodal metastasis
CCR9	Thymus-expressed chemokine (CCL25)	T, melanoma cells	Associated with melanoma small bowel metastases
CCR10	CTACK (CCL27)	T (benign and malignant), melanoma cells	Preferential response of CLA+ T cells to CTACK in vitro; may be involved in T cell (benign as well as malignant) homing to epidermis, where CTACK is expressed; survival of melanoma is skin
CXCR1,2	IL-8 (CXCL8), MGSA/GRO (CXCL1), ENA-78 (CXCL5)	N, NK, En, melanoma cells	Recruitment of neutrophils (eg, epidermis in psoriasis); may be involved in angiogenesis; melanoma growth factor
CXCR3	IP-10 (CXCL10), Mig (CXCL9), I-TAC (CXCL11)	T	Marker for Th1 cells and may be involved in T cell recruitment to epidermis in CTCL; includes arrest of activated T cells on stimulated endothelium
CXCR4	SDF-1, (CXCL12)	T, DC, En, melanoma cells	Major HIV-1 fusion coreceptor; involved in vascular formation; involved in melanoma metastasis to lungs
CX3CR1	Fractalkine (CX3CL1)	T, Mo, MC, NK	May be involved in adhesion on activated T cells, Mo, NK cells to activated endothelium

B, B cells; Ba, basophils; CLA, cutaneous lymphocyte-associated antigen; CTACK, cutaneous T cell attracting chemokine; DC, dendritic cells; En, endothelial cells; Eo, eosinophils; GRO, growth regulated oncogene; HIV, human immunodeficiency virus; IL-8, interleukin-8; I-TaC, interferon-inducible T-cell alpha chemoattractant; LARC, liver and activation-regulated chemokine (also known as MIP-3); MC, mast cell; MCP, monocyte chemoattractant protein; MDC, macrophage-derived chemokine; MGSA, melanoma growth stimulatory activity; Mig, monokine-induced by IFN-; MIP, macrophage inflammatory protein; Mo, monocytes; N, neutrophils; NK, natural killer cell; RANTES, regulated upon activation, normal T cell expressed and secreted; SDF, stromal-derived factor; SLC, secondary lymphoid-tissue chemokine; T, T cells; TARC, thymus and activation-regulated chemokine; Th1,2, T helper 1,2 cell.

in chemotactic migration. There is also evidence that binding of chemokine receptors results in the activation of other intracellular effectors, including Ras and Rho, phosphatidylinositol-3-kinase (PI[3]K).[74]

RhoA and protein kinase C appear to play a role in integrin affinity changes, and PI(3)K may be critical for changes in the avidity state of lymphocyte function-associated antigen 1 (LFA-1). Other proteins have been found that regulate the synthesis, expression, or degradation of GPCRs. For example, receptor-activity-modifying proteins (RAMPS) act as chaperones of seven transmembrane spanning receptors and regulate surface expression as well as the ligand specificity of chemokine receptors (see Fig. 12-8). Importantly, after chemokine receptors are exposed to appropriate ligands, they are frequently internalized, leading to an inability of the chemokine receptor to mediate further signaling. This downregulation of chemokine function, which has been termed "desensitization," occurs because of phosphorylation of Ser/Thr residues in the C-terminal tail by proteins termed GPCR kinases and subsequent internalization of the receptor (see Fig. 12-8). Desensitization may be an important mechanism for regulating the function of chemokine receptors by inhibiting cell migration as leukocytes arrive at the primary site of inflammation.

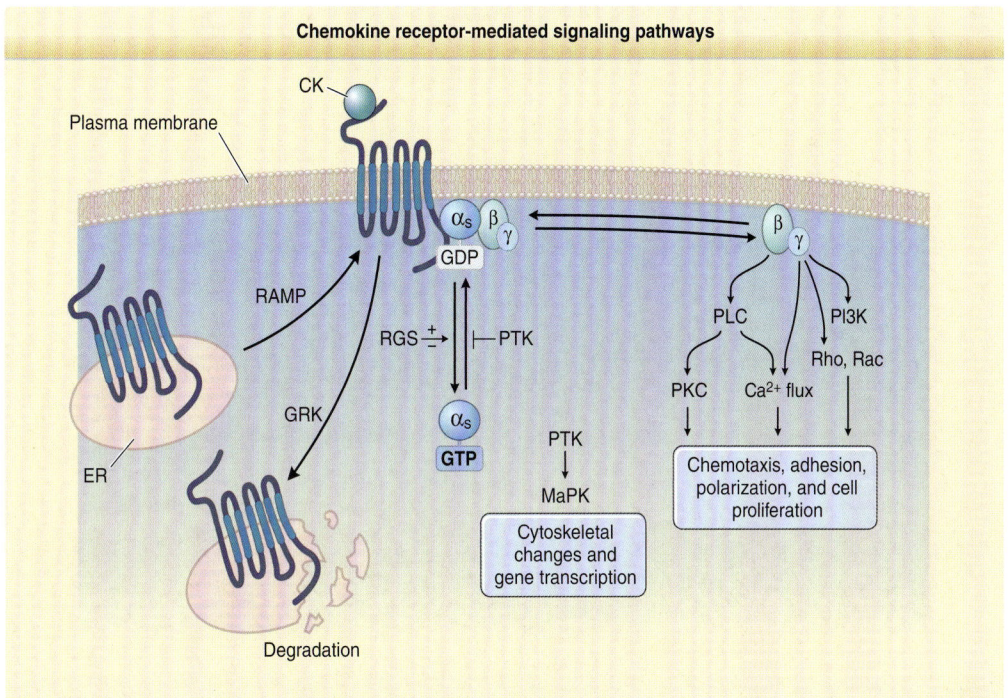

Figure 12-8 Chemokine receptor-mediated signaling pathways. CK, chemokine; DG, 1,2-diacylglycerol; ER, endoplasmic reticulum; GRK, G-protein coupled receptor kinase; IP3, inositol-1,4,5-triphosphate; MAPK, Mitogen activated protein kinase; PIP2, phosphatidylinositol-4,5-bisphosphate; PKC, protein kinase C; PLC, phospholipase C; PTK, protein tyrosine kinase(s); PTX, pertussis toxin; RAMP, receptor-activity-modifying protein; RGS, regulator of G-protein signaling.

CHEMOKINES AND CUTANEOUS LEUKOCYTE TRAFFICKING

Generally speaking, chemokines are thought to play at least three different roles in the recruitment of host defense cells, predominantly leukocytes, to sites of inflammation.[75] First, they provide the signal or signals required to cause leukocytes to come to a complete stop (ie, arrest) in blood vessels at inflamed sites such as skin. Second, chemokines have been shown to have a role in the transmigration of leukocytes from the luminal side of the blood vessel to the abluminal side. Third, chemokines attract leukocytes to sites of inflammation in the dermis or epidermis following transmigration. Keratinocytes and endothelial cells are a rich source of chemokines when stimulated by appropriate cytokines. In addition, chemokines and their receptors are known to play critical roles in the emigration of resident skin DCs (ie, LCs and dermal DCs) from the skin to draining LN via afferent lymphatic vessels, a process that is essential for the development of acquired immune responses.

This section is divided into three subsections. The first introduces basic concepts of how all leukocytes arrest in inflamed blood vessels before transmigration by introducing the multistep model of leukocyte recruitment. The second details mechanisms of T-cell migration, and the final subsection focuses on the mechanisms by which chemokines mediate the physiological migration of DCs from the skin to regional LNs.

THE MULTISTEP MODEL OF LEUKOCYTE RECRUITMENT

For leukocytes to adhere and migrate to peripheral tissues, they must overcome the pushing force of the vascular blood stream as they bind to activated endothelial cells at local sites of inflammation. According to the multistep or cascade model of leukocyte recruitment (Fig. 12-9), one set of homologous adhesion molecules termed *selectins* mediates the transient attachment of leukocytes to endothelial cells, and another set of adhesion molecules termed *integrins* and their receptors (*immunoglobulin superfamily members*) mediates stronger binding (ie, arrest) and transmigration.[76] The selectins (E-, L-, and P-selectins) are members of a larger family of carbohydrate-binding proteins termed lectins. The selectins bind their respective carbohydrate ligands located on protein scaffolds and thus mediate the transient binding or "rolling" of leukocytes on endothelial cells.

The skin-associated vascular selectin known as E-selectin is upregulated on endothelial cells by inflam-

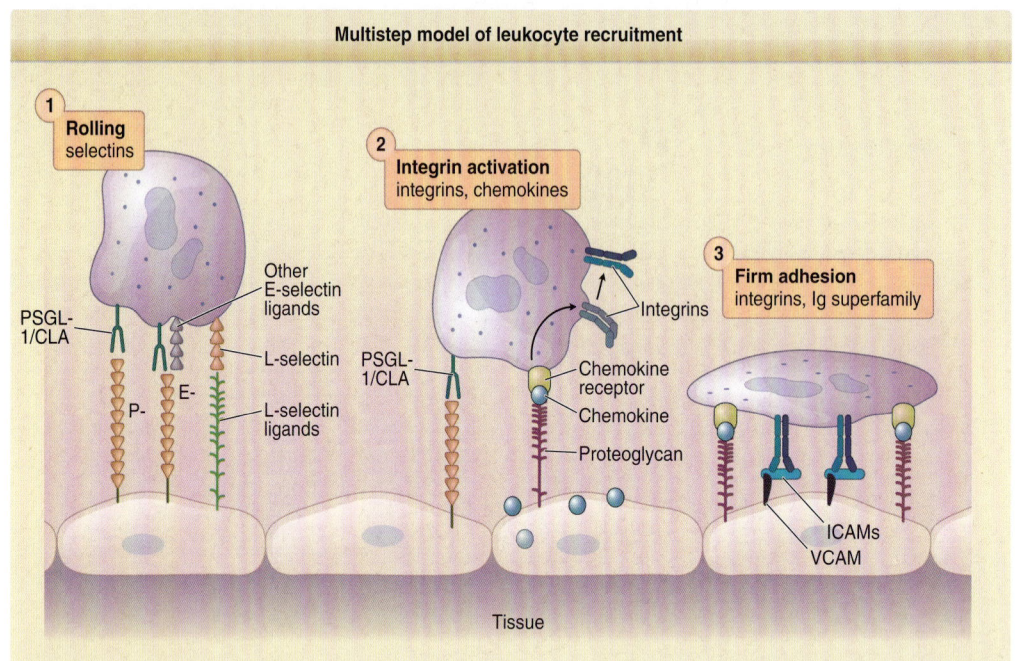

Figure 12-9 Multistep model of leukocyte recruitment. Leukocytes, pushed by the bloodstream, first transiently bind or "roll" on the surface of activated endothelial cells via rapid interactions with P-, E-, or L-selectin. Chemokines are secreted by endothelial cells and bind to proteoglycans that present the chemokine molecules to chemokine receptors on the surface of the leukocyte. After chemokine receptor ligation, intracellular signaling events lead to a change in the conformation of integrins and changes in their distribution on the plasma membrane, resulting in "integrin activation." These changes result in high-affinity and -avidity binding of integrins to endothelial cell intercellular adhesion molecules (ICAMs) and vascular cell adhesion molecule-1 (VCAM-1) in a step termed "firm adhesion," which is then followed by transmigration of the leukocyte between endothelial cells and into tissue.

matory cytokines such as TNF-α and binds to sialyl Lewis x-based carbohydrates. E-selectin ligands form distinct epitopes known as the cutaneous lymphocyte-associated antigen (CLA). CLA is expressed by 10% to 40% of memory T cells and has been suggested as a marker for skin-homing T cells.[77] At least two chemokine receptors (CCR10 and CCR4) show preferential expression in CLA+ memory T cells.[78,79] Although E-selectin is likely to be an important component of skin-selective homing, there is also evidence to suggest that L-selectin is involved in T-cell migration to skin.[80,81]

In the second phase of this model, leukocyte integrins such as those of the β_2 family must be "turned on" or activated from their resting state to bind to their counter receptors such as ICAM-1 that are expressed by endothelial cells. A vast array of data suggest that the binding of chemokines to leukocyte chemokine receptors plays a critical role in activating both β1 and β2 integrins.[74,82] Activation of chemokine receptors leads to a complex signaling cascade (see Fig. 12-9) that causes a conformational change in individual integrins that leads to increases in the affinity and avidity of individual leukocyte integrins for their ligands. Furthermore, later steps of migration (ie, transmigration or diapedesis) have been shown to be dependent on chemokines as well in specific cellular contexts.[83] In the case of neutrophils, their ability to roll on inflamed blood vessels likely depends on their expression of L-selectin and E-selectin ligands, while and arrest on activated endothelia likely depends on their expression of CXCR1 and CXCR2 as described later for wound healing. Integrin activation via chemokine-mediated signals appears to be more complex in T cells, which appear to use multiple chemokine receptors, and is described in more detail later.

CHEMOKINE-MEDIATED MIGRATION OF T CELLS

Antigen-inexperienced T cells are termed naïve and can be identified by expressing three cell surface proteins: CD45RA (an isoform of the pan-leukocyte marker), L-selectin, and the chemokine receptor CCR7. These T cells migrate efficiently to secondary LNs, where they may make contact with antigen-bearing DCs from the periphery. After being activated by DCs presenting antigen, T cells then express CD45RO, are termed "memory" T cells, and appear to express a variety of adhesion molecules and chemokine receptors, which facilitate their extravasation from blood vessels to inflamed peripheral tissue. A specific subset of CCR7−,

L-selectin memory T cells has been proposed to represent an effector memory T-cell subset that is ready for rapid deployment at peripheral sites in terms of their cytotoxic activity and ability to mobilize cytokines.[84]

Although chemokines are both secreted and soluble, the net positive charge on most chemokines allows them to bind to negatively charged proteoglycans such as heparin sulfate that are present on the luminal surface of endothelial cells, thus allowing them to be presented to T cells as they roll along the luminal surface (see Fig. 12-9). After ligand binding, chemokine receptors send intracellular signals that lead to increases in the affinity and avidity of T-cell integrins such as LFA-1 and very late antigen-4 (VLA-4) for their endothelial receptors ICAM-1 and VCAM-1, respectively.[85] Only a few chemokine receptors (CXCR4, CCR7, CCR4, and CCR6) are expressed at sufficient levels on resting peripheral blood T cells to mediate this transition. With activation and IL-2 stimulation, increased numbers of chemokine receptors (eg, CXCR3) are expressed on activated T cells, making them more likely to respond to other chemokines. In several different systems, inhibition of specific chemokines produced by endothelial cells or chemokine receptors found on T cells dramatically influences T-cell arrest in vivo and in vitro.[86]

CXCR3 serves as a receptor for chemokine ligands Mig, IP-10, and I-Tac. All three of these chemokines are distinguished from other chemokines by being highly upregulated by IFN-γ. Resting T cells do not express functional levels of CXCR3 but upregulate this receptor with activation and cytokines such as IL-2. When expressed on T cells, CXCR3 is capable of mediating arrest of memory T cells on activated endothelial cells.[87] The expression of its chemokine ligands is strongly influenced by the cytokine IFN-γ, which synergistically works with proinflammatory cytokines such as TNF-α to increase expression of these ligands by activated endothelial cells[87] and epithelial cells.

In general, activation of T cells by cytokines such as IL-2 is associated with the enhanced expression of chemokine receptors CCR1, CCR2, CCR5, and CXCR3. Just as Th1 and Th2 (T cell) subsets have different functional roles, it might have been predicted that these two subsets of T cells would express different chemokine receptors. Indeed, CCR4[88-90] and CCR3[91] are associated with Th2 cells in vitro, and Th1 cells are associated with CCR5 and CXCR3.[92]

In some instances, chemokine receptors may be regarded as functional markers that characterize distinct T helper cell subsets while also promoting their recruitment to inflammatory sites characterized by "allergic" or "cell-mediated" immune responses, respectively. When T cells are activated in vitro in the presence of Th1-promoting cytokines, CXCR3 and CCR5 appear to be highly expressed, but in the presence of Th2-promoting cytokines, CCR4, CCR8, and CCR3 expression predominates. In rheumatoid arthritis, a Th1-predominant disease, many infiltrating T cells express CCR5 and CXCR3,[93] but in atopic disease, CCR4 expressing T cells may be more frequent.[88] CCR6 has recently been described as a marker for a newly characterized T-helper subset, expressing the hallmark effector cytokines IL-17 and IL-22.[94] These so-called Th17 cells play a central role in the pathogenesis of psoriasis and other chronic inflammatory autoimmune diseases.[95] However, in normal skin, the majority of skin resident T cells also co-express CCR6, suggesting that CCR6 and CCL20 interactions regulate T-cell infiltration in the skin under inflammatory as well as homeostatic conditions.[96]

Although certain chemokine receptors characterize distinct T-cell subsets, flexible regulation of their expression may increase the migratory potential of circulating T cells to diverse tissues. For example, under some conditions, both Th1 and Th2 type T cells can express CCR4.[90] Similarly, Treg and Th17 cells share chemokines receptors with other T-cell lineages but may alter their chemokine receptor expression profiles, depending on the microenvironment in which they are activated.[97]

The epidermis is a particularly rich source of chemokines, including RANTES, MIP-3α (CCL20), macrophage chemotactic protein-1 (MCP-1), IP-10, IL-8, LARC, and thymus and activation-regulated chemokine (TARC), which likely contribute to epidermal T cell migration. Keratinocytes from patients with distinctive skin diseases appear to express unique chemokine expression profiles. For instance, keratinocytes derived from patients with atopic dermatitis synthesized mRNA for RANTES at considerably earlier time points in response to IL-4 and TNF-α in comparison with cells derived from healthy individuals and psoriatic patients.[98] Keratinocytes derived from psoriatic patients synthesized higher levels of IP-10 with cytokine stimulation as well as higher constitutive levels of IL-8,[98] a chemokine known to recruit neutrophils. IL-8 may contribute to the large numbers of neutrophils that localize to the suprabasal and cornified layers of the epidermis in psoriasis. IP-10 may serve to recruit activated T cells of the Th1 helper phenotype to the epidermis and has been postulated to have a role in the recruitment of malignant T cells to the skin in cutaneous T-cell lymphomas.[99]

CTACK/CCL27 is selectively and constitutively expressed in the epidermis, and its expression is only marginally increased under inflammatory conditions.[100] Interestingly, CTACK has been reported to preferentially attract CLA+ memory T cells in vitro[100] and has been demonstrated to play a role in the recruitment and function of skin-homing T cells in inflammatory disease models.[101,102]

CHEMOKINES IN THE TRAFFICKING OF DENDRITIC CELLS FROM SKIN TO REGIONAL LYMPH NODES

Antigen-presenting cells, including DCs of the skin, are critical initiators of immune responses and their trafficking patterns are thought to influence immunological outcomes. Their mission includes taking up antigen at sites of infection or injury and bringing these antigens to regional LNs, where they both present antigen and regulate the responses of T and B cells. Skin-resident DCs are initially derived from hematopoietic bone marrow progenitors[103] and migrate to skin during the late prenatal and newborn periods of life. Under resting (steady-state) conditions, homeostatic production by keratinocytes of CXCL14 (receptor unknown) may be involved in attracting CD14+ DC precursors to the basal layer of the epidermis.[104] Similarly, LCs as well as CD1c+ LC precursors are strongly chemoattracted to keratinocyte-derived CCL20.[105] Under inflammatory conditions, when skin-resident DC and LC leave the skin in large numbers, keratinocytes release a variety of chemokines, including CCL2 and CCL7 (via CCR2)[106] and CCL20 (via CCR6),[107] which may attract monocyte-like DC precursors to the epidermis to replenish the LC population.

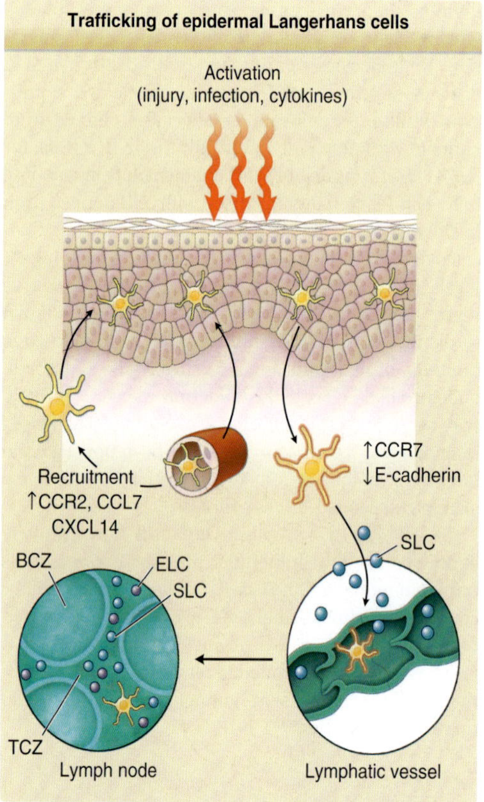

When activated by inflammatory cytokines (eg, TNF-α and IL-1β), LPS, or injury, skin DCs, including LCs, leave the epidermis, enter afferent lymphatic vessels, and migrate to draining regional LNs, where they encounter both naive and memory T cells. Chemokines guide the DCs on this journey. Activated DC specifically upregulate expression of CCR7, which binds to secondary lymphoid tissue chemokine (SLC/CCL21), a chemokine expressed constitutively by lymphatic endothelial cells.[108,109] SLC guides DC into dermal lymphatic vessels and helps retain them in SLC-rich regional draining LN (Fig. 12-10).[110]

Interestingly, naïve T cells also strongly express CCR7 and use this receptor to arrest on high endothelial venules.[111] The importance of the CCR7 pathway is demonstrated by LCs from CCR7 knockout mouse that demonstrate poor migration from the skin to regional LN[112] and by the observation that antibodies to SLC block migration of DC from the periphery to LNs.[108] Thus, CCR7 and its ligands facilitate the recruitment of at least two different kinds of cells—naïve T cells and DCs—to the LNs through two different routes under both inflammatory[112] and resting conditions.[110]

After DCs reach the LNs, they must interact with T cells to form a so-called "immunologic synapse" that is critical for T-cell activation. Activated DCs secrete a number of chemokines, including macrophage-derived chemokine (MDC),[113] which attracts T cells to the vicinity of DCs and promotes adhesion between the two cell types.[114,115] CCR5 (via CCL3/4) has also been identified as mediating recruitment of naive CD8+ T cells to aggregates of antigen-specific CD4+ T cells and DCs.[116] Therefore, chemokines orchestrate a complex series of migration patterns bringing both DCs and T cells to the confines of the LNs, where expression of chemokines by DC themselves appears to be a direct signal for binding of the T cell (see Fig. 12-10).

CHEMOKINES IN DISEASE

ATOPIC DERMATITIS

Atopic dermatitis is a prototypical Th2-mediated, allergic skin disease with multifactorial genetic and environmental factors involved in its pathogenesis. Although multiple chemokines have been associated with the atopic phenotype, the roles of CCR4 and CCR10 in atopic dermatitis have been particularly well documented.[117] Clinical data from humans as well as experimental data in the NC/Nga mouse model of atopic dermatitis suggest that the Th2-associated chemokine receptor, CCR4, in conjunction with its ligand, TARC/CCL17, may play a role in recruiting T cells to atopic skin. In patients with atopic dermatitis, CLA+CCR4+CCR10+ lymphocytes were found to be increased in the peripheral blood and in lesional skin compared with control participants.[88] Moreover, serum

Figure 12-10 Trafficking of epidermal Langerhans cells to regional lymph nodes. Langerhans cells are activated by a variety of stimuli, including injury, infectious agents, and cytokines such as interleukin-1α (IL-1α) and tumor necrosis factor-α (TNF-α). Having sampled antigens, the activated Langerhans cells (LCs) downregulate E-cadherin and strongly upregulate CCR7. Sensing the CCR7-ligand, SLC, produced by lymphatic endothelial cells, the LCs migrate into lymphatic vessels, passively flow to the lymph nodes, and stop in the T-cell zones (TCZ) that are rich in two CCR7 ligands, SLC and EBI1 ligand chemokine (ELC). Note that chemokines also contribute to the recruitment of LC under both resting and inflammatory conditions. BCZ, B-cell zones.

levels of TARC/CCL17 and CTACK/CCL27 in atopic dermatitis patients were significantly higher than concentrations found in healthy or psoriatic control participants and correlated with disease severity.[118]

CCL18, whose receptor is currently unknown, has been reported to be expressed at higher levels in the skin of patients with atopic disease compared with psoriasis.[119] CCL18 is produced by APCs and attracts CLA+ memory T cells to the skin.[120] Elevated levels of CCL18 can be found in the skin and sera of patients with atopic dermatitis but show a significant decrease after therapy.[121] Of note, CCL18 and another chemokine, CCL1 (produced by mast cells and endothelial cells), are elicited in volunteer skin after topical challenge with dust mite allergen and *Staphylococcal superantigen*.[119,122]

The recruitment of eosinophils to skin is a frequently observed finding in allergic skin diseases, including atopic dermatitis and cutaneous drug reactions, and likely is mediated by chemokines. Eotaxin/CCL11 was initially isolated from the bronchoalveolar fluid of guinea pigs after experimental allergic inflammation and binds primarily to CCR3, a receptor expressed by eosinophils,[123] basophils, and Th2 cells.[91] Injection of eotaxin into the skin promotes the recruitment of eosinophils, and antieotaxin antibodies delay the dermal recruitment of eosinophils in the late-phase allergic reaction in mouse skin.[124] Immunoreactivity and mRNA expression of eotaxin and CCR3 are both increased in lesional skin and serum of patients with atopic dermatitis but not in nonatopic controls.[125,126] Eotaxin has also been shown to increase proliferation of CCR3-expressing keratinocytes in vitro.[127] Finally, expression of eotaxin (and RANTES) by dermal endothelial cells has been correlated with the appearance of eosinophils in the dermis in patients with onchocerciasis that experience allergic reactions after treatment with ivermectin.[128] The observations above suggest that production of eotaxin and CCR3 may contribute to the recruitment of eosinophils and Th2 lymphocytes in addition to stimulating keratinocyte proliferation.

PSORIASIS

Psoriasis is characterized by hyperplasia of the epidermis (acanthosis) and a prominent dermal and epidermal inflammatory infiltrate, typically resulting in thickened, hyperkeratotic plaques. The inflammatory infiltrate of psoriatic skin is predominantly composed of Th1- and Th17-polarized memory T cells, as well as neutrophils, macrophages, and increased numbers of DCs.[129] As reviewed by others,[117] there is a growing body of evidence supporting a central role for chemokines in regulating the complex events leading to psoriatic skin inflammation. Chemokines, including CCL20[130] and CCL17,[78] mediate the arrest of effector memory T cells on endothelial cells that synthesize these chemokines.[131] In addition, both CCL17 and CCL20 can be synthesized by keratinocytes, possibly contributing to T-cell migration to the epidermis (Fig. 12-11).

Accumulating evidence strongly implicates pathogenetic Th17 cells, which strongly express CCR6, in the pathogenesis of psoriasis.[132] Th17 cells, their signature effector cytokines IL-17 and IL-22, as well as high levels of IL-23, a major growth and differentiation factor for Th17 cells, are abundant in psoriatic skin lesions.[133] Recent research suggests that CCR6 and its ligand, CCL20, are important mediators of psoriasis because both CCL20 as well as CLA+CCR6+ skin-homing Th17 cells are found in abundance in lesional psoriatic skin.[60,133] Moreover, CCR6-deficient mice failed to develop psoriasis-like inflammation[134] in response to intradermal IL-23 injections, a murine model for human psoriasis.[57] Interestingly, CCR6 was required for both T cell–dependent as well as T cell–independent skin inflammation in this model.[134]

Neutrophils found in the epidermis of psoriatic skin are probably attracted there by high levels of IL-8, which would act via CXCR1 and CXCR2. In addition to attracting neutrophils, IL-8 is an ELR+ CXC chemokine that is known to be angiogenic, and it may also attract endothelial cells. This may lead to the formation of the long tortuous capillary blood vessels in the papillary dermis that are characteristic of psoriasis. Moreover, keratinocytes also express CXCR2 and thus may be autoregulated by the expression of CXCR2 ligands in the skin. Of note, an IL-8/CXCL8-producing population of memory T cells that express CCR6 has been isolated from patients with acute generalized exanthematous pustulosis (AGEP), a condition induced most commonly by drugs (eg, aminopenicillins) and characterized by small intraepidermal or subcorneal sterile pustules.[135] Similar T cells have been isolated from patients with Behçet disease and pustular psoriasis.[136] It is possible that this subpopulation of T cells contributes to neutrophil accumulation in the stratum corneum (Munro abscesses) in psoriasis and other inflammatory skin disorders characterized by neutrophil-rich infiltrates in the absence of frank infection.

CANCER

Chemokines may play a role in tumor formation and immunity in several distinct ways, including the control of angiogenesis and the induction of tumor immune responses.[137] CXC chemokines that express a three-amino-acid motif consisting of glu-leu-arg (ELR) immediately preceding the CXC signature are angiogenic, but most non–ELR CXC chemokines, except SDF-1, are angiostatic. Interestingly, it is not clear that ELR− chemokines actually bind to chemokine receptors to reduce angiogenesis. It has been proposed that they act by displacing growth factors from proteoglycans. In any event, the balance between ELR+ versus ELR− chemokines is thought to contribute to the complex regulation of angiogenesis at tumor sites. IL-8, a prototypical ELR+ chemokine,

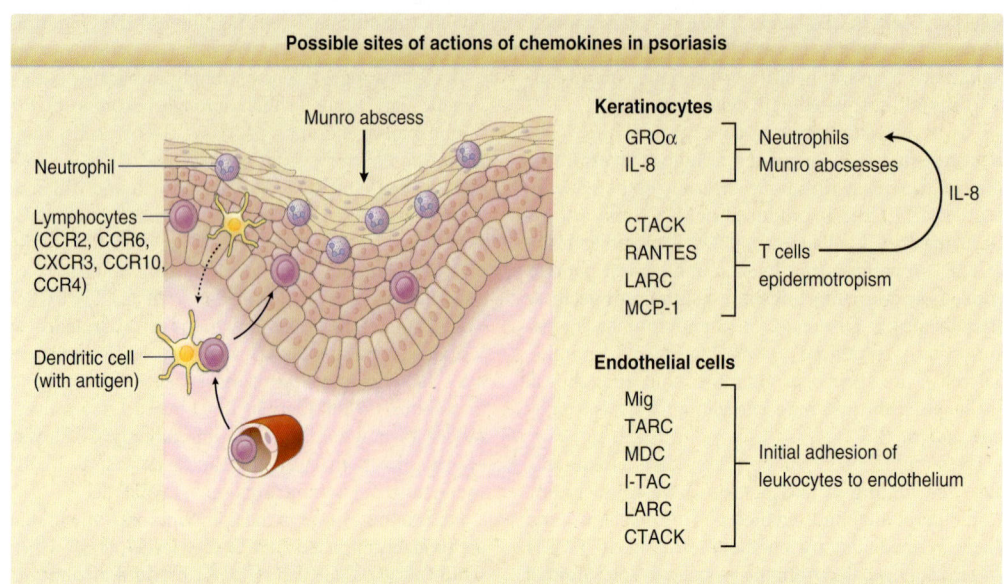

Figure 12-11 Possible sites of actions of chemokines in psoriasis. Chemokines attract both neutrophils (to form Munro abscesses) and lymphocytes via attachment to endothelial cells and then migration to the epidermis (epidermotropism). Specific chemokines tend to attract either neutrophils or lymphocytes but generally not both. A newly identified subset of T cells can secrete interleukin-8 (IL-8) and attract neutrophils in conditions such as acute generalized exanthematous pustulosis (AGEP). Dendritic cells may also secrete chemokines, attract T cells, and stimulate conjugate formation that activates T cells. Cutaneous T-cell-attracting chemokine (CTACK); growth-regulated oncogene-alpha (GRO-α); I-TAC, interferon-inducible T-cell alpha chemoattractant; LARC, liver and activation-regulated chemokine; MCP-1, macrophage chemotactic protein-1; MDC, macrophage-derived chemokine; Mig, monokine induced by gamma interferon; RANTES, regulated upon activation, normal T cell expressed and secreted; TARC, thymus and activation-regulated chemokine. (Adapted from Lonsdorf AS, Hwang ST. Chemokines. In: Goldsmith LA, Katz SI, Gilchrest BA, et al. *Fitzpatrick's Dermatology in General Medicine*, 8th ed. New York: McGraw-Hill; 2012:eFigure 12-3.1.)

can be secreted by melanoma cells and has been detected in conjunction with metastatic dissemination of this cancer,[138] which may be related to its ability to attract circulating tumor cells to primary tumors and to influence leukocyte and endothelial cell recruitment.[139,140] IL-8 may also act as an autocrine growth factor for melanoma[141] as well as several other types of cancer. Although CXCR1 and CXCR2 bind IL-8 in common, several other ELR+ CXC chemokines also bind to and activate CXCR2.

Tumors, including melanoma, have long been known to secrete chemokines that can attract a variety of leukocytes. The question arises as to why this is not deleterious to the tumor itself. Breast cancers, for instance, are known to secrete MCP-1, a chemokine that attracts macrophages through CCR2. Higher tissue levels of MCP-1 correlate with increasing number of macrophages within the tissue. Although chemokines secreted by tumor cells do lead to recruitment of immune cells, this does not necessarily lead to increased clearance of the tumor.[142]

Inflammatory cells such as macrophages may actually play a critical role in cancer invasion and metastasis. First, MCP-1 may increase expression of macrophage IL-4 through an autocrine feedback loop and possibly skew the immune response from Th1 to Th2. Interestingly, MCP-1–deficient mice show markedly reduced dermal fibrosis after dermal challenge with bleomycin, a finding of possible relevance to the pathogenesis of conditions such as scleroderma.[143] Second, macrophages may promote tumor invasion and metastasis.[144] The antitumor effects of specific chemokines may occur by a variety of mechanisms. ELR− CXCR3 ligands such as IP-10 are potently antiangiogenic and may act as downstream effectors of IL-12-induced, NK cell–dependent angiostasis.[145] Of note, some cancer cells can synthesize LARC, attracting immature DCs that express CCR6.[146] Experimentally, LARC has been transduced into murine tumors, where it attracts DCs in mice and suppresses tumor growth in experimental systems.[147] Last, chemokines produced by tumor cells may attract CD4+CD25+ Tregs that suppress host antitumor cytolytic T cells.[148]

Tumor metastasis is the most common cause of mortality and morbidity in cancer. With skin cancers such as melanoma, there is a propensity for specific sites such as brain, lung, and liver, as well as distant skin sites. Cancers may also metastasize via afferent lymphatics and eventually reach regional draining LNs. The discovery of nodal metastasis often portends a poor prognosis for the patient. In fact, the presence of nodal metastases is one of the most powerful negative predictors of survival in melanoma.[149]

Chemokines may play an important role in the site-specific metastases of cancers of the breast and

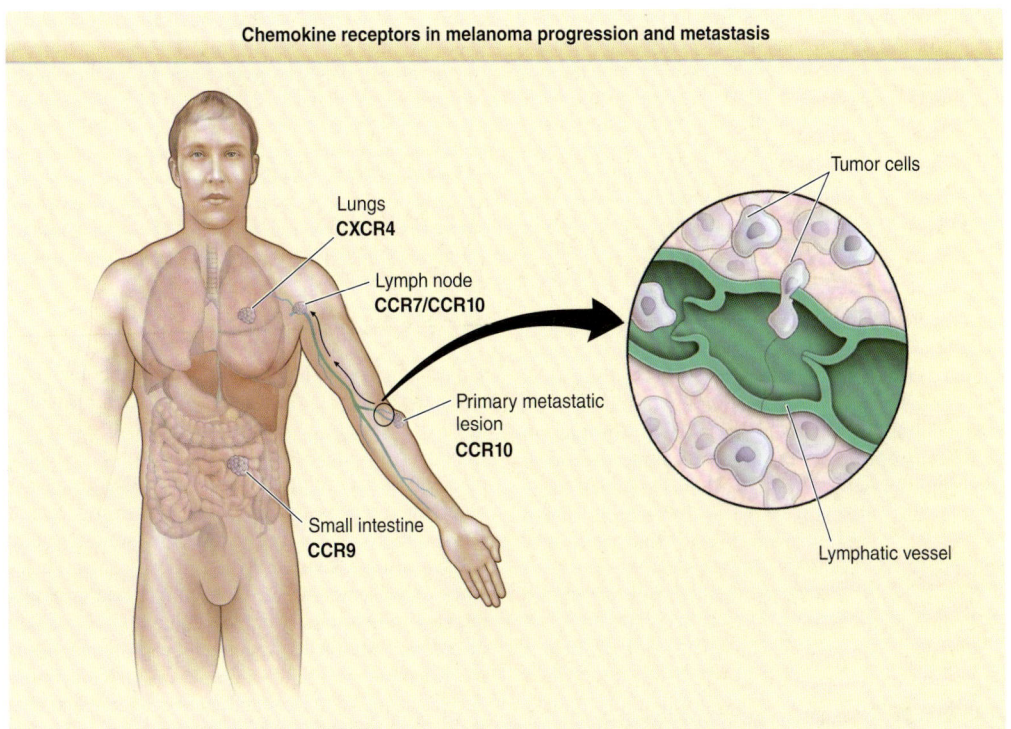

Figure 12-12 Chemokine receptors in melanoma progression and metastasis. Chemokine receptors play distinct roles in melanoma metastasis.[117] CCR10 may enhance survival of primary melanoma tumors and skin metastases. CCR7, CCR10, and, possibly CXCR4 may contribute to lymph node metastasis. CXCR4 appears to be involved in primary tumor development and metastasis at distant organ sites such as the lungs. CCR9 has been implicated in melanoma small bowel metastasis in patients.

of melanoma[150] (Fig. 12-12). Human breast cancer and melanoma lines express the chemokine receptors CXCR4 and CCR7, but normal breast epithelial cells and melanocytes do not appear to express these receptors.[151] CXCR4 is expressed in more than 23 different solid and hematopoietic cancers. Broad expression of this receptor may be due to its regulation by hypoxia, a condition common to growing tumors, via the hypoxia inducible factor-1α transcription factor.[152] Notably stromal fibroblasts within human cancers express the CXCR4 ligand, CXCL12, which stimulates tumor growth as well as angiogenesis.[153] In several different animals of breast cancer[151] and melanoma metastasis,[154] inhibition of CXCR4 with antibodies or peptides resulted in dramatically reduced metastases to distant organs. Expression of CCR7 by cancer cells, including gastric carcinoma and melanoma, appears to be critical for invasion of afferent lymphatics and LN metastasis. CCR7-transfected B16 murine melanoma cells were found to metastasize with much higher efficiency to regional LNs compared with control B16 cells after inoculation into the footpad of mice,[155] but CCR7 also directly stimulates primary B16 tumor development.[156] CCR9 may also play a role in melanoma metastasis to the small bowel, which shows high expression of the CCR9 ligand, CCL25.[157]

CCR10 is highly expressed by melanoma primary tumors[158] and is correlated with nodal metastasis in melanoma patients[159] and in experimental animal models.[158] Engagement of CCR10 by CTACK results in activation (via phosphorylation) of the phosphatidylinositol 3-kinase (PI3K) and Akt signaling pathways, leading to antiapoptotic effects in melanoma cells.[158] Because CTACK is constitutively produced by keratinocytes, it may act as a survival factor for both primary as well as secondary (metastatic) melanoma tumors that express CCR10. In fact, CCR10-activated melanoma cells become resistant to killing by melanoma antigen-specific T cells.[158] Interestingly, CCR4,[160] CXCR4,[161] and CCR10[162,163] have been implicated in the trafficking or survival of malignant T- (lymphoma) cells to skin. Thus, a limited number of specific chemokine receptors appear to play distinct, nonredundant roles in facilitating cancer progression and metastasis (summarized in Fig. 12-12).

INFECTIOUS DISEASES

Although chemokines and chemokine receptors may have evolved as a host response to infectious agents, recent data suggest infectious organisms may have coopted chemokine- or chemokine receptor–like molecules to their own advantage in selected instances. A variety of microorganisms express chemokine receptors, including US28 by cytomegalovirus and Kaposi sarcoma herpes virus (or HHV-8) GPCR. In the case of KSHV GPCR, this receptor is able to promiscuously bind several chemokines. More importantly, it is constitutively active and may work as a growth promoter in Kaposi sarcoma.[164]

The human immunodeficiency virus (HIV)-1, the causative agent of the acquired immunodeficiency syndrome (AIDS), is an enveloped retrovirus that enters cells via receptor-dependent membrane fusion. CD4 is the primary fusion receptor for all strains of HIV-1 and binds to HIV-1 proteins, gp120 and gp41. However, different strains of HIV-1 have emerged that preferentially use CXCR4 (T-tropic) or CCR5 (M-tropic) or either chemokine receptor as a coreceptor for entry. Although other chemokine coreceptors can potentially serve as coreceptors, most clinical HIV-1 strains are primarily dual tropic for either CCR5 or CXCR4.[165]

The discovery of a 32–base pair deletion (D32) in CCR5 in some individuals that leads to low levels of *CCR5* expression in T cells and DCs and correlates with a dramatic resistance to HIV-1 infection demonstrated a clear role for CCR5 in the pathogenesis of HIV-1 infection.[166] Interestingly, the frequency of Δ32 mutations in humans is surprisingly high, and the complete absence of CCR5 in homozygotes has only been associated with a more clinically severe form of sarcoidosis. Otherwise, these individuals are healthy. In fact, there is an association of less severe autoimmune diseases in patients with these mutations.[167]

LCs reside in large numbers in the genital mucosa and may be one of the first initial targets of HIV-1 infection.[168] Because infected (activated) LCs likely enter dermal lymphatic vessels and then localize to regional LNs as described earlier, the physiologic migratory pathway of LCs may also coincidentally lead to the transmission of HIV-1 to T cells within secondary lymphoid organs. CCR5 is expressed by immature or resting LCs in the epidermis and is the target of CCR5 analogs of RANTES that block HIV infection.[169] Already, an FDA-approved small molecule inhibitor of CCR5, maraviroc, is available for use in treatment of HIV disease and may show fewer adverse effects than certain reverse transcriptase inhibitors.[170] CXCR4 antagonists may also be of clinical utility with T- or dual-tropic viruses.[171] A newly described autosomal dominant genetic syndrome composed of *w*arts (human papilloma virus [HPV] associated), *h*ypogammaglobulinemia, *i*nfections, and *m*yelokathexis (WHIM) is the result of an activating mutation in the cytoplasmic tail of the CXCR4 receptor or in yet unidentified downstream regulators of CXCR4 function.[172,173] Bacterial infections are common because myelokathexis is associated with neutropenia and abnormal neutrophil morphology. The nearly universal presence of HPV infections associated with this syndrome can involve multiple common, as well as genital, wart subtypes and suggests a critical role for normal CXCR4 function in immunologic defense against this common human pathogen.

SOLUBLE MEDIATOR NETWORK: THERAPEUTIC IMPLICATIONS AND APPLICATIONS

This chapter has attempted to bring some degree of order and logic to the analysis of a field of human biology that continues to grow at a rapid rate. An appreciation of the underlying biology governing soluble mediators sheds light on the mechanisms of cutaneous tissue homeostasis. An imbalance in this careful orchestration of cytokines and chemokines can lead to chronic disease. As highlighted in this chapter, cytokines and chemokines are currently being clinically targeted to help treat patients with a number of skin disorders. Each of the aforementioned approaches is still relatively new and open to considerable future development. An understanding of cytokines and chemokines by clinicians of the future is likely to be central to effective patient care.

REFERENCES

1. Oppenheim JJ. Cytokines: past, present, and future. *Int J Hematol*. 2001;74:3-8.
2. Charo IF, Ransohoff RM. The many roles of chemokines and chemokine receptors in inflammation. *N Engl J Med*. 2006;354:610-621.
3. Bigazzi PE, Yoshida T, Ward PA, et al. Production of lymphokine-like factors (cytokines) by simian virus 40-infected and simian virus 40-transformed cells. *Am J Pathol*. 1975;80:69-78.
4. Luger TA, Stadler BM, Katz SI, et al. Epidermal cell (keratinocyte)-derived thymocyte-activating factor (ETAF). *J Immunol*. 1981;127:1493-1498.
5. Kupper TS. The activated keratinocyte: a model for inducible cytokine production by non-bone marrow-derived cells in cutaneous inflammatory and immune responses. *J Invest Dermatol*. 1990;94:146S-150S.
6. Albanesi C, Pastore S. Pathobiology of chronic inflammatory skin diseases: interplay between keratinocytes and immune cells as a target for anti-inflammatory drugs. *Curr Drug Metab*. 2010;11:210-227.
7. Mosmann TR, Coffman RL. TH1 and TH2 cells: different patterns of lymphokine secretion lead to different functional properties. *Annu Rev Immunol*. 1989;7:145-173.
8. O'Quinn DB, Palmer MT, Lee YK, et al. Emergence of the Th17 pathway and its role in host defense. *Adv Immunol*. 2008;99: 115-163.
9. Josefowicz SZ, Rudensky A. Control of regulatory T cell lineage commitment and maintenance. *Immunity*. 2009;30:616-625.
10. Rubtsov YP, Rudensky AY. TGFbeta signalling in control of T-cell-mediated self-reactivity. *Nat Rev Immunol*. 2007;7:443-453.

11. Rubtsov YP, et al. Regulatory T cell-derived interleukin-10 limits inflammation at environmental interfaces. *Immunity*. 2008;28:546-558.
12. Purwar R, et al. Robust tumor immunity to melanoma mediated by interleukin-9-producing T cells. *Nat Med*. 2012;18:1248-1253.
13. Vallabhapurapu S, Karin M. Regulation and function of NF-kappaB transcription factors in the immune system. *Annu Rev Immunol*. 2009;27:693-733.
14. Arend WP, Palmer G, Gabay C. IL-1, IL-18, and IL-33 families of cytokines. *Immunol Rev*. 2008;223:20-38.
15. Kawai T, Akira S. The role of pattern-recognition receptors in innate immunity: update on Toll-like receptors. *Nat Immunol*. 2010;11:373-384.
16. O'Shea JJ, Murray PJ. Cytokine signaling modules in inflammatory responses. *Immunity*. 2008;28:477-487.
17. Bachelez H, et al. Tofacitinib versus etanercept or placebo in moderate-to-severe chronic plaque psoriasis: a phase 3 randomised non-inferiority trial. *Lancet*. 2015;386:552-561.
18. Kennedy Crispin M, et al. Safety and efficacy of the JAK inhibitor tofacitinib citrate in patients with alopecia areata. *JCI Insight*. 2016;1:e89776.
19. Hornung T, et al. Remission of recalcitrant dermatomyositis treated with ruxolitinib. *N Engl J Med*. 2014;371:2537-2538,.
20. Kurtzman DJ, et al. Tofacitinib citrate for refractory cutaneous dermatomyositis: an alternative treatment. *JAMA Dermatol*. 2016;152:944-945.
21. Martinon F, Mayor A, Tschopp J. The inflammasomes: guardians of the body. *Annu Rev Immunol*. 2009;27:229-265.
22. Kupper TS. Immune and inflammatory processes in cutaneous tissues. Mechanisms and speculations. *J Clin Invest*. 1990;86:1783-1789.
23. Conti HR, et al. Th17 cells and IL-17 receptor signaling are essential for mucosal host defense against oral candidiasis. *J Exp Med*. 2009;206:299-311.
24. Ho AW, Shen F, Conti HR, et al. IL-17RC is required for immune signaling via an extended SEF/IL-17R signaling domain in the cytoplasmic tail. *J Immunol*. 2010;185:1063-1070.
25. Kovanen PE, Leonard WJ. Cytokines and immunodeficiency diseases: critical roles of the gamma(c)-dependent cytokines interleukins 2, 4, 7, 9, 15, and 21, and their signaling pathways. *Immunol Rev*. 2004;202:67-83.
26. Ma A, Koka R, Burkett P. Diverse functions of IL-2, IL-15, and IL-7 in lymphoid homeostasis. *Annu Rev Immunol*. 2006;24:657-679.
27. Simpson EL, Guttman-Yassky E, Beck LA, et al. Two phase 3 trials of dupilumab versus placebo in atopic dermatitis. *N Engl J Med*. 2016;375(24):2335-2348.
28. Mentink-Kane MM, Wynn TA. Opposing roles for IL-13 and IL-13 receptor alpha 2 in health and disease. *Immunol Rev*. 2004;202:191-202.
29. Soussi-Gounni A, Kontolemos M, Hamid Q. Role of IL-9 in the pathophysiology of allergic diseases. *J Allergy Clin Immunol*. 2001;107:575-582.
30. Parrot T, Allard M, Oger R, et al. IL-9 promotes the survival and function of human melanoma-infiltrating CD4(+) CD8(+) double-positive T cells. *Eur J Immunol*. 2016;46:1770-1782.
31. Leonard WJ, Zeng R, Spolski R. Interleukin 21: a cytokine/cytokine receptor system that has come of age. *J Leukoc Biol*. 2008;84:348-356.
32. Mehta DS, Wurster AL, Grusby MJ. Biology of IL-21 and the IL-21 receptor. *Immunol Rev*. 2004;202:84-95.
33. Wang YH, Ito T, Wang YH, et al. Maintenance and polarization of human TH2 central memory T cells by thymic stromal lymphopoietin-activated dendritic cells. *Immunity*. 2006;24:827-838.
34. Ziegler SF, Artis D. Sensing the outside world: TSLP regulates barrier immunity. *Nat Immunol*. 2010;11:289-293.
35. Geijsen N, Koenderman L, Coffer PJ. Specificity in cytokine signal transduction: lessons learned from the IL-3/IL-5/GM-CSF receptor family. *Cytokine Growth Factor Rev*. 2001;12:19-25.
36. Dranoff G. GM-CSF-based cancer vaccines. *Immunol Rev*. 2002;188:147-154.
37. Eager R, Nemunaitis J. GM-CSF gene-transduced tumor vaccines. *Mol Ther*. 2005;12:18-27.
38. Sonkoly E, Muller A, Lauerma AI, et al. IL-31: a new link between T cells and pruritus in atopic skin inflammation. *J Allergy Clin Immunol*. 2006;117:411-417.
39. Diveu C, Lelièvre E, Perret D, et al. GPL, a novel cytokine receptor related to GP130 and leukemia inhibitory factor receptor. *J Biol Chem*. 2003;278:49850-49859.
40. Mach N, Dranoff G. Cytokine-secreting tumor cell vaccines. *Curr Opin Immunol*. 2000;12:571-575.
41. Kastelein RA, Hunter CA, Cua DJ. Discovery and biology of IL-23 and IL-27: related but functionally distinct regulators of inflammation. *Annu Rev Immunol*. 2007;25:221-242.
42. Yoshida H, Miyazaki Y. Regulation of immune responses by interleukin-27. *Immunol Rev*. 2008;226:234-247.
43. Collison LW, Vignali DA. Interleukin-35: odd one out or part of the family? *Immunol Rev*. 2008;226:248-262.
44. Griffiths CE, Strober BE, van de Kerkhof P, et al. Comparison of ustekinumab and etanercept for moderate-to-severe psoriasis. *N Engl J Med*. 2010;362:118-128.
45. Theofilopoulos AN, Baccala R, Beutler B, et al. Type I interferons (alpha/beta) in immunity and autoimmunity. *Annu Rev Immunol*. 2005;23:307-336.
46. Ank N, West H, Paludan SR. IFN-lambda: novel antiviral cytokines. *J Interferon Cytokine Res*. 2006;26:373-379.
47. McInturff JE, Modlin RL, Kim J. The role of toll-like receptors in the pathogenesis and treatment of dermatological disease. *J Invest Dermatol*. 2005;125:1-8.
48. Saraiva M, O'Garra A. The regulation of IL-10 production by immune cells. *Nat Rev Immunol*. 2010;10:170-181.
49. Commins S, Steinke JW, Borish L. The extended IL-10 superfamily: IL-10, IL-19, IL-20, IL-22, IL-24, IL-26, IL-28, and IL-29. *J Allergy Clin Immunol*. 2008;121:1108-1111.
50. Sa SM, Valdez PA, Wu J, et al. The effects of IL-20 subfamily cytokines on reconstituted human epidermis suggest potential roles in cutaneous innate defense and pathogenic adaptive immunity in psoriasis. *J Immunol*. 2007;178:2229-2240.
51. He M, Liang P. IL-24 transgenic mice: in vivo evidence of overlapping functions for IL-20, IL-22, and IL-24 in the epidermis. *J Immunol*. 2010;184:1793-1798.
52. Eyerich S, Eyerich K, Pennino D, et al. Th22 cells represent a distinct human T cell subset involved in epidermal immunity and remodeling. *J Clin Invest*. 2009;119:3573-3585.
53. Fujita H, Nograles KE, Kikuchi T, et al. Human Langerhans cells induce distinct IL-22-producing CD4+ T cells lacking IL-17 production. *Proc Natl Acad Sci U S A*. 2009;106:21795-21800.
54. Feng XH, Derynck R. Specificity and versatility in tgf-beta signaling through Smads. *Annu Rev Cell Dev Biol*. 2005;21:659-693.

55. Varga J, Pasche B. Transforming growth factor beta as a therapeutic target in systemic sclerosis. *Nat Rev Rheumatol*. 2009;5:200-206.
56. Zaba LC, Cardinale I, Gilleaudeau P, et al. Amelioration of epidermal hyperplasia by TNF inhibition is associated with reduced Th17 responses. *J Exp Med*. 2007;204:3183-3194.
57. Zheng Y, Danilenko DM, Valdez P, et al. Interleukin-22, a TH17 cytokine, mediates IL-23-induced dermal inflammation and acanthosis. *Nature*. 2006;445:648-651.
58. Reich K, Papp KA, Griffiths CE, et al. An update on the long-term safety experience of ustekinumab: results from the psoriasis clinical development program with up to four years of follow-up. *J Drugs Dermatol*. 2012;11:300-312.
59. Kopp T, Riedl E, Bangert C, et al. Clinical improvement in psoriasis with specific targeting of interleukin-23. *Nature*. 2015;521:222-226.
60. Nograles KE, Zaba LC, Guttman-Yassky E, et al. Th17 cytokines interleukin (IL)-17 and IL-22 modulate distinct inflammatory and keratinocyte-response pathways. *Br J Dermatol*. 2008;159(5):1092-102.
61. Langley RG, Elewski BE, Lebwohl M, et al. Secukinumab in plaque psoriasis—results of two phase 3 trials. *N Engl J Med*. 2014;371:326-338.
62. Gordon KB, Blauvelt A, Papp KA, et al. Phase 3 trials of ixekizumab in moderate-to-severe plaque psoriasis. *N Engl J Med*. 2016;375:345-356.
63. Schafer PH, Parton A, Gandhi AK, et al. Apremilast, a cAMP phosphodiesterase-4 inhibitor, demonstrates anti-inflammatory activity in vitro and in a model of psoriasis. *Br J Pharmacol*. 2010;159:842-855.
64. Papp K, et al. Apremilast, an oral phosphodiesterase 4 (PDE4) inhibitor, in patients with moderate to severe plaque psoriasis: results of a phase III, randomized, controlled trial (Efficacy and Safety Trial Evaluating the Effects of Apremilast in Psoriasis [ESTEEM] 1). *J Am Acad Dermatol*. 2015;73:37-49.
65. Papp KA, Reich K, Leonardi CL, et al. Efficacy and safety of tofacitinib, an oral Janus kinase inhibitor, in the treatment of psoriasis: a Phase 2b randomized placebo-controlled dose-ranging study. *Br J Dermatol*. 2012;167:668-677.
66. Craiglow BG, King BA. Killing two birds with one stone: oral tofacitinib reverses alopecia universalis in a patient with plaque psoriasis. *J Invest Dermatol*. 2014;134:2988-2990.
67. Liu LY, Craiglow BG, Dai F, et al. Tofacitinib for the treatment of severe alopecia areata and variants: a study of 90 patients. *J Am Acad Dermatol*. 2017;76:22-28.
68. Van Belle AB, de Heusch M, Lemaire MM, et al. IL-22 is required for imiquimod-induced psoriasiform skin inflammation in mice. *J Immunol*. 2012;188:462-469.
69. Nograles KE, Zaba LC, Shemer A, et al. IL-22-producing "T22" T cells account for upregulated IL-22 in atopic dermatitis despite reduced IL-17-producing TH17 T cells. *J Allergy Clin Immunol*. 2009;123: 1244-1252 e1242.
70. Koreth J, Kim HT, Jones KT, et al. Efficacy, durability, and response predictors of low-dose interleukin-2 therapy for chronic graft-versus-host disease. *Blood*. 2016;128:130-137.
71. Zlotnik A, Yoshie O. Chemokines: a new classification system and their role in immunity. *Immunity*. 2000;12:121-127.
72. Bazan JF, Bacon KB, Hardiman G, et al. A new class of membrane-bound chemokine with a CX3C motif. *Nature*. 1997;385:640-644.
73. Jiang H, Kuang Y, Wu Y, et al. Pertussis toxin-sensitive activation of phospholipase C by the C5a and fMet-Leu-Phe receptors. *J Biol Chem*. 1996;271:13430-13434.
74. Constantin G, Majeed M, Giagulli C, et al. Chemokines trigger immediate $\beta 2$ integrin affinity and mobility changes. *Immunity*. 2000;13:759-769.
75. Homey B. Chemokines and inflammatory skin diseases. *Adv Dermatol*. 2005;21:251-277.
76. Springer TA. Traffic signals for lymphocyte recirculation and leukocyte emigration: the multistep paradigm. *Cell*. 1994;76:301-314.
77. Berg EL. The cutaneous lymphocyte antigen is a skin lymphocyte homing receptor for the vascular lectin endothelial cell-leukocyte adhesion molecule 1. *J Exp Med*. 1991;174:1461-1466.
78. Campbell JJ, Haraldsen G, Pan J, et al. The chemokine receptor CCR4 in vascular recognition by cutaneous but not intestinal memory T cells. *Nature*. 1999;400:776-780.
79. Homey B, Wang W, Soto H, et al. Cutting edge: the orphan chemokine receptor G protein-coupled receptor-2 (GPR-2, CCR10) binds the skin-associated chemokine CCL27 (CTACK/ALP/ILC). *J Immunol*. 2000; 164:3465-3470.
80. Lechleitner S, Kunstfeld R, Messeritsch-Fanta C, et al. Peripheral lymph node addressins are expressed on skin endothelial cells. *J Invest Dermatol*. 1999;113:410-414.
81. Hwang ST, Fitzhugh DJ. Aberrant expression of adhesion molecules by sézary cells: functional consequences under physiologic shear stress conditions. *J Invest Dermatol*. 2001;116:466-470.
82. Campbell JJ. Chemokines and the arrest of lymphocytes rolling under flow conditions. *Science*. 1998; 279:381-384.
83. Kawai T, Seki M, Hiromatsu K, et al. Selective diapedesis of Th1 cells induced by endothelial cell RANTES. *J Immunol*. 1999;163:3269-3278.
84. Sallusto F, Lenig D, Förster R, et al. Two subsets of memory T lymphocytes with distinct homing potentials and effector functions. *Nature*. 1999;401:708-712.
85. Sallusto F, Mackay CR. Chemoattractants and their receptors in homeostasis and inflammation. *Curr Opin Immunol*. 2004;16:724-731.
86. Hwang ST. Mechanisms of T-cell homing to skin. *Adv Dermatol*. 2001;17:211-241.
87. Piali L, Weber C, LaRosa G, et al. The chemokine receptor CXCR3 mediates rapid and shear-resistant adhesion-induction of effector T lymphocytes by the chemokines IP10 and Mig. *Eur J Immunol*. 1998;28:961-972.
88. Vestergaard C, Bang K, Gesser B, et al. A Th2 chemokine, TARC, produced by keratinocytes may recruit CLA+CCR4+ lymphocytes into lesional atopic dermatitis skin. *J Invest Dermatol*. 2000;115:640-646.
89. Imai T. Selective recruitment of CCR4-bearing Th2 cells toward antigen-presenting cells by the CC chemokines thymus and activation-regulated chemokine and macrophage-derived chemokine. *Int Immunol*. 1999;11:81-88.
90. Andrew DP, Ruffing N, Kim CH, et al. C-C chemokine receptor 4 expression defines a major subset of circulating nonintestinal memory T cells of both Th1 and Th2 potential. *J Immunol*. 2001;166:103-111.
91. Sallusto F. Selective expression of the eotaxin receptor CCR3 by human T helper 2 cells. *Science*. 1997;277:2005-2007.
92. Bonecchi R, Bianchi G, Bordignon PP, et al. Differential expression of chemokine receptors and chemotactic

responsiveness of type 1 T helper cells (Th1s) and Th2s. *J Exp Med*. 1998;187:129-134.
93. Qin S, Rottman JB, Myers P, et al. The chemokine receptors CXCR3 and CCR5 mark subsets of T cells associated with certain inflammatory reactions. *J Clin Invest*. 1998;101:746-754.
94. Steinman L. A brief history of TH17, the first major revision in the TH1/TH2 hypothesis of T cell–mediated tissue damage. *Nat Med*. 2007;13:139-145.
95. Lowes MA, Bowcock AM, Krueger JG. Pathogenesis and therapy of psoriasis. *Nature*. 2007;445:866-873.
96. Clark RA, Chong B, Mirchandani N, et al. The vast majority of CLA+ T cells are resident in normal skin. *J Immunol*. 2006;176:4431-4439.
97. Bromley SK, Mempel TR, Luster AD. Orchestrating the orchestrators: chemokines in control of T cell traffic. *Nat Immunol*. 2008;9:970-980.
98. Giustizieri ML, Mascia F, Frezzolini A, et al. Keratinocytes from patients with atopic dermatitis and psoriasis show a distinct chemokine production profile in response to T cell–derived cytokines. *J Allergy Clin Immunol*. 2001;107:871-877.
99. Sarris AH, Daliani D, Ulmer R, et al. Interferon-inducible protein 10 as a possible factor in the pathogenesis of cutaneous T-cell lymphomas. *Clin Cancer Res*. 1997;3:169-177.
100. Morales J, Homey B, Vicari AP, Het al. CTACK, a skin-associated chemokine that preferentially attracts skin-homing memory T cells. *Proc Natl Acad Sci U S A*. 1999;96:14470-14475.
101. Reiss Y, Proudfoot AE, Power CA, et al. CC chemokine receptor (CCR)4 and the CCR10 ligand cutaneous T cell–attracting chemokine (CTACK) in lymphocyte trafficking to inflamed skin. *J Exp Med*. 2001;194:1541-1547.
102. Homey B, Alenius H, Müller A, et al. CCL27–CCR10 interactions regulate T cell–mediated skin inflammation. *Nat Med*. 2002;8:157-165.
103. Katz SI, Tamaki K, Sachs DH. Epidermal Langerhans cells are derived from cells originating in bone marrow. *Nature*. 1979;282:324-326.
104. Schaerli P, Willimann K, Ebert LM, et al. Cutaneous CXCL14 targets blood precursors to epidermal niches for Langerhans cell differentiation. *Immunity*. 2005;23:331-342.
105. Dieu-Nosjean M-C, Massacrier C, Homey B, et al. Macrophage inflammatory protein 3α is expressed at inflamed epithelial surfaces and is the most potent chemokine known in attracting Langerhans cell precursors. *J Exp Med*. 2000;192:705-718.
106. Merad M, Manz MG, Karsunky H, et al. Langerhans cells renew in the skin throughout life under steady-state conditions. *Nat Immunol*. 2002;3:1135-1141.
107. Varona R, Villares R, Carramolino L, et al. CCR6-deficient mice have impaired leukocyte homeostasis and altered contact hypersensitivity and delayed-type hypersensitivity responses. *J Clin Invest*. 2001;107:R37-R45.
108. Saeki H, Moore AM, Brown MJ, et al. Cutting edge: secondary lymphoid-tissue chemokine (SLC) and CC chemokine receptor 7 (CCR7) participate in the emigration pathway of mature dendritic cells from the skin to regional lymph nodes. *J Immunol*. 1999;162:2472-2475.
109. Gunn MD, Tangemann K, Tam C, et al. A chemokine expressed in lymphoid high endothelial venules promotes the adhesion and chemotaxis of naive T lymphocytes. *Proc Natl Acad Sci U S A*. 1998;95:258-263.
110. Ohl L, Mohaupt M, Czeloth N, et al. CCR7 governs skin dendritic cell migration under inflammatory and steady-state conditions. *Immunity*. 2004;21:279-288.
111. Stein JV, Rot A, Luo Y, et al. The CC chemokine thymus-derived chemotactic agent 4 (Tca-4, secondary lymphoid tissue chemokine, 6ckine, exodus-2) triggers lymphocyte function–associated antigen 1–mediated arrest of rolling T lymphocytes in peripheral lymph node high endothelial venules. *J Exp Med*. 2000;191:61-76.
112. Förster R, Schubel A, Breitfeld D, et al. CCR7 coordinates the primary immune response by establishing functional microenvironments in secondary lymphoid organs. *Cell*. 1999;99:23-33.
113. Sallusto F, Palermo B, Lenig D, et al. Distinct patterns and kinetics of chemokine production regulate dendritic cell function. *Eur J Immunol*. 1999;29:1617-1625.
114. Tang HL. Chemokine up-regulation and activated T cell attraction by maturing dendritic cells. *Science*. 1999;284:819-822.
115. Wu M, Fang H, Hwang ST. Cutting edge: CCR4 mediates antigen-primed T cell binding to activated dendritic cells. *J Immunol*. 2001;167:4791-4795.
116. Castellino F, Huang AY, Altan-Bonnet G, et al. Chemokines enhance immunity by guiding naive CD8+ T cells to sites of CD4+ T cell–dendritic cell interaction. *Nature*. 2006;440:890-895.
117. Lonsdorf AS, Hwang ST, Enk AH. Chemokine receptors in T-cell-mediated diseases of the skin. *J Invest Dermatol*. 2009;129:2552-2566.
118. Kakinuma T, Nakamura K, Wakugawa M, et al. Thymus and activation-regulated chemokine in atopic dermatitis: serum thymus and activation-regulated chemokine level is closely related with disease activity. *J Allergy Clin Immunol*. 2001;107:535-541.
119. Pivarcsi A, Gombert M, Dieu-Nosjean MC, et al. CC chemokine ligand 18, an atopic dermatitis-associated and dendritic cell-derived chemokine, is regulated by staphylococcal products and allergen exposure. *J Immunol*. 2004;173:5810-5817.
120. Günther C1, Bello-Fernandez C, Kopp T, et al. CCL18 is expressed in atopic dermatitis and mediates skin homing of human memory T cells. *J Immunol*. 2005;174:1723-1728.
121. Park CO, Lee HJ, Lee JH, et al. Increased expression of CC chemokine ligand 18 in extrinsic atopic dermatitis patients. *Exp Dermatol*. 2008;17(1):24-9.
122. Gombert M, et al. CCL1-CCR8 interactions: an axis mediating the recruitment of T cells and Langerhans-type dendritic cells to sites of atopic skin inflammation. *J Immunol*. 2005;174:5082-5091.
123. Combadiere C, Ahuja SK, Murphy PM. Cloning and functional expression of a human eosinophil CC chemokine receptor. *J Biol Chem*. 1995;270:16491-16494.
124. Teixeira MM, Dieu-Nosjean MC, Winterberg F, et al. Chemokine-induced eosinophil recruitment. Evidence of a role for endogenous eotaxin in an in vivo allergy model in mouse skin. *J Clin Invest* 1997;100:1657-1666.
125. Yawalkar N, Uguccioni M, Schärer J, et al. Enhanced expression of eotaxin and CCR3 in atopic dermatitis. *J Invest Dermatol*. 1999;113:43-48.
126. Kaburagi Y, Shimada Y, Nagaoka T, et al. Enhanced production of CC-chemokines (RANTES, MCP-1, MIP-1α, MIP-1β, and eotaxin) in patients with atopic dermatitis. *Arch Dermatol Res*. 2001;293:350-355.

127. Petering H, Kluthe C, Dulkys Y, et al. Characterization of the CC chemokine receptor 3 on human keratinocytes. *J Invest Dermatol*. 2001;116:549-555.
128. Cooper PJ, Beck LA, Espinel I, et al. Eotaxin and RANTES expression by the dermal endothelium is associated with eosinophil infiltration after ivermectin treatment of onchocerciasis. *Clin Immunol*. 2000;95:51-61.
129. Prens E, Debets R, Hegmans J. T lymphocytes in psoriasis. *Clin Dermatol*. 1995;13:115-129.
130. Homey B, Dieu-Nosjean MC, Wiesenborn A, et al. Up-regulation of macrophage inflammatory protein-3 alpha/CCL20 and CC chemokine receptor 6 in psoriasis. *J Immunol*. 2000;164:6621-6632.
131. Fitzhugh DJ, Naik S, Caughman SW, et al. Cutting edge: C-C chemokine receptor 6 is essential for arrest of a subset of memory T cells on activated dermal microvascular endothelial cells under physiologic flow conditions in vitro. *J Immunol*. 2000;165:6677-6681.
132. Singh SP, Zhang HH, Foley JF, et al. Human T cells that are able to produce IL-17 express the chemokine receptor CCR6. *J Immunol*. 2007;180:214-221.
133. Blauvelt A. T-helper 17 Cells in psoriatic plaques and additional genetic links between IL-23 and psoriasis. *J Invest Dermatol*. 2008;128:1064-1067.
134. Hedrick MN, Lonsdorf AS, Shirakawa AK, et al. CCR6 is required for IL-23–induced psoriasis-like inflammation in mice. *J Clin Invest*. 2009;119:2317-2329.
135. Schaerli P, Britschgi M, Keller M, et al. Characterization of human T cells that regulate neutrophilic skin inflammation. *J Immunol*. 2004;173:2151-2158.
136. Keller M, Spanou Z, Schaerli P, et al. T cell-regulated neutrophilic inflammation in autoinflammatory diseases. *J Immunol*. 2005;175:7678-7686.
137. Schneider G, Salcedo R, Welniak L, et al. The diverse role of chemokines in tumor progression: [rospects for intervention [review]. *Int J Mol Med*. 2001;8(3):235-44.
138. Singh RK, Gutman M, Radinsky R, et al. Expression of interleukin 8 correlates with the metastatic potential of human melanoma cells in nude mice. *Cancer Res*. 1994;54:3242-3247.
139. Addison CL, Daniel TO, Burdick MD, et al. The CXC chemokine receptor 2, CXCR2, is the putative receptor for ELR+ CXC chemokine-induced angiogenic activity. *J Immunol*. 2000;165:5269-5277.
140. Kim M-Y, Oskarsson T, Acharyya S, et al. Tumor self-seeding by circulating cancer cells. *Cell*. 2009;139:1315-1326.
141. Schadendorf D, Möller A, Algermissen B, et al. IL-8 produced by human malignant melanoma cells in vitro is an essential autocrine growth factor. *J Immunol*. 1993;151:2667-2675.
142. Coussens LM, Werb Z. Inflammatory cells and cancer. *J Exp Med* 2001;193:F23-F26.
143. Ferreira AM, Takagawa S, Fresco R, et al. Diminished induction of skin fibrosis in mice with MCP-1 deficiency. *J Invest Dermatol*. 2006;126:1900-1908.
144. Lin EY, Nguyen AV, Russell RG, et al. Colony-stimulating factor 1 promotes progression of mammary tumors to malignancy. *J Exp Med*. 2001;193:727-740.
145. Yao L, Sgadari C, Furuke K, et al. Contribution of natural killer cells to inhibition of angiogenesis by interleukin-12. *Blood* 1999;93:1612-1621.
146. Bell D. In breast carcinoma tissue, immature dendritic cells reside within the tumor, whereas mature dendritic cells are located in peritumoral areas. *J Exp Med*. 1999;190:1417-1426.
147. Fushimi T, Kojima A, Moore MAS, et al. Macrophage inflammatory protein 3α transgene attracts dendritic cells to established murine tumors and suppresses tumor growth. *J Clin Invest*. 2000;105:1383-1393.
148. Curiel TJ, Coukos G, Zou L, et al. Specific recruitment of regulatory T cells in ovarian carcinoma fosters immune privilege and predicts reduced survival. *Nat Med*. 2004;10:942-949.
149. Balch CM, Soong SJ, Gershenwald JE, et al. Prognostic factors analysis of 17,600 melanoma patients: validation of the American Joint Committee on Cancer melanoma staging system. *J Clin Oncol*. 2001;19:3622-3634.
150. Kakinuma T. Chemokines, chemokine receptors, and cancer metastasis. *J Leukoc Biol*. 2006;79:639-651.
151. Muller A, Homey B, Soto H, et al. Involvement of chemokine receptors in breast cancer metastasis. *Nature* 2001;410:50-56.
152. Staller P, Sulitkova J, Lisztwan J, et al. Chemokine receptor CXCR4 downregulated by von Hippel–Lindau tumour suppressor pVHL. *Nature*. 2003;425:307-311.
153. Orimo A, Gupta PB, Sgroi DC, et al. Stromal fibroblasts present in invasive human breast carcinomas promote tumor growth and angiogenesis through elevated SDF-1/CXCL12 secretion. *Cell*. 2005;121:335-348.
154. Murakami T, Maki W, Cardones AR, et al. Expression of CXC chemokine receptor-4 enhances the pulmonary metastatic potential of murine B16 melanoma cells. *Cancer Res*. 2002;62:7328-7334.
155. Wiley HE, Gonzalez EB, Maki W, et al. Expression of CC chemokine receptor-7 and regional lymph node metastasis of B16 murine melanoma. *JNCI J Natl Cancer Inst*. 2001;93:1638-1643.
156. Fang L, Lee VC, Cha E, et al. CCR7 regulates B16 murine melanoma cell tumorigenesis in skin. *J Leukoc Biol*. 2008;84:965-972.
157. Letsch A, Keilholz U, Schadendorf D, et al. Functional CCR9 expression is associated with small intestinal metastasis. *J Invest Dermatol*. 2004;122:685-690.
158. Murakami T, Cardones AR, Finkelstein SE, et al. Immune evasion by murine melanoma mediated through CC chemokine receptor-10. *J Exp Med*. 2003;198:1337-1347.
159. Simonetti O, Goteri G, Lucarini G, et al. Potential role of CCL27 and CCR10 expression in melanoma progression and immune escape. *Eur J Cancer*. 2006;42:1181-1187.
160. Ferenczi K, Fuhlbrigge RC, Kupper TS, et al. Increased CCR4 expression in cutaneous T cell lymphoma. *J Invest Dermatol*. 2002;119:1405-1410.
161. Narducci MG. Skin homing of Sezary cells involves SDF-1-CXCR4 signaling and down-regulation of CD26/dipeptidylpeptidase IV. *Blood*. 2005;107:1108-1115.
162. Notohamiprodjo M, Segerer S, Huss R, et al. CCR10 is expressed in cutaneous T-cell lymphoma. *Int J Cancer*. 2005;115:641-647.
163. Sokolowska-Wojdylo M, Wenzel J, Gaffal E, et al. Circulating clonal CLA+ and CD4+ T cells in Sezary syndrome express the skin-homing chemokine receptors CCR4 and CCR10 as well as the lymph node-homing chemokine receptor CCR7. *Br J Dermatol*. 2005;152:258-264.
164. Arvanitakis L, Geras-Raaka E, Varma A, et al. Human herpesvirus KSHV encodes a constitutively active G-protein-coupled receptor linked to cell proliferation. *Nature*. 1997;385:347-350.

165. Locati M, Murphy PM. Chemokines and chemokine receptors: biology and clinical relevance in inflammation and AIDS. *Annu Rev Med*. 1999;50:425-440.
166. Liu R, Paxton WA, Choe S, et al. Homozygous defect in HIV-1 coreceptor accounts for resistance of some multiply-exposed individuals to HIV-1 infection. *Cell*. 1996;86:367-377.
167. Gerard C, Rollins BJ. Chemokines and disease. *Nat Immunol*. 2001;2:108-115.
168. Blauvelt A. The role of skin dendritic cells in the initiation of human immunodeficiency virus infection. *Am J Med*. 1997;102:16-20.
169. Kawamura T, Cohen SS, Borris DL, et al. Candidate microbicides block HIV-1 infection of human immature langerhans cells within epithelial tissue explants. *J Exp Med*. 2000;192:1491-1500.
170. Cooper DA, Heera J, Goodrich J, et al. Maraviroc versus efavirenz, both in combination with zidovudine-lamivudine, for the treatment of antiretroviral-naive subjects with CCR5-tropic HIV-1 infection. *J Infect Dis*. 2010;201(6):803-13.
171. Murakami T, Nakajima T, Koyanagi Y, et al. A small molecule CXCR4 inhibitor that blocks T cell line-tropic HIV-1 infection. *J Exp Med* 1997;186:1389-1393.
172. Hernandez PA, Gorlin RJ, Lukens JN, et al. Mutations in the chemokine receptor gene CXCR4 are associated with WHIM syndrome, a combined immunodeficiency disease. *Nat Genet*. 2003;34:70-74.
173. Diaz GA, Gulino AV. WHIM syndrome: a defect in CXCR4 signaling. *Curr Allergy Asthma Rep*. 2005;5:350-355.

Chapter 13 :: Basic Principles of Immunologic Diseases in Skin (Pathophysiology of Immunologic/Inflammatory Skin Diseases)
:: Keisuke Nagao & Mark C. Udey

第十三章
皮肤免疫性疾病发生的基本原理（免疫性/炎症性皮肤病的病理生理学）

中文导读

本章内容分为7节：①过敏性接触性皮炎；②药物反应；③特应性皮炎；④银屑病；⑤斑秃；⑥自身免疫性大疱病；⑦结论和未来方向。本章介绍了过敏性和炎症性皮肤病、自身免疫性疾病和药物反应的精选例子，详细了解导致免疫性/炎症性皮肤病的机制，将有助于开发毒性更低、更有效的治疗方法。

第一节过敏性接触性皮炎，介绍了过敏性接触性皮炎(ACD)是一种常见的炎症性皮肤疾病，其免疫学的病理生理学机制包括遗传易感性，半抗原诱导的接触超敏反应（CHS）。CD8+T细胞应该是ACD皮肤炎症的主要介质，但CD4+T细胞的激活可能是CD8+T细胞反应所必需的。

第二节药物反应，介绍了严重的皮肤不良反应(SCARs)是由药物引起的异常免疫反应，其免疫学的病理生理学机制包括遗传易感性、细胞毒性T细胞、嗜酸性粒细胞增多、药物类型、TCR结构和特异性的改变等，并介绍了目前的研究进展。

第三节特应性皮炎，介绍了特应性皮炎(AD)是一种常见的炎症性皮肤病，病理生理学机制包括Filaggrin基因功能缺失突变等、遗传因素、皮肤微生物群中金黄色葡萄球菌的菌群失调等。最后还介绍了目前治疗AD的生物制剂。

第四节银屑病，介绍了目前新的观点，认为银屑病是一种皮肤炎症非常明显的全身性疾病。对于其病理生理学基础的认识经历了几个阶段，首先发现淋巴细胞在银屑病发病机制中的关键作用，然后发现抗肿瘤坏死因子α拮抗药治疗银屑病的有效性，随后进一步明确了全新的T细胞亚群，IL-23/IL-17轴在银屑病中的相关性。

第五节斑秃，介绍了斑秃是以淋巴细胞为主的炎症。对于其病理生理学基础，编者提到了CD4+CD25-(辅助)T细胞与CD8+T细胞可促进疾病进展，而CD4+CD25+(调节性)T细胞与CD8+T细胞可防止疾病的发生、基因的多态性，是JAK和STAT转录因子的关键作用。但对于其病因探讨还有待进一步研究。

第六节自身免疫性大疱病，介绍了天疱疮和大疱性类天疱疮是研究最深入的两种自身免疫性大疱病。天疱疮患者的表皮Dsg3和Dsg1、大疱性类天疱疮患者的基底膜带BP180和BP230是主要的自身抗原。编者特别介绍了目前除糖皮质激素等治疗外，抗B细胞表达的细胞表面蛋白CD20单克隆抗体利妥昔单抗使得对自身免疫性大疱性疾病，特别是天疱疮的靶向治疗成为可能，最后还提到CAART细胞的替代方法，将会是治疗天疱疮（和其他自身抗体介导的疾病）的新的抗原特异性疗法，这些疗法将比目前治疗更安全和更有效。

第七节结论和未来方向，介绍了目前在银屑病和斑秃方面取得成功的方法，很可能在其他免疫性/炎症性皮肤病患者的研究中具有指导作用，成为将来治疗方法改进的基础。

〔粟 娟〕

> **AT A GLANCE**
>
> - Immunologic/inflammatory skin diseases result from inappropriate and frequently exaggerated responses to endogenous skin constituents or external stimuli and are orchestrated by leukocytes and nonleukocytes.
> - Disease pathogenesis is often incompletely understood, but select experimental models and skin diseases have provided insight into the pathogenesis of human immunologic/inflammatory skin diseases.
> - This chapter provides examples where disease pathogenesis is reasonably well understood and describes contemporary approaches that have resulted in improved understanding and, in some instances, improved therapy.

INTRODUCTION

The skin is a physical barrier that is vital for the maintenance of organismal homeostasis. It experiences, and reacts to, a constant barrage of external insults including environmental changes (heat extremes, changes in humidity, sunlight exposure, etc), allergens, toxic chemicals, and pathogenic microbes. In addition to keratinocytes, Merkel cells, melanocytes, fibroblasts, adipocytes, and vascular cells, recent studies document that skin harbors a community of resident leukocytes whose composition and activation status is tuned by commensal microbes. In aggregate, these leukocytes and nonleukocytes constitute a critically important immunologic interface between organism and other.

Immune responses involving skin are highly orchestrated. Appropriate immune responses are directed exclusively (or primarily) against external agents, they are sufficiently (but not excessively) vigorous and they are time-limited. Correspondingly, there are multiple mechanisms that promote and suppress immune and inflammatory reactions in skin. Inappropriate or dysregulated local or systemic responses against self-antigens, foreign antigens, or microbes that are associated with, or enter via, skin may result in skin diseases. Examples include allergic and inflammatory skin diseases, autoimmune diseases, and drug reactions. Selected examples of each of these disease categories will be discussed. Ultimately, detailed understanding of mechanisms that cause immunologic/inflammatory skin diseases will facilitate development of less toxic, more effective therapies.

ALLERGIC CONTACT DERMATITIS

Allergic contact dermatitis (ACD) is a common inflammatory skin condition caused by repeated exposures to haptens, typically low-molecular-weight chemicals and metals, which interact with endogenous proteins to form immunogenic (complete) antigens after entering skin. ACD can be acute or chronic, depending on the nature, dose, and frequency of allergen exposure. For example, after sensitization to urushiol (a lipid component of poison ivy sap), individuals predictably develop acute ACD after reexposure. In contrast, occupational ACD commonly results from long-term exposure to low doses of metal ions such as nickel or chromium. Topical or systemic corticosteroids are commonly prescribed for ACD, but avoiding reexposure to the relevant allergen is crucial for effective treatment. However, it is not uncommon for the offending allergen to be difficult to identify, particularly in patients with occupational ACD.

Individual susceptibility and/or familial predisposition to ACD has been observed in studies where haptens were used to sensitize human volunteers in controlled experiments. However, evidence suggesting that genetic susceptibility to ACD is important is not strong. HLA haplotype associations have been reported, but results of different studies are conflicting. Polymorphisms in genes including *ACE*, *TNFA*, and *IL16* have been described,[1-3] but the cohorts studied were small and the significance of these findings remains to be determined. A recent genomewide association studies (GWAS) performed in a Korean population with patch test–proven nickel allergy reported associations of SNPs in *Netrin-4* and *Pellino-1* with ACD.[4] Although the functional significance of these SNPs remains to be validated, the suggested involvement of Pellino-1 in ACD is interesting because Pellino-1 participates in toll-like receptor 4 (TLR4)–mediated signaling, a pathway known to be involved in nickel allergy. Possible explanations for conflicting results in different GWASs may relate to the diversity of chemicals that cause ACD and the varying genetic compositions of the populations selected for investigation.

Rodent models of ACD (hapten-induced contact hypersensitivity [CHS] responses) have been extensively studied. These studies have provided mechanistic insights into initial responses to allergen introduction and those that occur after subsequent challenge. In the laboratory, CHS is initiated by applying haptens to shaved mouse abdominal skin. Haptens are typically dissolved in mixtures of organic solvents that penetrate stratum corneum and are mildly irritating after topical application. Although initial exposures to haptens do not cause dermatitis, the innate immune system is engaged, leading to activation of antigen-presenting cells (APCs) that acquire or express complete antigens and subsequently stimulate allergen-specific memory T cells, completing the sensitization (afferent) phase (Fig. 13-1A). When haptens are subsequently applied to mouse ear skin, T cell–mediated dermatitis results (Fig. 13-1B). The intensities of the immune responses that ensue during this elicitation phase is quantitated by measuring ear thickness (ear swelling).

Initial exposures to haptens that commonly elicit ACD in patients signal via inflammasomes and/or toll-like receptors (TLRs); 2 major pathways involved in innate immunity. In the case of urushiol, skin cells are stimulated to release ATP and other danger-associated molecular patterns (DAMPs), as well as reactive oxygen species (ROS), which generates low-molecular-weight hyaluronic acid. These events lead to inflammasome activation, resulting in release of proinflammatory chemokines and cytokines including IL-1β, IL-18, and TNF-α.[5] The human contact allergen Ni^{2+} directly binds to human, but not mouse, TLR4.[6] Ni^{2+} is not an effective sensitizer in control mice, but TLR4-deficient mice that have been genetically engineered to express human TLR4 exhibit Ni^{2+}-induced CHS. After binding to TLR4, Ni^{2+} stimulates production of interferons, IL-1β and IL-18. Cr^{2+}, another metal ion and common contact allergen, stimulates the innate immune cells by engaging both TLRs and inflammasomes.[7] TLR-signaling mediates an initial priming event to induce pro-IL-1β synthesis, and activation of the inflammasome component NLRP3 via ROS leads to processing of pro-IL-1β into bioactive cytokine.

The frequently used experimental haptens TNCB, DNFB, oxazolone, and fluorescein isothiocyanate (FITC) also activate multiple immunologically relevant signaling pathways. Activation of inflammasomes is critical because mice that are individually deficient in inflammasome components (Asc, Card9 and Nalp3 or caspase-1) each exhibit impaired CHS responses.[8-10] Deficiency of MyD88, an adaptor molecule that is required for signaling by most TLRs, and simultaneous deficiency of TLR2 and TLR4 also lead to

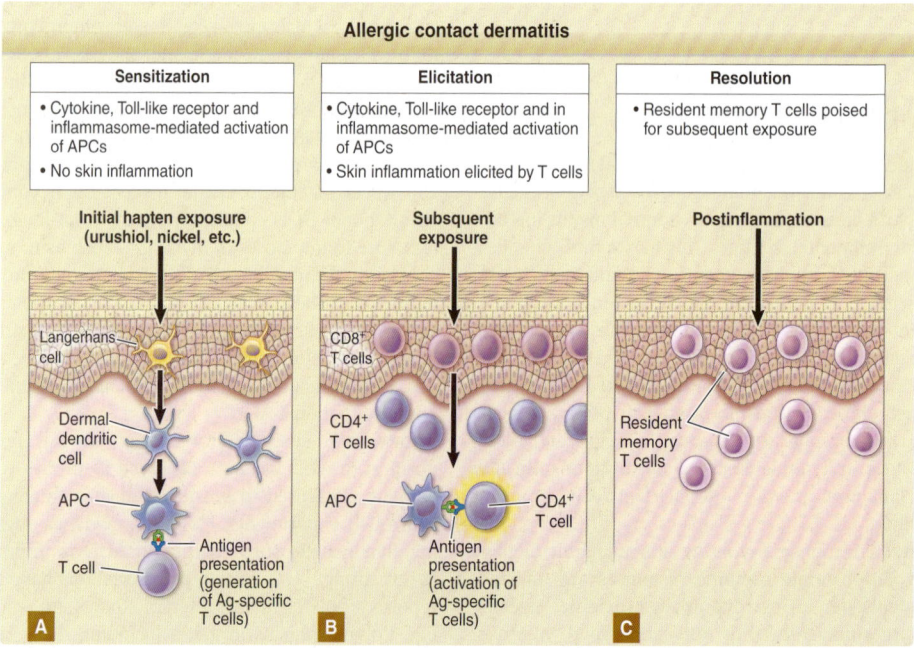

Figure 13-1 Phases of acute contact dermatitis/contact hypersensitivity. Initial exposure to haptens causes perterbations in the epidmeris, activating APCs to generate antigen-specific T cells (**A**). Subsequent exposure to the same hapten results in T cell–mediated inflammation in the skin (**B**). Resident memory T cells that are generated and distributed throughout the body surface are poised to cause inflammation on further encounters with the hapten (**C**).

impaired CHS responses in mice, indicating that TLRs play important roles.[11] Thus, epicutaneous application of contact sensitizers activates multiple pathways that result in an inflammatory milieu that activates APCs in skin and leads to expansion of antigen-specific T cells. These innate proinflammatory processes may originate in leukocytes and nonleukocytes, and are important upstream events that are required for contact sensitization.

Although Langerhans cells (LCs) have long been considered to be critically important APCs in CHS, evidence supporting this concept is not entirely convincing. Because haptens easily penetrate epidermis and reach the dermis, both LCs and dermal dendritic cells (DDCs) encounter contact allergens. Analysis of CHS responses in a mouse model in which LCs were constitutively depleted revealed enhanced CHS responses,[12] whereas 2 mouse models involving transient LC depletion exhibited unchanged or slightly reduced CHS responses.[13,14] Although different haptens were used in these latter studies and the timing of LC depletion also differed, none of these reports concluded that LCs were absolutely essential for CHS responses. DDCs have been demonstrated to contribute to CHS responses and may compensate for the loss of LCs in the experiments just described. Indeed, CD8α+ DCs and DDCs, but not LCs, contribute to CD8+ T-cell responses during antiviral responses.[15] It is possible that antigen-specific CHS responses are primarily dependent on DCs other than LCs. Another possibility is that immune responses to chemically distinct contact allergens involve different signaling pathways and/or even different leukocyte subpopulations. Recent studies propose that urushiol binds to CD1a, an MHC-related cell surface molecule that is expressed by LCs, and that CD1a-bound urushiol stimulates antigen-reactive T cells to release cytokines.[16] This may be an example in which LCs play a critical role in ACD because LCs preferentially form the complete antigen.

After activation, allergen-bearing DC migrate to skin-draining lymph nodes to initiate T-cell expansion and development of hapten-specific memory T cells (Fig. 13-1A). CD8+ T cells appear to be the primary mediators of skin inflammation in ACD, but CD4+ T-cell activation may be required for optimal CD8+ T-cell responses (Fig. 13-1B). CD8+ T cells accumulate not only in lesional and postlesional skin, but they also distribute to distant skin sites where they can persist locally as resident memory T cells (TRMs)[17] (Fig. 13-1C). After contact allergen exposure, antigen-activated naïve T cells undergo clonal expansion and differentiate into both TRM and central memory T cells.[18] TRMs mediate rapid CHS responses, whereas central memory T cells cause delayed responses. The existence of these distinct T-cell subpopulations explains why ACD can be induced in sensitized individuals after prolonged periods of time and why ACD frequently involves multiple skin sites. As is true in most T cell–mediated diseases, regulatory T cells are thought to play major roles in attenuation or termination of inflammation in CHS.

DRUG REACTIONS

Severe cutaneous adverse reactions (SCARs) are potentially life-threating conditions that are thought to be caused by aberrant immune responses that are elicited by drugs, and represent another example of immunologic/inflammatory skin diseases caused by external agents. SCARs include Stevens–Johnson syndrome (SJS), toxic epidermal necrolysis (TEN), and drug-induced hypersensitivity syndrome (DiHS) (or drug reaction eosinophilia with systemic symptoms [DRESS]).[19] Acute generalized exanthematous pustulosis is commonly included as SCAR, but is, in general, less severe than SJS/TEN and DiHS/DRESS.[19]

Prompt identification and discontinuation of offending drugs is critical for treatment of SCARs. SCARs have not been effectively modeled in experimental animals.

Evidence of genetic predisposition to SCARs and other drug eruptions has emerged in recent years. In cohorts of Han-Chinese patients, SJS/TEN that is caused by allopurinol and carbamazepine is strongly associated with the HLA haplotypes B*58:01[20] and B*15:02,[21] respectively. These studies indicate that HLA haplotypes predispose to SCARs and also demonstrate that the relationship between genotype and SJS/TEN susceptibility is drug-specific. Importantly, HLA haplotypes B*58:01 and B*15:02 are not associated with SJS/TEN in European or Japanese cohorts, indicating that genetic predispositions are dependent on ethnicity. Along these lines, dapsone hypersensitivity syndrome, a form of DiHS/DRESS, has been associated with the HLA-B*13:01 haplotype in Asians but not in Europeans and Africans.[22] The striking association of specific MHC Class I haplotypes with SCARs is consistent with the concept that T-cell receptor engagement on drug-specific CD8+ T cells is causal. Although genetic predisposition to SCARs in non-Asians is also likely, this has yet to be demonstrated.

Cytotoxic T cells can be readily detected in SJS/TEN lesions, suggesting that these cells are pathogenic. In early SJS, CD8+ T cells accumulate along the dermal–epidermal junction, causing interface dermatitis with keratinocyte apoptosis (Fig. 13-2) as is also observed in erythema multiforme. The involvement of CD8+ T cells in SJS/TEN is consistent with the GWAS data alluded to above, because CD8+ T cells recognize antigen epitopes that are associated with MHC Class I antigens. Fixed drug eruptions (FDEs) also feature CD8+ T cell–mediated interface dermatitis. In FDE, discrete erythema multiforme-like lesions predictably recur in previously involved locations after systemic drug administration. This phenomenon probably reflects the existence of clones of drug-reactive CD8+ resident memory T (TRM) cells that remain at sites of previous skin lesions where they are poised to respond if offending drugs are readministered. Indeed, persistence of CD8+ T cells can be detected in skin long after FRD lesions have resolved.[23]

Cytotoxic T cells responses are less prominent in DiHS/DRESS. Here patients present with

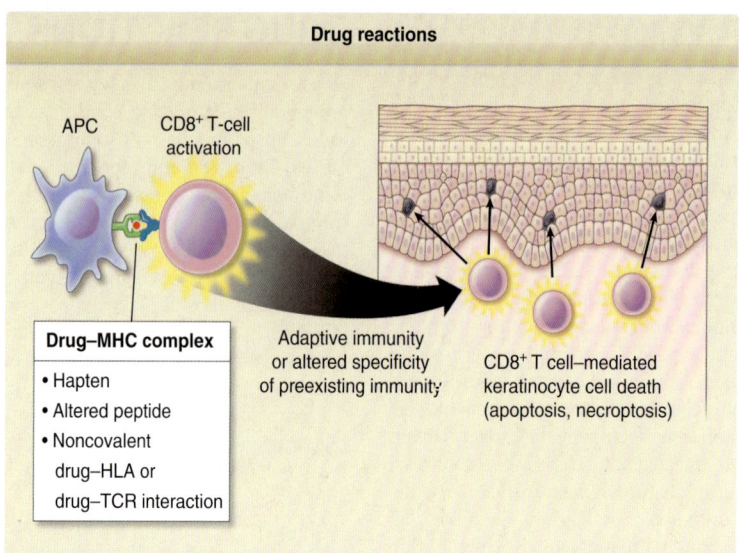

Figure 13-2 Immune-mediated mechanisms in drug hypersensitivity. Canonical or aberrant activation of T cells triggered by a culprit drug results in T cell–mediated keratinocyte cell death in severe drug reactions such as Stevens–Johnson syndrome and toxic epidermal necrolysis.

maculopapular or morbilliform lesions that may coalesce and become confluent. Peripheral eosinophilia is a hallmark feature of DiHS/DRESS, but the role of eosinophils in disease pathogenesis is uncertain. The presence of lymphadenopathy and appearance of atypical (activated) lymphocytes in peripheral blood suggests a T cell–mediated pathophysiology. Expansion of regulatory T cells may result in immunocompromise in the initial stage of DiHS/DRESS,[24] allowing reactivation of herpes virus infections, including human herpes viruses 6 and 7, Epstein–Barr (EB) virus, and cytomegalovirus. EB virus–specific CD8+ T cells are reported to be increased in the circulation and cause tissue damage in EB virus–infected tissues, including liver, that is typical of DiHS/DRESS.[25] B cells, which serve as a reservoir for EB virus, also may be targeted because patients frequently exhibit hypogammaglobinemia.

DiHS/DRESS patients exhibit immunologic abnormalities long after resolution of the acute phase and may develop autoimmune diseases such as Hashimoto thyroiditis, systemic lupus erythematosus, and Type I diabetes.[26] Accentuated immune responses against herpes viruses and the occurrence of autoimmune diseases suggest that breakdown of peripheral tolerance is a major contributor to DiHS/DRESS.

Drugs that cause SCARs are small molecules that are unlikely to be directly recognized by T cells. The nature of epitopes that are recognized and mechanisms that are responsible for their generation have not been delineated with certainty. Several models have been proposed[27] (Fig. 13-2). As is the case in CHS, drugs that cause SCARs may act like haptens, forming complete antigens by combining with endogenous proteins. Penicillins, for example, may bind to carrier proteins to form immunogenic neoantigens that may become targets of adaptive immunity. In abacavir hypersensitivity, the altered peptide model proposes that abacavir binds directly to the peptide-binding groove of HLA-B*57:01, thereby modifying the self-peptides that are presented, creating functionally abacavir-dependent neoantigens that can be recognized by CD8+ T cells. The pharmacologic interaction with immune receptors (p-i) concept posits that drugs bypass classic antigen-processing mechanisms and trigger immune responses through direct, noncovalent interactions with human leucocyte antigen (HLA) alleles and/or T-cell receptors (TCRs) that are expressed on cell surfaces. Activation of preexisting T cells via such mechanisms could explain why drug reactions occur within hours to few days in patients after initial exposure to causative drugs.

Finally, the altered TCR repertoire model proposes that drugs bind directly to TCRs and promote inappropriate T-cell reactivity to self-antigens. Using a T-cell clone isolated from a patient with a maculopapular drug eruption, it was shown that sulfamethoxazole binds to TCR containing Vβ20-1 variable domains. TCR–drug binding could induce a conformational change in the TCR that could alter TCR specificity. TCR VB-11-ISGSY was the predominant clonotype in carbamazepine-reactive T cells (those that proliferate and produce the cytotoxic molecule granulysin) from SJS/TEN in Taiwanese patients harboring HLA B*15:02. In these studies, activation of T cells by carbamazepine was inhibited by a blocking antibody against TCR VB-11, reinforcing the importance of TCR engagement in drug hypersensitivity.

Recent human studies have improved our understanding of the pathophysiology of drug reactions (Fig. 13-2), but much remains to be learned. Development of humanized mouse models in which mechanisms can be dissected in vivo may advance the field considerably.

ATOPIC DERMATITIS

Atopic dermatitis (AD) is a common inflammatory skin disease that is characterized by dry skin and eczematous dermatitis with severe itching. Classic AD arises in children and may be accompanied by the later onset of asthma, allergic rhinitis, and/or food allergies ("the atopic march") (Fig. 13-3). Serum levels of IgE and CCL17 (TARC), both of which are characteristic of Type 2 immune responses, are increased in AD. Other immune cells, including T helper Type 1 (Th1), Th17, and Th22 cells, likely mediate the dermatitis, however (Fig. 13-3). AD commonly remits in late childhood, but can recur later in life and persist for years thereafter. AD is routinely treated with combinations of topical steroids, immunosuppressives, and emollient creams but current therapies are inadequate. Anti-histamines are commonly prescribed, but unrelieved pruritus is a major clinical problem.

Combinations of endogenous and exogenous factors have long been suspected to be involved in AD pathogenesis but, until recently, causal factors had not been identified. The discovery that AD patients harbor loss-of-function mutations in the gene encoding the structural protein filaggrin provided compelling evidence that impairment of an epidermal structural protein contributes to AD pathogenesis.[28] GWAS have demonstrated that single-nucleotide polymorphisms (SNPs) in a number of other genes are also associated with AD.[29,30] Many of these genes are expressed in immune cells and/or pathways (eg, *IL2*, *IL6R*, *IL7RA*, and *IL18R1*), strongly suggesting that AD etiology is multifactorial. Importantly, GWASs involving genetically distinct patient cohorts have identified both overlapping and nonoverlapping gene associations, consistent with the clinical observations that AD symptoms and signs may differ depending on the patients' ethnicities, and supporting the concept that different genes may influence AD susceptibility in different patient populations.

Although GWASs identify candidate loci that may be involved in AD pathogenesis, SNPs may not result in functional alterations in gene function. Additionally, SNPs may be genetically linked to, but distinct from, genes that are actually involved in AD (linkage disequilibrium). Studies of rare genetic diseases that are caused by mutations in known genes may provide mechanistic insights if clinical features of these

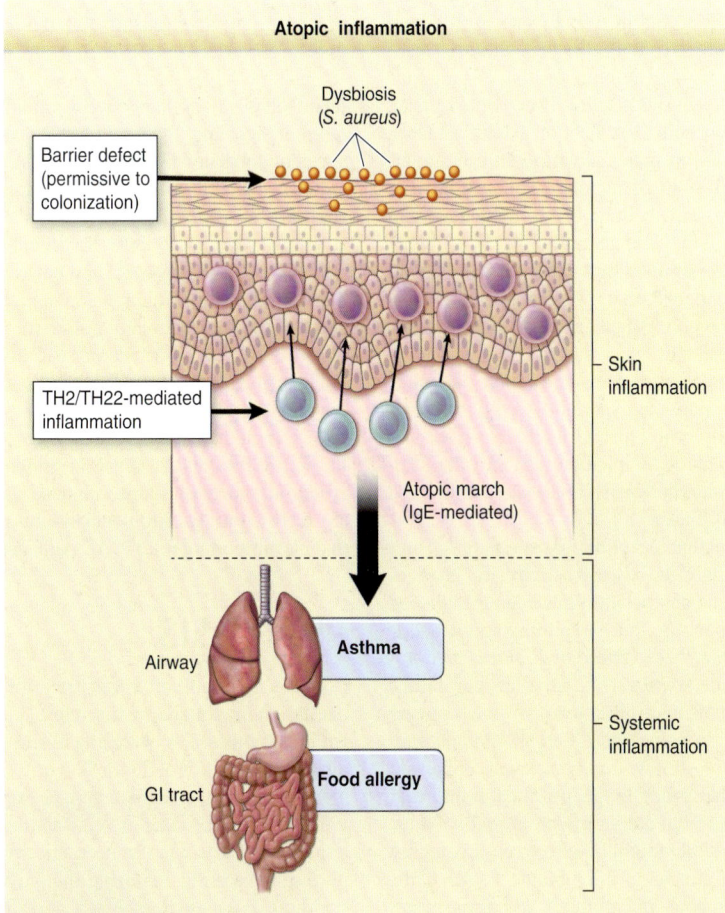

Figure 13-3 Barrier–microbiota–immune cell crosstalk in atopic dermatitis. Impaired barrier, altered microbiota, and accentuated immune responses cause local inflammation in the skin and may also lead to inflammation in distant organs.

diseases overlap with those of AD. For example, Netherton syndrome, a disease with eczematous dermatitis as a prominent feature, is caused by mutations in the cell surface protease inhibitor *SPINK5*.[31] Loss of *SPINK5* leads to increased activity of cell surface serine proteases that compromises the barrier function of the stratum corneum. Interestingly, *SPINK5* polymorphisms have been associated not with AD, but with elevated IgE levels in patients with AD.[32] Job syndrome (hyper IgE syndrome) is characterized by dermatitis and impaired Th17 responses leading to increased susceptibility to *Staphylococcus aureus* colonization or infection, and is caused by loss of function mutations in STAT3.[33] A *STAT3* SNP has been identified in classic AD,[30] suggesting that pathway dysregulation that occurs in Job syndrome might also contribute to AD. Mouse models that feature mutations of genes that are involved in genetic forms of human AD or that correspond to SNPs that are characteristic of AD could provide important mechanistic information that is relevant to patients.

Whereas asthma, allergic rhinitis, and food allergies are clearly IgE-mediated allergic diseases, the mechanisms that drive skin inflammation in AD are not well understood. Patch testing identifies allergens that cause contact dermatitis, but the utility of patch testing in AD patients is controversial, suggesting that skin inflammation that occurs in AD may not result from repetitive exposure to contact allergens. *S. aureus* commonly colonizes AD skin, but the role that this microbe plays in AD pathogenesis also has been controversial. Microbe detection and identification based on DNA sequencing has led to major advances in our understanding of the diversity of microbial communities that reside in human skin (collectively termed the "skin microbiome").[34] Using next-generation DNA sequencing, it has been determined that although only 20% to 30% of non-AD patients carry *S. aureus* as a commensal microbe, both the abundance and relative frequency of *S. aureus* representation in the skin microbiome is increased in AD patients, even when their disease is quiescent. When patients experience acute exacerbations of AD, staphylococci (primarily *S. aureus*) become predominant in the skin microbiome, indicating an intimate relationship between AD disease activity and staphylococcal dysbiosis.[35]

A mouse model that recapitulates aspects of AD and the relationship between disease activity and changes is skin microbiome composition has been established recently.[36] In this model, mice exhibited spontaneous microbial dysbiosis characterized by *S. aureus* predominance accompanied by severe eczematous dermatitis. Furthermore, cutaneous application of *S. aureus* caused eczema, whereas a commensal *Corynebacterium* species did not. Interestingly, *Corynebacterium* enhanced Th2 responses that promote IgE production and that may be relevant to the atopic march in AD patients. This suggests that AD might be effectively treated by manipulating the cutaneous microbiome. Bleach baths modify the cutaneous microbiome and thus represent a practical and cost-effective means of therapy, but mechanisms by which bleach baths control AD have yet to be characterized in detail. Because topical steroids can reverse microbial dysbiosis even in the absence of antibacterial therapy, both inflammation and microbial dysbiosis are likely to be important contributors in a vicious cycle that drives skin inflammation in AD.

The recent development of biologic agents or "biologics" allows selective targeting of mediators or cells, and the efficacy of these interventions can provide insight into the involvement of the targeted pathways in inflammatory skin diseases including AD. Omalizumab, a humanized monoclonal anti-IgE antibody, effectively treats asthma, food allergies and urticaria, but it has not been effective in AD.[37] Although this lack of efficacy may be attributed to the high serum levels of IgE in AD patients, an alternative conclusion is that skin inflammation in AD is not mediated by an IgE-dependent mechanism. Signaling pathways involving IL-4 and/or IL-13 also may be relevant in AD. Phase 3 trials document that dupilumab, which blocks IL-4 and IL-13 signaling by binding to IL-4Rα, is effective in AD.[38] The leukocytes that produce IL-4 and IL-13 in AD remain to be determined. Human and mouse Th2 cells are known to be major sources of IL-4, and murine innate lymphoid cells (lymphoid cells that lack conventional T-cell antigen receptors) have been identified as major sources of IL-13. The contribution of innate lymphoid cells to human AD will be assessed in future studies.

Small molecules that occupy the ATP-binding sites of Janus kinases (JAKs) are effective inhibitors of cytokine receptor signaling. JAK1 and JAK3 play critical roles in signaling mediated by the Th2 cytokines IL-3 and IL-13, as well as IL-7 and IL-15. These cytokines collectively support the maintenance of T lymphocytes, NK cells, and innate lymphoid cells. Tofacitinib and ruxolitinib inhibit both JAK1 and JAK3 and have activity in inflammatory diseases including rheumatoid arthritis, psoriasis and alopecia areata. In light of the efficacy of IL-4/IL-13 blockade and the association of IL-7 and IL-15 receptor polymorphisms in AD, JAK inhibitors may be useful in this patient population. Indeed, topical tofacitinib has been reported to improve Eczema Area and Severity Index (EASI) scores in a Phase IIa randomized trial in AD. Studies of newly developed targeted therapeutic agents are likely to provide additional insights into mechanisms that play important roles in AD pathogenesis.

PSORIASIS

Psoriasis is a common, recalcitrant inflammatory skin disease characterized by discrete plaques with adherent micaceous scales occurring at sites of predilection, including locations of minor skin trauma. Nail involvement is frequent, and characteristic arthritis ("psoriatic arthritis") can co-occur or occur in the absence of skin lesions. Psoriasis has not been effectively modeled in mice until recently, requiring that advances in understanding disease pathogenesis and developing effective therapies be driven by clinical research involving patients. Very recent work indicates that psoriasis is a systemic disease in which skin inflammation is dramatically evident, rather than a disease whose impact is restricted to skin.[39]

The histology of psoriatic lesions is typified by a thickened, hyperproliferative epidermis featuring markedly reduced basal keratinocyte transit times, abnormal keratinocyte differentiation, neutrophilic and lymphocytic inflammation, and prominent capillary loops that extend into the very superficial dermis. At various times, competing schools of thought espoused that psoriasis was caused by abnormalities in keratinocytes, immunocytes, and endothelial cells. The ability of antimetabolites (eg, methotrexate) and ultraviolet radiation (UVB or psoralen + UVA) to ameliorate aspects of the disease was consistent with the concept that keratinocyte growth was abnormal in psoriasis and that this might reflect intrinsic keratinocyte defects, but these interventions also have immunomodulatory properties.

The critical involvement of lymphocytes in psoriasis pathogenesis was convincingly demonstrated when increasingly selective therapies became available.[40] The calcineurin inhibitor cyclosporine is a remarkably effective antipsoriatic agent. The ability of high concentrations of cyclosporine to modulate keratinocyte growth and gene expression in vitro did not exclude keratinocytes as relevant targets in psoriatic patients with certainty, but follow-up clinical studies with the specific lymphocyte-depleting agents denileukin diftitox (an IL-2 receptor–directed cytotoxin) and alefacept (a CD2-binding LFA-3/Fc fusion protein) settled this question. Both of these agents were too toxic to be routinely administered to psoriatic patients because they have broad-spectrum antilymphocyte effects, but studies with increasingly selective immunomodulators have informed our understanding of psoriasis pathogenesis and identified effective therapeutics.

Improved treatment of psoriasis and more detailed understanding of psoriasis pathogenesis has developed in concert with the revolution in "biologic therapy." Although the anti-TNFα neutralizing antibody infliximab (one of the first widely used biologics) was first tested in patients with inflammatory bowel diseases,[41] improvement in skin lesions in patients with concurrent psoriatic led to formal testing of infliximab and demonstration of efficacy in patients with severe psoriasis vulgaris. TNFα is a primary proinflammatory cytokine with many sources, targets, and actions in skin and elsewhere, so initially it was not obvious why infliximab and other TNFα-targeting agents were particularly effective in patients with psoriasis.

The effectiveness of lymphocyte-depleting and lymphocyte-modulating agents in patients with psoriasis indicated that T cells and perturbations in cellular immunity were critical. Prior to the advent of biologics, atopic dermatitis was conceptualized as a Th2-predominant disease whereas psoriasis was thought to be Th1 mediated, with IFNγ as an important effector cytokine. Discovery of entirely new T cell subsets, especially Th17 cells that produce IL-17, opened an entirely new avenue for psoriasis research. TNFα is coproduced by dermal dendritic cells that also produce IL-23, a cytokine that is required for Th17-cell development. IL-23 is a heterodimeric protein composed of IL-23–specific p19 as well as p40, a polypeptide that is shared with the Th1-promoting cytokine IL-12. IL-17 promotes neutrophil-predominant inflammation and plays important roles in responses to microbial pathogens, in part because IL-17 modulates gene expression in keratinocytes leading to increased production of antimicrobial peptides, defensins, and other inflammatory mediators. TNFα augments the effects of IL-17 on keratinocytes.

TNFα, IL-23, and IL-17 production is elevated in lesional skin from patients with psoriasis, and effective treatment reduces the levels of these cytokines. The existence of an IL-17–dependent, TNFα-augmented feed-forward loop that amplifies inflammation in psoriatic lesions provides a construct for understanding why agents that antagonize TNFα signaling are efficacious in this disease. The relevance of the IL-23/IL-17 axis in psoriasis has been even more convincingly demonstrated in subsequent studies with increasingly selective therapeutics. Ustekinumab (anti-human p40) had dramatic effects in patients with psoriasis in pilot studies, and its efficacy has been borne out in subsequent, now long-term, Phase III studies. Because p40 is a polypeptide subunit that is shared by Th17-modulating IL-23 and Th1-modulating IL-12, effects of ustekinumab could not be definitively attributed to modulation of Th17 cells and Il-17.

The anti-IL-17A monoclonal antibodies secukiumab and ixekinumab are now FDA approved for use in patients with psoriasis because they are remarkably effective with rapid onset of action and frequently complete or almost complete responses, convincingly solidifying IL-17's critical role in psoriasis pathogenesis. Anti-IL-23 p19 monoclonal antibodies (including guselkumab) are also reported to be efficacious in psoriatic patients and may be commercially available soon. The utility of agents that target signaling of the Th17-cell product IL-22 that may cause acanthosis by acting directly on keratinocytes has yet to be demonstrated, but this approach may also have merit.

One unanswered question relates to the cellular source of IL-17 in psoriatic skin. Conventional T cells bearing antigen-specific receptors composed of α and β chains were presumed to be responsible, but the possible involvement of recently discovered innate lymphocytes must now be considered. Subsets of innate lymphocytes (termed ILC1, ILC2, and ILC3) have the capacity to produce T-cell cytokines (IFNγ, IL-5/IL-13, and IL-17, respectively) but do not recognize and are not activated by peptide antigens. These cells also do not need to proliferate to express effector function. The extent to which ILCs participate in psoriasis will require further study.

Another unanswered question relates to the aggressiveness with which psoriasis patients should be treated with biologic agents. As of this writing, studies have involved only patients with moderate to severe psoriasis. Several effective biologics have been remarkably well tolerated, but the cost of therapy is significant and cures or long-term remissions do not typically result. The discovery that patients with psoriasis have significant comorbidities, including cardiovascular disease,[42] and decreased life spans suggests that widespread use of systemic treatments might be appropriate. It is possible that biologics may have general health-promoting activities, even in patients with mild psoriasis. Additional clinical research will be required.

From a disease pathogenesis perspective, the major unanswered question in psoriasis relates to the nature of the initial triggering event(s) and the process(es) by which the IL-23/IL-17 axis becomes engaged. Related to this, identification of the source(s) of the lynchpin cytokine IL-17 is critical (see before). Increasingly large and sophisticated GWASs have been conducted with psoriasis patients over the past several decades in an effort to obtain mechanistic insights.[43] Despite that fact that currently identified susceptibility loci explain only a minor component of the genetic predisposition in psoriasis, some conclusions can be drawn. Genetic susceptibility loci in atopic dermatitis and psoriasis are largely nonoverlapping,[44] consistent with the concept that disease-causing mechanisms are distinct in these 2 disorders. GWASs of patients with differing ethnicities yield differing results, reaffirming that psoriasis is a complex multifactorial/multigenic disorder. GWASs of psoriasis variants (including pustular psoriasis and psoriatic arthritis) also highlight different genetic loci, as might be expected in studies of patients with such distinct clinical features.[45]

Most single nucleotide polymorphisms (SNPs) that have been linked to psoriasis occur in regions of the genome that do not encode proteins. Some genetic variants may occur in important gene regulatory regions or may influence gene expression indirectly via transcription of gene regulatory noncoding RNAs. However, it is likely that at least some (and perhaps most) SNPs are actually in linkage disequilibrium with the genetic alterations that are causative. Higher-resolution studies that involve more extensive genetic characterization (whole exome or whole genome sequencing, for example) and/or even larger numbers of patients may be additionally informative.

SNPs in the MHC Class I locus confer the largest amount of genetic risk in both European and Chinese psoriasis populations.[46] Other well-established genetic risk loci include the gene encoding endoplasmic reticulum aminopeptidase 1, genes encoding components of signaling pathways that are operative in innate immunity, and genes that influence the activity of the IL-23/IL-17 axis. There are rare examples of patients with causative mutations in individual genes of interest. These genes include *IL23R*, *CARD14* (a scaffolding protein that participates in NF*k*B signaling), and *IL36RN*. It is not difficult to incorporate linkage of psoriasis to genetic alterations in genes regulating innate immunity and/or the IL-23/IL-17 axis. Strong linkage of psoriasis to genetic alterations in the MHC Class I locus suggests that adaptive immunity and conventional T cells are also very important.

Modern concepts of psoriasis pathogenesis can easily incorporate conventional T cells, but the accepted importance of Th17 cells would predict that variants of interest would occur in the MHC Class II locus, rather than the MHC Class I locus. Despite this, it has been possible to identify MHC Class I–restricted IL-17–producing CD8+ T cells that react with melanocyte-derived ADAMTS-like protein 5 in some psoriatic patients.[47] In other studies, CD4+ and CD8+ T cells reactive with keratinocyte-derived antimicrobial peptide LL37 have been identified.[48] T cells producing IL-17 as well as IFNγ, IL-22, and IL-21 in response to LL37 are more prevalent in psoriatic patients than controls, and frequencies of antigen LL37-reactive T cells in peripheral blood correlate with disease severity. LL37 is an interesting protein antigen because it is more promiscuous with respect to MHC restriction than typical protein antigens. LL37/self DNA complexes are also potent inducers of IFNα/β production by accessory cells, so it is possible that the adjuvant properties of LL37 are also relevant to psoriasis. Undoubtedly, future studies will provide additional insights into early aspects of psoriasis pathogenesis.

ALOPECIA AREATA

Alopecia areata (AA) is an often chronic and disabling disease that is characterized by intermittent and/or long-lasting hair loss of varying severity that can occur in association with other autoimmune diseases including thyroiditis. The 3 major phenotypic variants are termed patchy, universalis (involving the entire scalp), and totalis (involving entire integument). Scalp biopsies obtained from the peripheries of expanding lesions feature lymphocyte-predominant inflammation and patients may respond to locally administered or systemic corticosteroids, both consistent with an immune-mediated etiology. Preferential association of lesional lymphocytes with anagen hair bulbs (Fig. 13-4), rather than the stem cell–containing bulge regions, is consistent with the characterization of AA as a nonscarring alopecia and the ability of skin that appears devoid of terminal hairs to "re-grow" apparently normal complements of hair in some instances.

AA is an example of a fascinating skin disease that has been studied for many years and that has only recently begun to reveal its secrets. Progress can be attributed to multidisciplinary studies of thousands of AA patients buttressed by work involving animal models. Interestingly, studies with patients and rodents have proceeded in parallel and results obtained have often been highly complementary.

Several animal models have been particularly informative.[49] One particular mouse, the C3H/HeJ mouse, develops inflammatory lesions that resemble AA with some regularity as it ages. This occurrence in mice and AA patients is thought to result from loss of "immune privilege" that is a property of normal hair follicles (HFs). The HF antigens that are targeted by lymphocytes and the mechanisms that protect HFs from immune-mediated damage under normal circumstances have not been completely characterized. Immune privilege may depend on low-level expression of MHC Class I and Class II antigens by HF

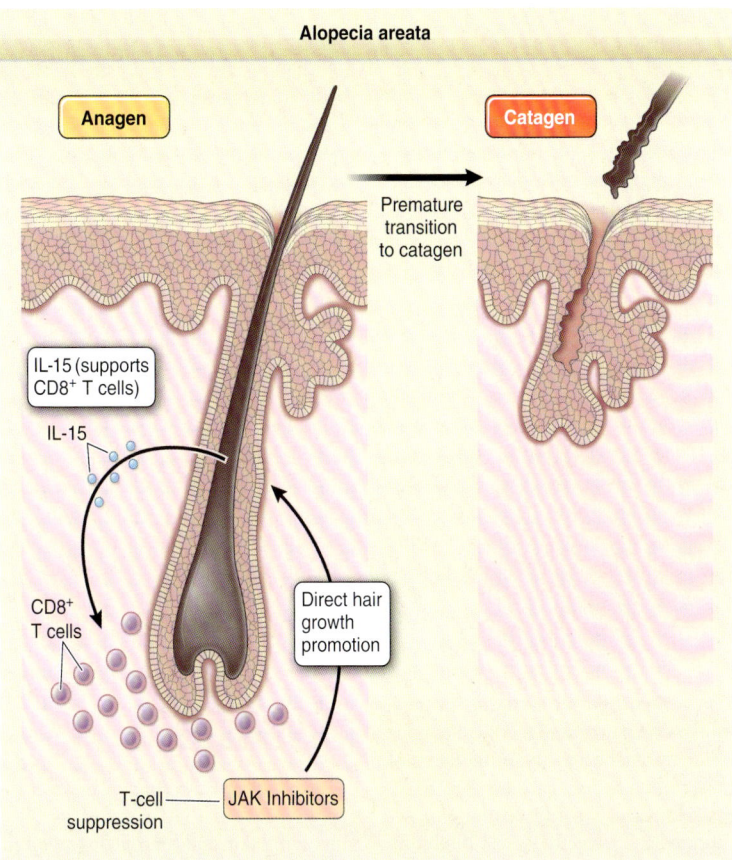

Figure 13-4 Mechanisms involved in alopecia areata. T cell–mediated inflammation in the bulb area induces premature catagen transition and leads to hair loss in alopecia areata. JAK inhibitors can reverse hair loss by suppressing inflammation and by directly acting on hair follicles to induce hair growth.

keratinocytes and local production of immunosuppressive cytokines and perhaps neuropeptides. The frequency of disease development in C3H/HeJ mice can be greatly enhanced by transferring lymphocytes from affected mice into disease-free mice, documenting the importance of lymphocytes in disease pathogenesis and providing an experimental platform with which to characterize the properties of pathogenic cells, potentially dissecting mechanisms that cause HF damage and test novel therapeutic interventions.

Studies in the C3H/HeJ mouse demonstrate that $CD8^+$ (cytotoxic) T cells and IFNγ are important effectors in this model,[50] inducing HF dystrophy and premature entry into catagen via mechanisms that are incompletely characterized (Fig. 13-4). The cytokine IL-15 is known to be important for $CD8^+$ T-cell induction and/or persistence, so it is not surprising that neutralization of IL-15 also attenuates AA activity. Coadministration of $CD4^+$ $CD25^-$ (helper) T cells with $CD8^+$ T cells promotes disease progression whereas coadministration of $CD4^+$ $CD25^+$ (regulatory) T cells with $CD8^+$ T cells prevents disease induction.

The use of xenograft models that involve placement of AA patient scalp skin or normal volunteer glabrous skin onto immunocompromised SCID or SCID beige mice followed by introduction of syngeneic or allogeneic human leukocytes locally or systemically serves as a bridge between studies of the C3H/HeJ mouse model and studies of AA patients. Adoptive transfer of leukocytes results in hair loss within the xenografts, resulting in an experimental system that may facilitate delineation of pathogenic mechanisms and trials of new therapies in a relevant preclinical model. Initial studies of mice engrafted with AA scalp documented the pathogenicity of intracutaneous $CD8^+$ T cells, but logistics limited the general utility of this approach. Attempts to substitute skin and leukocytes from normal volunteers for those from AA patients demonstrated that activated lymphocytes, including NK cells, from even normal individuals could induce AA-like hair loss from syngeneic or allogeneic skin after local injection. Although this "AA" model does not allow assessment of patient-specific factors, it has been used to characterize mechanisms that can lead to hair dystrophy and to screen for agents, including phosphodiesterase inhibitors and ion channel blockers, that may have utility in AA.

There are important physiologic differences between cutaneous immune systems and hair follicles in mice and humans and, as alluded to above, xenograft studies have significant limitations. Fortunately, using contemporary approaches, in recent years it has become possible to move from observational, correlative studies of limited scope to large-scale studies of AA patients who were initially hypothesis-generating and later hypothesis-testing. One important consequence is the identification of targeted therapies that can be expected to have a major impact on AA in the immediate future.

Initial GWASs involving >1000 AA patients and >3000 case controls identified a number of single-nucleotide polymorphisms (SNPs) that were disease-associated.[51] The location of these SNPs suggested the possible involvement of genes related to T cell–mediated immune responses (*CTLA4*, *ICOS*, *IL21/IL2*, *IL2RA*), NK cells (NKG2D ligand genes), as well as antigen presentation (HLA-DR/DQ genes). Subsequent GWASs and related studies have highlighted additional candidate genes that reinforce the importance of T-cell regulators and the role of HLA-DR (encoding MHC Class II antigens) as the dominant susceptibility locus.[52] In follow-up studies of the C3H/HeJ AA mouse model, the importance of CD8$^+$ NKG2D$^+$ T cells and the T-cell cytokines IFNγ, IL-2, and IL-15 was convincingly demonstrated.[50] Involvement of CD8$^+$ T cells, IFNγ and IL-15, in conjunction with studies of gene expression in lesional skin, suggested a critical role for JAKs and STAT (signal transducers and stimulators of transcription) transcription factors and the JAK/STAT pathway as a possible target for intervention. Subsequent studies indicated that selective JAK1 inhibitors have considerable activity in this model, whereas JAK3 inhibitors did not.

The best source of critical information regarding disease effector mechanisms and disease activity is involved tissue obtained from patients. Global transcriptional profiling of lesional skin is an unbiased and comprehensive way to gain insights into cells and proteins that are likely to be present at sites of disease activity. Patient- and animal model-derived samples can be subjected to analogous analyses, so results in these 2 settings can be easily compared. Recent studies of patients with patchy AA (AAP), AA universalis (AAU), and AA totalis (AAT) reinforce preexisting concepts and provide new insights as well.[53] Comparison of AA and normal cutaneous transcriptomes resulted in an AA gene expression signature with ~1000 elevated and ~1000 reduced transcripts in AA lesional skin as compared with controls. Principal components analysis indicated that the gene expression signatures of controls and AAP patients could be distinguished from those of AAU and AAT patients, while the gene expression profiles of AAU and AAT patients did not segregate. Highly represented transcripts in AA biopsies were attributable to the presence of CD8$^+$ T cells, chemokines involved in leukocyte trafficking, and IFNγ signaling (Th1-predominant inflammation). Generation of numerical scores that reflected the aggregate deviation of the gene expression signatures in AA biopsies from those of normal individuals confirmed that AAP patients could be differentiated from controls and AAU/AAT patients, and that profiles from AAU/AAT patients were more abnormal than AAP profiles. Because transcriptional profiling is a measure of ongoing physiologic activity, the latter result suggests that disease is active in AAU/AAT skin and perhaps even more active than in AAP skin. This result is not compatible with the concept that the AAU/AAT is end stage, that HFs are in irreversible catagen, and that antiinflammatory therapies cannot be of benefit in these recalcitrant AA variants.

Although the final solution of the AA puzzle is not yet available, complementary laboratory and clinical research has led to great progress. It is not yet possible to prospectively identify individuals who are at risk or to prevent disease development, but rational and effective targeted therapies are likely to be in widespread use soon. Indeed, recent Phase II studies document significant responses to JAK inhibitors in subpopulations of AA patients.[54,55] One can make the case that AA could be a "poster child" for immunologic/inflammatory skin diseases of uncertain etiology, and analogous laboratory and clinical research approaches could someday result in similar advances.

AUTOIMMUNE BLISTERING DISEASES

Autoimmune blistering diseases are chronic, debilitating diseases that manifest as blisters or erosions involving skin and/or mucous membranes. Some autoimmune blistering diseases are fatal if left untreated. Classification of these diseases is based on clinical features, including lesion distribution and gross and histologic morphology. Pemphigus and pemphigoid are the most common autoimmune blistering disorders. Pemphigus can additionally be subcategorized into pemphigus vulgaris (PV) and pemphigus foliaceous (PF). PV manifests with flaccid bullae or erosions involving mucous membranes and skin, whereas PF affects only the skin and presents with fragile blisters or superficial erosions. Bullous pemphigoid may manifest with urticarial lesions with subsequent development of tense bullae on skin and, much less commonly, erosions on mucous membranes. This stands in contradistinction to mucous membrane pemphigoid and epidermolysis bullosa acquisita, which feature primarily mucosal lesions and mucosal and cutaneous lesions, respectively.

Results from routine histology and direct or indirect immunofluorescence microscopy can provide important diagnostic information. The identification and characterization of autoantigens in blistering diseases, coupled with the demonstration that autoantibodies are pathogenic, have enabled development of novel diagnostic enzyme-linked immunosorbent assays (ELISAs) that detect circulating autoantibodies that react to corresponding autoantigens.

Pemphigus and bullous pemphigoid (BP) are the 2 most intensively studied autoimmune blistering diseases. Studies of patients' sera identified autoantibodies that react with the epidermis in the case of pemphigus patients and with the basement membrane zone in patients with bullous pemphigoid. The demosomal protein desmoglein 3 (Dsg3) is the major autoantigen targeted initially by antibodies in pemphigus vulgaris, and desmoglein 1 (Dsg1) is the primary autoantigen in pemphigus foliaceus.[56] PV patients typically develop anti-Dsg1 autoantibodies at some point after anti-Dsg3 autoantibodies appear. Dsg3 is a major component of desmosomes that mediate cell adhesion between keratinocytes in the lower layers of the epidermis, whereas Dsg1 is a major desmosomal protein expressed by superficial epidermal keratinocytes. The distribution of Dsg3 and Dsg1 in epidermis determines the locations of blister formation in PV and PF, and the sequence of appearance of oral and cutaneous lesions in PV. Because Dsg3, but not Dsg1, is expressed in oral and esophageal mucosae, mucosal involvement is observed in PV but not in PF. Other rare forms of pemphigus include IgA pemphigus, in which IgA autoantibodies against desmocollin 1 (another component of desmosomes), Dsg1, or Dsg3 cause disease, and paraneoplastic pemphigus, which is associated with autoantibodies against multiple desmosomal proteins as well as T cells that may contribute to epidermal–dermal interface destruction.[57]

BP is caused by IgG autoantibodies that react with components of hemidesmosomes, adhesive structures that mediate adhesion of basal keratinocytes to the basement membrane. Two major antigens are targeted in BP; collagen XVII (COL17, also known as BP180 or BPAG1) and the plakin family protein BP230 (BPAG2).[58] COL17 is expressed on cell surfaces and it is considered to be the major BP autoantigen. Although anti-BP230 antibodies also can be frequently detected in patients, the pathophysiologic role of anti-BP230 antibodies is uncertain because BP230 is an intracellular protein. Related diseases include pemphigoid gestationis and pemphgoid herpetiformis. Pemphigoid gestationis exhibits clinical features and autoantibody profiles that are identical to BP and develops only in pregnant women. Mucous membrane pemphigoid has been reported in patients with circulating antibodies reactive with COL17, BP230, laminin 5, laminin 6, Type VII collagen (COL7), laminin 5, laminin 6, and β4 integrins,[59] whereas epidermolysis bullosa acquisita is caused by anti-COL7 antibodies.[60]

Injection of human PV-derived IgG causes blister development in mice.[61] Studies involving recombinant Dsg3 and Dsg1, as well as engineered molecules in which the extracellular domains were exchanged, demonstrated that the anti-Dsg3 autoantibodies that cause skin blistering target N-terminal domains of Dsg3 (extracellular domains 1 and 2).[62,63] Generation of Dsg3 knockout (KO) mice allowed development of an active disease model for PV.[64] Dsg3-reactive T and B cells are generated when Dsg3 KO mice are immunized with recombinant Dsg3. When splenocytes from Dsg3-immune Dsg3 KO mice were transferred into Dsg3-sufficient mice, recipient mice developed skin and mucosal lesions and autoantibodies reactive with Dsg3. Formation of anti-Dsg3 autoantibodies by B cells in these mice is dependent on the presence of CD4+ T cells. Patients with PV and PF also harbor autoantibodies that react with antigens other than Dsg3 and Dsg1.[56,65] It is possible that these autoantibodies also contribute to pemphigus pathogenesis. Lesion formation is not thought to be complement-dependent, and anti-DSG antibodies may cause acantholysis by triggering intracellular signaling in keratinocytes.

In BP patients, the majority of anti-COL17 IgG autoantibodies target the NC16a domain.[66] In contrast to PV, passive transfer of IgG from BP patients does not cause disease in mice.[67] This may reflect varying amino acid sequences in the NC16A domains of COL17 in mice and humans. Supporting this, transgenic mice that express human COL17 do develop blisters after injection with IgG from BP patients.[68] Mechanisms that cause lesion formation in BP appear to be different from those that cause blisters in pemphigus patients. Complement (C3) deposition in the basement membrane zone is universal in BP. Passive transfer of rabbit anti-COL17 into mice causes blisters in normal mice, but not in complement-deficient mice, indicating a critical role for complement in BP lesion formation.[69] Consistent with this, passive transfer of recombinant Fab fragments of human anti-NC16a domain autoantibodies does not cause disease in human COL17-expressing transgenic mice.[66] Local complement activation in BP lesions attracts neutrophils in mice, and these cells are also thought to participate in blister formation, perhaps by producing metalloproteinases. Prominent tissue and peripheral blood eosinophilia also occurs in BP, and IgE autoantibodies can be detected in the sera and skin of a subset of BP patients, consistent with the concept that the immune mechanisms operative in BP are distinct from those in pemphigus.[66]

Autoimmune diseases develop when the immune system inappropriately attacks self-antigens. Central and peripheral tolerance, immune regulatory mechanisms acting in the thymus and peripheral organs, respectively, prevent the immune system from reacting against self in normal individuals. Mechanisms responsible for loss of tolerance in patients with autoimmune diseases have not been elucidated. However, the increased incidence of pemphigus (especially PF) in patients with thymoma suggests that impairment of central tolerance relates to the onset of pemphigus. Some patients with pemphigoid gestationis also develop autoimmune thyroiditis, suggesting that loss of tolerance may occur in these patients as well, and that both autoimmune diseases arise due to dysregulated immunity that occurs during pregnancy.

Autoimmune blistering diseases are commonly treated with systemic glucocorticoids with or without other immunosuppressive agents, including azathioprine, mycophenolate mofetil, and cyclophosphamide. The development of the monoclonal antibody rituximab has allowed targeted therapies for autoimmune bullous diseases, in particular pemphigus, that has redefined standard care of these diseases.[70,71] Rituximab binds the cell surface protein CD20 that is expressed by B cells. This leads to the depletion of both normal and autoreactive B cells in patients, and the possibility of prolonged remissions. Rituximab therapy is well tolerated, and its efficacy and safety as first line of therapy in combination with short-term corticosteroid has been recently demonstrated.[71]

A recent study reports development of an alternative approach involving chimeric autoantigen receptor (CAAR) T cells.[72] T cells are genetically modified to express Dsg3 that was engineered to activate T cells after surface crosslinking. When Dsg3-expressing CAAR T cells bind to B cells that express surface anti-Dsg3 IgG, the CAAR T cells are activated and they subsequently destroy Dsg3-reactive B cells. This strategy, or related strategies, may ultimately lead to novel antigen-specific therapies in pemphigus (and other autoantibody-mediated disorders) that are safer and more efficacious than those in use currently.

CONCLUSIONS AND FUTURE DIRECTIONS

This chapter summarizes our current understanding of the pathophysiology of several immunologic/inflammatory skin diseases. We have selected examples of diseases where our understanding is detailed. This list is short, whereas the list of immunologic/inflammatory skin diseases in which our understanding of disease pathogenesis is inadequate is long. Although studies of experimental animal models, in many cases, provide fundamental knowledge that is prerequisite for studies of humans, the efficiency with which studies of patients yield information that affects patient care is increasing. In the case of immunologic/inflammatory skin diseases, the advent of "low cost" GWAS and other genetic studies and the availability of biologic agents with exquisite specificity have been both timely and important. It seems likely that the types of approaches that have been successful in psoriasis and alopecia areata will have utility in studies of patients with other immunologic/inflammatory skin diseases if implemented with similar enthusiasm, and that improved therapies will result.

REFERENCES

1. Allen MH, Wakelin SH, Holloway D, et al. Association of TNFA gene polymorphism at position –308 with susceptibility to irritant contact dermatitis. *Immunogenetics*. 2000;51(3):201-205.
2. Nacak M, Erbagci Z, Buyukafsar K, et al. Association of angiotensin-converting enzyme gene insertion/deletion polymorphism with allergic contact dermatitis. *Basic Clin Pharmacol Toxicol*. 2007;101(2):101-103.
3. Reich K, Westphal G, König IR, et al. Association of allergic contact dermatitis with a promoter polymorphism in the IL16 gene. *J Allergy Clin Immunol*. 2003;112(6):1191-1194.
4. Kim DS, Kim DH, Lee H, et al. A genome-wide association study in Koreans identifies susceptibility loci for allergic nickel dermatitis. *Int Arch Allergy Immunol*. 2013;162(2):184-186.
5. Kaplan DH, Igyártó BZ, Gaspari AA. Early immune events in the induction of allergic contact dermatitis. *Nat Rev Immunol*. 2012;12(2):114-124.
6. Schmidt M, Raghavan B, Muller V, et al. Crucial role for human Toll-like receptor 4 in the development of contact allergy to nickel. *Nat Immunol*. 2010;11(9):814-819.
7. Adam C, Wohlfarth J, Haußmann M, et al. Allergy-inducing chromium compounds trigger potent innate immune stimulation via ROS-dependent inflammasome activation. *J Invest Dermatol*. 137(2):367-376.
8. Sutterwala FS, Ogura Y, Szczepanik M, et al. Critical role for NALP3/CIAS1/cryopyrin in innate and adaptive immunity through its regulation of caspase-1. *Immunity*. 2006;24(3):317-327.
9. Watanabe H, Gaide O, Pétrilli V, et al. Activation of the IL-1β-processing inflammasome is involved in contact hypersensitivity. *J Invest Dermatol*. 2007;127(8):1956-1963.
10. Antonopoulos C, Cumberbatch M, Dearman RJ, et al. Functional caspase-1 is required for Langerhans cell migration and optimal contact sensitization in mice. *J Immunol*. 2001;166(6):3672.
11. Martin SF, Dudda JC, Bachtanian E, et al. Toll-like receptor and IL-12 signaling control susceptibility to contact hypersensitivity. *J Exp Med*. 2008;205(9):2151.
12. Kaplan DH, Jenison MC, Saeland S, et al. Epidermal Langerhans cell-deficient mice develop enhanced contact hypersensitivity. *Immunity*. 2005;23(6):611-620.
13. Bennett CL, van Rijn E, Jung S, et al. Inducible ablation of mouse Langerhans cells diminishes but fails to abrogate contact hypersensitivity. *J Cell Biol*. 2005;169(4):569-576.
14. Kissenpfennig A, Henri S, Dubois B, et al. Dynamics and function of Langerhans cells In vivo: dermal dendritic cells colonize lymph node areas distinct from slower migrating Langerhans cells. *Immunity*. 2005;22(5):643-654.
15. Allan RS, Waithman J, Bedoui S, et al. Migratory dendritic cells transfer antigen to a lymph node-resident dendritic cell population for efficient CTL priming. *Immunity*. 2006;25(1):153-162.
16. Kim JH, Hu Y, Yongqing T, et al. CD1a on Langerhans cells controls inflammatory skin disease. *Nat Immunol*. 2016;17(10):1159-1166.
17. Jiang X, Clark RA, Liu L, et al. Skin infection generates non-migratory memory CD8+ T(RM) cells providing global skin immunity. *Nature*. 2012;483(7388):227-231.
18. Gaide O, Emerson RO, Jiang X, et al. Common clonal origin of central and resident memory T cells following skin immunization. *Nat Med*. 2015;21(6):647-653.
19. Duong TA, Valeyrie-Allanore L, Wolkenstein P, et al. Severe cutaneous adverse reactions to drugs. *Lancet*. 2017; 390(10106):1996-2011.
20. Hung S-I, Chung W-H, Liou L-B, et al. HLA-B*5801 allele as a genetic marker for severe cutaneous adverse reactions caused by allopurinol. *Proc Natl Acad Sci U S A*. 2005;102(11):4134-4139.
21. Chung W-H, Hung S-I, Hong H-S, et al. Medical genetics: a marker for Stevens-Johnson syndrome. *Nature*. 2004;428(6982):486.
22. Zhang FR, Liu H, Irwanto A, et al. HLA-B*13:01 and the dapsone hypersensitivity syndrome. *N Engl J Med*. 2013;369(17):1620-1628.
23. Shiohara T. Fixed drug eruption: pathogenesis and diagnostic tests. *Curr Opin Allergy Clin Immunol*. 2009;9(4):316-321.
24. Takahashi R, Kano Y, Yamazaki Y, et al. Defective regulatory T cells in patients with severe drug eruptions: timing of the dysfunction is associated with the pathological phenotype and outcome. *J Immunol*. 2009;182(12):8071.
25. Picard D, Janela B, Descamps V, et al. Drug reaction with eosinophilia and systemic symptoms (DRESS):

a multiorgan antiviral T cell response. *Sci Transl Med.* 2010;2(46):46ra62.
26. Kano Y, Tohyama M, Aihara M, et al. Sequelae in 145 patients with drug-induced hypersensitivity syndrome/drug reaction with eosinophilia and systemic symptoms: Survey conducted by the Asian Research Committee on Severe Cutaneous Adverse Reactions (ASCAR). *J Dermatol.* 2015;42(3):276-282.
27. Chung W-H, Wang C-W, Dao R-L. Severe cutaneous adverse drug reactions. *J Dermatol.* 2016;43(7):758-766.
28. Palmer CNA, Irvine AD, Terron-Kwiatkowski A, et al. Common loss-of-function variants of the epidermal barrier protein filaggrin are a major predisposing factor for atopic dermatitis. *Nat Genet.* 2006;38(4):441-446.
29. Hirota T, Takahashi A, Kubo M, et al. Genome-wide association study identifies eight new susceptibility loci for atopic dermatitis in the Japanese population. *Nat Genet.* 2012;44(11):1222-1226.
30. Paternoster L, Standl M, Waage J, et al; for the EArly Genetics & Lifecourse Epidemiology (EAGLE) eczema consortium. Multi-ancestry genome-wide association study of 21,000 cases and 95,000 controls identifies new risk loci for atopic dermatitis. *Nat Genet.* 2015;47(12):1449-1456.
31. Chavanas S, Bodemer C, Rochat A, et al. Mutations in SPINK5, encoding a serine protease inhibitor, cause Netherton syndrome. *Nat Genet.* 2000;25(2):141-142.
32. Hubiche T, Ged C, Benard A, et al. Analysis of SPINK 5, KLK 7 and FLG genotypes in a French atopic dermatitis cohort. *Acta Derm Venereol.* 2007; 87:499–505.
33. Holland SM, DeLeo FR, Elloumi HZ, et al. STAT3 Mutations in the hyper-IgE syndrome. *N Engl J Med.* 2007;357(16):1608-1619.
34. Grice EA, Kong HH, Conlan S, et al. Topographical and temporal diversity of the human skin microbiome. *Science.* 2009;324(5931):1190.
35. Kong HH, Oh J, Deming C, et al. Temporal shifts in the skin microbiome associated with disease flares and treatment in children with atopic dermatitis. *Genome Res.* 2012;22(5):850-859.
36. Kobayashi T, Glatz M, Horiuchi K, et al. Dysbiosis and *Staphyloccus aureus* colonization drives inflammation in atopic dermatitis. *Immunity.* 2015;42(4):756-766.
37. Krathen RA, Hsu S. Failure of omalizumab for treatment of severe adult atopic dermatitis. *J Am Acad Dermatol.* 2005;53(2):338-340.
38. Simpson EL, Bieber T, Guttman-Yassky E, et al. Two phase 3 trials of dupilumab versus placebo in atopic dermatitis. *N Engl J Med.* 2016;375(24):2335-2348.
39. Takeshita J, Grewal S, Langan SM, et al. Psoriasis and comorbid diseases. *J Am Acad Dermatol.* 2016;76(3):393-403.
40. Kim J, Krueger JG. Highly effective new treatments for psoriasis target the IL-23/Type 17 T cell autoimmune axis. *Annu Rev Med.* 2017;68(1):255-269.
41. Oh CJ, Das KM, Gottlieb AB. Treatment with anti-tumor necrosis factor alpha (TNF-alpha) monoclonal antibody dramatically decreases the clinical activity of psoriasis lesions. *J Am Acad Dermatol.* 2000;42(5 Pt 1):829-830.
42. Ogdie A, Yu Y, Haynes K, et al. Risk of major cardiovascular events in patients with psoriatic arthritis, psoriasis and rheumatoid arthritis: a population-based cohort study. *Ann Rheum Dis.* 2015;74(2):326.
43. Harden JL, Krueger JG, Bowcock A. The immunogenetics of psoriasis: a comprehensive review. *J Autoimmun.* 2015;64:66-73.
44. Baurecht H, Hotze M, Brand S, et al. Genome-wide comparative analysis of atopic dermatitis and psoriasis gives insight into opposing genetic mechanisms. *Am J Hum Genet.* 2014;96(1):104-120.
45. Stuart Philip E, Nair Rajan P, Tsoi Lam C, et al. Genome-wide association analysis of psoriatic arthritis and cutaneous psoriasis reveals differences in their genetic architecture. *Am J Hum Genet.* 2015;97(6):816-836.
46. Ray-Jones H, Eyre S, Barton A, et al. One SNP at a time: moving beyond GWAS in psoriasis. *J Invest Dermatol.* 2015;136(3):567-573.
47. Arakawa A, Siewert K, Stöhr J, et al. Melanocyte antigen triggers autoimmunity in human psoriasis. *J Exp Med.* 2015;212(13):2203.
48. Lande R, Botti E, Jandus C, et al. The antimicrobial peptide LL37 is a T-cell autoantigen in psoriasis. *Nat Commun.* 2014;5:5621.
49. Gilhar A, Schrum AG, Etzioni A, et al. Alopecia areata: animal models illuminate autoimmune pathogenesis and novel immunotherapeutic strategies. *Autoimmun Rev.* 2016;15(7):726-735.
50. Xing L, Dai Z, Jabbari A, et al. Alopecia areata is driven by cytotoxic T lymphocytes and is reversed by JAK inhibition. *Nat Med.* 2014;20(9):1043-1049.
51. Petukhova L, Duvic M, Hordinsky M, et al. Genome-wide association study in alopecia areata implicates both innate and adaptive immunity. *Nature.* 2010;466(7302):113-117.
52. Betz RC, Petukhova L, Ripke S, et al. Genome-wide meta-analysis in alopecia areata resolves HLA associations and reveals two new susceptibility loci. *Nat Commun.* 2015;6:5966.
53. Jabbari A, Cerise JE, Chen JC, et al. Molecular signatures define alopecia areata subtypes and transcriptional biomarkers. *EBioMedicine.* 2016;7:240-247.
54. Kennedy Crispin M, Ko JM, Craiglow BG, et al. Safety and efficacy of the JAK inhibitor tofacitinib citrate in patients with alopecia areata. *JCI Insight.* 2016;1(15):e89776.
55. Mackay-Wiggan J, Jabbari A, Nguyen N, et al. Oral ruxolitinib induces hair regrowth in patients with moderate-to-severe alopecia areata. *JCI Insight.* 2016;1(15):e89790.
56. Stanley JR, Amagai M. Pemphigus, bullous impetigo, and the staphylococcal scalded-skin syndrome. *N Engl J Med.* 2006;355(17):1800-1810.
57. Robinson ND, Hashimoto T, Amagai M, et al. The new pemphigus variants. *J Am Acad Dermatol.* 1999;40(5):649-671.
58. Bağcı IS, Horváth ON, Ruzicka T, et al. Bullous pemphigoid. *Autoimmun Rev.* 2017.
59. Neff AG, Turner M, Mutasim DF. Treatment strategies in mucous membrane pemphigoid. *Ther Clin Risk Manag.* 2008;4(3):617-626.
60. Woodley DT, Burgeson RE, Lunstrum G, et al. Epidermolysis bullosa acquisita antigen is the globular carboxyl terminus of type VII procollagen. *J Clin Invest.* 1988;81(3):683-687.
61. Anhalt GJ, Labib RS, Voorhees JJ, et al. Induction of pemphigus in neonatal mice by passive transfer of IgG from patients with the disease. *N Engl J Med.* 1982;306(20):1189-1196.
62. Amagai M, Stanley JR. Desmoglein as a target in skin disease and beyond. *J Invest Dermatol.* 2012;132(3, Part 2):776-784.
63. Futei Y, Amagai M, Sekiguchi M, et al. Use of domain-swapped molecules for conformational epitope

mapping of desmoglein 3 in pemphigus vulgaris. *J Invest Dermatol.* 2000;115(5):829-834.
64. Amagai M, Tsunoda K, Suzuki H, et al. Use of autoantigen-knockout mice in developing an active autoimmune disease model for pemphigus. *J Clin Invest.* 2000;105(5):625-631.
65. Ahmed AR, Carrozzo M, Caux F, et al. Monopathogenic vs multipathogenic explanations of pemphigus pathophysiology. *Exp Dermatol.* 2016;25(11):839-846.
66. Nishie W. Update on the pathogenesis of bullous pemphigoid: An autoantibody-mediated blistering disease targeting collagen XVII. *J Dermatol Sci.* 2014;73(3):179-186.
67. Liu Z, Diaz LA, Troy JL, et al. A passive transfer model of the organ-specific autoimmune disease, bullous pemphigoid, using antibodies generated against the hemidesmosomal antigen, BP180. *J Clin Invest.* 1993;92(5):2480-2488.
68. Nishie W, Sawamura D, Goto M, et al. Humanization of autoantigen. *Nat Med.* 2007;13(3):378-383.
69. Liu Z, Giudice GJ, Swartz SJ, et al. The role of complement in experimental bullous pemphigoid. *J Clin Invest.* 1995;95(4):1539-1544.
70. Joly P, Mouquet H, Roujeau J-C, et al. A single cycle of rituximab for the treatment of severe pemphigus. *N Engl J Med.* 2007;357(6):545-552.
71. Joly P, Maho-Vaillant M, Prost-Squarcioni C, et al. First-line rituximab combined with short-term prednisone versus prednisone alone for the treatment of pemphigus (Ritux 3): a prospective, multicentre, parallel-group, open-label randomised trial. *Lancet.* 2017;389(10083):2031-2040.
72. Ellebrecht CT, Bhoj VG, Nace A, et al. Reengineering chimeric antigen receptor T cells for targeted therapy of autoimmune disease. *Science.* 2016;353(6295):179.

Chapter 14 :: Skin Barrier
:: Akiharu Kubo & Masayuki Amagai

第十四章
皮肤屏障

中文导读

本章内容分为八节：①表皮屏障的比较生物学；②表皮的基本结构；③角质层；④紧密连接；⑤抗菌屏障；⑥新生儿表皮屏障；⑦抵御物理应力的屏障；⑧结论。

第一节表皮屏障的比较生物学，介绍了生物体屏障的差异，脂质双层细胞膜是单细胞生物体的基本屏障，多细胞生物的屏障为表皮或者上皮细胞膜。而且提到了高等生物的表皮表面被各种外部屏障所覆盖，提到的几个示例包括节肢动物的角质层，鱼类和两栖动物的黏液或者鸟类和哺乳动物的角质层等。

第二节表皮的基本结构，介绍了人表皮的组成。角质层起气液界面屏障的作用，下方的表皮细胞形成一个液-液界面屏障。表皮的持续周转使得附着在皮肤上的异物随着鳞片的每日脱落而被丢弃。

第三节角质层，介绍了人体皮肤角质层是人体表面最外层的屏障，起到双向屏障的作用，不仅可以防止外部分子和微生物向内渗透，而且还可以防止水和溶质向外泄漏。分别介绍了角质层的基本结构、角质细胞脂质膜的形成、角质层的脂质成分、桥粒、角蛋白细胞骨架与丝聚蛋白、丝聚蛋白降解与天然保湿因子、角质层的多域结构及透皮吸收等。

第四节紧密连接，介绍了紧密连接的结构是由质膜上的四个跨膜蛋白组成，其功能缺陷可能出现鱼鳞病等临床症状。接下来介绍了紧密连接屏障与膜间免疫介导细胞如朗格汉斯细胞之间的相互作用，提到了朗格汉斯细胞树突和角质形成细胞之间可形成了新的紧密连接，能够在不干扰紧密连接屏障功能的情况下摄取外部抗原。最后介绍了角质形成细胞形态对皮肤屏障动态平衡的影响。

第五节抗菌屏障，介绍了皮肤表面呈弱酸性，具有防止细菌生长的作用，进而介绍了皮肤表面的抗菌蛋白具有广泛的抗菌活性，放线菌素和β-防御素是皮肤的两种主要抗菌蛋白。皮肤表面的角质形成细胞是抗菌蛋白的主要来源。最后介绍了抗菌蛋白发挥抗菌屏障有多种作用机制。

第六节新生儿表皮屏障，介绍了足月新生儿出生时皮肤屏障发育良好，健康足月新生儿出生时经表皮失水等于或低于成人皮肤。而早产儿出生时表皮屏障较弱，真皮机械脆弱，新生儿皮肤受损的风险更大。

第七节抵御物理应力的屏障，介绍了表皮在抵御物理应力过程中的多种屏障方式，包括防止机械应力的物理结构、抵御紫外线的屏障、出汗以抵御热应激、热应激下的血管和血流控制。

第八节结论，总结皮肤直接暴露在外

部环境中，显示出特定物种的适应能力。皮肤科医生应该了解人类皮肤如何适应外部环境，以及这些适应是如何受疾病影响的。

〔粟　娟〕

AT-A-GLANCE

- One of the most important functions of the skin is to form a barrier between the organism and the external environment.
- The skin protects our bodies from physical damage caused by desiccation, physical stress, infection, overheating or heat loss, and ultraviolet (UV) irradiation.
- The skin is covered by the epidermis, a cornified, stratified epithelial cellular sheet that is equipped with a barrier formed by the stratum corneum and tight junctions.
- The stratum corneum is an air–liquid interface barrier on the body surface that prevents excessive water loss (inside–outside barrier) and the entry of harmful substances from the environment (outside–inside barrier).
- The stratum corneum barrier is composed of corneocytes and intercorneocyte water-impermeable lipid lamellae. Corneocytes are wrapped with cornified cell envelope and corneocyte lipid envelope and contain keratin filaments associated with filaggrin, which is degraded to natural moisturizing factors.
- The tight junctions seal the intercellular space between neighboring cells at the second layer in the stratum granulosum and form a liquid–liquid interface barrier that limits molecular movement through the paracellular pathway.
- Langerhans cells are located in the epidermis under the tight junction barrier in steady state but extend their dendrites to the outside tight junction barrier upon activation to capture external antigens at the tips of the dendrites.
- Antimicrobial peptides, lipids, the acidic pH of the stratum corneum, and continuous daily desquamation (daily detachment of dead skin cells) control the skin microbiota and protect us from infection by bacteria, yeasts, fungi, and viruses.
- UV light is reflected from the stratum corneum and absorbed by urocanic acid and melanin molecules, which protect genomic DNA from UV irradiation damage.
- Sweating, blood flow control, and heat storage in subcutaneous adipose tissue protect us from cold and overheating.

INTRODUCTION

The skin is the integument of vertebrates (Table 14-1). One of the key functions of the skin is to form a protective physical barrier between the body and the external environment. The limitation of molecular movement across the skin is largely dependent on the epidermis and especially the stratum corneum in mammals. The epidermis prevents the inward and outward passage of water, electrolytes, lipids, and proteins, as well as insults from chemicals, bacteria, fungi, virus, toxins, and allergens. Defects in the formation of the epidermal barrier cause various congenital diseases (Table 14-2).

The skin protects the body from various external stresses. In protecting from heat and cold stresses, the skin maintains the internal organs at a certain constant temperature by regulating blood flow, sweat production, thermal storage in the fat layer, and thermogenesis in brown fat cells. The skin protects the body from physical stresses through coordination of the rigid surface armor of the stratum corneum; keratin cytoskeleton; and cell adhesions between keratinocytes, epidermal–dermal junctions, and dermal collagen fibers; these are discussed in Chaps. 15 and 60. Furthermore, the epidermis reflects and absorbs ultraviolet (UV) radiation from the sun to protect the genomic DNA of cells; this is particularly important in preventing carcinogenesis, which is discussed in Chaps. 19 and 20. Skin appendages, such as sweat and sebaceous glands, hairs, and nails, also have physical and chemical barrier functions; these are discussed in Chaps. 6, 7, and 8, respectively.

The skin is also equipped with immunologic barriers to the innate and acquired immune systems. Antimicrobial proteins are a diverse group of proteins that form a chemical barrier against microorganisms on the surface of the epidermis. Toll-like receptors on keratinocytes detect pathogen-associated molecular patterns such as lipoprotein and peptidoglycans that are broadly shared by bacteria but distinguishable from host molecules and control the immune responses against the microorganisms. Dendritic cells within the skin govern the acquired immunologic and allergic responses to external insults. The mechanisms of acquired immunity that protect our skin are discussed in Chaps. 10 and 11.

TABLE 14-1
Short Commentary on Jargons
Integument
The tough outer protective layer of an animal or plant that demarcates the body from the external environment
Occlusive junction
Cell–cell adhesive junction that seals the intercellular space and controls paracellular molecular movement. Invertebrates and vertebrates have different occlusive junction structures. The occlusive junction of invertebrates is called a septate junction, and that of vertebrates is called a tight junction.
Comparative Biology
Comparative biology exploits natural variation and disparities among species or taxa to understand the patterns of life by investigating phylogenies, evolution, development, physiology, and genomics
Kelvin's Tetrakaidecahedron
Fourteen-sided polyhedron composed of eight hexagons and six squares, proposed in 1887 by William Thomson (Lord Kelvin) as the best shape for packing equal-sized cells together to fill the space using the minimal surface area of each cell[142]
Transepidermal Water Loss
The loss of water that passes from inside to outside a body through the epidermis. Measurement of transepidermal water loss is useful to evaluate the stratum corneum barrier as the elevation rates of transepidermal water loss are basically in proportion to the level of barrier damage or formation.

COMPARATIVE BIOLOGY OF THE EPIDERMAL BARRIER

The lipid bilayer cell membrane provides a fundamental barrier in unicellular organisms. The cell membrane compartmentalizes the cell from the external environment. Homeostasis of the cell is maintained within the compartment demarcated by the cell membrane in an energy-dependent manner. Because the lipid bilayer membrane is highly fragile, most unicellular organisms have an additional barrier structure outside of the cell membrane (ie, the cell wall) that functions as a type of armor (Fig. 14-1).

The body's barrier to multicellular organisms is analogous to its barrier to unicellular organisms. The cell membrane of unicellular organisms corresponds to the epidermis, which is the epithelial cellular sheet that delineates the surface of multicellular organisms (see Fig. 14-1). To form a barrier with a sheet of cells, prevention of the leakage of water and solutes through intercellular spaces is crucial. Thus, the intercellular spaces are sealed by occlusive junctions, such as septate junctions in arthropods and tight junctions in vertebrates (see Table 14-1). The epidermis is composed of a single layer of cells in cephalochordates and urochordates, but multilayered (stratified) cells in vertebrates (see Fig. 14-1). Because the epidermal cells are fragile when directly exposed to harsh external environmental factors, such as hypotonic fresh water, hypertonic sea water, or dry air, the surface of the epidermis of higher organisms is covered by various external barriers. Examples of these barriers include the cuticles of arthropods, tunics of tunicates, mucous of fish and amphibians, and cornified cell layer (stratum corneum) of adult amphibians, reptiles, birds, and mammals (see Fig. 14-1).[1]

BASIC STRUCTURE OF THE EPIDERMIS

The human epidermis is a stratified epithelial cellular sheet, the uppermost part of which is cornified to form the stratum corneum. The viable (enucleated) cell layers of the epidermis consist of the stratum basale (basal cell layer), stratum spinosum (spinous cell layer), and stratum granulosum (granular cell layer) (Fig. 14-2). The stratum granulosum consists of at least three layers of flattened granular cells.[2-5] From outside to inside, the layers are named SG1, SG2, and SG3, and tight junctions seal the intercellular spaces in the SG2 layer.[3,5] The stratum corneum consists of dead cornified cells (corneocytes) and functions as an air–liquid interface barrier. The intercellular spaces of the stratum corneum are filled with water-impermeable lipid lamellae. Under the stratum corneum, cells are immersed in a water environment. The extracellular water environment of the epidermis is divided into two parts by the tight junction barrier, which is a liquid–liquid interface barrier (see Fig. 14-2). To form the stratum corneum, the SG1 cells terminally differentiate into corneocytes by filling their intercellular spaces with lipid lamellae. The multilayered structure of the epidermis is maintained, and the epidermal cells are continuously turned over. Epidermal cells proliferate only in the basal layer, differentiate with detachment from the basement membrane, move upward, become flattened at the stratum granulosum, form a tight junction at the SG2 layer, lose the tight junction at the SG1 layer, terminally differentiate into corneocytes, and detach from the top of the cornified layer as squamous scales. Continuous turnover of the epidermis enables foreign substances attached to the skin to be discarded with the daily detachment of scales.

STRATUM CORNEUM

The stratum corneum of human skin is the outermost barrier of the body's surface. The stratum corneum in humans is approximately 10 to 20 μm thick and contains about 10 to 25 layers of cornified cells.[6] The stratum corneum is directly exposed to air and protects the inner cells from damage by desiccation. It acts as a two-way barrier to prevent not only inward penetration of external molecules and microorganisms but also outward leakage of water and solutes.

TABLE 14-2
Diseases and Their Animal Models Showing Aberrant Stratum Corneum

CLASSIFICATION	GENE	PROTEIN	FUNCTION	DISEASE NAME	MIM	REFERENCES	ANIMAL MODEL
Cornified envelope formation	LOR	Loricrin	Major component of cornified envelope	Vohwinkel syndrome with ichthyosis	604117	24	Mouse[153]
	TGM1	Transglutaminase 1	Protein crosslinking to form cornified envelope	ARCI1	242300	20	Mouse[16]
Cholesterol biosynthesis	NSDHL	NAD(P)H steroid dehydrogenase-like protein	C4 demethylase	CHILD syndrome	308050	34	Mouse[154]
	MSMO1	Methylsterol monooxygenase 1	Methylsterol monooxygenase	MCCPD	616834	33	—
Acylceramide biosynthesis	ELOVL4	Elongation of very-long-chain fatty acid–like 4	Elongation of very-long-chain fatty acids	ISQMR	614457	155	Mouse[156]
	CYP4F22	Cytochrome P450 4F22	γ-Hydroxylation of ultra-long-chain fatty acids	ARCI5	604777	157	—
	CERS3	Ceramide synthase 3	Catalyzing the linkage between a fatty acyl-CoA and a sphingoid base to produce ceramide	ARCI9	615023	158,159	Mouse[160]
	ABHD5	ABHD5/CGI58	ω-O-esterification of ceramide with linoleic acid	Chanarin-Dorfman syndrome	275630	161	—
	PNPLA1	Patatin-like phospholipase domain containing 1		ARCI10	615024	62	Dog[162]
	ALOX12B	Arachidonate 12-lipoxygenase type12R	Oxidation of linoleic acid in ceramide	ARCI2	242100	163	Mouse[164]
	ALOXE3	Arachidonate lipoxygenase 3		ARCI3	606545	163	Mouse[164]
Lipid transport	ABCA12	ATP-binding cassette A12	Lipid trafficking on the lamellar granule membrane	ARCI4A ARCI4B (Harlequin ichthyosis)	242500	26,27	Mouse[165]
Desquamation	ST14	Matriptase	Extracellular serine protease	ARCI11	602400	54	Mouse[166]
	SPINK5	LEKTI	Inhibitor of kallikrein proteases	Netherton syndrome	256500	55	Mouse[167,168]
Desmosomes and corneodesmosomes	CDSN	Corneodesmosin	Constituent of the corneodesmosome	Peeling skin syndrome 1	270300	56,57	Mouse[69]
	DSG1	Desmoglein1	Cell–cell adhesion molecule of the desmosome	SAM syndrome	615508	58	—
Filaggrin metabolism	FLG	Filaggrin	Bundling keratin filaments in the stratum corneum, source of natural moisturizing factors	Ichthyosis vulgaris (predisposed to atopic dermatitis)	146700	72,74	Mouse[75,170]
	CASP14	Caspase 14	Profilaggrin processing	ARCI12	617320	71	Mouse[67]
Tight junctions	CLDN1	Claudin-1	Cell–cell adhesion molecule of the tight junction	NISCH syndrome	607626	104	Mouse[102,103]

ABHD5, abhydrolase domain-containing 5; ARCI, autosomal recessive congenital ichthyosis; ATP, adenosine triphosphate; CGI58, comparative gene identification 58; CHILD syndrome, congenital hemidysplasia with ichthyosiform erythroderma and limb defects syndrome; CoA, coenzyme A; ISQMR, ichthyosis, spastic quadriplegia, and mental retardation; LEKTI, lymphoepithelial Kazal-type-related inhibitor; MCCPD, microcephaly, congenital cataract, and psoriasiform dermatitis; MIM, Mendelian Inheritance in Man; NISCH syndrome, neonatal ichthyosis-sclerosing cholangitis syndrome; SAM syndrome, severe dermatitis, multiple allergies and metabolic wasting syndrome.

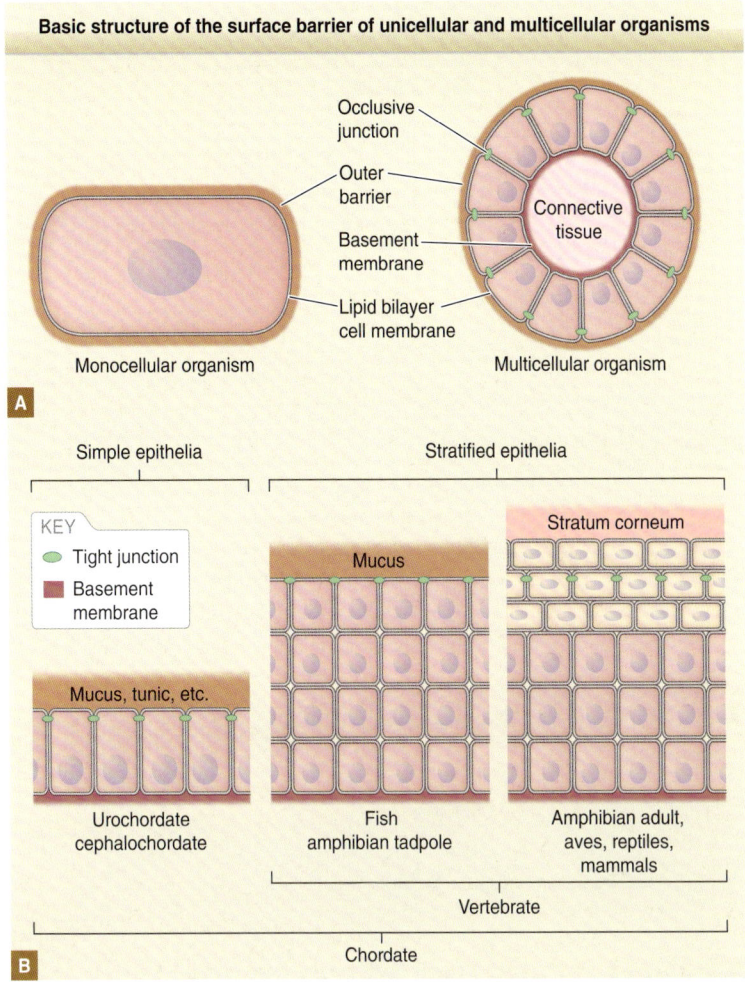

Figure 14-1 Basic structure of the surface barrier of unicellular and multicellular organisms. **A,** The lipid bilayer cell membrane is a basic diffusion barrier on the body surface of both monocellular organisms and multicellular organisms. In multicellular organisms, the intercellular spaces are sealed with occlusive junctions to limit leakage of the barrier through the paracellular pathway (see Fig. 14-9). In essence, both monocellular organisms and multicellular organisms are equipped with additional outer barriers (ie, a cell wall for monocellular organisms and mucus, cuticles, tunic matrix, or stratum corneum for multicellular organisms). **B,** Development of a stratified epithelium and stratum corneum were the two major evolutionary events in vertebrate skin. Under the outer barrier, tight junctions seal the intercellular spaces in vertebrates.

BASIC STRUCTURE OF THE STRATUM CORNEUM

The stratum corneum consists of stratified corneocytes and an intercorneocyte lipid-rich matrix (Fig. 14-3). The barrier function of the stratum corneum depends on both the protein-rich materials of the corneocytes and the intercellular lipid-rich matrix. Corneocytes are terminally differentiated dead keratinocytes that adhere to one another via proteinaceous cell–cell adhesion complexes called corneodesmosomes and the adhesive force of intercellular lipid lamellae (Fig. 14-4). On routine hematoxylin and eosin staining of paraffin-embedded skin sections, the stratum corneum shows a basket-weave structure, which may cause the stratum corneum to be mistaken for a porous structure that does not have a barrier function; the basket-weave structure is, in fact, an artifact of the processing of specimens. During paraffin removal using xylene, intercorneocyte lipid is extracted, and the intercellular lipid-dependent adhesion between corneocytes becomes weakened. Because the corneodesmosomes make the lateral adhesions between corneocytes more stable than the apicobasal adhesions, the corneocyte layers detach from one another while maintaining their lateral adhesions, resulting in the formation of a basket-weave structure in paraffin-embedded sections[7,8] (Fig. 14-5). Proper fixation and staining procedures reveal the tightly packed, well-organized structure of the stratum corneum in vertical sections of the skin[2,9] (see Fig. 14-5).

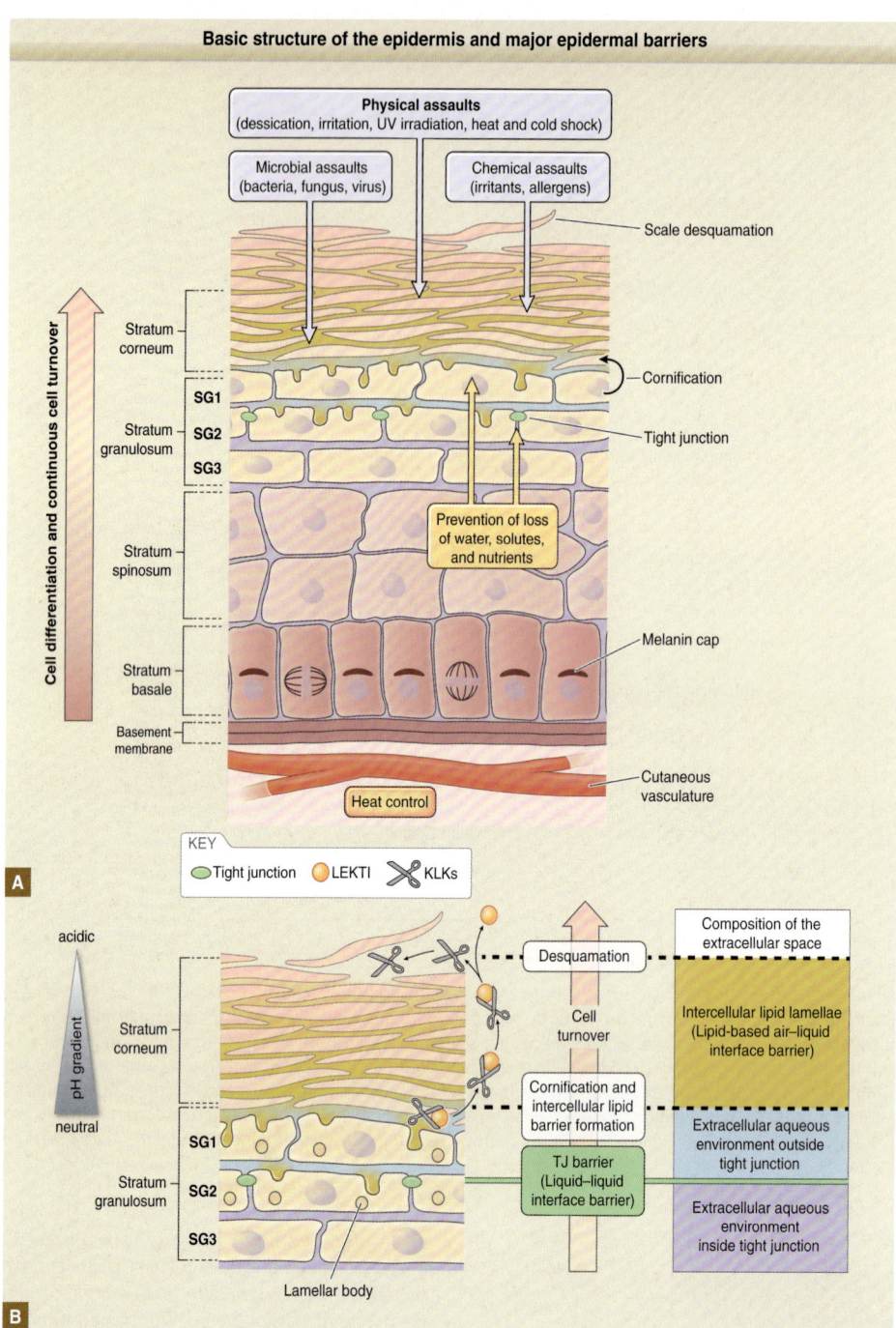

Figure 14-2 Basic structure of the epidermis and major epidermal barriers. **A,** Epidermal barriers protect the body against various outside-in physical, chemical, and microbial assaults in addition to inside-out leakage of water and solutes. Melanin caps protect the genomic DNA of basal cells from ultraviolet (UV) damage. Cells are continuously turned over to renew the epidermis and its barriers. At least three cell layers (SG1, SG2, and SG3 from outside to inside, respectively) exist in the stratum granulosum under the stratum corneum, where tight junctions (TJs) seal the intercellular spaces between the SG2 cells. **B,** Intercellular spaces are filled with lipids in, and with water under, the stratum corneum. The extracellular water environment is considered to be divided into two by the TJ barrier (extracellular space outside TJ barrier, *light blue*; extracellular space inside TJ barrier, *purple*). SG1 cells are ready to cornify at the outside TJ barrier. Contents of lamellar bodies (lipids, antimicrobial proteins, proteases, and protease inhibitors) are basically exocytosed from the apical surface of the SG2 cells to the outside TJ barrier. Kallikrein proteases (KLKs) are activated via the lower-pH-induced detachment of lymphoepithelial Kazal-type-related inhibitor (LEKTI) in the upper layers of the stratum corneum for desquamation. (Modified from Proksch E, Jensen J-M. Skin as an organ of protection. In: Goldsmith LA, Katz SI, Gilchrest BA, et al, eds. *Fitzpatrick's Dermatology in General Medicine*, 8th ed. New York: McGraw-Hill; 2012.)

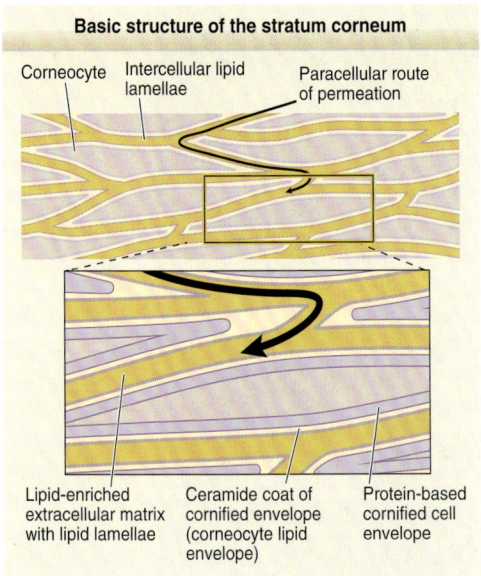

Figure 14-3 Basic structure of the stratum corneum. The stratum corneum comprises protein-based bricks (corneocytes) and lipid-based mortar (intercellular lipid lamellae). The surface of the corneocytes is coated with a thin layer of ceramide (lipid envelope). Details of how this structure is produced are shown in Fig. 14-6. (Modified from Proksch E, Jensen J-M. Skin as an organ of protection. In: Goldsmith LA, Katz SI, Gilchrest BA, et al, eds. *Fitzpatrick's Dermatology in General Medicine*, 8th ed. New York: McGraw-Hill; 2012.)

the entire inner surface of the plasma membrane.[10,17-19] Defects in transglutaminase 1 are known to cause congenital ichthyosis (see Table 14-2).[20]

Before the scaffold covers the inner surface of the plasma membrane, lamellar bodies are produced from the Golgi complex and become fused to the plasma membrane. The limiting membrane of the lamellar bodies is rich in acylceramides composed of omega-hydroxylated ultra-long-chain fatty acids. The fusion of the limiting membrane with the plasma membrane gradually increases the amount of acylceramides within the lipid bilayer of the plasma membrane. The acylceramides become covalently bound to the outer surface of the scaffold of the cornified envelope by the membrane-anchored form of transglutaminase 1.[21,22] The acylceramides eventually replace the plasma membrane, which is called the corneocyte lipid envelope[11,12] (see Fig. 14-6).

The involucrin-envoplakin-periplakin–based scaffold is further reinforced in the later stage of cornification. On the inner surface of the scaffold, loricrin molecules are translocated from the cytosol and covalently cross-linked onto the scaffold to build the cornified cell envelope. Loricrin, an insoluble protein that may contribute to the water resistance of the cornified cell envelope, eventually becomes the major component of the cornified cell envelope. Varying amounts of small proline-rich proteins with minor amounts of other proteins (eg, repetin, trichohyalin, cystatin A, elafin, and late envelope proteins) are also cross-linked to the inner surface of the cornified envelope.[23] Defects in loricrin are known to cause congenital ichthyosis (see Table 14-2).[24]

FORMATION OF A CORNIFIED CELL ENVELOPE AND CORNEOCYTE LIPID ENVELOPE

Granular layer cells terminally differentiate into corneocytes to form the stratum corneum. During cornification, a cornified cell envelope consisting of a 10-nm-thick layer of highly cross-linked insoluble proteins is formed beneath the plasma membrane,[10] and the lipid bilayer of plasma membrane is replaced by a 5-nm-thick layer of acylceramides, which is called corneocyte lipid envelope[11-13] (Fig. 14-6).

The formation of a cornified cell envelope and corneocyte lipid envelope is described as follows[14,15] (see Fig. 14-6). Envoplakin, periplakin, and involucrin expressed in granular layer cells associate with the inner surface of the plasma membrane in a calcium-dependent manner and are cross-linked to one another by transglutaminase 1.[16] Transglutaminase 1 also cross-links to other membrane-associated proteins and desmosomal proteins, fixing the cell junctions and associated cytoskeletons to the proteinaceous scaffold. The involucrin-envoplakin-periplakin–based scaffold eventually forms a monomolecular layer along

FORMATION OF THE LAMELLAE OF INTERCORNEOCYTE LIPIDS

Keratinocytes of the stratum granulosum develop a specific system of lamellar bodies that allow secretion of intercorneocyte lipid lamellae.[25] Lamellar bodies are produced from the Golgi complex and stored within the cytoplasm in SG3 cells as intracellular vesicles. Lamellar bodies are enriched in polar lipids, glycosphingolipids, free sterols, and phospholipids. ABCA12 functions in cellular lipid trafficking on the limiting membrane of lamellar bodies, in which severe defects cause Harlequin ichthyosis (see Table 14-2).[26,27] The lamellar bodies may also contain proteins, such as hydrolytic enzymes to modify lipids, corneodesmosins to modify corneodesmosomes, antimicrobial peptides, and proteases and protease inhibitors to control desquamation. The contents of the lamellar bodies are delivered into the extracellular milieu through exocytosis occurring via the apical cell membrane, most probably in the SG2 cells and SG1 cells, to fill the extracellular space surrounding the SG1 cells[28] (see Fig. 14-2).

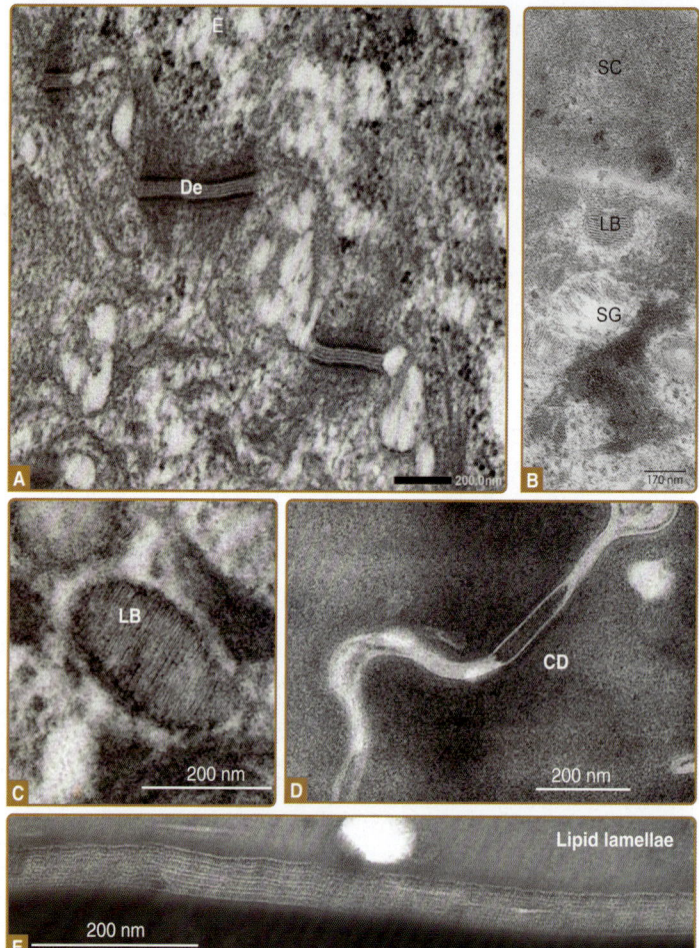

Figure 14-4 Major structures related to cornification, as seen under electron microscopy. **A,** Desmosomes (De) adhering to spinous layer cells. **B,** A lamellar body (LB) exocytosing its contents into the extracellular space at the apical surface of the SG1 cell. **C,** Contents of the lamellar body (LB) showing stripes of lipids. **D,** Corneodesmosomes (CD), cell–cell adhesion complexes between corneocytes. **E,** Intercellular lipid lamellae between corneocytes. (Images **C** and **E,** used with permission from Dr. Akemi Ishida-Yamamoto. Images **A** and **D,** used with permission from Dr. Toshihiro Nagai. Image **B** modified from Proksch E, Jensen J-M. Skin as an organ of protection. In: Goldsmith LA, Katz SI, Gilchrest BA, et al, eds. *Fitzpatrick's Dermatology in General Medicine,* 8th ed. New York: McGraw-Hill;2012.)

The lipids exocytosed from the lamellar bodies are subsequently organized into a characteristic lamellar structure that lies parallel to the cornified cell envelope during cornification of the SG1 cells (see Fig. 14-4). The covalently bound acylceramides of the corneocyte lipid envelope act as a scaffold allowing regular lamellar formation of the intercellular lipids (see Figs. 14-4 and 14-6).[22] After extrusion of the lamellar bodies into the extracellular spaces, the polar lipids are enzymatically converted into nonpolar products. Glycosphingolipids are hydrolyzed to generate ceramides, and phospholipids are converted into free fatty acids. These lipids form the intercellular lamellar component of the stratified lipid bilayer, a very dense structure packed into the interstices of corneocytes, thus forming a water-impermeable barrier.

LIPID COMPOSITION OF THE STRATUM CORNEUM

Intercellular lipids are indispensable in the formation of the permeability barrier of the stratum corneum. The major classes of lipids in the stratum corneum are cholesterol, free fatty acids, and ceramides.[29]

Cholesterol forms part of the plasma membrane in viable cell layers in the epidermis and part of the intercellular lipid lamellae in the stratum corneum. Whereas basal-layer keratinocytes are capable of resorbing cholesterol from the circulation, epidermal keratinocytes actively biosynthesize cholesterol and free fatty acids (Fig. 14-7). The majority of the cholesterol in the epidermis is synthesized

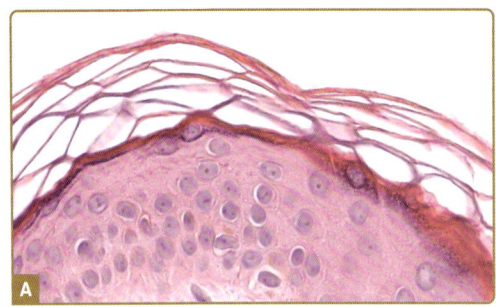

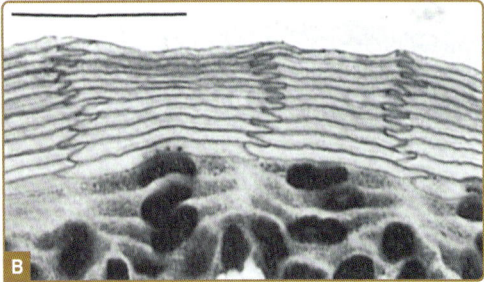

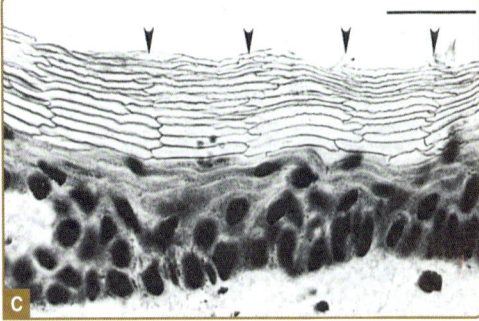

Figure 14-5 Morphology of the epidermis in cross-sections. **A,** Hematoxylin and eosin staining of paraffin-embedded section of human skin showing the basket weave–like pattern of the stratum corneum. **B,** Frozen section of hamster ear skin stained with methylene blue, expanded in an alkaline solution with a pH of 12 and showing a regular alignment of corneocytes. A remarkably ordered structure of flattened stratum granulosum cells and anucleate corneocytes can be seen. The corneocytes show a regular zigzag interdigitation pattern between cell columns. **C,** Frozen section of human abdominal skin stained with methylene blue and expanded in an alkaline solution showing partially regular alignment of corneocytes. (Image **B** from Mackenzie IC. Ordered structure of the epidermis. J Invest Dermatol. 1975;65:45-51, with permission; Image **C** from Mackenzie IC, Zimmerman K, Peterson L. The pattern of cellular organization of human epidermis. J Invest Dermatol. 1981;76:459-461, with permission. Copyright © The Society for Investigative Dermatology.)

in situ from acetyl coenzyme A (acetyl CoA).[30] The rate-limiting step in cholesterol biosynthesis is catalyzed by hydroxymethylglutaryl CoA (HMG CoA) reductase (see Fig. 14-7). Epidermal cholesterol biosynthesis is upregulated during barrier repair.[31] The cholesterol biosynthesis pathway in the epidermis is also important for the production of vitamin D.[32]

The metabolic intermediate of cholesterol biosynthesis, 7-dehydrocholesterol, is converted to previtamin D in a photolytic reaction by UVB radiation; this is followed by thermal isomerization to form vitamin D_3. Deficiency in the enzymes of NSDHL and MSMO1 corresponding to cholesterol biosynthesis causes inflammatory ichthyotic skin lesions through the accumulation of toxic intermediates in CHILD (congenital hemidysplasia with ichthyosiform erythroderma and limb defects) syndrome and MSMO1 deficiency, respectively[33-35] (see Table 14-2).

The skin contains free fatty acids, as well as fatty acids bound in triglycerides, phospholipids, glycosylceramides, and ceramides. Although biosynthesis of cholesterol originates from HMG-CoA, free fatty acid synthesis originates from malonyl-CoA produced from acetyl-CoA via acetyl-CoA carboxylase (see Fig. 14-7). Saturated and monounsaturated fatty acids are synthesized in the epidermis. However, not all fatty acids can be synthesized by the epidermis or the human body. Fatty acids unable to be produced by the human body are called essential fatty acids. Essential fatty acid deficiency (EFAD), caused by unusual diets or malabsorption in humans or experimentally induced in rodents, leads to rough, scaly, and erythematous skin with severe permeability barrier defects of the epidermis.[36,37]

Ceramides consist of long-chain amino alcohols, called sphingoid bases, linked to a fatty acid via an amide bond (see Fig. 14-7). Ceramides are synthesized by serine palmitoyltransferase and hydrolysis of both glucosylceramide and sphingomyelin in the epidermis. Whereas ceramides are a minor lipid component in the mammalian body (<10% of cholesterol or phospholipids), they are a major lipid component in the stratum corneum, accounting for 30% to 40% of lipids by weight.[29] Such a high ceramide content is only observed in the stratum corneum and not in the stratum granulosum, stratum spinosum, or stratum basale. This distribution indicates that ceramide biosynthesis is spatiotemporally controlled and highly activated in the uppermost keratinocytes under terminal differentiation to corneocytes.

Among the epidermal ceramides with marked molecular heterogeneity, acylceramide is essential not only for the formation of the corneocyte lipid envelope, as described earlier, but also for the proper organization of intercorneocyte lipid lamellae and thereby the barrier function of the stratum corneum.[38-42] Acylceramide is synthesized via esterification of omega-hydroxyceramide with linoleic acid. Acylceramide is an unusual ceramide, the N-acyl chain of which is composed of omega-hydroxylated ultra-long-chain fatty acids (see Fig. 14-7). It has been suggested that the ultra-long-chain fatty acid of acylceramide spans a bilayer of lipid lamellae to link the two membranes together in the lipid lamellae and thus serves as a molecular rivet to form stratified lipid lamellae.[43] Deficiencies of the biosynthesis pathway of acylceramide cause several types of congenital ichthyosis[44] (see Table 14-2).

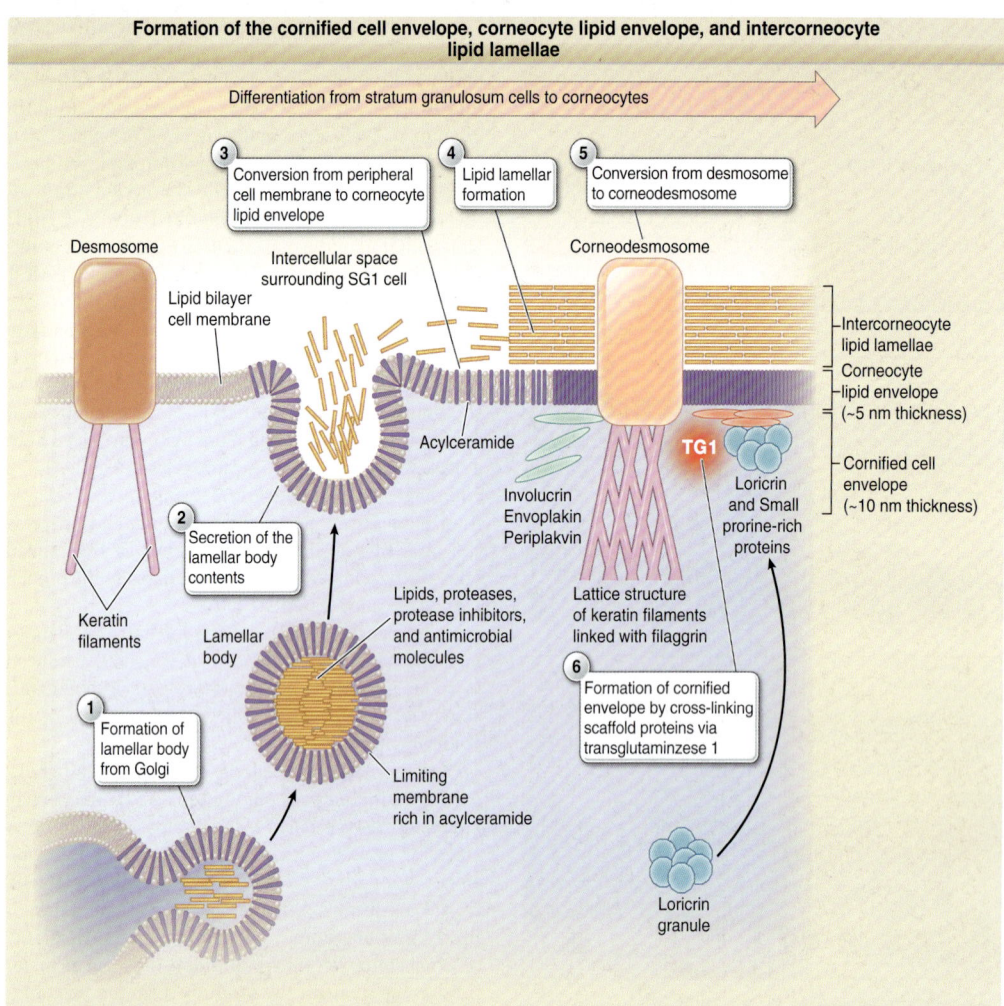

Figure 14-6 Formation of the cornified cell envelope, corneocyte lipid envelope, and intercorneocyte lipid lamellae. The time-dependent change of cornification (from SG2 cells via SG1 cells to corneocytes) is shown from left to right. A cornified cell envelope is formed beneath the lipid bilayer cell membrane via crosslinking of envoplakin, periplakin, and involucrin by transglutaminase 1 (TG1), which is further reinforced by loricrin in the later stage of cornification. Lamellar bodies exocytose their contents to the extracellular space outside tight junctions. The limiting membrane of the lamellar bodies contains a large number of acylceramides that replace the lipid bilayer cell membrane to form a corneocyte lipid envelope. As a result, the cornified cell envelope is coated by the corneocyte lipid envelope. The lipids exocytosed from lamellar bodies form the intercorneocyte lipid lamellae on the corneocyte lipid envelope to fill the intercellular space and form the water-resistant barrier of the stratum corneum. Corneodesmosin exocytosed from lamellar bodies is integrated into the desmosome, which is converted to the corneodesmosome. The lamellar bodies also exocytose proteases and protease inhibitors to control desquamation and antimicrobial proteins (see Fig. 14-12).

CORNEODESMOSOMES

Desmosomes are the major cell–cell adhesion structure in the granular, spinous, and basal cell layers. Corneodesmosin is secreted by lamellar bodies into the extracellular spaces surrounding the SG1 cells (see Figs. 14-2 and 14-6) and then integrated into the desmosomes, resulting in the formation of corneodesmosomes (ie, specific cell adhesion structures between corneocytes)[45] (see Fig. 14-4). Adhesion between corneocytes is dependent on both corneodesmosomes and intercellular lipid lamellae. Corneodesmosomes are degraded in the outer layers of the stratum corneum, and the outermost corneocytes are detached, one by one, from the top layer of the stratum corneum; this process is called desquamation.[46]

The major proteases involved in the degradation of corneodesmosomes are serine proteases belonging to the kallikrein group. Kallikreins 5, 7, and 14 are known to exist in the stratum corneum. These kallikreins are also secreted by lamellar bodies into the extracellular spaces surrounding the SG1 cells (see Fig. 14-2). Kallikreins are produced as inactive precursors and activated via proteolytic conversion by kallikreins themselves (autoactivation) or by matriptase, a transmembrane serine protease.[47,48] The protease activity

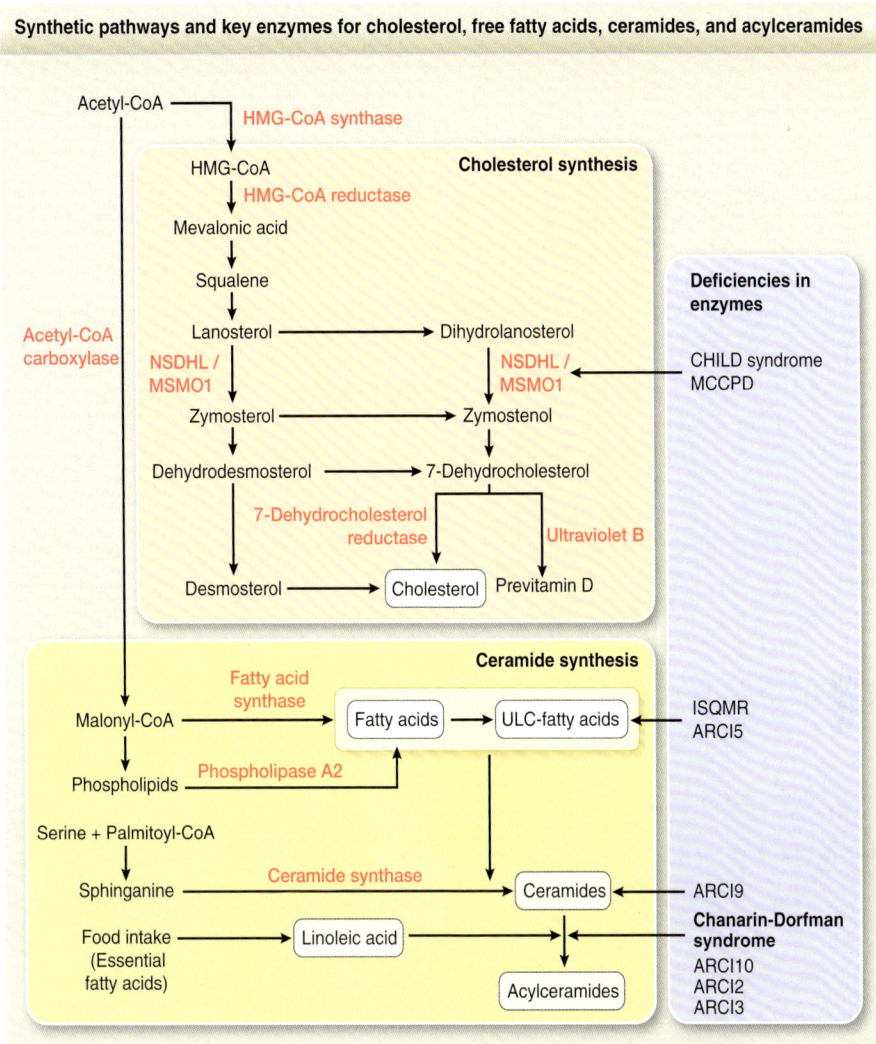

Figure 14-7 Synthetic pathways, key enzymes and deficiencies in the enzymes for cholesterol, free fatty acids, ceramides, and acylceramides. CoA, coenzyme A; HMG-CoA, hydroxymethylglutaryl CoA; CHILD syndrome, congenital hemidysplasia with ichthyosiform erythroderma and limb defects syndrome; MCCPD, microcephaly, congenital cataract, and psoriasiform dermatitis; ISQMR, ichthyosis, spastic quadriplegia, and mental retardation; ARCI, autosomal recessive congenital ichthyosis; NSDHL, NAD(P) dependent steroid dehydrogenase-like; MSMO1, methylsterol monooxygenase 1; ULC, ultra-long-chain.

of the activated kallikreins is thought to be inhibited by the direct binding of lymphoepithelial Kazal-type-related inhibitor (LEKTI), which is also secreted into the intercellular spaces via lamellar bodies.[49] The production of kallikreins as inactive precursors, and the inhibition of their protease activity by LEKTI, are considered to prohibit the degradation of corneodesmosomes in the lower layer of the stratum corneum and thus prevent premature desquamation.[50] LEKTI binding to kallikreins has been shown to be pH dependent. The lower pH of the intercellular spaces in the outer layers of the stratum corneum is thought to facilitate the dissociation of kallikreins from LEKTI and the kallikrein-dependent degradation of corneodesmosomes (see Fig. 14-2).[51-53] The outermost corneocytes eventually detach from the skin.

Congenital defects of matriptase induce congenital ichthyosis showing hyperkeratosis and impaired degradation of corneodesmosomes, probably caused by insufficient activation of kallikrein proteases.[54] In contrast, congenital defects of LEKTI induce Netherton syndrome, in which entire layers of the stratum corneum are prone to being peeled off, probably caused by the enhanced degradation of corneodesmosomes by kallikreins.[55] Such detachment of whole layers of the stratum corneum is also observed in the congenital defects of corneodesmosin or desmoglein 1[56-58] (see Table 14-2). Patients prone to total detachment of the stratum corneum are predisposed to various allergic conditions, probably via increased allergen penetration through the defective skin barrier and facilitation of percutaneous sensitization.[5,59]

KERATIN CYTOSKELETON AND FILAGGRIN

Filaggrin is the major protein of the stratum corneum. Various mutations in the filaggrin gene predispose patients to atopic eczema, allergic rhinitis, food allergies, and asthma complicated with eczema.[60-63]

In humans, filaggrin is expressed only in cornified stratified epithelia; therefore, it is expressed in skin but not in the esophagus or airways.[64] Profilaggrin is expressed in the stratum granulosum and forms intracellular aggregates known as keratohyalin granules. Under cornification, profilaggrin is processed by various proteases into mature filaggrin monomers[63] (Fig. 14-8). Filaggrin monomers bundle keratin

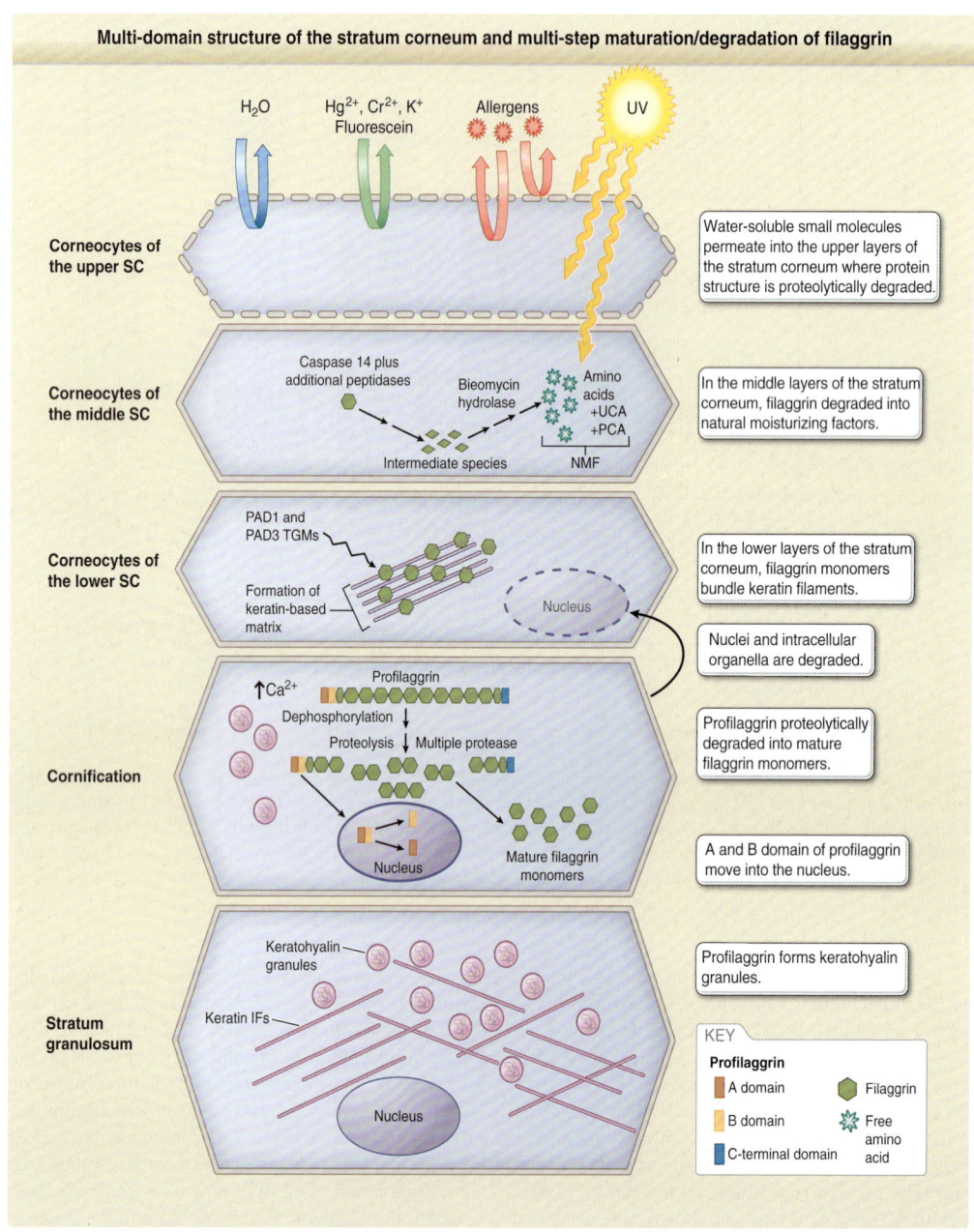

Figure 14-8 Multidomain structure of the stratum corneum and multistep maturation and degradation of filaggrin. The stratum corneum is thought to consist of at least three types of corneocytes undergoing different differentiation steps (corneocytes of the lower, middle, and upper stratum corneum). NMF, natural moisturizing factor; PAD, peptidylarginine deiminase; PCA, 2-pyrrolidone-5-carboxylic acid; IF, intermediate filament; SC, stratum corneum; TGM, transglutaminase; UCA, urocanic acid. (Modified from McAleer MA, Irvine AD. The multifunctional role of filaggrin in allergic skin disease. *J Allergy Clin Immunol.* 2013;131(2):280-291.)

intermediate filaments and may form a lattice structure in the lower layer of the stratum corneum.[65,66] The lattice structure can be observed under electron microscopy. In the later stage of cornification, keratin filaments bundled with filaggrin become cross-linked to the cornified cell envelope. The dead cornified cells lose most of their intracellular organelles and consist mostly of bundled intermediate filaments covalently attached to, and enclosed within, the cell envelope.

FILAGGRIN DEGRADATION AND NATURAL MOISTURIZING FACTORS

Filaggrin monomers bundle keratin filaments in the innermost layers of the stratum corneum. Because new corneocytes are continuously supplied at the bottom and old corneocytes are desquamated from the surface of the stratum corneum, each corneocyte gradually moves to the upper layers. During this upward movement of the corneocyte, intracellular filaggrin molecules are degraded into free amino acids and their derivatives by proteases, including caspase 14 and bleomycin hydrolase. Representative examples of the derivatives are trans-urocanic acid catalyzed from histidine by histidase and pyrrolidone carboxylic acid catalyzed from glutamine.[63,67-69] The natural moisturizing factors of the stratum corneum are composed primarily of these amino acids and their derivatives, together with lactic acid, urea, citrate, and sugars.[61,70] Deficiency of caspase 14 causes a defect in the proper degradation of filaggrin and the resultant phenotype of ichthyosis[71] (see Table 14-2).

Haploinsufficiency of filaggrin, because of various heterozygous mutations in the gene encoding filaggrin, causes ichthyosis vulgaris, a dry skin condition,[72] and predisposes patients to atopic dermatitis and various allergic diseases accompanied by eczema (eg, food allergy and asthma)[73,74] (see Table 14-2). The decrease in filaggrin induces a decrease in natural moisturizing factors, a disturbance of the lattice structure of the keratin filaments in the innermost layers of the stratum corneum, and a probable increase in the incidence of barrier breakage of the stratum corneum.[75] Such a weakness in the stratum corneum barrier may increase the chance of external allergens penetrating into the skin and the risk of percutaneous sensitization against various allergens. Most patients with severe stratum barrier defects, such as those with Netherton syndrome, have multiple allergies. In contrast, most patients who have mutations in the filaggrin gene basically develop ichthyosis vulgaris, and only some of these patients develop allergic diseases. This suggests that the barrier deficiency induced by filaggrin mutations is moderate and that the development of allergic diseases in these patients is modulated by various additional factors, such as genetic differences in immune reactions,[76] differences in the skin microbiota,[77-79] and environmental factors such as low air humidity[80] and air pollution.[81]

MULTIDOMAIN STRUCTURE OF THE STRATUM CORNEUM

Conventional cell biological analyses of the stratum corneum have been hampered by the insolubility of covalently cross-linked proteins. To overcome this difficulty, the stratum corneum has been analyzed by various special methods, such as cryoelectron microscopy, immunoelectron microscopy, Raman spectromicroscopy analysis, and time-of-flight secondary ion mass spectroscopy.[82-85] Based on the results of these analyses, the stratum corneum is considered to be divisible into several different parts with different characteristics, most likely into three parts (the upper, middle, and lower layers). For example, water-soluble small molecules soak in and out at the upper part of the stratum corneum, where the protein-based structure of the corneocytes is proteolytically degraded, and the corneocytes are thought to function as a sponge.[83,85] Further permeation of water-soluble small molecules into the middle part of the stratum corneum is rather limited, indicating that permeation barriers exist within the middle part of this structure.[83] The middle part of the stratum corneum also has a large potential to absorb and hold water, likely corresponding to the enrichment of natural moisturizing factors, which are mostly produced by the degradation of mature filaggrin.[63,82] The corneocytes of the lower part of the stratum corneum show an intracellular lattice structure of keratin filaments, integrated by mature filaggrin monomers, which is believed to contribute to the physical strength of the stratum corneum[84] (Fig. 14-9). The stratum corneum is a pile of "dead" corneocytes that lack any energy-dependent activities, such as adenosine triphosphate–dependent active transport, translation of proteins, and mRNA transcription. It is still largely unknown how the stratum corneum maintains homeostasis using the distinct features in its upper, middle, and lower layers.

PERCUTANEOUS ABSORPTION THROUGH THE STRATUM CORNEUM

Knowledge of how external molecules penetrate the epidermis is important not only for a better understanding of the pathogenesis of various skin diseases but also for the development of drug delivery for topical treatments. The paracellular route is a major pathway by which external molecules can penetrate the stratum corneum (see Fig. 14-3). Other routes of penetration into the skin are by the sebaceous glands or hair follicles, but the exact mechanisms of these pathways remain to be elucidated.[86]

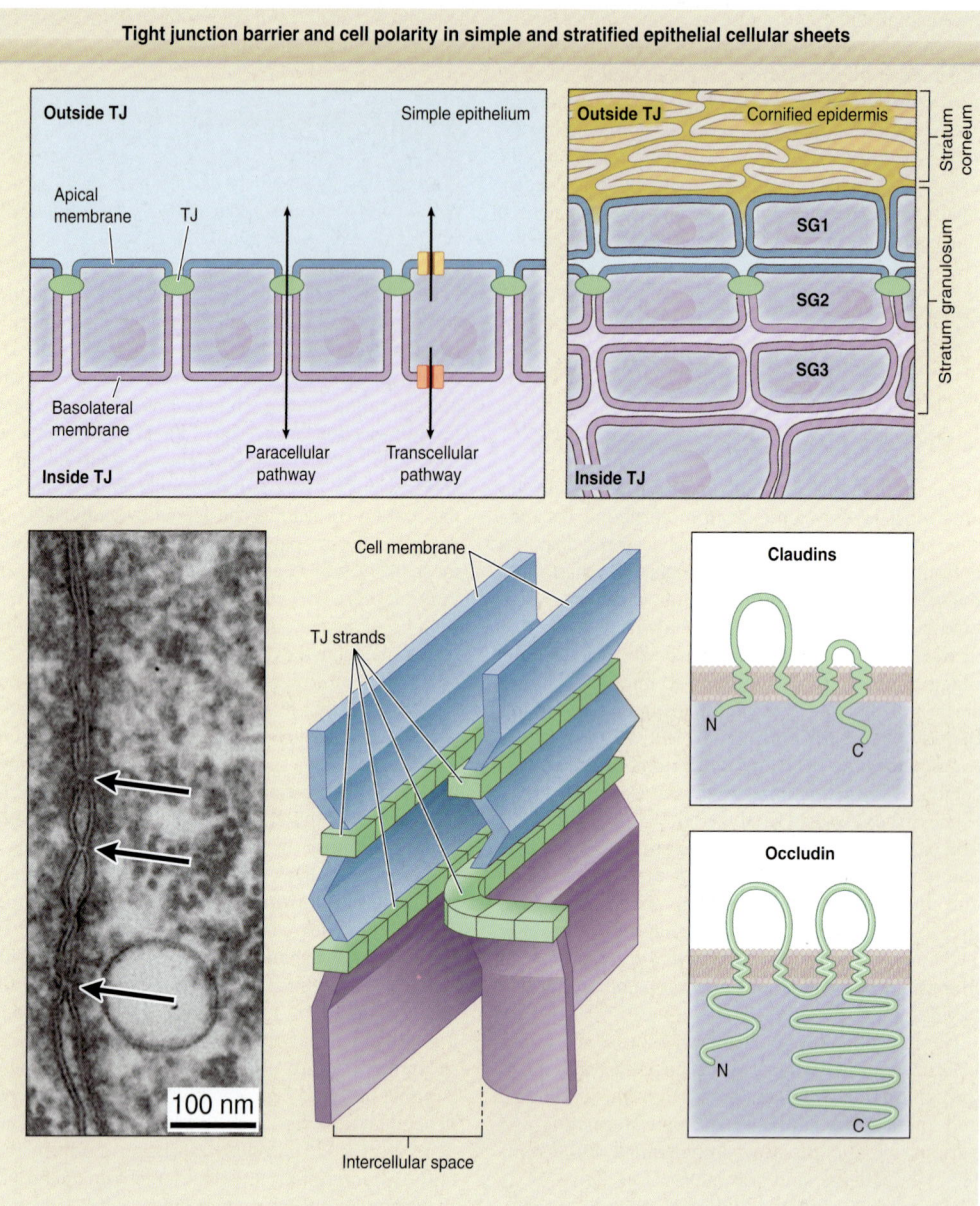

Figure 14-9 Tight junction (TJ) barrier in simple and stratified epithelial cellular sheets. The extracellular environment and plasma membrane are divided into two parts at the TJ barrier in simple epithelia. Solutes move between the two compartments via paracellular and transcellular pathways. In the epidermis, increasing evidence suggests that both the extracellular environment and plasma membrane are also divided into two parts at the TJ barrier formed between the SG2 cells, the extracellular environment outside and inside the TJ barrier, and the apical and basolateral cell membrane. In the electron micrograph (*left panel*), a TJ appears as a "kissing point" (*arrows*) where two plasma cell membranes face each other. The schematic shows the structure of TJ strands on the cell membrane and major transmembrane proteins of TJs. C, C-terminus; N, N-terminus. (Image used with permission from Dr. Hiroyuki Sasaki.)

Occlusive patches used in patch testing affect the intercorneocyte lipid lamellae and increase the permeation of solutes and solvents through the stratum corneum.[87] After passing through the stratum corneum, small molecules such as haptens can easily permeate the dermis, probably through the transcellular pathway (see Fig. 14-9). In contrast, large peptide antigens, such as the antigens of house dust mites or egg albumin, not only find it difficult to pass through the stratum corneum barrier but are also prohibited from further permeation into the skin by the tight junction barrier. Recent studies revealed that a defective stratum corneum barrier in early childhood is associated with the development of various allergic diseases, such as atopic dermatitis, allergic asthma, and food allergies, probably via enhanced antigen penetration through the stratum corneum and percutaneous sensitization.[74,88-91]

TIGHT JUNCTIONS

Multicellular organisms use epithelial cellular sheets to separate their body from the external environment or their organs from one another. Epithelia serve as selective permeability barriers to fluids that differ in chemical composition (Fig. 14-10). The occluding junctions are specialized intercellular adhesion complexes that are crucial for limiting molecular movement through the paracellular pathway (see Fig. 14-10) because they seal the intercellular spaces of the epithelial cellular sheets.[92] Tight junctions facilitate this barrier in vertebrates. In the gut of humans, for example, gut epithelia equipped with tight junction barriers separate body fluids from the fluid of the gut lumen.

consist of tight junction strands, which are mainly composed of four-transmembrane proteins of claudins on the plasma membrane that probably function as a zip lock to seal the adjacent plasma membrane, thereby forming a barrier against molecular movement through the paracellular pathway (see Fig. 14-9).[94,95] Other major components of tight junctions are the transmembrane proteins of occludin, junctional adhesion molecule A (JAM-A), tricellulin, and angulins, and the intracellular scaffold proteins of ZO-1, 2, and 3.[96,97] Tight junctions do not simply form an impermeable barrier but also serve as ion- and size-selective barriers that vary in tightness depending on the cell type and the composition of their structural adhesive molecules.[97-99]

STRUCTURE OF TIGHT JUNCTIONS

In simple epithelia, the tight junctions are located at the apical-most part of the apical junctional complex[93] (see Fig. 14-9). The apical junctional complex consists of tight junctions, beltlike adherens junctions, and desmosomes. The cell membrane is divided into two parts at the tight junctions—the apical cell membrane and basolateral cell membrane—both of which has a different composition of membranous proteins. Tight junctions

FUNCTION OF TIGHT JUNCTIONS

Observations of normal human trunk skin and mouse ear, abdominal, and back skin revealed that only the single-layer cells of the SG2 layer are equipped with tight junctions and show apical and basolateral cell membrane polarity in the epidermis (see Figs. 14-2 and 14-9).[100,101] The extracellular spaces of the epidermis are divided into two parts by the tight junction barrier.[5] The SG2 and SG1 cells secret various molecules (ie, lipids and proteases) via lamellar body secretions from

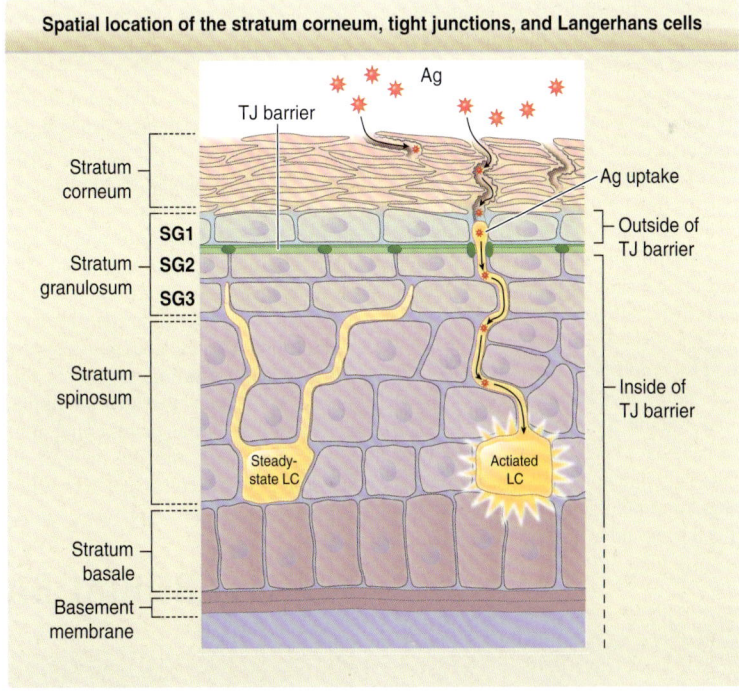

Figure 14-10 Spatial location of the stratum corneum, tight junctions (TJs), and Langerhans cells. SG2 cells form TJs (*closed circle* in *dark green*). SG1 cells are located outside the TJ barrier (*light blue*). In contrast, SG3 cells, spinous layer cells, and Langerhans cells are located inside the TJ barrier (*purple*). Dendrites of Langerhans cells in a steady state (*left yellow* cell) are located beneath the TJ but penetrate through the TJ barrier in their activated state (*right yellow* cell) to access to the outside TJ barrier. Antigen (Ag) uptake occurs from the tip of the dendrites (indicated by Ag uptake) at the outside TJ barrier.

their apical cell membrane into the extracellular spaces surrounding the SG1 cells, which are outside the tight junction barrier and are probably segregated from the environment inside the tight junction barrier (see Fig. 14-2).

A lack of claudin-1, a major claudin of the epidermis, causes leakage of the epidermal tight junction barrier and deficient formation of the stratum corneum barrier in mice, resulting in early neonatal death (probably caused by water loss from the body surface).[102] Decreased claudin-1 expression in mice induces an ichthyosis phenotype and skin inflammation.[103] A lack of claudin-1 in humans results in a very rare congenital disease called neonatal ichthyosis sclerosing cholangitis syndrome[104] (see Table 14-2). These observations indicate that a functional tight junction barrier is crucial for proper formation of the stratum corneum barrier and maintenance of epidermal homeostasis.

INTERACTION BETWEEN TIGHT JUNCTION BARRIERS AND INTRAEPIDERMAL IMMUNE-MEDIATED CELLS

Langerhans cells are antigen-presenting cells that are found in the epidermis and have multiple dendrites. They stay below the tight junction and project their dendrites upward in their steady state in both human and mice epidermis.[101,105] After activation, Langerhans cells extend their dendrites beyond the tight junction barrier and capture external antigens that penetrate through the stratum corneum (see Fig. 14-10). During this process, new tight junctions are formed between Langerhans cell dendrites and keratinocytes of the SG2 layer, enabling the uptake of external antigens without disturbing the barrier function of the tight junctions. The Langerhans cells migrate out from the epidermis, present the captured antigens to T cells in draining lymph nodes, and are considered to induce humoral immunity to the captured antigens.[101,106]

γ-δ T cells are a minor subpopulation of T cells that express T-cell receptor γ and δ. In the human epidermis, γ-δ T cells are rare; however, a large proportion of T cells are γ-δ T cells in mice epidermis.[107-110] The dendrites of γ-δ T cells have been shown to dock with the basal side of the tight junction-bearing cells in mice epidermis, forming immunologic synapses that polarize and anchor T cell projections at keratinocytes.[111]

SHAPE OF KERATINOCYTES FOR SKIN BARRIER HOMEOSTASIS

Corneocytes form according to a regular stacking structure, with regular zigzag interdigitation patterns between adjacent cell columns (see Fig. 14-5B). This regularly interdigitated stacking structure is most apparent in the skin of rodent ears but is also observed in the skin of other body regions in rodents, as well as in human skin.[112] Classic scanning electron microscopic studies of the skin surface corneocytes of the murine ear and a recent immunofluorescent microscopic study of the tight junction-bearing granular layer cells of the murine ear revealed that the basic shape of the cell is a flattened variation of Kelvin's tetrakaidecahedron (see Table 14-1) in the stratum corneum and stratum granulosum[4,113,114] (Fig. 14-11). The regular interdigitation pattern of the corneocytes is believed result from the regular interdigitated stacking of the flattened tetrakaidecahedron cells (see Figs. 14-5B and 14-11C). Computational simulation and in vivo imaging studies suggested that this regular structure is formed at the granular layer by transformation of the three-dimensional shape of cells supplied from the spinous layer, although the precise molecular mechanisms underlying the cell shape change are still unknown.[4,115-117] Only a single layer of cells (SG2 layer cells) form tight junctions at the apical edges of lateral cell–cell contacts. Therefore, tight junctions are formed at the edges of tetrakaidecahedron cells (see Fig. 14-11). When a tight junction-forming cell (an old cell) is replaced by a new cell located just beneath the old cell, the new cell first forms a new tight junction polygon beneath the old cell. Thus, each tight junction polygon becomes temporally double-edged during cell replacement (see Fig. 14-11). After that, the tight junction polygon of the old cells disappears, and eventually, the old cell is extruded to the outside of the tight junction barrier (the outside of the SG2 cell layer that forms the tight junction barrier). The temporal formation of the double-edged tight junction polygon at each cell turnover site maintains the homeostasis of the tight junction barrier.[4] The regular interdigitated stacking of the flattened tetrakaidecahedron cells enables not only the temporal formation of the double-edged tight junction polygon but also to maintain the spatial relationship between cells and desmosomal cell–cell adhesions during cell turnover that may be responsible the physical strength of the epidermis.[4] The molecular mechanisms that restrict tight junction-forming activity to the SG2 cell layer in the epidermis, the spatiotemporal regulation of cell turnover while maintaining tight junction barrier homeostasis, and the manner in which the tetrakaidecahedron cell shape is produced are currently unknown.

ANTIMICROBIAL BARRIER

ANTIMICROBIAL PROPERTY OF THE SKIN SURFACE

The skin constantly encounters microbial pathogens. Control of the skin microbiota is important to prevent bacterial and fungal infections. Continuous

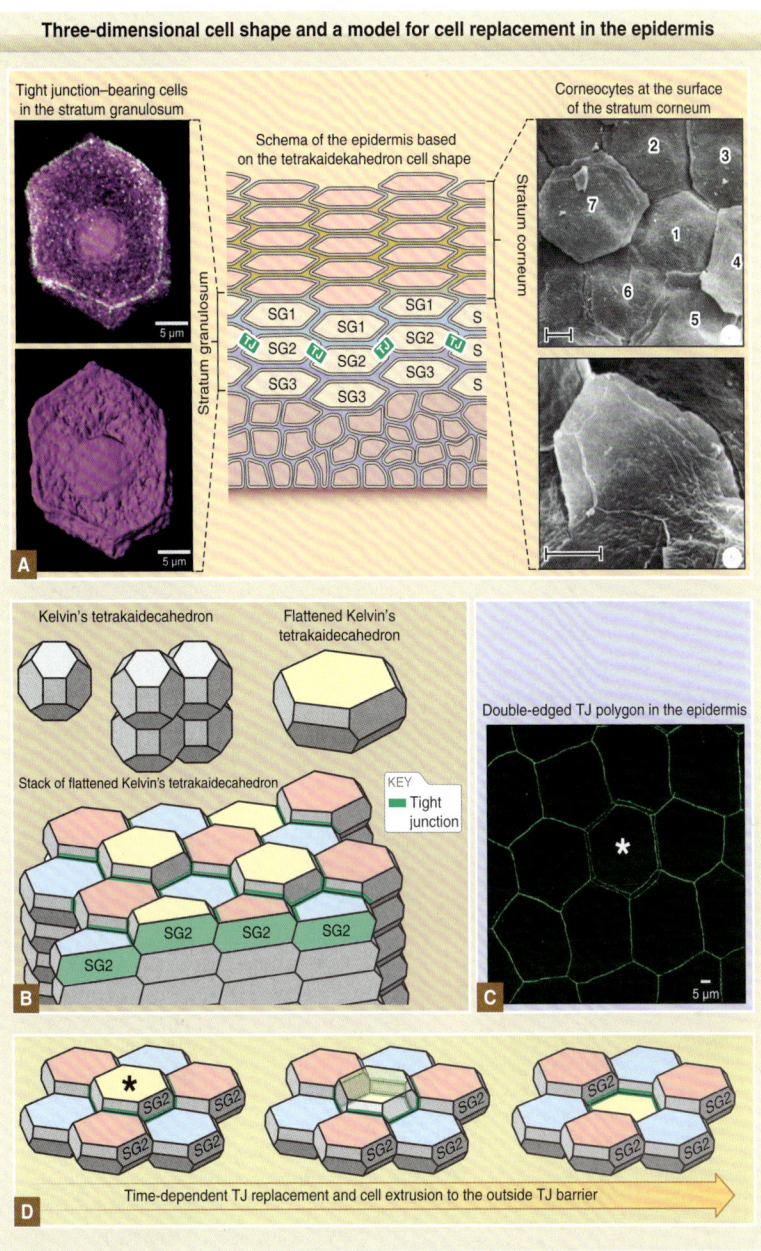

Figure 14-11 Three-dimensional cell shape of corneocytes and tight junction (TJ)–forming cells. **A,** Three-dimensional polyhedral shape of TJ-forming cells in immunofluorescent microscopic view (*left panel*) and the equivalent shape of corneocytes at the surface of the stratum corneum in scanning electron microscopic view (*right panel*) suggest that the basic shape of stratum granulosum cells and corneocytes is a flattened variation of Kelvin's tetrakaidecahedron. **B,** Kelvin's tetrakaidecahedron, flattened variation of Kelvin's tetrakaidecahedron, and regular interdigitated stacks of flattened Kelvin's tetrakaidecahedron cells. SG2 cells are displayed at the top of cell columns. Three different Z-axis positions of the SG2 cells are displayed in *yellow, pink,* and *blue* on the apical surface of the cells. Tight junctions (*green* edges) located at the apical edges of the cell-cell contact between SG2 cells. **C,** En face view of the TJs (green edges stained by anti-ZO-1 antibody) in mouse ear skin. Essentially, tight junction polygons are single edged. The double-edged polygon (*asterisk*) is the site where a new TJ polygon is formed to relocate a cell from inside to outside of the TJ barrier. **D,** Conceptual model for the formation of the double-edged TJ polygon (*asterisk*) during cell turnover from inside to outside of the TJ barrier. A new TJ polygon is formed beneath the *center yellow-colored cell* (*asterisk, left panel*), resulting in the formation of a double-edged polygon (*middle panel*). Then, the outer old polygon is degraded (*right panel*). The *center yellow-colored cell* in the left panel (*asterisk*) is relocated from inside the TJ barrier (*left panel*) to outside of the TJ barrier (*right panel*) after the temporal formation of the double-edged polygon (*middle panel*). (The scanning electron microscopic picture on the right side of Image **A,** is reproduced with permission of Springer Nature from Allen TD, Potten CS. Significance of cell shape in tissue architecture. *Nature*. 1976;264:545-547.) The immunofluorescent pictures of parts A and C and schemas in B and D are from Yokouchi M, Atsugi T, Logtestijn M, et al. Epidermal cell turnover across tight junctions based on Kelvin's tetrakaidecahedron cell shape. *Elife*. 2016;5:e19593.

turnover of epidermal cells by desquamation prohibits colonization of microorganisms on the skin. The physical properties of the skin surface itself prevents bacterial growth, that is, a low carbohydrate and water content and a weakly acidic pH (a pH of 5.6 to 6.4).[118-120] The weak acidic pH is due to various substances, such as free fatty acids secreted from sebaceous glands or derived from phospholipid hydrolysis in the stratum corneum, lactic acid secreted from derived from the eccrine glands, urocanic acid mostly derived from the degradation products of filaggrin, and metabolites produced by microorganisms.[121] The epidermis is also equipped with an active antimicrobial defense system comprising antimicrobial proteins (Table 14-3).

ANTIMICROBIAL PROTEINS ON THE SKIN SURFACE

Antimicrobial proteins are evolutionarily ancient innate immune effectors produced by almost all plants and animals.[122,123] Antimicrobial proteins show a broad antibacterial activity against both gram-positive and -negative bacteria; some even show antifungal or antiviral activity. The antimicrobial activity of most proteins occurs as a result of their unique structural characteristics, which enable disruption of the microbial membrane while leaving host cell membranes intact. These proteins also act as "alarmins" to alert host cells to react to injuries and microbial invasions.[124] Many proteins act as antimicrobial proteins/alarmins in the skin, including short proteins, such as β-defensins, cathelicidins, dermcidin, psoriasin, neuropeptides, and chemokines, and larger proteins, such as lysozymes, elastase, complement, and the S100 proteins. The variety of these antimicrobial proteins may reflect the complexity and long history of the microbial challenges at the skin surface.

The epithelial cells lining the surface of the intestine, respiratory tract, reproductive tract, and skin are the major source of antimicrobial proteins. Each epithelium has many characteristic antimicrobial proteins that are necessary for each microenvironment. Cathelicidins and β-defensins are the two major antimicrobial proteins of the skin and show a broad spectrum of antimicrobial activity in vivo.[125]

CELLS THAT PRODUCE ANTIMICROBIAL PROTEINS

Keratinocytes produce various antimicrobial proteins to defend the skin (Fig. 14-12). In particular, keratinocytes in the hair follicle constitutively produce cathelicidins and β-defensins at a higher level than the keratinocytes of the interfollicular epidermis, probably because the microenvironment of hair follicles facilitates bacterial colonization much more readily than that of the interfollicular epidermis. Secretory cells of the skin, such as those in the eccrine, apocrine, and sebaceous glands, secrete their own antimicrobial proteins and lipids and contribute to the antimicrobial activity of the skin surface. In the dermis, mast cells produce large amount of cathelicidins and store them within intracellular granules. After skin injuries, mast cells secrete cathelicidins to resist bacterial and viral infections.[126] Additionally, commensal bacteria produce their own antimicrobial proteins. For example, *Staphylococcus epidermidis*, the dominant commensal bacterium of the skin microbiota, produces several antimicrobial proteins.[127,128] These various antimicrobial proteins derived from host cells and microorganisms can modulate or regulate the composition of the skin microbiota.

TABLE 14-3
Antimicrobial Proteins on the Skin Surface

ANTIMICROBIAL PEPTIDES	EXPRESSION	FUNCTION
Human β-defensin 1	Epidermis	Antimicrobial activity against gram-negative bacteria Role in keratinocyte differentiation
Human β-defensin 2	Epidermis	Inducible by microbial components (*Pseudomonas aeruginosa, Staphylococcus aureus, Candida albicans*) Inducible by TNF-α IL-1 Antimicrobial activity against *Escherichia coli* and *P. aeruginosa* Weakly bacteriostatic against gram-positive bacteria
Human β-defensin 3	Epidermis	Induced by TNF-α and bacteria Bactericidal activity against Gram positive bacteria (*S. aureus* and vancomycin-resistant *Enterococcus faecium*)
Cathelicidin (LL-37)	Keratinocytes Mast cells Neutrophils Eccrine gland ductal cells	Vitamin D is a major inducer Antibacterial, antifungal, and antiviral activities Attracts mast cells and neutrophils
Psoriasin (S100A7)	Keratinocytes	Bacterial membrane permeability Bactericidal against *E. coli* Chemoattractant for CD4 cells and neutrophils
RNase 7	Stratum corneum	Broad spectrum antimicrobial activity (*S. aureus, Propionibacterium acnes, P. aeruginosa, E. coli, C. albicans*) Induced by IL-1β, IFN-γ, bacterial challenge

IFN, interferon; IL, interleukin; TNF-α, tumor necrosis factor-α.
From Modlin RL, Miller LS, Bangert C, et al. Innate and adaptive immunity in the skin. In: Goldsmith LA, Katz SI, Gilchrest BA, et al, eds. *Fitzpatrick's Dermatology in General Medicine*, 8th ed. New York: McGraw-Hill; 2012.

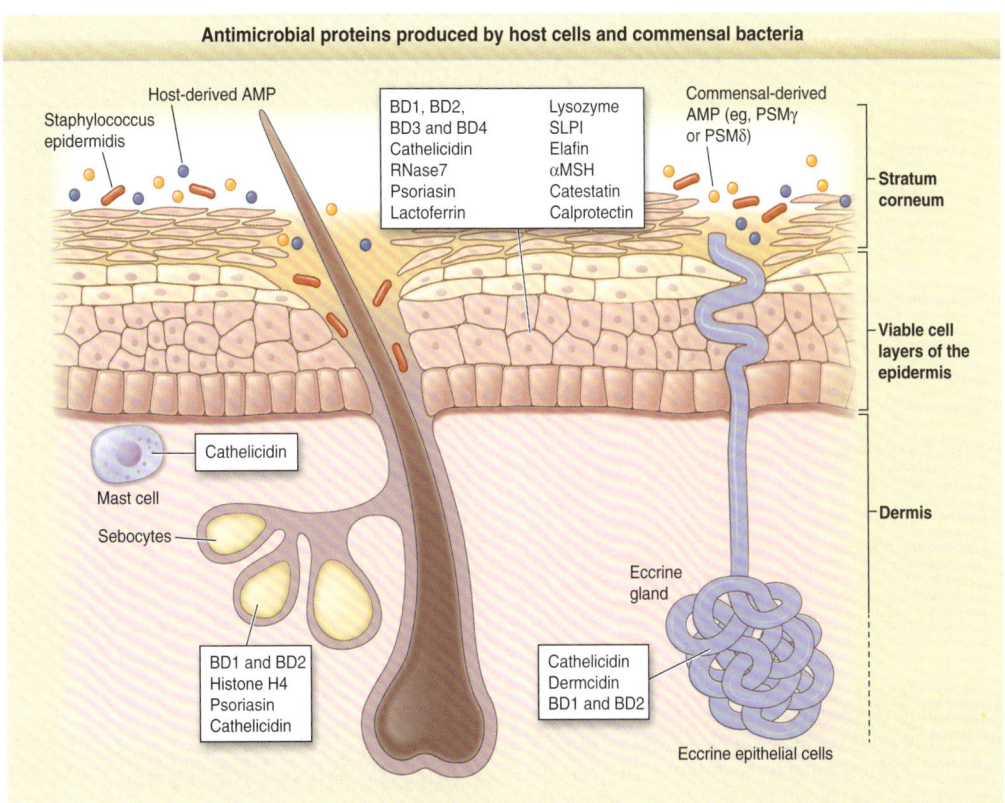

Figure 14-12 Antimicrobial proteins produced by host cells and commensal bacteria. AMP, antimicrobial proteins; BD, beta defencins; PSM, phenol soluble modulin; MSH, melanocyte-stimulating hormone; SLPI, secretory leukocyte protease inhibitor. (Adapted with permission from Springer Nature from Gallo RL, Hooper LV. Epithelial antimicrobial defence of the skin and intestine. *Nat Rev Immunol*. 2012;12:503.)

FUNCTIONS OF ANTIMICROBIAL PROTEINS

Antimicrobial proteins have various mechanisms of action[122,129,130]; many target the cell wall or cell membrane structure of microorganisms. For example, defensins and cathelicidins are usually cationic and interact with the bacterial membrane surface through electrostatic interactions. Some defensins form pores in the bacterial membrane to disrupt membrane integrity and promote bacterial lysis. Cathelicidins bind to bacterial membranes and promote membrane insertion and disruption. The mechanisms of action of several antimicrobial proteins remain unclear.

Increasing evidence indicates that some antimicrobial proteins modulate immune signaling through chemokine receptors and Toll-like receptors. Antimicrobial proteins not only stimulate chemokine and cytokine secretion from a variety of cell types but also use chemotactic activity to recruit leukocytes by direct or indirect mechanisms to modify the inflammatory response.[122,131-133] The chemotactic activities of different types of antimicrobial proteins are distinct from one another, and each recruits different types of cell. For example, LL-37, the human member of the cathelicidin family of antimicrobial peptides, recruits neutrophils, T cells, monocytes, and mast cells. LL-37 also induces keratinocytes through the mitochondrial antiviral signaling pathway to promote the production and secretion of interferon-β, which activates antiviral responses.[134] Toll-like receptors are transmembrane receptors for pattern recognition and are activated by the conserved structural pattern of microbial molecules, such as lipopolysaccharides, flagella, endotoxins, RNA, and DNA.[135] Toll-like receptor signaling is not restricted to such microbial molecules but can also be initiated by some antimicrobial proteins, allowing the immune cell responses to be modified.[136]

EPIDERMAL BARRIER OF NEWBORN SKIN

Full-term newborn babies have a well-developed and functional skin barrier at birth.[137] Although infant skin has a thinner stratum corneum with low levels of natural moisturizing factors and greater transepidermal water loss compared with adult skin, transepidermal water loss in healthy full-term newborns at birth is equal to or lower than that of adult skin (Table 14-4).[138-140]

TABLE 14-4
Similarities and Differences among Newborn, Infant, and Adult Skin

COMPOSITIONAL DIFFERENCES	PRETERM NEWBORN SKIN	FULL-TERM NEWBORN SKIN	INFANT SKIN	ADULT SKIN	REFERENCE
Epidermal surface	Lacking the stratum corneum (<24 wk of gestation) Lacking the vernix caseosa (<28 wk of gestation)	Coated by the vernix caseosa	Thin stratum corneum	Thick stratum corneum	137,140,171
Natural moisturizing factors	None or only in a few layers of the stratum corneum (<26 wk of gestation)	High in the vernix caseosa	Low in the stratum corneum	High in the stratum corneum	139,172
Surface pH	—	High	Low	Low	173-175
Sebum	—	—	Low (7-12 mo old)	High	176
Stratum corneum water content	—	—	High	Low	139
Dermal collagen fiber density	—	—	Low	High	140
Functional Differences					
Rate of water absorption	—	—	High	Low	139
Transepidermal water loss	Very high to high (depending on gestation period)	Low	High	Low	139

The stratum corneum is developed in utero under exposure to amniotic fluid, while extensive water exposure disrupts the stratum corneum barrier in adult skin. One putative mechanism for stratum corneum barrier development in utero is the formation of the fetal biofilm vernix caseosa, which coats the entire skin during the third (last) trimester.[141] The vernix caseosa is a complex mixture of water, proteins, and lipids; fetal corneocytes swollen with water are distributed throughout an amorphous mixture of lipids. The vernix protects the epidermis from amniotic fluid and facilitates formation of the stratum corneum beneath it. Vernix retention after birth, compared with vernix removal immediately after birth, has been reported to result in greater skin hydration and a lower skin surface pH at 24 hours after birth.[141] Moreover, vernix contains antimicrobial agents, including lysozyme and lactoferrin and exhibits antifungal and antibacterial activities.[142-144] This evidence implies value in retaining the vernix rather than removing it immediately after birth, as recommended by the World Health Organization.[145]

Unlike a full-term infant, a premature infant has a weak epidermal barrier and mechanically fragile dermis at birth. Babies born before 28 weeks of gestation lack the covering of the vernix. Newborns with very low birth weight have a greater risk of skin damage as a result of their insufficient skin barrier. Babies delivered at 25 weeks of gestation have only a few layers of the stratum corneum at birth and show transepidermal water loss of about 70 g/m²/hr.[146] The transepidermal water loss at birth in preterm newborns gradually decreases to about 7 g/m²/hr until 35 weeks' gestation, around which time the epidermal barrier becomes well developed in utero. The epidermal barrier continues to develop after birth, but the transepidermal water loss of extremely preterm infants is significantly higher than that of full-term infants even at 1 month after delivery.[146]

BARRIER AGAINST PHYSICAL STRESSES

PHYSICAL STRUCTURE PROTECTING AGAINST MECHANICAL STRESSES

The skin, which protects our body from various mechanical physical stimuli, consists of stripes of rigid and soft tissues, that is, the rigid stratum corneum, soft layers of keratinocytes, rigid collagenous tissue of the dermis, and soft cushion of the hypodermis (which is rich in adipocytes). Deficits in the physical strength, and defects in the border, of each stripe cause various diseases that lead to physical weakness, such as epidermolytic ichthyosis; simple, junctional, and dystrophic epidermolysis bullosa; and Ehlers-Danlos syndromes (see Chaps. 15, 47, 60, and 72).

BARRIERS AGAINST ULTRAVIOLET STRESSES

Reflection at the air–skin interface, absorption by trans-urocanic acid, and diffraction via keratin filaments aligned parallel to the skin surface limit the penetration of UV radiation into the stratum corneum. In the viable cell layer of the epidermis, melanin is the major factor that absorbs UV irradiation and protects genomic DNA from UV-induced damage. Although the upper layer cells of the epidermis may undergo greater DNA damage by UV irradiation than basal layer cells because of their location in the epidermis, the cells are tightly controlled in a nonproliferative state and are continuously eliminated from the epidermis via cell turnover, which prohibits tumorigenesis. In the proliferative basal layer cells, the damage to genomic DNA induced by UV irradiation is immediately repaired by DNA repair enzymes (see Chap. 130).

readily evaporate under fur, it is reasonable that hairy mammals do not use sweat to cool their body. In contrast, the furless skin of humans has a high density of eccrine sweat glands and enables effective cooling via water evaporation from the body surface. Interestingly, the density of eccrine glands and hair follicles are conversely determined by one transcription factor, *En1*, in the mouse footpad.[148]

SWEATING TO PROTECT AGAINST HEAT STRESSES

The skin is a protective organ against heat and cold stress and plays an important role in controlling body temperature. In humans, cooling is mainly achieved by the evaporation of water secreted from eccrine sweat glands. Thermoplegia tends to occur in patients with congenital and acquired anhidrosis or hypohidrosis. Human skin has the highest reported density of eccrine sweat glands among all mammals.[147] Most mammals have few sweat glands but have dense hairs covering their body. Because secreted sweat does not

VASCULATURE AND BLOOD FLOW CONTROL AGAINST HEAT STRESSES

Cooling and maintaining heat are, in part, dependent on the control of blood flow at the skin surface and countercurrent heat exchange between arteries and veins.[149,150] When the body temperature rises, skin surface blood vessels are dilated, and the skin appears red. The blood is cooled down via sweat evaporation and radiation-induced cooling on the skin surface (Fig. 14-13). In cold

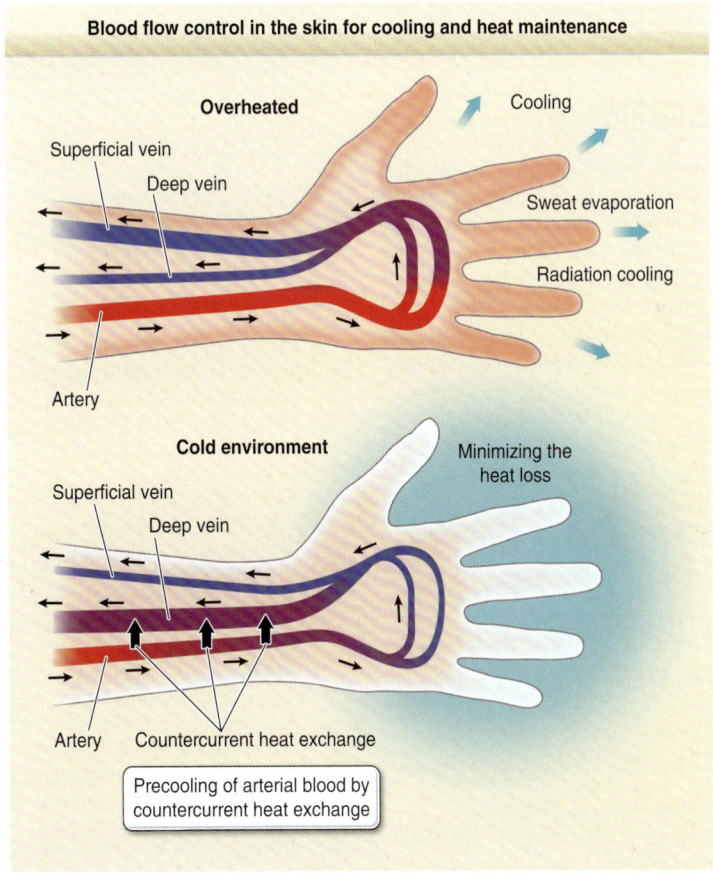

Figure 14-13 Blood flow control in the skin for cooling and heat maintenance. In a hot environment (upper panel), the superficial veins become dilated, and the blood in the superficial veins is mainly cooled via evaporation of eccrine sweat from the skin surface. In a cold environment (lower panel), the superficial veins contract, preventing heat loss from the blood. Countercurrent heat exchange between afferent arteries and dilated efferent deep veins precools the blood in the arteries before it reaches the superficial blood vessels, which also prevents heat loss from the skin surface.

air, the skin turns pale because blood vessels contract to decrease blood flow and minimize heat loss via radiation cooling. Therefore, the skin regulates blood flow at the skin surface to maintain homeostasis of the body temperature.

In the skin, arteries and veins run in close juxtaposition. Vascular countercurrent heat exchange between arteries and veins has been proposed as the mechanism by which the core body temperature is maintained under conditions of extreme cold or heat in homeothermic animals. For example, countercurrent heat exchange between afferent arteries and efferent veins in the legs of ducks prevents heat loss from the footpads, allowing ducks to paddle in icy water. In mouse skin, arteries and veins are aligned in close juxtaposition. Loss of the arteriovenous alignment in genetically engineered mice results in greater heat loss at the skin surface because warmer arterial blood reaches the skin surface without precooling via countercurrent heat exchange against the venous blood returned from the skin surface. The core body temperature decreases because of cooler venous blood returning to the body core.[151] These observations, together with measurements of the blood temperature in the arteries and veins of humans,[150] indicate that humans also use vascular countercurrent heat exchange to maintain the core body temperature under extreme conditions (see Fig. 14-13).

CONCLUSIONS

Skin, which is directly exposed to the external environment, shows species-specific adaptations, resulting in an amazing diversity among vertebrates and mammals and even among the human race and parts of the human body. It is important that dermatologists understand how human skin adapts to the external environment and how these adaptations are affected by disease. Skin is a complex superorgan consisting of the ectoderm, mesoderm, and skin microbiota. An integrated understanding of human skin, its microbiota, and the external environment that skin is exposed to is necessary for further investigation of normal skin function and of the molecular pathogenesis of various skin diseases; this will ultimately improve human health.

ACKNOWLEDGMENTS

The authors acknowledge the contributions of Ehrhardt Proksch and Jens-Michael Jensen, authors of Chap. 47, "Skin as an Organ of Protection," in the 8th edition of *Fitzpatrick's Dermatology in General Medicine*.

REFERENCES

1. Schempp C, Emde M, Wolfle U. Dermatology in the Darwin anniversary. Part 1: evolution of the integument. *J Dtsch Dermatol Ges*. 2009;7(9):750-757.
2. Mackenzie IC. Ordered structure of the epidermis. *J Invest Dermatol*. 1975;65(1):45-51.
3. Tsuruta D, Green KJ, Getsios S, et al. The barrier function of skin: how to keep a tight lid on water loss. *Trends Cell Biol*. 2002;12(8):355-357.
4. Yokouchi M, Atsugi T, Logtestijn M, et al. Epidermal cell turnover across tight junctions based on Kelvin's tetrakaidecahedron cell shape. *Elife*. 2016;5:e19593.
5. Kubo A, Nagao K, Amagai M. Epidermal barrier dysfunction and cutaneous sensitization in atopic diseases. *J Clin Invest*. 2012;122(2):440-447.
6. Potten CS. Epidermal cell production rates. *J Invest Dermatol*. 1975;65(6):488-500.
7. Haftek M, Callejon S, Sandjeu Y, et al. Compartmentalization of the human stratum corneum by persistent tight junction-like structures. *Exp Dermatol*. 2011;20(8):617-621.
8. Kitajima Y. Desmosomes and corneodesmosomes are enclosed by tight junctions at the periphery of granular cells and corneocytes, suggesting a role in generation of a peripheral distribution of corneodesmosomes in corneocytes. *J Dermatol Sci*. 2016;8(1):73-75.
9. Mackenzie JC. Ordered structure of the stratum corneum of mammalian skin. *Nature*. 1969;222(5196): 881-882.
10. Rice RH, Green H. The cornified envelope of terminally differentiated human epidermal keratinocytes consists of cross-linked protein. *Cell*. 1977;11(2):417-422.
11. Elias PM, Gruber R, Crumrine D, et al. Formation and functions of the corneocyte lipid envelope (CLE). *Biochim Biophys Acta*. 2014;1841(3):314-318.
12. Swartzendruber DC, Wertz PW, Madison KC, et al. Evidence that the corneocyte has a chemically bound lipid envelope. *J Invest Dermatol*. 1987;88(6):709-713.
13. Wertz PW, Downing DT. Covalently bound omega-hydroxyacylsphingosine in the stratum corneum. *Biochim Biophys Acta*. 1987;917(1):108-111.
14. Kalinin AE, Kajava AV, Steinert PM. Epithelial barrier function: assembly and structural features of the cornified cell envelope. *Bioessays*. 2002;24(9): 789-800.
15. Candi E, Schmidt R, Melino G. The cornified envelope: a model of cell death in the skin. *Nat Rev Mol Cell Biol*. 2005;6(4):328-340.
16. Matsuki M, Yamashita F, Ishida-Yamamoto A, et al. Defective stratum corneum and early neonatal death in mice lacking the gene for transglutaminase 1 (keratinocyte transglutaminase). *Proc Natl Acad Sci U S A*. 1998;95(3):1044-1049.
17. Ruhrberg C, Hajibagheri MA, Parry DA, et al. Periplakin, a novel component of cornified envelopes and desmosomes that belongs to the plakin family and forms complexes with envoplakin. *J Cell Biol*. 1997; 139(7):1835-1849.
18. Ruhrberg C, Hajibagheri MA, Simon M, et al. Envoplakin, a novel precursor of the cornified envelope that has homology to desmoplakin. *J Cell Biol*. 1996;134(3):715-729.
19. Simon M, Green H. Participation of membrane-associated proteins in the formation of the cross-linked envelope of the keratinocyte. *Cell*. 1984;36(4): 827-834.
20. Russell LJ, DiGiovanna JJ, Rogers GR, et al. Mutations in the gene for transglutaminase 1 in autosomal recessive lamellar ichthyosis. *Nat Genet*. 1995;9(3):279-283.
21. Marekov LN, Steinert PM. Ceramides are bound to structural proteins of the human foreskin

22. Nemes Z, Marekov LN, Fesus L, et al. A novel function for transglutaminase 1: attachment of long-chain omega-hydroxyceramides to involucrin by ester bond formation. *Proc Natl Acad Sci U S A.* 1999;96(15): 8402-8407.
23. Steven AC, Steinert PM. Protein composition of cornified cell envelopes of epidermal keratinocytes. *J Cell Sci.* 1994;107(2):693-700.
24. Ishida-Yamamoto A, McGrath JA, Lam H, et al. The molecular pathology of progressive symmetric erythrokeratoderma: a frameshift mutation in the loricrin gene and perturbations in the cornified cell envelope. *Am J Hum Genet.* 1997;61(3):581-589.
25. Freinkel RK, Traczyk TN. Lipid composition and acid hydrolase content of lamellar granules of fetal rat epidermis. *J Invest Dermatol.* 1985;85(4):295-298.
26. Akiyama M, Sugiyama-Nakagiri Y, Sakai K, et al. Mutations in lipid transporter ABCA12 in harlequin ichthyosis and functional recovery by corrective gene transfer. *J Clin Invest.* 2005;115(7):1777-1784.
27. Kelsell DP, Norgett EE, Unsworth H, et al. Mutations in ABCA12 underlie the severe congenital skin disease harlequin ichthyosis. *Am J Hum Genet.* 2005;76(5):794-803.
28. Elias PM, Cullander C, Mauro T, et al. The secretory granular cell: the outermost granular cell as a specialized secretory cell. *J Investig Dermatol Symp Proc.* 1998;3(2):87-100.
29. Feingold KR. Thematic review series: skin lipids. The role of epidermal lipids in cutaneous permeability barrier homeostasis. *J Lipid Res.* 2007;48(12): 2531-2546.
30. Wertz P. Biochemistry of human stratum corneum lipids. In: Elias PM, Feingold KR, eds. *Skin Barrier*, New York: Taylor and Francis; 2006:33-42
31. Proksch E, Elias PM, Feingold KR: Regulation of 3-hydroxy-3-methylglutaryl-coenzyme A reductase activity in murine epidermis. Modulation of enzyme content and activation state by barrier requirements. *J Clin Invest.* 1990;85(3):874-882.
32. Bikle DD. Vitamin D metabolism and function in the skin. *Mol Cell Endocrinol.* 2011;347(1-2):80-89.
33. He M, Kratz LE, Michel JJ, et al. Mutations in the human SC4MOL gene encoding a methyl sterol oxidase cause psoriasiform dermatitis, microcephaly, and developmental delay. *J Clin Invest.* 2011;121(3):976-984.
34. Konig A, Happle R, Bornholdt D, et al. Mutations in the NSDHL gene, encoding a 3beta-hydroxysteroid dehydrogenase, cause CHILD syndrome. *Am J Med Genet.* 2000;90(4):339-346.
35. Paller AS, van Steensel MA, Rodriguez-Martin M, et al. Pathogenesis-based therapy reverses cutaneous abnormalities in an inherited disorder of distal cholesterol metabolism. *J Invest Dermatol.* 2011; 131(11):2242-2248.
36. Kingery FA, Kellum RE. Essential fatty acid deficiency: histochemical changes in the skin of rats. *Arch Dermatol.* 1965;91 272-279.
37. Caldwell MD, Jonsson HT, Othersen HB Jr. Essential fatty acid deficiency in an infant receiving prolonged parenteral alimentation. *J Pediatr.* 1972;81(5):894-898.
38. Rabionet M, Gorgas K, Sandhoff R. Ceramide synthesis in the epidermis. *Biochim Biophys Acta.* 2014; 1841(3):422-434.
39. Elias PM, Williams ML, Holleran WM, et al. Pathogenesis of permeability barrier abnormalities in the ichthyoses: inherited disorders of lipid metabolism. *J Lipid Res.* 2008;49(4):697-714.
40. Breiden B, Sandhoff K. The role of sphingolipid metabolism in cutaneous permeability barrier formation. *Biochim Biophys Acta.* 2014;1841(3):441-452.
41. Uchida Y, Holleran WM. Omega-O-acylceramide, a lipid essential for mammalian survival. *J Dermatol Sci.* 2008;51(2):77-87.
42. Kihara A. Synthesis and degradation pathways, functions, and pathology of ceramides and epidermal acylceramides. *Prog Lipid Res.* 2016;63:50-69.
43. Wertz PW. Lipids and barrier function of the skin. *Acta Derm Venereol Suppl (Stockh).* 2000;208:7-11.
44. Akiyama M. Corneocyte lipid envelope (CLE), the key structure for skin barrier function and ichthyosis pathogenesis. *J Dermatol Sci.* 2017;88(1):3-9.
45. Serre G, Mils V, Haftek M, et al. Identification of late differentiation antigens of human cornified epithelia, expressed in re-organized desmosomes and bound to cross-linked envelope. *J Invest Dermatol.* 1991;97(6):1061-1072.
46. Furio L, Hovnanian A. When activity requires breaking up: LEKTI proteolytic activation cascade for specific proteinase inhibition. *J Invest Dermatol.* 2011;131(11):2169-2173.
47. Sales KU, Masedunskas A, Bey AL, et al. Matriptase initiates activation of epidermal pro-kallikrein and disease onset in a mouse model of Netherton syndrome. *Nat Genet.* 2010;42(8):676-683.
48. Brattsand M, Stefansson K, Lundh C, et al. A proteolytic cascade of kallikreins in the stratum corneum. *J Invest Dermatol.* 2005;124(1):198-203.
49. Ishida-Yamamoto A, Deraison C, Bonnart C, et al. LEKTI is localized in lamellar granules, separated from KLK5 and KLK7, and is secreted in the extracellular spaces of the superficial stratum granulosum. *J Invest Dermatol.* 2005;124(2):360-366.
50. Borgono CA, Michael IP, Komatsu N, et al. A potential role for multiple tissue kallikrein serine proteases in epidermal desquamation. *J Biol Chem.* 2007;282(6):3640-3652.
51. Deraison C, Bonnart C, Lopez F, et al. LEKTI fragments specifically inhibit KLK5, KLK7, and KLK14 and control desquamation through a pH-dependent interaction. *Mol Biol Cell.* 2007;18(9):3607-3619.
52. Descargues P, Deraison C, Bonnart C, et al. Spink5-deficient mice mimic Netherton syndrome through degradation of desmoglein 1 by epidermal protease hyperactivity. *Nat Genet.* 2005;37(1):56-65.
53. Yang T, Liang D, Koch PJ, et al. Epidermal detachment, desmosomal dissociation, and destabilization of corneodesmosin in Spink5-/- mice. *Genes Dev.* 2004;18(19):2354-2358.
54. Basel-Vanagaite L, Attia R, Ishida-Yamamoto A, et al. Autosomal recessive ichthyosis with hypotrichosis caused by a mutation in ST14, encoding type II transmembrane serine protease matriptase. *Am J Hum Genet.* 2007;80(3):467-477.
55. Chavanas S, Bodemer C, Rochat A, et al. Mutations in SPINK5, encoding a serine protease inhibitor, cause Netherton syndrome. *Nat Genet.* 2000;25(2): 141-142.
56. Israeli S, Zamir H, Sarig O, et al. Inflammatory peeling skin syndrome caused by a mutation in CDSN encoding corneodesmosin. *J Invest Dermatol.* 2011;131(3):779-781.
57. Oji V, Eckl KM, Aufenvenne K, et al. Loss of corneodesmosin leads to severe skin barrier defect, pruritus,

and atopy: unraveling the peeling skin disease. *Am J Hum Genet*. 2010;87(2):274-281.
58. Samuelov L, Sarig O, Harmon RM, et al. Desmoglein 1 deficiency results in severe dermatitis, multiple allergies and metabolic wasting. *Nat Genet*. 2013;45(10):1244-1248.
59. De Benedetto A, Kubo A, Beck LA. Skin barrier disruption: a requirement for allergen sensitization? *J Invest Dermatol*. 2012;132(3 Pt 2):949-963.
60. Bieber T. Atopic dermatitis. *N Engl J Med*. 2008;358(14):1483-1494.
61. Cabanillas B, Novak N. Atopic dermatitis and filaggrin. *Curr Opin Immunol*. 2016;42:1-8.
62. Brown SJ, McLean WH. One remarkable molecule: filaggrin. *J Invest Dermatol*. 2012;132(3 Pt 2):751-762.
63. Sandilands A, Sutherland C, Irvine AD, et al. Filaggrin in the frontline: role in skin barrier function and disease. *J Cell Sci*. 2009;122(9):1285-1294.
64. De Benedetto A, Qualia CM, Baroody FM, et al. Filaggrin expression in oral, nasal, and esophageal mucosa. *J Invest Dermatol*. 2008;128(6):1594-1597.
65. Norlen L, Al-Amoudi A. Stratum corneum keratin structure, function, and formation: the cubic rod-packing and membrane templating model. *J Invest Dermatol*. 2004;123(4):715-732.
66. Norlen L. Stratum corneum keratin structure, function and formation—a comprehensive review. *Int J Cosmet Sci*. 2006;28(6):397-425.
67. Denecker G, Hoste E, Gilbert B, et al. Caspase-14 protects against epidermal UVB photodamage and water loss. *Nat Cell Biol*. 2007;9(6):666-674.
68. Denecker G, Ovaere P, Vandenabeele P, et al. Caspase-14 reveals its secrets. *J Cell Biol*. 2008;180(3):451-458.
69. Kamata Y, Taniguchi A, Yamamoto M, et al. Neutral cysteine protease bleomycin hydrolase is essential for the breakdown of deiminated filaggrin into amino acids. *J Biol Chem*. 2009;284(19):12829-12836.
70. Elias PM. Stratum corneum defensive functions: an integrated view. *J Invest Dermatol*. 2005;125(2):183-200.
71. Kirchmeier P, Zimmer A, Bouadjar B, et al. Whole-exome-sequencing reveals small deletions in CASP14 in patients with autosomal recessive inherited ichthyosis. *Acta Derm Venereol*. 2017;96(7):102-104.
72. Smith FJ, Irvine AD, Terron-Kwiatkowski A, et al. Loss-of-function mutations in the gene encoding filaggrin cause ichthyosis vulgaris. *Nat Genet*. 2006;38(3):337-342.
73. Irvine AD, McLean WH, Leung DY. Filaggrin mutations associated with skin and allergic diseases. *N Engl J Med*. 2011;365(14):1315-1327.
74. Palmer CN, Irvine AD, Terron-Kwiatkowski A, et al. Common loss-of-function variants of the epidermal barrier protein filaggrin are a major predisposing factor for atopic dermatitis. *Nat Genet*. 2006;38(4):441-446.
75. Kawasaki H, Nagao K, Kubo A, et al. Altered stratum corneum barrier and enhanced percutaneous immune responses in filaggrin-null mice. *J Allergy Clin Immunol*. 2012;129(6):1538-1546 e1536.
76. Howell MD, Kim BE, Gao P, et al. Cytokine modulation of atopic dermatitis filaggrin skin expression. *J Allergy Clin Immunol*. 2007;120(1):150-155.
77. Nakamura Y, Oscherwitz J, Cease KB, et al. Staphylococcus delta-toxin induces allergic skin disease by activating mast cells. *Nature*. 2013;503(7476):397-401.
78. Kennedy EA, Connolly J, Hourihane JO, et al. Skin microbiome before development of atopic dermatitis: early colonization with commensal staphylococci at 2 months is associated with a lower risk of atopic dermatitis at 1 year. *J Allergy Clin Immunol*. 2017;139(1):166-172.
79. Kong HH, Oh J, Deming C, et al. Temporal shifts in the skin microbiome associated with disease flares and treatment in children with atopic dermatitis. *Genome Res*. 2012;22(5):850-859.
80. Sasaki T, Furusyo N, Shiohama A, et al. Filaggrin loss-of-function mutations are not a predisposing factor for atopic dermatitis in an Ishigaki Island under subtropical climate. *J Dermatol Sci*. 2014;76(1):10-15.
81. Hidaka T, Ogawa E, Kobayashi EH, et al. The aryl hydrocarbon receptor AhR links atopic dermatitis and air pollution via induction of the neurotrophic factor artemin. *Nat Immunol*. 2017;18(1):64-73.
82. Bouwstra JA, de Graaff A, Gooris GS, et al. Water distribution and related morphology in human stratum corneum at different hydration levels. *J Invest Dermatol*. 2003;120(5):750-758.
83. Kubo A, Ishizaki I, Kubo A, et al. The stratum corneum comprises three layers with distinct metal-ion barrier properties. *Sci Rep*. 2013;3:1731.
84. Manabe M, Sanchez M, Sun TT, et al. Interaction of filaggrin with keratin filaments during advanced stages of normal human epidermal differentiation and in ichthyosis vulgaris. *Differentiation*. 1991;48(1):43-50.
85. Bodde HE, Van den Brink I, Koerten HK, et al. Visualization of in vitro percutaneous penetration of mercuric chloride; transport through intercellular space versus cellular uptake through desmosomes. *J Control Release*. 1991;15:227-236.
86. Tran TN. Cutaneous drug delivery: an update. *J Investig Dermatol Symp Proc*. 2013;16(suppl 1):S67-S69.
87. Warner RR, Boissy YL, Lilly NA, et al. Water disrupts stratum corneum lipid lamellae: damage is similar to surfactants. *J Invest Dermatol*. 1999;113(6):960-966.
88. Lack G. Epidemiologic risks for food allergy. *J Allergy Clin Immunol*. 2008;121(6):1331-1336.
89. Lack G, Fox D, Northstone K, et al. Factors associated with the development of peanut allergy in childhood. *N Engl J Med*. 2003;348(11):977-985.
90. Brough HA, Liu AH, Sicherer S, et al. Atopic dermatitis increases the effect of exposure to peanut antigen in dust on peanut sensitization and likely peanut allergy. *J Allergy Clin Immunol*. 2015;135(1):164-170.
91. Brough HA, Simpson A, Makinson K, et al. Peanut allergy: effect of environmental peanut exposure in children with filaggrin loss-of-function mutations. *J Allergy Clin Immunol*. 2014;134(4):867-875 e861.
92. Furuse M, Tsukita S. Claudins in occluding junctions of humans and flies. *Trends Cell Biol*. 2006;16(4):181-188.
93. Axelrod J, Couchman J, De Rooij J, et al. Cell junctions and the extracellular matrix. In: Alberts B, Johnson A, Lewis J, et al, eds. *Molecular Biology of the Cell*, 6th ed. New York: Garland Science; 2014.
94. Suzuki H, Nishizawa T, Tani K, et al. Crystal structure of a claudin provides insight into the architecture of tight junctions. *Science*. 2014;344(6181):304-307.
95. Krause G, Protze J, Piontek J. Assembly and function of claudins: structure-function relationships based on homology models and crystal structures. *Semin Cell Dev Biol*. 2015;42:3-12.
96. Furuse M, Izumi Y, Oda Y, et al. Molecular organization of tricellular tight junctions. *Tissue Barriers*. 2014;2:e28960.
97. Itallie CMV, Anderson JM. Architecture of tight junctions and principles of molecular composition. *Semin Cell Dev Biol*. 2014;36:157-165.

98. Tsukita S, Furuse M. Claudin-based barrier in simple and stratified cellular sheets. *Curr Opin Cell Biol*. 2002;14(5):531-536.
99. Krug SM, Schulzke JD, Fromm M. Tight junction, selective permeability, and related diseases. *Semin Cell Dev Biol*. 2014;36:166-176.
100. Yoshida K, Yokouchi M, Nagao K, et al. Functional tight junction barrier localizes in the second layer of the stratum granulosum of human epidermis. *J Dermatol Sci*. 2013;71(2):89-99.
101. Kubo A, Nagao K, Yokouchi M, et al. External antigen uptake by Langerhans cells with reorganization of epidermal tight junction barriers. *J Exp Med*. 2009;206(13):2937-2946.
102. Furuse M, Hata M, Furuse K, et al. Claudin-based tight junctions are crucial for the mammalian epidermal barrier: a lesson from claudin-1-deficient mice. *J Cell Biol*. 2002;156(6):1099-1111.
103. Tokumasu R, Yamaga K, Yamazaki Y, et al. Dose-dependent role of claudin-1 in vivo in orchestrating features of atopic dermatitis. *Proc Natl Acad Sci U S A*. 2016;113(28):E4061-4068.
104. Hadj-Rabia S, Baala L, Vabres P, et al. Claudin-1 gene mutations in neonatal sclerosing cholangitis associated with ichthyosis: a tight junction disease. *Gastroenterology*. 2004;127(5):1386-1390.
105. Yoshida K, Kubo A, Fujita H, et al. Distinct behavior of human Langerhans cells and inflammatory dendritic epidermal cells at tight junctions in patients with atopic dermatitis. *J Allergy Clin Immunol*. 2014;134(4):856-864.
106. Ouchi T, Kubo A, Yokouchi M, et al. Langerhans cell antigen capture through tight junctions confers preemptive immunity in experimental staphylococcal scalded skin syndrome. *J Exp Med*. 2011;208(13):2607-2613.
107. Bos JD, Teunissen MB, Cairo I, et al. T-cell receptor gamma delta bearing cells in normal human skin. *J Invest Dermatol*. 1990;94(1):37-42.
108. Groh V, Porcelli S, Fabbi M, et al. Human lymphocytes bearing T cell receptor gamma/delta are phenotypically diverse and evenly distributed throughout the lymphoid system. *J Exp Med*. 1989;169(4):1277-1294.
109. Stingl G, Koning F, Yamada H, et al. Thy-1+ dendritic epidermal cells express T3 antigen and the T-cell receptor gamma chain. *Proc Natl Acad Sci U S A*. 1987;84(13):4586-4590.
110. Bonyhadi M, Weiss A, Tucker PW, et al. Delta is the Cx-gene product in the gamma/delta antigen receptor of dendritic epidermal cells. *Nature*. 1987;330(6148):574-576.
111. Chodaczek G, Papanna V, Zal MA, Zal T. Body-barrier surveillance by epidermal gammadelta TCRs. *Nat Immunol*. 2012;13(3):272-282.
112. Mackenzie IC, Zimmerman K, Peterson L. The pattern of cellular organization of human epidermis. *J Invest Dermatol*. 1981;76(6):459-461.
113. Allen TD, Potten CS. Significance of cell shape in tissue architecture. *Nature*. 1976;264(5586):545-547.
114. Menton DN. A minimum-surface mechanism to account for the organization of cells into columns in the mammalian epidermis. *Am J Anat*. 1976;145(1):1-22.
115. Honda H, Morita T, Tanabe A. Establishment of epidermal cell columns in mammalian skin: computer simulation. *J Theor Biol*. 1979;81(4):745-759.
116. Honda H, Tanemura M, Imayama S. Spontaneous architectural organization of mammalian epidermis from random cell packing. *J Invest Dermatol*. 1996;106(2):312-315.
117. Rompolas P, Mesa KR, Kawaguchi K, et al. Spatiotemporal coordination of stem cell commitment during epidermal homeostasis. *Science*. 2016;352(6292):1471-1474.
118. Grice EA, Segre JA. The skin microbiome. *Nat Rev Microbiol*. 2011;9(4):244-253.
119. Korting HC, Hubner K, Greiner K, et al. Differences in the skin surface pH and bacterial microflora due to the long-term application of synthetic detergent preparations of pH 5.5 and pH 7.0. Results of a crossover trial in healthy volunteers. *Acta Derm Venereol*. 1990;70(5):429-431.
120. Elias PM. The skin barrier as an innate immune element. *Semin Immunopathol*. 2007;29(1):3-14.
121. Ali SM, Yosipovitch G. Skin pH: from basic science to basic skin care. *Acta Derm Venereol*. 2013;93(3):261-267.
122. Gallo RL, Hooper LV. Epithelial antimicrobial defence of the skin and intestine. *Nat Rev Immunol*. 2012;12(7):503-516.
123. Schröder JM, Harder J. Antimicrobial skin peptides and proteins. *Cell Mol Life Sci*. 2006;63(4):469-486.
124. Li N, Yamasaki K, Saito R, et al. Alarmin function of cathelicidin antimicrobial peptide LL37 through IL-36γ induction in human epidermal keratinocytes. *J Immunol*. 2014;193(10):5140-5148.
125. Lai Y, Gallo RL. AMPed up immunity: how antimicrobial peptides have multiple roles in immune defense. *Trends Immunol*. 2009;30(3):131-141.
126. Di Nardo A, Yamasaki K, Dorschner RA, et al. Mast cell cathelicidin antimicrobial peptide prevents invasive group A Streptococcus infection of the skin. *J Immunol*. 2008;180(11):7565-7573.
127. Cogen AL, Yamasaki K, Muto J, et al. Staphylococcus epidermidis antimicrobial delta-toxin (phenol-soluble modulin-gamma) cooperates with host antimicrobial peptides to kill group A Streptococcus. *PLoS One*. 2010;5(1):e8557.
128. Nakatsuji T, Chen TH, Narala S, et al. Antimicrobials from human skin commensal bacteria protect against Staphylococcus aureus and are deficient in atopic dermatitis. *Sci Transl Med*. 2017;9(378):eaah4680.
129. Zhang LJ, Gallo RL. Antimicrobial peptides. *Curr Biol*. 2016;26(1):R14-R19.
130. Cullen TW, Schofield WB, Barry NA, et al. Gut microbiota. Antimicrobial peptide resistance mediates resilience of prominent gut commensals during inflammation. *Science*. 2015;347(6218):170-175.
131. Yang D, Chertov O, Oppenheim JJ. Participation of mammalian defensins and cathelicidins in antimicrobial immunity: receptors and activities of human defensins and cathelicidin (LL-37). *J Leukoc Biol*. 2001;69(5):691-697.
132. De Y, Chen Q, Schmidt AP, et al. LL-37, the neutrophil granule- and epithelial cell-derived cathelicidin, utilizes formyl peptide receptor-like 1 (FPRL1) as a receptor to chemoattract human peripheral blood neutrophils, monocytes, and T cells. *J Exp Med*. 2000;192(7):1069-1074.
133. Elssner A, Duncan M, Gavrilin M, Wewers MD. A novel P2X7 receptor activator, the human cathelicidin-derived peptide LL37, induces IL-1 beta processing and release. *J Immunol*. 2004;172(8):4987-4994.
134. Zhang LJ, Sen GL, Ward NL, et al. Antimicrobial peptide LL37 and MAVS signaling Drive interferon-beta production by epidermal keratinocytes during skin injury. *Immunity*. 2016;45(1):119-130.
135. Uematsu S, Akira S. Toll-like receptors (TLRs) and their ligands. *Handb Exp Pharmacol*. 2008;(183):1-20.

136. Funderburg N, Lederman MM, Feng Z, et al. Human-defensin-3 activates professional antigen-presenting cells via Toll-like receptors 1 and 2. *Proc Natl Acad Sci U S A*. 2007;104(47):18631-18635.
137. Visscher MO, Adam R, Brink S, et al. Newborn infant skin: physiology, development, and care. *Clin Dermatol*. 2015;33(3):271-280.
138. Kelleher MM, O'Carroll M, Gallagher A, et al. Newborn transepidermal water loss values: a reference dataset. *Pediatr Dermatol*. 2013;30(6):712-716.
139. Nikolovski J, Stamatas GN, Kollias N, et al. Barrier function and water-holding and transport properties of infant stratum corneum are different from adult and continue to develop through the first year of life. *J Invest Dermatol*. 2008;128(7):1728-1736.
140. Stamatas GN, Nikolovski J, Luedtke MA, et al. Infant skin microstructure assessed in vivo differs from adult skin in organization and at the cellular level. *Pediatr Dermatol*. 2010;27(2):125-131.
141. Visscher MO, Narendran V, Pickens WL, et al. Vernix caseosa in neonatal adaptation. *J Perinatol*. 2005;25(7):440-446.
142. Akinbi HT, Narendran V, Pass AK, et al. Host defense proteins in vernix caseosa and amniotic fluid. *Am J Obstet Gynecol*. 2004;191(6):2090-2096.
143. Tollin M, Bergsson G, Kai-Larsen Y, et al. Vernix caseosa as a multi-component defence system based on polypeptides, lipids and their interactions. *Cell Mol Life Sci*. 2005;62(19-20):2390-2399.
144. Marchini G, Lindow S, Brismar H, et al. The newborn infant is protected by an innate antimicrobial barrier: peptide antibiotics are present in the skin and vernix caseosa. *Br J Dermatol*. 2002;147(6):1127-1134.
145. World Health Organization Regional Office for the Western Pacific. *Newborn Care Until the First Week of Life: Clinical Practice Pocket Guide*. Manila, Republic of the Philippines; World Health Organization Regional Office for the Western Pacific; 2009.
146. Sedin G, Hammarlund K, Stromberg B. Transepidermal water loss in full-term and pre-term infants. *Acta Paediatr Scand Suppl*. 1983;305:27-31.
147. Lieberman DE. Human locomotion and heat loss: an evolutionary perspective. *Comprehensive Physiology*. 2015;5(1):99-117.
148. Kamberov YG, Karlsson EK, Kamberova GL, et al. A genetic basis of variation in eccrine sweat gland and hair follicle density. *Proc Natl Acad Sci U S A*. 2015;112(32):9932-9937.
149. Mitchell JW, Myers GE. An analytical model of the counter-current heat exchange phenomena. *Biophys J*. 1968;8(8):897-911.
150. Bazett H, Love L, Newton M, et al. Temperature changes in blood flowing in arteries and veins in man. *J Appl Physiol*. 1948;1(1):3-19.
151. Kidoya H, Naito H, Muramatsu F, et al. APJ regulates parallel alignment of arteries and veins in the skin. *Dev Cell*. 2015;33(3):247-259.
152. Thomson W. On the division of space with minimum partitional area. *Philos Mag*. 1887;24(151):503-514.
153. Koch PJ, de Viragh PA, Scharer E, et al. Lessons from loricrin-deficient mice: compensatory mechanisms maintaining skin barrier function in the absence of a major cornified envelope protein. *J Cell Biol*. 2000;151(2):389-400.
154. Liu XY, Dangel AW, Kelley RI, et al. The gene mutated in bare patches and striated mice encodes a novel 3beta-hydroxysteroid dehydrogenase. *Nat Genet*. 1999;22(2):182-187.
155. Aldahmesh MA, Mohamed JY, Alkuraya HS, et al. Recessive mutations in ELOVL4 cause ichthyosis, intellectual disability, and spastic quadriplegia. *Am J Hum Genet*. 2011;89(6):745-750.
156. Vasireddy V, Uchida Y, Salem N Jr, et al. Loss of functional ELOVL4 depletes very long-chain fatty acids (> or =C28) and the unique omega-O-acylceramides in skin leading to neonatal death. *Hum Mol Genet*. 2007;16(5):471-482.
157. Lefevre C, Bouadjar B, Ferrand V, et al. Mutations in a new cytochrome P450 gene in lamellar ichthyosis type 3. *Hum Mol Genet*. 2006;15(5):767-776.
158. Eckl KM, Tidhar R, Thiele H, et al. Impaired epidermal ceramide synthesis causes autosomal recessive congenital ichthyosis and reveals the importance of ceramide acyl chain length. *J Invest Dermatol*. 2013;133(9):2202-2211.
159. Radner FP, Marrakchi S, Kirchmeier P, et al. Mutations in CERS3 cause autosomal recessive congenital ichthyosis in humans. *PLoS Genet*. 2013;9(6):e1003536.
160. Rabionet M, Bayerle A, Jennemann R, et al. Male meiotic cytokinesis requires ceramide synthase 3-dependent sphingolipids with unique membrane anchors. *Hum Mol Genet*. 2015;24(17):4792-4808.
161. Lefevre C, Jobard F, Caux F, et al. Mutations in CGI-58, the gene encoding a new protein of the esterase/lipase/thioesterase subfamily, in Chanarin-Dorfman syndrome. *Am J Hum Genet*. 2001;69(5):1002-1012.
162. Grall A, Guaguere E, Planchais S, et al. PNPLA1 mutations cause autosomal recessive congenital ichthyosis in golden retriever dogs and humans. *Nat Genet*. 2012;44(2):140-147.
163. Jobard F, Lefevre C, Karaduman A, et al. Lipoxygenase-3 (ALOXE3) and 12(R)-lipoxygenase (ALOX12B) are mutated in non-bullous congenital ichthyosiform erythroderma (NCIE) linked to chromosome 17p13.1. *Hum Mol Genet*. 2002;11(1):107-113.
164. Epp N, Furstenberger G, Muller K, et al. 12R-lipoxygenase deficiency disrupts epidermal barrier function. *J Cell Biol*. 2007;177(1):173-182.
165. Yanagi T, Akiyama M, Nishihara H, et al. Harlequin ichthyosis model mouse reveals alveolar collapse and severe fetal skin barrier defects. *Hum Mol Genet*. 2008;17(19):3075-3083.
166. List K, Haudenschild CC, Szabo R, et al. Matriptase/MT-SP1 is required for postnatal survival, epidermal barrier function, hair follicle development, and thymic homeostasis. *Oncogene*. 2002;21(23): 3765-3779.
167. Furio L, de Veer S, Jaillet M, et al. Transgenic kallikrein 5 mice reproduce major cutaneous and systemic hallmarks of Netherton syndrome. *J Exp Med*. 2014;211(3):499-513.
168. Hewett DR, Simons AL, Mangan NE, et al. Lethal, neonatal ichthyosis with increased proteolytic processing of filaggrin in a mouse model of Netherton syndrome. *Hum Mol Genet*. 2005;14(2):335-346.
169. Leclerc EA, Huchenq A, Mattiuzzo NR, et al. Corneodesmosin gene ablation induces lethal skin-barrier disruption and hair-follicle degeneration related to desmosome dysfunction. *J Cell Sci*. 2009;122(15):2699-2709.
170. Presland RB, Boggess D, Lewis SP, et al. Loss of normal profilaggrin and filaggrin in flaky tail (ft/ft) mice: an animal model for the filaggrin-deficient skin disease ichthyosis vulgaris. *J Invest Dermatol*. 2000;115(6):1072-1081.

171. Chiou YB, Blume-Peytavi U. Stratum corneum maturation. A review of neonatal skin function. *Skin Pharmacol Physiol*. 2004;17(2):57-66.
172. Visscher MO, Utturkar R, Pickens WL, et al. Neonatal skin maturation—vernix caseosa and free amino acids. *Pediatr Dermatol*. 2011;28(2):122-132.
173. Yosipovitch G, Maayan-Metzger A, Merlob P, et al. Skin barrier properties in different body areas in neonates. *Pediatrics*. 2000;106(1 Pt 1):105-108.
174. Hoeger PH, Enzmann CC. physiology of the neonate and young infant: a prospective study of functional skin parameters during early infancy. *Pediatr Dermatol*. 2002;19(3):256-262.
175. Giusti F, Martella A, Bertoni L, et al. Skin barrier, hydration, and pH of the skin of infants under 2 years of age. *Pediatr Dermatol*. 2001;18(2):93-96.
176. Agache P, Blanc D, Barrand C, et al. Sebum levels during the first year of life. *Br J Dermatol*. 1980;103(6):643-649.

Chapter 15 :: Epidermal and Dermal Adhesion
:: Leena Bruckner-Tuderman & Aimee S. Payne

第十五章
表皮和真皮的黏附

中文导读

本章内容分为7节：①表皮黏附；②表皮-真皮黏附；③真皮细胞-基质黏附；④结论。将描述这些黏附结构的形态、分子和功能等方面。

第一节表皮黏附，介绍了桥粒是表皮的主要细胞黏附连接点，分为3个主要类别。接下来介绍了桥粒芯糖蛋白和桥粒芯胶蛋白是跨膜糖蛋白钙黏蛋白超家族的一部分，因其在天疱疮中的自身抗原的作用而被大家熟知。随后的观点认为所有的桥粒钙黏着蛋白都与人类自身免疫性、传染性和/或遗传性疾病相关。最后编者介绍了armadillo家族蛋白和斑蛋白中的各种蛋白的分布和功能等。

第二节表皮-真皮黏附，介绍了基底膜的结构和功能。基底膜超微结构为三层结构，在遏制肿瘤中尤其重要。接下来介绍了真皮-表皮交界处的超微结构，重点提到致密层作为表皮细胞附着的结构支架。本节还提到了半桥粒、锚定丝、致密层、锚定纤维等其他表皮-真皮黏附复合物。

第三节真皮细胞-基质黏附，介绍了真皮-表皮交界处与真皮乳头的细胞外基质是连续的，真皮的弹性和韧性等是由细胞外基质所获得，包含具有特定功能特性的胶原蛋白、弹性蛋白、糖蛋白和蛋白聚糖的结构网络。接下来介绍了细胞-基质相互作用可以调节细胞功能，包括发育、衰老和再生以及在诸如炎症和肿瘤中发挥作用。

第四节结论，总结了表皮和真皮的黏附为皮肤提供了抵抗环境影响的能力，这对于保护整个生物体免受机械、物理或微生物的侵害至关重要。表皮和真皮黏附的分子和功能细节研究取得了巨大的进展，将有助于设计罕见的遗传和常见的自身免疫黏附疾病的生物学治疗方法，还有助于了解皮肤衰老的生理过程。

〔粟 娟〕

AT-A-GLANCE

- The adhesive structures in the skin include desmosomes, focal adhesions, hemidesmosomes, basement membranes and dermal fibril networks.
- Desmosomes are primarily responsible for epidermal adhesion.
- The major components of desmosomes are the desmosomal cadherins (desmogleins and desmocollins), plakins (desmoplakin, envoplakin, and periplakin), and armadillo family proteins (plakoglobin and plakophilins).
- Hemidesmosomes are responsible for epidermal-dermal adhesion.
- The hemidesmosomal components comprise plakin homologs, integrins, and collagenous transmembrane proteins.
- All basement membranes contain collagen IV, laminins, nidogens, heparan sulfate proteoglycans, and fibulins.
- Functional specificity of basement membranes is provided by additional tissue-specific glycoproteins.
- In addition to their structural roles, desmosomes, hemidesmosomes, and the epidermal basement membrane are biologically active in cellular signaling.
- The dermal-epidermal junction is continuous with the extracellular matrix in the papillary dermis and thus attaches the epidermis with the dermis. The pliability and tenacity of the dermis are provided by a highly organized extracellular matrix that is also biologically active in cellular signaling.
- Mutations in the genes encoding the above proteins cause hereditary skin diseases, ranging from hypotrichosis and keratoderma to epidermolysis bullosa and Kindler syndrome.
- Protein components of desmosomes, hemidesmosomes, and epidermal basement membrane are targeted in autoimmune blistering diseases of the pemphigus or pemphigoid group.

INTRODUCTION

The cell–cell and cell–basement membrane adhesion in the epidermis, and the cell-matrix adhesion in the dermis provide the skin with its resistance against environmental influences; epidermal integrity is required for protection of the entire organism against mechanical, physical, or microbial insults. The major cellular structures involved are the desmosomes at cell–cell junctions in the epidermis and the hemidesmosome–basement membrane adhesion complexes and related structures at the dermal–epidermal junction. Ultrastructurally, the hemidesmosome closely resembles one-half of the desmosome; however, at the molecular level, these 2 structures are distinct. Both represent specifically organized assemblies of intracellular and transmembrane molecules. The desmosome anchors cytoskeletal filaments to cell–cell junctions, and the hemidesmosome anchors cytoskeletal filaments of basal epithelial cells to the basement membrane. Our knowledge of the desmosomal, hemidesmosomal, and basement membrane molecules has expanded drastically in recent years as a result of the great power of both molecular genetics and proteomics. After keratinocyte transmembrane proteins were initially identified as autoantigens in pemphigus and pemphigoid, a multitude of molecules have now been characterized at both protein and gene levels, and their expression, regulation, and functions have been discerned. The antigenic epitopes in different autoimmune blistering skin diseases have been carefully mapped and, as of this writing, mutations in at least 24 different genes have been shown to underlie heritable disorders of epidermal or epidermal–dermal adhesion in humans and mice. This chapter will describe the morphologic, molecular, and functional aspects of these adhesion structures.

EPIDERMAL ADHESION

ULTRASTRUCTURE OF DESMOSOMES

The desmosome (or *macula adherens*) is the major cell adhesion junction of the epidermis, serving to anchor apposing keratinocyte cell surface membranes to the intracellular keratin intermediate filament network. Desmosomes are present in almost all epithelial tissues, including the oropharynx, gut, liver, heart, lung, bladder, kidney, prostate, thymus, cornea, and CNS, although the desmosomal protein isoforms and intermediate filament proteins vary by cell type.[1] The primary role of desmosomes in epidermal cell adhesion is evidenced by the histologic findings in epidermal spongiosis, or intercellular edema, in which adjacent keratinocytes remain attached to each other only at desmosomal junctions (Fig. 15-1). These "intercellular bridges" served as the earliest description of desmosomes in tissues, their observation made possible with the advent of light microscopy in the 19th century.[2] The development of electron microscopy techniques in the mid-20th century allowed for higher resolution micrographs that revealed the ultrastructure of these intercellular junctions. Even in the 21st century, the desmosome still remains best defined by its electron micrographic appearance, with an electron-dense midline in the intercellular space halfway between apposing plasma membranes, sandwiched by 2 pairs of electron-dense cytoplasmic plaques (Fig. 15-2A).[3] The intercellular space between plasma membranes was called the *desmoglea* (from the Greek for "desmosomal glue"), because it was presumed to provide the adhesion that kept cells together.[4]

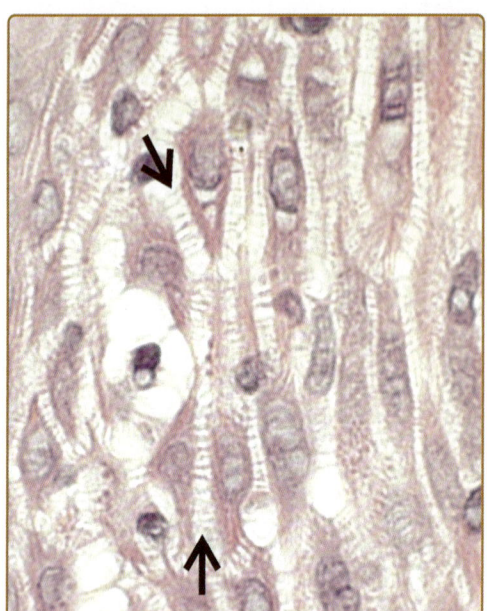

Figure 15-1 Desmosomes are the primary cell adhesion junction in the epidermis. Epidermal spongiosis, or intercellular edema due to inflammation, causes separation of keratinocytes, which remain attached by intercellular bridges representing desmosomal junctions (*arrows*). (Image used with permission from John Seykora, MD, PhD.)

STRUCTURE AND FUNCTION OF DESMOSOMAL PROTEINS

In anchoring the cell surface to the intermediate filament network, desmosomes create a 3-dimensional scaffolding of proteins that extend from the cell surface all the way to the nuclear envelope. This scaffolding is critical to stabilize epithelia in the face of shear stress or external trauma. Early morphologic studies led to the perception of the desmosome as a static structure, a "spot weld" functioning only to maintain intercellular adhesion.[5] Over the last 4 decades, the individual proteins comprising the desmosome have been biochemically characterized and cloned, shedding light on both the dynamic nature of the desmosome structure and the diversity of desmosomal protein function.

Desmosomal proteins fall into 3 major categories: (1) desmosomal cadherins (desmogleins and desmocollins), (2) armadillo family proteins (plakoglobin and plakophilins), and (3) plakins (desmoplakin, envoplakin, and periplakin). Additional proteins, such as corneodesmosin, kazrin, Perp, ninein, Lis1, Ndel1, and CLIP170, also have been localized to epidermal desmosomes.[6-10] Immunogold electron microscopy and cryoelectron tomography studies have further refined our understanding of how these molecular components of desmosomes are ordered within the desmosome ultrastructure[11,12] (Fig. 15-2B). The desmosomal cadherins are transmembrane proteins whose extracellular amino-terminal domains interact to form the trans-adhesive interface between cells, represented by the electron-dense midline of the desmoglea. Intracellularly, the outer dense plaque contains the desmosomal cadherin cytoplasmic tails, with plakoglobin and the desmoplakin amino-terminal domain bound approximately 20 nm from the plasma membrane, and plakophilin, approximately 10 nm from the plasma membrane. Approximately 40 to 50 nm from the plasma membrane, the desmoplakin carboxyl-terminus interacts with keratin intermediate filaments, producing the inner dense plaque. The biochemistry, expression pattern, and diseases of each desmosomal component are discussed in further detail next. Although the specific physiologic roles and pathophysiologic mechanisms affecting many of the desmosomal proteins remain under active investigation, current knowledge clearly indicates the importance of desmosomes and their components beyond just cell adhesion.

DESMOSOMAL CADHERINS

Desmogleins and desmocollins are part of the cadherin superfamily of transmembrane glycoproteins. Members of this superfamily, which includes the adherens junction protein E-cadherin, mediate calcium-dependent adhesion in a variety of epithelial tissues. In humans, there are 4 desmoglein (Dsg) isoforms and 3 desmocollin (Dsc) isoforms, each with varying expression patterns within and among epithelia.[13-15] Within normal human epidermis, Dsg1, Dsg4, and Dsc1 are expressed predominantly in the differentiated cells of the superficial epidermis, whereas Dsg2, Dsg3, Dsc2, and Dsc3 are expressed more strongly in the basal and/or suprabasal layers[16,17] (Fig. 15-3). Among different epithelial tissues, Dsg1 and Dsg3 expression are largely limited to stratified squamous epithelia in the skin and oropharynx, as well as thymic epithelial cells. Dsg3 is also strongly expressed in squamous cell carcinomas and other head and neck cancers, where it has been proposed as a potential molecular target for therapy.[18] Dsg2 is the major desmoglein isoform in most simple and transitional epithelia, as well as cardiac myocytes.[19] Dsg4 is prominent in desmosomes of the hair follicle, testis, and prostate.[20,21] The expression pattern of the human desmocollins is less well characterized. In normal tissues, Dsc1 expression is largely limited to skin and oral epithelia, whereas Dsc2 is more widely expressed in most desmosome-containing epithelia and is the only desmocollin isoform in cardiac tissue.[13] Dsc3, like Dsg3, is most strongly expressed in the stratified squamous epithelia of the skin and oropharynx,[22] although UniGene data suggest weaker expression in a variety of other epithelial tissues. Desmocollin switching has been described in colorectal cancer, with downregulation of Dsc2 and upregulation of Dsc1 and Dsc3.[23]

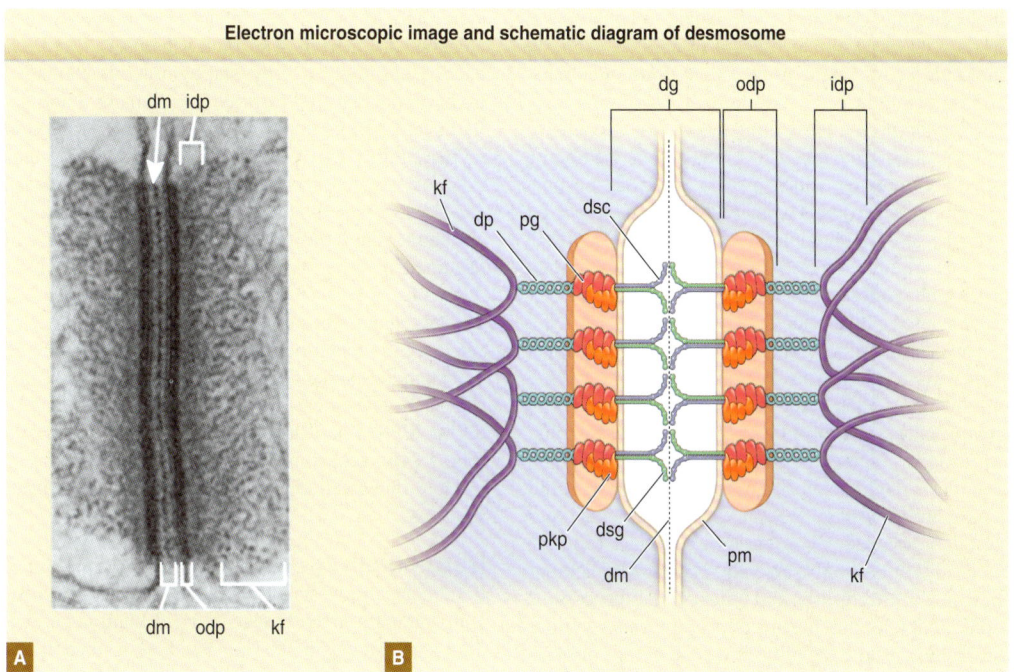

Figure 15-2 Electron microscopic image (**A**) and simplified schematic diagram (**B**) of a desmosome (drawing not to scale). Dg, desmoglea; dm, dense midline; dp, desmoplakin; dsc, desmocollin; dsg, desmoglein; idp, inner dense plaque; kf, keratin filaments; odp, outer dense plaque; pg, plakoglobin; pkp, plakophilins; pm, plasma membrane. (Electron micrograph used with permission from Kathleen Green and with permission of Elsevier, adapted from Yin T, Green KJ: Regulation of desmosome assembly and adhesion. *Semin Cell Develop Biol.* 2004;15:665.)

The extracellular domains of the desmosomal cadherins consist of 4 cadherin repeats plus an extracellular anchor domain, each separated by a calcium-binding motif. All cadherins are synthesized as preproteins, which include an amino-terminal signal sequence and propeptide. The propeptide is thought to prevent intracellular aggregation of newly synthesized cadherins within the secretory pathway of the cell. Proprotein convertases in the late Golgi network cleave the cadherin propeptide, thereby producing the mature adhesive protein.[24] Studies comparing the crystal structure of desmosomal cadherins, as well as the structure of desmosomes analyzed by cryo-electron tomography of vitreous sections compared with the solution structure of the classical cadherins, suggest common mechanisms of intercellular adhesion among the cadherin superfamily, in which a conserved amino-terminal tryptophan residue on one cadherin

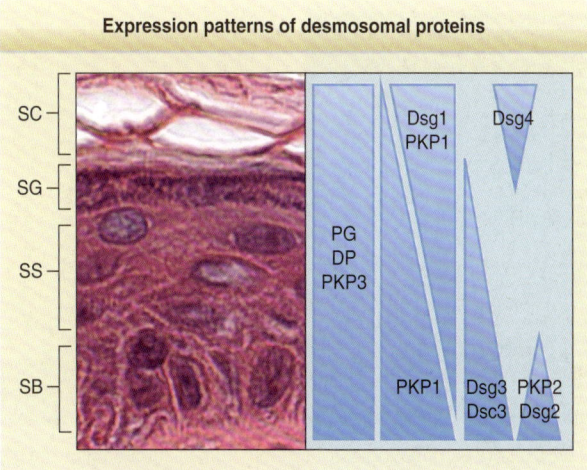

Figure 15-3 Expression patterns of desmosomal proteins in normal human epidermis. SC = stratum corneum, SG = stratum granulosum, SS = stratum spinosum, SB = stratum basale.

molecule interacts with a hydrophobic acceptor pocket in the first extracellular domain of another cadherin molecule on a neighboring cell to form the trans-adhesive interface.[25-28] Additionally, cadherins may participate in cis-adhesive interactions with cadherin molecules on the same cell through their membrane proximal domains, which may facilitate desmosome assembly. Desmosomal cadherins have been reported to engage in both homophilic (ie, Dsg–Dsg or Dsc–Dsc) and heterophilic (ie, Dsg–Dsc) interactions, although heterophilic interactions likely form the basis of epidermal intercellular adhesion.[28-31]

The cytoplasmic domains of the desmosomal cadherins are less conserved. Desmocollins have a full length "a" and a shorter "b" splice isoform. The cytoplasmic domains of desmoglein and desmocollin "a" isoforms bind plakoglobin, and some desmoglein and desmocollin isoforms may also directly bind plakophilins[32-34] (Fig. 15-2B). Increasing data suggest that desmosomal cadherins are not just adhesive molecules but may also actively regulate intracellular signaling, transcription, and other cellular processes.[1] Consistent with this, desmocollin 3-deficiency in mice causes embryonic lethality at day 2, before implantation, indicating a central role for desmocollin 3 in early tissue morphogenesis independent of its desmosomal adhesive function.[35]

In dermatology, the desmosomal cadherins are best known for their role as autoantigens in the immunobullous disease pemphigus (Chap. 52). The desmoglein 3 gene was originally discovered and cloned because it was the autoantigen in pemphigus vulgaris[36,37] (Fig. 15-4A). Since then, all of the desmosomal cadherins have been associated with human autoimmune, infectious, and/or genetic diseases (summarized below and in Table 15-1).

Desmoglein 1: Desmoglein 1 is the target of pathologic proteolytic cleavage in the infectious disorders bullous impetigo and staphylococcal scalded skin syndrome, as well as the inherited ichthyosis associated with Netherton syndrome (Chap. 47).[38,39] Cleavage of desmoglein 1 by staphylococcal exfoliative toxin occurs between extracellular domains 3 and 4.[40] Pathogenic autoantibodies to desmoglein 1 are found in pemphigus foliaceus, mucocutaneous pemphigus vulgaris, and paraneoplastic pemphigus (Chaps. 52 and 53). Most pathogenic pemphigus foliaceus autoantibodies bind the first 2 extracellular domains of desmoglein 1, overlapping sites that are critical for desmoglein intermolecular adhesion.[41-43] Desmoglein 1 is also targeted in some cases of immunoglobulin A pemphigus (intraepidermal neutrophilic-type; Chap. 57).[44] Autosomal dominant mutations causing haploinsufficiency of desmoglein 1 result in palmoplantar keratoderma (PPK; Chap. 49). The PPK is classically striate (Fig. 15-4B), occurring at sites of greatest trauma or friction, but focal and diffuse forms also have been described.[45-47]

Desmoglein 2: Desmoglein 2 has been implicated in human cardiovascular disease as a cause of autosomal dominant arrhythmogenic right ventricular cardiomyopathy (ARVC).[48] The lack of skin phenotypes in affected patients indicates that desmoglein 2 is not required for epidermal adhesion, likely due to compensatory adhesion from other more highly expressed epidermal desmosomal cadherin isoforms.

Desmoglein 3: Desmoglein 3 is the target of pathogenic autoantibodies in mucosal and mucocutaneous pemphigus vulgaris and paraneoplastic pemphigus (Chaps. 52 and 53). Most pathogenic autoantibodies in pemphigus vulgaris target the amino-terminal extracellular (EC1-2) domains of desmoglein 3, which are involved in trans- and cis-adhesion.[41,49-51] Because desmoglein 3 deficiency in mice phenotypically resembles autoimmunity to desmoglein 3 in mucosal pemphigus vulgaris with oral suprabasal erosions, pemphigus autoantibodies are thought to cause

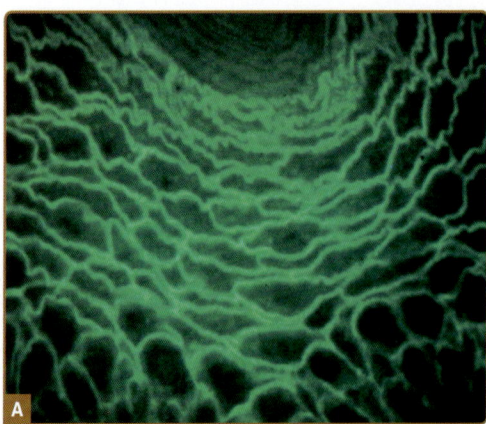
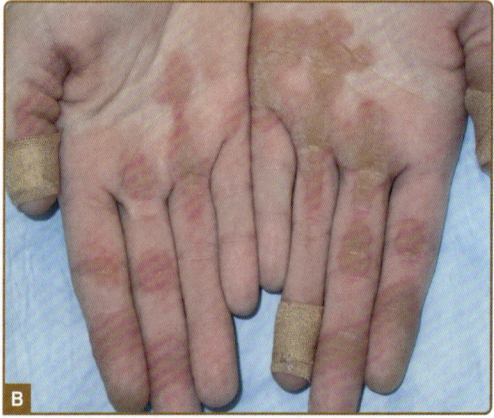

Figure 15-4 Desmosomal proteins are pathophysiologic targets in human autoimmune and genetic diseases. **A,** Indirect immunofluorescence on monkey esophagus with pemphigus serum that contains autoantibodies to desmoglein 3. The cell surface–intercellular pattern staining is diagnostic of pemphigus. **B,** Striate palmoplantar keratoderma is associated with haploinsufficiency of desmoglein 1 or desmoplakin.

TABLE 15-1
Desmosomal Targets in Human Disease

	DESMOSOME COMPONENT	AUTOIMMUNE TARGET	GENETIC TARGET
Desmosomal cadherins	Desmoglein 1[a]	Pemphigus foliaceus, pemphigus vulgaris, IgA pemphigus (intraepidermal neutrophilic-type)	Striate PPK (AD)
	Desmoglein 2		ARVC (AD)
	Desmoglein 3	Pemphigus vulgaris, paraneoplastic pemphigus, IgA pemphigus (intraepidermal neutrophilic-type)	
	Desmoglein 4	Pemphigus foliaceus,[b] pemphigus vulgaris[b]	Hypotrichosis (AR); Monilethrix (AR)
	Desmocollin 1	IgA pemphigus (subcorneal pustular dermatosis-type)	
	Desmocollin 2		ARVC (AR and AD)
	Desmocollin 3	Pemphigus vulgaris	Hypotrichosis (AR)
Desmosomal plaque proteins	Desmoplakin I/II	Paraneoplastic pemphigus	Striate PPK (AD); Carvajal syndrome (AR): diffuse PPK, wooly hair, left ventricular cardiomyopathy; lethal acantholytic epidermolysis bullosa (AR); skin fragility–wooly hair syndrome (AR): PPK, wooly hair, nail dystrophy
	Other plakins[c]	Paraneoplastic pemphigus	
	Plakoglobin		Naxos disease: diffuse PPK, wooly hair, ARVC (AR)
	Plakophilin 1		Skin fragility and ectodermal dysplasia (AR)
	Plakophilin 2		ARVC (AD)
Stratum corneum desmosome protein	Corneodesmosin		Hypotrichosis simplex of the scalp (AD)

[a]Also targeted by exfoliative toxin in bullous impetigo and staphylococcal scalded-skin syndrome and hyperactive serine proteases in Netherton syndrome.
[b]Desmoglein 4 immunoreactivity is due to cross-reactivity with desmoglein 1 in pemphigus sera.
[c]Including envoplakin, periplakin, and bullous pemphigoid antigen 1.
AD, autosomal dominant; AR, autosomal recessive; ARVC, arrhythmogenic right ventricular cardiomyopathy; PPK, palmoplantar keratoderma.

loss of desmosomal cadherin function.[52] More recent research has focused on signaling pathways activated after binding of pemphigus vulgaris autoantibodies to keratinocytes, as several biochemical inhibitors have been shown to prevent blistering in a neonatal mouse passive transfer model[53] (discussed in further detail in Chap. 52). Desmoglein 3 is also targeted in some cases of immunoglobulin A pemphigus (intraepidermal neutrophilic-type; Chap. 57).[54]

Desmoglein 4: Desmoglein 4 mutations have been described in rare autosomal recessive forms of hypotrichosis and monilethrix.[55-58] One patient demonstrated transient scalp erosions during the first 2 weeks of life. Most of the mutations in Dsg4 are frameshift or nonsense mutations that would be predicted to lead to haploinsufficiency, although missense mutations also have been reported.[59] Desmoglein 4 immunoreactivity can be observed in pemphigus vulgaris and pemphigus foliaceus sera,[58] but subsequent studies have attributed this to cross-reactivity from Dsg1 autoantibodies.[60]

Desmocollin 1: Desmocollin 1 is the target of autoantibodies in subcorneal pustular dermatosis-type immunoglobulin A pemphigus[61] (Chap. 57).

Desmocollin 2: Like desmoglein 2, desmocollin 2 is mutated in both autosomal dominant and recessive forms of ARVC, with no epidermal phenotype in affected patients.[62,63]

Desmocollin 3: Desmocollin 3 mutations were found in one Pakistani kindred with autosomal recessive hypotrichosis.[64] Autoantibodies to desmocollin 3 also have been found in pemphigus vulgaris patients, particularly those with vegetative lesions.[65-67]

PLAKOGLOBIN

Plakoglobin (also known as γ-catenin) directly binds the cytoplasmic tails of the desmogleins and desmocollin "a" isoforms, as well as E-cadherin, the major transmembrane protein of adherens junctions in epidermal keratinocytes.[68,69] It is expressed throughout all layers of the epidermis and is ubiquitously expressed in all epithelia. Plakoglobin, like plakophilin, is a member of the armadillo gene family, characterized by a conserved protein structure with head and tail domains that flank multiple homologous arm repeats.[70] Various domains of plakoglobin modulate its binding to the desmosomal cadherins.[71-73] Other domains bind to desmoplakin, thus linking desmogleins and desmocollins to desmoplakin.[74] Plakoglobin can also localize to the nucleus, where it may modulate gene transcription by TCF/LEF family members.[75,76] Although most depictions of the desmosome show both plakoglobin and plakophilin binding to desmoplakin, biochemical studies suggest that these interactions are mutually exclusive.[77] Likely, the armadillo family proteins play more dynamic roles in recruitment of desmosomal proteins to the plaque, similar to α-catenin in adherens junctions.[78,79]

Plakoglobin mutations result in Naxos disease, an autosomal recessive syndrome of diffuse PPK, wooly hair, and arrhythmogenic right ventricular cardiomyopathy, the latter of which may present in late childhood to adolescence.[80] Plakoglobin mutations also have been identified in patients with isolated cutaneous disease with normal heart development,[81] as well as in a patient with lethal congenital epidermolysis bullosa.[82]

DESMOPLAKIN

Desmoplakin exists in 2 RNA splice variants, desmoplakin I and II.[83,84] It is unknown whether different isoforms perform different cellular functions, although human disease mutations suggest that desmoplakin I is required for normal desmosomal function.[85] Desmoplakin is part of the plakin gene family,[86] which includes the hemidesmosomal proteins bullous pemphigoid antigen 1 and plectin, as well as envoplakin and periplakin. Similar to other desmosomal components, desmoplakin is a modular protein, with different modules fulfilling different functions. The central part of one desmoplakin molecule coils around the central part of another to form a rod-like center. The amino-terminal head domain binds to plakoglobin,[74] and the carboxyl-terminal tail binds to keratin.[87] Therefore, desmoplakin provides the major link between the keratin filaments and the desmosomal plaque. Desmoplakin also plays a critical role in development independent of its function in desmosomes, as desmoplakin-null mice die early in embryogenesis at E6.5, before desmosomes are formed.[88]

A broad range of desmoplakin mutations have been associated with human disease, leading to variable phenotypic combinations of PPK (striate or diffuse), dilated cardiomyopathy (left or right), wooly hair, nail abnormalities, and/or skin blisters.[59] Haploinsufficiency of desmoplakin leads to autosomal dominant striate PPK.[89] Autosomal recessive mutations in desmoplakin were described in 3 Ecuadorian families with Carvajal syndrome, consisting of diffuse PPK, wooly hair, and arrhythmogenic left ventricular cardiomyopathy.[90] A Naxos-like syndrome of PPK, wooly hair, and ARVC occurs with the p.R1267X nonsense mutation, which affects only the desmoplakin I splice isoform, indicating that desmoplakin II is not sufficient to restore normal desmosomal function in epidermis.[85] Lethal acantholytic epidermolysis bullosa (widespread epidermolysis, generalized alopecia, anonychia, and neonatal teeth) was attributed to compound heterozygous mutations in desmoplakin that caused loss of the desmoplakin tail.[91] Additionally, desmoplakin autoantibodies are observed in paraneoplastic pemphigus sera (Chap. 53).

PLAKOPHILINS

Plakophilins, like plakoglobin, can localize both to the plasma membrane as well as the nucleus, although their function outside of desmosomal adhesion is not well characterized. Plakophilins directly bind to desmoplakin, and may also directly bind keratins and some desmosomal cadherins, which is thought to aid in clustering and lateral stability of the desmosomal plaque.[32,33,77] Plakophilin 1 also associates with the eukaryotic translation initiation factor eIF4A1 in the mRNA cap complex, where it functions to regulate translation and cell proliferation.[92] Plakophilin 1 and 3 are both expressed throughout the epidermis, although plakophilin 1 is more predominant in basal compared to superficial epidermal keratinocytes, and plakophilin 2 is only expressed in the basal epidermal layer (Fig. 15-3).[93-95]

Mutations in plakophilin 1 cause ectodermal–dysplasia–skin fragility syndrome, suggesting a role for plakophilin 1 in epidermal morphogenesis as well as adhesion.[96] Plakophilin 2 mutations are the most common cause of autosomal dominant ARVC.[97,98] Currently, there are no known human diseases associated with plakophilin 3.

OTHER DESMOSOMAL PROTEINS

Envoplakin and *periplakin* are desmosomal plaque proteins expressed in the superficial layers of the epidermis. Both proteins incorporate into the corneodesmosomes of the stratum corneum. Mice deficient in envoplakin, periplakin, and involucrin do not demonstrate adhesion defects, but instead show impaired desquamation and epidermal barrier function.[99] Envoplakin and periplakin autoantibodies are characteristic of paraneoplastic pemphigus sera (Chap. 53).

Corneodesmosin is a secreted glycoprotein that incorporates into corneodesmosomes and is also expressed in the inner root sheath of the hair follicle. Heterozygous mutations in corneodesmosin are associated with an autosomal dominant hypotrichosis simplex of the scalp.[100] Loss of cohesion in the inner root sheath and aggregates of proteolytically cleaved corneodesmosin around the hair follicle are observed in scalp biopsies of affected patients.

EPIDERMAL–DERMAL ADHESION

STRUCTURAL AND FUNCTIONAL CHARACTERISTICS OF BASEMENT MEMBRANES

Basement membranes underlie epithelial and endothelial cells and separate them from each other or from the adjacent stroma. Another form of basement membrane surrounds smooth muscle or nerve cells. The physiologic functions of basement membranes are diverse: in the various organ systems they provide support for differentiated cells, maintain tissue architecture during remodeling and repair, and, in some cases, acquire specialized functions, including the ability to serve as selective permeability barriers (eg, the glomerular basement membrane or the blood–brain barrier) or acquire strong adhesive properties, like the basement membrane at the dermal–epidermal junction, or that surrounding smooth muscle cells, which provide the tissues resistance against shearing forces.[101,102] All of these characteristics are also used during development and differentiation of multicellular organisms (Table 15-2).

Ultrastructurally, basement membranes most often appear as trilaminar structures, consisting of a central electron-dense region, known as the *lamina densa*, adjacent on either side to an apparently less-dense area, known as the *lamina lucida*. The lamina lucida directly abuts the plasma membranes of the adherent cells. The relative size of each of these regions varies in different tissues, among the basement membranes of the same tissue at different ages, and as a consequence of diseases. Basement membranes serve as substrates for the attachment of cells and fix their polarity.[103] Their continuity throughout the various organ systems stabilizes the tissue orientations and provides a template for orderly repair after injury. Major disruptions in the basement membrane result in the formation of scar tissue and the loss of function in that area.

TABLE 15-2
Major Functions of Basement Membranes

- Scaffold for tissue organization and template for tissue repair.
- Selective permeability barriers. The renal basement membranes serve for the ultrafiltration of plasma, and other basement membranes also demonstrate selective filtration.
- Physical barriers between different types of cells or between cells and their underlying extracellular matrix.
- Firmly link an epithelium to its underlying matrix or to another cell layer and provide polarity.
- Regulate cellular functions.

Different basement membranes contain both common and unique components. All share a basic network structure to which specific macromolecules have been appended. These molecules are responsible for the specialized functions of different basement membranes. The basic constituents of these structures are collagen IV, laminins, nidogens, and heparan sulfate proteoglycans, although the isoforms, the polypeptide subunits, and their individual structures vary among species.[101-104]

Basement membranes provide physical separation between epithelia and their underlying extracellular matrices. This barrier is especially important in the containment of tumors. With the exception of certain cells of the immune system, nonmalignant cells seldom cross a basement membrane. In contrast, malignant cells employ multiple mechanisms to migrate through the basement membranes. Different basement membrane components and their receptors mediate the tumor-cell binding, and the basement membrane dissolution can occur by diverse mechanisms, including metalloproteases produced by the tumor cell.[105] The absence of distinguishable basement membranes in tumor biopsies is used as an indicator of malignancy. These observations underline the importance of the basal lamina as an obstacle to cell migration.

By binding biologically active signaling molecules, basement membranes regulate a multitude of biologic events. The constituent proteoglycans can bind growth factors that can be released from the complexes. Thus, the basement membranes are potent regulators of cell adhesion and migration, cytoskeleton and cell form, cell division, differentiation and polarization, and apoptosis.[103]

ULTRASTRUCTURE OF THE DERMAL-EPIDERMAL JUNCTION

The dermal–epidermal junction is an example of a highly complex form of basement membrane,[104,106] which underlies the basal cells and extends into the upper layers of the dermis (Fig. 15-5A). This basement membrane is continuous along the epidermis and skin appendages, including sweat glands, hair follicles, and sebaceous glands. The dermal–epidermal junction can be divided into 3 distinct zones.[107] The first zone contains the keratin filament–hemidesmosome complex of the basal cells and extends through the lamina lucida to the lamina densa. The plasma membranes of the basal cells in this region contain numerous electron-dense plates known as hemidesmosomes. The intracellular architecture of the basal cells are maintained by keratin intermediate filaments, 7 to 10 nm in diameter, that course through the basal cells and insert into the desmosomes and hemidesmosomes. External to the plasma membrane is a 25- to 50-nm-wide lamina lucida that

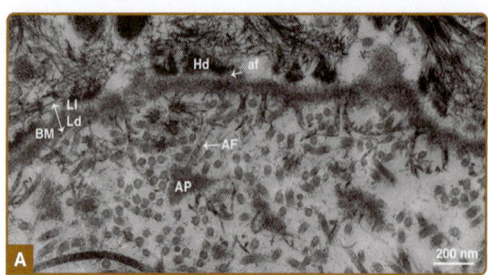 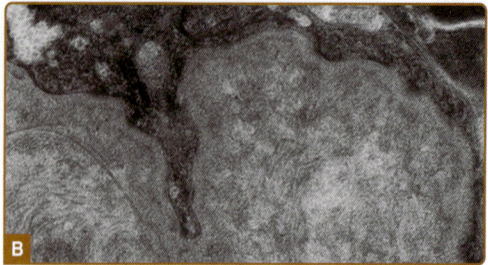

Figure 15-5 **A,** Ultrastructure of the human dermal–epidermal junction as visualized by transmission electron microscopy after standard fixation and embedding protocols. af, anchoring filament; AF, anchoring fibril; AP, anchoring plaque; BM, basement membrane; Hd, hemidesmosome; Ld, lamina densa; Ll, lamina lucida. (Bar = 200 nm.) **B,** Ultrastructure of the human dermal–epidermal junction by transmission electron microscopy following protocols using high-pressure fixation and embedding techniques. Note the dense character of both the basement membrane and the subjacent papillary dermis. Anchoring filaments, anchoring fibrils, and anchoring plaques are not distinguishable. (Both images used with permission from Douglas R. Keene, MD, Shriners Hospital, Portland, Oregon.)

contains anchoring filaments, 2 to 8 nm in diameter, originating in the plasma membrane and inserting into the lamina densa. The anchoring filaments can be seen throughout the lamina lucida but they are concentrated in the regions of the hemidesmosomes. Thus, they appear to secure the epithelial cells to the lamina densa.

The existence of the lamina lucida in vivo has been questioned.[108] When the ultrastructure of the basement membrane is evaluated after high-pressure preservation techniques, the lamina densa appears intimately associated with the epithelial cell surface. When the dermal–epidermal junction is similarly prepared, no distinct lamina lucida is seen (Fig. 15-5B). This suggests that the lamina lucida may result from shrinkage of the cell surface away from the lamina densa due to dehydration. The appearance of anchoring filaments spanning the lamina lucida may then result from the firm attachment of constituents of the lamina densa at the hemidesmosome that is subsequently pulled from the lamina densa by shrinkage. Regardless of its actual occurrence in vivo, the evaluation of the lamina lucida by standard electron microscopy techniques has allowed identification of specific structures that would otherwise have been difficult to detect. In addition, the morphologic term *lamina lucida* remains practical in the scientific communication and continues to be used.

The second zone, the lamina densa, appears as an electron-dense amorphous structure 20 to 50 nm in width. At high magnification, it has a granular–fibrous appearance. The major molecular components of the lamina densa are collagen IV, nidogens, perlecan, and laminins, which can polymerize to networks of variable thickness.[109]

The sublamina densa contains 2 readily distinguishable microfibrillar structures. *Anchoring fibrils* appear as condensed fibrous aggregates 20 to 75 nm in diameter[110] with, at high resolution, a cross-striated banding pattern (Fig. 15-5A). The length of the anchoring fibril is difficult to measure because of its random orientation in relation to the plane of the section, but is estimated to be approximately 600 to 700 nm. The ends of the fibrils appear less tightly packed, giving a somewhat frayed appearance. The proximal end inserts into the lamina densa, and the distal end is integrated into the fibrous network of the dermis. Many of the anchoring fibrils originating at the lamina densa loop back into the lamina densa in a horseshoe-like manner. Anchoring fibrils are primarily aggregates of collagen VII.[110]

Fibrillin-containing *microfibrils*, 10 to 12 nm in diameter, are also localized in the sublamina densa region. These are elastic-related fibers, because *elastic fibers* of the dermis are formed from microfibrillar and amorphous components.[111,112] In the papillary dermis, the microfibrils insert into the basal lamina perpendicular to the basement membrane and extend into the dermis, where they gradually merge with the elastic fibers to form a plexus parallel to the dermal–epidermal junction.

In summary, the ultrastructure of the dermal–epidermal junction strongly suggests that the lamina densa functions as a structural scaffold for the attachment of the epidermal cells at one surface, secured by anchoring filaments extending from the lamina densa to the hemidesmosomes. The latter also serve as insertion points for intracellular keratin filaments that form scaffolding for the basal cells. On the opposite surface, the extracellular matrix suprastructures of the dermis are firmly attached to the lamina densa. The interaction of collagen-containing dermal fibers with the lamina densa appears to be mediated by the anchoring fibrils. The elastic system of the dermis inserts directly into the basal lamina via the microfibrils. Thus, the dermal–epidermal junction provides a continuous series of attachments between the reticular dermis and the cytoskeleton of the basal cells. These observations suggest 4 major functions for the epidermal basement membrane: (1) a structural foundation for the secure attachment and polarity of the epidermal basal cells; (2) a barrier separating the epidermis and the dermis; (3) firm attachment of the dermis to the epidermis through a continuous system of structural elements; and (4) modification of cellular functions, such as organization of the cytoskeleton, differentiation, or rescue from apoptotic signaling via outside-in signaling mechanisms.

BIOCHEMICAL COMPOSITION OF THE BASEMENT MEMBRANE

Basement membranes contain collagenous and noncollagenous glycoproteins and proteoglycans. The collagens account for 40% to 65% of the total protein. All basement membranes contain certain isoforms of collagen IV, laminins, or nidogens, and heparan sulfate proteoglycans (Table 15-3). For example, the α3 chain of collagen IV is localized in the basement membrane of the kidney and lung, but not in those of the skin and blood vessels. In contrast, collagens VII and XVII are associated with the squamous epithelia of skin but not with the glomerular and alveolar basement membranes. In addition, many other tissue-specific components are found in basement membranes,[104,113] and the differences in macromolecular composition are responsible for morphologic and functional variance of basement membranes.

UBIQUITOUS COMPONENTS OF BASEMENT MEMBRANES

Collagen IV is a heterotrimer of 3 α chains.[113] Collagen IV molecules in different basement membranes contain genetically distinct but structurally homologous α chains. The α1 and α2 chains are ubiquitous, but the α3, α4, α5, and α6 chains show restricted distribution among tissues.[104,114] The chain organization and discriminatory interactions between the NC-1 domains govern network assembly in the basement membranes (Fig. 15-6).[114] The 6 chains of collagen IV are distributed in 3 major networks—(1) α1–α2, (2) α3–α4–α5, and (3) α1–α2–α5–α6—whose chain composition is determined by the NC-l domains. Two networks, namely, the α1–α2-containing and α3–α4–α5-containing networks, exist in the glomerular basement membrane. Smooth muscle basement membranes have an α1–α2–α5–α6-containing network in addition to the classic α1–α2 network. Within the dermal–epidermal junction, the α1–α2-containing collagen IV network dominates, but the α1–α2–α5–α6-containing network is also likely to be present.[104,114]

TABLE 15-3
Ubiquitous Components of Basement Membranes

- Collagen IV
- Laminins
- Nidogens
- Heparan sulfate proteoglycans
- Fibulins

Mutations in the genes encoding the α1 and α2 chains cause pathologies in different organs, ranging from eye, brain, and muscle defects to small-vessel disease, which often underlies ischemic strokes and intracerebral hemorrhages and to the HANAC (hereditary angiopathy with nephropathy, aneurysms, and muscle cramps) syndrome.[104,113] Interestingly, despite the ubiquitous presence of the α1 and α2 chains of collagen IV in basement membranes, aberrations do not occur in all basement membranes, suggesting varying tissue-specific roles for collagen IV. Structural aberrations in the genes encoding the α3, α4, α5, and α6 chains cause different forms of Alport syndrome, a genetic disease characterized by nephritis and deafness.[113] The α3(IV) chain is the antigen recognized by the circulating autoantibodies in the Goodpasture syndrome.[113]

Laminins are very large glycoproteins within the lamina lucida/lamina densa of all basement membranes.[115] Three types of subunit chains have been designated α, β, and γ chains, and each laminin is a trimeric aggregate of one α, β, and γ chain. The trimers have semirigid and extended structures, which appear as an asymmetric cross in rotary shadowing electron microscopy. The long arm of the cross is approximately 125 nm in length; the short arms are variable. Each laminin molecule contains globular and rod-like domains that have been individually implicated in various functions, such as aggregation with itself and with other components of the lamina densa (Fig. 15-7), cell attachment and spreading, neurite outgrowth, or cellular differentiation.[103,115,116] The C-terminal laminin-type globular (LG) domain of the α chain, at the foot of the long arm of the laminin cross, harbors the binding site for integrins.[115]

As of this writing, 16 laminin isoforms have been identified.[115] These represent different trimeric combinations of 5 distinct α chains, 3 β chains, and 3 γ chains. Historically, laminins were named as *laminin-1* to *laminin-15*, in the order of their discovery, but this classification had grown quite impractical, with the need to memorize the numbers. The current, simplified nomenclature is based on the chain composition and the number of each α, β, and γ chain (Table 15-4). For example, the classic "prototype" laminin-1, with α chain composition α1β1γ1, is now called *laminin 111*. The major laminin of the epidermal basement membrane, the previous laminin-5, with α chain composition α3β3γ2, is now called *laminin 332*.[115,116] Laminin 511 is present in the basement membrane of the epidermis and the hair follicles, where it is believed to be involved in dermal–epidermal communication, developmental signaling, and stem cell functions.[116,117] The β3 chain is involved in epithelial adhesion. The γ2 chain is found only in laminin 332 in the skin. The γ3 chain, a component of laminins 423 and 523, binds nidogens and is localized in basement membrane zones of adult and embryonic brain, kidney, skin, muscle, and testis. The functions of all laminins are not yet fully understood, but by interacting with integrins and other cell surface components, laminins control cellular activities such

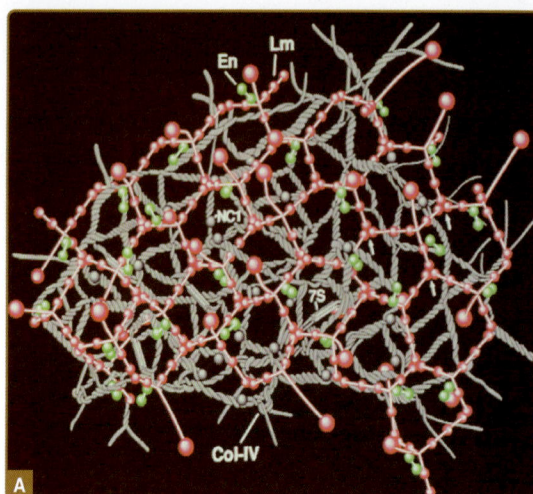 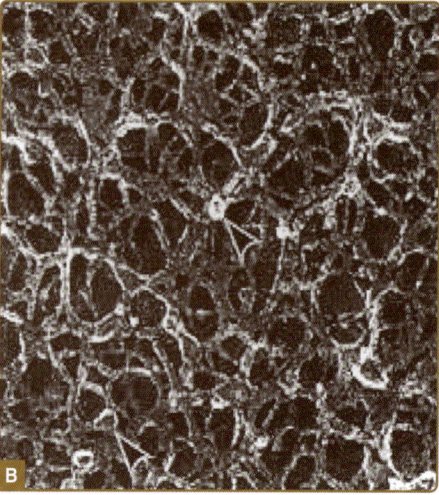

Figure 15-6 **A,** Representation of the networks formed by the ubiquitous components of the basement membranes. Monomeric collagen IV (Col-IV) self-assembles into dimers and tetramers that further aggregate into a complex lattice. Laminins self-polymerize into networks. Perlecan can oligomerize in vitro, and the glycosaminoglycan side chains interact with the Col-IV framework. Nidogen is thought to bind components of all 3 networks and also fibulins. Therefore, nidogen plays a central role as a stabilizer of the lamina densa framework. Individual molecules are not drawn to scale. (Drawing used with permission from Peter Yurchenco, MD, Robert Wood Johnson Medical School, Piscataway, NJ, USA.) **B,** Rotary shadowing image of a quick-freeze, deep-etch replica of Col-IV polymers. The replica shows an extensive, branching, and anastomosing network with occasional globular structures (*arrowhead*), which can be visualized as a model for the structure of the lamina densa. (Image B, used with permission from Toshihiko Hayashi, PhD, University of Tokyo, Japan.)

as adhesion, migration, proliferation, and polarity in a wide variety of organs.[116]

Several human congenital diseases are caused by mutations in the laminin chains.[115,118] For example, mutations in the α3, β3, or γ2 chains underlie junctional epidermolysis bullosa, and mutations in the α2 chain cause congenital muscular dystrophy and a significant decrease in the amount of basement membrane surrounding muscle cells.[119] The absence of the basement membrane leads to progressive degeneration of the muscle due to cell death. Therefore, the prediction is that laminins, and basement membranes in general, are required to prevent apoptosis by the cell types they support.[103,115,119]

Two nidogens, nidogen 1 and 2, are distinct gene products. Both are relatively small molecules, which bind laminins at a specific site within the γ1 and the γ3 chain,[104] but also collagen IV, perlecan, and fibulins. Nidogens may act as connecting elements between the collagen IV and laminin networks and integrate other basement membrane components into this specialized extracellular matrix. Targeted ablation of nidogens in mice showed that their loss has no effect on basement membrane formation per se, but severe defects of the lung and the heart[120] that are not compatible with life. Interestingly, despite the ubiquitous presence of nidogens in basement membranes, aberrations did not occur in all basement membranes, suggesting distinct roles for nidogens in different basement membranes.[104]

Another class of ubiquitous integral basement membrane constituents are the proteoglycans. Three proteoglycans are characteristically present in vascular and epithelial basement membranes: (1) perlecan, (2) agrin, and (3) collagen XVIII.[121-123] They consist of a core protein of various lengths, and carry primarily heparan sulfate side chains. Perlecan represents a complex multidomain proteoglycan with enormous dimensions and a number of posttranslational modifications. Knockout mice lacking perlecan exhibited abnormalities in many tissues, including basement membranes, and embryonic lethality. The basement membranes deteriorated in regions under increased mechanical stress, manifesting as lethal cardiac abnormalities and skin blistering.[122] Agrin is a major heparan sulfate proteoglycan of neuromuscular junctions and renal tubular basement membranes.[122] Collagen XVIII is considered to be a hybrid collagen–proteoglycan in various organs. In collagen XVIII–deficient mice, basement membranes were altered and pathologies have been observed in different organs.[123] The proteoglycans can interact with several other molecules and are believed to contribute to the overall architecture of the basement membrane as well as provide tissue-specific functions. The high sulfate content makes them highly negatively charged and hydrophilic, and the charge density is responsible for providing the selective permeability of the glomerular basement membrane.[121]

Syndecans are transmembrane heparan sulfate proteoglycans present on most cell types, including basal keratinocytes of the epidermis. The extracellular domains have affinity for laminins and, presumably through these interactions, they engage in outside-in signaling and regulate cellular processes rang-

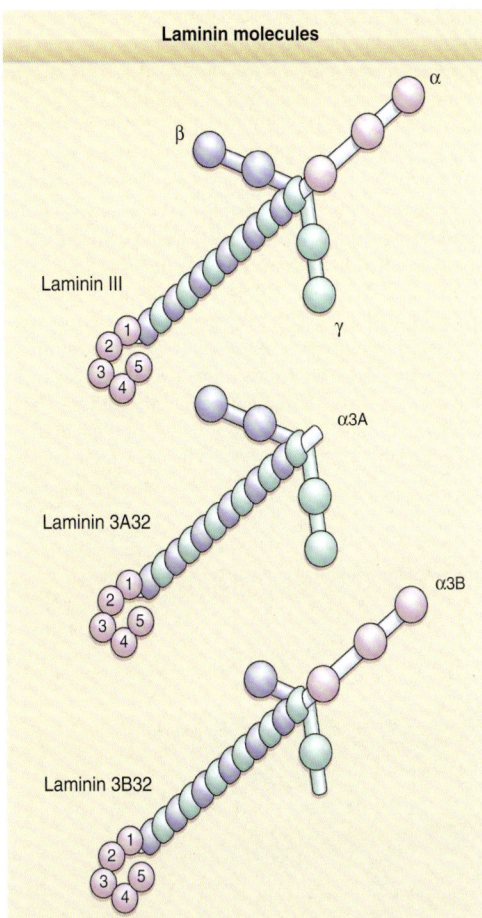

Figure 15-7 A schematic representation of laminin molecules. Each laminin is a heterotrimer of an α, a β, and a γ chain. On the top, the classic prototype laminin 111 consisting of α1β1γ1 chains is shown. The N-terminal short arm of each chain is free, the long C-termini fold to a coiled-coil and form the long arm. The distal C-terminus of the α chain contains 5 globular LG domains, which harbor the integrin-binding site. Laminin 332 exists in 2 forms, 3A32 and 3B32. These represent splice variants of the α chain, the short variant is 3A and the "full length" chain 3B. The N-termini of the β3 and γ2 chains are proteolytically processed to yield mature laminin 332.

TABLE 15-4
Most Common Laminin Isoforms[a]

NAME	CHAIN COMPOSITION	TISSUE DISTRIBUTION
Laminin 111	α1β1γ1	Developing epithelia
Laminin 121	α1β2γ1	Myotendinous junction
Laminin 211	α2β1γ1	Muscle, nerves
Laminin 213	α2β1γ3	Muscle
Laminin 221	α2β2γ1	Neuromuscular junction, glomerulus
Laminin 3A11	α3β1γ1	Stratified epithelia
Laminin 3A21	α3β2γ1	Amnion, maybe other stratified epithelia
Laminin 3A32	α3β3γ2	Stratified epithelia
Laminin 3B32	α3β3γ2	Stratified epithelia, uterus, lung
Laminin 411	α4β1γ1	Endothelia, nerves, smooth muscle, adipose tissue
Laminin 421	α4β2γ1	Endothelia, neuromuscular junction, smooth muscle, glomerulus, adipose tissue
Laminin 423	α4β2γ3	Retina, CNS, kidney, testis
Laminin 511	α5β1γ1	Mature epithelia and endothelia, smooth muscle
Laminin 521	α5β2γ1	Mature epithelia and endothelia, smooth muscle, neuromuscular junction, glomerulus
Laminin 523	α5β2γ3	Retina, CNS, muscle, kidney

[a]See Durbeej M: Laminins. *Cell Tissue Res.* 2010;339:259-268.

ing from growth factor signaling, cell adhesion, and cytoskeletal organization, to infection of cells with microorganisms.[124]

Fibulins are a family of highly conserved, calcium-binding extracellular matrix proteins. They are located in vessel walls, basement membranes, and microfibrillar structures and they have overlapping binding sites for a variety of ligands, both basement membrane proteins and components of the interstitial connective tissues.[104] Therefore, fibulins are believed to function as intermolecular bridges that stabilize the supramolecular organization of extracellular matrix structures, such as elastic fibers and basement membranes. Genetic defects of the genes encoding fibulin 4 and 5 cause different forms of cutis laxa.

EPIDERMAL-SPECIFIC BASEMENT MEMBRANE COMPONENTS

The dermal–epidermal junction of skin is an excellent example of specific divergence in basement membrane structure. The structural components of hemidesmosomes, anchoring filaments, and anchoring fibrils in the basement membrane zone are quite well characterized.[104,106,107,109,110] A diagram depicting the relative locations of the proteins found at the dermal–epidermal junction is shown in Fig. 15-8. These proteins are listed in Table 15-5 and discussed in the following sections.

HEMIDESMOSOMES

Ultrastructurally, the hemidesmosome closely resembles one-half of the desmosome at cell–cell junctions in the epidermis. However, the components of these 2 structures are distinct.[125] The 230-kDa bullous pemphigoid antigen 1, or BP230 is a protein with homology to plakins, which bind intermediate filaments. It is the major component of the hemidesmosomal inner dense plaque. Ablation of BP230 is associated with epidermolysis bullosa simplex in mice and humans.[106,118] The 180-kDa bullous pemphigoid antigen 2, BP180 and the major antigen in bullous pemphigoid (Fig. 15-9), is a transmembrane collagen known as *collagen XVII*, where the collagenous domain is extracellular.[126] The intracellular ligands of collagen XVII are plectin, BP230 and β4 integrin, and the extracellular ligands α6 integrin and laminin 332.[127] The 120-kDa ectodomain of collagen XVII is shed from the cell surface by proteinases of the ADAM (a disintegrin-like and metalloproteinase-containing) family through cleavage within the juxtamembranous NC-16 domain (Fig. 15-10).[126] Mutations in collagen XVII cause junctional epidermolysis bullosa (Chap. 60), indicating that it stabilizes interactions of basal keratinocytes with the basement membrane.[118] Collagen XVII is also known to regulate functions of hair follicle and melanocyte stem cells,[128] explaining why ablation of the mouse *Col17a1* gene resulted in moderate skin blistering, dental anomalies, and graying and loss of hair.[128] Plectin, another plakin homolog, is also a component of the hemidesmosome.[125] However, its tissue distribution is not limited to hemidesmosome-containing basement membranes. Mutations of plectin result in epidermolysis bullosa simplex with progressive muscular dystrophy and, in some cases, epidermolysis bullosa simplex with pyloric atresia,[118] indicating a role for plectin in the stability of cell–basement membrane adhesion in a variety of tissues. One key component of the hemidesmosome is the integrin α6β4.[125] It has a high affinity

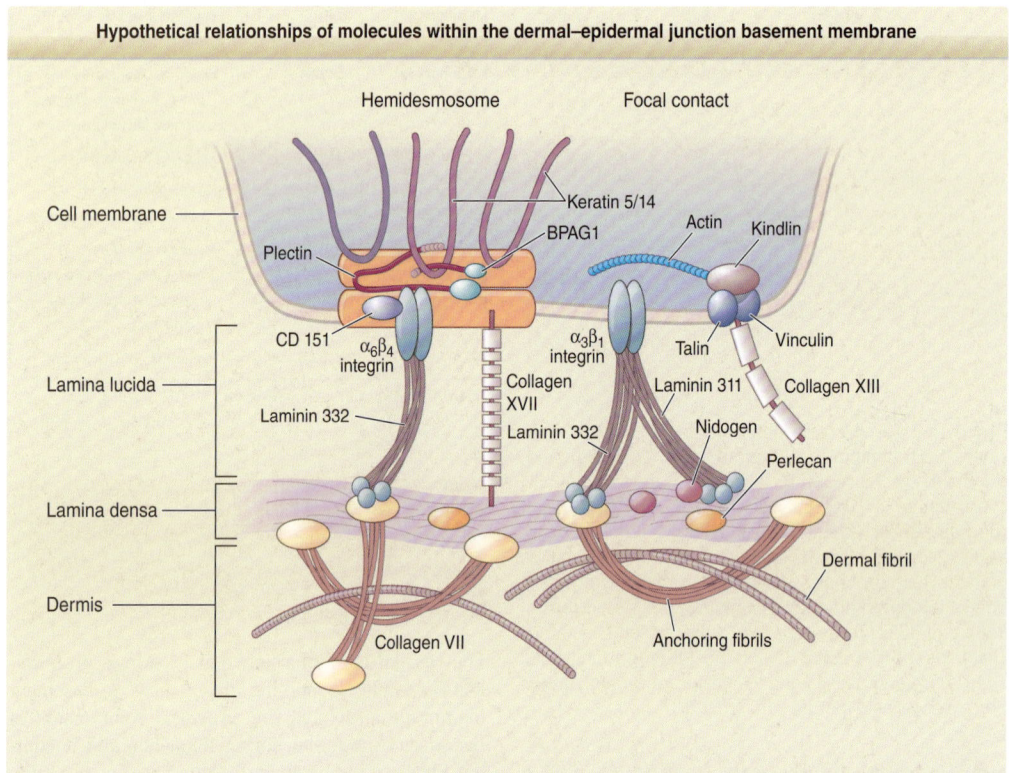

Figure 15-8 Model of the hypothetical relationships of molecules within the dermal–epidermal junction basement membrane. The illustration depicts laminin 332 as the bridge between the transmembrane hemidesmosomal integrin α6β4 and the collagen VII NC-1 domain. The tight binding of laminin 332 to α6β4 and to collagen VII provides the primary resistance to frictional forces. The transmembrane collagen XVII also participates in this stabilization, because its extracellular domain also binds laminin 332. Within the epithelial cell, the transmembrane elements bind the proteins of the hemidesmosomal dense plaque, bullous pemphigoid antigen (BPAG)1 and plectin, which then associate with the keratins. Collagen XVII binds BPAG1, integrin α6β4, and plectin, and integrin α6β4 binds plectin. The laminin 332–311 complex is shown within the basement membrane between hemidesmosomes, bound by integrin α3β1, and associated with the intracellular proteins kindlin-1, talin, and vinculin. This complex presumably maintains basement membrane stability. In vitro, integrin α3β1, kindlin-1, talin, and vinculin, and another transmembrane collagen, type XIII, are localized to the focal contacts, which may function as the link between the basement membrane and the epithelial cortical actin network. In the lamina densa, collagen IV and perlecan networks are stabilized by nidogen. Anchoring fibrils are secured to the lamina densa by the NC-1 domain of collagen VII. The fibrils project into the dermis and either terminate in anchoring plaques or loop back to the lamina densa. The anchoring fibril network binds dermal fibrils, thus securing the adhesion of the lamina densa to the papillary dermis. None of the molecules is drawn to scale.

TABLE 15-5
Hemidesmosomal and Basement Membrane Zone (Bmz) Targets in Skin Disease

	HEMIDESMOSOME/BMZ COMPONENT	AUTOIMMUNE TARGET	GENETIC TARGET
Cytoskeletal proteins	Keratin 5 and 14		EBS
Hemidesmosomal plaque proteins	Bullous pemphigoid antigen 1/BP230	BP	EBS
	Plectin	BP, CP	EBS-MD
			JEB-PA
Other intracellular adhesion complex proteins	Kindlin-1		KS
Hemidesmosomal transmembrane components	Collagen XVII/BP180	BP, CP, LAD, PG	JEB-non-Herlitz
	α6β4 integrin	BP, CP	JEB-PA
	CD151		Pretibial EB, nephritis, deafness, β-thalassemia minor
Anchoring filament proteins	Laminin 332	CP	JEB-Herlitz
			JEB–non-Herlitz
	Ectodomain of collagen XVII	LAD, BP	JEB–non-Herlitz
Anchoring fibril proteins	Collagen VII	EBA	DEB

BP, bullous pemphigoid (Chap. 54); CP, cicatricial pemphigoid (Chap. 55); DEB, dystrophic; EB (Chap. 60 for all); EB, epidermolysis bullosa; EBA, EB acquisita (Chap. 56); EBS, EB simplex; EBS–MD, EBS with muscular dystrophy; JEB, junctional EB; JEB–PA, JEB with pyloric atresia; KS, Kindler syndrome; LAD, linear immunoglobulin A dermatosis (Chap. 58); PG, pemphigoid gestationis.

for laminin 332 and is essential to integration of the hemidesmosome with the underlying basement membrane. Mutations in either the α6 or β4 chains result in junctional epidermolysis bullosa associated with pyloric atresia.[118]

A member of the widely expressed cell surface transmembrane proteins of the tetraspanin family, CD151, is also a component of the hemidesmosome. It forms

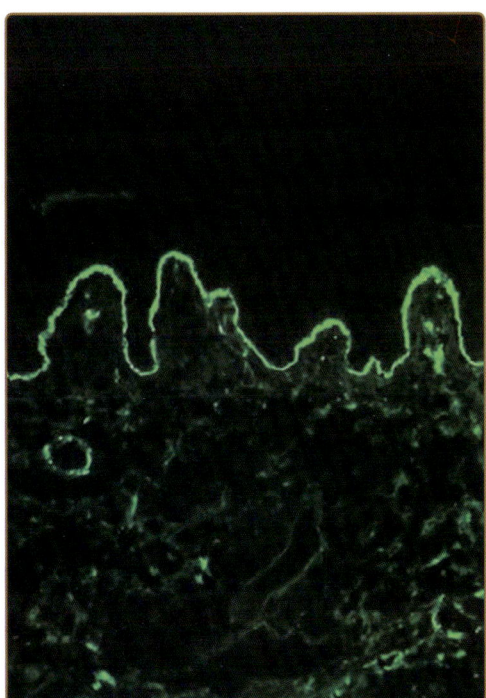

Figure 15-9 Indirect immunofluorescence staining of human skin with a pemphigoid serum that contains autoantibodies to collagen XVII.

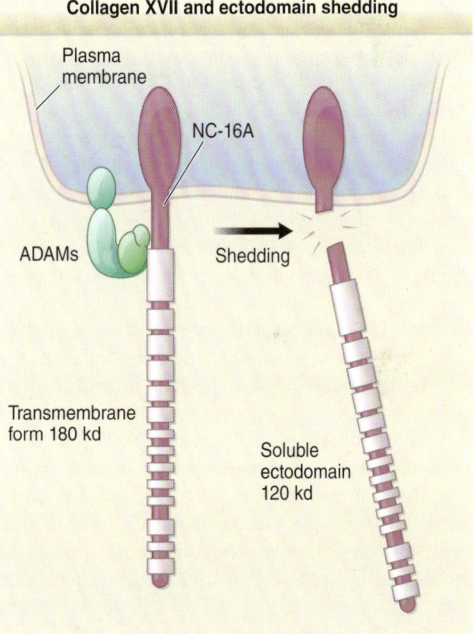

Figure 15-10 Schematic representation of collagen XVII and its ectodomain shedding. Collagen XVII is a hemidesmosomal transmembrane protein with an intracellular N-terminus. The extracellular C-terminus (ectodomain) contains several collagenous subdomains (*light pink*) and intervening noncollagenous sequences (*purple*). The ectodomain can be shed from the cell surface by proteinases of the ADAMs (a disintegrin-like and metalloproteinase-containing) family, themselves transmembrane proteins. Thus, the 180-kDa full-length molecule yields a shorter soluble ectodomain of 120 kDa. The 180-kDa full-length molecule is the classic bullous pemphigoid antigen-2, and the ectodomain is the 120-kDa linear immunoglobulin A (IgA) dermatosis antigen. Further degradation of the *C*-terminus of the ectodomain results in the 97-kDa linear IgA dermatosis antigen.

complexes with α3β1 and α6β4 integrins at the basolateral surface of basal keratinocytes and stabilizes their functions.[129] A very rare human genetic condition delivered indirect information on the functions of CD151. In addition to the expression of CD151 in several tissues like the kidney and the skin, its gene also encodes the MER2 blood group antigen on erythrocytes. MER2-negative patients presented with hereditary nephritis, sensorineural deafness, pretibial epidermolysis bullosa, and β-thalassemia minor.[117] These symptoms suggest that CD151 is important for the assembly of the basement membrane in the kidney, skin, and inner ear and plays a role in erythropoiesis.

OTHER EPIDERMAL–DERMAL ADHESION COMPLEXES

In addition to the hemidesmosomal components, other adhesion molecules are known to be present at the basolateral aspect of basal keratinocytes, for example, integrin α3β1, the receptor for the laminin 332–311 complex in the basement membrane between the hemidesmosomes, and another transmembrane collagen, type XIII.[118] Because these proteins are localized to focal contacts in vitro, together with vinculin and talin, they are predicted to function as the link between the basement membrane and the epithelial cortical actin network.[130] Mutations in the integrin α3 gene cause a rare systemic disorder with interstitial lung disease, nephrotic syndrome, and epidermolysis bullosa.[131] An intracellular component of this complex, kindlin-1,[132] is mutated in the Kindler syndrome,[118] a disorder with skin blistering in infancy, progressive poikiloderma, sun sensitivity, and skin cancer. In the epidermis, kindlin-1 has important functions in β1 integrin–mediated outside-in signaling that regulates cell–matrix adhesions, cell migration, and polarity.[132] Thus, kindlin-1 is necessary for the stability of the dermal–epidermal junction and that, in addition to hemidesmosomes, tethering the actin cytoskeleton to cell–matrix adhesions offers alternative means to anchor basal epithelial cells to the basement membrane.

ANCHORING FILAMENTS

The anchoring filaments contain laminin 332 and the ectodomain of collagen XVII, 2 ligands that interact with each other.[115,127] The ectodomain of collagen XVII, which protrudes from the plasma membrane into the lamina lucida, has a loop structure consistent with its role as an anchoring filament protein.[133] Laminin 332 is a disulfide-bonded complex of α3, β3, and γ2 chains. The 2 splice variants of the α3 chain, α3A and α3B, associate with the α3 and γ2 chains to form laminin 3A32 and 3B32 (Fig. 15-7).[115,116] The individual chains are considerably truncated relative to other laminin chains, and this truncation is reflected in the loss of the structures equivalent to the short arms of other laminins. Additionally, the α3 and γ2 chains are proteolytically processed after secretion from the keratinocyte, further trimming the short arms.[115] The C-terminus of the α chain, longer than that of the β and γ chains, comprises 5 globular LG modules, LG1 through LG5, which interact with cell surface receptors. The α3β1 and α6β4 integrins have affinity for the LG1-3 domains, whereas the LG4-5 tandem has affinity for syndecans and β-dystroglycan on the keratinocyte surface.[115] The LG4-5 modules are proteolytically cleaved in most laminins, a process that may modulate interactions with cell surface receptors.[115] Laminin 332 binds to laminin 311 (α3β1γ1) and to the NC-1 domain of collagen VII and to the distal ectodomain of collagen XVII.[115,116] Genetic evidence demonstrates that laminin 332 is essential in keratinocyte adhesion, as null mutations in any of its component α3, β3, or γ2 chains result in severe junctional epidermolysis bullosa[118] (Chap. 60). The severity of the laminin 332 null phenotype indirectly emphasizes its functional importance in bridging the hemidesmosomes and the anchoring fibrils.

EPITHELIAL LAMINA DENSA

The basement membrane beneath and between the hemidesmosomes contains the α1–α2-chain containing collagen IV network, probably some α1–α2–α5–α6-chain containing collagen IV network, as well as nidogen, perlecan, and α3- and α5-chain containing laminins.[104,113-115] The laminin α3 chain can associate with the β1 and γ1 chains of laminin 311, which has the unique property of forming disulfide-bonded dimers with laminin 332. The major α3-containing laminin in the lamina densa between hemidesmosomes is probably the laminin 332–311 complex.[115] As the laminin α3 chain is a ligand for integrin α3β1 present between hemidesmosomes, binding of the laminin 332–311 complex to the intracellular actin cytoskeleton is likely to be mediated by this integrin. This is consistent with observations in mice and in humans[131] in which mutations of the integrin α3 chain cause loss of the basement membrane between hemidesmosomes but not beneath them. The N-termini of laminin 332 bind to collagen VII, the main component of the anchoring fibrils in the sublamina densa that, in turn, binds tightly to collagen I containing fibrils so that anchoring filaments and fibrils are connected to each other and to the dermis.[134] The laminin 332–311 complex and laminin 511 (α5β1γ1) contain a γ1 chain and can therefore bind nidogens and the collagen IV network.[104,115] Further, nidogen 1 and fibulin 1 and 2 are ligands for the laminin γ2 chain.[104,115] These interactions are important for the integration of laminin 332 into the extracellular matrix before the maturation of the γ2 chain, as a substantial portion of N-terminus of the γ2 chain is cleaved in human adult skin. Yet another link, which strengthens dermal–epidermal cohesion, is provided by molecular interactions between perlecan within the lamina densa and fibrillin 1 in the microfibrils.[109]

ANCHORING FIBRILS

Collagen VII is the major component of the anchoring fibrils.[110,135] The collagen VII molecule is distinguished from other collagens in that it has a very long triple-helical domain, 450 nm in length. Globular domains exist at both ends of the triple helix, the N-terminal domain NC-1 is very large. The smaller C-propeptide, NC-2, is believed to facilitate the formation of the antiparallel, centrosymmetric dimers, before it is removed by the metalloproteinase bone morphogenetic protein 1[135] to yield a mature collagen VII. The dimers are covalently crosslinked through disulfide bonds at the carboxyl terminus, and they aggregate laterally to form the anchoring fibrils. The fibrils are further stabilized by tissue transglutaminase, which catalyzes the formation of covalent crosslinks.[135]

The NC-1 domain of collagen VII binds to laminin 332 and collagen IV within the lamina densa.[104,115] The triple-helical domains of an antiparallel collagen VII dimer make the length of the anchoring fibril. It extends perpendicularly from the lamina densa and either loops back into the lamina densa or inserts into the dermis.[110] The anchoring fibril network forms a scaffold that entraps large numbers of dermal fibrils and binds them through covalent crosslinks between collagen VII and collagen I,[134] thus securing the lamina densa to the subjacent dermis. In the acquired form of epidermolysis bullosa, epidermolysis bullosa acquisita (Chap. 56), and in bullous systemic lupus erythematosus (Chap. 61), autoantibodies target mainly the NC-1 domain of collagen VII.

Mutations in *COL7A1*, the gene encoding collagen VII, result in dystrophic epidermolysis bullosa (Chap. 60). Almost 1000 *COL7A1* mutations have been found in both recessive and dominant forms of dystrophic epidermolysis bullosa (Fig. 15-11), and the spectrum of biologic and clinical phenotypes is very broad.[118] In mouse models, deficiency of collagen VII recapitulated the clinical and morphologic characteristics of recessive dystrophic epidermolysis bullosa in humans.[136] These mice have been useful for testing of molecular therapy strategies for dystrophic epidermolysis bullosa. Cell-, gene-, and protein-based therapy approaches all have been tested.[137,138] Recently, repositioned small molecule drugs have shown promise as disease-modifying therapies.[139]

DERMAL CELL-MATRIX ADHESION

THE EXTRACELLULAR MATRIX OF THE DERMIS

The dermal–epidermal junction is continuous with the extracellular matrix in the papillary dermis and thus attaches the epidermis with the dermis. The pliability, elasticity, and tenacity of the dermis are provided by a highly organized extracellular matrix that contains structural networks of collagens, elastin, glycoproteins, and proteoglycans with specific functional properties.[140,141] Between the networks, the space is filled by a molecularly complex amorphous matrix that binds water. Beside their structural functions, both the fibrillar and the extrafibrillar matrix are biologically active in that they bind growth factors and cytokines, interact with cells, and regulate their functions.[140,141]

Recent proteomics studies have identified a multitude of matrix molecules and extended our knowledge about their aggregate structures and functional interactions.[142-144] A particular characteristic of extracellular matrix molecules is adhesiveness, and resident skin cells, inflammatory cells, tumor cells, and even microorganisms can adhere to them.[130] Through receptor-mediated interactions, matrix suprastructures or their fragments guide cellular functions under normal skin homeostasis, growth, and regeneration, but also under pathologic conditions such as in tumors.[145] In the following, the major protein families of the dermal extracellular matrix are delineated; for more detailed information, the reader is referred to recent reviews that provide comprehensive descriptions of the structure and functions of the extracellular matrix in the skin and other tissues.[111,112,140-144,146,147]

Collagens, a family of 28 different collagen types, are the most abundant proteins in the dermis and represent 75% of its dry weight and 20% to 30% of its volume.[140] All collagen molecules have a basic structure of 3 α-chains, which have glycine (Gly) as every third amino acid, and thus a typical sequence of (Gly-X-Y)n. During biosynthesis, the nascent α-chains undergo posttranslational modifications

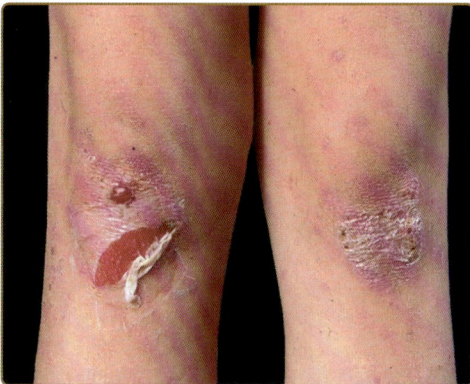

Figure 15-11 Skin fragility and blistering in dystrophic epidermolysis bullosa. Functional deficiency of collagen VII as a result of mutations in the *COL7A1* gene leads to trauma-induced separation of the epidermis and the dermis. The blister roof is below the lamina densa, leading to scar formation on healing of the blisters.

and are folded into a triple helix.[148] In a tissue-specific manner, different collagen types assemble into distinct fibrils or networks containing mixtures of several collagens and/or proteoglycans or glycoproteins that have specialized functions. In the dermis, the classic, cross-banded fibrils recognizable in the electron microscope contain collagen I, III, V, XII, and XIV. In contrast, collagen VI polymerizes into microfibrils. Other collagens are needed to provide cohesion of the epidermis or the vascular structures with the dermal extracellular matrix, for example, collagens VII, XIII, XVII, and XXIII in the epidermal basement membrane zone or collagens VIII, XV, and XVIII in the vascular basement membrane zone. Collagens have earlier been believed to be extremely stable and static structures, but it has recently become clear that collagen turnover is mediated by both control of synthesis and by an intricate catabolic network of proteinases and their inhibitors.[149]

Elastin provides dermal elasticity. Elastin molecules are rich in repetitive hydrophobic sequences and are highly crosslinked. The crosslinks between several individual molecules provide for both elasticity and insolubility of the elastic fibers. Characteristically, the fibers can be stretched by 100% or more, and still return to their original form. The main components of elastic fibers are elastin (90%) and microfibrils, which attach the fibers to the surrounding structures.[111,140] The microfibrils extend from the basement membrane into the papillary dermis, where they gradually merge with the elastic fiber plexus parallel to the dermal–epidermal junction, which appears to be continuous with the elastic fibers deep within the reticular dermis. A major component of the microfibrils is fibrillin, a family of very large glycoproteins, but they also contain or associate with other proteins, such as microfibril-associated glycoproteins (MAGPs), latent TGF-β-binding proteins (LTBPs), fibulins, EMILIN-1, and in the papillary dermis, collagen XVI.[112,150] Fibrillin 1 interacts with perlecan to attach the microfibrils to the basement membrane at the dermal–epidermal junction. Apart from guiding elastin fibril assembly and imparting tissue integrity, fibrillins and LTBPs serve as regulators of cell signaling in the dermis by controlling bioavailability of TGF-$β_1$. LTBPs contain multiple proteinase-sensitive sites, providing the means to solubilize the large latent complex from the dermal matrix.[112] Fibrillin can also bind to another group of signaling molecules, the bone morphogenetic proteins (BMPs). Thus, fibrillin/LTBP can target activatable TGF-β or BMPs into distinct matrix or cellular sites.

The dermal fibril networks and cells are embedded in an amorphous extrafibrillar matrix that binds water and provides the tautness of the skin. It contains proteoglycans, glycoproteins, and hyaluronic acid, which are molecularly and structurally diverse, highly organized, and biologically active.[121,140,146] Glycosaminoglycans are negatively charged polysaccharides that can bind large amounts of ions and water. They bind to different proteins to form proteoglycans with variable number, type, and length of the glycosaminoglycan chains. Four different proteoglycan-bound glycosaminoglycans are known: chondroitin sulfate, dermatan sulfate, keratan sulfate, and heparan sulfate. Versican is a major proteoglycan in the dermis, it is associated with elastic fibers and forms huge complexes with hyaluronic acid, which provides the skin with its tautness.[151] Hyaluronic acid is a ubiquitous glycosaminoglycan without protein core, a giant polysaccharide composed of N-acetylglucosamine/glucuronic acid disaccharides. Perlecan is the major heparan sulfate proteoglycan of basement membranes that can sequester and present growth factors to their receptors.[122] Collagen XVIII, a hybrid collagen/proteoglycan, is found in epidermal and vascular basement membranes in the skin.[123] Small leucine-rich proteoglycans, such as decorin and biglycan, have multiple functions; for example, they bind to collagen fibrils and regulate their assembly, they bind TGF-β, and are connected to immune reactions by signaling through toll-like receptors.[152] Syndecans are transmembrane and glypicans membrane–anchored heparan sulfate proteoglycans, which control cell adhesion to the matrix and interact with multiple extracellular proteins, including growth factors, and thereby regulate cell functions.[140]

CELL–MATRIX INTERACTIONS REGULATE CELLULAR FUNCTIONS

The extracellular matrix is in constant crosstalk with fibroblasts and other cell types in the dermis and guides their functions during development, aging, and regeneration, but also under pathologic conditions such as inflammation and tumorigenesis. Matrix molecules can influence a wide range of cellular events, ranging from cytoskeletal organization to cell differentiation, adhesion and migration, and apoptosis.[141,153-155] The cells in the dermis use different receptors to receive signals from the extracellular matrix, including integrins, cell surface proteoglycans, and transmembrane collagens. The family of $β_1$ integrins represents the most common class of matrix receptors.[130] The α-subunit of the integrin determines the ligand specificity, but the affinity and the specificity seem to vary.[145,153] The outside-in-signaling can occur via different mechanisms. Cues from the extracellular matrix can induce receptor clustering on the cell surface and thus induce cytoplasmic complex formation between the receptors and linker molecules that bind to the cytoskeleton and thus modulate cell shape. Activation of different receptors by the extracellular matrix can also induce signaling via several signal transduction pathways, for example, the focal adhesion kinase (pp[125]FAK)– or microtubule-associated protein (MAP) kinase-pathways that regulate transcription, cell proliferation, or differentiation.[145] Recently, it has become clear that cells also sense and react to the stiffness of the surrounding extracellular matrix. Integrins mediate the mechanosensation through binding dynamics of different integrin types, activation of stretch-activated ion channels, or unfolding of mechanosensitive proteins in focal adhesion complexes.[130] In turn, the stiffness of the dermal extracellular matrix is determined by the molecular and suprastructural composition of the collagen, elastin, and microfibrillar networks and the extrafibrillar matrix and its water content.[156,157] All these matrix–cell interactions regulate cell functions and are highly relevant not only under physiologic conditions but also in pathologically altered dermis in, for example, fibrosis or tumor stroma.[158] For detailed information on this topic, the reader is referred to excellent recent reviews.[146,147,150,153,156]

CONCLUSIONS

The epidermis and the dermal-epidermal junction are continuous with the extracellular matrix in the papillary dermis. The cell–cell and cell–basement membrane adhesion in the epidermis, and the cell–matrix adhesion in the dermis secure the attachment of the 2 skin layers and provide the skin with its resistance against environmental influences. The integrity of these adhesion structures is essential for protection of the entire organism against mechanical, physical, or microbial insults. This is indirectly demonstrated by human disorders in which cutaneous adhesion structures are targeted by either genetic mutations or by pathogenic antibodies that perturb the functions of the target proteins, such as in epidermolysis bullosa or pemphigus. Tremendous advances have recently been made in discerning the molecular and functional details of epidermal and dermal adhesion and in understanding the molecular pathology of skin fragility. This knowledge will facilitate the design of biologically valid therapeutic approaches not only for rare genetic and common autoimmune adhesion disorders but also for physiologic processes such as skin aging.

ACKNOWLEDGMENTS

The authors gratefully acknowledge the contribution of Thomas Krieg, Monique Aumailley, Manuel Koch, Mon-Li Chu, and Jouni Uitto, the authors of Chap. 63 in the 8th edition of this textbook. The contents of the chapter have been used as a basis for the section "Dermal Cell-Matrix Adhesion".

REFERENCES

1. Getsios S, Huen AC, Green KJ. Working out the strength and flexibility of desmosomes. *Nat Rev Mol Cell Biol*. 2004;5:271-281.
2. Calkins CC, Setzer SV. Spotting desmosomes: the first 100 years. *J Invest Dermatol*. 2007;127(suppl):E2-E3.
3. Staehelin LA. Structure and function of intercellular junctions. *Int Rev Cytol*. 1974;39:191-283.
4. Gorbsky G, Steinberg MS. Isolation of the intercellular glycoproteins of desmosomes. *J Cell Biol*. 1981; 90:243-248.
5. Staehelin LA, Hull BE. Junctions between living cells. *Sci Am*. 1978;238:140-152.
6. Jonca N, Guerrin M, Hadjiolova K, et al. Corneodesmosin, a component of epidermal corneocyte desmosomes, displays homophilic adhesive properties. *J Biol Chem*. 2002;277:5024-5029.
7. Groot KR, Sevilla LM, Nishi K, et al. Kazrin, a novel periplakin-interacting protein associated with desmosomes and the keratinocyte plasma membrane. *J Cell Biol*. 2004;166:653-659.
8. Ihrie RA, Marques MR, Nguyen BT, et al. Perp is a p63-regulated gene essential for epithelial integrity. *Cell*. 2005;120:843-856.
9. Lechler T, Fuchs E. Desmoplakin: an unexpected regulator of microtubule organization in the epidermis. *J Cell Biol*. 2007;176:147-154.
10. Sumigray KD, Chen H, Lechler T. Lis1 is essential for cortical microtubule organization and desmosome stability in the epidermis. *J Cell Biol*. 2011;194: 631-642.
11. North AJ, Bardsley WG, Hyam J et al. Molecular map of the desmosomal plaque. *J Cell Sci*. 1999; 112:4325-4336.
12. Al-Amoudi A, Castano-Diez D, Devos DP, et al. The three-dimensional molecular structure of the desmosomal plaque. *Proc Natl Acad Sci U S A*. 2011;108: 6480-6485.
13. Koch PJ, Goldschmidt MD, Zimbelmann R, et al. Complexity and expression patterns of the desmosomal cadherins. *Proc Natl Acad Sci U S A*. 1992;89: 353-357.
14. Arnemann J, Sullivan KH, Magee AI, King IA, Buxton RS. Stratification-related expression of isoforms of the desmosomal cadherins in human epidermis. *J Cell Sci*. 1993;104:741-750.
15. Wu H, Stanley JR, Cotsarelis G. Desmoglein isotype expression in the hair follicle and its cysts correlates with type of keratinization and degree of differentiation. *J Invest Dermatol*. 2003;120:1052-1057.
16. Wang LH, Katube K, Jiang WW, et al. Immunohistochemical distribution patter of desmocollin 3, desmocollin 1 and desmoglein 1,2 in the pemphigus of oral mucosa and skin. *Oral Med Pathol*. 2000;5:87-94.
17. Mahoney MG, Hu Y, Brennan D, et al. Delineation of diversified desmoglein distribution in stratified squamous epitheli: implications in diseases. *Exp Dermatol*. 2006;15:101-109.
18. Chen YJ, Chang JT, Lee L, et al. DSG3 is overexpressed in head neck cancer and is a potential molecular target for inhibition of oncogenesis. *Oncogene*. 2007;26: 467-476.
19. Schafer S, Koch PJ, Franke WW. Identification of the ubiquitous human desmoglein, Dsg2, and the expression catalogue of a subfamily of desmosomal cadherins. *Exp Cell Res*. 1994;211:391-399.
20. Whittock NV, Bower C. Genetic evidence for a novel human desmosomal cadherin, desmoglein 4. *J Invest Dermatol*. 2003;120:523-530.
21. Bazzi H, Getz A, Mahoney MG, et al. Desmoglein 4 is expressed in highly differentiated keratinocytes and trichocytes in human epidermis and hair follicle. *Differentiation*. 2006;74:129-140.
22. King IA, Sullivan KH, Bennett R Jr, et al. The desmocollins of human foreskin epidermis: identification and chromosomal assignment of a third gene and

23. Khan K, Hardy R, Haq A, et al. Desmocollin switching in colorectal cancer. *Br J Cancer*. 2006;95:1367-1370.
24. Posthaus H, Dubois CM, Muller E. Novel insights into cadherin processing by subtilisin-like convertases. *FEBS Lett*. 2003;536:203-208.
25. Shapiro L, Fannon AM, Kwong PD, et al. Structural basis of cell-cell adhesion by cadherins. *Nature*. 1995;374:327-337.
26. Boggon TJ, Murray J, Chappuis-Flament S, et al. C-cadherin ectodomain structure and implications for cell adhesion mechanisms. *Science*. 2002;296:1308-1313.
27. Al-Amoudi A, Diez DC, Betts MJ, et al. The molecular architecture of cadherins in native epidermal desmosomes. *Nature*. 2007;450:832-837.
28. Harrison OJ, Brasch J, Lasso G, et al. Structural basis of adhesive binding by desmocollins and desmogleins. *Proc Natl Acad Sci U S A*. 2016;113:7160-7165.
29. Amagai M, Karpati S, Klaus-Kovtun V, et al. The extracellular domain of pemphigus vulgaris antigen (desmoglein 3) mediates weak homophilic adhesion. *J Invest Dermatol*. 1994;102:402-408.
30. Chitaev NA, Troyanovsky SM. Direct Ca2+-dependent heterophilic interaction between desmosomal cadherins, desmoglein and desmocollin, contributes to cell-cell adhesion. *J Cell Biol*. 1997;138:193-201.
31. Marcozzi C, Burdett ID, Buxton RS, et al. Coexpression of both types of desmosomal cadherin and plakoglobin confers strong intercellular adhesion. *J Cell Sci*. 1998;111:495-509.
32. Hatzfeld M, Haffner C, Schulze K, et al. The function of plakophilin 1 in desmosome assembly and actin filament organization. *J Cell Biol*. 2000;149:209-222.
33. Bonné S, Gilbert B, Hatzfeld M, et al. Defining desmosomal plakophilin-3 interactions. *J Cell Biol*. 2003;161:403-416.
34. Tucker DK, Stahley SN, Kowalczyk AP. Plakophilin-1 Protects Keratinocytes from Pemphigus Vulgaris IgG by Forming Calcium-Independent Desmosomes. *J Invest Dermatol*. 2014;134(4):1033-1043.
35. Den ZN, Cheng X, Merchad-Sauvage M, et al. Desmocollin 3 is required for pre-implantation development of the mouse embryo. *J Cell Sci*. 2006;119:482-489.
36. Koch PJ, Walsh MJ, Schmelz M, et al. Identification of desmoglein, a constitutive desmosomal glycoprotein, as a member of the cadherin family of cell adhesion molecules. *Eur J Cell Biol*. 1990;53:1-12.
37. Amagai M, Klaus-Kovtun V, Stanley JR. Autoantibodies against a novel epithelial cadherin in pemphigus vulgaris, a disease of cell adhesion. *Cell*. 1991;67:869-877.
38. Amagai M, Matsuyoshi N, Wang ZH, et al. Toxin in bullous impetigo and staphylococcal scalded-skin syndrome targets desmoglein 1. *Nat Med*. 2000;6:1275-1277.
39. Descargues P, Deraison C., Bonnart C, et al. Spink5-deficient mice mimic Netherton syndrome through degradation of desmoglein 1 by epidermal protease hyperactivity. *Nat Genet*. 2004;37:56-65.
40. Hanakawa Y, Schechter N, Lin C, et al. Molecular mechanisms of blister formation in bullous impetigo and staphylococcal scalded skin syndrome. *J Clin Invest*. 2002;110:53-60.
41. Sekiguchi M, Futei Y, Fujii Y, et al. Dominant autoimmune epitopes recognized by pemphigus antibodies map to the N-terminal adhesive region of desmogleins. *J Immunol*. 2001;167:5439-5448.
42. Li N, Aoki V, Hans-Filho G, et al. The role of intramolecular epitope spreading in the pathogenesis of endemic pemphigus foliaceus (fogo selvagem). *J Exp Med*. 2003;197:1501-1510.
43. Chan PT, Ohyama B, Nishifuji K, et al. Immune response towards the amino-terminus of desmoglein 1 prevails across different activity stages in nonendemic pemphigus foliaceus. *Br J Dermatol*. 2010;162:1242-1250.
44. Karpati S, Amagai M, Liu WL, et al. Identification of desmoglein 1 as autoantigen in a patient with intraepidermal neutrophilic IgA dermatosis type of IgA pemphigus. *Exp Dermatol*. 2000;9:224-228.
45. Rickman L, Simrak D, Stevens HP, et al. N-terminal deletion in a desmosomal cadherin causes the autosomal dominant skin disease striate palmoplantar keratoderma. *Hum Mol Genet*. 1999;8:971-976.
46. Keren H, Bergman R, Mizrachi M, et al. Diffuse nonepidermolytic palmoplantar keratoderma caused by a recurrent nonsense mutation in DSG1. *Arch Dermatol*. 2005;141:628.
47. Milingou M, Wood P, Masouye I, et al. Focal palmoplantar keratoderma caused by an autosomal dominant inherited mutation in the desmoglein 1 gene. *Dermatology*. 2006;212:117-122.
48. Pilichou K, Nava A, Basso C, et al. Mutations in desmoglein-2 gene are associated with arrhythmogenic right ventricular cardiomyopathy. *Circulation*. 2006;113:1171-1179.
49. Payne AS, Ishii K, Kacir S, et al. Genetic and functional characterization of human pemphigus vulgaris monoclonal autoantibodies isolated by phage display. *J Clin Invest*. 2005;115:888-899.
50. Di Zenzo G, Di Lullo G, Corti D, et al. Pemphigus autoantibodies generated through somatic mutations target the desmoglein-3 cis-interface. *J Clin Invest*. 2012;122:3781-3790.
51. Ohyama B, Nishifuji K, Chan PT, et al. Epitope spreading is rarely found in pemphigus vulgaris by large-scale longitudinal study using desmoglein 2-based swapped molecules. *J Invest Dermatol*. 2012;132:1158-1168.
52. Koch PJ, Mahoney MG, Ishikawa H, et al. Targeted disruption of the pemphigus vulgaris antigen (desmoglein 3) gene in mice causes loss of keratinocyte cell adhesion with a phenotype similar to pemphigus vulgaris. *J Cell Biol*. 1997;137:1091-1102.
53. Sharma P, Mao X, Payne AS. Beyond steric hindrance: the role of adhesion signaling pathways in the pathogenesis of pemphigus. *J Dermatol Sci*. 2007;48:1-14.
54. Wang J, Kwon J, Ding X, et al. Nonsecretory IgA1 autoantibodies targeting desmosomal component desmoglein 3 in intraepidermal neutrophilic IgA dermatosis. *Am J Pathol*. 1997;150:1901-1907.
55. Schaffer JV, Bazzi H, Vitebsky A, et al. Mutations in the desmoglein 4 gene underlie localized autosomal recessive hypotrichosis with monilethrix hairs and congenital scalp erosions. *J Invest Dermatol*. 2006;126:1286-1291.
56. Shimomura Y, Sakamoto F, Kariya N, et al. Mutations in the desmoglein 4 gene are associated with monilethrix-like congenital hypotrichosis. *J Invest Dermatol*. 2006;126:1281-1285.
57. Zlotogorski A, Marek D, Horev L, et al. An autosomal recessive form of monilethrix Is caused by mutations in DSG4: clinical overlap with localized

57. autosomal recessive hypotrichosis. *J Invest Dermatol.* 2006;126:1292-1296.
58. Kljuic A, Bazzi H, Sundberg JP, et al. Desmoglein 4 in hair follicle differentiation and epidermal adhesion: evidence from inherited hypotrichosis and acquired pemphigus vulgaris. *Cell.* 2003;113:249-260.
59. Lai-Cheong JE, Arita K, McGrath JA. Genetic diseases of junctions. *J Invest Dermatol.* 2007;127:2713-2725.
60. Nagasaka T, Nishifuji K, Ota T, et al. Defining the pathogenic involvement of desmoglein 4 in pemphigus and staphylococcal scalded skin syndrome. *J Clin Invest.* 2004;114:1484-1492.
61. Hashimoto T, Kiyokawa C, Mori O, et al. Human desmocollin 1 (Dsc1) is an autoantigen for the subcorneal pustular dermatosis type of IgA pemphigus. *J Invest Dermatol.* 1997;109:127-131.
62. Heuser A, Plovie ER, Ellinor PT, et al. Mutant desmocollin-2 causes arrhythmogenic right ventricular cardiomyopathy. *Am J Hum Genet.* 2010;79:1081-1088.
63. Simpson MA, Mansour S, Ahnood D, et al. Homozygous mutation of desmocollin-2 in arrhythmogenic right ventricular cardiomyopathy with mild palmoplantar keratoderma and woolly hair. *Cardiology.* 2009;113:28-34.
64. Ayub M, Basit S, Jelani M, et al. A homozygous nonsense mutation in the human desmocollin-3 (DSC3) gene underlies hereditary hypotrichosis and recurrent skin vesicles. *Am J Hum Genet.* 2009;85:1-6.
65. Hisamatsu Y, Amagai M, Garrod DR, et al. The detection of IgG and IgA autoantibodies to desmocollins 1-3 by enzyme-linked immunosorbent assays using baculovirus-expressed proteins, in atypical pemphigus but not in typical pemphigus. *Br J Dermatol.* 2004;151:73-83.
66. Mao X, Nagler AR, Farber SA, et al. Autoimmunity to desmocollin 3 in pemphigus vulgaris. *Am J Pathol.* 2010;177:2724-2730.
67. Rafei D, Muller R, Ishii N, et al. IgG autoantibodies against desmocollin 3 in pemphigus sera induce loss of keratinocyte adhesion. *Am J Pathol.* 2011;178:718-723.
68. Cowin P, Kapprell HP, Franke WW, et al. Plakoglobin: a protein common to different kinds of intercellular adhering junctions. *Cell.* 1986;46:1063-1073.
69. Korman NJ, Eyre RW, Klaus-Kovtun V, et al. Demonstration of an adhering-junction molecule (plakoglobin) in the autoantigens of pemphigus foliaceus and pemphigus vulgaris. *N Engl J Med.* 1989;321:631-635.
70. Peifer M, Berg S, Reynolds AB. A repeating amino acid motif shared by proteins with diverse cellular roles. *Cell.* 1994;76:789-791.
71. Chitaev NA, Leube RE, Troyanovsky RB, et al. The binding of plakoglobin to desmosomal cadherins: patterns of binding sites and topogenic potential. *J Cell Biol.* 1996;133:359-369.
72. Wahl JK, Sacco PA, McGranahan-Sadler TM, et al. Plakoglobin domains that define its association with the desmosomal cadherins and the classical cadherins: identification of unique and shared domains. *J Cell Sci.* 1996;109(pt 5):1143-1154.
73. Witcher LL, Collins R, Puttagunta S, et al. Desmosomal cadherin binding domains of plakoglobin. *J Biol Chem.* 1996;271:10904-10909.
74. Kowalczyk AP, Bornslaeger EA, Borgwardt JE, et al. The amino-terminal domain of desmoplakin binds to plakoglobin and clusters desmosomal cadherin-plakoglobin complexes. *J Cell Biol.* 1997;139:773-784.
75. Williams BO, Barish GD, Klymkowsky MW, et al. A comparative evaluation of beta-catenin and plakoglobin signaling activity. *Oncogene.* 2000;19:5720-5728.
76. Williamson L, Raess NA, Caldelari R, et al. Pemphigus vulgaris identifies plakoglobin as key suppressor of c-Myc in the skin. *EMBO J.* 2006;25:3298-3309.
77. Bornslaeger EA, Godsel LM, Corcoran CM, et al. Plakophilin 1 interferes with plakoglobin binding to desmoplakin, yet together with plakoglobin promotes clustering of desmosomal plaque complexes at cell-cell borders. *J Cell Sci.* 2001;114:727-738.
78. Drees F, Pokutta S, Yamada S, et al. Alpha-catenin is a molecular switch that binds E-cadherin-beta-catenin and regulates actin-filament assembly. *Cell.* 2005;123:903-915.
79. Yamada S, Pokutta S, Drees F, et al. Deconstructing the cadherin-catenin-actin complex. *Cell.* 2005;123:889-901.
80. McKoy G, Protonotarios N, Crosby A, et al. Identification of a deletion in plakoglobin in arrhythmogenic right ventricular cardiomyopathy with palmoplantar keratoderma and woolly hair (Naxos disease). *Lancet.* 2000;355:2119-2124.
81. Cabral RM, Liu L, Hogan C, et al. Homozygous mutations in the 5' region of the JUP gene result in cutaneous disease but normal heart development in children. *J Invest Dermatol.* 2010;130(6):1543-150.
82. Pigors M, Kiritsi D, Krumpelmann S, et al. Lack of plakoglobin leads to lethal congenital epidermolysis bullosa: a novel clinico-genetic entity. *Hum Mol Genet.* 2011;20:1811-1819.
83. Mueller H, Franke WW. Biochemical and immunological characterization of desmoplakins I and II, the major polypeptides of the desmosomal plaque. *J Mol Biol.* 1983;163:647-671.
84. Green KJ, Parry DAD, Steinert PS, et al. Structure of the human desmoplakins. Implications for function in the desmosomal plaque. *J Biol Chem.* 1990;265:2603-2612.
85. Uzumcu A, Norgett EE, Dindar A, et al. Loss of desmoplakin isoform I causes early onset cardiomyopathy and heart failure in a Naxos-like syndrome. *J Med Genet.* 2006;43:e05.
86. Green KJ, Virata MLA, Elgart GW, et al. Comparative structural analysis of desmoplakin, bullous pemphigoid antigen and plectin: members of a new gene family involved in organization of intermediate filaments. *Int J Biol Macrobiol.* 1992;14:145-153.
87. Stappenbeck TS, Green KJ. The desmoplakin carboxyl terminus coaligns with and specifically disrupts intermediate filament networks when expressed in cultured cells. *J Cell Biol.* 1992;116:1197-1209.
88. Gallicano GI, Kouklis P, Bauer C, et al. Desmoplakin is required early in development for assembly of desmosomes and cytoskeletal linkage. *J Cell Biol.* 1998;143:2009-2022.
89. Armstrong DK, McKenna KE, Purkis PE, et al. Haploinsufficiency of desmoplakin causes a striate subtype of palmoplantar keratoderma. *Hum Mol Genet.* 1999;8:143-148.
90. Carvajal-Huerta L. Epidermolytic palmoplantar keratoderma with wooly hair and dilated cardiomyopathy. *J Am Acad Dermatol.* 1998;39:418-421.
91. Jonkman MF, Pasmooij AMG, Pasmans SGMA, et al. Loss of desmoplakin tail causes lethal acantholytic epidermolysis bullosa. *Am J Hum Genet.* 2005;77:653-660.

92. Wolf A, Krause-Gruszczynska M, Birkenmeier O, et al. Plakophilin 1 stimulates translation by promoting eIF4A1 activity. *J Cell Biol.* 2010;188:463-471.
93. Schmidt A, Langbein L, Rode M, et al. Plakophilins 1a and 1b: widespread nuclear proteins recruited in specific epithelial cells as desmosomal plaque components. *Cell Tissue Res.* 1997;290:481-499.
94. Schmidt A, Langbein L, Pratzel S, et al. Plakophilin 3—a novel cell-type-specific desmosomal plaque protein. *Differentiation.* 1999;64:291-306.
95. Mertens C, Kuhn C, Moll R, et al. Desmosomal plakophilin 2 as a differentiation marker in normal and malignant tissues. *Differentiation.* 1999;64:277-290.
96. McGrath JA, McMillan JR, Shemanko CS, et al. Mutations in the plakophilin 1 gene result in ectodermal dysplasia/skin fragility syndrome. *Nat Genet.* 1997;17:240-244.
97. Gerull B, Heuser A, Wichter T, et al. Mutations in the desmosomal protein plakophilin-2 are common in arrhythmogenic right ventricular cardiomyopathy. *Nat Genet.* 2004;36:1162-1164.
98. van Tintelen JP, Entius MM, Bhuiyan ZA, et al. Plakophilin-2 mutations are the major determinant of familial arrhythmogenic right ventricular dysplasia/cardiomyopathy. *Circulation.* 2006;113:1650-1658.
99. Sevilla LM, Nachat R, Groot KR, et al. Mice deficient in involucrin, envoplakin, and periplakin have a defective epidermal barrier. *J Cell Biol.* 2007;179:1599-1612.
100. Levy-Nissenbaum E, Betz RC, Frydman M, et al. Hypotrichosis simplex of the scalp is associated with nonsense mutations in CDSN encoding corneodesmosin. *Nat Genet.* 2003;34:151-153.
101. Timpl R. Macromolecular organization of basement membranes. *Curr Opin Cell Biol.* 1996;8(5):618-624.
102. Glentis A, Gurchenkov V, Matic Vignjevic D. Assembly, heterogeneity, and breaching of the basement membranes. *Cell Adh Migr.* 2014;8(3):236-245.
103. Yurchenco PD. Basement membranes: cell scaffoldings and signaling platforms. *Cold Spring Harb Perspect Biol.* 2011;3(2). pii: a004911.
104. van Agtmael T, BrucknerTuderman L. Basement membranes and human disease. *Cell Tissue Res.* 2010;339:167-188.
105. Kelley LC, Lohmer LL, Hagedorn EJ, et al. Traversing the basement membrane in vivo: a diversity of strategies. *J Cell Biol.* 2014;204(3):291-302.
106. Has C, Nyström A. Epidermal basement membrane in health and disease. *Curr Top Membr.* 2015;76:117-170.
107. Eady RA, McGrath JA, McMillan JR. Ultrastructural clues to genetic disorders of skin: the dermal epidermal junction. *J Invest Dermatol.* 1994;103(5 suppl):13S-18S.
108. Goldberg M, Escaig-Haye F. Is the lamina lucida of the basement membrane a fixation artifact? *Eur. J Cell Biol.* 1986;42:365-368.
109. Behrens DT, Villone D, Koch M, et al. The epidermal basement membrane is a composite of separate laminin- or collagen IV-containing networks connected by aggregated perlecan, but not by nidogens. *J Biol Chem.* 2012;287(22):18700-18709.
110. Keene DR, Sakai LY, Lunstrum GP, et al. Collagen VII forms an extended network of anchoring fibrils. *J Cell Biol.* 1987;104:611-621.
111. Baldwin AK, Simpson A, Steer R, et al. Elastic fibres in health and disease. *Expert Rev Mol Med.* 2013;15:e8.
112. Sengle G, Sakai LY. The fibrillin microfibril scaffold: a niche for growth factors and mechanosensation? *Matrix Biol.* 2015;47:3-12.
113. Mao M, Alavi MV, Labelle-Dumais C, et al. Type IV collagens and basement membrane diseases: cell biology and pathogenic mechanisms. *Curr Top Membr.* 2015;76:61-116.
114. Cummings CF, Pedchenko V, Brown KL, et al. Extracellular chloride signals collagen IV network assembly during basement membrane formation. *J Cell Biol.* 2016;213(4):479-494.
115. Yurchenco PD. Integrating activities of laminins that drive basement membrane assembly and function. *Curr Top Membr.* 2015;76:1-30.
116. Domogatskaya A, Rodin S, Tryggvason K. Functional diversity of laminins. *Annu Rev Cell Dev Biol.* 2012;28:523-553.
117. Wegner J, Loser K, Apsite G, et al. Laminin α5 in the keratinocyte basement membrane is required for epidermal-dermal intercommunication. *Matrix Biol.* 2016;56:24-41.
118. Has C, Bruckner-Tuderman L. The genetics of skin fragility. *Annu Rev Genomics Hum Genet.* 2014;15:245-268.
119. Durbeej M. Laminin-α2 chain-deficient congenital muscular dystrophy: pathophysiology and development of treatment. *Curr Top Membr.* 2015;76:31-60.
120. Bader BL, Smyth N, Nedbal S, et al. Compound genetic ablation of nidogen 1 and 2 causes basement membrane defects and perinatal lethality in mice. *Mol Cell Biol.* 2005;25:6846-6856.
121. Iozzo RV, Schaefer L. Proteoglycan form and function: a comprehensive nomenclature of proteoglycans. *Matrix Biol.* 2015;42:11-55.
122. McCarthy KJ. The basement membrane proteoglycans perlecan and agrin: something old, something new. *Curr Top Membr.* 2015;76:255-303.
123. Seppinen L, Pihlajaniemi T. The multiple functions of collagen XVIII in development and disease. *Matrix Biol.* 2011;30(2):83-92.
124. Chung H, Multhaupt HA, Oh ES, et al. Syndecans and their crucial roles during tissue regeneration. *FEBS Lett.* 2016;590(15):2408-2417.
125. Walko G, Castañón MJ, Wiche G. Molecular architecture and function of the hemidesmosome. *Cell Tissue Res.* 2015;360(3):529-544.
126. Franzke CW, Bruckner-Tuderman L, Blobel CP. Shedding of collagen XVII/BP180 in skin depends on both ADAM10 and ADAM9. *J Biol Chem.* 2009;284:23386-23396.
127. Nishie W, Kiritsi D, Nyström A, et al. Dynamic interactions of epidermal collagen XVII with the extracellular matrix: laminin 332 as a major binding partner. *Am J Pathol.* 2011;179(2):829-837.
128. Matsumura H, Mohri Y, Binh NT, et al. Hair follicle aging is driven by transepidermal elimination of stem cells via COL17A1 proteolysis. *Science.* 2016;351(6273):aad4395.
129. Karamatic Crew V, Burton N, Kagan A, et al. CD151, the first member of the tetraspanin (TM4) superfamily detected on erythrocytes, is essential for the correct assembly of human basement membranes in kidney and skin. *Blood.* 2004;104:2217-2223.
130. Heisenberg CP, Fässler R. Cell-cell adhesion and extracellular matrix: diversity counts. *Curr Opin Cell Biol.* 2012;24(5):559-561.

131. Has C, Spartà G, Kiritsi D, et al. Integrin α3 mutations with kidney, lung, and skin disease. *N Engl J Med.* 2012;366(16):1508-1514.
132. Rognoni E, Ruppert R, Fässler R. The kindlin family: functions, signaling properties and implications for human disease. *J Cell Sci.* 2016;129(1):17-27.
133. Nonaka S, Ishiko A, Masunaga T, et al. The extracellular domain of BPAG2 has a loop structure in the carboxy terminal flexible tail in vivo. *J Invest Dermatol.* 2000;115:889-892.
134. Villone D, Fritsch A, Koch M, et al. Supramolecular interactions in the dermo-epidermal junction zone: collagen VII in anchoring fibrils tightly bind to fibrillar collagen I. *J Biol Chem.* 2008;283:24506-24513.
135. Bruckner-Tuderman L. Dystrophic epidermolysis bullosa: pathogenesis and clinical features. *Dermatol Clin.* 2010;28:107-114.
136. Nyström A, Velati D, Mittapalli VR, et al. Collagen VII plays a dual role in wound healing. *J Clin Invest.* 2013;123(8):3498-3509.
137. Uitto J, Bruckner-Tuderman L, Christiano AM, et al. Progress toward treatment and cure of epidermolysis bullosa: summary of the DEBRA International research symposium EB2015. *J Invest Dermatol.* 2016;136(2):352-358.
138. Nyström A, Bornert O, Kühl T. Cell therapy for basement membrane-linked diseases. *Matrix Biol.* 2017;57-58:124-139.
139. Nyström A, Thriene K, Mittapalli V, et al. Losartan ameliorates dystrophic epidermolysis bullosa and uncovers new disease mechanisms. *EMBO Mol Med.* 2015;7(9):1211-1228.
140. Nyström A, Bruckner-Tuderman L. Biology of the extracellular matrix. In: Bolognia JL, Jorizzo JL, Schaffer JV, eds. *Dermatology.* 4th ed. Philadelphia, PA: Elsevier; 2018.
141. Mouw JK, Ou G, Weaver VM. Extracellular matrix assembly: a multiscale deconstruction. *Nat Rev Mol Cell Biol.* 2014;15(12):771-785.
142. Küttner V, Mack C, Rigbolt KT, et al. Global remodelling of cellular microenvironment due to loss of collagen VII. *Mol Syst Biol.* 2013;9:657.
143. Naba A, Clauser KR, Ding H, et al. The extracellular matrix: tools and insights for the "omics" era. *Matrix Biol.* 2016;49:10-24.
144. Randles MJ, Humphries MJ, Lennon R. Proteomic definitions of basement membrane composition in health and disease. *Matrix Biol.* 2017;57-58:12-28.
145. Eckes B, Krieg T, Wickström SA. Role of integrin signalling through integrin-linked kinase in skin physiology and pathology. *Exp Dermatol.* 2014;23(7):453-456.
146. Lee DH, Oh JH, Chung JH. Glycosaminoglycan and proteoglycan in skin aging. *J Dermatol Sci.* 2016;83(3):174-181.
147. Eckes B, Nischt R, Krieg T. Cell-matrix interactions in dermal repair and scarring. *Fibrogenesis Tissue Repair.* 2010;3:4.
148. Myllyharju J, Kivirikko KI. Collagens, modifying enzymes and their mutations in humans, flies and worms. *Trends Genet.* 2004;20:33-43.
149. Kühl T, Mezger M, Hausser I, et al. Collagen VII half-life at the dermal-epidermal junction zone: implications for mechanisms and therapy of genodermatoses. *J Invest Dermatol.* 2016;136(6):1116-1123.
150. Zeyer KA, Reinhardt DP. Fibrillin-containing microfibrils are key signal relay stations for cell function. *J Cell Commun Signal.* 2015;9(4):309-325.
151. Wight TN, Kang I, Merrilees MJ. Versican and the control of inflammation. *Matrix Biol.* 2014;35:152-161.
152. Chen S, Birk DE. The regulatory roles of small leucine-rich proteoglycans in extracellular matrix assembly. *FEBS J.* 2013;280(10):2120-2137.
153. Winograd-Katz SE, Fässler R, Geiger B, et al. The integrin adhesome: from genes and proteins to human disease. *Nat Rev Mol Cell Biol.* 2014;15(4):273-288.
154. Starke J, Wehrle-Haller B, Friedl P. Plasticity of the actin cytoskeleton in response to extracellular matrix nanostructure and dimensionality. *Biochem Soc Trans.* 2014;42(5):1356-1366.
155. Wolf K, Friedl P. Extracellular matrix determinants of proteolytic and non-proteolytic cell migration. *Trends Cell Biol.* 2011;21(12):736-744.
156. Wen JH, Vincent LG, Fuhrmann A, et al. Interplay of matrix stiffness and protein tethering in stem cell differentiation. *Nat Mater.* 2014;13(10):979-987.
157. Irianto J, Pfeifer CR, Xia Y, et al. SnapShot: mechanosensing matrix. *Cell.* 2016;165(7):1820-1820.e1.
158. Andrews JP, Marttala J, Macarak E, et al. Keloids: the paradigm of skin fibrosis-pathomechanisms and treatment. *Matrix Biol.* 2016;51:37-46.

Chapter 16 :: Microbiome of the Skin
:: Heidi H. Kong

第十六章
皮肤微生物组学

中文导读

本章内容分为3节：①定义皮肤微生物组学研究；②皮肤微生物组学的组成；③结论。本章介绍了皮肤微生物组的概念，皮肤微生物组的主要成分，以及皮肤微生物与宿主之间的一些相互作用，主要强调对健康人和疾病患者的人体皮肤中的常驻微生物组进行独立培养的研究。

第一节定义皮肤微生物组学研究，介绍了研究皮肤微生物的方法已经从培养发展到微生物DNA测序。目前出现了新的概念微生物组学，被定义为在特定生态系统中存在的所有微生物，其研究不是研究孤立的细菌或真菌分离物，而是指对整个皮肤微生物群落的研究。接下来介绍了皮肤微生物组学研究设计非常重要。最后介绍了微生物组学研究的挑战。

第二节皮肤微生物组学的组成，介绍了目前已经证明皮肤上存在共生菌和病原体，皮肤是一个多样化的栖息地。从宏观上来说，不同的皮肤解剖区域通常与某些细菌和真菌有关。从微观上看，微观结构导致不同的微环境，可以影响皮肤微生物的组成。接下来介绍了皮肤细菌群落的基因组学研究，皮肤真菌群落的基因组学研究，皮肤病毒群落的基因组学研究。

第三节结论，介绍了目前微生物组学的研究中针对肠道微生物组的研究大大超过了皮肤微生物组学的研究，因为肠道菌群可能会影响皮肤病。跨研究领域的合作努力和技术进步对于揭开这些疾病的复杂性以及与人类微生物群的潜在关系至关重要，期望开发潜在的预防或治疗干预措施。

〔粟　娟〕

AT-A-GLANCE

The microbes on skin are:
- Bacteria, fungi, viruses.
- Healthy vs pathogenic.

Human skin hosts a variety of commensal and pathogenic microbes, including bacteria, fungi, and viruses. The most common methods to study skin microbes are traditionally based on cultivation techniques, especially to help diagnose infections. Koch's postulates for linking a causative microbial agent to a disease represent a familiar and fundamental paradigm for understanding host–microbial interactions. Beyond the classical roles of infection-causing microbes, studies continue to examine how microbes may interact with the host as commensal symbionts and potentially contribute as pathobionts to noninfectious inflammatory diseases, such as atopic dermatitis or psoriasis, and in neoplasms, such as Merkel cell carcinoma. Ongoing research investigating host–microbial interactions increasingly uses multiple different concepts and methods to provide insights into human skin microbes.

One basic approach to exploring the symbionts and pathobionts among skin microbes is to initially determine the composition of the microbes that reside on human skin. A challenge of relying solely on cultivation methods is the difficulty in selecting the optimal culturing methods to capture the entire microbial community of human skin; some microbes may flourish under generic culture conditions, yet other microbes can require specific nutrients or special conditions. The advances in scientific methods and genomic sequencing technologies have enabled a more global culture-independent examination of the skin's complex communities of microbes.[1] Deeper study of the composition and the associated functions of the multitude of microbes residing on human skin may help uncover the roles of skin microbes in health and disease.

The constant exposure of human skin to surrounding environments presents innumerable potential interactions with such things as dust particles, humidity, clothing, emollients, other people, and pets. As a result, a rapidly growing number of studies are examining the microbiome of living organisms, the built environment, and inanimate objects that come into contact with human skin or skin debris, as well as the many potential interventions (eg, antibiotics, hygiene products, probiotics) that may alter the human skin microbiome.[2-18] This chapter introduces the concept of the skin microbiome, the major constituents of the cutaneous microbiome, and some of the interactions between skin microbes and the host, primarily highlighting culture-independent studies of the resident microbiome of human skin in healthy individuals and dermatologic disorders.

DEFINING SKIN MICROBIOME STUDIES

FROM CULTURING TO GENOMICS

Based on standard culturing methods, it is well-known that human skin harbors various microbes. Because many skin diseases are associated with microbes, the field of dermatology has been instrumental in investigating the composition of cultured bacteria and fungi on human skin and in exploring host–microbial interactions.[19-23] These culture-based studies have defined some of the basic tenets of skin microbes that continue to hold true decades later, including the presence of *Cutibacterium* (formerly *Propionibacterium*) and *Malassezia* (formerly *Pityrosporum*) on many individuals. An early example is Mary J. Marples' fundamental body of work on skin ecology including illustrations of scaled models of the body (homunculi) with relative distributions of skin microbes and physiologic features.[20] Pillsbury, Kligman, Noble, Somerville, Maibach, and many colleagues used cultivation methods to contribute significantly to the general understanding of the microbiology of skin in disease states and in healthy individuals.[19,20,24-28]

In addition to studying isolates cultivated from skin, advancements in scientific technologies have provided methods to study human skin microbes. By sequencing microbial DNA present within a sample, it is possible to eliminate initial culturing of a sample that could potentially skew the resultant findings on the composition of skin microbes. The reduced cost and increased access of sequencing have facilitated the investigations into the human microbiome. The term *microbiome* has been defined as all the microorganisms, their genomes, and the surrounding environmental conditions present in a particular ecosystem such as skin.[29] Thus, rather than studying solitary bacterial or fungal isolates, skin microbiome investigations refer to studies of the global cutaneous microbial communities. Of note, because standard microbiome studies are based on the DNA present within a sample, these methods cannot distinguish whether the DNA was from a dead or living organism and from a resident or transient microbe. Therefore, microbiome research can complement cultivation methods to collect isolates that can be used in mechanistic studies and other -omic methods that examine the genes that are actively expressed (transcriptomics) or what proteins are present (proteomics). Additionally, existing laboratory strains of microbes are repeatedly propagated and may have different biologic properties than microbes cultivated directly from patients.

The National Institutes of Health Common Fund launched the Human Microbiome Project in 2008 to catalyze the growth in microbiome research, bringing together multidisciplinary fields to explore the skin, gut, oral, vaginal, and nasal microbiomes in patients and healthy volunteers. In addition to developing protocols for study design, sample processing, sequencing, and analysis, the Human Microbiome Project has provided a reference database of human microbiome sequences.[30-32] Advances in newer sequencing methods and other omic techniques, as well as the novel approaches to interrogate the host organism, continue to expand the abilities to examine human microbes.

GENERAL SEQUENCING METHODS OF MICROBIOME STUDIES

Based on the most established methods of microbial sequencing, which were extensively developed by environmental microbial ecologists, many of the human microbiome studies have often focused on bacteria, similar to cultivation-based investigations.

Bacteria, along with cyanobacteria, are prokaryotes which have the 16S ribosomal RNA (rRNA) gene. The 16S rRNA is part of the 30S ribosomal subunit and is evolutionarily conserved because of its essential function. By focusing on the 16S rRNA gene for sequencing, investigators can target all the bacteria present within a sample without depending on the ability to cultivate these microbes.[33] There is sufficient variation among the 16S rRNA genes that enables taxonomic identification of the individual bacterial members of a given ecosystem, from soil to oceans and dental plaque to skin. With the widespread use of the 16S rRNA target gene, there are large established databases of 16S rRNA gene sequences that can be used as reference databases to taxonomically identify sequences originating from human samples. However, the nomenclature used to define a distinct bacterial entity differs between the fields of genomics and clinical microbiology. Genomic studies define a specific bacterial taxa based on the percent similarity of the genome, whereas traditional microbiology originally defined a distinct species based on morphologic, biochemical, and/or physiologic characteristics.[34] This distinction is important, particularly from a clinician's perspective, because genus- and species-level identification of a microorganism has clinical implications. Microbial genomics can provide a deeper understanding of what defines a "species" and potentially how it relates to human disease. Initial human microbiome studies used a method of sequencing (Sanger sequencing) to sequence all 9 hypervariable regions of the 16S rRNA gene, but technologic developments in sequencing methods (see Chap. 18) rely on sequencing fewer hypervariable regions of the 16S rRNA gene at a faster pace and cheaper cost, but at the expense of less-complete genomic information.

Fungi are also clinically important. Investigations about fungi have included studies regarding the roles in human infections/diseases, production of active metabolites, and influence on bacterial growth. Similar to the application of genomic sequencing of bacteria, studies have used molecular methods to study the "mycobiome". Unlike the universal use of the 16S rRNA gene as a marker gene in bacterial studies, the marker genes selected in mycobiome studies have included either a single region or combined regions targeting the 18S rRNA gene, the 28S rRNA gene, and/or the internal transcribed spacer (ITS) regions within fungal genomes.[35-39] The use of different marker genes in mycobiome studies with the resultant development of different fungal sequence reference databases, as well as the availability of relatively fewer fungal genomes than bacterial genomes, have hindered the ability to compare across studies. However, the clinical relevance of skin fungi in dermatologic disorders, and intriguing studies examining interactions between bacteria and fungi, highlight the importance of exploring the skin mycobiome.[35,37,40,41]

Studies of the human virome have been notably fewer in number than bacterial studies. The heterogeneity of viral genomes creates challenges in genomically capturing the potential breadth (ie, single-stranded and double-stranded DNA and RNA viruses) of the human virome. Genomics-based studies typically focus on DNA-only viruses or specific groups of viruses (eg, human papillomaviruses or polyomaviruses),[42-49] highlighting some of the limitations of marker gene–based studies.

Simultaneously sequencing multiple microbial kingdoms within a single skin sample requires shotgun metagenomic sequencing, which is quite complex from the processing and computational standpoints. Shotgun metagenomic sequencing is performed initially by shearing and sequencing all DNA present within a sample rather than focusing only on sequencing marker genes such as 16S or 18S rRNA genes. Thus, shotgun metagenomic sequencing can provide additional information beyond the identification of microbes within 1 kingdom (eg, bacteria), such that the functional genetic potential of the resident microbes is also sequenced and analyzed.[30,31,43,44] The limitations of shotgun metagenomic sequencing include the higher costs and the analytical challenges. The ability to sequence has outpaced the important research into the function and biology of genes. As a result, there is incomplete knowledge of the functions of many genes, and a large proportion of resultant sequences from metagenomic sequencing studies are classified as unknown functions. Although sequencing can provide tremendous insights into human–microbial interactions, further investigations into the basic sciences to understand mechanisms of genes (and gene expression and proteins) are fundamental and critical to understanding the clinical relevance of the human skin microbiome.

SKIN MICROBIOME STUDY DESIGN

Similar to other areas of human research, study design can significantly affect the quality of the resultant findings in skin microbiome studies. Due to the sensitivity of microbiome studies related to potential confounders and contamination, with skin in particular, reviews and commentaries on important considerations for human microbiome studies have been published to emphasize the importance of careful study design (Fig. 16-1).[50-53] Studies that examine multiple body sites have demonstrated that the human microbiome varies based on the specific body site: gut, skin, oral, nares, and vaginal.[30,31,54] Of all the body sites evaluated in published studies, the skin is comprised of the most diverse communities of bacteria.[30,54] This capacity to host a relatively wide variety of microbes is likely linked to the range of microenvironments present in human skin, which have been classified in some studies based on the physiologic skin features of moist, dry, and sebaceous.[43,44,55] Similar to the body site–specificity

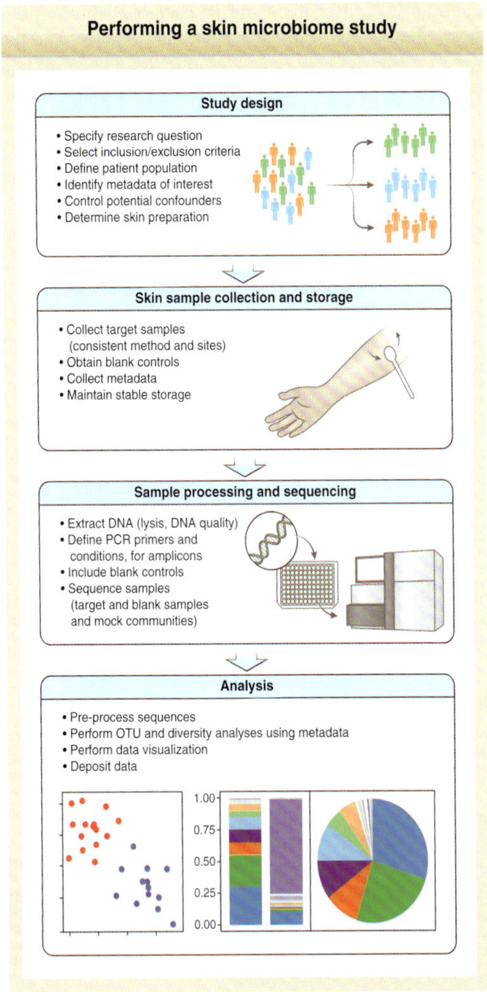

Figure 16-1 Performing a skin microbiome study. The general principles for a skin microbiome study of study design, sample collection and storage, sample processing and sequencing, and analysis with examples of data visualization are outlined. OTU, operational taxonomic unit; PCR, polymerase chain reaction. (From Kong HH, Andersson B, Clavel T, et al. Performing skin microbiome research: a method to the madness. *J Invest Dermatol.* 2017;137(3):561-568, with permission.)

of microbial communities observed across the gut, skin, oral, nasal, and vaginal communities, the skin microbiomes are also highly specific to the particular anatomical region of skin under investigation.

Skin samples can be collected via premoistened swab, superficial scraping, biopsy, tape strip, and/or cup scrub from defined anatomical regions.[53] Then DNA is isolated from the clinical samples. The type of DNA preparation and sequencing depends on whether the focus is on a particular kingdom of interest (ie, bacteria or fungi) or shotgun metagenomics. The sequencing reads are processed bioinformatically to enable subsequent analysis of the composition, diversity, and similarities of the microbial communities based on clinical metadata.

A major challenge in studying the microbiome of the skin is the presence of a low microbial biomass, or small amount of organic matter, leading to limited quantities of DNA. In contrast, other body regions, including the gut and oral cavity, contain large amounts of microbial DNA. The relatively low amounts of microbial DNA on skin result in samples that can be easily contaminated. For example, a small fixed amount of contaminant DNA would be a larger proportion of the microbial DNA isolated from a skin sample as compared to the microbial DNA collected from a stool sample. Because of the high risk of contamination in skin microbiome studies, appropriate negative and positive controls have been recommended for sample collection, sample processing, and sequencing.[50,52,53]

With microbiome sequencing, it is difficult to quantitatively determine microbial bioburden (number of microbes). Culture-based studies use colony-counting and other methods to compare the relative bioburden of microbes present in one sample versus another. Microbiome studies typically measure results in relative proportions or percentages. Additionally, most genomic studies and analyses cannot distinguish whether microbes are dead or alive. If contamination is ruled out and microbiome sequencing identifies microbial reads (sequences), some of the microbial DNA may be from dead organisms. However, more sophisticated analyses of metagenomic data may allow inference of whether particular microbes were proliferating at the time of sampling in comparison to other microbes.[56]

Although genomic sequencing can provide culture-independent taxonomic and metagenomic information on the microbial communities present on skin, additional studies on mechanism often require use of microbial isolates. Because two strain isolates that are classified as the same species (eg, methicillin-sensitive *Staphylococcus aureus* and methicillin-resistant *S. aureus*) can exhibit different biologic effects, collecting clinically relevant strains in parallel with microbiome studies may optimally inform subsequent functional studies.

COMPOSITION OF THE SKIN MICROBIOME

The existing knowledge of skin microbes is based on extensive work from many investigators, demonstrating the presence of both commensals and pathogens on skin including *Staphylococcus epidermidis, S. aureus, Cutibacterium acnes, Corynebacterium* spp., and *Pseudomonas aeruginosa*.[20,22,57-62] A common finding from many culture-based studies is that the skin is a diverse habitat from both macroscopic and microscopic perspectives.[63] Macroscopically, different anatomical regions (eg, forehead vs palm, flexural folds vs dorsal surfaces) are typically associated with certain bacteria and fungi. This topographical variation in skin microbes is also observed microscopically with regards to the biodiversity and localization of cutaneous microbes or microbial DNA. The surface of the skin is composed of ridges, creases, and appendageal openings and ducts. Each of these microscopic structures (eg, hair follicles, eccrine/apocrine glands, sebaceous glands) are distributed in different proportions over the skin surface, resulting in distinct microenvironments that can harbor and influence the composition of skin microbes.[63,64] For example, bacteria can break down sebum produced by sebaceous glands and the fatty substance excreted by apocrine sweat glands into byproducts. Given the microscopic topography, studies into host–cutaneous microbial interactions have examined both the different skin structures and the different layers of skin.[63,65,66]

GENOMICS STUDIES OF SKIN BACTERIAL COMMUNITIES

The early genomics-based studies focused on healthy skin and examined a single anatomical area of skin in healthy individuals, demonstrating skin microbes are more diverse than the most commonly recognized bacteria (eg, staphylococci, *Corynebacterium*, *Cutibacterium*) identified through culture-based studies and highlighting different methods for skin sample collection.[37,67,68] Additional studies of healthy volunteers examined multiple skin sites, including skin regions that are sites of predilection for dermatoses, including atopic dermatitis and psoriasis.[54,55] These studies showed that different skin sites harbored distinct populations of bacteria (site specificity). Even though the skin microbiome is site-specific, bacterial communities in different skin sites can share similar features based on the microenvironment of the anatomical skin site (eg, sebaceous areas, moist skin creases, dry flat surfaces).[14,43,55] Consistent with findings from culture-based studies, highly sebaceous sites (eg, forehead, retroauricular crease) were predominated by *C. acnes*. Sites that included flexural or moist folds (eg, antecubital fossa, inguinal crease) harbored bacterial species that can grow favorably in humid conditions (eg, *Corynebacterium* spp. and *Staphylococcus* spp.).[69,70] The flat surfaces of skin-hosted populations of bacteria demonstrated greater variability between study subjects as compared to sebaceous and moist skin sites. These findings highlighted the diversity and similarities of skin bacterial communities from specific anatomic regions over the human skin surface.

To further define the spatial and temporal variability of the skin microbiome, investigators studied the skin bacterial communities based on right and left symmetry, within an individual and between different individuals over time. Although the entire skin surface of a single healthy individual is comprised of multiple different skin bacterial communities, bilateral and symmetrical skin sites analyzed in healthy individuals, with the exception of hands, generally demonstrated highly similar skin microbiomes.[54,55,67,71] Because skin sites are often exposed to different surfaces and environments, potential alterations in the skin microbiome in response to specific exposures and over time have been evaluated in several studies. Examining shifts of the skin bacterial communities after exposure to bacterial communities from different skin sites (forehead and forearm) and the tongue shows that some skin sites (eg, forehead) can revert back to the originally observed bacterial communities faster than other skin sites (eg, forearm).[54] Studies have also examined the effects of hygiene practices on the skin microbiome. The elapsed time since the last handwashing affected the skin bacterial communities: some bacteria (eg, Staphylococceae, Streptococcaceae) were relatively more abundant on hands that were recently washed as compared to other bacteria (eg, Propionibacteriaceae) that were relatively more abundant with longer time intervals since the last handwashing.[71] Alteration or usage of hygiene products is associated with changes in the skin microbiome diversity in some healthy populations,[14] but not in others.[13] Studies examining the longitudinal variation in human skin bacterial communities using both 16S rRNA gene sequencing[55] and shotgun metagenomics sequencing[44,72] show that the skin bacterial communities can remain relatively stable up to 2 years after initial sampling. This stability of skin bacterial communities is specific to the particular skin site, as well specific to each individual,[44,72] and may be more likely influenced by the host environment, including global geographic location, than noncutaneous body sites.[73-76]

The largest human microbiome studies have focused on surveys of healthy young and middle-aged adults[30,31,77] with fewer studies examining the skin microbiome in children or the elderly. General changes in skin among different age groups are well-known,[78] and cultivation studies show that skin bacterial communities shift based on the age or sexual maturity of individuals.[20,22,26,79] Although the skin of neonates is considered sterile prior to birth, the skin is thought to quickly acquire skin microbes. In the skin microbiome studies of infants and young children that have been performed,[80-84] the bacterial diversity of skin has been observed to be low shortly after birth. The skin microbiome in neonates soon after delivery resembles maternal vaginal communities if born vaginally, and maternal skin communities if delivered by cesarean section.[15,82] By the second day of life, the site specificity of skin bacterial communities is observable.[83] Similar to culture-based studies, microbiome studies show that the skin bacterial communities in neonates, infants, and young children are distinct from more sexually mature children and adults, particularly at certain skin sites.[80,81,83,84] The skin microbiomes in older adults have been less frequently studied but may also demonstrate differences when comparing to younger individuals.[85] Skin physiology, including sebum production and hydration levels, may influence the composition of bacterial communities on skin.[86,87]

With the increase in skin microbiome studies, there has been an expansion of the cutaneous disorders under investigation using genomic sequencing of skin bacteria (Table 16-1). Based on common clinical observations and the considerable literature examining the link between atopic dermatitis and high frequency of *S. aureus* colonization and infections,[19,88] several genomic studies have more closely investigated the role of the microbiome in atopic dermatitis patients.[83,89-93] Questions remain whether the skin dysbiosis with increased staphylococci (*S. aureus* and, in some studies, *S. epidermidis*) observed in atopic dermatitis affects the development and/or worsening of atopic dermatitis or is a consequence of eczematous skin providing an environment conducive to staphylococcal growth. Several murine and in vitro studies suggest skin bacteria can elicit exacerbation of skin inflammation,[94-98] and one study showed topical application of *S. aureus* was associated with more-severe dermatitis.[99] However, human studies remain more challenging to study directly. If the murine studies that show that skin bacteria can modulate the developing skin immune system early in life correspond to what may occur in human skin,[100] longitudinal investigations of birth cohorts may provide a unique ability to examine skin microbes prior to the development of atopic dermatitis.[83]

Prior studies in psoriasis patients identified cocci in skin lesions,[101] isolated *S. aureus*,[28,102] and linked streptococci to psoriasis.[101,103] Consequently, microbial genomic techniques have been used to analyze the skin microbes in psoriatic skin lesions.[37,104-108] Some have identified increased relative abundances of the phylum Proteobacteria in psoriatic skin lesions as compared to controls.[105,108] Whereas the association between atopic dermatitis and staphylococci in microbiome studies is more consistently observed, the features of the skin microbiome in psoriasis are less defined.

In many cultivation studies, *C. acnes* frequently has been linked with acne.[109,110] As a result, several sequencing studies examined the skin microbiome in acne patients and identified different strains of *C. acnes* in individuals with acne as compared to controls.[111-115] However, the question of the role of *C. acnes* in acne causation remains unresolved[116-118] and continues to be an active area of investigation.

In addition to atopic dermatitis, psoriasis, and acne, other dermatologic conditions have been studied using microbiome methods. These studies include general atopy,[119] bacterial infections,[120,121] body odor,[122] dandruff,[39] diabetic wounds,[123-125] ichthyosis vulgaris,[126] melanoma and melanocytic nevi,[127] mycosis fungoides,[128] vitiligo,[129] and eczematous dermatitis related to primary immunodeficiency syndromes.[130,131] Distinctive patterns of skin microbiomes have been observed in several of these investigations, and further work is needed to elucidate the mechanism of the relationships between host and cutaneous microbiomes.

GENOMICS STUDIES OF SKIN FUNGAL COMMUNITIES

Conditions that favor the growth of bacteria may not optimally culture fungal organisms. Cultivation studies focused on isolating fungi from healthy human skin have isolated predominantly *Malassezia*, including *Malassezia globosa, Malassezia restricta,* and *Malassezia sympodialis*.[20,132,133] Even among the species within the genus *Malassezia*, some species grow more quickly than others.[134] As a result of the heterogeneity in optimal cultivation conditions, a comprehensive culture-based evaluation of the relative composition of skin microbes, particularly fungi, can be quite challenging. As genomics-based studies are cultivation-independent, microbiome methods can provide a global examination of microbial constituents in a given sample. Similar to culture-based studies,[20,133] genomics-based fungal studies in healthy individuals demonstrate that *Malassezia* spp. predominate in most skin sites,[35,37,41,135,136] except on feet.[35,135] Additionally, these studies show that the predominant species of *Malassezia* can vary based on the location on the skin surface.[35,135] Mycobiome studies showed *M. restricta* was predominant on the head and facial areas of healthy adult volunteers and *M. globosa* was predominant on truncal areas of skin in the same subjects. Other skin sites evaluated demonstrated mixed communities of *Malassezia*. In the studies examining fungal communities of feet, non-*Malassezia* fungi (eg, *Aspergillus, Cryptococcus, Epicoccum, Rhodotorula*) predominated.[35,135]

The topographical distribution of skin fungi likely reflects the heterogeneity of the many microenvironments of the human skin surface and the abilities of various fungal species to adapt to a particular skin region. As the predominant skin fungi, *Malassezia* isolates from skin have been studied and are known to lack the fatty synthase gene. Thus, *Malassezia* spp. are lipid-dependent and generally require lipid supplements for growth in the laboratory. Genomic differences have been identified among multiple different *Malassezia* species, particularly in the lipase and phos-

TABLE 16-1
Skin Microbiome Findings in Dermatologic Disorders[a]

SKIN DISEASE	SKIN MICROBIOME FINDINGS
Acne	Different strains of *Cutibacterium acnes* associated with acne patients versus controls; staphylococci are also associated with acne patients.
Atopic dermatitis	Increased relative abundances of *Staphylococcus aureus* and *Staphylococcus epidermidis* observed in flared skin; different *S. aureus* clonal strains associated with atopic dermatitis; higher fungal diversity associated with atopic dermatitis as compared to controls.
Diabetic skin and wounds	Bacterial communities in diabetic skin are less diverse; diabetic wounds associated with staphylococci and some fungi.
Primary immunodeficiency syndrome-associated dermatitis	Higher numbers of different fungi with increased *Aspergillus* and *Candida*.
Psoriasis	Lesional skin associated with decreased bacterial diversity; higher fungal diversity observed in psoriasis versus controls.

[a]Examples of microbiome findings described in patients with several dermatologic disorders.

pholipase gene content.[137] The variation in lipid profiles across different skin regions could account for the preferences of certain species of *Malassezia* found in some skin sites as compared to other sites.[138,139]

As observed in microbiome studies examining skin bacterial communities, fungal skin communities also differ depending on the age of the individual. Younger individuals are typically colonized by *Malassezia* less frequently and in lower abundances than in adults; however, colonization rates increase as individuals age during puberty and adulthood (Fig. 16-2).[134,140,141] These cultivation-based results were similar to a ITS1-based mycobiome study in which healthy preadolescent subjects between the ages of 8 and 13 years had low relative abundances of *Malassezia* and higher fungal diversity than healthy adults.[142] This has been attributed to the lipid-dependence of *Malassezia* and the increased sebaceous gland activity and sebum production in the skin of pubertal and adult individuals.[40] Additional differences are also observed in the predominant species of *Malassezia* in the skin of healthy children and more sexually mature individuals. Both culture-based and culture-independent methods show that adults have lower relative abundances of *M. globosa* and higher relative abundances of *M. restricta*. In contrast, children typically have higher relative abundances of *M. restricta* among the *Malassezia* spp. observed in their skin.[35,40,135] This distinction may be based on the variability in the lipid preferences of different *Malassezia* species.[137,142,143]

Interestingly, the high relative abundance of *Malassezia* spp. in postpubertal individuals corresponds to the higher frequency of tinea versicolor in adults, and the higher relative abundances of non-*Malassezia* fungi in the skin of prepubertal children corresponds to the higher prevalence of tinea capitis and tinea corporis in pediatric populations.[144-146] Whether mycobiome differences across different age ranges is directly linked with the predilection of dermatophyte infections in certain ages is unknown.[40] Mycobiome studies have also been performed in several dermatologic disorders, including psoriasis[37,147] and atopic dermatitis.[41] However, additional research is required to investigate whether the skin mycobiome influences dermatologic diseases.

GENOMICS STUDIES OF SKIN VIRAL COMMUNITIES

Skin viruses are of significant clinical interest because of the dermatologic diseases associated with viruses, including verruca vulgaris (human papillomaviruses), herpes labialis (herpes simplex viruses), and Merkel cell carcinoma (Merkel cell polyomavirus). Because studying cultured viruses requires use of living cells known to be infected by the viruses of interest, the application of sequencing could be used to facilitate investigations of cutaneous viruses. A major challenge of virome research is the lack of a marker gene common to all viruses, as compared to the 16S rRNA gene used for bacteria or the 18S rRNA/ITS1/28S rRNA genes used for fungi. Because DNA sequencing technology is more well-established than RNA sequencing, cutaneous virome studies have generally focused on DNA viruses and bacteriophages.

Shotgun metagenomic sequencing has been used to examine the healthy human skin virome.[42-46,49] The most common DNA viruses observed include bacteriophages, papillomaviruses, polyomaviruses, and circoviruses. The most common bacteriophages are those linked with *Cutibacterium* and *Staphylococcus*, which corresponds to the known presence of these bacterial genera in skin.[42-45] The populations of papillomaviruses observed in the microbiomes studies include both known human papillomaviruses and previously unknown papillomaviruses. With growing interest in human skin polyomaviruses after identification of the Merkel cell polyomavirus in Merkel cell carcinomas,[148] Merkel cell polyomavirus and other human polyomaviruses have been found in the skin of healthy individuals[149,150] and in some patients with skin diseases.[151-153] Unlike the site-specific predominance of bacterial and fungal communities observed in skin microbiome studies, the relative abundances of cutaneous viruses can vary widely over the skin surface within and between healthy individuals. Additionally, the stability of skin viral communities can fluctuate over time within the same person.[44] The application of culture-independent sequencing technologies will improve the ability to study skin viruses and potential links to dermatologic disorders.

CONCLUSIONS

A notable driver in the increase in human microbiome studies is the interest in the gut microbiome and the research examining the potential links to human disorders such as inflammatory bowel disorders, *Clostridium difficile* colitis, diabetes, cardiovascular diseases, and cancer immunotherapies. In addition, the promising therapeutic outcomes with the use of fecal microbiota transplantation in patients with refractory and debilitating *C. difficile* colitis has spawned significant enthusiasm in gut microbiome investigations. With the relative ease in collecting sufficient microbial DNA from the high microbial biomass in stool, gut microbiome studies significantly outnumber investigations of the skin microbiome.

Although the majority of human microbiome studies have focused on single body sites (gut, oral, vaginal, nares, or skin), human diseases, including those in the realm of dermatology, can be systemic disorders such as vitiligo and other autoimmune disorders, psoriasis and the links to psoriasis arthritis and cardiovascular disorders, or pyoderma gangrenosum and inflammatory bowel disease. Thus, there may be instances in which the gut bacteria may affect skin diseases, or skin bacteria may affect distal body sites. Noncutaneous microbiome studies have been performed in patients with der-

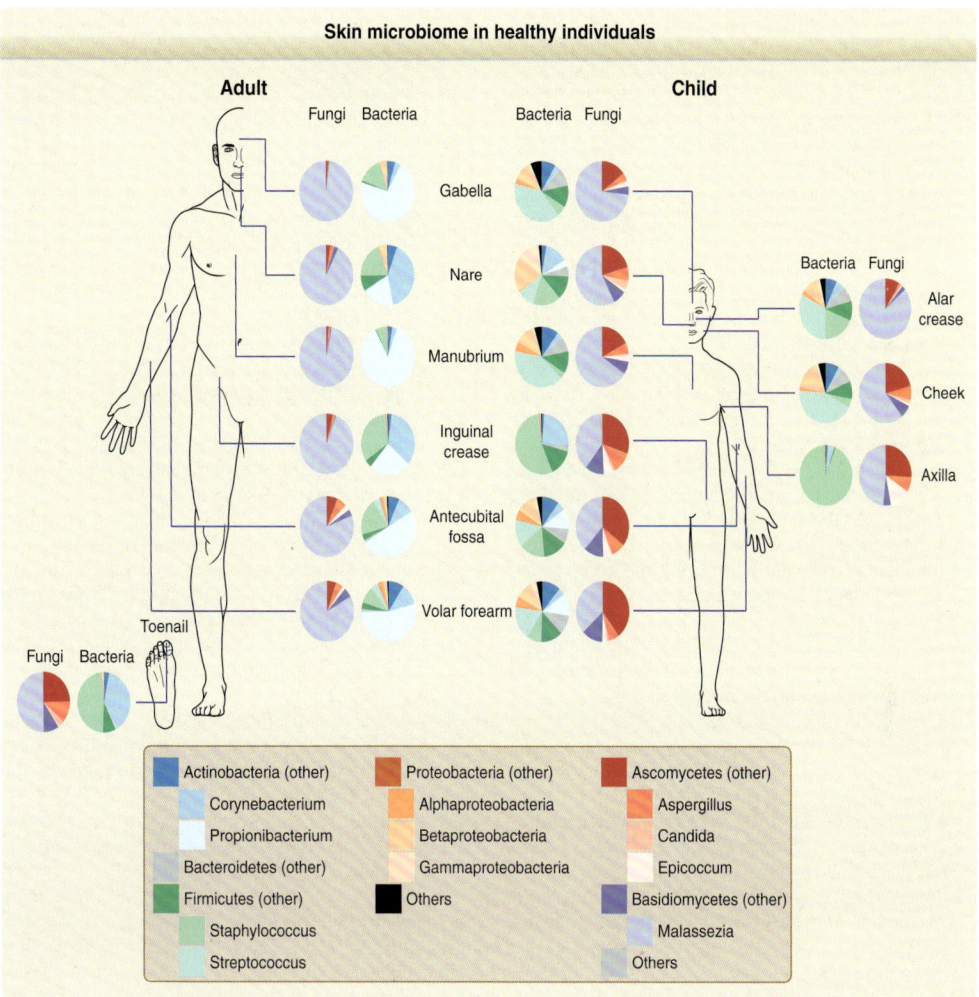

Figure 16-2 Skin microbiome in healthy individuals. The composition of skin bacterial and fungal communities from different anatomical regions in healthy adults are less diverse than in healthy children. (Figure derived from sequencing data from Jo et al.[40] and Findley et al.[35])

matologic conditions, including psoriasis/psoriatic arthritis[154] and atopic dermatitis.[155] These and other studies highlight the complexity of human disease and a major reason for the United States' National Institutes of Health Common Fund (the funder of the Human Microbiome Project) to bring together diverse areas of research from clinical medicine to basic research and from microbiology,[156] biochemistry, and molecular biology to -omics[157-159] and computational and systems biology, to jointly tackle these research challenges. Collaborative efforts across research fields and advances in technologies will be critical in unraveling the complexity of these diseases and the potential relationships with the human microbiome.

Some of the goals of investigating the skin microbiome are to determine how the microbial communities influence human health and disease and to potentially develop preventive or therapeutic interventions. To date, there remain significant gaps in both what is defined as a "healthy" skin microbiome and the understanding of the possible biologic links between the presence/absence and/or relative abundances of skin microbes and human health and disease. Although the therapeutic successes of fecal microbiota transplantation for *C. difficile* colitis has generated tremendous optimism for similar therapies for dermatologic conditions, enthusiasm has been tempered by the gaps in what is known about the skin microbiome and the factors that control the balance between commensalism and pathogenicity. Additional research will be fundamental to our ability to harness the power of the human skin microbiome.

REFERENCES

1. Dekio I, Hayashi H, Sakamoto M, et al. Detection of potentially novel bacterial components of the human skin microbiota using culture-independent molecular profiling. *J Med Microbiol*. 2005;54(pt 12):1231-1238.
2. Ross AA, Neufeld JD. Microbial biogeography of a university campus. *Microbiome*. 2015;3:66.

3. Shin H, Pei Z, Martinez KA 2nd, et al. The first microbial environment of infants born by C-section: the operating room microbes. *Microbiome*. 2015;3:59.
4. Wood M, Gibbons SM, Lax S, et al. Athletic equipment microbiota are shaped by interactions with human skin. *Microbiome*. 2015;3:25.
5. Bik HM, Maritz JM, Luong A, et al. Microbial community patterns associated with automated teller machine keypads in New York City. *mSphere*. 2016; 1(6):e00226.
6. Hsu T, Joice R, Vallarino J, et al. Urban transit system microbial communities differ by surface type and interaction with humans and the environment. *mSystems*. 2016;1(3):e00018.
7. Lax S, Smith DP, Hampton-Marcell J, et al. Longitudinal analysis of microbial interaction between humans and the indoor environment. *Science*. 2014;345(6200):1048-1052.
8. Fierer N, Lauber CL, Zhou N, et al. Forensic identification using skin bacterial communities. *Proc Natl Acad Sci U S A*. 2010;107(14):6477-6481.
9. Miletto M, Lindow SE. Relative and contextual contribution of different sources to the composition and abundance of indoor air bacteria in residences. *Microbiome*. 2015;3:61.
10. Song SJ, Lauber C, Costello EK, et al. Cohabiting family members share microbiota with one another and with their dogs. *Elife*. 2013;2:e00458.
11. Chase J, Fouquier J, Zare M, et al. Geography and location are the primary drivers of office microbiome composition. *mSystems*. 2016;1(2):e00022.
12. Abeles SR, Jones MB, Santiago-Rodriguez TM, et al. Microbial diversity in individuals and their household contacts following typical antibiotic courses. *Microbiome*. 2016; 4(1):39.
13. Two AM, Nakatsuji T, Kotol PF, et al. The cutaneous microbiome and aspects of skin antimicrobial defense system resist acute treatment with topical skin cleansers. *J Invest Dermatol*. 2016;136(10):1950-1954.
14. Perez Perez GI, Gao Z, Jourdain R, et al. Body site is a more determinant factor than human population diversity in the healthy skin microbiome. *PLoS One*. 2016;11(4):e0151990.
15. Dominguez-Bello MG, De Jesus-Laboy KM, Shen N, et al. Partial restoration of the microbiota of cesarean-born infants via vaginal microbial transfer. *Nat Med*. 2016;22(3):250-253.
16. Afshinnekoo EC, Meydan C, Chowdhury S, et al. Geospatial resolution of human and bacterial diversity with city-scale metagenomics. *Cell Syst*. 2015;1(1):72-87.
17. Misic AM, Davis MF, Tyldsley AS, et al. The shared microbiota of humans and companion animals as evaluated from Staphylococcus carriage sites. *Microbiome*. 2015;3:2.
18. Robertson CE, Baumgartner LK, Harris JK, et al. Culture-independent analysis of aerosol microbiology in a metropolitan subway system. *Appl Environ Microbiol*. 2013;79(11):3485-3493.
19. Leyden JJ, Marples RR, Kligman AM. Staphylococcus aureus in the lesions of atopic dermatitis. *Br J Dermatol*. 1974;90(5):525-530.
20. Marples M. *The Ecology of the Human Skin*. Springfield, IL: Charles C Thomas; 1965.
21. Nizet V, Ohtake T, Lauth X, et al. Innate antimicrobial peptide protects the skin from invasive bacterial infection. *Nature*. 2001;414(6862):454-457.
22. Noble WC, Somerville DA. Microbiology of human skin. In: Rook AH, ed. *Major Problems in Dermatology*. Vol 2. 2nd ed. London, UK: WB Saunders; 1974:341.
23. Sanford JA, Gallo RL. Functions of the skin microbiota in health and disease. *Semin Immunol*. 2013;25(5): 370-377.
24. Pillsbury DM, Nichols AC. Bacterial flora of the normal and infected skin; an evaluation of various methods of performing skin cultures. *J Invest Dermatol*. 1946;7(6):365-373.
25. Evans CA, Smith WM, Johnston EA, et al. Bacterial flora of the normal human skin. *J Invest Dermatol*. 1950;15(4):305-324.
26. Somerville DA. The normal flora of the skin in different age groups. *Br J Dermatol*. 1969;81(4):248-258.
27. Marples RR, Downing DT, Kligman AM. Control of free fatty acids in human surface lipids by Corynebacterium acnes. *J Invest Dermatol*. 1971;56(2):127-131.
28. Aly R, Maibach HE, Mandel A. Bacterial flora in psoriasis. *Br J Dermatol*. 1976;95(6):603-606.
29. Marchesi JR, Ravel J. The vocabulary of microbiome research: a proposal. *Microbiome*. 2015;3:31.
30. Human Microbiome Project Consortium. Structure, function and diversity of the healthy human microbiome. *Nature*. 2012;486(7402):207-214.
31. Human Microbiome Project Consortium. A framework for human microbiome research. *Nature*. 2012; 486(7402):215-221.
32. Aagaard K, Petrosino J, Keitel W, et al. The Human Microbiome Project strategy for comprehensive sampling of the human microbiome and why it matters. *FASEB J*. 2013;27(3):1012-1022.
33. Woese CR, Fox GE. Phylogenetic structure of the prokaryotic domain: the primary kingdoms. *Proc Natl Acad Sci U S A*. 1977;74(11):5088-5090.
34. Konstantinidis KT, Tiedje JM. Genomic insights that advance the species definition for prokaryotes. *Proc Natl Acad Sci U S A*. 2005;102(7):2567-2572.
35. Findley K, Oh J, Yang J, et al. Topographic diversity of fungal and bacterial communities in human skin. *Nature*. 2013;498(7454):367-370.
36. Khot PD, Ko DL, Fredricks DN. Sequencing and analysis of fungal rRNA operons for development of broad-range fungal PCR assays. *Appl Environ Microbiol*. 2009;75(6):1559-1565.
37. Paulino LC, Tseng CH, Strober BE, et al. Molecular analysis of fungal microbiota in samples from healthy human skin and psoriatic lesions. *J Clin Microbiol*. 2006;44(8):2933-2941.
38. Sugita T, Yamazaki T, Makimura K, et al. Comprehensive analysis of the skin fungal microbiota of astronauts during a half-year stay at the International Space Station. *Med Mycol*. 2016;54(3):232-239.
39. Wang L, Clavaud C, Bar-Hen A, et al. Characterization of the major bacterial-fungal populations colonizing dandruff scalps in Shanghai, China, shows microbial disequilibrium. *Exp Dermatol*. 2015;24(5):398-400.
40. Jo JH, Deming C, Kennedy EA, et al. Diverse human skin fungal communities in children converge in adulthood. *J Invest Dermatol*. 2016;136(12): 2356-2363.
41. Zhang E, Tanaka T, Tajima M, et al. Characterization of the skin fungal microbiota in patients with atopic dermatitis and in healthy subjects. *Microbiol Immunol*. 2011;55(9):625-632.
42. Hannigan GD, Meisel JS, Tyldsley AS, et al. The human skin double-stranded DNA virome: topographical and temporal diversity, genetic enrichment, and

dynamic associations with the host microbiome. *MBio*. 2015;6(5):e01578-15.
43. Oh J, Byrd AL, Deming C, et al. Biogeography and individuality shape function in the human skin metagenome. *Nature*. 2014;514(7520):59-64.
44. Oh J, Byrd AL, Park M, et al. Temporal stability of the human skin microbiome. *Cell*. 2016;165(4):854-866.
45. Foulongne V, Sauvage V, Hebert C, et al. Human skin microbiota: high diversity of DNA viruses identified on the human skin by high throughput sequencing. *PLoS One*. 2012;7(6):e38499.
46. Wylie KM, Mihindukulasuriya KA, Zhou Y, et al. Metagenomic analysis of double-stranded DNA viruses in healthy adults. *BMC Biol*. 2014;12:71.
47. Bzhalava D, Muhr LS, Lagheden C, et al. Deep sequencing extends the diversity of human papillomaviruses in human skin. *Sci Rep*. 2014;4:5807.
48. Deng Q, Li J, Pan Y, et al. Prevalence and associated risk factors of human papillomavirus in healthy skin specimens collected from rural Anyang, China, 2006-2008. *J Invest Dermatol*. 2016;136(6):1191-1198.
49. Ma Y, Madupu R, Karaoz U, et al. Human papillomavirus community in healthy persons, defined by metagenomics analysis of human microbiome project shotgun sequencing data sets. *J Virol*. 2014;88(9):4786-4797.
50. Goodrich JK, Di Rienzi SC, Poole AC, et al. Conducting a microbiome study. *Cell*. 2014;158(2):250-262.
51. Lauber CL, Zhou N, Gordon JI, et al. Effect of storage conditions on the assessment of bacterial community structure in soil and human-associated samples. *FEMS Microbiol Lett*. 2010;307(1):80-86.
52. Weiss S, Amir A, Hyde ER, et al. Tracking down the sources of experimental contamination in microbiome studies. *Genome Biol*. 2014;15(12):564.
53. Kong HH, Andersson B, Clavel T, et al. Performing skin microbiome research: a method to the madness. *J Invest Dermatol*. 2017;137(3):561-568.
54. Costello EK, Lauber CL, Hamady M, et al. Bacterial community variation in human body habitats across space and time. *Science*. 2009;326(5960):1694-1697.
55. Grice EA, Kong HH, Conlan S, et al. Topographical and temporal diversity of the human skin microbiome. *Science*. 2009. 324(5931):1190-1192.
56. Korem T, Zeevi D, Suez J, et al. Growth dynamics of gut microbiota in health and disease inferred from single metagenomic samples. *Science*. 2015;349(6252):1101-1106.
57. Kligman AM, Leyden JJ, McGinley KJ. Bacteriology. *J Invest Dermatol*. 1976;67(1):160-168.
58. Lai Y, Di Nardo A, Nakatsuji T, et al. Commensal bacteria regulate toll-like receptor 3-dependent inflammation after skin injury. *Nat Med*. 2009;15(12):1377-1382.
59. Leyden JJ, McGinley KJ, Nordstrom KM, et al. Skin microflora. *J Invest Dermatol*. 1987;88(3)(suppl):65s-72s.
60. Marples MJ. The normal flora of the human skin. *Br J Dermatol*. 1969;81(suppl 1):2-13.
61. Cogen AL, Nizet V, Gallo RL. Skin microbiota: a source of disease or defence? *Br J Dermatol*. 2008;158(3):442-455.
62. Chiller K, Selkin BA, Murakawa GJ. Skin microflora and bacterial infections of the skin. *J Investig Dermatol Symp Proc*. 2001;6(3):170-174.
63. Kong HH. Skin microbiome: genomics-based insights into the diversity and role of skin microbes. *Trends Mol Med*. 2011;17(6):320-328.
64. Grice EA, Segre JA. The skin microbiome. *Nat Rev Microbiol*. 2011;9(4):244-253.
65. Puhvel SM, Reisner RM, Amirian DA. Quantification of bacteria in isolated pilosebaceous follicles in normal skin. *J Invest Dermatol*. 1975;65(6):525-531.
66. Nakatsuji T, Chiang HI, Jiang SB, et al. The microbiome extends to subepidermal compartments of normal skin. *Nat Commun*. 2013;4:1431.
67. Gao Z, Tseng CH, Pei Z, et al. Molecular analysis of human forearm superficial skin bacterial biota. *Proc Natl Acad Sci U S A*. 2007;104(8):2927-2932.
68. Grice EA, Kong HH, Renaud G, et al. A diversity profile of the human skin microbiota. *Genome Res*. 2008;18(7):1043-1050.
69. Ogawa T, Katsuoka K, Kawano K, et al. Comparative study of staphylococcal flora on the skin surface of atopic dermatitis patients and healthy subjects. *J Dermatol*. 1994;21(7):453-460.
70. Hartmann AA. Effect of occlusion on resident flora, skin-moisture and skin-pH. *Arch Dermatol Res*. 1983;275(4):251-254.
71. Fierer N, Hamady M, Lauber CL, et al. The influence of sex, handedness, and washing on the diversity of hand surface bacteria. *Proc Natl Acad Sci U S A*. 2008;105(46):17994-17999.
72. Flores GE, Caporaso JG, Henley JB, et al. Temporal variability is a personalized feature of the human microbiome. *Genome Biol*. 2014;15(12):531.
73. Bashan A, Gibson TE, Friedman J, et al. Universality of human microbial dynamics. *Nature*. 2016;534(7606):259-262.
74. Clemente JC, Pehrsson EC, Blaser MJ, et al. The microbiome of uncontacted Amerindians. *Sci Adv*. 2015;1(3):e1500183.
75. Leung MH, Wilkins D, Lee PK. Insights into the pan-microbiome: skin microbial communities of Chinese individuals differ from other racial groups. *Sci Rep*. 2015;5:11845.
76. Hospodsky D, Pickering AJ, Julian TR, et al. Hand bacterial communities vary across two different human populations. *Microbiology*. 2014;160(pt 6):1144-1152.
77. Qin J, Li R, Raes J, et al. A human gut microbial gene catalogue established by metagenomic sequencing. *Nature*. 2010;464(7285):59-65.
78. Lee MM. Physical and structural age changes in human skin. *Anat Rec*. 1957;129(4):473-493.
79. Leyden JJ, McGinley KJ, Mills OH, et al. Age-related changes in the resident bacterial flora of the human face. *J Invest Dermatol*. 1975;65(4):379-381.
80. Capone KA, Dowd SE, Stamatas GN, et al. Diversity of the human skin microbiome early in life. *J Invest Dermatol*. 2011;131(10):2026-2032.
81. Costello EK, Carlisle EM, Bik EM, et al. Microbiome assembly across multiple body sites in low-birth-weight infants. *MBio*. 2013;4(6):e00782-13.
82. Dominguez-Bello MG, Costello EK, Contreras M, et al. Delivery mode shapes the acquisition and structure of the initial microbiota across multiple body habitats in newborns. *Proc Natl Acad Sci U S A*. 2010;107(26):11971-11975.
83. Kennedy EA, Connolly J, Hourihane JO, et al. Skin microbiome before development of atopic dermatitis: Early colonization with commensal staphylococci at 2 months is associated with a lower risk of atopic dermatitis at 1 year. *J Allergy Clin Immunol*. 2017;139(1):166-172.
84. Oh J, Conlan S, Polley EC, et al. Shifts in human skin and nares microbiota of healthy children and adults. *Genome Med*. 2012;4(10):77.

85. Ying S, Zeng DN, Chi L, et al. The influence of age and gender on skin-associated microbial communities in urban and rural human populations. *PLoS One*. 2015;10(10):e0141842.
86. Mukherjee S, Mitra R, Maitra A, et al. Sebum and hydration levels in specific regions of human face significantly predict the nature and diversity of facial skin microbiome. *Sci Rep*. 2016;6:36062.
87. Si J, Lee S, Park JM, et al. Genetic associations and shared environmental effects on the skin microbiome of Korean twins. *BMC Genomics*. 2015;16:992.
88. Aly R, Maibach HI, Shinefield HR. Microbial flora of atopic dermatitis. *Arch Dermatol*. 1977;113(6):780-782.
89. Chng KR, Tay AS, Li C, et al. Whole metagenome profiling reveals skin microbiome-dependent susceptibility to atopic dermatitis flare. *Nat Microbiol*. 2016;1(9):16106.
90. Gonzalez ME, Schaffer JV, Orlow SJ, et al. Cutaneous microbiome effects of fluticasone propionate cream and adjunctive bleach baths in childhood atopic dermatitis. *J Am Acad Dermatol*. 2016;75(3):481-493 e8.
91. Kong HH, Oh J, Deming C, et al. Temporal shifts in the skin microbiome associated with disease flares and treatment in children with atopic dermatitis. *Genome Res*. 2012;22(5):850-859.
92. Seite S, Flores GE, Henley JB, et al. Microbiome of affected and unaffected skin of patients with atopic dermatitis before and after emollient treatment. *J Drugs Dermatol*. 2014;13(11):1365-1372.
93. Shi B, Bangayan NJ, Curd E, et al. The skin microbiome is different in pediatric versus adult atopic dermatitis. *J Allergy Clin Immunol*. 2016;138(4):1233-1236.
94. Nakatsuji T, Chen TH, Two AM, et al. *Staphylococcus aureus* exploits epidermal barrier defects in atopic dermatitis to trigger cytokine expression. *J Invest Dermatol*. 2016;136(11):2192-2200.
95. Laouini D, Kawamoto S, Yalcindag A, et al. Epicutaneous sensitization with superantigen induces allergic skin inflammation. *J Allergy Clin Immunol*. 2003;112(5):981-987.
96. Nakamura Y, Oscherwitz J, Cease KB, et al. *Staphylococcus* delta-toxin induces allergic skin disease by activating mast cells. *Nature*. 2013;503(7476):397-401.
97. Brauweiler AM, Goleva E, Leung DY. Th2 cytokines increase *Staphylococcus aureus* alpha toxin-induced keratinocyte death through the signal transducer and activator of transcription 6 (STAT6). *J Invest Dermatol*. 2014;134(8):2114-2121.
98. Kaesler S, Skabytska Y, Chen KM, et al. *Staphylococcus aureus*-derived lipoteichoic acid induces temporary T-cell paralysis independent of toll-like receptor 2. *J Allergy Clin Immunol*. 2016;138(3):780-790 e6.
99. Kobayashi T, Glatz M, Horiuchi K, et al. Dysbiosis and *Staphylococcus aureus* colonization drives inflammation in atopic dermatitis. *Immunity*. 2015; 42(4):756-766.
100. Scharschmidt TC, Vasquez KS, Truong HA, et al. A wave of regulatory T cells into neonatal skin mediates tolerance to commensal microbes. *Immunity*. 2015;43(5):1011-1021.
101. Fry L, Baker BS, Powles AV, et al. Is chronic plaque psoriasis triggered by microbiota in the skin? *Br J Dermatol*. 2013;169(1):47-52.
102. Noble WC, Savin JA. Carriage of *Staphylococcus aureus* in psoriasis. *Br Med J*. 1968;1(5589):417-418.
103. Norrlind R. Psoriasis following infections with hemolytic streptococci. *Acta Derm Venereol*. 1950;30(1):64-72.
104. Martin R, Henley JB, Sarrazin P, et al. Skin microbiome in patients with psoriasis before and after balneotherapy at the Thermal Care Center of La Roche-Posay. *J Drugs Dermatol*. 2015;14(12):1400-1405.
105. Alekseyenko AV, Perez-Perez GI, De Souza A, et al. Community differentiation of the cutaneous microbiota in psoriasis. *Microbiome*. 2013;1(1):31.
106. Gao Z, Tseng CH, Strober BE, et al. Substantial alterations of the cutaneous bacterial biota in psoriatic lesions. *PLoS One*. 2008;3(7):e2719.
107. Statnikov A, Alekseyenko AV, Li Z, et al. Microbiomic signatures of psoriasis: feasibility and methodology comparison. *Sci Rep*. 2013;3:2620.
108. Fahlen A, Engstrand L, Baker BS, et al. Comparison of bacterial microbiota in skin biopsies from normal and psoriatic skin. *Arch Dermatol Res*. 2012;304(1):15-22.
109. Kirschbaum JO, Kligman AM. The pathogenic role of *Corynebacterium acnes* in acne vulgaris. *Arch Dermatol*. 1963;88:832-833.
110. Marples RR, McGinley KJ, Mills OH. Microbiology of comedones in acne vulgaris. *J Invest Dermatol*. 1973;60(2):80-83.
111. Kang D, Shi B, Erfe MC, et al. Vitamin B12 modulates the transcriptome of the skin microbiota in acne pathogenesis. *Sci Transl Med*. 2015;7(293):293ra103.
112. Liu J, Yan R, Zhong Q, et al. The diversity and host interactions of Propionibacterium acnes bacteriophages on human skin. *ISME J*. 2015;9(9):2078-2093.
113. Marinelli LJ, Fitz-Gibbon S, Hayes C, et al. *Propionibacterium acnes* bacteriophages display limited genetic diversity and broad killing activity against bacterial skin isolates. *MBio*. 2012;3(5):e00279-12.
114. Bek-Thomsen M, Lomholt HB, Kilian M. Acne is not associated with yet-uncultured bacteria. *J Clin Microbiol*. 2008;46(10):3355-3360.
115. Fitz-Gibbon S, Tomida S, Chiu BH, et al. *Propionibacterium acnes* strain populations in the human skin microbiome associated with acne. *J Invest Dermatol*. 2013;133(9):2152-2160.
116. Christensen GJ, Scholz CF, Enghild J, et al. Antagonism between *Staphylococcus epidermidis* and *Propionibacterium acnes* and its genomic basis. *BMC Genomics*. 2016;17:152.
117. Numata S, Akamatsu H, Akaza N, et al. Analysis of facial skin-resident microbiota in Japanese acne patients. *Dermatology*. 2014;228(1):86-92.
118. Yu Y, Champer J, Agak GW, et al. Different *Propionibacterium acnes* phylotypes induce distinct immune responses and express unique surface and secreted proteomes. *J Invest Dermatol*. 2016;136(11):2221-2228.
119. Hanski I, von Hertzen L, Fyhrquist N, et al. Environmental biodiversity, human microbiota, and allergy are interrelated. *Proc Natl Acad Sci U S A*. 2012;109(21):8334-8339.
120. Horton JM, Gao Z, Sullivan DM, et al. The cutaneous microbiome in outpatients presenting with acute skin abscesses. *J Infect Dis*. 2015;211(12):1895-1904.
121. van Rensburg JJ, Lin H, Gao X, et al. The human skin microbiome associates with the outcome of and is influenced by bacterial infection. *MBio*. 2015;6(5):e01315-15.
122. Troccaz M, Gaia N, Beccucci S, et al. Mapping axillary microbiota responsible for body odours using a culture-independent approach. *Microbiome*. 2015; 3(1):3.
123. Gardner SE, Hillis SL, Heilmann K, et al. The neuropathic diabetic foot ulcer microbiome is associated with clinical factors. *Diabetes*. 2013;62(3):923-930.

124. Redel H, Gao Z, Li H, et al. Quantitation and composition of cutaneous microbiota in diabetic and nondiabetic men. *J Infect Dis*. 2013;207(7):1105-1114.
125. Gontcharova V, Youn E, Sun Y, et al. A comparison of bacterial composition in diabetic ulcers and contralateral intact skin. *Open Microbiol J*. 2010;4:8-19.
126. Zeeuwen PL, Ederveen TH, van der Krieken DA, et al. Gram-positive anaerobe cocci are underrepresented in the microbiome of filaggrin-deficient human skin. *J Allergy Clin Immunol*. 2017;139(4):1368-1371.
127. Salava A, Aho V, Pereira P, et al. Skin microbiome in melanomas and melanocytic nevi. *Eur J Dermatol*. 2016;26(1):49-55.
128. Dereure O, Cheval J, Du Thanh A, et al. No evidence for viral sequences in mycosis fungoides and Sezary syndrome skin lesions: a high-throughput sequencing approach. *J Invest Dermatol*. 2013;133(3):853-855.
129. Ganju P, Nagpal S, Mohammed MH, et al. Microbial community profiling shows dysbiosis in the lesional skin of vitiligo subjects. *Sci Rep*. 2016;6:18761.
130. Oh J, Freeman AF, NISC Comparative Sequencing Program, et al. The altered landscape of the human skin microbiome in patients with primary immunodeficiencies. *Genome Res*. 2013;23(12):2103-2114.
131. Smeekens SP, Huttenhower C, Riza A, et al. Skin microbiome imbalance in patients with STAT1/STAT3 defects impairs innate host defense responses. *J Innate Immun*. 2014;6(3):253-262.
132. Gueho E, Midgley G, Guillot J. The genus *Malassezia* with description of four new species. *Antonie Van Leeuwenhoek*. 1996;69(4):337-355.
133. Aspiroz C, Moreno LA, Rezusta A, et al. Differentiation of three biotypes of *Malassezia* species on human normal skin. correspondence with *M. globosa, M. sympodialis* and *M. restricta. Mycopathologia*. 1999;145(2):69-74.
134. Sugita T, Suzuki M, Goto S, et al. Quantitative analysis of the cutaneous *Malassezia* microbiota in 770 healthy Japanese by age and gender using a real-time PCR assay. *Med Mycol*. 2010;48(2):229-233.
135. Zhang E, Tanaka T, Tsuboi R, et al. Characterization of *Malassezia* microbiota in the human external auditory canal and on the sole of the foot. *Microbiol Immunol*. 2012;56(4):238-244.
136. Leung MH, Chan KC, Lee PK. Skin fungal community and its correlation with bacterial community of urban Chinese individuals. *Microbiome*. 2016;4(1):46.
137. Wu G, Zhao H, Li C, et al. Genus-wide comparative genomics of *Malassezia* delineates its phylogeny, physiology, and niche adaptation on human skin. *PLoS Genet*. 2015;11(11):e1005614.
138. Michael-Jubeli R, Bleton J, Baillet-Guffroy A. High-temperature gas chromatography-mass spectrometry for skin surface lipids profiling. *J Lipid Res*. 2011;52(1):143-151.
139. Warren R, Wertz PW, Kirkbride T, et al. Comparative analysis of skin surface lipids of the labia majora, inner thigh, and forearm. *Skin Pharmacol Physiol*. 2011;24(6):294-299.
140. Faergemann J, Fredriksson T. Age incidence of *Pityrosporum orbiculare* on human skin. *Acta Derm Venereol*. 1980;60(6):531-533.
141. Gupta AK, Kohli Y. Prevalence of *Malassezia* species on various body sites in clinically healthy subjects representing different age groups. *Med Mycol*. 2004;42(1):35-42.
142. Yamamoto A, Serizawa S, Ito M, et al. Effect of aging on sebaceous gland activity and on the fatty acid composition of wax esters. *J Invest Dermatol*. 1987;89(5):507-512.
143. Pochi PE, Strauss JS, Downing DT. Age-related changes in sebaceous gland activity. *J Invest Dermatol*. 1979;73(1):108-111.
144. Havlickova B, Czaika VA, Friedrich M. Epidemiological trends in skin mycoses worldwide. *Mycoses*. 2008;51(suppl 4):2-15.
145. Seebacher C, Bouchara JP, Mignon B. Updates on the epidemiology of dermatophyte infections. *Mycopathologia*. 2008;166(5-6):335-352.
146. Kyriakis KP, Terzoudi S, Palamaras I, et al. Pityriasis versicolor prevalence by age and gender. *Mycoses*. 2006;49(6):517-518.
147. Takemoto A, Cho O, Morohoshi Y, et al. Molecular characterization of the skin fungal microbiome in patients with psoriasis. *J Dermatol*. 2015;42(2):166-170.
148. Feng H, Shuda M, Chang Y, et al. Clonal integration of a polyomavirus in human Merkel cell carcinoma. *Science*. 2008;319(5866):1096-1100.
149. Schowalter RM, Pastrana DV, Pumphrey KA, et al. Merkel cell polyomavirus and two previously unknown polyomaviruses are chronically shed from human skin. *Cell Host Microbe*. 2010;7(6):509-515.
150. Foulongne V, Dereure O, Kluger N, et al. Merkel cell polyomavirus DNA detection in lesional and nonlesional skin from patients with Merkel cell carcinoma or other skin diseases. *Br J Dermatol*. 2010;162(1):59-63.
151. Matthews MR, Wang RC, Reddick RL, et al. Viral-associated trichodysplasia spinulosa: a case with electron microscopic and molecular detection of the trichodysplasia spinulosa-associated human polyomavirus. *J Cutan Pathol*. 2011;38(5):420-431.
152. Nguyen KD, Lee EE, Yue Y, et al. Human polyomavirus 6 and 7 are associated with pruritic and dyskeratotic dermatoses. *J Am Acad Dermatol*. 2017;76(5):932-940.e3.
153. Stroh LJ, Gee GV, Blaum BS, et al. Trichodysplasia spinulosa-associated polyomavirus uses a displaced binding site on VP1 to engage sialylated glycolipids. *PLoS Pathog*. 2015;11(8):e1005112.
154. Scher JU, Ubeda C, Artacho A, et al. Decreased bacterial diversity characterizes the altered gut microbiota in patients with psoriatic arthritis, resembling dysbiosis in inflammatory bowel disease. *Arthritis Rheumatol*. 2015;67(1):128-139.
155. Song H, Yoo Y, Hwang J, et al. Faecalibacterium prausnitzii subspecies-level dysbiosis in the human gut microbiome underlying atopic dermatitis. *J Allergy Clin Immunol*. 2016;137(3):852-860.
156. Myles IA, Reckhow JD, Williams KW, et al. A method for culturing Gram-negative skin microbiota. *BMC Microbiol*. 2016;16:60.
157. Bouslimani A, Porto C, Rath CM, et al. Molecular cartography of the human skin surface in 3D. *Proc Natl Acad Sci U S A*. 2015;112(17):E2120-E2129.
158. Petras D, Nothias LF, Quinn RA, et al. Mass spectrometry-based visualization of molecules associated with human habitats. *Anal Chem*. 2016;88(22):10775-10784.
159. Arron ST, Dimon MT, Li Z, et al. High *Rhodotorula* sequences in skin transcriptome of patients with diffuse systemic sclerosis. *J Invest Dermatol*. 2014;134(8):2138-2145.

Chapter 17 :: Cutaneous Photobiology
:: Thomas M. Rünger

第十七章
皮肤光生物学

中文导读

本章内容分为5节：①紫外线和可见光辐射源；②光物理学、光化学和光生物学：电磁辐射与皮肤相互作用的原理；③皮肤对紫外线的反应；④皮肤对可见光和红外辐射的反应；⑤结论。介绍紫外线、可见光和红外线对皮肤的影响。对光物理、光化学和光生物过程的深入了解有助于了解皮肤暴露在这些类型的辐射下的临床表现，包括晒伤、晒黑、皮肤癌形成、光老化、光皮肤病以及对皮肤病的光治疗效果。

第一节紫外线和可见光辐射源，介绍了日光中UVA和UVB的特性。同时提到了人工光源，包括传统照明灯、工业应用灯、光疗灯、晒黑灯。临床上治疗炎症性皮肤病设计光的波长在311～312nm，不仅具有治疗效果，同时避免了导致晒伤但对治疗无效的较短波长的光。

第二节光物理学、光化学和光生物学：电磁辐射与皮肤相互作用的原理，介绍了光化学第一定律，也被称为格罗特苏-德雷珀定律，指出光必须首先被一种化学物质吸收，才能发生光化学反应。要使光子具有生物学上的相关结果，皮肤的光学因素和辐射的波长决定了光子在皮肤表面和皮肤内部反射和散射的数量和位置。

第三节皮肤对紫外线的反应，介绍了维生素D光生物学，详细讲述了维生素D的生物学功能。接下来介绍了紫外线对免疫系统的影响，既有促炎作用，又有抗炎作用。编者举例说明自身免疫性结缔组织疾病的诱导和触发以及炎症性皮肤病的光加重支持了促炎特性。然后介绍了不同波长的光在晒伤、晒黑、光疗的光生物学原理、光致癌的发生以及哪些波长的紫外线会导致皮肤癌、光老化等方面的作用及机制。

第四节皮肤对可见光和红外辐射的反应，介绍了目前对于可见光和红外辐射的影响研究较少，但越来越多的证据表明，这些物质对皮肤也有光生物效应。可见光会导致红斑和色素沉着。红外线与光老化和红斑有关。

第五节结论，介绍了UVR对皮肤唯一的积极影响，即维生素D的产生。但是因UVB、UVA、红外线和可见光的影响，光防护策略需要针对多种光进行。系统和局部抗氧化剂已经被用来减少紫外线、可见光和红外光诱导的氧化损伤，特别是氧化DNA损伤。2014年美国发布了预防皮肤癌的行动呼吁，其中就包括了防晒。

〔粟　娟〕

AT-A-GLANCE

- Radiation can only cause a photobiologic response, if it is first absorbed by a molecule (chromophore) in the skin.
- Understanding the photophysical, photochemical, and photobiologic effects of radiation exposure is helpful to understand the wavelength-dependent consequences, including burning, tanning, photodermatoses, formation of skin cancer, photoaging, and effects of phototherapy.
- Photoreactions have specific action spectra that depend on the absorption characteristics of various different intrinsic and extrinsic chromophores.
- Cutaneous vitamin D production is mediated by wavelengths within the UVB range. Optimal vitamin D blood levels are essential for good bone health and are increasingly associated with a myriad of other potential health benefits.
- Formation of DNA damage by ultraviolet radiation (UVR) mediates sunburning, tanning, and skin cancer formation.
- Skin cells are equipped with a number of damage response pathways that limit the negative impact of radiation exposure, including several different DNA repair mechanisms.
- Ultraviolet radiation–induced DNA damage can result in mutation formation. C to T and CC to TT mutations at dipyrimidine sites are highly characteristic for an induction by ultraviolet radiation and are called UV-signature mutations. Such UV-signature mutations are found in UV-induced skin cancers.
- Ultraviolet radiation has both pro- and antiinflammatory properties.
- Photoaging affects all compartments of the skin and is characterized by both clonal proliferative events and loss-of-function events.
- Photoaging is largely irreversible, possibly due in part to an UV-induced accumulation of undegradable abnormal proteins in the extra- and intracellular space.
- Exposure to visible light and infrared radiation also has photobiological consequences, including erythema, tanning, and degradation of extracellular matrix proteins.
- Rational phototherapy and photoprotection are based on these insights.

INTRODUCTION

As the outermost layer of the human body, skin is heavily exposed to damaging environmental agents, including different types of radiation (Table 17-1 and Fig. 17-1). Ionizing electromagnetic radiation, like, for example, x-rays or gamma rays, carries sufficient photon-energy to completely remove an electron from an atom or molecule (= ionization). Other types of ionizing radiation are alpha particles (2 protons and 2 neutrons) and beta particles (electrons). Alpha and beta particles are not part of the electromagnetic spectrum; they are energetic particles, as opposed to pure energy bundles (photons) of the electromagnetic radiation. Nonionizing radiation, which includes ultraviolet radiation (UVR), visible light, and infrared radiation, is able to move an electron to a higher energy state, but, in contrast to ionizing radiation, cannot remove an electron from atoms or molecules. Cutaneous photobiology is the science that studies the interaction of nonionizing radiation with skin. The term *light* is commonly reserved for wavelengths of the electromagnetic spectrum that are perceivable by the human eye: visible light.

Both ionizing and nonionizing radiation have detrimental effects on skin. Because during the development of life on earth, electromagnetic radiation has always been present, cells and organisms could only evolve with development of mechanisms that protect against the damaging effects of radiation. This chapter covers the effects of UVR, visible light, and infrared radiation on skin. Insights into the photophysical, photochemical, and photobiological processes help to understand clinical manifestations of skin exposure to these types of radiation, including sunburning, tanning, skin cancer formation, photoaging, photodermatoses, and phototherapeutic effects on skin diseases.

SOURCES OF ULTRAVIOLET AND VISIBLE RADIATION

SUNLIGHT

The shortest wavelength of solar electromagnetic radiation reaching the earth's surface is approximately 290 nm, although slightly shorter wavelengths are detected at higher altitudes. The filtering of UVC (100 to 290 nm) by the earth's atmosphere, in particular by ozone, is widely regarded a critical element in the development of life on earth, because the shorter wavelengths of UVR are highly damaging to animals and plants. The subdivisions of UVR (Table 17-1 and Fig. 17-1) and of the whole spectrum of electromagnetic radiation are rather arbitrary, and it is important to recognize that photophysical properties of photons do not change abruptly between the defined ranges, but rather gradually with changing wavelength. In general, energy decreases with increasing wavelength. For example, a 300-nm UVB photon has twice the energy of a 600-nm orange photon. The most commonly used subdivision of UVR is the one defined by the Commission Internationale de l'Eclairage, CIE, and sets 315 nm as the border between UVB and UVA. Other classifications use 320 nm. The defined threshold between ultraviolet and visible radiation is based on the properties of the human eye and its ability to sense radiation.

TABLE 17-1
Divisions and Subdivisions of Electromagnetic Radiation

NAME	WAVELENGTH RANGE	SUBDIVISION	WAVELENGTH RANGE
Ionizing Radiation			
Gamma-ray	10 fm-1 pm		
X-ray	1 pm-10 nm		
Vacuum ultraviolet	10 nm-200 nm		
Nonionizing Radiation			
Ultraviolet C	100 nm-290 nm		
Ultraviolet B	290 nm-315 nm		
Ultraviolet A	315 nm-400 nm	UVA2	315 nm-340 nm
		UVA1	340 nm-400 nm
Visible light	400 nm-760 nm	Violet	400 nm-450 nm
		Blue	450 nm-500 nm
		Green	500 nm-570 nm
		Yellow	570 nm-590 nm
		Orange	590 nm-610 nm
		Red	610 nm-760 nm
Infrared	760 nm-1 mm	IR-A	760 nm-1.4 mm
		IR-B	1.4 mm-3 mm
		IR-C	3 mm-1 mm
Microwaves and radio waves	>1 mm		

Some species, for example, birds, insects, and fish, can also see some UVA radiation.

The composition of solar radiation reaching the earth's surface varies with the time of the day because of changing angles of sunlight and with differences in the length solar radiation has to travel through the atmosphere. Shorter wavelengths of visible light (violet and blue) are more filtered by a longer passage through the atmosphere than longer wavelength of visible light (orange and red), resulting in redder light at sunrise and sunset, as compared to midday sunlight. Likewise, the longer wavelengths of UVR (UVA, 315 to 400 nm) penetrate matter better than UVB (280 to 315 nm). Therefore, the fraction of UVA relative to UVB increases with lower angles of solar radiation. At midday, natural sunlight contains about 50 times more UVA than UVB. Although both components are less abundant early or late in the day, the ratio between UVA and UVB increases with declining solar angles. Similarly, UVA can penetrate through window glass, but not UVB.

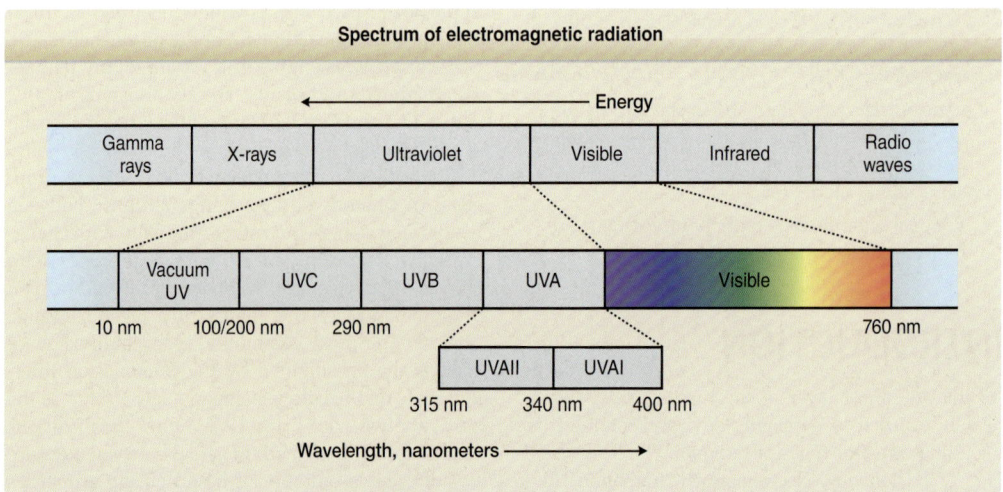

Figure 17-1 Spectrum of electromagnetic radiation divided into major wavelength regions and further subdivisions.

ARTIFICIAL SOURCES

There is a huge variety of different light sources that expose skin to visible, ultraviolet, and infrared radiation. These range from lamps used for conventional lighting purposes, for industrial applications, for phototherapy, and for tanning. Most of the light sources are designed to emit only the desired range of wavelength, for example, only visible light for lighting purposes. Nevertheless, some general lighting lamps sometimes emit small amounts of UVR, in particular fluorescent bulbs and halogen lamps. Unwanted wavelengths are often eliminated by filters. Fluorescent bulbs designed to emit UVR most often emit a broad range of wavelengths. For example, bulbs designed to emit UVA for photochemotherapy (PUVA) also emit some UVB, and those designed to emit UVB also emit some UVC. The Phillips TL01 fluorescent lamp has been a major advance in the design of UVB lamps for phototherapy, as it aligns its almost monochromatic emission at 311 to 312 nm, with therapeutic efficacy for inflammatory skin diseases, while avoiding shorter wavelengths that mostly cause sunburning, but are not effective for treatment.

PHOTOPHYSICS, PHOTOCHEMISTRY, AND PHOTOBIOLOGY: PRINCIPLES OF THE INTERACTION OF ELECTROMAGNETIC RADIATION WITH SKIN

For a photon to have biologically relevant consequences, a series of events must take place (Fig. 17-2). Optical factors of the skin and the wavelengths of the radiation determine how much and where a photon is reflected and scattered at the skin surface and within the skin. For ultraviolet and visible radiation, longer wavelengths penetrate matter better than shorter wavelengths. For example, UVA penetrates deeper into the dermis than UVB, of which only a small fraction penetrates deeper than the epidermis. UVC has the smallest penetration depth and in skin only reaches the stratum corneum and the upper layers of the epidermis (Fig. 17-3).

The first law of photochemistry, also known as the Grotthuß–Draper law, named after the chemists Freiherr Christian Johann Dietrich Theodor von Grotthuß and John William Draper, states that that light must first be absorbed by a chemical substance for a photochemical reaction to take place. A compound that absorbs radiation is called a chromophore. Each chromophore has a characteristic absorption spectrum, typically with one wavelength that is most likely to excite it (= absorption maximum) and a distribution of wavelengths that are less likely to do so. Well characterized chromophores in the skin are DNA

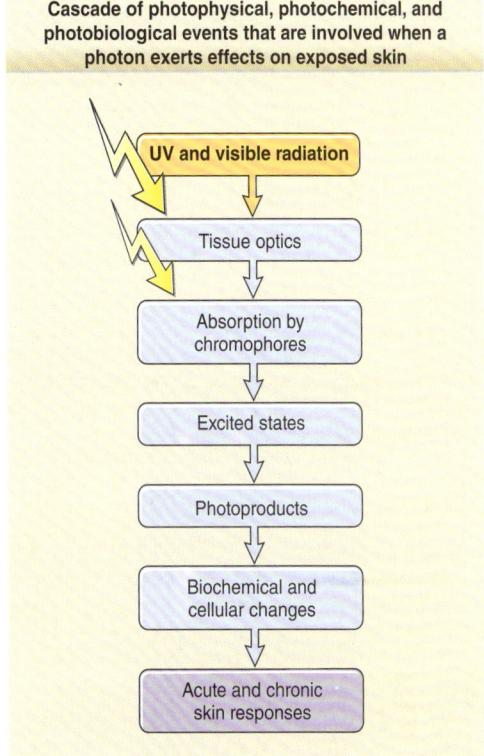

Figure 17-2 Series of photophysical, photochemical, and photobiological events that are required for a photon to have an effect on exposed skin.

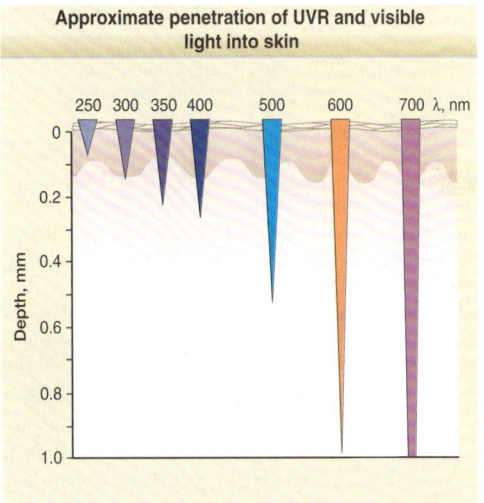

Figure 17-3 Approximate penetration of ultraviolet radiation and visible light into skin. λ = wavelength.

(absorption maximum at 260 nm), porphyrins (absorption maximum between 400 and 410 nm), and melanin (absorption maximum in the UVC range, but also very effectively excited by UVB and UVA) (Fig. 17-4).

When a chromophore in the ground state absorbs the energy of a photon, electrons are raised to a higher orbit.

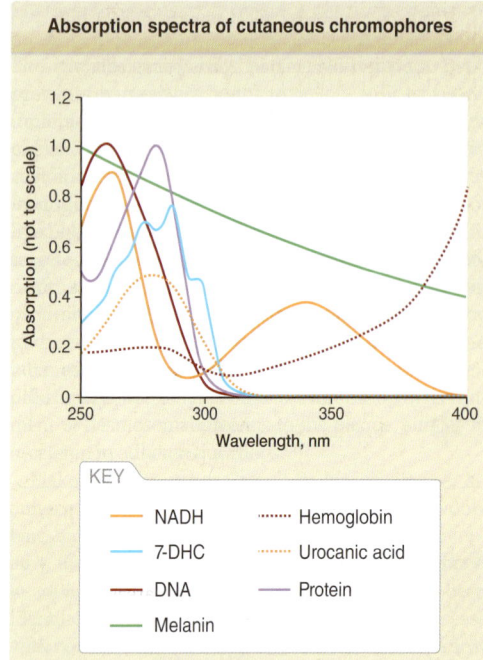

Figure 17-4 Absorption spectra of cutaneous chromophores absorbing ultraviolet radiation. Note that the relative amounts of UVR absorbed by these chromophores in skin depend on the heights of the absorption peak, the amount of each chromophore in skin, and the penetration of each wavelength into skin. For example, although the absorption maximum of naked DNA is at 260 nm, the most effective wavelengths to excite DNA in basal keratinocytes is 300 nm. This is because shorter wavelengths are absorbed and scattered in the stratum corneum and the upper layers of the epidermis and do not reach the basal keratinocytes as effectively. 7-DHC, 7-dihydrocholesterol; NADH, reduced nicotinamide adenine dinucleotide.

If this involves no change in spin, the excited state is called singlet state. If it also undergoes a change in spin, the excited state is called a triplet state (Fig. 17-5). Upon photoexcitation, a photochemical reaction can occur to form a new, different molecule called photoproduct. For example, previtamin D3 is a photoproduct of photoexcited 7-dehydrocholesterol and the cyclobutane pyrimidine dimer the photoproduct of excited DNA. The process in which energy from an excited chromophore is transferred to another molecules is called a photosensitized reaction. A typical photobiologically relevant photosensitized reaction is energy transfer of an excited chromophore, eg, porphyrin, to oxygen with production of singlet oxygen, which in turn then reacts with other substrates, eg, guanine DNA bases. Instead of forming a photoproduct, the excited chromophore can also return to its ground state with the release of energy as heat or emission of a photon as fluorescence. The wavelengths of fluorescence is always longer (=less energetic) than the exciting wavelength (Stokes Law). For example, on excitation of protoporphyrin IX with blue light, fluorescence is red light, which has a longer wavelength than blue light and is less energetic. The excited singlet state is short-lived and the resulting fluorescence occurs in nanoseconds. Triplet states are longer-lived, as long as seconds. The photon emission from return of triplet excited states to ground states is called phosphorescence, which have longer wavelengths than fluorescence.

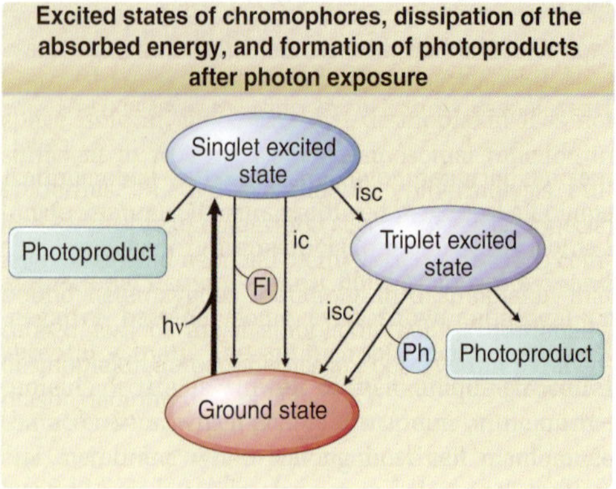

Figure 17-5 Excited states of chromophores, dissipation of the absorbed energy, and formation of photoproducts after exposure to photons of ultraviolet radiation and visible light. Fl, fluorescence; ic, internal conversion; isc, intersystem crossing; Ph, phosphorescence.

CUTANEOUS RESPONSES TO ULTRAVIOLET RADIATION

See Table 17-2.

VITAMIN D PHOTOBIOLOGY

FUNCTIONS OF VITAMIN D

Vitamin D regulates calcium and phosphorus metabolism. Its major role is to increase the flow of calcium into the bloodstream, by promoting absorption of calcium and phosphorus from the intestines, and reabsorption of calcium in the kidneys, thus enabling normal mineralization of bone and muscle function.

Vitamin D deficiency results in impaired bone mineralization that leads to bone softening diseases, rickets in children and osteomalacia in adults, and possibly contributes to osteoporosis.[1-3] Deficiency can arise from inadequate intake, inadequate sunlight exposure, disorders that limit its absorption, and conditions that impair conversion of vitamin D into active metabolites, such as liver or kidney diseases. Most vulnerable to low vitamin D levels are elders, individuals living at high latitudes with long winters, obese persons, and all individuals with dark skin pigmentation living at high latitudes.[4,5] Toxicity from excess vitamin D may manifest as hypercalciuria or hypercalcemia, the latter causing muscle weakness, apathy, headache, confusion, anorexia, irritability, nausea, vomiting, and bone

TABLE 17-2

Comparison of Cutaneous Responses to UVA and UVB

UVA	UVB
Immediate erythema	1000 × more erythemogenic than UVA; associated with sunburn
Immediate pigment darkening (within 20 minutes after UVR exposure)	Delayed melanogenesis (peaks at 3 days)
Major role in drug induced photosensitivity; contributes to carcinogenesis	Major role in carcinogenesis
Central role in photoaging	Role in photoaging
Penetrates down to deep dermis	Penetrates no deeper than the upper dermis
Not associated with vitamin D production	Role in vitamin D production
Penetrates window glass	Does not penetrate window glass
Immunosuppression	Immunosuppression

pain, and may lead to complications such as kidney stones and kidney failure. Chronic toxicity includes the aforementioned symptoms along with constipation, anorexia, abdominal cramps, polydipsia, polyuria, backache, and hyperlipidemia. Findings may also include calcinosis, followed by hypertension and cardiac arrhythmias (due to shortened refractory period). Although information about the effects of high doses of vitamin D is limited, 10,000 IU daily is considered a safe upper limit for adult intake. A chronic toxic dose is more than 50,000 IU/day in adults.

In addition to enhancing musculoskeletal health, vitamin D may also have an influence on the risk of a variety of other conditions, including cancer, cardiovascular disease, autoimmune disease, and infection. However, these effects remain a matter of significant controversy.[6-16]

There are 2 major sources of vitamin D, one is exogenous (diet) and the other is endogenous synthesis. When obtained from food or supplements, vitamin D is absorbed in the small intestine. Natural food sources rich in vitamin D include certain oily fish such as salmon, mackerel, tuna, herring, catfish, cod, sardines and eel, butter, margarine, yogurt, liver, liver oil, and egg yolks, but, at least in the United States, most dietary vitamin D comes from the fortification of foods like cereal, milk, and orange juice. Fortified milk, for example, typically provides 100 IU per 250-mL glass, or only a quarter of the estimated adequate daily intake for adults.

BIOCHEMICAL PATHWAY OF VITAMIN D PRODUCTION

As a result of UV exposure of the skin, provitamin D_3 (7-dehydrocholesterol, a precursor of cholesterol) is rapidly converted to previtamin D_3, which spontaneously isomerizes to vitamin D_3, entering the circulation on a binding protein and joining dietary D_2 (or ergocalciferol) and D_3 (cholecalciferol) absorbed from the gut (Fig. 17-6). Once reaching the liver, it is hydroxylated by the vitamin D 25-hydroxylase, a process that requires NADPH, O_2, and Mg^{2+}. The product 25-hydroxyvitamin D_3 (calcidiol) is stored in the hepatocytes until it is needed. On release into the plasma, it makes its way to the proximal tubules of the kidneys, where it is acted upon by 25(OH)D-1α-hydroxylase, an enzyme whose activity is increased by parathyroid hormone and low PO_4^{2-}. People with kidney disease may not be able to convert vitamin D to its active form. Following this conversion, 1,25-hydroxyvitamin D_3 (calcitriol) is released into the circulation, and by binding to a carrier protein in the plasma, vitamin D–binding protein (VDBP), it is transported to various target organs.

An action spectrum published by MacLaughlin et al. in 1982[17] shows that the most effective wavelengths to facilitate the photosynthesis of cutaneous vitamin D lie in the UVB range, with a peak at 297 nm, but the accuracy and validity of these data have been questioned more recently.[18] In tropical areas, adequate amounts of vitamin D_3 can be made in the skin with 10 to 15 minutes of biweekly sun exposure to the face, arms, and hands, or the back. Individuals with higher skin melanin content require more time in sunlight to produce the same amount of vitamin D as individuals with lower melanin content. It has been proposed that the evolutionary loss of pigment from human's African origin to the white race living in more northern, less sunny latitudes provided advantages with regard to vitamin D production and bone health in areas where the photoprotective effects of melanin were not as critical as in lower latitudes.[19] In today's lifestyles with increased indoor activity and wearing of more extensive clothing, vitamin D deficiency is often a particular problem in people of color who need more UVB exposure to produce the same amount of vitamin in the skin, as compared to more fair-skinned individuals.

It remains a matter of debate what are sufficient levels of vitamin D. These may be lower for the maintenance of bone health, and higher for the other, still controversial health benefits. Nevertheless, consistent photoprotection for the prevention of the deleterious effects of UVR exposure, can undoubtedly result in vitamin D deficiency.[20,21] Combining photoprotection with vitamin D supplementation therefore appears a wise choice, as dietary sources are often insufficient to maintain appropriate vitamin D levels.

EFFECTS ON THE IMMUNE SYSTEM

Several lines of observational evidence suggest that UV radiation has both proinflammatory and antiinflammatory properties. Proinflammatory properties are supported by observations of sunburning, elucidation of inflammatory photodermatoses, induction and triggering of autoimmune connective tissue dis-

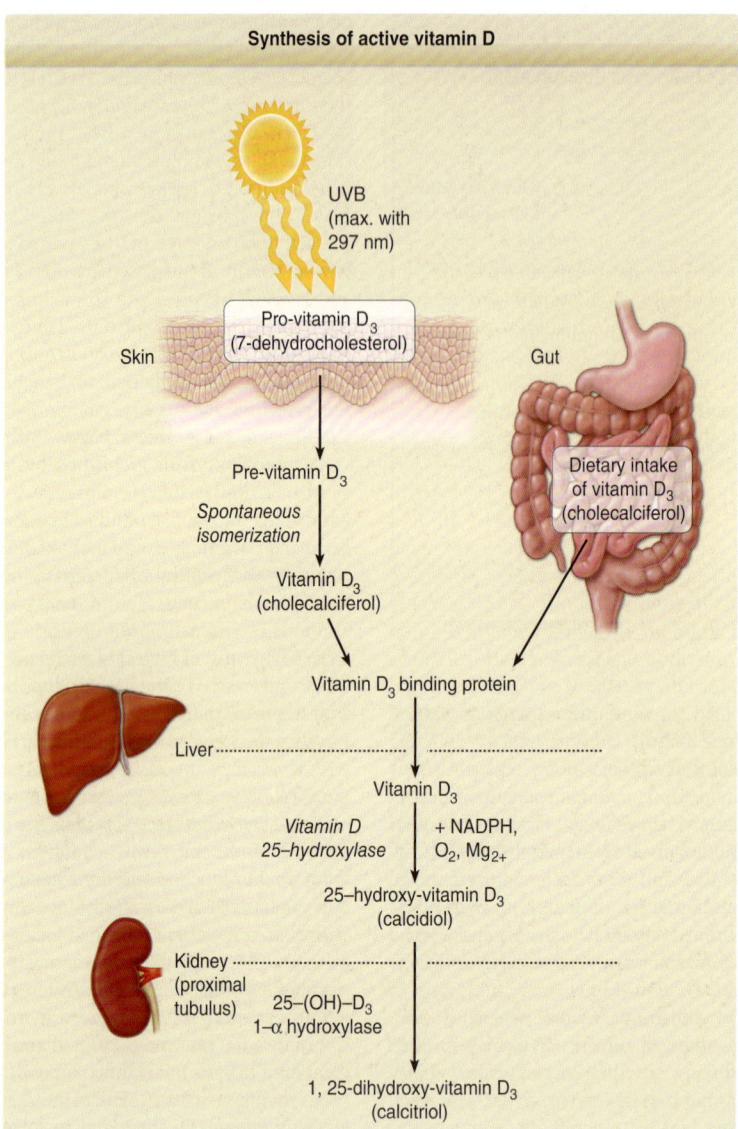

Figure 17-6 Synthesis of active vitamin D. The chromophore that absorbs UVB and initiates this pathway is 7-dehydrocholesterol. Its absorption maximum is 297 nm. The photoproduct of photoexcited 7-dehydrocholesterol is pre-vitamin D_3, which quickly isomerizes to vitamin D_3. See text for more details.

eases, and photoaggravation of inflammatory skin diseases in some patients. Antiinflammatory/immunosuppressive effects are supported by the observations of reactivation of labial herpes simplex with UVR exposure and efficacy of UV phototherapy for the treatment of inflammatory skin diseases. UVR has profound effects on the immune system, both locally at the sites of UV exposure and systemically. Currently, the immunostimulatory effects of UV radiation are thought to be mediated by innate immunity with release of proinflammatory mediators by skin-resident and nonresident cells (eg, serotonin, prostaglandins, IL-1, IL-6, IL-8, TNF-α), induction of antimicrobial peptides, and recruitment of neutrophils and lymphocytes.[22] The immunosuppressive effects are thought to be mediated by migration of Langerhans cells from the epidermis to regional lymph nodes, release of antiinflammatory mediators of skin-resident and nonresident cells (eg, IL-10, α-MSH), and induction of antigen-specific regulatory T cells (Fig. 17-7). However, the view of such a pro- versus antiinflammatory dichotomy is probably overly simplistic. Instead, a variety of individual factors are likely influencing the pro- and antiinflammatory responses, resulting in different balances between these two poles. For example, for most patients with psoriasis, exposure to UV radiation results in an improvement of skin lesions, which showcases the antiinflammatory properties of UVR. A small subset of patients, however, experience worsening of their psoriasis. This demonstrates that for patients with such photoaggravated psoriasis, the net result of UVR is proinflammatory. Another exam-

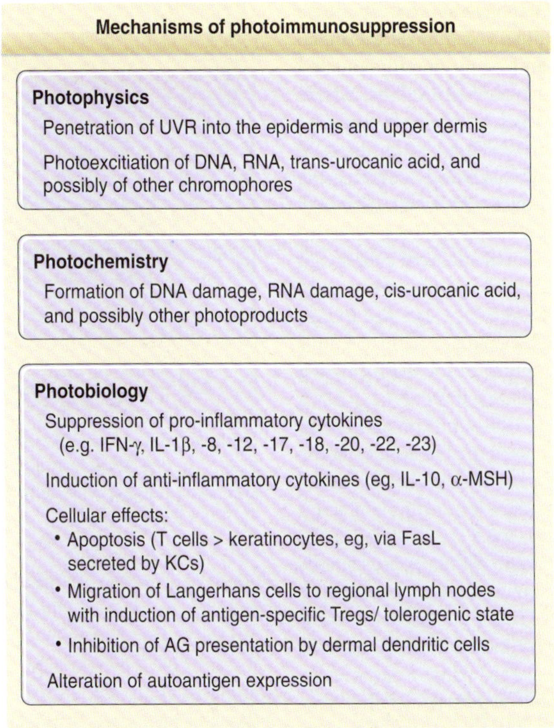

Mechanisms of photoimmunosuppression

Photophysics
Penetration of UVR into the epidermis and upper dermis
Photoexcitiation of DNA, RNA, trans-urocanic acid, and possibly of other chromophores

Photochemistry
Formation of DNA damage, RNA damage, cis-urocanic acid, and possibly other photoproducts

Photobiology
Suppression of pro-inflammatory cytokines
  (e.g. IFN-γ, IL-1β, -8, -12, -17, -18, -20, -22, -23)
Induction of anti-inflammatory cytokines (eg, IL-10, α-MSH)
Cellular effects:
 • Apoptosis (T cells > keratinocytes, eg, via FasL secreted by KCs)
 • Migration of Langerhans cells to regional lymph nodes with induction of antigen-specific Tregs/ tolerogenic state
 • Inhibition of AG presentation by dermal dendritic cells
Alteration of autoantigen expression

Figure 17-7 Mechanisms of photoimmunosuppression. Photoimmunosuppression is mediated by photoexcitation of chromophores, including DNA and trans-urocanic acid, formation of photoproduct (eg, cyclobutane pyrimidine dimers, cis-urocanic acid), and subsequently a range off immunologic endpoints. This cascade demonstrates a typical cascade of events following exposure of the skin to UVR, starting with photophysical responses (penetration of UVR into the skin and photoexcitation of chromophores), followed by photochemical reactions (production of photoproducts), and ultimately photobiologic consequences.

ple is the photodermatosis polymorphous light eruption, likely an inflammatory response to a UV-induced neoantigen. Patients with this condition have less UV-induced immunosuppression and are therefore more likely to develop this condition.[23] On the other hand, this provides them with some protection against photocarcinogenesis, likely due to a more robust immune-response to UV-induced tumor antigens.[24]

The beneficial effect of UV-induced immunosuppression is probably the prevention of autoimmune reactions against self-antigens unmasked by UV-induced cell damage. An example of a failure to prevent such autoimmune reactions is lupus erythematosus with not only aggravation of skin lesions, but also triggering of new lesions and even systemic flares after UV exposure. From animal experimentation, is has been well established that the immunosuppressive effects of UV radiation are not only local, meaning limited to UV-exposed skin, but systemic as well, affecting also nonexposed skin. These effects have been shown to be mediated by IL-10 and subsequent induction of regulatory T cells. The photoaggravation and phototriggering of lupus erythematosus can be regarded a failure to appropriately downregulate immune reactions. The downside of photo-immunosuppression is that it prevents the recognition of UV-induced tumor antigens and with that promotes photocarcinogenesis.

In addition to immunosuppression, UV radiation also induces long-lasting tolerance to antigens generated and/or unmasked following UV exposure. UV radiation can therefore be regarded a triple-edged sword for skin cancer development: it causes mutagenic DNA damage and not only inhibits the recognition of new tumor antigens but also induces tolerance against those. Chromophores of these effects on the immune system are DNA with formation of DNA damage, RNA with formation of RNA damage, urocanic acid with UV-induced isomerization from the trans- to the cis-isoform, and porphyrins that upon photoexcitation generate reactive oxygen species and subsequently change the redox potential of membrane lipids. Although most of the immunosuppressive effects are caused by UVB, UVA also has been shown to have similar effects.[25]

SUNBURNING

Sunburning (solar erythema) is clinically characterized by erythema and a burning sensation with pain (grade 1) and can progress to blister formation (grade 2), but does not progress to grade 3, at least not with solar available doses. It typically peaks 6 to 24 hours after sun exposure, followed by tanning and desquamation. Histologically, it is characterized by epidermal edema with spongiosis, few apoptotic keratinocytes (sunburn cells), depletion of Langerhans cells, vasodilation, and a mixed inflammatory infiltrate with lymphocytes and neutrophils. Action spectra for UV-induced erythema show that erythema formation peaks at 300 nm, which is within the UVB range, but then exponentially declines with increasing wavelength into the UVA range.[26] Although very high doses of UVA can induce erythema, nonphotosensitive individuals do not develop erythema from solar available doses of UVA. UVC, albeit not present in solar radiation reaching the earth's surface, can also induce sunburning. Because the erythema action spectrum is very similar to the action spectrum for the formation of directly UV-induced pyrimidine dimer type of DNA lesions, the chromophore for the sunburning reaction is thought to be DNA.[27,28] This is further supported by the observation that many patients with defects in the repair of this type of lesions (xeroderma pigmentosum) have acute photosensitivity with a decreased UVB minimal erythema dose[29,30] and similar observations from animal experimentation, where improvement of pyrimidine dimer repair reduces photosensitivity.[31,32] Exposed skin cells with UV-induced DNA damage switch on a variety of damage response pathways, some of which result in the secretion of either preformed (eg, serotonin and TNFα) or newly synthesized inflammatory mediators (eg, prostaglandins, nitric oxide, and neuropeptides).[33]

TANNING

Darkening of the skin (tanning) is a characteristic consequence of sunburning, but also can be observed without prior burning (Fig. 17-8). It peaks approximately 3 days after UVB exposure, and is histologically characterized by an increase in basal and suprabasal melanin in the epidermis. Sensitivity for sunburning and ability to tan varies greatly among the human race and has been categorized in skin phototypes (Table 17-3), based on baseline pigmentation, sensitivity to sunburning, and ability to tan. This classification scheme was developed by Thomas B. Fitzpatrick for white skin in 1975[34] and has since then been extended to darker skin types. In 2015, the computing industry standard Unicode has introduced Emoji modifiers to specify skin color based on Fitzpatrick's skin phototype scale to represent diversity, which underlines the pervasiveness of skin color perception even in popular culture. An individual's sensitivity to sunburning can be measured by determining the minimal erythema dose. This is the lowest dose that causes erythema in an individual, and it correlates, albeit poorly, with the clinically determined skin phototype.[35] The skin phototypes, which are based on acute responses to UVR, are also indicators for an individual's risk for long-term effects of UVR on skin, in particular photocarcinogenesis.

The fact that the action spectrum for tanning is almost identical to the action spectrum for the formation of DNA photoproducts[36,28] indicates that DNA is the chromophore for UVR-induced tanning, very

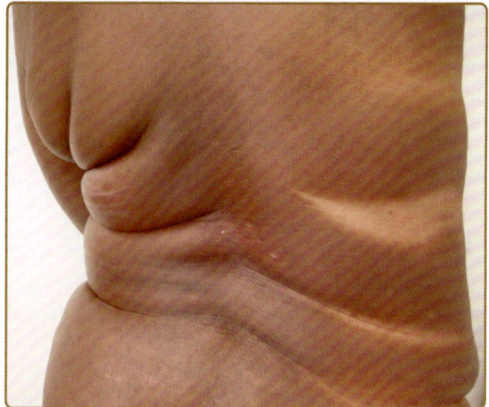

Figure 17-8 Tanning in a patient with nbUVB phototherapy. Note the lack of tanning in skin folds not exposed to UVR. This patient with skin phototype V did not have a sunburn prior to tanning.

similar to erythema formation (see above), and that cellular responses to DNA damage are critical to mediate the tanning response. The increased synthesis of melanin is dependent on the UV-induced induction and activation of p53, a central player in cellular DNA damage responses.[37-39] Melanin produced by melanocytes is transferred through an active process involving specialized motor-proteins to keratinocytes, where it is preferentially placed over the nuclei, forming a microparasol.[40] With this, the UV-absorbing properties of melanin shield the nuclei against the DNA-damaging effects of subsequent UV exposures. In response to the UV-induced inflammation (sunburning), the epidermal keratinocytes hyperproliferate, which results in thickening of the viable epidermis and of the stratum corneum. This thickening decreases penetration of UVR to the basal layer and with that also reduces formation of DNA damage and mutations in the skin's stem cells. These two protective mechanisms, increased pigmentation and skin thickening, together with molecular adaptations, including, for example, increased activity of DNA repair enzymes,

TABLE 17-3
Skin Phototypes

SKIN PHOTOTYPE	BURNING AND TANNING REACTIONS UPON SUN EXPOSURE	COLOR OF UNEXPOSED SKIN
I	Always burns, never tans	Pale white
II	Always burns, then tans	White
III	Sometimes burns, can tan without prior burn	White
IV	Usually does not burn, tans easily and deeply	White to light brown
V	Rarely burns, tans easily	Brown; moderately pigmented
VI	Burns only with very high UVR doses, tans	Dark brown to black; darkly pigmented

result in a several-fold increase of the erythema threshold.[41] In addition to this delayed tanning, which is mostly induced by UVB, there is also an immediate pigment darkening, which can be observed within 20 minutes after UVR exposure. The latter is mediated by oxidation and redistribution of existing melanin, is mostly induced by UVA, and provides much less, if any, protection against subsequent exposures.

PHOTOBIOLOGIC PRINCIPLES OF PHOTODERMATOSES

The above-mentioned requirement for an excitation of a chromophore before a photobiologic reaction can occur also applies to photo-induced or photo-triggered dermatoses. For some, the chromophores are known, for others not. For example, defects in the heme biosynthesis pathways result in the accumulation of toxic pathway intermediates and cause porphyrias. Defects at an early stage of the heme biosynthesis pathway result in accumulation of nonaromatic intermediates that do not act as chromophores/photosensitizers. These porphyrias are not characterized by phototoxic reactions in the skin, but affect other organs, including, for example, the liver (eg, acute intermittent porphyria). Defects at later stages of the heme biosynthesis pathway result in the accumulation of larger, aromatic intermediates that act as chromophores. On exposure to UVR or visible light, excitation of these chromophores cause a phototoxic reaction (eg, subepidermal blisters) that is mediated by an energy transfer from the excited chromophore to oxygen (photosensitized reaction) and formation of singlet oxygen (eg, in porphyria cutanea tarda or erythropoietic protoporphyria). The absorption maximum of these intermediates, for example, uroporphyrinogen in porphyria cutanea tarda and protoporphyrin in erythropoietic protoporphyria, is between 400 and 410 nm, at the border between UVA and visible blue light. Affected patients, therefore, need to protect themselves not only against UVA but also against visible light to prevent phototoxic reactions. Different cutaneous porphyrias present with different symptoms. This is likely due to differences in water solubility and subsequent difference in tissue distribution of the accumulated intermediates. The water-soluble uroporphyrinogen diffuses freely throughout the skin and induces most of its phototoxicity closest to the light source, at the epidermal junction, entailing blister formation. In erythropoietic protoporphyria, the much more lipophilic protoporphyrin remains in the endothelial lining and causes capillary damage with subsequent dermal necrosis and pain.

In drug-induced phototoxic and photoallergic dermatitis, the chromophore is a medication or a metabolite of the medication. Such photosensitizing medications are aromatic molecules that absorb within the UVA range. Therefore, phototoxic and photoallergic drug reactions are almost exclusively induced by UVA. Photo-phytodermatitis is a phototoxic reaction mediated by plant-based chromophores, namely furocoumarins. These molecules are related to psoralens and have an absorption maximum in the UVA range. Berloque dermatitis is also a phototoxic dermatitis, in which the chromophore is the perfume ingredient bergamot oil (5-methoxy psoralen).

Polymorphous light eruption and solar urticaria are likely heterogeneous conditions with regard to involved chromophores, as eliciting wavelength vary from patient to patient, ranging from UVB, to UVA, visible light, and possibly even infrared radiation.[42-44]

Diagnostic tools for the diagnosis of photodermatoses include determination of minimal erythema dose, separated for UVA and UVB (UVA-MED and UVB-MED), photopatch testing, and search for potential chromophores, for example, elevated porphyrins in blood, urine, and stool. Identification of the wavelength that elicit photodermatoses is important in tailoring appropriate photoprotection strategies for each individual patient.

PHOTOBIOLOGIC PRINCIPLES OF PHOTOTHERAPY

Therapeutic effects of electromagnetic radiation are used to treat a variety of skin diseases, either in combination with a photosensitizer, or without. For most phototherapy centers, psoriasis is the most common indication for phototherapy. In 1981, Parrish et al.[45] published an action spectrum for the therapeutic effects of UVR for the treatment of this inflammatory skin disease. No therapeutic effect in the UVC range or with 280 or 290 nm, a maximum effect at around 300 nm, and an exponential decline of therapeutic efficacy with increasing wavelengths from 300 nm to the UVA range is similar to the erythema action spectrum described above and overlaps with the action spectrum for the formation of pyrimidine dimer type of DNA damage in the basal layer of the epidermis.[27] This suggests that the chromophore that mediates the antipsoriasis therapeutic efficacy is DNA. At a time when psoriasis was mostly understood to be a condition that is driven by epidermal hyperproliferation, it was thought that UV-induced pyrimidine dimers would block replication of hyperproliferating keratinocytes and with that improve psoriasis. However, slowing of epidermal hyperproliferation has since then been shown to be a later effect of UVB on psoriasis lesions, not a primary therapeutic effect. Today, the therapeutic effects of UVB are thought to be mediated by the above-mentioned immunosuppressive effects. Although the exact mechanisms remain to be clarified, hyperproliferating activated T cells may be particularly prone to the cytotoxic, proapoptotic effects of UVB. Induction of immune-deviation, eg, with transformation of TH1 and TH17 lymphocytes to Tregs, may be involved.[46] Penetration of UVB is limited to the epidermis and the upper layers of the dermis, but it does not reach deeper levels of the dermis, which are often also infiltrated by immune cells in thick psoriatic plaques. It is also unclear whether skin-infiltrating lymphocytes or other immune cells are the primary target mediating efficacy of UVB phototherapy for psoriasis, or whether these are affected by signaling from UV-exposed keratinocytes.

The above-mentioned action spectrum for the therapeutic effects against psoriasis has led to the development of narrowband (nb) UVB phototherapy with bulbs that emit almost monochromatic UVB between 311 and 312 nm. This modality has been shown to be vastly more efficacious than the previously used broadband (bb) UVB phototherapy. This may be due to the avoidance of pro-erythemogenic short wavelengths of UVB (280-290 nm) that have no or only very little therapeutic efficacy and with that the ability to use significantly higher doses than with bbUVB. In addition, the higher proportion of UVB wavelengths penetrating deeper into the dermis may also facilitate a more effective reach of the target, the dermal inflammatory infiltrate. Today, nbUVB has replaced bbUVB not only for the treatment of psoriasis, but for all other UVB phototherapy indications as well, including, for example, atopic dermatitis, vitiligo, cutaneous T-cell lymphoma, etc. For these indications, the phototherapy mode of action is even less known than for psoriasis. The fact that nbUVB has been shown to be superior to bbUVB for all of these indications may suggest that the modes of action are similar to those in psoriasis. However, although the pathogenesis of these conditions is inflammatory in most of them, the exact inflammatory pathomechanisms are of course quite diverse. Much remains to learn how a single treatment modality, phototherapy with nbUVB, can improve such a diverse group of skin diseases.

Crude coal tar is a potent photosensitizer, making exposed skin very sensitive to UVR-induced erythema. At a time when bbUVB was only partially effective, the use of tar in combination with bbUVB was a common practice, for example, with the treatment regimen named of the first describer, William H. Goeckerman. Tar is a mixture of many different compounds, many of which have photosensitizing properties. With nbUVB being highly effective as a monotherapy, the use of tar as a photosensitizer has become an uncommon practice.

In contrast, photochemotherapy that combines either systemic or topical administration of psoralen with subsequent irradiation with UVA remains a common phototherapy modality, although it is much less used today than at the time before the introduction of nbUVB. Psoralens (the most commonly used one is 8-methoxy-psoralen) intercalate with DNA and on photoexcitation react with pyrimidine bases to form mono- and divalent inter- and intrastrand crosslinks. For PUVA treatment, the chromophore is 8-MOP and psoralen adducts the UVA-induced photoproducts. The absorption maxima of 8-MOP are at 248 and 301 nm, which are in the UVC and UVB range. However, the absorption curve is quite broad and UVA still effectively excites this molecule and also produces the crosslinks quite effectively. The photochemistry of 8-MOP is quite complex. Intercalated with DNA, the absorption maximum is 313 nm, and after the formation of a monoadduct, the absorption maximum shifts to 334 nm, which is in the UVA range. These crosslinks are complex DNA lesions that can only be repaired by DNA recombination, not by nucleotide excision repair, as pyrimidine dimers. Similar to the above-described earlier belief that the replication-blocking properties of UVB-induced DNA damage mediates antiproliferative and with that antipsoriatic effects, the same was suggested for PUVA-induced crosslinks.[47] As with UVB, this has since been refuted. The high efficacy of PUVA treatment may be explained by the deeper penetration of UVA into the dermis and its better reach to deeper inflammatory infiltrates. Because UVA is much less energetic and produces much less pyrimidine dimers than UVB, the addition of psoralen is likely required to bring UVA's DNA-damaging effects into the therapeutic range.

One way to circumvent the limited biologic effects of UVA is to just increase its dosing. This principle has been used for the development of high-dose UVA1 phototherapy without the use of a photosensitizer. This treatment has been shown to have some efficacy for the treatment of acute atopic dermatitis and for sclerosing conditions, for example, morphea. Chromophores that mediate this effect have not been identified, and the exact mode of action of this type of phototherapy also remains to be worked out.

Another mode of phototherapy that employs the use of a photosensitizer is photodynamic therapy (PDT). In the United States, the most commonly used agent to photosensitize skin for PDT is 5-amino-levulinic acid (5-ALA). However, 5-ALA is not the chromophore that mediates the therapeutic effects of PDT. Application of 5-ALA circumvents the rate-limiting step of 5-ALA synthesis of the heme biosynthesis pathway and results in an increase in the cellular content of protoporphyrin IX. This aromatic molecule has an absorption maximum at around 406 nm, the so-called Soret band. It is readily excited by such blue light, upon which it reacts with oxygen to form singlet oxygen. PDT with 5-ALA therefore uses blue light, and its effects are thought to be mediated by the cytotoxic effects of singlet oxygen. The destruction of premalignant and malignant skin neoplasms by PDT may be due to the complete destruction of premalignant or malignant cells, or, more likely, to the destruction of some of these cells with unmasking of tumor-antigens and subsequent immune-mediated destruction of others. At least partial tumor selectivity may be mediated by the more effective uptake of 5-ALA by premalignant and malignant cells.

There are a number of different treatment modalities for PDT, varying by the route of application, the nature of the photosensitizer, and the wavelengths used. In either case, the wavelengths used must be carefully chosen to not only match the absorption characteristics of the photosensitizer, but also to facilitate sufficient penetration. PDT with 5-ALA and blue light is limited by the depth of penetration of blue light. In Europe, the most commonly used skin-directed PDT modality uses methyl aminolevulinic acid (MAL) in combination with red light. MAL has the advantage of better uptake into cells because of its more lipophilic properties, as compared to 5-ALA. The resulting chromophore, however, is the same as with 5-ALA. Although protoporphyrin IX is most effectively excited by blue light, its absorption curve shows a few small peaks in the green, orange, yellow, and red light range (Q-bands), which still provide sufficient photoexcitation with red light. The combination of deeper penetration of MAL, as compared to 5-ALA with the deeper penetration of red light, as compared to blue light, may make this PDT modality more effective for thicker skin lesions, for example, infiltrating skin cancers.

PDT is not limited to regular, broad-spectrum sources of visible light but can also use monochromatic radiation from a variety of different laser sources, and research on the use of lasers for PDT is currently ongoing. Other modifications of current PDT practices involve the development of other photosensitizers with different photoabsorbing properties. The elegance of the current PDT, however, is that it uses a small molecule that is easily taken up into cells and then results in an increased production of the photosensitizer within the cell. This circumvents that problem that photoabsorbing molecules are usually larger and aromatic and are therefore less likely to be internalized by cells.

PHOTOCARCINOGENESIS

Chronic exposure of the skin to ultraviolet light increases the risk for a number of different cutaneous malignancies, including basal cell carcinoma, squamous cell carcinoma, malignant melanoma, and Merkel cell carcinoma. Photocarcinogenesis is the result of a chain of photophysical, photochemical, and photobiological events in UVR-exposed skin cells (Fig. 17-9).

FORMATION OF DNA DAMAGE AND MUTATIONS BY UVR

DNA has an absorption maximum at 260 nm, which is within the UVC range. UVB is still able to strongly excite DNA and penetrates deeper into the epidermis than UVC and therefore induces more photochemical reactions in the basal keratinocytes and in melanocytes. A critical consequence of directly UVR-induced photoexcitation of DNA is the formation of covalent chemical bindings between 2 adjacent pyrimidine bases, thymine and cytosine. There are 2 main types of such DNA photoproducts formed by UVR, cis-syn cyclobutane pyrimidine dimers (CPDs) and pyrimidine-pyrimidone photoproducts (6-4 PPs). Both types of dimers can form between any combination of thymine and cytosine—T:T, T:C, C:T, or C:C (Fig. 17-10).

Unrepaired CPDs or 6,4-pyrimidine–pyrimidone dimers impair DNA replication and can result in mispairing if not removed prior to cells entering the S-phase of the cell cycle for DNA replication. A mispairing results in the change of the DNA sequence, a mutation. Several types of such mutations are observed after UV exposure, but by far the most common ones

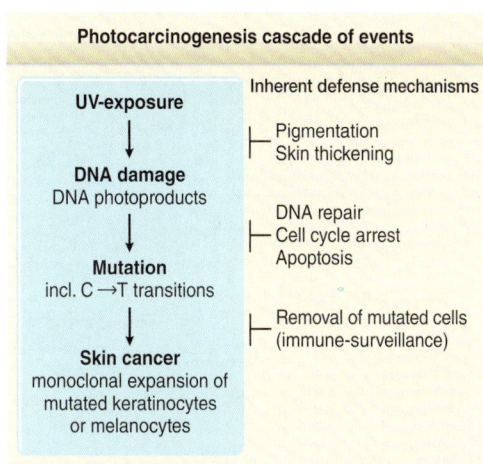

Figure 17-9 Photocarcinogenesis cascade of events. Exposure to UVR induces typical types of DNA damage, namely, cyclobutane pyrimidine dimers and 6,4-pyrimidine–pyrimidone photo-products. These often generate single and tandem base substitution mutations (C→T and CC→TT) at di-pyrimidine sites that are typical for UVR exposure and are therefore termed UV-signature mutations. With sufficient numbers of inactivating mutations in crucial genes (tumor suppressor genes), individual cells may undergo malignant transformation, clonally expand, and form skin cancers. Several inherent defense mechanisms counteract this chain of events.

are C → T base exchange mutations at sites of 2 adjacent pyrimidines (dipyrimidine sites) (Fig. 17-10). This mutation is the result of misincorporation of adenine opposite cytosine during replication of the photoproduct. Without UV exposure, for example, in noncutaneous tissues or tumors, such mutations are observed only rarely, and the C → T and the C:C → T:T tandem mutations at dipyrimidine sites have therefore been named UV signature mutations.[48] Once these mutations are formed, they remain for the life span of the affected cells and are also propagated during cell division. They can be considered the memory of a cell's lifetime exposure to UVR. Some authors use the term UVB signature mutations. However, this term is misleading, as they are also formed by UVA,[48,49] and should be avoided.

In squamous cell carcinomas and actinic keratoses, such UV signature mutations are found in the p53 gene,[48,50] in basal cell carcinomas in the genes of the sonic hedgehog signaling pathway (ptch, shh, smo) and in p53,[51] and in melanoma in the CDKN2A, PTEN, TERT promoter, and p53 genes,[52-55] demonstrating a molecular imprint of UVR as the transforming agent in tumor-specific gene mutations.

The best characterized mechanism of how UVR induces formation of pyrimidine dimers is via direct absorption of photons by DNA bases, with DNA itself acting as the chromophore (classic pathway; Fig. 17-11; left panel).

Recently, however, Premi et al.[56] (see also Brash[57]) described an alternative, melanin-dependent mechanism that likely contributes to pyrimidine dimer for-

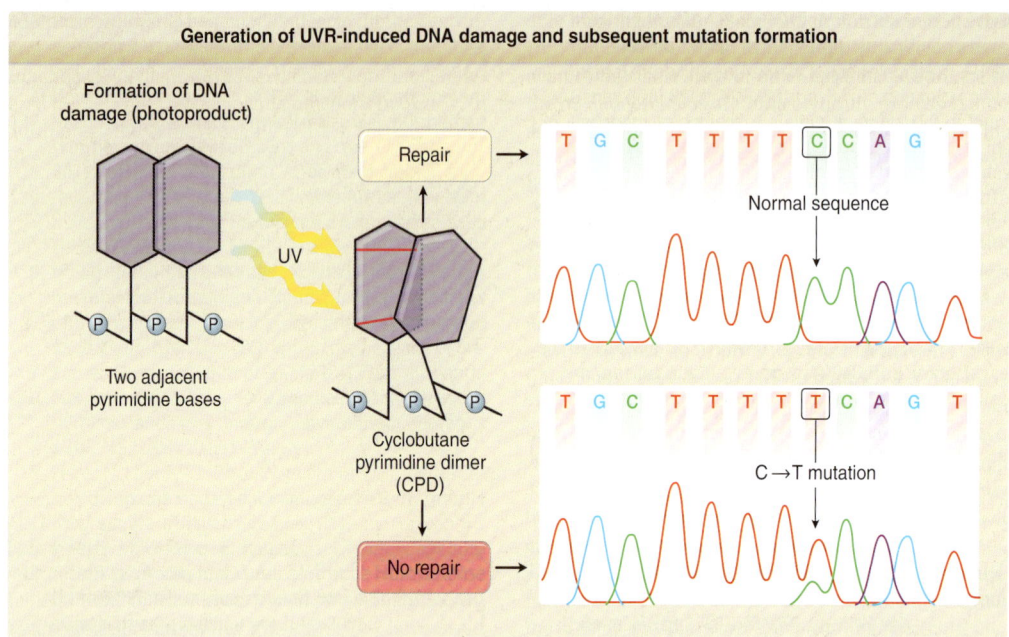

Figure 17-10 Example of UVR-induced generation of DNA damage and subsequent mutation. Upon direct excitation of the DNA molecule by UVR, adjacent pyrimidine bases (cytosine or thymine) may form covalent bonds between them, which leads to creation of pyrimidine dimers. The illustration shows an example in which 2 covalent bindings generate a tricyclic cyclobutane ring between 2 pyrimidines. Hence, this type of UV light–induced DNA damage is called a cyclobutane pyrimidine dimer, a common type of DNA photoproduct. The nucleotide excision repair DNA repair system functions to remove this damage, which results in the normal DNA sequence (upper box). If the damage is not repaired, this type of DNA photoproduct can lead to formation of a typical C→T single base substitution mutation (lower box). This is most likely to occur on replication of damaged DNA and misincorporation of adenine opposite the cytosine-containing photoproduct. An example of such a UV-signature mutation is shown on the right. Note that the mutation is located within a run of 7 pyrimidines, a common location for UV-signature mutations.

mation in melanocytes and in melanin-containing keratinocytes. They had observed formation of DNA photoproducts up to 3 hours after UV exposure, and then showed that the formation of these so-called "dark CPDs" is mediated by photoexcitation of melanin, in particular of pheomelanin, through formation of peroxynitrite from UV-induced nitric oxide and superoxide (melanin-dependent chemiexcitation pathway; Fig. 17-11; middle panel). With this, it appears that melanin is not only a photoprotector but may also contribute to cancer formation by increasing formation of DNA damage. This observation also provides an attractive explanation why UVA induces melanoma only in pigmented mice but not albino mice.[58]

The bystander effect describes the phenomenon that non-exposed cells in the vicinity of irradiated cells also demonstrate stress responses similar to exposed cells. UVA in particular has been shown to exert such a bystander effect in melanocytes, and long-lived UVR-induced radicals have been proposed to mediate it.[59,60] It is tempting to speculate that the long-lived peroxynitrite described by Premi et al.[56] could possibly not only generate "dark CPDs" in irradiated cells, but also in unirradiated bystander cells.

In addition to pyrimidine dimers, UVR can also induce oxidative DNA damage (oxidative pathway, Fig. 17-11; right panel), for example, through absorption of photons by other cellular chromophores and subsequent energy transfer to DNA (type I photosensitized reaction) or to molecular oxygen with formation of reactive oxygen species (ROS), which in turn react with DNA to form oxidative DNA base modifications (type II photosensitized reaction). Although UVB can generate some ROS, most of the oxidative DNA damage after exposure to natural sunlight is caused by UVA.[61,62] UVR-induced ROS are mostly singlet oxygen, but others, for example, hydrogen peroxide, the superoxide radical, and the hydroxyl radical also may be formed, albeit in much lower numbers. ROS-induced DNA damage involves predominantly guanine bases. Several such oxidative guanine lesions have been described after UVR exposure, of which 8-dihydro-8-oxoguanosine (8-oxoG) is the best studied.

During DNA replication, 8-oxoG mispairs with adenine, giving rise to G → T transversion mutations. Similarly, oxidation of a guanosine nucleotide can result in misincorporation opposite an adenine during replication, giving rise to A → C transversions. There is no notable increase of such mutations in UVR-induced cutaneous malignancies, and it remains a matter of debate how much oxidative DNA damage contributes to photocarcinogenesis.

An action spectrum for the formation of pyrimidine dimers and oxidative guanine base modifica-

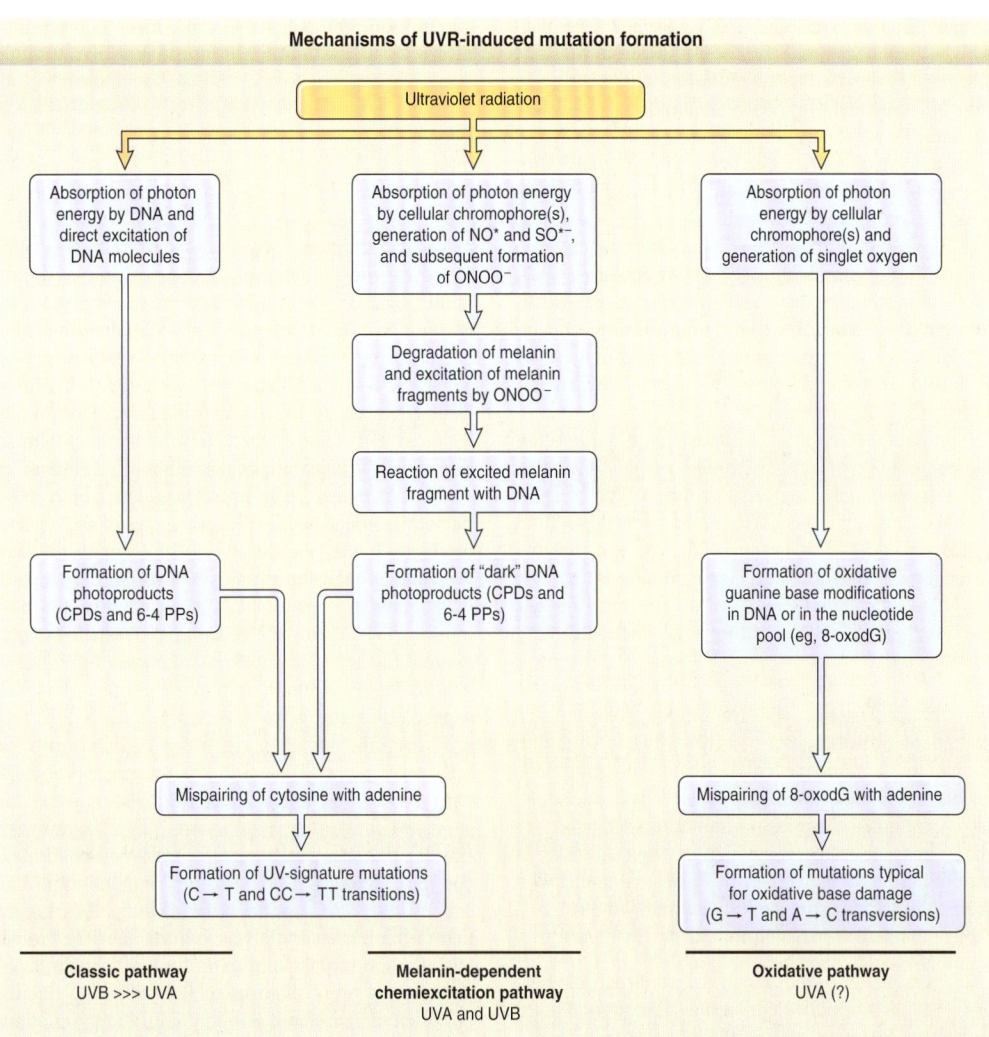

Figure 17-11 Mechanisms of UVR-induced mutation formation. In the classic pathway (left panel), adjacent pyrimidines react with each other and dimerize to form DNA photoproducts after direct excitation of DNA molecules by photons. The C → T and CC → TT UV-signature mutations may form at sites of DNA photoproducts by mispairing of cytosine(s) with adenine. Although 260 nm is the absorption maximum of DNA, UVB still strongly excites DNA and generates mutations through this pathway. UVA's ability to excite DNA is much weaker, but may still generate mutations via this mechanism. CPDs, cis-syn cyclobutane pyrimidine dimers; 6-4 PPs, pyrimidine (6-4) pyrimidone photoproducts.

The melanin-dependent chemiexcitation pathway (middle panel) was recently described by Premi et al.[56] It describes the formation of DNA photoproducts not by direct excitation of DNA, as in the classic pathway, but by energy transfer from excited melanin fragments to DNA, which involves nitric oxide (NO*), superoxide (SO*–), and peroxynitrite (ONOO–). This mechanism generates UV-signature mutations both after irradiation with UVA and with UVB, and contributes to mutation formation in melanocytes and melanin-containing keratinocytes.

The oxidative pathway (right panel) involves a photosensitized reaction with formation of singlet oxygen after excitation of a cellular chromophore other than DNA. Singlet oxygen then reacts with guanine either in DNA or in the nucleotide pool. A common oxidative base lesion is 8-oxo-7,8-dihydro-2′-deoxyguanosine (8-oxodG). By mispairing with adenine, G → T and A → C transversions can form. UVA has long been thought to contribute to UVR-induced mutation load through this mechanism. However, molecular evidence, in particular the low frequency of such transversions in melanomas, does not support a major role in the formation of skin cancer.

tions in mammalian cells shows gradually changing DNA-damaging capacity with increasing wavelengths from UVC, to UVB, UVA, and visible light.[62] Few pyrimidine dimers are formed by UVA, approximately 10,000-fold less than with UVB when comparing, for example, 360 nm with 300 nm. Even when considering the much higher abundance of UVA in natural sun, UVB is most likely generating the majority of solar radiation–induced pyrimidine dimers. Nevertheless, there is mounting evidence from both in vitro and in vivo mutation spectra that pyrimidine dimers are the most important premutagenic DNA lesions not only with UVB but also with UVA, and that oxidative DNA damage plays only a minor role in mutagenesis.[49,63]

One hypothesis we have brought forward to explain a higher rate of mutations at UVA-induced pyrimidine dimers, as compared to the mutation rate of the UVB-induced ones, is that UVA does not induce as robust a cellular DNA damage response as UVB, in particular with cell cycle arrest.[64] This may not be relevant for mutagenesis following exposure to broad-spectrum solar radiation, because with that the damage response can be evoked by the UVB component, which would also protect against mutagenesis at the few UVA-induced pyrimidine dimers. However, with exposures to pure UVA sources, as, for example, found with exposure to solar radiation through window glass or with use of tanning devices, UVA may be particularly mutagenic and carcinogenic.

Although oxygen radicals have been described following UVR exposure, we found no evidence that DNA double-strand breaks, a common type of DNA damage generated by such ROS, are formed by either UVB or UVA.[65,66] This is consistent with the fact that deletions or insertions, types of mutations that are commonly generated by DNA double-strand breaks, are not a common observation in UV-induced mutation spectra.

Upon accumulation of a sufficient number of mutations in specific genes (driver mutations), cells undergo malignant transformation. In this process, mutation formation is a random event. Usually, many mutations occur all over the genome of exposed cells to ultimately also accumulate the critical number of specific driver mutations. For example, the high mutagenic burden in melanoma was demonstrated by Pleasance et al.,[67] who were the first to report the full genomic sequence of a melanoma as compared to the normal sequence of a lymphoblast cell line from the same patient. Of 33,345 base substitution mutations observed in the melanoma, more than 70% were C → T UV-signature mutations. The predominance of this type of mutation that is otherwise rare in non-UV-exposed tumors is an impressive molecular account of a lifetime of sun exposure of a single melanocyte that has ultimately given rise to this melanoma. These data have since been confirmed in a large series of more than 300 melanomas, showing that a median of 77.7% of all mutations in melanoma are UV-signature mutations.[68] These data also show that the mean mutation rate in melanomas from sun-exposed sites is one of the highest of all cancers investigated in this way. This high burden of mutations with mostly C → T transitions again emphasizes the role of UVR's high mutagenic properties and its role in the pathogenesis of cutaneous melanoma.

A genetically distinct melanoma subtype presents most commonly on the face and in the elderly, but can also occur in other areas with heavily photodamaged skin. These melanomas on chronically sun-damaged skin (CSD melanomas) show an extremely high mutation burden (approx. 60 mutations/Mbase)[68,69] and often arise from an in situ melanoma termed lentigo maligna. Desmoplastic melanomas have an even higher mutation burden[70] and have a similar age and anatomic site distribution as CSD melanomas. Melanomas on sun-exposed skin without signs of chronic sun-induced damage (non-CSD melanomas) show a lower mutation burden of approximately 30 mutations/Mbase. The somatic mutations found in all of the above-mentioned melanoma subtypes show a clear UV signature, whereas mucosal and acral melanomas, which are not thought to be UVR-induced, do not. Non-CSD melanomas are most common on the lower legs in women and on the back in men.[71] At least in Western cultures, these areas tend to be photoprotected for long periods of time, for example, during winter, and are then exposed to the sun in the spring and summer, often suddenly and with subsequent sunburning. These types of melanoma therefore appear to be associated with sudden, intermittent high-dose UVR exposures of not sun-adapted skin.[72] Chronically UVR-exposed skin is characterized by an upregulation of anti-mutagenic mechanisms. The absence of such protective states in photoprotected skin, in combination with a relative inability of melanocytes to undergo apoptosis on high-dose UVR exposures has been suggested as an explanation for the induction of melanoma by intermittent UVR exposures[73] and may indicate the importance of cellular mechanisms that prevent formation of DNA damage and of mutations, and malignant transformation in chronically UVR-exposed skin (Fig. 17-9).

DNA REPAIR AND OTHER RESPONSES TO UVR-INDUCED DNA DAMAGE

DNA repair is an important cellular defense mechanism that prevents mutation formation at sites of DNA damage after UV exposure. However, it is not the only defense mechanism (Fig. 17-9). Most mutations are generated during replication of damaged DNA. Therefore, a damage-induced arrest in cell cycling, which allows more time for repair, is another important cellular damage response that prevents mutation formation.[64,74] Furthermore, programmed cell death (apoptosis) prevents the survival of cells with overwhelming DNA damage, and through that mechanism the frequency of cells with UV-induced mutations is also reduced. Other inherent defense mechanisms against the carcinogenic properties of UVR include increased melanogenesis and thickening of the epidermis and stratum corneum, which protect from future DNA damage, as well as removal of mutated cells through host immune responses. More than 100 DNA repair genes have been identified (http://sciencepark.mdanderson.org/labs/wood/DNA_Repair_Genes.html). The nucleotide excision repair (NER) pathway acts on DNA damaged by UVR, repairing CPDs and other photoproducts, as well as on DNA damaged by certain other carcinogens (such as benzo-[a]-pyrene). In NER, the damaged nucleotide is removed and replaced with undamaged DNA. A simplified schema of the NER system describing some of the many proteins that act in concert to repair UV-induced DNA damage is shown in Fig. 17-12. Defects in these repair genes can cause human diseases including xeroderma pigmentosum (XP), Cockayne syndrome (CS), and trichothiodystrophy (TTD) (Chap. 130). For instance, XP can be caused by a defect in any one of several genes involved in NER. Based on cell fusion experiments, cells/patients with defects in the same gene are considered to be in the same complementation group, and in different complementation groups if different genes are affected. If DNA repair in the fused cell is normalized, with the wildtype gene from each cell giving rise to a functional protein that is absent in the other cell, the cells "complement" each other and are in different complementation groups. Seven such complementation groups have been identified (XP-A to XP-G), which correspond with mutations in 7 distinct genes that can cause XP.

Transcribed genes are repaired faster than the rest of the genome. In the NER pathway, the first steps involving DNA damage recognition are different in nontranscribed (global genome NER) and transcribed genes (transcription-coupled NER). In nontranscribed genes and noncoding areas, which represent most of the genome, the *XPE* and *XPC* gene products bind to UV-damaged DNA, marking it for further processing. In contrast, DNA damage in transcribed genes appears to be sensed by a stalled RNA polymerase acting in conjunction with the CSA and CSB (CS complementation groups A and B) gene products. After the DNA damage recognition steps, global genome NER and transcription-coupled NER follow the same pathway (Fig. 17-12).

In XP, pronounced NER deficiencies confer a very high risk to develop nonmelanoma skin cancer and melanoma. More subtle variations in DNA repair capacity,

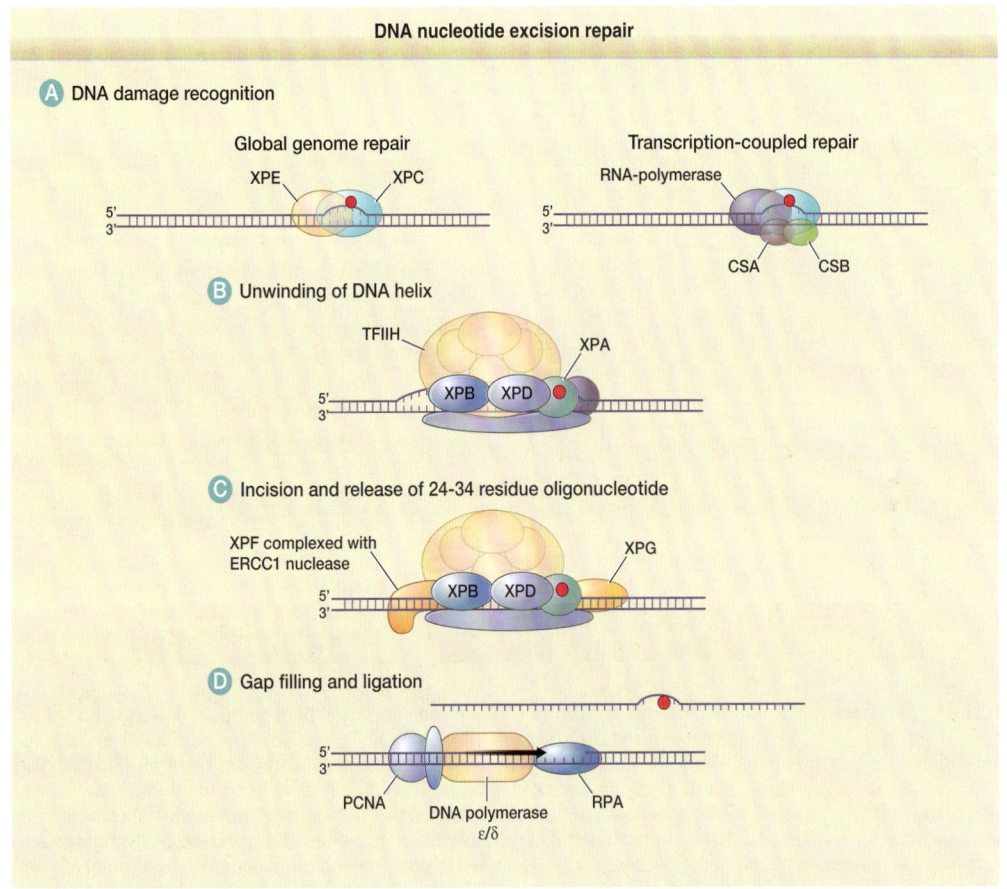

Figure 17-12 DNA nucleotide excision repair scheme. (A) Right: Damaged DNA in actively transcribed genes results in stalling of the RNA polymerase in a process that involves the CSA and CSB proteins. This serves as a signal to initiate transcription-coupled DNA repair. Left: Damaged DNA in the remainder of the genome is bound by the XPE and XPC gene products. This serves as a signal to initiate global genome repair. (B) A portion of the DNA, including the damage, is unwound by a complex of proteins including the XPB and XPD gene products. These proteins are also part of the 10-subunit basal transcription factor IIH (TFIIH). The XPA protein may stabilize the unwound DNA. (C) The XPF and XPG nucleases make single-strand cuts on either side of the damage, releasing a 24- to 34-residue segment of DNA. (D) The resulting gap is filled by DNA polymerase in a process that includes the proteins proliferating cell nuclear antigen (PCNA) and replication protein A (RPA). CSA, CSB, Cockayne syndrome complementation groups A and B; ERCC1, excision repair cross-complementing gene 1; LIG1, ligase 1; XPA, XPC, etc, xeroderma pigmentosum complementation groups A, C, etc.

for example, as a consequence of polymorphisms in NER genes or of an aging-related decline, also have been linked to an increased skin cancer risk.[75-78]

Oxidative base modifications are a simpler type of DNA damage than pyrimidine dimers, as they only involve chemical changes in a single DNA base. These lesions are processed by a different DNA repair pathway, called base excision repair.

Several cellular responses to DNA damage contribute to the maintenance of genome integrity by preventing mutation formation. These include cell cycle arrest, apoptosis (programmed cell death), and DNA repair. Because these responses need to be carefully orchestrated, there are many proteins involved in the signaling of DNA damage and in the regulation of cellular DNA damage responses. Different types of DNA-damaging agents and different types of DNA damage require different DNA damage responses. A simplified version of this complex pathway is presented in Fig. 17-13. As with defects in DNA repair genes, defects in many of these DNA damage–signaling genes (boxed in Fig. 17-13) are also implicated in hereditary disorders of genome instability, including, for example, ataxia telangiectasia, Fanconi anemia, familial breast cancer, Li-Fraumeni syndrome, and others (Chap. 130).

The tumor suppressor gene p53, often called the *guardian of the genome*, plays a pivotal role in regulating and orchestrating these responses and is mutated in many cancers, including cutaneous squamous cell carcinomas. Upstream regulators of p53 in the cellular DNA damage response pathway are ATM (ataxia telangiectasia mutated) and ATR (ataxia telangiectasia- and Rad3-related) genes. One of p53's several functions is the regulation of the cell cycle in response to DNA damage. After cell division (mitosis), cells have 23 pairs of chromosomes and are in the G_1 phase of the cell cycle. The chromosomes then replicate during

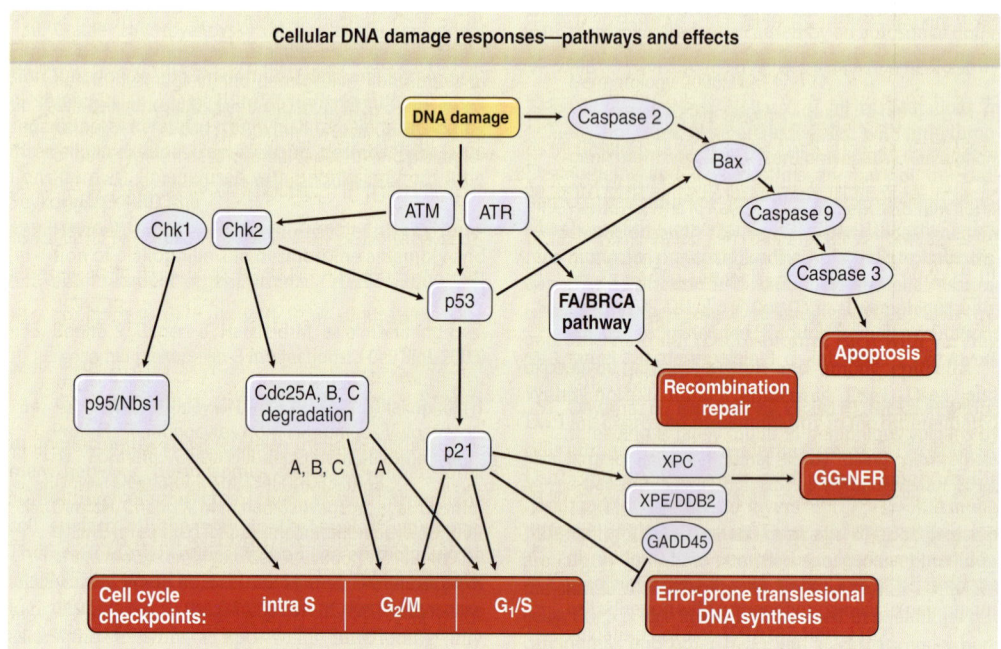

Figure 17-13 Signaling cascades that regulate apoptosis, DNA repair, translesional DNA synthesis, and activation of cell cycle checkpoints in response to UVR-induced DNA damage. This is a highly simplified diagram that depicts only the most important players in the intricate and interwoven DNA damage–signaling networks. The traditional thinking was that ATM (ataxia telangiectasia mutated gene) is activated (phosphorylated) in response to ionizing radiation (IR) and ATR (ataxia telangiectasia- and Rad3-related gene) in response to ultraviolet (UV) radiation, but newer data indicate that both are activated by IR and UV. ATM/ATR can activate (ie, phosphorylate) p53 either directly or indirectly through activation (phosphorylation) of Chk2 (an ATM target) or Chk1 (an ATR target). Through transcriptional activation of p21 and subsequent inhibition of cyclin-dependent kinases, which usually drive cells from the G1 into the S phase of the cell cycle, activated p53 activates the G1/S checkpoint (ie, arrests cells in G1). The G1/S checkpoint is also activated by Chk1/Chk2-induced phosphorylation and then degradation of Cdc25A and subsequent failure to activate cyclin-dependent kinases. Phosphorylation and subsequent degradation of Cdc25A, Cdc25B, and Cdc25C also mediate the G2/M arrest, as does p21. Intra–S phase arrest is mediated through activation (phosphorylation) of p95/Nbs1. p53 also induces global genome nucleotide excision repair (GG-NER) through transcriptional activation of XPC, XPE/p48, and GADD45. Translesional DNA synthesis has been shown to be downregulated by p53 via p21. Recombination repair is mediated through the Fanconi anemia (FA)/BRCA pathway, which in turn is dependent on ATR activation. The mitochondrial pathway of apoptosis is activated through activation of Bax by caspase 2 and p53, the initiator caspase 9, and the effector caspases 3, 6, and 7. Gene products that are defective in hereditary human diseases are boxed. DDB2, DNA damage binding protein 2; XPC, XPE, xeroderma pigmentosum complementation groups C and E.

DNA synthesis, or S phase, and as a result have twice the number of chromosomes (G_2 phase) just before mitosis (M phase). In response to damage, the cell may stop cycling (arrest) in specific cell cycle phases called *cell cycle checkpoints*. An important downstream effector in preventing cells from entering S phase (G_1/S checkpoint) is p21. p53 also induces NER by transcriptionally inducing XPC, XPE/p48, and GADD45.

If cells enter S phase with unrepaired DNA damage, or if cells are UV exposed during S phase, regular DNA polymerases stall at DNA photoproducts and detach from the DNA strand.[79] For these instances, cells are equipped with several specialized DNA polymerases for translesional DNA synthesis. DNA polymerase eta is one of these; it is specialized to bypass DNA photoproducts but may introduce mutations while doing so. It is mutated in XP variant patients, who are clinically indistinguishable from other XP patients with defects in NER (Chap. 130).[80,81] This demonstrates the importance of this second line of defense against the mutagenic and carcinogenic consequences of DNA photoproducts. p53 and p21 also downregulate the activity of this translesional DNA synthesis to maintain a low mutagenic activity at the price of reduced damage bypass.

If this translesional DNA synthesis fails, cells can use recombination repair to resolve stalled replication forks.[82] When invoked in response to damage from UV light, this third line of defense is mediated by activation of the Fanconi anemia/BRCA DNA damage response pathway.[65]

Apoptosis is a regulated physiologic process leading to cell death characterized by cell shrinkage, membrane blebbing, and DNA fragmentation. A group of cysteine proteases called *caspases* are central regulators of apoptosis. Triggers may be extrinsic or intrinsic to the cell (eg, DNA damage) and involve separate initiator caspases (eg, caspase 2 in response to DNA damage) but share the same downstream effector caspases.

Mutations in the p53 tumor suppressor gene are very commonly found in cutaneous squamous cell carcinomas and their precursors, actinic keratoses. In addition, chronically sun-exposed skin harbors many clonal proliferations of keratinocytes with p53 mutations, which are not detectable by macroscopic or microscopic abnormalities.[83] Loss of p53 function as a central regulator of antimutagenic responses entails a higher rate of mutation formation with subsequent UVR exposures. This so-called UV mutator phenotype is critical in the development of cutaneous squamous cell cancers, as it makes it much more likely that all the mutations necessary for complete malignant transformation of a single keratinocyte are accumulated with repeated UV exposures.[84]

WHICH WAVELENGTHS OF UVR CAUSE SKIN CANCER?

Although the carcinogenic properties of UVB have been well known for decades, UVA has long been considered harmless because of its inability to induce sunburning with solar available doses. However, it is now recognized that UVR is also damaging and carcinogenic in suberythemogenic doses and that UVA can induce cutaneous squamous cell carcinomas by itself in mice. Consequently, the WHO has classified UVA as an independent class I carcinogen.[85] The Utrecht-Philadelphia action spectrum for photocarcinogenesis in mice shows an exponential decline in carcinogenic efficacy in mice with increasing wavelengths from UVB to UVA.[86] Some of this decline is offset by the higher abundance of UVA in natural solar radiation. In addition, exposures to pure UVA by window glass–filtered solar radiation and in tanning parlors may significantly increase the contribution of UVA to photocarcinogenesis, as detailed above. Therefore, although it appears that UVB contributes more to photocarcinogenesis than UVA, the relative contributions of either one to a lifetime risk to develop nonmelanoma skin cancer remains unclear.

Several animal models have been used to answer the wavelengths question for melanoma. Ley[87] observed the induction of melanoma precursor lesions in the opossum with UVA, more than with UVB. However, no infiltrative melanomas could be induced. Setlow et al[88] used swordfish and observed that UVA induces melanomas more effectively than UVB. However, this observation could not be reproduced and the opposite result was reported by Mitchell et al.[89] DeFabo et al[90] used HGF/SF transgenic mice and observed melanoma induction only with UVB, but not with UVA. Later, the same group[58] observed that UVA does induce melanoma, but only in pigmented mice, not in the previously studied nonpigmented mice. With that, it appears that, at least in this mouse model, the presence of melanin is required for the induction of melanoma with UVA, but not with UVB, and that both wavelengths, UVA and UVB, can induce melanoma, but possibly via a different mechanism. It is very plausible that the recently described melanin-dependent chemiexcitation pathway for the generation of pyrimidine dimers and UV signature mutations (Fig. 17-11; middle panel) is that postulated alternative mechanism for melanomagenesis with UVA.

In addition, increases of melanoma risk with tanning parlor use provide further support for UVA being a particular risk factor for melanoma. Many studies have shown a significantly increased risk for melanoma subsequent to sunbed/sunlamp use,[91,92] including a large prospective cohort study in 106,379 women in Sweden and Norway, showing a relative melanoma risk of 1.42 to 2.58 with use of tanning devices.[93] A melanoma epidemic in Iceland with increasing rates of melanoma between 1990 and 2006, mainly in young women, also has been associated with increased tanning bed use.[94] Melanomas at usually covered sites, for example, skin in the sacral and pubic areas, also may be attributable to UVR exposure from sunbed use.[95] When a few decades ago it was increasingly recognized that UVB (280 to 315 nm) had skin-damaging effect, but UVA (315 to 400 nm) was still considered relatively safe, the tanning industry reduced the UVB output in their devices and claimed that a UVA-induced tan would be safe. This is why the increased melanoma risk with tanning bed use may support the role of UVA as a particular risk factor for melanoma. However, tanning machines differ widely in their spectral output.[96,97] Therefore, the increased melanoma risk with sunbed use also may be due to the UVB that is still emitted by tanning devices.

The ability to generate oxidative DNA lesions increases with increasing wavelengths from UVB to UVA and it has been hypothesized that such damage, in particular when induced by UVA, could play a role in melanomagenesis.[63] When contemplating this hypothesis, it is important to recognize that at least in fibroblasts and keratinocytes, UVA has been shown to produce more pyrimidine dimers than 8-oxodG.[98] Unlike an early report of a separate UVA signature mutation observed in transformed rodent cells,[99] the majority of UVA-induced mutations has later been shown to be C → T transitions, without a particular signal for a separate UVA signature mutation or a high rate of mutations typical for oxidative base modifications, both in vitro and in vivo.[100-103]

An attractive candidate for generation of oxidative stress on exposure to UVR in melanocytes is melanin. Melanin has been described to have some photosensitizing properties, in particular, the more reddish-colored pheomelanin.[104,105] Wang et al.[106,107] reported that, on irradiation with UVA, melanocytes generate more oxidative DNA damage, have less efficient repair of oxidative DNA damage, and produce more mutations. They proposed that oxidative DNA damage is a major driver in melanomagenesis. However, they did not sequence the UVA-induced mutations and with that did not provide ultimate proof that the UVA-induced mutations are indeed the G → T or A → C transversions that are typical for oxidative DNA damage. In addition, the above-mentioned mutation data from melanomas show only a small percentage of such mutations typical for oxidative DNA damage.[67,68] Taken together, there is no proof that oxidative DNA base lesions play a major role in UVR-induced mutation formation that drives melanoma.

In summary, the evidence supports that both UVB and UVA can induce melanoma, possibly through different mechanisms. However, the relative contribution to the overall melanoma risk of UVB and UVA remain unclear.

PHOTOAGING

Photoaging describes changes observed in chronically sun-exposed skin, whereas intrinsic aging of the skin describes changes that occur with advancing age without extrinsic damage from chronic sun exposure. Skin alterations with photoaging are observed in all compartments of the skin, including the epidermis, the pigmentary system, the dermal connective tissue, the vasculature, and the subcutaneous fat (Figs. 17-14 and 17-15).[108,109] Although subtle changes of photoaging can sometimes be observed in young individuals already, manifestations of photoaging are more common in older patients, indicating that skin changes of photoaging are typically superimposed on changes of intrinsic skin aging. Many manifestations of photoaging are also observed in intrinsically aged skin. This raises the question whether photoaging is solely an acceleration of the normal aging process by chronic photodamage. Table 17-4 lists typical manifestation of cutaneous photoaging. Symptoms that involve benign, premalignant, and malignant clonal proliferations of keratinocytes and melanocytes are associated with aging, as cancer in general is associated with aging. They are better classified as neoplastic events, rather than aging events. They are not observed in intrinsically aged, only in photoprotected, skin. The mechanisms that drive these events are described under section "Photocarcinogenesis".

In contrast, thinning of the epidermis, hypopigmentations, loss of dermal collagen, telangiectasias (as a consequence of a diminished extracellular matrix scaffold), and loss of subcutaneous fat are loss-of-function events (Table 17-4), which are also observed with intrinsic aging. Accelerated proliferative exhaustion by chronic photodamage is a likely mechanism for these features, which is consistent with the view that photoaging represents damage-accelerated aging.

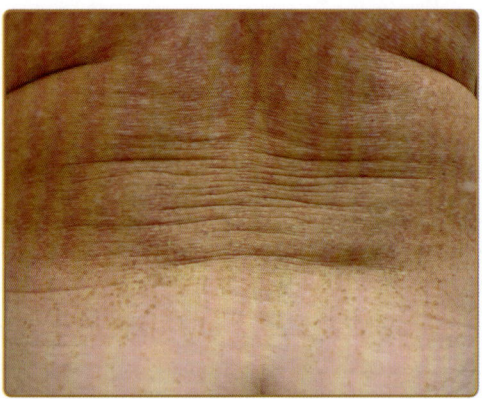 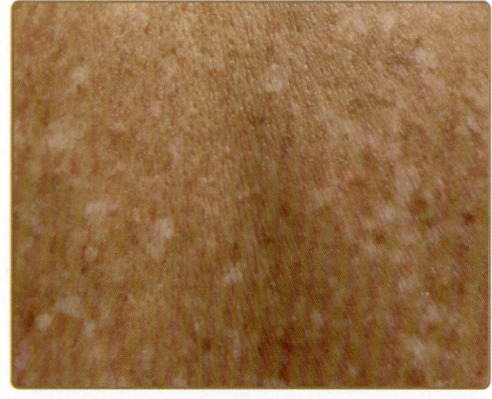

Figure 17-14 Pigmentary changes of photoaged skin include freckles, which are the result of clonal melanocyte proliferation events, and hypopigmentations, which are melanocyte loss-of-function events.

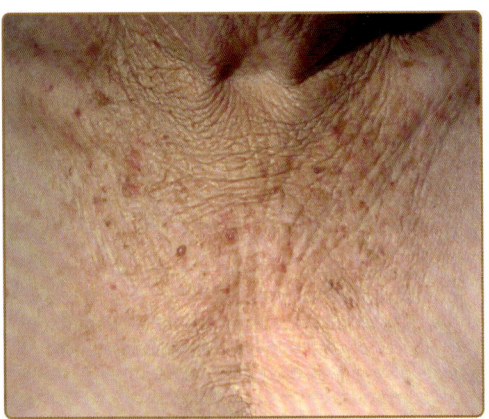

Figure 17-15 Deep wrinkling, in chronically photoaged skin due to actinic elastosis. Note the absence of such wrinkling in the more photoprotected areas on the lateral aspects of the chest.

The only nonproliferative feature of photoaged skin that is not observed in intrinsically aged skin is actinic elastosis, which is characterized by accumulation of fibrillary basophilic material in the upper and middermis. Clinically, it presents with yellowish thickening of the skin, sometimes nodular, loss of elasticity, and formation of deep wrinkles (Fig. 17-15). It is composed mainly of elastin and fibrillin, stains strongly with elastin stains, and can be degraded by elastase, but not collagenase. Elastin synthesis is upregulated following UV exposure,[110] but the UVR-induced influx of neutrophils, as seen, for example, in sunburned skin, also provides a mechanism for increased degradation via activity of elastase secreted by neutrophils. Following degradation of elastin in the extracellular space, dermal fibroblast internalize elastin fragments through receptor-mediated endocytosis to lysosomes for further degradation by the lysosomal protease cathepsin K.[111] Cathepsin K is upregulated by UVA to promote this intracellular clearing.[112] Aged fibroblasts do not upregulate cathepsin K in response to UVA, and it is hypothesized that this entails a failure to properly clear elastin fragments from the extracellular space and ultimately results in the accumulation of elastin with crosslinking to a large, abnormal macromolecule.[112] With this, actinic elastosis can be classified as a loss-of-function event. Actinic elastosis is largely irreversible, even with consistent photoprotection, which is most likely due to the fact that the large abnormal macromolecule has become undegradable. This is reminiscent of the intracellular accumulation of abnormal macromolecules and subsequent impairment of cellular function as a result of a failure to clear them from the cytoplasm via a mechanism called macroautophagy, which is an important mechanism how aged cells in general loose functions.[113]

Progerin is an abnormal splice variant of the nuclear membrane protein Lamin A. It is found in high concentrations in cells from patients with the premature aging syndrome Hutchinson Gilford progeria, but also accumulates in normally aging cells.[114,115] It interferes with many nuclear functions and ultimately results in cellular senescence and an aged cellular phenotype. This aging protein is induced by UVA via oxidative stress and induction of abnormal splicing.[116] This is yet another example how UVA in particular promotes an aging phenotype. As a result of a loss of a farnesylation site that allows degradation of lamin A, progerin is largely undegradable. This is a second example how exposure to UVA results in the accumulation of an undegradable protein that interferes with cell function. Although some of the effects of acute UVR-induced inflammation induce metabolic changes that may contribute to photoaging, for example, increased elastin synthesis, increased expression of matrix metalloproteinase (ie, collagenases), and decreased collagen synthesis, these should be reversible on cessation of UV exposure. The observation, however, is that changes of the extracellular matrix, which manifest as wrinkling and increased laxity of skin, are not reversible, may be explained by the accumulation of abnormal and undegradable proteins in the extra- and intracellular space. Although the contribution of oxidative DNA damage to photocarcinogenesis is unproven, UVA-induced oxidative stress is likely a central mediator in these loss-of-function events in photoaging. As ROS mediate senescence, for example, via the formation of progerin,[116] they probably entail an anticancer effect that counteracts the pro-carcinogenic effects of UVR. With this, antioxidants may prevent UVR-induced loss of function events of photoaging, but may in turn also promote photocarcinogenesis.

In addition to its specific roles in inducing a cellular aging phenotype with loss of cell functions, UVA also may be a particular culprit for the changes in the dermal extracellular matrix because of its deeper penetration into the dermis, as compared to UVB. However, UVB does affect metabolism in the deep dermis even

TABLE 17-4
Photoaging: Loss-of-Function Events and Clonal Proliferation Events

	LOSS OF FUNCTION	CLONAL PROLIFERATION
Epidermis		
Epidermal atrophy	✓	
Expansion of mutant clones		✓
Malignant transformation		✓
Pigmentary System		
Freckles/lentigines		✓
Hypopigmentations	✓	
Melanocytic nevi		✓
Malignant melanoma		✓
Dermal Connective Tissue		
Loss of collagen	✓	
Actinic elastosis	✓	
Vasculature		
Telangiectasias (loss of ECM scaffolding)	✓	
Subcutaneous Fat		
Loss of fat	✓	

without reaching into it. For example, the induction of matrix metalloproteinases in the dermis after irradiation with UVB has been shown to be mediated by a paracrine mechanism via excretion of inflammatory mediators from keratinocytes and signaling to dermal fibroblasts.[117-119] Further signaling into the subcutaneous fat may even mediate loss of subcutaneous fat as a feature of photoaging.[120]

CUTANEOUS RESPONSES TO VISIBLE LIGHT AND INFRARED RADIATION

In comparison to UVR, the effects of other types of nonionizing radiation of the electromagnetic spectrum, namely, visible light and infrared radiation (IR), have been studied much less. However, there is increasing evidence that these also have photobiological effects on the skin.

Visible light can induce erythema and pigmentation (immediate and delayed pigment darkening, in particular in darker skin types)[121,122] and some photodermatoses can sometimes also be elicited by visible light, including, for example, solar urticaria, chronic actinic dermatitis, and cutaneous porphyrias. Potential chromophores that absorb visible light and could be mediating these effects are porphyrins, melanin, β-carotene, riboflavin, bilirubin, and hemoglobin. In addition, the action spectra for the formation of pyrimidine dimer types of DNA damage and oxidative DNA base modification extend well into the range of visible light.[62] Although the mode of action of these effects is still only very incompletely understood, these insights have led to the development of visible light–based treatment devices, including, for example, intense pulsed light (IPL), lasers, and photodynamic therapy.

IR has been implicated in photoaging and in erythema ab igne.[123,124] IRA penetrates deep into the dermis and has profound effects on the gene expression profile of dermal fibroblasts, including, for example, the induction of matrix metalloproteinase. This may contribute to the loss of collagen fiber in chronically sun-exposed skin. Although infrared radiation alone does not appear to cause skin cancer, growth behavior may be affected, for example, via prevention of apoptosis.[125]

CONCLUSIONS

The only positive effect of UVR on skin, vitamin D production, is offset by a number of serious and potentially life-threatening detrimental effects that mandate effective photoprotection for prevention. Fortunately, the negative effect of photoprotection on vitamin D metabolism can easily be addressed with oral vitamin D supplementation.

From the described effects of UVB and UVA, is it clear that photoprotection strategies must include protection against both qualities. Fortunately, the Food and Drug Administration (FDA) of the US Department of Health and Human Services issued a final role on labeling and effectiveness testing of sunscreen drug products for nonprescription human use in 2011 that addresses such broad-spectrum protection. This new standard adds an in vitro measurement for broad-spectrum protection to include UVA. It uses the critical wavelength criterion originally suggested by Diffey et al, defining broad spectrum by a wavelength of at least 370 nm at which 90% of the area under the 290- to 400-nm absorbance curve is met.[126]

The recognition that IR and visible light can damage skin has given rise in efforts to extend photoprotection to these types of radiation.[127,128] Attempts to filter visible light will probably be hampered by poor acceptability, as such filters will be visible. There may be an opportunity to filter IR, but the development of such filters has only just begun.

Systemic and topical antioxidants have been advocated to reduce UVR-, visible light-, and IR-induced oxidative damage, in particular, oxidative DNA damage.[129] However, their protective effects against any of the above-mentioned endpoints have not been well established, or are marginal at best. In addition, the evidence that oxidative DNA damage might not contribute significantly to UVA-induced mutagenesis (as was previously thought) raises the question whether antioxidants provide any protection against skin cancer. Reactive oxygen species are not only damaging but also induce cellular responses that can protect against photocarcinogenesis, including, for example, induction of senescence through generation of the aging-associated protein called progerin.[116] This suggests that antioxidants may actually be promoting photocarcinogenesis, as already suggested for other types of cancer.

In 2014, the Surgeon General and the U.S. Department of Health and Human Services published a Call to Action to Prevent Skin Cancer. Stated goals include (1) increase opportunities for sun protection in outdoor settings; (2) provide individuals with the information they need to make informed, healthy choices about UV exposure; (3) promote policies that advance the national goal of preventing skin cancer; (4) reduce harms from indoor tanning; and (5) strengthen research, surveillance, monitoring, and evaluation related to skin cancer prevention.

When thinking about public awareness campaigns, it is important to recognize that sun-seeking and tanning device–seeking behavior is, at least in some individuals, associated with a pleasurable central nervous system effect.[130-132] Such features of addiction to UVR exposure are reminiscent of the addictive nature of nicotine that has made smoking cessation programs for lung cancer prevention difficult. The fact that anti-smoking campaigns have been able to overcome nicotine addiction and have resulted in a decline in smoking and consequently in lung cancer deaths are encouraging for efforts to reduce rates of nonmelanoma skin cancer and melanoma by addressing addictive tanning and sun seeking. The dermatologic community has the opportunity to make a huge impact on public health by supporting the Surgeon General's Call to Action.

ACKNOWLEDGMENTS

Parts of this chapter used significant portions of Chap. 90 of the previous edition of this book, "Fundamentals of Cutaneous Photobiology and Photoimmunology," written by Irene E. Kochevar, Charles R. Taylor, and Jean Krutmann. Other parts used elements of Chap. 110, "Genome Instability, DNA Repair, and Cancer," written by Thomas M. Rünger and Kenneth H. Kraemer.

REFERENCES

1. Hudec SM, Camacho PM. Secondary causes of osteoporosis. Endocr Pract. 2013;19:120.
2. Clemens TL, Adams JS, Henderson SL, et al. Increased skin pigment reduces the capacity of skin to synthesize vitamin D3. Lancet. 1982;1(8263):74.
3. Holick M. Vitamin D deficiency. N Engl J Med. 2007;357:266.
4. Norman AW. Sunlight, season, skin pigmentation, vitamin D and 25-hydroxyvitamin: integral components of the vitamin D endocrine system. Am J Clin Nutr. 1998;67:1108.
5. Libon F, Cavalier E, Nikkels AF. Skin color is relevant to vitamin D synthesis. Dermatology. 2013;227:250.
6. Chin K, Appel LJ, Michos ED. Vitamin D, calcium, and cardiovascular disease: A"D"vantageous or "D"etrimental? An era of uncertainty. Curr Atheroscler Rep. 2017;19:5.
7. Unholzer S, Rothmund A, Haen E. All-rounder vitamin D? Nervenarzt. 2017;88(5):489.
8. Sommer I, Griebler U, Kien C, et al. Vitamin D deficiency as a risk factor for dementia: a systematic review and meta-analysis. BMC Geriatr. 2017;17:16.
9. Hoel DG, Berwick M, de Gruijl FR, et al. The risks and benefits of sun exposure 2016. Dermatoendocrinol. 2016;8:e1248325.
10. Libman H, Malabanan AO, Strewler GJ, et al. Should we screen for vitamin D deficiency? Grand rounds discussion from Beth Israel Deaconess medical center. Ann Intern Med. 2016;165:800.
11. Yakoob MY, Salam RA, Khan FR, et al. Vitamin D supplementation for preventing infections in children under five years of age. Cochrane Database Syst Rev. 2016;11:CD008824.
12. Kopecky SL, Bauer DC, Gulati M, et al. Lack of evidence linking calcium with or without vitamin D supplementation to cardiovascular disease in generally healthy adults: a clinical guideline from the national osteoporosis foundation and the American Society for Preventive Cardiology. Ann Intern Med. 2016;165:867.
13. Trummer C, Pandis M, Verheyen N, et al. Beneficial effects of UV-radiation: vitamin D and beyond. Int J Environ Res Public Health. 2016;13:pii: E1028.
14. Wimalawansa SJ. Non-musculoskeletal benefits of vitamin D. J Steroid Biochem Mol Biol. 2018;175:60.
15. Bikle DD. Extraskeletal actions of vitamin D. Ann N Y Acad Sci. 2016;1376:29.
16. Reddy KK, Gilchrest BA. The role of vitamin D in melanoma prevention: evidence and hyperbole. J Am Acad Dermatol. 2014;71:1004.
17. MacLaughlin JA, Anderson RR, Holick MF. Spectral character of sunlight modulates photosynthesis of previtamin D3 and its photoisomers in human skin. Science. 1982;16:1001.
18. Norval M, Björn LO, de Gruijl FR. Is the action spectrum for the UV-induced production of previtamin D3 in human skin correct? Photochem Photobiol Sci. 2010;9:11.
19. Beleza S, Santos AM, McEvoy B, et al. The timing of pigmentation lightening in Europeans. Mol Biol Evol. 2013;30:24.
20. Kuwabara A, Tsugawa N, Tanaka K, et al. High prevalence of vitamin D deficiency in patients with xeroderma pigmentosum—a under strict sun protection. Eur J Clin Nutr. 2015;69:693.
21. Gentzsch S, Kern JS, Loeckermann S, et al. Iatrogenic vitamin D deficiency in a patient with Gorlin syndrome: the conundrum of photoprotection. Acta Derm Venereol. 2014;94:459.
22. Schwarz T, Beissert S. Milestones in photoimmunology. J Invest Dermatol. 2013;133:E7.
23. Palmer RA, Friedmann PS. Ultraviolet radiation causes less immunosuppression in patients with polymorphic light eruption than in controls. J Invest Dermatol. 2004;122:291.
24. Lembo S, Fallon J, O'Kelly P, et al. Polymorphous light eruption and skin cancer prevalence: is one protective against the other? Br J Dermatol. 2008;159:1342.
25. Halliday GM, Byrne SN, Damian DL. Ultraviolet A radiation: its role in immunosuppression and carcinogenesis. Semin Cutan Med Surg. 2011;30:214.
26. Schmalwieser AW, Wallisch S, Diffey B. A library of action spectra for erythema and pigmentation. Photochem Photobiol Sci. 2012;11:251.
27. Young AR, Chadwick CA, Harrison GI, et al. The similarity of action spectra for thymine dimers in human epidermis and erythema suggests that DNA is the chromophore for erythema. J Invest Dermatol. 1998;111:982.
28. Freeman SE, Hacham H, Gange RW, et al. Wavelength dependence of pyrimidine dimer formation in DNA of human skin irradiated in situ with ultraviolet light. Proc Natl Acad Sci U S A. 1989;86:5605.
29. Tamura D, DiGiovanna JJ, Khan SG, et al. Living with xeroderma pigmentosum: comprehensive photoprotection for highly photosensitive patients. Photodermatol Photoimmunol Photomed. 2014;30:146.
30. Kraemer KH, Lee MM, Scotto J. Xeroderma pigmentosum. Cutaneous, ocular, and neurologic abnormalities in 830 published cases. Arch Dermatol. 1987;123:241.
31. Wolf P, Yarosh DB, Kripke ML. Effects of sunscreens and a DNA excision repair enzyme on ultraviolet radiation-induced inflammation, immune suppression, and cyclobutane pyrimidine dimer formation in mice. J Invest Dermatol. 1993;101:523.
32. Ley RD. Photoreactivation of UV-induced pyrimidine dimers and erythema in the marsupial Monodelphis domestica. Proc Natl Acad Sci U S A. 1985;82:2409.
33. Clydesdale GJ, Dandie GW, Muller HK. Ultraviolet light induced injury: immunological and inflammatory effects. Immunol Cell Biol. 2001;79:547.
34. Fitzpatrick TB. Soleil et peau. Journal de Médecine Esthétique. 1975;2:33.
35. Youn JI, Oh JK, Kim BK, et al. Relationship between skin phototype and MED in Korean, brown skin. Photodermatol Photoimmunol Photomed. 1997;13:208.
36. Parrish JA, Jaenicke KF, Anderson RR. Erythema and melanogenesis action spectra of normal human skin. Photochem Photobiol. 1982;36:187.

37. Nylander K, Bourdon JC, Bray SE, et al. Transcriptional activation of tyrosinase and TRP-1 by p53 links UV irradiation to the protective tanning response. *J Pathol*. 2000;190:39.
38. Khlgatian MK, Eller M, Yaar M, et al. Tyrosinase expression is regulated by p53. *J Invest Dermatol*. 1999;112:548.
39. Cui R, Widlund HR, Feige E, et al. Central role of p53 in the suntan response and pathologic hyperpigmentation. *Cell*. 2007;128:853.
40. Byers HR, Dykstra SG, Boissel SJ. Requirement of dynactin p150(Glued) subunit for the functional integrity of the keratinocyte microparasol. *J Invest Dermatol*. 2007;127:1736.
41. Hexsel CL, Mahmoud BH, Mitchell D, et al. A clinical trial and molecular study of photoadaptation in vitiligo. *Br J Dermatol*. 2009;160:534.
42. Boonstra HE, van Weelden H, Toonstra J, et al. Polymorphous light eruption: a clinical, photobiologic, and follow-up study of 110 patients. *J Am Acad Dermatol*. 2000;42:199.
43. Du-Thanh A, Debu A, Lalheve P, et al. Solar urticaria: a time-extended retrospective series of 61 patients and review of literature. *Eur J Dermatol*. 2013;23:202.
44. de Gálvez MV, Aguilera J, Sánchez-Roldán C, et al. Infrared radiation increases skin damage induced by other wavelengths in solar urticaria. *Photodermatol Photoimmunol Photomed*. 2016;32:284.
45. Parrish JA, Jaenicke KF. Action spectrum for phototherapy of psoriasis. *J Invest Dermatol*. 1981;76:359.
46. Johnson-Huang LM, Suárez-Fariñas M, Sullivan-Whalen M, et al. Effective narrow-band UVB radiation therapy suppresses the IL-23/IL-17 axis in normalized psoriasis plaques. J Invest Dermatol. 2010;130:2654.
47. Gasparro FP. Psoralen photobiology: recent advances. *Photochem Photobiol*. 1996;63:553.
48. Brash DE. UV-signature mutations. *Photochem Photobiol*. 2015;91:15.
49. Rünger TM. C → T transition mutations are not solely UVB-signature mutations, because they are also generated by UVA. *J Invest Dermatol*. 2008;128:2138.
50. Wikondahl NM, Brash DE. Ultraviolet radiation induced signature mutations in photocarcinogenesis. *J Investig Dermatol Symp Proc*. 1999;4:6.
51. Jayaraman SS, Rayhan DJ, Hazany S, et al. Mutational landscape of basal cell carcinomas by whole-exome sequencing. *J Invest Dermatol*. 2014;134:213.
52. Hocker T, Tsao H. Ultraviolet radiation and melanoma: a systematic review and analysis of reported sequence variants. *Hum Mutat*. 2007;28:578.
53. Horn S, Figl A, Rachakonda PS, et al. TERT promoter mutations in familial and sporadic melanoma. *Science*. 2013;339:959.
54. Huang FW, Hodis E, Xu MJ, et al. Highly recurrent TERT promoter mutations in human melanoma. *Science*. 2013;339:957.
55. Rünger TM. Is UV-induced mutation formation in melanocytes different from other skin cells? *Pigment Cell Melanoma Res*. 2011;24:10.
56. Premi S, Wallisch S, Mano CM, et al. Photochemistry. Chemiexcitation of melanin derivatives induces DNA photoproducts long after UV exposure. *Science*. 2015;347:842.
57. Brash DE. UV-induced melanin chemiexcitation. A new mode of melanoma pathogenesis. *Toxicologic Pathol*. 2016;44:552.
58. Noonan FP, Zaidi MR, Wolnicka-Glubisz A, et al. Melanoma induction by ultraviolet A but not ultraviolet B radiation requires melanin pigment. *Nat Commun*. 2012;3:884.
59. Nishiura H, Kumagai J, Kashino G, et al. The bystander effect is a novel mechanism of UVA-induced melanogenesis. *Photochem Photobiol*. 2012;88:389.
60. Redmond RW, Rajadurai A, Udayakumar D, et al. Melanocytes are selectively vulnerable to UVA-mediated bystander oxidative signaling. *J Invest Dermatol*. 2014;134:1083.
61. Kvam E, Tyrell RM. Induction of oxidative DNA base damage in human skin cells by UV and near visible radiation. *Carcinogenesis*. 1997;18:2379.
62. Kielbassa C, Roza L, Epe B. Wavelength dependence of oxidative DNA damage induced by UV and visible light. *Carcinogenesis*. 1997;18:811.
63. Rünger TM, Kappes UP. Mechanisms of mutation formation with long-wave ultraviolet light (UVA). *Photodermatol Photoimmunol Photomed*. 2008;24:2.
64. Rünger TM, Farahvash B, Hatvani Z, et al. Comparison of DNA damage responses following equimutagenic doses of UVA and UVB: a less effective cell cycle arrest with UVA may render UVA-induced pyrimidine dimers more mutagenic than UVB-induced ones. *Photochem Photobiol Sci*. 2012;11:207.
65. Dunn J, Potter M, Rees A, et al. Activation of the Fanconi anemia/BRCA pathway and recombination repair in the cellular response to solar UV. *Cancer Res*. 2006;66:11140.
66. Rizzo JL, Dunn J, Rees A, et al. No formation of DNA double-strand breaks and no activation of recombination repair with UVA. *J Invest Dermatol*. 2011;131:1139.
67. Pleasance ED, Cheetham RK, Stephens PJ, et al. A comprehensive catalogue of somatic mutations from a human cancer genome. *Nature*. 2010;463:191.
68. Cancer Genome Atlas Network. Genomic classification of cutaneous melanoma. *Cell*. 2015;161:1681.
69. Krauthammer M, Kong Y, Bacchiocchi A, et al. Exome sequencing identifies recurrent mutations in NF1 and RASopathy genes in sun-exposed melanomas. *Nat Genet*. 2015;47:996.
70. Shain AH, Garrido M, Botton T, et al. Exome sequencing of desmoplastic melanoma identifies recurrent NFKBIE promoter mutations and diverse activating mutations in the MAPK pathway. *Nat Genet*. 2015;47:1194.
71. Gordon D, Gillgren P, Eloranta S, et al. Time trends in incidence of cutaneous melanoma by detailed anatomical location and patterns of ultraviolet radiation exposure: a retrospective population-based study. *Melanoma Res*. 2015;25:348.
72. Bodekær M, Philipsen PA, Petersen B, et al. Defining "intermittent UVR exposure." *Photochem Photobiol Sci*. 2016;15:1176.
73. Gilchrest BA, Eller MS, Geller AC, et al. The pathogenesis of melanoma induced by ultraviolet radiation. *N Engl J Med*. 1999;340:1341.
74. Rünger TM. How different wavelengths of the ultraviolet spectrum contribute to skin carcinogenesis: the role of cellular damage responses. *J Invest Dermatol*. 2007;127:2103.
75. Wei Q, Lee JE, Gershenwald JE, et al. Repair of UV light-induced DNA damage and risk of cutaneous malignant melanoma. *J Natl Cancer Inst*. 2003;95:308.
76. Blankenburg S, Konig IR, Moessner R, et al. Assessment of 3 xeroderma pigmentosum group C gene polymorphisms and risk of cutaneous melanoma: a case-control study. *Carcinogenesis*. 2005;26:1085.
77. Torres S M, Luo L, Lilyquist J, et al. DNA repair variants, indoor tanning, and risk of melanoma. *Pigment Cell Melanoma Res*. 2013;26:677.

78. Wei Q. Effect of aging on DNA repair and skin carcinogenesis: a minireview of population-based studies. *J Invest Dermatol Symp Proc.* 1998;3:19.
79. Woodgate R. A plethora of lesion-replicating DNA polymerases. *Genes Dev.* 1999;13:2191.
80. Masutani C, Kusumoto R, Yamada A, et al. The XPV (xeroderma pigmentosum variant) gene encodes human DNA polymerase eta. *Nature.* 1999;399(6737):700.
81. Johnson RE, Kondratick CM, Prakash S, et al. hRAD30 mutations in the variant form of xeroderma pigmentosum. *Science.* 1999;285:263.
82. Limoli CL, Giedzinski E, Cleaver JE. Alternative recombination pathways in UV-irradiated XP variant cells. *Oncogene.* 2005;24:3708.
83. Zhang W, Remenyik E, Zelterman D, et al. Escaping the stem cell compartment: sustained UVB exposure allows p53-mutant keratinocytes to colonize adjacent epidermal proliferating units without incurring additional mutations. *Proc Natl Acad Sci U S A.* 2001;98:13948.
84. Loeb LA. Cancer cells exhibit a mutator phenotype. *Adv Cancer Res.* 1998;72:25.
85. El Ghissassi F, Baan R, Straif K, et al. A review of human carcinogens—part D: radiation. *Lancet Oncol.* 2009;10:751.
86. de Gruijl FR, Sterenborg HJ, Forbes PD, et al. Wavelength dependence of skin cancer induction by ultraviolet irradiation of albino hairless mice. *Cancer Res.* 1993;53:53.
87. Ley RD. Ultraviolet radiation A-induced precursors of cutaneous melanoma in *Monodelphis domestica*. *Cancer Res.* 1997;57:3682.
88. Setlow RB, Grist E, Thompson K, et al. Wavelengths effective in induction of malignant melanoma. *Proc Natl Acad Sci U S A.* 1993;90:6666.
89. Mitchell DL, Fernandez AA, Nairn RS, et al. Ultraviolet A does not induce melanomas in a Xiphophorus hybrid fish model. *Proc Natl Acad Sci U S A.* 2010;107:9329.
90. De Fabo EC, Noonan FP, Fears T, et al. Ultraviolet B but not ultraviolet A radiation initiates melanoma. *Cancer Res.* 2004;64:6372.
91. Boniol M, Autier P, Boyle P, et al. Cutaneous melanoma attributable to sunbed use: systematic review and meta-analysis. *BMJ.* 2012;345:e4757.
92. Gallagher RP, Spinelli JJ, Lee TK. Tanning beds, sunlamps, and risk of cutaneous malignant melanoma. *Cancer Epidemiol Biomarkers Prev.* 2005;14:562.
93. Veierød MB, Weiderpass E, Thörn M, et al. A prospective study of pigmentation, sun exposure, and risk of cutaneous malignant melanoma in women. *J Natl Cancer Inst.* 2003;95:1530.
94. Autier P, Dore JF, Eggermont A, et al. Epidemiological evidence that UVA radiation is involved in the genesis of cutaneous melanoma. *Curr Opin Oncol.* 2011;23:189.
95. Higgins EM, Du Vivier AW. Possible induction of malignant melanoma by sunbed use. *Clin Exp Dermatol.* 1992;17:357.
96. Facta S, Fusette SS, Bonino A, et al. UV emissions from artificial tanning devices and their compliance with the European technical standard. *Health Phys.* 2013;104:385.
97. Gerber B, Mathys P, Moser M, et al. Ultraviolet emission spectra of sunbeds. *Photochem Photobiol.* 2002;76:664.
98. Courdavault S, Baudouin C, Charveron M, et al. Larger yield of cyclobutane dimers than 8-oxo-7,8-dihydroguanine in the DNA of UVA-irradiated human skin cells. *Mutat Res.* 2004;556:135.
99. Drobetsky EA, Turcotte J, Châteauneuf A. A role for ultraviolet A in solar mutagenesis. *Proc Natl Acad Sci U S A.* 1995;92:2350.
100. Ikehata H, Kawai K, Komura J, et al. UVA1 genotoxicity is mediatated not by oxidative damage but by cyclobutane pyrimidine dimers in normal mouse skin. *J Invest Dermatol.* 2008;128:2289.
101. Ikehata H, Higashi S, Nakamura S, et al. Action spectrum analysis of UVR genotoxicity for skin: the border wavelengths between UVA and UVB can bring serious mutation loads to skin. *J Invest Dermatol.* 2013;133:1850.
102. Rünger TM. Much remains to be learned about how UVR induces mutations. *J Invest Dermatol.* 2013;133:1717.
103. Rünger TM, Kappes UP. Mechanisms of mutation formation with long-wave ultraviolet light (UVA). *Photodermatol Photoimmunol Photomed.* 2008;24:2.
104. Kollias N, Sayre RM, Zeise L, et al. Photoprotection my melanin. *J Photochem Photobiol B.* 1991;9:135.
105. Micillo R, Panzella L, Koike K, et al. "Fifty Shades" of black and red or how carboxyl groups fine tune eumelanin and pheomelanin properties. *Int J Mol Sci.* 2016;17(5). pii: E746.
106. Wang HT, Choi BC, Tang MS. Melanocytes are deficient in repair of oxidative DNA damage and UV-induced photoproducts. *Proc Natl Acad Sci U S A.* 2010;107:12180.
107. Rünger TM. Is UV-induced mutation formation in melanocytes different from other skin cells? *Pigment Cell Melanoma Res.* 2011;24:10.
108. Poon F, Kang S, Chien A. Mechanisms and treatments of photoaging. *Photodermatol Photoimmunol Photomed.* 2014;31:65.
109. Gilchrest BA. Photoaging. *J Invest Dermatol.* 2013;133:E2.
110. Bernstein EF, Brown DB, Urbach F, et al. Ultraviolet radiation activates the human elastin promoter in transgenic mice: a novel in vivo and in vitro model of cutaneous photoaging. *J Invest Dermatol.* 1995;105:269.
111. Gan SD, Rünger TM. Dermal fibroblasts internalize elastin to lysosomes via the elastin-binding protein of the elastin-laminin receptor. *J Dermatol Sci.* 2011;61:60.
112. Codriansky KA, Quintanilla-Dieck MJ, Gan S, et al. Intracellular degradation of elastin by cathepsin K in skin fibroblasts—a possible role in photoaging. *Photochem Photobiol.* 2009;85:1356.
113. Saftig P, Eskelinen EL. Live longer with LAMP-2. *Nat Med.* 2008;14:909.
114. Eriksson M, Brown WT, Gordon LB, et al. Recurrent de novo point mutations in lamin A cause Hutchinson-Gilford progeria syndrome. *Nature.* 2003;423:293.
115. McClintock D, Ratner D, Lokuge M, et al. The mutant form of lamin A that causes Hutchinson-Gilford progeria is a biomarker of cellular aging in human skin. *PLoS One.* 2007;2:e1269.
116. Takeuchi H, Rünger TM. Longwave UV light induces the aging-associated progerin. *J Invest Dermatol.* 2013;133:1857.
117. Fagot D, Asselineau D, Bernerd F. Matrix metalloproteinase-1 production observed after solar-simulated radiation exposure is assumed by dermal fibroblasts but involves a paracrine activation through epidermal keratinocytes. *Photochem Photobiol.* 2004;79:499.

118. Yarosh D, Dong K, Smiles K. UV-induced degradation of collagen I is mediated by soluble factors released from keratinocytes. *Photochem Photobiol.* 2008;84:67.
119. Dong KK, Damaghi N, Picart SD, et al. UV-induced DNA damage initiates release of MMP-1 in human skin. *Exp Dermatol.* 2008;17:1037.
120. Li WH, Pappas A, Zhang L, et al. IL-11, IL-1alpha, IL-6, and TNF-alpha are induced by solar radiation in vitro and may be involved in facial subcutaneous fat loss in vivo. *J Dermatol Sci.* 2013;71:58.
121. Mahmoud BH, Hexsel CL, Hamzavi IH, et al. Effects of visible light on the skin. *Photochem Photobiol.* 2008;84:450.
122. Sklar LS, Almutawa F, Lim HW, et al. Effects of ultraviolet radiation, visible light, and infrared radiation on erythema and pigmentation: a review. *Photochem Photobiol Sci.* 2013;12:54.
123. Barolet D, Christiaens F, Hamblin MR. Infrared and skin: friend or foe. *J Photochem Photobiol B.* 2016;155:78.
124. Holzer AM, Athar M, Elmets CA. The other end of the rainbow: infrared and skin. *J Invest Dermatol.* 2010;130:1496.
125. Jantschitsch C, Weichenthal M, Maeda A, et al. Infrared radiation does not enhance the frequency of ultraviolet radiation-induced skin tumors, but their growth behaviour in mice. *Exp Dermatol.* 2011;20:346.
126. Diffey BL, Tanner PR, Matts PJ, et al. In vitro assessment of the broad-spectrum ultraviolet protection of sunscreen products. *J Am Acad Dermatol.* 2000;43:1024.
127. Grether-Beck S, Marini A, Jaenicke T, et al. Photoprotection of human skin beyond ultraviolet radiation. *Photodermatol Photoimmunol Photomed.* 2014;30:167.
128. Diffey B, Cadars B. An appraisal of the need for infrared radiation protection in sunscreens. *Photochem Photobiol Sci.* 2016;15:361.
129. Lim HW, Arellano-Mendoza MI, Stengel F. Current challenges in photoprotection. *J Am Acad Dermatol.* 2017;76(3S1):S91.
130. Aubert PM, Seibyl JP, Price JL, et al. Dopamine efflux in response to ultraviolet radiation in addicted sunbed users. *Psychiatry Res.* 2016;251:7.
131. Fell GL, Robinson KC, Mao J, et al. Skin β-endorphin mediates addiction to UV light. *Cell.* 2014;157:1527.
132. Robinson KC, Fisher DE. Tanning as a substance abuse. *Commun Integr Biol.* 2014;7(5):e971579.

Chapter 18 :: Genetics in Relation to the Skin
:: Etienne C. E. Wang, John A. McGrath, & Angela M. Christiano

第十八章
皮肤遗传学

中文导读

本章分为18节，介绍了与皮肤科医生临床相关的遗传学关键术语。

第一节人类皮肤基因组，介绍了新的基因组和蛋白质组数据库的出现正在逐渐改变位置克隆方法和传统的功能研究。新的技术，如全外显子组测序，将识别更多的单基因疾病，可根据患者特有的突变对其进行分类。最近，对罕见遗传性皮肤病的研究也使人们对更常见的多基因皮肤病的病理生理有了新的认识，这些新的信息对患者开发新的治疗方法和管理策略具有重要意义。

第二节人类基因组，介绍了人类基因组测序草图于2003年完成。除了编码蛋白质的基因外，还有许多编码未翻译的RNA分子的基因，包括转移RNA、核糖体RNA和micro-RNA基因。近年来大量基因组以外来自新RNA物种的形式在低水平转录，这些转录正在成为关键的调控分子，这增加了基因表达的表观遗传控制的复杂性。

第三节遗传和基因组数据库，介绍了人类基因组和其他基因组的大小和复杂性，以及来自基于群体的遗传研究和基因表达研究的海量数据集，计算能力已经成为整合和分析这些数据的越来越重要的因素。许多用于访问基因组数据的网络浏览器都是可用的，其中最有用的在表18-1中列出。这也将为制药公司和流行病学家提供有价值的参考数据集。

第四节染色体与基因结构，介绍了人类染色体由两条染色体臂组成，其命名分别为"p"和"q"。可以根据基因在给定染色体的DNA序列中跨越的碱基对范围进行绝对精确的定位。同时介绍了染色体臂中端粒、着丝粒的作用与功能。同时阐述了大多数染色体DNA含有散布着大小不一的非编码DNA片段的基因，基因的密度在染色体上差异很大，因此有基因密集的区域，或者是几乎没有功能基因的大片区域。

第五节基因表达，介绍了基因表达的过程，在很大程度上由基因的启动子元件决定。启动子的大小可以根据基因家族的不同或单个基因本身的不同而有很大的不同。并且介绍了启动子与基因启动子区域的结合导致转录机制的激活和RNA聚合酶Ⅱ对基因的转录，转录因子蛋白由启动子控制的基因编码，启动子受其他基因编码的其他转录因子的调控。

第六节寻找疾病基因，介绍了寻找致病基因有两个关键步骤。首先，必须确定与特定疾病相关的基因，其次，必须确定该基因内的致病突变。全外显子组测序再次给人类遗传学带来革命性的变化，不仅将对诊断产生影响，还将为未来的CRISPR/CAS9基因校正和诱导多潜能干细胞治疗等精确医学方法奠定基础。

第七节基因突变和多态性，介绍了基因突变和多态性的定义和功能。在人类基因组中，两个健康个体的遗传密码可能显示出许多与疾病或表型特征无关的序列差异。正常人群中的这种变化称为多态性。基因突变被定义为导致蛋白质化学成分改变的核苷酸序列的改变。

第八节孟德尔遗传病，介绍了大约有5000种人类单基因疾病，虽然其中大约2000种的分子基础已经确定，但了解遗传模式对于父母咨询未来的孩子是否有遗传风险是至关重要的。遗传方式主要有：①常染色体显性遗传；②常染色体隐性遗传；③X连锁显性遗传；④X连锁隐性遗传。

第九节染色体疾病，介绍了染色体数目或结构的畸变是很常见的，大多数会导致流产，但仍有活体分娩中染色体异常，频率约为0.6%。目前不仅可以用标准的细胞遗传学来检测，新的检测手段如SNP阵列和比较基因组杂交阵列等在临床应用中也已经非常广泛。

第十节线粒体疾病，介绍了细胞包含线粒体基因组，而且这些线粒体基因组只从个体的母亲遗传。线粒体DNA突变在体细胞中非常常见，从1988年首次报道了线粒体DNA的28个突变以来，目前超过250个致病性点突变和基因组重排被证明是许多肌肉疾病和神经退行性疾病的基础。但目前对线粒体基因组在健康和疾病中的相互作用知之甚少。

第十一节复杂疾病遗传学，介绍了全基因组关联研究（GWASs）已经成为绘制复杂疾病图的主要技术，目前已经对银屑病、特应性皮炎、白癜风和脱发进行了GWASs。提到了一个典型的GWAS设计包括从所选条件的表型良好的病例系列中收集DNA，最好是从种族同质的人群中收集DNA。

第十二节嵌合现象，介绍了具有不同遗传或染色体特征的混合细胞群体的存在导致表型多样性被称为嵌合体，包括单基因嵌合体、染色体嵌合体、功能性嵌合体和突变型嵌合体。本节最后提到了逆转嵌合体，也称天然基因治疗，证明是治疗遗传性皮肤病的可行方案。

第十三节组织相容性抗原疾病，介绍了人类白细胞抗原(HLA)分子具有高度多态性，每个位点都有许多等位基因，使免疫系统能够定义什么是外来的，什么是自己的，具有组织相容性。但遗传和流行病学数据表明这些分子与各种自身免疫性和慢性炎症性疾病的发病机制有关，如斑秃、银屑病、银屑病关节病等均与某些HLA单倍型的遗传有关。

第十四节表观遗传学，介绍了表观遗传的概念。疾病表型反映了特定基因型和环境相互作用的结果，生物化学、细胞、组织和有机体水平上的附加影响被称为表观遗传现象，参与到细胞周期调控、凋亡、细胞信号转导、肿瘤细胞侵袭、转移、血管生成和免疫识别。

第十五节遗传咨询，介绍了遗传咨询应包括：①解释家族史和病史以评估疾病发生或复发的机会；②关于遗传、检测、管理、预防、资源和研究的教育；③促进知情选择和对风险状况适应的咨询。

第十六节产前诊断，介绍了产前诊断的进展历程，从最初的胎儿皮肤活检，发展至超声波引导下胎儿皮肤活检，到针对各种基底膜成分的单克隆和多克隆抗体的引入，免疫组织化学实验发展，建立准确的诊断。到20世纪90年代初以来，胎儿皮肤活检逐渐被羊水细胞或绒毛样本中的胎儿DNA诊断筛查所取代。到目前体外受精的进展解决家族性线粒体疾病。

第十七节基因治疗与编辑，介绍了基因治疗领域可以以不同的方式细分。首先有针对隐性遗传病的治疗方法，再有治疗显性-隐性遗传疾病的基因抑制疗法。并提到了多种基因编辑和导入的方法，如siRNA抑制药离子导入、超声导入和微针等。

第十八节精准医学，概述了目前我们已经进入了一个预测性、预防性、个性化和参与性医学的新时代,在这个时代,每个患者的诊断将被分层到遗传和表观遗传学水平,治疗将专门针对这种独特的异常。这一新的方式有望让我们理解和解决治疗无效的遗传病患者。

〔粟 娟〕

AT-A-GLANCE

- 25% of monogenic gene disorders with known molecular mechanisms have skin manifestations.
- Skin disease may also arise from polygenic, complex inheritance, mosaicism, and chromosomal abnormalities.
- It is crucial for dermatologists to be up-to-date with new methods of genetic diagnosis and treatment (as well as their limitations).

THE HUMAN GENOME IN DERMATOLOGY

The completion of the Human Genome Project in 2003 coincided with the dawn of the Information or Digital Age. Having sequenced more than 3 billion base pairs (bp) of DNA, with identification of most of the estimated 25,000 genes in the entire human genome, this initiative provided ourselves with a treasure trove of information to make sense of the human body and its diseases. Although a few relatively small gaps remain, the near completion of the entire sequence of the human genome is having a huge impact on both the clinical practice of genetics and the strategies used to identify disease-associated genes. Laborious positional cloning approaches and traditional functional studies are gradually being transformed by the emergence of new genomic and proteomic databases.[1] Some of the exciting challenges that clinicians and geneticists now face are determining the function of these genes, defining disease associations and, relevant to patients, correlating genotype with phenotype. Nevertheless, many discoveries are already influencing how clinical genetics is practiced throughout the world, particularly for patients and families with rare, monogenic inherited disorders. The key benefits of dissection of the genome thus far have been the documentation of new information about disease causation, improving the accuracy of diagnosis and genetic counseling, and making DNA-based prenatal testing feasible.[2] Indeed, the genetic basis of more than 2000 inherited single gene disorders has now been determined, of which about 25% have a skin phenotype. Therefore, these "genodermatoses" have direct relevance to dermatologists and their patients, and newer technologies such as whole-exome sequencing will identify even more single-gene disorders and even allow us to classify them according to their patient-specific mutations.[3]

Recently, studies in rare inherited skin disorders have also led to new insight into the pathophysiology of more common polygenic skin disorders.[4] This new information is expected to have significant implications for the development of new therapies and management strategies for patients. Therefore, understanding the basic language and principles of clinical and molecular genetics has become a vital part of day-to-day practice for clinicians. The aim of this chapter is to provide an overview of key terminology in genetics that is clinically relevant to dermatologists.

THE HUMAN GENOME

Humans have a large complex genome packaged in the form of 46 chromosomes. These consist of 22 pairs of autosomes, numbered in descending order of size from the largest (chromosome 1) to the smallest (chromosome 22), in addition to two sex chromosomes, X and Y. Whereas females possess two copies of the X chromosome, males carry one X and one Y chromosome. The haploid genome consists of about 3.3 billion bp of DNA. Of this, only about 1.5% corresponds to protein-encoding exons of genes. Apart from genes and regulatory sequences, perhaps as much as 97% of the genome is of unknown function, often referred to as "junk" DNA. However, caution should be exercised in labeling the noncoding genome as "junk" because other unknown functions may reside in these regions. Much of the noncoding DNA is in the form of repetitive sequences, pseudogenes ("dead" copies of genes lost in recent evolution), and transposable elements of uncertain relevance. Although initial estimates for the number of human genes was in the order of 100,000, current predictions, based on the essentially complete genome sequence, are in the range of 20,000 to 25,000.[5] Surprisingly, therefore, the human genome is comparable in size and complexity to that of primitive organisms such as the fruit fly. However, it is thought that the generation of multiple protein isoforms from a single gene via alternate splicing of exons, each with a discrete function, is what contributes to increased complexity in higher organisms, including humans. In addition to protein-encoding genes, there are also many genes encoding untranslated RNA molecules, including transfer RNA, ribosomal RNA, and microRNA genes. MicroRNA is thought to be involved in the control of a large number of other genes through the RNA inhibition pathway. Recently, it has emerged that tracts of the genome are transcribed at low levels in the form of exotic new RNA species, including natural antisense RNA, long interspersed noncoding

TABLE 18-1
Websites for Accessing Human Genome Data

WEBSITE	URL
University of California, Santa Cruz	http://genome.ucsc.edu
National Center for Biotechnology Information	http://www.ncbi.nlm.nih.gov
ENSEMBL	http://www.ensembl.org
Online Mendelian Inheritance in Man	http://www.ncbi.nlm.nih.gov/entrez/query.fcgi?db=omim

RNA (lncRNA), and even competing endogenous RNAs (ceRNA). These transcripts are emerging as key regulatory molecules, which add level of complexity to the epigenetic control of gene expression. Thus, a much greater proportion of the genome is actively transcribed than was previously recognized, and this trend is likely to continue in the current "postgenome" era of human genetics.

The draft sequence of the human genome was completed in 2003. Subsequently, small gaps have been filled, and the sequence has now been extensively annotated in terms of genes, repetitive elements, regulatory sequences, polymorphisms, and many other features recognizable by in silico data mining methods informed, wherever possible, by functional analysis. This annotation process will continue for some time as more features are uncovered. The human genome data, and that for an increasing number of other species, is freely available on websites (Table 18-1). Some regions of the genome, particularly near the centromeres, consist of long stretches of highly repetitive sequences that are difficult or impossible to clone or sequence. These heterochromatic regions of the genome are unlikely to be sequenced and are thought to be structural in nature, mediating the chromosomal architecture required for cell division rather than contributing to heritable characteristics.

GENETIC AND GENOMIC DATABASES

Given the size and complexity of the human genome and other genomes now available, along with the massive datasets from population-based genetic studies and gene expression studies, computing power has become increasingly central to the integration and analysis of these data. Even storage and retrieval of the sequence data associated with mammalian genome require considerable computer power and memory, and even the assembly of the raw sequence of any mammalian genome would not have been feasible without computers. Many web browsers for accessing genome data are available, and the most useful of these are listed in Table 18-1. Each of these interfaces, which are the ones that the authors find most useful and user friendly, contains a wide variety of tools for analysis and searching of sequences according to keyword, gene name, protein name, and homology to DNA or protein sequence data.

The main source of historical, clinical, molecular, and biochemical data relating to human genetic diseases is the Online Mendelian Inheritance in Man (OMIM) (see Table 18-1). All recognized genetic diseases and nonpathogenic heritable traits, including common diseases with a genetic component, as well as all known genes and proteins, are listed and reviewed by OMIM number with links to PubMed. In the spirit of the Information Age and social media, the consumer genetics company 23andMe has democratized genomic sequencing and allowed the general public to take a peek into their own genetic makeup. Their business plan, although bringing up questions about privacy and patents (out of the scope of this chapter), will provide a valuable reference dataset for pharmaceutical companies and epidemiologists in the near future.

CHROMOSOME AND GENE STRUCTURE

Human chromosomes share common structural features (Fig. 18-1). All consist of two chromosomal arms, designated as "p" and "q." If the arms are of unequal length, the short arm is always designated as the "p" arm (for *petit*, the French word for small), and the other arm is named "q" (for the subsequent letter in the alphabet). Chromosomal maps to seek abnormalities are based on the stained, banded appearance of condensed chromosomes during metaphase of mitosis. During interphase, the uncondensed chromosomes are not discernible by normal microscopy techniques. Genes can now be located with absolute precision in terms of the range of base pairs that they span within the DNA sequence for a given chromosome. The bands are numbered from the centromere outward using a system that has evolved as increasingly discriminating chromosome stains, as well as higher resolution light microscopes, became available. A typical cytogenetic chromosome band is 17q21.2, within which the type I keratin genes reside (see Fig. 18-1). Type II keratins are similarly found in a cluster on the chromosome band 12q13.

The ends of the chromosomal arms are known as *telomeres*, and these consist of multiple tandem repeats of short DNA sequences. In germ cells and certain other cellular contexts, additional repeats are added to telomeres by a protein–RNA enzyme complex known as *telomerase*. During each round of cell division in somatic cells, one of the telomere repeats is trimmed off as a consequence of the DNA replication mechanism. By measuring the length of telomeres, the "age" of somatic cells, in terms of the number of times they have divided during the lifetime of the organism, can be determined. When the telomere length falls below a certain threshold, the cell undergoes senescence. Thus, telomeres contribute to an important biological clock function that removes somatic cells that have gone through too many rounds of replication and are at a high risk of accumulating mutations that could lead to tumorigenesis or other functional aberration.[6]

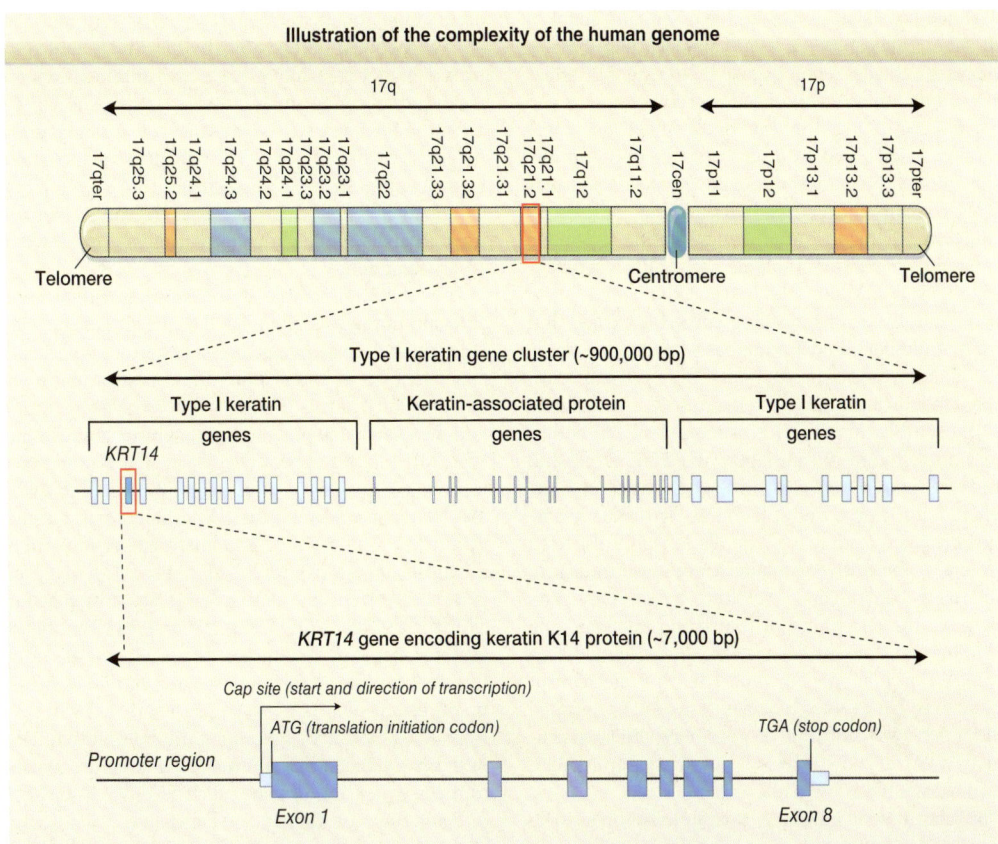

Figure 18-1 Illustration of the complexity of the human genome. At the top, the short (p) and long (q) arms of human chromosome 17 are depicted with their cytogenetic chromosome bands. One of these band regions, 17q21.2, is then highlighted to show that it is made up of approximately 900,000 base pairs (bp) and contains several genes, including 27 functional type I keratin genes. Part of this region is then further amplified to show one keratin gene, KRT14, encoding keratin 14, which is composed of eight exons.

The chromosome arms are separated by the centromere, which is a large stretch of highly repetitious DNA sequence. The centromere has important functions in terms of the movement and interactions of chromosomes. The centromeres of sister chromatids are where the double chromosomes align and attach during the prophase and anaphase stages of mitosis (and meiosis). The centromeres of sister chromatids are also the site of kinetochore formation. The latter is a multiprotein complex to which microtubules attach, allowing mitotic spindle formation, which ultimately results in pulling apart of the chromatids during anaphase of the cell division cycle.

The majority of chromosomal DNA contains genes interspersed with noncoding stretches of DNA of varying sizes. The density of genes varies widely across the chromosomes so that there are gene-dense regions or, alternately, large areas almost devoid of functional genes. An example of a comparatively gene-rich region of particular relevance to inherited skin diseases is the type I keratin gene cluster on chromosome band 17q21.2 (see Fig. 18-1). This figure also gives an idea of the sizes in base pairs of DNA of a typical chromosome and a typical gene located within it. This gene cluster spans about 900,000 bp of DNA and contains 27 functional type I keratin genes, several genes encoding keratin-associated proteins, and a number of pseudogenes (not shown). Because chromosome 17 is one of the smaller chromosomes, Fig. 18-1 starts to give some idea of the overall complexity and organization of the genome.

Protein-encoding genes normally consist of several exons, which collectively code for the amino acid sequence of the protein (or open reading frame). These are separated by noncoding introns. In human genes, few exons are much greater than 1000 bp in size, and introns vary from less than 100 bp to more than 1 million bp. A typical exon might be 100 to 300 bp in size. The KRT14 gene encoding keratin 14 (K14) protein is one of the genes in which mutations lead to epidermolysis bullosa (EB) simplex (see Chap. 60) and is illustrated in Fig. 18-1. KRT14 is contained within about 7000 bp of DNA and consists of eight modestly sized exons interspersed by seven small introns. Although all genes are present in all human cells that contain a nucleus, not every gene is expressed in all cells of tissues. For example, the KRT14 gene is only active in basal keratinocytes of the epidermis and other stratified epithelial tissues and is essentially silent in all other tissues. When a protein-encoding gene is expressed, the RNA polymerase II enzyme transcribes the coding strand of the gene, starting from the cap site and continuing to the end of the final exon, where various signals lead to termination of transcription. The initial RNA transcript, known as *heteronuclear RNA*, contains intronic as well as exonic sequences. This primary transcript undergoes splicing to remove the introns, resulting in the messenger RNA (mRNA) molecule.[7] In addition, the bases at the 5′ end (start) of the mRNA are chemically modified (capping) and a large number of adenosine bases are added at the 3′ end, known as the *poly-A tail*. These posttranscriptional modifications stabilize the mRNA and facilitate its transport within the cell. The mature mRNA undergoes a test round of translation, which, if successful, leads to the transport of the mRNA to the cytoplasm, where it undergoes multiple rounds of translation by the ribosomes, leading to accumulation of the encoded protein. If the mRNA contains a nonsense mutation, otherwise known as a *premature termination codon mutation*, the test round of translation fails, and the cell degrades this mRNA via the nonsense-mediated mRNA degradation pathway.[8] This is a mechanism that the cell has evolved to remove aberrant transcripts, and it may also contribute to gene regulation, particularly when very low levels of a particular protein are required within a given cell.

Splicing out of introns is a complex process. The genes of prokaryotes, such as bacteria, do not contain introns, so mRNA splicing is a process that is specific to higher organisms. In some more primitive eukaryotes, RNA molecules contain catalytic sequences known as *ribozymes*, which mediate the self-splicing out of introns without any requirement for additional factors. In mammals, splicing involves a large number of protein and RNA factors encoded by several genes. This allows another level of control over gene expression and facilitates alternative splicing of exons, so that a single gene can encode several functionally distinct variants of a protein. These isoforms are often differentially expressed in different tissues. In terms of the gene sequences important for splicing, a few base pairs at the beginning and at the end of an intron, known as the 5′ splice site (or splice donor site) and the 3′ splice site (or splice acceptor site), are crucial. A few other base pairs within the intron, such as the branch point site located 18 to 100 bp away from the 3′ end, are also critical. Mutations affecting any of the invariant residues of these splice sites lead to aberrant splicing and either complete loss of protein expression or generation of a highly abnormal protein.

The mRNA also contains two untranslated regions (UTR): (1) the 5′UTR upstream of the initiating ATG codon and (2) the 3′UTR downstream of the terminator (or stop codon, which can be TGA, TAA, or TAG). Whereas the 5′ UTR can and often does possess introns, the 3′UTR of more than 99% of mammalian genes does not contain introns. The nonsense-mediated mRNA decay pathway identifies mutant transcripts by means of assessing where the termination codon occurs in relation to introns. The natural stop codon is always followed immediately by the 3′UTR, which in turn does not normally possess any introns. If a stop codon occurs in an mRNA upstream of a site where an intron has been excised, this message is targeted for nonsense-mediated decay. The only genes that contain introns within their 3′UTR sequences are expressed at extremely low levels. This is one of the ways in which the cell can determine how much protein is made from a particular gene.

The structural complexity of genes is widely variable and not necessarily related to the size of the protein encoded. Some genes consist of only a single small exon, such as those encoding the connexin family of gap junction proteins. Such single exon genes are rapid and inexpensive to sequence routinely. In contrast, the type VII collagen gene, *COL7A1*, in which mutations lead to the dystrophic forms of EB (see Chap. 60), has 118 exons, meaning that 118 different parts of the gene need to be isolated and analyzed for molecular diagnosis of each dystrophic EB patient. The filaggrin gene (*FLG*) on chromosome 1, is the causative gene for ichthyosis vulgaris (see Chap. 47) and a susceptibility gene for atopic dermatitis (see Chap. 22) and has only three exons. However, the third exon of *FLG* is made up of repeats of a 1000-bp sequence and varies in size from 12,000 to 14,000 bp among different individuals in the population. This unusual gene structure makes routine sequencing of genes such as *COL7A1* or *FLG* difficult, time consuming, and expensive.

GENE EXPRESSION

Each specific gene is generally only actively transcribed in a subset of cells or tissues within the body. Gene expression is largely determined by the promoter elements of the gene. In general, the most important region of the promoter is the stretch of sequence immediately upstream of the cap site. This proximal promoter region contains consensus binding sites for a variety of transcription factors, some of which are general in nature and required for all gene expression, others are specific to particular tissue or cell lineage, and some are absolutely specific for a given cell type or stage of development or differentiation. The size of the promoter can vary widely according to gene family or between the individual genes themselves. For example, the keratin genes are tightly spaced within two gene clusters on chromosomes 12q and 17q, but these are exquisitely tissue specific in two different ways. First, these genes are only expressed in epithelial cells, and therefore their promoters must possess regulatory sequences that determine epithelial expression. Therefore, these regulatory elements are specific for cells of ectodermal origin. Second, these genes are expressed in very specific subsets of epithelial cells, so there must be a second level of control that specifies which epithelial cell layers express specific keratin genes. This is best illustrated in the hair follicle, where there are many different epithelial cell layers, each with a specific pattern of keratin gene expression (see Chap. 7).[9]

Transcription factors are proteins that either bind to DNA directly or indirectly by associating with other DNA-binding proteins. Binding of these factors to the promoter region of a gene leads to activation of the transcription machinery and transcription of the gene by RNA polymerase II. The transcription factor proteins are encoded by genes that are in turn controlled by promoters that are regulated by other transcription factors encoded by other genes. Thus, there are several tiers of control over gene expression in a given cell type, and the intricacies of this can be difficult to fully unravel experimentally. Nevertheless, by isolation of promoter sequences from genes of interest and placing these in front of reporter genes that can be assayed biochemically, such as firefly luciferase that can be assayed by light emission, the activity of promoters can be reproduced in cultured cells that normally express the gene. Combining such a reporter gene system with site-directed mutagenesis to make deletions or alter small numbers of base pairs within the promoter can help define the extent of the promoter and the important sequences within it that are required for gene expression. A variety of biochemical techniques, such as DNA footprinting, ribonuclease protection, electrophoretic mobility shift assays, or chromatin immunoprecipitation, can be used to determine which transcription factors bind to a particular promoter and help delineate the specific promoter sequences bound. Expression of reporter genes under the control of a cloned promoter in transgenic mice also helps shed light on the important sequences that are required to recapitulate the endogenous expression of the gene under study. Keratin promoters are unusual in that, generally, a small fragment of only 2000 to 3000 bp upstream of the gene can confer most of the tissue specificity. For this reason, keratin promoters are widely used to drive exogenous transgene expression in the various specific cellular compartments of the epidermis and its appendages for experiments to determine gene, cell, or tissue function.[10]

Some promoter or enhancer sequences act over very long distances. In some cases, sequences located millions of base pairs away, with several other genes in the intervening region, influence expression of a target gene over a distance. In some genetic diseases, mutations affecting such long-range promoter elements are now emerging. Newer techniques such as chromatin conformation capture (3C, and its next-generation iterations 4C/5C and Hi-C) allow researchers to interrogate DNA structure and regional assembly in order to identify such elements.[11,12] ATAC-seq (assay for transposase-accessible chromatin with high-throughput sequencing) is a technique that allows for distinguishing epigenetic marks in different tissues,[13,14] for example, diseased versus healthy tissues. In general, relatively few disease-causing mutations have been shown to involve promoters or enhancer elements, but this class of variation is probably greatly underrepresented because the sequences that are important for promoter activity are currently poorly characterized. Prediction of transcription factor binding sites by computer analysis is an area for further study. Pathogenic defects in microRNA or other noncoding regulatory RNA species have been postulated to contribute to autoimmunity, and their role in the pathogenesis of systemic immune disorders such as lupus erythematosus are underway.[15]

Techniques such as microarrays and RNA-sequencing have allowed researchers to study gene expression in diseased versus healthy tissues, which may have genetic, epigenetic, or environmental causes. Improvements in the accuracy, resolution, and computational analysis of these methods have allowed accurate readings down to a single cell, whereby tissue heterogeneity (whether innate or as a result of mosaicism) can be identified.

FINDING DISEASE GENES

In establishing the molecular basis of an inherited skin disease, there are two key steps. First, the gene linked to a particular disorder must be identified, and second, pathogenic mutations within that gene must be determined. Previously, diseases can be matched to genes either by genetic linkage analysis or by a candidate gene approach[16] and now additionally using whole-exome sequencing. Genetic linkage involves studying pedigrees of affected and unaffected individuals and isolating which bits of the genome are specifically associated with the disease phenotype. The goal is to identify a region of the genome that all the affected individuals—and none of the unaffected individuals—have in common; this region is likely to harbor the gene for the disorder, as well as perhaps other nonpathogenic neighboring genes that have been inherited by linkage disequilibrium. Traditionally, genome-wide linkage strategies make use of variably sized microsatellite markers scattered throughout the genome, although for recessive diseases involving consanguineous pedigrees, a more rapid approach may be to carry out homozygosity mapping using single nucleotide polymorphism (SNP) chip arrays. By contrast, the candidate gene approach involves first looking for a clue to the likely gene by finding a specific disease abnormality, perhaps in the expression (or lack thereof) of a particular protein or RNA, or from an ultrastructural or biochemical difference between the diseased and control tissues. Nevertheless, the genetic linkage and candidate gene approaches are not mutually exclusive and are often used in combination. For example, to identify the gene responsible for the autosomal recessive disorder lipoid proteinosis (see Chap. 72), genetic linkage using microsatellites was first used to establish a region of linkage on 1q21 that contained 68 genes.[17] The putative gene for this disorder, *ECM1* encoding extracellular matrix protein 1, was then identified by a candidate gene approach that searched for reduced gene expression (lack of fibroblast complementary DNA) in all these genes. A reduction in *ECM1* gene expression in lipoid proteinosis compared with control provided the clue to the candidate gene because there were no differences in any of the other patterns of gene expression. Ultrastructural and immunohistochemical analyses can also provide clues to underlying gene pathology. For example, loss of hemidesmosomal inner plaques noted on transmission electron microscopy and a complete absence of skin immunostaining for the 230-kDA bullous pemphigoid antigen (BP230) at the dermal–epidermal junction led to the discovery of loss-of-function mutations in the dystonin (*DST*) gene, which codes for BP230, in a new form of autosomal recessive EB simplex.[18]

Having identified a putative gene for an inherited disorder, the next stage is to find the pathogenic mutation(s). This can be done by sequencing the entire gene, a feat that is becoming easier as technologic advances make automated nucleotide sequencing faster, cheaper, and more accessible. However, the large size of some genes may make comprehensive sequencing impractical, and therefore initial screening approaches to identify the region of a gene that contains the mutation may be a necessary first step. There are many mutation detection techniques available to scan for sequence changes in cellular RNA or genomic DNA, and these include denaturing gradient gel electrophoresis, chemical cleavage of mismatch, single-stranded conformation polymorphism, heteroduplex analysis, conformation sensitive gel electrophoresis, denaturing high-performance liquid chromatography, and the protein truncation test.[19]

Whichever approach is taken, having identified a difference in the patient's DNA compared with the control sample, the next stage is to determine how this segregates within a particular family and whether it is pathogenic or not. Recently, great advances have been made in DNA sequencing technology, with the emergence of "next-generation sequencing" (NGS) technologies. Currently, whole-exome sequencing has become affordable enough to be routinely used to diagnoses rare genetic disorders. Novel de novo mutations can be identified in this way, even when neither biological parent harbors the mutation. This incredible new technology is set to revolutionize human genetics again, and in particular, will facilitate identification of mutated genes in small kindreds that are not tractable by genetic linkage methods. These advances will not only have an impact on diagnosis, but it will set a foundation for precision medicine approaches such as CRISPR/Cas9 (clustered regularly interspaced short palindromic repeats) gene correction and induced pluripotent stem cell (iPSC) therapies in the future.[20,21]

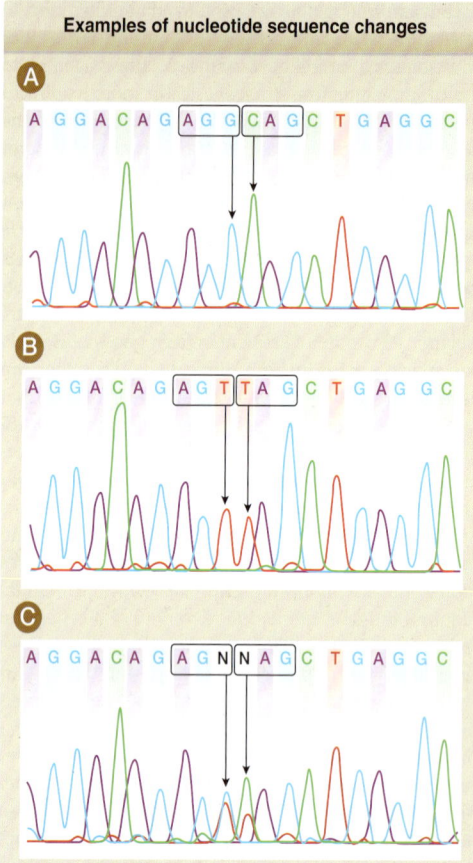

Figure 18-2 Examples of nucleotide sequence changes resulting in a polymorphism and a nonsense mutation. **A,** Two adjacent codons are highlighted. The AGG codon encodes arginine and the CAG codon encodes glutamine. **B,** The sequence shows two homozygous nucleotide substitutions. The AGG codon now reads AGT (ie, coding for serine rather than arginine). This is a common sequence variant in the normal population and is referred to as a *nonpathogenic missense polymorphism*. In contrast, the glutamine codon CAG now reads TAG, which is a stop codon. This is an example of a homozygous nonsense mutation. **C,** This sequence is from one of the parents of the subject sequenced in **B** and shows heterozygosity for both the missense polymorphism AGG > AGT and the nonsense mutation CAG > TAG, indicating that this individual is a carrier of both sequence changes.

GENE MUTATIONS AND POLYMORPHISMS

Within the human genome, the genetic code of two healthy individuals may show a number of sequence dissimilarities that have no relevance to disease or phenotypic traits. Such changes within the normal population are referred to as *polymorphisms* (Fig. 18-2). Indeed, even within the coding region of the genome, clinically irrelevant substitutions of 1 bp, known as *SNPs*, are common and occur approximately once every 250 bp.[22]

Frequently, these SNPs do not change the amino acid composition; for example, a C-to-T transition in the third position of a proline codon (CCC to CCT) still encodes for proline and is referred to as a *silent mutation*. However, some SNPs do change the nature of the amino acid; for example, a C-to-G transversion at the second position of the same proline codon (CCC to CGC) changes the residue to arginine. It then becomes necessary to determine whether a missense change such as this represents a nonpathogenic polymorphism or a pathogenic mutation. Factors favoring the latter include the sequence segregating only with the disease phenotype in a particular family, the amino acid change occurring within an evolutionarily conserved residue, the substitution affecting the function of the encoded protein (size, charge, conformation, and so on), and the nucleotide switch not being detectable in at least 100 ethnically matched control chromosomes. Nonpathogenic polymorphisms do not always involve single nucleotide substitutions; occasionally, deletions and insertions may also be nonpathogenic.

A mutation can be defined as a change in the nucleotide sequence that leads to a change in the chemical composition of a protein. A missense mutation changes one amino acid to another. Mutations may also be insertions or deletions of bases, the consequences of which will depend on whether this disrupts the normal reading frame of a gene or not, as well as nonsense mutations, which lead to premature termination of translation (see Fig. 18-2). For example, a single nucleotide deletion within an exon causes a shift in the reading frame, which usually leads to a downstream stop codon, thus giving a truncated protein, or often an unstable mRNA that is readily degraded by the cell. However, a deletion of three nucleotides (or multiples thereof) will not significantly perturb the overall reading frame, and the consequences will depend on the nature of what has been deleted. Nonsense mutations typically occur at CpG dinucleotides, where methylation of a cytosine nucleotide often occurs. Inherent chemical instability of this modified cytosine leads to a high rate of mutation to thymine. Where this alters the codon (eg, from CGA to TGA), it will change an arginine residue to a stop codon. Nonsense mutations usually lead to a reduced or absent expression of the mutant allele at the mRNA and protein levels. In the heterozygous state, this may have no clinical effect (eg, parents of individuals with generalized severe junctional EB are typically carriers of nonsense mutations in one of the laminin 332 genes but have no skin fragility themselves; see Chap. 60), but a heterozygous nonsense mutation in the desmoplakin gene, for example, can result in the autosomal dominant skin disorder, striate palmoplantar keratoderma (see Chap. 49). This phenomenon is referred to as *haploinsufficiency* (ie, half the normal amount of protein is insufficient for function).

Apart from changes in the coding region that result in frameshift, missense, or nonsense mutations, approximately 15% of all mutations involve alterations in the gene sequence close to the boundaries between the introns and exons, referred to as *splice site mutations*. This type of mutation may abolish the usual acceptor and donor splice sites that normally splice out the introns during gene transcription. The consequences of splice site mutations are complex; sometimes they lead to skipping of the adjacent exon, and other times they result in the generation of new mRNA transcripts through utilization of cryptic splice sites within the neighboring exon or intron.

Mutations within one gene do not always lead to a single inherited disorder. For example, mutations in the *ERCC2* gene may lead to xeroderma pigmentosum (type D), trichothiodystrophy, or cerebrofacioskeletal syndrome, depending on the position and type of mutation. Other transacting factors may further modulate phenotypic expression. This situation is known as *allelic heterogeneity*. Conversely, some inherited diseases can be caused by mutations in more than one gene (eg, generalized intermediate junctional EB; see Chap. 60) and can result from mutations in the *COL17A1, LAMA3, LAMB3,* or *LAMC2* genes. This is known as *genetic* (or *locus*) *heterogeneity*. In addition, the same mutation in one particular gene may lead to a range of clinical severity in different individuals. This variability in phenotype produced by a given genotype is referred to as the *expressivity*. If an individual with such a genotype has no phenotypic manifestations, the disorder is said to be *nonpenetrant*. Variability in expression reflects the complex interplay between the mutation, modifying genes, epigenetic factors, and the environment and demonstrates that interpreting what a specific gene mutation does to an individual involves more than just detecting one bit of mutated DNA in a single gene.

MENDELIAN DISORDERS

There are approximately 5000 human single-gene disorders and, although the molecular basis of approximately 2000 of these has been established, understanding the pattern of inheritance is essential for counseling prospective parents about the risk of having affected children. The four main patterns of inheritance are (1) autosomal dominant, (2) autosomal recessive, (3) X-linked dominant, and (4) X-linked recessive.

For individuals with an autosomal dominant disorder (Table 18-2), one parent is affected unless there has been a de novo mutation in a parental gamete. Males and females are affected in approximately equal numbers, and the disorder can be transmitted from generation to generation; on average, half the offspring will have the condition (Fig. 18-3). It is important to counsel affected individuals that the risk of transmitting the disorder is 50% for each of their children, and that this is not influenced by the number of previously affected or unaffected offspring. Any offspring that are affected will have a 50% risk of transmitting the mutated gene to the next generation, but for any unaffected offspring, the risk of the next generation being affected is negligible, providing that the partner does not have the autosomal dominant condition. Some

TABLE 18-2
Examples of Autosomal Dominant Disorders

AUTOSOMAL DOMINANT SKIN DISORDERS	AFFECTED GENE
Ichthyosis vulgaris[a]	FLG
Neurofibromatosis	NF1
Tuberous sclerosis	TSC1 or TSC2
Darier disease	ATP2A2
Hailey-Hailey disease	ATP2C1

[a]Semidominant.

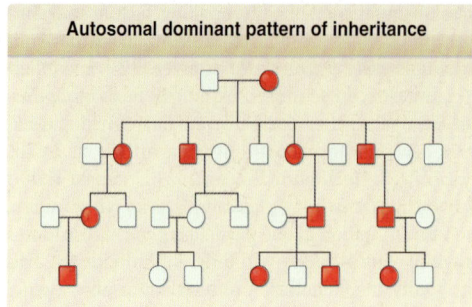

Figure 18-3 Pedigree illustration of an autosomal dominant pattern of inheritance. Key observations include the disorder affects both males and females; on average, 50% of the offspring of an affected individual will be affected; affected individuals have one normal copy and one mutated copy of the gene; and affected individuals usually have one affected parent, unless the disorder has arisen de novo. Importantly, examples of male-to-male transmission, seen here, distinguish this from X-linked dominant and are therefore the best hallmark of autosomal dominant inheritance. *Filled circles* indicate affected females; *filled squares* indicate affected males; and *unfilled circles* and *squares* represent unaffected individuals.

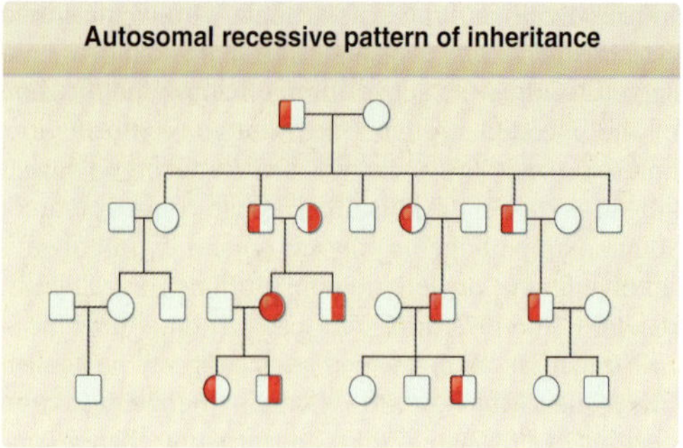

Figure 18-4 Pedigree illustration of an autosomal recessive pattern of inheritance. Key observations include the disorder affects both males and females, there are mutations on both inherited copies of the gene, the parents of an affected individual are both heterozygous carriers and are usually clinically unaffected, and autosomal recessive disorders are more common in consanguineous families. *Filled circle* indicates affected female; *half-filled circles* and *squares* represent clinically unaffected heterozygous carriers of the mutation; and *unfilled circles* and *squares* represent unaffected individuals.

dominant alleles can behave in a partially dominant fashion. The term *semidominant* is applied when the phenotype in heterozygous individuals is less than that observed for homozygous subjects. For example, ichthyosis vulgaris is a *semidominant* disorder in which the presence of one or two mutant profilaggrin gene (*FLG*) alleles can strongly influence the clinical severity of the ichthyosis.

In autosomal recessive disorders (Table 18-3), both parents are carriers of one normal and one mutated allele for the same gene, and, typically, they are phenotypically unaffected (Fig. 18-4). If both of the mutated alleles are transmitted to the offspring, this will give rise to an autosomal recessive disorder, the risk of which is 25%. If one mutated and one wild-type allele is inherited by the offspring, the child will be an unaffected carrier, similar to the parents. If both wild-type alleles are transmitted, the child will be genotypically and phenotypically normal with respect to an affected individual. If the mutations from both parents are the same, the individual is referred to as a *homozygote*, but if different parental mutations within a gene have been inherited, the individual is termed a *compound heterozygote*. For someone who has an autosomal recessive condition, be it a homozygote or compound heterozygote, all offspring will be carriers of one of the mutated alleles but will be unaffected because of inheritance of a wild-type allele from the other, clinically and genetically unaffected, parent. This assumes that the unaffected parent is not a carrier. Although this is usually the case in nonconsanguineous relationships, it may not hold true in first-cousin marriages or other circumstances when there is a familial interrelationship. For example, if the partner of an individual with an autosomal recessive disorder is also a carrier of the same mutation, albeit clinically unaffected, then there is a 50% chance of the offspring inheriting two mutant alleles and therefore also inheriting the same autosomal recessive disorder. This pattern of inheritance is referred to as *pseudodominant*.

In X-linked dominant inheritance (Table 18-4), both males and females are affected, and the pedigree pattern may resemble that of autosomal dominant inheritance (Fig. 18-5). However, there is one important difference. An affected male transmits the disorder to all his daughters and to none of his sons. X-linked dominant inheritance has been postulated as a mechanism in incontinentia pigmenti (see Chaps. 76 and 77), Conradi-Hünermann syndrome, and focal dermal hypoplasia (Goltz syndrome), conditions that are

TABLE 18-3
Examples of Autosomal Recessive Disorders

AUTOSOMAL RECESSIVE SKIN DISORDERS	AFFECTED GENE
Lamellar ichthyosis	TGM1
Xeroderma pigmentosum	XP-A to XP-G
Junctional epidermolysis bullosa	LAMA3, LAMB3, LAMC2
Kindler syndrome	FERMT1

TABLE 18-4
Examples of X-Linked Dominant Disorders

X-LINKED DOMINANT SKIN DISORDERS	AFFECTED GENE
Conradi-Hunermann-Happle syndrome	EBP
Incontinentia pigmenti	NEMO
Focal dermal hypoplasia	PORCN
X-linked dominant protoporphyria	ALAS2

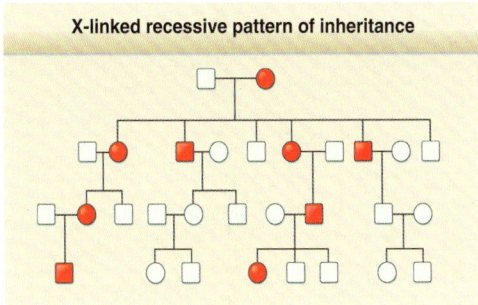

Figure 18-5 Pedigree illustration of an X-linked dominant pattern of inheritance. Key observations include affected individuals are either hemizygous males or heterozygous females, affected males will transmit the disorder to their daughters but not to their sons (no male-to-male transmission), affected females will transmit the disorder to half their daughters and half their sons, and some disorders of this type are lethal in hemizygous males and only heterozygous females survive. *Filled circles* indicate affected females; *filled squares* indicate affected males; and *unfilled circles* and *squares* represent unaffected individuals.

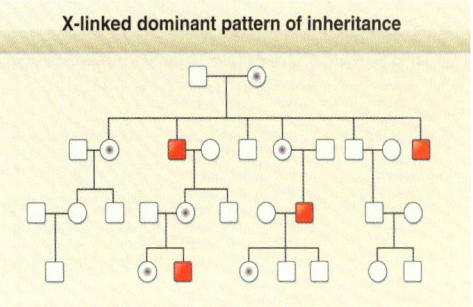

Figure 18-6 Pedigree illustration of an X-linked recessive pattern of inheritance. Key observations include usually affects only males but females can show some features because of lyonization (X-chromosome inactivation); transmitted through female carriers, with no male-to-male transmission; for affected males, all daughters will be heterozygous carriers; and female carrier will transmit the disorder to half her sons, and half her daughters will be heterozygous carriers. *Dots within circles* indicate heterozygous carrier females who may or may not display some phenotypic abnormalities; *filled squares* indicate affected males; and *unfilled circles* and *squares* represent unaffected individuals.

almost always limited to females. In most X-linked dominant disorders with cutaneous manifestations, affected males may be aborted spontaneously or die before implantation (leading to the appearance of female-to-female transmission). Most viable male patients with incontinentia pigmenti have a postzygotic mutation in *IKBKG* and no affected mother; occasionally, males with an X-linked dominant disorder have Klinefelter syndrome with an XXY genotype.

X-linked recessive conditions (Table 18-5) occur almost exclusively in males, but the gene is transmitted by carrier females, who have the mutated gene only on one X chromosome (heterozygous state). The sons of an affected male will all be normal (because their single X chromosome comes from their clinically unaffected mother) (Fig. 18-6). However, the daughters of an affected male will all be carriers (because all had to have received the single X chromosome from their father that carries the mutant copy of the gene). Some females show clinical abnormalities as evidence of the carrier state (eg, in hypohidrotic ectodermal dysplasia; see Chap. 131); the variable extent of phenotypic expression can be explained by Lyonization, the normally random process that inactivates either the wild-type or mutated X chromosome in each cell during the first weeks of gestation and all progeny cells.[23] Other carriers may not show manifestations because the affected region on the X chromosome escapes lyonization (as in recessive X-linked ichthyosis) or the selective survival disadvantage of cells in which the mutated X chromosome is activated (as in the lymphocytes and platelets of carriers of Wiskott-Aldrich syndrome; see section "Mosaicism").

CHROMOSOMAL DISORDERS

Aberrations in chromosome number or structure are common. They occur in about 6% of all conceptions, although most of these lead to miscarriage, and the frequency of chromosomal abnormalities in live births is about 0.6%. Approximately two thirds of these involve abnormalities in either the number of sex chromosomes or the number of autosomes; the remainder is chromosomal rearrangements. The number and arrangement of the chromosomes is referred to as the *karyotype*. The most common numerical abnormality is trisomy, the presence of an extra chromosome. This occurs because of nondisjunction, when pairs of homologous chromosomes fail to separate during meiosis, leading to gametes with an additional chromosome. Loss of a complete chromosome, monosomy, can affect the X chromosome but is rarely seen in autosomes because of nonviability. A number of chromosomal disorders are also associated with skin abnormalities, as detailed in Table 18-6.

Structural aberrations (fragility breaks) in chromosomes may be random, although some chromosomal regions appear more vulnerable. Loss of part of a

TABLE 18-5
Examples of X-Linked Recessive Disorders

X-LINKED RECESSIVE SKIN DISORDERS	AFFECTED GENE
Hypohidrotic ectodermal dysplasia	EDA, EDA1, HED
X-linked ichthyosis	STS
Wiskott-Aldrich syndrome	WAS
Fabry disease	GLA
Menkes syndrome	MNK

TABLE 18-6
Chromosomal Disorders with a Skin Phenotype

CHROMOSOMAL ABNORMALITY	SYNONYM	GENERAL FEATURES	SKIN MANIFESTATIONS
Trisomy 21	Down syndrome	Small head with flat face	1-10 year: dry skin, xerosis, lichenification
		Short and squat nose	10+ year: increased frequency of atopic dermatitis, alopecia areata, single crease in palm and fifth finger
		Ears small and misshapen	Other associations: skin infections, angular cheilitis, geographic tongue, blepharitis, red cheeks, folliculitis, seborrheic dermatitis, boils, onychomycosis, fine hypopigmented hair, vitiligo, delayed dentition and hypoplastic teeth, acrocyanosis, livedo reticularis, cutis marmorata, calcinosis cutis, palmoplantar keratoderma, pityriasis rubra pilaris, syringomas, elastosis perforans serpiginosa, anetoderma, hyperkeratotic form of psoriasis, collagenoma, eruptive dermatofibromas, urticaria pigmentosa, leukemia cutis, keratosis follicularis spinulosa decalvans
		Slanting palpebral fissures	
		Thickened eyelids	
		Eyelashes short and sparse	
		Shortened limbs, lax joints	
		Fingers short, sometimes webbed	
		Hypoplastic iris, lighter outer zone (Brushfield spots)	
Trisomy 18	Edwards syndrome	Severe mental deficiency	Cutis laxa (neck), hypertrichosis of forehead and back, superficial hemangiomas, abnormal dermatoglyphics, single palmar crease, hyperpigmentation, ankyloblepharon filiforme adnatum
		Abnormal skull shape	
		Small chin, prominent occiput	
		Low-set, malformed ears	
		"Rocker bottom" feet	
		Short sternum	
		Malformations of internal organs	
		Only 10% survive beyond first year	
Trisomy 13	Patau syndrome	Mental retardation	Vascular anomalies (especially on forehead)
		Sloping forehead because of forebrain maldevelopment (holoprosencephaly)	Hyperconvex nails
		Microphthalmia or anophthalmia	Localized scalp defects
		Cleft palate or cleft lip	Cutis laxa (neck)
		Low-set ears	Abnormal palm print (distal palmar axial triradius)
		"Rocker bottom" feet	
		Malformations of internal organs	
		Survival beyond 6 months is rare	
Chromosome 4, short arm deletion		Microcephaly	Scalp defects
		Mental retardation	
		Hypospadias	
		Cleft lip or cleft palate	
		Low-set ears, preauricular pits	

(Continued)

TABLE 18-6
Chromosomal Disorders with a Skin Phenotype (*Continued*)

CHROMOSOMAL ABNORMALITY	SYNONYM	GENERAL FEATURES	SKIN MANIFESTATIONS
Chromosome 5, short arm deletion		Mental retardation	Premature graying of hair
		Microcephaly	
		Cat-like cry	
		Low-set ears, preauricular skin tag	
Chromosome 18, long arm deletion		Hypoplasia of midface	Eczema in 25% of cases
		Sunken eyes	
		Prominent ear antihelix	
		Multiple skeletal and ocular abnormalities	
45 XO	Turner syndrome	Early embryonic loss; prenatal ultrasound findings of cystic hygroma, chylothorax, ascites and hydrops	Redundant neck skin and peripheral edema
		Short stature, amenorrhea	Webbed neck, low posterior hairline
		Broad chest, widely spaced nipples	Cutis laxa (neck, buttocks)
		Wide carrying angle of arms	Hypoplastic, soft upturned nails
		Low misshapen ears, high arched palate	Increased incidence of keloids
		Short fourth and fifth fingers and toes	Increased number of melanocytic nevi and halo nevi
		Skeletal abnormalities, coarctation of aorta	Failure to develop full secondary sexual characteristics
			Lymphatic hypoplasia or lymphedema
47 XXY	Klinefelter syndrome	No manifestations before puberty	May develop gynecomastia
		Small testes, poorly developed secondary sexual characteristics	Sparse body and facial hair
		Infertility	Increased risk of leg ulcers
		Tall, obese, osteoporosis	Increased incidence of systemic lupus erythematosus
48 XXYY		Similar to Klinefelter syndrome	Multiple cutaneous angiomas
			Acrocyanosis, peripheral vascular disease
47 XYY		Phenotypic males (tall)	Severe acne
		Mental retardation	
		Aggressive behavior	
49 XXXXY		Low birth weight	Hypotrichosis (variable)
		Slow mental and physical development	
		Large, low-set, malformed ears	
		Small genitalia	
Fragile X syndrome		Mental retardation	—
		Mild dysmorphism	
		Hyperextensible joints, flat feet	

chromosome is referred to as a *deletion*. If the deletion leads to loss of neighboring genes, this may result in a contiguous gene disorder, such as a deletion on the X chromosome giving rise to X-linked ichthyosis (see Chap. 47) and Kallmann syndrome. If two chromosomes break, the detached fragments may be exchanged, known as *reciprocal translocation*. If this process involves no loss of DNA, it is referred to as a *balanced translocation*. Other structural aberrations include duplication of sections of chromosomes, two breaks within one chromosome leading to inversion, and fusion of the ends of two broken chromosomal arms, leading to joining of the ends and formation of a ring chromosome. Chromosomal anomalies may be detected using standard metaphase cytogenetics but newer approaches, such as SNP arrays and comparative genomic hybridization arrays, can also be used for karyotyping. Array-based cytogenetic tools do not rely on cell division and are very sensitive in detecting unbalanced lesions as well as copy number-neutral loss of heterozygosity. These new methods have become commonplace in diagnostic genetics laboratories. A further possible chromosomal abnormality is the inheritance of both copies of a chromosome pair from just one parent (paternal or maternal), known as *uniparental disomy*.[24] Whereas *uniparental heterodisomy* refers to the presence of a pair of chromosome homologs, *uniparental isodisomy* describes two identical copies of a single homolog, and *meroisodisomy* is a mixture of the two. Uniparental disomy with homozygosity of recessive alleles is being increasingly recognized as the molecular basis for several autosomal recessive disorders, including junctional and dystrophic EB (see Chap. 60), resulting from this type of chromosomal abnormality. For certain chromosomes, uniparental disomy can also result in distinct phenotypes depending on the parental origin of the chromosomes, a phenomenon known as *genomic imprinting*.[25,26] This parent-of-origin, specific gene expression is determined by epigenetic modification of a specific gene or, more often, a group of genes, such that gene transcription is altered, and only one inherited copy of the relevant imprinted gene(s) is expressed in the embryo. This means that, during development, the parental genomes function unequally in the offspring. The most common examples of genomic imprinting are Prader-Willi (OMIM #176270) and Angelman (OMIM #105830) syndromes, which can result from maternal or paternal uniparental disomy for chromosome 15, respectively. Three phenotypic abnormalities commonly associated with uniparental disomy for chromosomes with imprinting are (1) intrauterine growth retardation, (2) developmental delay, and (3) short stature.[27]

MITOCHONDRIAL DISORDERS

In addition to the 3.3 billion bp nuclear genome, each cell contains hundreds or thousands of copies of a further 16.5-kb mitochondrial genome, which is inherited solely from an individual's mother. This closed, circular genome contains 37 genes, 13 of which encode proteins of the respiratory chain complexes; the other 24 genes generate 22 transfer RNAs and 2 ribosomal RNAs used in mitochondrial protein synthesis.[28] Mutations in mitochondrial DNA were first reported in 1988, and more than 250 pathogenic point mutations and genomic rearrangements have been shown to underlie a number of myopathic disorders and neurodegenerative diseases, some of which show skin manifestations, including lipomas, abnormal pigmentation or erythema, and hypo- or hypertrichosis.[29] Mitochondrial DNA mutations are very common in somatic mammalian cells, more than two orders of magnitude higher than the mutation frequency in nuclear DNA.[30] Mitochondrial DNA has the capacity to form a mixture of both wild-type and mutant DNA within a cell, leading to cellular dysfunction only when the ratio of mutated to wild-type DNA reaches a certain threshold. The phenomenon of having mixed mitochondrial DNA species within a cell is known as *heteroplasmy*. Mitochondrial mutations can induce or be induced by reactive oxygen species and may be found in or contribute to both chronologic aging and photoaging.[31] Somatic mutations in mitochondrial DNA have also been reported in several premalignant and malignant tumors, including malignant melanoma, although it is not yet known whether these mutations are causally linked to cancer development or simply a secondary bystander effect as a consequence of nuclear DNA instability. Conversely, adults with mitochondrial disorders have been reported to have an increased incidence of both benign (lipomas) and malignant neoplasms (eg, extramammary Paget disease, Bowen disease) of the skin,[32] suggesting a role for the mitochondrial genome in tissue and stem cell homeostasis. There is currently little understanding of the interplay between the nuclear and mitochondrial genomes in both health and disease. Nevertheless, it is evident that the genes encoded by the mitochondrial genome have multiple biologic functions linked to energy production, cell proliferation, and apoptosis.[33]

COMPLEX DISEASE GENETICS

For Mendelian disorders, identifying genes that harbor pathogenic mutations has become relatively straightforward, with hundreds of disease-associated genes being discovered through a combination of linkage, positional cloning, and candidate gene analyses. By contrast, for complex diseases, such as psoriasis and atopic dermatitis, these traditional approaches have been largely unsuccessful in mapping genes influencing the disease risk or phenotype because of low statistical power and other factors.[34,35] Complex diseases do not display simple Mendelian patterns of inheritance, although genes do have an influence, and close relatives of affected individuals may have an increased risk. To identify genes that contribute and influence susceptibility to complex traits, several stages may be necessary, including establishing a genetic basis for the disease in one or more populations, measuring the distribution of gene effects, studying statistical power using models, and carrying out marker-based mapping studies using linkage or association. It is possible to establish quantitative genetic models to estimate the heritability of a complex trait, as well as to predict the distribution of gene effects and to test whether one or more quantitative trait loci exist. These models can predict the power of different mapping approaches but often only provide approximate predictions. Moreover, low power often limits other strategies such as transmission analyses, association studies, and family-based association tests. In addition, and relevant to several studies on psoriasis, linkage disequilibrium observed in a sample of unrelated affected and normal individuals can also be used to fine-map a disease susceptibility locus in a candidate region.

In recent years, advances in the identification of many millions of SNPs across the entire genome, as well as major advances in gene chip technology that allows up to 2 million SNPs to be typed in a given individual for a few hundred dollars, coupled with high powered computation, have led to the current era of genome-wide association studies (GWASs).[36] This has become the predominant technology for mapping complex diseases, with GWASs having already been performed for psoriasis, atopic eczema, vitiligo, and alopecia areata, and GWASs for other dermatologic complex diseases are underway. A typical GWAS design involves collecting DNA from a well-phenotyped case series of the condition of choice, preferably from an ethnically homogenous population. Normally, 2000 or more cases are required versus 3000 ethnically matched population control participants. Correct clinical ascertainment of the cases is paramount, so GWASs represent a great opportunity for close cooperation between physicians and scientists. These 5000 or more individuals are genotyped for 500,000 to 2 million SNPs, generating billions of data points. For each SNP across the genome, a statistical test is performed and a P value derived. If an SNP is closely linked to a disease susceptibility gene, then a particular genotype will be greatly enriched in the case series compared with the general unselected population. The P values are plotted along each chromosome ("Manhattan plot"), and where disease susceptibility loci exist, there are clusters of strong association. Typically, P values of 10^{-10} or lower are indicative of a true locus, although this generally has to be replicated in a number of other case-control sets for confirmation. Although an SNP-based GWAS is currently the method of choice in mapping complex disease genetics, it has limitations. If a causative lesion in a susceptibility locus is very heterogeneous (ie, if there are multiple mutations or other changes that cause the susceptibility), then the locus will be difficult to pinpoint by GWAS. Furthermore, across the entire field of complex disease genetics, relatively few causative genes have emerged (the role of the filaggrin gene in atopic dermatitis being a notable exception). In the majority of cases, there is currently little clue about what defect the associated SNPs are linked to that actually causes the disease susceptibility. GWASs can be very useful in uncovering new disease pathways involved in disease pathogenesis at a population level because individual variants take longer to identify.

However, recently, a conventional genetics approach has revealed fascinating new insight into the pathophysiology of one particular complex trait, namely atopic dermatitis. This finding emanated from the discovery that the disorder ichthyosis vulgaris was due to loss-of-function mutations in the gene encoding the skin barrier protein filaggrin (see Chaps. 22 and 47).[37] To dermatologists, the clinical association between this condition and atopic dermatitis is well known, and the same loss-of-function mutations in filaggrin have subsequently been shown to be a major susceptibility risk factor for atopic dermatitis, as well as asthma associated with atopic dermatitis but not asthma alone.[4] This suggests that asthma in individuals with atopic dermatitis may be secondary to allergic sensitization, which develops because of the defective epidermal barrier that allows allergens to penetrate the skin to make contact with antigen-presenting cells. Indeed, transmission–disequilibrium tests have demonstrated an association between filaggrin gene mutations and extrinsic atopic dermatitis associated with high total serum immunoglobulin E levels and concomitant allergic sensitizations.[38] These recent data on the genetics of atopic dermatitis demonstrate how the study of a "simple" genetic disorder (ichthyosis) can also provide novel insight into a complex disease (atopic dermatitis). Therefore, Mendelian disorders may be useful in the molecular dissection of more complex traits.[39]

MOSAICISM

The presence of a mixed population of cells bearing different genetic or chromosomal characteristics leading to phenotypic diversity is referred to as *mosaicism*. There are several different types of mosaicism, including single gene, chromosomal, functional, and revertant mosaicism.[40] Multiple expression patterns are recognized.[41]

Mosaicism for a single gene, referred to as *somatic mosaicism*, indicates a mutational event occurring after fertilization. The earlier this occurs, the more likely it is that there will be clinical expression of a disease phenotype as well as involvement of gonadal tissue (gonosomal mosaicism), for example, when individuals with segmental neurofibromatosis subsequently have offspring with fully penetrant neurofibromatosis (see Chap. 135). However, in general, if the mutation occurs after generation of cells committed to germline formation, then the mosaicism will not involve the gametes, and the reproductive risk of transmission is negligible. *Gonosomal mosaicism* refers to involvement of both gonads and somatic tissue, but mosaicism can occur exclusively in gonadal tissue, referred to as *gonadal mosaicism*. Clinically, this may explain recurrences among siblings of autosomal dominant disorders such as tuberous sclerosis or neurofibromatosis, when neither parent has any clinical manifestations and gene screening using genomic DNA from peripheral blood samples yields no mutation. Segmental mosaicism for autosomal dominant disorders is thought to occur in one of two ways: either there is a postzygotic mutation with the skin outside the segment and genomic DNA being normal (type 1), or there is a heterozygous genomic mutation in all cells that is then exacerbated by loss of heterozygosity within a segment or along the lines of Blaschko (type 2). This pattern has been described in several autosomal dominant disorders, including Darier disease, Hailey-Hailey disease (see Chap. 50), superficial actinic porokeratosis (see Chap. 51), and tuberous sclerosis (see Chap. 136).

The lines of Blaschko (Fig. 18-7) were described more than 100 years ago; the pattern is attributed to the lines of migration and proliferation of epidermal cells during embryogenesis (ie, the bands of abnormal skin represent clones of cells carrying a mutation in a gene expressed in the skin).[42] Although attributed to the German dermatologist Alfred Blaschko, the literature records an almost simultaneous description of "the lines" by the American dermatologist Douglass Montgomery. Indeed, one of the clinical photographs in Montgomery's paper is illustrated as a diagram in Blaschko's work. Apart from somatic mutations (either in dominant disorders, such as epidermolytic ichthyosis [formerly called bullous congenital ichthyosiform erythroderma] leading to linear epidermolytic ichthyosis [epidermal nevus of the epidermolytic hyperkeratosis type] [see Chap. 47], or in conditions involving mutations in lethal dominant genes such as in McCune-Albright syndrome), mosaicism following Blaschko's lines is also seen in chromosomal mosaicism and functional mosaicism (random X-chromosome inactivation through Lyonization). Monoallelic expression on autosomes (with random inactivation of either the maternal or paternal allele) is also feasible and probably underdocumented.[43] Chromosomal mosaicism results from nondisjunction events that occur after fertilization. Clinically, this is found in the linear mosaic pigmentary disorders (hypomelanosis of Ito [see Chap. 77] and linear and whorled hyperpigmentation). It is important to point out that hypomelanosis of Ito is not a specific diagnosis but may occur as a consequence of several different chromosomal abnormalities that perturb various genes relevant to skin pigmentation, which has led to the term "pigmentary mosaicism" to describe this group of disorders.

Functional mosaicism relates to genes on the X chromosome because during embryonic development in females, one of the X chromosomes, either the maternal

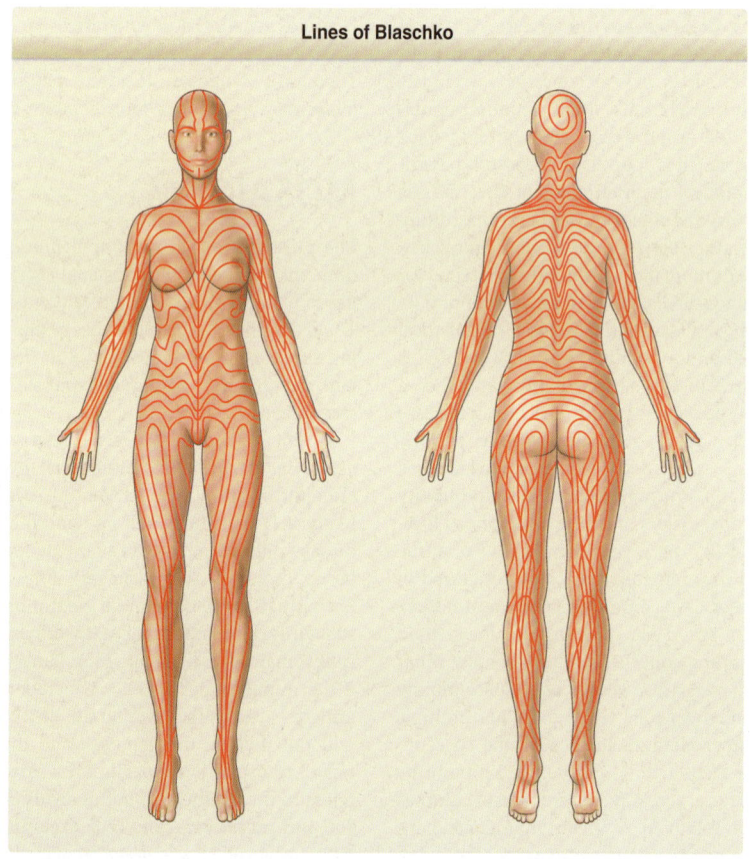

Figure 18-7 Lines of Blaschko.

or the paternal, is inactivated. For X-linked dominant disorders, such as focal dermal hypoplasia (Goltz syndrome) or incontinentia pigmenti (see Chaps. 76 and 77), females survive because of the presence of some cells in which the X chromosome without the mutation is active and able to function. For males, these X-linked dominant disorders are typically lethal unless associated with an abnormal karyotype (eg, Klinefelter syndrome; 47,XXY) or if the mutation occurs during embryonic development. For X-linked recessive conditions, such as X-linked recessive hypohidrotic ectodermal dysplasia (see Chap. 131), the clinical features are evident in hemizygous males (who have only one X chromosome), but females may show subtle abnormalities caused by mosaicism caused by X-inactivation, such as decreased sweating or reduced hair in areas of the skin in which the normal X is selectively inactivated. There are 1317 known genes on the X chromosome, and most undergo random inactivation but a small percentage (~27 genes on Xp, including the steroid sulfatase gene, and 26 genes on Xq) escape inactivation.

Revertant mosaicism, also known as *natural gene therapy*, refers to genetic correction of an abnormality by various different phenomena, including back mutations, intragenic crossovers, mitotic gene conversion, and second site mutations.[44,45] Indeed, multiple different correcting events can occur in the same patient. Such changes have been described in a few genes expressed in the skin, including the keratin 14, laminin 332, collagen XVII, collagen VII, and kindlin-1 (fermitin family homolog 1) genes in different forms of EB (Fig. 18-8; see Chap. 60) and in keratins 10 and 1 in ichthyosis with confetti (see Chap. 47). The clinical relevance of the conversion process depends on several factors, including the number of cells involved, how much reversal actually occurs, and at what stage in life the reversion takes place. Attempts have been made to culture reverted keratinocytes and graft them to unreverted sites,[46] a pioneering approach that may have therapeutic potential for some patients. Clinical success has also been reported using punch grafting of revertant mosaic skin (*LAMB3* gene correction) with sustained expression of the reversion at the grafted site.[47A] Newer protocols in provirus-mediated gene correction of keratinocyte stem cells have recently resulted in the successful replacement of significant amounts of epidermis in a severe case of junctional EB, providing further proof of concept that this is a feasible option for management of genetic skin diseases.[47B]

Apart from mutations in nuclear DNA, mosaicism can also be influenced by environmental factors, such as viral DNA sequences (retrotransposons) that can be incorporated into nuclear DNA, replicate, and activate or silence genes through methylation or demethylation. This phenomenon is known as *epigenetic mosaicism*; such events may be implicated in tumorigenesis but have not been associated with any genetic skin disorder.

HISTOCOMPATABILITY ANTIGEN DISEASE ASSOCIATION

Human leukocyte antigen (HLA) molecules are glycoproteins that are expressed on almost all nucleated cells. The HLA region is located on the short arm of chromosome 6, at 6p21, referred to as the *MHC*. There are three classic loci at HLA class I—(1) HLA-A, (2) HLA-B, and (3) HLA-Cw—and five loci at class II—(1) HLA-DR, (2) HLA-DQ, (3) HLA-DP, (4) HLA-DM, and (5) HLA-DO. The HLA molecules are highly polymorphic, with many alleles at each individual locus. Thus, allelic variation contributes to defining a unique "fingerprint" for each person's cells, which allows an individual's immune system to define what is foreign and what is self. The clinical significance of the HLA system is highlighted in human tissue transplantation, especially in kidney and bone marrow transplantation, where efforts are made to match at the HLA-A, -B, and -DR loci. Major histocompatibility (MHC) class I molecules, complexed to certain peptides, act as substrates for CD8+ T-cell activation, but MHC class II molecules on the surface of antigen-presenting cells display a range of peptides for recognition by the T-cell receptors of CD4+ T helper cells (see Chap. 11). Therefore, MHC molecules are central to effective adaptive immune responses.

Conversely, however, genetic and epidemiologic data have implicated these molecules in the pathogenesis of various autoimmune and chronic inflammatory diseases. Several skin diseases, such as alopecia areata (see Chap. 87), psoriasis (see Chap. 28), psoriatic arthropathy (central and peripheral), vitiligo, dermatitis herpetiformis, pemphigus, reactive arthritis syndrome (see Chap. 65), and Behçet disease (see Chap. 141), all show an association with inheritance of certain HLA haplotypes (ie, there is a higher incidence of these conditions in individuals and families with particular HLA alleles; Table 18-7). However, the molecular mechanisms by which polymorphisms in

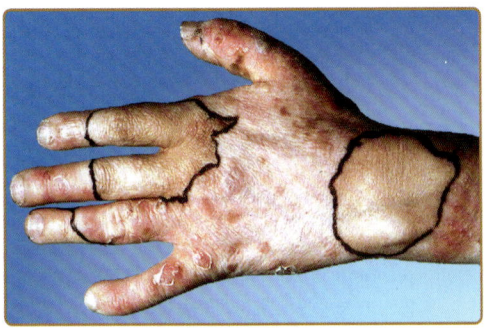

Figure 18-8 Revertant mosaicism in an individual with non-Herlitz junctional epidermolysis bullosa. The subject has loss-of-function mutations on both alleles of the type XVII collagen gene, *COL17A1*, but spontaneous genetic correction of the mutation in some areas has led to patches of normal-appearing skin (areas within black marker outline) that do not blister. (From Jonkman MF, Scheffer H, Stulp R, et al. Revertant mosaicism in epidermolysis bullosa caused by mitotic gene conversion. *Cell*. 1997;88:543, with permission. Copyright © Elsevier.)

TABLE 18-7
Diseases and HLA Haplotype

DISEASE	HLA HAPLOTYPE
Psoriasis	HLA cw6
Alopecia areata	HLA DWB1*03; HLA DR4; HLA DQ7[a]
Psoriatic arthropathy	HLA B27; HLA B7; HLA B13, BLA B16, HLA B38, HLA B39, HLA B17, HLA cw6
Dermatitis herpetiformis	HLA DQw2[b]
Pemphigus	HLA DR4, HLA DQ1
Reactive arthritis syndrome	HLA B27
Behcet disease	HLA B51
Increased risk for carbamazepine-induced SJS and TEN	HLA-B*1502

[a]Colombe BW, Lou CD, Price VH. The genetic basis of alopecia areata: HLA associations with patchy alopecia areata versus alopecia totalis and alopecia universalis. *J Investig Dermatol Symp Proc.* 1999;4(3):216-219.

[b]Hall MA, Lanchbury JS, PJ Ciclitira, et al. HLA Association with dermatitis herpetiformis is accounted for by a cis or transassociated DQ heterodimer. *Gut.* 1991;32(5):487-490.

SJS, Stevens-Johnson syndrome; TEN, toxic epidermal necrolysis.

HLA molecules confer susceptibility to certain disorders are still unclear. This situation is further complicated by the fact that, for most diseases, it is unknown which autoantigens (presented by the disease-associated MHC molecules) are primarily involved. For many diseases, the MHC class association is the main genetic association. Nevertheless, for most of the MHC-associated diseases, it has been difficult to unequivocally determine the primary disease-risk gene(s) because of the extended linkage disequilibrium in the MHC region. However, recent genetic and functional studies support the long-held assumption that common MHC class I and II alleles themselves are responsible for many disease associations, such as the HLA cw6 allele in psoriasis. Of practical clinical importance is the strong genetic association between certain HLA alleles and the risk of adverse drug reactions. For example, in Han Chinese and some other Asian populations, HLA-B*1502 confers a greatly increased risk of carbamazepine-induced Stevens-Johnson syndrome and toxic epidermal necrolysis (60- to 80-fold increase). Therefore, screening for HLA-B*1502 before starting carbamazepine in patients from high-risk populations is recommended or required by regulatory agencies.[48]

EPIGENETICS

Disease phenotypes reflect the result of the interaction between a particular genotype and the environment, but it is evident that some variation, for example, in monozygotic twins, is attributable to neither. Additional influences at the biochemical, cellular, tissue, and organism levels occur, and these are referred to as *epigenetic phenomena*.[49] Single genes are not solely responsible for each separate function of a cell. Genes may collaborate in circuits, be mobile, exist in plasmids and cytoplasmic organelles, and can be imported by nonsexual means from other organisms or as synthetic products. Epigenetic effects reflect chemical modifications to DNA that do not alter DNA sequence but instead affect the probability or level of gene transcription. Mammalian DNA methylation machinery is made up of two components: (1) DNA methyltransferases, which establish and maintain genome-wide DNA methylation patterns, and (2) the methyl-CpG-binding proteins, which are involved in scanning and interpreting the methylation patterns. Analysis of any changes in these processes is known as *epigenomics*.[50] Examples of modifications include direct covalent modification of DNA by methylation of cytosines and alterations in proteins that bind to DNA. Such changes may affect DNA accessibility to local transcriptional complexes as well as influencing chromatin structure at regional and genome-wide levels, thus providing a link between genome structure and regulation of transcription. Indeed, epigenome analysis is now being carried out in parallel with gene expression studies (eg, microarray studies or RNA sequencing) to identify genome-wide methylation patterns and profiles of all human genes. For example, there is considerable interindividual variation in cytosine methylation of CpG dinucleotides within the MHC region genes, and hypermethylation of the HLA-C promoter has been postulated to be an epigenetic marker for psoriasis.[51]

New sensitive and quantitative methylation-specific polymerase chain reaction-based assays can identify epigenetic anomalies in cancers such as melanoma.[52] DNA hypermethylation contributes to gene silencing by preventing the binding of activating transcription factors and by attracting repressor complexes that induce the formation of inactive chromatin structures. With regard to melanoma, such changes may impact on several biologic processes, including cell cycle control, apoptosis, cell signaling, tumor cell invasion, metastasis, angiogenesis, and immune recognition. A further but as yet unresolved issue is whether there is heritability of epigenetic characteristics. Likewise, it is unclear whether environmentally induced changes in epigenetic status, and hence gene transcription and phenotype, can be transmitted through more than one generation. Such a phenomenon might account for the cancer susceptibility of grandchildren of individuals who have been exposed to diethylstilbestrol, but this has not been proved.[53] However, germ line epimutations have been identified in other human diseases, such as colorectal cancers characterized by microsatellite instability and hypermethylation of the *MLH1* DNA mismatch repair gene, although the risk of transgenerational epigenetic inheritance of cancer from such a mutation is not well established and probably small. Over the course of an individual's lifespan, epigenetic mutations (affecting DNA methylation and histone modifications) may occur more frequently than DNA mutations, and it is expected that, over the next decade, the role of epigenetic phenomena in influencing phenotypic variation will gradually become better understood.[54] High-throughput methods of identifying differentially methylated sites in the genome has implicated epigenetics in the pathogenesis of diseases like schizophrenia,[55] obesity,[56] and type 2 diabetes mellitus.[57]

GENETIC COUNSELING

The National Society of Genetic Counselors (http://www.nsgc.org) has defined genetic counseling as "the process of helping people understand and adapt to the medical, psychological and familial implications of genetic contributions to disease." Genetic counseling should include (1) interpretation of family and medical histories to assess the chance of disease occurrence or recurrence, (2) education about inheritance, testing, management, prevention, resources, and research, and (3) counseling to promote informed choice and adaptation to the risk or condition.[58]

When the diagnosis of an inherited skin disease is established and the mode of inheritance is known, every dermatologist should be able to advise patients correctly and appropriately, although additional support from specialists in medical genetics is often necessary. Genetic counseling must be based on an understanding of genetic principles and on a familiarity with the usual behavior of hereditary and congenital abnormalities. It is also important to be familiar with the range of clinical severity of a particular disease, the social consequences of the disorder, the availability of therapy (if any), and the options for mutation detection and prenatal testing in subsequent pregnancies at risk for recurrence (one useful site is http://www.genetests.com).

A key component of genetic counseling is to help parents, patients, and families know about the risks of recurrence or transmission for a particular condition. This information is not only practical but often relieves guilt and can allay rather than increase anxiety. For example, it may not be clear to the person that he or she cannot transmit the given disorder. The unaffected brother of a patient with an X-linked recessive disorder such as Fabry disease (see Chap. 127), X-linked ichthyosis (see Chap. 47), Wiskott-Aldrich syndrome (see Chap. 132), or Menkes syndrome (see Chap. 85) need not worry about his children being affected or even carrying the abnormal allele, but he may not know this information.

Prognosis and counseling for conditions such as psoriasis in which the genetic basis is complex or still unclear is more difficult (see Chap. 28). Individuals can be advised, for example, that if both parents have psoriasis, the probability is 60% to 75% that a child will have psoriasis; if one parent and a child of that union have psoriasis, then the chance is 30% that another child will have psoriasis; and if two normal parents have produced a child with psoriasis, the probability is 15% to 20% for another child with psoriasis.[59] Ongoing discoveries in other diseases, such as melanoma, can also impact on genetic counseling. The identification of family-specific mutations in the *CDKN2A* and *CDK4* genes, as well as risk alleles in the *MC1R* and *OCA2* genes and other genetic variants allow for more accurate and informative patient and family consultations.[60]

The advent of NGS has also created new issues and dilemmas for genetic counseling. Notably, in sequencing whole exomes or genomes, the question has arisen what to do with incidental findings (ie, gene mutations not related to the phenotype that is being investigated) or variants of unknown significance. Currently, best practice guidelines dictate the need to act or pass on such collateral information only if the findings are "clinically actionable," although such policies are likely to change in the future. In addition, key governance concerns over storage and ownership of personal genomic data must be addressed.

PRENATAL DIAGNOSIS

In recent years, there has been considerable progress in developing prenatal testing for severe inherited skin disorders (Fig. 18-9). Initially, ultrastructural examination of fetal skin biopsies was established in a limited number of conditions. In the late 1970s, the first diagnostic examination of fetal skin was reported for epidermolytic hyperkeratosis (epidermolytic ichthyosis) and Herlitz (generalized severe) junctional EB (see Chap. 60).[61,62] These initial biopsies were performed with the aid of a fetoscope to visualize the fetus. However, with improvements in sonographic imaging, biopsies of fetal skin are now taken under ultrasound guidance. The fetal skin biopsy samples obtained during the early 1980s could be examined only by light microscopy and transmission electron microscopy. However, the introduction of a number of monoclonal and polyclonal antibodies to various basement membrane components during the mid-1980s led to the development of immunohistochemical tests to help complement ultrastructural analysis in establishing an accurate diagnosis, especially in cases of EB.[63] Fetal skin biopsies are taken during the midtrimester. For disorders such as EB, testing at 16 weeks' gestation is appropriate. However, for some forms of ichthyosis, the disease-defining structural pathology may not be evident at this time, and fetal skin sampling may need to be deferred until 20 to 22 weeks of development.

Nevertheless, since the early 1990s, as the molecular basis of an increasing number of genodermatoses has been elucidated, fetal skin biopsies have gradually been replaced by DNA-based diagnostic screening using fetal DNA from amniotic fluid cells or samples of chorionic villi; taken at 16 weeks' gestation for amniotic fluid and 10 to 12 weeks' for chorionic villus sampling (ie, at the end of the first trimester).[64,65] In addition, advances with in vitro fertilization and embryo micromanipulation have led to the feasibility of even earlier DNA-based assessment through preimplantation genetic diagnosis, an approach first successfully applied in 1990, for risk of recurrence of cystic fibrosis.[66] Successful preimplantation testing has also been reported for severe inherited skin disorders.[67]

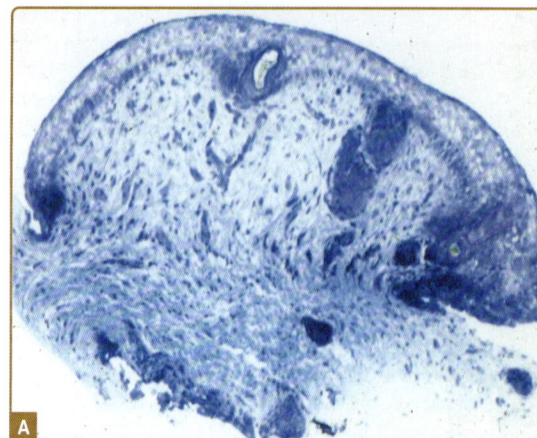
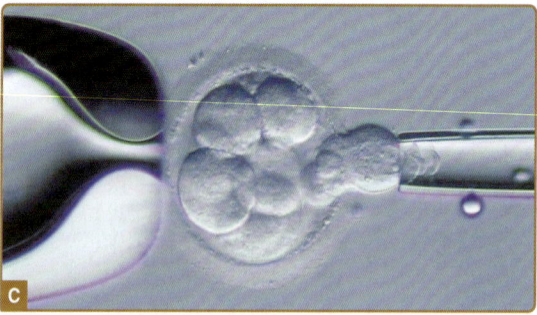
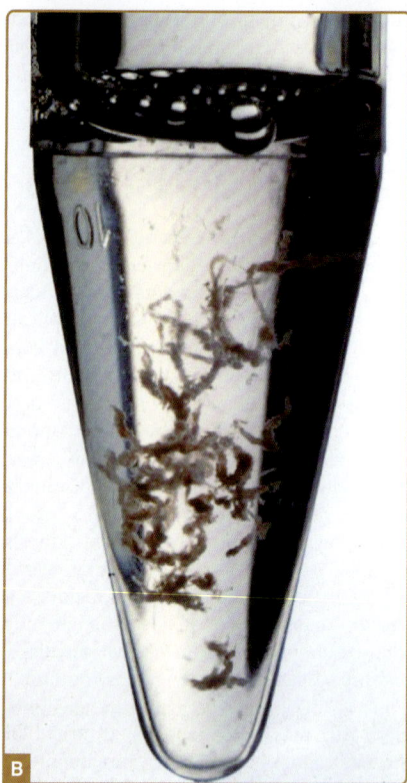

Figure 18-9 Options for prenatal testing of inherited skin diseases. **A,** Fetal skin biopsy, here shown at 18 weeks' gestation. **B,** Chorionic villi sampled at 11 weeks' gestation. **C,** Preimplantation genetic diagnosis. A single cell is being extracted from a 12-cell embryo using a suction pipette.

This is likely to become a more popular, though still technically challenging, option for some couples, in view of recent advances in amplifying the whole genome in single cells and the application of multiple linkage markers in an approach termed *preimplantation genetic haplotyping*.[68] This approach has been developed and applied successfully for generalized severe junctional EB.[69] For some disorders, alternative less invasive methods of testing are now also being developed, including analysis of fetal DNA or RNA from within the maternal circulation and the use of three-dimensional ultrasonography.

Advances in in vitro fertilization have also helped to address familial mitochondrial disorders, whereby the mothers carry mutations in the mitochondrial genome. The mother's nucleus, along with its genomic DNA, is transferred into a donated egg from another woman with healthy mitochondria, which is then fertilized by the father's sperm. This procedure, which results in three-parent families, was approved by the British Parliament in 2015 and is currently under consideration by the US Food and Drug Administration (FDA).

In the absence of effective treatment for many hereditary skin diseases at present, prenatal diagnosis can provide valuable information to couples at risk of having affected children, although detailed and supportive genetic counseling is also a vital element of all prenatal testing procedures.

GENE THERAPY AND EDITING

The field of gene therapy can be subdivided in different ways.[70] First, there are approaches aimed at treatment of recessive genetic diseases in which homozygous or compound heterozygous loss-of-function mutations lead to complete absence or complete functional ablation of a protein. These types of diseases are amenable to gene replacement therapy, and this form of gene therapy has tended to predominate because it is generally technically more feasible than treatment of dominant genetic conditions.[71] In dermatology, these include diseases such as lamellar ichthyosis (see Chap. 47), in which in most cases, there is hereditary absence of transglutaminase-1 activity in the outer epidermis, or the severe generalized form of recessive dystrophic EB, in which there is complete absence of type VII collagen expression due to recessive mutations.[72]

The second form of gene therapy, in broad terms, is aimed at treatment of dominant-negative genetic disorders and is known as *gene inhibition therapy*. Here, there is a completely different approach because these patients already carry one normal copy of the gene as well as one mutated copy. The disease occurs because an abnormal protein product produced by the mutant allele, dominant-negative mutant protein, binds to and inhibits the function of the normal protein produced by the wild-type allele. In these cases of dominant negative inheritance, where one normal allele is sufficient for skin function, suppression of expression of the dominant negative mutant allele should be therapeutically beneficial. Recent advances in gene editing have made this therapeutic option possible. Technologies such as TALENS (transcription activator-like effector nucleases) and CRISPR/Cas9 have enabled specific targeting and manipulation of the genome and have been used to disrupt the activity of mutant alleles. For example, using iPSCs to model dystrophic dominant EB (DDEB), the mutant collagen *COL7A1* allele has been successfully edited such that the truncated mutant protein underwent proteolysis, allowing the normal allele to function in its absence.[73] This method provides proof-of-concept for ex vivo therapies, whereby keratinocytes or fibroblasts would be obtained from a skin biopsy, edited to correct the genetic mutation, and then grafted onto or injected back into the patient.

Gene therapy approaches can also be broadly subdivided according to whether they involve in vivo or ex vivo strategies.[71] Using an in vivo approach, the gene therapy agent would be delivered directly to the patient's skin or another tissue. A disadvantage of the skin as a target organ for gene therapy is that it is a barrier tissue that is fundamentally designed to prevent entry of foreign nucleic acid in the form of viruses or other pathogenic agents. This is an impediment to in vivo gene therapy development but is not insurmountable because of developments in liposome technology and other methods for cutaneous macromolecule delivery.[74] In an ex vivo approach, a skin biopsy would be taken. Keratinocytes or fibroblasts would be expanded in culture, treated with the gene therapy agent, and then grafted onto or injected back into the patient. The skin is a good organ system for both these approaches because it is very accessible for in vivo applications. In addition, the skin can be readily biopsied, and cell culture and regrafting of keratinocytes can be adapted for ex vivo gene therapy. In the future, these methods will likely be used in combination with gene editing and iPSC approaches for gene correction.

Gene replacement therapy systems have been developed for lamellar ichthyosis (see Chap. 47) and the recessive forms of EB (see Chap. 60), among other diseases. These mostly consist of expressing the normal complementary DNA encoding the gene of interest from some form of gene therapy vector adapted from viruses that can integrate their genomes stably into the human genome. Therefore, such viral vectors can lead to long-term stable expression of the replacement gene.[75] Early studies tended to use retroviral vectors or adeno-associated viral vectors, but these have a number of limitations. For example, retroviruses only transduce dividing cells and therefore fail to target stem cells; consequently, gene expression is quickly lost because of turnover of the epidermis through keratinocyte differentiation. Furthermore, there have been some safety issues in small-scale human trials for both retroviral and adeno-associated viral vectors. Lentiviral vectors, derived from short integrating sequences found in a number of immunodeficiency viruses, have the advantage of being able to stably transduce dividing and nondividing cells, with close to 100% efficiency and at low copy number. These may be the current vectors of choice, but they also have potential problems because their preferred integration sites in the human genome are currently ill defined and may lead to concerns about safety. As a proof of concept, certain serotypes of adenovirus (eg, AAV-DJ) have been shown to mediate homologous recombination efficiently and accurately ex vivo in the treatment of generalized severe junction EB without the need for drug selection. A wide variety of other vectors are under development and testing, and it should become clear in future years which vectors are effective and safe for human use. Ultimately, like all novel therapeutics, animal testing can only act as a guide because the human genome is quite different and may react differently to foreign DNA integration, so that phase I, II, and III human trials or adaptations thereof will ultimately have to be performed to determine efficacy and safety. Currently, small-scale clinical trials are ongoing for junctional and dystrophic forms of EB and are planned for a number of other genodermatoses, mainly concentrating on the more severe recessive conditions.

Treatment of dominant-negative disorders received a great deal of attention with the discovery of the RNA inhibition pathway in humans and the finding that small synthetic double-stranded RNA molecules of 19 to 21 bp, known as *short inhibitory RNA* (siRNA), can efficiently inhibit expression of human genes in a sequence-specific, user-defined manner.[76,77] There is currently a focus on development of siRNA inhibitors to selectively silence mutant alleles in dominant-negative genetic diseases, such as the keratin disorders EB simplex and pachyonychia congenita (PC). The main obstacles in developing topical siRNA therapies are their rapid degradation and poor cellular uptake. Nanospheres and liposomes are methods that increase siRNA delivery across the stratum. To enhance cellular uptake of siRNA, nonviral methods such as iontophoresis, sonophoresis, and microneedling have been attempted.

In particular, significant progress has been made in PC in recent years. Following development of reporter gene methodology to rapidly screen many different siRNA species, two siRNAs were identified that could specifically and potently silence mutant keratin K6a mRNA differing from the wild-type mRNA by only a single nucleotide (ie, these siRNAs represent allele-specific gene silencing agents). Following a battery of preclinical studies in cells and animal models to show efficacy, the K6a mutation–specific siRNA was manufactured to Good Manufacturing Practice standards and was shown to have an excellent toxicity profile in rodents, as per a small molecule drug. This facilitated FDA approval for a double-blind split body phase 1b clinical trial in a single volunteer with PC. The trial was successful, with a number of objective measures showing statistically significant clinical improvement. This study, funded by the patient advocacy organization PC Project (http://www.pachyonychia.org), was the first in human siRNA trial using a mutation-specific gene silencing approach and only the fifth siRNA trial in humans. Together with newer gene editing technologies, this personalized medicine strategy gives hope for patients with dominant genodermatoses in which the mutant allele can be selectively targeted and future trials in EB simplex are currently in the planning stages.

PRECISION MEDICINE

We are currently at a point of convergence of the massive amounts of data obtained from population-level GWASs, patient-level whole-exome sequencing, RNA-Seq and microarray analyses, and even microbiome data, with exponential improvements in computing power and organized patient electronic health records. This gives us the opportunity to reconceptualize our dogma of diagnosis and treatment. We have entered a new era of Predictive, Preventive, Personalized and Participatory medicine, whereby each patient's diagnosis will be stratified down to the genetic and epigenetic level, and therapy will be specifically directed at this unique aberration. This new paradigm promises to allow us to understand and resolve treatment nonresponders and reorganize traditional classifications of disease, which have up till now been based on phenotype alone.

REFERENCES

1. Tsongalis GJ, Silverman LM. Molecular diagnostics: a historical perspective. *Clin Chim Acta*. 2006;369:188.
2. McGrath JA. Translational benefits from research on rare genodermatoses. *Australas J Dermatol*. 2004;45:89.
3. Takeichi T, Nanda A, Liu L, et al. Impact of next generation sequencing on diagnostics in a genetic skin disease clinic. *Exp Dermatol*. 2013;22(12): 825-831.
4. Palmer CNA, Irvine AD, Terron-Kwiatkowski A, et al. Common loss-of-function variants of the epidermal barrier protein filaggrin are a major predisposing factor for atopic dermatitis. *Nat Genet*. 2006;38:441.
5. Hsu F, Cui W, Vongsangnak W, et al. The UCSC known genes. *Bioinformatics*. 2006;22:1036.
6. Gilchrest BA, Eller MS. The tale of the telomere: implications for prevention and treatment of skin cancers. *J Investig Dermatol Symp Proc*. 2005;10:124.
7. Wessagowit V, Nalla VK, Rogan PK, et al. Normal and abnormal mechanisms of gene splicing and relevance to inherited skin diseases. *J Dermatol Sci*. 2005;40:73.
8. Amrani N, Sachs MS, Jacobson A. Early nonsense: mRNA decay solves a translational problem. *Nat Rev Mol Cell Biol*. 2006;7:415.
9. Rogers GE. Hair follicle differentiation and regulation. *Int J Dev Biol*. 2004;48:163.
10. Sinha S, Degenstein L, Copenhaver C, et al. Defining the regulatory factors required for epidermal gene expression. *Mol Cell Biol*. 2000;20:2543.
11. Barutcu AR, Fritz AJ, Zaidi SK, et al. C-ing the Genome: A Compendium of Chromosome Conformation Capture Methods to Study Higher-Order Chromatin Organization. *J Cell Physiol*. 2016;231(1):31-35.
12. Jakub JW, Grotz TE, Jordan P, et al. A pilot study of chromosomal aberrations and epigenetic changes in peripheral blood samples to identify patients with melanoma. *Melanoma Res*. 2015;25(5):406-411.
13. Buenrostro JD, Wu B, Chang HY, et al. ATAC-seq: a method for assaying chromatin accessibility genome-wide. *Curr Protoc Mol Biol*. 2015;109:21.29.1-9.
14. Bao X, Rubin AJ, Qu K, et al. A novel ATAC-seq approach reveals lineage-specific reinforcement of the open chromatin landscape via cooperation between BAF and p63. *Genome Biol*. 2015;16:284.
15. Miao CG, Yang YY, He X, et al. The emerging role of microRNAs in the pathogenesis of systemic lupus erythematosus. *Cell Signal*. 2013;25(9):1828-1836.
16. Ashton GH, McGrath JA, South AP. Strategies to identify disease genes. *Drugs Today (Barc)*. 2002;38:235.
17. Hamada T, McLean WH, Ramsay M, et al. Lipoid proteinosis maps to 1q21 and is caused by mutations in the extracellular matrix protein 1 gene (ECM1). *Hum Mol Genet*. 2002;11:833.
18. Groves RW, Liu L, Dopping-Hepenstal PJ, et al. A homozygous nonsense mutation within the dystonin gene coding for the coiled-coil domain of the epithelial isoform of BPAG1 underlies a new subtype of autosomal recessive epidermolysis bullosa simplex. *J Invest Dermatol*. 2010;130(6):1551-1557.
19. Whittock NV, Ashton GH, Mohammedi R, et al. Comparative mutation detection screening of the type VII collagen gene (COL7A1) using the protein truncation test, fluorescent chemical cleavage of mismatch, and conformation sensitive gel electrophoresis. *J Invest Dermatol*. 1999;113:673.
20. Webber BR, Osborn MJ, McElroy AN, et al. CRISPR/Cas9-based genetic correction for recessive dystrophic epidermolysis bullosa. *NPJ Regen Med*. 2016;1. pii: 16014.
21. Wu W, Lu Z, Li F, et al. Efficient in vivo gene editing using ribonucleoproteins in skin stem cells of recessive dystrophic epidermolysis bullosa mouse model. *Proc Natl Acad Sci U S A*. 2017;114(7):1660-1665.
22. Gunderson KL, Kuhn KM, Steemers FJ, et al. Whole-genome genotyping of haplotype tag single nucleotide polymorphisms. *Pharmacogenomics*. 2006;7:641.
23. Happle R. X-chromosome inactivation: role in skin disease expression. *Acta Paediatr Suppl*. 2006;95:16.
24. Kotzot D, Utermann G. Uniparental disomy (UPD) other than 15: phenotypes and bibliography updated. *Am J Med Genet*. 2005;136:287.
25. Millington GW. Genomic imprinting and dermatological disease. *Clin Exp Dermatol*. 2006;31:681.
26. Pauler FM, Barlow DP. Imprinting mechanisms—it only takes two. *Genes Dev*. 2006;20:1203.
27. Fowden AL, Sibley C, Reik W, et al. Imprinted genes, placental development and fetal growth. *Horm Res*. 2006;65:50.
28. Birch-Machin MA. The role of mitochondria in ageing and carcinogenesis. *Clin Exp Dermatol*. 2006;31:548.
29. Schapira AH. Mitochondrial disease. *Lancet* 368:70, 2006.
30. Todorov IN, Todorov GI. Multifactorial nature of high frequency of mitochondrial DNA mutations in somatic mammalian cells. *Biochemistry (Mosc)*. 74:962, 2009.
31. Birch-Machin MA, Swalwell H. How mitochondria record the effects of UV exposure and oxidative stress using human skin as a model tissue. *Mutagenesis*. 2010;25:101.
32. Finsterer, J, Frank M. Prevalence of neoplasms in definite and probable mitochondrial disorders. *Mitochondrion*. 2016;29:31-34.

33. Chan DC. Mitochondria: dynamic organelles in disease, aging, and development. *Cell*. 2006;125:1241.
34. Thornton-Wells TA, Moore JH, Haines JL. Genetics, statistics and human disease: analytical retooling for complexity. *Trends Genet*. 2004;20:640.
35. Morar N, Willis-Owen SA, Moffatt MF, et al. The genetics of atopic dermatitis. *J Allergy Clin Immunol*. 2006;118:24.
36. Manolio TA. Genomewide association studies and assessment of the risk of disease. *N Engl J Med*. 2010;363:166.
37. Smith FJD, Irvine AD, Terron-Kwiatkowski A, et al. Loss-of-function mutations in the gene encoding filaggrin cause ichthyosis vulgaris. *Nat Genet*. 2006;38:337.
38. Weidinger S, Illig T, Baurecht H. Loss-of-function variations within the filaggrin gene predispose for atopic dermatitis with allergic sensitizations. *J Allergy Clin Immunol*. 2006;118:214.
39. Antonarakis SE, Beckmann JS. Mendelian disorders deserve more attention. *Nat Rev Genet*. 2006;7:277.
40. Siegel DH, Sybert VP. Mosaicism in genetic skin disorders. *Pediatr Dermatol*. 2006;23:87.
41. Itin P, Burger B. Mosaic manifestations of monogenic skin diseases. *J Dtsch Dermatol Gen*. 2009;7:744.
42. Happle R. Transposable elements and the lines of Blaschko: a new perspective. *Dermatology*. 2002;204:4.
43. Happle R. Monoallelic expression on autosomes may explain an unusual form of pigmentary mosaicism: a historical case revisited. *Clin Exp Dermatol*. 2009;34:834.
44. Jonkman MF, Scheffer H, Stulp R, et al. Revertant mosaicism in epidermolysis bullosa caused by mitotic gene conversion. *Cell*. 1997;88:543.
45. Jonkman MF, Passmooij AM. Revertant mosaicism—patchwork in the skin. *N Engl J Med*. 2009;360:1680.
46. Gostynski A, Deviaene FC, Pasmooij AM, et al. Adhesive stripping to remove epidermis in junctional epidermolysis bullosa for revertant cell therapy. *Br J Dermatol*. 2009;161:444.
47a. Gostynski A, Pasmooij AM, Jonkman MF. Successful therapeutic transplantation of revertant skin in epidermolysis bullosa. *J Am Acad Dermatol*. 2014;70(1):98-101.
47b. Hirsch et al, *Nature*. Nov 2017. [PMID 29144448].
48. Chung WH, Hung SI, Chen YT. Genetic predisposition of life-threatening antiepileptic-induced skin reactions. *Expert Opin Drug Saf*. 2010;9:15.
49. Redei GP, Koncz C, Phillips JD. Changing images of the gene. *Adv Genet*. 2006;56:53.
50. Callinan PA, Feinberg AP. The emerging science of epigenomics. *Hum Mol Genet*. 2006;15:R95.
51. Chen M, Wang Y, Yao X, et al. Hypermethylation of HLA-C may be an epigenetic marker in psoriasis. *J Dermatol Sci*. 2016;83(1):10-16.
52. Howell PM Jr, Liu S, Ren S, et al. Epigenetics in human melanoma. *Cancer Control*. 2009;16:200.
53. Fenichel P, Brucker-Davis F, Chevalier N. The history of Distilbene(R) (Diethylstilbestrol) told to grandchildren—the transgenerational effect. *Ann Endocrinol (Paris)*. 2015;76(3):253-259.
54. Horstemke B. Epimutations in human disease. *Curr Top Microbiol Immunol*. 2006;310:45.
55. Alelu-Paz R, Carmona FJ, Sanchez-Mut JV, et al. Epigenetics in Schizophrenia: A Pilot Study of Global DNA Methylation in Different Brain Regions Associated with Higher Cognitive Functions. *Front Psychol*. 2016;7:1496.
56. Dick KJ, Nelson CP, Tsaprouni L, et al. DNA methylation and body-mass index: a genome-wide analysis. *Lancet*. 2014;383(9933):1990-1998.
57. Dayeh T, Volkov P, Salö S, et al. Genome-wide DNA methylation analysis of human pancreatic islets from type 2 diabetic and non-diabetic donors identifies candidate genes that influence insulin secretion. *PLoS Genet*. 2014;10(3):e1004160.
58. Resta RG. Defining and redefining the scope and goals of genetic counseling. *Am J Med Genet C Semin Med Genet*. 2006;142:269.
59. Capon F, Trembath RC, Barker JN. An update on the genetics of psoriasis. *Dermatol Clin*. 2004;22:339.
60. Newton-Bishop JA, Gruiss NA. Genetics: what advice for patients who present with a family history of melanoma. *Semin Oncol*. 2007;34(6):452-459.
61. Rodeck CH, Eady RA, Gosden CM. Prenatal diagnosis of epidermolysis bullosa letalis. *Lancet*. 1980;1:949.
62. Golbus MS, Sagebiel RW, Filly RA, et al. Prenatal diagnosis of congenital bullous ichthyosiform erythroderma (epidermolytic hyperkeratosis) by fetal skin biopsy. *N Engl J Med*. 1980;302:93.
63. Heagerty AH, Kennedy AR, Gunner DB, et al. Rapid prenatal diagnosis and exclusion of epidermolysis bullosa using novel antibody probes. *J Invest Dermatol*. 1986;86:603.
64. Christiano AM, Pulkkinen L, McGrath JA, et al. Mutation-based prenatal diagnosis of Herlitz junctional epidermolysis bullosa. *Prenat Diagn*. 1997;17:343.
65. Fassihi H, Eady RA, Mellerio JE, et al. Prenatal diagnosis for severe inherited skin disorders: 25 years' experience. *Br J Dermatol*. 2006;154:106.
66. Braude P, Pickering S, Flinter F, et al. Preimplantation genetic diagnosis. *Nat Rev Genet*. 2002;3:941.
67. Fassihi H, Grace J, Lashwood A, et al. Preimplantation genetic diagnosis of skin fragility-ectodermal dysplasia syndrome. *Br J Dermatol*. 2006;154:546.
68. Renwick PJ, Trussler J, Ostad-Saffari E, et al. Proof of principle and first cases using preimplantation genetic haplotyping—a paradigm shift for embryo diagnosis. *Reprod Biomed Online*. 2006;13:110.
69. Fassihi H, Liu L, Renwick PJ, et al. Development and successful clinical application of preimplantation genetic haplotyping for Herlitz junctional epidermolysis bullosa. *Br J Dermatol*. 2010;162(6):1330-1336.
70. Hengge UR. Progress and prospects of skin gene therapy: a ten year history. *Clin Dermatol*. 2005;23:107.
71. Ferrari S, Pellegrini G, Matsui T, et al. Gene therapy in combination with tissue engineering to treat epidermolysis bullosa. *Expert Opin Biol Ther*. 2006;6:367.
72. Khavari PA. Genetic correction of inherited epidermal disorders. *Hum Gene Ther*. 2000;11:2277.
73. Shinkuma S, Guo Z, Christiano AM. Site-specific genome editing for correction of induced pluripotent stem cells derived from dominant dystrophic epidermolysis bullosa. *Proc Natl Acad Sci U S A*. 2016;113(20):5676-5681.
74. Foldvari M, Kumar P, King M, et al. Gene delivery into human skin in vitro using biphasic lipid vesicles. *Curr Drug Deliv*. 2006;3:89.
75. Gagnoux-Palacios L, Hervouet C, Spirito F, et al. Assessment of optimal transduction of primary human skin keratinocytes by viral vectors. *J Gene Med*. 2005;7:1178.
76. Hickerson RP, Smith FJ, Reeves RE, et al. Single-nucleotide-specific siRNA targeting in a dominant-negative skin model. *J Invest Dermatol*. 2008;128:59.
77. Leachman SA, Hickerson RP, Schwartz ME, et al. First-in-human mutation targeted siRNA phase Ib trial of an inherited skin disorder. *Mol Ther*. 2010;18:442.

Chapter 19 :: Carcinogenesis and Skin
:: Kenneth Y. Tsai & Andrzej A. Dlugosz

第十九章
癌变与皮肤

中文导读

本章分为4节：①皮肤癌的发生；②人类皮肤癌的动物模型；③皮肤癌的治疗和预防；④结论。主要焦点是以非黑色素瘤皮肤癌为例介绍癌变的发生、病因、治疗和预防。

第一节皮肤癌发生，介绍了恶性肿瘤的发生有其特征性的表型改变，反映了从肿瘤发生到侵袭和转移所需的多种基因和表观遗传改变的获得，是癌症生物学的基本原则。肿瘤进展的驱动力包括DNA修复缺陷、肿瘤内的异质性等，此外也提到了癌症干细胞和肿瘤间的异质性，对于肿瘤治疗和表型的重要性。同时介绍了皮肤癌遗传学和人类皮肤癌的病因学研究。

第二节人类皮肤癌的动物模型，介绍了人类皮肤癌模型有皮肤癌基因工程小鼠模型、化学物质诱发啮齿动物皮肤癌、紫外线诱发啮齿动物皮肤癌，并详细介绍了其在研究中的应用。

第三节皮肤癌的治疗和预防，介绍了鉴于紫外线诱变在皮肤癌发展中的核心作用，限制阳光和其他紫外线来源的暴露在皮肤肿瘤预防中的重要作用。治疗主要是手术治疗，其次Hedgehog通路抑制药等也用于皮肤癌。

第四节结论，总结了对皮肤癌的临床和实验研究使人们对基底细胞癌和鳞状细胞癌的分子和细胞基础有了重要的了解，对其预防和治疗具有很好的指导意义。

〔粟 娟〕

AT-A-GLANCE

- The estimated annual incidence of skin carcinomas is at least twofold higher than that of all other cancers combined, making these cancers a major burden on the U.S. health care system and a source of significant morbidity and mortality.

- Most skin cancers arise because of mutations caused by ultraviolet radiation in sunlight, with chemical carcinogens, oncogenic viruses, and other factors contributing to the development of a smaller proportion of tumors.

- The convergence of evidence from epidemiology, inherited predisposition syndromes, cancer genetics, animal models, and most recently genomics have collectively revealed unprecedented insights into the key causative events that drive the development of basal cell carcinoma (BCC) and squamous cell carcinoma (SCC).

- BCC and SCC display markedly different dependencies on specific pathways: whereas BCC is almost exclusively a Hedgehog pathway—dependent tumor, SCC appears to rely on a more varied set of gene mutations and oncogenic signaling.

- The accessibility of skin and the ability to model cancer development in animals has been highly useful in identifying the components and functions of key oncogenic signaling pathways, facilitating development of targeted therapeutics, and uncovering general principles of cancer biology.

INTRODUCTION

It was estimated that in 2017, there would be 87,110 new cases of invasive melanoma and 74,680 new cases of melanoma in situ.[1] Precise incidence data are not available for basal cell carcinoma (BCC) and cutaneous squamous cell carcinoma (SCC) because these tumors are not typically reported to cancer registries, but based on Medicare datasets, the total number of nonmelanoma skin cancers in 2006 was estimated at 4,013,890 cases (2,463,567 individuals) and in 2012 at 5,434,193 cases (affecting 3,315,554 individuals).[2] Another study, using data from the Medical Expenditure Panel Survey, estimated the number of individuals treated annually for nonmelanoma skin cancers at 3,090,442 (based on data from 2002 to 2006) and 4,301,338 (based on 2007 to 2011 data), with annual treatment costs up from $2.7 to $4.8 billion, respectively.[3] The combined incidence of BCC and SCC is thus likely to be at least twofold higher than that of all other cancers combined, which is estimated at 1,688,780 for 2017.[1] Only a small fraction of patients with BCC or SCC will die because of their cancer, but the high frequency of these malignancies nonetheless results in an estimated 2000 deaths per year, according to the American Cancer Society, and most cases are SCC. Although much less common than nonmelanoma skin cancer, melanoma has a continually rising death rate now estimated at 9730 per year.[1]

Although they are rarely lethal, nonmelanoma skin cancers cause considerable cosmetic morbidity because they frequently arise on sun-exposed sites such as the face. Understanding the etiology and pathogenesis of these malignancies is thus a significant public health goal, and development of mechanism-based, nondeforming therapies is urgently needed. The high prevalence of skin tumors, their external location, and well-defined preneoplastic lesions (for SCC and melanoma) all provide an excellent opportunities for studying the factors regulating cutaneous cancer induction in humans. Qualities that facilitate the study of human skin cancers have also been useful in establishing relevant animal models. Advances in molecular genetics, keratinocyte cell culture, and development of genetically altered mice and reconstructed human skin models have greatly facilitated the analysis of basic mechanisms of cutaneous carcinogenesis. The main focus in this chapter is on general aspects of cutaneous carcinogenesis using nonmelanoma skin cancers as illustrative examples, with more detailed discussion of specific cutaneous malignancies presented in other chapters.

CUTANEOUS CARCINOGENESIS

GENERAL PRINCIPLES

The majority of malignant tumors arise through a stepwise process marked by characteristic phenotypic changes that reflect the acquisition of multiple genetic and epigenetic alterations needed to drive tumorigenesis from its inception through to invasion and metastasis. This basic tenet of cancer biology holds true for SCC (Fig. 19-1), but the pathogenesis of BCC provides a notable exception to this rule: precursor lesions have not been identified, metastases are extremely rare, and uncontrolled activation of a single oncogenic pathway may be sufficient for BCC tumorigenesis.[4] Established cancers exhibit fundamental alterations in behavior that distinguish them from the normal tissues in which they arise. These differences include a reduced requirement for growth stimuli, impaired responses to growth inhibitory and differentiation signals, alterations in apoptosis, delayed or blocked senescence, angiogenesis, the capacity for invasion and metastasis, metabolic reprogramming, and the ability to evade elimination by the immune system[5] (Fig. 19-2). Although one or more of these abnormalities can be detected at different stages of tumor progression and may thus be seen in premalignant lesions, all are typically present in advanced cancers.

A driving force underlying neoplastic progression is defective DNA repair,[6] which enables the accumulation of mutations involving oncogenes and tumor

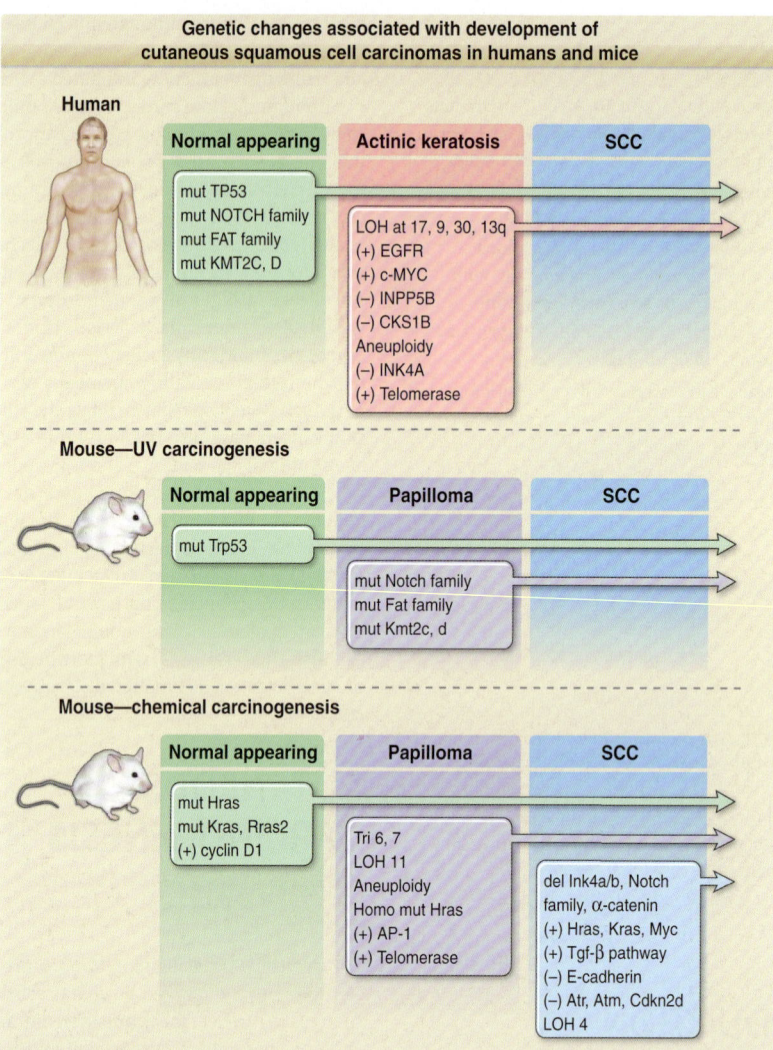

Figure 19-1 Molecular and genetic changes associated with development of cutaneous squamous cell carcinomas (SCCs) in humans and mice. The multistage evolution of cutaneous SCC in humans is depicted schematically with frequently associated genetic changes. Whereas single base mutations in early lesions frequently are characteristic of ultraviolet light-induced damage, later changes are associated with genomic instability. Increased activity of telomerase (deletion of inhibitor) or epidermal growth factor receptor (EGFR) tyrosine kinase (gene amplification) may also result from epigenetic changes. Similar changes are observed in ultraviolet (UV)-driven mouse models of cutaneous SCC.
In chemically induced mouse cutaneous SCC, the multistage evolution to invasive tumors in this model is highly ordered both temporally and genetically. Operationally defined stages include initiation, promotion, and progression. Ras mutations are characteristic of chemical mutagens used to initiate tumor formation. Early upregulation of cyclin D1 and later upregulation of transforming growth factor (TGF)-β1 occur through epigenetic mechanisms and appear to be important components of carcinogenesis. Note that most events occur early in the progression sequence in UV-induced tumors (eg, TP53 mutations), but in chemical carcinogenesis, most events occur late and often do not bear the signatures of the original mutagen. It should be noted that the data are derived from many different sources and reflect a panoply of technologies used to survey these changes.

suppressor genes that contribute to the observed aberrations in tumor cell function. In the past, uncovering the molecular basis of cancers relied on genetic linkage studies to identify the chromosomal locus which segregates with tumor phenotypes in cancer susceptibility syndromes or the use functional screens to identify genes from tumor cells that can drive neoplastic transformation in culture. However, the recent development of rapid and affordable next-generation sequencing technology, which can be used to screen for mutations in the coding portions of genes (exome sequencing) or the entire genome, has revolutionized the approach to identifying mutations that may drive cancer and serve as targets for therapeutic intervention through "personalized oncology."[7] Although some changes in cell function are cell-autonomous and can be studied in purified populations of tumor cells, others depend on various additional cell types in the

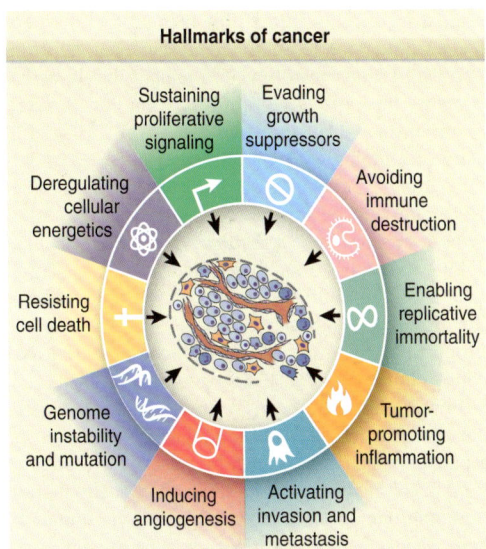

Figure 19-2 Hallmarks of cancer. Cancer cells acquire multiple properties distinguishing them from normal cells, including protection from cell death, sustained proliferation, evasion of growth inhibitory signals, the ability to invade and metastasize, immortalization, and induction of angiogenesis. More recently recognized properties important for tumorigenesis include deregulation of cellular energetics, immune evasion, genomic instability, and stimulation of inflammation. (Modified from Hanahan D, Weinberg RA. Hallmarks of cancer: the next generation. *Cell.* 2011;144(5):646-674.)

tumor microenvironment that participate in the development and progression of cancer in intact organisms, including inflammatory cells, cancer-associated fibroblasts, nerves, blood vessels and lymphatics, and other components of tumor stroma.[8]

Many tumors exhibit intratumor heterogeneity,[9] which may be apparent at multiple levels. Molecular heterogeneity provides a driving force for neoplastic progression, selecting for outgrowth of cells that have acquired mutations conferring a proliferative or survival advantage and the ability to invade and metastasize. Biochemical heterogeneity occurs when subsets of tumor cells exhibit distinct oncogenic signaling properties and behavior, driven by regional differences in secreted growth factors or other microenvironmental factors.

Perhaps the most striking example of heterogeneity is the presence of a small subset of stem cell–like tumor cells, called *cancer stem cells*, in at least some tumor types. According to the cancer stem cell hypothesis, tumors contain a small number of self-renewing stem cells that produce transient-amplifying and differentiating progeny that constitute the overwhelming majority of cells in a tumor (reviewed by Nassar and coworkers[10]) (Fig. 19-3), reflecting the hierarchical organization of cell lineages in normal tissues. Cancer stem cells are also called *tumor-initiating cells* because they are functionally defined by their ability, when purified and tested in small numbers or even as single cells, to reform a tumor in cell transplantation experiments. Tumor cells that are not cancer stem cells, in contrast, fail to produce tumors even when tested in relatively large numbers.[10] This functional characterization generally requires that cancer stem cells possess a unique marker profile that enables them to be isolated from a heterogeneous population of tumor cells. Although the cancer stem cell concept was initially established in work centered on acute myeloid leukemia,[11] results of many subsequent studies support the existence of a hierarchical organization of tumor-initiating cells and progeny in many, but not all, solid tumors. Cancer stem cell populations have been described in SCC (reviewed by Nassar and coworkers[10]) and BCC.[12]

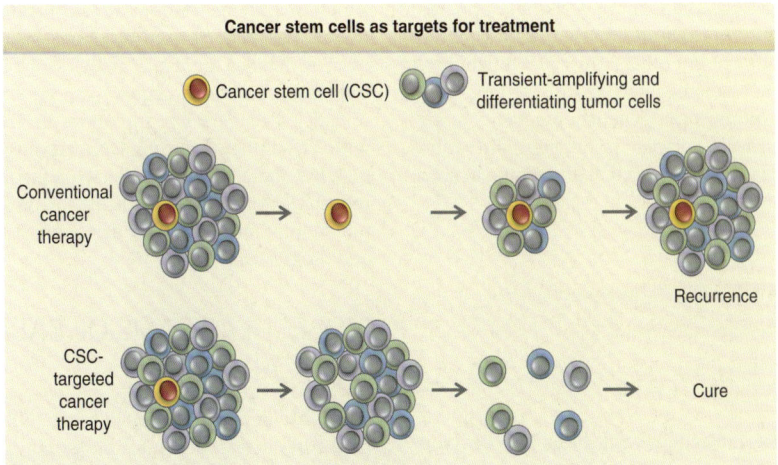

Figure 19-3 Cancer stem cells as targets for treatment. Representation of tumor mass containing a putative cancer stem cell (CSC) with its transient-amplifying and differentiating progeny that make up the bulk of the tumor. Treatment with conventional therapy may lead to rapid tumor regression, but if residual CSCs are present, tumors may recur after treatment is stopped. In contrast, CSC-targeted therapy may lead to a slower response, but after tumor cells regress, recurrence is unlikely if the CSC population has been eliminated. A hierarchical organization of CSCs and transiently amplifying progeny has been described in many, but not all, tumor types.

The cancer stem cell concept has important clinical implications because therapies that effectively kill cancer stem cells may lead to cures by eliminating the key cell population from which all remaining cells in a tumor arise. In contrast, treatments that target non–stem cells representing most of a tumor's mass may lead to striking tumor regression, but this is eventually followed by tumor recurrence because of outgrowth from remaining cancer stem cells (see Fig. 19-3). Although there are technical limitations to some of the assays used to ascertain "stemness" of isolated cancer cells, the cancer stem cell concept has been validated in multiple mouse models, and selective targeting of cancer stem cells is being pursued in an attempt to treat cancer more effectively.[13] The success of this approach will depend in part on whether transient-amplifying or differentiating tumor cells possess sufficient plasticity to revert back to a stem cell–like population after effective depletion of the original cancer stem cell pool.

An additional general property of cancers is intertumor heterogeneity. This includes phenotypic differences between tumors of the same type that are not necessarily related to malignant progression but are sufficient to justify classification into distinct morphologic categories, for example, superficial, nodular, and morpheaform subtypes of BCC. One explanation for intertumor heterogeneity is based on the notion that transformation of different cell populations produces different tumor subtypes, so a tumor's cell of origin is a key determinant of its ultimate phenotype. For example, mouse modeling suggests that oncogenic activation of the Hedgehog pathway in an epidermal basal cell may produce superficial BCC, but nodular BCCs may arise from responsive cell populations within hair follicle epithelium.[14] Experimental evidence from other tumor types supports the concept that different cells of origin give rise to distinct tumor subtypes.[15] Another example of intertumor heterogeneity is the disparate growth rates of histologically similar tumor types. This can be strikingly apparent in BCC patients, for example, in whom some nodular tumors are indolent but others grow at a much faster rate. Intertumor heterogeneity in this setting could be explained by intrinsic (genetic, epigenetic, or signaling) or extrinsic (microenvironmental) alterations that provide a growth or survival advantage to some tumors but not others.

regulators of cell proliferation or inhibitors of apoptosis. Conversion to an oncogene can occur through point mutations resulting in a constitutively active protein, through DNA amplification, or through chromosomal translocations that link a highly active promoter with the proto-oncogene. The latter two mechanisms cause increased or inappropriate expression of a proto-oncogene and may alter growth regulation of a responsive normal cell. Less common mechanisms implicated in cancer entail fusion of the coding domains of two genes, producing a novel, chimeric molecule with oncogenic properties[16] or mutations in non-coding DNA that control the expression of oncogenes.[17]

Tumor suppressor genes normally function to negatively regulate cell proliferation, cause apoptosis, repair damaged DNA, or induce cellular differentiation. In contrast to oncogenes, which typically require that only one allele undergo activation via mutation, both alleles of a tumor suppressor gene must be inactivated to promote tumor development. Frequently, inactivating point mutations occur in one copy of a tumor suppressor gene, and the remaining normal copy is lost through a process of chromosomal missegregation during mitosis that leads to loss of heterozygosity. However, mutations in noncoding DNA[17] could also lead to functionally significant reductions in expression of tumor suppressor genes. In addition, altered expression of long noncoding RNAs could influence tumorigenesis by affecting signaling pathways at multiple levels.[18]

Which oncogenes and tumor suppressors contribute to development of cutaneous neoplasms? Considerable insight into the genetic basis of sporadic skin cancers has come from the identification of specific genes that underlie hereditary skin tumor syndromes.[19] The importance of DNA as a target for carcinogenesis was strongly supported by the discovery of defects in DNA repair genes in skin cancer–prone patients with xeroderma pigmentosum (see later) and several other dermatoses characterized by photosensitivity.[20] Moreover, a detailed genomic analysis of 500 metastatic tumors from various primary cancers has uncovered unanticipated germline mutations in 12.2% of cases, with 75% of them affecting DNA repair genes.[21] Taken together, these findings underscore the importance of robust DNA repair mechanisms for preventing accumulation of mutations that drive cancer development and progression.

GENETICS OF SKIN CANCER

GENERAL CONCEPTS

Studies on the molecular basis of cancer development have revealed two main classes of genes, oncogenes and tumor suppressor genes, that play a key role in the pathogenesis of cancer. An oncogene is any gene that can transform normal cells in culture and induce cancer in animals. Most oncogenes are derived from proto-oncogenes, which generally encode proteins that function as critical positive

MOLECULAR BASIS OF BASAL CELL CARCINOMA

Patients with nevoid BCC syndrome (NBCCS) are at a markedly increased risk for developing BCCs, which arise at a younger age and appear in greater numbers than in the general population. Patients with NBCCS are also predisposed to the development of a pediatric brain tumor arising in the cerebellum, medulloblastoma, as well as a variety of other defects throughout the body, including bifid ribs, calcified falx cerebri, odontogenic keratocysts, frontal bossing, palmar pits, and bifid ribs.²² Some of these structural abnormalities must have taken place during fetal development, suggesting that the genetic alteration in NBCCS influences tissue or organ formation during embryogenesis, as well as cancer development after birth. The discovery that NBCCS is caused by germline mutations disrupting the *PTCH1* gene,²³,²⁴ which encodes a key component of the Hedgehog signaling pathway, is in keeping with this idea. Physiologic Hedgehog signaling plays an important role in patterning and morphogenesis of various organs and tissues during development and contributes to tissue homeostasis and regeneration postnatally; in contrast, uncontrolled activation of the Hedgehog pathway (Fig. 114-1), caused by mutations affecting *PTCH1* or other Hedgehog pathway components (Table 114-1), is tightly associated with BCC development both in NBCCS patients and the general population[25-27] (see Chap. 111). Because deregulated activation of the Hedgehog pathway is detected in essentially all BCCs and pathway activation has been shown to be sufficient for BCC development and required for tumor maintenance, it was believed that pharmacologic inhibitors of this pathway may be useful in the medical management of BCC. This has proven to be the case in a significant proportion of patients with advanced or metastatic BCC treated with Hedgehog pathway inhibitors, as discussed later and in Chap. 111.

Despite the pivotal role of deregulated Hedgehog signaling in BCC development, next-generation sequencing studies have uncovered additional potential driver mutations in genes encoding MYCN, PPP6C, STK19, LATS1, PIK3CA, RAS proteins, with loss-of-function mutations and missense mutations in *PTPN14*, *RB1*, and *FBXW7*.[28] Additional studies will be needed to determine the functional significance of these genetic alterations and others[27] on BCC biology and treatment response.

MUTATIONS AND MOLECULAR DRIVERS IN SQUAMOUS CELL CARCINOMA

In contrast to BCC, the identification of pivotal genetic events that drive the development of cutaneous SCC has been somewhat complicated by the fact that no inherited cancer syndromes exclusively predispose to cutaneous SCC, and there is no high-frequency oncogenic driver analogous to mutant *BRAF* in melanoma. As a result, the key evidence implicating specific genetic alterations in SCC development has been pieced together through characterization of high-risk clinical scenarios, molecular analysis of animal models, genomics, and proteomics.

Three rare inherited syndromes have highlighted the importance of environmental influences, specific clinical scenarios, and pathways that drive SCC development. Xeroderma pigmentosum, characterized by extreme photosensitivity and stark acceleration in the onset of skin cancer, is associated with a nearly 10,000-fold increased risk of skin cancer before the age of 20 years.[29] The key unifying defect, caused by recessive inactivation of genes distributed across eight complementation groups, results in the lack of nucleotide excision repair, which is required for removing mutagenic DNA photoproducts caused by ultraviolet (UV) radiation. Recessive dystrophic epidermolysis bullosa is a skin fragility disorder caused by loss-of-function mutations in *COL7A1*, which results in subepidermal blistering, nonhealing wounds, and a high predisposition to SCC. The chronic scarring that results predisposes to SCC, which are clinically difficult to manage and frequently fatal.[30] Finally, heterozygous germline inactivation of transforming growth factor (TGF)-βR1 results in a susceptibility to keratoacanthomas as part of Smith-Ferguson syndrome[31] and indeed, inactivation of TGF-βR signaling more globally is associated with typical SCC development.[32] Additional genodermatoses and genes linked to SCC development are listed in Table 112-1.

By using the two-stage chemical carcinogenesis approach in mice (see later), Balmain and colleagues pioneered the molecular genetic analysis of tumor development in this classical skin cancer model and identified mutated *Hras* as the primary oncogenic driver of tumors in this model[33] 1 year after its isolation as the first human oncogene.[34] By 1991, recurrent *TP53* mutations had been identified in human SCC corresponding to hotspot sites in the DNA-binding domain and bearing characteristic C → T transitions attributed to UV exposure.[35,36]

Next-generation DNA sequencing has now provided extensive insight into the genetic lesions that may drive cutaneous SCC development. Although many of these reports are from primary tumors, some series of metastatic lesions has been reported now as well.[37-41] The mutational spectrum across the exome is, as expected, strongly dominated by C → T transitions and UV signature mutations and is overwhelmingly represented by the inactivation of tumor suppressor genes, with very few highly recurrent mutations. Taken across published exome and targeted sequencing efforts, the most frequently mutated tumor suppressor genes are *TP53*, *CDKN2A*, *NOTCH* family members, atypical cadherin *FAT* family members, the histone methyltransferases *KMT2C* and *KMT2D*, and *KNSTRN*.[37-42] The panoply of sample sources, sequencing methodologies and analysis pipelines makes direct comparisons difficult, but additional potential tumor suppressors include *CASP8*, *CREBBP*, and *CARD11*.[43] Mutant *HRAS* is observed in up to 20% of SCC in one series.[38] Amplifications in *MYC* and *EGFR* as well as loss of *CKS1B* and *INPP*5A have also been reported in cutaneous SCC.[44-47]

Importantly, these data also show striking similarities to SCC arising in other sites. Because stratified squamous epithelia form interfaces with the environment, these tissues are frequent sites of interaction with carcinogens. *TP53* mutations occur at more than 70% frequency across all SCCs; *NOTCH* family genes are mutated in more than 70% of cutaneous SCC (cuSCC), 20% of oral head and neck SCC (HNSCC), 13% of lung SCC, and 10% of esophageal SCC, and SOX2 amplification is a common lineage-specific driver of SCC.[48] Coupled with previous results, this shows that SCCs from diverse sites share deep molecular commonalities, including alterations in global gene expression and in *TP53*, *TP63*, *NOTCH* family, and *SOX2* signaling. There is less published transcriptomic and proteomic data, although the correspondence to carcinogen-induced SCC holds prominently for HNSCC and lung SCC. Transcriptional profiling implicates transcription factors downstream of wingless-related integration site (WNT), β-catenin, and ERK (extracellular signal-regulated kinase) signaling.[37,48] Emerging literature also implicates multiple microRNAs in the development of SCC (reviewed by Konicke and coworkers[49]). Several have been implicated in multiple contexts with tumor-promoting and tumor-suppressive functions in proliferation, apoptosis, and migration.

Reverse-phase protein array-based interrogation of canonical cancer pathways showed upregulation of ERK and mTOR (mammalian target of rapamycin) pathway signaling across the progression sequence of SCC development.[50] The importance of ERK pathway signaling has also been reflected in two clinical scenarios involving drug-induced SCC: BRAF (v-raf murine sarcoma viral oncogene homolog B) inhibition used for melanoma and smoothened (SMO) inhibition used for BCC. It was observed in the initial clinical trials with the first Food and Drug Administration–approved BRAF inhibitor, vemurafenib, that approximately 22% of treated melanoma patients developed SCC or keratoacanthoma-like lesions; this adverse effect is less frequently observed with the more potent BRAF inhibitors dabrafenib and encorafenib.[51] Mechanistically, this has been attributed to both paradoxical ERK signaling resulting from the aberrant drug-induced hyperactivation of MEK (mitogen activated protein/extracellular signal-related kinase kinase)/ERK signaling in the context of wild-type *BRAF*,[52,53] often in the context of oncogenic mutant *HRAS*,[54] and to the suppression of apoptosis that occurs as a result of off-target suppression of c-Jun-N-terminal kinase (JNK) signaling.[55] Accordingly, the concomitant use of MEK with BRAF inhibitors almost completely suppresses the emergence of these SCCs.[51] Interestingly, the long-term treatment of BCCs with the SMO inhibitor vismodegib has occasionally been associated with the evolution of treated tumors to a SCC morphology that is associated with drug resistance and activation of ERK signaling.[56,57] Collectively, these data strongly implicate ERK signaling as an important pathway in SCC. This has also been validated in a UV-driven preclinical model in which MEK inhibition has potent therapeutic and chemopreventative effects.[58]

ETIOLOGY OF HUMAN SKIN CANCER

PHOTOCARCINOGENESIS

Ultraviolet radiation (UVR) in sunlight is the primary etiologic agent for all skin cancers, and thus UVR is the major carcinogen in the human environment. The powerful carcinogenic activity of UVR is attributable to its ability to damage DNA and cause mutations, its capacity to clonally expand incipient neoplastic cells whose altered signaling pathways provide a survival advantage in the face of UV-induced cytotoxicity, its ability to induce reactive oxygen species (ROS), and its activity as an immune suppressant. The association of UVR with skin cancer is so strongly supported by clinical, epidemiologic, and experimental data that it represents perhaps the most clear-cut etiologic factor in human malignancy.

UV light is a complete carcinogen and chronic exposure alone is sufficient to induce skin cancers. The process begins with carcinogen exposure, DNA damage, and the progressive acquisition of mutations. Clonal expansion occurs at least partially because of selection for these mutations, increasing the target size for further damage. The combination of these changes with key microenvironmental and immunologic consequences of UV exposure collectively drive tumor development.[59] In addition to environmental or occupational exposures, patients with various dermatoses are treated with UVR. The vast majority of experience in assessing the resulting risk for skin cancer has been in the context of psoriasis phototherapy. This risk was best established for psoralen and ultraviolet A light (PUVA) therapy in a prospective study with 20 years of follow-up initiated by Stern and colleagues, in which the risk of SCC was more than 100-fold higher and the risk of BCC was more than 11-fold higher.[60] The data on narrowband UVB has been largely confined to retrospective analyses, which suggest that there is no elevated risk of skin cancer; however, these studies are additionally limited by shorter follow-up.

ULTRAVIOLET RADIATION-INDUCED DNA DAMAGE AND REPAIR

DNA Photoproducts: The first molecular step in sunlight-induced carcinogenesis occurs when UVB photons induce DNA photoproducts (see Fig. 19-4). UVB and UVC tend to be absorbed at the 5–6 double bond of pyrimidines (thymine and cytosine). If two adjacent pyrimidines are activated, the resulting open bonds cross-react, creating a cyclobutane pyrimidine dimer (CPD). The most frequent is TT, but TC, CT, and CC cyclobutane dimers are also made. A single bond between the 6 position of one pyrimidine and the exocyclic group of the other instead creates a pyrimidine (6–4) pyrimidone photoproduct [(6–4)PP][61] most frequently TC. Both photoproducts distort the DNA helix and are recognized by DNA repair enzymes. Although there is 20-fold more UVA than UVB in sunlight, UVA requires up to 1000-fold greater doses for some of its biological effects such as DNA damage and minimal erythemal doses at 300 nm (UVB) and at 360 nm (UVA) for skin type II are 25 mJ/cm^2 and 32,000 mJ/cm^2, respectively.[62] UVB induces 500 photolesions per 10^6 normal bases per J/cm^2 in human skin.[63]

Ultraviolet Radiation—Induced Mutations: A CPD can lead to a mutation in two ways (Fig. 19-5). When the lesion is copied during DNA replication, the

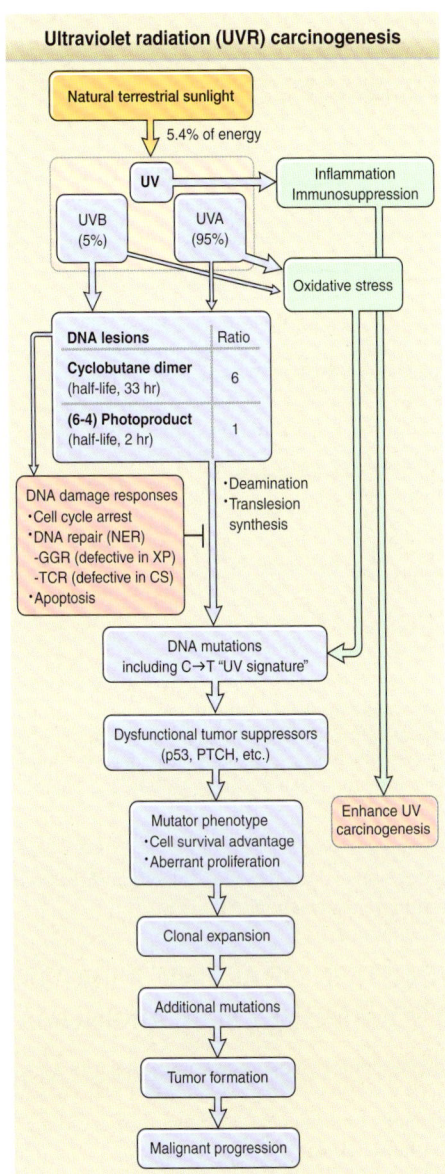

Figure 19-4 Ultraviolet radiation (UVR) carcinogenesis. UVR induces two major DNA lesions at dipyrimidine sites: cyclobutane pyrimidine dimers (CPDs) and pyrimidine (6–4) pyrimidone photoproducts [(6–4)PPs]. Ratio given [6 CPDs per 1 (6–4)PP] is that induced by simulated sunlight. UVB accounts for only 5% of UVR (~0.3% of all terrestrial sunlight energy) but produces the majority of UV-induced DNA lesions. Cells respond to UVR-induced DNA damage by activating DNA damage signaling pathways and inducing cell cycle arrest. Damaged DNA is repaired by nucleotide excision repair (NER). Unrepaired DNA lesions lead to genetic mutations through deamination or error-prone translesion synthesis. Unrepaired cytosine-containing CPDs contribute to UV signature mutation: C→T transition. Mutations in genes responsible for carcinogenesis confer a mutator phenotype including resistance to apoptosis. This expands the pool of clones susceptible to further damage and increases the potential for transformation. CS, Cockayne syndrome; GGR, global genome repair; PTCH, PATCHED1; TCR, transcription coupled repair; XP, xeroderma pigmentosum.

DNA polymerase may read a damaged cytosine as a thymine and insert an adenine opposite it. At the next round of replication, the polymerase correctly inserts thymine across from adenine, resulting in a C → T substitution. Alternatively, CPDs accelerate spontaneous deamination of their cytosines to uracil, resulting in the same change. Although the TT CPD is the most common photoproduct, the addition of A across damaged T bases by DNA polymerase eta causes no mutations. If two adjacent cytosines mutate, the result is CC → TT. This distinctive pattern of mutation, C → T in which the C lies next to another pyrimidine, including CC → TT, is unique to UVR and is called the *UV signature mutation.*[64]

Signature mutations provide a tool for deducing the original carcinogen from mutations found in tumors.[64,65] Nearly all experimentally created UVB or UVC mutations are located at adjacent pyrimidines, and about two thirds are signature mutations. The remaining third, typically G → T and T → C substitutions or small insertions or deletions, are caused by UV but probably arise indirectly by ROS. G → T transversion can be caused by incorporation of adenine opposite 8-hydroxy-2'-deoxyguanosine (see Fig. 19-5), a common oxidative DNA lesion. Because this oxidative class of damage can be caused by many carcinogens, these mutations do not reveal whether their source was UVB, UVA, tobacco smoke, or intracellular oxidative phosphorylation. However, tumors carrying classic UV signature mutations must also contain UV-induced oxidative mutations. UVA weakly induces UVB signature mutations by photosensitization but generates oxidation-like mutations and T → G changes, which have been proposed to be a UVA fingerprint.[61]

Recently, a chemically distinct pathway of UV-induced CPD generation was discovered.[66] In this mechanism, UV-induced generation of the ROS peroxynitrite was found to interact with melanin, resulting in chemiexcitation of electrons in melanin to extremely high-energy states, analogous to reactions that culminate in bioluminescence. However, instead of generating light, these excited electrons can directly interact with DNA, resulting in continuous CPD formation hours after UVA or UVB exposure has ceased, so-called "dark CPDs." Importantly, these dark CPDs account for more than half of CPDs in melanocytes after UV exposure. This discovery suggests that any source of ROS can potentially generate CPDs and that the kinetics of CPD generation by this mechanism may offer an opportunity for novel chemoprevention strategies beyond blocking UV exposure.[66]

MUTATION BURDEN AND CLONAL DYNAMICS IN SKIN

The repeated exposure of skin to UVR over a lifetime represents an enormous collective DNA damage burden. Indeed, initial reports dating back to 1996 showed that clones of keratinocytes aberrantly expressing stable (and therefore likely mutated) p53 could be detected in whole-mounted skin.[67,68] These

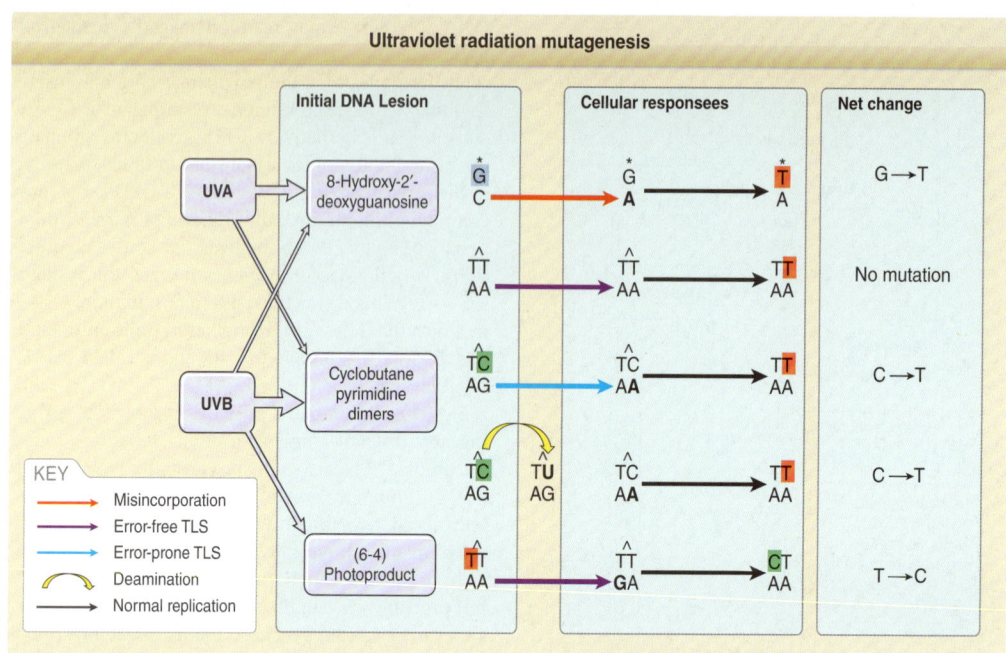

Figure 19-5 Ultraviolet radiation mutagenesis: how replication through unrepaired DNA lesions leads to DNA mutation. Cyclobutane pyrimidine dimers (CPDs) are the most relevant for ultraviolet (UV) mutagenesis and are primarily induced by UVB. Error-free translesion synthesis (TLS) adds adenines opposite CPDs, leaving thymine dimers unaffected but causing UV signature C→T transitions in cytosine dimers, which may also result from deamination. The (6–4) photoproduct induced by UVB and 8-hydroxy-2′-deoxyguanosine primarily induced by UVA are mutagenic but relatively rare.

TP53-mutant clones have also been identified in UV-exposed mouse skin.

Recently, targeted and whole-exome sequencing have shown that chronically UV-exposed clinically and histologically normal-appearing epidermis harbors about five mutations per megabase of DNA[37,69] (Fig. 19-6), a remarkably high mutational load that exceeds that of many human cancers. Indeed, skin cancers have the highest mutational loads of any human cancer reported with the possible exception of mismatch repair-deficient colon carcinomas. To be identified at all by existing DNA sequencing methodologies, there must be clones of cells bearing identical mutations of sufficient quantity to be reliably detectable at a given sequencing depth. Therefore, the extent of UV-induced mosaicism in epidermis is likely to be even greater than reported.

Although the presence of clones is interpreted as evidence of positive selection for specific mutations,[69] the frequency distribution of clone sizes suggests that clones can also spontaneously arise without the need for such selection.[70] In the case of *TP53*, it is clear that although *TP53* mutations compromise apoptosis, continued UV exposure is necessary for a selective advantage for these mutations to manifest themselves in the form of expanding clones, presumably through the inhibition or killing of surrounding normal keratinocytes. Deep sequencing of *TP53*-mutant clones in archival samples of UV-exposed human skin showed that many subclonal mutations in genes associated with SCCs are present, suggesting the widespread existence of keratinocyte patches highly predisposed to transformation.[71]

EVOLUTION OF ACTINIC KERATOSES TO SQUAMOUS CELL CARCINOMA

Estimates of the rate of progression of AK to SCC range from 0.6% at 1 year to 2.6% in 4 years.[72] At the genomic level, many of the key mutated genes observed in SCC and irradiated skin are also found in AK.[37,71] There have been no consistently identified transcriptional differences between AK and SCC. Instead, the molecular profiles of most AKs are largely indistinguishable from those of well-differentiated invasive SCC, suggesting that chemoprevention targeted to heavily mutagenized UV-exposed skin may be more effective.

VIRAL CARCINOGENESIS

GENERAL FEATURES

Virus-associated cancers comprise up to 10% of all human malignancies, including several that arise in skin: Kaposi sarcoma; SCC (arising in epidermodysplasia verruciformis patients and a small fraction of immunosuppressed individuals); and Merkel cell carcinoma[73] (see Table 19-1). DNA viruses have

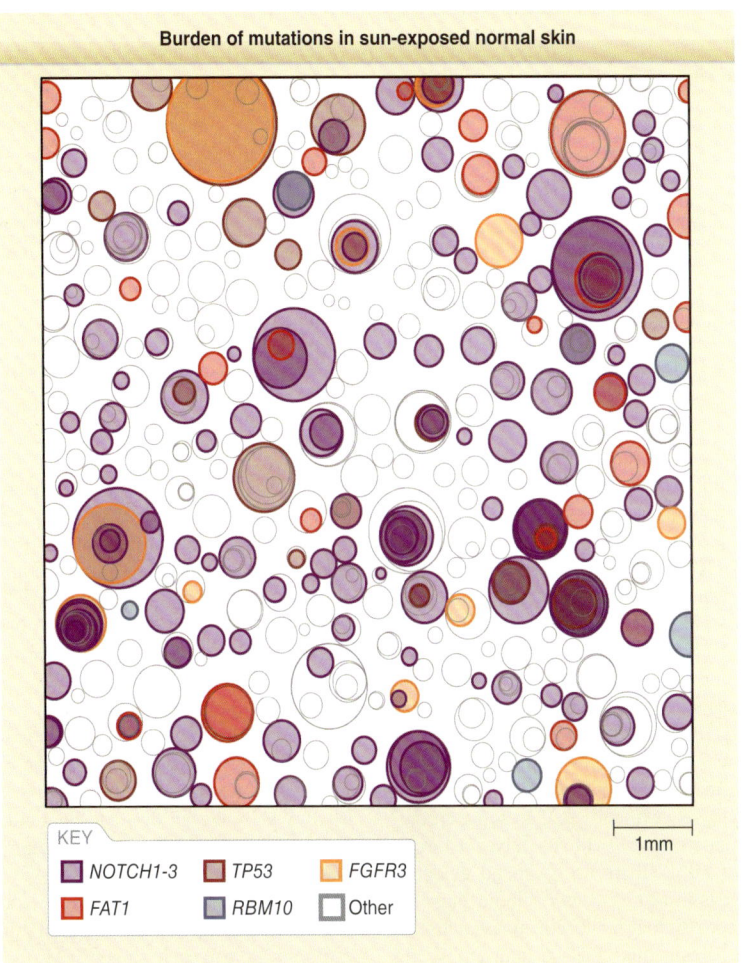

Figure 19-6 Graphical representation of mutant clone sizes in normal skin linked to specific genes implicated in SCC development. The plot represents estimated physical sizes of clones of epidermal cells based on the proportion of DNA sequences bearing a recurrent mutation and knowledge of skin biopsy sizes. Hundreds of clones bearing recurrently mutated cancer-relevant genes are found within a 1-cm² patch of epidermis. Some mutations are inferred to represent subclones within larger clones (overlapping circles); however, bulk sequencing precludes definitive spatial mapping. (Adapted from Martincorena I, Roshan A, Gerstung M, et al. Tumor evolution. High burden and pervasive positive selection of somatic mutations in normal human skin. *Science*. 2015;348(6237):880-886.[69] Reprinted with permission from AAAS.)

evolved highly effective mechanisms, in permissive host cells, for replicating their genomes, synthesizing capsid proteins, and assembling infectious viral particles during their normal, vegetative life cycles. Because of their small size, viruses cannot produce the full complement of proteins needed for DNA replication; instead, viral "early proteins" needed during early stages of the viral life cycle hijack the host cell cycle machinery to replicate the viral genome. After primary infection, most viruses are kept in check by the host immune system with minimal evidence of productive infection. Immunosuppression can lead to viral reactivation and disease, which may reflect lysis of host cells that accumulate large numbers of viral particles.

Viral infection typically precedes cancer development by many years, and only a small subset of infected individuals develop cancer, frequently in the setting of systemic immunosuppression or impaired immune surveillance. Viral transformation is a dead end for viruses because it is usually associated with integration of viral DNA into the host cell genome in a manner that precludes viral genome replication and completion of the viral life cycle but allows for persistent expression of early viral proteins that drive cellular transformation by targeting key host cell signaling proteins.[74] Thus, viral oncoproteins contribute to cancer by dysregulating many of the same proteins and pathways that are altered by exposure to UV light or other mutagens in sporadic cancers.

HUMAN PAPILLOMAVIRUSES

More than 200 types of human papillomaviruses (HPVs) have been identified and grouped into five genera, with the alpha and beta HPV types most closely linked to

TABLE 19-1
Virus-Induced Human Skin Tumors

VIRUS	VIRUS TYPE	SIZE	GENOME	TRANSMISSION	SKIN TUMOR TYPE (S)	OTHER TUMORS
HPV (high-risk alpha subtypes)[a]	Papillomavirus	55 nm	dsDNA (~8 kb)	Sexual contact	SCC (anogenital)	Cervical, head, and neck
KSHV (HHV8)	Herpes virus	180–200 nm	dsDNA (~165 kb)	Body fluids, tissue	Kaposi sarcoma	Primary effusion lymphoma, multicentric Castleman disease
MCPyV	Polyomavirus	45 nm	dsDNA (5.3 kb)	?	MCC	?

[a]See text for discussion of beta human papillomavirus (HPV) and cutaneous squamous cell carcinoma (SCC).

dsDNA, double-stranded DNA; HHV8, human herpesvirus-8; KSHV, Kaposi sarcoma–associated herpesvirus; MCC, Merkel cell carcinoma; MCPyV, Merkel cell polyomavirus.

cancer.[75] Some alpha HPVs infect skin and cause warts, but others infect mucosal surfaces, with low-risk HPVs producing benign lesions (condylomata) and high-risk HPVs, typically HPV16 or 18, associated with malignancy (cervical cancer, most anorectal cancers, and a sizeable fraction of genital and oropharyngeal cancers). Infection by high-risk alpha HPVs is relatively common in young, sexually active individuals, but the infection is cleared via the immune system in most individuals. Beta HPVs have been linked to development of cutaneous warts and SCC in individuals with epidermodysplasia verruciformis and may play a role in the pathogenesis of cutaneous SCC in some chronically immunosuppressed individuals.[76] Nevertheless, unlike the alpha HPVs, there has been no evidence for viral transcripts in skin cancers,[37,77] indicating that beta HPVs are not required for tumor maintenance. A hit-and-run mechanism that posits a temporally and functionally restricted requirement for HPV gene transcription is still compatible with a causal role but is difficult to demonstrate definitively. The early genes E6 and E7 from high-risk alpha HPVs drive tumorigenesis by binding and degrading the tumor suppressors TP53 and RB1, respectively. In contrast, beta HPVs influence other oncogenic effectors and processes to drive cancer, leading to deficient double-strand DNA repair, impaired apoptosis, disrupted epithelial differentiation, and altered NOTCH and TGF-β signaling.[78]

HUMAN POLYOMAVIRUSES

Human polyomavirus (PyV) infections are ubiquitous. The great majority of adults harbor serologic evidence of infection by multiple human PyVs occurring at an early age followed by establishment of subclinical, persistent infection because of the presence of episomal viral DNA in the nucleus of the host cell.[79] Viral reactivation and productive infection, which requires viral genome replication and packaging into infectious virions, can occur in immunosuppressed individuals and cause clinically evident disease.[79] For example, BKPyV is associated with development of posttransplant nephropathy and hemorrhagic cystitis, and JCPyV causes progressive multifocal leukoencephalopathy.

Several PyVs have been isolated from human skin, and some are associated with distinctive skin disorders, including pruritic and dyskeratotic dermatoses (HPyV6 and HPyV7) and the hair follicle disorder trichodysplasia spinulosa (TSPyV).[80] In nearly all cases, these conditions arise in immunosuppressed hosts and are associated with productive infection, leading to accumulation of a large numbers of virions in affected cells. Merkel cell PyV (MCPyV) is also present in normal human skin but is not associated with any known skin disorders linked to productive viral infection. MCPyV is, however, detected in about 80% of Merkel cell carcinomas, which are rare but aggressive neuroendocrine malignancies that arise in skin (see Chap. 113). MCPyV viral DNA was found to be clonally integrated in MCCs,[81] strongly suggesting that this virus plays an important role at early stages of MCC development in virus-positive tumors.

Given the strong evidence pointing to a causal role for MCPyV in MCC, much effort has gone into investigating the transforming potential of the MCPyV early gene products large T and small T antigens (LTAg, sTAg). Historically, LTAg from a simian polyomavirus, SV40, has been used extensively to study fundamental aspects of cancer because of its potent ability to transform cells in cell culture and produce tumors in experimental animals.[82] The transforming properties of SV40 LTAg have been attributed largely to its ability to disrupt the functions of both TP53 and RB1, identifying these two tumor suppressors as key targets for viral oncogenesis. In contrast to LTAg, SV40 sTAg alone is not a potent oncogene, although it may contribute to LTAg-driven transformation. Intriguingly, the contribution of MCPyV TAgs to transformation appears reversed relative to that of SV40 in that sTAg appears to be the main oncogenic driver both in vitro and in vivo.[83,84] Current studies in this area include work aimed at better defining the contributions of sTAg and LTAg to MCC development, identifying key TAg-driven changes in host cells and interacting proteins and pathways that contribute to tumorigenesis, and uncovering the MCC cell of origin.

CHEMICAL CARCINOGENESIS

Also implicated in the development of a relatively small proportion of human skin cancers are various chemicals, as a result of environmental, occupational, or medicinal exposures (Table 19-2). In 1775, Sir Percivall Pott[85] attributed the increased incidence of scrotal cancer in chimney sweeps to repeated exposure to soot. This report provided the first link between an occupational exposure and the development of cancer as well as the first example of chemical carcinogenesis. The National Toxicology Program's 14th Report on Carcinogens (http://ntp.niehs.nih.gov/go/roc14), released in 2016, lists 248 substances as either known (62 substances) or reasonably anticipated (186 substances) to be human carcinogens. Although most of these are chemicals, the list also includes physical agents (eg, ionizing and UVR) and infectious agents (eg, Kaposi sarcoma–associated herpesvirus and MCPyV), discussed earlier. Although not yet listed, the antifungal voriconazole has been linked to an increased incidence of SCCs in immunosuppressed patients.[86] Mechanisms by which chemicals cause cancer reveal striking similarities to those uncovered for UVR-induced cancer, including DNA damage, selective cytotoxicity, and immunosuppression.

OTHER CARCINOGENIC STIMULI

Ionizing radiation (IR) had been used to treat a variety of skin disorders, including acne and tinea capitus as well as malignant tumors. Interestingly the excess risk of skin cancer associated with IR exposure is almost exclusively confined to BCC and has been documented in atomic bomb survivors, radiologists, miners, and children treated for tinea capitis.[87] Childhood exposure has been associated with a significantly increased risk of BCC with a latency of over 20 years, particularly in fair-complected individuals, suggesting a strong interactions between UV and IR exposures.[88] Epidemiologically, pilots are highly exposed to cosmic IR, which is associated with a 3-fold elevated risk of BCC and 3.5-fold elevated risk of melanoma.[89]

Chronic wounds have long been recognized clinically as a risk factor for skin cancer, particularly SCC. Marjolin ulcers refer to skin cancers that arise in sites of chronic ulcers or scars, most often caused by burns[90] and most often occurring on the lower extremities and scalp. Several series detailing long-term follow-up conclude that more than 77% of these cancers are associated with burns, almost 90% of tumors are SCC, and the average interval from initial injury to tumor development was 37 years.[91,92] These SCCs are highly

TABLE 19-2
Agents Identified as Known Human Skin Carcinogens[a]

CLASS	AGENT	EXPOSURE	SKIN TUMOR TYPE(S)	OTHER TUMORS
Chemical	Arsenic	Contaminated drinking water, occupational, iatrogenic	Arsenical keratoses, SCC, BCC	Lung, digestive tract, liver, bladder, kidney, lymphatic, hematopoietic
Chemical	Azathioprine	Iatrogenic	SCC	Non-Hodgkin lymphoma, mesenchymal tumors, hepatobiliary carcinoma
Chemical	Coal tar, coal tar pitches	Occupational, iatrogenic	SCC	Lung, bladder, kidney, digestive tract, leukemia
Chemical	Coke-oven emissions	Occupational	not specified	Bladder, respiratory tract, kidney (possibly prostate, colon, and pancreas)
Chemical	Cyclosporine A	Iatrogenic	SCC	Lymphoma
Physical	Ionizing radiation	Iatrogenic, atomic bomb blast	SCC, BCC, (possibly melanoma, after childhood exposure)	Leukemia, thyroid, breast, lung, liver, salivary gland, stomach, colon, bladder, ovary, central nervous system, angiosarcoma (possibly lymphoma after childhood exposure)
Chemical	8-Methoxypsoralen	PUVA therapy	SCC, BCC, melanoma	None reported
Chemical	Mineral oils	Occupational	SCC	Gastrointestinal, sinonasal, bladder cancer (possibly lung, rectal, oral, and pharyngeal)
Chemical	Soots	Occupational	SCC	Lung, prostate, bladder, esophageal, lymphatic, hematopoietic (possibly liver)
Physical	Solar radiation; broad-spectrum UVR	Occupational (farmers, electric arc welders), recreational, indoor tanning	SCC, BCC, melanoma	None reported

[a]Information obtained primarily from the 14th Report on Carcinogens (2016), National Toxicology Program. Viral agents that cause human skin cancers are listed in Table 19-1.
BCC, basal cell carcinoma; PUVA, psoralen and ultraviolet A light; SCC, squamous cell carcinoma; UVR, ultraviolet radiation.

aggressive, resulting in nodal involvement in more than 30% of cases and distant metastases in more than 11%.[93]

ANIMAL MODELS OF HUMAN SKIN CANCER

GENETICALLY ENGINEERED MOUSE MODELS OF SKIN CANCER

SQUAMOUS CELL CARCINOMA MOUSE MODELS

Genetically engineered mouse models have enabled close focus on specific genetic events now known to be critical for SCC. Given the identification of activating *Hras* mutations in nearly all squamous papillomas and carcinomas arising during chemical carcinogenesis in mouse skin (see later), early transgenic mouse studies used oncogenic forms of *Hras* to establish the central role of sustained Hras-driven signaling in initiation and progression of squamous neoplasia. Expression of the *Hras* oncogene in skin led to development of either benign squamous papillomas or invasive SCC, depending on which cell populations were engineered to express the transgene. Only benign papillomas developed in mice with *Hras* expression targeted to interfollicular epidermis, and these required either wounding or treatment with a tumor promoter, but expression of the same oncogene in hair follicle epithelia that included stem cells led to spontaneous SCC development.[94,95] These types of studies established the utility of genetically engineered mouse models for studying the genetic and cellular basis of skin tumors.

With these initial models serving as a foundation, numerous subsequent studies explored the contribution of various other genes and pathways to squamous tumor development.[96-99] Skin-targeted expression of TGF-α or other growth factors or receptors that activate the Ras pathway also lead to squamous tumors. Expression of components of the cell cycle machinery, including E2F1, cyclin D1, and Cdk4, could also contribute to SCC development, progression, or both. Transgenic overexpression of protein kinase C (PKC) isozymes, which are key regulators of epidermal differentiation and other cellular processes, leads to development of squamous papillomas and carcinomas (PKC-α) or less differentiated SCCs that rapidly metastasized to regional lymph nodes (PKC-ε). Spontaneous or carcinogen-induced tumor formation in genetically modified mice has revealed genes and pathways that appear to be important in skin cancer induction but would not have been apparent from hereditary cancer syndromes or analysis of human skin cancers. Targeting of *Myc* to differentiating cells in transgenic mice permits proliferation in this normally postmitotic compartment and produces an actinic keratosis–like phenotype, and basal cell targeting of *Myc* using a Keratin 5 promoter yields spontaneous tumors. Mice carrying a deletion in *c-fos* developed *v-ras*[Ha]–driven papillomas, but malignant progression to SCC was blocked. Multiple additional molecules and pathways have been implicated in SCC development through transgenic mouse modeling or recombinant human skin studies, including Smad2, Smad4, Stat3, PKC delta, PKC eta, Rac1, Pak1, Atf3, Sos, mTOR, TGF-β, Akt, Src, Fyn, and NF-κB (nuclear factor kappa B).[96-100]

The simultaneous inactivation of *Rb1* and *Trp53* in epidermis is sufficient to induce SCC in mice,[101] consistent with the ability of high-risk HPV E6 and E7 expression to cause SCC in skin.[102] Experiments using genetic ablation of the two most frequently mutated genes in SCC, *Notch1* and *Trp53*, have implicated important pathways in tumor suppression, differentiation, proliferation, and stromal interactions. Removal of *Trp53* in mice dramatically accelerates tumor induction with both chemical and UV carcinogenesis models.[96] Epidermis-specific removal of *Notch1* dramatically enhances carcinogenesis in the DMBA (7,12-dimethylbenz[a]-anthracene)/TPA (12-O-tetradecanoylphorbol-13-acetate) model resulting in both BCC and SCC induction.[103] When removed in mosaic fashion, it was subsequently shown that *Notch1* inactivation in skin resulted in non–cell-autonomous effects, resulting in an inflammatory woundlike phenotype, specifically acting in tumor promotion.[104] The most dramatic example of this was seen in mice lacking the *CSL* gene, a vital component of Notch signaling, solely in mesenchymal cells, including dermal fibroblasts. Remarkably, these mice spontaneously developed multifocal SCC without the need for any initiating or promoting agent,[105] demonstrating how simply disrupting Notch signaling between the mesenchyme and overlying epithelia is sufficient for tumorigenesis.

BASAL CELL CARCINOMA MOUSE MODELS

The discovery of *PTCH1* mutations in NBCCS patients and either *PTCH1* or *SMO* mutations in sporadic BCCs set the stage for studies directly testing the involvement of the Hedgehog pathway in BCC tumorigenesis. Skin-targeted mouse models developed to either express Hedgehog signaling activators (SHH, SMO, GLI1, GLI2), or delete Hedgehog signaling repressors (PTCH1, SUFU) reliably produce BCCs or BCC-like tumors in genetically engineered mice (reviewed in [4,106]) (see Chap. 111). In addition to providing in vivo evidence strongly supporting a central role for deregulated Hedgehog signaling in BCC development, these models have yielded valuable insights into the requirement for sustained Hedgehog signaling in tumor maintenance; established the importance of tissue and cellular context, as well as Hedgehog signaling levels, during BCC tumorigenesis; uncovered functionally significant interactions with other signaling pathways; and have provided powerful models for preclinical studies.

Cellular Origins of Skin Cancer: Historically,

the cell of origin of human skin tumors was inferred from histopathology and the phenotypic characteristics of tumor cells. The undifferentiated appearance of BCC tumor cells pointed to a potential origin from the epidermal basal layer or hair follicle outer root sheath. In addition, the resemblance of early-stage BCCs to embryonic hair germs and consistent expression of the outer root sheath marker keratin 17, coupled with the absence of typical BCCs on palmar and plantar skin that is devoid of pilosebaceous units, were taken as evidence supporting a hair follicle origin for BCC. SCCs, on the other hand, harbor cells that undergo terminal differentiation to form squames resembling cells in the cornified layer of epidermis, leading to the assertion that SCCs are more likely to be derived from epidermis than hair follicles. Although these observations provide a useful starting point, they assume that the phenotype of a tumor cell faithfully reflects the cell type from which it originated.

Experimental studies in mice have yielded insight into cell populations within skin that can give rise to nonmelanoma skin cancers. These studies are frequently performed by activating expression of a putative oncogene or deleting a tumor suppressor gene in specific cell populations and assessing tumor development over time. This approach typically requires breeding at least two different genetically engineered mouse models to generate bitransgenic mice carrying (1) a Cre recombinase–inducible oncogene or Cre-excisable tumor suppressor gene and (2) a hormone-activatable form of Cre recombinase expressed in specific cell types.[107] Treating these bitransgenic mouse models with hormone activates Cre recombinase in defined cell types at a specific time, leading to activation of the dormant oncogene or excision of the tumor suppressor gene. For modeling SCC, inducible expression of oncogenic *Hras* or *Kras* is frequently combined with deletion of the *Trp53* tumor suppressor gene; for modeling BCC, Hedgehog pathway oncogenes are activated or tumor suppressor genes are deleted. By combining different mouse models to target specific cell types, investigators have examined the tumorigenic potential of oncogenic drivers in hair follicle stem cells, transient-amplifying hair follicle and other progenitor cells, or interfollicular epidermal basal cells.[106-108]

From these types of experiments, several general conclusions can be drawn regarding the potential cells of origin of SCC and BCC and the importance of cellular and tissue context in tumorigenesis. Hair follicle stem cells appear to be uniquely sensitive to invasive SCC development driven by oncogenic *Kras* combined with *Trp53* deletion, with tumors progressing to advanced stages of development with a spindle cell morphology. Using the same set of oncogenic drivers, transiently amplifying hair matrix cells are completely resistant to tumor development, and interfollicular epidermal cells form either benign squamous papillomas or SCC, depending on the targeting strategy.[107,108] These studies also showed that although SCCs readily develop from follicle stem cells during the transition from the resting phase of the hair cycle (telogen) to active growth (anagen), they are largely resistant to SCC development when quiescent, in telogen.

Genetic-based models have also provided insight into the potential cell of origin of BCC but have yielded some conflicting results.[106,107,109] Initial studies showed that BCCs preferentially arose from interfollicular epidermis or from hair follicle stem cells that migrated into epidermis after wounding, but subsequent studies using a different oncogenic driver showed that BCCs could arise from follicle stem cells as well as several progenitor populations, with superficial BCCs arising from interfollicular epidermis and nodular tumors from hair follicle epithelia. Similar to *Kras+/Trp53*-deficient SCC, development of nodular BCCs was potentiated by activation of the hair cycle, establishing the importance of tissue context in driving tumorigenesis. Moreover, the magnitude of Hedgehog signaling activity was a critical determinant of tumor phenotype, with low-level signaling producing basaloid hamartomas and high-level signaling yielding nodular tumors. Taken together, these studies underscore the importance of a tumor's cell of origin in defining whether or not a tumor will develop, and if it does, its specific phenotype.

CHEMICALLY INDUCED SKIN CANCER IN RODENTS

The classical model of chemical carcinogenesis in skin has been studied for over 70 years and has proven to be a profoundly useful model for studying separable steps of tumor initiation, progression, and metastasis.[97] In the most commonly used incarnation of the model, the carcinogen DMBA is applied initially, metabolized into a potent mutagen, and causes activating *Hras* mutations, most often at Q61 with over 90% frequency. Subsequent repeated application of tumor promoters, most commonly the phorbol ester TPA, results in highly reproducible tumor induction in terms of latency, multiplicity, incidence, and progression. Other tumor promoters can be used, including UVR, okadaic acid, and physical wounding.[97] The dominant driver of these tumors is mutant *Hras*, which can undergo subsequent amplification. In this regard, one important contrast with human SCC is the early requirement for *ras* mutation as enforced by DMBA exposure, with the emergence of *Trp53* mutations later.[110] In humans, *TP53* mutations occur very early and *RAS* mutations are detected less commonly.[37-41] Nevertheless, the literature associated with this model mirrors the rise of the genetic paradigm of cancer because nearly every major cancer-related pathway has been investigated using this platform, particularly in conjunction with genetically engineered mouse models. These include the TP53, INK4A-RB1-E2F, TGF-β, PI3K/AKT, STAT3, mTOR, and COX2 pathways, as well as multiple receptor tyrosine kinases, including EGFR (epidermal growth factor receptor) family members.[96,97] In addition, the model has been critically important in elucidating important downstream effectors of RAS in cancer.[96]

ULTRAVIOLET LIGHT–INDUCED RODENT SKIN CANCER

The most frequently used rodent model for UV-induced skin cancers has been the immunocompetent Hairless mouse, an outbred strain that lacks a functional Hairless (*Hr*) gene. These mice undergo one round of anagen soon after birth, after which point follicles degenerate into cystic structures.[111] The lack of hair obviates the need to shave the mice repeatedly and allows for consistent UV exposure over time. Although *Hr* gene function is implicated in NF-κB signaling[112] and adipogenesis,[113] the function of *Hr* in cancer is not completely understood. In terms of acquired mutations in the tumors, this model is significantly more faithful to the human condition than the DMBA/TPA model.[114] UV irradiation has also been used in more common strains such as C57BL/6 with varying degrees of susceptibility to carcinoma, the SENCAR strain being among the most sensitive. Although highly informative, UV-driven mouse models have suffered somewhat from a lack of uniformity in the spectra, dose, and irradiances used across groups and strains. Some of this is unavoidable and caused by technical limitations in reproducing spectra across different light sources.

Nevertheless, many important conclusions have been drawn from experiments with UV-driven models. *Trp53* mutations occur early, and as in chronically irradiated human skin, *Trp53* mutant clones are observed.[115] Tumors exhibit very high mutational burdens with a median of 155 mutations per megabase in a series of 18 SCCs.[114] Other mutations observed in tumors include *Notch* family members, *Ink4a*, and relatively rare mutations in *ras* and recurrent chromosomal alterations are seen that map to corresponding syntenic regions on human 3p, 11p, and 9q.[114,116-121]

As with the chemical carcinogenesis approach, many studies have focused on specific pathways, combining UV exposure with transgenic mouse models. Bypassing UV-induced apoptosis, as regulated by *Trp53*, *Survivin*, *Bcl2*, and *E2f-1*, has been shown to be necessary for full tumor susceptibility.[122-126] Some of the same regulators implicated in chemical carcinogenesis are also known to be important in UV-driven models, including the COX-2, mTOR, AKT, and ERK pathways.[127-131] Cross-species analysis with human SCC has also been performed using UV-driven models implicating WNT, β-catenin, and ERK pathways, as well as several microRNAs, including miR-21 and miR-31.[37]

TREATMENT AND PREVENTION OF SKIN CANCER

The most effective approach to reducing cancer-associated morbidity and mortality is prevention, and given the central role of UV-driven mutagenesis in skin cancer development, efforts aimed at effectively limiting exposure to sunlight and other UV sources, such as tanning beds, are likely to have a major impact on overall skin tumor development. Federal legislation restricting use of tanning beds by minors in nearly all US states is thus predicted to have a major beneficial effect at reducing skin cancer incidence in the future.[132] Various approaches to chemoprevention may also play an important role in reducing the number of SCCs,[133,134] with encouraging results presented for nicotinamide in a randomized phase 3 trial in high-risk patients, which showed a 20% and 30% reduction of BCC and SCC, respectively, at 3 months, and 11% fewer actinic keratoses.[135]

Although most skin cancers can be effectively treated with surgery, a deeper understanding of the molecular basis of these cancers may provide unique opportunities for targeting key oncogenic drivers for prevention or nonsurgical treatment. For example, because nearly all BCCs appear to be caused by unrestrained Hedgehog signaling, systemic Hedgehog pathway inhibition can be effective in treating patients with locally advanced or metastatic BCC, although side effects are common, drug resistance can develop, and tumors may recur after stopping therapy.[136] In addition to causing regression of preexisting tumors, systemic Hedgehog pathway inhibitors effectively block development of new BCCs in patients with Gorlin syndrome.[137] These findings suggest that regular use of a topical inhibitor, if effective at blocking oncogenic Hedgehog signaling, may be useful for BCC prevention in high-risk patients. Although this is an exciting possibility for patients with BCC, it seems unlikely that a single targeted therapeutic could be similarly useful for prevention of SCC tumors because multiple oncogenic alterations are engaged to variable degrees in SCC development.

CONCLUSIONS

Extensive clinical and experimental study of skin cancers has yielded important insights into the molecular and cellular basis of both BCC and SCC; led to the development of mechanism-based, targeted therapy for BCC; uncovered key molecular similarities between SCCs arising in skin and several other organs; provided powerful platforms for studying multistep cancer development using highly tractable mouse models of chemical and UV-driven carcinogenesis, as well as genetically engineered models; and shed light on fundamental aspects of tumor genetics and cancer biology that are relevant to understanding tumorigenesis in other organs. Continued progress in understanding the pathogenesis of BCC and SCC is likely to lead to new approaches to preventing and treating these extremely common malignancies.

ACKNOWLEDGMENTS

We regret not being able to include citations to all relevant articles, given the space restrictions. We appreciate previous authors' contributions to some of the material included in the current chapter, including Drs. Masaoki Kawasumi, Paul Nghiem, Timothy Heffernan, Douglas Brash, Adam Glick, and Stuart Yuspa.

REFERENCES

1. Siegel RL, Miller KD, Jemal A. Cancer Statistics, 2017. *CA Cancer J Clin*. 2017;67(1):7-30.
2. Rogers HW, Weinstock MA, Feldman SR, et al. Incidence estimate of nonmelanoma skin cancer (keratinocyte carcinomas) in the US population, 2012. *JAMA Dermatol*. 2015;151(10):1081-1086.
3. Guy GP Jr, Machlin SR, Ekwueme DU, et al. Prevalence and costs of skin cancer treatment in the U.S., 2002-2006 and 2007-2011. *Am J Prev Med*. 2015;48(2):183-187.
4. Wong SY, Dlugosz AA. Basal cell carcinoma, Hedgehog signaling, and targeted therapeutics: the long and winding road. *J Invest Dermatol*. 2014;134(e1):E18-22.
5. Hanahan D, Weinberg RA. Hallmarks of cancer: the next generation. *Cell*. 2011;144(5):646-674.
6. Jeggo PA, Pearl LH, Carr AM. DNA repair, genome stability and cancer: a historical perspective. *Nat Rev Cancer*. 2016;16(1):35-42.
7. Roychowdhury S, Chinnaiyan AM. Translating cancer genomes and transcriptomes for precision oncology. *CA Cancer J Clin*. 2016;66(1):75-88.
8. Quail DF, Joyce JA. Microenvironmental regulation of tumor progression and metastasis. *Nat Med*. 2013;19(11):1423-1437.
9. McGranahan N, Swanton C. Clonal heterogeneity and tumor evolution: past, present, and the future. *Cell*. 2017;168(4):613-628.
10. Nassar D, Blanpain C. Cancer stem cells: basic concepts and therapeutic implications. *Ann Rev Pathol*. 2016;11:47-76.
11. Lapidot T, Sirard C, Vormoor J, et al. A cell initiating human acute myeloid leukaemia after transplantation into SCID mice. *Nature*. 1994;367(6464):645-648.
12. Colmont CS, Benketah A, Reed SH, et al. CD200-expressing human basal cell carcinoma cells initiate tumor growth. *Proc Natl Acad Sci U S A*. 2013;110(4):1434-1439.
13. Batlle E, Clevers H. Cancer stem cells revisited. *Nat Med*. 2017;23(10):1124-1134.
14. Grachtchouk M, Pero J, Yang SH, et al. Basal cell carcinomas in mice arise from hair follicle stem cells and multiple epithelial progenitor populations. *J Clin Invest*. 2011;121(5):1768-1781.
15. Sutherland KD, Visvader JE. Cellular mechanisms underlying intertumoral heterogeneity. *Trends Cancer*. 2015;1(1):15-23.
16. Kumar-Sinha C, Kalyana-Sundaram S, Chinnaiyan AM. Landscape of gene fusions in epithelial cancers: seq and ye shall find. *Genome Med*. 2015;7:129.
17. Piraino SW, Furney SJ. Beyond the exome: the role of non-coding somatic mutations in cancer. *Ann Oncol*. 2016;27(2):240-248.
18. Lin C, Yang L. Long Noncoding RNA in cancer: wiring signaling circuitry. *Trends Cell Biol*. 2018 Apr;28(4):287-301. doi: 10.1016/j.tcb.2017.11.008. Epub 2017 Dec 20.
19. Jaju PD, Ransohoff KJ, Tang JY, et al. Familial skin cancer syndromes: increased risk of nonmelanotic skin cancers and extracutaneous tumors. 2016 Mar;74(3):437-451; quiz 452-4. doi: 10.1016/j.jaad.2015.08.073.
20. Giordano CN, Yew YW, Spivak G, et al. Understanding photodermatoses associated with defective DNA repair: syndromes with cancer predisposition. *J Am Acad Dermatol*. 2016;75(5):855-870.
21. Robinson DR, Wu YM, Lonigro RJ, et al. Integrative clinical genomics of metastatic cancer. *Nature*. 2017;548(7667):297-303.
22. Kimonis VE, Goldstein AM, Pastakia B, et al. Clinical manifestations in 105 persons with nevoid basal cell carcinoma syndrome. *Am J Med Genet*. 1997;69(3):299-308.
23. Hahn H, Wicking C, Zaphiropoulous PG, et al. Mutations of the human homolog of Drosophila patched in the nevoid basal cell carcinoma syndrome. *Cell*. 1996;85(6):841-851.
24. Johnson RL, Rothman AL, Xie J, et al. Human homolog of patched, a candidate gene for the basal cell nevus syndrome. *Science*. 1996;272(5268):1668-1671.
25. Barakat MT, Humke EW, Scott MP. Learning from Jekyll to control Hyde: Hedgehog signaling in development and cancer. *Trends Mol Med*. 2010;16(8):337-348.
26. Petrova R, Joyner AL. Roles for Hedgehog signaling in adult organ homeostasis and repair. *Development*. 2014;141(18):3445-3457.
27. Pellegrini C, Maturo MG, Di Nardo L, et al. Understanding the molecular genetics of basal cell carcinoma. *Int J Mol Sci*. 2017 Nov; 18(11):2485.
28. Bonilla X, Parmentier L, King B, et al. Genomic analysis identifies new drivers and progression pathways in skin basal cell carcinoma. *Nat Genet*. 2016;48(4):398-406.
29. DiGiovanna JJ, Kraemer KH. Shining a light on xeroderma pigmentosum. *J Invest Dermatol*. 2012;132 (3 Pt 2):785-796.
30. Kim M, Murrell DF. Update on the pathogenesis of squamous cell carcinoma development in recessive dystrophic epidermolysis bullosa. *Eur J Dermatol*. 2015;25(suppl 1):30-32.
31. Goudie DR, D'Alessandro M, Merriman B, et al. Multiple self-healing squamous epithelioma is caused by a disease-specific spectrum of mutations in TGFBR1. *Nat Genet*. 2011;43(4):365-369.
32. Cammareri P, Rose AM, Vincent DF, et al. Inactivation of TGFbeta receptors in stem cells drives cutaneous squamous cell carcinoma. *Nat Commun*. 2016;7:12493.
33. Balmain A, Pragnell IB. Mouse skin carcinomas induced in vivo by chemical carcinogens have a transforming Harvey ras oncogene. *Nature*. 1983;303:72-74.
34. Parada LF, Tabin CJ, Shih C, et al. Human EJ bladder carcinoma oncogene is homologue of Harvey sarcoma virus ras gene. *Nature*. 1982;297(5866):474-478.
35. Brash DE, Rudolph JA, Simon JA, et al. A role for sunlight in skin cancer: UV-induced p53 mutations in squamous cell carcinoma. *Proc Natl Acad Sci U S A*. 1991;88(22):10124-10128.
36. Pierceall WE, Mukhopadhyay T, Goldberg LH, et al. Mutations in the p53 tumor suppressor gene in human cutaneous squamous cell carcinomas. *Mol Carcinog*. 1991;4(6):445-449.
37. Chitsazzadeh V, Coarfa C, Drummond JA, et al. Cross-species identification of genomic drivers of squamous cell carcinoma development across preneoplastic intermediates. *Nat Commun*. 2016;7:12601.
38. Pickering CR, Zhou JH, Lee JJ, et al. Mutational landscape of aggressive cutaneous squamous cell carcinoma. *Clin Cancer Res*. 2014;20(24):6582-6592.

39. Li YY, Hanna GJ, Laga AC, et al. Genomic analysis of metastatic cutaneous squamous cell carcinoma. *Clin Cancer Res.* 2015;21(6):1447-1456.
40. Wang NJ, Sanborn Z, Arnett KL, et al. Loss-of-function mutations in Notch receptors in cutaneous and lung squamous cell carcinoma. *Proc Natl Acad Sci U S A.* 2011;108(43):17761-17766.
41. South AP, Purdie KJ, Watt SA, et al. NOTCH1 mutations occur early during cutaneous squamous cell carcinogenesis. *J Invest Dermatol.* 2014;134(10):2630-2638.
42. Lee CS, Bhaduri A, Mah A, et al. Recurrent point mutations in the kinetochore gene KNSTRN in cutaneous squamous cell carcinoma. *Nat Genet.* 2014;46(10):1060-1062.
43. Watt SA, Purdie KJ, den Breems NY, et al. Novel CARD11 Mutations in human cutaneous squamous cell carcinoma lead to aberrant NF-kappaB regulation. *Am J Pathol.* 2015;185(9):2354-2363.
44. Salgado R, Toll A, Alameda F, et al. CKS1B amplification is a frequent event in cutaneous squamous cell carcinoma with aggressive clinical behaviour. *Genes Chromosomes Cancer.* 2010;49(11):1054-1061.
45. Sekulic A, Kim SY, Hostetter G, et al. Loss of inositol polyphosphate 5-phosphatase is an early event in development of cutaneous squamous cell carcinoma. *Cancer Prev Res (Phila).* 2010;3(10):1277-1283.
46. Toll A, Salgado R, Yebenes M, et al. MYC gene numerical aberrations in actinic keratosis and cutaneous squamous cell carcinoma. *Br J Dermatol.* 2009;161(5):1112-1118.
47. Toll A, Salgado R, Yebenes M, et al. Epidermal growth factor receptor gene numerical aberrations are frequent events in actinic keratoses and invasive cutaneous squamous cell carcinomas. *Exp Dermatol.* 2010;19(2):151-153.
48. Dotto GP, Rustgi AK. Squamous cell cancers: a unified perspective on biology and genetics. *Cancer Cell.* 2016;29(5):622-637.
49. Konicke K, Lopez-Luna A, Munoz-Carrillo JL, et al. The microRNA landscape of cutaneous squamous cell carcinoma. *Drug Discovery Today.* 2018 Apr;23(4):864-870. doi: 10.1016/j.drudis.2018.01.023. Epub 2018 Jan 6.
50. Einspahr JG, Calvert V, Alberts DS, et al. Functional protein pathway activation mapping of the progression of normal skin to squamous cell carcinoma. *Cancer Prev Res (Phila).* 2012;5(3):403-413.
51. Menzies AM, Kefford RF, Long GV. Paradoxical oncogenesis: are all BRAF inhibitors equal? *Pigment Cell Melanoma Res.* 2013;26(5):611-615.
52. Hatzivassiliou G, Song K, Yen I, et al. RAF inhibitors prime wild-type RAF to activate the MAPK pathway and enhance growth. *Nature.* 2010;464(7287):431-435.
53. Poulikakos PI, Zhang C, Bollag G, et al. RAF inhibitors transactivate RAF dimers and ERK signalling in cells with wild-type BRAF. *Nature.* 2010;464(7287):427-430.
54. Su F, Viros A, Milagre C, et al. RAS mutations in cutaneous squamous-cell carcinomas in patients treated with BRAF inhibitors. *N Engl J Med.* 2012;366(3):207-215.
55. Vin H, Ojeda SS, Ching G, et al. BRAF inhibitors suppress apoptosis through off-target inhibition of JNK signaling. *eLife.* 2013;2:e00969.
56. Ransohoff KJ, Tang JY, Sarin KY. Squamous Change in Basal-Cell Carcinoma with Drug Resistance. *N Engl J Med.* 2015;373(11):1079-1082.
57. Zhao X, Ponomaryov T, Ornell KJ, et al. RAS/MAPK Activation drives resistance to Smo inhibition, metastasis, and tumor evolution in Shh pathway-dependent tumors. *Cancer Res.* 2015;75(17):3623-3635.
58. Adelmann CH, Truong KA, Liang RJ, et al. MEK Is a therapeutic and chemopreventative target in squamous cell carcinoma. *J Invest Dermatol.* 2016;136(9):1920-1924.
59. Valejo Coelho MM, Matos TR, Apetato M. The dark side of the light: mechanisms of photocarcinogenesis. *Clin Dermatol.* 2016;34(5):563-570.
60. Archier E, Devaux S, Castela E, et al. Carcinogenic risks of psoralen UV-A therapy and narrowband UV-B therapy in chronic plaque psoriasis: a systematic literature review. *J Eur Acad Dermatol Venereol.* 2012;26(suppl 3):22-31.
61. Cadet J, Mouret S, Ravanat JL, et al. Photoinduced damage to cellular DNA: direct and photosensitized reactions. *Photochem Photobiol.* 2012;88(5):1048-1065.
62. Young AR, Chadwick CA, Harrison GI, et al. The similarity of action spectra for thymine dimers in human epidermis and erythema suggests that DNA is the chromophore for erythema. *J Invest Dermatol.* 1998;111(6):982-988.
63. Mouret S, Baudouin C, Charveron M, et al. Cyclobutane pyrimidine dimers are predominant DNA lesions in whole human skin exposed to UVA radiation. *Proc Natl Acad Sci U S A.* 2006;103(37):13765-13770.
64. Brash DE. UV signature mutations. *Photochem Photobiol.* 2015;91(1):15-26.
65. Alexandrov LB, Nik-Zainal S, Wedge DC, et al. Signatures of mutational processes in human cancer. *Nature.* 2013;500(7463):415-421.
66. Premi S, Wallisch S, Mano CM, et al. Photochemistry. Chemiexcitation of melanin derivatives induces DNA photoproducts long after UV exposure. *Science.* 2015;347(6224):842-847.
67. Ziegler A, Jonason AS, Leffell DJ, et al. Sunburn and p53 in the onset of skin cancer. *Nature.* 1994;372(6508):773-776.
68. Jonason AS, Kunala S, Price GJ, et al. Frequent clones of p53-mutated keratinocytes in normal human skin. *Proc Natl Acad Sci. U S A.* 1996;93(24):14025-14029.
69. Martincorena I, Roshan A, Gerstung M, et al. Tumor evolution. High burden and pervasive positive selection of somatic mutations in normal human skin. *Science.* 2015;348(6237):880-886.
70. Simons BD. Deep sequencing as a probe of normal stem cell fate and preneoplasia in human epidermis. *Proc Natl Acad Sci U S A.* 2016;113(1):128-133.
71. Albibas AA, Rose-Zerilli MJJ, Lai C, et al. Subclonal evolution of cancer-related gene mutations in p53 immunopositive patches in human skin. *J Invest Dermatol.* 2018;138(1):189-198.
72. Criscione VD, Weinstock MA, Naylor MF, et al. Actinic keratoses: natural history and risk of malignant transformation in the Veterans Affairs Topical Tretinoin Chemoprevention Trial. *Cancer.* 2009;115(11):2523-2530.
73. Schiller JT, Lowy DR. Virus infection and human cancer: an overview. *Recent Results Cancer Res.* 2014;193:1-10.
74. Mesri EA, Feitelson MA, Munger K. Human viral oncogenesis: a cancer hallmarks analysis. *Cell Host Microbe.* 2014;15(3):266-282.
75. Schiffman M, Doorbar J, Wentzensen N, et al. Carcinogenic human papillomavirus infection. *Nat Rev Dis Primers.* 2016;2:16086.
76. Meyers JM, Munger K. The viral etiology of skin cancer. *J Invest Dermatol.* 2014;134(e1):E29-E32.
77. Arron ST, Ruby JG, Dybbro E, et al. Transcriptome sequencing demonstrates that human papillomavirus

is not active in cutaneous squamous cell carcinoma. *J Invest Dermatol*. 2011;131(8):1745-1753.
78. Galloway DA, Laimins LA. Human papillomaviruses: shared and distinct pathways for pathogenesis. *Curr Opin Virol*. 2015;14:87-92.
79. Imperiale MJ, Jiang M. Polyomavirus persistence. *Ann Rev Virol*. 2016;3(1):517-532.
80. Moens U, Krumbholz A, Ehlers B, et al. Biology, evolution, and medical importance of polyomaviruses: an update. *Infect Genet Evol*. 2017;54:18-38.
81. Feng H, Shuda M, Chang Y, et al. Clonal integration of a polyomavirus in human Merkel cell carcinoma. *Science*. 2008;319(5866):1096-1100.
82. Atkin SJ, Griffin BE, Dilworth SM. Polyoma virus and simian virus 40 as cancer models: history and perspectives. *Semin Cancer Biol*. 2009;19(4):211-217.
83. Wendzicki JA, Moore PS, Chang Y. Large T and small T antigens of Merkel cell polyomavirus. *Curr Opin Virol*. 2015;11:38-43.
84. Liu W, MacDonald M, You J. Merkel cell polyomavirus infection and Merkel cell carcinoma. *Curr Opin Virol*. 2016;20:20-27.
85. Pott P. Cancer scrotic. In: *Chirurgical Observations Relative to the Cataract, the Polypus of the Nose, the Cancer of the Scrotum, the Different Kinds of Ruptures, and the Mortification of the Toes and Feet*. London: Hawes, Clarke, and Collins; 1775:63.
86. Williams K, Mansh M, Chin-Hong P, et al. Voriconazole-associated cutaneous malignancy: a literature review on photocarcinogenesis in organ transplant recipients. *Clin Infect Dis*. 2014;58(7):997-1002.
87. Li C, Athar M. Ionizing radiation exposure and basal cell carcinoma pathogenesis. *Radiat Res*. 2016;185(3):217-228.
88. Kleinerman RA. Cancer risks following diagnostic and therapeutic radiation exposure in children. *Pediatr Radiol*. 2006;36(suppl 2):121-125.
89. Gudmundsdottir EM, Hrafnkelsson J, Rafnsson V. Incidence of cancer among licenced commercial pilots flying North Atlantic routes. *Environ Health*. 2017;16(1):86.
90. Bazalinski D, Przybek-Mita J, Baranska B, et al. Marjolin's ulcer in chronic wounds - review of available literature. *Contemp Oncol (Pozn)*. 2017;21(3):197-202.
91. Karasoy Yesilada A, Zeynep Sevim K, Ozgur Sucu D, et al. Marjolin ulcer: clinical experience with 34 patients over 15 years. *J Cutan Med Surg*. 2013;17(6):404-409.
92. Oruc M, Kankaya Y, Sungur N, et al. Clinicopathological evaluation of Marjolin ulcers over two decades. *Kaohsiung J Med Sci*. 2017;33(7):327-333.
93. Shen R, Zhang J, Zhang F, et al. Clinical characteristics and therapeutic analysis of 51 patients with Marjolin's ulcers. *Exp Ther Med*. 2015;10(4):1364-1374.
94. Brown K, Strathdee D, Bryson S, et al. The malignant capacity of skin tumours induced by expression of a mutant H-ras transgene depends on the cell type targeted. *Curr Biol*. 1998;8:516-524.
95. Bailleul B, Surani MA, White S, et al. Skin hyperkeratosis and papilloma formation in transgenic mice expressing a ras oncogene from a suprabasal keratin promoter. *Cell*. 1990;62:697-708.
96. Huang PY, Balmain A. Modeling cutaneous squamous carcinoma development in the mouse. *Cold Spring Harbor Perspect Med*. 2014;4(9):a013623.
97. Abel EL, Angel JM, Kiguchi K, et al. Multi-stage chemical carcinogenesis in mouse skin: fundamentals and applications. *Nat Protoc*. 2009;4(9):1350-1362.
98. Ratushny V, Gober MD, Hick R, et al. From keratinocyte to cancer: the pathogenesis and modeling of cutaneous squamous cell carcinoma. *J Clin Invest*. 2012;122(2):464-472.
99. Amberg N, Holcmann M, Glitzner E, et al. Mouse models of nonmelanoma skin cancer. *Methods Mol Biol*. 2015;1267:217-250.
100. Khavari PA. Modelling cancer in human skin tissue. *Nat Rev Cancer*. 2006;6(4):270-280.
101. Martinez-Cruz AB, Santos M, Lara MF, et al. Spontaneous squamous cell carcinoma induced by the somatic inactivation of retinoblastoma and Trp53 tumor suppressors. *Cancer Res*. 2008;68(3):683-692.
102. Lambert PF, Pan H, Pitot HC, et al. Epidermal cancer associated with expression of human papillomavirus type 16 E6 and E7 oncogenes in the skin of transgenic mice. *Proc Natl Acad Sci U S A*. 1993;90(12):5583-5587.
103. Nicolas M, Wolfer A, Raj K, et al. Notch1 functions as a tumor suppressor in mouse skin. *Nat. Genet*. 2003;33(3):416-421.
104. Demehri S, Turkoz A, Kopan R. Epidermal Notch1 loss promotes skin tumorigenesis by impacting the stromal microenvironment. *Cancer Cell*. 2009;16(1):55-66.
105. Hu B, Castillo E, Harewood L, et al. Multifocal epithelial tumors and field cancerization from loss of mesenchymal CSL signaling. *Cell*. 2012;149(6):1207-1220.
106. Kasper M, Jaks V, Hohl D, et al. Basal cell carcinoma—molecular biology and potential new therapies. *J Clin Invest*. 2012;122(2):455-463.
107. Blanpain C. Tracing the cellular origin of cancer. *Nat Cell Biol*. 2013;15(2):126-134.
108. Lowry WE, Flores A, White AC. Exploiting mouse models to study Ras-induced cutaneous squamous cell carcinoma. *J Invest Dermatol*. 2016;136(8):1543-1548.
109. White AC, Lowry WE. Refining the role for adult stem cells as *Cancer Cells* of origin. *Trends Cell Biol*. 2015;25(1):11-20.
110. Nassar D, Latil M, Boeckx B, et al. Genomic landscape of carcinogen-induced and genetically induced mouse skin squamous cell carcinoma. *Nat Med*. 2015;21(8):946-954.
111. Benavides F, Oberyszyn TM, VanBuskirk AM, et al. The hairless mouse in skin research. *J Dermatol Sci*. 2009;53(1):10-18.
112. Kim H, Casta A, Tang X, et al. Loss of hairless confers susceptibility to UVB-induced tumorigenesis via disruption of NF-kappaB signaling. *PLoS One*. 2012;7(6):e39691.
113. Kumpf S, Mihlan M, Goginashvili A, et al. Hairless promotes PPARgamma expression and is required for white adipogenesis. *EMBO Rep*. 2012;13(11):1012-1020.
114. Knatko EV, Praslicka B, Higgins M, et al. Whole-exome sequencing validates a preclinical mouse model for the prevention and treatment of cutaneous squamous cell carcinoma. *Cancer Prev Res (Phila)*. 2017;10(1):67-75.
115. Remenyik E, Wikonkal NM, Zhang W, et al. Antigen-specific immunity does not mediate acute regression of UVB-induced p53-mutant clones. *Oncogene*. 2003;22(41):6369-6376.
116. Ashton KJ, Weinstein SR, Maguire DJ, et al. Chromosomal aberrations in squamous cell carcinoma and solar keratoses revealed by comparative genomic hybridization. *Arch Dermatol*. 2003;139(7):876-882.
117. Dworkin AM, Tober KL, Duncan FJ, et al. Chromosomal aberrations in UVB-induced tumors of

118. Khan SG, Mohan RR, Katiyar SK, et al. Mutations in ras oncogenes: rare events in ultraviolet B radiation-induced mouse skin tumorigenesis. *Mol Carcinog.* 1996;15(2):96-103.
119. Popp S, Waltering S, Holtgreve-Grez H, et al. Genetic characterization of a human skin carcinoma progression model: from primary tumor to metastasis. *J Invest Dermatol.* 2000;115(6):1095-1103.
120. Soufir N, Queille S, Mollier K, et al. INK4a-ARF mutations in skin carcinomas from UV irradiated hairless mice. *Mol Carcinog.* 2004;39(4):195-198.
121. van Kranen HJ, de Gruijl FR, de Vries A, et al. Frequent p53 alterations but low incidence of ras mutations in UV-B-induced skin tumors of hairless mice. *Carcinogenesis.* 1995;16(5):1141-1147.
122. Brash DE. Roles of the transcription factor p53 in keratinocyte carcinomas. *Br J Dermatol.* 2006;154(suppl 1): 8-10.
123. Grossman D, Kim PJ, Blanc-Brude OP, et al. Transgenic expression of survivin in keratinocytes counteracts UVB-induced apoptosis and cooperates with loss of p53. *J Clin Invest.* 2001;108(7):991-999.
124. Knezevic D, Zhang W, Rochette PJ, et al. Bcl-2 is the target of a UV-inducible apoptosis switch and a node for UV signaling. *Proc Natl Acad Sci U S A.* 2007;104(27):11286-11291.
125. Raj D, Brash DE, Grossman D. Keratinocyte apoptosis in epidermal development and disease. *J Invest Dermatol.* 2006;126(2):243-257.
126. Wikonkal NM, Remenyik E, Knezevic D, et al. Inactivating E2f1 reverts apoptosis resistance and cancer sensitivity in Trp53-deficient mice. *Nat Cell Biol.* 2003;5(7):655-660.
127. Bermudez Y, Stratton SP, Curiel-Lewandrowski C, et al. Activation of the PI3K/Akt/mTOR and MAPK signaling pathways in response to acute solar-simulated light exposure of human skin. *Cancer Prev Res (Phila).* 2015;8(8):720-728.
128. Dickinson SE, Janda J, Criswell J, et al. Inhibition of Akt enhances the chemopreventive effects of topical rapamycin in mouse skin. *Cancer Prev Res (Phila).* 2016;9(3):215-224.
129. Einspahr JG, Bowden GT, Alberts DS, et al. Cross-validation of murine UV signal transduction pathways in human skin. *Photochem Photobiol.* 2008; 84(2):463-476.
130. Kim JE, Roh E, Lee MH, et al. Fyn is a redox sensor involved in solar ultraviolet light-induced signal transduction in skin carcinogenesis. *Oncogene.* 2016;35(31): 4091-4101.
131. Lee MH, Lim DY, Kim MO, et al. Genetic ablation of caspase-7 promotes solar-simulated light-induced mouse skin carcinogenesis: the involvement of keratin-17. *Carcinogenesis.* 2015;36(11):1372-1380.
132. Madigan LM, Lim HW. Tanning beds: impact on health, and recent regulations. *Clin Dermatol.* 2016; 34(5):640-648.
133. Soltani-Arabshahi R, Tristani-Firouzi P. Chemoprevention of nonmelanoma skin cancer. *Facial Plast Surg.* 2013;29(5):373-383.
134. Chen AC, Halliday GM, Damian DL. Non-melanoma skin cancer: carcinogenesis and chemoprevention. *Pathology.* 2013;45(3):331-341.
135. Chen AC, Martin AJ, Choy B, et al. A phase 3 randomized trial of nicotinamide for skin-cancer chemoprevention. *N Engl J Med.* 2015;373(17):1618-1626.
136. Basset-Seguin N, Sharpe HJ, de Sauvage FJ. Efficacy of Hedgehog pathway inhibitors in Basal cell carcinoma. *Mol Cancer Ther.* 2015;14(3):633-641.
137. Tang JY, Mackay-Wiggan JM, Aszterbaum M, et al. Inhibiting the hedgehog pathway in patients with the basal-cell nevus syndrome. *N Engl J Med.* 2012;366(23):2180-2188.

Chapter 20 :: Pigmentation and Melanocyte Biology
:: Stephen M. Ostrowski & David E. Fisher

第二十章
色素沉着和黑素细胞生物学

中文导读

本章分5节：①人皮肤黑素细胞的解剖、超微结构和分布；②黑素细胞的形成、迁移和存活；③黑素与黑素小体；④人体色素沉着变异的调控；⑤结论。

第一节人皮肤黑素细胞的解剖、超微结构和分布，介绍了黑素细胞与角质形成细胞混合存在于表皮的基底层，主要超微结构特征是黑素小体。根据黑素细胞的位置分为毛囊间黑素细胞、毛囊黑素细胞、肢端黑素细胞、皮肤外黑素细胞。

第二节黑素细胞的形成、迁移和存活，介绍了黑素细胞完全来源于高度迁移和多能的神经嵴群体。神经嵴细胞沿着两条路径迁移，一条是体节和外胚层之间的背外侧路径，另一条是腹内侧路径。神经嵴细胞迁移到其靶部位，形成多种细胞类型。转录因子已被证明在黑素细胞存活中起着关键作用。黑素成细胞和黑素细胞表达的受体及其同源生长因子配体对黑素细胞的产生和维持存活也很重要。

第三节黑素与黑素小体，介绍了黑素有两种形式，真黑素和褐黑素，黑素合成发生在黑素小体中。黑素合成使人类皮肤的色素沉着，提供了对紫外线引起的晒伤和DNA损伤的保护。随后介绍了黑素小体是溶酶体相关的细胞器，仅存在于黑素细胞和视网膜色素上皮中。它们是黑素合成和储存的主要场所。最后介绍了黑素小体的生物发生和运输，以及黑素向角质形成细胞的转移。

第四节人体色素沉着变异的调控，介绍了基因变异、紫外线辐射会引起色素沉着，受MSH-MC1R-MITF途径的调控。此外调节人类群体色素变化的其他因素：如TYR、TYRP1、SLC45A2和OCA2编码等。

第五节结论，总结了无论是黑色素瘤皮肤癌还是非黑色素瘤皮肤癌，未来的研究有望确定改善皮肤癌的预防策略。

〔栗 娟〕

AT-A-GLANCE

- Development of Melanocytes
  - Melanocytes are derived from neural crest lineage
  - Transcription factors (MITF, SOX10, PAX3) and signaling pathways (KIT, EDNRB) that are important for development, migration, and survival of melanocytes also play key roles in melanoma
- Function of melanocytes
  - Key function of melanocytes is to synthesize melanin and transfer to surrounding keratinocytes
  - Melanocytes can produce brown/black melanin (eumelanin) or orange/yellow melanin (pheomelanin)
  - The melanosome, a specialized lysosome-related organelle, is the site of melanin synthesis and storage
- Regulation of human pigmentation
  - Common human variants in melanocortin 1 receptor (MC1R) lead to the "red hair phenotype"—red hair, fair skin, inability to tan, and increased melanoma risk
  - MC1R signals to the MITF transcription factor to regulate pigmentation and sun-tanning

ANATOMY, ULTRASTRUCTURE, AND DISTRIBUTION OF MELANOCYTES IN HUMAN SKIN

HISTOLOGY

Melanocytes are melanin-synthesizing cells of dendritic morphology located within the basal layer of the epidermis, the hair bulb, and the outer root sheath of hair follicles. The dendritic morphology of melanocytes is not appreciable by light microscopy, but can be appreciated by immunohistochemistry (Fig. 20-1). Melanocytes contain oval nuclei slightly smaller than that of surrounding keratinocytes. Processing artifact often leaves a clear halo of cytoplasm when hematoxylin and eosin (H&E)–stained sections are viewed.

Melanocytes exist admixed with keratinocytes in the basal layer of the epidermis (Fig. 20-1). Within the epidermis, melanocytes are present at about 1/10th the number of keratinocytes.[3] On H&E-stained sections, there are very few visible melanin granules in the basal layer of light-skinned individuals. However, in persons with darker skin types, melanin granules are visible throughout all layers of the epidermis, including the stratum corneum. Special stains can be used to better visualize melanin. Silver stains such as the Fontana-Mason and Warthin-Starry stains rely on the ability of melanin to become impregnated with silver, causing intensely black precipitate in the tissue on reduction.[4,5] It has been reported that silver stains react with melanocytes from eumelanotic, but not pheomelanotic, skin tissue.[6] The oxidation of the substrate dopa to insoluble, black melanin (dopa reaction), reflects tyrosinase activity occurring in melanosomes.[7]

Immunohistologic identification of melanocytes using antibodies directed against tyrosinase, MITF, and Melan-A/Mart1 allows identification of melanocytes in paraffin-embedded tissues as well as melanoma.[8,9] Although less specific for the melanocyte lineage, antibodies directed against S100 protein have long been used with great sensitivity to detect melanocytes and melanomas.[10] Immunostaining with antibody HMB-45 (directed against gp100/PMEL17) is negative in normal adult melanocytes but offers additional specificity for examination of melanocytic neoplasms.[11] MITF protein is a transcription factor that was shown to regulate the expression of several immunohistochemical markers, including tyrosinase, Melan-A/Mart1, and HMB-45/gp100/PMEL17.[12]

INTRODUCTION

Melanocytes are specialized cells of the epidermis and hair follicle whose primary function is to synthesize and transfer melanin to adjacent keratinocytes. Melanin synthesis occurs in a specialized organelle, the melanosome; proper melanosome biogenesis and trafficking are required for normal pigmentation. Melanocyte numbers are similar in individuals of different racial backgrounds, and instead differences of pigmentation are a result of the amount and quality of melanin in the skin, in large part driven by variability in the number, size, distribution, and function of melanosomes within keratinocytes.[1,2] Analysis of mutations in mice and humans (Table 20-1) that cause pigmentation defects have allowed the identification of key regulators of melanocyte development, survival, and function. Many of these same genes play critical roles in the pathogenesis of melanoma.

TABLE 20-1
Genetic Hypopigmentation and Hyperpigmentation Disorders Caused by Mutations in Genes Important for Melanocyte Development and Biology

DISORDER	GENE MUTATION	CLINICAL FEATURES
Hypopigmentation disorders		
Ocular albinism (OA1)	GPR143	Reduced pigmentation of iris and retina; photosensitivity; decreased visual acuity; nystagmus; strabismus; misrouting of optic nerve
Oculocutaneous albinism		Cutaneous albinism (pigmentary dilution of skin and hair)
		Ocular albinism (see above)
▪ OCA1	TYR	OCA1A: tyrosinase-negative (severe) albinism (complete loss of tyrosinase function)
		OCA1B: tyrosinase-positive (mild to moderate) albinism
▪ OCA2	OCA2	"Brown" albinism
▪ OCA3	TYRP1	"Rufous" albinism
▪ OCA4	SLC45A2/MATP	Variable degrees of albinism
Waardenburg Syndrome		Piebaldism, congenital deafness, heterochromia irides, synophrys, broad nasal root, dystopia canthorum
▪ WS1	PAX3	Classic type
▪ WS2	MITF	Lacks dystopia canthorum
	SNAI2	
▪ WS3	PAX3	Limb abnormalities (hypoplasia, syndactyly)
▪ WS4	SOX10	Hirschsprung disease
	EDN3	
	EDNRB	
Tietz syndrome	MITF	Tyrosinase-positive cutaneous albinism; deafness; eyebrow hypoplasia
Piebaldism	cKIT	Depigmented forelock and abdominal skin
Hermansky-Pudlak syndrome (HPS)		Tyrosinase-positive oculocutaneous albinism (melanosome dysfunction)
		Bleeding diathesis (platelet granule dysfunction)
		Interstitial pulmonary fibrosis (HPS 1,2,4), granulomatous colitis (HPS 1,4), renal failure (rare), cardiomyopathy (rare) (caused by ceroidal lipofuscin accumulation in lysosomes)
		Neutropenia and cytotoxic T-cell dysfunction (HPS2)
▪ HPS1	HPS1 (BLOC-3)	
▪ HPS2	AP3B1 (AP-3)	
▪ HPS3	HPS3 (BLOC-2)	
▪ HPS4	HPS4 (BLOC-3)	
▪ HPS5	HPS5 (BLOC-2)	
▪ HPS6	HPS6 (BLOC-2)	
▪ HPS7	DTNBP1 (BLOC-2)	
▪ HPS8	BLOC1S3 (BLOC-1)	
▪ HPS9	BLOC1S6 (BLOC-1)	
Chediak-Higashi syndrome	LYST	Tyrosinase-positive oculocutaneous albinism (melanosome dysfunction)
		Bleeding diathesis (platelet granule dysfunction)
		Progressive neurologic dysfunction (mechanism unknown)
		Severe immunodeficiency (NK cell, cytotoxic T cell, neutrophil dysfunction)
		Lymphomalike syndrome (overwhelming infiltration of organs by defective white blood cells)
		Giant lysosome-related organelles (these large granules are visible within leukocytes in peripheral blood smear)
Griscelli Syndrome		Pigmentary dilution of skin and hair (clumping of melanin within melanocytes)
		Neurologic abnormalities (GS1)
		Immunodeficiency (GS2)
▪ GS1	MYO5A	
▪ GS2	RAB27A	
▪ GS3	MLPH	
Hyperpigmentation disorders		
Familial progressive hyperpigmentation (FPH)	KITLG	Generalized patches of hyperpigmentation of skin and mucous membranes without systemic symptoms
Familial progressive hyper- and hypopigmentation (FPPH)	KITLG	Diffuse hyperpigmented and hypopigmented patches without systemic symptoms. Variable penetrance

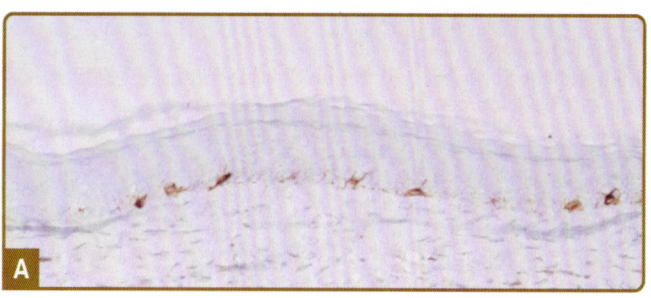
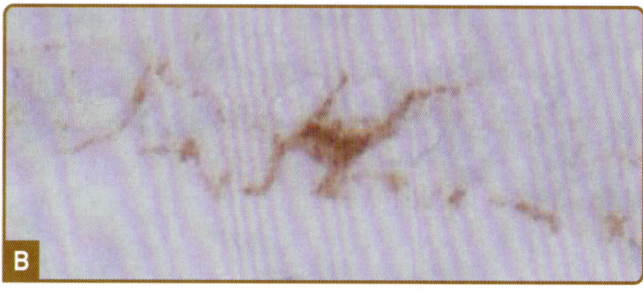

Figure 20-1 Melan-A/Mart1 immunostaining of melanocytes. **A,** Immunohistochemistry using antibody directed against Melan-A identifies melanocytes admixed with keratinocytes in the basal layer of epidermis. **B,** Higher-power magnification demonstrates the dendritic morphology of melanocytes. (Images used with permission from Dr. Roberto Novoa, Stanford University.)

ULTRASTRUCTURE

Unlike keratinocytes, melanocytes do not possess desmosomes or tonofilaments. Where they adjoin the basement membrane, melanocytes demonstrate structures resembling the hemidesmosomes of basal keratinocytes.[13] The key ultrastructural feature of the melanocyte is the melanosome, a round to oval-shaped membrane-enveloped organelle. Melanosomes containing primarily eumelanin (eumelanosomes) can be classified into 4 stages based on morphology, correlating to increasing stages of melanosome maturation (stage I to IV)[14-16] (Fig. 20-2). Stage I melanosomes are round, approximately 0.3 μm in diameter, and contain small intraluminal vesicles reminiscent of multivesicular bodies of the early endosomal compartment. Stage II melanosomes are oval in shape and are approximately 0.5 μm in diameter and exhibit deposition of a parallel fibrillar matrix. Stage I and stage II melanosomes are not melanized. Stage III melanosomes demonstrate deposition of pigment along the filaments, whereas stage IV melanosomes are fully melanized, with the electron-dense melanin completely obscuring the underlying structures (Fig. 20-2). Overall, melanosomes containing primarily pheomelanin (pheomelanosomes) exhibit similar ultrastructural stages of maturation with late stage III and IV pheomelanosomes exhibiting melanization obscuring underlying structures. However, pheomelanosomes are smaller, retain a rounded morphology at all stages, and contain a disorganized and less dense filament network.[16-18]

DISTRIBUTION OF MELANOCYTES

INTERFOLLICULAR MELANOCYTES AND THE EPIDERMAL MELANIN UNIT

In human interfollicular skin (defined as epidermal locations between hair follicles), melanocytes are admixed with keratinocytes at the basal layer of the epidermis. Cutaneous interfollicular melanocytes are present at highest density in the facial and genital skin, and at lower density in the skin of the trunk and extremities.[1,19] Chronic, sun-exposed skin contains up to a 2-fold higher number and an increase in the size and activity of the melanocytes as compared to adjacent sun-protected skin.[20,21] Thus, the differences in pigmentation following sun-induced hyperpigmentation (tanning) are predominantly due to altered pigment synthesis per melanocyte, rather than major alterations in melanocyte numbers. Similarly, there is little variation in melanocyte numbers between individuals of different skin phototypes. The key determinant of skin pigmentation is not melanocyte density but instead the increased ability of melanocytes from darker-skinned persons to synthesize and transfer brown-black eumelanin.[1]

Melanin synthesis by melanocytes and subsequent transfer of melanin to adjacent keratinocytes is required for normal pigmentation. The term "epidermal melanin unit" was first coined by Fitzpatrick to

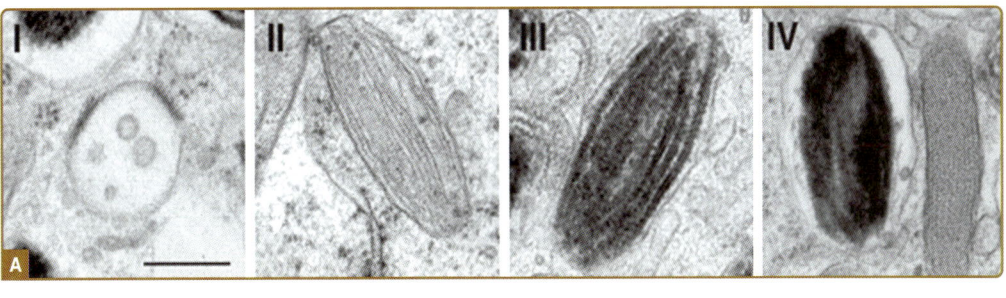

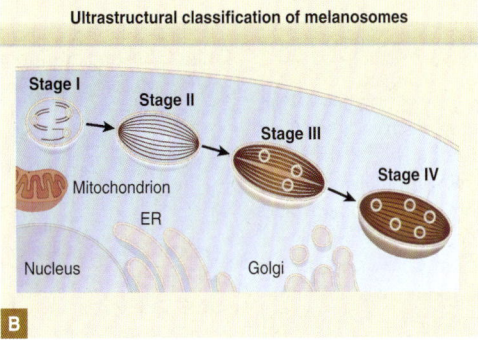

Figure 20-2 Ultrastructural classification of melanosomes. **A,** Selected images of stage I, II, III, and IV melanosomes from MNT-1 melanoma cells. High-pressure freezing of cells and freeze substitution was utilized by these authors to optimize ultrastructural preservation. (Scale bars: 200 nm.) (Used with permission from Hurbain I, et al. Electron tomography of early melanosomes: implications for melanogenesis and the generation of fibrillar amyloid sheets. *Proc Natl Acad Sci* 105(50):19726-31. Copyright (2008) National Academy of Sciences, U.S.A.) **B,** Schematic versions of the electron microscopy images.

describe this fundamental multicellular interaction.[22] Histologically, the epidermal melanin unit is characterized by a melanocyte and each of the keratinocytes that it physically contacts. Each melanocyte contacts and delivers melanin to approximately 40 keratinocytes, irrespective of anatomical location, via direct contacts with the melanocyte's protruding dendrites.

It has long been known that epidermal repigmentation during vitiligo occurs around hair follicles, suggesting that epidermal melanocytes can be regenerated from a "reservoir" of melanocyte stem cells (McSCs) of the hair follicle.[23,24] After depletion of interfollicular melanocytes in a transgenic mouse model, melanocytes were seen to be repopulated by hair follicle–derived McSCs.[25] Recent studies from mouse models have demonstrated that after wounding or UVB irradiation, hair follicle McSCs migrate before proliferation to populate the interfollicular epidermis.[26] However, the signaling pathways that guide the differentiation, survival, quiescence, and migration of McSCs to the epidermis are only beginning to emerge, and include Wnt, Endrb, transforming growth factor beta (TGFβ), and MC1R signaling.[26-29] Although most epidermal melanocytes are derived from hair follicle–resident McSCs, some epidermal melanocytes may have other origins. Recent studies in zebrafish and mice have shown that differentiated epidermal melanocytes retain the ability to proliferate in vivo.[30,31] Under the pathologic circumstance of nerve injury, Schwann cells may undergo dedifferentiation to generate ectopic melanocytes.[32]

FOLLICULAR MELANOCYTES

Within the hair follicle, the melanocyte population varies by the stage of the hair cycle. Similar to epithelial stem cells, melanocyte stem cells (McSCs) reside within the permanent bulge/secondary hair germ (sHG) area of the hair follicle and maintain a quiescent state during telogen.[25] During the anagen phase of the hair cycle, the McSCs become activated via Wnt signaling, proliferate, and give rise to differentiated melanocytes.[33] These melanocytes migrate to the bulb of the hair follicle and undergo maturation by early to mid-anagen. Differentiated melanocytes then produce and transfer melanin to the surrounding keratinocytes throughout anagen, ultimately resulting in pigmentation of the hairs. Differentiated melanocytes of the hair bulb undergo apoptosis during late catagen in step with the degenerating lower hair follicle, while the McSC population persists through each hair cycle.[34] Gradual loss of McSCs occurs with age, suggesting that age-dependent hair graying seen in humans and mice is the result of incomplete maintenance of the hair follicle McSC cell pool.[35] The demise of these follicular McSCs appears to involve their "inappropriate" differentiation and pigmentation within the stem cell niche (bulge region)—a phenomenon that temporally precedes their apoptotic cell death. Follow-up studies have shown that triggers of DNA damage such as ionizing radiation can accelerate this process of aberrant McSC differentiation and hair graying.[36]

ACRAL MELANOCYTES

Melanocytes also exist in the hairless acral surfaces of palms and soles. Recently, the lower permanent portion of the eccrine gland has been demonstrated as a niche for McSCs of the acral epidermis.[37] It has been hypothesized that acral melanoma is derived from this McSC population. Correspondingly, acral melanomas are diagnosed with high sensitivity and specificity as a result of their preferential pigmentation of the eccrine-rich ridges of the dermatoglyphs.[38]

EXTRACUTANEOUS MELANOCYTES

Neural crest–derived melanocytes exist in other areas of the body including the mucosa, cochlea, uvea, leptomeninges, and heart. Of note, retinal pigment epithelium cells synthesize melanin and form melanosomes, but these cells are derived from neuroectoderm and are developmentally unrelated to the neural crest/melanocyte lineage. The roles of melanocytes in extracutaneous sites are diverse. In addition to contributing to pigment variation of the iris, ocular melanin protects against UV radiation, and darker eye pigmentation is associated with decreased incidence of age-related macular degeneration.[39] The role of melanocytes in the CNS is unclear, but autoimmunity directed against melanocytes in Vogt–Koyanagi–Harada syndrome can lead to severe CNS inflammation. In the cochlea of the ear, melanocytes are located in and required for the normal development and function of the stria vascularis layer, a nonsensory structure required for normal hearing. Defects of the stria vascularis explain the sensorineural deafness that is found, in addition to pigmentation defects, in human patients with Waardenburg and Tietz syndromes.[40,41] Dysfunction of cardiac melanocytes predispose to arrhythmias in a mouse model.[42] Mouse studies have suggested that different signaling pathways govern the development of cutaneous versus extracutaneous melanocytes.[43] Similarly, activation of distinct biologic pathways drive the pathogenesis of ocular, cutaneous, and acral lentiginous subtypes of melanomas.[44]

FORMATION, MIGRATION, AND SURVIVAL OF THE MELANOCYTE

Melanocytes are derived from the neural crest lineage. Although traditionally melanocytes were thought to migrate only along the dorsolateral migration pathway, recent evidence has demonstrated the importance of a second wave of melanocytes derived from Schwann cell precursors that migrate along developing nerves in the ventromedial migratory pathway.[32] Evidence from mouse coat color mutants and human patients with pigmentation syndromes (Table 20-1) has allowed identification of many genes required for melanocyte formation, migration, and survival. Many of these same factors play pivotal roles in the pathogenesis of melanoma.

DIFFERENTIATION AND MIGRATION OF MELANOCYTES FROM THE NEURAL CREST

Melanocytes are exclusively derived from the highly migratory and multipotent neural crest population, as first demonstrated by seminal xenotransplantation experiments in chick embryos.[45,46] The neural crest is a transient cell population that forms at the margin of the early forming neural tube. Neural crest cells migrate along one of 2 defined migratory pathways, a dorsolateral pathway between the somites and the ectoderm and a ventromedial pathway. Neural crest cells migrate to their target sites and give rise to multiple cell types including melanocytes, craniofacial cartilage and bone, secretory endocrine cells, smooth muscles of heart and great vessels, peripheral sensory and autonomic neurons, enteric neurons, and peripheral glia.

Decades of experimental evidence supported a model in which melanocyte precursors, termed melanoblasts, delaminate from the neural tube and follow the dorsolateral pathway between the ectoderm and the somites to reach the skin, whereas the ventrolateral pathway was thought to be used only by neural crest cells specified to the neuronal and glial lineages.[47] However, a recent study has demonstrated that a significant percentage of skin melanocytes are derived from Schwann cell precursors that travel the ventromedial pathway along the developing nerve sheath. The ventromedial-derived melanocytes then detach from the nerve before migrating to the epidermis (Fig. 20-3).[32]

The development and specification of melanoblasts along the dorsolateral pathway has been well characterized in mice. Melanoblasts appear to become specified prior to or early after delamination from the neural tube. The master melanocyte transcription factor, MITF, is first expressed in melanoblasts shortly after exit from the neural tube at embryonic day 10.5-11 (E10.5-11). Immediately after delamination from the neural tube, melanoblasts move to the migration staging area (MSA) (E11.5), a structure between the neural tube and somites where melanoblasts pause before traveling upon the dorsolateral migration pathway (E12.5).[48] Other markers of melanoblast specification such as the melanogenic enzymes Dct and TYRP1 are expressed at this stage.[49] Melanoblasts then migrate laterally through the dermis, and at E12.5-13.5 melanoblasts enter the epidermis in a synchronous wave.[50] The mechanisms underlying homing and migration of melanocytes to the epidermis are incompletely understood. At around E15.5, clusters of epidermal melanoblasts migrate and populate the hair follicles. Melanocytes express the key melanogenic enzyme

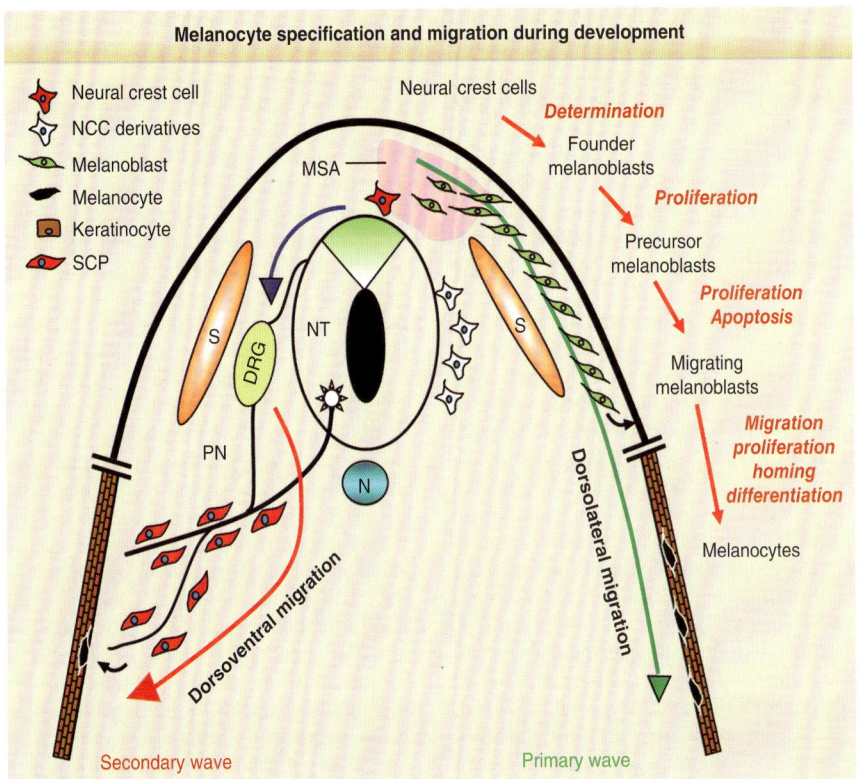

Figure 20-3 Melanocyte specification and migration during development. Upon exiting the neural tube, melanoblast precursors stall in the migration staging area (MSA), then move between the somites (S) and the ectoderm to migrate along the dorsolateral pathway (*green arrow*). Schwann cell precursors (SCPs) move through the dorsoventral pathway (*blue arrow*) in between the somites (S) and the neural tube (NT). A second wave of melanocytes (*red arrow*) arises from the SCPs. (From Bonaventure J, Domingues MJ, Larue L. Cellular and molecular mechanisms controlling the migration of melanocytes and melanoma cells. *Pigment Cell Melanoma Res*. 26(3):316-25, with permission. Copyright © 2013 John Wiley & Sons.)

tyrosinase by E14.5 and display pigmentation by E16.5. In mice, interfollicular epidermal melanocytes disappear during early postnatal life, while this population persists in humans.[51]

Though there is evidence of melanoblast specification at early developmental stages, there is controversy over whether neural crest cells and more specified precursors, such as melanoblasts, retain multipotency and give rise to multiple cell types. In vitro evidence suggests that migratory neural crest cells can give rise to multiple neural crest cell derivatives.[52,53] Similarly, melanoblasts and differentiated melanocytes isolated from the skin can exhibit multipotency when placed in culture.[54,55] Although the in vivo multipotency of neural crest cells has long been subject of debate, recent genetic lineage–tracing studies have provided exciting evidence that in vivo most premigratory and migratory neural crest cells give rise to multiple cell types, demonstrating that neural crest cells previously thought to be specified to a certain fate likely retain developmental plasticity.[56,57] This same plasticity may play an important role in the development of melanoma. In a zebrafish model, melanocytes reactivate markers of neural crest progenitors at the earliest stages of cancerous transformation.[58]

FACTORS THAT REGULATE MELANOCYTE DEVELOPMENT, SURVIVAL, AND MIGRATION

Characterization of mutations causative of mouse and human genetic pigmentary disorders (Table 20-1) has allowed the identification of networks of genes that are important for melanocyte formation, migration, and survival. Transcription factors have been shown to play a key role in directing the specification of neural crest precursors to the melanocyte fate. Receptors expressed by melanoblasts and melanocytes and their cognate growth factor ligands also are important for establishment and maintenance of the melanocyte fate. Many of these different factors also play key roles in the pathogenesis of melanoma.

TRANSCRIPTION FACTORS

MITF: Microphthalmia-associated transcription factor (MITF) is a basic helix-loop-helix leucine-zipper (bHLHzip) transcription factor first identified as the gene mutated in *microphthalmia* mice, which, in addition to defects in retinal pigment epithelium, osteoclasts, and mast cells, exhibit loss of melanocytes of the skin and inner ear.[59] Soon after, germline mutations in MITF were identified in humans with Waardenburg syndrome type 2a, characterized by pigmentation defects and hearing loss.[60] The molecular characterization of MITF revealed a gene encoding multiple isoforms, each with a variable first exon spliced to common downstream exons 2-9.[61] The melanocyte-specific isoform (m-MITF) is downstream of promoter elements that specify transcription only in melanocytes, whereas other isoforms are generally more ubiquitously expressed.[62] The regulation of the promoter of m-MITF has been well characterized and MITF is positively regulated by other transcription factors important for neural crest development including SOX10 and PAX3 (Fig. 20-4). The developmental roles of these factors are vividly illustrated by the phenotypic consequences of their germline disruption, as occurs in the sensorineural deafness and pigmentation syndromes known as Waardenburg syndrome types 1 through 4. Of these factors, MITF (in particular the melanocyte-specific isoform m-MITF) is most lineage selective in specifying melanocyte differentiation, whereas SOX10 and PAX3 regulate expression of other lineages, including certain muscle groups and enteric ganglia/neurons. Correspondingly, mutation of MITF results in prominent pigment cell–related phenotypes whereas mutations of SOX10 and PAX3 produce pigment cell defects as well as certain nonpigmentary phenotypes (such as megacolon for SOX10).

MITF has been shown to be required for the survival, proliferation and differentiation of melanocytes. At the molecular level, MITF binds to specific E-box sequences containing the core hexanucleotide consensus element CA[C/T]GTG which is present in promoters or enhancers of numerous pigmentation-related genes.[63] Through recognition of this element, MITF drives expression of genes regulating melanin synthesis and melanosome biogenesis, including tyrosinase, TYRP1, DCT, PMEL17/silver, MLANA, and Rab27a, proliferation genes such as Cyclin-Dependent Kinase 2 (CDK2), whose genomic location is so close to PMEL17 that both are uniquely coregulated by MITF in the melanocyte lineage, and survival genes such as the antiapoptotic factors B-cell lymphoma 2 (BCL2) and BCL2a1.[64-66] MITF acts as an oncogene and is amplified in a subset of melanoma.[67] It is also subject to recurrent activating germline or sporadic mutation.[68] Activity of MITF is regulated posttranslationally by phosphorylation, ubiquitination, and sumoylation (Fig. 20-4). Sumoylation of MITF mildly reduces its transcriptional activity at genes containing multiple MITF-binding sites.[69] The E318K MITF polymorphism found at low frequency in European, North American, and Australian populations is associated with significantly increased melanoma risk, an effect likely mediated by disruption of a consensus MITF sumoylation site.[68]

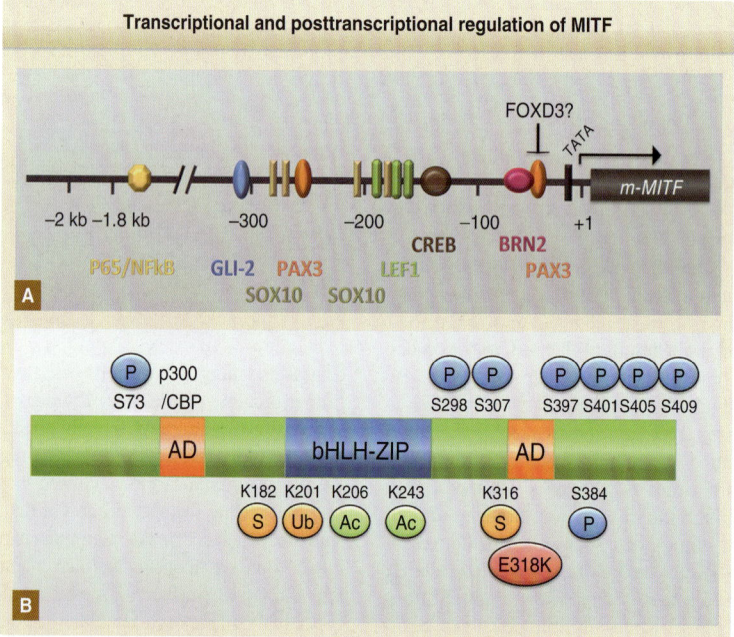

Figure 20-4 Transcriptional and posttranscriptional regulation of MITF. **A,** The proximal melanocyte-specific MITF (m-MITF) promoter contains binding sites for transcription factors, including SOX10, PAX3, CREB, and LEF1. Negative regulators of the m-MITF promoter include Brn2 and FOXD3. **B,** MITF is posttranslationally modified by several mechanisms, including phosphorylation (P), sumoylation (S), and ubiquitination (Ub). Kit signals via ERK to phosphorylate MITF at Serine 73 to positively regulate MITF activity. Sumoylation of K316 negatively regulates MITF; K316 sumoylation site is disrupted by E318K mutation. (Adapted from Wellbrock C, Arozarena I. Microphthalmia-associated transcription factor in melanoma development and MAP-kinase pathway targeted therapy. *Pigment Cell Melanoma Res.* 2015;28(4):390-406.)

PAX3: Paired Box 3 (PAX3) is a transcription factor critical for development of the neural tube.[70] PAX3 is one of the earliest markers of the neural crest, and PAX3 mutation in mice, in addition to pigmentation defects, results in abnormalities of neural crest derivatives of the sensory and sympathetic ganglia, Schwann cells, and cardiac neural crest.[71] PAX3 was subsequently found to be mutated in human Waardenburg syndrome types 1 and 3 (hearing loss, pigmentation defect, arm and hand developmental defects).[72] Pigmentation defects caused by mutation of PAX3 may be explained by a defect in melanoblast proliferation during development.[73] PAX3 has been shown to be a positive regulator of the MITF promoter in melanocytes and melanoma.[74,75]

SOX10: SRY-Box 10 (SOX10) is a transcription factor first identified as being mutated in Waardenburg type IV (Waardenburg plus megacolon) and is required for development of neural, glial, and melanocyte neural crest lineages.[76,77] SOX10 is first expressed in premigratory neural crest cells, and loss of SOX10 during development leads to complete absence of melanoblasts.[78] Recent studies using transgenic mouse models and human melanoma cell lines have demonstrated that SOX10 function is required for survival of postnatal melanocytes, melanocyte stem cells, nevi, and melanoma.[79,80] SOX10 likely mediates many of its effects on melanocyte and melanoma survival through regulation of MITF expression.[81]

SOX2: The transcription factor SOX2 plays key roles in stem cell maintenance and is one of 4 transcriptions factors required for reprogramming of somatic cells to induced pluripotent stem cells.[82] SOX2 has recently been shown play a role in specifying the melanocyte lineage during development. SOX2 binds and represses the MITF promoter. Gradual downregulation of SOX2 in Schwann cell precursors allows increased expression of MITF and emergence of the melanocyte population.[83] SOX2 also has been shown to downregulate MITF in cultured human melanocytes and human melanoma.[84]

FoxD3: Forkhead Box D3 (FoxD3) is a transcription factor that is upregulated early during neural crest development and is important for establishing the neural crest lineage. Loss of FoxD3 early in development leads to the loss of most neural crest–derived structures.[85] During later stages of neural crest development, FoxD3 acts to modulate specification of neural crest derivatives. FoxD3 actively represses MITF to favor the Schwann cell fate whereas downregulation of FoxD3 favors the melanocyte fate.[86]

GROWTH FACTOR SIGNALING

Ednrb: Endothelin receptor type B (Ednrb) is a G-protein–coupled receptor that activates several signaling pathways, including include protein kinase C (PKC), mitogen-activated protein kinase (MAPK) and cAMP/PKA. Ednrb agonists, the endothelins, are encoded by 3 genes: Endothelin 1 (Edn1), Edn2, and Edn3. Although all 3 endothelins can bind Ednrb with similar efficiency, and Edn1 has been shown to initiate melanogenesis in cultured melanocytes, Edn3 seems to be the important ligand during melanocyte development. In humans, Ednrb mutation results in Hirschsprung disease, whereas Edn3 mutation results in Waardenburg plus megacolon, suggesting roles in the development of melanocytes as well as other neural crest derivatives.[87,88] Although it does not seem to be required for the initial specification of melanoblasts, Ednrb has been shown to be required mainly for proper melanoblast migration.[89,90] Activation of Endothelin signaling also has been shown to induce melanocyte proliferation and skin pigmentation.[91,92]

c-Kit: The receptor tyrosine kinase c-Kit and the cognate Kit ligand (KITLG) (also known as Steel factor or stem cell factor/SCF) play important roles during melanocyte development. KITLG exists in transmembrane and soluble forms and in the skin is produced by endothelial cells and keratinocytes.[93] In humans, the heterozygous mutation of c-Kit results in piebaldism, which is characterized by a depigmentation of the forelock and abdominal skin.[94] Mutation of c-Kit or KITLG in mice results in loss of melanocytes.[95,96] Although c-Kit signaling does not appear to be necessary for the specification of melanoblasts, on c-Kit deficiency, the melanoblasts soon disappear after migration from the neural tube.[97]

c-Kit also plays important roles in regulating survival and differentiation/pigmentation of mature melanocytes. Blocking antibodies to c-Kit in human skin explants or adult mouse skin results in loss of melanocytes.[98,99] Conversely, KITLG injection to human skin explants increased the number, dendricity, and melanogenesis of melanocytes. Recently, polymorphism in KITLG has been shown to cause familial progressive pigmentation (FPH) and familial progressive hyper- and hypopigmentation (FPPH), 2 conditions that share the feature of enlarging hyperpigmented patches corresponding to increased melanization without change in melanocyte number.[100,101] Activating mutations and amplification of c-Kit drive the progression of a subset of acral lentiginous, mucosal, and lentigo maligna melanomas.[102] Whereas c-KIT signaling has been shown to cause MAPK-dependent phosphorylation and activation of MITF, additional mechanisms by which KIT signaling affects melanocyte survival and differentiation are poorly understood.[103]

Wnt/α-Catenin: β-Catenin is an evolutionarily conserved protein that plays key roles in developmental signaling. The multiprotein membrane destruction complex, consisting of APC, Axin1/2, and GSK3β, target β-catenin for phosphorylation and ubiquitin-dependent degradation. Canonical Wnt signaling involves binding of a Wnt family ligand to a Frizzled family receptor, which signals through Dishevelled to inhibit the membrane destruction complex, allowing for β-catenin to enter the nucleus and interact with LEF/TCF family transcription factors to activate gene transcription. Experimental evidence supports that activating β-catenin, at least during a certain window of melanoblast migration, leads to increased proliferation and differentiation of melanocytes.[104,105] Mechanistically, β-catenin-LEF/TCF complexes have been shown to transcriptionally regulate MITF in cultured melanocytes and melanoma cells.[106] β-Catenin pathway activation also potentiates melanoma formation and metastasis in mouse models.[107,108]

Neuregulin/ErbB2/ErbB3: It has recently been reported that some melanocytes are derived from Schwann cell precursors that travel along the ventral migratory pathway.[32] The ErbB2/ErbB3 heterodimer tyrosine kinase receptor controls Schwann cell proliferation, migration, and myelination. The ligand for this receptor, neuregulin, promotes the Schwann cell fate and represses the melanocyte fate. Loss of ErbB3 or neuregulin during development decreases the number of Schwann cells and increases the number of ventrally migrated melanocytes.[32] Other signals that regulate the formation of Schwann cell–derived melanocytes during embryonic development remain to be identified.

REGULATION OF MELANOCYTE MOTILITY AND MIGRATION

Rac1: Rac1 belongs to the Rho superfamily of GTPases. Similar to other Rho GTPases, Rac1 exhibits an active conformation when bound to GTP and has well known roles in cellular migration through regulation of the actin cytoskeleton.[109] When Rac1 is deleted from melanoblasts during mouse development, melanoblasts migrate less efficiently as a result of impairment of Scar/WAVE and Arp2/3 actin regulatory complexes.[110] However, Rac1-deficient melanoblasts are still able to cross the dermal–epidermal junction and home normally to hair follicles. Recurrent activating mutations in Rac1 have been found in 9% of sun-exposed melanomas.[111] Mutation of PREX2, a guanine nucleotide exchange factor (GEF), occurs frequently in human melanomas, and these mutations may promote melanoma through activation of Rac1.[112] Loss of function of PREX1, another Rac-specific GEF, impairs melanoblast migration and melanoma metastasis in a mouse model.[113]

MELANIN AND THE MELANOSOME

There are 2 forms of melanin, eumelanin and pheomelanin, that are both derived from the precursor tyrosine. Tyrosinase converts tyrosine to dopaquinone and is a key enzyme regulating both eumelanogenesis and pheomelanogenesis. Melanin synthesis occurs in the melanosome, a specialized lysosome-related organelle. Human skin pigmentation requires both the biogenesis of melanosomes and delivery of melanogenic proteins and enzymes to the melanosome, as well as proper trafficking of the melanosome to the keratinocyte.

STRUCTURE AND FUNCTION OF MELANIN

Eumelanin (brown/black) and pheomelanin (yellow/orange) represent the 2 main forms of melanin in humans and other mammals. Eumelanin is a macromolecule composed of polymers of 5,6-dihydroxyindole (DHI; insoluble in strong alkali, black) and the carboxylate form 5,6-dihydroxyindole-2-carboxylic acid (DHICA; partially soluble in strong alkali, lighter black/brown).[114] Pheomelanin is a complex macromolecule formed by oxidation and polymerization of sulfur-containing cysteinyldopa. Pheomelanin is highly soluble in alkali.[114] The solubility of melanin may be clinically relevant, as it has been suggested that melanin degradation products can escape the melanosome and enter the nucleus to contribute to DNA damage.[115]

Pigmentation of human skin offers protection against UV-induced sunburn and DNA damage.[116-118] Skin pigmentation also protects against UV-induced skin cancer in humans, as evidenced by increased risk of nonmelanoma skin cancer in patients with albinism and lighter/fair-skinned individuals, and decreased skin cancer risk in human populations of darker skin types.[117,119] Similarly, skin pigmentation inhibits UV-induced carcinogenesis in animal models.[120,121] Melanin, and in particular eumelanin, can shield against UV radiation, though it has been demonstrated that pigmented skin or dispersed melanosomes offer only a relatively low sun protection factor (SPF).[122] Thus, melanin may have other functions in protecting against UV-induced damage. In line with this, eumelanin has been shown to scavenge UV-induced reactive oxygen species (ROS) to minimize UV damage.[123]

Pheomelanin, on the other hand, not only has decreased shielding property against UV radiation, but evidence also suggests that pheomelanin may act as a pro-oxidant. Several studies have shown that UVA reacts with purified pheomelanin to generate free radicals.[124,125] It also has been demonstrated that ROS generated by UVA interacts with pheomelanin, and to a lesser extent eumelanin, leading to melanin degradation products that induce cyclobutane pyrimidine dimer (CPD) formation long after UV exposure has ended—the so-called dark CPD. CPDs were previously thought to only be caused by immediate and direct photochemical interaction of UV with DNA, and this new mechanism could explain melanocyte-specific CPD formation that is exacerbated by the presence of pheomelanin.[115] In addition, a recent study demonstrated that in a melanoma-prone BRAF (V600E) genetically engineered mouse model, the presence of Mc1r dysfunction (the "red hair, fair skin" phenotype) was associated with significantly increased risk of melanoma in the *absence* of UV, and correlated with increased ROS in the skin of pheomelanotic mice. This effect was abrogated by introduction of a tyrosinase loss-of-function mutation (albino-redheads), suggesting that elevated melanoma risk in the red-haired background was indeed traceable to the pheomelanin synthesis pathway. These data suggest the existence of both UV-mediated and

UV-independent mechanisms through which pheomelanin contributes to melanoma formation, presumably via ROS-mediated DNA damage, to promote melanoma.[126] Recent data in humans have corroborated the murine findings, showing that melanoma risk is higher in red-haired/fair-skinned individuals even after normalization/correction for UV exposure, as defined by a set of UV damage indicators.[127,128]

MELANIN SYNTHESIS

TYROSINASE AND OTHER MELANOGENIC ENZYMES

The first step in the synthesis of both eumelanin and pheomelanin is oxidation of tyrosine to dopaquinone by the enzyme tyrosinase. Tyrosinase was first isolated from mushroom in 1895, and tyrosinase activity was first demonstrated in normal human skin by Fitzpatrick et al in 1950.[129] Tyrosinase requires binding of copper for proper function, and delivery of copper to the melanosome by ATP7A transporter is required for normal tyrosinase function.[130]

Two tyrosine-related proteins (TYRP), TYRP1 and TYRP2/Dopachrome tautomerase (DCT), show significant homology to tyrosinase and play key roles in melanogenesis. As discussed below, these proteins have distinct catalytic functions in eumelanin synthesis downstream of tyrosinase. In addition, TYRP1 and DCT complex with tyrosinase and have been shown to be important for proper trafficking and stabilization of tyrosinase.[131] Defects of tyrosinase, TYRP1, and DCT cause oculocutaneous albinism in humans. Two other genes mutated in human albinism, *OCA2* (P-protein) and *SCL45a2* (MATP, AIM, "underwhite" mutant) encode transporters whose functions are not clearly determined, but seem to be important for proper tyrosinase trafficking and melanosome maturation.[132-135]

EUMELANOGENESIS

Dopaquinone spontaneously undergoes intramolecular cyclization to form cyclodopa. Cyclodopa then undergoes redox exchange with a second molecule of dopaquinone to form dopachrome and dopa.[136] Dopachrome spontaneously decarboxylates to form DHI (less soluble, black) and DHICA (more soluble, lighter black/brown). Although the uncatalyzed reaction favors DHI formation, the presence of the (DCT) protein favors production of DHICA.[137] DHI and DHICA are then oxidized and polymerized to form eumelanin. TYRP1 exhibits DHICA-oxidase activity, promoting incorporation of DHICA into eumelanin (Fig. 20-5).[138]

PHEOMELANOGENESIS

Nonenzymatic addition of sulfhydryl groups to dopaquinone results in the formation of 5-*S*-cysteinaldopa and 2-*S*-cysteinaldopa. Cysteine serves as a major source of sulfhydryl groups, with the other source being glutathione. It has been shown that cysteinaldopa synthesis predominates in the presence of cysteine, whereas in cultured cells high tyrosine and/or low cysteine favor eumelagenesis.[139-141] Cysteinaldopa then undergoes redox exchange with dopaquinone to produce cysteinaldopaquinones. Oxidation and cyclization of cysteinaldopaquinones is followed by dehydration, rearrangement, and decarboxylation to form benzothiazole intermediates. The benzothiazole intermediates then polymerize to form pheomelanin (Fig. 20-5).

THE MELANOSOME

Melanosomes are lysosome-related organelles that exist only in melanocytes and retinal pigment epithelium. They are the main sites of synthesis and storage of melanin. Mutations in human disease syndromes that result in melanosome dysfunction, causing hypopigmentation in addition to dysfunction of other lysosome-related organelles, have resulted in identification of pathways involved in melanosome biogenesis.

STRUCTURE OF THE MELANOSOME

As described above, melanosomes have been classified by electron microscopy into morphologic stages that correspond to degree of maturation. As melanosomes mature, the key ultrastructural feature is the appearance of the parallel fibrillar network; PMEL (also known as gp100 or silver) is a pigment cell–specific protein that has been shown to be the main component of these structures. The intraluminal vesicles of stage I melanosomes have been shown to be the first site of PMEL deposition. The transmembrane PMEL protein is cleaved within the stage I and II melanosomes by the beta-site APP-cleaving enzyme 1 (BACE1) to release intraluminal amyloidogenic fragments with the capability to oligomerize.[142] The PMEL protein represents a remarkable setting in which protein aggregation, mediated by amyloid-related interactions, participate in a physiologic process: organization and deposition of melanin pigments within the melanosome organelles. Stage II melanosomes are identified by increased organization of PMEL amyloid into visible proteinaceous fibrils, which push the intraluminal vesicles outward to fuse with the melanosome membrane. 3D electron microscopy has shown that the fibrils visible on EM sections actually represent parallel sheets.[143,144] Stage III melanosomes become increasingly pigmented as melanogenic enzymes are delivered and melanin synthesis proceeds. Stage IV melanosomes are fully pigmented, and tyrosinase activity and melanin synthesis has ceased. Pheomelanosomes also have been characterized ultrastructurally in humans and other mammals, and are smaller, spherical in shape, with a granular and microvesicular, rather than fibrillar, matrix, and with microgranular and spotty melanization.[16,18] Although it is tempting to contrast pheomelanotic melanosomes

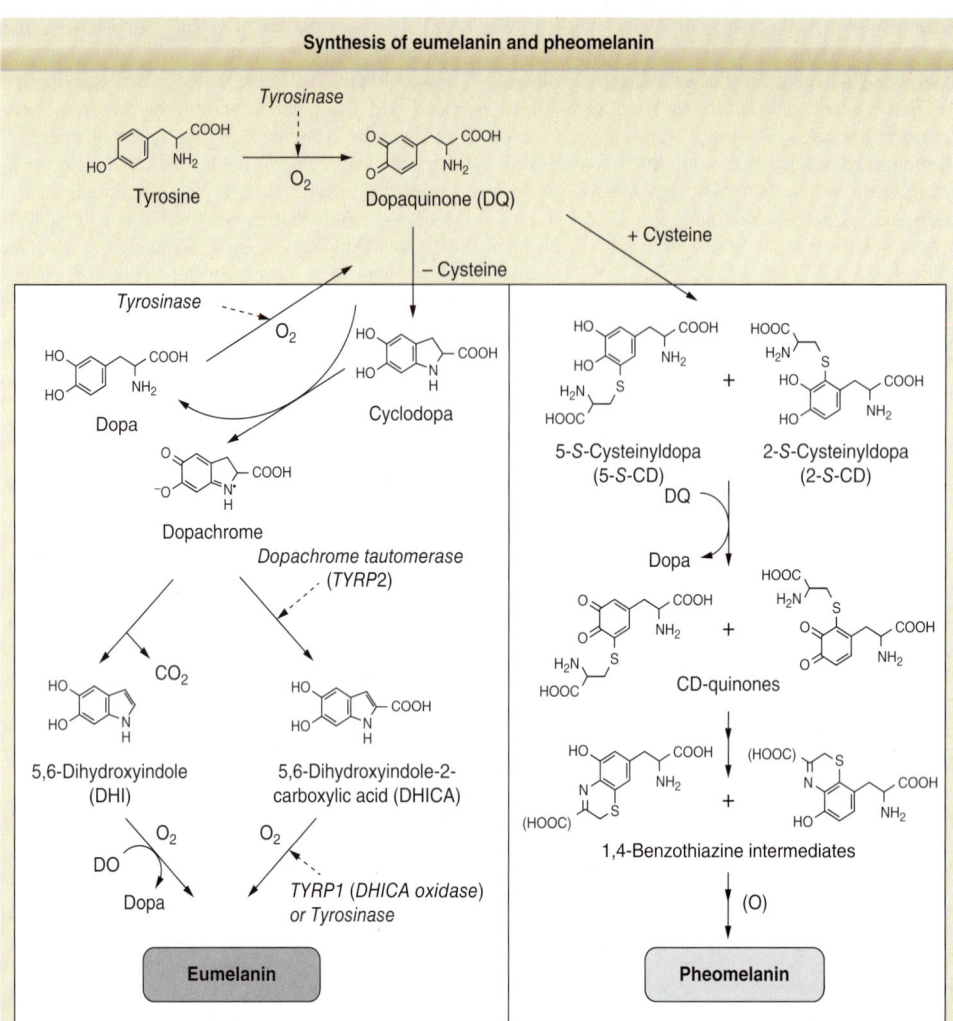

Figure 20-5 Synthesis of eumelanin and pheomelanin. Tyrosinase (TYR) is needed to generate dopaquinone (DQ) from tyrosine. DQ is the common precursor of eumelanin and pheomelanin. The enzymes tyrosinase-related protein1 (TYRP1) and TYRP2/dopachrome tautomerase are also involved in eumelanin synthesis. (From Ito S, Wakamatsu K. Chemistry of mixed melanogenesis-pivotal roles of dopaquinone. *Photochem Photobiol.* 84(3):582-92, with permission. Copyright © 2007 John Wiley & Sons.)

as differing primarily in the specific melanin species (pheomelanin vs eumelanin), it is important to recall that other melanosomal constituents also differ in the setting of MC1R variants associated with red hair, because MITF resides downstream of MC1R and regulates the expression of pigment enzymes as well as numerous melanosomal factors including PMEL, tyrosinase, TRP1, and DCT.[145]

MELANOSOME BIOGENESIS AND TRAFFICKING

Although melanosomes express some lysosomal proteins and derive from the endosomal pathway, they require unique sorting and trafficking pathways for their formation.[146] Newly synthesized PMEL traffics to the plasma membrane, and then is transferred via the endosomal pathway to the early melanosome compartment.[147] However, the exact membrane trafficking events that allow specification of the early melanosome as a distinct compartment are not well understood. Stage I melanosomes, though they are accessible to endocytosis tracing compounds and morphologically resemble early multivesicular bodies derived from the endosomal pathway, seem to form independently of the endosomal sorting complex required for transport (ESCRT) machinery needed for the classical multivesicular body pathway.[148]

Melanogenic enzymes are delivered to stage II melanosomes after the fibrillar PMEL network has been deposited, allowing melanin synthesis to begin. It has been recently shown that the recycling endosome compartment plays a key role in delivery of cargoes (tyrosinase, TYRP1, DCT) to the maturing melanosome. The recycling endosome compartment is composed of interconnected and functionally distinct tubular networks that originate from early endosomes, and transport cargoes along microtubule tracks.[149] Mutations of any of the 10 genes encoding components of the BLOC-1, BLOC-2, BLOC-3, and AP-3 protein complexes have been long known to be responsible for Hermansky-Pudlak syndrome, a heterogeneous group of disorders characterized by hypopigmentation due to melanosome dysfunction in addition to platelet dysfunction, immunodeficiency, and lung fibrosis due to abnormalities of other lysosome-related organelles. Although the mechanism by which BLOC and AP3 complexes act in melanosome- and lysosome-related organelle biogenesis has long been unclear, they have recently been shown to play critical roles in the delivery of melanosomal cargoes in recycling endosomes.

Dysfunction of BLOC complexes cause accumulation of TYRP1 and other melanogenic enzymes within the endosomal compartment, leading to pigmentary abnormalities.[150] Recently, it has been shown that BLOC1 coordinates the action of microtubule- and actin-dependent machineries to allow proper formation and stabilization of recycling endosomal tubules required for transfer of cargoes to melanosomes.[149,151] BLOC-2 acts to properly direct recycling endosomal tubular transport intermediates to maturing melanosomes to promote melanogenic cargo deliery.[152] AP-3 is also important for sorting cargo proteins bound for melanosomes, and in different scenarios can act in concert with or independently of BLOC complexes.[153,154]

The final step in the delivery of cargo to melanosomes is the fusion of cargo-containing vesicle and tubules with the developing melanosome. This process has been shown to involve SNARE proteins that are required for membrane fusion. It has been recently shown that VAMP7 is the SNARE responsible for BLOC-1-dependent delivery of TYRP1 to the melanosome.[155] BLOC-3 is required for the subsequent recycling of VAMP7 after delivery of cargo to the melanosome, suggesting a novel mechanism by which BLOC-3 dysfunction causes pigmentation deficits[155] (Fig. 20-6).

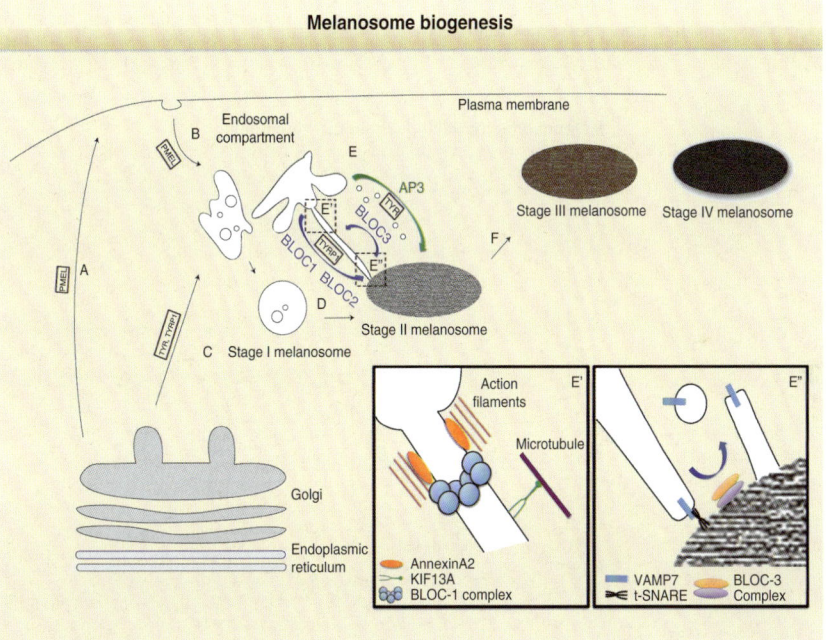

Figure 20-6 Melanosome biogenesis. The endosomal compartment plays a key role in melanosome biogenesis. (A) PMEL protein is largely delivered to the plasma membrane followed by (B) endocytosis to the endosomal compartment and then to early melanosomes. PMEL processing leads to fibril formation within the melanosome. (C) Other melanogenic enzymes such as TYR and TYRP1 are delivered to the endosomal compartment via the Golgi network. (D) Early stage I melanosomes resemble early endosomes but through unknown mechanisms are specified as a distinct compartment. These melanosomes then undergo maturation through stages II to IV. (E) Melanogenic cargoes such as TYR and TYRP1 are transferred from the early endosome/sorting endosomal compartment to stage II/III melanosomes (TYR) via an AP-3-dependent/BLOC-independent vesicular pathway or (TYRP1) via BLOC-dependent transport through recycling endosome tubules. Inset E' BLOC-1 is required for early elongation of recycling endosome tubules on the actin cytoskeleton and for KIF13A-dependent sustained elongation along microtubules. BLOC-2 then targets these carriers specifically to the melanosome. Inset E'' VAMP7 is the t-SNARE required for fusion of the recycling endosome with the melanosome, allowing delivery of TYRP1 and other melanogenic cargoes. BLOC-3 is required for recycling of VAMP7 back to the recycling endosome.z. (F) After melanogenic cargo has been delivered, melanin synthesis takes place, leading to further maturation of melanosomes.

TRANSFER OF MELANOSOMES TO KERATINOCYTES

Stage IV melanosomes are first transferred to the dendrite tips by kinesin-mediated microtubule-dependent anterograde transport.[156,157] Dynein-mediated retrograde transport of melanosomes away from the melanocyte dendrites has been reported, and the balance of anterograde/retrograde transport may modulate melanosomal distribution after UV expsoure.[157,158] Once the melanosomes reach the actin-rich peripheral dendrite tips, the melanosome is "captured" by a receptor complex to promote peripheral accumulation and eventual transfer to the keratinocyte.[157] The GTPase Rab27a is incorporated into the melanosome membrane by a hydrophobic geranylgeranyl tail. Although Rab membrane association is intimately linked to GTP/GDP cycling, the mechanisms underlying specific targeting of Rab27a to the melanosome membrane are unknown.[159] The adapter protein melanophilin (Mlph) binds Rab27a and serves as a linker to the actin-binding motor protein MyosinVa (MyoVa), allowing transport and retention of melanosomes on the actin cytoskeleton.[160] Disruption of any component of this receptor complex leads to inefficient transfer of melanosomes to surrounding keratinocytes, and mutations in Rab27a, Mlph, and MyoVa have been identified in human patients with Griscelli syndrome (partial albinism and immunodeficiency)[161-163] (Fig. 20-7).

Once accumulated at the dendrite tips, the melanosomes can be transferred to neighboring keratinocytes. Several models have been proposed to mediate this transfer and are supported in varying degrees by experimental evidence. These models include cytophagocytosis, membrane channel, shedding-phagocytosis, and exocytosis models (Fig. 20-8). Several recent papers have given stronger support to the shedding-phagocytosis model, whereby the melanocyte sheds small plasma membrane–bound vesicles containing groups of melanosomes, which are then phagocytosed by the neighboring keratinocyte.[164,165]

Interestingly, activation of some keratinocyte-signaling pathways increases melanosome transfer. Keratinocyte growth factor (KGF), a fibroblast growth factor family member, promotes phagocytosis and transfer of melanosomes from melanocytes to keratinocytes.[166] Protease-activated receptor-2 (PAR2) activation increases phagocytosis and melanosome uptake by keratinocytes.[167] Interestingly, PAR2 expression and activity are highest in keratinocytes derived from those with darker skin type, suggesting a role in regulation of human pigmentation variation.[168]

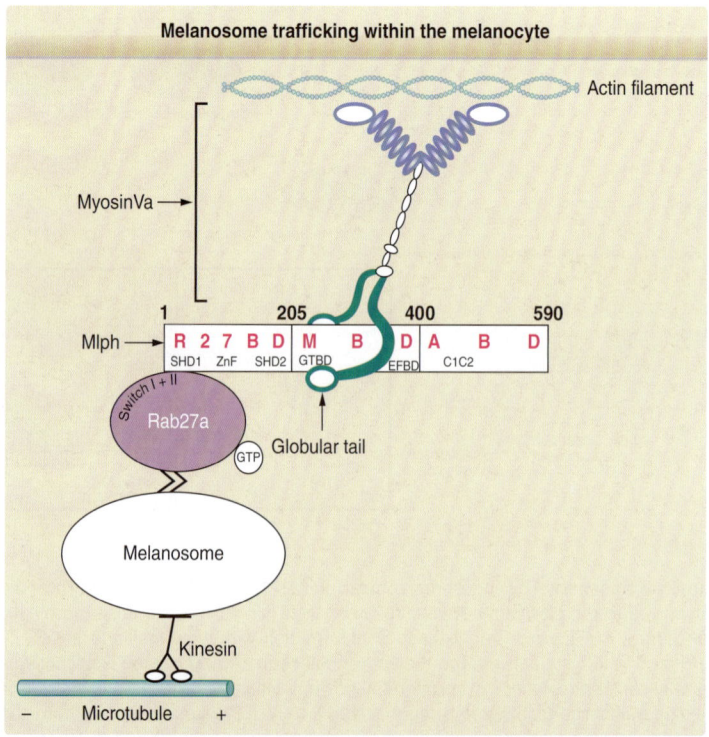

Figure 20-7 Melanosome trafficking within the melanocyte. In melanocytes, activated Rab27a localizes to the surface of mature melanosomes that have been delivered to the cell periphery on microtubules via the motor protein kinesin. On arrival to the cell periphery, melanophilin binds directly to Rab27a. Finally, MyoVa is recruited to the Rab27a–Mlph complex through a direct interaction between the MyoVa globular tail and Mlph. The stable Rab27a–Mlph–MyosinVa complex captures the melanosomes in the actin-rich dendritic tips, a necessary step for retention of the melanosome in the periphery before transfer of melanosomes to the surrounding keratinocytes. (Adapted from Van Gele M, Dynoodt P, Lambert J. Griscelli syndrome: a model system to study vesicular trafficking. *Pigment Cell Melanoma Res*. 2009;22(3):268-82, with permission. Copyright © 2009 John Wiley & Sons.)

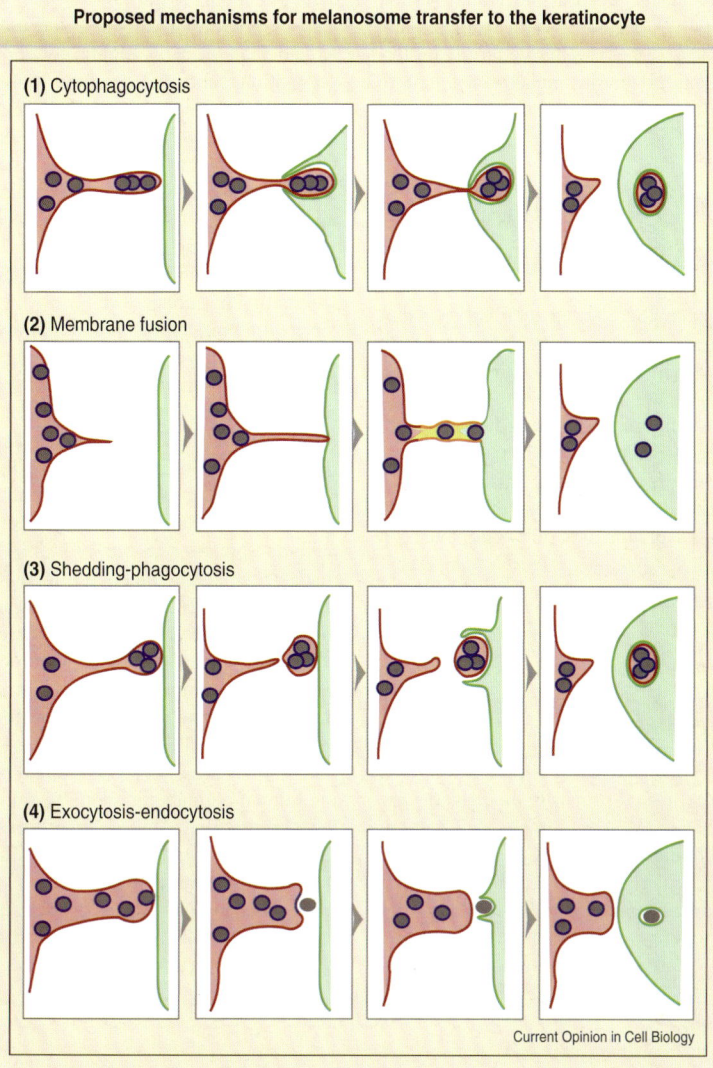

Figure 20-8 Proposed mechanisms for melanosome transfer to the keratinocyte. Cytophagocytosis model—the dendrite tip containing melanosomes is directly phagocytosed by the keratinocyte (KC) membrane. Membrane fusion model—the dendrite tip fuses with the KC membrane forming a channel through which melanosomes are trafficked. Shedding-phagocytosis model—the dendrite tip containing melanosomes buds off and is then engulfed by the KC. Exocytosis-endocytosis—individual melanosomes are exocytosed and then endocytosed by the KC. The limiting membrane of the melanosome (*blue*), the plasma membrane of the melanocyte (*red*), and the plasma membrane of the keratinocyte (*green*). (From Wu X, Hammer JA. Melanosome transfer: it is best to give and receive. *Curr Opin Cell Biol*. 2014;29:1-7, with permission. Copyright © Elsevier.)

TRAFFICKING AND DEGRADATION OF MELANOSOMES WITHIN THE KERATINOCYTE

After transfer to the keratinocyte, melanosomes are transferred by dynein-mediated retrograde transport to a perinuclear location ("nuclear capping") to protect basal keratinocytes from UV-induced DNA damage.[169] It has long been known that although the number of melanocytes does not differ between individuals of different skin types, the number, size, and distribution of melanosomes within keratinocytes shows marked racial variability.[2,170,171] Although melanosomes are primarily situated over the nucleus in all skin types, in light-skinned individuals, melanosomes are smaller, and are grouped in membrane-enclosed clusters of 4 to 8 melanosomes, whereas in darker-skinned individuals, melanosomes are larger, more numerous, and are distributed individually.[2,172] In cell culture, the skin type of the donor keratinocytes regulates the distribution of phagocytosed melanosomes.[173,174]

After localization over the nucleus of basal keratinocytes, melanosomes are thought to be degraded during the keratinocyte terminal differentiation process, as in corneocytes melanosome structures are only rarely identified, even in individuals of the darkest skin types.[175] Several recent studies have demonstrated that keratinocytes derived from darker-skinned individuals degrade melanosomes more slowly, possibly through impairment of autophagy mediated degradation[176,177]

REGULATION OF HUMAN PIGMENTATION VARIATION

In humans and mice, there are genetic variants that favor eumelanogenesis over pheomelanogenesis. In addition, pigmentation can be induced by UV radiation. It has been shown that both the eumelanin/pheomelanin "switch" and UV-induced tanning are regulated by the MSH-MC1R-MITF pathway. The MC1R pathway also regulates other important functions of melanocytes. Other factors that regulate variations in pigmentation of human populations have been recently identified.

MSH-MC1R-MITF PATHWAY

MC1R SIGNALING

Melanocortin 1 receptor (MC1R) is a G-protein–coupled receptor (GPCR) expressed primarily by melanocytes. Similar to other GPCRs, MC1R is composed of 7 alpha-helical transmembrane domains. MC1R signaling has been shown to play a critical role in determining if a melanocyte produces predominantly eumelanin or pheomelanin. It was first discovered that inactivating mutation of *MC1R* was responsible for the reddish coat color phenotype in mice with mutation at the *extension* locus.[178] Soon after, Valverde and colleagues demonstrated that *MC1R* is highly polymorphic in human populations, and that common loss-of-function variants of *MC1R* are associated with the "red hair phenotype" characterized by red hair, fair skin, and inability to tan.[179] Activating mutations that cause constitutive activation of MC1R lead to darkening of coat color in mice.[178]

MC1R signaling is highly regulated by extracellular ligands. The canonical agonist for MC1R is α-melanocyte stimulating hormone (α-MSH). α-MSH is a key regulator of vertebrate pigmentation that was first shown by Lerner and Fitzpatrick to induce pigmentation when injected into human skin.[180] α-MSH is derived from proteolytic processing of its precursor proopiomelanocortin (POMC) (Fig. 20-9). Cleavage of POMC also generates other important signaling ligands, including β-endorphin and ACTH. Human patients with *POMC* gene mutation, in addition to endocrine dysfunction mediated by loss of action of MSH/POMC at MC4R, display the red hair phenotype, mediated by decreased signaling at MC1R.[181] Agouti protein acts as an antagonist (formally described as a "reverse agonist" that can suppress even ligand-independent activity) of MC1R signaling. Activating mutations of agouti leads to increased pheomelanin production and red-blond hair in the mouse.[182,183] Although a role for the homologous human protein agouti signal protein (ASIP) in regulating human pigmentation long remained unidentified, recent studies have linked variants in *ASIP* to skin sensitivity to sun, freckling and red hair, and skin cancer in human populations.[184,185]

As a G coupled protein receptor, it has been demonstrated that MC1R is coupled to the heterotrimeric G protein. Upon activation of MC1R, the Gαs subunit

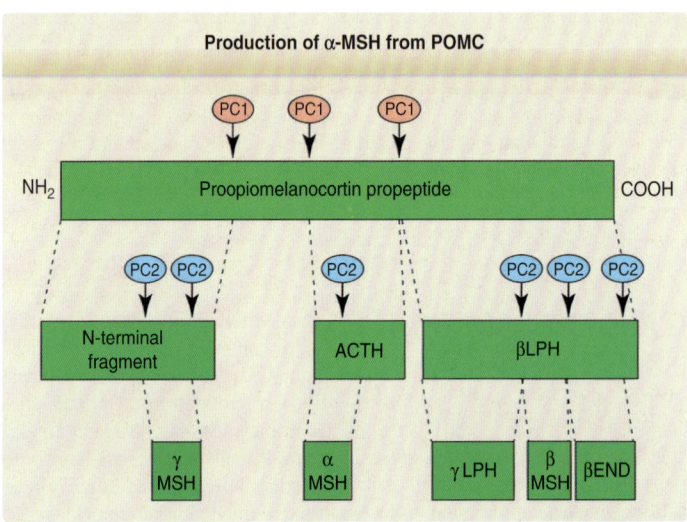

Figure 20-9 Production of α-MSH from POMC. Proopiomelanocortin (POMC) protein is cleaved into by a pair of serine protease pro-protein convertases, PC1 and PC2. PC1 cleaves POMC into 4 subunits, including an N-terminal region from which γ-MSH is derived, adrenocorticotropic hormone (ACTH), and β-lipotropin (β-LPH). α-MSH overlaps with the first 13 amino acids of ACTH and is generated by PC2 cleavage. (From Wolf Horrell EM, Boulanger MC, D'Orazio JA. Melanocortin 1 receptor: structure, function, and regulation. *Front Genet*. 2016 May 31;7:95, with permission.)

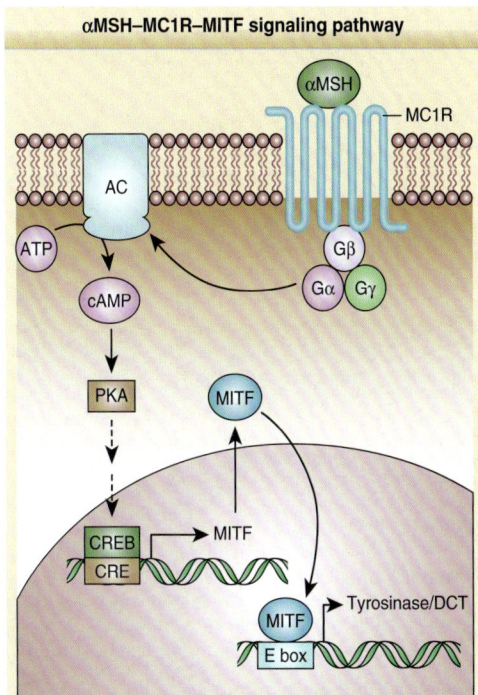

Figure 20-10 αMSH–MC1R–MITF signaling pathway. αMSH binds the melanocortin-1 receptor (MC1R), leading to G-protein activation of adenylyl cyclase. Adenylyl cyclase catalyzes the conversion of cytoplasmic ATP to cyclic AMP (cAMP). Increased intracellular cAMP activates protein kinase A (PKA), which then translocates to the nucleus to phosphorylate the CREB (cAMP-responsive-element binding protein) family of transcription factors. Phosphorylated CREB proteins induce expression of genes, including MITF. MITF binds to the conserved E boxes to induce activation of the expression of pigmentation genes such as tyrosinase and DCT. (Adapted by permission from Springer Nature: Chin L. The genetics of malignant melanoma: lessons from mouse and man. *Nat Rev Cancer*. 3(8)559-70. Copyright © 2003.)

UV-INDUCED TANNING AND THE MC1R PATHWAY

Human pigmentation is categorized into constitutive and inducible responses. Inducible pigmentation after UV exposure (sun tanning) has 2 components that are wavelength dependent. Immediate tanning occurs within minutes to hours after sun exposure, and is mainly a response to UVA radiation. It is most noticeable in darker-skinned individuals and is mediated by oxidation and redistribution of existing melanin. Delayed tanning is mainly a response to UVB and shorter-wavelength UVA radiation and peaks at about 3 days to 1 week after sun exposure. Histologically, delayed tanning is characterized by a modest increase in the number of epidermal melanocytes, increased melanocyte dendricity and transfer of melanosome to keratinocytes, and greater melanization of individual melanosomes.[188] Overall, these factors make delayed tanning much more protective against subsequent sun exposure than immediate tanning.[189]

The inability of individuals with MC1R variants to tan after UV exposure, and the well-known ability of MSH to stimulate pigmentation long suggested a role of the MSH/MC1R pathway in regulation of UV-induced tanning. Studies in mouse models have helped to elucidate the exact nature of this interaction.[121,190] UV radiation of keratinocytes stimulates expression of POMC in a p53 dependent manner (Fig. 20-11). This leads to increased production of α-MSH from the keratinocyte, stimulation of MC1R signaling on the melanocyte, and activation of MITF and melanogenesis (Fig. 20-11). Importantly, in mice with MC1R receptor mutation that have red hair and inability to tan, stimulation of the downstream cAMP/PKA/MITF pathway by application of topical forskolin leads to increased epidermal pigmentation and protection against UV-induced carcinogenesis.[121] This suggests that the pigmentary pathways downstream of a defective MC1R remain intact, providing an opportunity for features of the "red hair phenotype," such as risk of sunburn and melanoma, to be pharmacologically reversed with development of appropriate topical agents.

Another mechanism involved in UV-induced tanning involves the TGFβ pathway. TGFβ1 produced by keratinocytes negatively regulates MITF. UV radiation of keratinocytes decreases TGFβ1 production, ultimately resulting in increased MITF pathway stimulation and increased melanogenesis.[75]

ROLE OF MC1R IN MELANOMAGENESIS

Hypomorphic MC1R variants, in addition to promoting red hair, are strong risk factors for development of human melanoma, leading to a 2- to 4-fold increased melanoma risk. MC1R variants promote pheomelanogenesis and fair skin, suggesting that decreased UV shielding may be responsible for increased melanoma risk.[191,192] However, melanoma risk is enhanced

dissociates and stimulates adenylyl cyclase activity, resulting in formation of the second messenger cyclic AMP (cAMP) from ATP (Fig. 20-10). cAMP binds to and activates protein kinase A (PKA). PKA phosphorylates and activates the transcription factor CREB. CREB binds to target DNA sequences, including those in the m-MITF promoter, increasing transcription of MITF and ultimately resulting in upregulation of MITF target genes related to melanogenesis (Fig. 20-10). Stimulation of MITF by other pathways also has been shown to increase melanogenesis. Phosphodiesterase D4 (PDED4) is transcriptionally activated by MITF in melanocytes and serves as a negative feedback regulator that degrades cAMP. Inhibition of PDED4 activates MITF expression and stimulates pigmentation in red-haired mice, toward dark brown/black melanin.[186] PPAR-gamma coactivator (PGC)-1alpha and PGC-1beta are transcriptional coactivators primarily involved in oxidative metabolism that have been shown to stimulate melanogenesis through upregulation of MITF.[187]

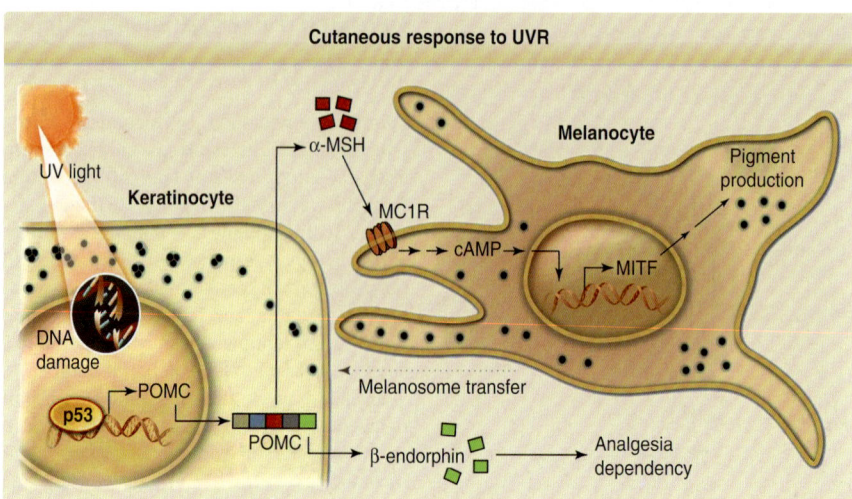

Figure 20-11 Cutaneous response to UVR. Tanning involves p53 activation in keratinocytes in response to UVR-induced DNA damage, leading to p53-mediated upregulation of proopiomelanocortin (POMC). Posttranslational cleavage of POMC produces β-endorphin and α-MSH. Secreted α-MSH stimulates MC1R on adjacent melanocytes, resulting in melanin synthesis and eventual transfer of melanin-containing vesicles (melanosomes) to keratinocytes. Chronic UVR results in elevated circulating β-endorphin levels, leading to analgesia and physical dependence. (Reprinted with permission from AAAS: Lo JA, Fisher DE. The melanoma revolution: from UV carcinogenesis to a new era in therapeutics. *Science*. 2014;346(6212):945-9.)

by MC1R variants even when controlling for degree of skin pigmentation, and missense variants of M1CR less strongly associated to the red hair phenotype still increase melanoma risk, suggesting that other mechanisms must play a role in the increased melanoma risk.[179,193] As discussed above, pheomelanin itself may play an important role in increasing melanoma risk through generation of ROS via UV-dependent and/or UV-independent mechanisms.

Recently, several other cancer-related pathways regulated by MC1R have been identified. MC1R signaling promotes the DNA nucleotide excision repair (NER) pathway, and defective NER may be a cause of the increased risk of melanoma in MC1R variant populations.[194] In support of this hypothesis, melanomas derived from patients with MC1R polymorphism harbor increased numbers of mutations.[195] Wildtype MC1R also protects the tumor suppressor PTEN from UVB-induced degradation. A recent study supports a mechanism whereby increased UVB-mediated PTEN degradation in MC1R-deficient melanocytes promotes melanoma formation.[196]

OTHER FACTORS REGULATING HUMAN PIGMENTATION

In recent years, population genetics studies have identified genetic variants that are associated with variation of skin pigmentation, hair color, and eye color in human populations. Many of these genes, such as *MC1R*, *ASIP*, and *KITLG*, play known roles in melanocyte signaling, and others such as *TYR*, *TYRP1*, *SLC45A2*, and *OCA2* encode genes known to be critical for melanin synthesis.[197,198] However, many novel genes also have been identified. A variant of *SLC24A5* is nearly ubiquitous in European populations and correlates with lighter skin color in other populations.[199,200] *SLC24A5* encodes a putative cation exchanger that is essential for normal pigmentation in cell culture and animal models.[156,201] *TPCN2* variants are associated with hair color variation, and *TPCN2* encodes a cation channel thought to regulate pigmentation through regulating melanosome pH and size.[184,202] Variants of the *Interferon Regulatory Factor 4* (*IRF4*) gene play a key role in regulating human pigmentation, and IRF4 has been shown to act with MITF to stimulate the transcription of tyrosinase.[203,204] Several studies have linked the transcription factor basonuclin 2, a transcription factor known to regulate pigmentation in zebrafish, to human pigmentation variation (BNC2).[205-207]

CONCLUSIONS

Melanocytes are neural crest derived cells that comprise a minority of epidermal cells, but impose major phenotypic changes to the appearance and functionality of skin. They synthesize pigment both constitutively and in response to environmental triggers, and participate in extensive intercellular signaling pathways that regulate production of pigment and often the final disposition of pigment in keratinocytes or the hair matrix. UV protection that is provided by melanocytes is mostly attributable to eumelanin species, whereas pheomelanin and its synthetic pathway not only lack strong UV protection but even contribute to elevated oxidative stress and measurably increased carcinogenicity. Future studies will hopefully identify opportunities to improve on strategies for skin cancer prevention—both for melanoma and non-melanoma skin cancers. Strategies exist which can effectively shield UV species (as in broad spectrum UV filters in sunscreens). Other approaches may attempt to rescue eumelanin synthesis either through use of MSH peptides (or their analogs), or through small molecules that rescue eumelanogenesis downstream of MC1R, in skin from individuals with MC1R variants (ie light skin). Given the fact that skin cancers are among the few human malignancies for which a key carcinogen has been identified, it is hoped that these mechanistic insights may lead to improvements in prevention of skin cancer as well as general photodamage in humans.

REFERENCES

1. Staricco RJ, Pinkus H. Quantitative and qualitative data on the pigment cells of adult human epidermis. *J Invest Dermatol.* 1957;28(1):33-45.
2. Szabo G, Gerald AB, Pathak MA, et al. Racial differences in the fate of melanosomes in human epidermis. *Nature.* 1969;222(5198):1081-1082.
3. Cochran AJ. The incidence of melanocytes in normal human skin. *J Invest Dermatol.* 1970;55(1):65-70.
4. Warkel RL, Luna LG, Helwig EB. A modified Warthin-Starry procedure at low pH for melanin. *Am J Clin Pathol.* 1980;73(6):812-815.
5. Barbosa AJ, Castro LP, Margarida A, et al. A simple and economical modification of the Masson-Fontana method for staining melanin granules and enterochromaffin cells. *Stain Technol.* 1984;59(4):193-196.
6. Cleffmann G. Agouti pigment cells in situ and in vitro. *Ann N Y Acad Sci.* 1963;100:749-761.
7. Bloch B. Das problem der pigmentbildung in der Haut. *Arch Derm Syphilol.* 1917;124:129-208.
8. Jungbluth AA, Iversen K, Coplan K, et al. T311—an anti-tyrosinase monoclonal antibody for the detection of melanocytic lesions in paraffin embedded tissues. *Pathol Res Pract.* 2000;196(4):235-242.
9. King R, Weilbaecher KN, McGill G, et al. Microphthalmia transcription factor. A sensitive and specific melanocyte marker for MelanomaDiagnosis. *Am J Pathol.* 1999;155(3):731-738.
10. Nakajima T, Watanabe S, Sato Y, et al. Immunohistochemical demonstration of S100 protein in malignant melanoma and pigmented nevus, and its diagnostic application. *Cancer.* 1982;50(5):912-918.
11. Gown AM, Vogel AM, Hoak D, et al. Monoclonal antibodies specific for melanocytic tumors distinguish subpopulations of melanocytes. *Am J Pathol.* 1986;123(2):195-203.
12. Du J, Miller AJ, Widlund HR, et al. MLANA/MART1 and SILV/PMEL17/GP100 are transcriptionally regulated by MITF in melanocytes and melanoma. *Am J Pathol.* 2003;163(1):333-343.
13. Tarnowski WM. Ultrastructure of the epidermal melanocyte dense plate. *J Invest Dermatol.* 1970; 55(4):265-268.
14. Moyer FH. In: Smelser GK, ed. *The Structure of the Eye.* New York: Academic Press Inc; 1961.
15. Toshima S, Moore GE, Sandberg AA. Ultrastructure of human melanoma in cell culture. Electron microscopy studies. *Cancer.* 1968;21(2):202-216.
16. Moyer FH. Genetic variations in the fine structure and ontogeny of mouse melanin granules. *Am Zool.* 1966;6(1):43-66.
17. Slominski A, Tobin DJ, Shibahara S, et al. Melanin pigmentation in mammalian skin and its hormonal regulation. *Physiol Rev.* 2004;84(4):1155-1228.
18. Jimbow K, Ishida O, Ito S, et al. Combined chemical and electron microscopic studies of pheomelanosomes in human red hair. *J Invest Dermatol.* 1983;81(6):506-511.
19. Szabo G. The number of melanocytes in human epidermis. *Br Med J.* 1954;1(4869):1016-1017.
20. Gilchrest BA, Blog FB, Szabo G. Effects of aging and chronic sun exposure on melanocytes in human skin. *J Invest Dermatol.* 1979;73(2):141-143.
21. Hendi A, Brodland DG, Zitelli JA. Melanocytes in long-standing sun-exposed skin: quantitative analysis using the MART-1 immunostain. *Arch Dermatol.* 2006;142(7):871-876.
22. Fitzpatrick TB, Breathnach AS. The Epidermal Melanin Unit System [in German]. *Dermatol Wochenschr.* 1963;147:481-489.
23. Ortonne JP, MacDonald DM, Micoud A, et al. PUVA-induced repigmentation of vitiligo: a histochemical (split-DOPA) and ultrastructural study. *Br J Dermatol.* 1979;101(1):1-12.
24. Ortonne JP, Schmitt D, Thivolet J. PUVA-induced repigmentation of vitiligo: scanning electron microscopy of hair follicles. *J Invest Dermatol.* 1980;74(1):40-42.
25. Nishimura EK, Jordan SA, Oshima H, et al. Dominant role of the niche in melanocyte stem-cell fate determination. *Nature.* 2002;416(6883):854-860.
26. Chou WC, Takeo M, Rabbani P, et al. Direct migration of follicular melanocyte stem cells to the epidermis after wounding or UVB irradiation is dependent on Mc1r signaling. *Nat Med.* 2013;19(7):924-929.
27. Yamada T, Hasegawa S, Inoue Y, et al. Wnt/beta-catenin and kit signaling sequentially regulate melanocyte stem cell differentiation in UVB-induced epidermal pigmentation. *J Invest Dermatol.* 2013; 133(12):2753-2762.
28. Takeo M, Lee W, Rabbani P, et al. EdnrB governs regenerative response of melanocyte stem cells by crosstalk with Wnt signaling. *Cell Rep.* 2016;15(6):1291-1302.
29. Nishimura EK, Suzuki M, Igras V, et al. Key roles for transforming growth factor beta in melanocyte stem cell maintenance. *Cell Stem Cell.* 2010;6(2):130-140.
30. Taylor KL, Lister JA, Zeng Z, et al. Differentiated melanocyte cell division occurs in vivo and is promoted by mutations in Mitf. *Development.* 2011;138(16): 3579-3589.
31. Glover JD, Knolle S, Wells KL, et al. Maintenance of distinct melanocyte populations in the interfollicular epidermis. *Pigment Cell Melanoma Res.* 2015;28(4):476-480.
32. Adameyko I, Lallemend F, Aquino JB, et al. Schwann cell precursors from nerve innervation are a cellular origin of melanocytes in skin. *Cell.* 2009;139(2):366-379.
33. Rabbani P, Takeo M, Chou W, et al. Coordinated activation of Wnt in epithelial and melanocyte stem cells initiates pigmented hair regeneration. *Cell.* 2011;145(6):941-955.
34. Sharov A, Tobin DJ, Sharova TY, et al. Changes in different melanocyte populations during hair follicle involution (catagen). *J Invest Dermatol.* 2005;125(6): 1259-1267.
35. Nishimura EK, Granter SR, Fisher DE. Mechanisms of hair graying: incomplete melanocyte stem cell maintenance in the niche. *Science.* 2005;307(5710):720-724.
36. Inomata K, Aoto T, Binh NT, et al. Genotoxic stress abrogates renewal of melanocyte stem cells by triggering their differentiation. *Cell.* 2009;137(6):1088-1099.

37. Okamoto N, Aoto T, Uhara H, et al. A melanocyte–melanoma precursor niche in sweat glands of volar skin. *Pigment Cell Melanoma Res*. 2014;27(6):1039-1050.
38. Oguchi S, Saida T, Koganehira Y, et al. Characteristic epiluminescent microscopic features of early malignant melanoma on glabrous skin. A videomicroscopic analysis. *Arch Dermatol*. 1998;134(5):563-568.
39. Mitchell P, Wang JJ, Foran S, et al. Five-year incidence of age-related maculopathy lesions: the Blue Mountains Eye Study. *Ophthalmology*. 2002;109(6):1092-1097.
40. Ni C, Zhang D, Beyer LA, et al. Hearing dysfunction in heterozygous Mitf(Mi-wh)/+ mice, a model for Waardenburg syndrome type 2 and Tietz syndrome. *Pigment Cell Melanoma Res*. 2013;26(1):78-87.
41. Shibata S, Miwa T, Wu HH, et al. Hepatocyte growth factor-c-MET signaling mediates the development of nonsensory structures of the mammalian cochlea and hearing. *J Neurosci*. 2016;36(31):8200-8209.
42. Levin MD, Lu MM, Petrenko NB, et al. Melanocyte-like cells in the heart and pulmonary veins contribute to atrial arrhythmia triggers. *J Clin Invest*. 2009;119(11):3420-3436.
43. Aoki H, Yamada Y, Hara A, et al. Two distinct types of mouse melanocyte: differential signaling requirement for the maintenance of non-cutaneous and dermal versus epidermal melanocytes. *Development*. 2009;136(15):2511-2521.
44. Curtin JA, Fridlyand J, Kageshita T, et al. Distinct sets of genetic alterations in melanoma. *N Engl J Med*. 2005;353(20):2135-2147.
45. Rawles ME. Origin of pigment cells from the neural crest in the mouse embryo. *Physiol Zool*. 1947;20(3):248-266.
46. Dorris F. The production of pigment by chick neural crest in grafts to the 3-day limb bud. *J Exp Zool*. 1939;80(2):315-345.
47. Serbedzija GN, Fraser SE, Bronner-Fraser M. Pathways of trunk neural crest cell migration in the mouse embryo as revealed by vital dye labelling. *Development*. 1990;108(4):605-612.
48. Weston JA. Sequential segregation and fate of developmentally restricted intermediate cell populations in the neural crest lineage. *Curr Top Dev Biol*. 1991;25:133-153.
49. Opdecamp K, Nakayama A, Nguyen MT, et al. Melanocyte development in vivo and in neural crest cell cultures: crucial dependence on the Mitf basic-helix-loop-helix-zipper transcription factor. *Development*. 1997;124(12):2377-2386.
50. Yoshida H, Kunisada T, Kusakabe M, et al. Distinct stages of melanocyte differentiation revealed by analysis of nonuniform pigmentation patterns. *Development*. 1996;122(4):1207-1214.
51. Hirobe T. Histochemical survey of the distribution of the epidermal melanoblasts and melanocytes in the mouse during fetal and postnatal periods. *Anat Rec (Hoboken)*. 1984;208(4):589-594.
52. Stemple DL, Anderson DJ. Isolation of a stem cell for neurons and glia from the mammalian neural crest. *Cell*. 1992;71(6):973-985.
53. Baroffio A, Dupin E, Le Douarin NM. Clone-forming ability and differentiation potential of migratory neural crest cells. *Proc Natl Acad Sci U S A*. 1988;85(14):5325-5329.
54. Dupin E, Glavieux C, Vaigot P, et al. Endothelin 3 induces the reversion of melanocytes to glia through a neural crest-derived glial-melanocytic progenitor. *Proc Natl Acad Sci U S A*. 2000;97(14):7882-7887.
55. Motohashi T, Yamanaka K, Chiba K, et al. Unexpected multipotency of melanoblasts isolated from murine skin. *Stem Cells*. 2009;27(4):888-897.
56. Baggiolini A, Varum S, Mateos JM, et al. Premigratory and migratory neural crest cells are multipotent in vivo. *Cell Stem Cell*. 2015;16(3):314-322.
57. Singh AP, Dinwiddie A, Mahalwar P, et al. Pigment cell progenitors in zebrafish remain multipotent through metamorphosis. *Dev Cell*. 2016;38(3):316-330.
58. Kaufman CK, Mosimann C, Fan ZP, et al. A zebrafish melanoma model reveals emergence of neural crest identity during melanoma initiation. *Science*. 2016;351(6272):aad2197.
59. Hodgkinson CA, Moore KJ, Nakayama A, et al. Mutations at the mouse microphthalmia locus are associated with defects in a gene encoding a novel basic-helix-loop-helix-zipper protein. *Cell*. 1993;74(2):395-404.
60. Tassabehji M, Newton VE, Read AP. Waardenburg syndrome type 2 caused by mutations in the human microphthalmia (MITF) gene. *Nat Genet*. 1994;8(3):251-255.
61. Yasumoto K, Amae S, Udono T, et al. A big gene linked to small eyes encodes multiple Mitf isoforms: many promoters make light work. *Pigment Cell Res*. 1998;11(6):329-336.
62. Fuse N, Yasumoto K, Suzuki H, et al. Identification of a melanocyte-type promoter of the microphthalmia-associated transcription factor gene. *Biochem Biophys Res Commun*. 1996;219(3):702-707.
63. Aksan I, Goding CR. Targeting the microphthalmia basic helix-loop-helix-leucine zipper transcription factor to a subset of E-box elements in vitro and in vivo. *Mol Cell Biol*. 1998;18(12):6930-6938.
64. McGill GG, Horstmann M, Widlund HR, et al. Bcl2 regulation by the melanocyte master regulator Mitf modulates lineage survival and melanoma cell viability. *Cell*. 2002;109(6):707-718.
65. Haq R, Yokoyama S, Hawryluk EB, et al. BCL2A1 is a lineage-specific antiapoptotic melanoma oncogene that confers resistance to BRAF inhibition. *Proc Natl Acad Sci U S A*. 2013;110(11):4321-4326.
66. Du J, Widlund HR, Horstmann MA, et al. Critical role of CDK2 for melanoma growth linked to its melanocyte-specific transcriptional regulation by MITF. *Cancer Cell*. 2004;6(6):565-576.
67. Garraway LA, Widlund HR, Rubin MA, et al. Integrative genomic analyses identify MITF as a lineage survival oncogene amplified in malignant melanoma. *Nature*. 2005;436(7047):117-122.
68. Yokoyama S, Woods SL, Boyle GM, et al. A novel recurrent mutation in MITF predisposes to familial and sporadic melanoma. *Nature*. 2011;480(7375):99-103.
69. Miller AJ, Levy C, Davis IJ, et al. Sumoylation of MITF and its related family members TFE3 and TFEB. *J Biol Chem*. 2005;280(1):146-155.
70. Epstein DJ, Vekemans M, Gros P. Splotch (Sp2H), a mutation affecting development of the mouse neural tube, shows a deletion within the paired homeodomain of Pax-3. *Cell*. 1991;67(4):767-774.
71. Conway SJ, Henderson DJ, Copp AJ. PAX3 is required for cardiac neural crest migration in the mouse: evidence from the splotch (Sp2H) mutant. *Development*. 1997;124(2):505-514.
72. Tassabehji M, Read AP, Newton VE, et al. Waardenburg's syndrome patients have mutations in the human homologue of the Pax-3 paired box gene. *Nature*. 1992;355(6361):635-636.

73. Hornyak TJ, Hayes DJ, Chiu LY, et al. Transcription factors in melanocyte development: distinct roles for Pax-3 and Mitf. *Mech Dev*. 2001;101(1-2):47-59.
74. Smith MP, Brunton H, Rowling EJ, et al. Inhibiting drivers of non-mutational drug tolerance is a salvage strategy for targeted melanoma therapy. *Cancer Cell*. 2016;29(3):270-284.
75. Yang G, Li Y, Nishimura EK, et al. Inhibition of PAX3 by TGF-beta modulates melanocyte viability. *Mol Cell*. 2008;32(4):554-563.
76. Pingault V, Bondurand N, Kuhlbrodt K, et al. SOX10 mutations in patients with Waardenburg-Hirschsprung disease. *Nat Genet*. 1998;18(2):171-173.
77. Britsch S, Goerich DE, Riethmacher D, et al. The transcription factor SOX10 is a key regulator of peripheral glial development. *Genes Dev*. 2001;15(1):66-78.
78. Potterf SB, Mollaaghababa R, Hou L, et al. Analysis of SOX10 function in neural crest-derived melanocyte development: SOX10-dependent transcriptional control of dopachrome tautomerase. *Dev Biol*. 2001;237(2):245-257.
79. Shakhova O, Zingg D, Schaefer SM, et al. SOX10 promotes the formation and maintenance of giant congenital naevi and melanoma. *Nat Cell Biol*. 2012;14(8):882-890.
80. Harris ML, Buac K, Shakhova O, et al. A dual role for SOX10 in the maintenance of the postnatal melanocyte lineage and the differentiation of melanocyte stem cell progenitors. *PLoS Genet*. 2013;9(7):e1003644.
81. Verastegui C, Bille K, Ortonne JP, et al. Regulation of the microphthalmia-associated transcription factor gene by the Waardenburg syndrome type 4 gene, SOX10. *J Biol Chem*. 2000;275(40):30757-30760.
82. Yu J, Vodyanik MA, Smuga-Otto K, et al. Induced pluripotent stem cell lines derived from human somatic cells. *Science*. 2007;318(5858):1917-1920.
83. Adameyko I, Lallemend F, Furlan A, et al. SOX2 and Mitf cross-regulatory interactions consolidate progenitor and melanocyte lineages in the cranial neural crest. *Development*. 2012;139(2):397-410.
84. Cimadamore F, Shah M, Amador-Arjona A, et al. SOX2 modulates levels of MITF in normal human melanocytes, and melanoma lines in vitro. *Pigment Cell Melanoma Res*. 2012;25(4):533-536.
85. Teng L, Mundell NA, Frist AY, et al. Requirement for Foxd3 in the maintenance of neural crest progenitors. *Development*. 2008;135(9):1615-1624.
86. Nitzan E, Pfaltzgraff ER, Labosky PA, et al. Neural crest and Schwann cell progenitor-derived melanocytes are two spatially segregated populations similarly regulated by Foxd3. *Proc Natl Acad Sci U S A*. 2013;110(31):12709-12714.
87. Edery P, Attie T, Amiel J, et al. Mutation of the endothelin-3 gene in the Waardenburg-Hirschsprung disease (Shah-Waardenburg syndrome). *Nat Genet*. 1996;12(4):442-444.
88. Puffenberger EG, Hosoda K, Washington SS, et al. A missense mutation of the endothelin-B receptor gene in multigenic Hirschsprung's disease. *Cell*. 1994;79(7):1257-1266.
89. Shin MK, Levorse JM, Ingram RS, et al. The temporal requirement for endothelin receptor-B signalling during neural crest development. *Nature*. 1999;402(6761):496-501.
90. Lee HO, Levorse JM, Shin MK. The endothelin receptor-B is required for the migration of neural crest-derived melanocyte and enteric neuron precursors. *Dev Biol*. 2003;259(1):162-175.
91. Yada Y, Higuchi K, Imokawa G. Effects of endothelins on signal transduction and proliferation in human melanocytes. *J Biol Chem*. 1991;266(27):18352-18357.
92. Garcia RJ, Ittah A, Mirabal S, et al. Endothelin 3 induces skin pigmentation in a keratin-driven inducible mouse model. *J Invest Dermatol*. 2008;128(1):131-142.
93. Grabbe J, Welker P, Dippel E, et al. Stem cell factor, a novel cutaneous growth factor for mast cells and melanocytes. *Arch Dermatol Res*. 1994;287(1):78-84.
94. Giebel LB, Spritz RA. Mutation of the KIT (mast/stem cell growth factor receptor) protooncogene in human piebaldism. *Proc Natl Acad Sci U S A*. 1991;88(19):8696-8699.
95. Geissler EN, Ryan MA, Housman DE. The dominant-white spotting (W) locus of the mouse encodes the c-kit proto-oncogene. *Cell*. 1988;55(1):185-192.
96. Matsui Y, Zsebo KM, Hogan BL. Embryonic expression of a haematopoietic growth factor encoded by the Sl locus and the ligand for c-kit. *Nature*. 1990;347(6294):667-669.
97. Hou L, Panthier JJ, Arnheiter H. Signaling and transcriptional regulation in the neural crest-derived melanocyte lineage: interactions between KIT and MITF. *Development*. 2000;127(24):5379-5389.
98. Okura M, Maeda H, Nishikawa S, et al. Effects of monoclonal anti-c-kit antibody (ACK2) on melanocytes in newborn mice. *J Invest Dermatol*. 1995;105(3):322-328.
99. Grichnik JM, Burch JA, Burchette J, et al. The SCF/KIT pathway plays a critical role in the control of normal human melanocyte homeostasis. *J Invest Dermatol*. 1998;111(2):233-238.
100. Wang ZQ, Si L, Tang Q, et al. Gain-of-function mutation of KIT ligand on melanin synthesis causes familial progressive hyperpigmentation. *Am J Hum Genet*. 2009;84(5):672-677.
101. Amyere M, Vogt T, Hoo J, et al. KITLG mutations cause familial progressive hyper- and hypopigmentation. *J Invest Dermatol*. 2011;131(6):1234-1239.
102. Curtin JA, Busam K, Pinkel D, et al. Somatic activation of KIT in distinct subtypes of melanoma. *J Clin Oncol*. 2006;24(26):4340-4346.
103. Hemesath TJ, Price ER, Takemoto C, et al. MAP kinase links the transcription factor Microphthalmia to c-Kit signalling in melanocytes. *Nature*. 1998;391(6664):298-301.
104. Dunn KJ, Williams BO, Li Y, et al. Neural crest-directed gene transfer demonstrates Wnt1 role in melanocyte expansion and differentiation during mouse development. *Proc Natl Acad Sci U S A*. 2000;97(18):10050-10055.
105. Hari L, Miescher I, Shakhova O, et al. Temporal control of neural crest lineage generation by Wnt/beta-catenin signaling. *Development*. 2012;139(12):2107-2117.
106. Widlund HR, Horstmann MA, Price ER, et al. Beta-catenin-induced melanoma growth requires the downstream target Microphthalmia-associated transcription factor. *J Cell Biol*. 2002;158(6):1079-1087.
107. Delmas V, Beermann F, Martinozzi S, et al. Beta-catenin induces immortalization of melanocytes by suppressing p16INK4a expression and cooperates with N-Ras in melanoma development. *Genes Dev*. 2007;21(22):2923-2935.
108. Damsky WE, Curley DP, Santhanakrishnan M, et al. beta-catenin signaling controls metastasis in Braf-activated Pten-deficient melanomas. *Cancer Cell*. 2011;20(6):741-754.

109. Ridley AJ. Rho GTPase signalling in cell migration. *Curr Opin Cell Biol.* 2015;36:103-112.
110. Li A, Ma Y, Yu X, et al. Rac1 drives melanoblast organization during mouse development by orchestrating pseudopod-driven motility and cell-cycle progression. *Dev Cell.* 2011;21(4):722-734.
111. Krauthammer M, Kong Y, Ha BH, et al. Exome sequencing identifies recurrent somatic RAC1 mutations in melanoma. *Nat Genet.* 2012;44(9):1006-1014.
112. Lissanu Deribe Y, Shi Y, Rai K, et al. Truncating PREX2 mutations activate its GEF activity and alter gene expression regulation in NRAS-mutant melanoma. *Proc Natl Acad Sci U S A.* 2016;113(9):E1296-E1305.
113. Lindsay CR, Lawn S, Campbell AD, et al. P-Rex1 is required for efficient melanoblast migration and melanoma metastasis. *Nat Commun.* 2011;2:555.
114. Ozeki H, Ito S, Wakamatsu K, et al. Chemical characterization of hair melanins in various coat-color mutants of mice. *J Invest Dermatol.* 1995;105(3):361-366.
115. Premi S, Wallisch S, Mano CM, et al. Photochemistry. Chemiexcitation of melanin derivatives induces DNA photoproducts long after UV exposure. *Science.* 2015;347(6224):842-847.
116. Tadokoro T, Kobayashi N, Zmudzka BZ, et al. UV-induced DNA damage and melanin content in human skin differing in racial/ethnic origin. *FASEB J.* 2003;17(9):1177-1179.
117. Fleming ID, Barnawell JR, Burlison PE, et al. Skin cancer in black patients. *Cancer.* 1975;35(3):600-605.
118. Bykov VJ, Marcusson JA, Hemminki K. Effect of constitutional pigmentation on ultraviolet B-induced DNA damage in fair-skinned people. *J Invest Dermatol.* 2000;114(1):40-43.
119. Shapiro MP, Keen P, Cohen L, et al. Skin cancer in the South African Bantu. *Br J Cancer.* 1953;7(1):45-57.
120. Yamazaki F, Okamoto H, Miyauchi-Hashimoto H, et al. XPA gene-deficient, SCF-transgenic mice with epidermal melanin are resistant to UV-induced carcinogenesis. *J Invest Dermatol.* 2004;123(1):220-228.
121. D'Orazio JA, Nobuhisa T, Cui R, et al. Topical drug rescue strategy and skin protection based on the role of Mc1r in UV-induced tanning. *Nature.* 2006;443(7109):340-344.
122. Kaidbey KH, Agin PP, Sayre RM, et al. Photoprotection by melanin—a comparison of black and Caucasian skin. *J Am Acad Dermatol.* 1979;1(3):249-260.
123. Wang A, Marino AR, Gasyna Z, et al. Photoprotection by porcine eumelanin against singlet oxygen production. *Photochem Photobiol.* 2008;84(3):679-682.
124. Wenczl E, Van der Schans GP, Roza L, et al. (Pheo)melanin photosensitizes UVA-induced DNA damage in cultured human melanocytes. *J Invest Dermatol.* 1998;111(4):678-682.
125. Panzella L, Szewczyk G, d'Ischia M, et al. Zinc-induced structural effects enhance oxygen consumption and superoxide generation in synthetic pheomelanins on UVA/visible light irradiation. *Photochem Photobiol.* 2010;86(4):757-764.
126. dMitra D, Luo X, Morgan A, et al. An ultraviolet-radiation-independent pathway to melanoma carcinogenesis in the red hair/fair skin background. *Nature.* 2012;491(7424):449-453.
127. Wendt J, Rauscher S, Burgstaller-Muehlbacher S, et al. Human determinants and the role of melanocortin-1 receptor variants in melanoma risk independent of UV radiation exposure. *JAMA Dermatol.* 2016;152(7):776-782.
128. Roider EM, Fisher DE. Red hair, light skin, and UV-independent risk for melanoma development in humans. *JAMA Dermatol.* 2016;152(7):751-753.
129. Fitzpatrick TB, Becker SW Jr, Lerner AB, et al. Tyrosinase in human skin: demonstration of its presence and of its role in human melanin formation. *Science.* 1950;112(2904):223-225.
130. Setty SR, Tenza D, Sviderskaya EV, et al. Cell-specific ATP7A transport sustains copper-dependent tyrosinase activity in melanosomes. *Nature.* 2008;454(7208):1142-1146.
131. Kobayashi T, Hearing VJ. Direct interaction of tyrosinase with Tyrp1 to form heterodimeric complexes in vivo. *J Cell Sci.* 2007;120(pt 24):4261-4268.
132. Potterf SB, Furumura M, Sviderskaya EV, et al. Normal tyrosine transport and abnormal tyrosinase routing in pink-eyed dilution melanocytes. *Exp Cell Res.* 1998;244(1):319-326.
133. Costin GE, Valencia JC, Vieira WD, et al. Tyrosinase processing and intracellular trafficking is disrupted in mouse primary melanocytes carrying the underwhite (uw) mutation. A model for oculocutaneous albinism (OCA) type 4. *J Cell Sci.* 2003;116(pt 15):3203-3212.
134. Du J, Fisher DE. Identification of Aim-1 as the underwhite mouse mutant and its transcriptional regulation by MITF. *J Biol Chem.* 2002;277(1):402-406.
135. Newton JM, Cohen-Barak O, Hagiwara N, et al. Mutations in the human orthologue of the mouse underwhite gene (uw) underlie a new form of oculocutaneous albinism, OCA4. *Am J Hum Genet.* 2001;69(5):981-988.
136. Riley PA. The great DOPA mystery: the source and significance of DOPA in phase I melanogenesis. *Cell Mol Biol (Noisy-le-grand).* 1999;45(7):951-960.
137. Tsukamoto K, Jackson IJ, Urabe K, et al. A second tyrosinase-related protein, TRP-2, is a melanogenic enzyme termed DOPAchrome tautomerase. *EMBO J.* 1992;11(2):519-526.
138. Jimenez-Cervantes C, Solano F, Kobayashi T, et al. A new enzymatic function in the melanogenic pathway. The 5,6-dihydroxyindole-2-carboxylic acid oxidase activity of tyrosinase-related protein-1 (TRP1). *J Biol Chem.* 1994;269(27):17993-18000.
139. Land EJ, Riley PA. Spontaneous redox reactions of dopaquinone and the balance between the eumelanic and phaeomelanic pathways. *Pigment Cell Res.* 2000;13(4):273-277.
140. del Marmol V, Ito S, Bouchard B, et al. Cysteine deprivation promotes eumelanogenesis in human melanoma cells. *J Invest Dermatol.* 1996;107(5):698-702.
141. van Nieuwpoort F, Smit NP, Kolb R, et al. Tyrosine-induced melanogenesis shows differences in morphologic and melanogenic preferences of melanosomes from light and dark skin types. *J Invest Dermatol.* 2004;122(5):1251-1255.
142. Rochin L, Hurbain I, Serneels L, et al. BACE2 processes PMEL to form the melanosome amyloid matrix in pigment cells. *Proc Natl Acad Sci U S A.* 2013;110(26):10658-10663.
143. Berson JF, Harper DC, Tenza D, et al. Pmel17 initiates premelanosome morphogenesis within multivesicular bodies. *Mol Biol Cell.* 2001;12(11):3451-3464.
144. Hurbain I, Geerts WJ, Boudier T, et al. Electron tomography of early melanosomes: implications for melanogenesis and the generation of fibrillar amyloid sheets. *Proc Natl Acad Sci U S A.* 2008;105(50):19726-19731.

145. Jimbow K, Hua C, Gomez PF, et al. Intracellular vesicular trafficking of tyrosinase gene family protein in eu- and pheomelanosome biogenesis. *Pigment Cell Res.* 2000;13(suppl 8):110-117.
146. Raposo G, Tenza D, Murphy DM, et al. Distinct protein sorting and localization to premelanosomes, melanosomes, and lysosomes in pigmented melanocytic cells. *J Cell Biol.* 2001;152(4):809-824.
147. Theos AC, Berson JF, Theos SC, et al. Dual loss of ER export and endocytic signals with altered melanosome morphology in the silver mutation of Pmel17. *Mol Biol Cell.* 2006;17(8):3598-3612.
148. Theos AC, Truschel ST, Tenza D, et al. A lumenal domain-dependent pathway for sorting to intralumenal vesicles of multivesicular endosomes involved in organelle morphogenesis. *Dev Cell.* 2006;10(3):343-354.
149. Delevoye C, Heiligenstein X, Ripoll L, et al. BLOC-1 brings together the actin and microtubule cytoskeletons to generate recycling endosomes. *Curr Biol.* 2016;26(1):1-13.
150. Di Pietro SM, Falcon-Perez JM, Tenza D, et al. BLOC-1 interacts with BLOC-2 and the AP-3 complex to facilitate protein trafficking on endosomes. *Mol Biol Cell.* 2006;17(9):4027-4038.
151. Delevoye C, Hurbain I, Tenza D, et al. AP-1 and KIF13A coordinate endosomal sorting and positioning during melanosome biogenesis. *J Cell Biol.* 2009;187(2):247-264.
152. Dennis MK, Mantegazza AR, Snir OL, et al. BLOC-2 targets recycling endosomal tubules to melanosomes for cargo delivery. *J Cell Biol.* 2015;209(4):563-577.
153. Theos AC, Tenza D, Martina JA, et al. Functions of adaptor protein (AP)-3 and AP-1 in tyrosinase sorting from endosomes to melanosomes. *Mol Biol Cell.* 2005;16(11):5356-5372.
154. Sitaram A, Dennis MK, Chaudhuri R, et al. Differential recognition of a dileucine-based sorting signal by AP-1 and AP-3 reveals a requirement for both BLOC-1 and AP-3 in delivery of OCA2 to melanosomes. *Mol Biol Cell.* 2012;23(16):3178-3192.
155. Dennis MK, Delevoye C, Acosta-Ruiz A, et al. BLOC-1 and BLOC-3 regulate VAMP7 cycling to and from melanosomes via distinct tubular transport carriers. *J Cell Biol.* 2016;214(3):293-308.
156. Hara M, Yaar M, Byers HR, et al. Kinesin participates in melanosomal movement along melanocyte dendrites. *J Invest Dermatol.* 2000;114(3):438-443.
157. Wu X, Bowers B, Rao K, et al. Visualization of melanosome dynamics within wild-type and dilute melanocytes suggests a paradigm for myosin V function In vivo. *J Cell Biol.* 1998;143(7):1899-1918.
158. Byers HR, Yaar M, Eller MS, et al. Role of cytoplasmic dynein in melanosome transport in human melanocytes. *J Invest Dermatol.* 2000;114(5):990-997.
159. Pylypenko O, Goud B. Posttranslational modifications of Rab GTPases help their insertion into membranes. *Proc Natl Acad Sci U S A.* 2012;109(15):5555-5556.
160. Wu XS, Rao K, Zhang H, et al. Identification of an organelle receptor for myosin-Va. *Nat Cell Biol.* 2002;4(4):271-278.
161. Menasche G, Pastural E, Feldmann J, et al. Mutations in RAB27A cause Griscelli syndrome associated with haemophagocytic syndrome. *Nat Genet.* 2000;25(2):173-176.
162. Pastural E, Barrat FJ, Dufourcq-Lagelouse R, et al. Griscelli disease maps to chromosome 15q21 and is associated with mutations in the myosin-Va gene. *Nat Genet.* 1997;16(3):289-292.
163. Menasche G, Ho CH, Sanal O, et al. Griscelli syndrome restricted to hypopigmentation results from a melanophilin defect (GS3) or a MYO5A F-exon deletion (GS1). *J Clin Invest.* 2003;112(3):450-456.
164. Wu XS, Masedunskas A, Weigert R, et al. Melanoregulin regulates a shedding mechanism that drives melanosome transfer from melanocytes to keratinocytes. *Proc Natl Acad Sci U S A.* 2012;109(31):E2101-E2109.
165. Ando H, Niki Y, Ito M, et al. Melanosomes are transferred from melanocytes to keratinocytes through the processes of packaging, release, uptake, and dispersion. *J Invest Dermatol.* 2012;132(4):1222-1229.
166. Cardinali G, Ceccarelli S, Kovacs D, et al. Keratinocyte growth factor promotes melanosome transfer to keratinocytes. *J Invest Dermatol.* 2005;125(6):1190-1199.
167. Sharlow ER, Paine CS, Babiarz L, et al. The protease-activated receptor-2 upregulates keratinocyte phagocytosis. *J Cell Sci.* 2000;113 (pt 17):3093-3101.
168. Babiarz-Magee L, Chen N, Seiberg M, et al. The expression and activation of protease-activated receptor-2 correlate with skin color. *Pigment Cell Res.* 2004;17(3):241-251.
169. Byers HR, Maheshwary S, Amodeo DM, et al. Role of cytoplasmic dynein in perinuclear aggregation of phagocytosed melanosomes and supranuclear melanin cap formation in human keratinocytes. *J Invest Dermatol.* 2003;121(4):813-820.
170. Konrad K, Wolff K. Hyperpigmentation, melanosome size, and distribution patterns of melanosomes. *Arch Dermatol.* 1973;107(6):853-860.
171. Alaluf S, Atkins D, Barrett K, et al. Ethnic variation in melanin content and composition in photoexposed and photoprotected human skin. *Pigment Cell Res.* 2002;15(2):112-118.
172. Thong HY, Jee SH, Sun CC, et al. The patterns of melanosome distribution in keratinocytes of human skin as one determining factor of skin colour. *Br J Dermatol.* 2003;149(3):498-505.
173. Minwalla L, Zhao Y, Le Poole IC, et al. Keratinocytes play a role in regulating distribution patterns of recipient melanosomes in vitro. *J Invest Dermatol.* 2001;117(2):341-347.
174. Yoshida Y, Hachiya A, Sriwiriyanont P, et al. Functional analysis of keratinocytes in skin color using a human skin substitute model composed of cells derived from different skin pigmentation types. *FASEB J.* 2007;21(11):2829-2839.
175. Goldschmidt H, Raymond JZ. Quantitative analysis of skin color from melanin content of superficial skin cells. *J Forensic Sci.* 1972;17(1):124-131.
176. Ebanks JP, Koshoffer A, Wickett RR, et al. Epidermal keratinocytes from light vs. dark skin exhibit differential degradation of melanosomes. *J Invest Dermatol.* 2011;131(6):1226-1233.
177. Murase D, Hachiya A, Takano K, et al. Autophagy has a significant role in determining skin color by regulating melanosome degradation in keratinocytes. *J Invest Dermatol.* 2013;133(10):2416-2424.
178. Robbins LS, Nadeau JH, Johnson KR, et al. Pigmentation phenotypes of variant extension locus alleles result from point mutations that alter MSH receptor function. *Cell.* 1993;72(6):827-834.
179. Valverde P, Healy E, Jackson I, et al. Variants of the melanocyte-stimulating hormone receptor gene are associated with red hair and fair skin in humans. *Nat Genet.* 1995;11(3):328-330.

180. Lerner AB, McGuire JS. Effect of alpha- and beta-melanocyte stimulating hormones on the skin colour of man. *Nature*. 1961;189:176-179.
181. Krude H, Biebermann H, Luck W, et al. Severe early-onset obesity, adrenal insufficiency and red hair pigmentation caused by POMC mutations in humans. *Nat Genet*. 1998;19(2):155-157.
182. Duhl DM, Vrieling H, Miller KA, et al. Neomorphic agouti mutations in obese yellow mice. *Nat Genet*. 1994;8(1):59-65.
183. Voisey J, van Daal A. Agouti: from mouse to man, from skin to fat. *Pigment cell Res*. 2002;15(1):10-18.
184. Sulem P, Gudbjartsson DF, Stacey SN, et al. Two newly identified genetic determinants of pigmentation in Europeans. *Nat Genet*. 2008;40(7):835-837.
185. Gudbjartsson DF, Sulem P, Stacey SN, et al. ASIP and TYR pigmentation variants associate with cutaneous melanoma and basal cell carcinoma. *Nat Genet*. 2008;40(7):886-891.
186. Khaled M, Levy C, Fisher DE. Control of melanocyte differentiation by a MITF-PDE4D3 homeostatic circuit. *Genes Dev*. 2010;24(20):2276-2281.
187. Shoag J, Haq R, Zhang M, et al. PGC-1 coactivators regulate MITF and the tanning response. *Mol Cell*. 2013;49(1):145-157.
188. Tadokoro T, Yamaguchi Y, Batzer J, et al. Mechanisms of skin tanning in different racial/ethnic groups in response to ultraviolet radiation. *J Invest Dermatol*. 2005;124(6):1326-1332.
189. Coelho SG, Yin L, Smuda C, et al. Photobiological implications of melanin photoprotection after UVB-induced tanning of human skin but not UVA-induced tanning. *Pigment Cell Melanoma Res*. 2015;28(2):210-216.
190. Cui R, Widlund HR, Feige E, et al. Central role of p53 in the suntan response and pathologic hyperpigmentation. *Cell*. 2007;128(5):853-864.
191. Peles DN, Simon JD. The ultraviolet absorption coefficient of melanosomes decreases with increasing pheomelanin content. *J Phys Chem B*. 2010;114(29):9677-9683.
192. Peles DN, Simon JD. The UV-absorption spectrum of human iridal melanosomes: a new perspective on the relative absorption of eumelanin and pheomelanin and its consequences. *Photochem Photobiol*. 2012;88(6):1378-1384.
193. Raimondi S, Sera F, Gandini S, et al. MC1R variants, melanoma and red hair color phenotype: a meta-analysis. *Int J Cancer*. 2008;122(12):2753-2760.
194. Jarrett SG, Wolf Horrell EM, Christian PA, et al. PKA-mediated phosphorylation of ATR promotes recruitment of XPA to UV-induced DNA damage. *Mol Cell*. 2014;54(6):999-1011.
195. Robles-Espinoza CD, Roberts ND, Chen S, et al. Germline MC1R status influences somatic mutation burden in melanoma. *Nat Commun*. 2016;7:12064.
196. Cao J, Wan L, Hacker E, et al. MC1R is a potent regulator of PTEN after UV exposure in melanocytes. *Mol Cell*. 2013;51(4):409-422.
197. Kenny EE, Timpson NJ, Sikora M, et al. Melanesian blond hair is caused by an amino acid change in TYRP1. *Science*. 2012;336(6081):554.
198. Anno S, Abe T, Yamamoto T. Interactions between SNP alleles at multiple loci contribute to skin color differences between caucasoid and mongoloid subjects. *Int J Biol Sci*. 2008;4(2):81-86.
199. Lamason RL, Mohideen MA, Mest JR, et al. SLC24A5, a putative cation exchanger, affects pigmentation in zebrafish and humans. *Science*. 2005;310(5755):1782-1786.
200. Basu Mallick C, Iliescu FM, Mols M, et al. The light skin allele of SLC24A5 in South Asians and Europeans shares identity by descent. *PLoS Genet*. 2013;9(11):e1003912.
201. Ginger RS, Askew SE, Ogborne RM, et al. SLC24A5 encodes a trans-Golgi network protein with potassium-dependent sodium-calcium exchange activity that regulates human epidermal melanogenesis. *J Biol Chem*. 2008;283(9):5486-5495.
202. Ambrosio AL, Boyle JA, Aradi AE, et al. TPC2 controls pigmentation by regulating melanosome pH and size. *Proc Natl Acad Sci U S A*. 2016;113(20):5622-5627.
203. Han J, Kraft P, Nan H, et al. A genome-wide association study identifies novel alleles associated with hair color and skin pigmentation. *PLoS Genet*. 2008;4(5):e1000074.
204. Praetorius C, Grill C, Stacey SN, et al. A polymorphism in IRF4 affects human pigmentation through a tyrosinase-dependent MITF/TFAP2A pathway. *Cell*. 2013;155(5):1022-1033.
205. Visser M, Palstra RJ, Kayser M. Human skin color is influenced by an intergenic DNA polymorphism regulating transcription of the nearby BNC2 pigmentation gene. *Hum Mol Genet*. 2014;23(21):5750-5762.
206. Jacobs LC, Wollstein A, Lao O, et al. Comprehensive candidate gene study highlights UGT1A and BNC2 as new genes determining continuous skin color variation in Europeans. *Hum Genet*. 2013;132(2):147-158.
207. Lang MR, Patterson LB, Gordon TN, et al. Basonuclin-2 requirements for zebrafish adult pigment pattern development and female fertility. *PLoS Genet*. 2009;5(11):e1000744.

Chapter 21 :: Neurobiology of the Skin :: Sonja Ständer, Manuel P. Pereira, & Thomas A. Luger

第二十一章
皮肤神经生物学

中文导读

本章分5节：①皮肤神经系统；②瘙痒神经生物学；③神经系统在皮肤病中的作用；④瘙痒；⑤结论与展望。

第一节皮肤神经系统，介绍了皮肤神经的解剖、感觉神经的功能亚群，并提到了皮肤C类和A类纤维在瘙痒中的作用，灼热、疼痛、瘙痒、温暖和触觉是由C类纤维传递的。同时介绍了皮肤感觉神经的传出功能、自主神经功能以及脊髓在瘙痒及疼痛信号传导中的作用。

第二节瘙痒神经生物学，介绍了皮肤神经纤维配备的几个不同的受体类别，GPCRs、瞬时受体电位通道、细胞因子和Toll样受体主要存在于瘙痒感受器上。内皮素、细胞因子、白三烯、神经肽、5-羟色胺和前列腺素是已知导致瘙痒的介质。目前慢性瘙痒的病理生理机制尚不清楚，但急性瘙痒的机制更为明显。角质形成细胞、肥大细胞和炎症细胞在瘙痒的诱导和维持中起重要作用。

第三节神经系统在皮肤病中的作用，介绍了特应性皮炎、结节性痒疹、寻常型银屑病、酒渣鼻、带状疱疹、荨麻疹和伤口愈合是具有重要的神经源性成分的皮肤病。神经介质通过刺激成纤维细胞和角质形成细胞的产生以及血管生成来协助伤口愈合过程。神经肽具有刺激人肥大细胞和诱导荨麻疹的能力。感觉神经和肥大细胞表达Trp离子通道，该通道可由导致荨麻疹的温暖、寒冷和食物过敏原等因素触发。

第四节瘙痒，介绍了瘙痒的分型和临床表现及治疗方法、新药。推荐采用循序渐进的方法治疗慢性瘙痒。首先采取基本的措施，其次如果确定瘙痒来源，行针对性的治疗，若病因不明或靶向治疗不成功，建议进行对症局部治疗或全身治疗。此外，提出可以治疗瘙痒的新药有NK1R拮抗药、RPV1和酪氨酸受体激酶A、κ阿片受体激动药等。

第五节结论与展望，介绍了神经系统可以控制皮肤的动态平衡。神经调节药既可以促炎，也可以抗炎。总结了慢性瘙痒症可能病因非常多，除了采取基本的治疗措施，需对潜在疾病实施有针对性的治疗。针对各种靶点的拮抗药尤其是胆汁酸转运体抑制药治疗胆汁淤积性瘙痒具有巨大前景。

〔粟 娟〕

AT-A-GLANCE

- The nervous system of the skin has multiple functions:
  - Collecting and transmitting environmental information on touch, pain, pruritus and temperature to the brain.
  - Reacting to ligands that induce nerve activation by the antidromic release of neuropeptides and initiation of vascular and inflammatory reactions.
  - Communication with various skin cells, including those in the immune and endocrine systems.
  - Because of these, it also has a role in maintaining skin homeostasis and processes including thermoregulation, cell growth, inflammation, host defense mechanisms, apoptosis, and wound healing.
  - In pathological conditions, the nervous system is involved in the maintenance of pruritus, pain, and inflammatory skin diseases (eg, psoriasis vulgaris, atopic dermatitis).

INTRODUCTION

The skin has a dense sensory network enabling human beings to sense different ranges and qualities of pain, pruritus, mechanical stimuli (eg, touch and vibration), and temperature. These senses have a role in the nonverbal communication among humans and also serve as protective mechanisms as they organize sensations taken from the environment that are sent to the brain. The brain not only plays a critical role in the perception of these sensations but also in their interpretation as pleasant, unpleasant, dangerous, or harmless. The skin contains a dense cutaneous sensory and autonomic network designed to sense these stimuli that also communicates with surrounding skin cells and has a bidirectional communication network within the central nervous system (CNS). This complex network is known to play a central role in the development of chronic pain and, as recently discovered, also in chronic pruritus. The latter constitutes a novel research area and is a major focus of this chapter.

THE CUTANEOUS NERVOUS SYSTEM

ANATOMY OF CUTANEOUS NERVES

Barring the stratum corneum, the entirety of the human skin is innervated. The nerves that innervate the skin, apart from the face, consist of cutaneous branches of musculocutaneous nerves that segmentally arise from the spinal nerves. Branches of trigeminal nerves in the facial tissue are responsible for its innervation. At the dermal subcutaneous junction, the primary nerve trunks enter the subcutaneous fat tissue and divide, forming a branching network. This nerve plexus supplies the vasculature, adnexal structures, and encapsulated sensory nerves (eg, Pacinian corpuscles). The nerve fibers subsequently rearrange into small nerve bundles, which, together with the blood and lymphatic vessels, form a network of interlaced nerves both beneath and within the epidermis (Fig. 21-1).[1,2] Sensory and autonomic nerve fibers constitute cutaneous nerve fibers. Afferent impulses are conducted from the periphery of sensory nerves to cell bodies in the dorsal root ganglia (DRG) and to the trigeminal ganglion in the face. Because of their unipolar nature, one branch of a cutaneous sensory neuron's single axon extends from their cell body towards the periphery, and the other extends toward the CNS. Sensory innervation is arranged into well-defined segments called dermatomes; however, an overlapping innervation can possibly occur. The skin is innervated by autonomic nerves in a dissimilar manner: a sequential two-neuron pathway is built between preganglionic fibers of spinal nerves that synapse with postganglionic fibers before innervating the target organ such as skin glands, blood vessels, and arrector pili muscles.[3]

The free nerve endings of sensory nerve fibers are found in the epidermis and papillary dermis (Fig. 21-2). Region-specific differences concerning the nerve fiber innervation density and specificity can be observed from the proximal to distal parts of the body. Specific structures (eg, the hair disk ie, an epithelial thickening around hair follicles) and encapsulated endings, such as the Ruffini and Pacinian corpuscles, as well as Meissner and Krause corpuscles, are equipped with sensory nerves and are able to sense different types of mechanical stimuli (vibration, pressure, and so on). Sensory nerves in the epidermis are in close vicinity to keratinocytes, melanocytes, Langerhans cells, and Merkel cells. Electron and confocal microscopy have

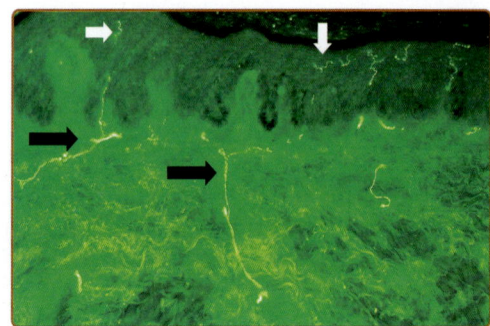

Figure 21-1 Skin nerve fibers (immunostaining with protein gene product 9.5). Dermal nerves (*black arrows*) are myelinated and thicker than intraepidermal nerves (*white arrows*). Dermal nerves from branches enter the epidermis and innervate all vital epidermal layers except the stratum corneum.

demonstrated that intraepidermal neurons are in contact with keratinocytes due to their slight invagination into keratinocyte cytoplasm. The keratinocytes' adjacent plasma membranes have been found to be slightly thickened, similar to postsynaptic membrane specializations in nervous tissues.[4,5] Autonomic nerves, in contrast to sensory nerves, do not innervate the mammalian epidermis.

FUNCTIONAL SUBGROUPS OF SENSORY NERVES

An array of physiological and pathophysiological functions in the skin is influenced by both sensory and autonomic nerves, including embryogenesis, vessel function regulation (vasoconstriction, vasodilation), body temperature and subsidiary mechanisms (eccrine and apocrine gland and erector pili activity), the perception of physical, chemical and biological stimuli on the skin's surface, epidermal barrier function modulation, nerve development, inflammation, immune defenses, and wound healing. Cutaneous nerves perform said functions with the assistance of afferent (pruritus detection, pain, touch, temperature, and so on) and efferent (neuropeptide release in the skin) mechanisms. The epidermis and peripheral nervous system serve as the skin's sensory forefront. Cutaneous nerves transmit essential information to the CNS following contact or injury by parasites and their toxins, allergens, chemicals, ultraviolet radiation, pH alterations, and stress. These are considered to be the skin's natural protective mechanisms and are normally accompanied by a reaction such as an increased focus on the affected skin area, as well as scratching or the need to restrain oneself. The transmitted information can, at various CNS levels, be modulated to include the brain, spinal cord, autonomic neurons, and DRG..[6,7]

Cutaneous nerves and their respective mediators impact normal cutaneous biological processes such as postnatal skin homeostasis and prenatal skin development. The pathophysiology of a variety of systemic

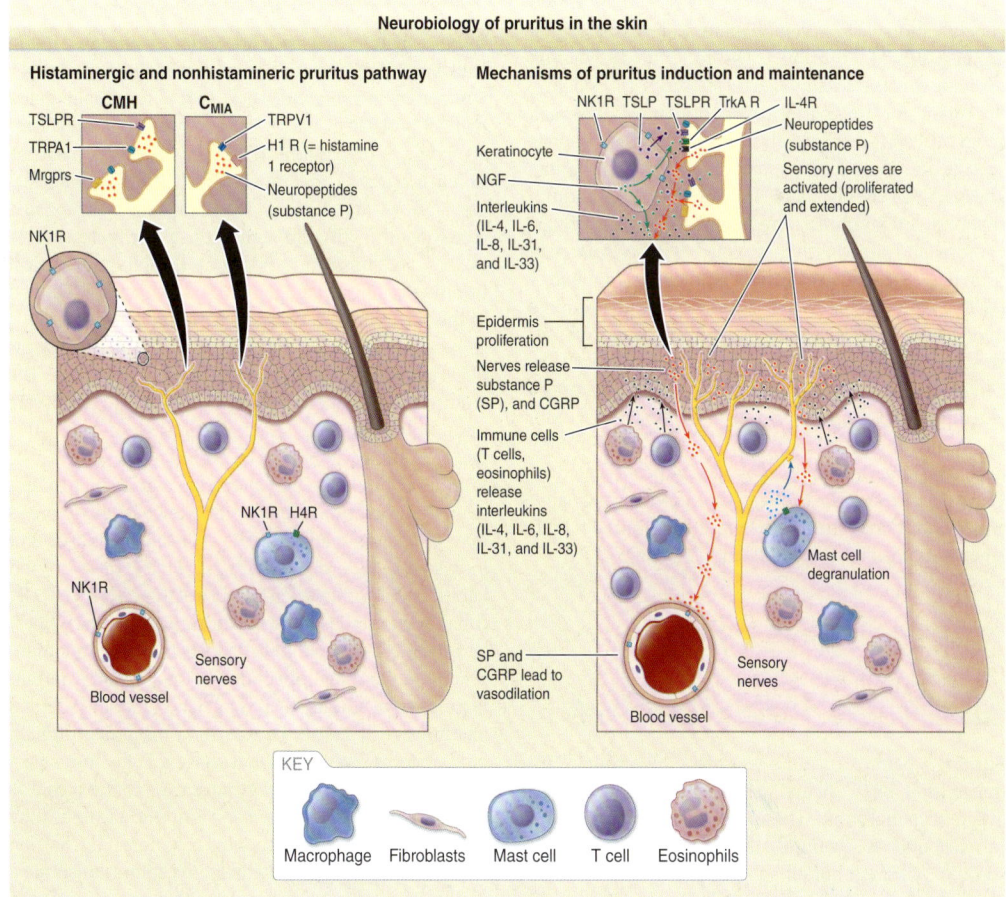

Figure 21-2 Cutaneous nerve system in normal and diseased skin. **A,** Normal skin. **B,** Pruritus. CGRP, calcitonin gene-related peptide; CMH, C mechano-heat sensitive; C_{MIA}, C mechano-insensitive afferences; H4R, Histamine 4 Receptor; IL, interleukin; Mrgprs, Mas-related G-protein coupled receptors; NGF, nerve growth factor; NK1R, neurokinin-1 receptor; TrkA, Tropomyosin receptor kinase A; TRPA1, Transient receptor potential ankyrin 1; TRPV1, transient receptor potential vanilloid 1; TSLP, thymic stromal lymphopoietin; TSLPR, thymic stromal lymphopoietin receptor.

and skin diseases, ranging from chronic pruritus to chronic pain syndromes, are additionally affected by cutaneous nerves. It is suspected that interactions between the peripheral nervous system and CNS are involved in thermoregulation and the pathophysiology of various skin diseases, including psoriasis, atopic dermatitis and acne, wound healing, and hair loss and regrowth.

As a stress response to external or endogenous stimuli, pathophysiological and physiological processes are modulated by autonomic nerves, forming an essential communicative link with the endocrine, immune, and vascular systems.

Contingent upon the extent of their myelination, the function of cutaneous sensory nerves can be assigned to various groups, including conduction velocity, response to trophic stimuli (eg, glial cell line–derived neurotrophic factor and nerve growth factor), and neuropeptide and neuroreceptor expression: (1) Aβ sensory fibers, myelinated to a moderate degree (6 to 12 μm nerve fiber diameter) and able to stimulate touch receptors; (2) Aδ fibers, which have a thin myelin coating (1 to 5 μm diameter) and exhibit an intermediate conduction velocity (4 to 30 m/sec), as well as mediate cold and quick pain sensations and pressure; and (3) unmyelinated, thin (0.2 to 1.5 μm diameter), slow-conducting C fibers (0.5 to 2.0 m/sec). The receptor distribution of these diverse sensory nerve subtypes is evidently important for the performance of various thermal, chemical, and mechanical functions and sensations such as burning, pruritus, pain, prickling, and stinging. The $Na_v1.8$ (SNS/PN3) and $Na_v1.9$ (SNS/SNS2) sodium channels, for example, are expressed by peptidergic neurons and are closely associated with certain pain subtypes. The transient receptor potential vanilloid 1 (TRPV1) ion channel is expressed by C and Aδ nerve fiber classes.[8] TRPV1 belongs to a group of thermosensors that are expressed on keratinocytes and sensory nerves. These thermosensors perceive diverse ranges of temperature, ranging from cold (TRPA1 and TRPM8) to warmth and heat (TRPV1 to TRPV4). Furthermore, heat, pain, and pruritus are also able to be mediated by TRPV1 activation. The CNS can thus discern the quality and localization of incoming signals transmitted by different neurons thanks to this complex system.

ROLE OF CUTANEOUS C AND A FIBERS IN PRURITUS

Burning, pain, pruritus, warmth, and touch are transmitted by C fibers, which are organized into different subgroups. These polymodal nociceptors can respond to chemical, mechanical, and thermal stimuli,[9] although not all subgroups are able to sense the full range of said stimuli. Two subgroups of C fibers that perform as pruriceptors mediate pruritus, of which one subgroup responds to histamine signaling through phospholipase-β3 (PLCβ3) and the ion channel TRPV1. This same subgroup, called C_{MIA} (C mechano-insensitive afferences), is insensitive to mechanical stimuli. The second C fiber subgroup is responsive to pruritic stimuli such as cowhage. They are named CMH (C mechano-heat sensitive) because of their responsiveness to heat and mechanical stimuli. Recent studies suggest that Aδ fibers can, upon activation of several pruritogens, also transmit pruritus (Fig. 21-3). Although these subgroups of pruritus-transmitting cutaneous nerves have been validated in humans, other molecular signatures of pruritus-transmitting subpopulations of nerves have been identified in animals, and mostly on the spinal level, such as with the recent discovery of gastrin-releasing peptide (GRP)/GRP receptor and natriuretic polypeptide B (Nppb), and its corresponding receptor, natriuretic peptide receptor A (Npra), as well as somatostatin and neurons expressing the receptor tyrosine kinase Ret.[10,11]

EFFERENT FUNCTION OF CUTANEOUS SENSORY NERVES

More than 20 neuropeptides, among them substance P (SP), neurotensin, neurokinin A (NKA), vasoactive intestinal peptide (VIP), calcitonin gene-related peptide (CGRP), pituitary adenylate cyclase-activating polypeptide (PACAP), peptide histidine isoleucine amide, neuropeptide Y (NPY), somatostatin (SST), dynorphin, β-endorphin, encephalin, secretoneurin, thyroid-stimulating hormone (TSH), melanocyte-stimulating hormone (MSH), and corticotropin-releasing hormone (CRH), have been identified in the skin, either in sensory nerves or other cells such as keratinocytes. Cytoplasmic vesicles store neuropeptides in unstimulated cutaneous sensory nerves. The antidromic activation of the peptidergic C_{MIA} fibers can, upon stimulation, generate the release of vasoactive neuropeptides (eg, SP and CGRP). Their release can, as a result of autocrine and paracrine signaling, produce neurogenic inflammation by initiating vasodilation and mast cell degranulation. Nerve fibers are thus capable of influencing epidermal growth, cytokine expression, and keratinocyte proliferation because of this efferent effect.[12] It has been established that unmyelinated nerve fibers and mast cells have a direct connection and communication via these neuropeptides in the papillary dermis. Experimental studies have established that intradermal injections of SP cause the release of histamine through binding to its receptor on mast cells, thereby inducing a pruritogenic effect. However, it remains controversial as to whether this same connection is applicable to healthy human skin.[13] G protein–coupled receptors (GPCRs), ion channels, and particular cytokine receptors constitute a variety of neuropeptide receptors that are expressed in different cutaneous cells and are thus targets of released neuropeptides. In addition, keratinocytes, Merkel cells, microvascular endothelial cells, leukocytes, and fibroblasts are cutaneous cells that release neuropeptides

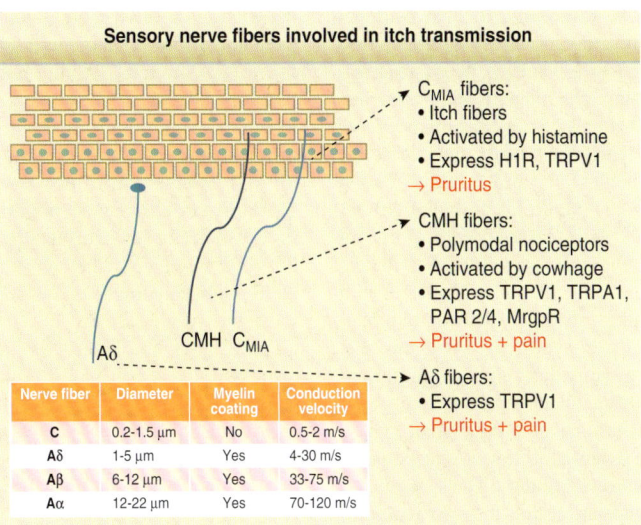

Figure 21-3 Sensory nerve fibers involved in itch transmission. C and Aδ fibers are responsible for peripheral itch transmission. Two subgroups of C fibers have been identified. Intraepidermal mechano-insensitive afferences (C_{MIA}) are activated by histamine via the TRPV1 ion channel, and mechano-heat sensitive C-fibers (CMH) respond to cowhage and express TRPV1, TRPA1, PAR2 2/4, and Mas-related G protein–coupled receptors (Mrgprs). CMH fibers also act as polymodal nociceptors. Recently, the role of Aδ fibers, which also express TRPV1, has been acknowledged in itch transmission. Properties of peripheral nerve fibers are shown in the table. (Table from Chuquilin M, Alghalith Y, Fernandez KH. Neurocutaneous disease: Cutaneous neuroanatomy and mechanisms of itch and pain. *J Am Acad Dermatol*. 2016;74:197-212, with permission. Copyright © American Academy of Dermatology.)

under certain physiological and pathophysiological circumstances. Endopeptidases (ie, neutral endopeptidase, endothelin converting enzyme, and angiotensin-converting enzyme) are widely expressed in the skin, degrade the neuropeptides, and terminate neuropeptide-induced inflammatory and immune responses.

Neuropeptides and their high affinity receptors are essential for retaining and restoring tissue integrity, as well as regulating the skin's pathophysiological conditions. As a result, it has become apparent that a greater understanding of the skin and nervous systems' complex interactions can provide improved therapeutic approaches to skin diseases in the future. Current information demonstrates that the skin's neuronal network has a vital role in influencing a diverse range of physiological and pathophysiological functions, including host defense, inflammation, pruritus, pain, burning, wound healing, and perhaps cancer (eg, by means of modulating angiogenesis).

AUTONOMIC NERVES

Autonomic nerves, compared to sensory nerves, represent a smaller fraction of cutaneous nerve fibers. Autonomic nerve fibers in human skin are seldom derived from parasympathetic neurons but are instead nearly entirely composed of sympathetic neurons. These nerve fibers innervate arteriovenous anastomoses, blood vessels, apocrine glands, lymphatic vessels, erector pili muscles, eccrine glands, and hair follicles and are strictly distributed throughout the dermis. Autonomic nerves induce their effects primarily through releasing classic neurotransmitters (eg, acetylcholine and noradrenaline) and, to a lesser extent, certain neuropeptides, including VIP, NPY, and atrial natriuretic peptide.

The cutaneous autonomic nervous system influences the function of sweat glands and thus regulates body temperature, water modulation, and the maintenance of electrolyte balance in many organs. Noradrenaline, NPY, or both is released by sympathetic nerve fibers to innervate arteriovenous anastomoses, arterioles, and venous sinusoids, resulting in vasoconstriction. Parasympathetic nerve fibers, in contrast, mediate vasodilation via activation of the venous sinusoids. The release of acetylcholine and VIP or peptide histidine methionine assists in this process. Sensory and autonomic nerve fibers are closely associated with dermal blood vessels. These vessels not only synthesize neuropeptides but also express receptors for neuropeptides. The seemingly most innervated regions consist of arterial sections of the arteriovenous anastomoses, arteries, capillaries, metarterioles, and precapillary sphincters. Considerable increases in the skin's blood flow provide the necessary quantity of convective heat loss during heat illness and physical activity. Reflex cutaneous vasoconstriction is necessary to hinder excessive heat dispersion during exposure to cold temperatures. Sensory nerves are essential for vasodilation. Oppositely, neuropeptides composed of sympathetic neurons (eg, NPY) mediate vasoconstriction, thus adopting a key role in several processes, including thermoregulation, the control of blood flow during inflammation and tumorigenesis, and endothelial and smooth muscle cell activation. Both cell types have been found to be responsive to both neuronal modulation in inflammatory diseases (eg, atopic dermatitis) and host defense mechanisms, neovascularization, and wound healing. The function of the apocrine, sebaceous, and sweat glands, as well as the pilosebaceous unit, is modulated by the sensory and autonomic nerves. Autonomic nerves are, under certain pathophysiological conditions, implicated in hyperhidrosis and hypohidrosis and play a pathological role in congenital diseases (eg, progressive segmental hypohidrosis and congenital sensory neuropathy type IV) and a host of other conditions, including diabetic neuropathy, complex regional pain syndrome, syringomyelia, and dysfunction after sympathectomy. It is important to note that through upregulation of the corresponding receptors during trauma or inflammation, Ciber nociceptors have the potential to develop responsiveness to adrenergic neurotransmitters. The sensory and autonomic nervous systems are thus proven to communicate and interact with diseases on a molecular level.

SPINAL CORD

Ascending afferent and descending inhibitory neurons, as well as interneurons, constitute the complex neuroanatomy of the spinal cord and, principally, the circuitry transmitting pruritus and pain signals. Pruritus transmission has been primarily studied in animal models and through clinical observations of affected patients. Both methods have provided valuable information on pruritus mechanisms in humans. The spinal cord's spinothalamic tract and other common ascending sensory pathways are shared in both pruritus and pain.[6] Many functions in pruritus and pain processing differ, although both symptoms share several mechanisms and their neuroanatomy.[14] κ-opioids are known to be analgesic and antipruritic. Although μ-opioids (eg, morphine) are also analgesic, they can potentially induce pruritus. Recent studies have used animal models to discover more about the neurotransmitters involved in spinal and trigeminal pruritus transmission. These studies have put particular emphasis on the gastrin-releasing peptide receptor (GRPR) and neurokinin-1 receptor (SP receptor; NK1R).[6] It was found that GRPR and MOR1D, a μ-opioid receptor isoform, are considerably colocalized in the superficial spinal cord and that the GRPR antagonist eradicated morphine-induced scratching. These findings were established with experiments on mice and suggest that there is a specific spinal pathway reserved for pruritus. Other substances currently under evaluation include glutamate and its effects on the AMPA/kainate receptor, natriuretic polypeptide B (Nppb) and its receptor Npra, and somatostatin and the receptor tyrosine kinase Ret. Interestingly, it is speculated that Nppb is released from primary afferent pruriceptors to excite second-order spinal interneurons. Thus, a chain of spinal neurons and interneurons may possibly play a role in cascading pruritus transmission or inhibition, depending on the discharged mediators. The correct knowledge of this process would permit the establishment of novel therapeutic targets for those with pruritus. Although this information requires adaptation for humans with chronic pruritus, these experimental data are promising and represent the first step toward better understanding the complex physiological mechanisms of pruritus. The mechanisms behind scratching are also of great importance. While a patient scratches her or his pruritus, the pruritus is relieved. It is thus speculated whether scratching triggers interneurons modulating pain, which have the potential to inhibit systems conducting pruritus transmission. μ-opioid and κ-opioid receptors are both believed to be expressed and involved with interneurons mediating pruritus. Systemic treatments with μ-antagonists (eg, naltrexone and naloxone) and κ-agonists (nalfurafine) may control various forms of chronic pruritus, including cholestatic and uremic pruritus.

NEUROBIOLOGY OF PRURITUS

To better identify environmental stimuli, cutaneous nerve fibers come equipped with several different receptor classes. Primarily GPCRs, transient receptor potential (TRP) channels, and cytokine and toll-like receptors (TLRs) are those found primarily on pruriceptors. GPCR does not directly result in the production of an action potential but is conjoined to TRP channels via intracellular signaling pathways. The activation of TRP channels, with a sufficient ion influx, allows for the generation of action potentials.[15,16] Histamine, for example, activates H1 receptors on the C_{MIA}, beginning activation of phospholipase Cβ3 (PLCβ3) and an intracellular signal cascade (Table 21-1). This results in TRPV1 activation and allows for an influx of ions, therefore producing an action potential.[15] Many of these signaling cascades have recently been detected in pruriceptors and are relevant for pruritus research. Mas-related GPCRs (Mrgprs) share a connection to thymic stromal lymphopoietin (TSLP) receptors and have been identified amongst the mechanisms of chloroquine-induced and atopic pruritus. Mrgprs are known to induce pruritus via the cold sensory receptor TRPA1 in CMH fibers. These fibers can be selectively activated with cowhage, a cysteine protease appearing in spicules of the plant *Mucuna pruriens*.

Nowadays, cowhage and histamine are often adopted for use in experimental pruritus studies on humans. Cowhage is thought to act via protease-activated receptors (PARs) 2 and 4 located in CMH fibers. Recent studies have suggested that a functional overlapping of the PARs and Mrgprs is likely and propose that Mrgprs activation is related to the effects of cowhage.[17] The human cysteine protease cathepsin S and cowhage are highly homologous. Under certain pathological conditions, cathepsin S is induced in keratinocytes by γ interferon. It also has a role in the pruritus associated with atopic dermatitis and seborrheic dermatitis[18,19] and binds to PAR and Mrgprs. The responses to pruritus, however, share a greater link with Mrgprs in mice. TSLP, which is released by keratinocytes in atopic dermatitis, is upregulated through activation of PARs in keratinocytes. In summary, the functions of PARs and Mrgprs remain unclear, although both appear to have a role in pruritus induction.[17]

Research efforts to learn more about these have proven fruitful within the past few years. Several different pruritogens have recently been identified, and experts' knowledge on the molecular mechanisms of pruritus is continuously growing. Endothelin, cytokines (eg, interleukins [ILs] 6, 8, 31, and 33), leukotrienes, neuropeptides (SP, CGRP), serotonin, and prostaglandins are examples of mediators that are known to cause pruritus either directly via neuroreceptor activation or indirectly via upregulation of ligands targeting nerves and nerve fiber sensitization (see Table 21-1). IL-31 is a protein that has received a moderate amount of attention for its elevated levels in both the lesioned skin and serum of patients with atopic dermatitis and is also known to activate the IL-31 receptor (IL-31R). An IL-31RA subunit and oncostatin M receptor subunit constitute the heterodimeric IL-31 receptor (IL-31R). Its corresponding antibody was found to quickly diminish pruritus in affected patients.[20,21] Furthermore, IL-31 is released by inflammatory cells (eg, T cells, including Th2 cells in atopic dermatitis and eosinophils). It is suspected that a line of communication between eosinophils and keratinocytes exists in pruritic inflammatory skin diseases. TLR3, TLR4 and TLR7 are TLRs that serve as innate sensors in the immune system and thought to have a role in pruritus. They are expressed in DRGs, peripheral sensory nerves, spinal glial cells, and superficial dorsal horn neurons and are colocalized with GRP, ion channels, and Mrgprs. Experiments conducted with knockout mice have demonstrated that TLRs promote pruritus transmission[22,23] caused by multiple pruritogens such as chloroquine, endothelin-1, imiquimod, and Mrgpr agonists; however, they do not directly induce pruritus. TLR3 in the DRG, for example, intensifies TRPV1 activity and thereby boosts histamine-induced pruritus signal transduction.

The pathophysiology of chronic pruritus in humans remains unclear; however, the mechanisms of acute pruritus are much more evident. It can be assumed that complex mechanisms in the skin and CNS contribute to the development of chronic pruritus and lead to a peripheral sensitization of cutaneous nerves, central sensitization, impaired interneuron function, and descending inhibitory neurons at the spinal level. In summary, recent experimental animal models of certain diseases suggest a clinical role of certain pruritogens in inflammatory skin diseases and systemic pruritus. In most cases, however, this remains to be clinically validated in humans.

TABLE 21-1
Neurobiology of Pruritus: Mediators, Corresponding Receptors, and Assumed Clinical Role

MEDIATOR	NEURORECEPTOR	GENERATION OF ACTION POTENTIAL ON C FIBERS VIA	ASSUMED CLINICAL ROLE IN PRURITUS
Histamine	Histamin1 receptor	TRPV1	Urticaria
	Histamine 4 receptor on Th2 cells: increased production of IL-31	—	Atopic dermatitis
Cathepsin S	Mas-related G protein–coupled receptors (Mrgprs)	TRPA1	Atopic dermatitis, seborrheic dermatitis
Thymic stromal lymphopoietin (TSLP)	TSLP receptor (heterodimeric receptor composed of TSLP receptor chain and IL-7 receptor alpha chain)	TRPA1	Atopic dermatitis, allergic asthma
Serotonin	5-HT7	TRPA1	Atopic dermatitis, prurigo nodularis? (increased serum levels), cholestatic pruritus?, uremic pruritus?
	5-HT2	TRPV4	
Endothelin	Endothelin-1 receptor	TRPA1	Atopic dermatitis, prurigo nodularis
Substance P	Neurokinin-1 receptor (NK1R) on keratinocytes, mast cells, endothelia cells; release of pruritogenic mediators	—	Atopic dermatitis, eczema, prurigo nodularis, psoriasis vulgaris
Interleukin-31 (IL-31)	IL-31 receptor (IL-31R) (heterodimeric receptor of IL-31RA subunit and oncostatin M receptor subunit)		Atopic dermatitis, prurigo nodularis, cutaneous T-cell lymphoma, familial primary localized cutaneous amyloidosis, urticaria (serum), mastocytosis (serum)
Unknown	Toll-like receptors (TLRs) on sensory nerves, dorsal root ganglia, spinal glia cells	TRPV1	Dry skin
Autotaxin/ lysophosphatidic acid (LPA)	LPA receptor	TRPV1 (A fibers)	Cholestatic pruritus
Bile acids	TGR5 receptor	TRPA1	Cholestatic pruritus

Keratinocytes, mast cells, and inflammatory cells play important roles in the induction and maintenance of pruritus. Interestingly, the cutaneous neuroanatomy is also altered in pruritic diseases. Researchers discovered that overexpression of IL-31 in transgenic mice caused pruritic skin. IL-31 was found to influence the cutaneous nerve anatomy and induce dermal nerve elongation and branching. It might also be a factor contributing to the cutaneous hyperinnervation attributed to atopic dermatitis. In humans, this might be due to disproportionate nerve elongation (eg, nerve growth factor [NGF]) and nerve repulsion factors (eg, semaphorin 3A) produced by keratinocytes.[24] The hyperinnervation of dermal nerves has been confirmed for chronic pruritus and prurigo nodularis. The intraepidermal nerves penetrating the basal membrane are reduced in numbers, which might be caused by scratching.[25] This neuroanatomical imbalance of intraepidermal nerves (caused by scratching) and dermal nerves (caused by pruritic mediators released by keratinocytes and inflammatory cells) thus clearly carries significance for the function and induction of pruritus.

ROLE OF THE NERVOUS SYSTEM IN SKIN DISEASES

Atopic dermatitis, prurigo nodularis, psoriasis vulgaris, rosacea, herpes zoster, urticaria, and wound healing represent a small number of several dermatoses with a vital neurogenic component (besides pruritus induction). Although the peripheral nervous system modulates inflammatory responses, neuronal mediators assist in the wound healing process by managing fibroblast and keratinocyte production, as well as angiogenesis. It has been known for several years that neuropeptides possess the ability to stimulate human mast cells and induce urticaria. Chronic spontaneous urticaria and, to a lesser extent, pressure urticaria exhibit increased SP levels and CGRP-induced wheal and flare reactions. Sensory nerves and mast cells express TRP ion channels that can be triggered by factors such as warmth, cold, and food allergens resulting in urticaria.

A subset of sensory neurons expressing the TRPV1 and Nav1.8 affirmed the neurogenic components involved in the pathophysiology of psoriasis and are crucial for facilitating the psoriatic inflammatory response. IL-23–producing dermal dendritic cells have been found to be in close connection to these TRPV1/Nav 1.8 positive nociceptors. Upon selective pharmacological or genetic ablation of the nociceptors, the dermal dendritic cells failed to produce IL-23 and thereby to initiate the psoriasiform skin inflammation.[26] This link seems to be clinically relevant because topical capsaicin application (depleting neuropeptides from sensory nerves and destroying superficial sensory nerves) can lead to significant improvement of psoriasis.[27] Novel topical formulations with liposomes containing capsaicin were recently developed for this indication.[28]

The skin's nervous system plays an important part in various processes, including wound healing. Several neuropeptides secreted by sensory and autonomic nerve fibers are essential to the different phases of wound healing,[29] including neurotrophin-3 (eg, nerve regeneration), CGRP (eg, angiogenesis), brain-derived neurotrophic factor (BDNF; eg, wound contraction and epithelialization), NGF (eg, nerve regeneration and fibroblast differentiation into myofibroblasts), and SP (eg, collagen maturation and remodeling).

PRURITUS

CLASSIFICATION AND CLINICAL MANIFESTATION

Pruritus, the most common symptom in dermatology, is listed by the World Health Organization's Global Burden of Disease study as one of the 50 most frequent interdisciplinary symptoms.[30,31] If present for longer than 6 weeks, pruritus is considered chronic. It is estimated that one-fifth of the global population has chronic pruritus, with a substantial number of these affected individuals having a highly impaired quality of life.[32]

The distinction between acute and chronic pruritus is not merely academic. Although the cause of acute pruritus is often easy to identify (eg, a reaction to an allergen or an episode of urticaria) and easily treated, this is not the case for chronic pruritus.[33] Complex processes, including peripheral and central sensitization involving a plethora of neuromodulators and receptors at all levels of the nervous system, are believed to take place, explaining the persistence of pruritus even after the original cause has been eliminated.[34]

Because pruritus is a highly complex symptom potentially arising from many different clinical diseases, a systematic diagnostic approach is decisive for its clinical management. A clinical classification system developed by the International Forum for the Study of Itch (IFSI) divides chronic pruritus patients into groups according to their skin condition (Fig. 21-4).[33] Patients may present with pruritus on inflamed skin (IFSI group I), on seemingly normal skin (IFSI group II), or accompanied by chronic scratch lesions (IFSI group III) (Fig. 21-5). This classification system has diagnostic relevance. For instance, although skin biopsies for histological examinations may be useful in further characterizing possible dermatoses in patients with inflamed skin or those with chronic scratch lesions, laboratory workups to investigate possible systemic or neurologic conditions gain relevance in patients with pruritus on normal skin or with chronic scratch lesions (Fig. 21-4).[33]

It is useful to group the patient into an etiological category upon taking their medical history and performing a physical, laboratory and radiological examination. This greatly aids in planning a therapeutic strategy. The IFSI has proposed a classification of chronic pruritus into categories composed of skin diseases and systemic, neurological, or somatoform conditions as causative

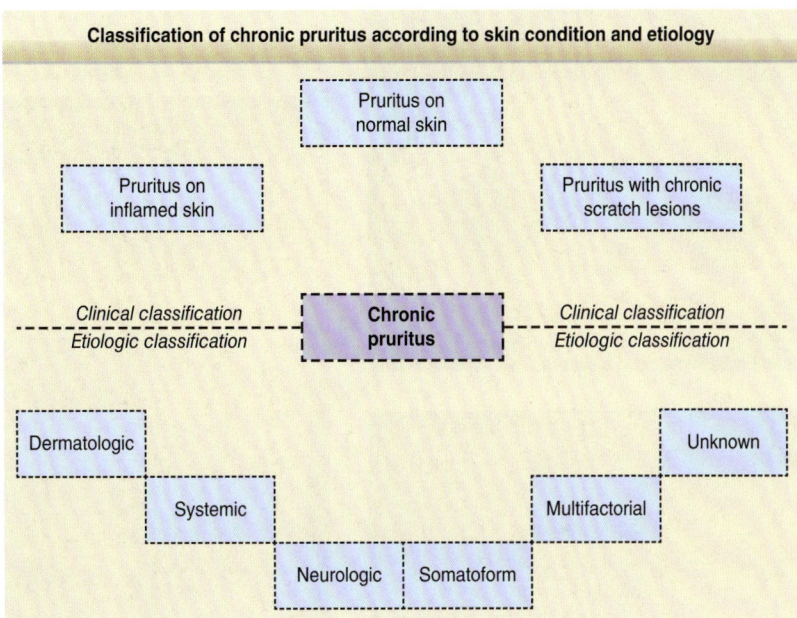

Figure 21-4 Classification of chronic pruritus according to skin condition and etiology by the International Forum for the Study of Itch.

entities for chronic pruritus (see Fig. 21-4). Noteworthy multiple causes may be present in the same patient (multifactorial pruritus), or no cause may be identifiable (pruritus of unknown origin).[33]

THERAPEUTIC APPROACH

A step-by-step approach is recommended for the treatment of chronic pruritus (Fig. 21-6). Elementary measures such as the consequent use of emollients to prevent xerosis or the avoidance of allergens and potentially irritating substances should be adopted regardless of the cause for the pruritus. Ointments containing antipruritic compounds, such as urea, menthol, and polidocanol should be recommended to patients. Additionally, antihistamines have proven symptom relief for various pruritic diseases and may be prescribed even before the etiology is discovered.[35]

If the origin of the pruritus can be determined, the physician should prepare a targeted therapy, for instance, immunosuppressive drugs (eg, cyclosporine) for atopic dermatitis, gabapentinoids for neuropathic pruritus, and antidepressants (eg, paroxetine) for paraneoplastic pruritus.

If the etiology remains unknown or the targeted therapy is unsuccessful, a symptomatic topical or systemic therapy (or both) is recommended. The topical use of calcineurin inhibitors may be useful when dealing with inflammatory conditions, and capsaicin has shown efficacy in many disorders such as neuropathic and aquagenic pruritus. Local anesthetics can be used for notalgia paraesthetica. Antidepressants are systemic agents useful for pruritus of various origins, and naltrexone may help against cholestatic and nephrogenic pruritus. Many other drugs have been used in the treatment of pruritus of various origins and can be consulted in the available guidelines.[36]

Chronic pruritus frequently leads to accompanying disorders, including sleep disturbances, depression, and anxiety. These should be treated from an early stage to mitigate a decrease in quality of life and prevent their development into a chronic condition. The use of hypnotic substances, sedating antidepressant drugs, and relaxation techniques should be discussed with the patient. Consultation with a psychosomatic specialist should be encouraged in case of mental factors.

If the mechanisms have become chronic, the pruritus may persist even after elimination of the original cause. Peripheral and central processes in the nervous system are believed to be responsible for this phenomenon.[34,37] Therapeutically, centrally acting drugs may be necessary in blocking these pathophysiological mechanisms. Another aspect to consider is the itch-scratch cycle that may develop after a prolonged period with a pruritic condition. Patients feel the urge to scratch and display an automatic scratching behavior even though the pruritus is no longer present. Behavioral therapies are useful in these cases and should be discussed with the patients.

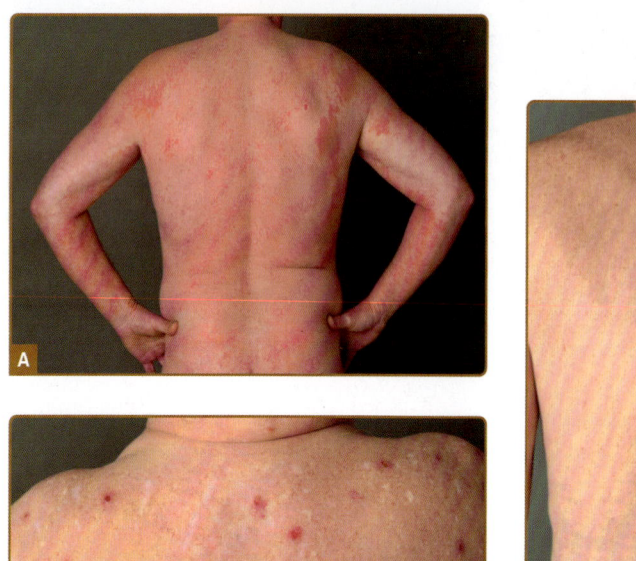
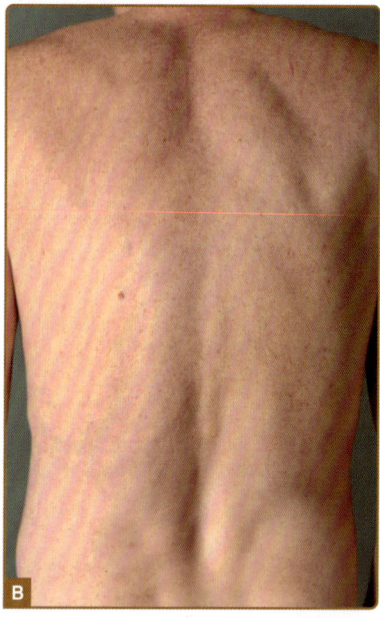
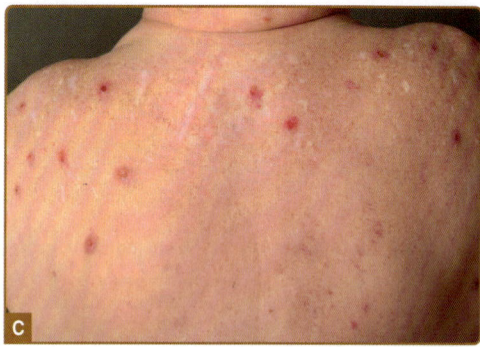

Figure 21-5 Clinical presentation of chronic pruritus. Patients with chronic pruritus may present with inflamed skin (**A**), normal-appearing skin (**B**), or chronic scratch lesions (**C**). **A,** A 58-year-old man with atopic dermatitis. **B,** A 45-year-old man with cholestatic pruritus after liver transplant. **C,** A 60-year-old man with chronic prurigo with underlying advanced renal insufficiency.

NEW DRUGS

As described earlier in this chapter, new mediators, receptors, and pathways have been identified in recent years, leading to novel antipruritic compounds.

In inflammatory conditions (eg, atopic dermatitis), NK1R antagonists led to a significant reduction of scratching behavior in a mouse model of atopic dermatitis,[38] and off-label use in patients with

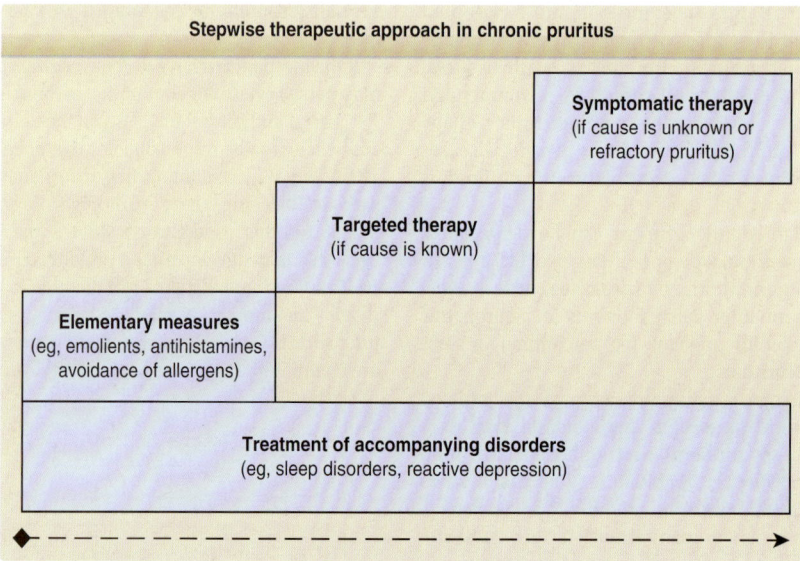

Figure 21-6 Stepwise therapeutic approach in chronic pruritus.

chronic pruritus has shown promising symptomatic improvement.[39] Phase II clinical trials testing both topical and systemic NK1R antagonist compounds are underway, targeting not only inflammatory dermatoses but also prurigo nodularis, cutaneous T-cell lymphoma, and epidermolysis bullosa. Another drug class of interest targeting inflammatory dermatoses is the antibody blocking the IL-31 receptor. IL-31 receptor antagonists showed promising findings in studies on atopic dermatitis and are currently being tested in further clinical trials.[40] Topical agents targeting TRPV1 and the tyrosine receptor kinase A, a nerve growth factor receptor, are also being developed.

For pruritus arising from systemic diseases, κ-opioid receptor agonists have shown antipruritic efficacy in patients with uremic pruritus,[41,42] and bile acid transporter inhibitors are promising drugs in the treatment of cholestatic pruritus.

Randomized controlled trials are thus greatly needed for the rapid approval of promising new antipruritic agents.

SUMMARY AND PERSPECTIVES

The nervous system alters cutaneous functions in many ways. Under certain physiological conditions, it can also lead to the control of skin homeostasis; however, neuromodulators can both aggravate (proinflammatory) or mitigate (antiinflammatory) disease development under pathophysiological conditions. The skin's bidirectional capability within the peripheral nervous system and CNS is vital for skin homeostasis and disease states, as observed in inflammation, pain, and pruritus. Recent findings have enhanced our knowledge of the molecular mechanisms that regulate the functions of neuromodulators, their receptors, and controlling enzymes. Proteomics, genomics, metabolics, and the molecular imaging of neuronal structures are modern techniques that provide intriguing insights into this complex network comprised of the skin, nerves, and immune system during inflammation, chronic pain, pruritus, and tumorigenesis. Chronic pruritus is highly prevalent and can considerably impair one's quality of life. A systematic diagnostic approach is necessary because of its abundance of possible etiologies. In addition to adopting basic therapeutic measures consisting of emollient application to prevent xerosis and avoiding allergies, it is recommended to implement a targeted therapy of the underlying disease, if possible. Novel agents are currently in development in clinical and preclinical trials. Neurokinin-1 receptor antagonists, IL-31 receptor antagonists, and other agents targeting the TRPV1 constitute a group of interesting new agents for treatment of inflammatory dermatoses. κ-opioid receptor agonists, partly with μ-opioid receptor antagonist properties, are presently undergoing tests for use against uremic pruritus, and bile acid transporter inhibitors show great promise for cholestatic pruritus.

REFERENCES

1. Chuquilin M, Alghalith Y, Fernandez KH. Neurocutaneous disease: cutaneous neuroanatomy and mechanisms of itch and pain. *J Am Acad Dermatol*. 2016; 74(2):197-212.
2. Lloyd DM, McGlone FP, Yosipovitch G. Somatosensory pleasure circuit: from skin to brain and back. *Exp Dermatol*. 2015;24(5):321-324.
3. Wang N, Gibbons CH. Skin biopsies in the assessment of the autonomic nervous system. *Handb Clin Neurol*. 2013;117:371-378.
4. Chateau Y, Misery L. Connections between nerve endings and epidermal cells: are they synapses? *Exp Dermatol*. 2004;13(1):2-4.
5. Schwendinger-Schreck J, Wilson SR, Bautista DM. Interactions between keratinocytes and somatosensory neurons in itch. *Handb Exp Pharmacol*. 2015;226:177-190.
6. Akiyama T, Carstens E. Neural processing of itch. *Neuroscience*. 2013;250:697-714.
7. Boulais N, Misery L. The epidermis: a sensory tissue. *Eur J Dermatol*. 2008;18(2):119-127.
8. Wilson SR, Bautista DM. Frontiers in neuroscience: role of transient receptor potential channels in acute and chronic itch. In: Carstens E, Akiyama T, eds. *Itch: Mechanisms and Treatment*. Boca Raton, FL: CRC Press/Taylor & Francis Group; 2014.
9. Ringkamp M, Meyer R. Frontiers in neuroscience: pruriceptors. In: Carstens E, Akiyama T, eds. *Itch: Mechanisms and Treatment*. Boca Raton, FL: CRC Press/Taylor & Francis Group; 2014.
10. Stantcheva KK, Iovino L, Dhandapani R, et al. A subpopulation of itch-sensing neurons marked by Ret and somatostatin expression. *EMBO Rep*. 2016;17(4): 585-600.
11. Akiyama T, Carstens E. Frontiers in neuroscience: spinal coding of itch and pain. In: Carstens E, Akiyama T, eds. *Itch: Mechanisms and Treatment*. Boca Raton, FL: CRC Press/Taylor & Francis Group; 2014.
12. Hsieh ST, Lin WM. Modulation of keratinocyte proliferation by skin innervation. *J Invest Dermatol*. 1999;113(4):579-586.
13. Weidner C, Klede M, Rukwied R, et al. Acute effects of substance P and calcitonin gene-related peptide in human skin—a microdialysis study. *J Invest Dermatol*. 2000;115(6):1015-1020.
14. Stander S, Schmelz M. Chronic itch and pain—similarities and differences. *Eur J Pain*. 2006;10(5):473-478.
15. Garibyan L, Rheingold CG, Lerner EA. Understanding the pathophysiology of itch. *Dermatol Ther*. 2013; 26(2):84-91.
16. Bautista DM, Wilson SR, Hoon MA. Why we scratch an itch: the molecules, cells and circuits of itch. *Nat Neurosci*. 2014;17(2):175-182.
17. Reddy VB, Sun S, Azimi E, et al. Redefining the concept of protease-activated receptors: cathepsin S evokes itch via activation of Mrgprs. *Nat Commun*. 2015;6:7864.
18. Viode C, Lejeune O, Turlier V, et al. Cathepsin S, a new pruritus biomarker in clinical dandruff/seborrhoeic dermatitis evaluation. *Exp Dermatol*. 2014;23(4):274-275.
19. Kim N, Bae KB, Kim MO, et al. Overexpression of cathepsin S induces chronic atopic dermatitis in mice. *J Invest Dermatol*. 2012;132(4):1169-1176.
20. Nemoto O, Furue M, Nakagawa H, et al. The first trial of CIM331, a humanized anti-human IL-31 receptor A antibody, for healthy volunteers and patients with atopic dermatitis to evaluate safety, tolerability and

pharmacokinetics of a single dose in a randomised, double-blind, placebo-controlled study. *Br J Dermatol*. 2016;174(2):296-304.
21. Feld M, Garcia R, Buddenkotte J, et al. The pruritus- and TH2-associated cytokine IL-31 promotes growth of sensory nerves. *J Allergy Clin Immunol*. 2016;138(2):500-8.e24.
22. Taves S, Ji RR. Itch control by Toll-like receptors. *Handb Exp Pharmacol*. 2015;226:135-150.
23. Liu T, Xu ZZ, Park CK, et al. Toll-like receptor 7 mediates pruritus. *Nat Neurosci*. 2010;13(12):1460-1462.
24. Tominaga M, Takamori K. Frontiers in neuroscience: sensitization of itch signaling: itch sensitization-nerve growth factor, semaphorins. In: Carstens E, Akiyama T, eds. *Itch: Mechanisms and Treatment*. Boca Raton, FL: CRC Press/Taylor & Francis Group; 2014.
25. Haas S, Capellino S, Phan NQ, et al. Low density of sympathetic nerve fibers relative to substance P-positive nerve fibers in lesional skin of chronic pruritus and prurigo nodularis. *J Dermatol Sci*. 2010;58(3):193-197.
26. Riol-Blanco L, Ordovas-Montanes J, Perro M, et al. Nociceptive sensory neurons drive interleukin-23-mediated psoriasiform skin inflammation. *Nature*. 2014;510(7503):157-161.
27. Boyd K, Shea SM, Patterson JW. The role of capsaicin in dermatology. *Prog Drug Res*. 2014;68:293-306.
28. Gupta R, Gupta M, Mangal S, et al. Capsaicin-loaded vesicular systems designed for enhancing localized delivery for psoriasis therapy. *Artif Cells Nanomed Biotechnol*. 2016;44(3):825-834.
29. Ashrafi M, Baguneid M, Bayat A. The role of neuromediators and innervation in cutaneous wound healing. *Acta Derm Venereol*. 2016;96(5):587-594.
30. Kopyciok ME, Stander HF, Osada N, et al. prevalence and characteristics of pruritus: a one-week cross-sectional study in a German dermatology practice. *Acta Derm Venereol*. 2016;96(1):50-55.
31. Hay RJ, Johns NE, Williams HC, et al. The global burden of skin disease in 2010: an analysis of the prevalence and impact of skin conditions. *J Invest Dermatol*. 2014;134(6):1527-1534.
32. Stander S, Schafer I, Phan NQ, et al. Prevalence of chronic pruritus in Germany: results of a cross-sectional study in a sample working population of 11,730. *Dermatology*. 2010;221(3):229-235.
33. Stander S, Weisshaar E, Mettang T, et al. Clinical classification of itch: a position paper of the International Forum for the Study of Itch. *Acta Derm Venereol*. 2007;87(4):291-294.
34. Ikoma A, Steinhoff M, Stander S, et al. The neurobiology of itch. *Nat Rev Neurosci*. 2006;7(7):535-547.
35. Yosipovitch G, Bernhard JD. Clinical practice. Chronic pruritus. *N Engl J Med*. 2013;368(17):1625-1634.
36. Weisshaar E, Szepietowski JC, Darsow U, et al. European guideline on chronic pruritus. *Acta Derm Venereol*. 2012;92(5):563-581.
37. Stander S, Weisshaar E, Luger TA. Neurophysiological and neurochemical basis of modern pruritus treatment. *Exp Dermatol*. 2008;17(3):161-169.
38. Ohmura T, Hayashi T, Satoh Y, et al. Involvement of substance P in scratching behaviour in an atopic dermatitis model. *Eur J Pharmacol*. 2004;491(2-3):191-194.
39. Stander S, Siepmann D, Herrgott I, et al. Targeting the neurokinin receptor 1 with aprepitant: a novel antipruritic strategy. *PLoS One*. 2010;5(6):e10968.
40. Kasutani K, Fujii E, Ohyama S, et al. Anti-IL-31 receptor antibody is shown to be a potential therapeutic option for treating itch and dermatitis in mice. *Br J Pharmacol*. 2014;171(22):5049-5058.
41. Inui S. Nalfurafine hydrochloride to treat pruritus: a review. *Clin Cosmet Investig Dermatol*. 2015;8:249-255.
42. Wikstrom B, Gellert R, Ladefoged SD, et al. Kappa-opioid system in uremic pruritus: multicenter, randomized, double-blind, placebo-controlled clinical studies. *J Am Soc Nephrol*. 2005;16(12):3742-3747.

Dermatitis PART 3

第三篇 皮炎

Chapter 22 :: Atopic Dermatitis
:: Eric L. Simpson, Donald Y. M. Leung, Lawrence F. Eichenfield, & Mark Boguniewicz

第二十二章
特应性皮炎

中文导读

本章共分为10节：①前言；②诊断标准；③流行病学；④临床表现；⑤病因与发病机制；⑥诊断；⑦鉴别诊断；⑧病程与预后；⑨治疗；⑩预防。全面阐述了特应性皮炎（AD）的历史背景、临床特征、诊断标准及其防治方法。

第一节介绍特应性皮炎术语的历史演变，指出特应性皮炎应是该病最常用的名称。

第二节简单介绍了AD的几个主要诊断标准，如Hanifin-Rajka诊断标准为AD的第一个综合性诊断标准，也是AD诊断的金标准。另外，还简述了英国工作组标准、美国皮肤科学会诊断标准的来源和诊断价值。

第三节介绍了AD的患病率、经济负担、年龄、性别和种族差异，指出AD是全球主要的公共卫生问题，环境因素在疾病发生中起了重要作用。

第四节从皮肤表现（包括急性、亚急性和慢性湿疹样损害的形态、部位）、非皮肤表现（包括特应性并发症和对心理、社会影响两方面）、并发症（感染、眼部并发症、手部皮炎、剥脱性皮炎）三个方面详细介绍了AD的临床表现。

第五节介绍了遗传、免疫和环境因素相互作用对AD发病的影响。详细阐述了皮肤屏障功能降低、遗传、免疫病理、细胞因子驱动的皮肤炎症、表皮分化复合体免疫效应在AD发病机制中的作用和意义，并介绍了导致AD瘙痒的分子基础。

第六节介绍了AD的诊断主要基于临床表

现和病史，以现有的诊断标准为参考。AD的辅助检查包括实验室检查、病理学检查、影像学检查、IgE抗体检测或血清特异性IgE抗体检测等。尚需排除与湿疹相关的免疫缺陷的实验室检查，以及活检、影像学检查在AD临床中的意义。

第七节介绍了需要与AD鉴别的疾病，包括许多炎症性皮肤病、免疫缺陷、皮肤恶性肿瘤、遗传性疾病、感染性疾病等可能与AD有类似的症状和体征。

第八节介绍了AD的病程和预后。预测持续疾病进程的危险因素包括疾病严重程度、晚期发病，FLG或FLG-2的基因突变基因和早期变态反应致敏。

第九节介绍了AD的治疗方案，指出成功的AD治疗需要采取系统的、多管齐下的方法。对于常规治疗无效的患者，可能需要其他抗炎药和免疫调节药。在以下方面进行了详细讲述：健康教育、证实和去除刺激因素（特异性过敏原、传染原和情绪应激等激发因素）、局部治疗（润肤剂、外用糖皮质激素、外用钙调磷酸酶抑制药、PDE4抑制药、焦油制剂）、光疗、系统治疗（IL-4/IL-13单抗、糖皮质激素、环孢素、MTX）、其他治疗（包括干扰素、奥马珠单抗、过敏原免疫治疗、益生菌、中医中药等）。

第十节从如何预防发生过敏、益生菌的作用等方面，介绍了目前对AD预防措施的研究进展。

〔李　捷〕

AT-A-GLANCE

- Atopic dermatitis (AD) has a prevalence peak of 15% to 20% in early childhood in industrialized countries.
- AD has variable rates of remission, with many patients continuing or recurring with symptoms into adulthood.
- AD is a chronic or chronically relapsing disorder with major features of:
  - Pruritus
  - Eczematous dermatitis (acute, subacute, or chronic) with typical morphology and age-specific patterns
  - Facial and extensor involvement in infancy
  - Flexural eczema or lichenification in children and adults
  - Commonly associated with the following:
    - Personal or family history of atopy (allergic rhinitis, asthma, atopic dermatitis)
    - Xerosis or skin barrier dysfunction
    - Immunoglobulin E reactivity
- Pathogenesis driven by skin barrier defects (most importantly in the *FLG* gene), environmental effects and alterations in immunologic responses in T cells, antigen processing, inflammatory cytokines, host defense proteins, allergen sensitivity, and infection.

INTRODUCTION

Atopic dermatitis (atopic eczema, AD) is a chronic inflammatory skin disease primarily beginning in childhood with a variable natural course. Itch is the hallmark symptom of the disease, often unrelenting in severe cases, and leads to sleep disturbance and excoriated, infection-prone skin. Patients with AD often additionally have atopic comorbidities such as allergic asthma and allergic rhinitis and experience a significantly impaired quality of life.

DEFINITIONS AND HISTORICAL PERSPECTIVE

NOMENCLATURE

The term *atopic dermatitis* was first coined in 1933 by Sulzberger and Wise and replaced early terms corresponding to probable AD such as tinea *muquese, porrigo larvalis,* and *Hebra's prurigo.* The term *atopy* was first introduced by Coca and Cooke in 1923 to describe the tendency toward developing allergic hypersensitivity manifested by asthma and hayfever.[1] The term *atopi* is derived from the Greek word *atopos* meaning "without place," reflecting the mysterious pathogenic underpinnings of allergic hypersensitivity disease. Wise and Sulzberger coined the term *atopic dermatitis* in 1933 to describe recurring eczematous skin disease found in patients with a family history of atopic disease.[2]

Importantly, they noted that patients with AD may not have a personal history of other atopic disease. Since this seminal paper, several groups attempted to rename the disease primarily to differentiate AD that has concomitant immunoglobulin E (IgE) sensitization from AD without sensitization, such as *atopiform dermatitis* and *nonatopic eczema*. A recent systematic review reveals *atopic dermatitis* to be the most commonly used name for the disease and proposed the universal use of this term for AD.[3] The authors of that paper discourage the use of less specific terms such as *eczema*, which is a morphological term and includes contact and other eczematous conditions.

DIAGNOSTIC CRITERIA

Significant advancement of our understanding of the disease could not be made without a proper disease definition. Early work by luminaries in AD, such as Rajka, Lobitz, and Hanifin, paved the way for the first comprehensive diagnostic criteria for AD—the Hanifin-Rajka criteria.[4] The major criteria have been validated and remain the gold standard for AD diagnosis. Similar to AD nomenclature, numerous attempts have been made to refine and shorten the original criteria to make them more useful in clinical practice. The UK Working Party Criteria were developed using modern statistical methods and represent a distilled set of the original criteria useful for population-based epidemiologic study.[5] The American Academy of Dermatology consensus diagnostic criteria for pediatric AD are a useful and clinician-friendly guide to AD diagnosis, although no formal validation studies have been published.[6]

EPIDEMIOLOGY

Since the 1960s, there has been a more than threefold increase in the prevalence of AD.[2] AD is a major public health problem worldwide, with a prevalence in children of 10% to 20% in the United States, Northern and Western Europe, urban Africa, Japan, Australia, and other industrialized countries.[3] The Global Disease Burden project ranks "dermatitis," which includes AD, as the highest ranking skin disease in regards to total global disability burden.[7] The prevalence of AD in adults is less clear, but recent studies estimate the prevalence to be between 3% to 7% in the United States, Germany, and Japan.[8-10] The International Study of Asthma and Allergies in Childhood (ISAAC) Phase Three study confirmed that AD is a disease with high prevalence worldwide, affecting patients in both developed and developing countries.[4] There is also an observed female preponderance for AD, with an overall female-to-male ratio of 1.3 to 1.0. Racial and ethnic differences in prevalence also exist with African Americans having a higher prevalence of the disease in the United States.[11]

Wide variations in prevalence have been observed within countries inhabited by similar ethnic groups, suggesting that environmental factors are critical in determining disease expression. Several studies reveal lower prevalence rates in rural settings compared with urban centers within the same country.[12] Other risk factors reported to be associated with AD include exposure to airborne pollution, use of hard water, increased income and education both in whites and blacks, obesity, and increased use of antibiotics.[13-17] Climate may also play a role in disease expression with lower humidity and lower ultraviolet (UV) areas displaying higher prevalence rates.[18] Climatic factors and pollution levels may also influence symptoms and flares of the disease.[19]

CLINICAL FEATURES

CUTANEOUS FINDINGS

Acute eczematous lesions are characterized by erythematous papulovesicles, often with pinpoint crusting or frank weeping. More subacute to chronic lesions often display scale, excoriation, and lichenification. Patients with AD may present with only one stage of eczematous lesions, but most often patients have a mixture of both acute and chronic lesions in multiple areas of the body simultaneously or even in the same lesion. Individual eczematous lesions of AD cannot be readily distinguished clinically or histologically from lesions found in other eczematous conditions such as allergic contact dermatitis or nummular dermatitis. Patients with darker skin tones often present with follicular accentuation, flat-topped papules in lichenified areas, and a tendency toward hyperpigmentation in inflamed areas, which can be very distressing for patients. Rarely, patients may also experience a vitiligo-like depigmentation in involved areas that is difficult to distinguish from topical steroid-induced pigment loss.

The distribution of eczematous lesions vary according to the patient's age (Fig. 22-1) and disease activity. During infancy, the AD is generally more acute and primarily involves the face (Fig. 22-2), the scalp, and the extensor surfaces of the extremities (Fig. 22-3).[20] The diaper area is usually spared. In older children and in those who have long-standing skin disease, the patient develops the chronic form of AD with lichenification and localization of the rash to the flexural folds of the extremities (Fig. 22-4). AD may subside as the patient grows older, leaving an adult with skin that is prone to itching and inflammation when exposed to exogenous irritants. Chronic hand eczema may be the primary manifestation of AD in many adults (Fig. 22-5). At least one third of patients will have clinical features of filaggrin deficiency such as ichthyosis vulgaris, keratosis pilaris, and hyperlinear palms. These clinical features are associated with genetic defects encoding the filaggrin protein and can identify patients who have a more severe disease course and allergic comorbidities.[21] Other less specific but common associated features of AD are listed in Table 22-1. Other specific skin conditions associated with AD include vitiligo and alopecia areata.[22]

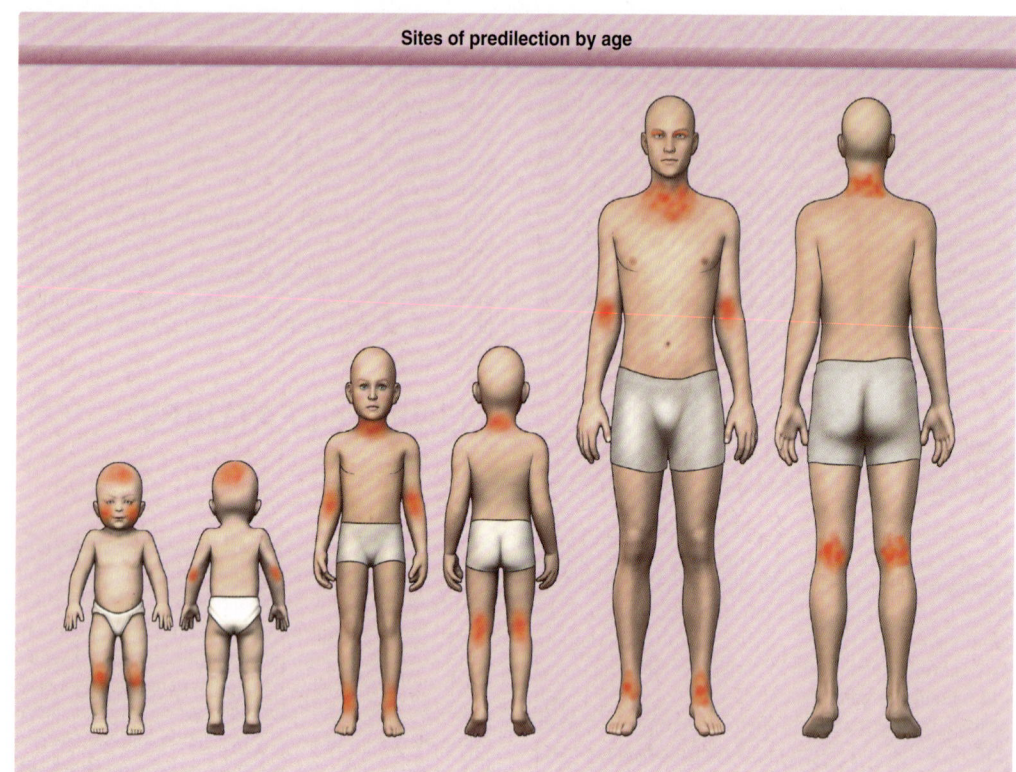

Figure 22-1 Atopic dermatitis progression and distribution: infancy, older childhood, and adulthood.

NONCUTANEOUS FINDINGS

ATOPIC COMORBIDITIES

There is growing recognition that patients with AD carry a large burden of comorbid conditions. Patients with AD often show signs of T helper 2 (Th2) immune activation, including high levels of total and specific serum IgE, eosinophilia, and a predisposition toward allergic comorbidities. Large population-based studies reveal patients with AD have a higher prevalence of

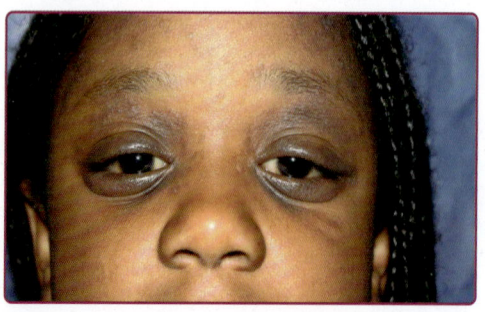

Figure 22-2 Edematous, erythematous eyelids with lichenification and hyperpigmentation in an adolescent with atopic dermatitis. Note the infraocular (Dennie-Morgan) folds.

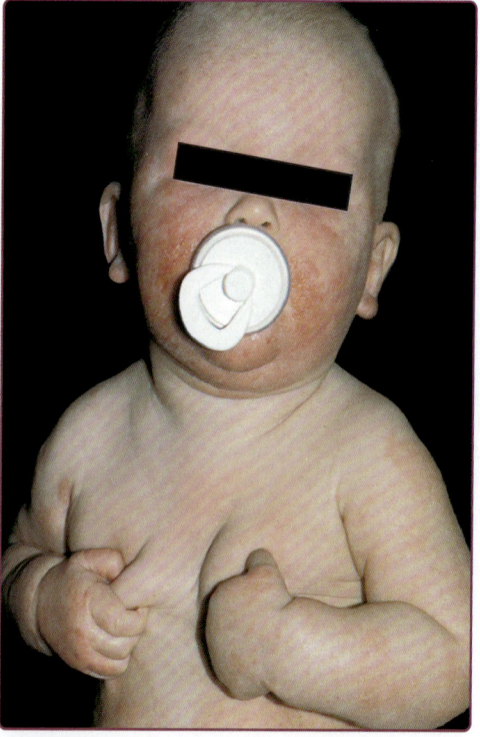

Figure 22-3 Itching infant with atopic dermatitis. (Used with permission from Oholm Larsen, MD.)

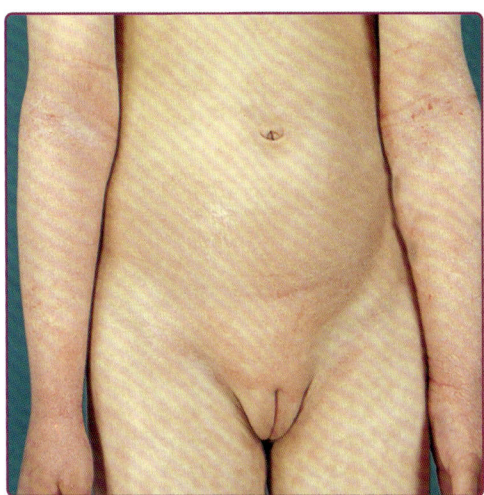

Figure 22-4 Childhood atopic dermatitis with lichenification of antecubital fossae and generalized severely pruritic eczematous plaques.

food allergy, asthma, and allergic rhinitis. The severity of the skin disease correlates with both the risk and severity of the comorbidity.[23] AD is often the first atopic disease to develop, but the diseases can occur in any order and in any combination.[24] For example, allergic sensitization may occur before or after AD development[25] but does develop in up to 80% of patients. Large collaborative efforts to integrate clinical cohort and "omics" data are underway and suggest Th2-driven pathobiological pathways underlie the multimorbidity seen in AD.[26] There are no studies as of yet demonstrating treatment of the skin alone has a positive impact on allergic comorbidities or whether prevention of AD can halt the development of other atopic diseases ("atopic march").

PSYCHOSOCIAL IMPACT

Numerous studies in pediatric populations and adults reveal AD, especially moderate to severe disease,

TABLE 22-1
Features of Atopic Dermatitis

Major Features
Pruritus
Rash on face, extensors, or both in infants and young children
Lichenification in flexural areas in older children
Tendency toward chronic or chronically relapsing dermatitis
Personal or family history of atopic disease: asthma, allergic rhinitis, atopic dermatitis

Other Common Findings
Dryness
Dennie-Morgan folds (accentuated lines or grooves below the margin of the lower eyelid)
Allergic shiners (darkening beneath the eyes)
Facial pallor
Pityriasis alba
Keratosis pilaris
Ichthyosis vulgaris
Hyperlinearity of palms and soles
White dermatographism (white line appears on skin within 1 minute of being stroked with a blunt instrument)
Conjunctivitis
Keratoconus
Anterior subcapsular cataracts
Elevated serum immunoglobulin E
Immediate skin test reactivity

profoundly impacts the emotional and psychological well-being of a patient. Children with AD display more emotional and behavioral problems compared with normal control participants.[27] Population-based studies also find a higher prevalence of attention-deficit hyperactivity disorder (ADHD), anxiety, conduct disorder, and autism in children with AD compared with children without AD.[28] Children with more severe disease appear to be particularly at risk. The risk of ADHD in both children and adults appears to be mediated by sleep disturbance, a common consequence of pruritus in AD.[29]

Anxiety and depression are commonly found comorbidities in adult patients with AD. Between 43% and 57% of patients met thresholds on the Hospital Anxiety and Depression Scale for probable anxiety or depression in phase 3 clinical trials for AD.[30] Effective antiinflammatory therapy appeared to alleviate both anxiety and depression symptoms in a significant proportion of adults during these trials.

COMPLICATIONS

BACTERIAL INFECTION

Superficial *Staphylococcus aureus* infections are by far the most common infection found in AD. *S. aureus* colonizes skin lesions in more than 70% of patients with AD with more severe AD having higher rates of colonization.[31,32] Studies conflict regarding the prevalence of methicillin-resistant *S. aureus* (MRSA) in this population but does not appear to be higher than

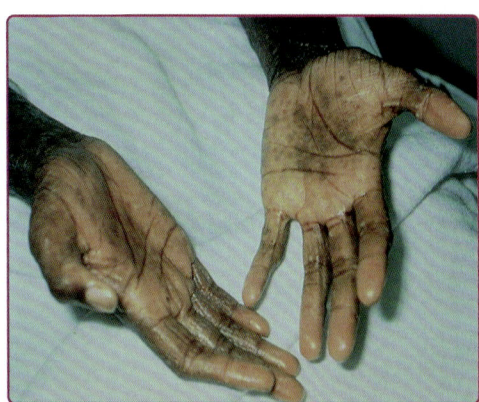

Figure 22-5 Typical papules, vesicles, and erosions seen in atopic hand dermatitis.

background colonization rates. Few studies address the rate of true infection from *S. aureus*, in contrast to colonization. One study from Japan found almost a twofold increase in impetigo in children with AD compared with non-AD control participants.[33] The rate of serious infections from *S. aureus* is also not well characterized in patients with AD, but there are reports in the literature of endocarditis, osteomyelitis, and septicemia.[34]

Both skin barrier and immune deficits found in AD may explain the propensity to colonization and infection. Inflamed skin increases the expression of fibronectin and fibrinogen, which are *S. aureus* binding sites.[35] The elevated pH and disrupted barrier from excoriation seen in AD skin promotes *S. aureus* growth. Antimicrobial peptide expression is also blunted in these patients, thought to be secondary to the inhibitory effect of type 2 cytokines.[36,37] Type 2 cytokines also augment the killing effect of *S. aureus* toxins on keratinocytes.[38] Blockade of type 2 cytokines in AD appears to reduce skin infections in AD.[39]

S. aureus colonization likely contributes to skin inflammation; *S. aureus* toxins activate antigen presenting cells and increase T-cell cutaneous lymphocyte antigen (CLA) expression. Flares of AD correspond to shifts in the microbiome toward larger proportions of *S. aureus* representation.[40] Antibiotic treatment of clinically uninfected skin, however, has not been found to reduce AD severity.[41] The use of dilute sodium hypochlorite baths (bleach baths) appears to improve AD severity, but it is uncertain if this is through antiinflammatory and barrier effects rather than antimicrobial ones.[42]

The decision to treat a *S. aureus* infection is not straightforward. It is often difficult to distinguish acute crusted AD or excoriation from *S. aureus* impetiginization, and culturing of lesions does not help in distinguishing between colonization and infection. Culturing is recommended, however, to help guide antibiotic therapy and identify MRSA strains. MRSA has become an increasingly important pathogen in patients with AD.[43] Erosive plaques, honey-colored crusting, folliculitis, and persistent or multiple tender pustules are indicators of clinically relevant secondary bacterial skin infection in which antibiotic use would be indicated. Interestingly, topical steroids alone reduce *S. aureus* counts illustrating the role inflammation plays in *S. aureus* susceptibility.

VIRAL INFECTION

Patients with AD display an increased susceptibility to common warts and exaggerated clinical presentations to other viral infections such molluscum contagiosum. The most serious virally mediated complication is eczema herpeticum (EH). After an incubation period of 5 to 12 days, multiple itchy, vesiculopustular lesions erupt in a disseminated pattern; vesicular lesions are umbilicated, tend to cluster, and often become hemorrhagic and crusted (Fig. 22-6). Punched-out and extremely painful erosions result. These lesions may coalesce to large, denuded, and bleeding areas that can extend over the entire body and be fatal in some cases.

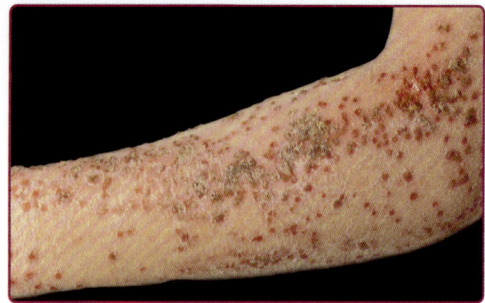

Figure 22-6 Eczema herpeticum. Typical vesicles and crusting in a patient with disseminated disease.

Defects in interferon pathways may explain why some patients develop this potentially devastating complication.[44]

Although smallpox infections have been eradicated worldwide since the late 1970s, threats of bioterrorism (with smallpox and other infectious agents) have forced nations to reconsider their policies toward initiating vaccination programs. In AD patients, smallpox vaccination (or even exposure to vaccinated individuals) (see Chap. 166) may cause a severe widespread eruption (eczema vaccinatum) that appears very similar to EH. Thus, in patients with AD, vaccination is contraindicated unless there is a clear risk of smallpox. In addition, decisions regarding vaccination of family members should take into consideration the potential of eczema vaccinatum in household contacts.

Exaggerated responses to coxsackie virus have also been reported in patients with AD that may resemble EH and has been termed eczema coxsackium.[45] Children present with hand and foot vesicles or papules that resemble typical hand, foot, and mouth disease, but lesions tend to be more severe and hemorrhagic and involve additional areas involved with eczema. Despite the sometimes dramatic presentation, the skin rash resolves with no negative sequelae.

FUNGAL INFECTION

It is unclear whether superficial fungal infections are more common in atopic individuals. There has been particular interest in the role of *Malassezia sympodialis* (*Pityrosporum ovale* or *Pityrosporum orbiculare*) in AD. *M. sympodialis* is a lipophilic yeast (see Chaps. 160 and 161) commonly present in the seborrheic areas of the skin. IgE antibodies against *Malassezia furfur* are commonly found in AD patients and most frequently in patients with head and neck dermatitis.[46] Although there are some case reports of improvement of head and neck AD with antifungal therapy, controlled trials are needed to determine the efficacy of targeting fungi in AD in this subset of patients.

OCULAR PROBLEMS

Eye complications associated with severe AD can lead to significant morbidity. Eyelid dermatitis and chronic blepharitis are commonly associated with AD and may result in visual impairment from corneal scarring. Atopic keratoconjunctivitis is usually bilateral and can have disabling symptoms that include itching, burning, tearing, and copious mucoid discharge. Vernal conjunctivitis is a severe bilateral recurrent chronic inflammatory process associated with papillary hypertrophy or cobblestoning of the upper eyelid conjunctiva. It usually occurs in younger patients and has a marked seasonal incidence, often in the spring. The associated intense pruritus is exacerbated by exposure to irritants, light, or sweating. Keratoconus is a conical deformity of the cornea believed to result from chronic rubbing of the eyes in patients with AD and allergic rhinoconjunctivitis. Cataracts were reported in the early literature to occur in up to 21% of patients with severe AD. However, it is unclear whether this was a primary manifestation of AD or the result of the extensive use of systemic and topical glucocorticoids, particularly around the eyes. Indeed, more recent studies suggest that routine screening for cataracts in patients with AD may not be productive unless there is concern about potential side effects from steroid therapy.

HAND DERMATITIS

Patients with AD often develop nonspecific, irritant hand dermatitis. It is frequently aggravated by repeated wetting and by washing of the hands with harsh soaps, detergents, and disinfectants. Atopic individuals with occupations involving wet work are prone to develop an intractable hand dermatitis in the occupational setting, which is a common cause of occupational disability. Less frequently, patients with AD may also develop a recurring chronic palmar or palmoplantar vesicular dermatitis.

EXFOLIATIVE DERMATITIS

Patients with extensive skin involvement may develop exfoliative dermatitis (see Chap. 21). This is associated with generalized redness, scaling, weeping, crusting, systemic toxicity, lymphadenopathy, and fever. Although this complication is rare, it is potentially life threatening. It is usually caused by superinfection, for example, with toxin-producing *S. aureus* or herpes simplex infection, continued irritation of the skin, or inappropriate therapy. In some cases, the withdrawal of topical or systemic glucocorticoids used to control severe AD may be a precipitating factor for exfoliative erythroderma.

ETIOLOGY AND PATHOGENESIS

OVERVIEW

Atopic dermatitis is a complex familial transmitted skin disease caused by interactions among genetic, immune, and environmental risk factors.[47] The interindividual variation of these factors compound the heterogeneity of mechanisms leading to AD. AD often occurs in association with asthma, allergic rhinitis, and food allergy. As such, AD may be considered part of a systemic disorder. Genetic and mechanistic studies suggest that two major biologic pathways are responsible for AD: epidermal dysfunction and altered innate or adaptive immune responses to microbes, allergens, stress, and irritants. Discovery of key pathogenic pathways and their associated biomarkers represents an active area of investigation required for the discovery of novel drugs or biologics that will effectively treat severe AD unresponsive to standard medications.

DECREASED SKIN BARRIER FUNCTION

Atopic dermatitis is associated with decreased in skin barrier function caused by the downregulation of cornified envelope genes (eg, keratin, filaggrin, and loricrin), reduced ceramide levels, increased endogenous proteolytic enzyme activity, and enhanced transepidermal water loss.[48] Addition of soap and detergents to the skin raises its pH, thereby increasing activity of endogenous proteases, leading to further breakdown of epidermal barrier function. The epidermal barrier may also be damaged by scratching, exposure to exogenous proteases from house dust mites, and *S. aureus*. This is worsened by the lack of certain endogenous protease inhibitors in atopic skin. These epidermal changes likely contribute to increased allergen absorption into the skin and microbial colonization. Because epicutaneous sensitization to allergen results in higher level allergic immune responses, decreased skin barrier function could act as a site for allergen sensitization and predispose such children to the development of food allergy and respiratory allergy.

GENETICS

More than 80 genes have been associated with AD.[43,49] Of these genes, loss-of-function mutations involving the epidermal barrier protein filaggrin have been most consistently replicated to be a major predisposing factor for AD in European whites and Asians. Of note, the filaggrin gene is found on chromosome 1q21, which contains genes (including involucrin, loricrin, and S100 calcium binding proteins) in the epidermal differentiation complex (EDC), known to be expressed during terminal differentiation of the epidermis. Gene profiling studies have demonstrated downregulation of genes encoding proteins involved in epidermal differentiation, including multiple skin barrier proteins and antimicrobial peptides required for host defense in AD.[50] Candidate gene approaches have also implicated variants in the *SPINK5* gene, which is expressed in the uppermost epidermis, where its product, LEKT1, inhibits two serine proteases involved in desquamation and inflammation (stratum corneum tryptic enzyme and stratum corneum chymotryptic enzyme). Stratum corneum tryptic enzyme and stratum corneum tryptic enzyme expression is increased in AD, suggesting that an imbalance of protease versus protease inhibitor activity may contribute to atopic skin inflammation. Other skin barrier genes that have been implicated in AD include LAMA3, TMEM79, filaggrin-2 (FLG2), Late Cornified Envelope-like Proline-rich 1 (LELP1), and claudin-1 (CLDN1). The relative importance of different skin barrier genes and immune responses may vary by race.[51] It is interesting, for example, that FLG mutations have currently not been consistently found in African populations; however, loss-of-function mutations in FLG2 are associated with increased risk in African Americans.[49]

These observations establish a key role for impaired skin barrier function in the pathogenesis of AD because impaired skin barrier formation allows increased transepidermal water loss, and importantly, increased attachment and entry of allergens and chemicals from the environment, resulting in skin inflammatory responses.[47] It is important to note that filaggrin mutations and likely other mutations affecting the skin barrier can occur in normal healthy individuals, patients with ichthyosis vulgaris who do not have significant skin inflammation, and only a minority of individuals with AD have filaggrin gene mutations. This suggests that factors other than skin barrier gene mutations are also required for the development of AD.

Atopic dermatitis has also been associated with variation of genes involved in innate and adaptive immunity, interleukin-1 (IL-1) family signaling, regulatory T cells, vitamin D pathway, and nerve growth factor pathway.[43] Thus, a combination of various genetic factors may influence the development of different AD phenotypes. Patients with filaggrin null mutations often have early onset of AD, severe eczema, and high-level allergen sensitization and develop asthma later in childhood (ie, the so-called atopic march).[48,49] In patients with AD susceptible to EH (ADEH+), filaggrin mutations occur in combination with transcriptomic signatures in peripheral blood mononuclear cells (PBMCs) that are distinct from AD without a history of AD (ADEH-). In a recent report, it was demonstrated that unstimulated ADEH+ and ADEH- PBMC had similar transcriptomes.[52] However, after stimulation with herpes simplex virus (HSV), PBMCs from ADEH+ had distinct transcriptomic profiles compared with ADEH-, with striking downregulation of antiviral cytokines, including both type I and type III INFs. These results are indicative of defective innate immune responses in ADEH+ subjects.

Atopic dermatitis is a complex trait that involves interactions between multiple gene products requiring environmental factors and the immune response, leading to a final clinical phenotype. Chromosome 5q31-33 contains a clustered family of functionally related cytokine genes—IL-3, IL-4, IL-5, IL-13, and granulocyte macrophage colony-stimulating factor involved in generation of IgE, eosinophilia, and allergic inflammation. Gain-of-function mutations in the alpha subunit of the IL-4 receptor, IL-4, and IL-13 has been significantly associated with AD, providing a rationale for the use of biologicals that interfere with the IL-4 receptor signaling pathway.[30] A significant association has also been observed between *TSLP* gene polymorphisms and AD supporting further evidence for the importance of Th2 polarization in this disease.[53]

IMMUNOPATHOLOGY OF ATOPIC DERMATITIS

Based on clinical appearance and duration of illness, AD skin can be characterized as nonlesional AD, acute AD lesions (3 or fewer days after onset), and chronic skin lesions (>3 days' duration). Nonlesional AD skin may not be normal but characterized by mild epidermal hyperplasia and a sparse perivascular T-cell infiltrate. Dendritic antigen-presenting cells (eg, Langerhans cells (LCs), inflammatory dendritic epidermal cells [IDECs], macrophages) in lesional and, to a lesser extent, in nonlesional skin of AD exhibit surface-bound immunoglobulin E molecules. In acute lesions, there is epidermal spongiosis with an increased infiltration of activated memory T cells bearing the skin-homing CLA. Eosinophils, basophils, and neutrophils are rare. Mast cells are in various stages of degranulation.

Chronic lichenified lesions are characterized by a hyperplastic epidermis with elongation of the rete ridges, prominent hyperkeratosis, and minimal spongiosis. There is an increased number of IgE-bearing LCs and in the epidermis, and macrophages dominate the dermal mononuclear cell infiltrate. Mast cells are increased in number but are fully granulated. Neutrophils are absent in AD skin lesions even in the setting of increased *S. aureus* colonization and infection. Increased numbers of eosinophils are observed in chronic AD skin lesions. Eosinophils are thought to contribute to allergic inflammation by the secretion of cytokines and mediators that augment allergic inflammation and induce tissue injury in AD through the production of reactive oxygen intermediates and release of toxic granule proteins.

CYTOKINE-DRIVEN ATOPIC DERMATITIS SKIN INFLAMMATION

Atopic skin inflammation is orchestrated by the local expression of proinflammatory cytokines.[47] A key difference between epidermal keratinocytes found in AD, as compared with normal, skin is the presence of thymic stromal lymphopoietin (TSLP) and IL-33 in AD epidermis. TSLP, along with IL-33, are key cytokines secreted by epithelial cells that induce dendritic cells to drive Th0 cells into the Th2 cell differentiation pathway. Nonlesional AD and acute AD skin lesions are predominantly associated with expression of IL-4, IL-5, IL-13, IL-25, IL-31, and IL-33 expression. These type 2 cytokines are present in all stages of AD and can be secreted by multiple cell types, including innate lymphoid type 2 cells, mast cells, and basophils, present in AD skin lesions. This contributes to substantial redundancy in allergic inflammation. As such, cytokine targeting, as opposed to cell targeting, is considered a more effective approach in the treatment of AD. The importance role of type 2 cytokines is that, in animal models, they can recapitulate elevated IgE responses, eosinophilia, skin barrier dysfunction, allergic skin inflammation, and itching observed in clinical AD.

Aside from Th2, other cytokine pathways are also activated during the evolution of AD. The IL-22–IL-17 pathway is of particular interest because it, along with IL-4 and IL-13, can inhibit terminal keratinocyte differentiation, including filaggrin expression. Because dendritic cell–derived, IL-23, enhances IL-22–IL-17 cell differentiation, all of these cytokines are being closely examined for their potential role in AD. It is interesting that IL-4 and IL-13 can enhance IL-23 production by dendritic cells. Furthermore, blockade of IL-4 and IL-13 pathway, leading to improvement in AD, is also associated with reduced IL-23 and IL-17 expression in AD skin.[54]

When acute AD become chronic AD skin lesions, there is an increase in Th1 cytokines such as INF-γ, which potentiates AD skin inflammation. It is noteworthy that experimental studies demonstrate pretreatment with IL-4 and IL-13 dampens responses to interferons and IL-17, suggesting that when the early AD lesion is exposed to IL-4 and IL-13, there is a long-lasting, persistent effect. A recent birth cohort study, however, demonstrated that TSLP could be detected in at-risk infants before the onset of AD, suggesting that the TSLP–Th2-ILC2 pathway plays a critical role in initiation of AD.[55] In chronic AD, there is an increased in IL-5, which is involved in eosinophil development and survival.

The skin-specific chemokine, cutaneous T cell–attracting chemokine (CTACK; CC chemokine ligand 27 [CCL27]), is highly upregulated in AD and preferentially attracts skin homing cutaneous lymphoid antigen (CLA)⁺ CC chemokine receptor 10⁺ (CCR10⁺) T cells into the skin. CCR4 expressed on skin homing CLA⁺ T cells can also bind to CCL17 on the vascular endothelium of cutaneous venules. Selective recruitment of CCR4-expressing Th2 cells is mediated by macrophage-derived chemokine and thymus and activation-regulated cytokine, both of which are increased in AD. The severity of AD has been linked to the magnitude of thymus and activation-regulated cytokine levels. In addition, chemokines such as fractalkine, IFN-γ–inducible protein 10, and monokine induced by IFN-γ are strongly upregulated in keratinocytes and result in Th1-cell migration toward epidermis, particularly in chronic AD. Increased expression of the CC chemokines, macrophage chemoattractant protein-4, eotaxin, and RANTES (regulated on activation normal T-cell expressed and secreted) contribute to infiltration of macrophages, eosinophils, and T cells into both acute and chronic AD skin lesions.

IMMUNE EFFECTS ON EPITHELIAL DIFFERENTIATION COMPLEX

The dry skin and increased transepidermal water loss in individuals with AD reflect the underlying skin barrier dysfunction and loss of natural moisturizing factors that play an important role in the pathogenesis of AD.[47] Only a minority of patients, however, have FLG null mutations. Other genetic variants in the EDC and tight junctions are even rarer. The majority of patients with AD likely have immune-mediated reduction in epidermal terminal differentiation, leading to decreased generation of various epidermal structural proteins, filaggrin breakdown products, epidermal lipids, and antimicrobial peptides. TSLP, IL-4, and IL-13 are the most potent cytokines downregulating filaggrin expression by keratinocytes. IL-17, IL-22, IL-25, and IL-33 can act synergistically with IL-4 and IL-13 to further downregulate expression of epidermal proteins and lipids. This combination of events along with activation of proteases and lipases creates defective epidermal barrier function and alters epidermal acidification and loss of moisturization in AD, thereby contributing to enhanced allergen and microbial penetration met by the host immune response and clinical appearance of AD. The critical role for immune activation in driving AD pathogenesis is supported by the observation that cyclosporin is highly effective in controlling severe AD and reverses the epidermal pathology.[56] Clinical studies demonstrating that blockade of IL-4 and IL-13 immune pathways is highly effective in reversing severe AD provides definitive data that in the majority of patients, cytokine activation drives atopic inflammation. Recent studies showing AD immune activation may differ in various races and according to age group suggests the importance of more precise stratification of immune responses with clinical AD subsets.[51]

BASIS OF PRURITUS IN ATOPIC DERMATITIS

Pruritus is a prominent feature of AD, manifested as cutaneous hyperreactivity and scratching after exposure to allergens, changes in humidity, excessive sweating, and low concentrations of irritants. Control of pruritus is important because mechanical injury from scratching can induce proinflammatory cytokine and chemokine release, leading to a vicious scratch–itch cycle, perpetuating the AD skin rash. The mechanisms of pruritus in AD are poorly understood. Allergen-induced release of histamine from skin mast cells is not an exclusive cause of pruritus in AD because H_1 antihistamines do not appear to control the itch of AD.[57,58] Recent studies demonstrating a potential role for H_4 receptors in skin pathobiology, however, suggests that histamine may play a contributory role. The observation, however, that treatment with topical corticosteroids (TCs) and calcineurin inhibitors is effective at reducing pruritus suggests that the inflammatory cells play an important role in pruritus. Molecules that have been implicated in pruritus include T cell–derived cytokines such as IL-31, stress-induced neuropeptides, proteases such as proteases that can act on protease-activated receptors, eicosanoids, and eosinophil-derived proteins.

DIAGNOSIS

The diagnosis of AD is based on a clinical assessment and guided by the criteria discussed previously. A diagnosis of AD is made only after other conditions such as psoriasis, scabies infestation, seborrheic dermatitis, or contact dermatitis have been considered and ruled out, if necessary, with additional testing. AD not responding to routine skin care or topical antiinflammatory therapy or skin lesions that are atypical in morphology or distribution should prompt the clinician to consider additional diagnoses such as T-cell lymphoma, nutritional deficiencies, or metabolic syndromes. Patients with a history of sinopulmonary infections, severe skin infections, erythroderma, or failure to thrive should be evaluated for immunodeficiency syndromes.

SUPPORTIVE STUDIES

LABORATORY TESTING

Routine potassium hydroxide microscopic evaluation can be used to rule out cutaneous fungal infections that may mimic AD. Mineral oil examination for scabies is warranted if burrows are present or vesicles are present on the palms and soles in infants. If the clinical picture suggests allergic contact dermatitis may be present (eg, atypical distribution, refractory disease), patch testing is warranted.

Atopic dermatitis guidelines of care from the American Academy of Dermatology do not recommend routine allergy testing for AD because many patients with AD have detectable antigen-specific IgE to foods and airborne and environmental allergens, especially those with severe disease.[59] History-directed skin prick testing or serum-specific IgE antibody testing may be performed to confirm a true type I food allergy if a patient reports a history of immediate-type hypersensitivity symptoms (eg, urticaria, lip swelling, abdominal pain). The Food Allergy Expert Panel sponsored by the National Institute of Allergy and Infectious Disease defined allergy as an "adverse health event"; thus, patients should not be labeled as "allergic" solely based on sensitization alone.[60] In patients with AD, positive allergy test results (in the absence of controlled food challenges) poorly predict true type I allergic responses.[61] There remains limited evidence that removal of allergens from the diet or environment improves AD outcomes.[62,63] Thompson and Hanifin noted that proper AD control with routine therapy reduces parental concern regarding diet as a contributory factor in AD.[64] The Food Allergy Expert Panel suggests that children younger than 5 years old with moderate to severe AD be considered for food allergy evaluation for milk, egg, peanut, wheat, and soy if at least one of the following conditions is met: (1) the child has persistent AD despite optimized management and topical therapy or (2) the child has a reliable history of an immediate reaction after ingestion of a specific food.[60]

Laboratory studies to rule out immunodeficiency associated with eczema include a complete blood count with differential for white blood cell count; lymphocyte phenotyping for T cells, B cells, and natural killer cells; and lymphocyte proliferation assays as well as genomic DNA analysis for pathogenic variants in genes resulting in severe combined deficiency (eg, *IL2RG, ADA, IL7R*), Omenn syndrome (hypomorphic mutations in *RAG1/RAG2* genes) or hyper-IgE (HIE) syndrome (eg, *STAT3, DOCK8, SPINK5, TYK2*). Small platelets seen on peripheral blood smear are characteristic of Wiskott-Aldrich syndrome. Both elevated serum IgE levels and elevated circulating blood eosinophils can be seen in a number of diseases besides AD, including HIE syndrome but also some immunodeficiencies. Zinc levels to rule out zinc deficiency should be obtained on fasting morning blood and corrected for any concomitant low albumin level.

PATHOLOGY

Biopsy of AD lesions with hematoxylin and eosin staining (Table 22-2) will not allow differentiation among various eczematous processes such as nummular dermatitis or allergic contact dermatitis because all eczematous processes show spongiotic dermatitis on histopathology. Biopsy is helpful to rule out cutaneous T-cell lymphomas (see Chap. 119) and should reveal epidermotropic neoplastic T cells with hyperconvoluted cerebriform nuclei and intraepidermal Pautrier microabscess formation. T-cell receptor gene rearrangement studies will demonstrate clonal rearrangement. Biopsies may not be diagnostic for Sézary syndrome, and diagnostic criteria include an absolute Sezary cell count of 1000 cells/mm³ or greater in peripheral blood, increased CD4/CD8 ratio greater than 10 on flow cytometry analysis, or circulating T-cell clone detected by cytogenetic methods. Histopathology of psoriasis shows characteristic changes that depend on the stage of evolving lesion—initial, developing, or mature (see Chap. 28).

IMAGING

Imaging is not recommended in AD diagnosis except when ruling out specific immunodeficiencies. Chest radiographs will reveal an absent thymus in most forms of severe combined immunodeficiency as well as pulmonary infiltrates from infectious complications.

TABLE 22-2
Histopathology Comparison for Nonlesional Atopic Dermatitis, Acute Atopic Dermatitis, and Chronic Atopic Dermatitis

NONLESIONAL ATOPIC DERMATITIS	ACUTE ATOPIC DERMATITIS (<3 DAYS)	CHRONIC SKIN LESIONS (>3 DAYS)
Mild epidermal hyperplasia, sparse perivascular infiltrate	Epidermal spongiosis, increased inflammatory infiltrate	Hyperplastic epidermis with elongated rete ridges, prominent hyperkeratosis, minimal spongiosis
Langerhans cells, inflammatory dendritic epidermal cells, macrophages	Mast cells (degranulating); rare eosinophils, basophils, and neutrophils	Langerhans cells, mast cells (fully granulated), neutrophils absent, increased eosinophils

Chest radiographs or computed tomography scans may reveal extensive infiltrates, cyst-forming pneumonias, and occasionally fungal lesions in HIE syndrome.

DIFFERENTIAL DIAGNOSIS

Because AD is currently not defined by a unique diagnostic biomarker, a number of inflammatory skin diseases, immunodeficiencies, skin malignancies, genetic disorders, infectious diseases, and infestations may share symptoms and signs with AD (Table 22-3). These should be considered in the initial evaluation of a patient presenting with an eczematous rash but also if a patient with a diagnosis of AD is not responding to appropriate therapy. Infants presenting in the first year of life with failure to thrive, diarrhea, a generalized scaling erythematous rash, and recurrent cutaneous or systemic infections should be evaluated for severe combined immunodeficiency syndrome. Omenn syndrome, caused by mutations in *RAG1* and *RAG2* as well as several other genes, is an autosomal recessive severe combined immunodeficiency that can present with an erythrodermic rash, as well as elevated IgE, eosinophilia, diarrhea, lymphadenopathy, hepatosplenomegaly, and susceptibility to infections.[65] The dermatitis can be eczematous though with pachydermia. Other immunodeficiency with eczematous rash includes immune dysregulation, polyendocrinopathy, enteropathy X-linked (IPEX) syndrome.[66] IPEX results from mutations of *Foxp3*, a gene located on the X chromosome that encodes a DNA-binding protein required for development of regulatory T cells. Besides dermatitis, patients typically present with a recalcitrant enteropathy, as well as autoimmune features such as type 1 diabetes, thyroiditis, hemolytic anemia, or thrombocytopenia. Wiskott-Aldrich syndrome is an X-linked recessive disorder characterized by an eczematous rash associated with thrombocytopenia along with variable abnormalities in humoral and cellular immunity and severe bacterial infections.

Hyper-IgE syndrome caused by *STAT3* mutations is an autosomal dominant multisystem disorder characterized by recurrent deep-seated bacterial infections, including cutaneous cold abscesses and pneumonias with pneumatocele formation due to *S. aureus*.[67] Although *S. aureus* is an important pathogen in this disorder, infection with other bacteria, including gram-negative species (eg, *Pseudomonas aeruginosa*) and nontuberculous mycobacteria and fungi (eg, *Aspergillus*) may occur, including invasive disease. STAT3 is an essential transcription factor for Th17 T-cell development, and because Th17 T cells play an essential role in protecting against *Candida* spp., patients with mutations in *STAT3* are susceptible to chronic mucocutaneus candidiasis. In infancy, patients may present with a papulopustular eruption of the face and scalp. Other features of HIE syndrome include skeletal abnormalities with coarse facial features and prominent frontal bossing, dental anomalies with retained primary teeth, bone fractures, and osteoporosis. Despite elevated serum IgE levels, patients usually are not atopic. Patients with mutations in the gene encoding dedicator of cytokinesis 8 protein (*DOCK8*) have an immunodeficiency that accounts for most cases of autosomal recessive HIE.[68] These patients have an eczematous dermatitis with recurrent viral infections, including some with central nevous system involvement. Patients may present with recalcitrant warts secondary to human papilloma virus, disseminated molluscum or recurrent herpes simplex infections. Malignancies, including squamous cell carcinomas and lymphomas, are an important cause of death in patients starting in the second decade of life. Another unique feature in patients with DOCK8 is that many have associated food allergies. Patients with tyrosine kinase 2 deficiency can also present with an eczematous rash with high serum IgE and recurrent cutaneous staphylococcal infections.[69]

TABLE 22-3
Differential Diagnosis of Atopic Dermatitis
Most Likely
Contact dermatitis (allergic and irritant)
Seborrheic dermatitis
Scabies
Psoriasis
Ichthyosis vulgaris
Keratosis pilaris
Dermatophytosis
Consider
Asteatotic eczema
Lichen simplex chronicus
Nummular dermatitis
Juvenile palmar-plantar dermatosis
Impetigo
Drug eruptions
Perioral dermatitis
Pityriasis alba
Photosensitivity disorders (hydroa vacciniforme, polymorphous light eruption, porphyrias)
Molluscum dermatitis
Less Common or Rare Disorders Predominant in Adolescents and Adults
Cutaneous T-cell lymphoma (mycosis fungoides or Sézary syndrome)
Human immunodeficiency virus–associated dermatosis
Lupus erythematosus
Dermatomyositis
Graft-versus-host disease
Pemphigus foliaceus
Dermatitis herpetiformis
Photosensitivity disorders (hydroa vacciniforme, polymorphous light eruption, porphyrias)
Less Common or Rare Disorders Predominant in Infants and Children
Metabolic or Nutritional
Phenylketonuria
Prolidase deficiency
Multiple carboxylase deficiency
Zinc deficiency (acrodermatitis enteropathica, prematurity, deficient breast milk zinc, cystic fibrosis)
Others: biotin, essential fatty acids, organic acidurias
Primary Immunodeficiency Disorders

Other diseases to consider in the differential diagnosis of AD include cutaneous T-cell lymphoma, especially in adults without a history of childhood eczema and without other atopic features.[70] Mycosis fungoides (discussed in Chap. 119) is the most common form of CTCL, Sézary syndrome is characterized by generalized erythroderma with lymphadenopathy and circulating malignant T cells (Sézary cells). Although contact dermatitis should be considered in the differential diagnosis of AD (see Chap. 24), contact allergy can also complicate AD, especially in patients whose AD appears to worsen with therapy, typically with TCs.[71] Allergic contact dermatitis complicating AD may appear as an acute flare of the underlying disease. Eczematous dermatitis has been also reported with human immunodeficiency virus infection as well as with a variety of infestations such as scabies. Other diseases that can be confused with AD include psoriasis, ichthyoses, and seborrheic dermatitis. Although psoriasis can typically be distinguished from AD based on characteristic clinical features (see Chap. 28), inverse (flexural) psoriasis or erythrodermic psoriasis may at times present more of a diagnostic challenge. Zinc deficiency can result from dietary deficiency; excessive losses with diarrhea; or chronic disease, including renal or hepatic as well as inadequate absorption associated with an inherited deficiency of the zinc carrier protein ZIP4 and can present with an eczematous rash with a perioral, acral, or perineal distribution.[72]

CLINICAL COURSE AND PROGNOSIS

Most AD starting in childhood is mild in severity, and a review of birth cohort studies found that 80% of cases remitted, at least temporarily, by 10 years of age.[73] Symptoms of AD, however, may persist or reemerge in adulthood. One primarily pediatric AD cohort found that more than 80% of patients prescribed calcineurin inhibitors reported persistent symptoms into adulthood.[74] Risk factors reported to be predictive of a persistent disease course include disease severity, later onset disease, genetic mutations in *FLG* or *FLG-2* genes, and early allergic sensitization.[75,76] It is not known whether early or aggressive treatment of AD alters the natural course. For occupational counseling, adults whose childhood AD has been in remission for a number of years may present with hand dermatitis, especially if daily activities require repeated hand wetting.

MANAGEMENT

OVERVIEW

Successful treatment of AD requires a systematic, multipronged approach that incorporates education about the disease state, skin hydration, pharmacologic therapy, and the identification and elimination of flare factors such as irritants, allergens, infectious agents, and emotional stressors (Fig. 22-7). Many factors lead to the symptom complex characterizing AD. Thus, treatment plans should be individualized to address each patient's skin disease reaction pattern, including the acuity of the rash, and the trigger factors that are unique to the particular patient. In patients refractory to conventional forms of therapy, alternative antiinflammatory and immunomodulatory agents may be necessary.

EDUCATION AS INTERVENTION

Education may be considered as a therapeutic intervention for the management of atopic dermatitis.[77]

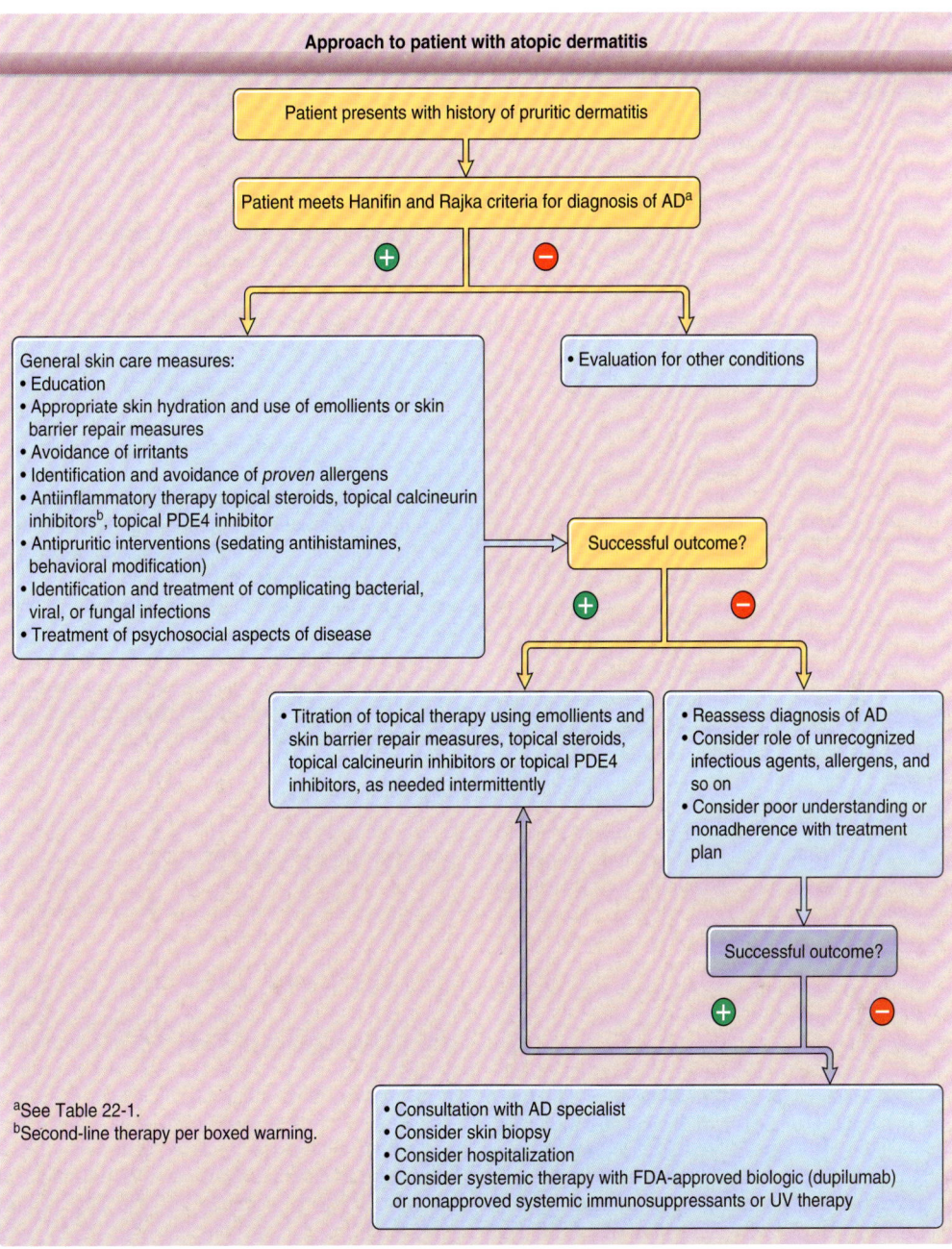

Figure 22-7 Approach to patient with atopic dermatitis (AD). FDA, Food and Drug Administration; PDE, phosphodiesterase; UV, ultraviolet.

Intensive disease education has been shown in randomized, controlled trials to improve subjective quality-of-life and objective eczema severity scores.[78] Intensive education may include comprehensive "center-based" patient/family teaching, written "handouts" and care plans, patient and family support groups, and internet-accessed media. Several resources available online are listed in Table 22-4.

IDENTIFICATION AND ELIMINATION OF TRIGGERS

GENERAL CONSIDERATIONS

Patients with AD are more susceptible to irritants than are unaffected individuals. Thus, it is important to identify and eliminate aggravating factors that trigger

TABLE 22-4
Online Resources for Patients with Atopic Dermatitis and Their Families

Coping Strategies and Support Groups
National Eczema Association (www.nationaleczema.org)
Under My Skin: A Kid's Guide to Atopic Dermatitis (www.undermyskin.com)

Specialized Atopic Dermatitis Care
American Academy of Dermatology EczemaNet (www.skincarephysicians.com/eczemanet/index.html)
The Eczema Center at Rady Children's Hospital (www.eczemacenter.org)
National Jewish Health (www.njc.org)
Northwestern University Eczema Care and Education Center (www.eczemacarecenter.com)

Information on Allergic Triggers
American Academy of Allergy, Asthma & Immunology (www.aaaai.org)
Food Allergy & Anaphylaxis Network (www.foodallergy.org)

---

the itch–scratch cycle. These include soaps or detergents, contact with chemicals, smoke, abrasive clothing, and exposure to extremes of temperature and humidity. Alcohol and astringents found in toiletries are drying. When soaps are used, they should have minimal defatting activity and a neutral pH or slightly acidic pH. New clothing may be laundered before wearing to decrease levels of formaldehyde and other added chemicals. Residual laundry detergent in clothing may be irritating. Using a liquid rather than powder detergent and adding a second rinse cycle facilitate removal of the detergent.

Recommendations regarding environmental living conditions should include temperature and humidity control to avoid problems related to heat, humidity, and perspiration. Every attempt should be made to allow children to be as normally active as possible. Certain sports, such as swimming, may be better tolerated than other sports involving intense perspiration, physical contact, or heavy clothing and equipment. Although UV light may be beneficial to some patients with AD, sunscreens should be used to avoid sunburn. However, because sunscreens can be irritants or allergens, care should be used to identify a nonirritating product.

SPECIFIC ALLERGENS

Foods and aeroallergens such as dust mites, animal danders, molds, and pollens have been demonstrated to exacerbate AD in some patients. In patients not responding to routine skin care and topical antiinflammatory therapies, potential allergens can be identified by taking a careful history, looking for immediate or anaphylactic clinical reactions that may trigger the itch–scratch cycle, and carrying out selective skin-prick tests or specific serum IgE levels. Negative skin test results or serum test results for allergen-specific IgE have a high predictive value for ruling out suspected allergens. Positive allergy testing results, on the other hand, poorly predicts adverse clinical reactions. Fleischer and colleagues performed food challenges on 125 children with AD who were labeled as having food allergy by allergy testing.[61] After oral food challenge, 84% to 93% of the foods being avoided were returned to the children's diet, when no immediate reactions were observed.

Elimination diets, which in some cases can be nutritionally deficient, are rarely, if ever, required. Even in patients with multiple positive skin test results, the majority of patients react to three or fewer foods on controlled challenge. In dust mite–allergic patients with AD, prolonged avoidance of dust mites has not been consistently found to result in improvement of their skin disease.[63] Avoidance measures include use of dust mite–proof encasings on pillows, mattresses, and box springs; washing bedding in hot water weekly; removing bedroom carpeting; and decreasing indoor humidity levels with air conditioning. Because there are many triggers contributing to the flares of AD, attention should be focused on identifying and controlling the flare factors that are important to the individual patient. Whereas infants and young children are more likely to have food allergies, older children and adults are more likely to be sensitive to environmental aeroallergens. Contact allergens have been increasingly recognized in AD. One study found that of children with relevant positive reactions, 34% had a diagnosis of AD.[77]

EMOTIONAL STRESSORS

Although emotional stress does not cause AD, patients often report it exacerbates the illness. AD patients often respond to frustration, embarrassment, or other stressful events with increased pruritus and scratching. Psychological evaluation or counseling should be considered in patients who have difficulty with emotional triggers or concomitant metal health conditions or symptoms contributing to difficulty in managing their disease. It may be especially useful in adolescents and young adults who consider their skin disease disfiguring. Relaxation, behavioral modification, or biofeedback may be helpful in patients with habitual scratching.[58]

INFECTIOUS AGENTS

Antistaphylococcal antibiotics are often needed in the treatment of patients who are infected with *S. aureus*. Cephalosporins or penicillinase-resistant penicillins (dicloxacillin, oxacillin, or cloxacillin) are usually beneficial for patients who are not colonized with resistant *S. aureus* strains. Because erythromycin-resistant *Staphylococci* are common, erythromycin and newer macrolide antibiotics are usually of limited utility. Topical antimicrobials such as mupirocin, fusidic acid, or more recently retapamulin offers some utility in the treatment of impetiginized lesions. A Cochrane analysis of interventions for impetigo found that topical mupirocin and topical fusidic acid are equal to or more effective than oral treatment for patients with limited disease and that fusidic acid and mupirocin are of similar efficacy.[79] Patients should be cautioned against using topical antibiotics in an "as-needed" manner that can lead to resistant organisms.

Use of neomycin topically can result in development of allergic contact dermatitis because neomycin is among the more common allergens causing contact dermatitis. In patients with extensive superinfection, a course of systemic antibiotics is most practical. MRSA may require culture and sensitivity testing to assist in appropriate antibiotic selection. Baths with dilute sodium hypochlorite (bleach) may also benefit AD patients with superinfected eczema, especially those with recurrent MRSA, although they can occasionally be irritating. Of note, a controlled study of twice-weekly bleach baths for 3 months showed clinical benefit, although skin colonization by *S. aureus* did not disappear even when combined with intranasal mupirocin 5 days each month.[80] Bleach baths may exert their beneficial effect on AD via antiinflammatory mechanisms rather than antimicrobial ones.[81]

Herpes simplex can provoke recurrent dermatitis and may be misdiagnosed as *S. aureus* infection or severe eczema. The presence of punched-out erosions, vesicles, or infected skin lesions that do not respond to oral antibiotics should initiate a search for herpes simplex. This can be diagnosed by polymerase chain reaction identification of herpes genetic material, Giemsa-stained Tzanck smear, or direct immunofluorescence of cells scraped from the vesicle base or viral culture. Antiviral treatment for cutaneous herpes simplex infections is of critical importance in the patient with widespread AD because life-threatening dissemination has been reported (EH). Acyclovir, 400 mg three times daily for 10 days or 200 mg four times daily for 10 days by oral administration (or an equivalent dosage of one of the newer antiherpetic medications), is useful in adults with herpes simplex confined to the skin. Intravenous treatment may be necessary for severe disseminated EH. The dosage should be adjusted according to weight in children.

Dermatophyte infections can complicate AD and may contribute to exacerbation of disease activity. Patients with dermatophyte infection or IgE antibodies to *Malassezia* spp. may benefit from a trial of topical or systemic antifungal therapy, although high-quality controlled studies are lacking.

PRURITUS

The treatment of pruritus in AD should be directed primarily at the underlying causes. Reduction of skin inflammation and dryness with topical glucocorticoids or nonsteroidal antiinflammatory drugs (NSAIDs) and skin hydration, respectively, often symptomatically reduce pruritus. Inhaled and ingested allergens should be eliminated if documented to cause an urticarial skin rash in controlled challenges. Systemic antihistamines act primarily by blocking the H_1 receptors in the dermis, thereby ameliorating histamine-induced pruritus. However, histamine is not the primary mediator of itch in AD skin, thus the relative lack of convincing evidence that antihistamines improve pruritus in AD.[80] Some antihistamines are also mild anxiolytics and may offer symptomatic relief through tranquilizing and sedative effects. Studies of newer, nonsedating antihistamines show variable results in the effectiveness of controlling pruritus in AD, although they may be useful in the subset of AD patients with concomitant urticaria or concurrent allergic rhinitis.

Because pruritus is usually worse at night, the sedating antihistamines, for example, hydroxyzine or diphenhydramine, may offer an advantage with their soporific side effects when used at bedtime. Doxepin hydrochloride has both tricyclic antidepressant and H_1- and H_2-histamine receptor-blocking effects. It can be used in doses of 10 to 75 mg orally at night or up to 75 mg twice daily in adult patients. If nocturnal pruritus remains severe, short-term use of a sedative or melatonin to allow adequate rest may be appropriate for some patients.[82] Treatment of AD with topical antihistamines is generally not recommended because of potential cutaneous sensitization. However, short-term (1-week) application of topical 5% doxepin cream has been reported to reduce pruritus without sensitization. Of note, sedation is a side effect of widespread application of doxepin cream, and allergic contact dermatitis has been reported.

TOPICAL THERAPY

EMOLLIENTS

Emollients represent the cornerstone of treatment for mild AD and serve as an important flare preventive therapy for all levels of disease severity. Patients with AD have abnormal skin barrier function with increased transepidermal water loss and decreased water content and dry skin (xerosis) contributing to disease morbidity by the development of microfissures and cracks in the skin. These microfissures may serve as portals of entry for skin pathogens, irritants, and allergens. *FLG* gene mutations or acquired filaggrin protein deficiencies caused by inflammation have also been shown to result in decreased epidermal levels of natural moisturizing factor.[83] AD xerosis can become aggravated during the dry winter months and in certain work environments.

The daily use of an effective emollient helps to restore and preserve the stratum corneum barrier, decreases the need for topical glucocorticoids and NSAIDs and improves outcomes. Moisturizers are available in the form of lotions, creams, or ointments. Some lotions and creams may be irritating because of added preservatives, solubilizers, and fragrances. Lotions with high water content may be drying because of an evaporative effect and provide few lipids to the skin. Thicker, bland emollients with high lipid content are preferred but are sometimes not well tolerated because of interference with the function of the eccrine sweat ducts and the induction of folliculitis or itching. In these patients, less occlusive agents should be used. Plain petrolatum is a common lipid base for effective emollients. Petrolatum intercalates into the stratum corneum and appears to upregulate skin barrier and antimicrobial peptide gene expression thought to be beneficial in AD.[84] The benefit of emollients with special additives, such as ceramides, is not clear, although one study found the use of a urea-containing moisturizer provided better clinical results than a standard emollient.[85]

Hydration, by baths or wet dressings, promotes transepidermal penetration of topical glucocorticoids. The optimal bathing regimen for patients with AD is not known, however, and recommendations vary by specialty. Kohn and colleagues found no differences in outcomes in patients applying TCs to wet skin compared with dry skin,[86] but the "soak and smear" method is often used in recalcitrant disease.[87] Wet dressings or "wet wraps" are recommended for use on severely affected or chronically involved areas of dermatitis refractory to therapy. However, overuse of wet dressings may result in maceration of the skin complicated by secondary infection. Wet dressings or baths also have the potential to promote drying and fissuring of the skin if not followed by topical emollient use. Thus, wet dressing therapy is reserved for poorly controlled AD and should be closely monitored by a physician.

TOPICAL ANTIINFLAMMATORY THERAPY

Topical Corticosteroids: According to AD treatment guidelines, TCs are the cornerstone of antiinflammatory treatment in AD.[88] Because of potential side effects, many health care practitioners use topical glucocorticoids only to control acute exacerbations of AD. However, studies suggest that after control of AD is achieved with a daily regimen of topical glucocorticoid, long-term control can be maintained in a subset of patients with scheduled intermittent applications of TCs, such as twice-weekly fluticasone, to areas that have healed but are prone to developing eczema.[89]

Patients should be carefully instructed in the use of topical glucocorticoids to avoid potential side effects. The potent fluorinated glucocorticoids should be avoided on the face, the genitalia, and the intertriginous areas. A low-potency glucocorticoid preparation is generally recommended for these areas and only used intermittently for long-term use. Patients should be instructed to apply topical glucocorticoids to their skin lesions and to use emollients on uninvolved skin. Failure of a patient to respond to topical glucocorticoids is sometimes partly caused by an inadequate supply or inadequate quantity of use. It is important to remember that it takes approximately 30 g of cream or ointment to cover the entire skin surface of an adult once. To treat the entire body twice daily for 2 weeks requires approximately 840 g (2 lb) of topical glucocorticoids.

There are seven classes of topical glucocorticoids, ranked according to their potency based on vasoconstrictor assays. Because of their potential side effects, the ultrahigh-potency glucocorticoids should be used daily or twice daily only for very short periods of time (usually 2 weeks) and in areas that are lichenified but not on the face or intertriginous areas. Midpotency glucocorticoids can be used for longer periods of time to treat chronic AD involving the trunk and extremities. Newer formulations of topical steroids include gel formulations without alcohol bases that moisturize skin, and solutions, oils, foams, and shampoos that may be useful on hair-bearing surfaces.

Factors that influence topical glucocorticoid potency and the risk of side effects include the molecular structure of the compound, the vehicle, the amount of medication applied, the duration of application, and occlusion, as well as host factors, including age, body surface area and weight, skin inflammation, anatomic location of treated skin, and individual differences in cutaneous or systemic metabolism. Side effects from topical glucocorticoids are directly related to the potency ranking of the compound and the length and frequency of use, so it is incumbent on the clinician to balance the need for a more potent steroid with the potential for side effects. In addition, ointments have a greater potential to occlude the epidermis, resulting in enhanced systemic absorption when compared with creams.

Side effects from topical glucocorticoids can be divided into local side effects and systemic side effects resulting from suppression of the hypothalamic–pituitary–adrenal axis. Local side effects include the development of striae, skin atrophy, perioral dermatitis, and acne rosacea. Prolonged daily use of TCs, especially on the face, can also lead to steroid withdrawal syndrome, a condition characterized by severe erythema, swelling, and burning upon TC discontinuation.[90] The potential for potent topical glucocorticoid to cause adrenal suppression is greatest in infants and young children. Several topical steroid formulations have been specifically tested for safety and received specific U.S. Federal Drug Administration (FDA) approval for use in younger children such as desonide hydrogel and nonethanolic foam, fluocinolone acetonide oil, and fluticasone 0.05% cream. Mometasone cream and ointment are approved for children aged 2 years and older.

Because normal-appearing skin in AD shows evidence of immunologic dysregulation and inflammation, the use of TCs as maintenance therapy to normal-appearing skin has been reported in several controlled studies.[91] After control of AD with a once-daily regimen was achieved, long-term control could be maintained with twice-weekly application of fluticasone to previously involved areas. Given recent insights into skin barrier and immunologic abnormalities and colonization of normal-appearing skin in AD by *S. aureus*, it is important to appreciate that "proactive therapy" is an attempt to control residual disease, not just application of an active drug to unaffected skin.

Topical Calcineurin Inhibitors: Topical tacrolimus and pimecrolimus have been developed as nonsteroidal immunomodulators.[68] Tacrolimus ointment 0.03% has been approved for intermittent treatment of moderate to severe AD in children aged 2 years and older, with tacrolimus ointment 0.1% approved for use in adults and children 16 years and older; pimecrolimus cream 1% is approved for treatment of patients aged 2 years and older with mild to moderate AD. Both drugs have proven to be effective with a good safety profile for treatment up to 4 years with tacrolimus ointment and up to 2 years with pimecrolimus cream. A frequently observed side effect with topical calcineurin inhibitors (TCIs) is a transient burning sensation of the skin. Importantly, treatment with TCIs is not associated with skin atrophy; thus, they are particularly useful for the treatment of areas such as the face and intertriginous regions. Three-times-weekly "proactive" maintenance therapy using tacrolimus ointment has also been reported in both adults and children with AD.[92]

Ongoing surveillance and recent reports have not shown a trend for increased frequency of viral superinfections, especially EH. TCIs carry an FDA black box warning for rare cases of skin malignancy and lymphoma have been reported with topical tacrolimus, although a systematic literature review showed a slightly higher risk of lymphoma in patients with AD, with severity appearing to be a risk factor but concluding that TCIs are unlikely to be a significant factor.[93] Importantly, a case-control study of a large database that identified a cohort of 293,253 patients with AD found no increased risk of lymphoma with the use of TCIs.[93] Margolis and colleagues found no increase in malignancy incidence rates with pimecrolimus cream in a study evaluating more than 26,000 person-years.[94]

Crisaborole: Crisaborole is a boron-based topical phosphodiesterase 4 (PDE4) inhibitor recently approved for the treatment of mild to moderate AD in patients older than the age of 2 years. PDE4 inhibition is thought to decrease proinflammatory cytokine production by key immune cells that drive chronic inflammatory skin disease. Two identically designed pivotal phase 3 trials revealed crisaborole 2% ointment resulted in clear or almost clear disease (plus a two-step improvement) in 31.4% to 32.8% in the active group compared with 18.0% to 25.4% in the vehicle control groups with these differences being statistically significant.[95] No significant adverse events emerged with 4% of patients experiencing burning. Crisaborole represents a safe and efficacious novel nonsteroidal option for the treatment of mild-moderate AD.

Tar Preparations: Coal tar preparations may have antipruritic and antiinflammatory effects on the skin, although not as pronounced as those of topical glucocorticoids. Newer coal tar products have been developed that are more acceptable with respect to odor and staining of clothes than some older products. Tar shampoos can be beneficial for scalp dermatitis and are often helpful in reducing the concentration and frequency of topical glucocorticoid applications. Tar preparations should not be used on acutely inflamed skin because this often results in skin irritation. Side effects associated with tars include folliculitis and photosensitivity. There is a theoretic risk of tar being a carcinogen based on observational studies of workers using tar components in their occupations; however, epidemiologic studies do not confirm similar outcomes when used topically.[83]

PHOTOTHERAPY

Natural sunlight is frequently beneficial to patients with AD. However, if the sunlight occurs in the setting of high heat or humidity, thereby triggering sweating and pruritus, it may be deleterious to patients. Broadband UVB, broadband UVA, narrowband UVB (311 nm), UVA-1 (340 to 400 nm), and combined UVAB phototherapy can be useful adjuncts in the treatment of AD. Investigation of the photoimmunologic mechanisms responsible for therapeutic effectiveness indicates that epidermal LCs and eosinophils may be targets of UVA phototherapy, with and without psoralen, but UVB exerts immunosuppressive effects via blocking of function of antigen-presenting LCs and altered keratinocyte cytokine production. Photochemotherapy with psoralen and UVA light may be indicated in patients with severe, widespread AD, although studies comparing it with other modes of phototherapy are limited. Short-term adverse effects with phototherapy may include erythema, skin pain, pruritus, and pigmentation. Long-term adverse effects include premature skin aging and cutaneous malignancies (see Chaps. 198 and 199 for detailed discussion of phototherapy and photochemotherapy, respectively).

HOSPITALIZATION

Patients with AD who appear erythrodermic or who have widespread severe skin disease resistant to outpatient therapy should be considered for hospitalization. In many cases, removing the patient from environmental allergens or emotional stresses, intense patient education, and assurance of compliance with therapy results in a sustained improvement in their AD. Clearing of the patient's skin during hospitalization also allows the patient to undergo patch testing or allergen skin testing and appropriately controlled provocative challenges to correctly identify or rule out exacerbating factors.

SYSTEMIC THERAPY

The decision to initiate systemic therapies should be based on overall disease severity, response to topical therapy, adherence to previous topical regimens, impact of the disease on the patient's quality of life, and understanding the patient's comorbidities and preferences. Before initiating systemic therapy, other diagnoses should be considered that can mimic or exacerbate AD such as cutaneous T-cell lymphoma, allergic contact dermatitis, scabies, or immunodeficiency syndrome. A biopsy or additional laboratory testing may be needed. What follows are discussions of oral and injectable medications previously studied or commonly used as systemic therapy in AD.[96] There are no specific guidelines or comparative effectiveness data to inform guidelines regarding the optimal first-line systemic treatment in AD nor is there a definitive algorithm for treatment.

DUPILUMAB

Dupilumab is a fully human monoclonal antibody targeting the IL-4 receptor alpha subunit. The IL-4 and IL-13 receptors share this subunit; thus, dupilumab blocks cytokine signaling through both of these receptors. Except for oral corticosteroids, dupilumab is the only FDA-approved systemic agent for the treatment of AD at this time. Dupilumab is dosed every other week and delivered as a subcutaneous injection. It is indicated for the treatment of adult patients with moderate to severe AD whose disease is not adequately controlled with topical prescription therapies or when those therapies are not advisable. In two identically designed phase 3 studies named SOLO 1 and SOLO 2, dupilumab resulted in 36% to 38% of patients reaching clear or almost clear skin after 16 weeks of treatment compared with 9% to 10% in the placebo, group which were statistically significant differences.[30] Signs of the disease as measured by the Eczema and Area Severity Index (EASI) reduced by 67% to 72%. Dupilumab treatment led to significant improvement in pruritus, quality of life, and clinically meaningful reductions in anxiety and depressive symptoms. SOLO 1 and 2 were designed as monotherapy, that is, without the concomitant use of TCs. A recent study evaluating the effects of dupilumab in combination with TCs found the addition of TCs to dupilumab to be safe and provides modest increased benefit over monotherapy.[97] This combination study named CHRONOS also evaluated outcomes with 1 year of continuous therapy showing a maintenance of benefit with longer term use.

To date, there appear to be few adverse effects of dupilumab therapy. Dupilumab does not appear to suppress normal immune responses. A recent analysis found skin infections are reduced with dupilumab treatment.[39] Vaccine responses to both T cell–dependent and T cell–independent vaccines were unchanged with treatment.[98] Injection site reactions (eg, pain on injection) and conjunctivitis are the most common drug-related adverse effects. The cause of the conjunctivitis is unclear, but it does not appear to be infectious, is usually mild to moderate in severity, and can improve with topical lubricants or antiinflammatory therapy and may spontaneously resolve.

SYSTEMIC GLUCOCORTICOIDS

The use of systemic glucocorticoids, such as oral prednisone, is rarely indicated in the treatment of patients with chronic AD but is commonly used by providers. Some patients and physicians prefer the use of systemic glucocorticoids to avoid the time-consuming skin care involving hydration and topical therapy. However, the dramatic clinical improvement that may occur with systemic glucocorticoids is frequently associated with a severe rebound flare of AD after the discontinuation of systemic glucocorticoids. Short courses of oral glucocorticoids may be appropriate for an acute exacerbation of AD while other treatment measures are being instituted. If a short course of oral glucocorticoids is given, it is important to taper the dosage and to begin intensified skin care, particularly with topical glucocorticoids and frequent bathing followed by application of emollients to prevent rebound flaring of AD.

CYCLOSPORINE

Cyclosporine is a potent immunosuppressive drug that acts primarily on T cells by suppressing cytokine transcription. The drug binds to cyclophilin, an intracellular protein, and this complex, in turn, inhibits calcineurin, a molecule required for initiation of cytokine gene transcription. Multiple studies demonstrate that both children and adults with severe AD, refractory to conventional treatment, can benefit from short-term cyclosporine treatment. Various oral dosing regimens have been recommended: whereas 5 mg/kg has generally been used with success in short- and long-term (1 year) use, some authorities advocate body weight–independent daily dosing of adults with 150 mg (low dose) or 300 mg (high dose) daily of cyclosporine microemulsion. Treatment with cyclosporine is associated with reduced skin disease and an improved quality of life (see Chap. 192 for further discussion). Discontinuation of treatment may result in rapid relapse of skin disease, although some patients may have sustained remission. Elevated serum creatinine or more significant renal impairment, hypertension, and drug–drug interactions are specific side effects of concern with cyclosporine use.

ANTIMETABOLITES

Methotrexate (MTX) is an antimetabolite with potent inhibitory effects on inflammatory cytokine synthesis and cell chemotaxis. MTX has been studied for both pediatric and adult AD patients with recalcitrant disease. One controlled study found MTX to provide an approximate 42% reduction in disease severity scores in adult patients, similar to the active comparator azathioprine.[99] A trial in children showed similar responses.[100] Side effects of MTX include hematologic abnormalities and hepatic toxicity. The long-term risk of occult hepatic toxicity with continued use of MTX is not known, and no guidelines exist regarding the role of liver biopsy or imaging in this patient population.

Mycophenolate mofetil is a purine biosynthesis inhibitor used as an immunosuppressant in organ transplantation, which has been used for treatment of refractory inflammatory skin disorders (see Chap. 192). Open-label studies report that short-term oral mycophenolate mofetil, 2 g/day, as monotherapy results in clearing of skin lesions in adults with AD resistant to other treatment, including topical and oral steroids and psoralen and UVA light. Similar results were previously reported in another open study of ten patients with a mean reduction in the SCORAD (SCORing Atopic Dermatitis) index of 68% in all 10 patients.[101] The drug was also found to be a reasonably useful flare prevention therapy after induction with cyclosporine.[102]

The drug has generally been well tolerated with the exception of one patient developing herpes retinitis that may have been secondary to this immunosuppressive agent. Hematologic toxicity has also been observed as have cases of progressive multifocal encephalopathy. The use of the drug during pregnancy has also been associated with pregnancy loss and congenital malformations.

Azathioprine is a purine analog with antiinflammatory and antiproliferative effects. It has been used for severe AD, and several controlled trials have been reported in adults and children with modest efficacy. Myelosuppression is a significant adverse effect. Thiopurine methyl transferase levels may predict individuals at risk.

OTHER THERAPIES

Interferon-γ: IFN-γ is known to suppress IgE responses and downregulate Th2 cell proliferation and function. Several studies of patients with AD, including a multicenter, double-blind, placebo-controlled trial and two long-term open trials, have demonstrated that treatment with recombinant human IFN-γ results in clinical improvement.[103] Reduction in clinical severity of AD correlated with the ability of IFN-γ to decrease total circulating eosinophil counts. Influenza-like symptoms are commonly observed side effects early in the treatment course.

Omalizumab: Omalizumab is a monoclonal antibody targeting IgE and is approved for allergic asthma and chronic urticarial. Even though elevated IgE is present in nearly all patients with AD, case reports of omalizumab's effect in AD were conflicting. A randomized controlled trial found no clinical effects of omalizumab on AD.[104] This study suggest IgE does not play a direct role in AD pathogenesis.

Allergen Immunotherapy: Unlike allergic rhinitis and extrinsic asthma, immunotherapy with aeroallergens has not proven to be efficacious in the treatment of AD. There are anecdotal reports of both disease exacerbation and improvement. A Cochrane review of 12 studies found limited evidence supporting their use in AD, although studies were of low quality.[105] Well-controlled studies are still required to determine the role for immunotherapy with this disease.

Extracorporeal Photopheresis: Extracorporeal photopheresis consists of the passage of psoralen-treated leukocytes through an extracorporeal UVA light system. Clinical improvement in skin lesions associated with reduced IgE levels has been reported in a few patients with severe, resistant AD who were treated with extracorporeal photopheresis and topical glucocorticoids. One study found the treatment to be comparable to daily 3 mg/kg cyclosporine.[106]

Probiotics: Several studies have shown perinatal administration of probiotics, especially *Lactobacillus rhamnosus* strain GG to prevent AD in at-risk children during the first 2 years of life. The efficacy of probiotics to treat AD is less clear. Probiotics are purported to deliver beneficial microbes to the gut of patients, establishing a bacterial milieu that reduces systemic inflammatory responses. A systematic review evaluating 12 trials including 781 participants of probiotic supplementation for AD found little beneficial effect.[107] A meta-analysis of seven trials showed no significant difference in eczema severity between probiotic and placebo groups. For both treatment and prevention, more research into subgroups of responders, length of treatment, strain of *Lactobacillus*, and mechanisms involved is clearly needed.

Chinese Herbal Medications: Several placebo-controlled clinical trials have suggested that patients with severe AD may benefit from treatment with traditional Chinese herbal therapy. However, the beneficial response of Chinese herbal therapy is often temporary, and effectiveness may wear off despite continued treatment. The possibility of hepatic toxicity, cardiac side effects, or idiosyncratic reactions remains a concern. The specific ingredients of the herbs also remain to be elucidated and some topical preparations have been found to be contaminated with corticosteroids. At present, Chinese herbal therapy for AD is considered investigational.

Oral Vitamin D: Vitamin D is thought to normalize immune responses and increase antimicrobial peptide expression in AD. A pilot randomized, double-blind, placebo-controlled study looked at the benefit of oral vitamin D supplementation in children with AD from February to March in Boston.[108] Eleven pediatric patients primarily with mild AD were treated with either vitamin D (1000 IU ergocalciferol) or placebo once daily for 1 month. Investigator Global Assessment (IGA) score improved in four of six subjects in the vitamin D group (80%) compared with one of five participants in the placebo group ($P = .04$). In addition, there was a greater reduction in EASI score in the vitamin D compared with the placebo group, although the difference was not statistically significant. In another small controlled study, 14 healthy participants and 14 participants with AD were supplemented with 4000 IU/day of oral vitamin D_3 (cholecalciferol) for 3 weeks.[109] Expression of the antimicrobial peptide cathelicidin was significantly increased in the skin biopsies of AD lesions compared with those in healthy skin or uninvolved AD skin, suggesting a role for oral vitamin D in improving innate immune responses in patients with AD.

Since these promising early observations, two larger controlled trials have been performed. A study of 107 Mongolian children with winter-exacerbated AD confirmed previous findings and found a significant improvement in the supplemented children.[110] In contrast, a study in 60 adults found no clinical effect of vitamin D supplementation on epidermal antimicrobial expression or clinical scores measured by EASI.[111]

PREVENTION

Given the high prevalence and morbidity associated with AD, disease prevention represents the holy grail of AD research. For decades, allergen avoidance remained the primary approach to AD prevention with middling or conflicting results. Food avoidance in pregnant or lactating mothers proved dangerous and food avoidance in infancy likely promoted the development of food allergy. The Learning Early About Peanut Allergy study found early exposure of peanut, rather than delayed exposure, dramatically reduced peanut allergy at age 5 years.[112] The 2017 NIAID Expert Panel Addendum Guidelines on prevention of peanut allergy recommend that for children with severe eczema, egg allergy, or both, introduction of solid foods begins at 4 to 6 months of age, starting with solid food other than peanuts, so that the child can demonstrate the ability to consume solid food without evidence of nonspecific signs and symptoms that could be confused with IgE-mediated food allergy.[113] A practical consideration for applying this guideline at 4 to 6 months of age is that that infants visit their health care providers for well-child evaluations and infant immunizations at this time. This provides an opportunity for eczema evaluation and, if needed, referral to a specialist for peanut allergy evaluation. Allergy testing in children with severe eczema or egg allergy should be strongly considered before the first peanut protein feeding. The use of hydrolyzed formula for AD prevention has shown a positive effect in studies, including persistence of effect in the German Infant and Nutrition study. A recent Cochrane review, however, concluded that there was no convincing evidence of hydrolyzed formula for the prevention of AD in high-risk infants.[114] Probiotics supplements appear to have a protective effect on AD development when delivered both pre- and postnatally.[115] The exact strains, dosing, and timing of the intervention is not standardized, nor is the mechanism of action understood. Protecting the skin barrier with emollients early in life in high-risk infants also appears to be promising and reduced the incidence of AD by up to 50% in two small studies.[116,117] Larger studies of this approach to AD prevention are ongoing.

REFERENCES

1. Coca AF, Cooke RA. On the classification of the phenomena of hypersensitiveness. *J Immunol*. 1923;8(3):163-182.
2. Wise F, Sulzberger MB. Footnote on problem of eczema, neurodermatitis and lichenification. In: Wise F, Sulzberger MB, eds. *The 1933 Year Book of Dermatology and Syphilogy*. Chicago: The Year Book Publishers; 1933:38-39.
3. Kantor R, Thyssen J, Paller A, et al. Atopic dermatitis, atopic eczema, or eczema? A systematic review, meta-analysis, and recommendation for uniform use of "atopic dermatitis." *Allergy*. 2016;71(10):1480-1485.
4. Hanifin JM, Rajka G. Diagnostic features of atopic dermatitis. *Acta Derm Venereol (Stockh)*. 1980;92:44-47.
5. Williams HC, Burney PG, Pembroke AC, et al. The U.K. Working Party's Diagnostic Criteria for Atopic Dermatitis. III. Independent hospital validation. *Br J Dermatol*. 1994;131(3):406-416.
6. Eichenfield LF, Hanifin JM, Luger TA, et al. Consensus conference on pediatric atopic dermatitis. *J Am Acad Dermatol*. 2003;49(6):1088-1095.
7. Karimkhani C, Dellavalle RP, Coffeng LE, et al. Global Skin Disease Morbidity and Mortality: An Update From the Global Burden of Disease Study 2013. *JAMA Dermatol*. 2017;153(5):406-412.
8. Bergmann K-C, Heinrich J, Niemann H. Current status of allergy prevalence in Germany. *Allergo J Int*. 2016;25(1):6-10.
9. Saeki H, Tsunemi Y, Fujita H, et al. Prevalence of atopic dermatitis determined by clinical examination in Japanese adults. *J Dermatol*. 2006;33(11):817-819.
10. Silverberg JI, Hanifin JM. Adult eczema prevalence and associations with asthma and other health and demographic factors: a US population–based study. *J Allergy Clin Immunol*. 2013;132(5):1132-1138.
11. Shaw TE, Currie GP, Koudelka CW, et al. Eczema prevalence in the United States: data from the 2003 National Survey of Children's Health. *J Invest Dermatol*. 2011;131(1):67-73.
12. Schram ME, Tedja AM, Spijker R, et al. Is there a rural/urban gradient in the prevalence of eczema? A systematic review. *Br J Dermatol*. 2010;162(5):964-973.
13. Tsakok T, McKeever TM, Yeo L, et al. Does early life exposure to antibiotics increase the risk of eczema? A systematic review. *Br J Dermatol*. 2013;169(5):983-991.
14. Kabashima K, Otsuka A, Nomura T. Linking air pollution to atopic dermatitis. *Nat Immunol*. 2016;18(1):5-6.
15. Engebretsen KA, Bager P, Wohlfahrt J, et al. Prevalence of atopic dermatitis in infants by domestic water hardness and season of birth: cohort study. *J Allergy Clin Immunol*. 2017;139(5):1568-1574.e1561.
16. Uphoff E, Cabieses B, Pinart M, et al. A systematic review of socioeconomic position in relation to asthma and allergic diseases. *Eur Respir J*. 2015;46(2):364-374.
17. Zhang A, Silverberg JI. Association of atopic dermatitis with being overweight and obese: a systematic review and metaanalysis. *J Am Acad Dermatol*. 2015;72(4):606-616.e604.
18. Silverberg JI, Hanifin J, Simpson EL. Climatic factors are associated with childhood eczema prevalence in US. *J Invest Dermatol*. 2013;133(7):1752-1759.
19. Kim YM, Kim J, Han Y, et al. Short-term effects of weather and air pollution on atopic dermatitis symptoms in children: a panel study in Korea. *PLoS One*. 2017;12(4):e0175229.

20. Halkjaer LB, Loland L, Buchvald FF, et al. Development of atopic dermatitis during the first 3 years of life: the Copenhagen prospective study on asthma in childhood cohort study in high-risk children. *Arch Dermatol*. 2006;142(5):561-566.
21. Bremmer SF, Hanifin JM, Simpson EL. Clinical detection of ichthyosis vulgaris in an atopic dermatitis clinic: implications for allergic respiratory disease and prognosis. *J Am Acad Dermatol*. 2008;59(1):72-78.
22. Drucker AM, Thompson JM, Li WQ, et al. Incident alopecia areata and vitiligo in adult women with atopic dermatitis: Nurses' Health Study 2. *Allergy*. 2017;72(5):831-834.
23. Silverberg JI, Simpson EL. Association between severe eczema in children and multiple comorbid conditions and increased healthcare utilization. *Pediatr Allergy Immunol*. 2013;24(5):476-486.
24. Belgrave DC, Granell R, Simpson A, et al. Developmental profiles of eczema, wheeze, and rhinitis: two population-based birth cohort studies. *PLoS Med*. 2014;11(10):e1001748.
25. Lowe AJ, Abramson MJ, Hosking CS, et al. The temporal sequence of allergic sensitization and onset of infantile eczema. *Clin Exp Allergy*. 2007;37(4):536-542.
26. Anto JM, Bousquet J, Akdis M, et al. Mechanisms of the Development of Allergy (MeDALL): introducing novel concepts in allergy phenotypes. *J Allergy Clin Immunol*. 2017;139(2):388-399.
27. Chamlin SL. The psychosocial burden of childhood atopic dermatitis. *Dermatol Ther*. 2006;19(2):104-107.
28. Yaghmaie P, Koudelka CW, Simpson EL. Mental health comorbidity in patients with atopic dermatitis. *J Allergy Clin Immunol*. 2013;131(2):428-433.
29. Strom MA, Fishbein AB, Paller AS, et al. Association between atopic dermatitis and attention deficit hyperactivity disorder in U.S. children and adults. *Br J Dermatol*. 2016;175(5):920-929.
30. Simpson EL, Bieber T, Guttman-Yassky E, et al. Two phase 3 trials of dupilumab versus placebo in atopic dermatitis. *N Engl J Med*. 2016;375(24):2335-2348.
31. Tauber M, Balica S, Hsu CY, et al. Staphylococcus aureus density on lesional and nonlesional skin is strongly associated with disease severity in atopic dermatitis. *J Allergy Clin Immunol*. 2016;137(4):1272-1274.e1271-1273.
32. Totte JE, van der Feltz WT, Hennekam M, et al. Prevalence and odds of Staphylococcus aureus carriage in atopic dermatitis: a systematic review and meta-analysis. *Br J Dermatol*. 2016;175(4):687-695.
33. Hayashida S, Furusho N, Uchi H, et al. Are lifetime prevalence of impetigo, molluscum and herpes infection really increased in children having atopic dermatitis? *J Dermatol Sci*. 2010;60(3):173-178.
34. Patel D, Jahnke MN. Serious Complications from Staphylococcal aureus in atopic dermatitis. *Pediatr Dermatol*. 2015;32(6):792-796.
35. Cho SH, Strickland I, Boguniewicz M, et al. Fibronectin and fibrinogen contribute to the enhanced binding of Staphylococcus aureus to atopic skin. *J Allergy Clin Immunol*. 2001;108(2):269-274.
36. Howell MD, Boguniewicz M, Pastore S, et al. Mechanism of HBD-3 deficiency in atopic dermatitis. *Clin Immunol*. 2006;121(3):332-338.
37. Ong PY, Ohtake T, Brandt C, et al. Endogenous antimicrobial peptides and skin infections in atopic dermatitis. *N Engl J Med*. 2002;347(15):1151-1160.
38. Brauweiler AM, Goleva E, Leung DY. Th2 cytokines increase Staphylococcus aureus alpha toxin-induced keratinocyte death through the signal transducer and activator of transcription 6 (STAT6). *J Invest Dermatol*. 2014;134(8):2114-2121.
39. Drucker A, Fleming P. 282 Risk of skin infections with dupilumab for atopic dermatitis: systematic review and meta-analysis of randomized controlled trials. *J Invest Dermatol*. 2017;137(5):S48.
40. Kong HH, Oh J, Deming C, et al. Temporal shifts in the skin microbiome associated with disease flares and treatment in children with atopic dermatitis. *Genome Res*. 2012;22(5):850-859.
41. Bath-Hextall FJ, Birnie AJ, Ravenscroft JC, et al. Interventions to reduce Staphylococcus aureus in the management of atopic eczema: an updated Cochrane review. *Br J Dermatol*. 2010;163(1):12-26.
42. Knowlden S, Yoshida T, Perez-Nazario N, et al. 296 Bleach baths promote early induction of inflammatory pathway genes with no effect on skin bacterial dysbiosis in AD subjects. *J Invest Dermatol*. 2017;137(5):S50.
43. Paternoster L, Standl M, Waage J, et al. Multi-ancestry genome-wide association study of 21,000 cases and 95,000 controls identifies new risk loci for atopic dermatitis. *Nat Genet*. 2015;47(12):1449-1456.
44. Leung DY, Gao PS, Grigoryev DN, et al. Human atopic dermatitis complicated by eczema herpeticum is associated with abnormalities in IFN-gamma response. *J Allergy Clin Immunol*. 2011;127(4):965-973.e961-965.
45. Mathes EF, Oza V, Frieden IJ, et al. "Eczema coxsackium" and unusual cutaneous findings in an enterovirus outbreak. *Pediatrics*. 2013;132(1):e149-e157.
46. Bayrou O, Pecquet C, Flahault A, et al. Head and neck atopic dermatitis and malassezia-furfur-specific IgE antibodies. *Dermatology (Basel, Switzerland)*. 2005;211(2):107-113.
47. Leung DY, Guttman-Yassky E. Deciphering the complexities of atopic dermatitis: shifting paradigms in treatment approaches. *J Allergy Clin Immunol*. 2014;134(4):769-779.
48. Leung DY. Clinical implications of new mechanistic insights into atopic dermatitis. *Curr Opin Pediatr*. 2016;28(4):456-462.
49. Irvine AD, McLean WH, Leung DY. Filaggrin mutations associated with skin and allergic diseases. *N Engl J Med*. 2011;365(14):1315-1327.
50. Leung DY. New insights into atopic dermatitis: role of skin barrier and immune dysregulation. *Allergol Int*. 2013;62(2):151-161.
51. Leung DY. Atopic dermatitis: age and race do matter! *J Allergy Clin Immunol*. 2015;136(5):1265-1267.
52. Bin L, Edwards MG, Heiser R, et al. Identification of novel gene signatures in patients with atopic dermatitis complicated by eczema herpeticum. *J Allergy Clin Immunol*. 2014;134(4):848-855.
53. Wang IJ, Wu LS, Lockett GA, et al. TSLP polymorphisms, allergen exposures, and the risk of atopic disorders in children. *Ann Allergy Asthma Immunol*. 2016;116(2):139-145.e131.
54. Hamilton JD, Suarez-Farinas M, Dhingra N, et al. Dupilumab improves the molecular signature in skin of patients with moderate-to-severe atopic dermatitis. *J Allergy Clin Immunol*. 2014;134(6):1293-1300.
55. Kim J, Kim BE, Lee J, et al. Epidermal thymic stromal lymphopoietin predicts the development of atopic dermatitis during infancy. *J Allergy Clin Immunol*. 2016;137(4):1282-1285.e1281-1284.

56. Khattri S, Shemer A, Rozenblit M, et al. Cyclosporine in patients with atopic dermatitis modulates activated inflammatory pathways and reverses epidermal pathology. *J Allergy Clin Immunol.* 2014;133(6):1626-1634.
57. Klein PA, Clark RA. An evidence-based review of the efficacy of antihistamines in relieving pruritus in atopic dermatitis. *Arch Dermatol.* 1999;135(12):1522-1525.
58. van Zuuren EJ, Apfelbacher CJ, Fedorowicz Z, et al. No high level evidence to support the use of oral H1 antihistamines as monotherapy for eczema: a summary of a Cochrane systematic review. *Syst Rev.* 2014;3(1):25.
59. Sidbury R, Tom WL, Bergman JN, et al. Guidelines of care for the management of atopic dermatitis: section 4. Prevention of disease flares and use of adjunctive therapies and approaches. *J Am Acad Dermatol.* 2014;71(6):1218-1233.
60. Boyce JA, Assa'ad A, Burks AW, et al. Guidelines for the diagnosis and management of food allergy in the United States: report of the NIAID-sponsored expert panel. *J Allergy Clin Immunol.* 2010;126(6 suppl):S1-58.
61. Fleischer DM, Bock SA, Spears GC, et al. Oral food challenges in children with a diagnosis of food allergy. *J Pediatr.* 2011;158(4):578-583.e571.
62. Bath-Hextall F, Delamere FM, Williams HC. Dietary exclusions for established atopic eczema. *Cochrane Database Syst Rev.* 2008(1):Cd005203.
63. Nankervis H, Pynn EV, Boyle RJ, et al. House dust mite reduction and avoidance measures for treating eczema. *Cochrane Database Syst Rev.* 2015;1:Cd008426.
64. Thompson MM, Hanifin JM. Effective therapy of childhood atopic dermatitis allays food allergy concerns. *J Am Acad Dermatol.* 2005;53(2 Suppl 2):S214-219.
65. Fuchs S, Rensing-Ehl A, Pannicke U, et al. Omenn syndrome associated with a functional reversion due to a somatic second-site mutation in CARD11 deficiency. *Blood.* 2015;126(14):1658-1669.
66. Bin Dhuban K, Piccirillo CA. The immunological and genetic basis of immune dysregulation, polyendocrinopathy, enteropathy, X-linked syndrome. *Curr Opin Allergy Clin Immunol.* 2015;15(6):525-532.
67. Odio CD, Milligan KL, McGowan K, et al. Endemic mycoses in patients with STAT3-mutated hyper-IgE (Job) syndrome. *J Allergy Clin Immunol.* 2015;136(5):1411-1413.e1411-1412.
68. Aydin SE, Kilic SS, Aytekin C, et al. DOCK8 deficiency: clinical and immunological phenotype and treatment options—a review of 136 patients. *J Clin Immunol.* 2015;35(2):189-198.
69. Casanova JL, Holland SM, Notarangelo LD. Inborn errors of human JAKs and STATs. *Immunity.* 2012;36(4):515-528.
70. Jawed SI, Myskowski PL, Horwitz S, et al. Primary cutaneous T-cell lymphoma (mycosis fungoides and Sezary syndrome): part I. Diagnosis: clinical and histopathologic features and new molecular and biologic markers. *J Am Acad Dermatol.* 2014;70(2):205.e201-216; quiz 221-202.
71. Chen JK, Jacob SE, Nedorost ST, et al. A Pragmatic Approach to Patch Testing Atopic Dermatitis Patients: Clinical Recommendations Based on Expert Consensus Opinion. *Dermatitis.* 2016;27(4):186-192.
72. Corbo MD, Lam J. Zinc deficiency and its management in the pediatric population: a literature review and proposed etiologic classification. *J Am Acad Dermatol.* 2013;69(4):616-624.e611.
73. Kim JP, Chao LX, Simpson EL, et al. Persistence of atopic dermatitis (AD): a systematic review and meta-analysis. *J Am Acad Dermatol.* 2016;75(4):681-687.e611.
74. Margolis JS, Abuabara K, Bilker W, et al. Persistence of mild to moderate atopic dermatitis. *JAMA Dermatol.* 2014;150(6):593-600.
75. Margolis DJ, Apter AJ, Gupta J, et al. The persistence of atopic dermatitis and filaggrin (FLG) mutations in a US longitudinal cohort. *J Allergy Clin Immunol.* 2012;130(4):912-917.
76. Margolis DJ, Gupta J, Apter AJ, et al. Filaggrin-2 variation is associated with more persistent atopic dermatitis in African American subjects. *J Allergy Clin Immunol.* 2014;133(3):784-9.
77. Ahrens B, Staab D. Extended implementation of educational programs for atopic dermatitis in childhood. *Pediatr Allergy Immunol.* 2015;26(3):190-196.
78. Mason JM, Carr J, Buckley C, et al. Improved emollient use reduces atopic eczema symptoms and is cost neutral in infants: before-and-after evaluation of a multifaceted educational support programme. *BMC Dermatol.* 2013;13:7-5945-5913-5947.
79. Koning S, van der Sande R, Verhagen AP, et al. Interventions for impetigo. *Cochrane Database Syst Rev.* 2012;1:Cd003261.
80. Nankervis H, Thomas KS, Delamere FM, et al. Programme grants for applied research. In: *Scoping Systematic Review of Treatments for Eczema.* Southampton, United Kingdom: NIHR Journals Library, 2016.
81. Leung TH, Zhang LF, Wang J, et al. Topical hypochlorite ameliorates NF-kappaB-mediated skin diseases in mice. *J Clin Invest.* 2013;123(12):5361-5370.
82. Chang YS, Lin MH, Lee JH, et al. Melatonin supplementation for children with atopic dermatitis and sleep disturbance: a randomized clinical trial. *JAMA Pediatr.* 2016;170(1):35-42.
83. Mlitz V, Latreille J, Gardinier S, et al. Impact of filaggrin mutations on Raman spectra and biophysical properties of the stratum corneum in mild to moderate atopic dermatitis. *J Eur Acad Dermatol Venereol.* 2012;26(8):983-990.
84. Czarnowicki T, Malajian D, Khattri S, et al. Petrolatum: barrier repair and antimicrobial responses underlying this "inert" moisturizer. *J Allergy Clin Immunol.* 2015.
85. Akerstrom U, Reitamo S, Langeland T, et al. Comparison of moisturizing creams for the prevention of atopic dermatitis relapse: a randomized double-blind controlled multicentre clinical trial. *Acta Derm Venereol.* 2015;95(5):587-592.
86. Kohn LL, Kang Y, Antaya RJ. A randomized, controlled trial comparing topical steroid application to wet versus dry skin in children with atopic dermatitis (AD). *J Am Acad Dermatol.* 2016;75(2):306-311.
87. Hajar T, Hanifin JM, Tofte SJ, et al. Prehydration is effective for rapid control of recalcitrant atopic dermatitis. *Dermatitis.* 2014;25(2):56-59.
88. Eichenfield LF, Tom WL, Berger TG, et al. Guidelines of care for the management of atopic dermatitis: section 2. Management and treatment of atopic dermatitis with topical therapies. *J Am Acad Dermatol.* 2014;71(1):116-132.
89. Hanifin J, Gupta AK, Rajagopalan R. Intermittent dosing of fluticasone propionate cream for reducing the risk of relapse in atopic dermatitis patients. *Br J Dermatol.* 2002;147(3):528-537.

90. Hajar T, Leshem YA, Hanifin JM, et al. A systematic review of topical corticosteroid withdrawal ("steroid addiction") in patients with atopic dermatitis and other dermatoses. *J Am Acad Dermatol*. 2015;72(3):541-549. e542.
91. Schmitt J, von Kobyletzki L, Svensson A, et al. Efficacy and tolerability of proactive treatment with topical corticosteroids and calcineurin inhibitors for atopic eczema: systematic review and meta-analysis of randomized controlled trials. *Br J Dermatol*. 2011;164(2):415-428.
92. Paller AS, Eichenfield LF, Kirsner RS, et al. Three times weekly tacrolimus ointment reduces relapse in stabilized atopic dermatitis: a new paradigm for use. *Pediatrics*. 2008;122(6):e1210-1218.
93. Arellano FM, Wentworth CE, Arana A, et al. Risk of lymphoma following exposure to calcineurin inhibitors and topical steroids in patients with atopic dermatitis. *J Invest Dermatol*. 2007;127(4):808-816.
94. Margolis DJ, Abuabara K, Hoffstad OJ, et al. Association between malignancy and topical use of pimecrolimus. *JAMA Dermatol*. 2015;151(6):594-599.
95. Paller AS, Tom WL, Lebwohl MG, et al. Efficacy and safety of crisaborole ointment, a novel, nonsteroidal phosphodiesterase 4 (PDE4) inhibitor for the topical treatment of atopic dermatitis (AD) in children and adults. *J Am Acad Dermatol*. 2016;75(3):494-503. e494.
96. Roekevisch E, Spuls PI, Kuester D, et al. Efficacy and safety of systemic treatments for moderate-to-severe atopic dermatitis: a systematic review. *J Allergy Clin Immunol*. 2014;133(2):429-438.
97. Blauvelt A, de Bruin-Weller M, Gooderham M, et al. Long-term management of moderate-to-severe atopic dermatitis with dupilumab and concomitant topical corticosteroids (LIBERTY AD CHRONOS): a 1-year, randomised, double-blinded, placebo-controlled, phase 3 trial. *Lancet*. 2017 Jun 10;389(10086):2287-2303. doi: 10.1016/S0140-6736(17)31191-1. Epub 2017 May 4. PubMed PMID: 28478972.
98. Blauvelt A, Simpson EL, Tyring SK, et al. Dupilumab does not affect correlates of vaccine-induced immunity: a randomized, placebo-controlled trial in adults with moderate-to-severe atopic dermatitis. *J Am Acad Dermatol*. 2018 Aug 6. pii: S0190-9622(18)32351-X. doi: 10.1016/j.jaad.2018.07.048. [Epub ahead of print] PubMed PMID: 30092324.
99. Schram ME, Roekevisch E, Leeflang MM, et al. A randomized trial of methotrexate versus azathioprine for severe atopic eczema. *J Allergy Clin Immunol*. 2011;128(2):353-359.
100. El-Khalawany MA, Hassan H, Shaaban D, et al. Methotrexate versus cyclosporine in the treatment of severe atopic dermatitis in children: a multicenter experience from Egypt. *Eur J Pediatr*. 2013;172(3):351-356.
101. Neuber K, Schwartz I, Itschert G, Dieck AT. Treatment of atopic eczema with oral mycophenolate mofetil. *Br J Dermatol*. 2000;143(2):385-391.
102. Haeck IM, Knol MJ, Ten Berge O, et al. Enteric-coated mycophenolate sodium versus cyclosporin A as long-term treatment in adult patients with severe atopic dermatitis: a randomized controlled trial. *J Am Acad Dermatol*. 2011;64(6):1074-1084.
103. Chang TT, Stevens SR. Atopic dermatitis: the role of recombinant interferon-gamma therapy. *Am J Clin Dermatol*. 2002;3(3):175-183.
104. Heil PM, Maurer D, Klein B, et al. Omalizumab therapy in atopic dermatitis: depletion of IgE does not improve the clinical course–a randomized, placebo-controlled and double blind pilot study. *J Dtsch Dermatol Ges*. 2010;8(12):990-998.
105. Tam H, Calderon MA, Manikam L, et al. Specific allergen immunotherapy for the treatment of atopic eczema. *Cochrane Database Syst Rev*. 2016;2:Cd008774.
106. Koppelhus U, Poulsen J, Grunnet N, et al. Cyclosporine and extracorporeal photopheresis are equipotent in treating severe atopic dermatitis: a randomized cross-over study comparing two efficient treatment modalities. *Front Med (Lausanne)*. 2014;1:33.
107. Boyle RJ, Bath-Hextall FJ, Leonardi-Bee J, et al. Probiotics for treating eczema. *Cochrane Database Syst Rev*. 2008(4):Cd006135.
108. Sidbury R, Sullivan AF, Thadhani RI, et al. Randomized controlled trial of vitamin D supplementation for winter-related atopic dermatitis in Boston: a pilot study. *Br J Dermatol*. 2008;159(1):245-247.
109. Hata TR, Kotol P, Jackson M, et al. Administration of oral vitamin D induces cathelicidin production in atopic individuals. *J Allergy Clin Immunol*. 2008;122(4):829-831.
110. Camargo CA Jr, Ganmaa D, Sidbury R, et al. Randomized trial of vitamin D supplementation for winter-related atopic dermatitis in children. *J Allergy Clin Immunol*. 2014;134(4):831-835.e831.
111. Hata TR, Audish D, Kotol P, et al. A randomized controlled double-blind investigation of the effects of vitamin D dietary supplementation in subjects with atopic dermatitis. *J Eur Acad Dermatol Venereol*. 2014;28(6):781-789.
112. Du Toit G, Roberts G, Sayre PH, et al. Randomized trial of peanut consumption in infants at risk for peanut allergy. *N Engl J Med*. 2015;372(9):803-813.
113. Togias A, Cooper SF, Acebal ML, et al. Addendum guidelines for the prevention of peanut allergy in the United States: report of the National Institute of Allergy and Infectious Diseases-sponsored expert panel. *J Allergy Clin Immunol*. 2017;139(1):29-44.
114. Osborn DA, Sinn JK, Jones LJ. Infant formulas containing hydrolysed protein for prevention of allergic disease and food allergy. *Cochrane Database Syst Rev*. 2017;3:Cd003664.
115. Panduru M, Panduru NM, Salavastru CM, et al. Probiotics and primary prevention of atopic dermatitis: a meta-analysis of randomized controlled studies. *J Eur Acad Dermatol Venereol*. 2015;29(2):232-242.
116. Horimukai K, Morita K, Narita M, et al. Application of moisturizer to neonates prevents development of atopic dermatitis. *J Allergy Clin Immunol*. 2014;134(4):824-830.e826.
117. Simpson EL, Chalmers JR, Hanifin JM, et al. Emollient enhancement of the skin barrier from birth offers effective atopic dermatitis prevention. *J Allergy Clin Immunol*. 2014;134(4):818-823.

Chapter 23 :: Nummular Eczema, Lichen Simplex Chronicus, and Prurigo Nodularis
:: Jonathan I. Silverberg

第二十三章
钱币状湿疹、慢性单纯性苔藓和结节性痒疹

中文导读

本章共分为3节：①钱币状湿疹；②慢性单纯性苔藓；③结节性痒疹。分别介绍了这三种皮炎的流行病学、临床表现、病因和发病机制、鉴别诊断、并发症、病程、预后与治疗。

〔李 捷〕

AT-A-GLANCE

Nummular eczema:

- Also known as nummular dermatitis and discoid eczema.
- A chronic inflammatory skin disorder of unknown etiology.
- Papules and papulovesicles coalesce to form nummular plaques with oozing, crust, and scale.
- Most common sites of involvement are upper extremities in men and women, particularly the dorsal hands in women, and the lower extremities in men.
- Pathology may show acute, subacute, or chronic eczema.

Lichen simplex chronicus

- A chronic, severely pruritic disorder characterized by one or more lichenified plaques.
- Most common sites of involvement are scalp, nape of neck, extensor aspects of extremities, ankles, and anogenital area.
- Pathology consists of hyperkeratosis, hypergranulosis, psoriasiform epidermal hyperplasia, and thickened papillary dermal collagen.

Prurigo nodularis

- Also known as prurigo, picker's nodules, or nodular prurigo of Hyde.
- A pruritic disorder that runs a chronic course.
- Hyperkeratotic firm nodules vary in size from 0.5 to 3.0 cm and may be excoriated.
- Associations include atopic dermatitis and systemic causes of pruritus.
- Pathology consists of hyperkeratosis, hypergranulosis, psoriasiform epidermal hyperplasia, thickened papillary dermal collagen, and characteristic neural hypertrophy.

This chapter discusses the evaluation and management of *nummular dermatitis*, *lichen simplex chronicus*, and *prurigo nodularis*. These disorders are each associated with intense itch and characteristic morphologic findings. Each of these disorders may present in patients with atopic and contact dermatitis. However, these disorders often present in the absence of atopic disease and may be associated with underlying systemic disease.

NUMMULAR ECZEMA

Nummular eczema or *discoid eczema* is a morphologic term to describe coin-shaped plaques that may have multiple etiologies. The term was first coined by Devergie in 1857.[1] Nummular lesions are commonly observed in atopic dermatitis (AD), and may have a predilection for school-age children with AD[2,3] and adult-onset AD.[4] A large proportion of patients with nummular eczema have underlying allergic contact dermatitis.[5,6]

However, some use this term to describe a specific diagnosis, which excludes other common dermatoses presenting with nummular lesions.[7] The epidemiology of nummular eczema is not well-defined, in part owing to the different definitions used in studies. Prevalence estimates for nummular eczema were found to be 1 to 2 per 1000 population in studies of the populations of the U.S. in 1978[8] and Sweden in 1969.[7] Nummular eczema was encountered in 2.2% of dermatologic visits in Turkey in 2011-2012.[9] Nummular eczema is more common in adults, with multiple observed peak ages-of-onset at 15-25,[7,8,10] 50-59,[7,10] and 65-74 years.[7,8] Previous studies found conflicting results about whether nummular eczema is more common in adult males[7] or adult females.[8] No racial or ethnic predilection for nummular eczema has been demonstrated.

ETIOLOGY AND PATHOGENESIS

The pathogenesis of nummular eczema appears to be multifactorial. Many of the proposed triggers of nummular eczema overlap with those of AD, including atopy, xerosis, exogenous insult by irritants and/or allergens, microbiome, and infection. Nummular eczema does not appear to be consistently associated with atopy. Most studies found low or normal rates of personal (1.5% to 11%) and/or family history of atopy (2.5% to 15%).[7,11] However, a Thai study found high rates of personal (50%) and/or family history of atopy (38%).[10] One study found that patients with nummular eczema were less likely to have elevated immunoglobulin E (IgE) levels.[12]

Similar to AD, nummular eczema in elderly patients is associated with xerosis clinically and lower hydration of the stratum corneum.[13] Moreover, epidermal and dermal inflammation occurring in nummular eczema was found to be predominated by T cells with even higher T-cell counts compared to AD.[14] However, in contrast with AD, the water-barrier function of stratum corneum in nummular eczema appears to be normal.[13] Nummular eczema has been reported to be triggered by exposure to irritants[10,15-17] and environmental factors[10,18] and most commonly flares in the wintertime.[7,10,19] A role for environmental allergens, such as the house dust mite and *Candida albicans* has also been touted.[13]

A large subset of nummular eczema may be related to allergic contact dermatitis. Retrospective studies of patch testing results for patients with nummular eczema found that 32.5% to 50% had at least one positive allergen,[5,6,20] of which 12% to 67% were felt to be clinically relevant.[6,10,20] Patients may develop nummular eczema-like reactions to their topical medicaments.[21] Generalized nummular eczema may be caused by oral and/or topical exposures to allergens.[22]

Microbial colonization and/or infection may play a role in nummular eczema. Nummular eczema lesions have been repeatedly shown to be sterile.[23-25] However, patients with nummular eczema may have higher rates of colonization with *Staphylococcus aureus* and methicillin-resistant *S. aureus* in the nares and subungual space.[26] Extracutaneous foci of infection, including teeth, upper respiratory tract, and lower respiratory tract, were found in 68% of patients in one study.[15] A case series found that infections were present in 39% of nummular eczema patients, with dental caries and upper respiratory tract infections being most common.[10] However, no control groups were examined in these studies. One study compared the frequency of infections in patients with nummular eczema to a matched group of patients with psoriasis and chronic urticaria.[7] Nummular eczema was associated with higher rates of dental abscesses and paradental diseases than psoriasis, but not with pulmonary or nasal infections or elevated antistreptolysin titers.[7] In a series of 13 patients with generalized nummular eczema (without a history of atopic eczema), the skin disease completely improved after odontogenic infections were treated.[27]

Nummular eczema has been reported during therapy with medications, including isotretinoin,[28] gold,[29] combination therapy with interferon α-2b and ribavirin for hepatitis C,[30,31] and infliximab.[32] Mercury amalgam was implicated as a cause of nummular eczema in two patients.[33]

Emotional stress may be a common and clinically relevant trigger of nummular eczema.[10]

CLINICAL FINDINGS

Well-demarcated, coin-shaped plaques form from coalescing papules and papulovesicles. Often, studded or satellite papulovesicles appear at the periphery of an expanding central plaque and should not be confused with the satellitosis present in fungal or yeast infections. Pinpoint oozing and crusting eventuate, and are distinctive (Figs. 23-1 and 23-2). Crust may, however, cover the entire surface (Fig. 23-3). Plaques range from 1 to >3 cm in size. The surrounding skin is generally normal, but may be xerotic and/or have asteatotic

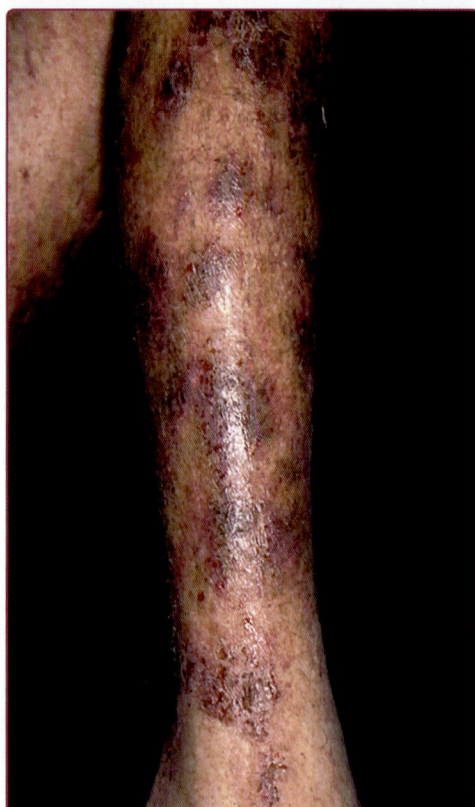

Figure 23-1 Nummular eczema. Coin-shaped plaques with pinpoint erosions and excoriations. (Image from Division of Dermatology, University of the Witwatersrand, Johannesburg, South Africa, with permission, from Professor D. Modi.)

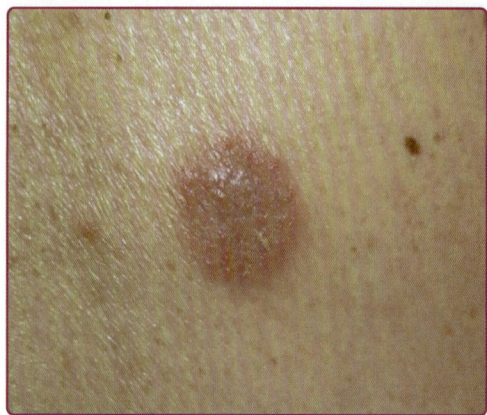

Figure 23-2 Nummular eczema. Single plaque showing pinpoint erosions and crusting.

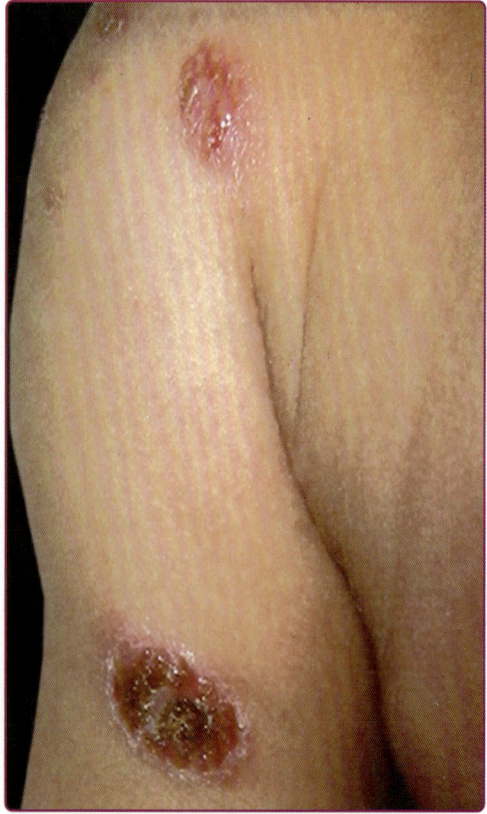

Figure 23-3 Nummular eczema in a child. Crusted plaques. (Used by permission of P. Lio, MD, Northwestern University's Feinberg School of Medicine, Chicago, IL.)

eczema lesions. Pruritus varies from minimal to severe and may be worse in the evening and during periods of relaxation. Central resolution may occur, leading to annular forms. Chronic plaques are dry, scaly, and lichenified. The classic distribution of lesions is the extensor aspects of the extremities, particularly the lower extremities.[7,10] Onset of nummular eczema peaks in the winter and troughs in the summer.[7,10]

LABORATORY TESTS

Nummular eczema is not consistently associated with atopy and serum IgE levels are not useful. Nummular eczema lesions are sterile and lesional bacterial cultures are not indicated, unless there is suspicion for a superimposed infection. Antistreptolysin-O titers are not useful.

SPECIAL TESTS

Patch testing is indicated in chronic recalcitrant cases to rule out underlying contact dermatitis. Previous studies found a variety of relevant positive allergens in patch testing, including nickel, chromates, and other metals; rubber; fragrances, formaldehyde, and other preservatives commonly found in cosmetics and personal care products; neomycin and other topical medicaments; and colophony.[6,10,20]

Skin biopsy and histopathologic examination may be needed to rule out other clinical entities, such as autoimmune blistering disorders and cutaneous T-cell lymphoma. Histopathologic changes are reflective of the stage at which the biopsy is performed. Acutely, there is spongiosis, with or without spongiotic microvesicles. In subacute plaques, there is parakeratosis, scale crust, epidermal hyperplasia, and spongiosis of the epidermis (Fig. 23-4). There is a mixed cell infiltrate in the dermis. Chronic lesions may resemble lichen simplex chronicus microscopically.

DIFFERENTIAL DIAGNOSIS

Table 23-1 outlines the differential diagnosis of nummular eczema.

COMPLICATIONS

Nummular eczema may be complicated by profound sleep disturbance owing to intense itch and secondary bacterial infection.

PROGNOSIS AND CLINICAL COURSE

Nummular eczema is associated with considerable quality-of-life impairment, particularly in more extensive disease.[10] Nummular eczema is often chronic, with either an intermittent or persistent course. One study found that nummular eczema persisted for up to 30 years, with a mean duration of 3.8 years; only 44% of patients were ever free of lesions.[10] Another study found that only 22% of nummular eczema patients were disease-free, 25% had some intermittent disease, and 53% were never free of lesions after 2 years of follow-up.[19] Recurrence at prior sites of involvement is a feature of the disease.[15]

TREATMENT

Topical corticosteroids are the mainstay of treatment. Lesions are often refractory to mid-potency topical corticosteroids and require superpotent topical corticosteroids. Topical calcineurin inhibitors, such as tacrolimus and pimecrolimus, and tar preparations also may be effective. Emollients can be added adjunctively if there is accompanying xerosis. Home humidifiers may be useful for patients with winter flares; however, there is no evidence to support this recommendation. Oral sedating antihistamines are useful to improve sleep when pruritus is severe. Oral antibiotics are indicated when secondary infection is present. For widespread involvement or lesions refractory to topical treatments, phototherapy with broadband or narrowband ultraviolet B or systemic treatment with corticosteroids, cyclosporine, methotrexate[34] and the like may be beneficial.

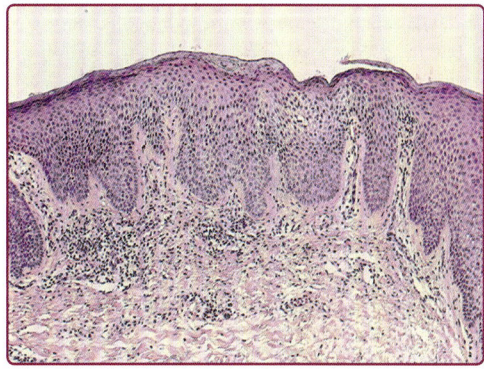

Figure 23-4 Histopathology of nummular eczema. Parakeratosis containing plasma and neutrophils (scale crust) and psoriasiform epidermal hyperplasia with spongiosis are present, with a superficial dermal perivascular infiltrate of lymphocytes, macrophages, and eosinophils.

LICHEN SIMPLEX CHRONICUS/PRURIGO NODULARIS

EPIDEMIOLOGY

Lichen simplex chronicus (LSC) and prurigo nodularis (PN) are phenotypes that are caused by repeated itching, scratching, and rubbing of the skin. They can be associated with multiple etiologies of dermatologic and/or systemic disease.[35] However, some use these terms (LSC and PN) to describe a specific diagnosis, which excludes other dermatologic disorders that present with these lesions, such as AD (ie, *nodular prurigo of Hyde*).[36,37] The epidemiology of LSC and PN is not well-defined, owing to scant studies and the different definitions used in the studies. Little is known about the descriptive epidemiology of PN. A retrospective

TABLE 23-1
Differential Diagnosis of Nummular Eczema

Most Likely
- Allergic contact dermatitis
- Stasis dermatitis
- Atopic dermatitis
- Tinea corporis

Consider
- Impetigo
- Psoriasis (longstanding plaques)
- Mycosis fungoides (longstanding plaques)
- Paget disease, when there is unilateral involvement of nipple/areola
- Bullous pemphigoid
- Pemphigus vulgaris
- Other nummular dermatoses:
  - Fixed-drug eruption
  - Pityriasis rotunda

Always Rule Out
- Tinea corporis

population-based study in Taiwan found the incidence of LSC to be 25 to 28 versus 17.8 per 10,000 person-years in those with versus those without a history of anxiety disorders.[38] A cross-sectional study found that LSC and PN were encountered in 3% and 2.1% of dermatology visits, respectively.[9] PN more commonly occurs in adults, but can occasionally affect children.[9,39,40] Patients with PN in the setting of AD have been found to have an earlier age of onset as compared to those without AD.[41] LSC may be more common in patients of Asian descent for reasons unknown.[42]

ETIOLOGY AND PATHOGENESIS

LSC is induced by rubbing and scratching, whereas prurigo nodules are induced by picking and scratching secondary to itch. Some authors suggest that PN is a form of LSC.[43,44] These two disorders may represent a spectrum of manifestations secondary to chronic itch.

Various factors incite itch in both disorders and not all are well understood. Both types of lesions are commonly found in patients with AD along with xerosis and other signs and symptoms of AD. Some studies found that patients with LSC and PN have high rates of atopic disease and/or a history of AD.[39,41,45,46] "Besnier prurigo" refers to the prurigo nodules seen in AD. Prurigo nodules may also occur in other dermatoses, such as contact dermatitis[47] and pemphigoid nodularis, a rare variant of bullous pemphigoid.[48,49] LSC may develop superimposed on other dermatoses, including contact dermatitis,[50-52] psoriasis, *Candida*, and tinea infections.[53]

There may be underlying systemic causes of pruritus in patients with PN and LSC without AD. These causes include renal insufficiency, hyper- or hypothyroidism, liver failure, hepatitides B and C viruses even without liver failure, HIV disease, *Helicobacter*, mycobacterial or parasitic infection, or an underlying hematologic or solid-organ malignancy, including Hodgkin disease, and gastric and bladder cancers.[54-59] PN also has been reported to occur in the setting of celiac disease and/or dermatitis herpetiformis.[60,61] A relationship between LSC, neuropathy, and radiculopathy has been suggested in a subset of patients.[35,62]

PN and LSC appear to have a bidirectional relationship with emotional and psychological factors. A retrospective population-based study in Taiwan found that persons with anxiety disorders had significantly higher risk of subsequently developing LSC.[38] On the other hand, patients with LSC and PN have higher rates of depression, anxiety, obsessive-compulsive disorder, and other psychological disorders.[39,63-67] One study found that 72% of patients thought that psychosocial problems were of relevance.[39]

The higher rates of psychological disorders may be partly a result of the detrimental effects of the chronic itchiness and sequelae of their skin disease.

Several pathways have been postulated for heightened perception to touch and itch in patients with LSC and PN. These include cellular and neurochemical changes at the level of cutaneous nerves in lesions, the spinal cord, and the central nervous system. PN lesions were found to have increased cutaneous nerve fibers (neural hyperplasia) and increased staining for the neuropeptides calcitonin gene-related peptide (CGRP) and substance P, but not tyrosine hydroxylase, vasoactive intestinal polypeptide, and the C-flanking region of neuropeptide Y.[68] Nerve growth factor is overexpressed in PN lesions and is implicated in the pathogenesis of cutaneous neural hyperplasia and upregulated expression of neuropeptides, such as CGRP and substance P.[69] CGRP and substance P may be modulators of itch and upregulate secretion of proinflammatory cytokines, including tumor necrosis factor alpha, interleukin (IL)-1 and IL-8 within lesional skin of PN.[68] Keratinocytes also express transient receptor potential cation channel subfamily V member 1 (TRPV1) channels, which play important roles in sensation of itch, heat and pain. TRPV1 receptors are greatly upregulated in PN.[70] IL-31 is produced by T cells and may be a direct inflammatory mediator of itch.[71] One study found that IL-31 levels were dramatically increased in PN lesions of atopic skin disease.[72] Neurotransmitters that affect mood, such as dopamine, serotonin, or opioid peptides, modulate perception of itch via descending spinal pathways.[73] Finally, environmental factors, such as heat, sweat, and irritation have been implicated in inducing itch in anogenital LSC.[53]

CLINICAL FINDINGS

HISTORY

Severe itching is the hallmark of LSC and PN. Itching may be paroxysmal, continuous, or sporadic, localized or diffuse. Itching may be described by patients as burning, stinging, or a creepy-crawly sensation akin to formication. Patients may not be aware of itching and scratching that occurs during sleep time. Patients may also develop habitual scratching or picking of lesions, even when they are not itchy. Itch is often triggered by sweating, heat, friction, extreme humidity or dryness, irritation from personal care products or clothing, and/or times of psychological distress.[53,54] LSC and PN are associated with moderate to severe quality-of-life impairment[74-77] and sexual dysfunction.[78]

CUTANEOUS LESIONS

In LSC, repeated rubbing and scratching gives rise to lichenified, dry, and scaly plaques with or without excoriations. Hyperpigmentation and hypopigmentation can be seen, particularly in patients with skin of color. The most common sites of involvement are the scalp, the nape of the neck, the ankles, the extensor aspects of the extremities, and the anogenital and vulvar regions.[79] The labia majora in women and the scrotum in men (Fig. 23-5) are the most common sites of genital involvement.[45] The upper inner thighs, groin, nipple, and areola also may be affected.[79]

Prurigo nodules are firm to hard on palpation, varying in size from 0.5 cm to >3.0 cm, and numbering from few to hundreds. The surface may be hyperkeratotic or crateriform. There is often overlying excoriation. Pruritus is usually severe. Limbs are affected in most cases, especially the extensor aspects (Fig. 23-6). The abdomen and sacrum were the next most common sites of involvement in one study.[39] Face and palms are rarely involved. Nodules may occur on any site that can be reached by the patient. There can be a characteristic "butterfly sign" with lesional sparing on the upper back. However, some patients may even develop nodules on hard-to-reach areas secondary to using back-scratchers, knives, forks, brushes, or other instruments to scratch. Nodules may persist for months to years and resolve with postinflammatory hyperpigmentation or hypopigmentation and scarring.

RELATED PHYSICAL FINDINGS

In patients with AD, the intervening skin is often lichenified and xerotic, and patients may have other

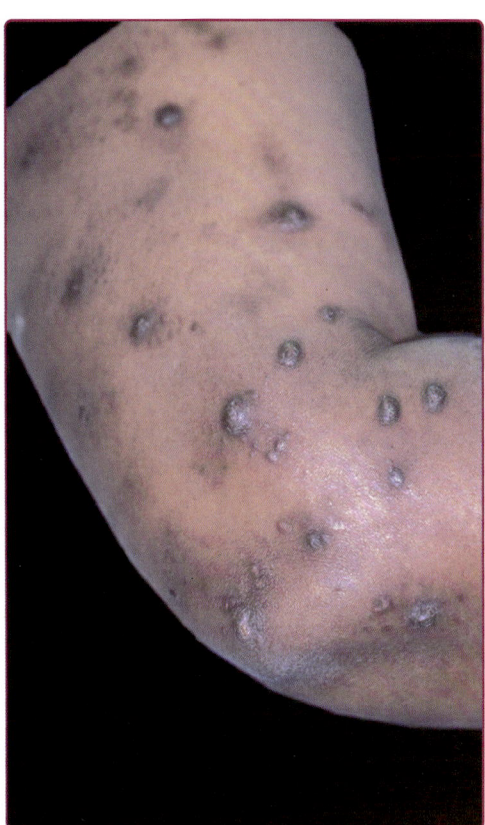

Figure 23-6 Prurigo nodularis. (Used by permission of Professor D. Modi, Division of Dermatology, University of the Witwatersrand, Johannesburg, South Africa.)

signs of atopy, such as Dennie-Morgan fold or palmar hyperlinearity. In nonatopic patients, cutaneous signs of underlying systemic disease or lymphadenopathy, signifying lymphoma, may be present.

LABORATORY TESTS

In patients with LSC or PN in whom an underlying systemic cause of pruritus is suspected, a complete blood count with differential and renal, liver, and thyroid function tests may be ordered. Testing for HIV, diabetes (fasting glucose and/or hemoglobin A1C) may be indicated.[35] A chest radiograph may be obtained to screen for lymphoma. The need for a more extensive evaluation should be individualized based on patient history and results of the aforementioned tests.

Additional testing for iron deficiency, erythrocyte sedimentation rate, gliadin antibody, zinc, cobalamin, total porphyrins, and stool examination for *Strongyloides stercoralis* may also be indicated. Ultrasound of the abdomen or lymph nodes may be indicated to rule out liver or kidney disease or lymphoma. Breath test for *Helicobacter*, lactose, and sorbitol intolerance may be indicated. Magnetic resonance imaging of the cervical

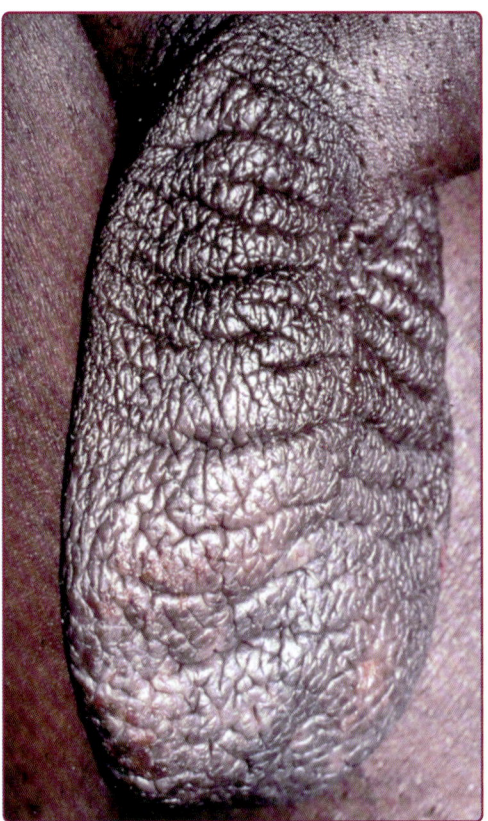

Figure 23-5 Lichen simplex chronicus of the scrotum: lichenification, hyperpigmentation, and hypopigmentation with excoriation. (Image from Division of Dermatology, University of the Witwatersrand, Johannesburg, South Africa, with permission, from Professor D. Modi.)

spinal column is called for if the patient has localized LSC or PN (eg, brachioradial distribution).

SPECIAL TESTS

On histopathologic sections, LSC shows varying degrees of hyperkeratosis with parakeratosis and orthokeratosis, hypergranulosis, and psoriasiform epidermal hyperplasia. The papillary dermis shows thickening of collagen with coarse collagen bundles and vertical streaks. There is a variable inflammatory infiltrate around the superficial vascular plexus with lymphocytes, histiocytes, and eosinophils. A biopsy may also reveal a primary pruritic disorder, such as psoriasis, that has led to secondary lichenification. Direct immunofluorescence may be needed to rule out autoimmune skin disease, such as bullous pemphigoid or dermatitis herpetiformis. Polymerase chain reaction testing for mycobacteria may be needed if histological investigation finds granulomatous inflammatory infiltrate.

The epidermal findings in PN are similar to LSC. The lesion is more papular with bulbous epidermal hyperplasia. Papillary dermal changes also resemble LSC. There may be cutaneous neural hypertrophy with thickened nerve bundles and an increase in nerve fibers by S-100 staining. This finding may not be seen in all cases.[80]

DIFFERENTIAL DIAGNOSIS

Tables 23-2 and 23-3 outline the differential diagnoses for LSC and PN, respectively.

COMPLICATIONS

Sleep studies show that disturbances in the sleep cycle in LSC are present. Non-rapid eye movement sleep is disturbed and patients have an increased arousal index (brief awakenings from sleep) caused by scratching.[81]

TABLE 23-2
Differential Diagnosis of Lichen Simplex Chronicus

Most Likely
- Lichenified atopic eczema
- Lichenified psoriasis
- Hypertrophic lichen planus

Consider
- Genital: extramammary Paget disease

Always Rule Out
- Vulva, perianally: underlying lichen sclerosus, human papillomavirus, or tinea cruris
- Scrotum: underlying human papillomavirus or tinea cruris

TABLE 23-3
Differential Diagnosis of Prurigo Nodularis

Most Likely
- Perforating disease
- Hypertrophic lichen planus
- Pemphigoid nodularis (bullous pemphigoid)
- Actinic prurigo
- Multiple keratoacanthomas
- Dermatitis herpetiformis

Consider
Nodular scabies
Dermatitis herpetiformis

Patients with LSC and PN have higher rates of depression, anxiety, obsessive-compulsive disorder, and other psychological disorders.[39,63-67]

A retrospective population-based cohort study found that patients with LSC had higher baseline rates of diabetes, hypertension, hyperlipidemia, cardiovascular disease, peripheral arterial disease, chronic kidney disease, depression, and anxiety, and an increased risk of developing erectile dysfunction.[78]

PROGNOSIS AND CLINICAL COURSE

Both diseases run a chronic course with persistence or recurrence of lesions. The mean duration of PN was found to be 77.5 months,[35] whereas that of anogenital LSC was found to be 30.6 months.[82] LSC and PN in association with systemic disease may have a more prolonged course than other etiologies.[35] The presence of PN in patients with renal pruritus is associated with more prolonged itch.[83] Exacerbations can occur in response to emotional stress and exogenous stimuli.

TREATMENT

Figure 23-7 outlines the stepwise management of LSC and PN. Treatment is aimed at interrupting the itch–scratch cycle. Both components should be addressed. Systemic causes of itch should be identified and addressed. In both conditions, first-line measures to control itch include potent topical corticosteroids as well as nonsteroidal antipruritic preparations such as menthol, phenol, or pramoxine. Emollients are an important adjunct, particularly for those patients with AD. Intralesional steroids, such as triamcinolone acetonide, given in varying concentrations according to the thickness of the plaque or nodule are beneficial. Topical tacrolimus has been successfully employed as a steroid-sparing agent, but may require application under occlusion to improve transcutaneous absorption. Sedating antihistamines, such as hydroxyzine, or tricyclic antidepressants, such as doxepin, may be used to

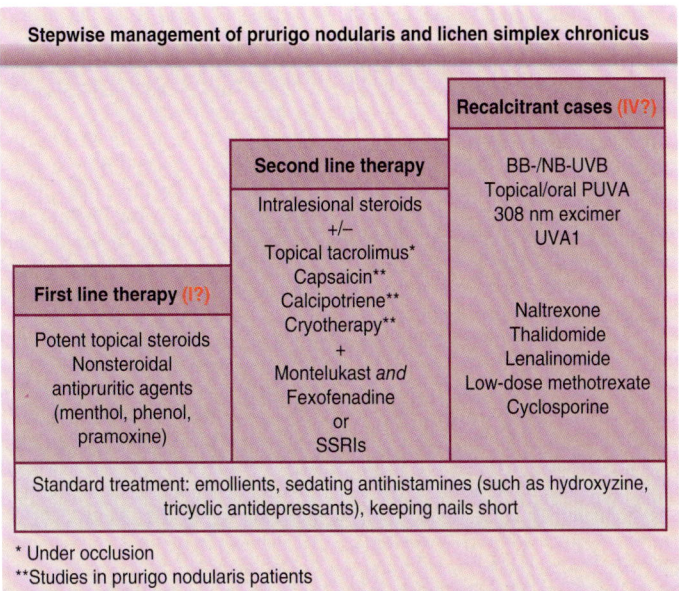

Figure 23-7 Stepwise management of prurigo nodularis and lichen simplex chronicus. BB, broadband; NB, narrowband; PUVA, psoralen and ultraviolet A; UVA, ultraviolet A; UVB, ultraviolet B.

abolish nighttime itch in both conditions. An open-label study of 9 patients with conventional therapy-resistant PN found that daily montelukast and fexofenadine was effective at reducing itch in 75% of patients.[84] Selective serotonin reuptake inhibitors have been recommended for relief of daytime pruritus or in patients with comorbid obsessive-compulsive disorder.[53]

Capsaicin, calcipotriene, and cryotherapy, with or without intralesional steroid injections, have all been successfully used in PN. Both broadband and narrowband ultraviolet B, as well as topical or oral psoralen and ultraviolet A (PUVA) show efficacy and are indicated in widespread cases. The 308-nm excimer monochromatic light, UVA1 phototherapy, and naltrexone were all effective in small series.[85-87] Thalidomide and lenalinomide,[88] low-dose methotrexate,[89] and cyclosporine[90] also are beneficial, albeit with some adverse effects reported.

The importance of avoiding scratching should be addressed with the patient. Nails should be kept short and mittens can be used to prevent scratching. Occlusive measures, such as plastic films, topical steroid impregnated tape, or Unna boots may be needed in widespread or refractory cases.

REFERENCES

1. Gross P. Nummular eczema: its clinical picture and successful therapy. *Arch Derm Syphilol*. 1941;44:1060-1077.
2. Julian-Gonzalez RE, Orozco-Covarrubias L, Duran-McKinster C, et al. Less common clinical manifestations of atopic dermatitis: prevalence by age. *Pediatr Dermatol*. 2012;29(5):580-583.
3. Krol A, Krafchik B. The differential diagnosis of atopic dermatitis in childhood. *Dermatol Ther*. 2006;19(2):73-82.
4. Kulthanan K, Boochangkool K, Tuchinda P, et al. Clinical features of the extrinsic and intrinsic types of adult-onset atopic dermatitis. *Asia Pac Allergy*. 2011;1(2):80-86.
5. Bonamonte D, Foti C, Vestita M, et al. Nummular eczema and contact allergy: a retrospective study. *Dermatitis*. 2012;23(4):153-157.
6. Krupa Shankar DS, Shrestha S. Relevance of patch testing in patients with nummular dermatitis. *Indian J Dermatol Venereol Leprol*. 2005;71(6):406-408.
7. Hellgren L, Mobacken H. Nummular eczema—clinical and statistical data. *Acta Derm Venereol*. 1969;49(2):189-196.
8. Johnson MT, Roberts J. Skin conditions and related need for medical care among persons 1-74 years. United States, 1971-1974. *Vital Health Stat 11*. 1978(212):i-v, 1-72.
9. Bilgili ME, Yildiz H, Sarici G. Prevalence of skin diseases in a dermatology outpatient clinic in Turkey. A cross-sectional, retrospective study. *J Dermatol Case Rep*. 2013;7(4):108-112.
10. Jiamton S, Tangjaturonrusamee C, Kulthanan K. Clinical features and aggravating factors in nummular eczema in Thais. *Asian Pac J Allergy Immunol*. 2013;31(1):36-42.
11. Carr RD, Berke M, Becker SW. Incidence of atopy in the general population. *Arch Dermatol*. 1964;89:27-32.
12. Krueger GG, Kahn G, Weston WL, et al. IgE levels in nummular eczema and ichthyosis. *Arch Dermatol*. 1973;107(1):56-58.
13. Aoyama H, Tanaka M, Hara M, et al. Nummular eczema: an addition of senile xerosis and unique cutaneous reactivities to environmental aeroallergens. *Dermatology*. 1999;199(2):135-139.
14. Bos JD, Hagenaars C, Das PK, et al. Predominance of "memory" T cells (CD4+, CDw29+) over "naive" T cells

(CD4+, CD45R+) in both normal and diseased human skin. *Arch Dermatol Res*. 1989;281(1):24-30.
15. Krogh HK. Nummular eczema. Its relationship to internal foci of infection. A survey of 84 case records. *Acta Derm Venereol*. 1960;40:114-126.
16. Denig NI, Hoke AW, Maibach HI. Irritant contact dermatitis. Clues to causes, clinical characteristics, and control. *Postgrad Med*. 1998;103(5):199-200, 207-198, 212-193.
17. Wilkinson DS. Discoid eczema as a consequence of contact with irritants. *Contact Dermatitis*. 1979;5(2):118-119.
18. Shenoi SD, Seth M. Environmental influence, atopy and contact sensitivity in nummular dermatitis. *Indian J Dermatol Venereol Leprol*. 1999;65(5):245.
19. Cowan MA. Nummular eczema. A review, follow-up and analysis of a series of 325 cases. *Acta Derm Venereol*. 1961;41:453-460.
20. Fleming C, Parry E, Forsyth A, et al. Patch testing in discoid eczema. *Contact Dermatitis*. 1997;36(5):261-264.
21. Caraffini S, Lisi P. Nummular dermatitis-like eruption from ethylenediamine hydrochloride in 2 children. *Contact Dermatitis*. 1987;17(5):313-314.
22. Morrow DM, Rapaport MJ, Strick RA. Hypersensitivity to aloe. *Arch Dermatol*. 1980;116(9):1064-1065.
23. Jadassohn J. *Dermatologie*. Wien, Austria: Verl. f. Medizin, Weidmann & Co.; 1938.
24. Rockl H. Studies on clinical manifestations and pathogenesis of microbial eczema. I [in German]. *Hautarzt*. 1955;6(12):532-537.
25. Török L. Über das Verhältnis des Ekzems zur artefiziellen Hautentzündung und zur Impetigo. *Dermatol Wochenschr*. 1923;76:273.
26. Kim WJ, Ko HC, Kim MB, et al. Features of *Staphylococcus aureus* colonization in patients with nummular eczema. *Br J Dermatol*. 2013;168(3):658-660.
27. Tanaka T, Satoh T, Yokozeki H. Dental infection associated with nummular eczema as an overlooked focal infection. *J Dermatol*. 2009;36(8):462-465.
28. Bettoli V, Tosti A, Varotti C. Nummular eczema during isotretinoin treatment. *J Am Acad Dermatol*. 1987;16(3, pt 1):617.
29. Wilkinson SM, Smith AG, Davis MJ, et al. Pityriasis rosea and discoid eczema: dose related reactions to treatment with gold. *Ann Rheum Dis*. 1992;51(7):881-884.
30. Shen Y, Pielop J, Hsu S. Generalized nummular eczema secondary to peginterferon alfa-2b and ribavirin combination therapy for hepatitis C infection. *Arch Dermatol*. 2005;141(1):102-103.
31. Moore MM, Elpern DJ, Carter DJ. Severe, generalized nummular eczema secondary to interferon alfa-2b plus ribavirin combination therapy in a patient with chronic hepatitis C virus infection. *Arch Dermatol*. 2004;140(2):215-217.
32. Delle Sedie A, Bazzichi L, Bombardieri S, et al. Psoriasis, erythema nodosum, and nummular eczema onset in an ankylosing spondylitis patient treated with infliximab. *Scand J Rheumatol*. 2007;36(5):403-404.
33. Adachi A, Horikawa T, Takashima T, et al. Mercury-induced nummular dermatitis. *J Am Acad Dermatol*. 2000;43(2, pt 2):383-385.
34. Roberts H, Orchard D. Methotrexate is a safe and effective treatment for paediatric discoid (nummular) eczema: a case series of 25 children. *Australas J Dermatol*. 2010;51(2):128-130.
35. Iking A, Grundmann S, Chatzigeorgakidis E, et al. Prurigo as a symptom of atopic and non-atopic diseases: aetiological survey in a consecutive cohort of 108 patients. *J Eur Acad Dermatol Venereol*. 2013;27(5):550-557.
36. Lezcano L, Di Martino Ortiz B, Rodriguez Masi M, et al. Prurigo nodularis [in Spanish]. *Arch Argent Pediatr*. 2008;106(5):446-449.
37. Vaidya DC, Schwartz RA. Prurigo nodularis: a benign dermatosis derived from a persistent pruritus. *Acta Dermatovenerol Croat*. 2008;16(1):38-44.
38. Liao YH, Lin CC, Tsai PP, et al. Increased risk of lichen simplex chronicus in people with anxiety disorder: a nationwide population-based retrospective cohort study. *Br J Dermatol*. 2014;170(4):890-894.
39. Rowland Payne CM, Wilkinson JD, McKee PH, et al. Nodular prurigo—a clinicopathological study of 46 patients. *Br J Dermatol*. 1985;113(4):431-439.
40. Doyle JA, Connolly SM, Hunziker N, et al. Prurigo nodularis: a reappraisal of the clinical and histologic features. *J Cutan Pathol*. 1979;6(5):392-403.
41. Tanaka M, Aiba S, Matsumura N, et al. Prurigo nodularis consists of two distinct forms: early-onset atopic and late-onset non-atopic. *Dermatology*. 1995;190(4):269-276.
42. Rein CR, Snider BL. Lichen simplex chronicus in Orientals. *AMA Arch Derm Syphilol*. 1952;66(5):612-617.
43. Besselmann A. Zur Kenntnis der Prurigo nodularis. *Arch Derm Syphilol*. 1932;166:212-225.
44. Shaffer B, Beerman H. Lichen simplex chronicus and its variants; a discussion of certain psychodynamic mechanisms and clinical and histopathologic correlations. *AMA Arch Derm Syphilol*. 1951;64(3):340-351.
45. Singh G. Atopy in lichen simplex (neurodermatitis circumscripta). *Br J Dermatol*. 1973;89(6):625-627.
46. Miyachi Y, Okamoto H, Furukawa F, et al. Prurigo nodularis. A possible relationship to atopy. *J Dermatol*. 1980;7(4):281-283.
47. Zelickson BD, McEvoy MT, Fransway AF. Patch testing in prurigo nodularis. *Contact Dermatitis*. 1989;20(5):321-325.
48. Dangel B, Kofler L, Metzler G. Nodular subtype of bullous pemphigoid. *J Cutan Med Surg*. 2016;20(6):570-572.
49. Al-Salhi W, Alharithy R. Pemphigoid nodularis. *J Cutan Med Surg*. 2015;19(2):153-155.
50. Chey WY, Kim KL, Yoo TY, et al. Allergic contact dermatitis from hair dye and development of lichen simplex chronicus. *Contact Dermatitis*. 2004;51(1):5-8.
51. Virgili A, Bacilieri S, Corazza M. Evaluation of contact sensitization in vulvar lichen simplex chronicus. A proposal for a battery of selected allergens. *J Reprod Med*. 2003;48(1):33-36.
52. Virgili A, Bacilieri S, Corazza M. Managing vulvar lichen simplex chronicus. *J Reprod Med*. 2001;46(4):343-346.
53. Lynch PJ. Lichen simplex chronicus (atopic/neurodermatitis) of the anogenital region. *Dermatol Ther*. 2004;17(1):8-19.
54. Lee MR, Shumack S. Prurigo nodularis: a review. *Australas J Dermatol*. 2005;46(4):211-218; quiz 219-220.
55. Seshadri P, Rajan SJ, George IA, et al. A sinister itch: prurigo nodularis in Hodgkin lymphoma. *J Assoc Physicians India*. 2009;57:715-716.
56. Lin JT, Wang WH, Yen CC, et al. Prurigo nodularis as initial presentation of metastatic transitional cell carcinoma of the bladder. *J Urol*. 2002;168(2):631-632.
57. Callen JP, Bernardi DM, Clark RA, et al. Adult-onset recalcitrant eczema: a marker of noncutaneous lymphoma or leukemia. *J Am Acad Dermatol*. 2000;43(2, pt 1):207-210.
58. Neri S, Raciti C, D'Angelo G, et al. Hyde's prurigo nodularis and chronic HCV hepatitis. *J Hepatol*. 1998;28(1):161-164.

59. Shelnitz LS, Paller AS. Hodgkin's disease manifesting as prurigo nodularis. *Pediatr Dermatol*. 1990;7(2):136-139.
60. Delfino M, Nino M, Delfino G, et al. Dermatitis herpetiformis and gluten-sensitive enteropathy in a patient with nodular prurigo. *J Eur Acad Dermatol Venereol*. 2002;16(1):88-89.
61. Francesco Stefanini G, Resta F, Marsigli L, et al. Prurigo nodularis (Hyde's prurigo) disclosing celiac disease. *Hepatogastroenterology*. 1999;46(28):2281-2284.
62. Solak O, Kulac M, Yaman M, et al. Lichen simplex chronicus as a symptom of neuropathy. *Clin Exp Dermatol*. 2009;34(4):476-480.
63. Konuk N, Koca R, Atik L, et al. Psychopathology, depression and dissociative experiences in patients with lichen simplex chronicus. *Gen Hosp Psychiatry*. 2007;29(3):232-235.
64. Bhatia MS, Gautam RK, Bedi GK. Psychiatric profile of patients with neurodermatitis. *J Indian Med Assoc*. 1996;94(12):445-446, 454.
65. Sanjana VD, Fernandez RJ. Lichen simplex chronicus—a psychocutaneous disorder? *Indian J Dermatol Venereol Leprol*. 1995;61(6):336-338.
66. Attah Johnson FY, Mostaghimi H. Co-morbidity between dermatologic diseases and psychiatric disorders in Papua New Guinea. *Int J Dermatol*. 1995;34(4):244-248.
67. Fried RG, Fried S. Picking apart the picker: a clinician's guide for management of the patient presenting with excoriations. *Cutis*. 2003;71(4):291-298.
68. Abadia Molina F, Burrows NP, Jones RR, et al. Increased sensory neuropeptides in nodular prurigo: a quantitative immunohistochemical analysis. *Br J Dermatol*. 1992;127(4):344-351.
69. Johansson O, Liang Y, Emtestam L. Increased nerve growth factor- and tyrosine kinase A-like immunoreactivities in prurigo nodularis skin—an exploration of the cause of neurohyperplasia. *Arch Dermatol Res*. 2002;293(12):614-619.
70. Stander S, Moormann C, Schumacher M, et al. Expression of vanilloid receptor subtype 1 in cutaneous sensory nerve fibers, mast cells, and epithelial cells of appendage structures. *Exp Dermatol*. 2004;13(3):129-139.
71. Stott B, Lavender P, Lehmann S, et al. Human IL-31 is induced by IL-4 and promotes TH2-driven inflammation. *J Allergy Clin Immunol*. 2013;132(2):446-454, e445.
72. Sonkoly E, Muller A, Lauerma AI, et al. IL-31: a new link between T cells and pruritus in atopic skin inflammation. *J Allergy Clin Immunol*. 2006;117(2):411-417.
73. Wallengren J. Prurigo: diagnosis and management. *Am J Clin Dermatol*. 2004;5(2):85-95.
74. Kouris A, Christodoulou C, Efstathiou V, et al. Comparative study of quality of life and obsessive-compulsive tendencies in patients with chronic hand eczema and lichen simplex chronicus. *Dermatitis*. 2016;27(3):127-130.
75. An JG, Liu YT, Xiao SX, et al. Quality of life of patients with neurodermatitis. *Int J Med Sci*. 2013;10(5):593-598.
76. Murota H, Kitaba S, Tani M, et al. Impact of sedative and non-sedative antihistamines on the impaired productivity and quality of life in patients with pruritic skin diseases. *Allergol Int*. 2010;59(4):345-354.
77. Kantor R, Dalal P, Cella D, et al. Impact of pruritus on quality of life: a systematic review. *J Am Acad Dermatol*. 2016;75(5):885-886.e4.
78. Juan CK, Chen HJ, Shen JL, et al. Lichen simplex chronicus associated with erectile dysfunction: a population-based retrospective cohort study. *PLoS One*. 2015;10(6):e0128869.
79. Novick NL. Unilateral, circumscribed, chronic dermatitis of the papillary-areolar complex: case report and review of the literature. *Mt Sinai J Med*. 2001;68(4-5):321-325.
80. Weigelt N, Metze D, Stander S. Prurigo nodularis: systematic analysis of 58 histological criteria in 136 patients. *J Cutan Pathol*. 2010;37(5):578-586.
81. Koca R, Altin R, Konuk N, et al. Sleep disturbance in patients with lichen simplex chronicus and its relationship to nocturnal scratching: a case control study. *South Med J*. 2006;99(5):482-485.
82. Rajalakshmi R, Thappa DM, Jaisankar TJ, et al. Lichen simplex chronicus of anogenital region: a clinico-etiological study. *Indian J Dermatol Venereol Leprol*. 2011;77(1):28-36.
83. Bohme T, Heitkemper T, Mettang T, et al. Clinical features and prurigo nodularis in nephrogenic pruritus [in German]. *Hautarzt*. 2014;65(8):714-720.
84. Shintani T, Ohata C, Koga H, et al. Combination therapy of fexofenadine and montelukast is effective in prurigo nodularis and pemphigoid nodularis. *Dermatol Ther*. 2014;27(3):135-139.
85. Saraceno R, Nistico SP, Capriotti E, et al. Monochromatic excimer light (308 nm) in the treatment of prurigo nodularis. *Photodermatol Photoimmunol Photomed*. 2008;24(1):43-45.
86. Rombold S, Lobisch K, Katzer K, et al. Efficacy of UVA1 phototherapy in 230 patients with various skin diseases. *Photodermatol Photoimmunol Photomed*. 2008;24(1):19-23.
87. Metze D, Reimann S, Beissert S, et al. Efficacy and safety of naltrexone, an oral opiate receptor antagonist, in the treatment of pruritus in internal and dermatological diseases. *J Am Acad Dermatol*. 1999;41(4):533-539.
88. Lim VM, Maranda EL, Patel V, et al. A review of the efficacy of thalidomide and lenalidomide in the treatment of refractory prurigo nodularis. *Dermatol Ther (Heidelb)*. 2016;6(3):397-411.
89. Spring P, Gschwind I, Gilliet M. Prurigo nodularis: retrospective study of 13 cases managed with methotrexate. *Clin Exp Dermatol*. 2014;39(4):468-473.
90. Siepmann D, Luger TA, Stander S. Antipruritic effect of cyclosporine microemulsion in prurigo nodularis: results of a case series. *J Dtsch Dermatol Ges*. 2008;6(11):941-946.

Chapter 24 :: Allergic Contact Dermatitis
:: Jake E. Turrentine, Michael P. Sheehan, & Ponciano D. Cruz, Jr.

第二十四章
变应性接触性皮炎

中文导读

本章共分为8节：①流行病学；②临床特征；③病因和发病机制；④诊断；⑤斑贴试验机制；⑥鉴别诊断；⑦病程和预后；⑧治疗。

第一节横向和纵向比较了变应性接触性皮炎（ACD）的发病率及年龄、性别、人种对ACD发病的影响。

第二节描述了急性、亚急性和慢性期ACD的皮肤表现和分布特点。描述了一些临床少见的ACD的非湿疹样临床表现，包括多形红斑样ACD、紫癜性ACD、苔藓样ACD、色素沉着性ACD、淋巴瘤样ACD。

第三节介绍了ACD是经典的细胞介导的（Ⅳ型）迟发型超敏反应，分为致敏阶段、激活阶段。

第四节详细介绍了诊断ACD的流程和要点，主要根据病史、临床表现和斑贴试验结果诊断ACD，必要时结合组织病理学检查。详细介绍了ACD的两种诊断算法：地形图方法和过敏原特异性方法。全面介绍了体表各部位的接触致敏物及其所致皮肤表现，并提出了对称性药物相关性间擦部及屈侧疹（SDRIFE）、过敏性接触性皮炎综合征的概念及其诊断标准。列出了一些已知的口服或静脉用药，这些药物可能导致先前致敏的患者的ACD再次激发全身。在"过敏原特异性方法"的描述中，对北美最常见的阳性且重要的斑贴试验过敏原做了说明。认为金属（镍、钴、铬等）是导致ACD的常见原因。并分别对防腐剂、香料、外用抗菌剂、对苯二胺、橡胶、外用类固醇引起的接触性皮炎做了阐述。

第五节详细介绍了斑贴试验的机制，包括以下几个方面：过敏原的选择、放置方法及时间长短、结果评估及判读、如何判定与临床的相关性、斑贴试验并发症以及系统免疫抑制药对斑贴试验的影响。

第六节介绍了ACD的鉴别诊断。

第七节介绍了ACD的病程与预后，指出其主要影响患者生活质量。

第八节介绍了ACD的诊断和治疗，指出主要根据病史、临床表现结合斑贴试验进行诊断。局部皮质类固醇是一线治疗，在严重或广泛爆发的情况下，通常需要口服泼尼松。

〔李　捷〕

AT-A-GLANCE

- Allergic contact dermatitis (ACD) is a cell-mediated (type IV), delayed type, hypersensitivity reaction caused by skin contact with an environmental allergen.
- Prior sensitization is required for allergy to develop.
- The clinical manifestation of ACD is an eczematous dermatitis. The acute phase is characterized by pruritus, erythema, edema, and vesicles, usually confined to the area of direct exposure. Recurrent contact to the causative allergen may lead to chronic disease, characterized by lichenified erythematous plaques with variable hyperkeratosis, fissuring, and pigmentary changes that may spread beyond the areas of direct exposure.
- Itch and swelling are key components of the history and may be clues to allergy.
- Patch testing is the diagnostic test of choice to identify causal allergens and is indicated for patients with persistent or recurrent dermatitis in whom ACD is suspected.
- Allergen avoidance is the mainstay of ACD treatment. Educating patients about avoiding the allergen and related substances, and providing suitable alternatives, are crucial to a good outcome.

The skin is a complex and dynamic organ that serves many purposes, among which is maintenance of a physical and immunologic barrier to the environment. Therefore, the skin is the first line of defense after exposure to a variety of chemicals. Allergic contact dermatitis (ACD) accounts for approximately 20% of new incident cases of *contact dermatitis* (irritant contact dermatitis accounts for the remainder).[1] ACD, as the name implies, is an adverse cutaneous inflammatory reaction caused by contact with a specific exogenous allergen to which a person was previously sensitized. More than 3700 chemicals are implicated as causal agents of ACD in humans.[2] Following contact with an allergen, the skin reacts immunologically so that in allergic individuals, such contact produces eczematous inflammation, which can range from a mild, short-lived condition to a severe, persistent, chronic disease, depending on the specific allergen and the amount, extent, and frequency of exposure. Appropriate allergen identification through proper epicutaneous patch testing improves quality of life as measured by standard tools,[3] as it allows for avoidance of the inciting allergen and possibly sustained remission from the potentially debilitating condition. Recognition of the presenting signs and symptoms, and appropriate patch testing, are crucial in the evaluation of a patient with suspected ACD.

EPIDEMIOLOGY

Several studies have investigated the prevalence of contact allergy in the general population and in unselected subgroups of the general population. In 2007, Thyssen and colleagues[4] performed a retrospective study that reviewed the main findings from previously published epidemiologic studies on contact allergy in unselected populations of all age groups and from publishing countries (mainly North America and Western Europe). Based on these heterogeneous published data collected between 1966 and 2007, the median prevalence of contact allergy to at least 1 allergen in the general population was 21.2%. Additionally, the study found that the most prevalent contact allergens in the general population were nickel, thimerosal, and fragrance mix. The prevalence of contact allergy to specific allergens differs among various countries[5-7] and the prevalence to specific allergens is not necessarily static, as prevalence is influenced by regional changes and developments, exposure patterns, regulatory standards, and societal customs and values.

AGE

Multiple studies have recognized contact dermatitis as an important and common cause of childhood dermatitis. Although ACD is equally as likely to develop in childhood as in adulthood,[8,9] the most common allergens identified differ between the age groups. While fragrance was an important sensitizer in all ages, certain studies, such as the 2001 Augsburg study based on adults 28 to 75 years of age, showed a significant increase in fragrance allergy with increasing age.[10] Similarly, a recent Danish study demonstrated the prevalence allergy to preservatives to be higher among those 41 to 60 years of age.[11]

GENDER

Because very few studies have looked at the induction of allergic contact sensitization in men and women under controlled circumstances, gender differences in the development of ACD are largely unknown. When the human repeat-insult patch-testing method was used to assess induction rates for 10 common allergens, women were more often sensitized to 7 of the 10 allergens studied.[12] With regard to frequency, Thyssen and colleagues found that the median prevalence of contact allergy among the general population was 21.8% in women versus 12% in men. Looking specifically at nickel sensitivity, the same study showed the prevalence to be much higher among women than men (17.1% in women vs 3% in men). This may be because pierced ears are a significant risk factor for development of nickel allergy,[13-17] and there was a higher prevalence of pierced ears in women in comparison with men (81.5% vs 12%) in the population studied.

RACE/ETHNICITY

The role of race, if any, in the development of ACD remains controversial. In one study examining North American Contact Dermatitis Group (NACDG) patch test results of 9624 patients (8610 [89.5%] white and 1014 [10.5%] black) between 1992 and 1998, there were no differences in the overall response rate to allergens. Although there were no differences in the overall response rates, white and black patients differed in the frequency of ACD to specific allergens. Although possibly related to genetic factors, ethnicity also may have determined exposure patterns and, therefore, influenced the difference in frequencies in the study.

CLINICAL FEATURES

CUTANEOUS FINDINGS

The classic presentation of ACD is a pruritic, eczematous dermatitis initially localized to the primary site of allergen exposure. Geometric, linear, or focal patterns of involvement are suggestive of an exogenous etiology. For example, ACD from plants such as poison ivy, poison oak, or poison sumac, typically presents as a linear or streaky array of erythematous papules and vesicles. Occasionally, the sensitizing substance in these plants, an oleoresin named *urushiol* may be aerosolized when the plants are burned, leading to a more generalized and severe eruption on exposed areas. Transfer of the resin from sources other than directly from the plant (such as clothes, pets, or hands) may result in rashes on unexpected sites (eg, genital involvement in a patient with poison ivy). Because the mechanism of allergen exposure influences the clinical presentation, relevant historic data gathered from thoughtful questioning may prove as useful as the distribution of the lesions.

Importantly, ACD will vary morphologically depending on the stage of the disease and severity of reaction. During the acute phase, lesions are marked by edema, erythema, and vesicle formation. Stronger allergens often result in vesicle formation, whereas weaker allergens often lead to papular lesion morphology, with surrounding erythema and edema. In the subacute phase, vesicular rupture leads to oozing, and scaly juicy papules associated with weeping and crusting dominate the clinical picture. Finally, the chronic phase is characterized by scaling, fissuring, and lichenification. A key symptom for ACD is pruritus, which seems to occur more typically than a symptom of a burning sensation.

Moreover, there are some noneczematous clinical variants of ACD (Table 24-1) that are infrequently observed.[18,19] *Erythema multiforme-like ACD* has been linked primarily to exotic woods, topical medicaments, and numerous miscellaneous chemicals. In contrast to true erythema multiforme, which typically presents on acral sites, lesions of erythema multiforme-like ACD are typically at the periphery site of contact with the allergen, fever is usually absent, and mucosal involvement is rare. *Purpuric ACD* is mainly observed on the lower legs and/or feet and has been reported with a wide variety of allergens, including rubber and textile dyes. *Lichenoid ACD* is considered a rare variant that can mimic lichen planus; it is associated with color developers and metallic dyes in tattoos. Also, oral lichenoid ACD from dental amalgams can resemble typical oral lichen planus. *Pigmented ACD* has been mainly described in Asian-ethnicity populations. It is linked to textile dyes, cosmetics, and fragrances. *Lymphomatoid ACD* is based only on histopathologic criteria (presence of significant dermal infiltrate displaying features of pseudolymphoma). Nonspecific clinical signs include erythematous plaques, sometimes very infiltrated, at

TABLE 24-1
Noneczematous Variants of Allergic Contact Dermatitis

	SITES/APPEARANCE	COMMON CAUSES
Erythema multiforme-like allergic contact dermatitis (ACD)	Occur at periphery of allergen application; systemic symptoms of erythema multiforme are absent.	Exotic woods, medicaments
Purpuric ACD	Lower legs	Rubber, textile dyes
Lichenoid ACD	Commonly oral mucosa	Color developers, metallic dyes in tattoos; dental amalgams (oral lichenoid ACD)
Pigmented ACD	Clothed portions of body, face may be involved (Riehl melanosis)	Textile dyes, cosmetics, and fragrances
Lymphomatoid ACD	Histologic criteria only	Metals, *para*-phenylenediamine, dimethylfumarate, *para*-tert-butylphenol resin

the site of application of the contact allergen. Allergens implicated in lymphomatoid ACD include metals (nickel and gold), *para*-phenylenediamine (hair dye), *para*-tert-butylphenol resin (glue), and dimethylfumarate (a mold inhibitor found in sachets within some furniture implicated in causing a previously severe epidemic of ACD).

ETIOLOGY AND PATHOGENESIS

ACD represents a classic cell-mediated (type IV), delayed hypersensitivity reaction. Type IV hypersensitivity reactions result from exposure and sensitization of a genetically susceptible host to an environmental allergen, followed by subsequent reexposure that triggers a complex inflammatory reaction. The resulting clinical picture is that of erythema, edema, and papulovesiculation, usually in the distribution of contact with the instigating allergen, and with pruritus as a major symptom.[20] To mount such a reaction, the individual must have sufficient contact with a sensitizing chemical, develop immunologic memory, and then have repeated contact with that substance later to elicit the immune response. This is an important distinction from irritant contact dermatitis in which sensitization is not required, and in which the intensity of the irritant inflammatory reaction is proportional to the dose (concentration and amount) of the irritant. By contrast, in ACD, even minute quantities of an allergen can elicit overt allergic reactions in a sensitized individual. There are two distinct phases in the development of ACD: the sensitization phase and the elicitation phase.[21]

SENSITIZATION PHASE

Unprocessed allergens are more correctly called haptens, which are typically small, lipophilic molecules with a low molecular weight (<500 daltons). Once a hapten penetrates the skin, it binds with epidermal carrier proteins to form a hapten–protein complex, which produces a complete antigen. Simultaneously, innate immunity is activated by keratinocyte release of several cytokines including interleukins 1, 8, and 18, tumor necrosis factor-α, and granulocyte-macrophage colony-stimulating factor.[22] Next, the antigen-presenting cells of the skin (Langerhans cells [LCs] and/or dermal dendritic cells), take up the hapten–protein complex ("the antigen") and express it on the cell surface on an human leukocyte antigen molecule. The antigen-presenting cell then migrates via lymphatics to regional lymph nodes where it presents the human leukocyte antigen complex to naïve antigen-specific T cells. These naïve T cells are then primed and differentiate into memory (effector) T cells, which expand clonally, acquire skin-specific homing antigens, and immigrate into circulation where they can act as effectors on target cells presenting the same antigen in the future.[23,24] The sensitization phase generally lasts 10 to 15 days and often is asymptomatic.[25] Subsequent exposure to the antigen (called *rechallenge*) leads to the elicitation phase and can occur via multiple routes, including transepidermal, subcutaneous, intravenous, intramuscular, inhalation, and oral ingestion.[26]

Of note, LCs have long been assumed to be the antigen-presenting cell responsible for inducing T cells in ACD, because of their abundance in the epidermis, easy accessibility to haptens, and strong antigen-presentation ability in vitro. However, recent studies reveal that depletion of LCs during the sensitization phase does not completely impair contact hypersensitivity responses.[27,28] Interestingly, it seems that CD1a+/CD141+ dermal dendritic cells may be the primary cells responsible for contact sensitization, although LCs may still play a role in some situations.[22,27,29] Furthermore, it is important to note that sensitization can stimulate both helper (Th) and cytotoxic (Tc) T cells. While the most important population of cells in allergic sensitization is the Th1/Tc1 subset (interferon-γ producing), induction of Th2 and Th17/Tc17 subsets has been described and may play a role in the sensitization phase of ACD.[28]

ELICITATION PHASE

During this phase, subsequent exposure to an allergen to which the patient is already sensitized leads to clinical disease. First, hapten exposure leads to low-grade nonspecific inflammation through cellular stress as well as activation of toll-like receptors and nucleotide-binding oligomerization domain-like receptors, leading to neutrophil recruitment and, subsequently, effector T-cell recruitment.[28] Once antigen-specific effector T cells are recruited into skin containing their target antigen, they interact with antigen-presenting cells (LCs and dermal dendritic cells) in a cluster around postcapillary venules. This cluster of immune cells previously was considered the *skin-associated lymphoid tissue* but is now called *inducible skin-associated lymphoid tissue* because the clusters of immune cells only appear when they are induced by inflammation, rather than in the steady state.[28,30] In response, the antigen-specific T cells amplify the specific immune response, releasing cytokines, including interferon-γ and tumor necrosis factor-α, which, in turn, recruit other inflammatory cells while stimulating macrophages and keratinocytes to release more cytokines.[31,32] An inflammatory response occurs as monocytes migrate into the affected area, mature into macrophages, and attract more T cells. The inflammatory response elicited typically lasts several weeks, and if allowed to run its natural course, it is thought that regulatory T cells are involved in suppression of the response. Interestingly, LCs may be involved in promoting the development of regulatory T cells that subsequently suppress the immune response in ACD, although the exact mechanisms are not yet clear.[22,28]

DIAGNOSIS

Any patient who presents with an eczematous dermatitis should be regarded as possibly having ACD. Additionally, one must consider contact allergy in patients with other types of dermatitis (eg, atopic) that is persistent and recalcitrant despite appropriate standard therapies, as well as in patients with erythroderma, or scattered generalized dermatitis.[33] Finally, it is important to avoid some commonly held misconceptions about ACD that can alter a physician's ability to recognize contact dermatitis. These were described by Marks and DeLeo[33] and include the following:

- ACD is not always bilateral even when the antigen exposure is bilateral (eg, shoe or glove allergy).
- Even when exposure to an allergen is uniform (eg, contact allergy to an ingredient of a cream that is applied on the entire face), eczematous manifestations are very often patchy.
- ACD can and does affect the palms and the soles.

The first step in the diagnosis of ACD is a careful medical and environmental exposure history. History taking should begin with a discussion of the present illness, focusing on the site(s) of onset and the topical agents used to treat the problem (including over-the-counter and prescription medications). A history of skin disease, atopy, and general health should be investigated routinely and followed by details of the usage of personal care products (soap, shampoo, conditioner, deodorant, lotions, creams, medications, hair styling products, etc.) and investigation of the patient's avocations or hobbies. The patient's occupation should be ascertained as well, and if it appears contributory, or there are potential allergenic exposures, then a thorough occupational history should be taken. Occupations requiring frequent hand washing, glove use, or chemical exposure should be prime suspects.

SUPPORTIVE STUDIES

Typically, ACD is diagnosed based on history, clinical examination, and patch test results. Occasionally, prior to determining that a dermatitis is of the allergic contact type, workup may include laboratory studies or skin biopsy. In these cases, a complete blood count may demonstrate eosinophilia or may be normal. Histologically, the presence of eosinophilic spongiosis and multinucleate dermal dendritic fibrohistiocytic cells is especially suggestive of ACD, when encountered in the presence of acanthosis, a lymphocytic infiltrate, dermal eosinophils, and hyperkeratosis.[34]

DIAGNOSTIC ALGORITHM

Independent of patch testing (discussed in "Patch-Testing Mechanics" below), the causative allergen(s) can rarely be identified by skillful analysis of the patient's exposure history and distribution of dermatitis. Most of the time, an exact cause cannot be identified based on history and examination alone, so one must develop a clinical approach that will guide patch testing. In the opinion of the authors, the two most useful approaches are a topographic approach (based on the distribution of dermatitis on the patient's skin) and an allergen-specific approach (based on knowledge of trends in dermatitis to specific allergens). Each of these approaches is reviewed in this section.

TOPOGRAPHIC APPROACH

Figure 24-1 identifies the allergens to consider based on skin lesion topography. Dermatitis distribution is often the single most important clue to the diagnosis of ACD. Typically, the area of greatest eczematous dermatitis is the area of greatest contact with the offending allergen(s). Location, in fact, can be one of the most valuable clues as to which chemical might be the culprit of a patient's ACD. For instance, an eczematous dermatitis in the periumbilical or infraumbilical area suggests contact allergy to metal snaps in jeans and belt buckles, whereas eczema distributed around the hairline and behind the ears suggests contact allergy to an ingredient(s) in hair products (hair dyes, shampoo, conditioners, styling products) (Fig. 24-2). Using the same rationale, eczema on the dorsum of the feet suggests contact allergy to products used to make shoe uppers—like leather, rubber, or dyes—whereas eczematous dermatitis on the weight-bearing surfaces of the feet suggests contact allergy to products used to make insoles/soles—like rubber and adhesive materials. Notably, facial, eyelid, lip, and neck patterns of dermatitis should always raise suspicion of a cosmetic-related contact allergy. However, for all these presentations, correct identification of the culprit chemical(s) will still require patch testing, as even the most astute and experienced clinician is, for the most part, unable to properly surmise the positive allergen(s) prior to testing. The pattern of dermatitis should be mainly used to determine whether or not to patch test, and which allergens and screening series to test.

Occasionally, the topographic approach does not hold, and the distribution can actually be misleading. This mainly refers to cases of ectopic ACD or airborne ACD. Ectopic ACD can follow 2 circumstances: *auto transfer*, in which the allergen is inconspicuously transferred to other body sites by the fingers, the classical example being nail lacquer dermatitis located on the eyelids or lateral aspects of the neck; and *heterotransfer*, in which the offending allergen is transferred to the patient by someone else (spouse, parent, etc.); this is described in the literature as connubial or consort ACD.

A discussion of allergens in the context of common patterns of presentation is briefly detailed below.

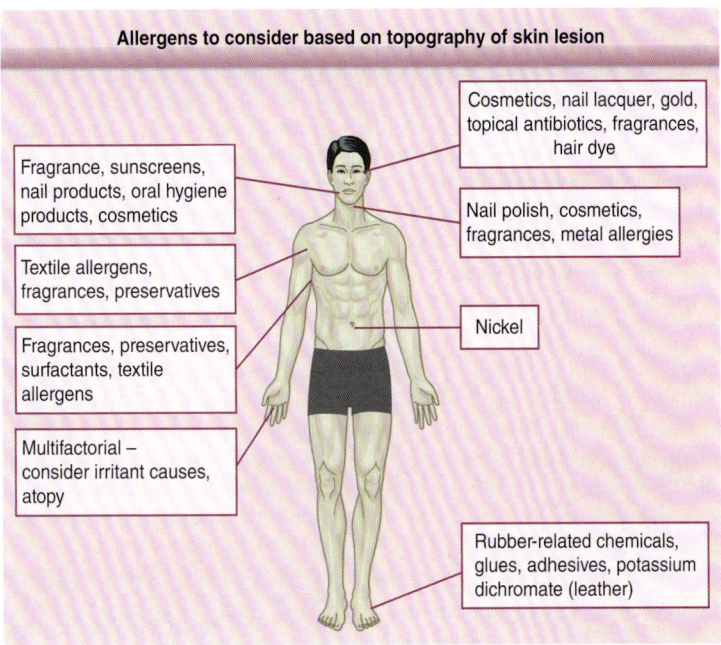

Figure 24-1 Allergens to consider based on topography of skin lesions.

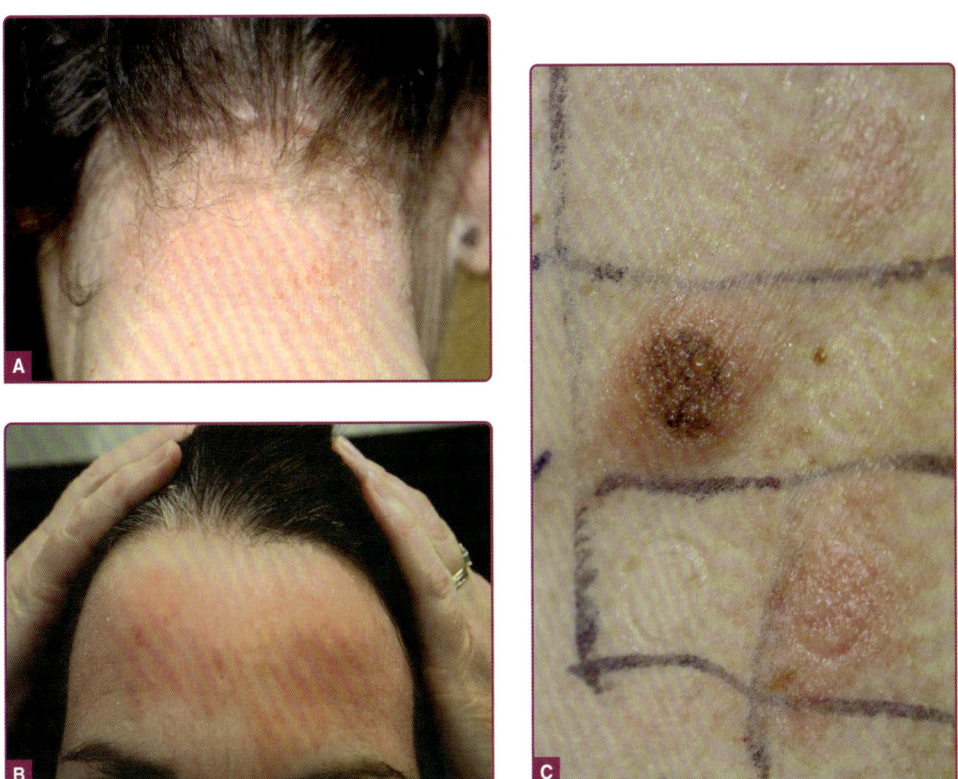

Figure 24-2 Allergic contact dermatitis to *para*-phenylenediamine. **A,** Notice the eczema on the distribution of the hairline and behind the ears. **B,** Dermatitis on the forehead where the bangs came in contact with the skin of the same patient. **C,** *para*-Phenylenediamine, the most frequent relevant allergen in hair dye, is a strong sensitizer.

FACE

The face is a common site for ACD. Among patients with facial dermatitis, women are more commonly affected than men, particularly by cosmetic-associated allergens such as fragrances, *para*-phenylenediamine (PPD), preservatives, and lanolin alcohols.[35] Allergens can be applied to the face directly, or inadvertently contacted from airborne or hand-to-face exposure. In addition to allergens found as ingredients in cosmetics, products used to apply them, such as cosmetic sponges, are also reported to produce facial dermatitis in rubber-sensitive patients.[36] A similar situation can be seen with nickel-plated objects such as eyelash curlers, tweezers, and bobby pins. Cellphones and accessories may also result in facial ACD. The prototypical presentation is that of a preauricular facial dermatitis in a nickel-allergic patient.[37]

SCALP

Scalp-applied allergens paradoxically show a predilection for causing dermatitis on nonscalp sites. Downstream anatomical sites, such as the face, eyelids, ears, neck, and hands, may show ACD while the scalp remains relatively uninvolved. This is likely secondary to regional differences affording the scalp a greater degree of epidermal barrier protection to potential allergens.[38] Nevertheless, patients exquisitely sensitive to certain chemicals in hair products, such as PPD or glyceryl monothioglycolate (GMT), may show a marked scalp reaction with edema and crusting. PPD is one of the most potent sensitizers known and is widely used as an ingredient in hair dyes. In general, PPD sensitization manifests on the face and scalp of female adult patients who had contact with a hair dye.[39-42] GMT is a chemical substance used in permanent wave solutions. Allergic sensitivity to GMT can manifest as intense scalp pruritus with scaling, edema, and crusting.[43]

EYELIDS

The eyelids are one of the most sensitive skin areas and are highly susceptible to irritants and allergens. This is likely a consequence of the thinness of the eyelid skin, as compared with other skin, and perhaps because the offending chemical may accumulate in eyelid folds. Transfer of small amounts of allergens used on the scalp, face, or hands can be enough to cause an eczematous reaction of the eyelids, while the primary sites of contact remain unaltered. Similarly, volatile agents may affect the eyelids first and exclusively, causing airborne eyelid contact dermatitis. Sources of contact dermatitis of the eyelids include cosmetics such as mascara, eyeliner and eye shadow, adhesive in fake eyelashes, and nickel and rubber in eyelash curlers. Furthermore, marked edema of the eyelids is often a feature of hair-dye dermatitis.[44] As mentioned earlier, eyelids are also known for being a typical site for "ectopic contact dermatitis" caused by ingredients found in nail lacquer, such as tosylamide formaldehyde resin, the chemical added to nail varnish to facilitate adhesion of the varnish to the nail and epoxy resin, also added to some nail polishes. Topical antibiotics (like bacitracin and neomycin) and certain metals (such as gold[45]) can also cause eyelid contact dermatitis. In fact, in the 2007 NACDG analysis of contact allergens associated with eyelid dermatitis,[46] gold was the most common allergen, accounting for isolated eyelid dermatitis. Notably, it has been observed that upon contact with hard particles such as titanium dioxide (used to opacify facial cosmetics, and in sunscreens as a physical blocker of ultraviolet light), gold found in jewelry may abrade, resulting in the release of gold particles that can then make contact with facial and eyelid skin, causing dermatitis.[47] Aside from gold, fragrances and preservatives are the main cosmetic allergens to cause isolated eyelid dermatitis.[48] ACD caused by allergens found in ophthalmic medicaments should also be considered. The most frequent allergens in ophthalmic preparations are the preservative phenylmercuric acetate and antibiotics.[49] Benzalkonium chloride is another preservative that is frequently used in ophthalmic preparations, and a potential irritant and allergen.[50]

LIPS

According to a NACDG study, approximately one-third of patients with isolated cheilitis—without other areas of dermatitis—are typically found to have an allergen as a contributing factor.[51,52] Allergic contact cheilitis has been reported to result from the use of a wide array of products, including cosmetics such as lip balms, lipsticks, lip glosses, moisturizers, sunscreens, nail products, and oral hygiene products (mouthwashes, toothpastes, dental floss; Fig. 24-3).[53-55] Allergic contact cheilitis has a marked female predominance, with most studies reporting a range of 70.7% to 90% female patients.[56] This is likely explained by the assumption that women wear more cosmetics and lip products than men. Most studies have reported fragrance allergens (such as fragrance mix and *Myroxylon*

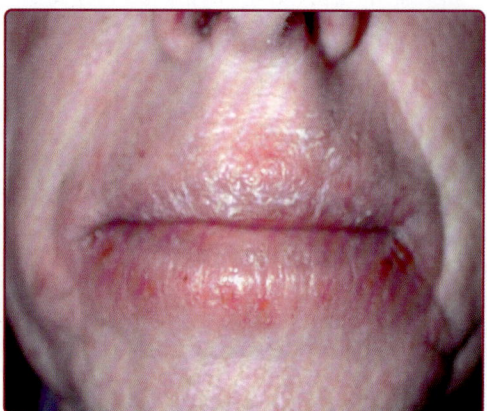

Figure 24-3 Allergic contact cheilitis. Fragrances and flavorings are among the most common causes of contact allergy in patch-tested patients with cheilitis.

pereirae [balsam of Peru]) as the most common cause of contact allergy in patch-tested patients with cheilitis.[57] Of note, some uncommonly reported allergens, namely, benzophenone-3 and gallates, may be relevant to a dermatitis localized to the lips. Benzophenone-3 (oxybenzone), a major constituent of many sunscreens, is also a common ingredient in many lip products and is increasingly reported as a culprit for allergic contact cheilitis.[58,59] Gallates are antioxidants used in waxy or oily products such as lip balms, lipsticks, and lip glosses.[60] Patch testing directly to the patient's lip cosmetics can be of particular usefulness in the evaluation of isolated cheilitis. It is also important to consider wind instruments as a cause of perioral ACD in musicians.

NECK

The neck is also a highly reactive site for ACD. Cosmetics applied to the face, scalp, or hair often initially affect the neck. Nail polish ingredients (tosylamide formaldehyde resin and epoxy resin) are common culprits in this region.[61] Furthermore, as a cultural practice, perfumes are typically sprayed on the neck. In a fragrance-sensitized individual, the practice of repeated application of fragrances to the anterior neck may result in the appearance of a dermatitic plaque on the neck, which has been coined the *atomizer sign*.[62] Also, in this topographic area, metal allergy can manifest as chronic eczematous dermatitis from exposure to necklaces and jewelry clasps that contain nickel and/or cobalt.

TORSO

The differential diagnosis of an eczematous dermatitis affecting the torso can be broad. There is a multitude of potentially allergenic chemical exposures to consider if the diagnosis of ACD is entertained. The torso is typically exposed to fragrances, preservatives, surfactants, and other chemicals daily with the use of personal care products. Textile-associated chemicals may also provide a source of sensitization and elicitation of ACD. The primary potential textile allergens are disperse dyes and formaldehyde textile resins. In the past, formaldehyde textile resins contained large amounts of free formaldehyde, which led to many cases of ACD to clothing in the 1950s and 1960s.

Today, most textile finishes use modified dimethyloldihydroxyethylene urea. Blended fabrics labeled "wrinkle resistant" or "permanent press" are most likely to contain formaldehyde textile resins. Recent studies suggest that the amount of free formaldehyde in most garments today is likely below the threshold for the elicitation of dermatitis for all but the most sensitive patients.[63]

AXILLAE

Textile-associated allergens are implicated in causing ACD of the axillae. Heat, humidity, and friction may contribute to the leaching of textile resins and dyes. The prototypical presentation is an eczematous dermatitis affecting the axillary folds with relative sparing of the axillary vault.[64] The axillary region is also uniquely exposed to deodorants and antiperspirants. These products may contain high concentrations of fragrances[65] in addition to preservatives (eg, formaldehyde releasers, parabens).

HANDS AND FEET

Hand dermatitis is common and accounts for up to 80% of occupational skin disease. Certain occupations are at an increased risk for hand dermatitis, including health care workers, food handlers, and hairdressers. Hand dermatitis is most often multifactorial (eg, irritant exposure, atopy, pompholyx or chronic vesicular hand eczema, psoriasis, dermatophyte infection) adding to the complexity of both diagnosing and treating these patients. Clinical clues to an underlying component of ACD include pruritus, vesicular dermatitis affecting the finger tips, and destabilization of chronic dermatitis. Destabilization of chronic dermatitis refers to a change in treatment response, symptoms, or extent of a preexisting chronic dermatitis, and is a clue to the development of ACD. Chronic hand dermatitis in and of itself is an indication for patch testing. Similarly, the evaluation of foot dermatitis should include patch testing. The most common class of allergens to cause ACD of the feet are rubber-related chemicals (such as mercaptobenzothiazole, carbamates, thiurams, black rubber mix, and mixed dialkyl thioureas). Other allergens that need to be considered are glues and adhesives such as *p*-tert-butylphenol formaldehyde resin and potassium dichromate found in tanned leather. Footwear, such as socks and shoes, may also serve to retain topical medicaments (antibiotics, corticosteroids, antifungals) used on the feet and provide continued skin exposure over time.

MUCOUS MEMBRANES

ACD of the oral mucosa may present with contact stomatitis from dental metals, and ACD of the perianal area may be caused by sensitizing chemicals in proctologic preparations such as benzocaine.

SCATTERED GENERALIZED DISTRIBUTION

Patients with dermatitis in a scattered generalized distribution (SGD) can present a difficult diagnostic and therapeutic challenge. SGD is defined as involvement of more than 3 body sites or involvement of 3 body sites if the sites are trunk, arms, and legs. Patch testing is often an important part of the workup in refractory cases of SGD dermatitis. In 2008, Zug and NACDG colleagues[66] examined the yield of patch testing as well as the relevant allergens in patients with SGD rashes referred for patch testing. Of 10,061 patients studied during a period of 4 years, 14.9% were categorized as SGD. Interestingly, a higher incidence of SGD was seen in males and patients with a history of atopic dermatitis. Of the patients presenting with SGD rashes, 49% had at least 1 relevant positive patch test reaction. Preservatives, fragrances, propylene glycol, cocamidopropyl betaine, ethyleneurea melamine formaldehyde, and corticosteroids were among the more frequently relevant positive allergens.

SYSTEMIC CONTACT DERMATITIS

Systemic exposure to an allergen in a sensitized patient with the subsequent development of a cutaneous delayed hypersensitivity reaction is termed *systemic contact dermatitis* (SCD).[67] Sensitization typically occurs with cutaneous exposure as with other forms of ACD. There are multiple routes of exposure for the elicitation of SCD—subcutaneous, intravenous, intramuscular, inhalation, and oral ingestion. By definition, there is no occurrence of topical skin contact to the allergen in SCD.

The clinical presentation of SCD can be complex with a high degree of variability. The simplest presentation seen is a localized recall reaction where the dermatitis occurs at the site of prior topical sensitization. The other end of the spectrum would be erythrodermic SCD. The term "baboon syndrome" was introduced in 1984 to describe a specific dermatologic response to a systemic contact allergen in which erythema of the buttocks and upper inner thighs was seen resembling the red rump of baboons.[68] Mercury, nickel, and ampicillin were the first described causative agents.[69] Over time use of the term *baboon syndrome* has broadened to include cases of drug-induced erythema of the buttocks and upper inner thighs in which previous cutaneous sensitization has not occurred. This is a deviation from the strict definition of SCD, and some have advocated for a change in nomenclature to *drug-related baboon syndrome* with or without previous cutaneous exposure to reflect the difference in pathogenic mechanisms.[69] Others have suggested the term *symmetrical drug-related intertriginous and flexural exanthema* as a more precise term which by definition denotes a specific cutaneous adverse drug reaction in which previous cutaneous sensitization is not a necessary condition. Table 24-2 shows the diagnostic criteria for symmetrical drug-related intertriginous and flexural exanthema.[69] The term *allergic contact dermatitis syndrome* has been proposed to encompass all cutaneous reactions that share the commonality of sensitization occurring through cutaneous exposure. These reactions can be further delineated based on the extent of dermatitis and route of exposure driving the elicitation phase (Table 24-3).[18] Table 24-4 lists some known oral or IV medications which may cause systemic reactivation of ACD in patients previously sensitized to related allergens by direct skin contact.[70-73]

A few specific examples of SCD are worth noting. Dietary nickel and balsam of Peru are associated with dyshidrosiform hand eczema.[74] The major constituents of balsam of Peru (cinnamic acid, cinnamyl cinnamate, benzyl benzoate, benzoic acid, benzyl alcohol, and esterified polymers of coniferyl alcohol) are naturally derived and have a significant number of natural cross-reactors. Tomatoes, citrus peel/zest, chocolate, ice cream, wine, beer, dark-colored sodas, and spices such as cinnamon, cloves, curry, and vanilla are potential cross-reactors with balsam of Peru.[75] Consumption of these foods may result in a systemic reactivation of ACD in some patients allergic to balsam of Peru. Salam and Fowler drew attention to the potential for dietary triggers to induce SCD in patients sensitive to balsam of Peru. In their study, almost half of the participants with a positive patch test to balsam of Peru noted clinical improvement in their dermatitis on a balsam of Peru elimination diet.

TABLE 24-2
Diagnostic Criteria for SDRIFE

1. Exposure to a systemically administered drug either at the first or repeated dose.
2. Sharply demarcated erythema of the gluteal/perianal area and/or V-shaped erythema of the inguinal/perigenital area.
3. Involvement of at least one other intertriginous/flexural localization.
4. Symmetry of affected areas.
5. Absence of systemic signs or symptoms.

SDRIFE, symmetrical drug-related intertriginous and flexural exanthema. From Hausermann P, Harr TH, Bircher AJ. Baboon syndrome resulting from systemic drugs: is there strife between SDRIFE and allergic contact dermatitis syndrome? *Contact Dermatitis* 2004;51:297-310, with permission. Copyright © 2004 John Wiley & Sons.

TABLE 24-3
Allergic Contact Dermatitis Syndrome

Stage 1: Localized allergic contact dermatitis
Stage 2: Regional dissemination of allergic contact dermatitis
Stage 3A: Generalized or distant involvement of allergic contact dermatitis
Stage 3B: Systemic exposure resulting in systemic contact dermatitis

Data from Lachapelle JM. The spectrum of diseases for which patch testing is recommended. Patients who should be investigated. In: Lachapelle JM, Maibach HI, eds. *Patch Testing/Prick Testing. A Practical Guide*. Berlin, Germany: Springer Verlag; 2003:11.

TABLE 24-4
Systemic Drugs That Can Cause Systemic Reactivation of Allergic Contact Dermatitis

CONTACT ALLERGEN[a]	RELATED DRUG WITH POTENTIAL TO CAUSE SYSTEMIC REACTIVATION OF ALLERGIC CONTACT DERMATITIS
Ethylenediamine dihydrochloride (stabilizer infrequently found in skin care products)	Aminophylline Piperazine antihistamines: hydroxyzine, cetirizine, levocetirizine and meclizine
Thiuram (rubber antioxidant)	Tetraethyl thiuram disulfide (generic name: disulfiram)
Thimerosal (mercury-derived preservative)	Piroxicam

[a]To which a patient had previously become sensitized by direct, topical application of the contact allergen to the skin.

ALLERGEN-SPECIFIC APPROACH

Optimal management of ACD requires knowledge of specific allergens, their sources, and the mechanisms by which individuals are exposed to the allergens. What follows are brief descriptions of the most commonly positive and important patch test allergens in North America.

METALS

Metals are a common cause of ACD. Nickel is the most frequently patch test-positive allergen worldwide, with sensitization rates that hover mostly in the range of 18% to 30%.[76]

Nickel: Nickel is an ubiquitous metal found in a variety of objects that get in contact with the skin, including costume jewelry, suspenders, zippers, button snaps, belt buckles, eyeglasses frames, cell phones, nickel-containing coins, and keys.[77] High rates of sensitization to nickel have been ascribed in women to ear piercing at an early age and in both men and women to the rising trend in piercings of other body parts.[77] Classic nickel dermatitis presents as an eruption on the earlobes, the neckline, the wrist, or the periumbilical area, which are commonly exposed to nickel-containing jewelry and to button snaps, zippers, and belt buckles. Facial dermatitis caused by nickel has also been reported to musical instruments and to cell phones.[37]

Nickel and other metals in implantable medical devices are implicated as a source of sensitization and cause of complications from local and systemic inflammation resulting from such allergy in metal-sensitive individuals. While fully confirmed cases of joint replacement failure associated with nickel or other metal sensitivity are rare, and arthroplasty prostheses uncommonly cause problems in nickel-sensitive patients, the true relevance of metal allergy in the failure of metal orthopedic implants and cardiovascular devices has yet to be fully elucidated.[78] Existing publications have largely been retrospective and can thus only suggest a possible association of metal allergy with implant failure rather than determine causation.[79] Moreover, eczematous reactions related temporally to joint replacements, stents, pacemakers, or other implants continue to be reported, albeit infrequently. With sustained use of metal implants as medical devices, we are likely to see a rise in cases referred for patch testing to help adjudicate the relevance of metal allergy. Preoperatively, patch testing may guide the choice of implants based on allergy to ingredients; postoperatively, it may help diagnose the cause of complications.[80]

To prevent development of nickel sensitivity, the European Union, in 1994, regulated the amount of nickel that may be released from objects with direct and prolonged skin contact to ≤0.5 μg nickel/cm^2/week; in 2014 this restriction was strengthened to ≤0.2 μg nickel/cm^2/week for items inserted as pierced body parts. Among Danish women, the prevalence of nickel allergy decreased from 28% in 1985 to 17% in 2007.[81] The American Academy of Dermatology and the American Contact Dermatitis Society favor enacting similar legislation in the United States.

Spot tests containing dimethylgloxime are available commercially to detect the presence of nickel, with nickel concentrations >1:10,000 (or >0.44 μg/cm^2) producing a pink precipitate on a white cotton swab and the intensity of this color read-out increasing with nickel concentration.

Cobalt: Cobalt is often added to other metals to increase the overall strength of an alloy. Cobalt is a common contaminant in nickel ores and thus frequently found in nickel compounds.[82] As with nickel, most sensitization exposures result from contact with jewelry, clothing snaps, buckles, coins, keys, and other metal objects. Like nickel, cobalt can be found in prosthetic joint replacements and dental alloys. Cobalt is also often used in ceramics, paints, and tattoos to impart a blue color. On jewelry, this blue color confers a darker appearance to alloys containing cobalt.[83] Cobalt is an ingredient of multivitamins containing vitamin B_{12} or cyanocobalamine.[84]

Cobalt often produces a pseudopurpuric appearance on patch testing in the absence of erythema or edema. This is not a positive patch test reaction, but rather an irritant effect from deposition of cobalt within eccrine glands.[78] Concomitant patch test positivity to nickel and cobalt is a common occurrence, most likely from cosensitization to both allergens. Avoidance of nickel-plated objects is a practical way of managing ACD to cobalt.

Similar to the dimethylgloxime test for nickel, a spot test using 2-nitroso-1-naphthol-4-sulfonic acid was created to detect cobalt. In contrast to the pink readout from the dimethylgloxime test for nickel, the spot test for cobalt yields a yellow-orange color in the presence of cobalt.[83]

Other Metals: Chromium (potassium chromate in patch tests) has been long-considered the classic marker for allergy to leather goods and to wet cement. However, cobalt is also a relevant marker for allergy to both leather and cement.[83] Gold is a controversial allergen as it can often give produce a positive patch test but fail to meet standards for relevance. Conversely, gold frequently manifests extremely delayed hypersensitivity that runs the risk of being interpreted as negative in patch tests that are only read less than 96 hours after application.

PRESERVATIVES

Preservative allergens include formaldehyde (and its releasers) as well as non-formaldehyde-releasing preservatives.

Formaldehyde and Formaldehyde Releasers: Formaldehyde is a colorless gas with preservative and disinfectant properties. Even though formaldehyde and formaldehyde-like agents have a broad range of uses as glues, biocides, and photographic developing agents, these chemicals are now rarely used in personal care products because of their potent sensitization capacity.[85] Instead manufacturers have replaced formaldehyde with other preservatives to prolong the microbe-free shelf life of their products. These substitutes for formaldehyde can be sorted into agents that can release formaldehyde (formaldehyde releasers) and those that do not. Formaldehyde-releasing preservatives include 2-bromo-2-nitropropane-1,3-diol (bronopol), diazolidinyl urea (Germall II), DMDM hydantoin (Glydant), imidazolidinyl urea (Germall I), quaternium-15, and tris-nitromethane (Tris Nitro).[86] Of these preservatives, quaternium-15 is the most common cosmetic allergen.[87-89]

Note that formaldehyde-containing resins are linked to 2 other forms of ACD. The first form involves the glues, toluene sulfonamide formaldehyde resin or tosylamide (used in artificial nails) and *p*-tert butylphenol formaldehyde resin (used in shoes and other garments). The second form involves use of formaldehyde derivatives to make wrinkle-free or permanent-press fabrics and clothing.

Nonreleasers of Formaldehyde: The 2 major preservatives in this category are methyldibromoglutaronitrile/phenoxyethanol (MDGN/PE) also known as *Euxyl K400* and methylchloroisothiazolinone/methylisothiazolinone (MCI/MI) also known as *Kathon CG*. Because of their high propensity for causing ACD, both of these preservatives have been banned from use in cosmetics in Europe.[90] However cosmetics produced outside the European Union and toiletries sold elsewhere may contain them. Most allergic reactions to these preservatives originate from personal care products such as creams, lotions, wet wipes, liquid soaps, and medicated tissue and toilet paper containing the allergens. Also note that, because of peculiarities related to concentrations of allergens, optimal testing may require assaying both the combined allergen pairs (*Euxyl K400* and *Kathon CG*) as well as their individual components (MDGN or PE; MCI or MI), as patch tests to only the former can miss reactions to specific allergens.

FRAGRANCES

Fragrances are aromatic compounds that impart a scent. Fragrances can be natural (from botanical or animal products) or synthetic in origin. Up to 4% of the general population are allergic to fragrances,[91,92] making these chemicals among the top causes of ACD to personal care products, with typical sites of involvement including the face and hands, behind the ears, and the neck and axillae, yielding a scattered but generalized distribution of eczematous dermatitis.[93,94] Among the main substances used by most patch test groups for screening are *M. pereirae*, *fragrance mix I* (mixture of 8 fragrance allergens), and *fragrance mix II* (6 additional allergens).[95] It is estimated that *M. pereirae* can identify up to 50% of fragrance-allergic individuals.[96] Fragrance allergens are found in many cosmetics, perfumes, pharmaceutical preparations, toothpastes, and mouthwashes, as well as in scents and flavorings for foods and drinks. Fragrance allergens can be included in skin-care products without being labeled as fragrances if they are not used primarily as fragrances but as neutralizers of unwanted scents within the merchandise.[95]

TOPICAL ANTIBIOTICS

Although there are several topical antibiotics, the 2 most commonly implicated in ACD are neomycin and bacitracin.

Neomycin: Neomycin is a member of the aminoglycoside family of antibiotics commonly used in topical formulations to prevent and treat skin, ear, and eye infections. At least 1% of the general population is allergic to neomycin, with sensitization rates as high as 10% in North America.[97] This latter high rate is most likely a result of the presence of neomycin in numerous over-the-counter preparations, especially in combination with polymyxin and bacitracin as a "triple antibiotic" cream or ointment.[98] Patients at higher risk include those with stasis dermatitis and leg ulcers, anogenital dermatitis, and otitis externa. Because antibiotic preparations are applied to already damaged skin, ACD to neomycin is not always easily recognized as it often presents as persistence or worsening of a preexisting dermatitis.[99] It may also mimic cellulitis, for which the clue for ACD is itching rather than pain. Occupational dermatitis involving the hands can occur in nurses, physicians, pharmacists, dentists, and veterinarians.[100]

Bacitracin: Like neomycin, bacitracin is a topical antibiotic frequently used for postoperative and general wound care by both the medical profession and the general public as it is readily available in over-the-counter preparations. Not only can bacitracin cause ACD, but it has been reported in association with urticarial reactions and even, rarely, anaphylaxis.[101] Despite its high prevalence as an allergen, bacitracin is not included in the currently available T.R.U.E. (thin-layer rapid-use epicutaneous) test series. Interestingly, many patients show simultaneous sensitivity to bacitracin and neomycin, although the 2 substances are not chemically related, thereby indicating cosensitization (rather than coreactivity) to both substances.[102]

PARA-PHENYLENEDIAMINE

PPD is an oxidizing agent used as a permanent hair dye. Both consumers and hairdressers are at risk for sensitization. Interestingly, ACD to PPD often spares the scalp, while presenting as dermatitis on thinner skin of the face, eyelids, and neck.[103] Once oxidized, PPD is no longer allergenic, so that dyed hair itself does not pose further risk of allergic stimulation. This is in contrast to permed or waved hair, in which the allergen, GMT, persists in its ability to cause ACD in a sensitized individual long after the allergen has been exposed to the air (eg, from contaminated sites in a hair salon). Table 24-5 lists other allergens commonly associated with hair care. PPD can cross-react with other *para*-amino–group chemicals such as *para*-aminobenzoic acid, sulfonylureas, hydrochlorothiazide, benzocaine, procainamide, and certain azo and aniline dyes.[104,105] Additionally, PPD has gained notoriety as an adulterant added to natural henna for temporary tattoos; it darkens the henna tattoo.[106,107]

RUBBER

Rubber allergens can be classified into chemicals associated with processing of natural latex derived from the proteinaceous sap of the rubber tree (*Hevea brasiliensis*) and synthetic rubber that is unrelated to latex. Latex is a common cause of immediate-type hypersensitivity mediated by latex protein-specific immunoglobulin E. Rarely, latex itself can also cause ACD, but it is the accelerator and vulcanizing chemicals (carbamates, mercaptobenzothiazole, thiuram) and dyes (PPD) used to convert latex into commercial products (gloves, condoms, automobile tires) that are the principal causes of ACD to rubber. From a general perspective, individuals allergic to either the rubber accelerator/vulcanizer chemicals (or to latex itself) can safely use Vicryl gloves, which are safer than nitrile gloves (in lieu of latex gloves). From an epidemiologic perspective, ACD to synthetic rubber is a lesser but growing problem, with these new forms of rubber (dialkyl thioureas, neoprene, polyurethane) being incorporated into athletic clothing and equipment as well as daily wear.

TOPICAL STEROIDS

ACD to topical steroids is uncommon but important to consider, especially in patients whose dermatitis is unimproved or worsens despite treatment with topical steroids. On the other hand, allergy to a steroid-containing preparation is frequently due to components other than the steroid (eg, propylene glycol or preservatives). In the absence of real evidence from patch testing, desoximethasone ointment is the safest topical steroid from an allergic standpoint. The currently available T.R.U.E. Test series includes 3 markers for topical steroid allergy, namely tixocortol pivalate, budesonide, and hydrocortisone-17-butyrate. Table 24-6 lists the 5 classes of steroids based on chemical structure, the patch test allergen marker for each class, and cross reactions. The least-allergenic steroids belong to class C, as exemplified by desoximethasone.

PATCH-TESTING MECHANICS

ALLERGEN SELECTION AND PLACEMENT

Patch testing remains the gold standard for identification of the allergen or allergens causing ACD. The T.R.U.E. Test (SmartPractice, Hillerod Denmark) was introduced in 1995 and is an epicutaneous patch test system that is approved by the U.S. Food and Drug Administration for use in the diagnosis of ACD in persons 18 years of age and older. The T.R.U.E. test originally contained 23 allergens and 1 control; today, it consists of 3 panels with a total of 35 allergens plus 1 blank control. Expanded patch testing with other commercially available allergens, patch testing with patient items, and patch testing in pediatric patients remains off-label but is considered standard practice in the diagnosis of ACD. Among the 30 most frequently positive allergens found by the NACDG the T.R.U.E. test is missing the following 9 allergens: fragrance mix II, lanolin, iodopropynyl butylcarbamate, cinnamal, carmine, propylene glycol, oleamidopropyl betaine, 2-hydroxyethyl methacrylate, compositae, propolis.[76] It is challenging to quantify the sensitivity of the T.R.U.E. test system, but there is consensus that patch testing with a greater number of allergens increases the sensitivity.[108-112] A previous study noted that less than one-third of patch test patients would have all their allergens completely identified if only a standard series of 28 allergens was used,[113] thus highlighting the need for expanded patch testing in many patients.

Patch testing with the T.R.U.E. test, commercially available standardized allergens, or a patient's personal care products generally follows a standard closed-test protocol. With this protocol the allergens are placed on the back under occlusion, removed at 48 hours, and a final delayed read is performed at 72 or 96 hours. Many patch testers will perform a preliminary or early read at the 48-hour visit, but it is important to allow time after patch test removal for tape irritation to subside prior to performing a read. An interval of 20 minutes is usually sufficient. Certain situations call for an extended reading time up to 7 to 10 days out. Metals, antibiotics, and corticosteroids are notable allergens which may produce a delayed reaction. This protocol differs from the repeat open application test or use test in which a substance is applied to the cubital fossa twice a day for 1 to 3 weeks to simu-

TABLE 24-5
Hair Product Allergens

Hair dyes	*p*-Phenylenediamine
	p-Toluenediamine sulfate
	Azo dyes
Bleaching agents	Ammonium persulfate
Waving agents	Glyceryl thioglycolate
Relaxer/Straightening agents	Sodium hydroxide
Shampoos and conditioners	Fragrances
	Preservatives

TABLE 24-6 Steroid Allergens

STRUCTURAL CLASS	PATCH-TEST ALLERGEN	CROSS-REACTIONS	MEMBERS
A	Tixocortol-21-pivalate	D2	Hydrocortisone valerate Cloprednol Fludrocortisone Prednisone
B	Budesonide	D2 (budesonide specifically)	Triamcinolone Amcinonide Desonide Fluocinolone Halcinonide Procinonide
C	—	—	Desoximethasone Betamethasone Clocortolone Dexamethasone Fluocortolone pivalate Rimexolone
D1	Clobetasol	? D2	Clobetasol Alclometasone Betamethasone valerate Diflorasone Fluocortolone hexanoate Mometasone
D2	Hydrocortisone-17-butyrate	A & budesonide	Hydrocortisone-17-butyrate Prednicarbate

late real life use. The repeat open application test can be useful for testing leave-on personal care products. A semiopen patch test protocol can be useful if testing to liquid products with irritant potential. Here the test substance or dilutions of the test substance are applied to the skin surface covering a 1 cm² area. The liquid is allowed to evaporate and dry. Excess material can be removed with a cotton swab. The completely dry skin is then covered with hypoallergenic tape and readings are performed at standard time intervals as noted above.

GRADING AND INTERPRETING RESULTS

At each test reading, it is traditional to note the results as positive, negative, questionable, or irritant. Positive results are also given a grade based on the strength of the reaction. The International Contact Dermatitis Research Group recommends using the grading scale for positive patch test reactions outlined by Wilkinson and colleagues,[114] which is a + to +++ scoring system, where + represents a weak nonvesicular reaction but with palpable erythema, ++ represents a strong (edematous or vesicular) reaction, and +++ represents an extreme (bullous or ulcerative) reaction (Fig. 24-4). Very weak or questionable reactions where there is only faint or macular (nonpalpable) erythema are recorded by a question mark (which is +/− in the Wilkinson system), and irritant reactions are recorded as "IR." Irritant patch test reactions have varied findings that are related to the nature and the concentration of the irritant[115] and are classically described as (a) erythematous reactions limited to the site of application of the chemical, with sharp, well-delineated margins; discretely scaly (may look "chapped") and usually not edematous. Among the patch test allergens, fragrance mix, cocamidopropyl betaine, iodopropynyl butylcarbamate, glutaraldehyde, and thiuram

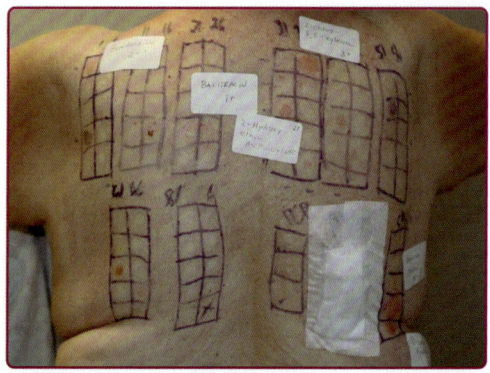

Figure 24-4 Patch-test grading. This patient had multiple relevant positive patch tests. Bacitracin, chloroxylenol, and 2-hydroxyethyl methacrylate are relevant to this patient's severe dermatitis, but are not allergens on the currently available commercial screening series.

mix are identified as the most common allergens to produce such marginal irritant reactions. (b) Purpuric reactions with petechial hemorrhage, which are seen in approximately 5% of patients tested to cobalt chloride. This is sometimes referred as *punctate purpura of cobalt* and should always be interpreted as an irritant reaction. Pustular reactions indicate an irritant reaction and are most commonly encountered with metallic salts such as potassium dichromate, cobalt, nickel, gold, and copper. Individuals with an atopic diathesis may show pustular irritant reactions more frequently. Other allergens in which marginal reactions should be interpreted with caution given their mild irritant potential include the preservatives formaldehyde, benzalkonium chloride, and iodopropynyl butylcarbamate; the rubber allergen carba mix, fragrance chemicals such as fragrance mix I and propolis (bee glue); the foaming agent cocamidopropyl betaine; and the emulsifiers oleamidopropyl dimethylamine and triethanolamine. It is important to mention that even paying close attention to the aforementioned morphologic features, irritant reactions are still difficult to interpret, and the morphology of the patch test response can still be a confusing guide to whether the response is allergic or irritant. When morphology is not enough, it is advisable to keep in mind that in general when the patch test reaction is sufficiently strong, an irritant reaction will be early appearing (during the first reading), and promptly resolving (often times the reaction is not as strong or sometimes not even present during the second reading). In contrast, a strong allergic reaction usually spreads, is more slowly disappearing, and is more clearly eczematous. The irritant pattern is often described as *decrescendo*, while the allergic pattern is *crescendo*.

Of note, the evaluation of positive reactions may be slightly more difficult in darker skin types (Fitzpatrick types V and VI), as erythema may not be as obvious, posing the risk of overlooking a mild positive allergic reaction. However, the edema and papules/vesicles are usually obvious and palpable; consequently, palpation of the patch test site can help detect allergic reactions in patients with darker skin types. Additionally, the darker the skin type, the more difficult it is to mark the patch test site after removal. For very dark skin, a florescent marking ink is probably best (such as a yellow highlighter), and the markings can subsequently be located by a Wood light in a darkened room at the time of patch test reading.[116]

ASSIGNING CLINICAL RELEVANCE

A positive patch test indicates a state of cutaneous sensitization to a particular allergen but does not equate to the diagnosis of ACD. A good example of this point is thimerosal. This mercuric preservative is unique in the sense that it commonly causes positive patch test reactions but very seldom does thimerosal allergy account for the patient's dermatitis. Most allergic patients presumably have been sensitized to the thimerosal present in vaccines, but have no clinical disease associated with this allergen.[117] Establishing the relevance of a positive patch test result is a critical and challenging part of patch testing. Often preliminary relevance is assigned at the time of the final patch test reading with final relevance given *retrospectively* at a later followup visit when the dermatitis has cleared after avoidance measures were implemented. Relevance is deemed to be definitive if a use test with a suspected item is positive or a patch test of a suspected object or product is positive. Current relevance is possible if the allergen is among the chemicals a patient is exposed to and can be upgraded to probable if the distribution of the dermatitis is consistent with exposure to that particular allergen. Past relevance is designated if there is a history of dermatitis in association with previous exposure to the particular allergen but to which the patient is no longer exposed. An example is a patient who is patch test-positive to neomycin who reports a rash with prior use of over-the-counter antibiotic ointments but has had no further difficulties following avoidance of products containing neomycin. Doubtful relevance is designated when there is no identifiable exposure source or if the clinical history and presentation do not fit with exposure to a particular allergen.

COMPLICATIONS OF PATCH TESTING

Patch testing is considered a safe diagnostic procedure and unwanted effects are seldom encountered. The most common side effects are expected, such as itching at the site of a positive test reaction, and irritation or pruritus from tape application. Less commonly described effects include postinflammatory pigmentary changes, infections, scarring, persistent patch test reactions, induction of flares of dermatitis, sensitization to the tested allergen, and, rarely, anaphylaxis.[118] Postinflammatory hypopigmentation or hyperpigmentation can occur, with hyperpigmentation being more likely in darkly pigmented persons; it typically fades with time and the use of topical corticosteroids. Exposure to sunlight or artificial ultraviolet light immediately following removal of patch tests, especially to fragrance materials, can lead to hyperpigmentation of the patch test site in relation to allergen-related photosensitivity. Infection is typically mild impetiginization of the patch test site with *Staphylococcus aureus*, although other infections can occur. Scarring is most likely when patients develop bullous reactions; patients who are prone to keloids can develop keloids at these sites. Patch test reactions that persist for more than 1 month (>30 days) are considered persistent patch test reactions; this occurs most commonly from gold salts in a gold-sensitive patient (Fig. 24-5). Induction

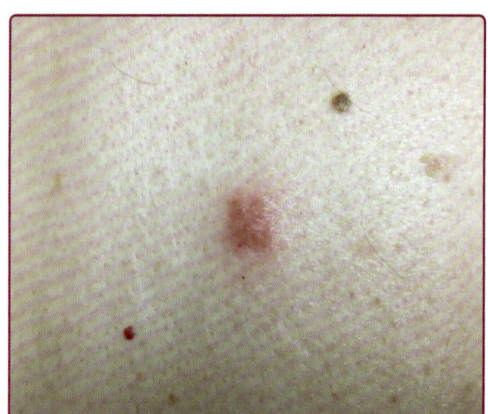

Figure 24-5 Persistent patch test reaction to gold. This patient demonstrated sensitivity to gold during patch testing, and presented back to the clinic 3 months later stating that the patch test reaction had not resolved. The patient was treated with intralesional triamcinolone.

of a dermatitis flareup at the original site of an existing or preexisting dermatitis (that was caused by the positive patch test allergen) can also occur. This can be minimized by testing patients free of any current active dermatitis, if possible. Also, a positive patch test reaction in a patient who has active psoriasis or lichen planus may reproduce these dermatoses at the patch test sites (as a *Koebner phenomenon*), during the weeks following patch testing.[119] Although the risk of active sensitization during patch testing is low, it is most common to strong sensitizers, such as PPD. It typically presents as a "new reaction" noticed by the patient 10 to 21 days after patch testing, when initial patch test readings are negative at 48- and 96-hour readings.[118,120] Sometimes this can be difficult to distinguish from a delayed reaction (such as with gold or topical steroids). Anaphylaxis is an exceedingly rare side effect of patch testing that may occur with allergens known to cause a type I (immediate) hypersensitivity reaction, such as bacitracin, neomycin, ammonium persulfate (most often reported), latex, formaldehyde, and penicillin.[118]

COMPLICATIONS FROM FAILURE TO PATCH TEST

The greatest hazard is failure to patch test appropriate patients with dermatitis. Such omission potentially dooms the patient to repeated episodes of avoidable contact dermatitis. In 2004, the American Academy of Dermatology and the Society of Investigative Dermatology studied the burden of skin disease and estimated that 72 million people in the United States suffer from ACD.[121] It is the third most common reason for patients to seek consultation with a dermatologist, accounting for 9.2 million visits in 2004 alone. Likewise, in that same year, primary care physicians received 5 million visits for unexplained dermatitis or eczema.[122] Although many of these patients will respond readily to standard treatments, others will demonstrate recalcitrant eczema. It has been estimated that approximately 16% of all chronic eczema patients would benefit from patch testing,[123] and clinical experience suggests this number may be much larger. Based on the figures above, it could be estimated that approximately 2.2 million patients each year in the United States would benefit from patch testing.

PATCH TESTING AND SYSTEMIC IMMUNOSUPPRESSIVE AGENTS

Because systemic drugs that suppress T-cell responses will suppress patch test responses, it is ideal for patch testing to be performed on patients who are not under the influence of these medications (like prednisone and cyclosporine). However, there may be circumstances when it is not possible to stop the immunosuppressive drug. In such cases, the next best option is to reduce the dose of the potentially confounding medication to a minimum to avoid false-negative patch test results.

DIFFERENTIAL DIAGNOSIS

The differential diagnosis of ACD includes a wide range of inflammatory skin disorders (Table 24-7).[124,125]

CLINICAL COURSE AND PROGNOSIS

It is difficult to assess the actual prognosis of ACD because there is no standardized instrument for such evaluation. The disruption of work, ability to return to work, and improvement of dermatitis with time are among outcome measures that have been studied in patients with ACD. Newer study designs have aimed to capture the increasingly important outcome measure of health-related quality of life.[126] When different quality-of-life assessment tools have been applied to populations of patients with ACD, it has been demonstrated that ACD negatively impacts quality of life significantly. Holness and colleagues[127] found that pain, itching, embarrassment, work interference, and sleep difficulties were the most significant effects in quality of life of their patch test population. Kadyk and colleagues[128] found the greatest impact on emotions, followed by symptoms, functioning, and occupational impact. Similarly, Woo and colleagues[129] reported that patients with the final diagnosis of ACD had a mean baseline quality of life equal to that of patients

TABLE 24-7
Differential Diagnosis of Allergic Contact Dermatitis

DIAGNOSIS	DIAGNOSTIC CLUES
Irritant contact dermatitis (ICD)	Physical findings can be indistinguishable clinically; in general, there is an absence of vesiculation (only very strong irritants produce vesicles) and burning exceeds itching. Does not spread beyond the area of contact with continued exposure.
Atopic dermatitis	Distribution of skin findings can be helpful; atopic patients can and do develop contact allergies. Worsening disease can indicate new contact allergy development.
Nummular dermatitis (ND)	Widespread ACD can assume this pattern in certain patients; nonetheless, the classical morphology of coin-shaped, well-demarcated plaques on the legs, dorsal hands, and extensor surfaces favors ND.
Seborrheic dermatitis	Greasy and scaly papulosquamous plaques usually located in the hair-bearing regions, glabella, and nasolabial folds.
Asteatotic eczema	Parchment-like patches with no edema or vesiculation on the lower legs. May have appearance of dry river bed.
Stasis dermatitis	Papulosquamous plaques with dyschromia located on the shins and medial surfaces of the lower legs, with presence of concomitant varicosities.
Pompholyx and/or dyshidrotic eczema psoriasis	Deep-seated vesicles on palms, soles, sides of the fingers, and volar edges. When it presents in its classic form, diagnosis can be straightforward, however, when the lesions are few and limited to the hands and/or feet differentiation can be more difficult. Classical location and predominance in areas of trauma (Koebnerization) can be helpful as well as the presence (if any) of concomitant arthritis.
Mycosis fungoides (MF) (patch/plaque stage cutaneous T-cell lymphoma)	The well-demarcated, atrophic, poikilodermatous, scaly patches and plaques of MF are usually found in non–sun-exposed areas of the skin, such as the trunk, breasts, hips, and buttocks (bathing suit distribution).

experiencing hair loss and psoriasis. Zug and colleagues[130] found that patients referred for patch testing were severely affected by frustration, reported feeling annoyed, and had a great concern about the persistence of their skin problem. Notably, hand involvement is strongly predictive of a negative impact on quality of life. Similarly, the extent of the disease[131] and the duration of symptoms before diagnosis are both correlated with a poor prognosis and recalcitrant disease.[132] Some studies, however, have associated increased patient knowledge with an improved prognosis.[133,134] Much of this information is extrapolated from data regarding occupational contact dermatitis.

MANAGEMENT

Identification of the offending allergen and its avoidance are the goals of diagnosis and treatment of ACD.[135] These goals can be achieved by a thorough history and physical examination that lead to patch testing of the appropriate allergens, relevant counseling tailored to the individual patient's circumstances, and effort by the patient to avoid the causative agent(s). Currently, there are 2 databases that can help patients avoid their allergens by providing lists of alternative products; these are the Contact Allergen Management Program (CAMP)[136] and the Contact Allergen Replacement Database (CARD).[137]

For a localized acute flare of ACD resulting from unintentional or inadvertent allergen exposure, topical corticosteroids are the first-line treatment and are typically required for 2 to 3 weeks of use to prevent rebound. In cases of severe or widespread eruptions, a 3-week taper of oral prednisone is usually needed; the typical oral-dosing regimen is 1 mg/kg/day for 1 week, followed by tapering weekly, for a total of 3 to 4 weeks.

ACKNOWLEDGMENTS

We thank the prior authors, Mari Paz Castanedo-Tardan, MD, and Kathryn A. Zug, MD, for providing us the framework for revising and updating this chapter.

REFERENCES

1. Mark BJ, Slavin RG. Allergic contact dermatitis. *Med Clin North Am*. 2006;90(1):169-185.
2. Cohen D, Moore M. Occupational skin disease. In: Rom WM, Markowitz S, eds. *Environmental and Occupational Medicine*. 4th ed. Philadelphia, PA: Lippincott-Williams & Wilkins; 2007:617.
3. Rajagopalan R, Anderson R. Impact of patch testing on dermatology-specific quality of life in patients with allergic contact dermatitis. *Am J Contact Dermat*. 1997;8(4):215-221.
4. Thyssen JP, Linneberg A, Menné T, et al. The epidemiology of contact allergy in the general population–prevalence and main findings. *Contact Dermatitis*. 2007;57(5):287-299.
5. Mirshahpanah P, Maibach HI. Relationship of patch test positivity in a general versus an eczema population. *Contact Dermatitis*. 2007;56(3):125-130.
6. Schnuch A, Uter W, Geier J, et al. Epidemiology of contact allergy: an estimation of morbidity employing the clinical epidemiology and drug-utilization research (CE-DUR) approach. *Contact Dermatitis*. 2002;47(1):32-39.

7. Uter W, Gefeller O, Giménez-Arnau A, et al. Characteristics of patients patch tested in the European Surveillance System on Contact Allergies (ESSCA) network, 2009-2012. *Contact Dermatitis*. 2015;73(2):82-90.
8. Fernandez Vozmediano JM, Armario Hita JC. Allergic contact dermatitis in children. *J Eur Acad Dermatol Venereol*. 2005;19(1):42-46.
9. Zug KA, McGinley-Smith D, Warshaw EM, et al. Contact allergy in children referred for patch testing: North American Contact Dermatitis Group data, 2001-2004. *Arch Dermatol*. 2008;144(10):1329-1336.
10. Schäfer T, Böhler E, Ruhdorfer S, et al. Epidemiology of contact allergy in adults. *Allergy*. 2001;56(12):1192-1196.
11. Thyssen JP, Engkilde K, Lundov MD, et al. Temporal trends of preservative allergy in Denmark (1985-2008). *Contact Dermatitis*. 2010;62(2):102-108.
12. Jordan WP, King SE. The development of allergic contact dermatitis in females during the comparison of two predictive patch tests. *Contact Dermatitis*. 1977;3(1):19-26.
13. Larsson-Stymne B, Widström L. Ear piercing—a cause of nickel allergy in schoolgirls? *Contact Dermatitis*. 1985;13(5):289-293.
14. Dotterud LK, Falk ES. Metal allergy in north Norwegian schoolchildren and its relationship with ear piercing and atopy. *Contact Dermatitis*. 1994;31(5):308-313.
15. Mattila L, Kilpelainen M, Terho EO, et al. Prevalence of nickel allergy among Finnish university students in 1995. *Contact Dermatitis*. 2001;44(4):218-223.
16. Jensen CS, Lisby S, Baadsgaard O, et al. Decrease in nickel sensitization in a Danish schoolgirl population with ears pierced after implementation of a nickel-exposure regulation. *Br J Dermatol*. 2002;146(4):636-642.
17. Dotterud LK, Smith-Sivertsen T. Allergic contact sensitization in the general adult population: a population-based study from Northern Norway. *Contact Dermatitis*. 2007;56(1):10-15.
18. Lachapelle J-M, Maibach HI. *Patch Testing and Prick Testing*. Springer Science + Business Media; 2003.
19. Bonamonte D, Foti C, Vestita M, et al. Noneczematous contact dermatitis. *ISRN Allergy*. 2013;2013:361746.
20. De Groot AC. Allergic contact dermatitis. In: Marks R, ed. *Eczema*. London, UK: Martin Dunitz; 1992:104.
21. Mozzanica N. Pathogenetic aspects of allergic and irritant contact dermatitis. *Clin Dermatol*. 1992;10(2):115-121.
22. Mowad CM, Anderson B, Scheinman P, et al. Allergic contact dermatitis: patient diagnosis and evaluation. *J Am Acad Dermatol*. 2016;74(6):1029-1040.
23. Riemann H, Schwarz T, Grabbe S. Pathomechanisms of the elicitation phase of allergic contact dermatitis [in German]. *J Dtsch Dermatol Ges*. 2003;1(8):613-619.
24. Janeway CE, Travers P, Walport M, et al. *Immunobiology: The Immune System in Health and Disease*. 6th ed. New York, NY: Garland Science Publishing; 2005.
25. Saint-Mezard P, Krasteva M, Berard F, et al. Allergic contact dermatitis. In: Bos JD, ed, *Cutaneous Immunology and Clinical Immunodermatology*. 3rd ed. Informa UK Limited; 2004:593-613.
26. Veien NK. Ingested food in systemic allergic contact dermatitis. *Clin Dermatol*. 1997;15(4):547-555.
27. Bennett CL, van Rijn E, Jung S, et al. Inducible ablation of mouse Langerhans cells diminishes but fails to abrogate contact hypersensitivity. *J Cell Biol*. 2005;169(4):569-576.
28. Honda T, Kabashima K. Novel concept of iSALT (inducible skin-associated lymphoid tissue) in the elicitation of allergic contact dermatitis. *Proc Jpn Acad Ser B Phys Biol Sci*. 2016;92(1):20-28.
29. Wang L, Bursch LS, Kissenpfennig A, et al. Langerin expressing cells promote skin immune responses under defined conditions. *J Immunol*. 2008;180(7):4722-4727.
30. Streilein JW. Skin-associated lymphoid tissues (SALT): origins and functions. *J Invest Dermatol*. 1983;80(suppl):12s-16s.
31. Saint-Mezard P, Berard F, Dubois B, et al. The role of CD4+ and CD8+ T cells in contact hypersensitivity and allergic contact dermatitis. *Eur J Dermatol*. 2004;14(3):131-138.
32. Elsaie ML, Olasz E, Jacob SE. Cytokines and Langerhans cells in allergic contact dermatitis. *G Ital Dermatol Venereol*. 2008;143:195.
33. Marks, James G., DeLeo VA. *Contact and Occupational Dermatology*. St Louis, MO: Mosby-Year Book; 1992.
34. Wildemore JK, Junkins-Hopkins JM, James WD. Evaluation of the histologic characteristics of patch test confirmed allergic contact dermatitis. *J Am Acad Dermatol*. 2003;49(2):243-248.
35. Schnuch A, Szliska C, Uter W, et al. Facial allergic contact dermatitis. Data from the IVDK and review of the literature [in German]. *Hautarzt*. 2009;60(1):13-21.
36. Furman D, Fisher AA, Leider M. Allergic eczematous contact-type dermatitis caused by rubber sponges used for the application of cosmetics. *J Invest Dermatol*. 1950;15(3):223-231.
37. Corazza M, Minghetti S, Bertoldi AM, et al. Modern electronic devices: an increasingly common cause of skin disorders in consumers. *Dermatitis*. 2016;27(3):82-89.
38. O'Goshi K, Iguchi M, Tagami H. Functional analysis of the stratum corneum of scalp skin: studies in patients with alopecia areata and androgenetic alopecia. *Arch Dermatol Res*. 2000;292(12):605-611.
39. Chan Y-C, Ng S-K, Goh C-L. Positive patch-test reactions to *para*-phenylenediamine, their clinical relevance and the concept of clinical tolerance. *Contact Dermatitis*. 2001;45(4):217-220.
40. Katugampola RP, Statham BN, English JSC, et al. A multicentre review of the hairdressing allergens tested in the UK. *Contact Dermatitis*. 2005;53(3):130-132.
41. Patel S, Basketter DA, Jefferies D, et al. Patch test frequency to *p*-phenylenediamine: follow up over the last 6 years. *Contact Dermatitis*. 2007;56(1):35-37.
42. Duarte I, Fusaro M, Lazzarini R. Etiology of *para*-phenylenediamine sensitization: hair dye and other products. *Dermatitis*. 2008;19(6):342.
43. Parsons LM. Glyceryl monothioglycolate. *Dermatitis*. 2008;19(6):E51-E52.
44. Castanedo-Tardan MP, Zug KA. Patterns of cosmetic contact allergy. *Dermatol Clin*. 2009;27(3):265-280.
45. Fowler J. Gold allergy in North America. *Am J Contact Dermat*. 2001;12(1):3-5.
46. Rietschel RL, Warshaw EM, Sasseville D, et al. Common contact allergens associated with eyelid dermatitis: Data from the North American Contact Dermatitis Group 2003-2004 study period. *Dermatitis*. 2007;18(2):78-81.
47. Nedorost S, Wagman A. Positive patch-test reactions to gold: patients' perception of relevance and the

role of titanium dioxide in cosmetics. *Dermatitis*. 2005;16(02):067.
48. Guin JD. Eyelid dermatitis: experience in 203 cases. *J Am Acad Dermatol*. 2002;47(5):755-765.
49. Landeck L, John SM, Geier J. Periorbital dermatitis in 4779 patients-patch test results during a 10-year period. *Contact Dermatitis*. 2013;70(4):205-212.
50. Wentworth AB, Yiannias JA, Davis MD, et al. Benzalkonium chloride: a known irritant and novel allergen. *Dermatitis*. 2016;27(1):14-20.
51. Lim SW, Goh CL. Epidemiology of eczematous cheilitis at a tertiary dermatological referral centre in Singapore. *Contact Dermatitis*. 2000;43(6):322-326.
52. Zoli V, Silvani S, Vincenzi C, et al. Allergic contact cheilitis. *Contact Dermatitis*. 2006;54(5):296-297.
53. Fisher AA. Contact stomatitis, glossitis and cheilitis. *Otolaryngol Clin North Am*. 1974;7(3):827-843.
54. Ophaswongse S, Maibach HI. Allergic contact cheilitis. *Contact Dermatitis*. 1995;33(6):365-370.
55. Francalanci S, Sertoli A, Giorgini S, et al. Multicentre study of allergic contact cheilitis from toothpastes. *Contact Dermatitis*. 2000;43(4):216-222.
56. Freeman S, Stephens R. Cheilitis: analysis of 75 cases referred to a contact dermatitis clinic. *Dermatitis*. 1999;10(4):198-200.
57. Strauss RM, Orton DI. Allergic contact cheilitis in the United Kingdom: a retrospective study. *Dermatitis*. 2003;14(2):75-77.
58. Aguirre A, Izu R, Gardeazahal J, et al. Allergic contact cheilitis from a lipstick containing oxybenzone. *Contact Dermatitis*. 1992;27(4):267-267.
59. Schram SE, Glesne LA, Warshaw EM. Allergic contact cheilitis from benzophenone-3 in lip balm and fragrance/flavorings. *Dermatitis*. 2007;18(4):221-224.
60. Serra-Baldrich E, Puig LL, Arnau AG, et al. Lipstick allergic contact dermatitis from gallates. *Contact Dermatitis*. 1995;32(6):359-360.
61. Lazzarini R, Duarte I, de Farias DC, et al. Frequency and main sites of allergic contact dermatitis by nail varnish. *Dermatitis*. 2008;19(6):319-322.
62. Jacob SE, Castanedo-Tardan MP. A diagnostic pearl in allergic contact dermatitis to fragrances: the atomizer sign. *Cutis*. 2008;82(5):317-318.
63. De Groot AC, Le Coz CJ, Lensen GJ, et al. Formaldehyde-releasers: relationship to formaldehyde contact allergy. Part 2. Formaldehyde-releasers in clothes: durable press chemical finishes. *Contact Dermatitis*. 2010;63(1):1-9.
64. Cohen D, Hatch KL, Maibach H, et al. Clothes make the (wo)man: diagnosis and management of clothing dermatitis. *Dermatitis*. 2001;12(4):229-231.
65. Heisterberg MV, Menné T, Andersen KE, et al. Deodorants are the leading cause of allergic contact dermatitis to fragrance ingredients. *Contact Dermatitis*. 2011;64(5):258-264.
66. Zug KA, Rietschel RL, Warshaw EM, et al. The value of patch testing patients with a scattered generalized distribution of dermatitis: retrospective cross-sectional analyses of North American Contact Dermatitis Group data, 2001 to 2004. *J Am Acad Dermatol*. 2008;59(3):426-431.
67. Jacob SE, Zapolanski T. Systemic contact dermatitis. *Dermatitis*. 2008;19(1):9-15.
68. Andersen KE, Hjorth N, Menné T. The baboon syndrome: systemically-induced allergic contact dermatitis. *Contact Dermatitis*. 1984;10(2):97-100.
69. Hausermann P, Harr T, Bircher AJ. Baboon syndrome resulting from systemic drugs: is there strife between SDRIFE and allergic contact dermatitis syndrome? *Contact Dermatitis*. 2004;51(5-6):297-310.
70. Kitamura K, Osawa J, Ikezawa Z, et al. Cross-reactivity between sensitivity to thimerosal and photosensitivity to piroxicam in guinea pigs. *Contact Dermatitis*. 1991;25(1):30-34.
71. Walker SL, Ferguson JE. Systemic allergic contact dermatitis due to ethylenediamine following administration of oral aminophylline. *Br J Dermatol*. 2004;150(3):594-594.
72. Cusano F, Ferrara G, Crisman G, et al. Clinicopathologic features of systemic contact dermatitis from ethylenediamine in cetirizine and levocetirizine. *Dermatology*. 2006;213(4):353-355.
73. Lerbaek A, Menné T, Knudsen B. Cross-reactivity between thiurams. *Contact Dermatitis*. 2006;54(3):165-168.
74. Veien NK, Hattel T, Justesen O, et al. Oral challenge with metal salts (II). Various types of eczema. *Contact Dermatitis*. 1983;9(5):407-410.
75. Salam TN, Fowler JF. Balsam-related systemic contact dermatitis. *J Am Acad Dermatol*. 2001;45(3):377-381.
76. Warshaw EM, Maibach HI, Taylor JS, et al. North American Contact Dermatitis Group patch test results. *Dermatitis*. 2015;26(1):49-59.
77. Goldenberg A, Vassantachart J, Lin EJ, et al. Nickel allergy in adults in the US. *Dermatitis*. 2015;26(5):216-223.
78. Basko-Plluska JT, Thyssen JP, Schalock, PC. Cutaneous and systemic hypersensitivity reactions to metallic implants. *Dermatitis*. 2011;22(2):65-79.
79. Schram SE, Warshaw EM, Laumann A. Nickel hypersensitivity: a clinical review and call to action. *Int J Dermatol*. 2010;49(2):115-125.
80. Schalock PC, Thyssen JP. Patch testers' opinions regarding diagnostic criteria for metal hypersensitivity reactions to metallic implants. *Dermatitis*. 2013;24(4):183-185.
81. Thyssen JP, Johansen JD, Carlsen BC, et al. Prevalence of nickel and cobalt allergy among female patients with dermatitis before and after Danish government regulation: a 23-year retrospective study. *J Am Acad Dermatol*. 2009;61(5):799-805.
82. Brant WT. *The Metallic Alloys: A Practical Guide for the Manufacture of All Kinds of Alloys, Amalgams, and Solders, Used by Metal-workers: Together with Their Chemical and Physical Properties and Their Application in the Arts and Industries*. London, UK: Henry Cary Baird; 1896.
83. Fowler JF. Cobalt. *Dermatitis*. 2016;27(1):3-8.
84. Marks JG, Elsner P, Deleo VA. Standard allergens. *Contact & Occupational Dermatology*. Elsevier BV St. Louis, MO; 2002:65-139.
85. Biebl KA, Warshaw EM. Allergic contact dermatitis to cosmetics. *Dermatol Clin*. 2006;24(2):215-232.
86. Sasseville D. Hypersensitivity to preservatives. *Dermatol Ther*. 2004;17(3):251-263.
87. Eiermann HJ, Larsen W, Maibach HI, et al. Prospective study of cosmetic reactions: 1977-1980. *J Am Acad Dermatol*. 1982;6(5):909-917.
88. Adams RM, Maibach HI, Adams RM, et al. A five-year study of cosmetic reactions. *J Am Acad Dermatol*. 1985;13(6):1062-1069.
89. de Groot AC. Contact allergy to cosmetics: causative ingredients. *Contact Dermatitis*. 1987;17(1):26-34.
90. Johansen JD, Veien N, Laurberg G, et al. Decreasing trends in methyldibromo glutaronitrile contact allergy–following regulatory intervention. *Contact*

91. Larsen WG. How to test for fragrance allergy. *Cutis*. 2000;65(1):39-41.
92. Schnuch A, Uter W, Geier J, et al. Contact allergy to farnesol in 2021 consecutively patch tested patients. Results of the IVDK. *Contact Dermatitis*. 2004;50(3):117-121.
93. de Groot AC, Frosch PJ. Adverse reactions to fragrances. *Contact Dermatitis*. 1997;36(2):57-86.
94. Tomar J, Jain VK, Aggarwal K, et al. Contact allergies to cosmetics: testing with 52 cosmetic ingredients and personal products. *J Dermatol*. 2005;32(12): 951-955.
95. Cheng J, Zug KA. Fragrance allergic contact dermatitis. *Dermatitis*. 2014;25(5):232-245.
96. Larsen WG. Perfume dermatitis. *J Am Acad Dermatol*. 1985;12(1):1-9.
97. Zug KA, Warshaw EM, Fowler JF Jr, et al. Patch-test results of the North American Contact Dermatitis Group 2005-2006. *Dermatitis*. 2009;20(3):149-160.
98. Sasseville D. Neomycin. *Dermatitis*. 2010;21(1):3-7.
99. Andersen KE, White IR, Goossens A. Allergens from the standard series. In: Frosch PJ, Menne T, Lepoittevin JP, eds. *Contact Dermatitis*. Berlin, Germany: Springer; 2006:453.
100. Phillips, DK. Neomycin sulfate. In: Guin JD, ed. *Practical Contact Dermatitis*. New York, NY: McGraw-Hill; 1995: 167.
101. Katz BE, Fisher AA. Bacitracin: a unique topical antibiotic sensitizer. *J Am Acad Dermatol*. 1987;17(6): 1016-1024.
102. Sood A, Taylor JS. Bacitracin: Allergen of the year. *Am J Contact Dermat*. 2003;14(1):3-4.
103. Zapolanski T; Jacob SE. para-Phenylenediamine. *Dermatitis*. 2008;19(3):E20-E21.
104. Arroyo MP. Black henna tattoo reaction in a person with sulfonamide and benzocaine drug allergies. *J Am Acad Dermatol*. 2003;48(2):301-302.
105. Sornin de Leysat C, Boone M, Blondeel A, et al. Two cases of cross-sensitivity in subjects allergic to paraphenylenediamine following ingestion of Polaroril. *Dermatology*. 2003;206(4):379-380.
106. Chung W-H, Chang Y-C, Yang L-J, et al. Clinicopathologic features of skin reactions to temporary tattoos and analysis of possible causes. *Arch Dermatol*. 2002;138(1):88-92.
107. Neri I, Guareschi E, Savoia F, et al. Childhood allergic contact dermatitis from henna tattoo. *Pediatr Dermatol*. 2002;19(6):503-505.
108. Belsito DV. Patch testing with a standard allergen ("screening") tray: rewards and risks. *Dermatol Ther*. 2004;17(3):231-239.
109. Cohen DE, Brancaccio R, Andersen D, et al. Utility of a standard allergen series alone in the evaluation of allergic contact dermatitis: a retrospective study of 732 patients. *J Am Acad Dermatol*. 1997;36(6):914-918.
110. Larkin A. The utility of patch tests using larger screening series of allergens. *Am J Contact Dermat*. 1998;9(3):142-145.
111. Katsarma G, Gawkrodger DJ. Suspected fragrance allergy requires extended patch testing to individual fragrance allergens. *Contact Dermatitis*. 1999;41(4): 193-197.
112. Hoeck UL. More T.R.U.E Test allergens are needed. *J Am Acad Dermatol*. 2005;52(3):538.
113. Patel D, Belsito DV. The detection of clinically relevant contact allergens with a standard screening tray of 28 allergens. *Contact Dermatitis*. 2012;66(3):154-158.
114. Wilkinson DS, Fregert S, Magnusson B, et al. Terminology of contact dermatitis. *Acta Derm Venereol*. 1970;50(4):287-292.
115. Foussereau J, Benezra C, Maibach HI. *Occupational Contact Dermatitis: Clinical and Chemical Aspects*. Copenhagen, Denmark: Munkgaard; 1982.
116. Cronin E. *Contact Dermatitis*. Edinburgh, UK: Churchill Livingston; 1980.
117. Suneja T, Belsito DV. Thimerosal in the detection of clinically relevant allergic contact reactions. *J Am Acad Dermatol*. 2001;45(1):23-27.
118. Mowad CM, Anderson B, Scheinman P, et al. Allergic contact dermatitis: patient management and education. *J Am Acad Dermatol*. 2016;74(6):1043-1054.
119. Weiss G, Shemer A, Trau H. The Koebner phenomenon: review of the literature. *J Eur Acad Dermatol Venereol*. 2002;16(3):241-248.
120. Jensen CD, Paulsen E, Andersen KE. Retrospective evaluation of the consequence of alleged patch test sensitization. *Contact Dermatitis*. 2006;55(1):30-35.
121. Bickers DR, Lim HW, Margolis D, et al. The burden of skin diseases: 2004. *J Am Acad Dermatol*. 2006;55(3):490-500.
122. Stern RS. Dermatologists and office-based care of dermatologic disease in the 21st century. *J Investig Dermatol Symp Proc*. 2004;9(2):126-130.
123. Rietschel RL. Is patch testing cost-effective? *J Am Acad Dermatol*. 1989;21(4):885-887.
124. Freedman S. Diagnosis and differential diagnosis. In: Adams RM, ed. *Adams: Occupational Skin Disease*. 3rd ed. Philadelphia, PA: W.B. Saunders; 1999:189.
125. Rietschel RL. Clues to an accurate diagnosis of contact dermatitis. *Dermatol Ther*. 2004;17(3):224-230.
126. Skoet R, Zachariae R, Agner T. Contact dermatitis and quality of life: a structured review of the literature. *Br J Dermatol*. 2003;149(3):452-456.
127. Linn Holness D. Results of a quality of life questionnaire in a patch test clinic population. *Contact Dermatitis*. 2001;44(2):80-84.
128. Kadyk DL, Hall S, Belsito DV. Quality of life of patients with allergic contact dermatitis: an exploratory analysis by gender, ethnicity, age, and occupation. *Dermatitis*. 2004;15(03):117.
129. Woo PN, Hay IC, Ormerod AD. An audit of the value of patch testing and its effect on quality of life. *Contact Dermatitis*. 2003;48(5):244-247.
130. Zug KA, Aaron DM, Mackenzie T. Baseline quality of life as measured by Skindex-16+5 in patients presenting to a referral center for patch testing. *Dermatitis*. 2009;20(1):21-28.
131. Veien NK, Hattel T, Laurberg G. Hand eczema: causes, course, and prognosis II. *Contact Dermatitis*. 2008;58(6):335-339.
132. Adisesh A, Meyer JD, Cherry NM. Prognosis and work absence due to occupational contact dermatitis. *Contact Dermatitis*. 2002;46(5):273-279.
133. Holness DL, Nethercott JR. Is a worker's understanding of their diagnosis an important determinant of outcome in occupational contact dermatitis? *Contact Dermatitis*. 1991;25(5):296-301.
134. Kalimo K, Kautiainen H, Niskanen T, et al. "Eczema school" to improve compliance in an occupational dermatology clinic. *Contact Dermatitis*. 1999;41(6): 315-319.
135. Jacob SE, Castanedo-Tardan MP. Pharmacotherapy for allergic contact dermatitis. *Expert Opin Pharmacother*. 2007;8(16):2757-2774.

136. American Contact Dermatitis Society. Contact Allergen Management Program. http://acdscamp.org/. Accessed June 19, 2016.

137. Contact Allergen Replacement Database (CARD). 2008. http://contactallergy.com/index.html. Accessed June 29, 2016.

Chapter 25 :: Irritant Dermatitis
:: Susan T. Nedorost

第二十五章
刺激性皮炎

中文导读

本章共分为10节：①定义；②历史回顾；③流行病学；④临床表现；⑤病因与发病机制；⑥并发症；⑦诊断；⑧鉴别诊断；⑨临床病程与预后；⑩治疗。全面介绍了刺激性皮炎的流行病学、诊断、治疗与预后。

第一节介绍了"皮炎""刺激性皮炎""真皮损伤导致的瘢痕""手部皮炎"的定义和不同点。

第二节回顾了刺激性接触性皮炎概念的由来和发展，比较了刺激性接触性皮炎和变应性接触性皮炎的区别。

第三节介绍了气候、性别、AD、特异性暴露史（职业暴露/非职业暴露）等危险因素对刺激性皮炎发病的影响。

第四节介绍了刺激性皮炎的临床表现，指出表皮破坏是刺激性皮炎的主要表现，且皱褶部位更明显。

第五节介绍了刺激性皮炎的病因与发病机制，主要描述了危险因素：潮湿工作、香料、手套，并阐述了发病的三个步骤。

第六节介绍了刺激性皮炎的并发症。分别对过敏性接触性皮炎、弱过敏原的免疫反应、食物过敏进行了阐述和说明。

第七节介绍了刺激性皮炎的诊断，指出需进行斑贴试验以排除过敏性接触性皮炎的成分。还可检测表皮失水（TEWL），必要时结合组织病理学和影像学检查来诊断。

第八节介绍了需要与刺激性皮炎相鉴别的疾病，最主要需与变应性接触性皮炎进行鉴别。

第九节介绍了刺激性皮炎的临床病程与预后。

第十节介绍了刺激性皮炎的治疗，详细叙述了防护措施（隔离霜、防护手套、润肤剂等）及其使用方法，以及对该病的早期预防和早期筛查。并着重指出筛查可以减轻疾病的社会负担，但最终只有随着治疗的进展和对预防并发症的方法加深了解，才能减轻疾病负担。

〔李　捷〕

AT-A-GLANCE

- Irritant dermatitis from wet-to-dry cycling is common in cold seasons.
- Decreasing the duration and frequency of contact with irritants may improve symptoms of irritant contact dermatitis (as opposed to allergic contact dermatitis which requires complete avoidance to clear).
- Innate immune signals from irritant dermatitis predispose to allergic dermatitis (allergic contact and atopic dermatitis).
- Emollients accelerate recovery and may help prevent the complication of allergic dermatitis in infants.
- Emollients used on normal skin over long intervals may predispose to irritant dermatitis.
- Hardening, or disappearance of symptoms, often occurs with continued irritant exposure without any treatment.
- Future understanding of ways to promote hardening could reduce the impact of allergic contact dermatitis and atopic disease which complicate irritant dermatitis.

INTRODUCTION

Irritant contact dermatitis is sometimes encountered as a primary diagnosis, but it is most important for its critical role in predisposing to atopic and allergic contact dermatitis.

When acute irritant dermatitis is the sole diagnosis, patients are often able to self-diagnose. There is obvious temporal relationship because irritant dermatitis manifests within hours of the causative exposure, and resolves within days of cessation of exposure. In contrast, allergic contact dermatitis may manifest days after exposure and persist for weeks. Consequently, accurate self-diagnosis of contact dermatitis is more common with irritant contact dermatitis than allergic contact dermatitis. The combination of straightforward self-diagnosis and shorter duration makes the presentation of irritant dermatitis for dermatologic consultation less common than that of allergic contact dermatitis.

T cells produce the inflammation of atopic and allergic contact dermatitis as part of the adaptive immune response. The adaptive response is influenced by upstream innate immune response. Irritant dermatitis provides the innate immune signals that predispose to allergic contact and atopic dermatitis. Therefore, the importance of irritant contact dermatitis is less recognition and treatment as a primary diagnosis, but its role in downstream dermatitis mediated by the adaptive immune response. Study of barrier disruption and the resulting innate immune signals should help us develop strategies to prevent irritant dermatitis so as to prevent more severe and disabling allergic and atopic dermatitis.

DEFINITIONS

Dermatitis is an inflammatory disruption of the epidermis related to physical or immunologic provocation. Dermatitis and eczema are often used interchangeably.[1] Dermatitis appears as spongiosis histologically. There is impairment of the barrier functions of the skin, which results in increased transepidermal water loss.

As Fig. 25-1 illustrates, dermatitis is usually multifactorial. Irritant dermatitis results in barrier disruption which may predispose to higher concentrations of bacteria and yeast, and these microorganisms may stimulate immune response.[2-4] Immune signals from barrier disruption also predispose to allergic contact dermatitis to chemical antigens,[5] as discussed later in "Complications."

Irritant dermatitis begins with damage to keratinocytes, which then release danger signals that promote recruitment of inflammatory cells. In severe cases, necrotic keratinocytes are evident.

Irritant dermatitis is caused by physical damage to the epidermis and is temporally more immediate after provocation than the delayed hypersensitivity response leading to allergic contact dermatitis. Many variables influence expression of irritant dermatitis including climate and season, occlusion, frequency of exposure to the irritant, and concentration of the irritant.

Dermal injury producing scarring can result from corrosive chemicals that coagulate protein and cause cutaneous scars. Corrosive chemicals are not further discussed in this chapter. Irritant chemicals by definition do not cause scarring when in contact with the skin for less than 4 hours.[6] Rarely, scarring can result from secondary infection of dermatitis, but not from uncomplicated dermatitis.

Hand dermatitis is a common site for irritant contact dermatitis. Repeated wetting and drying of the skin causes fissuring, especially if drying is rapid because of low ambient humidity.

Contact with an allergen often results in allergic contact hand dermatitis complicating irritant contact dermatitis. Consequently, the definition of pure irritant contact dermatitis is one of exclusion. Irritant hand dermatitis has been defined as "A documented exposure of the hands to an irritant, which is quantitatively likely to cause contact dermatitis. No relevant contact allergy (no current exposure to allergens to which the patient has reacted positive in patch test)."[7]

HISTORICAL PERSPECTIVE

In the past, homemakers did more wet work, such as washing dishes by hand, and were often diagnosed with "dishpan hands." Today, irritant dermatitis in its pure

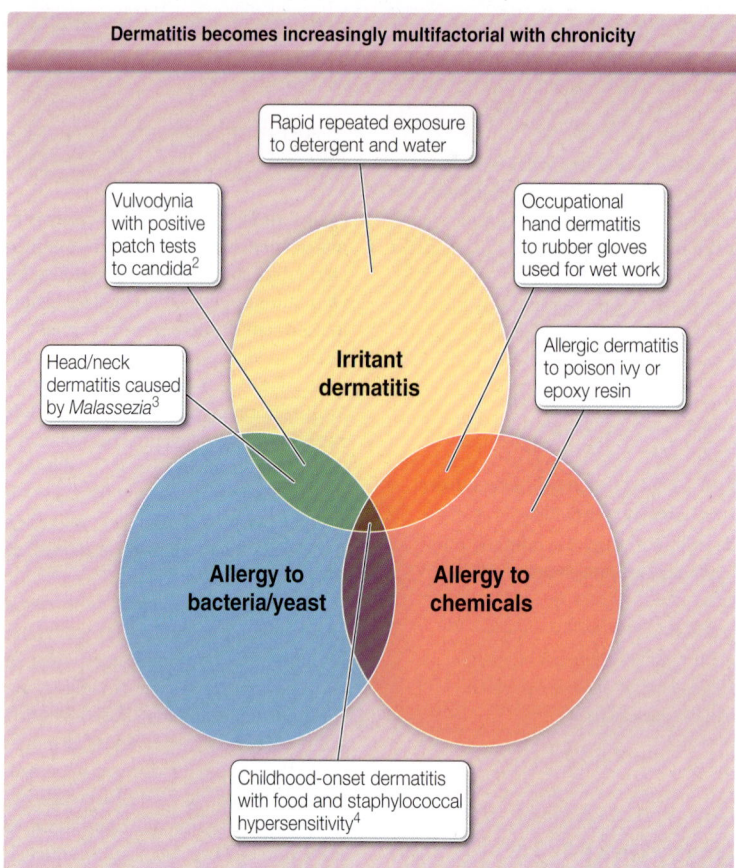

Figure 25-1 Irritant dermatitis leads to barrier disruption that promotes immune response to bacteria and yeast, as well as to chemicals in contact with the skin. Dermatitis often results from a combination of causative factors. Examples are shown here for various combinations of causative factors.

form is commonly described as "chapping" or rough, cracked, sore skin. Compared to prior decades, this more commonly occurs from frequent hand hygiene as required for health care workers, or from exposure to wind and cold during outdoor sports and exercise.

Patient history is very helpful when distinguishing acute irritant dermatitis from acute allergic contact dermatitis. When chronic, irritant and allergic contact dermatitis cannot reliably be differentiated clinically or histologically. A detailed clinical history and often patch testing are required to diagnosis allergic contact dermatitis (Table 25-1).

The classification of hand dermatitis as purely irritant may depend on the absence of relevant positive patch tests to indicate allergic contact dermatitis. The percentage of cases identified as irritant varies between clinics as the number of patch tests used varies. Many cases are classified as irritant hand dermatitis with allergic or atopic hand dermatitis.[7]

The lack of a diagnostic test for irritant dermatitis makes it very difficult to comment on prevalence over time.[8] Irritant contact dermatitis in its pure form is probably a less-common reason for presentation to a dermatologist now than in the past. This may be because of decreased prevalence resulting from technology reducing the amount of wet work required for homemaking, or improved patient access to medical information, and/or improved formulations of products such as emollients and diapers.

EPIDEMIOLOGY

CLIMATE

Climate influences the rapidity of wet-to-dry cycles. In low ambient humidity, water evaporates rapidly causing uneven surface change, whereas slow drying in higher humidity conditions results in a smoother surface. Irritant contact dermatitis can occur from cumulative irritancy from wet-to-dry cycles with or without exposure to irritant chemicals, including detergents and solvents. Wet-to-dry cycles are a common cause of irritant dermatitis in the setting of genetic predisposition to impaired barrier, as in atopic dermatitis where perioral chapping occurs in infants from drooling. Occupational hand dermatitis in the setting of wet work is more common in cold seasons when humidity indoors is low.[9]

TABLE 25-1
Comparison of the Symptoms of Allergic Contact Dermatitis and Irritant Contact Dermatitis

		IRRITANT CONTACT DERMATITIS	ALLERGIC CONTACT DERMATITIS
Margination and site	Acute	Sharp, strictly confined to the site of exposure	Spreading from site of exposure to **the periphery**; usually tiny papules; may become generalized
	Chronic	Ill-defined	Ill-defined, spreads
Evolution	Acute	**Rapid** (few hours after exposure)	**Not so rapid** (12-72 hours after exposure)
Causative agents		**Dependent on concentration of agent and state of skin barrier**; occurs only above threshold level	**Relatively independent of amount applied**, usually very low concentrations sufficient, but depends on degree of sensitization
Incidence		**May occur in practically everyone**	**Occurs only in the sensitized**

From Wolff K, Johnson R, Saavedra AP, Roh EK. *Fitzpatrick's Color Atlas and Synopsis of Clinical Dermatology*, 8th ed. New York, NY: McGraw-Hill; 2017, Table 2-3, p. 29, with permission.

GENDER

Women are more likely than men to have hand dermatitis, presumably because of greater wet work exposure. Occupational hand dermatitis is often multifactorial, with both an irritant and an allergic contact component, for example, in hairdressers and machinists.[10] Women reported more itching compared to men in one large study where the severity of hand dermatitis was similar in men and women.[11]

Frequency of hand washing is a risk factor for irritant hand dermatitis. Women are more likely than men to perform higher-risk wet tasks such as hairdressing, and are more likely to wash their hands frequently when away from work.[11] Irritant hand dermatitis increased coincident with campaigns to improve hand hygiene in health care workers to decrease hospital-acquired infections.[12]

ATOPIC DERMATITIS

Some people with atopic dermatitis have a genetic barrier defect. In some racial cohorts, this is caused by a mutation leading to defective filaggrin, which weakens the protein milieu that binds corneocytes together in the stratum corneum and decreases natural moisturizing factor.[13] In a study comparing patients with atopic dermatitis to healthy controls, the atopic dermatitis patients had greater reactivity to the irritant detergent sodium lauryl sulfate,[14] and in a prospective study of workers evaluated for irritant contact dermatitis, atopic patients were more likely to discontinue work.[15]

In contrast, in a population of health care workers with no history of dermatitis severe enough to warrant physician evaluation, a history of childhood flexural dermatitis did not predispose to lower the irritancy threshold to various concentrations of sodium lauryl sulfate, although irritant response to sodium lauryl sulfate did correlate with development of wintertime irritant hand dermatitis.[16] The latter observation suggests that there are individual risk factors for irritant hand dermatitis in addition to atopic dermatitis in a population of healthy hospital workers.

SPECIFIC EXPOSURES

OCCUPATIONAL EXPOSURES

In the setting of dermatologic consultation for occupational hand dermatitis, allergic contact dermatitis may be more commonly diagnosed than irritant contact dermatitis.[17] Irritant contact dermatitis is more commonly diagnosed than allergic contact dermatitis[10] in studies where larger numbers of workers are assessed. The greater prevalence of irritant dermatitis in the working population compared to the dermatologic consultation cohort may reflect the relative ease of self-diagnosing irritant contact dermatitis, and its comparative lesser severity compared to allergic contact dermatitis, such that many workers do not seek medical consultative care for irritant contact dermatitis.

Table 25-2 lists common irritants by occupation. These are rarely important diagnostically, as patients self-identify and avoid most irritants. Water—from wet work, drooling, and sweating—is the most important irritant that provokes irritant dermatitis leading to allergic contact and atopic dermatitis because it is difficult to avoid.

Oil dermatitis occurs in workers whose hands and forearms have prolonged contact with oil and who may develop a type of irritant dermatitis characterized by perifollicular papules and pustules.[18] Workers exposed to oil often use solvents to remove oil from the skin that further aggravates the irritant dermatitis.

Plants and *insects* less commonly cause irritant dermatitis, but when they do cause irritant dermatitis, it may appear in areas other than the hands. An example is an outbreak of irritant dermatitis from blister beetles in Thai military recruits.[19]

Fiberglass dermatitis can cause irritant contact or airborne irritant dermatitis. Airborne irritant dermatitis is characterized by eyelid and other flexural involvement of exposed skin.[20]

TABLE 25-2
Irritants Encountered in Various Occupations

CONDITION	IRRITANT
Agriculture workers	Artificial fertilizers, disinfectants, pesticides, cleaners, gasoline, diesel oil, plants, and grains
Artists	Solvents, clay, plaster
Automobile and aircraft industry workers	Solvents, cutting oils, paints, hand cleansers
Bakers and confectioners	Flour, detergents
Bartenders	Detergents, wet work
Bookbinders	Solvents, glues
Butchers	Detergents, meat, waste
Cabinet makers and carpenters	Glues, detergents, thinners, solvents, wood preservatives
Cleaners	Detergents, solvents, wet work
Coal miners	Dust (coal, stone), wet conditions
Construction workers	Cement
Cooks and caterers	Detergents, vegetable juices, wet work
Dentists and dental technicians	Detergents, hand cleansers, wet work
Dry cleaners	Solvents
Electricians	Soldering fluxes
Electroplaters	Acids, alkalis
Floor-layers	Solvents
Florists and gardeners	Manure, artificial fertilizers, pesticides, wet work
Hairdressers	Permanent wave solutions, shampoos, bleaching agents, wet work
Hospital workers	Detergents, disinfectants, foods, wet work
Homemakers	Detergents, cleansers, foods, wet work
Jewelers	Detergents, solvents
Mechanics	Oils, greases, gasoline, diesel fuel, cleaners, solvents
Metal workers	Cutting oils, solvents, hand cleansers
Nurses	Disinfectants, detergents, wet work
Office workers	Solvents (photocopiers, adhesives)
Painters	Solvents, thinners, wallpaper adhesives, hand cleansers
Photography industry workers	Solvents, wet work
Plastics workers	Solvents, acids, styrene, oxidizing agents
Printers	Solvents
Rubber workers	Solvents, talc, zinc stearate, uncured rubber
Shoemakers	Solvents
Tannery workers	Acids, alkalis, reducing and oxidizing agents, wet work
Textile workers	Fibers, bleaching agents, solvents
Veterinarians and slaughterhouse workers	Disinfectants, wet work, animal entrails and secretions

Wet work (water or water plus detergent) is the most common occupational irritant.
From What occupations are at risk? OSH Answers, Canadian Centre for Occupational Health and Safety (CCOHS), October 15, 2008. https://www.ccohs.ca/oshanswers/diseases/dermatitis.html. Reproduced with the permission of CCOHS, 2016.

NONOCCUPATIONAL EXPOSURES

Table 25-3 shows common irritants encountered outside of work. *Medicaments* may cause irritation, which is commonly seen with the use of retinoids and benzoyl peroxide.

Diaper rash is another common example of irritant dermatitis that can occur with wet-to-dry cycles and irritation from stool. Irritant diaper dermatitis has decreased with use of superabsorbent and less-occlusive disposable diapers.[21]

EXPOSURE TO RUBBING OR STRETCHING THE SKIN

Friction from sporting equipment, such as shin guards, rubbing against skin can cause irritant dermatitis. The

TABLE 25-3 Common Irritants
Solvents including water
Detergents
Disinfectants
Anti-wrinkle medicaments

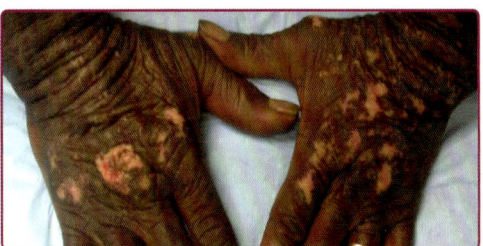

Figure 25-2 Thickened skin with pigment changes in areas of chronic friction on the dorsal hands caused by occupation. This is an exception to the usual finding of accentuation in flexural areas, because the frictional exposure was to the dorsal surface of the hands only.

friction is worsened by perspiration, and the resulting dermatitis may be complicated by allergic contact dermatitis to rubber chemicals or textile dyes in the shin guard. Athletes may also develop contact dermatitis from dye in clothing that reaches skin as a result of liberation from the fabric by perspiration and friction. Testing to materials obtained from the patient's own sporting equipment in addition to relevant commercial patch test series increases the sensitivity of patch testing for allergic contact dermatitis caused by sporting equipment.[22,23] Irritant dermatitis may be mitigated by use of powder that absorbs perspiration and reduces friction.

Friction blisters are an acute skin injury that can be occupational or avocational, such as from raking leaves.

Stasis dermatitis occurs when swollen lower legs experience barrier disruption caused by stretching. Lymphatic obstruction accentuates inflammation in mice when challenged with the irritant croton oil. When challenged with the sensitizer dinitrofluorobenzene, mice with lymphatic obstruction had more swelling than those without, but also had lower levels of the inflammatory signals interferon-γ, tumor necrosis factor-α, and the chemokines CXCL9 and CXCL10 than did mice without lymphatic obstruction, suggesting that the increased swelling is a consequence of fluid retention rather than accentuated allergic contact dermatitis.[24]

CLINICAL FEATURES

CUTANEOUS FINDINGS

Epidermal disruption is the primary finding in irritant dermatitis, as opposed to allergic contact dermatitis which displays proportionately more dermal inflammatory infiltrate. Irritant contact dermatitis is characterized by redness, fissuring, oozing, and pain. Figure 25-2 shows chronic irritant contact dermatitis with epidermal thickening and pigment change. Figure 25-3 shows an irritant patch test created by applying sodium lauryl sulfate 2.5% under occlusion. Note that there is scorched appearing skin surface without much induration. Irritant dermatitis, like this patch test, usually demonstrates more epidermal than dermal inflammation. As Fig. 25-4 shows, severe acute irritant dermatitis can also produce blisters.

Allergic contact dermatitis can occur with irritant dermatitis and is more likely to present with the symptoms of itch and more likely to demonstrate induration.

Figure 25-5 shows an allergic patch test result. Note that there is more induration than epidermal change.

FLEXURAL ACCENTUATION

Flexural accentuation is an important sign of irritant dermatitis. Common areas for irritant dermatitis are folds in the eyelid, neck, antecubital fossae, volar wrist, and intertriginous regions.

In the cases of irritant hand dermatitis and of diaper rash, irritant dermatitis is more apparent in finger webs and creases (Fig. 25-6) and intertriginous folds, respectively, where irritants concentrate, and is worsened by increased pH from soaps and feces, respectively. Irritant cleansers cause predominantly flexural dermatitis where the concentration of irritant is highest because of occlusion.[25] Figure 25-7 shows flexural accentuation of acute dermatitis in a patient who inadvertently applied a cleanser, mistaking it for an emollient, to the entire surface of both legs.

Retinoid dermatitis also preferentially involves folds such as the nasolabial fold. This is often noted several days after starting cutaneous application, as retinoids

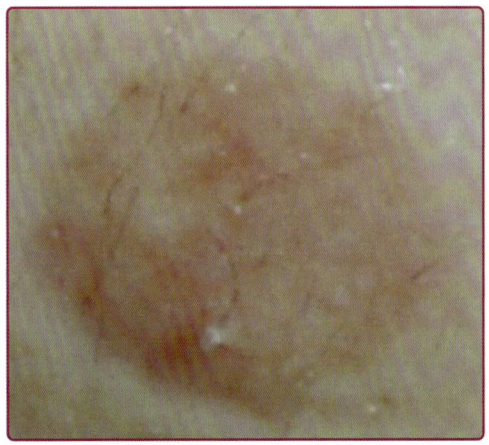

Figure 25-3 Irritant dermatitis from a patch test with sodium lauryl sulfate. Note the scorched appearance of the skin with more surface change than papules.

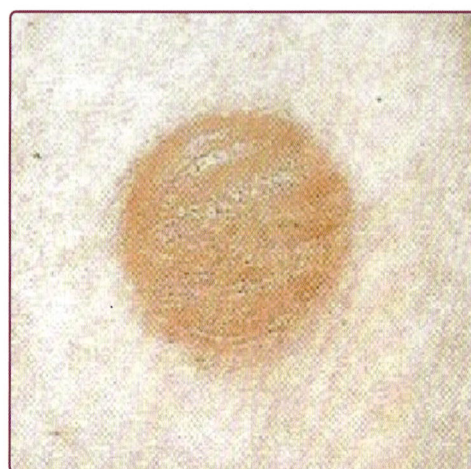

Figure 25-4 Bullous irritant patch test response with blister but no surrounding induration.

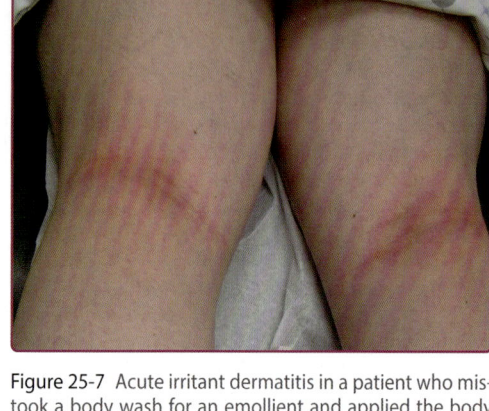

Figure 25-7 Acute irritant dermatitis in a patient who mistook a body wash for an emollient and applied the body wash at bedtime. The patient awoke with inflammation primarily in the flexural areas despite application to the entire leg.

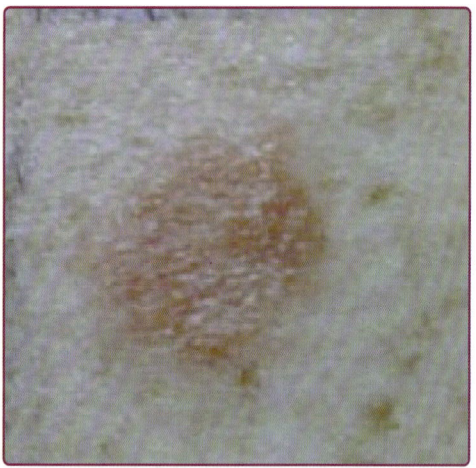

Figure 25-5 Allergic dermatitis from a patch test to gold; there are multiple papules and an indurated base.

produce a delayed irritant reaction.[26] Figure 25-8 shows irritant dermatitis on the neck in a patient who began applying tretinoin daily to the neck after tolerating long-term use on the face.

NONCUTANEOUS FINDINGS

Hand dermatitis, which always has an irritant component, is associated with anxiety and obsessive-compulsive traits, but not with depression, compared to healthy controls.[27] Contact dermatitis leads to substantial costs and lower work productivity in adults, which may lead to financial harm.[28]

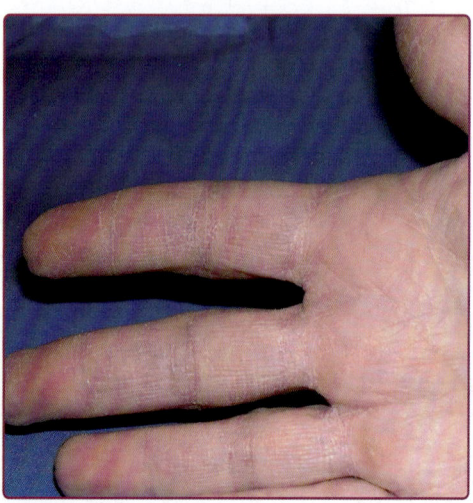

Figure 25-6 Mild wintertime irritant dermatitis in a health care worker. Note the accentuation of the chapping in the flexural areas.

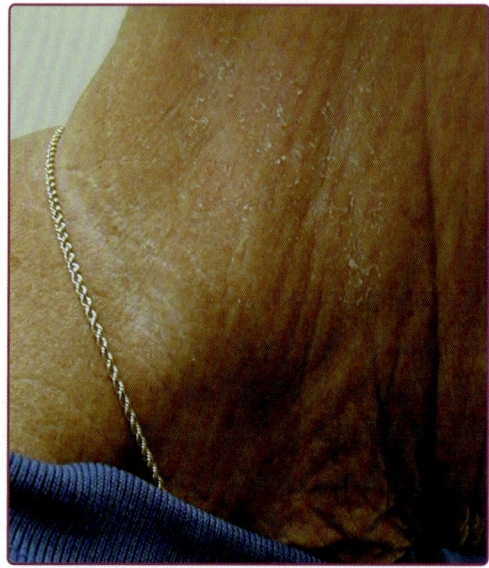

Figure 25-8 Topical retinoid-induced irritant dermatitis on the neck.

ETIOLOGY AND PATHOGENESIS

RISK FACTORS

WET WORK, DETERGENTS, AND GLOVES

Occupational hand dermatitis is common in wet workers. Irritation from water is synergistic with irritation from detergent. Solvent exposure is also synergistic with detergent exposure.[29]

Glove use can protect skin from water and detergents, but perspiration or leakage of moisture around the cuff can occlude moisture under the glove causing maceration from perspiration. Rapid drying of the retained moisture when the glove is removed causes even more damage to the epidermis. Figure 25-9 shows a patient with underlying hand dermatitis who aggravated the dermatitis by wearing occlusive gloves.

In healthy human controls with no history of atopic dermatitis who were exposed to repeated half-hour intervals of water occlusion over 4 days, the detergent sodium lauryl sulfate and the alcohol *n*-propanol both caused more irritation at the test sites than they did on previously unoccluded skin. The detergent was more irritating than the alcohol solution by visual inspection of the skin, measure of transepidermal water loss, and measured decrease in natural moisturizing factor levels.[30] A review of the effects of glove occlusion similarly concluded that using waterproof gloves predisposed the skin to more-severe irritation from detergents used for hand hygiene.[31]

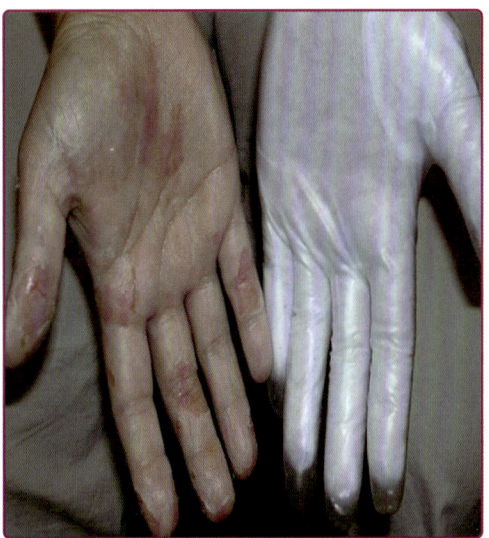

Figure 25-9 Irritant macerated dermatitis from wearing a wet cotton glove under an occlusive glove.

ATOPIC DERMATITIS

Filaggrin mutations are associated with early-onset dermatitis,[32] which is often considered to be "atopic dermatitis." As children become more active, flexural areas develop frictional irritant dermatitis, which leads to allergic contact dermatitis in many cases. Patch testing should be considered in cases of chronic flexural dermatitis.[33]

PATHOGENESIS

STEP 1: EPIDERMAL INSULT

The barrier function of the epidermis can be diminished by solvents that remove lipids from the upper epidermal layers, or by desiccation of the stratum corneum from repeated rapid drying. Genetic factors, such as filaggrin mutations, lower the threshold for epidermal damage to include even minor friction.

STEP 2: DANGER SIGNALS

Damaged keratinocytes release danger signals termed *alarmins* that are analogous to pathogen associated molecular patterns that defend against infections. Examples of candidate alarmins include defensins and uric acid, which may be operative in psoriasis and other inflammatory skin diseases in addition to dermatitis. In fact, the signals from epidermal trauma that drive koebnerization in psoriasis may be different than those in dermatitis and may explain the differences in downstream cytokines that explain the inverse relationship between psoriasis and autoimmune disease and allergic dermatitis.[34]

These danger signals can bind toll-like receptors and promote inflammatory pathways such as nuclear factor-κB that link to the adaptive immune response leading to allergic dermatitis.[35]

STEP 3: POTENTIAL FOR ALLERGIC SENSITIZATION

Chemical allergens and microorganisms stimulate the innate immune system, and toll-like receptors play an important role in mediating both irritant and subsequent allergic contact dermatitis.[36]

Irritant dermatitis predisposes to allergic sensitization to antigens that would not normally cause allergic contact dermatitis on noninflamed skin.

Potent sensitizers that can cause allergy on previously noninflamed skin are dependent on their inherent irritant properties. Athymic mice, as an example of intact innate response without adaptive response, mount a neutrophil response and some diminished T-helper (Th)1/Th2 cell response to the sensitizer oxazolone, while FcγR knockout mice, as an example of intact adaptive response without innate response, have a greatly diminished response when sensitized and rechallenged with oxazolone.[37]

COMPLICATIONS

ALLERGIC CONTACT DERMATITIS

Allergic contact dermatitis is dependent on irritant dermatitis either in the context of previously inflamed skin or the inherent irritant properties of the sensitizer. Toll-like receptors in a mouse model trigger an innate response that begins the education of the adaptive immune response[36] and are well-positioned to initiate an inflammatory response to microorganisms on the skin.

IMMUNE RESPONSE TO LESS-POTENT ALLERGENS, INCLUDING THE MICROBIOME

Childhood-onset dermatitis, also known as atopic dermatitis, is associated with inflammatory responses to common organisms such as *Staphylococcus aureus*, *Malassezia sympodialis*, and *Alternaria*. These organisms may exist as part of a biofilm that concentrates microorganisms and their antigens and may lead to an allergic-like immunologic response to these organisms.[38] Figure 25-10 shows a positive patch test to *M. sympodialis* yeast in a patient with adult-onset dermatitis of the neck and upper torso (Fig. 25-11).

The immune response to microbial allergens is distinct from allergic contact dermatitis to potent conventional sensitizers that function as their own irritants on normal-appearing skin. Weakly potent antigens such as propylene glycol, defined as negative in the guinea pig local lymph node assay,[39] are more likely to cause contact allergy in patients with barrier disruption triggering "danger signals." In general, patients with ongoing innate immune signals from either genetic barrier dysfunction or wet work become sensitized to less potent allergens as measured by the local lymph node assay.[40]

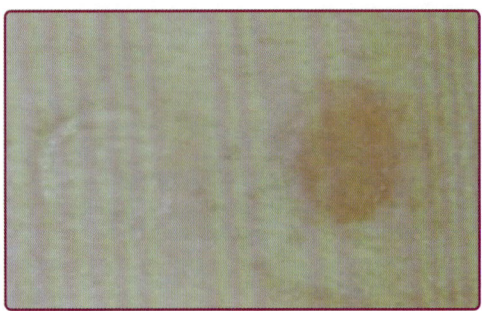

Figure 25-10 Positive patch test to *Malassezia sympodialis* yeast in an adult patient with dermatitis of the anterior axillary line and neck.

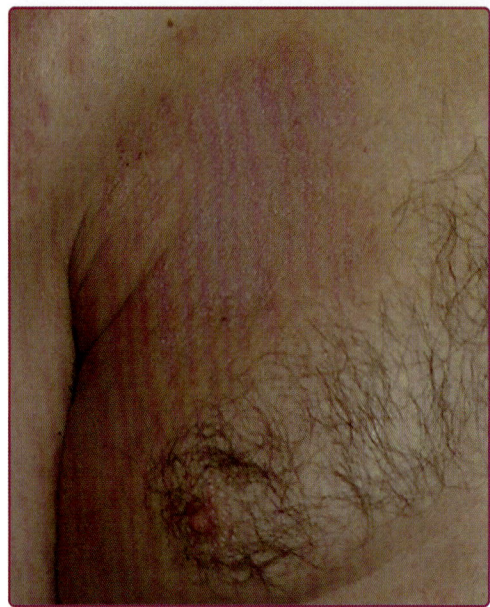

Figure 25-11 Distribution of dermatitis seen in patients with sensitivity to *Malassezia sympodialis*.

Patients without preexisting irritant dermatitis are more likely to become sensitized to potent antigens that likely create their own innate signal, such as poison ivy. Innate signal from disrupted skin barrier, together with the irritant signal of a potent antigen, may drive dendritic cells into the dermis and promote immunologic tolerance.[41] This is consistent with the observation that patients with atopic dermatitis are less likely to exhibit dermatitis to the potent allergen in poison ivy that is also a strong irritant.

FOOD ALLERGY

Infants with irritant dermatitis around the mouth from drooling are at risk for allergic contact sensitization from food contact with the inflamed skin. Foods are generally weak allergens and do not sensitize noninflamed skin. If initial food exposure is on mucosa, tolerance develops.[42] This likely explains the higher incidence of peanut allergy in the Unites States where initial peanut exposure is often by self-feeding peanut butter as opposed to the 10-fold lower incidence Israel where initial exposure is to soft baked peanut bambas, which are placed into the mouth directly.

Patients with atopic dermatitis often, but not always, have only a transient Th1 response to cutaneous contact sensitization. This might explain the tendency for atopic dermatitis to improve as children get older. These patients also develop a more persistent Th2 skewed response[43] that might contribute to the atopic march. Figure 25-12 shows the typical perioral inflammation seen with infantile dermatitis that can be complicated by contact sensitization and food allergy

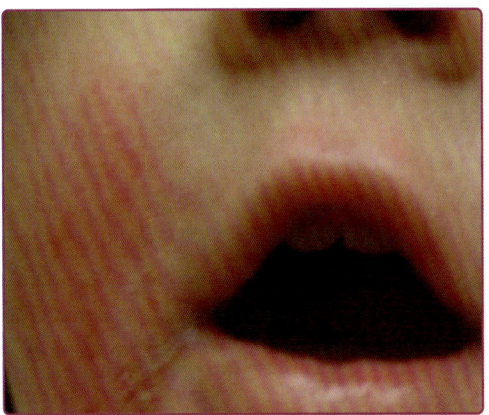

Figure 25-12 Infantile dermatitis that likely began as irritant dermatitis from drooling and in this case was complicated by allergic contact dermatitis to an emollient cream confirmed by patch testing.

with delayed and immediate type hypersensitivity (the atopic march).

Although there is no prospective study to confirm the recommendation, new foods should logically be introduced when there is no perioral irritant dermatitis and fed with an infant feeding spoon directly into the mouth rather than being self-fed, which results in substantially more skin contact.

DIAGNOSIS

SUPPORTIVE STUDIES

PATCH TESTING

Patch testing is needed to exclude a component of allergic contact dermatitis. Sensitivity of patch testing is dependent on obtaining a detailed history of personal and occupational exposures and then testing to all potential allergens based on this history. Occupational exposures almost always require specialty patch test series tailored to occupation, and often require dilution of the worker's own products to an appropriate patch test concentration and vehicle.

LABORATORY TESTING

Transepidermal water loss (TEWL) is a measure of the ability of the skin to maintain homeostasis of fluids in the body. In addition to the stratum corneum, tight junctions between living keratinocytes contribute to skin barrier function and provide defense between microbial pathogens and their ligands including toll-like receptors.[44] TEWL is a measure of barrier function and increased TEWL indicates increased permeability to antigens.[45] TEWL is not routinely tested in clinical practice but is used in research studies of irritant contact dermatitis.

PATHOLOGY

All forms of dermatitis show intercellular edema, or spongiosis, of the epidermis. In the acute phase, there is more fluid which correlates with the clinical presence of vesicles, bullae, and crusting. With chronicity, the stratum corneum exhibits hyperkeratosis, and there is less spongiosis. Figure 25-13 shows the features of subacute dermatitis. In very chronic dermatitis, there is even less spongiosis, no crusting, and elongation of the rete ridges in the epidermis and dermal fibrosis.

IMAGING

Confocal microscopy has been studied to help differentiate irritant from allergic contact dermatitis in vivo, but this is not currently used in practice.[46]

DIAGNOSTIC ALGORITHM

Diagnosis of irritant dermatitis begins with a detailed history of potential irritants, temporal course of symptoms, and examination for evidence of flexural accentuation. In patients with severe inflammation and itch, allergic contact dermatitis needs to be investigated with appropriate testing.

An example is shown in Table 25-4 for a patient with complaint of itching and redness of the hands after wearing rubber gloves for wet work where irritant contact dermatitis, contact urticaria, and allergic contact dermatitis are considered. Contact urticaria to latex is an example of a contact allergen that is more common in atopic patients and where the allergic contact sensitization has a more persistent Th2 than Th1 response.

DIFFERENTIAL DIAGNOSIS

Irritant dermatitis occasionally mimics other inflammatory dermatoses such as the "mechanic's hands"

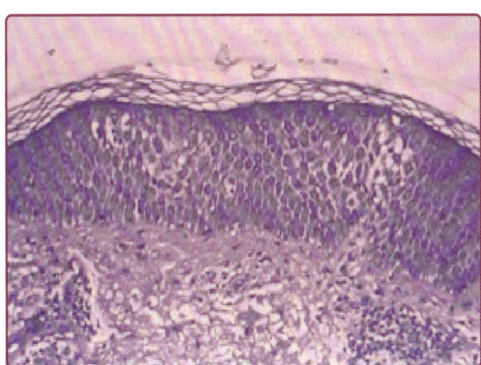

Figure 25-13 Subacute spongiotic dermatitis as seen in irritant and in allergic contact dermatitis.

TABLE 25-4
Example of Differential Diagnosis Including Irritant Dermatitis Caused by Gloves

	TIMING	TEST	COUNSELING
Contact urticaria	Itchy hives begin within minutes of exposure and resolves within hours; when chronic, skin findings may resemble dermatitis	Skin prick to latex glove or antigen specific immunoglobulin E (sensitivity 50%-90%); if negative, 15-minute wear test of latex finger cot[47]	Avoid latex if positive
Allergic contact dermatitis to rubber[a]	Itchy dermatitis begins hours to days after exposure and resolves over weeks	Patch test to a series including rubber accelerators and antioxidants, and to pieces of glove as is	Avoid natural and synthetic rubber gloves containing allergens; use vinyl or allergen-free chemically resistant gloves depending on exposure needs
Irritant contact dermatitis exacerbated by occlusive gloves	Inflammation begins within hours and resolves within days of glove avoidance; becomes more chronic over time	If patch tests are negative, proceed with counseling for irritant dermatitis, but consider the possibility of an allergen not patch tested	Wear cotton under occlusive gloves; change gloves frequently; reduce exposure to hand washing

[a]Irritant dermatitis is often the precursor of allergic dermatitis, such that counseling for irritant dermatitis is usually appropriate in addition to counseling for confirmed allergic dermatitis.

TABLE 25-5
Examples of Allergens Speculated to Be Most Likely to Cause Sensitization Based on the Type and Severity of Preexisting Irritant Contact Dermatitis

TYPE OF PREEXISTING IRRITATION	EXAMPLE	POTENCY OF ALLERGEN	EXAMPLE OF ALLERGENS
Normal skin or subclinical decreased irritancy threshold	Positive patch test to low concentration sodium lauryl sulfate[48]	Strong	Poison ivy; epoxy resin
Moderate	Irritant hand dermatitis from wet work[40]	Medium	Rubber chemicals; formaldehyde-releasing preservatives
Severe	Infantile perioral dermatitis from drooling in cold season[49]	Weak	Foods; vitamin E; propylene glycol

sign seen in dermatomyositis (see Chap. 62).

The more common clinical dilemma is differentiating irritant dermatitis as the sole explanation for cutaneous inflammation as opposed to irritant dermatitis complicated by allergic disorder. The allergens that cause sensitization depend on the type and degree of irritant dermatitis that is present at the time of sensitization. More research in this area is needed to develop appropriate patch test series. Table 25-5 demonstrates the concept.

The likelihood of sensitization to a moderate to highly potent antigen may be greater in patients with a subclinically decreased irritancy threshold as detected by response to a low concentration patch test to sodium lauryl sulfate.[48] Wet workers are more likely to be sensitized to moderately potent allergens such as rubber accelerators.[40] The prevalence of eczema and food allergy is higher in children born in autumn or winter months,[49] supporting the relationship between climate and irritant dermatitis caused by drooling and sensitization to food on inflamed skin. However, maternal immune factors related to season may also contribute to prevalence of eczema based on immune markers in cord blood that vary by season.[50]

Patch test series are currently grouped by commonality of exposure rather than skin condition at time of sensitization, which is often not known. As discussed in the section "Immune Response to Less Potent Allergens", strong sensitizers function as their own irritant and can sensitize noninflamed skin. Most allergens on standard screening series are strong or medium potency allergens and therefore fail to detect the weaker potency allergens that sensitize patients with preexisting severe irritant contact dermatitis. As a result, allergic contact dermatitis caused by weakly potent allergens in the setting of irritant contact dermatitis is not well studied and the prevalence as well as recommendations for type and frequency of patch testing are not established.

CLINICAL COURSE AND PROGNOSIS

HARDENING

Irritant dermatitis often resolves despite continued exposure to the irritant; this is known as *harden-*

ing. The process is incompletely understood, which makes it difficult to know which patients will go on to develop chronic irritant hand dermatitis.[51] In a prospective experiment, participants challenged with repeated higher concentrations of sodium lauryl sulfate were more likely to harden than those challenged with lower concentrations or distilled water. Only about half of all participants hardened. Those who hardened and those who did not had similar measurements of hyperkeratosis and ceramide content of the stratum corneum.[52]

This area represents a tremendous knowledge gap. Hardening is the ideal response to unavoidable chronic irritant exposure. Understanding how to promote hardening could reduce the impact of allergic complications of irritant dermatitis including allergic contact dermatitis and atopic diseases.

MANAGEMENT

INTERVENTIONS

TOPICAL PREWORK PRODUCTS

British standards for occupational contact dermatitis suggest that the term *prework cream* replace *barrier cream* to avoid the suggestion that creams can replace more effective barrier equipment such as protective gloves.[53] These creams, designed for application prior to irritant exposure, may be modestly effective in some circumstances. A systematic review of barrier creams revealed considerable variation in methodology. The reviewers point out that participants were often tested on the forearm or back, rather than the hand, which is the most frequently affected site. Friction and multiple flexures on the hands may increase the risk of irritation at this site.[54] Barrier creams may not be applied in the same quantity in the workplace as in the studies. Barrier creams were more effective for preventing irritation from the detergent sodium lauryl sulfate and the alkaline sodium hydroxide than against the solvent toluene.[55]

MEDICATIONS

Given the weak evidence for the most commonly used treatments, avoidance of irritants is the best treatment option.

Although not clearly effective for prevention of hand dermatitis, use of emollients is recommended for treatment of hand dermatitis, even though some emollients appear to increase the penetration of allergen and irritants, and it is not clear which emollients are best in specific settings.[56] Only some emollients, usually with high lipid content, including petrolatum, accelerate barrier repair in experimentally induced irritant and allergic contact dermatitis.[57]

Topical corticosteroids are frequently used, but chronic use may impair barrier function by thinning the epidermis.[26] Topical immunomodulators may be of some benefit but are not consistently more effective than vehicle alone.[26]

Although rarely needed for purely irritant dermatitis, phototherapy and systemic immunosuppressive medications are often used for multifactorial dermatitis, such as hand dermatitis. Alitretinoin is considered second-line therapy for chronic hand dermatitis in Europe,[56] but is not available in the United States as of 2018.

COUNSELING

There is weak evidence that nurse-led counseling improves disease severity, but not quality of life, in patients with contact dermatitis of the hands.[58] Patients may increasingly prefer technology-assisted counseling, such as by telemedicine, as opposed to travel to a clinic, although traveling to a clinic is still needed for diagnostic testing, including patch testing.

Decreasing the frequency of exposure may allow a worker to continue with their job.[59] Alcohol-based hand sanitizers should substitute for hand washing whenever allowed, especially in cold seasons when indoor heating lowers ambient humidity.[56]

Gloves: Avoidance of irritants, including use of water-resistant gloves for wet work, is the best strategy to prevent and treat irritant dermatitis. In people without other irritant factors, that is, no history of childhood onset dermatitis to suggest genetically impaired barrier function, no use of irritant chemicals at work, infrequent wet work, occlusive gloves are well tolerated. However, occlusion alone can cause inflammation in skin that is already irritated.[60] Figure 25-14 shows a patient with atopic dermatitis where polyethylene film alone applied to the skin for 24 hours caused visible inflammation as did the adjacent 3 patch tests to sodium lauryl sulfate.

Occlusive gloves should be used for wet work but only worn for the shortest time possible. In persons with preexisting irritant dermatitis, cotton gloves are recommended under occlusive gloves if the duration of glove usage is longer than 10 minutes.[56]

People who itch with occlusion often also report itching with perspiration. The same factors that contribute to irritant dermatitis under gloves also cause irritation under bandages that mimic allergic contact dermatitis to adhesive.[61]

Patients who itch with occlusion generally prefer foam, lotion, or cream vehicles for topical products as they find ointments to cause itching.

TREATMENT ALGORITHM

Dermatitis should be treated as soon as it is recognized, as chronic dermatitis has a worse prognosis than acute dermatitis. All irritants should be avoided for weeks beyond visual recovery. There was lowered irritancy threshold lasting longer than 10 weeks after visual

Figure 25-14 Inflammation from a rectangular piece of polyethylene film applied to atopic skin for 24 hours and compared to 3 round chambers containing sodium lauryl sulfate applied to the same subject for 24 hours.

recovery from experimentally induced dermatitis from sodium lauryl sulfate applied 15 times to forearm skin over 3 weeks.[62]

The British guidelines for occupational contact dermatitis suggest referral to a dermatologist knowledgeable about patch testing for occupational contact dermatitis if there is no improvement 3 months after initial evaluation for dermatitis and if there is suspicion for allergic contact dermatitis or changes to job duties are contemplated.[53]

PREVENTION OF IRRITANT DERMATITIS

A systematic review published in 2010 found no significant evidence to prove efficacy of gloves, barrier creams, emollients, or worker education programs in preventing occupational irritant hand dermatitis.[63]

Barrier creams were discussed in the section "Topical Pre-Work Products" earlier. There are studies that show some emollients may provide some degree of prevention when used prior to developing dermatitis rather than as intervention for dermatitis. A study of normal volunteers who washed their hands 15 times daily with an antiseptic soap to mimic hand hygiene in health care workers found that 3 of 5 emollients decreased visible irritation and TEWL compared to no emollient.[64]

Duration of application prior to exposure may influence the degree to which it provides protection from an irritant. An emollient applied 15 minutes prior to exposure to sodium lauryl sulfate (SLS) prevented irritation as measured by TEWL, but daily use of the same emollient increased irritation after sodium lauryl sulfate exposure. This suggests that hydrated skin may be more susceptible to irritants and that prolonged use of emollients may actually increase the risk of irritant contact dermatitis.[65]

PREVENTION OF COMPLICATIONS

In regard to prevention of atopic dermatitis as a complication of irritant dermatitis resulting from genetic barrier deficits, a randomized controlled trial of daily application of emollients in infants from 3 weeks to 6 months of age showed a significant benefit in favor or emollients compared to no emollients. Thirteen percent of the control group used emollients despite randomization to the nonemollient group, and the authors did not comment on seasonal comparability of the control groups during this year-long study in cities in Oregon and the United Kingdom. Cream-based emollients were favored by parents in this study over oil- and ointment-based emollients.[66]

Another study of daily versus occasional application of petroleum jelly to infants from birth to 32 weeks of age showed lower incidence of dermatitis in the daily application group, but no significant decrease in sensitization to egg white as measured by antigen-specific immunoglobulin E to egg at 32 weeks of life.[67]

Prevention of both irritant contact dermatitis and its complications is understudied as discussed in the section "Clinical Course and Prognosis" on hardening. We do not know the components of emollients least likely to cause allergic contact dermatitis in various populations, the ideal pH of emollients, or the effect of various types of emollients on potentially inflammatory components of the microbiome.

SCREENING

Screening with a questionnaire to assess risk factors and visual assessment of health care worker's hands in Toronto revealed a 72% prevalence of mostly mild and some moderate hand dermatitis. Risk factors included handwashing frequency and duration of wearing gloves, but not age or gender.[68]

Screening may help identify early cases of irritant hand dermatitis, which is important because there is a delay in obtaining diagnostic patch testing from onset of symptoms ranging from 2 to 5 years. The delay is attributable to patient factors including hope that the condition will go away and anxiety over obtaining care, and to access, with most patients seeing a primary care physician first and then waiting for an appointment with dermatologist and then again after referral to a patch test expert.[69]

Given the association between chronicity and poor prognosis, screening may reduce societal burden of disease. However, reduced burden of disease will occur only with advances in treatment and improved understanding of ways to prevent complications.

REFERENCES

1. Smith SM, Nedorost ST. "Dermatitis" defined. *Dermatitis.* 2010;21(5):248-250.
2. Ramirez De Knott HM, McCormick TS, Offertory S, et al. Cutaneous hypersensitivity to *Candida albicans* in idiopathic vulvodynia. *Contact Dermatitis.* 2005;53(4):214-218.

3. Ramirez de Knott HM, McCormick TS, Kalka K, et al. Cutaneous hypersensitivity to *Malassezia sympodialis* and dust mite in adult atopic dermatitis with a textile pattern. *Contact Dermatitis*. 2006;54(2):92-99.
4. Nakamura Y, Oscherwitz J, Cease KB, et al. *Staphylococcus* δ-toxin induces allergic skin disease by activating mast cells. *Nature*. 2013;503(7476):397-401.
5. McFadden JP. Inflammatory skin diseases and "danger" signalling: time to take centre stage? *Br J Dermatol*. 2014;171(1):7-8.
6. Tovar R, Leikin JB. Irritants and corrosives. *Emerg Med Clin North Am*. 2015;33(1):117-131.
7. Agner T, Aalto-Korte K, Andersen KE, et al; European Environmental and Contact Dermatitis Research Group. Classification of hand eczema. *J Eur Acad Dermatol Venereol*. 2015;29(12):2417-2422.
8. Friis UF, Menné T, Schwensen JF, et al. Occupational irritant contact dermatitis diagnosed by analysis of contact irritants and allergens in the work environment. *Contact Dermatitis*. 2014;71(6):364-370.
9. Tupker R, Pinnagoda J, Coenraads P, et al. Susceptibility to irritants: a role of barrier function, skin dryness, and history of atopic dermatitis. *Br J Dermatol*. 1990;123(2):199-205.
10. Cahill JL, Williams JD, Matheson MC, et al. Occupational skin disease in Victoria, Australia. *Australas J Dermatol*. 2016;57(2):108-114.
11. Mollerup A, Veien NK, Johansen JD. An analysis of gender differences in patients with hand eczema—everyday exposures, severity, and consequences. *Contact Dermatitis*. 2014;71(1):21-30.
12. Stocks SJ, McNamee R, Turner S, et al. The impact of national-level interventions to improve hygiene on the incidence of irritant contact dermatitis in healthcare workers: changes in incidence from 1996 to 2012 and interrupted times series analysis. *Br J Dermatol*. 2015;173(1):165-171.
13. Kezic S, Kemperman PM, Koster ES, et al. Loss-of-function mutations in the filaggrin gene lead to reduced level of natural moisturizing factor in the stratum corneum. *J Invest Dermatol*. 2008;128(8):2117-2119.
14. Bandier J, Carlsen BC, Rasmussen MA, et al. Skin reaction and regeneration after single sodium lauryl sulfate exposure stratified by filaggrin genotype and atopic dermatitis phenotype. *Br J Dermatol*. 2015;172(6):1519-1529.
15. Landeck L, Visser M, Skudlik C, et al. Clinical course of occupational irritant contact dermatitis of the hands in relation to filaggrin genotype status and atopy. *Br J Dermatol*. 2012;167(6):1302-1309.
16. Callahan A, Baron E, Fekedulegn D, et al. Winter season, frequent hand washing, and irritant patch test reactions to detergents are associated with hand dermatitis in health care workers. *Dermatitis*. 2013;24(4):170-175.
17. Coman G, Zinsmeister C, Norris P. Occupational contact dermatitis: workers' compensation patch test results of Portland, Oregon, 2005-2014. *Dermatitis*. 2015;26(6):276-283.
18. Chew A, Maibach H. Occupational issues of irritant contact dermatitis. *Int Arch Occup Environ Health*. 2003;76(5):339-346.
19. Suwannahitatorn P, Jatapai A, Rangsin R. An outbreak of *Paederus* dermatitis in Thai military personnel. *J Med Assoc Thai*. 2014;97(suppl 2):S96-S100.
20. Lárraga-Piñones G, Heras-Mendaza F, Conde-Salazar L. Occupational contact dermatitis in the wind energy industry. *Actas Dermosifiliogr*. 2012;103(10):905-909.
21. Tüzün Y, Wolf R, Bağlam S, et al. Diaper (napkin) dermatitis: a fold (intertriginous) dermatosis. *Clin Dermatol*. 2015;33(4):477-482.
22. Marzario B, Burrows D, Skotnicki S. Contact dermatitis to personal sporting equipment in youth. *J Cutan Med Surg*. 2016;20(4):323-326.
23. Powell D, Ahmed S. Soccer shin guard reactions: allergic and irritant reactions. *Dermatitis*. 2010;21(3):162-166.
24. Sugaya M, Kuwano Y, Suga H, et al. Lymphatic dysfunction impairs antigen-specific immunization, but augments tissue swelling following contact with allergens. *J Invest Dermatol*. 2012;132(3, pt 1):667-676.
25. Segal R, Eskin-Schwartz M, Trattner A, et al. Recurrent flexural pellagroid dermatitis: an unusual variant of irritant contact dermatitis. *Acta Derm Venereol*. 2015;95(1):116-117.
26. Ale IS, Maibach HI. Irritant contact dermatitis. *Rev Environ Health*. 2014;29(3):195-206.
27. Kouris A, Armyra K, Christodoulou C, et al. Quality of life, anxiety, depression and obsessive-compulsive tendencies in patients with chronic hand eczema. *Contact Dermatitis*. 2015;72(6):367-370.
28. Saetterstrøm B, Olsen J, Johansen JD. Cost-of-illness of patients with contact dermatitis in Denmark. *Contact Dermatitis*. 2014;71(3):154-161.
29. Schliemann S, Schmidt C, Elsner P. Tandem repeated application of organic solvents and sodium lauryl sulphate enhances cumulative skin irritation. *Skin Pharmacol Physiol*. 2014;27(3):158-163.
30. Angelova-Fischer I, Stilla TR, Kezic S, et al. Barrier function and natural moisturizing factor levels after cumulative exposure to short-chain aliphatic alcohols and detergents: results of occlusion-modified tandem repeated irritation test. *Acta Derm Venereol*. 2016;96(7):880-884.
31. Tiedemann D, Clausen ML, John SM, et al. Effect of glove occlusion on the skin barrier. *Contact Dermatitis*. 2016;74(1):2-10.
32. Rupnik H, Rijavec M, Korošec P. Filaggrin loss-of-function mutations are not associated with atopic dermatitis that develops in late childhood or adulthood. *Br J Dermatol*. 2015;172(2):455-461.
33. Jacob SE, Goldenberg A, Nedorost S et al Flexural eczema versus atopic dermatitis. *Dermatitis*. 2015;26(3):109-115.
34. Engebretsen KA, Thyssen JP. Skin barrier function and allergens. *Curr Probl Dermatol*. 2016;49:90-102.
35. Bianchi ME. DAMPs, PAMPs and alarmins: all we need to know about danger. *J Leukoc Biol*. 2007;81(1):1-5.
36. Nakamura N, Tamagawa-Mineoka R, Ueta M, et al. Toll-like receptor 3 increases allergic and irritant contact dermatitis. *J Invest Dermatol*. 2015;135(2):411-417.
37. Zhang L, Tinkle SS. Chemical activation of innate and specific immunity in contact dermatitis. *J Invest Dermatol*. 2000;115(2):168-176.
38. Hammond MI, Chandra J, Retuerto M, et al. "Skin Microbiome in Atopic Dermatitis: Interactions Between Bacteria (*Staphylococcus*) and Fungi (*Alternaria*)" poster. Society for Investigative Dermatology Annual Meeting; Scottsdale, AZ; 2016 (manuscript in submission).
39. Gerberick GF, Robinson MK, Ryan CA, et al. Contact allergenic potency: correlation of human and local lymph node assay data. *Am J Contact Dermat*. 2001;12(3):156-161.
40. Kohli N, Nedorost S. Inflamed skin predisposes to sensitization to less potent allergens. *J Am Acad Dermatol*. 2016;75(2):312-317.e1.

41. Lee HY, Stieger M, Yawalkar N, et al. Cytokines and chemokines in irritant contact dermatitis. *Mediators Inflamm*. 2013;2013:916497.
42. Wennergren G. What if it is the other way around? Early introduction of peanut and fish seems to be better than avoidance. *Acta Paediatr*. 2009;98(7):1085-1087.
43. Newell L, Polak ME, Perera J, et al. Sensitization via healthy skin programs Th2 responses in individuals with atopic dermatitis. *J Invest Dermatol*. 2013;133(10):2372-2380.
44. Brandner JM, Zorn-Kruppa M, Yoshida T, et al. Epidermal tight junctions in health and disease. *Tissue Barriers*. 2015;3(1-2):e974451.
45. Kasemsarn P, Bosco J, Nixon RL. The role of the skin barrier in occupational skin diseases. *Curr Probl Dermatol*. 2016;49:135-143.
46. Bohaty B, Fricker C, Gonzalez S, et al. Visual and confocal microscopic interpretation of patch tests to benzethonium chloride and benzalkonium chloride. *Skin Res Technol*. 2012;18:272-277.
47. Burkhart C, Schloemer J, Zirwas M. Differentiation of latex allergy from irritant contact dermatitis. *Cutis*. 2015;96(6):369-371, 401.
48. Schwitulla J, Brasch J, Löffler H, et al. Skin irritability to sodium lauryl sulfate is associated with increased positive patch test reactions. *Br J Dermatol*. 2014;171(1):115-123.
49. Tanaka K, Matsui T, Sato A, et al. The relationship between the season of birth and early-onset food allergies in children. *Pediatr Allergy Immunol*. 2015;26(7):607-613.
50. Thysen AH, Rasmussen MA, Kreiner-Møller E, et al. Season of birth shapes neonatal immune function. *J Allergy Clin Immunol*. 2016;137(4):1238-1246.
51. Watkins SA, Maibach HI. The hardening phenomenon in irritant contact dermatitis: an interpretative update. *Contact Dermatitis*. 2009;60(3):123-130.
52. Park SY, Kim JH, Cho SI, et al. Induction of a hardening phenomenon and quantitative changes of ceramides in stratum corneum. *Ann Dermatol*. 2014;26(1):35-42.
53. Adisesh A, Robinson E, Nicholson PJ, et al; Standards of Care Working Group. U.K. standards of care for occupational contact dermatitis and occupational contact urticaria. *Br J Dermatol*. 2013;168(6):1167-1175.
54. Mostosi C, Simonart T. Effectiveness of barrier creams against irritant contact dermatitis. *Dermatology*. 2016;232(3):353-362.
55. Schliemann S, Petri M, Elsner P. Preventing irritant contact dermatitis with protective creams: influence of the application dose. *Contact Dermatitis*. 2014;70(1):19-26.
56. Diepgen TL, Andersen KE, Chosidow O, et al. Guidelines for diagnosis, prevention and treatment of hand eczema—short version. *J Dtsch Dermatol Ges*. 2015;13(1):77-85.
57. Held E, Lund H, Agner T. Effect of different moisturizers on SLS-irritated human skin. *Contact Dermatitis*. 2001;44(4):229-234.
58. Mollerup A, Veien NK, Johansen JD. Effectiveness of the healthy skin clinic—a randomized clinical trial of nurse-led patient counselling in hand eczema. *Contact Dermatitis*. 2014;71(4):202-214.
59. Lurati AR. Occupational risk assessment and irritant contact dermatitis. *Workplace Health Saf*. 2015;63(2):81-87.
60. Fartasch M. Wet work and barrier function. *Curr Probl Dermatol*. 2016;49:144-151.
61. Smith SM, Zirwas MJ. Nonallergic reactions to medical tapes. *Dermatitis*. 2015;26(1):38-43.
62. Choi JM, Lee JY, Cho BK. Chronic irritant contact dermatitis: recovery time in man. *Contact Dermatitis*. 2000;42(5):264-269.
63. Bauer A, Schmitt J, Bennett C, et al. Interventions for preventing occupational irritant hand dermatitis. *Cochrane Database Syst Rev*. 2010;(6):CD004414.
64. Williams C, Wilkinson SM, McShane P, et al. A double-blind, randomized study to assess the effectiveness of different moisturizers in preventing dermatitis induced by hand washing to simulate healthcare use. *Br J Dermatol*. 2010;162(5):1088-1092.
65. Held E, Sveinsdóttir S, Agner T. Effect of long-term use of moisturizer on skin hydration, barrier function and susceptibility to irritants. *Acta Derm Venereol*. 1999;79(1):49-51.
66. Simpson EL, Chalmers JR, Hanifin JM, et al. Emollient enhancement of the skin barrier from birth offers effective atopic dermatitis prevention. *J Allergy Clin Immunol*. 2014;134(4):818-823.
67. Horimukai K, Morita K, Narita M, et al. Application of moisturizer to neonates prevents development of atopic dermatitis. *J Allergy Clin Immunol*. 2014;134(4):824-830.e6.
68. Nichol K, Copes R, Spielmann S, et al. Workplace screening for hand dermatitis: a pilot study. *Occup Med (Lond)*. 2016;66(1):46-49.
69. Nurmohamed S, Bodley T, Thompson A, et al. Health care utilization characteristics in patch test patients. *Dermatitis*. 2014;25(5):268-272.

Chapter 26 :: Seborrheic Dermatitis
:: Dae Hun Suh

第二十六章
脂溢性皮炎

中文导读

本章共分为6节：①临床特征；②病因和发病机制；③诊断；④鉴别诊断；⑤临床病程和预后；⑥治疗。

第一节介绍了脂溢性皮炎（SD）的临床特征，包括患病率、影响因素、皮损形态、分布部位、症状等。还介绍了婴儿脂溢性皮炎（ISD）、落屑性红皮病、石棉状糠疹、HIV相关SD的临床特点和病因。

第二节介绍了SD的病因和发病机制，主要涉及炎症与免疫反应、微生物效应、脂质与宿主易感性、表皮过度增殖、神经递质转运异常。

第三节介绍了SD的诊断，主要依靠临床诊断。指出皮肤镜检查能够详细识别形态结构，这对于诊断头皮的SD尤其有用。

第四节介绍了SD的鉴别诊断，如银屑病、特应性皮炎。

第五节介绍了SD的临床病程和预后，指出其多为慢性复发性，ISD可自然消失。

第六节介绍了SD的治疗，具体讲述了各种治疗手段的使用方法和价值，指出SD一线治疗的主要建议是局部用药，包括皮质类固醇、钙调神经磷酸酶抑制药、抗真菌药等。

〔李 捷〕

AT-A-GLANCE

- Seborrheic dermatitis is a common inflammatory skin disease affecting various age groups.
- Erythematous, greasy, scaling patches and plaques appear on scalp, face, ears, chest, and intertriginous areas.
- Severe forms, like generalized erythroderma, rarely occur.
- Etiology is unclear but may be related to abnormal immune mechanism, *Malassezia*, sebaceous glands, and individual susceptibility.
- Treatment is based on symptomatic control.

Seborrheic dermatitis (SD) is clinically characterized by erythematous, scaly patches on sebaceous gland–rich sites, including scalp, face, upper trunk, and intertriginous areas.[1] The affected areas present as various appearances from mild pinkish and sometimes greasy scaling to solid adherent crusts. Patients with this condition complain of discomfort, with symptoms of itching and burning, and also have some serious cosmetic problems, leading to psychosocial distress that has a negative impact on their quality of life.[2] SD arises in all races and ethnic groups and has a worldwide distribution, but a higher incidence and more-severe forms are observed in AIDS patients and individuals with certain neurologic conditions, such as Parkinson disease.[3]

CLINICAL FEATURES

GENERAL FEATURES

SD usually appears as a chronic and relapsing pattern in adolescents and young adults when the activity of sebaceous glands increases from hormonal effects, with the incidence increasing in patients with older than 50 years of age.[4] SD can also affect babies as young as age 2 weeks with peak incidence at 3 months of age, which is called *infantile seborrheic dermatitis* (ISD; Fig. 26-1). The overall prevalence of SD in general population is between 2.35% and 11.30%, depending on the study.[5] A male predominance is observed in all ages without any racial or regional predilection. SD is often influenced by a seasonal impact. It becomes more common and severe in the cold and dry climates, whereas it may be mitigated by sun exposure. However, several cases induced by treatment of psoralen plus ultraviolet A (PUVA) therapy have been reported.[6]

The symptoms of SD are mainly chronic, persistent, and recurrent. The red, flaking, and greasy lesions of scalp and face are easily observed, particularly on nasolabial folds (Fig. 26-2); eyebrows, upper eyelid, forehead, postauricular areas (Fig. 26-3); external audi-

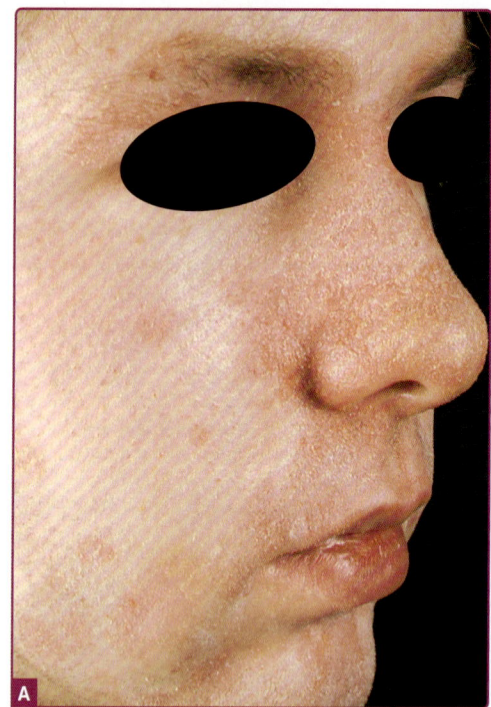

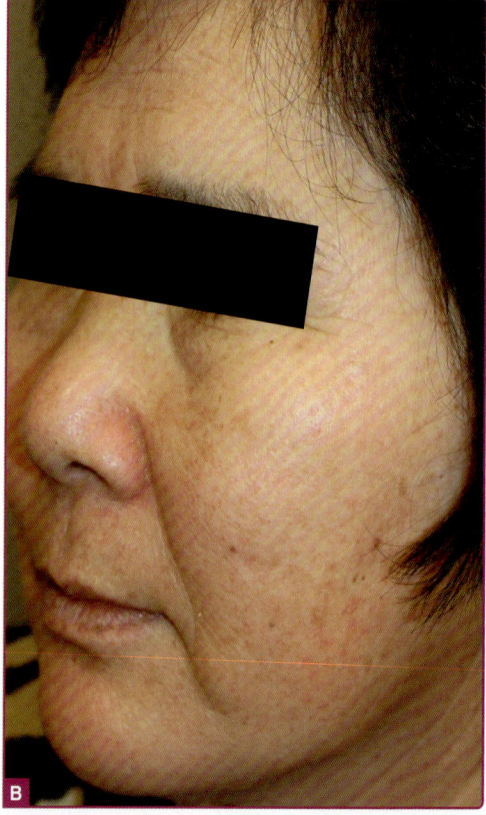

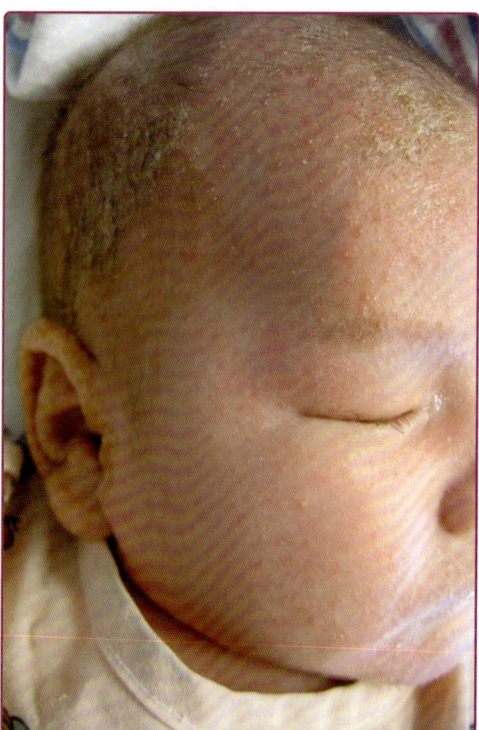

Figure 26-1 Cradle cap or infantile seborrheic dermatitis. (Photo contributed by University of North Carolina Department of Dermatology. From Tintinalli JE, et al. Rashes in infants and children. In Tintinalli JE, et al. *Tintinalli's Emergency Medicine: A Comprehensive Study Guide.* 8th ed. New York, NY: McGraw-Hill Education; 2016:934-952, Fig. 141-30.)

Figure 26-2 Seborrheic dermatitis with involvement of (**A**) nasolabial folds, cheeks, eyebrows, and nose in white person and (**B**) nasolabial folds in a person of Asian descent.

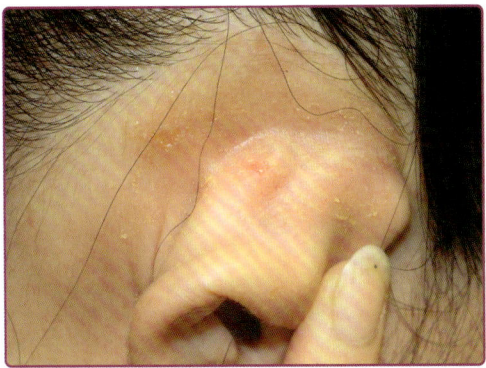

Figure 26-3 Seborrheic dermatitis of the postauricular area.

tory canal and auricle (Fig. 26-4), with generally symmetrical distribution. SD can appear in other sites, such as occiput and neck. When the sternal area on the chest (Fig. 26-5), upper back (Fig. 26-6), and umbilicus are involved, petaloid or arcuate lesions with fine pink scale can be seen. In contrast, intertriginous areas, including inguinal and axillary regions, show less scale, making SD easily confusable with intertrigo. However, variations of these clinical appearances are common. Scalp involvement is more common in the male patient, in the patient with long disease duration, and in the patient with a history of acne.[1] The severity of SD varies from mild erythema and pruritus to severe, oily, thick scale with a burning or tingling sensation. Some patients with SD also may present with *Pityrosporum* folliculitis and blepharitis. *Pityrosporum* folliculitis typically manifests as a diffuse papulopustular eruption with peripheral erythema on the trunk and arises more in immunocompromised patients. Seborrheic blepharitis usually appears as a type of anterior blepharitis, inducing flaking and scaling on the eyelids and creating uncomfortable, irritating problems.

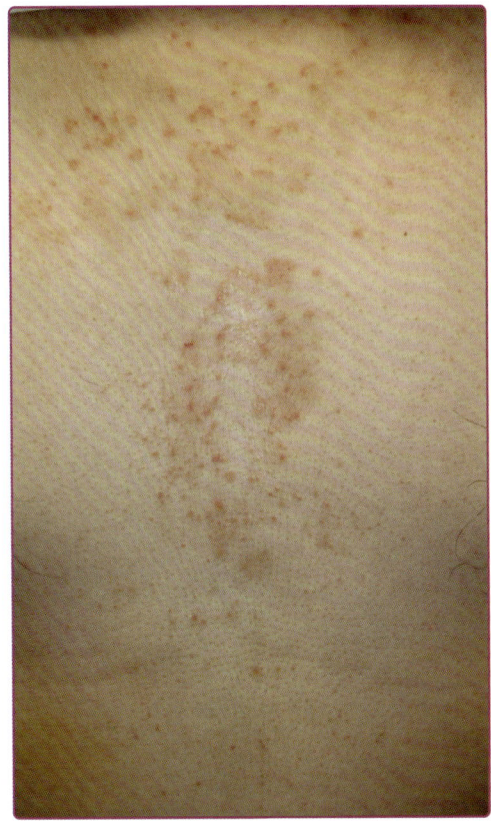

Figure 26-5 Seborrheic dermatitis of the chest.

Characteristically, ISD has a relatively different feature in contrast with SD in older ages. The nonpruritic skin eruption generally affects the frontal or vertex areas (or both areas) of the scalp and the central areas of the face with dry, thick, adherent, and flaking scale, and may be accompanied

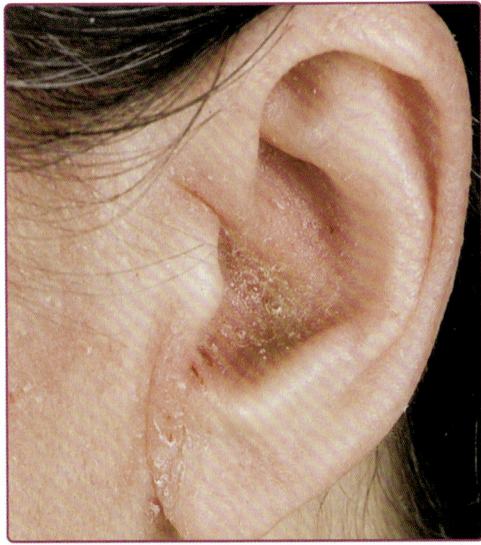

Figure 26-4 Seborrheic dermatitis of the ear: external canal, concha bowl, and auricle.

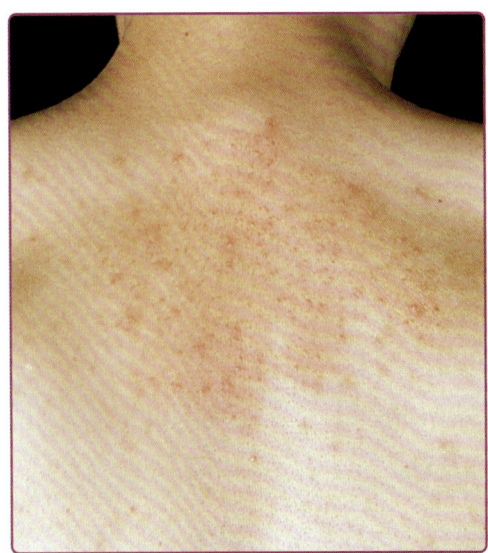

Figure 26-6 Seborrheic dermatitis of the upper back.

by erythematous rash on intertriginous folds of the trunk and extremities (Fig. 26-7). The extensive involvement of the scalp, commonly called "cradle cap," is one of the typical appearances observed in ISD. ISD normally resolves spontaneously within the first 6 to 12 months of life. Extensive and serious conditions should be differentiated from immunosuppressed status.

LEINER DISEASE

The term *Leiner disease* was first introduced by Carl Leiner in 1908, to describe infants with desquamative erythroderma, sparse hair, frequent loose stools, and failure to thrive.[7] Later, Miller reported other patients with similar clinical features who had generalized SD. Miller also found a lack of opsonization by the serum of the patients.[8] Since Miller's findings it has become clear that Leiner disease is an umbrella phenotype rather than a single-disease entity, and a variety of immunologic defects have been identified.[9] Congenital or acquired deficiencies of C3, C5, and phagocytic activity results in defective opsonization of yeast and bacteria. Association of Leiner disease and Netherton syndrome was also suggested.[9] Secondary bacterial infection can bring death to a Leiner disease patient, so appropriate treatment, such as IV hydration, temperature regulation, and antibiotics, is essential. Infusion of fresh-frozen plasma or whole blood can be beneficial in supplementing the deficient factors in a hereditary form of Leiner's disease.[8] The prognosis of Leiner disease depends on the nature of the underlying immunologic abnormality of the patients.

PITYRIASIS AMIANTACEA

Asbestos-like scalp, called pityriasis amiantacea, was first described by Alibert in 1832. Pityriasis amiantacea is also called tinea asbestina, tinea amiantacea, keratosis follicularis amiantacea, and porrigo amiantacea. Pityriasis amiantacea is an inflammatory condition of the scalp that is characterized by large plates of thick, silvering scale firmly adherent to both the scalp and hair tufts (Fig. 26-8). This can be a localized or diffuse condition, and is attributed to diffuse hyperkeratosis and parakeratosis with follicular keratosis surrounding each hair with a sheath of corneocytes and debris. It is more common in females and it may occur at any age, often without evident causes. Alopecia, which is generally reversible but is sometimes cicatricial, is a common feature of pityriasis amiantacea.[10] Concomitant secondary bacterial infection, mostly *Staphylococcus aureus*, may result in scarring alopecia, so early and appropriate treatment is necessary. The most frequent skin diseases associated with pityriasis amiantacea are psoriasis (35%) and eczematous conditions like SD and atopic dermatitis (34%). Of pediatric patients with pityriasis amiantacea, lesions in 2% to 15% develop into typical psoriasis.[11] Pityriasis amiantacea may also manifest as a complication of lichen planus, lichen simplex chronicus, superficial fungal, or pyogenic infection, or as an adverse effect of molecu-

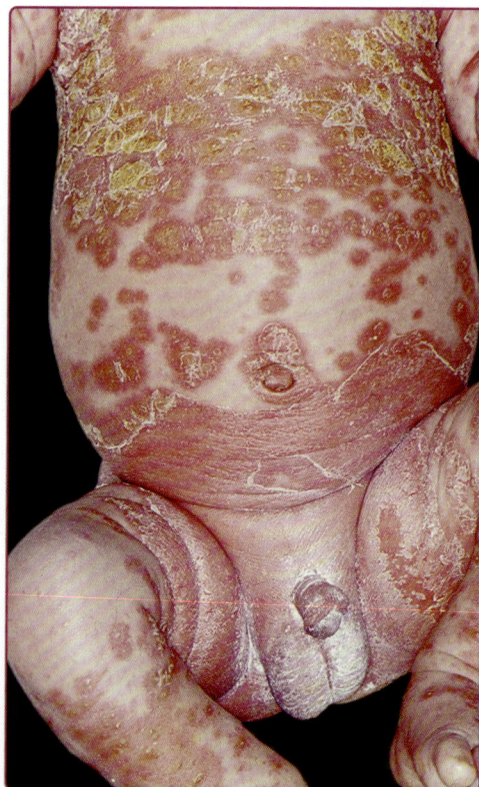

Figure 26-7 Seborrheic dermatitis in an infant. Widespread pattern of seborrheic dermatitis with psoriasiform lesions on the trunk and groin.

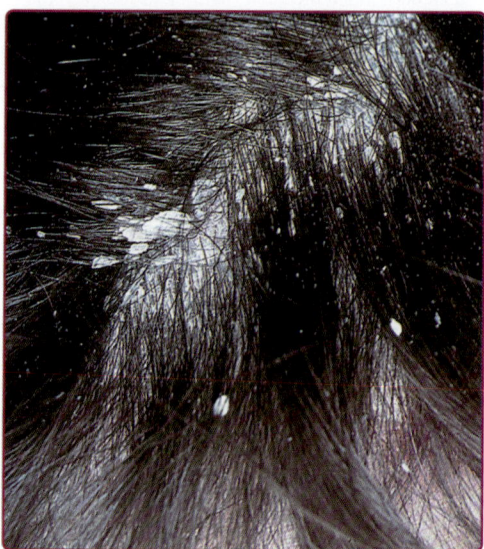

Figure 26-8 Pityriasis amiantacea. Masses of sticky silvery scales adhere to the scalp and cause matting of hairs they surround.

larly targeted therapy such as vemurafenib.[12,13] In these cases, therapy should be directed toward the underlying etiology.

ASSOCIATIONS OF HIV AND AIDS

SD arises in more extensive and refractory patterns in up to 83% of HIV-seropositive and AIDS patients (Fig. 26-9).[4] The initial clinical symptom may appear as a butterfly-like rash seen in systemic lupus erythematosus. SD is associated with reduction of T-cell function, and gets worse as the CD4+ lymphocyte count decreases, making SD an indicator for evaluating the progression of AIDS.[14]

ETIOLOGY AND PATHOGENESIS

Many studies to uncover the pathogenesis of SD in adult and adolescent patients have been conducted, but the etiology has not been clearly identified yet. Multifactorial causes, including several endogenous and exogenous predisposing factors, are associated with SD. The role of sebaceous glands in pathogenesis of SD is notable considering time and lesional distribution of SD. The immunologic status of patients or the susceptibility to SD can be an important factor because SD is much more seen in those with certain underlying diseases such as AIDS and Parkinson disease. *Malassezia* may also be one of the causes of SD as antifungal medications are effective. The relationship of the SD lesions with seasonal fluctuations or sun exposure implies that multiple exogenous factors can contribute to the development of SD.

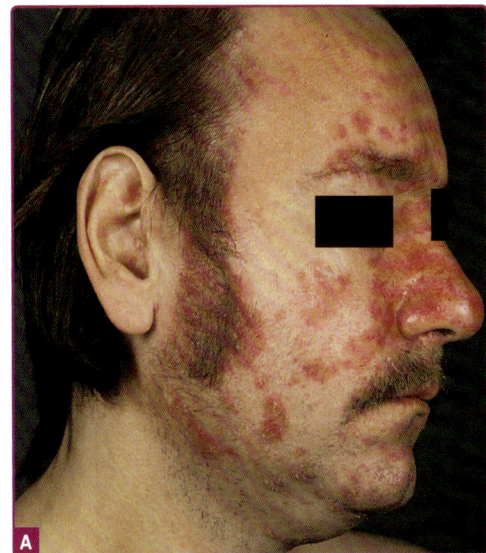

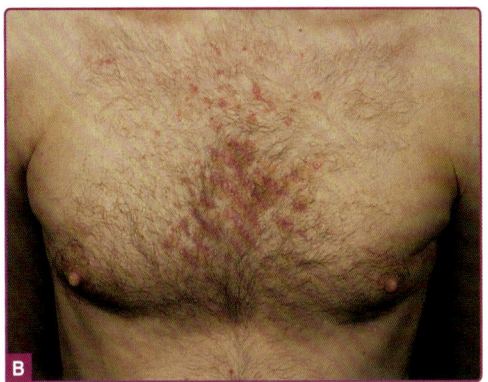

Figure 26-9 Wide spread unusual distribution pattern of seborrheic dermatitis in a patient with AIDS. **A,** Moist patches on the centrofacial region, beard, and scalp. **B,** Moist lesions on the chest. In patients with AIDS, seborrheic dermatitis responds poorly to conventional therapy.

IMMUNE RESPONSE AND INFLAMMATION

The immune component may be important in the pathogenesis of SD because SD is much more common in immunosuppressed patients. The DBA/2 2C TCR transgenic mouse, which has a defect in expression of CD4+ and CD8+ cells owing to the lack of T-cell progenitor thymocytes, exhibited SD-like eruptions.[15] Several studies have focused on the cellular immunity and humoral immunity in SD, but there are some controversies. One study showed a normal CD4+-to-CD8+ ratio, whereas another study demonstrated a decreased CD4+-to-CD8+ ratio in 68% of patients.[16] A decrease in the number of B cells in 28% of patients and a rise of the number of natural killer cells in 48% of patients were reported. In addition, 60% of patients showed an increase in CD8+ cells and 70% of patients showed a diminished CD4+-to-CD8+ ratio.

Also, it was stated that SD patients had an increased production of immunoglobulin (Ig) A and IgG antibodies in serum.[16] However, there was no change in the total amount of antibodies against *Malassezia* in SD, suggesting that changes to the antibodies are not likely linked with *Malassezia*.[17] The alteration of inflammatory cytokines in patients with SD has been demonstrated by immunohistochemical studies. The production of interleukin (IL)-1α, IL-1β, IL-4, IL-12, tumor necrosis factor-α, and interferon (IFN)-γ was increased in the lesions compared with the normal skin.[18] Significantly increased IL-1RA–to–IL-1α and IL-1RA–to–IL-8 ratios, as well as overproduction of histamine, were also shown to occur in SD when compared with healthy controls.[19] An investigation of gene expression by DNA microarrays in 15 patients with dandruff showed the reciprocal expression of induced inflammatory genes and repressed lipid metabolism genes compared with nondandruff individuals.[20] The expression of induced inflammatory genes was distinctly observed in uninvolved skin of the patients as well, indicating the presence of predisposing factors related to inflammation in patients with SD. Furthermore, inflammation induced by oxidative stress through reactive oxygen species may have a potential role in the pathogenesis of SD.[21]

MICROBIAL EFFECTS

Malassezia, normal flora that inhabits human skin, is suggested to be important in SD. This opinion is based on the evidences that the common lesions of SD are related to the distribution of sebaceous glands where *Malassezia* preferentially colonizes, and that antifungal medications have therapeutic effects on SD. A decline in the number of *Malassezia* by use of antifungal agents corresponds with the relief of the symptoms.[4] Moreover, pityriasis versicolor and *Pityrosporum* folliculitis, induced by *Malassezia*, are commonly accompanied by SD. However, there is a lack of difference in *Malassezia* counts between patients with SD and healthy individuals. In addition, a mycelial form of *Malassezia*, a pathogenic form observed in pityriasis versicolor, has not been detected in SD.[17] These facts propose a complex causative role of *Malassezia* for SD. The prevalence and types of the most predominant *Malassezia* species found on SD lesions differ among studies, countries, or parts of body, but *Malassezia globosa* and *Malassezia restricta* are considered to be the most important of the 14 *Malassezia* species identified.[4,22] The complete genome sequences of *M. globosa* and *M. restricta* have been determined and these genomes encode lipase and phospholipase, making the species lipophilic or lipid-dependent.[23] The primary role of these enzymes is to metabolize lipid into fatty acids to produce fungal cell walls responsible for virulence, including invasion and dissemination.[24] Not all *M. globosa* or *M. restricta* strains were found in SD, implying that there may exist specific strains capable of causing the disease.[25] Also, an increased amount of *Malassezia furfur* was observed in patients with SD versus healthy controls.[26] The high concentration of *M. furfur* can disturb protective skin barriers and induce inflammation. *Malassezin*, generated by *M. furfur* or *M. restricta*, can serve as agonists to aryl hydrocarbon receptor, which is involved in the differentiation of T-helper 17 cells and the mediation of contact sensitivity.[27]

LIPID AND HOST SUSCEPTIBILITY FACTORS

Several analyses of skin surface lipids in patients with SD or dandruff have shown alterations in those irrespective of HIV status.[28] These findings were not consistent with one another, but they introduced the causative relationship between SD and the composition of skin surface lipids. Specifically, irritating free fatty acids, such as oleic acid produced by lipase of *M. globosa*, could mediate dandruff-like flaking in the dandruff-susceptible individuals with SD but not in nonsusceptible individuals.[29] Individual susceptibility is considered to be associated with a disrupted epidermal barrier that allows penetration of the irritating metabolites. The process for *Malassezia* to reach the aryl hydrocarbon receptor in the granular and spinous layers also may depend on such defective skin character. This host susceptibility factor could explain the lack of a positive correlation between the number of *Malassezia* and the severity of dandruff.

EPIDERMAL HYPERPROLIFERATION

Increased epidermal turnover in SD, which is also shown in psoriasis, implicates SD in a disorder of hyperproliferation, and *Malassezia* can be considered as one of the incidental outcomes derived from the phenomenon. SD resembles psoriasis in many aspects, both clinically and histologically, and it is sometimes difficult to differentiate the two diseases even after a skin biopsy. There are case reports that keratolytics and antiinflammatory medications were successful in the treatment of the patients with SD whose treatment with amphotericin B had failed.[30] This alteration of epidermis may be related with the increased activity of calmodulin and explains the basis of use of cytostatic medications such as azelaic acid.[31]

NEUROTRANSMITTER ABNORMALITIES

SD expressed in Parkinson disease has been thought to result from the elevated levels of sebum allowing the proliferation of *Malassezia*. Bilateral seborrhea observed in unilateral parkinsonism suggests the changes of sebum levels are presumably triggered by endocrine effects rather than neurotrophic effects. It may be associated with an increased circulating α-melanocyte–stimulating hormone in Parkinson disease.[32] Because the severity of SD in Parkinson disease does not correlate with the sebum excretion rate, the sebum accumulation by facial immobility may play a key role. Administration of levodopa can clinically improve the skin symptoms by reducing the sebum production or secretion by restoring the production of melanocyte-stimulating hormone-inhibiting factor. The prevalence of SD is also increased in patients with other neurologic disorders, including mood disorder, Alzheimer disease, syringomyelia, epilepsy, cerebrovascular infarcts, postencephalitis, mental retardation, poliomyelitis, quadriplegia, trigeminal nerve injury, and alcoholism. Indoor lifestyle with less sunlight exposure and hygiene status of the patients may function in this association.[4]

OTHER FACTORS

Low humidity and cold temperatures worsen SD, especially in the winter and early spring. Facial trauma (eg, scratching) and PUVA therapy also are aggravating factors.[6] Multiple drugs can lead to SD-like eruptions, including griseofulvin, cimetidine, lithium, methyldopa, arsenic, gold, auranofin, aurothioglucose, buspirone, chlorpromazine, ethionamide, haloperidol, IFN-α, phenothiazines, stanozolol, thiothixene, psoralen, methoxsalen, and trioxsalen. The SD-like dermatitis also appears in patients with zinc deficiency (acrodermatitis enteropathica and acrodermatitis enteropathica–like conditions) or biotin deficiency, but the skin eruptions do not respond to zinc or biotin supplementation.[33] It is noted that the familial form of SD was reported in an Israeli Jewish family of Moroccan descent, which was caused by autosomal dominant genetic mutation (ZNF750) encoding a zinc finger protein (C2H2).[34]

DIAGNOSIS

The diagnosis of SD remains a clinical one, based on SD's characteristic morphology and patterns. Dermoscopy enables the detailed identification of morphologic structures, which is especially helpful in diagnosing SD of the scalp. The typical magnified vascular patterns observed by dermoscopy are twisted loop, red dots and globules, and glomerular vessels in scalp psoriasis, but arborizing vessels and atypical red vessels in SD.[35] A skin biopsy is not routinely required, but may be useful when the diagnosis is unclear. The various histopathologic features can be observed depending on the different stages of the disease: acute, subacute, and chronic. Acute and subacute SD may exhibit slight to moderate spongiotic dermatitis with mild psoriasiform hyperplasia, folliculocentric crust containing scattered neutrophils at the tips of the follicular opening, orthokeratosis with focal parakeratosis, and superficial perivascular lymphohistiocytic infiltration. Chronic SD shows a more intense pattern of the foregoing features with minimal spongiosis and markedly dilated superficial vessels. However, the histopathologic picture in chronic cases is sometimes similar to those of psoriasis, and careful attention should be paid to the histopathology reading. HIV-associated SD is histologically distinctive from the ordinary SD, showing very severe patterns such as extensive parakeratosis, leukoexocytosis, necrosis of keratinocytes, and superficial perivascular infiltrate of plasma cells (Table 26-1).[36] Lesion scraping for a potassium hydroxide preparation can be beneficial to confirm the diagnosis of accompanied *Pityrosporum* folliculitis. It should be kept in mind that SD can simultaneously occur with other dermatoses. When SD occurs in infants, the classic diagnostic criteria suggested by Beare and Rook can be used in diagnosing ISD. It is composed of early onset (before 6 months of age); erythematous and scaling rash distributed in the scalp, diaper, or flexural areas; and the relative absence of pruritus.[37] Involvement of the diaper area alone is considered as a characteristic sign favoring a psoriasiform type of ISD. Above all, the clinician should remember that there is not a characteristic pathognomonic feature or laboratory test to establish the accurate diagnosis of SD.

DIFFERENTIAL DIAGNOSIS

Several diseases should be considered in the differential diagnosis of SD (Tables 26-2 and 26-3), especially as ISD is easily confused with atopic dermatitis, psoriasis, histiocytosis, and scabies; sometimes it is impossible to distinguish among these diseases in infants younger than 3 months of age. Checking family history and pruritus and taking certain laboratory tests including serum IgE levels and multiple allergen stimulation tests may give a clue to whether it is atopic dermatitis or ISD. When the skin eruption arises solely on the scalp, an involvement of frontal hair lines is a distinctive feature for scalp psoriasis.[38] Langerhans cell histiocytosis, previously called Letterer-Siwe disease has more generally purpuric lesions and tends to desquamate on the scalp and ulcerate on the folds and the mucosal areas. Severe itching that includes the palms and soles suggests scabies. Intertrigo, contact dermatitis, neonatal erythroderma, and multiple carboxylase deficiency should also be excluded in infants.[39]

CLINICAL COURSE AND PROGNOSIS

Generally SD in adolescents or adults has a chronic and recurrent relapsing course. Consequently, the primary goal of treatment should be control of symptoms like pruritus, erythema, and scales, rather than cure of dis-

TABLE 26-1

Histopathologic Differences between Classic Seborrheic Dermatitis and AIDS-Associated Seborrheic Dermatitis

CLASSIC SEBORRHEIC DERMATITIS	AIDS-ASSOCIATED SEBORRHEIC DERMATITIS
Epidermis	
Limited parakeratosis	Widespread parakeratosis
Rare necrotic keratinocytes	Many necrotic keratinocytes
No interface obliteration	Focal interface obliteration with clusters of lymphocytes
Prominent spongiosis	Sparse spongiosis
Dermis	
Thin-walled vessels	Many thick-walled vessels
Rare plasma cells	Increased plasma cells
No leukocytoclasis	Focal leukocytoclasis

From Soeprono FF, Schinella RA, Cockerell CJ, Comite SL. Seborrheic-like dermatitis of acquired immunodeficiency syndrome. A clinicopathologic study. *J Am Acad Dermatol.* 1986;14(2):242-248, with permission.

ease. Also, patients should be informed that they need to prepare for a future re-outbreak and avoid aggravating factors of SD. However, ISD has a benign, self-limited course; ISD spontaneously disappears by 6 to 12 months of age. Severe exacerbation with exfoliating dermatitis may occur, albeit rarely, but its prognosis is usually favorable. ISD does not progress to adulthood.

MANAGEMENT

Basically, using emollients (eg, mineral oil, vegetable oil, or petroleum jelly) can help improve symptoms such as scales. Soft rubbing with a brush or comb aids removing thick, adherent scales, but aggressive scraping should be avoided because it can induce further inflammation. The main recommendations for the first-line treatment of SD are topical medications, including corticosteroids, calcineurin inhibitors, antifungal drugs, and keratolytics. In the case of topical corticosteroids, mild-potency formulations are recommended to be used first because of their cutaneous adverse effects and frequent rebound phenomena. Treatment with corticosteroids is highly effective for reducing erythema, scaling, and pruritus rapidly, resulting in total clearance more often than placebo.[40] Topical calcineurin inhibitors (tacrolimus and pimecrolimus) manifest good effects on SD by blocking calcineurin, thus preventing both inflammatory cytokines and a signaling pathway in T-lymphocyte cells. No difference between topical calcineurin inhibitors and topical corticosteroids in total clearance was identified in short-term trials.[40] There is no risk of telangiectasia and skin atrophy, so topical calcineurin inhibitors are recommended

TABLE 26-2
Site-Specific Differential Diagnosis of Seborrheic Dermatitis

Scalp[a]	Psoriasis, atopic dermatitis, impetigo, tinea capitis[a] (mimics dandruff in children)
Face	Psoriasis, rosacea, contact dermatitis, impetigo, discoid lupus, sarcoid (petaloid type in African Americans), drug-induced photosensitivity
Ear canal	Psoriasis, contact dermatitis
Eyelids	Atopic dermatitis, psoriasis, *Demodex folliculorum* infestation
Chest, back	Pityriasis rosea, tinea versicolor, subacute cutaneous lupus, psoriasis vulgaris
Groin, buttock	Intertrigo (fungal, *Candida*, erythrasma), glucagonoma, extramammary Paget disease, zinc deficiency
Intertriginous	Inverse psoriasis, candidiasis, erythrasma, contact dermatitis, tinea intertrigo, Langerhans cell histiocytosis (Letterer-Siwe disease in infants)
Generalized[b]	Scabies, secondary syphilis, pemphigus foliaceus, pemphigus erythematosus, Leiner disease (infants), drug eruption
Erythrodermic[c]	Psoriasis, contact dermatitis, pityriasis rubra pilaris, drug eruption, mycosis fungoides (Sézary syndrome), lichen planus, chronic actinic dermatitis, HIV, Hodgkin disease, paraneoplastic syndrome, leukemia cutis

[a]Diffuse scalp dermatitis or inflammatory alopecia in children warrants fungal culture, potassium hydroxide preparation.
[b]Widespread truncal types warrant scabies prep and rapid plasma reagin to rule out syphilis.
[c]Erythrodermic type should be biopsied.

TABLE 26-3
Comparison of Infantile Seborrheic Dermatitis with Differential Diagnoses

INFANTILE SEBORRHEIC DERMATITIS	"NAPKIN" PSORIASIS	ATOPIC DERMATITIS	LETTERER-SIWE DISEASE
Occurs in the first few weeks to 3 months	Onset at 3 months	Onset within first 2 months of life, most within the first year	Occurs in newborns; other types of Langerhans cell histiocytosis (LCH) may occur between 1 and 3 years of age
Self-limited, regresses spontaneously	Self-limited	Severity decreases with age	Fatal if untreated; other variants of LCH have differing prognoses
Vertex scalp most commonly affected	Diaper commonly affected; scalp and face may be affected	Face primarily involved	Trunk and scalp involved
Adherent, yellow-brown, greasy scale	Macerated, shiny erythema on diaper region	Intensely pruritic, erythematous papules with excoriation, vesicles and serous exudate; skin appears dry	Slightly raised, rose-yellow papules on trunk that may crust and ulcerate
Face, neck, trunk, and extremities may be affected with intertriginous sites affected (axillae, groin); isolated diaper lesions more suggestive of seborrheic dermatitis	Similarly extensive involvement, but less scaling on intertriginous sites; diaper region primarily affected	Forearms and shins (extensors) often affected, axillae are spared; diaper area usually spared	Extensive involvement with moist erythematous plaques and petechial lesions on intertriginous areas; scalp involvement similar to seborrheic dermatitis

for application to the susceptible regions instead of topical corticosteroids. There are no studies comparing the efficacy of tacrolimus with pimecrolimus in SD. Maintenance therapy with topical calcineurin inhibitors may be useful in preventing the relapse or exacerbation, but their long-term safety has not been verified. Based on the presumed etiologic roles of *Malassezia*, ketoconazole has been the most heavily investigated topical agent for SD. Several randomized studies have demonstrated that 1% to 2% ketoconazole significantly lowers and improves the severity of SD versus placebo, achieving an equal remission rate with corticosteroids, with nearly 44% fewer adverse events.[41] The use of 1% ciclopirox also improved skin symptoms. In single studies for evaluating the short-term efficacy of clotrimazole and miconazole, those had almost equivalent impacts on SD compared with corticosteroids.[41] Other topical antifungal agents, such as bifonazole, terbinafine, fluconazole, and zinc pyrithione, are also likely to be useful.[4] Dandruff or pityriasis simplex capillitii may be treated by shampoos containing zinc pyrithione, selenium sulfide, ketoconazole, salicylic acid, ciclopirox, and coal tar. Lithium seems to have an antiinflammatory role inhibiting the release of arachidonic acid and restricting availability of free fatty acids essential for the growth of *Malassezia*.[42] Topical lithium has shown good results in total clearance both in HIV-negative patients and in AIDS-associated SD. Topical sulfur, propylene glycol, metronidazole, and benzoyl peroxide wash have also been used. Seborrheic blepharitis should be managed by long-term eyelid hygiene with warm compresses, followed by proper topical antibiotics and topical corticosteroid to reduce the bacterial load and marked inflammation, respectively.[43] Aluminum acetate solution can be used to decrease the symptoms of seborrheic otitis externa. In cases refractory to topical treatment, systemic therapies can be prescribed for uncontrolled multiple widespread lesions and severe cases. Low doses of systemic glucocorticoids may be used for a short period. Patients should know that SD can be controlled but not eradicated. SD patients treated by glucocorticoids should be informed of the side effects and rebound flares that occur after discontinuation of glucocorticoids. Oral antifungals may be tried for severe and refractory cases. Itraconazole, fluconazole, and pramiconazole have been used with various regimens.[44] For example, itraconazole 200 mg/day for the first 7 days of the month for several months is a regimen used to get clinical improvement. The daily administration of isotretinoin 0.1 to 0.5 mg/kg also may be effective in severe cases.

The basic principle of treatment is the same for infants. When ISD involves the diaper areas, the use of superabsorbent disposable diapers with frequent changes prevents the aggravation of the symptoms.[45] Soap and alcohol-containing compounds are not recommended in cleaning the diaper lesions. Topical medications having antifungal and antiinflammatory activities are effective choices that have a high clinical cure rate. A mild-potency steroid, such as 1% hydrocortisone, is preferred but used with caution because of its adverse effects. In more refractory cases, a mid-potency topical steroid, such as 0.1% betamethasone valerate, may be required but usable only for a short time. Keratolytic agents, including salicylic acid and selenium sulfide are dangerous to neonates because of the possibility of its percutaneous absorption. Lotion containing 0.025% licochalcone, an extract from *Glycyrrhiza inflata*, was shown to have a similar effect compared to 1% hydrocortisone.[46] If secondary infection with fungi or bacteria is accompanied, appropriate systemic drugs should be prescribed. Dietary controls and vitamin supplementation are not beneficial in ISD.

Many researchers have proposed various alternative methods to treat SD as well, in preparation for the antifungal resistance and the adverse effects of existing therapies. Homogeneous mixture of biodegradable elements, such as urea, propylene glycol, and lactic acid, was shown to be highly effective in treatment of SD of the scalp.[47] Tea tree oil, derived from nature, was found to be of benefit in improving severity, pruritus, and greasiness in a randomized single-blind study. The antifungal property of tee tree oil, mostly to *M. furfur*, was established in an in vitro study.[48] Narrow-band ultraviolet B phototherapy was confirmed as an additional choice and to be both safe and effective in an open-label prospective study. Its role in SD may be associated with its immunomodulatory and antiinflammatory function.[49]

ACKNOWLEDGMENTS

The author acknowledges the contributions of Chris D. Collins, MD, FAAD, and Chad Hivnor, MD, the former authors of this chapter, and thanks Jungyoon Moon, MD, for his devoted assistance.

REFERENCES

1. Park SY, Kwon HH, Min S, Yoon JY, et al. Clinical manifestation and associated factors of seborrheic dermatitis in Korea. *Eur J Dermatol*. 2016;26(2):173-176.
2. Szepietowski JC, Reich A, Wesołowska-Szepietowska E, et al. Quality of life in patients suffering from seborrheic dermatitis: influence of age, gender and education level. *Mycoses*. 2009;52(4):357-363.
3. Arsic Arsenijevic VS, Milobratovic D, Barac AM, et al. A laboratory-based study on patients with Parkinson's disease and seborrheic dermatitis: the presence and density of Malassezia yeasts, their different species and enzymes production. *BMC Dermatol*. 2014;14:5.
4. Gupta A, Bluhm R. Seborrheic dermatitis. *J Eur Acad Dermatol Venereol*. 2004;18(1):13-26.
5. Misery L, Rahhali N, Duhamel A, et al. Epidemiology of dandruff, scalp pruritus and associated symptoms. *Acta Derm Venereol*. 2013;93(1):80-81.
6. Naldi L, Rebora A. Clinical practice. Seborrheic dermatitis. *N Engl J Med*. 2009;360(4):387-396.
7. Dhar S, Banerjee R, Malakar R. Neonatal erythroderma: diagnostic and therapeutic challenges. *Indian J Dermatol*. 2012;57(6):475-478.

8. Schwartz RA, Janusz CA, Janniger CK. Seborrheic dermatitis: an overview. *Am Fam Physician*. 2006; 74(1):125-130.
9. Ong C, O'Toole EA, Ghali L, et al. LEKTI demonstrable by immunohistochemistry of the skin: a potential diagnostic skin test for Netherton syndrome. *Br J Dermatol*. 2004;151(6):1253-1257.
10. Verardino GC, Azulay-Abulafia L, Macedo PM, et al. Pityriasis amiantacea: clinical-dermatoscopic features and microscopy of hair tufts. *An Bras Dermatol*. 2012; 87(1):142-145.
11. Abdel-Hamid IA, Agha SA, Moustafa YM, et al. Pityriasis amiantacea: a clinical and etiopathologic study of 85 patients. *Int J Dermatol*. 2003;42(4):260-264.
12. Lacouture ME, Duvic M, Hauschild A, et al. Analysis of dermatologic events in vemurafenib-treated patients with melanoma. *Oncologist*. 2013;18(3):314-322.
13. Belum VR, Rosen AC, Jaimes N, et al. Clinico-morphological features of BRAF inhibition–induced proliferative skin lesions in cancer patients. *Cancer*. 2015;121(1):60-68.
14. Nnoruka EN, Chukwuka JC, Anisuiba B. Correlation of mucocutaneous manifestations of HIV/AIDS infection with CD4 counts and disease progression. *Int J Dermatol*. 2007;46(s2):14-18.
15. Oble DA, Collett E, Hsieh M, et al. A novel T cell receptor transgenic animal model of seborrheic dermatitis-like skin disease. *J Invest Dermatol*. 2005;124(1): 151-159.
16. Dessinioti C, Katsambas A. Seborrheic dermatitis: etiology, risk factors, and treatments: facts and controversies. *Clin Dermatol*. 2013;31(4):343-351.
17. Sandström Falk MH, Tengvall Linder M, Johansson C. The prevalence of *Malassezia* yeasts in patients with atopic dermatitis, seborrhoeic dermatitis and healthy controls. *Acta Derm Venereol*. 2005;85(1):17-23.
18. Faergemann J, Bergbrant IM, Dohse M, et al. Seborrhoeic dermatitis and *Pityrosporum (Malassezia)* folliculitis: characterization of inflammatory cells and mediators in the skin by immunohistochemistry. *Br J Dermatol*. 2001;144(3):549-556.
19. Kerr K, Schwartz JR, Filloon T, et al. Scalp stratum corneum histamine levels: novel sampling method reveals association with itch resolution in dandruff/seborrhoeic dermatitis treatment. *Acta Derm Venereol*. 2011;91(4):404-408.
20. Mills KJ, Hu P, Henry J, et al. Dandruff/seborrhoeic dermatitis is characterized by an inflammatory genomic signature and possible immune dysfunction. *Br J Dermatol*. 2012;166(Suppl2):33-40.
21. Emre S, Metin A, Demirseren DD, et al. The association of oxidative stress and disease activity in seborrheic dermatitis. *Arch Dermatol Res*. 2012;304(9):683-687.
22. Tanaka A, Cho O, Saito M, et al. Molecular characterization of the skin fungal microbiota in patients with seborrheic dermatitis. *J Clin Exp Dermatol Res*. 2014;5(6):239.
23. Xu J, Saunders CW, Hu P, et al. Dandruff-associated *Malassezia* genomes reveal convergent and divergent virulence traits shared with plant and human fungal pathogens. *Proc Natl Acad Sci U S A*. 2007;104(47): 18730-18735.
24. Patino-Uzcategui A, Amado Y, Cepero de Garcia M, et al. Virulence gene expression in *Malassezia* spp from individuals with seborrheic dermatitis. *J Invest Dermatol*. 2011;131(10):2134-2136.
25. Hiruma M, Cho O, Hiruma M, et al. Genotype analyses of human commensal scalp fungi, *Malassezia globosa*, and *Malassezia restricta* on the scalps of patients with dandruff and healthy subjects. *Mycopathologia*. 2014;177(5-6):263-269.
26. Tajima M, Sugita T, Nishikawa A, et al. Molecular analysis of *Malassezia* microflora in seborrheic dermatitis patients: comparison with other diseases and healthy subjects. *J Invest Dermatol*. 2008;128(2):345-351.
27. Gaitanis G, Magiatis P, Stathopoulou K, et al. AhR ligands, malassezin, and indolo[3,2-b]carbazole are selectively produced by *Malassezia furfur* strains isolated from seborrheic dermatitis. *J Invest Dermatol*. 2008;128(7):1620-1625.
28. De Luca C, Valacchi G. Surface lipids as multifunctional mediators of skin responses to environmental stimuli. *Mediators Inflamm*. 2010;2010:321494.
29. DeAngelis YM, Gemmer CM, Kaczvinsky JR, et al. Three etiologic facets of dandruff and seborrheic dermatitis: *Malassezia* fungi, sebaceous lipids, and individual sensitivity. *J Invest Dermatol Proc*. 2005;10(3):295-297.
30. Hay RJ. *Malassezia*, dandruff and seborrhoeic dermatitis: an overview. *Br J Dermatol*. 2011;165(suppl 2):2-8.
31. Donovan M, Ambach A, Thomas-Collignon A, et al. Calmodulin-like skin protein level increases in the differentiated epidermal layers in atopic dermatitis. *Exp Dermatol*. 2013;22(12):836-837.
32. Mastrolonardo M, Diaferio A, Logroscino G. Seborrheic dermatitis, increased sebum excretion, and Parkinson's disease: a survey of (im)possible links. *Med Hypotheses*. 2003;60(6):907-911.
33. Trüeb RM. Serum biotin levels in women complaining of hair loss. *Int J Trichology*. 2016;8(2):73.
34. Birnbaum RY, Zvulunov A, Hallel-Halevy D, et al. Seborrhea-like dermatitis with psoriasiform elements caused by a mutation in ZNF750, encoding a putative C2H2 zinc finger protein. *Nat Genet*. 2006;38(7):749-751.
35. Kim GW, Jung HJ, Ko HC, et al. Dermoscopy can be useful in differentiating scalp psoriasis from seborrhoeic dermatitis. *Br J Dermatol*. 2011;164(3):652-656.
36. Soeprono FF, Schinella RA, Cockerell CJ, et al. Seborrheic-like dermatitis of acquired immunodeficiency syndrome. A clinicopathologic study. *J Am Acad Dermatol*. 1986;14(2):242-248.
37. Alexopoulos A, Kakourou T, Orfanou I, et al. Retrospective analysis of the relationship between infantile seborrheic dermatitis and atopic dermatitis. *Pediatr Dermatol*. 2014;31(2):125-130.
38. Kibar M, Aktan Ş, Bilgin M. Dermoscopic findings in scalp psoriasis and seborrheic dermatitis; two new signs; signet ring vessel and hidden hair. *Indian J Dermatol*. 2015;60(1):41.
39. Carlo G, Ramon G. Infantile seborrhoeic dermatitis. In: Alan I, Peter H, Albert Y. *Harper's Textbook of Pediatric Dermatology*. 3rd ed. Oxford, UK: Wiley-Blackwell; 2011:35.1-35.8.
40. Kastarinen H, Oksanen T, Okokon EO, et al. Topical anti-inflammatory agents for seborrhoeic dermatitis of the face or scalp. *Cochrane Database Syst Rev*. 2011;(5):CD009446.
41. Okokon EO, Verbeek JH, Ruotsalainen JH, et al. Topical antifungals for seborrhoeic dermatitis. *Cochrane Database Syst Rev*. 2015;(5):CD008138.
42. Mayser P, Schulz S. Precipitation of free fatty acids generated by *Malassezia*—a possible explanation for the positive effects of lithium succinate in seborrhoeic dermatitis. *J Eur Acad Dermatol Venereol*. 2016;30(8):1384-1389.

43. Pflugfelder SC, Karpecki PM, Perez VL. Treatment of blepharitis: recent clinical trials. *Ocul Surf*. 2014;12(4):273-284.
44. Gupta AK, Richardson M, Paquet M. Systematic review of oral treatments for seborrheic dermatitis. *J Eur Acad Dermatol Venereol*. 2014;28(1):16-26.
45. Tüzün Y, Wolf R, Bağlam S, et al. Diaper (napkin) dermatitis: a fold (intertriginous) dermatosis. *Clin Dermatol*. 2015;33(4):477-482.
46. Wananukul S, Chatproedprai S, Charutragulchai W. Randomized, double-blind, split-side comparison study of moisturizer containing licochalcone vs. 1% hydrocortisone in the treatment of infantile seborrhoeic dermatitis. *J Eur Acad Dermatol Venereol*. 2012;26(7):894-897.
47. Emtestam L, Svensson Å, Rensfeldt K. Treatment of seborrhoeic dermatitis of the scalp with a topical solution of urea, lactic acid, and propylene glycol (K301): results of two double-blind, randomised, placebo-controlled studies. *Mycoses*. 2012;55(5):393-403.
48. Pazyar N, Yaghoobi R, Bagherani N, et al. A review of applications of tea tree oil in dermatology. *Int J Dermatol*. 2013;52(7):784-790.
49. Gambichler T, Breuckmann F, Boms S, et al. Narrow-band UVB phototherapy in skin conditions beyond psoriasis. *J Am Acad Dermatol*. 2005;52(4):660-670.

Chapter 27 :: Occupational Skin Diseases*
:: Andy Chern, Casey M. Chern, & Boris D. Lushniak

第二十七章

职业性皮肤疾病

中文导读

　　本章共分为7节：①前言；②流行病学；③职业性接触性皮炎；④接触性荨麻疹与速发型接触反应；⑤其他职业性皮肤疾病；⑥职业性皮肤病的诊断；⑦治疗。全章介绍了职业性皮肤病的临床类型、病因、诊断与防治。

　　第一节介绍了职业性皮肤病的疾病背景、对其认知的历史演变、暴露类别、常见的职业性皮肤疾病的临床类型。

　　第二节介绍了职业性皮肤病的流行病学，指出职业性皮肤病以自然资源和采矿业的发病率为最高，其次是教育和卫生服务业。

　　第三节介绍了职业性接触性皮炎的定义和分类，主要包括刺激性接触性皮炎和变应性接触性皮炎，分别介绍了其定义及病因、临床表现及分类以及主要的职业接触性过敏原。

　　第四节介绍了接触性荨麻疹与速发型接触反应（包括非免疫性接触性荨麻疹、免疫性接触性荨麻疹和未确定机制所致荨麻疹）的病因、诊断流程和临床特征。

　　第五节介绍了其他职业性皮肤疾病的分类，根据暴露因素分类可分为化学暴露因素所致职业性皮肤疾病、机械暴露因素（如摩擦、压力、撞击和振动等）所致职业性皮肤疾病、物理暴露因素［如极端温度、离子和非离子辐射（紫外线）等］所致职业性皮肤疾病、生物学因素（细菌、真菌、病毒感染）所致职业性皮肤疾病，并详述了其背景和临床表现。

　　第六节介绍了职业性皮肤病的诊断，指出斑贴试验是诊断变应性接触性皮炎的金标准，在评估接触性皮炎时帮助确定职业性皮肤病的病因至关重要。皮肤点刺试验（SPT）是用于识别IgE介导的速发型超敏反应（例如免疫接触性荨麻疹）的变态反应试验。详述了以上两种检测方法的意义和应用。简单介绍了其他检测方法如血清特异性IgE检测、氢氧化钾（KOH）、皮肤活检和重金属检测。

　　第七节介绍了职业性皮肤病的治疗，提出大多数职业性皮肤病是可以预防的，因此应该对患者进行适当的预防措施教育。还要了解职业性皮肤病的危险因素如年龄、性别、种族和遗传学因素等，以预防职业性皮肤病的发生。并提倡从以下4个方面，包括危害识别、剂量反应关系、暴露评估和风险特征对暴露工人进行健康风险评估。

〔李　捷〕

AT-A-GLANCE

- Occupational skin diseases are the second most common occupational illness accounting for approximately 15% of occupational illnesses.
- The vast majority of occupational skin diseases are occupational contact dermatoses (irritant contact dermatitis and allergic contact dermatitis), with approximately 80% of cases occurring on the hands.
- Workers in the natural resources and mining, manufacturing, and education and health services have the highest rates of reported skin diseases and disorders.
- Occupational exposures (ultraviolet radiation and chemical carcinogens) can have a significant role in skin cancer development, which is a major public health concern.
- Personal protective equipment should be the last consideration in addressing occupational skin hazards.

INTRODUCTION

BACKGROUND

Occupational skin diseases (OSDs) are a category of skin conditions caused or aggravated primarily by workplace factors. Occupational skin diseases are common and also contribute to significant economic costs. An estimate as high as $1 billion is associated with the burden of workplace skin diseases in the US annually.[1,2] In addition, OSDs may have unique implications. Federal agencies such as the Occupational Safety and Health Administration (OSHA) have mandated criteria for recording occupationally related injuries and illnesses by the employer, and the determination of work-relatedness may result in the involvement of a workers' compensation system. Thus, a thorough knowledge of contributing factors to OSDs is vital for the timely treatment and prevention of these skin conditions to return patients and employees back to work.

HISTORICAL PERSPECTIVE

Occupational skin diseases have existed throughout history. Even in antiquity, the Roman poet Virgil (70-19 BCE) described the cutaneous manifestations of *Bacillus anthracis* exposure in sheepmen.[3] However, it was centuries later that the Italian physician Bernardino Ramazzini (1633-1714), recognized as "the Father of Occupational Medicine," would document his pioneering observations of various occupational diseases in *De Morbis Artificum Diatriba* (Diseases of Workers). In regard to OSDs, Ramazzini observed leg ulcers in fishermen, fissures and inflammation of the hands in laundrywomen, and skin eruptions in grain workers among others.[4] Although Ramazzini described associations between occupation and disease, further work identifying the causal relationship between the 2 has been the impetus for labor laws and reform. One classic example was the identification of scrotal cancer in chimney sweepers by Sir Percivall Pott (1714-1788), a British surgeon. Pott recognized that chronic exposure to soot (polycyclic aromatic hydrocarbons) lodged in the rugae led to scrotal cancer; and, in 1788, Pott's work led to the first of many Chimney Sweeps Acts passed in Britain.[5]

EXPOSURE CLASSIFICATION

The etiology of occupational injuries and illnesses, including OSDs, can be classified by the following exposures:

- Chemical: organic and inorganic compounds, elemental substances
- Mechanical: friction, pressure, vibration
- Physical: ionizing and nonionizing radiation, thermal stress
- Biologic: bacteria, viruses, fungi, parasites, insects, plants, animals

The vast majority of OSDs are attributed to chemical agents; however, mechanical, physical, and biologic exposures must be considered in the differential diagnoses as multiple concurrent exposures can often occur in the workplace.

OCCUPATIONAL DISEASE SPECTRUM

Of all the work-related dermatologic diseases, occupational contact dermatitis (OCD) comprises 90% to 95% of OSDs.[6] The remaining 5% to 10% of OSD cases consist of a wide variety of diseases. Some of these include immunologic and nonimmunologic contact urticaria, occupational skin cancers, vibration white

---

*Disclaimer: The contents of this publication are the sole responsibility of the authors and do not necessarily reflect the views, opinions or policies of the Uniformed Services University of the Health Sciences (USUHS), the Department of Defense (DoD), or the Departments of the Army, Navy, or Air Force. Mention of trade names, commercial products, or organizations does not imply endorsement by the U.S. Government.

finger, and infections. Table 27-1 lists common categories of OSDs.

EPIDEMIOLOGY

In the United States, the Bureau of Labor Statistics (BLS) publishes annual data on occupational injuries and illnesses. Among private industry, nonfatal occupational injuries and illnesses accounted for nearly 3 million cases in 2014. Nonfatal occupational illnesses only consisted of 4.9% of the total cases, but of these, 15.2% were skin diseases.[7] The distribution of nonfatal occupational illness cases is depicted in Fig. 27-1.

Additionally, the rate of reported OSDs declined in 2014 among all industries from the previous year from 3.2 to 2.6 cases per 10,000 full-time workers.[7] However, limitations in BLS epidemiologic data may considerably underestimate the true incidence of OSDs by as much as 10 to 50 times.[2,8] Moreover, BLS categorizes wounds and bruises separately under injuries, which is not reflected in the aforementioned rates. In comparison, several studies of European countries including those with active nationwide notification programs for OCD reported incidence rates between 5 and 19 cases per 10,000 full-time workers per year for OCD alone.[9-13]

When comparing OSD among industries in the United States, education and health services accounted for the highest total skin disease cases (6100) followed by the manufacturing industry (4400) in 2014.[7] However, the highest incidence rate occurred in the natural resources and mining industries. With only 1000 total cases, natural resources and mining had an incidence rate of 5.5 cases per 10,000 full-time workers, with education and health services following behind with 4 cases per 10,000 full-time workers.[7] The total distribution of OSDs by industry is demonstrated in Fig. 27-2.

The total cases of OSD has declined over the last decade, and a corresponding decline in the incidence of OSD cases involving days away from work also has been observed, potentially reflecting not only better prevention measures but improved early management.[14] In 2014, among all OSDs, skin infections resulted in the longest duration away from work (median = 6 days) while wounds and bruises had the highest incidence rate involving days away from work (9.1 cases per 10,000 full-time workers).[7]

OCCUPATIONAL CONTACT DERMATITIS

Occupational contact dermatitis refers to any irritation of the skin arising from direct exposure to an exogenous agent and can be further divided into 2 general categories based on exposure, etiology, and pathophysiology of the resulting skin disease. These are irritant contact dermatitis (ICD) and allergic contact dermatitis (ACD). Occupations at increased risk for OCD are listed in Table 27-2.

Specifically, ICD results from a nonimmunologic reaction to a chemical, physical, or mechanical irritation of the skin causing cutaneous inflammation via a direct cytotoxic effect from an agent. Anyone may develop an ICD, and those with compromised skin barrier such as atopic dermatitis, xerosis, or light colored skin are at higher risk.[15]

In contrast, ACD is a reaction to a substance by a type IV, delayed hypersensitivity reaction. This cell-mediated, immune reaction requires prior sensitization to an allergen, which is usually a low-molecular weight chemical that acts as a hapten. Only a small percentage of people will develop ACD after contact from various haptens. For perspective, more than 57,000 chemicals have been known to cause skin irritation (ICD), whereas only about 3700 chemicals have been identified as true skin allergens.[16] Table 27-3 provides a comparison of ICD and ACD characteristics. As would be expected, the vast proportion of OCD occur on the hands (80%).[16]

IRRITANT CONTACT DERMATITIS

BACKGROUND

Irritant contact dermatitis occurs when the normal epidermal barrier is disrupted by an irritant and is often concentration or duration dependent, with no previous substance exposure necessary to elicit an effect. Effects may be visible within minutes to a few hours. Wet work tasks have been identified as the most common occupational exposure leading to contact dermatitis though other frequent causes include exposure to soaps, petroleum products, cutting oils, coolants, and solvents (Fig. 27-3).[21] The exposed hands are the most commonly involved sites for ICD given their interaction with the environment and opportunities for irritant exposure. Though there is no readily available diagnostic test for ICD, a careful history in addition to the patient's clinical presentation are usually sufficient in making the diagnosis.

CLINICAL FEATURES

Irritant contact dermatitis, unlike ACD, is not a distinct clinical entity. The clinical pictures of ICD is dependent on time-effect and dose relationship.[22] For instance, a severe acute response to a strong noxious irritant may present with necrosis or ulceration, whereas chronic lesions often present with lichenification, scaling, hyperpigmentation, or fissuring.

TABLE 27-1
Common Occupational Skin Diseases

	ORGANISM	OCCUPATION	TREATMENT
Bacterial Infections			
Impetigo, cellulitis, furuncles, and abscesses	*Staphylococcus* sp., *Streptococcus* sp.	Meat packers, construction workers, farm workers, nurses, athletes, hairdressers, manicurists	Topical: mupirocin 2%, retapamulin 1%, fusidic acid 1%; Systemic agents: dicloxacillin, cephalexin, erythromycin, clindamycin, TMP-SMX[a]
Anthrax	*Bacillus anthracis*	Workers in contact with goat hair, wool, hides	Penicillin, doxycycline (naturally occurring anthrax); Fluoroquinolone (suspected weaponized anthrax)
Fish tank granuloma	*Mycobacterium marinum*	Fisherman, fish market worker	Doxycycline, ethambutol, minocycline, rifampicin
Erysipeloid	*Erysipelothrix rhusiopathiae*	Fishermen, butchers, farmers, veterinary surgeons, poultry dressers	Penicillin, ampicillin, ceftriaxone, fluoroquinolone
Pitted keratolysis	*Corynebacterium* sp.	Barefooted laborers, soldiers, miners	Prophylactic measures; benzoyl peroxide cleanser; topical clindamycin, erythromycin solutions, miconazole, fusidic acid
Brucellosis	*Brucella* sp.	Slaughterhouse workers, farmers, veterinarians, meat packers, livestock breeders, laboratory workers.	Doxycycline combined with streptomycin OR gentamicin OR rifampin
Tularemia	*Francisella tularensis*	Laboratory workers, farmers, veterinarians, sheep workers, hunters, cooks, meat handlers, landscapers	Aminoglycoside, fluoroquinolone, doxycycline
Fungal and Yeast Infections[b]			
Tinea pedis	*Trichophyton rubrum; E. floccosum, T. mentagrophytes/interdigitale*	Miners, military personnel, athletes, laborers	Topical: allylamines, imidazoles; Systemic agents: terbinafine, itraconazole, fluconazole
Candida, other yeast infections	*Candida albicans*	Waitresses, bartenders, food handlers	Topical: imidazoles, nystatin; Systemic agents: fluconazole
Other superficial mycoses	*Trichophyton verrucosum*	Exposure to cattle, farm buildings, and straw	Topical: allylamines, imidazoles; Systemic agents: terbinafine, itraconazole, fluconazole)
	Trichophyton mentagrophytes/interdigitale	Cattle, domestic animal exposure	Topical: allylamines, imidazoles; Systemic agents: terbinafine, itraconazole, fluconazole
	Microsporum canis	Domestic animals, esp. cats	Systemic agents: terbinafine, itraconazole, fluconazole
	Microsporum nanum	Pigs	Topical: imidazoles[c]
	Sporothrix schenckii	Gardeners, forestry workers, nursery workers, miners, farmers	Systemic agents: itraconazole, terbinafine
Deep mycoses	*Histoplasma capsulatum*	Workers with exposure to demolition, excavation activities	Systemic agents: itraconazole; amphotericin B
	Chromoblastomycosis	Farmers, outdoor workers	Systemic agents: itraconazole, terbinafine, amphotericin B
	Phaeohyphomycosis	Farmers, outdoor workers	Surgical excision
	Eumycetoma	Farmers, outdoor workers	Itraconazole, voriconazole
Viral Infections			
Herpetic whitlow	Herpes simplex virus	Dental workers	Acyclovir, valacyclovir, famciclovir
Orf/ecthyma contagiosum	Parapoxvirus	Veterinarians, sheep herders, farmers	Supportive care, antibiotic coverage if secondary infection is suspected
Pseudocowpox/milker's nodule	Paravaccinia virus	Farmers, veterinarians, fresh meat handlers	Symptomatic treatment; surgical curettage for large lesions
Human papilloma virus	Human papilloma virus (HPV)-7	Butchers	Destructive modalities (cryotherapy, curettage, electrodessication), podophyllotoxin, topical 5-fluorouracil, cantharidin, caustics and acids, imiquimod

[a] Dose and duration, as well as antibiotic option dependent on clinical manifestation of the infection, sites affected, and methicillin-sensitivity of the causative organism.
[b] Dose and duration of treatment are dependent on the clinical manifestation of the infection, as well as the sites affected.
[c] Roller JA, Westblom TU. Microsporum nanum infection in hog farmers. *J Am Acad Dermatol.* 1986;15(5 Pt 1):935-939.

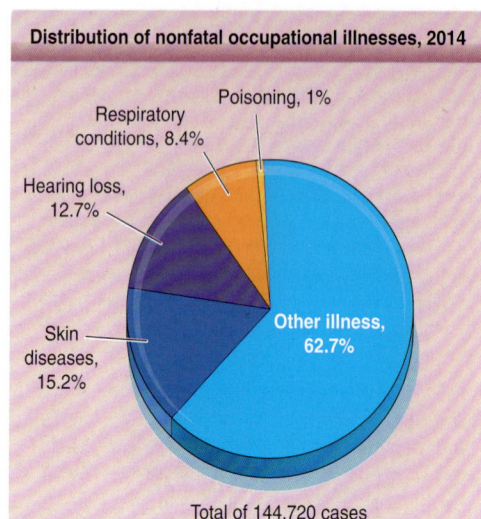

Figure 27-1 Distribution of nonfatal occupational illnesses. Distribution of nonfatal occupational illness cases by category of illness; private industry; 2014. Less than 5% of injury and illness cases reported among the private industry establishments in 2014 were illnesses. More than 60% of illness cases were categorized as "all other illnesses," which includes such things as repetitive motion cases and other systemic diseases and disorders. (Data from U.S. Bureau of Labor Statistics: 2014 Survey of Occupational Injuries & Illnesses.)

ICD presentations may be categorized as follows, although no standard case definition exists for the spectrum of ICD[16,23]:

- Acute
- Irritant reaction
- Cumulative
- Traumatic
- Asteatotic dermatitis
- Pustular and acneiform
- Subjective

Even with these categories, it is important to recognize that ICD and ACD can both have similar clinical manifestations as acute, subacute, and chronic skin conditions.

Acute Irritant Contact Dermatitis:
Acute ICD manifests when the skin is exposed to a potent irritant or caustic chemical from an accident at work. The irritant reaction quickly reaches a peak, then starts to heal; this is called a *decrescendo phenomenon*. Because of the short lag time (minutes to hours after exposure) and the clear association between exposure and skin symptoms, the diagnosis can be easily made. However, it may be difficult when the patient is unaware of an exposure, and consequently, an acute ACD should be considered in the differential diagnosis. Because acute ACD is a delayed sensitization reaction, it is characterized by the *crescendo phenomenon* that is a transient increase of symptom intensity despite removal of the allergen.

Symptoms of acute ICD include burning, soreness, and stinging of the skin. These lesions are restricted to the areas where the irritant damages the skin, which may result in erythema, edema, bullae, or necrosis with sharply demarcated borders. An asymmetric pattern may hint at an exogenous cause.

Acute ICD has a good prognosis with appropriate and symptomatic management. Acids and alkaline

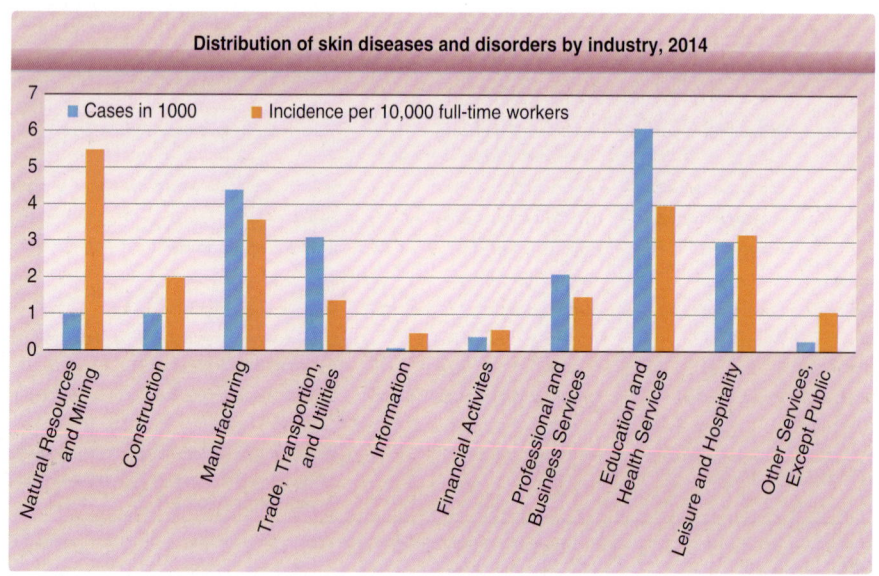

Figure 27-2 Distribution of skin diseases and disorders by industry. Distribution of skin diseases or disorders by private industry; 2014. Natural resources and mining excludes farms with fewer than 11 employees. Data for mining include establishments not governed by the Mine Safety and Health Administration rules and reporting, such as those in Oil and Gas Extraction and related support activities. (Data from U.S. Bureau of Labor Statistics: 2014 Employer-Reported Workplace Injuries & Illnesses.)

TABLE 27-2
Occupations at Increased Risk for Irritant and Allergic Contact Dermatitis

OCCUPATION	IRRITANTS	ALLERGENS
Agricultural workers	Fertilizers, germicides, dust, diesel, gasoline, oils, pesticides, plants, solvents, wet-work	Pesticides, animal feeds, barley and oats, fungicides, germicidal products, cement, plants, veterinary medications, wood dust, preservatives, wool
Bakers	Acids, flour, spices, soaps and detergents, oven cleaners, essential oils, yeast, enzymes	Ammonium persulfate; benzoyl peroxide; dyes; essential oils; enzymes; flavors; flour; some fruits
Construction workers	Acids, fibrous glass, concrete, solvents, hand cleaners	Cement, chromium, chromium compounds, cobalt, epoxy resins, nickel, resins, rubber allergens, wood dust
Cooks	Wet work, soaps and detergents, vegetable and fruit juices, raw meat and fish, spices, sugar and flour, heat	Flavors and spices, formaldehyde, garlic, sodium metabisulfite (antioxidant for vegetables)
Cosmetologists	Soaps and detergents, bleaches, solvents, permanent wave solutions, shampoos, wet-work	Dyes, amine-based products including parphenylene diamine, glyceryl monothioglycolate (perming solution), rosin, preservatives, rubber allergens, ethylmethacrylate, methylmethacrylate
Dentists and dental technicians	Wet work, adhesives (epoxy and cyanoacrylates), essential oils, orthodontic plasters, amalgam mixtures, solvents	Dental impression material, eugenol, anesthetics, mercury, disinfectants, methacrylates, latex, rubber accelerators
Florists	Wet work, soaps and detergents, fertilizers, herbicides, pesticides, mechanical and chemical plant irritants	Plants, pesticides, insecticides
Health care workers	Wet work, soaps and detergents, alcohol, ethylene oxide, medications	Latex gloves, anesthetics, antibiotics and antiseptics, phenothiazines, formaldehyde, glutaraldehyde, chloroxylenol
Housekeepers	Wet work, soaps and detergents, cleaners, polishes, oven cleaners, disinfectants	Potassium dichromate, preservatives, rubber accelerators, latex
Machinists	Solvents, coolants, cutting oils, degreasers, acids, corrosion inhibitors, heat, soaps and detergents, metal filings and swarf	Additives/preservatives in cutting fluids, chromium, nickel
Automobile mechanics	Abrasive skin cleaners, diesel, gasoline, greases, oils, solvent, transmission fluid, motor oils	Chromium, cobalt, epoxy resin; nickel
Painters	Paints, solvents, adhesives, paint removers, paintbrush cleaners, soaps and detergents	Turpentine, thinners, chromium, formaldehyde, epoxy products, polyester resins

are the most frequent potent culprits giving rise to an acute ICD. A common example can be seen in construction workers developing chemical burns when alkaline concrete fluid spills into work boots or soaks through garments.[24] Also, several agents causing chemical burns warrant brief mention as they require more specific therapies. These agents are summarized in Table 27-4.

Irritant Reaction Contact Dermatitis:
Irritant reaction contact dermatitis is a subclinical irritant dermatitis in workers whose hands are

TABLE 27-3
Comparison of ICD and ACD

	IRRITANT	ALLERGIC
Onset	Within minutes for strong irritants, up to days/weeks with weak irritants	Within 24-96 h in sensitized individuals
Resolution	Improves after 3-6 weeks away from exposure	May improve within days after exposure; some cases persist
Histology	Spongiotic dermatitis	Spongiotic dermatitis
Mechanism	Nonimmune, sensitization not required; epidermal barrier disruption, epidermal cellular damage, pro-inflammatory mediators released from keratinocytes[17-19]	Immune-mediated, sensitization required; Antigen-activated primed T cells; sensitization phase typically takes 10-14 d[20]
Agent	Concentration dependent	Not concentration dependent
Atopy	Predisposition	Variable
Diagnosis	Clinical	Patch testing

Modified from Belsito DV. Occupational contact dermatitis: etiology, prevalence, and resultant impairment/disability. *J Am Acad Dermatol.* 2005;53:303-313.

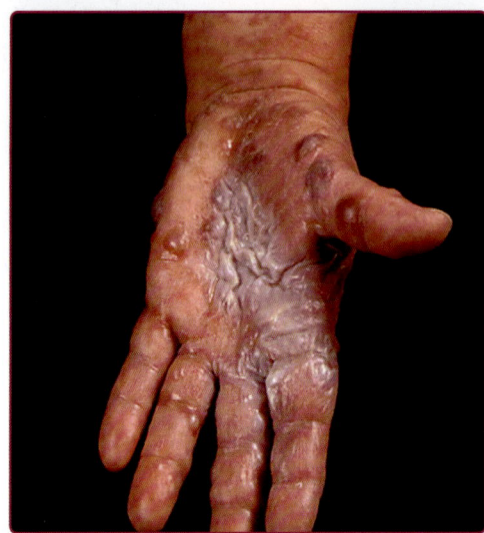

Figure 27-3 Acute irritant contact dermatitis on the hand caused by an industrial solvent. There is massive blistering on the palm.

excessively wet, including hairdressers, bartenders, and metal workers. On the hands, scaling and erythema are first identified under rings before spreading over fingers to hands and forearms. The thinner skin of the dorsum of the hand is usually affected, though irritants can also cause vesiculation resembling pompholyx. Frequently, irritant reaction contact dermatitis heals spontaneously with hardening of the skin, but may progress to cumulative irritant dermatitis.

Cumulative Irritant Contact Dermatitis:
Cumulative ICD is a consequence of multiple sub-threshold insults to the skin with insufficient time between insults to allow complete restoration of the skin barrier function.[28] It may result from the frequent repetition of one agitating factor but is more commonly the result of a variety of stimuli, each beginning before recovery from the foregoing stimulant. Clinical symptoms develop only when the damage exceeds an individually determined *manifestation threshold*. Patients with sensitive skin (ie, atopics) have a decreased irritant threshold or a prolonged restoration time, leading to earlier development of cumulative ICD. The threshold is not a fixed value for an individual but may decrease with disease progression. Therefore, in patients with cumulative ICD, even limited irritant exposure may sustain the condition. Cumulative ICD is associated with weak irritants rather than potent irritants with exposures occurring not only at work but also at home. The link between exposure and disease is frequently not obvious to the patient, and therefore, the diagnosis may be considerably delayed. These patients often complain of pruritus and pain due to fissuring of the hyperkeratotic skin with notable lichenification and chapping. In contrast to acute irritant dermatitis, the lesions are less sharply demarcated (Fig. 27-4).

Traumatic Irritant Contact Dermatitis:
Traumatic ICD may arise after acute skin trauma, such as lacerations, burns, or acute ICD. The latter is seen frequently after use of harsh cleansers, and inquiring if patients have cleansed their skin with strong soaps or detergents is warranted. The

TABLE 27-4
Selected Chemical Burns That Require Unique Therapies

CHEMICAL	TREATMENT BASICS (THEN TRANSPORT TO HOSPITAL EMERGENCY DEPARTMENT FOR FURTHER EVALUATION AND TREATMENT)
Burning metal fragments of sodium, potassium, and lithium	Extinguish with Class D fire extinguisher (containing sodium chloride, sodium carbonate or graphite base) or with sand; cover with mineral oil; extract metal particles mechanically[a]
Hydrofluoric acid	Flush with running water; then administer calcium gluconate gel (2.5%) followed by intralesional injection, if needed
White phosphorus	Remove particles mechanically; wash with soap and water; then apply copper ($CuSO_4$) sulfate in water for several minutes, remove black copper phosphide, and wash with water. Vigorous water irrigation and removal of phosphorus particles mechanically; the use of a Wood lamp (ultraviolet light) results in the fluorescing of the white phosphorus and may facilitate its removal. A brief rinse with 1% copper sulfate solution may be helpful. Copper sulfate combines with phosphorus to form a dark-copper phosphide coating on the particles that makes them easier to see and debride, and also impedes further oxidation. However, copper sulfate can cause hemolysis and hemoglobinuria, and should be used with caution.[25] More recently Kaushik and Bird recommend vigorous water washing rather than using copper sulfate.[26]
Phenolic compounds	Decontaminate with undiluted 200- to 400-Da molecular weight polyethylene glycol (PEG), which can be located in the chemical section of hospital pharmacies, followed by copious water irrigation. Isopropanol or glycerol may be substituted if PEG is not available.[27] Initial soap and water washing followed by treatment with polyethylene glycol 300 or 400 or ethanol (10%) in water.
Bromine or iodine	Wash frequently with soap and water followed by treatment with 5% sodium thiosulfate.

[a]Use of water to extinguish burning metal fragments is contraindicated because of the formation of highly alkaline hydroxides.

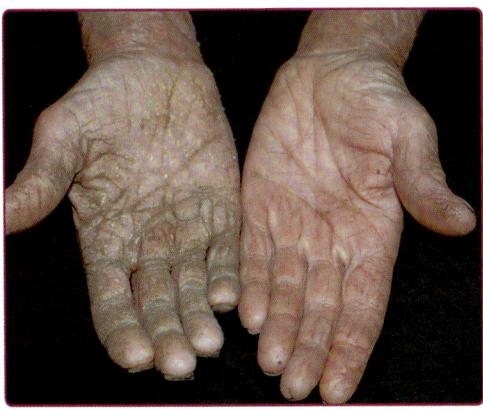

Figure 27-4 Irritant contact dermatitis in a construction worker who works with cement. Note the hyperkeratosis, scaling, and fissuring. There is also minimal postulation. Note that right (dominant working) hand is more severely affected than left hand.

ALLERGIC CONTACT DERMATITIS

BACKGROUND

Although it has been widely reported that 80% of all OCD cases are caused by ICD, there is broad variation in the distribution of ACD versus ICD among reports of OCD in the literature.[16,33] For instance, the North American Contact Dermatitis Group (NACDG) reported significantly more occupational ACD (60%) than ICD (32%).[34] A myriad of reasons may contribute to the disparate rates and include differences in the types of industries being studied in a geographical area, the age and sex distribution of evaluated patients, selection biases inherent among patients referred to tertiary dermatologic centers, the ability of the health care provider to fully assess the worker by patch testing, and existing national regulations and notification systems.[35]

CLINICAL FEATURES

Clinically, both ICD and ACD can have similar manifestations of pruritus, pain, erythema, swelling, xerosis, formation of wheals or blisters as well as lichenification. They both can manifest as an acute, subacute, or chronic condition. Health care workers are reported to be one of the most commonly affected professions with identified allergens, including glutaraldehyde, formaldehyde, quaternium-15, and thiuram mix.[36] Other professions frequently affected include machinists, construction workers, homemakers/house cleaners, food handlers, custodians, stock handlers, cosmetologists, and laboratory technicians (Fig. 27-5).[35] Major occupational contact allergens are listed in Table 27-5.

syndrome is characterized by eczematous lesions and delayed healing. Continued use of the irritant may cause the condition to persist, and full resolution may not occur for many months after discontinuation of exposure. When warranted, harsh soaps should be replaced by an appropriate soap. Soap is used to emulsify an unwanted material on the skin. Typically, a specific cleanser for the substance that is to be removed can be identified and should be "harmless" yet effective.

Asteatotic Dermatitis: Also known as exsiccation eczematid ICD, asteatotic eczema, winter dermatitis, or eczema craquelé, asteotoic dermatitis is a unique variant seen predominantly in elderly individuals with a history of extensive usage of soaps and cleansing products.[29] This leads to dry-appearing skin with ichthyosiform scaling, and patients experiencing intense pruritus. It is a condition mainly occurring in low-humidity, winter months.[30]

Pustular and Acneiform Irritant Contact Dermatitis: Pustular and acneiform ICD result from exposure to specific irritants such as croton oil, mineral oils, tars, greases, and naphthalenes. This syndrome should always be considered when acneiform lesions develop in postadolescent patients who never had teenage acne. The pustules are sterile and transient.

Subjective Irritant Contact Dermatitis: Although not well understood, subjective ICD is characterized by the lack of objective clinical signs as individuals complain of a sensation of burning or stinging (sensory irritation) after contact with certain chemicals.[31] Though no visible cutaneous irritation is generally observed, these reactions are usually dose-related and have been observed with chemicals such as lactic acid, which can be found in cosmetic products.[32]

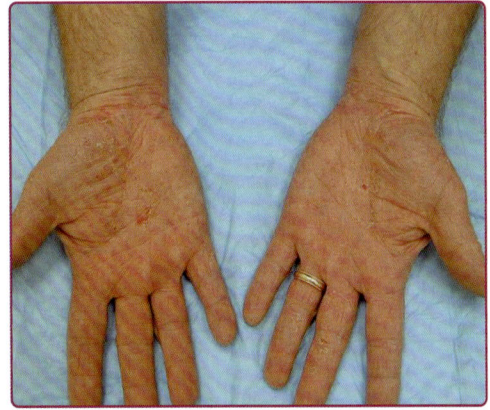

Figure 27-5 Hand dermatitis due to mercaptobenzothiazole in corrosion inhibitors at work and subsequent use of nitrile gloves containing mercaptobenzothiazole.

CONTACT URTICARIA AND IMMEDIATE CONTACT REACTIONS

Contact urticaria (CU) is a transient wheal and flare reaction from direct contact with a chemical or protein agent. Lesions appear within minutes to an hour and resolve within hours after exposure. Contact urticaria is categorized as either nonimmune-mediated or immune-mediated.[38] Additionally, CU of uncertain mechanism also has been recognized and demonstrates features of both nonimmune and immune-mediated CU.

NONIMMUNOLOGIC CONTACT URTICARIA

BACKGROUND AND CLINICAL FEATURES

Nonimmunologic contact urticaria (NICU), though less well understood in regard to pathogenesis, is caused by a wide array of agents in exposed individuals who develop a reaction without previous sensitization. Nonimmunologic contact urticaria is the most common type of contact urticaria, remains localized, and is less severe than immunologic contact urticaria (ICU) reactions. Additionally, in contrast to ICU, NICU reactions are not inhibited by H-1 antihistamines, but oral or topical nonsteroidal anti-inflammatory medications are effective, suggesting a role of prostaglandins in the pathogenesis of these lesions.[39] Classification of NICU agents are reviewed in Table 27-6.[40]

IMMUNOLOGIC CONTACT URTICARIA

BACKGROUND AND CLINICAL FEATURES

Immunologic contact urticaria (ICU) is a type I hypersensitivity reaction mediated by allergen-specific immunoglobulin E (IgE) and seen in individuals previously exposed to the specific agent. Atopic individuals are particularly at risk. ICU can spread beyond the cutaneous localized contact point and the level of spread is categorized in a staging system presented in Table 27-7.[41]

Contact urticaria from latex gloves is the prototypical example of ICU. Beginning in the early 1980s, a combination of factors including the use of latex gloves for universal precautions in light of the increasing prevalence of HIV and viral hepatitis contributed to an alarming number of individuals with type I hypersensitivity from latex rubber.[42] As the natural rubber latex (NRL) allergy epidemic was identified in the United States and Europe, various organizations and agencies recommended several prevention strategies, including reduction of protein content in gloves (to reduce allergenicity) and providing latex-free alternatives, which helped reduce the incidence of latex allergies.[43,44] Apart

TABLE 27-5

Most Frequently Reported Occupational Skin Allergens[37]

Cobalt
Chromate
Cosmetics and fragrances
Epoxies
Nickel
Plants
Preservatives
Resins
Acrylics

TABLE 27-6

Classification of Nonimmunologic Contact Urticaria Exposures

CATEGORIES	EXAMPLES
Animals	Caterpillars, arthropods, corals
Foods	Pepper, mustard, thyme
Fragrances and flavorings	Cinnamic aldehyde, balsam of Peru, cinnamic acid
Medicaments	Witch hazel, benzocaine, camphor
Metals	Cobalt
Plants	Nettles, seaweed
Preservatives and disinfectants	Benzoic acid, formaldehyde, sorbic acid
Miscellaneous	Butyric acid, pine oil, turpentine

Data from Basketter D, Lahti A. Immediate contact reactions. In: Johansen DJ, Frosch JP, Lepoittevin JP, eds. *Contact Dermatitis*. 5th ed. Berlin: Springer; 2011:137-153.

TABLE 27-7

Staging System for Immunologic Contact Urticaria

STAGING SYSTEM	
Stage 1	Localized urticaria, dermatitis, or nonspecific symptoms (itching, tingling, burning, etc.)
Stage 2	Generalized urticaria
Stage 3	Urticaria *and* rhinoconjunctivitis, asthma, or GI symptoms
Stage 4	Anaphylaxis

Adapted from Wang CY, Maibach HI. Immunologic contact urticaria—the human touch. *Cutan Ocul Toxicol*. 2013;32:154-160.

from health care workers, occupations commonly affected by ICU from NRL include kitchen workers, cleaners, others who wear NRL, as well as those with occupations involved in manufacturing rubber bands, surgical gloves, and latex dolls. It is important to note that NRL products can also cause a type IV hypersensitivity reaction (ie, ACD) mostly attributed to NRL additives, which accounts for the majority of allergic reactions (>80%) to NRL.[45,46]

Furthermore, virtually any food is capable of eliciting an ICU response and is the second most common cause of ICU. Foods such as potato, carrot, apple, tomato, shellfish, seafood, and meats are well documented, and recent literature has highlighted the problem of wheat allergens among bakers.[41] Additional causes include preservatives, fragrances, disinfectants, antibiotics, topical medications, epoxy resin hardeners, formaldehyde in clothing, several woods, and birch pollen.

CONTACT URTICARIA OF UNCERTAIN MECHANISM

BACKGROUND AND CLINICAL FEATURES

This type of reaction may occur with substances that produce a CU and a generalized histamine-type reaction but lacks a direct or immunologic basis for the reaction. It is most commonly caused by ammonium persulfate in bleaching hair boosters and typically has a sudden onset characterized by erythema, edema, severe pruritus, urticaria, and occasionally syncope with wheezing and dyspnea.

OTHER OCCUPATIONAL SKIN DISEASES BY EXPOSURE CATEGORIES

CHEMICAL EXPOSURES

A significant proportion of chemical exposures result in OCD. However, there are also several exposures that lead to unique skin manifestations such as acne.

ACNE

Background and Clinical Features: Different forms of acne have been observed in several work settings associated with certain chemical exposures. Machinists with skin exposed to industrial or cutting oils can develop oil acne not only in oil-soaked clothing regions but in other areas exposed to potential airborne oil mists.[47] Additionally, coal tar plant workers, roofers, and road and construction workers exposed to coal tar oils, creosote, and pitch can develop comedonal acne particularly on the face and malar regions.[48] These compounds also contain polycyclic aromatic hydrocarbons (PAH), which are carcinogenic as well.

Exposures to certain dioxins, naphthalenes, biphenyls, dibenzofurans, azobenzenes, and azoxybenzenes also have been associated with one of the more notable forms of acne, chloracne.[49] Chloracne from these chemical exposures are typically characterized by multiple closed comedones and straw-colored cysts primarily over the malar crescents and retroauricular folds that may also involve the neck, trunk extremities, buttocks, scrotum, and penis. Specifically, a potent inducer of chloracne includes 2,3,7,8-tetrachlorodibenzo-*p*-dioxin (TCDD), which was a contaminant in some batches of Agent Orange used during the Vietnam War as well as a by-product in other industrial processes.

MECHANICAL EXPOSURES

The skin is exposed to various forms of mechanical insults on a daily basis, and numerous occupations involving repetitive tasks may lead to mechanical trauma of the skin. Friction, pressure, pounding, and vibration of the skin may create changes ranging from calluses and blisters to myositis, tenosynovitis, osseous injury, nerve damage, lacerations, shearing of tissue, or abrasions. Lacerations, abrasions, tissue disruption, and blisters additionally pave the way for secondary infection by bacteria, or less often, fungi, parasites, and viruses. Though the skin is well adapted to cope with such insults, the time allowed for adaptation determines the reaction of the skin. The effects on the skin manifestations induced by the trauma are modified by age, gender, humidity, sweating, nutritional status, infection, preexisting skin disease, as well as genetic and racial factors.[50]

Certain occupations are prone to having distinct mechanically induced skin dermatoses. For instance, musicians may develop lesions in areas of chronic rubbing specific to the instrument being played (harpist's finger, fiddler's neck, guitar nipple, cellist's chest, flautist's chin). Athletes who experience repetitive trauma while running or shearing forces from quick changes in directional movements may develop black heel or *talon noir* as well as blisters and jogger's toe. A relatively new group of skin disorders has been described with prolonged computer use with either repetitive trauma (mousing callus) or prolonged pressure (computer palms).[51] Fiberglass may cause a mechanical irritation by penetration into the skin in those who work with the man-made fibers, often causing a pruritic eruption that may resemble scabies. Plants may also induce mechanical irritant dermatitis from delicate hairs (trichromes) or hairs with barbs (glochids). The irritation is caused by both the mechanical action of the oxalate crystal and subsequent penetration of plant toxin or enzyme into the skin.[52] Onycholysis has been reported from repetitive pressure leading to total or partial anoxia of the distal finger tips in housewives and slaughter house workers who skin cattle.[53,54]

The use of vibration-producing tools can induce painful vascular spasms in the fingers and hands known as white finger or vibration-induced white finger (VWF), which is a secondary type of Raynaud phenomenon.[55] In addition to neurovascular, soft tissue, fibrous, and bone injury to the hands and forearms, workers who use pneumatic riveters, chippers, chainsaws, drills, and hammers are at greater risk of suffering from VWF, especially in cold climates. Vibration frequencies between 30 and 300 Hz are most strongly associated with VWF and smoking is a known risk factor. Continued improvements in design of modern equipment has helped to reduce vibration and decrease the prevalence of these symptoms.

In today's society with increasing automation, less frequent manual operation of tools, and better protective gear, mechanically induced occupational skin lesions have greatly decreased in prevalence.[30]

PHYSICAL EXPOSURES

Physical agents such as extremes in temperatures, ionizing, and nonionizing radiation are well-known causes of occupational skin disease.

THERMAL STRESS

Background and Clinical Features: Heat may cause burns, hyperhidrosis, erythema, and telangiectasias. Workers in hot environments such as farmers and construction workers may develop miliaria in areas of chronic rubbing with clothing, leading to symptoms of pruritus, papule formation, and even a small risk of heat exhaustion due to an inability to maintain normal homeostasis through sweating. Relief may be obtained with wearing loose clothing and cooling the skin. Erythema ab igne also has been observed in repeated, prolonged exposure to heat and in those using laptops on their laps for extensive periods of time. In addition, preexisting skin conditions and diseases may be aggravated by heat exposure, such as rosacea, herpes simplex, and acne vulgaris.

Work-related burn injuries often result in hospitalizations with extensive treatment. Hot grease burns may be seen in kitchen workers, roofers may incur hot tar burns, and flammable and explosive liquids are known to cause most industry-related burns. Specific occupations are associated with higher rates of burn injuries, with welders having the highest incidence rates for all burn injuries.[56] Cooks, laborers, food service workers, mechanics, and nurse aides are also occupations at higher risk. One report noted that almost one third of all hospitalized burn injuries were work-related, highlighting the impact of this occupational hazard.[57]

Cold exposure may lead to Raynaud phenomenon. Frostbite is another common cold injury that may be seen affecting acral body surface areas such as the nose, ears, fingers, and toes of firemen, construction workers, postal workers, and military personnel. Individuals engaged in winter sports, refrigeration workers, icemakers, liquefied gas makers, ski patrolmen, and mountain rescue workers are also at risk.

IONIZING AND NONIONIZING RADIATION

Background and Clinical Features: Occupational skin cancers are more common than generally recognized, although it is difficult to obtain an accurate estimate of their prevalence. Ultraviolet radiation (UV), both natural and artificial, is the most important cause for all types of skin cancer to include melanoma, squamous cell carcinoma, and basal cell carcinoma.[58] It is estimated that avoiding this risk factor alone could prevent more than 3 million cases of skin cancer each year.[59]

Occupational skin cancer is characterized by long induction periods, often decades, with the first manifestations often not seen until many years after the occupational exposure.[60] Outdoor workers, loosely defined as individuals who work outdoors for 3 or more hours on a typical workday, are at high risk of harmful UV exposure and development of skin cancer.[61] These may include workers in industries such as agriculture, building and construction, fishing, transport, and landscaping as well as physical education teachers and police officers.

Other professions at risk include pilots and cabin attendants. A meta-analysis identified twice the rate of melanoma in pilots and cabin crew compared with the general population.[62] Because UV radiation is recognized to increase by 10% to 12% for every 1000 m in elevation, airline crews have the potential for increased UV exposure by as much as 2 to 3 times at cruising altitude.[63] One study identified that pilots and cabin crew flying for approximately 56 minutes at cruising altitude receive the same amount of UV-A as that from a 20-minute tanning bed session.[64]

As 90% of squamous cell carcinoma and basal cell carcinoma and two-thirds of melanomas may be attributed to excessive UV radiation exposure, the aim of primary skin cancer prevention is to limit UV radiation exposure.[60] Three measures successful in the prevention of skin cancer in outdoor workers include regular use of sunscreen, protection from direct UV radiation by suitable clothing, and changes in behavior with awareness of health and diseases resulting from exposure to UV radiation. Even with recommended strategies to use protective measures such as wide-brimmed hats, long-sleeve shirts and pants, sunscreen, and avoiding peak UV times (10 AM to 3 PM), many studies have shown inadequate use of sun protection measures by outdoor workers.[65] An Australian study of construction workers discovered that only 10% of workers were using adequate sun protective measures.[66] This highlights the continued need for an increase in skin cancer awareness and safe sun practices in individuals with high levels of work-related UV radiation exposure.

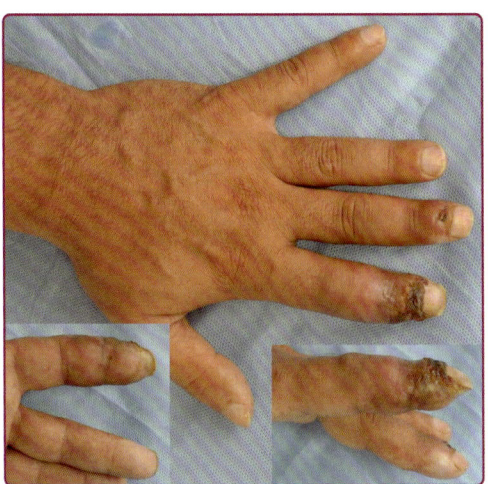

Figure 27-6 Finger injury from overexposure to an industrial gamma radiation source. (From Sahin C, Cesur C, Sever C, Eren F. Finger injury from over-exposure to an industrial gamma radiation source. *Burns*. 2015;41:e8-e10, with permission. Copyright © Elsevier.)

To determine the role of the workplace in the development of skin cancer and actinic skin damage, one must take into consideration not only detailed occupational history with job descriptions from earliest worker employment but also nonoccupational activities, hobbies, and outdoor recreational pursuits from a worker's past.

Ionizing radiation, such as X-rays, can also cause skin cancer, primarily squamous cell carcinoma and less often basal cell carcinoma. High levels of acute exposure may lead to acute radiation dermatitis observed as erythema, itching, and cutaneous inflammation. Higher doses may manifest as skin blisters, hemorrhage, and even necrosis (Fig. 27-6). Delayed sequelae from exposure may result in chronic radiation dermatitis with skin atrophy, abnormal pigmentation, keratinization disorders, increasing sclerosis, telangiectasias, hair loss, and xerosis due to loss of sebaceous glands. Ionizing radiation sources may be found in a wide range of occupational settings, and examples include health care facilities, nuclear weapon production facilities, nuclear reactors and their support facilities, and various manufacturing settings.[67]

BIOLOGIC EXPOSURES

BACKGROUND

A number of infectious agents are responsible for occupational skin disease, especially in occupations that involve contact with animals. With greater awareness and implementation of public health measures, many historically prominent infections have greatly diminished in the general population. However, certain infectious agents are still observed in at-risk occupational groups such as health care workers, military personnel, farmers, and forestry workers. These infections, in turn, may affect the productivity of a worker and ultimately the employer when conditions favor disease transmission.

BACTERIAL INFECTIONS

Staphylococcus and Streptococcus: Staphylococci and streptococci are gram-positive bacteria that can contaminate minor lacerations, burns, puncture wounds, or abrasions leading to impetigo, cellulitis, furuncles, and abscesses. Though all occupations may be at risk, they are prevalent in meat packers, construction workers, farm workers, and those working in close contact with other infected individuals, for example, nurses, athletes, hairdressers, and manicurists. Epidemics of methicillin-resistant *Staphylococcus aureus* infections that have been difficult to control have been documented in professional football players in the United States.[68]

Anthrax: Anthrax, though endemic in parts of Africa and Asia, is rare in the United States and predominantly a cutaneous infection (Woolsorter disease) found in occupations in which workers handle imported goat hair, wool, and hides contaminated with the spores from the bacterium *Bacillus anthracis*.[69] Only 49 anthrax-related epidemiologic investigations were conducted by the U.S. Centers for Disease Control and Prevention between 1950 and 2001, with most involving agricultural settings or textile mills.[70] Because of the highly infectious nature of its spores and recent world events including the 2001 bioterrorism anthrax attacks in the United States, *Bacillus anthracis* is also considered a high-priority pathogen by several U.S. government agencies for its potential as a bioterrorist agent.

Fish Tank Granuloma: *Mycobacterium marinum* is an acid-fast, nontuberculous mycobacterium that was first isolated in 1926 from salt water fish carcasses in the Philadelphia aquarium.[71] It is responsible for fish tank granuloma (also known as swimming pool granuloma), a distinct infection presenting as a warty nodule or plaque usually at a point of trauma, often 6 weeks after exposure. Individuals with fish- or water-based occupations and hobbies are most at risk. Vectors of the infection include fresh or salt water fish, shellfish, snails, water fleas, or dolphins.[72,73]

Erysipeloid (Fish-Handler Disease): The gram-positive bacterium *Erysipelothrix rhusiopathiae* is responsible for the acute infection of erysipeloid, which is almost always an occupational disease. Human infection is associated with handling of decaying animal products such as fish, shellfish, mammals, and poultry. Infection occurs when a worker has a predisposing insult to the skin, such as an abrasion or cut that allows entry of the bacteria. A localized sharply demarcated bright red to violaceous infection, often involving the hands, then ensues. Occupations at risk include fisherman, butchers, farmers, veterinary surgeons, and poultry dressers.[74]

Pitted Keratolysis: Pitted keratolysis is a rather common dermatologic condition caused by gram-positive bacterium (usually *Corynebacterium* species) that infects the stratum corneum of the plantar skin, leading to malodor, hyperhidrosis, and sliminess of the skin. Though well documented among bare-footed laborers, such as paddy farmers in the tropics, it is also observed in soldiers, miners, and laborers as a result of occlusive, protective shoe-wear that creates a warm and moist environment for the bacteria. Because of pain while marching and walking, the condition may cause reduced operational deployability when observed in military personnel.[75] A study of 144 US Marine volunteers in combat in Vietnam during monsoon months discovered that 49% of soldiers were affected with this condition.[76]

Brucellosis: Brucellosis is a worldwide zoonosis caused by gram-negative bacterium of the genus *Brucella* that is primarily a disease of animals in which humans are an accidental host.[77] Occupationally, the disease is contracted through inhalation of contaminated aerosols, contact with conjunctival mucosa, or entry of bacteria through cuts in the skin as a result of contact with infected animals or their products.[78] Occupations at highest risk include slaughterhouse workers, farmers, veterinarians, meat packers, livestock breeders, and laboratory workers. Nonoccupational sources of exposure include ingestion of infected milk or milk products. Brucellosis is a multisystem disease that presents with symptoms such as fevers, night sweats, myalgia, weight loss, and arthralgia but has a propensity for more serious chronicity. Skin manifestations are generally infrequent and have been reported to affect anywhere from 1% to 14% of those infected.[79] Cutaneous findings of brucellosis are often nonspecific, and findings include disseminated papular and nodular eruptions, nodosum-like erythema, extensive purpura, diffuse macular and papular rash, chronic ulcerations, and abscesses.[80]

Tularemia: Tularemia is a potentially severe zoonosis caused by *Francisella tularensis*, a gram-negative bacterium transmitted by ticks, fleas, deerflies, as well as by ingestion, inhalation, or direct contact with infected tissues. The most common presentation of tularemia is the ulceroglandular form, where an ulcer arises at the site of inoculation and regional lymphadenopathy develops. The more severe, though less common, pneumonic form may develop after inhalation of the bacteria. Historically, tularemia has been reported among laboratory workers, farmers, veterinarians, sheep workers, hunters, cooks, and meat handlers; however, recent literature supports an increased risk in landscapers, particularly for the pneumonic form of the disease. Health care workers in tularemia-endemic areas should consider a diagnosis of tularemia in landscapers who have fever or pneumonia.[81]

FUNGAL AND YEAST INFECTIONS

A wide variety of mycoses may be responsible for occupational dermatoses including most kinds of dermatophytoses, candidiasis, and even deep mycoses. Tinea pedis is a common infection of the general population but certain workers are at even greater risk of infection as a result of humid, occlusive footwear such as miners, military personnel, athletes, and laborers.[25] Zoophilic dermatophytes such as *Trichophyton verrucosum* are associated with cattle, farm buildings, and straw; *Trichophyton mentagrophytes* may be transmitted by cattle and domestic animals; *Microsporum canis* is identified in domestic animals, especially cats; and, *Microsporum nanum* may be found in pigs.[26,27,82] Thus, occupations at risk for these zoophilic dermatophytes include slaughterhouse workers, veterinarians, farmers, and pet shop workers.

Bartenders, waitresses, and food handlers are prone to developing candida skin infections as a result of their wet work, which provides a favorable environment for the yeast in macerated skin near the nails and between the digits. Prevention is key through proper drying of the skin and wearing protective gloves.

Inoculation of *Sporothrix schenckii* via puncture wounds from thorns, splinters, sticks, and sphagnum moss can lead to sporotrichosis. Those at risk include gardeners, forestry workers, nursery workers, miners, and farmers. Since the late 1990s, there has been an epidemic of sporotrichosis associated with transmission by cats in Rio de Janeiro, Brazil, thus adding veterinarians as an at-risk occupation.[83]

Other subcutaneous and deep mycoses known to be responsible for OSDs include histoplasmosis, with at-risk occupations being construction workers and farmers who participate in demolition, soil-disrupting activities, and excavation in endemic areas. Chromoblastomycosis, phaeohyphomycosis, and eumycetoma (Madura foot) are subcutaneous mycoses that are all acquired as a result of penetrating trauma to the skin.[84] Farmers and outdoor workers are most at risk for these chronic and challenging mycoses.

VIRAL INFECTIONS

Herpes Simplex Virus: The high prevalence and infectious nature of herpes simplex virus (HSV) makes it an occupational hazard among health care workers, particularly for dental practices, where HSV can be easily spread by direct (lip) or indirect (finger) contact, especially when a lesion is present in the patient.[85]

Orf (Ecthyma Contagiosum): Orf, or ecthyma contagiosum, is a zoonotic infection caused by a parapoxvirus that commonly infects sheep and goats and is transmitted to humans through contact with infected animals or fomites. Veterinarians, sheep herders, and farmers are most at risk, though it has been reported in children after visiting petting zoos and livestock fairs.[86]

Pseudocowpox (Milker Nodule): Milker nodule, also known as pseudocowpox, is an occupational viral infection transmitted by direct contact from infected cows' udders to farmers, veterinarians, and also fresh meat handlers. Painful nodules similar to orf develop on exposed sites, become crusted, and then spontaneously resolve. Prevention consists of treating the cows' mastitis as well as using preventive measures such as gloves, soap, water, and disinfectants before and after handling these animals.[87]

Human Papilloma Virus: Viral warts causes by human papilloma virus (HPV) have been well documented in butchers and meat and fish handlers. Though these warts may be due to many different serotypes of HPV, HPV-7 (Butcher wart virus) is almost exclusive to this group of workers.[88] Recent innovations in dermatology as well as other medical specialties in the treatment of HPV-induced diseases have brought up questions regarding the controversial nature of the risk of nasopharyngeal HPV in health care personnel. However, a recent study supports a low HPV transmission risk of oral and nasal HPV in employees performing CO_2-laser evaporation of genital warts or loop electrode excision procedure (LEEP) of cervical dysplasia by gynecologists, though more studies are likely needed to further assess this relatively new occupational risk.[89]

Bloodborne Pathogens: The 3 bloodborne viruses that are known to pose a serious occupational threat to health care workers include hepatitis B virus (HBV), hepatitis C virus (HCV), and HIV. Although infections by these bloodborne pathogens generally do not exhibit acute skin findings, untreated and prolonged viral burden may have skin manifestations as well as other systemic dysfunctions. Acquisition of infection from body fluids and accidental puncture wounds are known routes of risk to health care personnel. Though safer needle devices for performing procedures and universal infection control precautions are in place, they will not completely eliminate the risk, and prophylactic treatment will remain an important component of prevention efforts.[90]

DIAGNOSIS OF OCCUPATIONAL SKIN DISEASES

PATCH TESTING AND ALLERGIC CONTACT DERMATITIS

Patch testing is the gold standard in diagnosing ACD and is pivotal in helping to determine the etiology of OSDs when assessing contact dermatitis. Early evaluation and diagnosis of ACD has been associated with decreased health care costs and improved disease course and quality of life of the patient.[91] Taking a careful exposure and occupational history is pivotal in guiding appropriate selection of allergens to be tested. Testing is performed using commercially prepared allergens, which are mixed in petrolatum or water and sold in individual syringes or vials. Allergens are grouped in series, such as the rubber, metals, glues and adhesives series, or by profession, such as the dental, hairdressers', or bakers' series. The TRUE Test® is a prepackaged, ready-to-apply kit that now consists of 3 adhesive panels of 35 allergens and allergen mixes that are reported to be responsible for the majority of cases of ACD. The North American Contact Dermatitis Group (NACDG) standard screening tray includes a greater range of allergens and is also widely used among other commercially available series.

It may be necessary to test products from the workplace, as not all allergens may be included in the panel used. However, a basic principle is to never test an unknown substance or test with known irritants such as solvents, cements, and soaps. Patch testing should be performed by a trained provider, who has access to a wide range of allergens for testing purposes and experience in interpreting results. The successful management of ACD requires a meticulous and dedicated physician who is able to not only recognize and treat the skin disease but also has an understanding of the ramifications of the results in regard to the patient's occupation and potential legal aspects of workers' compensation boards.

SKIN PRICK TESTING AND CONTACT URTICARIA

In contrast to patch testing, skin prick testing (SPT) is an allergy test used for the identification of IgE-mediated immediate hypersensitivity reactions (eg, immunologic contact urticaria). The skin prick introduces a small amount of allergen into the epidermis eliciting a localized response in the form of a wheal and erythema at the site of testing when positive. In regard to OCD, the test is used to help make a diagnosis when contact urticaria is suspected. Conventionally, it is also used for diagnosing other type I immediate hypersensitivity reactions in patients with rhinoconjunctivitis, asthma, atopic eczema, and food allergy. Specifically for ICU, a diagnostic algorithm is illustrated in Fig. 27-7. Of note, alternatives similar to SPT include scratch testing and scratch-chamber testing, which may be used for non-standardized allergens because routine use in place of SPT is not recommended.[92]

RADIOALLERGOSORBENT TESTING AND CONTACT URTICARIA

Blood tests may be used to help measure the amount of allergen-specific antibodies present in the blood and guide the diagnosis in regards to an allergy. For instance, the radioallergosorbent test (RAST) measures serum-specific IgE, though it has become outdated and is now often replaced with the more sensitive enzyme-linked immunosorbent assay (ELISA) tests that do not require radioactivity. In 2010 the United States

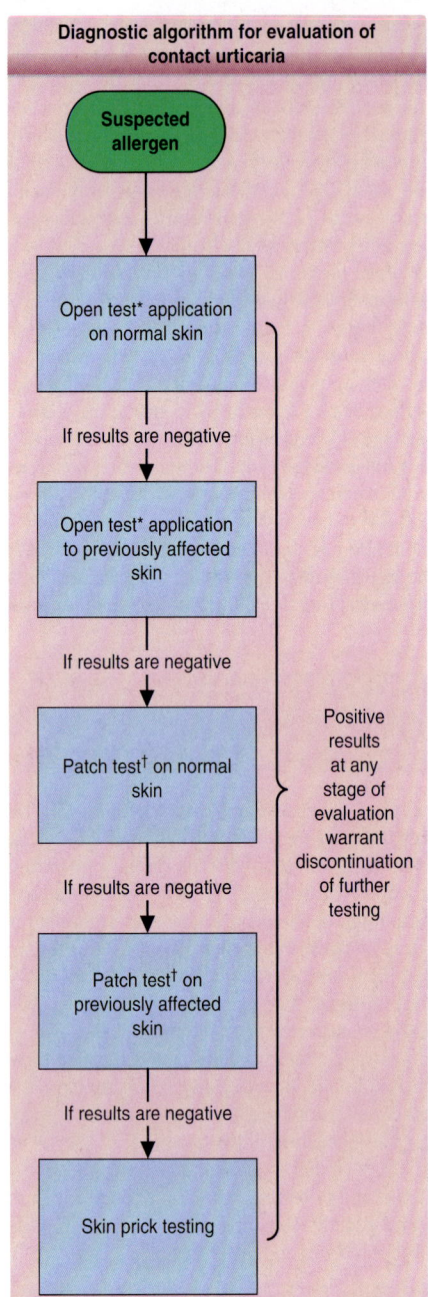

Figure 27-7 Diagnostic algorithm for evaluation of contact urticaria.[92,93,94] *Open test: application of the substance in a vehicle (petrolatum, ethanol, water) is applied over a 3 × 3-cm area and usually read at 20-, 40-, and 60-min intervals. Immunologic contact urticaria usually presents earlier (15-20 min), whereas nonimmunologic contact urticaria may be delayed (45-60 min) after application. †Patch should be removed after 15-20 min after application and interpreted at similar intervals to the open test.[38] Appropriate resuscitation equipment and medications should be readily available when testing for contact urticaria.

National Institute of Allergy and Infectious Diseases recommended that the RAST measurements of specific IgE for the diagnosis of allergy be abandoned in favor of testing with more sensitive fluorescence enzyme-labeled assays.[95]

OTHER DIAGNOSTIC TESTING

Depending on the potential exposure based on occupational history and clinical examination, other diagnostic modalities may be used to make a definitive diagnosis. Common procedures in nonoccupational settings such as skin scraping with potassium hydroxide (KOH) preparation and skin biopsies can similarly be utilized in the occupational setting.

In addition, several other biomonitoring methods may be employed particularly for certain occupational exposures. For example, exposure to arsenic can be detected in the blood, hair, nails, and urine; however, measuring arsenic in the urine provides the most reliable indicator of exposure. In addition, when measuring arsenic in the urine, it is important to request speciation to determine the specific amounts of organic versus inorganic arsenic. Inorganic arsenic, elemental arsenic, and arsine gas are the toxic forms leading to adverse health effects. Organic arsenic (eg, arsenobetaine), on the other hand, is relatively benign and can be found in seafood, which can significantly elevate total arsenic levels up to 72 hours after ingesting a seafood meal.

Furthermore, although beryllium sensitization can be detected through patch testing, laboratory testing of the blood is also commonly used in the occupational setting. The beryllium lymphocyte proliferation test (Be-LPT) exposes the separated white blood cells drawn from a venipuncture to a beryllium solution and measures the proliferation of these white blood cells. In one large study of more than 12,000 individuals, the sensitivity and specificity of the Be-LPT were 68.3% and 96.9%, respectively.[96] Identifying sensitization to beryllium is paramount because sensitized workers can develop chronic beryllium disease (CBD), a permanent and potentially progressive granulomatous restrictive lung disease. Observational studies suggest that early treatment of clinically apparent CBD is associated with improved pulmonary function, radiographic findings, respiratory symptoms, and functional status.[97] When beryllium sensitization is initially suspected, additional testing in conjunction with temporary or permanent work restriction may be recommended.

MANAGEMENT

Treatment of OSDs is dependent on the initial cause and is practically the same as that for skin diseases of nonoccupational origin. Identifying the specific cause(s) of the patient's disease and outlining the appropriate steps to avoid exposure and recurrences is an important role to be played by the provider. As most occupational skin disorders are preventable, patients should be educated on the appropriate preventive measures. Employers should work with their employees to mitigate hazards through the hierarchy of controls (Fig. 27-8), with the last resort for prevention being protective clothing and topical barriers, if practical. Ideally, medical providers and occupationally related disciplines including industrial hygiene should work with employers to eliminate or substitute known hazards. However, if elimination or substitution is unrealistic, engineering controls should be considered that protect workers through physically isolating hazardous processes. Other methods to help reduce exposure include administrative controls, which include alterations in work cycles to decrease exposure time to hazards.

RISK FACTORS

Understanding risk factors for OSDs is important for potential prevention of disease. Risk factors may be endogenous and beyond the control of the individual, such as age, gender, race and genetics. Or, risk factors may be exogenous and potentially modifiable, including specific occupations and duties, work practices and environment, experience level of the worker, and protective measures used.

In regard to age, reports have indicated that older individuals have reduced reactivity to irritants.[98] However, research on age and development of ACD is less clear, with studies showing mixed results.[99] Several studies have also shown that occupational ICD is seen more commonly in females. At the same time, many epidemiologic assessments may be biased by chemical exposure patterns and specific gender-related occupations, which may give a perception that females are more reactive to irritants than males, and this difference is not necessarily supported by direct comparative testing.[98] Females may be more predisposed to developing ACD, but again, this is likely related to exposure patterns and not to intrinsic skin characteristics.[100] Racial differences in dermatologic response to chemical agents also have been described, with some evidence that Asian skin may be more reactive and black skin less reactive than white skin.[101]

Increasing research on genetic factors has found genetic susceptibility markers associated with ICD and ACD. For ICD and ACD, alterations in production of pro-inflammatory cytokines interleukin (IL)-1alpha, IL-1beta, IL-8, tumor necrosis factor (TNF-alpha), and anti-inflammatory IL-1 have been associated with increased risk.[102] Additionally, mutations in the filaggrin gene have been shown to affect skin barrier functions and contribute to the development of atopic dermatitis and potential susceptibility towards contact dermatitis. Maceration and other skin disease that disrupt the skin barrier can enhance penetration of both irritants and allergens. Atopic dermatitis is known to increase the susceptibility of skin to irritants but not to allergens.[102] Consequently, workers with atopic skin disease are more likely to develop OSDs when also exposed to wet work conditions (defined as exposure of skin to liquid for more than 2 hours per day, use of occlusive gloves for more than 2 hours per day, or frequent handwashing).[103] And studies of polymorphisms in genes encoding for metabolic enzymes, such as N-acetyltransferases, suggest a role in developing ACD.[102]

Certain industries and occupations also appear to pose a higher risk of developing occupational dermatoses. Based on the 2010 *Occupational Health Supplement* of the National Health Interview Survey (NHIS) that sampled 17,524 adults who had worked in the preceding 12 months, the period prevalence of occupational dermatitis was highest in arts, entertainment, and recreation (12.6%) followed by health care and social assistance (12.5%) and accommodation and food services (12.4%) industries after adjusting for age, sex, and race/ethnicity.[104] Similarly, occupational categories (defined by the Standard Occupational Classification) identified with the highest prevalence of reported dermatitis included life, physical, and social sciences (18.2%) and art, design, entertainment, sports, and media (15.1%).[104] In contrast, the overall prevalence rate among the surveyed current/recent workers for dermatitis was 9.8%.

Other exogenous risk factors beyond industry and occupation may include chemical concentration, exposure duration, and use of personal protective equipment (PPE). The use of PPE, including gloves and clothing, can often limit hazardous exposures; however, if used improperly, it may actually increase permeation and penetration of irritants and allergens. Furthermore, the PPE itself may directly irritate the skin or contain allergens (eg, latex gloves), so correct

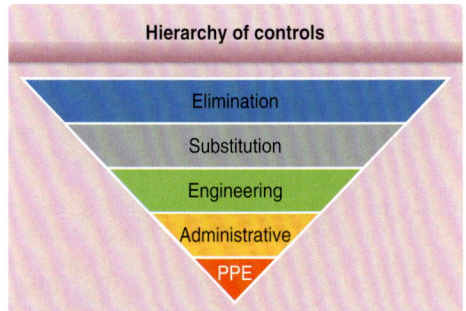

Figure 27-8 Hierarchy of controls. The hierarchy of controls highlights the major categories of mitigating hazards. The most protective to least protective are (1) complete elimination of the hazard, (2) substitution to a nonhazardous or lesser hazardous substance, (3) engineering controls to prevent exposure to the employee, (4) administrative controls to limit the duration of potential exposure, and (5) donning personal protective equipment (PPE).

use of PPE is paramount. Although handwashing is generally encouraged, excessive hygiene measures and use of soaps and detergents can lead to ICD.

HEALTH RISK ASSESSMENT

Although occupational dermatologic hazards exist in many workplaces, the risks to workers are often variable and depend on a multitude of factors. In the occupational environment, this probability is evaluated through a methodical approach known as a health risk assessment. Health risk assessments encompass 4 main components: (1) hazard identification, (2) dose-response relationship, (3) exposure assessment, and (4) risk characterization.

HAZARD IDENTIFICATION

The initial step to identify workplace hazards should incorporate knowledge from industries involving similar work practices and recognize potential injuries and illnesses that can result from related exposures. Hazardous chemicals, in particular, legally require Safety Data Sheets (SDSs, formerly known as Material Safety Data Sheets [MSDSs]), which display not only chemical properties but also adverse health effects, protective equipment necessary for safe handling, and first aid measures for acute exposure treatment among others.[105] Employers must have SDSs readily available to employees for all hazardous chemicals in the workplace.

DOSE-RESPONSE RELATIONSHIP

The dose-response assessment helps delineate relative threshold concentrations of an exposure that results in adverse health effects. For many OCDs, the adverse effects are often dose-dependent with exposure. However, it is important to recognize health conditions (eg, atopic dermatitis) that can contribute to adverse health effects (eg, ICD) at lower exposure doses.

EXPOSURE ASSESSMENT

Because not all OCDs are purely from direct dermal exposures, careful assessment should be taken to determine the potential routes of exposure in the particular workplace. The work task duration and frequency should also be noted as adverse health effects can not only be dose-dependent but time-dependent as well. Furthermore, monitoring is often performed since certain toxic substances have legal permissible exposure limits (PELs) enforced by OSHA. One important caveat is that PELs do not necessarily represent safe limits. The National Institute for Occupational Safety and Health (NIOSH) and American Conference of Governmental Industrial Hygienists (ACGIH) provide recommended exposure limits that are based on adverse health effects.

RISK CHARACTERIZATION

By analyzing the collected data from hazard identification, dose-response assessments, and exposure evaluations, an overall level of risk can be assigned to the evaluated hazards. Some assessors use a risk matrix incorporating toxicity and probability of exposure to determine risk level, but regardless of the method, a safe margin of error should be in place to buffer a higher risk hazard misclassified in a lower risk category.

Ultimately, risk characterization also allows recommendations on control measures, if necessary, which may include substitution of chemicals, changes in ventilation, addition of local exhaust, alterations in work cycles, and donning of PPE.

REFERENCES

1. Kalia S, Haiducu ML. The burden of skin disease in the United States and Canada. *Dermatol Clin.* 2012;30(1):5-18, vii.
2. Mathias CG. The cost of occupational skin disease. *Arch Dermatol.* 1985;121(3):332-334.
3. Sternbach G. The history of anthrax. *J Emerg Med.* 2003;24(4):463-467.
4. Martin C, Meachen GN, Martin SC. *The Urologic and Cutaneous Review: Technical Supplement.* Vol 3. St. Louis, MO: Philmar Company; 1915.
5. Herr HW. Percivall Pott, the environment and cancer. *BJU Int.* 2011;108(4):479-481.
6. Lushniak BD. Occupational contact dermatitis. *Dermatol Ther (Heidelb).* 2004;17(3):272-277.
7. Bureau of Labor Statistics (BLS). Nonfatal Occupational Injuries and Illnesses. http://www.bls.gov/iif/.
8. Lushniak BD. The importance of occupational skin diseases in the United States. *Int Arch Occup Environ Health.* 2003;76(5):325-330.
9. Dickel H, Kuss O, Blesius CR, et al. Occupational skin diseases in Northern Bavaria between 1990 and 1999: a population-based study. *Br J Dermatol.* 2001;145(3):453-462.
10. Diepgen TL, Coenraads PJ. The epidemiology of occupational contact dermatitis. *Int Arch Occup Environ Health.* 1999;72(8):496-506.
11. Halkier-Sorensen L. Occupational skin diseases. *Contact Dermatitis.* 1996;35(1)(suppl):1-120.
12. Mathias CG, Sinks TH, Seligman PJ, et al. Surveillance of occupational skin diseases: a method utilizing workers' compensation claims. *Am J Ind Med.* 1990;17(3):363-370.
13. Meyer JD, Chen Y, Holt DL, et al. Occupational contact dermatitis in the UK: a surveillance report from EPIDERM and OPRA. *Occup Med (Lond).* 2000;50(4):265-273.

14. Emmett EA. Occupational contact dermatitis, I: incidence and return to work pressures. *Am J Contact Dermat.* 2002;13(1):30.
15. Agner T. An experimental study of irritant effects of urea in different vehicles. *Acta Derm Venereol Suppl.* 1992;177:44-46.
16. Belsito DV. Occupational contact dermatitis: etiology, prevalence, and resultant impairment/disability. *J Am Acad Dermatol.* 2005;53(2):303-313.
17. Smith HR, Basketter DA, McFadden JP. Irritant dermatitis, irritancy and its role in allergic contact dermatitis. *Clin Exp Dermatol.* 2002;27(2):138-146.
18. Weltfriend S, Ramon M, Maibach HI. *Dermatotoxicology.* 6th ed. Boca Raton, FL: CRC Press; 2004.
19. Wigger-Alberti W, Elsner P. Contact dermatitis due to irritation. *Handbook of Occupational Dermatology.* Berlin: Springer; 2000:99-110.
20. Tan CH, Rasool S, Johnston GA. Contact dermatitis: allergic and irritant. *Clin Dermatol.* 2014;32(1):116-124.
21. Caroe TK, Ebbehoj N, Agner T. A survey of exposures related to recognized occupational contact dermatitis in Denmark in 2010. *Contact Dermatitis.* 2014;70(1):56-62.
22. Patil S, Maibach HI. Effect of age and sex on the elicitation of irritant contact dermatitis. *Contact Dermatitis.* 1994;30(5):257-264.
23. Iliev D, Elsner P. Clinical irritant contact dermatitis syndromes. *Immunol Allergy Clin North Am.* 1997;17(3):365-375.
24. Skogstad M, Levy F. Occupational irritant contact dermatitis and fungal infection in construction workers. *Contact Dermatitis.* 1994;31(1):28-30.
25. Kamihama T, Kimura T, Hosokawa JI, et al. Tinea pedis outbreak in swimming pools in Japan. *Public Health.* 1997;111(4):249-253.
26. Agnetti F, Righi C, Scoccia E, et al. *Trichophyton verrucosum* infection in cattle farms of Umbria (Central Italy) and transmission to humans. *Mycoses.* 2014;57(7):400-405.
27. Khosravi AR, Mahmoudi M. Dermatophytes isolated from domestic animals in Iran. *Mycoses.* 2003;46(5-6):222-225.
28. Malten KE. Thoughts on irritant contact dermatitis. *Contact Dermatitis.* 1981;7(5):238-247.
29. Seyfarth F, Schliemann S, Antonov D, et al. Dry skin, barrier function, and irritant contact dermatitis in the elderly. *Clin Dermatol.* 2011;29(1):31-36.
30. Kanerva L, Elsner P, Wahlberg J, et al. *Handbook of Occupational Dermatology.* New York: Springer Science & Business Media; 2013.
31. Green BG. Measurement of sensory irritation of the skin. *Am J Contact Derm.* 2000;11(3):170-180.
32. Robinson MK, Perkins MA. Evaluation of a quantitative clinical method for assessment of sensory skin irritation. *Contact Dermatitis.* 2001;45(4):205-213.
33. Holness DL. Characteristic features of occupational dermatitis: epidemiologic studies of occupational skin disease reported by contact dermatitis clinics. *Occup Med.* 1994;9(1):45-52.
34. Rietschel RL, Mathias CG, Fowler JF Jr, et al. Relationship of occupation to contact dermatitis: evaluation in patients tested from 1998 to 2000. *Am J Contact Derm.* 2002;13(4):170-176.
35. Kucenic MJ, Belsito DV. Occupational allergic contact dermatitis is more prevalent than irritant contact dermatitis: a 5-year study. *J Am Acad Dermatol.* 2002;46(5):695-699.
36. Suneja T, Belsito DV. Occupational dermatoses in health care workers evaluated for suspected allergic contact dermatitis. *Contact Dermatitis.* 2008;58(5):285-290.
37. Nicholson PJ, Llewellyn D, English JS. Evidence-based guidelines for the prevention, identification and management of occupational contact dermatitis and urticaria. *Contact Dermatitis.* 2010;63(4):177-186.
38. McFadden J. Immunologic contact urticaria. *Immunol Allergy Clin North Am.* 2014;34(1):157-167.
39. Lahti A. Non-immunologic contact urticaria. *Acta Derm Venereol Suppl.* 1980;60:1-49.
40. Basketter D, Lahti A. Immediate contact reactions. In: Johansen DJ, Frosch JP, Lepoittevin JP, eds. *Contact Dermatitis.* 5th ed. Berlin: Springer; 2011:137-153.
41. Wang CY, Maibach HI. Immunologic contact urticaria—the human touch. *Cutan Ocul Toxicol.* 2013;32(2):154-160.
42. Christopher CN. Latex allergy: a real problem. *Med J Aust.* 1996;165(8):460.
43. Cohen DE, Scheman A, Stewart L, et al. American Academy of Dermatology's position paper on latex allergy. *J Am Acad Dermatol.* 1998;39(1):98-106.
44. Kahn SL, Podjasek JO, Dimitropoulos VA, et al. Natural rubber latex allergy. *Dis Mon.* 2016;62(1):5-17.
45. Heese A, van Hintzenstern J, Peters KP, et al. Allergic and irritant reactions to rubber gloves in medical health services. Spectrum, diagnostic approach, and therapy. *J Am Acad Dermatol.* 1991;25(5, pt 1):831-839.
46. von Hintzenstern J, Heese A, Koch HU, et al. Frequency, spectrum and occupational relevance of type IV allergies to rubber chemicals. *Contact Dermatitis.* 1991;24(4):244-252.
47. Bjorkner BE. Industrial airborne dermatoses. *Dermatol Clin.* 1994;12(3):501-509.
48. Adams BB, Chetty VB, Mutasim DF. Periorbital comedones and their relationship to pitch tar: a cross-sectional analysis and a review of the literature. *J Am Acad Dermatol.* 2000;42(4):624-627.
49. Taylor JS. Environmental chloracne: update and overview. *Ann N Y Acad Sci.* 1979;320:295-307.
50. Kligman AM. The chronic effects of repeated mechanical trauma to the skin. *Am J Ind Med.* 1985;8(4-5):257-264.
51. Goksugur N, Cakici H. A new computer-associated occupational skin disorder: Mousing callus. *J Am Acad Dermatol.* 2006;55(2):358-359.
52. Epstein W. House and garden plants. In: Jackson E, Goldner R, eds. *Irritant Contact Dermatitis.* New York: Marcel Dekker; 1990:127-165.
53. Menne T, Roed-Petersen J, Hjorth N. Pressure onycholysis in slaugtherhouse workers. *Acta Derm Venereol Suppl (Stockh).* 1985;120:88-89.
54. Sharquie IK, Al-Faham M, Karhoot JM, et al. Housewife onycholysis. *Saudi Med J.* 2005;26(9):1439-1441.
55. Olsen N. Diagnostic aspects of vibration-induced white finger. *Int Arch Occup Environ Health.* 2002;75(1-2):6-13.
56. Islam SS, Nambiar AM, Doyle EJ, et al. Epidemiology of work-related burn injuries: experience of a state-managed workers' compensation system. *J Trauma.* 2000;49(6):1045-1051.
57. Rossignol AM, Locke JA, Boyle CM, et al. Epidemiology of work-related burn injuries in Massachusetts requiring hospitalization. *J Trauma.* 1986;26(12):1097-1101.

58. American Cancer Society. Cancer Facts & Figures 2016. http://www.cancer.org/research/cancerfactsstatistics/cancerfactsfigures2016/. Published 2016.
59. American Cancer Society. Cancer Facts & Figures 2014. http://www.cancer.org/acs/groups/content/@research/documents/webcontent/acspc-042151.pdf. Published 2014.
60. Diepgen TL, Fartasch M, Drexler H, et al. Occupational skin cancer induced by ultraviolet radiation and its prevention. *Br J Dermatol.* 2012;167(suppl 2):76-84.
61. Horsham C, Auster J, Sendall MC, et al. Interventions to decrease skin cancer risk in outdoor workers: update to a 2007 systematic review. *BMC Res Notes.* 2014;7:10.
62. Sanlorenzo M, Wehner MR, Linos E, et al. The risk of melanoma in airline pilots and cabin crew: a meta-analysis. *JAMA Dermatol.* 2015;151(1):51-58.
63. Blumthaler M, Ambach W, Ellinger R. Increase in solar UV radiation with altitude. *J Photochem Photobiol B.* 1997;39(2):130-134.
64. Sanlorenzo M, Vujic I, Posch C, et al. The risk of melanoma in pilots and cabin crew: UV measurements in flying airplanes. *JAMA Dermatol.* 2015;151(4):450-452.
65. Kutting B, Drexler H. UV-induced skin cancer at workplace and evidence-based prevention. *Int Arch Occup Environ Health.* 2010;83(8):843-854.
66. Gies P, Wright J. Measured solar ultraviolet radiation exposures of outdoor workers in Queensland in the building and construction industry. *Photochem Photobiol.* 2003;78(4):342-348.
67. Occupational Safety and Health Administration. Safety and health topics: ionizing radiation. https://www.osha.gov/SLTC/radiationionizing/. Published 2016.
68. Kazakova SV, Hageman JC, Matava M, et al. A clone of methicillin-resistant *Staphylococcus aureus* among professional football players. *N Engl J Med.* 2005;352(5):468-475.
69. Marks JG Jr, Elsner P, Deleo VA. *Contact & Occupational Dermatology.* 3rd ed. St. Louis, MO: Mosby; 2002.
70. Bales ME, Dannenberg AL, Brachman PS, et al. Epidemiologic response to anthrax outbreaks: field investigations, 1950-2001. *Emerg Infect Dis.* 2002;8(10):1163-1174.
71. Ang P, Rattana-Apiromyakij N, Goh CL. Retrospective study of *Mycobacterium marinum* skin infections. *Int J Dermatol.* 2000;39(5):343-347.
72. Bonamonte D, De Vito D, Vestita M, et al. Aquarium-borne *Mycobacterium marinum* skin infection. Report of 15 cases and review of the literature. *Eur J Dermatol.* 2013;23(4):510-516.
73. Huminer D, Pitlik SD, Block C, et al. Aquarium-borne *Mycobacterium marinum* skin infection. Report of a case and review of the literature. *Arch Dermatol.* 1986;122(6):698-703.
74. Fidalgo SG, Wang Q, Riley TV. Comparison of methods for detection of *Erysipelothrix* spp. and their distribution in some Australasian seafoods. *Appl Environ Microbiol.* 2000;66(5):2066-2070.
75. van der Snoek EM, Ekkelenkamp MB, Suykerbuyk JC. Pitted keratolysis; physicians' treatment and their perceptions in Dutch army personnel. *J Eur Acad Dermatol Venereol.* 2013;27(9):1120-1126.
76. Gill KA Jr, Buckels LJ. Pitted keratolysis. *Arch Dermatol.* 1968;98(1):7-11.
77. American Academy of Pediatrics. Brucellosis. In: Kimberlin D, Brady M, Jackson M, Long S, eds. *Red Book: 2015 Report of the Committee on Infectious Diseases.* Elk Grove Village, IL: American Academy of Pediatrics; 2015:268-270.
78. Cutler SJ, Whatmore AM, Commander NJ. Brucellosis—new aspects of an old disease. *J Appl Microbiol.* 2005;98(6):1270-1281.
79. Metin A, Akdeniz H, Buzgan T, et al. Cutaneous findings encountered in brucellosis and review of the literature. *Int J Dermatol.* 2001;40(7):434-438.
80. Milionis H, Christou L, Elisaf M. Cutaneous manifestations in brucellosis: case report and review of the literature. *Infection.* 2000;28(2):124-126.
81. Feldman KA, Stiles-Enos D, Julian K, et al. Tularemia on Martha's Vineyard: seroprevalence and occupational risk. *Emerg Infect Dis.* 2003;9(3):350-354.
82. Roller JA, Westblom TU. Microsporum nanum infection in hog farmers. *J Am Acad Dermatol.* 1986;15(5, pt 1):935-939.
83. Barros MB, de Almeida Paes R, Schubach AO. *Sporothrix schenckii* and Sporotrichosis. *Clin Microbiol Rev.* 2011;24(4):633-654.
84. Garnica M, Nucci M, Queiroz-Telles F. Difficult mycoses of the skin: advances in the epidemiology and management of eumycetoma, phaeohyphomycosis and chromoblastomycosis. *Curr Opin Infect Dis.* 2009;22(6):559-563.
85. Lewis MA. Herpes simplex virus: an occupational hazard in dentistry. *Int Dent J.* 2004;54(2):103-111.
86. Human orf virus infection from household exposures—United States, 2009-2011. *MMWR Morb Mortal Wkly Rep.* 2012;61(14):245-248.
87. Leavell UW Jr, Phillips IA. Milker's nodules. Pathogenesis, tissue culture, electron microscopy, and calf inoculation. *Arch Dermatol.* 1975;111(10):1307-1311.
88. Orth G, Jablonska S, Favre M, et al. Identification of papillomaviruses in butchers' warts. *J Invest Dermatol.* 1981;76(2):97-102.
89. Kofoed K, Norrbom C, Forslund O, et al. Low prevalence of oral and nasal human papillomavirus in employees performing CO_2-laser evaporation of genital warts or loop electrode excision procedure of cervical dysplasia. *Acta Derm Venereol.* 2015;95(2):173-176.
90. Gerberding JL. Management of occupational exposures to blood-borne viruses. *N Engl J Med.* 1995;332(7):444-451.
91. Kadyk DL, McCarter K, Achen F, et al. Quality of life in patients with allergic contact dermatitis. *J Am Acad Dermatol.* 2003;49(6):1037-1048.
92. Kim E, Maibach H. Changing paradigms in dermatology: science and art of diagnostic patch and contact urticaria testing. *Clin Dermatol.* 2003;21(5):346-352.
93. Nijhawan RI, Jacob SE. The role of patch testing in contact urticaria. *J Am Acad Dermatol.* 2008;59(2):354-355.
94. von Krogh G, Maibach HI. The contact urticaria syndrome—an updated review. *J Am Acad Dermatol.* 1981;5(3):328-342.
95. Boyce JA, Assa'ad A, Burks AW, et al. Guidelines for the diagnosis and management of food allergy in the United States: report of the NIAID-sponsored expert panel. *J Allergy Clin Immunol.* 2010;126(6)(suppl):S1-S58.
96. Stange AW, Joseph Furman F, Hilmas DE. The beryllium lymphocyte proliferation test: Relevant issues in beryllium health surveillance. *Am J Ind Med.* 2004;46(5):453-462.
97. Balmes JR, Abraham JL, Dweik RA, et al. An official American Thoracic Society statement: diagnosis and management of beryllium sensitivity and chronic

beryllium disease. *Am J Respir Crit Care Med.* 2014;190(10):e34-e59.
98. Robinson MK. Population differences in acute skin irritation responses. Race, sex, age, sensitive skin and repeat subject comparisons. *Contact Dermatitis.* 2002;46(2):86-93.
99. Zhai H, Meier-Davis SR, Cayme B, et al. Allergic contact dermatitis: effect of age. *Cutan Ocul Toxicol.* 2012;31(1):20-25.
100. Modjtahedi BS, Modjtahedi SP, Maibach HI. The sex of the individual as a factor in allergic contact dermatitis. *Contact Dermatitis.* 2004;50(2):53-59.
101. Modjtahedi SP, Maibach HI. Ethnicity as a possible endogenous factor in irritant contact dermatitis: comparing the irritant response among Caucasians, blacks, and Asians. *Contact Dermatitis.* 2002;47(5):272-278.
102. Kezic S, Visser MJ, Verberk MM. Individual susceptibility to occupational contact dermatitis. *Ind Health.* 2009;47(5):469-478.
103. Chew AL, Maibach HI. Occupational issues of irritant contact dermatitis. *Int Arch Occup Environ Health.* 2003;76(5):339-346.
104. Luckhaupt SE, Dahlhamer JM, Ward BW, et al. Prevalence of dermatitis in the working population, united states, 2010 National Health Interview Survey. *Am J Ind Med.* 2013;56(6):625-634.
105. Occupational Safety and Health Administration. Hazard Communication. 29 CFR 1910.1200(g). Washington, DC: Occupational Safety and Health Administration; 2012.

Psoriasiform Disorders   PART 4

第四篇　银屑病样皮肤疾病

Chapter 28 :: Psoriasis
:: Johann E. Gudjonsson & James T. Elder

第二十八章

银屑病

中文导读

本章介绍了银屑病的流行病学、临床特征、病因和发病机制、诊断、鉴别诊断、临床病程及预后、治疗。银屑病根据临床特征可分为各种亚型，临床诊断通常基于临床特征，病理检查可以用于难以诊断的银屑病。银屑病的治疗方法主要包括局部和系统治疗，本章介绍了治疗银屑病不同类型药物的剂量、安全性、有效性等，也列出了对特殊人群如育龄期妇女和妊娠妇女的治疗方案，为临床应用提供了依据。

〔朱　武〕

AT-A-GLANCE

- Worldwide occurrence; affects 2% to 3% of Americans; prevalence ranges from 0.1% to 3% in various populations.
- A chronic disorder with polygenic predisposition combined with triggering environmental factors such as trauma, infection, or medication.
- Erythematous scaly papules and plaques; pustular and erythrodermic eruptions occur.
- Most common sites of involvement are the scalp, elbows, knees, hands, feet, trunk, and nails.

- Psoriatic arthritis occurs in 10% to 25% of patients; pustular and erythrodermic forms may be associated with fever.
- Pathology of fully developed lesions is characterized by uniform elongation of the rete ridges, with dilated blood vessels, thinning of the suprapapillary plate, and intermittent parakeratosis. Epidermal and perivascular dermal infiltrates of lymphocytes, with neutrophils occasionally in aggregates in the epidermis.

INTRODUCTION

DEFINITION

Psoriasis is a common, immunologically mediated, inflammatory disease characterized by skin inflammation, epidermal hyperplasia, and increased risk of a painful and destructive arthritis as well as cardiovascular morbidity and psychosocial challenges. The economic and health burden of this constellation of pathologies is very substantial, yet its cause remains unknown.

HISTORICAL PERSPECTIVE

More than 2000 years ago, Hippocrates used the terms *psora* and *lepra* for conditions that can be recognized as psoriasis. Later, Celsus (ca. 25 BC) described a form of impetigo that was interpreted by Robert Willan (1757–1812) as being psoriasis. Willan separated two diseases as psoriasiform entities, a discoid lepra Graecorum and a polycyclic confluent psora leprosa, which later was called *psoriasis*. In 1841, the Viennese dermatologist Ferdinand von Hebra (1816–1880) unequivocally showed that Willan's lepra Graecorum and psora leprosa were one disease that had caused much confusion because of differences in the size, distribution, growth, and involution of lesions.

EPIDEMIOLOGY

PREVALENCE

Psoriasis is universal in occurrence. However, its reported prevalence in different populations varies considerably, from 0.91% in the United States to 8.5% in Norway.[1] The prevalence of psoriasis is lower in Asians, and in an examination of more than 25,000 Andean Indians, not a single case was seen.[2] Psoriasis appears to be equally common in males and females.

AGE OF ONSET

Psoriasis may begin at any age, but it is uncommon before the age of 10 years. It is most likely to appear between the ages of 15 and 30 years. Possession of certain human leukocyte antigen (HLA) class I antigens, particularly HLA-Cw6, is associated with an earlier age of onset and with a positive family history. This finding led Henseler and Christophers[3] to propose that two different forms of psoriasis exist: type I, with age of onset before 40 years and HLA associated, and type II, with age of onset after 40 years, although many patients do not fit into this classification.

GENETIC EPIDEMIOLOGY

The concordance rate for psoriasis in monozygotic twins ranges from 35% to 73%.[4] This variability and the fact that these rates do not approach 100% support a role for environmental factors. Thus, the mode of inheritance for psoriasis is best described as multifactorial (ie, polygenic plus environmental factors). Interestingly, the overall prevalence of psoriasis,[1] and the concordance of psoriasis in both monozygotic and dizygotic twins decreases with decreasing distance from the equator. These observations suggest that ultraviolet (UV) light exposure may be a major environmental factor interacting with genetic factors in psoriasis.

CLINICAL FEATURES

CUTANEOUS FINDINGS

PLAQUE-TYPE PSORIASIS

The classic lesion of psoriasis is a well-demarcated, raised, red plaque with a white scaly surface (Fig. 28-1). Lesions can vary in size from pinpoint papules to plaques that cover large areas of the body. Under the scale, the skin has a glossy homogeneous erythema, and bleeding points appear when the scale is removed, traumatizing the dilated capillaries below (the Auspitz sign) (Fig. 28-2). Psoriasis tends to be a symmetric eruption, and symmetry is a helpful feature in establishing a diagnosis. Unilateral involvement can occur, however. The psoriatic phenotype may present a changing spectrum of disease expression even within the same patient.

The Koebner phenomenon (also known as the *isomorphic response*) is the traumatic induction of psoriasis on nonlesional skin; it occurs more frequently during flares of disease and is an all-or-none phenomenon (ie, if psoriasis occurs at one site of injury, it will occur at all sites of injury) (Fig. 28-3). The Koebner reaction usually occurs 7 to 14 days after injury, and from 25% to 75% of patients may develop trauma-related Koebner phenomenon at some point during their disease.

Psoriasis vulgaris is the most common form of psoriasis, seen in approximately 90% of patients. Red, scaly, symmetrically distributed plaques are characteristically localized to the extensor aspects of the extremities; particularly the elbows and knees, along with scalp, lower lumbosacral, buttocks, and genital involvement (see Fig. 28-1). Other sites of predilection include the umbilicus and the intergluteal cleft. The extent of involvement varies widely from patient to patient. Lesions may extend laterally and become circinate because of the confluence of several plaques (psoriasis gyrata). Occasionally, there is partial central clearing, resulting in ringlike lesions (annular psoriasis) (Fig. 28-4). This is usually associated with lesional clearing and portends a good prognosis. Other clini-

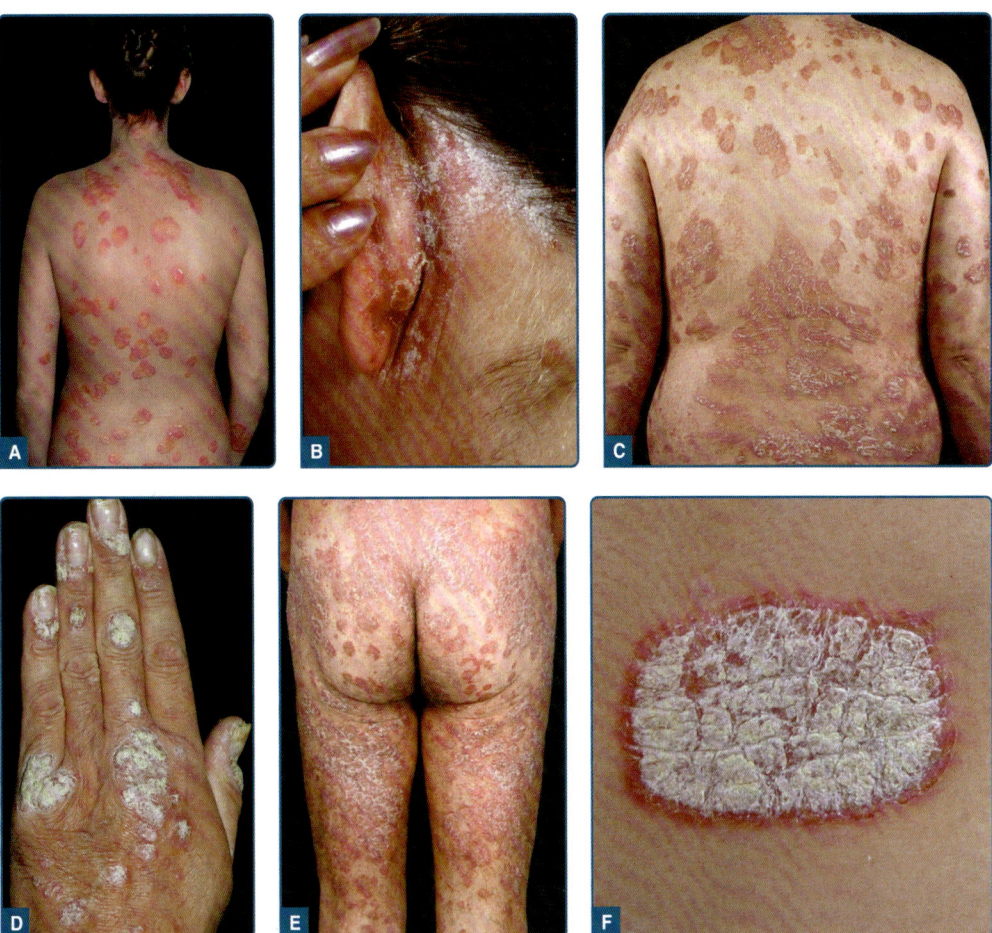

Figure 28-1 **A–F.** Chronic plaque psoriasis located at typical sites. Note the marked symmetry of the lesions. (Used with permission from Dr. Johann Gudjonsson and Mr. Harrold Carter.)

cal variants of plaque psoriasis have been described depending on the morphology of the lesions, particularly those associated with gross hyperkeratosis (see Fig. 28-4). *Rupioid psoriasis* refers to lesions in the shape of a cone or limpet. *Ostraceous psoriasis*, an infrequently used term, refers to a ringlike, hyperkeratotic concave lesion, resembling an oyster shell. Finally, *elephantine psoriasis* is an uncommon form characterized by thickly scaling, large plaques, usually on the lower extremities. A hypopigmented ring (Woronoff ring) surrounding individual psoriatic lesions may occasionally be seen and is usually associated with treatment, most commonly UV radiation or topical corticosteroids (see Fig. 28-4). The pathogenesis of the Woronoff ring is not well understood but may result from inhibition of prostaglandin synthesis.

GUTTATE (ERUPTIVE) PSORIASIS

Guttate psoriasis (from the Latin *gutta*, meaning "a drop") is characterized by eruption of small (0.5–1.5 cm in diameter) papules over the upper trunk and proximal extremities (Fig. 28-5). It typically manifests at an early age and as such is found frequently in young adults. This form of psoriasis has the strongest association to HLA-Cw6,[5] and streptococcal throat infection frequently precedes or is concomitant with the onset or flare of guttate psoriasis.[6] However, antibiotic treatment has not been shown to be beneficial or to shorten the disease course.[7] Patients with a history of chronic plaque psoriasis may develop guttate lesions, with or without worsening of their chronic plaques.

SMALL PLAQUE PSORIASIS

Small plaque psoriasis resembles guttate psoriasis clinically but can be distinguished by its onset in older patients, by its chronicity, and by having somewhat larger lesions (typically 1–2 cm) that are thicker and scalier than in guttate disease. It is said to be a common adult-onset presentation of psoriasis in Korea and other Asian countries.[8]

INVERSE PSORIASIS

Psoriasis lesions may be localized in the major skin folds, such as the axillae, the genitocrural region, and the neck. Scaling is usually minimal or absent,

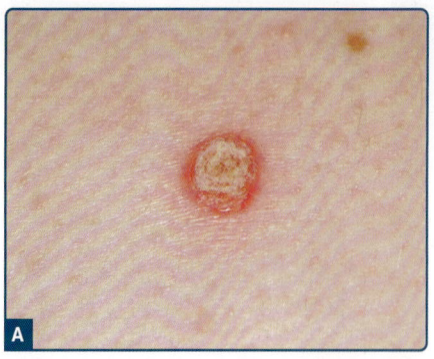
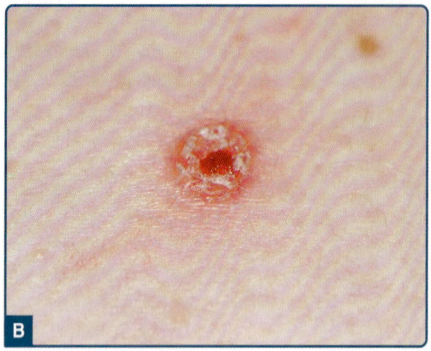

Figure 28-2 **A,** Auspitz sign. **B,** Note the point of bleeding after the scale is removed. (Used with permission from Dr. Johann Gudjonsson and Ms. Laura Vangoor.)

and the lesions show a glossy sharply demarcated erythema, which is often localized to areas of skin-to-skin contact (Fig. 28-6). Sweating is impaired in affected areas.

ERYTHRODERMIC PSORIASIS

Psoriatic erythroderma affects all body sites, including the face, hands, feet, nails, trunk, and extremities (Fig. 28-7). Although all the symptoms of psoriasis are present, erythema is the most prominent feature, and scaling is different compared with chronic stationary psoriasis. Instead of thick, adherent, white scale, there is superficial scaling. Patients with erythrodermic psoriasis lose excessive heat because of generalized vasodilatation, and this may cause hypothermia. Patients may shiver in an attempt to raise their body temperature. Psoriatic skin is often hypohidrotic because of occlusion of the sweat ducts, and there is an attendant risk of hyperthermia in warm climates. Lower extremity edema is common secondary to vasodilation and loss of protein from the blood vessels into the tissues. High-output cardiac failure and impaired hepatic and renal function may also occur. Psoriatic erythroderma has a variable presentation, but two forms are thought to exist. In the first form, chronic plaque psoriasis may worsen to involve most or all of the skin surface, and patients remain relative responsive to therapy. In the second form, generalized erythroderma may present suddenly and

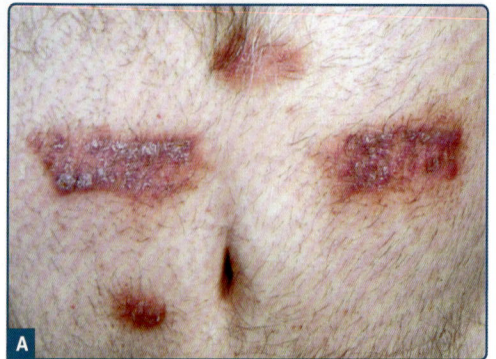
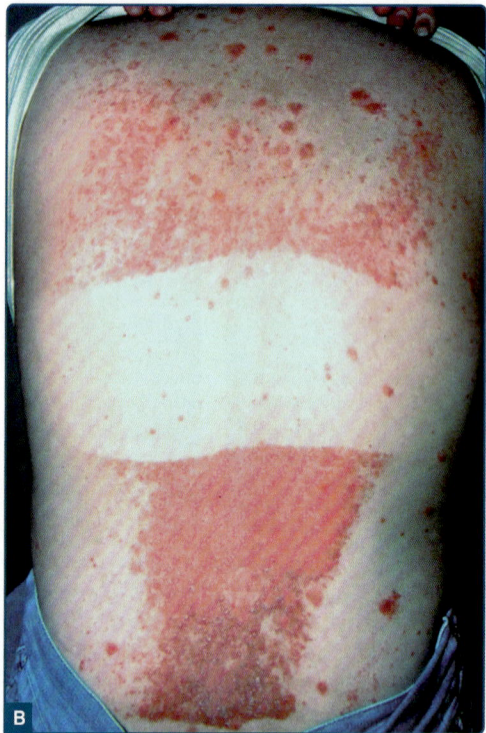

Figure 28-3 Koebner phenomenon. **A,** Psoriasis appearing in keratome biopsy sites 4 weeks after biopsy. **B,** Flare of psoriasis on the back after a sunburn. Note sparing of sun-protected areas. (Image **A,** used with permission from Mr. Harrold Carter. Image **B,** used with permission from Dr. James Rasmussen.)

unexpectedly or result from nontolerated external treatment (eg, UVB, anthralin), thus representing a generalized Koebner reaction. Generalized pustular psoriasis (see later) may revert to erythroderma with diminished or absent pustule formation. Occasional diagnostic problems may arise in differentiating psoriatic erythroderma from other causes.

PUSTULAR PSORIASIS

Several clinical variants of pustular psoriasis exist: generalized pustular psoriasis (von Zumbusch type),

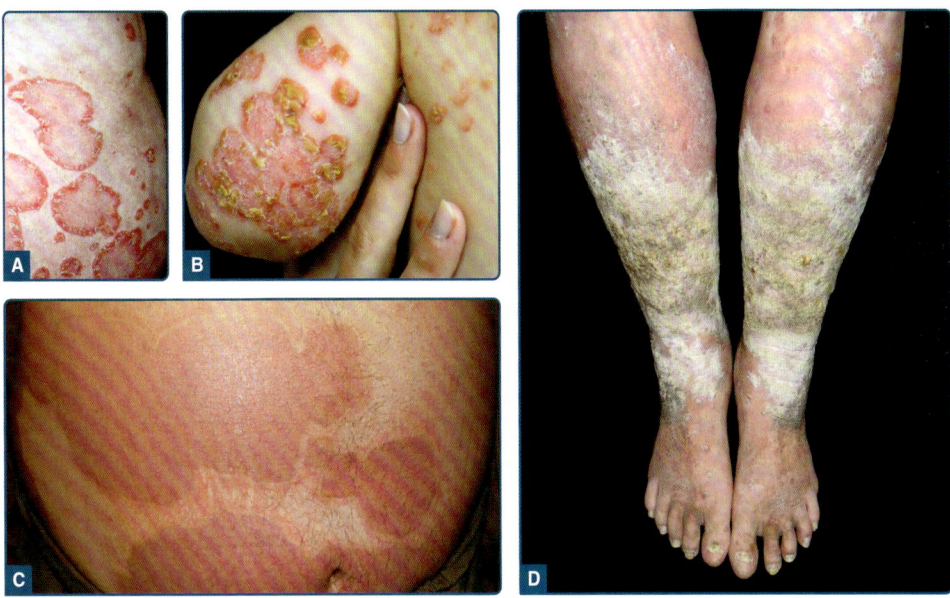

Figure 28-4 Unusual forms of plaque-type psoriasis. **A,** Annular psoriasis on the flank. **B,** Rupioid psoriasis in an infant. Note the cone-shaped lesions. **C,** Psoriatic patient undergoing modified Goeckerman therapy (ultraviolet B light, coal tar, and topical steroid), demonstrating Woronoff rings. **D,** Elephantine psoriasis of the lower extremities. Note psoriatic involvement of toenails. (Used with permission from Dr. Johann Gudjonsson, Mr. Harrold Carter, and Ms. Laura Vangoor.)

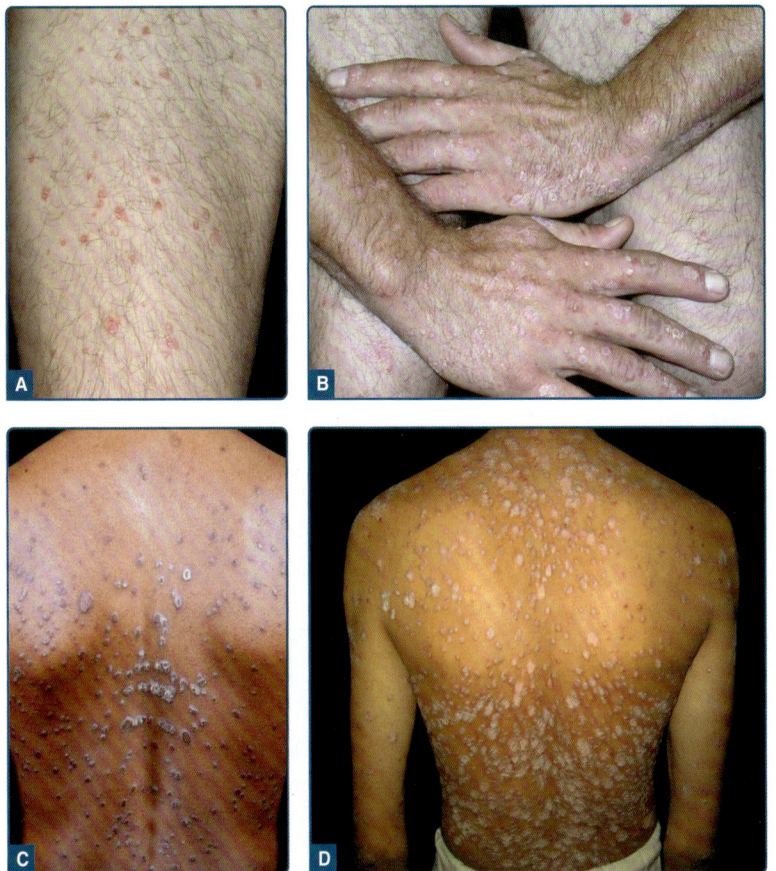

Figure 28-5 Guttate psoriasis, involving the thigh (**A**), hands (**B**), and back (**C** and **D**). The patient in **D** went on to develop chronic plaque psoriasis. (Used with permission from Drs. Johann Gudjonsson and Trilokraj Tejasvi, Mr. Harrold Carter, and Ms. Laura Vangoor.)

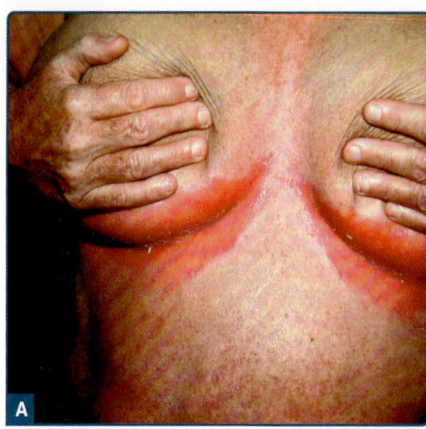
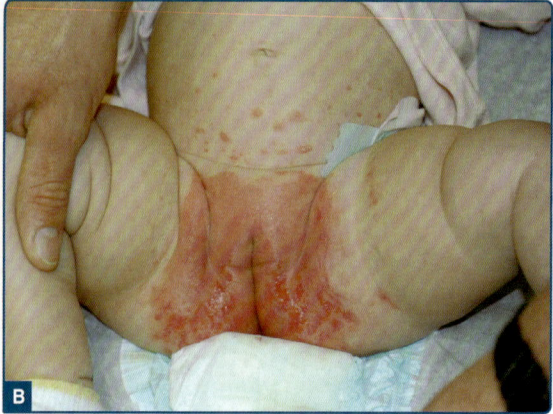

Figure 28-6 Flexural psoriasis. **A,** Well-demarcated, beefy-red, shiny plaques. **B,** Infant with "napkin psoriasis." (Used with permission from Dr. Johann Gudjonsson and Mr. Harrold Carter.)

annular pustular psoriasis, impetigo herpetiformis, and two variants of localized pustular psoriasis—pustulosis palmaris et plantaris and acrodermatitis continua of Hallopeau. In children, pustular psoriasis can be complicated by sterile, lytic lesions of bones and can be a manifestation of the SAPHO syndrome (synovitis, acne, pustulosis, hyperostosis, osteitis).

Generalized Pustular Psoriasis (von Zumbusch): This is a distinctive acute variant of psoriasis that is usually preceded by other forms of the disease. Attacks are characterized by fever that lasts several days and a sudden generalized eruption of sterile pustules 2 to 3 mm in diameter (Fig. 28-8). The pustules are disseminated over the trunk and extremities, including the nail beds, palms, and soles. The pustules usually arise on highly erythematous skin, first as patches (see Fig. 28-8) and then become confluent as the disease becomes more severe. With prolonged disease, the fingertips may become

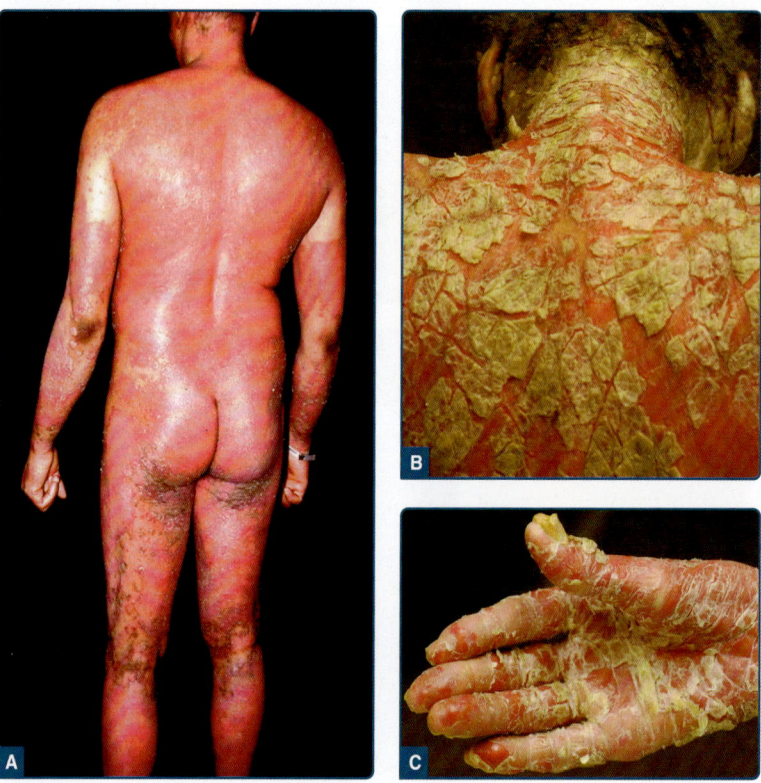

Figure 28-7 Erythrodermic psoriasis. **A,** This patient rapidly developed near-complete involvement and complained of fatigue and malaise. Note the islands of sparing. **B** and **C,** This patient had total-body involvement with marked hyperkeratosis and desquamation. (Used with permission from Mr. Harrold Carter and Dr. Johann Gudjonsson.)

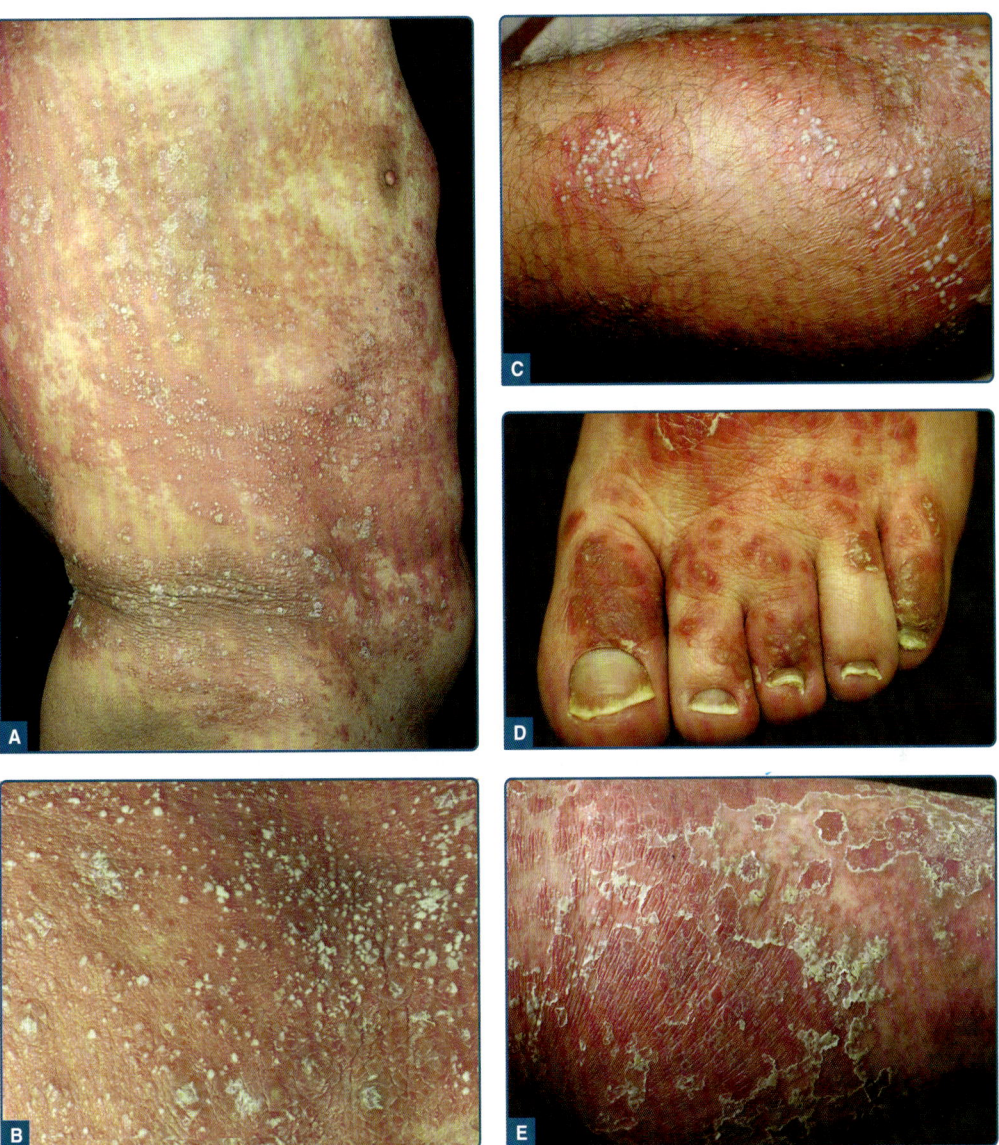

Figure 28-8 Pustular psoriasis. **A** and **B,** von Zumbusch-type generalized pustular psoriasis. Note the tiny pustules, 1 to 2 mm in diameter, on erythematous skin. **C** and **D,** localized pustular psoriasis of the leg and foot, respectively. **E,** Resolving pustular psoriasis. Note the extensive areas of desquamation. (C–E used with permission from Dr. Johann Gudjonsson, Dr. Trilokraj Tejasvi, and Neena Khanna.)

atrophic. The erythema that surrounds the pustules often spreads and becomes confluent, leading to erythroderma. Characteristically, the disease occurs in waves of fevers and pustules. The cause of generalized psoriasis von Zumbusch type is unknown. Various provoking agents include infections, irritating topical treatment (Koebner phenomenon), and withdrawal of oral corticosteroids.[9] This form of psoriasis is usually associated with prominent systemic signs and can potentially have life-threatening complications such as hypocalcemia, bacterial superinfection, sepsis, and dehydration. Severe pustular psoriasis can be difficult to control and requires a potent treatment regimen with rapid onset of action to avoid life-threatening complications.

Exanthematic Pustular Psoriasis: Exanthematic pustular psoriasis tends to occur after a viral infection and consists of widespread pustules with generalized plaque psoriasis. However, unlike the von Zumbusch pattern, there are no constitutional symptoms, and the disorder tends not to recur. There is an overlap between this form of pustular psoriasis and acute generalized exanthematous pustulosis, a type of drug eruption.

Annular Pustular Psoriasis: Annular pustular psoriasis is a rare variant of pustular psoriasis. It usually presents in an annular or circinate form. Lesions may appear at the onset of pustular psoriasis, with a tendency to spread and form enlarged rings, or they may develop during the course of generalized pustular psoriasis. The characteristic features are pustules on a ringlike erythema that sometimes resembles erythema annulare centrifugum. Identical lesions are found in patients with impetigo herpetiformis, an entity defined by some as a variant of pustular psoriasis occurring in pregnancy. Onset in pregnancy is usually early in the third trimester and persists until delivery. It tends to develop earlier in subsequent pregnancies. Impetigo herpetiformis is often associated with hypocalcemia.[9] There is usually no personal or family history of psoriasis.

Pustulosis Palmaris et Plantaris: Palmoplantar pustular psoriasis (PPPP) is a rare variant of pustular psoriasis that is localized to the palms and soles. It may coexist with chronic plaque psoriasis with approximately 27% of patients having concomitant chronic plaque psoriasis.[10] It differs from chronic plaque psoriasis both in terms of genetic predisposition[11] and transcriptional changes.[12] Therefore, many authors make a distinction between palmoplantar pustulosis (PPP) and PPPP, in which chronic plaque psoriasis is present, although the lesions of PPPP and PPP are indistinguishable by themselves both clinically and transcriptionally.[12] Pustulosis palmaris et plantaris is more common in females (about 78%) with a median age of onset of 47 years.[10] Psoriatic arthritis (PsA) can be seen with pustulosis palmaris et plantaris, with a prevalence of 13% to 25%.[10] Smoking is strongly associated with pustulosis palmaris et plantaris, and about 80% of patients are tobacco smokers at the time of presentation.[10]

Acrodermatitis Continua of Hallopeau: Acrodermatitis continua of Hallopeau, also known as dermatitis repens, is an extremely rare localized sterile pustular eruption of the fingers and toes.[13] It typically involves the distal portions of the fingers and toes and may occur after minor trauma or infection. Pustules often coalesce to form lakes of pus and nail loss is common. Over time, sclerosis of the underlying soft tissues and osteolysis of the distal phalanges may occur. Similar to pustulosis palmaris et plantaris, it is more common in middle-aged women. Evolution of acrodermatitis continua into generalized pustular psoriasis has been described.[13]

SEBOPSORIASIS

A common clinical entity, sebopsoriasis presents with erythematous plaques with greasy scales localized to seborrheic areas (scalp, glabella, nasolabial folds, perioral and presternal areas, and intertriginous areas). In the absence of typical findings of psoriasis elsewhere, distinction from seborrheic dermatitis is difficult. Sebopsoriasis may represent a modification of seborrheic dermatitis by the genetic background of psoriasis and is relatively resistant to treatment. Although an etiologic role of *Pityrosporum* remains unproven, antifungal agents may be useful.

NAPKIN PSORIASIS

Napkin psoriasis usually begins between the ages of 3 and 6 months and first appears in the diaper (napkin) areas as a confluent red area with appearance a few days later of small red papules on the trunk that may also involve the limbs. These papules have the typical white scales of psoriasis. The face may also be involved with red scaly eruption. Unlike other forms of psoriasis, the rash responds readily to treatment and tends to disappear after the age of 1 year.

LINEAR PSORIASIS

Linear psoriasis is quite rare. The psoriatic lesion presents as linear lesion most commonly on the limbs but may also be limited to a dermatome on the trunk. This may be an underlying nevus, possibly an inflammatory linear verrucous epidermal nevus (ILVEN) because these lesions resemble linear psoriasis both clinically and histologically. The existence of a linear form of psoriasis distinct from ILVEN is controversial.

NAIL CHANGES

Nail changes are frequent in psoriasis, being found in up to 40% of patients,[14] and are rare in the absence of skin disease elsewhere. Nail involvement increases with age, with duration and extent of disease, and with the presence of PsA. Several distinct changes have been described and can be grouped according to the portion of the nail that is affected (Table 28-1). Nail pitting is one of the commonest features of psoriasis, involving the fingers more often than the toes (Fig. 28-9). Pits range from 0.5 to 2.0 mm in size and can be single or multiple. The proximal nail matrix forms the dorsal

TABLE 28-1
Nail Changes in Psoriasis

NAIL SEGMENT INVOLVED	CLINICAL SIGN
Proximal matrix	Pitting, onychorrhexis, Beau's lines
Intermediate matrix	Leukonychia
Distal matrix	Focal onycholysis, thinned nail plate, erythema of the lunula
Nail bed	"Oil drop" sign or "salmon patch," subungual hyperkeratosis, onycholysis, splinter hemorrhages
Hyponychium	Subungual hyperkeratosis, onycholysis
Nail plate	Crumbling and destruction plus other changes secondary to the specific site
Proximal and lateral nail folds	Cutaneous psoriasis

Modified from Del Rosso JQ, et al. Dermatologic diseases of the nail unit. In: Scher RK, Daniel CR, eds. *Nails: Therapy, Diagnosis, Surgery*, 2nd ed. Philadelphia: WB Saunders; 1997; with permission. Copyright © Elsevier.

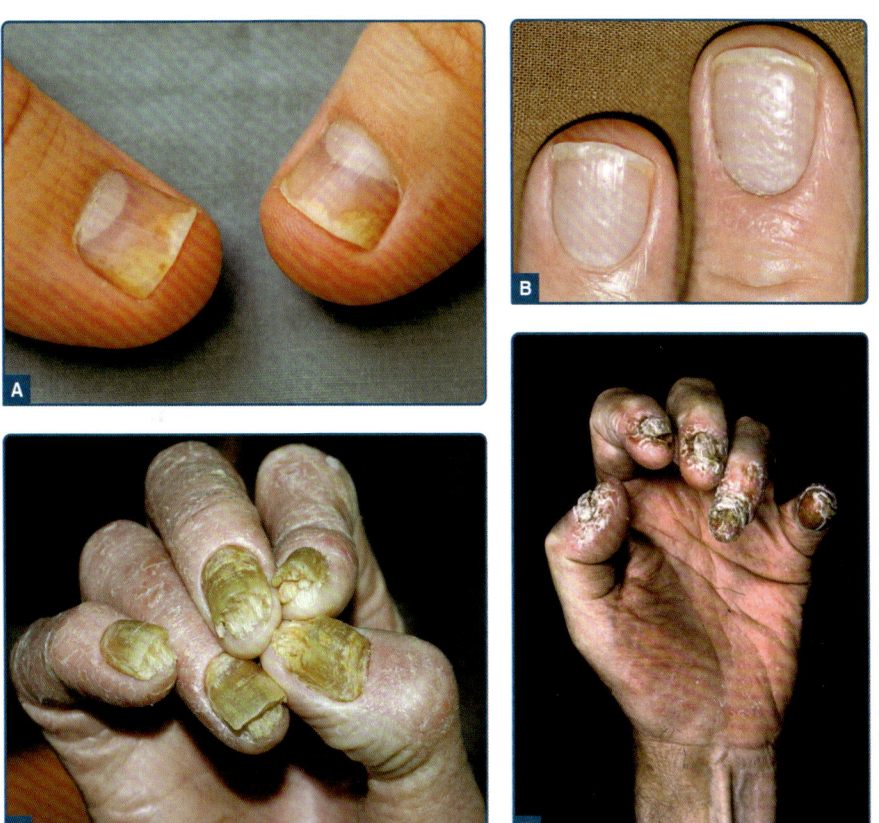

Figure 28-9 Nail psoriasis. **A,** Distal onycholysis and oil drop spotting. **B,** Nail pitting. **C,** Subungual hyperkeratosis. **D,** Onychodystrophy and loss of nails in a patient with psoriatic arthritis. (Used with permission from Dr. Johann Gudjonsson, Dr. Allen Bruce, and Mr. Harrold Carter.)

(superficial) portion of the nail plate, and psoriatic involvement of this region results in pitting caused by defective keratinization. Other alterations in the nail matrix resulting in deformity of the nail plate (onychodystrophy) include leukonychia, crumbling nail, and red spots in the lunula. Onychodystrophy has a stronger association with PsA than other nail changes.[14] Oil spots and salmon patches are translucent, yellow-red discolorations observed beneath the nail plate often extending distally toward the hyponychium caused by psoriasiform hyperplasia, parakeratosis, microvascular changes, and trapping of neutrophils in the nail bed.[15] Unlike pitting, which is also seen in alopecia areata and other disorders, oil spotting is considered to be nearly specific for psoriasis. Splinter hemorrhages result from capillary bleeding underneath the thin suprapapillary plate of the psoriatic nail bed. Subungual hyperkeratosis is caused by hyperkeratosis of the nail bed and is often accompanied by onycholysis (separation of the nail plate from the nail bed), which usually involves the distal aspect of the nail. Anonychia is total loss of the nail plate. Although nail changes are rarely seen in the localized pustular variant of pustulosis palmaris et plantaris, anonychia can be seen in other forms of pustular psoriasis.

HAIR AND SEBACEOUS GLANDS

Alopecia is not a common observation in scalp psoriasis clinically; however, both scarring and non-scarring forms of scalp alopecia have been reported (reviewed by Rittie and coworkers[16]). A recent study of nonscalp psoriasis demonstrated that psoriasis plaques have markedly fewer visible hairs than adjacent uninvolved or normal skin, without loss of hair shafts, and suggested that this might be related to sebaceous gland atrophy, which is profound in psoriasis.[16]

NONCUTANEOUS FINDINGS

GEOGRAPHIC TONGUE

Geographic tongue, also known as *benign migratory glossitis* or *glossitis areata migrans*, is an idiopathic inflammatory disorder resulting in the local loss of filiform papillae. The condition usually presents as asymptomatic erythematous patches with serpiginous borders, resembling a map. These lesions characteristically have a migratory nature. Geographic tongue has been postulated to be an oral variant of psoriasis because these lesions show several histologic features of psoriasis, including acanthosis, clubbing of the rete ridges, focal parakeratosis, and neutrophilic infiltrate. Although the prevalence of geographic tongue is increased in psoriatic patients, this is a relatively common condition that is seen in many nonpsoriatic individuals, so its relationship to psoriasis needs further clarification.

PSORIATIC ARTHRITIS

Arthritis is a common extracutaneous manifestation of psoriasis seen in up to 40% of patients. It has a strong genetic component, and several overlapping subtypes exist. This condition is discussed in Chap. 65.

COMPLICATIONS

CARDIOVASCULAR MORBIDITY

Patients with psoriasis have an increased morbidity and mortality from cardiovascular events, particularly those with severe and long duration of psoriasis skin disease.[17] Risk of myocardial infarction is particularly elevated in younger patients with severe psoriasis,[18] and vascular inflammation as detected by ^{18}F-fluorodeoxyglucose–positron emission tomography computed tomography (PET/CT) correlates directly with the extent of cutaneous involvement.[19] In a recent study of 1.3 million German health care recipients, metabolic syndrome was 2.9-fold more frequent among patients with psoriasis, and the most common diagnoses were hypertension (35.6% in psoriasis vs 20.6% in control participants) and hyperlipidemia (29.9% vs 17.1%).[20] Patients with psoriasis have also been shown to be at increased risk for rheumatoid arthritis (RA), Crohn's disease, and ulcerative colitis[20] as well as Hodgkin's lymphoma and cutaneous T-cell lymphoma.[21]

PSYCHOSOCIAL RAMIFICATIONS

Psoriasis is emotionally disabling, carrying with it significant psychosocial difficulties. Emotional difficulties arise from concerns about appearance, resulting in lowered self-esteem, social rejection, guilt, embarrassment, emptiness, sexual problems, and impairment of professional ability.[22] The presence of pruritus and pain can aggravate these symptoms. Psychological aspects can modify the course of illness; in particular, feeling stigmatized can lead to treatment noncompliance and worsening of psoriasis. Likewise, psychological stress can also lead to depression and anxiety. The prevalence of suicidal ideation and depression in patients with psoriasis is higher than that reported in people with other medical conditions and the general population. A comparative study reported reduction in physical and mental functioning comparable with that seen in cancer, arthritis, hypertension, heart disease, diabetes, and depression.[23] According to one survey, 79% of patients with severe psoriasis reported a negative impact on their lives.[24]

ETIOLOGY AND PATHOGENESIS

DEVELOPMENT OF LESIONS

Detailed light, electron microscopic, immunohistochemical, and molecular studies of involved and uninvolved skin of newly appearing and established psoriatic lesions provide a useful framework for relating the many cellular events that take place in a psoriatic lesion. They are illustrated schematically in Fig. 28-10 and with actual photomicrographs in Fig. 28-11. The normal-appearing skin of psoriatic patients has long been known to manifest subclinical morphologic and biochemical changes, particularly involving lipid biosynthesis.[25] In the initial pinhead-sized macular lesions, there is marked edema, and mononuclear cell infiltrates are found in the upper dermis,[26] usually confined to the area of one or two papillae. The overlying epidermis soon becomes spongiotic, with focal loss of the granular layer. The venules in the upper dermis dilate and become surrounded by a mononuclear cell infiltrate. Similar findings have been described in early macules and papules of psoriasis and in the uninvolved skin of guttate psoriasis.[27] The clinical margins of somewhat larger lesions (0.5–1.0 cm) manifest doubling of epidermal thickness, increased metabolic activity of epidermal cells, and increased mast cells and dermal macrophages with increased mast cell degranulation, as well as increased dermal T cells and dendritic cells (DCs). Toward the center of these evolving lesions, there are increasing bandlike epidermal thickness, parakeratosis, and capillary elongation, as well as perivascular infiltration of lymphocytes and macrophages without exudation into the epidermis. Squamous cells manifest enlarged extracellular spaces with only a few desmosomal connections, and parakeratosis is typically mounded or spotty. More mature lesions of psoriasis manifest uniform elongation of rete ridges, with thinning of the epidermis overlying the dermal papillae.[25] Epidermal mass is increased three to five times, and many more mitoses are observed, frequently above the basal layer. About 10% of basal keratinocytes are cycling in normal skin, but this value rises to 100% in lesional psoriatic skin.[28] Widening of the extracellular spaces between keratinocytes persists but is less prominent than in developing lesions and is more uniform than the typical spongiosis of eczematous skin lesions. The tips of the rete ridges are often clubbed or fused with adjacent ones, with thin, elongated, edematous papillae containing dilated, tortuous capillaries. Parakeratosis, with accompanying loss of the granular layer, is often horizontally confluent but may alternate with orthokeratosis. The inflammatory infiltrate around the

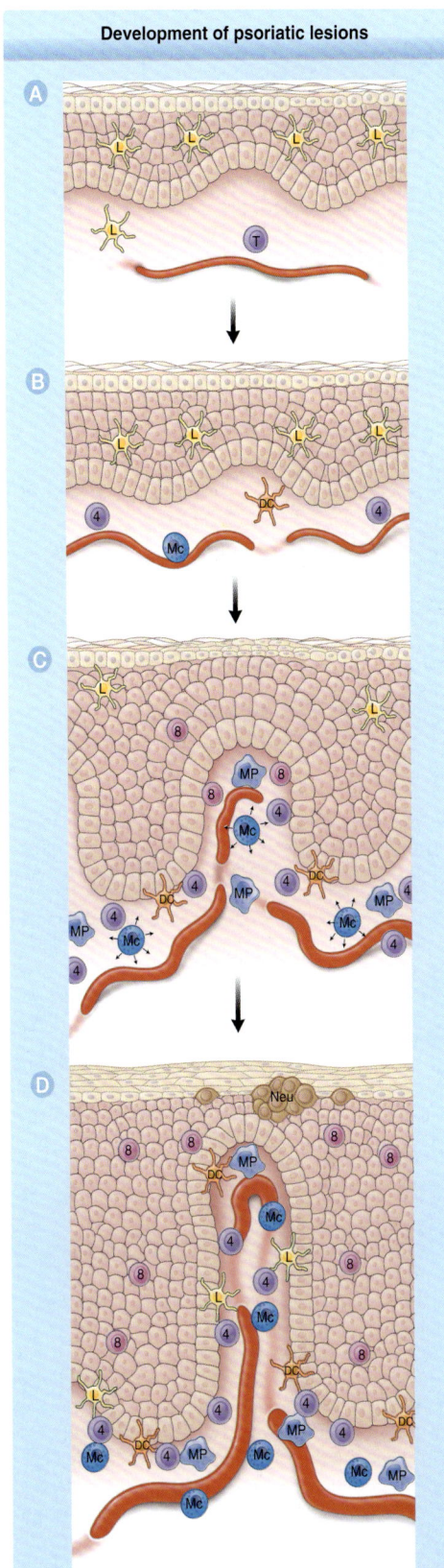

Development of psoriatic lesions

blood vessels in the papillary dermis becomes more intense but still consists of lymphocytes, macrophages, DCs, and mast cells. Unlike the initial lesion and the transitional zone, lymphocytes are observed in the epidermis of the mature lesion. Neutrophils exit from the tips of a subset of dermal capillaries (the "squirting papillae"), leading to their accumulation in the overlying parakeratotic stratum corneum (Munro's microabscesses) and, less frequently, in the spinous layer (spongiform pustules of Kogoj). Collections of serum can also be seen in the epidermis and stratum corneum.[25]

IMMUNOPATHOGENESIS OF PSORIASIS

LYMPHOCYTES

T cells play an essential role in psoriasis as demonstrated in 1996, when it was shown that psoriasis could be induced by injecting activated autologous T cells into uninvolved psoriatic skin transplanted onto severe combined immunodeficient mice.[29] Early studies suggested that at least some T-cell responses are antigen specific because oligoclonal expansions of both CD4+ and CD8+ T cells have repeatedly been identified in psoriatic lesions.[30] However, more recent studies using

Figure 28-10 Development of psoriatic lesions. Normal skin from a healthy individual (**A**) contains epidermal Langerhans cells, scattered immature dendritic cells (D), and skin-homing memory T cells (T) in the dermis. Normal-appearing skin from a psoriatic individual (**B**) manifests slight capillary dilatation and curvature and a slight increase in the numbers of dermal mononuclear cells and mast cells (Mcs). A slight increase in epidermal thickness may be present. The transition zone of a developing lesion (**C**) is characterized by progressive increases in capillary dilatation and tortuosity, numbers of mast cells, macrophages (MPs), and T cells and mast cell degranulation (*arrowheads*). In the epidermis, there are increasing thickness with increasingly prominent rete pegs, widening of the extracellular spaces, transient dyskeratosis, spotty loss of the granular layer, and parakeratosis. Langerhans cells (L) begin to exit the epidermis, and inflammatory dendritic epidermal cells (I) and CD8+ T cells (8) begin to enter the epidermis. The fully developed lesion (**D**) is characterized by fully developed capillary dilatation and tortuosity with a 10-fold increase in blood flow, numerous macrophages underlying the basement membrane, and increased numbers of dermal T cells (mainly CD4+) making contact with maturing dermal dendritic cells (D). The epidermis of the mature lesion manifests markedly increased (~10-fold) keratinocyte hyperproliferation extending to the lower suprabasal layers, marked but not necessarily uniform loss of the granular layer with overlying compaction of the stratum corneum and parakeratosis, increased numbers of CD8+ T cells, and accumulation of neutrophils in the stratum corneum (Munro's microabscesses).

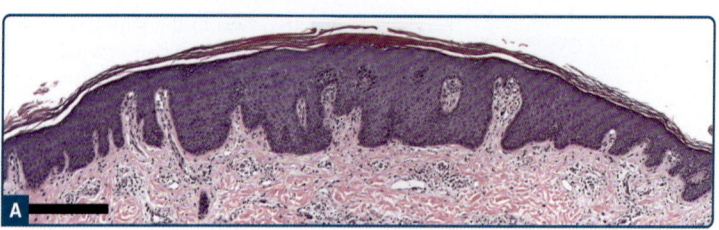
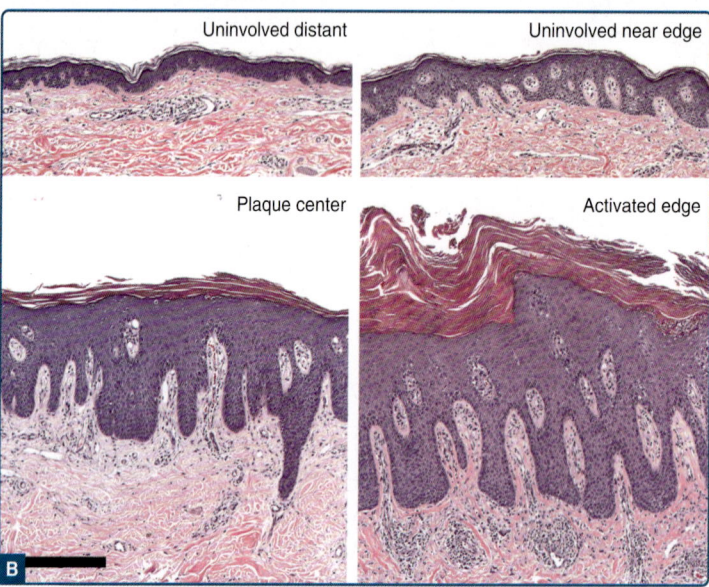

Figure 28-11 Histopathology of psoriasis. **A,** Pinpoint papule of psoriasis. In the transition from the edges to the center of the lesion, note progressive thickening of epidermis with elongation of rete pegs, increasing dilation and tortuosity of vessels, and increasing mononuclear cell infiltrate. Also note the transition from basket-weave to compact stratum corneum with loss of granular layer in the center of the lesion. (Four-mm punch biopsy, hematoxylin and eosin, scale bar, 100 μM.) **B,** Comparison of uninvolved versus involved skin. Four 4-mm biopsies were taken from the same individual sampled in A on the same day. "Uninvolved distant" skin was taken from the upper back 30 cm from the nearest visible lesion of psoriasis. The "uninvolved near edge" skin was taken 0.5 cm from the edge of a 20-cm plaque, which had been present for several years, according to the patient. "Center plaque" skin was taken from a relatively inactive (less red and scaly) area in the center of this plaque. "Involved edge" skin was taken from an active (more red and scaly) area about 1 cm inside the edge of the same plaque. In comparing "uninvolved distant" with "uninvolved near-edge" skin, note that the latter manifests increased thickness and early elongation of the rete pegs, dilation and early tortuosity of blood vessels, and increased numbers of mononuclear cells in the upper dermis, many of which are in a perivascular location. In this patient, "uninvolved near-edge" skin also manifests an increased frequency of dyskeratotic keratinocytes, a finding that has been noted previously at the periphery of psoriatic lesions.[53] In comparing less active with more active areas of the plaque, note that the more active area manifests increased dermal mononuclear infiltrate, increased hyperkeratosis and parakeratosis, and Munro microabscesses. (Four-mm punch biopsies, hematoxylin and eosin, scale bar, 100 μM.)

deep T-cell receptor (TCR) sequencing indicate most of the T cells in normal, uninvolved and lesional psoriatic skin are polyclonal with approximately equal diversity[31] and thus may accumulate in response to the cytokine environment of the lesion. There is virtually no evidence for B-cell involvement or antibody-mediated processes in psoriasis. The best-characterized T cells are the CD4+ and CD8+ subsets. Predominantly of the memory phenotype (CD45RO+), these cells express the cutaneous lymphocyte antigen, a ligand for E-selectin, which is selectively expressed on skin capillaries and therefore provides them with access to the skin.[32] Whereas CD8+ T cells are predominantly located in the epidermis, CD4+ T cells are predominantly located in the upper dermis. Epidermal T cells, particularly CD8+ cells, appear to have a critical role in development of psoriatic plaques as either blocking the entry of these cells into the epidermis,[33] or neutralization of CD8+ T cells[34] prevents development of psoriasis in a xenograft model.

The cytokine profile of psoriatic lesions is rich in interferon (IFN)-γ, indicative of T helper 1 (Th1) polarization of CD4+ cells, and T cytotoxic 1 (Tc1) polarization of CD8+ cells (Fig. 28-12). Two other subsets of CD4+ T cells, stimulated by interleukin (IL)-23 and characterized by production of IL-17 (Th17, ~20% of T cells) or IL-22 (Th22, ~15% of T cells), have been shown to play a major role in maintaining chronic inflammation in psoriasis[35] (Fig. 28-13) as well as other autoinflammatory conditions. In addition to IFN-γ–producing Tc1 cells, CD8+ T-cells producing IL-17 (Tc17) and IL-22 (Tc22) are found in psoriasis, most of which localize to

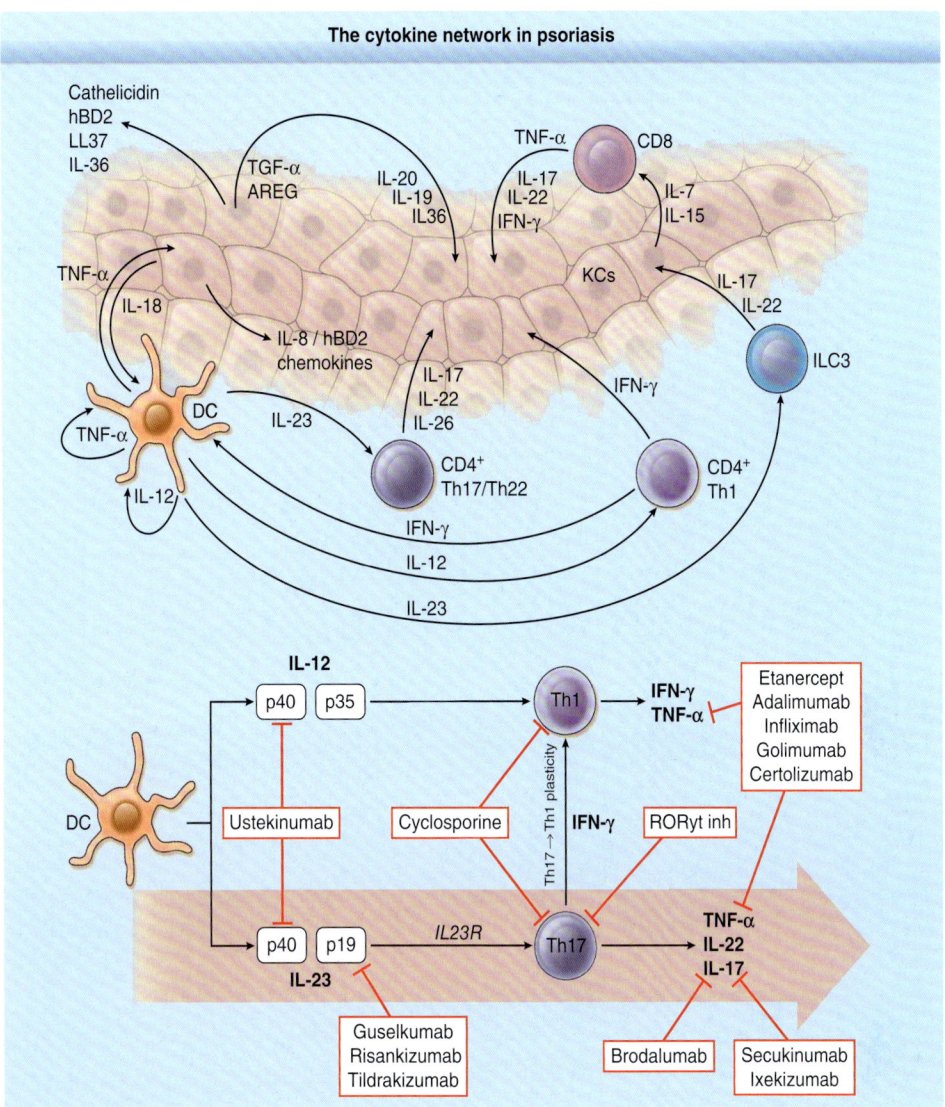

Figure 28-12 The cytokine network in psoriasis. Interferon (IFN)-γ is produced by T helper (Th) 1 cells and tumor necrosis factor (TNF)-α is produced by activated T cells and dendritic cells (DCs). IFN-γ amplifies the production of interleukin (IL)-23 by DC. In turn, IL-23 maintains and expands subsets of CD4+ T cells, called Th 17 and Th22 cells, which are characterized by production of IL-17 and IL-22, respectively. ILC3 also contribute to IL-17 in psoriatic skin. CD8+ T cells are predominantly found in the epidermis, and their entry into the epidermis is necessary for lesion development. IL-17, TNF-α, IFN-γ, and IL-22 synergistically promote activation of the innate keratinocyte defense response involving secretion of antimicrobial peptides such as human-β-defensin 2 (hBD-2), cathelicidin (LL37), IL-8 and other chemokines, and growth factors such as transforming growth factor (TGF)-α, amphiregulin (AREG), IL-19, and IL-20. Keratinocytes also produce IL-7 and IL-15, which influence the survival and turnover of CD8+ T cells; IL-18, which via IL-12 causes DCs to further increase the production of IFN-γ by T-cells; and IL-36 family cytokines, which attracts leukocytes, including neutrophils. Notably, the majority of available systemic therapeutic agents that have shown high therapeutic efficacy in psoriasis target the IL-12–Th1 and IL-23–Th17 axes.

the epidermis. These T-cell subsets have considerable functional plasticity and conversions of Tc17 to Tc1 and Th17 to Th1 have been described. Regulatory T cells (Tregs) suppress immune responses in an antigen-specific fashion and are responsible not only for downregulating successful responses to pathogens but also for the maintenance of immunologic tolerance. Several different populations of Tregs exist, but the best characterized one is the CD4+ CD25+ subset.[36] Tregs manifest impaired inhibitory function and failure to suppress effector T-cell proliferation in psoriasis.[37] Other "unconventional" lymphocytes implicated in the pathogenesis of psoriasis include natural killer (NK) cells, NK-T cells, γδ T-cells, mucosal-associated invariant T (MAIT) cells, and innate lymphoid cells (ILCs). These populations also represent important sources of IL-17, IFN-γ, tumor necrosis factor (TNF), and other cytokines.[38,39]

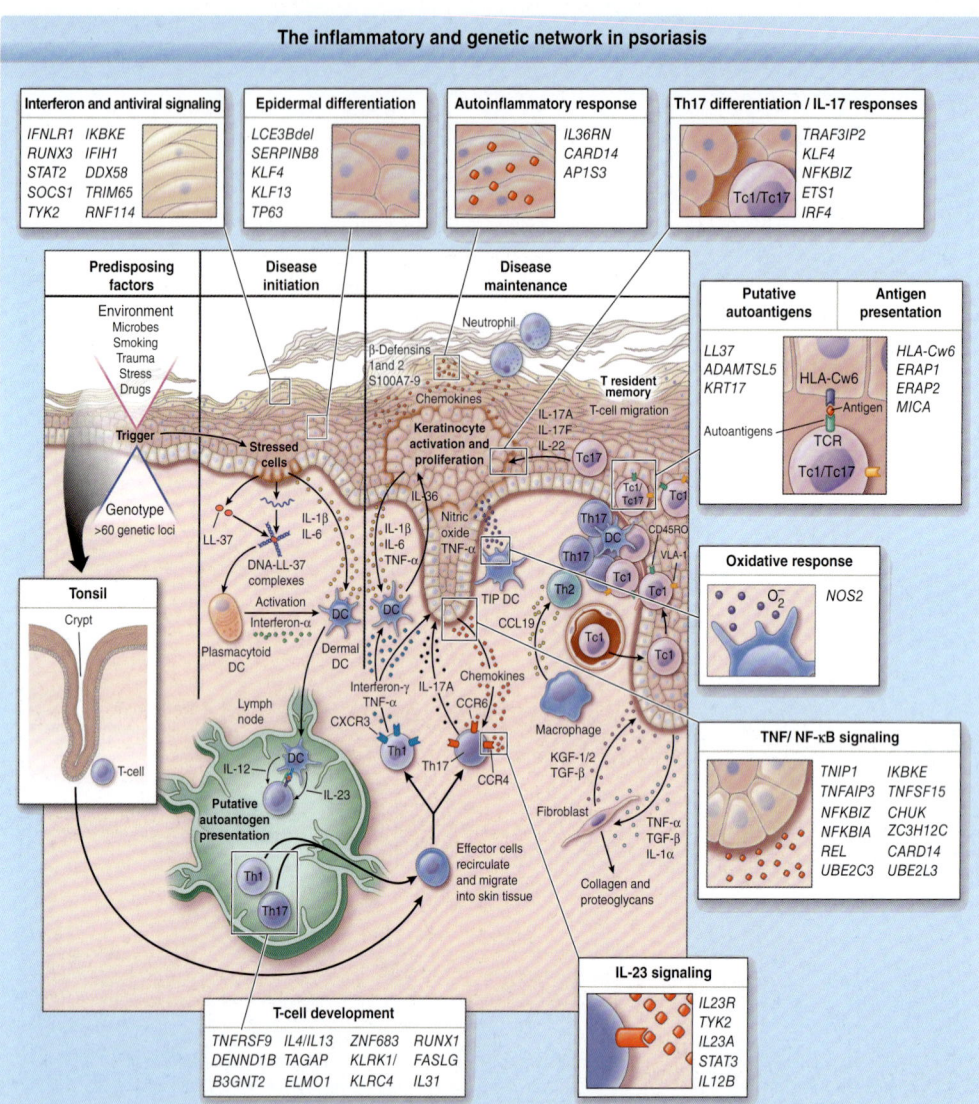

Figure 28-13 The inflammatory and genetic network in psoriasis. Psoriasis is initiated and maintained by interactions between intrinsic genetic susceptibility factors and external environmental factors, with the cutaneous immune system playing a central role. Initiation (triggering) of psoriasis lesions can occur in the skin (Koebnerization) or in the tonsils (streptococcal pharyngitis). In the context of environmental challenge, dendritic cells (DCs) are activated by "danger signals" released by damaged keratinocytes such as nucleic acids, S100 proteins, cathelicidins, and β-defensins; microbial products such as bacterial lipopolysaccharide; and proinflammatory cytokines such as interleukin (IL)-1, IL-36, and IL-8 induced in damaged keratinocytes. Through secretion of the key cytokines IL-12 and IL-23, activated DCs drive polarization and expansion of "T1" (T helper [Th] 1 and Tc1), "T17" (Th17 and Tc17) lymphocytes, which acquire skin-homing properties. Activated T1 and T17 cells secrete pro-inflammatory mediators including interferon (IFN)-γ, tumor necrosis factor (TNF)-α, IL-22, and IL-17, which act in a synergistic manner to amplify keratinocyte responses in the vicinity of the initial insult. To this end, keratinocytes increase their production of inflammatory mediators, including IL-1, IL-36, and a large number of chemokines, including IL-8 (CXCL8), CXCL9, and CXCL10. Cytokine-activated keratinocytes also release larger amounts of the various "danger signals" such as S100 proteins, cathelicidins, and β-defensins, many of which also have antimicrobial and chemotactic properties. This amplified inflammatory circuit recruits in chemotaxis and recruitment other inflammatory cells, including macrophages, DC, neutrophils, and other T-cell subsets, which act in synergy to maintain the disease process. Injured keratinocytes also produce growth factors such as TGF-α, amphiregulin (AREG), fibroblast growth factor (FGF), and nerve growth factor (NGF) to promote structural integrity, as well as T-cell growth factors, including IL-7 and IL-15. Key aspects of this process, which continue to be topics of active investigation, include the role of specific antigens in initiation versus maintenance of psoriasis and the mechanism of psoriatic epidermal hyperplasia. As indicated in the highlighted boxes, genetic variation influences multiple steps in this process, including INF and antiviral signaling, epidermal response, IL-23 signaling, cellular responses to IL-17 and TNF via NF-κB and other intracellular signaling pathways, autoinflammatory response, oxidative responses, and antigen presentation, T-cell development. Details on the role of specific candidate genes in this process can be found in Table 28-2.

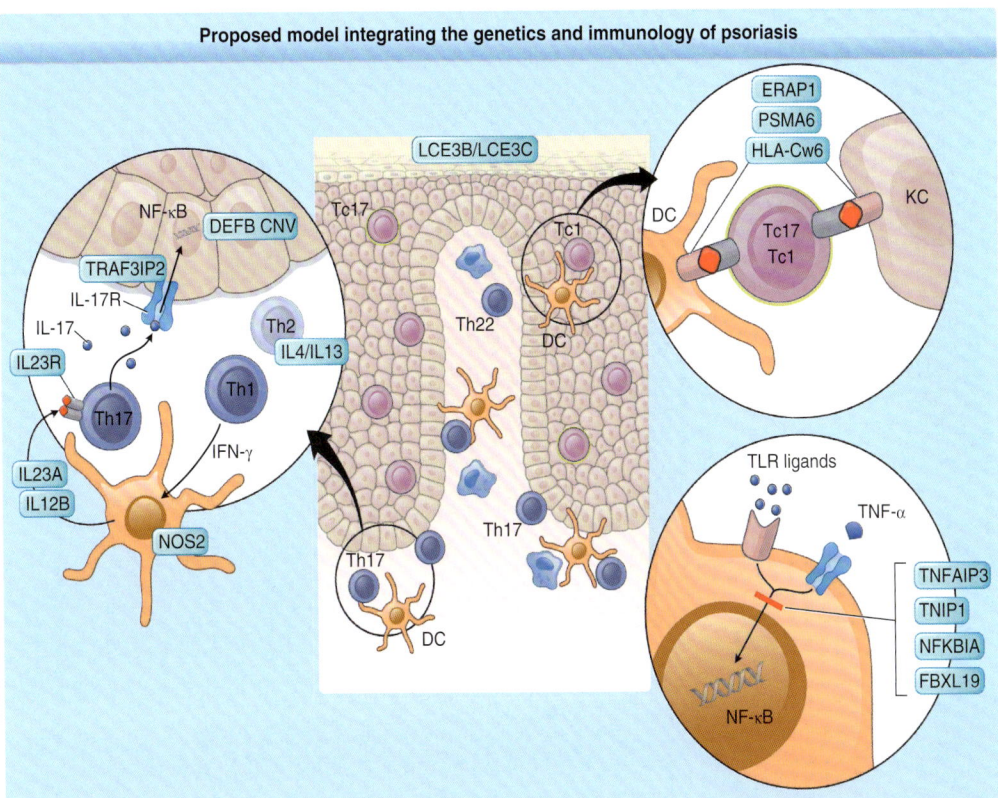

Figure 28-14 Proposed model integrating the genetics and immunology of psoriasis. Whereas the majority of the CD8+ T-cells (*green*) are located in the epidermis, CD4+ T cells (*purple*) predominate in the dermis along with antigen-presenting cells and dendritic cells (DCs) (*blue*) and macrophages (Mɸs) (*orange*). Confirmed association signals are indicated by the likely candidate genes they contain. Not all known psoriasis loci are depicted in this figure; please see text and Table 28-2 for additional details. Th, T helper; TLR, toll-like receptor. (Adapted from Nair RP et al. Psoriasis bench to bedside: genetics meets immunology. *Arch Dermatol.* 2009;145(4):462-464, with permission. Copyright © 2009 American Medical Association. All rights reserved.)

MYELOID CELLS

T cells in psoriatic lesions are in constant communication with DCs, which have a role in both the priming of adaptive immune responses and the induction of self-tolerance (see Chap. 11; Fig. 28-13). Several subsets of DCs have been defined, and many of these are found in markedly increased numbers within psoriatic lesions.[40] However, the specific role of each subset is still somewhat unclear. As noted earlier, macrophages are prominent in developing psoriasis lesions, with neutrophils appearing somewhat later. Studies in a mouse model that was used to implicate macrophages suggested that neutrophils may be unnecessary for lesional development.[41] However, neutrophils are likely to play a major role in pustular psoriasis by amplifying the local inflammatory reaction through secretion of proteases such as cathepsin G, elastase, and proteinase-3. These proteases are capable of processing inactive IL-36 family cytokines (IL-36α, IL-36β, and IL-36γ) secreted by keratinocytes into their active forms. When activated, IL-36 cytokines are strong activators of keratinocytes, leading to secretion of chemotactic proteins, particularly neutrophil chemokines, thereby amplifying and sustaining the inflammatory process.

KERATINOCYTES

Comprising the bulk of the epidermis and its appendages, keratinocytes are a major producer of proinflammatory cytokines, chemokines, and growth factors, as well as other inflammatory mediators such as eicosanoids and mediators of innate immunity such as cathelicidins, defensins, and S100 proteins. Psoriatic keratinocytes are engaged in an alternative pathway of keratinocyte differentiation called *regenerative maturation*.[42] Regenerative maturation is activated in response to immunologic stimulation. Besides keratinocytes, other skin-resident cell types, such as endothelial cells and fibroblasts, are also likely participants in the pathogenic process.[40]

GENETICS OF PSORIASIS

In recent years, many genetic variants contributing to psoriasis susceptibility have been identified, initially through linkage studies and more recently through genome-wide association studies (GWAS). An overview of the major genetically-implicated pathways in psoriasis is provided in Fig. 28-14, and a list of genetic loci identified to date is provided in Table 28-2.

TABLE 28-2
Genetic Susceptibility Loci in Psoriasis

CANDIDATE GENE(S)	CHROMOSOME REGION	EUROPEAN ORIGIN	CHINESE ORIGIN	PMID	FUNCTION
TNFRSF9	1p36.23	•		23143594, 26626624	Inhibits proliferation of activated T lymphocytes and induces programmed cell death
MTHFR	1p36.22		•	25854761	Required for homocysteine remethylation to methionine
IFNLR1	1p36.11	•	•	23143594, 23897274	Forms a receptor complex with IL-10 receptor β; interacts with IFN-λ family members IL28A, IL28B, and IL29
RUNX3	1p36.11	•		23143594	TF required for development of IFN-γ–producing pathogenic Th17 cells through binding with T-bet
ZNF683	1p36.11		•	25854761	TF expressed in quiescent and long-lived effector-type CD8+ T cells. Its function in human T cells seems adapted to lifelong, periodic pathogen challenges.
IL23R	1p31.3	•	•	19169254, 25854761	Subunit of the IL-23 receptor that pairs with IL12Rβ1 to initiate IL-23 signaling; associates with TYK2 and JAK2 and binds to STAT3 in a ligand-dependent manner
LRRC7	1p31.1	•		25939698	Brain-expressed leucine-rich repeat protein found in the postsynaptic density; contains a PDZ domain near its C-terminus
FUBP1	1p31.1	•		28301294	Encodes a single-stranded DNA-binding protein that binds to multiple DNA elements and has 3′-5′ helicase activity
PTPN22	1p13.2	•		25923216	Encodes a lymphoid-specific intracellular phosphatase regulating CBL function in the TCR signaling pathway; also associated with T1D, RA, SLE, vitiligo, and Graves disease
LCE3A-D	1q21.3	•	•	19169253, 19169255, 20953190	LCE genes are expressed in differentiated keratinocytes. LCE3 genes are upregulated in psoriatic skin and after skin injury.
AIM2	1q23.1		•	25854761	Encodes a cytoplasmic sensor that recognizes dsDNA of microbial or host origin and assembles inflammasomes, which cleave the proinflammatory cytokines pro–IL-1β and pro–IL-18α
FASLG	1q24.3	•		28537254	Encodes Fas ligand (CD95), a transmembrane protein of the TNF family. Fas ligand–receptor interactions regulate inflammation via apoptosis and promotion of inflammatory responses.
DENND1B	1q31.3	•		25651891	Guanine nucleotide exchange factor for the endosomal small GTPase RAB35, linking RAB35 with the clathrin machinery
IKBKE	1q32.1	•		28537254	Encodes IKKε, essential for regulation of antiviral signaling. Activated downstream of cytosolic RNA/DNA sensors and mediates activation of TFs, including IRF3, IRF7, and NF-κB.
REL	2p16.1	•		20953190, 22170493	Encodes c-Rel, a member of the NF-κB family with an important role in B-cell survival and proliferation. Mice lacking both REL and RELA in KC develop a psoriasiform dermatitis.
B3GNT2	2p15	•		23143594	Encodes a member of the β-1,3-N-acetylglucosaminyl transferase family. Deficiency results in hyperactivation of lymphocytes.
IL1RL1	2q12.1		•	25854761	Encodes a member of the IL1 receptor family induced by proinflammatory stimuli and involved in helper T cell function; associated with atopic dermatitis in Oriental populations

Gene	Locus		PMID	Description
IFIH1	2q24.2		20953190, 23143594, 25006012	Encodes a DEAD box protein upregulated in response to treatment with IFN-β; variation in *IFIH1* is associated with type 1 diabetes, vitiligo, SLE, and UC
PLCL2	3p24.3	•	25939698	Encodes a phospholipase C-like protein; associated with primary biliary cirrhosis, MS, and RA
NFKBIZ	3q12.3	•	25939698	NFKBIZ: encodes IκBz, which is an TRAF3IP2-dependent IL-17 target gene in mice and humans
CASR	3q21.1	•	25854761	Encodes a GPCR expressed in the parathyroid gland, which senses calcium concentration and modifies PTH secretion; plays a key role in mineral homeostasis and KC differentiation
GPR160	3q26.2	•	25854761	Associated with stroke in Japanese population
TP63	3q28		25903422	Encodes a member of the p53 family of TFs; essential for epidermal development in mice; mutations associated with ectodermal dysplasia, cleft lip or palate, and others; epidermal overexpression results in an AD-like phenotype
NFKB1	4q24		25006012	Encodes a 105-kD Rel-specific transcription inhibitor that is processed to a 50-kD DNA binding subunit of NF-κB; activated by cytokines, oxidants, UV light, and bacterial or viral products
CARD6	5p13.1		25939698	Encodes a microtubule-associated protein that interacts with RIPKs and modulates signaling pathways converging on NF-κB
ZFYVE16	5q14.1		25854761	Encodes an endosomal protein that regulates membrane trafficking; scaffold protein in the TGF-β pathway
ERAP1, LNPEP	5q15	•	20953187, 20953190, 23143594	Both genes encode endoplasmic reticulum aminopeptidases involved in trimming HLA class I-binding peptide precursors for antigen presentation. ERAP1 acts as a monomer or ERAP1/2 heterodimer. Epistasis with HLA class I in AS and Behçet disease.
IL13, IL4	5q31.1		19169254, 25903422	Cytokines with overlapping functions produced by Th2 cells. *IL3*, *IL5*, *IL4*, and *CSF2* form a gene cluster on chromosome 5q.
TNIP1	5q33.1		19169254, 20953187	Encodes an A20-binding protein involved in autoimmunity and tissue homeostasis through regulation of NF-κB activation; associated with myasthenia gravis, systemic sclerosis, and SLE
IL12B	5q33.3	•	17236132, 19169254, 19169255, 20953186, 20953190	Encodes the p40 a subunit of IL-12, a cytokine that acts on T and NK cells; expressed by DCs and activated macrophages, IL-12 is an essential inducer of Th1 development that protects against intracellular pathogens; associated with MS, CD, UC, and AS
PTTG1	5q33.3	•	20953187	Encodes an APC substrate involved in sister chromatid separation
IRF4	6p25.3		23143594	Encodes a TF that regulates IL17A promoter activity and Th17-mediated colitis in vivo; stabilizes the Th17 phenotype through IL-21; associated with pigmentation, RA, lymphoma, leukemia, and schizophrenia
CDKAL1	6p22.3	•	26626624	Encodes a member of the methylthiotransferase family of unknown function; variation associated with T2D, BMI, and CD
HLA-C, HLA-B, HLA-A, HLA-DR	6p21.33	•	19169254, 19169255, 19680446, 20953190, 25087609	HLA-B and HLA-C present antigens to CD8⁺ T cells. HLA-C is a ligand for KIRs on NK cells. Conditional analysis demonstrates associations with multiple HLA loci. Amino acid 45 at HLA-B distinguishes between PsC and PsA.
TRAF3IP2	6q21	•	20953186, 20953188, 20953190	Interacts with TRAF proteins and I-κB kinase and MAPK to activate NF-κB TFs that mediate innate immunity

(*Continued*)

TABLE 28-2
Genetic Susceptibility Loci in Psoriasis (Continued)

CANDIDATE GENE(S)	CHROMOSOME REGION	EUROPEAN ORIGIN	CHINESE ORIGIN	PMID	FUNCTION
TNFAIP3	6q23.3	•		19169254, 23143594	Rapidly induced by TNF; encodes an ubiquitin-editing enzyme involved in cytokine-regulated responses; inhibits NF-κB activation and TNF-induced apoptosis
TAGAP	6q25.3	•		23143594	Encodes a protein activating a Rho GTPase for T-cell activation; mutations are associated with RA, celiac disease, and MS
CCDC129	7p14.3		•	25854761	Encodes coiled-coil domain containing protein 129 involved in receptor binding
ELMO1	7p14.1	•		23143594	An engulfment and cell motility protein that promotes phagocytosis and cell migration; associated with glioma cell invasion and diabetic nephropathy
CSMD1	8p23.2		•	20953187	A postulated tumor suppressor of squamous cell carcinomas
DDX58	9p21.1	•		23143594	Encodes a protein with a caspase recruitment domain and RNA helicase motif; recognizes dsRNA; controls immune responses
KLF4	9q31.2	•		23143594	A transcription factor that regulates p53 in G1-to-S phase transition after DNA damage; necessary for skin barrier function
TNFSF15	9q32			28973304	Induced by TNF and IL-1α; its product activates NF-κB and MAPKs; induces apoptosis; inhibits endothelial cell proliferation
ZNF365	10q21.2	•			Zinc finger protein; mutations are associated with uric acid-induced nephrolithiasis
CAMK2G	10q22.2	•		25939698	Encodes the γ chain of a serine/threonine, Ca(2+)/calmodulin-dependent protein kinase
ZMIZ1	10q22.3	•		22482804	Regulates transcription factors, such as androgen receptor, Smad3/4, and p53
PTEN, KLLN	10q23.31	•		28537254	PTEN: tumor suppressor that negatively regulates the AKT/PKB signaling pathway KLLN: nuclear protein that increases S phase arrest and apoptosis and is upregulated by p53
CHUK	10q24.31	•		28537254	A serine/threonine protein kinase that activates NF-κB via degradation of its inhibitor IκBα
ZNF143	11p15.4		•	25854761	Zinc finger protein transcriptional activator that initiates RNA polymerase activity
RPS6KA4, PRDX5	11q13.1	•		22482804	RPS6KA4: serine/threonine kinase that phosphorylates CREB1, ATF1, and histone H3 to regulate genes involved in inflammation PRDX5: a protective antioxidant enzyme
FOSL1	11q13.1	•		25854761	Regulates cell proliferation and differentiation via interactions with other AP-1 family members
ZC3H12C	11q22.3	•		23143594	Encodes a protein that inhibits TNF-induced endothelial cell activation
ETS1	11q24.3	•		23143594	TF with activator and repressor activity; plays a role in stem cell development, cell aging, and tumorigenesis
CD27	12p13.3		•	25006012	Encodes a member of the TNF receptor superfamily required for T-cell immunity; LAG3 encodes a ligand for MHC class II receptors that is related to CD4
KLRK1, KLRC4	12p13.2	•		28537254	Transmembrane receptors that can activate NK and T cells; targeted in immune disorder and cancer treatment

Gene	Locus		PubMed ID	Description
IL23A, STAT2	12q13.3		19169254	IL23A: encodes p19 subunit of IL-23, which acts on memory CD4+ T cells to induce STAT4 and IFN-γ STAT2: transcriptional activator; complexes with STAT1 in response to IFN
BRAP, MAPKAPK5	12q24.12	•	29553248	BRAP: sequesters BRCA1 to the cytoplasm MAPKAPK5: tumor suppressor activated by MAPKs in response to cell stress and inflammatory cytokines; phosphorylates HSP27
IL31	12q24.31	•	29046191	Produced by Th2 T cells; acts on keratinocyte and epithelial cells; may regulate allergic dermatoses and other allergic diseases
GJB2	13q12.11		20953187	A gap junction protein, also known as a connexin 26; mutations of this gene account for more than half of recessive deafness cases
COG6	13q14.11	•	25903422	Encodes a subunit of the conserved oligomeric Golgi complex
LINC00330	13q14.2	•	25903422	Long intergenic noncoding RNA 330; function unknown
UBAC2	13q32.3	•		UBA domain-containing 2, implicated in Behçet disease
NFKBIA, PSMA6	14q13.2	•	20953189, 20953190, 24070858	NFKBIA: moves between cytoplasm and nucleus to inhibit NF-κB; mutations associated with ectodermal dysplasia with T-cell immunodeficiency PSMA6: encodes a proteasomal subunit involved in cleavage of MHC class I peptides
SYNE2	14q23.2		25854761	A nuclear outer membrane protein that binds cytoplasmic F-actin to secure the nucleus to the cytoskeleton and maintain its structural integrity
RP11-61O1.1	14q32.2	•		Noncoding gene of unknown function
KLF13	15q13.3	•	27041562	A transcription factor containing three zinc finger DNA-binding domains?; regulates HPV life cycle in keratinocytes
SOCS1	16p13.13	•	23143594	A cytokine-induced negative feedback inhibitor of STAT signaling
FBXL19, PRSS53	16p11.2	•	20953189	FBXL19: an E3 ubiquitin ligase that ubiquitinates IL1RL1 for degradation PRSS53: encodes a protein with serine-type endopeptidase activity
NOS2	17q11.2		20953189	Encodes an iNOS that is markedly overexpressed in psoriasis lesions
IKZF3	17q12	•	25006012	Encodes a TF in the Ikaros family; controls proliferation and differentiation of B cells; functions in chromatin remodeling
STAT3, STAT5A/B	17q21.2	•	23143594	STAT3, STAT5A, STAT5B: transcription factors involved in cell growth, apoptosis, and immunoregulation
TRIM65	17q25.1	•	28031478	TRIM65: tripartite motif containing 65; deactivates p53 through ubiquitination and is upregulated in lung carcinoma; essential for MDA5-mediated innate immunity
TMC6	17q25.3		25854761	An integral membrane protein of the endoplasmic reticulum; one of two genes causing epidermodysplasia verruciformis, a disease with increased susceptibility to HPV and SCC
CARD14	17q25.3	•	23143594, 24212883	A caspase recruitment domain-containing protein of the MAGUK family, members of which act as scaffold proteins in cell adhesion, cell polarity, and signal transduction; interacts with BCL10 to activate NF-κB and promote apoptosis

(Continued)

TABLE 28-2
Genetic Susceptibility Loci in Psoriasis (Continued)

CANDIDATE GENE(S)	CHROMOSOME REGION	EUROPEAN ORIGIN	CHINESE ORIGIN	PMID	FUNCTION
PTPN2	18p11.21	•		18923449	Encodes a protein tyrosine phosphatase with a highly conserved catalytic motif; serves as a signaling molecule to regulate cell growth, differentiation, mitosis, and oncogenesis
POLI, STARD6, MBD2	18q21.2	•		23143594	POLI: DNA polymerase involved in DNA repair and in mutation of immunoglobulin genes STARD6: homologous to STAR proteins involved in sterol transport MBD2: methyl-CpG binding protein that can repress or activate transcription
SERPINB8	18q22.1			20953187	Protease inhibitor-8, a member of the ov-serpin subfamily; serpins play a role in complement activation, fibrinolysis, coagulation, migration, apoptosis, and tumor suppression
TYK2	19p13.2	•		20953190, 23143594	Belongs to the JAK family of tyrosine kinases that propagate inflammatory signals; functions in IFN-mediated antiviral immunity; linked to hyper-IgE syndrome
ILF3, CARM1	19p13.2	•		23143594	ILF3: A dsRNA binding protein that regulates gene expression via mRNA stabilization CARM1: A arginine methyltransferase that acts on histones to regulate gene expression
FUT2	19q13.33	•		22482804	Encodes the galactoside 2-L-fucosyltransferase enzyme involved in production of H antigen precursor for the ABO blood group
ZNF816	19q13.41		•	20953187	Encodes a zinc finger protein with TF activity
RNF114, SNAI1	20q13.13	•		18364390, 23143594	RNF114: ubiquitin-protein ligase that degrades the inhibitor of CDKN1A to induce G1-to-S phase transition SNAI1: zinc finger transcriptional repressor involved in mesodermal development
IFNGR2	21q22.11		•	25854761	Non–ligand-binding β chain of IFN-γ receptor; mutations result in susceptibility to mycobacterial disease
RUNX1	21q22.12	•		25903422	The α subunit of core binding factor, which plays a role in hematopoietic development; leads to leukemia via chromosomal translocation
YDJC, UBE2L3	22q11.21	•		22482804, 23143594	YDJC: deacetylates carbohydrates in the breakdown of oligosaccharide UBE2L3: ubiquitin-conjugating enzyme that ubiquitinates p53, c-FOS, and p105.

AD, atopic dermatitis; AKT, serine/threonine kinase 1; AP-1, activator protein-1; APC, anaphase-promoting complex; AS, ankylosing spondylitis; ATF1, activating transcription factor-1; BMI, body mass index; CBL, Casitas B-lineage Lymphoma; CD, Crohn's disease; CREB1, cAMP responsive element binding protein 1; DC, dendritic cell; dsDNA, double-stranded DNA; GPCR, G-protein coupled receptor; HLA, human leukocyte antigen; HPV, human papillomavirus; IKKε, I-κB kinase epsilon; IL, interleukin; IFN, interferon; iNOS, inducible nitric oxide synthase; JAK, Janus kinase; KC, keratinocyte; KIR, killer immunoglobulin-like receptor; LCE, late cornified envelope; MAGUK, membrane-associated guanylate kinase; MAPK, mitogen-activated protein kinase; MHC, major histocompatibility complex; MS, multiple sclerosis; NF-κB, nuclear factor kappa B; NK, natural killer; PDZ, post-synaptic density, Dlg1, and ZO-1 protein; PKB, protein kinase B; PsA, psoriatic arthritis; PsC, purely cutaneous psoriasis; RA, rheumatoid arthritis; REL, proto-oncogene c-REL; RELA, proto-oncogene, NF-κB subunit; RIP, receptor-interacting kinase; SCC, squamous cell carcinoma; SLE, systemic lupus erythematosus; STAT, signal transducer and activator of transcription; T1D, type 1 diabetes; T2D, type 2 diabetes; TCR, T-cell receptor; TF, transcription factor; TGF, transforming growth factor; Th, T helper; TNF, tumor necrosis factor; TRAF, TNF receptor-associated factor; TYK2, tyrosine kinase 2; UC, ulcerative colitis; UV, ultraviolet; RIPKs, receptor-interacting protein kinase.

MAJOR HISTOCOMPATIBILITY COMPLEX GENES

Overall, the major histocompatibility complex (MHC) accounts for the bulk of the overall genetic risk for psoriasis. Thus, although 63 currently known European-origin signals explain 28% of the genetic heritability of psoriasis, MHC signals alone contribute 11.2% of the 28%, or about 40% of the detectable heritability.[43] The major genetic signal for psoriasis in the MHC is *HLAC*0602*, which encodes HLA-Cw6 protein.[44,45] HLA-Cw6 presents antigens to CD8+ T cells, which are MHC class I restricted and comprise about 80% of the T cells in the epidermis of psoriatic lesions (Fig. 28-15). CD8+ T cells selectively traffic to the epidermis because they express integrin α1β1, which binds to Type IV basement membrane collagen[33] as well as integrin αEβ7, which binds to keratinocyte E-cadherin.[46] Functionally, epidermal invasion by CD8+ T cells correlates with lesional development in a xenograft model of psoriasis.[47] Further emphasizing the importance of MHC class I antigen presentation, several other MHC class I risk variants are associated with psoriasis independently of HLA-Cw6 in both European-origin[45] and Chinese populations.[48] The fact that oligoclonal T-cell expansions are found in CD8+ T-cells in psoriatic skin[30] suggests that in the epidermis, CD8+ T cells "interrogate" peptides bound to HLA-Cw6 on the surface of dendritic antigen-presenting cells (APCs) and expand in response to one or more specific antigens (see Figs. 28-14 and 28-15).

The nature of these antigens remains a topic of active investigation. Besides candidate antigens described in previous editions of this chapter, three recent publications have implicated additional candidate autoantigens in psoriasis, including the antimicrobial protein LL37,[49] neolipid antigens generated by mast cell phospholipase and presented by the MHC-like class I

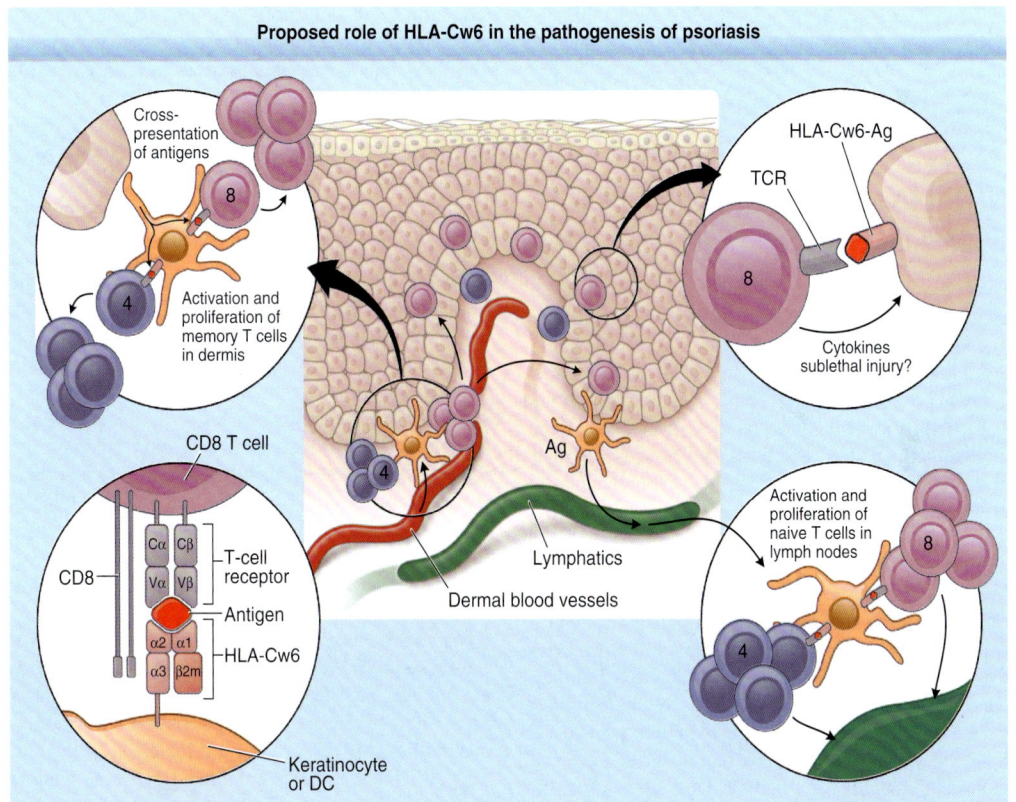

Figure 28-15 Proposed role of HLA-Cw6 in the pathogenesis of psoriasis. Antigen (Ag) in the binding pocket of human leukocyte antigen (HLA)-Cw6 interacts with a T-cell receptor (TCR). The role of HLA-Cw6 in psoriasis is likely to be twofold. HLA-Cw6 is active in cross-presenting peptides on the surface of dendritic cells (DCs), allowing activation and clonal expansion of antigen-specific CD8+ T cells. This process is dependent on CD4+ T-cell help for cross-presentation of intracellular antigens and is likely to happen both in the dermis (activation of resident memory T cells) and local lymph nodes (activation of naïve T cells). Subsequently, the activated CD8+ T cells are able to migrate into the epidermis, where they encounter HLA-Cw6 on the surface of DCs or keratinocytes presenting those same pathogenic peptides. Because these T cells express perforin, they may directly damage keratinocytes in the traditional cytotoxic manner. Activated CD8+ T cells may also trigger the local release soluble factors, including cytokines, chemokines, eicosanoids, and innate immune mediators, which could further increase local inflammation and stimulate keratinocyte proliferation.

antigen-presenting protein CD1a,[50] and the melanocyte antigen ADAMTSL5. Of these, the ADAMTSL5 antigen is of genetic interest because it is presented specifically by HLA-Cw6.[51] Of note, recent immunohistochemical data suggest that expression of ADAMTSL5 may not be limited to melanocytes.[52] Although much remains to be learned about specific autoantigens, the observations that multiple HLA alleles are implicated genetically and that expanded TCR rearrangements are usually oligoclonal in nature suggest that multiple autoantigens may be involved in the pathogenesis of psoriasis.

CD4+ T cells predominate in the dermis of psoriasis lesions and are also clonally expanded in psoriasis. CD4+ T cells are also required for the development of psoriasis lesions from uninvolved skin in a xenograft model.[53] This is consistent with the identification of genetic signals in the MHC class II region in both European-origin[45] and Chinese[48] populations. Although CD4+ and CD8+ memory T cells can traffic among the skin, lymph nodes, and blood, increasing evidence indicates that when initially activated in the cutaneous environment, they spend most of their time in the skin site at which they were activated, as resident memory T cells.[32] This would be consistent with the behavior of psoriatic plaques, which tend to recur in the same body sites after therapeutic or spontaneous improvement.

NON-MAJOR HISTOCOMPATIBILITY COMPLEX GENES

Over the past decade, GWAS have identified 86 genomic regions that are associated with psoriasis at genome-wide significance (see Table 28-2). Eleven of the 86 known psoriasis risk loci are shared by European and Chinese populations, 55 loci have been established for Europeans only, and 20 loci have been established for Chinese only. Sixteen loci have also been established as susceptibility loci for PsA and 12 for purely cutaneous psoriasis.[45,54,55] Perhaps surprisingly, most of the genetic signals identified in psoriasis thus far do not affect the structure of a protein and instead are regulatory in nature.[43] Moreover, because of topologic looping of DNA in chromatin, the regulatory signals affected by genetic variation may lie at a substantial distance from the causal gene being regulated. Thus, the "candidate genes" listed in Table 28-2 cannot simply be assumed to be the causal genes underlying the observed associations. However, there is strong bioinformatic evidence indicating that the genes underlying these psoriasis genetic signals are disproportionately involved in immunity and host defense, including functions such as lymphocyte differentiation and regulation, type I IFN and pattern recognition, nuclear factor kappa B (NF-κB) signaling, and response to viruses and bacteria.[43] Correspondingly, psoriasis signals are enriched in regulatory elements active in several T-cell subsets, including CD8+ T cells, and CD4+ T-cell subsets, including T_h0, T_h1, and T_h17.[43] Thus, there can be little doubt that "psoriasis genes" are involved in various aspects of immunity and host defense even if many of them remain to be formally identified. Most of the non-MHC associations identified thus far fall into several interconnected functional axes: IL-23–IL-17 signaling, interferon signaling, NF-κB signaling, DC–macrophage function, and keratinocyte responses (see Fig. 28-14 and Table 28-2).

IL-23–IL-17 Signaling: Three strong regions of association map near genes involved in IL-23 signaling: *IL12B* (encoding the p40 subunit of IL-23 and IL-12), *IL23A* (encoding the p19 subunit of IL-23), and *IL23R* (encoding a subunit of the IL-23 receptor). These associations are further supported by the impressive efficacy of biologics targeting the p40 subunit common to IL-12 and IL-23[56] as well as the p19 subunit,[57] which is unique to IL-23. IL-23 signaling promotes the survival and expansion of IL-17–expressing T-cells, which protect epithelia against microbial pathogens.[58] Ankylosing spondylitis (AS) is another HLA class I–associated autoimmune disorder that is clinically associated with inflammatory bowel disease[59] and genetically associated with *IL23R*.[60] PsA shares a number of clinical similarities with AS, and is genetically associated with *IL12B*, *IL23A*, and *IL23R* (see Chap. 65). Other candidate genes relevant to this signaling axis include *TRAF3IP2* encoding Act1; a ubiquitin ligase coupling IL-17 receptors to downstream signaling pathways; *RUNX3*, which encodes a transcription factor (TF) required for development of Th17 cells; *NFKBIZ*, a TF whose expression is stimulated by IL-17 via Act1[61]; and *IRF4*, encoding a TF that regulates *IL-17A* promoter activity.

Interferon Signaling: Although the *IFNG* gene does not itself map to a psoriasis susceptibility region, its product IFN-γ is secreted by activated Th1 cells and stimulates DC to produce IL-23.[62] This may explain why Th1 and Th17 cells are co-localized in psoriasis lesions and many other sites of inflammation.[62] Another psoriasis susceptibility region contains the *IL4* and *IL13* genes. In addition to biasing T-cell differentiation away from Th1 and toward Th2, IL-4 inhibits Th17 cell development.[63] Moreover, treatment of psoriasis with IL-4 resulted in significant clinical improvement by selective silencing of IL-23 in APCs.[64] Other psoriasis genetic signals suggest involvement of Type I IFN signaling in disease pathogenesis, including associations with *DDX58* encoding RIG-I and *IFIH1* encoding MDA5. Each of these proteins bind viral nucleic acids and activate the mitochondrial antiviral signaling protein (MAVS), leading ultimately to activation of type I IFNs and IFN-stimulated genes as well as NF-κB.[65] *TYK2* encodes Tyk2, which also prominently involved in downstream type I IFN signaling and mediates responses to several other cytokines.[66]

NF-φB Signaling: Several psoriasis-associated genomic regions contain genes involved with controlling signaling through the TF NF-κB. TNF-α is a major activator of NF-κB signaling, and these associations are clinically reinforced by the dramatic therapeutic response of psoriasis to anti-TNF biologicals (see Treatment). *TNFAIP3* and *TNIP1*, respectively, encode

A20 and ABIN-1, which interact with each other to regulate the ubiquitin-mediated destruction of IKKγ/NEMO, a central nexus of NF-κB signaling.[67] *TNFAIP3* is genetically associated with RA, and both *TNFAIP3* and *TNIP1* are associated with systemic lupus erythematosus (SLE). The polymorphisms implicated in RA and SLE show no association with psoriasis, suggesting that each of these diseases is driven by different variants of the *TNFAIP3* gene. *CHUK* encodes IKK-α, which activates NF-κB via degradation of IκBα, and *NFKBIA* encodes IκBα, which inhibits NF-κB signaling by sequestering it in the cytoplasm. Other notable candidate genes in this category include *FASLG* encoding Fas ligand (CD95), a transmembrane protein of the TNF family; *REL* and *NFKB1*, both of which encode members of the NF-κB family; *TNFSF15* encoding TL1, a TNF-inducible cytokine that activates NF-κB; *IKBKE* encoding IKK-ε, which functions downstream of viral sensors to activate NF-κB; and *CARD14* encoding CARMA2, which activates NF-κB via interactions with BCL10. Notably, *CARD14* has been identified as the causative gene in the *PSORS2* locus, initially identified in a large pedigree by linkage analysis.[68]

Dendritic Cell and Macrophage Function: Besides the MHC, two other regions of association contain genes whose products function in antigen presentation: *PSMA6*, which encodes a proteasomal subunit involved in MHC class I antigen processing, and *ERAP1*, an IFN-γ–inducible aminopeptidase that trims peptides for optimal binding to the MHC class I peptide groove. Macrophages and inflammatory DCs are major sources of IL-23, TNF-α and inducible nitric oxide synthetase (iNOS). Psoriasis risk variants are present in *NOS2* (encoding iNOS) and *ZC3H12C* encoding the zinc-finger protein MCPIP3, both of which are important for macrophage function.

Keratinocyte Responses: Although the TNF-α and IL-23–Th17 axes described above converge strongly at a physiological level to stimulate production of innate inflammatory mediators such as hBD2 by keratinocytes,[69] relatively few psoriasis-associated regions contain genes that are thought to function primarily in keratinocytes. The most well-established association is an insertion-deletion (indel) polymorphism of the late cornified envelope genes *LCE3B* and *LCE3C*, which was independently discovered in European-origin[70] and Chinese[71] populations. Located in the epidermal differentiation complex (EDC), these genes are expressed very late in keratinocyte terminal differentiation and are markedly overexpressed in psoriasis, wound healing, and epidermal stress.[72] Notably, the *LCE3B/3C* indel is associated with cutaneous psoriasis but not with PsA.[54] Another psoriasis risk variant resides near the *KLF4* gene, which is a TF required for establishment of skin barrier function. *TRAF3IP2*- and *NFKBIZ* –encoded proteins are known to function in IL-17 responses of epidermal cells, and several genes implicated in the pathogenesis of generalized or PPPP are primarily expressed in the epidermis, including *IL36RN*, *AP1S3*, and *CARD14*.

OTHER RISK FACTORS

OBESITY

It has been demonstrated that obese individuals are more likely to present with severe psoriasis. However, obesity does not appear to have a role in defining the onset of psoriasis.[73]

SMOKING

Heavy smoking (>20 cigarettes daily) has been associated with more than a twofold increased risk of severe psoriasis.[74] Unlike obesity, smoking appears to have a role in the onset of psoriasis.[73]

INFECTIONS

An association between streptococcal throat infection and guttate psoriasis has been repeatedly confirmed. Streptococcal throat infections have also been demonstrated to exacerbate preexisting chronic plaque psoriasis,[75] and tonsillectomy has been shown to lead to long-term improvement in psoriasis,[76] particularly in HLA-Cw6 carriers.[77] Severe exacerbation of psoriasis can be a manifestation of HIV infection. The prevalence of psoriasis in HIV infection is no higher than in the general population, indicating that this infection is not a trigger for psoriasis but rather a modifying agent. Psoriasis is increasingly more severe with progression of immunodeficiency but can remit in the terminal phase. This paradoxical exacerbation of psoriasis may be caused by loss of Tregs and increased activity of the CD8 T-cell subset.[78] Psoriasis exacerbation in HIV disease may be effectively treated with antiretroviral therapy. Psoriasis has also been associated with hepatitis C infection.

DRUGS

Medications that exacerbate psoriasis include antimalarials, β blockers, lithium, nonsteroidal antiinflammatory drugs (NSAIDs), IFNs-α and -γ, imiquimod, angiotensin-converting enzyme inhibitors, and gemfibrozil. Imiquimod acts on plasmacytoid dendritic cells (pDCs) and stimulates IFN-α production, which then strengthens both innate and Th1 immune responses.[79] Exacerbations and onset of psoriasis have been described in patients receiving TNF inhibitor therapy. The majority of these patients have PPP, but about one third develop chronic plaque psoriasis.[80] New-onset psoriasis has also been described after the anti-IL-6 treatment tocilizumab. Lithium has been proposed to cause exacerbation by interfering with calcium release within keratinocytes, whereas β blockers are thought to interfere with intracellular cyclic adenosine monophosphate levels.[81] The mechanisms by which the remaining medications exacerbate psoriasis are largely unknown.

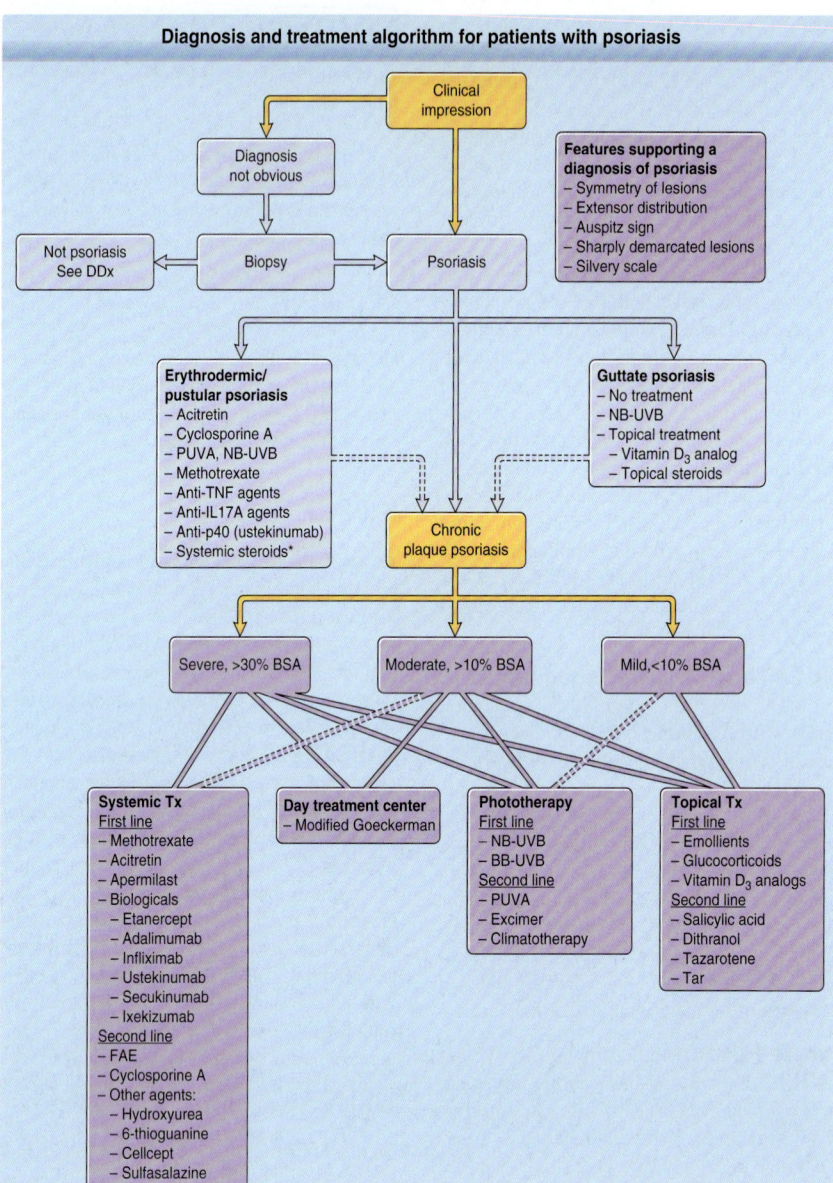

Figure 28-16 Diagnosis and treatment algorithm for patients with psoriasis. The diagnosis of psoriasis is usually based on clinical features. In the few cases in which clinical history and examination is not diagnostic, biopsy is indicated to establish the correct diagnosis. The majority of psoriasis cases fall into three major categories; guttate, erythrodermic/pustular, and chronic plaque, of which the latter is by far the most common. Guttate psoriasis is often a self-limited disease with spontaneous resolution within 6 to 12 weeks. In mild cases of guttate psoriasis, treatment may not be needed, but with widespread disease, ultraviolet B (UVB) phototherapy in association with topical therapy is very effective. Erythrodermic/pustular psoriasis is often associated with systemic symptoms and necessitates treatment with fast-acting systemic medications. The most commonly used drug for erythrodermic and pustular psoriasis is acitretin. In occasional cases of pustular psoriasis, systemic steroids may be indicated (*asterisk*). *Dotted arrows* indicate that guttate, erythrodermic, and pustular forms often evolve into chronic plaque psoriasis. Therapeutic choices for chronic plaque psoriasis are typically based on the extent of the disease. Among the main treatment regimens (topical treatment, phototherapy, day treatment centers, and systemic treatments), first- and second-line modalities are indicated by the *solid* and *dashed lines*, respectively. Individuals with conditions that limit their activities, including painful palmoplantar involvement and psoriatic arthritis, may require more potent treatments irrespective of the extent of affected body surface area. Likewise, psychological issues and the impact on quality of life should be taken into consideration. Within each treatment regimen, first-line and second-line choices are grouped. Cyclosporin A is not considered a first-line long-term systemic treatment because of its side effects, but short-term treatment can be helpful for induction of remission. If patients have incomplete response to or are unable to tolerate individual first-line systemic medications, combination regimens, rotational treatments, or use of biologic therapies should be considered. BB-UVB, broadband UVB; BSA, body surface area; DDx, differential diagnosis; FAE, fumaric acid ester; NB-UVB, narrowband UVB; PUVA, psoralen and ultraviolet A light; tx, therapy.

DIAGNOSIS

An algorithm for the diagnosis and treatment of psoriasis is presented in Fig. 28-16.

PATHOLOGY

Although histopathologic examination is rarely necessary to make the diagnosis of psoriasis, it can be helpful in difficult cases. The histopathologic manifestations of guttate and chronic plaque psoriasis have already been described (see Development of Lesions).

LABORATORY TESTING

Laboratory abnormalities in psoriasis are usually not specific and may not be performed in all patients. In severe psoriasis vulgaris, generalized pustular psoriasis, and erythroderma, a negative nitrogen balance can be detected, manifested by a decrease of serum albumin. Patients with psoriasis manifest altered lipid profiles, even at the onset of their skin disease.[82] Whether these differences in lipid profile can explain or are contributing to an increased incidence of cardiovascular events in psoriasis remains to be seen. The serum uric acid is elevated in up to 50% of patients and is mainly correlated with the extent of lesions and the activity of disease. There is an increased risk of developing gouty arthritis. Serum uric acid levels usually normalize after therapy. Markers of systemic inflammation, including C-reactive protein, α_2-macroglobulin, and erythrocyte sedimentation rate, can be increased. However, such elevations are rare in chronic plaque psoriasis uncomplicated by arthritis. Increased serum immunoglobulin (Ig) A levels and IgA immune complexes, as well as secondary amyloidosis, have also been observed in psoriasis, and the latter carries a poor prognosis.

DIFFERENTIAL DIAGNOSIS

A schema for the differential diagnosis of psoriasis is presented in Table 28-3.

CLINICAL COURSE AND PROGNOSIS

NATURAL HISTORY

It is useful to determine the age at onset and the presence or absence of a family history of psoriasis because a younger age of onset and positive family

TABLE 28-3
Differential Diagnosis of Psoriasis

PSORIASIS VULGARIS	GUTTATE	ERYTHRODERMIC	PUSTULAR
Most Likely	**Most Likely**	**Most Likely**	**Most Likely**
• Discoid/nummular eczema	• Pityriasis rosea	• Drug-induced erythroderma	• Impetigo
• Cutaneous T-cell lymphoma (CTCL)	• Pityriasis lichenoides chronica	• Eczema	• Superficial candidiasis
• Tinea corporis	• Lichen planus	• CTCL or Sézary syndrome	• Reactive arthritis syndrome
Consider	**Consider**	• Pityriasis rubra pilaris	• Superficial folliculitis
• Pityriasis rubra pilaris	• Small plaque parapsoriasis		**Consider**
• Seborrheic dermatitis	• Pityriasis lichenoides et varioliformis acuta		• Pemphigus foliaceus
• Subacute cutaneous lupus erythematosus	• Lichen planus		• Immunoglobulin A pemphigus
• Erythrokeratoderma (the fixed plaques of keratoderma variabilis or progressive symmetric erythrokeratoderma	• Drug eruption		• Sneddon-Wilkinson disease (subcorneal pustular dermatosis)
	Always Rule Out		• Migratory necrolytic erythema
	• Secondary syphilis		• Transient neonatal pustular melanosis
• Inflammatory linear verrucous epidermal nevus			• Acropustulosis of infancy
• Hypertrophic lichen planus			• Acute generalized exanthematous pustulosis
• Lichen simplex chronicus			
• Contact dermatitis			
• Chronic cutaneous lupus erythematosus/discoid lupus erythematosus			
• Hailey-Hailey disease (flexural)			
• Intertrigo (flexural)			
• *Candida* infection (flexural)			
Always Rule Out			
• Bowen disease or squamous cell carcinoma in situ			
• Extramammary Paget disease			

history have been associated with more widespread and recurrent disease.[3,14] In addition, the physician should inquire about the prior course of the disease because major differences exist between "acute" and "chronic" disease. In the latter form, lesions may persist unchanged for months or even years, but acute disease shows sudden outbreak of lesions within a short time (days). Likewise, patients have great variability in regard to relapses. Some patients have frequent relapses occurring weekly or monthly, but others have more stable disease with only occasional recurrence. The frequently relapsing patients tend to develop more severe disease with rapidly enlarging lesions covering significant portions of the body surface[83] and may require more rigorous treatment than those with more stable disease. The physician should also inquire about joint complaints. Although osteoarthritis is extremely common and can coexist with psoriasis, a history of onset of joint symptoms before the fourth decade or a history of warm, swollen joints should raise the suspicion of PsA (see Chap. 65). Guttate psoriasis is often a self-limited disease, lasting from 12 to 16 weeks without treatment. It has been estimated that one third to two thirds of these patients later develop the chronic plaque type of psoriasis.[84] In contrast, chronic plaque psoriasis is in most cases a lifelong disease, manifesting at unpredictable intervals. Spontaneous remissions, lasting for variable periods of time, may occur in the course of psoriasis in up to 50% of patients. The duration of remission ranges from 1 year to several decades. Erythrodermic and generalized pustular psoriasis have a poorer prognosis, with the disease tending to be severe and persistent.

TABLE 28-4
Topical Treatments for Psoriasis[83]

	TOPICAL STEROIDS	VITAMIN D ANALOGUES	TAZAROTENE	CALCINEURIN INHIBITORS
Mechanism of action	Bind to glucocorticoid receptors, inhibiting the transcription of many different AP-1– and NF-κB–dependent genes, including IL-1 and TNF-α	Bind to vitamin D receptors, influencing the expression of many genes; promote keratinocyte differentiation	Metabolized to tazarotenic acid, its active metabolite, which binds to retinoic acid receptors; normalizes epidermal differentiation, exhibits a potent antiproliferative effect, and decreases epidermal proliferation	Bind to FKBP and inhibit calcineurin, decreasing the activation of the transcription factor, NF-AT, with resultant decrease in cytokine transcription, including IL-2
Dosing	10,000-fold range of potency; high-potency steroids are applied to affected areas twice daily for 2–4 wk and then intermittently (weekends)	Calcipotriene, 0.005%, to affected areas twice daily; often used alternating with topical steroids (ie, vitamin D analogues on weekdays; topical steroids on weekends)	Available in 0.05% and 0.1% formulations, both as cream and gels; apply every night to affected area	Application to affected areas twice daily
Efficacy	Very effective as short-term treatment	Efficacy is increased by combination with topical steroids; can be combined with various other therapies	Efficacy is increased by combination with topical steroids	Effective for treatment of facial and flexural psoriasis but minimally for chronic plaque psoriasis
Safety	Suppression of the hypothalamic–pituitary–adrenal axis (higher risk in children); atrophy of the epidermis and dermis; formation of striae; tachyphylaxis	Development of irritation at the site of application is common; isolated reports of hypercalcemia in patients who applied excessive quantities	When used as monotherapy, significant proportion of patients develop irritation at the site of application	Burning sensation at the site of application; case reports of development of lymphoma
Contraindications	Hypersensitivity to the steroid, active skin infection	Hypercalcemia, vitamin D toxicity	Pregnancy, hypersensitivity to tazarotene	Use only with caution for treatment of children younger than 2 yr of age
Remarks and long-term use	Long-term use increases risk of side effects	Calcipotriol is well tolerated and continues to be clinically effective with minimum of adverse effects in long-term use	Combination of steroid with tazarotene may reduce atrophy seen with superpotent topical steroids; if added during phototherapy, the UV doses should be reduced by one third	Because of anecdotal reports of association with malignancy, this class of medications recently received a black-box warning by the FDA
Pregnancy Category	C	C	X	C

AP, activator protein; FDA, Food and Drug Administration; FKBP, FK506-binding protein; IL, interleukin; NF-AT, nuclear factor of activated T cells; NF-κB, nuclear factor kappa B; UV, ultraviolet.

TABLE 28-5
Phototherapy of Psoriasis[87]

	NARROWBAND UVB (NB-UVB; 310–331 NM)	BROADBAND UVB (BB-UVB)	PSORALEN AND UVA LIGHT (PUVA)	EXCIMER LASER (308 NM)
Dosing	Dosage based on either the Fitzpatrick skin type or MED; determine MED; initial treatment at 50% of MED followed by three to five treatments weekly; lubricate before treatment Treatments 1–20: increase by 10% of initial MED Treatments ≥21: increase as ordered by physician Maintenance therapy after >95% clearance: once a week for 4 wk; keep dose the same once every two weeks for 4 weeks; decrease dose by 25% once every 4 weeks, 50% of highest dose	The dosage may be administered according to the Fitzpatrick skin type; initial treatment at 50% of MED followed by three to five treatments weekly Treatments 1–10: increase dose by 25% of initial MED Treatments 11–20: increase by 10% of initial MED Treatments ≥21: increase as ordered by physician	Dose based on MPD is recommended; if MPD testing is impractical, a regimen based on skin type may be used Initial dose: 0.5–2.0 J/cm^2, depending on skin type (or MPD) Treat twice weekly, increments of 40% per week until erythema, and then maximum 20% per week No further increments when 15 J/cm^2 is reached	The dose of energy delivered is guided by the patient's skin type and thickness of plaque; further doses are adjusted based on response to treatment or development of side effects; treatment usually given twice weekly
Efficacy	>70% improvement in a split-body study after 4 wk of treatment; 9 of 11 patients showed clearance; more effective than BB-UVB	47% improvement in a split-body study after 4 wk; only 1 of 11 patients showed clearance	Induces remission in 70%–90% of patients; less convenient than NB-UVB but may be more effective	High response rates In one study, 85% of patients showed ≥90% improvement in PASI after an average 7.2 wk of treatment; another study showed >75% improvement in 72% of patients in an average of 6.2 treatments
Safety	Photodamage, polymorphic light eruption, increased risk of skin aging and skin cancers but lower than that for PUVA	Photodamage, polymorphic light eruption, increased risk of skin aging and skin cancers	Photodamage, premature skin aging, increased risk of melanoma and non-melanoma skin cancers, ocular damage; eye protection required with oral psoralens	Erythema, blisters, hyperpigmentation, and erosions; long-term side effects not yet clear but likely similar to NB-UVB
Contraindications	Absolute: photosensitivity disorders Relative: photosensitizing medications, melanoma, and nonmelanoma skin cancers	Absolute: photosensitivity disorders Relative: photosensitizing medications, melanoma, and nonmelanoma skin cancers	Absolute: light-sensitizing disorder, lactation, melanoma Relative: age <10 yr, pregnancy, photosensitizing medications, nonmelanoma skin cancers, severe organ dysfunction	Absolute: photosensitivity disorders Relative: photosensitizing medications, melanoma, and nonmelanoma skin cancers
Remarks	Effective as a monotherapy, but coal tar (Goeckerman regimen), anthralin (Ingram regimen), or systemic therapies may increase effectiveness in resistant cases	Coal tar (Goeckerman regimen), anthralin (Ingram regimen), or systemic therapies may increase effectiveness in resistant cases	<200 total treatments (or <2000 J/cm^2 UVA) are recommended; combination with oral retinoids can reduce cumulative UVA exposure	Normal skin is spared from unnecessary radiation exposure because therapy is selectively directed toward lesional skin.

MED, minimal erythema dose; MPD, minimal phototoxic dose; PASI, Psoriasis Area and Severity Index; UVA, ultraviolet A; UVB, ultraviolet B.

MANAGEMENT

GENERAL CONSIDERATIONS

Figure 28-16 is an algorithm showing recommended treatments for various forms of psoriasis.

A broad spectrum of antipsoriatic treatments, both topical and systemic, is available for the management of psoriasis. As detailed in Tables 28-4 to 28-7, it is notable that most, if not all, of these treatments are immunomodulatory. When choosing a treatment regimen (see Fig. 28-16), it is important to reconcile the extent and the measurable severity of

TABLE 28-6
Systemic Treatments for Psoriasis[96-98]

	CYCLOSPORIN A	METHOTREXATE	ACITRETIN	FUMARIC ACID ESTERS
Mechanism of action	Binds cyclophilin, and the resulting complex blocks calcineurin, reducing the effect of the NF-AT in T cells, resulting in inhibition of IL-2 and other cytokines	Blocks dihydrofolate reductase, leading to inhibition of purine and pyrimidine synthesis; also blocks AICAR transformylase, leading to accumulation of antiinflammatory adenosine	Binds to retinoic acid receptors; may contribute to improvement by normalizing keratinization and proliferation of the epidermis	Interferes with intracellular redox regulation, inhibiting NF-κB translocation; skews the T-cell response toward a Th2-like pattern
Dosing	High-dose approach: 5 mg/kg/day; then tapered. Low-dose approach: 2.5 mg/kg/day; increased every 2–4 wk up to 5 mg/kg/day; tapering is recommended on discontinuation	Start with a test dose of 2.5 mg and then gradually increase dose until a therapeutic level is achieved (average range, 10–15 mg weekly; maximum, 25–30 mg weekly)	Initiate at 25–50 mg/day and escalate and titrate to response	Initiate at low dose and escalate dose weekly; after treatment response is achieved, the dose should be individually adjusted; maximum dose, 1.2 g/day
Efficacy	Very effective; ≤90% of patients achieve clearance or marked improvement	May reduce the severity of psoriasis by at least 50% in >75% of patients	Modestly effective as monotherapy	80% mean reduction in PASI
Safety	Nephrotoxicity, HTN, immunosuppression; increased risk of malignancy if before PUVA	Hepatotoxicity; chronic use may lead to hepatic fibrosis; fetal abnormalities or death, myelosuppression, pulmonary fibrosis, severe skin reactions; rarely, severe opportunistic infections	Hepatotoxicity, lipid abnormalities, fetal abnormalities or death, alopecia, mucocutaneous toxicity, hyperostosis	GI symptoms, including diarrhea; flushing ± headaches; lymphopenia, acute renal failure
Monitoring	BP; obtain baseline CBC, CMP, magnesium, uric acid, lipids, UA; repeat tests every 2–4 wk; then every month along with BP	Baseline CBC and LFTs; monitor CBC and LFTs weekly until target dose is achieved; then every 4–8 wk[a%]; liver biopsy every 1.5 g (high risk) to every 3.5–4.0 g (low risk) of cumulative dose or use procollagen III assay	Baseline LFTs, CBC, lipids, pregnancy test; repeat LFTs, CBC, lipids every week for 1 mo and then every 4 wk; pregnancy test every month for women; spinal radiography if symptoms	Baseline CBC, CMP, UA; repeat tests every month for the first 6 mo and bimonthly thereafter
Contraindications	Absolute: uncontrolled HTN, abnormal renal function, history or current malignancy	Absolute: pregnancy, lactation, bone marrow dysfunction, alcohol abuse. Relative: hepatic dysfunction, hepatitis, renal insufficiency, severe infections, reduced lung function	Absolute: pregnancy during or within 3 years after termination of acitretin, breastfeeding	Absolute: patients with chronic disease of the GI tract or renal disease; pregnant or lactating women; malignancy (or history of)
Remarks and long-term use	Intermittent short-course treatments appear to be safer than chronic long-term use	With appropriate monitoring, long-term use appears to be safe	Retinoids have been combined with PUVA and occasionally with UVB in an attempt to minimize the side effects and to improve therapeutic response	Not approved by the FDA for psoriasis but widely used in Europe; new formulations may reduce risk of GI symptoms
Pregnancy Category	C	X	X	C

Chapter 28 :: Psoriasis

	HYDROXYUREA	6-THIOGUANINE	MYCOPHENOLATE MOFETIL	SULFASALAZINE
Mechanism of action	Inhibits ribonucleotide diphosphate reductase, which converts ribonucleotides to deoxyribonucleotides, thus selectively inhibiting DNA synthesis in proliferating cells	Purine analog that interferes with purine biosynthesis, thereby inducing cell cycle arrest and apoptosis	A noncompetitive inhibitor of inosine monophosphate dehydrogenase, blocking de novo purine biosynthesis; selectively cytotoxic for cells that rely on de novo purine synthesis (ie, lymphocytes)	Antiinflammatory agent; inhibits 5-lipoxygenase, molecular mechanism unclear
Dosing	500 mg/day; increased to 1.0–1.5 g/day based on response and tolerance	Starting dose is 80 mg twice weekly, with 20-mg increments every 2–4 weeks; maximum dose, 160 mg three times weekly	Doses often initiated at 500– 750 mg twice a day and then increased to 1.0–1.5 g twice a day	Starting dose: 500 mg three times a day. If tolerated after 3 days, increase dose to 1 g three times a day. If tolerated after 6 wk, increase dose to 1 g four times a day.
Efficacy	In a study of 85 patients with extensive chronic plaque psoriasis, 61% had satisfactory remission	A small retrospective cohort study demonstrated >90% improvement in ≤80% of patients	Appears to be only moderately effective for treatment of psoriasis	Appears to be moderately effective treatment for severe psoriasis
Safety	Bone marrow suppression, macrocytosis; teratogenicity and mutagenicity; dermatologic side effects: lichen planus–like eruptions, exacerbation of postirradiation erythema, leg ulcers, and dermatomyositis changes	Bone marrow suppression; GI complaints, including nausea and diarrhea; hepatic dysfunction; instances of hepatoveno-occlusive disease have been reported	GI, including constipation, diarrhea, nausea and vomiting, bleeding; myelosuppression, leukopenia; headaches, HTN, peripheral edema; infectious disease, lymphoma	Headache, nausea and vomiting, which occur in approximately one third of patients; rashes, pruritus, and hemolytic anemia (associated with G6PD deficiency)
Monitoring	Baseline CBC, CMP, LFTs; repeat baseline tests weekly for 4 wk; then every 2–4 wk for at least 12 wk; then repeat tests every 3 mo; hold dosage if WBC count <2.5 × 10⁹/L, platelet count is <100 × 10⁹/L, or severe anemia	Baseline CBC, CMP, LFTs; repeat baseline tests weekly during dose escalation and then every 2 wk; hold if WBC count ≤ 4.0 × 10⁹/L, platelet count is <125 × 10⁹/L, or hemoglobin <110 g/L	Baseline CBC and CMP; repeat laboratory tests weekly × 6 wk, then every 2 wk × 2 mo, and then monthly; monitor BP	Baseline CBC, CMP, and G6PD; repeat CBC and CMP weekly for 1 mo, then every 2 wk for 1 mo, then monthly for 3 mo, and then every 3 mo
Contraindications	Absolute: prior bone marrow depression (leukopenia, thrombocytopenia, anemia), pregnancy, lactation. Relative: renal abnormalities	Absolute: patients with inherited deficiency of thiopurine methyltransferase enzyme have increased risk of myelosuppression; liver toxicity; pregnancy	Absolute: patients with severe infections, malignancy	Absolute: hypersensitivity to sulfasalazine, sulfa drugs, salicylates, intestinal or urinary obstruction, porphyria; precaution in patients with G6PD deficiency
Remarks and long-term use	Limited experience with long-term treatment	Patients have been effectively maintained on treatment for ≤33 mo	Limited experience with long-term treatment	Limited experience with long-term treatment
Pregnancy Category	D	D	C	B

(Continued)

TABLE 28-6
Systemic Treatments for Psoriasis[91-93] (Continued)

	APREMILAST	TOFACITINIB
Mechanism of action	Inhibits PDE4	Inhibit the tyrosine kinases JAK1 and JAK3, with lesser inhibitory effect on JAK2
Dosing	Dose escalation from 10 mg to 30 mg twice a day in the first week and then 30 mg twice a day thereafter	5 mg twice-a-day dosing; 10 mg twice-a-day dosing is currently being assessed in clinical trials
Efficacy	In a study of 274 treated patients, 28.8% and 55.5% of patients achieved PASI-75 and PASI-50 response at week 16, respectively	In a study of 1861 patients, 5 mg twice-a-day dosing led to approximately 55% and 30% PASI-75 and PASI-90 response, respectively, and 10 mg twice-a-day dosing had approximately 70% and 45% PASI-75 and PASI-90 responses, respectively (week 28)
Safety	Worsening depression; nausea, diarrhea; mild weight loss (5%–10%) has been described	Bone marrow suppression; infections, particularly upper respiratory tract infections and nasopharyngitis; diarrhea
Monitoring	No laboratory monitoring is required	Baseline CBC, CMP, LFTs, lipids; repeat baseline tests monthly; lymphocyte count <500 cell/mm³, ANC <500 cells/mm³, discontinue drug; if ANC between 500 and 1000 cells/mm³ or Hgb decrease >2 g/dL or <8 g/dL interrupt dosing until ANC >1000 cell/mm³ or Hgb has normalized
Contraindications	Absolute: known hypersensitivity to apremilast Relative: depression	Absolute: do not initiate in patients with lymphocyte count <500 cell/mm³, ANC <1000 cells/mm³, or Hgb <9g/dL Relative: infections, risk of GI perforations, history of malignancy and lymphoproliferative disease
Remarks and long-term use		FDA approval for psoriasis and PsA pending
Pregnancy Category	C	C

AICAR, 5-Aminoimidazole-4-carboxamide ribonucleotide; ANC, absolute neutrophil count; BP, blood pressure; CBC, complete blood cell count; CMP, comprehensive metabolic panel; FDA, Food and Drug Administration; G6PD, glucose-6-phosphate dehydrogenase; GI, gastrointestinal; HTN, hypertension; IL, interleukin; JAK, Janus kinase; LFTs, liver function tests; NF-AT, nuclear factor of activated T cells; NF-κB, nuclear factor kappa B; PDE, phosphodiesterase; PUVA, psoralen and ultraviolet A light; Th, T helper; UA, urinalysis; UV, ultraviolet; WBC, white blood cell.

TABLE 28-7
Biologic Treatments for Psoriasis

	USTEKINUMAB	ETANERCEPT	INFLIXIMAB	ADALIMUMAB	SECUKINUMAB	IXEKIZUMAB
Mechanism	Binds p40 (the common subunit of IL-12 and IL-23); blocks Th1 and Th17 differentiation and proliferation	Human recombinant, soluble TNF-α receptor; binds TNF-α and neutralizes its activity	Chimeric monoclonal antibody that has high specificity, affinity, and avidity for TNF-α	Fully human recombinant monoclonal antibody that specifically targets TNF-α	Fully human recombinant monoclonal antibody that specifically targets IL-17A	Humanized monoclonal antibody that specifically targets IL-17A
Dosing	SC injections; weight-based dosing. Individuals weighing <100 kg (220 lb): 45 mg. Individuals weighing >100 kg: 90 mg. Injections at wk 0 and 4 and then every 12 wk	25- to 50-mg injections SC twice weekly; commonly given as 50 mg twice weekly for 12 wk followed by 50 mg weekly. For pediatric patients, recommended dosing is 0.8 mg/kg weekly with a maximum of 50 mg per week	IV infusions over 2 hr; 5–10 mg/kg at weeks 0, 2, and 6	Initial dose of 80 mg followed by 40 mg given every other week starting 1 week after the initial dose	150- to 300-mg injections at weeks 0, 1, 2, 3, and 4 (loading dose) followed by injections every 4 wk	160-mg injection at week 0 followed by 80 mg at weeks 2, 4, 6, 8, 10, and 12; then 80 mg every 4 wk
Efficacy	PASI-75 at 12 wk, 67%; 71%–78% at wk 28	PASI-75 at 12 wk, 34% and at 24 wk, 44% for the 25-mg twice-weekly vs 49% and 59% for 50-mg twice-weekly dosing	PASI-75 at 10 wk, 82% (5 mg/kg) and 91% (10 mg/kg); at wk 26 (after a single course), 57% of patients maintained PASI-50, and 50% maintained PASI-75	PASI-75 at 16 wk, 71%	PASI-75 at week 12 in the range of 77%–82%; PASI-90 52%–59% and PASI-100 24%–29% for 300-mg dosing	PASI-75 at week 12 achieved in 87% of patients; PASI-90 in 68% and PASI-100 in 38% of patients
Safety	Serious infections, increased risk of malignancy, reversible posterior leukoencephalopathy syndrome; live vaccinations not recommended	Serious infections, exacerbation of MS, pancytopenia, malignancy, worsening congestive heart failure; lupus-like symptoms (anti-dsDNA positive); live vaccinations should not be given	Infusion-related reactions, infections, worsening of MS, malignancy, or lymphoproliferative disease, worsening heart failure; lupus-like symptoms (anti-dsDNA positive); live vaccinations should not be given	Injection site reactions, infections, lupus-like syndrome, worsening heart failure, cytopenias, neurologic events; live vaccinations should not be given	Infections, particularly nasopharyngitis; exacerbation of IBD; hypersensitivity reactions; patients should not receive live vaccines while on treatment	Infections; hypersensitivity reactions; exacerbation of IBD
Monitoring	Baseline PPD/QuantiFERON-TB Gold	Baseline PPD/QuantiFERON-TB Gold	Baseline PPD/QuantiFERON-TB Gold	Baseline PPD/QuantiFERON-TB Gold	Baseline PPD/QuantiFERON-TB Gold	Baseline PPD/QuantiFERON-TB Gold
Long-term administration	Clinical trials have established safety up to 76wk; appears to be similar to TNF-α inhibitors	PASI response continues to increase to wk 24; large databases in patients with other immunologic diseases indicate relative safety	As intermittent therapy; large databases in patients with other immunologic diseases indicate relative safety	Similar to other TNF-α inhibitors	Clinical trials have shown maintenance of efficacy beyond 52 wk of treatment	Clinical trials have shown maintenance of efficacy beyond 60 wk of treatment
Pregnancy Category	B	B	B	B	B	B

dsDNA, double-stranded DNA; IBD, inflammatory bowel disease; IL, interleukin; IV, intravenous; LFA, lymphocyte function–associated antigen; MS, multiple sclerosis; PASI-50, 50% improvement in Psoriasis Area and Severity Index; PASI-75, 75% improvement in Psoriasis Area and Severity Index; PPD, purified protein derivative (of tuberculin); SC, subcutaneous; TNF, tumor necrosis factor.

TABLE 28-8
Treatment of Women of Childbearing Potential and During Pregnancy

- Special caution needs to be exercised when treating women of childbearing potential and during pregnancy.
- Medications such as methotrexate and oral retinoids should be avoided or used with extreme caution and then only along with appropriate contraception.
- In selected cases, isotretinoin rather than acitretin may be the preferred agent because of its much shorter half-life.
- Because methotrexate is fetotoxic and an abortifacient and retinoids are potent teratotoxins, the use of these agents is absolutely contraindicated in pregnancy.
- Many women experience improvement or remission during periods of pregnancy, thus decreasing the need for the more potent agents.
- If treatment is needed, emollients and other topical agents are first-line agents, often in association with ultraviolet B phototherapy.
- Many of the topical agents, such as topical steroids and calcipotriene, are Pregnancy Category C agents, and caution should be exercised with their use.
- Several of the biologic agents are Pregnancy Category B and can be used in pregnancy. Likewise, cyclosporin A may be considered because it is Pregnancy Category C and is nonteratogenic.
- Systemic psoralen and ultraviolet A light has been used on occasion in selected cases and appears to be safe.

the disease with the patient's own perception of his or her disease. One study found that 40% of patients felt frustrated with the ineffectiveness of their current therapies, and 32% reported that treatment was not aggressive enough.[24] As psoriasis is a chronic condition, it is important to know the safety of a treatment during long-term use. In most treatments, the duration of a treatment is restricted because of the cumulative toxicity potential of an individual treatment, and in some instances, treatment efficacy may diminish with time (tachyphylaxis). Some treatments, such as calcipotriol, methotrexate (MTX), and acitretin, can be regarded as appropriate for continuous use.[85] These treatments maintain efficacy and have low cumulative toxicity potential. In contrast, topical corticosteroids, dithranol, tar, photo(chemo) therapy, and cyclosporin are not indicated for continuous chronic use, and combinatorial or rotational treatments[85] are suggested. However, patients with stable chronic plaque psoriasis who respond well to local treatments may not require a change of treatment.[85] In cases of itchy or pruritic psoriasis, treatments with an irritative potential, such as dithranol, vitamin D_3 analogues, and photo(chemo) therapy, should be used cautiously; treatments with potent antiinflammatory effects, such as topical corticosteroids, are more appropriate.[85] In patients with erythrodermic and pustular psoriasis, treatments with an irritant potential should be avoided, and acitretin, MTX, or short-course cyclosporin are the treatments of first choice.[85] See Table 28-8 for special considerations in the treatment of women of childbearing potential.

TOPICAL TREATMENTS

See Table 28-4.

Most cases of psoriasis are treated topically.[86] Because topical treatments are often cosmetically unacceptable and time consuming to use, noncompliance is on the order of 40%.[87] In most cases, ointment formulations are more effective than creams but are less cosmetically acceptable. For many patients, it is worth prescribing both cream and ointment formulations—cream for use in the morning and ointment for nighttime. Topical agents are also used adjunctively for resistant lesions in patients with more extensive psoriasis and who are concurrently being treated with either UV light or systemic agents.[88] It is worth noting that around 400 g of a topical agent is required to cover the entire body surface of an average-sized adult when used twice daily for 1 week.

CORTICOSTEROIDS

Glucocorticoids exert many, if not all, of their myriad effects by stabilizing and causing nuclear translocation of glucocorticoid receptors, which are members of the nuclear hormone receptor superfamily. Topical glucocorticoids are commonly first-line therapy in mild to moderate psoriasis and in sites such as the flexures and genitalia, where other topical treatments can induce irritation. Improvement is usually achieved within 2 to 4 weeks, with maintenance treatment consisting of intermittent applications (often restricted to the weekends). Tachyphylaxis to treatment with topical corticosteroids is a well-established phenomenon in psoriasis. Long-term topical corticosteroids may cause skin atrophy, telangiectasia, striae (Fig. 28-17), and adrenal suppression. Another concern is that when topical steroids are discontinued, patients may reflare, sometimes worse than it was before treatment.[88] This class of agents is discussed in detail in Chap. 184.

VITAMIN D_3 AND ANALOGUES

Vitamin D exerts its actions by binding to the vitamin D receptor, another member of the nuclear hormone receptor superfamily. Vitamin D_3 acts to regulate cell growth, differentiation, and immune function, as well as calcium and phosphorous metabolism. Vitamin D has been shown to inhibit the proliferation of keratinocytes in culture and to modulate epidermal differentiation. Furthermore, vitamin D inhibits production of several proinflammatory cytokines by psoriatic T-cell clones, including IL-2 and IFN-γ. Analogues of vitamin D that have been used for the treatment of skin diseases are calcipotriene, (calcipotriol), tacalcitol, and maxacalcitol. In short-term studies, potent topical corticosteroids were found to be superior to calcipotriene. When compared with short-contact anthralin or 15% coal tar, calcipotriene was the more effective agent. The efficacy of calcipotriene is not reduced with long-term treatment. Calcipotriene applied twice daily is more effective than once-

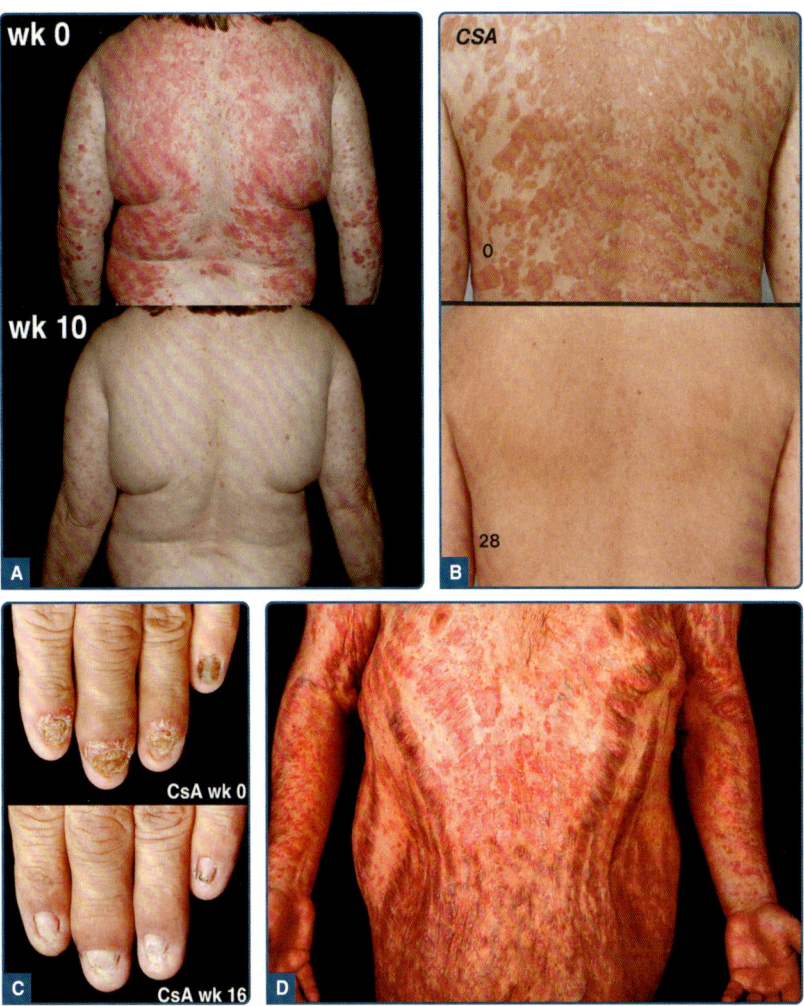

Figure 28-17 Positive and negative outcomes of psoriasis treatment. **A,** Near-complete improvement of psoriasis after 10 weeks of infliximab therapy. **B,** Marked improvement after 28 days of oral cyclosporin A (CsA) treatment. **C,** Marked reduction in nail dystrophy after 16 weeks of CsA treatment. **D,** Severe atrophy with striae distensae after several years of treatment with potent topical steroid creams. (Images used with permission from Mr. Harrold Carter.)

daily use. Hypercalcemia is the only major concern with the use of topical vitamin D preparations. When the amount used does not exceed the recommended 100 g/week, calcipotriene can be used with a great margin of safety. Vitamin D analogues are often used in combination with or in rotation with topical corticosteroids in an effort to maximize therapeutic effectiveness while minimizing steroid-related skin atrophy.

ANTHRALIN (DITHRANOL)

Dithranol (1,8-dihydroxy-9-anthrone) is a naturally occurring substance found in the bark of the araroba tree in South America. It can also be synthesized from anthrone. Dithranol is made up in a cream, ointment, or paste. Dithranol is approved for the treatment of chronic plaque psoriasis. Its most common use has been in the treatment of psoriasis, particularly on plaques resistant to other therapies. It can be combined with UVB phototherapy with good results (the Ingram regimen). Most common side effects are irritant contact dermatitis and staining of clothing, skin, hair, and nails. Anthralin possesses antiproliferative activity on human keratinocytes along with potent antiinflammatory effects. Classic anthralin therapy starts with low concentrations (0.05%–0.1%) incorporated in petrolatum or zinc paste and given once daily. To prevent auto-oxidation, salicylic acid (1% to 2%) should be added. The concentration is increased weekly in individually adjusted increments up to 4% until the lesions resolve. Scalp psoriasis should be treated with great caution as anthralin can stain hair purple to green.

COAL TAR

The use of tar to treat skin diseases dates back nearly 2000 years. In 1925, Goeckerman introduced the use of crude coal tar and UV light for the treatment of psoriasis. Its mode of action is not understood, and because of its inherent chemical complexity, tar is not pharmacologically standardized. It was recently suggested that carbazole, a coal-derived chemical, is the main active ingredient in tar.[89] Coal tar can be compounded in creams, ointments, and pastes at concentrations of 5% to 20%. It is often combined with salicylic acid (2%–5%), which by its keratolytic action leads to better absorption of the coal tar. Occasionally, patients become sensitized, and a folliculitis may occur. Furthermore, it has an unwelcome smell and appearance and can stain clothing. Coal tar is carcinogenic.

TAZAROTENE

Tazarotene is a third-generation retinoid for topical use that reduces mainly scaling and plaque thickness, with limited effectiveness on erythema. It is thought to act by binding to retinoic acid receptors. It is available in 0.05% and 0.1% gels, and a cream formulation has been developed. When this drug is used as a monotherapy, a significant proportion of patients develop local irritation. Efficacy of this drug can be enhanced by combination with mid- to high-potency glucocorticoids or UVB phototherapy. When used in combination with phototherapy, it lowers the minimal erythema dose (MED) for both UVB and UVA. It has been recommended that UV doses be reduced by at least one third if tazarotene is added to phototherapy.

TOPICAL CALCINEURIN INHIBITORS

See Chap. 192.

Tacrolimus (FK-506) is a macrolide antibiotic, derived from the bacteria *Streptomyces tsukubaensis*, which, by binding to immunophilin (FK506 binding protein), creates a complex that inhibits calcineurin, thus blocking both T-lymphocyte signal transduction and IL-2 transcription. Pimecrolimus is also a calcineurin inhibitor and works in a manner similar to tacrolimus. In a study of 70 patients with chronic plaque psoriasis treated with topical tacrolimus, there was no improvement beyond that seen for placebo. However, for treatment of inverse and facial psoriasis, these agents appear to provide effective treatment.[90] The main side effect of these medications is a burning sensation at application site. Anecdotal reports of lymph node or skin malignancy require further evaluation in controlled studies, and these drugs currently carry a U.S. Food and Drug Administration (FDA) "black box warning."

SALICYLIC ACID

Salicylic acid is a topical keratolytic agent. Its mechanism of action includes reduction of keratinocyte adhesion and lowering the pH of the stratum corneum, which results in reduced scaling and softening of the plaques, thereby enhancing absorption of other agents. Therefore, salicylic acid is often combined with other topical therapies such as corticosteroids and coal tar. Topical salicylic acid decreases the efficacy of UVB phototherapy,[88] and systemic absorption can occur, particularly in patients with abnormal hepatic or renal function and when applied to more than 20% of the body surface area. No placebo-controlled studies have been performed to verify the efficacy and safety of salicylic acid as a monotherapy.

BLAND EMOLLIENTS

Between treatment periods, skin care with emollients should be performed to avoid dryness. Emollients reduce scaling, may limit painful fissuring, and can help control pruritus. They are best applied immediately after bathing or showering. The addition of urea (up to 10%) is helpful to improve hydration of the skin and remove scaling of early lesions. The use of liberal bland emollients over a thin layer of topical prescription treatments improves hydration while minimizing treatment costs.

PHOTOTHERAPY

See Table 28-5 and Chap. 198.

Phototherapy of psoriasis with artificial light sources dates back to 1925 when Goeckerman introduced a combination of topical crude coal tar and subsequent UV irradiation. In the 1970s, it was shown that broadband UVB radiation alone, if given in doses that produce a faint erythematous reaction, could clear the milder clinical forms of psoriasis. Major steps forward were the introduction of photochemotherapy with psoralen and UVA light (PUVA) in the 1970s and narrowband UVB (311–313 nm) in the 1980s.[91]

The mechanism of action of phototherapy appears to involve selective depletion of T cells, predominantly those that reside in the epidermis.[78] The mechanism of depletion may involve apoptosis, accompanied by a shift from a Th1 to a Th2 response in lesional skin.

ULTRAVIOLET B LIGHT

Ultraviolet B (UVB) light is in the range of 290-320 nm. The initial therapeutic UVB dose lies at 50% to 75% of the MED. Treatments are given two to five times per week. Because peak UVB erythema appears within 24 hours of exposure, increments can be performed at each successive treatment. The objective is to maintain a minimally perceptible erythema as a clinical indicator of optimal dosing. Treatments are given until total remission is reached or until no further improvement can be obtained with continued treatment.[92] The main side effects of UVB phototherapy are summarized in Chap. 198.

Narrowband (312 nm) UVB (NB-UVB) phototherapy is superior to conventional broadband UVB with respect to both clearing and remission times. Although early studies found NB-UVB to be as effective as

PUVA, a controlled trial found that PUVA was more effective, albeit less convenient.[93] On clearing, treatment is either discontinued, or patients are subjected to maintenance therapy for 1 or 2 months. During this period, the frequency of UVB treatments is reduced while maintaining the last dose given at the time of clearing.[91,92] Systemic drugs, such as retinoids, increase the efficacy of UVB light, particularly in patients with chronic and hyperkeratotic plaque–type psoriasis.

PSORALEN AND ULTRAVIOLET A LIGHT

PUVA is the combined use of psoralens (P) and long-wave UVA radiation. The combination of drug and radiation results in a therapeutic effect, which is not achieved by the single component alone. Remission is induced by repeated controlled phototoxic reactions. A detailed account of PUVA therapy and its short- and long-term side effects is to be found in Chap. 199.

EXCIMER LASER

See Chap. 208.

Supraerythemogenic fluences of UVB and PUVA are known to result in faster clearing of psoriasis; however, the limiting factor for the use of such high fluences lies with the intolerance of the uninvolved surrounding skin as psoriatic lesions can often withstand much higher UV exposures. The monochromatic 308-nm excimer laser can deliver such supraerythemogenic doses of light (up to 6 MED, usually in the range of 2–6 MEDs) focally to lesional skin. The dosing is guided by the patients' skin type and thickness of the plaque with subsequent doses based on the response to therapy or development of side effects.[92] In a study on 124 patients, 72% of study participants achieved at least 75% clearing in an average of 6.2 treatments delivered twice weekly.[94] This treatment is commonly used for patients with stable recalcitrant plaques, particularly of the elbows and knees.

CLIMATIC THERAPY

It is well known that going to a sunny climate can improve psoriasis, although a small proportion of patients actually deteriorate. Patients should be warned not to overexpose themselves in the first few days because sunburn may progress to psoriasis (Koebner phenomenon). The best-studied effects are from the Dead Sea area,[95] and the therapeutic effects may be attributed, at least partially, to its unique climate. Because it is situated 400 m below sea level, the evaporation of the sea forms an aerosol that stays in the atmosphere above the sea and surrounding beaches. This aerosol screens out the majority of the UVB rays but not the UVA. This mixture of UV light appears to be sufficient to clear psoriasis but without sunburn. Thus, patients can stay on the shores of the Dead Sea for long periods of time with a greatly reduced risk of sunburn. This treatment is carried out over a period of 3 to 4 weeks, and improvements comparable to NB-UVB or PUVA treatments are observed. The main disadvantages are time and expense.

SYSTEMIC ORAL AGENTS[96-98]

See Table 28-6.

METHOTREXATE

Methotrexate is highly effective for chronic plaque psoriasis and is also indicated for the long-term management of severe forms of psoriasis, including psoriatic erythroderma and pustular psoriasis.[96] For mechanisms of action, see Chap. 190. When first used for the treatment of psoriasis, MTX was thought to act directly to inhibit epidermal hyperproliferation via inhibition of dihydrofolate reductase (DHFR). However, it was found to be effective at much lower doses (0.1–0.3 mg/kg/wk) in the management of psoriasis, PsA, and other inflammatory conditions such as RA. At these concentrations, MTX inhibits the in vitro proliferation of lymphocytes but not proliferation of keratinocytes. It is now thought that the main mechanism of antiinflammatory action of MTX is inhibition of (AICAR [5-aminoimidazole-4-carboxamide ribonucleotide] transformylase), an enzyme involved in purine metabolism. This leads to accumulation of extracellular adenosine, which has potent anti-inflammatory activities.[99] Consistent with a DHFR-independent mechanism of action, concomitant administration of folic acid (1–5 mg/day) reduces certain side effects, such as nausea and megaloblastic anemia, without diminishing the efficacy of anti-psoriatic treatment. The very long half-life of MTX may account for its efficacy after weekly administration and may help to explain why its onset of action is rather slow (therapeutic effects usually require 4–8 weeks to become evident). MTX is renally excreted and should therefore not be administered to patients with impairment in renal function because MTX side effects are generally dose related. Short-term toxicity and long-term concerns are discussed in Chap. 190. Recent guidelines[98] suggest that patients be divided into two separate groups based on their risk factors for liver injury: The low risk patients follow the American College of Rheumatology guidelines and are not asked to undergo liver biopsy until they have reached a cumulative MTX dose of 3.5 to 4.0 g. In contrast, patients with one or more risk factors continue to follow the previous, more stringent guidelines requiring baseline liver biopsy either before treatment or after 2 to 6 months of treatment and then at each cumulative MTX dose of 1.0 to 1.5 g.[98] The risk factors include current or past alcohol consumption, persistent abnormalities of liver function enzymes, personal, or family history of liver disease, exposure to hepatotoxic drugs or chemicals, diabetes mellitus, hyperlipidemia, and obesity. Some groups have recommended the use of amino terminal type III procollagen peptide assay for screening of liver fibrosis. Another well-known side effect of MTX is myelosuppression, especially pancytopenia, which usually occurs in the setting of folate deficiency. Leucovorin calcium (folinic acid) is the only antidote for the hematologic toxicity of MTX. When an overdose is suspected, an immediate leucovorin dose of 20 mg should be given parenterally or orally, and subsequent doses should be given every 6 hours. Pneumonitis can develop, and mucosal and skin ulcerations have also been reported in patients treated with MTX. Discontinuation of MTX treatment is required in the event of hepatotoxicity, hematopoietic suppression, active infections, nausea, and pneumonitis. MTX is also teratogenic and should therefore not be prescribed for women who are pregnant or breastfeeding. Several classes of drugs, including NSAIDs and sulfonamides, may interact with MTX to increase toxicity.

ACITRETIN

Acitretin is a second-generation, systemic retinoid that has been approved for the treatment of psoriasis since 1997 and is discussed in Chap. 185. The clinical forms most responsive to etretinate or acitretin as monotherapy include generalized pustular and erythrodermic psoriasis.[100] Acitretin induces clearance of psoriasis in a dose-dependent fashion. Overall, higher starting doses appeared to clear psoriasis faster. The mechanism of action of retinoids for psoriasis is not fully understood. The optimal initial dose of acitretin for psoriasis is reported at 25 mg/day, with a maintenance dose of 20 to 50 mg/day. Adverse effects, such as hair loss and paronychia, occur more frequently with higher initial dose (ie, ≥50 mg/day). Most patients relapse within 2 months after discontinuing etretinate or acitretin. Acitretin should be discontinued if liver dysfunction, hyperlipidemia, or diffuse idiopathic hyperostosis develops.

APREMILAST

Apremilast is a small-molecule inhibitor of phosphodiesterase (PDE)-4, which degrades cyclic adenosine monophosphate (cAMP) intracellularly. The inhibition of PDE4 increases intracellular levels of cAMP resulting in increased activity of the TF CREB (cAMP response element-binding protein), while inhibiting NF-κB signaling. To reduce risk of gastrointestinal (GI) symptoms the drug is titrated over a period of 1 week, starting at 10-mg dosing at day 1 and ending in 30-mg twice-a-day dosing on day 6, which is maintained for the duration of treatment. Adverse effects include GI symptoms such as diarrhea, nausea, and headaches. Worsening of depression has been described, and the drug should be used with caution in individuals with history of depression or suicidal thoughts or behaviors.

TOFACITINIB

Tofacitinib is an oral Janus kinase (JAK) inhibitor. Janus kinases are a family of four tyrosine kinases (JAK1, JAK2, JAK3, and TYK2) and have a role in downstream signaling of multiple proinflammatory cytokines, including IL-2, IL-4, IL-9, IL-13, IL-21, type I and II IFN signaling, IL-6, and to a lesser extent IL-12 and IL-23.[101] At the time of this writing, tofacitinib is only approved for RA, but several clinical trials in psoriasis have been completed using either 5 mg twice a day or 10 mg twice a day.[102,103] Patients should be screened for tuberculosis before initiation, and patients need to be monitored for changes in hemoglobin, leukopenias, or lipid abnormalities. Increased incidences of viral infections, particularly herpes zoster, have been reported in patients with RA taking tofacitinib.

CYCLOSPORIN A

Cyclosporin A (CsA) is a neutral cyclic undecapeptide derived from the fungus *Tolypocladium inflatum gams*. Its mechanism of action and side effects are discussed in Chap. 192. The only formulation approved for treatment of psoriasis is available as an oral solution or in capsules. It is highly effective for cutaneous psoriasis and can also be effective for nail psoriasis (see Fig. 28-9). CsA is particularly useful in patients who present with widespread, intensely inflammatory, or frankly erythrodermic psoriasis. The dosage ranges from 2 to 5 mg/kg/day. Because the nephrotoxic effects of CsA are largely irreversible, CsA treatment should be discontinued if kidney dysfunction or hypertension occurs. CsA-induced hypertension may be treated with calcium antagonists such as nifedipine. The most common adverse effects noted in patients using CsA for short periods of time are neurologic, including tremors, headache, paresthesia, or hyperesthesia. Long-term treatment of psoriasis with low-dose CsA was found to increase risk of nonmelanoma skin cancers. However, unlike organ transplant patients treated with higher doses of CsA, there is little or no increased risk of lymphoma.

FUMARIC ACID ESTERS

Fumaric acid was first reported in 1959 to be beneficial in the systemic treatment of psoriasis[104] and is licensed in Germany for the treatment of psoriasis. Because fumaric acid itself is poorly absorbed after oral intake, esters are used for treatment. The esters are almost completely absorbed in the small intestine, and dimethylfumarate is rapidly hydrolyzed by esterases to monomethylfumarate, which is regarded as the active metabolite. The mode of action in psoriasis is not fully understood.[104] Patients with severe concomitant disease, chronic disease of the GI tract, chronic kidney disease, or with bone marrow disease leading to leukocytopenias or leukocyte dysfunction should not be treated. Likewise, pregnant or lactating women and patients with malignant disease (including positive history of malignancy) should be excluded from treatment. Prolonged therapy (up to 2 years) to prevent relapse in psoriasis patients with high disease activity is possible. Another therapeutic option is short-course intermittent therapy. Fumaric acid esters (FAEs) are given until a major improvement is achieved and are then withdrawn. If a patient remains lesion-free during prolonged treatment, the FAE dose should be gradually decreased to reach the individual's threshold.[104] Therapy with FAEs can be stopped abruptly because rebound phenomena have not been observed.

SULFASALAZINE

Sulfasalazine is an uncommonly used systemic agent in the management of psoriasis. In the only prospective double-blind study on the efficacy of sulfasalazine in psoriasis, moderate effects were seen, with 41% of the patients showing marked improvement, 41% with moderate improvement, and 18% with minimal improvement after 8 weeks of treatment.[105]

SYSTEMIC STEROIDS

See Chap. 184

In general, systemic steroids should not be used in the routine care of psoriasis. When systemic steroids are used, clearance of psoriasis is rapid, but the disease usually breaks through, requiring progressively higher doses to control symptoms. If withdrawal is attempted, the disease tends to relapse promptly and may rebound in the form of erythrodermic and pustular psoriasis. However, systemic steroids may have a role in the management of persistent, otherwise uncontrollable, erythroderma and in fulminant generalized pustular psoriasis (von Zumbusch type) if other drugs are ineffective.

MYCOPHENOLATE MOFETIL

See Chap.192

Mycophenolate mofetil is a prodrug of mycophenolic acid, an inhibitor of inosine-5′-monophosphate dehydrogenase. Mycophenolic acid depletes guanosine nucleotides preferentially in T and B lymphocytes and inhibits their proliferation, thereby suppressing cell-mediated immune responses and antibody formation. The drug is usually well tolerated with few side effects. Few studies have been done on this medication for psoriasis, but in a prospective open-label trial on 23 patients with dosage between 2 to 3 g/day, a 24% reduction of the Psoriasis Area and Severity Index (PASI) was seen after 6 weeks, with 47% improvement at 12 weeks.

6-THIOGUANINE

6-Thioguanine is a purine analog that has been highly effective for psoriasis. Apart from bone marrow suppression, GI complaints, including nausea and diarrhea, can occur, and elevation of liver function test results is common.[96] Isolated instances of hepatic veno-occlusive disease have been reported.

HYDROXYUREA

Hydroxyurea is an antimetabolite that has been shown to be effective as monotherapy, but nearly 50% of patients who achieve marked improvement develop bone marrow toxicity with leukopenia or thrombocytopenia. Megaloblastic anemia is also common but rarely requires treatment.[96] Cutaneous reactions affect most patients treated with hydroxyurea, including leg ulcers, which are the most troublesome.[106]

BIOLOGIC TREATMENTS

See Table 28-7 and Chap. 193.

Based on the continuous progress in psoriasis research and advances in molecular biology, a new class of agents—targeted biologic therapies—has emerged. These agents are designed to block specific molecular steps important in the pathogenesis of psoriasis or have been transferred to the psoriasis arena after being developed for other inflammatory diseases. Currently, three types of biologics are approved or are in development for psoriasis: (1) recombinant human cytokines, (2) fusion proteins, and (3) monoclonal antibodies, which may be fully human, humanized or chimeric. Because of the risk of the development of antibodies to mouse sequences, humanized or fully human antibodies are preferred for clinical use.

Using internationally acknowledged safety and efficacy endpoints, the overall utility and benefit of biologics have been demonstrated based on the percentage of patients achieving at least a 50% improvement in PASI (PASI-50), a 75% improvement in PASI (PASI-75), the impact of treatment on quality of life, and safety and tolerability. Many of these agents have antipsoriatic activity roughly comparable to that of MTX and lack its risk of hepatotoxicity. However, they are far more expensive and carry risks of immunosuppression, infusion reactions, and antibody formation, and their long-term safety remains to be evaluated. In the opinion of the authors, use of biologic agents should be reserved for treatment of moderate to severe psoriasis that is either unresponsive to MTX or in patients for whom the use of MTX is contraindicated.

TUMOR NECROSIS FACTOR-α ANTAGONISTS

The clinical application of TNF antagonists in inflammatory diseases has exploded on the clinical realm in a manner reminiscent of the discovery of the activity of corticosteroids. TNF-α is a homotrimeric protein that exists in both transmembrane and soluble forms, the latter resulting from proteolytic cleavage and release. It is still unclear which form is more important in mediating its proinflammatory activities or the relative importance of the two p55- and p75-kd TNF-α–binding receptors. Currently, five anti-TNF biologics are available in the United States. Infliximab is a chimeric monoclonal antibody that has high specificity, affinity, and avidity for TNF-α. An example of an excellent treatment outcome with infliximab is shown in Fig. 28-17. Etanercept is a human recombinant, soluble, TNF-α receptor-Fc IgG fusion protein that binds TNF-α and neutralizes its activity. Adalimumab and golimumab are fully human recombinant IgG1 monoclonal antibodies and specifically targets TNF-α. Certolizumab pegol is a polyethylene glycol (PEG) Fab' fragment of a humanized TNF inhibitor monoclonal antibody. The pegylation is thought to reduce immunogenicity of the drug and prolongs serum half-life without compromising activity. Currently, golimumab and certolizumab pegol are only FDA approved for PsA. Clinical trials have shown that each of these agents is well tolerated and appears suitable for long-term use in chronic plaque psoriasis. However, like all the targeted biologic therapies, they carry risks of immunosuppression.

Clinical studies have found infliximab and adalimumab to be slightly more effective than etanercept in the treatment of psoriasis. It is likely that the differential effects of these agents are associated with selectivity in their ability to perturb these receptor–ligand interactions. It is known that infliximab, adalimumab, golimumab, and etanercept bind TNF differently; whereas infliximab and adalimumab bind to both soluble and membrane-bound TNF, etanercept binds primarily to soluble TNF. Binding to membrane-bound TNF can induce a dose-dependent increase in apoptosis of T cells, but the relevance of this mechanism in psoriasis has not been evaluated. New onset of psoriasis has been described several times in patients on these agents for other conditions such as Crohn disease or RA. These paradoxical reactions are characterized by increased production of IFN-α.[107]

INTERLEUKIN-12 AND INTERLEUKIN-23 ANTAGONISTS

Ustekinumab is a human monoclonal antibody that binds the shared p40 subunit of IL-12 and IL-23 and prevents interaction with their receptors. This treatment blocks IL-12, which is critical for Th1 differentiation, but its inhibitory effect on IL-23 may be more important. As described earlier, IL-23 supports chronic inflammation mediated by Th17 and Th22 cells. Clinical studies have found ustekinumab to be slightly more effective than etanercept in the treatment of psoriasis,[108] but direct comparison with infliximab or adalimumab has not been reported.

Several agents specifically targeting the p19 subunit of IL-23 are currently in development and appear to be highly effective, consistent with a key role for IL-23 in psoriasis pathogenesis.[57,109,110]

INTERLEUKIN-17A ANTAGONISTS

Two IL-17A antagonists are currently approved for the treatment of psoriasis. Secukinumab is a fully human antibody, and ixekizumab is a humanized antibody that binds and neutralizes IL-17A. IL-17A is a critical cytokine in the pathogenesis of psoriasis, and biologics targeting IL-17A are among the most effective drugs available for the treatment of psoriasis.[111-113] Brodalumab, a fully human antibody targeting the IL-17 receptor α chain, is also highly effective[114] and has recently been FDA approved for use in psoriasis after screening for depression and suicidal ideation.

COMBINATION TREATMENTS

Combination treatment may increase efficacy and reduce side effects, so it may result in a more substantial improvement, or alternatively, may permit reduced doses to reach the same improvement as compared with monotherapy.[85] Data on combination of biologics with other systemic or topical agents are not yet widely available, but some combinations commonly used in the treatment of inflammatory arthritides, such as a combination of MTX and anti-TNF agents, may be appropriate for treatment of recalcitrant psoriatic disease.

TREATMENT OF PALMOPLANTAR PUSTULAR PSORIASIS

Palmoplantar pustular psoriasis (including PPP and PPPP) tends to be difficult to treat and is often unresponsive to treatments used for chronic plaque psoriasis. Given its rarity, randomized controlled trials are lacking. Phototherapy, cyclosporine, and topical steroids are the treatments with the most well-documented efficacy.[115] Tonsillectomy has been used to treat pustulosis palmaris et plantaris, and in a cohort of 116 Japanese patients, clinical improvement was seen in 109 (94%).[116] Notably, given its strong association with smoking, smoking cessation provides substantial clinical improvement.[117]

PREVENTION

There is no known prevention for psoriasis.

REFERENCES

1. Parisi R, Symmons DP, Griffiths CE, et al. Global epidemiology of psoriasis: a systematic review of incidence and prevalence. *J Invest Dermatol*. 2013;133(2):377-385.
2. Raychaudhuri SP, Farber EM. The prevalence of psoriasis in the world. *J Eur Acad Dermatol Venereol*. 2001;15(1):16-17.
3. Henseler T, Christophers E. Psoriasis of early and late onset: characterization of two types of psoriasis vulgaris. *J Am Acad Dermatol*. 1985;13(3):450-456.
4. Lonnberg AS, Skov L, Skytthe A, et al. Heritability of psoriasis in a large twin sample. *Br J Dermatol*. 2013;169(2):412-416.
5. Mallon E, Bunce M, Savoie H, et al. HLA-C and guttate psoriasis. *Br J Dermatol*. 2000;143(6):1177-1182.
6. Telfer NR, Chalmers RJ, Whale K, et al. The role of streptococcal infection in the initiation of guttate psoriasis. *Arch Dermatol*. 1992;128(1):39-42.
7. Chalmers RR, O'Sullivan T, Owen CC, et al. A systematic review of treatments for guttate psoriasis. *Br J Dermatol*. 2001;145(6):891-894.
8. Kim J, Oh CH, Jeon J, et al. Molecular phenotyping small (Asian) versus large (western) plaque psoriasis shows common activation of IL-17 pathway genes but different regulatory gene sets. *J Invest Dermatol*. 2016;136(1):161-172.
9. Baker H, Ryan TJ. Generalized pustular psoriasis. A clinical and epidemiological study of 104 cases. *Br J Dermatol*. 1968;80(12):771-793.
10. Becher G, Jamieson L, Leman J. Palmoplantar pustulosis—a retrospective review of comorbid conditions. *J Eur Acad Dermatol Venereol*. 2015;29(9):1854-1856.
11. Asumalahti K, Ameen M, Suomela S, et al. Genetic analysis of PSORS1 distinguishes guttate psoriasis and palmoplantar pustulosis. *J Invest Dermatol*. 2003;120(4):627-632.
12. Bissonnette R, Suarez-Farinas M, Li X, et al. Based on molecular profiling of gene expression, palmoplantar pustulosis and palmoplantar pustular psoriasis are highly related diseases that appear to be distinct from psoriasis vulgaris. *PLoS One*. 2016;11(5):e0155215.
13. Kim KH, Kim HL, Suh HY, et al. A case of acrodermatitis continua accompanying with osteolysis and atrophy of the distal phalanx that evolved into generalized pustular psoriasis. *Ann Dermatol*. 2016;28(6):794-795.
14. Gudjonsson JE, Karason A, Runarsdottir EH, et al. Distinct clinical differences between HLA-Cw*0602 positive and negative psoriasis patients—an analysis of 1019 HLA-C- and HLA-B-typed patients. *J Invest Dermatol*. 2006;126(4):740-745.
15. Kvedar JC, Baden HP. Nail changes in cutaneous disease. *Semin Dermatol*. 1991;10(1):65-70.
16. Rittie L, Tejasvi T, Harms PW, et al. Sebaceous gland atrophy in psoriasis: an explanation for psoriatic alopecia? *J Invest Dermatol*. 2016;136(9):1792-1800.
17. Henseler T, Christophers E. Disease concomitance in psoriasis. *J Am Acad Dermatol*. 1995;32(6):982-986.
18. Gelfand JM, Neimann AL, Shin DB, et al. Risk of myocardial infarction in patients with psoriasis. *JAMA*. 2006;296(14):1735-1741.
19. Naik HB, Natarajan B, Stansky E, et al. Severity of psoriasis associates with aortic vascular inflammation detected by FDG PET/CT and neutrophil activation in a prospective observational study. *Arterioscler Thromb Vasc Biol*. 2015;35(12):2667-2676.
20. Augustin M, Reich K, Glaeske G, et al. Co-morbidity and age-related prevalence of psoriasis: analysis of health insurance data in Germany. *Acta Derm Venereol*. 2010;90(2):147-151.
21. Gelfand JM, Shin DB, Neimann AL, et al. The risk of lymphoma in patients with psoriasis. *J Invest Dermatol*. 2006;126(10):2194-2201.
22. Fortune DG, Richards HL, Griffiths CE. Psychologic factors in psoriasis: consequences, mechanisms, and interventions. *Dermatol Clin*. 2005;23(4):681-694.
23. Rapp SR, Feldman SR, Exum ML, et al. Psoriasis causes as much disability as other major medical diseases. *J Am Acad Dermatol*. 1999;41(3 Pt 1):401-407.
24. Krueger G, Koo J, Lebwohl M, et al. The impact of psoriasis on quality of life: results of a 1998 National Psoriasis Foundation patient-membership survey. *Arch Dermatol*. 2001;137(3):280-284.
25. Braun-Falco O. Dynamics of growth and regression in psoriatic lesions: alterations in the skin from normal into a psoriatic lesion, and during regression of psoriatic lesions. In: Farber EM, Cox AJ, eds. *Psoriasis: Proceedings of the International Symposium, Stanford University, 1971*. Stanford, CA: Stanford University Press; 1971:215-237.
26. Christophers E, Parzefall R, Braun-Falco O. Initial events in psoriasis: quantitative assessment. *Br J Dermatol*. 1973;89(4):327-334.
27. Brody I. Alterations of clinically normal skin in early eruptive guttate psoriasis. *J Cutan Pathol*. 1978;5:219-233.
28. Wright NA, Camplejohn RS, eds. *Psoriasis: Cell Proliferation*. Edinburgh: Churchill Livingstone; 1983.
29. Wrone-Smith T, Nickoloff BJ. Dermal injection of immunocytes induces psoriasis. *J Clin Invest*. 1996;98(8):1878-1887.
30. Chang JC, Smith LR, Froning KJ, et al. CD8+ T cells in psoriatic lesions preferentially use T-cell receptor V beta 3 and/or V beta 13.1 genes. *Proc Natl Acad Sci U S A*. 1994;91(20):9282-9286.
31. Harden JL, Hamm D, Gulati N, et al. Deep sequencing of the T-cell receptor repertoire demonstrates polyclonal T-cell infiltrates in psoriasis. *F1000Res*. 2015;4:460.
32. Clark RA. Resident memory T cells in human health and disease. *Sci Transl Med*. 2015;7(269):269rv261.
33. Conrad C, Boyman O, Tonel G, et al. Alpha1beta1 integrin is crucial for accumulation of epidermal T cells and the development of psoriasis. *Nat Med*. 2007;13(7):836-842.
34. Di Meglio P, Villanova F, Navarini AA, et al. Targeting CD8(+) T cells prevents psoriasis development. *J Allergy Clin Immunol*. 2016;138(1):274-276, e276.
35. Zaba LC, Cardinale I, Gilleaudeau P, et al. Amelioration of epidermal hyperplasia by TNF inhibition is associated with reduced Th17 responses. *J Exp Med*. 2007;204(13):3183-3194.
36. Beissert S, Schwarz A, Schwarz T. Regulatory T cells. *J Invest Dermatol*. 2006;126(1):15-24.
37. Sugiyama H, Gyulai R, Toichi E, et al. Dysfunctional blood and target tissue CD4+CD25high regulatory T cells in psoriasis: mechanism underlying unrestrained pathogenic effector T cell proliferation. *J Immunol*. 2005;174(1):164-173.
38. Laggner U, Di Meglio P, Perera GK, et al. Identification of a novel proinflammatory human skin-homing Vgamma9Vdelta2 T cell subset with a potential role in psoriasis. *J Immunol*. 2011;187(5):2783-2793.

39. Teunissen MB, Munneke JM, Bernink JH, et al. Composition of innate lymphoid cell subsets in the human skin: enrichment of NCR(+) ILC3 in lesional skin and blood of psoriasis patients. *J Invest Dermatol.* 2014;134(9):2351-2360.
40. Lowes MA, Suarez-Farinas M, Krueger JG. Immunology of psoriasis. *Annu Rev Immunol.* 2014;32:227-255.
41. Stratis A, Pasparakis M, Rupec RA, et al. Pathogenic role for skin macrophages in a mouse model of keratinocyte-induced psoriasis-like skin inflammation. *J Clin Invest.* 2006;116(8):2094-2104.
42. Mansbridge JN, Knapp AM, Strefling AM. Evidence for an alternative pathway of keratinocyte maturation in psoriasis from an antigen found in psoriatic but not normal epidermis. *J Invest Dermatol.* 1984;83(4):296-301.
43. Tsoi LC, Stuart PE, Tejasvi T, et al. Large-scale meta-analysis identifies 18 novel psoriasis susceptibility loci. *Nat Commun.* 2017;8:15382.
44. Nair RP, Stuart PE, Nistor I, et al. Sequence and haplotype analysis supports HLA-C as the psoriasis susceptibility 1 gene. *Am J Hum Genet.* 2006;78(5):827-851.
45. Okada Y, Han B, Tsoi LC, et al. Fine mapping major histocompatibility complex associations in psoriasis and its clinical subtypes. *Am J Hum Genet.* 2014;95(2):162-172.
46. Rottman JB, Smith TL, Ganley KG, et al. Potential role of the chemokine receptors CXCR3, CCR4, and the integrin alphaEbeta7 in the pathogenesis of psoriasis vulgaris. *Lab Invest.* 2001;81(3):335-347.
47. Boyman O, Hefti HP, Conrad C, et al. Spontaneous development of psoriasis in a new animal model shows an essential role for resident T cells and tumor necrosis factor-alpha. *J Exp Med.* 2004;199(5):731-736.
48. Zhou F, Cao H, Zuo X, et al. Deep sequencing of the MHC region in the Chinese population contributes to studies of complex disease. *Nat Genet.* 2016;48(7):740-746.
49. Lande R, Botti E, Jandus C, et al. The antimicrobial peptide LL37 is a T-cell autoantigen in psoriasis. *Nat Commun.* 2014;5:5621.
50. Cheung KL, Jarrett R, Subramaniam S, et al. Psoriatic T cells recognize neolipid antigens generated by mast cell phospholipase delivered by exosomes and presented by CD1a. *J Exp Med.* 2016;213(11):2399-2412.
51. Arakawa A, Siewert K, Stohr J, et al. Melanocyte antigen triggers autoimmunity in human psoriasis. *J Exp Med.* 2015;212(13):2203-2212.
52. Bonifacio KM, Kunjravia N, Krueger JG, et al. Cutaneous expression of A disintegrin-like and metalloprotease domain containing thrombospondin type 1 motif-like 5 (ADAMTSL5) in psoriasis goes beyond melanocytes. *J Pigment Disord.* 2016;3(3).
53. Nickoloff BJ, Wrone-Smith T. Injection of pre-psoriatic skin with CD4+ T cells induces psoriasis. *Am J Pathol.* 1999;155(1):145-158.
54. Stuart PE, Nair RP, Tsoi LC, et al. Genome-wide association analysis of psoriatic arthritis and cutaneous psoriasis reveals differences in their genetic architecture. *Am J Hum Genet.* 2015;97(6):816-836.
55. Bowes J, Budu-Aggrey A, Huffmeier U, et al. Dense genotyping of immune-related susceptibility loci reveals new insights into the genetics of psoriatic arthritis. *Nat Commun.* 2015;6:6046.
56. Krueger GG, Langley RG, Leonardi C, et al. A human interleukin-12/23 monoclonal antibody for the treatment of psoriasis. *N Engl J Med.* 2007;356(6):580-592.
57. Kopp T, Riedl E, Bangert C, et al. Clinical improvement in psoriasis with specific targeting of interleukin-23. *Nature.* 2015;521(7551):222-226.
58. Bettelli E, Oukka M, Kuchroo VK. T(H)-17 cells in the circle of immunity and autoimmunity. *Nat Immunol.* 2007;8(4):345-350.
59. Thomas GP, Brown MA. Genetics and genomics of ankylosing spondylitis. *Immunol Rev.* 2010;233(1):162-180.
60. Reveille JD, Sims AM, Danoy P, et al. Genome-wide association study of ankylosing spondylitis identifies non-MHC susceptibility loci. *Nat Genet.* 2010;42(2):123-127.
61. Johansen C, Mose M, Ommen P, et al. IkappaBzeta is a key driver in the development of psoriasis. *Proc Natl Acad Sci U S A.* 2015;112(43):e5825-5833.
62. Kryczek I, Bruce AT, Gudjonsson JE, et al. Induction of IL-17+ T cell trafficking and development by IFN-gamma: mechanism and pathological relevance in psoriasis. *J Immunol.* 2008;181(7):4733-4741.
63. Mills KH. Induction, function and regulation of IL-17-producing T cells. *Eur J Immunol.* 2008;38(10):2636-2649.
64. Guenova E, Skabytska Y, Hoetzenecker W, et al. IL-4 abrogates T(H)17 cell-mediated inflammation by selective silencing of IL-23 in antigen-presenting cells. *Proc Natl Acad Sci U S A.* 2015;112(7):2163-2168.
65. Wu J, Chen ZJ. Innate immune sensing and signaling of cytosolic nucleic acids. *Annu Rev Immunol.* 2014;32:461-488.
66. Kreins AY, Ciancanelli MJ, Okada S, et al. Human TYK2 deficiency: mycobacterial and viral infections without hyper-IgE syndrome. *J Exp Med.* 2015;212(10):1641-1662.
67. Mauro C, Pacifico F, Lavorgna A, et al. ABIN-1 binds to NEMO/IKKgamma and co-operates with A20 in inhibiting NF-kappaB. *J Biol Chem.* 2006;281(27):18482-18488.
68. Jordan CT, Cao L, Roberson ED, et al. PSORS2 is due to mutations in CARD14. *Am J Hum Genet.* 2012;90(5):784-795.
69. Chiricozzi A, Nograles KE, Johnson-Huang LM, et al. IL-17 induces an expanded range of downstream genes in reconstituted human epidermis model. *PLoS One.* 2014;9(2):e90284.
70. de Cid R, Riveira-Munoz E, Zeeuwen PL, et al. Deletion of the late cornified envelope LCE3B and LCE3C genes as a susceptibility factor for psoriasis. *Nat Genet.* 2009;41(2):211-215.
71. Zhang XJ, Huang W, Yang S, et al. Psoriasis genome-wide association study identifies susceptibility variants within LCE gene cluster at 1q21. *Nat Genet.* 2009;41(2):205-210.
72. Niehues H, van Vlijmen-Willems IM, Bergboer JG, et al. Late cornified envelope (LCE) proteins: distinct expression patterns of LCE2 and LCE3 members suggest non-redundant roles in human epidermis and other epithelia. *Br J Dermatol.* 2016;174(4):795-802.
73. Herron MD, Hinckley M, Hoffman MS, et al. Impact of obesity and smoking on psoriasis presentation and management. *Arch Dermatol.* 2005;141(12):1527-1534.
74. Fortes C, Mastroeni S, Leffondre K, et al. Relationship between smoking and the clinical severity of psoriasis. *Arch Dermatol.* 2005;141(12):1580-1584.
75. Gudjonsson JE, Thorarinsson AM, Sigurgeirsson B, et al. Streptococcal throat infections and exacerbation of chronic plaque psoriasis: a prospective study. *Br J Dermatol.* 2003;149(3):530-534.

76. Thorleifsdottir RH, Eysteinsdottir JH, Olafsson JH, et al. Throat infections are associated with exacerbation in a substantial proportion of patients with chronic plaque psoriasis. *Acta Derm Venereol.* 2016;96(6):788-791.
77. Thorleifsdottir RH, Sigurdardottir SL, Sigurgeirsson B, et al. HLA-Cw6 homozygosity in plaque psoriasis is associated with streptococcal throat infections and pronounced improvement after tonsillectomy: a prospective case series. *J Am Acad Dermatol.* 2016; 75(5):889-896.
78. Gudjonsson JE, Johnston A, Sigmundsdottir H, et al. Immunopathogenic mechanisms in psoriasis. *Clin Exp Immunol.* 2004;135(1):1-8.
79. Nestle FO, Conrad C, Tun-Kyi A, et al. Plasmacytoid predendritic cells initiate psoriasis through interferon-{alpha} production. *J Exp Med.* 2005;202(1):135-143.
80. Ko JM, Gottlieb AB, Kerbleski JF. Induction and exacerbation of psoriasis with TNF-blockade therapy: a review and analysis of 127 cases. *J Dermatolog Treat.* 2008:1-8.
81. O'Brien M, Koo J. The mechanism of lithium and beta-blocking agents in inducing and exacerbating psoriasis. *J Drugs Dermatol.* 2006;5(5):426-432.
82. Mallbris L, Granath F, Hamsten A, et al. Psoriasis is associated with lipid abnormalities at the onset of skin disease. *J Am Acad Dermatol.* 2006;54(4):614-621.
83. Christophers E. Psoriasis—epidemiology and clinical spectrum. *Clin Exp Dermatol.* 2001;26(4):314-320.
84. Martin BA, Chalmers RJ, Telfer NR. How great is the risk of further psoriasis following a single episode of acute guttate psoriasis? *Arch Dermatol.* 1996;132(6):717-718.
85. van de Kerkhof PC. Therapeutic strategies: rotational therapy and combinations. *Clin Exp Dermatol.* 2001;26(4):356-361.
86. Lebwohl M, Ali S. Treatment of psoriasis. Part 1. Topical therapy and phototherapy. *J Am Acad Dermatol.* 2001;45(4):487-498; quiz 499-502.
87. Richards HL, Fortune DG, O'Sullivan TM, et al. Patients with psoriasis and their compliance with medication. *J Am Acad Dermatol.* 1999;41(4):581-583.
88. Menter A, Korman NJ, Elmets CA, et al. Guidelines of care for the management of psoriasis and psoriatic arthritis. Section 3. Guidelines of care for the management and treatment of psoriasis with topical therapies. *J Am Acad Dermatol.* 2009;60(4):643-659.
89. Arbiser JL, Govindarajan B, Battle TE, et al. Carbazole is a naturally occurring inhibitor of angiogenesis and inflammation isolated from antipsoriatic coal tar. *J Invest Dermatol.* 2006;126(6):1396-1402.
90. Martin Ezquerra G, Sanchez Regana M, Herrera Acosta E, et al. Topical tacrolimus for the treatment of psoriasis on the face, genitalia, intertriginous areas and corporal plaques. *J Drugs Dermatol.* 2006;5(4):334-336.
91. Honigsmann H. Phototherapy for psoriasis. *Clin Exp Dermatol.* 2001;26(4):343-350.
92. Menter A, Korman NJ, Elmets CA, et al. Guidelines of care for the management of psoriasis and psoriatic arthritis: section 5. Guidelines of care for the treatment of psoriasis with phototherapy and photochemotherapy. *J Am Acad Dermatol.* 2010;62(1):114-135.
93. Yones SS, Palmer RA, Garibaldinos TT, et al. Randomized double-blind trial of the treatment of chronic plaque psoriasis: efficacy of psoralen-UV-A therapy vs narrowband UV-B therapy. *Arch Dermatol.* 2006;142(7):836-842.
94. Asawanonda P, Anderson RR, Chang Y, et al. 308-nm excimer laser for the treatment of psoriasis: a dose-response study. *Arch Dermatol.* 2000;136(5):619-624.
95. Halevy S, Sukenik S. Different modalities of spa therapy for skin diseases at the Dead Sea area. *Arch Dermatol.* 1998;134(11):1416-1420.
96. Lebwohl M, Ali S. Treatment of psoriasis. Part 2. Systemic therapies. *J Am Acad Dermatol.* 2001;45(5):649-661; quiz 662-644.
97. Pathirana D, Ormerod AD, Saiag P, et al. European S3-guidelines on the systemic treatment of psoriasis vulgaris. *J Eur Acad Dermatol Venereol.* 2009;23 (suppl 2):1-70.
98. Menter A, Korman NJ, Elmets CA, et al. Guidelines of care for the management of psoriasis and psoriatic arthritis: section 4. Guidelines of care for the management and treatment of psoriasis with traditional systemic agents. *J Am Acad Dermatol.* 2009;61(3):451-485.
99. Cronstein BN, Naime D, Ostad E. The antiinflammatory effects of methotrexate are mediated by adenosine. *Adv Exp Med Biol.* 1994;370:411-416.
100. Lee CS, Koo J. A review of acitretin, a systemic retinoid for the treatment of psoriasis. *Expert Opin Pharmacother.* 2005;6(10):1725-1734.
101. Krueger J, Clark JD, Suarez-Farinas M, et al. Tofacitinib attenuates pathologic immune pathways in patients with psoriasis: a randomized phase 2 study. *J Allergy Clin Immunol.* 2016;137(4):1079-1090.
102. Papp KA, Krueger JG, Feldman SR, et al. Tofacitinib, an oral Janus kinase inhibitor, for the treatment of chronic plaque psoriasis: long-term efficacy and safety results from 2 randomized phase-III studies and 1 open-label long-term extension study. *J Am Acad Dermatol.* 2016;74(5):841-850.
103. Bachelez H, van de Kerkhof PC, Strohal R, et al. Tofacitinib versus etanercept or placebo in moderate-to-severe chronic plaque psoriasis: a phase 3 randomised non-inferiority trial. *Lancet.* 2015;386(9993):552-561.
104. Mrowietz U, Christophers E, Altmeyer P. Treatment of severe psoriasis with fumaric acid esters: scientific background and guidelines for therapeutic use. The German Fumaric Acid Ester Consensus Conference. *Br J Dermatol.* 1999;141(3):424-429.
105. Gupta AK, Ellis CN, Siegel MT, et al. Sulfasalazine improves psoriasis. A double-blind analysis [see comments]. *Arch Dermatol.* 1990;126(4):487-493.
106. Kirby B, Gibson LE, Rogers S, et al. Dermatomyositis-like eruption and leg ulceration caused by hydroxyurea in a patient with psoriasis. *Clin Exp Dermatol.* 2000;25(3):256-257.
107. de Gannes GC, Ghoreishi M, Pope J, et al. Psoriasis and pustular dermatitis triggered by TNF-{alpha} inhibitors in patients with rheumatologic conditions. *Arch Dermatol.* 2007;143(2):223-231.
108. Griffiths CE, Strober BE, van de Kerkhof P, et al. Comparison of ustekinumab and etanercept for moderate-to-severe psoriasis. *N Engl J Med.* 2010;362(2):118-128.
109. Krueger JG, Ferris LK, Menter A, et al. Anti-IL-23A mAb BI 655066 for treatment of moderate-to-severe psoriasis: safety, efficacy, pharmacokinetics, and biomarker results of a single-rising-dose, randomized, double-blind, placebo-controlled trial. *J Allergy Clin Immunol.* 2015;136(1):116-124.
110. Gordon KB, Duffin KC, Bissonnette R, et al. A phase 2 trial of guselkumab versus adalimumab for plaque psoriasis. *N Engl J Med.* 2015;373(2):136-144.
111. Langley RG, Elewski BE, Lebwohl M, et al. Secukinumab in plaque psoriasis—results of two phase 3 trials. *N Engl J Med.* 2014;371(4):326-338.

112. Gordon KB, Blauvelt A, Papp KA, et al. Phase 3 trials of ixekizumab in moderate-to-severe plaque psoriasis. *N Engl J Med*. 2016;375(4):345-356.
113. Griffiths CE, Reich K, Lebwohl M, et al. Comparison of ixekizumab with etanercept or placebo in moderate-to-severe psoriasis (UNCOVER-2 and UNCOVER-3): results from two phase 3 randomised trials. *Lancet*. 2015;386(9993):541-551.
114. Lebwohl M, Strober B, Menter A, et al. Phase 3 studies comparing brodalumab with ustekinumab in psoriasis. *N Engl J Med*. 2015;373(14):1318-1328.
115. Sevrain M, Richard MA, Barnetche T, et al. Treatment for palmoplantar pustular psoriasis: systematic literature review, evidence-based recommendations and expert opinion. *J Eur Acad Dermatol Venereol*. 2014;28(suppl 5):13-16.
116. Takahara M. Clinical outcome of tonsillectomy for palmoplantar pustulosis and etiological relationship between palmoplantar pustulosis and tonsils. *Adv Otorhinolaryngol*. 2011;72:86-88.
117. Michaelsson G, Gustafsson K, Hagforsen E. The psoriasis variant palmoplantar pustulosis can be improved after cessation of smoking. *J Am Acad Dermatol*. 2006;54(4):737-738.

Chapter 29 :: Pityriasis Rubra Pilaris
:: Knut Schäkel

第二十九章
毛发红糠疹

中文导读

本章介绍了毛发红糠疹的流行病学、临床特征、病因和发病机制、诊断、鉴别诊断、临床病程及预后、治疗。根据发病年龄、临床病程和预后将毛发红糠疹分为典型成人型、不典型成人型、典型幼年型、幼年局限型、非典型幼年型五类，与HIV感染相关时可分为第六类毛发红糠疹，本章介绍了不同类型的临床表现，并提出因临床表现易与银屑病混淆需重点鉴别，而目前对毛发红糠疹的治疗依赖于小样本病例的治疗经验。

〔朱　武〕

AT-A-GLANCE

- A rare inflammatory papulosquamous dermatosis, often self-limiting within a few years.
- The disease is subclassified into 6 types, including both hereditary and acquired forms.
- The hereditary form of pityriasis rubra pilaris is linked to CARD14 gain-of-function mutations, the cause of the acquired forms is unknown.
- Typical features are follicular hyperkeratotic papules that coalesce into scaly, reddish-orange–colored plaques, which may progress to erythroderma with well-demarcated islands of normal skin.
- Distinguishing pityriasis rubra pilaris from psoriasis poses a major diagnostic challenge, particularly in the early phases of the disease.
- Histopathologic examination reveals hyperkeratosis, alternating parakeratosis and orthokeratosis in a checkerboard pattern, with focal acantholytic dyskeratosis.
- The most successful treatment options are systemic retinoids, methotrexate, and photochemotherapy (psoralen and ultraviolet A). In recent years, biologics blocking tumor necrosis factor-α and interleukins-12 and -12p40 were shown to be effective.

Pityriasis rubra pilaris (PRP) is a rare, inflammatory skin disease of juvenile or adult onset with distinctive clinical features and a self-limiting or chronic evolution.

EPIDEMIOLOGY

The exact prevalence of PRP is not known. It accounts for approximately 1 in 5000 new patients presenting with skin disease in Great Britain.[1] In India this is approximately 1 in 50,000 patients (pityriasis rubra pilaris in Indians.) The disease occurs in all races with an equal male-to-female ratio.[2]

CLINICAL FEATURES

PRP comprises different entities and most cases are sporadic and have an unknown etiology. Approximately 6.5% of cases of PRP are familial[3-5] and linked to CARD14 mutations.[6] In 1980, Griffiths proposed classifying PRP into 5 types based on age of onset, clinical course, and prognosis. A sixth, HIV-associated, category was added in later years (Table 29-1).[2]

Type I (classic adult) is the most common subtype and occurs in more than 50% of all cases. Characteristically, type I PRP starts with erythematous macules

TABLE 29-1
Classification Scheme of Pityriasis Rubra Pilaris[a]

TYPE	DESCRIPTION	% OF CASES	CLINICAL CHARACTERISTICS	DISTRIBUTION	COURSE
I	Classic adult	>50	Erythroderma with islands of normal skin ("nappes claires"), follicular hyperkeratosis, waxy diffuse palmoplantar keratoderma	Generalized, beginning on the head and neck, then spreading caudally	Often resolves within an average period of 3 years
II	Atypical adult	5	Combination of follicular hyperkeratosis and ichthyosiform lesions on the legs, sparse scalp hair	Generalized	Long duration (>20 years)
III	Classic juvenile	10	Similar to type I but appears in years 1 or 2 of life	Generalized	Often resolves within an average period of 1–2 years
IV	Circumscribed juvenile	25	Prepubertal children; well-demarcated scaly, erythematous plaques on the elbows and knees, resembling localized psoriasis	Localized	Uncertain, some cases clear in the late teens
V	Atypical juvenile, associated with CARD14 mutations	5	Begins in first few years, accounts for most familial cases; follicular hyperkeratosis, scleroderma-like appearance of the hands and feet	Generalized	Chronic course, improvement with retinoids but relapses when stopped
VI	HIV-associated	NA[b]	Similar to type I with variable beginning; associated with acne conglobata, hidradenitis suppurativa and lichen spinulosus	Generalized	May respond to antiretroviral triple therapy

[a]Types I to V are according to Griffiths.[2]
[b]Data not available.

forming patches and with follicular hyperkeratotic papules on the upper half of the body (Figs. 29-1A and 29-2). As the disease evolves, a yellow-orange, scaling dermatitis often spreads to a generalized erythroderma over a period of 2 to 3 months (Fig. 29-3). A diagnostic hallmark of PRP is the presence of sharply demarcated

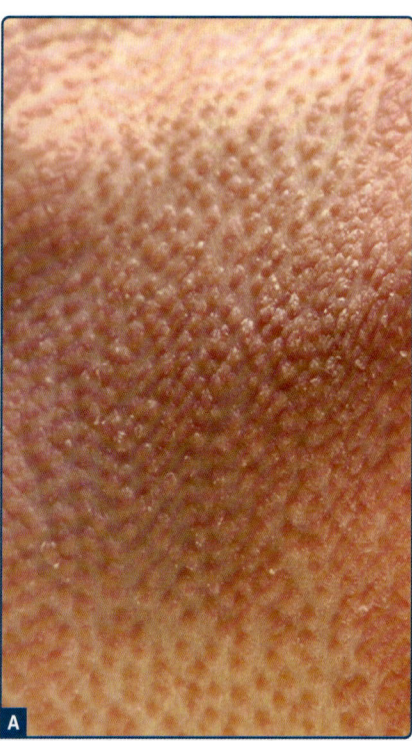
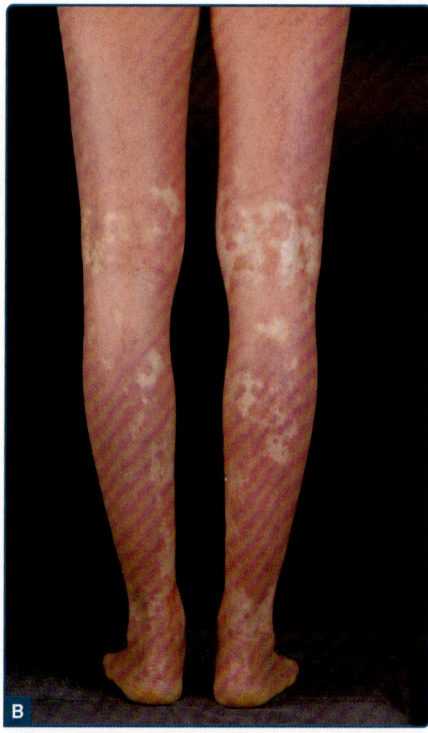

Figure 29-1 **A,** Follicular papules and **B,** islands of normal skin "nappes claires" in pityriasis rubra pilaris.

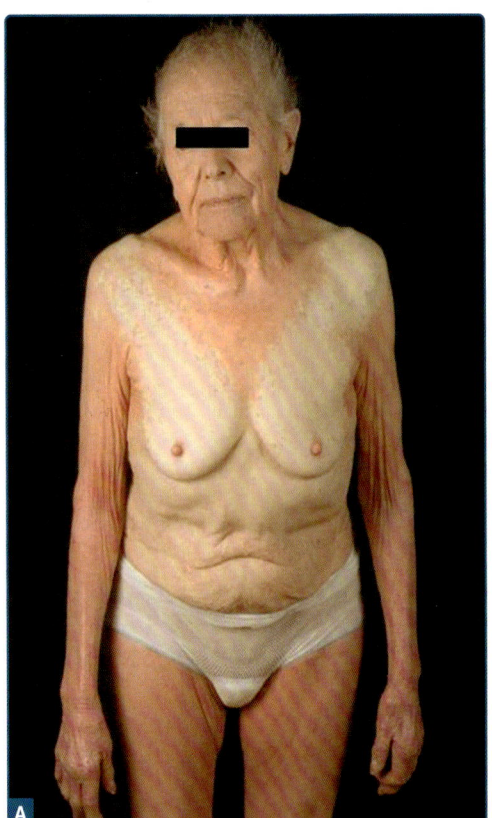

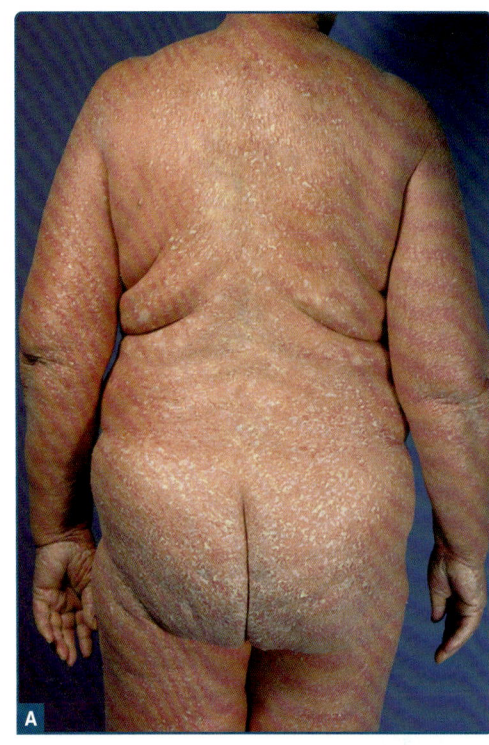

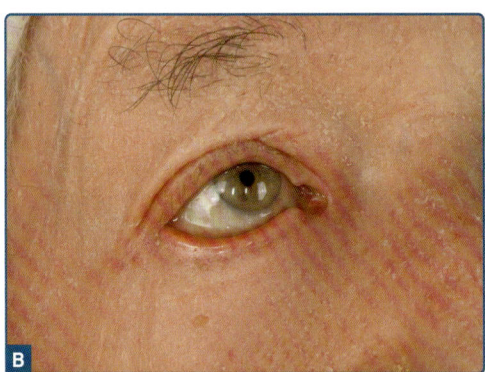

Figure 29-2 Classic adult type I pityriasis rubra pilaris presenting with monomorphic regions of affected skin, sharp margins, diffuse alopecia (**A**), and ectropion (**B**).

islands of unaffected skin ("nappes claires"; Fig. 29-1B). Frequently patients develop a waxy, diffuse, yellowish keratoderma of the palms and soles (Fig. 29-4).[7] Nail changes are common in these patients and include nail plate thickening, splinter hemorrhages, and subungual hyperkeratosis. In patients with uniform facial involvement, ectropion frequently develops (Fig. 29-2B).

Type II (atypical adult) PRP describes an variant, which affects 5% of PRP patients. It is characterized by its atypical morphologic picture and a long duration of more than 20 years. The clinical picture resembles ichthyosiform scaling, areas of follicular hyperkerato-

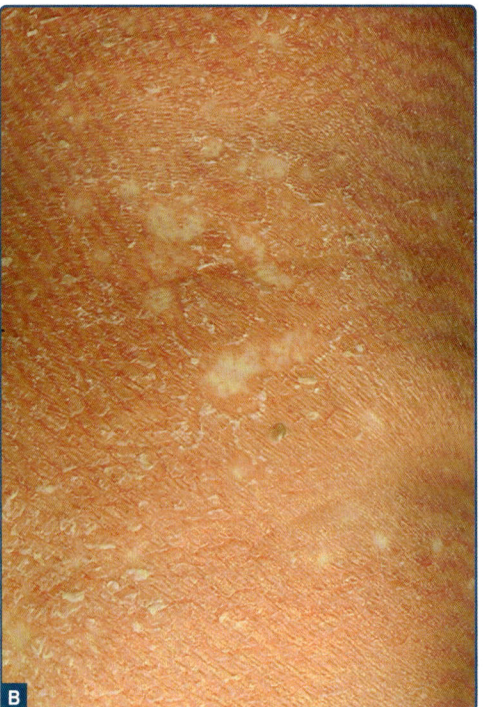

Figure 29-3 Erythrodermic patient (classic adult type I, as in Fig. 29-2) with psoriasiform scaling (**A**) and island of normal skin (**B**).

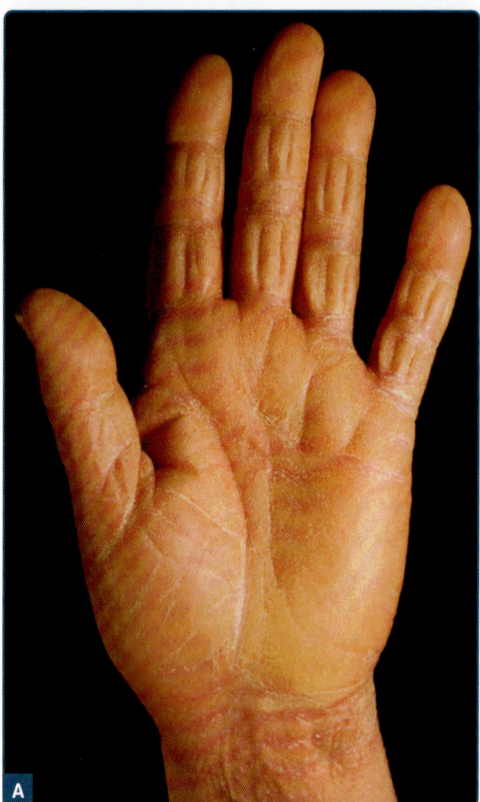
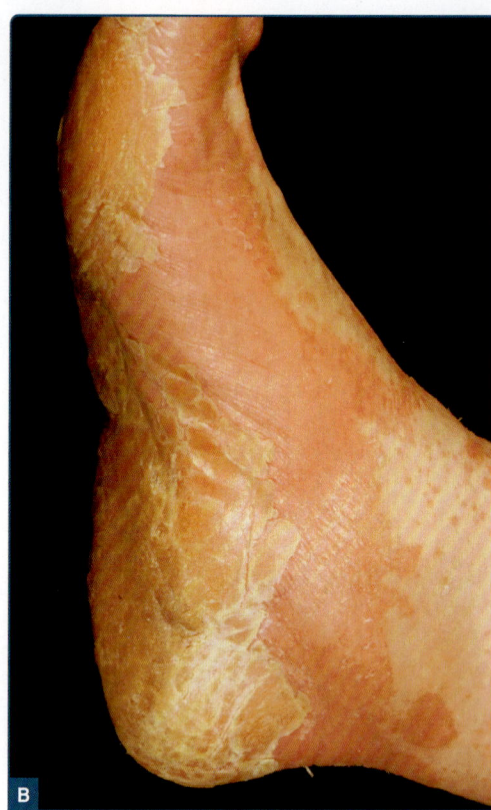

Figure 29-4 Palmar (**A**) and plantar (**B**) "waxy" keratoderma in pityriasis rubra pilaris.

sis, and sparseness of the scalp hair. The cephalocaudal progression observed in type I is missing, and there is less tendency for the patients to develop erythroderma.

Type III (classic juvenile) is the clinical counterpart of type I PRP in children. It affects 10% of PRP patients, with the onset usually between the ages of 5 and 10 years.[1] The clinical course may be shorter with clearing after 1 year (Fig. 29-5).

Type IV (circumscribed juvenile) affects approximately 25% of patients. This type usually manifests in prepubertal children and young adults. It is characterized by well-demarcated hyperkeratotic erythematous plaques on the elbows and knees, resembling localized psoriasis (Fig. 29-6). These lesions do not progress to the more widespread classical type. Palmoplantar keratoderma is characteristic for type IV PRP, but may also be absent.[8] The 3-year remission rate is 32%.

Type V (atypical juvenile) PRP occurs in 5% of patients and is characterized by an early age of onset and a chronic course. Most patients of the familial PRP belong

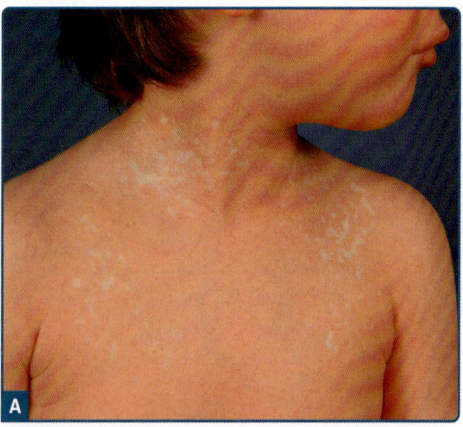
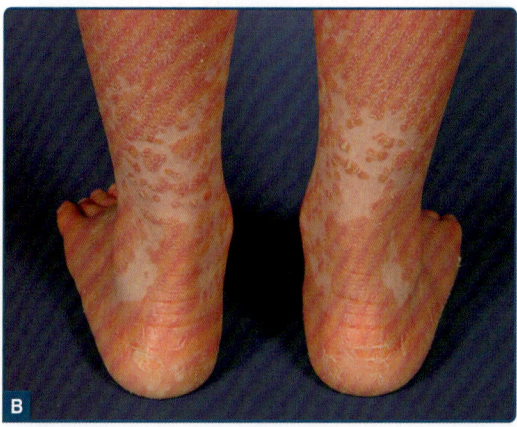

Figure 29-5 Classic juvenile pityriasis rubra pilaris type III. **A**, Confluence of lesions leads to erythroderma. **B**, Characteristic scattered islands of unaffected skin are evident.

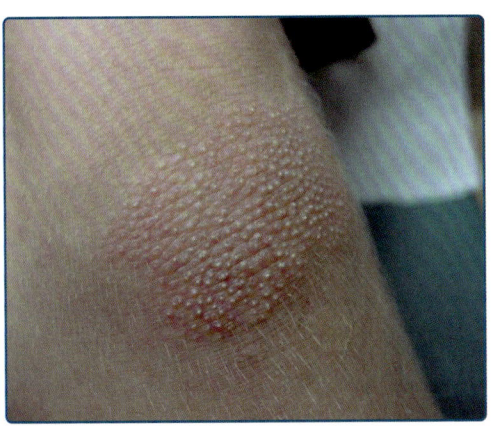

Figure 29-6 Circumscribed juvenile pityriasis rubra pilaris type IV. Well-demarcated hyperkeratotic erythematous plaques are found on the elbows and knees mimicking psoriasis.

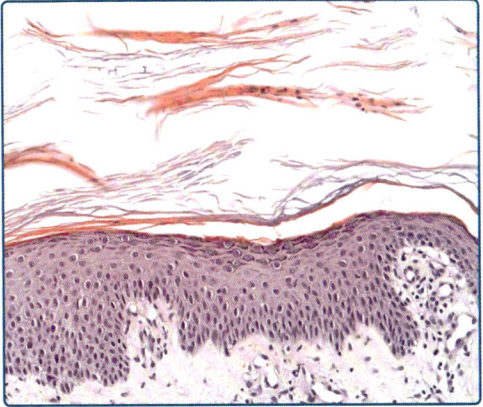

Figure 29-7 Histopathologic features of pityriasis rubra pilaris. Hyperkeratosis, alternating parakeratosis and orthokeratosis in a checkerboard pattern, with focal acantholytic dyskeratosis.

to this category. These patients were recently shown to harbor a gain-of-function mutation in the CARD14 gene encoding the Caspase Recruitment Domain family member 14 (CARD14).[6] It manifests as hyperkeratotic follicular lesions. Some patients present with scleroderma-like features affecting hands and feet.

The *type VI* (HIV-associated) variant was proposed by Miralles and colleagues.[9] These HIV-associated cases manifest with follicular papules and prominent follicular plugging. The symmetrically distributed lesions of the extensor surfaces frequently progress to erythroderma. Additional manifestations include acne conglobata, hidradenitis suppurativa, and lichen spinulosus.

ASSOCIATIONS OF PITYRIASIS RUBRA PILARIS

There is an association of PRP with HIV infections, proposed as type VI PRP. In some cases, manifestation of PRP was the first sign of HIV infection,[10] and clinical responses occurred with antiretroviral therapy.[11] Multiple associations with infections, malignancies, or autoimmune diseases have been noticed, but may occur rather fortuitously.

ETIOLOGY AND PATHOGENESIS

The etiology and pathogenesis of sporadic PRP remain elusive. Pathogenic mechanisms associated with infection, such as upper respiratory tract infection and HIV infection, were proposed. In type V PRP, gain-of-function mutations in the CARD14 gene linked to autosomal dominant inheritance have been identified. CARD14 is expressed in the skin and encodes the caspase recruitment domain family member 14, a known activator of nuclear factor-κB signaling. Accordingly, CARD14 levels were increased in affected individuals with PRP, and p65 was found to be activated in the skin. CARD14 mutations also have been described in familial psoriasis.[12] A study of 48 patients with PRP type I identified 12.5% of patients as having CARD14 putative mutations.[13] A second study of 61 patients with sporadic PRP did not observe CARD14 mutations.[14] Hence, CARD14 mutations may be rare in sporadic cases, and alternate mechanisms may be responsible for activation of the nuclear factor-κB signaling observed in these patients.[13]

In lesional PRP skin samples from a single patient successfully treated with the anti-IL-12/IL-23 antibody ustekinumab, upregulated expression levels were found for most proinflammatory innate cytokines, including tumor necrosis factor (TNF), IL-6, IL-12, IL-23, and IL-1β. Among adaptive T-cell cytokines, an increase of TH1 cytokines and, in particular, TH17 cytokines IL-17A, IL-17F, and IL-22 was seen.[15] Based on these findings, PRP may now be classified as a papulosquamous disease that results from abnormal activation of different inflammatory pathways. Even though PRP and psoriasis have overlapping clinical symptoms, the clinical and histopathologic features of the 2 diseases are distinct. PRP often affects the face, has the typical salmon-colored appearance, presents with classical islands of healthy skin over the trunk, distinct areas of follicular hyperkeratosis, and a waxy palmoplantar keratoderma (see Fig. 29-4). Although psoriasis-associated nail changes are missing, nail plates may be hypertrophic. The histologic picture of psoriasis with hypogranulosis, elongation of the rete ridges, vascular dilation, a high frequency of neutrophils manifesting as intraepidermal Munro microabscesses is not shared with PRP, which presents with histologic features such as alternating horizontal and vertical parakeratosis and orthokeratosis, hypergranulosis, thickening of the rete ridges, follicular hyperkeratosis, lack of neutrophilic infiltration, and limited vascular dilatation (Fig. 29-7).

Nevertheless, differentiation between PRP and psoriasis can be difficult in individual cases.

DIAGNOSIS

PRP is typically a clinical diagnosis based on the characteristic skin lesions and the age of onset. Psoriasis is an important differential diagnosis. Initial manifestations of the scalp may mimic seborrheic dermatitis. A biopsy should be taken and helps differentiating PRP from psoriasis.

DIFFERENTIAL DIAGNOSIS

Table 29-2 outlines the differential diagnosis of pityriasis rubra pilaris.

CLINICAL COURSE, PROGNOSIS MANAGEMENT

Classic adult type I PRP frequently resolves within 3 years. Reoccurrence was observed after periods of subclinical disease in up to 20% of cases. Classic juvenile type III commonly resolves within 1 to 2 years. A less-favorable prognosis for remission is reported for the atypical variants types II and IV, although some cases of type IV improve in the patient's late teens. Type V PRP, which is associated with CARD14 mutations, has little or no tendency to resolve spontaneously.

PRP responds hesitantly to topical and classic systemic treatment regimens, which makes finding an effective therapy for PRP challenging. As PRP is an infrequent disease of unpredictable duration, conducting double-blind, placebo-controlled studies addressing the value of individual systemic treatment strategies are difficult. Published treatment recommendations rely on results from small case series and individual cases. From the patient's point of view, corticosteroids, and salicylic acid in combination with oral retinoids, methotrexate, and tumor necrosis factor (TNF) inhibitors were regarded as most helpful.[16] A growing number of reports demonstrate the role of biologics targeting TNF-α, interleukin (IL)-12/IL-23p40 or anti-IL-17 as a valuable second-line treatment option.

TOPICAL TREATMENT

Local treatment options for PRP regularly do not suffice to control the disease and are used as an adjunct to systemic therapy. As in psoriasis, classical keratolytic treatment is used where hyperkeratosis is the leading sign. To dampen the local inflammatory response, topical corticosteroids are often initially employed and may be followed by topical calcineurin inhibitors. Furthermore, vitamin D_3 analogs for the inhibition of various aspects of cutaneous inflammation and epidermal proliferation with enhancement of normal keratinization are successfully used for the treatment of PRP. However, percutaneous resorption of vitamin D analogs restricts treatment to no more than 30% of body surface.

SYSTEMIC TREATMENT

So far, there is no systemic therapy that works for all patients with PRP. Finding a successful therapy for the individual patient can be a challenging task. Oral retinoids generally serve as the first-line therapy in patients with PRP. They block the proliferation of keratinocytes and reduce hyperkeratosis. Acitretin and isotretinoin (1-2 mg/kg/day)[17] are effective; good responses to alitretinoin also have been reported. In a substantial proportion of patients, disease manifests at an early age. Although isotretinoin is proven to be effective in prepubertal patients, oral retinoids can induce premature closure of epiphyses or hyperostosis, and should be used with caution. Teratogenicity is another important concern in oral retinoid therapy. Teratogenicity is also a known adverse effect of methotrexate, the second most used drug for the treatment of PRP. In severe cases, methotrexate can be combined with oral retinoids.

Psoralen and ultraviolet A (PUVA) alone or in combination with oral retinoids (RE-PUVA) is another efficient treatment option. In addition, narrowband ultraviolet B (UVB) or broadband UVB can be successful. However, because PRP can be aggravated by UV light,[18-20] phototesting should be performed before initiating UV treatment.

Some authors report about beneficial effects of fumaric acid esters.[21,22] The phosphodiesterase 4-inhibitor apremilast also may be a treatment option.[23]

As an alternative treatment, anti–TNF-α, anti–IL-12/IL-23p40 (ustekinumab), and anti-IL17 have been used with good results. There are more than 30 published cases of patients with adult PRP type I

TABLE 29-2
Differential Diagnosis of Pityriasis Rubra Pilaris

Most Likely
Localized
- Psoriasis
- Ichthyosis
- Seborrheic dermatitis of the scalp

Generalized
- Psoriasis
- Erythrokeratoderma

Consider
Localized
- Follicular eczema
- Lichen planus acuminatus
- Keratosis pilaris

Generalized
- Pityriasis lichenoides chronica
- Ichthyosiform erythroderma

Always Rule Out
- Generalized (therapy-resistant cases)
- HIV infection
- Cutaneous T-cell lymphoma

TABLE 29-3
Treatment Options for Pityriasis Rubra Pilaris

First Line

Topical
- Emollients (water-in-oil emulsion)
- Keratolytics (salicylic acid, urea)
- Vitamin D_3 (calcipotriol)

Systemic
- Retinoids (0.5-0.75 mg/kg acitretin/day)
- Methotrexate (10-25 mg weekly or higher)
- Antiretroviral therapy (HIV-associated variant)

Second Line

Topical
- Glucocorticoids (medium to high potency)
- Vitamin A analogs (tazarotene)

Physical
- Photochemotherapy (topical or systemic PUVA)
- UVA1 phototherapy
- UVB (narrowband) phototherapy
- UVB phototherapy
- Extracorporeal photopheresis

Systemic
- TNF-α antagonists
- Anti-IL-12/IL-23p40 ustekinumab
- Anti-IL17
- Azathioprine (100-150 mg/day)
- Fumaric acid esters
- Cyclosporine (5 mg/kg/day)
- Apremilast

---

successfully treated with anti-TNF.[24,25] Interestingly, ustekinumab was effective in a number of patients with PRP type I,[26-30] in a patient with a CARD14 mutation (type V),[30] but not in a patient with type IV PRP.[31] An underreporting of negative results when treatment outcomes are published as individual case reports should be considered.

In some patients with PRP, extracorporeal photopheresis has been used with success. Evidence for the use of cyclosporine, glucocorticosteroids, or azathioprine is low.

PRP associated with HIV infection has responded to triple antiretroviral therapy.[32]

Table 29-3 lists the current therapeutic options (including drug doses) for PRP used in adults and children.

REFERENCES

1. Griffiths WA. Pityriasis rubra pilaris. *Clin Exp Dermatol.* 1980;5:105-112; Sehgal VN, Jain MK, Mathur RP. Br J Dermatol. 1989 Dec;121(6):821-822.
2. Griffiths WA. Pityriasis rubra pilaris—an historical approach. 2. Clinical features. *Clin Exp Dermatol.* 1976;1:37-50.
3. Vasher M, Smithberger E, Lien MH, et al. Familial pityriasis rubra pilaris: report of a family and therapeutic response to etanercept. *J Drugs Dermatol.* 2010;9:844-850.
4. Thomson MA, Moss C. Pityriasis rubra pilaris in a mother and two daughters. *Br J Dermatol.* 2007;157:202-204.
5. Sehgal VN, Srivastava G. (Juvenile) Pityriasis rubra pilaris. *Int J Dermatol.* 2006;45:438-446.
6. Fuchs-Telem D, Sarig O, van Steensel MA, et al. Familial pityriasis rubra pilaris is caused by mutations in CARD14. *Am J Hum Genet.* 2012;91:163-170.
7. Clayton BD, Jorizzo JL, Hitchcock MG, et al. Adult pityriasis rubra pilaris: a 10-year case series. *J Am Acad Dermatol.* 1997;36:959-964.
8. Caldarola G, Zampetti A, De Simone C, et al. Circumscribed pityriasis rubra pilaris type IV. *Clin Exp Dermatol.* 2007;32:471-472.
9. Miralles ES, Nunez M, De Las Heras ME, et al. Pityriasis rubra pilaris and human immunodeficiency virus infection. *Br J Dermatol.* 1995;133:990-993.
10. Sanchez-Regana M, Fuentes CG, Creus L, et al. Pityriasis rubra pilaris and HIV infection: a part of the spectrum of HIV-associated follicular syndrome. *Br J Dermatol.* 1995;133:818-819.
11. Misery I, Faure M, Claidy A. Pityriasis rubra pilaris and human immunodeficiency virus infection—type 6 pityriasis rubra pilaris? *Br J Dermatol.* 1996;135:1008-1009.
12. Jordan CT, Cao L, Roberson ED, et al. Rare and common variants in CARD14, encoding an epidermal regulator of NF-kappaB, in psoriasis. *Am J Hum Genet.* 2012;90:796-808.
13. Li Q, Jin Chung H, Ross N, et al. Analysis of CARD14 polymorphisms in pityriasis rubra pilaris: activation of NF-kappaB. *J Invest Dermatol.* 2015;135:1905-1908.
14. Eytan O, Qiaoli L, Nousbeck J, et al. Increased epidermal expression and absence of mutations in CARD14 in a series of patients with sporadic pityriasis rubra pilaris. *Br J Dermatol.* 2014;170:1196-1198.
15. Feldmeyer L, Mylonas A, Demaria O, et al. Interleukin 23-helper T cell 17 axis as a treatment target for pityriasis rubra pilaris. *JAMA Dermatol.* 2017 Apr 1;153(4):304-308. doi: 10.1001/jamadermatol.2016.5384
16. Ross NA, Chung HJ, Li Q, et al. Epidemiologic, clinicopathologic, diagnostic, and management challenges of pityriasis rubra pilaris: a case series of 100 patients. *JAMA Dermatol.* 2016;152:670-675.
17. Borok M, Lowe NJ. Pityriasis rubra pilaris. Further observations of systemic retinoid therapy. *J Am Acad Dermatol.* 1990;22:792-795.
18. Evangelou G, Murdoch SR, Palamaras I, et al. Photoaggravated pityriasis rubra pilaris. *Photodermatol Photoimmunol Photomed.* 2005;21:272-274.
19. Iredale HE, Meggitt SJ. Photosensitive pityriasis rubra pilaris. *Clin Exp Dermatol.* 2006;31:36-38.
20. Yaniv R, Barzilai A, Trau H. Pityriasis rubra pilaris exacerbated by ultraviolet B phototherapy. *Dermatology.* 1994;189:313.
21. Klein A, Coras B, Landthaler M, et al. Off-label use of fumarate therapy for granulomatous and inflammatory skin diseases other than psoriasis vulgaris: a retrospective study. *J Eur Acad Dermatol Venereol.* 2012;26:1400-1406.
22. Coras B, Vogt TH, Ulrich H, et al. Fumaric acid esters therapy: a new treatment modality in pityriasis rubra pilaris? *Br J Dermatol.* 2005;152:388-389.
23. Krase IZ, Cavanaugh K, Curiel-Lewandrowski C. Treatment of refractory pityriasis rubra pilaris with novel phosphodiesterase 4 (PDE4) inhibitor apremilast. *JAMA Dermatol.* 2016;152:348-350.
24. Garcovich S, Di Giampetruzzi AR, Antonelli G, et al. Treatment of refractory adult-onset pityriasis rubra pilaris with TNF-alpha antagonists: a case series. *J Eur Acad Dermatol Venereol.* 2010;24:881-884.
25. Petrof G, Almaani N, Archer CB, et al. A systematic review of the literature on the treatment of pityriasis

rubra pilaris type 1 with TNF-antagonists. *J Eur Acad Dermatol Venereol*. 2013;27: e131-e135.
26. Di Stefani A, Galluzzo M, Talamonti M, et al. Long-term ustekinumab treatment for refractory type I pityriasis rubra pilaris. *J Dermatol Case Rep*. 2013;7:5-9.
27. Byekova Y, Sami N. Successful response of refractory type I adult-onset pityriasis rubra pilaris with ustekinumab and acitretin combination therapy. *J Dermatol*. 2015;42:830-831.
28. Ruiz Villaverde R, Sanchez Cano D. Successful treatment of type 1 pityriasis rubra pilaris with ustekinumab therapy. *Eur J Dermatol*. 2010;20:630-631.
29. Wohlrab J, Kreft B. Treatment of pityriasis rubra pilaris with ustekinumab. *Br J Dermatol*. 2010;163:655-656.
30. Chowdhary M, Davila U, Cohen DJ. Ustekinumab as an alternative treatment option for chronic pityriasis rubra pilaris. *Case Rep Dermatol*. 2015;7:46-50.
31. Eytan O, Sarig O, Sprecher E, et al. Clinical response to ustekinumab in familial pityriasis rubra pilaris caused by a novel mutation in CARD14. *Br J Dermatol*. 2014;171:420-422.
32. Gonzalez-Lopez A, Velasco E, Pozo T, et al. HIV-associated pityriasis rubra pilaris responsive to triple antiretroviral therapy. *Br J Dermatol*. 1999;140:931-934.

Chapter 30 :: Parapsoriasis and Pityriasis Lichenoides
:: Stefan M. Schieke & Gary S. Wood

第三十章
副银屑病和苔藓样糠疹

中文导读

本章共分为2节：①副银屑病；②苔藓样糠疹。

第一节介绍了副银屑病，指出副银屑病分类包括大斑块型副银屑病（LPP）、小斑块型副银屑病（SPP）以及急慢性苔藓样糠疹，本节主要介绍了LPP和SPP的流行病学、临床特征、合并症、病因和病理生理机制、诊断、病理学、鉴别诊断、临床病程及预后、治疗。本节详细介绍了LPP和SPP的临床表现及病理特征，并指出LPP与皮肤淋巴瘤相关，可以被视为皮肤淋巴瘤的临床良性末端，在临床中需要定期监测。

第二节介绍了苔藓样糠疹，分别为急性痘疮样苔藓样糠疹（PLEVA）、慢性苔藓样糠疹（PLC），本节介绍了PLEVA和PLC的流行病学、临床特征、病因和发病机制、诊断、鉴别诊断、临床病程及预后、治疗。PLC和PLEAV在临床和病理上表现为连续性过程，部分患者可同时或先后出现PLC和PLEAV，严重的病例可以发展为发热坏死溃疡性苔藓样糠疹（PLUH）或发热性坏死溃疡性穆-哈病（FUMHD），仅少数可进展为皮肤淋巴瘤。

〔朱 武〕

PARAPSORIASIS

AT-A-GLANCE

- Also known as parapsoriasis en plaques.
- Parapsoriasis occurs worldwide and affects mainly adults.
- Large-plaque parapsoriasis (LPP) and small-plaque parapsoriasis (SPP) are recognized.
- Large and small "plaque" lesions actually present as flat patches rather than infiltrated plaques.
- Lesions are chronic and favor non–sun-exposed skin; LPP may be poikilodermatous.
- Pathology consists of superficial, mostly CD4+ T-cell infiltrate; dominant clonality is more common in LPP than in SPP.
- LPP appears to exist on a continuum with patch-stage mycosis fungoides (MF) and progresses to overt MF at a rate of approximately 10% per decade.
- SPP has minimal risk of progression to overt MF in the experience of most experts.
- Treatment options include topical corticosteroids; ultraviolet B irradiation, and psoralen and ultraviolet A irradiation; excimer laser; and topical cytotoxic drugs.

The term *parapsoriasis* was coined originally by Brocq in 1902.[1] As Table 30-1 shows, the currently accepted classification of parapsoriasis includes large- and small-plaque forms of parapsoriasis en plaques (often referred to simply as parapsoriasis) as well as acute and chronic forms of pityriasis lichenoides (known today as pityriasis lichenoides et varioliformis acuta [PLEVA] and pityriasis lichenoides chronica [PLC], respectively).[2] Pityriasis lichenoides was first described in 1894 by Neisser[3] and Jadassohn.[4] In 1899, Juliusberg delineated the chronic form and named it PLC.[5] Mucha redescribed the acute form in 1916 and distinguished it from the chronic form.[6] Habermann named the acute variant PLEVA in 1925.[7] Mucha-Habermann disease is synonymous with PLEVA. Some authors regarded lymphomatoid papulosis as a variant of pityriasis lichenoides, whereas others considered it to be a separate disease (see below). Lymphomatoid papulosis is discussed in Chap. 119 as part of the spectrum of CD30+ cutaneous lymphoproliferative disorders.

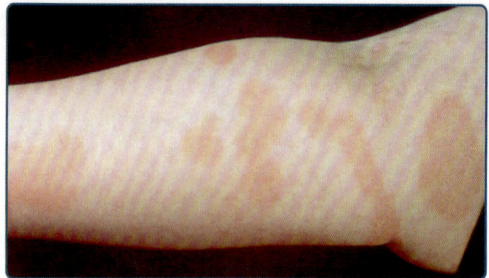

Figure 30-1 Large-plaque parapsoriasis. Irregularly shaped patches of variable size on the arm of a 16-year-old girl.

EPIDEMIOLOGY

Large-plaque parapsoriasis (LPP) and small-plaque parapsoriasis (SPP) are, in general, diseases of middle-aged and older people, with a peak incidence in the fifth decade. Occasionally, lesions arise in childhood and may be associated with pityriasis lichenoides. SPP shows a definite male predominance of approximately 3:1. LPP is probably more common in males, but the difference is not as striking as in SPP. Both occur in all racial groups and geographic regions.

CLINICAL FEATURES

CUTANEOUS FINDINGS

LPP lesions are either oval or irregularly shaped patches or very thin plaques that are asymptomatic or mildly pruritic. They are usually well marginated but may also blend imperceptibly into the surrounding skin. The size is variable, but typically most lesions are larger than 5 cm, often measuring more than 10 cm in diameter. Lesions are stable in size and may increase in number gradually. They are found mainly on the "bathing trunk" and flexural areas (Fig. 30-1). Extremities and the upper trunk, especially the breasts in women, also may be involved. They are light red-brown or salmon pink, and their surface is covered with small and scanty scales. Lesions may appear finely wrinkled—"cigarette paper" wrinkling. Such lesions exhibit varying degrees of epidermal atrophy. Telangiectasia and mottled pigmentation also are observed when the atrophy becomes prominent (Fig. 30-2). This triad of atrophy, mottled pigmentation, and telangiectasia defines the term *poikiloderma* or *poikiloderma atrophicans vasculare*, which also may be seen in other conditions (Table 30-2).

Retiform parapsoriasis refers to a rare variant of LPP that presents as an extensive eruption of scaly macules

TABLE 30-1
Classification of Parapsoriasis

1. Parapsoriasis en plaques
   A. Large-plaque parapsoriasis; variants: poikilodermatous, retiform
   B. Small-plaque parapsoriasis; variant: digitate dermatosis
2. Pityriasis lichenoides
   A. Pityriasis lichenoides chronica (Juliusberg)
   B. Pityriasis lichenoides et varioliformis acuta (Mucha-Habermann)

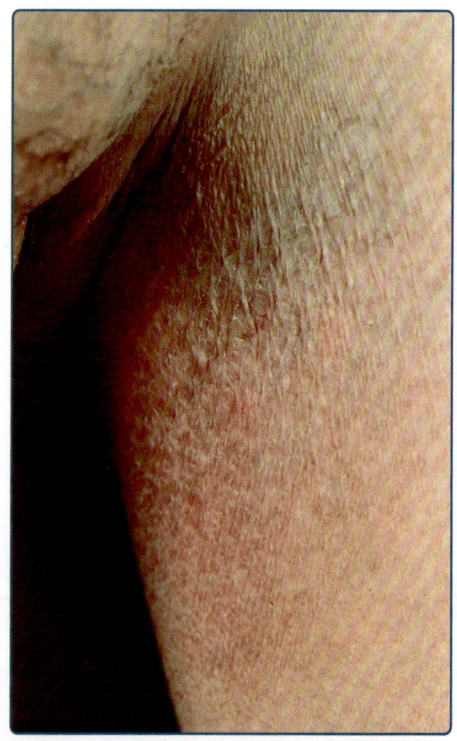

Figure 30-2 Large-plaque parapsoriasis. Poikilodermatous variant.

TABLE 30-2
Differential Diagnosis of Poikiloderma
- Large-plaque parapsoriasis - Dermatomyositis - Lupus erythematosus - Chronic radiation dermatitis - Bloom syndrome - Rothmund-Thomson syndrome - Dyskeratosis congenita - Xeroderma pigmentosum

and papules in a net-like or zebra-stripe pattern that eventually becomes poikilodermatous (Fig. 30-3).

SPP, synonymously referred to as chronic superficial dermatitis, characteristically occurs as round or oval discrete patches or very thin plaques, mainly on the trunk (Fig. 30-4). The lesions measure less than 5 cm in diameter; they are asymptomatic and covered with fine, moderately adherent scales. The general health of the patient is unaffected. A distinctive variant with lesions of a finger shape, known as digitate dermatosis,[8] has yellowish or fawn-colored lesions (Fig. 30-5). It follows lines of cleavage of the skin and gives the appearance of a hug that left fingerprints on the trunk. The long axis of these lesions often measures greater than 5 cm. Recently, several cases of hypopigmented SPP have been described, which possibly represent a new variant of parapsoriasis.[9] Digitate lesions with a yellow hue were referred to in the past as xanthoerythrodermia perstans.[2]

COMPLICATIONS

LPP can be associated with other forms of parapsoriasis and overt cutaneous lymphomas as detailed elsewhere in this chapter. Both LPP and SPP occasionally can develop areas of impetiginization secondary to excoriation. Data from a recent Danish cohort study suggests that parapsoriasis and mycosis fungoides are associated with an increased risk for cardiovascular disease such as acute myocardial infarction and stroke, as well as increased risk for subsequent hematologic and nonhematologic malignancies and increased mortality.[10,11]

ETIOLOGY AND PATHOGENESIS

It is likely that a complete understanding of the pathogenesis of parapsoriasis will develop with our understanding of the pathogenesis of both chronic dermatitis and mycosis fungoides (MF), because parapsoriasis appears to bridge these disorders. The T cells that mediate most inflammatory skin diseases belong to the skin-associated lymphoid tissue (SALT).[12] These T cells express the cutaneous lymphocyte-associated antigen and traffic between the skin and the T-cell domains of peripheral lymph nodes via the lymphatics and bloodstream. MF (see Chap. 119) is a neoplasm of SALT T cells. Sensitive polymerase chain reaction–based

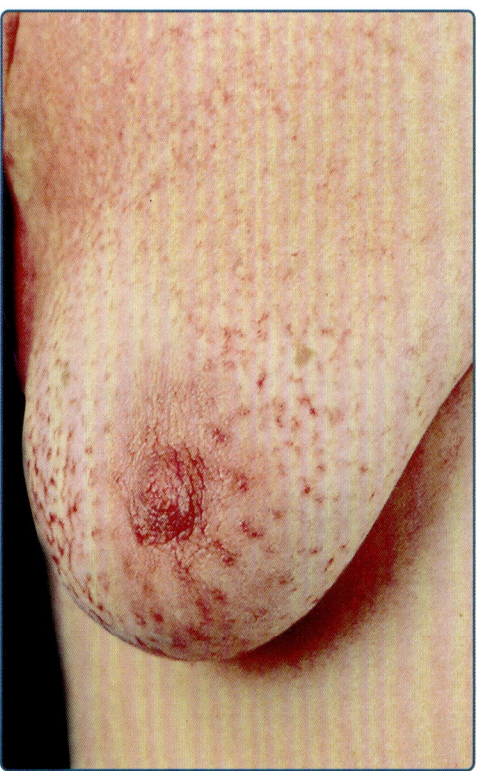

Figure 30-3 Large-plaque parapsoriasis. Retiform variant.

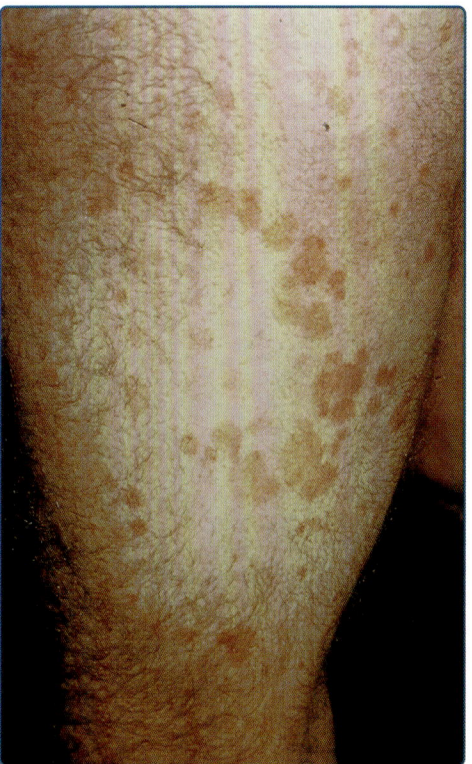

Figure 30-4 Small-plaque parapsoriasis. Small, discrete patches less than 5 cm in diameter.

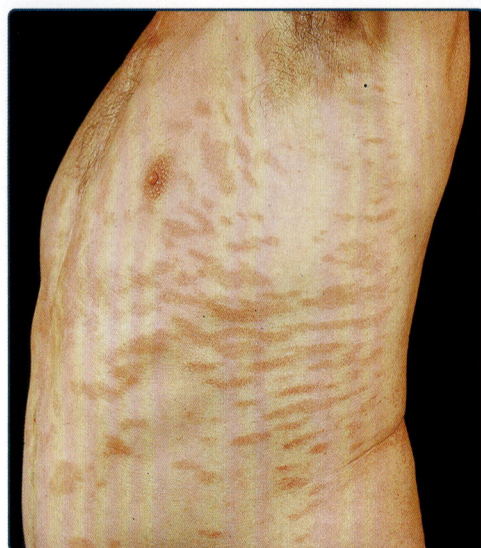

Figure 30-5 Small-plaque parapsoriasis. Digitate dermatosis variant. Typical "fingerprint" patches on the flank. Note that their length often exceeds 5 cm.

tumor clonality assays have underscored the SALT nature of MF tumor clones by showing that they can continue to traffic after neoplastic transformation,[13] and can even participate in delayed-type hypersensitivity reactions to contact allergens.[14] This implies that rather than being a skin lymphoma per se, MF is actually a SALT lymphoma, that is, a malignancy of a T-cell circuit rather than of one particular tissue. Trafficking of MF tumor cells has been detected even in patients with very early stage disease whose lesions were consistent clinicopathologically with LPP.[13,15] Therefore, it can be said that at least in some cases LPP is a monoclonal proliferation of SALT T cells that have the capacity to traffic between the skin and extracutaneous sites.

This view is also supported by the presence of structural and numerical chromosomal abnormalities in the peripheral blood mononuclear cells of patients with LPP.[16] In this context, LPP can be regarded as the clinically benign end of the MF disease spectrum, which eventuates in transformed large cell lymphoma at its malignant extreme. To say that these diseases belong to the same disease spectrum is not to say that they are biologically equivalent disorders. To lump them all together simply as "MF" would be to ignore their distinctive clinicopathologic features, which are likely due to genetic and/or epigenetic differences, such as the *p53* gene somatic mutations observed in some cases of large-cell transformation of MF.[17] It is likely that several such differences separate these clinicopathologically defined disorders in a stepwise fashion analogous to the sequential acquisition of somatic mutations that occurs in the colon cancer disease spectrum as colonic epithelial cells progress through normal, hyperplastic, in situ carcinoma, invasive carcinoma, and metastatic carcinoma stages.

A unifying feature of the parapsoriasis group of diseases is that all of them appear to be cutaneous T-cell lymphoproliferative disorders: LPP,[12,18,19] SPP,[19] pityriasis lichenoides,[20,21] have all been shown to be monoclonal disorders in many cases. These relationships suggest that progression from LPP through the various stages of the MF disease spectrum is accompanied by an increasing gradient of dominant T-cell clonal density resulting from mutations that confer increasing growth autonomy to the neoplastic T-cell clone.[22] Interestingly, analysis of peripheral blood has demonstrated that clonal T cells are often detectable in patients with LPP/early MF[19] or SPP,[19,23] which again supports the systemic SALT nature of these "primary" skin disorders.

Dominant clonality as seen in the parapsoriasis disease group, follicular mucinosis, pagetoid reticulosis, and certain other disorders does not equate to clinical malignancy. In fact, most patients with these diseases experience a benign clinical course, and in some cases the disease resolves completely. In addition, other types of chronic cutaneous T-cell infiltrates sometimes exhibit dominant clonality, including primary (idiopathic) erythroderma and nonspecific chronic spongiotic dermatitis. This has given rise to the concept of clonal dermatitis,[15,24] originally described in the context of clonal nonspecific chronic spongiotic dermatitis but later expanded to include other nonlymphomatous cutaneous T-cell infiltrates that harbor occult monoclonal T-cell populations. Several cases of clonal dermatitis, some of which have progressed to MF, have been identified.[15,24] We suspect that for each disease with a potential for progression to MF, the principal risk may reside in the subset showing clonal dermatitis, because this is the subset in which dysregulation has begun to occur.

Figure 30-6 depicts the postulated relationships among MF, clonal dermatitis, and selected types of chronic dermatitis. Each of the entities shown is postulated to be at risk for MF through a clonal dermatitis intermediate. In this model, MF becomes the final common pathway for the clonal evolution of neoplastic T cells emerging from the polyclonal SALT T-cell populations present in each of the various precursor diseases.

Various viruses including human herpesvirus-8 have been proposed to play a role in the pathogenesis of MF. None has been substantiated thus far.[25,26]

DIAGNOSIS

LPP is distinguished from SPP by the larger size, asymmetric distribution, and irregular shape of its lesions, which are less discrete and often poikilodermatous. LPP may be clinically and histopathologically indistinguishable from the patch stage of MF. Both LPP and SPP are readily distinguished from more advanced infiltrated plaques of MF because parapsoriasis lesions are, by definition, not thicker than patches or at most very thin plaques. This is so because the English equivalent of the French term plaques is patches, that is, lesions that are essentially flat and devoid of induration or palpable infiltration. Failure to appreciate this important distinction has led to considerable confusion and misuse of the terms LPP and SPP by some

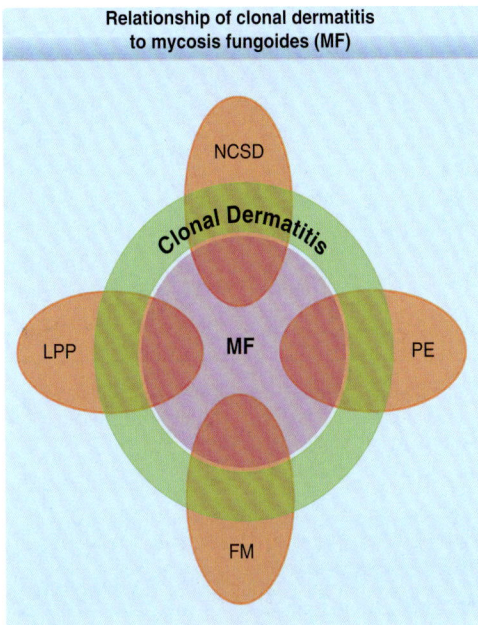

Figure 30-6 The relationship of clonal dermatitis to mycosis fungoides (MF) and various types of chronic dermatitis. The proportions of each entity that represent clonal dermatitis and MF vary with each disease and are not drawn to scale. FM, follicular mucinosis; LPP, large-plaque parapsoriasis; NCSD, nonspecific chronic spongiotic dermatitis; PE, primary erythroderma.

TABLE 30-3
Algorithm for the Diagnosis of Patch-Stage Mycosis Fungoides (4 Points Are Required)[a]

PARAMETER	2 POINTS	1 POINT
Clinical:	Any two	Any one
Persistent, progressive patches and plaques ±		
Non–sun-exposed distribution		
Variation in size and shape		
Poikiloderma		
Histopathologic:	Both	Either
Superficial dermal T-cell infiltrate ±		
Epidermotropism		
Nuclear atypia		
Immunopathologic:	Not applicable	Any one
CD2, CD3, or CD5 <50%		
CD7 <10%		
Epidermal–dermal discordance		
Molecular biologic:	Not applicable	Present
Dominant T-cell clonality		

[a]Note: Epidermotropism implies the lack of significant spongiosis (intraepidermal lymphoid cells associated with spongiosis is termed *exocytosis* rather than *epidermotropism*). Discordance refers to differential antigen expression between the epidermis and dermis, as opposed to the biopsy specimen as a whole.

From Pimpinelli N, Olsen EA, Santucci M, et al. Defining early mycosis fungoides. *J Am Acad Dermatol.* 2005;53(6):1053-1063, with permission. Copyright © American Academy of Dermatology.

individuals. These designations more appropriately might be thought of as large-patch parapsoriasis and small-patch parapsoriasis.

The degree to which LPP is differentiated from early MF depends primarily on the histopathologic criteria used to diagnose the latter disorder. Unfortunately, there are no universally accepted minimal criteria for the diagnosis of MF; however, Table 30-3 presents one set proposed by the International Society for Cutaneous Lymphoma.[27] This algorithm is based on a holistic integration of clinical, histopathologic, immunopathologic, and clonality data. It differs significantly from many prior approaches because it does not rely solely on histopathologic features.[28] Assuming that histopathologic examination does not disclose features diagnostic of some other dermatosis, these criteria allow lesions to be classified as either patch-stage MF or not. For the practical purposes of clinical management, patients presenting clinically with patch lesions whose features result in a score of 4 points or more are considered to have unequivocal MF. Obviously, the more liberal the criteria, the more cases could be considered to be MF. However, there will always be some cases that fail to meet any specific set of criteria, and the designation LPP is a useful term to apply to them because it guides treatment and followup and conveys an understanding that the risk of dying from lymphoma is small.

SPP, when it presents with its distinctive digitate dermatosis lesions parallel to skin lines in a truncal distribution, stands out from other types of parapsoriasis. Individual SPP lesions may show some superficial resemblance to PLC.

Sometimes patients with MF may exhibit small patches of disease at presentation; however, these lesions typically have histopathologic features at least consistent with MF and generally are associated with larger, more classic lesions of MF elsewhere on the skin. They also may show poikilodermatous features not seen in SPP. Furthermore, the presence of well-developed, moderate to thick, small plaques, as seen in some MF patients, is incompatible with the diagnosis of SPP because the latter disorder includes only lesions that are no more than patches or very thin plaques. It is also important to recognize that partially treated or early relapsing lesions of MF may show only nonspecific features that should not be taken as evidence of a pathogenetic link to SPP or any other dermatosis.

PATHOLOGY

In early LPP lesions, the epidermis is mildly acanthotic and slightly hyperkeratotic with spotty parakeratosis. The dermal lymphocytic infiltrate tends to be perivascular and scattered (Fig. 30-7). In the more advanced lesions one observes an interface infiltrate with definite epidermotropism. These invading lymphocytes may

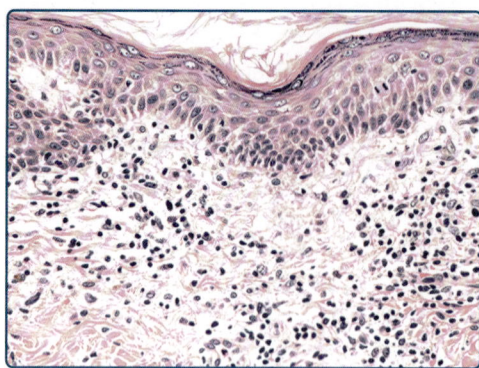

Figure 30-7 Large-plaque parapsoriasis. Mildly hyperkeratotic and focally parakeratotic epidermis with moderately dense superficial perivascular infiltrate. Lymphoid cells are mostly small, cytologically normal lymphocytes, and there is focal single-cell epidermotropism. (Used with permission from Helmut Kerl, MD.)

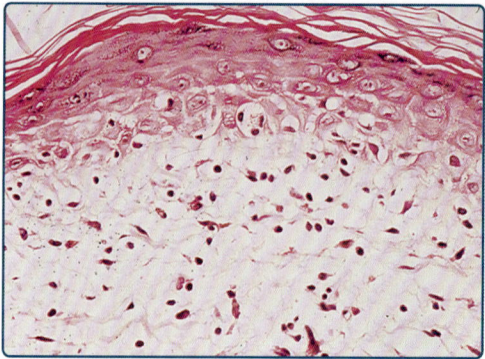

Figure 30-8 Large-plaque parapsoriasis. Atrophic variant. Sparse superficial lymphoid infiltrate with mild epidermotropism and epidermal atrophy.

be scattered singly or in groups, sometimes associated with mild spongiosis. In addition, the poikilodermatous lesions show atrophic epidermis, dilated blood vessels, and melanophages (Fig. 30-8). Immunohistologic studies reveal similar features in LPP and early MF, including a predominance of CD4+ T-cell subsets, frequent CD7 antigen deficiency, and widespread epidermal expression of Class II human leukocyte antigen D-related (HLA-DR).[18,29,30]

SPP exhibits mild spongiotic dermatitis with focal areas of hyperkeratosis, parakeratosis, scale crust, and exocytosis. In the dermis, there is a mild superficial perivascular lymphohistiocytic infiltrate and dermal edema (Fig. 30-9). There is no progression of the histologic features with time. Immunohistologic studies reveal a predominantly CD4+ T-cell infiltrate with nonspecific features resembling those seen in various types of dermatitides.

DIFFERENTIAL DIAGNOSIS

The clinical and/or histopathologic differential diagnosis of LPP also includes those collagen vascular diseases and genodermatoses exhibiting poikilodermatous features, lichenoid drug eruptions, secondary syphilis, chronic radiodermatitis, and occasionally several other diseases tabulated in Table 30-4. These generally can be distinguished by their associated clinical findings.

SPP is distinguished from psoriasis by the absence of the Auspitz sign (see Chap. 28), micaceous scale, nail pits, and typical psoriatic lesions involving the scalp, elbows, and knees. Histologically, its mild spongiotic dermatitis and absence of other characteristic features distinguish it from PLC, psoriasis, and several of the other entities listed in Table 30-4. Clinical features are also important, such as the herald patch of pityriasis rosea and the papulovesicular coin-shaped patches favoring the lower extremities in nummular dermatitis.

CLINICAL COURSE AND PROGNOSIS

Both LPP and SPP may persist for years to decades with little change in appearance, either clinically or histopathologically. Approximately 10% to 30% of cases of LPP progress to overt MF.[2,31,32] In this context, LPP represents the clinically benign end of the MF disease spectrum, with transformation to large cell lymphoma at the opposite extreme. The rare retiform variant is said to progress to overt MF in most cases.[2]

In contrast to LPP with its malignant potential, SPP is a clinically benign disorder in the experience of most experts. Patients with this disease as defined in this chapter rarely develop overt MF.[33] Despite this fact and what most observers consider to be its nonspecific histopathologic features, some authors favor lumping SPP within the MF disease spectrum as a very early, nonprogressive variant.[34,35] A few studies report progression from SPP to MF in approximately 10% of cases, but may have used different criteria than described in this chapter.[31-33]

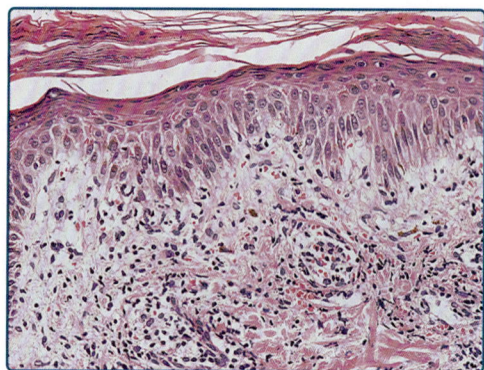

Figure 30-9 Small-plaque parapsoriasis. Superficial perivascular lymphoid infiltrate, mild spongiosis, parakeratosis, and focal scale crust.

MANAGEMENT

Patients with SPP should be reassured and may forego treatment. The disease may be treated with emollients, topical tar preparations, topical corticosteroids, and/or broadband or narrowband ultraviolet B (UVB) phototherapy (Table 30-5).[36] Response to therapy is variable. Patients should initially be examined every 3 to 6 months and subsequently every year to ensure that the character of the process is stable. LPP requires more aggressive therapy: high-potency topical corticosteroids with phototherapy such as broadband UVB, narrowband UVB, low-dose ultraviolet A (UVA)1,[36] or psoralen and UVA (PUVA). The goal of treatment is to suppress the disorder to prevent possible progression to overt MF. Other methods of treatment, such as topical nitrogen mustard, have been used successfully.[37] Localized lesions may respond to excimer laser (308 nm).[38] The patient should be examined carefully every 3 months initially and every 6 months to 1 year subsequently for evidence of progression. Repeated multiple biopsies of suspicious lesions should be performed. Cases that satisfy the clinicopathologic criteria for early MF can be treated with broadband UVB, narrowband UVB, PUVA, topical nitrogen mustard, topical bexarotene gel, topical imiquimod, or topical carmustine (BCNU). Electron-beam radiation therapy generally is reserved for more advanced, infiltrated lesions of MF.

TABLE 30-4
Differential Diagnosis of Large-Plaque Parapsoriasis (LPP) and Small-Plaque Parapsoriasis (SPP)

Most Likely
- LPP
  - Tinea corporis
  - Plaque-type psoriasis
  - Contact dermatitis
  - Subacute cutaneous lupus erythematosus
- SPP
  - Nummular dermatitis
  - Pityriasis rosea
  - Plaque and guttate psoriasis
  - Pigmented purpuric dermatoses
  - Pityriasis lichenoides chronica

Consider
- LPP
  - Xerotic dermatitis
  - Atopic dermatitis
  - Dermatomyositis
  - Drug eruption
  - Erythema dyschromicum perstans
  - Pigmented purpuric dermatoses
  - Early inflammatory morphea
  - Atrophoderma of Pasini–Pierini
  - Erythema annulare centrifugum
  - Pityriasis rubra pilaris
  - Genodermatoses with poikiloderma
  - Chronic radiodermatitis
- SPP
  - Tinea versicolor
  - Seborrheic dermatitis
  - Drug eruption

Always Rule Out
- LPP
  - Mycosis fungoides
- SPP
  - Mycosis fungoides
  - Secondary syphilis

TABLE 30-5
Treatment of Large-Plaque Parapsoriasis and Small-Plaque Parapsoriasis

First Line
- Emollients
- Topical corticosteroids
- Topical tar products
- Sunbathing
- Broadband UVB phototherapy
- Narrowband UVB phototherapy
- Low-dose ultraviolet A1 (UVA1) phototherapy

Second Line
(Mainly for large-plaque parapsoriasis cases considered to be early mycosis fungoides)
- Topical bexarotene
- Topical imiquimod
- Psoralen and UVA phototherapy
- Topical mechlorethamine
- Topical carmustine (BCNU)
- Excimer laser (308 nm)

PITYRIASIS LICHENOIDES

AT-A-GLANCE

- PLEVA and PLC represent opposite ends of a disease spectrum; both entities and intermediate forms can coexist.
- All forms are characterized by spontaneously resolving, temporally overlapping crops of papules.
- PLEVA papules last for weeks and may develop crusts, vesicles, pustules, or ulcers.
- PLC papules persist for months and develop scales.
- All forms contain interface, cytotoxic T-cell infiltrates with variable epidermal destruction.
- In PLEVA, CD8+ cells predominate.
- In PLC, CD8+ or CD4+ cells predominate.
- Dominant T-cell clonality can be detected in all forms, more often in PLEVA than in PLC.
- Treatment depends on severity and ranges from topical steroids, systemic antibiotics, UV irradiation, and psoralen and UVA to systemic immunosuppressants.

EPIDEMIOLOGY

Pityriasis lichenoides affects all racial and ethnic groups in all geographic regions.[39,40] It is more common in children and young adults but can affect all ages with seasonal variation in onset favoring fall and winter. There is a male predominance of 1.5:1 to 3:1. PLC is 3 to 6 times more common than PLEVA.

CLINICAL FEATURES

CUTANEOUS FINDINGS

PLC and PLEVA exist on a clinicopathologic continuum.[2,28] Therefore, individual patients may exhibit a mixture of acute and chronic lesions sequentially or concurrently. In addition, lesions representing clinical or histopathologic intergrades between the extremes may also occur at any time.

Lesions are often asymptomatic but can be pruritic or burning, especially in the more acute cases. PLC typically presents as recurrent crops of erythematous scaly papules that spontaneously regress over several weeks to months (Fig. 30-10). PLEVA manifests as recurrent crops of erythematous papules that develop crusts, vesicles, pustules, or erosions before spontaneously regressing within a matter of weeks (Fig. 30-11). The more severe ulcerative variant is known as pityriasis lichenoides with ulceronecrosis and hyperthermia (PLUH) or febrile ulceronecrotic Mucha–Habermann disease (FUMHD). It presents as purpuric papulonodules with central ulcers up to a few centimeters in diameter (Fig. 30-12). Some researchers have proposed

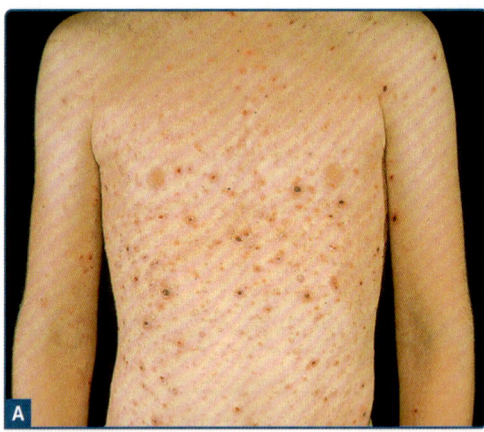
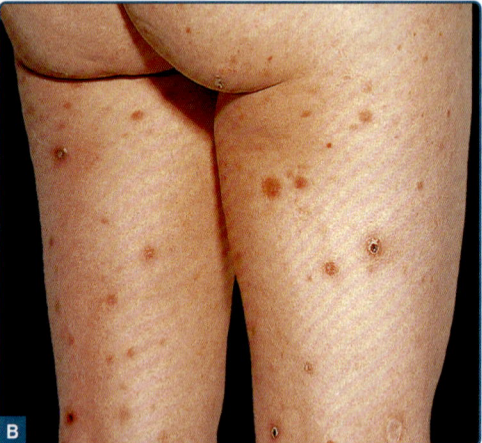
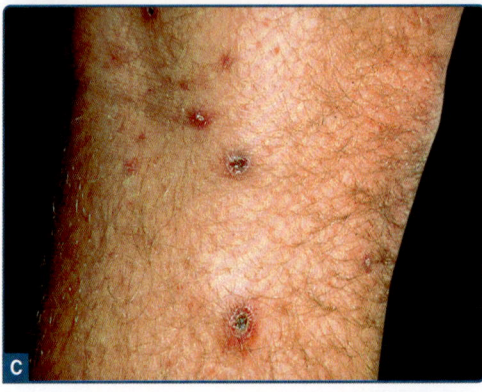

Figure 30-11 Pityriasis lichenoides et varioliformis acuta. **A,** Adolescent with multiple erythematous papules and crusted lesions in various stages of evolution. **B,** Larger papulovesicular and hemorrhagic, crusted lesions in an adult. Note varioliform scars adjacent to active lesions on posterior thigh and leg. **C,** Pustules, crusts, and necrotic-centered papules with erythematous, indurated base.

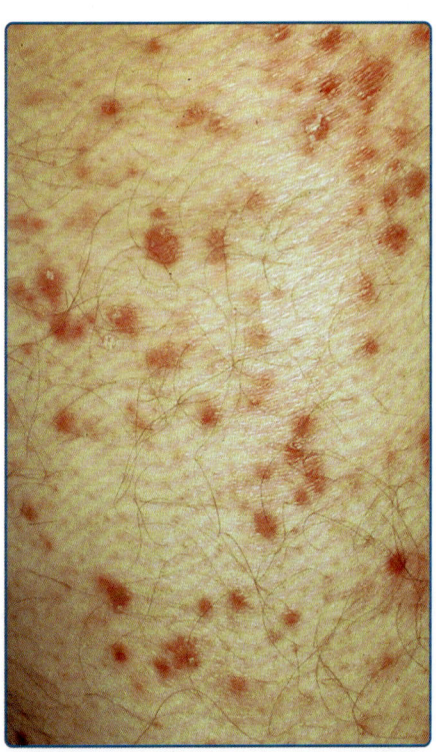

Figure 30-10 Pityriasis lichenoides chronica. Polymorphous appearance ranging from early erythematous papules to scaling brown-red lesions and tan-brown involuting, flat papules, and macules.

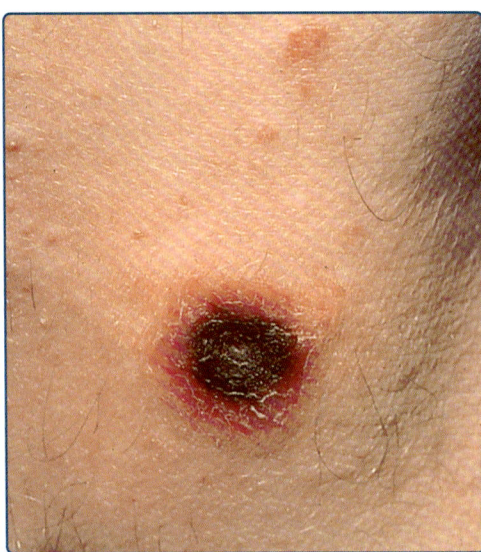

Figure 30-12 Pityriasis lichenoides, ulceronecrotic, hyperacute variant. Large necrotic eschar with halo erythema developing in febrile patient with antecedent pityriasis lichenoides et varioliformis acuta.

that this severe variant is actually an overt T-cell lymphoma.[31] Pityriasis lichenoides lesions tend to concentrate on the trunk and proximal extremities, but any region of the skin, even mucous membranes, can be involved. Rare regional or segmental lesion distributions have been described,[41] as has rare conjunctival nodular inflammation.[42] Although there are usually numerous coexistent lesions, occasionally only a small number of lesions will be present at any one time. All forms of pityriasis lichenoides can result in postinflammatory hypopigmentation or hyperpigmentation. Chronic lesions can resolve with postinflammatory hypopigmentation, sometimes presenting as idiopathic guttate hypomelanosis. Chronic lesions rarely lead to scars. In contrast, acute lesions result in deeper dermal injury and consequently often resolve leaving varioliform (smallpox-like) scars. The presence of lesions in various stages of evolution imparts a polymorphous appearance that is characteristic of pityriasis lichenoides.

COMPLICATIONS

Secondary infection is the most common complication of pityriasis lichenoides. PLEVA may be associated with low-grade fever, malaise, headache, and arthralgia. Patients with PLUH or FUMHD can develop high fever, malaise, myalgia, arthralgia, gastrointestinal, and central nervous system symptoms which can occasionally be fatal.[43] PLC is associated uncommonly with LPP in children.[44] Despite their sometimes dominant T-cell clonal nature, PLC and PLEVA are largely considered clinically benign disorders without significant linkage to lymphomas or other malignancies, although very rare cases of progression to MF have been described.[33]

ETIOLOGY AND PATHOGENESIS

The etiology of pityriasis lichenoides is unknown. Several cases have been associated with infectious agents such as *Toxoplasma gondii*,[45] Epstein-Barr virus,[46] cytomegalovirus,[46] varicella-zoster virus,[47] parvovirus B19,[46,48] human herpesvirus-8,[49] and HIV.[50] At least 1 case was linked with each of the following: estrogen–progesterone therapy, chemotherapy drugs, radiocontrast iodide, and influenza vaccine.[51-54] Recently, 3 cases linked to β-hydroxy-β-methylglutaryl-coenzyme A (HMG-CoA) reductase inhibitors have been described with 1 case suggestive of recurrent cutaneous eruptions upon reexposure.[55] It is uncertain whether these agents are actively involved in disease pathogenesis or merely coincidental bystanders; however, several cases associated with toxoplasmosis have cleared fairly quickly in response to specific therapy.[45] A 10-fold higher level of maternal keratinocytes have been reported in the epidermis of children with pityriasis lichenoides compared to controls.[56]

Immunohistologic studies show a reduction in CD1a+ antigen-presenting dendritic (Langerhans) cells within the central epidermis of pityriasis lichenoides lesions.[57] Keratinocytes and endothelial cells are HLA-DR+, which suggests activation by T-cell cytokines.[57] CD8+ T cells expressing the cytotoxic proteins (TIA-1) and granzyme B predominate in PLEVA, whereas CD4+ T cells predominate in PLC. Some of the T cells in PLC express FoxP3 suggestive of a regulatory T-cell phenotype.[49] Dominant T-cell clonality has been demonstrated in about half of PLEVA cases and a minority of PLC cases.[20,57,58] In aggregate, these findings raise the possibility that pityriasis lichenoides is a variably clonal cytotoxic memory T-cell lymphoproliferative response to one or more foreign antigens. Deposition of immunoglobulin M, C3, and fibrin in and around blood vessels and along the dermal–epidermal junction in early acute lesions suggests a possible concomitant humoral immune response, although this could be a secondary phenomenon.

The relationship of pityriasis lichenoides to lymphomatoid papulosis remains controversial because of overlapping clinical, histopathologic, and molecular features.[28,57,59,60] Common features include dominant T-cell clonality and spontaneous resolution of papular, predominantly lymphoid lesions. Furthermore, individual lesions with the clinicopathologic characteristics of either pityriasis lichenoides or lymphomatoid papulosis can coexist in the same patient, either concurrently or serially. It remains to be determined whether this can be explained as an artifact of sampling lymphomatoid papulosis lesions at various stages of their evolution. The presence of large CD30+ atypical lymphoid cells is the hallmark of lymphomatoid papulosis (at least types A and C). Furthermore, these cells are typically CD4+ and often lack 1 or more mature T-cell antigens, such as CD2, CD3, and CD5. These features serve to distinguish lymphomatoid papulosis from pityriasis lichenoides. Although occasional CD30+ cells can be seen in a wide variety of dermatoses, the presence of any appreciable number should favor lymphomatoid papulosis over pityriasis lichenoides as a matter of definition. It may be that the "PLC-PLEVA" and "lymphomatoid papulosis–CD30+ anaplastic large cell lymphoma" disease spectra are intersecting rather than overlapping entities; that is, although pityriasis lichenoides is a distinct cutaneous T-cell disorder, it is possible that it may sometimes serve as fertile soil for the development of the CD30+ T-cell clone characteristic of lymphomatoid papulosis.

Occasional CD30+ lymphoid cells and occasional atypical lymphoid cells may be seen as a nonspecific finding in many cutaneous lymphoid infiltrates. The presence of appreciable numbers of these cells is not consistent with classic pityriasis lichenoides and should raise concern for the lymphomatoid papulosis–CD30+ anaplastic large cell lymphoma disease spectrum. However, a recently described CD30+ variant of PLEVA illustrates the potential diagnostic confusion of some cases of pityriasis lichenoides with lymphomatoid papulosis and once more highlights the potential pathogenetic overlap between the two entities.[61] Other immunohistologic features and the clonality of pityriasis lichenoides are discussed above in "Etiology and Pathogenesis" under "Pityriasis Lichenoides."

DIAGNOSIS

Miscellaneous nonspecific abnormalities in blood test results occur but are of little practical value. Leukocytosis and a decreased CD4-to-CD8 ratio can occur.

PATHOLOGY

As with the morphology of the clinical lesions, pityriasis lichenoides can exhibit a range of histopathologic features encompassing acute, chronic, and intermediate lesional variants (Figs. 30-13 and 30-14). All cases of pityriasis lichenoides contain an interface dermatitis that is denser and more wedge shaped in the acute lesions. The infiltrate is composed mainly of lymphocytes with a variable admixture of neutrophils and histiocytes. There is exocytosis, parakeratosis, and extravasation of erythrocytes. Epidermal damage ranges from intercellular and extracellular edema in less severe cases to extensive keratinocyte necrosis, vesicles, pustules, and ulcers. The acute variants can exhibit lymphocytic vasculitis with fibrinoid degeneration of blood vessel walls.

DIFFERENTIAL DIAGNOSIS

The differential diagnosis of pityriasis lichenoides includes many papular eruptions (Table 30-6). Those that develop crusts, vesicles, pustules, or ulcers are grouped with PLEVA, whereas those that form predominantly scaly papules are grouped with PLC. Most of them can be excluded based on history and typical clinicopathologic features. A few, such as secondary syphilis and virus-associated lesions, can also be excluded based on serologic tests. Among the most challenging diseases to distinguish from pityriasis lichenoides are lymphomatoid papulosis and macular or papular variants of MF.[60] As detailed earlier, the presence of large atypical lymphoid cells (often CD30+) usually differentiates lymphomatoid papulosis from pityriasis lichenoides. Macular or papular variants of MF are rare. They exhibit classic histopathologic features of MF, including small atypical epidermotropic lymphoid cells with convoluted nuclei and a band-like superficial dermal lymphoid infiltrate.

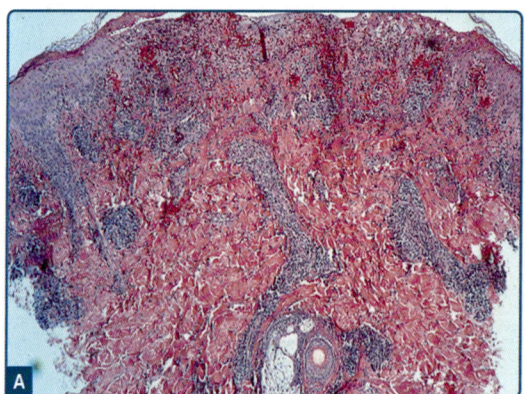
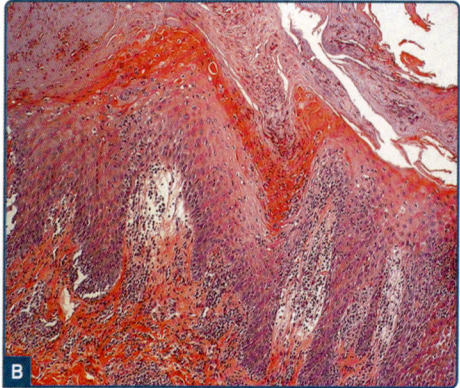

Figure 30-13 Pityriasis lichenoides et varioliformis acuta. **A,** Ulcerated papule with epidermal necrosis, hemorrhage, and superficial and deep perivascular lymphocytic infiltrate. Hematoxylin and eosin (H&E) stain. **B,** Parakeratosis and crust with marked spongiosis and epidermal necrosis. Lymphocyte exocytosis and basal hydropic changes. H&E stain.

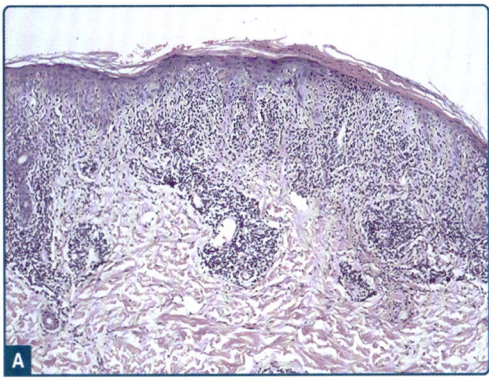 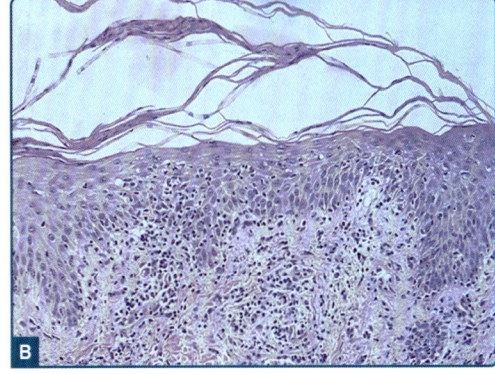

Figure 30-14 Pityriasis lichenoides] chronica. **A,** Compact parakeratosis, lymphocytic exocytosis, occasional eosinophilic necrotic keratinocytes, edema, and diffuse lymphocytic infiltrate localizing to epidermal–dermal interface and perivascular sites within the dermis. Hematoxylin and eosin (H&E) stain. **B,** Parakeratosis, spongiosis, and a predominant mononuclear cell infiltrate in the epidermis and dermis with papillary edema. H&E stain.

CLINICAL COURSE AND PROGNOSIS

Pityriasis lichenoides has a variable clinical course characterized by recurrent crops of lesions that spontaneously resolve. The disorder may resolve spontaneously within a few months or, less commonly, persist for years. PLEVA usually has a shorter duration than PLC. Although the conclusion was not confirmed by subsequent investigation, one report suggested that the duration of pityriasis lichenoides in children correlated better with its clinical distribution than with the relative abundance of acute and chronic lesions, which often coexisted.[62] From longest to shortest duration, the distribution of lesions ranged from peripheral (distal extremities) to central (trunk) to diffuse.

MANAGEMENT

The mainstay of traditional therapy has been a combination of topical corticosteroids and phototherapy (Table 30-7). Systemic antibiotics, such as tetracyclines, erythromycin, and azithromycin, are used primarily for their antiinflammatory rather than antibiotic effects.[63,64] Cases with minimal disease activity may not require any

TABLE 30-6
Differential Diagnosis of Pityriasis Lichenoides et Varioliformis Acuta (PLEVA) and Pityriasis Lichenoides Chronica (PLC)

Most Likely
- PLEVA
  - Arthropod bites, stings, infestations
  - Leukocytoclastic vasculitis
  - Viral exanthem (eg, varicella-zoster, herpes simplex)
- PLC
  - Pityriasis rosea
  - Drug eruption
  - Guttate psoriasis

Consider
- PLEVA
  - Folliculitis
  - Rickettsiosis
  - Erythema multiforme
  - Dermatitis herpetiformis
- PLC
  - Spongiotic dermatitis, papular variant
  - Small-plaque parapsoriasis
  - Lichen planus
  - Gianotti-Crosti syndrome

Always Rule Out
- PLEVA
  - Lymphomatoid papulosis
  - Secondary syphilis
- PLC
  - Lymphomatoid papulosis
  - Mycosis fungoides (papular variant)
  - Secondary syphilis

TABLE 30-7
Treatment of Pityriasis Lichenoides et Varioliformis Acuta and Pityriasis Lichenoides Chronica

First Line
- Topical corticosteroids
- Antibiotics (erythromycin 500 mg PO 2-4 × daily[64]; tetracycline 500 mg PO 2-4 × daily,[66] minocycline 100 mg PO twice daily; azithromycin 500 mg PO on day 1 and 250 mg PO on days 2-5 bimonthly[65])
- Phototherapy (sunbathing, UVB, UVA + UVB, narrowband UVB[68,69])

Second Line
- Topical tacrolimus[70]
- Prednisone (60/40/20 mg PO taper, 5 days each)[71]
- Methotrexate (10-25 mg PO weekly)[72]
- Phototherapy (UVA1[73], psoralen + UVA[69])
- Cyclosporine (2.5-4 mg/kg/day total dose divided into twice-daily PO doses; use the minimum)[74]
- Retinoids (eg, acitretin 25-50 mg PO daily)
- Photodynamic therapy[66]
- Bromelain (pineapple extract)[67]

treatment. Photodynamic therapy has been used successfully for PLC.[65] The more acute the clinical course and the more severe the individual lesions, the more systemic therapy is indicated. Methotrexate is often effective in relatively low doses. Calcineurin inhibitors and retinoids may also be beneficial. Severe cases of PLEVA and PLUH often require systemic corticosteroids or similar drugs to gain control of systemic symptoms. Topical and systemic antibiotics may be needed to treat secondary infections complicating ulcerated skin lesions. These agents are often selected initially to cover Gram-positive pathogens, but subsequent use should be guided by culture results. Bromelain, a pineapple extract, cleared PLC lesions in 8 of 8 cases.[66]

REFERENCES

1. Brocq L. *Les Parapsoriasis, par L. Brocq*. Paris, France: Masson; 1902.
2. Lambert WC, Everett MA. The nosology of parapsoriasis. *J Am Acad Dermatol*. 1981;5(4):373-395.
3. Neisser A. Zur Frage der lichenoiden Eruptionen. *Verh Dtsch Dermatol Ges*. 1894;4:495.
4. Jadassohn J. Uber ein eigenartiges psoriasiformes und lichenoides Exanthem. *Verh Dtsch Dermatol Ges*. 1894;4:524.
5. Juliusberg F. Uber die Pityriasis lichenoides chronica (psoriasiform lichenoides exanthem). *Arch Dermatol Syph*. 1899;50:359.
6. Mucha V. Uber einen der Parakeratosis variegata (Unna) bzw, Pityriasis lichenoides chronica nahestehenden eigentumlichen Fall. *Arch Dermatol Syph*. 1916;123:586.
7. Habermann R. Uber die akut verlaufende, nekrotisierende Unterart der Pityriasis lichenoides (Pityriasis lichenoides et varioliformis acuta). *Dermatol Ztschr*. 1925;45:42.
8. Hu CH, Winkelmann RK. Digitate dermatosis. A new look at symmetrical, small plaque parapsoriasis. *Arch Dermatol*. 1973;107(1):65-69.
9. El-Darouti MA, Fawzy MM, Hegazy RA, et al. Hypopigmented parapsoriasis en plaque, a new, overlooked member of the parapsoriasis family: a report of 34 patients and a 7-year experience. *J Am Acad Dermatol*. 2012;67(6):1182-1188.
10. Lindahl LM, Heide-Jørgensen U, Pedersen L, et al. Risk of acute myocardial infarction or stroke in patients with mycosis fungoides and parapsoriasis. *Acta Derm Venereol*. 2016;96(4):530-534.
11. Lindahl LM, Fenger-Grøn M, Iversen L. Subsequent cancers, mortality, and causes of death in patients with mycosis fungoides and parapsoriasis: a Danish nationwide, population-based cohort study. *J Am Acad Dermatol*. 2014;71(3):529-535.
12. Bos J, ed. *Skin Immune System*. Boca Raton, FL: CRC Press; 1990.
13. Veelken H, Wood GS, Sklar J. Molecular staging of cutaneous T-cell lymphoma: evidence for systemic involvement in early disease. *J Invest Dermatol*. 1995;104(6):889-894.
14. Veelken H, Sklar JL, Wood GS. Detection of low-level tumor cells in allergic contact dermatitis induced by mechlorethamine in patients with mycosis fungoides. *J Invest Dermatol*. 1996;106(4):685-688.
15. Wood GS. Analysis of clonality in cutaneous T cell lymphoma and associated diseases. *Ann N Y Acad Sci*. 2001;941:26-30.
16. Karenko L, Hyytinen E, Sarna S, et al. Chromosomal abnormalities in cutaneous T-cell lymphoma and in its premalignant conditions as detected by G-banding and interphase cytogenetic methods. *J Invest Dermatol*. 1997;108(1):22-29.
17. Li G, Chooback L, Wolfe JT, et al. Overexpression of p53 protein in cutaneous T cell lymphoma: relationship to large cell transformation and disease progression. *J Invest Dermatol*. 1998;110(5):767-770.
18. Kikuchi A, Naka W, Harada T, et al. Parapsoriasis en plaques: its potential for progression to malignant lymphoma. *J Am Acad Dermatol*. 1993;29(3):419-422.
19. Klemke CD, Dippel E, Dembinski A, et al. Clonal T cell receptor gamma-chain gene rearrangement by PCR-based GeneScan analysis in the skin and blood of patients with parapsoriasis and early-stage mycosis fungoides. *J Pathol*. 2002;197(3):348-354.
20. Shieh S, Mikkola DL, Wood GS. Differentiation and clonality of lesional lymphocytes in pityriasis lichenoides chronica. *Arch Dermatol*. 2001;137(3):305-308.
21. Dereure O, Levi E, Kadin ME. T-Cell clonality in pityriasis lichenoides et varioliformis acuta: a heteroduplex analysis of 20 cases. *Arch Dermatol*. 2000;136(12):1483-1486.
22. Wood GS. Lymphocyte activation in cutaneous T-cell lymphoma. *J Invest Dermatol*. 1995;105(suppl 1):105S-109S.
23. Muche JM, Lukowsky A, Heim J, et al. Demonstration of frequent occurrence of clonal T cells in the peripheral blood but not in the skin of patients with small plaque parapsoriasis. *Blood*. 1999;94(4):1409-1417.
24. Siddiqui J HD, Misra M, Wood GS. Clonal dermatitis: a potential precursor of CTCL with varied clinical manifestations. *J Invest Dermatol*. 1997;108:584.
25. Amitay-Laish I, Sarid R, Ben-Amitai D, et al. Human herpesvirus 8 is not detectable in lesions of large plaque parapsoriasis, and in early-stage sporadic, familial, and juvenile cases of mycosis fungoides. *J Am Acad Dermatol*. 2012;66(1):46-50.
26. Kreuter A, Bischoff S, Skrygan M, et al. High association of human herpesvirus 8 in large-plaque parapsoriasis and mycosis fungoides. *Arch Dermatol*. 2008;144(8):1011-1016.
27. Pimpinelli N, Olsen EA, Santucci M, et al. Defining early mycosis fungoides. *J Am Acad Dermatol*. 2005;53(6):1053-1063.
28. Wood G. *The Benign and Malignant Cutaneous Lymphoproliferative Disorders Including Mycosis Fungoides*. Baltimore, MD: Williams and Wilkins; 2001.
29. Wood GS, Michie SA, Durden F, et al. Expression of class II major histocompatibility antigens by keratinocytes in cutaneous T cell lymphoma. *Int J Dermatol*. 1994;33(5):346-350.
30. Lindae ML AE, Hoppe RT, Wood GS. Poikilodermatous mycosis fungoides and atrophic large plaque parapsoriasis exhibit similar abnormalities of T cell antigen expression. *Arch Dermatol*. 1988;124:366-372.
31. Vakeva L, Sarna S, Vaalasti A, et al. A retrospective study of the probability of the evolution of parapsoriasis en plaques into mycosis fungoides. *Acta Derm Venereol*. 2005;85(4):318-323.
32. Bernier C, Nguyen JM, Quéreux G, et al: CD13 and TCR clone: markers of early mycosis fungoides. *Acta Derm Venereol*. 2007;87(2):155-159.
33. Sibbald C, Pope E. Systematic review of cases of cutaneous T-cell lymphoma transformation in pityriasis

lichenoides and small plaque parapsoriasis. *Br J Dermatol.* 2016;175(4):807-809.
34. King-Ismael D, Ackerman AB. Guttate parapsoriasis/digitate dermatosis (small plaque parapsoriasis) is mycosis fungoides. *Am J Dermatopathol.* 1992;14(6):518-530, discussion 531-515.
35. Burg G, Dummer R. Small plaque (digitate) parapsoriasis is an "abortive cutaneous T-cell lymphoma" and is not mycosis fungoides. *Arch Dermatol.* 1995;131(3):336-338.
36. Aydogan K, Yazici S, Balaban Adim S, et al. Efficacy of low-dose ultraviolet A-1 phototherapy for parapsoriasis/early-stage mycosis fungoides. *Photochem Photobiol.* 2014;90(4):873-877.
37. Lindahl LM, Fenger-Gron M, Iversen L. Topical nitrogen mustard therapy in patients with mycosis fungoides or parapsoriasis. *J Eur Acad Dermatol Venereol.* 2013;27(2):163-168.
38. Gebert S, Raulin C, Ockenfels HM, et al. Excimer-laser (308 nm) treatment of large plaque parapsoriasis and long-term follow-up. *Eur J Dermatol.* 2006;16(2):198-199.
39. Wahie S, Hiscutt E, Natarajan S, et al. Pityriasis lichenoides: the differences between children and adults. *Br J Dermatol.* 2007;157(5):941-945.
40. Bowers S, Warshaw EM. Pityriasis lichenoides and its subtypes. *J Am Acad Dermatol.* 2006;55(4):557-572, quiz 573-556.
41. Cliff S, Cook MG, Ostlere LS, et al. Segmental pityriasis lichenoides chronica. *Clin Exp Dermatol.* 1996;21(6):464-465.
42. Verhamme T, Arnaout A, Ayliffe WH. Limbal and bulbar inflammatory nodules in a patient with pityriasis lichenoides et varioliformis acuta. *Bull Soc Belge Ophtalmol.* 2008; (307):13-18.
43. Cozzio A, Hafner J, Kempf W, et al. Febrile ulceronecrotic Mucha-Habermann disease with clonality: a cutaneous T-cell lymphoma entity? *J Am Acad Dermatol.* 2004;51(6):1014-1017.
44. Samman PD. The natural history of parapsoriasis en plaques (chronic superficial dermatitis) and prereticulotic poikiloderma. *Br J Dermatol.* 1972;87(5):405-411.
45. Nassef NE, Hammam MA. The relation between toxoplasmosis and pityriasis lichenoides chronica. *J Egypt Soc Parasitol.* 1997;27(1):93-99.
46. Chuh AA. The association of pityriasis rosea with cytomegalovirus, Epstein-Barr virus and parvovirus B19 infections—a prospective case control study by polymerase chain reaction and serology. *Eur J Dermatol.* 2003;13(1):25-28.
47. Cho E, Jun HJ, Cho SH, et al. Varicella-zoster virus as a possible cause of pityriasis lichenoides et varioliformis acuta. *Pediatr Dermatol.* 2014;31(2):259-260.
48. Nanda A, Alshalfan F, Al-Otaibi M, et al. Febrile ulceronecrotic Mucha-Habermann disease (pityriasis lichenoides et varioliformis acuta fulminans) associated with parvovirus infection. *Am J Dermatopathol.* 2013;35(4):503-506.
49. Kim JE, Yun WJ, Mun SK, et al. Pityriasis lichenoides et varioliformis acuta and pityriasis lichenoides chronica: comparison of lesional T-cell subsets and investigation of viral associations. *J Cutan Pathol.* 2011;38(8):649-656.
50. Griffiths JK. Successful long-term use of cyclosporin A in HIV-induced pityriasis lichenoides chronica. *J Acquir Immune Defic Syndr Hum Retrovirol.* 1998;18(4):396-397.
51. Wood GS, Strickler JG, Abel EA, et al. The immunohistology of pityriasis lichenoides et varioliformis acuta and pityriasis lichenoides chronica: evidence for their interrelationship with lymphomatoid papulosis. *J Am Acad Dermatol.* 1987;16:559-570.
52. Jowkar F, Namazi MR, Bahmani M, et al. Triggering of pityriasis lichenoides et varioliformis acuta by radiocontrast iodide. *J Dermatolog Treat.* 2008;19(4):249-250.
53. Kawamura K, Tsuji T, Kuwabara Y. Mucha-Habermann disease-like eruptions due to Tegafur. *J Dermatol.* 1999;26(3):164-167.
54. Castro BA, Pereira JM, Meyer RL, et al. Pityriasis lichenoides et varioliformis acuta after influenza vaccine. *An Bras Dermatol.* 2015;90(3)(suppl 1):181-184.
55. Massay RJ, Maynard AA. Pityriasis lichenoides chronica associated with use of HMG-CoA reductase inhibitors. *West Indian Med J.* 2012;61(7):743-745.
56. Khosrotehrani K, Guegan S, Fraitag S, et al. Presence of chimeric maternally derived keratinocytes in cutaneous inflammatory diseases of children: the example of pityriasis lichenoides. *J Invest Dermatol.* 2006;126(2):345-348.
57. Magro C, Crowson AN, Kovatich A, et al. Pityriasis lichenoides: a clonal T-cell lymphoproliferative disorder. *Hum Pathol.* 2002;33(8):788-795.
58. Weiss LM, Wood GS, Ellisen LW, et al. Clonal T-cell populations in pityriasis lichenoides et varioliformis acuta (Mucha-Habermann disease). *Am J Pathol.* 1987;126(3):417-421.
59. Vonderheid EC, Kadin ME, Gocke CD. Lymphomatoid papulosis followed by pityriasis lichenoides: a common pathogenesis? *Am J Dermatopathol.* 2011;33(8):835-840.
60. Vonderheid EC, Kadin ME, Telang GH. Commentary about papular mycosis fungoides, lymphomatoid papulosis and lymphomatoid pityriasis lichenoides: more similarities than differences. *J Cutan Pathol.* 2016;43(4):303-312.
61. Kempf W, Kazakov DV, Palmedo G, et al. Pityriasis lichenoides et varioliformis acuta with numerous CD30(+) cells: a variant mimicking lymphomatoid papulosis and other cutaneous lymphomas. A clinicopathologic, immunohistochemical, and molecular biological study of 13 cases. *Am J Surg Pathol.* 2012;36(7):1021-1029.
62. Rongioletti F, Rivara G, Rebora A. Pityriasis lichenoides et varioliformis acuta and acquired toxoplasmosis. *Dermatologica.* 1987;175(1):41-44.
63. Piamphongsant T. Tetracycline for the treatment of pityriasis lichenoides. *Br J Dermatol.* 1974;91(3):319-322.
64. Hapa A, Ersoy-Evans S, Karaduman A. Childhood pityriasis lichenoides and oral erythromycin. *Pediatr Dermatol.* 2012;29(6):719-724.
65. Skinner RB, Levy AL. Rapid resolution of pityriasis lichenoides et varioliformis acuta with azithromycin. *J Am Acad Dermatol.* 2008;58(3):524-525.
66. Fernandez-Guarino M, Harto A, Reguero-Callejas ME, et al. Pityriasis lichenoides chronica: good response to photodynamic therapy. *Br J Dermatol.* 2008;158(1):198-200.
67. Massimiliano R, Pietro R, Paolo S, et al. Role of bromelain in the treatment of patients with pityriasis lichenoides chronica. *J Dermatolog Treat.* 2007;18(4):219-222.
68. Brazzelli V, Carugno A, Rivetti N, et al. Narrowband UVB phototherapy for pediatric generalized pityriasis lichenoides. *Photodermatol Photoimmunol Photomed.* 2013;29(6):330-333.
69. Farnaghi F, Seirafi H, Ehsani AH, et al. Comparison of the therapeutic effects of narrow band UVB vs. PUVA in patients with pityriasis lichenoides. *J Eur Acad Dermatol Venereol.* 2011;25(8):913-916.

70. Simon D, Boudny C, Nievergelt H, et al. Successful treatment of pityriasis lichenoides with topical tacrolimus. *Br J Dermatol.* 2004;150(5):1033-1035.
71. Maekawa Y, Nakamura T, Nogami R. Febrile ulceronecrotic Mucha-Habermann's disease. *J Dermatol.* 1994;21(1):46-49.
72. Griffith-Bauer K, Leitenberger SL, Krol A. Febrile ulceronecrotic Mucha-Habermann disease: two cases with excellent response to methotrexate. *Pediatr Dermatol.* 2015;32(6):e307-e308.
73. Pinton PC, Capezzera R, Zane C, et al. Medium-dose ultraviolet A1 therapy for pityriasis lichenoides et varioliformis acuta and pityriasis lichenoides chronica. *J Am Acad Dermatol.* 2002;47(3):410-414.
74. Uzoma MA, Wilkerson MG, Carr VL, et al. Pentoxifylline and cyclosporine in the treatment of febrile ulceronecrotic Mucha-Habermann disease. *Pediatr Dermatol.* 2014;31(4):525-527.

Chapter 31 :: Pityriasis Rosea
:: Matthew Clark & Johann E. Gudjonsson

第三十一章

玫瑰糠疹

中文导读

本章介绍了玫瑰糠疹的流行病学、临床特征、病因和发病机制、诊断、实验室检验、组织病理学、鉴别诊断、临床病程及预后、治疗。玫瑰糠疹发病可能与人类疱疹病毒HHV-7和/或HHV-6相关，典型表现常可见母斑，子斑分布与皮纹平行，易于诊断，而不典型玫瑰糠疹诊断存在挑战。实验室检查及病理检查多无特异性，大多数可不需特异性治疗，大环内酯类抗生素及阿昔洛韦可能有治疗效果。

〔朱　武〕

AT-A-GLANCE

- Common self-limited papulosquamous eruption typically lasting 5 to 8 weeks.
- Occurs worldwide in all races and age groups, with peak incidence between the ages of 10 and 35 years.
- Classically begins as an isolated 3- to 5-cm oval plaque on the trunk with a collarette of fine scale just inside the periphery, which plaque is called a *herald patch*.
- This is followed by a secondary eruption of similar appearing but smaller lesions on the trunk and proximal extremities, usually with their long axis along the lines of cleavage.
- Many atypical variants exist in contrast to the pattern described above.
- Pityriasis rosea can have associated systemic symptoms and pruritus, but many cases are asymptomatic.
- Etiology is unknown, but it is thought to be a viral exanthem most likely related to infection or reactivation of human herpesvirus (HHV)-6 and/or HHV-7.
- Usually only supportive treatment and reassurance is needed, but for severe cases acyclovir may hasten recovery and lessen symptoms.

In 1860, Gibert first used the term *pityriasis rosea* (PR), meaning pink (rosea) scales (pityriasis).[1] PR is most common in teenagers and young adults, and is likely a viral exanthema currently thought to be related to primary infection or reactivation of human herpesvirus (HHV)-6 (HHV-6) and/or HHV-7.[2-6] PR is fairly common, self-limited, and not associated with long-term sequelae. It classically begins as an isolated 3- to 5-cm oval plaque on the trunk with a collarette of fine scale just inside the periphery, which plaque is called a *herald patch*. This lesion is then followed by a secondary eruption of similar appearing but smaller lesions most prominently on the trunk and proximal extremities, usually with their long axis along the lines of cleavage in what is often described as a "Christmas tree" pattern. However, there are many atypical presentations of the herald patch distribution, secondary eruption morphology, and overall rash distribution. PR is commonly asymptomatic, but pruritus and systemic flu-like symptoms may be present. Often only supportive treatment and patient education are needed for management, but in cases with a widespread eruption, severe pruritus, or significant systemic symptoms acyclovir may be beneficial.

EPIDEMIOLOGY

PR has a worldwide distribution and is found in all races. One institution in the United States found the incidence to be 0.16% (~160 cases per 100,000 person-years).[7] Studies in other countries report incidences ranging from 0.75% to 1.17%.[8,9] A recent publication combined many of the PR epidemiologic studies from around the world and reported an incidence of 0.64 per 100 dermatologic patients.[10] In some studies PR was found to be more common in colder months,[7,9] but other studies show no significant seasonal variation.[2,11] Studies have demonstrated clustering of cases supporting the hypothesis of an infectious etiology.[12,13] There is a slight female preponderance at 1.39:1.[10] The peak incidence of PR occurs between the ages of 10 and 35 years, but cases have been reported ranging in age from 3 months to 83 years.[7,9,10,14] Relapse is thought to be rare, ranging from 1.8% to 3.7%.[7,15]

CLINICAL FEATURES

HISTORY

Classic PR typically begins with a solitary lesion on the trunk or less commonly an extremity known as a herald patch. This lesion typically remains isolated on average for 2 weeks in adults and 4 days in children, after which time it is followed by the onset of a secondary eruption of morphologically similar but smaller lesions on the trunk and proximal extremities. The eruption may be preceded by various prodromal symptoms such as malaise, nausea, headache, gastrointestinal, and upper respiratory symptoms. The incidence of these prodromal symptoms varies in the literature from 5% to 69%.[14,16] These symptoms can also occur during the eruption. Pruritus is severe in 25%, mild to moderate in 50%, and absent in 25% of patients.[17]

In contrast to classic PR, Drago and colleagues have reported several variants of PR, such as in pediatric patients (<10 years of age), relapsing, and a persistent form.[15,17-20] The relapsing form of PR generally consists of single episode of relapse within 1 year of the initial episode, although multiple relapses have been reported. In this variant, the secondary episodes generally lack a herald patch, are shorter lived, and consist of fewer and more localized lesions than the initial eruption. The persistent form of PR, is defined as having the eruption last for greater than 12 weeks without interruption. It commonly has a herald patch, and oral manifestations are thought to be more common than in classic PR. When PR presents in the pediatric population it often has a different clinical course compared to classic PR. Thus, the time between the presentation of the herald patch and the secondary eruption is shorter, often lasting only 4 days, in contrast to the more typical 2-week interval. In addition, the average overall duration of the eruption tends to be shorter and on average lasts approximately 16 days.[19] Lastly, PR is reported to occur more frequently in pregnant women than in the general population, but otherwise PR during pregnancy presents in a manner similar to classic PR.

CUTANEOUS FINDINGS

The initial classic herald patch presents as a well-demarcated, thin, oval to round plaque that is usually pink, rose colored, erythematous, or, less commonly, hyperpigmented. It frequently has a slightly depressed center and fine collarette of scale within the periphery of the lesion (Figs. 31-1 and 31-2). It most commonly occurs on the trunk (50%) followed by the extremities and neck.[2] Atypical locations such as the dorsal feet, face, scalp, and genitalia have been reported. This lesion enlarges over several days usually reaching a diameter greater than 3 cm with a range of 2 to 10 cm. The incidence of the herald patch is reported to be anywhere from 12% to 94%, but is thought to be present in approximately 80% of the cases. Multiple herald patches have been observed with an incidence of 5% (Fig. 31-3). The herald patch may appear concurrently with the more generalized eruption or, less commonly, be the sole manifestation of the disease.[2,14]

The secondary eruption commonly begins approximately 2 weeks following the onset of the herald

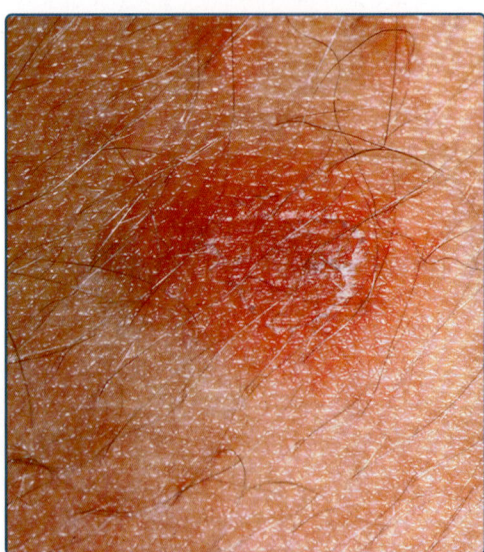

Figure 31-1 A typical primary plaque (herald patch) of pityriasis rosea, demonstrating an oval shape and fine scale inside the periphery of the plaque.

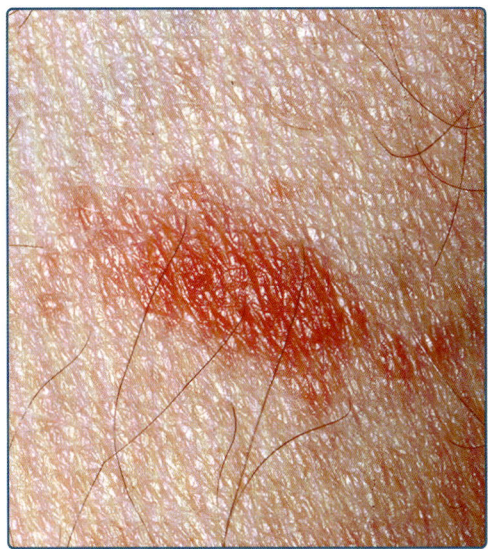

Figure 31-2 A nonscaly purpuric primary plaque (herald patch) of pityriasis rosea.

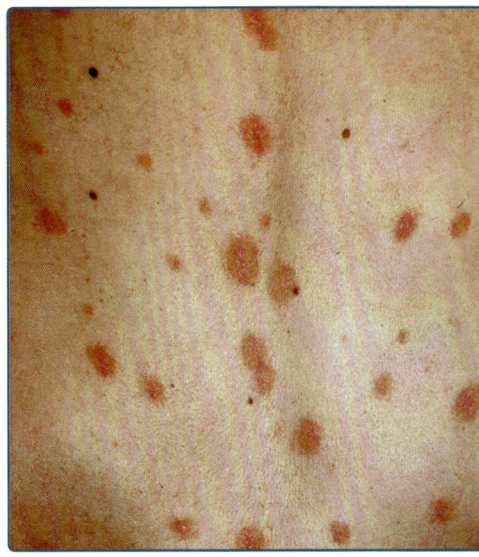

Figure 31-4 Typical distribution of secondary plaques along the lines of cleavage on the back in a Christmas tree pattern.

patch. However, this interval is described as ranging from a few hours to 3 months.[14] This secondary eruption is characterized by multiple, round-to-oval, 0.5- to 1.5-cm macules, papules, and plaques. These lesions are often light pink with a fine collarette of scale and resemble the herald patch in miniature. They are typically found bilaterally and symmetrically on the trunk and proximal extremities (Figs. 31-4 to 31-6). However, these lesions can extend to the distal extremities, and

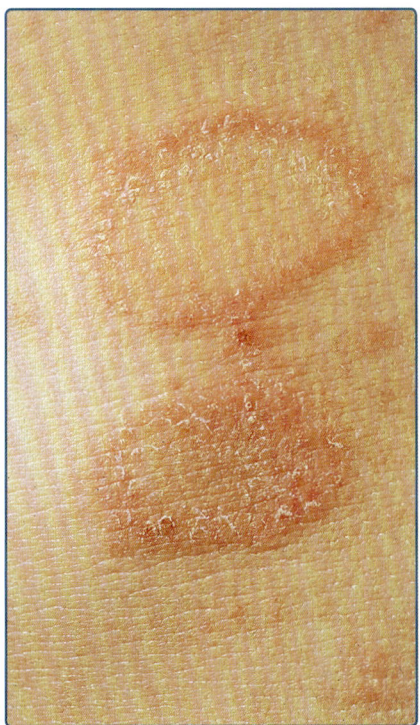

Figure 31-3 A double herald patch of pityriasis rosea.

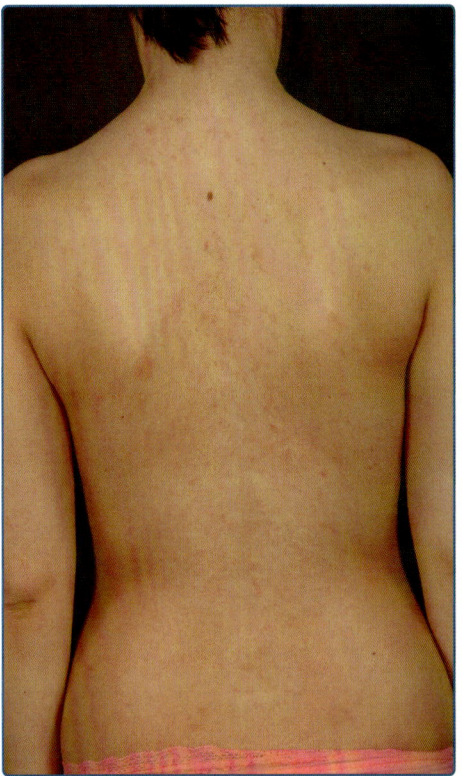

Figure 31-5 Typical distribution along the lines of cleavage and morphology of the secondary eruption on the back of a 23-week pregnant patient. (Used with permission from Dr. Thy Thy Do and Mr. Harrold Carter.)

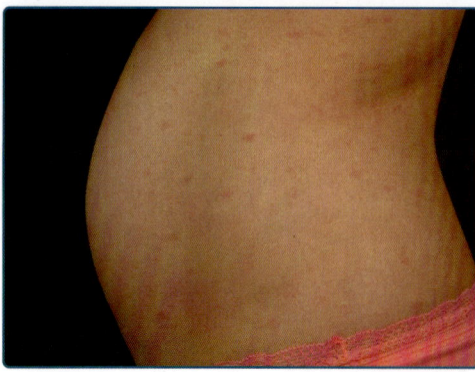

Figure 31-6 Typical distribution along the lines of cleavage and morphology of the secondary eruption on the flank and abdomen of a 23-week pregnant patient. (Used with permission from Dr. Thy Thy Do and Mr. Harrold Carter.)

can been found on the palms and soles. In the classic description, these lesions are aligned with their long axis parallel to lines of cleavage giving a "Christmas tree" distribution on the upper chest and back (Fig. 31-7). This secondary eruption usually occurs in crops every few days over the course of 2 weeks, where it reaches its maximum intensity. Rarely, the secondary eruption is confined to sun-protected skin; in other cases, it is found only on sun-exposed surfaces.[14]

Many different forms of atypical secondary lesions have been described, including eczematous, papular, follicular, vesicular, urticarial, pustular, and purpuric (Figs. 31-8 and 31-9).[2,14,17] These lesions may be the only manifestation of the secondary eruption or they may

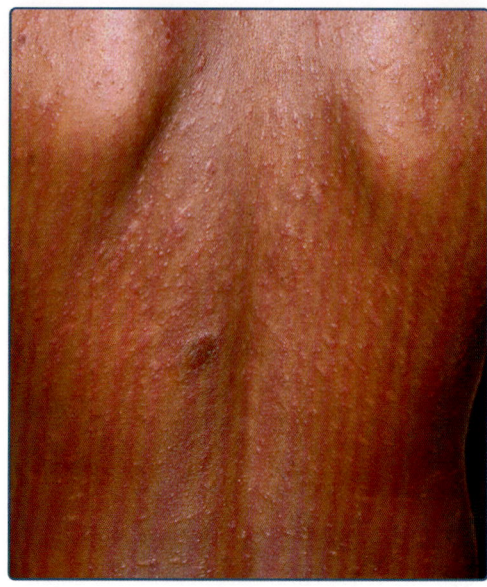

Figure 31-8 Vesicular pityriasis rosea, showing typical primary plaque and secondary papulovesicles. Note Christmas tree distribution.

occur admixed with other morphologies, including the classic type. The vesicular lesions may be arranged in a rosette and are more common in children and young adults.[2]

Mucosal lesions can occur with PR, and although these lesions are thought to be uncommon, they have been reported in up to 16% of patients with PR.[21] The oral lesions can have varying morphologies, including punctate hemorrhagic, ulcerative, erythematous macules, plaques, bullous, and annular lesions.[22] Ulcerations are thought to be the most common form. The oral lesions typically occur along with the cutaneous eruption.[2] Lymphadenopathy can also be associated with PR particularly when patients have associated flu-like symptoms.

There are several atypical variants of PR, such as unilateral, localized, and inverse, which make up approximately 20% of cases.[14] Localized PR is often limited to 1 truncal site, whereas unilateral PR does

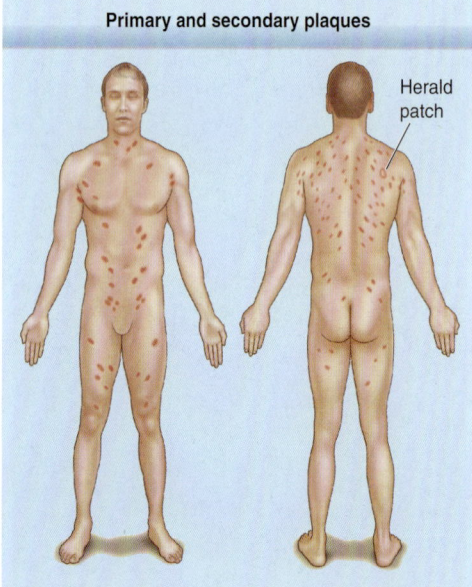

Figure 31-7 Schematic diagram of the primary plaque (herald patch) and the typical distribution of secondary plaques along the lines of cleavage on the trunk in a Christmas tree pattern.

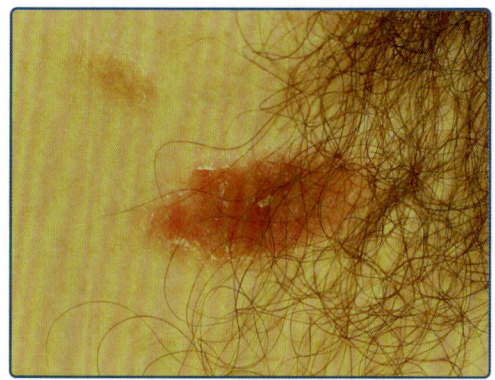

Figure 31-9 Purpuric pityriasis rosea.

not cross midline. Inverse PR, which is more common in children, is characterized by involvement of the body folds, face, and often distal extremities.[2,14] PR in a blaschkoid distribution or with prominent acral involvement has also been reported.[23,24]

COMPLICATIONS

PR is not associated with any long-term complications in otherwise healthy individuals. Systemic symptoms, when present, are transient. PR, mostly because of the uncertain etiology, length of disease recovery, and fear of progression, can be associated with the development of anxiety and depression in 30% of cases and does negatively impact quality of life.[25] PR in pregnancy deserves special mention as it may be associated with adverse outcomes. In one study where 38 women who developed PR during pregnancy were observed, 13% had a miscarriage; it was noted, however, that the miscarriage rate of the general population is approximately 10%.[26] Perhaps of more interest was that in the 8 cases where PR began before 15 weeks of gestation, 5 (62%) resulted in abortion. Of the 33 women who bore children in this study, 9 (27%) had a premature delivery, but none of the infants had birth defects, although hypotonia, weak motility, and hyporeactivity was noted in 6 cases (18%). Based on these findings, women who develop PR during pregnancy, particularly during the first trimester, should be followed carefully for the development of adverse events.

ETIOLOGY AND PATHOGENESIS

PR has long been thought to be caused by an infectious agent. This assumption is based on the findings of case clustering, possible seasonal variation, resemblance to other known exanthems, and the presence of prodromal symptoms in some patients. Over the years there have been numerous investigations into potential causative bacterial, fungal, and viral pathogens, all with largely negative results. However, in 1997, Drago and colleagues found HHV-7 DNA in peripheral blood mononuclear cells, skin, and cell-free plasma of patients with PR suggesting an association.[6] Since 1997, multiple studies have been done that support HHV-7 and/or HHV-6 as the likely cause of PR.[5,3,27-29] These studies demonstrated the presence of HHV-7, and to a lesser extent HHV-6 DNA and messenger RNA, in both lesional and nonlesional PR skin, in peripheral blood mononuclear cells, and in plasma via real-time polymerase chain reaction, but not in controls. Furthermore serological studies using immunoglobulins M and G against HHV-7 and HHV-6 are in alignment with the findings above. All this evidence suggests PR may be related to infection with HHV-7 and, to a lesser extent, HHV-6. It is not clear if PR is caused by HHV-7 and/or HHV-6 primary infection, reactivation, or both. The hypothesis of reactivation is supported by the finding of 7 and HHV-6 DNA in saliva which is a known reservoir of these viruses and the usual mode of transmission.[28] However, the antibody profile found by Vag and colleagues was more consistent with primary infection.[29] It should be noted that there have also been various studies with results that failed to duplicate the findings of HHV-7 and/or HHV-6 DNA in PR patients, failed to show differences in patients with PR and controls, or, in some cases, found even higher prevalence of HHV-7 and HHV-6 DNA in control individuals.[30-35] There are numerous potential reasons for these discordant results. First, HHVs have a very high prevalence in the general population, making it hard to show differences in prevalence between disease states and healthy controls without large numbers. The prevalence of HHV-6 and HHV-7 seropositivity in healthy adults has been found to be 80% to 100%[36] and >85%,[37] respectively. Also complicating analysis is that HHV-7 may influence and even cause reactivation of latent HHV-6 with subsequent disappearance of active HHV-7 replication.[2,30] This could account for the varying percentages of HHV-7 and HHV-6 in the positive studies. Lastly, the varied findings may reflect that PR like other exanthems, such as Gianotti-Crosti syndrome, can be induced by multiple pathogens.[30]

Overall the pathogenesis of PR is poorly understood and if HHV-7 and HHV-6 are the etiologic agents the mechanisms by which they lead to the clinical findings seen in PR are not known. Several studies have looked into the immunologic aspects of PR. A review of the available literature shows that cell-mediated immunity is important in the pathogenesis of PR.[38] Specifically, one study demonstrated that the inflammatory infiltrate of PR was predominantly T cells with an increased CD4-to-CD8 ratio as well as an increased proportion of Langerhans cells, which are common findings in other inflammatory skin conditions thought to be driven by cell-mediated immunity. No significant difference was found between the herald patch and fully developed PR lesions.[39] Another study looking specifically at the cytokine profile of PR found increased interleukin-17, interferon-γ, vascular endothelial growth factor, and interferon-inducible protein-10 (CXCL10). Interleukin-17 and interferon-γ in particular were mentioned as evidence that the cytokine profile in PR was not specific for, but consistent with, a viral-induced disease process.[40] Lastly, an autoimmune pathogenesis for PR has been investigated, but to date no compelling autoantigens or supporting evidence has been found.[38]

DIAGNOSIS

The diagnosis of PR is usually clinical, and in the case of classic PR fairly straightforward. The various atypical presentations, however, can pose a diagnostic challenge. A set of clinical diagnostic criteria was proposed in 2003.[41,42] In these criteria, the patient had to have 3 essential features and at least 1 of 3 optional features. The 3 essential features were discrete circular or oval lesions, scaling on most lesions, and a peripheral collarette of scale with central clearance on at least 2 lesions. The optional criteria included a truncal and proximal limb distribution with less than 10% of lesions distal to the mid-upper-arm and mid-thighs, distribution of most lesions along the ribs, and a herald patch appearing at least 2 days before the eruption. They also proposed 3 exclusion features, including multiple small vesicles at the center of 2 or more lesions, most lesions on palmar or plantar skin surfaces, and clinical or serological evidence of secondary syphilis.

LABORATORY TESTING

Routine blood tests are typically normal in PR. Although various abnormalities, including leukocytosis and an elevated erythrocyte sedimentation rate may be found, blood tests are nonspecific. As such, blood tests are not needed nor are they recommended in the diagnosis of PR.

PATHOLOGY

The histologic features of PR are nonspecific and patients with the classic presentation often do not require skin biopsy as the diagnosis can confidently be made on clinical grounds alone. The epidermal changes seen include parakeratosis which may be focal, multifocal, or confluent; orthokeratosis; mild acanthosis; a thinned granular layer; and spongiosis often with some degree of lymphocyte exocytosis (Fig. 31-10). In the dermis there is typically a superficial perivascular lymphocytic infiltrate and variable extravasated red

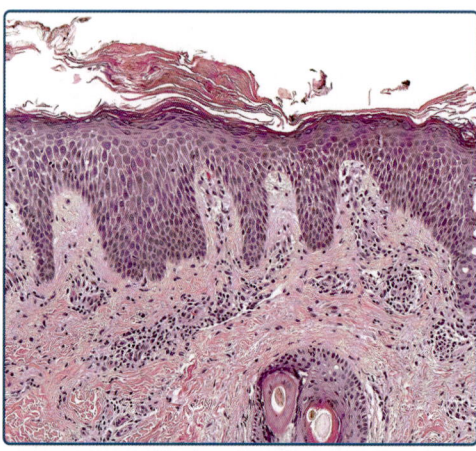

Figure 31-10 Typical epidermal changes seen in pityriasis rosea, including mounded parakeratosis with lift off, mild acanthosis, and spongiosis. (A 4-mm punch biopsy, hematoxylin and eosin stain, ×10 magnification, used with permission from Dr. Paul Harms.)

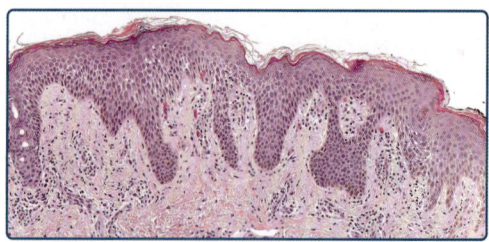

Figure 31-11 Biopsy that highlights the spongiosis, superficial perivascular lymphocytic infiltrate, and red blood cell extravasation typically seen in pityriasis rosea. (A 4-mm punch biopsy, hematoxylin and eosin stain, ×10 magnification, used with permission from Dr. Paul Harms.)

blood cells (Fig. 31-11).[39] The inflammatory infiltrate is predominantly composed of lymphocytes, neutrophils, histiocytes, and eosinophils can be seen.[2,43] There are no consistent differences in the histology of the herald patch versus the secondary lesion, but the herald patch may have a slightly deeper infiltrate with more acanthosis.[2]

DIFFERENTIAL DIAGNOSIS

Table 31-1 outlines the differential diagnosis of PR.

The differential diagnosis of PR includes various other papulosquamous disorders, including nummular eczema, guttate psoriasis, lichen planus, pityriasis lichenoides, tinea corporis, parapsoriasis, and

TABLE 31-1
Differential Diagnosis of Pityriasis Rosea

Most Likely
- *Tinea corporis:* Scale is usually at periphery of plaques, plaques usually not oval and distributed along lines of cleavage, positive potassium hydroxide (KOH) examination.
- *Nummular dermatitis:* Plaques are usually more circular than oval, there are no collarettes of scale, and tiny vesicles are common.
- *Guttate psoriasis:* Plaques are usually smaller than pityriasis rosea (PR) lesions and do not follow lines of cleavage; scales are thick and silvery. When in doubt, perform a biopsy.

Consider
- *Pityriasis lichenoides chronica:* More chronic with persistent crops of new lesions, more confluent scale, no herald patch, and more common on extremities.
- *Lichen planus:* More pruritic, chronic, and with distal extremity involvement. Scale may show classic Wickham striae.
- *Seborrheic dermatitis:* Look for characteristic face and scalp involvement.

Always Rule Out
- *Secondary syphilis:* History of primary chancre, no herald patch, lesions typically more widespread and classically involve palms and soles. Other features of secondary syphilis, such as condyloma lata, alopecia, mucous patches, and split papules, may be present. Usually there are more severe systemic complaints and lymphadenopathy. If there is any clinical concern, perform a serologic test for syphilis (eg, a rapid plasma reagin).
- *PR-like drug eruption:* See the text for an extensive list. A drug history is needed.

seborrheic dermatitis. Nummular eczema generally has more round than oval lesions, typically does not follow the lines of cleavage, and has a predilection for extensor extremities. Seborrheic dermatitis can have truncal lesions similar to PR, but they generally have corresponding lesions on the scalp and/or face. Although guttate psoriasis can be very difficult to distinguish from PR, it also does not follow the lines of cleavage, lacks a larger lesion that could mimic a herald patch, and has a thicker more confluent scale typical of psoriasis. Pityriasis lichenoides has a more chronic and relapsing course, lacks a herald patch, has lesions in various stages, and involves the extremities more than classic PR. Lichen planus is usually more pruritic and chronic than PR, lacks collarette of scale, has a more violaceous color, and often prominently involves the distal extremities. Dermatophyte infection is particularly difficult to distinguish from the herald patch, especially when it presents in the folds, making mycologic investigations, such as potassium hydroxide examination, necessary to distinguish dermatophyte infection from herald patch. Skin biopsy often can help to differentiate the above conditions from PR, particularly in the atypical forms of PR.

Another entity commonly in the differential of PR that deserves special mention is secondary syphilis. The rash produced by each of these entities can be identical. Certain features that favor a diagnosis of syphilis include oral lesions, involvement of the palms and soles, and persistent lymphadenopathy. However, as noted above, all these features can be seen in PR, requiring serologic tests, starting with a rapid plasma reagin, to differentiate syphilis from PR. Because of this, some clinicians advocate checking a rapid plasma reagin in every patient suspected of having PR. In addition, one can look for other features of secondary syphilis, such as split papules, a "moth-eaten" appearing alopecia, and condyloma lata.

Many medications are also reported to cause a PR-like eruption and there is some debate over whether these cases represent a separate entity or if PR might be drug induced in some instances. Medications reported to cause such eruptions include barbiturates, captopril, clonidine, gold, metronidazole, D-penicillamine, isotretinoin, levamisole, nonsteroidal antiinflammatory agents, omeprazole, and terbinafine.[2] PR or PR-like rashes also have been described from the tyrosine kinase inhibitor imatinib and the tumor necrosis factor inhibitor adalimumab.[44-46] The development of a PR-like eruption from adalimumab is of particular interest as this medication dampens the T-helper 1 cell response, which is key in the body's defense against viral infections, and could therefore predispose to both viral infection or reactivation. The drug-induced PR-like eruptions are very similar to classic PR in appearance, but don't resolve unless the offending agent is stopped, often leaving more marked hyperpigmentation and frequently transitioning to a more lichenoid morphology.[2] The histopathology of a drug-induced PR-like eruption is also more likely to show interface dermatitis, dyskeratotic keratinocytes, and eosinophils.

CLINICAL COURSE AND PROGNOSIS

PR typically self-resolves after an average of 45 days, but ranges from 2 weeks to 5 months have been reported.[2,17] As previously stated, eruptions lasting longer than 3 months may fit into the proposed category of persistent PR. Upon resolution the only sequela is typically postinflammatory hyperpigmentation or hypopigmentation. As with other inflammatory conditions this dyspigmentation is more common in individuals with a darker skin color. There are no other significant long-term clinical outcomes from PR. As stated above, recurrence can occur, but it is very uncommon. When recurrence does happen, it is usually only once and also does not have any long-term health consequences.

MANAGEMENT

INTERVENTIONS

As discussed, PR is self-limited and therefore no treatment is necessary in many cases. Also given that many cases of PR have minimal to no symptoms the benefits of any treatment must be weighed against the potential side effects of the intervention on a case-by-case basis. Counseling patients on the natural history of PR and reassurance regarding its self-limited nature is paramount given the anxiety often associated with PR. Although there is no good data to support their use topical steroids and antihistamines are safe and may be helpful for associated pruritus. The macrolide erythromycin has been reported to hasten the clearance of PR.[16] In addition, a 2007 Cochrane review found one small, good-quality study that demonstrated benefit from erythromycin.[47] However, subsequent studies evaluating the efficacy of the macrolide antibiotics erythromycin and azithromycin failed to show any benefit when compared to placebo.[48-50] Acyclovir also has been studied as a potential therapy for PR. Drago and colleagues initially found that treatment with high-dose acyclovir (800 mg 5 times daily) for 1 week led to a 78.6% rate of complete clearance at 2 weeks compared to only a 4.4% rate of complete clearance in the placebo group, but this study was not randomized and the investigators were not blinded.[51] Several subsequent trials have all shown that acyclovir at varying doses may hasten the resolution of the rash, improve associated pruritus, and, in some cases, improve associated systemic symptoms.[52-55] Therefore, given the low cost and good safety profile of acyclovir and its derivatives, these therapeutic agents may be reasonable to consider in PR patients, particularly in those with significant pruritus, an extensive rash, or significant systemic symptoms. It should be noted that the mechanism of action of acyclovir in the treatment of PR is unclear given that acyclovir's effect is dependent on thymidine kinase, an enzyme whose gene is not expressed by HHV-7.[2] Ultraviolet B phototherapy also is reported to have some benefit in PR clearance time, although results vary on whether or not it helps with the associated pruritus.[56,57]

PREVENTION

There is currently no data available on prevention of PR.

ACKNOWLEDGMENTS

The authors acknowledge the contributions of Andrew Blauvelt, the former author of this chapter.

REFERENCES

1. Gibert CM. *Traité Pratique Des Maladies de La Peau et de La Syphilis, Volume 2*. H. Plon, Paris, France; 1860.
2. Drago F, Broccolo F, Rebora A. Pityriasis rosea: an update with a critical appraisal of its possible herpesviral etiology. *J Am Acad Dermatol*. 2009;61(2):303-318.
3. Broccolo F, Drago F, Careddu AM, et al. Additional evidence that pityriasis rosea is associated with reactivation of human herpesvirus-6 and -7. *J Invest Dermatol*. 2005;124(6):1234-1240.
4. Rebora A, Drago F, Broccolo F. Pityriasis rosea and herpesviruses: facts and controversies. *Clin Dermatol*. 2010;28(5):497-501.
5. Canpolat Kirac B, Adisen E, Bozdayi G, et al. The role of human herpesvirus 6, human herpesvirus 7, Epstein-Barr virus and cytomegalovirus in the aetiology of pityriasis rosea. *J Eur Acad Dermatol Venereol*. 2009;23(1):16-21.
6. Drago F, Ranieri E, Malaguti F, et al. Human herpesvirus 7 in patients with pityriasis rosea. *Dermatology*. 1997;195(4):374-378.
7. Chuang T-Y, Ilstrup DM, Perry H, et al. Pityriasis rosea in Rochester, Minnesota, 1969 to 1978. *J Am Acad Dermatol*. 1982;7(1):80-89.
8. Nanda A, Al-Hasawi F, Alsaleh QA. A prospective survey of pediatric dermatology clinic patients in Kuwait: an analysis of 10,000 cases. *Pediatr Dermatol*. 1999;16(1):6-11.
9. Harman M, Aytekin S, Akdeniz S, et al. An epidemiological study of pityriasis rosea in the Eastern Anatolia. *Eur J Epidemiol*. 1998;14(5):495-497.
10. Chuh A, Zawar V, Sciallis GF, et al. Pityriasis rosea, Gianotti-Crosti syndrome, asymmetric periflexural exanthem, papular-purpuric gloves and socks syndrome, eruptive pseudoangiomatosis, and eruptive hypomelanosis: do their epidemiological data substantiate infectious etiologies? *Infect Dis Rep*. 2016;8(1):6418.
11. Harvell JD, Selig DJ. Seasonal variations in dermatologic and dermatopathologic diagnoses: a retrospective 15-year analysis of dermatopathologic data. *Int J Dermatol*. 2016;55(10):1115-1118.
12. Chuh AAT, Molinari N, Sciallis G, et al. Temporal case clustering in pityriasis rosea: a regression analysis on 1379 patients in Minnesota, Kuwait, and Diyarbakir, Turkey. *Arch Dermatol*. 2005;141(6):767-771.
13. Chuh AAT, Lee A, Molinari N. Case clustering in pityriasis rosea: a multicenter epidemiologic study in primary care settings in Hong Kong. *Arch Dermatol*. 2003;139(4):489-493.
14. Gonzalez LM, Allen R, Janniger CK, et al. Pityriasis rosea: an important papulosquamous disorder. *Int J Dermatol*. 2005;44(9):757-764.
15. Drago F, Ciccarese G, Rebora A, et al. Relapsing pityriasis rosea. *Dermatology*. 2014;229(4):316-318.
16. Sharma PK, Yadav TP, Gautam RK, et al. Erythromycin in pityriasis rosea: a double-blind, placebo-controlled clinical trial. *J Am Acad Dermatol*. 2000;42(2, pt 1):241-244.
17. Drago F, Ciccarese G, Rebora A, et al. Pityriasis rosea: a comprehensive classification. *Dermatology*. 2016;232(4):431-437.
18. Drago F, Broccolo F, Ciccarese G, et al. Persistent pityriasis rosea: an unusual form of pityriasis rosea with persistent active HHV-6 and HHV-7 infection. *Dermatology*. 2015;230(1):23-26.
19. Drago F, Ciccarese G, Broccolo F, et al. Pityriasis rosea in children: clinical features and laboratory investigations. *Dermatology*. 2015;231(1):9-14.
20. Gündüz O, Ersoy-Evans S, Karaduman A. Childhood pityriasis rosea. *Pediatr Dermatol*. 26(6):750-751.
21. Vidimos AT, Camisa C. Tongue and cheek: oral lesions in pityriasis rosea. *Cutis*. 1992;50(4):276-280.
22. Kay MH, Rapini RP, Fritz KA, et al. Oral lesions in pityriasis rosea. *Arch Dermatol*. 1985;121(11):1449.
23. Ang C-C, Tay Y-K. Blaschkoid pityriasis rosea. *J Am Acad Dermatol*. 2009;61(5):906-908.
24. Deng Y, Li H, Chen X. Palmoplantar pityriasis rosea: two case reports. *J Eur Acad Dermatol Venereol*. 2007;21(3):406-407.
25. Kaymak Y, Taner E. Anxiety and depression in patients with pityriasis rosea compared to patients with tinea versicolor. *Dermatol Nurs*. 2008;20(5):367-370, 377.
26. Drago F, Broccolo F, Zaccaria E, et al. Pregnancy outcome in patients with pityriasis rosea. *J Am Acad Dermatol*. 2008;58(5)(suppl 1):S78-S83.
27. Drago F, Malaguti F, Ranieri E, et al. Human herpes virus-like particles in pityriasis rosea lesions: an electron microscopy study. *J Cutan Pathol*. 2002;29(6):359-361.
28. Watanabe T, Kawamura T, Jacob SE, et al. Pityriasis rosea is associated with systemic active infection with both human herpesvirus-7 and human herpesvirus-6. *J Invest Dermatol*. 2002;119(4):793-797.
29. Vág T, Sonkoly E, Kárpáti S, et al. Avidity of antibodies to human herpesvirus 7 suggests primary infection in young adults with pityriasis rosea. *J Eur Acad Dermatol Venereol*. 2004;18(6):738-740.
30. Chuh AAT, Chan HHL, Zawar V. Is human herpesvirus 7 the causative agent of pityriasis rosea?—A critical review. *Int J Dermatol*. 2004;43(12):870-875.
31. Kempf W, Adams V, Kleinhans M, et al. Pityriasis rosea is not associated with human herpesvirus 7. *Arch Dermatol*. 1999;135(9):1070-1072.
32. Kempf W, Burg G. Pityriasis rosea—a virus-induced skin disease? An update. *Arch Virol*. 2000;145(8):1509-1520.
33. Kosuge H, Tanaka-Taya K, Miyoshi H, et al. Epidemiological study of human herpesvirus-6 and human herpesvirus-7 in pityriasis rosea. *Br J Dermatol*. 2000;143(4):795-798.
34. Wong WR, Tsai CY, Shih SR, et al. Association of pityriasis rosea with human herpesvirus-6 and human herpesvirus-7 in Taipei. *J Formos Med Assoc*. 2001;100(7):478-483.

35. Yasukawa M, Sada E, MacHino H, et al. Reactivation of human herpesvirus 6 in pityriasis rosea. *Br J Dermatol*. 1999;140(1):169-170.
36. Levy JA, Ferro F, Greenspan D, et al. Frequent isolation of HHV-6 from saliva and high seroprevalence of the virus in the population. *Lancet*. 1990;335(8697):1047-1050.
37. Ablashi DV, Berneman ZN, Kramarsky B, et al. Human herpesvirus-7 (HHV-7): current status. *Clin Diagn Virol*. 1995;4(1):1-13.
38. Guarneri F, Cannavó SP, Minciullo PL, et al. Pityriasis rosea of Gibert: immunological aspects. *J Eur Acad Dermatol Venereol*. 2015;29(1):21-25.
39. Neoh CY, Tan AWH, Mohamed K, et al. Characterization of the inflammatory cell infiltrate in herald patches and fully developed eruptions of pityriasis rosea. *Clin Exp Dermatol*. 2010;35(3):300-304.
40. Drago F, Ciccarese G, Broccolo F, et al. The role of cytokines, chemokines, and growth factors in the pathogenesis of pityriasis rosea. *Mediators Inflamm*. 2015;2015:438963.
41. Chuh A. Diagnostic criteria for pityriasis rosea: a prospective case control study for assessment of validity. *J Eur Acad Dermatol Venereol*. 2003;17(1):101-103.
42. Zawar V, Chuh A. Applicability of proposed diagnostic criteria of pityriasis rosea: Results of a prospective case-control study in India. *Indian J Dermatol*. 2013;58(6):439.
43. Hussein MRA, Abdel-Magid WM, Saleh R, et al. Phenotypical characteristics of the immune cells in allergic contact dermatitis, atopic dermatitis and pityriasis rosea. *Pathol Oncol Res*. 2009;15(1):73-79.
44. Rajpara SN, Ormerod AD, Gallaway L. Adalimumab-induced pityriasis rosea. *J Eur Acad Dermatol Venereol*. 2007;21(9):1294-1296.
45. Cho AY, Kim DH, Im M, et al. Pityriasis rosea-like drug eruption induced by imatinib mesylate (Gleevec). *Ann Dermatol*. 2011;23(suppl 3):S360-S363.
46. Verma P, Singal A, Sharma S. Imatinib mesylate-induced cutaneous rash masquerading as pityriasis rosea of gilbert. *Indian J Dermatol*. 2014;59(3):311-312.
47. Chuh AAT, Dofitas BL, Comisel GG, et al. Interventions for pityriasis rosea. *Cochrane Database Syst Rev*. 2007;(2):CD005068.
48. Rasi A, Tajziehchi L, Savabi-Nasab S. Oral erythromycin is ineffective in the treatment of pityriasis rosea. *J Drugs Dermatol*. 2008;7(1):35-38.
49. Pandhi D, Singal A, Verma P, et al. The efficacy of azithromycin in pityriasis rosea: a randomized, double-blind, placebo-controlled trial. *Indian J Dermatol Venereol Leprol*. 2014;80(1):36.
50. Amer A, Fischer H. Azithromycin does not cure pityriasis rosea. *Pediatrics*. 2006;117(5):1702-1705.
51. Drago F, Vecchio F, Rebora A. Use of high-dose acyclovir in pityriasis rosea. *J Am Acad Dermatol*. 2006;54(1):82-85.
52. Das A, Sil A, Das NK, et al. Acyclovir in pityriasis rosea: An observer-blind, randomized controlled trial of effectiveness, safety and tolerability. *Indian Dermatol Online J*. 2015;6(3):181-184.
53. Ganguly S. A randomized, double-blind, placebo-controlled study of efficacy of oral acyclovir in the treatment of pityriasis rosea. *J Clin Diagn Res*. 2014;8(5):YC01-YC04.
54. Noormohammadpour P, Toosi S, Hosseinpour A, et al. The comparison between the efficacy of high dose acyclovir and erythromycin on the period and signs of pityriasis rosea. *Indian J Dermatol*. 2010;55(3):246.
55. Rassai S, Feily A, Sina N, et al. Low dose of acyclovir may be an effective treatment against pityriasis rosea: a random investigator-blind clinical trial on 64 patients. *J Eur Acad Dermatol Venereol*. 2011;25(1):24-26.
56. Jairath V, Mohan M, Jindal N, et al. Narrowband UVB phototherapy in pityriasis rosea. *Indian Dermatol Online J*. 6(5):326-329.
57. Leenutaphong V, Jiamton S. UVB phototherapy for pityriasis rosea: a bilateral comparison study. *J Am Acad Dermatol*. 1995;33(6):996-999.

Lichenoid and Granulomatous Disorders

PART 5

第五篇　苔藓样皮炎和肉芽肿性皮炎

Chapter 32 :: Lichen Planus
:: Aaron R. Mangold & Mark R. Pittelkow

第三十二章
扁平苔藓

中文导读

　　本章介绍了扁平苔藓的病理生理、流行病学史、临床特点、诊断和治疗。在临床特点方面主要介绍了扁平苔藓所累及的器官，并着重介绍了该病的皮肤表现，也介绍了扁平苔藓一些特殊类型的临床特点。诊断方面：详细阐述了扁平苔藓的临床特点以及组织病理、免疫荧光的特点，也配了图片说明。对于鉴别诊断列出了表格说明。治疗上，介绍了扁平苔藓及变异性扁平苔藓的治疗方法，包括系统治疗和局部治疗，为本病提供了全面的诊疗参考。

〔李芳芳〕

AT-A-GLANCE

- Lichen planus is an idiopathic T cell–mediated process without a clear autoantigen.
- The worldwide prevalence of lichen planus is approximately 1%.
- The lesions are well-marginated, flat-topped, red-violet polygonal papules.
- The distribution is symmetrical and grouped lesions affect the flexural aspects of the arms and legs.
- Variants are based on configuration, morphology of lesion, and site of involvement.
- Histology shows basal keratinocyte damage with a lymphocyte-rich interface reaction.

INTRODUCTION

Lichen planus (Greek *leichen*, "tree moss"; Latin *planus*, "flat") is a common inflammatory condition that can affect any ectodermal-derived tissue. Both Hebra and Erasmus Wilson described a similar inflammatory papulosquamous eruption, lichen ruber and lichen planus, respectively, which likely represented the same entity.[1] Weyl and Wickham elaborated upon the morphology of lichen planus, and Gougerot and Burnier described disease involvement of mucosal sites.[2-4] Although no single feature of lichen planus is a sine qua non, classic lichen planus is typified clinically by "the four Ps"—(1) purple, (2) polygonal, (3) pruritic, and (4) papules—and histologically by a brisk lymphocytic interface reaction.

PATHOGENESIS

The pathogenesis of lichen planus is unknown. Many contributing factors are implicated and include infectious, immune, metabolic, and genetic causes. It is evident that specific immunologic mechanisms control the development of lichen planus. T cell–mediated pathologic alterations involving proinflammatory and counterregulatory mechanisms function in the pathogenesis of lichen planus. No consistent alterations in immunoglobulins have been shown in lichen planus, and humoral immunity most likely is a secondary response in immunopathogenesis. Cell-mediated immunity, on the other hand, plays a major role in lichen planus. One consistent feature of lichen planus is CD4-positive T-helper (CD4-Th) cells in the dermis despite disease chronicity and CD8-positive T-cytotoxic (CD8-Tc) cells in close proximity to damaged basal keratinocytes.[5] Based on these observations and insights from other lichenoid tissue reactions (LTRs), such as graft-versus-host-disease (GVHD), modern theories encompass three major stages: antigen recognition, lymphocyte activation, and keratinocyte apoptosis. A fourth stage, resolution, is a new and emerging facet of the disease to further understand the pathogenesis of lichen planus.

ANTIGEN RECOGNITION

The CD8-Tc cell is the effector cell of lichen planus; however, the initial antigen recognition and CD8-Tc stimulation may be driven by the initial interaction between the CD4-Th cell with the Langerhans cell (LC). The targeted antigen(s) and trigger(s) for lichen planus remains unknown. However, in other similar diseases, such as lichenoid GVHD, the target antigens are alloantigens. In oral disease, a lichen planus–specific antigen associated with major histocompatibility complex (MHC) class I on keratinocytes has been reported.[6] It is unknown if this antigen is unique to oral lichen planus and if this antigen is an autoreactive peptide or an exogenous antigen. Circulating antibodies have also been identified in multiple studies without a clear target antigen.[7,8] A small but significant population of CD 56–positive CD 16–negative natural killer (NK) cells are observed early in the disease course of lichen planus.[9] These cells express chemokine receptor-3 (CXCR-3) and chemokine (c-c) motif ligand (CCL) -5 and -6 and release interferon-γ (IFN-γ) and tumor necrosis factor-α (TNF-α).[9] Taken together, NK cells may migrate to the site of inflammation and provide an early stimulating signal for the recruitment of CD4-Th and CD8-Tc cells.

The CD4-Th population is localized to the dermis with scattered cells in the epidermis. CD4-Th cells colocalize with the LCs. LCs are the principal antigen-presenting cells of the epidermis and they upregulate MHC class II receptors in lichenoid disease, which allows for an interaction between CD4-Th cells and keratinocytes.[10] In particular, CD4-positive LCs are seen in close approximation with the HLA-DR–positive keratinocytes.[11] In addition, the CD4-Th cells have restricted V-β gene expression, which suggests antigen-specific oligoclonal T-cell expansion.[12,13] Upon costimulation by LCs, CD4-Th cells release inflammatory cytokines, including IFN-γ, which leads to CD8-Tc activation and additional oligoclonal expansion.[14] Taken together, these findings suggest an integral role of LCs, keratinocytes, and CD4 T helper cells in antigen presentation as well as the initiation and propagation of the Th1 response via the production of IFN-γ.

The nature of antigenic stimulation is not known. Contact sensitizers such as metals could act as haptens and elicit an immunologic response. Enhanced lymphocyte reactivity to inorganic mercury, a component of dental amalgam, has been found in patients with oral LTRs. Low-grade chronic exposure to mercury, and possibly to other metals such as gold, may stimulate a lymphocytic reaction that manifests as lichen planus. A list of contact chemicals and drugs that can elicit lichenoid reactions is discussed in the section "Drug-Induced Lichen Planus." With more widespread use of biologics, specifically TNF-α inhibitors, for the treatment of various chronic inflammatory diseases, cases of TNF-α associated LTRs have been identified and implicate dysregulated cytokine production, including the upregulation of type I IFN.[15] Microbial mediators in the development of lichen planus have elicited recurring debate. Although provocative, no conclusive evidence has molecularly linked lichen planus to any of the following infections or colonization: syphilis, herpes simplex virus 2, human immunodeficiency virus (HIV), amebiasis, chronic bladder infections, hepatitis C virus (HCV), *Helicobacter pylori*, or human papillomavirus (HPV).

LYMPHOCYTE ACTIVATION

As mentioned in the prior section, following antigen recognition, CD8-Tc cells are activated and undergo oligoclonal expansion. A cascade of both pro- and antiinflammatory cytokines is released, including interleukin (IL)-2, -4, and -10; IFN-γ; TNF-α; and transforming growth factor-β1 (TGF-β1).[16,17] In lichen planus, the balance between lymphocyte activation, downregulation, and the cytokine milieu determines the disease phenotype.

IFN-γ plays a central role in lichen planus. IFN-γ induces the expression of inflammatory chemokines such as chemokine ligand (CXCL)-9, -10, and -11.[18-20] CXCR-3, their matching receptor, is predominantly expressed on the surface of IFN-γ–producing CD4-Th cells.[19-22] Peroxisome-proliferator-activated receptor γ (PPARγ) inhibits CXCL-10 and -11, and its loss may be an underlying driver result in scarring alopecia.[23,24] IFN-γ increases peripheral blood mononuclear cell (PBMC) binding to HLA-DR–positive keratinocytes.[19] Intercellular adhesion molecule 1 and vascular cell adhesion molecule expression is also enhanced by IFN-γ.[21] Therefore, IFN-γ is fundamentally involved in the upregulation of cellular adhesion molecules and subsequent migration of lymphocytes to the dermal–epidermal junction (DEJ).[25,26]

KERATINOCYTE APOPTOSIS

CD8-Tc cells are likely the terminal effector cells in lichen planus. They colocalize with apoptotic keratinocytes and have in vitro cytotoxic activity against autologous keratinocytes.[6,27] The cytotoxic effects of the CD8-Tc cells can be inhibited by blockade of the MHC class I domain.[6] The exact mechanism of apoptosis in lichen planus remains unknown. The possible mechanisms include granzyme B release, TNF-α–TNF-α R1 receptor interaction, and Fas–Fas-L interaction. Granzyme B and granulysin are expressed at 100- to 200-fold higher levels in lichen planus relative to normal skin.[28] Granzyme B, excreted by CD8-Tc cells, activates caspase-3 and promotes apoptosis.[29] TNF-α upregulates the expression of matrix metalloproteinase-9 (MMP-9) in lesional T lymphocytes of oral lichen planus and leads to disruption of the basement membrane and damage to basilar keratinocytes.[30] MMP-9 levels correlate with the phenotype, with high levels correlating with ulcerative disease.[31] Taken together, MMP-9 likely disrupts the basement membrane homeostasis, blocking normal cell survival signaling and leads to apoptosis and cell death. Fas–Fas-L expression is elevated in oral lichen planus, correlates with disease progression, and likely contributes to apoptosis of keratinocytes.[32-34]

RESOLUTION

Lichen planus tends to be a self-resolving disease; however, there is a paucity of research into the resolution phase of disease. T-regulatory cells are seen in oral lichen planus and correlate with disease subtype and activity.[35,36] Studies in acute GVHD have shown the central role of T-regulatory cells in disrupting dendritic cell (DC) and allogeneic T-cell interactions[37] and prevents disease development. DCs have a complex role in lichen planus and are involved in T-cell migration, as well as, the modulation of inflammatory signals.[38,39] Fas-L, granzyme B, and perforin can be expressed by keratinocytes, allowing for apoptosis of lymphocytes.[40,41] Further understanding of the resolution phase of LTRs should lead to development of novel targeted therapies.

GENETIC AND EPIGENETIC REGULATION

The immune system targets various naturally occurring, but potentially deleterious, antigens (ie, viruses and bacteria, malignant cells, and exogenous contactants).[42] However, the generation of an immune response to exogenous antigens poses a risk for the development of cross-reactivity to self-antigens.[43,44] Genetic polymorphisms have been implicated in the risk of development of lichen planus, including HLA, immune signaling molecules and receptors (IFN-γ, TNF-α, TNF-α R2, IL-4, IL-6, and IL-18), oxidative stress, prostaglandin E_2 synthesis, formation of transglutaminase, thyroid hormone synthesis, prothrombin, and nuclear factor kappa B (NF-κB) as well as epigenetic regulation of genes by micro-RNA (miRNA)-146a and -155.[45] These polymorphisms may regulate the activity of proinflammatory mediators and lead to aberrant signaling. Gene expression profiling of lichen planus, identified the expression of the CXCR-3 ligand, CXCL-9, as the most specific marker for lichen planus.[46] In addition, keratinocytes were confirmed as a source of type I IFNs (-α and -β).[46]

EPIDEMIOLOGY

The exact incidence and prevalence of lichen planus are unknown. Additionally, most large, epidemiologic studies of lichen planus focus on the prevalence of oral disease or cutaneous disease and few include the ectodermal (skin, hair, nail, and mucous membranes) spectrum of lichen planus. Therefore, the 1% prevalence of lichen planus in the general population should be interpreted with caution.[47] The prevalence of lichen planus varies geographically with a range from 0.1% to 4%. Nearly two thirds of cases of lichen planus present between the ages of 30 and 60 years with a peak onset between 55 and 74 years.[48] lichen planus is less common at the extremes of age. There is no clear sexual or racial predilection in lichen planus; however, the age of onset is earlier in women.[47-49]

Childhood lichen planus accounts for only 1% to 5% of the total lichen planus cases in the general population. In Pacific Indians, childhood lichen planus is more common and accounts for nearly 20% of all cases.[50] In the United States, childhood lichen planus may be slightly more common in African Americans. Much like adult lichen planus, there is no clear sexual predilection in childhood lichen planus. The peak onset of disease is between 8 and 12 years of age.[50-53]

Fewer than 100 cases of familial lichen planus have been reported. However, a strong family history has been reported in 1.5% of adult cases and 3.8% of pediatric cases.[50,54] Familial forms are characterized by early onset, widespread and often erosive or ulcerative disease, mucosal involvement, and frequent relapses.[55,56] The atypical nature of familial lichen planus has led some to consider it a unique dermatosis. Multiple HLA haplotypes have been reported in familial lichen planus, including HLA-B27, Aw19, -B18, and -Cw8. In nonfamilial cases, HLA-A3, -A5, -A28, -B8, -B16, and Bw35 are more common.[57] HLA-B8 is more common in patients with oral lichen planus alone, and HLA-Bw35 is more common with cutaneous lichen planus alone.

CLINICAL FEATURES

Although lichen planus most commonly involves the skin and oral mucosa, any ectodermal-derived tissue may be affected, including hair, nails, internal and external genitalia, eyes, and esophagus. For this reason, a detailed history and physical examination is required to guide appropriate therapy, referrals, and monitoring. The skin lesions of lichen planus typically develop over the course of weeks. The disease duration is dependent on the location of the lesions, lesion morphology, and histologic pattern.

CUTANEOUS FINDINGS

The classic cutaneous lesions of lichen planus are well-marginated, dull red-violet, flat-topped, polygonal papules. The papules are grouped and often coalesce into plaques. Wickham striae, fine, white and adherent reticulate scale, are noted in well-developed lesions (Fig. 32-1). Wickham striae are highly characteristic in lichen planus and are more easily visualized with dermoscopy. The characteristic clinical and dermoscopic features of lichen planus correlate with the characteristic histological findings of lichen planus. Wickham striae correlate with orthokeratosis, epidermal thickening, and an increased granular layer. The dull red-violet color correlates with the combination of vascular dilation and pigment incontinence. The lesions of lichen planus are often symmetrically distributed over the over the extremities. The most common areas of involvement are the flexural wrists, arms, and legs. The proximal thighs, trunk, and neck are other common sites of involvement. Involvement of the face and palms are atypical for classic lichen planus. Inverse lichen planus (discussed below) commonly involves the axillae, groin, and inframammary region.

Lichen planus tends to be extremely pruritic. The degree of pruritus appears to directly correlate with the extent of involvement with the most symptomatic disease in generalized lichen planus. One major exception is hypertrophic lichen planus, which often affects limited areas, such as the lower extremities, and is extremely pruritic.

In the acute setting, lichen planus exhibits an isomorphic (Koebner) phenomenon in which trauma induces disease (Fig. 32-2). This phenomenon is now explained by trauma-induced exposure of plasmacytoid DCs to endogenous peptides, such as cathelicidin LL-37, and endogenous antigens, such as DNA and RNA, which stimulate the release of type I IFNs (-α and -β), which propagates disease.[58] Lichen planus usually heals with postinflammatory

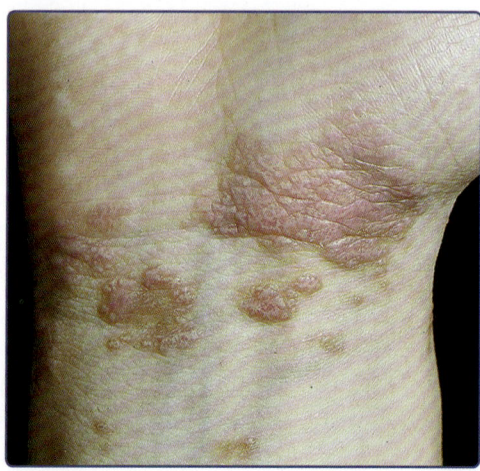

Figure 32-1 Lichen planus. Flat-topped, polygonal, sharply defined papules of violaceous color, grouped and confluent. The surface is shiny and reveals fine white lines (Wickham striae). Note the hyperpigmentation of resolving lesions. (Used with permission from Mayo Foundation for Medical Education and Research, all rights reserved.)

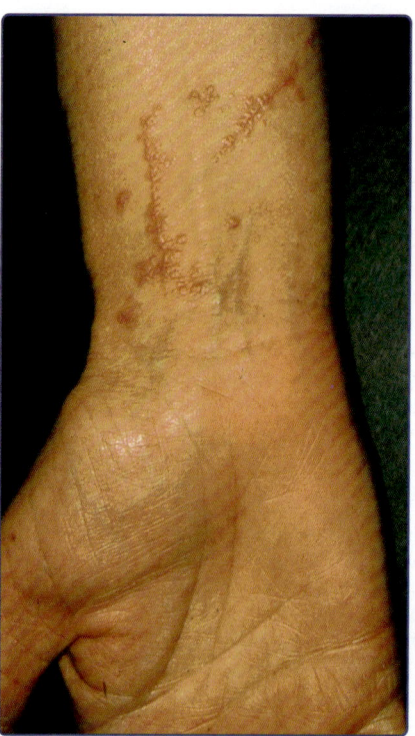

Figure 32-2 Koebnerization. Linear pattern with a Koebner response adjacent to clustered papules on the flexural wrist. (Used with permission from Mayo Foundation for Medical Education and Research, all rights reserved.)

hyperpigmentation, which is more common in darker skinned individuals. Hypopigmentation is uncommon in lichen planus, and its presence should prompt consideration of an alternative diagnosis.

Frequent reports of childhood lichen planus have come from the Indian subcontinent.[50-52] The explanation of such a phenomenon may be multifactorial, including genetic susceptibility, infectious exposure, and social stigma associated with pigmentary changes. In support of the social implications of pigmentary changes, the largest study of childhood lichen planus in the United States found a predominance in African American children.[53] The clinical and histological features of childhood lichen planus are similar to adult lichen planus with skin and oral involvement in 42% to 60% and 17% to 30% of cases, respectively.[50-53] However, hair involvement and nail involvement is rare in 2% to 6% and 0% to 19% of cases, respectively.[50-53]

CLINICAL VARIANTS

Many variations in the clinical presentation of lichen planus have been described and are most easily categorized by the configuration of lesions, the morphologic appearance, and the site of involvement (Table 32-1). Although there may be significant variation in the presentation of specific subtypes of lichen planus, there are often morphological clues of an LTR. The underlying mechanisms driving these clinical variants are unknown; however, akin to psoriasis, these variations are likely caused by genetic polymorphisms and environmental stimuli.

CONFIGURATION

Annular Lichen Planus: Annular lesions occur in approximately 10% of lichen planus and commonly develop as an arcuate grouping of individual papules of lichen planus that coalesce to form a ring or expand centrifugally with a central clearing. Annular lesions are more common on the penis and scrotum (Fig. 32-3). Additionally, large lesions often appear annular because of central resolution and hyperpigmentation with an active, raised rim. Actinic lichen planus is seen in subtropical zones on sun-exposed, dark-skinned young adults and children, is frequently annular in shape.

Linear, Blaschkoid, and Zosteriform Lichen Planus: Papules of lichen planus may develop in a linear pattern secondary to trauma. Rarely, in fewer than 0.2% of lichen planus cases, the eruption may follow lines of Blaschko. Similar to other segmental diseases, the etiology is thought to be related to postzygotic, somatic mutations in susceptibility-associated genes.[59] Zosteriform and linear lichen planus were thought to be the same disease; however, a recent study of zosteriform lichen planus found varicella zoster antigens exclusively in zosteriform lichen planus suggesting either a viral trigger of disease or an isotopic response related to underlying resident memory cells.[60] Therefore, the term *linear lichen planus* should only be used when dermatomal lines are not followed. It is important to differentiate linear and zosteriform lichen

TABLE 32-1
Clinical Subtypes of Lichen Planus

SUBTYPES	MOST COMMON SITES OF INVOLVEMENT
Cutaneous Lichen Planus	
Actinic	Sun-exposed areas
Annular	Male genitalia, intertriginous areas
Atrophic	Predominantly on lower extremities, may occur on other areas of the body
Erosive	Soles of the feet
Guttate	Trunk
Hypertrophic	Anterior legs, ankles, interphalangeal joints
Linear	Lower extremities
Follicular	Trunk and proximal extremities
Papular	Flexural surfaces
Bullous	Feet
Pigmentosus	Sun-exposed areas
Pigmentosus inversus	Intertriginous and flexural areas
Nail	Fingernails > toenails
Palmoplantar	Malleoli Palms Soles
Lichen planopilaris	Classic: vertex scalp Frontal fibrosing alopecia Graham-Little-Piccardi-Lasseur syndrome
Mucosal Lichen Planus	
Oral	
Reticular	Buccal mucosa and mucobuccal folds
Atrophic	Attached gingiva
Hypertrophic	Buccal mucosa
Erosive	Lateral and ventral tongue Buccal mucosa
Bullous	Posterior and inferior areas of the buccal mucosa
Plaque-like	Dorsum of tongue and buccal mucosa
Vulvovaginal	Vaginal introitus, clitoral hood, labia minora, labia majora, vagina
Esophageal	Proximal esophagus Proximal and distal esophagus Distal esophagus
Special Forms	
Drug induced	Sun-exposed areas, lacks oral involvement
Lichen planus–lupus erythematosus overlap	Distal extremities, sun exposed
Lichen planus pemphigoides	Extremities

Adapted with permission from Gorouhi F, Davari P, Fazel N. Cutaneous and mucosal lichen planus: a comprehensive review of clinical subtypes, risk factors, diagnosis, and prognosis. *Scientific World Journal.* 2014;2014:742826.

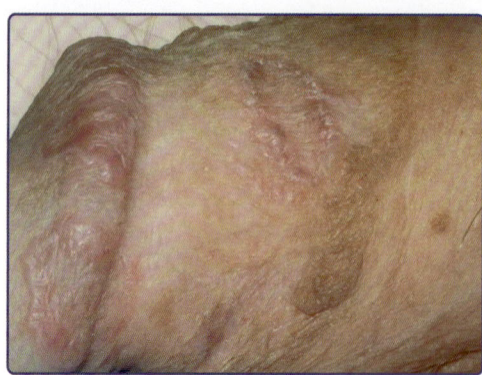

Figure 32-3 Annular lichen planus. Violaceous, annular lesions involving the corona and body of the penis. (Used with permission from Mayo Foundation for Medical Education and Research, all rights reserved.)

planus from other segmental diseases, including lichen striatus, linear epidermal nevus, inflammatory linear and verrucal epidermal nevus, linear psoriasis, and linear Darier disease.

MORPHOLOGY OF LESIONS

Hypertrophic Lichen Planus: Hypertrophic lichen planus occurs most commonly on the anterior shins and interphalangeal joints (Fig. 32-4). Additionally, hypertrophic lichen planus tends to be highly pruritic, refractory to treatment, and associated with relapse. The primary lesions are thickened, elevated, purple-red, hyperkeratotic plaques and nodules. Verrucal lesions may develop, which can simulate keratinocyte carcinomas, rupioid psoriasis, rupioid syphilis, reactive arthropathy, and cutaneous lupus erythematosus. The lesions of hypertrophic lichen planus may show follicular accentuation, elevation, and chalk-like scale. Chronic venous insufficiency is commonly among individuals with hypertrophic lichen planus.

Atrophic Lichen Planus: The atrophic variant of lichen planus is characterized by oligo-lesional disease with well-marginated, blue-white papules or plaques with central atrophy.[49] Early lesions are often a few millimeters in diameter but may coalesce into larger plaques. Atrophic lichen planus is most common on the proximal lower extremity and trunk. The two clinical entities in the differential diagnosis are lichen sclerosus et atrophicus and mycosis fungoides (MF). The histopathology may be subtle and has led some to believe that atrophic lichen planus occurs in late-stage resolved disease and is not a true variant of lichen planus.

Vesiculobullous Lichen Planus: Vesiculobullous lesions in lichen planus are rare. They occur secondary to an exuberant inflammatory response and an exaggerated Max-Joseph space. This is in contrast to lichen planus pemphigoides, which has classic lesions of lichen planus separated from lesions of bullous pemphigoid and positive bullous pemphigoid

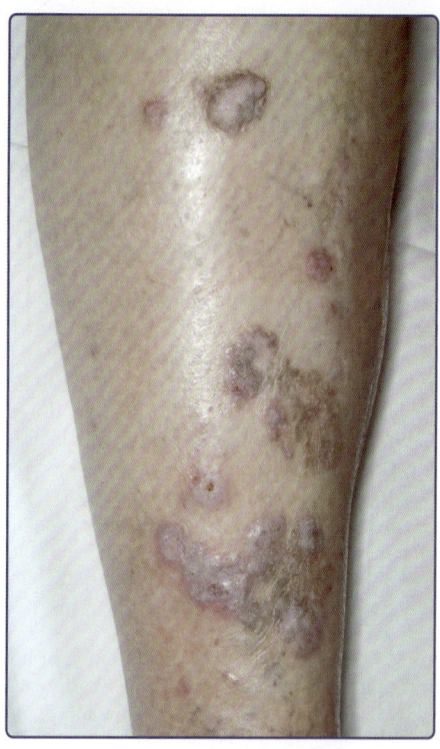

Figure 32-4 Hypertrophic lichen planus. Well-marginated, acanthotic and papillomatous, dull-violet plaques are noted over the anterior shin. Areas of postinflammatory hyperpigmentation as well as superficial varicosities, signifying venous stasis, are noted. (Used with permission from Mayo Foundation for Medical Education and Research, all rights reserved.)

antibodies (BP 180 and 230) and immunofluorescence. Vesiculobullous lesions on the skin are more common on the lower extremities (Fig. 32-5) and tend to occur in acute flares of lichen planus. The disease course is similar to that of classic lichen planus. Oral vesiculobullous disease is often symptomatic and leads to erosion and ulceration.

Erosive and Ulcerative Lichen Planus: Erosive and ulcerative cutaneous disease is more common on the feet (Fig. 32-6) and oral cavity and is associated with significant pain and scarring.[61] Patients often

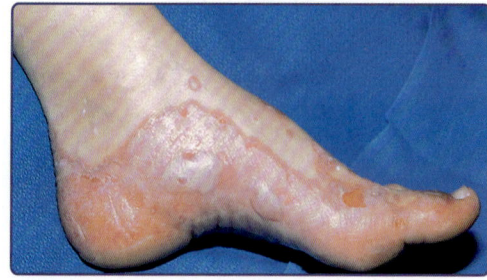

Figure 32-5 Vesiculobullous lichen planus. Vesicles and bullae with violaceous-erythematous papules and plaques on the foot. (Used with permission from Mayo Foundation for Medical Education and Research, all rights reserved.)

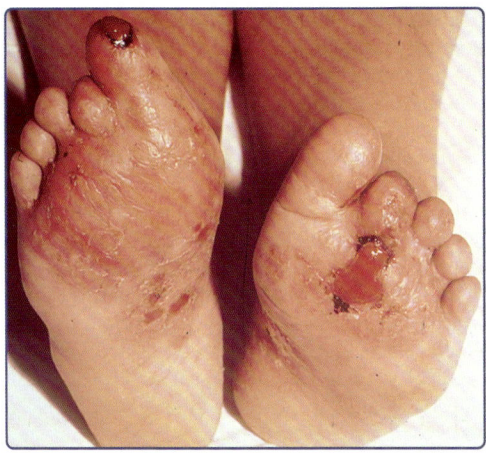

Figure 32-6 Erosive–ulcerative lichen planus. Erosions, ulcers, and granulation tissue and scarring of toes, interdigital web spaces, and soles. (Used with permission from Mayo Foundation for Medical Education and Research, all rights reserved.)

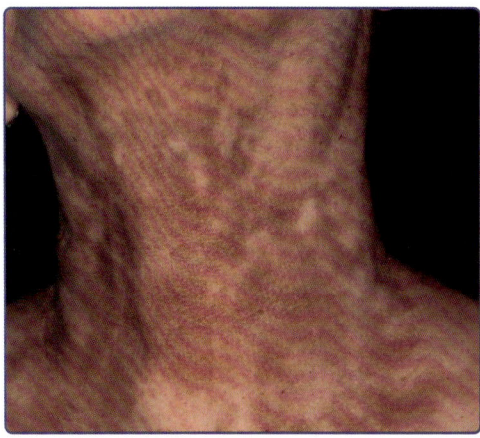

Figure 32-7 Lichen planus pigmentosus. Multiple, well-marginated, hyperpigmented, dark-brown macules located along the neck, with sparing of the face. The macules coalesce to form a slightly retiform pattern. This patient had involvement of the intertriginous regions and negative patch testing results. (Used with permission from Mayo Foundation for Medical Education and Research, all rights reserved.)

have other ectodermal involvement, which aids in the diagnosis. Scarring alopecia and loss of the toenails are common. Squamous cell carcinoma (SCC) has been described in chronic lesions of ulcerative oral lichen planus.

Follicular Lichen Planus: Follicular lichen planus may occur alone or in association with other cutaneous or mucosal forms of lichen planus.[62] Follicular lichen planus occurs most commonly on the scalp and occurs in three distinct variants, including lichen planopilaris, frontal fibrosing alopecia, and Gram-Little-Piccardi-Lassueur syndrome (GLPLS) (see the discussion of lichen planus of the scalp). Rare reported cases of lichen planus follicularis tumidus, which is characterized clinically by pruritic, red-violet pseudo-tumoral facial and posterior auricular plaques with yellow cysts.[63] Lichen planus follicularis tumidus cases often have signs of lichen planus elsewhere. The diagnosis of lichen planus follicularis tumidus should be made with caution and folliculotropic MF, and cutaneous lupus erythematosus should be considered in the differential diagnosis.

Lichen Planus Pigmentosus: Lichen planus pigmentosus is characterized by hyperpigmented, dark-brown macules in sun-exposed and flexural folds (Fig. 32-7). Lichen planus pigmentosus is more common in darker skinned individuals. Histologically, there are epidermal atrophy, a lymphocyte poor LTR, and pigment incontinence. Lichen planus pigmentosus and ashy dermatosis, or erythema dyschromicum perstans, have significant overlapping features and likely represent a phenotypic spectrum based on genetic and environmental factors.

Actinic Lichen Planus: Actinic lichen planus was first described in subtropical countries.[64] Actinic lichen planus affects young individuals of Middle Eastern descent and is most common in the spring and summer months.[65-68] There is a predilection for the face; however, the dorsal hands, arms, and nape of the neck are also affected.[68] The primary lesions are annular well-marginated, hyperpigmented brown-violet, flat-topped, plaques with a slightly rolled border.[66] The lesions are minimally symptomatic, and more classic lesions of lichen planus may be seen in non–photo-exposed areas. The histopathology is characterized by a more brisk LTR relative to lichen planus pigmentosus, vacuolar changes, and pigment incontinence.[68]

SITE OF INVOLVEMENT

Lichen Planus of the Scalp: Lichen planopilaris, or follicular lichen planus, is a distinct clinical and histologic entity with a female predominance. There are three distinct follicular variants of lichen planus on the scalp, including lichen planopilaris, frontal fibrosing alopecia, and GLPLS. In classic lichen planopilaris, individual keratotic follicular papules form plaques on the scalp with associated scarring alopecia. Classic lichen planopilaris affects the vertex scalp and consists of diffuse erythema with perifollicular hyperkeratosis and livid erythema (Fig. 32-8A).[69] Dermoscopy can aid in the diagnosis of early scarring lichen planopilaris. Dermoscopic features of lichen planopilaris include absence of follicular opening, cicatricial white patches, peripilar casts and perifollicular scale, blue-gray dots, perifollicular erythema, and polytrichia (two or three hairs) (Fig. 32-8B).[70] Most active lesions are found within the hair-bearing areas at the edge of the alopecic patch. The scarring alopecia may be unilesional or multifocal with severe cases resulting in near-total scalp involvement. Lichen planopilaris, as well as frontal fibrosing alopecia and GLPLS, often has a significant psychological impact on affected individuals.

Frontal fibrosing alopecia was once considered an uncommon condition characterized by progressive frontotemporal recession caused by inflammatory destruction of the hair follicles (Fig. 32-8C). Up to 75% of women with frontal fibrosing alopecia report concomitant loss of the eyebrows, which tends to be noninflammatory.[71] The number of cases of frontal fibrosing alopecia has increased dramatically in recent years. Leave-on facial products, including sunscreen, and positive patch test results to fragrances are more common in individuals with frontal fibrosing alopecia.[72] Frontal fibrosing alopecia is more common in postmenopausal women but can occur in younger women as well. The disease is characterized by slow progression of frontal hairline recession over years.

GLPLS is a rare subtype characterized by cicatricial alopecia of the scalp, nonscarring alopecia of the axilla and groin, and follicular papules on the trunk and extremities.[73]

Pseudopelade of Brocq is a rare clinical syndrome of scarring alopecia and fibrosis, in which distinct pathologic features are absent. It is generally accepted that pseudopelade of Brocq is the end stage of follicular fibrosis caused by a primary inflammatory dermatosis such as lichen planus, lupus erythematosus, pustular scarring forms of folliculitis, fungal infections, scleroderma, and sarcoidosis.

Mucosal Lichen Planus: Lichen planus can affect any mucosal surface and most commonly involves the mouth or genitalia. Its prevalence is estimated at approximately 1% of the adult population.[47] Oral involvement occurs in approximately 60% to 70% of patients with lichen planus and may be the only manifestation in 20% to 30% of patients.[49,54,74-76] Multiple types of oral lichen planus have been described, including reticular, plaque-like, atrophic, papular, erosive or ulcerative, and bullous forms (Fig. 32-9). The reticular form of oral lichen planus is the most common and is often asymptomatic. The buccal mucosa is the most common site of involvement followed by the tongue and gingiva. Erosive and ulcerative oral lichen planus is most on the tongue, is extremely painful, and thus is commonly reported in the literature.[77] Gingival involvement may take the form of gingival stomatitis or desquamative gingivitis and is the sole manifestation in 8% of oral lichen planus. On the other hand, oral lichen planus is the most common cause of desquamative gingivitis, accounting for 75% of cases.[78]

Oral lichenoid reactions (OLRs) are similar clinically and histologically to oral lichen planus; however, with an identifiable cause. Differentiating these two entities clinically is often difficult. OLRs are usually seen on the buccal mucosa adjacent to amalgam dental fillings (Fig. 32-10).[79] Patch tests frequently show positive reactions to mercury, gold, and other metals.[80-82] Interestingly, patients with an OLR, no cutaneous lichen planus, and negative patch test results often improve with removal of amalgams.[83] This brings into question if amalgams are a bona fide hapten response or represent a special site irritant reaction, which leads to koebnerization.[84,85]

A unique lichenoid eruption has been described on the tongues of individuals with HIV. This reaction is

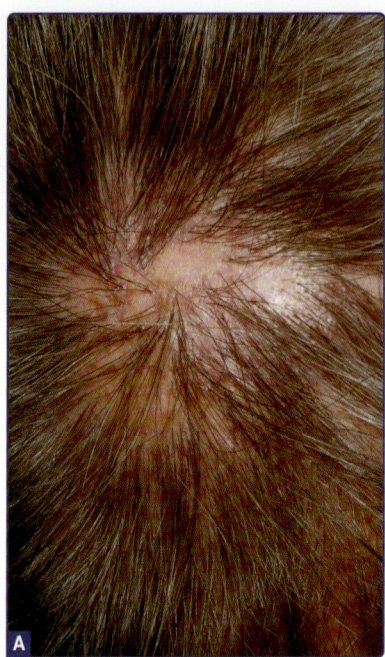

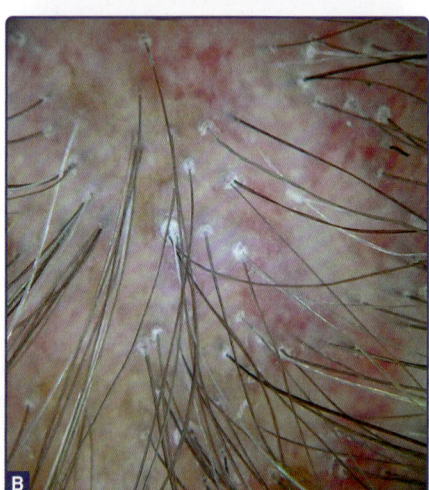

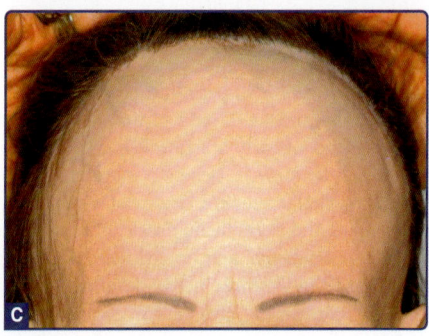

Figure 32-8 Follicular lichen planus. Lichen planopilaris. **A,** Posterior scalp scarring alopecia with perifollicular erythema and scaling. **B,** Dermoscopy showing white scarred patches, peripilar casts, perifollicular scale and erythema, and polytrichia. Frontal fibrosing alopecia. **C,** Frontal scalp with scarring alopecia, perifollicular erythema, and scaling. Note the complete loss of the eyebrows bilaterally.

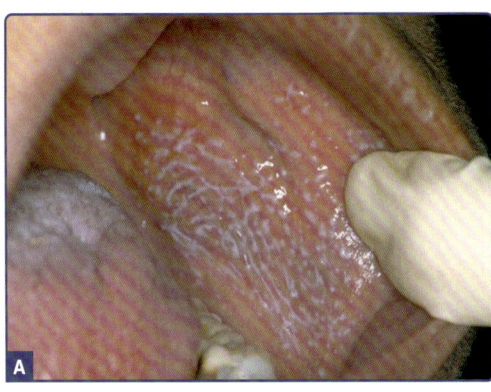
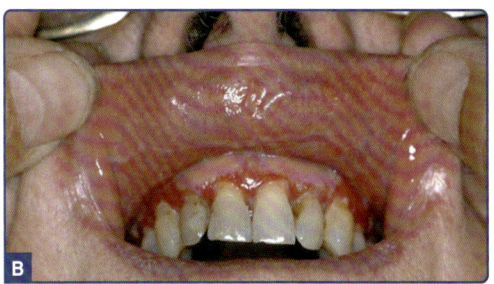

Figure 32-9 Mucosal lichen planus. **A,** Reticulate oral lichen planus with the typical lace-like, whitish reticulated pattern of oral lesions is seen on the buccal mucosa. **B,** Erosive oral lichen planus with painful erosions on the gingiva. (Used with permission from Mayo Foundation for Medical Education and Research, all rights reserved.)

characterized by bilateral reticular keratotic or atrophic changes of the buccal mucosa and lichenoid atrophic patches over the dorsal tongue.[86] The eruption usually follows zidovudine or ketoconazole intake and may therefore represent a unique drug hypersensitivity in the setting of immunosuppression.

Esophageal lichen planus is rare and most often affects the proximal esophagus. Esophageal lichen planus is most common in middle-aged women.[87] Nearly all cases of esophageal lichen planus have preceding or concomitant oral lichen planus.[88] Clinical clues of progressive dysphagia and odynophagia in the setting of oral lichen planus should prompt a gastroenterology referral for endoscopy. Endoscopic findings can include lacy white papules, pinpoint erosions, desquamation, pseudomembranes, and stenosis. Esophageal stricture is common and often requires multiple dilations. Histologically, esophageal lichen planus shows parakeratosis, epithelial atrophy, and lack of hypergranulosis.[87] Esophageal lichen planus often requires systemic immunosuppression with oral corticosteroids. Malignant transformation has been described; therefore, regular surveillance with gastroenterology is required.[87,89]

Male genitalia are involved in 25% of cases of lichen planus (see Fig. 32-3). The glans penis is most commonly affected with annular lesions. Anal lesions of mucosal lichen planus present with leukokeratosis, hyperkeratosis, fissuring, and erosions (Fig. 32-11). Vulvar and vaginal lichen planus is present in 25% to 60% of patients with oral lichen planus.[74,90] Erosive and atrophic disease is most commonly reported in the literature. Clinically, the condition is often asymptomatic unless erosions develop, and then burning, itching, pain, and abnormal discharge become common.[91] Clinical examination often shows patches of leukoplakia or erythroplakia, sometimes with erosions, and occasionally, as a more generalized desquamative vaginitis. Vaginal adhesions and labial agglutination may result. Vulvovaginal gingival syndrome is a distinct triad of vulvar, vaginal, and gingival disease. Vulvovaginal gingival syndrome is characterized by erythema and erosions of the gingivae and tongue and desquamation and erosions of vulva and vagina.[92]

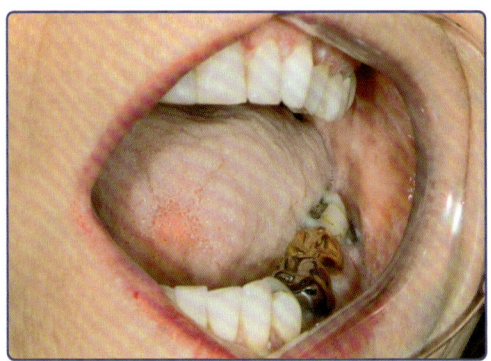

Figure 32-10 Oral lichenoid tissue reaction. Reticulate oral lichenoid eruption with typical lace-like, reticulated pattern concentrated along the lower buccal mucosa and in close approximation to the underlying dental amalgams. (Used with permission from Mayo Foundation for Medical Education and Research, all rights reserved.)

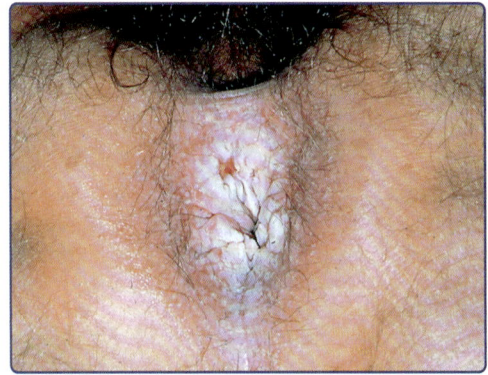

Figure 32-11 Mucosal lichen planus. Perianal leuko- and hyperkeratosis with hypertrophic, folded violaceous epithelium, fissures, and a healing biopsy site. (Used with permission from Mayo Foundation for Medical Education and Research, all rights reserved.)

Other cutaneous sites of involvement include skin (40%), scalp (20%), nails (13%), and esophagus (15%).[93] Vulvovaginal gingival syndrome is associated with significant long-term sequelae with nearly 90% of individuals developing fibrosis and stricture.[93] Class II HLA DBQ1*0201 allele has been found in 80% of individuals with vulvovaginal gingival syndrome with a relative risk of 3.71.[93] Given the multifocal involvement and chronic nature of vulvovaginal gingival syndrome, early institution of aggressive topical and systemic immunosuppression as well as a multidisciplinary approach is needed for optimal outcomes.

Conjunctival lichen planus may manifest as cicatricial conjunctivitis. Histologically, irregular thickening with reduplication of the basement membrane is seen. Conjunctival lichen planus often a diagnostic challenge with significant overlap with cicatricial pemphigoid. In cases with severe oral and ocular disease and a lichenoid infiltrate on biopsy, one should also consider paraneoplastic autoimmune multiorgan syndrome and paraneoplastic and cicatricial pemphigoid in the differential diagnosis. Direct immunofluorescence, indirect immunofluorescence, and serologies for autoantibodies are often helpful to distinguish conjunctival lichen planus from cicatricial pemphigoid and paraneoplastic autoimmune multiorgan syndrome.[94,95] Long-term sequelae include corneal scarring, symblepharon, blindness, and lacrimal duct stenosis.[96]

Otic lichen planus is another rare manifestation of lichen planus affecting the external auditory canal and the tympanic membrane. Otic lichen planus is more common in women, often has concomitant disease at multiple body sites, and can lead to progressive hearing loss.[97] Otic lichen planus should be considered in the differential diagnosis in a patient with mucosal or cutaneous lichen planus with persistent, unexplained otorrhea or external auditory canal stenosis.

Lichen Planus of the Nails: Nail involvement occurs in 10% to 15% of lichen planus patients.[98] Lichen planus limited to the nails is uncommon and, in many cases, is followed by the development of more typical cutaneous or mucosal lesions of lichen planus. Nail involvement in children with lichen planus is rare and affects approximately 5%.[50-53] There are three major forms of nail lichen planus: classic nail lichen planus (described later) (Fig. 32-12A), 20-nail dystrophy (Fig. 32-12B), and idiopathic atrophy of the nails. The most common findings of nail lichen planus are diffuse nail involvement with thinning, longitudinal ridging, and distal nail splitting (onychoschizia). Other findings include onycholysis, longitudinal striation with a "sandpaper-like quality" (onychorrhexis), subungual hyperkeratosis, and atrophic or absent nail plates (anonychia). Dermoscopy can aid in the early diagnosis of nail lichen planus because early nail pitting may be present before the development of more classic disease.[99] Disease with prominent inflammation can result in nail loss and scarring. Pterygium or forward growth of the eponychia with adherence to the proximal nail plate is a classic finding in nail lichen planus involving the matrix. Dorsal pterygium is an

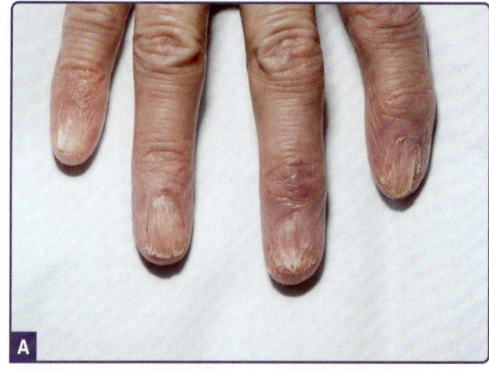

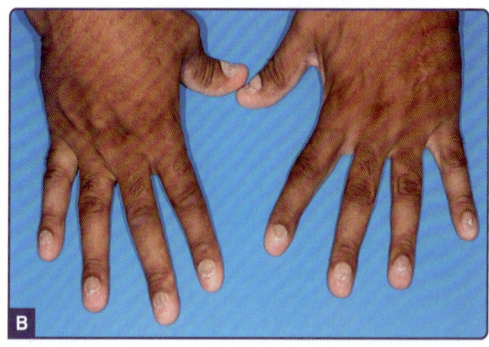

Figure 32-12 Nail lichen planus. **A,** Classic nail lichen planus showing longitudinal ridging and splitting of all nails (onychorrhexis) with distal splitting (onychoschizia). Additionally, the third finger shows dorsal pterygium at the lateral aspect of the nail bed with loss of the nail (anonychia). **B,** Twenty-nail dystrophy showing longitudinal ridging of all nails (trachyonychia) and atrophic nails. (Used with permission from Mayo Foundation for Medical Education and Research, all rights reserved.)

irreversible process and, if present as the primary clinical findings, will likely not improve with treatment. Involvement of the nail bed results in elevation of the nail plate and nail splitting. Trachyonychia, or uniform roughness of the nails, often affects all 20 nails and follows an indolent course. Idiopathic atrophy of the nails is characterized by an abrupt onset and rapidly progressive thinning of the nails with subsequent loss and scarring with or without dorsal pterygium. The latter two forms of nail lichen planus are more common in children.[100] The differential diagnosis of isolated nail lichen planus includes psoriasis, alopecia areata, atopic dermatitis, and rarely immunobullous diseases.

Inverse Lichen Planus: The inverse pattern of lichen planus is rare and is characterized by red-brown, discrete papules and flat-topped plaques. Inverse lichen planus commonly affects the flexural areas, including the axillae, inframammary region, and groin. The antecubital and popliteal areas may be rarely involved. The findings of inverse lichen planus are often isolated and involvement of other ectodermal-derived tissues is uncommon. Inverse lichen planus has been most commonly reported in whites, Asians, and recently Tunisians.[101] Unlike lichen planus pigmentosus, there is an absence of involvement in sun-exposed areas, and some prefer the term *lichen planus pigmentosus inversus*.

Palmoplantar Lichen Planus: Palmoplantar lichen planus is a rare, difficult-to-diagnose form of lichen planus. Approximately 25% of individuals with palmoplantar lichen planus have other areas of cutaneous involvement, most commonly on the anterior shin and malleoli in those with plantar disease.[102] Palmoplantar lichen planus is characterized by pruritic, red-purple, scaly plaques with or without hyperkeratosis. Because of the thickness of palmar and plantar skin, Wickham striae are absent. Four patterns of palmoplantar lichen planus are seen: plaque type, punctate, diffuse keratoderma, and ulcerated. Lesions are commonly seen on the internal plantar arch on the feet (see Fig. 32-5) and the thenar and hypothenar eminence on the hands (Fig. 32-13). Yellow, compact keratotic papules or papulonodules are seen on the lateral margins of the fingers and hand surfaces. Involvement of the fingertips is uncommon and, if present, raises the possibility of a primary or concomitant dermatitis. The lesions often appear callus-like with a faint purple hue and an inflammatory halo. The differential diagnosis includes psoriasis, warts, calluses, porokeratosis, hyperkeratotic dermatitis or eczema, tinea, or secondary syphilis.

SPECIAL FORMS

Drug-Induced Lichen Planus: Lichen planus–like or lichenoid drug eruptions are a group of cutaneous reactions identical or similar to lichen planus. Lichenoid drug eruptions have been reported after ingestion, contact, or inhalation of certain chemicals (Table 32-2).[103] They may be localized or generalized with eczematous papules and plaques. The degree of desquamation is variable. They often manifest with hyperpigmentation and alopecia. Wickham striae are rare. The eruption is often symmetrical on the trunk and extremities with less common flexural involve-

TABLE 32-2
Agents Inducing Lichen Planus and Lichenoid Drug Eruptions

Most Likely
- Gold salts
- β-Blockers
- Antimalarials
- Diuretics (thiazides, furosemide, spironolactone)
- Penicillamine
- Immune checkpoint inhibitors (pembrolizumab, nivolumab, ipilimumab)

Less Likely
- Angiotensin-converting inhibitors
- Calcium channel blockers
- Sulfonylurea
- Nonsteroidal antiinflammatory drugs
- Ketoconazole
- Tetracycline
- Phenothiazine
- Sulfasalazine
- Carbamazepine
- Lithium
- Antituberculosis agents
- Iodides
- Radiocontrast media
- Radiotherapy
- Antipsoriatic therapy: etanercept, infliximab, adalimumab
- TNFα inhibitors (etanercept, infliximab, adalimumab, certolizumab)

Contact Inducers of Lichen Planus
- Color film developers
- Dental restoration materials
- Musk ambrette
- Nickel
- Gold

Photo Inducers of Lichen Planus and Lichenoid Drug Eruption
- 5-Fluorouracil
- Carbamazepine, chlorpromazine, diazoxide
- Ethambutol
- Pyritinol
- Quinine
- Quinidine
- Tetracycline
- Thiazide
- Furosemide

Inducers of Oral Lichen Planus and Lichenoid Drug Eruption
- Allopurinol
- Angiotensin-converting inhibitors
- Cyanamide
- Dental restoration materials
- Mercury, silver, gold
- Ketoconazole
- Nonsteroidal antiinflammatory drugs
- Penicillamines
- Sulphonylureas
- Interferon-α and ribavirin

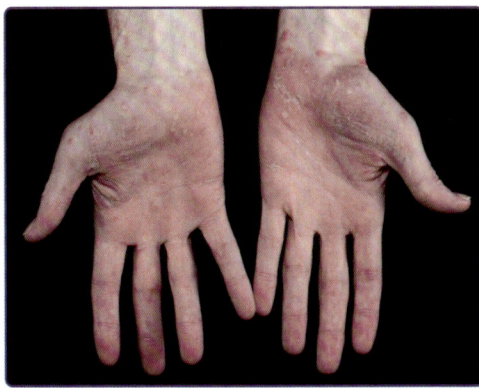

Figure 32-13 Palmar lichen planus. Callus-like keratotic papules with a faint purple hue and an inflammatory halo are concentrated over the thenar and hypothenar eminence bilaterally. Note the relative sparing of the distal fingertips. (Used with permission from Mayo Foundation for Medical Education and Research, all rights reserved.)

ment (Fig. 32-14). Involvement of the mucous membranes is rare and is associated with specific drugs and chemicals. A photodistributed pattern is implicated with specific drugs and chemicals as well. One new class of drugs with a high rate of lichenoid drug eruption is immune checkpoint inhibitors, ipilimumab, pembrolizumab, and nivolumab, which target CTLA-4

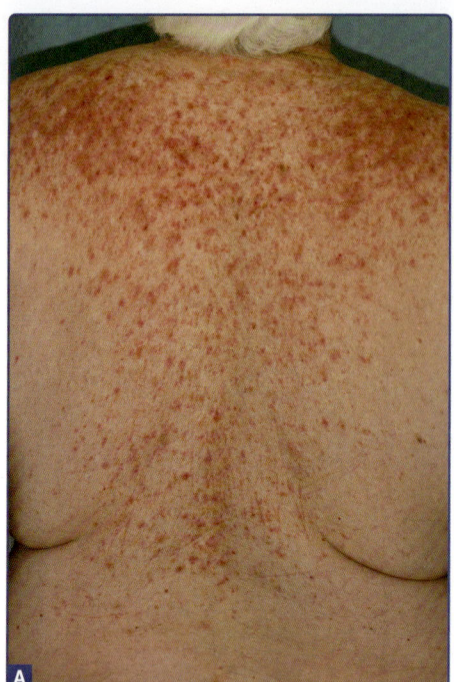

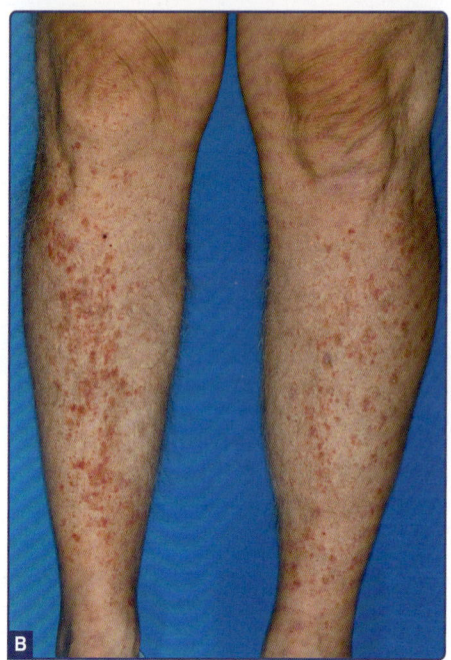

Figure 32-14 Lichenoid drug eruption. **A,** and **B,** Symmetrical, generalized, eczematous papules and plaques over the trunk and anterior shins. Wickham striae are absent, and there is sparing of the flexural surfaces. (Used with permission from Mayo Foundation for Medical Education and Research, all rights reserved.)

The time of onset depends on the dosage, host response, previous exposure, and concomitant drugs. The resolution of the lichenoid drug eruption is variable, and most resolve in 3 to 4 months. Exceptions are gold-induced lichenoid drug eruption, which can require years for resolution. For many drugs, the severity and extent of disease affect the rate of clearance. Occasionally, the lichenoid drug eruption may intermittently recur. Genetic susceptibility is likely important, especially in recurrent cases and cases involving immune-modulating drugs, such as INF-α, ipilimumab, pembrolizumab, and nivolumab.

Lichenoid contact dermatitis may result from contact with compounds such as color film developers, dental restorations, amalgams (silver, mercury, gold), and aminoglycosides (see "Mucosal Lichen Planus").[106,107] Oral lichenoid eruptions are most commonly related to dental restorations metals such as mercury, silver, and gold.[79-81,108]

Lichen Planus–Lupus Erythematosus Overlap: This rare variant of lichen planus is characterized by features of lichen planus and lupus erythematosus.[109,110] Lesions of lichen planus–lupus erythematosus overlap are red-violet, atrophic patches and plaques with hypopigmentation, telangiectasia, and minimal scale. The dorsal aspect of the extremities, specifically the hands and nails, are most commonly affected and patients often develop anonychia (Fig. 32-15). Classic features of lichen planus and lupus erythematosus are absent. Some individuals go on to

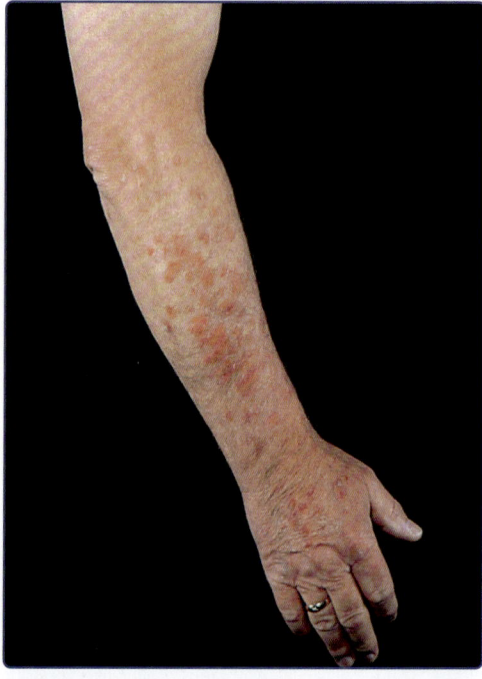

Figure 32-15 Lichen planus–lupus erythematosus overlap syndrome. Lichenoid lesions over the dorsal hand and forearm. Direct immunofluorescence showed evidence of lupus erythematous. (Used with permission from Mayo Foundation for Medical Education and Research, all rights reserved.)

and programmed cell death-1. Lichenoid drug eruptions are some of the most common side effects with this drug class, affecting 17% of patients.[104,105]

The latency period for the development of a lichenoid drug eruption varies from months to more than 1 year.

develop systemic lupus erythematosus. Laboratory studies may find a weakly positive antinuclear antibody, and traditional histology and immunofluorescence show overlapping features of lichen planus and lupus erythematosus. The disease course of lichen planus–lupus erythematosus overlap is often prolonged and refractory to treatment.

Lichen Planus Pemphigoides: Lichen planus pemphigoides has features of lichen planus and bullous pemphigoid (Fig. 32-16). The pathogenesis is unclear but is believed to result from the liquefactive degeneration of keratinocytes caused by a brisk LTR and the subsequent exposure of autoantigens, which result in antibody formation. Some have argued that lichen planus pemphigoides is simply lichen planus and bullous pemphigoid in coexistence. However, there are key clinical and serologic features that differentiate true lichen planus pemphigoides from concomitant lichen planus and bullous pemphigoid. First, lichen planus commonly affects individuals in the fifth to seventh decades of life and bullous pemphigoid most commonly after the seventh decade, but lichen planus pemphigoides is most common in younger individuals in the four to fifth decades of life. Additionally, lichen planus pemphigoides blisters may occur on top of lichenoid lesions as well as normal-appearing skin.

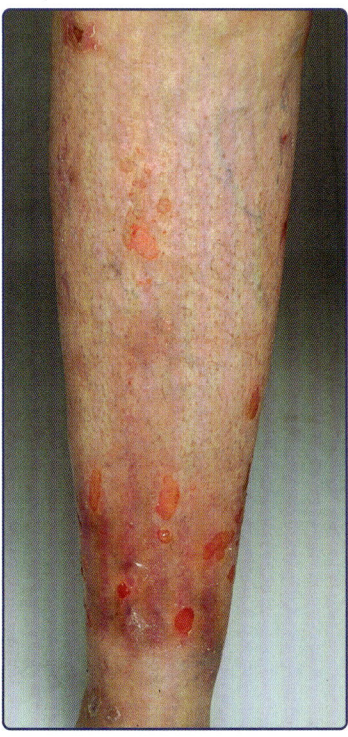

Figure 32-16 Lichen planus pemphigoides. Erythema, erosions, and bullae over the distal shin with histology showing a lichenoid tissue reaction and direct immunofluorescence showing features of bullous pemphigoid. Indirect immunofluorescence result also was positive. (Used with permission from Mayo Foundation for Medical Education and Research, all rights reserved.)

The prognosis of lichen planus pemphigoides is good and is response to conventional therapy.[111] Last, the Medical College of Wisconsin domain 4 (MCW-4) of bullous pemphigoid antigen 180 (BPAG180) appears to be unique for lichen planus pemphigoides.[112] The major consideration in the differential diagnosis is bullous lichen planus, which can be differentiated on serologies and immunofluorescence. Drug-induced lichen planus pemphigoides has been described.[113]

Keratosis Lichenoides Chronica (Nekam Disease): Keratosis lichenoides chronica (KLC), or Nekam disease, is a rare dermatosis that has distinct clinical and histologic features. Clinically, KLC is distinct from lichen planus and is characterized by lichenoid, keratotic papules and plaques in a seborrheic distribution with characteristic linear or reticulate pattern.[114] Additional sites of involvement include the palms and soles. The individual lesions tend to be folliculo- and infundibulocentric. The eruption is often asymptomatic and refractory to treatment. Histologically, KLC is characterized by a brisk LTR and often shows parakeratosis with neutrophils in the crust.[115] The diagnosis of KLC should be made with caution because other diseases such as lichen planus, lichen simplex, and lupus erthematosus (LE) may manifest a similar reaction pattern.[115]

Lichenoid Graft versus Host Disease: Chronic GVHD is traditionally considered that occurring 100 days after transplant and may manifest as a dermatitic, sclerodermoid, or lichenoid eruption, which can be indistinguishable from lichen planus. A newer consensus definition of GVHD focuses in on both clinical and chronological features, including classic acute GVHD, persist, recurrent, or late-onset acute GVHD occurring after 100 days, classic chronic GVHD, and overlap syndromes.[116] GVHD is caused by immunocompetent donor cells attacking fast dividing tissue such as the liver, gastrointestinal tract, and skin.

Although the mechanism is incompletely understood, the various forms of GVHD appear to be pathogenically distinct. Because there is a better understanding of GVHD relative to lichen planus and a clear driver of an autoantigen stimulating an allogeneic immune response, we will discuss the mechanism briefly. Whereas acute GVHD is driven by Th2 cytokine signaling, chronic GVHD is driven by Th1/Th17 signaling and increased numbers of IFN-γ– and IL-17–producing cytotoxic CD8-positive T cells.[117] Supporting this theory, mice deficient of IL-17 receptors are unable to develop GVHD.[118] Additionally, exciting new research with therapeutic potential points to the possible role of IL-17 blockade in the transdifferentiation of Th17 cells into CD4-positive T-regulatory cells.[119] Similar targets may be useful in refractory lichen planus.

Clinically, lichenoid GVHD is characterized by classic lichenoid papules with prominent follicular involvement of the head and neck as well as oral involvement.[120] Onycholysis and cicatricial alopecia may be prominent features. Histopathologically, lichenoid GVHD is often indistinguishable from lichen planus; however, satellite cell necrosis, plasma cells, and eosinophils may be subtle clues to the diagnosis.[121]

Lichenoid Keratosis: Lichenoid keratosis often consists of a single, nonpruritic, brown to red, scaling flat-topped plaque on sun-exposed skin of the extremities.[122] Lichenoid keratosis is easily differentiated clinically from lichen planus. These lesions can be histologically identical to lichen planus; however, they may have some differentiating features such as parakeratosis or a remnant lentigo, seborrheic keratosis, or actinic keratosis.

Lichenoid Dermatitis: Lichenoid dermatitis describes a reaction pattern with nonclassic lichenoid features as well as spongiosis. A study of 62 patients with lichenoid dermatitis had an alternative diagnoses with further clinical, serologic, and histopathological analysis. The differential diagnosis of lichenoid dermatitis includes dermatitis, drug eruption, lupus erythematosus, lichen planus, and cutaneous T-cell lymphoma.[123] Additional features, specifically granuloma formation, expand the differential diagnosis to include drug eruptions (including pseudolymphoma in 31%), hepatobiliary disease, endocrinopathy (diabetes mellitus and thyroiditis), rheumatoid arthritis, Crohn disease, and infection (in 28%).[124]

RELATED FINDINGS

See Table 32-3.

Lichen planus is associated with liver diseases such as autoimmune chronic active hepatitis, primary biliary cirrhosis (PBC), and postviral chronic, active hepatitis. The association of PBC is observed regardless of the use of penicillamine. Hepatitis C virus (HCV) and lichen planus are associated in certain endemic regions (East and Southeast Asia, South America, the Middle East, and Southern Europe) but not in others (North America, South Asia, and Africa).[125,126] The prevalence of HCV is 16% to 29% in southern European patients with lichen planus.[127,128] In patients with oral lichen planus and liver disease, there are significantly higher rates of HCV in selected populations (78% versus 3%). There is no clear association of HCV with pure cutaneous lichen planus.[129] There may be specific unidentified genetic factors contributing to this co-occurrence because large studies on HCV have not found lichen planus to be a common finding.[130] The heterogeneity of HCV and oral lichen planus may be related to the human leukocyte antigen-DR6 (HLA-DR6) haplotype, which is found in endemic regions of both diseases.[131,132] There is no strong link between hepatitis B virus (HBV) and lichen planus.[133]

Patients with lichen planus have been reported to have higher rates of dyslipidemia and to harbor more cardiac risk factors than healthy individuals.[134-136] Metabolic syndrome appears to be more common in individuals with oral lichen planus.[137] Thyroid dysfunction, most commonly hypothyroidism, is found in up to 34% of patients with lichen planopilaris.[138] Lichen sclerosus et atrophicus is seen in up to 16% of patients with oral lichen planus; however, there is no associated risk of oral lichen planus in individuals with lichen sclerosus et atrophicus.[90,139] Recent population studies have found an association between lichen planus and autoimmune diseases, including systemic lupus erythematosus, Sjögren disease, dermatomyositis, vitiligo, and alopecia areata, in the Taiwanese population.[140] Cases of lichen planus in association with internal malignancy may represent a manifestation of paraneoplastic autoimmune multiorgan syndrome.

MALIGNANT TRANSFORMATION

There has been considerable controversy as to whether oral lichen planus inherently harbors malignant potential.[77,141] It is currently believed that the risk of malignant transformation is low. Risk factors that increase the likelihood of developing oral cancer are long-standing disease, erosive or atrophic types, tobacco use, and possibly esophageal involvement. Additionally, oncogenic subtypes of HPV, including type 16, are more common in oral lichen planus and may account, in part, for the malignancy risk.[142] The reported rates of SCC development have varied: 0.8% of oral lichen planus in the United States, 1.9% in the United Kingdom, 0.6% in China, and 1% in the Swedish population.[77,143-145] The majority of these cases are in situ carcinoma or with a microinvasive pattern. The most common site for cancer is the tongue (Fig. 32-17) followed by the buccal mucosa, gingiva, and, rarely, the lip. Clinically, the lesions appear as indurated, nonhealing ulcers or exophytic lesions with a keratotic surface. Red atrophic plaques could also be seen and often correlate with in situ disease. Advanced cases may result in nodal metastases and even death. No overall increased risk of malignancy has been observed in cutaneous lichen planus.[145] There are rare case reports of cutaneous SCC arising in long-standing

TABLE 32-3
Diseases Commonly Associated with Lichen Planus

Hepatitis C virus
Autoimmune chronic active hepatitis
Primary biliary cirrhosis
Postviral chronic, active hepatitis
Dyslipidemia
Metabolic syndrome
Hypothyroidism[a]
Lichen sclerosus et atrophicus[b]
Systemic lupus erythematosus
Sjögren disease
Dermatomyositis
Vitiligo
Alopecia areata

[a]Lichen planopilaris.
[b]Oral lichen planus.

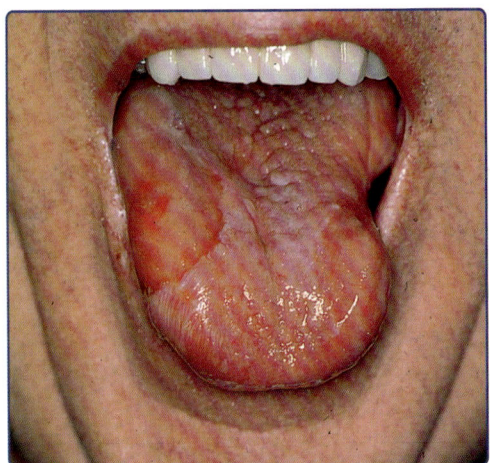

Figure 32-17 Lichen planus and squamous cell carcinoma (SCC). Long-standing oral lichen planus with scarring of the tongue. Well-circumscribed erythroplakia and erosions of the right lateral tongue was biopsied and confirmed SCC. (Used with permission from Mayo Foundation for Medical Education and Research, all rights reserved.)

TABLE 32-4
Laboratory Tests to Consider for Lichen Planus
Complete blood count
Patch testing[a]
Lipid panel
Thyroid function tests[b]
Antithyroid peroxidase antibodies
Antithyroglobulin antibodies
Hepatitis C virus testing[c]

[a]Particularly for oral lichen planus.
[b]For lichen planopilaris.
[c]For endemic areas; oral lichen planus.

lesions of lichen planus. Risk factors include: hypertrophic or verrucous lichen planus, location on the lower extremity, a history of arsenic or x-ray exposure, and long-standing disease (average, 12 years).[145]

DIAGNOSIS

The diagnosis of lichen planus is largely clinical. However, in cases with atypical or overlapping clinical features, a histopathologic diagnosis may be required. In cases of vesiculobullous disease or erosive disease, immunofluorescence (DIF), indirect immunofluorescence (IIF), and enzyme-linked immunosorbent assay (ELISA), may be needed to differentiate from immunobullous diseases. Laboratory testing is not required and is largely focused in upon associated morbidities and should be part of age-specific screening for risk reduction of diseases such as thyroid and cardiac disease.

SUPPORTIVE STUDIES

LABORATORY TESTING

See Table 32-4.

No specific abnormalities of laboratory analyses are seen in lichen planus. The total white blood cell count and lymphocytes may be decreased. This could be related to cytokine activation and local trafficking of cells to skin or other tissue compartments.

In cases of oral disease, allergic contact dermatitis should be ruled out because oral contact stomatitis can appear identical to lichen planus.[80,146-148] Sensitivity to mercury, gold, chromate, flavoring agents, acrylate, and thimerosal are common sensitizers. Avoidance of these clinically relevant sensitizers results in amelioration of disease.

Dyslipidemia is more common in patients with lichen planus compared with control participants and should be tested as part of normal, preventative care.[134,135,137,149] Additionally, in cases of lichen planopilaris, one should consider testing for associated thyroid abnormalities, including thyroid-stimulating hormone, antithyroid peroxidase antibodies, and antithyroglobulin antibodies.[138]

HCV testing is controversial in lichen planus and testing should be considered in those with oral disease, risk factors for HCV (elevated liver function, intravenous drug use, a history of blood transfusion prior to 1992, and high risk sexual behaviors) as well as those in endemic areas (East and Southeast Asia, South America, the Middle East, and Southern Europe) having a prevalence of greater than 7%.[150]

PATHOLOGY

The two major pathologic findings in lichen planus are basal epidermal keratinocyte damage and a lichenoid-interface lymphocytic reaction. Classic changes are seen in established cutaneous lesions.[151] Classic lichen planus is characterized by a dense, continuous, and band-like lymphohistiocytic infiltrate at the DEJ (Fig. 32-18). The heavy infiltrate can result in effacement of the DEJ. Parakeratosis and eosinophils are absent. The epidermal changes include hyperkeratosis, wedge-shaped areas of hypergranulosis, and elongation of rete ridges that resemble a sawtooth pattern. Multiple apoptotic cells or colloid-hyaline (Civatte) bodies are seen at the DEJ. Eosinophilic colloid bodies are present in the papillary dermis. Eosinophils are absent in classic lichen planus and are seen in two thirds of lichenoid drug eruptions and are seen in significant numbers in 20.6% of cases of hypertropic lichen planus.[152-154] Melanin pigmentation is invariably present and is more pronounced in older, waning lesions in dark-skinned individuals and lichen planus pigmentosus. Separation of the epidermis in small clefts (Max Joseph cleft formation) is seen in 20% of cases.

Late disease is characterized by an atrophic epidermis, effacement of the rete ridges, occasional colloid

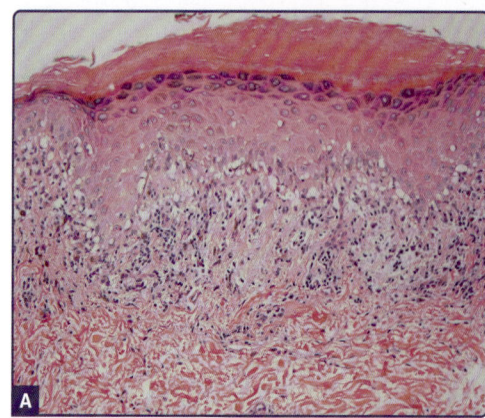
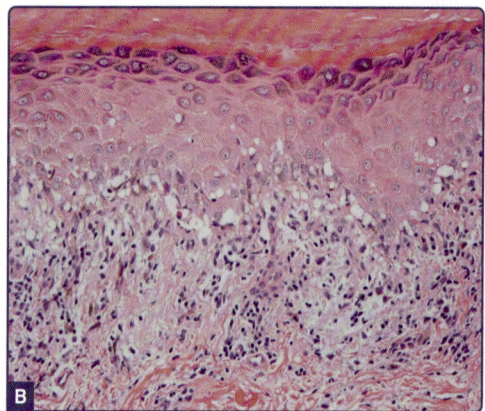

Figure 32-18 Lichen planus. **A,** The characteristic findings of lichen planus with compact orthohyperkeratosis, wedge-shaped hypergranulosis, sawtoothed rete ridges, and a lichenoid infiltrate. (Hematoxylin and eosin [H&E] × 100.) **B,** Dense, lichenoid lymphocytic infiltrate with scattered apoptotic keratinocytes and pigment incontinence. A small Max-Joseph space is noted centrally. (H&E × 200.) (Photo contributors: David J. DiCaudo, MD and Steven A. Nelson, MD. Used with permission from Mayo Foundation for Medical Education and Research, all rights reserved.)

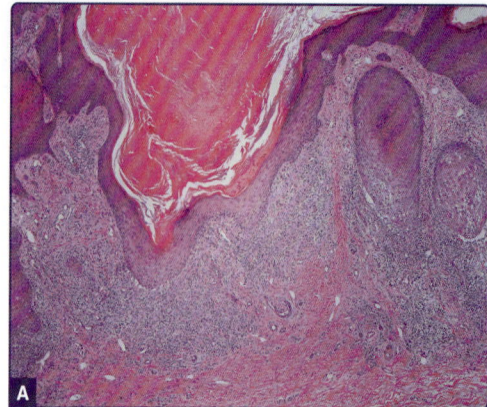
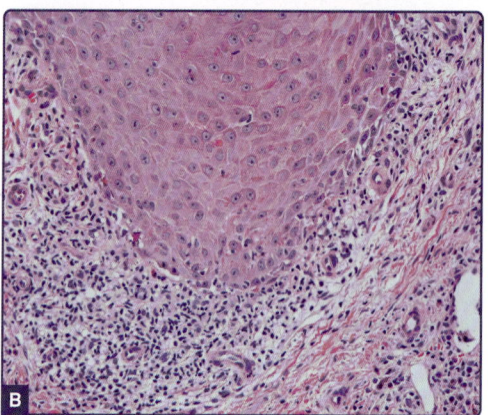

Figure 32-19 Hypertrophic lichen planus. **A,** The characteristic findings of hypertrophic lichen planus with hyperkeratosis, acanthosis, and papillomatosis. (Hematoxylin and eosin [H&E] × 40.) **B,** Dense, lichenoid lymphocytic infiltrate with scattered apoptotic keratinocytes and eosinophils. (H&E × 200.) (Photo contributors: David J. DiCaudo, MD and Steven A. Nelson, MD. Used with permission from Mayo Foundation for Medical Education and Research, all rights reserved.)

bodies, dermal fibrosis, and melanophages. When few colloid bodies are present, distinguishing from poikiloderma may be very difficult.

Hypertrophic lichen planus is characterized by hyperkeratosis, acanthosis, papillomatosis, and thickened collagen bundles in the dermis (Fig. 32-19). Hypertrophic lichen planus can be mistaken for SCC; therefore, good clinical pathological correlation is needed to avoid inappropriate treatment.[155] As mentioned earlier, eosinophils are more commonly seen in hypertrophic lesions.[152]

Mucosal lesions tend to have less specific changes, and genital disease can often be inconclusive. Parakeratosis and an absent granular layer are common at mucosal sites, and plasma cells are often prominent.

Lichen planopilaris is characterized by a perifollicular, lymphohistiocytic inflammatory reaction with perifollicular fibrosis, scarring, and follicular atrophy. The initial inflammation is at the level of the isthmus and infundibulum and spares the lower segment.[156]

DIF studies are focused on oral disease and show a positive finding in 62% to 75% of cases with numerous apoptotic cells at the DEJ (60%) staining with immunoglobulin M (IgM) and, occasionally, with IgG and IgA (Fig. 32-20).[157] Shaggy deposition of fibrinogen at the DEJ is seen in 55% to 70% of cases.[157,158] The criterion for lichen planus requires basement membrane zone fibrinogen and colloid bodies with one or more conjugate(s) (Mayo Clinic criteria).[157] Multiple immunoglobulin (IgG, A, and M) conjugates and granular, basilar deposition of immunoglobulins are more common in LE, and the diagnosis of lichen planus should be suspect when multiple conjugates are present.[159] DIF of oral lichen planus (sensitivity of 61% and specificity of 96%) is inferior to both hematoxylin and eosin (sensitivity of 84% and specificity of 93%) and clinical impression (sensitivity of 74% and specificity of 87%).[157] These findings emphasize the importance of clinical examination and routine histology in classic lichen planus. DIF has a role in atypical disease and is a

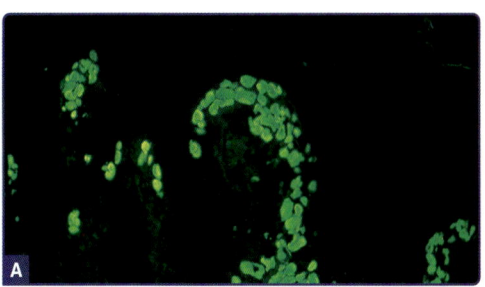

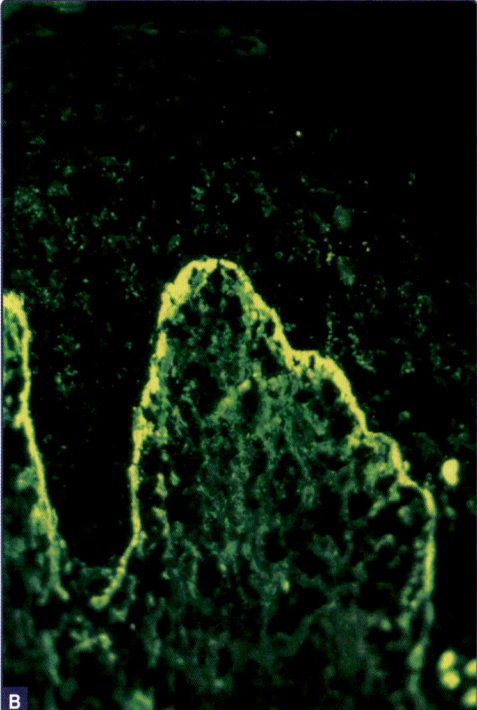

Figure 32-20 Lichen planus. Direct immunofluorescence. **A,** Fibrinogen/fibrin, shaggy pattern at the dermal–epidermal junction. **B,** Numerous immunoglobulin M-positive cytoids at the dermal–epidermal junction. (Used with permission from Mayo Foundation for Medical Education and Research, all rights reserved.)

prerequisite for the diagnosis of ulcerative and vesiculobullous lichen planus variants.

The location of the biopsy is critically important in lichen planus and varies by lichen planus subtype. The optimal location for biopsy of cutaneous lichen planus is on the proximal trunk with avoidance of the distal extremities.[158] Dermoscopic-driven biopsies of lichen planopilaris showing the key features of perifollicular erythema and scaling led to definitive diagnosis in 95% of cases.[160] Biopsies for nail disease should be guided by dermoscopy and should focus on the underlying structures involved. The presence of trachyonychia and pitting should guide a matrix biopsy, chromonychia, nail plate fragmentation, splinter hemorrhage, onycholysis, and subungual debris should guide a nail bed biopsy.[99] For DIF, the highest sensitivity is on the mouth floor and the ventral side of the tongue. The oral biopsy specimen for DIF may be taken up to 1 cm from the lesion (including glabrous skin) without a decrease in sensitivity and should not be split.[158,161,162]

DIFFERENTIAL DIAGNOSIS

The differential diagnosis of lichen planus is quite broad. A more practical approach is to look at the age of the individual, morphology of the primary lesion, and site of involvement (Table 32-5).

CLINICAL COURSE AND PROGNOSIS

Most cutaneous lichen planus resolves within one to 2 years and may be associated with relapses. Recurrence is seen in up to 20% of cases but is more common in generalized cutaneous disease.[54,163] The duration of disease depends on the extent and site of involvement. In general, generalized disease tends to resolve more quickly. Disease duration, in ascending order, is generalized cutaneous, nongeneralized cutaneous,

---

TABLE 32-5
Differential Diagnosis of Lichen Planus

Morphology and Age

Classic: psoriasis, lichenoid drug eruption, lichen simplex chronicus, chronic cutaneous lupus, graft-versus-host disease, secondary syphilis, pityriasis rosea, mycosis fungoides

Annular: granuloma annulare, tinea corporis

Linear: nevus unius lateris, lichen striatus, linear epidermal nevus, psoriasis, Darier disease

Hypertrophic: lichen simplex chronicus, prurigo nodularis, lichen amyloidosis, Kaposi sarcoma, squamous cell carcinoma, psoriasis

Atrophic: lichen sclerosus, cutaneous lupus erythematosus, poikiloderma, mycosis fungoides, morphea

Vesiculobullous: lichen planus pemphigoides, epidermolysis bullosa pruriginosa, pemphigus vulgaris, bullous pemphigoid, bullous amyloidosis

Follicular: lichen nitidus, lichen spinulosa, follicular psoriasis, pityriasis rubra pilaris

Childhood: lichen nitidus, lichen striatus, pityriasis lichenoides, papular acrodermatitis of childhood, annular lichenoid dermatitis of youth, mycosis fungoides, frictional lichenoid eruption

Special Sites

Nail: psoriasis, onychomycosis, alopecia areata, atopic dermatitis

Genital: psoriasis, seborrheic dermatitis, fixed drug eruption

Palms and soles: secondary syphilis, erythema multiforme

Scalp: cicatricial alopecia, lupus erythematosus, inflammatory folliculitis, alopecia areata, cicatricial pemphigoid, keratosis follicularis spinulosa decalvans

Mucosal: pemphigus vulgaris, cicatricial pemphigoid, bullous pemphigoid, epidermolysis bullosa acquisita, paraneoplastic autoimmune multiorgan syndrome or paraneoplastic pemphigus, candidiasis, lupus erythematosus, leukokeratosis, secondary syphilis, traumatic patches, chronic ulcerative stomatitis, erythema multiforme

cutaneous and mucosal, mucosal, hypertrophic, and lichen planopilaris.[164] The mean duration of oral disease is 5 years, and hypertrophic and scalp disease are often unremitting. In higher Fitzpatrick skin types, postinflammatory changes manifest as significant, persistent pigmentary abnormalities.

TREATMENT

The treatment of lichen planus is challenging and discouraging for both physicians and patients. Because of its ability to affect multiple ectodermal-derived tissues, lichen planus may require a multidisciplinary approach with dermatologists, dentists, gynecologists, and occasionally otolaryngologists, gastroenterologists, and ophthalmologists. The goal of therapy is to minimize morbidity and improve the patient's quality of life. Treatment options and the potential risks of therapy should be weighed against the extent and severity of disease. Potentially exacerbating drugs should be discontinued, trauma minimized, and microbial overgrowth reduced.

The basic concepts in the treatment of lichen planus have remained largely unchanged over the past decade. The therapies are mainly divided into skin-directed and systemic agents. The therapies for various ectodermal tissues are also similar. Nearly all of these agents act in a manner to suppress the immune response. To date, there are no disease-specific medications for lichen planus. However, Janus kinase (JAK) inhibitors target CD8-Tc cells and represent a potential, disease-specific treatment of lichenoid diseases, including lichen planus.[165] JAK inhibitors have been successful in treating refractory dermatomyositis, alopecia areata, and vitiligo.[166-168] This section provides a brief overview of the general approach to therapy for lichen planus and its variants of lichen planus.

CUTANEOUS LICHEN PLANUS

SKIN-DIRECTED THERAPIES

Topical Corticosteroids: Despite few clinical trials, high-potency topical corticosteroids are considered first-line therapy for limited cutaneous lichen planus. Occlusion may be necessary to increase penetration in cases of hypertrophic lichen planus. The sole randomized controlled trial in cutaneous lichen planus comparing calcipotriene to betamethasone valerate (twice daily for 12 weeks) found no difference between treatments.[169] If no response is observed with twice daily application for 2 to 4 weeks, changing to a higher potency corticosteroid or intralesional injections should be considered.[170]

Topical Calcineurin Inhibitors: There are no trials using topical calcineurin inhibitors in cutaneous lichen planus. However, clinical data in oral lichen planus suggest that topical calcineurin inhibitors may be the most effective topical therapy for lichen planus. Application of tacrolimus 0.1% ointment is as effective as 0.05% clobetasol.[171] Because of cost, topical calcineurin inhibitors are a second-line topical agent and are often used in conjunction with topical steroids in refractory cases of limited cutaneous lichen planus. The combination of topical corticosteroids and calcineurin inhibitors often allows one to taper topical corticosteroids and minimize the possibility of steroid atrophy.

Intralesional Corticosteroids: Intralesional corticosteroids (5 to 10 mg/mL injected on a monthly basis) can be highly effective in resistant and hypertrophic lichen planus. However, one should use caution to prevent excessive trauma to avoid Koebnerization. Because of the risk of relapse, intralesional corticosteroids should always be combined with topical therapy or an additional corticosteroid-sparing agent.

Phototherapy: Phototherapy has been used successfully in many inflammatory diseases of the skin. Ultraviolet B (UVB) exposure of dendritic cells (DCs) impairs their interaction with T cells, alters cytokine expression, and leads to T-cell suppression and apoptosis.[172,173] UVB three times weekly until remission with taper after remission over 3 to 6 weeks has a 70% remission rate, and 85% of the patients remained in remission at 34 months.[174] A short course of oral corticosteroids in combination with UV light therapy is highly effective for generalized cutaneous lichen planus. Narrow-band UVB (311 nm) is as effective in lichen planus and has largely supplanted UVA, psoralen plus UVA (PUVA), and UVB phototherapy.[175]

SYSTEMIC THERAPIES

Systemic medications are often needed for severe, more protracted lichen planus. Oral corticosteroids are often first systemic treatments. Second-line, corticosteroid-sparing agents are sulfasalazine, metronidazole, acitretin, antimalarials (hydroxychloroquine and chloroquine), methotrexate, mycophenolate mofetil (MMF), and azathioprine (less preferred second-line agent). Because of its side effect profile, cyclosporine is considered a third-line corticosteroid-sparing agent. Within the second-line agents, particular agents are more effective for specific variants of lichen planus, which is outlined later. In general, drugs that target lymphocytes more specifically (methotrexate, MMF, and azathioprine) are of higher utility in refractory and ulcerative disease, but drugs acting indirectly on lymphocytes (sulfasalazine and metronidazole) or cellular differentiation (acitretin) are more effective for generalized disease and hypertrophic disease, respectively.

Systemic Corticosteroids: Systemic corticosteroids for cutaneous lichen planus have only been reported in one study with a 90% response rate and 32% relapse rate at 6 months.[176] Lichen planus is often responsive to 0.3 mg/kg to 1 mg/kg of oral prednisone within 4 to 6 weeks of treatment and requires a

4- to 6-week taper. In our clinical experience, systemic corticosteroids are highly effective and serve a role in attaining rapid disease control but are associated with high rates of relapse upon discontinuation. Therefore, oral should always be combined with topical therapy or an additional corticosteroid-sparing agent. Long-term monotherapy with oral corticosteroids is not recommended.

Sulfasalazine: Sulfasalazine (initial dose, 1 g/day with an increase every 3 days by 0.5 g to a maximum of 2.5 g/day) has the highest level of evidence of efficacy for lichen planus with an 83% improvement in skin lesions of generalized lichen planus and a 91% improvement in itch at 6 weeks in the therapy group.[177,178] Agranulocytosis and elevated liver function tests can occur with sulfasalazine; therefore, it is important to monitor these laboratory tests during drug initiation.

Metronidazole: An open-labeled study of oral metronidazole (250 mg three times daily for 12 weeks) showed a 74% response rate at 3 months of follow-up.[179] Alternate dosing (500 mg twice daily for 20 to 60 days) has also been reported to be successful.[180] In our experience, metronidazole is more effective in generalized cutaneous lichen planus. Because of its side effect profile, metronidazole is often considered the first-line nonimmunosuppressive systemic agent; however, one should caution patients as well as monitor for possible sensory peripheral neuropathy.[181]

Acitretin: A double-blind, placebo-controlled trial of acitretin (30 mg/day for 8 weeks) showed marked improvement in 64% of individuals.[182] Mucocutaneous side effects and hyperlipidemia were common. In our experience, acitretin is highly effective for hypertrophic lichen planus. Topical retinoids are of limited value in cutaneous lichen planus.

Antimalarials: Chloroquine has been reported effective in cutaneous lichen planus.[183,184] Hydroxychloroquine has been reported effective in oral lichen planus, lichen planopilaris, and actinic lichen planus.[185-190] However, given its favorable side effect profile, hydroxychloroquine (200 to 400 mg [up to 6.5 mg/kg ideal body weight] for 6 to 12 months) is often used as a second-line agent in cutaneous lichen planus and the first-line agent in actinic lichen planus.

Methotrexate: Methotrexate has been shown to be of benefit for more recalcitrant disease as well as in specific forms of disease, including hypertrophic lichen planus and lichen planopilaris. Recent, nonrandomized, prospective data have shown methotrexate (15 to 20 mg weekly for 4 to 24 weeks) to be highly efficacious with complete responses in 58% to 91% of cases.[191-193] Methotrexate is useful and cost effective and is a preferred second-line systemic agent.

Mycophenolate Mofetil and Azathioprine: Both oral MMF and azathioprine are used commonly in refractory cutaneous lichen planus. MMF, 2 to 3 g/day in divided doses is effective in refractory cases; however, the clinical responses are delayed and adjuvant oral corticosteroids are often required during initiation.[194] Azathioprine has been reported effective in refractory lichen planus; however, because of its suppressive effects on T and B lymphocytes and its tolerability issues, we reserve this as a less preferred second-line agent.[195]

Cyclosporine: Cyclosporine has been reported effective at doses of 3 to 10 mg/kg/day; however, lower doses of 1.0 mg/kg/day to 2.5 mg/kg/day are likely to achieve disease remission.[196] Frequent relapses of lichen planus after discontinuation of cyclosporine, as well as its long-term side effects, limit its use in chronic lichen planus.

Other Therapies: TNF-α inhibitors, apremilast, trimethoprim–sulfamethoxazole, griseofulvin, itraconazole, terbinafine, tetracyclines, laser, IFN, alitretinoin, thalidomide, and low-dose heparin have also been reported.

ORAL LICHEN PLANUS

The cornerstone of treatment in oral lichen planus is good oral hygiene with regular professional dental cleanings.[197] Minimizing other exacerbating factors such as contact allergens, drug reactions, reducing oral microbes, and minimizing trauma can reduce disease severity as well as frequency of flares. Replacement of dental amalgams and gold dental restorations can be beneficial, even in patients with negative patch testing results.[84,85] Gingival lesions may respond less favorably. However, removal and restoration should be individualized based on the severity of disease as well as the index of suspicion of the level of involvement of the metal or prosthesis.

SKIN-DIRECTED THERAPIES

Topical Corticosteroids: Topical steroids are first-line therapy in oral lichen planus with overall clinical responses on the order of 70% to 80%. The use of occlusive materials, such as Orabase, may alleviate pain associated with ulcerative lesions. Although few direct comparisons between topical corticosteroids in lichen planus exist, the most beneficial are likely: 0.1% triamcinolone acetonide in Orabase, 0.025% to 0.05% clobetasol-17-propionate in Orabase, and 0.1% fluocinonide gel.[198,199] However, only clobetasol and fluocinonide have demonstrated a clear benefit over placebo.[200] Higher potency corticosteroids as well as more occlusive preparations lead to faster healing times.[201-203] However, the clinician and patient must weigh the benefit of an occlusive ointment or Orabase with the difficulty of application and potential for noncompliance. In general, topical corticosteroids should be applied two to six times daily based on the severity of disease. One therapeutic approach is to initiate high to ultrapotent steroid gel three times daily after meals to all affected areas followed by tacrolimus ointment twice daily. The corticosteroids are tapered every 2 to 4 weeks to a maintenance dose of two to three times weekly, and tacrolimus is continued twice daily.

The major complications of topical corticosteroids are fungal infections and, in general, higher rates of fungal infections are seen with more potent topical corticosteroids. Therefore, concomitant therapy with oral chlorhexidine gluconate mouthwash, topical anticandidal medications, or prophylactic oral fluconazole is recommended.[202,204]

Topical Calcineurin Inhibitors: Pimecrolimus 1% cream is effective in curing the erosive lesions of oral lichen planus but is ineffective at symptomatic control.[198,205] Meta-analysis has found tacrolimus 0.1% ointment one to four times daily to be more effective than clobetasol propionate ointment.[198] Cyclosporine in various preparations has been found to be less effective than both clobetasol and triamcinolone.[198,206] Because of cost, commercially available calcineurin inhibitors and increasing restrictions on compounding, we would recommend topical cyclosporine as a third-line topical agent. Transient burning with usage of topical calcineurin inhibitors is common and overlap therapy with topical corticosteroids may alleviate the burning sensation.

Retinoids: Topical tretinoin 0.05% to 0.1% gel applied twice daily may be effective in oral lichen planus; however, because of issues of irritation, this is a third-line topical agent and is often used in conjunction with topical corticosteroids.[207,208]

Intralesional Corticosteroids: Intralesional triamcinolone 0.5 mL of 40 mg/mL on a weekly basis for 4 weeks is effective in oral lichen planus.[209] More dilute concentrations, 10 mg/mL, injected every 1 to 4 weeks, in conjunction with topical corticosteroids, is highly effective. However, because of the discomfort of injection and few well-controlled studies, intralesional therapies are reserved after exhausting topical therapies.

SYSTEMIC THERAPIES

The approach to systemic therapies in oral lichen planus is similar to that of cutaneous disease. A few exceptions are the larger reported series of MMF and hydroxychloroquine in refractory oral lichen planus, the efficacy and dual benefit of oral acitretin, and the high levels of iatrogenic candida infections. In general, the hierarchy of therapy is the same; however, one should always consider the increased risk of oral SCC in erosive and refractory oral lichen planus and more heavily weigh the risks of immunosuppression against the benefits of disease control. Based on this, drugs such as acitretin, with its antiproliferative effects, and less immunosuppressive agents such as hydroxychloroquine and methotrexate are preferred.

Oral Corticosteroids: Systemic steroids are one of the most effective treatment for oral lichen planus and can provide rapid improvement in acute exacerbations. However, there are no randomized clinical trials for systemic corticosteroids. Both clinical experience as well as prospective studies indicates that oral corticosteroids 1.5 to 2 mg/kg tapered over 3 to 6 weeks are highly effective.[210,211] Based on evidence in other erosive and blistering dermatologic diseases, doses greater than 1 mg/kg of corticosteroids add little clinical benefit and dramatically increase side effects. Studies using pulsed betamethasone, 5 mg on 2 consecutive days weekly for 3 months, showed a more rapid response but no clear long-term advantage over topicals.[212] Oral therapy should be done concomitantly with topical therapy or systemic steroid-sparing agents because patients often flare upon discontinuation. Oral candidiasis is a common complication of oral corticosteroids, and prophylaxis should be used.

Oral Retinoids: Oral acitretin is effective in oral lichen planus; one study of severe lichen planus found that 30 mg/day for 8 weeks resulted in remission in two thirds of cases.[182] Acitretin can be effective at lower doses of 25 mg 3 to 7 days per week; however, oral lichen planus often recurs after the discontinuation of therapy; therefore, adjuvant topical therapy is often necessary. In a pilot study, oral alitretinoin dosed at 30 mg/day for up to 24 weeks reduced the severity of disease by 50% in 4 of 10 patients with severe oral lichen planus.[213]

Antimalarials: Hydroxychloroquine (200 to 400 mg [up to 6.5 mg/kg ideal body weight] for 6 months) is effective as a monotherapy in oral lichen planus.[186] Despite its long half-life, improvement in erythema and pain may be seen within 1 to 2 months and reduction in erosions in 3 to 6 months.[186]

Methotrexate: Methotrexate at 2.5 to 7.5 mg weekly with adjuvant topical therapies is effective for severe, refractory oral lichen planus.[214] Based on reports in cutaneous lichen planus and in clinical practice, 10 to 15 mg weekly is more efficacious without an increase in side effects. The benefits of methotrexate can be seen within 4 to 8 weeks of initiation. Both methotrexate and MMF are first choices as a corticosteroid-sparing agent. Whereas MMF and methotrexate are preferred with erosive disease, oral retinoids are preferred with noneroded and hyperkeratotic disease. Given its low cost and relatively fast onset, methotrexate is often our preferred second-line systemic agent.

Mycophenolate Mofetil: MMF at 2 to 3 g/day in divided doses led to remission in 6 of 10 patients with severe oral lichen planus.[215] Of note, the clinical improvement of oral lichen planus using MMF can be gradual, often over 3 to 6 months, and adjuvant topical or oral corticosteroids are often necessary. Because of its tolerability and safety, MMF is considered a second-line systemic agent.

Cyclosporine: Cyclosporine has been reported effective in a report of two patients.[196] The dosages of cyclosporine are outlined in the prior section on cutaneous lichen planus therapies. Because of its long-term side effect profile and because there is no clear evidence that cyclosporine is superior to methotrexate or MMF in oral lichen planus, it is a third-line systemic agent.

Other Therapies: Additional therapies have been reported, including mesalazine, antibiotics, hydroxychloroquine, griseofulvin, thalidomide, and azathioprine, as well as parenteral alefacept, extracorporeal photopheresis, laser therapy, and PUVA therapy have all been reported as efficacious. However, these therapies often have attendant side effects or do not show clear efficacy. They are reserved as third-line corticosteroid-sparing therapies, and the risks and benefits of therapy should be considered before institution.

LICHEN PLANOPILARIS AND FRONTAL FIBROSING ALOPECIA

There are no randomized controlled trials in lichen planopilaris and only one controlled study. Therefore, many of the therapies in lichen planopilaris are based on expert opinion.[216] Lichen planopilaris has three major subtypes; however, for therapeutic purposes, they will be divided into lichen planopilaris and frontal fibrosing alopecia. These clinically distinct entities also appear to be responsive to different therapies.[217] When considering therapeutic modalities, the psychosocial effects of irreversible, scarring alopecia should be taken into account. Although the pathogenesis of lichen planopilaris is unknown, there is destruction of the bulge region, which leads to scarring. Recent studies have indicated a deficiency of PPARγ, which may lead to loss of immune privilege and scarring alopecia.[24] However, targeting of PPARγ with pioglitazone has shown mixed results with cessation of disease progression in 14% to 73% of cases.[218,219]

LICHEN PLANOPILARIS

Skin-Directed Therapies: First-line therapies for lichen planopilaris are mid to high potency topical corticosteroids with an average 53% response rate.[156,217,220] There are only limited data to determine the efficacy of topical calcineurin inhibitors, but its efficacy in cutaneous and oral lichen planus makes it common second-line topical therapy.

Systemic Therapies: Hydroxychloroquine (6.5 mg/kg of ideal body weight for 6 to 12 months) is the second most commonly used drug and showed a good response in 23% of cases.[185,217] There have been several negative studies using hydroxychloroquine, and there is good evidence that although clinical evidence of inflammation is decreased, progressive scarring of follicles continues.[216] Based on these findings, we advocate against hydroxychloroquine as a monotherapy. Oral corticosteroids at 1 mg/kg/day for 15 days with taper over 4 months and cyclosporine 300 mg/day for 3 to 5 months are the third most commonly used drugs with a good response in 60% of cases.[156,217,220,221] However, because of its side effect profile, cyclosporine has been largely supplanted by methotrexate and MMF. Relapse is common upon discontinuation of these medicines; therefore, topicals or intralesional therapy should be used concomitantly. A commonly used combinational regimen of oral doxycycline 100 mg twice daily, MMF 2 to 3 g/day, and intralesional steroids 10 mg/mL monthly basis had marked improvement in one third of cases in 6 to 12 months.[220,222-224]

Therapeutic Approach: One approach is superpotent topical corticosteroids, clobetasol, twice daily for 1 month, daily for 3 months, and every other day for 3 months.[221] Intralesional corticosteroids, hydroxychloroquine, and doxycycline (often in combination) can be added if there is no effect at 1 to 3 months, recognizing that hydroxychloroquine monotherapy is ineffective. Other immunosuppressive agents can then be added in severe, refractory, and rapidly progressive cases, including prednisone in combination with methotrexate or MMF, and cyclosporine monotherapy may be used with the above skin-directed therapies.

FRONTAL FIBROSING ALOPECIA

Skin-Directed Therapies: High-potency topical corticosteroids have been shown to be ineffective in frontal fibrosing alopecia, for 93% of cases, but intralesional corticosteroids (10 to 20 mg/mL injected every 3 to 6 months) led to partial improvement in 60% of cases.[217,221,225,226]

Systemic Therapies: Oral 5 α-reductase inhibitors, such as finasteride (2 mg to 5 mg/day dose for 12–18 months) or dutasteride (0.5 mg every 1 to 7 days) for 12 months), are most commonly used and most effective drugs, and they result in a good response in 45% to 47% of cases.[217,225,227-230] The largest study of frontal fibrosing alopecia to date found that androgenetic alopecia (AGA) was concurrently present in 40% of the women and 67% of the men.[226] Therefore, the benefit seen with antiandrogens may be due to the component of AGA. Hydroxychloroquine has been reported effective in approximately 30% of cases; however, many of the studies had concomitant topical therapy with immune modulators and minoxidil.[71,217] Other reported therapies (eg, systemic prednisone, hormone replacement, topical calcineurin inhibitors, topical minoxidil, cyclosporine, and MMF) have only been reported in small series and have highly variable response rates.

Therapeutic Approach: Based on the above evidence, many hair experts will use as first-line therapy an oral 5-αreductase inhibitor, intralesional corticosteroids, and occasionally topical minoxidil. For severe, rapidly progressive cases, corticosteroids in combination with MMF or methotrexate and cyclosporine monotherapy may be used in conjunction with these therapies.

NAIL LICHEN PLANUS

Nail lichen planus can be extremely difficult to treat, and 20-nail dystrophy and atrophic nails are often non-responsive. The goal of therapy should be to reduce the number of inflammatory cells within the nail and to prevent irreversible pterygium. A therapeutic approach should be very similar to cutaneous lichen planus. Ultrapotent topical and intralesional corticosteroids (5 to 10 mg/mL injected on a weekly basis) are first-line therapies. Systemic therapies should be reserved for cases manifesting significant compromise of function and causing debilitating pain. Additional therapies such as hydroxychloroquine has also been reported.[187]

ACKNOWLEDGMENTS

Steven A Nelson, MD, David J DiCaudo, and Collin Costello

REFERENCES

1. Wilson E. On leichen planus. *J Cutan Med Surg*. 1869; 3(10):117-132.
2. Weyl A. Bemerkungen zum lichen planus. *Dtsch Med Wochenschr*. 1885;11:624-626.
3. Wickham L. Sur un signe pathognomonique du lichen de Wilson (lichen plan) Stries et ponctuations grisatres. *Ann Dermatol Syphiligr (Paris)*. 1895;6:517-520.
4. Gougerot H, Burnier R. Lichen plan du col uterin, accompagnant un lichen plan jugal et un lichen plan stomacal: lichen plurimuqueux sans lichen cutane. *Bull Soc Fr Dermatol Syphiligr*. 1937;44:637-640.
5. Shiohara T, Moriya N, Tanaka Y, et al. Immunopathologic study of lichenoid skin diseases: correlation between HLA-DR-positive keratinocytes or Langerhans cells and epidermotropic T cells. *J Am Acad Dermatol*. 1988; 18(1 Pt 1):67-74.
6. Sugerman PB, Satterwhite K, Bigby M. Autocytotoxic T-cell clones in lichen planus. *Br J Dermatol*. 2000; 142(3):449-456.
7. Parodi A, Cozzani E, Massone C, et al. Prevalence of stratified epithelium-specific antinuclear antibodies in 138 patients with lichen planus. *J Am Acad Dermatol*. 2007;56(6):974-978.
8. de la Faille-Kuyper EH, de la Faille HB. An immunofluorescence study of lichen planus. *Br J Dermatol*. 1974; 90(4):365-371.
9. Carbone T, Nasorri F, Pennino D, et al. CD56 highCD16-NK cell involvement in cutaneous lichen planus. *Eur J Dermatol*. 2010;20(6):724-730.
10. McCartan BE, Lamey PJ. Expression of CD1 and HLA-DR by Langerhans cells (LC) in oral lichenoid drug eruptions (LDE) and idiopathic oral lichen planus (LP). *J Oral Pathol Med*. 1997;26(4):176-180.
11. Farthing PM, Matear P, Cruchley AT. Langerhans cell distribution and keratinocyte expression of HLADR in oral lichen planus. *J Oral Pathol Med*. 1992; 21(10):451-455.
12. Kawamura E, Nakamura S, Sasaki M, et al. Accumulation of oligoclonal T cells in the infiltrating lymphocytes in oral lichen planus. *J Oral Pathol Med*. 2003;32(5):282-289.
13. Zhou XJ, Savage NW, Sugerman PB, et al. TCR V beta gene expression in lesional T lymphocyte cell lines in oral lichen planus. *Oral Dis*. 1996;2(4):295-298.
14. Fayyazi A, Schweyer S, Soruri A, et al. T lymphocytes and altered keratinocytes express interferon-gamma and interleukin 6 in lichen planus. *Arch Dermatol Res*. 1999;291(9):485-490.
15. Seneschal J, Milpied B, Vergier B, et al. Cytokine imbalance with increased production of interferon-alpha in psoriasiform eruptions associated with antitumour necrosis factor-alpha treatments. *Br J Dermatol*. 2009; 161(5):1081-1088.
16. Lodi G, Scully C, Carrozzo M, Griffiths M, et al. Current controversies in oral lichen planus: report of an international consensus meeting. Part 1. Viral infections and etiopathogenesis. *Oral Surg Oral Med Oral Pathol Oral Radiol Endod*. 2005;100(1):40-51.
17. Meller S, Gilliet M, Homey B. Chemokines in the pathogenesis of lichenoid tissue reactions. *J Invest Dermatol*. 2009;129(2):315-319.
18. Tensen CP, Flier J, Van Der Raaij-Helmer EM, et al. Human IP-9: A keratinocyte-derived high affinity CXC-chemokine ligand for the IP-10/Mig receptor (CXCR3). *J Invest Dermatol*. 1999;112(5):716-722.
19. Cole KE, Strick CA, Paradis TJ, et al. Interferon-inducible T cell alpha chemoattractant (I-TAC): a novel non-ELR CXC chemokine with potent activity on activated T cells through selective high affinity binding to CXCR3. *J Exp Med*. 1998;187(12):2009-2021.
20. Farber JM. Mig and IP-10: CXC chemokines that target lymphocytes. *J Leukoc Biol*. 1997;61(3):246-257.
21. Kim CH, Rott L, Kunkel EJ, et al. Rules of chemokine receptor association with T cell polarization in vivo. *J Clin Invest*. 2001;108(9):1331-1339.
22. Szabo SJ, Sullivan BM, Stemmann C, et al. Distinct effects of T-bet in TH1 lineage commitment and IFN-gamma production in CD4 and CD8 T cells. *Science*. 2002;295(5553):338-342.
23. Marx N, Mach F, Sauty A, et al. Peroxisome proliferator-activated receptor-gamma activators inhibit IFN-gamma-induced expression of the T cell-active CXC chemokines IP-10, Mig, and I-TAC in human endothelial cells. *J Immunol*. 2000;164(12):6503-6508.
24. Karnik P, Tekeste Z, McCormick TS, et al. Hair follicle stem cell-specific PPARgamma deletion causes scarring alopecia. *J Invest Dermatol*. 2009;129(5): 1243-1257.
25. Groves RW, Ross EL, Barker JN, et al. Vascular cell adhesion molecule-1: expression in normal and diseased skin and regulation in vivo by interferon gamma. *J Am Acad Dermatol*. 1993;29(1):67-72.
26. Bennion SD, Middleton MH, David-Bajar KM, et al. In three types of interface dermatitis, different patterns of expression of intercellular adhesion molecule-1 (ICAM-1) indicate different triggers of disease. *J Invest Dermatol*. 1995;105(1 suppl):71S-79S.
27. Khan A, Farah CS, Savage NW, et al. Th1 cytokines in oral lichen planus. *J Oral Pathol Med*. 2003;32(2):77-83.
28. Ammar M, Mokni M, Boubaker S, et al. Involvement of granzyme B and granulysin in the cytotoxic response in lichen planus. *J Cutan Pathol*. 2008;35(7):630-634.
29. Quan LT, Tewari M, O'Rourke K, et al. Proteolytic activation of the cell death protease Yama/CPP32 by granzyme B. *Proc Natl Acad Sci U S A*. 1996;93(5): 1972-1976.
30. Zhou XJ, Sugerman PB, Savage NW, et al. Matrix metalloproteinases and their inhibitors in oral lichen planus. *J Cutan Pathol*. 2001;28(2):72-82.

31. Mazzarella N, Femiano F, Gombos F, et al. Matrix metalloproteinase gene expression in oral lichen planus: erosive vs. reticular forms. *J Eur Acad Dermatol Venereol.* 2006;20(8):953-957.
32. Neppelberg E, Johannessen AC, Jonsson R. Apoptosis in oral lichen planus. *Eur J Oral Sci.* 2001;109(5):361-364.
33. Shen LJ, Ruan P, Xie FF, et al. [Expressions of Fas/FasL and granzyme B in oral lichen planus and their significance]. *Di Yi Jun Yi Da Xue Xue Bao.* 2004;24(12):1362-1366.
34. Dekker NP, Lozada-Nur F, Lagenaur LA, et al. Apoptosis-associated markers in oral lichen planus. *J Oral Pathol Med.* 1997;26(4):170-175.
35. Pereira JS, Monteiro BV, Nonaka CF, et al. FoxP3(+) T regulatory cells in oral lichen planus and its correlation with the distinct clinical appearance of the lesions. *Int J Exp Pathol.* 2012;93(4):287-294.
36. Tao XA, Xia J, Chen XB, et al. FOXP3 T regulatory cells in lesions of oral lichen planus correlated with disease activity. *Oral Dis.* 2010;16(1):76-82.
37. Lin KL, Fulton LM, Berginski M, et al. Intravital imaging of donor allogeneic effector and regulatory T cells with host dendritic cells during GVHD. *Blood.* 2014;123(10):1604-1614.
38. Shiohara T, Moriya N, Saizawa KM, et al. Role of Langerhans cells in epidermotropism of T cells. *Arch Dermatol Res.* 1988;280(1):33-38.
39. Gueiros LA, Gondak R, Jorge Junior J, et al. Increased number of Langerhans cells in oral lichen planus and oral lichenoid lesions. *Oral Surg Oral Med Oral Pathol Oral Radiol.* 2012;113(5):661-666.
40. Arnold R, Seifert M, Asadullah K, et al. Crosstalk between keratinocytes and T lymphocytes via Fas/Fas ligand interaction: modulation by cytokines. *J Immunol.* 1999;162(12):7140-7147.
41. Berthou C, Michel L, Soulie A, et al. Acquisition of granzyme B and Fas ligand proteins by human keratinocytes contributes to epidermal cell defense. *J Immunol.* 1997;159(11):5293-5300.
42. Wenzel J, Tuting T. An IFN-associated cytotoxic cellular immune response against viral, self-, or tumor antigens is a common pathogenetic feature in "interface dermatitis." *J Invest Dermatol.* 2008;128(10):2392-2402.
43. Kurts C. Cross-presentation: inducing CD8 T cell immunity and tolerance. *J Mol Med.* 2000;78(6):326-332.
44. Platzer B, Stout M, Fiebiger E. Antigen cross-presentation of immune complexes. *Front Immunol.* 2014;5:140.
45. Gorouhi F, Davari P, Fazel N. Cutaneous and mucosal lichen planus: a comprehensive review of clinical subtypes, risk factors, diagnosis, and prognosis. *ScientificWorldJournal.* 2014;2014:742826.
46. Wenzel J, Peters B, Zahn S, et al. Gene expression profiling of lichen planus reflects CXCL9+-mediated inflammation and distinguishes this disease from atopic dermatitis and psoriasis. *J Invest Dermatol.* 2008;128(1):67-78.
47. McCartan BE, Healy CM. The reported prevalence of oral lichen planus: a review and critique. *J Oral Pathol Med.* 2008;37(8):447-453.
48. Axell T, Rundquist L. Oral lichen planus—a demographic study. *Community Dent Oral Epidemiol.* 1987;15(1):52-56.
49. Boyd AS, Neldner KH. Lichen planus. *J Am Acad Dermatol.* 1991;25(4):593-619.
50. Pandhi D, Singal A, Bhattacharya SN. Lichen planus in childhood: a series of 316 patients. *Pediatr Dermatol.* 2014;31(1):59-67.
51. Kanwar AJ, De D. Lichen planus in childhood: report of 100 cases. *Clin Exp Dermatol.* 2010;35(3):257-262.
52. Sharma R, Maheshwari V. Childhood lichen planus: a report of fifty cases. *Pediatr Dermatol.* 1999;16(5):345-348.
53. Walton KE, Bowers EV, Drolet BA, et al. Childhood lichen planus: demographics of a U.S. population. *Pediatr Dermatol.* 2010;27(1):34-38.
54. Altman J, Perry HO. The variations and course of lichen planus. *Arch Dermatol.* 1961;84:179-191.
55. Singal A. Familial mucosal lichen planus in three successive generations. *Int J Dermatol.* 2005;44(1):81-82.
56. Copeman PW, Tan RS, Timlin D, et al. Familial lichen planus. Another disease or a distinct people? *Br J Dermatol.* 1978;98(5):573-577.
57. La Nasa G, Cottoni F, Mulargia M, et al. HLA antigen distribution in different clinical subgroups demonstrates genetic heterogeneity in lichen planus. *Br J Dermatol.* 1995;132(6):897-900.
58. Wenzel J, Scheler M, Proelss J, et al. Type I interferon-associated cytotoxic inflammation in lichen planus. *J Cutan Pathol.* 2006;33(10):672-678.
59. Batra P, Wang N, Kamino H, et al. Linear lichen planus. *Dermatol Online J.* 2008;14(10):16.
60. Mizukawa Y, Horie C, Yamazaki Y, et al. Detection of varicella-zoster virus antigens in lesional skin of zosteriform lichen planus but not in that of linear lichen planus. *Dermatology.* 2012;225(1):22-26.
61. Schepis C, Siragusa M, Lentini M. Erosive lichen planus: two uncommon cases. *Acta Derm Venereol.* 2008;88(3):268-270.
62. Gunduz K, Sacar T, Inanir I, et al. Flexural follicular lichen planus. *Clin Exp Dermatol.* 2009;34(7):e297-298.
63. Jimenez-Gallo D, Albarran-Planelles C, Linares-Barrios M, et al. Facial follicular cysts: a case of lichen planus follicularis tumidus? *J Cutan Pathol.* 2013;40(9):818-822.
64. Katzenellenbogen I. Lichen planus actinicus (lichen planus in subtropical countries). *Dermatologica.* 1962;124:10-20.
65. Bouassida S, Boudaya S, Turki H, et al. [Actinic lichen planus: 32 cases]. *Ann Dermatol Venereol.* 1998;125(6-7):408-413.
66. Dammak A, Masmoudi A, Boudaya S, et al. [Childhood actinic lichen planus (6 cases)]. *Arch Pediatr.* 2008;15(2):111-114.
67. Denguezli M, Nouira R, Jomaa B. [Actinic lichen planus. An anatomoclinical study of 10 Tunisian cases]. *Ann Dermatol Venereol.* 1994;121(8):543-546.
68. Salman SM, Kibbi AG, Zaynoun S. Actinic lichen planus. A clinicopathologic study of 16 patients. *J Am Acad Dermatol.* 1989;20(2 Pt 1):226-231.
69. Meinhard J, Stroux A, Lunnemann L, et al. Lichen planopilaris: epidemiology and prevalence of subtypes—a retrospective analysis in 104 patients. *J Dtsch Dermatol Ges.* 2014;12(3):229-235, 229-236.
70. Duque-Estrada B, Tamler C, Sodre CT, et al. Dermoscopy patterns of cicatricial alopecia resulting from discoid lupus erythematosus and lichen planopilaris. *An Bras Dermatol.* 2010;85(2):179-183.
71. Samrao A, Chew AL, Price V. Frontal fibrosing alopecia: a clinical review of 36 patients. *Br J Dermatol.* 2010;163(6):1296-1300.
72. Aldoori N, Dobson K, Holden CR, et al. Frontal fibrosing alopecia: possible association with leave-on facial skin care products and sunscreens; a questionnaire study. *Br J Dermatol.* 2016;175(4):762-767.

73. Abbas O, Chedraoui A, Ghosn S. Frontal fibrosing alopecia presenting with components of Piccardi-Lassueur-Graham-Little syndrome. *J Am Acad Dermatol.* 2007;57(2 Suppl):S15-18.
74. Eisen D. The evaluation of cutaneous, genital, scalp, nail, esophageal, and ocular involvement in patients with oral lichen planus. *Oral Surg Oral Med Oral Pathol Oral Radiol Endod.* 1999;88(4):431-436.
75. Silverman S Jr, Gorsky M, Lozada-Nur F. A prospective follow-up study of 570 patients with oral lichen planus: persistence, remission, and malignant association. *Oral Surg Oral Med Oral Pathol.* 1985;60(1):30-34.
76. Andreasen JO. Oral lichen planus. 1. A clinical evaluation of 115 cases. *Oral Surg Oral Med Oral Pathol.* 1968;25(1):31-42.
77. Eisen D. The clinical features, malignant potential, and systemic associations of oral lichen planus: a study of 723 patients. *J Am Acad Dermatol.* 2002;46(2):207-214.
78. Lo Russo L, Fierro G, Guiglia R, et al. Epidemiology of desquamative gingivitis: evaluation of 125 patients and review of the literature. *Int J Dermatol.* 2009;48(10):1049-1052.
79. Cobos-Fuentes MJ, Martinez-Sahuquillo-Marquez A, Gallardo-Castillo I, et al. Oral lichenoid lesions related to contact with dental materials: a literature review. *Med Oral Patol Oral Cir Bucal.* 2009;14(10):e514-520.
80. Yiannias JA, el-Azhary RA, Hand JH, et al. Relevant contact sensitivities in patients with the diagnosis of oral lichen planus. *J Am Acad Dermatol.* 2000;42(2 Pt 1):177-182.
81. Rogers RS 3rd, Bruce AJ. Lichenoid contact stomatitis: is inorganic mercury the culprit? *Arch Dermatol.* 2004;140(12):1524-1525.
82. Scalf LA, Fowler JF Jr, Morgan KW, et al. Dental metal allergy in patients with oral, cutaneous, and genital lichenoid reactions. *Am J Contact Dermat.* 2001;12(3):146-150.
83. Dunsche A, Kastel I, Terheyden H, et al. Oral lichenoid reactions associated with amalgam: improvement after amalgam removal. *Br J Dermatol.* 2003;148(1):70-76.
84. Ibbotson SH, Speight EL, Macleod RI, et al. The relevance and effect of amalgam replacement in subjects with oral lichenoid reactions. *Br J Dermatol.* 1996;134(3):420-423.
85. Smart ER, Macleod RI, Lawrence CM. Resolution of lichen planus following removal of amalgam restorations in patients with proven allergy to mercury salts: a pilot study. *Br Dent J.* 1995;178(3):108-112.
86. Ficarra G, Flaitz CM, Gaglioti D, et al. White lichenoid lesions of the buccal mucosa in patients with HIV infection. *Oral Surg Oral Med Oral Pathol.* 1993;76(4):460-466.
87. Chandan VS, Murray JA, Abraham SC. Esophageal lichen planus. *Arch Pathol Lab Med.* 2008;132(6):1026-1029.
88. Harewood GC, Murray JA, Cameron AJ. Esophageal lichen planus: the Mayo Clinic experience. *Dis Esophagus.* 1999;12(4):309-311.
89. Chryssostalis A, Gaudric M, Terris B, et al. Esophageal lichen planus: a series of eight cases including a patient with esophageal verrucous carcinoma. A case series. *Endoscopy.* 2008;40(9):764-768.
90. Belfiore P, Di Fede O, Cabibi D, et al. Prevalence of vulval lichen planus in a cohort of women with oral lichen planus: an interdisciplinary study. *Br J Dermatol.* 2006;155(5):994-998.
91. Kennedy CM, Galask RP. Erosive vulvar lichen planus: retrospective review of characteristics and outcomes in 113 patients seen in a vulvar specialty clinic. *J Reprod Med.* 2007;52(1):43-47.
92. Eisen D. The vulvovaginal-gingival syndrome of lichen planus. The clinical characteristics of 22 patients. *Arch Dermatol.* 1994;130(11):1379-1382.
93. Setterfield JF, Neill S, Shirlaw PJ, et al. The vulvovaginal gingival syndrome: a severe subgroup of lichen planus with characteristic clinical features and a novel association with the class II HLA DQB1 0201 allele. *J Am Acad Dermatol.* 2006;55(1):98-113.
94. Thorne JE, Jabs DA, Nikolskaia OV, et al. Lichen planus and cicatrizing conjunctivitis: characterization of five cases. *Am J Ophthalmol.* 2003;136(2):239-243.
95. Hahn JM, Meisler DM, Lowder CY, et al. Cicatrizing conjunctivitis associated with paraneoplastic lichen planus. *Am J Ophthalmol.* 2000;129(1):98-99.
96. Webber NK, Setterfield JF, Lewis FM, et al. Lacrimal canalicular duct scarring in patients with lichen planus. *Arch Dermatol.* 2012;148(2):224-227.
97. Sartori-Valinotti JC, Bruce AJ, Krotova Khan Y, et al. A 10-year review of otic lichen planus: the Mayo Clinic experience. *JAMA Dermatol.* 2013;149(9):1082-1086.
98. Tosti A, Peluso AM, Fanti PA, et al. Nail lichen planus: clinical and pathologic study of twenty-four patients. *J Am Acad Dermatol.* 1993;28(5 Pt 1):724-730.
99. Nakamura R, Broce AA, Palencia DP, et al. Dermatoscopy of nail lichen planus. *Int J Dermatol.* 2013;52(6):684-687.
100. Tosti A, Piraccini BM, Cambiaghi S, et al. Nail lichen planus in children: clinical features, response to treatment, and long-term follow-up. *Arch Dermatol.* 2001;137(8):1027-1032.
101. Mohamed M, Korbi M, Hammedi F, et al. Lichen planus pigmentosus inversus: a series of 10 Tunisian patients. *Int J Dermatol.* 2016.
102. Sanchez-Perez J, Rios Buceta L, Fraga J, Garcia-Diez A. Lichen planus with lesions on the palms and/or soles: prevalence and clinicopathological study of 36 patients. *Br J Dermatol.* 2000;142(2):310-314.
103. Ellgehausen P, Elsner P, Burg G. Drug-induced lichen planus. *Clin Dermatol.* 1998;16(3):325-332.
104. Voskens CJ, Goldinger SM, Loquai C, et al. The price of tumor control: an analysis of rare side effects of anti-CTLA-4 therapy in metastatic melanoma from the ipilimumab network. *PLoS One.* 2013;8(1):e53745.
105. Hwang SJ, Carlos G, Wakade D, et al. Cutaneous adverse events (AEs) of anti-programmed cell death (PD)-1 therapy in patients with metastatic melanoma: a single-institution cohort. *J Am Acad Dermatol.* 2016;74(3):455-461 e451.
106. Brancaccio RR, Cockerell CJ, Belsito D, et al. Allergic contact dermatitis from color film developers: clinical and histologic features. *J Am Acad Dermatol.* 1993;28(5 Pt 2):827-830.
107. Lembo G, Balato N, Patruno C, et al. Lichenoid contact dermatitis due to aminoglycoside antibiotics. *Contact Dermatitis.* 1987;17(2):122-123.
108. Raap U, Stiesch M, Reh H, et al. Investigation of contact allergy to dental metals in 206 patients. *Contact Dermatitis.* 2009;60(6):339-343.
109. Copeman PW, Schroeter AL, Kierland RR. An unusual variant of lupus erythematosus or lichen planus. *Br J Dermatol.* 1970;83(2):269-272.

110. Romero RW, Nesbitt LT Jr, Reed RJ. Unusual variant of lupus erythematosus or lichen planus. Clinical, histopathologic, and immunofluorescent studies. *Arch Dermatol.* 1977;113(6):741-748.
111. Zaraa I, Mahfoudh A, Sellami MK, et al. Lichen planus pemphigoides: four new cases and a review of the literature. *Int J Dermatol.* 2013;52(4):406-412.
112. Zillikens D, Caux F, Mascaro JM, et al. Autoantibodies in lichen planus pemphigoides react with a novel epitope within the C-terminal NC16A domain of BP180. *J Invest Dermatol.* 1999;113(1):117-121.
113. Ben Salem C, Chenguel L, Ghariani N, et al. Captopril-induced lichen planus pemphigoides. *Pharmacoepidemiol Drug Saf.* 2008;17(7):722-724.
114. Konstantinov KN, Sondergaard J, Izuno G, et al. Keratosis lichenoides chronica. *J Am Acad Dermatol.* 1998;38(2 Pt 2):306-309.
115. Boer A. Keratosis lichenoides chronica: proposal of a concept. *Am J Dermatopathol.* 2006;28(3):260-275.
116. Filipovich AH, Weisdorf D, Pavletic S, et al. National Institutes of Health consensus development project on criteria for clinical trials in chronic graft-versus-host disease: I. Diagnosis and staging working group report. *Biol Blood Marrow Transplant.* 2005;11(12):945-956.
117. Bruggen MC, Klein I, Greinix H, et al. Diverse T-cell responses characterize the different manifestations of cutaneous graft-versus-host disease. *Blood.* 2014;123(2):290-299.
118. Nakae S, Komiyama Y, Nambu A, et al. Antigen-specific T cell sensitization is impaired in IL-17-deficient mice, causing suppression of allergic cellular and humoral responses. *Immunity.* 2002;17(3):375-387.
119. Gagliani N, Amezcua Vesely MC, Iseppon A, et al. Th17 cells transdifferentiate into regulatory T cells during resolution of inflammation. *Nature.* 2015;523(7559):221-225.
120. Aractingi S, Chosidow O. Cutaneous graft-versus-host disease. *Arch Dermatol.* 1998;134(5):602-612.
121. Shulman HM, Cardona DM, Greenson JK, et al. NIH Consensus development project on criteria for clinical trials in chronic graft-versus-host disease: II. The 2014 Pathology Working Group Report. *Biol Blood Marrow Transplant.* 2015;21(4):589-603.
122. Kim HS, Park EJ, Kwon IH, et al. Clinical and histopathologic study of benign lichenoid keratosis on the face. *Am J Dermatopathol.* 2013;35(7):738-741.
123. Oliver GF, Winkelmann RK, Muller SA. Lichenoid dermatitis: a clinicopathologic and immunopathologic review of sixty-two cases. *J Am Acad Dermatol.* 1989;21(2 Pt 1):284-292.
124. Magro CM, Crowson AN. Lichenoid and granulomatous dermatitis. *Int J Dermatol.* 2000;39(2):126-133.
125. Shengyuan L, Songpo Y, Wen W, et al. Hepatitis C virus and lichen planus: a reciprocal association determined by a meta-analysis. *Arch Dermatol.* 2009;145(9):1040-1047.
126. Halawani M. Hepatitis C virus genotypes among patients with lichen planus in the Kingdom of Saudi Arabia. *Int J Dermatol.* 2014;53(2):171-177.
127. Imhof M, Popal H, Lee JH, et al. Prevalence of hepatitis C virus antibodies and evaluation of hepatitis C virus genotypes in patients with lichen planus. *Dermatology.* 1997;195(1):1-5.
128. Mignogna MD, Lo Muzio L, Favia G, et al. Oral lichen planus and HCV infection: a clinical evaluation of 263 cases. *Int J Dermatol.* 1998;37(8):575-578.
129. del Olmo JA, Pascual I, Bagan JV, et al. Prevalence of hepatitis C virus in patients with lichen planus of the oral cavity and chronic liver disease. *Eur J Oral Sci.* 2000;108(5):378-382.
130. Cheng Z, Zhou B, Shi X, et al. Extrahepatic manifestations of chronic hepatitis C virus infection: 297 cases from a tertiary medical center in Beijing, China. *Chin Med J (Engl).* 2014;127(7):1206-1210.
131. Carrozzo M, Brancatello F, Dametto E, et al. Hepatitis C virus-associated oral lichen planus: is the geographical heterogeneity related to HLA-DR6? *J Oral Pathol Med.* 2005;34(4):204-208.
132. Carrozzo M, Francia Di Celle P, Gandolfo S, et al. Increased frequency of HLA-DR6 allele in Italian patients with hepatitis C virus-associated oral lichen planus. *Br J Dermatol.* 2001;144(4):803-808.
133. Mahboob A, Haroon TS, Iqbal Z, et al. Prevalence of hepatitis B surface antigen carrier state in patients with lichen planus—report of 200 cases from Lahore, Pakistan. *J Ayub Med Coll Abbottabad.* 2007;19(4):68-70.
134. Saleh N, Samir N, Megahed H, et al. Homocysteine and other cardiovascular risk factors in patients with lichen planus. *J Eur Acad Dermatol Venereol.* 2013.
135. Arias-Santiago S, Buendia-Eisman A, Aneiros-Fernandez J, et al. Cardiovascular risk factors in patients with lichen planus. *Am J Med.* 2011;124(6):543-548.
136. Ozlu E, Karadag AS, Toprak AE, et al. Evaluation of cardiovascular risk factors, haematological and biochemical parameters, and serum endocan levels in patients with lichen planus. *Dermatology.* 2016;232(4):438-443.
137. Baykal L, Arica DA, Yayli S, et al. Prevalence of metabolic syndrome in patients with mucosal lichen planus: a case-control study. *Am J Clin Dermatol.* 2015;16(5):439-445.
138. Atanaskova Mesinkovska N, Brankov N, Piliang M, et al. Association of lichen planopilaris with thyroid disease: a retrospective case-control study. *J Am Acad Dermatol.* 2014;70(5):889-892.
139. Saunders H, Buchanan JA, Cooper S, et al. The period prevalence of oral lichen planus in a cohort of patients with vulvar lichen sclerosus. *J Eur Acad Dermatol Venereol.* 2010;24(1):18-21.
140. Chung PI, Hwang CY, Chen YJ, et al. Autoimmune comorbid diseases associated with lichen planus: a nationwide case-control study. *J Eur Acad Dermatol Venereol.* 2015;29(8):1570-1575.
141. Mignogna MD, Lo Muzio L, Lo Russo L, et al. Clinical guidelines in early detection of oral squamous cell carcinoma arising in oral lichen planus: a 5-year experience. *Oral Oncol.* 2001;37(3):262-267.
142. Syrjanen S, Lodi G, von Bultzingslowen I, et al. Human papillomaviruses in oral carcinoma and oral potentially malignant disorders: a systematic review. *Oral Dis.* 2011;17 Suppl 1:58-72.
143. Ingafou M, Leao JC, Porter SR, et al. Oral lichen planus: a retrospective study of 690 British patients. *Oral Dis.* 2006;12(5):463-468.
144. Xue JL, Fan MW, Wang SZ, et al. A clinical study of 674 patients with oral lichen planus in China. *J Oral Pathol Med.* 2005;34(8):467-472.
145. Sigurgeirsson B, Lindelof B. Lichen planus and malignancy. An epidemiologic study of 2071 patients and a review of the literature. *Arch Dermatol.* 1991;127(11):1684-1688.
146. Allen CM, Blozis GG. Oral mucosal reactions to cinnamon-flavored chewing gum. *J Am Dent Assoc.* 1988;116(6):664-667.

147. Gunatheesan S, Tam MM, Tate B, et al. Retrospective study of oral lichen planus and allergy to spearmint oil. *Australas J Dermatol.* 2012;53(3):224-228.
148. Lomaga MA, Polak S, Grushka M, et al. Results of patch testing in patients diagnosed with oral lichen planus. *J Cutan Med Surg.* 2009;13(2):88-95.
149. Dreiher J, Shapiro J, Cohen AD. Lichen planus and dyslipidaemia: a case-control study. *Br J Dermatol.* 2009;161(3):626-629.
150. Lapane KL, Jakiche AF, Sugano D, et al. Hepatitis C infection risk analysis: who should be screened? Comparison of multiple screening strategies based on the National Hepatitis Surveillance Program. *Am J Gastroenterol.* 1998;93(4):591-596.
151. Ellis FA. Histopathology of lichen planus based on analysis of one hundred biopsy specimens. *J Invest Dermatol.* 1967;48(2):143-148.
152. Alomari A, McNiff JM. The significance of eosinophils in hypertrophic lichen planus. *J Cutan Pathol.* 2014;41(4):347-352.
153. Lage D, Juliano PB, Metze K, et al. Lichen planus and lichenoid drug-induced eruption: a histological and immunohistochemical study. *Int J Dermatol.* 2012;51(10):1199-1205.
154. Van den Haute V, Antoine JL, Lachapelle JM. Histopathological discriminant criteria between lichenoid drug eruption and idiopathic lichen planus: retrospective study on selected samples. *Dermatologica.* 1989;179(1):10-13.
155. Tan E, Malik R, Quirk CJ. Hypertrophic lichen planus mimicking squamous cell carcinoma. *Australas J Dermatol.* 1998;39(1):45-47.
156. Mehregan DA, Van Hale HM, Muller SA. Lichen planopilaris: clinical and pathologic study of forty-five patients. *J Am Acad Dermatol.* 1992;27(6 Pt 1):935-942.
157. Helander SD, Rogers RS 3rd. The sensitivity and specificity of direct immunofluorescence testing in disorders of mucous membranes. *J Am Acad Dermatol.* 1994; 30(1):65-75.
158. Kulthanan K, Jiamton S, Varothai S, et al. Direct immunofluorescence study in patients with lichen planus. *Int J Dermatol.* 2007;46(12):1237-1241.
159. Schiodt M, Holmstrup P, Dabelsteen E, et al. Deposits of immunoglobulins, complement, and fibrinogen in oral lupus erythematosus, lichen planus, and leukoplakia. *Oral Surg Oral Med Oral Pathol.* 1981; 51(6):603-608.
160. Miteva M, Tosti A. Dermoscopy guided scalp biopsy in cicatricial alopecia. *J Eur Acad Dermatol Venereol.* 2013; 27(10):1299-1303.
161. Sano SM, Quarracino MC, Aguas SC, et al. Sensitivity of direct immunofluorescence in oral diseases. Study of 125 cases. *Med Oral Patol Oral Cir Bucal.* 2008; 13(5):E287-291.
162. Mutasim DF, Adams BB. Immunofluorescence in dermatology. *J Am Acad Dermatol.* 2001;45(6):803-822; quiz 822-804.
163. Schmidt H. Frequency, duration and localization of lichen planus. A study based on 181 patients. *Acta Derm Venereol.* 1961;41:164-167.
164. Daoud MS, Pittelkow MR. Lichen planus. In: Goldsmith L, Katz SI, Gilchrest AS, P et al, eds. *Fitzpatrick's Dermatology in General Medicine*, 8th ed. New York, NY: McGraw-Hill; 2012.
165. Okiyama N, Furumoto Y, Villarroel VA, et al. Reversal of CD8 T-cell-mediated mucocutaneous graft-versus-host-like disease by the JAK inhibitor tofacitinib. *J Invest Dermatol.* 2014;134(4):992-1000.
166. Kurtzman DJ, Wright NA, Lin J, et al. Tofacitinib citrate for refractory cutaneous dermatomyositis: an alternative treatment. *JAMA Dermatol.* 2016;152(8): 944-945.
167. Hornung T, Janzen V, Heidgen FJ, et al. Remission of recalcitrant dermatomyositis treated with ruxolitinib. *N Engl J Med.* 2014;371(26):2537-2538.
168. Harris JE, Rashighi M, Nguyen N, et al. Rapid skin repigmentation on oral ruxolitinib in a patient with coexistent vitiligo and alopecia areata (AA). *J Am Acad Dermatol.* 2016;74(2):370-371.
169. Theng CT, Tan SH, Goh CL, et al. A randomized controlled trial to compare calcipotriol with betamethasone valerate for the treatment of cutaneous lichen planus. *J Dermatol Treat.* 2004;15(3):141-145.
170. Bjornberg A, Hellgren L. Betamethasone-I7, 2I-dipropionate ointment: an effective topical preparation in lichen ruber planus. *Curr Med Res Opin.* 1976; 4(3):212-217.
171. Samycia M, Lin AN. Efficacy of topical calcineurin inhibitors in lichen planus. *J Cutan Med Surg.* 2012; 16(4):221-229.
172. Wachter T, Averbeck M, Hara H, et al. Induction of CD4+ T cell apoptosis as a consequence of impaired cytoskeletal rearrangement in UVB-irradiated dendritic cells. *J Immunol.* 2003;171(2):776-782.
173. Gibbs NK, Norval M. Photoimmunosuppression: a brief overview. *Photodermatol Photoimmunol Photomed.* 2013;29(2):57-64.
174. Pavlotsky F, Nathansohn N, Kriger G, et al. Ultraviolet-B treatment for cutaneous lichen planus: our experience with 50 patients. *Photodermatol Photoimmunol Photomed.* 2008;24(2):83-86.
175. Wackernagel A, Legat FJ, Hofer A, et al. Psoralen plus UVA vs. UVB-311 nm for the treatment of lichen planus. *Photodermatol Photoimmunol Photomed.* 2007; 23(1):15-19.
176. Pitche P, Saka B, Kombate K, et al. [Treatment of generalized cutaneous lichen planus with dipropionate and betamethasone disodium phosphate: an open study of 73 cases]. *Ann Dermatol Venereol.* 2007;134 (3 Pt 1):237-240.
177. Omidian M, Ayoobi A, Mapar MA, et al. Efficacy of sulfasalazine in the treatment of generalized lichen planus: randomized double-blinded clinical trial on 52 patients. *J Eur Acad Dermatol Venereol.* 2010; 24(9):1051-1054.
178. Bauza A, Espana A, Gil P, et al. Successful treatment of lichen planus with sulfasalazine in 20 patients. *Int J Dermatol.* 2005;44(2):158-162.
179. Rasi A, Behzadi AH, Davoudi S, et al. Efficacy of oral metronidazole in treatment of cutaneous and mucosal lichen planus. *J Drugs Dermatol.* 2010;9(10): 1186-1190.
180. Buyuk AY, Kavala M. Oral metronidazole treatment of lichen planus. *J Am Acad Dermatol.* 2000;43(2 Pt 1): 260-262.
181. Zivkovic SA, Lacomis D, Giuliani MJ. Sensory neuropathy associated with metronidazole: report of four cases and review of the literature. *J Clin Neuromuscul Dis.* 2001;3(1):8-12.
182. Laurberg G, Geiger JM, Hjorth N, et al. Treatment of lichen planus with acitretin. A double-blind, placebo-controlled study in 65 patients. *J Am Acad Dermatol.* 1991;24(3):434-437.
183. Ayres S, 3rd, Ayres S Jr. Chloroquine in treatment of lichen planus and other dermatoses. *J Am Med Assoc.* 1955;157(2):136-138.

184. Pirila V, Helanen S. Trial of chloroquine in the treatment of lichen planus. *Acta Derm Venereol.* 1958; 38(3):194-197.
185. Chiang C, Sah D, Cho BK, et al. Hydroxychloroquine and lichen planopilaris: efficacy and introduction of Lichen Planopilaris Activity Index scoring system. *J Am Acad Dermatol.* 2010;62(3):387-392.
186. Eisen D. Hydroxychloroquine sulfate (Plaquenil) improves oral lichen planus: an open trial. *J Am Acad Dermatol.* 1993;28(4):609-612.
187. Mostafa WZ. Lichen planus of the nail: treatment with antimalarials. *J Am Acad Dermatol.* 1989;20(2 Pt 1): 289-290.
188. Ramirez P, Feito M, Sendagorta E, et al. Childhood actinic lichen planus: successful treatment with antimalarials. *Australas J Dermatol.* 2012;53(1): e10-13.
189. Rivas-Tolosa N, Requena C, Llombart B, et al. Antimalarial drugs for the treatment of oral erosive lichen planus. *Dermatology.* 2016;232(1):86-90.
190. Schewach-Millet M, Skpiro D, Sofer E. Actinic lichen planus: treatment with antimalarials. *J Am Acad Dermatol.* 1990;22(2 Pt 1):325.
191. Hazra SC, Choudhury AM, Khondker L, et al. Comparative efficacy of methotrexate and mini pulse betamethasone in the treatment of lichen planus. *Mymensingh Med J.* 2013;22(4):787-797.
192. Kanwar AJ, De D. Methotrexate for treatment of lichen planus: old drug, new indication. *J Eur Acad Dermatol Venereol.* 2013;27(3):e410-413.
193. Turan H, Baskan EB, Tunali S, et al. Methotrexate for the treatment of generalized lichen planus. *J Am Acad Dermatol.* 2009;60(1):164-166.
194. Frieling U, Bonsmann G, Schwarz T, et al. Treatment of severe lichen planus with mycophenolate mofetil. *J Am Acad Dermatol.* 2003;49(6):1063-1066.
195. Verma KK, Sirka CS, Khaitan BK. Generalized severe lichen planus treated with azathioprine. *Acta Derm Venereol.* 1999;79(6):493.
196. Ho VC, Gupta AK, Ellis CN, et al. Treatment of severe lichen planus with cyclosporine. *J Am Acad Dermatol.* 1990;22(1):64-68.
197. Holmstrup P, Schiotz AW, Westergaard J. Effect of dental plaque control on gingival lichen planus. *Oral Surg Oral Med Oral Pathol.* 1990;69(5):585-590.
198. Davari P, Hsiao HH, Fazel N. Mucosal lichen planus: an evidence-based treatment update. *Am J Clin Dermatol.* 2014;15(3):181-195.
199. Ungphaiboon S, Nittayananta W, Vuddhakul V, et al. Formulation and efficacy of triamcinolone acetonide mouthwash for treating oral lichen planus. *Am J Health Syst Pharm.* 2005;62(5):485-491.
200. Voute AB, Schulten EA, Langendijk PN, et al. Fluocinonide in an adhesive base for treatment of oral lichen planus. A double-blind, placebo-controlled clinical study. *Oral Surg Oral Med Oral Pathol.* 1993; 75(2):181-185.
201. Rödström P, Hakeberg M, Jontell M, et al. Erosive oral lichen planus treated with clobetasol propionate and triamcinolone acetonide in Orabase: a double-blind clinical trial. *J Dermatol Treat* 1994;5(1): 7-10.
202. Carbone M, Conrotto D, Carrozzo M, et al. Topical corticosteroids in association with miconazole and chlorhexidine in the long-term management of atrophic-erosive oral lichen planus: a placebo-controlled and comparative study between clobetasol and fluocinonide. *Oral Dis.* 1999;5(1):44-49.
203. Lo Muzio L, della Valle A, Mignogna MD, et al. The treatment of oral aphthous ulceration or erosive lichen planus with topical clobetasol propionate in three preparations: a clinical and pilot study on 54 patients. *J Oral Pathol Med.* 2001;30(10):611-617.
204. Lodi G, Tarozzi M, Sardella A, et al. Miconazole as adjuvant therapy for oral lichen planus: a double-blind randomized controlled trial. *Br J Dermatol.* 2007; 156(6):1336-1341.
205. Lodi G, Carrozzo M, Furness S, Thongprasom K. Interventions for treating oral lichen planus: a systematic review. *Br J Dermatol.* 2012;166(5):938-947.
206. Conrotto D, Carbone M, Carrozzo M, et al. Ciclosporin vs. clobetasol in the topical management of atrophic and erosive oral lichen planus: a double-blind, randomized controlled trial. *Br J Dermatol.* 2006;154(1): 139-145.
207. Kar HK, Parsad D, Gautam RK, et al. Comparison of topical tretinoin and betamethasone in oral lichen planus. *Indian J Dermatol Venereol Leprol.* 1996;62(5): 304-305.
208. Giustina TA, Stewart JC, Ellis CN, et al. Topical application of isotretinoin gel improves oral lichen planus. A double-blind study. *Arch Dermatol.* 1986;122(5): 534-536.
209. Lee YC, Shin SY, Kim SW, et al. Intralesional injection versus mouth rinse of triamcinolone acetonide in oral lichen planus: a randomized controlled study. *Otolaryngol Head Neck Surg.* 2013;148(3):443-449.
210. Lodi G, Scully C, Carrozzo M, et al. Current controversies in oral lichen planus: report of an international consensus meeting. Part 2. Clinical management and malignant transformation. *Oral Surg Oral Med Oral Pathol Oral Radiol Endod.* 2005;100(2):164-178.
211. Carbone M, Goss E, Carrozzo M, et al. Systemic and topical corticosteroid treatment of oral lichen planus: a comparative study with long-term follow-up. *J Oral Pathol Med.* 2003;32(6):323-329.
212. Malhotra AK, Khaitan BK, Sethuraman G, et al. Betamethasone oral mini-pulse therapy compared with topical triamcinolone acetonide (0.1%) paste in oral lichen planus: a randomized comparative study. *J Am Acad Dermatol.* 2008;58(4):596-602.
213. Kunz M, Urosevic-Maiwald M, Goldinger SM, et al. Efficacy and safety of oral alitretinoin in severe oral lichen planus—results of a prospective pilot study. *J Eur Acad Dermatol Venereol.* 2016;30(2):293-298.
214. Jang N, Fischer G. Treatment of erosive vulvovaginal lichen planus with methotrexate. *Australas J Dermatol.* 2008;49(4):216-219.
215. Wee JS, Shirlaw PJ, Challacombe SJ, et al. Efficacy of mycophenolate mofetil in severe mucocutaneous lichen planus: a retrospective review of 10 patients. *Br J Dermatol.* 2012;167(1):36-43.
216. Sperling LC, Nguyen JV. Commentary: treatment of lichen planopilaris: some progress, but a long way to go. *J Am Acad Dermatol.* 2010;62(3):398-401.
217. Racz E, Gho C, Moorman PW, et al. Treatment of frontal fibrosing alopecia and lichen planopilaris: a systematic review. *J Eur Acad Dermatol Venereol.* 2013; 27(12):1461-1470.
218. Mesinkovska NA, Tellez A, Dawes D, et al. The use of oral pioglitazone in the treatment of lichen planopilaris. *J Am Acad Dermatol.* 2015;72(2):355-356.
219. Spring P, Spanou Z, de Viragh PA. Lichen planopilaris treated by the peroxisome proliferator activated receptor-gamma agonist pioglitazone: lack of lasting

improvement or cure in the majority of patients. *J Am Acad Dermatol.* 2013;69(5):830-832.
220. Chieregato C, Zini A, Barba A, et al. Lichen planopilaris: report of 30 cases and review of the literature. *Int J Dermatol.* 2003;42(5):342-345.
221. Assouly P, Reygagne P. Lichen planopilaris: update on diagnosis and treatment. *Semin Cutan Med Surg.* 2009; 28(1):3-10.
222. Cho BK, Sah D, Chwalek J, et al. Efficacy and safety of mycophenolate mofetil for lichen planopilaris. *J Am Acad Dermatol.* 2010;62(3):393-397.
223. Cevasco NC, Bergfeld WF, Remzi BK, et al. A case-series of 29 patients with lichen planopilaris: the Cleveland Clinic Foundation experience on evaluation, diagnosis, and treatment. *J Am Acad Dermatol.* 2007; 57(1):47-53.
224. Spencer LA, Hawryluk EB, English JC 3rd. Lichen planopilaris: retrospective study and stepwise therapeutic approach. *Arch Dermatol.* 2009;145(3):333-334.
225. Moreno-Ramirez D, Camacho Martinez F. Frontal fibrosing alopecia: a survey in 16 patients. *J Eur Acad Dermatol Venereol.* 2005;19(6):700-705.
226. Vano-Galvan S, Molina-Ruiz AM, Serrano-Falcon C, et al. Frontal fibrosing alopecia: a multicenter review of 355 patients. *J Am Acad Dermatol.* 2014;70(4): 670-678.
227. Georgala S, Katoulis AC, Befon A, et al. Treatment of postmenopausal frontal fibrosing alopecia with oral dutasteride. *J Am Acad Dermatol.* 2009;61(1): 157-158.
228. Katoulis A, Georgala, Bozi E, et al. Frontal fibrosing alopecia: treatment with oral dutasteride and topical pimecrolimus. *J Eur Acad Dermatol Venereol.* 2009; 23(5):580-582.
229. Ladizinski B, Bazakas A, Selim MA, et al. Frontal fibrosing alopecia: a retrospective review of 19 patients seen at Duke University. *J Am Acad Dermatol.* 2013; 68(5):749-755.
230. Tosti A, Piraccini BM, Iorizzo M, et al. Frontal fibrosing alopecia in postmenopausal women. *J Am Acad Dermatol.* 2005;52(1):55-60.

Chapter 33 :: Lichen Nitidus and Lichen Striatus
:: Aaron R. Mangold & Mark R. Pittelkow

第三十三章

光泽苔藓和线状苔藓

中文导读

本章共分为2节：①光泽苔藓；②线状苔藓。分别介绍了这两种疾病的流行病学史、病因及病理生理机制、临床特点、组织病理学、诊断和治疗。

〔李芳芳〕

AT-A-GLANCE

- Lichen nitidus consists of small, glistening, monomorphic, flesh-colored to pink or reddish-brown papules of unknown etiology.
- On histopathology, lichen nitidus has a distinct, circumscribed infiltrate of lymphocytes, histiocytes, and giant cells in papillary dermis directly beneath a thinned epidermis.
- With lichen nitidus, there is no association with systemic disease.

LICHEN NITIDUS

EPIDEMIOLOGY

The epidemiology of lichen nitidus is unknown. Lichen nitidus does not show a clear racial or sexual predilection and is more common in children and young adults.[1] The true prevalence is unknown; however, an early clinical experience reported from the early 1900s estimated lichen nitidus to be approximately 34 cases per 100,000 African American individuals.[2] At the Mayo Clinic, the ratio of biopsies of lichen nitidus to lichen planus is 1.7 per 100. Assuming a prevalence of 1% in lichen planus and that the rates of biopsy of lichen planus and lichen nitidus are similar, this would imply a prevalence of approximately 17 cases per 100,000.

ETIOLOGY AND PATHOGENESIS

Once considered a tuberculoid reaction, lichen nitidus is currently regarded as an idiopathic lichenoid tissue reaction with distinctive clinical and histologic features.[3] The relationship between lichen nitidus and lichen planus is debated.[4] The coexistence of both diseases in some patients, the development of lichen planus after generalized lichen nitidus, and the clinical similarities to small papules of lichen planus support the view that lichen nitidus is a variant of lichen planus.[5] However, most clinicians and researchers favor the separation of these two diseases as distinct entities based on both clinical and immunologic differences and distinctive histologic changes.[6,7] Table 33-1 summarizes some of these differences and similarities. One common theory is that exogenous antigens and allergens stimulate epidermal and dermal antigen-presenting cells (eg, Langerhans cells) to activate a cell-mediated response, initiate lymphocyte accumulation, and form discrete inflammatory papules. Large numbers of Langerhans cells in the infiltrate supports this theory.[4,6] After antigen stimulation occurs, the cytokine milieu produced by the inflammatory infiltrate may

TABLE 33-1
Comparison of Features between Lichen Nitidus and Lichen Planus

	LICHEN NITIDUS	LICHEN PLANUS
Incidence	Rare	Common
Lesion		
Size	Usually 1-2 mm	Variable, usually larger
Shape	Round	Polygonal
Color	Flesh, pink, red-brown	Erythematous to violaceous
Wickham striae	Absent	Present
Mucosal changes	Rare	Variably present
Pruritus	Uncommon	Usually present, marked
Histopathology		
Hyperkeratosis	Variable and focal	Usually present
Parakeratosis	Mostly present	Not found
Infiltrate	Most commonly three papillary bodies	Bandlike, extends through many rete ridges
Lymphocytes	Variable	Vast majority of cells
Histiocytes	Almost always present	Almost none
Giant cells	Occasional	None
Dyskeratotic	Occasional	Very common
Immunopathology		
Cytoids	Usually negative	Immunoglobulin M and other conjugates
Basement membrane	Usually negative	Fibrinogen, other conjugates
Immunohistochemistry		
CD4+ lymphocytes	Majority of cells (less than lichen planus)	Majority of cells
CD68+ cells	Common	Uncommon

lead to T-helper type 2 (Th2) cell polarization, which results in superficial dermal granulomas in the appropriate genetic background.[8] Functional impairment in cellular immunity has been reported in lichen nitidus with anergic responses to antigen stimulations and the documentation of photo-induced lichen nitidus in association with HIV.[8-10]

Interestingly, in the case of anergy, the recovery of a normal antigen response was associated with disease resolution. Similarly, the induction of allergic contact dermatitis by the topical application of dinitrochlorobenzene in a patient with lichen nitidus cleared the eruption, presumably by altering the cellular immunity, cellular infiltration, and cytokine expression.[8] Rare cases of lichen nitidus have been associated with atopic dermatitis, Crohn disease, and juvenile chronic arthritis.[11-15] A rare familial presentation of lichen nitidus has been reported, although no genetic factors of the disease have been identified.[16-18]

CLINICAL FINDINGS

Lichen nitidus is composed of multiple 1- to 2-mm, discrete, smooth, round, skin-colored papules. Individual lesions may be umbilicated with a glistening appearance (Fig. 33-1). Scale may be present and can be elicited by rubbing the surface of the papules. Occasionally, in pruritic, generalized lichen nitidus (Fig. 33-2), the papules are grouped, and an isomorphic or Koebner phenomenon (12% of cases) is observed.[19] Lesions may occur anywhere over the skin surface; however, the most frequent sites of predilection (in descending order of frequency) are the trunk (Fig. 33-3), genitalia, face, neck, hands, and lower extremities.[1] There are rare reports of linear, Blaschkoid, generalized, and actinic disease.[20-28]

Less common sites of involvement include: mucous membranes, nails, palms (Fig. 33-4), and soles.[1,29] Palmoplantar involvement is more common in older individuals, most commonly involves the central palm, and has several morphologic variants that range from pinpoint papules, pompholyx, and keratoderma.[29-34] Minute keratotic spicules, or central plugs, on the central, palmar surfaces can help distinguish palmar lichen nitidus from lichen planus. The papules may extend to the dorsa of the extremities. Nail abnormalities may be associated with palmar disease and usually manifest as longitudinal, beaded ridging, and terminal splitting with or without irregular pitting.[34] Rare clinical morphological variants include vesicular, hemorrhagic-purpuric, and spinous-follicular[35-39] (Table 33-2). The hemorrhagic-purpuric lesions are common on the palms and distal extremities.[40-42]

Actinic lichen nitidus appears most commonly in dark-skinned individuals in areas of significant sun exposure, such as the face and arms. It can recur with repetitive exposure to the sun and often shows a seasonal pattern.[22,23] The term *summertime lichenoid actinic eruption* is reported in the literature but is less descriptive, clinically and histologically, because it could include actinic lichen planus.[43] Cases of actinic

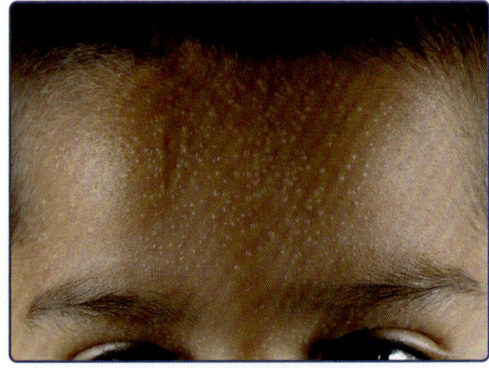

Figure 33-1 Lichen nitidus. Multiple 1- to 2-mm, discrete, smooth, round, skin-colored papules over the forehead. Individual lesions have a glistening appearance. (Used with permission of Mayo Foundation for Medical Education and Research, all rights reserved.)

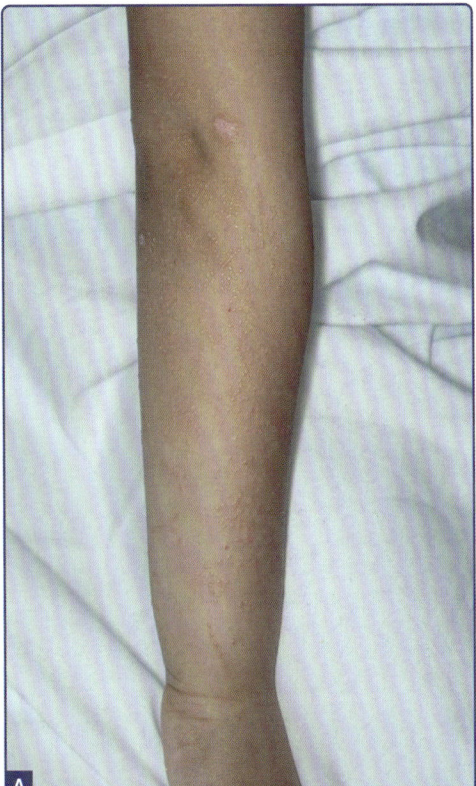

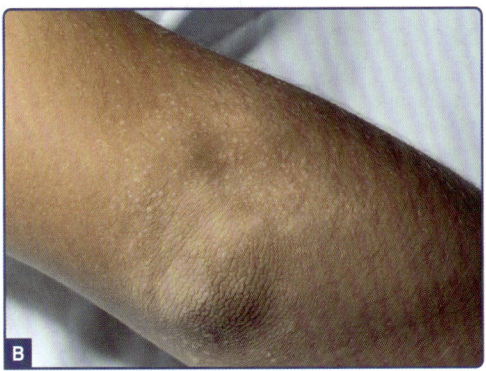

Figure 33-2 Lichen nitidus. **A,** Multiple, smooth flesh-colored to pink papules over the dorsal forearm showing isomorphic or Koebner phenomenon with linearly grouped papules over sites of excoriation. **B,** Similar appearing rash in a darker skinned individual. (Used with permission of Mayo Foundation for Medical Education and Research, all rights reserved.)

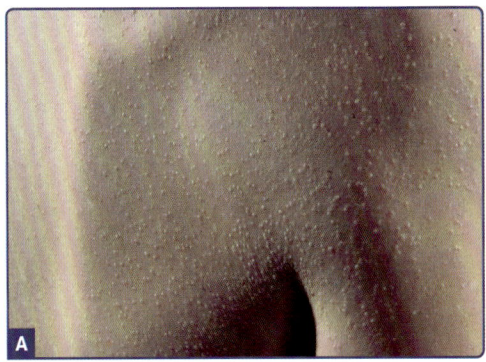

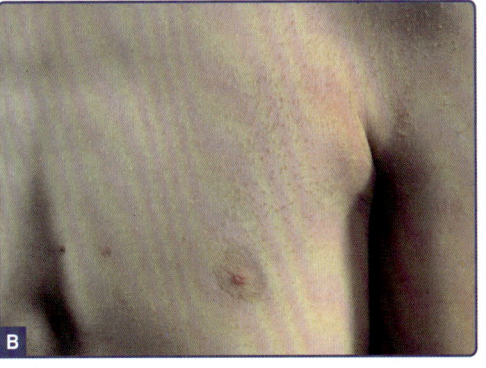

Figure 33-3 Lichen nitidus. **A,** Multiple monomorphic, dome-shaped papules over upper back, shoulder, and arm. Side lighting, as performed here, enhances visualization of the lesions. **B,** Individual papules, flesh- to pink-colored over the chest and arm and coalescing over the anterior axilla. (Used with permission of Mayo Foundation for Medical Education and Research, all rights reserved.)

lichen nitidus can be differentiated from other frictional lichenoid eruptions based on histology because the former should have typical histologic features of lichen nitidus, but and the latter is likely a manifestation of atopic dermatitis or polymorphous light eruption.[22,43-47]

Lichen nitidus is usually asymptomatic; however, pruritus is present in approximately 12% of cases and may be intense in fewer than 5%.[1] No constitutional symptoms or systemic abnormalities are associated with lichen nitidus.

PATHOLOGY

The histologic features of lichen nitidus are distinctive. A focused, dense infiltrate "ball" of lymphocyte, histiocytes, and foreign body or Touton-type giant cells are immediately below the epidermis with elongation of the rete ridges, expansion of the papillary dermis, and the apparent embracement by neighboring rete ridges forming the "claw" (Fig. 33-5). The classic "ball and claw" pattern, with involvement of up to three dermal papillae, is seen in 90% of cases.[1] Plasma cells and eosinophils are rare. The overlying epidermis is thinned in up to 90% of cases and demonstrates central parakeratosis without hypergranulosis in up to 56% of cases.[1] There are minimal hydropic degeneration, few dyskeratotic cells, and rare clefting and the dermal–epidermal junction (DEJ). Colloid bodies are rarely seen (10% of cases).[1,4]

Unique histologic features may be seen with clinical variants. Palmar lesions may show a deep parakeratotic plug. Perforating lesions tend to occur in areas of friction and may have transepidermal elimination of the inflammatory infiltrate.[48,49] Purpuric or hemorrhagic lesions are associated with capillary wall degeneration and red blood cell extravasation.[41]

TABLE 33-2
Rare Forms of Lichen Nitidus

SITE OF INVOLVEMENT	CLINICAL VARIANT
Generalized	Actinic
Palmar	Vesicular
Plantar	Hemorrhagic
Linear or Blaschkoid	Spinous follicular
Nail involvement	Perforating
	Purpuric

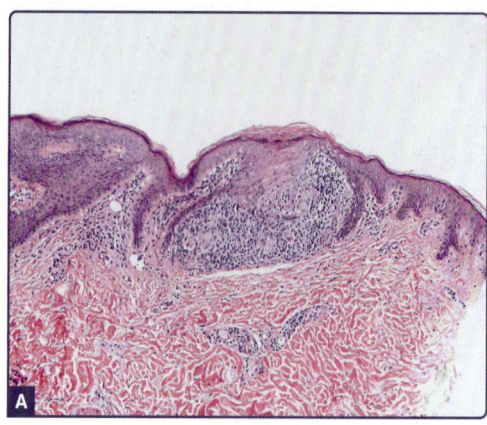

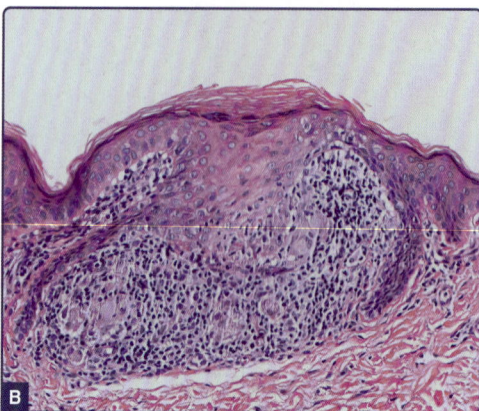

The majority of the cells in the infiltrate are T lymphocytes (CD4+ cells predominate over CD8+), Langerhans cells (S100+, CD1+), and macrophages-histiocytes (CD14+, CD68+).[4,6,50] Results of direct immunofluorescence examination of lichen nitidus are usually negative.[7]

DIFFERENTIAL DIAGNOSIS

Differential diagnosis of lichen nitidus is summarized in Table 33-3.

PROGNOSIS

Lichen nitidus is typically a focal, asymptomatic, chronic inflammatory reaction that eventually resolves

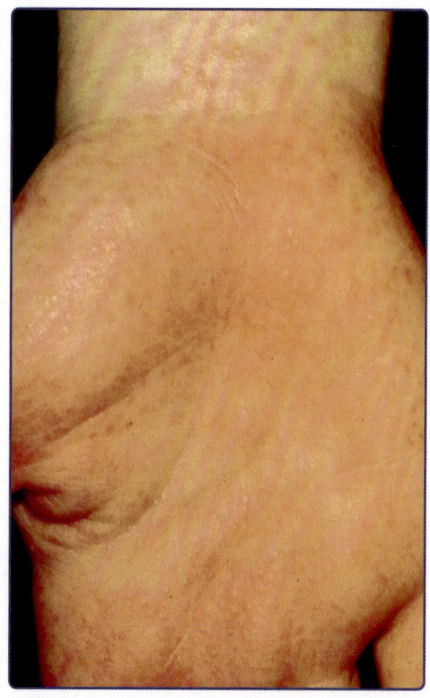

Figure 33-4 Lichen nitidus. Extensive wrist and palmar involvement with development of hyperkeratotic lesions. (Used with permission of Mayo Foundation for Medical Education and Research, all rights reserved.)

Figure 33-5 Lichen nitidus. **A,** Typical small, well-circumscribed lesion occupying only a couple of dermal papillae. Note the clawlike epidermal lateral borders. (Hematoxylin and eosin × 200.) **B,** Distinctive, circumscribed infiltrate of papillary dermis situated directly beneath thinned epidermis. Many histiocytes mingle with lymphocytes that are enveloped by bordering rete ridges. Central hyperkeratosis, epidermal thinning, and finger-like extensions of the epidermis. (Hematoxylin and eosin × 200.) (Photo contributors: David J. DiCaudo, MD and Steven A. Nelson, MD. Used with permission from Mayo Foundation for Medical Education and Research, all rights reserved.)

spontaneously within 1 year in two thirds of patients or, less frequently, over a few years.[1] Rarely, the eruption may persist indefinitely. Palmoplantar disease may be associated with a more chronic course.[29] New lesions may continue to develop as older lesions resolve. Lesions heal without scar formation or pigmentary abnormalities.

TREATMENT

Lichen nitidus is often asymptomatic and self-limiting, and most patients do not require treatment. However, treatment may be warranted in patients with protracted pruritus (in fewer than 5% of all cases), a generalized pattern, or lesions in cosmetically sensi-

TABLE 33-3
Differential Diagnosis of Lichen Nitidus
Most Likely
▪ Lichen planus
▪ Larger, polymorphic lesions located on flexural wrist, arms, and legs
▪ Dermoscopy shows dotted and linear vessels with whitish lines
▪ Highly pruritic
▪ CD8 lymphocytes predominate
▪ No granulomatous inflammation or parakeratosis
▪ Direct immunofluorescence (DIF) often positive with immunoglobulin binding to cytoid bodies and shaggy deposition of fibrinogen
▪ Psoriasis
▪ Plaques have silvery scale
▪ Dermoscopy shows even dotted vessels throughout with white scale
▪ Verruca plana
▪ Limited, asymmetric involvement
▪ Variable in size
▪ Verrucous surface
▪ Dermoscopy shows filiform structures or red dots and globular vessels with an even colored background
▪ Keratosis pilaris
▪ Commonly seen on the cheeks, lateral arms, and lateral hips
▪ Strong atopic diathesis
▪ Persistent disease
▪ Dermoscopy shows perifollicular scaling with keratotic plug formation, peripilar casts, and perifollicular erythema
▪ Absence of lichenoid and granulomatous infiltrate on biopsy
Consider
▪ Lichen spinulosus
▪ Papular eczema
▪ Follicular atopic dermatitis
▪ Frictional lichenoid eruption
▪ Molluscum contagiosum
▪ Lichen scrofulosorum
▪ Lichenoid syphilitic lesions
▪ Bowenoid papulosis
▪ Sarcoidosis
▪ Phrynoderma
▪ Lichen amyloidosis
▪ Papular mucinosis
▪ Darier disease
▪ Type II and IV pityriasis rubra pilaris

loratadine, may be used as alternatives.[57] Systemic treatments beyond antihistamines are rarely indicated and should be reserved for more symptomatic and cosmetically disfiguring disease. In general, a therapeutic approach similar to lichen planus (see Chap. 32) with targeting of lymphocytes in aggressive and atypical disease (using prednisone or low-dose cyclosporine) and safe, less targeted therapies for specific subtypes of disease (eg, acitretin in hyperkeratotic palmar disease).[33] A short course of low-dose oral glucocorticoids (prednisone 0.3 mg/kg) may hasten resolution of more extensive, generalized, or symptomatic disease.[26] Oral corticosteroids are most successful when combined with skin-directed therapies such as topical steroids or phototherapy.

Additional systemic and skin-directed therapies have been reported and are summarized in Table 33-4. Caution is advised when considering these therapies, and the potential harm of treatment should be weighed against the relatively benign nature of lichen nitidus. When appropriate, the medications that can be considered include antituberculous medications (note: a pediatric case had a positive purified protein derivative test result),[58] low-molecular-weight heparin,[59] low-dose cyclosporine (note: concomitant atopic dermatitis),[15] and oral itraconazole (note: included lichen planus or lichen nitidus).[60] Future therapeutic modalities to consider, based on mechanistic activity, include tumor necrosis factor-α inhibitors in cases with significant granuloma formation, as well as methotrexate, mycophenolate mofetil, azathioprine, and Janus kinase inhibitors in severe, refractory cases with more marked lichenoid infiltrate.

LICHEN STRIATUS

EPIDEMIOLOGY

AT-A-GLANCE

- Lichen striatus is a rare, idiopathic, papular eruption that usually resolves in 6 to 12 months.
- Lichen striatus occurs most commonly in children aged 3 to 5 years, on the limbs, and in females.
- In lichen striatus, the eruption is characterized by the sudden onset of flat-topped, 1- to 3-mm, pink, tan, or hypopigmented papules in a linear configuration or Blaschkoid distribution.
- Lichen striatus is associated with an atopic diathesis.
- The prognosis for lichen striatus is good.

tive areas.[1,27,28] For most cases of lichen nitidus, topical therapies are appropriate. Mid- to high-potency topical corticosteroids are first-line topical treatments for lichen nitidus. Tacrolimus ointment is a second-line topical treatment on the body and a first-line treatment for facial and intertriginous disease.[19,51,52] Psoralen plus ultraviolet A (PUVA) has been successfully used for generalized and palmar disease; however, this has largely been supplanted by narrowband ultraviolet B, which is a safer and effective alternative.[53-56]

In cases of pruritus, oral antihistamines are a first-line systemic agent. Astemizole has been reported in the literature; however, other sedating antihistamines, such as diphenhydramine, and nonsedating antihistamines, such as fexofenadine, cetirizine, and

Lichen striatus was first described in 1898 by Balzer and Merier as "lichenoid trophoneurosis."[61] Lichen striatus, is a rare, idiopathic, linear dermatosis that most commonly affects individuals younger than the age of

TABLE 33-4
Treatment of Lichen Nitidus

	TOPICAL	PHYSICAL	SYSTEMIC
First-line treatment	Topical steroids	Narrowband UVB (generalized)	Antihistamines (pruritus)
	Sun protection (actinic)		
Second-line treatment	Topical tacrolimus (first-line treatment on the face or intertriginous areas and second-line treatment elsewhere)	UVA and UVB (generalized)	Oral steroids, 0.3 mg/kg/day (generalized and symptomatic)
		Local PUVA (palmar)	Oral retinoids (acitretin) (palmar)
			Low-dose cyclosporine, 4 mg/kg/day (generalized and symptomatic)
Third-line treatment		PUVA (generalized)	Itraconazole (generalized)
			Antituberculous agents (isoniazid) (positive PPD result)
			Enoxaparin (generalized)

PPD, purified protein derivative; PUVA, psoralen plus ultraviolet A; UVA, ultraviolet A; UVB, ultraviolet B.

18 years with a mean age of onset between 3 and 5 years of age.[62-64] The true incidence and prevalence of lichen striatus is unknown. This self-limited dermatosis is common in females (2–3:1) and occurs most frequently on the limbs.[63-65] Up to 60% of individuals with lichen striatus have a personal of family history of atopy.[63]

ETIOLOGY AND PATHOGENESIS

The etiology of lichen striatus is incompletely understood; however, the Blaschko-linear pattern suggests somatic mosaicism. Postzygotic, somatic mutations of keratinocytes may lead to the development of altered antigens that migrate along lines of Blaschko and can trigger an immune response. Immune tolerance develops to these endogenous autoantigens. External precipitants have been implicated in the loss of tolerance and triggering an immune response. Possible precipitating factors include environmental stressors, drugs (specifically interferon), vaccines (bacillus Calmette–Guérin), viral antigens, hypersensitivity, and skin injury.[63,64,66,67] External triggers are supported by rare cases of simultaneous onset of lichen striatus in related and unrelated siblings.[68-71] Seasonal variation, with higher onset and clustered outbreaks of lichen striatus in the spring and summer months, support an infective etiology.[64,72] Viral infections have the ability to mediate a cell-mediated responses that could act as potential triggers.[73] For example, in linear lichen planus, herpes virus DNA has been detected within lesions.[74] Similar antigenic stimuli have not been found in lichen striatus.

CLINICAL FEATURES

Lichen striatus, a type of Blaschko linear acquired inflammatory skin eruption (BLAISE), is characterized by the sudden onset (days to weeks) of flat-topped, 1- to 3-mm, pink, tan, or hypopigmented papules in a linear configuration or Blaschkoid distribution (Figs. 33-6 and 33-7).[63,75] Individual lesions may have scale. Bilateral and parallel eruptions have been reported.[63] Pruritus is present in 5% to 34% of cases and are more common in atopic individuals and adults.[62,63,65,76] The

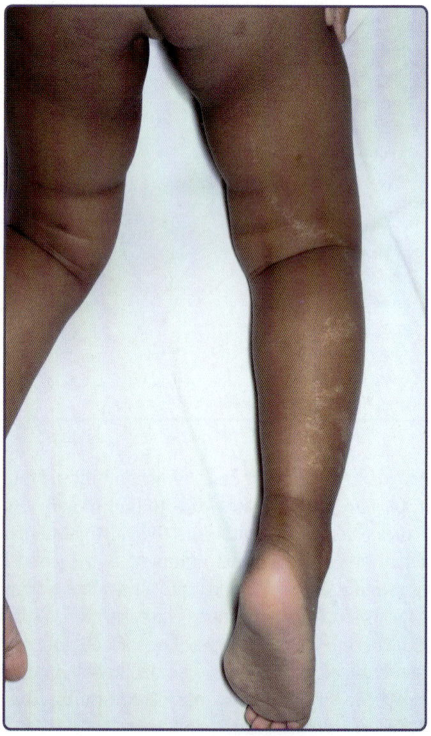

Figure 33-6 Lichen striatus. Multiple flat-topped, 1-t to 3-mm pink papules in a linear configuration or Blaschkoid distribution in a dark-skinned individual. (Used with permission of Mayo Foundation for Medical Education and Research, all rights reserved.)

most common locations on the body are the extremities (75% to 77%) and the trunk (9% to 21%).[62,65] Less commonly, the face (3% to 13%) and nails (2.6%) can be involved.[63-65] More extensive disease is seen in adults, and these cases often appear to have concomitant dermatitis.[76] Nail involvement is uncommon and may lead to longitudinal ridging, onycholysis, splitting, fraying, and loss of the nail plate.[63,77,78] With treatment, the nail changes tend to be reversible.[77]

PATHOLOGY

The histologic features of lichen striatus are variable, and biopsies are rarely performed (10% of cases).[63,64] The classic pathologic findings include hyperkeratosis, focal parakeratosis, mild spongiosis with a lichenoid tissue reaction and exocytosis, keratinocyte necrosis, and perivascular and appendageal lymphocytic infiltrate (Fig. 33-8).[62] The superficial lichenoid dermatitis and deep lymphocytic infiltrate of lichen striatus are seen in almost all cases.[62] Nonspecific findings are more common in early and late-stage disease. Histologic mimickers include lichen planus, lupus erythematosus, graft-versus-host-disease,

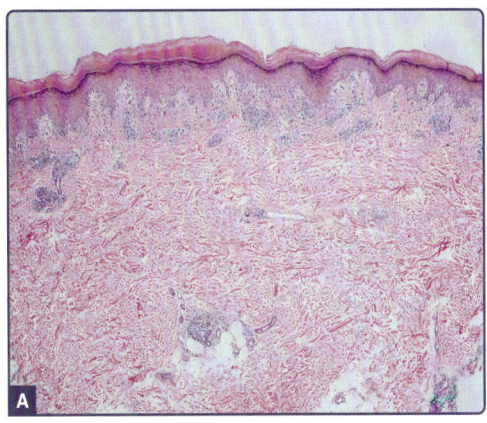

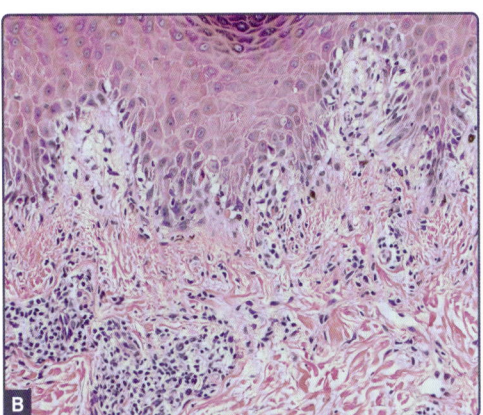

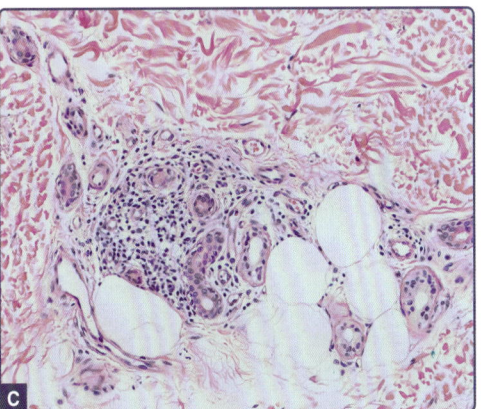

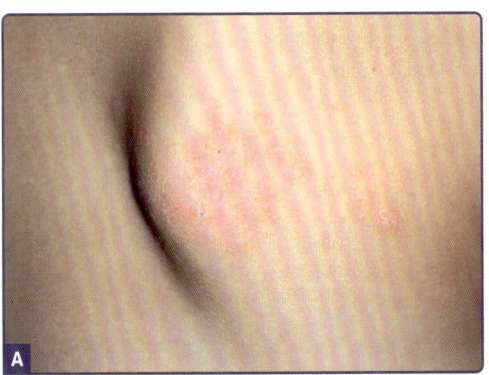

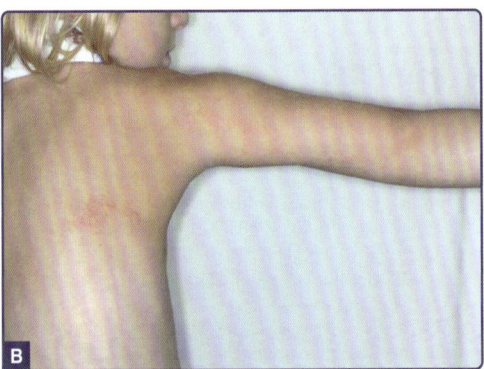

Figure 33-7 Lichen striatus. **A,** Discrete, 1- to 3-mm pink and tan papules coalescing into larger plaques over the right scapula with a linear orientation. **B,** Pink and tan papules and plaques following the lines of Blaschko. (Used with permission of Mayo Foundation for Medical Education and Research, all rights reserved.)

Figure 33-8 Lichen striatus. **A,** Hyperkeratosis, mild spongiosis, and lichenoid tissue reaction with perivascular and appendageal lymphocytic infiltrate. (Hematoxylin and eosin × 40.) **B,** Mild spongiosis, vacuolar lichenoid tissue reaction, clusters of necrotic keratinocytes, pigment incontinence, and perivascular lymphocytic infiltrate. (Hematoxylin and eosin × 200) **C,** Perieccrine lymphocytic infiltrate. (Hematoxylin and eosin × 200). (Photo contributors: David J. DiCaudo, MD and Steven A. Nelson, MD. Used with permission from Mayo Foundation for Medical Education and Research, all rights reserved.)

lichen planopilaris, mycosis fungoides, syphilis, and atypical dermatitis. Langerhans cells are decreased overall; however, intraepidermal vesicles containing them along with T lymphocytes can be seen in 23% to 45% of cases.[62,79] In clinical practice, vesicles are rarely seen, indicating that atypical cases are more likely to be biopsied. Plasma cells, eosinophils, and multinucleate giant cells are seen in 22%, 19%, and 2% of cases, respectively.[62] CD8 cells are the predominant infiltrate at the DEJ, and CD4 cells are located in the dermis and perivascular area.[79,80] Dermal macrophages are common, and colloid bodies may be seen in up to half of cases.

DIFFERENTIAL DIAGNOSIS

The differential diagnosis of lichen striatus is summarized in Table 33-5.

PROGNOSIS AND TREATMENT

Lichen striatus is a self-limited disease with a mean duration of approximately 6 to 12 months.[63] Relapse is rare. Postinflammatory hypopigmentation is seen in up to 50% of cases but is self-limited, and lesions heal without scarring.[75] In general, treatment and laboratory testing are not necessary. For symptomatic control of pruritus, low to medium-potency topical steroids may be used as a first-line topical.[63] With facial involvement or disease refractory to topical corticosteroids, the topical calcineurin inhibitors tacrolimus and pimecrolimus are an effective alternative.[81] The use of topical calcineurin inhibitors for up to 6 weeks often results in significant improvement.[51,76] With nail involvement; topical corticosteroids and calcineurin inhibitors combined with intralesional corticosteroids (5 mg/mL of triamcinolone) improved six of seven cases.[77] Oral antihistamines may be helpful in cases of more generalized itch or in cases of sleep disruption.

ACKNOWLEDGMENTS

Steven A. Nelson, MD, David J. DiCaudo, and Collin Costello.

TABLE 33-5
Differential Diagnosis of Lichen Striatus

Most Likely
- Linear lichen planus
  - Patients are older
  - More violaceous primary lesion and may have other areas of involvement
  - Highly pruritic
  - Brisk lichenoid tissue reaction without periadnexal or perieccrine involvement
  - DIF often positive with Immunoglobulin binding to cytoid bodies and shaggy deposition of fibrinogen
- Inflammatory linear verrucous epidermal nevus
  - Occurs in children
  - Clinically appears psoriasis-like
  - Highly pruritic
  - Most resolve by adulthood
  - Psoriasiform changes on histopathology with alternating ortho- and parakeratosis
- Blaschkitis
  - Patients are older
  - Papular eruption, tends to be truncal, and has multiple streaks
  - Often has features of concomitant dermatitis
  - Often resolves in days to weeks
  - Relapse if common

Consider
- Linear psoriasis
- Linear Darier disease
- Linear porokeratosis
- Linear lichen nitidus
- Incontinentia pigmenti

REFERENCES

1. Lapins NA, Willoughby C, Helwig EB. Lichen nitidus. A study of forty-three cases. *Cutis*. 1978;21(5):634-637.
2. Hazen HH. Syphilis and skin diseases in the American Negro: personal observations. *Arch Dermatol Syphilol*. 1935;31(3):316-323.
3. Barber HW. Case of lichen nitidus (pinkus) or tuberculide licheniforme et nitida (Chatellier). *Proc R Soc Med*. 1924;17(Dermatol Sect):39.
4. Smoller BR, Flynn TC. Immunohistochemical examination of lichen nitidus suggests that it is not a localized papular variant of lichen planus. *J Am Acad Dermatol*. 1992;27(2 Pt 1):232-236.
5. Di Lernia V, Piana S, Ricci C. Lichen planus appearing subsequent to generalized lichen nitidus in a child. *Pediatr Dermatol*. 2007;24(4):453-455.
6. Wright AL, McVittie E, Hunter JA. An immunophenotypic study of lichen nitidus. *Clin Exp Dermatol*. 1990;15(4):273-276.
7. Waisman M, Dundon BC, Michel B. Immunofluorescent studies in lichen nitidus. *Arch Dermatol*. 1973;107(2):200-203.
8. Kano Y, Otake Y, Shiohara T. Improvement of lichen nitidus after topical dinitrochlorobenzene application. *J Am Acad Dermatol*. 1998;39(2 Pt 2):305-308.
9. Berger TG, Dhar A. Lichenoid photoeruptions in human immunodeficiency virus infection. *Arch Dermatol*. 1994; 130(5):609-613.
10. Maeda M. A case of generalized lichen nitidus with Koebner's phenomenon. *J Dermatol*. 1994;21(4):273-277.
11. Magro CM, Crowson AN. Lichenoid and granulomatous dermatitis. *Int J Dermatol*. 2000;39(2):126-133.
12. Kano Y, Shiohara T, Yagita A, et al. Erythema nodosum, lichen planus and lichen nitidus in Crohn's disease: report of a case and analysis of T cell receptor V gene

expression in the cutaneous and intestinal lesions. *Dermatology*. 1995;190(1):59-63.
13. Wanat KA, Elenitsas R, Chachkin S, et al. Extensive lichen nitidus as a clue to underlying Crohn's disease. *J Am Acad Dermatol*. 2012;67(5):e218-220.
14. Bercedo A, Cabero MJ, Garcia-Consuegra J, et al. Generalized lichen nitidus and juvenile chronic arthritis: an undescribed association. *Pediatr Dermatol*. 1999;16(5):406-407.
15. Lestringant GG, Piletta P, Feldmann R, et al. Coexistence of atopic dermatitis and lichen nitidus in three patients. *Dermatology*. 1996;192(2):171-173.
16. Marks R, Jones EW. Familial lichen nitidus. The simultaneous occurrence of lichen nitidus in brothers. *Trans St Johns Hosp Dermatol Soc*. 1970;56(2):165-167.
17. Kato N. Familial lichen nitidus. *Clin Exp Dermatol*. 1995;20(4):336-338.
18. Leung AK, Ng J. Generalized lichen nitidus in identical twins. *Case Rep Dermatol Med*. 2012;2012:982084.
19. Dobbs CR, Murphy SJ. Lichen nitidus treated with topical tacrolimus. *J Drugs Dermatol*. 2004;3(6):683-684.
20. Francoeur CJ Jr, Frost M, Treadwell P. Generalized pinhead-sized papules in a child. Generalized lichen nitidus. *Arch Dermatol*. 1988;124(6):935, 938.
21. Kanwar AJ, Kaur S. Lichen nitidus actinicus. *Arch Dermatol*. 1999;135(6):714.
22. Hussain K. Summertime actinic lichenoid eruption, a distinct entity, should be termed actinic lichen nitidus. *Arch Dermatol*. 1998;134(10):1302-1303.
23. Kanwar AJ, Kaur S. Lichen nitidus actinicus. *Pediatr Dermatol*. 1991;8(1):94-95.
24. Petrozzi JW, Shmunes E. Linear lichen nitidus. *Cutis*. 1970;6(10):1109-1112.
25. Aravind M, Do TT, Cha HC, et al. Blaschkolinear acquired inflammatory skin eruption, or blaschkitis, with features of lichen nitidus. *JAAD Case Rep*. 2016;2(2):102-104.
26. Chen W, Schramm M, Zouboulis CC. Generalized lichen nitidus. *J Am Acad Dermatol*. 1997;36(4):630-631.
27. Soroush V, Gurevitch AW, Peng SK. Generalized lichen nitidus: case report and literature review. *Cutis*. 1999;64(2):135-136.
28. Rallis E, Verros C, Moussatou V, et al. Generalized purpuric lichen nitidus. Report of a case and review of the literature. *Dermatol Online J*. 2007;13(2):5.
29. Cakmak SK, Unal E, Gonul M, et al. Lichen nitidus with involvement of the palms. *Pediatr Dermatol*. 2013;30(5):e100-101.
30. Weiss RM, Cohen AD. Lichen nitidus of the palms and soles. *Arch Dermatol*. 1971;104(5):538-540.
31. Qian G, Wang H, Wu J, et al. Different dermoscopic patterns of palmoplantar and nonpalmoplantar lichen nitidus. *J Am Acad Dermatol*. 2015;73(3):e101-103.
32. Thibaudeau A, Maillard H, Croue A, et al. [Palmoplantar lichen nitidus: a rare cause of palmoplantar hyperkeratosis]. *Ann Dermatol Venereol*. 2004;131(8-9):822-824.
33. Park SH, Kim SW, Noh TW, et al. A case of palmar lichen nitidus presenting as a clinical feature of pompholyx. *Ann Dermatol*. 2010;22(2):235-237.
34. Munro CS, Cox NH, Marks JM, et al. Lichen nitidus presenting as palmoplantar hyperkeratosis and nail dystrophy. *Clin Exp Dermatol*. 1993;18(4):381-383.
35. Jetton RL, Eby CS, Freeman RG. Vesicular and hemorrhagic lichen nitidus. *Arch Dermatol*. 1972;105(3):430-431.
36. Madhok R, Winkelmann RK. Spinous, follicular lichen nitidus associated with perifollicular granulomas. *J Cutan Pathol*. 1988;15(4):245-248.
37. Summe HS, Greenlaw SM, Deng A, et al. Generalized spinous follicular lichen nitidus with perifollicular granulomas. *Pediatr Dermatol*. 2013;30(3):e20-21.
38. MacDonald AJ, Drummond A, Chui D, Holmes S. Lichen nitidus and lichen spinulosus or spinous follicular lichen nitidus? *Clin Exp Dermatol*. 2005;30(4):452-453.
39. Park JS. Lichen nitidus and lichen spinulosus or spinous follicular lichen nitidus? A second case. *Clin Exp Dermatol*. 2011;36(5):557-558.
40. Ikenberg K, Pflugfelder A, Metzler G, et al. Thirty-year history of palmar eruptions: a quiz. Palmar purpuric lichen nitidus. *Acta Derm Venereol*. 2011;91(1):108-109.
41. Endo M, Baba S, Suzuki H. Purpuric lichen nitidus. *Eur J Dermatol*. 1998;8(1):54-55.
42. Coulson IH, Marsden RA, Cook MG. Purpuric palmar lichen nitidus—an unusual though distinctive eruption. *Clin Exp Dermatol*. 1988;13(5):347-349.
43. Bedi TR. Summertime actinic lichenoid eruption. *Dermatologica*. 1978;157(2):115-125.
44. Isaacson D, Turner ML, Elgart ML. Summertime actinic lichenoid eruption (lichen planus actinicus). *J Am Acad Dermatol*. 1981;4(4):404-411.
45. Sardana K, Goel K, Garg VK, et al. Is frictional lichenoid dermatitis a minor variant of atopic dermatitis or a photodermatosis. *Indian J Dermatol*. 2015;60(1):66-73.
46. Menni S, Piccinno R, Baietta S, et al. Sutton's summer prurigo: a morphologic variant of atopic dermatitis. *Pediatr Dermatol*. 1987;4(3):205-208.
47. Patrizi A, Di Lernia V, Ricci G, et al. Atopic background of a recurrent papular eruption of childhood (frictional lichenoid eruption). *Pediatr Dermatol*. 1990;7(2):111-115.
48. Bardach H. Perforating lichen nitidus. *J Cutan Pathol*. 1981;8(2):111-116.
49. Yoon TY, Kim JW, Kim MK. Two cases of perforating lichen nitidus. *J Dermatol*. 2006;33(4):278-280.
50. Nakamizo S, Egawa G, Miyachi Y, et al. Accumulation of S-100+ CD1a+ Langerhans cells as a characteristic of lichen nitidus. *Clin Exp Dermatol*. 2011;36(7):811-812.
51. Sorgentini C, Allevato MA, Dahbar M, et al. Lichen striatus in an adult: successful treatment with tacrolimus. *Br J Dermatol*. 2004;150(4):776-777.
52. Park J, Kim JI, Kim DW, et al. Persistent generalized lichen nitidus successfully treated with 0.03% tacrolimus ointment. *Eur J Dermatol*. 2013;23(6):918-919.
53. Do MO, Kim MJ, Kim SH, et al. Generalized lichen nitidus successfully treated with narrow-band UVB phototherapy: two cases report. *J Korean Med Sci*. 2007;22(1):163-166.
54. Nakamizo S, Kabashima K, Matsuyoshi N, et al. Generalized lichen nitidus successfully treated with narrowband UVB phototherapy. *Eur J Dermatol*. 2010;20(6):816-817.
55. Randle HW, Sander HM. Treatment of generalized lichen nitidus with PUVA. *Int J Dermatol*. 1986;25(5):330-331.
56. Kim YC, Shim SD. Two cases of generalized lichen nitidus treated successfully with narrow-band UV-B phototherapy. Int *J Dermatol*. 2006;45(5):615-617.

57. Vaughn RY, Smith JG Jr. The treatment of lichen nitidus with astemizole. *J Am Acad Dermatol*. 1990;23(4 Pt 1): 757-758.
58. Kubota Y, Kiryu H, Nakayama J. Generalized lichen nitidus successfully treated with an antituberculous agent. Br *J Dermatol*. 2002;146(6):1081-1083.
59. Cholongitas E, Kokolakis G, Giannikaki E, et al. Persistent generalized lichen nitidus successfully treated with enoxaparin sodium. *Am J Clin Dermatol*. 2008;9(5): 349-350.
60. Libow LF, Coots NV. Treatment of lichen planus and lichen nitidus with itraconazole: reports of six cases. *Cutis*. 1998;62(5):247-248.
61. Balzer F, Mercier R. Trophoneurose lichenoid en bande linéare sur le trajet du nerve petit sciatique. *Ann Dermatol Syphiol*. 1898;9:258.
62. Zhang Y, McNutt NS. Lichen striatus. Histological, immunohistochemical, and ultrastructural study of 37 cases. *J Cutan Pathol*. 2001;28(2):65-71.
63. Patrizi A, Neri I, Fiorentini C, et al. Lichen striatus: clinical and laboratory features of 115 children. *Pediatr Dermatol*. 2004;21(3):197-204.
64. Kennedy D, Rogers M. Lichen striatus. *Pediatr Dermatol*. 1996;13(2):95-99.
65. Taniguchi Abagge K, Parolin Marinoni L, et al. Lichen striatus: description of 89 cases in children. *Pediatr Dermatol*. 2004;21(4):440-443.
66. Zaki SA, Sanjeev S. Lichen striatus following BCG vaccination in an infant. *Indian Pediatr*. 2011;48(2): 163-164.
67. Mask-Bull L, Vangipuram R, Carroll BJ, et al. Lichen striatus after interferon therapy. *JAAD Case Rep*. 2015; 1(5):254-256.
68. Kanegaye JT, Frieden IJ. Lichen striatus: simultaneous occurrence in siblings. Pediatrics. 1992;90(1 Pt 1): 104-106.
69. Patrizi A, Neri I, Fiorentini C, et al. Simultaneous occurrence of lichen striatus in siblings. *Pediatr Dermatol*. 1997;14(4):293-295.
70. Smith SB 3rd, Smith JB, Ellis LE, et al. Lichen striatus: simultaneous occurrence in two nonrelated siblings. *Pediatr Dermatol*. 1997;14(1):43-45.
71. Racette AJ, Adams AD, Kessler SE. Simultaneous lichen striatus in siblings along the same Blaschko line. *Pediatr Dermatol*. 2009;26(1):50-54.
72. Sittart JA, Pegas JR, Sant'Ana LA, et al. [Lichen striatus. Epidemiologic study]. *Med Cutan Ibero Lat Am*. 1989; 17(1):19-21.
73. Muller CS, Schmaltz R, Vogt T, et al. Lichen striatus and blaschkitis: reappraisal of the concept of blaschkolinear dermatoses. Br *J Dermatol*. 2011;164(2):257-262.
74. Mizukawa Y, Horie C, Yamazaki Y, et al. Detection of varicella-zoster virus antigens in lesional skin of zosteriform lichen planus but not in that of linear lichen planus. *Dermatology*. 2012;225(1):22-26.
75. Taieb A, el Youbi A, Grosshans E, et al. Lichen striatus: a Blaschko linear acquired inflammatory skin eruption. *J Am Acad Dermatol*. 1991;25(4):637-642.
76. Campanati A, Brandozzi G, Giangiacomi M, et al. Lichen striatus in adults and pimecrolimus: open, off-label clinical study. Int *J Dermatol*. 2008;47(7):732-736.
77. Kim M, Jung HY, Eun YS, et al. Nail lichen striatus: report of seven cases and review of the literature. *Int J Dermatol*. 2015;54(11):1255-1260.
78. Tosti A, Peluso AM, Misciali C, et al. Nail lichen striatus: clinical features and long-term follow-up of five patients. *J Am Acad Dermatol*. 1997;36(6 Pt 1): 908-913.
79. Gianotti R, Restano L, Grimalt R, et al. Lichen striatus—a chameleon: an histopathological and immunohistological study of forty-one cases. *J Cutan Pathol*. 1995; 22(1):18-22.
80. Zhou Y, Yu ZZ, Peng J, et al. Lichen striatus versus linear lichen planus: a comparison of clinicopathological features, immunoprofile of infiltrated cells, and epidermal proliferation and differentiation. *Int J Dermatol*. 2016; 55(4):e204-210.
81. Fujimoto N, Tajima S, Ishibashi A. Facial lichen striatus: successful treatment with tacrolimus ointment. Br *J Dermatol*. 2003;148(3):587-590.

Chapter 34 :: Granuloma Annulare :: Julie S. Prendiville

第三十四章
环状肉芽肿

中文导读

本章对环状肉芽肿从以下几个方面进行了阐述：流行病学史、临床特点、病因及病理生理机制、环状肉芽肿与系统性疾病的关系、组织病理学、治疗和预后。本章重点介绍了该病的临床特点，描述了环状肉芽肿变异的类型：局限型、全身型、皮下型、穿通型和播散型。并图文并茂地描述了不同类型环状肉芽肿的皮损特点和临床表现，比如局限型环状肉芽肿最常见的形式是环状或弧形病变。在诊断方面，以表格的形式列出了鉴别诊断以及一些排除诊断。

〔李芳芳〕

AT-A-GLANCE

- Granuloma annulare is a relatively common disorder. The exact prevalence is unknown, but it occurs more often in children and young adults.
- A localized ring of beaded papules on the extremities is typical; generalized, subcutaneous, perforating, and patch subtypes also occur.
- The cause of granuloma annulare is unknown, and the pathogenesis is poorly understood.
- Pathologic features consist of granulomatous inflammation in a palisaded or interstitial pattern associated with varying degrees of connective tissue degeneration and mucin deposition.
- Most localized cases resolve spontaneously within 2 years.

Granuloma annulare is a benign self-limited disease that was first described by Colcott-Fox in 1895 and Radcliffe-Crocker[1] in 1902.

EPIDEMIOLOGY

Granuloma annulare is a relatively common disorder.[2] It occurs in all age groups but is rare in infancy.[2-4] The localized annular and subcutaneous forms occur more frequently in children and young adults. The generalized or disseminated variant is more common in adults. Many studies report a female preponderance,[2] but some have found a higher frequency in males.[5] Granuloma annulare does not favor a particular race or geographic area.

Most cases of granuloma annulare are sporadic. Occasional familial cases are described with occurrence in twins, siblings, and members of successive generations.[2,6,7] Attempts to identify an associated human leukocyte antigen subtype have yielded disparate results in different population groups.

CLINICAL FEATURES

HISTORY

The typical history is of one or more papules with centrifugal enlargement and central clearing. These annular lesions are often misdiagnosed as tinea corporis and treated unsuccessfully with topical antifungal agents. Subcutaneous nodules may raise suspicion about malignancy or rheumatoid disease.

Granuloma annulare is usually asymptomatic. Mild pruritus may be present, but painful lesions are rare. Nodular lesions on the feet may cause discomfort from footwear. Cosmesis is often a concern for adolescent and adult patients, particularly with generalized disease.

CUTANEOUS FINDINGS

Clinical variants of granuloma annulare include the localized, generalized, subcutaneous, perforating, and patch types. Linear granuloma annulare, a follicular pustular form, papular umbilicated lesions in children, and giant plaques have also been described. There is overlap among the different variants, and more than one morphologic type may coexist in the same patient.

LOCALIZED TYPE

The most common form of granuloma annulare is an annular or arcuate lesion. It may be skin colored, erythematous, or violaceous. It usually measures 1 to 5 cm in diameter.[2] The annular margin is firm to palpation and may be continuous or consist of discrete or coalescent papules in a complete or partial circle (Fig. 34-1). The epidermis is usually normal, but surface markings may be attenuated over individual papules. Within the annular ring, the skin may have a violaceous or pigmented appearance. Solitary firm papules or nodules may also be present. Papular lesions on the fingers may appear umbilicated.

The dorsal hands and feet, ankles, lower limbs, and wrists are the sites of predilection (see Figs. 34-1 and 34-2). Less commonly, lesions occur at other sites, including the eyelids. The palms and soles are occasionally involved. Localized annular lesions may coexist with the subcutaneous or patch forms.

GENERALIZED TYPE

The generalized form of granuloma annulare is said to comprise 8% to 15% of cases.[8] The majority of patients are adults, but it may also be seen in childhood. Unlike in localized disease, the trunk is frequently involved in addition to the neck and extremities. The face, scalp, palms, and soles may also be affected.

Generalized granuloma annulare presents as widespread papules (Fig. 34-3A), some of which coalesce to form small annular plaques or larger discolored patches with raised arcuate and serpiginous margins (see Fig. 34-3B). Lesions may be skin colored, pink, violaceous, tan, or yellow. An annular or nonannular morphology may predominate. A generalized form of perforating granuloma annulare has also been described.

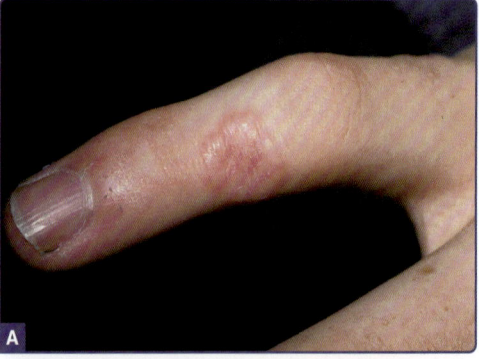
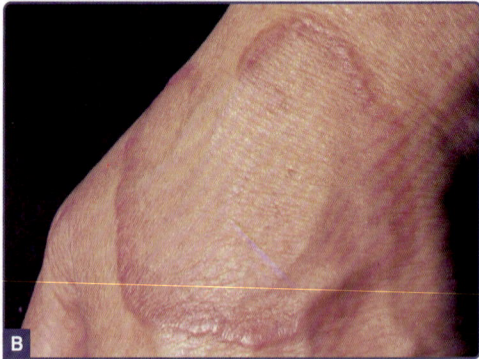

Figure 34-1 **A,** Typical annular lesion of granuloma annulare on a finger. **B,** A larger annular lesion of granuloma annulare on the dorsum of the hand.

SUBCUTANEOUS TYPE

The subcutaneous form of granuloma annulare occurs predominantly in children[9,10] but is also described in adult patients. It is characterized by firm to hard, usually asymptomatic nodules located in the deep dermis and subcutaneous tissues. They may extend to underlying muscle, and nodules on

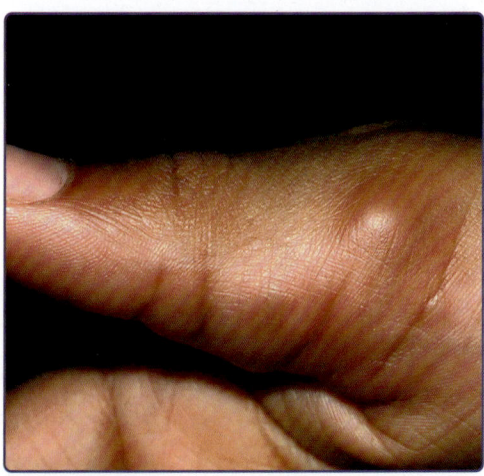

Figure 34-2 Localized granuloma annulare with nodule on the hand of a child.

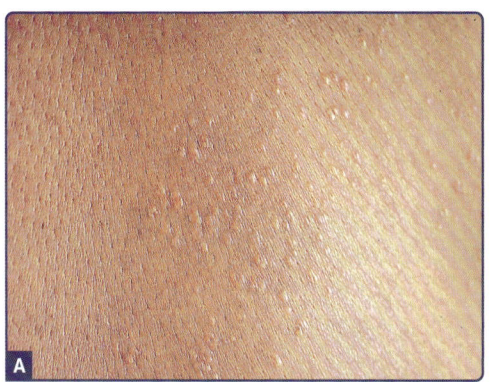

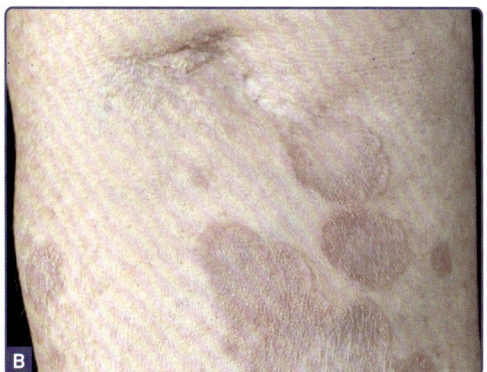

Figure 34-3 A, Generalized granuloma annulare. Small papular lesions that are too small to exhibit annular configuration. **B,** Multiple annular lesions on the lower arm.

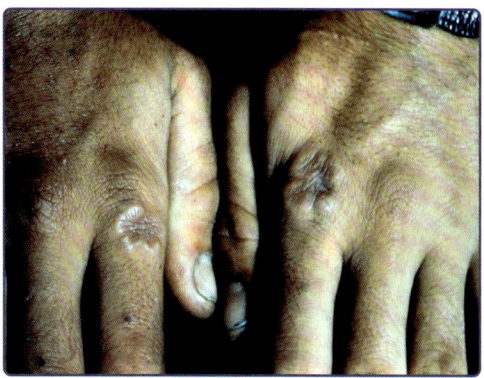

Figure 34-4 Granuloma annulare on the knuckles of a dark-skinned patient. (Image used with permission from the Graham Library of Wake Forest Department of Dermatology.)

the scalp and orbit are often adherent to the underlying periosteum.

Individual lesions measure from 6 mm to 3.5 cm in diameter. They are distributed most often on the anterior lower legs in a pretibial location. Other sites of predilection are the ankles, dorsal feet, buttocks, and hands. Nodules on the scalp, eyelids, and orbital rim may present a diagnostic challenge. Subcutaneous granuloma annulare may also be found on the penis.

PERFORATING TYPE

The perforating type of granuloma annulare is a rare variant characterized by transepidermal elimination of the necrobiotic collagen. It may be localized, usually to the dorsal hands and fingers (Fig. 34-4), or generalized over the trunk and extremities. It has been described on the ears, on the scrotum, and within herpes zoster scars and tattoos. Superficial small papules develop central umbilication or crusting, and there may be discharge of a creamy fluid. Lesions heal with atrophic or hyperpigmented scars. In one series, 24% of patients complained of pruritus and 21% of pain. Papular umbilicated granuloma annulare on the hands of children and a generalized follicular pustular type of granuloma annulare may be clinical variants.

PATCH TYPE

Macular lesions that present as erythematous, red-brown, or violaceous patches without an annular rim are reported in adult women.[11] An arcuate dermal erythema is also observed.

NONCUTANEOUS FINDINGS

Most patients with granuloma annulare are healthy and have no other abnormal physical findings. Arthralgia is reported in association with painful lesions on the hands.[12] Granuloma annulare–like skin lesions and joint disease characterize a multisystem disorder described as interstitial granulomatous dermatitis with arthritis.[13]

Oral involvement has been observed in HIV-associated disease.[14]

ETIOLOGY AND PATHOGENESIS

The etiology of granuloma annulare is unknown, and the pathogenesis is poorly understood. Most cases occur in otherwise healthy children. A variety of predisposing events and associated systemic diseases is reported, but their significance is unclear. It is possible that granuloma annulare represents a phenotypic reaction pattern with many different initiating factors.

PREDISPOSING EVENTS

Nonspecific mild trauma is considered a possible triggering factor because of the frequent location of lesions on the distal extremities of children. An early study of subcutaneous granuloma annulare found a history of trauma in 25% of children,[2] but this observation has not been replicated. Trauma is also a suspected factor in auricular lesions. Granuloma annulare has occurred after a bee sting, a cat bite, and an octopus bite, and insect bite reactions have also been implicated.[2] There is a report of perforating granuloma annulare in long-standing tattoos. Widespread lesions have developed after waxing-induced pseudofolliculitis and erythema multiforme minor and in association with systemic sarcoidosis.[2,15] Severe uveitis without other evidence of sarcoidosis has occurred in a few patients with granuloma annulare.[16-18]

INFECTIONS AND IMMUNIZATIONS

There are several reports of the development of granuloma annulare within herpes zoster scars, sometimes many years after the active infection. It is also described after chickenpox. Generalized, localized, and perforating forms of granuloma annulare may occur in association with HIV infection. Adenovirus was isolated from a lesion in one HIV-positive patient. Epstein-Barr virus was excluded as a causative agent in these cases. However, in other instances, generalized granuloma annulare has been linked to viral infections, including Epstein-Barr virus infection, chronic hepatitis B, and hepatitis C. Vaccinations for tetanus, diphtheria toxoid, and hepatitis B vaccination have been implicated as triggering factors, although vaccination sites were spared in one case of generalized granuloma annulare.[19]

Lesions compatible with granuloma annulare may occur in patients with active tuberculosis. There are also reports of granuloma annulare after tuberculin skin tests and bacille Calmette–Guérin immunization. Evidence of *Borrelia burgdorferi* infection was detected in two reports, but this association was not confirmed in a serologic study. A case in which chronic relapsing granuloma annulare flared during scabies infestation was attributed to the Koebner phenomenon.[20]

SUN EXPOSURE

Granuloma annulare with a predilection for sun-exposed areas and seasonal recurrence has been described. Photosensitive granuloma annulare has been observed in patients with HIV infection.[14] Generalized disease after psoralen plus ultraviolet A (UVA) light therapy is reported, but it is of note that phototherapy and PUVA phototherapy have been used to treat generalized granuloma annulare.[21-23]

Actinic granuloma, also known as *annular elastolytic giant cell granuloma*, develops on photodamaged skin and is believed to represent a granulomatous reaction to actinic elastosis.[24] Its relationship to granuloma annulare is debated.

DRUGS

Granuloma annulare–like drug reactions are reported for gold therapy and treatment with allopurinol, diclofenac, quinidine, intranasal calcitonin, topiramate, amlodipine, and thalidomide.[25] There are also reports of an association with adalimumab, infliximab, etanercept, efalizumab, and vemurafinib.[22,23,25]

An interstitial granulomatous drug reaction linked to the use of angiotensin-converting enzyme inhibitors, calcium channel blockers, and other medications is considered a distinct entity but may mimic granuloma annulare.[26,27]

PATHOGENIC MECHANISMS

The pathogenic mechanisms that result in foci of altered connective tissue surrounded by a granulomatous inflammatory infiltrate are not understood. Proposed mechanisms include (1) a primary degenerative process of connective tissue initiating granulomatous inflammation, (2) a lymphocyte-mediated immune reaction resulting in macrophage activation and cytokine-mediated degradation of connective tissue, and (3) a subtle vasculitis or other microangiopathy leading to tissue injury.[28-30]

SYSTEMIC DISORDERS AND GRANULOMA ANNULARE

DIABETES MELLITUS AND THYROID DISEASE

Development of granuloma annulare in patients with diabetes mellitus is extensively documented. Whether this is a true relationship has long been debated. The link is primarily with type 1 insulin-dependent diabetes, but cases are also reported with type 2 non–insulin-dependent disease. Localized and generalized as well as subcutaneous nodular and perforating forms of granuloma annulare have been observed. Granuloma annulare rarely predates the onset of diabetes. The histopathologic similarity between granuloma annulare and necrobiosis lipoidica diabeticorum and the coexistence of both conditions in occasional diabetic patients suggest a true association. However, most patients with granuloma annulare do not have diabetes mellitus. Studies attempting to establish a causal correlation have yielded conflicting results.[22]

Granuloma annulare has also occurred in a number of patients with thyroiditis, hypothyroidism, and thyroid adenoma.[22]

MALIGNANCY

An association between granuloma annulare and malignancy in adult patients is reported primarily with Hodgkin and non-Hodgkin lymphoma, including mycosis fungoides, Lennert lymphoma, B-cell disease, T-cell leukemia and lymphoma, and angioblastic T-cell lymphoma. It is reported less commonly with myeloid leukemias and with solid tumors, particularly of the breast. The skin lesions of cutaneous lymphoma and other hematologic malignancies can mimic granuloma annulare both clinically and histopathologically. It may be difficult to distinguish whether they represent true granuloma annulare with atypical lymphocytes or cutaneous lymphoma obscured by a granulomatous infiltrate.[31,32]

DYSLIPIDEMIA

An increased prevalence of dyslipidemia has been reported in patients with granuloma annulare.[32] This was more commonly found in generalized granuloma annulare, particularly in cases with an annular morphology.

LABORATORY TESTS

A diagnosis of localized granuloma annulare is made on clinical examination, and further evaluation is rarely indicated. Biopsy to obtain a specimen for histopathologic examination is necessary when the presentation is atypical, when lesions are symptomatic, and when the diagnosis is otherwise in doubt. Histopathologic analysis may be required to confirm a diagnosis of generalized granuloma annulare or subcutaneous nodular disease on the head and orbital region.

HISTOPATHOLOGIC FINDINGS

The diagnosis is best made at low magnification. Changes are usually observed in the upper and middle dermis, although any part of the dermis or subcutis can be involved. The characteristic histopathologic finding is a lymphohistiocytic granuloma associated with varying degrees of connective tissue degeneration and mucin deposition. The inflammatory infiltrate may have a palisaded or interstitial pattern or a mixture of both patterns.[33-35] Occasionally, a sarcoid-like pattern with large epithelioid histiocytes is seen.

The typical appearance is of single or multiple foci of inflammation with a central core of altered collagen (necrobiosis) surrounded by a wall of palisaded histiocytes (Fig. 34-5). The necrobiotic centers are usually oval, slightly basophilic, devoid of nuclei, and marked by a loss of definition of the collagen bundles and diminished or absent elastic tissue fibers. Stains for mucin and lipid often give positive results.[36]

An interstitial, nonpalisaded pattern of inflammation with histiocytes infiltrating among fragmented collagen bundles may be predominant, particularly in the generalized form. This interstitial pattern is also observed in the absence of apparent connective tissue change. Stains for mucin may be helpful in detecting connective tissue alteration within the infiltrate.

Lymphocytes are admixed with histiocytes in the granuloma and in a perivascular distribution. Multinucleated giant cells may be present but are not as

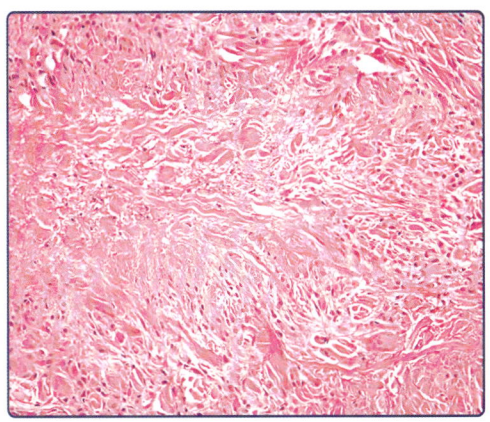

Figure 34-5 Palisading granulomatous inflammation surrounding degenerating collagen within the dermis. (Hematoxylin and eosin stain, ×200.) (Used with permission from Dr. Richard Crawford.)

numerous as in actinic granuloma.[37] Neutrophils and eosinophils are occasionally seen, but plasma cells are rare. Evidence of vascular reactivity includes variable endothelial cell swelling, red cell extravasation, fibrin, leukocytoclasis, and neutrophilic infiltration in blood vessel walls. When leukocytoclastic vasculitis or nuclear debris is a prominent finding, a diagnosis of palisaded neutrophilic and granulomatous dermatitis of immune complex disease should be considered.[38]

In subcutaneous granuloma annulare (Fig. 34-6), the foci of necrobiosis are larger and lie within the deep dermis and subcutaneous fat. They may be distinguished from rheumatoid nodules by the presence of mucin in the necrobiotic zone. Central ulceration and communication between the area of necrobiosis and the surface are characteristic of perforating granuloma annulare (Fig. 34-7). Examination of serial sections may be necessary to demonstrate the necrobiotic plug. An interstitial pattern of inflammation with diffuse necrobiosis is reported in the patch type of granuloma annulare. Palisaded granulomas have also been observed in macular lesions.

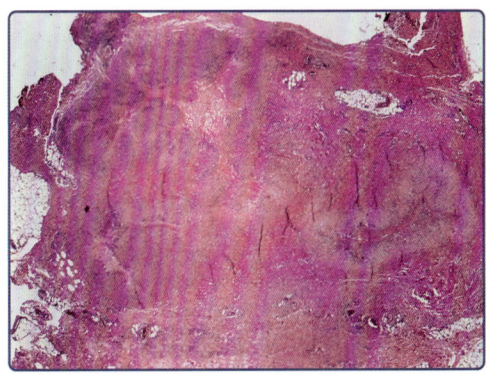

Figure 34-6 Subcutaneous granuloma annulare pathology. (Used with permission from the Graham Library of Wake Forest Department of Dermatology.)

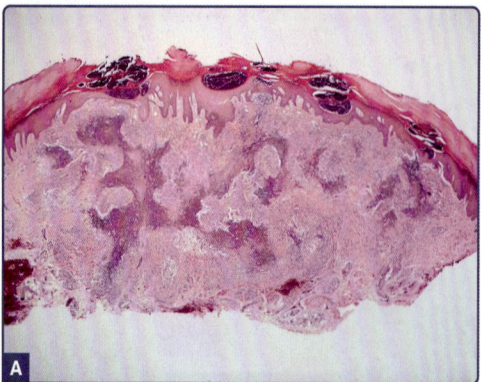

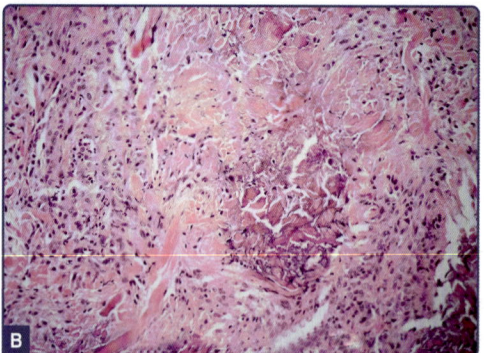

Figure 34-7 A and **B,** Histopathology of perforating granuloma annulare. (Used with permission from the Graham Library of Wake Forest Department of Dermatology.)

Immunofluorescence testing may show deposition of fibrin, immunoglobulin (Ig) M, and C3 as a variable finding around vessel walls or at the basement membrane zone; IgM cytoid bodies are also reported.[39] Immunohistochemistry may be useful to confirm the histiocytic nature of equivocal disease. Ultrastructural changes in the connective tissue and capillaries have been described.[40]

SPECIAL TESTS

A diagnosis of granuloma annulare is made clinically or by skin biopsy. Special investigations are usually not necessary. Further evaluation to rule out systemic disease such as infection, sarcoidosis, or malignancy may be required in atypical cases of granuloma annulare. Investigation for endocrine disease is indicated if the patient has signs or symptoms of diabetes or thyroid dysfunction. Lipid studies may be considered in the evaluation of generalized granuloma annulare.[32]

Imaging studies may be performed in subcutaneous granuloma annulare when the clinical features are not recognized or when the presentation is atypical with rapid enlargement or pain. Radiographs show a nonspecific soft tissue mass without calcification or bone involvement. Ultrasonographic examination reveals a hypoechoic area in the subcutaneous tissues.[41,42]

TABLE 34-1

Differential Diagnosis of Granuloma Annulare

Annular Type

Consider
- Tinea corporis
- Subacute cutaneous lupus erythematosus
- Neonatal lupus erythematosus
- Annular lichen planus
- Acute febrile neutrophilic dermatosis
- Erythema chronicum migrans
- Actinic granuloma/annular elastolytic giant cell granuloma
- Necrobiosis lipoidica diabeticorum

Rule Out
- Infections (eg, tuberculosis, atypical mycobacteria, syphilis)
- Interstitial granulomatous dermatitis with arthritis
- Interstitial granulomatous drug reaction
- Annular sarcoidosis
- Lymphoma

Generalized Type

Consider
- Lichen planus
- Lichen nitidus
- Molluscum contagiosum

Rule Out
- Lichenoid and granulomatous dermatitis of acquired immunodeficiency syndrome
- Infections (eg, tuberculosis, atypical mycobacteria, syphilis)
- Sarcoidosis
- Blau syndrome (familial granulomatous arthritis, skin eruption, and uveitis)
- Interstitial granulomatous drug reaction
- Lymphoma

Subcutaneous Type

Consider
- Erythema nodosum
- Dermoid cyst
- Rheumatoid nodules

Rule Out
- Epithelioid sarcoma
- Benign or other malignant tumors
- Deep infections

Perforating Type

Consider
- Molluscum contagiosum
- Insect bites
- Pityriasis lichenoides
- Perforating collagenosis and other perforating disorders
- Foreign body granuloma
- Papulonecrotic tuberculid
- Palisaded neutrophilic and granulomatous dermatitis of immune complex disease

Patch Type

Consider
- Morphea
- Erythema annulare centrifugum
- Parapsoriasis

Rule Out
- Lymphoma

Magnetic resonance imaging shows a mass with indistinct margins, isointense or slightly hyperintense to muscle with T1-weighted images and with a heterogeneous but predominantly high signal intensity on T2-weighted images.[41,43]

DIFFERENTIAL DIAGNOSIS

See Table 34-1.

TREATMENT

The usual treatment options include awaiting spontaneous resolution, topical steroids, and intralesional steroids. These and various other therapies of anecdotal benefit are summarized in Table 34-2. Most treatment recommendations are based on single case reports and small cases series, and there are no controlled studies.[21-23,44-47]

CLINICAL COURSE AND PROGNOSIS

Most cases of localized granuloma annulare resolve spontaneously without sequelae. Lesions may clear within a few weeks or persist for several years. The majority disappear within 2 years. Recurrent lesions may develop months or even years later, frequently at the same site. Generalized granuloma annulare often runs a more protracted course. Perforating granuloma annulare results in scarring. There are a number of reports of anetoderma or middermal elastolysis following generalized granuloma annulare and annular elastolytic giant cell granuloma.[48,49] One case of generalized granuloma annulare in a photosensitive distribution healed with scarring and milia formation.[50]

TABLE 34-2
Treatment Options for Granuloma Annulare

- Await spontaneous resolution
- Apply topical corticosteroid with or without occlusion
- Administer intralesional triamcinolone 2.5 mg/mL

Anecdotal Reports of Benefit
- Topical
  - Tacrolimus 0.1% ointment
  - Pimecrolimus cream
  - Imiquimod 5% cream[a]
- Intralesional
  - Interferon-γ
  - Interferon-β
  - Sterile water or saline
- Systemic
  - Antimalarials
  - Retinoids
  - Antibiotics[b]
  - Corticosteroids
  - Cyclosporine
  - Zileuton with vitamin E
  - Fumaric acid esters
  - Pentoxifylline
- Hydroxyurea, chlorambucil, niacinamide, potassium iodide, dapsone
  - Etanercept[c]
  - Infliximab[c]
  - Efalizumab[c]
  - Adalimumab[c]
- Other
  - Phototherapy[d]
  - Photodynamic therapy
  - Fractional photothermolysis
- Skin biopsy
  - Cryotherapy
  - Pulsed dye, Excimer, Nd:YAG or CO_2 laser

[a]Application of 5% imiquimod cream has been reported to worsen granuloma annulare in a child.
[b]Triple antibiotic regimen (rifampicin, ofloxacin, minocycline), doxycycline, antituberculosis therapy.
[c]Development of granuloma annulare has been reported during therapy with etanercept, infliximab, and adalimumab.
[d]Narrowband ultraviolet B, ultraviolet A1, psoralen plus ultraviolet A.
Nd:YAG, neodymium-doped yttrium aluminum garnet.

REFERENCES

1. Radcliffe Crocker H. Granuloma annulare. *Br J Dermatol*. 1902;14:1.
2. Muhlbauer JE. Granuloma annulare. *J Am Acad Dermatol*. 1980;3:217.
3. De Aloe G, Risulo M, Sbano P, et al. Congenital subcutaneous granuloma annulare. *Pediatr Dermatol*. 2005;22:234.
4. Choi J-C, Bae J-Y, Cho S, et al. Generalized perforating granuloma annulare in an infant. *Pediatr Dermatol*. 2003;20:2.
5. Martinon-Torres F, Martinon-Sanchez JM, Martinon-Sanchez F. Localized granuloma annulare in children: a review of 42 cases. *Eur J Paediatr*. 1999;158:866.
6. Friedman SJ, Winkelmann RK. Familial granuloma annulare. *J Am Acad Dermatol*. 1987;16:600.
7. Abrusci V, Weiss E, Planas G. Familial perforating granuloma annulare. *Int J Dermatol*. 1988;27:126.
8. Dabski K, Winkelmann RK. Generalized granuloma annulare: clinical and laboratory findings in 100 patients. *J Am Acad Dermatol*. 1989;20:39.
9. Grogg KL, Nascimento AG. Subcutaneous granuloma annulare in childhood: clinicopathologic features in 34 cases. *Pediatrics*. 2001;107:e42.
10. Felner EI, Steinberg JB, Weinberg AG. Subcutaneous granuloma annulare: a review of 47 cases. *Pediatrics*. 1997;100:965.
11. Mutasim DF, Bridges AG. Patch granuloma annulare: clinicopathologic study of 6 patients. *J Am Acad Dermatol*. 2000;42:417.
12. Brey NV, Malone J, Callen JP. Acute-onset, painful acral granuloma annulare. *Arch Dermatol*. 2006;142:49.
13. Long D, Thiboutot DM, Majeski JT, et al. Interstitial granulomatous dermatitis with arthritis. *J Am Acad Dermatol*. 1996;34:957.
14. Cohen PR. Granuloma annulare: a mucocutaneous condition in human immunodeficiency virus-infected patients. *Arch Dermatol*. 1999;135:1404.
15. Ehrich EW, McGuire JL, Kim YH. Association of granuloma annulare with sarcoidosis. *Arch Dermatol*. 1992;128:855.

16. van Kooij B, van Dijk MC, de Boer J, et al. Is granuloma annulare related to intermediate uveitis with retinal vasculitis? *Br J Ophthalmol*. 2003;87:763.
17. Brey NV, Purkiss TJ, Sehgal A, et al. Association of inflammatory eye disease with granuloma annulare? *Arch Dermatol*. 2008;144:803.
18. Arekapudi S, Whitfield K, Morrison D. Panuveitis associated with granuloma annulare in a child. *J Pediatr Ophthalmol Strabismus*. 2009;46:45.
19. Huilgol SC, Liddell K, Black MM. Generalized granuloma annulare sparing vaccination sites. *Clin Exp Dermatol*. 1995;20:51.
20. Wilsmann-Theis D, Wenzel J, Gerdsen R, et al. Granuloma annulare induced by scabies. *Acta Derm Venereol*. 2003;83:318.
21. Pavlovsky M, Samuelov L, Sprecher E, et al. NB-UVB phototherapy for generalized granuloma annulare. *Dermatol Ther*. 2016; 29:152.
22. Thornsberry LA, English JC. Etiology, diagnosis, and therapeutic management of granuloma annulare: an update. *Am J Clin Dermatol*. 2013;14:279.
23. Keimig EL. Granuloma annulare. *Dermatol Clin*. 2015; 33(3):315-29.
24. O'Brien JP, Regan W. Actinically degenerate elastic tissue is the likely antigenic basis of actinic granuloma of the skin and of temporal arteritis. *J Am Acad Dermatol*. 1999;40:214.
25. Lee SB, Weide B, Ugurel S, et al. Vemurafenib-induced granuloma annulare. *J Dtsch Dermatol Ges*. 2016;14:305.
26. Magro CM, Crowson AN, Schapiro BL. The interstitial granulomatous drug reaction. A distinctive clinical and pathological entity. *J Cutan Pathol*. 1998;25:72.
27. Perrin C, Lacour J-P, Castanet J, et al. Interstitial granulomatous drug reaction with a histological pattern of interstitial granulomatous dermatitis. *Am J Dermatopathol*. 2001;23:295.
28. Dahl MV. Speculations on the pathogenesis of granuloma annulare. *Australas J Dermatol*. 1985;26:49.
29. Mempel M, Musette P, Flaguel B, et al. T-cell receptor repertoire and cytokine pattern in granuloma annulare: defining a particular type of cutaneous granulomatous inflammation. *J Invest Dermatol*. 2002;118:957.
30. Fayyazi A, Schweyer S, Eichmeyer B, et al. Expression of IFNγ, coexpression of TNFα and matrix metalloproteinases and apoptosis of T lymphocytes and macrophages in granuloma annulare. *Arch Dermatol* Res. 2000;292:384.
31. Jouary T, Beylot-Barry M, Bergier B, et al. Mycosis fungoides mimicking granuloma annulare. *Br J Dermatol*. 2002;146:1102.
32. Wu H, Barusevicius A, Lessin SR. Granuloma annulare with mycosis fungoides-like distribution and palisaded granulomas of CD-68-positive histiocytes. *J Am Acad Dermatol*. 2004;51:39.
33. Friedmann-Birnbaum R, Weltfriend S, Munichor M, et al. A comparative histopathologic study of generalized and localized granuloma annulare. *Am J Dermatopathol*. 1989;11:144.
34. Stefanaki K, Tsivitanidou-Kakourou T, Stefanaki C, et al. Histological and immunohistochemical study of granuloma annulare and subcutaneous granuloma annulare in children. *J Cutan Pathol*. 2007;34:392.
35. Dabski K, Winkelmann RK. Generalized granuloma annulare: histopathology and immunopathology. A systematic review of 100 cases and comparison with localized granuloma annulare. *J Am Acad Dermatol*. 1989;20:28.
36. Schulman JM, LeBoit P. Adipophilin expression in necrobiosis lipoidica, granuloma annulare, and sarcoidosis. *Am J Dermatopathol*. 2015;37:203.
37. Al-Hoqail IA, Al-Ghamdi AM, Martinka M, et al. Actinic granuloma is a unique and distinct entity: a comparative study with granuloma annulare. *Am J Dermatopathol*. 2002;24:209.
38. Chu P, Connolly MK, LeBoit PE. The histopathologic spectrum of palisaded neutrophilic and granulomatous dermatitis in patients with collagen vascular disease. *Arch Dermatol*. 1994;130:1278.
39. Stefanaki K, Tsivitanidou Kakourou T, Sefananaki C, et al. Histological and immunohistochemical study of granuloma annulare and subcutaneous granuloma annulare in children. *J Cutan Pathol*. 2007;34:392.
40. Hanna WM, Moreno-Merlo F, Andrighetti L. Granuloma annulare: an elastic tissue disease? Case report and literature review. *Ultrastructural Pathol*. 1999;23:33.
41. Chung S, Frush DP, Prose NP, et al. Subcutaneous granuloma annulare: MR imaging features in six children and literature review. *Radiology*. 1999;210:845.
42. Stenzel M, Voss U, Mutze S, et al. A pretibial lump in a toddler—sonographic findings in subcutaneous granuloma annulare. *Ultraschall Med*. 2010;31:68.
43. Navarro OM, Laffan EE, Ngan B-Y. Pediatric soft-tissue tumors and pseudotumors: MR imaging features with pathologic correlation. *Radiographics*. 2009;29:887.
44. Lukacs J, Schliemann S, Elsner P. Treatment of generalized granuloma annulare—a systematic review. *J Eur Acad Dermatol Venereol*. 2015;29:1467.
45. Min MS, Lebwohl M. Treatment of recalcitrant granuloma annulare with adalimumab. *J Am Acad Dermatol*. 2016;74:127.
46. Simpson B, Foster S, Ku JH, et al. Triple antibiotic combination therapy may improve but not resolve granuloma annulare. *Dermatol Ther*. 2014;27:343.
47. Verne SH, Kennedy J, Falto-Aizpurua LA, et al. Laser treatment of granuloma annulare: a review. *Int J Dermatol*. 2016;55:376.
48. Kang HS, Paek JO, Lee MW, et al. Anetoderma developing in generalized granuloma annulare in an infant. *Ann Dermatol*. 2014;26:283.
49. Sanyal S, Hejmadi R, Taibjee SM. Granuloma annulare resolving with features of mid-dermal elastolysis. *Clin Exp Dermatol*. 2009;34:e1017.
50. Gass JK, Todd PM, Rytina E. Generalized granuloma annulare in a photosensitive distribution resolving with scarring and milia formation. *Clin Exp Dermatol*. 2009;34:e53.

Chapter 35 :: Sarcoidosis
:: Richard Marchell

第三十五章

结节病

中文导读

本章主要介绍了结节病的流行病学史、临床特点、诊断和治疗。着重介绍了该病的临床特点。从皮肤表现和皮肤外表现两个方面介绍了该病的特点并提到了一些特异性皮损和非特异性皮损。在诊断方面：结节病是一种排他性诊断，需要临床结合病理结果，并排除其他能够产生类似组织学或临床表现的疾病。因为结节病是一种累及多器官的全身性疾病。孤立的皮肤肉芽肿不应被认为是结节病，单个器官系统出现非干酪样肉芽肿并不能确定为结节病的诊断，必须努力排除其他诊断。同时文中介绍了结节病的肺部影像学分期。

〔李芳芳〕

AT-A-GLANCE

- Sarcoidosis is a multisystem disease characterized by granulomatous inflammation of unknown etiology commonly occurring in the lung and the skin, but any organ system can be affected.
- The type of cutaneous lesion may suggest prognosis. Lupus pernio lesions are associated with chronic disease course and scarring. Erythema nodosum lesions portend an acute self-resolving course.
- Specific lesions of sarcoidosis have a varied clinical morphology, including macules, papules, plaques, nodules, and ulcerations.
- Topical, systemic, and intralesional corticosteroids are the mainstay of therapy.
- Patients initially diagnosed with cutaneous sarcoidosis should get baseline testing to look for deleterious systemic disease, including a physical examination; neurologic review of systems; a chest radiograph; an electrocardiogram; pulmonary function tests; urine analysis; complete blood count; comprehensive metabolic panel; serum calcium level; tuberculosis screening; and an ophthalmologic examination.

Sarcoidosis is a multisystem disease characterized by granulomatous inflammation. It is theorized to be a disease of hyperactivation of the immune system, but its etiology is unknown.

HISTORICAL PERSPECTIVE

Although the lungs are the organs most commonly afflicted, sarcoidosis was actually first described in the late 1800s because of its skin manifestations. Boeck reported a case of "multiple benign sarkoid of the skin" as he believed the skin lesions resembled sarcomas but were benign.[1]

EPIDEMIOLOGY

Sarcoidosis occurs worldwide and may affect all ages and races. Disease onset is most common in the third decade of life and is slightly higher in women.[2] Sarcoidosis has a higher incidence with greater distance from the equator. The highest prevalence of sarcoidosis is found in whites in Denmark and Sweden, and in persons of African descent in the United States.[3] In the United States, the lifetime risk of sarcoidosis is 2.4%

in African Americans and 0.85% in whites.[3] The incidence rate of sarcoidosis in the United States is 17.8 per 100,000 for African Americans and 8.1 per 100,000 for whites; the prevalence rate is 141.8 per 100,000 for African Americans and 49.8 per 100,000 for white individuals.[4] The highest prevalence is in African American women (178.5 per 100,000).[4] African Americans tend to have more severe symptomatic disease. African Americans are more likely to have extrapulmonary disease,[5] require treatment,[6] and have a lower rate of clinical recovery[7,8] than whites.

CLINICAL FEATURES

Table 35-1 summarizes the variable presentations of sarcoidosis.

CUTANEOUS FINDINGS

With the advent of penicillin, sarcoidosis has replaced syphilis as the great mimicker for dermatologists. The diverse variety of cutaneous sarcoidosis is bewildering. Almost all primary morphologies have been reported, including macules, papules, patches, plaques, and nodules. Alopecia occurs with scalp involvement and nail changes also occur. Epidermal changes of scaling, telangiectasia, and atrophy exist. Cutaneous lesions of sarcoidosis may occur before, coincident with, or after systemic involvement. Classically, lesions are divided into two categories: specific and nonspecific. Specific lesions have granulomatous inflammation histologically similar to the pattern seen in sarcoid lesions in other organs. Nonspecific skin findings are reactive and do not exhibit sarcoidal granulomas.

SPECIFIC CUTANEOUS LESIONS

Despite the diversity in appearance, there are several clinical presentations of specific lesions that are typical of cutaneous sarcoidosis.

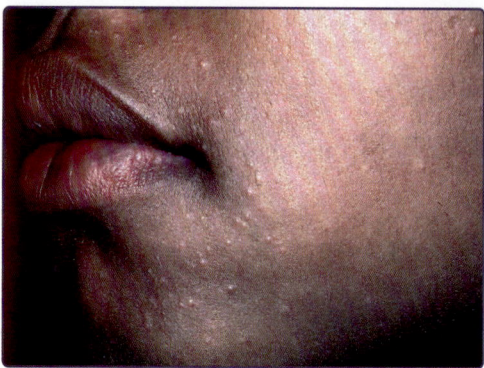

Figure 35-1 Perioral papular lesions.

Papules and Plaques: The most common presentation is the papular form (Figs. 35-1 and 35-2). These firm 1- to 5-mm papules often have a translucent red-brown or yellow-brown color. The yellow-brown coloration as reminiscent of "apple jelly" and is accentuated with the pressing of a glass slide to the skin (diascopy) (Fig. 35-3). In addition to the color change, the granulomatous lesions have a nodular quality that is appreciated with diascopy. The apple jelly appearance and nodules is not pathognomonic for sarcoidosis, as other granulomatous skin conditions, including lupus vulgaris and granuloma annulare, may exhibit similar diascopic properties. However, dermoscopy may prove useful in distinguishing the cutaneous granulomas of sarcoidosis from necrobiotic granulomas. Even after therapy, dermoscopic findings of pink homogenous background, translucent orange areas, fine white scaling, and scar-like depigmentation are significantly associated with cutaneous sarcoidosis compared to necrobiosis lipoidica, granuloma annulare, and rheumatoid nodules.[9]

Epidermal changes may or may not be present (Figs. 35-4 and 35-5), but the lesions often have a waxy appearance, which reflects mild epidermal atrophy. Papular lesions occur most commonly on the face and neck, with a predilection for periorbital skin. Typically the papular lesions are asymptomatic without pain or pruritus; the most common complaint is cosmetic disfigurement.

TABLE 35-1
Variable Presentations of Sarcoidosis

	CLINICAL MANIFESTATIONS
Lupus pernio	Symmetric, violaceous, indurated plaques and nodules on nose, earlobes, cheeks, and digits
Mikulicz syndrome	Sarcoidal granulomas on mucosal surface and tongue, with bilateral enlargement of the lacrimal, parotid, sublingual, and submandibular glands
Darier-Roussy sarcoid	Presents as persistent subcutaneous nodules that may be tender or painless; occurs on extremities
Lofgren syndrome	Erythema nodosum with bilateral hilar adenopathy, arthralgia, and fever; often the presenting manifestation of sarcoidosis
Heerfordt syndrome	Fever, parotid gland enlargement, facial palsy, and anterior uveitis

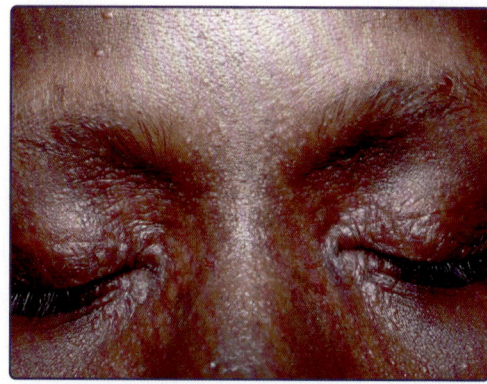

Figure 35-2 Periorbital papular lesions.

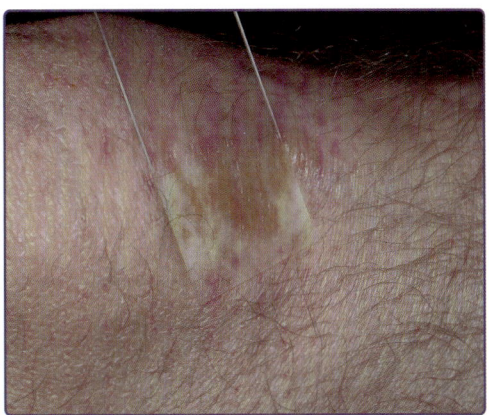

Figure 35-3 Diascopy revealing "apple-jelly" coloration.

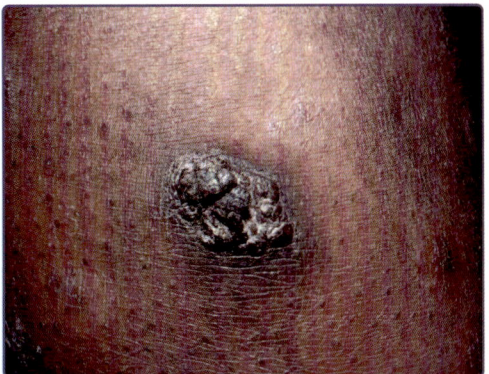

Figure 35-4 Scaling plaque. Despite being a disease that is characterized by granulomas in the dermis epidermal changes such as psoriasiform scale occur.

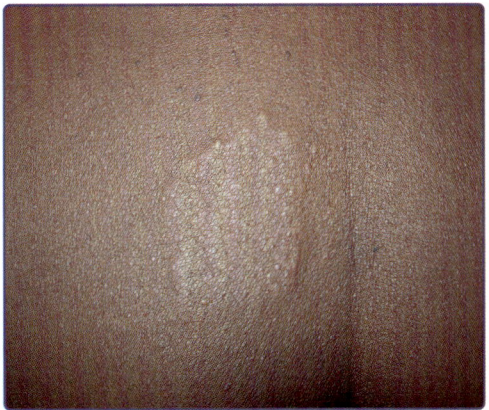

Figure 35-5 Dermal plaque. Notice there are no epidermal changes in this example of cutaneous sarcoidosis.

Plaques, both annular and nonannular, and nodules may develop from papular lesions and may retain the translucent yellow-brown coloration (Fig. 35-6).

Lupus Pernio: Lupus pernio describes the relatively symmetric, violaceous, indurated plaques and nodules occurring on the nose, earlobes, cheeks, and digits (Figs. 35-7 and 35-8). The name *lupus pernio* is a misnomer preserved from the erroneous notion that these lesions might be related to lupus vulgaris and cold injury when lupus pernio was first described by Besnier in the 19th century. This distinctive clinical variant is associated with a higher incidence of systemic involvement and upper respiratory tract disease.[10] Lupus pernio lesions may directly extend into the nasal sinus, leading to epistaxis, nasal crusting, and sine bone involvement. Angiolupoid lesions are pink and violaceous papules and plaques with prominent telangiectasias that usually occur on the face; they are often considered a variant of lupus pernio.

Scar Sarcoid: Cutaneous sarcoidosis occurs preferentially within scar tissue, at traumatized skin sites, and around embedded foreign material such as silica and tattoo ink (Fig. 35-9). Scars become inflamed and infiltrated with sarcoidal granulomas. Inflammation of old scars may precede or parallel systemic disease activity. Infiltrated scars may be tender or pruritic and the only finding of a patient with significant systemic involvement. The presence of sarcoidal granulomas surrounding foreign material does not establish the diagnosis of sarcoidosis, nor does foreign material in the presence of granulomas exclude the diagnosis.

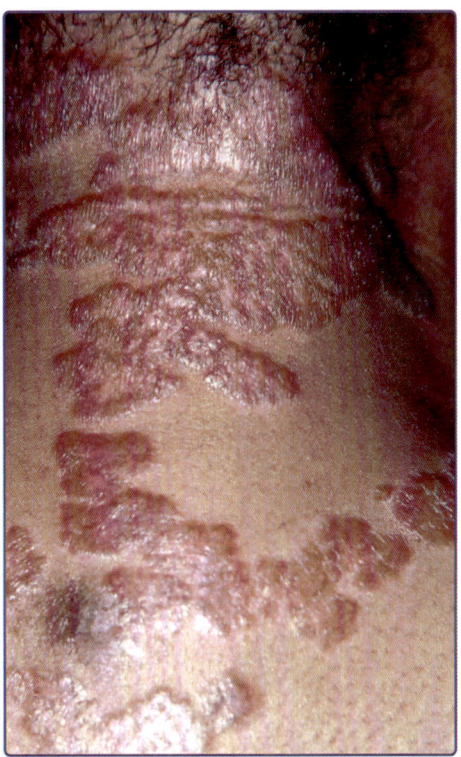

Figure 35-6 Plaques on neck.

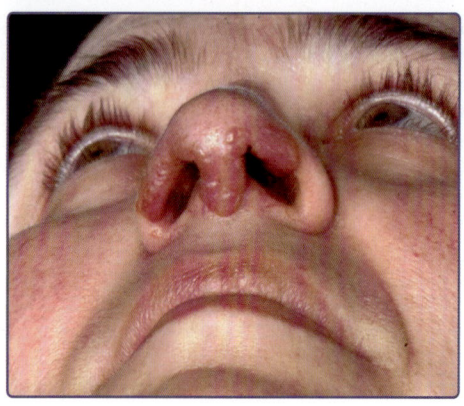

Figure 35-7 Lupus pernio along the nasal rim. This patient also had sarcoidosis of the upper respiratory tract (SURT).

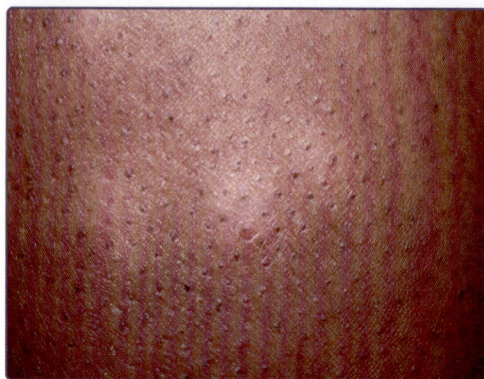

Figure 35-10 Hypopigmented macules.

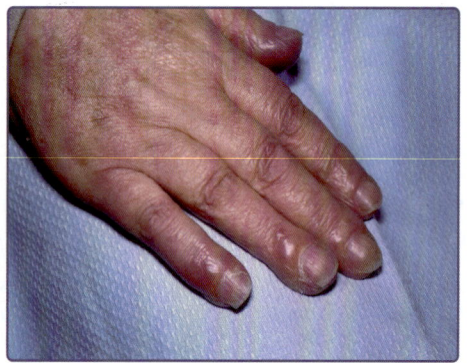

Figure 35-8 Lupus pernio of the digits.

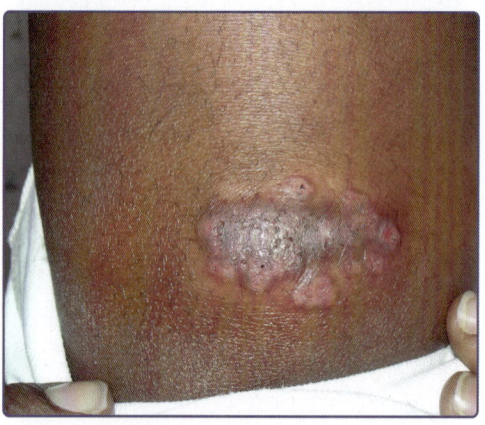

Figure 35-9 Scar sarcoid arising in an excision site.

Subcutaneous Nodules (Darier-Roussy Sarcoid): Rarely, sarcoidosis can present as persistent subcutaneous nodules (Darier-Roussy sarcoid).[11] The nodules may be tender or painless, and preferentially occur on the extremities.

Hypopigmented Areas: Lesions appearing to be hypopigmented macules occur primarily in darkly pigmented persons (Fig. 35-10). However, upon careful palpation, induration can usually be appreciated in the areas that have granulomatous inflammation histologically. Some hypopigmented truly macular areas likely reflect postinflammatory pigment alteration as well.

Alopecia: Alopecia, both scarring and nonscarring, may occur with cutaneous lesions on hair-bearing skin such as the face and scalp. Annular plaques may have alopecia centrally. The reversibility is dependent on the degree of fibrosis and destruction of the hair follicle.

Nail Findings: Nail plate deformation and discoloration occur rarely including clubbing, subungual hyperkeratosis, and nail plate destruction. Granulomas in the nail matrix or adjacent bone lead to nail changes.

Mucous Membranes: Sarcoidal granulomas may cause papules and plaques of the mucosal surface and tongue. Infiltration of the gingiva causing "strawberry gums" mimicking Wegner granulomatosis may occur. Sarcoidosis is one cause of Mikulicz syndrome, the bilateral enlargement of the lacrimal, parotid, sublingual, and submandibular glands.

Additional Cutaneous Findings: A myriad of additional clinical presentations have also been reported. These include ichthyosis,[12] erythroderma,[13] ulcerations[14] (Fig. 35-11), morphea-form plaques,[15] lichen nitidus-like papules,[16] folliculitis-like lesions,[17] psoriasiform plaques,[18] gyrate erythema,[19] verrucous lesions,[17] faint erythema, genital lesions,[20,21] palmar erythema,[22] discoid lupus-like plaques,[23] lower-extremity edema,[24] lesions mimicking tuberculoid leprosy, areas mimicking polymorphous light eruptions,[17] and pustular lesions.[17]

NONSPECIFIC CUTANEOUS LESIONS

Erythema nodosum is the main nonspecific cutaneous manifestation of sarcoidosis. Erythema nodosum with bilateral hilar adenopathy, arthralgia, and fever is frequently the initial manifestation of sarcoidosis (Lofgren syndrome). These patients tend to have an acute form of sarcoidosis with eventual resolution.

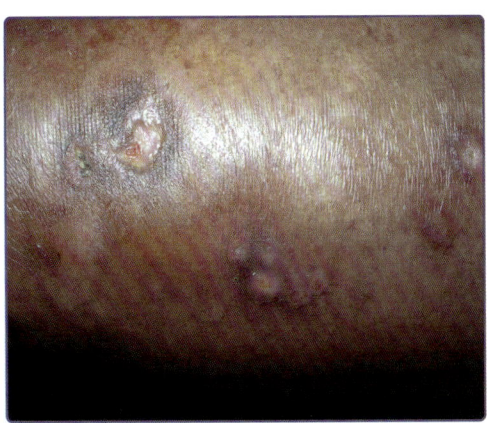

Figure 35-11 Ulcerative lesions on the leg.

Other nonspecific cutaneous manifestations of sarcoidosis are much less common. The neutrophilic dermatoses, Sweet disease and pyoderma gangrenosum, have been reported. Most patients with pyoderma gangrenosum have concomitant erythema nodosum.[25] Nonspecific erythematous eruptions resembling viral exanthems or drug reaction without histologic evidence of granulomas occur very rarely with acute sarcoidosis. Additionally, patients with sarcoidosis may have pruritus without granulomatous inflammation leading to prurigo nodules.[26] Erythema multiforme had been regularly cited as a nonspecific cutaneous manifestation of sarcoidosis,[17] but reports of histologically proven erythema multiforme with interface dermatitis are virtually nonexistent in the literature,[27,28] and any association is more likely coincidental. Erythroderma and nonspecific lower-extremity edema have been described as both specific and nonspecific lesions of sarcoidosis.[24,26,29,30]

NONCUTANEOUS FINDINGS

Sarcoidosis is a multisystemic disease by definition and essentially all organ systems can be involved. However, symptoms are often lacking and diagnosis of systemic involvement is commonly found incidentally on routine testing, such as a chest radiograph.

PULMONARY SARCOIDOSIS

The lung is the most common organ involved with sarcoidosis. Findings on pulmonary examination are usually absent, and patients are usually asymptomatic. Dyspnea, cough, chest pain, hypoxemia, and wheezing may occur. Sarcoid lesions directly infiltrate the parenchyma of the lungs, which can lead to pulmonary fibrosis. Fibrotic disease can lead to pulmonary hypertension and chronic *Aspergillus* infection. Additionally, lesions distort the airways and cause an obstructive lung disease. Pulmonary function tests are more likely to be abnormal when chest radiographs reveal abnormal lung parenchyma, but also may be abnormal without parenchymal findings.

OCULAR SARCOIDOSIS

The eyes are involved in at least 25% of sarcoidosis patients and involvement can be vision threatening.[31] Patients may initially be asymptomatic warranting routine ophthalmologic examination.[32] Redness, burning, itching, and dryness are the most common symptoms when present. Any portion of the eye may be involved with uveitis being most common. Lacrimal gland enlargement may occur (Fig. 35-12). Uveitis can lead to glaucoma and cataracts. Other manifestations include conjunctivitis, lacrimal gland involvement leading to keratoconjunctivitis sicca (dry eyes), and optic neuritis. Optic neuritis may rapidly lead to vision loss. Heerfordt syndrome, which includes fever, parotid gland enlargement, facial palsy, and anterior uveitis, is a classic presentation of sarcoidosis.[2]

CARDIAC SARCOIDOSIS

Clinical evidence of cardiac involvement is found in only 5% of sarcoidosis patients, but myocardial granulomas have been found in approximately 25% of patients at time of autopsy.[33] Most clinical problems

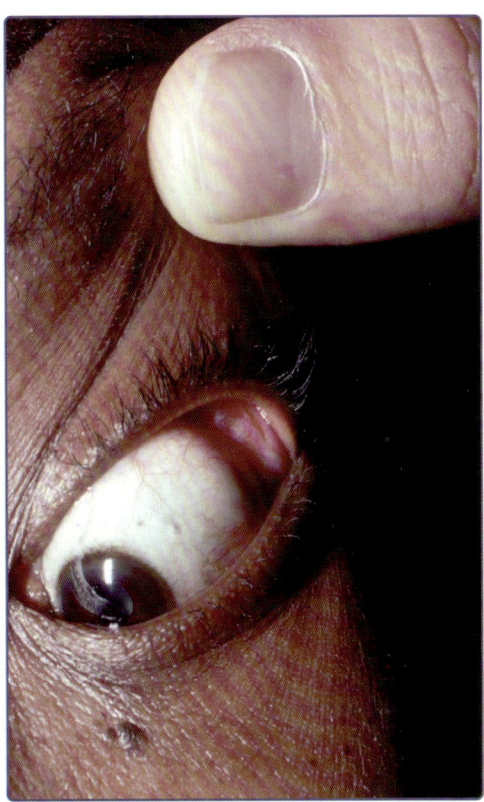

Figure 35-12 Lacrimal gland enlargement in a patient with sarcoidosis.

are related to cardiac arrhythmias or left ventricular dysfunction.[34] Sudden death may occur. Congestive heart failure may result when the myocardium is massively infiltrated with granulomas. An electrocardiogram is recommended for every patient diagnosed with sarcoidosis.

NEUROSARCOIDOSIS

Any portion of the central or peripheral nervous system may be affected. Neurosarcoidosis has a predilection for the base of the brain, and cranial neuropathies are the most common manifestation.[35] The facial nerve is the most frequently involved. Mass lesions may develop in the brain or spinal cord. Aseptic meningitis and peripheral neuropathy can occur.

RENAL SARCOIDOSIS

The kidneys may be affected by direct granulomatous inflammation or by nephrolithiasis resulting from hypercalcemia. Activated sarcoidal macrophages have increased 1α-hydroxylase activity. This converts 25-hydroxyvitamin D to 1,25-dihydroxyvitamin D, the active form of the vitamin, resulting in hypercalcemia, hypercalciuria, and nephrolithiasis.[36]

HEPATIC SARCOIDOSIS

Liver involvement is common but rarely causes any clinically relevant signs or symptoms. Histologic evidence of sarcoidal granulomas is common and the liver can be a good site to biopsy to confirm the diagnosis. An increase in serum alkaline phosphatase occurs in approximately 33% of patients,[37] but does not mandate treatment. Treatment is reserved for patients with significant symptoms (hepatosplenomegaly, abdominal pain, pruritus), evidence of synthetic dysfunction, or hyperbilirubinemia. Rarely, primary biliary cirrhosis-type disease and portal hypertension may develop.[38]

OTHER ORGANS

The sinuses and upper airway are commonly involved with sarcoidosis, a condition known as sarcoidosis of the upper respiratory tract. Nasal sarcoidosis of the upper respiratory tract is often associated with lupus pernio and may cause severe epistaxis and nasal crusting. Sarcoidosis may involve the spleen, and may be associated with reduction in any blood cell line. Splenic sequestration and bone marrow involvement may lead to leukopenia. Thrombocytopenia may result from bone marrow involvement, splenic sequestration, or from an idiopathic thrombocytopenic purpura-like syndrome related to hypergammaglobulinemia often seen in patients with sarcoidosis.[39]

ETIOLOGY AND PATHOGENESIS

Sarcoidosis is triggered by exposure to an antigen(s) with hyperactivity of the cell-mediated immune system leading to granulomatous inflammation. Presumably antigen-presenting cells, such as macrophages, recognize, process, and present the processed sarcoid-inducing antigen to CD4+ T cells of the T-helper (Th)1 subtype. The processed antigen is presented to these lymphocytes via human leukocyte antigen (HLA) class II molecules on the antigen-presenting cells that have undergone enhanced expression from exposure to the sarcoidosis antigen and possibly interferon gamma (IFN-γ).[40,41] These activated macrophages produce interleukin (IL)-12 which induces lymphocytes to shift toward a Th1 profile and causes T lymphocytes to secrete IFN-γ. These activated T cells release IL-2 and chemotactic factors that recruit monocytes and macrophages to the site of disease activity. IL-2 and other cytokines also expand various T-cell clones. IFN-γ further activates macrophages and transforms them into giant cells.[40] Tumor necrosis factor (TNF)-α, IL-2, and other cytokines may also be important in stimulating macrophages (Fig. 35-13). There is also evidence that CD4+ T cells of the Th17 subtype and Th17 cytokines also may play a role in the development of the lesions.[42] The identity of the putative antigen(s) triggering the immunologic cascade is unknown. Infectious agents and environmental antigens and have been investigated.

RISK FACTORS

Infectious agents such as mycobacteria,[43] *Propionibacterium acnes*,[44] and *Chlamydia*[45] are associated with sarcoidosis. However, patients with sarcoidosis improve with immunosuppressive agents, which argues against a purely infectious etiology. Mineral dusts, including silica, iron,[46] and titanium,[47] are associated with sarcoidosis. Firefighters and persons with wood burning stoves are documented as having an increased risk of developing sarcoidosis.[48,49] Lifelong nonsmokers are more likely to develop the disease[50] than smokers.

Genetics play a major role in determining susceptibility to sarcoidosis. Relatives of an affected person are more likely to develop disease than is the general population.[51] Numerous studies in various ethnic groups show a relationship between HLA antigens and the development of disease, protection from disease, good prognosis, bad prognosis, acute disease, chronic disease, and various phenotypic expressions of sarcoidosis. Additionally, mutations in genes related to the immune system, including those encoding TNF, lymphotoxin α, and the IL-23 receptor, are associated with different presentations of sarcoidosis,

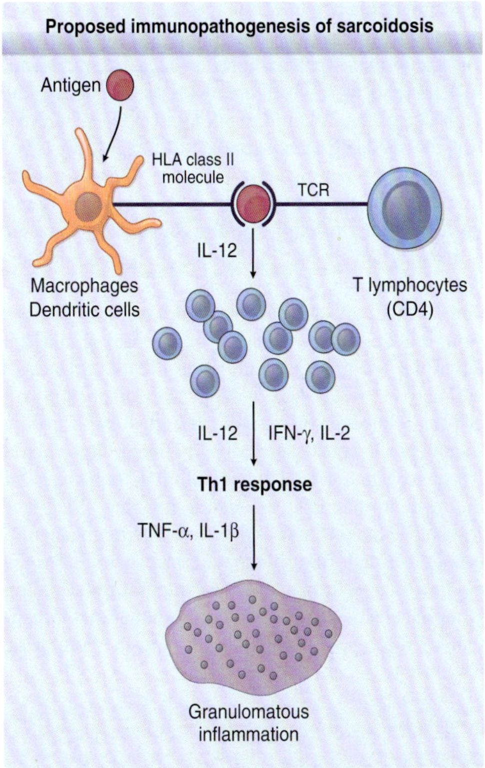

Figure 35-13 Proposed immunopathogenesis of sarcoidosis. An antigen, presently unknown, is engulfed and processed by an antigen-presenting cell (macrophage or dendritic cell). The processed antigen is presented to a T-cell receptor (TCR) of a T lymphocyte via an HLA class II molecule. Once the HLA receptor and TCR have bound the processed antigen, numerous lymphokines and cytokines of the T-helper cell subtype 1 (Th1) class are released that lead to T-cell proliferation, recruitment of monocytes, and eventual granuloma formation. A few of these lymphokines and cytokines are shown, with those released by the antigen-presenting cells on the left and those released by lymphocytes on the right. IFN, interferon; IL, interleukin; TNF, tumor necrosis factor.

including erythema nodosum, cardiac sarcoidosis, and uveitis.[52-55]

The interplay of antigenic and genetic risk factors suggests that there may be multiple causes of sarcoidosis. Perhaps patients have to experience a specific interaction between one or several exposures and be genetically programmed to one or several immunologic responses. Each putative antigen may be associated with a specific HLA class II molecule and T-cell receptor and/or other polymorphisms of the many molecules of the human immune system.

DIAGNOSIS

The diagnosis of sarcoidosis requires a compatible clinical picture, histologic demonstration of noncaseating granulomas, and exclusion of other diseases capable of producing similar histology or clinical features. As sarcoidosis is a diagnosis of exclusion, the diagnosis can never be confirmed with 100% certainty.[56] Often the diagnosis is assumed when the clinical presentation is typical for the disease and is not explained by an alternative cause.

The presence of noncaseating granulomas in a single organ system does not conclusively establish the diagnosis of sarcoidosis because sarcoidosis is, by definition, a systemic disease that involves multiple organs.[57] Isolated skin granulomas should not be assumed to represent sarcoidosis, and efforts must be made to exclude alternative diagnoses. Although confirmation of sarcoidosis requires proof of granulomatous involvement in at least 2 separate organs, histologic confirmation is not necessarily required in the second organ.[58]

Certain disease presentations are so specific for the diagnosis of sarcoidosis (eg, Lofgren syndrome, Heerfordt syndrome, and asymptomatic bilateral hilar adenopathy) that the diagnosis may be accepted without a tissue biopsy. For example, asymptomatic bilateral hilar lymphadenopathy noted on chest radiograph is relatively specific for sarcoidosis.

Some clinical, imaging, and laboratory tests are recommended when a diagnosis of sarcoidosis is considered. These tests screen for involvement of various organ systems (Table 35-2).

A physical examination and routine ophthalmologic examination should be performed in addition to testing. A history to assess for risk of other granulomatous diseases by occupational and environmental (eg,

TABLE 35-2
Recommended Initial Evaluation of Patients with Sarcoidosis

- History (occupational and environmental exposure, symptoms)
- Physical examination
- Posteroanterior chest radiograph
- Pulmonary function tests: spirometry, DL_{CO}, and KL_{CO}
- Peripheral blood counts: white blood cells, red blood cells, platelets
- Serum chemistries: calcium, liver enzymes (alanine aminotransferase, aspartate aminotransferase, alkaline phosphatase), creatinine, and blood urea nitrogen
- Urine analysis
- Electrocardiogram
- Routine ophthalmologic examination
- Tuberculin skin test

DL_{CO}, diffusing capacity of lung for carbon monoxide; KL_{CO}, diffusing capacity per liter alveolar volume.
Adapted with permission of the American Thoracic Society. Copyright © 2017 American Thoracic Society. Originally from American Thoracic Society/European Respiratory Society: Statement on sarcoidosis. Joint Statement of the American Thoracic Society (ATS), the European Respiratory Society (RS) and the World Association of Sarcoidosis and Other Granulomatous Diseases (WASOG) adopted by the ATS Board of Directors and the ERS Executive Committee, February 1999. *Am J Respir Crit Care Med.* 1999;160:736. The *American Journal of Respiratory and Critical Care Medicine* is an official journal of the American Thoracic Society.

exposure to tuberculosis, endemic fungi, and beryllium exposure) should be performed.

LABORATORY TESTING

Recommended tests to evaluate for system disease include pulmonary function tests, complete blood count, comprehensive metabolic panel, urine analysis, electrocardiogram, and tuberculosis testing (QuantiFERON-TB gold tuberculosis assay or tuberculin skin test).

The epithelioid cell of the sarcoidal granuloma secretes angiotensin-converting enzyme.[59] Consequently, serum angiotensin-converting enzyme (SACE) levels reflect the total granuloma burden in sarcoidosis. However, elevated SACE levels are insufficiently specific for the diagnosis of sarcoidosis to rest on it alone, and insufficiently sensitive to exclude the diagnosis.[60] SACE levels are elevated in all granulomatous diseases, including infectious ones. Initial SACE levels are not different between patients who deteriorate and those who improve,[61] so they should not be used to determine treatment. Serial SACE levels may be useful for monitoring the course of sarcoidosis, but this test is not presently routinely used.

IMAGING

A posteroanterior chest radiograph is abnormal in more than 90% of patients with sarcoidosis. Staging of pulmonary radiographs is as follows:

Stage 0: normal
Stage I: bilateral hilar and/or paratracheal adenopathy
Stage II: adenopathy with pulmonary infiltrates
Stage III pulmonary infiltrates only
Stage IV: pulmonary fibrosis

Bilateral hilar adenopathy is noted in 50% to 85% of cases. Pulmonary parenchymal infiltrates are seen in 25% to 60% of cases. Asymptomatic hilar adenopathy on chest radiograph almost always represent sarcoidosis.[62] It has been suggested that histologic confirmation of sarcoidosis may not be required in asymptomatic patients provided the physical examination, complete blood count, and routine blood tests are all normal and there is no prior history of malignancy.[63] Although chest computed tomography reveals more thoracic disease than can be appreciated on chest radiography, there is insufficient evidence that computed tomography has a clinical role in the management of pulmonary sarcoidosis.[64] Characteristic round, punched out, lytic, cystic lesions may be found in radiographs of the hands and feet.

The mechanism of gallium-67 uptake in sarcoidosis is incompletely understood. It is thought that inflammatory processes cause hyperemia and increased capillary permeability of gallium. Gallium also accumulates in macrophages and, to a lesser extent, in T lymphocytes, which are major participants in the granulomatous inflammation of sarcoidosis. Sarcoidosis may cause gallium uptake in thoracic and extrathoracic sites, although typically not in areas of skin involvement. Gallium scanning has not been found useful for monitoring the clinical course of sarcoidosis, but it may have a role in identifying organs with sarcoid involvement. The presence of panda sign (bilateral lacrimal and parotid gland uptake) and lambda sign (bilateral hilar and right paratracheal uptake) on gallium-67 scanning is highly specific for sarcoidosis and may obviate the need for invasive diagnostic procedures. However, these signs are both positive in only a small percentage of sarcoidosis patients. Organ activity has been detected by gadolinium enhancement on nuclear magnetic resonance imaging. Magnetic resonance imaging is useful in detecting neurosarcoidosis and monitoring therapeutic response. Fluorodeoxyglucose positron emission tomography scanning is more sensitive in revealing granulomatous inflammation than gallium-67 scanning and in monitoring response to treatment.[65,66]

PATHOLOGY

The epithelioid granuloma of sarcoidosis usually contains a compact collection of mononuclear phagocytes. The granulomas typically are surrounded by a paucity of lymphocytes ("naked granulomas"), but varying degrees of lymphocytic inflammation may be present (Fig. 35-14). Epithelioid cells, which are themselves transformed monocytes, are commonly present within the sarcoidal granuloma. Multinucleated giant cells of the Langerhans type result from the fusion of epithelioid cells. Although central fibrinoid necrosis is not uncommon, gross necrosis is not a characteristic feature of sarcoid granulomas and suggests

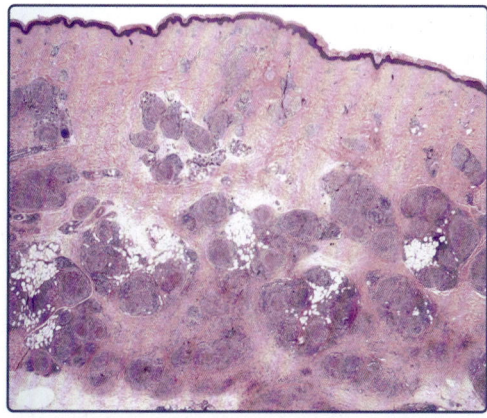

Figure 35-14 Histology of cutaneous sarcoidosis with "naked" granulomas.

an alternative diagnosis, such as tuberculosis, fungal infection, or vasculitis.[59] Mycobacterial and fungal diseases must always be considered as alternative diagnoses; therefore, stains and cultures for mycobacteria and fungi should be routinely performed. Reaction to foreign bodies such as beryllium, tattoo pigment, and paraffin can have similar histologic findings. Although there are often distinguishing features from sarcoidosis, granuloma annulare, necrobiosis lipoidica, rheumatoid nodules, cheilitis granulomatosa, and annular elastolytic giant cell granuloma may have cutaneous granulomas and are in the differential diagnosis. A clinically important aspect of the pathology of sarcoidosis involves the development of fibrosis. Dense bands of fibroblasts may encase the ball-like granulomas. This fibrotic response can produce tissue destruction and organ dysfunction that cannot be successfully reversed with therapy.

DIAGNOSTIC ALGORITHM

Figure 35-15 shows an algorithm for diagnosing whether a patient has sarcoidosis.

DIFFERENTIAL DIAGNOSIS

Granulomatous syphilis, granulomatous cutaneous T-cell lymphoma, annular elastotic giant cell granuloma, fungal infections, Blau syndrome, granuloma annulare, lupus vulgaris, atypical mycobacterial infections, foreign-body reactions (eg, tattoo, soft-tissue fillers, ruptured hair follicles/cyst), rheumatoid nodules, necrobiosis lipoidica, cheilitis granulosa, and granulomatous rosacea are in the differential diagnosis. Histologic findings are very different, but clinically, syndromes with multiple adnexal tumors, amyloidosis of the skin, and cutaneous xanthomas may resemble cutaneous sarcoidosis (Table 35-3).

CLINICAL COURSE AND PROGNOSIS

The granulomatous inflammation of sarcoidosis can remit spontaneously or with therapy. Therefore, the general prognosis of sarcoidosis is good.[57] Pulmonary sarcoidosis resolves, improves, or stabilizes in 60% to 90% of patients without treatment.[67] Remissions often occur within the first 6 months after diagnosis, although it may take 2 to 5 years.[68] The prognosis is generally favorable for liver and peripheral lymph node sarcoidosis as well. Skin lesions may resolve with or without scarring or pigmentary changes.

The development of fibrosis causes almost all significant impairment from sarcoidosis. This is probably the result of hyalinization of granulomatous inflammation. Host response and inadequate treatment may be to blame for the propensity for a brisk fibrotic response. In addition to permanent scarring of the skin from fibrosis, cutaneous lesions may ulcerate or destroy adjacent bone and cartilage. Lupus pernio lesions most commonly leave permanent scarring and destruction.

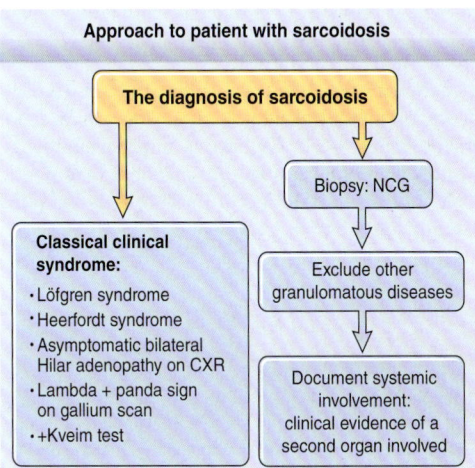

Figure 35-15 Approach to patient with sarcoidosis. Diagnostic algorithm. Usually the diagnosis is made by following the pathway on the right: A tissue biopsy demonstrates noncaseating granulomatous inflammation with a compatible clinical picture, alternative causes of granulomatous inflammation are excluded (including tuberculosis), and there is clinical evidence of systemic (multiorgan) granulomatous inflammation. On occasion, the diagnosis can be assumed without biopsy confirmation if the clinical presentation is very specific for sarcoidosis. These clinical presentations are listed on the left side of the pathway. CXR, chest radiograph; NCG, noncaseating granulomas.

TABLE 35-3
Differential Diagnosis for Cutaneous Sarcoidosis

Histologic and Clinically Similar Conditions
- Deep fungal infections can be granulomatous and clinically resemble sarcoid like blastomycosis, histoplasmosis and others
- Annular elastotic giant cell granuloma
- Granuloma annulare
- Lupus vulgaris
- Atypical mycobacterial infection
- Cheilitis granulosa
- Foreign-body reactions (eg, tattoo, soft-tissue fillers, ruptured hair follicles/cyst)
- Rheumatoid nodules
- Necrobiosis lipoidica
- Granulomatous rosacea
- Cutaneous Crohn disease
- Blau syndrome
- Granulomatous syphilis
- Granulomatous cutaneous T-cell lymphoma
- Melkersson-Rosenthal syndrome

Clinically Similar Conditions Without Similar Histologic Findings
- Amyloidosis of the skin
- Cutaneous xanthomas
- Syndromes with multiple adnexal tumors and/or dermal tumors (eg, Cowden syndrome, Brooke-Spiegler)

In the United States, three-fourths of the sarcoidosis deaths are related to pulmonary involvement. Sarcoidosis of the heart and central nervous system accounts for most of the remaining deaths.[69]

There is no current laboratory tests or radiologic findings that can reliably predict the outcome of sarcoidosis. Skin lesions are not a reliable indicator of prognosis, but several useful associations have been documented. Patients with cutaneous lesions area more likely to have chronic systemic sarcoidosis than patients without skin involvement.[70] Erythema nodosum with fever and arthralgia portends a good prognosis.[71] Patients with Lofgren syndrome have a more than 80% rate of spontaneous remission, generally within 4 to 6 weeks.[2] Lupus pernio indicates chronic disease and is associated with upper respiratory tract involvement, pulmonary fibrosis, and bony cysts.[2] African descent, higher stage chest radiograph (greater than stage I), age older than 40 years, splenic involvement, disease duration longer than 2 years, and forced vital capacity less than 1.5 L are associated with a worse prognosis.[57]

MANAGEMENT

Sarcoidosis often spontaneously remits, and therapy may be associated with significant side effects. Consequently, monitoring patients for development of progressive irreversible damage is a reasonable strategy. Clinicians should treat cutaneous sarcoidosis when the lesions are cosmetically unacceptable for the patient or they are scarring and infiltrative as in lupus pernio. Other appropriate reasons to initiate therapy include pulmonary symptoms, worsening pulmonary function, neurologic involvement, ocular involvement, symptomatic cardiac disease, evidence of hepatic synthetic dysfunction, and splenomegaly.

THERAPY DIRECTED AT THE SKIN

Cutaneous sarcoidosis, including lupus pernio, may be improved with prolonged application (at least 2 weeks) of class I topical steroids such as clobetasol ointment. Intralesional injections of triamcinolone (strength 3 to 10 mg/mL) are more effective. Both therapies can cause skin atrophy and hypopigmentation. Topical tacrolimus may be effective for skin disease and does not pose the same adverse effects, but is not generally as effective.[72,73]

SYSTEMIC CORTICOSTEROIDS

Systemic corticosteroids are the most reliable immediate initial therapy for sarcoidosis. Treatment of cutaneous disease is usually initiated with 40 to 60 mg/day of prednisone equivalent with tapering of therapy over a month to doses of 10 to 20 mg/day. The recommended initial dose of pulmonary sarcoidosis is 20 to 40 mg of prednisone equivalent/day.[74] Cardiac and neurologic sarcoidosis may require higher initial doses, up to 60 to 80 mg of prednisone equivalent/day.[74] The corticosteroid dosage typically is tapered 0.1 to 0.2 mg/kg over a few months.[74] It is unusual for pulmonary disease to require a maintenance dose of more than 15 mg of prednisone equivalent/day, but cutaneous, cardiac, and neurologic disease may require higher doses. An attempt should be made to taper the dose within 9 to 12 months of the initiation of therapy.[74] Life-threatening arrhythmias are an exception to this rule, and placement of an internal defibrillators may be indicated.[75-77]

If patients cannot be successfully weaned from corticosteroids, a variety of immunosuppressive medications can be used as steroid-sparing agents. Most immunosuppressive are inadequate as monotherapy. Table 35-4 lists the appropriate doses for treatment of sarcoidosis.

METHOTREXATE

Methotrexate is the most studied steroid-sparing agent. The drug requires careful monitoring of liver function tests and blood cell counts. Folic acid can be given in conjunction with methotrexate to alleviate side effects. Patients with sarcoidosis may develop cirrhosis, even if their liver function tests are normal. Liver biopsies should be considered in patients after 1 to 2 g of total therapy. Typical doses of methotrexate for cutaneous disease are 10 to 25 mg/week. Cutaneous improvement may be noted within 1 month, but maximal therapeutic benefit often does not occur until at least 6 months after the initiation of treatment.

ANTIMALARIALS HYDROXYCHLOROQUINE/CHLOROQUINE

Antimalarial drugs are useful for sarcoidosis affecting the joints and skin, and hypercalcemia.[78,79] Antimalarial agents area not highly effective for pulmonary disease, and often take several months to be effective. Chloroquine has a higher potential of causing retinal damage than hydroxychloroquine, but patients taking either drug must have regular ophthalmologic exams. Hemolytic anemia may occur and patients with glucose-6 phosphate dehydrogenase deficiency may have a higher rate of anemia, but with usual dermatologic doses the deficiency is not an absolute contraindication for usage of hydroxychloroquine.

TABLE 35-4
Sarcoid Medical Therapy

AGENT	DOSE/COMMENT
Topical steroids and intralesional steroids	Localized skin lesions Class I ultrapotent steroids (eg, clobetasol 0.05% ointment) BID for 2-4 weeks then BIW Intralesional triamcinolone 2.5-10.0 mg/mL
Topical tacrolimus	Tacrolimus 0.1% ointment BID Localized skin lesions
Systemic corticosteroids	Prednisone (or equivalent) 20-40 mg/day then taper Consider higher doses for cardiac, neurologic involvement
Methotrexate	10-25 mg/week Monitor complete blood count, liver function tests >1.5 g cumulative dose consider liver biopsy or procollagen III peptide testing Consider adjunctive folate 1 mg/day
Hydroxychloroquine	200-400 mg/day Yearly ophthalmologic screening
Chloroquine	250-1000 mg/day Yearly ophthalmologic screening
Tetracycline	Minocycline 200 mg/day Doxycycline 200 mg/day Primarily for nonlupus pernio skin disease
Broad-spectrum antibiotics	CLEAR (combined levofloxacin, 500 mg/day; ethambutol, 25 mg/kg/day up to 1200 mg; azithromycin, 250 mg/day; and rifampin, 10 mg/kg/day or up to 300 mg/day) for 8 weeks
Infliximab	5 mg/kg IV q6weeks Screening/monitoring for tuberculosis Consider adjunctive low-dose methotrexate to prevent antidrug antibody formation
Adalimumab	40 mg weekly beginning at week 4 following a 160-mg dose at week 0 and an 80-mg dose at week 2
Pentoxifylline	400 mg TID
Leflunomide	100 mg/day for 3 days loading, then 10 mg/day; can increase to 20 mg/day; monitor complete blood count and liver function tests
Thalidomide	50-200 mg/day QHS dosing as sedating Peripheral neuropathy common monitoring necessary
Melatonin	20 mg/day for 1 year then 10 mg/day for 1 year QHS dosing
Cyclophosphamide	500-1000 mg IV q3-4weeks; monitor complete blood count and urinalysis; stop if hematuria develops Reserved for life-threatening disease because of carcinogenicity

CYCLOPHOSPHAMIDE

Cyclophosphamide is effective for many forms of sarcoidosis. However, because of its significant side-effect profile, including carcinogenic potential, cyclophosphamide is reserved for severe or potentially life-threatening disease.

ANTIBIOTICS

Minocycline and doxycycline (doses of 100 mg twice daily) have been reported to improve skin sarcoidosis in case series. These drugs may take up to 2 years to be effective.[80] Tetracyclines modify the immune response by suppressing activity of macrophages and T lymphocytes.[81] Several months of the CLEAR (combined levofloxacin, 500 mg/day; ethambutol, 25 mg/kg/day up to 1200 mg; azithromycin, 250 mg/day; and rifampin, 10 mg/kg/day or up to 300 mg/day) regimen has also shown some effectiveness, and clinical trials are currently ongoing to better assess the usefulness of this regimen.[82]

TUMOR NECROSIS FACTOR ANTAGONISTS

TNF is a cytokine that is secreted in macrophages associated with sarcoidal granulomas.[18] Antagonists of TNF have been shown to be useful for the treatment of sarcoidosis. Pentoxifylline,[83] thalidomide,[84] infliximab,[85] and adalumimab[85] are the most studied. Infliximab appears to be particularly useful for the treatment of lupus pernio,[86] and it may be superior to the other TNF antagonists, as a study of etanercept failed to show benefit for sarcoidal uveitis.[87] Paradoxically, administration of these drugs for other conditions has been rarely associated with the development of sarcoidosis.[88]

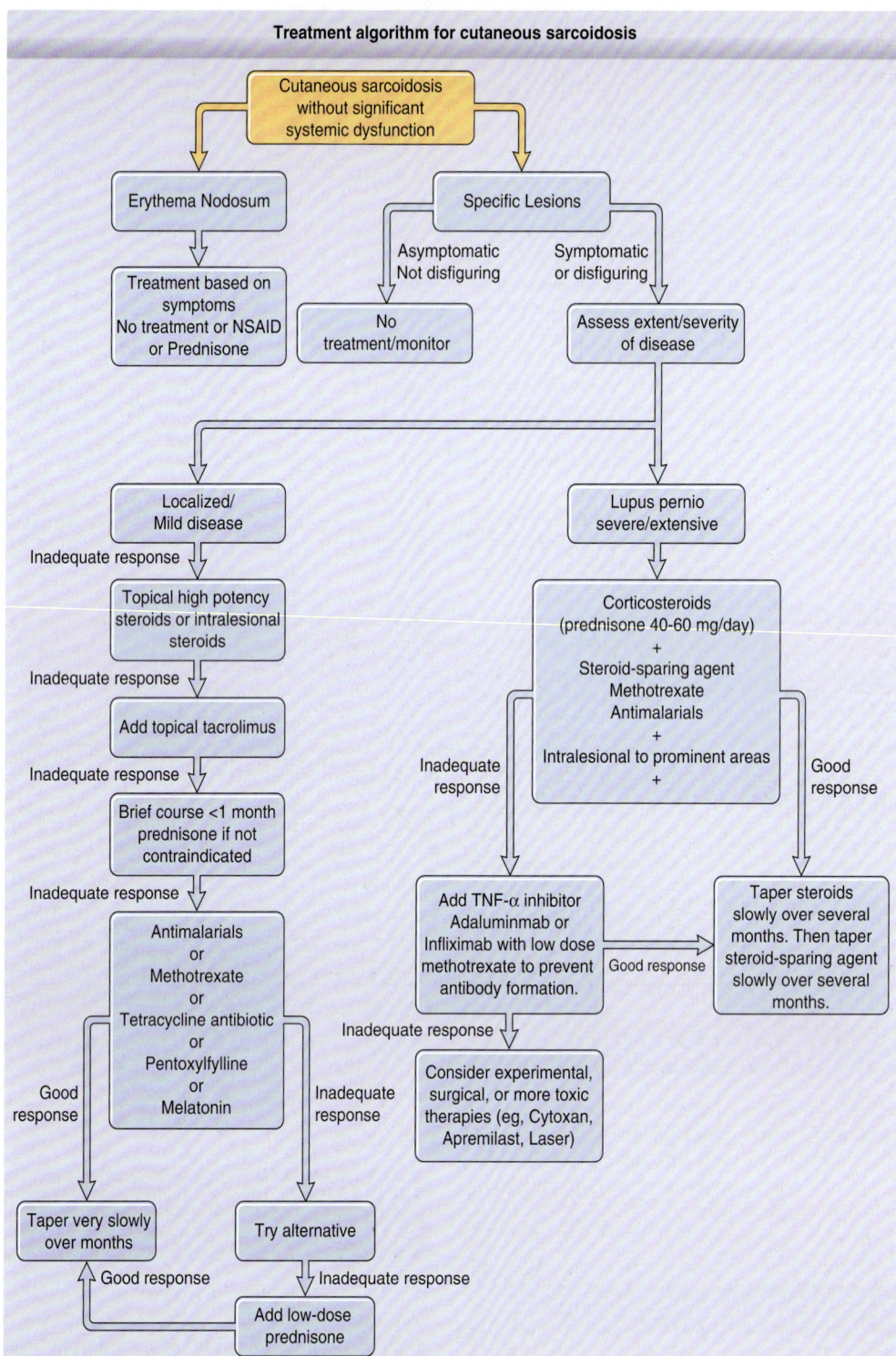

Figure 35-16 Treatment algorithm for cutaneous sarcoidosis.

OTHER AGENTS

Azothioprine,[89] mycophenolate mofetil,[90] leflunomide,[91] and cyclosporine[92] have been reported to be useful for the treatment of systemic sarcoidosis in small case series. Melatonin,[93] allopurinol,[94] isotretinoin,[95] and fumaric acid esters[96] have been reported to be effective for cutaneous sarcoidosis.

PROCEDURES

Phototherapy and photodynamic therapy have been used to mitigate cutaneous sarcoidosis.[97] Electrodessication, pulse-dye laser, carbon dioxide laser therapy, and reconstructive surgical procedures have all been used successfully to improve the cosmetic disfigurement of cutaneous disease.

TREATMENT ALGORITHM

Figure 35-16 presents a treatment algorithm for cutaneous sarcoidosis.

PREVENTION/SCREENING

Prevention and screening for this elusive disease are not currently practical or available.

ACKNOWLEDGMENTS

Thanks to Marc Judson, MD for his continued guidance in all things related to sarcoidosis.

REFERENCES

1. Boeck C. Multiple benign sarcoid of the skin. *J Cutan Genitourinary Dis.* 1899;17:543.
2. American Thoracic Society/European Respiratory Society: Statement on sarcoidosis. Joint Statement of the American Thoracic Society (ATS), the European Respiratory Society (RS) and the World Association of Sarcoidosis and Other Granulomatous Diseases (WASOG) adopted by the ATS Board of Directors and the ERS Executive Committee, February 1999. *Am J Respir Crit Care Med.* 1999;160:736.
3. Rybicki BA, Major M, Popovich J Jr, et al. Racial differences in sarcoidosis incidence: a 5-year study in a health maintenance organization. *Am J Epidemiol.* 1997;145(3):234-241.
4. Baughman RP, Field S, Costabel U, et al. Sarcoidosis in America. Analysis based on health care use. *Ann Am Thorac Soc.* 2016;13(8):1244-1252.
5. Baughman RP, Teirstein AS, Judson MA, et al; Case Control Etiologic Study of Sarcoidosis (ACCESS) research group. Clinical characteristics of patients in a case control study of sarcoidosis. *Am J Respir Crit Care Med.* 2001;164(10, pt 1):1885-1889.
6. Gottlieb JE, Israel HL, Steiner RM, et al. Outcome in sarcoidosis: the relationship of relapse to corticosteroid therapy. *Chest.* 1997;111(3):623-631.
7. Westney GE, Judson MA. Racial and ethnic disparities in sarcoidosis: from genetics to socioeconomics. *Clin Chest Med.* 2006;27:453.
8. Judson MA, Baughman RP, Thompson BW, et al; ACCESS Research Group. Two year prognosis of sarcoidosis: the ACCESS experience. *Sarcoidosis Vasc Diffuse Lung Dis.* 2003;20(3):204-211.
9. Ramadan S, Hossam D, Saleh MA. Dermoscopy could be useful in differentiating sarcoidosis from necrobiotic granulomas even after treatment with systemic steroids. *Dermatol Pract Concept.* 2016;6(3):17-22.
10. Spiteri MA, Matthey F, Gordon T, et al. Lupus pernio: a clinico-radiological study of thirty-five cases. *Br J Dermatol.* 1985;112(3):315-322.
11. Ando M, Miyazaki E, Hatano Y, et al. Subcutaneous sarcoidosis: a clinical analysis of nine patients. *Clin Rheumatol.* 2016;35(9):2277-2281.
12. Cather JC, Cohen PR. Ichthyosiform sarcoidosis. *J Am Acad Dermatol.* 1999;40(5, pt 2):862-865.
13. Greer KE, Harman LE Jr, Kayne AL. Unusual cutaneous manifestations of sarcoidosis. *South Med J.* 1977;70(6):666-668.
14. Albertini JG, Tyler W, Miller OF 3rd. Ulcerative sarcoidosis case report and review of the literature. *Arch Dermatol.* 1997;133(2):215-219.
15. Burov EA, Kantor GR, Isaac M. Morpheaform sarcoidosis: report of three cases. *J Am Acad Dermatol.* 1998;39(2, pt 2):345-348.
16. Okamoto H, Horio T, Izumi T. Micropapular sarcoidosis simulating lichen nitidus. *Dermatologica.* 1985;170(5):253-255.
17. Elgart ML. Cutaneous sarcoidosis: definitions and types of lesions. *Clin Dermatol.* 1986;4:35.
18. Vega ML, Abrahams J, Keller M. Psoriasiform sarcoidosis: collision of two entities or expression of one common pathogenesis? *J Clin Aesthet Dermatol.* 2016;9(4) 55-57.
19. Altomare GF, Capella GL, Frigerio E. Sarcoidosis presenting as erythema annulare centrifugum. *Clin Exp Dermatol.* 1995;20(6):502-503.
20. McLaughlin SS, Linquist AM, Burnett JW. Cutaneous sarcoidosis of the scrotum: A rare manifestation of systemic disease. *Acta Derm Venereol.* 2002;82(3):216-217.
21. Klein PA, Appel J, Callen JP. Sarcoidosis of the vulva: a rare cutaneous manifestation. *J Am Acad Dermatol.* 1998;39(2, pt 1):281-283.
22. Cliff S, Hart Y, Knowles G, et al. Sarcoidosis presenting as palmar erythema. *Clin Exp Dermatol.* 1998;23(3):123-124.
23. Harman KE, Setterfield JF, Shirlaw PJ, et al. Clinicopathological case 1: mucous membrane pemphigoid, epidermolysis bullosa acquisita and linear immunoglobulin A disease. *Clin Exp Dermatol.* 2003;28(4):461-462.
24. Ramanan AV, Denning DW, Baildam EM. Cutaneous childhood sarcoidosis—a rare disease refractory to treatment. *Rheumatology (Oxford).* 2003;42(12):1570-1571.
25. Dadban A, Hirschi S, Sanchez M, et al. Association of Sweet's syndrome and acute sarcoidosis: report of a

case and review of the literature. *Clin Exp Dermatol.* 2008;34(2):189-191.
26. Callen JP. Sarcoidosis. In: Callen JP, Jorizzo JL, Bolognia J, et al, eds. *Dermatological Signs of Internal Disease*, 3rd ed. Barcelona Spain: Saunders Elsevier Science; 2003:257.
27. Beacham BE, Schuldenfrei J, Julka SS. Sarcoidosis presenting with erythema multiforme-like cutaneous lesions. *Cutis.* 1994;33(5):461-463.
28. Carswell WA. A case of sarcoidosis presenting with erythema multiforme. *Am Rev Respir Dis.* 1972;106:462.
29. Kumar S. Bilateral ankle edema with bilateral iritis. *Clin Rheumatol.* 2006;26(7):1145-1147.
30. Tomada F, Oda Y, Takata M, et al. A rare case of sarcoidosis with bilateral leg lymphedema as an initial symptom. *Am J Med Sci.* 1999;318(6):413-414.
31. Ohara K, Judson MA, Baughman RP, et al. Clinical aspects of ocular sarcoidosis. *Eur Respir J Monogr.* 2005;10:188.
32. Liu D, Birnbaum AD. Update on sarcoidosis. *Curr Opin Ophthalmol.* 2015;26(6):512-516.
33. Silverman KJ, Hutchins GM, Bulkley BH. Cardiac sarcoid: a clinicopathologic study of 84 unselected patients with systemic sarcoidosis. *Circulation.* 1978;58(6): 1204-1211.
34. Birnie DH, Nery PB, Ha AC, et al. Cardiac sarcoidosis. *J Am Coll Cardiol.* 2016;68(4):411-421.
35. Hebel R, Dubaniewicz-Wybieralska M, Dubaniewicz A. Overview of neurosarcoidosis: recent advances. *J Neurol.* 2015;262(2):258-267.
36. Singer FR. Abnormal calcium homeostasis in sarcoidosis. *N Engl J Med.* 1986;315:755.
37. Vatti R, Sharma OP. Course of asymptomatic liver involvement in sarcoidosis: the role of therapy in selected cases. *Sarcoidosis Vasc Diffuse Lung Dis.* 1997;14(1):73-76.
38. Devaney K, Goodman ZD, Epstein MS, et al. Hepatic sarcoidosis: clinicopathologic features in 100 patients. *Am J Surg Pathol.* 1993;17(12):1272-1280.
39. Sharma OP. Sarcoidosis of the upper respiratory tract: selected cases emphasizing diagnostic and therapeutic difficulties. *Sarcoidosis Vasc Diffuse Lung Dis.* 2002;19:227.
40. Costabel U. Sarcoidosis: clinical update. *Eur Respir J.* 2001;18(suppl 32):56s.
41. Newman LS, Rose CS, Maier LA. Sarcoidosis. *N Engl J Med.* 1997;336(17):1224-1234.
42. Chiarchiaro J, Chen BB, Gibson KF. New molecular targets for the treatment of sarcoidosis. *Curr Opin Pulm Med.* 2016;22(5):515-521.
43. Saboor SA, Johnson NM, McFadden J. Detection of mycobacterial DNA in sarcoidosis and tuberculosis with polymerase chain reaction. *Lancet.* 1992; 339(8800):1012-1015.
44. Ishige I, Usui Y, Takemura T, et al. Quantitative PCR of mycobacterial and propionibacterial DNA in lymph nodes of Japanese patients with sarcoidosis. *Lancet.* 1999;354(9173):120-123.
45. Gaede KI, Wilke G, Brade L, et al. Anti-Chlamydophila immunoglobulin prevalence in sarcoidosis and usual interstitial pneumoniae. *Eur Respir J.* 2002; 19(2):267-274.
46. Rybicki BA, Amend KL, Maliarik MJ, et al. Photocopier exposure and risk of sarcoidosis in African-American sibs. *Sarcoidosis Vasc Diffuse Lung Dis.* 2004;21(1): 49-55.
47. Kucera GP, Rybicki BA, Kirkey KL, et al. Occupational risk factors for sarcoidosis in African-American siblings. *Chest.* 2003;123(5):1527-1535.
48. Kajdasz DK, Lackland DT, Mohr LC, et al. A current assessment of various rurally-linked exposures as potential risk factors for sarcoidosis. *Ann Epidemiol.* 2001;11(2):111-117.
49. Presant DJ, Dhala A, Goldstein A, et al. The incidence, prevalence, and severity of sarcoidosis in New York City firefighters. *Chest.* 1999;116(5):1183-1193.
50. Newman LS, Rose CS, Bresnitz EA, et al. A case control etiologic study of sarcoidosis: Environmental and occupational risk factors. *Am J Respir Crit Care Med.* 2004;170(12):1324-1330.
51. Rybicki BA, Iannuzzi MC, Frederick MM, et al. Familial aggregation of sarcoidosis. A case-control etiologic study of sarcoidosis (ACCESS). *Am J Respir Crit Care Med.* 2001;164(11):2085-2091.
52. Gialafos E, Triposkiadis F, Kouranos V, et al. Relationship between tumor necrosis factor-α (TNFA) gene polymorphisms and cardiac sarcoidosis. *In Vivo.* 2014;28(6):1125-1129.
53. Thompson IA, Liu B, Sen HN, et al. Association of complement factor H tyrosine 402 histidine genotype with posterior involvement in sarcoid-related uveitis. *Am J Ophthalmol.* 2013;155(6):1068-1074.
54. McDougal KE, Fallin MD, Moller DR, et al; ACCESS Research Group. Variation in the lymphotoxin-alpha/ tumor necrosis factor locus modifies risk of erythema nodosum in sarcoidosis. *J Invest Dermatol.* 2009;129(8): 1921-1926.
55. Kim HS, Choi D, Lim LL, et al. Association of interleukin 23 receptor gene with sarcoidosis. *Dis Markers.* 2011;31(1):17-24.
56. Judson MA. The diagnosis of sarcoidosis. *Clin Chest Med.* 2008;29:415-427.
57. Judson MA, Baughman RP. Sarcoidosis. In: Baughman RP, DuBois RM, Lynch JP, eds. *Diffuse Lung Disease, A Practical Approach*. London, UK: Arnold Publishers; 2004:109.
58. Judson MA, Baughman RP, Teirstein AS, et al. Defining organ involvement in sarcoidosis: the ACCESS proposed instrument. ACCESS Research Group. A Case Control Etiologic Study of Sarcoidosis. *Sarcoidosis Vasc Diffuse Lung Dis.* 1999;16(1):75-86.
59. Sheffield EA. Pathology of sarcoidosis. *Clin Chest Med.* 1997;18:741.
60. Studdy PR, James DG. The specificity and sensitivity of serum angiotensin-converting enzyme in sarcoidosis and other diseases: experiences in 12 centers in six different countries. In: Chertien J, Marsac J, Saltiel JC, eds. *Sarcoidosis*. Paris, France: Pergamon Press; 1983:332.
61. Finkel R, Teirstein AS, Levine R, et al. Pulmonary function tests, serum angiotensin-converting enzyme levels, and clinical findings as prognostic indicators in sarcoidosis. *Ann N Y Acad Sci.* 1986;465:665-671.
62. Winterbauer RH, Belic N, Moores KD. A clinical interpretation of bilateral hilar adenopathy. *Ann Intern Med.* 1973;78(1):65-71.
63. Lynch JP 3rd, Kazerooni EA, Gay SE. Pulmonary sarcoidosis. *Clin Chest Med.* 1997;18(4):755-785.
64. Maña J, Teirstein AS, Mendelson DS, et al. Excessive thoracic computed tomographic scanning in sarcoidosis. *Thorax.* 1995;50(12):1264-1266.
65. Teirstein AS, Machac J, Almeida O, et al. Results of 188 whole-body fluorodeoxyglucose positron emission tomography scans in 137 patients with sarcoidosis. *Chest.* 2007;132(6):1949-1953.
66. Tavee JO, Stern BJ. Neurosarcoidosis. *Clin Chest Med.* 2015;36 (4):643-656.

67. Sones M, Israel HL. Course and prognosis of sarcoidosis. *Am J Med*. 1960;29:84-93.
68. Mañá J, Salazar A, Manresa F. Clinical factors predicting persistence of activity in sarcoidosis: A multivariate analysis of 193 cases. *Respiration*. 1994;61(4):219-225.
69. Huang CT, Heurich AE, Sutton AL, et al. Mortality in sarcoidosis: a changing pattern of the causes of death. *Eur J Respir Dis*. 1981;62(4):231-238.
70. Yanardağ H, Pamuk ON, Karayel T. Cutaneous involvement in sarcoidosis: analysis of the features in 170 patients. *Respir Med*. 2003;97(8):978-982.
71. Neville E, Walker AN, James DG. Prognostic factors predicting the outcome of sarcoidosis: an analysis of 818 patients. *Q J Med*. 1983;52(208):525-533.
72. Gutzmer R, Völker B, Kapp A, et al. Successful topical treatment of cutaneous sarcoidosis with tacrolimus [in German]. *Hautarzt*. 2003;54(12):1193-1197.
73. Katoh N, Mihara H, Yasuno H. Cutaneous sarcoidosis successfully treated with topical tacrolimus. *Br J Dermatol*. 2002;147(1):154-156.
74. Judson MA. Corticosteroids in sarcoidosis. *Rheum Dis Clin North Am*. 2016;42(1):119-135.
75. Yazaki Y, Isobe M, Hiroe M, et al; Central Japan Heart Study Group. Prognostic determinants of long-term survival in Japanese patients with cardiac sarcoidosis treated with prednisone. *Am J Cardiol*. 2001;88(9):1006-1010.
76. Mezaki T, Chinushi M, Washizuka T, et al. Discrepancy between inducibility of ventricular tachycardia and activity of cardiac sarcoidosis—requirement of defibrillator implantation for the inactive stage of cardiac sarcoidosis. *Intern Med*. 2001;40(8):731-735.
77. Smedema J, Snoep G, van Kroonenburgh MP, et al. Cardiac involvement in patients with pulmonary sarcoidosis assessed at two university medical centers in the Netherlands. *Chest*. 2005;128(1):30-35.
78. Siltzbach LE, Teirstein AS. Chloroquine therapy in 43 patients with intrathoracic and cutaneous sarcoidosis. *Acta Med Scand Suppl*. 1964;425:302-308.
79. Adams JS, Diz MM, Sharma OP. Effective reduction in the 1,25-dihydroxyvitamin D and calcium concentration in sarcoidosis-associated hypercalcemia with short-course chloroquine therapy. *Ann Intern Med*. 1989;111(5):437-438.
80. Bachelez H, Senet P, Cadranel J, et al. The use of tetracyclines for the treatment of sarcoidosis. *Arch Dermatol*. 2001;137(1):69-73.
81. Thong YH, Ferrante A. Effect of tetracycline treatment on immunological responses in mice. *Clin Exp Immunol*. 1980;39(3):728-732.
82. Drake WP, Richmond BW, Oswald-Richter K, et al. Effects of broad-spectrum antimycobacterial therapy on chronic pulmonary sarcoidosis. *Sarcoidosis Vasc Diffuse Lung Dis*. 2013;30(3):201-211.
83. Zabel P, Entzian P, Dalhoff K, et al. Pentoxifylline in treatment of sarcoidosis. *Am J Respir Crit Care Med*. 1997;155(5):1665-1669.
84. Baughman RP, Judson MA, Teirstein AS, et al. Thalidomide for chronic sarcoidosis. *Chest*. 2002;122(1):227-232.
85. Saketkoo LA, Baughman RP. Biologic therapies in the treatment of sarcoidosis. *Expert Rev Clin Immunol*. 2016;12(8):817-825.
86. Stagaki E, Mountford WK, Lackland DT, et al. The treatment of lupus pernio: the results of 116 treatment courses in 54 patients. *Chest*. 2009;135(2):468-476.
87. Baughman RP, Lower EE, Bradley DA, et al. Etanercept for refractory ocular sarcoidosis: Results of a double-blind randomized trial. *Chest*. 2005;128(2):1062.
88. Toussirot E, Aubin F. Paradoxical reactions under TNF-α blocking agents and other biologic agents given for chronic immune-mediate diseases: an analytical and comprehensive overview. *RMD Open*. 2016;2(2):e000239.
89. Lewis SJ, Ainslie GM, Bateman ED. Efficacy of azathioprine as second-line treatment in pulmonary sarcoidosis. *Sarcoidosis Vasc Diffuse Lung Dis*. 1999;16(1):87-92.
90. Kouba DJ, Mimouni D, Rencic A, et al. Mycophenolate mofetil may serve as a steroid-sparing agent for sarcoidosis. *Br J Dermatol*. 2003;148(1):147-148.
91. Baughman RP, Lower EE. Leflunomide for chronic sarcoidosis. *Sarcoidosis Vasc Diffuse Lung Dis*. 2004;21(1):43-48.
92. Stern BJ, Schonfeld SA, Sewell C, et al. The treatment of neurosarcoidosis with cyclosporine. *Arch Neurol*. 1992;49(10):1065-1072.
93. Pignone AM, Rosso AD, Fiori G, et al. Melatonin is a safe and effective treatment for chronic pulmonary and extrapulmonary sarcoidosis. *J Pineal Res*. 2006;41(2) 95-100.
94. Voelter-Mahlknecht S, Benez A, Metzger S, et al. Treatment of subcutaneous sarcoidosis with allopurinol. *Arch Dermatol*. 1999;135(12):1560-1561.
95. Georgiou S, Monastirli A, Pasmatzi E, et al. Cutaneous sarcoidosis: complete remission after oral isotretinoin therapy. *Acta Derm Venereol*. 1998;78(6):457-459.
96. Breuer K, Gutzmer R, Völker B, et al. Therapy of noninfectious granulomatous skin diseases with fumaric acid esters. *Br J Dermatol*. 2005;152(6):1290-1295.
97. Karrer S, Abels C, Wimmershoff MB, et al. Successful treatment of cutaneous sarcoidosis using topical photodynamic therapy. *Arch Dermatol*. 2002;138(5):581-584.

Neutrophilic, Eosinophilic, and Mast Cell Disorders

第六篇　中性粒细胞、嗜酸性粒细胞、肥大细胞相关性疾病

PART 6

Chapter 36 :: Sweet Syndrome
:: Philip R. Cohen & Razelle Kurzrock

第三十六章
Sweet综合征

中文导读

本章从疾病的历史及流行病学史、临床表现、病因及发病机制、诊断及治疗七个方面全面讲述了Sweet综合征。在临床表现上，本文除了介绍该病的常见表现外，还介绍了几种特殊表现。在诊断上，本章先从Sweet综合症等一些临床特点出发，分析了其诊断标准的建立和修订历程。在治疗上，本章认为Sweet综合征的一线治疗还是药物治疗，通过表格列出了一线和二线治疗的主要药物以及使用剂量。

〔李芳芳〕

AT-A-GLANCE

- Sweet syndrome, also referred to as acute febrile neutrophilic dermatosis, is characterized by a constellation of symptoms and findings: the acute onset of fever, neutrophilia, tender erythematous skin lesions that typically show mature neutrophils in the upper dermis, and—after initiation of systemic corticosteroids—a prompt improvement of both symptoms and lesions.

- Extracutaneous manifestations of Sweet syndrome can include cardiovascular, central nervous system, gastrointestinal, hepatic, musculoskeletal, ocular, oral, otic, pulmonary, renal, and splenic organs.

- Infection of the upper respiratory tract and/or gastrointestinal tract, inflammatory bowel disease, and pregnancy may be associated with classical Sweet syndrome.

- In individuals with previously undiagnosed or relapsing hematologic malignancies and solid tumors, malignancy-associated Sweet syndrome may occur as a cutaneous paraneoplastic syndrome.

- The onset of the dermatosis in patients following the initiation of certain medications—drug-induced Sweet syndrome—is most commonly associated with granulocyte colony-stimulating factor.

- The pathogenesis of Sweet syndrome remains to be established; cytokines—directly or indirectly—may have an important etiologic role.

- Corticosteroids, potassium iodide, and colchicine are the first-line oral systemic agents for treating Sweet syndrome.

- Indomethacin, clofazimine, cyclosporine, and dapsone are the second-line oral systemic agents for treating Sweet syndrome.

- Localized Sweet syndrome lesions may be effectively treated with the topical application of high-potency corticosteroids or intralesional corticosteroids.

DEFINITION

Sweet syndrome (also known as acute febrile neutrophilic dermatosis) is typically characterized by the acute onset of pyrexia and painful cutaneous lesions that are composed of a dense dermal inflammatory infiltrate of mature neutrophils. Neutrophilia is also frequently present. Both the condition-associated symptoms and the dermatosis-related lesions promptly resolve after initiation of treatment with systemic corticosteroids.[1]

HISTORICAL PERSPECTIVE

Dr. Robert Douglas Sweet, originally described acute febrile neutrophilic dermatosis in the August–September 1964 issue of the *British Journal of Dermatology*. He summarized the cardinal features of "a distinctive and fairly severe illness" that had been encountered in 8 women during the 15-year period from 1949 to 1964. In Dr. Sweet's department, the condition was originally referred to as the Gomm-Button disease "in eponymous honor of the first two patients" with the disease. Subsequently, this acute febrile neutrophilic dermatosis has become best known by the eponym "Sweet syndrome."[1-3]

EPIDEMIOLOGY

Numerous individuals with Sweet syndrome have been reported. There is no racial predilection and the distribution of Sweet syndrome cases is worldwide.[1] The dermatosis may present in various clinical settings: classical, malignancy-associated, and drug-induced (Tables 36-1 and 36-2).[4-7]

CLINICAL FEATURES

HISTORY

Patients with Sweet syndrome may appear dramatically ill. Fever and leukocytosis often accompany the skin eruption. However, the skin disease can be concurrently present with the fever for the entire episode of the dermatosis or follow the fever by several days to weeks. Other Sweet syndrome associated symptoms include arthralgia, general malaise, headache, and myalgia (Table 36-3).[1]

CUTANEOUS FINDINGS

LESION MORPHOLOGY

Sweet syndrome cutaneous lesions typically appear as tender, red or purple-red, papules or nodules. The skin eruption can present as either a single lesion or multiple—often asymmetrically distributed—lesions (Fig. 36-1). The transparent, vesicle-like appearance of the lesions, described as an "illusion of vesiculation," results from the pronounced edema in the upper dermis (Fig. 36-2). Central clearing may result in annular or arcuate patterns in the later stages; indeed, these lesions can appear targetoid. In patients with malignancy-associated Sweet syndrome, the lesions may appear bullous, become ulcerated, and/or mimic the morphologic features of pyoderma gangrenosum. Over a period of days to weeks, the lesions enlarge; subsequently, they may coalesce and form irregular sharply bordered plaques (Fig. 36-3). The lesions usually resolve without scarring—either spontaneously or after treatment. In one-third to two-thirds of patients, the lesions are associated with recurrent episodes of Sweet syndrome.[1]

TABLE 36-1
Diagnostic Criteria for Classical Sweet Syndrome versus Drug-Induced Sweet Syndrome

CLASSICAL[a]	DRUG-INDUCED[b]
(1) Abrupt onset of painful erythematous plaques or nodules	(A) Abrupt onset of painful erythematous plaques or nodules
(2) Histopathologic evidence of a dense neutrophilic infiltrate without evidence of leukocytoclastic vasculitis	(B) Histopathologic evidence of a dense neutrophilic infiltrate without evidence of leukocytoclastic vasculitis
(3) Pyrexia >38°C (100.4°F)	(C) Pyrexia >38°C (100.4°F)
(4) Association with an underlying hematologic (most commonly acute myelogenous leukemia) or visceral malignancy (most commonly carcinomas of the genitourinary organs, breast, and gastrointestinal tract), inflammatory disease (Crohn disease and ulcerative colitis), or pregnancy, *or* preceded by an upper respiratory (streptococcosis) or gastrointestinal (salmonellosis and yersiniosis) infection or vaccination	(D) Temporal relationship between drug ingestion and clinical presentation, *or* temporally related recurrence after oral challenge
(5) Excellent response to treatment with systemic corticosteroids or potassium iodide	(E) Temporally related resolution of lesions after drug withdrawal or treatment with systemic corticosteroids
(6) Abnormal laboratory values at presentation (3 of 4): erythrocyte sedimentation rate >20 mm/h; positive C-reactive protein; >8000/μL leukocytes; >70% neutrophils	

[a]The presence of both major criteria (1 and 2), and 2 of the 4 minor criteria (3, 4, 5, and 6) is required to establish the diagnosis of classical Sweet syndrome; the patients with malignancy-associated Sweet syndrome are included with the patients with classical Sweet syndrome in this list of diagnostic criteria.
[b]All 5 criteria (A, B, C, D, and E) are required for the diagnosis of drug-induced Sweet syndrome.
Adapted with permission from Walker DC, Cohen PR: Trimethoprim-sulfamethoxazole-associated acute febrile neutrophilic dermatosis: case report and review of drug induced Sweet's syndrome. *J Am Acad Dermatol*. 1996;34:918-923. Copyright 1996, American Academy of Dermatology, Inc., Mosby-Year Book, Inc., St. Louis, MO.

TABLE 36-2
Medications Associated with Drug-Induced Sweet Syndrome

Abacavir	Interleukin-2
Abatacept	Ipilimumab
Aceclofenac	Isotretinoin
Acyclovir	Ketoconazole
Adalimumab	Lamivudine
All-*trans*-retinoic acid	Lenalidomide
Amoxicillin	Levonorgestrel/ethinyl estradiol (Triphasil)
Amoxapine	Levonorgestrel-releasing intrauterine system (Mirena)
Azacitidine	Lithium
Azathioprine	Lopinavir
Benzylthiouracil	Minocycline
Bortezomib	Mitoxantrone
Carbamazepine	Nitrofurantoin
Celecoxib	Norfloxacin
Chloroquine	Ofloxacin
Ciprofloxacin	Omeprazole
13-*Cis* retinoic acid	Orphenadrine citrate
Citalopram	Pegfilgrastim
Clindamycin	Perphenazine
Clozapine	Phenylbutazone
Contraceptives	Piperacillin/tazobactam
Cyclooxygenase-2 inhibitor	Propylthiouracil
Diazepam	Quinupristin/dalfopristin
Diclofenac	Radiocontrast agent
Doxycycline	Riboflavin
Efavirenz	Ritonavir
Erythropoietin	Ruxolitinib
Esomeprazole	Stavudine
Etanercept	Sulfa
Furosemide	Sulfasalazine
Granulocyte colony-stimulating factor	Ticagrelor
Granulocyte-macrophage colony-stimulating factor	Topotecan
Hydralazine	Trimethoprim-sulfamethoxazole
Imatinib mesylate	Triphasil
Infliximab	Vemurafenib
Interferon alpha (pegylated)	Vorinostat
Interferon beta-1b	

CUTANEOUS PATHERGY AND ISOTOPIC RESPONSE

A dermatosis-associated feature of Sweet syndrome is cutaneous pathergy. This form of skin hypersensitivity occurs when Sweet syndrome skin lesions appear at sites of cutaneous trauma such as prior biopsies, injections, intravenous catheter placement, scalding, and venipuncture. They also include sites of insect bites and cat scratches, areas that have received radiation therapy, and places that have been contacted by sensitizing antigens or henna tattoo.[1,7,8]

The dermatologic eponym "Wolf's isotopic response" describes the occurrence of a new skin disorder at the site of another unrelated and already healed skin disease. Sweet syndrome has presented in this manner: lesions affecting a lymphedematous leg or postmastectomy arm and a bullous variant of Sweet syndrome on the side of the cheek and neck where a herpes zoster infection previously occurred in a 75-year-old man.[9-11]

In addition, lesions have been photodistributed or localized to the site of a prior phototoxic reaction (sunburn) in some Sweet syndrome patients.[12]

TABLE 36-3
Clinical Features in Patients with Sweet Syndrome

	CLINICAL FORM			
CHARACTERISTIC	CLASSICAL (%)[a]	HEMATOLOGIC MALIGNANCY (%)[a]	SOLID TUMOR (%)[a]	DRUG-INDUCED (%)[b]
Epidemiology				
Women	80	50	59	71
Prior upper respiratory tract infection	75-90	16	20	21
Recurrence[c]	30	69	41	67
Clinical Symptoms				
Fever[d]	80-90	88	79	100
Musculoskeletal involvement	12-56	26	34	21
Ocular involvement	17-72	7	15	21
Lesion Location				
Upper extremities	80	89	97	71
Head and neck	50	63	52	43
Trunk and back	30	42	33	50
Lower extremities	Infrequent	49	48	36
Oral mucous membranes	2	12	3	7
Laboratory Findings				
Neutrophilia[e]	80	47	60	38
Elevated erythrocyte sedimentation rate[f]	90	100	95	100
Anemia[g]	Infrequent	82	83	100
Abnormal platelet count[h]	Infrequent	68	50	50
Abnormal renal function[i]	11-50	15	7	0

[a]Percentages for classical, hematologic malignancy, and solid-tumor-associated Sweet syndrome adapted with permission from Cohen PR, Kurzrock R: Sweet's syndrome and cancer. Clin Dermatol. 1993;11:149-157. Copyright 1993, Elsevier Science Publishing Co., Inc., New York, NY.
[b]Percentages for drug-induced Sweet syndrome adapted with permission from Walker DC, Cohen PR: Trimethoprim-sulfamethoxazole-associated acute febrile neutrophilic dermatosis: case report and review of drug induced Sweet's syndrome. J Am Acad Dermatol. 1996;34:918-923. Copyright 1996, American Academy of Dermatology, Inc., Mosby-Year Book, Inc., St. Louis, MO.
[c]Recurrence following oral rechallenge testing in the patients with drug-induced Sweet syndrome.
[d]Temperature greater than 38°C (100.4°F).
[e]Neutrophil count greater than 6000 cells/μL.
[f]Erythrocyte sedimentation rate greater than 20 mm/h.
[g]Hemoglobin less than 13 g/dL in men and less than 12 g/dL in women.
[h]Platelet count less than 150,000/μL or greater than 500,000/μL.
[i]This includes hematuria, proteinuria, and renal insufficiency.

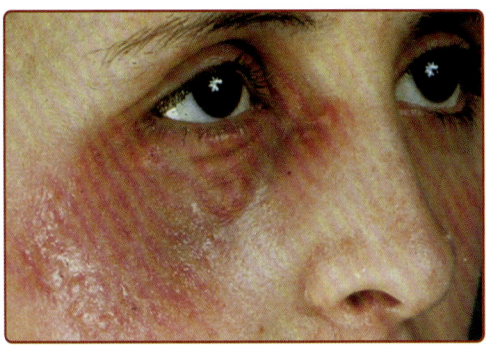

Figure 36-1 Unilateral lesions of Sweet syndrome around the eye and upper lip consisting of plaques and pseudovesicular papules suggesting herpes simplex.

PUSTULAR DERMATOSIS

Sweet syndrome can present as a pustular dermatosis. The lesions appear as tiny pustules on the tops of the red papules or erythematous-based pustules. Some of the patients previously described as having the "pustular eruption of ulcerative colitis" are perhaps more appropriately included in this clinical variant of Sweet syndrome.[13,14]

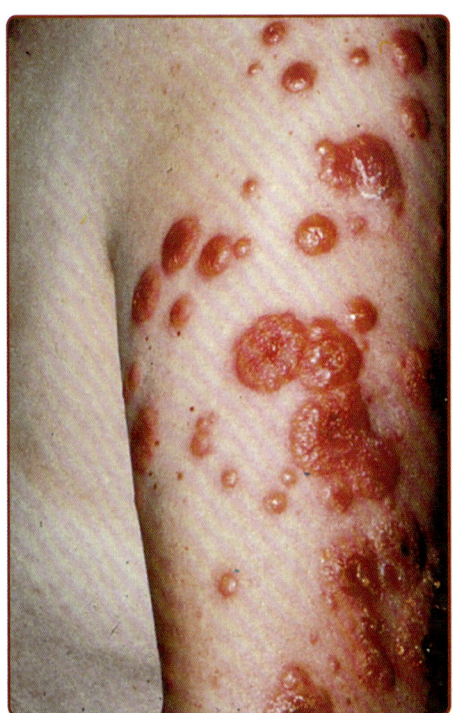

Figure 36-2 Multiple confluent papules and plaques of Sweet syndrome that at first sight give the illusion of vesiculation but are solid on palpation. (From Hönigsmann H, Kempter R, Wolff K. Acute febrile neurophilic dermatosis [Sweet's syndrome]—report of two cases [author's transl] [in German]. *Wien Klin Wochenschr.* 1979;91(24):842-847, with permission.)

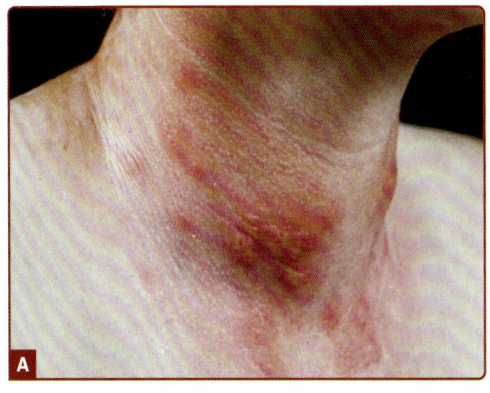

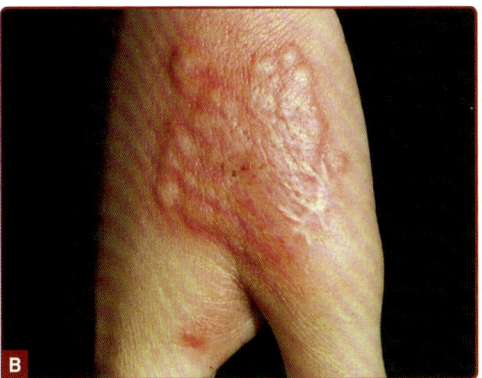

Figure 36-3 Acute febrile neutrophilic dermatosis. Typical lesion consisting of coalescing, plaque-forming papules. **A,** Bright-red lesions on the neck. **B,** Lesion on the dorsum of the right hand exhibiting the "relief of a mountain range" feature. (From Hönigsmann H, Wolff K. Acute febrile neutrophilic dermatosis [Sweet's syndrome]. In Wolff K, Winkelmann RK, eds. *Major Problems in Dermatology.* Vol 10, Vasculitis. London, UK: Lloyd-Luke; 1980:307, with permission.)

NEUTROPHILIC DERMATOSIS OF THE DORSAL HANDS

A localized, pustular variant of Sweet syndrome, when the clinical lesions are predominantly restricted to the dorsal hands, is described as "neutrophilic dermatosis of the dorsal hands" or "pustular vasculitis of the dorsal hands." In these individuals, the lesions are similar to those of Sweet syndrome in morphology and rapid resolution after systemic corticosteroids and/or dapsone therapy was initiated. Many of patients with this form of the disease also had concurrent oral mucosa, arm, leg, back, and/or face lesions.[2,15]

SUBCUTANEOUS PANNICULITIS

Subcutaneous Sweet syndrome lesions usually present as erythematous, tender dermal nodules on the extremities. The lesions mimic erythema nodosum when they are located on the legs. One study reported findings of panniculitis in 80% of patients in which the hypodermis was affected. Therefore, even in a patient with biopsy-confirmed Sweet syndrome, tissue evaluation of one or more new dermal nodules may be necessary to establish the correct diagnosis as Sweet syndrome can present concurrently or sequentially with erythema nodosum.[3,8,15-17]

HISTIOCYTOID VARIANT

Histiocytoid Sweet syndrome was initially described by Requena et al. in 2005. The skin lesion morphology is similar to that of idiopathic Sweet syndrome. However, the dermal infiltrate is composed of mononuclear cells with a histiocytic appearance—representing immature myeloid cells.[18]

This variant of Sweet syndrome is often associated with malignancy. Drug-induced histiocytoid Sweet syndrome has also been observed in patients receiving bortezomib.[18,19]

GIANT CELLULITIS-LIKE VARIANT

A morphologically distinctive clinical variant of Sweet syndrome, characterized by relapsing widespread giant lesions, is giant cellulitis-like Sweet syndrome. In 2013, it was originally reported in 3 morbidly obese individuals. In 2014, 2 additional patients were described, and in 2015, a sixth patient with concurrent histiocytoid Sweet syndrome was reported.[18,20-22]

Giant cellulitis-like Sweet syndrome has been observed in 5 women and 1 man, ranging in age from 48 years to 72 years (median = 61 years). The upper leg and buttocks were the most common locations of their skin lesions (Fig. 36-4). Most of the patients (66%) were obese and half of the patients had cancer.[18,20-22]

NECROTIZING VARIANT

Necrotizing Sweet syndrome is a new variant of neutrophilic dermatosis that mimics necrotizing fasciitis. It clinically presents as the rapid onset of edematous, erythematous, warm cutaneous lesions. An infectious etiology for the lesions is absent. Biopsy shows a deep-tissue neutrophilic infiltration and soft-tissue necrosis.[23]

NONCUTANEOUS FINDINGS

POTENTIAL ORGANS

The bones, central nervous system, ears, eyes, kidneys, intestines, liver, heart, lung, mouth, muscles, and spleen can be sites of extracutaneous manifestations of Sweet syndrome (Table 36-4).[1,7]

BONE INVOLVEMENT

In children, dermatosis-related sterile osteomyelitis has been reported.[1]

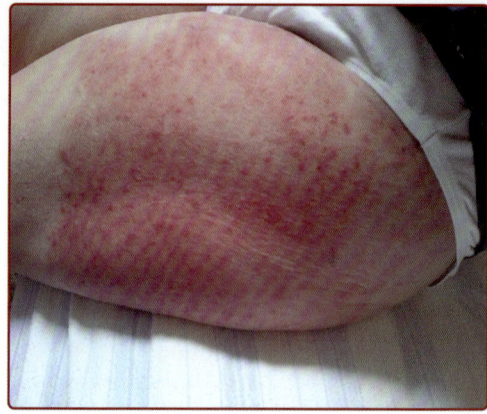

Figure 36-4 Histiocytoid giant cellulitis Sweet syndrome presenting as an erythematous plaque on the left lateral thigh of a 72-year-old woman who had an unclassified myelodysplastic syndrome/myeloproliferative disorder. (From So JK, Carlos CA, Frucht CS, et al. Histiocytoid giant cellulitis-like Sweet's syndrome: case report and review of the literature. *Dermatol Online J.* 2015;21(3):4, with permission.)

CARDIAC INVOLVEMENT

Sweet syndrome-associated cardiovascular involvement may occur in children. A 22-month-old white boy with Sweet syndrome developed postinflammatory elastolysis and Takayasu arteritis. Cardiovascular involvement resulting from elastolysis of the heart and aorta occurred in 3 children who were ages 17 months, 16 months, and 7 months; 2 of the patients died.[24,25]

Cardiovascular involvement, including coronary artery occlusion, occurred in a 43-year-old man with Sweet syndrome.[26]

CENTRAL NERVOUS SYSTEM INVOLVEMENT

A wide variety of neurologic symptoms have been observed in neuro-Sweet disease. This rare variant of the dermatosis, which can affect regions of the central nervous system, was originally proposed by Hisanaga et al. in 1999. Neuro-Sweet disease, in a 72-year-old man, presented with self-remitting and reversible parkinsonism. In a 49-year-old man, optic nerve involvement with panuveitis was reported. Bilateral endogenous endophthalmitis with chorioretinitis arising from nontuberculous mycobacterial infection occurred in a 47-year-old Thai woman with underlying Sweet syndrome. Radiation therapy-induced neuro-Sweet disease was described in a 67-year-old woman with oral squamous cell carcinoma.[27-30]

OCULAR INVOLVEMENT

Ocular manifestations of Sweet syndrome may be the presenting feature of the condition. In classical Sweet syndrome, the incidence of ocular involvement (such

TABLE 36-4
Extracutaneous Manifestations of Sweet Syndrome

Bone	Acute sterile arthritis; arthralgias; focal aseptic osteitis; pigmented villonodular synovitis; sterile osteomyelitis (chronic recurrent multifocal osteomyelitis)
Central nervous system	Acute benign encephalitis; aseptic meningitis; brain single-photon emission computed tomography (SPECT) abnormalities; brainstem lesions; cerebrospinal fluid abnormalities; computerized axial tomography abnormalities; electroencephalogram abnormalities; encephalitis; Guillain-Barré syndrome; idiopathic hypertrophic cranial pachymeningitis; idiopathic progressive bilateral sensorineural hearing loss; leukoencephalopathy; magnetic resonance imaging abnormalities; neurologic symptoms; "neuro-Sweet disease"; pareses of central origin; polyneuropathy; psychiatric symptoms
Ears	Tender red nodules and pustules that coalesced to form plaques in the external auditory canal and the tympanic membrane
Eyes	Blepharitis; chemosis; conjunctival erythematous lesions with tissue biopsy showing neutrophilic inflammation; conjunctival hemorrhage; conjunctivitis; dacryoadenitis; episcleritis; glaucoma; iridocyclitis; iritis; limbal nodules; ocular congestion; periocular swelling; peripheral ulcerative keratitis; retinal vasculitis; scleritis; uveitis
Kidneys	Mesangiocapillary glomerulonephritis; urinalysis abnormalities (hematuria and proteinuria)
Intestines	Intestine with extensive and diffuse neutrophilic inflammation; neutrophilic ileal infiltrate; pancolitis (culture-negative)
Liver	Hepatic portal triad with neutrophilic inflammation; hepatic serum enzyme abnormalities; hepatomegaly
Heart	Aortic stenosis (segmental); aortitis (neutrophilic and segmental); cardiomegaly; coronary artery occlusion; heart failure; myocardial infiltration by neutrophils; vascular (aorta, brachiocephalic trunk and coronary arteries) dilatation
Lung	Bronchi (main stem) with red-bordered pustules; bronchi with neutrophilic inflammation; pleural effusion showing abundant neutrophils without microorganisms; chest roentgenogram abnormalities; corticosteroid-responsive culture-negative infiltratives; pulmonary tissue with neutrophilic inflammation
Mouth	Aphthous-like superficial lesions (buccal mucosa, tongue); bullae and vesicles (hemorrhagic: labial and gingival mucosa); gingival hyperplasia; necrotizing ulcerative periodontitis; nodules (necrotic: labial mucosa); papules (macerated: palate and tongue); pustules (individual and grouped: palate and pharynx); swelling (tongue); ulcers (buccal mucosa and palate)
Muscles	Magnetic resonance imaging (T1-weighted and T2-weighted) abnormalities: high signal intensities caused by myositis and fasciitis; myalgias (in up to half of the patients with idiopathic Sweet syndrome); myositis (neutrophilic); tendinitis; tenosynovitis
Spleen	Aseptic abscess; splenomegaly.

From Cohen PR, Kurzrock R. Sweet's syndrome revisited: a review of disease concepts. *Int J Dermatol.* 2003;42:761-778, with permission.

as conjunctivitis) is variable. However, in the malignancy-associated and drug-induced forms of the dermatosis it is uncommon.[1]

ORAL INVOLVEMENT

Mucosal ulcers of the mouth are uncommon in patients with classical Sweet syndrome. However, they occur more frequently in Sweet syndrome patients with hematologic disorders. The oral lesions—similar to extracutaneous manifestations of Sweet syndrome occurring at other sites—typically resolve after initiation of treatment with systemic corticosteroids.[1]

OTIC INVOLVEMENT

In a 65-year-old woman with a 10-year history of Sweet syndrome, a rapid, profound loss of hearing was reported; bilateral, progressive sensorineural hearing loss after a severe exacerbation of Sweet syndrome had been diagnosed 7 years prior.[31]

SPLEEN INVOLVEMENT

Spleen and lymph node involvement was preceded by parvovirus B19 infection in a 45-year-old white woman with Sweet syndrome.[32]

COMPLICATIONS

Complications may occur in Sweet syndrome patients. They can either be directly related to the mucocutaneous lesions or indirectly related to the Sweet syndrome-associated conditions. Antimicrobial therapy may be necessary if the skin lesions become secondarily infected. Reappearance of the dermatosis may herald the unsuspected discovery that the cancer has recurred in patients with malignancy-associated Sweet syndrome. Disease-specific treatment may be warranted for systemic manifestations of Sweet syndrome-related conditions such as inflammatory bowel disease, sarcoidosis, and thyroid disease.[1,7]

ETIOLOGY AND PATHOGENESIS

ASSOCIATED CONDITIONS

ASSOCIATED DISEASES

Several conditions have been observed to occur either before, concurrent with, or following the diagnosis of Sweet syndrome (Table 36-5). Behçet disease, cancer, erythema nodosum, infections, inflammatory bowel

TABLE 36-5
Sweet Syndrome and Associated Conditions

Probably bona fide associated conditions
- Cancer: hematologic malignancies (most commonly acute myelogenous leukemia) and solid tumors (most commonly carcinomas of the genitourinary organs, breast, and gastrointestinal tract)
- Infections: most commonly of the upper respiratory tract (streptococcosis) and the gastrointestinal tract (salmonellosis and yersiniosis)
- Inflammatory bowel disease: Crohn disease and ulcerative colitis
- Medications: most commonly granulocyte colony-stimulating factor
- Pregnancy
- Vaccinations (bacille Calmette-Guérin [BCG] and influenza)

Possibly bona fide associated conditions
- Behçet disease
- Erythema nodosum
- Relapsing polychondritis
- Rheumatoid arthritis
- Sarcoidosis
- Thyroid disease: Grave disease and Hashimoto thyroiditis

Validity of associated conditions remains to be established
- α₁-Antitrypsin deficiency
- Antineutrophilic cytoplasmic antibody–associated vasculitis
- Ankylosing spondylitis
- Anti–factor VIII inhibitor
- Antiphospholipid syndrome
- Aortitis (Takayasu arteritis)
- Aplastic anemia
- Autoimmune disorders: cholangitis, dermatomyositis, lupus erythematosus (subacute and systemic), pemphigus vulgaris, and Sjögren syndrome
- Autologous stem cell transplant
- Bronchiolitis obliterans and organizing pneumonia
- Chemical fertilizer
- Chronic fatigue syndrome
- Chronic recurrent multifocal osteomyelitis
- Celiac disease
- Cirrhosis (cryptogenic)
- Common bile duct and intrahepatic duct stones
- Congenital dyserythropoietic anemia
- Congenital neutropenia (Kostmann syndrome)
- Cutis laxa (acquired, Marshall syndrome)
- Differentiation syndrome
- Dressler syndrome (postmyocardial infarction syndrome)
- End-stage renal disease
- Eosinophilic granuloma
- Familial Mediterranean fever
- Fanconi anemia
- Glycogen storage disease (type Ib)
- Granuloma annulare
- Hemophagocytic syndrome
- Immunoglobulin A nephropathy (Berger disease)
- Immunizing agent (BCG vaccination and flu)
- Immunodeficiency diseases: chronic granulomatous disease, common variable immunodeficiency, complement deficiency, HIV infection, and primary T-cell immunodeficiency disease
- Infections: *Anaplasma phagocytophilum*, bartholinitis, bronchitis, *Campylobacter* spp., *Capnocytophaga canimorsus*, *Chlamydia*, *Chlamydophila pneumoniae*, cholangitis, cholecystitis, coccidioidomycosis, cytomegalovirus, dermatophyte, *Entamoeba histolytica*, Epstein-Barr virus, *Francisella tularensis*, *Helicobacter pylori*, hepatitis (acute or chronic hepatitis B, autoimmune, cholestatic, chronic active, hepatitis C, and prior hepatitis A), herpes simplex, herpes zoster, histoplasmosis, HIV, leprosy, leptospirosis, lymphadenitis (not otherwise specified and subacute necrotizing), mycobacteria avium, chelonae, nontuberculous, and tuberculous, otitis media, pancreatitis, parvovirus B19, *Pasteurella multocida* bronchitis, *Penicillium* spp., *Pneumocystis carinii* pneumonia, pyelonephritis, sporotrichosis, *Staphylococcus aureus*, *Staphylococcus epidermidis* (methicillin-resistant), subacute bacterial endocarditis, tonsillitis, toxoplasmosis, tuberculosis, tularemias (glandular), ureaplasmosis, urinary tract, and vulvovaginitis
- Kidney transplantation
- Kikuchi disease
- Malabsorption
- Microscopic polyangiitis
- Mid-dermal elastolysis
- POEMS syndrome (*polyneuropathy, organomegaly, endocrinopathy, M protein, and skin changes*)
- Postoperative (pneumonectomy)
- Psoriasis vulgaris
- Rhinosinusitis
- Sialadenitis
- Still disease
- Takayasu arteritis
- Thermal injury
- Transient acantholytic dermatosis (Grover disease)
- Ureter obstruction
- Urticaria (chronic)
- Urticaria pigmentosa
- Wegner granulomatosis
- Welding burns

disease, pregnancy, relapsing polychondritis, rheumatoid arthritis, sarcoidosis, and thyroid disease may be etiologically related to the development of Sweet syndrome. The association between Sweet syndrome and other conditions remains to be established.[1]

Sweet syndrome associated with differentiation syndrome (an inflammatory reaction with increased capillary permeability that occurs in up to 25% of patients with acute promyelocytic leukemia treated with all-*trans*-retinoic acid) was suspected in a 50-year-old man with acute promyelocytic leukemia who underwent chemotherapy with idarubicin and all-*trans*-retinoic acid.[33] The histiocytoid variant of Sweet syndrome is associated not only with medications, but also with several other conditions, including autoimmune diseases, infections and inflammation, inflammatory bowel disease, and malignancy (Table 36-6).[18] Giant cellulitis-like Sweet syndrome was associated with obesity (4 of 6 patients) and malignancy (3 of 6 patients): hematologic dyscrasia (multiple myeloma or myelodysplastic syndrome/myeloproliferative disorder) and breast cancer (Table 36-7).[18,20-22]

ASSOCIATED NEUTROPHILIC DERMATOSES

The unifying characteristic of neutrophilic dermatoses of the skin and mucosa is an inflammatory infiltrate of mature polymorphonuclear leukocytes.

> **TABLE 36-6**
> **Conditions and Drugs Associated with Histiocytoid Sweet Syndrome**
>
> **Autoimmune diseases**
> - Positive lupus erythematosus serologies
> - Relapsing polychondritis
> - Rheumatoid arthritis
> - Systemic lupus erythematosus
>
> **Infections/inflammation**
> - Conjunctivitis
> - Methicillin-resistant *Staphylococcus aureus* (pneumonia)
> - Parotitis
> - Sinusitis
>
> **Inflammatory bowel disease**
> - Crohn disease
> - Ulcerative colitis
>
> **Malignancies**
> - Acute myelogenous leukemia
> - Breast carcinoma
> - Chronic lymphocytic leukemia
> - Chronic monocytic leukemia
> - Chronic myelogenous leukemia
> - Hodgkin lymphoma
> - Leukemia cutis (from acute myelomonocytic leukemia)
> - Lymphoma
> - Monoclonal gammopathy of undetermined significance
> - Multiple myeloma
> - Myelodysplastic syndrome
> - Myelodysplastic syndrome/myeloproliferative disorder
> - Renal carcinoma
>
> **Medications**
> - Azacitidine
> - Azathioprine
> - Bortezomib
> - Cox-2 inhibitor
> - Decitabine
> - Trimethoprim-sulfamethoxazole
>
> **Other conditions**
> - Diabetes mellitus
> - Erythema nodosum
> - Eyelid edema
> - Familial Mediterranean fever
> - Glomerulonephritis
> - Hypertension
> - Immunosuppression
> - None
> - Polyarteritis nodosa
> - Pregnancy
>
> From So JK, Carlos CA, Frucht CS, et al. Histiocytoid giant cellulitis-like Sweet's syndrome: case report and review of the literature. *Dermatol Online J*. 2015;21(3):4 with permission.

Concurrent or sequential occurrence either of erythema elevatum diutinum, neutrophilic eccrine hidradenitis, pyoderma gangrenosum, subcorneal pustular dermatosis, and/or vasculitis with Sweet syndrome has been observed. These conditions can display similar clinical and pathologic features; however, the location of the neutrophilic infiltrate helps differentiate them.[2,3,34,35]

CONCURRENT LEUKEMIA CUTIS

Sweet syndrome may present as either a paraneoplastic syndrome (signaling the initial discovery of an unsuspected malignancy), a drug-induced dermatosis (following treatment with either all-*trans*-retinoic acid, bortezomib, granulocyte colony-stimulating factor (G-CSF), or imatinib mesylate), or a condition whose skin lesions concurrently demonstrate leukemia cutis in patients with hematologic disorders. The most frequent hematologic dyscrasias associated with leukemia cutis (characterized by abnormal neutrophils) and Sweet syndrome (consisting of mature polymorphonuclear leukocytes) being present in the same skin lesion are acute myelocytic leukemia and acute promyelocytic leukemia. Other associated hematologic disorders that have been associated with concurrent Sweet syndrome and leukemia cutis include myelodysplastic syndrome and either chronic myelogenous leukemia or myelogenous leukemia not otherwise specified.[1,7]

One of the hypotheses to explain concurrent Sweet syndrome and leukemia cutis in the same lesion is "secondary" leukemia cutis; in patients with "secondary" leukemia cutis, the circulating immature myeloid precursor cells are innocent bystanders that have been recruited to the skin as the result of an inflammatory oncotactic phenomenon stimulated by the Sweet syndrome lesions. Another possibility is the occurrence of "primary" leukemia cutis. In patients with "primary" leukemia cutis, the leukemic cells within the skin constitute the bonified incipient presence of a specific leukemic infiltrate. Finally, in patients with "primary" leukemia cutis who were being treated with G-CSF, it is possible that the atypical cells of leukemia cutis developed into mature neutrophils of Sweet syndrome as a result of G-CSF therapy-induced differentiation of the sequestered leukemia cells.[1]

SYSTEMIC INFLAMMATORY RESPONSE SYNDROME

Sweet syndrome can occur with systemic inflammatory response syndrome. A 76-year-old man with Sweet syndrome-associated pulmonary involvement also experienced systemic inflammatory response syndrome. Sepsis refers to systemic inflammatory response syndrome caused by infection. Yet, this man's systemic inflammatory response syndrome was attributed to Sweet syndrome because his cultures were persistently negative.[36,37]

PATHOGENESIS

The pathogenesis of Sweet syndrome remains to be definitively established and may be multifactorial.

TABLE 36-7
Characteristics of Patients with Giant Cellulitis-Like Sweet Syndrome

AS	SYMPTOMS	WBC (cells/uL)	OTHER LABS	ASSOC DIS	TX	RESPONSE	REF
62M	Fever Malaise	10.6+	ANA– CRP+	Ob MM	Amox Pred	No effect from antibiotics; good response from oral prednisone	20 C1
48F	Fever Malaise	24+	CRP+	Ob	Pred	Good control	20 C2
54F	Fever	4.1	Creat+ TC–	Ob PBC Si	Pred	Excellent	21
60F^	Fever	10.3	TC–	–	Col Pred Dap	Response, but recurrence on colchicine and prednisone; excellent response to dapsone and prednisone	22
68F	Fever Malaise	11.3+	CRP+ TC–	Br Ob	Surg Top	Transient improvement then recurrence with topical corticosteroid; remission after surgical treatment of breast carcinoma	20 C3
72F	Fever Foot pain	73.5+	LDH+ TC–	MDS/MPD	Top	Excellent	18

The site of skin lesions and (number of patients) were: lower extremity (6 patients) [18,20 (cases 1,2, and 3), 21,22]; trunk (5 patients) [18,20 (cases 1 and 2), 21,22]; buttock (3 patients) [20 (cases 1 and 2), 21]; upper extremity (2 patients) [20 (case 2), 21]; and head and neck (1 patients).[21]

Negative; ^, patient was in her "60's"; +, elevated; Amox, amoxicillin/clavulanic acid; ANA, antinuclear antibody; AS, age (in years) and sex; Assoc dis, associated disease; Br, breast carcinoma; Col, colchicine; CR, current report; Creat, serum creatinine; CRP, C-reative protein; Dap, dapsone; F, female; LDH, lactate dehydrogenase; M, male; MDS/MPD, myelodysplastic/myeloproliferative disorder; MM, multiple myeloma; Ob, obesity; PBC, primary biliary cirrhosis; Pred, prednisone; Ref, reference; Si, sicca syndrome; Surg, surgical treatment of breast carcinoma; TC, tissue culture; Top, topical corticosteroid; Tx, treatment; WBC, white blood cell.

From So JK, Carlos CA, Frucht CS, et al. Histiocytoid giant cellulitis-like Sweet's syndrome: case report and review of the literature. Dermatol Online J. 2015;21(3):4 with permission.

ANIMAL MODELS

Animal models of Sweet syndrome have been described. An alteration in the gene encoding protein tyrosine phosphatase nonreceptor type 6—originally found in a mouse with clinical and histopathologic characteristics resembling Sweet syndrome—appears to be involved in the pathogenesis of certain subsets of neutrophilic dermatoses, including Sweet syndrome. In a female standard poodle dog (after treatment with the nonsteroidal antiinflammatory drug firocoxib) and in multiple dogs (temporally associated with the administration of carprofen) a condition presenting as a sterile neutrophilic dermatosis, and similar to Sweet syndrome, has been observed; subsequent examination also revealed extracutaneous involvement of the esophagus, heart, lungs, and tarsus (joint space and synovium). In addition, a sterile neutrophilic dermatosis of the skin—similar to Sweet syndrome—has been described in a female Dachshund; the condition responded rapidly to corticosteroid therapy.[38-40]

BACTERIAL, VIRAL, OR TUMOR ANTIGENS

A hypersensitivity reaction to an eliciting bacterial, viral, or tumor antigen may elicit Sweet syndrome. The accompanying fever and peripheral leukocytosis suggests the possibility of a septic process. Indeed, in patients with classic Sweet syndrome, a febrile upper respiratory tract bacterial infection or tonsillitis may precede skin lesions by 1 to 3 weeks. Also, Sweet syndrome patients with *Yersinia enterocolitica* intestinal infection have improved with systemic antibiotics.[1]

FAMILIAL MEDITERRANEAN FEVER

The systemic manifestations of familial Mediterranean fever resemble those of Sweet syndrome. Indeed, the simultaneous occurrence of both conditions has been observed. In addition, the causative gene mutation for familial Mediterranean fever was detected in a patient with chronic myelogenous leukemia-associated Sweet syndrome. Hence, these conditions may have a similar pathogenesis.[7]

HUMAN LEUKOCYTE ANTIGEN SEROTYPES

A 5-week-old Japanese girl with Sweet syndrome and non-B54 types of human leukocyte antigen was reported. She is one of the youngest patients reported with the dermatosis. The potential importance of genetic background in association with Sweet syndrome is suggested by this observation.[41]

CYTOKINES

Circulating autoantibodies, dermal dendrocytes, immune complexes and leukotactic mechanisms have all been postulated to contribute to the pathogenesis of Sweet syndrome. The immunoreactivity of several cytokines (interleukin [IL]-1, IL-8, IL-17, and tumor necrosis factor-α), inflammatory cell markers (CD3, CD163, and myeloperoxidase), metalloproteinases (metalloproteinase-2 and metalloproteinase-9), and vascular endothelial growth factor have displayed significantly higher values in the lesional skin of patients with Sweet syndrome from non-Sweet syndrome individuals or patients with other neutrophilic dermatoses. The observation of a 48-year-old white woman with coexisting Sweet syndrome, Hashimoto thyroiditis, and psoriasis suggests the possibility of a CD4+ T-cell dysfunction in the pathogenesis of the dermatosis. Complement does not appear to be essential to the disease process. Antibodies to neutrophilic cytoplasmic antigens have been demonstrated in some patients; however, these are thought to represent an epiphenomenon.[1,42,43]

The development of Sweet syndrome symptoms and lesions may—directly and/or indirectly—be caused by cytokines. A patient with myelodysplastic syndrome-associated Sweet syndrome demonstrated elevated serum levels of G-CSF and IL-6; the individual was not receiving the drugs. An infant with classical Sweet syndrome had detectable levels of intraarticular synovial fluid granulocyte-macrophage colony-stimulating factor (GM-CSF). Compared to dermatosis patients with inactive Sweet syndrome, a study demonstrated that the serum G-CSF level was significantly higher in individuals with active Sweet syndrome. And, in a patient with acute myelogenous leukemia-associated Sweet syndrome and neutrophilic panniculitis, the level of endogenous G-CSF was closely associated with Sweet syndrome disease activity.[1,7,17]

IMMUNOHISTOCHEMICAL STUDIES

Significantly elevated levels of helper T-cell type 1 cytokines (IL-2 and interferon-gamma [IFN-γ]) and normal levels of a helper T-cell type 2 cytokine (IL-4) in the sera of Sweet syndrome patients have been observed in immunohistochemical studies. Serial measurements of cerebral spinal fluid IL-6, IFN-γ, IL-8, and interferon-inducible protein-10 were elevated as compared to levels in control subjects with neurologic disorders and also correlated with total cerebral spinal fluid cell counts in a patient with neuro-Sweet disease presenting with recurrent encephalomeningitis. This data suggests an important role of the helper T-cell type 1 cell (whose cytokines include IFN-γ and interferon-inducible protein-10) and IL-8 (a specific neutrophil chemoattractant) in the pathogenesis of neuro-Sweet disease. Other studies postulated that cytokine release into the dermis accounted for decreased epidermal staining for IL-1 and IL-6. In summary, G-CSF, GM-CSF, IFN-γ, IL-1, IL-3, IL-6, and IL-8 are potential cytokine candidates in the pathogenesis of Sweet syndrome.[1,7,12,17]

PHOTOSENSITIVITY

Photosensitivity may play a role in the pathogenesis of Sweet syndrome. Experimental induction of Sweet syndrome has been elicited by phototesting. Also, in a woman who was receiving trimethoprim-sulfamethoxazole, photodrug-associated Sweet syndrome developed in sun-exposed areas. Although the mechanism of pathogenesis is unknown, one hypothesis suggests an isomorphic Koebner reaction. Another postulated theory associates ultraviolet-B radiation with neutrophil activation and epidermal production of tumor necrosis factor-α and IL-8.[12,44-46]

DIAGNOSIS

DIAGNOSTIC CRITERIA

In 1986, diagnostic criteria for classical or idiopathic Sweet syndrome were proposed by Su and Liu. They were modified in 1994 by von den Driesch (see Table 36-1). Infection (upper respiratory tract or gastrointestinal tract), inflammatory bowel disease, or pregnancy may be associated with Sweet syndrome. A seasonal preference for the onset of Sweet syndrome for either autumn or spring has been observed.[7,12,47]

Classical Sweet syndrome most commonly occurs in women; onset appears between the ages of 30 years and 60 years. Yet, classical Sweet syndrome has also been observed in younger adults and children. Brothers who developed the dermatosis at 10 and 15 days of age are the youngest Sweet syndrome patients. In the neonatal period, the appearance of Sweet syndrome in the first 6 weeks of life often heralds a serious underlying disorder, thus requiring a thorough investigation for the associated condition.[48,49]

It is appropriate to distinguish the classical form of Sweet syndrome from the malignancy-associated variant of this condition as there is a temporal association with the discovery or relapse of cancer and the onset or recurrence of many Sweet syndrome cases. A comprehensive review of 66 pediatric Sweet syndrome patients observed an associated hematologic malignancy in 44% of 30 children between 3 years and 18 years of age. In adults, malignancy-associated Sweet syndrome is most often associated with acute myelogenous leukemia and does not have a female predominance. Carcinomas of the genitourinary organs, breast, and gastrointestinal tract are the most frequently occurring cancers in Sweet syndrome patients with dermatosis-related solid tumors.[1,7,47,50]

In 1996, Walker and Cohen established the criteria for drug-induced Sweet syndrome (see Table 36-1). G-CSF is the most frequently observed agent associated with this variant of the dermatosis. However, other medications are also implicated in eliciting drug-induced Sweet syndrome (Fig. 36-5; see Table 36-2).[7,10,18,33,51-55]

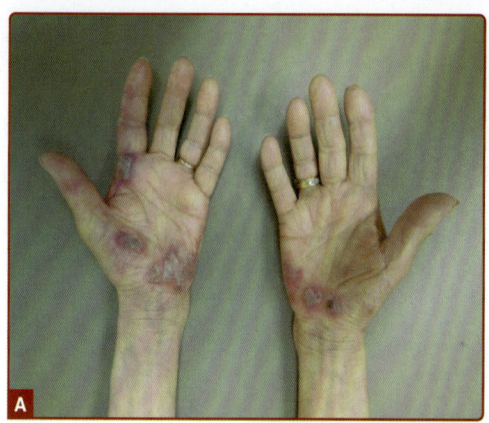
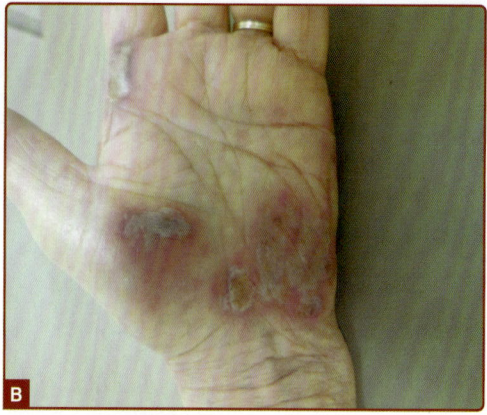
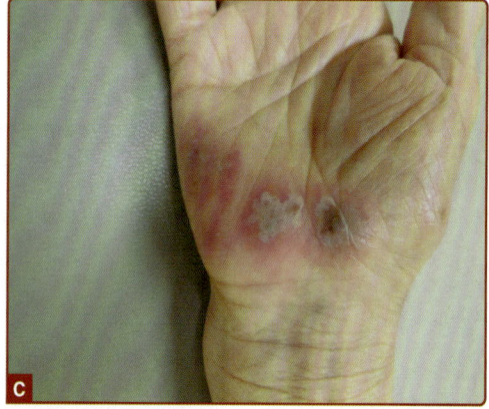

Figure 36-5 Distant (**A**) and closer (**B** and **C**) views of the left (**B**) and right (**C**) palms of an 86-year-old woman with proton pump inhibitor–induced Sweet syndrome. The painful erythematous-based pustules and pseudovesicular violaceous plaques on her hands appeared within 6 hours after she took an initial dose of esomeprazole. Previously, she had developed similar hand lesions on day 8 of omeprazole, which resolved after a short course of oral prednisone. (From Cohen PR. Proton pump inhibitor-induced Sweet's syndrome: report of acute febrile neutrophilic dermatosis in a woman with recurrent breast cancer. *Dermatol Pract Concept*. 2015;5:113-119, published under a Creative Commons Attribution License [http://creativecommons.org/licenses/by-nc/3.0/], with permission.)

SUPPORTIVE STUDIES

LABORATORY TESTING

A complete blood cell count with leukocyte differential and platelet count, evaluation of acute-phase reactants (such as the erythrocyte sedimentation rate or C-reactive protein), serum chemistries (evaluating hepatic function and renal function), and an urinalysis should be performed. As there appears to be a bona fide association between thyroid disease and Sweet syndrome, it is also reasonable to perform a serologic evaluation of thyroid function.[1]

Peripheral leukocytosis with neutrophilia and an elevated erythrocyte sedimentation rate and are the most consistent laboratory findings in Sweet syndrome. However, in patients with biopsy-confirmed Sweet syndrome, leukocytosis is not always present. For example, in some of the patients with malignancy-associated Sweet syndrome, anemia, neutropenia, and/or abnormal platelet counts may be observed.[1]

Urinalysis abnormalities (hematuria and proteinuria) and hepatic serum enzyme elevation may be observed in patients with kidney and liver involvement. Abnormalities in cerebrospinal fluid analysis may be observed in patients with central nervous system involvement.[1,7]

PATHOLOGY

When the diagnosis of Sweet syndrome is suspected, evaluation of a lesional skin biopsy is helpful. As the pathologic findings of Sweet syndrome are similar to those observed in cutaneous lesions caused by infectious agents, lesional tissue should also be submitted for bacterial, fungal, mycobacterial, and, possibly, viral cultures.[1]

Characteristically, a diffuse infiltrate of mature neutrophils is present in the papillary and upper reticular dermis (Fig. 36-6). However, the inflammatory infiltrate can also involve the epidermis or adipose tissue. In contrast to the infiltrate of mature neutrophils typically seen in Sweet syndrome, histiocytoid Sweet syndrome is characterized by a dermal infiltrate composed

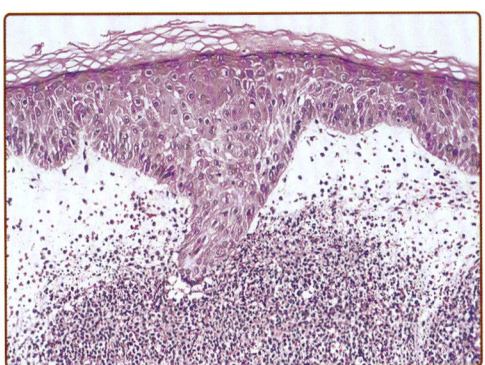

Figure 36-6 Histopathologic presentation of acute febrile neutrophilic dermatosis (Sweet syndrome) demonstrates massive edema of the papillary dermis and a dense diffuse infiltrate of mature neutrophils throughout the upper dermis (hematoxylin and eosin stain). (From Cohen PR, Holder WR, Tucker SB, et al. Sweet's syndrome in patients with solid tumors. *Cancer.* 1993;72:2723-2731, with permission. Copyright © 2006 John Wiley & Sons.)

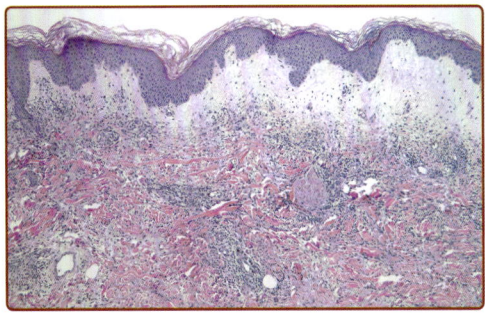

Figure 36-7 An intermediate magnification view of the histopathologic presentation of histiocytoid giant cellulitis Sweet syndrome shows prominent superficial dermal edema with a perivascular and interstitial inflammatory dermal infiltrate consisting of histiocytoid and immature granulocytic cells admixed with lymphocytes, eosinophils, and occasional neutrophils. (From So JK, Carlos CA, Frucht CS, et al. Histiocytoid giant cellulitis-like Sweet's syndrome: case report and review of the literature. *Dermatol Online J.* 2015;21(3):4, with permission.)

of immature granulocytes that are histiocytic mononuclear cells (Fig. 36-7). Morphologically, the small cells of histiocytoid Sweet syndrome appear similar to neutrophils; however, they stain for CD15, CD43, CD45 (LCA), CD68, HAM56, lysozyme, and MAC 387—thereby identifying a monocytic-histiocytic profile (Fig. 36-8).[7,18]

The inflammation in the dermis is typically dense and diffuse. However, it can also be perivascular. In addition, the dermal inflammation can demonstrate "secondary" changes of leukocytoclastic vasculitis; these changes are considered to be an epiphenomenon and not representative of a "primary" vasculitis.[2]

Exocytosis of neutrophils into the epidermis can result in neutrophilic spongiotic vesicles or subcorneal pustules. The condition is referred to as "subcutaneous Sweet syndrome" when the neutrophils are located either entirely or partially in the subcutaneous fat.[1,3]

The spectrum of pathologic changes described in cutaneous lesions of Sweet syndrome has expanded; it now includes concurrent leukemia cutis, vasculitis, and variability of the composition or the location of the inflammatory infiltrate. Edema in the dermis, swollen endothelial cells, dilated small blood vessels, and fragmented neutrophil nuclei (referred to as karyorrhexis or leukocytoclasia) may also be present (Fig. 36-9). However, the overlying epidermis is normal and fibrin deposition or neutrophils within the vessel walls (changes of "primary" leukocytoclastic vasculitis) are usually absent.[1,2]

The inflammatory infiltrate of Sweet syndrome lesions may also contain lymphocytes or histiocytes. In some patients with either idiopathic or drug-induced or malignancy-associated Sweet syndrome, the cutaneous lesions contain eosinophils. In some of the Sweet syndrome patients with hematologic disorders, abnormal neutrophils (leukemia cutis)—in addition to mature neutrophils—comprise the dermal infiltrate.[56-58]

Extracutaneous sites can also show pathologic findings of Sweet syndrome. They often, appear as sterile neutrophilic inflammation in the involved organ. These changes have been observed in the aorta, bones, intestines, liver, lungs, and muscles of patients with Sweet syndrome.[1,7]

IMAGING

Abnormalities on brain single-photon emission computed tomography, computerized axial tomography, electroencephalograms, and magnetic resonance imaging may be observed in patients with central nervous system involvement. In a 62-year-old man with Sweet syndrome, magnetic resonance imaging findings of dermatosis-associated neutrophilic fasciitis and musculoskeletal involvement were reported. Pleural effusions and corticosteroid-responsive culture-negative infiltrates on their chest roentgenograms may be noted in patients with pulmonary involvement.[1,59]

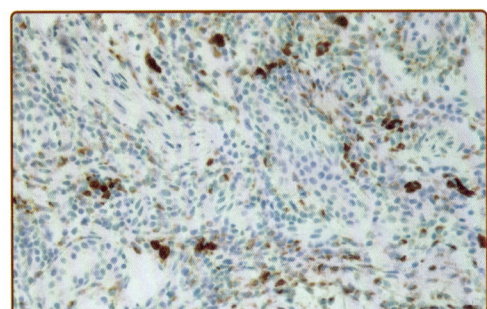

Figure 36-8 A high magnification view of the immunoperoxidase staining of the skin biopsy from the histiocytoid giant cellulitis Sweet syndrome shows positive staining of the CD68 (a histiocyte marker) cells comprising the dermal infiltrate. (From So JK, Carlos CA, Frucht CS, et al. Histiocytoid giant cellulitis-like Sweet's syndrome: case report and review of the literature. *Dermatol Online J.* 2015;21(3):4, with permission.)

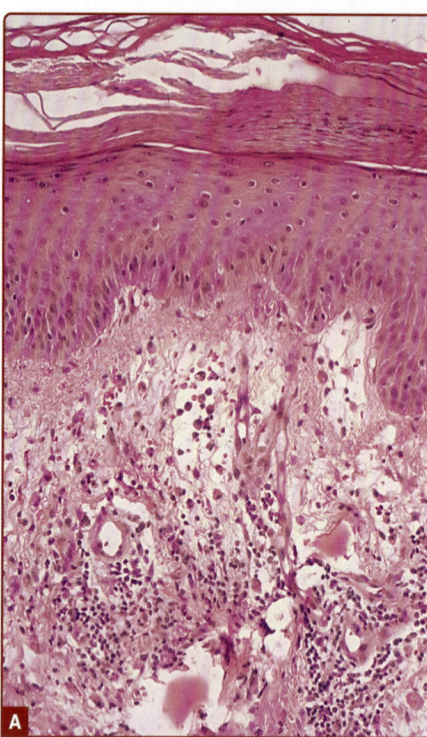 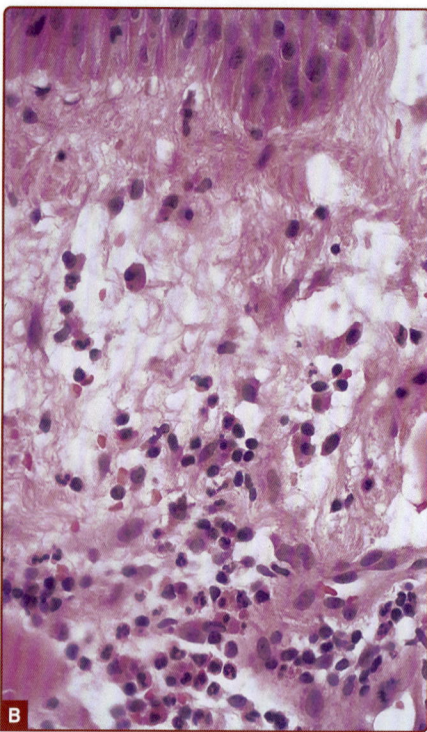

Figure 36-9 Characteristic histopathologic features of Sweet syndrome are observed at low (**A**) and high (**B**) magnification: papillary dermal edema, swollen endothelial cells, and a diffuse infiltrate of predominantly neutrophils with leukocytoclasia, yet no evidence of vasculitis (hematoxylin and eosin stain). (From Cohen PR, Holder WR, Rapini RP. Concurrent Sweet's syndrome and erythema nodosum: a report, world literature review and mechanism of pathogenesis. *J Rheumatol.* 1992;19:814-820, with permission.)

DIFFERENTIAL DIAGNOSIS

CLINICAL DIFFERENTIAL DIAGNOSIS

The skin and mucosal lesions of Sweet syndrome mimic those of other conditions (Table 36-8). The clinical differential diagnosis of Sweet syndrome includes infectious and inflammatory disorders, neoplastic conditions, reactive erythemas, vasculitis, other cutaneous conditions, and other systemic diseases.[1,7,47]

Patients with Behçet disease, similar to those with Sweet syndrome, may develop lesions at sites of trauma. An important differentiator between Sweet syndrome and Behçet disease is human leukocyte antigen analysis. In Japan, the B51 marker is significantly higher in Behçet disease, whereas the B54 marker is more frequently associated with Sweet syndrome.[60]

Other conditions in the clinical differential diagnosis of Sweet syndrome include azathioprine hypersensitivity reaction, chronic atypical neutrophilic dermatosis with lipodystrophy and elevated temperature (CANDLE) syndrome, and gemcitabine-associated Sweet syndrome-like eruptions. In addition, not only cellulitis and other infections, but also periodic syndromes (such as familial Mediterranean fever) can be included in the differential diagnosis of giant cellulitis-like Sweet syndrome. Therefore, biopsy of the skin lesion for histology, as well as tissue cultures, should be considered in individuals for whom this variant of Sweet syndrome is suspected.[18,61-63]

HISTOLOGIC DIFFERENTIAL DIAGNOSIS

The histologic differential diagnosis of Sweet syndrome includes conditions microscopically characterized by either neutrophilic dermatosis or neutrophilic panniculitis (Table 36-9). Because the pathologic changes associated with Sweet syndrome are similar to those observed in an abscess or cellulitis, culture of lesional tissue for bacteria, fungi, and mycobacteria should be considered to rule out infection. Leukemia cutis not only mimics the dermal changes of Sweet syndrome, but can potentially occur within the same skin lesion as Sweet syndrome; however, in contrast to the mature polymorphonuclear neutrophils found in Sweet syndrome, the dermal infiltrate in leukemia cutis consists of malignant immature leukocytes.[1,3,7]

The pathologic changes in the adipose tissue of subcutaneous Sweet syndrome lesions can be found either in the lobules, the septae, or both. Therefore, condi-

TABLE 36-8
Clinical Differential Diagnosis of Sweet Syndrome (Lane)

- Acral erythema
- Azathioprine hypersensitivity reaction
- Bacterial sepsis
- Behçet disease
- Bowel bypass syndrome
- Cellulitis
- Chloroma
- Chronic atypical neutrophilic dermatosis with lipodystrophy and elevated temperature (CANDLE) syndrome
- Dermatomyositis
- Drug eruptions
- Erysipelas
- Erythema elevatum diutinum
- Erythema multiforme
- Erythema nodosum
- Familial Mediterranean fever
- Gemcitabine-associated Sweet syndrome-like eruptions
- Granuloma faciale
- Halogenoderma
- Leprosy
- Leukemia cutis
- Leukocytoclastic vasculitis
- Lupus erythematosus
- Lymphangitis
- Lymphoma
- Metastatic tumor
- Neutrophilic eccrine hidradenitis
- Panniculitis
- Periarteritis nodosa
- Pyoderma gangrenosum
- Rheumatoid neutrophilic dermatitis
- Rosacea fulminans
- Schnitzler syndrome
- Syphilis
- Systemic mycosis
- Thrombophlebitis
- Tuberculosis
- Urticaria
- Viral exanthem

Adapted from Cohen PR, Kurzrock R: Sweet's syndrome and cancer. *Clin Dermatol.* 1993;11:149-157. Copyright © Elsevier.

tions characterized by a neutrophilic lobular panniculitis also need to always be considered and ruled out.[1,3]

The pathologic differential diagnosis of histiocytoid Sweet syndrome includes leukemia cutis and other inflammatory dermatoses histopathologically characterized by histiocytes interstitially arranged between dermal collagen bundles such as interstitial type of granuloma annulare, interstitial granulomatous dermatitis with arthritis, and methotrexate-induced rheumatoid papules.[18]

Arthropod bite reaction has also mimicked the pathologic changes observed in Sweet syndrome. Unrelated to the use of medication, the presence of eosinophils in Sweet syndrome may range from rare to abundant. Although a dense inflammatory infiltrate of neutrophils is characteristic of Sweet syndrome, sites of arthropod bites with abundant eosinophils and some neutrophils may be misinterpreted as the dermatosis.[16,64]

CLINICAL COURSE AND PROGNOSIS

In some patients with classical Sweet syndrome, the symptoms and lesions of the dermatosis eventually resolved without any therapeutic intervention. However, the lesions may persist for weeks to months. Successful management of the cancer occasionally results in clearing of the related dermatosis in patients with malignancy-associated Sweet syndrome. Similarly, spontaneous improvement and subsequent resolution

TABLE 36-9
Histologic Differential Diagnosis of Sweet Syndrome

- Abscess/cellulitis: Positive culture for infectious agent
- Arthropod bite reaction: History of exposure to arthropods
- Bowel (intestinal) bypass syndrome: History of jejunal-ileal bypass surgery for morbid obesity
- Erythema elevatum diutinum: Erythematous asymptomatic plaques often located on the dorsal hands and elbows; younger lesions have microscopic features of leukocytoclastic vasculitis, whereas older lesions have dermal fibrosis and mucin
- Granuloma faciale: Yellow-to-red-to-brown indurated asymptomatic facial plaques; there is a grenz zone of normal papillary dermis beneath which there is a dense diffuse inflammatory infiltrate of predominantly neutrophils (with microscopic features of leukocytoclastic vasculitis) and numerous eosinophils
- Halogenoderma: Neutrophilic dermal infiltrate with necrosis and pseudoepitheliomatous hyperplasia with intraepidermal abscesses; history of ingestion of bromides (leg lesions), iodides (facial lesions), or topical fluoride gel to teeth during tumor radiation therapy to face
- Leukemia cutis: Dermal infiltrate consists of immature neutrophils
- Leukocytoclastic vasculitis: Vessel wall destruction—extravasated erythrocytes, fibrinoid necrosis of vessel walls, karyorrhexis, and neutrophils in the vessel wall
- Lobular neutrophilic panniculitides: In addition to subcutaneous Sweet syndrome, these include α_1-antitrypsin deficiency syndrome, factitial panniculitis (secondary to the presence of iatrogenic or self-induced foreign bodies), infectious panniculitis (secondary to either a bacterial, fungal, mycobacterial, or protozoan organism), pancreatic panniculitis, rheumatoid arthritis–associated panniculitis
- Neutrophilic eccrine hidradenitis: Neutrophils around eccrine glands, often in patients with acute myelogenous leukemia receiving induction chemotherapy
- Neutrophilic urticarial dermatosis: An urticarial eruption demonstrating perivascular and interstitial neutrophilic infiltrate with intense leukocytoclasia, but without vasculitis and without dermal edema, that is often associated with a systemic disease such as Schnitzler syndrome, adult-onset Still disease, lupus erythematosus, and the hereditary autoinflammatory fever syndromes
- Pyoderma gangrenosum: Ulcer with overhanging, undermined violaceous edges
- Rheumatoid neutrophilic dermatitis: History of rheumatoid arthritis, nodules, and plaques

Adapted from Cohen PR: Paraneoplastic dermatopathology: cutaneous paraneoplastic syndromes. *Adv Dermatol.* 1995;11:215-252.

of the syndrome typically follows discontinuation of the associated medication in patients with drug-induced Sweet syndrome. In some of the patients who had associated tonsillitis, solid tumors, or renal failure, surgical intervention resulted in the resolution of Sweet syndrome.[1,7,12,47]

Following either spontaneous remission or therapy-induced clinical resolution, Sweet syndrome may recur. The duration of remission between recurrent episodes of the dermatosis is variable. In cancer patients, the reappearance of dermatosis-associated symptoms and lesions may represent a paraneoplastic syndrome that is signaling the return of the previously treated malignancy. Sweet syndrome recurrences are more common in this patient population.[1,7,47]

MANAGEMENT

MEDICATIONS

FIRST-LINE TREATMENTS

The therapeutic mainstay for Sweet syndrome is systemic corticosteroids (Table 36-10). Improvement of the symptoms and resolution of the mucocutaneous lesions promptly results after initiation of therapy. In patients with refractory disease, daily pulse methylprednisolone administered intravenously may be necessary. For treating localized Sweet syndrome lesions, topical (such as 0.05% clobetasol propionate) or intralesional (such as triamcinolone acetonide at a dose between 3.0 mg/cc and 10.0 mg/cc) corticosteroids may be effective.[1,7,12,17,34]

Other first-line systemic treatments for Sweet syndrome are potassium iodide and colchicine (see Table 36-10). Potential drug-induced side effects of potassium iodide include vasculitis and hypothyroidism. Gastrointestinal symptoms such as diarrhea, abdominal pain, nausea and vomiting are potential adverse effects from colchicine that may improve after lowering the daily dose of the drug.[1,7,34]

SECOND-LINE TREATMENTS

Indomethacin, clofazimine, cyclosporine, and dapsone are second-line systemic agents for Sweet syndrome (see Table 36-10). They have all been used as monotherapy after first-line therapies have failed or in the initial management of the patient. In addition, either as a corticosteroid-sparing agent or with other drugs, cyclosporine and dapsone have been used in combination therapy.[1,7,34]

ANTIBIOTICS

In some patients, Sweet syndrome lesions have improved after receiving systemic antibiotics. These patients not only include individuals with *Staphylococcus aureus* secondarily impetiginized lesions treated with an antimicrobial agent to which their bacterial strain is susceptible and patients with inflammatory bowel disease treated with metronidazole, but also persons with dermatosis-related *Yersinia* or *Chlamydia* infection treated with either doxycycline, minocycline, or tetracycline.[1,7,34]

TABLE 36-10
Systemic Treatments for Sweet Syndrome

LINE	MEDICATION	DOSE
First	Prednisone	1 mg/kg/day (usually ranging from 30 mg-60 mg) as a single, oral, morning dose. Within 4-6 weeks, taper dose to 10 mg/day; however some patients may require 2-3 months of treatment or intravenous therapy.
	Methylprednisolone sodium succinate	Intravenously administered (up to 1000 mg/day) over 1 or more hours, daily for 3-5 days. This is followed by a tapering oral dose of corticosteroid or another immunosuppressant agent.
	Potassium iodide	Administered orally as 300 mg enteric-coated tablets, TID (for a daily dose of 900 mg) or as a saturated solution (1 g/mL of water) of potassium iodide (SSKI; also referred to as Lugol's solution), beginning at a dose of 3 drops TID (9 drops/day = 450 mg/day) and increasing by 1 drop TID, typically to a final dose of 21 drops/day (1050 mg) to 30 drops/day (1500 mg).[a]
	Colchicine	Administered orally at a dose of 0.5 mg TID (for a daily dose of 1.5 mg).
Second	Indomethacin	Administered at an oral daily dose of 150 mg for 7 days, and then 100 mg/day for 14 days.
	Clofazimine	Administered orally at a daily dose of 200 mg for 4 weeks, and then 100 mg/day for 4 weeks.
	Cyclosporine	Administered as monotherapy or as a second-line agent (after failure of first-line therapy or as a corticosteroid-sparing agent). Initial oral daily dose ranges from 2 mg/kg/day to 4 mg/kg/day to 10 mg/kg/day.
	Dapsone	Administered as either monotherapy or in combination therapy. Initial oral dose ranges from 100 mg/day to 200 mg/day; the latter dose is either administered as a single dose or divided into 2 equal doses.

[a]When a "standard" medicine dropper (which dispenses 20 drops per mL) is used, 1 drop = 0.05 mL (or 50 mg when the concentration of potassium iodide is 1000 mg/mL).

From Cohen PR, Kurzrock R: Sweet's syndrome revisited: a review of disease concepts. *Int J Dermatol.* 2003;42:761-778, with permission.

OTHER AGENTS

In addition, predominantly in case reports, effective treatment of Sweet syndrome also has been described with other drugs, such as antineoplastic therapies (azacitidine, chlorambucil, cyclophosphamide, and rituximab), danazol, etretinate, hepatitis therapy, immunoglobulin, IFN-α, and tumor necrosis factors antagonists (adalimumab, etanercept, infliximab, and thalidomide).[7,34,51,65,66] Anakinra (an IL-1 receptor antagonist) in combination with oral prednisone was promptly effective in resolving the symptoms, and subsequently the clinical lesions, of Sweet syndrome in a patient with longstanding disease that was refractory to other therapies; it also resulted in dramatic clinical and biologic improvement in a 66-year-old man who had a 5-year history of Sweet syndrome that was refractory to various conventional treatments.[67,68] Pentoxifylline was hypothesized to be beneficial for treating Sweet syndrome; however, when used as monotherapy, it was not found to be efficacious.[2] Some of the drugs used for the treatment of Sweet syndrome, such as azacitidine, minocycline, and the tumor necrosis factor-inhibitors adalimumab, etanercept, infliximab, and lenalidomide, also have been observed to elicit the condition.[1,7,34,55]

MALIGNANCY WORKUP

In 1993, Cohen and Kurzrock proposed recommendations for the initial malignancy workup in newly diagnosed Sweet syndrome patients without a prior cancer. Their recommendations were based on the neoplasms that had concurrently been present or subsequently developed in previously cancer-free Sweet syndrome patients and the age-related recommendations of the American Cancer Society for early detection of cancer in asymptomatic persons. The recommendations included: (a) a detailed medical history; (b) a complete physical examination, including: (i) examination of the thyroid, lymph nodes, oral cavity, and skin; (ii) digital rectal examination; (iii) breast, ovary, and pelvic examination in women; and (iv) prostate and testicle examination in men; (c) laboratory evaluation: (i) carcinoembryonic antigen level; (ii) complete blood cell count with leukocyte differential and platelet count; (iii) pap test in women; (iv) serum chemistries; (v) stool guaiac slide test; (vi) urinalysis; and (vii) urine culture; and (d) other screening tests: (i) chest roentgenograms; (ii) endometrial tissue sampling in either menopausal women or women with a history of abnormal uterine bleeding, estrogen therapy, failure to ovulate, infertility, or obesity; and (iii) sigmoidoscopy in patients older than 50 years of age. Cohen and Kurzrock also suggested that it was reasonable to check a complete blood cell count with leukocyte differential and platelet count every 6 to 12 months as the initial appearance of dermatosis-related skin lesions had been reported to precede the diagnosis of a Sweet syndrome–associated hematologic malignancy by as long as 11 years.[1,47]

REFERENCES

1. Cohen PR. Sweet's syndrome—a comprehensive review of an acute febrile neutrophilic dermatosis. *Orphanet J Rare Dis.* 2007;2:34.
2. Cohen PR. Skin lesions of Sweet syndrome and its dorsal hand variant contain vasculitis: an oxymoron or an epiphenomenon? *Arch Dermatol.* 2002;138:400-403.
3. Cohen PR. Subcutaneous Sweet's syndrome: a variant of acute febrile neutrophilic dermatosis that is included in the histologic differential diagnosis of neutrophilic panniculitis. *J Am Acad Dermatol.* 2005;52:927-928.
4. Amouri M, Masmoudi A, Ammar M, et al. Sweet's syndrome: a retrospective study of 90 cases from a tertiary care center. *Int J Dermatol.* 2016;55(9):1033-1039.
5. Villarreal-Villarreal CD, Ocampo-Candiani J, Villarreal-Martinez A. Sweet syndrome: a review and update. *Actas Dermosifiliogr.* 2016;107:369-378.
6. Rochet NM, Chavan RN, Cappel MA, et al. Sweet syndrome: clinical presentation, associations, and response to treatment in 77 patients. *J Am Acad Dermatol.* 2013; 69:557-564.
7. Anzalone CL, Cohen PR. Acute febrile neutrophilic dermatosis (Sweet's syndrome). *Curr Opin Hematol.* 2013;20:26-35.
8. Qiao J, Wang Y, Bai J, et al. Concurrence of Sweet's syndrome, pathergy phenomenon and erythema nodosum-like lesions. *An Bras Dermatol.* 2015;90: 237-239.
9. Chu CH, Cheng YP, Kao HL, et al. Lymphedema-associated neutrophilic dermatosis: two cases of localized Sweet syndrome on the lymphedematous lower limbs. *J Dermatol.* 2016;43(9):1062-1066.
10. Ainechi S, Carlson JA. Neutrophilic dermatosis limited to lipo-lymphedematous skin in a morbidly obese woman on dasatinib therapy. *Am J Dermatopathol.* 2016;38:e22-e26.
11. Endo Y, Tanioka M, Tanizaki H, et al. Bullous variant of Sweet's syndrome after herpes zoster virus infection. *Case Rep Dermatol.* 2011;3:259-262.
12. Walker DC, Cohen PR. Trimethoprim-sulfamethoxazole-associated acute febrile neutrophilic dermatosis: case report and review of drug-induced Sweet's syndrome. *J Am Acad Dermatol.* 1996;34:918-923.
13. Sommer S, Wilkinson SM, Merchant WJ, et al. Sweet's syndrome presenting as palmoplantar pustulosis. *J Am Acad Dermatol.* 2000;42:332-334.
14. Sarkany RPE, Burrows NP, Grant JW, et al. The pustular eruption of ulcerative colitis: a variant of Sweet's syndrome [letter]. *Br J Dermatol.* 1998;138:365-366.
15. Kaur S, Gupta D, Garg B, et al. Neutrophilic dermatosis of dorsal hands. *Indian Dermatol Online J.* 2015;6(1):42-45.
16. Rochael MC, Pantaleão L, Vilar EA, et al. Sweet's syndrome: study of 73 cases, emphasizing histopathological findings. *An Bras Dermatol.* 2011;86:702-707.
17. Cohen PR, Holder WR, Rapini RP. Concurrent Sweet's syndrome and erythema nodosum: a report, world literature review and mechanism of pathogenesis. *J Rheumatol.* 1992;19:814-820.
18. So JK, Carlos CA, Frucht CS, et al. Histiocytoid giant cellulitis-like Sweet's syndrome: case report and review of the literature. *Dermatol Online J.* 2015;21(3):4.
19. Ghoufi L, Ortonne N, Ingen-Housz-Oro S, et al. Histiocytoid Sweet syndrome is more frequently associated with myelodysplastic syndromes than the

classical neutrophilic variant: a comparative series of 62 patients. *Medicine (Baltimore)*. 2016;95:e3033.
20. Surovy AM, Pelivani N, Hegyi I, et al. Giant cellulitis-like Sweet Syndrome, a new variant of neutrophilic dermatosis. *JAMA Dermatol*. 2013;149:79-83.
21. Kaminska EC, Nwaneshiudu AI, Ruiz de Luzuriaga A, et al. Giant cellulitis-like Sweet syndrome in the setting of autoimmune disease. *J Am Acad Dermatol*. 2014;71:e94-e95.
22. Koketsu H, Ricotti C, Kerdel FA. Treatment of giant cellulitis-like Sweet syndrome with dapsone. *JAMA Dermatol*. 2014;150:457-459.
23. Kroshinsky D, Alloo A, Rothschild B, et al. Necrotizing Sweet syndrome: a new variant of neutrophilic dermatosis mimicking necrotizing fasciitis. *J Am Acad Dermatol*. 2012;67(5):945-954.
24. Ma EH, Akikusa JD, Macgregor D, et al. Sweet's syndrome with postinflammatory elastolysis and Takayasu arteritis in a child: a case report and literature review. *Pediatr Dermatol*. 2012;29(5):645-650.
25. Timmer-DE Mik L, Broekhuijsen-VAN Henten DM, Oldhoff JM, et al. Acquired cutis laxa in childhood Sweet's syndrome. *Pediatr Dermatol*. 2009;26:358-360.
26. Acikel S, Sari M, Akdemir R. The relationship between acute coronary syndrome and inflammation: a case of acute myocardial infarction associated with coronary involvement of Sweet's syndrome. *Blood Coagul Fibrinolysis*. 2010;21:703-706.
27. Wallett A, Newland K, Foster-Smith E. Radiation therapy-induced neuro-Sweet disease in a patient with oral squamous cell carcinoma. *Australas J Dermatol*. 2017;58(2):e51-e53.
28. Niwa F, Tokuda T, Kimura M, et al. Self-remitting and reversible parkinsonism associated with neuro-Sweet disease. *Intern Med*. 2010;49:1201-1204.
29. Lobo AM, Stacy R, Cestari D, et al. Optic nerve involvement with panuveitis in Sweet syndrome. *Ocul Immunol Inflamm*. 2011;19:167-170.
30. Sinawat S, Yospaiboon Y, Sinawat S. Bilateral endogenous endophthalmitis in disseminated NTM infection: a case report. *J Med Assoc Thai*. 2011;94:632-636.
31. Cheng S, da Cruz M. Sweet's disease and profound, bilateral, sensorineural hearing loss. *J Laryngol Otol*. 2010;124:105-107.
32. Fortna RR, Toporcer M, Elder DE, et al. A case of sweet syndrome with spleen and lymph node involvement preceded by parvovirus B19 infection, and a review of the literature on extracutaneous sweet syndrome. *Am J Dermatopathol*. 2010;32:621-627.
33. Solana-Lopez G, Llamas-Velasco M, Concha-Garzon MJ, et al. Sweet syndrome and differentiation syndrome in a patient with acute promyelocytic leukemia. *World J Clin Cases*. 2015;3:196-198.
34. Cohen PR. Neutrophilic dermatoses. a review of current treatment options. *Am J Clin Dermatol*. 2009;10:301-312.
35. Ajili F, Souissi A, Bougrine F, et al. Coexistence of pyoderma gangrenosum and sweet's syndrome in a patient with ulcerative colitis. *Pan Afr Med J*. 2015;21:151.
36. Vanourny J, Swick BL. Sweet syndrome with systemic inflammatory response syndrome. *Arch Dermatol*. 2012;148:969-970.
37. Shugarman IL, Schmit JM, Sbicca JA, et al. Easily missed extracutaneous manifestation of malignancy-associated Sweet's syndrome: systemic inflammatory response syndrome. *J Clin Oncol*. 2011;29(24):e702-e705.
38. Nesterovitch AB, Gyorfy Z, Hoffman MD, et al. Alteration in the gene encoding protein tyrosine phosphatase nonreceptor type 6 (PTPN6/SHP1) may contribute to neutrophilic dermatoses. *Am J Pathol*. 2011;178:1434-1441.
39. Johnson CS, May ER, Myers RK, et al. Extracutaneous neutrophilic inflammation in a dog with lesions resembling Sweet's Syndrome. *Vet Dermatol*. 2009;20:200-205.
40. Gains MJ, Morency A, Sauvé F, et al. Canine sterile neutrophilic dermatitis (resembling Sweet's syndrome) in a Dachshund. *Can Vet J*. 2010;51:1397-1399.
41. Omoya K, Naiki Y, Kato Z, et al. Sweet's syndrome in a neonate with non-B54 types of human leukocyte antigen. *World J Pediatr*. 2012;8:181-184.
42. Marzano AV, Cugno M, Trevisan V, et al. Inflammatory cells, cytokines and matrix metalloproteinases in amicrobial pustulosis of the folds and other neutrophilic dermatoses. *Int J Immunopathol Pharmacol*. 2011;24451-24460.
43. Saeed M, Brown GE, Agarwal A, et al. Autoimmune clustering: sweet syndrome, Hashimoto thyroiditis, and psoriasis. *J Clin Rheumatol*. 2011;17:76-78.
44. Pai VV, Gupta G, Athanikar S, et al. Photoinduced classic sweet syndrome presenting as hemorrhagic bullae. *Cutis*. 2014;93:E22-E24.
45. Meyer V, Schneider SW, Bonsmann G, et al. Experimentally confirmed induction of Sweet's syndrome by phototesting. *Acta Derm Venereol*. 2011;91:720-721.
46. Natkunarajah J, Gordon K, Chow J, et al. Photoaggravated Sweet's syndrome. *Clin Exp Dermatol*. 2010;35:18-19.
47. Cohen PR, Kurzrock R. Sweet's syndrome and cancer. *Clin Dermatol*. 1993;11:149-157.
48. Parsapour K, Reep MD, Gohar K, et al. Familial Sweet's syndrome in 2 brothers, both seen in the first 2 weeks of life. *J Am Acad Dermatol*. 2003;49:132-138.
49. Gray PE, Bock V, Ziegler DS, et al. Neonatal Sweet syndrome: a potential marker of serious systemic illness. *Pediatrics*. 2012;129:e1353-e1359.
50. Kazmi SM, Pemmaraju N, Patel KP, et al. Characteristics of Sweet syndrome in patients with acute myeloid leukemia. *Clin Lymphoma Myeloma Leuk*. 2015;15:358-363.
51. Calixto R, Menezes Y, Ostronoff M, et al. Favorable outcome of severe, extensive, granulocyte colony-stimulating factor-induced, corticosteroid-resistant Sweet's syndrome treated with high-dose intravenous immunoglobulin. *J Clin Oncol*. 2014;32(5):e1-e2.
52. McNally A, Ibbetson J, Sidhu S. Azathioprine-induced Sweet's syndrome: a case series and review of the literature. *Australas J Dermatol*. 2017;58(1):53-57.
53. Cohen PR. Proton pump inhibitor-induced Sweet's syndrome: report of acute febrile neutrophilic dermatosis in a woman with recurrent breast cancer. *Dermatol Pract Concept*. 2015;5:113-119.
54. Yorio JT, Mays SR, Ciurea AM, et al. Case of vemurafenib-induced Sweet's syndrome. *J Dermatol*. 2014;41:817-820.
55. Kalai C, Brand R, Yu L. Minocycline-induced Sweet syndrome (acute febrile neutrophilic dermatosis). *J Am Acad Dermatol*. 2012;67:e289-e291.
56. Vignon-Pennamen MD, Jullard C, Rybojad M, et al. Chronic recurrent lymphocytic Sweet's syndrome as a predictive marker of myelodysplasia: a report of 9 cases. *Arch Dermatol*. 2006;142:1170-1176.
57. Kakaletsis N, Kaiafa G, Savo[poulos C, et al. Initially lymphocytic Sweet's syndrome in male patients with myelodysplasia: a distinguished clinicopathological

entity? Case report and systematic review of the literature. *Acta Haematol.* 2014;132:220-225.
58. Soon CW, Kirsch IR, Connolly AJ, et al. Eosinophilic-rich acute febrile neutrophilic dermatosis in a patient with enteropathy-associated T-cell lymphoma, type 1. *Am J Dermatopathol.* 2016;38(9):704-708.
59. Gaeta M, Mileto A, Musumeci O, et al. MRI findings of neutrophilic fasciitis in a patient with acute febrile neutrophilic dermatosis (Sweet's syndrome). *Skeletal Radiol.* 2011;40:779-782.
60. Takahama H, Kanbe T. Neutrophilic dermatosis of the dorsal hands: a case showing HLA B54, the marker of Sweet's syndrome. *Int J Dermatol.* 2010;49:1079-1080.
61. Bidinger JJ, Sky K, Battafarano DF, Henning JS. The cutaneous and systemic manifestations of azathioprine hypersensitivity syndrome. *J Am Acad Dermatol.* 2011;65:184-191.
62. Cavalcanate MF, Brunelli JB, Miranda CC, et al. CANDLE syndrome: chronic atypical neutrophilic dermatosis with lipodystrophy and elevated temperature—a rare case with a novel mutation. *Eur J Pediatr.* 2016;175:735-740.
63. Martorell-Calatayud A, Requena C, Sanmartin O, et al. Gemcitabine-associated sweet syndrome-like eruption. *J Am Acad Dermatol.* 2011;65:1236-1238.
64. Battistella M, Bourrat E, Fardet L, et al. Sweet-like reaction due to arthropod bites: a histopathologic pitfall. *Am J Dermatopathol.* 2012;34:442-445.
65. Hashemi SM, Fazeli SA, Vahedi A, et al. Rituximab for refractory subcutaneous Sweet's syndrome in chronic lymphocytic leukemia: a case report. *Mol Clin Oncol.* 2016;4:436-440.
66. Agarwal A, Barrow W, Selim MA, et al. Refractory subcutaneous Sweet syndrome treated with adalimumab. *JAMA Dermatol.* 2016;152(7):842-844.
67. Delluc A, Limal N, Puechal X, et al. Efficacy of anakinra, an IL1 receptor antagonist, in refractory Sweet syndrome. *Ann Rheum Dis.* 2008;67:278-279.
68. Kluger N, Gil-Bistes D, Guillot B, et al. Efficacy of anti-interleukin-1 receptor antagonist anakinra (Kineret) in a case of refractory Sweet's syndrome. *Dermatology.* 2011;222:123-127.

Chapter 37 :: Pyoderma Gangrenosum
:: Natanel Jourabchi & Gerald S. Lazarus

第三十七章
坏疽性脓皮病

中文导读

本章从疾病的历史及流行病学史、临床表现、病因及发病机制、诊断及治疗七个方面全面讲述坏疽性脓皮病（PG）。首先对PG进行了疾病定义以及流行病学的介绍，随后提到了PG多伴随一些系统性疾病，尤其是炎症性肠病。本章重点介绍了PG的临床特征。介绍了PG可以分为溃疡型、水疱型、脓疱型、浅表肉芽肿型四种类型。并对这四种类型给出了详细的图文介绍，让大家对于PG的皮损表现有一个直观的了解。在诊断方面，本章具体介绍了该病的诊断标准。

〔李芳芳〕

AT-A-GLANCE

- Pyoderma gangrenosum (PG) is an uncommon, neutrophilic inflammatory skin condition, which classically presents as a painful nodule, plaque, or pustule that enlarges and breaks down to form a progressively enlarging ulcer with raised, undermined, violaceous borders and a surrounding zone of erythema. Healing PG lesions develop a cribriform appearance.

- PG tends to occur and recur in areas of trauma because of the pathergic phenomenon, where trauma or irritation can induce flaring of PG.

- PG most often occurs in association with systemic inflammation, and most reported cases have an associated underlying disease (such as inflammatory bowel disease, monoclonal gammopathy, hematologic disease, inflammatory arthritis, malignancy, hidradenitis suppurativa, etc); however, PG may precede these disorders. PG has also been reported in association with genetic mutations and syndromes, such as the pyogenic arthritis, pyoderma gangrenosum, and acne (PAPA) syndrome, or without an identifiable underlying disease.

- PG most commonly presents as the classic ulcerative variant, but may also arise as bullous, pustular, or vegetative variants. Clinical features of different variants sometimes overlap in individual patients but usually one variant dominates the clinical picture.

- There is no laboratory test or investigation that establishes the diagnosis of PG with certainty. The histopathologic findings are not diagnostic but can be supportive of the diagnosis of PG in the appropriate clinical setting and are essential to rule out alternative diagnoses.

- Specified criteria (see "Diagnostic Algorithm" section) suggest the diagnosis of PG, but other conditions (particularly infection, vascular disease, and malignancy) must be excluded.

- The mainstays of management are systemic immunosuppressive agents together with appropriate local and topical therapy.

- Classic ulcerative PG is a chronic condition. Complete healing usually requires months of treatment; maintenance therapy is necessary in many and relapses are common. Significant morbidity and mortality are experienced by patients with ulcerative and bullous PG.

DEFINITIONS

Pyoderma gangrenosum (PG) is an uncommon, chronic, neutrophilic inflammatory skin condition, with the classic ulcerative variant typically presenting initially as a painful nodule, plaque, or pustule that enlarges and breaks down to form a progressively enlarging ulcer with raised, undermined, violaceous borders and a surrounding zone of erythema.[1,2] The lesions are commonly very painful, develop a cribriform appearance with healing, and tend to occur and recur in areas of trauma in up to 50% of cases.[1,2] PG is believed to occur in association with systemic inflammation, and most reported cases are associated with autoinflammatory or hematologic conditions, and typically respond to immune suppression.[1,3-5] PG most commonly presents as the classic ulcerative variant, but may also present as bullous, pustular, or vegetative variants. Unless otherwise specified, when we refer to PG in this text, we are referring to the classic ulcerative variant.

EPIDEMIOLOGY

PG is estimated to affect up to 10 cases per million people per year, and represents up to 3% of chronic leg ulcer cases, but may occur anywhere on the body. PG has been reported in people of all ages; most cases, however, present in the second to sixth decades of life, with a possible female predominance.[2,6]

DISEASE ASSOCIATIONS

Up to 70% of reported PG cases are associated with a known underlying systemic disease, such as inflammatory bowel disease (IBD), monoclonal gammopathy, hematologic disease, inflammatory arthritis, malignancy, hidradenitis suppurativa, and others, even though PG may precede these disorders. PG also has been associated with genetic mutations, as part of a genetic syndrome such as the pyogenic arthritis, PG, and acne (PAPA) syndrome, or without an identifiable underlying disorder.[7]

Nearly one-third of PG cases are associated with IBD, with similar frequency of both Crohn disease and ulcerative colitis (UC), although most of the Crohn disease cases have colonic involvement.[3,8] Paraproteinemia (monoclonal gammopathy) is seen in 10% of PG cases,[9] most commonly immunoglobulin A monoclonal gammopathy.[10] Hematologic malignancy has been seen in up to 7% of PG cases, with the most common subtype reported being acute myeloid leukemia, and most cases of leukemia being preceded by an hematologic abnormality such as myelodysplastic syndrome.[1,11] Myeloproliferative diseases, such as polycythemia vera,[12] essential thrombocythemia,[13] and myelofibrosis (agnogenic myeloid metaplasia),[14,15] as well as leukemoid reaction,[16] also have been associated with PG. There also have been fewer reports of PG associated with Hodgkin and non-Hodgkin lymphomas, cutaneous T-cell lymphoma, and solid neoplasms originating in the breast, ovaries, bladder, prostate, colon, carcinoid, and bronchus,[9,17] although the significance of these less-frequent associations is less certain.

There also are reports of medications inducing PG, including several cases of PG associated with granulocyte colony-stimulating factor (G-CSF), which resolved after G-CSF was discontinued.[18]

CLINICAL FEATURES

CUTANEOUS FINDINGS

PG can be classified morphologically as being (a) ulcerative, (b) bullous, (c) pustular, or (d) vegetative. Although some patients may show more than 1 variant (eg, isolated pustular lesions frequently occur in patients with ulcerative PG), usually 1 variant of PG dominates the clinical picture and the patient should be classified accordingly.

Ulcerative PG is the most common and originally described variant of PG. The most common initial clinical lesion in a patient with ulcerative PG is an intensely painful erythematous papule, pustule, or nodular furuncle (these lesions are usually single but may be multiple). They erupt on apparently normal-looking skin, with the most common site being the leg. The enlarging initial lesion develops a surrounding zone of erythema that extends into the surrounding skin. As it enlarges, the center degenerates, necroses, and erodes, converting it into an eroding ulcer (Fig. 37-1), the development of which is accompanied by an alarming increase in pain. The ulcer often has a bluish/violaceous undermined edge and the base is covered with purulent necrotic material. Ulcerative PG may erode deeply with exposure of muscle or tendon in some cases.[1,2] PG can also occur at the site of trauma or surgery (Fig. 37-2), which is known as the pathergic phenomenon, where trauma or irritation can induce exaggerated flaring of PG.[1,2]

Bullous PG (sometimes called *atypical PG*) presents as a painful, rapidly expanding superficial inflammatory blister that quickly erodes. In the early acute stage, the bullous nature of the lesion is evident, but because the roof of the blister necroses rapidly, close inspection of the border of established lesions is necessary to reveal its bullous nature (Fig. 37-3). Bullous PG is commonly associated with hematologic disease and most often appears on the upper limbs.[19] This variant of PG may show clinical and histologic overlap with Sweet syndrome (one of the neutrophilic dermatoses which is itself often associated with hematologic disease).

Pustular PG (also called the *pustular eruption of IBD*) is a generalized eruption that occurs almost exclusively in the setting of an exacerbation of acute IBD (usually UC). Its onset is dramatic, with the rapid development

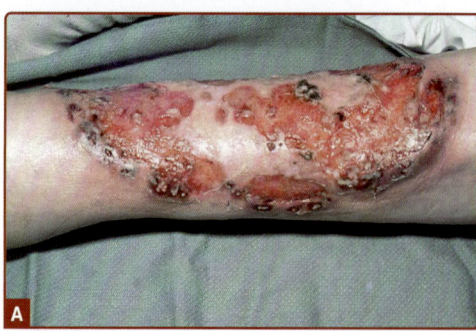
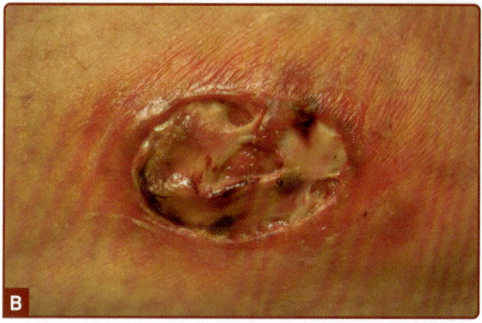

Figure 37-1 **A, B,** Established lesion of classic ulcerative pyoderma gangrenosum showing well-defined ulceration, undermining, and surrounding zone of erythema.

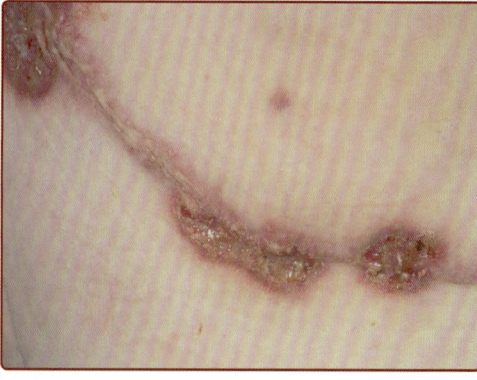

Figure 37-2 Pathergic pyoderma gangrenosum lesions occurring along a thoracotomy scar site. Note central ulceration, violaceous borders, and peripheral rim of erythema.

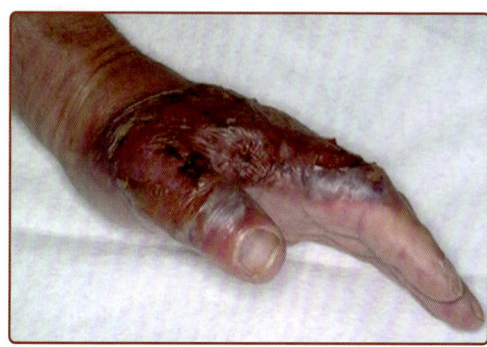

Figure 37-3 Bullous pyoderma gangrenosum lesion showing collapsed roof of blister and superficial erosive quality of the subsequent ulceration.

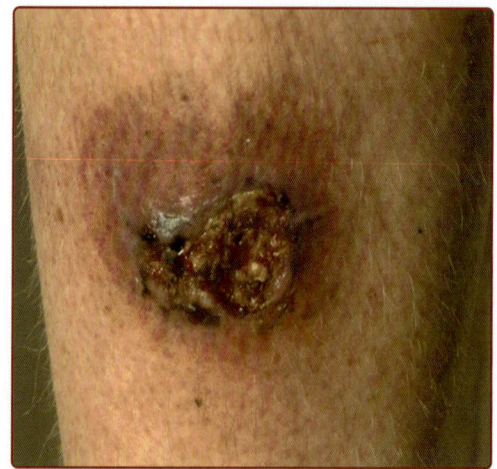

Figure 37-4 Vegetative pyoderma gangrenosum—an indolent area of chronic inflammation and ulceration that was present for months.

of multiple, large, circular-to-oval, painful pustules on the trunk and, to a lesser extent, the face and limbs. Control of this eruption is difficult without controlling the bowel disease, which may require resection of diseased bowel in some cases.[1,2]

Vegetative PG (or *superficial granulomatous pyoderma*) usually presents as a single furunculoid nodule, abscess, plaque, or superficial ulcer, typically on the trunk (Fig. 37-4). In contrast to the other variants, this uncommon variant is gradual in its onset, mild in the discomfort it generates, and not usually associated with the presence of systemic disease. This form of PG is usually more responsive to localized or mild forms of systemic therapy than the other variants.[20]

Postoperative and *parastomal* PG are considered to be examples of ulcerative PG demonstrating the pathergic phenomenon.[1,2]

NONCUTANEOUS FINDINGS

As the majority of PG cases are associated with, or precede, a concurrent underlying systemic disease, a thorough history and physical examination is mandatory with a particular search for clinical and biologic markers of IBD, inflammatory arthritis, hematologic disease (monoclonal gammopathy and other dyscrasias), hematologic malignancy, and internal malignancy. Additionally, The clinician should be aware that sterile neutrophilic infiltration of internal organs (lung, bone joints, CNS, cardiovascular system, intraabdominal viscera, eye) can occur in association with or even precede the onset of cutaneous PG.[21]

COMPLICATIONS

Active or poorly controlled cutaneous PG causes significant morbidity, including severe pain, loss of mobility, anemia of chronic disease, and complications from therapeutic interventions. Many of the treatments for PG must be administered for many months and may have significant side effects. For example, corticosteroids can induce or worsen diabetes, cyclosporine can induce or worsen renal dysfunction, and immunotherapy can lead to immunocompromise, which increases risk for infection by both common and atypical microorganisms. Consequently, close monitoring and followup of patients is necessary.

Care must be taken to avoid trauma to the skin and elective surgery should be undertaken with caution because of the possibility of inducing new PG lesions through the pathergic phenomenon. Additionally, lack of recognition of the neutrophilic infiltration of internal organs in PG can lead to unnecessary surgical procedures.[1,22]

ETIOLOGY AND PATHOGENESIS

The etiology of PG is unknown, its pathogenesis is poorly understood, and the mechanisms of its pathophysiology likely differ depending on the associated underlying contributory disease. The factors predisposing to, inciting, and regulating these abnormalities are likely multifactorial, including genetic predisposition, paraimmune and/or paraneoplastic phenomena,[7] which may cause increased sensitivity to, or increased activity of, the immune response and inflammation.

Interestingly, PG occurs in association with a broad spectrum of diseases, and yet they all lead to or associate with the common phenotype of PG, lending to the hypothesis that these diseases somehow converge on inflammatory pathways leading to aberrant neutrophil activity and function.[23] Despite this similarity, there is variation in reports of the association between the disease activity of PG and that of the underlying disease state. In the setting of IBD, PG activity classically has been associated with the inflammatory process in the bowel. According to the systematic review of Agarwal et al,[8] which included 60 patients, of whom 35 (58%) had active IBD and only 9 (15%) had inactive IBD at PG diagnosis (16 (27%) with IBD activity unspecified). While some have reported no apparent association between exacerbations of bowel disease with worsening of the skin lesions,[24,25] there are multiple reports demonstrating healing of PG following therapy for the diseased bowel. Powell et al[12] reported a case series where PG lesions improved in all of 9 patients with UC following total proctocolectomy, and Talansky et al[26] reported prompt PG skin healing within 2 months after resection of diseased bowel in 3 patients with severe ileocolitis, 1 with severe UC and 1 with moderate UC. Notably, there also has been a case of PG reported in a patient with UC 10 years after proctocolectomy,[9] which raises the question of whether there was any remaining diseased bowel.

Improvement of bullous PG has been reported after treatment and remission of acute myeloid leukemia,[27] which may be partially explained by the presence of a leukemic cell infiltrate consisting of atypical myeloblasts discovered within a PG skin sample from a patient with acute myeloid leukemia.[28] Complete recovery of PG has been reported after successful treatment of underlying hairy cell leukemia with cladribine.[29] Successful treatment of refractory PG associated with renal cell carcinoma has been reported with ustekinumab, but only after excision of the carcinoma.[30]

INFLAMMATORY MEDIATORS AND ABERRANT NEUTROPHIL ACTIVITY

T cells may be important in the development of PG through various mechanisms, including cytokine signaling and antigenic stimulus,[31] and are likely involved in some of the of the observed aberrant neutrophil activity. Marzano et al[32] looked at lesional skin biopsies from 21 patients with PG and found wound edge infiltrates of predominately CD3+ T cells and CD163+ macrophages, along with increased tumor necrosis factor-α (TNF-α), interleukin (IL)-8 (potent neutrophil chemotactic agent), IL-17 (proinflammatory cytokine; stimulates the expression of IL-8 and G-CSF), matrix metalloproteinase (MMP)-2/MMP-9 (collagenase mediating tissue damage) in the wound bed.

Based on the presence of a lymphocytic infiltrate at the active advancing border of PG lesions, it has been postulated that lymphocytic antigen activation occurs with cytokine release and neutrophil recruitment. This may take place not only in the skin but also in other tissues, such as the lung, intestine, and joints.[33] Neutrophils are thought to play a significant role in PG based on the prominent neutrophil-rich dermal infiltrate in PG pathology specimens, and PG response to antineutrophil medications like dapsone. Multiple studies have reported abnormalities in neutrophil chemotaxis, signaling, and trafficking in patients with PG.[4,34,35] These neutrophil abnormalities, and the predominance of neutrophils on histology, also give PG a place among the broader spectrum of neutrophilic dermatoses, which include Sweet syndrome (acute febrile neutrophilic dermatosis), Behçet disease, dermatitis herpetiformis, and neutrophilic eccrine hidradenitis. Besides dermal neutrophilia, other common features these conditions share include an associated underlying disorder, similarities in treatment, and a tendency for pathergy, in some more than others (PG, Sweets, Behçet, dermatitis herpetiformis).[7]

TNF-α plays an important role in production of proinflammatory cytokines, including IL-1, IL-6, IL-8, and interferon-γ, and has been shown to stimulate and enhance neutrophil degranulation and superoxide production.[36-38] TNF-α, IL-6, and soluble IL-2 receptor elevation has been reported in a patient with PG, with serum levels correlating with ulcer activity.[39] In addition to being increased in PG, IL-8 also has been shown to cause similar ulceration in human skin xenografts transfected with recombinant human IL-8.[40] Guenova et al[41] found elevated expression of IL-23 by polymerase chain reaction in a PG lesion compared with normal skin, which is significant because IL-23 plays an important role in driving inflammation associated with IL-17 production and neutrophil recruitment. Additionally, patients with the PAPA syndrome and some variants have been found to have increased production of IL-1β and IL-18.[42,43]

GENETICS

Uncovering genetic associations with PG is important as it can provide a better understanding of the pathophysiology of PG and help elucidate new targets for treatment. PG has been reported in association with systemic diseases, genetic mutations and syndromes, or in isolation. The systematic review of syndromes and genetic mutations associated with PG by DeFilippis et al[44] included 823 cases of PG, and revealed 31 (3.8%) cases of PAPA syndrome and its variants, 2 (0.2%) patients with mutations in Janus kinase (JAK) 2, 3 (0.4%) patients with mutations in methylenetetrahydrofolate reductase (MTHFR) who developed PG-like ulcerations, and 14 (1.7%) familial cases with no specific reported mutations, in addition to cases associated with IBD, polyarthritis, and hematologic disease.

The PAPA syndrome, which is an autosomal dominant disorder, has been linked to mutations in the proline-serine-threonine phosphatase interacting protein 1(*PSTPIP1*; also known as CD2 antigen-binding protein 1 [*CD2BP1*]) gene on chromosome 15q, encoding PSTPIP1, which binds to pyrin and regulates the inflammasome. Mutations in *PSTPIP1* lead to decreased inhibition of the inflammasome and increased production of IL-1β and IL-18, which can result in the inflammation seen with PAPA.[42,43]

Variations of the PAPA syndrome have been described in the literature, including PAPASH syndrome (pyogenic sterile arthritis, PG, cystic acne, and hidradenitis suppurativa), which results from an E277D missense mutation in the *PSTPIP1* gene,[45] PASH syndrome (PG, acne, and suppurative hidradenitis), which results from an increased CCTG microsatellite repeat in the promoter region of PSTPIP1,[46] as well as other variations.

JAKs are intracellular tyrosine kinases that are needed for cell differentiation, proliferation, and apoptosis. Mutations in JAKs can cause inflammatory and myeloproliferative disorders, and also have been associated with cases of PG. Interestingly, the pathway is activated by G-CSF and TNF-α, as well as ILs and interferons.[44]

Some specific genetic loci linked to IBD susceptibility have been found to correlate with the development of PG.[47] Weizman et al[47] reviewed 5756 patients with IBD using genome-wide association data and described several genes associated with susceptibility to IBD that were significantly associated with PG, including *IL8RA* (a mediator of neutrophil migration), *MUC17*, *MMP24*, *WNK2*, *DOCK9*, *PRDM1*, and *NDIFIP1*,[22] in addition to other genetic loci associated with IBD and PG, such as *GPBAR1*, *TIMP3*, and *TRAF31P2*.[44]

HORMONAL INFLUENCES

There are reports of premenstrual flares associated with several dermatologic conditions such as hidradenitis suppurativa and acne vulgaris; the medical literature describes a positive role of estrogen and a negative role of androgens, or androgen receptor activation, in cutaneous wound healing. Jourabchi et al[48] reported a case of PG with premenstrual flares that was controlled with use of a combined oral contraceptive and antiandrogen (ethinyl estradiol/drospirenone).[48] Interestingly, hidradenitis suppurativa and acne are known to occur with PG in some patients, suggesting a related pathophysiologic mechanism. Additionally, PG, hidradenitis suppurativa, and acne have some other overlapping features, including elevated IL-17 and TNF-α in lesional skin, and positive response to TNF-α inhibitors.[22,49,50]

DIAGNOSIS

PG is currently diagnosed clinically and, very importantly, after excluding other potential causes for the skin manifestations (especially infectious causes such as atypical mycobacteria and deep fungal infections) as no specific serologic, histologic, or genetic markers have yet been found.

DIAGNOSTIC ALGORITHM

Because there are no specific diagnostic tests for PG, the following criteria are proposed to help make the diagnosis of PG, which requires the fulfillment of both major criteria and at least 2 minor criteria:[1,3,7,22]

1. Major criteria:
   a. Sudden onset of a painful lesion with the characteristic morphology described in "Cutaneous Findings" section in a patient who does not have fever, significant toxemia, or relevant drug intake.
   b. Histopathologic exclusion of significant vasculitis, malignancy, and infective organisms by special histologic studies/stains and negative tissue cultures, as well as exclusion of significant vascular stasis/occlusion by appropriate studies.
2. Minor criteria that are supportive of the diagnosis are as follows:

a. Occurrence in an individual with systemic disease, as described in "Disease Associations" section.
b. Classic histologic PG findings. (Note: In patients who have received systemic corticosteroids, the presence of neutrophils may be blunted and mononuclear cells may instead predominate.)
c. Rapid reduction of pain and inflammation on initiation of high-dose systemic corticosteroid therapy and rapid ulcer healing response to high-dose systemic corticosteroid therapy with a 50% decrease in ulcer size within 1 month.
d. History suggestive of pathergy or a clinical finding of cribriform scarring.

Providers must be aware that many patients may present months or years after initial development of skin manifestations, while taking or having tried various medications, including systemic corticosteroids or other immunosuppressants, and consequently may not present with the classic clinical findings or diagnostic criteria. Consequently, obtaining a detailed history is crucial to making the appropriate diagnosis.

SUPPORTIVE STUDIES

HISTOPATHOLOGIC STUDIES AND INFECTIOUS STAINS AND CULTURES

The histopathologic changes in the skin are not diagnostic but can be highly suggestive of PG. Pathologic changes must be considered in view of the total clinical picture. The microscopic changes that are seen depend on (a) the clinical variant of PG (ulcerative, bullous, pustular, or vegetative), (b) the timing of the biopsy, and (c) the site of the biopsy relative to the inflammatory process.

An incisional wedge skin biopsy should be taken from the edge of the PG lesion, taking care to sample a portion of normal skin progressing through the border into the area of active inflammation, to allow the various histologic patterns to be discerned. The excised tissue should then be divided with one section (fresh tissue) sent for bacterial culture, mycobacterial culture with smear, and fungal culture with microscopy, and the other portion sent in formalin for histologic evaluation requesting hematoxylin and eosin preparation with periodic acid–Schiff, Giemsa, Fite, Gram, and other stains considered relevant. If an incisional biopsy is not possible, two 4-mm punch biopsies may be performed instead. Immunofluorescence studies may show positive perivascular staining in lesional skin, which may be secondary to profound inflammation; it is not required for diagnostic purposes and can be omitted unless vasculitis is suspected in the differential diagnosis. Because PG can be complicated by secondary infection with the organisms mentioned above, nonhealing PG or recurring PG should be rebiopsied to exclude superimposed infection.

The location of the biopsy within the lesion is particularly important as biopsies taken from the center of established lesions may have different findings from biopsies taken from peripheral skin. A marked perivascular lymphocytic infiltration may be seen in biopsies taken from the "zone" or area of erythema that surrounds active lesions of ulcerative PG. Lymphocytes may be seen to infiltrate vessel walls with intramural and intravascular fibrin deposition indicative of vascular damage (sometimes called *lymphocytic vasculitis*). Abscess formation with intense dermal neutrophilic infiltration may extend to the panniculus and areas of tissue necrosis, dominating the histologic findings in biopsies taken from central areas of ulcerative PG lesions. Leukocytoclasis is not a prominent finding and although occasionally evidence of leukocytoclastic vasculitis is seen close to the necrotic center, this is a minor feature and considered secondary to the intense inflammatory changes rather than the primary event. Histologic examination of lesional skin from a patient with bullous PG will show a subepidermal or intraepidermal bulla with overlying epidermal necrosis and marked upper dermal edema with prominence of neutrophils. Biopsy of pustular PG will show a dense dermal neutrophilic infiltration (often centered about a follicle) with subepidermal edema and infiltration of neutrophils into the epidermis with subcorneal aggregations. Vegetative PG is characterized histologically by the presence of pseudoepitheliomatous hyperplasia, sinus tract formation, and the presence of palisading granulomas in the setting of focal dermal neutrophilic abscesses.[3,7,38]

LABORATORY TESTING

All patients with PG should have these tests performed: full blood cell count with differential white cell count; complete metabolic panel; erythrocyte sedimentation rate; autoantibody screen (including antinuclear antibodies, anti-Ro/La antibodies); rheumatoid factor; antiphospholipid antibody screen; antineutrophilic cytoplasmic antibodies; serum protein electrophoresis and immunofixation studies; and chest radiography.

VASCULAR STUDIES

All patients with leg ulcers should have venous reflux studies performed to rule out significant venous insufficiency and deep venous thrombosis, in addition to ankle/toe brachial index studies to rule out ischemia as an underlying cause for the ulceration.

OTHER INVESTIGATIONS

In most patients, the following additional tests may are warranted: endoscopy (upper and/or lower gastrointestinal) to rule out often-associated IBD; careful examination of peripheral blood morphology when indicated, and if any abnormality is found, bone marrow aspirate examination should be performed; ultrasound of abdomen (including liver/spleen/aorta); and computed tomography for visualization of the thorax, abdomen, and pelvis. Figure 37-5 outlines other directed investigations.

DIFFERENTIAL DIAGNOSIS

The differential diagnosis to be considered in a patient with PG is extensive.[51] Different variants of PG (ulcerative, bullous, vegetative, pustular) suggest alternative diagnoses, and the occurrence of PG at certain cutaneous sites raises further diagnostic issues for the clinician, as shown in Table 37-1.

CLINICAL COURSE AND PROGNOSIS

The prognosis depends on the PG variant; the age and sex of the patient; presence of underlying systemic disease and other comorbid conditions; and the type, dosage, and duration of therapy required to bring the disease under control. Classic ulcerative PG is a chronic recurrent disease with a significant morbidity and mortality. Patients with this variant who are older than 65 years of age and male

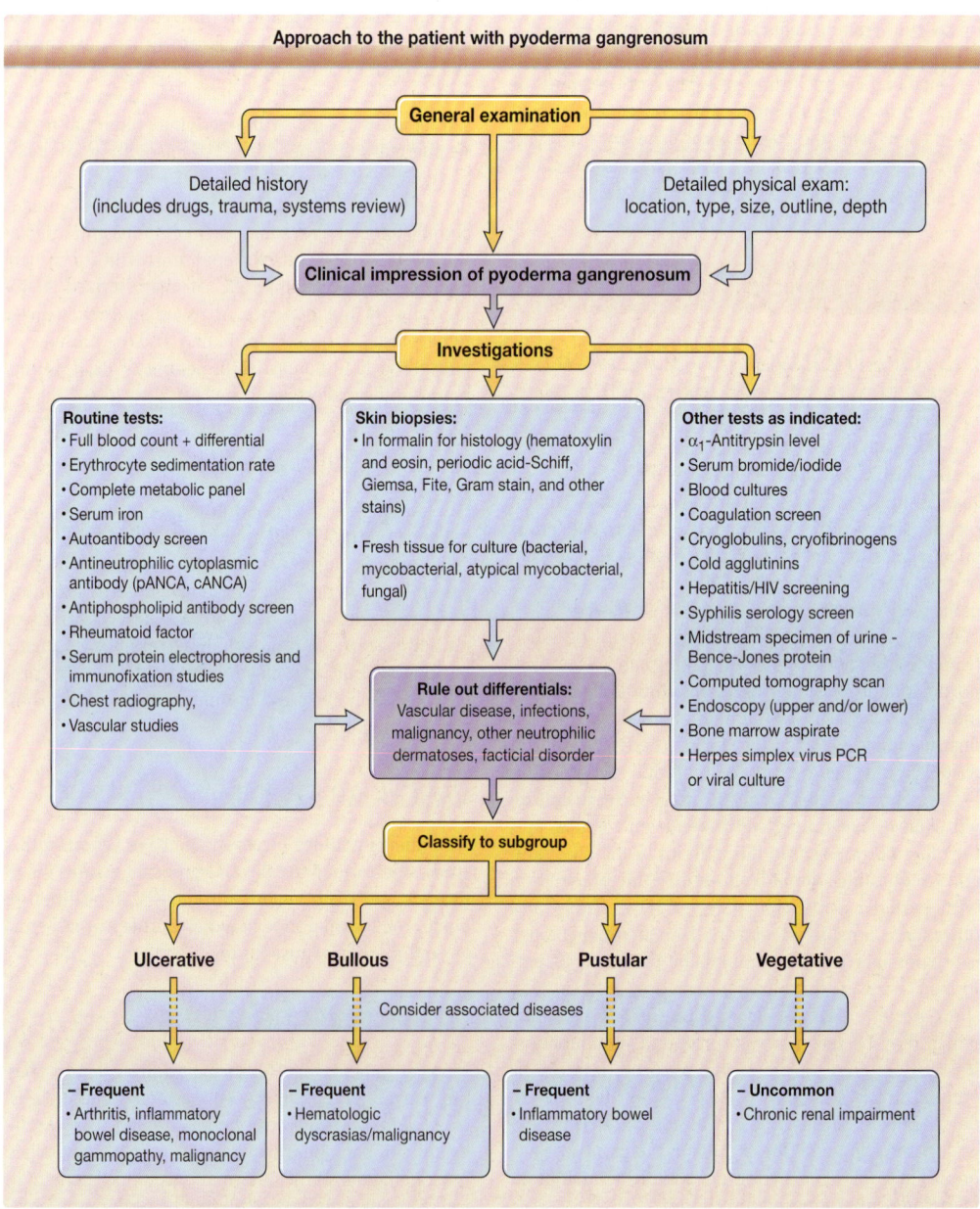

Figure 37-5 Approach to the patient with pyoderma gangrenosum. cANCA, cytoplasmic antineutrophil cytoplasmic antibody; pANCA, perinuclear antineutrophil cytoplasmic antibody; PCR, polymerase chain reaction.

TABLE 37-1
Differential Diagnosis of Pyoderma Gangrenosum

VARIANT SPECIFIC

Ulcerative pyoderma gangrenosum (PG)
Most Likely
- Vascular
  - Venous stasis ulceration
  - Vasculopathy
  - Arterial occlusive disease
  - Vasculitis
  - Antiphospholipid–antibody syndrome
- Infection
  - Bacterial (ecthyma gangrenosum)
  - Mycobacterial/atypical mycobacterial (eg, *Mycobacterium chelonae, Mycobacterium marinum*)
  - Deep fungal infection (eg, North American blastomycosis, sporotrichosis, *Aspergillus, Cryptococcus*)

Consider
- Infection
  - Tertiary syphilitic ulcer
  - Amebiasis
  - Viral (herpes simplex)
- Drugs (eg, hydroxyurea, halogenoderma)
- Other
  - Dermatitis artefacta
  - Calciphylaxis
  - Necrotizing insect bite (eg, brown recluse spider)
  - Malignant rheumatoid disease (with high-titer rheumatoid factor and depressed complement levels)
  - Cutaneous involvement of malignancy process (eg, lymphoma, leukemia cutis)

Bullous PG
Most Likely
- Infection
  - Bacterial (cellulitis/impetigo)
  - Viral (especially in immunocompromised)
  - Fungal (eg, mucormycosis in persons with diabetes)
- Other
  - Sweet syndrome/Behçet disease

Consider
- Bullous dermatoses
  - Erythema multiforme
- Other
  - Insect/arthropod bite

Pustular PG
Most Likely
- Infection
  - Bacterial/viral/fungal
- Vasculitis
  - Pustular vasculitis

Consider
- Other
  - Pustular psoriasis
  - Sneddon-Wilkinson disease
  - Pustular drug eruption
  - Bowel bypass syndrome

SITE SPECIFIC[a]

Parastomal
Most Likely
- Dermatoses
  - Irritant/allergic contact dermatitis
  - Other (eg, psoriasis, eczema)
- Infection
  - Bacterial (*Staphylococcus/Streptococcus*)/cellulitis
  - Fungal (*Candida*)
- Other
  - Extraintestinal inflammatory
  - Bowel disease
  - Malignancy

Postsurgical Wounds
Most Likely
- Infection
  - Bacterial/cellulitis
  - Mycobacterial/atypical mycobacterial
  - Fungal (eg, mucormycosis)
- Breakdown
  - Suture allergy
  - Mechanical

Consider
- Necrotizing fasciitis
- Malignancy

Perineum
Most Likely
- Infection
  - Bacterial/viral infection (herpes simplex virus, Epstein-Barr virus, cytomegalovirus)
  - Fournier gangrene
- Other
  - Hidradenitis suppurativa
  - Extraintestinal Crohn disease
  - Squamous cell/extramammary Paget disease

Consider
- Infection
  - Syphilis
  - Lymphogranuloma venereum/granuloma inguinale
  - Leishmaniasis
- Other
  - Dermatitis artefacta
  - Behçet disease

Vegetative PG
Most Likely
- Infection
  - Bacterial/viral/fungal
  - Mycobacterial/atypical mycobacterial
  - Leishmaniasis

Consider
- Blastomycosis-like pyoderma
- Dermatitis artefacta/malignancy
- Pyoderma vegetans
- Other
  - Dermatitis artefacta

[a]The differential diagnosis of lower-limb PG is essentially that delineated for variant-specific ulcerative PG.

patients seem to have a worse prognosis. Patients with vegetative PG generally have a good prognosis, and compared to classic PG, vegetative PG lesions are more likely to heal without the use of oral corticosteroids.[20] Parastomal PG has a good prognosis, often responding to topical or intralesional steroid therapy. Patients with pustular PG often have complete remission of their cutaneous lesions if the severe IBD that usually accompanies this variant is controlled. Patients with bullous PG who have an associated hematologic disorder have a poor prognosis. The onset of bullous PG in a patient with stable polycythemia rubra vera has been reported to herald the onset of leukemic change.[30,38,52]

MANAGEMENT

APPROACH TO MANAGEMENT

Understanding the context in which PG is occurring is crucial in deciding on proper treatment approach. The unpredictable nature of PG and its variable aggressiveness in individual patients necessitate a flexible approach to treatment. Therapeutic agents must be adapted to the patient's physiologic state (pregnancy, old age, renal disease, diabetes, immunosuppressed status, etc) and also with their underlying associated disease state. Although the course of the underlying disease does not always correlate with PG flares, its treatment can result in improvement of PG. Systemic steroids and/or cyclosporine may be effective in controlling PG regardless of the underlying disease state, but PG often requires combination therapy and multiple medication trials to achieve healing, and in these cases the underlying disease state should be used to help guide medication selection and treatment approach.

Adequate rest, efficient pain relief, and appropriate therapy for any comorbidities (venous stasis disease, diabetes, congestive heart failure with fluid overload, etc) that affect healing are also pivotal in the overall management strategy of a patient with PG. If other systemic illnesses are present, close collaboration with an internal medicine specialist and pertinent subspecialty physicians is needed.

MEDICATIONS

Definitive treatment guidelines for PG do not exist, partly because PG associated with different underlying diseases seems to behave differently, and also because there is a paucity of data in the literature. Approach to treatment is based on directed therapeutic immunomodulation to decrease inflammation and promote healing. Choice of treatment depends on the severity of the PG, and when possible should also attempt to treat the patient's underlying condition (eg, infliximab for patients with IBD and methotrexate for patients with rheumatoid arthritis).

Mild PG with small shallow ulcers or a plaque of vegetative PG may respond to topical class I corticosteroids (clobetasol propionate 0.05%), intralesional corticosteroids, or a calcineurin inhibitor such as tacrolimus 0.1%, with twice-a-day application.

First-line therapy for more severe or extensive PG is systemic glucocorticoids. We typically begin treatment at 1 to 2 mg/kg of oral prednisone daily, with a maximum dose of 150 mg/day. For very aggressive disease, intravenous pulse methylprednisone 1 g/day for 3 to 5 days can be helpful as initial therapy, followed by daily oral glucocorticoids.[1,53,54] Response to systemic glucocorticoids is typically rapid, typically halting progression within 1 to 2 weeks. Because long-term therapy is associated with significant adverse effects, slow glucocorticoid taper should begin once progression of PG has stopped. Simultaneously beginning a steroid-sparing adjunctive agent (eg, cyclosporine, dapsone, infliximab) can help prevent flares while tapering.[1]

Oral cyclosporine is an alternative first-line treatment for patients who cannot tolerate systemic glucocorticoids and is also used as adjunctive therapy. A multicenter, parallel group, observer blind, randomized, controlled trial comparing oral prednisolone 0.75 mg/kg/day with cyclosporine 4 mg/kg/day for PG found comparable effectiveness between the 2 groups.[55] Adverse effects include renal toxicity and hypertension, which must be monitored, and recommended time course for treatment is less than 1 year.[55,56]

Systemic glucocorticoids and cyclosporine are rapid acting, which makes them ideal for initial therapy, whereas some of the other therapies can take weeks for therapeutic effect and are better suited as adjunctive or maintenance therapy, especially for severe cases. It is not uncommon for severe cases of PG to require combination therapy to control the condition while minimizing side effects from therapy. Table 37-2 outlines additional therapies. Note that most of these medications require specific baseline laboratory test results, close monitoring for adverse effects, care to prevent drug interactions, and caution for immunosuppression.

Maintenance therapy should be continued until there is complete wound healing and then slowly tapered off. In addition, patients with ulcerative PG have a significant risk of relapse, so long-term followup is required, and some patients require long-term maintenance therapy.

UNRESPONSIVE PYODERMA GANGRENOSUM AND TREATMENT CONSIDERATIONS

When PG is not responding to treatment, or if healing stalls, the provider must reassess the case:

1. Is there an uncontrolled comorbidity (eg, venous stasis, vascular ischemia, diabetes) that is inhibiting wound healing and needs to be addressed?
2. Is there a new superimposed infection that needs workup and treatment? And if so, should another biopsy be performed for pan-culture?

TABLE 37-2
Treatment Options for Pyoderma Gangrenosum

MEDICATION	ADULT DOSING	LIKELY MECHANISM
Very Severe Disease		
Methylprednisolone pulse (initial treatment)	1 g/day IV for 3-5 days[a]	Blocks promoter sites of proinflammatory genes, such as IL-1α and IL-1β; inhibits synthesis of almost all known cytokines; impairs neutrophil migration; reduces circulating T cells[52,57]
Severe Disease		
Prednisone (first line)	1 mg/kg/day PO	Blocks promoter sites of proinflammatory genes, such as IL-1α and IL-1β; inhibits synthesis of almost all known cytokines; impairs neutrophil migration; reduces circulating T cells[52,57]
Cyclosporine (first line)	3-5 mg/kg/day PO	Calcineurin inhibitor on T cells, causing reduced transcriptional activation of genes for IL-2, TNF-α, IL-3, IL-4, CD40L, G-CSF, and interferon-γ[52,58,59]
Adjunctive Therapy		
Minocycline	100 mg twice daily PO	Suppresses neutrophil migration/chemotaxis, matrix metalloproteinases, and cytokine release (TNF-α, IL-6, IL-1β), and inhibits T-cell activation and proliferation[52,60]
Dapsone	50-200 mg/day PO	Inhibits neutrophil myeloperoxidase; suppresses IL-8 and TNF-α[52,61]
Mycophenolate mofetil	500 mg to 1.5 g twice daily PO	Inhibits inosine monophosphate dehydrogenase and de novo protein synthesis, thereby inhibiting T-cell and B-cell proliferation; also suppresses leukocyte recruitment[52,62]
Azathioprine	Max of 2.0-2.5 mg/kg/day PO	Synthetic purine analog derived from 6-mercaptopurine disrupts nucleic acid synthesis and interferes with T-cell activation and function[52,63]
Methotrexate	Initial test dose of 5 mg PO, gradually increasing weekly by 2.5-5.0 mg as needed, up to max dose of 30 mg/week	Folate antimetabolite that targets T cells, inhibiting dihydrofolate reductase and thymidylate synthetase, decreasing T-cell proliferation and migration, in addition to inducing adenosine release, which suppresses neutrophil oxidative activity, chemotaxis, and suppresses production of TNF-α, IL-6, IL-8, IL-12[52,64]
Biologics[b]	Infliximab: 5 mg/kg IV at weeks 0, 2, 6, followed by infusions every 6-8 weeks Etanercept: 50 mg twice weekly for 3 months, followed by 50 mg weekly Adalimumab: load with 80 mg SC, followed by 40 mg SC every 1-2 weeks Ustekinumab: weight ≤100 kg: 45 mg at 0 and 4 weeks, and then every 12 weeks weight >100 kg: 90 mg at 0 and 4 weeks, and then every 12 weeks	Infliximab: monoclonal Ab against TNF-α; binds soluble and membrane bound TNF-α and blocks its interaction with cell-surface receptors[22,52,65] Etanercept: fusion protein; binds soluble TNF-α and blocks its interaction with cell-surface receptors[22,52,65] Adalimumab: monoclonal Ab against TNF-α; binds soluble and membrane bound TNF-α and blocks its interaction with cell-surface receptors[22,52,65] Ustekinumab: IgG₁ monoclonal antibody; binds to the p40 subunit of both IL-12 and IL-23, blocking its interaction with cell-surface receptors, interfering with T-cell activation, and expression of TNF-α, IL-8, and other cytokines[52,65]
Thalidomide[c]	50-300 mg/day	Inhibits TNF-α, chemotaxis of monocytes and leucocytes, and inhibits phagocytosis by neutrophils[44,52,65]
Severe, Refractory PG, or Those With Significant Contraindications to Other Treatment Options		
Intravenous immune globulin	2 g/kg/cycle per month IV divided over 3 consecutive days	Suppression or neutralization of cytokines; blockade of leukocyte adhesion molecules; alterations in regulatory T cells and inhibition of the proinflammatory Th17 pathway[52,65,66]

[a]Followed by daily oral prednisone.
[b]Consider for severe PG in IBD (except etanercept, which is not helpful for IBD), rheumatoid arthritis, or hidradenitis suppurativa.
[c]Consider for severe PG in myelodysplastic syndrome.
Ab, antibody; G-CSF, granulocyte colony-stimulating factor; Ig, immunoglobulin; IL, interleukin; PO, per os (by mouth); SC, subcutaneously; Th, T-helper cell; TNF, tumor necrosis factor.

3. Is there a better, more directed medication that should be tried?

In patients with refractory or difficult-to-treat PG, genetic analysis can be considered and may help identify better directed therapy. DeFilippis et al[44] reviewed the published literature regarding syndromes and genetic mutations associated with PG, and found that PG responded to different treatments depending on the underlying disease process. For example, cases with the PAPA syndrome and variants with increased IL-1β improved with the anti–IL-1β monoclonal antibody canakinumab, the IL-1 receptor antagonist anakinra, and TNF-α inhibitors, whereas a case of polycythemia vera with JAK2 mutation responded to the JAK1/JAK2 inhibitor ruxolitinib, and PG-like cases with MTHFR mutations (whose pathway relies on vitamins B_6, B_9, and B_{12}) improved with B-vitamin therapy.[44]

WOUND CARE

The location, morphology, size, and depth of each lesion should be recorded (with photography) on presentation and subsequent review to help monitor course. The cutaneous lesions of PG are usually extremely tender so cleansing should be carried out daily with tepid sterile saline or a mild antiseptic solution. Silver sulfadiazine 1% cream is usually soothing when applied to the ulcerated lesions of PG and may facilitate granulation tissue formation while also inhibiting bacterial growth. A nonadhesive dressing should be applied over the lesion and held in place with a crêpe elasticized bandage wrapped firmly, but not tightly, over it. Some patients, particularly those with superficial lesions, obtain significant relief with the use of hydrocolloid dressings, which can be left on for 2 to 3 days and "melt" into the lesion. Careful instruction to the patient and nurse is important to ensure compliance and to avoid the use of irritants such as chemical desloughing agents, caustics (such as silver nitrate), or dressings such as gauze impregnated with soft paraffin and/or antibacterial agents that may adhere to the ulcer base. A variety of bacteria may be cultured from the wound surface, but these usually represent contaminants and directed antibiotic therapy is not required unless there are clinical signs of incipient cellulitis around the wound.

PROCEDURES

Debridement must not be performed aggressively and skin grafting should be avoided if possible because of pathergy and the risk of inducing new PG lesions at the donor sites. Cultured tissue allografts/autografts and the use of bovine collagen matrix have been reported to be useful in patients in whom the disease is controlled but re-epithelialization incomplete.[67]

COUNSELING

The patient should be given realistic expectations of the speed of recovery likely in this disease. Thus, although lesions develop and evolve within days, the healing process can take weeks to months.

PREVENTION/SCREENING

A patient who has had a history of PG should be advised to avoid trauma to the skin as there is the possibility of precipitating a new lesion through the pathergic phenomenon. If such patients have to undergo surgery, they should have close supervision by a dermatologist of their postoperative course. Patients with a history of aggressive PG may warrant a course of systemic steroids during and for a period (2 weeks or longer) postoperatively to prevent the development of new PG lesions, and subcuticular sutures should be used where possible. Patients with a history of PG and Crohn disease who are to have an ileostomy should be warned about the possible development of parastomal PG lesions, and to try to avoid irritation to the area to help prevent pathergy.

ACKNOWLEDGMENTS

We give special thanks to the authors of the prior version of this chapter, Frank C. Powell, Bridget C. Hackett, and Daniel Wallach.

REFERENCES

1. Ahronowitz I, Harp J, Shinkai K. Etiology and management of pyoderma gangrenosum: a comprehensive review. *Am J Clin Dermatol*. 2012;13:191-211.
2. Ruocco E, Sangiuliano S, Gravina AG, et al. Pyoderma gangrenosum: an updated review. *J Eur Acad Dermatol Venereol*. 2009;23:1008-1017.
3. Powell FC, Su WP, Perry HO. Pyoderma gangrenosum: classification and management. *J Am Acad Dermatol*. 1996;34:395-409.
4. Adachi Y, Kindzelskii AL, Cookingham G, et al. Aberrant neutrophil trafficking and metabolic oscillations in severe pyoderma gangrenosum. *J Invest Dermatol*. 1998;111:259-268.
5. Hickman JG, Lazarus GS. Pyoderma gangrenosum: a reappraisal of associated systemic diseases. *Br J Dermatol*. 1980;102:235-237.
6. Korber A, Klode J, Al-Benna S, et al. Etiology of chronic leg ulcers in 31,619 patients in Germany analyzed by an expert survey. *J Dtsch Dermatol Ges*. 2011;9:116-121.
7. Su WP, Davis MD, Weenig RH, et al. Pyoderma gangrenosum: clinicopathologic correlation and proposed diagnostic criteria. *Int J Dermatol*. 2004;43:790-800.
8. Agarwal A, Andrews JM. Systematic review: IBD-associated pyoderma gangrenosum in the biologic era, the response to therapy. *Aliment Pharmacol Ther*. 2013;38:563-572.
9. Cox NH, Peebles-Brown DA, MacKie RM. Pyoderma gangrenosum occurring 10 years after proctocolectomy for ulcerative colitis. *Br J Hosp Med*. 1986;36:363.
10. Powell FC, Schroeter AL, Su WP, et al. Pyoderma gangrenosum and monoclonal gammopathy. *Arch Dermatol*. 1983;119:468-472.
11. Duguid CM, O'Loughlin S, Otridge B, et al. Paraneoplastic pyoderma gangrenosum. *Australas J Dermatol*. 1993;34:17-22.
12. Powell FC, Schroeter AL, Su WP, et al. Pyoderma gangrenosum: a review of 86 patients. *Q J Med*. 1985;55:173-186.
13. Stanojevic N, Mai C. It starts with a dog scratch. *J Hosp Med*. 2010;5:494-495.
14. Callen JP, Dubin HV, Gehrke CF. Recurrent pyoderma gangrenosum and agnogenic myeloid metaplasia. *Arch Dermatol*. 1977;113:1585-1586.
15. Caughman W, Stern R, Haynes H. Neutrophilic dermatosis of myeloproliferative disorders. Atypical forms of

15. pyoderma gangrenosum and Sweet's syndrome associated with myeloproliferative disorders. *J Am Acad Dermatol*. 1983;9:751-758.
16. Ryu J, Naik H, Yang FC, et al. Pyoderma gangrenosum presenting with leukemoid reaction: a report of 2 cases. *Arch Dermatol*. 2010;146:568-569.
17. Shahi V, Wetter DA. Pyoderma gangrenosum associated with solid organ malignancies. *Int J Dermatol*. 2015;54:e351-e357.
18. Ross HJ, Moy LA, Kaplan R, et al. Bullous pyoderma gangrenosum after granulocyte colony-stimulating factor treatment. *Cancer*. 1991;68:441-443.
19. Bennett ML, Jackson JM, Jorizzo JL, et al. Pyoderma gangrenosum. A comparison of typical and atypical forms with an emphasis on time to remission. Case review of 86 patients from 2 institutions. *Medicine (Baltimore)*. 2000;79:37-46.
20. Kim RH, Lewin J, Hale CS, et al. Vegetative pyoderma gangrenosum. *Dermatol Online J*. 2014;20.
21. Field S, Powell FC, Young V, et al. Pyoderma gangrenosum manifesting as a cavitating lung lesion. *Clin Exp Dermatol*. 2008;33:418-421.
22. Braswell SF, Kostopoulos TC, Ortega-Loayza AG. Pathophysiology of pyoderma gangrenosum (PG): an updated review. *J Am Acad Dermatol*. 2015;73:691-698.
23. Butler D, Shinkai K. What do autoinflammatory syndromes teach about common cutaneous diseases such as pyoderma gangrenosum? A commentary. *Dermatol Clin*. 2013;31:427-435.
24. Vidal D, Puig L, Gilaberte M, et al. Review of 26 cases of classical pyoderma gangrenosum: clinical and therapeutic features. *J Dermatolog Treat*. 2004;15:146-152.
25. Menachem Y, Gotsman I. Clinical manifestations of pyoderma gangrenosum associated with inflammatory bowel disease. *Isr Med Assoc J*. 2004;6:88-90.
26. Talansky AL, Meyers S, Greenstein AJ, et al. Does intestinal resection heal the pyoderma gangrenosum of inflammatory bowel disease? *J Clin Gastroenterol*. 1983;5:207-210.
27. Fox LP, Geyer AS, Husain S, et al. Bullous pyoderma gangrenosum as the presenting sign of fatal acute myelogenous leukemia. *Leuk Lymphoma*. 2006;47:147-150.
28. Rafael MR, Fernandes CM, Machado JM, et al. Pyoderma gangrenosum or leukaemia cutis? *J Eur Acad Dermatol Venereol*. 2003;17:449-451.
29. Tombak A, Aygun S, Serinsoz E, et al. Complete recovery of pyoderma gangrenosum after successful treatment of underlying hairy cell leukemia with cladribine. *Korean J Intern Med*. 2015;30:739-741.
30. Cosgarea I, Lovric Z, Korber A, et al. Successful treatment of refractory pyoderma gangrenosum with ustekinumab only after excision of renal cell carcinoma. *Int Wound J*. 2016;13(5):1041-1042.
31. Brooklyn TN, Williams AM, Dunnill MG, et al. T-cell receptor repertoire in pyoderma gangrenosum: evidence for clonal expansions and trafficking. *Br J Dermatol*. 2007;157:960-966.
32. Marzano AV, Cugno M, Trevisan V, et al. Role of inflammatory cells, cytokines and matrix metalloproteinases in neutrophil-mediated skin diseases. *Clin Exp Immunol*. 2010;162:100-107.
33. Wallach D, Vignon-Pennamen MD. From acute febrile neutrophilic dermatosis to neutrophilic disease: forty years of clinical research. *J Am Acad Dermatol*. 2006;55:1066-1071.
34. Nerella P, Daniela A, Guido M, et al. Leukocyte chemotaxis and pyoderma gangrenosum. *Int J Dermatol*. 1985;24:45-47.
35. Shore RN. Pyoderma gangrenosum, defective neutrophil chemotaxis, and leukemia. *Arch Dermatol*. 1976;112:1792-1793.
36. Berkow RL, Wang D, Larrick JW, et al. Enhancement of neutrophil superoxide production by preincubation with recombinant human tumor necrosis factor. *J Immunol*. 1987;139:3783-3791.
37. Klebanoff SJ, Vadas MA, Harlan JM, et al. Stimulation of neutrophils by tumor necrosis factor. *J Immunol*. 1986;136:4220-4225.
38. Stewart RJ, Marsden PA. Biologic control of the tumor necrosis factor and interleukin-1 signaling cascade. *Am J Kidney Dis*. 1995;25:954-966.
39. Montoto S, Bosch F, Estrach T, et al. Pyoderma gangrenosum triggered by alpha2b-interferon in a patient with chronic granulocytic leukemia. *Leuk Lymphoma*. 1998;30:199-202.
40. Oka M, Berking C, Nesbit M, et al. Interleukin-8 overexpression is present in pyoderma gangrenosum ulcers and leads to ulcer formation in human skin xenografts. *Lab Invest*. 2000;80:595-604.
41. Guenova E, Teske A, Fehrenbacher B, et al. Interleukin 23 expression in pyoderma gangrenosum and targeted therapy with ustekinumab. *Arch Dermatol*. 2011;147:1203-1205.
42. Wise CA, Gillum JD, Seidman CE, et al. Mutations in CD2BP1 disrupt binding to PTP PEST and are responsible for PAPA syndrome, an autoinflammatory disorder. *Hum Mol Genet*. 2002;11:961-969.
43. Farasat S, Aksentijevich I, Toro JR. Autoinflammatory diseases: clinical and genetic advances. *Arch Dermatol*. 2008;144:392-402.
44. DeFilippis EM, Feldman SR, Huang WW. The genetics of pyoderma gangrenosum and implications for treatment: a systematic review. *Br J Dermatol*. 2015;172:1487-1497.
45. Marzano AV, Trevisan V, Gattorno M, et al. Pyogenic arthritis, pyoderma gangrenosum, acne, and hidradenitis suppurativa (PAPASH): a new autoinflammatory syndrome associated with a novel mutation of the PSTPIP1 gene. *JAMA Dermatol*. 2013;149:762-764.
46. Braun-Falco M, Kovnerystyy O, Lohse P, et al. Pyoderma gangrenosum, acne, and suppurative hidradenitis (PASH)—a new autoinflammatory syndrome distinct from PAPA syndrome. *J Am Acad Dermatol*. 2012; 66:409-415.
47. Weizman A, Huang B, Berel D, et al. Clinical, serologic, and genetic factors associated with pyoderma gangrenosum and erythema nodosum in inflammatory bowel disease patients. *Inflamm Bowel Dis*. 2014;20:525-533.
48. Jourabchi N, Rhee SM, Lazarus GS. Premenstrual flares of pyoderma gangrenosum controlled with use of a combined oral contraceptive and antiandrogen (ethinyl estradiol/drospirenone). *Br J Dermatol*. 2016;174:1096-1097.
49. Kelhala HL, Palatsi R, Fyhrquist N, et al. IL-17/Th17 pathway is activated in acne lesions. *PLoS One*. 2014; 9:e105238.
50. Schlapbach C, Hanni T, Yawalkar N, et al. Expression of the IL-23/Th17 pathway in lesions of hidradenitis suppurativa. *J Am Acad Dermatol*. 2011;65:790-798.
51. Weenig RH, Davis MD, Dahl PR, et al. Skin ulcers misdiagnosed as pyoderma gangrenosum. *N Engl J Med*. 2002;347:1412-1418.
52. Patel F, Fitzmaurice S, Duong C, et al. Effective strategies for the management of pyoderma gangrenosum:

a comprehensive review. *Acta Derm Venereol.* 2015;95:525-531.
53. Prystowsky JH, Kahn SN, Lazarus GS. Present status of pyoderma gangrenosum. Review of 21 cases. *Arch Dermatol.* 1989;125:57-64.
54. Johnson RB, Lazarus GS. Pulse therapy. Therapeutic efficacy in the treatment of pyoderma gangrenosum. *Arch Dermatol.* 1982;118:76-84.
55. Ormerod AD, Thomas KS, Craig FE, et al. Comparison of the two most commonly used treatments for pyoderma gangrenosum: results of the STOP GAP randomised controlled trial. *BMJ.* 2015;350:h2958.
56. Matis WL, Ellis CN, Griffiths CE, et al. Treatment of pyoderma gangrenosum with cyclosporine. *Arch Dermatol.* 1992;128:1060-1064.
57. Oppong E, Cato AC. Effects of glucocorticoids in the immune system. *Adv Exp Med Biol.* 2015;872:217-233.
58. Kutlubay Z, Erdogan BC, Engin B, et al. Cyclosporine in dermatology. *Skinmed.* 2016;14:105-109.
59. Amor KT, Ryan C, Menter A. The use of cyclosporine in dermatology: part I. *J Am Acad Dermatol.* 2010;63:925-946; quiz 47-48.
60. Perret LJ, Tait CP. Non-antibiotic properties of tetracyclines and their clinical application in dermatology. *Australas J Dermatol.* 2014;55:111-118.
61. Wozel G, Blasum C. Dapsone in dermatology and beyond. *Arch Dermatol Res.* 2014;306:103-124.
62. Orvis AK, Wesson SK, Breza TS Jr, et al. Mycophenolate mofetil in dermatology. *J Am Acad Dermatol.* 2009;60:183-199; quiz 200-202.
63. Patel AA, Swerlick RA, McCall CO. Azathioprine in dermatology: the past, the present, and the future. *J Am Acad Dermatol.* 2006;55:369-389.
64. Chan ES, Cronstein BN. Molecular action of methotrexate in inflammatory diseases. *Arthritis Res.* 2002;4:266-273.
65. Fathi R, Armstrong AW. The role of biologic therapies in dermatology. *Med Clin North Am.* 2015;99:1183-1194.
66. Dourmishev LA, Guleva DV, Miteva LG. Intravenous Immunoglobulins: mode of action and indications in autoimmune and inflammatory dermatoses. *Int J Inflam.* 2016;2016:3523057.
67. de Imus G, Golomb C, Wilkel C, et al. Accelerated healing of pyoderma gangrenosum treated with bioengineered skin and concomitant immunosuppression. *J Am Acad Dermatol.* 2001;44:61-66.

Chapter 38 :: Subcorneal Pustular Dermatosis (Sneddon-Wilkinson Disease)
:: Franz Trautinger & Herbert Hönigsmann

第三十八章

角层下脓疱病

中文导读

本章全面讲述了角层下脓疱病的历史及流行病学史、临床表现、病因及发病机制、诊断及治疗。在临床特点上，予以图文并茂的方式介绍了该病的典型临床和病理表现。在诊断上，以表格的方式介绍了相关疾病的鉴别诊断，并详细说明了鉴别要点。首选治疗是氨苯砜，每日剂量为50～150mg，但是起效较慢。此外，维生素A、光化疗、紫外光B、秋水仙碱、环孢素等也有效。值得注意的是糖皮质激素疗效欠佳。

〔李芳芳〕

AT-A-GLANCE

- A rare condition with worldwide occurrence.
- A chronic, recurrent, neutrophilic disorder with a benign course, frequently associated with various forms of immune dysfunction (most commonly immunoglobulin [Ig] A monoclonal gammopathy).
- Occurrence of intraepidermal deposits of IgA indicates a relationship with IgA pemphigus.
- Crops of flaccid, coalescing pustules; often in annular or serpiginous patterns.
- Usually distributed symmetrically in the axillae, groins, submammary, the flexor aspects of the limbs, and on the abdomen.
- Pathology: subcorneal pustules filled with polymorphonuclear leukocytes.

Subcorneal pustular dermatosis (SPD) is a rare, chronic, recurrent, pustular eruption characterized histopathologically by subcorneal pustules that contain abundant neutrophils. The condition was originally described in 1956 by Sneddon and Wilkinson,[1] who separated SPD from other previously unclassified pustular eruptions. Until 1966, when the first comprehensive review appeared, more than 130 cases had been reported, but not all fulfilled the clinical and histopathologic criteria required for this diagnosis.[2] A considerable number of additional cases have since appeared in the literature, and a subtype with intraepidermal deposits of immunoglobulin (Ig) A directed against desmocollin 1 has been recognized.[3] Today, these cases are usually classified as SPD-type IgA pemphigus, and it is a matter of debate whether the finding of epidermal IgA deposits defines a subset of SPD or a pemphigus variant that is otherwise indistinguishable from "classic" SPD.

EPIDEMIOLOGY

There is no racial predilection. Most of the reported cases have been in whites, but the disease also has been observed in Africans, Japanese, and Chinese. The condition is more common in women and in persons older than 40 years of age, but SPD may occur at any age.[2] A pustular eruption that is clinically and histologically similar to the human disease, which also responds to dapsone treatment, has been observed in dogs.[4]

ETIOLOGY AND PATHOGENESIS

The cause of SPD is unknown. Cultures of the pustules consistently do not reveal bacterial growth. The role of trigger mechanisms such as preceding or concomitant infections, although repeatedly discussed, has remained speculative. Immunologic mechanisms have been implicated in the pathogenesis and in a subset of patients, whose disease clinically resembled SPD, intraepidermal IgA deposits have been detected. Some of these patients also had circulating IgA antibodies against the same sites within the epidermis. Desmocollin 1 and in a single case also desmocollins 2 and 3 have been described as autoantigens in these cases, and the disease has been classified as a pemphigus variant (SPD-type IgA pemphigus; see Chap. 57).[3,5-7]

The occasional association of SPD with certain other diseases may represent more than a mere coincidence. Increased serum IgA has been detected in a number of patients, and the disease has been reported to occur in cases of IgA-paraproteinemia and IgA multiple myeloma.[8-12] In addition, SPD is associated with pyoderma gangrenosum,[13,14] ulcerative colitis,[15] and Crohn disease.[16] Whether or not the coexistence of these conditions reflects common pathogenetic mechanisms remain to be clarified, but an additional common denominator linking these disorders is their response to sulfone and sulfonamide therapy.

Further associations reported to date include IgG paraproteinemia,[17,18] CD30+ anaplastic large cell lymphoma,[19] marginal zone lymphoma,[20] non–small cell lung cancer,[21] apudoma,[22] rheumatoid arthritis,[23,24] systemic lupus erythematodes,[25] hyperthyroidism,[26] *Mycoplasma pneumoniae*,[27,28] and *Coccidioides immitis* infection.[29]

CLINICAL FINDINGS

The primary lesions are small, discrete, flaccid pustules, or vesicles that rapidly turn pustular and usually arise in crops within a few hours on clinically normal or slightly erythematous skin (Fig. 38-1). In dependent regions, pus characteristically accumulates in the lower half of the pustule (Fig. 38-1B); as the pustules usually have the tendency to coalesce, they often, but not always, form annular, circinate, or bizarre serpiginous patterns. After a few days, the pustules rupture and dry up to form thin, superficial scales and crusts, closely resembling impetigo. Peripheral spreading and central healing leave polycyclic, erythematous areas in which new pustules arise as others disappear

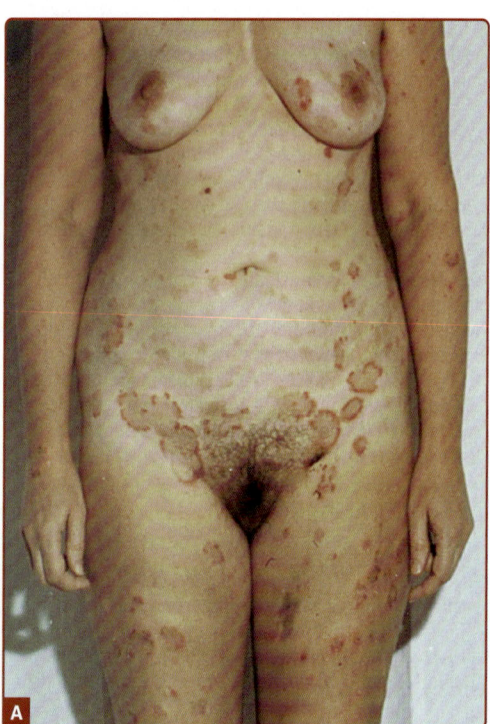
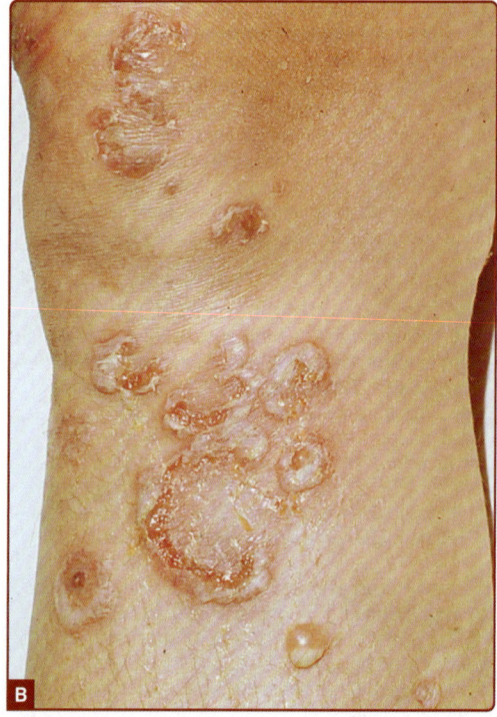

Figure 38-1 Subcorneal pustular dermatosis. **A,** Typical distribution. Note accentuated involvement of groin and abdomen. Hyperpigmented macules mark previously affected areas. **B,** Close-up showing coalescence of pustules, which form annular and circinate patterns. Lesions of different developmental stages are seen side by side. At the lower right, newly formed pustule with characteristic hypopyon formation.

(Fig. 38-1A). There is no atrophy or scarring, but an occasional brownish hyperpigmentation may mark previously affected sites. Variable intervals of quiescence, lasting from a few days to several weeks, may be followed by the sudden development of new lesions. The eruptions tend to occur symmetrically, affecting mainly the axillae, groin, abdomen, submammary areas, and the flexor aspects of the limbs. In rare cases, the face,[30] palms, and soles[31] may be involved. Scalp and mucous membranes invariably remain free of lesions. Episodic itching and burning represent subjective symptoms in a small number of patients, but there are no systemic symptoms or abnormalities in routine laboratory parameters.

TABLE 38-1
Differential Diagnosis of Subcorneal Pustular Dermatosis

- Bacterial impetigo
- Dermatitis herpetiformis
- Pemphigus foliaceus
- Subcorneal pustular dermatosis-type immunoglobulin A pemphigus
- Pustular psoriasis
- Necrolytic migratory erythema
- Acute generalized exanthematous pustulosis

HISTOPATHOLOGY

The hallmark of the disease is a strictly subcorneal pustule filled with polymorphonuclear leukocytes,[1] with only an occasional eosinophils.[2] Acantholysis is not involved in pustule formation, but a few acantholytic cells may be found in older lesions (secondary acantholysis). Surprisingly, the epidermal layers underlying the pustule exhibit little pathology, and, apart from a variable number of migrating leukocytes, there is little evidence of spongiosis or cytolytic damage to the epidermal cells. The dermis contains a perivascular infiltrate composed of neutrophils and rarely mononuclear cells and eosinophils (Fig. 38-2).

Direct immunofluorescence is usually negative. Upon detection of IgA in a pemphigus-like intercellular pattern (with or without the presence of circulating IgA antibodies directed against desmocollin 1) patients should be diagnosed as SPD-type IgA pemphigus (see Ethiology and Pathogenesis earlier).

DIFFERENTIAL DIAGNOSIS

Table 38-1 outlines the differential diagnosis of SPD. An early localized eruption of SPD may be clinically and histologically indistinguishable from impetigo, but the distribution pattern of the lesions, the absence of bacteria in the pustules, and the ineffectiveness of antibiotic therapy suggest the correct diagnosis. Dermatitis herpetiformis is highly pruritic, affects primarily the extensor surfaces, and has subepidermal vesicles with granular IgA deposits in the dermal papillary tips. Pemphigus foliaceus has acantholysis and a typical immunofluorescence pattern. IgA pemphigus of the SPD-type is only distinguishable through positive findings in direct and indirect immunofluorescence. Generalized pustular psoriasis (von Zumbusch type) presents with systemic symptoms (fever, malaise, leukocytosis), and spongiform pustules within the epidermis. The necrolytic migratory eruption of glucagonoma syndrome can be differentiated by its distribution, lack of actual pustule formation, erosions of the lips and oral mucosa, and, histologically, necrobiosis of the upper epidermis. Biochemically, hyperglycemia and excess levels of glucagon are diagnostic. Acute generalized exanthematous pustulosis is widespread with an acute febrile onset and histologically exhibits spongiform subcorneal and intraepidermal pustules sometimes with leukocytoclastic vasculitis.

PROGNOSIS AND CLINICAL COURSE

SPD is a benign condition. Without treatment, attacks recur over many years and remissions are variable, lasting from a few days to several weeks. Despite the protracted course the general health of the patient is usually not impaired. However, one of our own cases who had SPD, pyoderma gangrenosum, and IgA paraproteinemia of more than 20 years' duration died of septicemia with staphylococcal abscesses in the lungs, liver, and spleen.

TREATMENT

The drug of choice is dapsone (Table 38-2) in a dose of 50 to 150 mg daily. The response is slower and

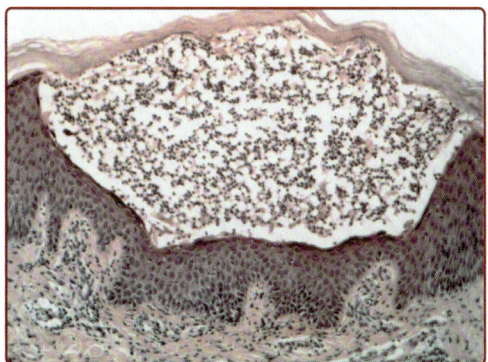

Figure 38-2 Subcorneal pustular dermatosis. Strictly subcorneal pustule filled with polymorphonuclear leukocytes, with the underlying epidermal layers exhibiting only slight edema and some migrating leukocytes. There is a mild inflammatory infiltrate around dermal blood vessels.

TABLE 38-2		
Treatments for Subcorneal Pustular Dermatosis		
First line	Dapsone	50-150 mg/day
	Corticosteroids	As required
Second line (anecdotally reported beneficial responses)	Retinoids, photochemotherapy, ultraviolet B, colchicine, cyclosporine, infliximab, etanercept	

less dramatic than in dermatitis herpetiformis, but complete remission is most often obtained. In some patients, the treatment may be withdrawn after several months, although in others it may have to be continued for years; the minimal effective dose to suppress disease should be determined in these patients with a chronic course. Systemic corticosteroids are less effective, although they can suppress generalized flares when given in high doses. Responses to retinoids, photochemotherapy, ultraviolet B, colchicine, cyclosporine, and topical tacalcitol (1α-24R-dihydroxyvitamin D_3) have been anecdotally reported.[32-35] More recently, anti–tumor necrosis factor-α therapy has been successfully used in single cases. Infliximab was described to induce rapid responses in 3 recalcitrant cases, with 1 patient relapsing despite continuing treatment.[25,36,37] In 2 patients, etanercept was able to induce almost complete continuing remissions for 7 and 22 months, as monotherapy or in combination with acitretin, respectively.[38] In 1 reported case of IgA myeloma-associated SPD long-lasting remission of both conditions was achieved with melphalan and autologous stem cell transplantation.[12]

REFERENCES

1. Sneddon IB, Wilkinson DS. Subcorneal pustular dermatosis. *Br J Dermatol*. 1956;68:385-394.
2. Wolff K. Ein Beitrag zur Nosologie der subcornealen pustulösen Dermatose (Sneddon-Wilkinson). *Arch Klin Exp Dermatol*. 1966;224(3):248-267.
3. Robinson ND, Hashimoto T, Amagai M, et al. The new pemphigus variants. *J Am Acad Dermatol*. 1999;40(5):649-671.
4. Kalaher KM, Scott DW. Subcorneal pustular dermatosis in dogs and in human beings: Comparative aspects. *J Am Acad Dermatol*. 1990;22:1023-1028.
5. Hashimoto T, Kiyokawa C, Mori O, et al. Human desmocollin 1 (Dsc1) is an autoantigen for the subcorneal pustular dermatosis type of IgA pemphigus. *J Invest Dermatol*. 1997;109(2):127-131.
6. Duker I, Schaller J, Rose C, et al. Subcorneal pustular dermatosis-type IgA pemphigus with autoantibodies to desmocollins 1, 2, and 3. *Arch Dermatol*. 2009;145(10):1159-1162.
7. Geller S, Gat A, Zeeli T, et al. The expanding spectrum of IgA pemphigus: a case report and review of the literature. *Br J Dermatol*. 2014;171(3):650-656.
8. Takata M, Inaoki M, Shodo M, et al. Subcorneal pustular dermatosis associated with IgA myeloma and intraepidermal IgA deposits. *Dermatology*. 1994;189:111-114.
9. Vaccaro M, Cannavo SP, Guarneri B. Subcorneal pustular dermatosis and IgA lambda myeloma: a uncommon association but probably not coincidental. *Eur J Dermatol*. 1999;9(8):644-646.
10. Stone MS, Lyckholm LJ. Pyoderma gangrenosum and subcorneal pustular dermatosis: clues to underlying immunoglobulin A myeloma. *Am J Med*. 1996;100:663-664.
11. Espana A, Gimenez-Azcarate A, Ishii N, et al. Anti-desmocollin 1 autoantibody negative subcorneal pustular dermatosis-type IgA pemphigus associated with multiple myeloma. *Br J Dermatol*. 2015;172(1):296-298.
12. von dem Borne PA, Jonkman MF, van Doorn R. Complete remission of skin lesions in a patient with subcorneal pustular dermatosis (Sneddon-Wilkinson disease) treated with anti-myeloma therapy: association with disappearance of M-protein. *Br J Dermatol*. 2017;176(5):1341-1344.
13. Scerri L, Zaki I, Allen BR. Pyoderma gangrenosum and subcorneal pustular dermatosis, without monoclonal gammopathy. *Br J Dermatol*. 1994;130:398-399.
14. Kohl PK, Hartschuh W, Tilgen W, et al. Pyoderma gangrenosum followed by subcorneal pustular dermatosis in a patient with IgA paraproteinemia. *J Am Acad Dermatol*. 1991;24:325-328.
15. Miyakawa K, Miyamoto R, Baba S, et al. Vesiculopustular dermatosis with ulcerative colitis. Concomitant occurrence of circulating IgA anti-intercellular and anti-basement membrane zone antibodies. *Eur J Dermatol*. 1995;5:122-124.
16. Delaporte E, Colombel JF, Nguyen Mailfer C, et al. Subcorneal pustular dermatosis in a patient with Crohn's disease. *Acta Derm Venereol*. 1992;72(4):301-302.
17. Lutz ME, Daoud MS, McEvoy MT, et al. Subcorneal pustular dermatosis: a clinical study of ten patients. *Cutis*. 1998;61(4):203-208.
18. Kavala M, Karadag AS, Zindanci I, et al. A case of subcorneal pustular dermatosis with IgG monoclonal gammopathy of undetermined significance: a rare association. *Int J Dermatol*. 2015;54(12):e551-e553.
19. Guggisberg D, Hohl D. Intraepidermal IgA pustulosis preceding a CD30+ anaplastic large T-cell lymphoma. *Dermatology*. 1995;191(4):352-354.
20. Ratnarathorn M, Newman J. Subcorneal pustular dermatosis (Sneddon-Wilkinson disease) occurring in association with nodal marginal zone lymphoma: a case report. *Dermatol Online J*. 2008;14(8):6.
21. Buchet S, Humbert P, Blanc D, et al. Pustulose sous-cornee associee a un carcinome epidermoide du poumon. *Ann Dermatol Venereol*. 1991;118(2):125-128.
22. Villey MC, Ehrsam E, Marrakchi S, et al. Apudoma and subcorneal pustular dermatosis (Sneddon-Wilkinson disease). *Dermatology*. 1992;185(4):269-271.
23. Roger H, Thevenet JP, Souteyrand P, et al. Subcorneal pustular dermatosis associated with rheumatoid arthritis and raised IgA: simultaneous remission of skin and joint involvements with dapsone treatment. *Ann Rheum Dis*. 1990;49:190-191.
24. Butt A, Burge SM. Sneddon-Wilkinson disease in association with rheumatoid arthritis. *Br J Dermatol*. 1995;132(2):313-315.
25. Naretto C, Baldovino S, Rossi E, et al. The case of SLE associated Sneddon-Wilkinson pustular disease successfully and safely treated with infliximab. *Lupus*. 2009;18(9):856-857.

26. Taniguchi S, Tsuruta D, Kutsuna H, et al. Subcorneal pustular dermatosis in a patient with hyperthyroidism. *Dermatology*. 1995;190:64-66.
27. Winnock T, Wang J, Suys E, et al. Vesiculopustular eruption associated with *Mycoplasma pneumoniae* pneumopathy. *Dermatology*. 1996;192:73-74.
28. Bohelay G, Duong TA, Ortonne N, et al. Subcorneal pustular dermatosis triggered by *Mycoplasma pneumoniae* infection: a rare clinical association. *J Eur Acad Dermatol Venereol*. 2015;29(5):1022-1025.
29. Iyengar S, Chambers CJ, Chang S, et al. Subcorneal pustular dermatosis associated with *Coccidioides immitis*. *Dermatol Online J*. 2015;21(8).
30. Lotery HE, Eedy DJ, McCusker G. Subcorneal pustular dermatosis involving the face. *J Eur Acad Dermatol Venereol*. 1999;12(3):230-233.
31. Haber H, Wells GC. Subcorneal pustular dermatosis of the soles. *Br J Dermatol*. 1959;71:253.
32. Bauwens M, De-Coninck A, Roseeuw D. Subcorneal pustular dermatosis treated with PUVA therapy. A case report and review of the literature. *Dermatology*. 1999;198(2):203-205.
33. Marliere V, Beylot-Barry M, Beylot C, et al. Successful treatment of subcorneal pustular dermatosis (Sneddon-Wilkinson disease) by acitretin: report of a case. *Dermatology*. 1999;199(2):153-155.
34. Cameron H, Dawe RS. Subcorneal pustular dermatosis (Sneddon-Wilkinson disease) treated with narrowband (TL-01) UVB phototherapy. *Br J Dermatol*. 1997;137(1):150-151.
35. Orton DI, George SA. Subcorneal pustular dermatosis responsive to narrowband (TL-01) UVB phototherapy. *Br J Dermatol*. 1997;137(1):149-150.
36. Voigtlander C, Luftl M, Schuler G, et al. Infliximab (antitumor necrosis factor alpha antibody): a novel, highly effective treatment of recalcitrant subcorneal pustular dermatosis (Sneddon-Wilkinson disease). *Arch Dermatol*. 2001;137(12):1571-1574.
37. Bonifati C, Trento E, Cordiali Fei P, et al. Early but not lasting improvement of recalcitrant subcorneal pustular dermatosis (Sneddon-Wilkinson disease) after infliximab therapy: relationships with variations in cytokine levels in suction blister fluids. *Clin Exp Dermatol*. 2005;30(6):662-665.
38. Berk DR, Hurt MA, Mann C, et al. Sneddon-Wilkinson disease treated with etanercept: report of two cases. *Clin Exp Dermatol*. 2009;34(3):347-351.

Chapter 39 :: Autoinflammatory Disorders
:: Takashi K. Satoh & Lars E. French

第三十九章
自身炎症性疾病

中文导读

本章共分为15节：①周期性综合症（CAPS）；②施尼茨勒综合征；③缺乏IL-1受体拮抗剂(DIRA)；④缺乏IL-36受体拮抗剂；⑤card14介导的脓疱性银屑病/银屑病；⑥家族性地中海热；⑦高免疫球蛋白血症伴周期性发热综合征/甲羟戊酸激酶缺乏；⑧肿瘤坏死因子受体相关周期综合征；⑨A20单倍体综合征；⑩Otulipenia/otulin相关的自身炎症综合征；⑪慢性非典型中性粒细胞性皮肤病伴脂肪营养不良和高温综合征/蛋白酶体相关的自身炎症综合征；⑫布劳综合征/早发结节病；⑬化脓性关节炎、坏疽性脓皮病、痤疮综合征；⑭马吉德综合征；⑮滑膜炎、痤疮、脓疱病、骨肥厚和骨炎综合征。每种疾病均从流行病学史、临床特点，涉及的基因以及诊断等方面进行介绍。本章重点介绍了自身炎症性疾病的临床特点和已知的发病机制(表39-1)。这些疾病大多表现为反复发热，可累及皮肤、关节、胃肠道、骨骼和浆膜表面，类似传染病、胶原血管疾病或恶性疾病。

〔李芳芳〕

AUTOINFLAMMATORY DISORDERS

AT-A-GLANCE

- Autoinflammatory disorders are caused by dysregulation of the innate immune system.
- Although many of the symptoms of autoinflammatory disorders, such as fever, skin lesions, and joint pain, mimic infection, the inflammation is sterile.
- Interleukin (IL)-1 plays a prominent role in a large subset of monogenic autoinflammatory disorders.
- Monogenic autoinflammatory disorders typically present in childhood but sometimes occur neonatally.
- Monogenic autoinflammatory disorders are mostly inherited in an autosomal-recessive or autosomal-dominant pattern, but there are a considerable number of sporadic cases.
- Characteristic skin eruptions are associated with a number of these disorders, including neutrophilic urticarial skin lesions, pustulosis, cellulitis-like skin lesions, erythematous and maculopapular eruptions. Skin lesions can be the sole remarkable disease manifestation in some disorders.
- Specific treatments exist, including IL-1 antagonists for cryopyrin-associated periodic syndromes (CAPS), Schnitzler syndrome, and deficiency of the interleukin (IL)-1 receptor antagonist (DIRA), and colchicine for familial Mediterranean fever (FMF). IL-1 antagonists have also been used with variable efficacy in FMF and hyperimmunoglobulinemia D with periodic fever syndrome (HIDS)/mevalonate kinase deficiency (MKD).
- An online database for autoinflammatory mutations is available at Infevers (http://fmf.igh.cnrs.fr/ISSAID/infevers/).

CRYOPYRIN-ASSOCIATED PERIODIC SYNDROMES

AT-A-GLANCE

- Cryopyrin-associated periodic syndromes (CAPS) are rare autosomal dominant disorders.
- CAPS are caused by gain of function mutations in NLRP3, the gene encoding NLRP3, also known as cryopyrin.
- Gain-of-function mutations in NLRP3 lead to inflammasome activation and subsequent abnormal interleukin (IL)-1β secretion.
- The spectrum of CAPS includes the familial cold autoinflammatory syndrome (FCAS; OMIM [Online Mendelian Inheritance in Man] #120100), Muckle-Wells syndrome (MWS; OMIM #191900), and the chronic infantile neurologic cutaneous and articular syndrome (CINCA; OMIM #607115), also known as neonatal-onset multisystem inflammatory disease (NOMID).
- The inheritance pattern in FCAS and MWS is familial whereas CINCA/NOMID cases are sporadic as a result of the severe phenotype that precludes reproduction.
- Urticarial skin lesions are a common characteristic feature in CAPS, and usually the first sign of disease.
- Clinical features include urticarial skin lesions, recurrent fever, arthralgia, conjunctivitis (FCAS, MWS, CINCA/NOMID); progressive hearing loss, amyloidosis, headache, progressive vision loss (MWS, CINCA/NOMID); and severe arthropathy, mental retardation and bone overgrowth (CINCA/NOMID).
- Histology of lesional skin reveals neutrophil-rich perivascular inflammation in the superficial dermis and mid-dermis. There is no evidence of vascular destruction or vasculitis.
- IL-1 antagonists are very effective and the standard of care in treating CAPS.

This chapter focuses on the clinical aspects and known pathogenesis of autoinflammatory disorders (Table 39-1). Most of these disorders present with recurrent fevers and involvement of the skin, the joints, the gastrointestinal tract, the bones, and serosal surfaces that mimic infectious disease, collagen-vascular disease, or malignant disease. Autoinflammatory disorders are, however, diseases of the innate immune system, characterized by recurrent episodes of systemic inflammation without the usual hallmarks of autoimmunity such as high autoantibody titers and the presence of antigen-specific T cells.[1,2] Although a delay in diagnosis is unfortunately common because of their rarity, the characteristic clinical features can help the clinician to make a diagnosis, which is confirmed by genetic testing.

EPIDEMIOLOGY

Cryopyrin-associated periodic syndromes (CAPS), also known as cryopyrinopathies, are a group of inherited inflammatory disorders caused by autosomal dominant gain-of-function mutations in NLRP3 (the gene encoding NLRP3, also known as cryopyrin).[3,4] The spectrum of CAPS includes the familial cold autoinflammatory syndrome (FCAS; OMIM #120100),[5] Muckle-Wells syndrome (MWS; OMIM #191900),[6] and the chronic infantile neurologic cutaneous and articular syndrome (CINCA; OMIM #607115),[7] also known

TABLE 39-1
Autoinflammatory Disorders

PATHOGENESIS	DISEASE	GENE	INHERITANCE PATTERN	PROTEIN	FLARE/FEVER PATTERN	INVOLVED ORGAN(S)
IL-1 mediated	CAPS:					
	FCAS	NLRP3/CIAS1	AD	NLRP3/Cryopyrin	<24 h	Skin, eyes, joints
	MWS	NLRP3/CIAS1	AD	NLRP3/Cryopyrin	24-48 h	Skin, eyes, joints, inner ears, meninges
	NOMID	NLRP3/CIAS1	AD/de novo	NLRP3/Cryopyrin	Continuous	Skin, eyes, joints, inner ears, meninges, bones
	Schnitzler syndrome	NLRP3/CIAS1[a]	De novo	NLRP3/Cryopyrin	Variable	Skin, bones, joints, blood (IgM gammopathy)
	DIRA	IL1RN	AR	IL-1 receptor antagonist	Continuous	Skin, bones, lungs (rare), vasculitis (rare)
Partially IL-1 mediated	FMF	MEFV	AR/AD[b]	Pyrin	1-3 days	Skin, joints, peritoneum, pleura
	HIDS/MKD	MVK	AR	Mevalonate kinase	3-7 days	Skin, mucosa, eyes, joints, prominent lymph nodes
	PAPA syndrome	PSTPIP1/CD2BP1	AD	PSTPIP1	Common	Skin, joints
	SAPHO syndrome	–	–	–	Uncommon	Skin, joints, bones
IL-36 mediated	DITRA	IL36RN	AR	IL-36 receptor antagonist	Common	Skin
Partially IL-36 mediated	CAMPS/PSORS2	CARD14	AD	CARD14	Variable	Skin
Other pathways	TRAPS	TNFRSF1A	AD	TNF receptor 1	1-4 weeks	Skin, eyes, joints, peritoneum, pleura
	HA20	TNFAIP3	AD	A20/TNFAIP3	Common	Skin, mucosa, eyes, joints, vasculitis, GI tract
	Otulipenia/ORAS	OTULIN	AR	OTULIN	Weeks	Skin, joints, muscles, lymph nodes, GI tract
	CANDLE/PRAAS	PSMB8	AR	PSMB8	Variable	Skin, joints, muscles, lymph nodes
	BS/EOS	NOD2/CARD15	AD/de novo	NOD2/CARD15	Uncommon	Skin, eyes, joints
	Majeed syndrome	LPIN2	AR	Lipin-2	Weeks-months	Skin, bones, periosteum, blood (anemia)

[a]Some patients have been shown to bear mosaicism of *NLRP3* mutations.
[b]AD is less common than AR in FMF.
AD, autosomal dominant; AR, autosomal recessive; BS, Blau syndrome; CAMPS, CARD14-mediated pustular psoriasis; CANDLE, chronic atypical neutrophilic dermatosis with lipodystrophy and elevated temperature; CAPS, cryopyrin-associated periodic syndromes; DIRA, deficiency of the IL-1 receptor antagonist; DITRA, deficiency of the IL-36 receptor antagonist; EOS, early-onset sarcoidosis; FCAS, familial cold autoinflammatory syndrome; FMF, familial Mediterranean fever; HA20, haploinsufficiency of A20; HIDS, hyperimmunoglobulinemia D with periodic fever syndrome; IgM, immunoglobulin M; IL, interleukin; MKD, mevalonate kinase deficiency; MWS, Muckle-Wells syndrome; NOMID, neonatal onset multisystem inflammatory disease; ORAS, OTULIN-related autoinflammatory syndrome; PAPA, pyogenic sterile arthritis, pyoderma gangrenosum, and acne; PRAAS, proteasome-associated autoinflammatory syndrome; PSORS2, Psoriasis 2; PSTPIP1, proline-serine-threonine phosphatase interacting protein 1; SAPHO, synovitis, acne, pustulosis, hyperostosis, and osteitis; TNF, tumor necrosis factor; TRAPS, TNF receptor-associated periodic syndrome.

as neonatal-onset multisystem inflammatory disease (NOMID). Periodic fever and urticarial skin lesions are the common clinical hallmarks, but FCAS, MWS, and CINCA/NOMID have certain distinctive clinical characteristics that differentiate these CAPS within a spectrum of increasing severity: FCAS being on the mild, and CINCA/NOMID on the severe end of the spectrum (Table 39-2).

The prevalence of CAPS is estimated to be between 1 and 2 individuals per 1,000,000 people in Europe, the United States and Japan. While the inheritance pattern in FCAS and MWS is usually familial, CINCA/NOMID is sporadic owing to the severe phenotype of untreated individuals and consequent inability to reproduce.

ETIOLOGY AND PATHOGENESIS

NLRP3 belongs to the NLRs (NOD-like receptors) family of cytoplasmic pattern recognition receptors. NLRP3 can form a multiprotein complex called the *inflammasome* together with adaptor proteins, and subsequently activate caspase-1, an enzyme that cleaves pro-interleukin (IL)-1β to its active form.[8] Gain-of-function mutations in *NLRP3* associated with CAPS lead to constitutive activation of caspase-1 and subsequent abnormal IL-1β secretion.[9,10]

CLINICAL FEATURES

Urticarial skin lesions are the common characteristic features in all forms of CAPS and are usually the first sign of disease (Fig. 39-1A). They resemble common urticaria at first glance because the smooth, slightly elevated erythematous lesions (wheals) are migratory and skin returns to its normal appearance without residual pigmentation. The symptoms, however, tend to be atypical for common urticaria because lesions are usually nonpruritic or only slightly itchy and not associated with any particular sensation; some patients describe sensations of stinging, burning, and tightness. Unlike in common urticaria, urticarial skin lesions in CAPS are unresponsive to antihistamines. Histologically, the urticarial skin lesions are characterized by a neutrophilic-rich dermal perivascular inflammatory infiltrate (Fig. 39-1B).

FCAS is the mildest condition of CAPS. The main clinical features are urticarial skin lesions and low-grade fever of short duration that develop usually 1 to 2 hours after exposure to cold temperature.[11] Attacks are more common in winter and can occur upon exposure to cold outside temperatures and cold air-conditioned rooms. The ice-cube provocation test is negative for the urticaria. Systemic cold exposure is needed to trigger an intense episode. The flares tend to be brief, typically lasting less than 24 hours, and can also include arthralgia, conjunctivitis, headaches, nausea, and fatigue. The arthralgia mostly affects the hands, knees, and ankles. The attacks usually begin in infancy and early childhood.

Patients with MWS or CINCA/NOMID typically present with urticarial skin lesions at birth or within hours of birth, although some patients present first symptoms later. MWS was originally described as a triad of urticaria, deafness, and amyloidosis. Inflammatory episodes in MWS can be frequent and random, and are only variably triggered by cold. Most attacks last 24 to 48 hours but can also be continuous. Patients with MWS commonly have fevers, urticarial skin lesions, arthralgia, and headache that reflects aseptic meningitis. Progressive sensory neural hearing loss often appears clinically during the second to third decade of life. Conjunctivitis and uveitis also can be present.

TABLE 39-2
Clinical Characteristics of CAPS

	FCAS	MWS	CINCA/NOMID
Severity	Mild	Moderate	Severe
Duration of clinical signs	<24 h	1-2 days or subcontinuous	Continuous with variable exacerbations
Triggers	Cold induced	None	None
Fever	Recurrent	Recurrent	Continuous
Skin manifestations	Cold-induced urticarial skin lesions	Urticarial skin lesions	Urticarial skin lesions
Joint involvement	Arthralgias, stiffness	Arthralgias, arthritis	Deforming arthropathy
Neurologic involvement	None	None	Chronic aseptic meningitis
Eye involvement	Conjunctivitis	Conjunctivitis, uveitis	Conjunctivitis, uveitis, optic neuritis, papilledema
Auditory involvement	None	Sensorineural hearing loss	Sensorineural hearing loss
Amyloidosis	Rare	Frequent	Frequent

CINCA, chronic infantile neurologic cutaneous and articular syndrome; FCAS; familial cold autoinflammatory syndrome; MWS, Muckle-Wells syndrome; NOMID, neonatal onset multisystem inflammatory disease.

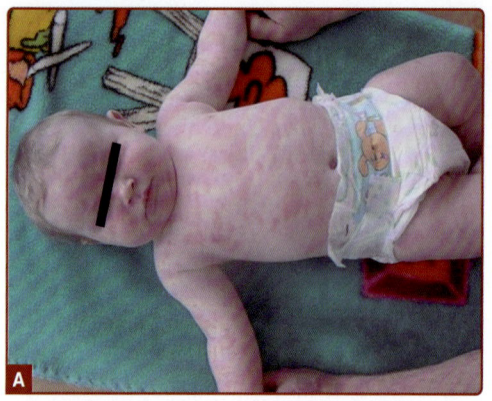

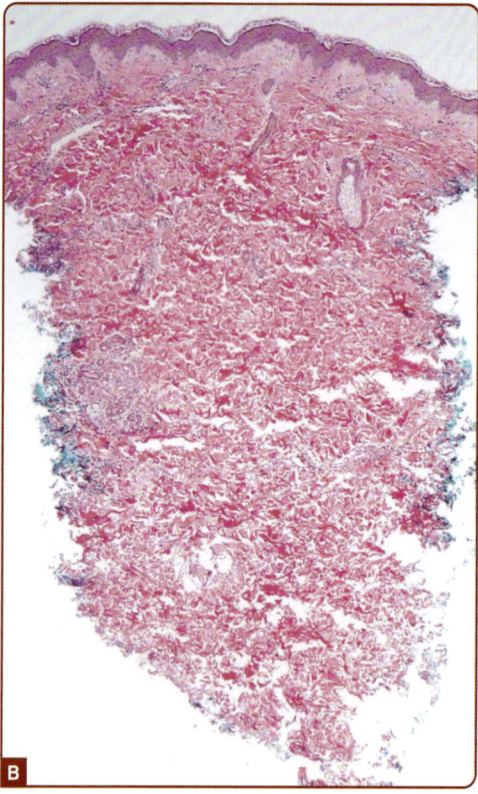

Figure 39-1 Cryopyrin-associated periodic syndromes (CAPS). **A,** Urticarial skin lesions in a 2-month-old baby with Muckle-Wells syndrome. (From Wolff K, Johnson R, Saavedra AP. *Fitzpatrick's Color Atlas and Synopsis of Clinical Dermatology*, 7th ed. New York, NY: McGraw-Hill; 2013. Used with permission from Drs. Klemens Rappersberger and Christian Posch.) **B,** Histology of the skin. Histologic examination reveals a predominant perivascular neutrophilic infiltrate without vasculitis, dilated superficial dermal capillaries, and dermal edema.

elevated CNS pressure causes chronic papilledema, which can lead to serious loss of vision. Sensory neural hearing loss develops typically within the first year of life.[9] Also, patients develop characteristic long-bone epiphyseal overgrowth and short stature, and amyloidosis develops after years of chronic inflammation.[12]

DIAGNOSIS

The initial diagnosis of CAPS relies heavily on the patients' history and it should be considered in patients presenting with recurrent episodes of fever, urticarial skin lesions, joint pain, and inflammation of the eyes, without evidence of infection or autoimmune disease. Positive family history is not always evident. A delay in the diagnosis is, unfortunately, common, and initial diagnoses of viral infection or allergy are usually considered. Elevated levels of blood acute-phase reactants such as C-reactive protein (CRP), erythrocyte sedimentation rate (ESR), and serum amyloid A (SAA) are typically present, especially during attacks, but can remain elevated to some extent even between episodes although at lower levels. Marked leukocytosis, especially neutrophilia, and mild anemia are also observed. Eosinophilia can variably be present.

Skin biopsy of an urticarial skin lesion can contribute to making the diagnosis of CAPS. The histologic features are the same for FCAS, MWS, and CINCA/NOMID, and characterized by a dermal perivascular infiltration of neutrophils in the superficial dermis and mid-dermis. There is no evidence of vascular destruction or vasculitis, and the epidermis is usually intact (see Fig. 39-1B).

Careful CNS assessment is useful in CINCA/NOMID. Elevated cerebrospinal fluid pressure and leukocytosis, predominantly with neutrophils but without any evidence of infection, are present. High-resolution gadolinium-enhanced MRI can show enhancement of the leptomeninges and cochlea. Radiographs of the long bones reveal epiphyseal overgrowth that is characteristic and unique to CINCA/NOMID.[12]

Diagnostic confirmation is achieved by genetic testing for *NLRP3* mutations. Although almost all patients with FCAS and MWS are mutation-positive, not all CINCA/NOMID patients who meet the phenotypic classification have a detectable mutation. Some mutation-negative patients have *NLRP3* mosaicism, which cannot be detected by conventional genetic analyses.[13] Consequently, a negative genetic test does not exclude the diagnosis of CAPS and it is important to consider genetic results in the context of the patient's symptoms.

DIFFERENTIAL DIAGNOSIS

FCAS may be confused with acquired cold urticaria, a more common condition. Acquired cold urticaria does not present with fever or arthralgia, and the skin lesions

Patients with CINCA/NOMID tend to have persistent inflammation and, in most cases, infants have diffuse erythema and fever at birth. Chronic aseptic meningitis is common, and without treatment with IL-1 antagonists, patients typically develop progressive brain atrophy and cognitive impairment. Conjunctivitis and uveitis starts shortly after birth and respond to antihistamines. Urticarial skin lesions at birth may be misdiagnosed as a benign newborn eruption. CINCA/NOMID patients can present more dramatically, mimicking neonatal sepsis or congenital "TORCH" (toxoplasmosis, other infections, rubella virus, cytomegalovirus, and herpes simplex virus) infections. Systemic juvenile idiopathic arthritis (sJIA, also called Still disease), a subtype of chronic childhood arthritis with daily fever episodes and evanescent erythematous macular skin lesions, needs to be considered in the differential diagnosis. Epiphyseal overgrowth of long bones in CINCA/NOMID can be differentially diagnosed as benign or malignant bone tumors.

CLINICAL COURSE AND PROGNOSIS

CAPS is a lifelong disease and the clinical course and prognosis greatly depends on the disease phenotype. Long-term prognosis of FCAS is good and clinical manifestations primarily affect quality of life. In MWS and CINCA/NOMID, however, early diagnosis and treatment can significantly improve the clinical course and prognosis, by reducing cumulative organ damage resulting from chronic inflammation and thus preventing severe complications. In untreated MWS individuals, the long-term prognosis is usually affected by amyloidosis, impaired renal function, and deafness. In CINCA/NOMID patients, the long-term prognosis depends on the severity of neurologic and joint involvement, as well as renal function. Hearing loss usually develops in the first decade of life, accompanied by mental retardation, progressive vision loss, and severe physical disabilities resulting from bone overgrowth and the development of joint contractures.[14]

MANAGEMENT

A large majority of patients with FCAS, MWS, and CINCA/NOMID respond dramatically to IL-1 antagonists with rapid and sustainable resolution of clinical symptoms and complete normalization of inflammatory markers such as CRP and SAA under continuous treatment. Anakinra (Kineret, a recombinant IL-1 receptor antagonist) was the first drug used to treat CAPS.[15-17] This biologic competitively inhibits the binding of IL-1α and IL-1β to the IL-1 receptor and is administered daily as a subcutaneous injection. Dosing is variable, with higher doses required to control more severe disease. Typically, 0.5 to 1.5 mg/kg/day of anakinra are sufficient to suppress disease activity in FCAS patients, but 6 to 10 mg/kg/day may be needed to treat CINCA/NOMID.[16] Anakinra can pass through the blood–brain barrier and improves aseptic meningitis and ocular and cochlear inflammation in CINCA/NOMID.

IL-1 antagonist therapy should be continued for life, and optimally started as early as possible so as to minimize irreversible neurologic complications. There are also two longer-acting IL-1 antagonists. Rilonacept (Arcalyst), also known as IL-1 Trap, is a dimeric fusion protein comprised of the extracellular domain of the human IL-1 receptor fused to the Fc domain of human immunoglobulin (Ig) G_1, that binds and neutralizes IL-1.[18] Its half-life is 8.6 days and it is administered as a weekly subcutaneous injection at 160 mg (a dose for an adult). Canakinumab (Ilaris) is a human monoclonal antibody specific for IL-1β, with a mean half-life of 26 days that is usually administered every 8 weeks at 150 mg (a dose for an adult) via subcutaneous injection.[19] Rilonacept and canakinumab have been approved by the U.S. Food and Drug Administration (FDA) for the treatment of FCAS and MWS and canakinumab by many countries including within the EU, Switzerland, and Japan, but not the United States, for CINCA/NOMID. All 3 drugs are generally well tolerated without significant limiting side effects.

SCHNITZLER SYNDROME

AT-A-GLANCE

- Schnitzler syndrome is a rare, late-onset inflammatory disease considered as a sporadic acquired autoinflammatory disorder.
- Some Schnitzler syndrome patients have been shown to have mosaicism of *NLRP3* mutations.
- Recurrent urticarial skin lesions, fever, bone pain and arthralgias are common manifestations, sharing many features with CAPS.
- Coexistence of a monoclonal IgM gammopathy is a diagnostic feature, and patients may develop a lymphoproliferative disorder.

EPIDEMIOLOGY

Schnitzler syndrome is a rare late-onset inflammatory disease characterized by recurrent fever, urticarial skin lesions, arthritis and lymphadenopathy accompanied by IgM gammopathy.[20,21] Patients present with the first symptoms typically around 50 years of age or older. Approximately 300 cases of Schnitzler syndrome have been reported worldwide.

ETIOLOGY AND PATHOGENESIS

The exact cause of Schnitzler syndrome is still a matter of investigation but it is now considered to be a

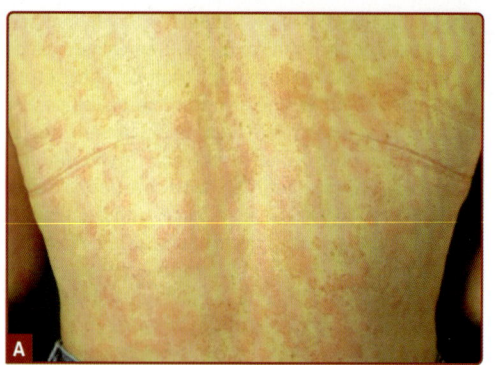
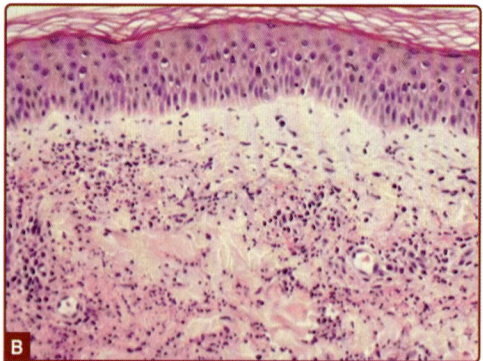
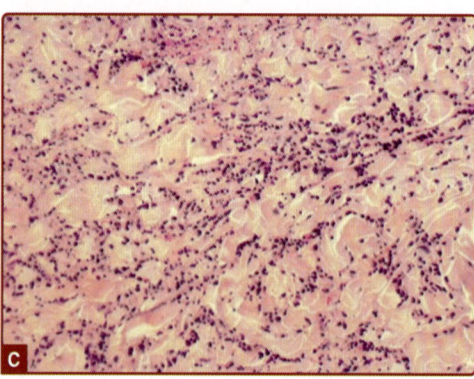

Figure 39-2 Schnitzler syndrome. **A,** Urticarial skin lesions in a patient with Schnitzler syndrome. **B,** Histology of the skin. A neutrophilic infiltrate of the dermis without vasculitis. **C,** Significant neutrophilic infiltrate with interstitial dispersion and leukocytoclasia. (From Lipsker D. The Schnitzler syndrome. *Orphanet J Rare Dis.* 2010;5:38, with permission.)

CLINICAL FEATURES

There are strong clinical similarities between Schnitzler syndrome and CAPS.[20] Recurrent urticarial skin lesions are usually the first sign of Schnitzler syndrome and can precede the other symptoms for years (Fig. 39-2A). The lesions are usually nonpruritic or only slightly itchy, resolve within 24 to 48 hours, and, invariably, antihistamines are ineffective. The frequency of urticarial skin changes ranges from daily to a few episodes per year. The histology reveals a neutrophilic infiltrate of the perivascular and interstitial dermis with intact epidermis and no signs of vasculitis, consistent with CAPS (Fig. 39-2B and C). The second most common symptom is intermittent fever, which can rise above 40°C (104°F). Many patients develop bone pain and arthralgias. Bone lesions can be observed on imaging studies. Lymphadenopathy and hepatosplenomegaly can also be seen.

Elevated CRP and ESR are typically present. Leukocytosis, usually neutrophilia, and mild anemia are also observed. Monoclonal gammopathy, mostly IgMκ light chain, is seen in 85% of Schnitzler syndrome patients, which is a characteristic feature of the syndrome and distinguishes it from CAPS.

DIAGNOSIS

The diagnosis of Schnitzler syndrome relies heavily on a combination of clinical, laboratory and radiologic findings. It should be considered in patients with recurrent episodes of urticarial skin lesions, fever, and bone and joint pain without evidence of infection or autoimmune disease.

The presence of a monoclonal IgM gammopathy helps the diagnosis. Detection of mosaicism in *NLRP3* by standard Sanger sequencing is difficult and next-generation sequencing provides the opportunity for scrutinizing genetic susceptibility. An immediate and marked response to anakinra or canakinumab is supportive of the diagnosis.

DIFFERENTIAL DIAGNOSIS

Schnitzler syndrome shares many features with CAPS, notably chronic systemic inflammation, which includes urticarial skin lesions and fever. Onset age would be a distinguishing factor from CAPS but not the absence of *NLRP3* mutation as some CAPS patients are also mutation-negative. Urticarial vasculitis should be excluded. Urticarial vasculitis usually presents with nonpruritic urticarial skin lesions persisting for more than 24 hours, arthralgia, fever, leukocytosis, and elevated CRP and ESR. Skin biopsy of urticarial vasculitis shows fibrinoid necrosis of vessel walls with fibrin extravasation, which is not observed in Schnitzler syndrome. Other differentials include cryoglobulinemia,

sporadic acquired autoinflammatory disorder. It has been reported that peripheral blood mononuclear cells taken from patients release increased amounts of IL-1β spontaneously and in response to lipopolysaccharide. Some Schnitzler syndrome patients have been shown to have a mosaicism of *NLRP3* mutations exclusively in the myeloid lineage.[20]

acquired C1 inhibitor deficiency, adult-onset Still disease, and hyperimmunoglobulinemia D with periodic fever syndrome (HIDS).

CLINICAL COURSE AND PROGNOSIS

Schnitzler syndrome follows a chronic course. Amyloidosis may develop and become a serious complication. Approximately 10% to 20% of patients with Schnitzler syndrome develop a lymphoproliferative disorder such as Waldenström macroglobulinemia and B-cell lymphoma. The prevalence rate for lymphoproliferative disorders is close to that observed in patients with monoclonal IgM gammopathies of undetermined significance. The overall prognosis of Schnitzler syndrome depends on the possible evolution to lymphoproliferative disorder.

MANAGEMENT

The urticarial skin legions of Schnitzler syndrome are resistant to antihistamines. Nonsteroidal antiinflammatory drugs (NSAIDs) and corticosteroids are reported to provide variable relief from fever, bone pain, and arthralgias, but not urticarial lesions. Both anakinra and canakinumab can induce a complete remission in more than 90% of Schnitzler syndrome cases. Symptoms recur within 1 to several days upon withdrawal of anakinra.

DEFICIENCY OF THE IL-1 RECEPTOR ANTAGONIST

AT-A-GLANCE

- Deficiency of the IL-1 receptor antagonist (DIRA) is a rare autosomal recessive disorder (OMIM #612852).
- DIRA is caused by mutations in *IL1RN*, the gene coding IL-1Ra.
- Mutations in *IL1RN* lead to complete absence or dysfunction of IL-1Ra and thus to unopposed and hyperactive IL-1 signaling.
- Pustular skin eruption, oral mucosal lesions, joint swelling, and bone inflammation are common manifestations.
- Cutaneous manifestation can vary widely from normal skin with pustules to generalized severe pustulosis or ichthyosiform lesions.
- IL-1–targeted therapy with recombinant IL-1Ra is very effective.

EPIDEMIOLOGY

Deficiency of the IL-1Ra (DIRA; OMIM #612852) is a very rare autosomal recessive inherited disease caused by mutations in *IL1RN*.[22,23] The mutations in *IL1RN* are founder mutations and the carrier frequencies of identified founder mutations in Newfoundland and Puerto Rico are estimated to be 0.2% and 1.3%, respectively.[22] Reported patients so far originated from Brazil, Canada, Lebanon, Netherlands, Puerto Rico, and Turkey. Heterozygous carriers are asymptomatic.

ETIOLOGY AND PATHOGENESIS

The IL-1Ra encoded by the *IL1RN* gene functions as a negative endogenous regulator of IL-1 signaling by competitively binding to IL-1R and preventing the activities of IL-1α and IL-1β. Mutations in *IL1RN* lead to complete absence or dysfunction of IL-1Ra and thus to unopposed hyperactive IL-1 signaling.

CLINICAL FEATURES

DIRA clinically manifests as perinatal to several months of age-onset pustular skin eruption, with oral mucosal lesions, failure to gain weight and painful joint swelling. Fetal distress was present in 6 of 10 reported patients before birth. Characteristic radiographic findings include balloon-like widening of the anterior rib ends, periosteal elevation of multiple long bones, and multifocal osteolytic lesions. High fever is not a typical feature in DIRA.

Cutaneous pustulosis can range from normal skin with rare individual pustules to discrete crops of pustules, generalized severe pustulosis, or ichthyosiform lesions (Fig. 39-3A).[22-24] Oral mucosal vesicular lesions or aphthous ulcers are seen early in life in some patients, but do not seem to recur later in life. Nail changes, including onychomadesis and pits, also can be seen. Histologically, the epidermal changes in DIRA are characterized by the presence of intraepidermal neutrophils and neutrophilic pustules. Marked papillary dermal edema is commonly present and may be associated with subepidermal vesiculation. An intense neutrophilic inflammatory infiltrate is present throughout the dermis and may extend to involve the superficial subcutis. Changes of frank vasculitis are absent in most patients; however, vasculitis was observed in the connective and fat tissue adjacent to bone in 1 patient.

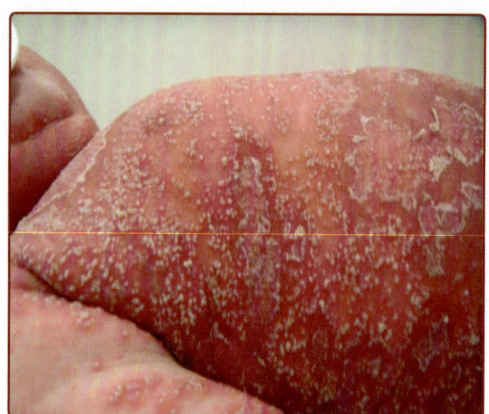

Figure 39-3 Deficiency of the IL-1 receptor antagonist (DIRA). Small pustules over erythematous patches on the skin of a child with DIRA. (From Jesus AA, Osman M, Silva CA, et al. A novel mutation of IL1RN in the deficiency of interleukin-1 receptor antagonist syndrome: description of two unrelated cases from Brazil. *Arthritis Rheum.* 2011;63(12):4007-4017, with permission. Copyright © 2011 John Wiley & Sons.)

DIAGNOSIS

DIRA may be initially erroneously diagnosed as infectious osteomyelitis because of the significant bone inflammation, but the bone and blood cultures are negative and symptoms are unresponsive to antibiotics. Although DIRA and CINCA/NOMID share certain clinical similarities, patients with DIRA typically do not show urticarial skin lesions or neurologic inflammation, such as aseptic meningitis, cochlear inflammation, and mental retardation, which are seen in CINCA/NOMID. Genetic testing to identify the mutation of *IL1RN* gene confirms the diagnosis of DIRA.

CLINICAL COURSE AND PROGNOSIS

Failure to recognize the disease and treat it appropriately with recombinant IL-1Ra leads to the development of a severe inflammatory response syndrome and neonatal death from multiorgan failure.

MANAGEMENT

Treatment with recombinant IL-1Ra (anakinra, brand name Kineret), which substitutes the missing functional IL-1Ra protein, results in rapid and dramatic clinical improvement.[22,23,25] Patients with DIRA need to be treated with anakinra for life. Long-term consequences of anakinra therapy in these patients are not yet well-defined.

DEFICIENCY OF THE IL-36 RECEPTOR ANTAGONIST

AT-A-GLANCE

- Deficiency of the IL-36 receptor antagonist (DITRA) is a rare autosomal recessive disorder (OMIM #614204).
- DITRA is caused by mutations in *IL36RN*, the gene coding IL-36 receptor antagonist (IL-36Ra).
- Lack of the negative regulator IL-36Ra leads to aberrant IL-36 signaling and subsequent overproduction of IL-8, a strong neutrophil chemoattractant, in keratinocytes.
- Although DITRA was originally described in patients with familial generalized pustular psoriasis (GPP), mutations in *IL36RN* have been reported in rare cases of sporadic GPP.
- DITRA typically presents as recurrent flares of a generalized erythematopustular skin eruption of sudden onset, accompanied by high fever.
- Onset of disease is during childhood in many cases, but can occur during adulthood.
- Viral or bacterial infections, medications, menstruation, pregnancy, and withdrawal of retinoid therapy can trigger the disease.

EPIDEMIOLOGY

Deficiency of the IL-36 receptor antagonist (DITRA; OMIM #614204) is a rare autosomal recessive disorder caused by homozygous or compound heterozygous mutations in *IL36RN*.[26,27] This gene was identified as one of the causative genes of familial generalized pustular psoriasis (GPP). Mutations in *IL36RN* are also found in certain sporadic cases of GPP. DITRA is termed as a monogenic form of GPP caused by *IL36RN* mutation. The disease onset mostly commences during childhood but can occur during adulthood. Interestingly, *IL36RN* mutations are also associated with some cases of localized pustular psoriasis such as palmoplantar pustulosis (PPP) and acrodermatitis continua of Hallopeau.

ETIOLOGY AND PATHOGENESIS

IL36RN encodes the IL-36 receptor antagonist (IL-36Ra) that antagonizes all 3 proinflammatory cytokines that belong to the IL-36 family: IL-36α, IL-36β, and IL-36γ. IL-36Ra is primarily expressed in keratinocytes in the skin. Lack of the negative regulator IL-36Ra causes aberrant IL-36 signaling and subsequent IL-8 production by keratinocytes, the latter being a strong chemoattractant for neutrophils.

CLINICAL FEATURES

DITRA typically presents as recurrent and sudden onset of flares of a generalized erythematopustular skin eruption (Fig. 39-4A-D), accompanied by high fever (40-42°C [104-107.6°F]), neutrophilia, and elevated hepatic acute-phase proteins. The disease flares are thought to be triggered by viral or bacterial infections, medications (eg, amoxicillin), menstruation, pregnancy, and withdrawal of retinoid therapy. Withdrawal of systemic corticosteroids can precipitate or worsen GPP but little is known concerning this phenomenon in DITRA. The frequency of flares varies from patient to patient, and in some patients the disease manifests itself as chronic erythematous plaques without pustules. No joint involvement is observed in DITRA, but nail dystrophy can occur. DITRA can be a life-threatening disease owing to severe complications resulting from the repeated flares of prominent systemic inflammation. Skin histology demonstrates neutrophil infiltration in the upper epidermis forming spongiform pustules of Kogoj with acanthosis (Fig. 39-4E).[28]

DIAGNOSIS

DITRA is diagnosed by genetic testing revealing *IL36RN* mutation in GPP patients. GPP is often suspected clinically and confirmed by skin biopsy and laboratory tests, including neutrophilia, elevated acute-phase reactants, and absence of bacterial infection. DITRA can occur in GPP patients with or without psoriasis vulgaris, but more frequently in the absence of psoriasis vulgaris.

DIFFERENTIAL DIAGNOSIS

Differential diagnosis includes bacterial impetigo, subcorneal pustular dermatosis (Sneddon-Wilkinson disease), impetigo herpetiformis, and acute generalized exanthematous pustulosis. Acute generalized exanthematous pustulosis is a severe adverse drug reaction that is widespread with an acute febrile onset, usually not recurrent, and histologically exhibits spongiform subcorneal and intraepidermal pustules. Of note, some acute generalized exanthematous pustulosis patients also have mutations in *IL36RN*.

MANAGEMENT

The optimal treatment for DITRA has not been established yet, but IL-1 and IL-17 antagonists are reported to have efficacy. Recombinant IL-36Ra, if and when available, would be expected to be a valuable therapy.

CARD14-MEDIATED PUSTULAR PSORIASIS/ PSORIASIS 2

AT-A-GLANCE

- CARD14-mediated pustular psoriasis (CAMPS)/psoriasis 2 (PSORS2) is a rare autosomal dominant disorder (OMIM #602723).
- CAMPS/PSORS2 is caused by gain-of-function mutations in *CARD14*.
- Gain-of-function mutations in *CARD14* lead to aberrant mitogen-activated protein kinase activity and nuclear factor-kappa B signaling, resulting in overproduction of IL-8 and IL-36γ.
- Patients with CAMPS/PSORS2 have various symptoms of psoriasis, including symptoms of plaque and pustular psoriasis.

EPIDEMIOLOGY

CARD14-mediated pustular psoriasis (CAMPS; OMIM #602723), also known as psoriasis 2 (PSORS2), is an autosomal dominant disorder caused by gain-of-function mutations in *CARD14* (also called *CARMA2*). Causative mutations in *CARD14* were described in 1 family of European decent, in 1 family of Taiwanese descent and in a Haitian child. Interestingly, some *CARD14* variants also predispose to psoriasis, and other *CARD14* mutations can cause familial pityriasis rubra pilaris (OMIM #173200).

ETIOLOGY AND PATHOGENESIS

CARD14 is primarily expressed in epidermal keratinocytes. CARD14 has multifactorial functions and activates the mitogen-activated protein kinase and nuclear factor-kappa B (NF-κB) signaling pathways. CAMPS/PSORS2-associated mutations are known to upregulate NF-κB activity.[29] This results in increased transcription of genes encoding psoriasis-associated

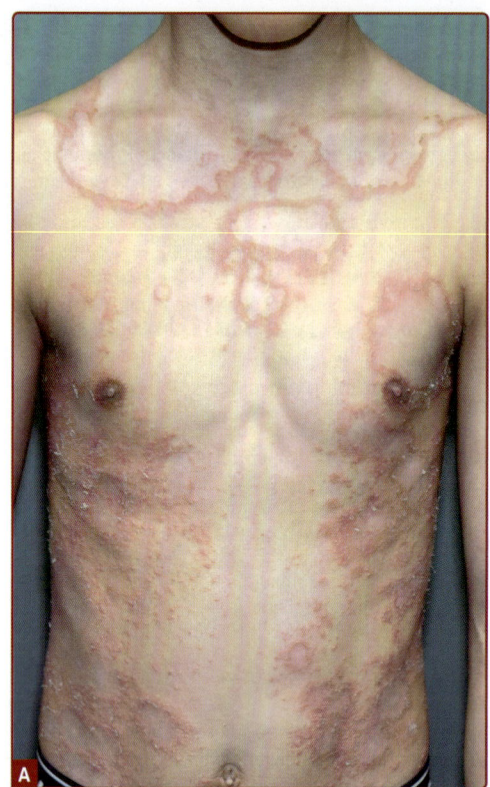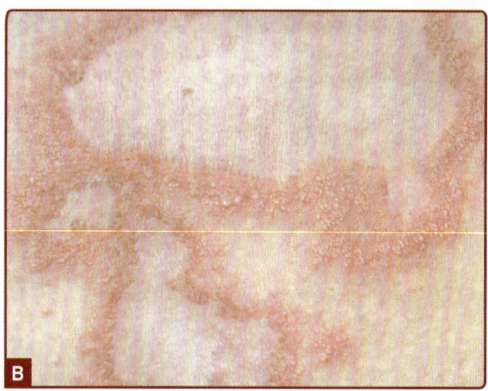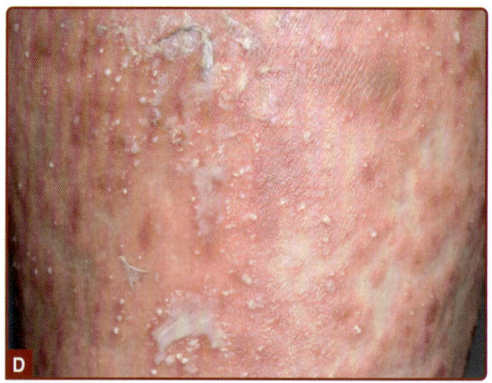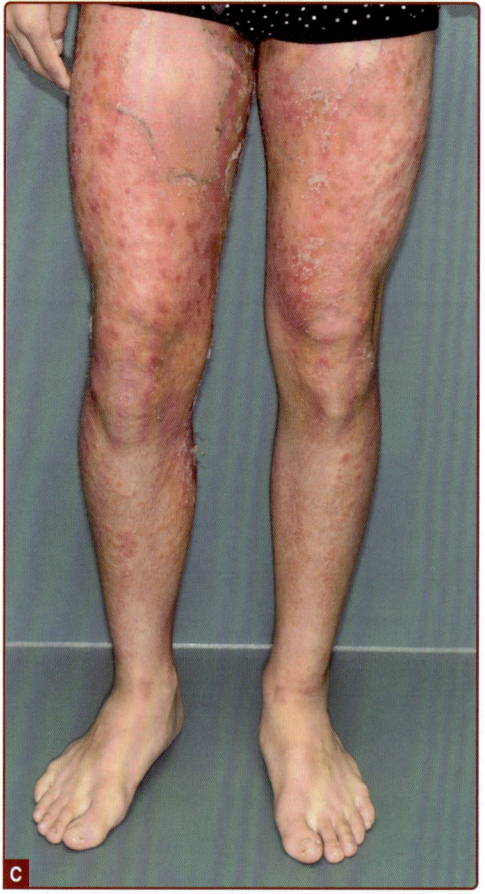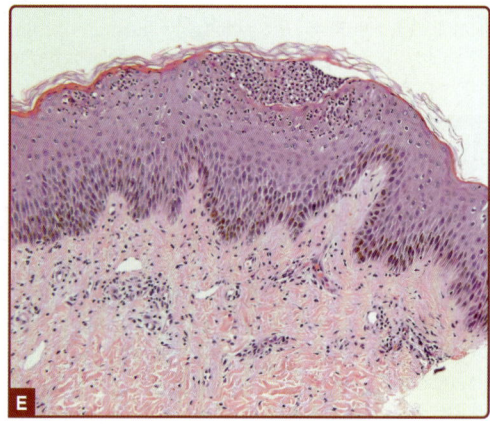

Figure 39-4 Deficiency of the IL-36 receptor antagonist (DITRA). **A** and **B**, Photographs of circinate erythema, accompanied by miliary pustules on his trunk, which enlarged over several weeks. **C** and **D**, Photographs of generalized pustular psoriasis, which developed in 2 months after the appearance of circinate erythema, accompanied by a high fever, edema, pustules, and yellow-green lakes of pus. **E**, Histopathologic examination showing spongiform pustules of Kogoj. (From Koike Y, Okubo M, Kiyohara T, et al. Granulocyte and monocyte apheresis can control juvenile generalized pustular psoriasis with mutation of IL36RN. *Br J Dermatol*. 2017;177(6):1732-1736, with permission. Copyright © 2017 John Wiley & Sons.)

cytokines and chemokines, including IL-8, IL-36γ, and C-C motif chemokine ligand 20 (CCL20) in keratinocytes.

CLINICAL FEATURES

Patients with CAMPS/PSORS2 can show various symptoms of common psoriasis, including plaque psoriasis and pustular psoriasis (Fig. 39-5).[30]

MANAGEMENT

Management remains to be defined, but one case of CAMPS/PSORS2 has been reported to be successfully treated with the IL-12/IL-23 antagonist ustekinumab.

FAMILIAL MEDITERRANEAN FEVER

AT-A-GLANCE

- Familial Mediterranean fever (FMF) is the most common and the first genetically characterized monogenic autoinflammatory disorder (OMIM #249100).
- FMF is caused by mutations in *MEFV*, the gene encoding pyrin.
- FMF is autosomal recessively inherited in most cases, but there is a less-common autosomal dominant form of FMF caused by mutations in *MEFV* (OMIM #134610).
- Mutations in *MEFV* lead to pyrin-inflammasome activation and subsequent abnormal IL-1β secretion.
- FMF is characterized by recurrent febrile attacks associated erysipelas-like skin lesions, peritonitis, pleuritis, and synovitis. These attacks last for 1 to 3 days.
- Erysipelas (cellulitis)-like skin lesions are a characteristic cutaneous feature of FMF.
- Histopathology of erysipelas-like skin lesions shows edema of the superficial dermis and a perivascular and interstitial neutrophilic infiltrate without vasculitis.
- Colchicine is very effective in preventing attacks and minimizing progression of amyloidosis.

EPIDEMIOLOGY

Familial Mediterranean fever (FMF; OMIM #249100) is an autosomal recessive disease characterized by recurrent attacks of fever and serosal inflammation.[31,32] FMF can affect individuals of any ethnic origin but the rates are highest in certain Mediterranean populations of Armenian, Sephardic-Jewish, Arabic, and Turkish ancestry. Of 200 people in these ethnic groups, 1 may develop the disease; 80% of cases are diagnosed before 10 years of age, and 90% before 20 years of age.

ETIOLOGY AND PATHOGENESIS

The gene responsible for FMF is the Mediterranean fever *(MEFV)* gene that encodes pyrin.[31,32] Pyrin is expressed predominantly in the cytoplasm of cells of myeloid lineage including neutrophils, along with synovial fibroblasts and dendritic cells. Pyrin can form an inflammasome together with adaptor proteins and subsequently activate caspase-1. Mutations in *MEFV* are thought to be gain-of-function mutations even though the homozygous or compound heterozygous mutations are required for inducing inflammation (gene–dosage effect is expected). Of note, there is a less-common autosomal dominant form of FMF caused by mutations in *MEFV* (OMIM #134610). Aberrant pyrin activity results in uncontrolled production of IL-1β. Pyrin is associated with microtubules and the microtubule-disrupting drug colchicine inhibits pyrin-inflammasome activation, as well as the neutrophil phagocytosis and chemotaxis.

CLINICAL FEATURES

FMF is characterized by recurrent short febrile attacks associated with peritonitis, pleuritis, synovitis and erysipelas-like skin lesions. Erysipelas-like skin lesions are well-demarcated, warm, tender, swollen, red skin lesions observed mainly on the front of the lower legs between the ankle and the knee, on the dorsum of the foot, or in the ankle region (Fig. 39-6A).[33,34] Typically, these attacks last for 1 to 3 days and occur randomly, from once per week to once in several months. Patients are completely well between the attacks. Cold exposure, fatigue, emotional stress, and menstruation may trigger an attack. Histopathology of the skin shows edema of the superficial dermis and a perivascular and interstitial neutrophilic infiltrate without vasculitis (Fig. 39-6B).

In infants, particularly children younger than age 2 years, fever alone can be the initial presenting symptom and typically progresses to include the other more specific symptoms by the age of 5 years,[35] which may

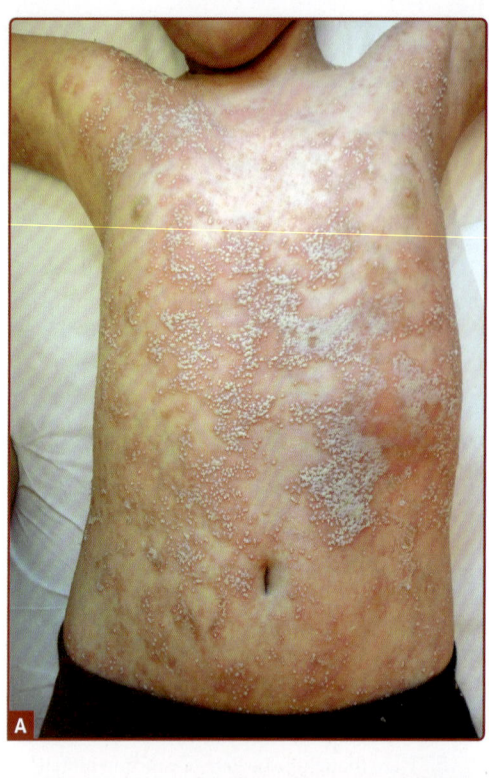
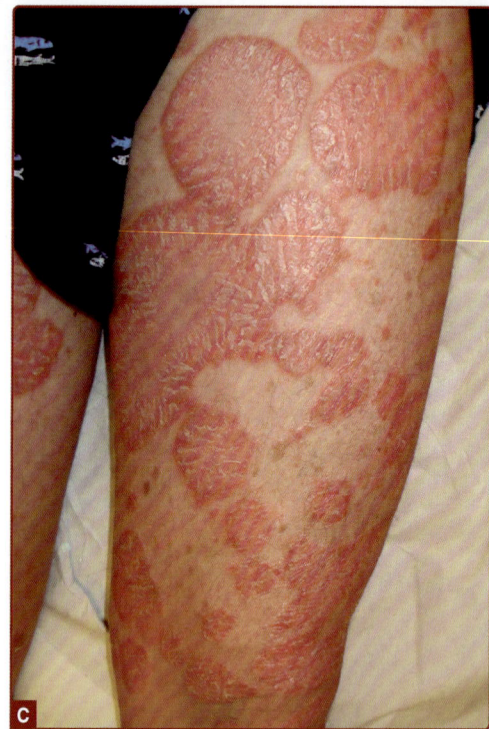
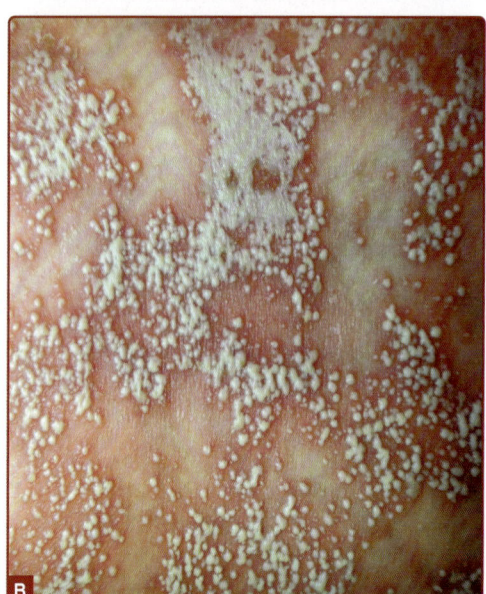
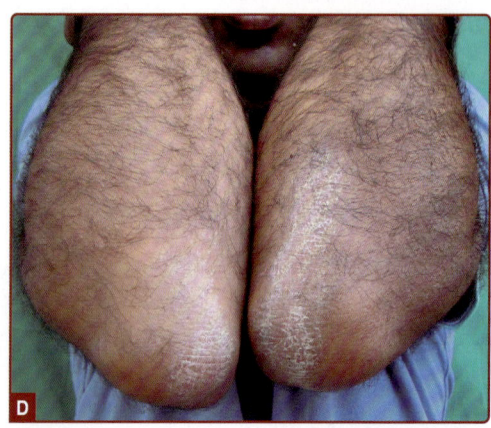
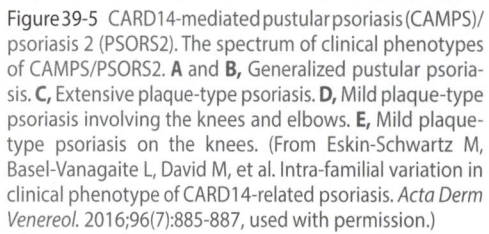
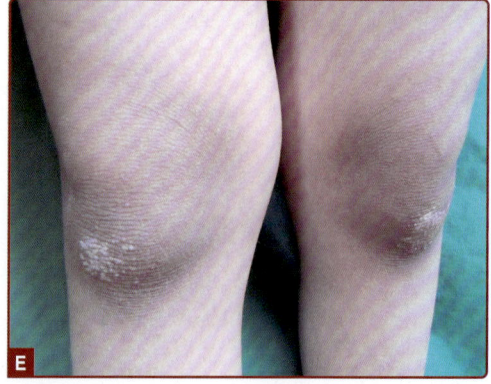

Figure 39-5 CARD14-mediated pustular psoriasis (CAMPS)/psoriasis 2 (PSORS2). The spectrum of clinical phenotypes of CAMPS/PSORS2. **A** and **B,** Generalized pustular psoriasis. **C,** Extensive plaque-type psoriasis. **D,** Mild plaque-type psoriasis involving the knees and elbows. **E,** Mild plaque-type psoriasis on the knees. (From Eskin-Schwartz M, Basel-Vanagaite L, David M, et al. Intra-familial variation in clinical phenotype of CARD14-related psoriasis. *Acta Derm Venereol.* 2016;96(7):885-887, used with permission.)

be further complicated by the development of amyloidosis. Symptomatic pericarditis during the attacks may occur but is rare,[36,37] and echocardiography reveals small, clinically nonsignificant effusions that can be present during attacks.

DIAGNOSIS

The diagnosis of FMF relies mainly on clinical findings and it should be suspected in individuals with recurrent episodes of fever-associated erysipelas-like skin lesions and abdominal, pleural, and joint pain lasting 1 to 3 days. An increase in ESR, CRP, SAA, and fibrinogen, and low-grade neutrophilia are commonly observed during episodes.[38] Genetic testing for *MEFV* mutations provides confirmation in many patients, but not all patients bear identifiable mutations in *MEFV*. Clinicians should interpret all laboratory results in the context of the clinical situation.

DIFFERENTIAL DIAGNOSIS

The differential diagnosis varies depending on the patient's predominant clinical features. In patients with peritonitis, acute appendicitis may be suspected. In patients with joint pain and erythematous skin lesions, sJIA (Still disease) can be considered. However, sJIA has a daily fever pattern that does not resolve after several days. Spontaneous resolution of fever is a clue to the diagnosis of FMF. Erysipelas-like skin lesions can be the presenting feature of FMF and may be misdiagnosed as infectious erysipelas or cellulitis. FMF also needs to be distinguished from other familial fever syndromes including tumor necrosis factor receptor-associated periodic syndrome (TRAPS), HIDS, and CAPS.

CLINICAL COURSE AND PROGNOSIS

FMF is a lifelong disease and, as of this writing, cannot be cured. The symptoms and severity vary among affected individuals. The most-severe complication is secondary amyloidosis, which can lead to renal failure, a major cause of mortality in patients with FMF.[38] There is a poor correlation between the severity or frequency of attacks and the extent of amyloidosis. Patients can present with renal amyloidosis as the first and only manifestation of FMF. The use of colchicine markedly decreases the incidence of amyloidosis.

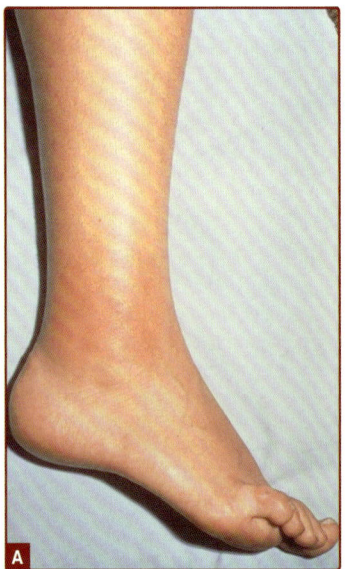
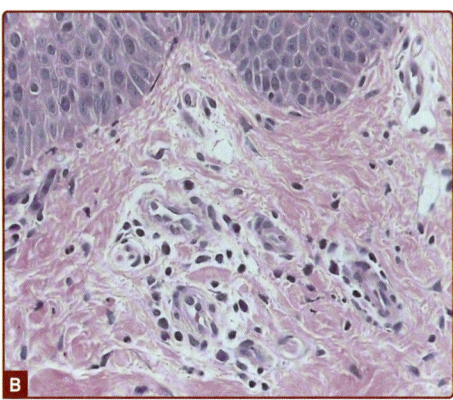

Figure 39-6 Familial Mediterranean fever (FMF). **A,** Erysipelas-like skin lesion on the right ankle showing sharply demarcated, swollen, bright erythematous skin. (From Azizi E, Fisher BK. Cutaneous manifestations of familial Mediterranean fever. *Arch Dermatol*. 1976;112(3):364-66, with permission. Copyright © 1976 American Medical Association. All rights reserved.) **B,** Histology of erysipelas-like skin lesion showing a perivascular inflammatory infiltrate in the superficial dermis.

MANAGEMENT

Colchicine is primarily effective in preventing attacks, minimizing subclinical inflammation between attacks and preventing the development and progression of amyloidosis.[39] Colchicine is recommended in all patients regardless of the frequency and intensity of attacks. Some patients do not have improvement with colchicine and some do not tolerate the drug mainly because of its gastrointestinal side effects. Elderly patients and those with renal impairment treated with colchicine may develop myopathy or neuropathy.[40] In these cases, IL-1 antagonists, including canakinumab (human anti–IL-1β monoclonal antibody), are the second-line therapy.

HYPERIMMUNOGLOBULINEMIA D WITH PERIODIC FEVER SYNDROME/MEVALONATE KINASE DEFICIENCY

AT-A-GLANCE

- Hyperimmunoglobulinemia D with periodic fever syndrome (HIDS)/mevalonate kinase deficiency (MKD) is a rare autosomal recessive disorder (OMIM #260920).
- HIDS/MKD is caused by mutations in *MVK*, the gene coding mevalonate kinase that is involved in many cellular functions via cholesterol and isoprenoid biosynthesis.
- Mutations of *MVK* lead to reduced mevalonate kinase enzyme activity, which results in the production of IL-1β via a complex mechanism.
- Mevalonic aciduria (OMIM #610377) is a severe and fatal form of HIDS/MVK in which the enzyme activity of mevalonate kinase is below 1%.

- Attacks manifest as high, spiking fever accompanied with abdominal pain, diarrhea, vomiting, headache, joint pain, cervical lymphadenopathy, skin lesions, and in 50% of patients oral aphthous ulcers with or without genital ulceration.
- Most common skin lesions are widespread erythematous macules and papules.
- Typically, these attacks last 3 to 7 days, cease spontaneously, and recur every 4 to 8 weeks.
- Since 2016 specific therapy is available and FDA-approved for HIDS: anti–IL-1 therapy with canakinumab.

EPIDEMIOLOGY

Hyperimmunoglobulinemia D with periodic fever syndrome (HIDS; OMIM #260920)/mevalonate kinase deficiency (MKD) is an inherited disease characterized by recurrent attacks of fever, abdominal pain, and skin lesions. HIDS can affect individuals of any ethnic origin but the incidence is much higher in The Netherlands, where 1 in 350 people carry the recessive gene mutation, and the north of France.[41,42] Patients with HIDS typically present clinical initial symptoms during the first year of life.

ETIOLOGY AND PATHOGENESIS

HIDS is an autosomal recessive disorder caused by mutations in the *MVK* gene, which encodes mevalonate kinase, an enzyme involved in many cellular functions via cholesterol and isoprenoid biosynthesis.[41-43] In HIDS, the gene mutations result in reduced enzyme activity, ranging from 1% to 10% of normal levels, and subsequent overproduction of IL-1β via a complex mechanism.[44,45] Mevalonic aciduria (OMIM #610377), a more severe form of MKD with enzyme activity below 1%, is fatal at an early age.[46,47]

CLINICAL FEATURES

Attacks manifest as high, spiking fever preceded by chills accompanied by abdominal pain, diarrhea, vomiting, headache, joint pain, cervical lymphadenopathy, and skin lesions.[48] Episodes last 3 to 7 days, recover spontaneously, and recur every 4 to 8 weeks, although the interval between attacks can vary significantly even in the same patient. Onset is usually before the age of 5 years. The flares are generally triggered by immunizations, trauma including surgery or physical and emotional stress.

There is no specific cutaneous manifestation of HIDS, but more than 80% of patients have skin lesions during an acute attack.[48,49] Widespread erythematous macules and papules are the most common, followed in frequency by urticaria, annular erythema, erythematous nodules, and petechiae (Fig. 39-7). Acral lesions occur more frequently than truncal lesions. Half of patients may also have oral aphthous ulcers with or without genital ulceration. Skin biopsies typically demonstrate a nonspecific perivascular lymphocytic infiltrate with some neutrophils.

The more-severe form of MKD mevalonic aciduria is clinically characterized by periodic fever, severe neurologic impairment, severe growth retardation, and early death.

DIAGNOSIS

The diagnosis of HIDS is usually suspected clinically, but the definitive diagnosis is made by genetic testing. Laboratory investigations during attacks show elevated ESR, CRP, and neutrophilic leukocytosis. This may persist at lower levels between attacks but laboratory tests can normalize completely. The most typical finding is the consistently elevated serum IgD level, although approximately 20% of patients can have normal levels; 80% of HIDS patients present with increased IgA levels as well. Increased IgD levels alone is not specific for HIDS and can be found in other autoinflammatory diseases, including FMF and TRAPS. The presence of oral aphthous ulcers in patients with recurrent fever episodes should lead to consideration of HIDS diagnosis.

DIFFERENTIAL DIAGNOSIS

The differential diagnosis includes other causes of recurrent severe abdominal pain such as appendicitis or of periodic fever. FMF, which also presents with recurrent fever and abdominal pain, is sometimes indistinguishable. The effectiveness of colchicine in FMF can greatly help in making a correct diagnosis. Other autoinflammatory diseases, including TRAPS and MWS, should be eliminated. Oral and genital ulceration frequently seen in HIDS can lead to the misdiagnosis of Behçet disease (BD), but BD is rarely present in infants and has other diagnostic features such as uveitis and bipolar aphthosis.

CLINICAL COURSE AND PROGNOSIS

Long-term prognosis of HIDS is good and patients rarely suffer from serious physical complications of the disease, with the one exception of amyloidosis.

Amyloidosis is quite rare in HIDS and all affected patients have an over 20 year-long history of attacks.

MANAGEMENT

The goal of management is to alleviate symptoms and improve quality of life. No one specific treatment for HIDS exists.[50] NSAIDs alleviate the severity and duration of fever in most patients. In patients refractory to NSAIDs, oral glucocorticoids are beneficial in reducing severity of attacks when given at the onset of an attack. Colchicine is not effective in HIDS. Anakinra (recombinant IL-1Ra) also has been successful in some cases as has the tumor necrosis factor (TNF)-α inhibitor etanercept. Canakinumab (human anti–IL-1β monoclonal antibody) has been used successfully in an increasing number of cases of HIDS. Canakinumab is longer-acting than anakinra and is administered subcutaneously every 4 to 8 weeks. Canakinumab became the first FDA-approved biologic treatment for patients with HIDS in 2016.[51]

TUMOR NECROSIS FACTOR RECEPTOR-ASSOCIATED PERIODIC SYNDROME

AT-A-GLANCE

- TRAPS is a rare autosomal dominant disorder (OMIM #142680).
- TRAPS is caused by mutations in *TNFRSF1A*, the gene coding TNF receptor-1 (TNFR1).
- The mechanism by which the mutations in *TNFRSF1A* cause TRAPS is not well understood.
- Although attacks typically last for 3 weeks and recur every 6 weeks, duration and frequency vary greatly among individuals.
- The episodes usually occur spontaneously, but infection, minor injury, stress, or exercise may be triggers.
- Attacks are characterized by recurrent episodes of high-grade fever, myalgia, serositis, periorbital edema, conjunctivitis, and skin lesions.
- Various types of skin lesions occur, most frequently erythematous patches and plaques that can be migratory and associated with underlying myalgia.
- Histopathology of skin lesions is nonspecific, characterized by a perivascular dermal infiltrate of lymphocytes and monocytes.

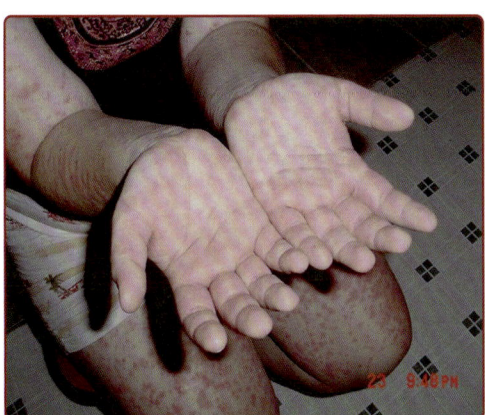

Figure 39-7 Hyperimmunoglobulinemia D with periodic fever syndrome (HIDS)/mevalonate kinase deficiency (MKD). Erythematous macules and papules distributed over both palms, arms, legs, and trunk (not shown) during an attack of HIDS/MKD. (From Takada K, Aksentijevich I, Mahadevan V, et al. Favorable preliminary experience with etanercept in two patients with the hyperimmunoglobulinemia D and periodic fever syndrome. *Arthritis Rheum.* 2003;48:2645-2651. Copyright © 2003 by the American College of Rheumatology. Reprinted with permission of Wiley-Liss, Inc., a subsidiary of John Wiley & Sons, Inc.)

EPIDEMIOLOGY

TNF receptor-associated periodic syndrome (TRAPS; OMIM #142680) is an autosomal dominant disease with episodes of recurrent fever, abdominal, chest, and muscle pain, and skin lesions that typically last for 3 weeks.[52] TRAPS was first described in a family of Irish-Scottish background and initially termed *familial Hibernian fever*. This disease has now been seen in almost all ethnic groups. TRAPS is the second most common known inherited periodic fever syndrome following FMF. More than 1000 patients have been diagnosed worldwide. About half of the patients with TRAPS have no family history. Most patients present before the age of 10 years, but approximately 10% of patients present after the age of 30 years.

ETIOLOGY AND PATHOGENESIS

TRAPS is caused by mutations of the *TNFRSF1A* gene that encodes the TNF receptor-1 (TNFR1).[52] TNFR1 is expressed on leukocytes and endothelial cells. TNFR1 is the main mediator of signaling by TNF-α and it can signal via 2 distinct pathways that lead to either apoptosis via caspase activation or to inflammation via activation of NF-κB. The pathogenic mechanism by which *TNFRSF1A* mutations lead to the autoinflammatory phenotype of TRAPS is not well understood. Several mechanisms have been proposed, including impaired TNFR shedding from the cell membrane, reduced ligand binding and defective apoptotic signaling. A murine knock-in model suggests that mutations in *TNFRSF1A* result in abnormal TNFR1 oligomerization, which sensitizes cells to stimuli such as lipopolysaccharide, resulting in enhanced activation of mitogen-activated protein kinases and increased synthesis of proinflammatory cytokines.[53]

CLINICAL FEATURES

Patients with TRAPS present recurrent episodes of high-grade fever with chills that typically last for 3 weeks. The duration and frequency of the episodes varies greatly among affected individuals. The fever can last from a few days to a few months. The frequency of recurrence can range from every 6 weeks to every few years. Occasionally, the patient may have no fevers for years. The episodes usually occur spontaneously, but infection, minor injury, stress, or exercise may be triggers. During episodes of fever, patients with TRAPS can present additional symptoms. Abdominal pain with nausea, vomiting, and diarrhea caused by sterile peritonitis are common. Most patients experience myalgia resulting from a monocytic fasciitis with a sensation of deep cramping that is migratory from the torso and the proximal limb toward the distal arms and legs. Headaches, serositis, monoarticular arthritis, and conjunctivitis are also observed.

Various types of skin lesions occur in TRAPS, including discrete erythematous macules and papules, erythematous patches, edematous or urticarial plaques, aphthous ulcers, and periorbital edema with conjunctivitis, some of which are migratory and associated with underlying myalgia (Fig. 39-8).[54,55] The foregoing symptoms can greatly vary both between and within individuals. Histologically, skin lesions in TRAPS are nonspecific, characterized by a perivascular dermal infiltrate of lymphocytes and monocytes.

DIAGNOSIS

The diagnosis of TRAPS relies mainly on clinical findings when recurrent long-lasting febrile attacks occur accompanied by abdominal pain and the characteristic migratory muscle pain with overlying skin lesions. Elevated levels of ESR, CRP, SAA, fibrinogen, and leukocytosis are typically present during attacks. Serum levels of soluble TNF receptor superfamily 1A may be low. The diagnosis of TRAPS is confirmed by genetic testing, but a rare mutation negative TRAPS-like phenotype also has been reported in familial and sporadic cases.

DIFFERENTIAL DIAGNOSIS

The differential diagnosis of TRAPS includes other diseases characterized by periodic fever such as FMF, HIDS, sJIA (Still disease), BD, and MWS. Fever attacks are usually longer in TRAPS than in other autoinflammatory diseases, such as FMF, HIDS, and MWS. HIDS

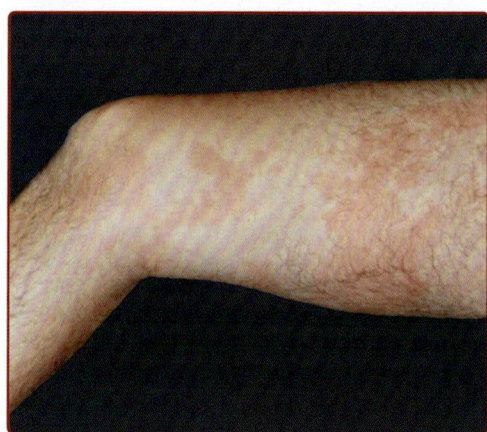

Figure 39-8 Tumor necrosis factor receptor-associated periodic syndrome (TRAPS). Migratory erythematous eruption on the right leg of a patient with TRAPS.

often presents with lymphadenopathy, which is not present in TRAPS or FMF.

CLINICAL COURSE AND PROGNOSIS

With age, fever attacks may decrease in intensity and become more chronic. Approximately 10% to 15% of TRAPS cases will suffer from amyloidosis as a consequence of tissue deposition of SAA. Renal deposition of SAA leads to proteinuria and can progress to renal failure.

MANAGEMENT

NSAIDs help relieve symptoms. High-dose corticosteroids are often effective but sustained usage is associated with known side effects. The TNF-α inhibitor etanercept is an effective treatment in some patients but it can trigger severe episodes of inflammation.[56] Recent evidence suggest that anakinra (recombinant IL-1Ra) and canakinumab (human anti–IL-1β monoclonal antibody) are more effective and provide optimal control of the inflammatory manifestations over the long term.[57,58] The FDA approved canakinumab for the treatment of TRAPS in 2016.

HAPLOINSUFFICIENCY OF A20

AT-A-GLANCE

- Haploinsufficiency of A20 (HA20) is a rare autosomal dominant disorder (OMIM #616744).
- HA20 is caused by loss-of-function mutations in *TNFAIP3* gene, the gene encoding A20/TNFAIP3.
- Mutant A20/TNFAIP3 proteins act through haploinsufficiency. Mutant A20/TNFAIP3 leads to increased K63 ubiquitination and increased NF-κB–dependent proinflammatory cytokines.
- The symptoms of HA20 are indistinguishable from BD, a genetically complex disorder with early adult onset.

EPIDEMIOLOGY

Haploinsufficiency of A20 (HA20; OMIM #616744) is a rare autosomal dominant disorder characterized by features indistinguishable from BD, which is thought to result from a combination of common genetic variants with low effect. HA20 is thus considered as a part of the BD spectrum.[59-61] Reported cases so far originate from Europe, Turkey, and Japan. The percentage of BD patients that can be explained by HA20 remains to be determined.

ETIOLOGY AND PATHOGENESIS

HA20 is caused by loss-of-function mutations in *TNFAIP3* gene. TNFAIP3, also known as A20, is an ubiquitin-editing enzyme that targets K63-linked ubiquitin chains and negatively regulates both the NF-κB signaling pathway and the NLRP3-inflammasome. Mutant A20/TNFAIP3 proteins act through haploinsufficiency and increase NF-κB–dependent proinflammatory cytokines.[59,60] Interestingly, in addition to BD, *TNFAIP3* has been identified as a susceptibility locus in many chronic inflammatory disorders including rheumatoid arthritis, systemic lupus erythematosus, and inflammatory bowel disease.[60]

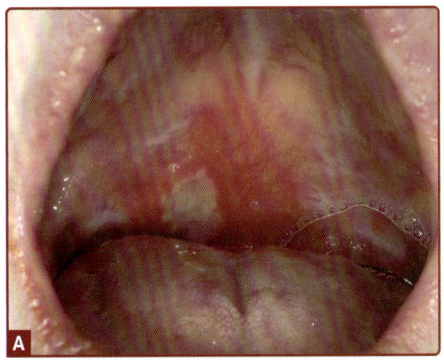
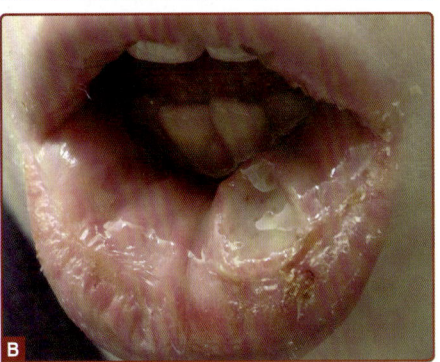

Figure 39-9 HA20. **A** and **B,** Recurrent oral ulcers. (Reprinted by permission from Springer Nature: Zhou Q, Wang H, Schwartz DM, et al. Loss-of-function mutations in TNFAIP3 leading to A20 haploinsufficiency cause an early-onset autoinflammatory disease. *Nat Genet.* 2016;48(1): 67-73. Copyright © 2016.)

CLINICAL FEATURES

Symptoms of HA20 start in childhood or early adulthood. Clinical manifestations of HA20 resemble BD, presenting with fevers, bipolar ulceration of mucosal surfaces, particularly in the oral and genital areas, skin lesions, uveitis, and polyarthritis. The skin lesions include erythematous papules, pseudofolliculitis, erythema nodosum-like lesions, and pathergy (Fig. 39-9).[59-61] These patients may also develop retinal vasculitis, gastrointestinal ulcers, and CNS vasculitis. Autoantibodies to nuclear antigens, ribonucleoprotein, double-stranded DNA, and the lupus anticoagulant can be found.[59]

DIAGNOSIS

The diagnosis is based on clinical findings and genetic testing for *TNFAIP3* gene mutations.

MANAGEMENT

Colchicine is effective in some patients with HA20 but not in all patients. TNF-α antagonists and IL-1R antagonists are reported to work with variable efficacy.[59-61] Future investigations are needed.

OTULIPENIA/OTULIN-RELATED AUTOINFLAMMATORY SYNDROME

AT-A-GLANCE

- Otulipenia/OTULIN-related autoinflammatory syndrome (ORAS) is a rare autosomal recessive disorder (OMIM #617099).
- Otulipenia/ORAS is caused by loss-of-function mutations in *OTULIN*.
- Mutant OTULIN leads to increased linear ubiquitination and elevated NF-κB–dependent proinflammatory transcripts.
- Patients suffer from early-onset severe systemic inflammation, including prolonged fever, rash, arthralgia, diarrhea, and progressive lipodystrophy.
- Relapsing nodular panniculitis with neutrophil infiltrate are typically observed.
- Otulipenia/ORAS can be treated with TNF-α inhibitor.

EPIDEMIOLOGY

The epidemiology of otulipenia/OTULIN-related autoinflammatory syndrome (ORAS) (OMIM #617099) is not known. Six patients have been reported and they are offspring of consanguineous relations. Two are of Turkish descent and one of Pakistani descent.[62,63]

ETIOLOGY AND PATHOGENESIS

Otulipenia/ORAS is inherited in an autosomal recessive fashion and caused by loss-of-function mutations in the *OTULIN* (also known as *GUMBY/FAM105B*) gene. OTULIN is a deubiquitinase that negatively regulates the NF-κB signaling pathway by cleaving linear ubiquitin chains, whereas A20 deubiquitinase does so by cleaving K63 ubiquitin chains. The mutant OTULIN is less stable and active, leading to activation of the NF-κB pathway and increased expression of proinflammatory transcripts in immune cells, particularly in myeloid cells.

CLINICAL FEATURES

Within days to months after birth, patients present with severe systemic inflammation, manifesting with prolonged fever, rash, arthralgia, diarrhea, progressive lipodystrophy, and developmental delay. Relapsing nodular panniculitis with neutrophil infiltrate and erythematous and pustular rash are observed in the skin. Skin biopsy demonstrates neutrophilic dermatitis and panniculitis. One patient showed septal panniculitis with vasculitis of small-sized and medium-sized blood vessels.

MANAGEMENT

Otulipenia/ORAS can be treated with TNF-α inhibitor. According to the literature, 3 patients treated with TNF-α inhibitor responded well. Variable or no efficacies have been reported with systemic steroids and anakinra (IL-1Ra). Two of 6 patients, neither of whom were treated with TNF-α inhibitor, died at the ages of 1 and 5 years old from pneumococcal septicemia, and acute renal failure and pulmonary edema, respectively.

CHRONIC ATYPICAL NEUTROPHILIC DERMATOSIS WITH LIPODYSTROPHY AND ELEVATED TEMPERATURE SYNDROME/PROTEASOME-ASSOCIATED AUTOINFLAMMATORY SYNDROME

AT-A-GLANCE

- Chronic atypical neutrophilic dermatosis with lipodystrophy and elevated temperature (CANDLE)/proteasome-associated autoinflammatory syndrome (PRAAS) is a rare autosomal recessive disorder (OMIM #256040).
- CANDLE/PRAAS is caused by homozygous or compound heterozygous mutations in *PSMB8*.
- Mutant PSMB8 results in dysregulated proteasome activity and increased interferon signaling.
- Recurrent fever, pernio-like and nodular erythema-like eruptions, long, clubbed fingers, and progressive lipodystrophy are characteristic features.

EPIDEMIOLOGY

Chronic atypical neutrophilic dermatosis with lipodystrophy and elevated temperature (CANDLE)/proteasome-associated autoinflammatory syndrome (PRAAS) is a rare inflammatory disease characterized by early-onset recurrent fever, pernio-like and nodular erythema-like eruptions, and lipomuscular atrophy.[64] This disorder was first reported in 1939 and has been described under different terms in the past, such as: Nakajo-Nishimura syndrome (OMIM #256040); joint contractures, muscle atrophy, hepatomegaly, splenomegaly, microcytic anemia, and panniculitis-induced lipodystrophy syndrome (OMIM #256040); Japanese autoinflammatory syndrome with lipodystrophy (OMIM #256040); and CANDLE syndrome (OMIM #256040). The discovery of *PSMB8* mutations in these disorders unified them within 1 spectrum of disease, also referred to as PRAAS. Approximately 60 cases have been reported in Japanese, white, Spanish, Hispanic, Jewish, and Bangladeshi families.

ETIOLOGY AND PATHOGENESIS

Autosomal recessive homozygous or compound heterozygous mutations in the proteasome subunit β8 (*PSMB8*) gene cause disorders in most cases. Of note, digenic inheritance of *PSMB8* with additional mutations of proteasome subunits including *PSMA3*, *PSMB4*, *PSMB9*, and proteasome maturation protein (*POMP*) was reported.[65] These mutations variably affect proteasome assembly and maturation, leading to an accumulation of ubiquitinated and oxidized proteins in the cell. This cell stress causes increased production of type I interferon and reactive oxygen species, resulting in a vicious cycle of increased interferon signaling.

CLINICAL FEATURES

Signs and symptoms of CANDLE/PRAAS generally develop during the first year of life. Common clinical features include recurrent fever and pernio-like and nodular erythema-like eruptions that last for a few days or weeks. Later during infancy, patients develop long, clubbed fingers and toes with joint contractures and progressive lipomuscular atrophy mainly in the face and upper limbs. (Refer to Fig. 74-2 A-E.) Other variable features include periorbital erythema and edema, myositis, short statue, lymphadenopathy, hepatosplenomegaly, and basal ganglia calcification.

DIAGNOSIS

Chronic anemia and an elevated CRP and ESR are typically present. Variable hypergammaglobulinemia and elevation of IgG, IgE, IgA, and IgM are present in the serum of CANDLE/PRAAS patients. Autoimmune features, including antinuclear antibody and other autoantibodies are also variable.

The common histologic feature of pernio-like and nodular erythema-like eruptions is a dense dermal infiltration of mononuclear cells, histiocytes, eosinophils, and neutrophils in the perivascular and interstitial areas of dermis and subcutaneous fat. There is no evidence of leukocytoclastic vasculitis.

Diagnostic confirmation is achieved by genetic testing for *PSMB8*.

CLINICAL COURSE AND PROGNOSIS

CANDLE/PRAAS is a lifelong disease with fluctuation in disease severity. Life expectancy can be reduced as a result of systemic inflammation. Quality of life is often hampered by recurrent episodes of severe inflammation and reduced activity.

MANAGEMENT

There is no effective treatment to date for CANDLE/PRAAS. Systemic steroids can temporally improve pernio-like and nodular erythema-like eruptions, but they often return after tapering. Lipodystrophy usually remains unchanged with systemic steroids. Various antirheumatic and immunosuppressant drugs, including anakinra (IL-1Ra), tocilizumab (IL-6Ra), TNF-α inhibitor, methotrexate, hydroxychloroquine, azathioprine, cyclosporine, and tacrolimus, have no effect or result in only transient clinical improvement.

BLAU SYNDROME/EARLY-ONSET SARCOIDOSIS

AT-A-GLANCE

- Blau syndrome (BS; OMIM #186580) is a rare autosomal dominant disorder; early-onset sarcoidosis (EOS; OMIM #609464) is a sporadic form of Blau syndrome.
- BS/EOS are caused by mutations in *NOD2*, the gene encoding NOD2.
- The mechanism by which the gain-of-function mutations in *NOD2* cause BS/EOS is unknown.
- Granulomatous dermatitis is typically the first sign of BS/EOS, occurring before 4 years of age.
- Histopathology is characterized by noncaseating granulomas composed of histiocytes and multinucleated giant cells located in the upper dermis.
- Characteristic arthritis (articular synovitis and tenosynovitis) and uveitis are common, but disease activity varies greatly among individuals.

EPIDEMIOLOGY

Blau syndrome (BS; OMIM #186580) and early-onset sarcoidosis (EOS; OMIM #609464) are rare inflammatory disorders that primarily affect the skin, joints, and eyes.[66] Although previously considered as distinct entities, BS and EOS are now recognized as familial and sporadic phenotypes of the same granulomatous disease.[67,68] BS is inherited in an autosomal dominant fashion and classically presents before the age of 4 years as a triad of granulomatous dermatitis, arthritis, and uveitis. The incidence and prevalence of BS/EOS is unknown.

ETIOLOGY AND PATHOGENESIS

BS/EOS is a monogenic disease resulting from gain-of-function mutations in *NOD2* (also known as *CARD15*). NOD2 is one of the NLRs, a family of cytoplasmic pattern recognition receptors.[69] NOD2 is mainly expressed in the cytoplasm of monocytes, macrophages, granulocytes, and dendritic cells. NOD2 recognizes muramyl dipeptide, a cell wall component of both Gram-positive and Gram-negative bacteria. This leads to activation of downstream transcriptional factors (NF-κB and mitogen-activated protein kinase) and secretion of inflammatory cytokines. The mechanism by which the gain-of-function mutations in *NOD2* induce BS/EOS is largely unknown.

CLINICAL FEATURES

Granulomatous dermatitis is typically the first sign of BS/EOS.[70,71] The skin lesions are asymptomatic, slightly scaly, discrete, yellowish to brown-red flat-topped papules on the trunk and extremities, observed in more than 90% of patients, classically children before the age of 4 years (Fig. 39-10A). Histologically, noncaseating granulomas composed of periodic acid-Schiff–positive histiocytes and multinucleated giant cells located in the upper dermis are characteristic (Fig. 39-10B). Bilateral hilar lymphadenopathy, often present in sarcoidosis, is absent in BS/EOS patients. Approximately 95% of patients have arthritis, which usually becomes clinically apparent within the first decade of life.[72] Arthritis in BS/EOS has a characteristic phenotype of chronic, symmetrical, and mostly painless polyarthritis that manifests as intraarticular synovitis and tenosynovitis (Fig. 39-10C). Joint range of motion is relatively preserved but impairment of physical function can occur. An insidious granulomatous iridocyclitis and posterior uveitis can develop into panuveitis. The usual ophthalmologic complaints are photophobia, blurred vision, and ocular pain. Eye involvement is usually bilateral and significant visual loss is observed in 20% to 30% of the affected individuals.

DIAGNOSIS

Diagnosis relies greatly on the demonstration of noncaseating granulomas in biopsies from skin, eye, and/or synovium of affected joints. Diagnostic confirmation is achieved by genetic testing for *NOD2* mutations. Familial history is a key element in defining BS. Musculoskeletal ultrasound is a useful diagnostic tool for detecting characteristically affected joints, as well as monitoring disease activity.[72]

DIFFERENTIAL DIAGNOSIS

Some children with BS/EOS may be misdiagnosed as sJIA (Still disease) because of similar clinical symptoms and disease course.

CLINICAL COURSE AND PROGNOSIS

BS/EOS is a chronic and progressive disease, but disease activity may fluctuate over time. A large spectrum of disease severity exists. Uveitis can be the most difficult manifestation to treat and is the main cause of long-term complications.

MANAGEMENT

Evidence concerning the optimal treatment for BS/EOS is lacking. Low-dose corticosteroid therapy is generally satisfactory during the quiescent stage. Systemic corticosteroids, immunosuppressants and biologics, mostly TNF antagonists,[73] are often combined to control both uveitis and arthritis. Methotrexate can be effective in suppressing arthritis and allowing corticosteroid tapering. IL-1 antagonists have been used with variable clinical outcomes.

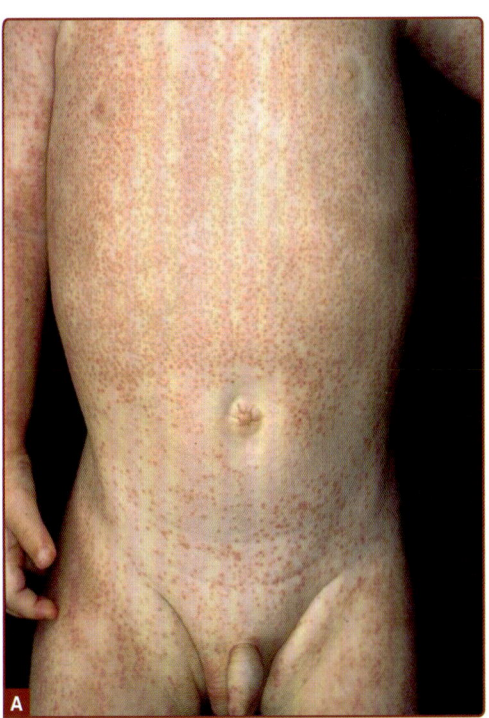
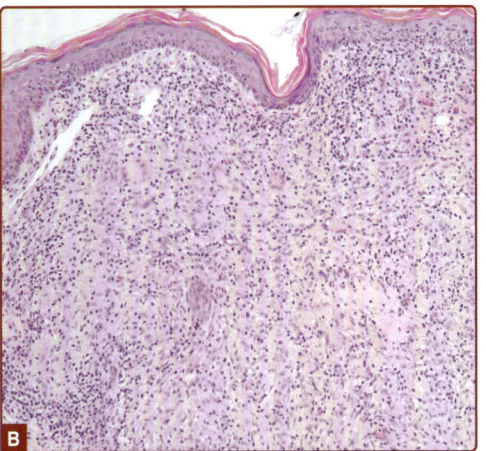
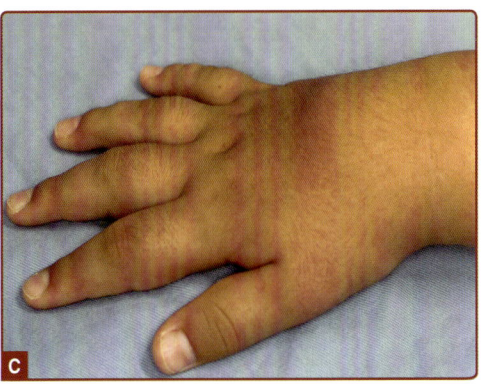

Figure 39-10 Blau syndrome (BS)/early-onset sarcoidosis (EOS). **A,** Generalized orange-brownish asymptomatic lichenoid papules at the age of 12 months. (From Stoevesandt J, Morbach H, Martin TM, et al. Sporadic Blau syndrome with onset of widespread granulomatous dermatitis in the newborn period. *Pediatr Dermatol.* 2010;27(1):69-73, with permission. Copyright © 2010 John Wiley & Sons.) **B,** Histology of the skin. A noncaseating epithelioid granulomas in the dermis accompanied by some multinucleated giant cells. (From Kambe N, Nishikomori R, Kanazawa N. The cytosolic pattern-recognition receptor Nod2 and inflammatory granulomatous disorders. *J Dermatol Sci.* 2005;39(2):71-80, with permission. Copyright © Elsevier.) **C,** The characteristic polyarthritis involves a thick granulomatous intraarticular synovitis and tenosynovitis, causing a boggy appearance in fingers and wrists. (From Ikeda K, Kambe N, Satoh T, et al. Preferentially inflamed tendon sheaths in the swollen but not tender joints in a 5-year-old boy with Blau syndrome. *J Pediatr.* 2013;163(5):1525.e1, with permission. Copyright © Elsevier.)

PYOGENIC ARTHRITIS, PYODERMA GANGRENOSUM, AND ACNE SYNDROME

AT-A-GLANCE

- Pyogenic arthritis, pyoderma gangrenosum, and acne (PAPA) syndrome is a rare autosomal dominant disorder (OMIM #604416).
- PAPA syndrome is caused by mutations in *PSTPIP1*, the gene encoding PSTPIP1 (proline-serine-threonine phosphatase interacting protein 1).
- PSTPIP1 can interact with pyrin, mutations of which cause FMF. Although mutant PSTPIP1 has been proposed to have increased binding to pyrin and thus induce overproduction of IL-1β via the inflammasome, the exact molecular pathogenesis of PAPA syndrome remains unclear.
- Pyoderma gangrenosum, severe nodulocystic acne, and pyogenic arthritis are the clinical features.
- Cutaneous manifestations present at the time of puberty.
- Although TNF-α antagonists and IL-1Ra have shown efficacy in some patients, the treatment of PAPA syndrome remains challenging.

EPIDEMIOLOGY

Pyogenic arthritis, pyoderma gangrenosum, and acne syndrome (PAPA syndrome; OMIM #604416) is a rare pleiotropic autoinflammatory disorder characterized by early onset of recurrent sterile arthritis with neutrophilic infiltrates, with variable skin involvement including pyoderma gangrenosum and severe nodulocystic acne in adolescence and beyond.[74]

ETIOLOGY AND PATHOGENESIS

PAPA syndrome is an autosomal dominant disease caused by mutations in the *PSTPIP1* gene, previously known as *CD2BP1*.[74] Proline-serine-threonine phosphatase interacting protein 1 (PSTPIP1) is primarily expressed on hematopoietic cells and involved in the regulation of the actin cytoskeleton. PSTPIP1 has been demonstrated to interact with pyrin, the protein encoded by the *MEFV* gene, mutations of which cause FMF.[75] It is proposed that mutant PSTPIP1 has increased binding to pyrin, leading to overproduction of IL-1β via inflammasome activation. However, colchicine, which can inhibit the pyrin-inflammasome activation and is an effective remedy for FMF, is ineffective in treating PAPA syndrome. To understand the exact role of PSTPIP1 in PAPA syndrome, further studies are needed.

CLINICAL FEATURES

The clinical manifestations of this disorder include sterile pyogenic arthritis, pyoderma gangrenosum, and nodulocystic acne.[74] Arthritis begins in the first decade of life and is progressively destructive. The inflammatory episodes often begin unprovoked or after minor trauma, leading to neutrophil-rich purulent synovial inflammation. Patients with arthritis sometimes require aspiration, intraarticular corticosteroids, or drainage. During episodes of arthritis patients may present with fever. The cutaneous symptoms, pyoderma gangrenosum and severe acne, develop at the time of puberty. Pyoderma gangrenosum presents as poorly healing ulcers with typical undermined edges (Fig. 39-11). It often occurs at sites of injury and can manifest in a multifocal fashion on the entire skin surface. Severe nodulocystic acne affects most individuals with PAPA syndrome to a variable degree. Nodulocystic acne can cause scarring if untreated. Fever is rarely observed.

DIAGNOSIS

The diagnosis of PAPA syndrome should be suspected in individuals with relapsing sterile arthritis, cutaneous ulcer formation, and severe acne. Laboratory investigations during attacks show elevated acute phase reactants. The diagnosis is confirmed by genetic testing for *PSTPIP1*.

DIFFERENTIAL DIAGNOSIS

sJIA (Still disease), FMF, synovitis, acne, pustulosis, hyperostosis, and osteitis (SAPHO) syndrome, and Majeed syndrome should be excluded. The autosomal dominant hereditary pattern in PAPA syndrome can help in suspecting the diagnosis.

CLINICAL COURSE AND PROGNOSIS

Typically, the symptoms get milder with age. However, the long-term prognosis is not well known because of the rarity of the disease. Joint destruction can be the main cause of long-term complications.

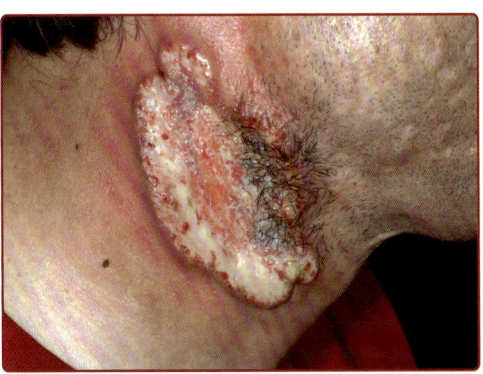

Figure 39-11 Pyogenic arthritis, pyoderma gangrenosum, and acne (PAPA) syndrome. Pyoderma gangrenosum of the neck in PAPA syndrome. (From Brenner M, Ruzicka T, Plewig G, et al. Targeted treatment of pyoderma gangrenosum in PAPA (pyogenic arthritis, pyoderma gangrenosum and acne) syndrome with the recombinant human interleukin-1 receptor antagonist anakinra. *Br J Dermatol.* 2009;161(5):1199-1201, with permission. Copyright © 2009 John Wiley & Sons.)

MANAGEMENT

The treatment of PAPA syndrome is challenging as the response to therapy varies greatly between patients. In the case of severe pyogenic arthritis, drainage of synovial fluid along with intraarticular steroid injections can help relieve pain. High-dose corticosteroids work well on arthritis and pyoderma gangrenosum, but often worsen the acne and their sustained usage can lead to cumulative side effects. TNF-α antagonist (etanercept) and IL-1Ra (anakinra) therapy have been reported to be effective in some patients with PAPA syndrome.[76,77] Further clinical evidence is, however, required.

MAJEED SYNDROME

AT-A-GLANCE

- Majeed syndrome is a rare autosomal recessive disorder (OMIM #609628).
- Majeed syndrome is caused by mutations of the *LPIN2* gene, the gene encoding lipin-2.
- The mechanism by which *LPIN2* mutation causes Majeed syndrome is not well understood.
- The symptom triad of Majeed syndrome is chronic recurrent multifocal osteomyelitis (CRMO), congenital dyserythropoietic anemia (CDA), and neutrophilic dermatosis resembling Sweet syndrome.

EPIDEMIOLOGY

Majeed syndrome (OMIM #609628) is a rare autosomal recessive disorder characterized by the triad of chronic recurrent multifocal osteomyelitis (CRMO), congenital dyserythropoietic anemia (CDA), and neutrophilic dermatosis.[78] To date, only a small number of families from the Middle East have been identified to harbor the mutation.[79]

ETIOLOGY AND PATHOGENESIS

Majeed syndrome is caused by mutations of the *LPIN2* gene that encodes lipin-2.[79] Lipin-2 is thought to be involved in glycerolipid biosynthesis, controlling inflammation and cell division, but the physiologic role of lipin-2 remains only partially understood. Mutations in the *LPIN2* gene alter the structure and function of lipin-2. Homozygotes and compound heterozygotes of nonsense and missense mutations have been identified.

CLINICAL FEATURES

CRMO begins in infancy or early childhood with recurrent episodes of pain and joint swelling. These symptoms typically persist into adulthood and can lead to short stature and joint contractures. CDA presents as hypochromic, microcytic anemia during the first year of life and ranges from mild to transfusion dependent. Most people with Majeed syndrome also develop neutrophilic dermatosis, resembling Sweet syndrome with unknown onset age and frequency. Patients can also develop erythematous plaques, psoriasis, and pustulosis. Histology of skin lesions shows dermal neutrophilic infiltration with papillary dermal edema similar to that observed in Sweet syndrome without histologic evidence of vasculitis.

DIAGNOSIS

The diagnosis is based on clinical findings and genetic testing for *LPIN2* gene mutations. Radiographs show osteolytic lesions with surrounding sclerosis. Bone biopsies are necessary to exclude infectious osteomyelitis. Bone and blood cultures are typically sterile.

DIFFERENTIAL DIAGNOSIS

The differential diagnosis includes DIRA, PAPA syndrome, SAPHO syndrome, and infectious osteomyelitis, as well as bone tumors.

CLINICAL COURSE AND PROGNOSIS

Majeed syndrome is a lifelong disease and long-term outcome is poor. The clinical course and prognosis greatly depends on the severity of clinical manifestations, particularly on the severity of anemia and disease complications, including contractures and diffuse muscle atrophy.

MANAGEMENT

CRMO can be treated with NSAIDs, or corticosteroids if nonresponsive to NSAIDs. Two Majeed syndrome patients who failed to improve with the TNF inhibitor etanercept reportedly responded dramatically to IL-1 blockade by anakinra or canakinumab.[80] CDA can be treated with red blood cell transfusion if clinically indicated. Neutrophilic dermatosis resembling Sweet syndrome can be treated by a short course of oral corticosteroids.

SYNOVITIS, ACNE, PUSTULOSIS, HYPEROSTOSIS, AND OSTEITIS SYNDROME

AT-A-GLANCE

- Synovitis, acne, pustulosis, hyperostosis, and osteitis (SAPHO) syndrome is an inflammatory disorder characterized by recurrent neutrophilic cutaneous and osteoarticular manifestations.
- PPP and severe acne are the most frequent cutaneous manifestations.
- The major osteoarticular manifestations are painful oligoarthritis and osteitis, mainly affecting the anterior chest wall.
- The treatment of SAPHO syndrome remains a challenge. Anakinra has shown promising effect in case reports.

EPIDEMIOLOGY

Synovitis, acne, pustulosis, hyperostosis, and osteitis (SAPHO) syndrome is an inflammatory disorder characterized by recurrent neutrophilic cutaneous and osteoarticular involvement. The onset of SAPHO syndrome has been often described in middle-aged adults, but it can occur at any age, including childhood. The annual prevalence is estimated at 1 in 10,000 persons in whites and 0.00144 in 100,000 persons in Japan,[81] but it may be higher as it is an an underrecognized condition with a variety of clinical presentations.

ETIOLOGY AND PATHOGENESIS

The etiology of SAPHO syndrome is considered as multifactorial, including genetic, environmental and immunologic components. Some familial cases have been reported but most cases are sporadic. IL-1 involvement in the pathogenesis of SAPHO syndrome has been proposed based on a few case reports[82,83] and needs to be defined.

CLINICAL FEATURES

SAPHO syndrome typically presents with neutrophilic skin lesions and osteoarticular manifestations, and usually these manifestations appear within 2 years of each other.[81] The most frequent skin manifestation in SAPHO syndrome is PPP, followed by severe acne, including acne conglobata, acne fulminans, or hidradenitis suppurativa.[84] Less-frequent manifestations include pustular psoriasis and psoriasis vulgaris (Fig. 39-12). The most common osteoarticular manifestations of SAPHO syndrome include oligoarthritis affecting sternocostal and sternoclavicular joints, sacroiliac joints, knees, and ankles, and osteitis affecting the anterior chest wall, such as the sternum, clavicle, and ribs, presenting with pain, tenderness, and sometimes swelling over the affected areas. Imaging with conventional radiography, ultrasonography, CT, MRI, and bone scintigraphy is useful to detect and evaluate osteoarticular involvement. Bone biopsy reveals abscesses, known as sterile osteomyelitis, progressively replaced by sclerotic bone trabeculae and marrow fibrosis in the later stages.

DIAGNOSIS

Making a diagnosis of SAPHO syndrome is challenging because not all symptoms are always present at the same time. The diagnosis is mainly based on clinical, radiologic, and histologic findings, which vary according to the duration of the disease.

DIFFERENTIAL DIAGNOSIS

During the early stage, infectious osteomyelitis and bone tumors, such as Ewing sarcoma and osteoblastoma, should be excluded. SAPHO syndrome can

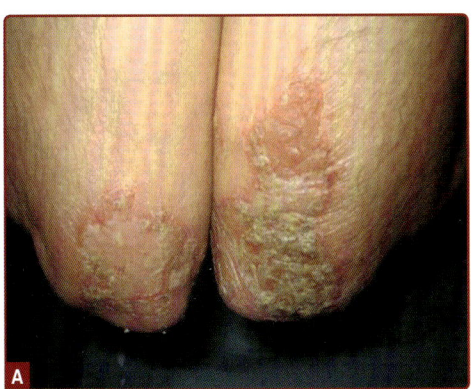
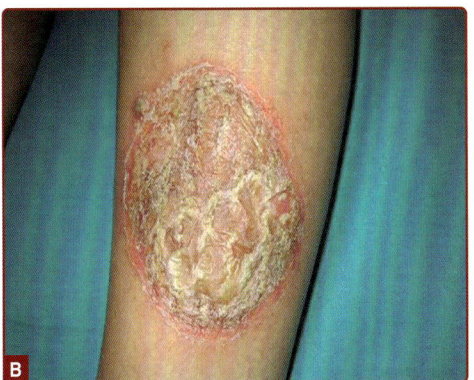
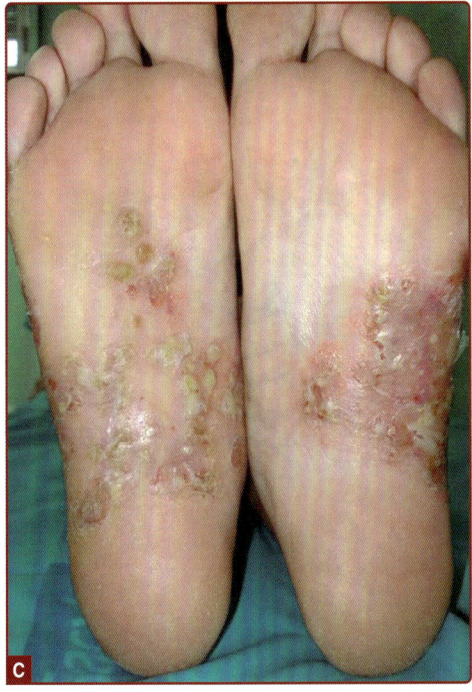

Figure 39-12 Synovitis, acne, pustulosis, hyperostosis, and osteitis (SAPHO) syndrome. **A** and **B**, Well-delineated erythematous plaques with pustular component yellowish scabs on elbows and leg. **C**, Erythematous lesions with deep pustules on the soles of both feet. (From Sáez-Martín LC, Gómez-Castro S, Román-Curto C, et al. Etanercept in the treatment of SAPHO syndrome. *Int J Dermatol*. 2015;54(6):e206-e208, with permission. Copyright © 2015 John Wiley & Sons.)

share several features with psoriatic arthritis, but the skin manifestation of severe acne and radiographic signs of osteitis with hyperostosis are not typical of psoriatic arthritis. Psoriatic nail dystrophy has not been reported in patients with SAPHO syndrome. In the pediatric cases, the differential diagnosis includes Langerhans cell histiocytosis, DIRA, PAPA syndrome, and Majeed syndrome.

CLINICAL COURSE AND PROGNOSIS

The disease is usually chronic, with alternating periods of remission and relapse, except for a minority of patients with spontaneous resolution of symptoms. Although complications such as impairment of bone and joint function can develop, patients with SAPHO syndrome have a favorable prognosis in general.

MANAGEMENT

The treatment of SAPHO syndrome is mainly symptomatic. NSAIDs are generally considered as the first line of treatment. Intraarticular and systemic corticosteroids are transiently effective in the majority of patients. PPP and pustular psoriasis usually respond well to topical corticosteroids and psoralen and ultraviolet A therapy. Oral antibiotics such as doxycycline are used to treat severe acne with limited efficacy. Bisphosphonates are sometimes very effective for bone lesions because they inhibit bone resorption and turnover. For unresponsive or refractory cases, TNF-α antagonists have been used and have demonstrated a marked amelioration of bone, joint, and skin manifestations. In some cases, however, paradoxical flares and recurrence of skin lesions can be seen. Promising therapeutic effects have been shown in case reports with the IL-1Ra anakinra.[83]

ACKNOWLEDGMENTS

The authors thank Chyi-Chia Richard Lee, MD, PhD, and Raphaela Goldbach-Mansky, MD, MHS, for their contributions to this chapter in previous editions.

REFERENCES

1. Masters SL, Simon A, Aksentijevich I, et al. Horror autoinflammaticus: the molecular pathophysiology of autoinflammatory disease (*). *Annu Rev Immunol*. 2009;27:621-668.
2. Kastner DL, Aksentijevich I, Goldbach-Mansky R. Autoinflammatory disease reloaded: a clinical perspective. *Cell*. 2010;140(6):784-790.
3. Hoffman HM, Mueller JL, Broide DH, et al. Mutation of a new gene encoding a putative pyrin-like

protein causes familial cold autoinflammatory syndrome and Muckle-Wells syndrome. *Nat Genet.* 2001;29(3):301-305.
4. Feldmann J, Prieur AM, Quartier P, et al. Chronic infantile neurological cutaneous and articular syndrome is caused by mutations in CIAS1, a gene highly expressed in polymorphonuclear cells and chondrocytes. *Am J Hum Genet.* 2002;71(1):198-203.
5. Kile RL and Rusk HA. A case of cold urticaria with an unusual family history. *JAMA Dermatol.* 1940;114: 1067-1068.
6. Muckle TJ. The 'Muckle-Wells' syndrome. *Br J Dermatol.* 1979;100(1):87-92.
7. Prieur AM, Griscelli C. Arthropathy with rash, chronic meningitis, eye lesions, and mental retardation. *J Pediatr.* 1981;99(1):79-83.
8. Martinon F, Burns K, Tschopp J. The inflammasome: a molecular platform triggering activation of inflammatory caspases and processing of proIL-beta. *Mol Cell.* 2002;10(2):417-426.
9. Goldbach-Mansky R, Dailey NJ, Canna SW, et al. Neonatal-onset multisystem inflammatory disease responsive to interleukin-1beta inhibition. *N Engl J Med.* 2006;355(6):581-592.
10. Gattorno M, Tassi S, Carta S, et al. Pattern of interleukin-1beta secretion in response to lipopolysaccharide and ATP before and after interleukin-1 blockade in patients with CIAS1 mutations. *Arthritis Rheum.* 2007;56(9):3138-3148.
11. Johnstone RF, Dolen WK, Hoffman HM. A large kindred with familial cold autoinflammatory syndrome. *Ann Allergy Asthma Immunol.* 2003;90(2):233-237.
12. Hill SC, Namde M, Dwyer A, et al. Arthropathy of neonatal onset multisystem inflammatory disease (NOMID/CINCA). *Pediatr Radiol.* 2007;37(2):145-152.
13. Tanaka N, Izawa K, Saito MK, et al. High incidence of NLRP3 somatic mosaicism in patients with chronic infantile neurologic, cutaneous, articular syndrome: results of an International Multicenter Collaborative Study. *Arthritis Rheum.* 2011;63(11):3625-3632.
14. Neven B, Prieur AM, Quartier dit Maire P. Cryopyrinopathies: update on pathogenesis and treatment. *Nat Clin Pract Rheumatol.* 2008;4(9):481-489.
15. Hawkins PN, Lachmann HJ, McDermott MF. Interleukin-1-receptor antagonist in the Muckle-Wells syndrome. *N Engl J Med.* 2003;348(25):2583-2584.
16. Neven B, Marvillet I, Terrada C, et al. Long-term efficacy of the interleukin-1 receptor antagonist anakinra in ten patients with neonatal-onset multisystem inflammatory disease/chronic infantile neurologic, cutaneous, articular syndrome. *Arthritis Rheum.* 2010;62(1):258-267.
17. Kullenberg T, Lofqvist M, Leinonen M, et al. Long-term safety profile of anakinra in patients with severe cryopyrin-associated periodic syndromes. *Rheumatology (Oxford).* 2016;55(8):1499-1506.
18. Hoffman HM, Throne ML, Amar NJ, et al. Efficacy and safety of rilonacept (interleukin-1 Trap) in patients with cryopyrin-associated periodic syndromes: results from two sequential placebo-controlled studies. *Arthritis Rheum.* 2008;58(8):2443-2452.
19. Lachmann HJ, Kone-Paut I, Kuemmerle-Deschner JB, et al. Use of canakinumab in the cryopyrin-associated periodic syndrome. *N Engl J Med.* 2009;360(23):2416-2425.
20. de Koning HD. Schnitzler's syndrome: lessons from 281 cases. *Clin Transl Allergy.* 2014;4:41.
21. Lipsker D. The Schnitzler syndrome. *Orphanet J Rare Dis.* 2010;5:38.
22. Aksentijevich I, Masters SL, Ferguson PJ, et al. An autoinflammatory disease with deficiency of the interleukin-1-receptor antagonist. *N Engl J Med.* 2009;360(23): 2426-2437.
23. Reddy S, Jia S, Geoffrey R, et al. An autoinflammatory disease due to homozygous deletion of the IL1RN locus. *N Engl J Med.* 2009;360(23):2438-2444.
24. Jesus AA, Osman M, Silva CA, et al. A novel mutation of IL1RN in the deficiency of interleukin-1 receptor antagonist syndrome: description of two unrelated cases from Brazil. *Arthritis Rheum.* 2011;63(12):4007-4017.
25. Schnellbacher C, Ciocca G, Menendez R, et al. Deficiency of interleukin-1 receptor antagonist responsive to anakinra. *Pediatr Dermatol.* 2013;30(6):758-760.
26. Marrakchi S, Guigue P, Renshaw BR, et al. Interleukin-36-receptor antagonist deficiency and generalized pustular psoriasis. *N Engl J Med.* 2011;365(7):620-628.
27. Onoufriadis A, Simpson MA, Pink AE, et al. Mutations in IL36RN/IL1F5 are associated with the severe episodic inflammatory skin disease known as generalized pustular psoriasis. *Am J Hum Genet.* 2011;89(3):432-437.
28. Koike Y, Okubo M, Kiyohara T, et al. Granulocyte and monocyte apheresis can control juvenile generalized pustular psoriasis with mutation of IL36RN. *Br J Dermatol.* 2017 177(6):1732-1736.
29. Jordan CT, Cao L, Roberson ED, et al. PSORS2 is due to mutations in CARD14. *Am J Hum Genet.* 2012;90(5):784-795.
30. Eskin-Schwartz M, Basel-Vanagaite L, David M, et al. Intra-familial variation in clinical phenotype of CARD14-related psoriasis. *Acta Derm Venereol.* 2016;96(7): 885-887.
31. Ancient missense mutations in a new member of the RoRet gene family are likely to cause familial Mediterranean fever. The International FMF Consortium. *Cell.* 1997;90(4):797-807.
32. French FMF Consortium. A candidate gene for familial Mediterranean fever. *Nat Genet.* 1997;17(1):25-31.
33. Azizi E, Fisher BK. Cutaneous manifestations of familial Mediterranean fever. *Arch Dermatol.* 1976;112(3):364-366.
34. Barzilai A, Langevitz P, Goldberg I, et al. Erysipelas-like erythema of familial Mediterranean fever: clinicopathologic correlation. *J Am Acad Dermatol.* 2000;42(5, pt 1): 791-795.
35. Padeh S, Livneh A, Pras E, et al. Familial Mediterranean fever in the first two years of life: a unique phenotype of disease in evolution. *J Pediatr.* 2010;156(6):985-989.
36. Zimand S, Tauber T, Hegesch T, et al. Familial Mediterranean fever presenting with massive cardiac tamponade. *Clin Exp Rheumatol.* 1994;12(1):67-69.
37. Kees S, Langevitz P, Zemer D, et al. Attacks of pericarditis as a manifestation of familial Mediterranean fever (FMF). *Q J Med.* 1997;90(10):643-647.
38. Lachmann HJ, Sengul B, Yavuzsen TU, et al. Clinical and subclinical inflammation in patients with familial Mediterranean fever and in heterozygous carriers of MEFV mutations. *Rheumatology (Oxford).* 2006;45(6): 746-750.
39. Zemer D, Revach M, Pras M, et al. A controlled trial of colchicine in preventing attacks of familial Mediterranean fever. *N Engl J Med.* 1974;291(18):932-934.
40. Kuncl RW, Duncan G, Watson D, et al. Colchicine myopathy and neuropathy. *N Engl J Med.* 1987;316(25): 1562-1568.
41. Houten SM, Kuis W, Duran M, et al. Mutations in MVK, encoding mevalonate kinase, cause hyperimmunoglobulinaemia D and periodic fever syndrome. *Nat Genet.* 1999;22(2):175-177.
42. Drenth JP, Cuisset L, Grateau G, et al. Mutations in the gene encoding mevalonate kinase cause hyper-IgD

43. Cuisset L, Drenth JP, Simon A, et al. Molecular analysis of MVK mutations and enzymatic activity in hyper-IgD and periodic fever syndrome. *Eur J Hum Genet*. 2001;9(4):260-266.
44. Frenkel J, Rijkers GT, Mandey SH, et al. Lack of isoprenoid products raises ex vivo interleukin-1beta secretion in hyperimmunoglobulinemia D and periodic fever syndrome. *Arthritis Rheum*. 2002;46(10):2794-2803.
45. Mandey SH, Kuijk LM, Frenkel J, et al. A role for geranylgeranylation in interleukin-1beta secretion. *Arthritis Rheum*. 2006;54(11):3690-3695.
46. Hoffmann G, Gibson KM, Brandt IK, et al. Mevalonic aciduria—an inborn error of cholesterol and nonsterol isoprene biosynthesis. *N Engl J Med*. 1986;314(25):1610-1614.
47. Schafer BL, Bishop RW, Kratunis VJ, et al. Molecular cloning of human mevalonate kinase and identification of a missense mutation in the genetic disease mevalonic aciduria. *J Biol Chem*. 1992;267(19):13229-13238.
48. van der Hilst JC, Bodar EJ, Barron KS, et al. Long-term follow-up, clinical features, and quality of life in a series of 103 patients with hyperimmunoglobulinemia D syndrome. *Medicine (Baltimore)*. 2008;87(6):301-310.
49. Drenth JP, Boom BW, Toonstra J, et al. Cutaneous manifestations and histologic findings in the hyperimmunoglobulinemia D syndrome. International Hyper IgD Study Group. *Arch Dermatol*. 1994;130(1):59-65.
50. Simon A, Drewe E, van der Meer JW, et al. Simvastatin treatment for inflammatory attacks of the hyperimmunoglobulinemia D and periodic fever syndrome. *Clin Pharmacol Ther*. 2004;75(5):476-483.
51. Kostjukovits S, Kalliokoski L, Antila K, et al. Treatment of hyperimmunoglobulinemia D syndrome with biologics in children: review of the literature and Finnish experience. *Eur J Pediatr*. 2015;174(6):707-714.
52. McDermott MF, Aksentijevich I, Galon J, et al. Germline mutations in the extracellular domains of the 55 kDa TNF receptor, TNFR1, define a family of dominantly inherited autoinflammatory syndromes. *Cell*. 1999;97(1):133-144.
53. Simon A, Park H, Maddipati R, et al. Concerted action of wild-type and mutant TNF receptors enhances inflammation in TNF receptor 1-associated periodic fever syndrome. *Proc Natl Acad Sci U S A*. 2010;107(21):9801-9806.
54. Toro JR, Aksentijevich I, Hull K, et al. Tumor necrosis factor receptor-associated periodic syndrome: a novel syndrome with cutaneous manifestations. *Arch Dermatol*. 2000;136(12):1487-1494.
55. Nakamura M, Kobayashi M, Tokura Y. A novel missense mutation in tumour necrosis factor receptor superfamily 1A (TNFRSF1A) gene found in tumour necrosis factor receptor-associated periodic syndrome (TRAPS) manifesting adult-onset Still disease-like skin eruptions: report of a case and review of the Japanese patients. *Br J Dermatol*. 2009;161(4):968-970.
56. Nedjai B, Hitman GA, Quillinan N, et al. Proinflammatory action of the antiinflammatory drug infliximab in tumor necrosis factor receptor-associated periodic syndrome. *Arthritis Rheum*. 2009;60(2):619-625.
57. Gattorno M, Pelagatti MA, Meini A, et al. Persistent efficacy of anakinra in patients with tumor necrosis factor receptor-associated periodic syndrome. *Arthritis Rheum*. 2008;58(5):1516-1520.
58. Gattorno M, Obici L, Cattalini M, et al. Canakinumab treatment for patients with active recurrent or chronic TNF receptor-associated periodic syndrome (TRAPS): an open-label, phase II study. *Ann Rheum Dis*. 2017;76(1):173-178.
59. Zhou Q, Wang H, Schwartz DM, et al. Loss-of-function mutations in TNFAIP3 leading to A20 haploinsufficiency cause an early-onset autoinflammatory disease. *Nat Genet*. 2016;48(1):67-73.
60. Shigemura T, Kaneko N, Kobayashi N, et al. Novel heterozygous C243Y A20/TNFAIP3 gene mutation is responsible for chronic inflammation in autosomal-dominant Behçet's disease. *RMD Open*. 2016;2(1):e000223.
61. Ohnishi H, Kawamoto N, Seishima M, et al. A Japanese family case with juvenile onset Behçet's disease caused by TNFAIP3 mutation. *Allergol Int*. 2017;66(1):146-148.
62. Zhou Q, Yu X, Demirkaya E, et al. Biallelic hypomorphic mutations in a linear deubiquitinase define otulipenia, an early-onset autoinflammatory disease. *Proc Natl Acad Sci U S A*. 2016;113(36):10127-10132.
63. Damgaard RB, Walker JA, Marco-Casanova P, et al. The deubiquitinase OTULIN is an essential negative regulator of inflammation and autoimmunity. *Cell*. 2016;166(5):1215-1230 e1220.
64. Kanazawa N. Nakajo-Nishimura syndrome: an autoinflammatory disorder showing pernio-like rashes and progressive partial lipodystrophy. *Allergol Int*. 2012;61(2):197-206.
65. Brehm A, Liu Y, Sheikh A, et al. Additive loss-of-function proteasome subunit mutations in CANDLE/PRAAS patients promote type I IFN production. *J Clin Invest*. 2015;125(11):4196-4211.
66. Blau EB. Familial granulomatous arthritis, iritis, and rash. *J Pediatr*. 1985;107(5):689-693.
67. Miceli-Richard C, Lesage S, Rybojad M, et al. CARD15 mutations in Blau syndrome. *Nat Genet*. 2001;29(1):19-20.
68. Kanazawa N, Okafuji I, Kambe N, et al. Early-onset sarcoidosis and CARD15 mutations with constitutive nuclear factor-kappaB activation: common genetic etiology with Blau syndrome. *Blood*. 2005;105(3):1195-1197.
69. Inohara N, Nunez G. NODs: intracellular proteins involved in inflammation and apoptosis. *Nat Rev Immunol*. 2003;3(5):371-382.
70. Schaffer JV, Chandra P, Keegan BR, et al. Widespread granulomatous dermatitis of infancy: an early sign of Blau syndrome. *Arch Dermatol*. 2007;143(3):386-391.
71. Stoevesandt J, Morbach H, Martin TM, et al. Sporadic Blau syndrome with onset of widespread granulomatous dermatitis in the newborn period. *Pediatr Dermatol*. 2010;27(1):69-73.
72. Ikeda K, Kambe N, Satoh T, et al. Preferentially inflamed tendon sheaths in the swollen but not tender joints in a 5-year-old boy with Blau syndrome. *J Pediatr*. 2013;163(5):1525 e1521.
73. Milman N, Andersen CB, Hansen A, et al. Favourable effect of TNF-alpha inhibitor (infliximab) on Blau syndrome in monozygotic twins with a de novo CARD15 mutation. *APMIS*. 2006;114(12):912-919.
74. Wise CA, Gillum JD, Seidman CE, et al. Mutations in CD2BP1 disrupt binding to PTP PEST and are responsible for PAPA syndrome, an autoinflammatory disorder. *Hum Mol Genet*. 2002;11(8):961-969.
75. Shoham NG, Centola M, Mansfield E, et al. Pyrin binds the PSTPIP1/CD2BP1 protein, defining familial Mediterranean fever and PAPA syndrome as disorders in the same pathway. *Proc Natl Acad Sci U S A*. 2003;100(23):13501-13506.
76. Stichweh DS, Punaro M, Pascual V. Dramatic improvement of pyoderma gangrenosum with infliximab

in a patient with PAPA syndrome. *Pediatr Dermatol.* 2005;22(3):262-265.
77. Brenner M, Ruzicka T, Plewig G, et al. Targeted treatment of pyoderma gangrenosum in PAPA (pyogenic arthritis, pyoderma gangrenosum and acne) syndrome with the recombinant human interleukin-1 receptor antagonist anakinra. *Br J Dermatol.* 2009;161(5):1199-1201.
78. Majeed HA, Kalaawi M, Mohanty D, et al. Congenital dyserythropoietic anemia and chronic recurrent multifocal osteomyelitis in three related children and the association with Sweet syndrome in two siblings. *J Pediatr.* 1989;115(5, pt 1):730-734.
79. Ferguson PJ, Chen S, Tayeh MK, et al. Homozygous mutations in LPIN2 are responsible for the syndrome of chronic recurrent multifocal osteomyelitis and congenital dyserythropoietic anaemia (Majeed syndrome). *J Med Genet.* 2005;42(7):551-557.
80. Herlin T, Fiirgaard B, Bjerre M, et al. Efficacy of anti-IL-1 treatment in Majeed syndrome. *Ann Rheum Dis.* 2013;72(3):410-413.
81. Rukavina I. SAPHO syndrome: a review. *J Child Orthop.* 2015;9(1):19-27.
82. Colina M, Pizzirani C, Khodeir M, et al. Dysregulation of P2X7 receptor-inflammasome axis in SAPHO syndrome: successful treatment with anakinra. *Rheumatology (Oxford).* 2010;49(7):1416-1418.
83. Wendling D, Prati C, Aubin F. Anakinra treatment of SAPHO syndrome: short-term results of an open study. *Ann Rheum Dis.* 2012;71(6):1098-1100.
84. Saez-Martin LC, Gomez-Castro S, Roman-Curto C, et al. Etanercept in the treatment of SAPHO syndrome. *Int J Dermatol.* 2015;54(6):e206-e208.

Chapter 40 :: Eosinophilic Diseases
:: Hideyuki Ujiie & Hiroshi Shimizu

第四十章
嗜酸性粒细胞疾病

中文导读

本章介绍了皮肤疾病中嗜酸性粒细胞的作用以及其可能引起的皮肤病。提到嗜酸性粒细胞可以在许多皮肤疾病的皮肤活检标本中看到，但对任何皮肤病都不是特异性的。嗜酸性粒细胞是少数几种疾病的典型组织学模式的重要组成部分，包括以下几种：血管淋巴样增生伴嗜酸性粒细胞增多、放射性皮炎、嗜酸性脓疱性毛囊炎、新生儿中毒性红斑、口腔黏膜嗜酸性溃疡、嗜酸性血管炎、面部肉芽肿、嗜酸性粒细胞增多综合症、色素失禁、木村病、嗜酸性增多性皮炎、嗜酸性蜂窝织炎。在后续文中对上述疾病的发病机制、临床特点、诊断以及鉴别诊断做了详细的描述。各类疾病的皮肤表现还给出了相应病例的图片，给予了读者更为直观的感受。

〔李芳芳〕

REGULATION OF THE PRODUCTION AND ACTIVATION OF EOSINOPHILS

AT-A-GLANCE

- Eosinophils are bone marrow–derived cells that circulate transiently and normally account for up to 6% (up to 600/mm^3) of circulating blood leukocytes.

- Eosinophils primarily are tissue-dwelling cells, but only in certain tissues in humans, with an average tissue life span of 2 to 5 days that may be increased with eosinophil survival factors for up to 14 days.

- As proinflammatory cells, the presence of eosinophils within most tissues is associated with pathologic states that include infections, allergic reactions and atopic diseases, fibrotic disorders, reactive eosinophilias, and hypereosinophilic syndromes.

- Eosinophils play a role in innate and adaptive immune responses, which may explain why they are present in normal, noninflamed tissues such as the gastrointestinal tract and lymphoid tissues.

- This section reviews the biologic actions of eosinophils with particular focus on what controls eosinophil production, activation, and tissue trafficking.

- Pharmacologic manipulation of eosinophil inflammation is possible as new, more specific strategies are emerging.

ONTOGENY AND DEVELOPMENT

Eosinophils develop in the bone marrow from multi-potential, stem cell–derived CD34+ myeloid progenitor cells in response to eosinophilopoietic cytokines and growth factors (Fig. 40-1). They are released into the circulation as mature cells.[1-3] Important stimulatory cytokines and growth factors for eosinophils include interleukin (IL)-3, granulocyte-macrophage colony-stimulating factor (GM-CSF), and IL-5. Activated T cells likely are the principal sources of IL-3, GM-CSF, and IL-5 that induce eosinophil differentiation in bone marrow. However, depending on pathogenic stimuli, eosinophilopoietic cytokines may be released by other cell types, including mast cells, macrophages, natural killer cells, endothelial cells, epithelial cells, fibroblasts, and even eosinophils, themselves.[4] IL-3 and GM-CSF are pluripotent cytokines that have effects on other hematopoietic lineages. IL-5 is the most selective eosinophil-active cytokine, but it is relatively late acting. Although it is both necessary and sufficient for eosinophil differentiation, IL-5 demonstrates maximum activity on the IL-5 receptor (IL-5R)–positive eosinophil progenitor pool that first is expanded by earlier acting pluripotent cytokines such as IL-3 and GM-CSF[4]; expression of the high-affinity IL-5R is a prerequisite for eosinophil development. Exodus from the bone marrow also is regulated by IL-5. IL-3 and GM-CSF, along with IL-5, promote survival, activation, and chemotaxis of eosinophils through binding to receptors that have a common β chain (CD131) with IL-5R, and unique α chains.

INTERACTIONS OF EOSINOPHILIC FACTORS AND CYTOKINES AND INTRACELLULAR SIGNALING

The interactions of eosinophilopoietic factors with their receptors stimulate a cascade of complex biochemical events through signal transduction. Signaling events progress in 4 steps: (a) juxtamembranous signaling in which membrane-anchored tyrosine kinases and lipid kinases are activated; (b) signal interfacing which serves to transduce juxtamembranous signals to cytosolic signals; (c) mobile signaling in which cytosolic signaling molecules translocate from the receptor site to other cellular compartments including the nucleus, mitochondria, and cytoskeleton; and (d) transcription activation resulting from nuclear translocation and initiation of gene transcription. Studies show the pivotal role of IL-5 in immune responses involving eosinophils through receptor-driven signaling.[5] IL-5 binds to the α chain of the IL-5R and induces recruitment of the common β (βc) chain to IL-5R. Janus kinase (JAK) 2 tyrosine kinase is constitutively associated with IL-5Rα, and JAK1 tyrosine kinase with IL-5Rβc; both are activated with IL-5 binding as part of the juxtamembranous step. Adaptor proteins, *src* homologs and collagen (Shc), SH2-containing phosphatase-2 (SHP-2), growth factor receptor-bound protein 2 (Grb2), Vav, and lipid kinases, phosphatidylinositol 3-kinase, function in the interfacing step. The activation of JAK2 and signal transducer and activator of transcription (STAT) 5 is essential for IL-5–dependent signal transduction. The Ras guanosine triphosphatase–extracellular signal-regulated kinase and also known as Ras–mitogen-activated protein kinase pathway, in addition to the JAK2-STAT5 pathway, is important in IL-5 signaling in the mobile step. The JAK-STAT and Ras–mitogen-activated protein kinase pathways converge at various levels in IL-5 signaling of eosinophils. Multiple other interactive signal transduction pathways induce and regulate gene expression for eosinophil growth, development, activation, and survival.[6]

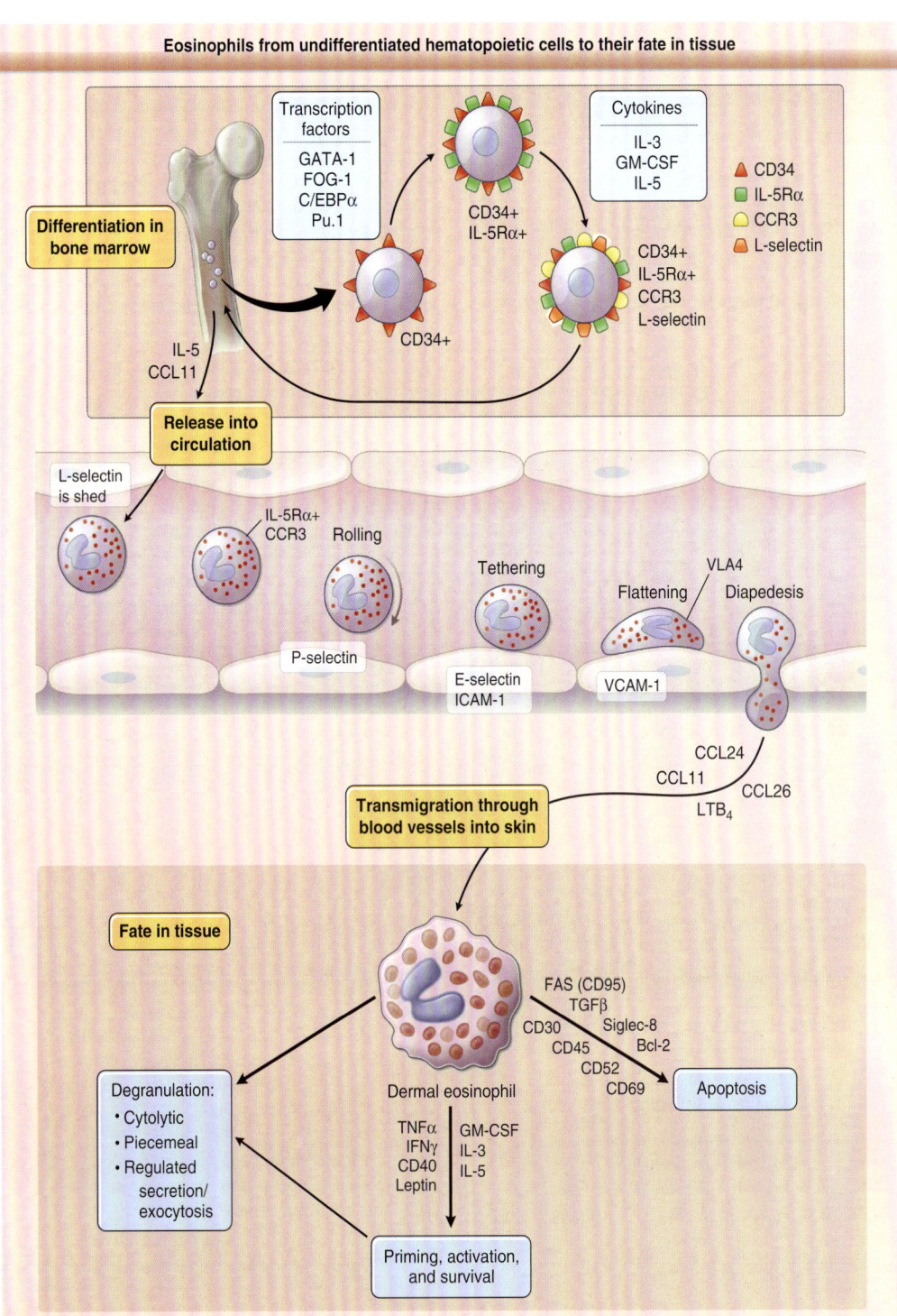

Figure 40-1 The progression of eosinophils from undifferentiated hematopoietic cells to their fate in tissue. The image depicts the eosinophil's life from differentiation in the bone marrow to vascular transmigration to its fate in tissue with key factors noted. GM-CSF, granulocyte-macrophage colony-stimulating factor; ICAM, intercellular adhesion molecule; IFN, interferon; IL, interleukin; LTB_4, leukotriene B_4; TGF, transforming growth factor; TNF, tumor necrosis factor; VCAM, vascular cell adhesion molecule.

EOSINOPHIL ULTRASTRUCTURE AND GRANULE CONTENT

Figure 40-2 shows the products of eosinophils and localization of granule proteins.

Mature eosinophils are 12 to 17 μm in diameter and, therefore, slightly larger than neutrophils. They typically have a bilobed nucleus with highly condensed peripheral chromatin. Eosinophils have distinctive cytoplasmic granules, demonstrated by their staining properties with acidic dyes such as eosin, and by their unique electron microscopy appearance. These specific or secondary granules are composed of an electron-dense core and a less-electron-dense matrix, the core being a crystalline lattice by electron microscopy. In cross section, the eosinophil contains approximately 30 of these membrane-bound, core-containing, secondary granules.[1] Five highly basic proteins are found within the granules: (a) major basic protein (MBP)-1, (b) MBP-2, (c) eosinophil-derived neurotoxin (EDN) also known as ribonuclease (RNase)2, (d) eosinophil

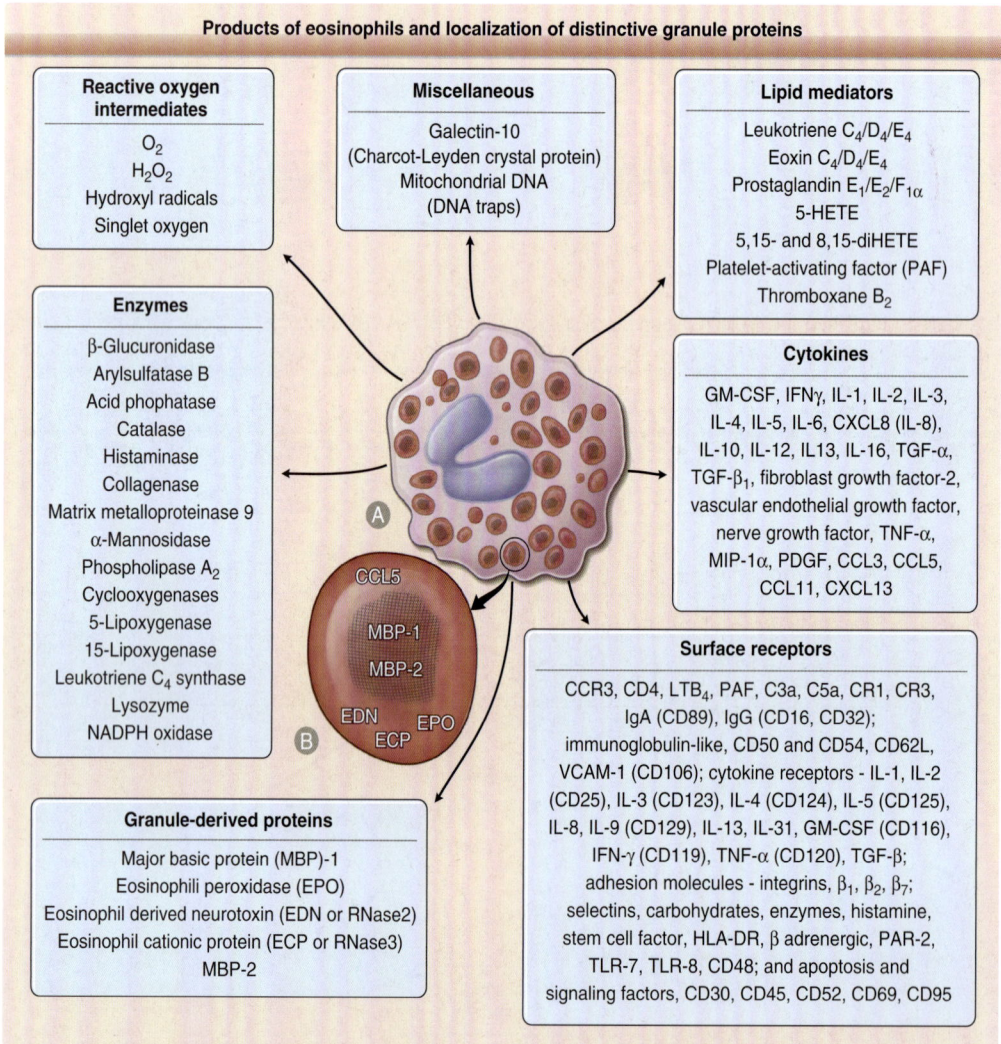

Figure 40-2 The products of eosinophils and localization of distinctive granule proteins. Eosinophils produce myriad products, including toxic granule proteins, which implicate their role in disease pathogenesis. The characteristic eosinophil granules are coarse and, as their name implies, eosinophilic upon staining with eosin. Distinctive granule proteins are localized to core and matrix portions of the specific cytoplasmic granules. **A,** An intact dermal eosinophil with its distinctive granules and typical bilobed nucleus. **B,** Characteristic specific (secondary) eosinophil granule with electron dense crystalline core and radiolucent matrix showing localization of distinctive granule proteins. GM-CSF, granulocyte-macrophage colony-stimulating factor; HETE, hydroxyeicosatetraenoic acid; HLA-DR, human leukocyte antigen-D related; IFN, interferon; Ig, immunoglobulin; IL, interleukin; MIP, macrophage inflammatory protein; NADPH, nicotinamide adenine dinucleotide phosphate; PDGF, platelet-derived growth factor; TGF, transforming growth factor; TLR, Toll-like receptor; TNF, tumor necrosis factor.

cationic protein (ECP) also known as RNase3, and (e) eosinophil peroxidase (EPO). Several other types of proteins are found in secondary granules and include enzymes, cytokines, growth factors, and chemokines. Eosinophils contain 3 other types of cytoplasmic granules, referred to as (a) primary granules, (b) small granules, and (c) secretory vesicles. Primary granules are of variable size, round, uniformly dense, present in 1 to 3 per electron microscopy cross section, and more common in immature eosinophilic promyelocytes. These granules may contain Charcot-Leyden crystal protein (also known as galectin-10), which also can be found in neutrophils[7]; Charcot–Leyden crystals are characteristically found in asthmatic sputum and in feces from patients with helminth infections or eosinophilic gastroenteritis. Small granules contain acid phosphatase and arylsulfatase and are present at 2 to 8 per electron microscopy cross section. Secretory vesicles, also referred to as tubulovesicular structures or microgranules, are characterized by their small, dumbbell-shaped appearance and their albumin content. They are the most abundant granules in number, with approximately 160 per electron microscopy cross section. Normal eosinophils contain varying numbers of non–membrane-bound lipid bodies, which are the principal stores of arachidonic acid. Lipid bodies also contain the enzymes, cyclooxygenase, 5- and 15-lipoxygenase, which are required to synthesize prostaglandins, leukotrienes (LTs), and eoxins, and are increased in activated eosinophils.[1]

BIOLOGIC FUNCTIONS

In mammals, such as the mouse and humans, the eosinophil is released as a mature cell into the circulation from the bone marrow, but is present in the blood only transiently, ranging from 8 to 18 hours. Eosinophils comprise a small portion, normally 6% or less, of circulating leukocytes. They are primarily tissue-dwelling cells, but only in certain tissues in humans, with an average tissue life span of 2 to 5 days. This may be prolonged by cytokines that increase eosinophil survival for up to 14 days. Under normal circumstances, a balance exists between bone marrow production and release of eosinophils, their time in circulation, and their entrance into tissues. Changes in any one of the compartments causes an increase or decrease in circulating and tissue eosinophils. Eosinophilia in blood or tissue or both is associated with helminthiasis, allergic hypersensitivity, and other pathologic conditions. In humans, bone marrow, spleen, lymph node, thymus, and gastrointestinal tract from the stomach through the colon, sparing the esophagus, are the only tissues in which eosinophils normally reside.[8] Furthermore, the gastrointestinal tract is the only organ other than bone marrow in which extracellular eosinophil granule protein deposition is observed even under homeostatic conditions. Eosinophils and their granule proteins are found in the lamina propria in normal gastrointestinal tract and are not found in Peyer patches or epithelium. Eosinophils in the lamina propria are reported to be able to induce the differentiation of regulatory T cells by producing transforming growth factor (TGF)-β_1 and all-*trans* retinoic acid.[9] The recruitment of eosinophils to the gastrointestinal, thymic, uterine, and mammary tissues is under the control of the CC chemokine, CCL11.[10,11] Eosinophils can also respond to tissue-damage signals and promote tissue remodeling. One study showed that eosinophils can migrate to areas of tissue injury or necrosis though the high-mobility group box-1 protein (HMGB1) released from necrotic cells and the receptor for advanced glycation end products expressed on eosinophils.[12] Moreover, it is proposed that eosinophils may play a role in the repair of gastric mucosal tissue during *Helicobacter pylori* infection.[13]

Once eosinophils enter tissues, most do not recirculate. Several possible mechanisms exist for removal of tissue eosinophils, including shedding of the cells across mucosal surfaces into the lumen of the intestinal or respiratory tract, engulfment of apoptotic eosinophils by macrophages, and lysis or degranulation with cellular degeneration. In various inflammatory conditions, including those affecting the skin, striking numbers of free granules and/or eosinophil granule protein deposition are present in the absence of intact eosinophils.[1] Isolated eosinophil granules express extracellular domains for interferon (IFN)-γ receptor and CCR3 and, upon stimulation, respond independently as organelles by releasing ECP.[14]

ROLE OF EOSINOPHILS IN IMMUNE FUNCTION

Shortly after their discovery by Paul Ehrlich in 1879, eosinophils were observed in association with helminth infections. Theories have been promulgated that eosinophils are important for host defense against parasites spawning numerous studies.[15] For example, in vitro studies demonstrated that eosinophils are cytotoxic to large nonphagocytosable organisms, such as multicellular helminthic parasites. Eosinophils bind to host-derived immunoglobulins and complement components on the surface of their targets (so-called antibody- or complement-) dependent cytotoxicity. They also bind to carbohydrate ligands expressed on parasites, such as the LewisX-related molecules, and cell adhesion molecules similar to selectins. Eosinophils are activated to release their granule products with deposition of these biologically active proteins in and around the parasites causing disruption of the parasite's integument and, ultimately, death of the organism. The granule proteins have different effects. ECP produces fragmentation and disruption whereas MBP-1 produces a distinctive ballooning detachment of the tegumental membrane, and EDN is active only at high concentrations, causing crinkling of the tegumental membrane.[16]

However, in murine models in which blood, marrow, and tissue eosinophilia is largely abolished by neutralizing IL-5 activity, the intensities of primary or secondary parasitic infection are unchanged, indicating that eosinophils have little or no role in parasitic host defense in these models.[1] The results must be interpreted cautiously because mouse and human eosinophils have functional differences, and mice are not natural hosts of many of the parasites tested experimentally.

Eosinophils also release cytotoxic granule proteins onto the surface of fungal organisms and into the extracellular milieu in fungal infections. Eosinophils kill fungi in a contact-dependent manner. Eosinophils adhere to the fungal cell wall component, β-glucan, via a $β_2$-integrin surface molecule, CD11b.[17] Eosinophils do not express other common fungal receptors, such as dectin-1 and lactosylceramide, and, specifically, do not react with chitin. However, chitin, which is a polymer that confers structural rigidity to fungi, helminths, crustaceans, and insects, induces accumulation of eosinophils in tissues through production of LTB_4 in mice.[18] Eosinophils also are activated by fungal organisms that release proteases, such as *Alternaria*, through protease-activated receptors (PARs). For example, fungal aspartate protease activates eosinophils through PAR-2, thereby mediating the innate responses of eosinophils to certain fungi.[19]

As a granulocyte, the eosinophil is capable of phagocytosing and killing bacteria and other small microbes in vitro, but eosinophils cannot effectively defend against bacterial infections when neutrophil function is deficient. Nevertheless, investigations reveal that eosinophils may have a role in innate immunity against bacteria using a unique mechanism, DNA trap.[20] Eosinophils rapidly release mitochondrial DNA when exposed to bacteria, a complement component, C5a, or CCR3 ligands. The traps contain eosinophil granule proteins, ECP and MBP, and have antimicrobial effects. In the extracellular space, the granule proteins and mitochondrial DNA form structures that bind and kill bacteria both in vitro and in vitro. Eosinophils, unlike neutrophils, do not undergo cell death as part of this process. This may be an important innate immune response, particularly in mucosal epithelium.[20]

Eosinophils may have other roles in immune responses as well. Through major histocompatibility complex class II expression and IL-1α production, they can function as antigen-presenting cells for a variety of viral, parasitic, and microbial antigens, including staphylococcal superantigens, and allergens.[21,22] Eosinophils are recruited to secondary lymphoid structures to promote the proliferation of effector T cells, even though they are unable to affect naïve T cells.[23] Eosinophils, as sources of cytokines, influence T-cell–dependent responses.[1] In keeping with the prominence of eosinophils in allergic disorders, eosinophils are involved in T-cell polarization favoring T-helper (Th)2 by promoting Th1 apoptosis in addition to their influence via cytokine expression.[21,24-27]

Interestingly, it is also reported that eosinophils play a role in helminth parasite-elicited protection against autoimmunity, as observed in a mouse model of multiple sclerosis.[28]

In allograft rejection, a number of studies have demonstrated the diagnostic and prognostic value of eosinophils, especially in the acute rejection of allografts.[29,30] On the other hand, a recent study indicated that a lower eosinophil count in peripheral blood predicts adverse prognosis of allograft rejection in heart transplant patients.[31] Further investigation into these possible roles of eosinophils and their mechanisms in acute allograft rejection is warranted.

ROLE OF EOSINOPHILS IN DISEASE

The activities of eosinophil-derived products include direct cytotoxic effects on structural cells and microbes, increased vascular permeability, procoagulant effects, innate immune responses to some parasites, viruses, fungi, and tumor cells, enhancement of leukocyte migration, amplification of effector T-cell responses, and, possibly, mammary gland development. Collectively, these varied biologic actions provide the pathophysiologic basis for the signs and symptoms observed in eosinophil-associated diseases.

Eosinophils in lymph nodes and spleen are especially increased after allergen exposures or microbial insults.[32,33] In allergic inflammation, the involvement of eosinophils is promoted by the stimulation of thymic stromal lymphopoietin, a cytokine that is mainly secreted by epithelial cells in response to allergens or other environmental stimuli.[34-36] Eosinophils have been found in several cancers, particularly in lymphomas, leukemias, and colon cancer. Clinical studies indicate that certain tumors associated with tissue and/or peripheral eosinophilia have a more favorable prognosis,[37] whereas in other tumors, such as nodular sclerosing Hodgkin disease, Sézary syndrome, and gastric carcinomas, they are thought to confer a poor prognosis. In Sézary syndrome, the tumor cells produce IL-5 and, therefore, are responsible for the eosinophilia, which is a reflection of tumor burden.[38] Where eosinophilia is a good prognostic factor, eosinophils are considered to be part of an effective host response to the tumor.[39,40]

EOSINOPHIL CONSTITUENTS AND THEIR ACTIVITIES

The eosinophil contains and produces myriad factors that implicate its role in inflammation and tissue destruction and remodeling (see Fig. 40-2).[41] Products released by eosinophils include chemoattractants, colony-stimulating factors, and endothelial-activating cytokines. In addition to toxic cationic proteins from specific granules and oxidative products released into tissues following activation, these factors include arachidonic acid–derived lipids, hydrolytic enzymes, neuropeptides, colony-stimulating factors, and cytokines/chemokines that facilitate further leukocyte recruitment to sites of inflammation (see Fig. 40-2). Surface molecule expression is important in all aspects of eosinophil biology, from promoting growth and differentiation to eosinophil trafficking into tissue to activation and/or priming of the cells to senescence. Numerous membrane factors are expressed on eosinophils that further direct eosinophil biologic effects.

EOSINOPHIL GRANULE PROTEINS

Among the products of eosinophils that are most damaging to the host are the specific granule's cationic proteins. Knowledge of their biologic actions provides insight into their functions in human disease. Once deposited, the granule proteins persist in tissues for extended times—EPO for 1 week, ECP for 2 weeks, EDN for 2.5 weeks, and MBP-1 for 6 weeks.[42] Each of these proteins induces direct tissue damage to both host cells, including myocytes, endothelium, neurons, epithelium, and smooth muscle, and microbes. All 4 of the cationic granule proteins (EPO, ECP, EDN, and MBP-1) likely contribute to the edema observed in skin diseases because of their vasodilatory effects, with contribution from mast cells and basophil histamine release by MBP-1.[43] Eosinophil granule proteins stimulate various cells in addition to mast cells and basophils, including neutrophils and platelets. Nodules, eosinophilia, rheumatism, dermatitis, and swelling (NERDS), episodic angioedema with eosinophilia (Gleich syndrome), urticaria, eosinophilic cellulitis (Wells syndrome), and insect bite reactions demonstrate variable degrees of edema that are probably explained, at least in part, by this mechanism. Eosinophil granule proteins injected into skin produce lesions, including dose-dependent wheal-and-flare reactions by MBP and ulcerations by ECP and EDN.[44,45]

MAJOR BASIC PROTEIN

MBP comprises the crystalloid core of the specific eosinophil granule. It was so named because it accounts for a major portion (approximately 55% in guinea pig) of the eosinophil granule protein and has a high isoelectric point (calculated at greater than pH 11) that is so strongly basic it cannot be measured accurately. It is now known that MBP is expressed as 2 homologs, MBP-1 and MBP-2, coded by different genes on chromosome 11. MBP-1 directly damages helminths and also lethally damages mammalian cells and tissues, examples of which are its ability to cause exfoliation of bronchial epithelial cells and to kill tumor cells. MBP-1 exerts its effects by increasing cell membrane permeability through surface charge interactions leading to disruption of the cell-surface lipid bilayer. MBP-1 and MBP-2, but none of the other eosinophil granule proteins, stimulate histamine and LTC_4 release from human basophils. Furthermore, MBP-1 and MBP-2 stimulate neutrophils, inducing release of superoxide, lysozyme, and IL-8. MBP-1 and EPO are potent platelet agonists causing release of 5-hydroxytryptamine and promoting clotting.

EOSINOPHIL PEROXIDASE

EPO is highly basic, pI 10.8, localized in the matrix of the specific eosinophil granule and is a key participant in generating reactive oxidants and free radical species in activated eosinophils. EPO consists of a heavy chain and a light chain encoded with a prosequence. Although MBP is present in the highest molar concentration in eosinophil granules, EPO, by weight, is the most abundant protein constituting approximately 25% of the specific eosinophil granule's total protein mass. EPO kills numerous microorganisms in the presence of hydrogen peroxide, generated by eosinophils and other phagocytes, and halide. This combination of products also initiates mast cell secretion. EPO binding to microbes, including *Staphylococcus aureus*, greatly potentiates their killing by phagocytes. EPO-coated tumor cells are spontaneously lysed by activated macrophages.

EOSINOPHIL CATIONIC PROTEIN AND EOSINOPHIL-DERIVED NEUROTOXIN

ECP (or RNase3) and EDN (or RNase2) are homologous proteins with sequence identity in 37 of 55 amino acid residues. ECP also has neurotoxic activity. ECP and EDN play a role in viral host defense to RNA viruses.[46-48] EDN induces the migration and maturation of dendritic cells.[49] It also is an endogenous ligand of Toll-like receptor 2 (TLR2) and can activate myeloid dendritic cells by triggering the Toll-like receptor 2–myeloid differentiation factor 88 signaling pathway.[27] Based on its ability to serve as a chemoattractant and activator of dendritic cells along with enhancing antigen-specific Th2-biased immune responses, EDN functions as an alarmin, alerting the adaptive immune system to preferentially enhance antigen-specific Th2 responses.[27]

LIPID MEDIATORS

Lipid bodies in eosinophils are storage sites for arachidonic acids. Eosinophils produce several arachidonic acid metabolites, including cysteinyl LTs from the 5-lipoxygenase pathway (LTC_4, LTD_4, and LTE_4) and thromboxanes and prostaglandins (PGs) from the cyclooxygenase pathway (thromboxane B_2, PGE_2, and $PGF_1\alpha$).[50,51]

CYTOKINES

Eosinophils are a considerable source of growth factors and regulatory and proinflammatory cytokines and chemokines.[1,52] The various growth factors produced by eosinophils include TGF-α, TGF-β, fibroblast growth factor (FGF)-2, vascular endothelial growth factor, nerve growth factor, and platelet-derived growth factor (PDGF)-β. There is evidence that these growth factors induce stromal fibrosis and basement membrane thickening at sites of chronic eosinophilic inflammation including nasal polyps, asthmatic airways and, likely, in certain skin disorders, such as atopic dermatitis.[1] Another group of cytokines produced by eosinophils modulates other immune cells and includes tumor necrosis factor (TNF)-α, macrophage inflammatory protein-1α (CCL3), IL-1α, IL-2, IL-3, IL-4, IL-5, IL-6, CXCL8 (IL-8), IL-10, IL-12, IL-13, IL-16, GM-CSF, and IFN-γ.[52] Additional chemokines produced by eosinophils are CXCL13 (B-lymphocyte chemoattractant factor), CCL5 (regulated on activation, normal T cells expressed and secreted [RANTES]), and CCL11, in addition to CCL3 and CXCL8. All these cytokines are constitutively produced in low levels in resting eosinophils and induced in inflammatory conditions with activation of eosinophils by engagement of receptors with immunoglobulins, complement and cytokines, including those produced by eosinophils, themselves, in an autocrine manner. Notably, eosinophils produce the 3 principal cytokines involved in their own growth and differentiation—IL-3, IL-5, and GM-CSF—as well as CCL5 and CCL11, the chemokines important in their own chemotaxis. In summary, the eosinophil-derived cytokines may function in both an autocrine and paracrine fashion and likely have pathophysiologic relevance.

SURFACE EXPRESSION

Eosinophils express numerous receptors and other factors on their surface membranes through which they communicate with the extracellular environment, but no single surface protein is uniquely expressed on eosinophils. These receptors have been identified either by flow cytometry or by functional assays, and can be grouped as follows: chemotactic factor and complement receptors, including chemokine, LT, and platelet-activating factor (PAF); immunoglobulin supergene family member receptors, including immunoglobulins; cytokine receptors; adhesion molecule receptors; receptors involved in apoptosis; and miscellaneous receptors and surface factors. Eosinophil membrane proteins are promising targets for therapeutic modulation of eosinophil effects (see "Pharmacologic Manipulation" below).

CHEMOTACTIC FACTOR AND COMPLEMENT RECEPTORS

Chemotactic factors are important in orchestrating cellular trafficking to sites of inflammation as well as physiologic homing (eg, eosinophils to gastrointestinal tract). The eosinophil has receptors for many chemotactic agents, including LTB_4, PAF, bacterial products (N-formyl-methionyl-leucyl-phenylalanine), and the complement anaphylatoxins C3a and C5a. Eosinophils express complement receptor (CR)1 (CD35), a receptor for C1q that also binds C4b, C3b, and iC3b, and CR3 (Mac-1, CD11b/CD18) in addition to receptors for C3a and C5a. These are important receptors in eosinophil effector functions. The binding of chemokines to their respective receptors mediates many biologic effects, which, in addition to cell shape change and migration, includes cell activation, receptor internalization, induction of the respiratory burst with generation of toxic oxygen metabolites, and transient activation of integrin adhesiveness. The chemotaxins listed above have potent effects on eosinophils but are nonselective in that they are active on other leukocytes. Because many eosinophil-associated diseases are characterized by tissue eosinophil infiltration with little or no neutrophil infiltration, the identification of the CCR3 receptor and its ligands was an important breakthrough in discovering eosinophil-selective chemotaxins.[53] Specific members of the chemokine family are critical for the cellular trafficking of eosinophils. The major ligands of CCR3, CCL5, CCL11, CCL13 (monocyte chemotactic protein-4), CCL24 (eotaxin-2), and CCL26 (eotaxin-3) play a critical role in both the homeostatic and inflammation-induced recruitment of eosinophils to tissue sites.[54,55]

IMMUNOGLOBULIN GENE SUPERFAMILY MEMBER RECEPTORS

Many of the studies of eosinophil functions, including phagocytosis, antigen-dependent cytotoxicity, oxygen metabolism, LTC_4 production, and eosinophil survival, have been performed using immunoglobulin (Ig) G-coated targets. Among eosinophil surface receptors for the Ig family members, the most highly expressed receptor is FcγRII (CD32), which binds aggregated IgG, particularly of the subclasses IgG_1 and IgG_3. The binding of IgG to this receptor may be important in eosinophil degranulation in parasitic and allergic diseases, along with other eosinophil functions.[1] Freshly isolated eosinophils express only FcγRII (CD32) of the IgG receptors, but eosinophils can be stimulated by cytokines, particularly IFN-γ, to express FcγRI (CD64) and FcγRIII (CD16), as well as to augment FcγRII (CD32) expression.

Intercellular adhesion molecule (ICAM)-1 (CD54) and ICAM-3 (CD50) are members of Ig superfamily expressed on eosinophils and are likely important in leukocyte–leukocyte and leukocyte–tissue cell adhesion through leukocyte function-associated antigen-1 ($\alpha_L\beta_2$; CD11a/CD18) as its counterligand (see Fig. 40-1).

CYTOKINE RECEPTORS

Cytokine receptors are present at low levels on the surfaces of eosinophils. Receptors for IL-3 (CD123), IL-5 (CD125), and GM-CSF (CD116) are readily detected and, all share a common β chain (CD132). Eosinophil activation has been observed by a variety of other cytokines through presumed and/or detected receptors. These include stem cell factor (c-kit receptor; CD117), IFN-γ (CD119), TNF-α (CD120), IL-4 (CD124), IL-9 (CD129 and CD132), IL-13 (gp65), IL-2 (CD25), IL-31, and TGF-β receptors. Many of these receptors are for cytokines that eosinophils produce, providing further evidence that they have autocrine functions.

ADHESION MOLECULE RECEPTORS

Adhesion molecule receptors are expressed on the eosinophil cell surface to mediate trafficking to and within tissues, and for general cell–cell interactions.[56] These receptors fall into three groups: (a) Ig superfamily, (b) selectins and their glycoprotein counterligands, and (3) integrins. L-selectin (CD62L) and P-selectin glycoprotein ligand-1 (PSGL-1, CD162) are expressed at high levels on eosinophils, whereas E-selectin ligands, as an example, sialyl–Lewis-X (CD15s), are expressed at very low levels. P-selectin together with PSGL-1 is the most important selectin pair in eosinophil migration into tissues.

Eosinophils express a variety of integrins (β_1, β_2, and β_7) on their surface, which facilitate their adhesion to extracellular matrix proteins, vascular cellular adhesion molecule (VCAM)-1 (CD106) on activated endothelium, or ICAM-1 present on resting or activated epithelium and activated endothelium. Integrins are composed of 2 subunits that exist as noncovalently associated heterodimers, with α and β subunits. The β_1 integrins expressed on eosinophils include $\alpha_4\beta_1$ (very late antigen [VLA]-4), which binds to VCAM-1 found on activated endothelium and the extracellular matrix protein, fibronectin. Eosinophil adhesion to fibronectin induces the autocrine production of eosinophil-activating survival cytokines, IL-3, IL-5, and GM-CSF.

RECEPTORS INVOLVED IN APOPTOSIS

Eosinophils express several "death receptors," which are involved in apoptotic pathways, such as Fas receptor (CD95), Siglec-8, CD30, CD45, Campath (CD52), and CD69, along with important intracellular regulators of eosinophil apoptosis, such as the members of the B-cell leukemia/lymphoma (Bcl)-2 and inhibitor of apoptosis families.[57] Diseases characterized by eosinophilia likely result, in part, from delayed or defective apoptotic pathways allowing accumulation and persistence of eosinophils in blood and/or tissues.

FACTORS WORKING TOGETHER

The various products elaborated by eosinophils in response to receptor activation do not necessarily function independently but often act in concert to mediate their biologic effects. For example, the release of TGF-α, TGF-β, FGF-2, vascular endothelial growth factor, matrix metalloproteinase-9, and inhibitors of matrix metalloproteinases from activated eosinophils collectively induce fibroblast proliferation and extracellular matrix protein production. Eosinophils contribute factors of their own and influence factor production from other cells; for example, eosinophil mediators induce platelet release of TGF-β. After intradermal eosinophil infiltration, there is production of extracellular proteins, including tenascin and procollagen 1, as well as myofibroblast formation.[58] Eosinophil-induced fibrosis is observed in the lungs and heart of patients with hypereosinophilic syndrome, in and around organs in other fibrosing/sclerosing disorders, and in the skin of patients with eosinophilic fasciitis (Shulman syndrome), eosinophilia–myalgia syndrome, and toxic oil syndrome.[59] Eosinophil granule proteins, MBP-1 and EDN, along with other neuroactive mediators produced by eosinophils, such as nerve growth factor, vasoactive intestinal peptide, and substance P, likely affect nerve physiology. In fact, eosinophils and eosinophil granule proteins are often observed in close proximity to nerve endings.[60,61] Eosinophil-induced nerve dysfunction is likely an important part of the gastric dysmotility observed in subjects with food allergies, the dysfunction of vagal muscarinic M2 receptors observed in patients with asthma, and may also contribute to itch along with other physiologic aberrations in atopic dermatitis and other cutaneous diseases.[61,62] Collectively, the eosinophil's response to surface factors determines its role in health and disease.

TISSUE TRAFFICKING

The selective recruitment of eosinophils into sites of inflammation results from interactions among eosinophil-activating cytokines, chemokine-inducing cytokines, and endothelial-activating cytokines (see Fig. 40-1). Similar to other leukocytes, selectin, integrin, and Ig gene superfamily members contribute to the signaling involved in eosinophil trafficking. In particular, eosinophils constitutively express the integrin, VLA-4, which interacts with its ligand, VCAM-1, induced on endothelial cells by cytokines, especially Th2 cytokines (IL-4 and IL-13).[63] After movement through vessels, eosinophils adhere to extracellular matrix proteins. Here, surface factors, such as CD11b/CD18 (Mac-1), bind to fibrous proteins such as fibronectin, laminin, and collagen, and, not only determine where eosinophils will reside, but likely prolong their survival.[64] In this regard, the CD11b/CD18 (Mac-1) integrin is also critical for eosinophil effector functions, including degranulation.[65]

EOSINOPHIL-ACTIVATING CYTOKINES

Eosinophil-activating cytokines can be produced by many cell types in addition to T cells and mast cells, including keratinocytes, endothelial cells, and monocytes, along with eosinophils, themselves. The eosinophil-activating cytokines, IL-3, IL-5, GM-CSF, and others, enhance chemotactic responses, in addition to multiple other effects on eosinophils, such as promoting maturation, cell survival, and LT production.[66]

ENDOTHELIAL-ACTIVATING CYTOKINES

During eosinophil migration, at least 3 types of endothelial activations occur. The first is the expression of P-selectin, which occurs when Weibel-Palade bodies in endothelial cells are transported to the cell surface rapidly after exposure to histamine, LTs, and a host of other inflammatory mediators. Expression of P-selectin on the endothelial cell surface initiates leukocyte rolling, via CD162 (PSGL-1), which is the important initial step before firm adhesion and transendothelial migration. A second type of endothelial activation is that induced by nonspecific activators such as IL-1 and TNF-α. These cytokines stimulate endothelial expression of E-selectin, ICAM-1, and VCAM-1, to which eosinophils firmly adhere, or "tether." They also induce production of chemokines by endothelial cells. The third type of endothelial activation is that induced by IL-4 and IL-13. These cytokines selectively induce VCAM-1, which is centrally involved in the recruitment of VLA-4–positive cells, including eosinophils, basophils, and lymphocytes, into sites of allergic inflammation.

CHEMOKINES

The transition from rolling to firm adherence is substantially increased by CCR3 ligands, the CC chemokines. Induction of the expression of chemokines by activated endothelial cells results in higher levels of chemokines on or near the endothelial surface, which transiently affect β_1-integrin and β_2-integrin avidity, resulting in firm adhesion of the eosinophil to the endothelial cell. However, chemokines produced by structural cells such as fibroblasts, smooth muscle cells, and epithelium probably are more important in directing migration and activation of eosinophils within tissues than those expressed on endothelial cells.[67]

Tissue chemokine expression forms a gradient signal that guides eosinophils into tissue. CCL11 guides eosinophils into tissue locations in which eosinophils are normally present, thymus, uterus, mammary gland, and gastrointestinal tract.[68] In Th2 disorders, Th2 cytokines induce chemokine expression. In skin, IL-4, IL-13, and TNF-α stimulate CCL11, CCL24, and CCL26 production from mast cell and lymphocyte sources, as well as from fibroblasts (CCL11 and CCL26) and keratinocytes (CCL26).[69] As in eosinophilic esophagitis, CCL26 may be important in atopic dermatitis in which serum CCL26 levels correlate with disease activity.[70]

Arachidonic acid metabolites, particularly, the cysteinyl LTs, LTC_4, LTD_4, and LTE_4, and PGD_2, are involved in eosinophil trafficking as evidenced by the observations that LT receptor antagonists reduce blood and lung eosinophilia and that mice, depleted of LTB_4 receptors, have markedly reduced lung eosinophilia after allergen exposure. Eosinophil, basophil, and Th2 cell recruitment occurs, to some extent, through CRTH2 (CD294), the high-affinity PGD_2 type 2 receptor.

ACTIVATION OF EOSINOPHILS

Various inflammatory mediators activate eosinophils. In addition to cytokines, TNF-α, GM-CSF, IL-3, and IL-5, the inflammatory mediators include complement components, C3a and C5a, lipid mediators, LTC_4 and PAF, and chemokines, as well as engagement of IgA and IgG Fc receptors. IL-33 regulates eosinophils in the mechanisms of allergic inflammatory response. Nuclear factor κB and mitogen-activated protein kinase pathways are activated upon IL-33 ligation to receptors on eosinophils, promoting the cell surface expression of CD11b and ICAM-1 and the production of proinflammatory cytokines such as IL-6, IL-8, and IL-13.[30,71] Eosinophil differentiation from CD117+ hematopoietic progenitor cells is directly induced by IL-33 in an IL-5-dependent manner.[72]

CD11b/CD18 (Mac-1)-dependent cellular adhesion is a critical component for degranulation and superoxide production induced by GM-CSF and PAF eosinophil activation and likely is an in vitro mechanism that results from eosinophil contact with stromal cells and/or proteins.[73] Members of the CC chemokine subfamily (CCL5, CCL7 [MCP-3], CCL11, CCL13 [MCP-4], and CCL24) that bind to the chemokine receptor, CCR3, also potently activate eosinophils. Activated eosinophils develop a number of phenotypic changes, including a reduction in granules, vacuolization, and an expansion of their cytoplasm, leading to a reduction in cell density and are referred to as *hypodense*. The number of hypodense cells predicts allergic disease severity. A cell-surface marker that distinguishes hypodense from normodense eosinophils has not been identified, but there are several surface markers with enhanced expression on in vitro or in vitro–activated or hypodense cells: α_M integrin (CD11b), α_X integrin (CD11c), FcγRIII (CD16), hyaluronic acid receptor (CD44), ICAM-1 (CD54), CD69, and HLA-DR (human leukocyte antigen-D related).[74]

Upon recruitment and activation in tissues, eosinophils have various effects as detailed in previous sections. In tissues, eosinophils release granule contents into their extracellular space via 3 mechanisms: piecemeal degranulation, regulated secretion (also referred to as regulated exocytosis), and cytolytic degranulation.

PHARMACOLOGIC MANIPULATION

Eosinophil-associated disease is a term that, strictly speaking, refers to diseases in which eosinophil numbers or eosinophil granule protein levels (or other eosinophil products) are associated with disease activity. This term encompasses multiple heterogeneous disorders, including skin diseases, in which targeting eosinophils and/or their products is a therapeutic goal. Many available treatments reduce eosinophil numbers, thereby inhibiting eosinophilic inflammation, including glucocorticoids, calcineurin inhibitors, IFN-α, IFN-γ, LT antagonists, myelosuppressive/cytotoxic drugs, and, possibly, antihistamines. However, none is specific for eosinophils. It is only in recent years that selective and direct reduction of eosinophils has been achieved, and these therapies have provided new insight into disease pathogenesis.[75]

Among the nonselective drugs for eosinophil reduction, glucocorticoids generally are very effective. The immediate (within 3 hours) reduction in circulating eosinophils observed after systemic administration of glucocorticoids likely occurs as a consequence of sequestration into extramedullary organs (liver, spleen, and lymph node), as has been shown in rodents. Glucocorticoids affect eosinophil infiltration into tissues by 4 mechanisms: sequestration into lymphoid tissues, induction of eosinophil apoptosis, reduction of eosinophil production by bone marrow, and alterations in the production of the cytokines/chemokines important in eosinophil trafficking.[76-78] Glucocorticoids suppress the production of several cytokines important for the induction of adhesion molecules on endothelial cells, including IL-1, TNF-α, IL-4, and IL-13, and the release of eosinophil-active chemokines, including CCL5, CCL7, and CCL11. Unfortunately, "steroid resistance" develops in some patients, and long-term administration of glucocorticoids is associated with limiting side effects.

Calcineurin antagonists, such as cyclosporine, tacrolimus, and pimecrolimus, broadly inhibit T-cell cytokine release, including those that specifically induce eosinophilic inflammation (IL-4, IL-5, and GM-CSF). They also decrease the expression of CCL5, CCL11, and IL-5 with associated decreased tissue eosinophilia as has been shown in atopic dermatitis.[79] Mammalian target of rapamycin (mTOR) inhibitors, including rapamycin, have direct effects on eosinophils, decreasing eosinophil granule protein release after IL-5 activation.[80] The use of these therapeutic agents are limited by their side effects, including immunosuppression, as well as other metabolic effects that may be in part genetically determined.[81]

Several myelosuppressive drugs, including hydroxyurea, vincristine sulfate, cyclophosphamide, methotrexate, 6-thioguanine, 2-chlorodeoxyadenosine and cytarabine combination therapy, pulsed chlorambucil, and etoposide, may be beneficial in eosinophil-associated disease alone or as steroid-sparing agents. Hydroxyurea has been particularly effective in decreasing circulating eosinophil numbers.

In myeloproliferative hypereosinophilic syndrome (chronic eosinophilic leukemia) with the *FIP1L1-PDGFRA* mutation that codes for a tyrosine kinase, imatinib mesylate, a tyrosine kinase inhibitor, is approved for the treatment of chronic myelogenous leukemia and the hypereosinophilic syndrome, and has produced rapid, complete or near-complete remissions.[82] Patients who have features of myeloproliferative hypereosinophilic syndrome (HES) but who lack *FIP1L1-PDGFRA* still may respond to imatinib.[83]

Alemtuzumab is a monoclonal antibody to CD52 that is used to deplete CD52+ lymphocytes in the treatment of chronic (B-cell) lymphocytic leukemia and T-cell lymphoma. Eosinophils, but not neutrophils, also express CD52, and alemtuzumab has been useful in treating patients with refractory HES, including those with abnormal T cells,[84-86] but has serious limiting side effects from cytopenias, infusion reactions and infections.

Mepolizumab is the first humanized monoclonal antibody against IL-5. It has proved effective in inhibiting eosinophilia and in reducing asthma exacerbation rates.[87]

Benralizumab is an anti–IL-5 receptor α (IL-5Rα) humanized monoclonal antibody. This therapy produced reduced eosinophilia in a dose-dependent manner in a Phase I trial on persons with asthma.[88] As other eosinophilopoietic factors may circumvent the requirement for IL-5 in some cases, targeting IL-5Rα is considered to be more effective in reducing eosinophils than therapies directed at IL-5 itself.[89]

Both IFN-α and IFN-γ may be therapeutically beneficial in eosinophil-associated disease by inhibiting eosinophil degranulation and inflammatory mediator release. IFN-α may be better tolerated than IFN-γ and is used as a steroid-sparing agent predominantly in patients with lymphocytic variant HES, but also may be useful in myeloproliferative variant HES.[90,91]

EOSINOPHILS IN CUTANEOUS DISEASES

AT-A-GLANCE

- Eosinophils may be seen in skin biopsy specimens from a broad range of cutaneous diseases but are not pathognomonic for any dermatosis.

- Eosinophils are an important component of the characteristic histologic pattern in a limited number of diseases, including the following:
  - Angiolymphoid hyperplasia with eosinophilia.
  - Eosinophilic, polymorphic, and pruritic eruption associated with radiotherapy.
  - Eosinophilic pustular folliculitis.
  - Erythema toxicum neonatorum.
  - Eosinophilic ulcer of the oral mucosa.
  - Eosinophilic vasculitis.
  - Granuloma faciale.
  - Hypereosinophilic syndromes.
  - Incontinentia pigmenti.
  - Kimura disease.
  - Pachydermatous eosinophilic dermatitis.
  - Wells syndrome (eosinophilic cellulitis).

- Clinical reaction patterns with eosinophil involvement include diseases in which eosinophils probably play a pathogenic role and are a component of the histologic pattern, but are not essential for diagnosis.

- Evidence for involvement of eosinophils in cutaneous diseases is provided by observation of intact eosinophils in lesional tissue sections and/or by immunostains for their toxic granule proteins, which are deposited in tissues.

Eosinophils have myriad inflammatory activities that implicate them in disease.[41,54,92] Peripheral blood eosinophilia and/or tissue infiltration by eosinophils occur in a variety of common and unusual diseases, including those of infectious, immunologic, and neoplastic etiologies. Organ-specific eosinophil disorders occur in the skin, lung, and gastrointestinal tract.[93-95] Eosinophils are conspicuous in tissue sections stained with hematoxylin and eosin because of their intense avidity for eosin dye. Common dermatoses associated with eosinophils in lesional tissues include arthropod bites and drug eruptions. Parasitic infections, especially those caused by ectoparasites and helminthes, typically have a marked host response with eosinophilia.[33,96] Autoimmune blistering diseases, such as bullous pemphigoid and the various forms of pemphigus, often have prominent eosinophil infiltration, including histologic presentation as eosinophilic spongiosis.[97,98] Infiltration of eosinophils in the subcutaneous tissues, so-called eosinophilic panniculitis, is not a specific diagnosis but rather is seen to a variable degree in diverse entities.[99,100] Eosinophils may be found in Langerhans cell histiocytosis,[101] cutaneous epithelial neoplasms,[102] and lymphoproliferative disorders.[103] Although eosinophils constitute one of the histologic features in numerous cutaneous diseases, eosinophil infiltration represents a criterion for histologic diagnosis in relatively few entities (Table 40-1).

TABLE 40-1
Eosinophils in Cutaneous Diseases

- Diseases characterized by tissue eosinophils
  - Angiolymphoid hyperplasia with eosinophilia
  - Eosinophilic, polymorphic, and pruritic eruption associated with radiotherapy
  - Eosinophilic pustular folliculitis
    - Classical (Ofuji disease)
    - Infantile/neonatal
    - HIV-associated
  - Erythema toxicum neonatorum
  - Eosinophilic ulcer of oral mucosa
    - Granuloma faciale
    - Hypereosinophilic syndromes
    - Kimura disease
    - Pachydermatous eosinophilic dermatitis
    - Wells syndrome (eosinophilic cellulitis)
- Diseases typically associated with tissue eosinophils
  - Arthropod bites and sting reactions
  - Bullous dermatoses
    - Pemphigoid
    - Pemphigus
    - Incontinentia pigmenti
  - Dermatoses of pregnancy
  - Drug reactions
    - DRESS (drug rash with eosinophilia and systemic symptoms)/drug hypersensitivity syndrome
    - Interstitial granulomatous drug reaction
  - Histiocytic diseases
    - Langerhans cell histiocytosis
    - Juvenile xanthogranuloma
  - Parasitic diseases/infestations
  - Urticaria and angioedema
  - Eosinophilic granulomatosis with polyangiitis
- Histologic patterns defined by eosinophils
  - Eosinophilic spongiosis
    - Acute dermatitis
      - Allergic contact dermatitis
    - Arthropod bite
    - Immunobullous diseases
      - Pemphigoid
      - Pemphigus
    - Incontinentia pigmenti
  - Eosinophilic panniculitis
    - Arthropod bite
    - Erythema nodosum
    - Gnathostomiasis
    - Injection granuloma
    - Vasculitis
    - Wells syndrome
- Eosinophils of doubtful, limited, or no value in histologic diagnosis
  - Drug reaction versus graft-versus-host disease
  - Granuloma annulare
  - Interstitial granulomatous dermatitis
  - Neoplasms
    - Lymphoproliferative disorders (except hypereosinophilic syndrome types)
    - Keratoacanthoma

The absence, presence, or number of eosinophils in skin biopsy specimens is often of limited value in reliably choosing among differential diagnoses with different and potentially important implications for clinical management, such as drug reaction versus acute graft-versus-host disease.[104,105] Eosinophils play a role in certain categories of clinical reactions, particularly those characterized by edema.[43] The degree of tissue eosinophil granule protein deposition in such diseases, that exhibit relatively few or no intact eosinophils, suggests that the pathogenic influence of eosinophils may be unrelated to their numbers in tissues. The degree of cutaneous eosinophil infiltration should be taken in the context of other clinical features, other histologic features, and knowledge that its diagnostic power has limitations.[106] However, eosinophils do have potent biologic activities, particularly imparted by their distinctive granules, and eosinophils may play a pathogenic role in the absence of identifiable cells in tissues.

HYPEREOSINOPHILIC SYNDROMES

AT-A-GLANCE

- Spectrum of entities defined by criteria (Table 40-2).
- Cutaneous lesions are common and may be the presenting sign.
- Two major HES subtypes and several variants.
  - Lymphocytic HES characterized by T-cell clones that produce IL-5.
  - Variant HES subtypes may evolve into lymphocytic HES.
    - Organ-restricted.
    - Associated with specific disorders such as eosinophilic granulomatosis with polyangiitis (formerly known as Churg-Strauss syndrome).
    - Undefined with benign, complex, and episodic presentations.
  - Myeloproliferative HES associated with a deletion on chromosome 4 that produces a tyrosine kinase fusion gene *Fip1-like 1*/PDGFRα or other mutation associated with eosinophil clonality.
    - Responsive to imatinib.
    - Severely debilitating mucosal ulcers portend a grim prognosis unless HES is treated.
    - Overlap with mastocytosis.
    - Familial HES variant, family history of documented persistent eosinophilia of unknown cause.
- Associated embolic events constitute a medical emergency.
- Eosinophilic endomyocardial disease occurs in HES and in patients with prolonged peripheral blood eosinophilia from any cause.

HES consists of a spectrum of disorders that occur worldwide and span all age groups. More than 90% of patients with myeloproliferative HES and the mutant gene are males, but lymphocytic HES shows equal gender distribution. The relative frequencies of these subtypes are unknown, although up to 25% of HES patients may have lymphocytic HES. Rare familial cases have been reported. A miniepidemic of eosinophilic esophagitis, a subtype of overlap HES with organ-restricted disease, emerged over the last decade with prevalence estimates as high as 1:2500 among children and 1:4000 among adults.[107,108]

CLINICAL FEATURES

Patients satisfying HES diagnostic criteria (see Table 40-2) present with signs and symptoms related to the organ systems infiltrated by eosinophils.[109-111] HES often presents with skin lesions that may be the only manifestations of HES.[112-114] Pruritic erythematous macules, papules, plaques, wheals, or nodules are present in more than 50% of patients.[115] CD3– CD4+ lymphocytic HES patients exhibit a particularly high prevalence of skin manifestation, as high as 94%.[116] Lesions may involve the head, trunk, and extremities. Urticaria and angioedema occur in all HES subtypes and are characteristic of certain variant subtypes. Erythema annulare centrifugum,[117] bullous pemphigoid,[118] lymphomatoid papulosis,[119] livedo reticularis, purpura and/or other signs of vasculitis,[120-123] Wells syndrome (eosinophilic cellulitis),[124,125] and multiple other mucocutaneous manifestations[126] may be found in patients with HES (Table 40-3). The complications are mostly hematologic, cardiovascular, pulmonary, and neurologic.[127]

In myeloproliferative HES, the usual presenting complex includes fever, weight loss, fatigue, malaise, skin lesions, and hepatosplenomegaly.[111,128-130] Mucosal ulcers of the oropharynx or anogenital region

TABLE 40-2
Revised Diagnostic Criteria for Hypereosinophilic Syndromes[148]

1. Blood eosinophilia >1500 eosinophils/mm³ on at least 2 separate determinations or evidence of prominent tissue eosinophilia associated with symptoms and marked blood eosinophilia.
2. Exclusion of secondary causes of eosinophilia, such as parasitic or viral infections, allergic diseases, drug-induced or chemical-induced eosinophilia, hypoadrenalism, and neoplasms.

Original Criteria[289]
- Peripheral blood eosinophilia of at least 1500 eosinophils/mm³.
  - Longer than 6 months; or
  - Less than 6 months with evidence of organ damage.
- Signs and symptoms of multiorgan involvement.
- No evidence of parasitic or allergic disease or other known causes of peripheral blood eosinophilia.

TABLE 40-3
Mucocutaneous Manifestations in Hypereosinophilic Syndrome

- Angioedema
- Bullae (bullous pemphigoid)
- Dermographism
- Digital gangrene
- Eczema
- Eosinophilic cellulitis (Wells syndrome)
- Erosions
- Erythema
- Erythema annulare centrifuge
- Erythroderma
- Excoriations
- Livedo reticularis
- Lymphomatoid papulosis
- Macules
- Mucosal ulcers (oral and genital)
- Nail-fold infarctions
- Necrosis
- Nodules
- Papules
- Patches
- Pruritus
- Purpura
- Raynaud phenomenon
- Splinter hemorrhages
- Ulcers
- Urticaria
- Vasculitis

Modified from Leiferman KM, Gleich GJ, Peters MS. Dermatologic manifestations of the hypereosinophilic syndromes. *Immunol Allergy Clin North Am.* 2007;27(3):415-441, and Stetson CL, Leiferman, KM. Eosinophilic dermatoses. In: Bolognia JL, Jorizzo JL, Rapini RP, et al, eds. *Dermatology.* 2nd ed. St. Louis, MO: Mosby; 2008:369-378.

(Fig. 40-3) are also seen. Cardiac disease occurs frequently.[131] Eosinophils adhere to endocardium and release granule proteins onto endothelial cells, thrombus formation follows, and, finally, subendocardial fibrosis with restrictive cardiomyopathy occurs. Mitral or tricuspid valvular insufficiency results from tethering of chordae tendineae.[131] Cardiac abnormalities that are essentially identical to those of HES but are confined to the intramural regions can occur without appreciable peripheral blood eosinophilia.[132,133] Splinter hemorrhages and/or nail-fold infarcts may herald the onset of thromboembolic disease. The central and peripheral nervous system, lungs, and, rarely, kidneys may be affected.[111] Patients with myeloproliferative HES frequently present with clinical features resembling those of chronic myelogenous leukemia and, depending on the classification, are regarded as having chronic eosinophilic leukemia. Although chromosomal abnormalities characterize this subtype and the disease may evolve into definite leukemia, the relatively mature nature of the eosinophils and lack of evidence for clonal expansion may preclude such classification.

Lymphocytic HES commonly is associated with severe pruritus, eczema, erythroderma, urticaria, and angioedema, as well as lymphadenopathy and, rarely, endomyocardial fibrosis.[134]

Eosinophilic granulomatosis with polyangiitis is a variant HES subtype. Other variant HES subtypes include Gleich syndrome,[44] in which eosinophil counts fluctuate with extreme angioedema.

ETIOLOGY AND PATHOGENESIS

Eosinophils are implicated as the cause of most end-organ damage in all HES subtypes.[41,75] Clinical improvement usually parallels a decrease in eosinophil count. Patients with lymphocytic HES have abnormal T-cell clones with unusual surface phenotypes, including CD3+ CD4– CD8– and CD3– CD4+. These T cells display activation markers, such as CD25, and secrete Th2 cytokines, including high levels of IL-5.[134,135] An 800-kilobase deletion on chromosome band 4q12 that codes for a tyrosine kinase has been found in myeloproliferative HES.[136] Patients with this *FIP1L1-PDGFRA* gene mutation form a distinct subset of HES, with cardiomyopathy and endomyocardial fibrosis, that responds to imatinib. Patients in this HES subset have elevated serum tryptase levels and increased atypical spindle-shaped mast cells in

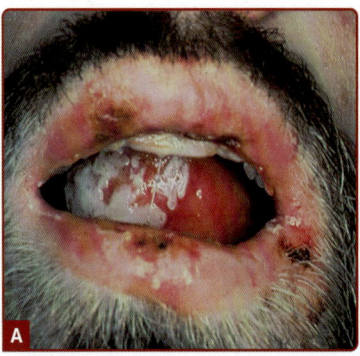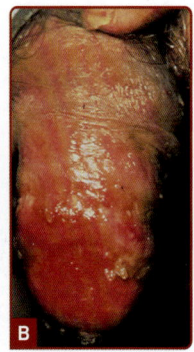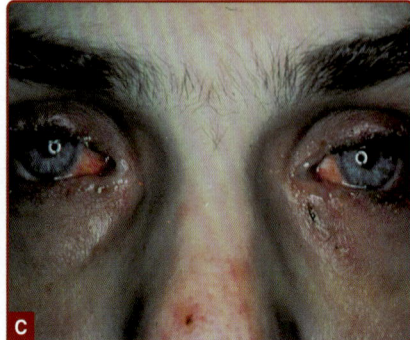

Figure 40-3 Hypereosinophilic syndrome. Mucosal erosions and ulcers of the mouth (**A**) and glans penis (**B**); conjunctival irritation (**C**).

bone marrow.[137-139] Although they do not have clinical manifestations of systemic mastocytosis or exhibit all its immunologic markers, these patients satisfy criteria for mastocytosis.[140] The *FIP1L1-PDGFRA* gene is detected in mast cells,[141] eosinophils, neutrophils, and mononuclear cells. Many HES patients also have marked neutrophilia, likely caused by the aberrant gene in the neutrophil lineage. Thus, alteration of several cell lines probably contributes to the pathogenesis of myeloproliferative HES.[142,143] Myeloproliferative HES with abnormalities of *PDGFRB* and *FGFR1*, other well-characterized variants of myeloproliferative HES, has the potential to progress to aggressive myeloid malignancies.[144] Therefore, it is recommended to assess other translocations in patients with negative *PDGFRA* screening. Multiple other chromosomal abnormalities have been identified in myeloproliferative HES, including translocations, partial and complete chromosomal deletions, and trisomies 8, 15, and 21. Myeloproliferative HES with documented mutations also is known as chronic eosinophilic leukemia. The World Health Organization has an updated 2008 classification scheme for myeloid disorders and eosinophilia.[145,146] The etiology of the other HES variants is not well understood, although patients in several HES subtypes, including with episodic angioedema and eosinophilia (Gleich syndrome)[44] and the NERDS syndrome,[147] have developed T-cell clones.[148]

DIAGNOSIS

A key criterion for diagnosis is marked peripheral blood eosinophilia (see Table 40-2).[109,149-151] Other causes of eosinophilia, including allergic and parasitic diseases, should be excluded. Tests to detect organ involvement, particularly measurement of liver enzyme levels, are important. Because eosinophilic endomyocardial disease can develop in any patient with prolonged peripheral blood eosinophilia, patients should undergo periodic echocardiography along with close observation for signs of thromboembolism. Increased serum levels of IgE are often present in lymphocytic HES, and levels of vitamin B_{12} and tryptase may be increased in myeloproliferative HES. The Chic2 fluorescent in situ hybridization assay detects the deletion that produces the *FIP1L1-PDGFRA* gene product and should be performed, because patients with this mutation respond to treatment with imatinib.[139,141] Alternatively, the mutant gene can be detected by a polymerase chain reaction assay. Both tests are available commercially. In patients who lack the fusion gene, testing for other clonal cytogenetic abnormalities or abnormal clonal T-cell populations is warranted.[137] Cytoflow of peripheral blood lymphocytes and immunophenotyping of tissue lymphocytes should be performed for the diagnosis of lymphocytic HES and repeated periodically to detect transformation from a variant HES type to lymphocytic HES or to T-cell lymphoma.[134] Table 40-4 an HES evaluation assessment scheme for patients with eosinophilia.

The cutaneous histopathologic features of HES vary with the type of lesion. Skin biopsy specimens from urticarial lesions resemble idiopathic urticaria, with generally mild, nonspecific perivascular and interstitial infiltration of lymphocytes, eosinophils, and, occasionally, neutrophils. Immunostaining reveals

TABLE 40-4
Evaluation of Patients with Eosinophilia

- History
- Attention to travel (parasite exposure)
- Ingestants (drugs, health foods, food supplements, and food allergy)
    - Close contacts with itch (ectoparasites)
- Physical examination
    - Cutaneous features (see Table 40-3)
    - Cardiovascular signs
        - Murmur of mitral insufficiency
        - Nails for splinter hemorrhage (medical emergency)
    - Hepatosplenomegaly
    - Lymphadenopathy
- Laboratory studies
    - Repeated complete blood counts with differentials
    - Cytogenetics for chromosomal abnormalities to include
        - *FIP1L1-PDGFRA* (*CHIC2* gene) deletional mutation
        - T-cell subsets for clonality by cytoflow/T-cell receptor gene rearrangement
    - B-cell clonality analyses
    - Inflammatory and immunologic markers
        - Erythrocyte sedimentation rate
        - C-reactive protein
        - Rheumatoid factor
        - Antiproteinase 3 and antimyeloperoxidase (cytoplasmic antineutrophil cytoplasmic antibody and perinuclear antineutrophil cytoplasmic antibody)
        - IgE level
        - Strongyloides IgG antibody
        - IL-5 serum level
    - Metabolic parameters
        - Liver function tests to include aspartate aminotransferase and alanine aminotransferase
        - Renal function tests to include creatinine, blood urea nitrogen and urinalysis for protein and sediment
        - Muscle enzymes to include creatine phosphokinase and aldolase
        - B_{12} serum level
        - Mast cell/basophil tryptase (protryptase) level
        - Coagulation factors
    - Troponin (before initiation of imatinib treatment)
    - Serum protein analyses
        - Serum protein electrophoresis
        - Quantitative immunoglobulins
        - Immunofixation electrophoresis for monoclonal proteins
- Imaging tests
    - Echocardiography
    - Computerized tomography of chest, abdomen, and pelvis
- Gastrointestinal endoscopy, as indicated
- Pulmonary function tests, as indicated
- Bone marrow aspirate and biopsy with staining for tryptase and reticulum (myelofibrosis)
- Tissue biopsy of skin and/or other accessible affected organs
    - Histologic examination
    - Direct immunofluorescence for immunobullous disease
    - Immunostaining for eosinophil granule proteins

Modified from Gleich GJ, Leiferman KM. The hypereosinophilic syndromes: current concepts and treatments. *Br J Haematol*. 2009;145(3):271-85, with permission. Copyright © 2009 Blackwell Publishing Ltd.

extensive deposition of eosinophil granule proteins, in the absence of intact eosinophils, in episodic angioedema with eosinophilia,[44] HES with mucosal ulcers,[45] and in synovial tissues in NERDS.[147] Other than in eosinophilic granulomatosis with polyangiitis, vasculitis only rarely is associated with HES.[120-122]

DIFFERENTIAL DIAGNOSIS

Table 40-5 outlines the differential diagnosis of HES.

Clinically, parasitic infections and infestations may closely resemble HES.[152] A history of travel to endemic areas or certain dietary exposure implicates helminthiasis. Along with eosinophilia, total serum IgE levels higher than 500 IU/mL commonly are found in helminthic infections. Examination of stool samples for ova and parasites and serologic testing for *Strongyloides* antibodies should be performed. In patients with isolated urticarial plaques with or without angioedema, the differential diagnosis includes common and persistent urticaria,[153,154] but demonstration of multiorgan involvement supports HES. HES with episodic angioedema may resemble hereditary angioedema clinically, although patients with hereditary angioedema often have a family history of the disease rarely have the markedly elevated eosinophil counts that characterize HES, and may be distinguished by complement abnormalities. Pruritic eczematous lesions of lymphocytic HES may resemble those of atopic dermatitis, contact dermatitis, drug reaction, fungal infection, and T-cell lymphoma. There are multiple diseases in the differential diagnosis of patients with orogenital ulcers,[129] including those associated with thrombosis, such as Behçet syndrome, Crohn disease, ulcerative colitis, and Reiter syndrome. Others considerations are recurrent aphthous stomatitis, immunobullous diseases, erythema multiforme, lichen planus, herpes simplex infection, and syphilis.

CLINICAL COURSE, PROGNOSIS, AND MANAGEMENT

Myeloproliferative HES with mucosal lesions portend an aggressive clinical course; death is likely within 2 years of presentation if the disorder is untreated.[129,155] In contrast to myeloproliferative HES, lymphocytic HES generally follows a benign course, and T-cell clones can remain stable for years. Patients should be observed closely and regarded as having premalignant or malignant T-cell proliferation, because the disease may evolve into lymphoma, especially in CD3– CD4+ T-cell populations.[156]

During the decade or more after diagnosis, HES may evolve into acute leukemia and, less commonly, is associated with B-cell lymphomas. The overall 5-year survival rate for HES patients is 80%; congestive heart failure from the restrictive cardiomyopathy of eosinophilic endomyocardial disease is a major cause of death, followed by sepsis.

The goal of treatment is to relieve symptoms and improve organ function while keeping peripheral blood eosinophils at 1000 to 2000/mm^3 and minimizing treatment side effects (Fig. 40-4). Recent reviews have delineated evaluation and management of HES.[29,70-72,77,82,128,149-151] Corticosteroids are one of the most commonly used and most effective therapeutic agents in the treatment of HES.[116] They are considered the first-line therapy in patients without the gene mutation, once *Strongyloides* infection has been excluded.[157] Approximately 70% of patients will respond, with peripheral eosinophil counts returning to normal. Patients with elevated thymus and activation-regulated chemokine (TARC) and with lymphocytic HES have particularly favorable responses to steroid therapy.[89,110,158] Patients for whom glucocorticoid monotherapy fails have a worse prognosis generally; in such cases, or when long-term side effects become problematic, other treatments should be used. Myeloproliferative HES is responsive to imatinib.[159] In patients with the mutant gene *FIP1L1-PDGFRA*, administration of imatinib mesylate is indicated and usually induces hematologic remission, but endomyocardial disease may worsen during the first several days of treatment. Troponin levels should be monitored before and during imatinib therapy.[160,161] To improve cardiac function, glucocorticoids should be given before and with initiation of imatinib therapy. Imatinib resistance can develop.[162-164] Effective treatment of HES in imatinib-responsive patients results in improvement of associated conditions, including cardiac involvement with endocarditis[165] and myelofibrosis,[166] and skin disease with bullous pemphigoid.[118] Patients who have features of myeloproliferative HES but who lack *FIP1L1-PDGFRA* still may respond to imatinib.[83] IFN-α has been beneficial in treating myeloid and lymphocytic HES.[90,91] In one patient, loss of the *FIP1L1-PDGFRA* mutation after several years of IFN-α therapy was

TABLE 40-5
Differential Diagnosis of Hypereosinophilic Syndrome

- Parasitic infection
- Ectoparasitic infestation
- Urticaria
- Hereditary angioedema
- Atopic dermatitis
- Contact dermatitis
- Drug reaction
- Fungal infection
- Mycosis fungoides
- Sézary syndrome
- Behçet syndrome
- Crohn disease
- Ulcerative colitis
- Reiter syndrome
- Recurrent aphthous stomatitis
- Erythema multiforme
- Lichen planus
- Immunobullous disease
- Herpes simplex infection
- Syphilis

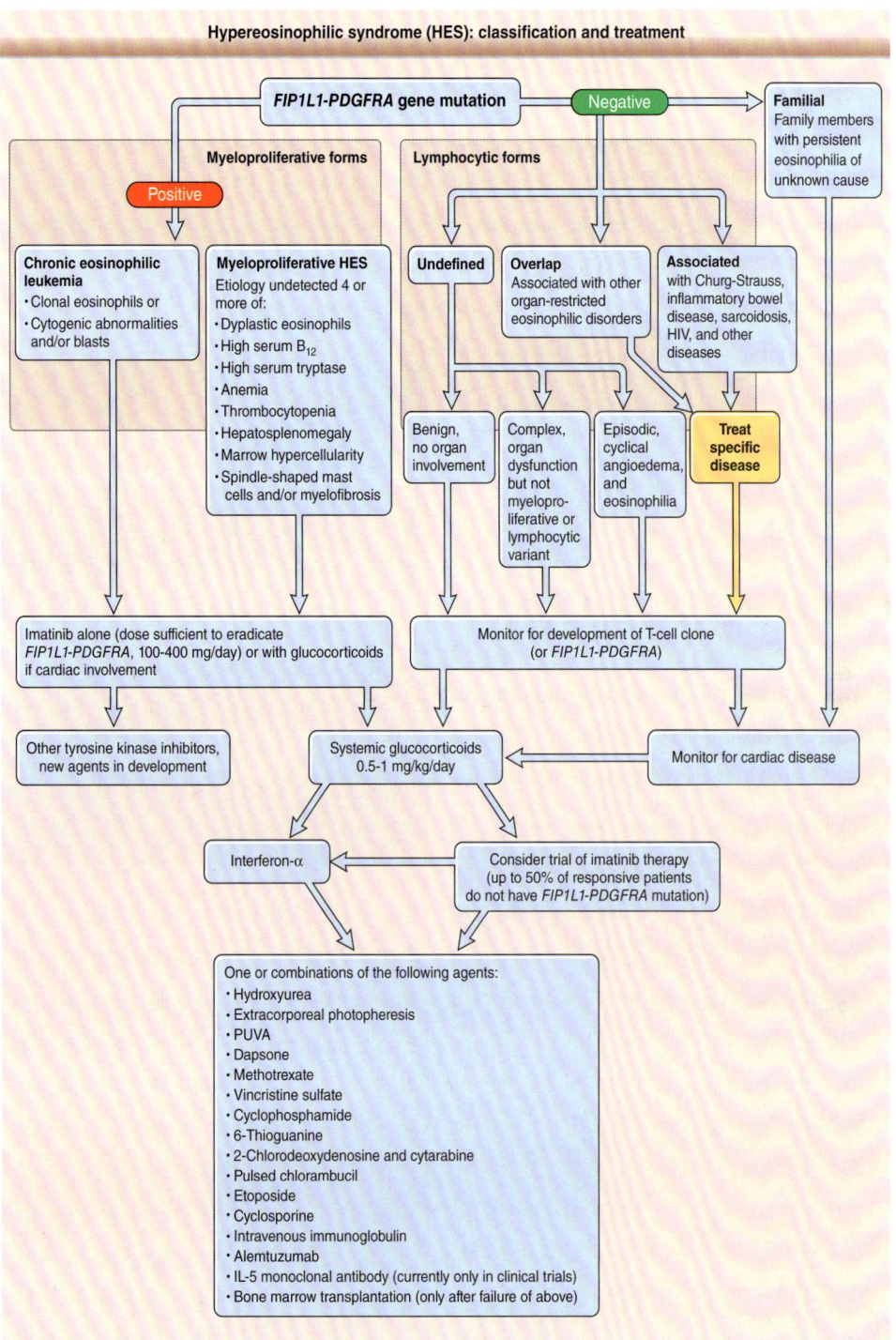

Figure 40-4 Hypereosinophilic syndrome (HES): classification and treatment. Provisional classification consists of myeloproliferative, lymphocytic and familial forms of HES. Chronic eosinophilic leukemia with clonal eosinophilia and myeloproliferative HES with features of the disease but without proof of clonality are included in the myeloproliferative forms of HES; HES with eosinophil hematopoietin-producing T cells with or without a documented T-cell clone constitute the lymphocytic forms of HES. Further HES classification refinement is expected in the near future from a multidisciplinary consensus compendium that is in preparation. *FIP1L1-PDGFRA*, Fip1-like 1 gene/platelet-derived growth factor receptor-α gene; IL-5, interleukin 5; PUVA, psoralen plus ultraviolet A phototherapy. (Information from Roufosse F, Weller PF. Practical approach to the patient with hypereosinophilia. *J Allergy Clin Immunol.* 2010;126(1):39-44; Klion AD. Approach to the therapy of hypereosinophilic syndromes. *Immunol Allergy Clin North Am.* 2007;27(3):551-556; and Stetson CL, Leiferman KM. Eosinophilic dermatoses. In: Bolognia JL, Jorizzo JL, Rapini RP, et al. *Dermatology*. 2nd ed. St. Louis, MO: Mosby; 2008:369-378.)

associated with complete remission.[167] Extracorporeal photopheresis alone or in combination with IFN-α or other therapies represent additional therapeutic options. Other treatments for HES with reported benefit include hydroxyurea, dapsone, vincristine sulfate, cyclophosphamide, methotrexate, 6-thioguanine, 2-chlorodeoxyadenosine and cytarabine combination therapy, pulsed chlorambucil, etoposide, cyclosporine, intravenous Ig, and psoralen plus ultraviolet A phototherapy.[168] Refractory disease may respond to infliximab (anti–TNF-α)[169] or alemtuzumab (anti-CD52),[84-86] as well as to bone marrow and peripheral blood stem cell allogeneic transplantation.[170,171] Two monoclonal antibodies against human IL-5 (mepolizumab and reslizumab) are associated with clinical improvement and reductions in peripheral blood and dermal eosinophils, particularly in patients with lymphocytic HES.[172-176] Treatments targeting IL-5 have provided new insights into understanding eosinophil-associated disease.[75]

WELLS SYNDROME

AT-A-GLANCE

- Single or multiple lesions commonly located on the extremities or trunk.
- Lesions may be painful or pruritic.
- Associated with general malaise but uncommonly with fever.
- Edematous and erythematous lesions evolve into plaques with violaceous borders.
- Blisters may be a prominent feature.
- Multiple recurrences.
- Peripheral blood eosinophilia common.
- Histologic pattern characterized by dermal infiltration with eosinophils, and flame figures surrounded by histiocytes.
- Systemic glucocorticoids usually therapeutic.

CLINICAL FEATURES

Cutaneous edema was the common clinical thread in the first 4 cases reported by Wells.[177] After prodromal burning or itching, lesions begin with erythema and edema (Fig. 40-5A), sometimes in the form of annular or arcuate plaques or nodules (Fig. 40-5B). Over a period of days, they evolve into large edematous plaques with violaceous borders. Bullae may develop.[178-181] Individual lesions gradually change from bright red to brown-red and then to blue-gray or greenish-gray, resembling morphea (Fig. 40-5C). Less-common clinical presentations include papules, vesicles (Fig. 40-6), and hemorrhagic bullae. The cutaneous lesions may be single or multiple and may be located at any site, but typically involve the extremities and, less often, the trunk.[182] The most frequent systemic complaint in patients with Wells syndrome is malaise; fever occurs in a minority of cases. Some patients have

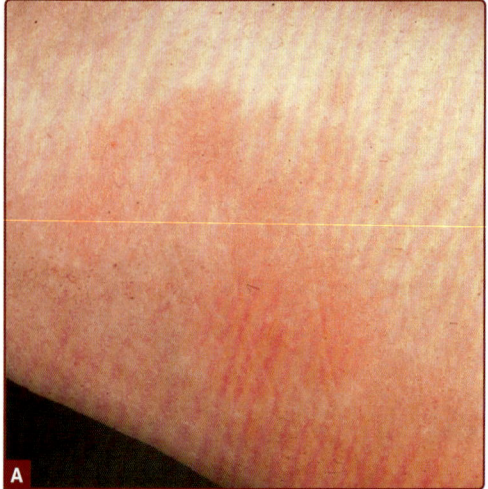
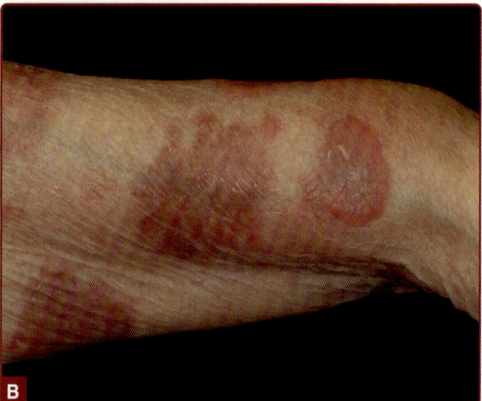
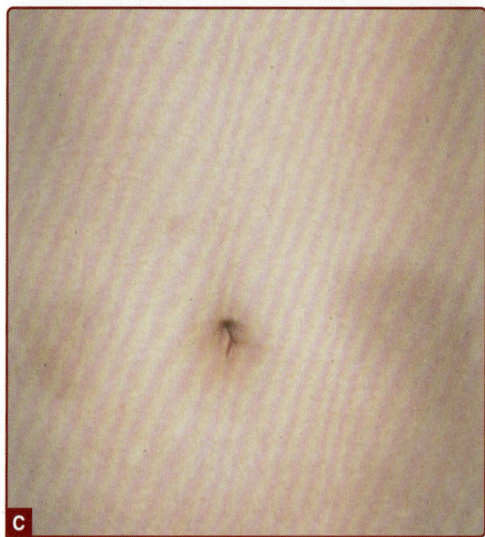

Figure 40-5 Wells syndrome. **A,** Early lesion with erythema and edema. **B,** An arcuate plaques and pigmentation. **C,** Late lesion resembling morphea.

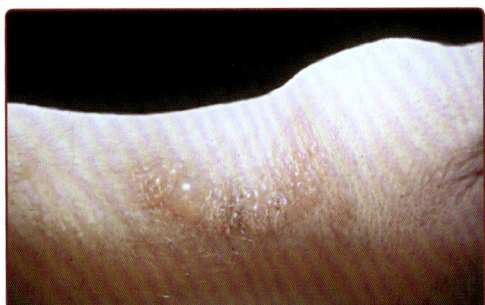

Figure 40-6 Familial Wells syndrome. Plaques with erythema, edema, vesicles, and bullae resembling acute dermatitis or pemphigoid. (From Davis MD, Brown AC, Blackston RD, et al. Familial eosinophilic cellulitis, dysmorphic habitus, and mental retardation. *J Am Acad Dermatol.* 1998;38(6, pt 1):919-928, with permission. Copyright © American Academy of Dermatology.)

TABLE 40-6
Conditions Associated with Wells Syndrome and/or Flame Figures

- Arthropod bite
- Ascariasis
- Bronchogenic carcinoma
- Eosinophilic granulomatosis with polyangiitis
- Colonic adenocarcinoma
- Dental abscess
- Dermographism
- Drug reaction
- Eczema
- Eosinophilic fasciitis
- Eosinophilic pustular folliculitis
- Herpes gestationis
- Herpes simplex infection
- HIV
- Hymenoptera sting
- Hypereosinophilic syndrome
- Immunobullous diseases
- Mastocytoma
- Molluscum contagiosum
- Myeloproliferative diseases
- Onchocerciasis
- Vaccinations
- Tinea
- Toxocariasis
- Urticaria
- Ulcerative colitis
- Varicella

an associated underlying disorder such as hematologic or nonhematologic malignancies.

ETIOLOGY AND PATHOGENESIS

The etiology and pathogenesis of Wells syndrome is unclear. A nonspecific hypersensitivity reaction in response to exogenous and/or endogenous stimuli is regarded as the important pathomechanism.[183] Some cases appear to be idiopathic, while many others suggest a triggering event, such as insect bites, viral or bacterial infections, and drugs and vaccines. The association with an underlying disorder, such as a malignancy, also has been reported.

DIAGNOSIS

Peripheral blood eosinophilia is observed in approximately 50% of patients. Skin lesions histologically are characterized by diffuse dermal infiltration with eosinophils, histiocytes, and foci of amorphous and/or granular material associated with connective tissue fibers, which Wells termed *flame figures*.[177] In the early stages, there also is dermal edema. Later, histiocytes palisade around flame figures. Vasculitis is usually absent.[184] In addition to 8 patients with the syndrome, the 1979 report of Wells and Smith includes 9 patients with the typical histologic features of eosinophilic cellulitis but in association with a variety of clinical diagnoses, including pemphigoid, eczema, and tinea.[185] This and subsequent reports of flame figures in lesions from patients with a wide spectrum of diseases (Table 40-6) indicate that the flame figure is characteristic for, but not diagnostic of, Wells syndrome.[186] When examined for eosinophil granule MBP by immunofluorescence, flame figures show bright extracellular staining (Fig. 40-7), indicating that extensive eosinophil degranulation has occurred.[187]

DIFFERENTIAL DIAGNOSIS

Table 40-7 outlines the differential diagnosis of Wells syndrome.

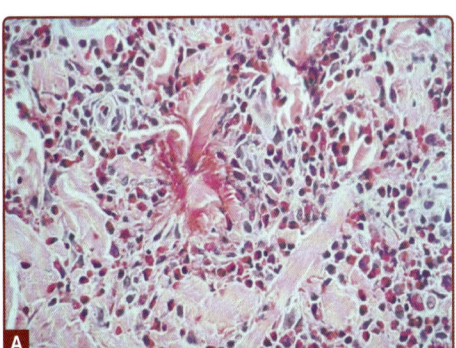

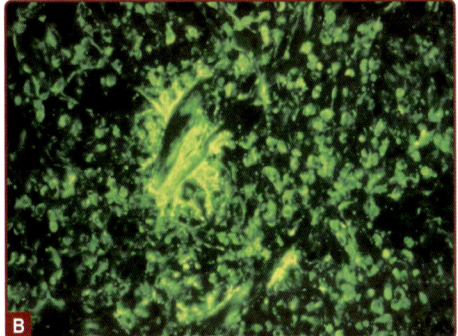

Figure 40-7 Flame figure in familial Wells syndrome. **A,** Hematoxylin and eosin–stained section. **B,** Eosinophil granule major basic protein immunostain (of serial section to **A**) shows extensive granule protein deposition localized to the flame figure. (Original magnification ×400.)

TABLE 40-7
Differential Diagnosis of Wells Syndrome
• Urticaria
• Erysipelas
• Acute cellulitis
• Pemphigoid
• Morphea

Urticaria, erysipelas, and acute cellulitis should be considered in the differential diagnosis of the early stages of Wells syndrome (see Fig. 40-5A). Later, plaques may resemble morphea (see Fig. 40-5C). The presence of blisters may suggest pemphigoid (see Fig. 40-6). Flame figures are the hallmark of Wells syndrome, but, because they have been identified in biopsy specimens from other dermatoses (see Table 40-6), they are not alone sufficient for the diagnosis. However, a diagnosis of Wells syndrome in the absence of flame figures should be met with skepticism, even in the presence of dermal infiltration with eosinophils and histiocytes.[186]

CLINICAL COURSE, PROGNOSIS, AND MANAGEMENT

Wells syndrome resolves without scarring, usually within weeks to months, but multiple recurrences are common. Lesions usually improve dramatically after administration of systemic glucocorticoids, and tapering of steroid dose over 1 month is well tolerated in most patients. Recurrences or persistent cases can be effectively maintained with low-dose (5 mg) alternate-day prednisone.[188] For patients who fail to respond, or who experience relapse often enough to raise concerns about the long-term side effects of systemic glucocorticoid therapy, other options, such as minocycline, dapsone, griseofulvin, and antihistamines, may be beneficial. Cyclosporine and IFN-α also have been used with success. For treatment of mild disease, topical glucocorticoids may be sufficient. It also can be beneficial to treat the underlying condition or triggering factor.[189-191]

ANGIOLYMPHOID HYPERPLASIA WITH EOSINOPHILIA (EPITHELIOID HEMANGIOMA)

AT-A-GLANCE

- Kimura disease (KD) occurs mainly in Asian males; angiolymphoid hyperplasia with eosinophilia (ALHE) occurs in all races, with a female predominance.
- KD is found in a younger age group than ALHE.

- Both ALHE and KD are characterized by recurrent dermal and/or subcutaneous lesions, primarily of the head and neck area.
    - ALHE lesions tend to be smaller, more superficial, and more numerous than those of KD.
    - KD tends to involve subcutaneous tissues, regional lymph nodes, and salivary glands.
- ALHE may be painful, pruritic, or pulsatile, whereas KD is generally asymptomatic.
- Peripheral blood eosinophilia present in both diseases.
- Increased IgE levels are found only in KD.
- Renal disease is associated only with KD (reported incidence of 10% to 20%).
- Histopathologic features:
    - Dominant feature of KD is lymphoid proliferation, often with germinal centers, whereas ALHE is characterized by vascular proliferation with numerous large epithelioid or histiocytoid endothelial cells.
    - Fibrosis is characteristic of KD and is limited or absent in ALHE.
    - Inconspicuous to numerous eosinophils in ALHE.
    - Eosinophil abscesses may occur in KD.

Angiolymphoid hyperplasia with eosinophilia (ALHE) occurs in both males and females, but there is a slight female predominance. Patients are generally in the third to fifth decade of life. In contrast to Kimura disease (KD), which develops mainly in Asian males at puberty, ALHE has no racial predilection.

CLINICAL FEATURES

ALHE shows a predilection for the head and neck area, including the ears,[192] and is characterized by solitary, few, or multiple, sometimes grouped, erythematous, violaceous, or brown papules, plaques, or nodules of the dermis and/or subcutaneous tissues (Fig. 40-8). Lesions may be associated with pruritus or pain, or may pulsate. Although they are confined to the skin in most patients, mucosal involvement may occur.[193]

ETIOLOGY AND PATHOGENESIS

The pathogenesis of ALHE is unknown, but it has been considered a vascular proliferation arising in response to or in association with underlying vascular malformation. There is a history of trauma in some cases. ALHE has been reported to occur in pregnancy, which implies that sex hormones may be a factor in its development.[194] ALHE also has developed in patients with T-cell clonality, which suggests that it may be an early or low-grade T-cell lymphoma and further highlights a relationship between T cells and eosinophils, particularly T cells with the Th2 phenotype.[195,196]

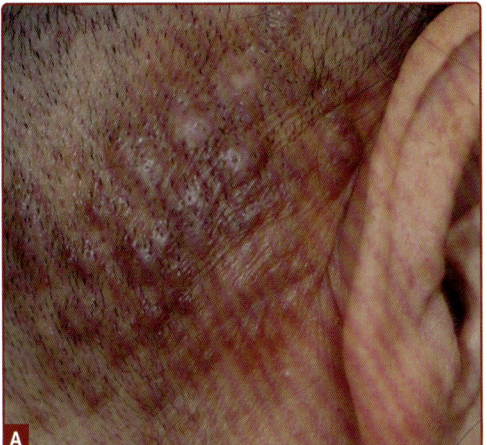

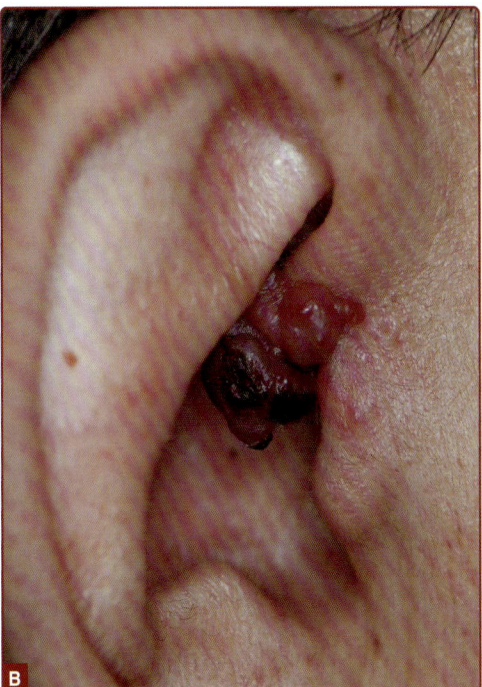

Figure 40-8 Angiolymphoid hyperplasia with eosinophilia. **A,** Multiple grouped brown nodules. **B,** Reddish papules.

TABLE 40-8
Differential Diagnosis of Angiolymphoid Hyperplasia with Eosinophilia

- Kimura disease
- Pyogenic granuloma
- Epithelioid hemangioendothelioma
- Epithelioid angiosarcoma
- Kaposi sarcoma

proliferation," which provided evidence that these lesions may represent a form of arteriovenous shunt.[198] The stroma typically is myxoid, and fibrosis is minimal or absent. Mast cells may be a component of the histologic picture.

DIFFERENTIAL DIAGNOSIS

Table 40-8 outlines the differential diagnosis of ALHE.

KD also develops preferentially on the head and neck area, especially around the ears. It is characterized by solitary or multiple brownish plaques or intracutaneous and/or subcutaneous masses (Fig. 40-9). The lesions are generally asymptomatic, but they can be pruritic. Atopic disease may be associated. Lesions of ALHE generally are smaller, more superficial, and more numerous than those of KD, and often are symptomatic. Patients with KD also show peripheral blood eosinophilia and increased IgE levels. The dominant histologic feature is lymphoid proliferation, often with germinal centers with prominent infiltration of eosinophils. Fibrosis is characteristic, and eosinophil abscesses may occur. Although lymphoid follicles may occur in ALHE, they represent the dominant characteristic of KD (Table 40-9), and although KD may exhibit some vascularity, it lacks the large epithelioid endothelial cells that are a key feature of ALHE (Table 40-9). ALHE should be distinguished from a variety of benign and malignant vascular proliferations, including pyogenic granuloma, epithelioid hemangioendothelioma, and

DIAGNOSIS

Approximately 20% of patients have peripheral blood eosinophilia; IgE levels are unremarkable. There is no association with renal disease. The dominant histologic feature is a well-defined area, in the dermis and/or subcutis, of prominent vascular proliferation with large epithelioid or histiocytoid endothelial cells that contain abundant eosinophilic cytoplasm, often with cytoplasmic vacuoles. There are variable numbers of eosinophils and lymphocytes,[197] with an occasional finding of lymphoid nodules. In their report of 116 patients with ALHE, Olsen and Helwig found 53 cases in which "an arterial structure" appeared to be associated with venules or "was the area of endothelial

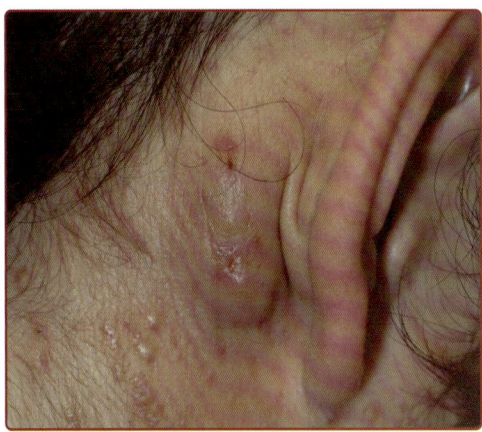

Figure 40-9 Kimura disease. Solitary brownish nodules and multiple papules.

TABLE 40-9
Comparison of Angiolymphoid Hyperplasia with Eosinophilia and Kimura Disease

	ALHE	KD
Gender	Typically middle-aged females	Predominantly young-adult Asian males
Symptoms	Pruritus, pain, pulsation	Asymptomatic
Lesion type and location	Small and superficial, with overlying erythema; head and neck region	Large, mainly subcutaneous; overlying skin normal; head and neck region; may involve regional lymph nodes and salivary glands
Lymphoid follicles	Uncommon	Prominent lymphoid follicles with germinal centers
Vascular proliferation	Prominent vascular proliferation with large epithelioid/histiocytoid endothelial cells; evidence of underlying vascular malformation may be evident	Some stromal vascularity with unremarkable endothelial cells
Fibrosis	Absent or limited	Prominent
Serum immunoglobulin E level	Normal	Increased
Nephropathy	Absent	Present in up to 20% of patients

Kaposi sarcoma—all of which lack a noticeable eosinophil infiltrate. Although it is nonspecific, the dermoscopic finding of ALHE with polymorphous vascular pattern may be helpful in differential diagnosis from other vascular tumors.[199]

CLINICAL COURSE, PROGNOSIS AND MANAGEMENT

ALHE tends to be chronic and nonremitting over months to years. Intervention is dictated in part by the number, location, size of lesions, and the patient's general health.[200] Patients with solitary or a few small lesions may benefit from excision or Mohs surgery,[201] but there may be recurrence at the surgical site (Fig. 40-10). A variety of other treatment modalities have been used with success, including systemic and intralesional glucocorticoid administration, IFN-α therapy,[202] cryotherapy,[203] laser therapy,[204] and topical application of tacrolimus.[205]

KIMURA DISEASE

Table 40-10 outlines the differential diagnosis of KD.

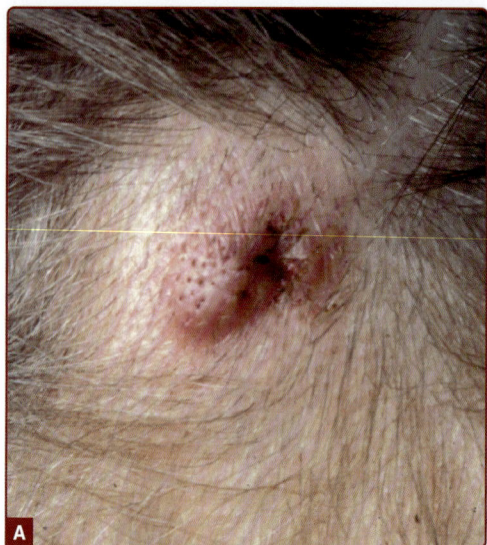
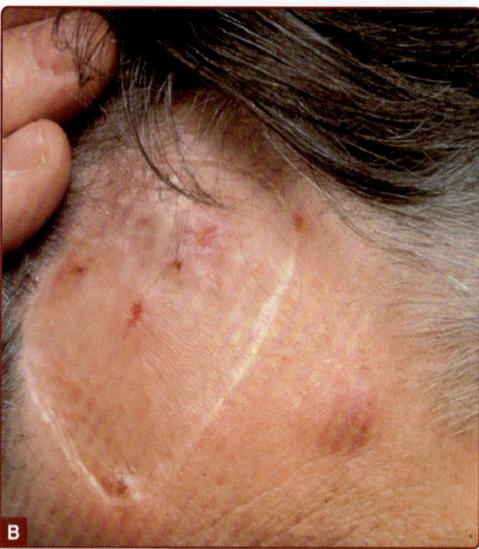

Figure 40-10 Angiolymphoid hyperplasia with eosinophilia. **A,** Forehead nodule. **B,** Recurrence of lesions in skin graft and adjacent sites 6 years after surgical removal of lesion in **A**.

MANAGEMENT

Surgical excision is the treatment of choice when feasible in patients with a single or a limited number of nodules, but lesions may recur.[206,207] Other therapeutic options include systemic glucocorticoids, cyclosporine, and radiation therapy.[208,209] The presence of renal disease may influence or dictate the therapeutic regimen.

TABLE 40-10
Differential Diagnosis of Kimura Disease

- Angiolymphoid hyperplasia with eosinophilia
- Lymphoma

The finding of PDGF-α and c-kit in tissues from KD patients suggests that imatinib or another tyrosine kinase inhibitor may be effective in the disease.[210]

EOSINOPHILIC PUSTULAR FOLLICULITIS

AT-A-GLANCE

- Three clinical types that are characterized by follicular papules and pustules, and may involve the head, trunk, and extremities.
- Classic eosinophilic pustular folliculitis (Ofuji disease).
  - Typically occurs in Japanese patients, who have chronic, recurrent follicular pustules, with a tendency to form circinate plaques, in a seborrheic distribution.
- Eosinophilic pustular folliculitis associated with immunosuppression.
  - Most often occurs in patients with human immunodeficiency virus infection, who have severely pruritic papules of the face and upper trunk.
- Eosinophilic pustular folliculitis of infancy/neonatal period.
  - Follicular pustules of the scalp.
- Tendency for recurrences and chronicity (except eosinophilic pustular folliculitis of infancy).
- Characterized by follicular and perifollicular eosinophil infiltration.
- Associated with peripheral blood eosinophilia.

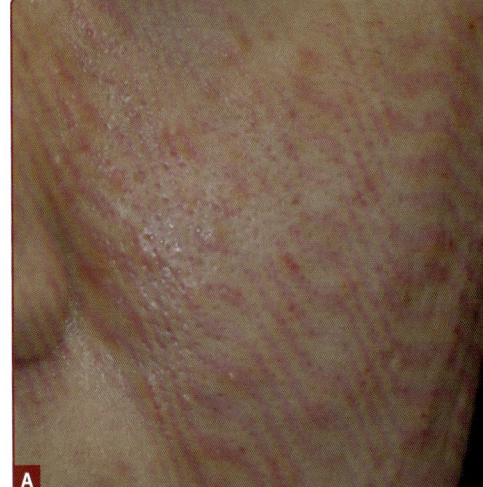

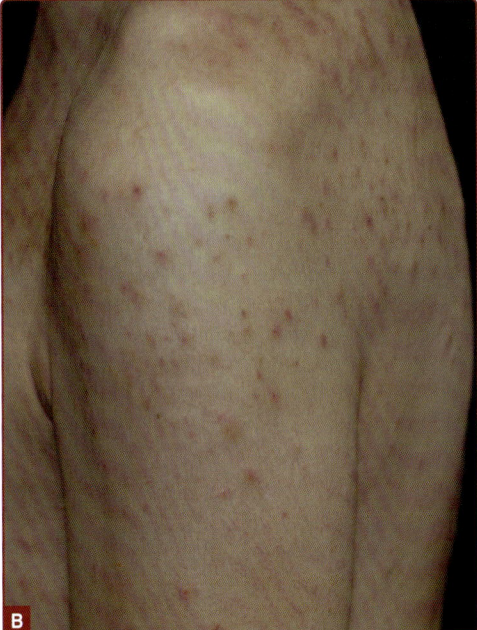

Figure 40-11 Eosinophilic pustular folliculitis. **A,** Itchy reddish papules and pustules on the cheek. **B,** An HIV-associated case with itchy red papules on the upper arm, shoulder, and back.

CLINICAL FEATURES

At present, eosinophilic pustular folliculitis (EPF) is divided into 3 variants: classical EPF, immunosuppression-associated EPF, and infantile EPF.[211] Immunosuppression-associated EPF may be subdivided into an HIV-associated type and a malignancy-associated type.[212-214] Classical EPF presents as recurrent crops or clusters of follicular papules and pustules, which may form an annular pattern and usually resolve in 7 to 10 days (Fig. 40-11A). Lesions predominantly involve the face and trunk but also may affect the extremities, with involvement of the palms and soles in approximately 20% of patients.[215] In infantile type of EPF, lesions typically are located on the scalp, but also may be found on the face and extremities. In some neonates who have pustular eruptions that clinically resemble EPF and typically have peripheral blood eosinophilia, the disorder may be classified more appropriately under the term *eosinophilic pustulosis* because the cutaneous infiltrates are not folliculocentric.[216] In contrast, HIV-associated EPF tends to manifest as extremely pruritic discrete follicular papules, typically involving the head and neck and often the proximal extremities (Fig. 40-11B). Rosenthal et al emphasized the urticarial quality of such lesions.[217]

ETIOLOGY AND PATHOGENESIS

The etiology of EPF remains unknown. The occasional association with HIV infection suggests the possible contribution of immunocompromised status to the development of EPF. Interestingly, some cases of HIV-associated EPF develop lesions after starting highly active anti-retroviral therapy (HAART), indicating that

EPF may occur as a result of immune reconstitution rather than immunodeficiency in these HAART-treated cases.[218-220] Drugs,[221,222] parasitic or viral infections,[223,224] and pregnancy[225,226] are also reported as possible factors related to EPF. The higher expression of ICAM-1 and leukocyte function-associated antigen-1 on the follicular epithelium, and VCAM-1 around hair follicles in EPF lesions, suggest that these molecules are relevant to the selective migration of eosinophils and lymphocytes to the hair follicles in EPF.[227] One study demonstrated that an interaction between PGD_2 and a chemoattractant receptor-homologous molecule expressed on T-helper type 2 (CRTH2) cells may be involved in the pathogenesis of classical EPF and that indomethacin may exert its therapeutic effect by reducing CRTH2 expression, as well as by inhibiting PGD_2 synthesis.[228]

DIAGNOSIS

Patients suspected of having EPF should be evaluated for underlying immune deficiency, particularly HIV infection. Peripheral blood eosinophilia is a component of all 3 types of EPF. TARC is reported to be elevated in serum and to correlate with peripheral blood eosinophilia.[229] Although patients with classical EPF usually have eosinophilia with leukocytosis, HIV-positive patients often exhibit eosinophilia with lymphopenia. Low CD4+ T-cell counts and high IgE levels are typical of HIV-associated EPF.[217] Elevated serum IgE is uncommon in infantile EPF.[230] Histologically, the most striking feature is the infiltration of eosinophils into hair follicles and perifollicular areas, sometimes with follicular damage. The infiltrates also may contain lymphocytes and neutrophils, and may be perivascular as well as follicular.[231] Flame figures can also be observed in infantile EPF.[230] Follicular mucinosis has been noted in association with EPF[232]; however, T-cell clonality is not observed in EPF-associated follicular mucinosis.[233]

DIFFERENTIAL DIAGNOSIS

Table 40-11 outlines the differential diagnosis of EPF.
Folliculitis secondary to bacterial or fungal infection must be kept in mind, particularly in immunosuppressed patients. Based on the distribution of lesions, seborrheic dermatitis should be considered, when there is head and neck involvement, and palmar–plantar pustular psoriasis may also be included in the differential diagnosis when there is hand and foot involvement. Acneiform eruption, rosacea, and lupus miliaris disseminatus faciei may resemble EPF. Erythema toxicum neonatorum, acropustulosis, and acne neonatorum also should be considered in infants. Follicular mucinosis usually is clinically and histologically distinguishable from EPF. One of the most important differential diagnoses is cutaneous T-cell lymphoma, which can resemble EPF both clinically and histopathologically.[212]

CLINICAL COURSE, PROGNOSIS, AND MANAGEMENT

The infantile type of EPF has a good prognosis, whereas classical and HIV-associated EPF are characterized by recurrences. Postinflammatory pigmentation may be seen as lesions resolve, but scarring does not occur.

Topical glucocorticoids and topical calcineurin inhibitors generally are the first approach to the treatment of all types of EPF. Topical tacrolimus is helpful for facial lesions.[234] Nonsteroidal antiinflammatory drugs, particularly indomethacin, also are recommended as first-line therapy; clinical improvement may be observed within 2 weeks and is associated with a decrease in peripheral blood eosinophil counts.[235-237] Ultraviolet light therapy (ultraviolet B or psoralen and ultraviolet A) may be beneficial. Topical permethrin, systemic retinoids, systemic glucocorticoids, cyclosporine, itraconazole, metronidazole, cetirizine, minocycline, dapsone, and IFNs have been tried with success.[235,236] Antiretroviral treatment that results in increased CD4 cell counts often is associated with improvement in HIV-associated EPF. The first-line treatment of infantile EPF is observation or topical steroid therapy. Infantile EPF tends to resolve spontaneously within several years and usually shows good response to topical steroids.[230]

TABLE 40-11
Differential Diagnosis of Eosinophilic Pustular Folliculitis

- Folliculitis, bacterial or fungal
- Seborrheic dermatitis
- Palmar–plantar pustular psoriasis
- Acne, including acne neonatorum
- Erythema toxicum neonatorum
- Acropustulosis
- Follicular mucinosis

PAPULOERYTHRODERMA OF OFUJI

AT-A-GLANCE

- Papuloerythroderma tends to occur in elderly males.
- The lesions are usually pruritic.
- Erythroderma-like eruptions formed by confluent flat-topped, red-to-brown papules are characteristic.
- The unique sparing of the abdominal skin folds is termed *deck-chair sign*.

(Continued)

AT-A-GLANCE (Continued)

- Approximately 20% of cases are associated with hematologic or visceral malignancies.
- Papuloerythroderma may progress to cutaneous T-cell lymphoma.
- The majority of cases are associated with peripheral blood eosinophilia.
- Ultraviolet treatment and corticosteroids are usually effective; however, the disorder is sometimes refractory to treatment.

CLINICAL FEATURES

Papuloerythroderma of Ofuji was described as a distinctive pattern of erythroderma by Ofuji in 1984.[238] Many cases occur in elderly males, especially in the eighth or ninth decades. Itchy erythroderma-like eruptions formed by the coalescence of flat-topped, red-to-brown papules with a cobblestone appearance is characteristic (Fig. 40-12).[239] It affects the limbs and trunk; the face and flexures are usually spared. The characteristic sparing of the abdominal skin folds is called *deck-chair sign*. Mucous membranes, hair, and nails are always spared. Palmoplantar keratoderma and dermatopathic lymphadenopathy are reported in approximately 20% of patients.[239] Approximately 20% of cases with papuloerythroderma are associated with hematologic neoplasms such as non-Hodgkin lymphoma and leukemia or visceral malignancies including gastric, colon, and prostate carcinomas.[240-243]

ETIOLOGY AND PATHOGENESIS

The pathogenesis of papuloerythroderma is unknown. It remains controversial whether it is an independent clinical entity or a unique manifestation of an underlying disorder. Malignancy, atopic diathesis, infections and drug intake are reported to be possible causes of papuloerythroderma. Several findings (eosinophil infiltration of the lesional skin and occasional association of atopic diathesis) suggest a role for T lymphocytes polarized toward the Th2 phenotype in the pathogenesis of papuloerythroderma, although the target antigens of those T lymphocytes are unclear. It is reported that the percentages of circulating CCR4+ CD4+ Th2 cells are higher than those of CXCR3+ CD4+ Th1 cells in patients with drug-induced papuloerythroderma.[244] A recent study demonstrated that the percentages of IL-4–producing, IL-13–producin, and IL-22–producing CD4+ and CD8+ T cells were significantly higher in the circulations of patients with papuloerythroderma than in the circulations of healthy controls. In addition, the expression of both cutaneous lymphocyte antigen and CCR4 was markedly upregulated in those cells. These findings suggest that skin-homing Th2/Th22 cells may contribute to the pathogenesis of papuloerythroderma.[245]

DIAGNOSIS

Characteristic flat-topped, red-to-brown confluent papules and the deck-chair sign are highly diagnostic, although the deck-chair sign is observed in other erythrodermas, such as psoriasis and atopic dermatitis.[243,246] Peripheral eosinophilia is detected in more than 80% of patients.[239] Lymphocytopenia and increased serum IgE are sometimes observed. Histopathology shows nonspecific spongiotic dermatitis-like patterns, that is, acanthosis, spongiosis, and infiltration of lymphocytes, histiocytes, and variable amounts of eosinophils distributed in the mid-upper dermis and around microvessels, which resemble chronic dermatitis.[239]

DIFFERENTIAL DIAGNOSIS

Typical papuloerythroderma can be distinguished from other erythrodermas by its characteristic clinical appearance. Some cases show histologic findings of cutaneous T-cell lymphoma such as mycosis fungoides.[247,248] It was also reported that papuloerythroderma progressed to cutaneous T-cell lymphoma.[246] As it can be associated with atopic diathesis, malignancies, infections, and drugs,[239] underlying complications must be examined.

CLINICAL COURSE, PROGNOSIS, AND MANAGEMENT

Papuloerythroderma tends to be chronic over years and non–self-limiting. Oral prednisolone is effective in the majority of cases. Ultraviolet treatment alone or in combination with oral and topical corticosteroids is reported to be very efficient.[242] Etretinate,[249] cyclosporine,[250] and IFN[251] are also reported as effective for papuloerythroderma. However, papuloerythroderma is frequently refractory to treatment.

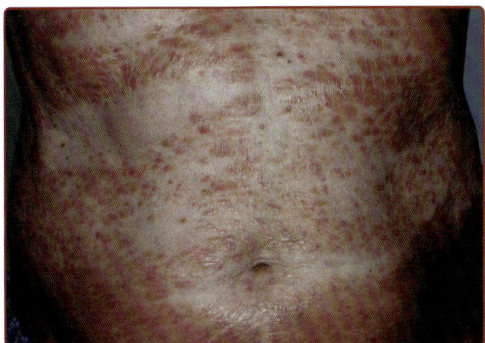

Figure 40-12 Papuloerythroderma of Ofuji. Flat-topped red-to-brown papules with a cobblestone appearance on the abdomen. The sparing of the skin folds, called *deck-chair sign*, is seen.

GRANULOMA FACIALE

AT-A-GLANCE

- Granuloma faciale is an uncommon inflammatory dermatosis characterized clinically by reddish brown papules and plaques primarily involving the face.
- The pathology shows changes of a chronic leukocytoclastic vasculitis with a mixed infiltrate containing eosinophils, extensive perivascular fibrin deposition, and dermal fibrosis.
- Etiology is unknown.

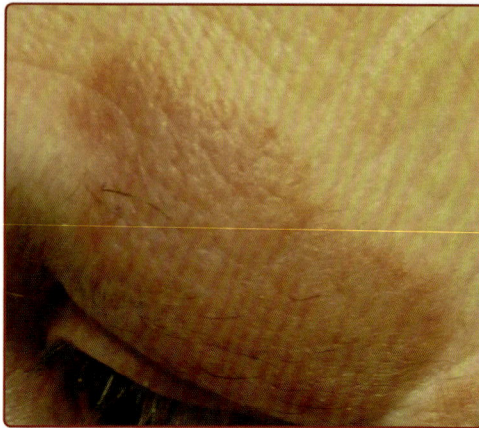

Figure 40-14 Granuloma faciale. Single plaque on the temple showing prominent follicular ostia and central dell.

Granuloma faciale occurs predominantly in adult men and women. There is a slight male predominance, and mean age at presentation is 52 years.[252,253] Granuloma faciale can occur in individuals of any race; however, it is more common in whites.

CLINICAL FEATURES

Granuloma faciale is characterized by solitary papules, plaques, or nodules. The lesions are typically asymptomatic red, brown, or violaceous plaques that are soft, smooth, and well circumscribed, often showing follicular accentuation and telangiectasia (Figs. 40-13 and 40-14). The prominent follicular openings sometimes show a "peau d'orange" appearance. Ulceration is rare. Lesions are most common on the face. Sites of predilection include the nose, preauricular area, cheeks, forehead, eyelids, and ears.[252,254] Rarely, patients may present with multiple lesions or lesions on the trunk or extremities. Extrafacial lesions have been reported both as isolated findings and in conjunction with facial lesions. Lesions are typically asymptomatic; however, patients may complain of tenderness, burning, or pruritus.[252] Photoexacerbation of lesions has been reported.[255] It is rarely associated with systemic disease.[256]

ETIOLOGY AND PATHOGENESIS

The etiology of granuloma faciale is unknown. The disease can be considered a localized chronic fibrosing vasculitis.[257] Immunofluorescence studies have revealed deposition of immunoglobulins and complement factors in the vessel walls consistent with a type III immunologic response, marked by deposition of circulating immune complexes surrounding superficial and deep blood vessels.[258,259] However, other authors have described negative results with immunofluorescence.[254]

DIAGNOSIS

An extensive laboratory evaluation is not required. Peripheral blood eosinophilia is occasionally detected. The diagnosis may be established by a combination of clinical findings and confirmatory tissue biopsy results. A punch biopsy that includes the full thickness of the dermis is recommended. Histologic examination shows a normal-appearing epidermis, which may be separated from the underlying inflammatory infiltrate by a narrow grenz zone (Fig. 40-15). Within the dermis is a dense and diffuse infiltrate of lymphocytes, plasma cells, eosinophils, and neutrophils with evidence of leukocytoclasis (Fig. 40-16). The inflammatory infiltrate surrounds the blood vessels, which show evidence of fibrin deposition. In later stages, the perivascular fibrin deposition becomes extensive and dominates the histologic picture. Deposition of hemosiderin may contribute to the brown color seen clinically. Electron microscopy studies confirm the presence of an extensive eosinophilic infiltrate with Charcot–Leyden crystals and numerous histiocytes filled with lysosomal vesicles; however, cases with few

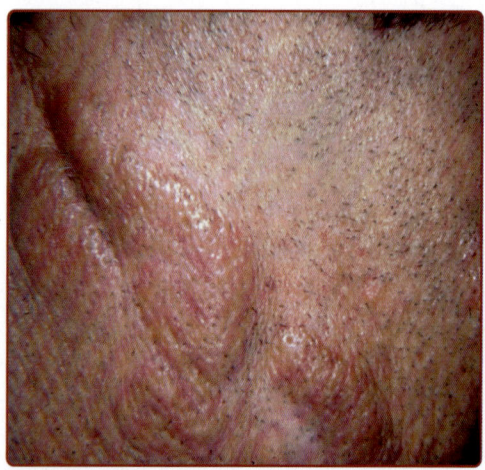

Figure 40-13 Granuloma faciale. Raised edematous plaques on cheek showing prominent follicular ostia.

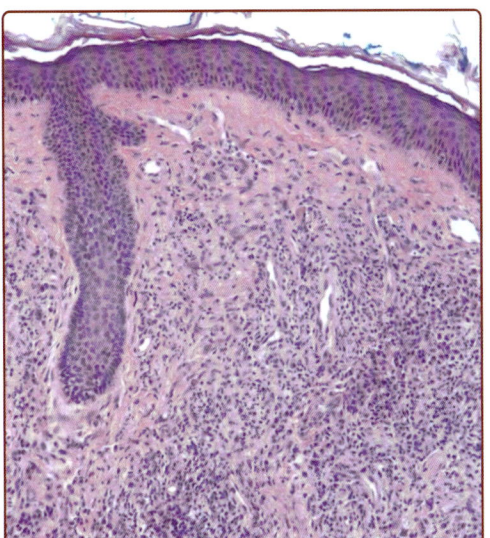

Figure 40-15 Granuloma faciale. This low-power histologic section shows a mixed infiltrate of lymphocytes, histiocytes, neutrophils, plasma cells, and eosinophils. There is sparing of a narrow grenz zone between the inflammatory infiltrate and the overlying epidermis.

eosinophils in the infiltrate have also been described.[260] Immunoglobulins, fibrin, and complement can be found deposited along the dermal–epidermal junction in a granular pattern and around blood vessels by direct immunofluorescence.[258] Recently, dermoscopy has come to be used for assisting the diagnosis. It reveals a translucent white-gray or pink background intermingled with whitish streaks and elongated telangiectasias. The finding of dilated follicular openings, which are more evident under dermoscopy, is of value in the differential diagnosis.[261]

DIFFERENTIAL DIAGNOSIS

The clinical differential diagnosis for granuloma faciale includes discoid lupus erythematosus, polymorphous light eruption, fixed drug eruption, benign lymphocytic infiltrate of Jessner, lymphoma cutis, pseudolymphoma, sarcoidosis, granuloma annulare, tinea faciei, insect bite reaction, xanthogranuloma, mastocytoma, actinic keratosis, basal cell carcinoma, Langerhans cell histiocytosis, and rosacea (Table 40-12). The diagnosis can be reliably made by histologic examination. Absence of serologic evidence of lupus erythematosus helps differentiate these lesions from the lesions of discoid lupus erythematosus. The primary histologic differential diagnosis is erythema elevatum diutinum (EED). Both diseases represent chronic forms of fibrosing small vessel vasculitis and may be related. However, there are several clinical and histologic differences. EED is characterized by multiple lesions, primarily located on extensor surfaces of the extremities in a symmetric acral distribution. The trunk and face are typically spared in EED. Histologically, both show a chronic fibrosing vasculitis.[262] However, a grenz zone of normal collagen beneath the epidermis is not typical of EED. Eosinophils and plasma cells are more prominent in granuloma faciale, whereas

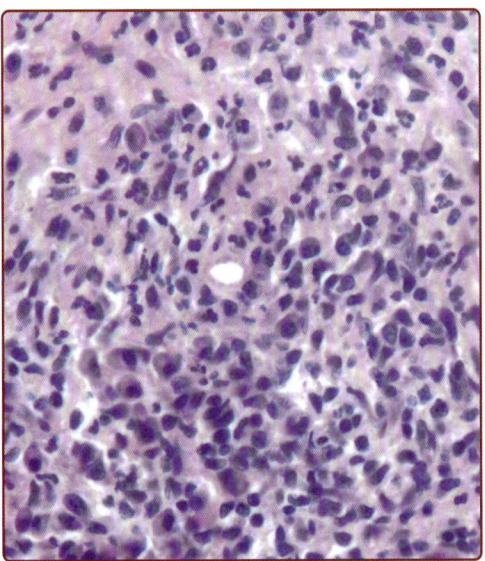

Figure 40-16 Granuloma faciale. This histologic section shows perivascular deposition of fibrin and a mixed infiltrate of lymphocytes, neutrophils, and eosinophils.

TABLE 40-12
Differential Diagnosis of Granuloma Faciale

Most Likely
- Face
  - Sarcoidosis
  - Benign lymphocytic infiltrate of Jessner
  - Rosacea
- Extrafacial
  - Erythema elevatum diutinum

Consider
- Face
  - Discoid lupus erythematosus
  - Lymphoma cutis
  - Angiolymphoid hyperplasia with eosinophilia
  - Tinea faciei
  - Actinic keratosis
  - Basal cell carcinoma
  - Xanthogranuloma
  - Mastocytoma
- Extrafacial
  - Granuloma annulare
  - Benign lymphocytic infiltrate of Jessner
  - Fixed drug eruption

Always Rule Out
- Face
  - Discoid lupus erythematosus
- Trunk
  - Erythema elevatum diutinum

neutrophils are more frequently found in EED. EED may be associated with systemic conditions, primarily monoclonal gammopathies, and shows an excellent response to dapsone.[263,264] The histologic and clinical differential may also include ALHE. However, the lesions of ALHE contain blood vessels with prominent "hobnail" endothelial cells that protrude into the vascular lumina rather than perivascular fibrin deposition. One case of tinea faciei caused by *Trichophyton rubrum* has been described with clinical and histologic changes consistent with granuloma faciale.[265]

CLINICAL COURSE, PROGNOSIS, AND MANAGEMENT

Granuloma faciale tends to be chronic and rarely resolves spontaneously. Lesions may be present for weeks or months. It is usually resistant to treatment and tends to relapse after treatment.

A variety of medical and surgical therapies have been used in the treatment of granuloma faciale (Table 40-13). Because of the small number of patients involved, randomized trials to evaluate these treatments are lacking. Resistance to therapy and cosmetic complications should be discussed with the patient before initiation of therapy. Topical and intralesional steroids have been administered with modest improvement.[252,266] Cryosurgery has been applied with effective results.[267,268] Because the disease is known to be a variant of chronic leukocytoclastic vasculitis, dapsone 25 to 100 mg/day has been used with benefit in a number of patients.[269,270] Topical tacrolimus ointment 0.1% also has been used with success.[271] Surgical excision may be an option for small lesions. Lesions of granuloma faciale have been treated with a variety of medical lasers. In multiple studies using pulsed-dye lasers at 585 to 595 nm, clinical improvement has been demonstrated.[272-275] A carbon dioxide laser also has been applied with varying success.[276] The use of an argon laser resulted in total resolution of the granuloma faciale with subsequent scarring. The lesions in 2 patients were reported to respond to the potassium-titanyl-phosphate 532-nm laser in combination with tacrolimus ointment 0.1%.[277] Case studies suggest a beneficial effect of tacrolimus ointment,[278,279] as well as pimecrolimus cream 1%.[279]

CLINICAL REACTION PATTERNS WITH EOSINOPHIL INVOLVEMENT

There are a variety of diseases in which eosinophils may be present in cutaneous lesions, with or without associated peripheral blood eosinophilia, but either the histologic pattern is unremarkable or eosinophils are not critical for the histologic diagnosis of the given entity (see Table 40-1). In many of these dermatoses, the eosinophil loses its morphologic integrity after disruption through cytolysis and is not identifiable histologically.[280] However, toxic granule proteins and other inflammatory eosinophil products are deposited in skin, persist for extended periods of time, and cause tissue effects.[42,45] Clinical reaction patterns associated with eosinophil involvement include edema, chronic dermatitis/pruritus (eg, atopic dermatitis and prurigo nodularis), drug reactions, blisters (eg, pemphigoid), fibrosis, and vasculitis. Eosinophils may be observed in a variety of cutaneous and extracutaneous neoplasms.

EOSINOPHILIC FASCIITIS

Eosinophilic fasciitis usually presents with pain, erythema, edema, and induration of the extremities, as well as peripheral blood eosinophilia and hypergammaglobulinemia.[281] Contractures and rippling of the skin may develop. Groove sign is a characteristic finding of eosinophilic fasciitis, consisting of a depression along the course of the superficial veins that is more marked upon elevation of the affected limb.[282] There is infiltration of lymphocytes, plasma cells, mast cells, and eosinophils, as well as increased thickness of the fascia.

EOSINOPHILIA-MYALGIA SYNDROME

Eosinophilia-myalgia syndrome, historically related to ingestion of certain lots of L-tryptophan,[283] is characterized by marked peripheral eosinophilia, disabling generalized myalgias, pneumonitis, myocarditis, neuropathy, encephalopathy, and fibrosis,[284] a constellation of features that are similar to but distinguishable from eosinophilic fasciitis.[285,286] Cutaneous abnormalities of eosinophilia-myalgia syndrome include edema, pruritus, a faint erythematous rash, hair loss, and *peau d'orange* or morphea-like skin lesions.[287] Lungs, heart, and nervous system may be affected.[288] There is a prominent inflammatory infiltrate in the perimysium and fascia, and striking evidence of eosinophil granule protein deposition in skin and around muscle bundles.[283]

TABLE 40-13
Treatments for Granuloma Faciale

	TOPICAL	PHYSICAL	SYSTEMIC
First-line therapy	Topical corticosteroids	Cryotherapy Intralesional steroids Pulsed-dye laser	Dapsone, 50-100 mg/day
Second-line therapy	Topical tacrolimus ointment	Surgical excision	

ACKNOWLEDGMENTS

The author gratefully acknowledges the following researchers for their valuable contributions: Kristin M. Leiferman, Lisa A. Beck, and Gerald J. Gleich for the section "Regulation of the Production and Activation of Eosinophils"; Kristin M. Leiferman and Margot S. Peters for the section "Eosinophils in Cutaneous Diseases" (excluding the section "Granuloma Faciale"); and David A. Mehregan and Darius R. Mehregan for parts of "Granuloma Faciale."

REFERENCES

1. Kita H, Adolphson CR, Gleich GJ: Biology of eosinophils. In: Adkinson NF Jr, Yunginger JW, Busse WW, et al, eds. *Middleton's Allergy: Principles and Practice*. 6th ed. Philadelphia, PA: Mosby; 2003:305-332.
2. Blanchard C, Rothenberg ME: Biology of the eosinophil. *Adv Immunol*. 2009;101:81-121.
3. Hogan SP, Rosenberg HF, Moqbel R, et al. Eosinophils: biological properties and role in health and disease. *Clin Exp Allergy*. 2008;38(5):709-750.
4. Ackerman SJ, Bochner BS. Mechanisms of eosinophilia in the pathogenesis of hypereosinophilic disorders. *Immunol Allergy Clin North Am*. 2007;27(3):357-375.
5. Adachi T, Alam R. The mechanism of IL-5 signal transduction. *Am J Physiol*. 1998;275(3, pt 1):C623-C633.
6. Kouro T, Takatsu K. IL-5- and eosinophil-mediated inflammation: from discovery to therapy. *Int Immunol*. 2009;21(12):1303-1309.
7. Abedin MJ, Kashio Y, Seki M, et al. Potential roles of galectins in myeloid differentiation into three different lineages. *J Leukoc Biol*. 2003;73(5):650-656.
8. Kato M, Kephart GM, Talley NJ, et al. Eosinophil infiltration and degranulation in normal human tissue. *Anat Rec*. 1998;252(3):418-425.
9. Chen HH, Sun AH, Ojcius DM, et al. Eosinophils from murine lamina propria induce differentiation of naïve T cells into regulatory T cells via TGF-β1 and retinoic acid. *PloS One*. 2015;10:e0142881.
10. Zhang J, Lathbury LJ, Salamonsen LA. Expression of the chemokine eotaxin and its receptor, CCR3, in human endometrium. *Biol Reprod*. 2000;62(2):404-411.
11. Gouon-Evans V, Pollard JW. Eotaxin is required for eosinophil homing into the stroma of the pubertal and cycling uterus. *Endocrinology*. 2001;142(10):4515-4521.
12. Lotfi R, Herzog GI, DeMarco RA, et al. Eosinophils oxidize damage-associated molecular pattern molecules derived from stressed cells. *J Immunol*. 2009;183:5023-5031.
13. Prevete N, Rossi FW, Rivellese F, et al. *Helicobacter pylori* HP (2-20) induces eosinophil activation and accumulation in superficial gastric mucosa and stimulates VEGF-alpha and TGF-beta release by interaction with formyl-peptide receptors. *Int J Immunopathol Pharmacol*. 2013;26:647-662.
14. Neves JS, Perez SA, Spencer LA, et al. Eosinophil granules function extracellularly as receptor-mediated secretory organelles. *Proc Natl Acad Sci U S A*. 2008;105(47):18478-18483.
15. Butterworth AE: The eosinophil and its role in immunity to helminth infection. *Curr Top Microbiol Immunol*. 1977;77:127-168.
16. Ackerman SJ, Gleich GJ, Loegering DA, et al. Comparative toxicity of purified human eosinophil granule cationic proteins for schistosomula of *Schistosoma mansoni*. *Am J Trop Med Hyg*. 1985;34(4):735-745.
17. Yoon J, Ponikau JU, Lawrence CB, et al. Innate antifungal immunity of human eosinophils mediated by a beta 2 integrin, CD11b. *J Immunol*. 2008;181(4):2907-2915.
18. Reese TA, Liang HE, Tager AM, et al. Chitin induces accumulation in tissue of innate immune cells associated with allergy. *Nature*. 2007;447(7140):92-96.
19. Matsuwaki Y, Wada K, White TA, et al. Recognition of fungal protease activities induces cellular activation and eosinophil-derived neurotoxin release in human eosinophils. *J Immunol*. 2009;183(10):6708-6716.
20. Yousefi S, Gold JA, Andina N, et al. Catapult-like release of mitochondrial DNA by eosinophils contributes to antibacterial defense. *Nat Med*. 2008;14(9):949-953.
21. Shi HZ, Humbles A, Gerard C, et al. Lymph node trafficking and antigen presentation by endobronchial eosinophils. *J Clin Invest*. 2000;105(7):945-953.
22. Shi HZ. Eosinophils function as antigen-presenting cells. *J Leukoc Biol*. 2004;76(3):520-527.
23. van Rijt LS, Vos N, Hijdra D, et al. Airway eosinophils accumulate in the mediastinal lymph nodes but lack antigen-presenting potential for naive T cells. *J Immunol*. 2003;171(7):3372-3378.
24. Kita H. The eosinophil: a cytokine-producing cell? *J Allergy Clin Immunol*. 1996;97(4):889-892.
25. Lacy P, Moqbel R. Eosinophil cytokines. *Chem Immunol*. 2000;76:134-155.
26. MacKenzie JR, Mattes J, Dent LA, et al. Eosinophils promote allergic disease of the lung by regulating CD4(+) Th2 lymphocyte function. *J Immunol*. 2001;167(6):3146-3155.
27. Yang D, Chen Q, Su SB, et al. Eosinophil-derived neurotoxin acts as an alarmin to activate the TLR2-MyD88 signal pathway in dendritic cells and enhances Th2 immune responses. *J Exp Med*. 2008;205(1):79-90.
28. Finlay CM, Stefanska AM, Walsh KP, et al. Helminth products protect against autoimmunity via innate type 2 cytokines IL-5 and IL-33, which promote eosinophilia. *J Immunol*. 2016;196:703-714.
29. Le Moine A, Surquin M, Demoor FX, et al. IL-5 mediates eosinophilic rejection of MHC class II-disparate skin allografts in mice. *J Immunol*. 1999;163:3778-3784.
30. Long H, Liao W, Wang L, et al. A player and coordinator: the versatile roles of eosinophils in the immune system. *Transfus Med Hemother*. 2016;43(2):96-108.
31. Arbon KS, Albers E, Kemna M, et al. Eosinophil count, allergies, and rejection in pediatric heart transplant recipients. *J Heart Lung Transplant*. 2015;34:1103-1111.
32. Adamko D, Lacy P, Moqbel R. Eosinophil function in allergic inflammation: from bone marrow to tissue response. *Curr Allergy Asthma Rep*. 2004;4(2):149-158.
33. Klion AD, Nutman TB. The role of eosinophils in host defense against helminth parasites. *J Allergy Clin Immunol*. 2004;113(1):30-37.
34. Kato A, Favoreto S Jr, Avila PC, et al. TLR3 and Th2 cytokine-dependent production of thymic stromal lymphopoietin in human airway epithelial cells. *J Immunol*. 2007;179:1080-1087.
35. Allakhverdi Z, Comeau MR, Jessup HK, et al. Thymic stromal lymphopoietin is released by human epithelial cells in response to microbes, trauma, or inflammation and potently activates mast cells. *J Exp Med*. 2007;204:2553-2558.

36. Hui CC, Rusta-Sallehy S, Asher I, et al. The effects of thymic stromal lymphopoietin and IL-3 on human eosinophil-basophil lineage commitment: relevance to atopic sensitization. *Immun Inflamm Dis.* 2014;2:44-55.
37. Ellyard JI, Simson L, Parish CR. Th2-mediated antitumour immunity: friend or foe? *Tissue Antigens.* 2007;70(1):1-11.
38. Tancrède-Bohin E, Ionescu MA, de La Salmonière P, et al. Prognostic value of blood eosinophilia in primary cutaneous T-cell lymphomas. *Arch Dermatol.* 2004;140(9):1057-1061.
39. Takanami I, Takeuchi K, Gika M. Immunohistochemical detection of eosinophilic infiltration in pulmonary adenocarcinoma. *Anticancer Res.* 2002;22(4):2391-2396.
40. Nielsen HJ, Hansen U, Christensen IJ, et al. Independent prognostic value of eosinophil and mast cell infiltration in colorectal cancer tissue. *J Pathol.* 1999;189(4):487-495.
41. Gleich GJ. Mechanisms of eosinophil-associated inflammation. *J Allergy Clin Immunol.* 2000;105(4):651-663.
42. Davis MD, Plager DA, George TJ, et al. Interactions of eosinophil granule proteins with skin: limits of detection, persistence, and vasopermeabilization. *J Allergy Clin Immunol.* 2003;112(5):988-994.
43. Leiferman KM, Peters MS, Gleich GJ. The eosinophil and cutaneous edema. *J Am Acad Dermatol.* 1986;15(3):513-517.
44. Gleich GJ, Schroeter AL, Marcoux JP, et al. Episodic angioedema associated with eosinophilia. *N Engl J Med.* 1984;310(25):1621-1626.
45. Plager DA, Davis MD, Andrews AG, et al. Eosinophil ribonucleases and their cutaneous lesion-forming activity. *J Immunol.* 2009;183(6):4013-4020.
46. Rosenberg HF, Domachowske JB. Eosinophils, eosinophil ribonucleases, and their role in host defense against respiratory virus pathogens. *J Leukoc Biol.* 2001;70(5):691-698.
47. Rosenberg HF, Dyer KD, Domachowske JB. Respiratory viruses and eosinophils: exploring the connections. *Antiviral Res.* 2009;83(1):1-9.
48. Rosenberg HF, Dyer KD, Domachowske JB. Eosinophils and their interactions with respiratory virus pathogens. *Immunol Res.* 2009;43(1-3):128-137.
49. Yang D, Chen Q, Rosenberg HF, et al. Human ribonuclease A superfamily members, eosinophil-derived neurotoxin and pancreatic ribonuclease, induce dendritic cell maturation and activation. *J Immunol.* 2004;173(10):6134-6142.
50. Bandeira-Melo C, Woods LJ, Phoofolo M, et al. Intracrine cysteinyl leukotriene receptor-mediated signaling of eosinophil vesicular transport-mediated interleukin-4 secretion. *J Exp Med.* 2002;196(6):841-850.
51. Bandeira-Melo C, Bozza PT, Weller PF. The cellular biology of eosinophil eicosanoid formation and function. *J Allergy Clin Immunol.* 2002;109(3):393-400.
52. Spencer LA, Szela CT, Perez SA, et al. Human eosinophils constitutively express multiple Th1, Th2, and immunoregulatory cytokines that are secreted rapidly and differentially. *J Leukoc Biol.* 2009;85(1):117-123.
53. Daugherty BL, Siciliano SJ, DeMartino JA, et al. Cloning, expression, and characterization of the human eosinophil eotaxin receptor. *J Exp Med.* 1996;183(5):2349-2354.
54. Rothenberg ME, Hogan SP. The eosinophil. *Annu Rev Immunol.* 2006;24:147-174.
55. Oliveira SH, Lukacs NW. The role of chemokines and chemokine receptors in eosinophil activation during inflammatory allergic reactions. *Braz J Med Biol Res.* 2003;36(11):1455-1463.
56. Tachimoto H, Ebisawa M, Bochner BS. Cross-talk between integrins and chemokines that influences eosinophil adhesion and migration. *Int Arch Allergy Immunol.* 2002;128(suppl 1):18-20.
57. Simon HU. Molecules involved in the regulation of eosinophil apoptosis. *Chem Immunol Allergy.* 2006;91:49-58.
58. Munitz A, Levi-Schaffer F. Eosinophils. "New" roles for "old" cells. *Allergy.* 2004;59(3):268-275.
59. Noguchi H, Kephart GM, Colby TV, et al. Tissue eosinophilia and eosinophil degranulation in syndromes associated with fibrosis. *Am J Pathol.* 1992;140(2):521-528.
60. Costello RW, Jacoby DB, Gleich GJ, et al. Eosinophils and airway nerves in asthma. *Histol Histopathol.* 2000;15(3):861-868.
61. Durcan N, Costello RW, McLean WG, et al. Eosinophil-mediated cholinergic nerve remodeling. *Am J Respir Cell Mol Biol.* 2006;34(6):775-86.
62. Steinhoff M, Neisius U, Ikoma A, et al. Proteinase-activated receptor-2 mediates itch: a novel pathway for pruritus in human skin. *J Neurosci.* 2003;23(15):6176-6180.
63. Bochner BS, Schleimer RP. The role of adhesion molecules in human eosinophil and basophil recruitment. *J Allergy Clin Immunol.* 1994;94(3, pt 1):427-438; quiz 439.
64. Pazdrak K, Young TW, Stafford S, et al. Cross-talk between ICAM-1 and granulocyte-macrophage colony-stimulating factor receptor signaling modulates eosinophil survival and activation. *J Immunol.* 2008;180(6):4182-4190.
65. Wardlaw A. Eosinophil trafficking: new answers to old questions. *Clin Exp Allergy.* 2004;34(5):676-679.
66. Rosenberg HF, Phipps S, Foster PS. Eosinophil trafficking in allergy and asthma. *J Allergy Clin Immunol.* 2007;119(6):1303-1310, quiz 1311-1312.
67. Lee SC, Brummet ME, Shahabuddin S, et al. Cutaneous injection of human subjects with macrophage inflammatory protein-1 alpha induces significant recruitment of neutrophils and monocytes. *J Immunol.* 2000;164(6):3392-3401.
68. Mishra A, Hogan SP, Lee JJ, et al. Fundamental signals that regulate eosinophil homing to the gastrointestinal tract. *J Clin Invest.* 1999;103(12):1719-1727.
69. Igawa K, Satoh T, Hirashima M, et al. Regulatory mechanisms of galectin-9 and eotaxin-3 synthesis in epidermal keratinocytes: possible involvement of galectin-9 in dermal eosinophilia of Th1-polarized skin inflammation. *Allergy.* 2006;61(12):1385-1391.
70. Kagami S, Kakinuma T, Saeki H, et al. Significant elevation of serum levels of eotaxin-3/CCL26, but not of eotaxin-2/CCL24, in patients with atopic dermatitis: serum eotaxin-3/CCL26 levels reflect the disease activity of atopic dermatitis. *Clin Exp Immunol.* 2003;134(2):309-313.
71. Suzukawa M, Koketsu R, Iikura M, et al. Interleukin-33 enhances adhesion, CD11b expression and survival in human eosinophils. *Lab Invest.* 2008;88:1245-1253.
72. Stolarski B, Kurowska-Stolarska M, Kewin P, et al. IL-33 exacerbates eosinophil-mediated airway inflammation. *J Immunol.* 2010;185:3472-3480.
73. Horie S, Kita H. CD11b/CD18 (Mac-1) is required for degranulation of human eosinophils induced

74. Matsumoto K, Appiah-Pippim J, Schleimer RP, et al. CD44 and CD69 represent different types of cell-surface activation markers for human eosinophils. *Am J Respir Cell Mol Biol.* 1998;18(6):860-866.
75. Bochner BS, Gleich GJ. What targeting eosinophils has taught us about their role in diseases. *J Allergy Clin Immunol.* 2010;126(1):16-25, quiz 26-27.
76. Schwiebert LM, Beck LA, Stellato C, et al. Glucocorticosteroid inhibition of cytokine production: relevance to antiallergic actions. *J Allergy Clin Immunol.* 1996;97(1, pt 2):143-152.
77. Schleimer RP, Bochner BS. The effects of glucocorticoids on human eosinophils. *J Allergy Clin Immunol.* 1994;94(6, pt 2):1202-1213.
78. Umland SP, Schleimer RP, Johnston SL. Review of the molecular and cellular mechanisms of action of glucocorticoids for use in asthma. *Pulm Pharmacol Ther.* 2002;15(1):35-50.
79. Park CW, Lee BH, Han HJ, et al. Tacrolimus decreases the expression of eotaxin, CCR3, RANTES and interleukin-5 in atopic dermatitis. *Br J Dermatol.* 2005;152(6):1173-1181.
80. Meng Q, Ying S, Corrigan CJ, et al. Effects of rapamycin, cyclosporine A, and dexamethasone on interleukin 5-induced eosinophil degranulation and prolonged survival. *Allergy.* 1997;52(11):1095-1101.
81. Bai JP, Lesko LJ, Burckart GJ. Understanding the genetic basis for adverse drug effects: the calcineurin inhibitors. *Pharmacotherapy.* 2010;30(2):195-209.
82. Klion AD. Approach to the therapy of hypereosinophilic syndromes. *Immunol Allergy Clin North Am.* 2007;27(3):551-560.
83. Cools J, DeAngelo DJ, Gotlib J, et al. A tyrosine kinase created by fusion of the PDGFRA and FIP1L1 genes as a therapeutic target of imatinib in idiopathic hypereosinophilic syndrome. *N Engl J Med.* 2003;348(13):1201-1214.
84. Pitini V, Teti D, Arrigo C, et al. Alemtuzumab therapy for refractory idiopathic hypereosinophilic syndrome with abnormal T cells: a case report. *Br J Haematol.* 2004;127(5):477.
85. Sefcick A, Sowter D, Dasgupta E, et al. Alemtuzumab therapy for refractory idiopathic hypereosinophilic syndrome. *Br J Haematol.* 2004;124(4):558-559.
86. Wagner LA, Speckart S, Cutter B, et al. Treatment of FIP1L1/PDGFRA-negative hypereosinophilic syndrome with alemtuzumab, an anti-CD52 antibody. *J Allergy Clin Immunol.* 2009;123(6):1407-1408.
87. Walsh G. Mepolizumab-based therapy in asthma: an update. *Curr Opin Allergy Clin Immunol.* 2015;15:392-396.
88. Wechsler ME, Fulkerson PC, Bochner BS, et al. Novel targeted therapies for eosinophilic disorders. *J Allergy Clin Immunol.* 2012;130:563-571.
89. Cogan E, Roufosse F. Clinical management of the hypereosinophilic syndromes. *Expert Rev Hematol.* 2012;5(3):275-290.
90. Butterfield JH. Interferon treatment for hypereosinophilic syndromes and systemic mastocytosis. *Acta Haematol.* 2005;114(1):26-40.
91. Butterfield JH. Treatment of hypereosinophilic syndromes with prednisone, hydroxyurea, and interferon. *Immunol Allergy Clin North Am.* 2007;27(3):493-518.
92. Leiferman KM. A current perspective on the role of eosinophils in dermatologic diseases. *J Am Acad Dermatol.* 1991;24(6, pt 2):1101-1112.
93. Simon D, Wardlaw A, Rothenberg ME. Organ-specific eosinophilic disorders of the skin, lung, and gastrointestinal tract. *J Allergy Clin Immunol.* 2010;126(1):3-13.
94. Zuo L, Rothenberg ME. Gastrointestinal eosinophilia. *Immunol Allergy Clin North Am.* 2007;27(3):443-455.
95. Wechsler ME. Pulmonary eosinophilic syndromes. *Immunol Allergy Clin North Am.* 2007;27(3):477-492.
96. Kephart GM, Andrade ZA, Gleich GJ. Localization of eosinophil major basic protein onto eggs of *Schistosoma mansoni* in human pathologic tissue. *Am J Pathol.* 1988;133(2):389-396.
97. Emmerson RW, Wilson-Jones E. Eosinophilic spongiosis in pemphigus. A report of an unusual histological change in pemphigus. *Arch Dermatol.* 1968;97(3):252-257.
98. Crotty C, Pittelkow M, Muller SA. Eosinophilic spongiosis: a clinicopathologic review of seventy-one cases. *J Am Acad Dermatol.* 1983;8(3):337-343.
99. Winkelmann RK, Frigas E. Eosinophilic panniculitis: a clinicopathologic study. *J Cutan Pathol.* 1986;13(1):1-12.
100. Adame J, Cohen PR. Eosinophilic panniculitis: diagnostic considerations and evaluation. *J Am Acad Dermatol.* 1996;34(2, pt 1):229-234.
101. Trocme SD, Baker RH, Bartley GB, et al. Extracellular deposition of eosinophil major basic protein in orbital histiocytosis X. *Ophthalmology.* 1991;98(3):353-356.
102. Quaedvlieg PJ, Creytens DH, Epping GG, et al. Histopathological characteristics of metastasizing squamous cell carcinoma of the skin and lips. *Histopathology.* 2006;49(3):256-264.
103. Butterfield JH, Kephart GM, Banks PM, et al. Extracellular deposition of eosinophil granule major basic protein in lymph nodes of patients with Hodgkin's disease. *Blood.* 1986;68(6):1250-1256.
104. Weaver J, Bergfeld WF. Quantitative analysis of eosinophils in acute graft-versus-host disease compared with drug hypersensitivity reactions. *Am J Dermatopathol.* 2010;32(1):31-34.
105. Marra DE, McKee PH, Nghiem P. Tissue eosinophils and the perils of using skin biopsy specimens to distinguish between drug hypersensitivity and cutaneous graft-versus-host disease. *J Am Acad Dermatol.* 2004;51(4):543-546.
106. Romero LS, Kantor GR. Eosinophils are not a clue to the pathogenesis of granuloma annulare. *Am J Dermatopathol.* 1998;20(1):29-34.
107. Rothenberg ME. Eosinophilic gastrointestinal disorders (EGID). *J Allergy Clin Immunol.* 2004;113(1):11-28, quiz 29.
108. Noel RJ, Putnam PE, Rothenberg ME. Eosinophilic esophagitis. *N Engl J Med.* 2004;351(9):940-941.
109. Roufosse F, Weller PF. Practical approach to the patient with hypereosinophilia. *J Allergy Clin Immunol.* 2010;126(1):39-44.
110. Ogbogu PU, Bochner BS, Butterfield JH, et al. Hypereosinophilic syndrome: a multicenter, retrospective analysis of clinical characteristics and response to therapy. *J Allergy Clin Immunol.* 2009;124(6):1319-1325.e3.
111. Sheikh J, Weller PF. Clinical overview of hypereosinophilic syndromes. *Immunol Allergy Clin North Am.* 2007;27(3):333-355.
112. Roufosse F, Simonart T, Cogan E. Skin lesions as the only manifestation of the idiopathic hypereosinophilic syndrome. *Br J Dermatol.* 2001;144(3):639.
113. Offidani A, Bernardini ML, Simonetti O, et al. Hypereosinophilic dermatosis: skin lesions as the only

113. manifestation of the idiopathic hypereosinophilic syndrome? *Br J Dermatol*. 2000;143(3):675-677.
114. Barna M, Kemeny L, Dobozy A. Skin lesions as the only manifestation of the hypereosinophilic syndrome. *Br J Dermatol*. 1997;136(4):646-647.
115. Kazmierowski JA, Chusid MJ, Parrillo JE, et al. Dermatologic manifestations of the hypereosinophilic syndrome. *Arch Dermatol*. 1978;114(4):531-535.
116. Curtis C, Ogbogu P. Hypereosinophilic syndrome. *Clin Rev Allergy Immunol*. 2016;50(2):240-251.
117. Miljkovic J, Bartenjev I: Hypereosinophilic dermatitis-like erythema annulare centrifugum in a patient with chronic lymphocytic leukaemia. *J Eur Acad Dermatol Venereol*. 2005;19(2):228-231.
118. Hofmann SC, Technau K, Müller AM et al. Bullous pemphigoid associated with hypereosinophilic syndrome: Simultaneous response to imatinib. *J Am Acad Dermatol*. 2007;56(suppl 5):S68-S72.
119. McPherson T, Cowen EW, McBurney E, et al. Platelet-derived growth factor receptor-alpha-associated hypereosinophilic syndrome and lymphomatoid papulosis. *Br J Dermatol*. 2006;155(4):824-826.
120. Jang KA, Lim YS, Choi JH, et al. Hypereosinophilic syndrome presenting as cutaneous necrotizing eosinophilic vasculitis and Raynaud's phenomenon complicated by digital gangrene. *Br J Dermatol*. 2000;143(3):641-644.
121. Kim SH, Kim TB, Yun YS, et al. Hypereosinophilia presenting as eosinophilic vasculitis and multiple peripheral artery occlusions without organ involvement. *J Korean Med Sci*. 2005;20(4):677-679.
122. Ito K, Hara H, Okada T, et al. Hypereosinophilic syndrome with various skin lesions and juvenile temporal arteritis. *Clin Exp Dermatol*. 2009;34(5):e192-e195.
123. Hayashi M, Kawaguchi M, Mitsuhashi Y, et al. Case of hypereosinophilic syndrome with cutaneous necrotizing vasculitis. *J Dermatol*. 2008;35(4):229-233.
124. Tsuji Y, Kawashima T, Yokota K, et al. Wells' syndrome as a manifestation of hypereosinophilic syndrome. *Br J Dermatol*. 2002;147(4):811-812.
125. Bogenrieder T, Griese DP, Schiffner R, et al. Wells' syndrome associated with idiopathic hypereosinophilic syndrome. *Br J Dermatol*. 1997;137(6):978-982.
126. Leiferman KM, Gleich GJ, Peters MS. Dermatologic manifestations of the hypereosinophilic syndromes. *Immunol Allergy Clin North Am*. 2007;27(3):415-441.
127. Weller PF, Bubley GJ. The idiopathic hypereosinophilic syndrome. *Blood*. 1994;83(10):2759-2779.
128. Klion AD, Bochner BS, Gleich GJ, et al. Approaches to the treatment of hypereosinophilic syndromes: A workshop summary report. *J Allergy Clin Immunol*. 2006;117(6):1292-1302.
129. Leiferman KM, Gleich GJ. Hypereosinophilic syndrome: case presentation and update. *J Allergy Clin Immunol*. 2004;113(1):50-58.
130. Vandenberghe P, Wlodarska I, Michaux L, et al. Clinical and molecular features of FIP1L1-PDFGRA (+) chronic eosinophilic leukemias. *Leukemia*. 2004;18(4):734-742.
131. Ogbogu PU, Rosing DR, Horne MK III. Cardiovascular manifestations of hypereosinophilic syndromes. *Immunol Allergy Clin North Am*. 2007;27(3):457-475.
132. Fuzellier JF, Chapoutot L, Torossian PF. Mitral valve repair in idiopathic hypereosinophilic syndrome. *J Heart Valve Dis*. 2004;13(3):529-531.
133. Blauwet LA, Breen JF, Edwards WD, et al. Atypical presentation of eosinophilic endomyocardial disease. *Mayo Clin Proc*. 2005;80(8):1078-1084.
134. Roufosse F, Cogan E, Goldman M. Lymphocytic variant hypereosinophilic syndromes. *Immunol Allergy Clin North Am*. 2007;27:389-413.
135. Roufosse F, Cogan E, Goldman M. Recent advances in pathogenesis and management of hypereosinophilic syndromes. *Allergy*. 2004;59(7):673-689.
136. Gotlib J, Cools J, Malone JM 3rd, et al. The FIP1L1-PDGFRalpha fusion tyrosine kinase in hypereosinophilic syndrome and chronic eosinophilic leukemia: implications for diagnosis, classification, and management. *Blood*. 2004;103(8):2879-2791.
137. Bain BJ, Fletcher SH. Chronic eosinophilic leukemias and the myeloproliferative variant of the hypereosinophilic syndrome. *Immunol Allergy Clin North Am*. 2007;27(3):377-388.
138. Gleich GJ, Leiferman KM. The hypereosinophilic syndromes: still more heterogeneity. *Curr Opin Immunol*. 2005;17(6):679-684.
139. Pardanani A, Brockman SR, Paternoster SF, et al. FIP1L1-PDGFRA fusion: prevalence and clinicopathologic correlates in 89 consecutive patients with moderate to severe eosinophilia. *Blood*. 2004;104(10):3038-3045.
140. Tefferi A, Pardanani A, Li CY. Hypereosinophilic syndrome with elevated serum tryptase versus systemic mast cell disease associated with eosinophilia: 2 distinct entities? *Blood*. 2003;102(8):3073-3074, author reply 3074.
141. Pardanani A, Ketterling RP, Brockman SR, et al. CHIC2 deletion, a surrogate for FIP1L1-PDGFRA fusion, occurs in systemic mastocytosis associated with eosinophilia and predicts response to imatinib mesylate therapy. *Blood*. 2003;102(9):3093-3096.
142. Yamada Y, Rothenberg ME, Lee AW, et al. The FIP1L1-PDGFRA fusion gene cooperates with IL-5 to induce murine hypereosinophilic syndrome (HES)/chronic eosinophilic leukemia (CEL)-like disease. *Blood*. 2006;107(10):4071-4079.
143. Yamada Y, Cancelas JA. FIP1L1/PDGFR alpha associated systemic mastocytosis. *Int Arch Allergy Immunol*. 2010;152(suppl 1):101-105.
144. Tefferi A, Gotlib J, Ardanani A. Hypereosinophilic syndrome and clonal eosinophilia: point-of-care diagnostic algorithm and treatment update. *Mayo Clin Proc*. 2010;85(2): 158-164.
145. Vardiman JW, Thiele J, Arber DA, et al. The 2008 revision of the World Health Organization (WHO) classification of myeloid neoplasms and acute leukemia: rationale and important changes. *Blood*. 2009;114(5):937-951.
146. Tefferi A, Thiele J, Vardiman JW. The 2008 World Health Organization classification system for myeloproliferative neoplasms: order out of chaos. *Cancer*. 2009;115(17):3842-3847.
147. Butterfield JH, Leiferman KM, Gleich GJ. Nodules, eosinophilia, rheumatism, dermatitis and swelling (NERDS): a novel eosinophilic disorder. *Clin Exp Allergy*. 1993;23(7):571-580.
148. Simon HU, Rothenberg ME, Bochner BS, et al. Refining the definition of hypereosinophilic syndrome. *J Allergy Clin Immunol*. 2010;126(1):45-49.
149. Klion A. Hypereosinophilic syndrome: current approach to diagnosis and treatment. *Annu Rev Med*. 2009;60:293-306.
150. Gleich GJ, Leiferman KM. The hypereosinophilic syndromes: current concepts and treatments. *Br J Haematol*. 2009;145(3):271-285.
151. Tefferi A, Gotlib J, Pardanani A. Hypereosinophilic syndrome and clonal eosinophilia: point-of-care

152. Nutman TB. Evaluation and differential diagnosis of marked, persistent eosinophilia. *Immunol Allergy Clin North Am*. 2007;27(3):529-549.
153. Lee JS, Loh TH, Seow SC, et al. Prolonged urticaria with purpura: the spectrum of clinical and histopathologic features in a prospective series of 22 patients exhibiting the clinical features of urticarial vasculitis. *J Am Acad Dermatol*. 2007;56(6):994-1005.
154. Amano H, Nagai Y, Ishikawa O. Persistent urticaria characterized by recurrent lasting urticarial erythema with histological features of prominent perivascular eosinophilic infiltration. *Clin Exp Dermatol*. 2009;34(5):e14-e17.
155. Leiferman KM, O'Duffy JD, Perry HO, et al. Recurrent incapacitating mucosal ulcerations. A prodrome of the hypereosinophilic syndrome. *JAMA*. 1982;247(7):1018-1020.
156. Pardanani A, Ketterling RP, Li CY, et al. FIP1L1-PDGFRA in eosinophilic disorders: prevalence in routine clinical practice, long-term experience with imatinib therapy, and a critical review of the literature. *Leuk Res*. 2006;30(8): 965-970.
157. Scowden EB, Schaffner W, Stone WJ. Overwhelming strongyloidiasis: an unappreciated opportunistic infection. *Medicine (Baltimore)*. 1978;57(6):527-544.
158. de Lavareille A, Roufosse F, Schmid-Grendelmeier P, et al. High serum thymus and activation-regulated chemokine levels in the lymphocytic variant of the hypereosinophilic syndrome. *J Allergy Clin Immunol*. 2002;110:476-479.
159. Simon HU, Cools J. Novel approaches to therapy of hypereosinophilic syndromes. *Immunol Allergy Clin North Am*. 2007;27(3):519-527.
160. Pitini V, Arrigo C, Azzarello D, et al. Serum concentration of cardiac troponin T in patients with hypereosinophilic syndrome treated with imatinib is predictive of adverse outcomes. *Blood*. 2003;102(9):3456-3457, author reply 3457.
161. Sato Y, Taniguchi R, Yamada T, et al. Measurement of serum concentrations of cardiac troponin T in patients with hypereosinophilic syndrome: a sensitive non-invasive marker of cardiac disorder. *Intern Med*. 2000;39(4):350.
162. Burgess MR, Sawyers CL. Treating imatinib-resistant leukemia: the next generation targeted therapies. *ScientificWorldJournal*. 2006;6:918-930.
163. O'Hare T, Corbin AS, Druker BJ. Targeted CML therapy: controlling drug resistance, seeking cure. *Curr Opin Genet Dev*. 2006;16(1):92-99.
164. Simon D, Salemi S, Yousefi S, et al. Primary resistance to imatinib in Fip1-like 1-platelet-derived growth factor receptor alpha-positive eosinophilic leukemia. *J Allergy Clin Immunol*. 2008;121:1054-1056.
165. Rotoli B, Catalano L, Galderisi M, et al. Rapid reversion of Loeffler's endocarditis by imatinib in early stage clonal hypereosinophilic syndrome. *Leuk Lymphoma*. 2004;45(12):2503-2507.
166. Klion AD, Robyn J, Akin C, et al. Molecular remission and reversal of myelofibrosis in response to imatinib mesylate treatment in patients with the myeloproliferative variant of hypereosinophilic syndrome. *Blood*. 2004;103(2):473-478.
167. Cervetti G, Galimberti S, Carulli G, et al. Imatinib therapy in hypereosinophilic syndrome: a case of molecular remission. *Leuk Res*. 2005;29(9):1097-1098.
168. Tefferi A. Modern diagnosis and treatment of primary eosinophilia. *Acta Haematol*. 2005;114(1):52-60.
169. Taverna JA, Lerner A, Goldberg L, et al. Infliximab as a therapy for idiopathic hypereosinophilic syndrome. *Arch Dermatol*. 2007;143(9):1110-1112.
170. Halaburda K, Prejzner W, Szatkowski D, et al. Allogeneic bone marrow transplantation for hypereosinophilic syndrome: long-term follow-up with eradication of FIP1L1- PDGFRA fusion transcript. *Bone Marrow Transplant*. 2006;38(4):319-320.
171. Ueno NT, Anagnostopoulos A, Rondón G, et al. Successful non-myeloablative allogeneic transplantation for treatment of idiopathic hypereosinophilic syndrome. *Br J Haematol*. 2002;119(1):131-134.
172. Walsh GM. Reslizumab, a humanized anti-IL-5 mAb for the treatment of eosinophil-mediated inflammatory conditions. *Curr Opin Mol Ther*. 2009;11(3):329-336.
173. Klion AD, Law MA, Noel P, et al. Safety and efficacy of the monoclonal anti-interleukin-5 antibody SCH55700 in the treatment of patients with hypereosinophilic syndrome. *Blood*. 2004;103(8):2939-2941.
174. Rothenberg ME, Klion AD, Roufosse FE, et al. Treatment of patients with the hypereosinophilic syndrome with mepolizumab. *N Engl J Med*. 2008;358(12):1215-1228.
175. Plotz SG, Simon HU, Darsow U, et al. Use of an anti-interleukin-5 antibody in the hypereosinophilic syndrome with eosinophilic dermatitis. *N Engl J Med*. 2003;349(24):2334-2339.
176. Boucher RM, Gilbert-McClain L, Chowdhury B. Hypereosinophilic syndrome and mepolizumab. *N Engl J Med*. 2008;358(26):2838-2839, author reply 2839-2840.
177. Wells GC. Recurrent granulomatous dermatitis with eosinophilia. *Trans St Johns Hosp Dermatol Soc*. 1971;57:46-56.
178. Gilliam AE, Bruckner AL, Howard RM, et al. Bullous "cellulitis" with eosinophilia: case report and review of Wells' syndrome in childhood. *Pediatrics*. 2005;116(1):e149-e155.
179. Ling TC, Antony F, Holden CA, et al. Two cases of bullous eosinophilic cellulitis. *Br J Dermatol*. 2002;146(1):160-161.
180. Utikal J, Peitsch WK, Kemmler N, et al. Bullous eosinophilic cellulitis associated with ulcerative colitis: Effective treatment with sulfasalazine and glucocorticoids. *Br J Dermatol*. 2007;156(4):764-766.
181. Katoulis AC, Bozi E, Samara M, et al. Idiopathic bullous eosinophilic cellulitis (Wells' syndrome). *Clin Exp Dermatol*. 2009;34(7):e375-e376.
182. Moossavi M, Mehregan DR. Wells' syndrome: a clinical and histopathologic review of seven cases. *Int J Dermatol*. 2003;42(1):62-67.
183. Arca E, Köse O, Karslioğlu Y, et al. Bullous eosinophilic cellulitis succession with eosinophilic pustular folliculitis without eosinophilia. *J Dermatol*. 2007;34:80-85.
184. Sinno H, Lacroix JP, Lee J, et al. Diagnosis and management of eosinophilic cellulitis (Wells' syndrome): a case series and literature review. *Can J Plast Surg*. 2012;20:91-97.
185. Wells GC, Smith NP: Eosinophilic cellulitis. *Br J Dermatol*. 1979;100(1):101-109.
186. Leiferman KM, Peters MS. Reflections on eosinophils and flame figures: where there's smoke there's not necessarily Wells syndrome. *Arch Dermatol*. 2006;142(9):1215-1218.
187. Peters MS, Schroeter AL, Gleich GJ. Immunofluorescence identification of eosinophil granule major

188. Coldiron BM, Robinson JK. Low-dose alternate-day prednisone for persistent Well's syndrome. *Arch Dermatol.* 1989;125:1625-1626.
189. Ludwig RJ, Grundmann-Kollmann M, Holtmeier W, et al. Herpes simplex virus type 2-associated eosinophilic cellulitis (Wells' syndrome). *J Am Acad Dermatol.* 2003;48(5 suppl):S60-S61.
190. Sakaria SS, Ravi A, Swerlick R, et al. Wells' syndrome associated with ulcerative colitis: a case report and literature review. *J Gastroenterol.* 2007;42:250-252.
191. Chung CL, Cusack CA. Wells syndrome: an enigmatic and therapeutically challenging disease. *J Drugs Dermatol.* 2006;5:908-911.
192. Effat KG. Angiolymphoid hyperplasia with eosinophilia of the auricle: progression of histopathological changes. *J Laryngol Otol.* 2006;120(5):411-413.
193. Suzuki H, Hatamochi A, Horie M, et al. A case of angiolymphoid hyperplasia with eosinophilia (ALHE) of the upper lip. *J Dermatol.* 2005;32(12):991-995.
194. Zarrin-Khameh N, Spoden JE, Tran RM. Angiolymphoid hyperplasia with eosinophilia associated with pregnancy: a case report and review of the literature. *Arch Pathol Lab Med.* 2005;129(9):1168-1171.
195. Gonzalez-Cuyar LF, Tavora F, Zhao XF, et al. Angiolymphoid hyperplasia with eosinophilia developing in a patient with history of peripheral T-cell lymphoma: evidence for multicentric T-cell lymphoproliferative process. *Diagn Pathol.* 2008;3:22.
196. Chen JF, Gao HW, Wu BY, et al. Angiolymphoid hyperplasia with eosinophilia affecting the scrotum: a rare case report with molecular evidence of T-cell clonality. *J Dermatol.* 2010;37(4):355-359.
197. Helander SD, Peters MS, Kuo TT, et al. Kimura's disease and angiolymphoid hyperplasia with eosinophilia: new observations from immunohistochemical studies of lymphocyte markers, endothelial antigens, and granulocyte proteins. *J Cutan Pathol.* 1995;22(4):319-326.
198. Olsen TG, Helwig EB. Angiolymphoid hyperplasia with eosinophilia. A clinicopathologic study of 116 patients. *J Am Acad Dermatol.* 1985;12(5, pt 1):781-796.
199. Rodríguez-Lomba E, Avilés-Izquierdo JA, Molina-López I, et al. Dermoscopic features in 2 cases of angiolymphoid hyperplasia with eosinophilia. *J Am Acad Dermatol.* 2016;75(1):e19-e21.
200. Cheney ML, Googe P, Bhatt S, et al. Angiolymphoid hyperplasia with eosinophilia (histiocytoid hemangioma): evaluation of treatment options. *Ann Otol Rhinol Laryngol.* 1993;102(4, pt 1):303-308.
201. Miller CJ, Ioffreda MD, Ammirati CT. Mohs micrographic surgery for angiolymphoid hyperplasia with eosinophilia. *Dermatol Surg.* 2004;30(8):1169-1173.
202. Rampini P, Semino M, Drago F, et al. Angiolymphoid hyperplasia with eosinophilia: successful treatment with interferon alpha 2b. *Dermatology.* 2001;202(4):343.
203. Cooper SM, Dawber RP, Millard P. Angiolymphoid hyperplasia with eosinophilia treated by cryosurgery. *J Eur Acad Dermatol Venereol.* 2001;15(5):489-490.
204. Angel CA, Lewis AT, Griffin T, et al. Angiolymphoid hyperplasia successfully treated with an ultralong pulsed dye laser. *Dermatol Surg.* 2005;31(6):713-716.
205. Mashiko M, Yokota K, Yamanaka Y, et al. A case of angiolymphoid hyperplasia with eosinophilia successfully treated with tacrolimus ointment. *Br J Dermatol.* 2006;154(4):803-804.
206. Yuen HW, Goh YH, Low WK, et al. Kimura's disease: a diagnostic and therapeutic challenge. *Singapore Med J.* 2005;46(4):179-183.
207. Takeishi M, Makino Y, Nishioka H, et al. Kimura disease: diagnostic imaging findings and surgical treatment. *J Craniofac Surg.* 2007;18(5):1062-1067.
208. Wang YS, Tay YK, Tan E, et al. Treatment of Kimura's disease with cyclosporine. *J Dermatolog Treat.* 2005;16(4):242-244.
209. Abuel-Haija M, Hurford MT. Kimura disease. *Arch Pathol Lab Med.* 2007;131(4):650-651.
210. Sun QF, Xu DZ, Pan SH, et al. Kimura disease: review of the literature. *Intern Med J.* 2008;38(8):668-672.
211. Takamura S, Teraki Y. Eosinophilic pustular folliculitis associated with hematological disorders: a report of two cases and review of Japanese literature. *J Dermatol.* 2016;43(4):432-435.
212. Fujiyama T, Tokura Y. Clinical and histopathological differential diagnosis of eosinophilic pustular folliculitis. *J Dermatol.* 2013;40(6):419-423.
213. Soeprono FF, Schinella RA. Eosinophilic pustular folliculitis in patients with acquired immunodeficiency syndrome. Report of three cases. *J Am Acad Dermatol.* 1986;14(6):1020-1022.
214. Lambert J, Berneman Z, Dockx P, et al. Eosinophilic pustular folliculitis and B-cell chronic lymphatic leukaemia. *Dermatology.* 1994;189(suppl 2):58-59.
215. Takematsu H, Nakamura K, Igarashi M, et al. Eosinophilic pustular folliculitis. Report of two cases with a review of the Japanese literature. *Arch Dermatol.* 1985;121(7):917-920.
216. Asgari M, Leiferman KM, Piepkorn M, et al. Neonatal eosinophilic pustulosis. *Int J Dermatol.* 2006;45(2):131-134.
217. Rosenthal D, LeBoit PE, Klumpp L, et al. Human immunodeficiency virus-associated eosinophilic folliculitis. A unique dermatosis associated with advanced human immunodeficiency virus infection. *Arch Dermatol.* 1991;127(2):206-209.
218. Long H, Zhang G, Wang L, et al. Eosinophilic skin diseases: a comprehensive review. *Clin Rev Allergy Immunol.* 2016;50(2):189-213.
219. Katoh M, Nomura T, Miyachi Y, et al. Eosinophilic pustular folliculitis: a review of the Japanese published works. *J Dermatol.* 2013;40:15-20.
220. Rajendran PM, Dolev JC, Heaphy MR Jr, et al. Eosinophilic folliculitis: before and after the introduction of anti-retroviral therapy. *Arch Dermatol.* 2005;141:1227-1231.
221. Mizoguchi S, Setoyama M, Higashi Y, et al. Eosinophilic pustular folliculitis induced by carbamazepine. *J Am Acad Dermatol.* 1998;38:641-643.
222. Laing ME, Laing TA, Mulligan NJ, et al. Eosinophilic pustular folliculitis induced by chemotherapy. *J Am Acad Dermatol.* 2006;54:729-730.
223. Opie KM, Heenan PJ, Delaney TA, et al. Two cases of eosinophilic pustular folliculitis associated with parasitic infestations. *Australas J Dermatol.* 2003;44:217-219.
224. Gul U, Kilic A, Demiriz M. Eosinophilic pustular folliculitis: the first case associated with hepatitis C virus. *J Dermatol.* 2007;34:397-399.
225. Kus S, Candan I, Ince U, et al. Eosinophilic pustular folliculitis (Ofuji's disease) exacerbated with pregnancies. *J Eur Acad Dermatol Venereol.* 2006;20:1347–1348.
226. Mabuchi T, Matsuyama T, Ozawa A. Case of eosinophilic pustular folliculitis associated with pregnancy. *J Dermatol.* 2011;38:1191-1193.

227. Teraki Y, Konohana I, Shiohara T, et al. Eosinophilic pustular folliculitis (Ofuji's disease). Immunohistochemical analysis. *Arch Dermatol*. 1993;129:1015-1019.
228. Satoh T, Shimura C, Miyagishi C, et al. Indomethacin-induced reduction in CRTH2 in eosinophilic pustular folliculitis (Ofuji's disease): a proposed mechanism of action. *Acta Derm Venereol*. 2010;90:18-22.
229. Murayama T, Nakamura K, Tsuchida T. Eosinophilic pustular folliculitis with extensive distribution: correlation of serum TARC levels and peripheral blood eosinophil numbers. *Int J Dermatol*. 2015;54(9):1071-1074.
230. Hernández-Martín Á, Nuño-González A, Colmenero I, et al. Eosinophilic pustular folliculitis of infancy: a series of 15 cases and review of the literature. *J Am Acad Dermatol*. 2014;68:150-155.
231. McCalmont TH, Altemus D, Maurer T, et al. Eosinophilic folliculitis. The histologic spectrum. *Am J Dermatopathol*. 1995;17(5):439-446.
232. Buezo GF, Fraga J, Abajo P, et al. HIV-Associated eosinophilic folliculitis and follicular mucinosis. *Dermatology*. 1998;197(2):178-180.
233. Lee MW, Lee DP, Choi JH, et al. Failure to detect clonality in eosinophilic pustular folliculitis with follicular mucinosis. *Acta Derm Venereol*. 2004;84(4):305-307.
234. Kabashima K, Sakurai T, Miyachi Y. Treatment of eosinophilic pustular folliculitis (Ofuji's disease) with tacrolimus ointment. *Br J Dermatol*. 2004;151(4):949-950.
235. Ellis E, Scheinfeld N. Eosinophilic pustular folliculitis: a comprehensive review of treatment options. *Am J Clin Dermatol*. 2004;5(3):189-197.
236. Fukamachi S, Kabashima K, Sugita K, et al. Therapeutic effectiveness of various treatments for eosinophilic pustular folliculitis. *Acta Derm Venereol*. 2009;89(2):155-159.
237. Ota T, Hata Y, Tanikawa A, et al. Eosinophilic pustular folliculitis (Ofuji's disease): indomethacin as a first choice of treatment. *Clin Exp Dermatol*. 2001;26(2):179-181.
238. Ofuji S, Furukawa F, Miyachi Y, et al. Papuloerythroderma. *Dermatologica*. 1984;169:125-130.
239. Torchia D, Miteva M, Hu S, et al. Papuloerythroderma 2009: two new cases and systematic review of the worldwide literature 25 years after its identification by Ofuji et al. *Dermatology*. 2010;220(4):311-320.
240. Ofuji S. Papuloerythroderma. *J Am Acad Dermatol*. 1990;22(4):697.
241. Schepers C, Malvehy J, Azón-Masoliver A. Papuloerythroderma of Ofuji: a report of 2 cases including the first European case associated with visceral carcinoma. *Dermatology*. 1996;193:131-135.
242. Bech-Thomsen N, Thomsen K. Ofuji's papuloerythroderma: a study of 17 cases. *Clin Exp Dermatol*. 1998;23:79-83.
243. Bettoli V, Pizzigoni S, Borghi A, et al. Ofuji papuloerythroderma: a reappraisal of the deck-chair sign. *Dermatology*. 2004;209:1-4.
244. Sugita K, Kabashima K, Nakamura M, et al. Drug-induced papuloerythroderma: Analysis of T-cell populations and a literature review. *Acta Derm Venereol*. 2009;89:618-622.
245. Teraki Y, Inoue Y. Skin-homing Th2/Th22 cells in papuloerythroderma of Ofuji. *Dermatology*. 2014;228:326-331.
246. Pal S, Haroon TS. Erythroderma: a clinicoetiologic study of 90 cases. *Int J Dermatol*. 1998;37:104-107.
247. Shah M, Reid WA, Layton AM. Cutaneous T-cell lymphoma presenting as papuloerythroderma—a case and review of the literature. *Clin Exp Dermatol*. 1995;20:161-163.
248. Suh KS, Kim HC, Chae YS, et al. Ofuji papuloerythroderma associated with follicular mucinosis in mycosis fungoides. *J Dermatol*. 1998;25:185-189.
249. Fujii K, Kanno Y, Ohgo N. Etretinate therapy for papuloerythroderma. *Eur J Dermatol*. 1999;9:610-613.
250. Sommer S, Henderson CA. Papuloerythroderma of Ofuji responding to treatment with cyclosporin. *Clin Exp Dermatol*. 2000;25:293-295.
251. Ota M, Sato-Matsumura KC, Sawamura D, et al. Papuloerythroderma associated with hepatitis C virus infection. *J Am Acad Dermatol*. 2005;52(suppl 1):61-62.
252. Radin DA, Mehregan DR. Granuloma faciale: distribution of the lesions and review of the literature. *Cutis*. 2003;72:213.
253. Marcoval J, Moreno A, Peyr J. Granuloma faciale: a clinicopathological study of 11 cases. *J Am Acad Dermatol*. 2004;51:269.
254. Ortonne N, Wechsler J, Bagot M, et al. Granuloma faciale: a clinicopathologic study of 66 patients. *J Am Acad Dermatol*. 2005;53(6):1002-1009.
255. Johnson WC, Higdon RS, Helwig EB. Granuloma faciale. *Arch Dermatol*. 1959;79:42.
256. Dowlati B, Firooz A, Dowlati Y. Granuloma faciale: successful treatment of nine cases with a combination of cryotherapy and intralesional corticosteroid injection. *Int J Dermatol*. 1997;36:548.
257. Carlson JA, LeBoit PE. Localized chronic fibrosing vasculitis of the skin: an inflammatory reaction that occurs in settings other than erythema elevatum diutinum and granuloma faciale. *Am J Surg Pathol*. 1997;21:698.
258. Nieboer C, Kalsbeek GL. Immunofluorescence studies in granuloma eosinophilicum faciale. *J Cutan Pathol*. 1978;5:68.
259. Barnadas MA, Curell R, Alomar A. Direct immunofluorescence in granuloma faciale: a case report and review of literature. *J Cutan Pathol*. 2006;33:508-511.
260. Schnitzler L, Verret JL, Schubert B. Granuloma faciale: ultrastructural study of three cases. *J Cutan Pathol*. 1977;4:123.
261. Teixeira DA, Estrozi B, Ianhez M. Granuloma faciale: a rare disease from a dermoscopy perspective. *An Bras Dermatol*. 2013;88(6)(suppl 1):97-100.
262. Sangueza OP, Pilcher B, Martin Sangueza J. Erythema elevatum diutinum: a clinicopathological study of eight cases. *Am J Dermatopathol*. 1997;19:214.
263. Roustan G, Sánchez Yus E, Salas C, et al. Granuloma faciale with extrafacial lesions. *Dermatology*. 1999;198(1):79-82.
264. Crowson AN, Mihm MC Jr, Magro CM. Cutaneous vasculitis: a review. *J Cutan Pathol*. 2003;30:161.
265. Frankel DH, Soltani K, Medenica MM, et al. Tinea of the face caused by *Trichophyton rubrum* with histologic changes of granuloma faciale. *J Am Acad Dermatol*. 1988;18(2, pt 2):403-406.
266. Maillard H, Grognard C, Toledano C, et al. Granuloma faciale: efficacy of cryosurgery in two cases [in French]. *Ann Dermatol Venereol*. 2000;127(1):77-79.
267. Zacarian SA. Cryosurgery effective for granuloma faciale. *J Dermatol Surg Oncol*. 1985;11:11.
268. Goldner R, Sina B. Granuloma faciale: the role of dapsone and prior irradiation on the cause of the disease. *Cutis*. 1984;33:478.
269. van de Kerkhof PC. On the efficacy of dapsone in granuloma faciale. *Acta Derm Venereol*. 1994;74:61.

270. Mitchell D. Successful treatment of granuloma faciale with tacrolimus. *Dermatol Online J.* 2004;10:23.
271. Cheung ST, Lanigan SW. Granuloma faciale treated with the pulsed dye laser: a case series. *Clin Exp Dermatol.* 2005;30:373.
272. Welsh JH, Schroeder TL, Levy, ML. Granuloma faciale in a child successfully treated with the pulsed dye laser. *J Am Acad Dermatol.* 1999;41:351.
273. Ammirati CT, Hruza GJ. Treatment of granuloma faciale with the 585-nm pulsed dye laser. *Arch Dermatol.* 1999;135:903.
274. Chatrath V, Rohrer TE. Granuloma faciale successfully treated with long-pulsed tunable dye laser. *Dermatol Surg.* 2002;28:527.
275. Elston DM. Treatment of granuloma faciale with the pulsed dye laser. *Cutis.* 2000;65:97.
276. Ludwig E, Allam JP, Bieber T, et al. New treatment modalities for granuloma faciale. *Br J Dermatol.* 2003;149(3):634-637.
277. Pérez-Robayna N, Rodríguez-García C, González-Hernández S, et al. Successful response to topical tacrolimus for a granuloma faciale in an elderly patient. *Dermatology.* 2009;219(4):359-360.
278. Patterson C, Coutts I. Granuloma faciale successfully treated with topical tacrolimus. *Australas J Dermatol.* 2009;50:217-219.
279. Ertam I, Ertekin B, Unal I, et al. Granuloma faciale: is it a new indication for pimecrolimus? A case report. *J Dermatolog Treat.* 2006;17(4):238-240.
280. Cheng JF, Ott NL, Peterson EA, et al. Dermal eosinophils in atopic dermatitis undergo cytolytic degeneration. *J Allergy Clin Immunol.* 1997;99(5):683-692.
281. Antic M, Lautenschlager S, Itin PH. Eosinophilic fasciitis 30 years after—what do we really know? Report of 11 patients and review of the literature. *Dermatology.* 2006;213(2):93-101.
282. Pinal-Fernandez I, Callejas-Moraga EL, Roade-Tato ML, et al. Groove sign in eosinophilic fasciitis. *Lancet.* 2014;384(9956):1774.
283. Hertzman PA, Blevins WL, Mayer J, et al. Association of the eosinophilia-myalgia syndrome with the ingestion of tryptophan. *N Engl J Med.* 1990;322(13):869-873.
284. Mori Y, Kahari VM, Varga J. Scleroderma-like cutaneous syndromes. *Curr Rheumatol Rep.* 2002;4(2):113-122.
285. Varga J, Griffin R, Newman JH, et al. Eosinophilic fasciitis is clinically distinguishable from the eosinophilia-myalgia syndrome and is not associated with L-tryptophan use. *J Rheumatol.* 1991;18(2):259-263.
286. Varga J, Kahari VM. Eosinophilia-myalgia syndrome, eosinophilic fasciitis, and related fibrosing disorders. *Curr Opin Rheumatol.* 1997;9(6):562-570.
287. Uitto J, Varga J, Peltonen J, et al. Eosinophilia-myalgia syndrome. *Int J Dermatol.* 1992;31(4):223-228.
288. Martin RW, Duffy J, Engel AG, et al. The clinical spectrum of the eosinophilia-myalgia syndrome associated with L-tryptophan ingestion. Clinical features in 20 patients and aspects of pathophysiology. *Ann Intern Med.* 1990;113(2):124-134.
289. Chusid MJ, Dale DC, West BC, et al. The hypereosinophilic syndrome: analysis of fourteen cases with review of the literature. *Medicine (Baltimore).* 1975;54(1):1-27.

Chapter 41 :: Urticaria and Angioedema
Michihiro Hide, Shunsuke Takahagi, & Takaaki Hiragun

第四十一章
荨麻疹和血管性水肿

中文导读

本章主要介绍了荨麻疹和血管性水肿的定义、流行病学史、临床特点、发病机制、诊断和治疗。对于荨麻疹的临床特点主要从皮肤表现和非皮肤表现两个方面介绍。在皮肤表现中，介绍了普通荨麻疹和血管性水肿的区别。并特别强调了血管性水肿常累及的部位，以及会引起疼痛，较少引起瘙痒。而荨麻疹病人一般瘙痒剧烈。同时，还介绍了不同荨麻疹的风团类型，持续的时间，以及出现血管性水肿的可能性。在非皮肤表现中，主要提到的是胃肠道不适，呼吸系统以及循环系统的症状。随后还提到了荨麻疹的并发症是自身免疫性皮肤病，本章以表格的形式介绍了荨麻疹的不同亚型，以及不同类型荨麻疹的临床特点。同时还总结了不同类型荨麻疹的风团出现的概率。在治疗上，介绍了EAACI指南中一线至四线治疗方法及药物。除了常用的抗组胺药物外，氨苯砜、甲氨蝶呤、他克莫司等药物对于荨麻疹有一定的效果，但是并不能改变荨麻疹的自然过程达到完全治愈。本章还介绍了孕妇等一些特殊人群的治疗。

〔李芳芳〕

AT-A-GLANCE

- Urticaria is defined as a skin disorder characterized by local transient skin or mucosal edema (wheal) and an area of redness (erythema) that typically accompany itchy sensations and diminish within 1 day.

- Symptoms may occur either spontaneously (spontaneous or idiopathic urticaria) or in response to specific stimuli, such as physical stimuli or sweating (the increase of body core temperature).

- Mast cells and their histamine being released either spontaneously or in response to various stimuli play a crucial role in the pathogenicity of urticaria.

- Spontaneous or idiopathic urticaria is the subtype of urticaria that most patients experience.

- Autoantibodies against immunoglobulin (Ig) E or the high-affinity IgE receptor (FcεRI) that activate mast cells and basophils and induce histamine release may be detected in up to half of patients with chronic spontaneous or idiopathic urticaria (type II autoimmunity).

- A certain population of patients may develop angioedema mediated by bradykinin rather than histamine.

- Infections, stress, fatigue, and drugs, especially nonsteroidal antiinflammatory drugs and angiotensin-converting enzyme inhibitors, may cause or aggravate urticaria or angioedema.

- However, the mechanism of mast cell activation or the exacerbation of urticaria by various factors, except for exogenous antigens and autoantibodies, remains largely unknown.

- Nonsedative second-generation antihistamines are the mainstay of pharmaceutical therapy.

- Omalizumab, anti-IgE antibody, or immunosuppressive medications may be taken for the treatment of urticaria and angioedema that is refractory to antihistamines even at high doses.

INTRODUCTION

DEFINITIONS

Urticaria is defined as a skin disorder characterized by local transient skin or mucosal edema (wheal) and an area of redness (erythema) that typically accompany itchy sensations and diminish within a day. Angioedema is a local and transient skin or mucosal edema that develops in deep tissues mostly without itching but may accompany pain or burning sensations. Both wheals and angioedema may develop together in one patient, but either one may develop exclusively in individual patients. Whereas the term *urticaria* is used as an entity of disease, *angioedema* may mean either disease or eruption. Either wheals and angioedema or both may appear as a symptom of other disease entities, such as anaphylaxis (either wheals or angioedema), autoinflammatory syndromes (wheals), mastocytosis (wheals known as Darier sign) or hereditary angioedema (HAE; angioedema). The international guidelines advocated by the European Academy of Allergy and Clinical Immunology (EAACI)/Global Allergy and Asthma European Network (GA²LEN)/European Dermatology Forum (EDF)/World Allergy Organization (WAO) (EAACI guideline) define urticaria as a disease characterized by the development of wheals (hives), angioedema, or both and distinguishes urticaria from medical conditions in which wheals, angioedema, or both can occur as a symptom, such as a skin prick test, anaphylaxis, autoinflammatory syndromes, or HAE (bradykinin-mediated angioedema).[1]

HISTORICAL PERSPECTIVE

The school of Hippocrates first described the association of urticaria with nettles and insect bites.[2] Stinging nettle (*Urtica dioica*) contains histamine-, serotonin-, and acetylcholine-containing fluids inside the spicules and causes contact urticaria-like symptoms.[3] Therefore, the name "nettles" frequently appeared in several languages until the middle of the 19th century. The word "urticaria" was first used in 1792 by Johann Peter Frank to describe the disease.[2] In 1878, Paul Ehrlich first described aniline-positive cells in connective tissues and named them "Mastzellen (well-fed cells)."[4] In 1910, Henry Dale clarified the physiological role of histamine on smooth muscle.[5] In 1913, Hans Eppinger showed that wheals, erythema, and pain developed at sites of local injections of histamine.[6] In 1937, Daniel Bovet[7] developed antihistamine, which became the mainstay of treatment for urticaria. In 1953, James F. Riley showed that mast cells are the main source of histamine in the skin.[8] In 1966, Kimishige Ishizaka identified immunoglobulin (Ig) E and clarified its role in type I hypersensitivity, the pathological mechanism of allergic urticaria.[9]

EPIDEMIOLOGY

Studies in Europe reported the lifetime prevalence (prevalence during the whole lifetime until the investigation) of urticaria as around 8% to 10%.[10-12] Hellgren found a point prevalence (prevalence at the time of the investigation) of around 0.1% in the total population of Sweden,[13] and more recently, Gaig and coworkers reported a point prevalence of 0.6% in the Spanish population.[14] The reason for such large variations in the prevalence among reports is unclear, but possible explanations include differences in the methods employed, definition of urticaria, and geographical and cultural characteristics. Many cases of urticaria that diminish within a few weeks or develop on just a single or a few occasions may be overlooked and not included in some survey results.

Chronic spontaneous urticaria (CSU) and inducible urticarias, including physical urticaria, cholinergic urticaria, and contact urticaria, that persist for more than 6 weeks can be grouped as "nonacute" or "chronic" urticaria. One study of the prevalence of CSU with the classification recommended by the EAACI guidelines found a prevalence of 0.8% in a 1-year period in Germany.[12] Statistical analysis of patients with nonacute urticaria suggests that 66% to 93% have CSU, 4% to 33% a physical urticaria, and 1% to 7% have cholinergic urticaria.[15-18] A limitation of many studies is that they give no information about how they evaluate combinations of multiple subtypes of urticaria. In fact, as many as half of patients with CSU may also have other types of urticaria.[19] In addition, CSU can be further divided into that with concomitant angioedema, that without angioedema and that with recurrent angioedema without wheals. The available data suggest that whereas 33% to 67% of all patients with CSU exhibit wheals and angioedema, 29% to 65% exhibit only wheals and 1% to 13% only angioedema.[20] Differences in prevalence by race or ethnic group are unknown, but data are scarce.[20]

Regarding sex, the majority of studies show that women have urticaria nearly twice as often as men do.[10,12,13-15,17,18,20-27] This is true not only for CSU but also for many other types of urticaria. Among patients with CSU, the prevalence of a positive autologous serum skin test (ASST) result was reported to be higher in women than in men.[28]

The peak age of CSU patients is between 20 and 40 years in most studies.[16,17,21,23,27,29] A survey of office-based practices for all types of urticaria in the United States reported a bimodal age distribution in patients aged birth to 9 years and 30 to 40 years.[30] The first peak may represent the predominance of acute spontaneous urticaria, allergic urticaria (urticarial reactions), and cholinergic urticaria in children.

Few data are available concerning the relationship between prevalence of urticaria and socioeconomic status, education, ethnic background or place of residence. A German study showed that people with a high socioeconomic status and those who live in larger cities are more likely to have urticaria.[11] However, the deviations were too small to conclude whether the results reflect true variations in prevalence or just differences in disease awareness. Other studies failed to show a difference in the prevalence of urticaria with regard to education, occupation, income, place of residence, and ethnic background.[10,12,14,31]

CLINICAL FEATURES

CUTANEOUS FINDINGS

Circumscribed, raised, usually pruritic, and evanescent areas of edema that involve the superficial portion of the dermis are known as wheals. A wheal may appear mostly reddish but could also be whitish, especially when edema is significant. Edema that extends into the deep dermis or subcutaneous and submucosal layers is known as angioedema.

Urticaria and angioedema may occur in any location together or individually. Angioedema commonly affects the face, especially the eyelids and lips, or a portion of the extremities (Fig. 41-1E). It may be painful but not pruritic and may last for several days. Involvement of the lips, cheeks, and periorbital areas is common, but angioedema also may affect the tongue, pharynx, or larynx. The individual lesions of urticaria arise suddenly, rarely persist for longer than 24 to 36 hours, and may continue to recur for indefinite periods. Most wheals, but not angioedema, are highly pruritic. The size, shape, and color of wheals are quite variable. Wheals on the eyelids and lips and those in the deep dermis in delayed pressure urticaria (DPU) may be difficult to be distinguished from angioedema. Certain subtypes of urticaria have characteristic morphologies. Spontaneous urticarias (acute and chronic) may involve large, small, flowerlike, or annular wheals, and they are usually heterogeneous (Fig. 41-2). The heterogeneity of wheals in size and shape is one of the characteristics of spontaneous urticaria. In severe cases of spontaneous urticaria, wheals may accompany purpura, lasting for a few days. In such cases, urticarial vasculitis should be excluded. In most cases of physical urticarias, wheals develop diffusely within the affected areas (Figs. 41-1A, 41-1B, and 41-1D), but wheals of cholinergic, adrenergic, and aquagenic urticaria are usually small (<5 mm) and disseminated in the provoked area of the skin (Fig. 41-1C). The duration of individual wheals is long in spontaneous urticarias and deep pressure urticaria and shorter in physical urticarias.[32] The development of angioedema is rare in physical urticaria but may be observed in cholinergic urticaria.[33-35]

NONCUTANEOUS FINDINGS

During urticarial attacks, patients often feel discomfort of the stomach and intestine. Infections of the gastrointestinal tract may induce urticaria and vice versa. Pharyngeal edema can be seen in angioedema, especially bradykinin-induced angioedema.[36] Certain kinds of urticarias, especially inducible ones such as allergic urticaria, and cholinergic urticaria, may develop into anaphylaxis. Anaphylaxis is defined as "a serious, life-threatening generalized or systemic hypersensitivity reaction" and "a serious allergic reaction that is rapid in onset and might cause death."[37] It mostly, but not always, affects the skin (urticarial rash) and respiratory (dyspnea) and circulatory systems (low blood pressure, syncope). Severe cases of physical urticaria may also include systemic symptoms such as headache, dizziness, syncope, wheezing, and nausea.

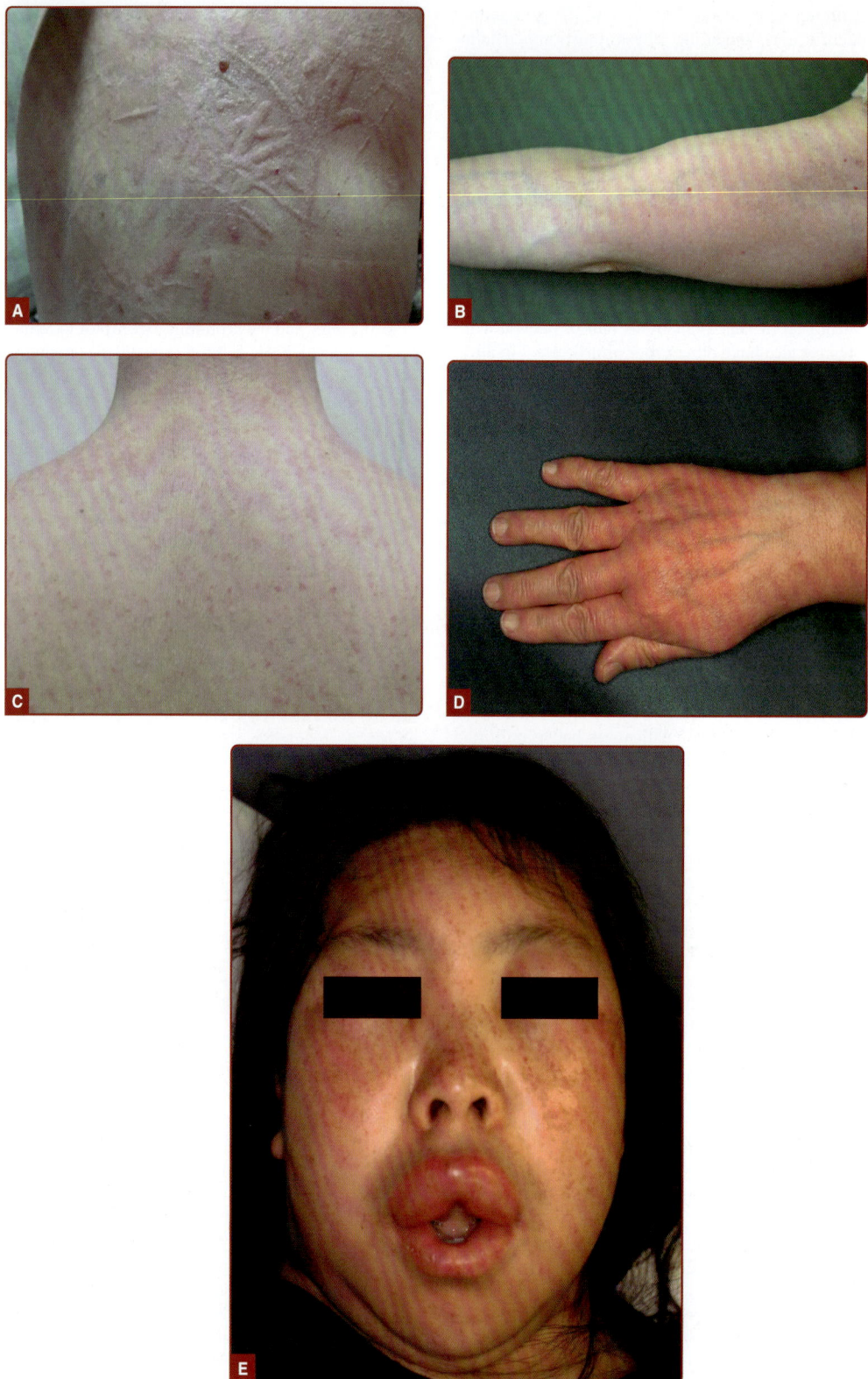

Figure 41-1 Clinical presentation of symptomatic dermographism (**A** and **B**), cholinergic urticaria evoked by exercise (**C**), local contact urticaria evoked by immersion in hot water (**D**), and hereditary angioedema (**E**).

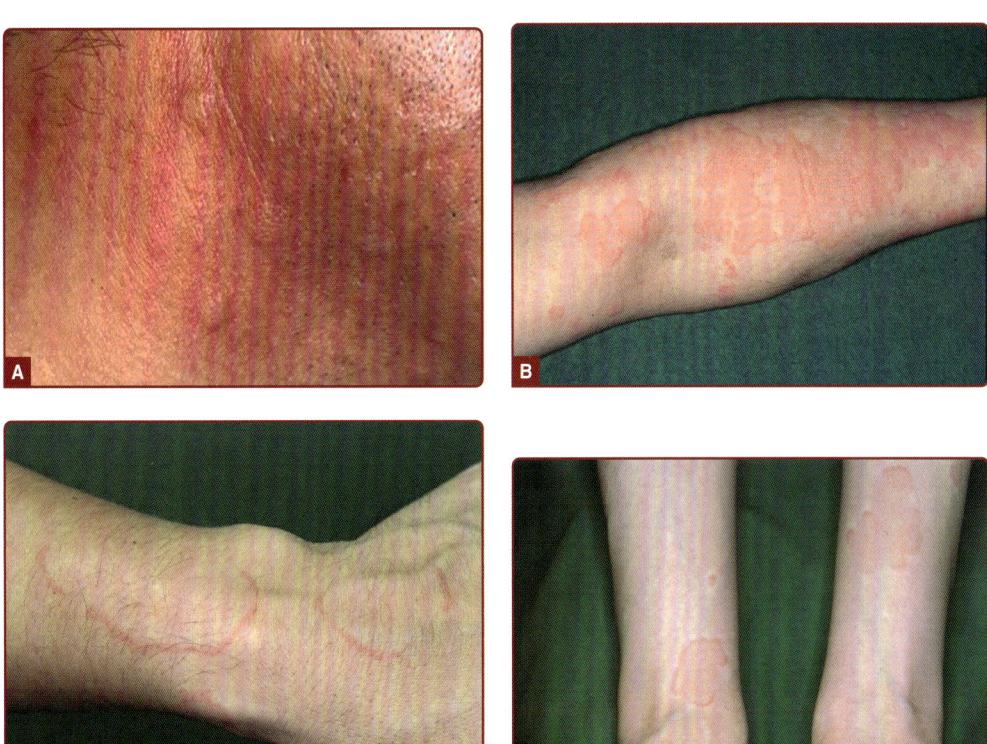

Figure 41-2 Clinical presentation of acute urticaria (**A**), chronic spontaneous urticaria (CSU) (**B**), CSU with an annular shape (**C**), and CSU with a flower shape (**D**). (Images **A, B,** and **D,** reproduced from *JDA*. 2012;122(11):2627-2634, with permission.)

COMPLICATIONS

AUTOIMMUNE THYROID DISEASES

The association between CSU and thyroid autoimmunity has been reported in many studies. The frequency of thyroid autoantibodies in patients with CSU is significantly higher than those in control participants.[38,39] The frequency of overt and subclinical thyroid dysfunction was also significantly higher than those of a control Spanish population.[39] A subgroup of patients with CSU who possess IgE antibodies against thyroid peroxidase (TPO) might evoke autoallergic degranulation of mast cells.[40]

OTHER AUTOIMMUNE DISEASES

Patients with CSU exhibit autoimmune diseases other than thyroid autoimmunity. Especially female patients with CSU were reported to have a significantly higher incidence of rheumatoid arthritis, Sjögren syndrome, celiac disease, type I diabetes mellitus, and systemic lupus erythematosus (SLE).[41]

SUBTYPES OF URTICARIA

Because there is a large variation in features in urticaria, not only in the pathogenesis but also in terms of management, urticaria has been classified by its various aspects, such as duration, trigger and mode of induction, and underlying causes. The international consensus meeting held in 2013 for making the EAACI guidelines reached a consensus for standard classification. This classification divides urticaria into acute and chronic at 6 weeks from the onset. Chronic urticaria is further classified into spontaneous urticaria and inducible urticaria. The latter is induced by physical stimuli and includes physical urticaria (cold urticaria, DPU, heat urticaria, solar urticaria, symptomatic dermographism, vibratory angioedema), cholinergic urticaria, and contact urticaria (Table 41-1). This classification has been maintained in the guideline updated in 2018.[1] In daily practice, wheals or angioedema may also develop as a reaction to certain stimuli or as a symptom of other disease entities. This chapter describes various subtypes of urticaria that require treatment or management in clinical practice even if they are not included in the EAACI guideline. Morphological characteristics of urticaria subtypes are summarized in Table 41-2.

TABLE 41-1
Recommended Diagnostic Tests in Frequent Urticarial Subtypes

TYPES	SUBTYPES	ROUTINE DIAGNOSTIC TESTS (RECOMMENDED)	EXTENDED DIAGNOSTIC PROGRAMME[a] (BASED ON HISTORY) FOR IDENTIFICATION OF UNDERLYING CAUSES OR ELICITING FACTORS AND FOR RULING OUT POSSIBLE DIFFERENTIAL DIAGNOSES IF INDICATED
Spontaneous urticaria	Acute spontaneous urticaria	None	None[b]
	CSU	Differential blood count. ESR and/or CRP	Avoidance of suspected triggers (eg, drugs); Conduction of diagnostic tests for (in no preferred order): (i) infectious diseases (eg, *Helicobacter pylori*); (ii) functional auto-antibodies (eg, autologous skin serum test); (iii) thyroid gland disorders (thyroid hormones and auto-antibodies); (iv) allergy (skin tests and/or allergen avoidance test, eg, avoidance diet); (v) concomitant CIndU, see below; (vi) severe systemic diseases (eg, tryptase); (vii) other (eg, lesional skin biopsy)
Inducible urticaria	Cold urticaria	Cold provocation and threshold test[c,d]	Differential blood count and ESR or CRP, rule out other diseases, especially infections[e]
	Delayed pressure urticaria	Pressure test and threshold test[c,d]	None
	Heat urticaria	Heat provocation and threshold test[c,d]	None
	Solar urticaria	UV and visible light of different wavelengths and threshold test[c]	Rule out other light-induced dermatoses
	Symptomatic dermographism	Elicit dermographism and threshold test[c,d]	Differential blood count, ESR or CRP
	Vibratory angioedema	Test with vibration, for example, Vortex or mixer[d]	None
	Aquagenic urticaria	Provocation testing[d]	None
	Cholinergic urticaria	Provocation and threshold testing[d]	None
	Contact urticaria	Provocation testing[d]	None

[a]Depending on suspected cause.
[b]Unless strongly suggested by patient history, for example allergy.
[c]All tests are carried out with different levels of the potential trigger to determine the threshold.
[d]For details on provocation and threshold testing, refer to Magerl M, Altrichter S, Borzova E, et al. The definition, diagnostic testing, and management of chronic inducible urticarias? The EAACI/GA2LEN/EDF/UNEV consensus recommendations 2016 update and revision.
[e]For further info, refer to Maurer M. Cold urticaria. In: Saini SS, Callen J, editors. UpToDate. Boston, MA: Wolters Kluwer Health; 2014.
ESR, erythrocyte sedimentation rate; CRP, C-reactive protein.
From Zuberbier T, Aberer W, Asero R, et al. The EAACI/GA(2) LEN/EDF/WAO Guideline for the definition, classification, diagnosis, and management of urticaria: the 2017 revision and update. *Allergy*. 2018;73:1393-1414, with permission. Copyright © 2018 EAACI and John Wiley and Sons.

SPONTANEOUS URTICARIA

Spontaneous urticaria is defined as urticaria that occurs spontaneously almost every day without any apparent cause or trigger. The name "idiopathic urticaria" has also been used for the same entity for a long time, but the use of "spontaneous" urticaria has been recommended by the EAACI guidelines and endorsed by many relevant societies.[1] The major skin manifestation is wheals, and they may be accompanied by angioedema in up to half of patients.[20] In some cases, only angioedema may appear. Compared with superficial wheals, angioedema occurs less frequently, such as every few days, weeks, or months, and the symptoms of angioedema last longer than a day, usually for a few days. The shape, size, and duration of individual wheals are highly variable and heterogeneous as described in the Cutaneous Findings in the section of "Clinical Features" and Fig. 41-2. Flowerlike or annular-shaped wheals are characteristic of this subtype of urticaria. Although symptoms may be very severe and disabling, they are mostly nonlethal. There is no qualitative difference between acute spontaneous urticaria and CSU, but acute forms tend to be more severe. Cutaneous manifestations of urticarial vasculitis and autoinflammatory syndromes may resemble long-lasting wheals observed in this type of urticaria.

SYMPTOMATIC DERMOGRAPHISM

Symptomatic dermographism, also called as urticaria factitia, dermographic urticaria, mechanical urticaria, or simply dermographism, is the most common subtype among the physical urticarias. Symptomatic dermographism is characterized by itching or burning skin

TABLE 41-2
Characteristics of Wheals Observed in Subtypes of Urticaria

	SPONTANEOUS URTICARIA TYPE (POLYMORPHIC)	ANNULAR TYPE, PRUPURIC LESION	CHOLINERGIC TYPE (SMALL (<5 MM) AND DISSEMINATED)	LINEAR TYPE	LOCALIZED PROVOKED AREA TYPE	MUCOSAL TYPE
Spontaneous urticaria	+++	++	+			none to ++[a]
Type I allergy mediated and many drug-induced urticarias	++				++	none to ++[a]
Cold, solar, heat, and deep pressure urticarias					+++	none to ±[c]
Symptomatic dermographism (mechanical urticaria)				+++	++	none to ±[c]
Cholinergic, aquagenic, and adrenergic urticarias			+++		none to ++[a]	none to +[b]
Angioedema						+++

[a] A spectrum from none to ++.
[b] A spectrum from none to +.
[c] A spectrum from non to ±.

sensations and the development of pruritic wheals and flare in areas exposed to shearing forces on the skin. The shape of wheals and erythema is mostly liner or consists of liner elements because of the forms of eliciting stimuli (see Fig. 41-1A). However, a widespread flare with vague margins may develop when patients extensively scratch the skin (see Fig. 41-1B). In rare and severe cases of symptomatic dermographism, erythematous lines may accompany punctate wheals characteristic of cholinergic urticaria (*cholinergic dermographism*).[42] Wheals and itch of this urticaria subtype develop shortly after the stimuli and disappear approximately within 30 minutes in most cases. In certain cases of DPU, wheals of symptomatic dermographism may return in the same site or newly develop 3 to 6 hours after stimulation and persist for up to 48 hours (*delayed dermographism*).[43] In some rare cases, wheals may be markedly augmented when the skin is chilled (*cold-dependent dermographism*).[44] There is a case report of this subtype urticaria developing in the genital region during sexual intercourse.[45]

COLD URTICARIA

Cold urticaria is a physical urticaria being characterized by the appearance of wheals and flare in response to cold. In most cases, local skin contact with a cold substance induces wheals and flare in the area of cold contact (*cold contact urticaria*). The cutaneous appearance of wheals and flare is typically flat and widely spread but may also be punctate. Itching and wheals of the skin occur within minutes and persist up to 1 hour. In severe cases, the mouth and pharynx may swell after drinking cold liquid. Patients with cold urticaria may also develop anaphylactic symptoms, including palpitations, headache, wheezing, and loss of consciousness, and drowning may occur after cold water bathing. In rare cases, erythematous edematous and deep swelling may appear 9 to 18 hours after cold challenge (*delayed cold urticaria*).[46]

In cases of *systemic cold urticaria*, widespread wheals and flare develop in response to cooling of the core body temperature, not by the local exposure to cold.[47] Systemic cold urticaria may be either idiopathic or secondary to underlying diseases. Patients with *familial cold urticaria syndrome* develop erythematous macules and infrequent wheals associated with burning and pruritus on exposure to cold; this is now classified as a subtype of *cryopyrin-associated periodic syndrome (CAPS)*, an autosomal dominant inherited disease which is associated with a genetic mutation of *NLRP3 (CIAS1)*. It may include headaches, conjunctivitis, and arthralgias. The average delay between cold exposure and onset of symptoms is 2.5 hours, and the average duration of an episode is 12 hours.[48] More recently, a new mutation in *PLCG2*, encoding phospholipase $C\gamma_2$, with gain of function has been identified in families with a dominantly inherited complex of cold-induced urticaria, antibody deficiency, and susceptibility to infection and autoimmunity.[49] Patients with these hereditary disorders do not develop wheals and flare in response to the local ice-cube test (see the "Diagnosis" section).

HEAT URTICARIA

Heat urticaria is a rare subtype of physical urticaria characterized by wheals and flare that develop within minutes after local heat exposure to the skin and disappear within a few hours at the longest (see Fig. 41-1D). In contrast to cholinergic urticaria that involves small punctate eruptions in response to conditions that elicit sweating, patients with heat urticaria develop wheals and flare that spread in the area of skin exposed to heat, regardless of the core body temperature or sweating.

SOLAR URTICARIA

Solar urticaria is a rare subtype of physical urticaria characterized by wheals and flare that develop within minutes after local exposure of the skin to certain wavelengths of light. The urticarial lesions usually resolve within hours but may accompany headache, syncope, dizziness, wheezing, and nausea. The shape of skin eruptions in solar urticaria is consistent with the area exposed to the light of an eliciting wavelength. There may be widespread wheals, flare, or punctate redness but not the small wheals observed in cholinergic urticaria. The face and hands may develop fewer lesions than skin areas that are usually covered by clothes because of hardening due to chronic exposure to sunlight.

DELAYED PRESSURE URTICARIA

Delayed pressure urticaria is characterized by deep dermal wheals that appear in a continuously compressed region with a latency of 30 minutes or several hours after the release of the compression. The wheals last for several hours or up to 3 days and may be accompanied by a burning sensation or pain rather than the itching often seen with CSU.[50] DPU may develop by itself but may often be accompanied by CSU.[51]

VIBRATORY URTICARIA AND ANGIOEDEMA

Vibratory urticaria and angioedema is a rare subtype of physical urticaria characterized by cutaneous swelling developing immediately at the site of contact with vibratory stimuli, such as jogging, vigorous toweling, or using lawnmowers.[52] Recently, the missense mutation of *ADGRE2* has been reported to be associated with familial vibratory urticaria with autosomal dominant inheritance.[53]

AQUAGENIC URTICARIA

Aquagenic urticaria is a rare subtype of urticaria induced by local skin exposure to water. The eruptions are induced regardless of the temperature of the water. This characteristic of aquagenic urticaria helps differentiate it from cold urticaria and heat urticaria, which may also be induced by skin exposure to water at certain temperatures. Aquagenic urticaria is characterized by small wheals, resembling eruptions of cholinergic urticaria, but wheals in this urticaria subtype are generally fewer in number as compared with eruptions of cholinergic urticaria. They are usually surrounded by wide flares. Pruritus without a wheal and flare reaction developing after exposure to water is classified as aquagenic pruritus of a different disease entity.[54]

CHOLINERGIC URTICARIA

Cholinergic urticaria is a distinct subtype of urticaria induced by stimuli that cause sweating and distinctive for its small urticarial eruptions. Cholinergic urticaria is more common in children, adolescents, and young adults. Stimuli can be physical exercise, a hot temperature environment, or emotional or gustatory excitation. The eruptions are punctate 1- to 4-mm wheals or red spots with or without surrounding flare (see Fig. 41-1C). In severe cases, the eruptions may become confluent, generalized urticaria and even develop into anaphylaxis.[35,55,56] In rare cases, such lesions may accompany angioedema (*cholinergic angioedema*).[34,57] A case of angioedema that developed in response to exercise without punctate wheals or erythema was also reported.[58] Of note, most patients who develop angioedema are female and have an associated atopic diathesis or sweat allergy.[57,58] Cholinergic urticaria is usually pruritic but may be painful or sting, especially at the time when eruptions are developing. The wheal and flare reaction usually develops within 30 minutes and completely disappears within a few hours.

Cholinergic urticaria must be differentiated from exercise-induced urticaria and anaphylaxis, which is induced by exercise but not by passive warming. Certain cases of cholinergic urticaria may be evoked by systemic cold stimuli (*cold cholinergic urticaria*). Such cases should be differentiated from familial cold urticaria. Pruritus without wheals induced by conditions that elicit sweating has also been described (*cholinergic pruritus*).[59]

A substantial proportion of patients with cholinergic urticaria may also have atopic dermatitis and show type I hypersensitivity against human sweat.[60] The major antigen in sweat has been identified as MGL_1304, a protein produced and released by *Malassezia globosa* on human skin.[61,62] Another subset of patients with cholinergic urticaria have partial impairment of sweat production.[63] Most patients with this type of cholinergic urticaria complain of pain rather than itching, especially in winter.[35]

CONTACT URTICARIA

Contact urticaria is classified as a subtype of inducible urticaria characterized by immediate development of a wheal and flare reaction at the site of contact with specific substances. It may be either immunologic (IgE mediated) or nonimmunologic. The wheal and flare usually appears within 30 minutes and completely disappears within a few hours and may also develop into generalized urticaria and even anaphylaxis. Cold urticaria, heat urticaria, and aquagenic urticaria are also induced by contact with a substance with corresponding physical characteristics but are usually not included in this category. Cases in which oral edema and discomfort are the main symptoms, induced by contact of the oral mucosa with certain foods, are called as *oral allergy syndrome* (OAS).[64]

URTICARIAL VASCULITIS

Urticarial vasculitis is characterized by recurrent urticarial lesions that last for more than 24 hours, leaving pigmentation and demonstrating histopathologic evidence of leukocytoclastic vasculitis. Shapes of wheals and flare observed in urticarial vasculitis are similar to those observed in spontaneous urticaria and may be indistinguishable from those of CSU with long-lasting wheals. Patients with urticarial vasculitis may also develop livedo reticularis, Raynaud phenomenon, and angioedema.[65-69]

URTICARIAL REACTIONS AND SYMPTOMS OF OTHER SYSTEMIC DISEASE ENTITIES

Wheal Developing from Skin Test: Wheals and flare may develop in response to intracutaneous injection of histamine or antigen. However, these reactions are usually not included in urticaria as a disease entity.

Hereditary Angioedema: Hereditary angioedema is a disease entity characterized by recurrent angioedema based on a hereditary etiology. Symptoms of HAE may develop anywhere in the body, especially in the skin, gastrointestinal tract and airway, and be extremely severe. This may be clinically indistinguishable from angioedema secondary to idiopathic mechanisms (see Fig. 41-1E). Importantly, those with HAE do not develop superficial wheals. Patients with HAE may be complicated with urticaria, but it is very rare.

Anaphylaxis: Wheal and flare is the most frequent sign observed in anaphylaxis. Anaphylaxis is induced by either allergic or nonallergic mechanisms and includes systemic symptoms beyond involvement of the skin.

Darier Sign: This is a wheal and flare reaction induced by scratching a lesion of mastocytosis. Nonlesional skin does not produce such a reaction.

ETIOLOGY AND PATHOGENESIS

The common feature of urticaria is a rapid and transient vasodilation and extravasation of plasma into cutaneous or mucosal tissues accompanied by itch sensory nerve activation. These reactions are mostly explained by degranulation of cutaneous mast cells, which release histamine and other vasoactive mediators, including arachidonic acid metabolites, such as prostaglandins and leukotrienes. The crucial role of mast cells in urticaria has been proven by histologic observations of mast cell degranulation in the lesional skin of wheals, the increase of local histamine concentration in skin fluid or plasma of urticarial lesions, and the clinical efficacy of antihistamines for more than half of patients with CSU.[20] Indeed, type I hypersensitivity against exogenous antigens may well explain such reactions in allergic urticaria. However, the mechanism of mast cell activation and its relationship to various underlying diseases in other types of urticaria are largely unclear.

TYPE I HYPERSENSITIVITY

Mast cells play a pivotal role in type I hypersensitivity reactions via the high-affinity IgE receptors (FcεRI) and antigen-specific IgE (Fig. 41-3). Crosslinking of FcεRI leads to the activation of numerous signaling molecules, SYK, LAT, PLCγ, and PKC, and finally results in degranulation with release of preformed mediators such as histamine and newly synthesized ones such as arachidonic acid metabolites, platelet-activating factor, and proinflammatory cytokines.[63] Patients who possess antigen-specific IgE may respond to antigens that reach cutaneous mast cells via various pathways such as ingestion, inhalation, or skin exposure. If patients are exposed daily to the causative antigen, urticaria may be chronic.[70] Otherwise, urticaria developing through this mechanism appears as episodic or acute urticaria. Certain dietary antigens that take time to be absorbed, such as poly-γ-glutamine contained in fermented soybeans and gel-fish, may cause symptoms after a few hours or even later.[71,72] However, in most cases, urticaria symptoms develop in 15 minutes to 1 hour after the antigen exposure. Many studies suggest that the population of patients who develop urticaria because of clinically apparent, classical type I allergy against exogenous antigens, such as food and drugs, is less than 10% of the whole population of patients with urticaria.[73,74]

Recently, it has been proven that approximately two thirds of patients with cholinergic urticaria are sensitized by antigens in human sweat. Such patients show positive

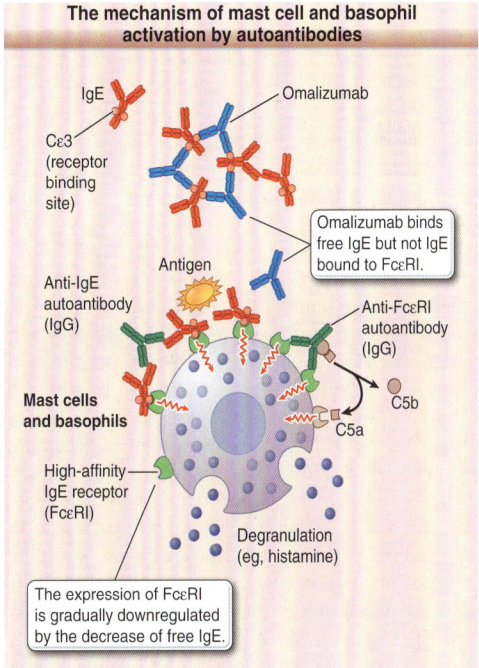

Figure 41-3 The pathogenesis of autoimmune urticaria and the proposed mechanism of action of omalizumab for autoimmune urticaria. FcεRI, the high-affinity immunoglobulin E receptor; Ig, immunoglobulin.

reactions in skin testing with autologous sweat and histamine release testing using their basophils and purified human sweat.[60,61] The major antigen of human sweat for these reactions has been identified as MGL_1304, a 17-kD protein produced and released by *M. globosa*.[62]

AUTOIMMUNE MECHANISM

An autoimmune diathesis in CSU was initially suspected because of the increased incidence of antithyroid antibodies, including antimicrosomal (peroxidase) and antithyroglobulin IgG autoantibodies, as seen in patients with Hashimoto disease.[75]

It is now known that one third to half of patients with CSU possess functional IgG autoantibodies against IgE[76] or the high-affinity IgE receptors (FcεRI)[77] that release histamine from mast cells and basophils.[78] Autoantibodies against IgE crosslink IgE together with FcεRI to which the IgE bind. In cases with autoantibodies against FcεRI, they directly bind to and crosslink FcεRI without IgE. In a certain population of patients, IgE bound to FcεRI competes with the autoantibodies against FcεRI (see Fig. 41-3). The histamine-releasing (basophil-activating) activity of the autoantibodies against FcεRI is partially, if not fully, dependent on the activation the classical complement cascade.[79,80] The presence of these autoantibodies may be screened using ASST and proven with the histamine release test using sera of the patients and basophils obtained from healthy individuals.[81]

Patients with CSU and a positive ASST result might be more intractable and reveal more severe symptoms than those with a negative ASST result.[82] A recent study revealed that the time to respond to treatment with omalizumab for patients with a positive ASST result is longer than for those with a negative ASST.[83]

The involvement of autoantigens that bind to IgE has also been suggested both in CSU and inducible urticarias.[78] Recently, the mechanism of autoimmunity involving tissue antigens recognized by IgE and that mentioned above involving IgE/FcεRI recognized by IgG have been proposed to be classified as type I and type II autoimmunities, respectively.[78] The involvement of type I autoimmunity has been suggested based on passive transfer of the sensitization using sera of patients or skin tests with human skin extracts.[84-93] In solar urticaria, there is evidence that an antigen on the skin may become evident on irradiation with light of crucial wavelengths followed by complement activation.[94-96] Histamine release from skin tissue specimens biopsied from a patient with cold urticaria in response to cooling and rewarming suggests the presence of a pathogenic molecule in the skin that is sufficient to activate mast cells.[97] However, no solid molecules have been identified to date.

Autoantibodies, either IgG or IgE against thyroid antigens, such as thyroglobulin and TPO, may be detected in patients with CSU. However, they are mostly not related to abnormalities of thyroid function, and the therapeutic effect of thyroxin on urticaria with normal thyroid functions is controversial.[98] Furthermore, the continuous presence of autoantibodies or autoantigens cannot explain diurnal and local occurrence of wheals observed in spontaneous urticaria. Thus, no autoantigens have been identified that explain the entire clinical picture of urticaria in each patient. Nevertheless, recently observed rapid effects of omalizumab, anti-IgE antibody, on both spontaneous and physical urticarias suggest the involvement of endogenous antigens that bind to IgE in the pathogenesis of various, if not all, types of urticaria.[99] Studies of some patients with physical urticaria suggested the involvement of abnormal IgE that change confirmation in response to physical stimuli and activate mast cells.[100]

In a subtype of urticarial vasculitis with hypocomplementemia, IgG autoantibody against C1q is identified (*hypocomplementemic urticarial vasculitis syndrome*).[66]

PSEUDOALLERGY

Nonallergic hypersensitivity to dietary pseudoallergens, including naturally occurring food ingredients such as salicylates and biogenous amines, food additives, and continuous use of oral or topical nonsteroidal antiinflammatory drugs (NSAIDs), may be relevant as a cause or a precipitating or aggravating factor for CSU. Because the mechanism of urticaria provoked by pseudoallergens remains unclear, strict exclusion and subsequent provocation testing with a suspected substance are necessary for the diagnosis.[32] For a diagnosis of food pseudoallergy, a 3-week pseudoallergen-free diet may be followed by well-motivated patients. The increased sensitivity of patients with CSU to histamine in the diet (histamine intolerance) has been suggested.[101] In fact, high concentrations of histamine produced in scombroid (histidine-rich fish) by bacteria-derived histidine-decarboxylase may cause anaphylactic reactions even in apparently normal individuals (scombroid poisoning).[102] Moreover, symptoms of some patients with CSU may be improved by the avoidance of pseudoallergens and histamine in the diet. However, the efficacy of such diet restriction in the management of CSU is still controversial.[103] Although many reports suggest that food additives aggravate chronic urticaria, they may be based on self-reporting[22] or on the improvement in symptoms from stringent pseudoallergen-free diets.[104] In a double-blind, placebo-controlled study, only 19% of patients responded to a provocation test with individual pseudoallergens, but the symptoms of 73% of patients ceased or were greatly reduced on the pseudoallergen-free diet. Red wines may contain vasoactive amines, including histamine, which could aggravate urticaria, but symptoms poorly correlate with histamine content.[105] Notably, pseudoallergy may not be simply diagnosed based on a patient's history.[101] Thus, dietary factors, including pseudoallergens and histamine, are likely involved in the cause of CSU to some extent, but none of them by themselves may explain the mechanisms of direct mast cell activation.

COAGULATION SYSTEM

In patients with CSU, especially those with severe symptoms, the levels of plasma coagulation markers, such as prothrombin fragment 1+2 (PF_{1+2}), fibrin degradative products (FDPs), and D-dimer, are higher than those in healthy control participants. They correlate with disease severity and return to normal levels with remission or control of symptoms by treatments.[106-110] Moreover, an increased potential for blood coagulation is also observed to correlate with disease severity in CSU.[111,112] Furthermore, massive expression of tissue factors has been demonstrated in eosinophils in the lesions of CSU.[108] Alternatively, small amounts of histamine and lipopolysaccharides may synergistically induce the expression of tissue factors, which is sufficient to trigger the coagulation cascade on endothelial cells.[113] Activated coagulation factors, such as FVIIa, FXa, and thrombin, can activate protease-activating receptors (PARs) and may thus activate skin mast cells. In fact, medications that control coagulation and the fibrinolytic system, such as warfarin, nafamostat, and the combination of heparin and tranexamic acid, have been reported to be effective for cases of CSU.[114-117] However, no direct evidence of human mast cell activation by activated coagulation factors by themselves has been reported. Moreover, no clinically apparent thrombosis is observed in patients with urticaria. Thus, it is still not clear whether abnormalities in the coagulation pathway observed in CSU are causative or epiphenomena of increased vascular permeability.

UNDERLYING DISORDERS ASSOCIATED WITH INDUCIBLE URTICARIAS

Symptoms of inducible urticarias are induced by specific stimuli, including specific physical conditions, sweat induction, and contact with specific substances corresponding to physical urticarias, cholinergic urticaria, and contact urticaria, respectively. As mentioned earlier, specific IgE may link such stimuli and mast cells, resulting in allergic reactions in response to the stimuli. The other mechanisms that make patients sensitive to certain stimuli remains largely unknown. However, in limited cases of cold urticaria, solar urticaria, and vibratory angioedema, definitive causes may be identified by serologic or genetic analyses.

COLD URTICARIA

Most cases of local cold urticaria are considered to be primary cold urticaria. In this type, no relation to underlying causes or abnormal findings upon clinical examination are observed. In rare cases, cryoproteins, such as cryoglobulin and cryofibrinogen, may be identified, either idiopathically or in association with collagen vascular disease, chronic lymphatic leukemia, myeloma, or infectious disease, including infectious mononucleosis.[86,118,119] Hereditary systemic cold urticaria may be presented as a systemic inflammatory symptom caused by genetic mutations of *NLRP3 (CIAS1)* or *PLCG2* (see the "Cold Urticaria" section of Clinical Features).

SOLAR URTICARIA

The cause of solar urticaria is usually unknown, but a rare case can be diagnosed as caused by porphyrias and classified as type VI solar urticaria.[120,121]

VIBRATORY ANGIOEDEMA

Recently, a missense mutation in *ADGRE2* has been identified in patients with autosomal dominant vibratory urticaria and revealed to make mast cells sensitive to vibration in an IgE-independent manner.[53] The role of protein coded by *ADGRE2* in nonhereditary-type vibratory angioedema remains to be investigated.

NEUROLOGIC MECHANISM

It is a unique characteristic of mast cells in the skin or connective tissues that they respond to basic peptides, such as substance P, vasoactive intestinal peptide, somatostatin, neurokinin A and B, bradykinin, calcitonin gene-related peptide, and adrenocorticotropic hormone (ACTH).[122-125] They also express numerous receptors for ligands, including the above-mentioned neuropeptides and acetylcholine as well as Toll-like receptors.[63,78,126,127] Therefore, these neurotransmitters have been hypothesized to be triggers of mast cell activation in urticaria. However, the concentration required for a neuropeptide to induce histamine release is as high as 10^{-6} M,[128] and the mechanism of neuropeptide release in the skin is still unclear. Recently, excessive release of acetylcholine from the cholinergic nerve terminal to compensate for impaired sweat production by sweat glands in acquired idiopathic generalized anhidrosis was suggested as a mechanism of mast cell activation and the development of cholinergic urticaria observed in this disease.[63]

INFECTIONS

Acute infections by viruses and bacteria are known to be often associated with spontaneous urticaria, especially with the onset of acute urticaria in children and in transient aggravation of CSU.[129] Many studies have suggested chronic persistent infection by *Helicobacter pylori* as an important cause of CSU,[130] but its significance is disputed.[131,132] The relationship between many other kinds of infections and urticaria have not been substantiated.

STRESS AND FATIGUE

Many investigators have suggested a relationship between stress or fatigue and aggravation or elicitation of urticaria.[133] Patients with CSU were found to have higher levels of life event stress and perceived stress[134] and experienced stressful life events before the onset of the disease.[135-137] However, urticaria itself induces stress and impairs the quality of life (QOL) of patients. Moreover, the importance of psychological factors is difficult to scientifically evaluate. Depression and anxiety were found more frequently in patients with chronic urticaria in one study[138] but not in another.[139] Thus, it is controversial whether stress and fatigue should be included as underlying causes of urticaria. Nevertheless, with respect to QOL assessments, it is good clinical practice to ask patients with urticaria about their psychosomatic and psychiatric conditions.

OTHER ORGAN DISORDERS

In addition to infections and thyroid dysfunction, which have already been described, many other extracutaneous disorders such as collagen diseases and malignancies have been reported to underlie chronic urticaria. In some cases, the treatment of these disorders resulted in the remission of urticaria. However, reports are mostly anecdotal, and a large epidemiologic study denied the association between malignancies and chronic urticaria.[140] A retrospective population-based cohort study using data from the National Health Insurance research database in Taiwan reported an increased risk of hematologic malignancies.[141] With respect to physical urticaria, cryoglobulinemia was identified in several patients with cold contact urticaria (see the paragraph of "Cold Urticaria in Underlying Disorders Associated With Inducible Urticarias" in this section). However, in other cases, the relationship between these disorders and the pathogenesis of urticaria is largely unknown. Moreover, screening for malignant neoplasms as a routine test for urticaria is no longer recommended by the guidelines and consensus document.[1,142]

In cases of angioedema without wheals, myeloproliferative disorders and autoimmune disorders such as SLE may underlie the disease by consuming C1-hinhibitor (C1-INH) and developing autoantibodies against C1-INH, respectively, resulting in an overproduction of bradykinin[143] (Fig. 41-4).

OTHER FACTORS THAT MAY INDUCE OR AGGRAVATE URTICARIAL REACTIONS

Various factors are known to elicit or aggravate urticaria, which are mostly preexisting. They may be a cause of episodic or acute urticaria but not fundamental causes of chronic urticarias (Table 41-3). They should be carefully evaluated and avoided, if present.

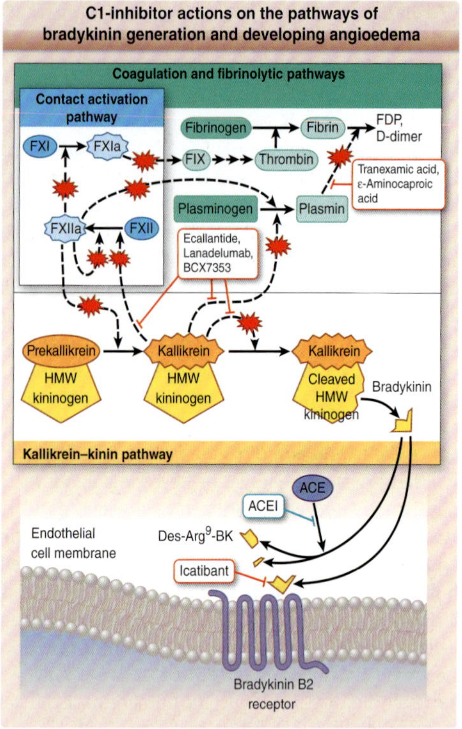

Figure 41-4 C1 inhibitor actions on pathways involved in bradykinin production. Points of inhibition by C1 inhibitor are shown by *red blasts*; other known mechanisms of pathway inhibition are also detailed. ACE, angiotensin-converting enzyme; ACEI, angiotensin-converting enzyme inhibitor; F, factor; FDP, fibrin degradative product; HMW, high molecular weight. (Information in this illustration was derived from Zuraw BL. Clinical practice. Hereditary angioedema. *N Engl J Med*. 2008;359:1027-1036.)

ASPIRIN AND OTHER NONSTEROIDAL ANTIINFLAMMATORY DRUGS

Aspirin and other NSAIDs, which inhibit cyclooxygenase (COX)-1, may induce or aggravate wheals and angioedema. These medications may also elicit respiratory symptoms (aspirin asthma). However,

TABLE 41-3
Potential Causes of Episodic or Acute Urticaria

Foods: allergens such as milk and eggs (for infants), nuts, seeds, fruits, and seafood (for adults) and pseudoallergens (food additives, salicylates, histamine, and other amines)

Drugs: antibiotics (β-lactams, vancomycin, polymyxin B), NSAIDs (oral, injection, topical), opioids, contrast media, opioids, ACE inhibitors (for angioedema)

Vaccines

Blood products: transfusions

Stings: bee, wasp venoms

Contactants: latex, chemicals

Inhalants: latex powder, chemicals

ACE, angiotensin-converting enzyme; NSAID, nonsteroidal antiinflammatory drug.

the development of skin symptoms and respiratory symptoms appears to be independent.[144,145] Food-dependent exercise-induced urticaria (FDEIA) may be aggravated or induced by aspirin or NSAIDs when administered with causative dietary elements even without exercise.[146,147] COX-2–selective NSAIDs tend to be safer than aspirin or other relatively potent COX-1 inhibitors. However, sensitivities of individual patients to NSAIDs are not necessarily correlated with their COX-1 inhibitory activities.[145]

SERUM SICKNESS

Several days to a few weeks after the administration of the offending agent, which could be not only heterologous serum, but also be certain drugs, urticaria may develop with fever, lymphadenopathy, myalgia, arthralgia, and arthritis. Symptoms are usually self-limited and last 4 to 5 days.[148,149]

BLOOD PRODUCTS

Urticaria may develop after the administration of blood products. It usually is the result of immune complex formation and complement activation.[149] Aggregated IgG may also be responsible for urticarial reactions.[149]

CONTRAST MEDIA

Contrast media may cause allergic reactions after its intravenous infusion. The prevalence of allergic reactions to iodinated contrast media (ICM) is estimated to be 0.05% to 0.1% of patients undergoing radiologic studies with ICM.[150] The application of nonionic dimeric ICM with higher physiological osmolality has decreased the number of immediate reactions occurring within 1 hour, but the prevalence of nonimmediate hypersensitivity reactions has increased in the past decade. Erythema and wheals with or without angioedema are the most common signs of immediate reactions, but delayed nonimmediate reactions may include a maculopapular rash.[150]

Most reactions are attributed to non-IgE mechanisms, but an IgE-mediated mechanism was also proven by positive skin testing or basophil activation testing in some cases.[150]

OTHER MAST CELL AND BASOPHIL ACTIVATORS

Opiate analgesics, polymyxin B, curare, D-tubocurarine, and vancomycin induce histamine release from mast cells or basophils, especially when given at high doses, and may cause urticaria or other cutaneous rashes upon the episode of administration.[149,151] On the other hand, angiotensin-converting enzyme (ACE) inhibitors do not cause release or production of mediators by themselves but inhibit degradation of bradykinin. Unlike most other medications, these may cause or aggravate angioedema after multiple administrations over a few days or longer after administration. These medications thus function as an underlying cause of angioedema rather than a direct stimulus (see Fig. 41-4).[143]

RISK FACTORS

Urticaria may occur at any age, and no difference in prevalence has been reported based on race or ethnic group. Women outnumber men by two to one with CSU. CSU may be associated with infections and autoimmune disorders, such as thyroid diseases and collagen diseases (see section "Complications in the Clinical Features"). However, the prevalence of urticaria in patients with these diseases is low, and thus they are not generally thought of as risk factors. Genetic analysis of a white population indicated a strong association between HLA-DR4 and patients with CSU with functional autoantibodies against IgE or FcεRI.[152] Cholinergic urticaria is often complicated by atopic dermatitis.[60] Urticaria mediated by an IgE mechanism, especially those caused by latex allergy and OAS, may be associated with an atopic diathesis. Health care workers, individuals with atopic dermatitis, and patients with spina bifida have a higher risk of developing latex allergy than other people.[153]

DIAGNOSIS

A characteristic feature of urticaria is the transient nature of individual eruptions. Therefore, the diagnosis of urticaria itself is not difficult. However, the diagnosis of subtypes of urticaria is necessary for proper management in individual patients. Laboratory tests and provocation tests should be performed based on careful history taking and inspection. Extensive laboratory investigations add little to making a final diagnosis.[154] The overall diagnostic algorithm recommended by the EAACI guidelines[1] is shown in Fig. 41-5.

HISTORY TAKING

A thorough and comprehensive history is essential for diagnosis and the elucidation of causative or aggravating factors. Because clinical examination findings for urticaria are highly variable and depend on the subtypes of urticaria, it is most important to narrow down the clinical diagnosis based on the history and physical examination before laboratory testing. Flares in disease activity during the evening to early morning is not specific but is a common feature of spontaneous urticaria. Wheals of inducible urticaria do not usually last for more than 4 hours, except for those of DPU. In some types of physical urticaria such as delayed dermographism[43] and delayed cold urticaria,[46] wheals may occur several hours after the stimuli, but the wheal does not last for long. Triggers; aggravating factors, if any; and the shape, size, and duration of

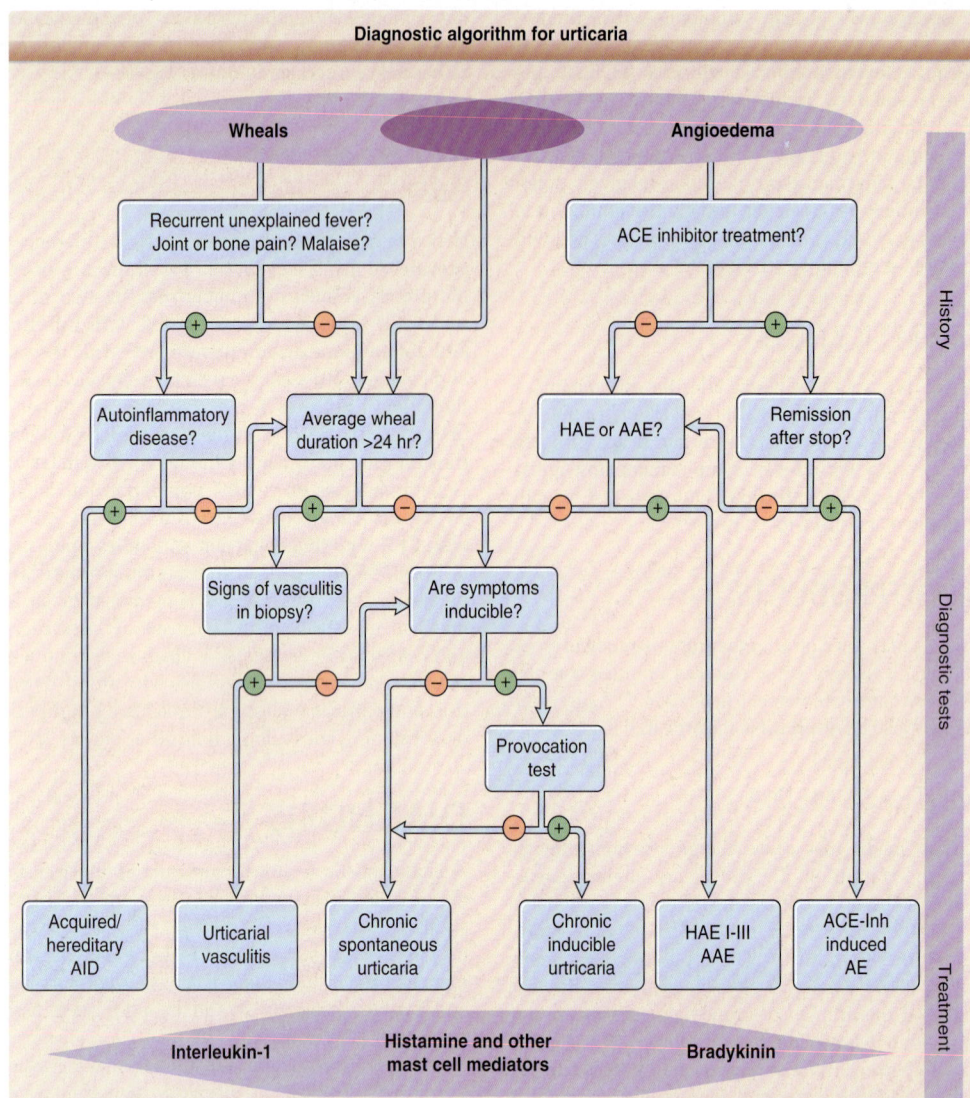

Figure 41-5 Diagnostic algorithm for urticaria. AAE, acquired angioedema due to C1-inhibitor deficiency; ACE-Inh, angiotensin-converting enzyme inhibitor; AE, angioedema; AID, auto-inflammatory disease; HAE, hereditary angioedema. (From Zuberbier T, Aberer W, Asero R, et al. The EAACI/GA(2) LEN/EDF/WAO Guideline for the definition, classification, diagnosis, and management of urticaria: the 2013 revision and update. *Allergy*. 2014;69:868-887, with permission. Copyright © 2014 John Wiley & Sons.)

individual wheals helps in diagnosing the subtype of urticaria (see section "Cutaneous Findings in the Clinical Features"). Urticarial vasculitis should be ruled out if individual wheals last for 24 hours or longer, especially with purpura. Mast cell–mediated angioedema (ie, non–bradykinin-mediated type) does not usually occur in the larynx. Bradykinin-mediated angioedema does not accompany superficial wheals.

LABORATORY TESTING

No routine laboratory testing is necessary or recommended for acute spontaneous urticaria. If a patient's history strongly suggests an allergic mechanism, prick tests and measurement of antigen-specific IgE are recommended. For CSU, a complete blood count, erythrocyte sedimentation rate, or C-reactive protein (CRP) is recommended. For further investigation, an extended diagnostic workup such as examination for *Helicobacter pylori*, Type I allergy, autoantibodies, and thyroid hormone may be undertaken. It is important, however, to note that the detection of a specific disorder may not always lead to an improvement in the symptoms of urticaria. Potential blood biomarkers in CSU to distinguish patients and control participants are D-dimer, CRP, matrix metalloproteinase-9, mean platelet volume (MPV), factor VIIa, prothrombin fragment 1+2 (PF1+2), tumor necrosis factor (TNF), dehydroepiandrosterone sulphate, and vitamin D.[155] Biomarkers reflecting disease severity in CSU are FDP, D-dimer, F1+2, CRP, interleukin-6 (IL-6), and MPV.[110,155]

Several factors, diseases, and conditions have been reported as underlying causes of urticaria. However, a systematic review of the laboratory investigations for chronic urticaria revealed that the number of diagnoses identified varied from 1% to 84% and was not related to the number of laboratory tests performed.[156] Therefore, extensive workups are not recommended for routine screening of the causes of urticarias unless suggested by the medical history or physical examination.[1] The recommended diagnostic tests corresponding to each urticaria subtype are summarized in Table 41-1.

DIAGNOSIS OF URTICARIA SUBTYPES

After thorough history taking and careful skin inspection, the following diagnostic tests should be considered based on tentative clinical diagnosis of urticaria subtype (see Table 41-1).

SPONTANEOUS URTICARIA

The diagnosis of spontaneous urticaria is made based on history and skin inspection. In addition to the spontaneous appearance of wheals of characteristic shape, diurnal variation and a long-lasting course of individual wheals may help make this diagnosis. For acute spontaneous urticaria, no routine laboratory tests are recommended, but the diseases and reactions listed in Table 41-4 should be differentiated. The presence of extracutaneous signs and symptoms and long-lasting eruptions, especially with purpura or epidermal change, such as dryness and desquamation, are important signs of different or complicated diseases. For such eruptions, a skin biopsy should help solidify the diagnosis.

The presence of IgG autoantibodies against IgE or FcεRI should be demonstrated by a histamine release assay using the patient's serum and basophils from healthy donors. This test may reveal the specificity of the autoantibodies against IgE, FcεRI, and degrees of their dependence on or competition with IgE for histamine release. However, this assay is somewhat cumbersome and requires special equipment, which has therefore limited its application. A solid phase assay, such as enzyme-linked immunosorbent assay, is relatively easy and quantitative but not specific.[79] Alternatively, skin reactions evoked by ASST[81] have been widely used as a screening test because of their relative simplicity and high sensitivity. In ASST, 0.05 mL of autologous serum is intradermally injected on the volar forearm skin along with normal saline and 10 μg/mL of histamine as the negative and positive controls, respectively.

SYMPTOMATIC DERMOGRAPHISM (MECHANICAL URTICARIA)

For the diagnosis of symptomatic dermographism, several instruments have been developed and used to determine the threshold of individual patients. The forearm is more suitable for this test than the abdomen, back, or pretibial areas. The result is considered positive if the patient shows a wheal and reports itching at the site of provocation at 36 g/mm^2 or less. A wheal response without itching on provocation at 60 g/mm^2 or higher indicates the less clinically significant simple dermographism.[32] Reactions of this subtype of urticaria and other inducible urticarias, except for DPU, should be evaluated 5 to 10 minutes after testing.

COLD CONTACT URTICARIA

Cold provocation is performed by applying a wrapped ice cube or cold water for 5 minutes. In this way, the threshold duration of cold application can be determined. The use of a thermoelectric element (TempTest)[157] can be used to determine the threshold by temperature.[32] These tests induce wheal formation in cold contact urticaria but not for systemic cold urticaria, in which patients develop widespread wheals in response to cooling of the core body temperature or to cold wind.[47,49]

Systemic cold urticaria should be differentiated from cold contact urticaria because it may be a manifestation of autoinflammatory disease (familial cold urticaria; see Cold Urticaria in section "Clinical Features").

HEAT URTICARIA

Provocation of heat contact urticaria is performed by applying hot metal, water, or a glass cylinder filled with hot water at 45°C to the skin of the volar forearm.

TABLE 41-4
Differential Diagnosis of Urticaria

Wheal-like Eruption
1. Insect bites
2. Erythema multiforme
3. Erythema nodosum
4. Drug eruptions
5. Adult-onset Still disease
6. Shiitake dermatitis (resembling dermographic urticaria)
7. Maculopapular cutaneous mastocytosis (urticaria pigmentosa)
8. Urticarial vasculitis
9. Cryopyrin-associated periodic syndromes
10. Schnitzler syndrome
11. Polymorphic eruption of pregnancy

Angioedema-like Eruption
1. Insect bites
2. Cellulitis
3. Erysipelas
4. Episodic angioedema with eosinophilia
5. Bradykinin-mediated angioedema (eg, HAE)
6. Well's syndrome
7. Cheilitis granulomatosa
8. Granulomatous blepharitis

HAE, hereditary angioedema.
Data from Zuberbier T, et al. *Allergy* 2014;69:868-87; Bernstein JA, Lang DM, Khan DA, et al. The diagnosis and management of acute and chronic urticaria: 2014 update. *J Allergy Clin Immunol.* 2014;133(5):1270-1277; and Hide M, et al. *Nihon Hifukagakkai Zasshi* 2011;121:1339-88.

The *TempTest*[157] used for cold contact urticaria may also be used for this type of urticaria. Cholinergic urticaria, solar urticaria, and aquagenic urticaria, which may also be associated with high temperatures or hot water, should be differentiated.

SOLAR URTICARIA

Solar urticaria should be differentiated from polymorphic light eruption. A provocation test for solar urticaria should be done on the buttock skin, but parts of the trunk that are usually covered by clothes can also be tested. The light source may be sunlight or a slide projector from a distance of 10 cm with or without filters or a monochromator (ultraviolet [UV] A or B, or visible light).[32]

DELAYED PRESSURE URTICARIA

Provocation may be performed by suspending a 7-kg weight on a 3-cm shoulder strap for 15 minutes or applying rods supported in a frame to the back, thighs, or forearm. Unlike the other inducible urticarias, the skin reaction should occur after a latent period, typically 2 to 4 hours after the pressure has been applied. Skin biopsies reveal an inflammatory infiltrate with prominent eosinophils but no vasculitis.[32]

VIBRATORY URTICARIA AND ANGIOEDEMA

The forearms are held on a flat plate placed on a vortex mixer that runs at between 780 and 1380 rpm for 10 minutes. The site of application should be assessed for swelling 10 minutes after testing.[32]

AQUAGENIC URTICARIA

Provocation is performed by attaching wet clothes at body temperature for 20 minutes. Wiping the test area with an organic solvent and challenging with saline instead of tap water may increase the reactivity.[1,32,158]

CHOLINERGIC URTICARIA

The diagnosis is established by an appropriate provocation test for the patient's age and general condition (eg, on a treadmill or stationary bicycle). To differentiate from exercise-induced anaphylaxis, a passive warming test should be done, recording core body temperature to achieve an increase of 1.0°C or more. Skin testing with intradermal injection of 0.1 mL of acetylcholine at 100 µg/mL may reinforce the diagnosis of cholinergic urticaria. The test result should be considered positive if the test site shows satellite wheals around the injection site. The specificity of this test seems to be high, but the sensitivity is approximately 30% to 50%.[32]

CONTACT URTICARIA

For the diagnosis of contact urticaria, the suspected substance is applied in its original form or as an extract on a normal looking area of the volar forearm or the upper back for 15 to 20 minutes. If this test result is negative, occlusive application is applied followed by a prick test. For patients with a history of severe symptoms, tests should be started with sufficiently diluted suspected substances. *In vitro* tests may also be used for contact urticaria from Type I allergy, such as latex allergy.[32]

URTICARIAL VASCULITIS

Urticaria-like eruptions that last for longer than 24 hours should be differentiated from urticarial vasculitis. Clinical features such as fevers, malaise, arthralgia, uveitis, diffuse glomerulonephritis, and obstructive and restrictive pulmonary disease may be diagnostically helpful, but histologic examination of a skin biopsy is essential for confirmation of the diagnosis.[67,159]

ANGIOEDEMA

Angioedema is diagnosed mostly by its clinical features, including localized mucosal or deep skin edema that is nonpitting and lasts for hours to a few days. If angioedema is induced by specific stimuli that are also known to induce superficial wheals or occurs together with wheals, it is likely mast cell mediated and is classified as a subtype of urticaria (see Table 41-1). If angioedema occurs spontaneously without wheals, a bradykinin-mediated mechanism should be carefully differentiated. Whereas mast cell–mediated spontaneous angioedema can be severe but is mostly nonlethal, bradykinin-mediated angioedema can be lethal.[143] The mechanisms of bradykinin production and degradation with related molecules are shown in Fig. 41-4.

Hereditary Angioedema: HAE is classified into three subtypes based on the condition of C1-INH.[143,160] Patients with type I lack C1-INH protein, but those with type II lack activity of C1-INH because of genetic point mutations. Type III, also called as HAE with normal C1-INH, is a rare subtype of HAE. Type III develops mostly in females, and a gain-of-function mutation of factor XII may be identified in some patients. Recently, new genetic mutations, one in an angiopoietin-1 gene and another in a plasminogen gene, were identified in families with type III HAE.[161,162] Whereas the levels of C1-INH activity and C4 are decreased in both type I and type II HAE, C1-INH protein concentration is low only in type I HAE. During attacks of HAE, coagulation markers, such as D-dimer, FDP and PF1+2 may increase.[163,164] Prodromal symptoms, such as erythema marginatum, may precede HAE attacks in up to 50% of patients.

Acquired Angioedema: Bradykinin-mediated angioedema may develop either by overconsumption of C1-INH caused by myeloproliferative diseases or because of the presence of autoantibodies against C1-INH. In the case of overconsumption of C1-INH, the level of C1q is decreased, as well as those of C1-INH and C4.

Angiotensin-Converting Enzyme Inhibitor–Induced Angioedema: ACE is a dipeptidylcarboxypeptidase that converts angiotensin I to angiotensin II and cleaves bradykinin. Therefore, its inhibitor, ACE inhibitor, used for the treatment of hypertension, inhibits degradation of bradykinin.

AUTOINFLAMMATORY SYNDROME

Autoinflammatory diseases are a diverse group of inherited conditions characterized by systemic inflammation in the absence of infection and are accompanied by a range of organ-specific manifestations.[165] Two of them, Schnitzler syndrome and cryopyrin-associated periodical syndrome (CAPS), are known to include urticaria-like symptoms.

Schnitzler Syndrome: Schnitzler syndrome is characterized by urticaria-like eruptions and monoclonal IgM or possibly IgG gammopathy accompanied by systemic symptoms such as fever and bone and muscle pain.[166,167] Its histology resembles an urticarial vasculitis or neutrophilic urticaria.

Cryopyrin Associated Periodical Syndrome: Familial cold-autoinflammatory syndrome, Muckle-Wells syndrome, and chronic infantile neurologic cutaneous articular syndrome may include an urticaria-like eruption. The eruption may be induced by exposure to cold but may also develop spontaneously and does not usually cause pruritus. Patients may develop periodic fever, arthralgia, amyloidosis, and nerve deafness. The common and crucial cause of these syndromes has been identified as gain-of-function mutations in *NLRP3 (CIAS1)*, resulting in overproduction of IL-1β.[168] Skin biopsy demonstrates neutrophil-dominant cell infiltration, but gene analysis is most definitive for making the diagnosis.

URTICARIA AND ANAPHYLAXIS INDUCED BY EXERCISE

Exercise may induce urticaria in patients with cholinergic urticaria and in patients with exercise-induced anaphylaxis. Some patients may develop urticaria and anaphylaxis regardless of food intake (exercise-induced anaphylaxis [EIA]), but others develop symptoms only when they exercise after eating certain foods (FDEIA). The demonstration of specific food allergen-reactive IgE in the serum may help but may not be sufficient for making the diagnosis of FDIEA.[146,147] The presence of anti–ω5-gliadine IgE in adults has been reported to be an exceptionally good marker for FDEIA caused by wheat in terms of both sensitivity and specificity.[169] An exercise challenge test is typically performed according to the protocol of Bruce and colleagues.[170] The sensitivity of provocation testing for FDEIA was reported to be up to 70%.[169]

EVALUATION OF DISEASE CONDITIONS

Urticaria and underlying conditions in patients with urticaria should be evaluated in both specific and comprehensive ways.

DISEASE SEVERITY

Disease severity of inducible urticarias may be evaluated according to the threshold for eliciting factors (see Table 41-1). For spontaneous urticaria and angioedema, questionnaire-based scores may be used. The urticaria activity score over 7 consecutive days (UAS7) is a unified and simple scoring system that records daily wheals and itching and has been validated in comparison with the Dermatology Life Quality Index (DLQI).[171] Disease activity of angioedema may be evaluated by a 4-week-long record of edema in terms of frequency, duration, subjective sensations, and disability of patients (Angioedema Activity Score [AAS]).[172]

For CSU, coagulation and fibrinolysis markers, such as D-dimer, FDP, PF1+2, and CRP, have been reported to reflect disease severity or activity (see Coagulation System in the section "Etiology and Pathogenesis"), but their sensitivities are low.[173] Serum levels of pro-inflammatory cytokines, such as IL-6, TNF, and IL-23, may also reflect disease activity in certain patients but are of doubtful usefulness.[32,174] Peripheral blood basopenia and low release of histamine from basophils may also be associated with disease activity,[175,176] but the value of these markers is at present confined to the research laboratory.[177]

QUALITY OF LIFE

CSU has a high overall impact on QOL as compared with other common dermatologic conditions,[178-180] The QOL of patients with superficial urticaria and that of patients with angioedema may be evaluated using the Chronic Urticaria Quality of Life Questionnaire (CU-Q2oL)[181] and Angioedema Quality of Life Questionnaire (AE-QoL),[182] respectively.[1]

CONTROL STATUS

The tools mentioned earlier—UAS-7, AAS, CU-Q2oL, and AE-QoL—may not adequately cover conditions of inducible urticarias and angioedema. More recently, an easy and comprehensive method of evaluation for all kinds of urticaria and angioedema has been developed. It is called the Urticaria Control Test (UCT), and it may be applied to all kinds of urticaria and angioedema.[183] The short version of the UCT asks only four retrospective questions about the patient's condition over the previous 4 weeks. These instruments have been translated and validated in many languages. The AAS, AE-QoL, and UCT are now available in various languages from Moxie GmbH, Berlin, Germany.[184]

PATHOLOGY

Pathological findings in urticaria consist of edema in the dermis and perivascular and interstitial infiltration of inflammatory cells. Inflammatory cells usually consist of lymphocytes, eosinophils, and neutrophils. Commonly, lymphocytes are dominant in the perivascular area, but eosinophils and neutrophils tend to have an interstitial distribution. A few reports revealed an increase in mast cells in perivascular areas and the interstitium of lesions,[185-187] but others did not.[188] The presence of basophils has been demonstrated with specific antibodies.[189] The degree of infiltration of these inflammatory cells varies according to subtypes of urticaria, individual variability, and the time from the onset of wheals (Figs. 41-6A to 41-6C). Detailed studies of infiltrated lymphocytes revealed that they are both Th_1 and Th_2, or Th_0 because they express IL-4, IL-5, and interferon (IFN)-γ.[190] Neutrophils and eosinophils exist in dermal capillaries, and this is considered as an early change in numerous inflammatory skin diseases, including urticarias. Infiltration of neutrophils is prominent especially in acute urticaria and physical urticarias. Urticaria or urticaria-like eruptions that persist for longer than a day and involve predominantly neutrophilic infiltration without apparent vasculitis may also be called neutrophilic urticaria, neutrophilic urticarial dermatosis, or urticaria-like neutrophilic dermatosis.[191-193] Similar changes may be observed in the skin lesions of CAPS and Schnitzler syndrome. Eosinophils may play a more important role than suggested by hematoxylin and eosin staining because extracellular eosinophil major basic protein is frequently

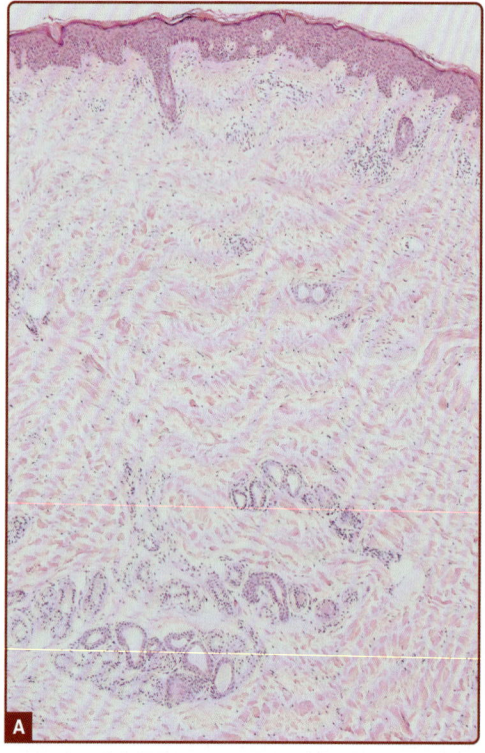

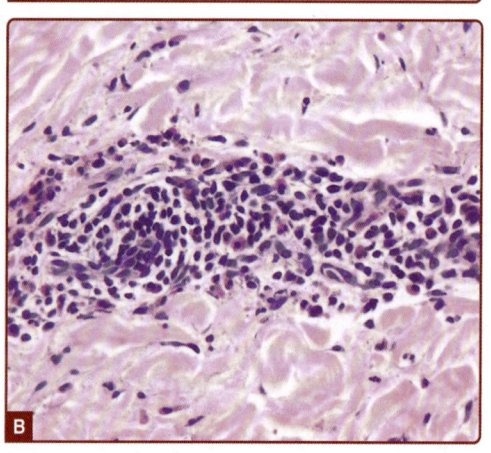

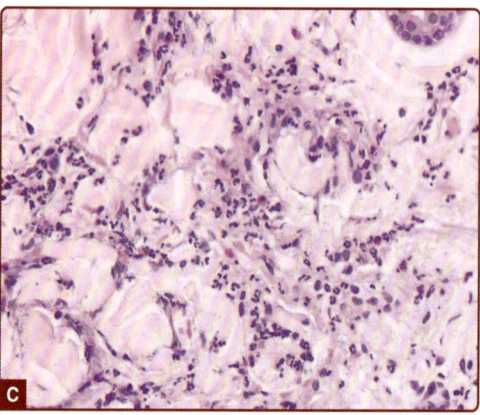

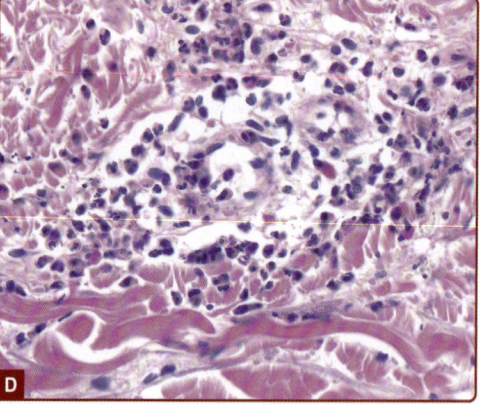

Figure 41-6 Histopathological presentation of urticaria. **A,** Edema of the dermis. **B,** Perivascular infiltration of lymphocytes and eosinophils. **C,** Neutrophilic urticaria. **D,** Urticarial vasculitis. (Reproduced from Shindo H. Histopathology of urticaria (Jinmashin No Byouri-Soshiki-Zou), In: Furue M, Hide M eds. *Hifuka Asset 16*. Tokyo, Japan: Nakayama-Shoten; 2013:62-70.)

deposited in spontaneous wheals.[194] Moderately dense infiltrates of eosinophils were observed in DPU.[51] These cellular changes correlated with moderate upregulation of the vascular endothelial adhesion molecules E-selectin, intercellular adhesion molecules 1, and vascular cell adhesion molecule 1 on perivascular cells.[195]

Urticaria with histologic evidence of vasculitis (*venulitis*) is defined as urticarial vasculitis (Fig. 41-6D). However, in clinical practice, it may sometimes be difficult to differentiate lesions of urticarial vasculitis from those of spontaneous urticaria when all histopathological features of vasculitis, including endothelial cell damage, fibrin deposition, leukocytoclasis, and erythrocyte extravasation, are not present in the skin specimen.[68] Moreover, a continuum of histologic changes between urticaria and urticarial vasculitis has been recognized in a series of patients with intermediate histologic features.[196,197] Some authors suggest that leukocytoclasis or fibrin deposition with or without erythrocyte extravasation may be sufficient for a diagnosis in difficult cases.[68]

IMAGING

Imaging examinations such as ultrasound, computed tomography (CT), or magnetic resonance imaging (MRI) are not required for ordinary urticarias. In cases of edema developing in pharyngeal and laryngeal areas or in the gastrointestinal tract, especially caused by bradykinin-mediated angioedemas, imaging tests might be useful or even essential. Patients with HAE may present with episodic swelling in various body parts, such as the face, neck, bowel, genitals, and extremities. Airway obstruction caused by edema of the larynx, oropharynx, and prevertebral soft tissue may cause suffocation, and this can be detected by endoscopy, radiographs, CT scans, and MRI examinations.[36,198] Patients may also have acute abdominal pain caused by swelling of the gastrointestinal tract. Imaging in such situations may be helpful to avoid unnecessary surgical interventions.[198]

DIAGNOSTIC ALGORITHM

A diagnosis of urticaria or angioedema (or both) should be made based on careful observation of the skin and history taking followed by clinical examination to confirm the diagnosis and evaluate disease severity. It is recommended not to perform extensive screening or workup without a known clinical diagnosis of an urticaria subtype.[1] The algorithm recommended by EAACI guidelines is shown in Fig. 41-5.

DIFFERENTIAL DIAGNOSIS

The diagnosis of urticaria is not difficult in most cases if suddenly appearing and transiently disappearing eruptions are confirmed by patient's history and clinical observations. Diseases that may manifest similar symptoms to urticaria and angioedema are listed in Table 41-4. Diseases that include wheals or angioedema should be differentiated by the presence of nonurticarial, mostly extracutaneous symptoms, such as fever and arthralgia.

CLINICAL COURSE AND PROGNOSIS

A study showed that most patients (85%) who had an acute spontaneous urticaria and began treatment within 1 week of disease onset improved shortly afterward. However, approximately 7% of this cohort continued to have symptoms for more than 1 year. Prolongation of disease activity tends to be seen among patients who required other medications in addition to a standard dose of antihistamine.[199] Other studies, albeit from specialized centers, indicate that most patients have CSU for more than 1 year.[14-18,22,200,201] Moreover, a considerable number of patients even seem to be affected for longer than 5 years. In some rare cases, urticaria may even last for up to 50 years.[200] A retrospective study using Kaplan-Meier methods of patients with CSU who visited a tertiary medical center revealed the estimated improved rates at 12 months, 24 months, and 60 months as 36.6%, 51.2%, and 66.1%, respectively.[201]

However, the reported time course is highly variable among studies. Reported remission rates at 1 year ranged from 20% to 80%. Among these studies, four factors appear to be associated with prolonged prognosis, namely, (1) initial disease severity, (2) presence of angioedema, (3) combination of CSU and physical urticaria(s), and (4) autoreactivity (positive ASST result).[20] A recent retrospective study showed that patients with CSU and positive ASST results responded more slowly to omalizumab than those with negative ASST results.[83]

MANAGEMENT

INTERVENTIONS

The treatment of urticaria and angioedema consists of two basic approaches. One is the identification and removal of the cause or factors that aggravate the condition. Another is the continuous use of antisymptomatic treatment with medications. For inducible urticaria, the avoidance of stimuli that induce symptoms is important, but in certain subtypes (solar urticaria, heat contact urticaria, cold contact urticaria, cholinergic urticaria, and urticaria induced by type I food allergy), repetitive exposure to slight stimuli may rather reduce the sensitivity of the patients (hardening or tolerance). Aggravating factors, if applicable for individual cases, should be removed to the extent possible (see section "Etiology and Pathogenesis" and Table 41-3). The algorithm of pharmaceutical treatment recommended by current guidelines[1] is essentially the same for all subtypes of chronic urticaria, except for bradykinin-mediated angioedema. In many cases of mast cell–mediated urticaria, especially in spontaneous urticaria, symptoms can be controlled to acceptable levels without identification of the cause. On the other hand, antihistamines, corticosteroids, and adrenaline are all ineffective for bradykinin-mediated angioedema.

MEDICATIONS

Medication should be taken continuously rather than an on-demand basis for both spontaneous urticaria and inducible urticaria patients who develop symptoms daily or almost daily.[1] However, if symptoms develop only occasionally, a schedule of medication use may be determined on a case-by-case basis. For HAE, three aims of medications should be considered based on the severity and frequency of the symptoms: on-demand therapy for emerging symptoms, short-term prophylaxis, and long-term prophylaxis.[143,160]

FIRST-LINE THERAPY

The second-generation nonsedating antihistamines are the mainstay of treatment for all kinds of mast cell–mediated urticaria. Generally, first-generation sedating antihistamines are no longer recommended. Although they appear to help with sleep at night, there may be carry-over effects of sedation in the morning and may cause paradoxical excitation or possibly epilepsy in children.

SECOND-LINE THERAPY

For intractable cases resistant to standard doses of antihistamines, increased dosing of antihistamines up to fourfold is recommended in EAACI guideline[202] and practice parameters by the American Academy of Allergy, Asthma and Immunology (AAAAI) and the American College of Allergy, Asthma and Immunology (ACAAI)[142] (American consensus document). Numerous reports have demonstrated the efficacy of high-dose antihistamines. Recently, a meta-analysis of using high dose antihistamines showed that this significantly improved control of pruritus but not wheal number.[203]

THIRD- AND FOURTH-LINE THERAPY

For cases in which high-dose antihistamines fail to achieve enough improvement, several additional therapies are recommended. The guideline published by the British Society for Allergy and Clinical Immunology (BSACI)[202] and the American consensus document[142] recommend adding antileukotrienes before the use of omalizumab and cyclosporine. However, EAACI guideline published in 2018 recommend adding omalizumab first as the third line therapy.[1] Systemic corticosteroids are recommended only to be used in limited circumstances, especially for severe symptoms in acute urticaria and acute aggravation of CSU. It should be noted that continuous use of corticosteroids (longer than 10 days) is not recommended because of the risk of side effects.[1,142,203] The treatment algorithms published in EAACI guidelines[1] and the American consensus document[142] are shown in Fig. 41-7.

The efficacy and safety of omalizumab, anti-IgE antibody, for the treatment of urticaria has been well studied, and it is now approved for the treatment of CSU in many countries.[204-206] The proposed mechanism of action of omalizumab is shown in Fig. 41-3. A recent meta-analysis of randomized controlled studies showed that a dosage of 300 mg/month is recommended for intractable CSU regardless of the levels of serum total IgE.[204] In theory, omalizumab inhibits circulating IgE and consequently decreases the number of FcεRI on mast cells and basophils. Although it takes 2 months or longer for omalizumab to decrease the number of cell surface FcεRI, the clinical effect of omalizumab on CSU may become apparent within 1 week.[100] Moreover, omalizumab is effective for virtually all subtypes of urticaria mediated by mast cells, including DPU and urticarial vasculitis,[99,207] although such usage is off label. A number of possible mechanisms have been hypothesized, but none of them so far can fully explain its effect on urticaria.[100]

EXCEPTIONAL CASES AND OTHER MEDICATIONS IN THE TREATMENT OF URTICARIA

In most cases of DPU and urticarial vasculitis, antihistamines are not effective. Systemic steroids or other immunosuppressive or modulatory agents may be necessary to suppress symptoms.[208] As supplementary or alternative treatments, the following may also be used in combination with antihistamines for refractory cases: histamine H2-blockers, dapsone (diaphenylsulfone, DDS), antifibrinolytics (tranexamic acid or ε-aminocaproic acid) especially for patients with angioedema, methotrexate, tacrolimus, hydroxychloroquine, intravenous immunoglobulin therapy, plasmapheresis, and narrow-band UVB.[1,209] However, evidence supporting the use of these medications is still weak, and reports are anecdotal. Moreover, most drugs have the potential for causing serious side effects. Most important, none of the pharmaceutical treatments mentioned has been proven to modify the natural course of urticaria in terms of achieving a cure. Therefore, it is important to consider a balance between the burden of symptoms and that of treatment.

Treatment of bradykinin-mediated HAE, as recommended in various guidelines and consensus documents,[143,160] is illustrated in Fig. 41-4. Icatibant, ecallantide, and purified or recombinant C1-INH are used for acute attacks. Purified or recombinant C1-INH, lanadelumab, and BCX7653 are used or are under development for use as prophylaxis. A few studies have reported the efficacy of icatibant for acute

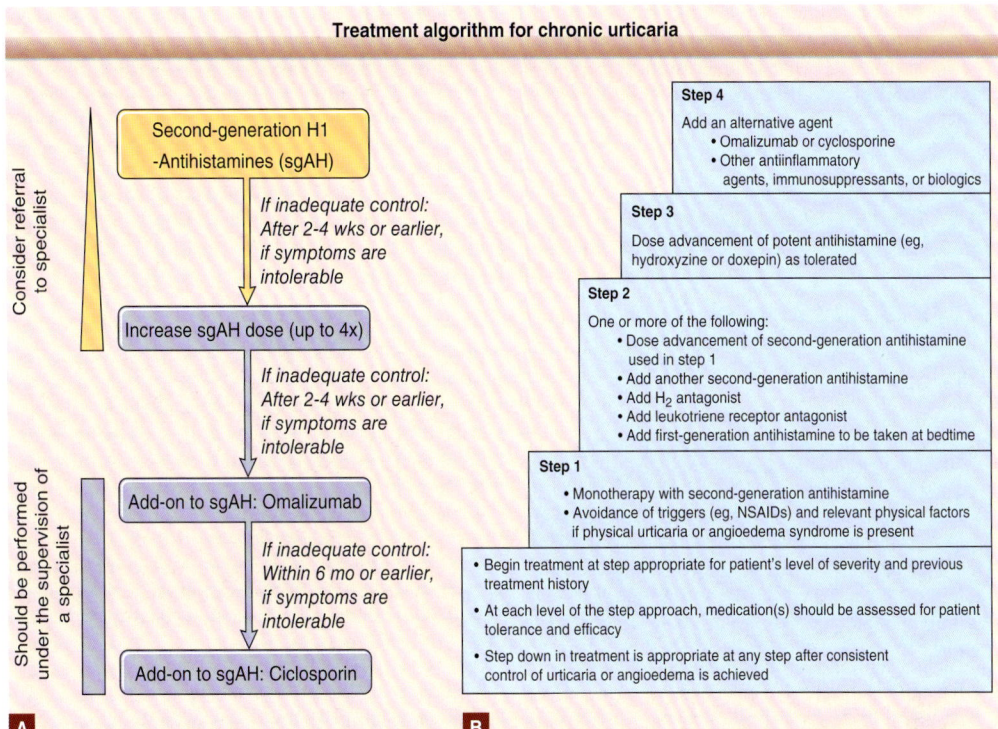

Figure 41-7 Treatment algorithm for chronic urticaria recommended by the European Academy of Allergy and Clinical Immunology/Global Allergy and Asthma European Network/European Dermatology Forum/World Allergy Organization (**A**) and that for chronic urticaria by the American Academy of Allergy, Asthma and Immunology and the American College of Allergy, Asthma and Immunology (**B**). NSAID, nonsteroidal antiinflammatory drug. (Image **A**, from Zuberbier T, Aberer W, Asero R, et al. The EAACI/GA(2) LEN/EDF/WAO Guideline for the definition, classification, diagnosis, and management of urticaria: the 2017 revision and update. *Allergy*. 2018;73:1393-1414, with permission. Copyright © 2018 EAACI and John Wiley and Sons. Image **B**, From Bernstein JA, Lang DM, Khan DA, et al. The diagnosis and management of acute and chronic urticaria: 2014 update. *J Allergy Clin Immunol*. 2014;133:1270-1277, with permission. Copyright © American Academy of Allergy, Asthma & Immunology.)

attacks of angioedema caused by ACE inhibitors,[210,211] although one study contradicted these findings.[212]

TREATMENT IN PEDIATRIC PATIENTS

The principle of treatment for children with urticaria is the same as for adults.[1] Dosing should follow the relevant manufacturer's recommendations.

TREATMENT IN PREGNANT AND LACTATING WOMEN

Use of any systemic treatment should generally be avoided in pregnant women, especially in the first trimester. Moreover, antihistamines cross the placenta. On the other hand, there is no reliable evidence that the medications listed in the algorithm of EAACI guideline are teratogenic. Thus, the same treatment principles and algorithm are suggested for both pregnant and lactating women with urticaria.[1] Among antihistamines, chlorphenamine is often chosen based on its long availability and safety record.[213] Current guidelines on urticaria support the use of cetirizine and loratadine desirably after the first trimester of pregnancy if the benefits of an antihistamine are considered to outweigh any risks of administration for an individual patient.[1,202]

COUNSELING

No particular methods have been established for urticaria, but patients with CSU may have substantial impairment of their QOL, as much as with ischemic heart disease.[214] Patients with hereditary diseases, such as HAE and autoinflammatory syndromes, should be offered qualified counseling as necessary.

TREATMENT ALGORITHM

The treatment algorithm recommended in EAACI guideline and the American consensus document are shown in Fig. 41-7.

PREVENTION AND SCREENING

There are no measures for preventing or screening for the development of urticaria. On the other hand, all family members of patients with HAE type I and type II who are older than 1 year old are recommended to undergo screening for the diagnosis of HAE. A case of a 9-year-old boy who died from the first attack of HAE has been reported.[215] Early diagnosis and preparation for attacks should reduce the risk.

REFERENCES

1. Zuberbier T, Aberer W, Asero R, et al. The EAACI/GA(2) LEN/EDF/WAO Guideline for the definition, classification, diagnosis, and management of urticaria: the 2017 revision and update. *Allergy*. 2018; 73(7):1393-1414.
2. Czarnetzki BM. History of urticaria. *Urticaria*. 1986:1-4.
3. Cummings AJ, Olsen M. Mechanism of action of stinging nettles. *Wilderness Environ Med*. 2011;22(2): 136-139.
4. Beaven MA. Our perception of the mast cell from Paul Ehrlich to now. *Eur J Immunol*. 2009;39(1): 11-25.
5. Dale HH, Laidlaw PP. The physiological action of β-iminazolylethylamine. *J Physiol*. 1910;41(5): 318-344.
6. Eppinger H. Über eine eigentümliche Hautkrankheit, hervorgerufen durch Ergamin. *Wien Med Wschr*. 1913; 63:1413-1416.
7. Bovet D. Introduction to antihistamine agents and antergan derivatives. 1950. *Ann N Y Acad Sci*. 50(9):1089-1126.
8. Riley JF, West GB. The presence of histamine in tissue mast cells. *J Physiol*. 1953;120(4):528-537.
9. Ishizaka K, Ishizaka T. Identification of IgE. *J Allergy Clin Immunol*. 2016;137(6):1646-1650.
10. Bakke P, Gulsvik A, Eide GE. Hay fever, eczema and urticaria in southwest Norway. Lifetime prevalences and association with sex, age, smoking habits, occupational airborne exposures and respiratory symptoms. *Allergy*. 1990;45(7):515-522.
11. Herrmann-Kunz E. Häufigkeit allergischer Krankheiten in Ost- und Westdeutschland. 1999;61(2):S100-S105.
12. Zuberbier T, Balke M, Worm M, et al. Epidemiology of urticaria: a representative cross-sectional population survey. *Clin Exp Dermatol*. 2010;35(8):869-873.
13. Hellgren L. The prevalence of urticaria in the total population. *Acta Allergol*. 1972;27(3):236-240.
14. Gaig P, Olona M, Munoz Lejarazu D, et al. Epidemiology of urticaria in Spain. *J Investig Allergol Clin Immunol*. 2004;14(3):214-220.
15. van der Valk PG, Moret G, Kiemeney LA. The natural history of chronic urticaria and angioedema in patients visiting a tertiary referral centre. *Br J Dermatol*. 2002; 146(1):110-113.
16. Kozel MM, Mekkes JR, Bossuyt PM, et al. Natural course of physical and chronic urticaria and angioedema in 220 patients. *J Am Acad Dermatol*. 2001; 45(3):387-391.
17. Kulthanan K, Jiamton S, Thumpimukvatana N, et al. Chronic idiopathic urticaria: prevalence and clinical course. *J Dermatol*. 2007;34(5):294-301.
18. Humphreys F, Hunter JA. The characteristics of urticaria in 390 patients. *Br J Dermatol*. 1998; 138(4):635-638.
19. Tanaka T, Kameyoshi Y, Hide M. [Analysis of the prevalence of subtypes of urticaria and angioedema]. *Arerugi*. 2006;55(2):134-139.
20. Maurer M, Weller K, Bindslev-Jensen C, et al. Unmet clinical needs in chronic spontaneous urticaria. A GA(2) LEN task force report. *Allergy*. 2011;66(3):317-330.
21. Quaranta JH, Rohr AS, Rachelefsky CS, et al. The natural history and response to therapy of chronic urticaria and angioedema. *Ann Allergy*. 1989;62(5):421-424.
22. Juhlin L. Recurrent urticaria: clinical investigation of 330 patients. *Br J Dermatol*. 1981;104(4):369-381.
23. Steinhardt MJ. Urticaria and angioedema—statistical survey of five hundred cases. *Ann Allergy*. 1954; 12(6):659-670.
24. Sabroe RA, Seed PT, Francis DM, et al. Chronic idiopathic urticaria: comparison of the clinical features of patients with and without anti-FcεRI or anti-IgE autoantibodies. *J Am Acad Dermatol*. 1999;40(3):443-450.
25. Nettis E, Dambra P, D'Oronzio L. Reactivity to autologous serum skin test and clinical features in chronic idiopathic urticaria. *Clin Exp Dermatol*. 2002;27(1):29-31.
26. Caproni M, Volpi W, Giomi B. Chronic idiopathic and chronic autoimmune urticaria: clinical and immunopathological features of 68 subjects. *Acta Derm Venereol*. 2004;84(4):288-290.
27. Giménez-Arnau AM, Ferrer M, Peter HJ, et al. Urticaria crónica: estudio etiológico prospectivo e importancia del síndrome autoinmune. *Actas Dermosifiliogr*. 2004;95(9):560-566.
28. Asero R. Sex differences in the pathogenesis of chronic urticaria. *J Allergy Clin Immunol*. 2003;111(2):425-426.
29. Champion R, Roberts S, Carpenter R, Roger J. Urticaria and angioedema: a review of 554 patients. *Br J Dermatol*. 1969;81(8):588-597.
30. Henderson RL Jr, Fleischer AB Jr, Feldman SR. Allergists and dermatologists have far more expertise in caring for patients with urticaria than other specialists. *J Am Acad Dermatol*. 2000;43(6):1084-1091.
31. Ferrer M. Epidemiology, healthcare, resources, use and clinical features of different types of urticaria. *J Investig Allergol Clin Immunol*. 2009;19(suppl 2):21-26.
32. Hide M, Hiragun M, Hiragun T. Diagnostic tests for urticaria. *Immunol Allergy Clin North Am*. 2014; 34(1):53-72.
33. Miyake M, Oiso N, Ishii K, et al. Angioedema associated with excessive sweating and sweat allergy. *J Dermatol*. 2017;44(4):e58-e59.
34. Washio K, Fukunaga A, Onodera M, et al. Clinical characteristics in cholinergic urticaria with palpebral angioedema: report of 15 cases. *J Dermatol Sci*. 2017;85(2):135-137.
35. Fukunaga A, Washio K, Hatakeyama M, et al. Cholinergic urticaria: epidemiology, physiopathology, new categorization, and management. *Clin Auton Res*. 2018;28(1):103-113.
36. Shibuya M, Takahashi N, Yabe M, et al. Hereditary angioedema as the cause of death from asphyxia: postmortem computed tomography study. *Allergol Int*. 2014;63(3):493-494.
37. Simons FE, Ardusso LR, Bilo MB, et al. World allergy organization guidelines for the assessment and management of anaphylaxis. *World Allergy Organ J*. 2011;4(2):13-37.
38. Pan XF, Gu JQ, Shan ZY. The prevalence of thyroid autoimmunity in patients with urticaria: a systematic review and meta-analysis. *Endocrine*. 2015;48(3):804-810.
39. Diaz-Angulo S, Lopez-Hoyos M, Munoz Cacho P, et al. Prevalence of thyroid autoimmunity in Spanish patients with chronic idiopathic urticaria: a case-control study involving 343 subjects. *J Eur Acad Dermatol Venereol*. 2016;30(4):692-693.

40. Altrichter S, Peter HJ, Pisarevskaja D, et al. IgE mediated autoallergy against thyroid peroxidase—a novel pathomechanism of chronic spontaneous urticaria? *PLoS One.* 2011;6(4):e14794.
41. Confino-Cohen R, Chodick G, Shalev V, et al. Chronic urticaria and autoimmunity: associations found in a large population study. *J Allergy Clin Immunol.* 2012;129(5):1307-1313.
42. Baughman RD, Jillson OF. Seven specific types of urticaria. With special reference to delayed persistent dermographism. *Ann Allergy.* 1963;21:248-255.
43. Warin RP. Clinical observations on delayed pressure urticaria. *Br J Dermatol.* 1989;121(2):225-228.
44. Kaplan AP. Unusual cold-induced disorders: cold-dependent dermatographism and systemic cold urticaria. *J Allergy Clin Immunol.* 1984;73(4):453-456.
45. Lambiris A, Greaves MW. Dyspareunia and vulvodynia are probably common manifestations of factitious urticaria. *Br J Dermatol.* 1997;136(1):140-141.
46. Back O, Larsen A. Delayed cold urticaria. *Acta Derm Venereol.* 1978;58(4):369-371.
47. Kivity S, Schwartz Y, Wolf R, et al. Systemic cold-induced urticaria—clinical and laboratory characterization. *J Allergy Clin Immunol.* 1990;85(1 Pt 1):52-54.
48. Hoffman HM, Wanderer AA, Broide DH. Familial cold autoinflammatory syndrome: phenotype and genotype of an autosomal dominant periodic fever. *J Allergy Clin Immunol.* 2001;108(4):615-620.
49. Ombrello MJ, Remmers EF, Sun G, et al. Cold urticaria, immunodeficiency, and autoimmunity related to PLCG2 deletions. *N Engl J Med.* 2012;366(4):330-338.
50. Nettis E, Colanardi MC, Soccio AL, et al. Desloratadine in combination with montelukast suppresses the dermographometer challenge test papule, and is effective in the treatment of delayed pressure urticaria: a randomized, double-blind, placebo-controlled study. *Br J Dermatol.* 2006;155(6):1279-1282.
51. Morioke S, Takahagi S, Iwamoto K, et al. Pressure challenge test and histopathological inspections for 17 Japanese cases with clinically diagnosed delayed pressure urticaria. *Arch Dermatol Res.* 2010;302(8):613-617.
52. Lawlor F, Black AK, Breathnach AS, et al. Vibratory angioedema: lesion induction, clinical features, laboratory and ultrastructural findings and response to therapy. *Br J Dermatol.* 1989;120(1):93-99.
53. Boyden SE, Desai A, Cruse G, et al. Vibratory urticaria associated with a missense variant in ADGRE2. *N Engl J Med.* 2016;374(7):656-663.
54. Heitkemper T, Hofmann T, Phan NQ, et al. Aquagenic pruritus: associated diseases and clinical pruritus characteristics. *J Dtsch Dermatol Ges.* 2010;8(10):797-804.
55. Kaplan AP, Natbony SF, Tawil AP, et al. Exercise-induced anaphylaxis as a manifestation of cholinergic urticaria. *J Allergy Clin Immunol.* 1981;68(4):319-324.
56. Sheffer AL, Soter NA, McFadden ER Jr, et al. Exercise-induced anaphylaxis: a distinct form of physical allergy. *J Allergy Clin Immunol.* 1983;71(3):311-316.
57. Grant RT. Observation on urticaria provoked by emotion, by exercise and by warming the body. *Clin Sci.* 1936;2:253-272.
58. Miyake M, Oiso N, Ishii K, et al. Angioedema associated with excessive sweating and sweat allergy. *J Dermatol.* 2017;44(4):e58-e59.
59. Berth-Jones J, Graham-Brown RA. Cholinergic pruritus, erythema and urticaria: a disease spectrum responding to danazol. *Br J Dermatol.* 1989;121(2):235-237.
60. Takahagi S, Tanaka T, Ishii K, et al. Sweat antigen induces histamine release from basophils of patients with cholinergic urticaria associated with atopic diathesis. *Br J Dermatol.* 2009;160(2):426-428.
61. Hiragun M, Hiragun T, Ishii K, et al. Elevated serum IgE against MGL_1304 in patients with atopic dermatitis and cholinergic urticaria. *Allergol Int.* 2014;63(1):83-93.
62. Hiragun T, Ishii K, Hiragun M, et al. Fungal protein MGL_1304 in sweat is an allergen for atopic dermatitis patients. *J Allergy Clin Immunol.* 2013;132(3):608-615.e604.
63. Tokura Y. New etiology of cholinergic urticaria. *Curr Probl Dermatol.* 2016;51:94-100.
64. Kashyap RR, Kashyap RS. Oral allergy syndrome: an update for stomatologists. *J Allergy (Cairo).* 2015;2015:543928.
65. Wisnieski JJ. Urticarial vasculitis. *Curr Opin Rheumatol.* 2000;12(1):24-31.
66. Grotz W, Baba HA, Becker JU, et al. Hypocomplementemic urticarial vasculitis syndrome: an interdisciplinary challenge. *Dtsch Arztebl Int.* 2009;106(46):756-763.
67. Zuberbier T, Maurer M. Urticarial vasculitis and Schnitzler syndrome. *Immunol Allergy Clin North Am.* 2014;34(1):141-147.
68. Monroe EW. Urticarial vasculitis: an updated review. *J Am Acad Dermatol.* 1981;5(1):88-95.
69. Black AK. Urticarial vasculitis. *Clin Dermatol.* 1999;17(5):565-569.
70. Takahagi S, Tanaka A, Iwamoto K, et al. Contact urticaria syndrome with IgE antibody against a cefotiam-unique structure, evoked by nonapparent exposure to cefotiam. *Clin Exp Dermatol.* 2017;42(5):527-531.
71. Inomata N, Chin K, Nagashima M, et al. Late-onset anaphylaxis due to poly (gamma-glutamic acid) in the soup of commercial cold Chinese noodles in a patient with allergy to fermented soybeans (natto). *Allergol Int.* 2011;60(3):393-396.
72. Inomata N, Chin K, Aihara M. Anaphylaxis caused by ingesting jellyfish in a subject with fermented soybean allergy: possibility of epicutaneous sensitization to poly-gamma-glutamic acid by jellyfish stings. *J Dermatol.* 2014;41(8):752-753.
73. Nettis E, Pannofino A, D'Aprile C, et al. Clinical and aetiological aspects in urticaria and angio-oedema. *Br J Dermatol.* 2003;148(3):501-506.
74. Champion RH. A practical approach to the urticarial syndromes—a dermatologist's view. *Clin Exp Allergy.* 1990;20(2):221-224.
75. Leznoff A, Sussman GL. Syndrome of idiopathic chronic urticaria and angioedema with thyroid autoimmunity: a study of 90 patients. *J Allergy Clin Immunol.* 1989;84(1):66-71.
76. Grattan CE, Francis DM, Hide M, et al. Detection of circulating histamine releasing autoantibodies with functional properties of anti-IgE in chronic urticaria. *Clin Exp Allergy.* 1991;21(6):695-704.
77. Hide M, Francis DM, Grattan CE, et al. Autoantibodies against the high-affinity IgE receptor as a cause of histamine release in chronic urticaria. *N Engl J Med.* 1993;328(22):1599-1604.
78. Kolkhir P, Church MK, Weller K, et al. Autoimmune chronic spontaneous urticaria: what we know and what we do not know. *J Allergy Clin Immunol.* 2017;139(6):1772-1781.e1771.

79. Kikuchi Y, Kaplan AP. Mechanisms of autoimmune activation of basophils in chronic urticaria. *J Allergy Clin Immunol*. 2001;107(6):1056-1062.
80. Ferrer M, Nakazawa K, Kaplan AP. Complement dependence of histamine release in chronic urticaria. *J Allergy Clin Immunol*. 1999;104(1):169-172.
81. Konstantinou GN, Asero R, Maurer M, et al. EAACI/GA(2)LEN task force consensus report: the autologous serum skin test in urticaria. *Allergy*. 2009;64(9):1256-1268.
82. Sanchez-Borges M, Caballero-Fonseca F, Capriles-Hulett A, et al. Factors linked to disease severity and time to remission in patients with chronic spontaneous urticaria. *J Eur Acad Dermatol Venereol*. 2017;31(6):964-971.
83. Gericke J, Metz M, Ohanyan T, et al. Serum autoreactivity predicts time to response to omalizumab therapy in chronic spontaneous urticaria. *J Allergy Clin Immunol*. 2017;139(3):1059-1061.e1051.
84. Sherman WB, Seebohm PM. Passive transfer of cold urticaria. *J Allergy*. 1950;21(5):414-424.
85. Samsoe-Jensen T. Cold urticaria; report of a case: passive transfer and in vitro experiments with skin cells. *Acta Derm Venereol*. 1955;35(2):107-110.
86. Houser DD, Arbesman CE, Ito K, et al. Cold urticaria. Immunologic studies. *Am J Med*. 1970;49(1):23-33.
87. Kaplan AP, Beaven MA. In vivo studies of the pathogenesis of cold urticaria, cholinergic urticaria, and vibration-induced swelling. *J Invest Dermatol*. 1976;67(3):327-332.
88. Horio T. Photoallergic urticaria induced by visible light. Additional cases and further studies. *Arch Dermatol*. 1978;114(12):1761-1764.
89. Newcomb RW, Nelson H. Dermographia mediated by immunoglobulin E. *Am J Med*. 1973;54(2):174-180.
90. Horiko T, Aoki T. Dermographism (mechanical urticaria) mediated by IgM. *Br J Dermatol*. 1984;111(5):545-550.
91. Murphy GM, Zollman PE, Greaves MW, et al. Symptomatic dermographism (factitious urticaria)—passive transfer experiments from human to monkey. *Br J Dermatol*. 1987;116(6):801-804.
92. Czarnetzki BM, Breetholt KH, Traupe H. Evidence that water acts as a carrier for an epidermal antigen in aquagenic urticaria. *J Am Acad Dermatol*. 1986;15(4 Pt 1):623-627.
93. Illig L, Heinicke A. [Pathogenesis of cholinergic urticaria. V. The pharmacologic reactivity of the Prausnitz-Kustner reaction and the origin of the antigen]. *Arch Klin Exp Dermatol*. 1967;230(1):34-47.
94. Gigli I, Schothorst AA, Soter NA, et al. Erythropoietic protoporphyria. Photoactivation of the complement system. *J Clin Invest*. 1980;66(3):517-522.
95. Lim HW, Perez HD, Poh-Fitzpatrick M, et al. Generation of chemotactic activity in serum from patients with erythropoietic protoporphyria and porphyria cutanea tarda. *N Engl J Med*. 1981;304(4):212-216.
96. Lim HW, Poh-Fitzpatrick MB, Gigli I. Activation of the complement system in patients with porphyrias after irradiation in vivo. *J Clin Invest*. 1984;74(6):1961-1965.
97. Kaplan AP, Garofalo J, Sigler R, et al. Idiopathic cold urticaria: in vitro demonstration of histamine release upon challenge of skin biopsies. *N Engl J Med*. 1981;305(18):1074-1077.
98. Kolkhir P, Metz M, Altrichter S, et al. Comorbidity of chronic spontaneous urticaria and autoimmune thyroid diseases: a systematic review. *Allergy*. 2017:1440-1460.
99. Metz M, Ohanyan T, Church MK, et al. Omalizumab is an effective and rapidly acting therapy in difficult-to-treat chronic urticaria: a retrospective clinical analysis. *J Dermatol Sci*. 2014;73(1):57-62.
100. Kaplan AP, Gimenez-Arnau AM, Saini SS. Mechanisms of action that contribute to efficacy of omalizumab in chronic spontaneous urticaria. *Allergy*. 2017;72(4):519-533.
101. Siebenhaar F, Melde A, Magerl M, et al. Histamine intolerance in patients with chronic spontaneous urticaria. *J Eur Acad Dermatol Venereol*. 2016.
102. Hungerford JM. Scombroid poisoning: a review. *Toxicon*. 2010;56(2):231-243.
103. Wagner N, Dirk D, Peveling-Oberhag A, et al. A Popular myth—low-histamine diet improves chronic spontaneous urticaria—fact or fiction? *J Eur Acad Dermatol Venereol*. 2017;31(4):650-655.
104. Zuberbier T, Chantraine-Hess S, Hartmann K, et al. Pseudoallergen-free diet in the treatment of chronic urticaria. A prospective study. *Acta Derm Venereol*. 1995;75(6):484-487.
105. Kanny G, Gerbaux V, Olszewski A, et al. No correlation between wine intolerance and histamine content of wine. *J Allergy Clin Immunol*. 2001;107(2):375-378.
106. Asero R. Plasma D-dimer levels and clinical response to ciclosporin in severe chronic spontaneous urticaria. *J Allergy Clin Immunol*. 2015;135(5):1401-1403.
107. Cugno M, Marzano AV, Asero R, et al. Activation of blood coagulation in chronic urticaria: pathophysiological and clinical implications. *Intern Emerg Med*. 2010;5(2):97-101.
108. Asero R, Tedeschi A, Coppola R, et al. Activation of the tissue factor pathway of blood coagulation in patients with chronic urticaria. *J Allergy Clin Immunol*. 2007;119(3):705-710.
109. Tedeschi A, Kolkhir P, Asero R, et al. Chronic urticaria and coagulation: pathophysiological and clinical aspects. *Allergy*. 2014;69(6):683-691.
110. Takahagi S, Mihara S, Iwamoto K, et al. Coagulation/fibrinolysis and inflammation markers are associated with disease activity in patients with chronic urticaria. *Allergy*. 2010;65(5):649-656.
111. Sakurai Y, Morioke S, Takeda T, et al. Increased thrombin generation potential in patients with chronic spontaneous urticaria. *Allergol Int*. 2015;64(1):96-98.
112. Takeda T, Sakurai Y, Takahagi S, et al. Increase of coagulation potential in chronic spontaneous urticaria. *Allergy*. 2011;66(3):428-433.
113. Yanase Y, Morioke S, Iwamoto K, et al. Histamine and Toll-like receptor ligands synergistically induce endothelial cell gap formation by the extrinsic coagulating pathway. *J Allergy Clin Immunol*. 2018;141(3):1115-1118.e7.
114. Mahesh PA, Pudupakkam VK, Holla AD, et al. Effect of warfarin on chronic idiopathic urticaria. *Indian J Dermatol Venereol Leprol*. 2009;75(2):187-189.
115. Parslew R, Pryce D, Ashworth J, et al. Warfarin treatment of chronic idiopathic urticaria and angio-oedema. *Clin Exp Allergy*. 2000;30(8):1161-1165.
116. Takahagi S, Shindo H, Watanabe M, et al. Refractory chronic urticaria treated effectively with the protease inhibitors, nafamostat mesilate and camostat mesilate. *Acta Derm Venereol*. 2010;90(4):425-426.
117. Asero R, Tedeschi A, Cugno M. Heparin and tranexamic acid therapy may be effective in treatment-resistant chronic urticaria with elevated d-dimer: a pilot study. *Int Arch Allergy Immunol*. 2010;152(4):384-389.

118. Costanzi JJ, Coltman CA Jr. Kappa chain cold precipitable immunoglobulin G (IgG) associated with cold urticaria. I. Clinical observations. *Clin Exp Immunol.* 1967;2(2):167-178.
119. Morais-Almeida M, Marinho S, Gaspar A, et al. Cold urticaria and infectious mononucleosis in children. *Allergol Immunopathol (Madr).* 2004;32(6):368-371.
120. Palma-Carlos AG, Palma-Carlos ML. Solar urticaria and porphyrias. *Eur Ann Allergy Clin Immunol.* 2005;37(1):17-20.
121. Goetze S, Elsner P. Solar urticaria. *J Dtsch Dermatol Ges.* 2015;13(12):1250-1253.
122. Yu Y, Blokhuis BR, Garssen J, et al. Non-IgE mediated mast cell activation. *Eur J Pharmacol.* 2016;778:33-43.
123. Theoharides TC. Neuroendocrinology of mast cells: challenges and controversies. *Exp Dermatol.* 2017;26(9):751-759.
124. Okabe T, Hide M, Koro O, et al. Substance P induces tumor necrosis factor-alpha release from human skin via mitogen-activated protein kinase. *Eur J Pharmacol.* 2000;398(2):309-315.
125. Okabe T, Hide M, Koro O, et al. The release of leukotriene B4 from human skin in response to substance P: evidence for the functional heterogeneity of human skin mast cells among individuals. *Clin Exp Immunol.* 2001;124(1):150-156.
126. Yu Y, Yip KH, Tam IY, et al. Differential effects of the Toll-like receptor 2 agonists, PGN and Pam3CSK4 on anti-IgE induced human mast cell activation. *PLoS One.* 2014;9(11):e112989.
127. Subramanian H, Gupta K, Ali H. Roles of Mas-related G protein-coupled receptor X2 on mast cell-mediated host defense, pseudoallergic drug reactions, and chronic inflammatory diseases. *J Allergy Clin Immunol.* 2016;138(3):700-710.
128. Weidner C, Klede M, Rukwied R, et al. Acute effects of substance P and calcitonin gene-related peptide in human skin—a microdialysis study. *J Invest Dermatol.* 2000;115(6):1015-1020.
129. Minciullo PL, Cascio A, Barberi G, et al. Urticaria and bacterial infections. *Allergy Asthma Proc.* 2014;35(4):295-302.
130. Federman DG, Kirsner RS, Moriarty JP, et al. The effect of antibiotic therapy for patients infected with Helicobacter pylori who have chronic urticaria. *J Am Acad Dermatol.* 2003;49(5):861-864.
131. Wedi B, Raap U, Kapp A. Chronic urticaria and infections. *Curr Opin Allergy Clin Immunol.* 2004;4(5):387-396.
132. Curth HM, Dinter J, Nigemeier K, et al. Effects of Helicobacter pylori eradication in chronic spontaneous urticaria: results from a retrospective cohort study. *Am J Clin Dermatol.* 2015;16(6):553-558.
133. Koblenzer CS. Psychosomatic concepts in dermatology. A dermatologist-psychoanalyst's viewpoint. *Arch Dermatol.* 1983;119(6):501-512.
134. Chung MC, Symons C, Gilliam J, et al. Stress, psychiatric co-morbidity and coping in patients with chronic idiopathic urticaria. *Psychol Health.* 2010;25(4):477-490.
135. Fava GA, Perini GI, Santonastaso P, et al. Life events and psychological distress in dermatologic disorders: psoriasis, chronic urticaria and fungal infections. *Br J Med Psychol.* 1980;53(3):277-282.
136. Malhotra SK, Mehta V. Role of stressful life events in induction or exacerbation of psoriasis and chronic urticaria. *Indian J Dermatol Venereol Leprol.* 2008;74(6):594-599.
137. Yang HY, Sun CC, Wu YC, et al. Stress, insomnia, and chronic idiopathic urticaria—a case-control study. *J Formos Med Assoc.* 2005;104(4):254-263.
138. Hashiro M, Okumura M. Anxiety, depression, psychosomatic symptoms and autonomic nervous function in patients with chronic urticaria. *J Dermatol Sci.* 1994;8(2):129-135.
139. Sheehan-Dare RA, Henderson MJ, Cotterill JA. Anxiety and depression in patients with chronic urticaria and generalized pruritus. *Br J Dermatol.* 1990;123(6):769-774.
140. Lindelof B, Sigurgeirsson B, Wahlgren CF, et al. Chronic urticaria and cancer: an epidemiological study of 1155 patients. *Br J Dermatol.* 1990;123(4):453-456.
141. Chen YJ, Wu CY, Shen JL, et al. Cancer risk in patients with chronic urticaria: a population-based cohort study. *Arch Dermatol.* 2012;148(1):103-108.
142. Bernstein JA, Lang DM, Khan DA, et al. The diagnosis and management of acute and chronic urticaria: 2014 update. *J Allergy Clin Immunol.* 2014;133(5):1270-1277.
143. Lang DM, Aberer W, Bernstein JA, et al. International consensus on hereditary and acquired angioedema. *Ann Allergy Asthma Immunol.* 2012;109(6):395-402.
144. Ameisen JC, Capron A. Aspirin-sensitive asthma. *Clin Exp Allergy.* 1990;20(2):127-129.
145. Inomata N, Osuna H, Yamaguchi J, et al. Safety of selective cyclooxygenase-2 inhibitors and a basic non-steroidal anti-inflammatory drug (NSAID) in Japanese patients with NSAID-induced urticaria and/or angioedema: comparison of meloxicam, etodolac and tiaramide. *J Dermatol.* 2007;34(3):172-177.
146. Harada S, Horikawa T, Ashida M, et al. Aspirin enhances the induction of type I allergic symptoms when combined with food and exercise in patients with food-dependent exercise-induced anaphylaxis. *Br J Dermatol.* 2001;145(2):336-339.
147. Asaumi T, Yanagida N, Sato S, et al. Provocation tests for the diagnosis of food-dependent exercise-induced anaphylaxis. *Pediatr Allergy Immunol.* 2016;27(1):44-49.
148. de Silva HA, Ryan NM, de Silva HJ. Adverse reactions to snake antivenom, and their prevention and treatment. *Br J Clin Pharmacol.* 2016;81(3):446-452.
149. Kaplan A. *Urticaria and Angioedema.* New York: McGraw-Hill Medical; 2012.
150. Rosado Ingelmo A, Dona Diaz I, Cabanas Moreno R, et al. Clinical practice guidelines for diagnosis and management of hypersensitivity reactions to contrast media. *J Investig Allergol Clin Immunol.* 2016;26(3):144-155.
151. Wood MJ. Comparative safety of teicoplanin and vancomycin. *J Chemother.* 2000;12(suppl 5):21-25.
152. O'Donnell BF, O'Neill CM, Francis DM, et al. Human leucocyte antigen class II associations in chronic idiopathic urticaria. *Br J Dermatol.* 1999;140(5):853-858.
153. Gawchik SM. Latex allergy. *Mt Sinai J Med.* 2011;78(5):759-772.
154. Kozel MM, Mekkes JR, Bossuyt PM, et al. The effectiveness of a history-based diagnostic approach in chronic urticaria and angioedema. *Arch Dermatol.* 1998;134(12):1575-1580.
155. Kolkhir P, Andre F, Church MK, et al. Potential blood biomarkers in chronic spontaneous urticaria. *Clin Exp Allergy.* 2017;47(1):19-36.
156. Kozel MM, Bossuyt PM, Mekkes JR, Bos JD. Laboratory tests and identified diagnoses in patients with physical and chronic urticaria and angioedema: A systematic review. *J Am Acad Dermatol.* 2003;48(3):409-416.

157. Magerl M, Abajian M, Krause K, et al. An improved Peltier effect-based instrument for critical temperature threshold measurement in cold- and heat-induced urticaria. *J Eur Acad Dermatol Venereol.* 2015;29(10):2043-2045.
158. Hide M, Yamamura Y, Sanada S, et al. Aquagenic urticaria: a case report. *Acta Derm Venereol.* 2000;80(2):148-149.
159. Soter NA, Austen KF, Gigli I. Urticaria and arthralgias as manifestations of necrotizing angiitis (vasculitis). *J Invest Dermatol.* 1974;63(6):485-490.
160. Maurer M, Magerl M, Ansotegui I, et al. The international WAO/EAACI guideline for the management of hereditary angioedema-The 2017 revision and update. *Allergy.* 2018;73(8):1575-1596.
161. Bafunno V, Firinu D, D'Apolito M, et al. Mutation of the angiopoietin-1 gene (ANGPT1) associates with a new type of hereditary angioedema. *J Allergy Clin Immunol.* 2018;141(3):1009-1017.
162. Bork K, Wulff K, Steinmuller-Magin L, et al. Hereditary angioedema with a mutation in the plasminogen gene. *Allergy.* 2018;73(2):442-450.
163. Cugno M, Zanichelli A, Bellatorre AG, et al. Plasma biomarkers of acute attacks in patients with angioedema due to C1-inhibitor deficiency. *Allergy.* 2009;64(2):254-257.
164. Iwamoto K, Morioke S, Yanase Y, et al. Tissue factor expression on the surface of monocytes from a patient with hereditary angioedema. *J Dermatol.* 2014;41(10):929-932.
165. Aksentijevich I, Zhou Q. NF-kappaB pathway in autoinflammatory diseases: dysregulation of protein modifications by ubiquitin defines a new category of autoinflammatory diseases. *Front Immunol.* 2017;8:399.
166. Krause K, Tsianakas A, Wagner N, et al. Efficacy and safety of canakinumab in Schnitzler syndrome: a multicenter randomized placebo-controlled study. *J Allergy Clin Immunol.* 2017;139(4):1311-1320.
167. Bhattacharyya J, Mihara K, Morimoto K, et al. Elevated interleukin-18 secretion from monoclonal IgM+ B cells in a patient with Schnitzler syndrome. *J Am Acad Dermatol.* 2012;67(3):e118-120.
168. de Torre-Minguela C, Mesa Del Castillo P, Pelegrin P. The NLRP3 and pyrin inflammasomes: implications in the pathophysiology of autoinflammatory diseases. *Front Immunol.* 2017;8:43.
169. Morita E, Kunie K, Matsuo H. Food-dependent exercise-induced anaphylaxis. *J Dermatol Sci.* 2007;47(2):109-117.
170. Bruce RA, Blackmon JR, Jones JW, et al. Exercising testing in adult normal subjects and cardiac patients. *Pediatrics.* 1963;32(suppl):742-756.
171. Mlynek A, Zalewska-Janowska A, Martus P, et al. How to assess disease activity in patients with chronic urticaria? *Allergy.* 2008;63(6):777-780.
172. Weller K, Groffik A, Magerl M, et al. Development, validation, and initial results of the Angioedema Activity Score. *Allergy.* 2013;68(9):1185-1192.
174. Rabelo-Filardi R, Daltro-Oliveira R, Campos RA. Parameters associated with chronic spontaneous urticaria duration and severity: a systematic review. *Int Arch Allergy Immunol.* 2013;161(3):197-204.
174. Metz M, Krull C, Maurer M. Histamine, TNF, C5a, IL-6, -9, -18, -31, -33, TSLP, neopterin, and VEGF are not elevated in chronic spontaneous urticaria. *J Dermatol Sci.* 2013;70(3):222-225.
175. Grattan CE, Dawn G, Gibbs S, et al. Blood basophil numbers in chronic ordinary urticaria and healthy controls: diurnal variation, influence of loratadine and prednisolone and relationship to disease activity. *Clin Exp Allergy.* 2003;33(3):337-341.
176. Eckman JA, Hamilton RG, Gober LM, et al. Basophil phenotypes in chronic idiopathic urticaria in relation to disease activity and autoantibodies. *J Invest Dermatol.* 2008;128(8):1956-1963.
177. Doong JC, Chichester K, Oliver ET, et al. Chronic idiopathic urticaria: systemic complaints and their relationship with disease and immune measures. *J Allergy Clin Immunol Pract.* 2017;5(5):1314-1318.
178. Lewis V, Finlay AY. 10 years experience of the Dermatology Life Quality Index (DLQI). *J Investig Dermatol Symp Proc.* 2004;9(2):169-180.
179. Maurer M, Staubach P, Raap U, et al. ATTENTUS, a German online survey of patients with chronic urticaria highlighting the burden of disease, unmet needs and real-life clinical practice. *Br J Dermatol.* 2016;174(4):892-894.
180. Murota H, Kitaba S, Tani M, et al. Impact of sedative and non-sedative antihistamines on the impaired productivity and quality of life in patients with pruritic skin diseases. *Allergol Int.* 2010;59(4):345-354.
181. Baiardini I, Giardini A, Pasquali M, et al. Quality of life and patients' satisfaction in chronic urticaria and respiratory allergy. *Allergy.* 2003;58(7):621-623.
182. Weller K, Groffik A, Magerl M, et al. Development and construct validation of the angioedema quality of life questionnaire. *Allergy.* 2012;67(10):1289-1298.
183. Weller K, Groffik A, Church MK, et al. Development and validation of the Urticaria Control Test: a patient-reported outcome instrument for assessing urticaria control. *J Allergy Clin Immunol.* 2014;133(5):1365-1372, 1372.e1361-1366.
184. GmbH M. Moxie. http://moxie-gmbh.de/medical-products/.
185. Natbony SF, Phillips ME, Elias JM, et al. Histologic studies of chronic idiopathic urticaria. *J Allergy Clin Immunol.* 1983;71(2):177-183.
186. Elias J, Boss E, Kaplan AP. Studies of the cellular infiltrate of chronic idiopathic urticaria: prominence of T-lymphocytes, monocytes, and mast cells. *J Allergy Clin Immunol.* 1986;78(5 Pt 1):914-918.
187. Nettis E, Dambra P, Loria MP, et al. Mast-cell phenotype in urticaria. *Allergy.* 2001;56(9):915.
188. Smith CH, Kepley C, Schwartz LB, et al. Mast cell number and phenotype in chronic idiopathic urticaria. *J Allergy Clin Immunol.* 1995;96(3):360-364.
189. Ito Y, Satoh T, Takayama K, et al. Basophil recruitment and activation in inflammatory skin diseases. *Allergy.* 2011;66(8):1107-1113.
190. Ying S, Kikuchi Y, Meng Q, et al. TH1/TH2 cytokines and inflammatory cells in skin biopsy specimens from patients with chronic idiopathic urticaria: comparison with the allergen-induced late-phase cutaneous reaction. *J Allergy Clin Immunol.* 2002;109(4):694-700.
191. Peters MS, Winkelmann RK. Neutrophilic urticaria. *Br J Dermatol.* 1985;113(1):25-30.
192. Winkelmann RK, Wilson-Jones E, Smith NP, et al. Neutrophilic urticaria. *Acta Derm Venereol.* 1988;68(2):129-133.
193. Levender MM, Silvers DN, Grossman ME. Urticaria-like neutrophilic dermatosis in association with IgA gammopathy: a new entity. *Br J Dermatol.* 2014;170(5):1189-1191.
194. Peters MS, Schroeter AL, Kephart GM, et al. Localization of eosinophil granule major basic protein in chronic urticaria. *J Invest Dermatol.* 1983;81(1):39-43.

195. Barlow RJ, Ross EL, MacDonald D, et al. Adhesion molecule expression and the inflammatory cell infiltrate in delayed pressure urticaria. *Br J Dermatol.* 1994;131(3):341-347.
196. Jones RR, Bhogal B, Dash A, et al. Urticaria and vasculitis: a continuum of histological and immunopathological changes. *Br J Dermatol.* 1983;108(6):695-703.
197. Phanuphak P, Kohler PF, Stanford RE, et al. Vasculitis in chronic urticaria. *J Allergy Clin Immunol.* 1980;65(6):436-444.
198. Gakhal MS, Marcotte GV. Hereditary angioedema: imaging manifestations and clinical management. *Emerg Radiol.* 2015;22(1):83-90.
199. Tanaka T, Hiragun M, Hide M, et al. Analysis of primary treatment and prognosis of spontaneous urticaria. *Allergol Int.* 2017;66(3):458-462.3.
200. Toubi E, Kessel A, Avshovich N, et al. Clinical and laboratory parameters in predicting chronic urticaria duration: a prospective study of 139 patients. *Allergy.* 2004;59(8):869-873.
201. Hiragun M, Hiragun T, Mihara S, et al. Prognosis of chronic spontaneous urticaria in 117 patients not controlled by a standard dose of antihistamine. *Allergy.* 2013;68(2):229-235.
202. Powell RJ, Leech SC, Till S, et al. BSACI guideline for the management of chronic urticaria and angioedema. *Clin Exp Allergy.* 2015;45(3):547-565.
203. Guillen-Aguinaga S, Jauregui Presa I, Aguinaga-Ontoso E, et al. Updosing nonsedating antihistamines in patients with chronic spontaneous urticaria: a systematic review and meta-analysis. *Br J Dermatol.* 2016;175(6):1153-1165.
204. Zhao ZT, Ji CM, Yu WJ, et al. Omalizumab for the treatment of chronic spontaneous urticaria: a meta-analysis of randomized clinical trials. *J Allergy Clin Immunol.* 2016;137(6):1742-1750.e1744.
205. Saini SS, Bindslev-Jensen C, Maurer M, et al. Efficacy and safety of omalizumab in patients with chronic idiopathic/spontaneous urticaria who remain symptomatic on H1 antihistamines: a randomized, placebo-controlled study. *J Invest Dermatol.* 2015;135(1):67-75.
206. Kaplan A, Ledford D, Ashby M, et al. Omalizumab in patients with symptomatic chronic idiopathic/spontaneous urticaria despite standard combination therapy. *J Allergy Clin Immunol.* 2013;132(1):101-109.
207. Fueyo-Casado A, Campos-Munoz L; Gonzalez-Guerra E, et al. Effectiveness of omalizumab in a case of urticarial vasculitis. *Clin Exp Dermatol.* 2017.
208. Kobza-Black A. Delayed pressure urticaria. *J Investig Dermatol Symp Proc.* 2001;6(2):148-149.
209. Berroeta L, Clark C, Ibbotson SH, et al. Narrow-band (TL-01) ultraviolet B phototherapy for chronic urticaria. *Clin Exp Dermatol.* 2004;29(1):97-98.
210. Bas M, Greve J, Stelter K, et al. A randomized trial of icatibant in ACE-inhibitor-induced angioedema. *N Engl J Med.* 2015;372(5):418-425.
211. Botnaru T, Robert A, Mottillo S. Icatibant compared to steroids and antihistamines for ACE-inhibitor-induced angioedema. *CJEM.* 2017;19(2):159-162.
212. Straka BT, Ramirez CE, Byrd JB, et al. Effect of bradykinin receptor antagonism on ACE inhibitor-associated angioedema. *J Allergy Clin Immunol.* 2016.
213. Grattan CE, Humphreys F. Guidelines for evaluation and management of urticaria in adults and children. *Br J Dermatol.* 2007;157(6):1116-1123.
214. O'Donnell BF, Lawlor F, Simpson J, et al. The impact of chronic urticaria on the quality of life. *Br J Dermatol.* 1997;136(2):197-201.
215. Bork K, Hardt J, Schicketanz KH, et al. Clinical studies of sudden upper airway obstruction in patients with hereditary angioedema due to C1 esterase inhibitor deficiency. *Arch Intern Med.* 2003;163(10):1229-1235.

Chapter 42 :: Mastocytosis
:: Michael D. Tharp

第四十二章
肥大细胞增生症

中文导读

　　本章主要从流行病学史和发病机制、临床特点、诊断和治疗等方面阐述了肥大细胞增生症。在临床特点方面，讲述了世界卫生组织对于肥大细胞增生症的分类。接着介绍了肥大细胞增生症的皮肤表现，主要从儿童和成人两个方面来讲。在诊断与鉴别诊断上，本章用流程图的形式了介绍了肥大细胞增生症的诊断流程。并给出了有皮肤临床表现和无皮肤临床表现的肥大细胞增生症的鉴别诊断。在治疗上本章提到肥大细胞增生症不能治愈，只能缓解。同时，对于一些反复发生危及生命的低血压患者建议随身携带肾上腺素以备紧急使用。

〔李芳芳〕

AT-A-GLANCE

MASTOCYTOSIS
- The hallmark of mastocytosis is a pathologic accumulation of mast cells in tissues.
- Mastocytosis occurs at any age but children are more commonly affected.
- Cutaneous findings consist of hyperpigmented macules, papules, or nodules, or a diffuse infiltration of the dermis.
- Most children only have skin involvement, whereas adults are more likely to have systemic disease.
- Mastocytosis is usually associated with somatic activating mutations of *c-kit* with the 816 codon mutation being most common.
- Many patients have few, if any, symptoms, but some experience varying degrees of flushing, pruritus, hypotension, nausea, dyspepsia, and diarrhea.
- Most common extracutaneous tissues involved are the bone marrow, liver, spleen, and lymph nodes.
- Some patients may develop an associated myeloproliferative or myelodysplastic disorder.
- No effective cure currently exists; treatment is focused on controlling symptoms

MAST CELLS
- Mast cells are derived from pluripotent stem cells.
- Stem cell factor is the ligand for KIT and is required for mast cell proliferation and survival.
- Mast cells release both preformed and newly generated mediators.

EPIDEMIOLOGY

Mastocytosis represents a group of disorders characterized by an abnormal accumulation of mast cells in one or more organs. Although the true incidence of this disease is unknown, most cases arise in children, with approximately 70% of cases occurring by 6 months of age and more than 90% occurring within the first 2 years of life.[1-5] Congenital mastocytosis is less common, representing approximately 18% to 31% of childhood cases.[2-4] The prevalence of childhood-onset mastocytosis is reported to range from 2.0 to 5.4 cases/1000 population.[1,2] The prevalence of adult-onset systemic mastocytosis (SM) in Denmark has been reported to be approximately 1/10,000 population over a 14-year period.[6] Mastocytosis has no gender preference, and it has been reported in all races.[5] While most mastocytosis patients have no family history, there are reports of more than 70 familial cases, including monozygotic twins, some of which were discordant for this disease.[7-9]

PATHOGENESIS

Mast cells arise from the bone marrow as agranular, undifferentiated, CD34+, KIT+ (CD117) pluripotent progenitor cells. After migrating into tissues, immature mast cells assume their typical granular morphology.[10] KIT, a Type III tyrosine kinase is the product of the protooncogene *c-kit* located on chromosome 4q12. This enzyme is expressed on mast cells, as well as melanocytes, primitive hematopoietic stem cells, primordial germ cells, and interstitial cells of Cajal and serves as the receptor for its ligand, stem cell factor (SCF). Crosslinking of KIT by SCF is essential for mast cell maturation. The gene for SCF is located on chromosome 12, and encodes a protein that localizes to the cell membrane.[10,11] Membrane-bound and a soluble forms of SCF exist, both of which are capable of inducing KIT activation. Soluble KIT is thought to arise from chymase-induced cleavage of the membrane bound form.[12] SCF is produced by bone marrow stromal cells, fibroblasts, keratinocytes, endothelial cells, as well as reproductive Sertoli and granulosa cells. Mature mast cells require SCF for survival.[11,12] Other cytokines that appear important in regulating mast cell growth and differentiation include interleukin-3 (IL-3), IL-4, IL-6, and IL-9 and interferon (IFN)-γ. IL-3 shares a number of signal transduction pathways with SCF, but has minimal direct effects on human mast cell proliferation except in early cultures. IL-4 enhances mast cell function when added to mature cultures. IL-6 increases mast cell mediator concentration[13] and IL-9 appears to increase the number of mast cells in culture.[14] In developing mast cells, IFN-γ inhibits mast cell proliferation and influences mast cell phenotype and function.[13]

Mutations in *c-kit* appear to play a central role in mastocytosis. Somatic mutations in codon 816 of *c-kit*, lead to amino acid substitutions (D816V, D816Y, D816F, D816I, and D816H), and cause constitutive activation of KIT, resulting in continued mast cell growth and development.[15,16] Mutations in this codon are most common in adults with mastocytosis, but also occur in childhood onset disease.[2,15,17] Among 50 children with this disorder, 42% had detectable mutations at codon 816 (exon 17), while another 42% had activating mutations in the extracellular and transmembrane regions of KIT (exons 8-11). The remaining 8 children reported in this study had no detectable *c-kit* mutations. There was no clear correlation between the extent of disease and the presence or absence of *c-kit* mutations among these 50 patients.[17] In another report of 22 children and adults with mastocytosis, 11 adult patients and 4 children had 816 activating mutations. Four other pediatric patients with typical lesions of urticaria pigmentosa (UP) lacked changes in this codon, and in 3 other children, an inactivating *c-kit* mutation (codon E839K) was detected.[15] Less common activating *c-kit* mutations, such asV560G, also have been characterized in some adult patients with mastocytosis,[15,16] as have severely truncated, inactive KITs (Table 42-1).[18] A transgenic mouse model of mastocytosis has been reported using the human activating D816V *c-kit* mutation.[19] The clinical expression of this disorder ranged from indolent mast cell hyperplasia to invasive mast cell tumors, even though genetically identical animals expressed the same D816V mutation. These clinical and investigative observations indicate that *c-kit* activating mutations play an important role in the development of mastocytosis. However, the finding of a varied clinical expression of mastocytosis in an animal model along with the fact that some children and adults with mastocytosis have no *c-kit* mutations or have inactivating *c-kit* mutations, strongly suggests that other, yet to be defined, factors influence the full clinical expression of this disease. Indeed, mutations in addition to *c-kit* have been identified in some adults with SM. These include the tumor-suppressor gene *TET2*, was well as *ASXL1, JAK2, SRSF2, DNMT3A, RUNX1,* and *CBL*, all of which may play a role in persistent and more aggressive disease.[20,21]

CLINICAL FINDINGS

CLASSIFICATION

Mastocytosis represents a disease spectrum characterized by a diverse phenotypic expression, along with

TABLE 42-1
c-Kit Mutations in Mastocytosis

Activating Mutations
D816V, D816Y, D816F, D816I, D816H, S849I, D835Y, N822I, D820G, V560G, V559I, A53D, D572A, F522C, K509I, S476I, C443Y, D419Y, del417-418, ITD 501-502, ITD 502-503, ITD 505-508

Inactivating Mutations
E839K, del exon 3-13

Increased Sensitivity to Stem Cell Factor
M541L

pathologic and genetic findings that affect prognosis. Table 42-2 represents the World Health Organization (WHO) classification of mastocytosis.[5] Cutaneous mastocytosis (CM) and indolent SM (ISM) represent the majority of patients with this disease. Most children have CM, which is manifested as UP (Fig. 42-1) or, less commonly, as mastocytomas (Fig. 42-2), or as diffuse CM (Fig. 42-3). SM occurs mostly in adults, and ISM is the most common form. Table 42-3 lists the criteria for SM. SM with an associated clonal hematologic non–mast-cell-lineage disease (SM-AHNMD) occurs almost uniquely in adults, and can be demonstrated, by examining the peripheral blood and bone marrow. Hematologic disorders associated with SM-AHNMD include myeloproliferative and myelodysplastic disorders, such as polycythemia rubra vera, chronic myeloid leukemia, chronic myelomonocytic leukemia, idiopathic myelofibrosis, chronic eosinophilic leukemia and the hypereosinophilic syndrome, acute and chronic lymphocytic leukemia, and non-Hodgkin and Hodgkin lymphoma. Patients with aggressive SM (ASM) frequently have evidence of impaired liver function, hypersplenism, and/or malabsorption, but they do not have a distinctive hematologic disorder or mast cell leukemia (MCL). Patients with ASM have rapidly increasing mast cell numbers and are difficult to manage medically.[5,22] MCL is rare and characterized by multiorgan failure, bone marrow smears demonstrating a greater than 20% mast cell population among the nucleated cell population. In the peripheral blood, mast cells are at least 10% of nucleated cells.[5,23] Both acute and chronic forms of MCL have been described; they are differentiated based on symptoms and organ involvement.[23] Mast cell sarcomas are rare; they have localized destructive growth, but distant spread is possible. Mast cells in these tumors are highly atypical and immature. Extracutaneous mastocytomas are extremely rare, usually localized to the lung, and consist of mature mast cells.[5,22,24,25]

CUTANEOUS LESIONS

UP was originally described in children and is the most common skin manifestation of childhood-onset CM. UP lesions in children appear as tan to brown papules and, less commonly, as macules, ranging in size from 1.0 to 2.5 cm in diameter (see Fig. 42-1). These lesions may be present at birth or arise during infancy. They frequently appear on the trunk and often spare the central face, scalp, palms, and soles. Cutaneous lesions in adults, on the other hand, are much smaller (approximately 5 mm or less in diameter) reddish-brown macules and papules (Fig. 42-4). On close lesion inspection, variable hyperpigmenta-

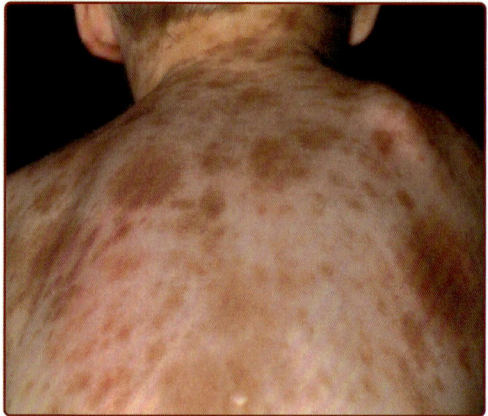

Figure 42-1 Urticaria pigmentosa in a child.

TABLE 42-2
World Health Organization Classification of Mastocytosis[a]

VARIANT TERM	ABBREVIATION	SUBVARIANTS	EXAMPLES
Cutaneous mastocytosis	CM		Urticaria pigmentosa Diffuse CM Mastocytoma of skin Telangiectasia macularis eruptiva perstans (TMEP)
Indolent systemic mastocytosis	ISM	Smoldering SM Isolated bone marrow mastocytosis	
Systemic mastocytosis with an associated clonal hematologic non–mast-cell-lineage disease	SM-AHNMD		Acute myelogenous leukemia Myelodysplastic syndrome Chronic myelomonocytic leukemia Chronic eosinophilic leukemia Non-Hodgkin lymphoma
Aggressive systemic mastocytosis	ASM	Acute vs chronic	
Mast cell leukemia	MCL		
Mast cell sarcoma	MCS		
Extracutaneous mastocytoma	ECM		

[a]For details of the WHO classification of mastocytosis, see Valent P, et al.[5]

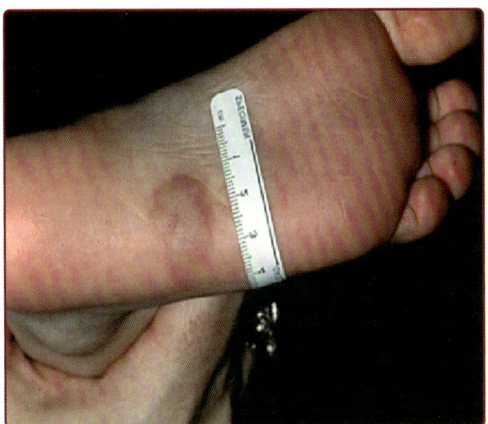

Figure 42-2 Mastocytoma on the sole of a child.

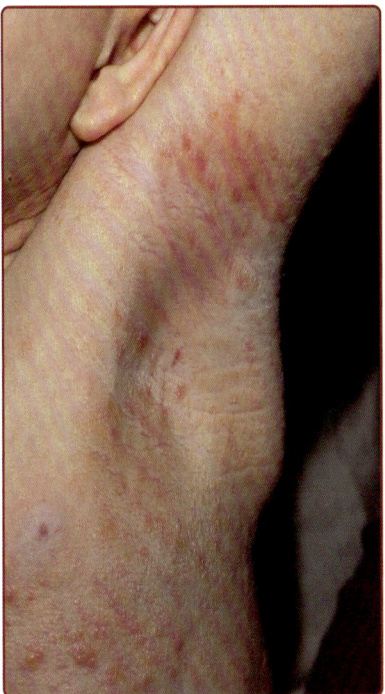

Figure 42-3 Diffuse cutaneous mastocytosis in a child.

TABLE 42-3
Diagnostic Criteria for Systemic Mastocytosis (Major and One Minor or Three Minor Criteria Are Needed)[a]

Major
- Multifocal dense infiltrates of mast cells in bone marrow and/or other extracutaneous organs

Minor
- More than 25% of the mast cells in bone marrow aspirate smears or tissue biopsy sections are spindle shaped or display atypical morphology.
- Detection of a codon 816 *c-kit* point mutation in blood, bone marrow, or lesional tissue.
- Mast cells in bone marrow, blood, or other lesional tissue expressing CD25 or CD2.
- Baseline total tryptase level greater than 20 ng/mL.

[a]For details of the WHO classification of mastocytosis, see Valent P, et al.[5]

tion and fine telangiectasias are detectable. In patients with Type I skin, these lesions may lack pigment and appear pink to red. Adult skin lesions are most numerous on the trunk and proximal extremities and appear less frequently on the face, distal extremities, or palms and soles. While adult lesions may appear and resolve over months in individual patients, their number usually increases over years. Most adults with ISM have cutaneous lesions, but skin involvement is less common in patients with more advanced forms of SM (SM-AHNMD, ASM, or MCL).[5,22,24,25]

Solitary mastocytomas are tan-brown nodules that occur in approximately 10% to 35% of children and frequently appear on the distal extremities (see Fig. 42-2). Their onset is generally before 6 months of age.[1-4] Scratching or rubbing skin lesions leads to urtication and erythema known as *Darier sign*. This reaction is readily demonstrated in childhood UP and mastocytomas, but often is less pronounced in adult skin lesions.[24-27] The difference in lesional skin reactivity between children and adults with CM is best explained by the observation that mast cell concentrations in mastocytomas and childhood UP are 150-fold and 40-fold greater than in normal skin, respectively, whereas the mast cell content in lesions of adult mastocytosis is only 8 times greater than normal controls.[27] Because trauma to mastocytomas is associated with systemic symptoms such as flushing and hypotension, vigorous scratching of UP lesions or mastocytomas is not advised.[1-4,24,26]

Diffuse CM (DCM) is seen almost exclusively in infants (see Fig. 42-3), although it may persist into adult life. The skin often has a peau d'orange appearance and yellowish-brown discoloration. Rarely, individual yellow-tan papules have been described; the individual yellow-tan papules are called *xanthelasmoidal mastocytosis*.[26,28] Dermographism with formation of hemorrhagic blisters can occur in the first months to years of life in children with DCM, but these blisters often resolve within several years, even though the DCM may persist (Fig. 42-5).[1-4,26] Telangiectasia macularis eruptiva perstans is rare, and is seen almost exclusively in adults. It appears as telangiectatic macules and patches without hyperpigmentation (Fig. 42-6). The Darier sign and pruritus are variable in patients with telangiectasia macularis eruptiva perstans.[24-26] Tumor-like growths also have been described in an adult mastocytosis patient in whose mast cells expressed the V560G *c-kit* mutation.[29]

RELATED CLINICAL FINDINGS

Most children with CM and adults with CM or ISM have few, if any, symptoms, but children with DCM are more likely to have skin and GI symptoms.[1,2] When

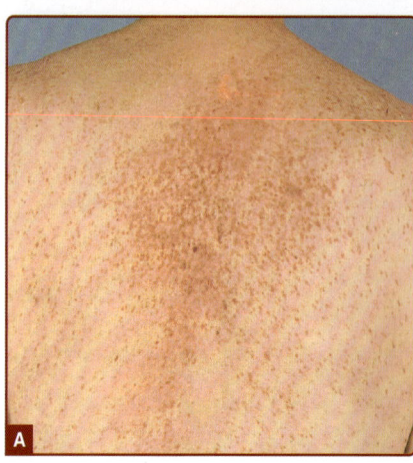 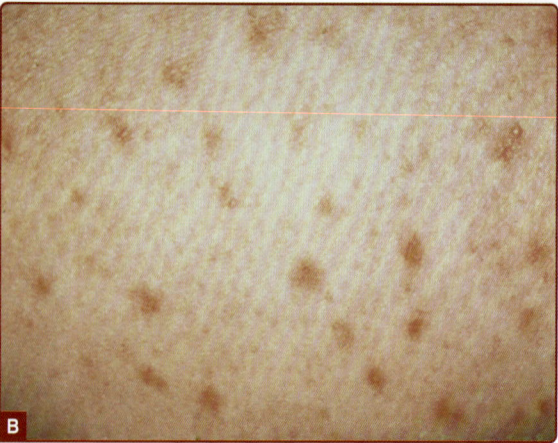

Figure 42-4 Typical red brown papules in an adult with indolent systemic mastocytosis. **A,** Hundreds of lentigo-like macules are seen on the back of this adult. If vigorously rubbed, these lesions will show urtication and become erythematous, raised, and pruritic. **B,** Close-up view of the macules.

symptoms occur, they are caused by the release of mast cell mediators, such as histamine, eicosanoids, and cytokines, and often involve several different organs (ie, skin and GI tract or skin and cardiovascular) (Table 42-4). Symptoms and signs of mastocytosis may include: pruritus, flushing, diarrhea, abdominal pain, nausea, bloating, vomiting, gastric reflux, palpitations, dizziness, and/or syncope. Of interest is the relative absence of pulmonary symptoms in mastocytosis patients. Complaints of fever, night sweats, malaise, weight loss, bone pain, epigastric distress, and problems with mentation (cognitive disorganization) often signal the presence of SM. Symptoms of mastocytosis can be exacerbated by exercise, heat, or local trauma to skin lesions (childhood UP and mastocytomas). In addition, alcohol, narcotics, salicylates, nonsteroidal antiinflammatory drugs (NSAIDs), polymyxin B, anticholinergics, and some systemic anesthetic agents may induce mast cell mediator release.[5,23-26] It has been suggested that anaphylaxis from hymenoptera stings may be more common in mastocytosis patients, but deaths associated with extensive mast cell mediator release are rare.[2,5,30]

Extracutaneous disease is extremely uncommon in children, but when present GI symptoms are the most frequent.[1,2,4] GI symptoms in adults ranges from 25% to 70%.[5,31,32] Diarrhea is the most common symptom and may result from gastric hypersecretion, increased motility, and/or malabsorption. Increased gastric acid secretion is likely a result of elevated histamine release, which may cause gastritis and peptic ulcer disease.[33] Malabsorption with associated diarrhea is limited to a subset of patients with usually more advanced disease. While hepatic disease in adults and children with ISM is rare, liver and spleen involvement, including portal hypertension and ascites associated with liver fibrosis, may occur in patients who have SM-AHNMD or ASM.[5,24,25,34] Splenomegaly, detected either clinically or by CT scan, has been reported in 50% to 60% of adult SM patients.[26,35] However, in 2 other studies, each with more than 140 adult mastocytosis patients, splenomegaly was observed in only 8% to 9% of cases.[36,37] Increased numbers of mast cells and eosinophils are frequently observed in the spleen, as are varying degrees of fibrosis and hematopoiesis. Lymph node enlargement is uncommon in most patients with

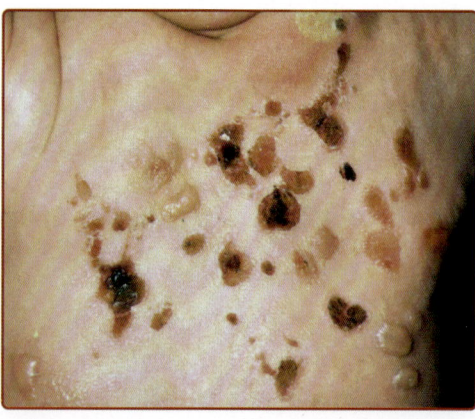

Figure 42-5 Bullous eruption on the back of a child with diffuse cutaneous mastocytosis.

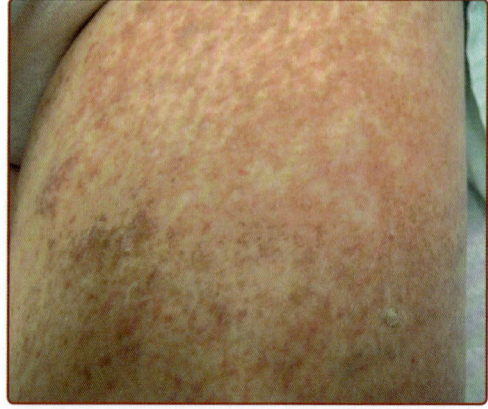

Figure 42-6 Telangiectasia macularis eruptive perstans.

ISM, but occurs in patients with more advanced disease. Among 58 SM patients, 15 (26%) had peripheral lymphadenopathy, whereas 11 (19%) had central nodal disease.[38] Anemia, leukopenia, thrombocytopenia, and eosinophilia also may occur in association with SM and suggest SM-AHNMD or ASM.[5,22,24,25]

Musculoskeletal pain affects 19% to 28% of mastocytosis patients. Skeletal lesions occur in patients with SM, but are rare in children with this disorder.[1,2,36,39,40] In one large study of 142 adults with mastocytosis, 40% had skeletal involvement.[36] Bony lesions may appear as radiopacities, radiolucencies, or a mixture of the two. The skull, spine, and pelvis are most commonly involved. In another study of 58 adult SM patients, 34 (57%) had diffuse bone involvement, whereas only 1(2%) had focal lesions.[39] In 199 ISM patients, disease-related lumbar spine osteoporosis was more frequently observed in men. The prevalence of vertebral fractures was 20% in men compared to 14% in women with mastocytosis. This observation has led to the recommendation to consider the diagnosis of mastocytosis in men with unexplained osteroporosis.[40]

Neuropsychiatric abnormalities have been reported, and include decreased attention span, memory impairment, headache, and irritability. Depression as a consequence of chronic disease or possibly mediated by mast cell mediators may occur.[41,42]

Information pertaining to pregnancy in mastocytosis is limited. However, there are numerous reports of successful, full-term deliveries in women with mast cell disease.[43,44] In a report of 45 pregnancies in 30 mastocytosis patients, 10 (22%) had worsening mast cell–related symptoms, whereas 15 (33%) experienced improved or resolved symptoms. Among the 45 newborns, only 7 were premature, had a low birthweight and/or suffered from respiratory distress. No fatal maternal or fetal outcomes were reported.[45]

LABORATORY TESTS

The diagnosis of mastocytosis is established by demonstrating increased numbers of mast cells in 1 or more organs. For patients with CM, mast cell infiltrates can be detected in a biopsy of lesional skin using special stains, such as toluidine (Fig. 42-7), Giemsa, or monoclonal antibodies that recognize mast cell tryptase or CD117 (KIT).[26,27,46] Biopsy specimens of normal-appearing skin from patients with mastocytosis have

TABLE 42-4
Selected Mast Cell Mediators

MEDIATORS	BIOLOGIC EFFECTS	POSSIBLE CONSEQUENCES
Preformed		
Histamine	Vasodilation, increased vascular permeability, gastric hypersecretion, bronchoconstriction	Hypotension, flushing, urticaria, abdominal pain (peptic, colic), nausea, vomiting, diarrhea, malabsorption CNS symptoms
Heparin	Anticoagulant, inhibition of platelet aggregation	Prolonged bleeding time Osteoporosis/osteopenia
Tryptase	Endothelial cell activation, fibrinogen cleavage, mitogenic for smooth muscle cells	Osteoporosis/osteopenia, disruption of cascade systems (clotting, etc)
Chymase	Converts angiotensin I to II, lipoprotein degradation	Hypertension Hyperpigmentation
	Cleaves membrane-bound stem cell factor	Skin mast cell accumulation (?)
Newly Synthesized		
Leukotrienes	Increased vascular permeability, bronchoconstriction, vasoconstriction	Bronchospasm, hypotension
Prostaglandins	Vasodilation, bronchoconstriction	Flushing, urticaria, hypotension CNS symptoms
Cytokines		
Stem cell factor	Growth and survival of mast cells, chemotaxis of KIT+ cells, melanogenesis	Mast cell hyperplasia, focal aggregates
Tumor necrosis factor-α	Activation of vascular endothelial cells, cachexia, fatigue	Weight loss, fever, fatigue
Transforming growth factor-β	Enhanced production of connective tissue components	Fibrosis
Interleukin (IL)-1	Activates fibroblasts, lymphocytes and increases neutrophils	Fibrosis, fever
IL-5	Eosinophil growth factor	Eosinophilia
IL-6	Growth and survival of mast cells	Fever, bone pain, osteoporosis/osteopenia
Granulocyte-macrophage colony-stimulating factor	Granulocyte and monocyte growth and activation	Eosinophilia

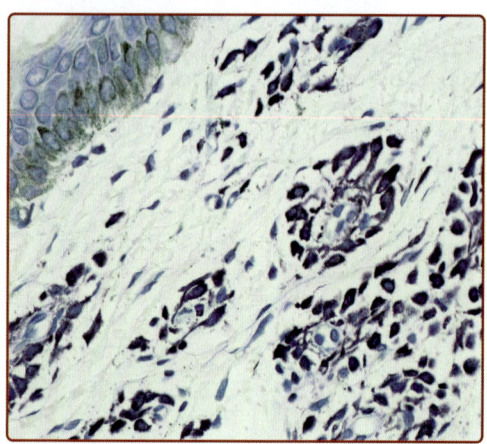

Figure 42-7 Histopathology of urticaria pigmentosa, toluidine blue stain.

normal concentrations of mast cells as determined by morphometrics, and thus are not helpful in establishing the diagnosis.[27]

Detection of circulating mast cell mediators and/or their metabolites can offer indirect evidence of mastocytosis, and their measurement may be useful in patients without cutaneous lesions. Two forms (α and β) of mast cell tryptase have been identified. α-Tryptase is elevated in patients with SM, with or without acute symptoms, whereas increased levels of β-tryptase can be detected both in mastocytosis patients and in allergic patients experiencing anaphylactic reactions. Total (α + β) serum tryptase levels are most commonly measured and correlate with the extent of mast cell disease.[47,48] In children, elevated serum tryptase levels correlate with more-extensive skin involvement and a greater number and severity of symptoms.[48] Of adult mastocytosis patients with total serum tryptase levels between 20 and 75 ng/mL, 50% had evidence of SM, whereas all patients with levels >75 ng/mL had proven systemic involvement.[47] Total serum tryptase levels of >20 ng/mL are currently considered abnormal and represent one of the minor criteria for SM (see Table 42-3).[5] Total serum tryptase levels also can provide an estimate of a patient's overall mast cell burden, and thus serial measurements in adults every 6 to 12 months may prove useful in following disease progression.

Determinations of urinary histamine metabolite levels may be worthwhile as a diagnostic test in patients without cutaneous lesions and in whom the diagnosis of mastocytosis is unclear. The major urinary metabolite of histamine, 1,4-methylimidazole acetic acid is often persistently elevated in SM patients and correlates with the extent of mast cell disease. Methylhistamine is next most common urinary histamine metabolite, and can be measured if 1,4-methylimidazole acetic acid levels are not available in commercial laboratories. Certain foods high in histamine content, such as spinach, eggplant, cheeses (eg, Parmesan, Roquefort, and blue), and red wines, can artificially elevate the levels of urinary histamine and its metabolites, and thus should be avoided during the collection process.[49]

Mast cells can induce bone changes that cause radiographically detectable lesions. Skeletal lesions occur more frequently in adult patients with SM, and are rare in children with this disorder.[1,26,36,40] In one large study of 142 adults with mastocytosis, 57 (40%) had skeletal involvement.[36] The proximal long bones, skull, spine, ribs, and pelvis are most commonly affected. Skeletal scintigraphy (bone scan) is more sensitive, but less specific, than routine radiographs for detecting and locating active lesions. Thus, radiographs of the skull, spine, and pelvis serve as a reasonable preliminary test for detecting bone involvement in mastocytosis patients.[36,40]

The bone marrow is often involved in patients with SM, and bone marrow biopsies are indicated for patients suspected of having more advanced disease (SM-AHNMD, ASM, MCL).[5,22] In a report of 71 adults with mastocytosis, 90% had increased numbers of spindle-shaped, bone marrow mast cells with focal perivascular, peritrabecular, and/or intertrabecular accumulations.[26] WHO criteria for SM have been defined and include the bone marrow findings of multifocal dense mast cell aggregates, atypical mast cell morphology, and the expression of CD2 and/or CD25 by bone marrow mast cells (see Table 42-3). A bone marrow biopsy in childhood-onset disease is not recommended unless there is evidence of systemic involvement as demonstrated by hepatosplenomegaly, lymphadenopathy, and/or unexplained peripheral blood abnormalities.[1,2,50] Mast cells in bone marrow biopsies are best identified by immunostaining with antitryptase (Fig. 42-8) or CD117 monoclonal antibodies as decalcification interferes with the effectiveness of metachromatic stains.[5,22]

Roentgenographic abnormalities of the GI tract fall into 3 major categories: (a) peptic ulcers; (b) abnormal mucosal patterns such as mucosal edema, multiple nodular lesions, coarsened mucosal folds, or multiple polyps; and (c) motility disturbances. A biopsy of the GI tract may be indicated for patients in

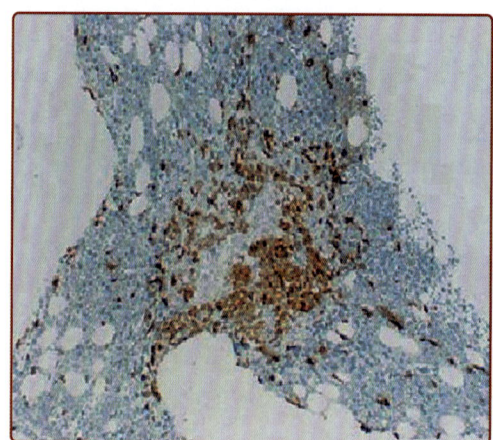

Figure 42-8 Classic mastocytosis bone marrow lesion (×100), tryptase stain.

whom the diagnosis of SM is suspected, but who lack skin lesions. Histologic sections of jejunal biopsies show moderate blunting of the villi and may show increased mast cell numbers in association with variable numbers of eosinophils.[22,26,31,51] Increased mast cells in bowel biopsies should always be correlated with other signs and symptoms of mastocytosis as these findings also have been reported in patients with irritable bowel syndrome and mast cell activation syndrome.[51]

Despite the infrequency of significant hepatic disease, liver function tests may be abnormal in up to 50% of SM patients.[26,39] Elevated serum IL-6 levels, soluble SCF receptor (CD117), and IL-2 receptor (CD25) levels are associated with SM, but their specificity is not established.[52]

The initial evaluation of a prepubertal child with mastocytosis generally does not require extensive testing if the history and physical examination do not indicate the presence of SM. In contrast, the presence of noncutaneous signs and symptoms or disease onset in adolescents or adults necessitates a complete blood count (CBC) with differential, liver function test, total serum tryptase level, and skeletal radiographs (Fig. 42-9 and see Table 42-4). While bone marrow biopsies have been recommended by some clinicians for all adult mastocytosis patients, it is the opinion of this author that this procedure is unnecessary for those with a normal CBC. Should the CBC become abnormal in an adult patient, however, then the cause of this abnormality should be investigated by examining the bone marrow.

DIFFERENTIAL DIAGNOSIS

Cutaneous lesions of childhood and adult mastocytosis are so characteristic, that they are rarely confused with other skin disorders. Because UP lesions may urticate, they could initially be mistaken for urticaria. However, individual urticaria lesions last only a few hours and lack the associated hyperpigmentation seen

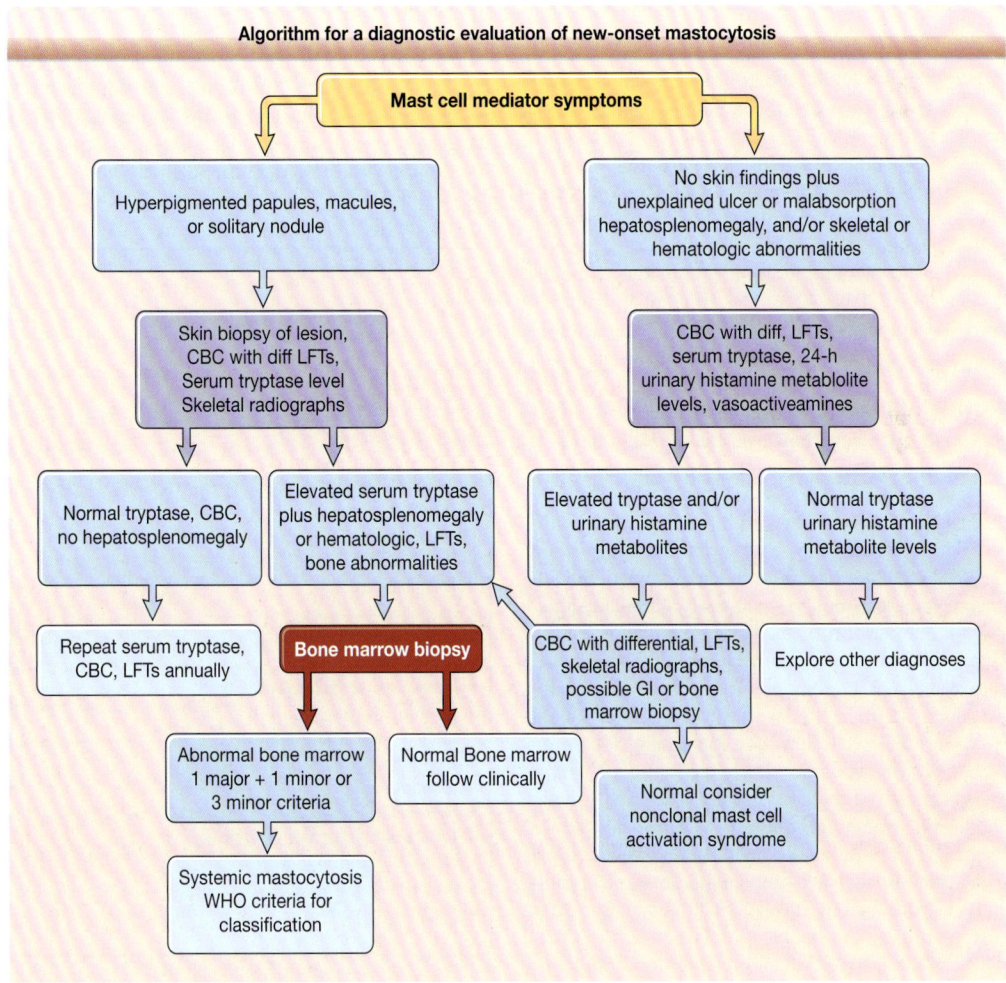

Figure 42-9 Algorithm for a diagnostic evaluation of new-onset mastocytosis (especially in adolescents and adults). CBC, complete blood cell count; LFT, liver function test; Tc, technetium; WHO, World Health Organization. For details of the WHO classification of mastocytosis, see Valent P, et al.[5]

TABLE 42-5
Differential Diagnosis of Cutaneous Mast Cell Disease
Most Likely
- Diffuse or localized red-brown papules/macules
- Urticaria
- Multiple nevi
- Langerhans cell histiocytosis
- Juvenile xanthogranulomas
- Nodular scabies
- Café-au-lait spots
- Multiple cutaneous lentiginosis
- Bullous lesions
- Linear immunoglobulin A dermatosis
- Bullous impetigo
- Epidermolysis bullosa
- Arthropod bite reaction
- Toxic epidermal necrolysis
- Incontinentia pigmenti
- Solitary papule or nodule
- Congenital nevus
- Juvenile xanthogranuloma
- Pseudolymphoma

in UP. Rarely, nodular scabies lesions have been confused with UP. Some childhood mastocytosis patients, especially those with DCM, may develop bullae, and, thus, the differential diagnosis for blistering diseases in infants such as bullous impetigo, bullous arthropod bites, linear immunoglobulin A bullous dermatosis, bullous pemphigoid, epidermolysis bullosa, toxic epidermal necrolysis, and incontinentia pigmenti should be considered (Table 42-5). The differential diagnosis of mastocytomas in children includes juvenile xanthogranulomas, Spitz nevi, pseudolymphomas, or, rarely, in resolving lesions, a café-au-lait macule. Adult UP lesions might initially appear as lentigines or atypical melanocytic nevi; however, they usually have an associated erythema (telangiectasia) not seen in these melanocytic lesions.

Mastocytosis should be suspected in patients without skin lesions if they have symptoms suggesting mast cell mediator release, and one or more of the following: hepatomegaly, splenomegaly, lymphadenopathy, and/or peripheral blood abnormalities as well as peptic ulcer disease, malabsorption, or unexplained osteoporosis or radiographic/bone scan abnormalities (Table 42-6). In the last few years, patients with nonclonal mast cell activation syndrome have been described. This condition is characterized by symptoms of mast cell mediator release, such as flushing, abdominal cramping, diarrhea, headache, and/or memory/concentration difficulties. However, these patients lack evidence of unregulated mast cell proliferation. Nonclonal mast cell activation syndrome has been reported more frequently in women who experience urticaria/angioedema, respiratory symptoms, have drugs as a trigger for their symptoms, and total serum tryptase levels <15 ng/mL.[53] In addition, these patients often respond to H_1 and H_2 antihistamines and leukotriene inhibitors.[53,54] Nonclonal mast cell activation syndrome must be differentiated from the broader term *mast cell activation disorder*, which also includes various forms of mastocytosis.[54] In patients with flushing, the diagnosis of a carcinoid tumor or pheochromocytoma should be considered. Mastocytosis patients, however, do not excrete increased amounts of 5-hydroxyindoleacetic acid, and patients with carcinoid tumor or pheochromocytoma do not have histologic evidence of mast cell proliferation or elevated serum tryptase levels.[24-26]

PROGNOSIS

Pediatric-onset cutaneous disease has a favorable prognosis with 45% to 68% of patients experiencing complete disease regression with a median followup of 15 to 20 years.[1,2] Children born of mothers with ISM reportedly are free of disease.[42,44] It has been postulated that children with activating *c-kit* mutations may represent those patients whose disease persists into adulthood; however, activating *c-kit* mutations, including D816V, have been identified in up to 84% of children with mastocytosis.[17] To date, there has been no correlation of disease severity or outcome in children who have *c-kit* mutations.[2,17] Most adults with skin lesions of mastocytosis have only CM or ISM, and rarely develop more advanced disease having a life expectancy commensurate with the general population. In a study of

TABLE 42-6
Differential Diagnosis of Systemic Mastocytosis without Skin Lesions[a]
Gastrointestinal
- Peptic ulcer disease
- Ulcerative colitis
- Gluten-sensitive enteropathy
- Hepatitis
- Parasitic disease
Nonclonal Mast Cell Activation Syndrome
- Cardiovascular
- Idiopathic anaphylaxis
- Intrinsic cardiac disease
- Endocrine
- Adrenal tumor
- Vasoactive intestinal polypeptide tumor
- Carcinoid syndrome
- Medullary thyroid carcinoma
- Gastrinoma
Neoplastic/Oncologic
- Hypereosinophilic syndrome
- Lymphoma
- Myeloma
- Histiocytosis
- Bone tumor metastases
- Paget disease of the bone

[a]Some forms of mast cell disease may not show cutaneous manifestations. These include aggressive systemic mastocytosis, mast cell leukemia, systemic mastocytosis with an associated clonal hematologic non–mast-cell-lineage disease, and isolated bone marrow mastocytosis.

145 adults with ISM, the cumulative probabilities of developing more advanced mast cell disease at 10 and 25 years were 1.7% and 8.4%, respectively.[37] Patients with ISM who have evidence of hepatosplenomegaly, lymphadenopathy and/or serum tryptase levels of >200 ng/mL have been referred to as smoldering SM. The prognosis of this group is not well defined but is believed to be less favorable than the ISM group.[5,22,37] Older patients who experience fading of their lesions continue to exhibit bone marrow lesions typical of their diagnosis, whether ISM or SM-AHNMD.[55] Patients with SM-AHNMD have a variable course, which is dependent on the prognosis of their hematologic disorder. One study suggests that SM-AHNMD patients who express a mutation in the *ASXL1* gene have a poorer overall survival than those who express wild-type *ASXL1*.[20] In patients with ASM, the mean survival is 2 to 4 years, but the prognosis may improve with aggressive symptomatic management. The prognosis for MCL is poor, with a mean survival of less than 1 year.[23,37] Additional poor prognostic findings in adult mastocytosis patients include detectable D816V mutations in non–mast cell populations, as well as the expression of one or more non–*c-kit* gene mutations (*TETS, SRSF2, ASXLI, ASCL1, RUNXI,* and *CBL*).[20,21]

TREATMENT

The management of patients with mastocytosis includes counseling patients about the pathophysiology of their disease, avoidance of factors that provoke mast cell mediator release, and management of symptoms associated with these released mediators (Tables 42-7 and 42-8). Mastocytosis patients should be cautioned to avoid potential mast cell degranulating agents such as ingested alcohol, anticholinergic preparations, aspirin, NSAIDs, narcotics, and polymyxin B sulfate. In addition, heat and friction can induce local or systemic symptoms and should be avoided whenever possible. A number of systemic anesthetic agents, including systemic lidocaine, D-tubocurarine, metocurine, etomidate, thiopental, succinylcholine hydrochloride (suxamethonium chloride), enflurane, and isoflurane, have been directly or indirectly implicated in precipitating symptoms of mastocytosis. Recent reports indicate that fentanyl, sufentanil, remifentanil, paracetamol, midazolam, propofol, ketamine, desflurane, sevoflurane, *cis*-atracurium, pancuronium, and vecuronium bromide are safe alternative systemic anesthetics for mastocytosis patients. It is recommended that mastocytosis patients undergoing general anesthesia be monitored postoperatively for 24 hours because delayed anaphylaxis can occur hours after surgery. In contrast to systemic anesthetics, local injections of lidocaine normally can be used safely in patients with mastocytosis unless there is a history of reaction.[56,57]

There is currently no generally recognized cure for mastocytosis, nor are there effective mast cell stabi-

TABLE 42-7
Treatment of Cutaneous Mastocytosis

	TOPICAL	SYSTEMIC
First line	Topical glucocorticoids	Avoidance of triggering factors such as heat, friction, or drugs $H_1 \pm H_2$ antihistamines
Second line	Psoralen and ultraviolet A light (adults only)	Leukotriene antagonists or 5-lipoxygenase inhibitor
	Pulsed-dye laser for adult-type skin lesions and telangiectasia macularis eruptiva perstans	Oral cromolyn sodium Ketotifen
Third line	Intralesional corticosteroids Surgical excision (mastocytoma)	Omalizumab

TABLE 42-8
Treatment of Noncutaneous Mastocytosis Symptoms

	GASTROINTESTINAL	CARDIOVASCULAR	MUSCULOSKELETAL	HEMATOLOGIC
First line	H_2 antihistamines, oral cromolyn (children)	H_1 and H_2 antihistamines Subcutaneous epinephrine (anaphylaxis)	Calcium supplement ± vitamin D supplement	2-Chlorodeoxyadenosine
Second line	Proton pump inhibitors	Oral glucocorticoids (prophylaxis)	Bisphosphonates	Systemic chemotherapy appropriate for hematologic disorder
	Leukotriene antagonist		Nonsteroidal antiinflammatory drugs with caution	
	Anticholinergics			
Third line	Omalizumab Oral glucocorticoids	Omalizumab	Omalizumab Oral glucocorticoids Local radiation to bony lesions	Allogeneic stem cell transplantation

Note: Cytoreductive therapy is restricted to patients with aggressive variants of mastocytosis (systemic mastocytosis with an associated clonal hematologic non–mast-cell-lineage disease, aggressive systemic mastocytosis, and mast cell leukemia).

lizing drugs. Thus, treatment of milder forms of this disorder is focused, in great part, on symptomatic relief. In children and adults who are asymptomatic, no therapy is needed. Chronic administration of H_1 antihistamines is often helpful in reducing cutaneous and GI symptoms.[22,45] The second-generation H_1 antihistamines, cetirizine, loratadine, and fexofenadine, have distinct advantages over first-generation antihistamines because they have longer half-lives and have more specific activity on the H_1 receptor.[58] Higher-than-recommended doses of combined H_1 antihistamines may be required for symptom control. For example, fexofenadine 360 mg in the morning and up to 40 mg of cetirizine at night may be necessary for alleviating histamine-related symptoms. Doxepin, a tricyclic antidepressant, has potent H_1 activity and can be used when H_1 antihistamines have been ineffective. This agent, however, can cause cardiac QT interval prolongation and should be used with caution in older patients as well as those with a history of cardiac arrhythmias, renal insufficiency, or hepatic disease.[57] Both ketotifen and azelastine, antihistamines with potential mast cell–stabilizing properties, appear to be most beneficial in relieving GI symptoms associated with mastocytosis, but neither drug offers a significant advantage over a standard antihistamines.[58,59] H_2 antihistamines (cimetidine, ranitidine, famotidine, or nizatidine) may be beneficial in patients with symptoms of gastric acid hypersecretion and malabsorption, but also may assist in controlling pruritus, flushing, and wheal formation when administered with an H_1 agent.[22,45,58] If GI symptoms persist with the use of H_2 antihistamines, proton pump inhibitors may be effective secondary treatments.[45,58]

Disodium cromoglycate (cromolyn sodium) may have some efficacy in the treatment of mastocytosis, particularly in relieving GI complaints in children, but may require higher-than-recommended doses. Cromolyn sodium, however, does not lower plasma or urinary histamine levels in patients with mastocytosis.[60] Low-dose aspirin (500 mg twice daily) has been used successfully in some patients to reduce flushing, tachycardia, and syncope. However, aspirin must be used with extreme caution in patients with a history of NSAID intolerance, as it may cause vascular collapse in some patients with mastocytosis and exacerbate peptic ulcer disease.[61] Leukotriene inhibitors antagonize cysteinyl leukotriene receptors, and have been reported effective in controlling symptoms of flushing, diarrhea, abdominal cramping, and wheezing in mastocytosis patients.[62,63]

Omalizumab is a monoclonal antibody against immunoglobulin E that has proven effective in reducing or eliminating symptoms of mastocytosis in adults who are recalcitrant to antihistamines and leukotriene inhibitors. Effective doses range from 150 to 450 mg/month. Although this monthly therapy has proven effective in managing symptoms from mast cell mediator release, it requires continued administration because it does not reduce mast cell proliferation.[64-66]

Potent topical glucocorticoids applied daily under occlusion for 8 to 12 weeks reduces the number of cutaneous lesions. However, this therapy is impractical for patients with diffuse skin involvement, and lesions of mastocytosis recur with discontinuation of therapy.[67] Oral glucocorticoids may have some efficacy in patients with malabsorption, bone disease, abdominal pain, recurrent anaphylaxis, and ascites; this medication, however, should be reserved for patients with advanced disease, and tapered to the lowest effective dose.[45,57,68] Osteoporosis should be treated with calcium and vitamin D supplementation along with bisphosphonates as needed to maintain normal bone density.[57,69]

Self-injectable epinephrine syringes should be prescribed for patients with a history of anaphylaxis. However, some experts recommend that all mastocytosis patients should carry preloaded epinephrine syringes with them regardless of their anaphylaxis history.[45,57] Patients prescribed epinephrine should be prepared to self-administer this drug, and have a plan for emergency management. If subcutaneous epinephrine is insufficient, intensive therapy for vascular collapse should be instituted in a hospital setting. Patients with recurrent episodes of anaphylaxis also should receive continuous H_1 and H_2 antihistamines to lessen the severity of attacks. Episodes of vascular collapse in mastocytosis patients may be spontaneous, but have also occurred after insect stings or after administration of iodinated contrast media. In the latter case, premedication with corticosteroids and antihistamines is recommended before such procedures.

Methoxypsoralen with ultraviolet A (PUVA) light can relieve pruritus and wheeling after 1 to 2 months of treatment.[70,71] However, pruritus usually recurs within 3 to 6 months after PUVA discontinuation. Pigmentation induced by PUVA also may camouflage lesions of UP in some adult patients; however, this benefit must be weighed against the increased risk of skin cancers associated with long-term treatment.

Cytoreductive therapy should be considered in patients with SM-AHNMD, ASM, MCL, or mast cell sarcoma. The risk-to-benefit ratio must be carefully considered because of the dose-limiting toxicities of the various drugs. IFN-α may be considered for advanced SM. In 2 studies, IFN-α was most efficacious in ameliorating the signs and symptoms of mast cell disease; however, improvement was only transitory.[72,73] 2-Chlorodeoxyadenosine is efficacious in more advanced SM patients with an overall response rate of approximately 55%.[73,74] Even though this drug appears to be the treatment of choice in patients with advanced mastocytosis, myelosuppression may limit its use.[74]

Splenectomy may improve survival in patients with ASM that have a poor prognosis.[75] Radiotherapy has been used to treat refractory bone pain in advanced disease.[76]

More recently, patients with advanced SM (SM-AHNMD, ASM, and MCL) have been treated with allogeneic hematopoietic stem cell transplantation. In a retrospective review of 57 mastocytosis patients treated with allogeneic hematopoietic stem cell transplantation, 16 (28%) had a complete remission, whereas 12 (21%) had stable disease. All 38 patients with SM-AHNMD achieved complete remission for a time; however, 10 experienced a relapse and 5 died of their associated clonal hematologic non–mast-cell-lineage disease. Patients with stable disease and SM-AHNMD had a better overall survival than those with progressing mastocytosis or MCL. The overall survival at 1 and 3 years for the entire treatment group was 62% and 55%, respectively.[77]

Targeting the tyrosine kinase KIT has been another important strategy for treating patients with mastocytosis. The first-generation tyrosine kinase inhibitor, imatinib, however, has proven ineffective in patients expressing KIT D816 because it is unable to inhibit this mutated receptor.[78,79] Imatinib, however, has been reported to cure a mastocytosis patient who expressed only normal (wild-type) *c-kit*.[80] Second-generation tyrosine kinase inhibitors, dasatinib and nilotinib, inhibit the in vitro growth of D816V-expressing mast cell lines. However, these agents also have been disappointing in their ability to reduce the signs or symptoms in SM patients with the D816 mutation.[81-83] The multikinase inhibitor midostaurin, which inhibits both wild-type and mutated *c-kit*, has been used in patients with advanced SM. Among 116 advanced SM patients receiving this agent, there were no complete remissions, but 53 patients had some response to therapy. Patients with SM-AHNMD had the best response rate (75%) in contrast to MCL patients who responded the least (50%). Unfortunately, these responses were limited in duration.[84] Taken together, these observations along with the clinical heterogeneity of mastocytosis, strongly suggest that other molecular abnormalities, in addition to *c-kit* mutations, play an important role in this disease. Thus it appears that more effective future therapies will be based on the identification of additional altered genes.

REFERENCES

1. Lange M, Niedoszytko M, Renke J, et al. Clinical aspects of paediatric mastocytosis: a review of 101 cases. *J Eur Acad Dermatol Venereol.* 2013;27:97.
2. Meni C, Bruneau J, Gorgin-Lavialle S, et al. Paediatric mastocytosis: a systematic review of 1747 cases. *Br J Dermatol.* 2015;172:642.
3. Caplan RM. The natural course of urticaria pigmentosa. *Arch Dermatol.* 1963;87:146.
4. Heide R, Tank B, Oranje AP. Mastocytosis in childhood. *Pediatr Dermatol.* 2002;19:375.
5. Valent P, et al. In: Jaffe ES, Harris NL, Stein H, et al, eds. *World Health Organization Classification of Tumours: Pathology and Genetics of Tumours of the Haematopoietic and Lymphoid Tissues.* Lyon, France: IARC Press; 2001.
6. Cohen SS, Skovbo S, Vestergaard H, et al. Epidemiology of systemic mastocytosis in Denmark. *Br J Haematol.* 2014;166:521.
7. Noto G, Pravata G. Arico M. Concordant urticaria pigmentosa in a couple of identical twins. A five-year follow up. *Acta Derm Venereol.* 1995;75:499.
8. Gay MW, Noojin RO, Finely WH. Urticaria pigmentosa discordant in identical twins. *Arch Dermatol.* 1970;102:29.
9. Cainelli T, Marchesi L, Pasquali F, et al. Monozygotic twins discordant for cutaneous mastocytosis. *Arch Dermatol.* 1983;119:1021.
10. Rottem M, Okada T, Goff JP, et al. Mast cells cultured from the peripheral blood of normal donors and patients with mastocytosis originate from a CD34+/FcεRI- cell population. *Blood.* 1994;84:2489.
11. Anderson DM, Lyman SD, Baird A, et al. Molecular cloning of mast cell growth factor, a hematopoietin that is active in both membrane bound and soluble forms. *Cell.* 1990;63:235.
12. Longley BJ, Tyrell L, Ma Y, et al. Chymase cleavage of stem cell factor yields a bioactive, soluble product. *Proc Natl Acad Sci U S A.* 1998;94:9017.
13. Kulka M, Metcalfe DD. High-resolution tracking of cell division demonstrates differential effects of TH1 and TH2 cytokines on SCF-dependent human mast cell production in vitro: correlation with apoptosis and Kit expression. *Blood.* 2005;105:592.
14. Lappalainen J, Lindstedt KA, Kovanen PT. A protocol for generating high numbers of mature and functional human mast cells from peripheral blood. *Clin Exp Allergy.* 2007;37:1404.
15. Longley BJ, Metcalfe DD, Tharp M, et al. Activating and dominant inactivating c-kit catalytic domain mutations in distinct clinical forms of human mastocytosis. *Proc Natl Acad Sci U S A.* 1999;96:1609.
16. Nagata H. kada T, Worobec A, et al. c-Kit mutation in a population of patients with mastocytosis. *Int Arch Allergy Immunol.* 1997;113:184.
17. Bodemer C, Hermine O, Pamerini F, et al. Pediatric mastocytosis is a clonal disease associated with D816V c-KIT mutations. *J Invest Dermatol.* 2010;130:804.
18. Ja CI, Tharp MD. Activating KIT mutations are not necessary for mastocytosis. *J Invest Dermatol.* 2016;136:S64.
19. Zappulla JP, Dubreuil P, Desbois S, et al. Mastocytosis in mice expressing human Kit receptor with the activating Asp816Val mutation. *J Exp Med.* 2005;202:1635.
20. Damaj G, Joris M, Chandesris O, et al. ASXL1 but not TET2 mutations adversely impact overall survival of patients suffering systemic mastocytosis with associated clonal hematologic non mast cell diseases. *PLoS One.* 2014;9:e85362.
21. Schwaab J, Schnittger S, Sotlar K, et al. Comprehensive mutational profiling in advanced systemic mastocytosis. *Blood.* 201;122:2460.
22. Valent P, Akin C, Sperr W, et al. Mastocytosis: pathology, genetics and current options for therapy. *Leuk Lymphoma.* 2005;46:35.
23. Valent P, Sotlar K, Sperr WR, et al. Refined diagnostic criteria and classification of mast cell leukemia (MCL) and myelomastocytic leukemia (MML): a consensus proposal. *Ann Oncol.* 2014;25:1691.
24. Theoharides T, Valent P, Akin C. Mast cells, mastocytosis and related disorders. *N Engl J Med.* 2015;373:163.
25. Carter MC, Metcalfe DD, Komarow HD. Mastocytosis. *Immunol Allergy Clin North Am.* 2014;34:1.
26. Sagher F, Even-Paz Z. *Mastocytosis and the Mast Cell*. Chicago, IL: Yearbook Medical; 1967.
27. Kasper CS, Freeman R, Tharp MD. Diagnosis of mastocytosis subsets using a morphometric point counting technique. *Arch Dermatol.* 1987;123:1017.

28. Nabavi NS, Nejad MH, Feli S, et al. Adult onset xanthelasmoid mastocytosis: report of a rare entity. *Indian J Dermatol.* 2016;61:468.
29. Kasprowicz S, Chan IJ, Tharp MD. Nodular mastocytosis. *Arch Dermatol.* 2006;55:347.
30. Dubois AD. Mastocytosis and hymenoptera allergy. *Curr Opin Allergy Clin Immunol.* 2004;4:291.
31. Jensen RT. Gastrointestinal abnormalities and involvement in systemic mastocytosis. *Hematol Oncol Clin North Am.* 2000;14:579.
32. Topar G, Staudacher C, Geisen F, et al. Urticaria pigmentosa: a clinical, hematopathologic and serologic study of 30 adults. *Am J Clin Pathol.* 1998;109:279.
33. Sokol H, Georgin-Lavialle S, Canioni D, et al. Gastrointestinal manifestations in mastocytosis: a study of 83 patients. *J Allergy Clin Immunol.* 2013;132:866.
34. Mican JM, Di Bisceglie Am, Fong TL, et al. Hepatic involvement in mastocytosis: clinicopathologic correlations in 41 cases. *Hepatology.* 1995;22:1163.
35. Metcalfe DD. The liver, spleen and lymph nodes in mastocytosis. *J Invest Dermatol.* 1991;96:45S.
36. Lanternier F, Cohen-Akenine A, Palmerini F, et al. Phenotypic and genotypic characteristics of mastocytosis according to the age of onset. *PLoS One.* 2008;3(4):e1906.
37. Escribano L, Alvarez-Twose I, Sanchez-Munoz L, et al. Prognosis in adult indolent systemic mastocytosis: a long-term study of the Spanish Network on Mastocytosis in a series of 145 patients. *J Allergy Clin Immunol.* 2009;124:514.
38. Travis WD, Li C-Y. Pathology of the lymph node and spleen in systemic mast cell disease. *Mod Pathol.* 1986;1:4.
39. Travis W, Li CY, Bergstralh EJ, et al. Systemic mast cell disease. *Medicine (Baltimore).* 1988;67:345
40. Rossini M, Zanotti R, Viapiana O, et al. Bone involvement and osteoporosis in mastocytosis. *Immunol Allergy Clin North Am.* 2014;34:383.
41. Rogers MP, Bloomingdale K, Murawski BJ, et al. Mixed organic brain syndrome as a manifestation of systemic mastocytosis. *Psychosom Med.* 1986;48:437.
42. Ciach K, Niedoszytko M, Abacjew-Chmylko A, et al. Pregnancy and delivery in patients with mastocytosis treated at the Polish center of European Competence Network on Mastocytosis (ECNM). *PLoS One.* 2016;11(1):e0146924.
43. Worobec AS, Akin C, Scott LM, et al. Mastocytosis complicating pregnancy. *Obstet Gynecol.* 2000;95:391.
44. Matito A, Alvarez-Twose I, Morgado JM, et al. Clinical Impact of pregnancy in mastocytosis: a study of the Spanish Network of Mastocytosis (REMA) in 45 cases. *Int Arch Allergy Immunol.* 2011;156:104.
45. Escribano L, Akin C, Castells M, et al. Mastocytosis: current concepts in diagnosis and treatment. *Ann Hematol.* 2002;81:677.
46. Akin C, Krishenbaum AS, Semere T, et al. Analysis of the surface expression of c-kit and occurrence of the c-kit Asp816Val activating mutation in T cells, B cells, and myelomonocytic cells in patients with mastocytosis. *Exp Hematol.* 2000;28:140.
47. Schwartz LB, Sakai K, Bradford TI, et al. The alpha form of human tryptase is the predominant type present in blood at baseline in normal subjects and is elevated in those with systemic mastocytosis. *J Clin Invest.* 1995;96:2702.
48. Alvarez-Twose I, Vano-Galvan S, Sanchez-Munoz L, et al. Increased serum baseline tryptase levels and extensive skin involvement are predictors for the severity of mast cell activation in children with mastocytosis. *Allergy.* 2012;67:813.
49. Keyzer JJ, de Monchy JG, van Doormall JJ, et al. Improved diagnosis of mastocytosis by measurement of urinary histamine metabolites. *N Engl J Med.* 1983;309:1603.
50. Uzzaman A. Maric, I, Noel P, et al. Pediatric-onset mastocytosis: a long term clinical follow up and correlation with bone marrow histology. *Pediatr Blood Cancer.* 2009;53:629.
51. Doyle LA, Sepehr GJ, Hamilton MJ, et al. A clinicopathologic study of 24 cases of systemic mastocytosis involving the gastrointestinal tract and assessment of mucosal mast cell density in irritable bowel syndrome and asymptomatic patients. *Am J Surg Pathol.* 2014;38:832.
52. Brockow K, Akin C, Huber M, et al. Levels of mast-cell growth factors in plasma and in suction skin blister fluid in adults with mastocytosis: correlation with dermal mast-cell numbers and mast-cell tryptase. *J Allergy Clin Immunol.* 2002;109:82.
53. Alvarez-Twose I, Gonzalez de Olano D, Sanchez-Munoz L, et al. Clinical, biological, and molecular characteristics of clonal mast cell disorders presenting with systemic mast cell activation symptoms. *J Allergy Clin Immunol.* 2010;125:1269.
54. Valent P. Mast cell activation syndromes: definition and classification. *Allergy.* 2013;68:417.
55. Brockow K, Scott LM, Worobec AS, et al. Regression of urticaria pigmentosa in adult patients with systemic mastocytosis: correlation with clinical patterns of disease. *Arch Dermatol.* 2002;138:785.
56. Konrad FM, Schroeder TH. Anaesthesia in patients with mastocytosis. *Acta Anaesthesiol Scand.* 2009;53;207.
57. Cardet JC, Akin C, Lee MJ, et al. Mastocytosis: update on pharmacotherapy and future directions. *Expert Opin Pharmacother.* 2013;14:2033.
58. Simons E, Akdis CA. Histamine and antihistamines. In: Busse W, Bochner B. Holgate S, et al, eds. *Middleton's Allergy: Principles and Practices.* Vol. 2. 7th ed. St. Louis, MO; Mosby; 2008:1517.
59. Kettelhut BV, Berkebile C, Bradely D, et al. A double-blind, placebo-controlled, crossover trial of ketotifen versus hydroxyzine in the treatment of pediatric mastocytosis [see comments]. *J Allergy Clin Immunol.* 1989;83:866.
60. Horan RF, Sheffer AL, Austen KF. Cromolyn sodium in the management of systemic mastocytosis. *J Allergy Clin Immunol.* 1990;85:852.
61. Butterfiedl JH. Survey of aspirin administration in systemic mastocytosis. *Prostaglandins Other Lipid Mediat.* 2009;88:122.
62. Tolar J, Tope, Neglia JP, et al. Leukotriene-receptor inhibition for the treatment of systemic mastocytosis. *N Engl J Med.* 2004;350:735.
63. Turner PJ, Kemp AS, Rogers M, et al. Refractory symptoms successfully treated with leukotriene inhibition in a child with systemic mastocytosis. *Pediatr Dermatol.* 2012;29:222.
64. Bell MC, Jackson DJ. Prevention of anaphylaxis related to mast cell activation syndrome with omalizumab. *Ann Allergy Asthma Immunol.* 2012;108:383.
65. Carter MC, Robyn JA, Bressler PB, et al. Omalizumab for the treatment of unprovoked anaphylaxis in patients with systemic mastocytosis. *J Allergy Clin Immunol.* 2007;119:1550.

66. Douglass JA, Carroll K, Voskamp A, et al. Omalizumab is effective in treating systemic mastocytosis in a non-atopic patient. *Allergy*. 2010;65:926.
67. Barton J, Lavker RM, Schechter NM, et al. Treatment of urticaria pigmentosa with corticosteroids. *Arch Dermatol*. 1985;121:1516.
68. Kurosawa M. Response to cyclosporin and low dose methylprednisone in aggressive systemic mastocytosis. *J Allergy Clin Immunol*. 1999;103:S412.
69. Lim AY, Ostor AJ, Love S, et al. Systemic mastocytosis; a rare cause of osteoporosis and its response to bisphosphonate treatment. *Ann Rheum Dis*. 2004;64:965.
70. Czarnetzki BM, Rosenbach T, Kolde G, et al. Phototherapy of urticaria pigmentosa: clinical response and changes of cutaneous reactivity, histamine and chemotactic leukotrienes. *Arch Dermatol Res*. 1985;277:105.
71. Vella Briffa D, Eady RA, James MP, et al. Photochemotherapy (PUVA) in the treatment of urticaria pigmentosa. *Br J Dermatol*. 1983;109:67.
72. Butterfield JH. Response of severe systemic mastocytosis to interferon alpha. *Br J Dermatol*. 1998;138:489.
73. Lim KH, Pardanani A, Butterfield JH, et al. Cytoreductive therapy in 108 adults with systemic mastocytosis: outcome analysis and response predication during treatment with interferon-alpha, hydroxyurea, imatinib mesylate or 2-chlorodeoxyadenosine. *Am J Hematol*. 2009;84:790.
74. Pardanani A, Hoffbrand AV, Butterfield JH, et al. Treatment of systemic mast cell disease with 2-chlorodeoxyadenosine. *Leuk Res*. 2004;28;127.
75. Friedman B, Darling G, Norton J, et al. Splenectomy in the management of systemic mast cell disease. *Surgery*. 1990;107:94.
76. Johnstone PA, Macan JM, Metcalfe DD, et al. Radiotherapy of refractory bone pain due to systemic mast cell disease. *Am J Clin Oncol*. 1994;17:328.
77. Ustun C, Reiter A, Scott BL, et al. Hematopoietic stem-cell transplantation for advanced systemic mastocytosis. *J Clin Oncol*. 2014;32:3264.
78. Akin C, Fumo G, Yavuz AS, et al. A novel form of mastocytosis associated with a transmembrane c-kit mutation and response to imatinib. *Blood*. 2004;103:3222.
79. Vega-Ruiz A, Cortes JE, Sever M, et al. Phase II study of imatinib mesylate as therapy for patients with systemic mastocytosis. *Leuk Res*. 2009;33;1481.
80. Valent P, Cerny-Reiterer S, Hoermann G, et al. Long-lasting complete response to imatinib in a patient with systemic mastocytosis exhibiting wild type KIT. *Am J Blood Res*. 2014;4:93.
81. Purtill D, Cooney J, Sinniah R, et al. Dasatinib therapy for systemic mastocytosis: four cases. *Eur J Haematol*. 2008;80;456.
82. Hochhaus A, Baccarani M, Giles FJ, et al. Nilotinib in patients with systemic mastocytosis: analysis of the phase 2, open-label, single-arm nilotinib registration study. *J Cancer Res Clin Oncol*. 2015;141:2047.
83. Verstovsek S, Tefferi, A, Cortes J, et al. Phase II study of dasatinib in Philadelphia chromosome-negative acute and chronic myeloid diseases, including systemic mastocytosis. *Clin Cancer Res*. 2008;14:3906.
84. Gotlib J, Kluin-Nelemans HC, George TI, et al. Efficacy and safety of midostaurin in advanced systemic mastocytosis. *N Engl J Med*. 2016;374:2530.

Reactive Erythemas

PART 7

第七篇　反应性红斑

Chapter 43 :: Erythema Multiforme
:: Jean-Claude Roujeau & Maja Mockenhaupt

第四十三章
多形红斑

中文导读

本章共分为8节：①前言；②流行病学；③临床表现；④病因与发病机制；⑤诊断；⑥鉴别诊断；⑦病程与预后；⑧临床管理。全面描述了多形红斑的背景知识、临床特征及治疗。

第一节介绍了历史上对多形红斑的定义、相关术语、分型和病因学认识上的演变与发展。

第二节介绍了多形红斑的发病率未知并说明了原因，指出了发生多形红斑的相关的危险因素。

第三节首先介绍了多形红斑的前驱症状、与单纯疱疹感染的关系。再详细描述了多形红斑的皮肤表现和非皮肤表现。还介绍了发热、咳嗽等全身表现及其各种并发症。

第四节介绍了多形红斑与感染的关系。指出HSV是最常见的原因，其他还可能有肺炎支原体、多种病毒（EBV、羊痘病毒、水痘-带状疱疹病毒、细小病毒B19、乙型肝炎病毒和丙型肝炎病毒）以及药物。阐述了多形红斑发生发展的机制。

第五节介绍了多形红斑的诊断主要基于临床表现和病史，以及多形红斑的诊断流程。当诊断不确定时，可结合皮肤活检和实验室检查，并详细描述了多形红斑的组织病理学改变。

第六节阐述了临床医生及时识别是否存在SJS（Stevens-Johnson综合征）及其病因的重要性（请参阅第44章）。

第七节描述了不同类型多形红斑的病程和预后，包括复发性、后遗症和合并症。

第八节介绍了糖皮质激素、免疫抑制药在多形红斑治疗中的价值，强调主要应该针对病因进行治疗并积极预防并发症。

〔李　捷〕

AT-A-GLANCE

- Erythema multiforme is a rare cutaneous or mucocutaneous eruption characterized by "target" lesions, predominantly on the face and extremities.
- The highest incidence was found in male children and young adults.
- It has a benign course but frequent recurrences, possible ocular complications.
- Most cases are related to infections (herpes simplex virus [HSV] and *Mycoplasma pneumoniae*). Medications are *not* a common cause, in contrast to the spectrum of drug-induced epidermal necrolysis (see Chap. 44) that are different diseases.
- Herpes-induced recurrences can be prevented by long-term use of anti-HSV medications. Thalidomide, mycophenolate mofetil, or both may be considered in recalcitrant, recurrent cases.

TABLE 43-1
Erythema Multiforme (EM) Subtypes

SUBTYPE	CLINICAL FEATURES	ASSOCIATED ETIOLOGY
EM minus (EMm)	Typical targets Acral skin and lip involvement No mucosal erosions	HSV, other infections
EM majus (EMM)	Typical targets Acral skin involvement Mucosal erosions	HSV, other infections
Atypical EMM	Giant targets Central distribution Prominent mucosal erosions	*Mycoplasma pneumoniae*, HSV
Mucosal EMM	No or minimal skin lesions Prominent mucosal erosions	*M. pneumoniae*
Continuous or persistent EM	Typical targets Acral skin involvement Few mucosal erosions Overlapping recurrences	HSV, idiopathic

HSV, herpes simplex virus.

INTRODUCTION

DEFINITIONS

Erythema multiforme (EM) is an acute mucocutaneous syndrome originally described by von Hebra in 1860 as *erythema exudativum multiforme*. It is defined by a distinctive clinical pattern (with consistent histopathology when done). The course is usually mild and self-limited but carries a risk of relapse. Based on the degree of mucous membrane involvement, EM is separated into EM minus (EMm, also called EM minor) if only the skin and lips are involved and EM majus (EMM, also called EM major) when mucous membranes are affected. Subtypes of EM are described in Table 43-1.

Historically, a variety of factors have contributed to a confusing nosology, especially with the concept of a so-called "EM spectrum" from EMm to Stevens-Johnson syndrome (SJS) and toxic epidermal necrolysis (TEN). The definition of EM in this chapter is based on the classification proposed 25 years ago by Bastuji-Garin and colleagues.[1] The principle of the classification was to consider SJS and TEN as severity variants of a process termed *epithelial necrolysis* (EN; see Chap. 44) and to separate them from EM. The validity of that classification has been established by several studies, especially the prospective international Severe Cutaneous Adverse Reactions study[2] and by recent series[3,4] showing that compared with SJS and TEN, EM cases have different demographic features, clinical presentation, severity, and causes.

The consensus classification was improved by German investigators by separation of EMM into *typical EMM* (typical targets on the extremities) and *atypical EMM* with more extensive distribution of atypical, larger targets, occasionally involving the skin around the mouth and the eyes, resulting in clown-like facies. The relevance of that subclassification was supported by the demonstration of younger age and more frequent association with *Mycoplasma pneumoniae* infection in cases of atypical EMM.[5]

Cases of mucosal disease with target lesions on the trunk are often diagnosed as SJS or *M. pneumoniae*–associated SJS, especially in the pediatric realm. However, we consider these cases EMM caused by *M. pneumoniae*. Other authors have proposed that mucocutaneous eruptions associated with *M. pneumoniae* are a distinct entity, termed *M. pneumoniae*-induced rash and mucositis (MIRM).[4] It is certainly true that EMM and the range of presentations of EN have to be differentiated, no matter what the cause. It is also true that typical EMM associated with herpes simplex virus (HSV) presents differently than atypical EMM associated with *M. pneumoniae*, but we do not consider atypical EMM a distinct entity.

Atypical EMM may present in a variety of forms, sometimes predominantly affecting the skin and sometimes predominantly affecting two or more mucosal sites. If only the mucous membranes are involved, making the correct diagnosis may be a challenge. In 1878, the ophthalmologist Fuchs described a patient with erosions of the eyes and mouth and a transient skin eruption. The term *Fuchs syndrome* (also called ectodermosis pluriorificialis) has been applied to such cases that share demographic and etiologic features with atypical EMM. The term *mucosal EMM*, a subset of atypical EMM, is now preferred.

Unfortunately, the International Classification of Diseases 10th Revision (ICD-10) did not incorporate these advances and uses the same code, L51.1, for SJS and bullous EM, and classifies TEN as L51.2 under the heading of EM (L51). Nonspecific codes maintain the confusion of a so-called "EM spectrum" despite the accumulation of evidence of different mechanisms, clinical presentations, severity, and causes of EM versus SJS-TEN.[2-4]

EPIDEMIOLOGY

EM is considered relatively common, but the true incidence is unknown. There is selection bias for severe cases requiring hospitalization in the medical literature; such cases are rare and occur in the range of 0.5 to 1 per million per year.[6] EMm is likely more frequent than EMM. Another obstacle to proper evaluation of incidence is the misdiagnosis of EM in patients with annular or figurate eruptions, including annular urticaria, serum sickness–like eruption, polymorphous maculopapular eruptions,[7] subacute cutaneous lupus erythematosus,[8] and even SJS or TEN.[7]

EM occurs in patients of all ages but is most prevalent in adolescents and young adults. There is a male preponderance (male:female ratio of 2 to 3:1). Recurrence happens in about 10% of patients with EMM and up to 30% in EMm, more frequently, but not exclusively, in HSV-associated cases.

There are no established associations of underlying disease with risk for EM. HIV infection and collagen vascular disorders increase the risk of SJS and TEN but not EM. Cases may occur in clusters, which supports a role for infectious agents. The incidence does not vary with ethnicity or geographic location.

Predisposing genes have been reported. A total of 66% of EM patients have HLA-DQB1*0301 allele compared with 31% of control participants.[9] However, this association has not translated into a meaningful clinical test or intervention.

CLINICAL FEATURES

HISTORY

Prodromal symptoms are absent in most cases. If present, they are usually mild, suggesting an upper respiratory infection (cough, rhinitis, low-grade fever). In EMM, fever higher than 38.5°C (101.3°F) is present in one third of cases.[2] Prior occurrences are reported in up to one third of patients and help make the correct diagnosis. The events of the preceding 3 weeks should be reviewed for clinical evidence of any precipitating agent, with a special focus on signs and symptoms of HSV and symptoms of respiratory infection or influenza-like illness.

In more than 70% of patients with recurrent EM, an episode of recurrent HSV infection precedes the skin lesions. The association with herpes labialis predominates over that with genital herpes or herpes in other locations. EM usually follows recurrent herpes but may also occur after primary HSV infection. The average interval is 7 days (range, 2–17 days). The duration of the lag period appears to be specific for individual patients. In a small number of patients, HSV recrudescence and EM may occur simultaneously. Not all episodes of EM are preceded by clinically evident HSV, and not all HSV episodes are followed by EM. Episodes of recurrent HSV infection may precede the development of HSV-related EM by years.

CUTANEOUS FEATURES

The skin eruption arises abruptly. In most patients, all lesions appear within 3 days, but in some, several crops follow each other during a single episode of EM. Often there are a limited number of lesions, but up to hundreds may form. Most occur in a symmetric, distribution on the extensor surfaces of the extremities (hands, feet, elbows, and knees), face, and neck and less frequently on the thighs, buttocks, and trunk. Lesions often first appear distally and then spread in a centripetal manner. Mechanical factors (Koebner phenomenon) and actinic factors (predilection for sun-exposed sites) appear to influence the distribution of lesions. Although patients occasionally report burning and itching, the eruption is usually asymptomatic.

The diversity in clinical pattern implied by the name *multiforme* is mainly related to the *features of single lesions*. Most lesions are usually very similar in a given patient at a given time. The typical target lesion is a highly regular, circular, wheal-like erythematous papule or plaque that persists for 1 week or longer (Fig. 43-1). It measures from a few millimeters to approximately 3 cm and may expand slightly over 24 to 48 hours. Although the periphery remains erythematous and edematous, the center becomes violaceous and dark; inflammatory activity may regress or relapse in the center, which gives rise to concentric rings of color (see Figs. 43-1 to 43-4). Often, the center turns purpuric or necrotic or transforms into a tense vesicle or bulla. The result is the classic target or iris lesion.

According to the current classification,[1,5] typical target lesions consist of at least three concentric components: (1) a dusky central disk or blister; (2) more peripherally, an infiltrated pale ring; and (3) an erythematous halo. Not all lesions of EM are typical; some display two rings only (raised atypical targets).

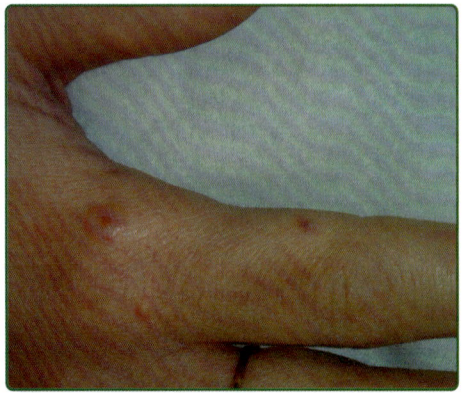

Figure 43-1 Mixture of typical targets and papules in a case of erythema multiforme.

However, all are infiltrated papules, in contrast to macules, which are the typical lesions in EN (SJS and TEN). In some patients with EM, most lesions are violaceous vesicles overlying a just slightly darker central portion, encircled by an erythematous margin (see Figs. 43-2 to 43-4). Larger lesions (Fig. 43-5) may have a central bulla and a marginal ring of vesicles (herpes iris of Bateman).

In most cases, EM affects well under 10% of the body surface area. In 88 hospital cases of EMM prospectively included in the Severe Cutaneous Adverse Reactions study, the median involvement was 1% of the body surface area.[2] The duration of an individual lesion is shorter than 2 weeks, but residual discoloration may remain for months. There is no scarring unless mechanical manipulation takes place.

NONCUTANEOUS FEATURES

Mucosal lesions are present in up to 70% of patients, most often limited to the oral cavity.

Predilection sites are the lips, on both the cutaneous and mucosal sides, nonattached gingivae, and the ventral side of the tongue. The hard palate is usually spared, as are the attached gingivae. On the cutaneous part of the lips, identifiable target lesions may be discernible (Fig. 43-6). In children and adolescents, lips and oral mucosa are often affected very severely both in cases caused by *M. pneumoniae* or by respiratory infections caused by unspecified infectious agents. On the mucosa proper, there are erosions with fibrinous deposits, and occasionally intact vesicles and bullae can be seen (Fig. 43-7). The process may rarely extend to the throat, larynx, and even the trachea and bronchi.

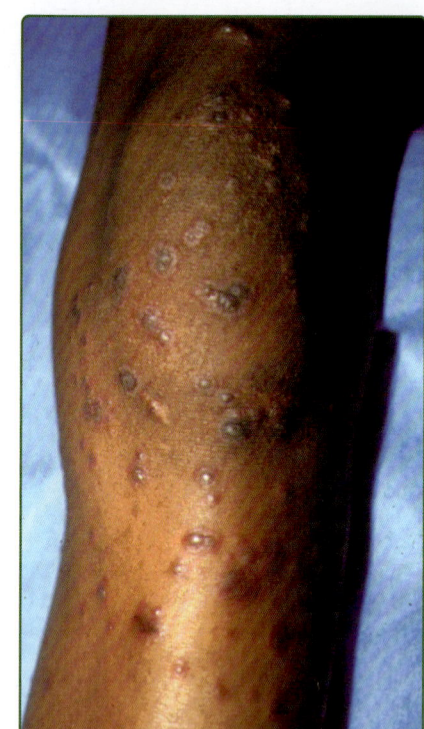

Figure 43-3 Typical targets around the knee.

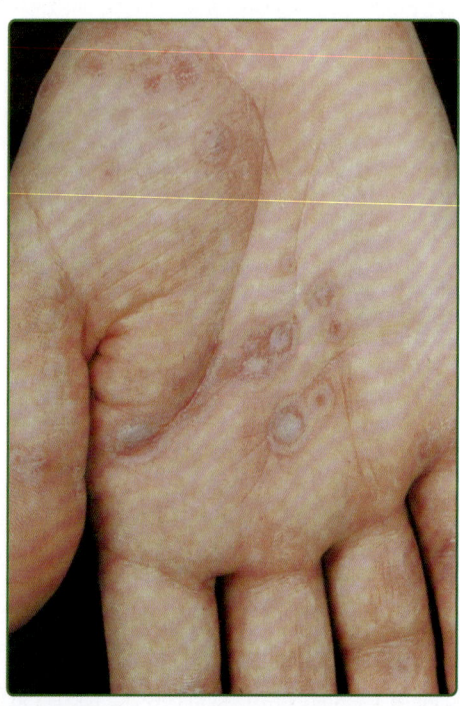

Figure 43-2 Typical target lesions on the palm.

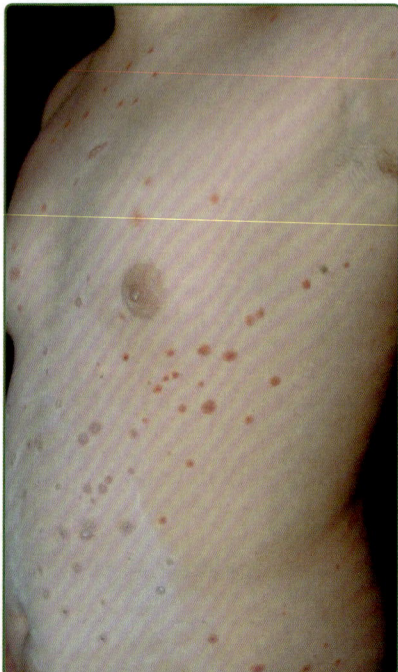

Figure 43-4 Disseminated targets on the trunk (atypical erythema multiforme majus).

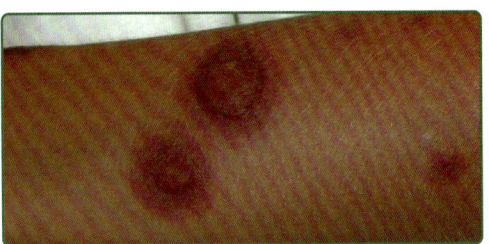

Figure 43-5 Giant targets on the arm (atypical erythema multiforme majus).

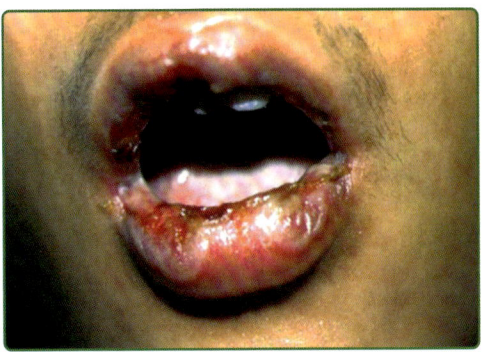

Figure 43-6 Involvement of the lips with a target pattern in erythema multiforme majus.

Eye involvement begins with pain and bilateral conjunctivitis in which vesicles and erosions can occur (Fig. 43-8). In children, ocular lesions appear to be more frequent and more severe in *M. pneumoniae*–associated cases.[10] The nasal, urethral, and anal mucosae also may be inflamed and eroded.

RELATED PHYSICAL FINDINGS

Fever and other constitutional symptoms are usually absent in EMm, and the noncutaneous physical examination is normal. Fever higher than 38.5°C (101.3°F) is present in one third of EMM cases. Mouth erosions may be painful enough to impair alimentation. The patient may be unable to close the mouth and constantly drools blood-stained saliva. Cervical lymphadenopathy is usually present in these patients. The pain of genital erosions may lead to reflex urinary retention. Cough and hypoxia may occur in *M. pneumoniae*–related cases.

COMPLICATIONS

In contrast to SJS, in which cutaneous lesions may progress to extensive detachment of the epidermis, there is no risk of "skin failure" or visceral involvement in EMM. Mouth erosions may impair oral alimentation. Reflex anuria from periurethral erosions rarely needs bladder catheterization. Severe ocular lesions leading to sequelae are rare but can occur, and ocular symptoms must be checked by an ophthalmologist in the acute phase of the disease and followed appropriately.[10]

ETIOLOGY AND PATHOGENESIS

Most cases of EM are related to infections (Table 43-2). HSV is the most common cause, principally in recurrent cases. Proof of causality of HSV is firmly established from clinical experience, epidemiology,[2] detection of HSV DNA in the lesions of EM,[11,12] and prevention of EM by suppression of HSV recurrences.[13] Clinically, a link with HSV can often be made. EM eruptions begin on average 7 days after HSV eruptions. The delay can be substantially shorter, especially with more recurrences. Not all symptomatic HSV recurrences are followed by EM, and asymptomatic ones can induce EM. Therefore, the causal link can be overlooked by both the patient and physician. HSV-1 is usually the cause, but HSV-2 can also induce EM.

M. pneumoniae is the second major cause of EM overall and the first in children.[5,14] In cases related to *M. pneumoniae*, the clinical presentation is often

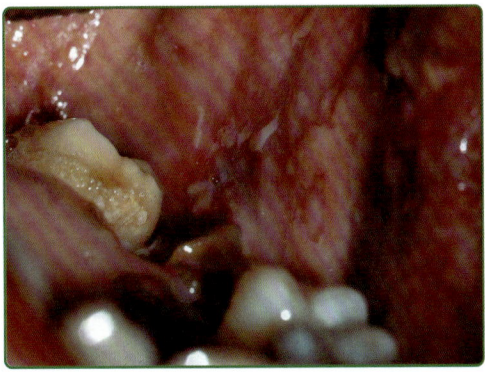

Figure 43-7 Oral erosions in erythema multiforme majus.

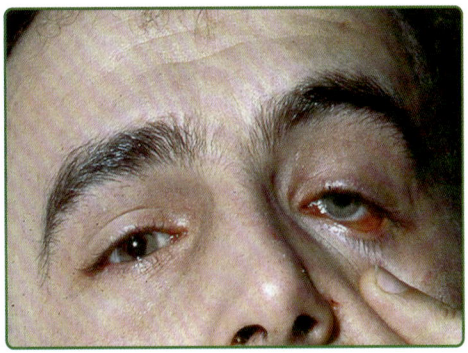

Figure 43-8 Conjunctivitis with erosions in erythema multiforme majus.

TABLE 43-2
Conditions Commonly Associated with Erythema Multiforme

Herpes simplex virus
Mycoplasma pneumoniae
Epstein-Barr virus
Orf
Varicella zoster virus
Parvovirus B19
Hepatitis B
Hepatitis C

atypical (giant targets, clown-like facial distribution) and more severe than in cases associated with HSV. The relationship to *M. pneumoniae* is often difficult to establish. Clinical and radiologic signs of atypical pneumonia can be mild, and *M. pneumoniae* is usually not directly detected. Polymerase chain reaction (PCR) testing of throat swabs, or bronchopulmonary lavage if performed, for *M. pneumoniae* is the most sensitive technique for diagnostic confirmation. Serologic results are considered diagnostic in the presence of IgM or IgA antibodies to *M. pneumoniae* in the acute phase or a more than twofold increase in IgG antibodies in paired serum samples obtained at onset and after 2 or 3 weeks. *M. pneumoniae*–related EM can recur.

Many other infections have been reported as causes of EM in individual cases or small series, but the evidence for causality of these other agents is only circumstantial. Published reports have implicated infection with EBV, Orf virus, varicella zoster virus, parvovirus B19, hepatitis B and C viruses, and a variety of other bacterial or viral infections. Immunization has been also implicated as a cause in children, but a spurious association can be suspected.

Drugs are also a reported cause of EM, although a true association is unlikely. Most reports of drug-associated EM actually deal with imitators,[7] for example, annular urticaria (also called urticaria multiforme)[15] or disseminated maculopapular eruptions with some lesions resembling targets (Fig. 43-9). EM-like dermatitis may also result from contact sensitization. These eruptions should be viewed as imitators of EM despite some clinical and histopathologic similarities. Literature reports of drug-associated EM also include typical cases of SJS or TEN, particularly under the moniker EMPACT syndrome (EM, phenytoin and cranial radiation therapy).[7] Such terms create more confusion on EM and minimize the potential severity of drug reactions.

Idiopathic cases are those in which neither HSV infection nor any other cause can be identified. These cases are fairly common in routine clinical circumstances. However, HSV has been found in situ by PCR in up to 40% of such presentations.[3] Some idiopathic cases respond to prophylactic antiviral treatment and are thus likely to have been triggered by asymptomatic HSV infection. Others are resistant and probably have another cause.

Another suspected variant of recurrent EMM was reported to be associated with desmoplakin I and II autoantibodies.[16] However, the presence of acantholysis in skin biopsies of such cases suggests a variant of pemphigus that clinically resembles EM. The recently reported efficacy of rituximab in such cases also supports this hypothesis.[17] Conversely, in a series of 54 cases of typical EMM, antiepidermal antibodies were not found.[18]

The underlying mechanisms of HSV-associated EM have been extensively investigated.[11,13,19,20] It is unknown whether similar mechanisms apply to EM from other causes.

Complete, infective HSV has never been isolated from lesions of HSV-associated EM, but the presence of HSV DNA in skin lesions has been reported in numerous studies using PCR assays. These studies demonstrated that keratinocytes contain viral DNA fragments that always include the viral polymerase (*Pol*) gene. HSV Pol DNA is located in basal keratinocytes and in the lower spinous cell layers, and viral Pol protein is synthesized. HSV-specific T cells, including cytotoxic cells, are recruited, and the virus-specific response is followed by a nonspecific inflammatory amplification by autoreactive T cells. The cytokines produced in these cells induce the delayed hypersensitivity–like appearance in histopathologic evaluation of biopsy sections of EM lesions.

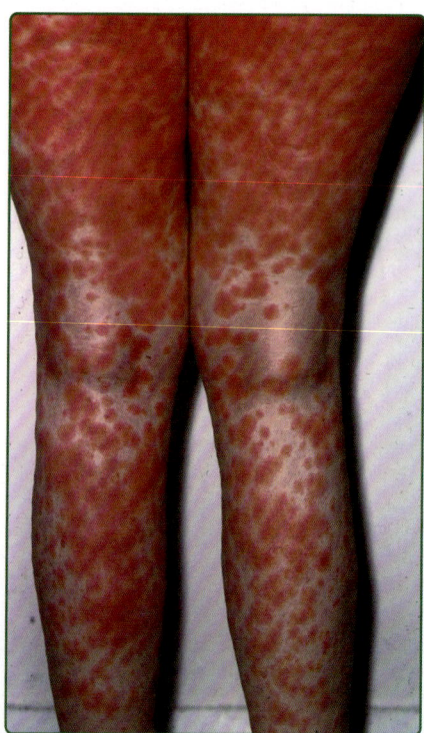

Figure 43-9 Figurate erythema in a case of "drug eruption" to amoxicillin, frequently and erroneously reported as drug-induced erythema multiforme.

HSV is present in the blood for a few days during an overt recurrence of herpes. If keratinocytes were infected from viremia, one would expect signs and symptoms of disseminated herpes rather than EM. Instead, HSV DNA is transported to the epidermis by monocytes, macrophages, and CD34+ Langerhans cell precursors harboring the skin-homing receptor cutaneous lymphocyte antigen that engulf the virus and fragment its DNA. Upregulation of adhesion molecules greatly increases binding of HSV-containing mononuclear cells to endothelial cells and contributes to the dermal inflammatory response. Upon reaching the epidermis, the cells transmit the viral polymerase gene *Pol* to keratinocytes. Viral genes may persist for a few months, but the synthesis and expression of the Pol protein will last for only a few days. This may explain the transient character of clinical lesions that are likely induced by a specific immune response to Pol protein and amplified by autoreactive cells. Effector cells are CD4 T lymphocytes with a restricted Vβ repertoire. Incomplete fragmentation of viral DNA, increased number of circulating CD34+ cells, or increased immune response to Pol protein characterize the small proportion of individuals with recurrent herpes infections who develop EM.

DIAGNOSIS

An approach to the diagnosis and management of EM is shown in Fig. 43-10. EM is usually diagnosed clinically. A skin biopsy and laboratory investigations are

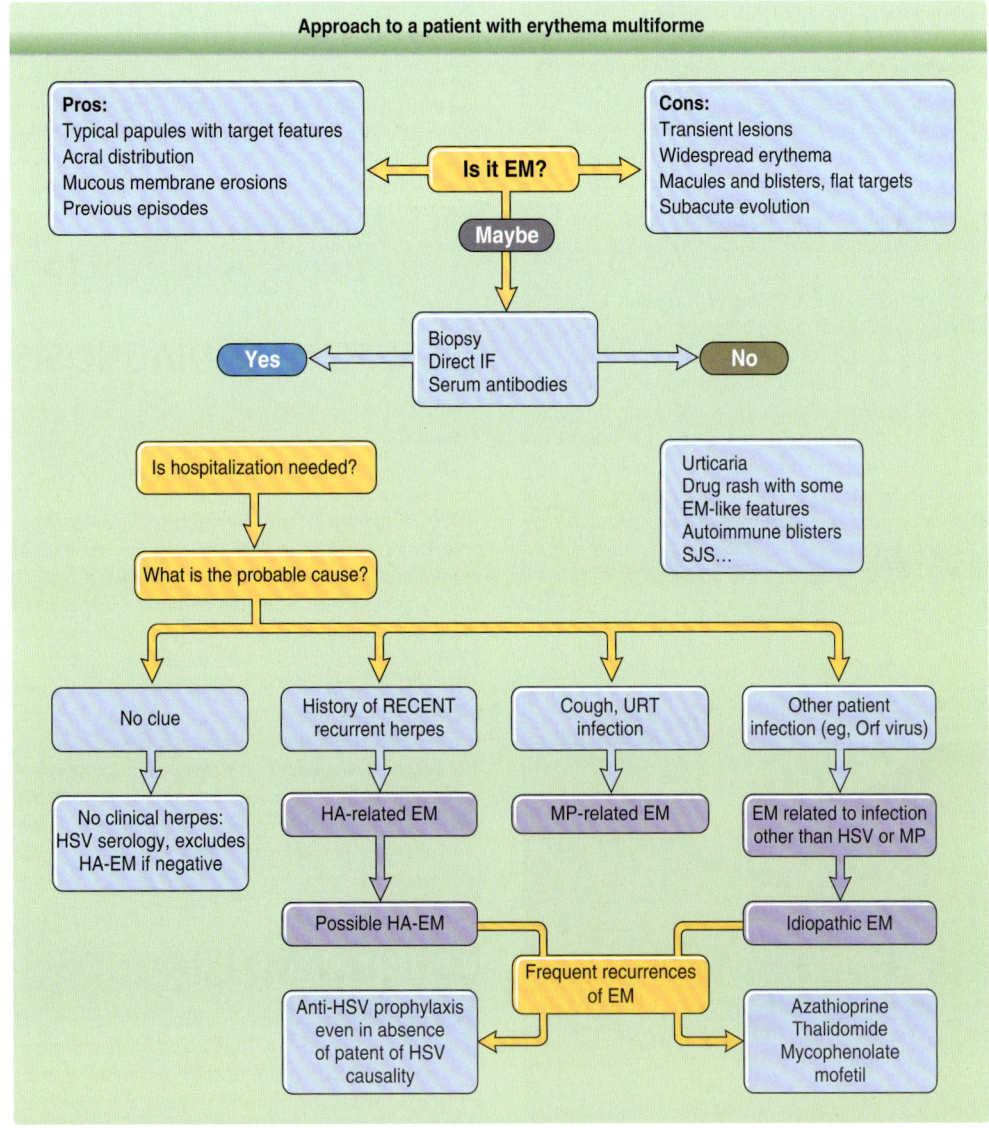

Figure 43-10 Approach to a patient with erythema multiforme (EM). ADR, adverse drug reaction; HA-EM, herpes-associated erythema multiforme; IF, immunofluorescence; MP, *Mycoplasma pneumoniae*; SJS, Stevens-Johnson syndrome; URT, upper respiratory tract.

useful when the diagnosis is not certain. After making the diagnosis, the need for hospitalization is considered. Admission is suggested for patients with EMM with oral lesions severe enough to impair drinking and feeding, when a diagnosis of SJS is suspected, or when severe constitutional symptoms are present. Establishing the underlying cause of EM is also part of the evaluation.

SUPPORTIVE STUDIES

LABORATORY

There are no specific laboratory tests for EM. In more severe cases, an elevated erythrocyte sedimentation rate, moderate leukocytosis, increased levels of acute-phase proteins, and mildly elevated liver aminotransferase levels may occur. Antidesmoplakin antibodies are not found.[18]

HISTOPATHOLOGY

Early lesions of EM exhibit lymphocyte accumulation at the dermal–epidermal interface with exocytosis into the epidermis, lymphocytes attached to scattered necrotic keratinocytes (satellite cell necrosis), spongiosis, vacuolar degeneration of the basal cell layer, and focal junctional and subepidermal cleft formation. Acantholysis is not a feature of EM. The papillary dermis may be edematous but principally contains a moderate to dense mononuclear cell infiltrate, which is more abundant in older lesions. The vessels are ectatic with swollen endothelial cells, and there may be extravasated erythrocytes and eosinophils. In advanced lesions, subepidermal blister formation may occur, but necrosis rarely involves the entire epidermis (Fig. 43-11). In late lesions, melanophages may be prominent. Immunofluorescence findings are negative or nonspecific.

The histopathologic appearance of EM lesions differs from that of EN, in which dermal inflammation is moderate to absent and epidermal necrosis is much more pronounced (see Chap. 44). Still, the histopathologic appearances are somewhat overlapping and often do not allow the distinction of EM from EN, especially if the sample is obtained from the bullous center of the lesion. The main reason for performing a biopsy in EM is to rule out other diagnoses, such as autoimmune blistering diseases, Sweet syndrome, and vasculitis.

UNDERLYING ETIOLOGY

In the presence of respiratory symptoms, a chest radiograph is indicated to evaluate for pneumonia, and PCR assay or serologic testing may help detect *M. pneumoniae* infection. In the case of recurrent EM, a link to HSV can be confirmed by evaluating preceding lesions of herpes labialis using HSV PCR, direct fluorescent antibodies, or viral culture. However, these studies are not useful when applied to the target lesions. Amplification of HSV *Pol* gene from biopsy samples of EM lesions is not done routinely. A negative result on serologic testing for HSV may be helpful only to exclude the possibility of herpes-association. The positive predictive value of the presence of HLA-DQB1*0301 is too low to have clinical value.

DIFFERENTIAL DIAGNOSIS

The differential diagnosis of EM is reviewed in Table 43-3.

The most important differential diagnosis, SJS, should be recognized promptly for three reasons: (1) the possibility of life-threatening complications, (2) the risk of progression to TEN, and (3) the need for urgent withdrawal of suspected causative drug(s) (see Chap. 44). Pain, constitutional symptoms, severe erosions of mucosae, rapid progression, and dusky or violaceous often confluent macules and blisters are alerting features.

In rare cases of EM affecting only mucous membranes, the diagnosis is especially difficult and often made when further bouts include a few skin lesions. The history is extremely important, especially related to infections and recurrence. Pemphigus, cicatricial pemphigoid, allergic or toxic contact stomatitis, toxic erosive stomatitis, aphthae, and lichen planus should be considered.

COURSE AND PROGNOSIS

EMm runs a mild course in most cases, and each individual attack subsides within 1 to 4 weeks. Recovery is complete, and there are usually no sequelae, except for transient skin discoloration. The ocular erosions of EMM may cause severe residual scarring of the eyes, especially in adults and in non–herpes-related cases.[21]

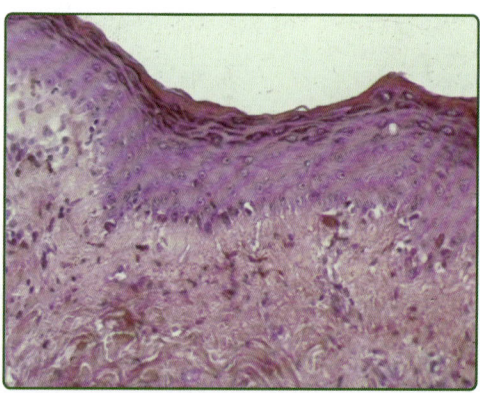

Figure 43-11 Histopathology of erythema multiforme.

TABLE 43-3
Differential Diagnoses of Erythema Multiforme (EM)

	MUCOUS MEMBRANE LESIONS	SKIN LESIONS PATTERN	HISTOPATHOLOGIC FINDINGS	LABORATORY TESTING	COURSE
Urticaria	No	Annular, circinate, blanching erythema Transient lesions (individual lesions last ≤24 hr)	Edema		More acute than EM
Maculopapular drug eruption	Rare (lips)	Widespread polymorphous, targetlike lesions, macules, papules, plaques	Most often nonspecific		
Lupus erythematosus ("Rowell syndrome")	Possible (mouth)	Face and thorax	Interface dermatitis Positive result of DIF ("lupus band")	Antinuclear antibodies present	Subacute
Paraneoplastic pemphigus	Always; tends to be severe	Large targetlike lesions, annular plaques EM-like lesion plus lichenoid papules Positive Nikolsky sign	Acantholysis, positive DIF	Antibodies present (not always)	Chronic
Cicatricial pemphigoid	Constant	Circinate erythematous patches	Subepidermal blister, positive DIF	Antibodies present	Chronic
Bullous pemphigoid (BP)/IgA-linear dermatosis	Possible in BP; rare in IgA-linear dermatosis	Bullae and crusts in different stages	Subepidermal blister, positive DIF	Antibodies present	Chronic (or relapsing)
Antidesmoplakin "EM majus"	Constant	EM-like lesions	Basal acantholysis, positive DIF	Antibodies present	Acute relapsing
Stevens-Johnson syndrome	Constant	Widespread small blisters Atypical targets, typically confluent Constitutional symptoms	Interface dermatitis, epidermal necrosis		Acute
Sweet syndrome (acute febrile neutrophilic dermatosis)	Rare	Erythematous papules and succulent plaques	Spongiosis with subcorneal vesicles and pustules	Neutrophilia	Acute

DIF, direct immunofluorescence testing; IgA, immunoglobulin A.

M. pneumoniae–related EMM may be associated with severe erosive bronchitis that may rarely lead to sequelae.[22]

Whatever the cause of EM, recurrences are common and may characterize the majority of cases. In reports of large series of patients with recurrent EM, the mean number of attacks was 6 per year (range, 2 to 36), and the mean total duration of disease was 6 to 9 years. In 33%, the condition persisted for more than 10 years.[23] Up to 50 recurrences have been described in a single patient. The severity of episodes in patients with recurrent EM is highly variable and unpredictable. The frequency of episodes and cumulative duration of disease are not correlated with the severity of attacks. The frequency and severity of recurrent EM tends to decrease spontaneously over time (after 2 years or longer), parallel with the improvement of recurring HSV infection when associated. In a substantial proportion of recurrent cases, a cause cannot be determined.[24] A small fraction of patients experience prolonged series of overlapping attacks of EM; this has been labeled *continuous EM* or *persistent EM*.[25] Persistent EM may be related to HSV but also to other viral infections, inflammatory bowel diseases, or malignancy.

MANAGEMENT

Based on retrospective series or small controlled trials, the use of systemic corticosteroids seems to shorten the duration of fever and eruption, especially swelling and pain of the mucosae but may increase the length of hospitalization because of complications. However, the methodology of most studies was poor, with small series often mixing the various forms of idiopathic and virus-associated EM and drug-induced SJS. The use of systemic corticosteroids can neither be recommended nor blamed.[20,26]

Administering anti-HSV drugs for the treatment of an established episode of postherpetic EM is useless.[27]

When symptomatic, patients with *M. pneumoniae* infection should be treated with antibiotics (macrolides in children; macrolides or quinolones in adults). There is no evidence indicating whether it improves the evolution of the associated EM. Therefore, when asymptomatic infection is diagnosed by PCR or serologic testing, treatment is not mandatory.

Liquid antacids, topical glucocorticoids, and local anesthetics relieve symptoms of painful mouth or genital erosions. In case of eye involvement, an ocular lubricant should be administered at least three times a day, and topical steroids may be recommended by the ophthalmologist. There are no specific studies on the use of amniotic membrane in EMM cases with eye involvement. However, a number of patients considered to have SJS who were treated successfully with amniotic grafts may have actually had EMM. Because the mucosal involvement is the same in EMM and SJS, grafting of amniotic membrane in EMM cases with severe eye involvement should be helpful.

PREVENTION

Continuous therapy with oral anti-HSV drugs is effective at preventing recurrences of herpes-associated EM, including some cases without clinical evidence of precipitating HSV.[13] Topical acyclovir therapy used in a prophylactic manner does not prevent recurrent herpes-associated EM.[28]

In a series of 65 patients with recurrent EM, 11 were treated with azathioprine when all other treatments had failed. Azathioprine was beneficial in all 11 patients.[23] Mycophenolate mofetil can be also useful.

Retrospective uncontrolled analyses of thalidomide therapy have indicated that it is moderately effective for the treatment of established EM.[29] Thalidomide is probably the most effective treatment of recurrent or persistent cases when anti-HSV drugs have failed.[30,31]

In one randomized controlled trial, levamisole appeared useful. Because agranulocytosis is a severe and not exceptional adverse effect, levamisole use is permitted in only a few countries. The benefit–risk ratio is probably too low to support its use in the treatment of EM.

REFERENCES

1. Bastuji-Garin S, Rzany B, Stern RS, S et al. A clinical classification of cases of toxic epidermal necrolysis, Stevens-Johnson syndrome and erythema multiforme. *Arch Dermatol*. 1993;129:92.
2. Auquier-Dunant A, Mockenhaupt M, Naldi L, et al. Correlations between clinical patterns and causes of erythema multiforme majus, Stevens-Johnson syndrome and toxic epidermal necrolysis. *Arch Dermatol*. 2002;138:1019.
3. Wetter DA, Camilleri RJ. Clinical, etiologic and histopathologic features of Stevens-Johnson syndrome during an 8-year period at Mayo Clinic. *Mayo Clin Proc*. 2010;85:131.
4. Canavan TN, Mathes EF, Frieden I, et al. Mycoplasma pneumoniae-induced rash and mucositis as a syndrome distinct from Stevens-Johnson syndrome and erythema multiforme: a systematic review. *J Am Acad Dermatol*. 2015;72:23.
5. Schröder W, Mockenhaupt M, Schlingmann J, et al. Clinical re-classification of severe skin reactions and evaluation of their etiology in a population-based registry. In: Victor N, et al, eds. *Medical Informatics, Biostatistics and Epidemiology for Efficient Health Care and Medical Research: Contributions from the 44th Annual Conference of the GMDS*. Heidelberg: Urban & Vogel; 1999:107-110.
6. Rzany B, Mockenhaupt M, Baur S, et al. Epidemiology of erythema exsudativum multiforme majus, Stevens-Johnson syndrome, and toxic epidermal necrolysis in Germany (1990-1992): structure and results of a population-based registry. *J Clin Epidemiol*. 1996;49:769.
7. Roujeau JC. Re-evaluation of "drug-induced" erythema multiforme in the medical literature. *Br J Dermatol*. 2016;175(3):650-651.
8. Bonciolini V, Antiga E, Caproni M, et al. Rowell syndrome. Does it exist? *Clin Exp Dermatol*. 2014;39:58.

9. Khalil I, Lepage V, Douay C, et al. HLA DQB1*0301 allele is involved in the susceptibility to erythema multiforme. *J Invest Dermatol.* 1991;97:697.
10. Moreau JF, Watson RS, Hartman ME, et al. Epidemiology of ophthalmologic disease associated with erythema multiforme, Stevens-Johnson syndrome, and toxic epidermal necrolysis in hospitalized children in the United States. *Pediatr Dermatol.* 2014;31:163.
11. Brice SL, Krzemien D, Weston WL, et al. Detection of simplex virus DNA in cutaneous lesions of erythema multiforme. *J Invest Dermatol.* 1989;93:183.
12. Ng PPL, Sun YJ, Tan HH, et al. Detection of Herpes simplex virus genomic DNA in various subsets of erythema multiforme by polymerase chain reaction. *Dermatology.* 2003;207:349.
13. Tatnall FM, Schofield JK, Leigh IM. A double-blind, placebo-controlled trial of continuous acyclovir therapy in recurrent erythema multiforme. *Br J Dermatol.* 1995;132:267.
14. Prindaville B, Newell BD, Nopper AJ, et al. Mycoplasma pneumoniae–associated mucocutaneous disease in children: dilemmas in classification. *Pediatr Dermatol.* 2014;6:670.
15. Starnes L, Patel T, Skinner RB. Urticaria multiforme—a case report. *Pediatr Dermatol.* 2011;28:436.
16. Foedinger D, Elbe-Bürger A, Sterniczky B, et al. Erythema multiforme associated human autoantibodies against desmoplakin I and II: biochemical characterization and passive transfer studies into newborn mice. *J Invest Dermatol.* 1998;111:503.
17. Hirsch G, Ingen-Housz-Oro S, Fite C, et al. Rituximab, a new treatment for difficult-to-treat chronic erythema multiforme major? Five cases. *J Eur Acad Dermatol Venereol.* 2016;30:1140.
18. Komorowski L, Mockenhaupt M, Sekula P, et al. Lack of a specific humoral autoreactivity in sera from patients with early erythema exsudativum multiforme majus. *J Invest Dermatol.* 2013;133:2799.
19. Kokuba H, Imafuku S, Burnett JW, et al. Longitudinal study of a patient with herpes-simplex-virus-associated erythema multiforme: viral gene expression and T cell repertoire usage. *Dermatology.* 1999;198: 233-242.
20. Ono F, Bhuvnesh K. Sharma BK, et al. CD34+ cells in the peripheral blood transport Herpes simplex virus DNA fragments to the skin of patients with erythema multiforme (HAEM). *J Invest Dermatol.* 2005;124:1215-1224.
21. Kunimi Y, Hirata Y, Aihara M, et al. Statistical analysis of Stevens-Johnson Syndrome caused by Mycoplasma pneumonia infection in Japan. *Allergol Int.* 2011;60;525-532.
22. Edwards C, Penny M, Newman J. Mycoplasma pneumoniae, Stevens-Johnson syndrome, and chronic obliterative bronchitis. *Thorax.* 1983;38:867.
23. Schofield JK, Tatnall FM, Leigh IM. Recurrent erythema multiforme: clinical features and treatment in a large series of patients *Br J Dermatol.* 1993;128:542.
24. Wetter DA, Davis MD. Recurrent erythema multiforme: Clinical characteristics, etiologic associations, and treatment in a series of 48 patients at Mayo Clinic, 2000 to 2007. *J Am Acad Dermatol.* 2010;62:45.
25. Chen CW, Tsai TF, Chen YF, et al. Persistent erythema multiforme treated with thalidomide. *Am J Clin Dermatol.* 2008;9:123.
26. Riley M, Jenner R. Towards evidence based emergency medicine: best BETs from the Manchester Royal Infirmary. Bet 2. Steroids in children with erythema multiforme. *Emerg Med J.* 2008;25:594.
27. Weston WL, Morelli JG. Herpes simplex virus-associated erythema multiforme in prepubertal children. *Arch Pediatr Adolesc Med.* 1997;151:1014.
28. Fawcett HA, Wansbrough-Jones MH, Clark AE, et al. Prophylactic topical acyclovir for frequent recurrent herpes simplex infection with and without erythema multiforme. *BMJ.* 1983;287:798.
29. Cherouati K, Claudy A, Souteyrand P, et al. Treatment by thalidomide of chronic multiforme erythema: its recurrent and continuous variants. A retrospective study of 26 patients [in French] *Ann Dermatol Venereol.* 1996;123:375.
30. Wu JJ, Huang DB, Pang KR, et al. Thalidomide: dermatological indications, mechanisms of action and side-effects. *Br J Dermatol.* 2005;153:254.
31. Lozada F. Levamisole ion the treatment of erythema multiforme; a double-blind trial in 14 patients. *Oral Surg Med Oral Pathol.* 1982;53:28.

Chapter 44 :: Epidermal Necrolysis (Stevens-Johnson Syndrome and Toxic Epidermal Necrolysis)
:: Maja Mockenhaupt & Jean-Claude Roujeau

第四十四章 表皮坏死松解症（Stevens–Johnson综合征和中毒性表皮坏死松解症）

中文导读

本章共分为11节：①前言；②流行病学；③病因学；④发病机制；⑤临床表现；⑥实验室检查；⑦鉴别诊断；⑧并发症；⑨病程和预后；⑩治疗；⑪预防。全面描述了表皮坏死松解症（主要包括Stevens-Johnson综合征和中毒性表皮坏死松解症）的病因、临床特征及其防治。

第一节介绍了Stevens–Johnson综合征（SJS）和中毒性表皮坏死松解症（TEN）是严重威胁生命的皮肤黏膜反应，其特征是表皮和黏膜上皮广泛坏死和剥离。

第二节介绍了SJS、TEN的发病率、死亡率和危险因素以及预后评分指标SCORTEN。

第三节指出药物是最重要的病因，并列出了导致SJS/TEN的"高风险"药物。

第四节介绍了细胞毒性细胞，包括自然杀伤性T细胞（NKT）和药物特异性CD8+ T淋巴细胞以及杀伤性效应分子、白细胞介素等多种免疫因子在SJS/TEN发病中的作用。

第五节介绍了表皮坏死皮肤病的诊断和处理流程。详细描述了SJS/TEN的皮肤表现，包括皮损形态特征、演变、尼氏征等，并重点讲述了内脏并发症包括消化道、肺、肾脏损害。

第六节介绍了实验室检查在评估病情严重程度、预后和日常临床管理中的重要性。通过检测动脉血气分析、血细胞计数、电解质、肝肾功能等监测内脏器官受累情况。还介绍了皮肤活检的重要性及表皮坏死的组织病理学表现。

第七节介绍了鉴别诊断，如需要与水痘、葡萄球菌烫伤性皮肤综合症、暴发性紫癜以及大疱性疾病等相鉴别。

第八节介绍了表皮坏死的后遗症，并详细描述了各并发症及后遗症的表现、治疗和预防。

第九节揭示了表皮坏死疾病的临床过程和预后，包括皮损演变、死亡率及影响预后的因素。

第十节总结了治疗方案的选择，包括系统治疗（补液、营养支持、护理、预防性抗凝治疗等）以及急性期特异性治疗［分别介绍了糖皮质激素治疗、大剂量静脉免疫球蛋白（IVIG）、环孢素、血浆置换术、抗肿瘤坏死因子抗体治疗的意义和价值〕。提出了后遗症治疗的进展。

第十一节中作者对SJS/TEN的一级预防和二级预防提出了方法和建议。

〔李 捷〕

AT-A-GLANCE

- Epidermal necrolysis is a rare life-threatening reaction mainly induced by medication.
- Widespread apoptosis of keratinocytes is provoked by the activation of a cell-mediated cytotoxic reaction and amplified by cytokines, mainly granulysin.
- Confluent purpuric and erythematous macules evolving to flaccid blisters and epidermal detachment often start on the upper trunk and spread to the limbs associated with mucous membrane involvement.
- Histopathology shows full-thickness necrosis of epidermis associated with mild mononuclear cell infiltrate.
- A dozen "high-risk" drugs account for half of cases.
- More than 20% of cases remain idiopathic or may be caused by infection.
- Early identification and withdrawal of suspect medication in drug-induced cases are essential for good patient outcomes.
- Treatment consists mainly of supportive care, but recent evidence suggests a significant benefit of immunomodulating treatment with cyclosporine.
- The death rate is high and increases with disease severity and age of the patient. The majority of survivors have long-lasting sequelae, needing systematic follow-up examinations.

INTRODUCTION

Stevens-Johnson syndrome (SJS) and toxic epidermal necrolysis (TEN) are acute life-threatening mucocutaneous reactions characterized by extensive necrosis and detachment of the epidermis and mucosal epithelium (Table 44-1). In 1922, Stevens and Johnson first reported two cases of disseminated cutaneous eruptions associated with an erosive stomatitis and severe ocular involvement.[1] In 1956, Lyell described patients with epidermal loss secondary to necrosis and introduced the term *toxic epidermal necrolysis*.[2] Because SJS and TEN share clinical pattern, histopathologic findings, etiology, risk factors, and mechanisms, they are considered as severity variants of one disease entity that differs only in the extent of skin detachment related to the body surface area.[3-5] Therefore, it seems more appropriate to use the designation *epidermal (or epithelial) necrolysis* for both, as proposed by Ruiz-Maldonado (acute disseminated epidermal necrosis)[6] and Lyell (exanthematic necrolysis).[7]

EPIDEMIOLOGY

Epidermal necrolysis (EN) is rare. The overall incidence of SJS and TEN was estimated at 1 to 6 cases per million person-years and 0.4 to 1.2 cases per million person-years, respectively.[8-10] Whereas incidences as high as 5 or 6 cases per million per year derive from medical databases not primarily designed for epidemiologic analysis of rare diseases,[11] incidences of 1 to 2 cases per million per year were calculated using population-based prospective case registry data.[12,13]

EN can occur at any age, but the risk increases with age leading to the highest incidence in older adults after 65 years of age.[14] Women are more frequently affected, showing a sex ratio of 0.6. Patients infected with HIV and to a lesser degree patients with collagen vascular disease and cancer are at increased risk.[15,16] The overall mortality rate associated with EN is 22% to 27%, varying from approximately 10% for SJS to almost 50% for TEN.[17-19] Increasing age, significant comorbidity, and greater extent of skin detachment correlate with poor prognosis. A prognosis score (SCORTEN) has been constructed for EN,[20] and its usefulness has been confirmed by several teams[21-24] (Table 44-2).

ETIOLOGY

The exact pathophysiology of EN is still unclear; however, drugs are the most important etiologic factors. More than 100 different drugs have been implicated,[25-31] but fewer than a dozen "high-risk" medications account for about half of cases in Europe (Table 44-3), as evidenced by two multinational case-control studies.[16,27-30] These high-risk drugs are antibacterial sulfonamides, aromatic antiepileptic drugs, allopurinol, oxicam nonsteroidal antiinflammatory drugs, lamotrigine, and nevirapine.[28-30] The risk seems confined to the first 8 weeks of treatment and most inducing medications revealed the first continuous

TABLE 44-1
Consensus Definition of Stevens-Johnson Syndrome/Toxic Epidermal Necrolysis[a]

CRITERION	EM MAJUS	SJS	SJS—TEN OVERLAP	TEN WITH MACULAE	TEN ON LARGE ERYTHEMA (WITHOUT SPOTS)
Skin detachment (%)	<10	<10	10–30	>30	>10
Typical target lesions	+	−	−	−	−
Atypical target lesions	Raised	Flat	Flat	Flat	−
Maculae	−	+	+	+	−
Distribution	Mainly limbs	Widespread	Widespread	Widespread	Widespread

[a]According to Bastuji-Garin et al.[3]
EM, erythema multiforme; SJS, Stevens-Johnson syndrome; TEN, toxic epidermal necrolysis.

exposure between 4 and 28 days before reaction onset.[28] Slow dose escalation decreases the rate of mild rashes to lamotrigine and nevirapine,[32,33] but there is no evidence that it decreases the risk of EN.[28,30] Oxcarbazepine, a 10-keto derivative of carbamazepine, which was considered to carry a lower risk, seems to significantly cross-react with carbamazepine.[34] Many nonsteroidal antiinflammatory drugs were suspected to be associated with EN, but there is a substantial difference in risk for EN among them, with oxicam derivatives showing the highest risk, acetic acid derivatives such as diclofenac a moderate, and propionic acid derivatives such as ibuprofen no increased risk.[16,28,35] A significant but much lower risk has also been reported for various groups of antibiotics such as cephalosporins, quinolones, tetracyclines, and aminopenicillins.[28] Corticosteroids were significantly associated with an increased relative risk, but confounding could not be

TABLE 44-2
SCORTEN: A Prognostic Scoring System for Patients with Epidermal Necrolysis

SCORTEN	
PROGNOSTIC FACTORS	POINTS
Age >40 yr	1
Heart rate >120 beats/min	1
Cancer or hematologic malignancy	1
Body surface area involved >10%	1
Serum urea level >10 mM	1
Serum bicarbonate level <20 mM	1
Serum glucose level >14 mM	1
Scorten	**Mortality rate (%)**
0–1	3.2
2	12.1
3	35.8
4	58.3
5	90

Data from Bastuji-Garin S, Fouchard N, Bertocchi M, et al: SCORTEN: A severity-of-illness score for toxic epidermal necrolysis. *J Invest Dermatol.* 2000;115:149.

TABLE 44-3
Drugs and Recommendations in Stevens-Johnson Syndrome/Toxic Epidermal Necrolysis[a]

Drugs with a high risk to induce SJS/TEN
Their use should be carefully evaluated, and they should be suspected promptly.
Allopurinol
Lamotrigine
Cotrimoxazole (and other antiinfective sulfonamides and sulfasalazine)
Carbamazepine
Nevirapine
NSAIDs (oxicam type, eg, meloxicam)
Phenobarbital
Phenytoin
An interval of 4–28 days between beginning of drug use and onset of the adverse reaction is most suggestive of an association between the medication and SJS/TEN.
When patients are exposed to several medications with high expected benefits, the timing of administration is important to determine which one(s) must be stopped and if some may be continued or reintroduced.
The risks of various antibiotics to induce SJS/TEN are within the same order of magnitude but substantially lower than the risk of antiinfective sulfonamides.
Valproic acid does not seem to have an increased risk for SJS/TEN in contrast to other antiepileptics.
Diuretics and oral antidiabetics with sulfonamide structure do not appear to be risk factors for SJS/TEN.

Drugs with a moderate (significant but substantially lower) risk for SJS/TEN
Cephalosporines
Macrolides
Quinolones
Tetracyclines
NSAIDs (acetic acid type, eg, diclofenac)

Drugs with no increased risk for SJS/TEN
Beta-blockers
ACE inhibitors
Calcium channel blockers
Thiazide diuretics (with sulfonamide structure)
Sulfonylurea antidiabetics (with sulfonamide structure)
Insulin
NSAIDs (propionic acid type, eg, ibuprofen)

[a]According to Mockenhaupt et al.[28]
ACE, angiotensin-converting enzyme; NSAID, nonsteroidal antiinflammatory drug; SJS, Stevens-Johnson syndrome; TEN, toxic epidermal necrolysis.

excluded.[28] Recent analysis of systematically ascertained registry data on EN using ALDEN (algorithm for causality assessment in EN)[36] in comparison with results of two case-control studies[16,28] revealed that over a period of more than 2 decades, the proportion of validated cases that could be explained by medications with a significant (high and moderate) risk was stable (65%–68%). For roughly one third of the cases, no patent drug cause could be identified, suggesting that many more cases than previously thought have to be considered as "non–drug related" or "idiopathic."[37] The role of infectious agents in the development of EN is much less prominent than for erythema multiforme (see Chap. 43).[5] However, cases of EN associated with *Mycoplasma pneumoniae* infection, viral disease, and immunization have been reported, particularly in children.[38] In many cases a clinical infection is present, but despite extensive laboratory workup, no specific viral or bacterial agent can be detected.[39] Cases of EN have been reported after bone marrow transplantation. Some are an extreme form of acute graft-versus-host disease (GVHD; see Chap. 129); others could be drug-induced. The relationship between EN and GVHD is difficult to assess because clinical and histologic skin features are often indistinguishable.[40] Lupus erythematosus (systemic LE or subacute cutaneous LE) is associated with an increased risk of EN.[16,28] In such cases, drug causality is often doubtful and necrolysis might be an extreme phenotype of cutaneous lupus. Therefore, erosive LE has to be considered as a differential diagnosis of EN.[41,42] Finally, radiotherapy in addition to treatment with antiepileptic drugs, such as phenytoin, phenobarbital, or carbamazepine, can trigger EN with lesions localized predominantly at sites of radiation treatment.[43,44]

PATHOGENESIS

Even if the precise sequence of molecular and cellular events is incompletely understood, several studies provided important clues to the pathogenesis of EN. The immunologic pattern of early lesions suggests a cell-mediated cytotoxic reaction against keratinocytes leading to massive apoptosis.[45,46] Immunopathologic studies have demonstrated the presence of cytotoxic cells, including natural killer T cells (NKT) and drug-specific CD8+ T lymphocytes in early lesions; monocytes and macrophages and granulocytes are also recruited.[47-49] CD94/NKG2C was identified as a killer effector molecule in patients with EN.[50] However, it is generally accepted that specific and nonspecific cytotoxic cells are too few within the lesions to explain full-thickness necrosis of extensive areas of the epidermis and mucous membranes. Amplification by cytokines has been suspected for years, especially for factors activating "death receptors" on cell membranes, especially antitumor necrosis factor (TNF) α and soluble Fas ligand (Fas-L).[47,51] In the past decade, it had been widely accepted that Fas-L was inducing the apoptosis of keratinocytes in EN,[51,52] despite partial evidence and discordant findings.[53-55] An important study has challenged this dogma by demonstrating the key role of granulysin in EN.[56] The cytolytic protein granulysin was present in the blister fluid of patients with EN at concentrations much higher than those of perforin, granzyme B, or Fas-L. At such concentrations, only granulysin, and to a much lesser degree perforin, were able to kill human keratinocytes in vitro; Fas-L was not. Furthermore, injection of granulysin in the dermis of normal mice resulted in clinical and histologic lesions of EN.[57] Recently, interleukin (IL)-15 could be demonstrated to be associated with severity and mortality in EN.[58] When combined, these results strongly suggest that the effector mechanisms of EN have been deciphered. Cytotoxic T cells develop and are usually specifically directed against the native form of the drug rather than against a reactive metabolite, contrarily to what has been postulated for many years. These cells kill keratinocytes directly and indirectly through the recruitment of other cells that release soluble death mediators, the principal being granulysin and probably also IL-15.[56-58]

These advances in understanding the final steps of the reaction point to inhibition of release or blockade of granulysin as major aims of therapeutic interventions.

Little is known on the initial and intermediate steps. We still do not understand why very few individuals develop a violent immune response to medications and why effector cells are especially directed to the skin and other epithelia. Actually, most drugs associated with a high risk for EN can also induce a variety of milder and more frequent reactions. Drug-specific CD8 cytotoxic T-lymphocytes were also found in milder skin like maculopapular eruption.[59] Hence, it is tempting to speculate on an abnormal regulation of immune response. Regulatory CD4+ CD25+ T cells have been demonstrated to be potentially important in the prevention of severe epidermal damage induced by reactive cytotoxic T lymphocytes in a mouse model of EN.[60] Similar regulatory cells may play a role in drug eruptions in humans.[61] Altered regulation of the immune response to medications in patients with EN could result from comorbidities that are frequent (eg, cancer, HIV infection, collagen vascular disease), from comedications (eg, corticosteroids), or from genetic background.

Genetic susceptibility plays an important role in the development of EN to a few "high-risk" medications. A strong association was observed in Han Chinese from Taiwan between the human leukocyte antigen HLA-B*1502 and EN induced by carbamazepine and between HLA-B*5801 and EN induced by allopurinol.[62,63] B*1502 association with carbamazepine-related cases was confirmed in several Southeast Asian countries[64,65] but not in Japan and Korea.[66,67] The association between carbamazepine-induced EN and HLA-B*1502 was not present in European patients without Asian ancestry.[68] On the other hand, HLA-B*5801 was confirmed to be associated with allopurinol-related EN in Japan[66] and Europe,[69] but the strength of association was lower than in Taiwan. A genome-wide association study on samples of European EN-patients confirmed the involvement of genetic variants located in the HLA region. No other locus reached genome-wide statistical significance in this large sample. If some loci outside HLA play a role in EN, their effect might be very small.[70]

CLINICAL FINDINGS

Even in cases requiring immediate referral to specialized wards, the dermatologist will have a specific role in the management of patients with EN (Fig. 44-1).

HISTORY

EN clinically most often begins with unspecific prodromal symptoms such as sore throat, runny nose, cough, headache, fever, and malaise preceding the mucocutaneous lesions by 1 to 3 days. They are followed by the appearance of erythematous macules and atypical targets of the skin that may be confluent and on which blisters occur. Burning or stinging of the eyes, pain when swallowing, or urinating progressively develop, heralding mucous membrane involvement. The majority of cases begin with nonspecific symptoms followed either first by mucous membrane or by cutaneous involvement, but some cases may start with the specific lesions of skin and mucosa. Whatever the initial symptoms are, their rapid progression, the addition of new signs, severe pain, and constitutional symptoms should alert one to the onset of a severe disease.

A common problem is the fact that medications taken to treat the prodromal symptoms are often accused to have caused the reaction. This mainly concerns antipyretics, analgesics, and secretolytics, sometimes summarized as "cough and cold medicines." When looking at the use of these medications more closely, they have usually been taken and tolerated before and were started after the onset of prodromal symptoms of EN ("protopathic bias"). Neither of these patterns is typical for exposure to medications causing EN, which have not been used previously and the exposure of which is the first continuous use started 4 weeks to 4 days before reaction onset. Furthermore, these substances do not belong to the drug groups for which epidemiologic studies have estimated an increased risk to induce EN.[28,39]

CUTANEOUS LESIONS

The eruption is initially symmetrically distributed on the face, the upper trunk, and the proximal part of limbs.[71] The distal portions of the arms as well as the legs are relatively spared, but the eruption can rapidly extend to the rest of the body within a few days and even within a few hours. The initial skin lesions are characterized by erythematous, dusky red, irregularly shaped purpuric macules, which progressively coalesce. Atypical target lesions with dark centers are often observed (Fig. 44-2A). Confluence of necrotic lesions leads to extensive and diffuse erythema. Nikolsky sign, or dislodgement of the epidermis by lateral pressure, is positive on erythematous zones (Figs. 44-3 and 44-4). At this stage, the lesions evolve to flaccid blisters, which spread with pressure and break easily (see Fig. 44-2B). The necrotic epidermis is easily detached at pressure points or by frictional trauma, revealing large areas of exposed, red, sometimes oozing dermis (see Figs. 44-2C and 44-2D). In other areas, epidermis may remain.

Patients are classified into one of three groups according to the total area in which the epidermis is detached or "detachable" (positive Nikolsky): (1) SJS, less than 10% of body surface area (BSA); (2) SJS–TEN overlap, between 10% and 30%; (3) TEN, more than 30% of BSA.[3,5] Correct evaluation of the extent of detachment is difficult, especially in zones with spotty lesions. It is helpful to remember that the surface of one hand (palm and fingers) represents a little less than 1% of the BSA.

MUCOUS MEMBRANE INVOLVEMENT

Mucous membrane involvement (nearly always on at least two sites) is observed in approximately 90% of cases and can precede or follow the skin eruption. It begins with erythema followed by painful erosions of the oral, ocular, genital, nasal, anal and sometimes

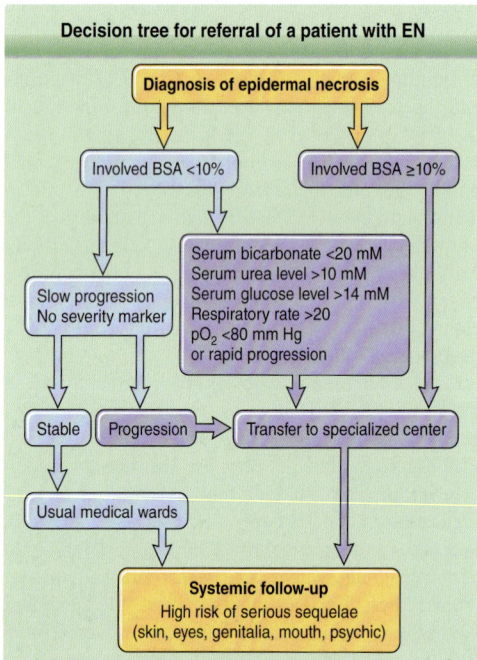

Figure 44-1 Decisional tree for referral of a patient with epidermal necrolysis. BSA, body surface area. (Adapted from Ellis MW. A case report and a proposed algorithm for the transfer of patients with Stevens-Johnson syndrome and toxic epidermal necrolysis to a burn center. *Mil Med.* 2002;167:701.)

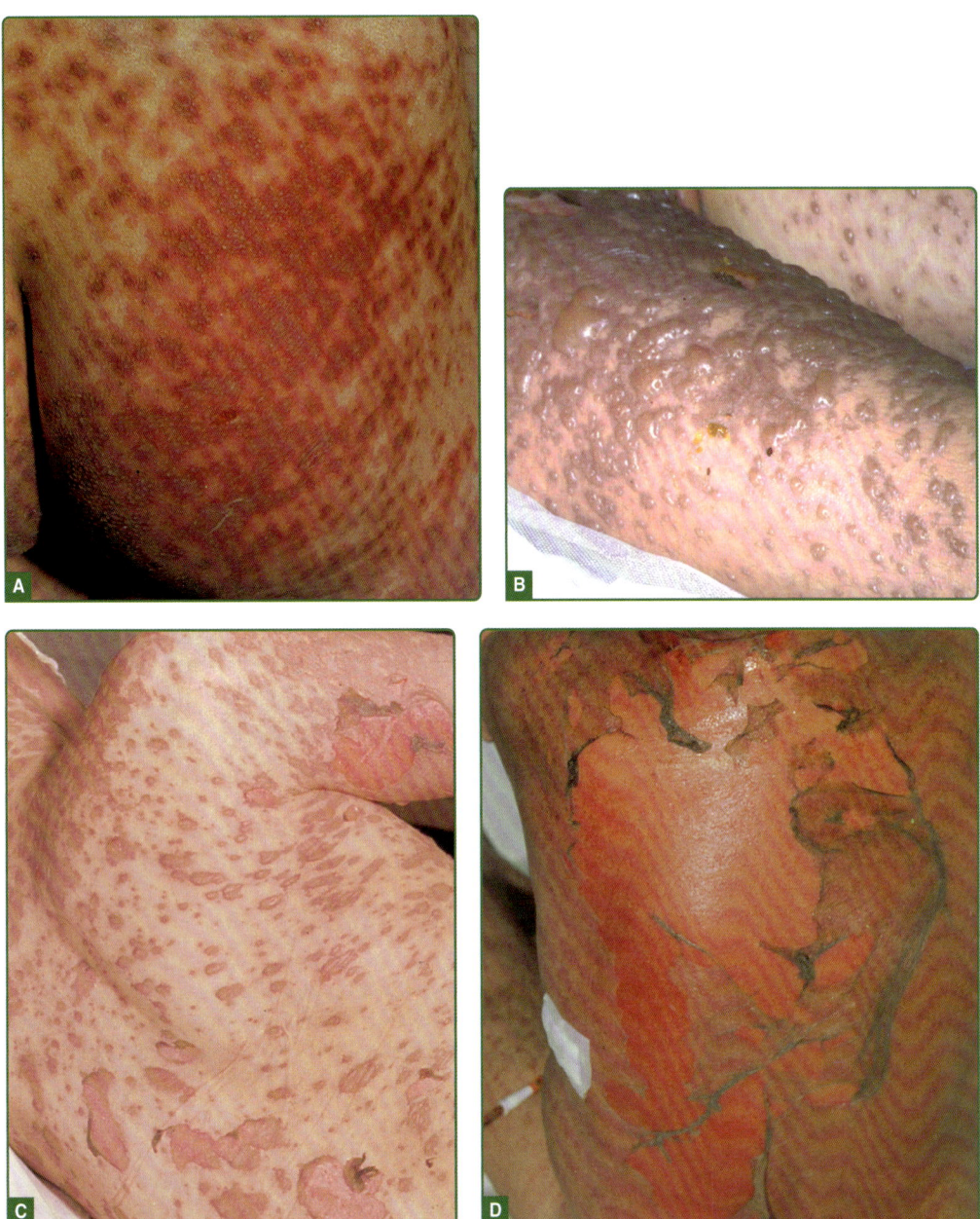

Figure 44-2 **A,** Early eruption. Erythematous dusky red macules (flat atypical target lesions) that progressively coalesce and show epidermal detachment. **B,** Early presentation with vesicles and blisters. Note the dusky color of blister roofs, strongly suggesting necrosis of the epidermis. **C,** Advanced eruption. Blisters and epidermal detachment have led to large confluent erosions. **D,** Full-blown epidermal necrolysis characterized by large erosive areas reminiscent of scalding.

tracheal or bronchial mucosa. This usually leads to impaired alimentation, photophobia, conjunctivitis, and painful micturition. The oral cavity and the vermilion border of the lips are almost invariably affected and feature painful hemorrhagic erosions coated by grayish white pseudomembranes and hemorrhagic crusts of the lips (Fig. 44-5). Approximately 80% of patients have conjunctival lesions,[72,73] mainly manifested by pain, photophobia, lacrimation, redness, and discharge. Severe forms may lead to epithelial defect and corneal ulceration, anterior uveitis, and purulent conjunctivitis. Synechiae between eyelids and conjunctiva often occur. There may be shedding of eyelashes (Fig. 44-5B). Genital erosions are frequent, often overlooked in women, and may lead to synechiae.[74,75]

SYSTEMIC INVOLVEMENT

EN is associated with high fever, pain, and weakness. Visceral involvement is also possible, particularly with

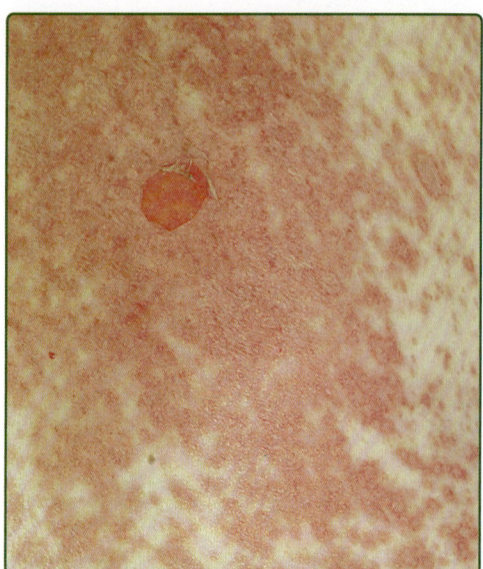

Figure 44-3 Early exanthematous phase with Nikolsky sign.

pulmonary and digestive complications. Early pulmonary complications occur in approximately 25% of patients and are essentially manifested by elevated respiratory rate and cough, which should prompt strict surveillance.[76,77] Bronchial involvement in EN is not correlated with the extent of skin lesions or with the offending agent. In most cases, chest radiographs are normal on admission but can rapidly reveal interstitial lesions that can progress to acute respiratory distress syndrome. In all reported cases, when acute respiratory failure developed rapidly after the onset of skin involvement, it was associated with poor prognosis. In the case of respiratory abnormalities, fiberoptic bronchoscopy may be useful to distinguish a specific epithelial detachment in the bronchi from an infectious pneumonitis, which has a much better prognosis.

Gastrointestinal tract involvement is less commonly observed, with epithelial necrosis of the esophagus, small bowel, or colon manifesting as profuse diarrhea with malabsorption, melena, and even colonic perforation.[78,79] Renal involvement has been reported. Proteinuria, microalbuminuria, hematuria, and azotemia are not rare. Proximal tubule damage can result from necrosis of tubule cells by the same process that destroys epidermal cells.[80] Glomerulonephritis is rare.[81]

LABORATORY TESTS

LABORATORY VALUES

There is no laboratory test to support the diagnosis of EN. Laboratory examinations are essential for evaluation of severity, prognosis, and daily management as for all life-threatening conditions in intensive care units (ICUs).

Evaluation of respiratory rate and blood oxygenation are among the first steps to take in the emergency department. Any alteration should be checked through measurement of arterial blood gas levels. Serum bicarbonate levels below 20 mM indicate a poor prognosis.[20] They usually result from respiratory alkalosis related to the specific involvement of bronchi and more rarely from metabolic acidosis.

Massive transdermal fluid loss is responsible for electrolyte imbalances, hypoalbuminemia, and hypoproteinemia, and mild and transient renal insufficiency and prerenal azotemia are common. Increased blood urea nitrogen level is one marker of severity. Anemia is common, and mild leukocytosis as well as thrombocytopenia may occur. Neutropenia is often considered to be an unfavorable prognostic factor but is too rare to have a significant impact on SCORTEN. Transient peripheral CD4+ lymphopenia is nearly always seen and is associated with decreased T-cell function. Mild elevation in levels of hepatic enzymes and amylase (most probably of salivary origin) are frequent but without impact on prognosis. A hypercatabolic state is responsible for inhibition of insulin secretion or insulin resistance, which results in hyperglycemia and occasionally overt diabetes. A blood glucose level above 14 mM may be a marker of severity.[20] Other abnormalities in laboratory values may occur, indicating involvement of other organs and complications such as sepsis.

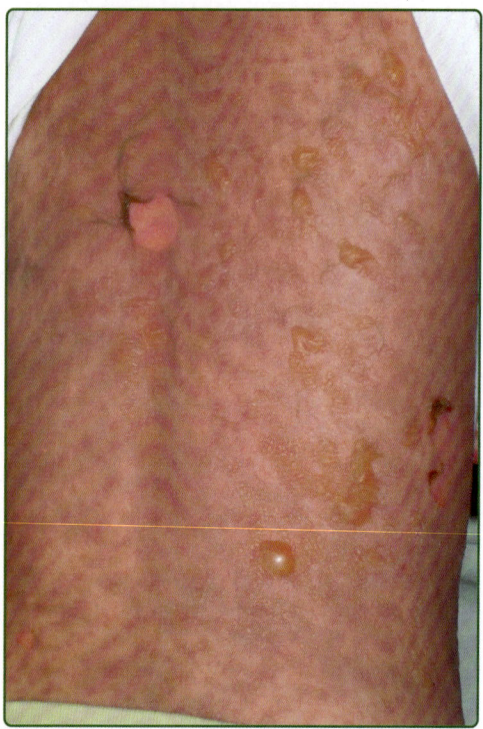

Figure 44-4 Blisters, erosions, and large areas of positive Nikolsky sign on the back of a patient with toxic epidermal necrolysis. One aim of local treatment is to protect "detachable" epidermis from being detached by using antishear dressings.

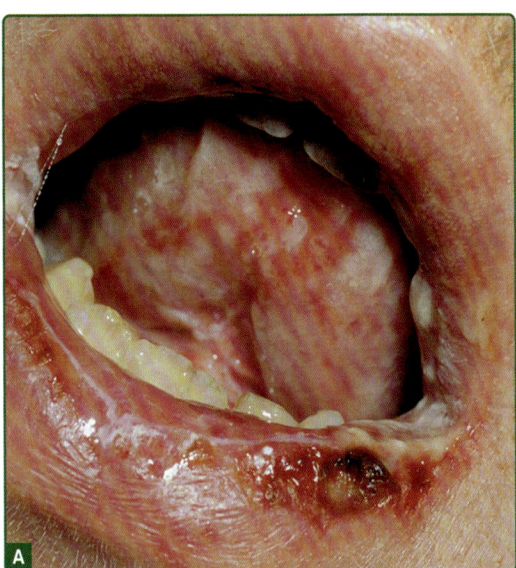 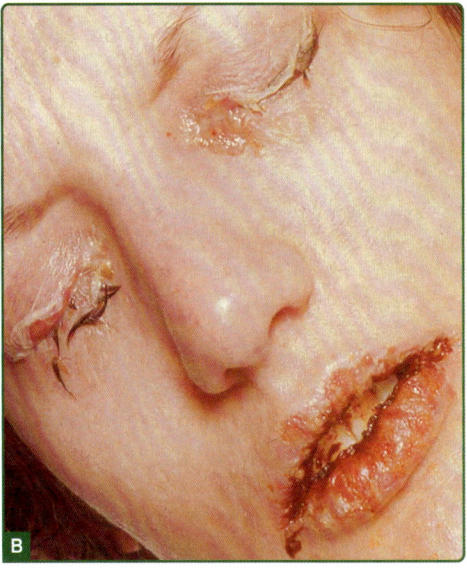

Figure 44-5 **A,** Extensive erosions and necroses of the lower lip and oral mucosa. **B,** Massive erosions covered by crusts on the lips. Note also shedding of the eyelashes.

HISTOPATHOLOGY

Skin biopsy for routine histologic and possibly immunofluorescence studies are strongly recommended, especially if there are alternative diagnoses to consider (see Fig. 44-3). The biopsy should be taken from a fresh lesion, preferably form the erythematous margin and not directly out of a blister because the latter carries the risk that epidermis and dermis are completely separated or partly lost. If similar lesions are present on the legs and elsewhere, the biopsy should preferentially not be taken from the legs below the knee. In the latter localization, changes could be superimposed by stasis dermatitis, complicating the correct histopathologic diagnosis.[82]

In the early stages, epidermal involvement is characterized by sparse apoptotic keratinocytes in the suprabasal layers (Fig. 44-6). In fully developed stages of the disease, when epidermal detachment and epidermolysis appear, in addition to the already mentioned changes subepidermal vesiculation secondary to extensive vacuolar alteration and confluent necrosis of keratinocytes develops.[82,83] Apoptosis of epithelial cells may involve sweat glands and hair follicles. A moderately dense mononuclear cell infiltrate of the papillary dermis is observed, mainly represented by lymphocytes, often CD8+ and macrophages.[83,84] Occasional eosinophilic granulocytes may be found. Variable numbers of extravasated erythrocytes are present. As the process develops rapidly, usually neither melanophages nor siderophages are found in the upper part of the dermis. The cornified layer remains unchanged. Results of direct immunofluorescence test are negative. Histopathology of involved mucous membranes show a similar pattern but are rarely performed.[85]

DIFFERENTIAL DIAGNOSIS

See Table 44-4.

Milder presentations of EN must be distinguished from erythema multiforme minus (without mucous membrane involvement) and majus (with mucous membrane involvement; EMM) (see Chap. 43). Early EN cases are often initially diagnosed as varicella, especially in children. The rapid progression of skin lesions and the severity of mucous membrane involvement should lead to considering potential EN.

The absence of mucous membrane involvement or its restriction to a single site must always raise the suspicion of an alternative diagnosis: staphylococcal scalded skin syndrome in infants but also in adults with septicemia; purpura fulminans in children and young adults; and acute generalized exanthematous pustulosis, phototoxicity, tension or pressure blisters in adults. Thermal burns are occasionally an issue when a transient loss of consciousness occurs as well as in small children or older adults in nursing homes.[71]

Linear immunoglobulin (Ig) A bullous disease and paraneoplastic pemphigus present with a less acute progression. Pathologic findings and a positive result on direct immunofluorescence testing are important for these diagnoses.

In all aspects, including pathology, generalized bullous fixed drug eruption (GBFDE) resembles EN. However, the distinction is worthwhile because GBFDE has a reputation for much better prognosis, probably because of the mild involvement of mucous membranes and the absence of visceral complications. Prior events, rapid onset after drug intake, and very large, well-demarcated blisters are the hallmarks of GBFDE.[86]

Toxic destruction of epithelia, whether through contact (fumigants) or ingestion (colchicine poisoning,

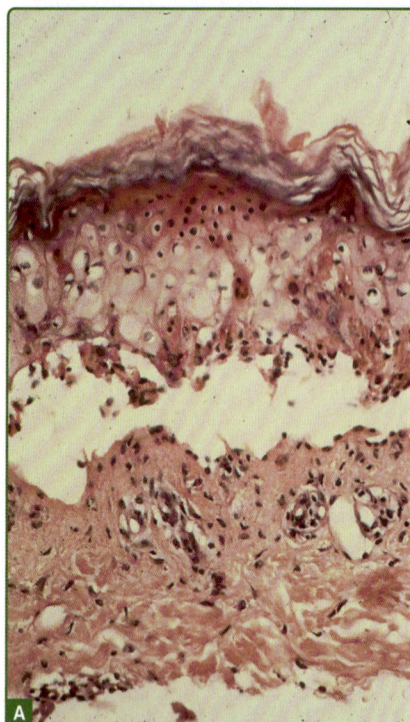 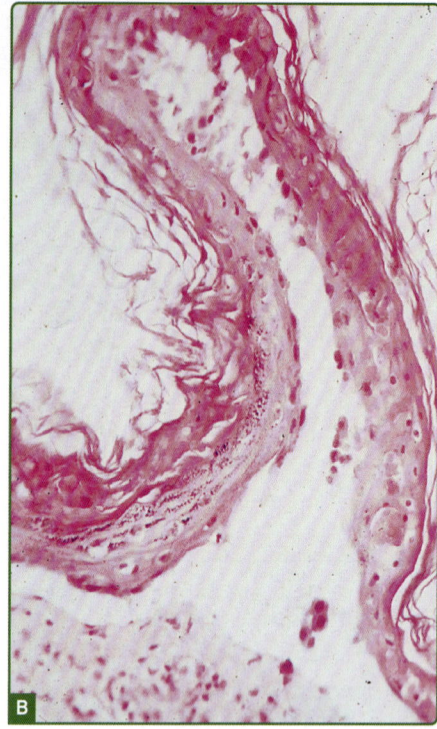

Figure 44-6 Histologic appearance of epidermal necrolysis. **A,** Eosinophilic necrosis of the epidermis in the peak stage, with little inflammatory response in the dermis. Note cleavage in the junction zone. **B,** The completely necrotic epidermis has detached from the dermis and folded like a sheet.

methotrexate overdose), may result in clinical features of EN but with skin erosions often predominating in the folds. In these rare cases, causality is generally obvious.

Overreporting of EN is common. It usually arises from confusion between desquamation and detachment of epidermis and between mucous membranes and periorificial skin. Because of such confusion, patients with a desquamative rash and scaly lips are not rarely diagnosed with and reported as having EN.

COMPLICATIONS AND SEQUELAE

During the acute phase, the most common complication of EN is sepsis. The epithelial loss predisposes these patients to infections, which are the main causes of mortality.[4,71] Central intravenous lines are a source for infection and should be avoided in favor of peripheral lines if possible. *Staphylococcus aureus* and *Pseudomonas* spp. are the most frequent pathogens, but about one third of positive blood cultures contain enterobacteriae not present on the skin, a finding that suggests bacterial translocation from gut lesions.[87] Multisystem organ failure and pulmonary complications are observed in more than 30% and 15% of cases, respectively.[88]

A very important advance in EN is the recent understanding that sequelae (Table 44-5) are more frequent and more severe than previously thought.[89] After the well-known risks of the acute stage, EN behaves as a chronic disease. More medical attention should be directed to that phase to better understand the

TABLE 44-4
Differential Diagnoses of Epidermal Necrolysis (EN)

Most Likely
- Limited EN (SJS)
  - Erythema multiforme majus
  - Varicella
- Widespread EN (SJS–TEN overlap and TEN)
  - Acute generalized exanthematous pustulosis
  - Generalized bullous fixed drug eruption

Consider
- Paraneoplastic pemphigus
- Linear IgA bullous disease
- Pressure blisters after coma
- Phototoxic reaction
- Graft-versus-host disease

Always Rule Out
- Staphylococcal scalded skin syndrome
- Thermal burns
- Skin necrosis from disseminated intravascular coagulation or purpura fulminans
- Chemical toxicity (eg, colchicine intoxication, methotrexate overdose)

IgA, immunoglobulin; EN, epidermal necrolysis; SJS, Stevens-Johnson syndrome; TEN, toxic epidermal necrolysis.

TABLE 44-5
Epidermal Necrolysis-Related Sequelae

Ophthalmic
- Chronic inflammation
- Fibrosis
- Entropion
- Trichiasis
- Symblepharon
- Alterations in vision
- Corneal ulcerations

Nails
- Dystrophy
- Permanent anonychia
- Ridging
- Pigmentary changes of the nail beds

Oral Mucosa
- Dryness
- Dysgeusia
- Late alterations of teeth

Vulvar or Vaginal
- Dyspareunia
- Vaginal dryness
- Genital adhesions

Other
- Esophageal strictures
- Intestinal strictures
- Urethral strictures
- Anal strictures
- Chronic lung disease

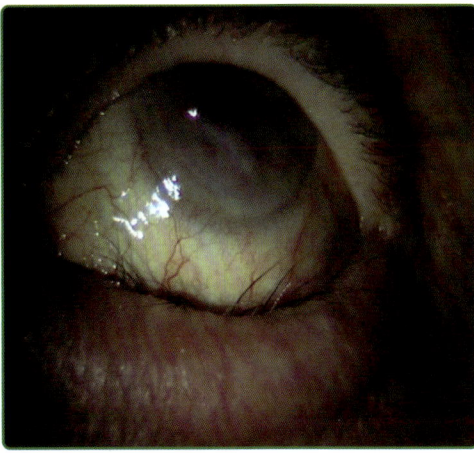

Figure 44-7 Late ocular complications of epidermal necrolysis. Note opaque corneal epithelium, neovessels, and irritating eyelashes on lower eyelids. (Used with permission from Julie Gueudry, MD, and Marc Muraine, MD, PhD, Hôpital Charles Nicolle, Rouen, France.)

frequency, mechanisms, and evolution of sequelae. Adequate management and prevention of sequelae are as important as saving the patient's life during the acute phase.

A large European cohort has found that 90% of patients who survived EN had sequelae 1 year after the acute stage of the disease, with a mean of three different problems per patient and an important negative impact on the quality of life for about half of them. A 5-year follow-up revealed similar data, demonstrating that many patients never got back to their normal activities before the reaction.[90] Symptoms suggesting posttraumatic stress disorder are not rare. Psychiatric consultation and psychological support have been considered to be helpful by affected patients and should be included into supportive care protocols. Late ophthalmic complications are reported in 20% to 75% of patients with EN, with a credible figure of about 50% (Fig. 44-7).[72,73,89] The relationship between the initial severity of ocular involvement and the development of late complications seems to be well established. However, late complications have also been observed in patients whose ocular involvement was considered to be mild during the acute stage of the disease. Late ophthalmic complications are mainly caused by functional alteration of the conjunctival epithelium with dryness and abnormal lacrimal film. This leads to chronic inflammation, fibrosis, entropion, trichiasis, and symblepharon. Long-term irritation and deficiency of stem cells in the limbus may result in metaplasia of corneal epithelium with painful ulcerations, scarring, and altered vision.[72]

Hypopigmentation and hyperpigmentation of the skin are most frequent sequelae; residual hypertrophic or atrophic scars rarely occur. Nail changes, including change in pigmentation of the nail bed, ridging, dystrophic nails, and permanent anonychia, occur in more than 30% of cases (Fig. 44-8). Mouth sequelae are present in about one third of patients who complain of dryness, altered taste, and late alterations of teeth.[91]

Vulvar and vaginal complications of EN are reported by about 25% of patients.[74] Dyspareunia is not rare and is related to vaginal dryness, itching, pain, and bleeding. Genital adhesions may lead to the requirement for surgical treatment.[75] Esophageal, intestinal, urethral, and anal strictures may also develop, although rarely. Chronic lung disease can be observed after EN, often attributed to bronchiolitis obliterans, and occasionally requiring lung transplantation.[77,92] Because these late complications and sequelae may develop insidiously, it is strongly suggested that all patients surviving EN

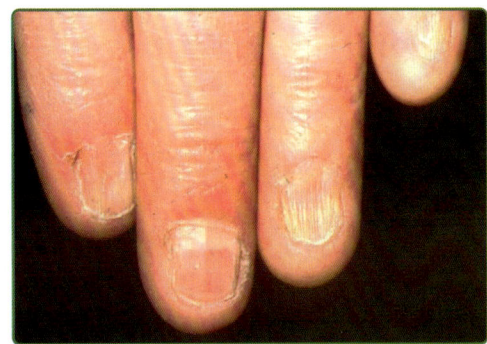

Figure 44-8 Abnormal regrowth of nails after epidermal necrolysis.

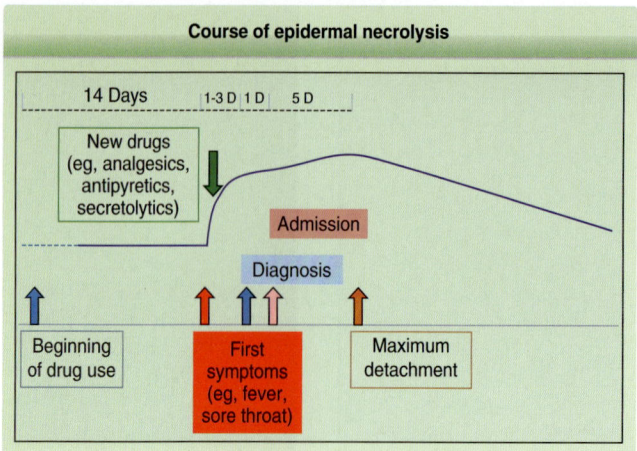

Figure 44-9 Course of epidermal necrolysis (EN). First symptoms of the reaction are unspecific like fever, sore throat, and reduced state of health (prodromal symptoms). Medications given for the prodromal symptoms are not associated with EN even if the first clear sign (mucosal involvement, macules) appears after their intake ("protopathic bias"; 1-3D). After admission the progression of EN to maximum skin detachment continues for up to 5 days (5D).

have a clinical follow-up a few weeks after discharge and 1 year later, including examination by an ophthalmologist and by other organ specialist(s) as indicated by abnormal signs and symptoms.

PROGNOSIS AND CLINICAL COURSE

The epidermal detachment progresses for 5 to 7 days (Figs. 44-9 and 44-10). Then patients enter a plateau phase, which corresponds to progressive reepithelialization. This can take a few days to a few weeks, depending on the severity of the disease and the prior general condition of the patient. During this period, life-threatening complications such as sepsis or systemic organ failure may occur. The overall mortality rate associated with EN is 22% to 27%, varying from approximately 10% for SJS to almost 50% for TEN,[17,18] but is highly dependent on the age of the patient and her or his underlying diseases. Thus, the mortality rate in children even with severe EN is very low compared with older adults. The prognosis is not affected by the cause of the reaction, whether drug or infection or unknown causality, type or dose of the responsible drug, or the presence of HIV infection (see Table 44-2).[16,20,71,88]

Prospective follow-up has shown an additional abnormally increased mortality rate in the 3-month period after hospital discharge, which seems to result from the negative impact of EN on prior severe chronic conditions, for example, malignancies (RegiSCAR, unpublished data).

TREATMENT

EN is a life-threatening disease that requires optimal management: early recognition and withdrawal of the offending drug(s) in drug-induced cases and supportive care in an appropriate hospital setting (Table 44-6).

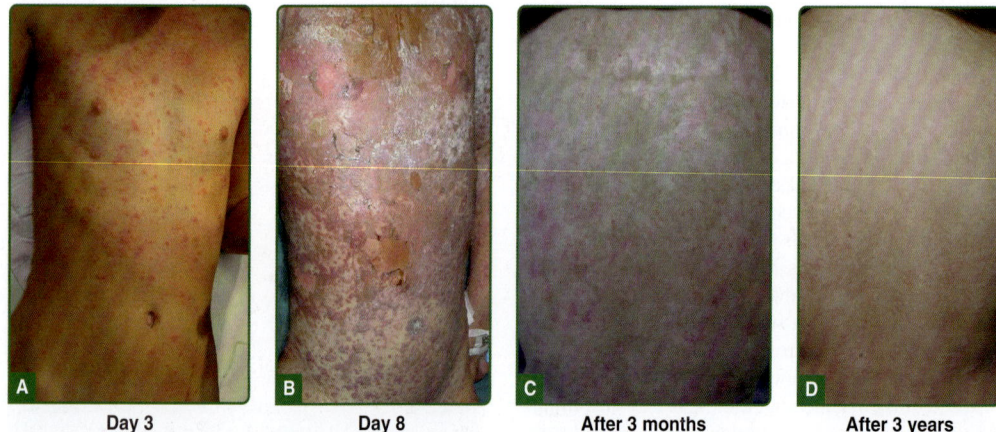

Figure 44-10 Clinical course of epidermal necrolysis (EN). Evolution at days 3 (**A**), 8 (**B**), 3 months (**C**), and 3 years (**D**) after onset of EN.

TABLE 44-6
Therapeutic Options in the Management of Epidermal Necrolysis[a]

1. Early recognition and immediate withdrawal of offending drugs(s)
2. Supportive treatment
   - Fluid replacement (preferably with a peripheral line)
   - Correct electrolyte imbalance
   - Early nutritional support (nasogastric tube)
   - Culture for skin, blood, and urine specimens
     - (Antibiotics only if bacterial infections are suspected)
   - Prophylactic anticoagulation
3. Skin care
   - Extensive debridement not recommended
4. Early ophthalmologic evaluation and care.
   - Use of preservative-free emollients, antiseptic eye drops, vitamin A

Mechanical disruption of early synechiae
5. Antifungal or antiseptic mouth rinse
6. Systemic steroids
   - Use is controversial

Medium doses for short periods (days rather than weeks) may be beneficial
7. Cyclosporine A
   - Early administration may halt the progression of skin detachment and increase survival
   - Dose: 3 mg/kg for 10 days
8. Anti-TNF monoclonal antibodies
   - Etanercept may be of benefit
   - Extreme caution is advised

[a]Specific treatment options for the acute phase of epidermal necrolysis (EN) are underlined. Although larger trials are still needed, recent evidence based on smaller studies has suggested these may be of benefit in the management of EN.
TFN, tumor necrosis factor.

Prompt withdrawal of offending agent(s) is associated with an increased rate of survival in patients with EN induced by drugs with short elimination half-lives.[93] At the same time, it is preferable to continue every important and nonsuspected medication. This is of medical benefit for the affected patient and may furthermore avoid reluctance of the patient's physicians to prescribe them in the future. In case of doubt, all not life-sustaining drugs should be stopped when initiated and administered within the previous 8 weeks.

SYMPTOMATIC TREATMENT

Only patients with limited skin involvement, a SCORTEN score of 0 or 1, and a disease that is not rapidly progressing can be treated in nonspecialized wards. Depending on the local or national facilities, patients who do not need intensive care may remain in dermatology units or hospitals (eg, in many European countries), others should be transferred to ICUs or burn centers.[94] Although recent studies suggest that immunomodulating treatment with cyclosporine (ciclosporin) could be beneficial (see later), supportive measures are most important.[18,88,95,96] Supportive care consists of maintaining hemodynamic equilibrium and preventing life-threatening complications. The aims are similar to those for the treatment of extensive burns.

EN is associated with significant fluid loss from erosions, which results in hypovolemia and electrolyte imbalance. Fluid replacement must be started as soon as possible and adjusted daily. Volumes of infusions are usually less than for burns of similar extent of skin detachment because interstitial edema is absent. Peripheral venous lines are preferred when possible because the sites of insertion of central lines are often involved in detachment of epidermis and prone to infection. The environmental temperature should be raised to 28°C to 30°C (82.4°F to 86°F). The use of an air-fluidized bed improves patient comfort.

Early nutritional support is preferentially provided by nasogastric tube to promote healing and to decrease the risk of bacterial translocation from the gastrointestinal tract. To reduce the risk of infection, aseptic and careful handing is required. Skin, blood, and urine specimens should be cultured for bacteria and fungi at frequent intervals. Prophylactic antibiotics are not indicated. Patients should receive antibiotics when clinical infection is suspected. Prophylactic anticoagulation should be provided during hospitalization.

We do not recommend extensive and aggressive debridement of necrotic epidermis in EN because the superficial necrosis is not an obstacle to reepithelialization and might even accelerate the proliferation of stem cells due to the inflammatory cytokines. This is the single noticeable divergence between authors of this chapter and the recommendations of US burn centers.[96] A few recent series suggest that debridement is necessary neither in superficial burns[97] nor in EN.[98,99] There is no standard policy on wound dressings and the use of antiseptics. It is a matter of experience for each center. Skillfulness on the part of specialized nurses, careful manipulation, and an aggressive protocol of prevention and treatment of pain are essential.

Eyes should be examined daily by an ophthalmologist. Preservative-free emollients, antibiotic or antiseptic eye drops, and vitamin A are often used every 2 hours in the acute phase, and mechanical disruption of early synechiae is indicated. Early graft of cryopreserved amniotic membrane has been proposed as capable to decrease the rate of severe eye sequelae.[72]

The mouth should be rinsed several times a day with antiseptic or antifungal solution.

SPECIFIC TREATMENT IN ACUTE STAGE

Because of the importance of immunologic and cytotoxic mechanisms, a large number of immunosuppressive and antiinflammatory therapies have been tried to halt the progression of the disease. The low prevalence of the disease makes randomized clinical trials hard to perform, so most publications on treatment are case reports and rather small case series.

CORTICOSTEROIDS

The use of systemic corticosteroids is still controversial. Some studies found that such therapy could prevent the extension of the disease when administered during the early phase, especially as intravenous pulses for a few days.[100] Other studies concluded that steroids did not stop the progression of the disease and were even associated with increased mortality and sepsis when administered for 2 to 3 weeks. Thus, systemic corticosteroids cannot be recommended as the mainstay treatment of EN,[96] but a large cohort study has suggested a benefit quoad vitam when steroids were given in a medium dose for a few days.[101] A recent systematic review revealed a beneficial effect on corticosteroids in the treatment of SJS and TEN. Although the potential effect on the progression of skin detachment could not be analyzed by that approach, the results on outcome (death versus survival) were favorable.[102]

INTRAVENOUS IMMUNOGLOBULINS

The proposal to use high-dose intravenous immunoglobulin (IVIG) was based on the hypothesis that Fas-mediated cell death can be abrogated by the anti-Fas activity present in commercial batches of normal human Ig.[51] Benefits have been claimed by several studies, mainly case compilations with patients included in more than one study and case reports[51,103-105] but refuted by several others.[22,101,106-108] The large cohort study published in 2008 comparing the treatment in 281 patients with EN could not demonstrate a beneficial effect of IVIG.[101] Thus, IVIG could not be considered the standard of care in recent years,[96] especially after the finding that the Fas-L—Fas pathway was not, or only marginally, involved in the mechanisms of EN.[56] The recent systematic review mentioned did not find a favorable effect of IVIG, neither on the study nor on the individual patient level.[102] Taking these findings into account, we conclude that IVIG should not be used to treat patients with EN.[109]

CYCLOSPORINE A

Cyclosporine is a powerful immunosuppressive agent associated with biologic effects that are theoretically useful in the treatment of EN: activation of T helper cells and cytokines; inhibition of CD8+ cytotoxic mechanisms; and antiapoptotic effect through inhibition of Fas-L, nuclear factor-κB, and TNF-α. Several case reports and series suggested the efficacy of cyclosporine A (CyA) in halting the progression of skin detachment in EN without worrisome side effects when administered early.[110,111] In the pilot study performed in the French Reference Center for EN, the initial dose of 3 mg of CyA per kilogram body weight was slowly tapered over 1 month (3 mg/kg body weight for 10 days followed by 2 mg/kg for 10 days and 1 mg/kg for 10 days).[111] However, in recent years, the protocol was modified to 3 mg/kg body weight for 10 days only, with the usual dose adjustment in cases with renal failure (personal communication). The recent systematic review of EN treatment also saw positive effects of CyA, but the number of studies and patients treated were too small to demonstrate a significant finding.[102] A recent study from Spain compared the treatments of EN in two large specialized units and concluded that the use of CyA was beneficial both in terms of halting disease progression and survival.[112]

These new studies are a real breakthrough concerning the immunomodulating treatment of EN. Because randomized double-blind, placebo-controlled trials are hardly feasible in rare and unexpectable conditions such as EN that may affect anyone at any time at any place, systematic surveillance of treatment modalities (eg, CyA use) is warranted.[109]

PLASMAPHERESIS OR HEMODIALYSIS

The rationale for using plasmapheresis or hemodialysis is to prompt the removal of the offending medication, its metabolites, or inflammatory mediators such as cytokines. A small series reported their efficacy and safety in treating EN.[113-116] However, considering the absence of evidence and the risks associated with intravascular catheters, these treatments cannot be recommended.

ANTI–TUMOR NECROSIS FACTOR AGENTS

Anti-TNF monoclonal antibodies have been successfully used to treat a few patients. Recently, a study comparing corticosteroids and etanercept reported improved clinical outcomes in patients with EN treated with the latter. Furthermore, decreased levels of TNF-α and granulysin were observed.[117] Nevertheless, because a prior randomized controlled trial of thalidomide, an anti-TNF agent, had to be interrupted because of significantly increased mortality,[118] extreme caution is suggested in the use of anti-TNF agents to treat EN.

TREATMENT OF SEQUELAE

Very promising treatments have now been developed for the ocular sequelae of EN, including gas-permeable scleral lenses[119,120] and grafting of autologous stem cells from contralateral limbus or mouth mucosa.[121,122] With the exception of ocular sequelae, the literature contains only case reports related to treating sequelae. Photoprotection and cosmetic lasers may help resolve the pigmentation changes on the skin, but specific studies do not exist. This also accounts for nail disorders caused by EN.

PREVENTION

Primary prevention is only feasible in populations where a strong association has been established between a simple genetic maker and the risk of EN.

That is the case for HLA-B*1502 and EN induced by carbamazepine in persons of Southeast Asian ancestry. The US Food and Drug Administration has issued the recommendation to test patients of Han Chinese and Thai origin for HLA-B*1502 before prescribing carbamazepine. In Taiwan, testing of HLA-B*1502 before prescription of carbamazepine has led to a substantial reduction of EN-cases.[123] In Hong Kong, however, the screening policy was associated with prevention of carbamazepine-induced EN without reducing the overall burden of EN induced by antiepileptic medication, likely because clinicians preferred drugs not requiring a genetic test but that may also induce EN.[124] In individuals of Han Chinese or Southeast Asian origin, alternative antiepileptic drugs can be carefully prescribed, although there may be an association of EN with phenytoin and HLA-B*1502 as well.[64] The present status of research on the pharmacogenetics of EN makes it rather unlikely to identify another genetic marker with such a clear and high association to be useful for primary prevention.[70]

Secondary prevention is important for patients who experienced EN and are reluctant to take any medication. The most important issue is to evaluate drug causality. In vitro tests or patch tests to medications occasionally can be useful in the exploration of drug allergy. When used in patients with EN, their sensitivity is low.[125,126] Careful inquiry into all exposures to medications in the few weeks preceding the onset of the reaction leads to the identification of a probable culprit drug in approximately 67% of cases. The most useful clinical criteria are duration of treatment before onset (typically 4 to 28 days), absence of prior intake, and use of a drug known for being associated with a high risk.[36]

The few published cases of recurrent SJS or TEN—and so-called recurrent cases of SJS that are actually cases of EMM—were always caused by inadvertent readministration of the same or a very closely related medication. Epidemiology and in vitro studies suggest that the list of possible cross-reactive medications is rather narrow, based on close chemical similarities. As an example, there is no evidence that patients who experienced EN in reaction to an antiinfective sulfonamide are at increased risk for reaction to sulfonamide-related diuretics or antidiabetic medications. Only antiinfectious sulfonamides and sulfasalazine should be contraindicated in this situation.

A list of the suspected medication(s) and molecules of the same biochemical structure must be given to the patient on a personal "allergy card" or "allergy passport." It may also be useful to provide a list of drugs of common use that cannot be suspected.

REFERENCES

1. Stevens AM, Johnson FC. A new eruptive fever associated with stomatitis and ophthalmia: report of two cases in children. *Am J Dis Child*. 1922;24:526.
2. Lyell A. Toxic epidermal necrolysis: an eruption resembling scalding of the skin. *Br J Dermatol*. 1956;68:355.
3. Bastuji-Garin S, Rzany B, Stern RS, et al. Clinical classification of cases of toxic epidermal necrolysis, Stevens-Johnson syndrome, and erythema multiforme. *Arch Dermatol*. 1993;129:92.
4. Lissia M, Mulas P, Bulla A, et al. Toxic epidermal necrolysis (Lyell's disease). *Burns*. 2010;36:152.
5. Auquier-Dunant A, Bastuji-Garin S, Revuz J, et al. Correlation between clinical patterns and causes of erythema multiforme majus, Stevens Johnson and toxic epidermal necrolysis. *Arch Dermatol*. 2002;138:1019.
6. Ruiz-Maldonado R. Acute disseminated epidermal necrosis types 1, 2, and 3: study of sixty cases. *J Am Acad Dermatol*. 1985;13:623.
7. Lyell A. Requiem for toxic epidermal necrolysis. *Br J Dermatol*. 1990;122:837.
8. Chan HL, Stern RS, Arndt KA, et al. The incidence of erythema multiforme, Stevens-Johnson syndrome, and toxic epidermal necrolysis: a population based study with particular reference to reactions caused by drugs among outpatients. *Arch Dermatol*. 1990;126:43.
9. Roujeau JC, Guillaume JC, Fabre JP, et al. Toxic epidermal necrolysis (Lyell syndrome). Incidence and drug etiology in France (1981–1985). *Arch Dermatol*. 1990;126:37.
10. Schöpf E, Stühmer A, Rzany B, et al. Toxic epidermal necrolysis and Stevens-Johnson syndrome. An epidemiologic study from West-Germany. *Arch Dermatol*. 1991;27:839-842.
11. Frey N, Jossi J, Bodmer M, et al. The epidemiology of Stevens-Johnson syndrome and toxic epidermal necrolysis in the UK. *J Invest Dermatol*. 2017;137(6):1240-1247.
12. Rzany B, Mockenhaupt M, Baur S, et al. Epidemiology of erythema exsudativum multiforme majus, Stevens-Johnson syndrome, and toxic epidermal necrolysis in Germany (1990-1992): structure and results of a population-based registry. *J Clin Epidemiol*. 1996;49:769.
13. Nägele D, et al. Incidence of Stevens-Johnson syndrome/toxic epidermal necrolysis: results of 10 years from the German Registry. *Pharmacoepidemiol Drug Safe*. 2017.
14. Mockenhaupt M, et al. Frequency and incidence of severe cutaneous adverse reactions in different age groups. *Pharmacoepidemiol Drug Safe*. 2011;20:34.
15. Rzany B, Mockenhaupt M, Stocker U, et al. Incidence of Stevens-Johnson syndrome and toxic epidermal necrolysis in patients with the acquired immunodeficiency syndrome in Germany. *Arch Dermatol*. 1993;129:1059.
16. Roujeau JC, Kelly JP, Naldi L, Ret al. Medication use and the risk of Stevens-Johnson syndrome or toxic epidermal necrolysis. *N Engl J Med*. 1995;333:1600.
17. Sekula P, Dunant A, Mockenhaupt M, et al. Comprehensive survival analysis of a cohort of patients with Stevens-Johnson syndrome and toxic epidermal necrolysis. *J Invest Dermatol*. 2013;133(5):1197-1204.
18. Paulmann M, Mockenhaupt M. Severe drug hypersensitivity reactions: clinical pattern, diagnosis, etiology and therapeutic options. *Curr Pharm Des*. 2017;22:6852-6861.
19. Risser J, Lewis K, Weinstock MA. Mortality of bullous skin disorders from 1979 through 2002 in the United States. *Arch Dermatol*. 2009;145:1005.

20. Bastuji-Garin S, Fouchard N, Bertocchi M, et al. SCORTEN: a severity-of-illness score for toxic epidermal necrolysis. *J Invest Dermatol*. 2000;115:149.
21. Trent JT, Kirsner RS, Romanelli P, et al. Use of the SCORTEN to accurately predict mortality in patients with toxic epidermal necrolysis in the United States. *Arch Dermatol*. 2004;140:890.
22. Brown KM, Silver GM, Halerz M, et al. Toxic epidermal necrolysis: does immunoglobulin make a difference? *J Burn Care Rehabil*. 2004;25:81.
23. Guégan S, Bastuji-Garin S, Poszepczynska-Guigné E, et al. Performance of the SCORTEN during the first five days of hospitalisation to predict the prognosis of epidermal necrolysis. *J Invest Dermatol*. 2006;126:272.
24. Cartotto R, Mayich M, Nickerson D, et al. SCORTEN accurately predicts mortality among toxic epidermal necrolysis patients treated in a burn center. *J Burn Care Res*. 2008;29:141.
25. Lyell A. Toxic epidermal necrolysis (the scalded skin syndrome): a reappraisal. *Br J Dermatol*. 1979;100:69.
26. Roujeau JC, Stern RS. Severe adverse cutaneous reactions to drugs. *N Engl J Med*. 1994;331:1272.
27. Rzany B, Correia O, Kelly JP, et al. Risk of Stevens-Johnson syndrome and toxic epidermal necrolysis during first weeks of antiepileptic therapy: a case control study. *Lancet*. 1999;353:2190.
28. Mockenhaupt M, Viboud C, Dunant A, et al. Stevens-Johnson syndrome and toxic epidermal necrolysis: assessment of medication risks with emphasis on recently marketed drugs. The EuroSCAR-study. *J Invest Dermatol*. 2008;128:35.
29. Halevy S, Ghislain PD, Mockenhaupt M, et al. Allopurinol is the most common cause of Stevens-Johnson syndrome and toxic epidermal necrolysis in Europe and Israel. *J Am Acad Dermatol*. 2008;58:25.
30. Fagot JP, Mockenhaupt M, Bouwes-Bavinck JN, et al. Nevirapine and the risk of Stevens Johnson syndrome or toxic epidermal necrolysis. *AIDS*. 2001;15:1843.
31. Mockenhaupt M, Messenheimer J, Tennis P, et al. Risk of Stevens-Johnson and toxic epidermal necrolysis in new users of antiepileptics. *Neurology*. 2005;64:1134.
32. Ketter TA, Wang PW, Chandler RA, et al. Dermatology precautions and slower titration yield low incidence of lamotrigine treatment-emergent rash. *J Clin Psychiatry*. 2005;66:642.
33. Warnock JK, Morris DW. Adverse cutaneous reactions to mood stabilizers. *Am J Clin Dermatol*. 2003;4:21.
34. Beran RG. Cross-reactive skin eruption with both carbamazepine and oxcarbazepine. *Epilepsia*. 1993;34:163.
35. Mockenhaupt M, Kelly JP, Kaufman D, et al. The risk of Stevens-Johnson syndrome and toxic epidermal necrolysis associated with nonsteroidal antiinflammatory drugs: a multinational perspective. *J Rheumatol*. 2003;30:2234.
36. Sassolas B, Haddad C, Mockenhaupt M, et al. ALDEN, an algorithm for assessment of drug causality in Stevens-Johnson syndrome and toxic epidermal necrolysis: comparison with case-control analysis. *Clin Pharmacol Ther*. 2010;88(1):60-68.
37. Mockenhaupt M, Dunant A, Paulmann M, et al. Drug causality in Stevens-Johnson syndrome/toxic epidermal necrolysis in Europe: analysis of 10 years RegiSCAR study. *Pharmacoepidemiol Drug Safe*. 2016; 25(Supp 3):3.
38. Fournier S, Bastuji-Garin S, Mentec H, et al. Toxic epidermal necrolysis associated with Mycoplasma pneumoniae infection. *Eur J Clin Microbiol Infect Dis*. 1995;14:558.
39. Paulmann M, Mockenhaupt M. Fever in Stevens-Johnson syndrome and toxic epidermal necrolysis in pediatric cases: laboratory work-up and antibiotic therapy. *Pediatr Infect Dis J*. 2017;36:513-515.
40. Stone N, Sheerin S, Burge S. Toxic epidermal necrolysis and graft versus host disease: a clinical spectrum but a diagnostic dilemma. *Clin Exp Dermatol*. 1999;24:260.
41. Ting W, Stone MS, Racila D, et al. Toxic epidermal necrolysis-like acute cutaneous lupus erythematosus and the spectrum of the acute syndrome of apoptotic pan-epidermolysis (ASAP): a case report, concept review and proposal for new classification of lupus erythematosus vesiculobullous skin lesions. *Lupus*. 2004;13:941.
42. Ziemer M, Kardaun SH, Liss Y, et al. Stevens-Johnson syndrome and toxic epidermal necrolysis in patients with lupus erythematosus: a descriptive study of 17 cases from a national registry and review of the literature. *Br J Dermatol*. 2012;166, 575-600.
43. Fleisher AB Jr, Rosenthal DI, Bernard SA, et al. Skin reactions to radiotherapy—a spectrum resembling erythema multiforme: case report and review of the literature. *Cutis*. 1992;49:35.
44. Wöhrl S, Loewe R, Pickl WF, et al. EMPACT syndrome. *J Dtsch Dermatol Ges*. 2005;3:39.
45. Correia O, Delgado L, Ramos JP, et al. Cutaneous T-cell recruitment in toxic epidermal necrolysis: further evidence of CD8+ lymphocyte involvement. *Arch Dermatol*. 1993;129:466.
46. Paul C, Wolkenstein P, Adle H, et al. Apoptosis as a mechanism of keratinocyte death in toxic epidermal necrolysis. *Br J Dermatol*. 1996;134:710.
47. Paquet P, Nikkels A, Arrese JE, et al. Macrophages and tumor necrosis factor alpha in toxic epidermal necrolysis. *Arch Dermatol*. 1994;130:605.
48. Le Cleach L, Delaire S, Boumsell L, et al. Blister fluid T lymphocytes during toxic epidermal necrolysis are functional cytotoxic cells which express human natural killer inhibitory receptors. *Clin Exp Immunol*. 2000;119:225.
49. Nassif A, Bensussan A, Dorothée G, et al. Drug specific cytotoxic T-cells in the skin lesions of a patient with toxic epidermal necrolysis. *J Invest Dermatol*. 2002;118:728.
50. Morel E, Escamochero S, Cabañas R, et al. CD94/NKG2C is a killer effector molecule in patients with Stevens-Johnson syndrome and toxic epidermal necrolysis. *J Allergy Clin Immunol*. 2010; 25, 3:703-710.
51. Viard I, Wehrli P, Bullani R, et al. Inhibition of toxic epidermal necrolysis by blockade of CD95 with human intravenous immunoglobulin. *Science*. 1998;282:490.
52. Abe R, Shimizu T, Shibaki A, et al. Toxic epidermal necrolysis and Stevens-Johnson syndrome are induced by soluble Fas Ligand. *Am J Pathol*. 2003;162:1515.
53. Berthou C, Michel L, Soulié A, et al. Acquisition of granzyme B and Fas ligand proteins by human keratinocytes contributes to epidermal cell defence. *J Immunol*. 1997;159:5293.
54. Nassif A, Moslehi H, Le Gouvello S, et al. Evaluation of the potential role of cytokines in toxic epidermal necrolysis. *J Invest Dermatol*. 2004;123:850.
55. Stur K, Karlhofer FM, Stingl G. Soluble FAS ligand: a discriminating feature between drug-induced skin eruptions and viral exanthemas. *J Invest Dermatol*. 2007;127:802.

56. Chung WH, Hung SI, Yang JY, et al. Granulysin is a key mediator for disseminated keratinocyte death in Stevens-Johnson syndrome and toxic epidermal necrolysis. *Nat Med*. 2008;14:1343.
57. Abe R, Yoshioka N, Murata J, et al. Granulysin as a marker for early diagnosis of the Stevens-Johnson syndrome. *Ann Intern Med*. 2009;151:514.
58. Su SC, Mockenhaupt M, Wolkenstein P, et al. Interleukin-15 is associated with severity and mortality in Stevens-Johnson syndrome/toxic epidermal necrolysis. *J Invest Dermatol*. 2017;137(5):1065-1073.
59. Kuechler PC, Britschgi M, Schmid S, et al. Cytotoxic mechanisms in different forms of T-cell-mediated drug allergies. *Allergy*. 2004;59:613.
60. Azukizawa H, Sano S, Kosaka H, et al. Prevention of toxic epidermal necrolysis by regulatory cells. *Eur J Immunol*. 2005;35:1722.
61. Takahashi R, Kano Y, Yamazaki Y, et al. Defective regulatory T cells in patients with severe drug eruptions: timing of the dysfunction is associated with the pathological phenotype and outcome. *J Immunol*. 2009;182:8071.
62. Chung WH, Hung SI, Hong HS, et al. Medical genetics: a marker for Stevens Johnson syndrome. *Nature*. 2004;428:486.
63. Hung SI, Chung WH, Liou LB, et al. HLA-B*5801 allele as a genetic marker for severe cutaneous adverse reactions caused by allopurinol. *Proc Natl Acad Sci U S A*. 2005;102:4134.
64. Locharernkul C, Loplumlert J, Limotai C, et al. Carbamazepine and phenytoin induced Stevens-Johnson syndrome is associated with HLA-B*1502 allele in Thai population. *Epilepsia*. 2008;49:2087.
65. Mehta TY, Prajapati LM, Mittal B, et al. Association of HLA-B*1502 allele and carbamazepine-induced Stevens-Johnson syndrome among Indians. *Indian J Dermatol Venereol Leprol*. 2009;75:579.
66. Kaniwa N, Saito Y, Aihara M, et al. HLA-B locus in Japanese patients with anti-epileptics and allopurinol-related Stevens-Johnson syndrome and toxic epidermal necrolysis. *Pharmacogenomics*. 2008;9:1617.
67. Chung WH, Hung SI, Chen YT. Genetic predisposition of life-threatening antiepileptic-induced skin reactions. *Expert Opin Drug Saf*. 2010;9:15.
68. Lonjou C, Thomas L, Borot N, et al. A marker for Stevens-Johnson syndrome: ethnicity matters. *Pharmacogenomics J*. 2006;6:265.
69. Lonjou C, Borot N, Sekula P, et al. A European study of HLA-B in Stevens-Johnson syndrome and toxic epidermal necrolysis related to five high-risk drugs. *Pharmacogenet Genomics*. 2008;18:99.
70. Genin E, Schumacher M, Roujeau JC, et al. Genome-wide association study of Stevens-Johnson syndrome and toxic epidermal necrolysis in Europe. *Orphanet J Rare Dis*. 2011;6:52.
71. Mockenhaupt M. Severe drug-induced skin reactions: clinical pattern, diagnostics and therapy. *J Dtsch Dermatol Ges*. 2009;7:142.
72. Shay E, Kheirkhah A, Liang L, et al. Amniotic membrane transplantation as a new therapy for the acute ocular manifestations of Stevens-Johnson syndrome and toxic epidermal necrolysis. *Surv Ophthalmol*. 2009;54:686.
73. Gueudry, Roujeau JC, Binaghi M, et al. Risk factors for the development of ocular complications of Stevens-Johnson syndrome and toxic epidermal necrolysis. *Arch Dermatol*. 2009;145:157.
74. Meneux E, Wolkenstein P, Haddad B, et al. Vulvovaginal involvement in toxic epidermal necrolysis: a retrospective study of 40 cases. *Obstet Gynecol*. 1998;91:283.
75. Mockenhaupt M, Ziemer M. Erythema multiforme majus, Stevens-Johnson syndrome, toxic epidermal necrolysis and graft-versus-host disease. In: Kirtschig G, Cooper S, eds. *Gynecologic Dermatology*., London: Medical Publishers; 2016:79-88.
76. Lebargy F, Wolkenstein P, Gisselbrecht M, et al. Pulmonary complications in toxic epidermal necrolysis: prospective clinical study. *Intensive Care Med*. 1997;23:1237.
77. McIvor RA, Zaidi J, Peters WJ, et al. Acute and chronic respiratory complications of toxic epidermal necrolysis. *J Burn Care Rehabil*. 1996;17:237.
78. Michel P, Joly P, Ducrotte P, et al. Ileal involvement in toxic epidermal necrolysis (Lyell syndrome). *Dig Dis Sci*. 1993;38:1938.
79. Carter FM, Mitchell CK. Toxic epidermal necrolysis—an unusual cause of colonic perforation. Report of a case. *Dis Colon Rectum*. 1993;36:773.
80. Blum L, Chosidow O, Rostoker G, et al. Renal involvement in toxic epidermal necrolysis. *J Am Acad Dermatol*. 1996;34:1088.
81. Krumlovsky FA, Del Greco F, Herdson PB, et al. Renal disease associated with toxic epidermal necrolysis (Lyell's disease). *Am J Med*. 1974;57:817.
82. Ziemer M, Mockenhaupt M. Severe drug-induced skin reactions: clinical pattern, diagnostics and therapy. In: Khopkar U, ed. *Skin Biopsy*. InTech-Open Access Publisher. 2011. http://www.intechopen.com/articles/show/title/severe-drug-induced-skin-reactions-clinical-pattern-diagnostics-and-therapy.
83. Rzany B, Hering O, Mockenhaupt M, et al. Histopathological and epidemiological characteristics of patients with erythema multiforme majus, Stevens-Johnson syndrome and toxic epidermal necrolysis. *Br J Dermatol*. 1996;135:6.
84. Quinn AM, Brown K, Bonish BK, et al. Uncovering histologic criteria with prognostic significance in toxic epidermal necrolysis. *Arch Dermatol*. 2005;141:683.
85. Williams GP, Mudhar HS, Leyland M. Early pathological features of the cornea in toxic epidermal necrolysis. *Br J Ophthalmol*. 2007;91:1129.
86. Lipowicz S, Sekula P, Ingen-Housz-Oro S, et al. Prognosis of generalized bullous fixed drug eruption: a case control study. *Br J Dermatol*. 2013;168(4):726-732.
87. de Prost N, Ingen-Housz-Oro S, Duong Ta, et al. Bacteremia in Stevens-Johnson syndrome and toxic epidermal necrolysis: epidemiology, risk factors, and predictive value of skin cultures. *Medicine (Baltimore)*. 2010;89:28.
88. Palmieri T, Greenhalgh DG, Saffle JR, et al. A multicenter review of toxic epidermal necrolysis treated in U.S. burn centers at the end of the twentieth century. *J Burn Care Rehabil*. 2002;23:87.
89. Haber J, Hopman W, Gomez M, et al. Late outcome in adult survivors of toxic epidermal necrolysis after treatment in burn center. *J Burn Care Rehabil*. 2005;26:33.
90. Paulmann M, Mockenhaupt M, Dunant A, et al. Stevens-Johnson syndrome and toxic epidermal necrolysis: long-term sequelae based on a 5-year follow-up analysis. *Pharmacoepidem Drug Safe*. 2017; 26(Supp 2):3.
91. Gaultier F, Rochefort J, Landru MM, et al. Severe and unrecognized dental abnormalities after drug-induced epidermal necrolysis. *Arch Dermatol*. 2009;145:1332.
92. Bakirtas A, Harmanci K, Toyran M, et al. Bronchiolitis obliterans: a rare chronic pulmonary complication

93. Garcia-Doval I, LeCleach L, Bocquet H, et al. Toxic epidermal necrolysis and Stevens-Johnson syndrome. Does early withdrawal of causative drugs decrease the risk of death? *Arch Dermatol*. 2000;136:323.
94. Ellis MW. A case report and a proposed algorithm for the transfer of patients with Stevens-Johnson syndrome and toxic epidermal necrolysis to a burn center. *Mil Med*. 2002;167:701.
95. Creamer D, Walsh SA, Dziewulski P, et al. U.K. guidelines for the management of Stevens-Johnson syndrome/toxic epidermal necrolysis in adults. *Br J Dermatol*. 2016;174, 1194-1227.
96. Endorf EW, Cancio LC, Gibran NS. Toxic epidermal necrolysis clinical guidelines. *J Burn Res*. 2008;29:706.
97. Lal S, Barrow RE, Wolf SE, et al. Biobrane improves wound healing in burned children without increased risk of infection. *Shock*. 2000;14:314.
98. Boorboor P, Vogt PM, Bechara FG, et al. Toxic epidermal necrolysis: use of Biobrane or skin coverage reduces pain, improves mobilisation and decreases infection in elderly patients. *Burns*. 2008;34:487.
99. Dorafshar AH, Dickie SR, Cohn AB, et al. Antishear therapy for toxic epidermal necrolysis: an alternative treatment approach. *Plast Reconstr Surg*. 2008;122:154.
100. Kardaun SH, Jonkman MF. Dexamethasone pulse therapy for Stevens-Johnson syndrome/toxic epidermal necrolysis. *Acta Derm Venereol*. 2007;87:144.
101. Schneck J, Fagot JP, Sekula P, et al. Effects of treatments on the mortality of Stevens-Johnson syndrome and toxic epidermal necrolysis: a retrospective study on patients included in the prospective EuroSCAR Study. *J Am Acad Dermatol*. 2008;58:33.
102. Zimmermann S, Sekula P, Venhoff M, et al. Systemic immunomodulating therapies for Stevens-Johnson syndrome and toxic epidermal necrolysis: a systematic review and meta-analysis. *JAMA Dermatol*. 2017;153(6):514-522.
103. Trent JT, Kirsner RS, Romanelli P, et al. Analysis of intravenous immunoglobulin for the treatment of toxic epidermal necrolysis using SCORTEN. *Arch Dermatol*. 2003;139:39.
104. Prins C, Kerdel FA, Padilla RS, et al. Treatment of toxic epidermal necrolysis with high-dose intravenous immunoglobulins. *Arch Dermatol*. 2003;139:26.
105. Stella M, Clemente A, Bollero D, et al. Toxic epidermal necrolysis (TEN) and Stevens-Johnson syndrome (SJS): experience with high-dose intravenous immunoglobulins and topical conservative approach. A retrospective analysis. *Burns*. 2007;33:452.
106. Bachot N, Revuz J, Roujeau JC. Intravenous immunoglobulin treatment for Stevens-Johnson and toxic epidermal necrolysis. *Arch Dermatol*. 2003;139:33.
107. Shortt R, Gomez M, Mittman N, et al. Intravenous immunoglobulin does not improve outcome in toxic epidermal necrolysis. *J Burn Care Rehabil*. 2004;25:246.
108. Faye O, Roujeau JC. Treatment of epidermal necrolysis with high-dose intravenous immunoglobulins (IVIG). Clinical experience to date. *Drugs*. 2005;65(15):2085-2090.
109. Roujeau JC, Mockenhaupt M, Guillaume JC, et al. New evidence supporting cyclosporine efficacy in epidermal necrolysis. *J Invest Dermatol*. 2017;137(10):2047-2049.
110. Arévalo JM, Lorente JA, González-Herrada C, et al. Treatment of toxic epidermal necrolysis with cyclosporine A. *J Trauma*. 2000;48:473.
111. Valeyrie-Allanore L, Wolkenstein P, Brochard L, et al. Pilot study of ciclosporin treatment for Stevens-Johnson syndrome and toxic epidermal necrolysis. *Br J Dermatol*. 2010;163(4):847-853.
112. González-Herrada C, Rodríguez-Martín S, Cachafeiro L, et al. Ciclosporin use in epidermal necrolysis is associated with an important mortality reduction: evidence from three different approaches. *J Invest Dermatol*. 2017;137(10):2092-2100.
113. Bamichas G, Natse T, Christidou F, et al. Plasma exchange in patients with toxic epidermal necrolysis. *Ther Apher*. 2002;6:225.
114. Chaidemenos GC, Chrysomallis F, Sombolos K, et al. Plasmapheresis in toxic epidermal necrolysis. *Int J Dermatol*. 1997;36:218.
115. Egan CA, Grant WJ, Morris SE, et al. Plasmapheresis as an adjunct treatment in toxic epidermal necrolysis. *J Am Acad Dermatol*. 1999;40:458.
116. Lissia M, Figus A, Rubino C. Intravenous immunoglobulins and plasmapheresis combined treatment in patients with severe toxic epidermal necrolysis: preliminary report. *Br J Plast Surg*. 2005;58:504.
117. Wang CW, Yang LY, Chen CB, et al. Randomized, controlled trial of TNF-α antagonist in CTL-mediated severe cutaneous adverse reactions. *J Clin Invest*. 2018;128(3):985-996.
118. Wolkenstein P, Latarjet J, Roujeau JC, et al. Randomised comparison of thalidomide versus placebo in toxic epidermal necrolysis. *Lancet*. 1998;352:1586.
119. Rosenthal P, Cotter J. The Boston Scleral Lens in the management of severe ocular surface disease. *Ophthalmol Clin North Am*. 2003;16:89.
120. Tougeron-Brousseau B, Delcampe A, Gueudry J, et al. Vision-related function after scleral lens fitting in ocular complications of Stevens-Johnson syndrome and toxic epidermal necrolysis. *Am J Ophthalmol*. 2009;148:852.
121. Daya SM, Ilari FA. Living related conjunctival limbal allograft for the treatment of stem cell deficiency. *Ophthalmology*. 2001;108:126.
122. Nishida K, Yamato M, Hayashida Y, et al. Corneal reconstruction with tissue engineered cell sheets composed of autologous oral epithelium. *N Engl J Med*. 2004;351:1187.
123. Chen P, Lin JJ, Lu CS, et al. Carbamazepine induced toxic effects and HLA-B*1502 screening in Taiwan. *N Engl J Med*. 2011;364:1126-1133.
124. Chen Z, Liew D, Kwan P. Effects of a HLA-B*15:02 screening policy on antiepileptic drug use and severe skin reactions. *Neurology*. 2014;83:2077-2084.
125. Barbaud A, Collet E, Milpied B. A multicentre study to determine the value and safety of drug patch tests for the three main classes of severe cutaneous adverse drug reactions. *Br J Dermatol*. 2013;3:555-562.
126. Kano Y, Hirahara K, Mitsuyama Y, et al. Utility of the lymphocyte transformation test in the diagnosis of drug sensitivity: dependence on its timing and the type of drug eruption. *Allergy*. 2007;62:1439.

Chapter 45 :: Cutaneous Reactions to Drugs
:: Kara Heelan, Cathryn Sibbald, & Neil H. Shear

第四十五章
药物所致皮肤反应

中文导读

本章共分为8节：①流行病学；②临床特征；③病因和发病机制；④诊断；⑤鉴别诊断；⑥临床病程和预后；⑦治疗；⑧预防。全面描述了药物所致皮肤反应的临床特征及其防治。

第一节介绍了不同人群药物性皮炎的发生率以及门诊和住院患者药物性皮炎的不同特点。

第二节按照皮损形态对各型药疹进行分类和阐述。首先介绍了临床最常见药疹——发疹型药疹皮疹的演变及发生发展过程、皮疹形态、鉴别诊断及常见致敏药物。接下来介绍了伴内脏损害的复杂药疹——超敏反应综合征（HSR）的临床特点及诱发因素。再依次介绍了荨麻疹样（药物诱导的IgE/非IgE介导的荨麻疹和血管性水肿、血清病样反应）、脓疱和痤疮样（痤疮型药疹、急性泛发性发疹性脓疱病）、大疱样（假卟啉症、药物诱导的线状IgA病、药物诱发的天疱疮、药物诱导的大疱性天疱疮）、SJS/TEN、固定型药疹、药物引起的色素沉着、药物诱导的苔藓样疹、药物诱导的皮肤假性淋巴瘤、药物性狼疮和皮肌炎、紫癜样疹（药物诱导的血管炎）、抗凝药物诱导的皮肤坏死、中性粒细胞性汗腺炎等多种药物性皮炎的临床特点、可能致敏药物、鉴别诊断。列举了与化疗相关的药物反应，总结了临床几种主要药疹的临床特征。

第三节，在这一部分中，非常详细地描述和总结了药物性皮炎的免疫性、非免疫性、遗传学等发病机制以及药物性皮炎发生的先天和获得性诱发因素。

第四节介绍了药疹的诊断要点，包括需要关注潜在的内脏损害，并总结了一些警示可能发生严重药物反应的临床特征，积极查找和分析病因。必要时可以结合斑贴试验、活检、嗜碱性粒细胞活化试验等检查以明确诊断或病因。

第五节介绍了需要与药物性皮炎相鉴别的疾病特征及其治疗。

第六节介绍了SJS/TEN的预后和评估量表SCORTEN在治疗中的应用价值。

第七节介绍了SJS/TEN的治疗，并强调需要根据药疹严重程度采取相应的处理措施。

第八节介绍了SJS/TEN的初级预防和二级预防。

〔李 捷〕

AT-A-GLANCE

- Drug-induced cutaneous eruptions are common.
- They range from common nuisance rashes to rare life-threatening diseases.
- The spectrum of clinical manifestations includes exanthematous, urticarial, pustular, and bullous eruptions.
- These reactions may mimic other cutaneous diseases such as acne, porphyria, lichen planus, and lupus.
- Fixed drug eruptions are usually solitary dusky macules that recur at the same site.
- Drug reactions may be limited solely to skin or may be part of a severe systemic reaction, such as drug hypersensitivity syndrome or toxic epidermal necrolysis.

Complications of drug therapy are a major cause of patient morbidity and account for a significant number of patient deaths.[1] Drug eruptions range from common nuisance eruptions to rare or life-threatening drug-induced diseases. Drug reactions may be solely limited to the skin, or they may be part of a systemic reaction, such as drug hypersensitivity syndrome or toxic epidermal necrolysis (TEN; see Chap. 44).

Drug eruptions are often distinct disease entities and must be approached systematically, like any other cutaneous disease. A precise diagnosis of the reaction pattern can help narrow possible causes, because different drugs are more commonly associated with different types of reactions.

EPIDEMIOLOGY

The incidence of cutaneous adverse drug reactions varies across populations. A systematic review of the medical literature, encompassing 9 studies, concluded that cutaneous reaction rates varied from 0% to 8%.[2] The risk in hospitalized patients ranges from 10% to 15%.[3] In a French cohort of hospitalized patients, the most common reactions were maculopapular (56%), with severe reactions in a minority (34%).[4]

Outpatient studies of cutaneous adverse drug reactions estimate that 2.5% of children who are treated with a drug, and up to 12% of children treated with an antibiotic, will experience a cutaneous reaction.[5] Elderly patients do not appear to have an increased risk of maculopapular exanthems, and may have a lower incidence of serious reactions.[6] Populations that may have an increased risk of drug reactions in hospital include patients with HIV, connective tissue disorders (including lupus erythematosus), non-Hodgkin lymphoma, and hepatitis.[7]

CLINICAL FEATURES

MORPHOLOGIC APPROACH TO DRUG ERUPTIONS

Although there are many presentations of cutaneous drug eruptions, the morphology of many cutaneous eruptions may be exanthematous, urticarial, blistering, or pustular. The extent of the reaction is variable. For example, once the morphology of the reaction has been documented, a specific diagnosis (eg, fixed drug eruption [FDE] or acute generalized exanthematous pustulosis [AGEP]) can be made. The reaction may also present as a systemic syndrome (eg, serum sickness–like reaction or hypersensitivity syndrome reaction). Fever is generally associated with such systemic cutaneous adverse drug reactions (ADRs).

EXANTHEMATOUS ERUPTIONS

Exanthematous eruptions, sometimes referred to as *morbilliform* or *maculopapular*, are the most common form of drug eruptions, accounting for approximately 95% of skin reactions (Fig. 45-1).[2] Simple exanthems are erythematous changes in the skin without blistering, pustulation, or associated systemic signs. The eruption typically starts on the trunk and spreads peripherally in a symmetric fashion. Pruritus is almost always

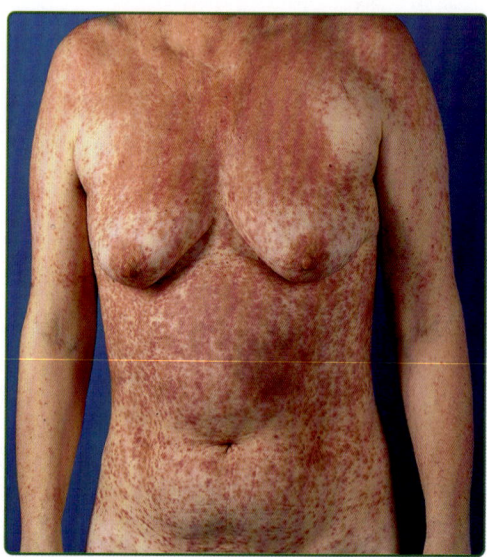

FIGURE 45-1 Exanthematous drug eruption: ampicillin. Symmetrically arranged, brightly erythematous macules and papules, which are discrete in some areas and confluent in others on the trunk and discrete on the extremities.

present. These eruptions usually occur within 1 week of initiation of therapy and may appear 1 or 2 days after drug therapy has been discontinued.[8] Resolution, usually within 7 to 14 days, occurs with a change in color from bright red to a brownish red, which may be followed by desquamation. The differential diagnosis in these patients includes an infectious exanthem (eg, viral, bacterial, or rickettsial), collagen vascular disease, and infections.

Exanthematous eruptions can be caused by many drugs, including β-lactams ("the penicillins"), sulfonamide antimicrobials, nonnucleoside reverse transcriptase inhibitors (eg, nevirapine), and antiepileptic medications. Studies show that drug-specific T cells play a major role in exanthematous, bullous, and pustular drug reactions.[9] In patients who have concomitant infectious mononucleosis, the risk of developing an exanthematous eruption while being treated with an aminopenicillin (eg, ampicillin) increases from 3% to 7% to 60% to 100%.[10] A similar drug–virus interaction has been observed in 50% of patients infected with HIV who are exposed to sulfonamide antibiotics.[11]

An exanthematous eruption in conjunction with fever and internal organ inflammation (eg, liver, kidney, CNS) signifies a more serious reaction, known as the *hypersensitivity syndrome reaction* (HSR), drug-induced hypersensitivity reaction, or drug reaction with eosinophilia and systemic symptoms (Table 45-1).[12] It occurs in approximately 1 in 3000 exposures to agents such as aromatic anticonvulsants, lamotrigine, sulfonamide

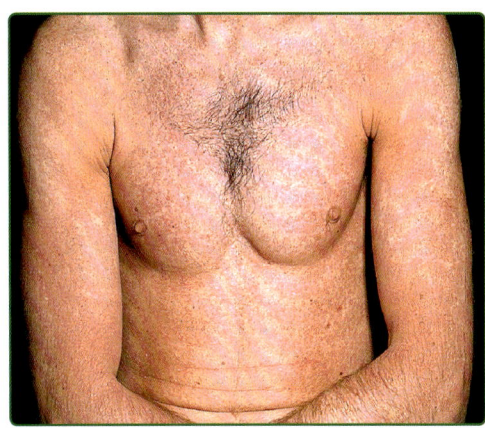

FIGURE 45-2 Drug hypersensitivity syndrome: phenytoin. Symmetric, bright red, exanthematous eruption, confluent in some sites; the patient had associated lymphadenopathy.

antimicrobials, dapsone, nitrofurantoin, nevirapine, minocycline, metronidazole, and allopurinol (Fig. 45-2). HSR occurs most frequently on first exposure to the drug, with initial symptoms starting 1 to 6 weeks after exposure. Fever and malaise are often the presenting symptoms. Atypical lymphocytosis with subsequent eosinophilia may occur during the initial phases of the reaction in some patients. Although most patients have an exanthematous eruption, more serious cutaneous manifestations may be evident (Fig. 45-3). Internal organ involvement can be asymptomatic.[13] Immune-mediated thyroid dysfunction is a possible long-term complication resulting in hyperthyroidism or hypothyroidism, and may not present until 3 to 12 months after the first symptoms appear.[14]

URTICARIAL ERUPTIONS

Urticaria is characterized by pruritic red wheals of various sizes. Individual lesions generally last for less than 24 hours, although new lesions can commonly

TABLE 45-1
Morphologic Classification

Category	Type	Description
Exanthematous	Simple	Exanthematous drug eruption
	Complex	Drug-induced hypersensitivity syndrome
Urticarial	Simple	Urticaria
	Complex	Serum sickness-like reaction
Pustular	Simple	Acneiform
	Complex	Acute generalized exanthematous pustulosis
Bullous	Simple	Pseudoporphyria
		Fixed drug eruption
	Complex	Drug-induced pemphigus
		Drug-induced bullous pemphigoid
		Drug-induced linear immunoglobulin A disease
		Stevens-Johnson syndrome
		Toxic epidermal necrolysis
Papulosquamous		Drug-induced subcutaneous lupus
		Drug-induced dermatomyositis
Purpuric		Drug-induced vasculitis
Lichenoid		Drug-induced lichenoid
Miscellaneous		Pseudolymphoma
		Neutrophilic eccrine hidradenitis

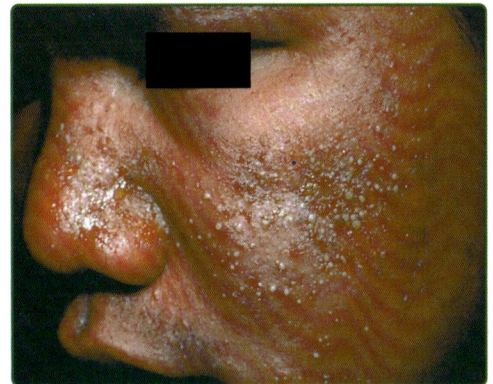

FIGURE 45-3 Hypersensitivity syndrome reaction, characterized by fever, a pustular eruption, and hepatitis, in a 23-year-old man after 18 days of treatment with minocycline.

develop. When deep dermal and subcutaneous tissues are also swollen, the reaction is known as *angioedema*. Angioedema is frequently unilateral and nonpruritic and lasts for 1 to 2 hours, although it may persist for 2 to 5 days.[15]

Urticaria and angioedema, when associated with drug use, are usually indicative of an immunoglobulin (Ig) E–mediated immediate hypersensitivity reaction. This mechanism is typified by immediate reactions to penicillin and other antibiotics (see Chap. 41). Signs and symptoms of IgE-mediated allergic reactions typically include pruritus, urticaria, cutaneous flushing, angioedema, nausea, vomiting, diarrhea, abdominal pain, nasal congestion, rhinorrhea, laryngeal edema, and bronchospasm or hypotension. Urticaria and angioedema can also be caused by non–IgE-mediated reactions that result in direct and nonspecific liberation of histamine or other mediators of inflammation.[8] Drug-induced non–IgE-mediated urticaria and angioedema are usually related to nonsteroidal antiinflammatory drugs (NSAIDs) and angiotensin-converting enzyme (ACE) inhibitors.[16]

Serum sickness–like reactions (see Table 45-1) are defined by the presence of fever, rash (usually urticarial), and arthralgias 1 to 3 weeks after initiation of drug therapy. Lymphadenopathy and eosinophilia may also be present; however, in contrast to true serum sickness, immune complexes, hypocomplementemia, vasculitis, and renal lesions are absent.

Cefaclor is associated with an increased relative risk of serum sickness–like reactions. The overall incidence of cefaclor-induced serum sickness–like reactions has been estimated to be 0.024% to 0.2% per course of cefaclor prescribed. In genetically susceptible hosts, a reactive metabolite is generated during the metabolism of cefaclor that may bind with tissue proteins and elicit an inflammatory response manifesting as a serum sickness–like reaction.[12]

Other drugs that have been implicated in serum sickness–like reactions are cefprozil, bupropion, minocycline, and rituximab[17] as well as infliximab.[18] The incidence of serum sickness–like reactions caused by these drugs is unknown.

PUSTULAR AND ACNEIFORM ERUPTIONS

Acneiform eruptions are associated with the use of iodides, bromides, adrenocorticotropic hormone, glucocorticoids, isoniazid, androgens, lithium, actinomycin D, and phenytoin. Drug-induced acne may appear in atypical areas, such as on the arms and legs, and is most often monomorphous. Comedones are usually absent. That acneiform eruptions do not affect prepubertal children indicates that previous hormonal priming is a necessary prerequisite. In cases in which the offending agent cannot be discontinued, topical tretinoin may be useful.[19]

An acneiform eruption occurs in the majority of patients taking epidermal growth factor receptor inhibitors (eg, gefitinib, erlotinib, cetuximab), with an incidence as high as 81.6%.[20] The eruption is characterized by pruritic follicular papules and pustules without comedones, and presents within 1 to 2 weeks of treatment initiation.[21] Concurrent cutaneous findings include paronychia, xerosis, and skin fissures. The eruption is dose dependent, with respect to both incidence and severity, and correlates with tumor response and overall survival.[15,22] Specific treatment alternatives include tetracyclines and low-dose isotretinoin.[21] Antihistamines (cetirizine, loratadine, hydroxyzine) and doxepin are helpful in targeting the associated pruritus. There is contradictory evidence for the benefit of tetracyclines for prophylaxis.[23,24]

AGEP is an acute febrile pustular eruption that occurs 24 to 48 hours after initiation of the implicated drug. It is characterized by small monomorphous nonfollicular sterile pustules concentrated on the trunk and intertriginous regions. Systemic features include leukocytosis with neutrophilia, fever, elevated liver enzymes with steatosis or hepatomegaly, renal insufficiency, and pleural effusions with hypoxemia (Fig. 45-4; see Table 45-1).[25] Generalized desquamation occurs after approximately 2 weeks. The estimated incidence of AGEP is approximately 1 to 5 cases per million per year. It is most commonly associated with β-lactam, macrolide and quinolone, antibiotics, anticonvulsants, sulfonamides, calcium channel blockers (diltiazem), and terbinafine.[26,27] Differential diagnosis includes pustular psoriasis, HSR with pustulation, subcorneal pustular dermatosis (Sneddon-Wilkinson disease), pustular vasculitis, or, in

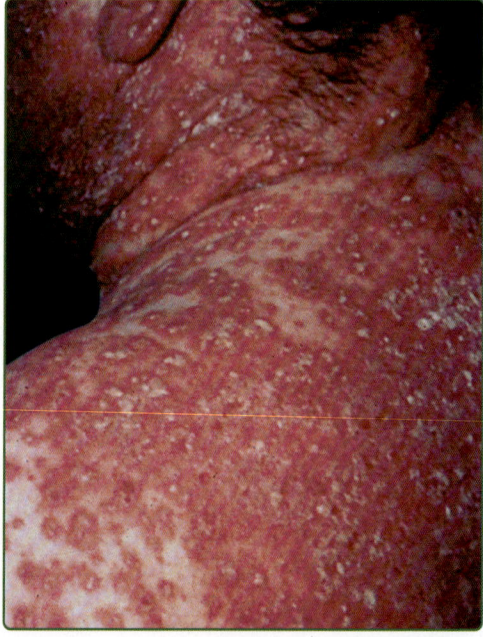

FIGURE 45-4 Acute generalized exanthematous pustulosis in a 48-year-old man who developed nonfollicular pustules and fever after 7 days of treatment with diltiazem.

severe cases of AGEP, TEN. The typical histopathologic analysis of AGEP lesions shows spongiform subcorneal and/or intraepidermal pustules, an often marked edema of the papillary dermis, and perivascular infiltrates with neutrophils and exocytosis of some eosinophils. Discontinuance of therapy is usually the extent of treatment necessary in most patients, although some patients may require the use of corticosteroids.

BULLOUS ERUPTIONS

Table 45-2 outlines the clinical features of selected cutaneous reactions to drugs.

PSEUDOPORPHYRIA

Pseudoporphyria is a cutaneous phototoxic disorder that can resemble either porphyria cutanea tarda in adults or erythropoietic protoporphyria in children but differs from these entities by the presence of normal porphyrin levels (see Chap. 124). Pseudoporphyria of the porphyria cutanea tarda variety is characterized by skin fragility, blister formation, and scarring in photodistribution. The other clinical pattern mimics erythropoietic protoporphyria and manifests as cutaneous burning, erythema, vesiculation, angular chicken pox–like scars, and waxy thickening of the skin. The eruption may begin within 1 day of initiation of therapy or may be delayed in onset for as long as 1 year. The course is prolonged in some patients, but most reports describe symptoms that disappear several weeks to several months after the offending agent is withdrawn. Because of the risk of permanent facial scarring, the implicated drug should be discontinued if skin fragility, blistering, or scarring occurs.[28] In addition, the use of broad-spectrum sunscreen and protective clothing should be recommended. Drugs that have been associated with pseudoporphyria include naproxen and other NSAIDs, diuretics, antibiotics (tetracycline, ciprofloxacin, ampicillin-sulbactam/cefepime), retinoids, cyclosporine, dapsone, oral contraceptive pills, amiodarone, and voriconazole.[29]

DRUG-INDUCED LINEAR IMMUNOGLOBULIN A DISEASE

Both idiopathic and drug-induced linear IgA disease (see Chap. 58) are heterogeneous in clinical presentation. Cases of the drug-induced type have morphologies resembling erythema multiforme, bullous pemphigoid, and dermatitis herpetiformis. The drug-induced disease may differ from the idiopathic entity in that mucosal or conjunctival lesions are less com-

TABLE 45-2
Clinical Features of Selected Cutaneous Reactions to Drugs

CLINICAL PRESENTATION	DRUG ERUPTION	TIME TO ONSET	FEVER	INTERNAL ORGAN INVOLVEMENT	ARTHRALGIA	LYMPHADENOPATHY	IMPLICATED DRUGS
Hypersensitivity syndrome reaction	Exanthem, exfoliative dermatitis, pustular eruptions, SJS-TEN	DRESS: 2-6 weeks, SJS-TEN: 1-3 weeks	Present	Present	Absent	Present	Aromatic anticonvulsants (eg, phenytoin, phenobarbital, carbamazepine), sulfonamide antibiotics, dapsone, minocycline, allopurinol, lamotrigine
Serum sickness–like reaction	Urticaria, exanthem		Present	Absent	Present	Present	Cefaclor, cefprozil, bupropion, minocycline, infliximab, rituximab
Drug-induced lupus	Usually absent		Present/absent	Present/absent	Present	Absent	Procainamide, hydralazine, isoniazid, minocycline, acebutolol
Drug-induced subacute cutaneous lupus erythematosus	Papulosquamous or annular cutaneous lesion (often photosensitive)	Variable	Absent	Absent	Absent	Absent	Thiazide diuretics, calcium channel blockers, ACE inhibitors
Acute generalized exanthematous pustulosis	Nonfollicular pustules on an edematous erythematous base	24-48 hours	Present	Present in ~20%	Absent	Absent	β Blockers, macrolide antibiotics, calcium channel blockers

Abbreviations: ACE, angiotensin-converting enzyme; DRESS, drug rash with eosinophilia and systemic symptoms; SJS, Stevens-Johnson syndrome; TEN, toxic epidermal necrolysis.

mon, spontaneous remission occurs once the offending agent is withdrawn, and immune deposits disappear from the skin once the lesions resolve. Drug-induced disease may present more commonly with erosions mimicking TEN, with a more severe clinical course and risk of sepsis and shock.[30] Time to onset is reported between 2 days to 4 weeks.

Biopsy specimens are necessary for diagnosis. Histologically, the 2 entities are similar. A study suggests that, as in the idiopathic variety, the target antigen is not unique in the drug-induced disease. Although 13% to 30% of patients with sporadic linear IgA have circulating basement membrane zone antibodies, these antibodies have not been reported in drug-induced cases.[31] In patients with linear IgA bullous disease proven by direct immunofluorescence, the index of suspicion of drug induction should be higher in cases with only IgA and no IgG in the basement membrane zone. Several drugs can induce linear IgA bullous dermatosis, the most frequently reported being vancomycin.[30,32]

DRUG-INDUCED PEMPHIGUS

Pemphigus may be considered as drug-induced or drug-triggered (ie, a latent disease that is unmasked by the drug exposure; see Chap. 57). Drug-induced pemphigus caused by penicillamine and other thiol-containing drugs (eg, piroxicam, captopril) tends to remit spontaneously in 35% to 50% of cases, presents as pemphigus foliaceus, has an average interval to onset of 1 year, and is associated with the presence of antinuclear antibodies in 25% of patients.

Most patients with nonthiol drug-induced pemphigus manifest clinical, histologic, immunologic, and evolutionary aspects similar to those of idiopathic pemphigus vulgaris with mucosal involvement and show a 15% rate of spontaneous recovery after drug withdrawal. Treatment of drug-induced pemphigus begins with drug cessation. Systemic glucocorticoids and other immunosuppressive drugs are often required until all symptoms of active disease disappear. Vigilant followup is required after remission to monitor the patient and the serum for autoantibodies to detect an early relapse.[16]

DRUG-INDUCED BULLOUS PEMPHIGOID

Drug-induced bullous pemphigoid (see Chap. 54) can encompass a wide variety of presentations, ranging from the classic features of large, tense bullae arising from an erythematous, urticarial base with moderate involvement of the oral cavity, through mild forms with few bullous lesions, to scarring plaques and nodules with bullae. Numerous medications have been reported to cause bullous pemphigoid, including diuretics (furosemide and spironolactone), ACE inhibitors, and antibiotics (penicillins and fluoroquinolones).[33] In contrast to patients with the idiopathic form, patients with drug-induced bullous pemphigoid are generally younger, and more commonly may have a positive Nikolsky sign, lesions on normal-appearing skin, target lesions on the palms and soles, involvement of the lower legs, and mucosal involvement.[33] In addition, the histopathologic findings are of a perivascular infiltration of lymphocytes with neutrophils and marked eosinophils, intraepidermal vesicles with foci of necrotic keratinocytes, thrombi in dermal vessels, and a possible lack of tissue-bound and circulating anti–basal membrane zone IgG.[34]

In the acute, self-limited condition, resolution occurs after the withdrawal of the culprit agent, with or without glucocorticoid therapy, and rarely recurs, unlike its idiopathic counterpart. In some patients, however, the drug may actually trigger the idiopathic form of the disease, with a more severe and persistent course.

STEVENS-JOHNSON SYNDROME AND TOXIC EPIDERMAL NECROLYSIS

(See Chap. 44)

Stevens-Johnson syndrome (SJS) and TEN or the SJS-TEN spectrum, represent variants of the same disease process. Differentiation between the 2 patterns depends on the nature of the skin lesions and the extent of body surface area involvement.

The understanding of the pathogenesis of severe cutaneous ADRs has expanded greatly. Various factors, including pharmacogenetic and immunogenic determinants, may influence the likelihood of a reaction and variability in innate and adaptive immunity may influence the clinical presentation.[35] In addition, the detection of drug-specific T-cell proliferation provides evidence that T cells are involved in severe skin rashes.[36]

FIXED DRUG ERUPTIONS

FDEs usually appear as solitary round or ovoid, erythematous, bright red or dusky red macules that may evolve into an edematous plaque; bullous-type lesions may be present. Widespread or generalized FDE may mimic TEN, but differs in its absence of systemic involvement and more marked hyperpigmentation.[37] FDEs are commonly found on the genitalia and in the perianal area, although they can occur anywhere on the skin surface (Figs. 45-5 and 45-6). A review of 59 cases suggested a sex-dependent pattern of distribution with women more commonly presenting with lesions on the hands and feet, and men on the genitalia.[38] Some patients may complain of burning or stinging, and others may have fever, malaise, and abdominal symptoms. FDE can develop from 30 minutes to 8 to 16 hours after ingestion of the medication. After the initial acute phase lasting days to weeks, residual grayish or slate-colored hyperpigmentation develops. On rechallenge, not only do the lesions recur in the same location, but also new lesions often appear.

More than 100 drugs have been implicated in causing FDEs (Table 45-3). A review of 134 cases at a single site highlighted NSAIDs, acetaminophen, and antibiotics as the most frequent culprits.[39] Another commonly

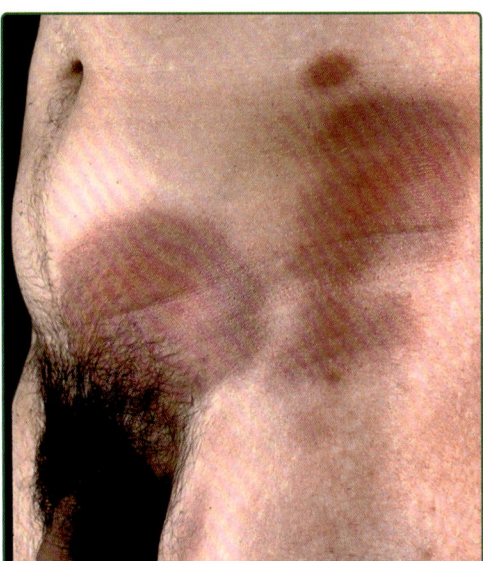

FIGURE 45-5 Fixed drug eruption. (From Wolff K, Johnson R, Saavedra AP, et al. *Fitzpatrick's Color Atlas and Synopsis of Clinical Dermatology*, 8th ed. New York, NY: McGraw-Hill; 2017, with permission, Fig. 23-7.)

TABLE 45-3
Drugs Implicated in Fixed Drug Eruptions

Nonsteroidal antiinflammatory agents (acetaminophen)
Antibiotics
    Tetracyclines (tetracycline, minocycline, doxycycline)
    Sulfonamides, other sulfa drugs
Metronidazole
Nystatin
Salicylates
Phenylbutazone, phenacetin
Barbiturates
Oral contraceptives
Quinine (including quinine in tonic water), quinidine
Phenolphthalein
Food coloring (yellow): in food or medications

cited trigger is pseudoephedrine. A haplotype linkage in trimethoprim-sulfamethoxazole–induced FDE has been documented.

A challenge or provocation test with the suspected drug may be useful in establishing the diagnosis. Patch testing at the site of a previous lesion yields a positive response in up to 43% of patients. Results of prick and intradermal skin tests may be positive in 24% and 67% of patients, respectively.[40,41] Food-initiated fixed eruptions also exist and are important to consider when assessing causation.

DRUG-INDUCED HYPERPIGMENTATION

Table 45-4 summarizes the main patterns of drug-induced hyperpigmentation, Table 45-5 outlines drug-induced nail hyperpigmentation, and Table 45-6 summarizes cytotoxic drug-induced skin pigmentation distribution patterns.

DRUG-INDUCED LICHENOID ERUPTIONS

Drug-induced lichen planus produces lesions that are clinically and histologically indistinguishable from those of idiopathic lichen planus (see Chap. 32); however, lichenoid drug eruptions often appear initially as eczematous with a purple hue and involve large areas of the trunk. Usually the mucous membranes and nails are not involved. Histologically, focal parakeratosis, focal interruption of the granular layer, cytoid bodies in the cornified and granular layers, the presence of eosinophils and plasma cells in the inflammatory infiltrate, and an infiltrate around the deep vessels favor a diagnosis of lichenoid drug eruption.[42] Photodistributed presentations may lack these specific features and be interchangeable with idiopathic lichen planus on histology.[43]

Many drugs, including β-blockers, penicillamine, and ACE inhibitors, especially captopril, reportedly produce this reaction. Lichen planus–like eruptions also have been reported with tumor necrosis factor (TNF)-α antagonists (infliximab, etanercept, and adalimumab) and antibodies to the immune checkpoint T-cell receptor programmed death (PD)-1 and PD-1 ligand.[44-46] The mean latent period is between 2 months

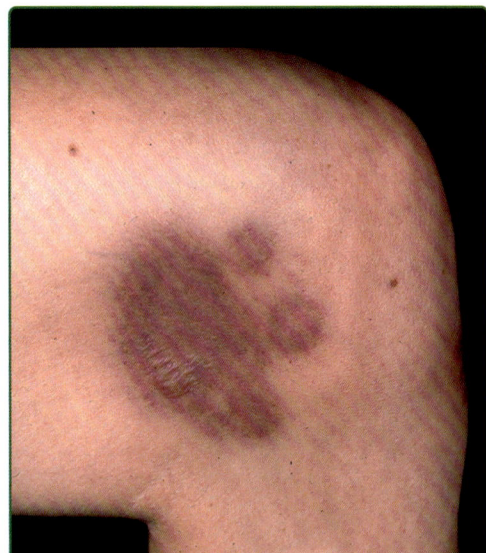

FIGURE 45-6 Fixed drug eruption: tetracycline. A well-defined plaque on the knee, merging with 3 satellite lesions. The large plaque exhibits epidermal wrinkling, a sign of incipient blister formation. This was the second such episode after ingestion of a tetracycline. No other lesions were present.

TABLE 45-4
Summary of the Main Patterns of Drug-Induced Hyperpigmentation

CAUSATIVE DRUG	DISTRIBUTION	HISTOLOGY
Nonsteroidal antiinflammatory drugs	Extremities, trunk, mucous membranes (fixed drug eruption)	Epidermal necrosis
Antimalarials	Nails, legs, head, rarely mucous membranes	Melanin, siderin deposition
Psychotropic drugs	Sun-exposed areas, sometimes blue-gray	Melanin and drug complexes within dermal macrophages
Amiodarone	Sun-exposed areas	Amiodarone and lipofuscin accumulation within dermal histiocytes
Cytotoxic drugs	Variable	Variable
Tetracyclines	Sun-exposed areas, acne scars, sites of previous inflammation, mucous membranes, internal organs	Cyclin, melanin, hemosiderin, lipofuscin accumulation
Silver	Skin (diffuse), nails, mucous membranes	Silver granule deposition within dermal histiocytes or free dermis
Gold	Sun-exposed areas, blue-gray	Deposits of gold granules within dermal histiocytes or free dermis

Adapted by permission from Springer: Dereure O. Drug-induced skin pigmentation. *Am J Clin Dermatol.* 2001;2(4):253-262. Copyright © 2001.

and 3 years for penicillamine, approximately 1 year for β-adrenergic blocking agents, and 3 to 6 months for ACE inhibitors. For anti-TNF treatments, the time to reaction is similar, with onset occurring between 3 weeks and 62 weeks, and for PD-1 and PD-1 ligand antibodies time to onset is several months. The latent period may be shortened if the patient has been previously exposed to the drug. Resolution usually occurs within 2 to 4 months. Rechallenge with the culprit drug has been attempted in a few patients, with reactivation of symptoms within 4 to 15 days.[46]

DRUG-INDUCED CUTANEOUS PSEUDOLYMPHOMA

Pseudolymphoma is a process that simulates lymphoma but has a benign behavior and does not meet the criteria for malignant lymphoma. Drugs are a well-known cause of both B-cell and T-cell cutaneous pseudolymphomas (see Chap. 120). Other possible triggers include foreign agents, such as insect bites, infections (eg, HIV), and idiopathic causes.[47] Medications that have been implicated

TABLE 45-5
Drug-Induced Nail Hyperpigmentation

CAUSATIVE DRUG	CLINICAL PATTERN OF PIGMENTATION
Antimalarials	Nail bed with transversal bands or diffuse pigmentation
Cytotoxic drugs: cisplatin, doxorubicin, idarubicin, fluorouracil, bleomycin, docetaxel, dacarbazine, and hydroxyurea (hydroxycarbamide)	Longitudinal or transverse pigmented bands or diffuse pigmentation, sometimes coexisting with leukonychia or onycholysis (docetaxel)
Silver	Longitudinal or diffuse
Phenothiazines	Diffuse
Zidovudine	Diffuse

Reprinted with permission from Springer: Dereure O. Drug-induced skin pigmentation. *Am J Clin Dermatol.* 2001;2(4):253-262. Copyright © 2001.

TABLE 45-6
Cytotoxic Drug-Induced Skin Pigmentation Distribution Patterns

CLINICAL PATTERN OF PIGMENTATION	CAUSATIVE DRUG
Diffuse	Busulfan, cyclophosphamide, methotrexate, hydroxyurea (hydroxycarbamide), procarbazine
Dorsal surfaces of extremities	Cisplatin, doxorubicin, mitoxantrone
Flexural areas, palmar and plantar surfaces	Ifosfamide, fluorouracil, tegafur, bleomycin, doxorubicin
Patchy	Cisplatin
On areas of trauma (electrocardiogram electrodes, occlusive dressing, friction)	Cyclophosphamide, fluorouracil, ifosfamide, topical carmustine, cisplatin, thiotepa, hydroxyurea (hydroxycarbamide), bleomycin, docetaxel
Serpentine supravenous pigmentation at infusion sites	Fotemustine, fluorouracil, vinorelbine, cisplatin, docetaxel, combination of cytarabine, asparaginase, mercaptopurine and cyclophosphamide
On previous tumoral areas	Mechlorethamine, cyclophosphamide, hydroxyurea
Postinflammatory	Combination of ifosfamide, cisplatin and etoposide (in intertriginous areas)
With photosensitivity	Fluorouracil, daunorubicin, doxorubicin
Flagellated	Fluorouracil, bleomycin
Reticulated	Fluorouracil

Reprinted with permission from Springer: Dereure O. Drug-induced skin pigmentation. *Am J Clin Dermatol.* 2001;2(4):253-262. Copyright © 2001.

include anticonvulsants (carbamazepine, phenytoin, valproic acid), ACE inhibitors, allopurinol, cyclosporine, levofloxacin, antihistamines, and analgesics.[48] Fluoxetine and other antidepressants may stimulate B-cell proliferation leading to a pseudolymphoma as a response to their suppressive effects on T cells.[49]

Anticonvulsant-induced pseudolymphoma generally occurs after 1 week to 2 years of exposure to the drug. Within 7 to 14 days of drug discontinuation, the symptoms usually resolve. The eruption often manifests as single lesions but can also be widespread erythematous papules, plaques, or nodules. Most patients also have fever, marked lymphadenopathy and hepatosplenomegaly, and eosinophilia. Mycosis fungoides–like lesions are also associated with these drugs.[50]

DRUG-INDUCED LUPUS AND DERMATOMYOSITIS

(See Chap. 61)

Drug-induced lupus is characterized by frequent musculoskeletal complaints, fever, weight loss, pleuropulmonary involvement in more than half of patients, and, in rare cases, renal, neurologic, or vasculitic involvement (see Table 45-1). Many patients have no cutaneous findings of lupus erythematosus. The most common serologic abnormality is positivity for antinuclear antibodies with a homogenous pattern. Although antihistone antibodies are seen in up to 95% of drug-induced lupus, they are not specific for the syndrome and are found in 50% to 80% of patients with idiopathic lupus erythematosus. Unlike in idiopathic lupus erythematosus, antibodies against double-stranded DNA are typically absent, whereas anti–single-stranded DNA antibodies are often present.[51] Genetic factors may also play a role in the development of drug-induced lupus. Human leukocyte antigen-D related (HLA-DR)-4 is present in 73% of the patients with hydralazine-induced lupus and in 70% of patients with minocycline-induced lupus.[52] Evidence now suggests that abnormalities during T-cell selection in the thymus initiate lupus-like autoantibody induction.[53]

Many drugs have been implicated in causing drug-induced lupus syndromes, especially hydralazine, procainamide, isoniazid, methyldopa, and minocycline.[54] The identification of minocycline as a cause of drug-induced lupus makes it important for dermatologists to recognize this syndrome. Minocycline-induced lupus typically occurs after 2 years of therapy. The patient presents with a symmetric polyarthritis. Hepatitis is often detected on laboratory evaluation. Cutaneous findings include livedo reticularis, painful nodules on the legs, and nondescript eruptions. Antihistone antibodies are seldom present.

In contrast, drug-induced subacute cutaneous lupus erythematosus (SCLE) is characterized by a papulosquamous or annular cutaneous lesion, which is often photosensitive, and absent or mild systemic involvement. Although it has been suggested that some of the implicated drugs may enhance photosensitivity in predisposed individuals leading to the eruption, this theory has not been proven. The clinical morphology and histopathology are indistinguishable from subacute cutaneous lupus erythematosus that is not drug-induced.[55] Circulating anti-Ro (Sjögren syndrome A) antibodies have also been identified in many patients.

The most common drugs associated with subacute cutaneous lupus erythematosus include terbinafine, thiazide diuretics, calcium channel blockers, and ranitidine.[55] The time course to onset of the eruption appears to be drug dependent, with an average of 5 weeks for terbinafine, 3 years for calcium channel blockers, and a range of 6 months to 5 years for thiazides.[55] The rash resolves after a few weeks with discontinuation of the offending drug, but anti-Ro antibodies may remain positive indefinitely.

Drug-induced dermatomyositis can present with the classic cutaneous findings in dermatomyositis, including a pruritic photodistributed papulosquamous exanthem. The majority of drug-induced cases have the pathognomonic heliotrope rash or Gottron papules.[56] In a review of 70 cases, muscular involvement (proximal muscle weakness or elevated muscle-derived enzymes) was present in 28 (40%) patients and pulmonary involvement in 8 patients (11%).[56] Both skin findings and myositis may clear after 2 months to 1 year of discontinuing the offending drug. The most common medications implicated are hydroxyurea, penicillamine, and β-hydroxy-β-methylglutaryl-coenzyme A (HMG-CoA) reductase inhibitors.[56] There are also reports of TNF-α-inhibitor–induced dermatomyositis.[57]

PURPURIC ERUPTIONS

Drug-induced vasculitis represents approximately 10% of the acute cutaneous vasculitides and usually involves small vessels (see Chap. 138). Drugs that are associated with vasculitis include propylthiouracil, hydralazine, granulocyte colony-stimulating factor, granulocyte-macrophage colony-stimulating factor, allopurinol, cefaclor, minocycline, penicillamine, phenytoin, isotretinoin, and anti-TNF agents, including etanercept, infliximab, and adalimumab.[45] More recent triggers have been rituximab and the cocaine adulterant levamisole.[58] The average interval from initiation of drug therapy to onset of drug-induced vasculitis is 7 to 21 days; in the case of rechallenge, lesions can occur in fewer than 3 days.[8]

The clinical hallmark of cutaneous vasculitis is palpable purpura, classically found on the lower extremities. Urticaria can be a manifestation of small-vessel vasculitis, with individual lesions remaining fixed in the same location for more than 1 day. Other features include hemorrhagic bullae, ulcers, nodules, Raynaud disease, and digital necrosis. The same vasculitic process may also affect internal organs, such as the liver, kidney, gut, and CNS, and can be potentially life threatening.[59]

Drug-induced vasculitis can be difficult to diagnose and is often a diagnosis of exclusion. In some cases, serologic testing has revealed the presence of perinuclear-staining antineutrophil cytoplasmic autoantibodies against myeloperoxidase. Unlike in antineutrophilic cytoplasmic antibody-associated vasculitides, antihistone and antiphospholipid antibodies can be seen.[60] Uniquely in levamisole-induced vasculitis, a common finding is both perinuclear and cytoplasmic antineutrophilic cytoplasmic antibody. Alternative causes for cutaneous vasculitis such as infection or autoimmune disease must be eliminated. Tissue eosinophilia may be an indicator of drug induction in cutaneous small-vessel vasculitis. Drug-induced vasculitis tends to have less progression to glomerulonephritis, better outcomes, and require less immunosuppressive treatment.[58] Most cases resolve with drug withdrawal alone, but systemic glucocorticoids may provide benefit.

ANTICOAGULANT-INDUCED SKIN NECROSIS

Anticoagulant-induced skin necrosis begins 3 to 5 days after initiation of treatment. The majority of cases of anticoagulant-induced skin necrosis (Fig. 45-7) have been attributed to coumarin congeners (bishydroxycoumarin, phenprocoumon, acenocoumarol, and warfarin). Early red, painful plaques develop in adipose-rich sites such as breasts, buttocks, and hips. These plaques may blister, ulcerate, or develop into necrotic areas. It is estimated that 1 in 10,000 persons who receive an anticoagulant is at risk of this adverse event. The incidence is 4 times higher in women, the majority of whom are obese, with a peak incidence in the sixth and seventh decades of life. Affected patients often have been given a large initial loading dose of warfarin in the absence of concomitant heparin therapy. An accompanying infection, such as pneumonia, viral infection, or erysipelas, may be seen in up to 25% of patients. An association with protein C and protein S deficiencies exists, but pretreatment screening is not warranted. An association with heterozygosity for factor V Leiden mutation has been reported.

The pathogenesis of this adverse event is the paradoxical development of occlusive thrombi in cutaneous and subcutaneous venules resulting from a transient hypercoagulable state. This results from the suppression of the natural anticoagulant protein C at a greater rate than the suppression of natural procoagulant factors.

Treatment involves the discontinuation of warfarin, administration of vitamin K, and infusion of heparin at therapeutic dosages. Fresh-frozen plasma and purified protein C concentrates have been used. Supportive measures for the skin are a mainstay of therapy. The morbidity rate is high; 60% of affected individuals require plastic surgery for remediation of full-thickness skin necrosis by skin grafting. These patients may be treated with warfarin in the future, but small dosages (2 to 5 mg daily) are recommended, with initial treatment under heparin coverage.[61,62]

NEUTROPHILIC ECCRINE HIDRADENITIS

Neutrophilic eccrine hidradenitis is a benign condition that has been described in patients with leukemia who are receiving chemotherapy (Table 45-7 identifies other chemotherapy-associated drug reactions). Cases have also been described in the absence of chemotherapy or drug triggers. It classically presents with dark erythematous to violaceous edematous plaques that can be asymptomatic or tender.[63] Lesions can occur on the face, including periorbitally, or on the trunk and extremities. It can mimic cellulitis, and is ultimately diagnosed based on histopathology demonstrating a neutrophilic infiltrate of the eccrine unit and necrosis of the eccrine coils and glands with dermal edema.[63] Antineutrophilic agents have been used successfully, including colchicine as treatment and dapsone prophylactically.[64,65]

ETIOLOGY AND PATHOGENESIS

ETIOLOGY

The list of implicated medications in adverse drug eruptions is exhaustive and includes all prescription and nonprescription substances, as well as naturopathic remedies, radiocontrast dyes, and illicit drugs.

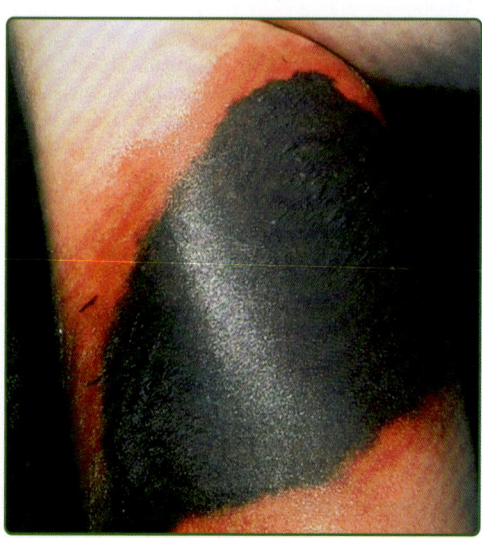

FIGURE 45-7 Skin necrosis in a patient after 4 days of warfarin therapy.

TABLE 45-7
Newer Chemotherapeutic Agents and Their Adverse Cutaneous Drug Reactions

CLASS	AGENTS	ADVERSE CUTANEOUS DRUG REACTIONS
Spindle inhibitor	Taxanes: docetaxel, paclitaxel	Hand–foot skin reaction; combined with sensory abnormalities: erythrodysesthesia; radiation recall urticaria, exanthems, mucositis, alopecia, nail changes; scleroderma-like changes on lower extremities; subacute cutaneous lupus erythematosus (SCLE), acute generalized exanthematous pustulosis (AGEP) and fixed drug reaction (paclitaxel)
Antimetabolites	Vinca alkaloids: vincristine, vinblastine, vinorelbine	Phlebitis, alopecia, acral erythema, extravasation reactions (including necrosis)
	Fludarabine	Serpentine supravenous hyperpigmentation, macular, papular exanthem, mucositis, acral erythema, paraneoplastic pemphigus, drug-induced SCLE
	Cladribine	Exanthem, toxic epidermal necrolysis (TEN)(?)
	Capecitabine	Hand–foot skin reaction, acral hyperpigmentation, palmoplantar keratoderma, pyogenic granuloma, inflammation of actinic keratoses
	Tegafur	Hand–foot skin reaction, acral hyperpigmentation; pityriasis lichenoides et varioliformis acuta, phototoxic reactions
	Gemcitabine	Mucositis, alopecia, maculopapular exanthem, radiation recall, linear immunoglobulin (Ig) A bullous dermatosis, pseudoscleroderma, lipodermatosclerosis, erysipelas-like plaques, pseudolymphoma, lymphomatoid papulosis
	Pemetrexed	Exanthema, radiation recall, urticarial vasculitis
Genotoxic agents	Carboplatin	Alopecia, hypersensitivity reaction (erythema, facial swelling, dyspnea, tachycardia, wheezing), palmoplantar erythema, facial flushing
	Oxaliplatin	Hypersensitivity reaction (see preceding); irritant extravasation reaction; radiation recall
	Liposomal doxorubicin	Acral erythema, palmoplantar erythrodysesthesia neutrophilic eccrine hidradenitis, hyperpigmentation (blue-gray), mucositis, alopecia, exanthems, radiation recall, ultraviolet light recall
	Liposomal daunorubicin	Alopecia, mucositis, extravasation reactions
	Idarubicin	Radiation recall; alopecia, acral erythema, mucositis, nail changes (transverse pigmented bands), extravasation reactions
	Topotecan	Maculopapular exanthem, alopecia, neutrophilic hidradenitis
	Irinotecan	Mucositis, alopecia, lichenoid reactions
Signal transduction inhibitors	Epidermal growth factor receptor (EGFR) antagonists: gefitinib, cetuximab, erlotinib, panitumumab	Papulopustular eruptions in seborrheic areas, erythematous plaques, telangiectasias; xerosis, paronychia; hair abnormalities (trichomegaly, curling, fragility). Usually start a week after initiation of drug. Can treat with topical antibiotics, retinoids (topical or systemic). Can also lead to paronychia, trichomegaly, leukocytoclastic vasculitis, urticaria, anaphylaxis and necrolytic migratory erythema
	Multikinase inhibitors: imatinib	Maculopapular exanthem (face, forearms, ankles), exfoliative dermatitis, graft-versus-host reaction-like reaction, erythema nodosum, vasculitis, Stevens-Johnson syndrome (SJS), AGEP; hypopigmentation, hyperpigmentation, darkening of hair, nail hyperpigmentation, lichen planus–like eruption (skin and oral mucosa), follicular mucinosis, pityriasis rosea–like eruption, Sweet syndrome, exacerbation of psoriasis, palmoplantar hyperkeratosis, porphyria cutanea tarda, primary cutaneous Epstein-Barr virus–related B-cell lymphoma
	Dasatinib and nilotinib	Localized and generalized erythema, maculopapular exanthem, mucositis, pruritus, exfoliation, alopecia, xerosis "acne," urticaria, panniculitis, Sweet syndrome
	Sorafenib and sunitinib	Rash/desquamation, hand–foot skin reaction, pain, alopecia, mucositis, xerosis, flushing edema, seborrheic dermatitis, yellow skin coloration (sunitinib, 1 week after starting drug), subungual splinter hemorrhages, pyoderma gangrenosum, squamous cell carcinoma (SCC) (KA-type), and eruptive melanocytic lesions (sorafenib)
Proteasome inhibitor	Bortezomib	Erythematous nodules and plaques, morbilliform exanthem, ulceration, vasculitis and Sweet syndrome
Immune modulators	Ipilimumab (CTLA-4 AB)	Immune-mediated side effects: macular and papular eruption, pruritus, hepatitis, vitiligo, hypothyroidism, enterocolitis, hepatitis, SJS-TEN
	Pembrolizumab and nivolumab (PD-1 receptor antibody)	Immune-mediated side effects: macular and papular eruption, pruritus, vitiligo, hypothyroidism, enterocolitis, hepatitis, mucositis
BRAF (v-raf murine sarcoma viral oncogene homolog B) inhibitors	Vemurafenib	Rash (68%), arthralgias, photosensitivity (42%), SCC (23%, most occur in first few months)
	Dabrafenib	Pyrexia, headaches, rash

From Wolff K, Johnson R, Saavedra AP, et al. *Fitzpatrick's Color Atlas and Synopsis of Clinical Dermatology*. 8th ed. New York, NY: McGraw-Hill; 2017, Table 23-7, with permission.

For this reason, in the evaluation of a patient with a history of a suspected ADR, it is important to obtain a detailed medication history. The morphology and systemic features of a presentation, as well as the time of onset with relation to the medication history, may provide guidance identifying the more-likely culprit medications. New drugs started within the preceding 3 months, especially those within 6 weeks, are potential causative agents for most cutaneous eruptions (exceptions include drug-induced lupus, drug-induced pemphigus, and drug-induced cutaneous pseudolymphoma), as are drugs that have been used intermittently.

PATHOGENESIS OF DRUG ERUPTIONS

Most cutaneous drug eruptions occur as a result of an immune-mediated reaction to a medication, and can involve IgE or IgG or lymphocytes (Table 45-8). The multiple possible reactions result in the heterogeneous spectrum of presentations. The immune system may target the native drug, its metabolic products, altered self, or a combination of these factors.[11] The specific pathogenesis of each presentation is described under "Clinical Features" section. Predisposing factors can be divided into constitutional and acquired factors (Table 45-9).

Constitutional factors include pharmacogenetic variation in drug-metabolizing enzymes and human leukocyte antigen (HLA) associations. Acetylator phenotype alters the risk of developing drug-induced lupus caused by hydralazine, procainamide, and isoniazid.

The formation of toxic metabolites of the aromatic anticonvulsants may play a pivotal role in the development of HSR.[66] In most individuals, the chemically reactive metabolites that are produced are detoxified by epoxide hydroxylases. If detoxification is defective, however, one of the metabolites may act as a hapten and initiate an immune response, stimulate apoptosis, or cause cell necrosis directly. Approximately 70% to 75% of patients who develop anticonvulsant HSR in response to one aromatic anticonvulsant show cross-reactivity to the other aromatic anticonvulsants. In addition, in vitro testing shows that there is a pattern of inheritance of HSR induced by anticonvulsants. Thus, counseling of family members and disclosure of risk is essential.

Sulfonamide antimicrobials are both sulfonamides (contain SO_2-NH_2) and aromatic amines (contain a benzene ring-NH_2). Aromatic amines can be metabolized to toxic metabolites, namely hydroxylamines and nitroso compounds.[67] In most people, the metabolite is detoxified. However, HSRs may occur in patients who either form excess oxidative metabolites

TABLE 45-9
Nonimmunologic Drug Reactions

Idiosyncrasy	Reactions resulting from hereditary enzyme deficiencies
Individual idiosyncrasy to a topical or systemic drug	Mechanisms not yet known
Cumulation	Reactions are dose dependent, based on the total amount of drug ingested; pigmentation caused by gold, amiodarone, or minocycline
Reactions caused by combination of a drug with ultraviolet irradiation (photosensitivity)	Reactions have a toxic pathogenesis but can also be immunologic in nature
Irritancy/toxicity of a topically applied drug	5-Fluorouracil, imiquimod
Atrophy by topically applied drug	Glucocorticoids

From Wolff K, Johnson R, Saavedra AP, et al. *Fitzpatrick's Color Atlas and Synopsis of Clinical Dermatology*. 8th ed. New York, NY: McGraw-Hill; 2017, Table 23-2, with permission.

TABLE 45-8
Immunologic Drug Reactions

TYPE OF REACTION	PATHOGENESIS	EXAMPLES OF CAUSATIVE DRUG	CLINICAL PATTERNS
Type I	Immunoglobulin (Ig) E-mediated; immediate-type immunologic reactions	Penicillin, other antibiotics	Urticaria/angioedema of skin/mucosa, edema of other organs, and anaphylactic shock
Type II	Drug + cytotoxic antibodies cause lysis of cells such as platelets or leukocytes	Penicillin, sulfonamides, quinidine, isoniazid	Petechiae resulting from thrombocytopenic purpura, drug-induced pemphigus
Type III	IgG or IgM antibodies formed to drug; immune complexes deposited in small vessels activate complement and recruitment of granulocytes	Immunoglobulins, antibiotics, rituximab, infliximab	Vasculitis, urticaria, serum sickness
Type IV	Cell-mediated immune reaction; sensitized lymphocytes react with drug, liberating cytokines, which trigger cutaneous inflammatory response	Sulfamethoxazole, anti-convulsants, allopurinol	Morbilliform exanthematous reactions, fixed drug eruption, lichenoid eruptions, Stevens-Johnson syndrome, toxic epidermal necrolysis

From Wolff K, Johnson R, Saavedra AP, et al. *Fitzpatrick's Color Atlas and Synopsis of Clinical Dermatology*. 8th ed. New York, NY: McGraw-Hill; 2017, Table 23-7, with permission.

or are unable to detoxify such metabolite. Because siblings and other first-degree relatives may be at an increased risk (perhaps as high as 1 in 4) of developing a similar adverse reaction, counseling of family members is essential.

Other aromatic amine-containing drugs, such as procainamide, dapsone, and acebutolol, may also be metabolized to chemically reactive compounds. It is recommended that patients who develop symptoms compatible with a sulfonamide-induced HSR avoid these aromatic amines, because the potential exists for cross-reactivity. However, cross-reactivity is much less likely to occur between sulfonamides antimicrobials and drugs that are not aromatic amines (eg, sulfonylureas, thiazide diuretics, furosemide, celecoxib, and acetazolamide).[68]

HLA class I molecules (HLA-A, HLA-B, HLA-C) present intracellular antigens to CD8+ T cells. Carriers of specific HLA class I alleles are associated with severe drug reactions: HLA-B*1502 with carbamazepine-induced SJS-TEN and phenytoin-induced SJS in Han Chinese, HLA-B*5801 with allopurinol-induced SJS-TEN, and HLA-B*5701 with abacavir drug hypersensitivity.

HLA class II molecules (HLA-DP, HLA-DQ, HLA-DR) present extracellular antigens to CD4+ T-helper cells. HLA-DR4 is significantly more common in individuals with hydralazine-related drug-induced lupus than in those with idiopathic systemic lupus erythematosus.[69] HLA factors may also influence the risk of reactions to nevirapine, abacavir, carbamazepine, and allopurinol.[70-72]

Many drugs associated with severe idiosyncratic drug reactions are metabolized by the body to form reactive, or toxic, drug products.[73] These reactive products comprise only a small proportion of a drug's metabolites and are usually rapidly detoxified. However, patients with drug hypersensitivity syndrome, TEN, and SJS resulting from treatment with sulfonamide antibiotics and the aromatic anticonvulsants (eg, carbamazepine, phenytoin, phenobarbital, primidone, and oxcarbazepine) show greater sensitivity in in vitro assessments to the oxidative, reactive metabolites of these drugs than do control subjects.[66]

Acquired factors also alter an individual's risk of drug eruption. Active viral infection and concurrent use of other medications alter the frequency of drug-associated eruptions. Reactivation of latent viral infection with human herpesvirus 6 also appears common in drug hypersensitivity syndrome, and may be partially responsible for some of the clinical features and/or course of the disease.[13,74] Active infection or reactivation of human herpesvirus 6 has been observed in patients who develop allopurinol HSR.[75] Viral infections may act as, or generate the production of, danger signals that lead to damaging immune responses to drugs, rather than immune tolerance.

Drug–drug interactions may also alter the risk of cutaneous eruption. Valproic acid increases the risk of severe cutaneous adverse reactions to lamotrigine, another anticonvulsant.[76] The basis of these interactions and reactions is unknown, but they may represent a combination of factors, including alterations in drug metabolism, drug detoxification, antioxidant defenses, and immune reactivity.

DIAGNOSIS

The iatrogenic disorders described here are distinct disease entities, although they may closely mimic many infective or idiopathic diseases. A drug cause should be considered in the differential diagnosis of a wide spectrum of dermatologic diseases, particularly when the presentation or course is atypical.

The diagnosis of a cutaneous drug eruption involves the precise characterization of reaction type. A wide variety of cutaneous drug-associated eruptions may also warn of associated internal toxicity (Table 45-10). Even the most minor cutaneous eruption should trigger a clinical review of systems, because the severity of systemic involvement does not necessarily mirror that of the skin manifestations. Hepatic, renal, joint, respiratory, hematologic, and neurologic changes should be sought, and any systemic symptoms or signs investigated. Fever, malaise, pharyngitis, and other systemic symptoms or signs should be investigated. A usual screen would include a full blood count, liver and renal function tests, and a urine analysis.

Skin biopsy should be considered for all patients with potentially severe reactions, such as those with systemic symptoms, erythroderma, blistering, skin tenderness, purpura, or pustulation, as well as in cases in which the diagnosis is uncertain. Some cutaneous reactions, such as FDE, are almost always due to drug therapy, and approximately 40–50%% of SJS-TEN cases are also drug related.[77] Other more common eruptions, including exanthematous or urticarial eruptions, have many nondrug causes.

There is no gold standard investigation for confirmation of a drug cause. Instead, diagnosis and assessment of cause involve analysis of a constellation of features, such as timing of drug exposure and reaction onset, course of reaction with drug withdrawal or continuation, timing and nature of a recurrent eruption on rechallenge, a history of a similar response to a cross-reacting medication, and previ-

TABLE 45-10
Clinical Features That Warn of a Potentially Severe Drug Reaction

- Systemic
  - Fever and/or other symptoms of internal organ involvement such as pharyngitis, malaise, arthralgia, cough, and meningismus
  - Lymphadenopathy
- Cutaneous
  - Evolution to erythroderma
  - Prominent facial involvement ± edema or swelling
  - Mucous membrane involvement (particularly if erosive or involving conjunctiva)
  - Skin tenderness, blistering or shedding
  - Purpura

ous reports of similar reactions to the same medication. Investigations to exclude nondrug causes are similarly helpful.

Several in vitro investigations can help confirm causation in individual cases, but their exact sensitivity and specificity remain unclear. Investigations include the lymphocyte toxicity and lymphocyte transformation assays.[78] The basophil activation test has been reported to be useful to evaluate patients with possible drug allergies to β-lactam antibiotics, NSAIDs, and muscle relaxants.[11] Penicillin skin testing with major and minor determinants is useful for confirmation of an IgE-mediated immediate hypersensitivity reaction to penicillin.[11] Patch testing has been used in patients with ampicillin-induced exanthematous eruptions, AGEP reactions,[79] and abacavir-induced hypersensitivity,[80] and in the ancillary diagnosis of FDEs. Patch testing has greater sensitivity if performed over a previously involved area of skin.

DIFFERENTIAL DIAGNOSIS

Table 45-11 summarizes drug eruptions mimicry.

CLINICAL COURSE AND PROGNOSIS

The course and outcome of drug-induced disease are influenced by both host and disease factors. The vast majority of simple drug exanthems are self-limited. In complicated exanthems, there can be significant morbidity and mortality related to systemic manifestations.

SJS-TEN is associated with the highest mortality. The SCORTEN (SCORe of TEN) is a scale that was developed to help assess severity and predict mortality, and is calculated within the first 24 hours of admission. The 7 criteria include age older than 40 years, laboratory indices (urea <10 mmol/L, glucose >14 mmol/L, bicarbonate <20 mEq/L), tachycardia (heart rate >140 beats per minute), presence of malignancy, and body surface area >10% at presentation.[81] Each criteria fulfilled is given a score of 1, with associated mortality ranging from 3% (1 point) to 90% (5 points).

Patients will have recurrence if exposed to the same medication, and in more systemic eruptions, the recurrence could be more severe and fatal. The recurrence rate in SJS-TEN may be as high as 20% as reported in a series of pediatric cases.[82]

Complex exanthems can also be associated with long-term complications. In SJS-TEN, scarring can affect multiple systems with resulting sequelae in skin (hyperpigmentation, eruptive nevi, alopecia, nail dystrophy), eyes (dry eyes, photophobia, trichiasis, symblepharon), genitalia (dyspareunia, urinary retention, dryness), and lungs (chronic bronchitis, bronchiectasis).[83] Immune-mediated thyroid disorders are a well-recognized complication of hypersensitivity syndromes and can present months after resolution of the exanthem.

MANAGEMENT

Treatment of SJS-TEN includes discontinuance of the suspected drug(s) and supportive measures, such as careful wound care, hydration, and nutritional support. The use of corticosteroids in the treatment of SJS and TEN is controversial.[84,85] Intravenous immunoglobulin (up to 4 g over 3 days) has been shown in some reports to halt progression of TEN, especially when intravenous immunoglobulin is started early. However, some studies have not found an improved outcome in

TABLE 45-11
Drug Eruptions Mimicry

CLINICAL PRESENTATION	PATTERN AND DISTRIBUTION OF SKIN LESIONS	MUCOUS MEMBRANE INVOLVEMENT	IMPLICATED DRUGS	TREATMENT
Stevens-Johnson syndrome	Atypical targets, widespread	Present	Aromatic anticonvulsants,[a] lamotrigine, sulfonamide antibiotics, allopurinol, piroxicam, dapsone	IVIg, cyclosporine, supportive care
Toxic epidermal necrolysis	Epidermal necrosis with skin detachment	Present	As above	IVIg, cyclosporine, supportive care
Pseudoporphyria	Skin fragility, blister formation in photodistribution	Absent	Tetracycline, furosemide, naproxen	Supportive care
Linear IgA disease	Bullous dermatosis	Present/absent	Vancomycin, lithium, diclofenac, piroxicam, amiodarone	Supportive care
Pemphigus	Flaccid bullae, chest	Present/absent	Penicillamine, captopril, piroxicam, penicillin, rifampin, propranolol	Supportive care
Bullous pemphigoid	Tense bullae, widespread	Present/absent	Furosemide, penicillamine, penicillins, sulfasalazine, captopril	Supportive care

Abbreviations: IgA, immunoglobulin A; IVIg, intravenous immunoglobulin.
[a]The aromatic anticonvulsants are phenytoin, carbamazepine, phenobarbital, oxcarbazepine, and primidone.

patients with TEN who are treated with intravenous immunoglobulin.[35] A newer study concluded that neither corticosteroids nor intravenous immunoglobulins had any significant effect on mortality in comparison to supportive care only.[86] Other treatment modalities include cyclosporine,[87] cyclophosphamide, and plasmapheresis. Patients who have developed a severe cutaneous ADR should not be rechallenged with the drug. Desensitization therapy with the medication may also be a risk.

Cutaneous drug eruptions do not usually vary in severity with dose. Less-severe reactions may abate with continued drug therapy (eg, transient exanthematous eruptions associated with commencement of a new HIV antiretroviral regimen). However, a reaction suggestive of a potentially life-threatening situation should prompt immediate discontinuation of the drug, along with discontinuation of any interacting drugs that may slow the elimination of the suspected causative agent. Although the role of corticosteroids in the treatment of serious cutaneous reactions is controversial, most clinicians choose to start prednisone at a dosage of 1 to 2 mg/kg/day when symptoms are severe. Antihistamines, topical corticosteroids, or both can be used to alleviate symptoms.[88] Resolution of the reaction over a reasonable time frame after the drug is discontinued is consistent with a drug cause but also occurs for many infective and other causes of transient cutaneous eruptions. Drug desensitization, also known as induction of drug tolerance, has been used primarily for IgE-mediated reactions caused by drugs such as penicillin or monoclonal antibodies such as rituximab and infliximab.[11,89] Patients should not be rechallenged or desensitized if they have suffered a potentially serious reaction.

PREVENTION

Cutaneous reactions to drugs are largely idiosyncratic and unexpected; serious reactions are rare. Once a reaction has occurred, however, it is important to prevent future similar reactions in the patient with the same drug or a cross-reacting medication. For patients with severe reactions, wearing a bracelet (eg, MedicAlert, www.medicalert.org) detailing the nature of the reaction is advisable, and patient records should be appropriate labeled.

Host factors appear important in many reactions. Some of these can be inherited, which places first-degree relatives at a greater risk than the general population for a similar reaction to the same or a metabolically cross-reacting drug. This finding appears to be important in SJS, TEN, and drug hypersensitivity syndrome.

Reporting reactions to the manufacturer or regulatory authorities is important. Postmarketing voluntary reporting of rare, severe, or unusual reactions remains crucial to enhance the safe use of pharmaceutical agents.

REFERENCES

1. Lazarou J, Pomeranz B, Corey P. Incidence of adverse drug reactions in hospitalized patients: a meta-analysis of prospective studies. *JAMA*. 1998;279:1200-1205.
2. Bigby M. Rates of cutaneous reactions to drugs. *Arch Dermatol*. 2001;137:765-770.
3. Thong BY, Tan TC. Epidemiology and risk factors for drug allergy. *Br J Clin Pharmacol*. 2011;71(5):684-700.
4. Fiszenson-Albala F, Auzerie V, Mahe E, et al. A 6-month prospective survey of cutaneous drug reactions in a hospital setting. *Br J Dermatol*. 2003;149(5):1018-1022.
5. Segal A, Doherty K, Leggott J, et al. Cutaneous reactions to drugs in children. *Pediatrics*. 2007;120:e1082-e1096.
6. Heng YK, Lim YL. Cutaneous adverse drug reactions in the elderly. *Curr Opin Allergy Clin Immunol*. 2015;15(4):300-307.
7. Hernandez-Salazar A, Rosales SP, Rangel-Frausto S, et al. Epidemiology of adverse cutaneous drug reactions. A prospective study in hospitalized patients. *Arch Med Res*. 2006;37(7):899-902.
8. Valeyrie-Allanore L, Sassolas B, Roujeau J. Drug-induced skin, nail and hair disorders. *Drug Saf*. 2007;30:1011-1030.
9. Schnyder B, Pichler W. Mechanisms of drug-induced allergy. *Mayo Clin Proc*. 2009;84:268-272.
10. Kerns D, Shira J, Go S. Ampicillin rash in children. *Am J Dis Child*. 1973;125:187-190.
11. Khan D, Solensky R. Drug Allergy. *J Allergy Clin Immunol*. 2010;125:S126-S137.
12. Kearns G, Wheeler J, Childress S, et al. Serum sickness-like reactions to cefaclor: role of hepatic metabolism and individual susceptibility. *J Pediatr*. 1994;125:805-811.
13. Eshki M, Allanore L, Musette P, et al. Twelve-year analysis of severe cases of drug reaction with eosinophilia and systemic symptoms. *Arch Dermatol*. 2009;145:67-72.
14. Gupta A, Eggo M, Uetrecht J, et al. Drug-induced hypothyroidism: the thyroid as a target organ in hypersensitivity reactions to anticonvulsants and sulfonamides. *Clin Pharmacol Ther*. 1992;51:56-67.
15. Liu HB, Wu Y, Lv TF, et al. Skin rash could predict the response to EGFR tyrosine kinase inhibitor and the prognosis for patients with non-small cell lung cancer: a systematic review and meta-analysis. *PLoS One*. 2013;8(1):e55128.
16. Ruocco V, Sacerdoti G. Pemphigus and bullous pemphigoid due to drugs. *Int J Dermatol*. 1991;30:307-312.
17. Todd D, Helfgott S. Serum sickness following treatment with rituximab. *J Rheumatol*. 2007;34:430-433.
18. Gamarra R, McGraw S, Drelichman VS, et al. Serum sickness-like reactions in patients receiving intravenous infliximab. *J Emerg Med*. 2006;30:41-44.
19. Remmer H, Falk W. Successful treatment of lithium-induced acne. *J Clin Psychiatry*. 1986;47:48.
20. Su X, Lacouture M, Jia Y, et al. Risk of hig-grade skin rash in cancer patients treated with cetuximab: an antibody against epidermal growth factor receptor: systemic review and meta-analysis. *Oncology*. 2009;77:124-133.
21. Macdonald JB, Macdonald B, Golitz LE, et al. Cutaneous adverse effects of targeted therapies: part I: inhibitors of the cellular membrane. *J Am Acad Dermatol*. 2015;72(2):203-218; quiz 219-220.
22. Cowen E. Epidermal growth factor receptor inhibitors: a new era of drug reactions in a new era of cancer therapy. *J Am Acad Dermatol*. 2007;56:514-517.

23. Jatoi A, Dakhil SR, Sloan JA, et al. Prophylactic tetracycline does not diminish the severity of epidermal growth factor receptor (EGFR) inhibitor-induced rash: results from the North Central Cancer Treatment Group (Supplementary N03CB). *Support Care Cancer.* 2011;19(10):1601-1607.
24. Scope A, Agero AL, Dusza SW, et al. Randomized double-blind trial of prophylactic oral minocycline and topical tazarotene for cetuximab-associated acne-like eruption. *J Clin Oncol.* 2007;25(34):5390-5396.
25. Hotz C, Valeyrie-Allanore L, Haddad C, et al. Systemic involvement of acute generalized exanthematous pustulosis: a retrospective study on 58 patients. *Br J Dermatol.* 2013;169(6):1223-1232.
26. Sidoroff A, Dunant A, Viboud C, et al. Risk factors for acute generalized exanthematous pustulosis (AGEP)-results of a multinational case-control study (EuroSCAR). *Br J Dermatol.* 2007;157(5):989-996.
27. Guevara-Gutierrez E, Uribe-Jimenez E, Diaz-Canchola M, et al. Acute generalized exanthematous pustulosis: report of 12 cases and literature review. *Int J Dermatol.* 2009;48:253-258.
28. Lang B, Finlayson L. Naproxen-induced pseudoporphyria in patients with juvenile rheumatoid arthritis. *J Pediatr.* 1994;124:639-642.
29. Beer K, Applebaum D, Nousari C. Pseudoporphyria: discussion of etiologic agents. *J Drugs Dermatol.* 2014;13(8):990-992.
30. Chanal J, Ingen-Housz-Oro S, Ortonne N, et al. Linear IgA bullous dermatosis: comparison between the drug-induced and spontaneous forms. *Br J Dermatol.* 2013;169(5):1041-1048.
31. Primka E, Liranzo E, Bergfeld W, et al. Amiodarone-induced linear IgA disease. *J Am Acad Dermatol.* 1994;31:809-811.
32. Panasiti V, Rossi M, Devirgiliis V, et al. Amoxicillin-clavulanic acid-induced linear immunoglobulin A bullous dermatosis: case report and review of the literature. *Int J Dermatol.* 2009;48:1006-1010.
33. Stavropoulos PG, Soura E, Antoniou C. Drug-induced pemphigoid: a review of the literature. *J Eur Acad Dermatol Venereol.* 2014;28(9):1133-1140.
34. Lee J, Downham T. Furosemide-induced bullous pemphigoid: case report and review of literature. *J Drugs Dermatol.* 2006;5:562-564.
35. Paquet P, Pierard G. New insights in toxic epidermal necrolysis (Lyell's syndrome): clinical considerationsk, pathobiology and targeted treatments revistied. *Drug Saf.* 2010;33:189-212.
36. Mockenhaupt M. Severe drug-induced skin reactions: clinical pattern, diagnostics and therapy. *J Dtsch Dermatol Ges.* 2009;7:142-160.
37. Patell RD, Dosi RV, Shah PC, et al. Widespread bullous fixed drug eruption. *BMJ Case Rep.* 2014;2014.
38. Brahimi N, Routier E, Raison-Peyron N, et al. A three-year-analysis of fixed drug eruptions in hospital settings in France. *Eur J Dermatol.* 2010;20(4):461-464.
39. Jung JW, Cho SH, Kim KH, et al. Clinical features of fixed drug eruption at a tertiary hospital in Korea. *Allergy Asthma Immunol Res.* 2014;6(5):415-420.
40. Barbaud A, Goncalo M, Bruynzeel D, et al. Guidelines for performing skin tests with drugs in the investigation of cutaneous adverse drug reactions. *Contact Dermatitis.* 2001;45:321-328.
41. Ozkaya E. Fixed drug eruption: state of the art. *J Drugs Dermatol.* 2008;6:181-188.
42. Lage D, Juliano PB, Metze K, et al. Lichen planus and lichenoid drug-induced eruption: a histological and immunohistochemical study. *Int J Dermatol.* 2012;51(10):1199-1205.
43. West AJ, Berger TG, LeBoit PE. A comparative histopathologic study of photodistributed and nonphotodistributed lichenoid drug eruptions. *J Am Acad Dermatol.* 1990;23(4, pt 1):689-693.
44. Schaberg KB, Novoa RA, Wakelee HA, et al. Immunohistochemical analysis of lichenoid reactions in patients treated with anti-PD-L1 and anti-PD-1 therapy. *J Cutan Pathol.* 2016;43(4):339-346.
45. Kerbleski J, Gottlieb A, SW. Dermatological complications and safety of anti-TNF treatments. *Gut.* 2009;58:1033-1039.
46. Halevy S, Shai A. Lichenoid drug eruptions. *J Am Acad Dermatol.* 1993;29:249-255.
47. Albrecht J, Fine L, Piette W. Drug-associated lymphoma and pseudolymphoma: recognition and management. *Dermatol Clin.* 2007;25:233-244.
48. Sarantopoulos GP, Palla B, Said J, et al. Mimics of cutaneous lymphoma: report of the 2011 Society for Hematopathology/European Association for Haematopathology workshop. *Am J Clin Pathol.* 2013;139(4):536-551.
49. Breza TS Jr, Zheng P, Porcu P, et al. Cutaneous marginal zone B-cell lymphoma in the setting of fluoxetine therapy: a hypothesis regarding pathogenesis based on in vitro suppression of T-cell-proliferative response. *J Cutan Pathol.* 2006;33(7):522-528.
50. Scheinfeld N. Impact of phenytoin therapy on the skin and skin disease. *Expert Opin Drug Saf.* 2004;3:655-665.
51. Antonov D, Kazandjieva J, Etugov D, et al. Drug-induced lupus erythematosus. *Clin Dermatol.* 2004;22:157-166.
52. Dunphy, Oliver M, Rands A, et al. Antineutrophil cytoplasmic antibodies and HLA class II alleles in minocycline-induced lupus-like syndrome. *Br J Dermatol.* 2000;142:461-467.
53. Rubin R. Drug-induced lupus. *Toxicology.* 2005;209:135-147.
54. Sarzi-Puttini P, Atzeni F, Capsoni F, et al. Drug-induced lupus erythematosus. *Autoimmunity.* 2005;38:507-518.
55. Lowe GC, Henderson CL, Grau RH, et al. A systematic review of drug-induced subacute cutaneous lupus erythematosus. *Br J Dermatol.* 2011;164(3):465-472.
56. Seidler AM, Gottlieb AB. Dermatomyositis induced by drug therapy: a review of case reports. *J Am Acad Dermatol.* 2008;59(5):872-880.
57. Klein R, Rosenbach M, Kim EJ, et al. Tumor necrosis factor inhibitor-associated dermatomyositis. *Arch Dermatol.* 2010;146(7):780-784.
58. Grau RG. Drug-induced vasculitis: new insights and a changing lineup of suspects. *Curr Rheumatol Rep.* 2015;17(12):71.
59. Justiniano H, Berlingeri-Ramos A, Sanchez J. Pattern analysis of drug-induced skin diseases. *Am J Dermatopathol.* 2008;30:352-369.
60. Radic M, Martinovic Kaliterna D, Radic J. Drug-induced vasculitis: a clinical and pathological review. *Neth J Med.* 2012;70(1):12-17.
61. Nazarian RM, Van Cott EM, Zembowicz A, et al. Warfarin-induced skin necrosis. *J Am Acad Dermatol.* 2009;61:325-332.
62. Bircher A, Harr T, Hohenstein L, et al. Hypersensitivity reactions to anticoagulant drugs: diagnosis and management options. *Allergy.* 2006;61:1432-1440.
63. Copaescu AM, Castilloux JF, Chababi-Atallah M, et al. A classic clinical case: neutrophilic eccrine hidradenitis. *Case Rep Dermatol.* 2013;5(3):340-346.

64. Shear NH, Knowles SR, Shapiro L, et al. Dapsone in prevention of recurrent neutrophilic eccrine hidradenitis. *J Am Acad Dermatol.* 1996;35(5, pt 2):819-822.
65. Belot V, Perrinaud A, Corven C, et al. Adult idiopathic neutrophilic eccrine hidradenitis treated with colchicine [in French]. *Presse Med.* 2006;35(10, pt 1):1475-1478.
66. Shear N, Spielberg S. Anticonvulsant hypersensitivity syndrome, in vitro assessment of risk. *J Clin Invest.* 1988;82:1826-1832.
67. Castrejon J, Berry N, El-Ghalesh S, et al. Stimulation of human T cells with sulfonamides and sulfonamide metabolites. *J Allergy Clin Immunol.* 2010;125:411-418.
68. Knowles S, Shapiro L, Shear N. Should celecoxib be contraindicated in patients who are allergic to sulfonamides? Revisiting the meaning of "sulfa" allergy. *Drug Saf.* 2001;24:239-247.
69. Batchelor J, Welsh K, Tinoco R, et al. Hydralazine-induced systemic lupus erythematosus: influence of HLA-DR and sex on susceptibility. *Lancet.* 1980;1:1107-1109.
70. Hung S, Chung W, Jee S, et al. Genetic susceptibility to carbamazepine-induced cutaneous adverse drug reactions. *Pharmacogenet Genomics.* 2006;16:297-306.
71. Dainichi T, Uchi H, Morol Y, et al. Stevens-Johnson syndrome, drug-induced hypersensitivity syndrome and toxic epidermal necrolysis caused by allopurinol in patients with a common HLA allele: what causes the diversity. *Dermatology.* 2007;215:86-88.
72. Tozzi V. Pharmacogenetics of antiretrovirals. *Antiviral Res.* 2010;85:190-200.
73. Uetrecht J. Is it possible to more accurately predict which drug candidates will cause idiosyncratic drug reactions? *Curr Drug Metab.* 2000;1:133-141.
74. Seishima M, Yamanaka S, Fujisawa T, et al. Reactivation of human herpesvirus (HHV) family members other than HHV-6 in drug-induced hypersensitivity syndrome. *Br J Dermatol.* 2006;155:344-349.
75. Chiou C, Yang L, Hung S, et al. Clinicopathological features and prognosis of drug rash with eosinophilia and systemic symptoms: a study of 30 cases in Taiwan. *J Eur Acad Dermatol Venereol.* 2008;22:1044-1049.
76. Sullivan J, Shear N. What are some of the lessons learnt from in vitro studies of severe unpredictable drug reactions? *Br J Dermatol.* 2000;142:205.
77. Auquier-Dunant A, Mockenhaupt M, Naldi L, et al. Correlations between clinical patterns and causes of erythema multiforme major, Stevens-Johnson syndrome and toxic epidermal necrolysis. *Arch Dermatol.* 2002;138:1019-1024.
78. Neuman M, Malkiewicz I, Shear N. A novel lymphocyte toxicity assay to assess drug hypersensitivity syndromes. *Clin Biochem.* 2000;33:517-524.
79. Barbaud A. Drug patch testing in systemic cutaneous drug allergy. *Toxicology.* 2005;209:209-216.
80. Shear N, LMilpied B, Bruynzeel D, et al. A review of drug patch testing and implications for HIV clinicians. *AIDS.* 2008;22:1-9.
81. Bastuji-Garin S, et al. SCORTEN: a severity-of-illness score for toxic epidermal necrolysis. *J Invest Dermatol.* 2000;115:149.
82. Finkelstein Y, Soon GS, Acuna P, et al. Recurrence and outcomes of Stevens-Johnson syndrome and toxic epidermal necrolysis in children. *Pediatrics.* 2011;128(4):723-728.
83. Downey A, Jackson C, Harun N, et al. Toxic epidermal necrolysis: review of pathogenesis and management. *J Am Acad Dermatol.* 2012;66(6):995-1003.
84. Tripathi J, Ditto A, Grammer L, et al. Corticosteroid therapy in an additional 13 cases of Stevens-Johnson syndrome: a total series of 67 cases. *Allergy Asthma Proc.* 2000;21:101-105.
85. Murphy J, Purdue G, Hunt J. Toxic epidermal necrolysis. *J Burn Care Rehabil.* 1997;18:417-420.
86. Schneck J, Fagot J, Sekula P, et al. Effects of treatments of the mortality of Stevens-Johnson syndrome and toxic epidermal necrolysis: a retrospective study on patients included in the prospective EuroSCAR study. *J Am Acad Dermatol.* 2008;58:33-40.
87. Arevalo J, Lorente J, Gonzalez-Herrada C, et al. Treatment of toxic epidermal necrolysis with cyclosporin A. *J Trauma.* 2000;48:473-478.
88. Drake L, Dinehart S, Farmer R, et al. Guidelines of care for cutaneous adverse drug reactions. *J Am Acad Dermatol.* 1996;35:458-461.
89. Brennan P, Bouza T, Hsu F, et al. Hypersensitivity reactions to mAbs: 105 desensitizations in 23 patients, from evaluation to treatment. *J Allergy Clin Immunol.* 2009;124:1259-1266.

Chapter 46 :: Erythema Annulare Centrifugum and Other Figurate Erythemas
:: Christine S. Ahn & William W. Huang

第四十六章
离心性环状红斑和其他形态红斑

中文导读

　　本章共分为4节：①离心性环状红斑；②游走性红斑；③环形红斑；④匐行性回状红斑。分别介绍了这四种反应性红斑的流行病学、临床特征、病因和发病机制、诊断、鉴别诊断、临床病程、预后和治疗。该类红斑为少见的炎症性超敏反应，以环形或多环形斑块为特征，伴有中央自愈倾向和外周鳞屑。好发于四肢和躯干。呈现复发和缓解交替的慢性过程。

〔李　捷〕

ERYTHEMA ANNULARE CENTRIFUGUM

AT-A-GLANCE

- Uncommon inflammatory hypersensitivity reaction characterized by annular or polycyclic plaques with central clearing and peripheral scale.
- Favors the extremities and trunk.
- Chronic condition that recurs and remits.
- Two histologic variants: superficial variant consists of spongiosis, parakeratosis, hyperkeratosis or basal vacuolar changes with a perivascular infiltrate, and deep variant consists of perivascular lymphocytic infiltrate concentrated in the upper dermis without any epidermal changes.
- Treatments include topical corticosteroids, vitamin D analogs, antibiotics, and antifungals.

The figurate or reactive erythemas encompass a variety of cutaneous eruptions that are characterized by erythematous lesions with annular, polycyclic, and/or arcuate configurations. The prototype of these disorders is erythema annulare centrifugum (EAC), which was a term first used by Darier in 1916 to describe an erythematous annular or polycyclic plaque that enlarged centrifugally with a trailing scale.[1] The classification of EAC and other figurate erythemas is controversial, with some authors believing that the superficial and deep forms of EAC represent distinct clinical entities, and others considering EAC to be a clinical reaction pattern rather than a specific clinicopathologic entity.[2]

EPIDEMIOLOGY

Although there is limited epidemiologic data on the prevalence of EAC, it is thought to be an uncommon disorder. Based on 4 clinicopathologic series in the literature that includes 202 patients, EAC exhibits no sex predilection and largely occurs in adults, with a peak incidence in the third and fourth decades.[2-5] EAC also has been described in infants and children.[6,7]

CLINICAL FEATURES

EAC presents in the skin as a pink papule that expands centrifugally, forming an annular or polycyclic plaque with central clearing. In the superficial variant, lesions are slightly elevated and demonstrate desquamation at the inner margin, also referred to as a "trailing scale" (Figs. 46-1 and 46-2). The deep variant of EAC has an indurated, firm border, often without prominent scaling. The most common symptom associated with EAC is pruritus, although it is often asymptomatic. Residual scarring is uncommon, although postinflammatory hyperpigmentation may occur after lesions resolve. The most frequent sites of involvement of EAC are the buttocks, thighs, and trunk. In a series of 66 cases, the most common sites of involvement were the lower extremities (36 cases, 48%) and trunk (22 cases, 28%). Upper extremities and head and neck involvement were less common, observed in 12 cases (16%) and 6 cases (8%), respectively. When categorized by the extent of involvement, 28 patients (58%) had lesions located on only one site, 19 patients (28%) on 2 sites, and 9 patients (14%) had generalized disease with 3 or more sites.[4]

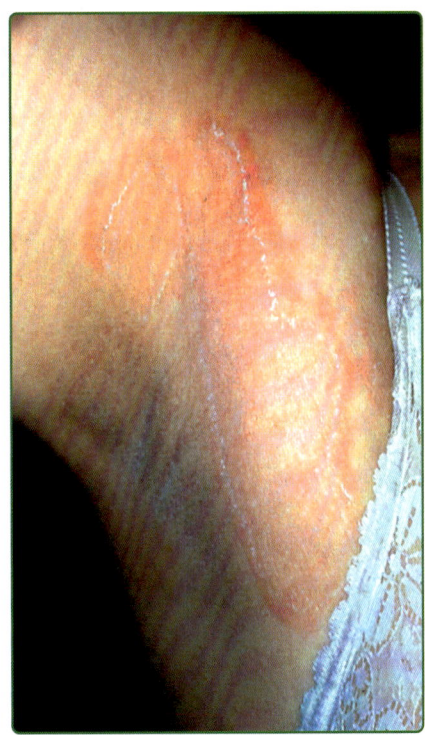

Figure 46-1 Superficial erythema annulare centrifugum. A large annular plaque with trailing scale behind the advancing erythematous edge.

ETIOLOGY AND PATHOGENESIS

The etiology of EAC is not fully understood. Although most cases are idiopathic, it has been suggested that EAC is a hypersensitivity reaction to an antigen, and has been linked to cutaneous or systemic infections, malignancy, drugs, certain disease states, and pregnancy.

RISK FACTORS

Although largely anecdotal, EAC has been observed in the setting of infections, malignancies, medications, pregnancy, and other systemic diseases in up to 72% of cases.[4] In one study, 40% of patients with EAC had a concomitant superficial dermatophyte infection, most commonly tinea pedis, and 13% had internal malignancies, including non-Hodgkin lymphoma and acute myelogenous leukemia.[4] In a separate review of 39 patients with EAC, 13 (33%) had associated conditions, with the most common being superficial dermatophyte infection 5 (13%), pregnancy 2 (5%), thyroid cancer 2 (5%), and medication use 2 (5%).[2]

Dermatophyte infections may be a risk factor for EAC. In cases associated with tinea pedis, lesions of EAC tend to resolve with treatment of the dermatophytosis.[2] In addition to dermatophytoses, EAC is associated with other cutaneous infections such as molluscum contagiosum and herpes zoster, as well as systemic infections, including Epstein-Barr virus and HIV.[8-10] Paraneoplastic erythema annulare centrifugum eruptions occur most commonly with lymphoprolifer-

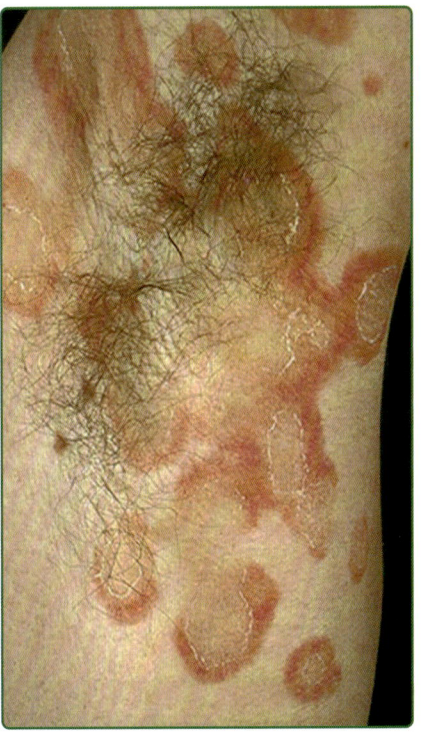

Figure 46-2 Superficial erythema annulare centrifugum. Multiple lesions demonstrated epidermal changes with a trailing scale. (Used with permission from Wilfried Neuse and Thomas Ruzicka, Düsseldorf, Germany.)

ative malignancies such as lymphomas and leukemias, and often precede the diagnosis of the underlying malignancy. It is thought to occur as a result of cytokine or tumor-associated factors as the clinical course tends to parallel the activity of the neoplasm, with resolution with treatment and recurrence with relapse of the malignancy.[11,12]

A wide of range of drugs are associated with EAC, including finasteride; azacitidine; pegylated interferon-α_{2a} and ribavirin in the treatment of hepatitis C; rituximab; ustekinumab; amitriptyline; and gold sodium thiomalate.[13-18] However, no specific drugs have been reported consistently to establish a true relationship. EAC also has been reported in the setting of some disease states, such as autoimmune hepatitis and systemic lupus erythematosus. In some cases, EAC can be the presenting sign of systemic disease.[19] In pregnant women, EAC tends to occur during the second and third trimesters, and typically remits spontaneously around the time of delivery without recurrence.[20,21]

DIAGNOSIS

The diagnosis of EAC is primarily a clinical diagnosis. Histopathologic examination can help differentiate EAC from other conditions that cause annular lesions and confirm the diagnosis. Other laboratory studies do not have a role in the diagnosis of EAC.

PATHOLOGY

EAC is characterized histologically by the presence of a dense perivascular infiltrate composed of lymphocytes, histiocytes, and occasional eosinophils. As a result of the well-demarcated distribution that tightly wraps around blood vessels, the infiltrate has been described as a "coat-sleeve" pattern. There are 2 distinct histologic patterns of EAC: superficial type and deep type. In the superficial type, epidermal changes that correspond to clinical findings are observed, which include parakeratosis, hyperkeratosis, spongiosis, and/or vacuolar degeneration. The perivascular infiltrates are more prominent in the upper dermis in the superficial type (Fig. 46-3). In the deep type, epidermal changes are absent or minimal, and there can be mild edema in the papillary dermis along with perivascular infiltrates involving vascular plexuses in both the upper and lower dermis.[2]

DIFFERENTIAL DIAGNOSIS

The differential diagnosis for EAC includes other annular erythematous lesions. It is important to rule out entities such as Lyme borreliosis, lupus erythematosus, and an underlying tumor or annular metastasis. See Table 46-1.

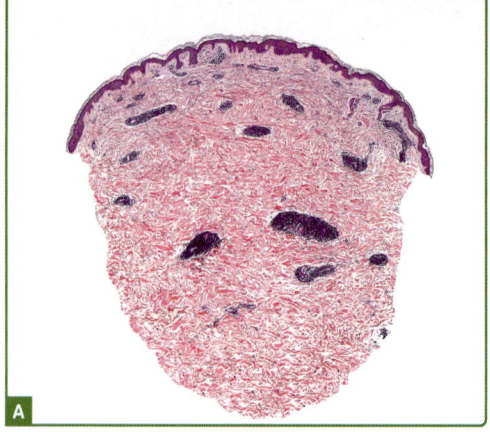
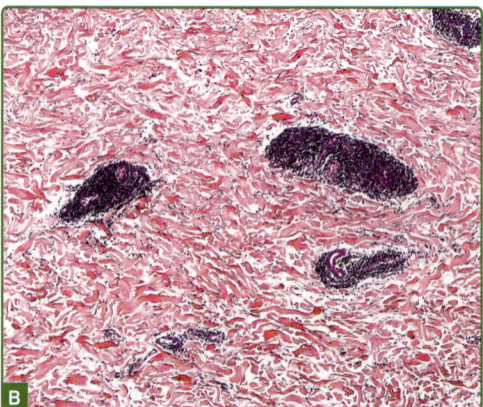
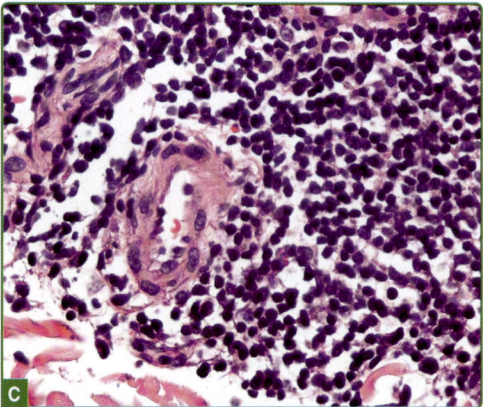

Figure 46-3 Erythema annulare centrifugum. **A,** Dense perivascular infiltrate in the superficial and med dermis. **B** and **C,** Lymphocytic infiltrate tightly wrapped around blood vessels in a "coat-sleeve" pattern.

CLINICAL COURSE AND PROGNOSIS

EAC is a chronic condition that tends to persist over several months to years, following a waxing and waning course. Some cases regress spontaneously, while others can be resistant to treatment. In a retrospective review

TABLE 46-1
Differential Diagnosis for Erythema Annulare Centrifugum
Erythema chronicum migrans
Annular subacute cutaneous lupus erythematosus
Annular urticaria
Erythema multiforme
Tinea corporis
Annular psoriasis
Mycosis fungoides

of 66 patients with EAC, the duration of disease was 2.8 years.[4] Among 27 patients with follow-up data, 13 (48%) of patients had an excellent response to treatment but 5 (18.5%) had persistent skin lesions that failed to improve after 1 year of treatment. Of these cases with poor response to treatment, almost all cases were superficial-type EAC. The average duration of continuous lesions of EAC was 4.75 months; although the deep-type lesions tended to be longer lasting, the recurrence rate was higher for superficial-type lesions.[2]

MANAGEMENT

Symptomatic EAC can be treated with topical corticosteroids, topical vitamin D analogs, and antihistamines if there is associated pruritus. Systemic corticosteroids clears lesions of EAC, but cessation of therapy can lead to rebound recurrence of disease. There are reports of antifungals and antibiotics such as fluconazole, erythromycin, and metronidazole being used successfully to treat EAC.

ERYTHEMA MIGRANS

AT-A-GLANCE

- Cutaneous manifestation of early localized Lyme disease that occurs at the site of the bite of *Ixodes* species ticks infected with *Borrelia burgdorferi*.
- Characterized by annular erythema that expands to create a "bull's-eye" appearance.
- Seen in 70% to 80% of individuals with Lyme disease.

Erythema migrans is an annular erythema that represents an early cutaneous manifestation of Lyme borreliosis, which is an infection caused by the spirochete *Borrelia burgdorferi*, transmitted through the bite of species of *Ixodes* ticks (see Chap. 179). Chapter 180 discusses other tick-borne diseases.

EPIDEMIOLOGY

Erythema migrans and Lyme disease are seen worldwide, but with a higher prevalence in parts of North America, central and eastern Europe, and eastern Asia. In the United States, it is the fifth most common nationally notifiable disease, with an estimated incidence of 7.9 cases per 100,000 population in 2014.[22] The incidence of Lyme disease is more heavily concentrated in areas endemic to the white-footed mouse and white-tailed deer, the natural hosts of *Ixodes* ticks. *Ixodes scapularis* is the primary vector responsible for Lyme disease in the northeastern, mid-Atlantic, and north-central US, whereas *Ixodes pacificus* is the primary vector in the Pacific coast. Approximately 96% of confirmed Lyme disease cases were reported from 14 states concentrated in the Northeast and upper Midwest in 2014, according to the Centers for Disease Control and Prevention.[22] Most cases of Lyme disease occur during the months of June, July, and August, and there is a bimodal distribution of incidence, with peaks between the ages of 5 and 19 years, and between 55 and 69 years.[1]

CLINICAL FEATURES

CUTANEOUS FINDINGS

The 3 stages of Lyme disease are early localized disease, early disseminated disease, and chronic disease. Erythema migrans occurs at the initial site of the tick bite and is a hallmark cutaneous finding of the first stage of Lyme disease. It is characterized by an erythematous expanding annular plaque with a central area of clearing, often described as a "bull's-eye" lesion (Fig. 46-4). The most common associated symptoms include warmth, pruritus, and pain, although it can

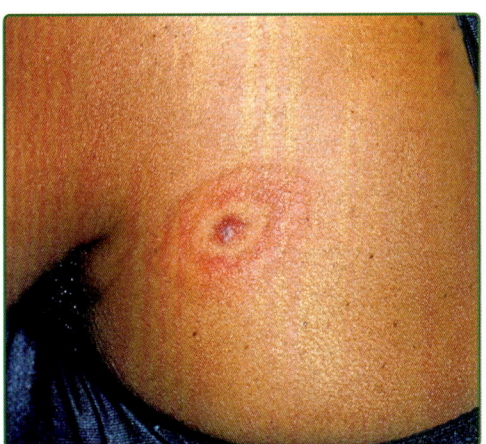

Figure 46-4 Erythema chronicum migrans. Erythematous bite site surrounded by an expanding red plaque, reminiscent of the bull's-eye of a target. (Used with permission from the collection of Dr. John L. Aeling.)

be asymptomatic. In some cases, erythema migrans can be vesicular. Primary lesions of erythema migrans occur in areas where tick bites are likely to occur and go unnoticed, such as the trunk, axillae, groin, and popliteal fossae. Lesions grow centrifugally and can grow at a rate of up to 3 cm per day.[1] At the time of presentation, the mean diameter of lesions of erythema migrans are 10 to 16 cm, depending on the site of involvement, with larger lesions found on the trunk and smaller lesions found on the lower extremities. Multiple lesions of erythema migrans can be seen in the setting of multiple tick bites or spirochetemia or lymphatic spread.

In most cases, ticks must be attached for at least 24 hours before bacteria is transmitted, and erythema migrans occurs at the site of the bite, approximately 7 to 14 days after tick detachment (range: 3 to 30 days). Approximately 70% to 80% of individuals infected with Lyme disease develop lesions of erythema migrans, and up to 45% of patients presenting with erythema migrans have spirochetemia.[1,23]

NONCUTANEOUS FINDINGS

In addition to erythema migrans, other signs and symptoms of early Lyme disease include regional lymphadenopathy, arthralgias, arthritis, myositis, pancarditis, facial palsy, conjunctivitis, and hepatitis.[1]

COMPLICATIONS

Complications of erythema migrans occur as a reflection of untreated Lyme disease. While the lesions of erythema migrans often resolve spontaneously over weeks to months, if untreated, patients can progress to the second stage of Lyme disease, which involves widespread spirochete dissemination with neurologic, rheumatologic, and cardiac involvement, and the third stage, with persistent neuroborreliosis, severe erosive arthritis, and acrodermatitis chronica atrophicans. Borrelial lymphocytoma is a benign reactive lymphoid hyperplasia that can occur in response to untreated *Borrelia* infections. Usually observed in the early disseminated stage of Lyme disease, it is rarely seen in the United States, as it is more associated with *Borrelia afzelii* and *Borrelia garinii*, which are causative organisms seen in Europe. Acrodermatitis chronica atrophicans, which is typical of chronic Lyme disease infection, is also seen more often in European populations, and is characterized by enlarging, edematous plaques on the distal extremities with a bluish-red hue that evolve into atrophic plaques.[1,23]

ETIOLOGY AND PATHOGENESIS

Erythema migrans occurs at the site of the bite of an *Ixodes* tick carrying a pathogenic strain of *B. burgdorferi*. *Ixodes* ticks acquire *B. burgdorferi* when feeding on an infected host, and the bacteria survive in a protected environment in the tick midgut epithelium because of the presence of surface lipoproteins outer-surface protein (Osp) A and OspB. Infected ticks then transmit *B. burgdorferi* to new hosts through the salivary glands. Another surface protein, OspC is involved in salivary gland invasion and plays an important role in the early colonization and infection of new hosts. OspC is thought to bind to Salp15, a tick salivary protein, which inhibits components of the host immune system.[1]

RISK FACTORS

Risk factors for erythema migrans are largely dependent on human behaviors that increase exposure to infected ticks, such as spending time outdoors in endemic areas and a lack of protective clothing. Other risk factors independent of modifiable behaviors include geographic location and seasonal patterns in tick activity.

DIAGNOSIS

The diagnosis of erythema migrans is made based on clinical presentation, signs and symptoms of Lyme disease, and a history of possible tick exposure. In some cases, laboratory tests and histopathologic examination can help confirm the diagnosis.

LABORATORY TESTING

The Centers for Disease Control and Prevention defines a 2-step process to support the diagnosis of Lyme disease. In the first step, enzyme immunoassay or indirect immunofluorescence assay is performed to detect antibodies. If positive or equivocal, a Western blot analysis is performed, which confirms the diagnosis if positive. Western blot analysis should not be performed without a positive or equivocal antibody test because of the risk for false-positive results.[22]

PATHOLOGY

The histologic features of erythema migrans are similar to those of other gyrate erythemas. Nonspecific findings of mild inflammatory infiltrates composed of lymphocytes and occasional eosinophils and plasma cells can be seen, concentrated around blood vessels. Silver stains such as the Warthin-Starry stain can be used to detect spirochetes in the skin, including *B. burgdorferi*.

DIFFERENTIAL DIAGNOSIS

The differential diagnosis for erythema migrans includes exaggerated arthropod bite reactions, cellulitis, erysipelas, and fixed drug eruptions. Another tick-borne disease, southern tick-associated rash illness, can present with a rash similar to erythema migrans.

CLINICAL COURSE AND PROGNOSIS

Erythema migrans can present with a single lesion or can progress to multiple lesions as the infection with *B. burgdorferi* becomes disseminated. The lesions of erythema migrans often resolve after weeks to months. In the absence of treatment, patients can develop signs and symptoms of early disseminated and chronic disseminated Lyme disease.

MANAGEMENT

MEDICATIONS

Treatment of erythema migrans with appropriate systemic antibiotics in the early stages of Lyme disease usually results in complete resolution. The most common antibiotics used to treat Lyme disease are doxycycline, amoxicillin, and cefuroxime. In disseminated and advanced disease with neurologic or cardiac involvement, intravenous antibiotics may be required. Empiric antibiotic treatment of individuals with tick bites is not recommended, as only 1% of individuals bitten by ticks in endemic areas develop Lyme disease.[1] Prophylaxis with a single dose of doxycycline is indicated to decrease the risk of developing Lyme disease only when the individual is from an endemic area, has been bitten by a tick identified as *I. scapularis*, has had tick attachment for longer than 36 hours, and prophylaxis can be started within 72 hours of tick removal.[22]

ERYTHEMA MARGINATUM

> **AT-A-GLANCE**
>
> - Cutaneous manifestation of rheumatic fever, occurring after pharyngeal infection with group A β-hemolytic streptococcus.
> - One of the major criteria of acute rheumatic fever.
> - Pink lesions that expand centrifugally that favor the trunk, axillae, and extremities, and spare the face.
> - Clinical course is independent of the underlying disease; lesions can persist after treatment of acute rheumatic fever.

Erythema marginatum, also known as erythema marginatum rheumaticum, is an annular, erythematous eruption that was first described in patients with rheumatic fever in 1831. Only seen in a minority of patients with acute rheumatic fever, erythema marginatum is a cutaneous manifestation that is one of the major American Heart Association criteria for rheumatic fever, which include carditis, migratory polyarthritis, Sydenham chorea, erythema marginatum, and subcutaneous nodules. Minor criteria are fever, arthralgias, and abnormal laboratory findings such as elevated erythrocyte sedimentation rate, C-reactive protein, or a prolonged PR interval on echocardiogram. The diagnosis of acute rheumatic fever is made when 2 major or 1 major and 2 minor criteria are met.[24]

EPIDEMIOLOGY

Acute rheumatic fever occurs as a complication of an antecedent pharyngeal infection with group A β-hemolytic streptococcus, seen in approximately 3% of untreated infections. The incidence of erythema marginatum is higher in developing countries, with a mean incidence of 19 cases per 100,000 population. In the United States and developed countries, the incidence of acute rheumatic fever is lower, ranging from 2 to 14 cases per 100,000 population. Although part of the major criteria, erythema marginatum is seen in fewer than 10% of patients with acute rheumatic fever. It occurs more often in children than in adults, with peak age of onset between 5 and 15 years.[25]

CLINICAL FEATURES

CUTANEOUS FINDINGS

Erythema marginatum classically presents as erythematous macules that spread to become annular or polycyclic patches or plaques. As the lesions expand centrifugally, there can be a central area of clearing. The borders of the lesions are often well demarcated. There are usually no epidermal changes present and the lesions are often asymptomatic. Lesions have a predilection for the trunk, axillae, and proximal extremities, and typically spare the face. Individual lesions of erythema marginatum tend to appear and disappear (Fig. 46-5), and may be more evident with hot showers or baths.

Subcutaneous nodules are another cutaneous finding that represents one of the major criteria of acute rheumatic fever. These are small and typically occur over bony prominences such as the wrists, elbows, knees, and ankles. They are seen more in patients with chronic, longstanding disease and are usually painless.

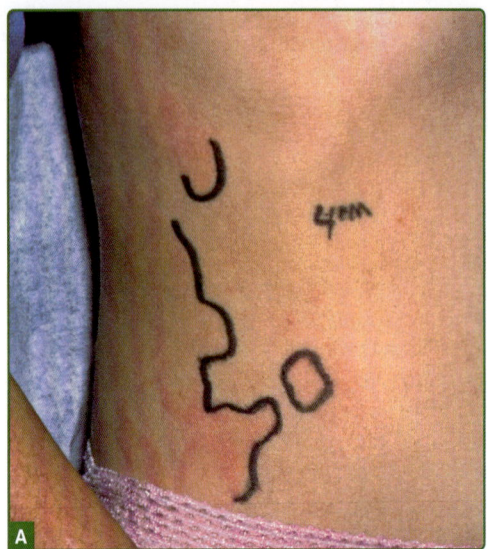
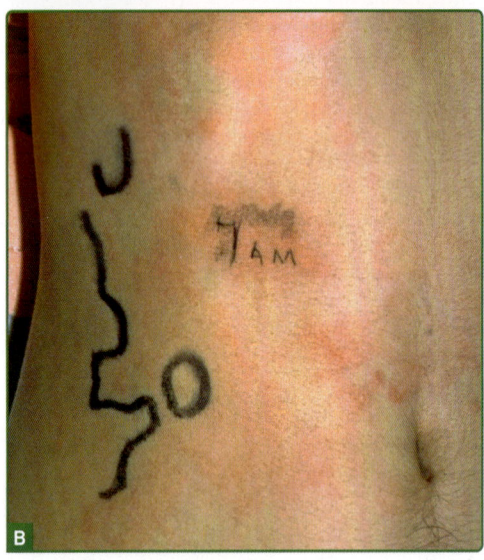

Figure 46-5 The transient nature of erythema marginatum. Polyclinic erythema that "migrated" over several hours. (Used with permission from the Fitzsimmons Army Medical Center Dermatology Archive.)

NONCUTANEOUS FINDINGS

Noncutaneous findings seen in association with erythema marginatum include migratory arthritis (usually involving the large joints), carditis, valvulitis, Sydenham chorea, fever, and arthralgias. In particular, erythema marginatum often occurs in conjunction with acute carditis.[24]

COMPLICATIONS

The complications of erythema marginatum are the sequelae of acute rheumatic fever, the most severe of which is rheumatic heart disease with valvular damage. Up to 50% of patients with carditis at the time of initial presentation go on to develop acquired valvular disease, most often involving calcification of the mitral valve, leading to mitral stenosis. A less-common complication associated with acute rheumatic fever is Jaccoud arthropathy, which is a chronic, painless arthropathy of the hands and feet.[24,25]

ETIOLOGY AND PATHOGENESIS

The exact mechanism by which the cutaneous lesions of erythema marginatum develop in acute rheumatic fever remains unknown. However, the pathogenesis of acute rheumatic fever is multifactorial, with pathogen triggers, molecular mimicry, and host genetic factors playing a role. Epitopes in human myosin, actin, tropomyosin, and other proteins also have been observed cross-reacting with group A streptococcal antigens.[25]

DIAGNOSIS

The diagnosis of erythema marginatum is a clinical one, based on the appearance of typical cutaneous findings and a history of acute rheumatic fever. Performing supportive studies to confirm the diagnosis of acute rheumatic fever can help confirm the diagnosis of erythema marginatum. Because of the nonspecific findings seen on histopathologic examination, skin biopsies do not have much of a role in diagnosing erythema marginatum.

LABORATORY TESTING

The diagnosis of streptococcal pharyngitis can be made through a positive throat culture, positive rapid streptococcal antigen test, or the presence of antistreptococcal antibodies such as antistreptolysin O antibody, antideoxyribonuclease B, streptokinase, and antihyaluronidase. Acute-phase reactants, such as C-reactive protein and erythrocyte sedimentation rate, are usually elevated and are part of the minor diagnostic criteria of acute rheumatic fever.[25]

PATHOLOGY

The histologic findings of erythema marginatum are nonspecific. Biopsy specimens usually demonstrate a patchy interstitial and perivascular infiltrate composed of neutrophils without evidence of vasculitis. Although these findings are not specific to erythema marginatum, a skin biopsy can help differentiate erythema marginatum from other clinical entities.

DIFFERENTIAL DIAGNOSIS

In addition to other gyrate erythemas, the main differential includes annular urticaria, annular erythema of infancy, and neutrophilic figurate erythema of infancy.

CLINICAL COURSE AND PROGNOSIS

Erythema marginatum follows an indolent clinical course that is independent of acute rheumatic fever. Even after the treatment of acute rheumatic fever, lesions of erythema marginatum may persist.

MANAGEMENT

No intervention is necessary for the treatment of erythema marginatum, apart from the treatment of the underlying acute rheumatic fever. Lesions of erythema marginatum are self-limited and eventually resolve spontaneously.

ERYTHEMA GYRATUM REPENS

AT-A-GLANCE

- Usually a paraneoplastic phenomenon.
- Characteristic wood grain appearance with multiple concentric rings.
- Thought to be an immune reaction caused by cross-reaction between tumor and skin antigens.
- Remits with treatment of the underlying malignancy.

Erythema gyratum repens is a figurate erythema with a distinctive clinical appearance that was historically considered to be strictly a paraneoplastic cutaneous phenomenon. Newer studies suggest that erythema gyratum repens can also occur abruptly without cause and in the setting of medication use.

EPIDEMIOLOGY

Erythema gyratum repens is a rare condition, with an unknown incidence. Approximately 70% to 80% of cases are associated with malignancy, with the most common being lung, breast, esophagus, and stomach neoplasms.[26] It is thought to primarily affect adults because of its link to malignancies, thus its distribution in the population, age of onset, and risk factors mirror those for underlying malignancies.

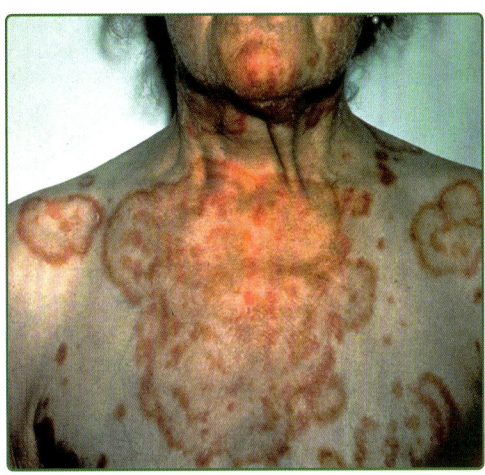

Figure 46-6 Erythema gyratum repens. Multiple annular lesions on a woman with underlying malignancy. (Used with permission from the Fitzsimmons Army Medical Center Dermatology Archive.)

CLINICAL FEATURES

Erythema gyratum repens features multiple, erythematous, annular lesions that advance at a rapid rate of up to 1 cm per day (Fig. 46-6). As the lesions spread, they form concentric rings that impart a "wood-grain" pattern. The epidermis often has a superficial scale at the edges, and patients often complain of pruritus. The onset of the lesions can occur from 1 year before to 1 year after the diagnosis of malignancy. Additional associated cutaneous findings can be seen, which include acquired ichthyosis and palmoplantar keratoderma.[26]

ETIOLOGY AND PATHOGENESIS

The etiology of erythema gyratum repens is not completely known, but it is suggested that it occurs as an immune reaction caused by the cross-reaction between tumor antigens and cutaneous antigens. In some cases, similar deposits of immunoglobulin G and C3 have been identified in the basement membrane zone of the skin and in the associated neoplasm, simultaneously.[27] The responsible antigens have not been identified but studies have shown an accumulation of Langerhans cells in the epidermis in lesions of erythema gyratum repens.

DIAGNOSIS

As a consequence of its distinctive clinical appearance, erythema gyratum repens can usually be diagnosed based on clinical appearance. The presence of a known malignancy can help support clinical suspicion, whereas the new diagnosis of erythema gyratum repens without a known malignancy should prompt the clinician to perform appropriate screening for a possible underlying neoplasm.

PATHOLOGY

Histopathologic features are nonspecific. Common epidermal changes include mild spongiosis, hyperkeratosis, and parakeratosis. Similar to other figurate erythemas, there is often a perivascular infiltrate composed of lymphocytes, histiocytes, and occasional eosinophils.

DIFFERENTIAL DIAGNOSIS

Table 46-2 outlines the differential diagnosis for erythema gyratum repens.

CLINICAL COURSE AND PROGNOSIS

The clinical course and prognosis of erythema gyratum repens parallels the course of the underlying malignancy.

MANAGEMENT

Treatment (Table 46-3) can involve symptomatic relief with topical corticosteroids. Resolution of skin lesions occurs with treatment of the underlying malignancy. In cases of relapse or metastases, erythema gyratum repens can recur.

TABLE 46-2
Differential Diagnosis for Erythema Gyratum Repens

- Figurate erythemas
  - Erythema annulare centrifugum
  - Erythema marginatum
- Erythrokeratoderma variabilis
- Psoriasis
- Pityriasis rubra pilaris
- Tinea corporis
- Tinea imbricate
- Mycosis fungoides
- Bullous pemphigoid
- Linear immunoglobulin A bullous dermatosis

ACKNOWLEDGMENTS

The authors would like to acknowledge Dr. Omar P. Sangueza for the contribution of histologic images to this chapter, and the contributions of Walter H.C. Burgdorf, the former author of this chapter.

REFERENCES

1. Darier J. De l'erythème annulaire centrifuge (erythema papulocirciné migrateur et chronique) et de quelque eruptions analogues. *Ann Dermatol Syphiligr (Paris)*. 1916;6:57-76.
2. Kim DH, Lee JH, Lee JY, et al. Erythema annulare centrifugum: analysis of associated diseases and clinical outcomes according to histopathologic classification. *Ann Dermatol*. 2016;28(2):257-259.
3. Weyers W, Diaz-Cascajo C, Weyers I. Erythema annulare centrifugum: results of a clinicopathologic study of 73 patients. *Am J Dermatopathol*. 2003;25(6):451-462.
4. Kim KJ, Chang SE, Choi JH, et al. Clinicopathologic analysis of 66 cases of erythema annulare centrifugum. *J Dermatol*. 2002;29(2):61-67.
5. Mahood JM. Erythema annulare centrifugum: a review of 24 cases with special reference to its association with underlying disease. *Clin Exp Dermatol*. 1983;8(4):383-387.
6. Kruse LL, Kenner-Bell BM, Mancini AJ. Pediatric erythema annulare centrifugum treated with oral fluconazole: a retrospective series. *Pediatr Dermatol*. 2016;33(5):501-506.
7. Bottoni U, Innocenzi D, Bonaccorsi P, et al. Erythema annulare centrifugum: report of a case with neonatal onset. *J Eur Acad Dermatol Venereol*. 2002;16(5):500-503.
8. Chu CH, Tuan PK, Yang SJ. Molluscum contagiosum-induced erythema annulare centrifugum. *JAMA Dermatol*. 2015;151(12):1385-1386.
9. Ohmori S, Sugita K, Ikenouchi-Sugita A, et al. Erythema annulare centrifugum associated with herpes zoster. *J UOEH*. 2012;34(3):225-229.
10. González-Vela MC, González-López MA, Val-Bernal JF, et al. Erythema annulare centrifugum in a HIV-positive patient. *Int J Dermatol*. 2006;45(12):1423-1425.
11. Chodkiewicz HM, Cohen PR. Paraneoplastic erythema annulare centrifugum eruption: PEACE. *Am J Clin Dermatol*. 2012;13(4):239-246.
12. Mu EW, Sanchez M, Mir A, et al. Paraneoplastic erythema annulare centrifugum eruption (PEACE). *Dermatol Online J*. 2015;21(12).
13. Gönül M, Külcü Çakmak S, Ozcan N, et al. Erythema annulare centrifugum due to pegylated interferon-α-2a plus ribavirin combination therapy in a patient with chronic hepatitis C virus infection. *J Cutan Med Surg*. 2014;18(1):65-68.
14. di Meo N, Stinco G, Fadel M, et al. Erythema annulare centrifugum in the era of triple therapy with boceprevir plus pegylated interferon α-2b and ribavirin for hepatitis C virus infection. *J Cutan Med Surg*. 2015;19(3):203-204.
15. Chou WT, Tsai TF. Recurrent erythema annulare centrifugum during ustekinumab treatment in a psoriatic patient. *Acta Derm Venereol*. 2013;93(2):208-209.
16. Al Hammadi A, Asai Y, Patt ML, et al. Erythema annulare centrifugum secondary to treatment with finasteride. *J Drugs Dermatol*. 2007;6(4):460-463.

TABLE 46-3
Summary for Erythema Annular Centrifugum and Other Figurate Erythemas

	EPIDEMIOLOGY	CLINICAL FEATURES	ETIOLOGY	RISK FACTORS AND ASSOCIATED CONDITIONS	HISTOLOGIC FINDINGS	PROGNOSIS	MANAGEMENT
erythema annular centrifugum (EAC)	Adults in 3rd or 4th decades	Pink papule that expands centrifugally; characteristic annular/polycyclic plaque with central clearing and trailing scale. Deep variants lack prominent scaling	Idiopathic; possibly a hypersensitivity reaction	Infections (dermatophyte), malignancies (non-Hodgkin lymphoma, acute myelogenous leukemia), medications, pregnancy	Dense perivascular infiltrate in a "coat sleeve" pattern	Chronic, with waxing and waning course. May regress spontaneously. Resolution of associated conditions (fungal infection, pregnancy) may lead to improvement	Topical corticosteroids, vitamin D analogs, antihistamines; treatment of underlying fungal infection, if present
Erythema migrans	Bimodal distribution: ages 5-19 years, and 55-69 years; occurs in 70%-80% of individuals infected with Lyme disease	Occurs at initial site of tick bite, with an erythematous expanding annular plaque with central clearing; "bull's-eye" lesion. May progress to multiple lesions	*Borrelia burgdorferi*; hallmark cutaneous finding of early Lyme disease	Dependent on exposure to infected ticks	Nonspecific inflammation; mild lymphocytic infiltrate with occasional eosinophils and plasma cells; Warthin-Starry stain may detect spirochetes	Lesions resolve spontaneously. Untreated Lyme disease can progress to systemic involvement	Doxycycline, amoxicillin, or cefuroxime
Erythema marginatum (also, erythema marginatum rheumaticum)	Children more commonly affected (peaks at age 5-15 years); seen in 3% of untreated group A β-hemolytic streptococcus infections	Erythematous macules that spread to become annular or polycyclic patches or plaques with central clearing. Predilection for trunk, axillae, proximal extremities	Cutaneous manifestation of acute rheumatic fever; molecular mimicry may play a role in cutaneous signs	Group A β-hemolytic streptococcus infection	Nonspecific; patchy interstitial and perivascular infiltrate composed of neutrophils	Indolent course; cutaneous findings are independent of rheumatic heart disease treatment	Acute rheumatic fever should be treated
Erythema gyratum repens	Rare. Adults most commonly affected; 70%-80% associated with malignancies	Multiple, erythematous, annular lesions with rapid rate of growth (1 cm per day). Characteristic "wood-grain" pattern or concentric rings. May be associated with acquired ichthyosis and palmoplantar keratoderma	May be caused by an immune reaction to the cross-reaction between tumor antigens and cutaneous antigens	Malignancies of the lung, breast, esophagus, and stomach	Nonspecific; mild spongiosis, hyperkeratosis, and parakeratosis	Resolves once underlying malignancy is treated. Course parallels underlying malignancy	Topical corticosteroids may provide symptomatic relief

17. Mendes-Bastos P, Coelho-Macias V, Moraes-Fontes MF, et al. Erythema annulare centrifugum during rituximab treatment for autoimmune haemolytic anaemia. *J Eur Acad Dermatol Venereol*. 2014;28(8):1125-1127.
18. García-Doval I, Peteiro C, Toribio J. Amitriptyline-induced erythema annulare centrifugum. *Cutis*. 1999; 63(1):35-36.
19. Chander R, Yadav P, Singh A, et al. Systemic lupus erythematosus presenting as erythema annulare centrifugum. *Lupus*. 2014;23(11):1197-1200.
20. Chiang CH, Lai FJ. Pregnancy-associated erythema annulare centrifugum. *J Formos Med Assoc*. 2015; 114(7):670-671.
21. Senel E, Gulec AT. Erythema annulare centrifugum in pregnancy. *Indian J Dermatol*. 2010;55(1):120-121.
22. Centers for Disease Control and Prevention. *Lyme Disease: Data and Statistics*. 2015. Accessed August 22, 2016. http://www.cdc.gov/lyme/stats/.
23. Bhate C, Schwartz RA. Lyme disease: part I. Advances and perspectives. *J Am Acad Dermatol*. 2011;64(4): 619-636.
24. Mullegger RR. Dermatological manifestations of Lyme borreliosis. *Eur J Dermatol*. 2004;14(5):296-309.
25. Burke RJ, Chang C. Diagnostic criteria of acute rheumatic fever. *Autoimmun Rev*. 2014;13(4-5):503-507.
26. Chakravarty SD, Zabriskie JB, Gibofsky A. Acute rheumatic fever and streptococci: the quintessential pathogenic trigger of autoimmunity. *Clin Rheumatol*. 2014; 33(7):893-901.
27. Rongioletti F, Fausti V, Parodi A. Erythema gyratum repens is not an obligate paraneoplastic disease: a systematic review of the literature and personal experience. *J Eur Acad Dermatol Venereol*. 2014;28(1):112-115.
28. Caux F, Lebbe C, Thomine E, et al. Erythema gyratum repens. A case studied with immunofluorescence, immunoelectron microscopy and immunohistochemistry. *Br J Dermatol*. 1994;131(1):102-107.

Disorders of Cornification

PART 8

第八篇 角化异常性疾病

Chapter 47 :: The Ichthyoses
:: Keith A. Choate & Leonard M. Milstone

第四十七章
鱼鳞病

中文导读

本章分15节：①前言；②分类；③临床表现；④遗传学；⑤病因和发病机制；⑥常用治疗方法；⑦寻常型鱼鳞病；⑧X连锁隐性鱼鳞病；⑨火棉胶婴儿和新生儿（ARCI）表现；⑩常染色体隐性遗传性先天性鱼鳞病；⑪角蛋白鱼鳞病；⑫连接蛋白紊乱；⑬剥脱性皮肤异常；⑭鱼鳞病综合征；⑮获得性鱼鳞病。

第一节前言，讲述了鱼鳞病名称源于希腊语中的horn，并介绍了鱼鳞病通常是由不同基因群的基因突变引起的，有些病例的诊断需要依赖基因检测。

第二节介绍了鱼鳞病的分类方法，本章的分类是2009年的基于遗传和病理生物学描述的分类，主要标准包括疾病是局限于皮肤（非综合征）还是影响皮肤和其他器官系统（综合征）、遗传方式和疾病病理生物学。

第三节介绍了有助于区别不同形式的鱼鳞病的几个表现，如发病年龄、出生时是否有火棉胶膜、是否有红皮病、是否有其他部位异常和附属器结构异常以及其他器官系统的受累。

第四节介绍了鱼鳞病的遗传方式有多种。目前多种产前分子诊断、植入前遗传学诊断已经成为可能。

第五节介绍了遗传性鱼鳞病的遗传学研究，揭示了上皮分化的核心途径，编码功能高度分化的蛋白质的一系列基因突变影响了正常角质形成细胞分化，导致鱼鳞病。但尚不清楚不同的缺陷如何导致相似的表型。

第六节介绍了目前针对遗传性鱼鳞病的治疗主要集中在水化、润滑和角质溶解，并介绍了常用的治疗药物及方法。

第七节至第十五节介绍了寻常型鱼鳞病是最常见的鱼鳞病，病情相对较轻，为常染色体显性遗传，而X连锁隐性鱼鳞病男性发病率为1/（1500~6000），是由类固醇硫酸酯酶缺乏导致。并详细介绍了寻常型鱼鳞病、X连锁隐性鱼鳞病、火棉胶婴儿和新生儿、常染色体隐性遗传性先天性鱼鳞病、角蛋白鱼鳞病、连接蛋白紊乱、剥脱性皮肤异常、鱼鳞病综合征、获得性鱼鳞病的临床表现、病因和发病机制、鉴别诊断、临床病程、预后和治疗。

〔粟　娟〕

AT-A-GLANCE

- The ichthyoses are a heterogeneous group of skin diseases characterized by generalized scaling, and often areas of thickened skin.
- Most types are inherited, and these usually present at birth or appear in childhood; however, some forms are acquired.
- Scales may vary in size, color, and body site.
- The may be accompanied by erythema, abnormalities in adnexal structures, and palmoplantar keratoderma.
- The may be associated with systemic findings, such as failure to thrive, increased susceptibility to infection, atopic dermatitis, neurosensory deafness, and neurologic and other disease.
- Histopathology is usually nonspecific with few notable exceptions.
- Early genetic testing can aid in the diagnosis and anticipation of potential systemic abnormalities.

The hallmark of ichthyosis is scale, which reflects altered differentiation of the epidermis. Because the Greek word for horn (scale) is *keras* and the Latin is *cornu*, in this chapter, the terms *epidermal differentiation*, *keratinization*, and *cornification* are used synonymously. The name *ichthyosis* is derived from the Greek *ichthys*, meaning "fish," and refers to the similarity in appearance of the skin to fish scale. Both inherited and acquired forms are found. Early reports of ichthyosis in the Indian and Chinese literature date back to several hundred years BC, and the condition was discussed by Willan in 1798.[1]

Ichthyosis can present at birth or develop later in life. It can occur as a disease limited to the skin or in association with abnormalities of other organ systems. A number of well-defined types of ichthyosis with characteristic features can be reliably diagnosed. However, because of the great clinical heterogeneity and the profound effect of the environment on scaling, a specific diagnosis can be challenging in certain patients and families without the aid of genetic testing.

INTRODUCTION

This chapter discusses the heterogeneous group of disorders known as the ichthyoses that share the common feature of generalized scaling and most commonly arise at birth or childhood but can be acquired later in life. Ichthyoses commonly result from genetic mutations in a diverse group of genes, including membrane transporters, lipid biosynthesis enzymes, and structural proteins, among many others. Ensuing epithelial barrier compromise, hyperproliferation, and hyperkeratosis become evident as scaling. Associated systemic abnormalities are often attributable to noncutaneous functions of mutant genes.

CLASSSIFICATION OF THE ICHTHYOSES

Siemens introduced genetic concepts into the ichthyoses.[2] Wells and Kerr classified the heritable ichthyoses[3] and separated X-linked recessive ichthyosis from ichthyosis vulgaris (IV).[4] Gassman developed the concept of retention versus hyperproliferation hyperkeratosis.[5] Van Scott, Frost, and Weinstein subsequently proposed a classification of the ichthyoses based on differences in rates of epidermal turnover, characterizing them as either disorders of epidermal hyperproliferation or disorders of prolonged retention of the stratum corneum.[6] Subsequently, Williams and Elias proposed a classification that lists the disorders of cornification in which clinical, genetic, or biochemical data suggest a distinct disease.[7]

Genetic investigation of the ichthyoses has revealed causative mutations in genes relevant to structural proteins, lipid biosynthesis, cell–cell communication, desquamation, and many other pathways and has, in many cases, provided insight into previously unknown determinants of epidermal homeostasis.[8] The advent of whole-exome sequencing (WES) has led to phenotypic expansion, and a new classification of the ichthyoses is evolving based not only on mutant genes but also on specific mutations. Knowing which gene is mutated and what the effects of a given mutation are enables understanding of disease pathobiology. Defining these disorders on the basis of common molecular processes leads to more rational approaches to understanding their pathophysiology and treatment. Inheritance patterns and common clinical features of selected hereditary ichthyoses are shown in Tables 47-1 to 47-3. Grouping these disorders according to the function of encoded proteins (Table 47-4) facilitates understanding of the clinical phenotypes in terms of underlying mechanism. However, further work is necessary to clearly understand how specific mutations result in clinical disease and to develop targeted therapeutic interventions.

In 2009, a consensus conference proposed a revised nomenclature and classification of the ichthyoses, which has replaced commonly used but varied descriptive terms with descriptors based on inheritance and pathobiology.[9] Primary criteria for classification included whether the disorder is limited to the skin (nonsyndromic) or affects the skin and other organ systems (syndromic), its mode of inheritance, and disease pathobiology. Thus, disorders previously referred to as harlequin ichthyosis, lamellar ichthyosis (LI), and congenital ichthyosiform erythroderma became autosomal recessive congenital ichthyosis (ARCI) and bullous ichthyosis, bullous congenital ichthyosiform erythroderma (BCIE), epidermolytic hyperkeratosis, and ichthyosis exfoliativa became epidermolytic ichthyosis (EI), among other updates.[9] Although likely to be further refined in coming years, 2009 consensus nomenclature will be used throughout this chapter.

CLINICAL PRESENTATION

Several features are useful in distinguishing different forms of ichthyosis. These include age of onset, presence of collodion membrane at birth, quality of scale, presence or absence of erythroderma, abnormalities in other parts of the skin (eg, thickened palms and soles, ectropion, eclabium) and adnexal structures (eg, alopecia or hair shaft abnormalities), and involvement of other organ systems. Among distinguishing features, the appearance of the surface of the skin can aid in diagnosis. Visible scaling may be seen in some patients, which can be distinguished by size, configuration, color, and adherence of scale, and there can be thickening of the skin with or without visible scale known as keratoderma. Thickening of the stratum corneum, evident either clinically or histologically, is termed *hyperkeratosis*. Light microscopic features are usually diagnostic in EI and can be helpful in selected ichthyoses (eg, Refsum disease, neutral lipid storage disease, acquired ichthyosis of sarcoidosis, and mycosis fungoides), but histopathologic examination may not be useful to distinguish other ichthyoses.[10] In many cases, the clinical diagnosis may be clarified by genetic analysis, although mutations are not always found. The development of ichthyosis in adulthood may be a marker of systemic disease.

GENETICS

Family history and a multigeneration pedigree may indicate the mode of inheritance. However, many autosomal dominant diseases (eg, EI) have a high frequency of spontaneous (also called *de novo*) mutation. Thus, the lack of a positive family history does not rule out autosomal dominant inheritance. Alternatively, the presence of parental consanguinity may suggest autosomal recessive inheritance. Distinguishing among autosomal dominant, de novo mutation, and autosomal recessive inheritance in pedigrees without prior affected individuals presents a unique clinical challenge in many cases. The advent of WES has permitted ascertainment of inheritance patterns, genetic diagnosis, and gene discovery in many cases.[11,12]

Prenatal molecular diagnosis has become possible. Alternative methods, including fetoscopy and fetal skin biopsy, are limited to later times in pregnancy, harbor a risk of fetal mortality, and are now rarely performed.[13] When it is possible to do prenatal diagnosis by molecular analysis of a fetal sample, it is optimally performed early in pregnancy. This can be done with chorionic villous sampling in the first trimester (10 to 12 weeks after last menstrual period) or by amniocentesis in the second trimester in disorders in which the underlying genetic defect is known and the specific mutation in the family has been identified.[14] Prenatal diagnosis by mutational analysis has been accomplished in a number of the ichthyoses. Preimplantation genetic diagnosis is a reasonable alternative and has been accomplished for many inherited disorders, including ARCI and EI.[15] The procedure requires that the couple undergo in vitro fertilization to obtain embryos. The embryos are then screened by molecular methods to detect the mutation that is segregating in the family. Only embryos that screen negative for the mutation are selected and then can be used for implantation in the uterus to achieve pregnancy. Noninvasive methods of molecular diagnosis (evaluation of fetal DNA circulating in the mother's blood) offer potential for the future.[16,17] For autosomal recessive disorders in which the mutation is known, carrier detection may be performed for at-risk relatives.

TABLE 47-1
Features of Selected Ichthyoses with Dominant Inheritance[a]

DIAGNOSIS	ONSET	CHARACTERISTIC CLINICAL FEATURES	ASSOCIATED FEATURES	GENE	PROTEIN	FUNCTION
Autosomal Semidominant						
Ichthyosis vulgaris (OMIM #146700)	Infancy or childhood	Fine or centrally tacked-down scale with superficial fissuring; relative flexural sparing, worse on lower extremities; hyperlinear palms and soles	Keratosis pilaris; atopy	FLG	Absence of filaggrin	Uncertain—may aggregate keratin filaments and be a precursor to stratum corneum humectants
Autosomal Dominant						
Epidermolytic ichthyosis (OMIM #113800)	Birth	Heterogeneous; may have verrucous, firm, hyperkeratotic (hystrix) spines, often linearly arrayed in flexural creases; blisters; may have erythroderma and/or palmar/plantar keratoderma	Frequent skin infections; characteristic pungent odor	KRT1, KRT10	Keratin 1 or 10	Structural protein abnormality leading to keratin intermediate filament dysfunction—epidermal fragility
Superficial epidermolytic ichthyosis (OMIM #146800)	Birth	Redness and blistering at birth; later develop hyperkeratosis, accentuated over flexures; mauserung (molting): collarette-like lesion where uppermost epidermis has been lost		KRT2	Keratin 2, which is expressed in superficial epidermis	As above for EI
Erythrokeratodermia variabilis (OMIM #133200)						
Generalized type	Birth	Generalized hyperkeratosis and figurate, migratory red patches	Red patches move over minutes to hours; may be triggered by changes in temperature	GJB3, GJB4, GJA	Connexin 30.3, 31, or 43; connexins form gap junction channels between cells	Abnormal intercellular communication
Localized type	Variable	Localized hyperkeratotic plaques with figurate, migratory red patches	Hyperkeratotic plaques may be induced by trauma; considerable intrafamilial variability			
Progressive symmetric erythrokeratoderma (OMIM #602036)	Shortly after birth	Erythematous, scaly plaques, symmetrically distributed over extremities, buttocks, and face; stabilize in early childhood; trunk tends to be spared		LOR, GJB4	Loricrin, connexin 30.3	Cornified envelope precursor, gap junction protein
Keratitis–ichthyosis–deafness (KID) syndrome Recessive has been reported (OMIM #148210)	Birth/infancy	Progressive corneal opacification; either mild generalized hyperkeratosis or discrete erythematous plaques, which may be symmetric; neurosensory deafness	Follicular hyperkeratosis, scarring alopecia, dystrophic nails, susceptibility to infection	GJB2	Connexin 26; connexins form gap junction channels between cells	Abnormal intercellular communication

[a]These are the predominant modes of inheritance.

EI, epidermolytic ichthyosis; OMIM, Online Mendelian Inheritance in Man.

TABLE 47-2
Features of Selected Ichthyoses with X-linked Inheritance[a]

DIAGNOSIS	ONSET	CHARACTERISTIC CLINICAL FEATURES	ASSOCIATED FEATURES	GENE	PROTEIN	FUNCTION
X-linked recessive ichthyosis (OMIM #308100)	Birth or infancy	Fine to large scales; comma-shaped corneal opacities on posterior capsule	Cryptorchidism; female carriers may have corneal opacities and delay of onset or progression of labor in affected pregnancies	STS	Steroid sulfatase	Lipid metabolism—abnormal cholesterol metabolism with accumulation of cholesterol sulfate
Chondrodysplasia punctata X-linked recessive (CDPX; (OMIM #302950)	Birth	May begin as erythroderma, linear or whorled atrophic areas or hyperkeratosis, alopecia, skeletal abnormalities, short stature	Cataracts, deafness	ARSE	Arylsulfatase E	Lipid metabolism—ill defined: failure of hydrolysis of sulfate ester bonds
X-linked dominant chondrodysplasia punctata (Conradi-Hünermann-Happle syndrome) (CDPX2) (OMIM #302960)	Birth	CIE at birth; clears and is replaced by linear hyperkeratosis, follicular atrophoderma and pigmentary abnormalities, and stippled calcifications on radiographs	Occurs almost exclusively in females; hair shaft abnormalities, short stature, cataracts	EBP	EBP, also known as 3β-hydroxysteroid-Δ^{8,7}-isomerase	Lipid metabolism—abnormal cholesterol biosynthesis
CHILD syndrome (OMIM #308050)	Birth	Congenital hemidysplasia, ichthyosiform erythroderma, limb defects	Occurs almost exclusively in females	NSDHL; EBP reported	NSDHL (3 β-hydroxysteroid dehydrogenase); EBP reported	Lipid metabolism—postsqualene cholesterol biosynthesis

[a]These are the predominant modes of inheritance.

CHILD, congenital hemidysplasia with ichthyosiform erythroderma and limb defects; CIE, congenital ichthyosiform erythroderma; EBP, emopamil-binding protein; NSDHL,= NAD(P)H steroid dehydrogenase-like protein; OMIM, Online Mendelian Inheritance in Man.

ETIOLOGY AND PATHOGENESIS

The epidermis undergoes a regular pattern of self-renewal. Its primary cell type, the keratinocyte, undergoes a regular pattern of differentiation to enable the skin to fulfil its role as a barrier to mechanical trauma and desiccation. The end product of differentiation is the stratum corneum, which is composed of terminally differentiated keratinocytes, corneocytes ("bricks"), surrounded by an intercellular matrix ("mortar") (see Chaps. 5 and 14). The corneocyte bricks are protein enriched, and the intercellular mortar is composed of hydrophobic, lipid-enriched membrane bilayers.[7]

The keratin-laden corneocytes are thought to be primarily responsible for the resilience and water retention properties of the stratum corneum, and the matrix forms most of the permeability barrier to water loss. The normal stratum corneum undergoes desquamation in an organized and invisible manner, with individual corneocytes separating from each other and shedding as single cells. Ichthyotic skin has an abnormal quality and quantity of scale, the barrier function of the stratum corneum is compromised, and there may be alterations in the kinetics of epidermal cell proliferation (see Chap. 5). The stratum corneum can be viewed as a compartment, with thickening of the stratum corneum being the result of cells entering the compartment at an increased rate, leaving (corneocyte desquamation) too slowly, or both.

The process of epidermal differentiation is complex and not completely understood. Defects in many different aspects and steps of this process can lead to a similar end result: abnormal stratum corneum and scale. Genetic investigation of inherited ichthyoses has revealed pathways central to epithelial differentiation. For example, mutations in genes that encode the suprabasal epidermal keratins, keratins 1 and 10, cause EI when they affect the highly conserved encoded rod domains necessary for polymerization of keratin intermediate filaments.[18-20] Mutations in the gene encoding transglutaminase-1, an enzyme that catalyzes the cross-linking of proteins and attachment of ceramides during the formation of corneocytes, are found in a large fraction of patients with autosomal recessive congenital ichthyosis.[21-23] Mutations in SPINK5, encoding a serine protease inhibitor, cause

TABLE 47-3
Features of Selected Ichthyoses with Autosomal Recessive Inheritance

DIAGNOSIS	ONSET	CHARACTERISTIC CLINICAL FEATURES	ASSOCIATED FEATURES	GENE	PROTEIN	FUNCTION OR FUNCTIONAL DEFECT
ARCI						
ARCI/LI	Birth; often collodion presentation	Large, platelike, brown scale over most of the body; accentuated on lower extremities; ectropion, eclabium, and alopecia, palmar/plantar involvement varies	Heat intolerance	See Table 47-4	See Table 47-4	See Table 47-4
ARCI/CIE		Fine, white scale; generalized erythroderma; palmar/plantar involvement varies				
Harlequin ichthyosis (OMIM #242500)	Birth	Markedly thickened skin with geometric, deep fissures; at birth survivors develop severe erythroderma	Restricted respiration, feeding; neonatal sepsis; often leads to neonatal death; failure to thrive	ABCA12	ATP-binding cassette, subfamily A, member 12	Lipid metabolism—membrane transport, abnormality of lipid metabolism
Ichthyosis prematurity syndrome (OMIM #608649)	Birth	Premature delivery of infants with erythrodermic, edematous, caseous scaling skin resembling excessive vernix caseosa, evolves into dry, scaly skin with follicular accentuation with signs of atopy	Respiratory distress, and transient peripheral eosinophilia; the respiratory signs resolve	FATP4 (SLC27)	Fatty acid transport protein 4	Lipid metabolism—fatty acid transport
Netherton syndrome (OMIM #256500)	Birth	Ichthyosis linearis circumflexa or similar to congenital ichthyosiform erythroderma; trichorrhexis invaginata	Atopy; high serum levels of IgE; may have aminoaciduria; failure to thrive	SPINK5	LEKTI (a serine protease inhibitor)	Protein metabolism—inhibits degradation of desmosomal proteins and perhaps filaggrin in stratum corneum.
Sjögren-Larsson syndrome (OMIM #270200)	Ichthyosis apparent at birth	Generalized fine to coarse hyperkeratosis; spastic diplegia; mental retardation; retinal glistening white dots	Short stature, seizures	FALDH (ALDH10, ALDH3A2)	Fatty aldehyde dehydrogenase	Lipid metabolism—fatty aldehyde metabolism

(Continued)

TABLE 47-3
Features of Selected Ichthyoses with Autosomal Recessive Inheritance (Continued)

DIAGNOSIS	ONSET	CHARACTERISTIC CLINICAL FEATURES	ASSOCIATED FEATURES	GENE	PROTEIN	FUNCTION OR FUNCTIONAL DEFECT
Refsum disease (OMIM #266500)	Ichthyosis develops years after birth	Progressive neurologic dysfunction; skeletal, cardiac, and renal abnormalities	Retinitis pigmentosa, elevated plasma phytanic acid	Most *PAHX*; *PEX 7* also reported (see RCPD below)	Phytanoyl-CoA hydroxylase (PhyH)	Peroxisome abnormality—deficiency of phytanic acid catabolism; results in phytanic acid accumulation.
Trichothiodystrophy (Tay syndrome; *PIBI(D)S*, *IBI(D)S*, *BI(D)S*) (OMIM #278730, OMIM #601675, OMIM #234050)	Some have ichthyosis, which may be apparent at birth; may have collodion presentation	Brittle hair, photosensitivity, short stature, ichthyosis, intellectual impairment, microcephaly, recurrent infections	Abnormally low sulfur content of hair.	Majority have defect in *ERCC2* (XPD). A few have mutations in *ERCC3* (XPB), *GTF2H5* (TTDA), or *TTDN1*.	Most XPD, XPB, TTDA, or TTDN1 in a few	Components of transcription factor TFIIH
Chanarin–Dorfman syndrome (neutral lipid storage disease; OMIM #275630)	Birth; may have collodion membrane	Generalized scaling, resembles CIE; variable extracutaneous involvement; cataracts, decreased hearing, psychomotor delay.	Severe pruritus; neurologic abnormalities; hepatic abnormalities; lipid droplets in circulating leukocytes	*ABHD5*	Abhydrolase domain-containing protein 5	Lipid metabolism—activates adipose-triglyceride lipase for lipolysis of triglycerides
Neonatal ichthyosis–sclerosing cholangitis syndrome (OMIM #6073718)	Birth	Neonatal cholestatic jaundice, mild ichthyosis with fine, white scales.	Scarring alopecia of the scalp and eyebrows, enamel dysplasia	*CLDN1*	Claudin 1	Abnormal tight junction
Multiple sulfatase deficiency (OMIM #272200)	Birth	Ichthyosis resembling X-linked recessive	Neurologic deterioration; skeletal abnormalities; facial dysmorphism	*SUMF1*	Cα-formylglycine generating enzyme	Generates catalytic residue in active site of eukaryotic sulfatases

ARCI, autosomal recessive congenital ichthyosis; CIE, congenital ichthyosiform erythroderma; IgE, immunoglobulin E; LI, lamellar ichthyosis; OMIM, Online Mendelian Inheritance in Man.

TABLE 47-4
Selected Ichthyoses Organized by Cellular Defect

DISEASE	INHERITANCE	GENE/PROTEIN	DISEASE	INHERITANCE	GENE/PROTEIN
Cytoskeleton					**Snare Protein**
Epidermolysis bullosa simplex	AD	KRT5,14/keratins 5,14	CEDNIK (cerebral dysgenesis, neuropathy, ichthyosis, and keratoderma)	AR	SNAP29/synaptosome associated protein 29
Dowling-Degos disease	AD	KRT5			
Galli-Galli disease	AD	KRT5	ARC (arthrogryposis-renal dysfunction-cholestasis)	AR	VSP33B/vacuolar protein sorting homologue B
Ichthyosis with confetti	AD	KRT10/KRT1			
Epidermolytic ichthyosis	AD	KRT1,10/keratins 1,10			**Metabolic Enzymes**
Ichthyosis bullosa of Siemens	AD	KRT2/keratin 2	X-linked ichthyosis	X-LR	STS/steroid sulfatase
Epidermolytic PPK	AD	KRT9/keratin 9	Tyrosinemia II (Richner-Hanhart)	AR	TAT/tyrosine aminotransferase
Pachyonychia congenita	AD	KRT6A,6B,16,17/keratins 6A,6B,16,17	Sjögren-Larsson	AR	ALDH3A2/fatty aldehyde dehydrogenase
Non-epidermolytic PPK	AD	KRT1, KRT16/keratins 1,16	Refsum	AR	PAXH/phytanoyl CoA hydroxylase
Naxos	AR	JUP/Junctional plakoglobin	Conradi-Hunermann	X-LD	EBP/3β-hydroxysterol δ7-isomerase
White sponge nevus	AD	KRT4,13/keratins 4,13			
Ichthyosis vulgaris	AD	FLG/filaggrin	CHILD (congenital hemidysplasia, ichthyosiform erythroderma and limb defects)	X-LD	EBP/3β-hydroxysterol δ7-isomerase NSDHL/ NAD(P) dependent steroid dehydrogenase-like
Cornified Envelope					
Lamellar ichthyosis	AR	TGM1/transglutaminase 1			
Bathing suit ichthyosis	AR	TGM1 temperature-sensitive mutation			
Keratoderma (Camissa)	AD	LOR/loricrin	Gaucher	AR	GBA/glucocerebrosidase B
Generalized peeling skin disease	AR	CDSN/corneodesmosin	Chanarin-Dorfman (neutral lipid storage)	AR	ABHD5/(CGI-58)
Membrane Transporters					
Darier disease	AD	ATP2A2/SERcalciumATPase	Neutral lipid storage with myopathy	AR	PNPLA2/patatin-like phospholipase domain-containing protein
Acrokeratosis verruciformis	AD	ATP2A2/SERcalciumATPase			
Hailey-Hailey disease	AD	ATP2C1	Autosomal recessive congenital ichthyosis	AR	ALOXE3/lipoxygenase 3 ALOX12B/12(R)-lipoxygenase E3 NIPAL4/magnesium transporter NIPA4 CYP4F22/cytochrome P450 family 4 subfamily F member 22 PNPLA1/patatin like phospholipase domain containing 1, CERS3/ceramide synthase 3, SDR9C7/short chain dehydrogenase/reductase family 9C, member 7, SULT2B1/sulfotransferase family 2B member 1
Ichthyosis with sclerosing cholangitis	AR	CLDN1/claudin-1			
Lamellar	AR	ABCA12			
Harlequin	AR	ABCA12			
Ichthyosis prematurity syndrome	AR	FATP4			
Cell Junction Proteins					
PPK with deafness (Vohwinkel)	AD	GJB2/Connexin 26			
Erythrokeratoderma variabilis	AD	GJB3/Connexin 31 GJB4/Connexin30.3			
Keratitis–ichthyosis–deafness (KID)	AD	GBJ2/Connexin 26			
Nonepidermolytic PPK (striate)	AD	DSP/desmoplakin			
	AR	DSP/desmoplakin	Self-improving collodion ichthyosis	AR	ALOX12B and ALOXE3
	AD	DSG1/desmoglein 1			

(Continued)

TABLE 47-4
Selected Ichthyoses Organized by Cellular Defect (*Continued*)

DISEASE	INHERITANCE	GENE/PROTEIN	DISEASE	INHERITANCE	GENE/PROTEIN
		Protease/Protease Inhibitors			**Secreted Proteins**
Papillon-Lefevre keratoderma	AR	*CTSC*/cathepsin C	Mal de Meleda keratoderma	AR	*SLURP1*/secreted Ly6/UPAR related protein 1
Ichthyosis linearis circumflexa (Netherton)	AR	*SPINK5*/serine protease inhibitor 5			**DNA Repair and Transcription**
			Trichothiodystrophy	AR	*ERCC2*/excision repair cross-complementation group 2
Ichthyosis follicularis/photophobia (IFAP)	X-LR	*MBTPS2*/membrane bound transcription factor peptidase, site 2			*GTF2H5*/general transcription factor IIH subunit 5
ARCI with hypotrichosis	AR	*ST14*/matriptase			*GTF2E2*/general transcription factor IIE subunit 2
		Proteasome			*ERCC3*/excision repair cross-complementation group 3
KLIK (keratosis linearis with ichthyosis congenita and sclerosing keratoderma)	AR	*POMP*/proteasome maturation protein			

AD, autosomal dominant; AR, autosomal recessive; ARCI, autosomal recessive congenital ichthyosis; CHILD, *congenital hemidysplasia, ichthyosiform erythroderma, and limb defects*; PPK X-LD, X-linked dominant; X-LR, X-linked recessive.

Netherton syndrome and confirm a role for proteolysis and protease inhibitors in normal epidermal differentiation.[24] Finally, mutations in *FLG* result in reduced or absent filaggrin and decreased moisture binding in the stratum corneum of patients with IV.[25] These cardinal examples highlight the observation that mutations in a host of genes encoding proteins with highly divergent functions affect normal keratinocyte differentiation and cause ichthyosis. It is yet unknown how defects in diverse processes result in similar phenotypes, although studies suggest that defects in the barrier may result in inflammation and hyperproliferation.[26,27] Furthermore, our evolving understanding of these mechanisms continues to clarify the multisystem, clinical phenotypes observed in several ichthyosiform disorders.

COMMON THERAPEUTIC APPROACHES

Current therapies for the inherited ichthyoses are symptomatic and focus on hydration, lubrication, and keratolysis.[28,29] Ichthyotic skin, even if thickened, has a decreased barrier function and increased transepidermal water loss. Because pliability of the stratum corneum is a function of its water content, hydration can soften the surface of the skin. In moist, humid climates, most ichthyoses improve. Moistening the skin with, for example, long baths can hydrate it. Well-hydrated areas of hyperkeratosis can more easily be thinned with mild abrasives (eg, sponges, buff puffs, pumice stones). Addition of bath oils or application of lubricants before drying can prolong the hydration and softening. Depending on the ichthyosis and environmental conditions, individual patients may prefer specific lubricating agents, which can take the form of lotions, creams, oils, ointments, or petrolatum. In dry climates and winter months, humidifiers can be used to create a more hospitable environment.

Keratolytic agents are used to enhance corneocyte desquamation and thereby remove scale and thin hyperkeratotic stratum corneum. There are many commercially available keratolytic creams and lotions containing urea, salicylic acid, or α-hydroxy acids (eg, lactic acid, glycolic acid). Urea may function by its capacity to bind water. Propylene glycol (40%–60% in water), with or without occlusion, can also be effective in scale removal. Occlusion can effectively increase skin hydration and facilitate desquamation; it can also enhance the effect of keratolytic agents. Special care should be taken when using extensive areas of occlusion with keratolytic agents and in individuals who may be heat intolerant. The markedly impaired barrier function in ichthyosis should be considered when using topical preparations over large areas of body surface. For example, widespread use of topical salicylic acid preparations can lead to significant absorption, intoxication (eg, nausea, tinnitus, dyspnea, hallucinations), and even death.[30] Children are at greater risk because they have a greater body surface area per unit weight than adults, a situation that effectively heightens the possibility of developing systemic toxicity from topicals. Although the use of topical retinoids in most of the ichthyoses appears to be safe,[31] the abnormal skin barrier should be considered when treating concomitant dermatoses in patients with ichthyosis. When using topical agents such as tacrolimus, pimecrolimus, or topical steroids, when increased systemic absorption has been observed, monitoring of serum levels may be necessary.[32]

Another risk to children is that in several types of ichthyosis nutritional requirements may be high, and inadequate nutrition can lead to failure to thrive. This was thought to be related to the large turnover of scale; however, recent studies suggest energy loss from impaired barrier function is the cause.[33]

Some patients with ichthyosis have decreased sweating with heat intolerance. It is important for the parents of a newborn with ichthyosis to be aware of the possibility of decreased sweating and to be attentive for signs of heat intolerance, such as flushing and lethargy, particularly during hot weather and, as the child grows, during exercise. Avoiding hot environments, carrying spray bottles with water to moisten the skin and cool it through evaporation, and cooling vests can minimize heat stress.

Systemic retinoid therapy with isotretinoin or acitretin (see Chap. 185) can induce dramatic improvement in many ichthyoses. The decision to initiate systemic retinoid therapy should be weighed carefully because after the drug is started, continued benefit usually requires chronic therapy. Retinoic acid metabolism–blocking agents, which increase endogenous retinoid levels, offer a possible alternative.[34]

Fungal infections are common, both of skin and nails, and are often undiagnosed because of the generalized scaling. A high index of suspicion can help diagnose tinea corporis, capitis, or versicolor when the only symptom may be localized pruritus (which is often intense) and the only sign a difference in the character of scale or a localized area of alopecia.

ICHTHYOSIS VULGARIS

Ichthyosis vulgaris (Online Mendelian Inheritance in Man [OMIM] #146700), the most common ichthyosis, is relatively mild. The disease was thought to be autosomal dominant, and a study of English school children found that 1 in 250 were affected.[4] Mutations in the gene encoding profilaggrin cause IV.[25] Profilaggrin contains multiple copies of filaggrin, which has various structural and biochemical functions during cornification. The inheritance pattern has been clarified to be semidominant; individuals who carry one mutated allele have a mild phenotype, but those with mutations in both profilaggrin alleles (homozygotes or compound heterozygotes for the mutations) (Fig. 47-1) manifest a severe clinical phenotype. In the Anglo-European population, the prevalence of clinical disease is as high as 1 in 80.[35,36]

CLINICAL FEATURES

Although infants usually have normal skin, the disease often manifests within the first year of life. The scale of IV is usually most prominent on the extensor surfaces of the extremities, with flexural sparing. The diaper area tends to be spared. There may be fine, white scales over large areas. Particularly on the lower extremities, which are often the most severely involved area, the scales may be centrally attached, with "cracking" (superficial fissuring through the stratum corneum) at the edges. This turning up at the edges can lead to the skin feeling rough.

ETIOLOGY AND PATHOGENESIS

Filaggrin is an epidermal protein involved in the aggregation of keratin intermediate filaments,[37] is an important component of the cornified envelope,[38] and helps retain moisture in the stratum corneum. Keratin filaments form a network, or cell matrix, that gives structural integrity to the epidermal keratinocytes. As keratinocytes mature into corneocytes, the keratin filaments collapse and are cross-linked to the cornified cell envelope. Filaggrin is synthesized as a high-molecular-weight precursor, profilaggrin, that contains multiple filaggrin molecules and is localized to keratohyalin granules. Biochemical studies of epidermis from patients with IV have shown absence of or decrease in filaggrin and its precursor, profilaggrin.[39,40] The association between IV and atopic dermatitis has been long appreciated on clinical grounds. Null mutations in the gene encoding profilaggrin (*FLG*) have now been shown to be a strong predisposing factor for atopic dermatitis in the Anglo-European population. A strong association is also found with individuals who have sensitivity to common allergens, allergic rhinitis, early-onset and persistent eczema, and asthma in the presence of atopic dermatitis.[35,41]

DIFFERENTIAL DIAGNOSIS

In some cases, it is difficult to distinguish mild IV from simple dry skin (xerosis). Evolving understanding of this very common condition is beginning to clarify how a spectrum of underlying mutations can cause the diverse clinical severity of dry skin from xerosis to severe IV. In addition, on the basis of skin findings alone, males with severe IV may be difficult to differentiate from those affected with X-linked recessive ichthyosis.[42,43] The histopathologic findings of IV are variable, and the characteristic orthohyperkeratosis and absent granular layer may only be seen in individuals with two abnormal alleles.

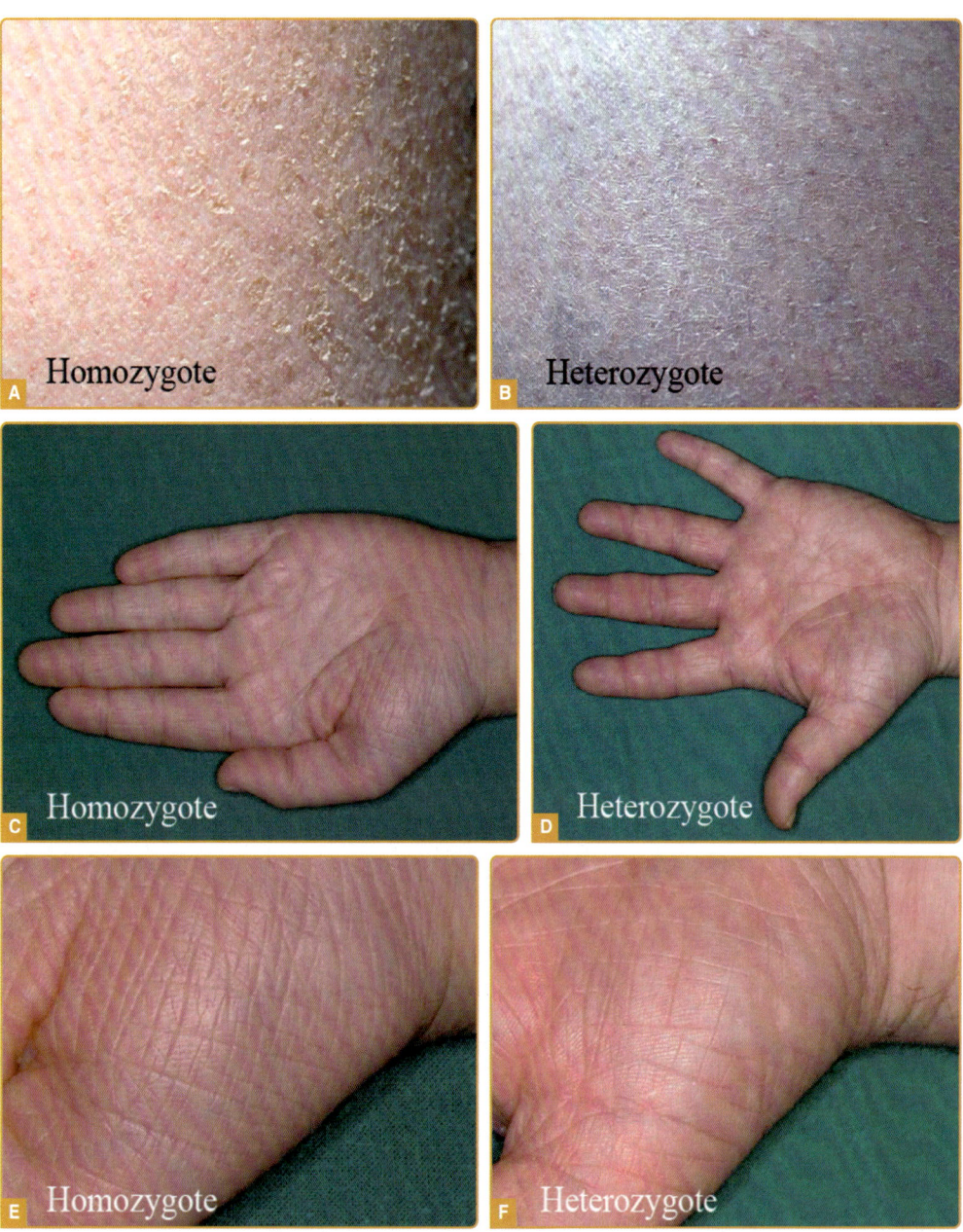

Figure 47-1 A–F, Ichthyosis vulgaris (*FLG* mutation). Small, centrally adherent scales generally spare intertriginous areas. Increased number and depth of palmar markings are usually noted.

CLINICAL COURSE, PROGNOSIS, AND MANAGEMENT

A number of other findings are commonly observed in association with IV.[42] Hyperlinear palms are usually present, and some patients may have palmar/plantar thickening approaching a keratoderma. Keratosis pilaris is common, even in individuals with mild IV, and usually involves the outside of the arms, extensor thighs, and buttocks. Even though IV is usually not considered a syndromic ichthyosis, atopy is also frequently observed and can manifest as hay fever, eczema, or asthma. These findings can confound an accurate diagnosis because hyperlinear palms and keratosis pilaris may be seen in atopic individuals who do not have IV. Rarely, individuals with IV may have hypohidrosis with heat intolerance. There is great variation in the severity of clinical manifestations among affected individuals in the same family. The condition usually worsens in climates that are dry and cold and improves in warm, humid environments, where the disease may clear dramatically. Most patients respond well to regular application of emollients, and use of α-hydroxy acids can reduce scaling when present.

X-LINKED RECESSIVE ICHTHYOSIS

In the 1960s, *X-linked recessive ichthyosis* (OMIM #308100) was distinguished clinically from other ichthyoses.[4] X-linked recessive ichthyosis occurs in approximately 1 in 1500 to 6000 males.[5,44] Steroid sulfatase (arylsulfatase C) deficiency causes XLI;[45,46] in 90% of cases, genetic deletion of the *STS* locus is causative.[47] The remainder are point mutations in *STS*.

CLINICAL FEATURES

Scaling may begin in the newborn period and is usually most prominent on the extensor surfaces, although there is significant involvement of the flexural areas. Although the extent and degree of scaling are variable, X-linked ichthyosis can usually be distinguished from IV on clinical criteria and inheritance pattern.[5,48] The latter tends to be associated with hyperlinear palms and soles, keratosis pilaris, and a family history of atopy. X-linked ichthyosis tends to have more severe involvement with larger scale (Fig. 47-2), and comma-shaped, corneal opacities may be present in half of adult patients.[49,50] Corneal opacities do not affect vision and may be present in female carriers. Affected males have an increased risk of cryptorchidism, and independently, they are at increased risk for the development of testicular cancer.[51]

ETIOLOGY AND PATHOGENESIS

Steroid sulfatase hydrolyzes sulfate esters, which include cholesterol sulfate and sulfated steroid hormones.[52] Sulfated fetal adrenal hormones undergo desulfation to estrogens, which are excreted in maternal urine. The absence of steroid sulfatase enzyme in the fetal placenta leads to low maternal urinary estrogens, and in some pregnancies, to a failure of labor to initiate or to progress normally. In males with X-linked recessive ichthyosis, steroid sulfatase enzyme activity is decreased or absent in many tissues, including epidermis, stratum corneum, leukocytes, and in cultured fibroblasts.[53] Carrier females have been found to have leukocyte steroid sulfatase levels intermediate between those observed in normal individuals and those in affected males.

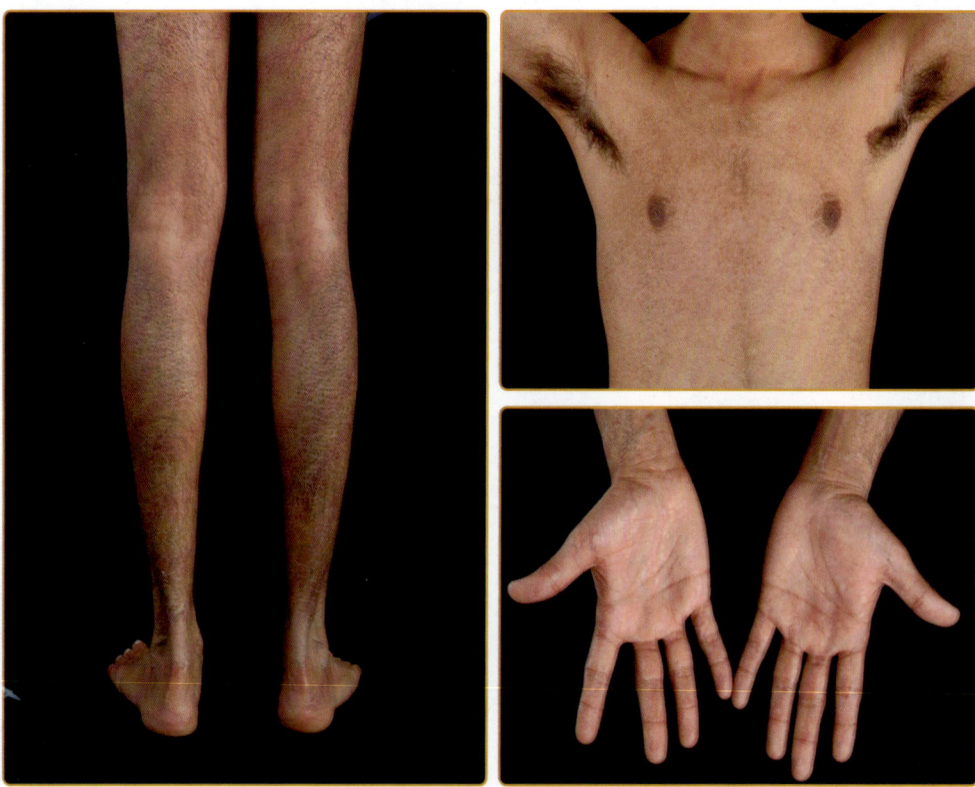

Figure 47-2 X-linked recessive ichthyosis (*STS* mutation). Small, centrally adherent, dark scales often involve sides of neck and face; they are less severe in flexures. Palms and soles show little to no involvement.

Cholesterol sulfate levels are elevated in the serum, epidermis, and scale.[54] Steroid sulfatase is one of a group of arylsulfatases located on chromosome Xp22. More than 90% of the mutations in X-linked ichthyosis are deletions that can often be detected by fluorescence in situ hybridization (FISH) or array-comparative genomic hybridization (CGH), available in many clinical laboratories. Confirmation of the diagnosis can also be made by finding an elevation in serum cholesterol sulfate levels.

In the epidermis, steroid sulfatase catalyzes the hydrolysis of cholesterol sulfate. Topical application of cholesterol sulfate in mice can induce a scaling disorder, further supporting the role of cholesterol sulfate hydrolysis in corneocyte desquamation. Cholesterol sulfate inhibits the proteases that degrade corneodesmosomes, resulting in inhibition of desquamation and a retention hyperkeratosis.[55]

DIAGNOSIS

Skin and eye findings, history of prolonged labor, and evidence of X-linked transmission enable diagnosis of XLI.[45,56] Notably, a significant fraction of patients now are recognized in utero through maternal screening that assesses levels of α-fetoprotein, human chorionic gonadotropin, and estriol. Because steroid sulfatase is necessary for placental estrogen production, triple screen results indicating low estriol are present in XLI pregnancies.[47] Because the majority of maternal urinary estrogens are derived from the fetal adrenal glands and are metabolized by the placenta, low levels can reflect fetal abnormalities or death, raising concern in parents. However, in XLI, low levels do not indicate severe fetal morbidity. Although skin biopsy is rarely done, histopathologic examination shows compact orthohyperkeratosis, acanthosis, papillomatosis, and a thickened granular layer. Many assays are available for the diagnosis of XLI, including FISH for *STS*, array-CGH, deletion and point mutation detection via next-generation sequencing, and enzymatic assays of steroid sulfatase function.

CLINICAL COURSE, PROGNOSIS, AND MANAGEMENT

Although in most cases, XLI is primarily a cutaneous disorder, genetic deletions that include *STS* and adjacent sulfatases explain the overlap syndromes involving chondrodysplasia punctata and X-linked ichthyosis.[57] The X-linked form of Kallmann syndrome, in which hypogonadotropic hypogonadism and anosmia are found, often with renal abnormalities, obesity, synkinesis (mirror image movements of the extremities), cleft palate, and spastic paraplegia, can also be seen in association with X-linked recessive ichthyosis as part of a contiguous gene deletion syndrome. Because of this and because of the association with testicular carcinoma, patients with X-linked recessive ichthyosis should be queried about anosmia and have periodic testicular examination.[44,58]

When scaling is prominent, long bathwater soaks with or without bicarbonate can aid in desquamation.[59] Emollients, including those with α-hydroxy acids or lactic acid, can aid in desquamation.

COLLODION BABY AND NEWBORN PRESENTATIONS

Most cases of ichthyosis, excluding IV and X-linked ichthyosis, present at birth with red, scaly skin. In the United States, the incidence of such cases is estimated to be 5 to 10 per 100,000 live births.[60] A fraction of these present with a collodion membrane, which is shed early in life with features of congenital ichthyosis or normal skin subsequently developing. Genotype is not the sole determinant of collodion baby presentation because many with the common genotypes associated with collodion membranes present with simply red scaly skin. No differences in the pathogenesis of these two newborn presentations of ichthyosis have been identified, and management is generally similar for both.

CLINICAL FEATURES

A *collodion baby* is born encased in a translucent, parchment-like membrane that is taut and may impair respiration and sucking. Birth can be premature, contributing to morbidity. During the first 2 weeks of life, the membrane breaks up and peels off and can leave fissures, with impairment of the barrier to infection and water loss (Fig. 47-3).

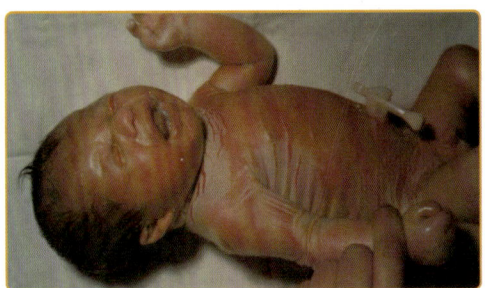

Figure 47-3 Collodion infant. The infant is 36 hours old and is covered with a macerated membrane that shows fissures; note ectropion and eclabium. The condition may develop over time into various clinical phenotypes, including autosomal recessive congenital ichthyosis and self-healing collodion baby.

TABLE 47-5
Disorders Associated with Collodion Membrane

Common
- Autosomal recessive congenital ichthyosis (lamellar ichthyosis, congenital ichthyosiform erythroderma, overlap)

Rare
- Ankyloblepharon-ectodermal dysplasia-cleft lip/palate (AEC) syndrome
- Chondrodysplasia punctata
- Gaucher disease
- Loricrin keratoderma
- Neutral lipid storage disease
- Self-healing collodion baby
- Sjögren–Larsson syndrome
- Trichothiodystrophy
- X-linked hypohidrotic ectodermal dysplasia

ETIOLOGY AND PATHOGENESIS

The in utero aqueous environment contributes to the development of the collodion presentation, which transforms into a wide spectrum of ichthyosis phenotypes as the child grows (Table 47-5). This is the usual presentation of ARCI and is less commonly seen in several other forms of ichthyosis and rarely Gaucher disease. In addition, an autosomal recessive, self-healing collodion phenotype has been described, in which the skin greatly clears within the first few weeks and transitions into mildly affected or normal skin.[61] Eleven Swedish and four Danish patients with a self-improving ichthyosis resulting in xerosis, hyperlinear palms, red cheeks, and anhidrosis were found to have mutations in *ALOX12B*, *ALOX3E*, or *TGM1*.[62]

CLINICAL COURSE, PROGNOSIS, AND MANAGEMENT

In caring for a collodion infant or other newborn with ichthyosis, consideration of a potentially increased risk of infection, difficulties in thermal regulation, and hypernatremic dehydration caused by increased transepidermal water loss is essential.[63] Newborn care should include careful monitoring for infection and of temperature, hydration, and electrolytes and measures to keep the peeling membrane soft and lubricated to facilitate flexibility and desquamation. Appropriate pain management and eye care should be used when indicated. These newborns usually benefit from a humidified incubator where the air is saturated with water; wet compresses followed by bland lubricants can be used to further hydrate the membrane and achieve maximum pliability.[64] Before spontaneous peeling of the collodion membrane, the thickened stratum corneum can dry and harden in areas such as the extremities and can constrict, leading to distal swelling, cyanosis, and rarely necrosis in some cases. Release of constricting bands via curettage or debridement can prevent complications.[65]

AUTOSOMAL RECESSIVE CONGENITAL ICHTHYOSIS

The term *autosomal recessive congenital ichthyosis* is used to describe a heterogeneous group of disorders that present at birth with generalized involvement of the skin. Autosomal recessive ichthyosis is rare and has been estimated to occur in about 1 in 300,000 persons.[5]

In older literature, *nonbullous congenital ichthyosiform erythroderma* (NCIE, also called *lamellar ichthyosis*, with autosomal recessive inheritance) was distinguished from BCIE (also called epidermolytic hyperkeratosis [EHK], with autosomal dominant inheritance) based on clinical appearance (bullae) and pattern of inheritance.[6,66] That the term LI was used interchangeably with NCIE and included a spectrum of phenotypes has led to some confusion. We also now understand that genotype alone does not determine whether the phenotype will be LI or CIE. Williams and Elias distinguished LI from NCIE (usually called *congenital ichthyosiform erythroderma*), a milder erythrodermic form, and these descriptors remain useful clinical descriptors in clinical practice.[67] In LI, one sees large, dark, platelike scales, and although infants may be red at birth, adults have little to no erythroderma (Figs. 47-4 to 47-6). In the more severe, classic presentation of LI, tautness of the facial skin leads to traction on the eyelids and lips, resulting in ectropion and eclabium. Scarring alopecia, most prominent at the periphery of the scalp, may be partly caused by traction at the hairline. In contrast, CIE has generalized redness and fine, white scales (eg, Figs. 47-7 and 47-9). Patients with classic CIE have little to no ectropion, eclabium, or alopecia. However, many patients do not fit neatly into these two clinical descriptions[68] in that they have features of both LI and CIE with a clinical phenotype intermediate between both disorders. Therefore, it can be useful to consider these two distinctive presentations as ends of a spectrum, between which lie a gradation of clinical phenotypes with variable degrees of erythema and coarseness of scale. Individual features such as collodion membrane (discussed earlier), ectropion, and alopecia can occur across the spectrum. Although attempts to refine the categorization of these disorders by biochemical and ultrastructural observations have failed to yield a consistent and replicable classification scheme, identification of the spectrum of specific molecular defects underlying these conditions may aid classification.[8] Identification of mutations has, so far, found ARCI to be caused by 10 different genes that are important for the formation of the intercellular lipid layer or the cornified envelope of keratinocytes, including *TGM1* (OMIM #191995), *ALOX12B*

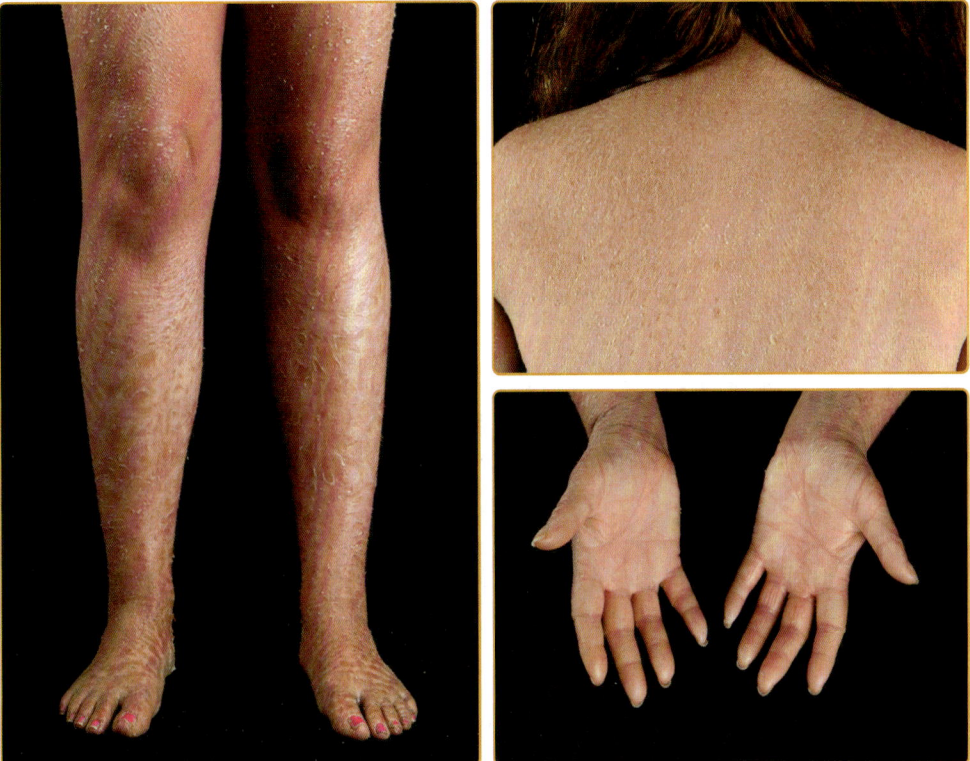

Figure 47-4 Autosomal recessive congenital ichthyosis (*TGM1* mutations, classic lamellar ichthyosis, moderate). Large dark scales are often most obvious over extensor extremities and forehead. Mild to moderate erythema and palmar-plantar keratoderma are usual. The severity of scale varies widely (see Fig. 47-6).

(OMIM #603741), *ALOXE3* (OMIM #607206), *NIPAL4* (OMIM #609383), *CYP4F22* (OMIM #611495), *ABCA12* (OMIM #607800), *PNPLA1* (OMIM #612121), *CERS3* (OMIM #615276), *SDR9C7* (OMIM #609767), and *SULT2B1* (OMIM #604125).

CLINICAL FEATURES

LAMELLAR ICHTHYOSIS PHENOTYPE

The LI phenotype of ARCI is apparent at birth, and the newborn usually presents encased in a collodion membrane (see Fig. 47-3). At this time, the skin may be red. Over time, the skin develops large, platelike scales, and most are centrally attached with raised borders. The scales tend to be largest over the lower extremities, where the large, platelike scales separated by superficial fissuring can lead to an appearance similar to that of a dry riverbed. During childhood and into adulthood, the degree of erythema may vary. Involvement of the palms and soles in LI is variable and ranges from minimal hyperlinearity to severe keratoderma. This phenotype is most often associated with mutations in *TGM1*, but even mutations in one gene result in a highly variable phenotype (see Figs. 47-4 to 47-6).

The lips and mucous membranes tend to be spared in LI, but the adnexal structures may be compromised by the adherent, firm scales. Thick stratum corneum on the scalp tends to encase hairs and in conjunction with the tautness of the skin may lead to a scarring alopecia, most marked at the periphery of the scalp. Hyperkeratosis interferes with normal sweat gland function, resulting in hypohidrosis, but the degree of impairment varies between patients. Some patients have severe heat intolerance and must be vigilant to avoid overheating.

Bathing suit ichthyosis is a subtype of LI in which affected individuals develop the scaling typical of LI but limited to the bathing suit area. The distribution correlates with warmer areas of skin. Decreased transglutaminase is found in these areas, and unique, temperature-sensitive mutations in *TGM1* have been identified in affected individuals.[69-72]

CONGENITAL ICHTHYOSIFORM ERYTHRODERMA PHENOTYPE

As with LI, the CIE phenotype of ARCI is apparent at birth, and the newborn usually presents with a taut, shiny, collodion membrane. After shedding of

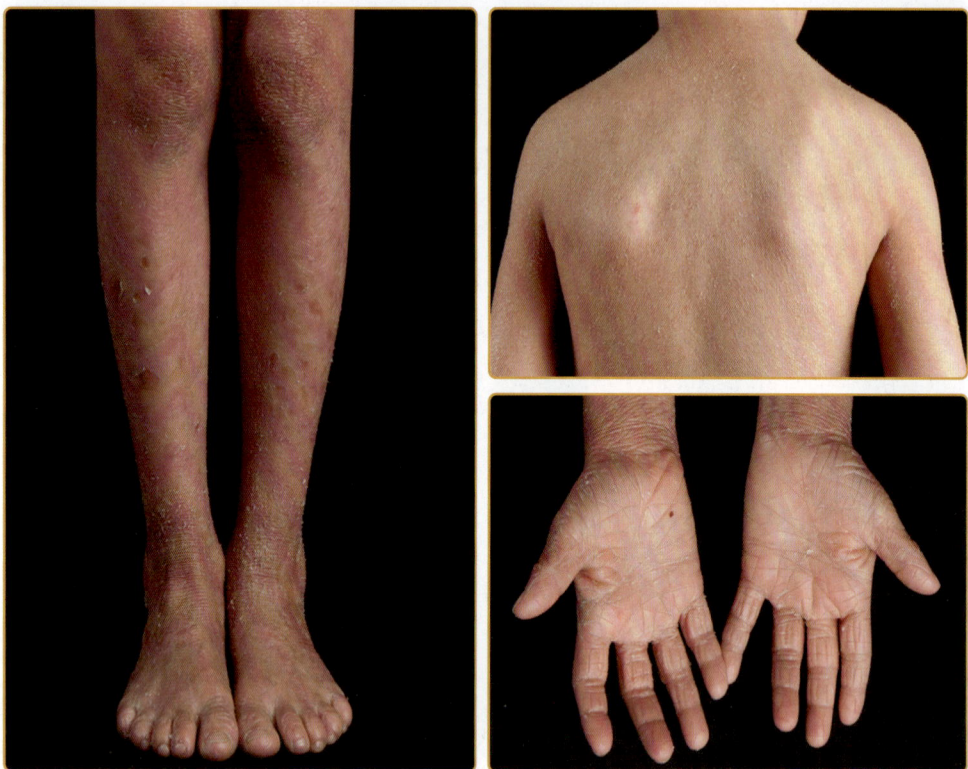

Figure 47-5 Autosomal recessive congenital ichthyosis (*TGM1* mutations, classic lamellar ichthyosis, mild). Large dark scales are often most obvious over extensor extremities and forehead. Mild to moderate erythema and palmar-plantar keratoderma are usual. Severity of scale varies widely (see Fig. 47-4).

the membrane, the skin of infants with CIE remains red, usually with a fine, white, generalized scale (see Figs. 47-7 and 47-8). On the lower legs, the scale may be larger and darker. In contrast to LI, the classic presentation of CIE may have little to no ectropion, eclabium, or alopecia. As in LI, there is a wide variation in the ability to sweat, and patients with CIE may have minimal sweating with severe heat intolerance. Mucous membranes are usually spared. Palm and sole involvement is variable. Nails may have ridging, but they are often spared. As with all the ichthyoses, dermatophyte infection of the skin and nails is common.

HARLEQUIN ICHTHYOSIS PHENOTYPE

A dramatic, severe, and sometimes fatal presentation of ichthyosis is that of *harlequin ichthyosis* (OMIM #242500) (Fig. 47-9). The child is often

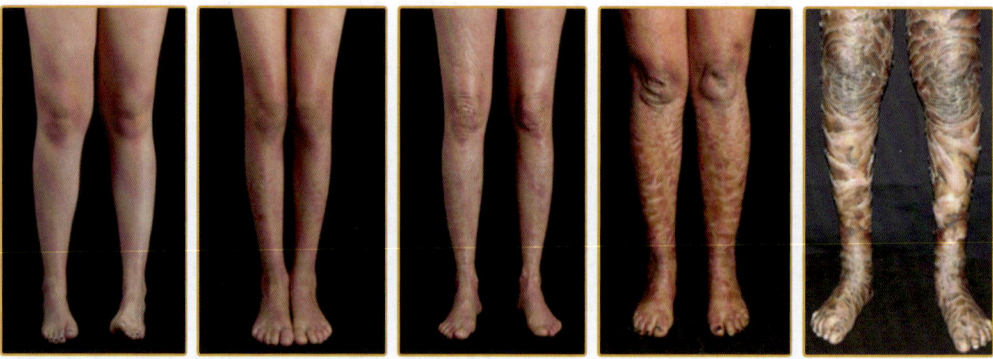

Figure 47-6 Severity spectrum for mutations in *TGM1*. Phenotypic variability is seen across individuals with the same mutation.

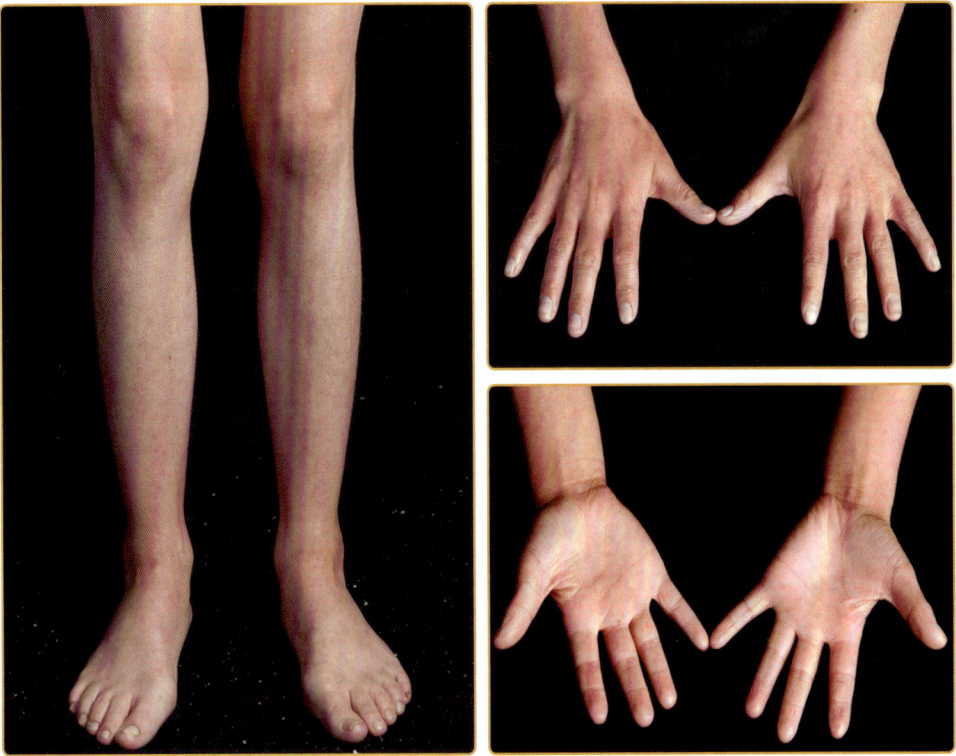

Figure 47-7 Autosomal recessive congenital ichthyosis (*ALOXE3* mutations). The volar and dorsal surfaces of hands and feet show exaggerated linear markings. Scale elsewhere, when present, is fine and white and overlies mild erythema.

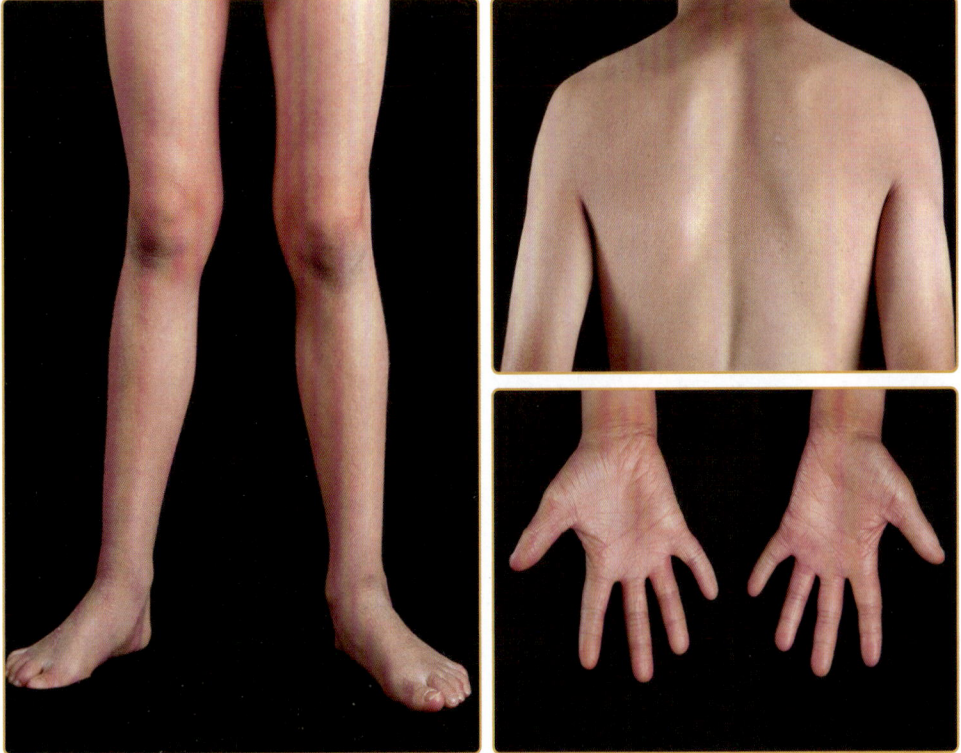

Figure 47-8 Autosomal recessive congenital ichthyosis (*ALOX12B* mutations). The volar and dorsal surfaces of hands and feet show increased linear markings. Scale elsewhere, when present, is fine and white and overlies mild erythema.

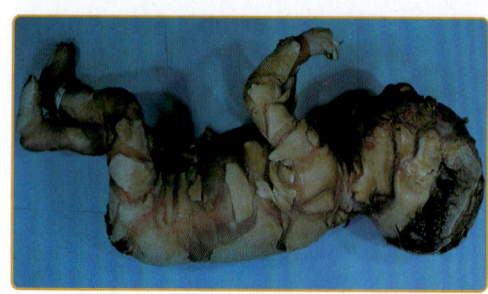

Figure 47-9 Harlequin infant. Harlequin ichthyosis. Note the rudimentary ears and the distorted appearance as a result of the thick "plates" of stratum corneum. This infant died a few days after birth.

premature and born with thick, shiny plates of stratum corneum separated by deep, red fissures that tend to form geometric patterns, as seen in the patched costumes of the harlequin clowns from the Italian Commedia dell'Arte dating from the 16th and 17th centuries. There are poorly developed or absent ears and marked ectropion and eclabium. The fingertips are tapered, and there is hyperconvexity of the nails. Uniformly fatal before 1980, a substantial fraction of patients with harlequin ichthyosis now survive with a persistent and severe erythroderma (Fig. 47-10).[65,73,74]

Netherton syndrome (OMIM #256500) is an autosomal recessive disorder featuring ichthyosis, a structural hair shaft abnormality, and atopy.[75] When present, a key finding is *ichthyosis linearis circumflexa* (ILC), a characteristic, polycyclic, serpiginous, migratory, double-edged scale at the margins of erythematous plaques (Fig. 47-11). Other patients, however, can present with a more severe erythroderma with or without ILC (Fig. 47-12). Histopathologic examination is not specific, but absent or thin stratum corneum is highly suggestive. Most patients have a specific hair shaft abnormality called *trichorrhexis invaginata*, in which the distal hair segment is telescoped into the proximal one, forming a ball-and-socket-like deformity on microscopic examination (Fig. 47-13). This is also known as "bamboo hair" and is caused by abnormal cornification of the internal root sheath. Hair from multiple areas should be examined because only 20% to 50% of hair may be affected; the characteristic abnormality may be more commonly observed on eyebrow hair.[76-78] The hair defects may not be detectable at birth and may disappear with age. Atopy-like diathesis may occur in these patients as atopic dermatitis, asthma, or severe food allergy (particularly to nuts) and marked elevations of serum immunoglobulin E. In some patients, generalized aminoaciduria, mild developmental delay, and impaired cellular immunity may also be present.[79]

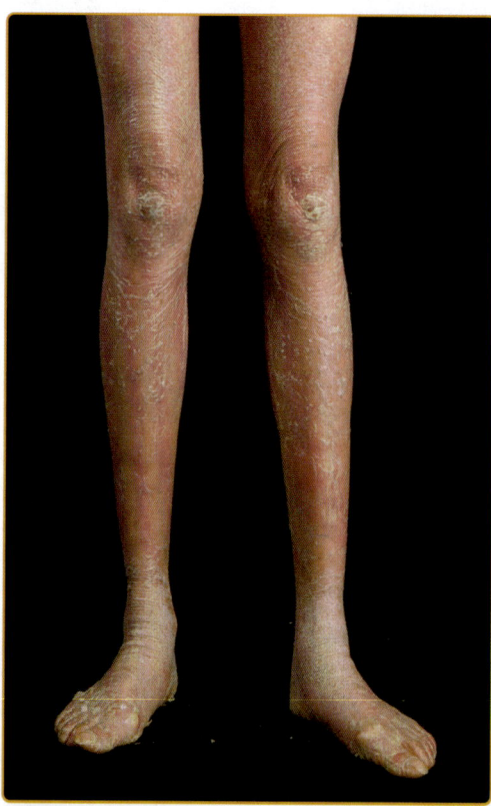

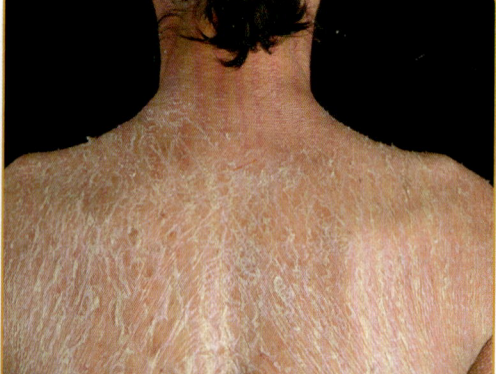

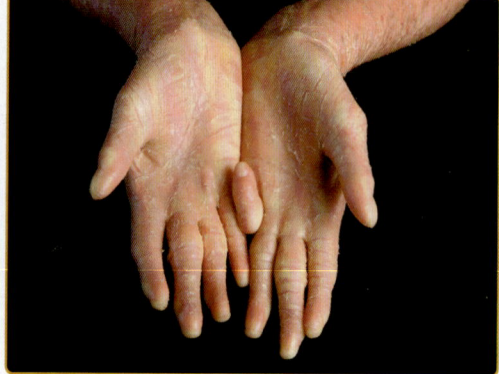

Figure 47-10 Autosomal recessive congenital ichthyosis (*ABCA12* mutations, moderate). Large flat scales and moderate generalized erythema. All digits are tapered.

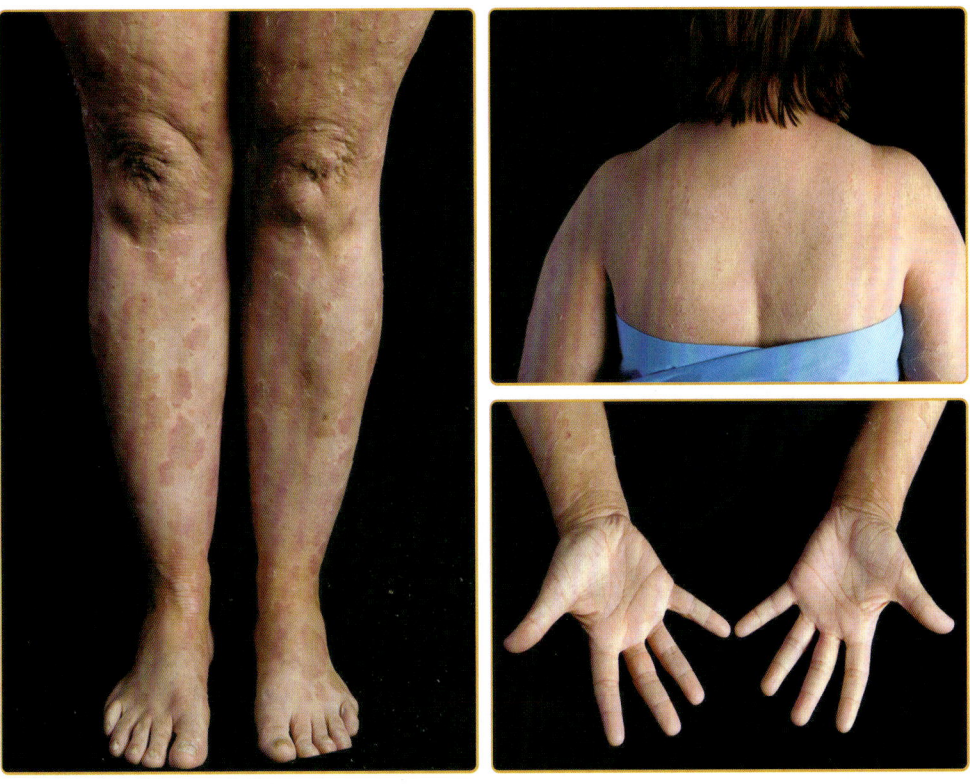

Figure 47-11 Netherton syndrome (*SPINK 5* mutation, ichthyosis linearis circumflexa predominant). Serpiginous, migrating scales peel away to reveal underling erythema. The palms and soles have mild to moderate keratoderma.

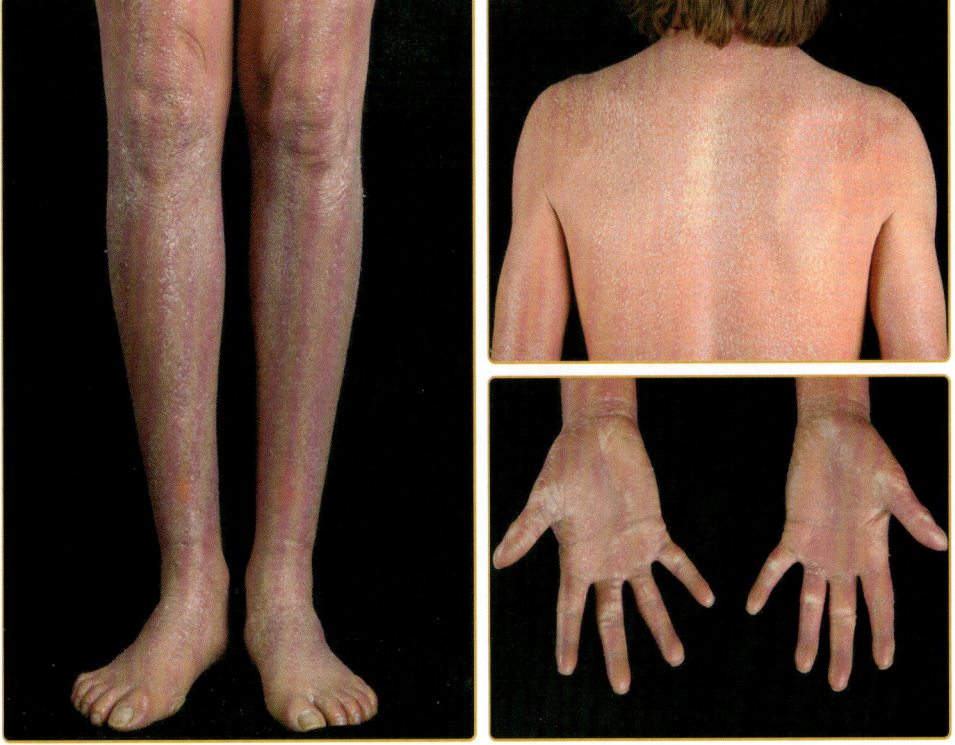

Figure 47-12 Netherton syndrome (*SPINK 5* mutation, erythroderma predominant). Small white scales cover areas of mild to severe generalized erythema. Serpiginous, peeling scales are often limited to areas around the ankles and wrists. The palms and soles have mild to moderate keratoderma.

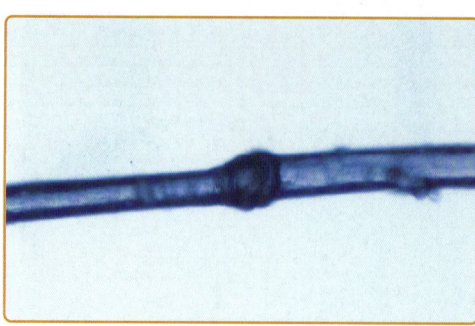

Figure 47-13 Netherton syndrome hair abnormalities. A small bamboo hair shaft shows features of trichorrhexis invaginata.

ETIOLOGY AND PATHOGENESIS

LAMELLAR ICHTHYOSIS AND CONGENITAL ICHTHYOSIFORM ERYTHRODERMA PHENOTYPES

The LI and CIE phenotypes represent a clinical spectrum, and mutations in many of the same genes underlie both phenotypes. A cardinal gene implicated in LI phenotypes is *TGM1*.[21,22] Even with this gene, there is great phenotypic variability (see Figs. 47-6 to 47-8). *TGM1* encodes transglutaminase 1; transglutaminases catalyze calcium-dependent cross-linking of proteins through the formation of ε-(γ-glutamyl)lysine isodipeptide bonds. During the formation of the stratum corneum, transglutaminase catalyzes the cross-linking of cellular proteins, including involucrin, loricrin, small proline-rich proteins, keratins, filaggrin, and others. The resulting protein complex is deposited on the inner side of the plasma membrane to form the cornified envelope. Transglutaminase also attaches ceramides secreted into the intercellular space by lamellar bodies to cornified envelope proteins, notably involucrin, and thereby is important in the formation of both the protein and lipid components of the stratum corneum.[80]

In a human skin–immunodeficient mouse xenograft model, transfer of a transglutaminase-1 gene into transglutaminase-1-deficient keratinocytes from LI patients resulted in normalization of transglutaminase expression and epidermal architecture in addition to restoration of cutaneous barrier function.[81] More recently, topical application of recombinant transglutaminase-1 in liposomes has been shown to normalize histology and function in murine xenografts.[82]

Autosomal recessive mutations in the genes encoding lipoxygenases *ALOXE3* (see Fig. 47-9) and *ALOX12B* (see Fig. 47-10) were found to cause CIE.[83] Lipoxygenases catalyze the formation of hydroperoxides from polyunsaturated fatty acids. In the skin, the products of *ALOXE3* and *ALOX12B* play a central role in the generated of oxidized ceramides, which are incorporated into the corneocyte lipid envelope.[84]

Altogether, mutations in 10 genes can cause ARCI phenotypes, and these include: *TGM1* (OMIM #190195), *ALOX12B* (OMIM #603741), *ALOXE3* (OMIM #*607206), *NIPAL4/Ichthyin*6 (OMIM #609383), *CYP4F22* (OMIM #611495), *ABCA12* (OMIM #607800), *PNPLA1* (OMIM #612121), *CERS3* (OMIM #615276), *SDR9C7* (OMIM #609767), and *SULT2B1* (OMIM #604125).

HARLEQUIN ICHTHYOSIS PHENOTYPE

Harlequin ichthyosis results from autosomal recessive inheritance of mutations in *ABCA12*, which codes for an adenosine triphosphate (ATP)-binding cassette (ABC) transporter involved in lamellar granule secretion and epidermal lipid transport. Whereas premature termination, loss-of-function mutations most commonly underlie harlequin ichthyosis,[85,86] missense mutations in *ABCA12* have been identified in individuals with less severe ARCI (see Fig. 47-14).[87,88] In harlequin ichthyosis, normal lamellar granules are not found; instead, there are small vesicles that lack internal structure. There is also no evidence of the lipid lamellae that form between granular and cornified cells as a result of discharge of lamellar granule contents into the intercellular space.[89]

Netherton syndrome has been found to be caused by mutations in *SPINK5*, a gene encoding LEKTI (lymphoepithelial Kazal-type related inhibitor).[24] LEKTI is a serine protease inhibitor that is predominantly expressed in epithelial and lymphoid tissues and may be important in the downregulation of inflammatory pathways. It inhibits the proteases that degrade the corneodesmosome, thus allowing premature desquamation. LEKTI polymorphisms are associated with common atopy and atopic dermatitis.[90,91] Early reports of Netherton syndrome recognized signs of reduced cellular immunity manifesting as viral warts and negative skin testing to microbial antigens. The danger of such defective cellular immunity was reinforced with the report of Folster-Holst and coworkers, who identified oncogenic human papillomavirus in a 28-year-old woman with vulvar condyloma that rapidly transformed to an aggressive squamous cell carcinoma.[92] In our experience, all adults with Netherton have papillomatous changes in intertriginous areas, but the role of papilloma viruses in the development of these lesions has not been established.

DIAGNOSIS

Clinical features and history are central to establishing a diagnosis in ARCI. Advances in genetic testing, either via research pathways (see section "Registry for Ichthyosis and Related Skin Disorders") or clinical laboratories, has allowed the rapid ascertainment of genetic diagnoses. These tests use next-generation sequencing of a panel of genes or a selected subset of genes assessed via exome sequencing. Genetic testing permits confirmation of diagnosis and counseling regarding potential disease comorbidities. Clinical features supporting phenotypes include the following:

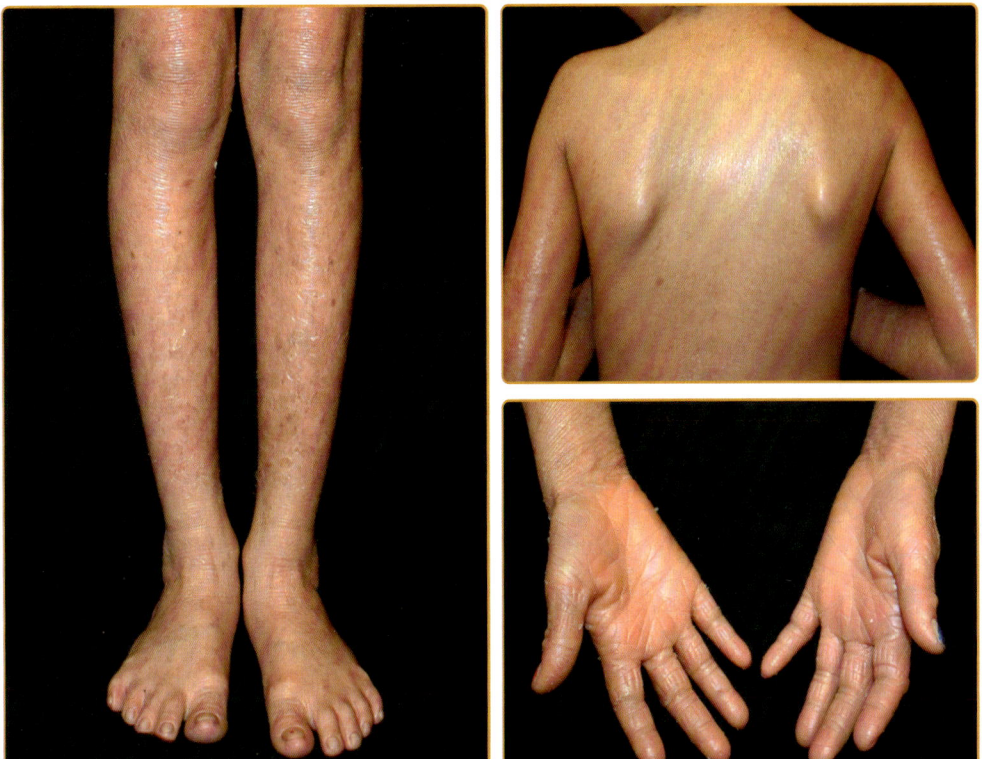

Figure 47-14 Autosomal recessive congenital ichthyosis (*ABCA12* mutation, mild). Scales on the shins are large, but those elsewhere are small on background of mild erythema. Moderate palmar keratoderma with increased linear markings and tapered fifth digit.

LI and CIE typically presents with a collodion membrane at birth that sheds to reveal either the thick, adherent scale of LI or the erythroderma and finer scale of CIE. Histopathologic examination rarely aids in the diagnosis of LI or CIE, with both disorders showing nonspecific acanthosis and hyperkeratosis.

Harlequin ichthyosis has a classical clinical presentation, with armorlike plates of scale and deep fissures present at birth which shed to reveal severe erythroderma and scaling.

Netherton syndrome presents with hair shaft abnormalities, with or without ILC or erythroderma, in the setting of atopic features. These clinical findings provide strong support for the diagnosis of Netherton syndrome.

CLINICAL COURSE, PROGNOSIS, AND MANAGEMENT

LAMELLAR ICHTHYOSIS AND CONGENITAL ICHTHYOSIFORM ERYTHRODERMA

Treatment with oral retinoids can improve or prevent some sequelae of these phenotypes. Patients frequently notice an increase in sweating, with improved heat tolerance. Although retinoid therapy can cause blepharitis or even conjunctivitis, it is usually well tolerated by patients with LI and CIE. Moreover, the ability of systemic retinoid (and in some cases, topical retinoid) therapy to decrease thick periocular scale can decrease the tendency to develop ectropion.[93] Nevertheless, patients with severe scaling and ectropion usually require careful eye maintenance. Because of the ectropion, the eyelids may fail to close fully, particularly during sleep; hydration with liquid tears during the day and ophthalmic lubricants at night can prevent exposure keratitis. Individuals with mutations in *ALOXE3* and *ALOX12B* tend to have less scaling that those with mutations in *TGM1* and, consistent with this observation, are findings in a recent study showing that ectropion is less common (35%) in CIE than in LI (57%).[94]

HARLEQUIN ICHTHYOSIS

Advances in neonatal intensive care, together with facilitating desquamation by judicious use of systemic retinoid therapy, have led to improvements in survival and to the use of the name "harlequin baby" rather than "harlequin fetus." These children are at risk during the neonatal period. Abnormal water loss through the skin and poor temperature regulation lead to risk of fluid and electrolyte imbalance.

The infants are also at risk for infection beginning in the skin but at the same time (because of poor temperature regulation) do not show the usual signs of infection. Normal respiration may be restricted by the taut skin. Treatment with systemic retinoids during the newborn period can facilitate desquamation of the membrane and is associated with improved outcomes.[73,95] Some infants and children have had failure to thrive and require tube feeding. After shedding of harlequin scale, erythroderma is prominent. In children and adults, topical and systemic retinoids can be helpful in the management of ectropion and hyperkeratosis.

NETHERTON SYNDROME

At birth, affected children may present with generalized erythroderma, and in some individuals, erythroderma persists throughout life with a phenotype on the LI–CIE spectrum of ARCI.[96] In others, erythroderma fades, and ILC ensues. Infants and children may have feeding problems, with poor absorption and failure to thrive.[97] Pruritus can be profound, and scratching can lead to lichenification at the flexures.

Tacrolimus ointment, a topical immunomodulator (see Chap. 192), is effective in common atopic dermatitis with minimal systemic absorption. However, Netherton syndrome is complicated by an abnormal skin barrier, allowing increased percutaneous absorption and associated risk for systemic toxic effects. This should be considered when using topical agents such as tacrolimus because monitoring of serum levels may be necessary[98] and topical steroids because iatrogenic Cushing syndrome has been reported.[32] Furthermore, topical and systemic retinoids should be avoided in patients with Netherton syndrome because they can further exacerbate the condition.

KERATINOPATHIC ICHTHYOSES

Keratinopathic ichthyoses result from mutations in genes encoding keratins, components of the intermediate filament network that are central to cellular structural integrity. Phenotypes falling within the keratinopathic ichthyosis spectrum include EI, superficial epidermolytic ichthyosis (SEI, ichthyosis bullosa of Siemens), ichthyosis hysterix Curth-Macklin, annular EI, and ichthyosis with confetti (IWC).

CLINICAL FEATURES

EPIDERMOLYTIC ICHTHYOSIS

In 1902, Brocq described bullous ichthyotic erythroderma and distinguished the blistering type from the nonblistering type of CIE.[99] The original description included three unrelated patients whose clinical manifestations varied. However, this was probably the first description of EI (OMIM #113800). The disease is named for the distinctive histopathologic features of vacuolar degeneration of the epidermal keratinocyte (ie, epidermal lysis) and associated hyperkeratosis. EI is also known as EHK and BCIE, earlier descriptive names signifying characteristic histopathologic changes or the blistering, neonatal presentation with subsequent scaling and redness, respectively.

EI is transmitted as an autosomal dominant trait with a prevalence of approximately 1 in 200,000 to 300,000 persons. There is a high frequency of spontaneous mutation, and as many as half of the patients have no family history.[10] The disease usually presents at birth with blistering, redness, and peeling and can be mistaken for epidermolysis bullosa or staphylococcal scalded skin on clinical examination (Fig. 47-15A). Because there is a high frequency of new mutations, the disease may be unexpected, and the diagnosis may be unknown. The newborn may require intensive care with fluid and electrolyte monitoring.

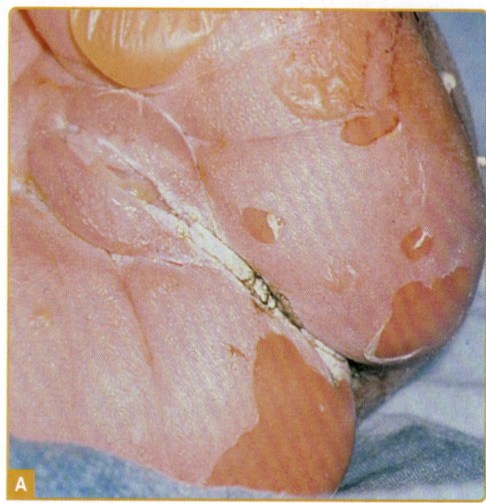

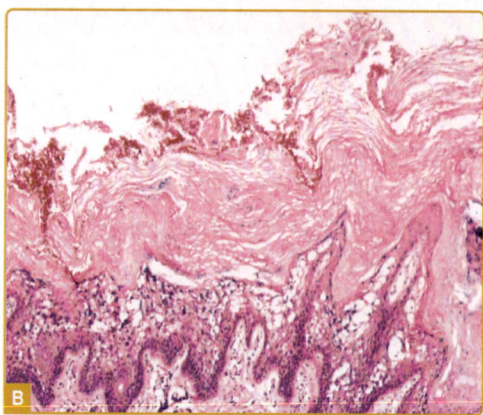

Figure 47-15 Epidermolytic ichthyosis infantile presentation. **A,** Newborn showing blistering and erosions. **B,** Epidermolytic ichthyosis histology. The stratum corneum is thickened (hyperkeratosis), and there is prominent vacuolar degeneration of suprabasilar epidermis most marked at the granular layer.

Specialized skin care can minimize blistering and enhance healing of erosions and may include lubrication to decrease friction and mechanical trauma, protective padding, and specialized wound dressings. Newborns with extensive erosions are prone to bacterial infection and sepsis, and carefully chosen topical and systemic antibiotics can minimize the extent of infection. With time, generalized hyperkeratosis may develop, which may or may not be associated with erythroderma. EI skin usually has a characteristic odor, thought to be related to superinfection by mixed flora. Histopathology shows a thickened stratum corneum and vacuolar degeneration of the upper epidermis, leading to the histologic term *EHK*. The vacuolar degeneration usually involves the upper epidermis and occasionally all of the suprabasilar keratinocytes. Granular cells exhibit dense, enlarged, irregularly shaped masses that appear to be keratohyalin granules (Fig. 47-15B).

All patients with EI have a characteristic corrugated scale that becomes accentuated in areas of body folds (Figs. 47-16 and 47-17). There is striking clinical heterogeneity in EI with phenotypes, including isolated, thick palmoplantar hyperkeratosis, generalized spiny scale, migratory patches of erythrokeratoderma, keratoderma with superficial peeling scale, and generalized exfoliative erythroderma.[100]

LINEAR ICHTHYOSIFORM ERYTHRODERMA

Linear EI, a variant of epidermal nevus, presents in a linear mosaic pattern caused by a postzygotic, spontaneous mutation during embryogenesis. Areas of hyperkeratosis alternating with normal skin are often distributed in streaks along Blaschko lines. These may be limited to a few streaks, often bounded by the midline, or there may be many stripes, with widespread, patchy involvement. Linear EI has been found to result from somatic mutations in *KRT1* and *KRT10* that are identical to those found in generalized disease.[101,102] If the mosaicism affected gonadal tissue, individuals with linear EI can transmit the mutation to offspring with resulting generalized EI.[103,104]

SUPERFICIAL EPIDERMOLYTIC ICHTHYOSIS

SIE (ichthyosis bullosa of Siemens) is a rare autosomal dominant genodermatosis. Patients are born with redness and blistering. The redness subsides over the subsequent weeks to months, and the skin develops corrugated hyperkeratosis, particularly over flexural areas (Fig. 47-18). In some areas, there may be a

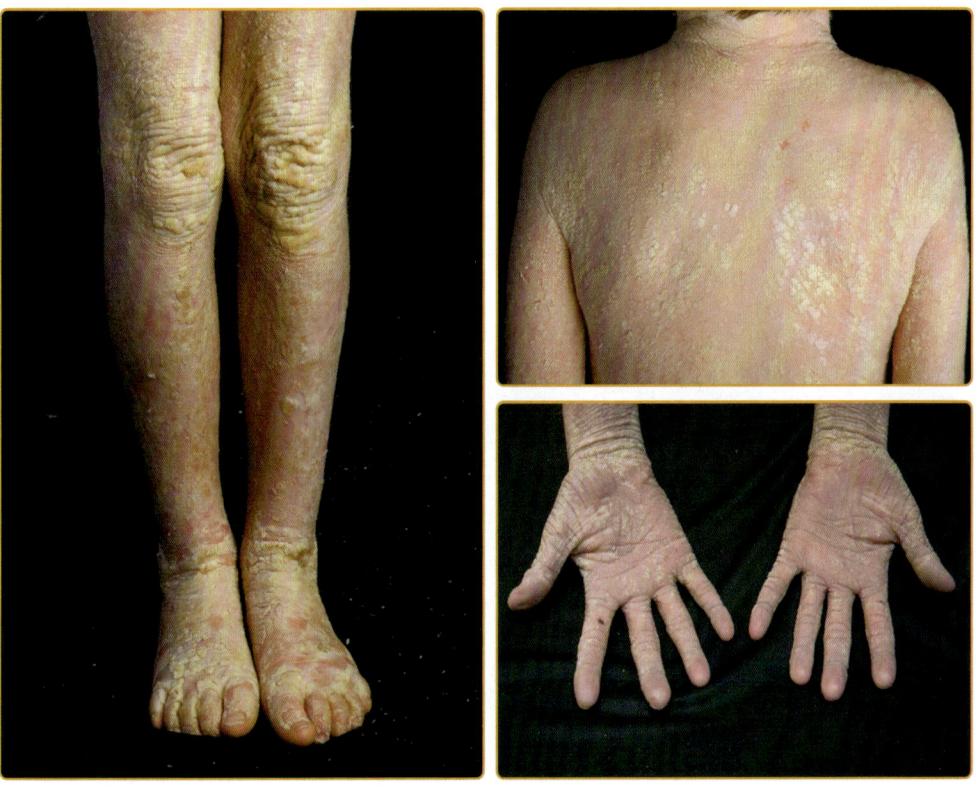

Figure 47-16 Epidermolytic ichthyosis (*KRT10* mutation). Generalized coarse, columnar scales often have a corrugated pattern over flexures. Scales unevenly desquamate from the underlying epidermis to reveal mild to moderate generalized erythema. Hyperkeratosis of the palms and soles is mild to moderate, and pseudoainhum occurs.

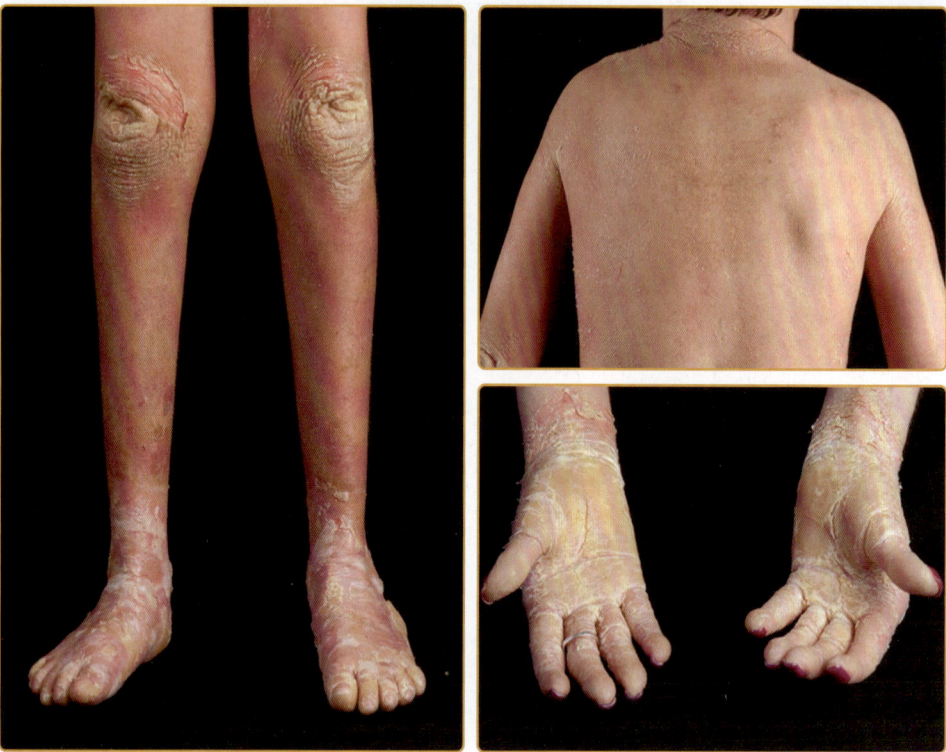

Figure 47-17 Epidermolytic ichthyosis (*KRT1* mutation). Generalized coarse, columnar scales often have a corrugated pattern over flexures. Scales unevenly desquamate from underlying epidermis to reveal mild to moderate generalized erythema. Hyperkeratosis of the palms and soles is often severe, and pseudoainhum occurs.

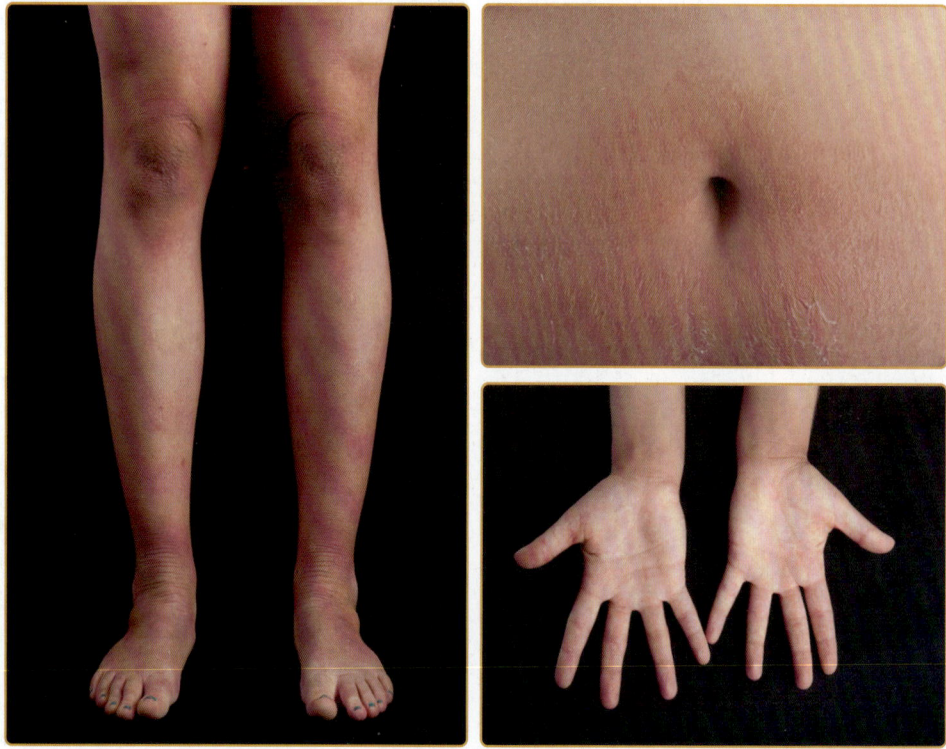

Figure 47-18 Epidermolytic ichthyosis (*KRT2* mutation). Smooth, mildly corrugated scale is generally accentuated at flexures or areas of mild friction. Circular or geometric areas of stratum corneum peeling are common. Erythema is mild, and the palms and soles are spared.

lichenified appearance to the skin. As with EI, the epidermis is fragile; however, the fragility is more superficial. This can result in loss of the uppermost epidermis (predominantly the stratum corneum), yielding a characteristic, collarette-like depressed area that has been described as "mauserung" (molting). Histologically, the epidermis shows hyperkeratosis and vacuolization similar to EHK but confined to the granular layer.[10] Mutations have been found in the gene encoding keratin 2, a differentiation keratin of the suprabasilar epidermis that is expressed in the more superficial epidermal layers.[105,106]

ANNULAR EPIDERMOLYTIC ICHTHYOSIS

Annular EI is a rare autosomal dominant disorder that presents at birth or within in the first few months of life with severe, intermittent scaling and blistering that resolves during puberty.[107,108] Residual, limited plaques with corrugated scale and erythema are seen primarily in flexural and intertriginous skin (Fig. 47-19). In some cases, explosive bouts of widespread erythema with blisters and pustules are seen.[109] Patients subsequently develop widespread, migratory, polycyclic, and annular scaling plaques. Light and electron microscopy reveals findings of EI. Mutations in *KRT10* and *KRT1* have been found.[109,110]

ICHTHYOSIS WITH CONFETTI

This rare disorder is also known as *ichthyosis variegata* and *congenital reticulated ichthyosiform erythroderma*, descriptive terms that fail to capture its clinical evolution over the course of life. IWC presents with congenital erythroderma, malformation of the auricle, and tapering of the digits which leads to the frequent clinical diagnosis of CIE. In childhood, palmoplantar keratoderma develops, and the severity ranges from mild to severe.[111] Most individuals with IWC develop small islands of normal-appearing skin beginning in childhood (Fig. 47-20), although later presentation has also been reported. Normal areas of skin have been shown to arise from loss of heterozygosity on chromosome 17q or 12q via mitotic recombination of disease-causing mutations in the genes encoding keratin 10 (*KRT10*) and keratin 1 (*KRT1*).[112-114] Histopathology shows a clear transition from affected epidermis to normal skin within white spots. In individuals with IWC caused by mutations in *KRT10*, bandlike parakeratosis, psoriasiform acanthosis and vacuolated, binuclear upper epidermal keratinocytes are seen, and electron microscopy shows perinuclear filament retraction and poor investment of desmosomes with intermediate filaments.[114] In individuals with IWC caused by mutations in *KRT1*, affected skin shows psoriasiform acanthosis, prominent keratohyalin granules, perinuclear vacuolization with rare binucleate cells, and thick

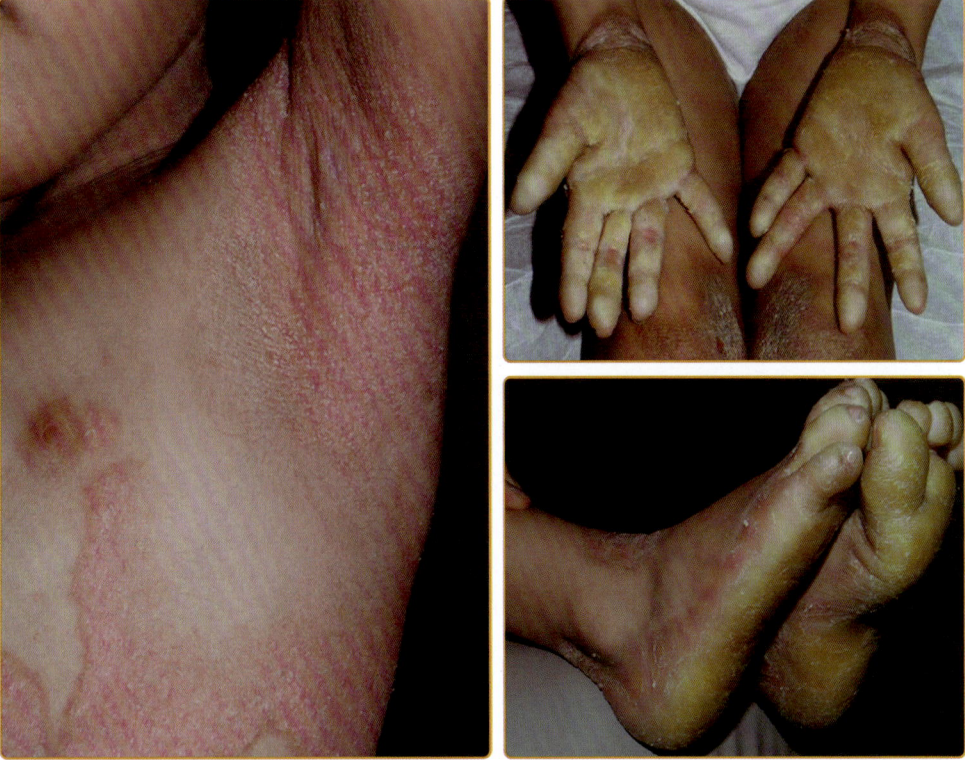

Figure 47-19 Epidermolytic ichthyosis, annular with PPK (*KRT1* mutation). Circumscribed erythematous plaques with coarse scale and a corrugated pattern accentuated at flexures. The palms and soles variably involved.

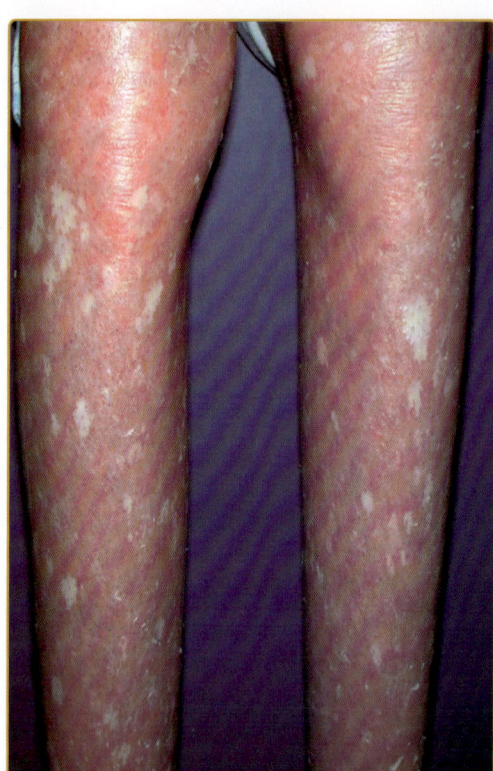
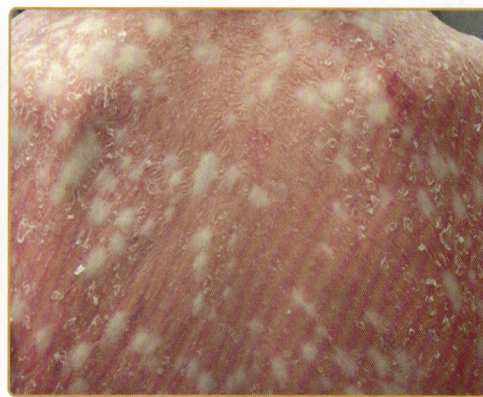
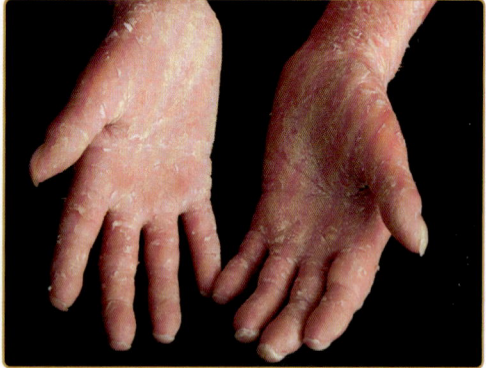

Figure 47-20 Ichthyosis with confetti (*KRT10* mutation). Phylloid (leaf-like) areas of normal skin on a background of mild to severe erythema and scale increase in number and size starting in the first decade of life. Palmar and plantar erythrokeratoderma vary from mild to severe. Contractures may occur at small and large joints.

hyperkeratosis, and electron microscopy shows perinuclear filament detachment.[113]

ETIOLOGY AND PATHOGENESIS

Within keratinocytes, keratin intermediate filaments form an elaborate network that confers structural stability to the cells. In the suprabasilar, differentiating keratinocytes of interfollicular epidermis, this network is primarily formed by keratins 1 and 10, which polymerize to form intermediate filaments. In the granular layer, keratin 2 partially replaces keratin 1 in intermediate filaments.

EPIDERMOLYTIC ICHTHYOSIS

On electron microscopic examination, clumping of filaments is observed to begin in the first suprabasal layer. These aggregated filaments are clumps of keratin intermediate filaments that contain the suprabasal keratins 1 and 10.[10,115] When expressed in keratinocytes, mutant keratins in EI and SEI aggregate and clump, with collapse of the intermediate filament network and ensuing cytolysis. Aggregates are cytotoxic, and mutations in *KRT10* have been shown to disrupt epidermal differentiation and formation of the lipid permeability barrier while inducing epidermal hyperproliferation.[116,117] Mutations in genes coding keratin 1, 2, or 10 have been identified in a number of EI kindreds.[118] In many cases, severe palmar/plantar involvement implies mutations in *KRT1*; this may reflect the "redundancy" of K9 (a keratin that occurs only in the suprabasal epidermis of palmar and plantar skin) and K10 in palmar/plantar epithelium. Mutations in *KRT9* have been found in families with epidermolytic PPK (Vörner) (see Chap. 48).[119]

ICHTHYOSIS WITH CONFETTI

IWC does not feature marked skin fragility, and electron microscopy shows no evidence of filament aggregates, though perinuclear filament retraction is seen. Expression of *KRT10* mutants in cells leads to intermediate filament network collapse and intranuclear accumulation of K10 within the nucleolus, and expression of *KRT1* mutants similarly leads to intermediate filament network collapse with intranuclear accumulation of K1.[112-114] Because all revertant spots arise from mitotic recombination and spots of normal skin increase in number and size over time, IWC *KRT1* and

KRT10 mutations appear to affect homologous recombination and confer selective advantage to normal keratinocytes.

DIAGNOSIS

Diagnosis combines clinical findings, histopathology, and genetic analysis. Clinical features can inform diagnosis. For examples, the appearance of white spots of normal skin in childhood suggests IWC, but a history of blistering at birth with less frequent blistering over time and histology showing epidermolysis and hypergranulosis suggests EI or SEI. Genetic testing permits precision in diagnosis, with mutations found in *KRT1*, *KRT10*, or *KRT2*.

CLINICAL COURSE, PROGNOSIS, AND MANAGEMENT

Although the neonatal presentation of widespread blistering can be dramatic in EI and SEI, in the first few weeks of life, hyperkeratosis becomes more prominent, and blisters become more localized to areas of friction. Areas of thick hyperkeratosis, which are not pliable and have a hard, rough surface, are prone to mechanical trauma. In patients with the hystrix type of porcupine-like hyperkeratosis, the rough surface causes high traction with objects moving across the skin surface, which tend to catch on the hyperkeratotic horn and peel it off. Topical agents such as lubricants and keratolytics can reduce the thickened, rough areas and help to minimize blistering and erosion. In contrast, patients with erythroderma and peeling, who do not have the thick areas of hyperkeratotic spines, have less need for keratolytics but still need lubricants. Acute exacerbations may occur from skin infections. Bacterial infection of the skin is common, often leads to enhanced blistering, and may require frequent therapy with topical and oral antibiotics. Dilute bleach baths aid in controlling bacterial odor and colonization, and bicarbonate baths can facilitate desquamation. Topical retinoids can reduce scaling locally,[120] and systemic retinoids can markedly reduce hyperkeratosis, decreasing grooming and bathing time.[121,122] Dosing must be slowly titrated because fragility can increase with higher doses, particularly in EI. For reasons that are not well understood, blistering and infection are less of a problem for adults than for children with EI.

CONNEXIN DISORDERS

Mutations in genes encoding connexins lead to erythrokeratoderma, and phenotypes include keratitis ichthyosis deafness syndrome and erythrokeratodermia variabilis et progressiva (EKVP). There are overlapping clinical features and phenotypic variability, even within kindreds, in these disorders.[123,124]

CLINICAL FEATURES

EKVP (OMIM #133200) represents a spectrum of phenotypes initially described as progressive symmetric erythrokeratodermia (PSEK) and erythrokeratodermia variabilis (EKV) but that have been found to have a common genetic basis.[125] The progressive symmetric erythrokeratodermia phenotype was first definitively described by Darier in 1911[126] and is characterized by well-demarcated, erythematous, hyperkeratotic plaques that are symmetrically distributed over the extremities and buttocks, and often the face[127] (Fig. 47-21). The trunk tends to be spared, but the palms and soles may be involved. The plaques appear shortly after birth, progress slowly during the first few years, and then stabilize in early childhood. The plaques usually remain stable in location and appearance but may undergo partial regression at puberty. The erythrokeratodermia variabilis phenotype was described by Mendes da Costa in 1925 as a rare disorder typically presenting at birth or during the first year of life.[128] Both generalized involvement (see Fig. 47-25) characterized by persistent, red-brown hyperkeratotic plaques and accentuated skin markings and localized involvement that is limited in extent and characterized by sharply demarcated, hyperkeratotic plaques that are symmetrically arrayed and remain relatively fixed for months to years have been described. Although many features are shared with PSEK, EKV also demonstrates sharply demarcated, migratory red patches that vary in size from a few to many centimeters. These geographic, figurate red patches appear or regress over minutes to hours; some individuals complain of burning at these sites, but they are asymptomatic in others. The red patches develop independently of the hyperkeratosis. Palmoplantar hyperkeratosis may be present, but hair and mucous membranes are unaffected. Histopathologic features include hyperkeratosis, acanthosis, papillomatosis, and capillary dilatation. Epidermis involved with severe papillomatosis and suprapapillary thinning may result in a "church spire" appearance. EKVP is inherited in an autosomal dominant pattern with incomplete penetrance and variable expressivity, although rare recessive cases have been described.[129]

KERATITIS-ICHTHYOSIS-DEAFNESS SYNDROME

KID syndrome (OMIM #148210) is a rare disorder characterized by keratitis (with progressive corneal opacification), ichthyosis, and deafness (neurosensory). Involvement of multiple ectodermal tissues qualifies KID syndrome as an ectodermal dysplasia. Most cases are compatible with autosomal dominant inheritance.

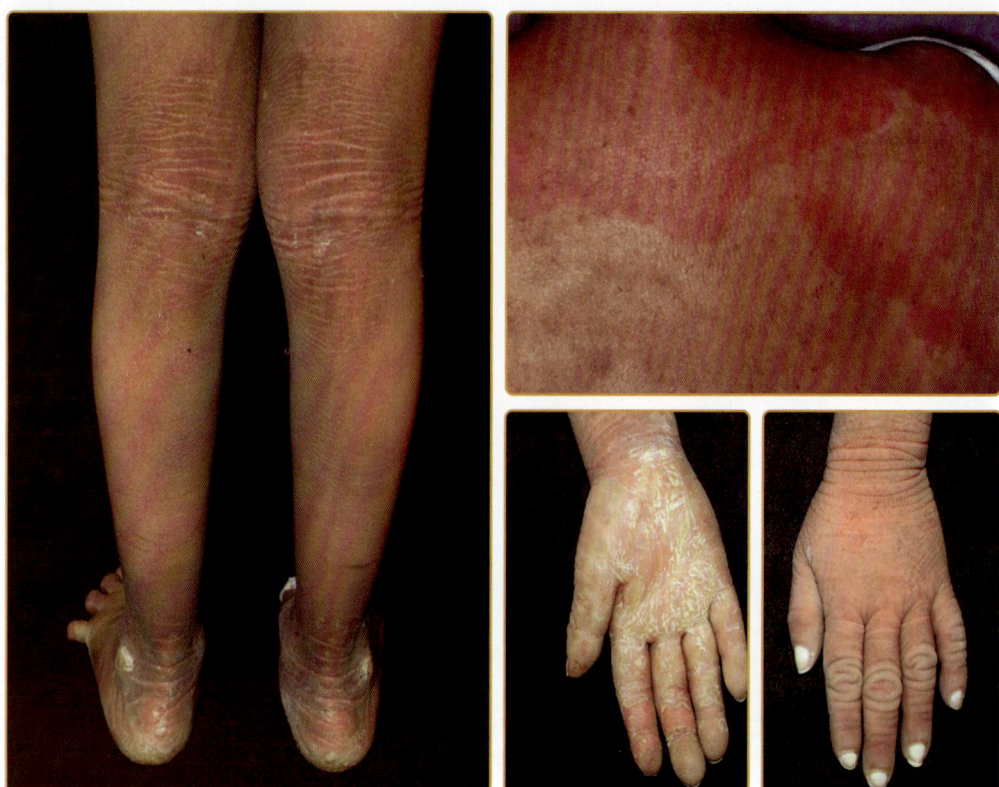

Figure 47-21 Erythrokeratoderma variabilis (*GJB3; GJB4; GJA1* mutations). Corrugated coarse plaques are usually accentuated in the flexures. Palm and sole involvement may be severe. Circumscribed erythematous patches may be fixed or evanescent.

The disease is characterized by discrete erythematous plaques, and there may be mild, generalized hyperkeratosis (Fig. 47-22). The distinctive plaques may have a discrete border and a verrucous appearance with crusting and may be conspicuously figurate and symmetric on the face. Furrowing about the mouth results in characteristic facies. There may be prominent follicular hyperkeratosis, which can result in a scarring alopecia of the scalp. "Leather-like" palmar/plantar keratoderma is almost always seen.[130] Descriptions of nail changes vary from absent, delayed appearance after birth, atrophic, or brittle to thickened, with loss of or "rough" cuticles, subungual hyperkeratosis, and leukonychia. The teeth may be small. Auditory evoked potential studies allow detection of the hearing deficit in infancy. Keratitis may develop.

ETIOLOGY AND PATHOGENESIS

ERYTHROKERATODERMIA VARIABILIS ET PROGRESSIVA

Mutations in *GJB3*, *GJB4*, and *GJA1*, the genes encoding connexin 31, 30.3, and 43, respectively, have been identified in kindreds with EKVP.[11,124,128,131,132] Connexins are a family of proteins that aggregate to form gap junctions that are important channels for intercellular communication. This intercellular signaling system is crucial for maintaining tissue homeostasis, growth control, development, and synchronized response of cells to stimuli. In the cell, connexins oligomerize to form homotypic or heterotypic hexameric connexons in the Golgi, which are transported to the cell membrane, where they can either function as nonjunctional hemichannels or dock with connexins in neighboring cells. Mutant connexins can show impaired intercellular communication through gap junctions and leakiness of hemichannels.[124] The critical deficit in causing the pathology has not been established.

KERATITIS–ICHTHYOSIS–DEAFNESS SYNDROME

Dominant mutations in *GJB2*, the gene encoding connexin 26, have been detected in sporadic cases and familial KID syndrome.[133] Functional studies of cells expressing mutated connexin 26 demonstrated failure of a fluorescent tracer to pass through gap junction channels to neighboring cells, consistent with disruption of intercellular communication.[124,133] Mutant connexin 26

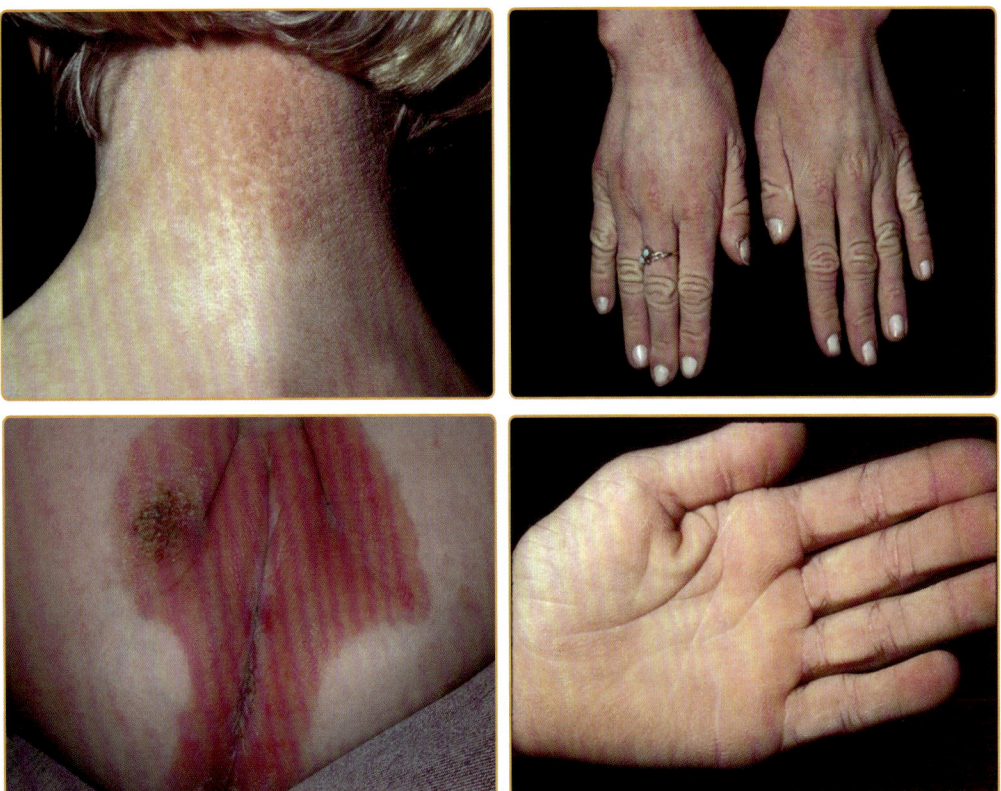

Figure 47-22 Keratitis ichthyosis deafness syndrome (*GJB2* mutation). Smooth or gritty columns of hyperkeratosis give the skin a pebbly or rough appearance and are most prominent at body folds, palms, and soles and around orifices. Erythema is usually mild. Bacterial and fungal infections are common.

also forms poor gap junctions and leaky heterotypic hemichannels with connexin 43.[134] Different mutations in the same gene (*GJB2*) encoding connexin 26 have also been found in a family with a mutilating palmoplantar keratoderma (Vohwinkel disease; see Chap. 48) and deafness (without ichthyosis).[135] The identification of mutations in the genes encoding a variety of connexin proteins has highlighted the role of connexin-mediated intercellular communication through gap junctions in the development and maintenance of ectodermal tissues. Connexins 26, 30, and 31 are expressed in the stratified epithelia of the cochlea and epidermis, and abnormalities in these proteins can cause sensorineural hearing impairment and skin disorders.[136]

CLINICAL COURSE, PROGNOSIS, AND MANAGEMENT

ERYTHROKERATODERMIA VARIABILIS ET PROGRESSIVA

Affected individuals frequently have normal skin at birth, and initial lesions present in infancy or childhood. Skin involvement can wax and wane over the course of an individual's life. Systemic retinoid treatment improves hyperkeratotic lesions and may also clear the figurate red patches when present. The hyperkeratotic skin lesions may be triggered by trauma to the skin, and the red patches may be triggered by a change in temperature.

KERATITIS ICHTHYOSIS DEAFNESS SYNDROME

Cutaneous severity can vary significantly in KID syndrome, particularly in the neonatal period. Keratitis and deafness are variably severe; when present, they may be progressive. Developmental brain defects, often asymptomatic, are common, and some recommend routine magnetic resonance imaging.[137] Affected individuals can have an increased susceptibility to bacterial, fungal, or viral infections.[138] Squamous cell carcinoma of the skin and tongue has also been reported.[139] In contrast to many other ichthyotic conditions, treatment of these patients with oral retinoids has been reported to be of little benefit and possibly to exacerbate the corneal neovascularization. The p.A88V and p.G45E mutations in *GJB2* are associated with neonatal lethality, primarily caused by respiratory failure.[140-143a]

PEELING SKIN DISORDERS

CLINICAL FEATURES

The *peeling skin syndromes* (PSSs; OMIM #270300) were initially described in case reports and were later classified into those with acral predominance, those that were generalized and noninflammatory, and those that were generalized and inflammatory. Skin peeling was often intermittent, and patients lacked the general hyperkeratosis seen in most ichthyoses. These few early cases made it clear that this was a very heterogeneous group of diseases. In the past 12 years, five recessive gene mutations have been reported from one to four families with findings described as PSSs.

The common clinical features included painless, easy peeling skin without scarring, exacerbation by friction and humidity, first appearance from the second day to mid-first decade of life. Many had itch, and some reportedly had cutaneous and systemic allergy.

ETIOLOGY AND PATHOGENESIS

Mutations in *CDSN*, which encodes corneodesmosin, cause inflammatory PSS with atopy, pruritus, and marked deficits in cutaneous barrier function, termed PSS1 (OMIM #270300).[144] Affected individuals have superficial exfoliation, ichthyosiform erythroderma, and frequent cutaneous infections in childhood. Corneodesmosin is a component of desmosomes and corneodesmosomes at the transition from cells of the stratum granulosum to the stratum corneum. Mutations in *CDSN* lead to loss of corneodesmosin expression, eliminating the adhesion between the upper epidermis and the stratum corneum and disrupting terminal differentiation. One consequence of defective differentiation is upregulation of kallikrein 5, a stratum corneum tryptic enzyme that further exacerbates the peeling skin phenotype.

Mutations in the gene coding for transglutaminase 5, a ubiquitously expressed transglutaminase with widespread expression in skin, have been identified in multiple kindreds with acral peeling skin, PSS2 (OMIM #609796).[145] Transglutaminase 5 is expressed in the granular layer of skin and is central to the formation of the cornified envelope, cross-linking structural proteins including involucrin, loricrin, filaggrin, and small proline-rich proteins. Failure to cross-link these proteins leads to shedding at the stratum corneum interface.

Autosomal recessive mutations in *CHST8*, which encodes N-acetylgalactosamine-4-O-sulfotransferase, an enzyme central to the production of sulfated glycosaminoglycans in the epidermis, have been found in a single kindred with PSS3 (OMIM #616265).[146] Affected individuals develop generalized white scaling after 5 years of age which is prominent on the extremities and peels easily. N-acetylgalactosamine-4-O-sulfotransferase functions in glycosylation of proteins central to epidermal differentiation and desquamation.

Autosomal recessive, loss of function mutations in *CSTA* which encodes cystatin A, a cysteine protease inhibitor expressed throughout the epidermis, have also been reported in kindreds with acral PSS, some with more generalized exfoliative ichthyosis, classified as PSS4 (OMIM #607936).[147-150] Cystatin A has a central role in desmosomal adhesion in basal layers of the epidermis, and peeling skin caused by *CSTA* mutations accordingly shows a deeper level of cleavage than is seen in individuals with mutations in *TGM5*.[149]

Autosomal recessive mutation in *SERPINB8*, which belongs to a large family of protease inhibitors, causes a noninflammatory PSS, PSS5 (OMIM #617115).

SYNDROMIC ICHTHYOSES

Syndromic ichthyoses feature moderate to severe extracutaneous involvement. A selection of syndromic ichthyoses will be described.

CHANARIN-DORFMAN SYNDROME

Chanarin-Dorfman syndrome (neutral lipid storage disease with ichthyosis; OMIM #275630) is an autosomal recessive disorder characterized by accumulation of triglycerides in the cytoplasm of keratinocytes, leukocytes, muscle, liver, fibroblasts, and other tissues with normal blood lipid levels. The resulting ichthyosis features generalized lamellar scales with variable erythema, and corrugated accentuation of hyperkeratosis in flexures is common (Fig. 47-23). An EKV-like presentation has been reported.[151] Presentation is often that of a collodion baby with ectropion and eclabium. Extracutaneous involvement, which is generally not as severe as in neutral lipid storage disease without ichthyosis caused by mutations in *PNPLA2*, is variable and may be mild, including cataracts, decreased hearing, hepatosplenomegaly with abnormal liver enzymes and fatty liver, psychomotor delay, myopathy with elevations in serum muscle enzymes, and neurologic abnormalities.

Histopathology of oil red O or Sudan III stains of frozen skin sections shows lipid droplets in dermal cells, in the basal layer (and to a lesser extent suprabasally), and in the acrosyringia of the eccrine ducts. Examination of peripheral blood smears shows lipid vacuoles within granulocytes, eosinophils, and monocytes, a feature that may also be present in carriers.[152] Mutations in the *ABHD5* gene have been identified.[153] ABHD5 belongs to a large family of proteins, most of which are enzymes, and appears to activate adipose-triglyceride lipase in the initial step in lipolysis of triglycerides. In the absence of ABHD5, triglycerides

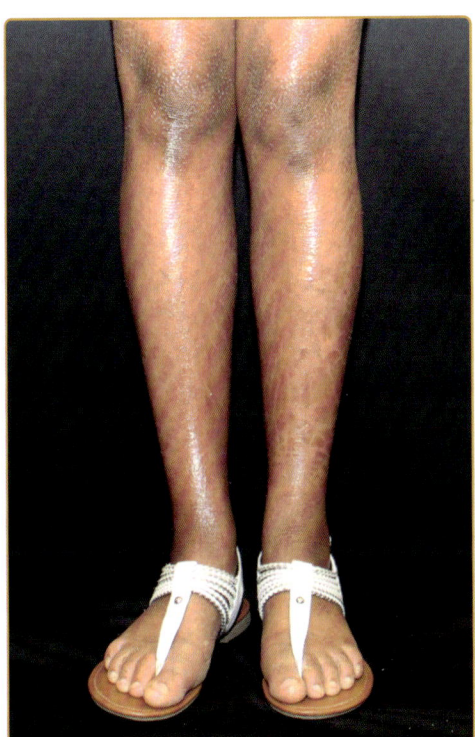
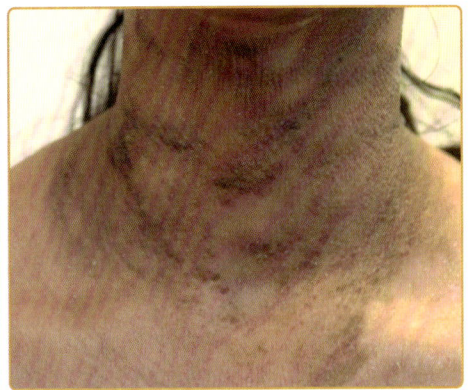
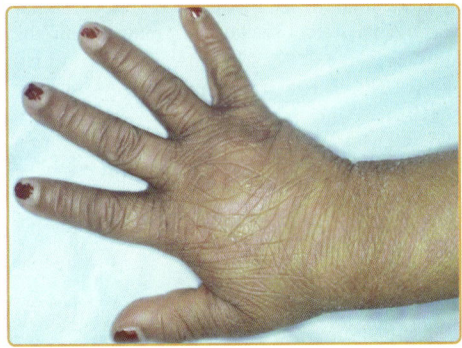

Figure 47-23 Autosomal recessive congenital ichthyosis (*ABHD5* mutations, Chanarin-Dorfman disease; neutral lipid storage disease). Dark scales may vary, in the same individual, from large and flat to small and columnar. Mild to moderate erythema and exaggerated r accentuated linear markings over dorsa of hands and feet are common.

accumulate in cells[154] and in lamellar bodies where, after secretion, they interfere with lipid lamellae formation in the stratum corneum, resulting in increased transepidermal water loss.[155]

CHILD SYNDROME

CHILD syndrome (OMIM #308050) is a rare disorder consisting of *c*ongenital *h*emidysplasia, *i*chthyosiform erythroderma, and *l*imb *d*efects, which is found almost exclusively in females. It is a mosaic disorder featuring red scaly plaques intermixed with normal skin on one side of the body with minimal contralateral involvement. There may be bands of normal skin on the affected side (Fig. 47-24). Limb defects occur ipsilateral to the ichthyosis and range from digital hypoplasia to agenesis of the extremity. There may be punctate calcification of cartilage. Unilateral hypoplasia can involve the central nervous system and cardiovascular, pulmonary, renal, endocrine, and genitourinary systems. The inheritance pattern is X-linked dominant, with the condition being lethal in males. X-inactivation of the mutant allele gives rise to normal skin in affected females. Most affected individuals have loss-of-function mutations in *NSDHL* (*N*AD[P]H *s*teroid *deh*ydrogenase-*l*ike protein) encoding a 3β-hydroxysteroid dehydrogenase.[156,157] NSDHL functions in the postsqualene cholesterol biosynthetic pathway, catalyzing

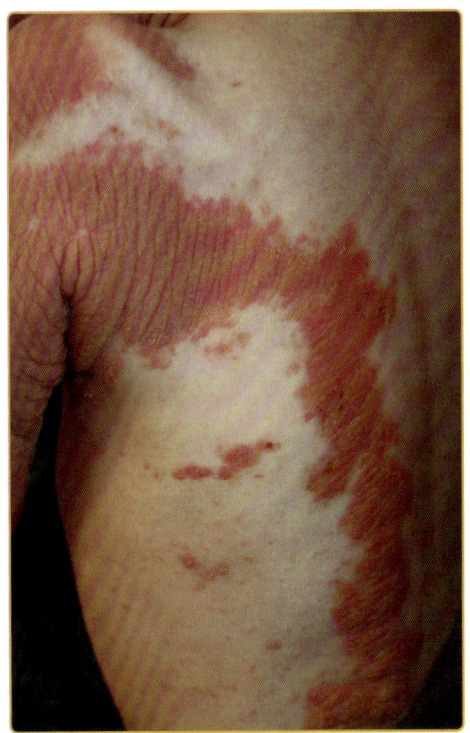

Figure 47-24 CHILD (congenital *h*emidysplasia, *i*chthyosiform erythroderma, and *l*imb *d*efects) syndrome. Linear stripes of erythrokeratoderma are present on the back.

intermediate steps in the conversion of lanosterol to cholesterol.[158] The disorder is related to X-linked dominant chondrodysplasia punctata caused by mutations in emopamil-binding protein (EBP), which also has skin and skeletal abnormalities, and one individual with a CHILD phenotype has been reported with an *EBP* mutation. EPB is downstream of NSDLH in the cholesterol synthetic pathway.

Pathogenesis-based therapy ameliorates the cutaneous findings in CHILD syndrome. Defects in NSDHL lead to a failure to synthesize cholesterol and accumulation of 4-methyl and 4,4-dimethol sterols to toxic levels. Phenotypic improvement of the skin findings in CHILD syndrome was achieved by topical application of cholesterol and lovastatin. This supplies the end product of cholesterol biosynthesis while blocking the pathway at the level of HMG CoA reductase, proximal to NSDHL, thereby preventing synthesis of toxic intermediates.[159]

CHONDRODYSPLASIA PUNCTATA

Chondrodysplasia punctata is a clinically and genetically diverse group of rare diseases, first described by Conradi, that share the features of stippled calcification of the epiphyses and skeletal changes resulting from abnormal deposition of calcium in the areas of enchondral bone formation during fetal development and early infancy. Clinical severity ranges from severe dwarfism and death during infancy to a radiographic abnormality that resolves over time leaving minor skeletal changes. Several forms also include ichthyosiform changes. An autosomal recessive (rhizomelic) type, and both X-linked dominant[160] and recessive forms[161] have been described.

RHIZOMELIC CHONDRODYSPLASIA PUNCTATA

Rhizomelic chondrodysplasia punctata (RCDP; OMIM #215100) is also known as peroxisomal biogenesis disorder complementation group 11 (CG11). It is an autosomal recessive, rare, multisystem developmental disorder characterized by dwarfism caused by symmetric shortening of the proximal long bones (ie, rhizomelia), specific radiologic abnormalities (ie, the presence of stippled calcifications of cartilage, vertebral body clefting), joint contractures, congenital cataracts, ichthyosis, and severe mental retardation. Skin changes are present in approximately 25% of patients. RCDP is a disorder of peroxisomes, membrane-bound multifunctional organelles found in all nucleated cells. Their functions vary with cell type and include a variety of pathways (eg, hydrogen peroxide–based respiration, fatty acid β-oxidation, and lipid and cholesterol synthesis) involving the synthesis and degradation of various compounds.

Hereditary human peroxisomal disorders are subdivided into disorders of peroxisome biogenesis, in which the organelle is not formed normally, and those involving a single peroxisomal enzyme. RCDP is caused by mutations in *PEX7*, a gene that encodes peroxin 7, a receptor required for targeting a subset of enzymes to peroxisomes.[162] Thus, it is a peroxisome biogenesis disorder characterized by loss of multiple peroxisomal metabolic functions.

X-LINKED RECESSIVE CHONDRODYSPLASIA PUNCTATA

X-linked recessive chondrodysplasia punctata (CDPX; OMIM #302950) can involve skin (linear or whorled atrophic or ichthyosiform hyperkeratosis, follicular atrophoderma, may begin as erythroderma), hair (coarse, lusterless, cicatricial alopecia), short stature and skeletal abnormalities, cataracts, and deafness. Curry and associates studied a family that had atypical ichthyosis and elevated cholesterol sulfate in two affected males and identified an X chromosomal deletion (Xp22) that included the gene for steroid sulfatase.[161] There is a cluster of arylsulfatase genes at this location. Mutations in *ARSE*, the gene encoding the enzyme arylsulfatase E, were found in five patients; however, it is possible that the disorder may also be caused by mutations in adjacent arylsulfatase genes.[163] The similarity to warfarin embryopathy suggests that warfarin embryopathy may be caused by drug-induced inhibition of the same enzyme.

X-LINKED DOMINANT CHONDRODYSPLASIA PUNCTATA

X-linked dominant chondrodysplasia punctata (CDPX2; Conradi-Hünermann-Happle syndrome, OMIM #302960) is characterized by a mosaic pattern of skin involvement along Blaschko lines caused by mosaic X-chromosome inactivation (lyonization). It occurs almost exclusively in females, with loss of the gene function hypothesized to be lethal to males.[164] Affected females have a normal life expectancy, and there may be increased disease expression in successive generations (anticipation). Occurrence in a male has been observed in association with a 47, XXY karyotype. Conradi-Hünermann-Happle syndrome presents at birth as a congenital ichthyosiform erythroderma that clears over months and is replaced by linear hyperkeratosis, follicular atrophoderma, and pigmentary abnormalities. Hair shaft abnormalities and cicatricial alopecia can also occur. Stippled calcifications are seen in radiographs of areas of endochondral bone formation during childhood but may no longer be visible after puberty. Stature may be short, with asymmetric shortening of the legs. Cataracts occur, usually asymmetrically, in about two thirds of patients. Histochemical staining for calcium may show calcifications within the epidermis, especially within hair follicles in young children, which may not be present in older children.[165] Mutations in the gene encoding the EBP cause the syndrome. EBP was first identified as a binding target for the drug emopamil, a calcium channel blocker. It was later found to be 3β-hydroxysteroid-δ8-δ7-isomerase that catalyses an intermediate step in the conversion of lanosterol to cholesterol.[160] Although this is another ichthyosis caused by abnormality in cholesterol synthesis, the pathophysiology of how this defect causes clinical manifestations is unclear.

ICHTHYOSIS FOLLICULARIS, ALOPECIA, AND PHOTOPHOBIA SYNDROME

Noninflammatory follicular hyperkeratosis, nonscarring alopecia, photophobia, and characteristic facies are seen in the X-linked recessive ichthyosis follicularis, alopecia, and photophobia syndrome (IFAP) syndrome (OMIM #308205, see Chap. 49). Less constant features include recurrent respiratory infections, nail abnormalities, angular cheilitis, keratotic plaques on the extensor surface of the extremities, inguinal hernia, cryptorchidism, short stature, seizures, and psychomotor developmental delay.[166] Mutations in the MBTPS2 gene cause this syndrome presumably by resulting in impaired cholesterol homeostasis and endoplasmic reticulum stress.[167]

ICHTHYOSIS PREMATURITY SYNDROME

Complications such as polyhydramnios in the second trimester of pregnancy occur in the ichthyosis prematurity syndrome (OMIM #608649), resulting in premature delivery of infants with erythrodermic, edematous, caseous scaling skin resembling excessive vernix caseosa, respiratory distress, and transient peripheral eosinophilia.[168] The respiratory signs, erythema, and skin changes resolve, leaving signs of atopy and dry, scaly skin with follicular accentuation more pronounced than is seen in keratosis pilaris. Mutations in the fatty acid transport protein 4 gene FATP4 (SLC27) cause this disorder.[169,170]

MULTIPLE SULFATASE DEFICIENCY

Multiple sulfatase deficiency (OMIM #272200) is a rare autosomal recessive disorder. Clinical features include neurologic deterioration, skeletal abnormalities, facial dysmorphism, and ichthyosis resembling that seen in X-linked steroid sulfatase deficiency. The disorder is a composite of the clinical features of both metachromatic leukodystrophy and a mucopolysaccharidosis. It is characterized by a deficiency of both lysosomal (arylsulfatases A and B) and microsomal (arylsulfatase C/steroid sulfatase of X-linked ichthyosis) arylsulfatases, resulting in the accumulation of sulfatides, glycosaminoglycans, sphingolipids, and steroid sulfates in tissues and body fluids.[171] The gene coding for sulfatase modifying factor 1 (SUMF1), which generates a unique amino acid derivative, C_α-formylglycine, necessary for catalytic activity of all sulfatases, is mutated in individuals with multiple sulfatase deficiency.[172,173]

REFSUM DISEASE

Refsum disease (heredopathia atactica polyneuritiformis; OMIM #266500) is a rare, progressive, degenerative disorder of lipid metabolism resulting from the failure to break down dietary phytanic acid and its subsequent accumulation in tissues. This autosomal recessive condition affects mostly Scandinavians and populations originating from Northern Europe. Clinical manifestations include retinitis pigmentosa, peripheral neuropathy, cerebellar ataxia, cranial nerve dysfunction (neural deafness, anosmia), miosis, electrocardiographic abnormalities, cardiomyopathy, renal tubular dysfunction, and skeletal abnormalities (epiphyseal dysplasia). Ichthyosis, which is variable, generally develops after the neurologic and ophthalmologic manifestations. Often there are small white scales over the trunk and extremities resembling IV. Routine hematoxylin and eosin histologic examination shows variably sized vacuoles in the epidermal basal and suprabasilar cells, which correspond to lipid accumulation seen with lipid stains of frozen sections.[174]

Phytanic acid (a 20-carbon, branched-chain fatty acid) is derived from a variety of dietary sources including dairy products, ruminant fats, and chlorophyll-containing foods, although chlorophyll-bound phytol cannot be absorbed in humans. The disease is caused by a deficiency of PhyH, a peroxisomal protein that catalyzes the α-oxidation of phytanic acid. PhyH deficiency leads to the accumulation of phytanic acid in the serum and tissues, where it substitutes for the fatty acids normally present. Although mutations in PAHX, the gene encoding PhyH, are responsible for most cases of Refsum disease, there is genetic heterogeneity.[175] The Refsum phenotype has been described in patients with mutations PEX7, the affected gene in RCDP (see earlier). Phytanic acid and other chlorophyll metabolites bind the retinoid X receptor (RXR), as does its natural ligand, 9-cis-retinoic acid, and they may be physiologically active in coordinating cellular metabolism through RXR-dependent signaling pathways. However, the role of RXR in the pathogenesis of Refsum disease is unclear. Refsum disease is distinguished from infantile Refsum disease, a fulminant generalized peroxisomal biogenesis disorder in which young children present with severe neurologic abnormalities, mental retardation, hepatomegaly, and dysmorphic features in addition to the other signs of adult Refsum disease.[176]

Refsum disease is a rare example of an ichthyosis whose pathophysiology was understood well enough before identification of the causative gene to make rational treatment recommendations. The diagnosis can be made by detection of elevated levels of plasma phytanic acid. In children who do not have elevated plasma levels of phytanic acid, the diagnosis may be made by measuring PhyH activity in cultured fibroblasts.[177] Treatment includes dietary restriction of foods containing phytanic acid and its precursors. In the clinical setting of a delayed onset of ichthyosis in association with neurologic impairment, this disorder should be considered because therapy can arrest progression.

SJÖGREN-LARSSON SYNDROME

In 1957, Sjögren and Larsson reported on 13 families from north Sweden with a syndrome of congenital ichthyosis, spastic paralysis, and mental retardation. Sjögren-Larsson syndrome (SLS; OMIM #270200) is a rare, autosomal recessive disorder that presents at birth with an ichthyosis that may range from fine scaling to generalized hyperkeratosis. Erythema may be present at birth but tends to gradually clear by 1 year of age. Collodion-like membranes are rarely seen. The ichthyosis manifests as fine scale, large scale, or thickening of the stratum corneum without scale. Pruritus is common. Thickened areas may be yellow to brown in color and have a lichenified appearance with accentuated skin markings (Fig. 47-25). The most involved areas are the sides and back of the neck, lower abdomen, and flexures. Hair, nails, and the ability to sweat are generally normal.[178] During the first 2 to 3 years, neurologic manifestations of spastic diplegia or tetraplegia and mental retardation develop and can be accompanied by speech defects and seizures. A characteristic ophthalmologic finding is the presence of glistening white dots in the macula of the retina. These occur after 1 year of age and may not be present in all patients.

SLS is caused by fatty alcohol:NAD oxidoreductase (FAO) deficiency. FAO is a complex enzyme with two separate proteins that sequentially catalyze the oxidation of fatty alcohol to fatty aldehyde and subsequently to fatty acid. Mutations found in the *ALDH3A2* gene confirmed the role for this enzyme in the cause of this disorder and the importance of this pathway for normal desquamation. *ALDH3A2* is a microsomal enzyme that catalyzes the oxidation of medium- and long-chain aliphatic aldehydes derived from metabolism of fatty alcohol, phytanic acid, ether glycerolipids, and

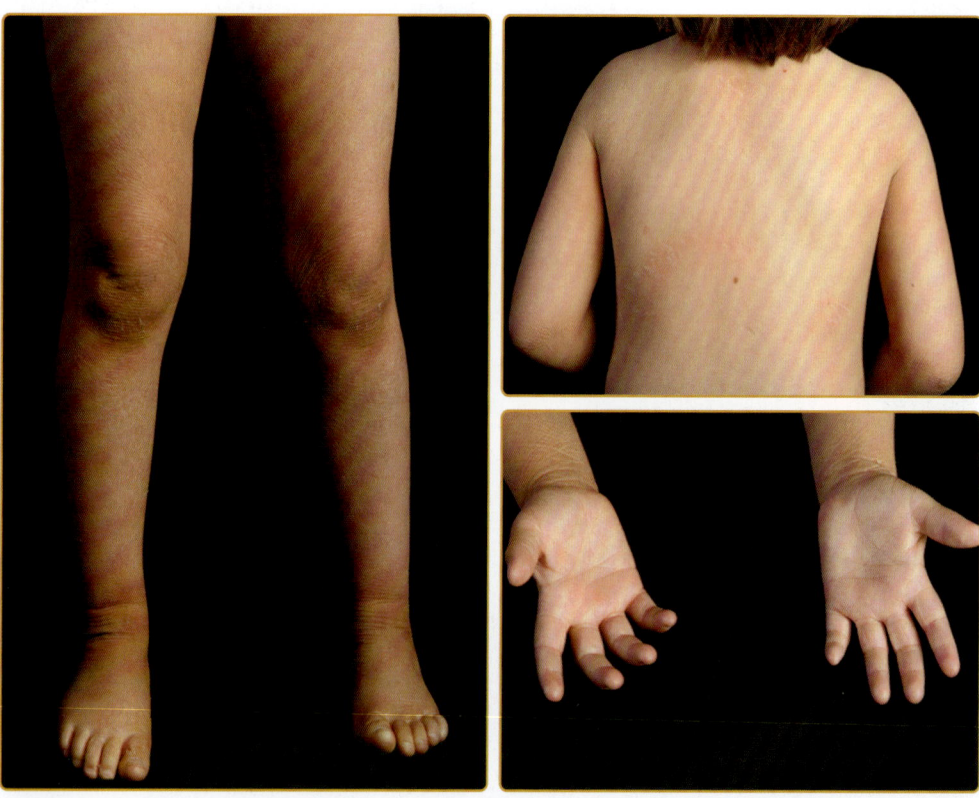

Figure 47-25 Autosomal recessive congenital ichthyosis, Sjögren-Larsson syndrome (*ALDH3A2* mutations). Generalized smooth hyperkeratosis *(keratoderma)* results in large adherent scales on extremities and accentuated linear surface markings. There is usually little erythema, but scratching produces fine white scale and erythema.

leukotriene B4.[179] The identification of decreased fibroblast FAO activity in a family with atypical cutaneous findings (lack of ichthyosis or discrete plaques rather than generalized ichthyosis) has expanded the spectrum of clinical phenotypes associated with abnormal FAO activity.[180]

TRICHOTHIODYSTROPHY

Trichothiodystrophy (TTD; OMIM #601675, also see Chap. 130) is an autosomal recessive disorder that includes a broad spectrum of clinical phenotypes linked by the characteristic features of sulfur deficient, brittle hair that exhibits alternating birefringence (tiger tail banding) when viewed under polarizing microscopy (Fig. 47-26).[181] The spectrum of clinical involvement is broad, ranging from only hair to severe multisystem abnormalities. A survey of 112 cases reported in the literature found ichthyosis (65%) as the most common skin finding followed by photosensitivity (42%). Of the patients with ichthyosis, about one third presented with a collodion membrane at birth. Erythroderma, when present at birth, usually decreases over weeks with evolution into a generalized ichthyosis, usually without erythema, which varies from small fine, scaling to large, dark yellow-brown hyperkeratosis (see Fig. 47-17B).[182,183] There may be flexural sparing and palmoplantar keratoderma. Nail findings are found in more than half of the patients and include dystrophic nails (ridging, splitting) (see Fig. 47-17A), hypoplasia, brittle nails, and koilonychia.[184] Ectropion usually does not occur. Photosensitivity can range from subtle to severe. Other common findings in TTD include intellectual impairment, short stature, microcephaly, characteristic facial features (protruding ears, micrognathia), recurrent infections, and cataracts.

A series of mnemonics have been used to describe the constellation of findings as BIDS (*b*rittle hair, *i*ntellectual impairment, *d*ecreased fertility, and *s*hort stature); patients who also have *i*chthyosis have been called IBIDS, and with the addition of *p*hotosensitivity, PIBI(D)S has been used.[185] However, these terms do not account for the other multisystem findings that are commonly present.

The majority of TTD patients with ichthyosis have a defect in the function or activity of TFIIH, a protein complex involved in DNA repair and transcription. Most mutations are in *ERCC2*. Other mutations affect *ERCC3*, *GTF2H5*, and *GTF2E2*. Two other genes causing TTD, *MPLKIP* and *RNF113A*, have not been associated with ichthyosis and their function is unknown.[186-190] Although many patients with

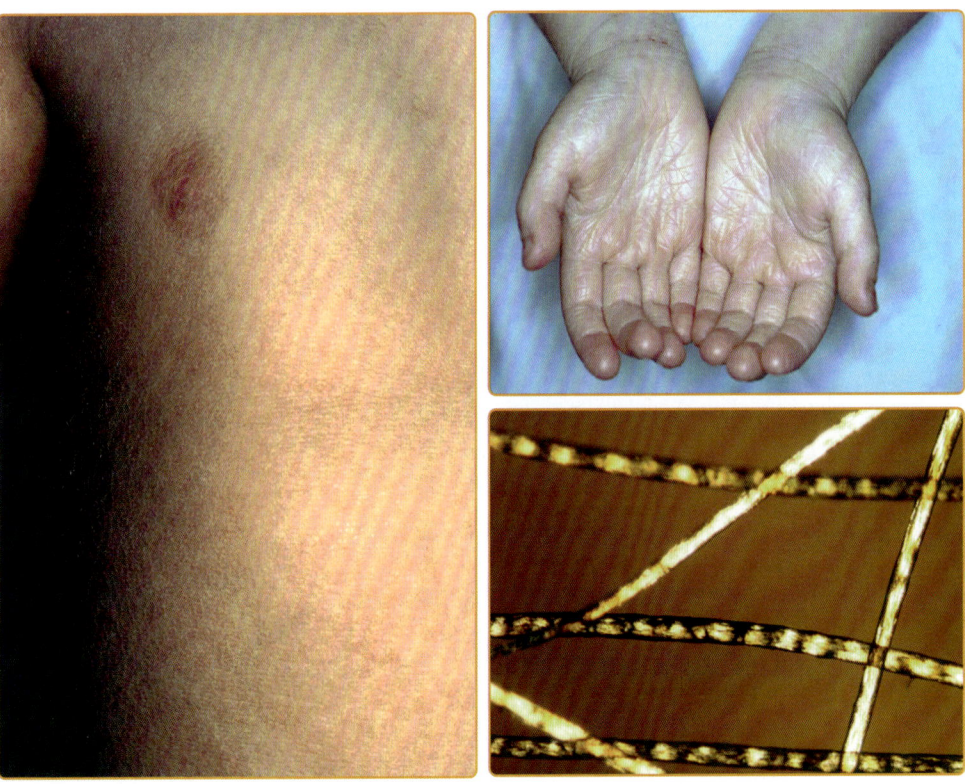

Figure 47-26 Autosomal recessive congenital ichthyosis, trichothiodystrophy (*ERCC2*, *ERCC3*, *GTF2H5*, *GTF2E2* mutations). Beyond the newborn period, there is usually very mild generalized hyperkeratosis and minimal erythema. Hair shows characteristic alternating birefringence in polarized light.

TTD have photosensitivity, in contrast to xeroderma pigmentosum, these photosensitive patients have not been observed to be at high risk for the development of skin cancer. Nucleotide excision repair is one normal cellular mechanism by which structural DNA damage (eg, ultraviolet-induced cyclobutane pyrimidine dimers) is removed and repaired (see Chaps. 20 and 134).

ACQUIRED ICHTHYOSIS

The development of ichthyosis in adulthood can be a manifestation of systemic disease and has been described in association with malignancies, drugs, endocrine and metabolic disease, malnutrition, HIV and other infections, and autoimmune conditions.[191-194] The granular layer is often attenuated in this disorder, and the scale often resembles to that seen in mild IV. Although Hodgkin disease is the most common malignancy reported with acquired ichthyosis, non-Hodgkin lymphomas and a variety of other malignancies have also been observed. Histology may be diagnostic in acquired ichthyosis associated with mycosis fungoides.[195] Skin involvement may follow the course of malignancy and clear with effective cancer treatment. Acquired ichthyosis is commonly seen in association with AIDS; ichthyotic or xerotic skin has been observed in up to 30% of patients with AIDS.[196] A study of HIV-1–positive intravenous drug users found acquired ichthyosis occurred only after profound helper T cell depletion, more frequently with coinfection with human T-cell leukemia or lymphoma virus type II, and suggested that it may be a marker for concomitant infection with both viruses.[197]

In acquired ichthyosis occurring in association with sarcoidosis, skin biopsy can be diagnostic, showing noncaseating granulomas in the dermis.[198] Acquired ichthyosis may be a marker of autoimmune disease, occurring with systemic lupus erythematosus, dermatomyositis, mixed connective tissue disease, and eosinophilic fasciitis.[199,200] It has been described in bone marrow transplant recipients, in whom it may be related to graft-versus-host disease.[201]

Although occurrence in association with cholesterol-lowering agents (nicotinic acid, triparanol) highlights the relationship between cholesterol metabolism and normal desquamation, acquired ichthyosis has been observed with a variety of drugs, including cimetidine, clofazimine, hydroxyurea, cholesterol-lowering agents, and others.[202,203] Kava is a psychoactive beverage made from the root of a pepper plant and used for thousands of years by Pacific Islanders. Heavy kava drinkers can acquire a reversible ichthyosiform eruption called kava dermopathy. In Western nations, kava is sold in health food stores as a relaxant.[204]

PITYRIASIS ROTUNDA

Sharply demarcated, round or oval scaly patches with hypo- or hyperpigmentation are seen in pityriasis rotunda. Although this uncommon disorder is usually acquired, occasional familial cases have been described.[205]

RETICULATED PAPILLOMATOSIS OF GOUGEROT AND CARTEAUD

Confluent and reticulated papillomatosis of Gougerot and Carteaud is an uncommon but distinctive acquired ichthyosiform dermatosis seen in young adults and characterized by persistent brown, scaly macules, papules, patches, and plaques. Lesions tend to be localized predominantly on the neck, upper trunk (intermammary and interscapular regions), and axillae, where they tend to be confluent and become reticulated towards the periphery. The lesions bear a clinical resemblance to tinea versicolor, a skin infection with *Pityrosporum* spp. A variety of treatment approaches have been reported, including topical (keratolytics, derivatives of vitamin A and D, antimicrobials) and systemic (antibiotics, retinoids) agents. Minocycline has been suggested as a first-line treatment; successful retreatment of recurrences supports the concept that this condition is an abnormal response to an infection or inflammation.[206,207]

RESOURCES

The Foundation for Ichthyosis and Related Skin Types (FIRST) (phone: 800-545-3286; http://www.firstskinfoundation.org; email: info@firstskinfoundation.org.) provides support and information for affected individuals, family members, friends, and health care provider.

The Genetic Testing Registry (https://www.ncbi.nlm.nih.gov/gtr/) provides disease reviews, genetic testing resources, and educational materials.

Online Mendelian Inheritance in Man, (http://www.ncbi.nlm.nih.gov/entrez/query.fcgi?db=OMIM) (trademark Johns Hopkins University), a catalog of human genes and genetic disorders, is a useful reference with links to additional resources.

The Registry for Ichthyosis and Related Disorders is a resource for investigators to improve diagnosis and treatment of these disorders (Yale University, Department of Dermatology, PO Box 208059, 333 Cedar Street, New Haven, CT 06510; email: ichthyosisregistry@yale.edu).

ACKNOWLEDGMENTS

The authors are grateful to Philip Fleckman and John J. DiGiovanna, who authored the prior version of this chapter and have provided text, tables, and photographs that appear here.

REFERENCES

1. Willan R. *On Cutaneous Diseases. [Pt. 1]*. Brown & Merritt, London: Kimber and Conrad; 1809:1798.
2. Siemens HW. Studies on the heredity of skin diseases XI ichthyosis congenita. *Archiv Fur Dermatologie Und Syphilis*. 1929;158(1):111-127.
3. Wells RS, Kerr CB. Genetic classification of ichthyosis. *Arch Dermatol*. 1965;92(1):1-6.
4. Wells RS, Kerr CB. Clinical features of autosomal dominant and sex-linked ichthyosis in an English population. *Br Med J*. 1966;1(5493):947-950.
5. Traupe H. The Ichthyoses: A Guide to Clinical Diagnosis, Genetic Counseling, and Therapy. Berlin; New York: Springer-Verlag; 1989.
6. Frost P, Van Scott EJ. Ichthyosiform dermatoses. Classification based on anatomic and biometric observations. *Arch Dermatol*. 1966;94(2):113-126.
7. Williams ML, Elias PM. Genetically transmitted, generalized disorders of cornification. The ichthyoses. *Dermatol Clin*. 1987;5(1):155-178.
8. Marukian NV, Choate KA. Recent advances in understanding ichthyosis pathogenesis. *F1000Res*. 2016;5.
9. Oji V, Tadini G, Akiyama M, et al. Revised nomenclature and classification of inherited ichthyoses: results of the First Ichthyosis Consensus Conference in Soreze 2009. *J Am Acad Dermatol*. 2010;63(4):607-641.
10. Ross R, DiGiovanna JJ, Capaldi L, et al. Histopathologic characterization of epidermolytic hyperkeratosis: a systematic review of histology from the National Registry for Ichthyosis and Related Skin Disorders. *J Am Acad Dermatol*. 2008;59(1):86-90.
11. Boyden LM, Craiglow BG, Zhou J, et al. Dominant de novo mutations in gja1 cause erythrokeratodermia variabilis et progressiva, without features of oculodentodigital dysplasia. *J Invest Dermatol*. 2015;135(6):1540-1547.
12. Boyden LM, Kam CY, Hernandez-Martin A, et al. Dominant de novo DSP mutations cause erythrokeratodermia-cardiomyopathy syndrome. *Hum Mol Genet*. 2016;25(2):348-357.
13. Fassihi H, McGrath JA. Prenatal diagnosis of epidermolysis bullosa. *Dermatol Clin*. 2010;28(2):231-237, viii.
14. Tabor A, Alfirevic Z. Update on procedure-related risks for prenatal diagnosis techniques. *Fetal Diagn Ther*. 2010;27(1):1-7.
15. Yanagi T, Akiyama M, Sakai K, et al. DNA-based prenatal exclusion of harlequin ichthyosis. *J Am Acad Dermatol*. 2008;58(4):653-656.
16. Meredith S, Kaposy C, Miller VJ, et al. Impact of the increased adoption of prenatal cfDNA screening on non-profit patient advocacy organizations in the United States. *Prenat Diagn*. 2016;36(8):714-719.
17. Buysse K, Beulen L, Gomes I, et al. Reliable noninvasive prenatal testing by massively parallel sequencing of circulating cell-free DNA from maternal plasma processed up to 24h after venipuncture. *Clin Biochem*. 2013;46(18):1783-1786.
18. Digiovanna JJ, Bale SJ. Epidermolytic hyperkeratosis—applied molecular-genetics. *J Invest Dermatol*. 1994;102(3):390-394.
19. Meibodi NT, Nahidi Y, Javidi Z. Epidermolytic hyperkeratosis in inflammatory linear verrucous epidermal nevus. *Indian J Dermatol*. 2011;56(3):309-312.
20. Mirza H, Kumar A, Craiglow BG, et al. Mutations affecting keratin 10 surface-exposed residues highlight the structural basis of phenotypic variation in epidermolytic ichthyosis. *J Invest Dermatol*. 2015;135(12):3041-3050.
21. Huber M, Rettler I, Bernasconi K, et al. Mutations of keratinocyte transglutaminase in lamellar ichthyosis. *Science*. 1995;267(5197):525-528.
22. Russell LJ, DiGiovanna JJ, Rogers GR, et al. Mutations in the gene for transglutaminase 1 in autosomal recessive lamellar ichthyosis. *Nat Genet*. 1995;9(3):279-283.
23. Fischer J. Autosomal recessive congenital ichthyosis. *J Invest Dermatol*. 2009;129(6):1319-1321.
24. Chavanas S, Bodemer C, Rochat A, et al. Mutations in SPINK5, encoding a serine protease inhibitor, cause Netherton syndrome. *Nat Genet*. 2000;25(2):141-142.
25. Smith FJ, Irvine AD, Terron-Kwiatkowski A, et al. Loss-of-function mutations in the gene encoding filaggrin cause ichthyosis vulgaris. *Nat Genet*. 2006;38(3):337-342.
26. Paller AS, Renert-Yuval Y, Suprun M, et al. An IL-17-dominant immune profile is shared across the major orphan forms of ichthyosis. *J Allergy Clin Immunol*. 2017;139(1):152-165.
27. Duckney P, Wong HK, Serrano J, et al. The role of the skin barrier in modulating the effects of common skin microbial species on the inflammation, differentiation and proliferation status of epidermal keratinocytes. *BMC Res Notes*. 2013;6:474.
28. Traupe H. Ichthyoses and related keratinization disorders. Management, clinical features and genetics. *Hautarzt*. 2004;55(10):931-941.
29. Fleckman P. Management of the ichthyoses. *Skin Therapy Lett*. 2003;8(6):3-7.
30. Germann R, Schindera I, Kuch M, et al. Life threatening salicylate poisoning caused by percutaneous absorption in severe ichthyosis vulgaris. *Hautarzt*. 1996;47(8):624-627.
31. Nguyen V, Cunningham BB, Eichenfield LF, et al. Treatment of ichthyosiform diseases with topically applied tazarotene: risk of systemic absorption. *J Am Acad Dermatol*. 2007;57(5 suppl):S123-125.
32. Borzyskowski M, Grant DB, Wells RS. Cushing's syndrome induced by topical steroids used for the treatment of non-bullous ichthyosiform erythroderma. *Clin Exp Dermatol*. 1976;1(4):337-342.
33. Moskowitz DG, Fowler AJ, Heyman MB, et al. Pathophysiologic basis for growth failure in children with ichthyosis: an evaluation of cutaneous ultrastructure, epidermal permeability barrier function, and energy expenditure. *J Pediatr*. 2004;145(1):82-92.
34. Verfaille CJ, Vanhoutte FP, Blanchet-Bardon C, et al. Oral liarozole vs. acitretin in the treatment of ichthyosis: a phase II/III multicentre, double-blind, randomized, active-controlled study. *Br J Dermatol*. 2007;156(5):965-973.
35. Palmer CN, Irvine AD, Terron-Kwiatkowski A, et al. Common loss-of-function variants of the epidermal barrier protein filaggrin are a major predisposing factor for atopic dermatitis. *Nat Genet*. 2006;38(4):441-446.
36. Brown SJ, Relton CL, Liao H, et al. Filaggrin haploinsufficiency is highly penetrant and is associated with increased severity of eczema: further delineation of the skin phenotype in a prospective

37. Dale BA, Holbrook KA, Steinert PM. Assembly of stratum corneum basic protein and keratin filaments in macrofibrils. *Nature*. 1978;276(5689):729-731.
38. Rice RH, Bradshaw KM, Durbin-Johnson BP, et al. Distinguishing ichthyoses by protein profiling. *PLoS One*. 2013;8(10):e75355.
39. Sybert VP, Dale BA, Holbrook KA. Ichthyosis vulgaris: identification of a defect in synthesis of filaggrin correlated with an absence of keratohyaline granules. *J Invest Dermatol*. 1985;84(3):191-194.
40. Sandilands A, Sutherland C, Irvine AD, et al. Filaggrin in the frontline: role in skin barrier function and disease. *J Cell Sci*. 2009;122(Pt 9):1285-1294.
41. van den Oord RA, Sheikh A. Filaggrin gene defects and risk of developing allergic sensitisation and allergic disorders: systematic review and meta-analysis. *BMJ*. 2009;339:b2433.
42. Mevorah B, Krayenbuhl A, Bovey EH, et al. Autosomal dominant ichthyosis and X-linked ichthyosis. Comparison of their clinical and histological phenotypes. *Acta Derm Venereol*. 1991;71(5):431-434.
43. Cuevas-Covarrubias SA, Kofman-Alfaro SH, Palencia AB, et al. Accuracy of the clinical diagnosis of recessive X-linked ichthyosis vs ichthyosis vulgaris. *J Dermatol*. 1996;23(9):594-597.
44. Hand JL, Runke CK, Hodge JC. The phenotype spectrum of X-linked ichthyosis identified by chromosomal microarray. *J Am Acad Dermatol*. 2015;72(4):617-627.
45. Marinkovic-Ilsen A, Koppe JG, Jobsis AC, et al. Enzymatic basis of typical X-linked ichthyosis. *Lancet*. 1978;2(8099):1097.
46. Shapiro LJ, Weiss R, Buxman MM, et al. Enzymatic basis of typical X-linked ichthyosis. *Lancet*. 1978;2(8093):756-757.
47. Fernandes NF, Janniger CK, Schwartz RA. X-linked ichthyosis: an oculocutaneous genodermatosis. *J Am Acad Dermatol*. 2010;62(3):480-485.
48. Merrett JD, Wells RS, Kerr CB, et al. Discriminant function analysis of phenotype variates in ichthyosis. *Am J Hum Genet*. 1967;19(4):575-585.
49. Jay B, Blach RK, Wells RS. Ocular manifestations of ichthyosis. *Br J Ophthalmol*. 1968;52(3):217-226.
50. Sever RJ, Frost P, Weinstein G. Eye changes in ichthyosis. *JAMA*. 1968;206(10):2283-2286.
51. Lykkesfeldt G, Bennett P, Lykkesfeldt AE, et al. Testis cancer. Ichthyosis constitutes a significant risk factor. *Cancer*. 1991;67(3):730-734.
52. Rose FA. Review: the mammalian sulphatases and placental sulphatase deficiency in man. *J Inherit Metab Dis*. 1982;5(3):145-152.
53. Epstein EH Jr, Williams ML, Elias PM. Steroid sulfatase, X-linked ichthyosis, and stratum corneum cell cohesion. *Arch Dermatol*. 1981;117(12):761-763.
54. Epstein EH Jr, Bonifas JM. Recessive X-linked ichthyosis: lack of immunologically detectable steroid sulfatase enzyme protein. *Hum Genet*. 1985;71(3):201-205.
55. Milstone LM. Epidermal desquamation. *J Dermatol Sci*. 2004;36(3):131-140.
56. Webster D, France JT, Shapiro LJ, et al. X-linked ichthyosis due to steroid-sulphatase deficiency. *Lancet*. 1978;1(8055):70-72.
57. Ballabio A, Zollo M, Carrozzo R, et al. Deletion of the distal short arm of the X chromosome (Xp) in a patient with short stature, chondrodysplasia punctata, and X-linked ichthyosis due to steroid sulfatase deficiency. *Am J Med Genet*. 1991;41(2):184-187.
58. Paige DG, Emilion GG, Bouloux PM, et al. A clinical and genetic study of X-linked recessive ichthyosis and contiguous gene defects. *Br J Dermatol*. 1994;131(5):622-629.
59. Milstone LM. Scaly skin and bath pH: rediscovering baking soda. *J Am Acad Dermatol*. 2010;62(5):885-886.
60. Milstone LM, Miller K, Haberman M, et al. Incidence of moderate to severe ichthyosis in the United States. *Arch Dermatol*. 2012;148(9):1080-1081.
61. Theiler M, Mann C, Weibel L. Self-healing collodion baby. *J Pediatr*. 2010;157(1):169-169;e161.
62. Vahlquist A, Bygum A, Ganemo A, et al. Genotypic and clinical spectrum of self-improving collodion ichthyosis: ALOX12B, ALOXE3, and TGM1 mutations in Scandinavian patients. *J Invest Dermatol*. 2010;130(2):438-443.
63. Ozturk A, Caksen H, Cetin N, et al. A retrospective study on 16 collodion babies. *Turk J Pediatr*. 1997;39(1):55-59.
64. Nguyen MA, Gelman A, Norton SA. Practical events in the management of a collodion baby. *JAMA Dermatol*. 2015;151(9):1031-1032.
65. Glick JB, Craiglow BG, Choate KA, et al. Improved management of harlequin ichthyosis with advances in neonatal intensive care. *Pediatrics*. 2017; 139(1).
66. Simpson JR. Congenital ichthyosiform erythrodermia. *Trans St Johns Hosp Dermatol Soc*. 1964; 50:93-104.
67. Williams ML, Elias PM. Heterogeneity in autosomal recessive ichthyosis. Clinical and biochemical differentiation of lamellar ichthyosis and nonbullous congenital ichthyosiform erythroderma. *Arch Dermatol*. 1985;121(4):477-488.
68. Bernhardt M, Baden HP. Report of a family with an unusual expression of recessive ichthyosis. Review of 42 cases. *Arch Dermatol*. 1986;122(4):428-433.
69. Jacyk WK. Bathing-suit ichthyosis. A peculiar phenotype of lamellar ichthyosis in South African blacks. *Eur J Dermatol*. 2005;15(6):433-436.
70. Oji V, Hautier JM, Ahvazi B, et al. Bathing suit ichthyosis is caused by transglutaminase-1 deficiency: evidence for a temperature-sensitive phenotype. *Hum Mol Genet*. 2006;15(21):3083-3097.
71. Hackett BC, Fitzgerald D, Watson RM, et al. Genotype-phenotype correlations with TGM1: clustering of mutations in the bathing suit ichthyosis and self-healing collodion baby variants of lamellar ichthyosis. *Br J Dermatol*. 2010;162(2):448-451.
72. Marukian NV, Hu RH, Craiglow BG, et al. Expanding the Genotypic spectrum of bathing suit ichthyosis. *JAMA Dermatol*. 2017;153(6):537-543.
73. Rajpopat S, Moss C, Mellerio J, et al. Harlequin ichthyosis: a review of clinical and molecular findings in 45 cases. *Arch Dermatol*. 2011;147(6):681-686.
74. Milstone LM, Choate KA. Improving outcomes for harlequin ichthyosis. *J Am Acad Dermatol*. 2013; 69(5):808-809.
75. Hurwitz S, Kirsch N, McGuire J. Reevaluation of ichthyosis and hair shaft abnormalities. *Arch Dermatol*. 1971;103(3):266-271.
76. Dev T, Raman Kumar M, Sethuraman G. Ichthyosis linearis circumflexa with bamboo hair: challenges in the diagnosis and management. *BMJ Case Rep*. 2017;2017.

77. Salodkar AD, Choudhary SV, Jadwani G, et al. Bamboo hair in Netherton's syndrome. *Int J Trichology.* 2009;1(2):143-144.
78. Ito M, Ito K, Hashimoto K. Pathogenesis in trichorrhexis invaginata (bamboo hair). *J Invest Dermatol.* 1984;83(1):1-6.
79. Renner ED, Hartl D, Rylaarsdam S, et al. Comel-Netherton syndrome defined as primary immunodeficiency. *J Allergy Clin Immunol.* 2009;124(3):536-543.
80. Nemes Z, Marekov LN, Fesus L, et al. A novel function for transglutaminase 1: attachment of long-chain omega-hydroxyceramides to involucrin by ester bond formation. *Proc Natl Acad Sci U S A.* 1999;96(15):8402-8407.
81. Choate KA, Medalie DA, Morgan JR, et al. Corrective gene transfer in the human skin disorder lamellar ichthyosis. *Nat Med.* 1996;2(11):1263-1267.
82. Aufenvenne K, Larcher F, Hausser I, et al. Topical enzyme-replacement therapy restores transglutaminase 1 activity and corrects architecture of transglutaminase-1-deficient skin grafts. *Am J Hum Genet.* 2013;93(4):620-630.
83. Jobard F, Lefevre C, Karaduman A, et al. Lipoxygenase-3 (ALOXE3) and 12(R)-lipoxygenase (ALOX12B) are mutated in non-bullous congenital ichthyosiform erythroderma (NCIE) linked to chromosome 17p13.1. *Hum Mol Genet.* 2002;11(1):107-113.
84. Munoz-Garcia A, Thomas CP, Keeney DS, et al. The importance of the lipoxygenase-hepoxilin pathway in the mammalian epidermal barrier. *Biochim Biophys Acta.* 2014;1841(3):401-408.
85. Akiyama M, Sugiyama-Nakagiri Y, Sakai K, et al. Mutations in lipid transporter ABCA12 in harlequin ichthyosis and functional recovery by corrective gene transfer. *J Clin Invest.* 2005;115(7):1777-1784.
86. Kelsell DP, Norgett EE, Unsworth H, et al. Mutations in ABCA12 underlie the severe congenital skin disease harlequin ichthyosis. *Am J Hum Genet.* 2005;76(5):794-803.
87. Sakai K, Akiyama M, Yanagi T, et al. ABCA12 is a major causative gene for non-bullous congenital ichthyosiform erythroderma. *J Invest Dermatol.* 2009;129(9):2306-2309.
88. Lefevre C, Audebert S, Jobard F, et al. Mutations in the transporter ABCA12 are associated with lamellar ichthyosis type 2. *Hum Mol Genet.* 2003;12(18):2369-2378.
89. Milner ME, O'Guin WM, Holbrook KA, Dale BA. Abnormal lamellar granules in harlequin ichthyosis. *J Invest Dermatol.* 1992;99(6):824-829.
90. Walley AJ, Chavanas S, Moffatt MF, et al. Gene polymorphism in Netherton and common atopic disease. *Nat Genet.* 2001;29(2):175-178.
91. Fortugno P, Furio L, Teson M, et al. The 420K LEKTI variant alters LEKTI proteolytic activation and results in protease deregulation: implications for atopic dermatitis. *Hum Mol Genet.* 2012;21(19):4187-4200.
92. Fölster-Holst R, Swensson O, Stockfleth E, et al. Comèl-Netherton syndrome complicated by papillomatous skin lesions containing human papillomaviruses 51 and 52 and plane warts containing human papillomavirus 16. *Br J Dermatol.* 1999;140(6):1139-1143.
93. Craiglow BG, Choate KA, Milstone LM. Topical tazarotene for the treatment of ectropion in ichthyosis. *JAMA Dermatol.* 2013;149(5):598-600.
94. Pigg MH, Bygum A, Ganemo A, et al. Spectrum of autosomal recessive congenital ichthyosis in Scandinavia: clinical characteristics and novel and recurrent mutations in 132 patients. *Acta Derm Venereol.* 2016;96(7):932-937.
95. Shibata A, Ogawa Y, Sugiura K, et al. High survival rate of harlequin ichthyosis in Japan. *J Am Acad Dermatol.* 2014;70(2):387-388.
96. Sprecher E, Tesfaye-Kedjela A, Ratajczak P, et al. Deleterious mutations in SPINK5 in a patient with congenital ichthyosiform erythroderma: molecular testing as a helpful diagnostic tool for Netherton syndrome. *Clin Exp Dermatol.* 2004;29(5):513-517.
97. Geyer AS, Ratajczak P, Pol-Rodriguez M, et al. Netherton syndrome with extensive skin peeling and failure to thrive due to a homozygous frameshift mutation in SPINK5. *Dermatology.* 2005;210(4):308-314.
98. Allen A, Siegfried E, Silverman R, et al. Significant absorption of topical tacrolimus in 3 patients with Netherton syndrome. *Arch Dermatol.* 2001;137(6):747-750.
99. Brocq L. *Erythrodermie congénitale ichthyosiforme avec hyperépidermotrophie, par L. Brocq. Ann Derm Syph.* Masson; 3:1-31,1902.
100. DiGiovanna JJ, Bale SJ. Clinical heterogeneity in epidermolytic hyperkeratosis. *Arch Dermatol.* 1994;130(8):1026-1035.
101. Paller AS, Syder AJ, Chan YM, et al. Genetic and clinical mosaicism in a type of epidermal nevus. *N Engl J Med.* 1994;331(21):1408-1415.
102. Uchiyama K, Nakanishi G, Fujimoto N, et al. Localized linear epidermolytic epidermal nevus of male genitalia with a recurrent keratin 10 mutation, p.Arg156His. *Eur J Dermatol.* 2013;23(4):557-558.
103. Nazzaro V, Ermacora E, Santucci B, et al. Epidermolytic hyperkeratosis: generalized form in children from parents with systematized linear form. *Br J Dermatol.* 1990;122(3):417-422.
104. Chassaing N, Kanitakis J, Sportich S, et al. Generalized epidermolytic hyperkeratosis in two unrelated children from parents with localized linear form, and prenatal diagnosis. *J Invest Dermatol.* 2006;126(12):2715-2717.
105. Rothnagel JA, Traupe H, Wojcik S, et al. Mutations in the rod domain of keratin 2e in patients with ichthyosis bullosa of Siemens. *Nat Genet.* 1994;7(4):485-490.
106. McLean WH, Morley SM, Lane EB, et al. Ichthyosis bullosa of Siemens—a disease involving keratin 2e. *J Invest Dermatol.* 1994;103(3):277-281.
107. Sahn EE, Weimer CE Jr, Garen PD. Annular epidermolytic ichthyosis: a unique phenotype. *J Am Acad Dermatol.* 1992;27(2 Pt 2):348-355.
108. Jha A, Taneja J, Ramesh V, et al. Annular epidermolytic ichthyosis: a rare phenotypic variant of bullous congenital ichthyosiform erythroderma. *Indian J Dermatol Venereol Leprol.* 2015;81(2):194-197.
109. Sybert VP, Francis JS, Corden LD, et al. Cyclic ichthyosis with epidermolytic hyperkeratosis: a phenotype conferred by mutations in the 2B domain of keratin K1. *Am J Hum Genet.* 1999;64(3):732-738.
110. Joh GY, Traupe H, Metze D, et al. A novel dinucleotide mutation in keratin 10 in the annular epidermolytic ichthyosis variant of bullous congenital ichthyosiform erythroderma. *J Invest Dermatol.* 1997;108(3):357-361.

111. Choate KA, Milstone LM. Phenotypic expansion in ichthyosis with confetti. *JAMA Dermatol.* 2015;151(1):15-16.
112. Lim YH, Qiu J, Saraceni C, et al. Genetic reversion via mitotic recombination in ichthyosis with confetti due to a KRT10 polyalanine frameshift mutation. *J Invest Dermatol.* 2016;136(8):1725-1728.
113. Choate KA, Lu Y, Zhou J, et al. Frequent somatic reversion of KRT1 mutations in ichthyosis with confetti. *J Clin Invest.* 2015;125(4):1703-1707.
114. Choate KA, Lu Y, Zhou J, et al. Mitotic recombination in patients with ichthyosis causes reversion of dominant mutations in KRT10. *Science.* 2010;330(6000):94-97.
115. Cheng J, Syder AJ, Yu QC, et al. The genetic basis of epidermolytic hyperkeratosis: a disorder of differentiation-specific epidermal keratin genes. *Cell.* 1992;70(5):811-819.
116. Li H, Torma H. Retinoids reduce formation of keratin aggregates in heat-stressed immortalized keratinocytes from an epidermolytic ichthyosis patient with a KRT10 mutation*. *Acta Derm Venereol.* 2013;93(1):44-49.
117. Fuchs E, Coulombe P, Cheng J, et al. Genetic bases of epidermolysis bullosa simplex and epidermolytic hyperkeratosis. *J Invest Dermatol.* 1994;103(5 suppl):25S-30S.
118. Hotz A, Oji V, Bourrat E, et al. Expanding the clinical and genetic spectrum of KRT1, KRT2 and KRT10 mutations in keratinopathic ichthyosis. *Acta Derm Venereol.* 2016;96(4):473-478.
119. Reis A, Hennies HC, Langbein L, et al. Keratin 9 gene mutations in epidermolytic palmoplantar keratoderma (EPPK). *Nat Genet.* 1994;6(2):174-179.
120. Ogawa M, Akiyama M. Successful topical adapalene treatment for the facial lesions of an adolescent case of epidermolytic ichthyosis. *J Am Acad Dermatol.* 2014;71(3):e103-105.
121. El-Ramly M, Zachariae H. Long-term oral treatment of two pronounced ichthyotic conditions: lamellar ichthyosis and epidermolytic hyperkeratosis with the aromatic retinoid, Tigason (RO 10-9359). *Acta Derm Venereol.* 1983;63(5):452-456.
122. Digiovanna JJ, Mauro T, Milstone LM, et al. Systemic retinoids in the management of ichthyoses and related skin types. *Dermatol Ther.* 2013;26(1):26-38.
123. Rogers M. Erythrokeratodermas: a classification in a state of flux? *Australas J Dermatol.* 2005;46(3):127-141; quiz 142.
124. Lilly E, Sellitto C, Milstone LM, et al. Connexin channels in congenital skin disorders. *Semin Cell Dev Biol.* 2016;50:4-12.
125. van Steensel MA, Oranje AP, van der Schroeff JG, et al. The missense mutation G12D in connexin30.3 can cause both erythrokeratodermia variabilis of Mendes da Costa and progressive symmetric erythrokeratodermia of Gottron. *Am J Med Genet A.* 2009;149A(4):657-661.
126. Darier MJ. Erythokeratodermia verruqueuse, symétrique et progressive. *Bull Soc Fr Dermatol Syphiligr.* 1911(22):252.
127. Ruiz-Maldonado R, Tamayo L, del Castillo V, et al. Erythrokeratodermia progressiva symmetrica: report of 10 cases. *Dermatologica.* 1982;164(2):133-141.
128. Richard G, Brown N, Rouan F, et al. Genetic heterogeneity in erythrokeratodermia variabilis: novel mutations in the connexin gene GJB4 (Cx30.3) and genotype-phenotype correlations. *J Invest Dermatol.* 2003;120(4):601-609.
129. Gottfried I, Landau M, Glaser F, et al. A mutation in GJB3 is associated with recessive erythrokeratodermia variabilis (EKV) and leads to defective trafficking of the connexin 31 protein. *Hum Mol Genet.* 2002;11(11):1311-1316.
130. Caceres-Rios H, Tamayo-Sanchez L, Duran-Mckinster C, et al. Keratitis, ichthyosis, and deafness (KID syndrome): review of the literature and proposal of a new terminology. *Pediatr Dermatol.* 1996;13(2):105-113.
131. Richard G, Smith LE, Bailey RA, et al. Mutations in the human connexin gene GJB3 cause erythrokeratodermia variabilis. *Nat Genet.* 1998;20(4):366-369.
132. Macari F, Landau M, Cousin P, et al. Mutation in the gene for connexin 30.3 in a family with erythrokeratodermia variabilis. *Am J Hum Genet.* 2000;67(5):1296-1301.
133. Richard G, Rouan F, Willoughby CE, et al. Missense mutations in GJB2 encoding connexin-26 cause the ectodermal dysplasia keratitis-ichthyosis-deafness syndrome. *Am J Hum Genet.* 2002;70(5):1341-1348.
134. Shuja Z, Li L, Gupta S, et al. Connexin26 mutations causing palmoplantar keratoderma and deafness interact with connexin43, modifying gap junction and hemichannel properties. *J Invest Dermatol.* 2016;136(1):225-235.
135. Maestrini E, Korge BP, Ocana-Sierra J, et al. A missense mutation in connexin26, D66H, causes mutilating keratoderma with sensorineural deafness (Vohwinkel's syndrome) in three unrelated families. *Hum Mol Genet.* 1999;8(7):1237-1243.
136. Richard G, Brown N, Smith LE, et al. The spectrum of mutations in erythrokeratodermias—novel and de novo mutations in GJB3. *Hum Genet.* 2000;106(3):321-329.
137. Todt I, Mazereeuw-Hautier J, Binder B, et al. Dandy-Walker malformation in patients with KID syndrome associated with a heterozygote mutation (p.Asp50Asn) in the GJB2 gene encoding connexin 26. *Clin Genet.* 2009;76(4):404-408.
138. Ma H, Liang P, Chen J, et al. Keratitis-ichthyosis-deafness syndrome accompanied by disseminated cutaneous fungal infection. *J Dermatol.* 2017.
139. Sakabe J, Yoshiki R, Sugita K, et al. Connexin 26 (GJB2) mutations in keratitis-ichthyosis-deafness syndrome presenting with squamous cell carcinoma. *J Dermatol.* 2012;39(9):814-815.
140. Esmer C, Salas-Alanis JC, Fajardo-Ramirez OR, et al. Lethal keratitis, ichthyosis, and deafness syndrome due to the A88V connexin 26 mutation. *Rev Invest Clin.* 2016;68(3):143-146.
141. Jonard L, Feldmann D, Parsy C, et al. A familial case of keratitis-ichthyosis-deafness (KID) syndrome with the GJB2 mutation G45E. *Eur J Med Genet.* 2008;51(1):35-43.
142. Huckstepp RT, Eason R, Sachdev A, et al. CO_2-dependent opening of connexin 26 and related beta connexins. *J Physiol.* 2010;588(Pt 20):3921-3931.
143. Huckstepp RT, id Bihi R, Eason R, et al. Connexin hemichannel-mediated CO_2-dependent release of ATP in the medulla oblongata contributes to central respiratory chemosensitivity. *J Physiol.* 2010;588(Pt 20):3901-3920.
143a. Lilly E, Bunick CG, Maley AM, et al. More than keratitis, ichthyosis and deafness: multisystem effects

of lethal GJB2 mutations. *J Amer Acad Dermatol*, in press.
144. Oji V, Eckl KM, Aufenvenne K, et al. Loss of corneodesmosin leads to severe skin barrier defect, pruritus, and atopy: unraveling the peeling skin disease. *Am J Hum Genet*. 2010;87(2):274-281.
145. Cassidy AJ, van Steensel MA, Steijlen PM, et al. A homozygous missense mutation in TGM5 abolishes epidermal transglutaminase 5 activity and causes acral peeling skin syndrome. *Am J Hum Genet*. 2005;77(6):909-917.
146. Cabral RM, Kurban M, Wajid M, et al. Whole-exome sequencing in a single proband reveals a mutation in the CHST8 gene in autosomal recessive peeling skin syndrome. *Genomics*. 2012;99(4):202-208.
147. Blaydon DC, Nitoiu D, Eckl KM, et al. Mutations in CSTA, encoding Cystatin A, underlie exfoliative ichthyosis and reveal a role for this protease inhibitor in cell-cell adhesion. *Am J Hum Genet*. 2011;89(4):564-571.
148. Pavlovic S, Krunic AL, Bulj TK, et al. Acral peeling skin syndrome: a clinically and genetically heterogeneous disorder. *Pediatr Dermatol*. 2012;29(3):258-263.
149. Muttardi K, Nitoiu D, Kelsell DP, et al. Acral peeling skin syndrome associated with a novel CSTA gene mutation. *Clin Exp Dermatol*. 2016;41(4):394-398.
150. Krunic AL, Stone KL, Simpson MA, et al. Acral peeling skin syndrome resulting from a homozygous nonsense mutation in the CSTA gene encoding cystatin A. *Pediatr Dermatol*. 2013;30(5):e87-88.
151. Pujol RM, Gilaberte M, Toll A, et al. Erythrokeratoderma variabilis-like ichthyosis in Chanarin-Dorfman syndrome. *Br J Dermatol*. 2005;153(4):838-841.
152. Srebrnik A, Tur E, Perluk C, et al. Dorfman-Chanarin syndrome. A case report and a review. *J Am Acad Dermatol*. 1987;17(5 Pt 1):801-808.
153. Lefevre C, Jobard F, Caux F, et al. Mutations in CGI-58, the gene encoding a new protein of the esterase/lipase/thioesterase subfamily, in Chanarin-Dorfman syndrome. *Am J Hum Genet*. 2001;69(5):1002-1012.
154. Yamaguchi T, Omatsu N, Matsushita S, et al. CGI-58 interacts with perilipin and is localized to lipid droplets. Possible involvement of CGI-58 mislocalization in Chanarin-Dorfman syndrome. *J Biol Chem*. 2004;279(29):30490-30497.
155. Demerjian M, Crumrine DA, Milstone LM, et al. Barrier dysfunction and pathogenesis of neutral lipid storage disease with ichthyosis (Chanarin-Dorfman syndrome). *J Invest Dermatol*. 2006;126(9):2032-2038.
156. Konig A, Happle R, Bornholdt D, et al. Mutations in the NSDHL gene, encoding a 3beta-hydroxysteroid dehydrogenase, cause CHILD syndrome. *Am J Med Genet*. 2000;90(4):339-346.
157. Bornholdt D, Konig A, Happle R, et al. Mutational spectrum of NSDHL in CHILD syndrome. *J Med Genet*. 2005;42(2):e17.
158. Avgerinou GP, Asvesti AP, Katsambas AD, et al. CHILD syndrome: the NSDHL gene and its role in CHILD syndrome, a rare hereditary disorder. *J Eur Acad Dermatol Venereol*. 2010;24(6):733-736.
159. Paller AS, van Steensel MA, Rodriguez-Martin M, et al. Pathogenesis-based therapy reverses cutaneous abnormalities in an inherited disorder of distal cholesterol metabolism. *J Invest Dermatol*. 2011;131(11):2242-2248.
160. Derry JM, Gormally E, Means GD, et al. Mutations in a delta 8-delta 7 sterol isomerase in the tattered mouse and X-linked dominant chondrodysplasia punctata. jderry@immunex.com. *Nat Genet*. 1999;22(3):286-290.
161. Curry CJ, Magenis RE, Brown M, et al. Inherited chondrodysplasia punctata due to a deletion of the terminal short arm of an X chromosome. *N Engl J Med*. 1984;311(16):1010-1015.
162. Braverman N, Steel G, Obie C, et al. Human PEX7 encodes the peroxisomal PTS2 receptor and is responsible for rhizomelic chondrodysplasia punctata. *Nat Genet*. 1997;15(4):369-376.
163. Franco B, Meroni G, Parenti G, et al. A cluster of sulfatase genes on Xp22.3: mutations in chondrodysplasia punctata (CDPX) and implications for warfarin embryopathy. *Cell*. 1995;81(1):15-25.
164. Happle R. X-linked dominant chondrodysplasia punctata. Review of literature and report of a case. *Hum Genet*. 1979;53(1):65-73.
165. Kolde G, Happle R. Histologic and ultrastructural features of the ichthyotic skin in X-linked dominant chondrodysplasia punctata. *Acta Derm Venereol*. 1984;64(5):389-394.
166. Bornholdt D, Atkinson TP, Bouadjar B, et al. Genotype-phenotype correlations emerging from the identification of missense mutations in MBTPS2. *Hum Mutat*. 2013;34(4):587-594.
167. Oeffner F, Fischer G, Happle R, et al. IFAP syndrome is caused by deficiency in MBTPS2, an intramembrane zinc metalloprotease essential for cholesterol homeostasis and ER stress response. *Am J Hum Genet*. 2009;84(4):459-467.
168. Lwin SM, Hsu CK, McMillan JR, et al. Ichthyosis prematurity syndrome: from fetus to adulthood. *JAMA Dermatol*. 2016;152(9):1055-1058.
169. Klar J, Schweiger M, Zimmerman R, et al. Mutations in the fatty acid transport protein 4 gene cause the ichthyosis prematurity syndrome. *Am J Hum Genet*. 2009;85(2):248-253.
170. Sobol M, Dahl N, Klar J. FATP4 missense and nonsense mutations cause similar features in ichthyosis prematurity syndrome. *BMC Res Notes*. 2011;4:90.
171. Kepes JJ, Berry A, 3rd, Zacharias DL. Multiple sulfatase deficiency: bridge between neuronal storage diseases and leukodystrophies. *Pathology*. 1988;20(3):285-291.
172. Dierks T, Schmidt B, Borissenko LV, et al. Multiple sulfatase deficiency is caused by mutations in the gene encoding the human C(alpha)-formylglycine generating enzyme. *Cell*. 2003;113(4):435-444.
173. Cosma MP, Pepe S, Annunziata I, et al. The multiple sulfatase deficiency gene encodes an essential and limiting factor for the activity of sulfatases. *Cell*. 2003;113(4):445-456.
174. Davies MG, Marks R, Dykes PJ, et al. Epidermal abnormalities in Refsum's disease. *Br J Dermatol*. 1977;97(4):401-406.
175. Jansen GA, Ofman R, Ferdinandusse S, et al. Refsum disease is caused by mutations in the phytanoyl-CoA hydroxylase gene. *Nat Genet*. 1997;17(2):190-193.
176. Jansen GA, Waterham HR, Wanders RJ. Molecular basis of Refsum disease: sequence variations in phytanoyl-CoA hydroxylase (PHYH) and the PTS2 receptor (PEX7). *Hum Mutat*. 2004;23(3):209-218.
177. Kitareewan S, Burka LT, Tomer KB, et al. Phytol metabolites are circulating dietary factors that

178. Jagell S, Liden S. Ichthyosis in the Sjogren-Larsson syndrome. *Clin Genet.* 1982;21(4):243-252.
179. Rizzo WB, Carney G. Sjogren-Larsson syndrome: diversity of mutations and polymorphisms in the fatty aldehyde dehydrogenase gene (ALDH3A2). *Hum Mutat.* 2005;26(1):1-10.
180. Nigro JF, Rizzo WB, Esterly NB. Redefining the Sjogren-Larsson syndrome: atypical findings in three siblings and implications regarding diagnosis. *J Am Acad Dermatol.* 1996;35(5 Pt 1):678-684.
181. Price VH, Odom RB, Ward WH, et al. Trichothiodystrophy: sulfur-deficient brittle hair as a marker for a neuroectodermal symptom complex. *Arch Dermatol.* 1980;116(12):1375-1384.
182. Happle R, Traupe H, Grobe H, et al. The Tay syndrome (congenital ichthyosis with trichothiodystrophy). *Eur J Pediatr.* 1984;141(3):47-152.
183. Jorizzo JL, Atherton DJ, Crounse RG, et al. Ichthyosis, brittle hair, impaired intelligence, decreased fertility and short stature (IBIDS syndrome). *Br J Dermatol.* 1982;106(6):705-710.
184. Faghri S, Tamura D, Kraemer KH, et al. Trichothiodystrophy: a systematic review of 112 published cases characterises a wide spectrum of clinical manifestations. *J Med Genet.* 2008;45(10):609-621.
185. Rebora A, Crovato F. PIBI(D)S syndrome—trichothiodystrophy with xeroderma pigmentosum (group D) mutation. *J Am Acad Dermatol.* 1987;16(5 Pt 1):940-947.
186. Nakabayashi K, Amann D, Ren Y, et al. Identification of C7orf11 (TTDN1) gene mutations and genetic heterogeneity in nonphotosensitive trichothiodystrophy. *Am J Hum Genet.* 2005;76(3):510-516.
187. Weeda G, Eveno E, Donker I, et al. A mutation in the XPB/ERCC3 DNA repair transcription gene, associated with trichothiodystrophy. *Am J Hum Genet.* 1997;60(2):320-329.
188. Corbett MA, Dudding-Byth T, Crock PA, et al. A novel X-linked trichothiodystrophy associated with a nonsense mutation in RNF113A. *J Med Genet.* 2015;52(4):269-274.
189. Marionnet C, Benoit A, Benhamou S, et al. Characteristics of UV-induced mutation spectra in human XP-D/ERCC2 gene-mutated xeroderma pigmentosum and trichothiodystrophy cells. *J Mol Biol.* 1995;252(5):550-562.
190. Stefanini M, Lagomarsini P, Arlett CF, et al. Xeroderma pigmentosum (complementation group D) mutation is present in patients affected by trichothiodystrophy with photosensitivity. *Hum Genet.* 1986;74(2):107-112.
191. Holzman SB, Durso SC. Nutritional deficiency and acquired ichthyosis. *J Gen Intern Med.* 2017.
192. Martin-Cascon M, Sanchez-Guirao AJ, Herranz-Marin MT. Paraneoplastic acquired ichthyosis in lung cancer. *Arch Bronconeumol.* 2015;51(11):609.
193. Sparsa A, Boulinguez S, Le Brun V, et al. Acquired ichthyosis with pravastatin. *J Eur Acad Dermatol Venereol.* 2007;21(4):549-550.
194. Patel N, Spencer LA, English JC 3rd, et al. Acquired ichthyosis. *J Am Acad Dermatol.* 2006;55(4):647-656.
195. Hodak E, Amitay I, Feinmesser M, et al. Ichthyosiform mycosis fungoides: an atypical variant of cutaneous T-cell lymphoma. *J Am Acad Dermatol.* 2004;50(3):368-374.
196. Goodman DS, Teplitz ED, Wishner A, et al. Prevalence of cutaneous disease in patients with acquired immunodeficiency syndrome (AIDS) or AIDS-related complex. *J Am Acad Dermatol.* 1987;17(2 Pt 1):210-220.
197. Kaplan MH, Sadick NS, McNutt NS, et al. Acquired ichthyosis in concomitant HIV-1 and HTLV-II infection: a new association with intravenous drug abuse. *J Am Acad Dermatol.* 1993;29(5 Pt 1):701-708.
198. Zhang H, Ma HJ, Liu W, et al. Sarcoidosis characterized as acquired ichthyosiform erythroderma. *Eur J Dermatol.* 2009;19(5):516-517.
199. Humbert P, Agache P. Acquired ichthyosis: a new cutaneous marker of autoimmunity. *Arch Dermatol.* 1991;127(2):263-264.
200. de la Cruz-Alvarez J, Allegue F, Oliver J. Acquired ichthyosis associated with eosinophilic fasciitis. *J Am Acad Dermatol.* 1996;34(6):1079-1080.
201. Spelman LJ, Strutton GM, Robertson IM, et al. Acquired ichthyosis in bone marrow transplant recipients. *J Am Acad Dermatol.* 1996;35(1):17-20.
202. Williams ML, Feingold KR, Grubauer G, et al. Ichthyosis induced by cholesterol-lowering drugs. Implications for epidermal cholesterol homeostasis. *Arch Dermatol.* 1987;123(11):1535-1538.
203. Kumar B, Saraswat A, Kaur I. Mucocutaneous adverse effects of hydroxyurea: a prospective study of 30 psoriasis patients. *Clin Exp Dermatol.* 2002;27(1):8-13.
204. Hannam S, Murray M, Romani L, et al. Kava dermopathy in Fiji: an acquired ichthyosis? *Int J Dermatol.* 2014;53(12):1490-1494.
205. Grimalt R, Gelmetti C, Brusasco A, et al. Pityriasis rotunda: report of a familial occurrence and review of the literature. *J Am Acad Dermatol.* 1994;31(5 Pt 2):866-871.
206. Petit A, Evenou P, Civatte J. Confluent and reticulated papillomatosis of Gougerot and Carteaud. Treatment by minocycline. *Ann Dermatol Venereol.* 1989;116(1):29-30.
207. Bruynzeel-Koomen CA, de Wit RF. Confluent and reticulated papillomatosis successfully treated with the aromatic etretinate. *Arch Dermatol.* 1984;120(9):1236-1237.

Chapter 48 :: Inherited Palmoplantar Keratodermas :: Liat Samuelov & Eli Sprecher

第四十八章 遗传性掌跖角化病

中文导读

本章分6节：①前言；②流行病学；③诊断；④鉴别诊断；⑤常用治疗方法；⑥遗传性掌跖角化病。

第一节前言，介绍了掌跖角化病(PPK)的分类方法，基于对临床和组织学特征评估进行分类，通常分为三种模式：弥漫性PPK、局灶性PPK、点状PPK。但随着大多数形式的遗传性PPK发病机制的破译，新的分类方案还包括了病因学。

第二节介绍了遗传性PPK部分患者可能不需要医疗干预或被误诊，实际患病率和发病率可能被低估。在近亲婚姻很普遍的国家或社区，遗传性PPK的发病率可能很高。

第三节诊断，介绍了目前结合临床和分子特征的算法可提高疾病诊断率，提出了一组新的算法包括皮肤表现、皮肤外表现、遗传模式，可达到最终诊断。

第四节介绍了掌跖过度角化可以是遗传性和获得性疾病的特征，获得性PPK需要与炎症性疾病、副肿瘤性角化病、皮肤淋巴瘤、化学和药物暴露、营养不良、更年期角化病和感染性疾病等相鉴别。遗传性PPK需要鉴别先天性角化不良、Rothmund-Thomson综合征和着色性干皮病等。

第五节介绍了PPK治疗主要目的是减轻临床表现，是用重点润肤剂和局部角质溶解制剂止痛、预防继发感染的治疗，也可采用各种助行器。重点介绍了维甲酸和外科治疗对PPK的作用。

第六节遗传性掌跖角化病，详细介绍了各种有/无皮肤外表现的弥漫性、局灶性及点状的掌跖角质病的临床特点、病因及发病机制、组织病理学及治疗等。

〔粟 娟〕

AT-A-GLANCE

- Inherited palmoplantar keratodermas (PPKs) are a heterogeneous group of genodermatoses characterized by hyperkeratosis of the palms and soles, with or without associated features. They are usually classified according to their morphology (diffuse, focal, punctate), mode of inheritance, and the presence or absence of extracutaneous features.
- Epidermolytic PPK (EPPK) is the most common form of diffuse keratoderma. It results from heterozygous mutations in *KRT9* (most cases) or *KRT1* (the minority of cases) encoding keratin 9 and keratin 1, respectively. Epidermolytic hyperkeratosis is seen on histology. A similar but milder phenotype of diffuse PPK is evident in nonepidermolytic PPK (NEPPK) Unna-Thost type, caused by heterozygous mutations in *KRT1*.
- Diffuse NEPPK with transgrediens may be observed in Greither syndrome and PPK Bothnia type caused by missense heterozygous mutations in *KRT1* and heterozygous gain-of-function mutations in *AQP5*, respectively. PPK Bothnia type also manifests with a white, spongy appearance of the palms and soles upon exposure to water.
- Mal de Meleda is a form of autosomal recessive, progressive, diffuse, mutilating PPK with transgrediens caused by biallelic mutations in *SLURP1*.
- Nagashima-type PPK is the most common type of PPK in the Asian population and is characterized by diffuse, transgrediens, nonprogressive, nonmutilating PPK. The palmoplantar skin assumes a typical whitish spongy appearance after water immersion. This form of PPK is caused by biallelic mutations in *SERPIN7* encoding a serine protease inhibitor.
- Olmsted syndrome, caused by mutations in *TRPV3* (autosomal dominant or autosomal recessive inheritance) or *MBTPS2* (X-linked recessive inheritance), is characterized by diffuse mutilating PPK with periorificial keratotic plaques.
- Heterozygous mutations in the gene *GJB2* encoding connexin 26 result in four genodermatoses featuring PPK and hearing impairment, including Vohwinkel syndrome (mutilating honeycomb-like PPK and starfish-shaped keratotic plaques), keratosis–ichthyosis–deafness (KID) syndrome (erythrokeratoderma, grainy PPK, abnormal ectodermal features, progressive keratitis, and recurrent infections), Bart-Pumphrey syndrome (honeycomb-like PPK, knuckle pads, and leukonychia), and PPK with deafness syndrome. A form of KID syndrome associated with congenital atrichia results from mutations in *GJB6* encoding Cx30.
- Loricrin keratoderma, caused by heterozygous frameshift mutations in *LOR* encoding loricrin, is a variant of Vohwinkel syndrome not associated with hearing impairment but featuring generalized ichthyosis.
- PPK with hearing impairment can also result from point mutations in the *MTTS1* gene encoding a mitochondrial transfer RNA.
- Hidrotic ectodermal dysplasia (Clouston syndrome) is a form of ectodermal dysplasia associated with diffuse PPK and nail and hair abnormalities caused by heterozygous mutations in *GJB6* encoding connexin 30.
- Huriez syndrome, an autosomal dominant inherited PPK with unknown etiology, is characterized by diffuse PPK, scleroatrophy, sclerodactyly, and occurrence of squamous cell carcinomas within atrophic skin.
- Papillon-Lefevre syndrome is an autosomal recessive disorder caused by mutations in the gene *CTSC* encoding cathepsin C. It is characterized by diffuse PPK with transgrediens and severe progressive periodontitis.
- Naxos disease (ND) and Carvajal syndrome (CS), caused by mutations in the genes *JUP* and *DSP* encoding plakoglobin and desmoplakin, respectively, are cardiocutaneous syndromes featuring PPK (diffuse in ND and striate in CS), woolly hair, and cardiomyopathy (right ventriculopathy in ND and mainly left ventricle involvement in CS).
- Striate PPK results from heterozygous nonsense or frameshift mutations in the genes encoding desmoglein 1, desmoplakin, and to a lesser degree keratin 1.
- Pachyonychia congenita is a group of rare autosomal dominant disorders caused by mutations in one of five keratin genes, including *KRT6A*, *KRT6B*, *KRT6C*, *KRT16*, or *KRT17* encoding keratins 6a, 6b, 6c, 16, and 17, respectively, known to be expressed in differentiated epithelial tissues. It manifests with focal painful PPK, thick dystrophic nails with a characteristic appearance, and associated features such as oral leukokeratosis, pilosebaceous cysts, and natal teeth.
- Howel-Evans syndrome is an autosomal dominant disorder featuring focal PPK and mucosal (particularly esophageal) squamous cell carcinomas with associated findings of follicular hyperkeratosis and oral leukokeratosis caused by heterozygous mutations in *RHBDF2*, encoding iRhom2, a protein known to play a role in epidermal growth factor receptor (EGFR) signaling.
- Richner-Hanhart syndrome is an autosomal recessive disease caused by mutations in the *TAT* gene encoding tyrosine aminotransferase, a hepatic cytosolic enzyme important for tyrosine and phenylalanine metabolism. It is characterized by

(Continued)

AT-A-GLANCE (Continued)

painful focal PPK, bilateral keratitis, and mental retardation.
- Punctate PPK (PPKP) type 1 is characterized by multiple, painful, yellow-brown hyperkeratotic papules on the palms and soles that most commonly appear during the first or second decades of life. It may result from mutations in one of two genes: *AAGAB* encoding p34 protein with resultant upregulation of EGFR or *COL14A1* encoding collagen type XIV α1. PPKP type 2 is characterized by skin-colored to yellow asymptomatic keratotic spines with histopathologic findings resembling cornoid lamella of porokeratosis. PPKP type 3 (acrokeratoelastoidosis of Costa) manifests with round to oval, white-yellow translucent papules with predilection to the thenar and hypothenar areas and pressure points with histopathologic findings of decreased elastic tissue and fragmented elastic fibers. The genes responsible for PPKP type 2 and 3 are still to be elucidated.
- Cole disease, characterized by punctate PPK, hypopigmented macules, and possible internal organs calcifications, is caused by mutations in *ENPP1* leading to impaired insulin signaling.
- Management of all forms of PPK focuses on topical treatments (mainly emollients and keratolytic agents), mechanical measures, methods to relieve pain or inhibit sweating, treatment of secondary infections, and various walking aids. Oral retinoids have been shown to be effective in several types of inherited PPK, and the development of more targeted therapeutic approaches is underway.

INTRODUCTION

The term *palmoplantar keratoderma (PPK)* refers to a group of potentially debilitating and clinically and genetically heterogeneous disorders of cornification which are clinically characterized by abnormal focal or diffuse thickening of the skin on the palms and soles. These disorders can occur as both acquired or inherited conditions. Inherited PPKs are characterized by familial occurrence and a relatively early age of onset in most cases. Genodermatoses associated with PPK are shown in Table 48-1, and several examples are presented in Fig. 48-1. This chapter focuses on inherited disorders in which PPK is a dominant feature.

Several classification systems of PPKs have been proposed. Originally, the classification was based on assessment of several clinical and histologic characteristics, including the specific morphology and pattern of palmoplantar hyperkeratosis, the extent of involvement (isolated PPK or syndromic PPK associated with ectodermal defects and/or extracutaneous manifestations), mode of inheritance (autosomal dominant, autosomal recessive, X-linked, mitochondrial), age of onset, and the presence or absence of epidermolysis on histology.[1-3] Three morphological patterns are usually distinguished: (1) diffuse PPK with uniform involvement of the entire palmoplantar surface; (2) focal PPK with localized hyperkeratosis predominantly on pressure points that is further subdivided into areata or nummular type (oval lesions, mainly on the plantar surface) and striate type (longitudinal hyperkeratotic lesions extending from the palms along the volar surface of the fingers associated with focal to diffuse thickening of the plantar skin); and (3) punctate PPK with multiple, discrete 1-mm to 1-cm round keratotic papules over the palms and soles. In addition, palmoplantar involvement may feature transgrediens (extension of hyperkeratosis onto the dorsal aspects of the fingers, toes, hands, feet, and flexor aspects of the wrists and heels) or mutilation caused by pseudoainhum (constricting bands around digits) formation.[4] With the deciphering of the pathogenesis of most forms of inherited PPKs, novel classification schemes include the etiology of the PPK in addition to morphological features.[2-6]

Elucidating the molecular disease mechanisms of PPKs has led to the discovery of new disorders and syndromes, providing new insights into the biological roles of epidermal structural components and paving the way for the development of novel, disorder-specific treatment modalities.[7-9]

EPIDEMIOLOGY

Although inherited PPKs are rare disorders when considered individually, their actual prevalence and incidence may be underestimated given the fact that mildly affected individuals do not require medical intervention or may be incorrectly diagnosed.[8,10] However, in several countries or communities in which consanguineous marriages are common, inherited PPKs may occur with high prevalence. In Northern Sweden, nonepidermolytic PPK (NEPPK) is characterized by a prevalence of 0.3% to 0.55%,[11] but in Northern Ireland, the prevalence of epidermolytic PPK (EPPK) was found to be 4.4 per 100,000 people.[12] In South India, a prevalence rate of 5.2 in 10,000 was documented with Unna-Thost syndrome being the most prevalent entity seen in approximately 38% of cases.[13] In general, EPPK is the most common form of diffuse keratoderma with a worldwide incidence of 2.2 to 4.4 per 100,000 live newborns.[1,14,15]

TABLE 48-1
Genodermatoses with Palmoplantar Keratoderma as an Associated Feature

	ENTITY WITH ASSOCIATED PALMOPLANTAR KERATODERMA
Ichthyoses	Autosomal recessive congenital ichthyosis (ARCI)
	Epidermolytic ichthyosis (Fig. 48-10A)
	Ichthyosis Curth-Macklin
	Keratosis linearis–ichthyosis congenital–keratoderma (KLICK) syndrome
	Trichothiodystrophy
	Chanarin-Dorfman syndrome
	Sjogren-Larsson syndrome
	Conradi-Hunermann-Happle syndrome (Fig. 48-10B)
	CEDNIK syndrome
	MEDNIK syndrome
	Ichthyosis prematurity syndrome
Erythrokeratodermias	Erythrokeratodermia variabilis
	Progressive symmetric erythrokeratodermia
Epidermolysis bullosa (EB)	EB simplex (localized and generalized severe)
	Recessive dystrophic epidermolysis bullosa
	Kindler syndrome
	Ectodermal dysplasia–skin fragility syndrome
Ectodermal dysplasias	Schopf-Schulz-Passarge syndrome
	Oculodentodigital dysplasia
	Odontoonychodermal dysplasia
	Naegeli-Franceschetti-Jadassohn syndrome
	Dermatopathia pigmentosa reticularis
	Autosomal recessive ectodermal dysplasia syndrome
Rasopathies	Costello syndrome
Others	Darier disease (see Fig. 48-10C)
	Acrokeratosis verruciformis of Hopf
	Cowden syndrome
	Epidermodysplasia verruciformis
	Pityriasis rubra pilaris
	Severe dermatitis, multiple allergies and metabolic wasting (SAM) syndrome
	Dyskeratosis congenita
	Keratosis follicularis spinulosa decalvans (KFSD)
	Ichthyosis follicularis congenital atrichia and photophobia syndrome (IFAP)
	Basal cell nevus syndrome (Gorlin syndrome)

CEDNIK, cerebral dysgenesis, neuropathy, ichthyosis, and keratoderma; MEDNIK, mental retardation, enteropathy, deafness, neuropathy, ichthyosis, keratodermia.

DIAGNOSIS

As briefly mentioned already, the past years have led to significant progress in our understanding of the pathogenesis of inherited PPKs. These advances can in turn be harnessed to facilitate the diagnosis of these conditions using algorithms integrating both clinical and molecular features. Fig. 48-2 depicts one such algorithm based on the use of four sets of data: (1) cutaneous findings including PPK morphology (eg, diffuse, focal, punctate, mutilating), hair (eg, woolly hair), or nail abnormalities, as well as features associated with other genodermatoses (eg, skin fragility); (2) extracutaneous findings (eg, periodontitis, deafness); (3) mode of inheritance (eg, autosomal dominant, autosomal recessive, mitochondrial inheritance); and (4) histopathologic findings such as epidermolytic hyperkeratosis, disadhesion of keratinocytes, or parakeratosis. Using this algorithm, almost forms of PPK can be assigned to one set of genes which should be sequenced to lead to the final diagnosis.

DIFFERENTIAL DIAGNOSIS

Palmoplantar hyperkeratosis may represent a feature of both inherited and acquired conditions. Acquired conditions listed in Table 48-2 usually occur later in life and include inflammatory disorders (eg, psoriasis, lichen planus, pityriasis rubra pilaris, chronic dermatitis, reactive arthritis), paraneoplastic keratoderma, cutaneous lymphoma, chemical and drug exposure, malnutrition, metabolic disorders (eg, hypothyroidism), keratoderma climactericum, and infectious diseases (eg, dermatophytes, scabies, verruca vulgaris and syphilis).[16]

Genodermatoses that feature PPK are listed in Table 48-1. Several distinctive characteristics can be shared by some of these diseases. For example, autoamputation of digits can accompany PPK in loricrin keratoderma (LK), Vohwinkel syndrome (VS), Olmsted syndrome (OS), Sybert PPK, mal-de-Meleda (MDM), PPK-Gamborg-Nielsen, and PPK congenital alopecia syndrome 2 (PPKCA2).[17,18] Other nonhereditary diseases that may cause constricting bands with or without hyperkeratosis include leprosy, tertiary syphilis, yaws, scleroderma, Raynaud syndrome, amniotic bands, ergotamine poisoning, spinal medulla tumors, syringomyelia, and scar formation from frostbite, burns, and trauma.[19]

PPK with transgrediens may be observed in LK, Nagashima type-PPK (NPPK), Greither disease, OS, Papillon-Lefevre syndrome (PLS). PPK with sensorineural hearing loss (SNHL) should raise the differential diagnosis of VS syndrome, keratitis–ichthyosis–deafness (KID) syndrome and other *GJB2*-associated diseases, or mitochondrial inherited-PPK with deafness.

Several syndromes are characterized by PPK associated with squamous cell carcinoma (SCC) within areas of abnormal keratinization (eg, Huriez and Unna-Thost syndromes). Other genodermatoses including

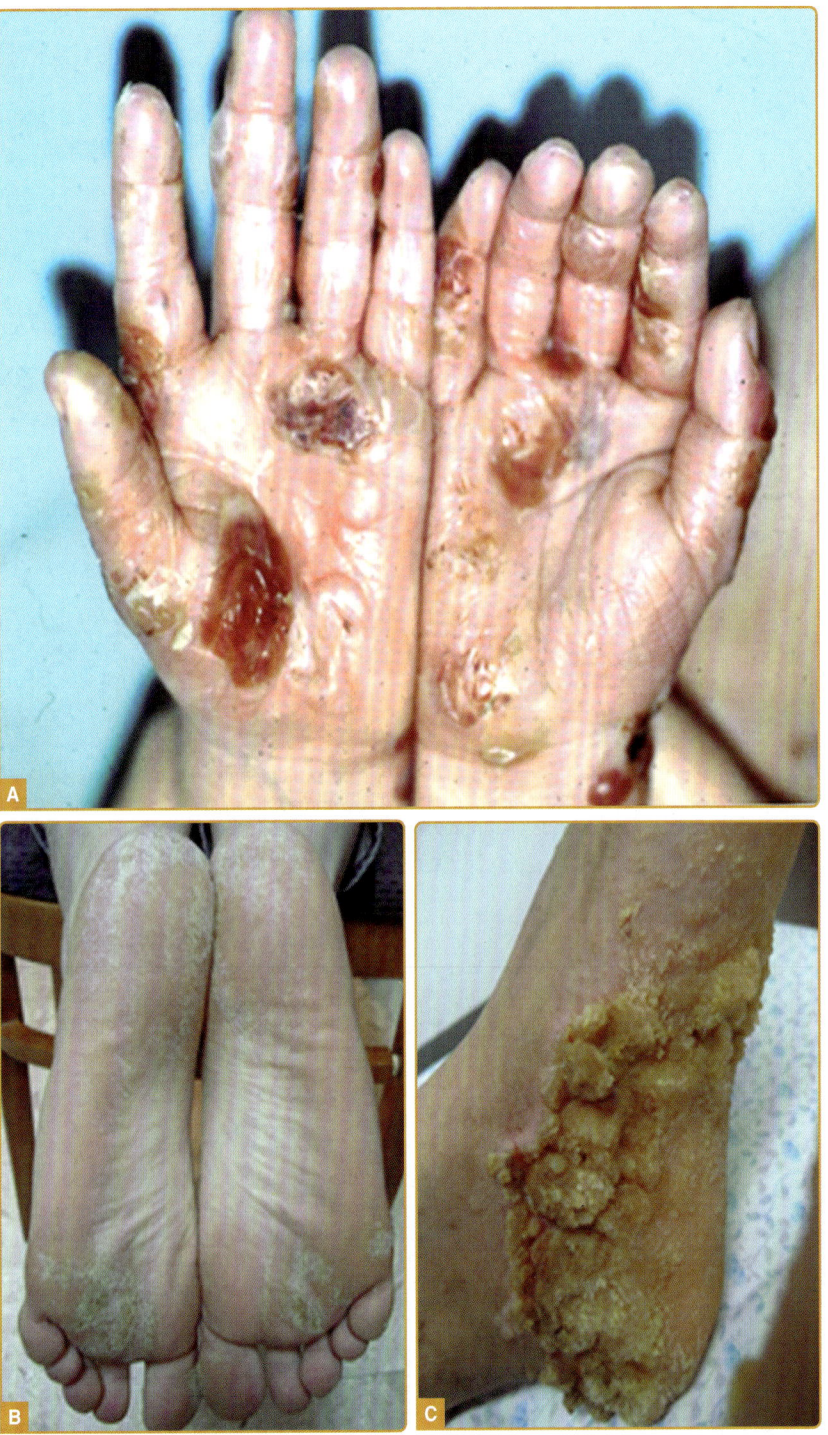

Figure 48-1 Genodermatoses with palmoplantar keratoderma as an associated feature. **A,** Diffuse palmar keratoderma with blisters in a patient with epidermolytic ichthyosis caused by *KRT1* mutation. **B,** Focal hyperkeratotic plantar plaques on weight-bearing areas in a patient with Conradi-Hunermann-Happle syndrome. **C,** Thick, yellow, hyperkeratotic plaques on plantar skin in a patient with Darier disease.

dyskeratosis congenita, Rothmund-Thomson syndrome, and xeroderma pigmentosum are associated with elevated absolute rates of SCC.

A few forms of PPKs feature gingival and dental anomalies (eg, OS, PLS, Haim-Munk syndrome, and Kindler syndromes).

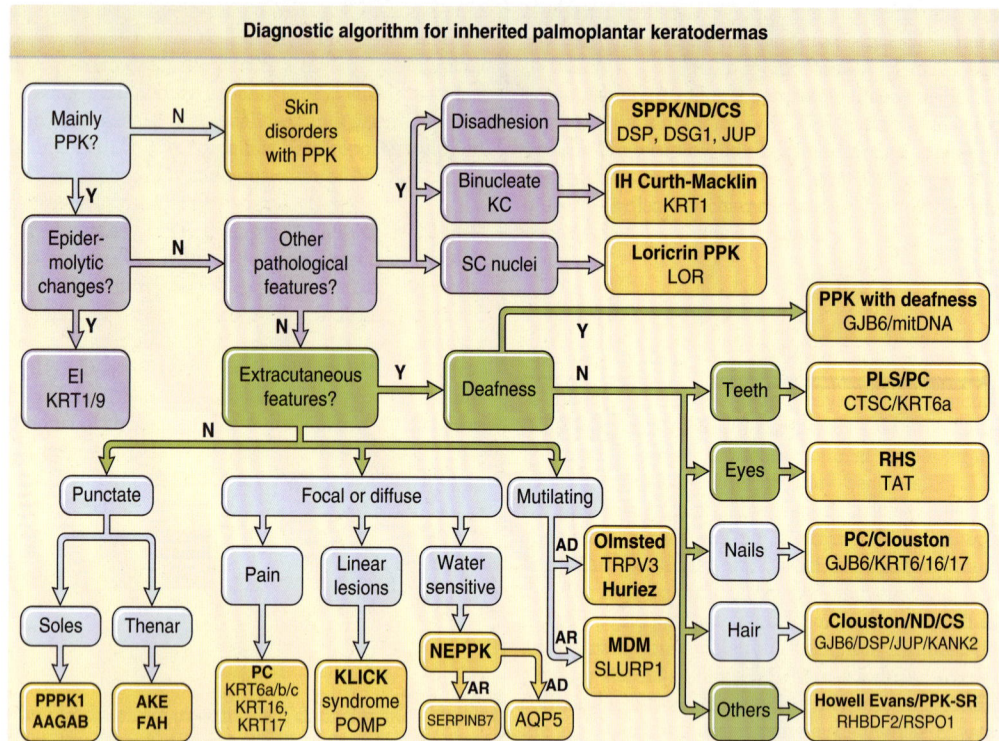

Figure 48-2 Diagnostic algorithm for inherited palmoplantar keratodermas (PPKs). Most patients with inherited PPK can be assigned to one gene based on four criteria: cutaneous findings, extracutaneous manifestations, mode of inheritance, and histopathologic findings. AAGAB, α-and γ-adaptin-binding protein P34; AKE, acrokeratoelastoidosis; AQP5, aquaporin 5; CS, Carvajal syndrome; CTSC, cathepsin C; DSG1, desmoglein 1; DSP, desmoplakin; EI, epidermolytic ichthyosis; FAH, focal acral hyperkeratosis; GJB6, gap junction protein β6; IH, ichthyosis hystrix; JUP, plakoglobin; KANK2, KN motif and ankyrin repeat domains 2; KC, keratinocytes; KLICK, Keratosis linearis–ichthyosis congenital–keratoderma; KRT, keratin; LOR, loricrin; MDM, mal de Meleda; ND, Naxos disease; NEPPK, nonepidermolytic palmoplantar keratoderma; PC, pachyonychia congenita; PLS, Papillon-Lefevre syndrome; POMP, proteasome maturation protein; PPK-SR, palmoplantar keratoderma with sex reversal; PPPK1, punctate palmoplantar keratoderma type I; RHBDF2, rhomboid 5 homolog 2; RHS, Richner-Hanhart syndrome; RSPO1, R-spondin 1; SC, stratum corneum; SERPINB7, serpin family B member 7; SLURP-1, secreted LY6/PLAUR domain containing 1; SPPK, striate palmoplantar keratoderma; TAT, tyrosine aminotransferase; TRPV3, transient receptor potential cation channel subfamily V member 3. (The authors acknowledge the contributions of Maurice van Steensel, Vinzenz Oji, Edel A. O'Toole, David Hansen, Mary Schwartz, and Frances Smith in the preparation of this figure.)

Wrinkling of palmoplantar skin may be a feature in aquagenic wrinkling of the palms with *CFTR* mutations, PPK Bothnia type with *AQP5* mutations, NPPK with *SERPINB7* mutations, and acrokeratoelastoidosis (AKE).

The differential diagnosis of punctate palmoplantar keratosis includes verruca vulgaris, corns over pressure points, porokeratosis punctate palmaris et plantaris, keratosis punctate of the palmar creases, Cole disease, Darier disease, Cowden disease, Gorlin syndrome, acrokeratosis verruciformis of Hopf, epidermodysplasia verruciformis, and arsenic exposure.[20-22]

PPK associated with sclerosis localized to dorsal hands and sclerodactyly may be a feature of Huriez syndrome, Unna-Thost syndrome (occasionally shows sclerodactyly or nail changes), PPKCA2, and palmoplantar hyperkeratosis with SCC of the skin and sex reversal. Systemic sclerosis may show similar features.

PPK with nail changes typical for pachyonychia congenita (PC) may be observed in Clouston syndrome caused by *GJB6* mutations (may show similar nail changes and painful keratoderma) or homozygous mutations in *FZD6*, encoding frizzled 6, a Wnt-signaling pathway receptor in the nail matrix, which was recently discovered as the cause of congenital nail dystrophy.[23] Dyskeratosis congenita manifest with features overlapping with PC, including nail dystrophy, PPK, hyperhidrosis, and oral leukoplakia. Onychomycosis should be excluded in cases of PPK with nail findings.

COMMON THERAPEUTIC APPROACHES

In general, the management of all forms of PPK is aimed at alleviating disease manifestations and focuses on mechanical measures, methods to relieve pain, treatment of secondary infections, and various

TABLE 48-2
Acquired Conditions Associated with Palmoplantar Hyperkeratosis and Other Features Resembling Palmoplantar Keratoderma
Inflammatory Skin Disorders
Palmoplantar psoriasis
Lichen planus
Pityriasis rubra pilaris
Chronic dermatitis
Reactive arthritis
Metabolic Disorders
Hypothyroidism, myxedema
Chronic lymphedema
Drugs and Chemical Exposures
Lithium, hydroxyurea, verapamil, bleomycin
Chemotherapeutic agents
Chlorinated hydrocarbon
Chronic arsenic exposure
Infectious Diseases
Dermatophytes
Scabies
Verruca vulgaris
Syphilis
Leprosy
Tuberculosis
Malignancies
Paraneoplastic keratoderma
Cutaneous lymphoma
Malnutrition
Miscellaneous
Keratoderma climactericum
Pitted keratolysis
Punctate porokeratosis

walking aids. Topical treatment includes the regular use of emollients and topical keratolytic formulations (eg, 10% to 20% salicylic acid or 35% to 70% propylene glycol combined with thick emollient), with occlusion if necessary. In addition, topical calcipotriol and topical tazarotene have been shown to be effective in EPPK and PLS, respectively.[24] Dermatophyte or bacterial secondary infections and hyperhidrosis should be diagnosed and treated aggressively to avoid disease aggravation. Soaking in water and mechanical removal of hyperkeratotic areas (eg, grooming and trimming) are additional therapeutic measures that may provide symptom relief. Pain can be relieved by orthotics or insoles, wicking socks, ventilated or cushioned footwear, and maintaining body weight to reduce repeated trauma to the feet and the tendency to develop callus and blisters.

ORAL RETINOIDS

Oral retinoids are usually effective. Low-dose, short-term, or intermittent therapy are sometimes recommended given the possible long-term side effects, the chronic nature of the condition, and the risk of aggravated skin fragility, which may exacerbate disease manifestation in several types of PPK. More specifically, systemic retinoids were shown to be effective in EPPK,[25] MDM,[26] VS, and LK[27-30] and in cases of OS,[31-34] Huriez syndrome,[35] punctate PPK 1,[36,37] and PLS (for both PPK and periodontopathy).[38-40] Systemic retinoids have been found to be effective in KID syndrome (for hyperkeratosis, dissecting cellulitis of the scalp, and cancer chemoprophylaxis), although some reports demonstrated only partial response and exacerbation of corneal neovascularization with isotretinoin.[28,41-46] Accordingly, a low starting dose of acitretin (0.5 mg/kg/day) or alitretinoin (10 mg/day) with gradual increase depending on response and tolerability is recommended.[47-49]

SURGICAL THERAPY

Surgical excision and grafting is an option in focal PPK and in cases associated with mutilation.[4,50] Specific surgical approaches are discussed later.

INHERITED PALMOPLANTAR KERATODERMAS

DIFFUSE PALMOPLANTAR KERATODERMAS WITHOUT EXTRACUTANEOUS FEATURES, DOMINANT INHERITANCE

EPIDERMOLYTIC PALMOPLANTAR KERATODERMA

Clinical Features: EPPK (Vörner type; Online Mendelian Inheritance in Man [OMIM] #144200), first described by Vörner in 1901, is an autosomal dominant disorder characterized by yellowish, diffuse PPK with erythematous sharp margins at the edge of the palms (Fig. 48-3A) and soles (Fig. 48-3B).[51] Most cases present at birth or during the first weeks of life, although appearance up to the third year of life has been reported. The initial presentation is palmoplantar erythema that starts at the margins of the palms and soles, extends toward the center, and subsequently becomes covered with thick scale and remains stable throughout life.[25,52] Transgrediens and hyperkeratotic lesions over the elbows, knees, and knuckle pads have been reported.[53-60] It may be complicated with painful fissures, hyperhidrosis, maceration, and secondary bacterial and fungal infections with an offending odor.[57] Digital mutilation with pseudoainhum and

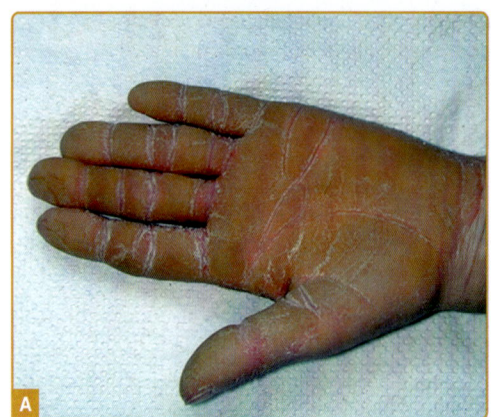

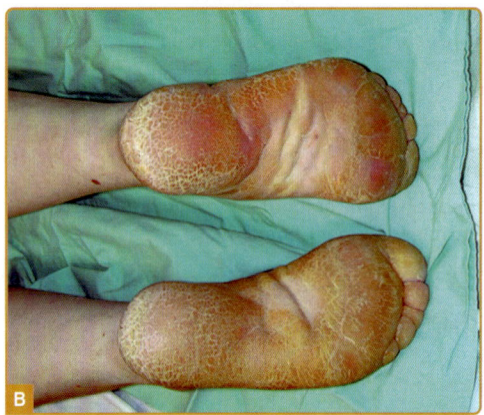

Figure 48-3 Epidermolytic palmoplantar keratoderma. Yellow, diffuse palmoplantar keratoderma with erythematous sharp margins at the edge of the palms (**A**) and soles (**B**). A heterozygous mutation in *KRT9* was identified in this patient.

camptodactyly has been reported.[59-62] In most cases, PPK is an isolated finding, although the rare occurrence of EPPK in association with leg ulcers, scleroderma, familial multiple carcinomas, and Ehlers-Danlos syndrome type III has been reported.[25,63-65]

Etiology and Pathogenesis: EPPK is an autosomal dominant genodermatosis caused by heterozygous mutations in *KRT9* encoding keratin 9.[66] Mutations in *KRT1* encoding keratin 1 have also been reported in association with EPPK in a minority of cases.[67-70]

Keratin 9 is a type I intermediate filament protein whose expression is confined to the suprabasal layers of the palmoplantar epidermis. Similar to all other keratins, KRT9 comprises three major domains: the head domain; the central α-helix rod domain, which is composed of four helical subsegments (1A, 1B, 2A, and 2B) that are interrupted by three nonhelical linker domains (L1, L12, and L2); and the tail domain.[71,72] Most *KRT9* mutations identified to date are located in the 1A or 2B segments of the α-helix rod domain, which are highly conserved in all keratin proteins and are essential for the formation of the keratin heterodimer and play a pivotal role in the congregation and stabilization of keratin intermediate filaments. Most causative genetic defects are missense or frameshift (small in-frame insertion–deletion) mutations acting in a dominant-negative manner. A mutational hotspot exists at codon 163 of *KRT9* (in the central α-helix rod domain) that encodes the amino acid arginine, which is often mutated to tryptophan, glutamine, or proline. p.Arg163Trp accounts for approximately 30% of all EPPK-causing mutations across different ethnic groups.[73,74]

Keratin 1 is a type II keratin expressed at the suprabasal cells committed to terminal differentiation that forms heterodimer with keratin 9 in palmoplantar epidermis and with keratin 10 in all other skin surfaces, including hair-bearing skin and other stratified orthokeratinized squamous epithelia.[6,75-77] The reported *KRT1* mutations in families with EPPK involve larger in-frame deletions affecting the helix boundary motifs of the rod domain,[68] different from the missense mutations in the same domains reported in epidermolytic ichthyosis (EI; see Chap. 47) and from frameshift mutations in the V2 domain that have been found in striate keratoderma and in ichthyosis hystrix Curth-Macklin.[78,79] Other mutations in *KRT1* that were associated with EPPK are gain-of-function (GOF) mutations at the beginning of the helix 1B domain of the central α-helical coiled-coil rod domain and an insertion of 18 amino acids in the 2B rod domain, emphasizing that mutations located more central in the rod domain of keratin 1 do not disrupt the function of filament assembly and stability as much as those in the helix initiation and termination sequence seen in EI cases.[67,70]

Pathology: Skin biopsies show compact orthohyperkeratosis, hypergranulosis, acanthosis, and epidermolytic hyperkeratosis manifested by perinuclear vacuolization of the keratinocytes and large irregularly-shaped keratohyaline granules located in the granular layers of the epidermis. Moreover, dyskeratosis manifested by intracytoplasmic and perinuclear eosinophilic homogenizations with round-oval eosinophilic inclusions were identified in involved epidermis corresponding to the intracytoplasmic aggregates and clumps of tonofilaments seen ultrastructurally.[3,80,81] More than one biopsy may be required to demonstrate epidermolytic changes and the typical histologic alterations of epidermolytic hyperkeratosis may be noticed in the acrosyringium.[25]

Ultrastructural findings include intracytoplasmic vacuolization in the upper spinous and granular cell layers; disruption and dispersion of the cellular organelles with indistinct cellular borders; intracytoplasmic dense aggregates of tonofilaments surrounding the nuclei; dense clumps of tonofilaments; abundant glycogen and ribosomes; detachment of tonofibrils from desmosomal plaques; large keratohyalin granules present from the mid malpighian layers; "composite" keratohyalin granules consisting of a homogeneous, relatively electron-lucent core; and dense peripheral deposits.[65,80,82-86]

Specific Treatments: Inhibition of *Krt9* mutant allele expression in a mouse model of EPPK using ribonucleic acid interference (RNAi)–based therapy has been demonstrated.[73] In addition, a transgenic mouse model of EPPK was treated with a mutant-specific short hairpin RNA (shRNA) that resulted in knockdown of the mutant protein with restoration of normal morphology and function of the skin.[87]

UNNA-THOST PALMOPLANTAR KERATODERMA

Clinical Features: Diffuse nonepidermolytic PPK (NEPPK, Unna-Thost type; OMIM #600962) is an autosomal dominant genodermatosis first described by Unna and Thost in 1880. Clinical features are similar to those of diffuse EPPK, although they are often milder, with presentation in the first few months of life. Onset during the third decade of life has been reported. NEPPK is characterized by diffuse, well-demarcated, yellowish, thick hyperkeratosis with an erythematous rim overlying the palms and soles. It tends to be smoother and waxier than EPPK, which is thicker and fissured.[4] Hyperhidrosis, as well as refractory secondary dermatophyte infections and pitted keratolysis leading to maceration and desquamation, are common findings seen more frequently in NEPPK than in EPPK.[88-91] In addition, the presence of hyperkeratosis around the umbilicus and the nipple with mild thickening and dryness of the knees and elbows has been reported.[92] Cases associated with atopic dermatitis[93] and verrucous carcinoma[94] have been described. Associations with acrocyanosis of the distal third of the extremities, clinodactyly of the fifth finger, and perianal or pericrural involvement have been reported.[95-97]

In general, EPPK and NEPPK show substantial clinical overlap, and histopathologic evaluation is often required to distinguish between them.

Etiology and Pathogenesis: Originally, Unna-Thost PPK was recognized as a nonepidermolytic form of diffuse PPK clinically resembling Vörner PPK. However, Kuster and coworkers investigated the original family reported by Unna and Thost and found epidermolytic hyperkeratosis on histology and identified a mutation located in the coil-1A domain at the beginning of the central rod domain of *KRT9*. This mutations is in close proximity to the mutation found in the original family reported by Vörner, suggesting that Unna-Thost and Vörner PPKs are the same entity.[57,98]

In a single family with diffuse NEPPK, a missense mutation was identified in the terminal V1 variable subdomain (nonhelical head domain) of keratin 1. In contrast with other reported *KRT1* mutations involving central domains important for filament assembly and stability that result in epidermolysis, this mutation is likely to be important for interactions of keratin filaments with other cellular components including the desmosomes.[92] This mutation results in distortion in keratinocytes shape and prevention of efficient distribution of lamellar body lipid material with impaired barrier formation.[99]

Another missense mutation in *KRT1* resulting in a mild phenotype has been identified in the 2B rod domain, again underscoring that mutations affecting the central part of the keratin 1 rod domain do not disrupt filament assembly to the same extent as mutations located at the initiation or termination motif of the helix sequence.[100]

Diffuse NEPPK, without other clinical features of PC, has been reported with heterozygous mutations in *KRT6c* and *KRT16*. The phenotype consists of diffuse PPK on the soles and focal hyperkeratosis on the palms. In cases of NEPPK when no pathogenic mutation is identified in *KRT1*, screening for *KRT6c* and *KRT16* mutations may be valuable.[101,102]

Pathology: Diffuse NEPPK shows nonspecific histopathologic findings, including hyperkeratosis, orthokeratosis, acanthosis, and either hyper- or hypogranulosis with no evidence of epidermolytic hyperkeratosis.[92,93] Close inspection and repeated biopsies are needed to exclude small foci of epidermolytic hyperkeratosis compatible with EPPK.

GREITHER SYNDROME

Clinical Features: Transgrediens et progrediens PPK (Greither syndrome; OMIM #133200) was originally described in 1952 by Greither.[103] Greither syndrome is an autosomal dominant disease with marked intra- and interfamilial variability. It characteristically starts to develop after the second year of life (although appearance soon after birth or later in childhood and adolescence has been documented). It is characterized by diffuse, thickened, scaly, yellowish PPK with an erythematous rim and transgrediens. The involvement of the skin over the Achilles tendon and gradual extension of patchy hyperkeratotic, erythematous, and hyperpigmented papules and plaques towards the shins, knees, thighs, knuckles, wrists, elbows, and flexural areas are typical.[95,103-107] Greither PPK tends to involute after the fifth decade of life. Hyperhidrosis is a common feature, and pitted keratolysis may be an associated finding. A case presenting as neonatal blistering and erythroderma, initially diagnosed as EI, has been reported.[77] An association with atopic dermatitis has been described.[108] A case of malignant melanoma arising on the hyperkeratotic sole of a patient with Greither PPK has been documented.[109] Severe cases of PPK may be complicated by spontaneous autoamputation and digit deformities.[110] Greither syndrome has been described in association with incontinentia pigmenti, acrocyanosis, and erythrokeratoderma variabilis in isolated cases.[104,111-113]

Sybert PPK is another form of progressive, diffuse, autosomal dominant PPK with transgrediens and autoamputation, however it manifests with more severe hyperkeratosis as compared to Greither PPK.[110]

Etiology and Pathogenesis: Greither syndrome is inherited in an autosomal dominant fashion and was shown to result from a missense mutation in *KRT1* affecting the helix initiation motif at the amino terminal end of the central rod domain of keratin 1,[108] a region known to be essential for effective filament assembly.[114] The causative gene for Sybert PPK has not been identified yet.

Pathology: The characteristic findings in Greither syndrome are acanthosis, marked hyperkeratosis, and hypergranulosis. A case with striking vacuolation of the superficial keratinocytes and numerous keratohyaline granules in the granular layer consistent with epidermolytic hyperkeratosis has been reported.[108] Moreover, focal depressions of the epidermis occupied by round foci of a compact orthokeratotic horny layer have been reported.[106] The described histopathologic findings in Sybert PPK are epidermal hyperplasia with hypergranulosis, parakeratosis, and orthokeratosis, as well as a sparse lymphocytic infiltrate in the papillary dermis. Ultrastructural studies revealed normal keratin filaments with abnormal structure and distribution of keratohyaline granules.[110]

LORICRIN KERATODERMA

Clinical Features: LK (mutilating keratoderma with ichthyosis, VS Camisa type; OMIM #604117) is a rare, autosomal dominant disorder. It features honeycomb-like PPK, starfish-like hyperkeratoses, prominent knuckle pads on the dorsal aspects of the hands, and pseudoainhum leading to autoamputation of the digits. These signs, when associated with hearing impairment, are referred to as VS (see later).[115] LK is a variant of VS reported by Camisa and Rossana in 1984 with no hearing impairment but with prominent generalized ichthyosis. The two essential clinical features for establishing the diagnosis are the characteristic honeycomb-like keratoderma and generalized ichthyosis, although the phenotype of LK is truly heterogeneous. LK manifests at birth or in early childhood and progresses gradually throughout adulthood. The clinical findings include moderate, generalized ichthyosiform dermatitis with dryness and fine scales affecting the trunk and extremities and hyperkeratosis localized to body folds with no evidence of erythema. Palmoplantar involvement is characterized by diffuse, symmetrical, well-demarcated transgrediens honeycomb-like PPK with an erythematous border (Fig. 48-4A),[27,116,117] although diffuse hyperkeratosis with no evidence of a honeycomb-like pattern may be seen. Knuckle pads, hyperkeratotic plaques on the dorsal parts of the hands, and pseudoainhum have been reported in LK pedigrees in varying frequencies,[117-124] and a collodion membrane may be seen at birth in approximately 35% of cases.[120,121,125] Association of LK with vitiligo, atopic dermatitis, neurodevelopmental delay, and microcephaly has been reported.[121,123]

Etiology and Pathogenesis: LK results from heterozygous frameshift insertion or deletion mutations in *LOR* which encodes loricrin. Loricrin is synthetized in the granular layer of the epidermis and then migrates to the cell periphery, where it is located beneath the plasma membrane and is crosslinked to other cytosolic proteins including involucrin, forming the cornified cell envelope (CCE).[30,117,119-121,123,125-130] Most mutations in *LOR* implicated in LK lead to a frameshift, delayed termination, and aberrant protein elongation. Experiments in transgenic mice suggest that *LOR* mutations exert a gain of function deleterious effect. The mutant loricrin forms arginine-rich nuclear localization sequences that "tag" a protein exposed on the cell surface for import into the cell nucleus by nuclear transport. The abnormal localization of loricrin in the nucleus alters nuclear/nucleolar functions, including nonribosomal RNA processing and growth factor signal transduction, and disrupts apoptotic processes in terminally differentiated keratinocytes.[124,126,131-134]

No clear genotype–phenotype correlation has been reported and variable intrafamilial disease severity has been reported.[117,120,121]

LK skin demonstrates abnormal epidermal permeability barrier function[130,131] similar to the skin barrier defects seen in various ichthyoses, including lamellar ichthyosis with transglutaminase-1 mutations.[135] Cell lines overexpressing mutant form of *LOR* demonstrated increased proliferation rate through activation of AKT-kinase with phosphorylation of ERK1/2, epidermal growth factor receptor (EGFR), and signal

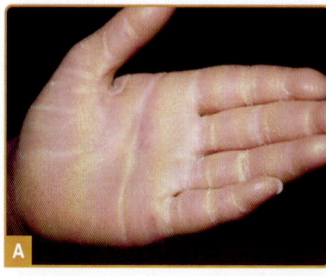
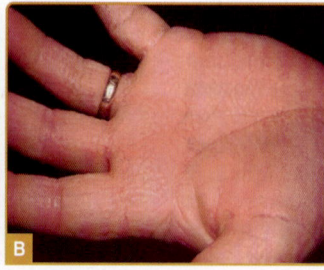
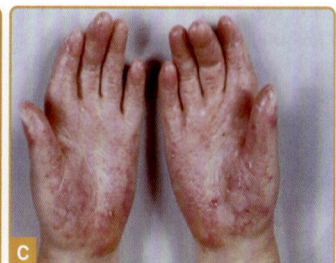

Figure 48-4 Rare forms of transgrediens palmoplantar keratoderma. **A,** A case of loricrin palmoplantar keratoderma with diffuse, well-demarcated, honeycomb-like palmoplantar keratoderma with an erythematous border. **B,** Vohwinkel syndrome with a "honeycomb-like" appearance **C,** Huriez syndrome. Diffuse, well-confined hyperkeratotic plaques over the palms. (Used with permission from Dr. Cameron Kennedy, Bristol Royal Infirmary, United Kingdom.)

transducer and activator of transcription 3 (STAT3) compared with cell lines expressing the wild-type loricrin.[136]

Pathology: Histopathologic features include hyperkeratosis, significant parakeratosis, acanthosis, hypergranulosis (although the granular later may appear normal), diffuse vacuolar changes, focal cytolytic changes, and necrotic suprabasal keratinocytes.[118] Ultrastructural findings consist of abundant keratohyaline granules, vacuolar changes and disruption of suprabasal keratinocytes, and deposition of electron-dense intranuclear inclusions within the granular layer that contain loricrin as shown by immunogold studies.[117,118]

PALMOPLANTAR KERATODERMA BOTHNIA TYPE

Clinical Features: PPK Bothnia type (PPKB; OMIM #600231) was first described in 1994 as an autosomal dominant form of diffuse NEPPK, which has a high prevalence (0.3% to 0.55%) in two provinces of the West and Northwest Gulf of Bothnia in Northern Sweden.[11] PPKB has been described also in a large pedigree of Chinese Han descent,[137] and a common founder mutation in the British population has been suggested.[138] PPKB clinically resembles Nagashima PPK (see later) and usually manifests during infancy or childhood with a diffuse, homogenous hyperkeratosis with a yellowish hue over the palms and soles that extends to the dorsal digits.[11] These patients, even with a barely detectable mild phenotype, demonstrate a typical white spongy appearance of affected areas upon exposure to water. Hyperhidrosis, maceration, and secondary fungal infections are common, as are abnormal nails (curved with ragged cuticles). In contrast to this condition, aquagenic wrinkling of the palms, which is often found in conjunction with cystic fibrosis (CF), is characterized by translucent whitish papules, excessive wrinkling, and palmar edema induced by brief exposure to water.[137,139,140]

Etiology and Pathogenesis: PPKB is an autosomal dominant disorder caused by GOF mutations in the gene *AQP5*, encoding water-channel protein aquaporin 5 (AQP5), first identified in 2013 by Blaydon and coworkers.[141]

Aquaporins are cell-membrane transporters that enable the osmotic movement of water across the cell membrane in many cell types. AQP5 is mostly found in the apical plasma membrane and is involved in the excretion of water from exocrine glands (salivary gland, lacrimal gland, and sweat gland); it is also expressed in epithelial cells of the lung and the cornea.[141] Of note, hypohidrosis in Sjogren syndrome has been associated with decreased expression of AQP5.[142] In normal palmoplantar skin, AQP5 is localized to the plasma membrane of keratinocytes of the stratum granulosum, and in PPKB lesions, AQP5 expression is retained. However, affected keratinocytes are subject to increased water uptake through the plasma membrane.[141]

It has been suggested from protein modeling studies that PPKB-causing mutations increase the diameter of the constriction point of the AQP5 water channel with a direct influence on AQP5 gating or water flow through the channel.[141] Aquagenic wrinkling of palms (transient edematous whitish plaques on the palms upon exposure to water and hyperhidrosis) has been associated with aberrant expression of AQP5 in sweat glands.[143] Activation of transient receptor potential vanilloid 4 (TRPV4) results in increased cytosolic calcium concentration essential for sweat secretion, although its overactivation in keratinocytes may result in apoptosis and hyperkeratosis as demonstrated in OS caused by *TRPV3* mutations.[144,145] Because TRPV4 and AQP5 are both expressed in eccrine sweat glands and keratinocytes,[141] it has been speculated that palmoplantar hyperhidrosis and hyperkeratosis in PPKB are a result of GOF effect of the AQP5–TRPV4 complex, indicating that PPKB is a skin channelopathy.[137] A possible disease mechanism for aquagenic wrinkling of the palms in patients with CF is dysfunction of the TRPV4 channels in keratinocytes, resulting in dysregulated water influx through eccrine ducts.[139]

Histopathology: Histopathologic findings are nonspecific and include orthohyperkeratosis and a mild lymphocytic infiltrate in the upper dermis.[137]

DIFFUSE PALMOPLANTAR KERATODERMA WITHOUT EXTRACUTANEOUS FEATURES, RECESSIVE INHERITANCE

MAL DE MELEDA

Clinical Features: MDM (OMIM #248300) is a rare autosomal recessive disorder initially described in patients native to the Croatian island of Meleda (Mljet). The diagnostic criteria for the disease were presented in 1969.[146] Since then, the disease has been described in other parts of the world, including the Middle East, Western Europe, and North Africa with higher prevalence in certain populations, mainly in the Mediterranean and Adriatic regions, because of a founder effect. A few cases have been reported in Taiwan, China, Japan, Indonesia, and India.[147-157]

The onset of the disease is during infancy or early childhood with diffuse transgressive yellowish waxy hyperkeratotic plaques outlined by a red scaly border over the palms (Fig. 48-5A) and soles

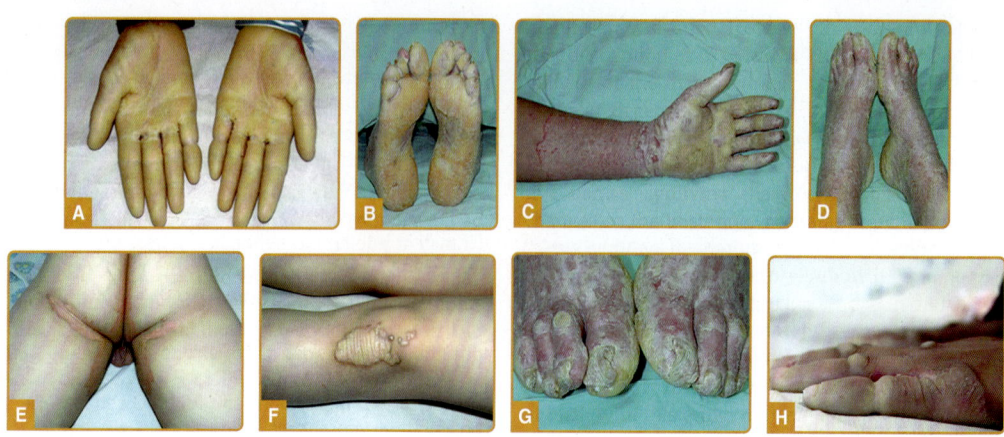

Figure 48-5 Mal de Meleda. Diffuse, yellow, waxy hyperkeratotic plaque outlined by a red, scaly border over the palms (**A**) and soles (**B**) with extension onto the dorsal surface of the hands and feet in a glove (**C**) and stocking (**D**) distribution. Involvement of the groin area (**E**), keratotic plaques over joints (**F**), nail abnormalities (**G**), and pseudoainhum (**H**) are associated findings.

(Fig. 48-5B) that are preceded by prominent and persistent erythema. The palmoplantar hyperkeratosis progresses with age and extends onto the dorsal surface of the hands and feet in a glove (Fig. 48-5C) and stocking (Fig. 48-5D) distribution, the flexor aspects of the wrists and ankles and over the Achilles tendon, forearms, elbows, and knees.[147,154] Involvement of the inguinal and groin regions (Fig. 48-5E) has been described.[147,148]

Additional features are knuckle pads, lichenoid or keratotic plaques over joints (Fig. 48-5F), perioral erythema, hyperhidrosis with superinfection, malodorous maceration and painful fissures, nail abnormalities (eg, koilonychia, clubbing, onycholysis, nail thickening, dystrophy and subungual hyperkeratosis) (Fig. 48-5G), sclerodactyly, and brachydactyly. Circumscribed hyperkeratotic plaques over the fingers and toes result in a cone-shaped appearance (Fig. 48-5H), digital constrictions, pseudoainhum, and progressive functional impairment with reduced mobility.[158-160]

Although penetrance is complete, phenotype varies with geographic origin and ethnic background. In addition, no clear genotype–phenotype correlation has been identified, and environmental factors (mechanical trauma and heat) seem to influence the disease course.[147,148,150,154] A case with no plantar involvement, a milder phenotype with slightly erythematous palmoplantar keratotic plaques, and an atypical appearance with multiple 2- to 5-mm keratolytic pits outlined by brownish red erythema over the palmoplantar surface (mainly plantar skin) have been described.[26,147,154] Cases with no evidence of transgrediens have been described.[151] Heterozygous carriers may manifest with mild diffuse PPK or smooth skin on the palms and soles with keratotic papules.[161]

Several cases of malignant melanoma (MM) arising in the hyperkeratotic lesions of patients with MDM have been described in the literature.[149,162,163] A case complicated by irregular hyperpigmented spots on palmoplantar skin and the appearance of Bowen disease on the sole in a patient have been reported.[164,165] Accordingly, periodic screening for MM and other neoplasms is warranted.

PPK Gamborg-Nielsen (PPK-GN; OMIM #244850), an autosomal recessive disorder first described in patients from the northernmost county of Sweden by Gamborg Nielsen in 1985, is considered by some as a milder form of MDM. It manifests with a similar phenotype but less severe diffuse palmoplantar hyperkeratosis and no nail deformities or distant keratosis, although knuckle pads and tapered fingers may be observed.[166-168]

Etiology and Pathogenesis: MDM is caused by biallelic mutations in the *SLURP1* gene (previously known as ARS component B), which contains three translated exons and encodes the lymphocyte antigen 6 /urokinase-type plasminogen activator receptor related protein-1 (SLURP-1), a member of the Ly-Upar superfamily of proteins that play a role in transmembrane signal transduction, cell activation, and cell adhesion.[148,169] SLURP-1 is considered a secreted epidermal neuromodulator that is likely to be essential for both epidermal homeostasis and inhibition of tumor necrosis factor (TNF)-α release by macrophages during wound healing.[170]

Genetic heterogeneity is suggested in MDM because families without a *SLURP1* mutation have been reported.[171,172]

PPK-GN has recently been shown to be an allelic variant of MDM. A homozygous mutation in *SLURP1*, c.43T>C, was identified in 14 individuals from northern Sweden, and compound heterozygous mutations, c.280T>A and c.43T>C, were identified in one individual from southern Sweden. The c.43T>C mutation had been previously reported in MDM,[168] supporting that PPK-GN is a mild variant of MDM and not a separate entity.[173]

SLURP-1 has been shown to be expressed in human skin, mainly in keratinocytes underlying the upper epidermal layers, and it has a role in maintaining the skin's physiologic and structural integrity. SLURP-1 upregulates the expression of transglutaminase 1, cytokeratin 10, and caspases 3 and 8 with resultant increased apoptotic activity which exceeds that of TNF-α. In addition, it regulates epidermal differentiation through cholinergic pathways.[174]

Moreover, SLURP-1 expression correlates with abnormal immune responses. Mutations in this gene resulted in defective T-cell activation responses,[149] and SLURP-1 increased acetylcholine synthesis in T cells and attenuated T-cell proliferation. These effects were abolished by a α7-nAChR antagonist, indicating that SLURP-1 modulates the functional development of T cells via α7-nAChR-mediated pathways.[175] Accordingly, patients with homozygous SLURP1 mutations are prone to viral infections and to the development of MM.[176] The higher incidence of MM in patients with MDM is not only attributable to defective T-cell activation and prolonged inflammation in hyperkeratotic skin[162,163] but may also result from defective apoptotic activity[177,178] and defective regulation of TNF-α release from macrophages.[179,180]

It has been suggested that SLURP-1 deficiency influences the efficiency of triglyceride hydrolysis in keratinocytes, an essential process for the formation of acylceramides important for the epidermal barrier.[181,182] It has been hypothesized that leakage of interstitial fluids into the stratum corneum and accumulation of triglyceride droplets in SLURP1-deficient skin are conditions favoring microorganism growth responsible for the malodorous skin of MDM.[181]

SLURP-1 may play a role in the pathogenesis of psoriasis. Its expression was upregulated in the skin of imiquimod-induced psoriasis in mice, and SLURP1 mRNA expression was significantly upregulated after stimulation with interleukin (IL)-22 which was completely suppressed by STAT3 inhibition. In addition, SLURP-1 significantly suppressed the growth of *Staphylococcus aureus*,[183] and it has been shown to regulate epithelialization and wound healing in both cutaneous and oral wounds.[184]

Pathology: The histologic features of MDM are hyperkeratosis, orthokeratosis, foci of parakeratosis, marked acanthosis, a more pronounced stratum lucidum, and a perivascular lymphohistiocytic infiltrate.[185] Electron microscopy findings are a less-abrupt-than-normal transition between the stratum granulosum and stratum corneum; normal intermediate filaments and corneodesmosomes; and nonspecific, irregularly shaped keratohyalin granules with a spongy appearance.[26] In palmoplantar sections from patients with MDM, as well as in their sweat, SLURP-1 was either absent or barely detectable. It has been suggested that SLURP-1 assessment in sweat collected by the standard pilocarpine procedure used for the diagnosis of CF may serve as a rapid screening test for MDM.[186]

NAGASHIMA-TYPE PALMOPLANTAR KERATODERMA

Clinical Features: Nagashima-type PPK (NPPK; OMIM #615598), is an autosomal recessive disorder first described by Nagashima in 1977. The disease was initially named Meleda-type PPK, but in 1989 the term NPPK (or keratosis palmoplantaris Nagashima) was coined to distinguish this form of PPK from true MDM, given its milder phenotype and on-progressive nature after puberty.[187,188] Most cases have been reported in Japan and China, and the estimated prevalence in those countries is 1.2 in 10,000 and 2.3 to 3.1 in 10,000, respectively,[189,190] making it the most common type of PPK in Asian populations. Several cases have been described outside East Asia with estimated prevalence rates of NPPK in non-Asian populations as low as 0.5 in 100,000,000.[189,191,192]

NPPK typically begins in the first years of life (from birth through the fourth year) and gradually progresses until puberty with no further progression thereafter. It is characterized by a diffuse, well-demarcated, erythematous palmoplantar hyperkeratosis that extends to the dorsal surfaces of the hands, feet, inner wrists, ankles, and Achilles tendon area. Involvement of the elbows and knees is common. A single case with involvement of the central lumbar area, cubital fossae, forearms, thighs, and popliteal fossae has been described.[193] Hyperkeratosis on the ears and toenail dystrophy (atrophic nail plates with fragile distal edges and spontaneous peeling) are rare features that have been reported in isolated cases.[194,195] It is frequently complicated by hyperhidrosis, superinfection by dermatophytes, a distinct odor, and maceration.[187,188,190-192] There is no evidence of constricting bands, spontaneous amputation, or flexion contractures in contrast to other more severe forms of autosomal recessive transgressive diffuse PPKs, such as MDM and PPK-GN.[188,192] In addition, patients with NPPK display a whitish spongy appearance within 10 minutes of water exposure specifically in the erythematous hyperkeratotic areas, suggesting enhanced water permeation into the stratum corneum in NPPK lesional skin.[189,190] A case of MM arising within the lesions of NPPK has been reported.[196]

Etiology and Pathogenesis: NPPK is caused by biallelic mutations in the gene *SERPINB7*, encoding serpin family B member 7 (SERPIN7), a cytoplasmic member of the serine protease inhibitor (serpin) superfamily. Most cases of NPPK are caused by loss-of-function (LOF) mutations resulting from aberrant splicing or premature stop codons with nonsense or frameshift mutations.[197] Compound heterozygosity for a missense founder mutation c.830C>T, resulting in proline to leucine in the highly conserved residue 277, resulted in NPPK phenotype with mislocalized SERPIN7 within corneocytes.[198]

A recurrent nonsense mutation in *SERPINB7*, c.796C>T, has been found to be prevalent in both Chinese and Japanese NPPK patients, probably reflecting a founder effect. Accordingly, it has been suggested that mutation screening for c.796C>T in *SERPINB7* can serve as a diagnostic strategy in the setting of Chinese and Japanese patients with diffuse, nonmutilating PPKs.[190,193,199]

Epidermal protease inhibitors, such as LEKTI, LEKTI-2, elafin, serpins, and cystatins, play a crucial role in maintaining epidermal homeostasis by inhibiting both endogenous proteases residing in the stratum granulosum and the stratum corneum and exogenous proteases from bacteria, fungi, viruses, pollen, and house dust mites that attack the epidermis.[200,201] Mutations affecting serpins can cause symptoms either by loss of protease inhibitory activity and uncontrolled protease activity or by aggregation of mutant serpins polymers in serpin-synthesizing cells with cell death and tissue damage (the "serpinopathies").

SERPINB7 has been shown to be distributed in the epidermis, especially in the stratum granulosum and upper part of the stratum corneum, with predominant cytoplasmic expression. In NPPK skin, SERPINB7 immunoreactivity is markedly diminished.[189] Although SERPINB7 is ubiquitously expressed in human epidermis, NPPK is limited to the hands, feet, knees, and elbows, suggesting that chronic exposure to mechanical stress may have a role in the development of NPPK and that SERPINB7 might inhibit mechanical stress-induced proteases and protect keratinocytes or corneocytes from protease-mediated cellular damage.[189]

The whitish spongy change upon water exposure in NPPK, similar to PPKB with *AQP5* mutations and aquagenic keratoderma with *CFTR* mutations has been suggested to result from enhanced water permeation into the damaged stratum corneum.

Pathology: Histopathologic findings in NPPK include orthohyperkeratosis with acanthosis, hypergranulosis, and a mild to moderate perivascular lymphocytic infiltrate in the upper dermis.[191,192,199] A predominance of CD4+ T cells with barely detectable CD20+ B cells was observed in dermal infiltrates.[202]

DIFFUSE INHERITED PALMOPLANTAR KERATODERMA WITH EXTRACUTANEOUS FEATURES, DOMINANT INHERITANCE

OLMSTED SYNDROME

Clinical Features: OS (OMIM #614594), first reported in 1927 by Olmsted,[203] is a rare disorder with a prevalence of less than 1 in 1,000,000. It usually appears at birth, during the neonatal period, or in early childhood, although appearance later in childhood has been described,[204] and progressively worsen over time. Both sexes are affected, although male patients comprise 60% of reported cases.[205] It is characterized by symmetric, sharply demarcated, diffuse PPK with yellowish-brown hyperkeratosis, painful fissures, and erythematous borders in association with periorificial keratotic plaques. These plaques may be restricted to the areas around the mouth, nostrils, ear meatus, anus, and perigenital region or may extend to involve nonperiorificial sites such as the neck, upper thorax, lower abdomen, arms, elbows, knees, thighs, and inguinal folds. The PPK typically starts focally and is distributed on the pressure points. It gradually extends to most of the surface of the palms and soles with thick hyperkeratotic plaques that eventually result in flexion deformity of the fingers, pseudoainhum, and spontaneous amputation of the digits or the hands. The PPK is typically painful and disabling, interfering with walking and daily activities. Cases with more focal or punctuate keratoderma, lacking pseudoainhum or significant periorificial keratotic lesions, have been reported.[204,206-209] Additional findings are severe pruritus with sleep disturbances, onychodystrophy (ridged and rough nails, onychogryphosis, leukonychia, onycholysis, paronychia, subungual hyperkeratosis, absence of nails), abnormal dentition (absence of premolar teeth, periodontal disease with premature teeth loss),[210,211] sweating abnormalities, oral leukokeratosis, hyperhidrosis, hyperkeratotic linear streaks, follicular keratosis, cheilitis, and ichthyotic lesions.[208,212-220] Hair abnormalities are common, although rare cases have normal hair, and include alopecia (diffuse, universal or patchy); hypotrichosis; and thinning, curly, woolly, coarse, and dry or easily broken hair. Microscopic findings of affected hair include pili torti, trichorrhexis nodosa, reduced pigment, longitudinal ridges, and transverse fractures of the hair shaft.[33,205,213,217-219] Sparse and thin eyebrows and eyelashes, madarosis, as well as trichomegaly were observed in OS.[206,214,221] Secondary bacterial and candidal infections,[216,222,223] SCC (verrucous carcinoma or its variant epithelioma cuniculatum), and MM can develop within the PPK.[224-227] A case associated with cone-shaped fingers and a sclerodactyly-like appearance overlapping with clinical features of Huriez syndrome has been described.[228] Extracutaneous manifestations are uncommon and include hearing loss,[211] ocular abnormalities (corneal dystrophy, inflamed lacrimal glands or ducts or meibomian gland dysfunction, chronic blepharitis),[214,216] short stature,[218,226] primary sclerosing cholangitis,[229] mental retardation,[203,230] joint laxity, ankyloses, osteopenia, and osteolysis.[145,203-205,211,218,223,226,231,232] Erythromelalgia[206,228,233] has been reported in several cases.

Etiology and Pathogenesis: Although most cases reported to date have been sporadic, familial cases with different modes of inheritance, including autosomal dominant, autosomal recessive and X-linked inheritance, have been reported. Autosomal dominant, semidominant, and autosomal recessive OS have been shown to be cause by mutations in the gene *TRPV3* encoding transient receptor potential vanilloid 3 (TRPV3),[145,206,221,232,233] and mutations in the gene *MBTPS2* encoding the membrane-bound transcription factor protease site 2 have been identified in X-linked recessive OS.[234] There is no clear genotype–phenotype correlation in OS.

Mutations in *TRPV3* are associated with persistence of basal keratins[208,235] and increased expression of Ki-67.[219,220] Keratinocytes expressing mutant TRPV3 are prone to cell death, and the epidermis of OS patients displays increased apoptotic cells compared with control participants.[145]

TRPV3 is highly expressed in keratinocytes and in the hair follicles (HFs), spinal cord, sensory neurons, brain, and cornea. It has an important role in epidermal barrier formation, regulation of hair growth, and modulation of pain sensation and pruritus, explaining the manifestations of OS.[236-240] TRPV3 activation increases intracellular Ca^{2+} concentration and is associated with transforming growth factor (TGF)-α/EGFR signaling, which is known to regulate epidermal differentiation.[241] The role of TRPV3 in mediating EGFR signaling in hair and skin barrier function was demonstrated using a *Trpv3* knockout mouse model that developed a wavy hair coat and curly whiskers in addition to red, dry, scaly skin at birth.[239] In addition, mice or rats carrying heterozygous mutations in *Trpv3* exhibited hair paucity and dermatitis.[242]

Mutations in *MBTPS2*, encoding a zinc metalloprotease essential for cholesterol homeostasis and endoplasmic reticulum (ER) stress response, have been reported in cases of OS with X-linked recessive inheritance.[234] Mutations in *MBTPS2* were first identified in ichthyosis follicularis atrichia photophobia (IFAP) syndrome[243] (see Chap. 49), which is allelic to X-linked recessive OS. A case with features of both OS and IFAP syndrome has been reported.[244]

There is no obvious clinical difference between OS patients carrying either *TRPV3* or *MBTPS2* mutations, and clinical variability is observed within the same family or among different patients harboring the same mutations, supporting a role for modifier genes, environmental effects, or epigenetic factors. Moreover, genetic heterogeneity is likely given the fact that some patients do not carry mutations in either *TRPV3* or *MBTPS2*.

Pathology: The histopathologic findings of OS are nonspecific and include psoriasiform epidermal hyperplasia, orthohyperkeratosis, focal parakeratosis, hypo- or hypergranulosis, acanthosis, and inflammatory infiltrates in the upper dermis, which may contain mast cells.[145,205,232] Epidermal vesicular degeneration has been reported.[228] Electron microscopy findings include large, coarse, densely packed bundles of tonofilaments in the keratinocytes of the mid Malpighian layer and increased numbers of coarse keratohyaline granules in the granular layer. Decreased number of pigment granules and absence of Langerhans cells were reported.[228]

Specific Treatments: Partial excision of palmoplantar keratosis or full-thickness excision with skin grafting has been performed with clinical improvement.[245] EGFR inhibitors have been shown to improve PPK,[246] and TRPV3 antagonists may be an effective treatment for patients harboring GOF mutations in the *TRPV3* gene.

CONNEXIN-ASSOCIATED PALMOPLANTAR KERATODERMAS: VOHWINKEL SYNDROME, KERATITIS–ICHTHYOSIS–DEAFNESS SYNDROME, BART-PUMPHREY SYNDROME, AND PALMOPLANTAR KERATODERMA WITH DEAFNESS

Clinical Features: VS (keratoderma hereditaria mutilans; OMIM #124500) was first reported in 1929 by Vohwinkel[115] and Wigley.[247] VS is characterized by a triad of diffuse, mutilating PPK with a "honeycomb-like" appearance (see Fig. 48-4B); "starfish-shaped" keratotic plaques on the dorsal hands, feet, and extensor surfaces; and fibrous constricting bands (pseudoainhum) at the interphalangeal joints of the hands and feet that result in autoamputation.[248] Most cases are also associated with high-frequency SNHL.[27,29,249-252] The disease is more common among white women. It tends to manifest in the neonatal period and progresses throughout life. Cases with PPK characterized by callosities at pressure points or striate lesions at sites of injury, suggesting an isomorphic phenomenon, have been reported.[250] The disease may be associated with generalized ichthyosis,[28] acanthosis nigricans,[253] cicatricial or nonscarring alopecia, nail anomalies, knuckle pads, bullous lesions on the soles,[249] and craniofacial anomalies (cleft lip and palate, microcephaly, and facial asymmetry).[27,29,249,250,254-257] The appearance of SCC and basal cell carcinoma (BCC) in the hyperkeratotic lesions has been reported.[28] Cases associated with deaf-mutism,[18] mental retardation,[258] spastic paraplegia with myopathy,[29] psychomotor developmental retardation, and epileptic seizures[259,260] have been reported.

KID syndrome (OMIM #148210; see Chap. 47) is the most severe cutaneous connexin disorder, involving epithelia of ectodermal origin (skin, appendages, nail, teeth) along with significant inner ear and cornea involvement.[261,262] Disease manifestations were first described in 1915, although the name KID syndrome was coined by Skinner and coworkers in 1981.[262,263] The disease manifests at birth or during infancy. Its cutaneous features are erythrokeratoderma with symmetrical, well-circumscribed hyperkeratotic plaques with a reticulated pattern, leather-like appearance, or diffuse furfuraceous scaling with underlying erythema and a relative predilection for the axillae and neck. Other manifestations include thickened skin with coarse-grained appearance or follicular hyperkeratosis without erythema. The characteristic PPK is diffuse and has a rough, stippled, or grainy appearance (Fig. 48-6). Chronic cheilitis and perleche are common. Associated findings are nail dystrophy, oral manifestations (leukokeratosis, deep fissures of the tongue, dental abnormalities including caries and delayed eruption of teeth, persistent oral mucosal papules), hypohidrosis, and heat intolerance. Numerous KID syndrome patients have sparse hair, and 10% to 23% have congenital atrichia.[261,264] Most patients develop

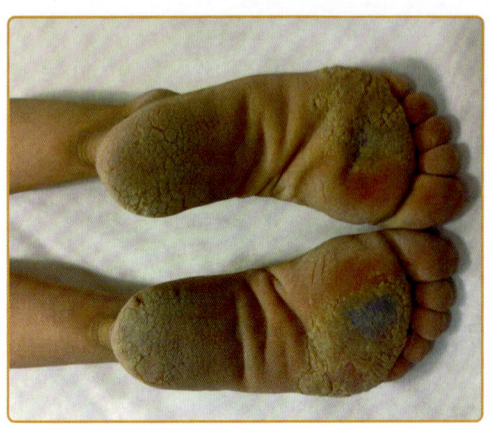

Figure 48-6 Keratitis–ichthyosis–deafness (KID) syndrome. Diffuse, hyperkeratotic, plantar keratoderma with the characteristic rough, stippled, and grainy appearance.

progressive keratitis that begins during childhood and may first manifest as photophobia. The keratitis is characterized by corneal inflammation, pain, and corneal neovascularization and may be associated with chronic blepharitis, conjunctivitis, keratoconjunctivitis sicca, and limbal defects and may cause progressive visual decline and blindness. Associated ophthalmologic features are loss of eyebrows and eyelashes, hyperkeratosis of the eyelids, trichiasis, early-onset cataract, and bilateral lacrimal punctal agenesis.[261,265-272] Conversely, cases with no evidence of ophthalmologic manifestations have been described.[273,274] In addition, patients with KID have congenital, bilateral, and severe SNHL, which is not progressive, compared with the corneal findings.[275] Patients are prone to mucocutaneous infections, mostly bacterial and candidal, which can be fatal in the neonatal period.[276,277] Viral infections (molluscum contagiosum and cytomegalovirus), recurrent pulmonary infiltrates, and recurrent otitis externa have been reported.[278,279] Patients are prone to developing benign cutaneous tumors, mainly trichilemmoma,[280-282] although isolated cases of multiple poromas and porokeratotic eccrine ostial and dermal duct nevus have been described.[283] Approximately 10% of affected individuals are reported to develop SCC of the skin (mainly acral sites and areas of chronic infection or inflammation) and tongue, apparently caused by p53 loss in the lesions.[41,261,268,269,278,280,284-287] SCCs may cause death in patients with KID given their aggressive phenotype and the tendency to develop multiple tumors.[280] In addition, single cases of an association with sebaceous carcinoma, peripheral T-cell non-Hodgkin lymphoma, malignant histiocytoma, and metastatic malignant pilar tumors have been reported.[271,281,288-290] An association between KID syndrome and hidradenitis suppurativa and dissecting cellulitis of the scalp has been described.[47,281,291,292] KID syndrome may result in death in infancy from severe infections or respiratory compromise.[276,293-295]

Bart-Pumphrey syndrome (BPS; OMIM #149200) is a rare, autosomal dominant disorder first described by Bart and Pumphrey in 1967. It is characterized by severe SNHL, PPK with a honeycomb-like appearance, knuckle pads, and leukonychia.[296-298] Hearing loss and knuckle pads are the most common findings; leukonychia and PPK are seen less frequently.[296,297,299-302] The PPK features diffuse, sharply demarcated thickening of the palmoplantar skin with a punctate, grainy surface reminiscent of VS. Striate appearance has been described as well.[302]

PPK and deafness (OMIM #148350) is an autosomal dominant condition in which PPK may be diffuse, transgrediens with fissures and underlying erythema or with a milder phenotype with skin fold accentuation over pressure points. Knuckle pads may be present. Hearing impairment may become apparent during infancy; is bilateral, prelingual, and slowly progressive; and affects high-frequency tones.[303-309]

Etiology and Pathogenesis: Gap junctions, which are formed by connexons, are intercellular junctions that facilitate and regulate the passage of water and small molecules between adjacent cells. The oligomerization of six connexins leads to the formation of a hemichannel called a connexon, and connexons of two opposing cells interact with each other through their extracellular portions to form a channel that is the basic unit of the gap junction. Connexins are expressed in a tissue and differentiation specific manner.[310-315] The epidermis, its appendages, and other ectoderm-derived epithelia of the inner ear and cornea share the expression of several connexin proteins, including Cx26, Cx30, Cx31, and Cx43. Cx43 is ubiquitously expressed in all epithelial cells of ectodermal origin, and similar to Cx26, it has been shown to play a role in wound healing.[316] The expression of Cx26 is limited to cochlear cells, corneal limbal cells, palmoplantar epidermis, around the openings of eccrine sweat glands and ducts, and in the inner and outer root sheath of human HFs. Cx26 expression is widely paralleled by the expression pattern of Cx30 (both share 76% amino acid identity).[317,318] In contrast to Cx30, which is prevalent in the upper differentiated layers of interfollicular epidermis, Cx26 is only expressed at low levels in palmoplantar epidermis but is strongly induced in response to wounding and in hyperproliferative diseases.[318-320] Cx26 is also expressed in epithelial supporting cells surrounding the sensory hair cells of the cochlea and in the fibrocytes lining the cochlear duct, where it mediates the recycling of potassium ions passing through the hair cells back to the endolymph during auditory transduction.[321,322]

GJB2 encodes Cx26. Recessive mutations producing complete loss of expression or function are the single most common cause of nonsyndromic SNHL in humans.[323] In addition, mutations in connexin genes are known to cause several inherited human disorders not associated with PPK or other dermatological abnormalities, including X-linked Charcot-Marie-Tooth disease (Cx32),[324] zonular pulverent cataract (Cx50),[325] and occulodentodigitaldysplasia (Cx43).[326] Moreover, several inherited genodermatoses result from heterozygous mutations in connexin genes (see Table 48-1 and Fig. 48-2).[250,327-329]

Connexins consist of four transmembrane domains, three cytoplasmic domains (the amino-terminus, a cytoplasmic loop and the carboxy terminus domains), and two extracellular loops. Both the N-terminal and C-terminal parts of the proteins are located in the cytoplasm. The membrane spanning and extracellular domains are highly conserved, and the main differences between connexins are found in their C-terminal tails.[311,330] Most dominant-negative *GJB2* mutations associated with hearing impairment and cutaneous involvement reported so far are located in the cytoplasmic N-terminal or in the first extracellular loop of Cx26, which is highly conserved among the connexins and is involved in the control of voltage gating, channel permeability, multimer assembly, and the interactions between connexons. Accordingly, mutations affecting the first extracellular domain may affect both protein transport and channel permeability.[311,317] In addition, different mutations in this domain result in different pathophysiological effects, such as blockage of conductance, dominant effect on wild-type Cx26, protein folding, and altered hemichannel structural stability, leading to a variable clinical phenotype. Moreover, co-oligomerization of different connexins into heteromeric connexons plays a role in the pathogenesis and in the dynamic nature of connexin-associated phenotypes, which are mostly caused by a dominant negative effect on intercellular communication.[311,331]

Most reported cases of VS result from the recurrent heterozygous missense mutation, p.Asp66His, in *GJB2* which results in an amino acid substitution from aspartic acid to histidine in a highly conserved residue of the first extracellular domain.[330] This mutation could selectively impair the ability of Cx26 to form heteromeric and homomeric connexons,[332] resulting in a change in charge or conformation of Cx26 with disruption of gating properties for certain molecules or ions.

Generalized knockout of *Gjb2* in mice is embryonic lethal (caused by placental insufficiency), but conditional *Gjb2* knockout in the mouse inner ear resulted in deafness.[333] Transgenic expression of a dominant-negative *Gjb2* mutation revealed a progressive degeneration of the sensory hair cells with the loss of the tunnel of Corti as a result of disturbed cortilymph homeostasis,[334] illustrating the essential role played by Cx26 in the auditory function in the inner ear. Transgenic mice expressing the p.Asp66His mutation exclusively in the suprabasal epidermis exhibited keratoderma with constriction bands on the tail, marked thickening of the epidermal cornified layers, and increased epidermal TUNEL staining, indicative of either excess apoptosis or premature terminal differentiation.[335] Premature keratinocyte death might induce compensatory basal cell proliferation, leading to the massive thickening of the stratum corneum.

Both autosomal dominant[41,43] and autosomal recessive[336] forms of KID syndrome have been described, although autosomal dominant inheritance is more common.[42,337] Cases with suggested parental germline mosaicism have been reported.[286,294,338] Most affected individuals harbor a recurrent missense mutation in *GJB2*, p.Asp50Asn, leading to replacement of aspartic acid in codon 50 with asparagine.[298,317,339-342] In addition, hystrix-like ichthyosis-deafness (HID) syndrome, which is allelic to KID syndrome,[343] has been reported to result from the p.Asp50Asn mutation and other *GJB2* missense mutations.[298] Asp50 is a pore-lining residue that is highly conserved among connexins and is crucial for gap junction formation and function; p.Asp50Asn results in intracellular expression of the mutant protein, suggesting altered trafficking to the plasma membrane and absence of gap junction plaques.[344,345] The mutation p.Gly45Glu has been identified in a fatal forms of KID syndrome.[294] All KID syndrome–causing mutations cluster in regions coding for the first extracellular domain and the cytoplasmic amino terminal domain of Cx26 and are predicted to alter the charge and structure of this domain, in contrast to nonsyndromic Cx26-associated mutations that are located along the protein.[314,317] Recent experiments in *Xenopus laevis* oocytes demonstrate that hemichannels formed by several Cx26 KID mutants are inhibited by mefloquine; mefloquine attenuated increased macroscopic membrane currents in primary mouse keratinocytes expressing the human Cx26 p.Gly45Glu mutation.[346]

A heterozygous mutation in *GJB6*, encoding Cx30, has been shown to result in KID syndrome as well. This mutation is predicted to alter the sequence and charge of the first transmembrane helix of Cx30 and was reported in a child with typical characteristics of KID syndrome, including follicular, spiny hyperkeratosis, congenital atrichia, and nail abnormalities.[264] A similar mutation had been implicated in Clouston syndrome (see later) without evidence for abnormal sweating, hearing, photophobia, and keratitis,[347] underscoring the profound influence of other genetic and epigenetic factors in modifying the clinical outcome of connexin disorders and emphasizing the phenotypic variability of *GJB6* mutations. It has been speculated that the unique phenotype of this patient is related to the presence of a homozygous polymorphism in *GJB2*.[264]

In BPS, two mutations involving the first extracellular domain of Cx26, p.N54K, and p.G59S have been reported, underscoring the importance of this domain in docking of connexin hemichannels and voltage gating.[299,302]

PPK with deafness results from heterozygous mutations in the *GJB2* gene clustered in or at the border of the first extracellular loop domain.[303-306] One of these dominant mutations, p.R75Q (c.224G>A), was described for the first time by Uyguner and coworkers in a Turkish family[305] and was reported in isolated deafness and in association with PPK.[348]

Pathology: Histopathologic manifestations of VS include compact hyperkeratosis; orthokeratosis; acanthosis; significant hypergranulosis with large, irregularly shaped keratohyaline granules; papillomatosis of the epidermis; and dermal fibrosis with a sparse perivascular lymphocytic infiltrate.[256,298,349] Ultrastructural findings are marked swollen mitochondria and increased numbers of desmosomes in the spinous and granular layers with corneocytes containing many membrane coating granules and lipid-like vacuoles.[349]

Skin biopsies obtain from PPK in KID syndrome may display epidermal hyperplasia, compact orthokeratotic hyperkeratosis, and focal parakeratosis. Hypogranulosis may be observed, although cases with a prominent granular layer have been reported, and swollen keratinocytes with slightly vacuolated cytoplasm are described. Keratotic plugging is a common feature. Inflammatory cells in the upper dermis may be evident, especially in cases of infection.[264,294,350]

Histopathologic findings in BPS are massive orthokeratotic hyperkeratosis, hypergranulosis, acanthosis, and papillomatosis. Epidermal gap junctions appear normal on electron microscopy.[302]

Specific Treatments: In VS, cross finger flap,[248] treatment with Z-plasty,[351] full-thickness excision of the constriction band with a full-thickness skin graft,[352] and a distant abdominal skin flap for fifth digit constriction bands[353] have been described. Reported treatments for the ocular manifestations of KID syndrome are keratolimbal allograft, keratoplasty and immunosuppression,[354] keratectomy,[43] topical corticosteroids and cyclosporine,[355] and bevacizumab has been shown to be effective in a single case.[356]

PALMOPLANTAR KERATODERMA–CONGENITAL ALOPECIA SYNDROME

Clinical Features: Two forms of PPK with congenital alopecia have been described. An autosomal dominant form has a milder phenotype (PPKCA1, Stevanovic type; OMIM #104100),[357-360] and the recessively inherited form is associated with pseudo-ainhum, sclerodactyly, contractures, and sometimes cataracts (PPKCA2, Wallis type; OMIM #212360).[257,361-363] Hair is normal or sparse at birth, and noncicatricial alopecia involving the scalp, body, or facial hair becomes apparent in early infancy. Trichorrhexis nodosa may be evident on hair microscopy. PPK develops in late infancy and is well-defined, focal or linear, nonmutilating, and transgrediens in the dominant cases. In the recessive cases, it features progressive thickening of the lateral and medial aspects of palms and soles with an erythematous rim and skin cracks that subsequently involve the dorsal fingers, resulting in contractures, pseudoainhum, and sclerodactyly. Associated findings are follicular plugging with ulerythema ophryogenes–like features; keratosis pilaris; and hyperkeratotic plaques over the ankles, elbows, and popliteal fossae, with multiple spiky, horn-like lesions reminiscent of ichthyosis hystrix and nail abnormalities (eukonychia, nail dystrophy).[364] Cataracts, meningocele, and unilateral deafness were reported in single cases.[257,358,361]

Etiology and Pathogenesis: PPKCA1 has been shown to result from a heterozygous missense mutation in the gene *GJA1*, encoding Cx43, which exerts a GOF effect on the Cx43 hemichannel. Cx43 is ubiquitously expressed in various organs, including the epidermis and HFs.[365,366]

PPKCA1 is allelic to oculodentodigital dysplasia (ODDD), which is characterized by craniofacial dysmorphism; dental, ophthalmologic, and limb abnormalities; and neurodegeneration, and is occasionally associated with PPK and hair and nail anomalies. In ODDD, most mutations result in retention of the mutant protein in the ER or decreased permeability of the channels with nonfunctional gap junctions.[326,367-369]

The responsible gene for PPKCA2 has not been identified yet.

Pathology: Hyperkeratotic plaques show orthohyperkeratosis with follicular plugging and perivascular lymphocytic infiltration in the papillary dermis.[364] Scanning electron microscopy of the hair shafts reveals multiple pits with cuticular weathering[364] or longitudinal grooves.[360]

HIDROTIC ECTODERMAL DYSPLASIA (CLOUSTON SYNDROME; SEE CHAP. 131)

Clinical Features: Hidrotic ectodermal dysplasia (HED, Clouston syndrome; OMIM #129500) was first described in 1895[370] and later by Clouston in families from Quebec.[371,372] HED is an autosomal dominant ectodermal dysplasia particularly common among the French-Canadian population because of a founder effect,[328] although it has been reported in several ethnic groups.[347,373-380] The main features of this condition include nail dystrophy, hair loss, and palmoplantar hyperkeratosis with normal sweat glands and teeth.[378,381,382]

Nail abnormalities are usually present; in nearly 30%, they are the only manifestation of the syndrome. They range from almost normal-appearing nails to short nails and anonychia.[371] Nail plate changes include thickening, brittleness, ridging, discoloration, splitting, onycholysis, and 20-nail dystrophy.[347,371,372,381] Paronychia and nail infections are common and may result in nail matrix destruction.[371,374,383] Hair abnormalities may be progressive and involve the scalp, facial, and body hair and include atrichia or hypotrichosis with brittle, fine, pale, or slow-growing hair.[384] PPK is diffuse with a velvet-like or cobblestoned appearance extending onto the fingertips and knuckles with fissures. In a large Han Chinese family, the hyperkeratosis of the palms and soles tended to worsen with time.[379] Cases of HED with nail changes resembling PC, either as a solitary finding or in association with alopecia but with no evidence of PPK have been reported.[385-387] Keratotic papules and plaques over the upper and lower extremities and discrete hyperpigmentation over digital joints have been described. Rare associations include strabismus, cataract and photophobia, hearing impairment, mental deficiency, and bone abnormalities (thickening of the skull, abnormal phalanges).[371,372,382,383,388-391]

Etiology and Pathogenesis: HED is caused by autosomal dominant heterozygous mutations in *GJB6*, encoding Cx30.[328] Cx30 is a 261–amino acid polypeptide consisting of four transmembrane domains, two extracellular domains, and three cytoplasmic domains similar to other connexins.[392,393] Cx30 is expressed in the epidermis (middle and upper spinous layers), HFs (outer root sheath, hair matrix), nails (nail matrix and nail bed), brain, and inner ear.[328,394-399]

A mouse model for HED carrying the p.A88V mutation in GJB6 demonstrates mild hyperkeratosis of palmoplantar skin, enlarged and hyperproliferative sebaceous glands, and altered hearing (both are not common features in HED).[400] In addition, this mutation resulted in significant apoptosis, possibly through leaky hemichannels.[401] It has been suggested that the leaky hemichannels resulting from the p.A88V mutation could stimulate proliferation through activation of Ca^{2+}-dependent kinases with altered gene expression or cell cycle reentry.[400]

Similar to other connexin disorders, HED is characterized by extensive clinical and genetic heterogeneity. A patient with clinical features of HED and ODD and extensive hyperkeratosis of the skin was found to have an heterozygous mutation, p.V41L, in GJA1 encoding Cx43, as well as a heterozygous sequence variant (P.R127H) in GJB2.[402] A Chinese patient with HED was found to carry two missense mutations, p.N14S in GJB6 and p.F191L in GJB2,[389] and a Japanese patient with HED associated with hearing impairment and photophobia was found to harbor a heterozygous missense mutations in GJB6 (p.Ala88Val) and a polymorphism in GJB2 (p.Val27Ile).[390]

In contrast to GJB2 mutations that result in skin symptoms and deafness, mutations in GJB6 typically result in skin manifestations with no evidence of hearing impairment. It is possible that Cx26 compensates for the absence of Cx30 in the inner ear and not in the skin, but Cx30 cannot completely compensate for the loss of Cx26 at both sites because mutant Cx26 exerts a dominant negative effect on other co-expressed connexins. However, a case of KID syndrome caused by a mutation in GJB6 and a case of HED with SNHL and photophobia have been reported; in addition, a p.T5M mutation in GJB6 results in dominant nonsyndromic hearing loss, suggesting that functional redundancy may be dependent on additional factors such as the location and nature of the causative mutations.[264,390,403]

Pathology: Hypotrichotic skin reveals normal epidermis, a normal distribution of eccrine and sebaceous glands, and absence or remnants of HFs.[347,379,384] PPK lesions reveal hyperkeratosis with irregular and reticulated acanthosis.[389]

HURIEZ SYNDROME

Clinical Features: Huriez syndrome (sclerotylosis; OMIM #181600) was first described by Huriez and coworkers in 1969 in two families from Northern France.[404] Since then, kindred from different ethnicities have been described, including Tunisian, Indian, German, English, Italian, and Japanese families.[405-411] Most cases are inherited in an autosomal dominant fashion, and several sporadic cases have been reported.[409,412] Huriez syndrome is characterized by diffuse PPK, scleroatrophy of the hands and fingers, occurrence of SCC within atrophic skin, and sclerodactyly leading to contractures. The disease is present at birth or appears in the first years of life and persists with no further progression. The PPK manifests as diffuse, yellowish-grey, nonerythematous, well-confined hyperkeratotic plaques mainly involving the palms with extension towards the fingers and accentuation of palmar creases (Fig. 48-4C). The soles are less frequently involved and usually show accentuation over pressure sites. A porokeratotic appearance has been described. Scleroatrophic changes include a pseudosclerodermoid appearance of the hands and digits with absence of dermatoglyphs and erythematous, atrophic appearance of the dorsal aspect of the hands, fingers, and tips of the fingers and toes with no evidence of Raynaud phenomenon. Associated findings are hypohidrosis and nail changes including hypoplasia, curving, onychorrhexis, koilonychia, longitudinal ridging, and clubbing. Manifestations reported in isolated cases are poikiloderma-like changes, distinctive small nodules on the fingers, and facial telangiectasia. Malignant degeneration starts with the occurrence of skin ulcers on the atrophic skin of the hands and development of SCC by the third to fourth decade of life. The estimated risk of SCC is 13%, a greater than 100-fold higher risk. These tumors tend to show poor differentiation with high rates of metastasis and a calculated mortality rate of 5%.[35,404,406-408,413,414] Cases associated with internal malignancies (gastric carcinoma, pharyngeal carcinoma) have been described, but internal malignancies do not seem to be more frequent in Huriez syndrome than in the general population.[35,404]

Etiology and Pathogenesis: The pathogenesis of Huriez syndrome and the mechanism involved in tumor formation are unknown. Previously, a linkage between Huriez syndrome and the certain blood groups has been reported[415]; however subsequent studies failed to confirm this finding.[35,407] Lee and coworkers mapped the gene to chromosome 4q23.[416] Loss of heterozygosity of 4q has been reported in the majority of SCCs originating from head and neck and in almost 50% of cases of cervical carcinoma. However, in the former, the region involved extends distal to the locus of Huriez syndrome with possible overlap on its centromeric end.[416]

Immunohistochemical and ultrastructural studies revealed an almost complete absence of epidermal Langerhans cells within involved skin.[405,406] Moreover, positive p53 staining (indicative of abnormal function of p53) was observed in atypical keratinocytes, suggesting that *p53* mutations may be responsible for the development of actinic keratoses and SCC in Huriez syndrome.[409]

Pathology: Skin biopsies obtained from PPK skin reveal marked acanthosis and papillomatosis, hypergranulosis with increased number of keratohyaline granules, and orthokeratotic hyperkeratosis. No abnormalities are observed in the dermis and sweat glands. In scleroatrophic regions, the epidermis shows hypergranulosis with orthokeratotic hyperkeratosis, dense collagen fibers in the reticular dermis, and thin elastic fibers. Sparse dermal mononuclear cell infiltrates may be seen.[35,405,409,412,413] A case with vacuolar degeneration of keratinocytes in the upper spinous layers has been reported.[411] Ultrastructural findings are dense bundles of tonofilaments throughout epidermal layers with abundant keratohyaline distributed in large clumps of irregular density. Areas of scleroatrophic skin show similar changes in tonofilaments and keratohyaline but with addition features of thinned oxytalan and elaunin fibers at the dermal–epidermal junction, irregular borders, and nonhomogeneous appearance of elastic fibers with evidence of elastic fibers engulfed by macrophages.[35]

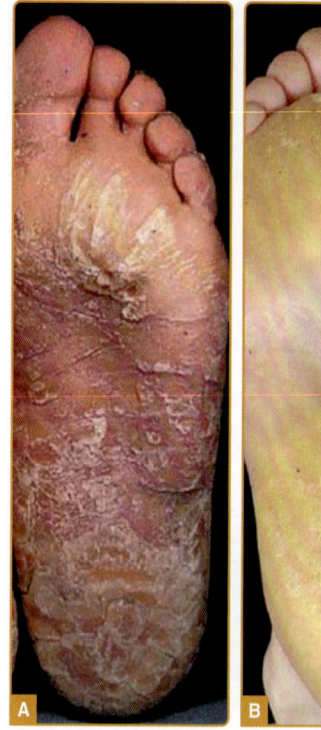
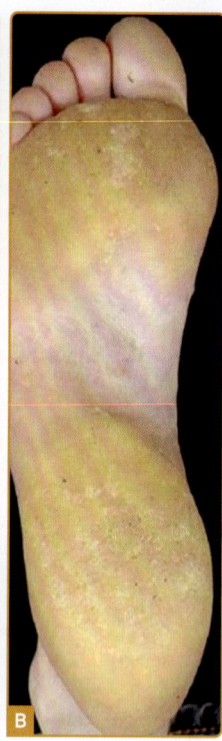

Figure 48-7 Plantar keratodermas of Papillon-Lefèvre and Howel-Evans syndromes. **A,** Diffuse keratoderma in Papillon-Lefèvre syndrome caused by mutation in cathepsin C. **B,** Howell-Evans syndrome showing focal, yellow, thick plaques localized to areas of pressure on the soles. (Part A used with permission from Barts and the London NHS Trust, United Kingdom.)

DIFFUSE INHERITED PALMOPLANTAR KERATODERMA WITH EXTRACUTANEOUS FEATURES, RECESSIVE INHERITANCE

PAPILLON-LEFEVRE SYNDROME

Clinical Features: PLS (OMIM #245000) is a rare, autosomal recessive disorder characterized by palmoplantar hyperkeratosis and severe progressive periodontitis, causing loss of primary and permanent teeth with periosteal changes of the alveolar bone.[417-420] Periodontal disease severity has been shown to peak in the teens and declines with age.[421] The estimated prevalence of PLS is 1 to 4 cases per 1 million people, and the carrier rate is 2 to 4 per 1000. There is no gender predilection, but consanguinity has been observed in approximately half of cases.[422,423] PPK may appear at birth or during the first months of life, although in most cases, both PPK and periodontitis develop between the sixth month and fourth year of life, often beginning with the eruption of the first teeth.[424] Of note, there is no correlation between the severity of the cutaneous and dental manifestations.[425] The PPK is characterized by diffuse, erythematous, sharply demarcated hyperkeratotic and scaly plaques on both palms and soles with transgrediens features extending onto the dorsal aspect of the hands and feet (Fig. 48-7A). It may be associated with hyperhidrosis, foul-smelling odor, and nail abnormalities (transverse grooving and fissuring). Atypical cases with late-onset periodontitis and palmoplantar lesions or cases with isolated PPK or periodontitis have been described.[426-429] Sharply demarcated, psoriasiform, hyperkeratotic plaques can be observed on the knees, elbows, and ankles, and a more widespread distribution resembling psoriasis has also been described.[38,423,425] Increased susceptibility to infections is typical; pyogenic skin infections as well as hepatic or cerebral abscesses and pneumonia have been reported.[423,430] PLS may be associated with intellectual disability and calcification of the dura mater. Isolated cases have been reported in association with growth retardation, infantile voice, and hypothyroidism, although these may not be directly related to the PLS phenotype.[38,420,423,431,432] An association with atopic diathesis and elevated immunoglobulin E (IgE) levels has been reported.[38,421,433,434] Acral lentiginous melanoma may be more common in PLS, at least among Japanese patients.[435]

Etiology and Pathogenesis: PLS results from LOF homozygous or compound heterozygous mutations in the gene *CTSC*, encoding cathepsin C (CTSC), also known as dipeptidyl peptidase I. More than 70 mutations have been reported from ethnically diverse populations; approximately half are homozygous missense mutations altering protein folding and function, 25% are nonsense, and nearly 25% are frameshift mutations.[38,420,436] PLS is allelic to Haim-Munk syndrome (HMS; OMIM #245010), a disorder described mostly in individuals from Cochin, India, characterized by the presence of pes planus, arachnodactyly, acroosteolysis, and onychogryphosis in addition to

PPK and periodontitis. Individuals with HMS do not have evidence of cerebral calcification and bacterial infections. Sulák and coworkers recently reported two Hungarian patients, one with PLS and one with HMS, who carry the same homozygous nonsense mutation in the *CTSC* gene,[437] supporting the notion that PLS and HMS are phenotypic variants of the same disease. PLS is also allelic to prepubertal periodontitis without skin manifestations.[438-440]

CTSC belongs to the papain superfamily of cysteine peptidases and is a tetrameric enzyme consisting of four identical subunits linked together by noncovalent bonds. It plays an important role in intracellular degradation of proteins and coordinates the zymogen activation of serine proteases in cells with immune or inflammatory function including neutrophils, mast cells, cytotoxic T cells, and natural killer cells.[441-446] The protein is expressed as a pro-proteinase in epithelial and myeloid cells, and a multistep process leads to its activation.[418,447] The *CTSC* mutations in patients with PLS are associated with loss of CTSC enzymatic protease activity; carriers of the mutations demonstrate reduced activity compared with control participants.[448] In has been shown that the absence of active CTSC in the urine serves as a strong and reliable indicator for PLS and allows screening for the disease in populations with a high frequency of consanguinity.[417]

Analysis of PLS patient neutrophils show that proteins normally found in the azurophilic granules (elastase, cathepsin G, proteinase 3) are completely absent in mature neutrophils but not in progenitor cells, indicating that *CTSC* mutations promotes protease degradation in mature immune cells. Because significant immunodeficiency is not evident in patients with PLS, neutrophil serine proteases are probably dispensable for human immunoprotection.[449]

Elevated IgE levels have been demonstrated in several cases of PLS, and the delayed resorption of the roots of primary teeth in hyper-IgE syndrome patients led to the suggestion that serum IgE may influence periodontal metabolism. This is supported by improvement in periodontal inflammation in PLS after a decline in IgE levels.[421] Moreover, a T helper (Th) 2 phenotype is evident in PLS with reduced levels of Th1 cells and interferon-γ and increased levels of IL-4.[434]

Pathology: Histopathology analysis in PLS reveal irregular hyperkeratosis, hypergranulosis, marked acanthosis, and perivascular lymphocytic and histiocytic infiltrate in the dermis.[39,428,434] Lipid-like vacuoles in corneocytes and granulocytes in addition to irregular keratohyalin granules and reduction in tonofilaments[39] are evident on electron microscopy.

NAXOS DISEASE

Clinical Features: Naxos disease (ND; OMIM #601214) is an autosomal recessive disease caused by mutations in *JUP* encoding plakoglobin (PG).[450] The disease was originally described in families from the Greek island of Naxos by Protonotarios and coworkers. Since then it has been reported in various ethnicities.[451-455]

The disease is characterized by a triad of diffuse PPK, cardiomyopathy, and woolly hair.[450,456,457] The woolly hair appears at birth and features sparse and brittle, sometimes hypopigmented hair. Hair abnormalities are seen in scalp, eyebrows, and axillary and pubic hair. PPK develops during the first year of life and is characterized by diffuse, well-demarcated, nontransgredient hyperkeratotic plaques over the palms and soles, which may be surrounded by an erythematous border. Other cutaneous features are hyperhidrosis and nail abnormalities. Arrhythmogenic right ventricular dysplasia/cardiomyopathy (ARVD/C) usually becomes symptomatic by adolescence with syncope being its first manifestation in most cases. Ventricular tachycardia and sudden death as a result of arrhythmia, which is a major cause of death in Naxos disease (one third of patients die prematurely with a mean age at death of 32 years), are common complications, and symptoms of right heart failure usually appear in the final stages. Left ventricular involvement may also be seen with further disease progression.[452,455,456,458-461]

Etiology and Pathogenesis: ND is an autosomal recessive disorder caused by biallelic mutations in *JUP* encoding PG. The most common reported mutation to date is a homozygous 2-bp deletion which results in a premature stop codon and expression of a truncated PG lacking 56 residues from the C-terminal domain of the protein.[450,454,456,462] Heterozygous carriers of that mutation usually have no skin or hair abnormalities, although woolly hair may be evident, and minor heart involvement has been documented in approximately 25% of cases.[456] Carriers of other mutations that result in residual PG expression display a milder phenotype of PPK, woolly hair, and skin fragility with no evidence of cardiomyopathy.[463] Interestingly, an autosomal dominant mutation with one amino acid insertion in the PG N-terminal domain has been described in cases of ARVC/C with no evidence of PPK or hair abnormalities.[464] Moreover, biallelic missense mutations in the *JUP* gene have been reported in association with PPK and ARVC/C similar to ND with universal alopecia instead of wooly hair.[465]

PG is a member of the armadillo protein family and a constituent protein in adherens and desmosomal junctions in many tissues, including heart muscle and epidermis. The intracellular tail of desmosomal cadherins (desmogleins and desmocollins) is connected to PG and plakophilins through armadillo repeat domains and amino-terminal head domains, respectively. These two armadillo proteins interact with desmoplakin, a plakin protein that links the desmosomal plaque to the keratin cytoskeleton.[466-471]

A Naxos-like phenotype (ARVC associated with severe left ventricular involvement, PPK, and woolly hair) is also associated with homozygous mutations in the gene *DSC2*, encoding the desmosomal cadherin desmocollin 2.[472] In addition, woolly hair and PPK similar to ND but with no evidence of cardiomyopathy are associated with a homozygous missense mutation in *KANK2*, encoding the steroid receptor coactivator interacting protein that controls activation of steroid receptors.[473]

Pathology: Palmoplantar skin reveals findings compatible with NEPPK.[450,457]

PALMOPLANTAR HYPERKERATOSIS WITH SQUAMOUS CELL CARCINOMA OF SKIN AND SEX REVERSAL SYNDROME

Clinical Features: Palmoplantar hyperkeratosis with SCC of skin and sex reversal (OMIM #610644) is an autosomal recessive disorder described in patients from Southern Italy. It is characterized by sclerodactyly, PPK associated with multiple cutaneous SCCs, early teeth loss caused by chronic periodontal disease, nail hypoplasia with longitudinal ridging, hypogenitalism (ambiguity of external genitalia), gynecomastia, hypospadias with altered plasma sex hormone levels (low testosterone and high follicle-stimulating hormone), and sex reversal (46,XX karyotype in a male phenotype). Associated findings are hypertriglyceridemia, laryngeal cancer, nodular testicular hyperplasia, bilateral cataracts, and bilateral optic nerve coloboma.[411,474,475] A similar presentation has been described in a case of true hermaphroditism with the presence of both ovarian and testicular tissue in a 46,XX woman.[476]

Etiology and Pathogenesis: This disorder results from homozygous mutations in the gene *RSPO1*, encoding R-spondin1. R-spondins are ligands interacting with Fzd–LRP receptor complexes important for β-catenin stabilization.[477] Keratinocytes isolated from the PPK revealed fibroblast-like morphology and larger intercellular spaces with inability to form stratified epidermal layers in organotypic cultures.[478]

Pathology: Palmoplantar skin reveals orthokeratotic hyperkeratosis compatible with NEPPK.[474]

DIFFUSE INHERITED PALMOPLANTAR KERATODERMA WITH EXTRACUTANEOUS FEATURES, MITOCHONDRIAL INHERITANCE

PALMOPLANTAR KERATODERMA WITH DEAFNESS

Clinical Features: The association of PPK and SNHL with a pattern of maternal inheritance caused by a mutation in the extrachromosomal mitochondrial genome (mtDNA) has been identified in several families originating from New Zealand, Japan, France, and Portugal. PPK appears during childhood (5 to 15 years of age) and is characterized by orange-yellow diffuse, well-demarcated, palmoplantar hyperkeratotic plaques with minimal to no erythema. It predominantly involves pressure points and may progress gradually. Although less common, extension onto the dorsal aspects of the hands and feet with a honeycomb-like pattern has been reported, and keratotic plaques over the knees, elbows, and Achilles tendon may be observed. PPK may also be rather focal, resembling calluses, and may involve only plantar skin. Clearing of PPK during pregnancy has been described. Hearing impairment may start in infancy but usually appears by 5 years of age and is bilateral, mild to severe, and may be progressive. Incomplete penetrance is common and is higher for hearing loss (60%) than for skin manifestations (37%). Both sexes are equally affected.

Etiology and Pathogenesis: All affected individuals harbor a common homoplasmic point mutation (c.A7445G) in the mitochondrial transfer RNA (tRNA) encoding the *MTTS1* gene.[479-481] This mutation results in a significant decrease in serine tRNA level with abnormal processing of mitochondrial mRNA and proteins.[482]

Pathology: PPK shows orthokeratotic hyperkeratosis, focal parakeratosis, acanthosis, and focal hypogranulosis.[479-481] Ultrastructural findings are large keratohyaline granules with bundles of tonofilaments not attached to desmosomes and located at the periphery of the nucleus.[479,481]

FOCAL INHERITED PALMOPLANTAR KERATODERMA WITHOUT EXTRACUTANEOUS FEATURES, DOMINANT INHERITANCE

STRIATE PALMOPLANTAR KERATODERMA

Clinical Features: Striate palmoplantar keratoderma (SPPK) is a rare autosomal dominant disorder that may result from mutations in *DSP*, *DSG1*, or *KRT1* encoding desmoplakin, desmoglein 1, or keratin 1, respectively. SPPK is characterized by linear, thickened, hyperkeratotic plaques over the palms that extend along the volar aspect of the digits (Fig. 48-8A) and by circumscribed areas of skin thickening on the soles (Fig. 48-8B). The disease initially presents during the first or second decade of life and is typically exacerbated by manual labor. Nail abnormalities may

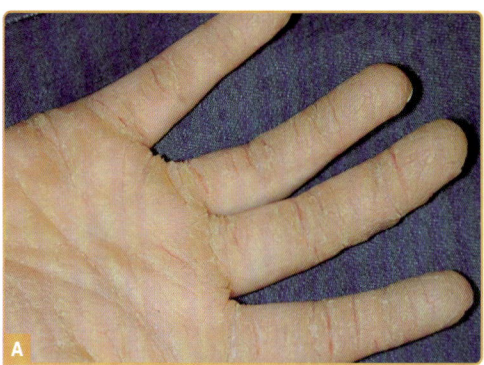 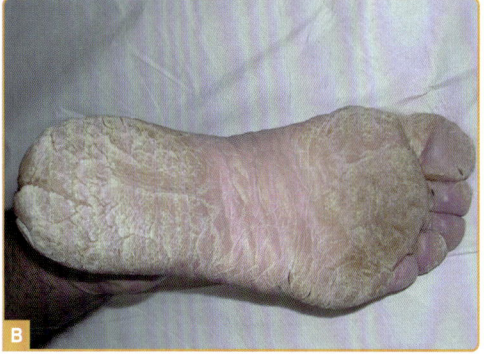

Figure 48-8 Focal palmoplantar keratoderma with *DSG1* mutation. Linear, thickened, hyperkeratotic plaques on the palms which extend along the volar aspect of the digits (**A**) and circumscribed areas of hyperkeratotic plaques on the soles (**B**).

rarely be observed (onycholysis, discoloration) and hyperkeratotic plaques over the knees, ankles, knuckle and toe pads, and dorsal aspect of the digits and toes have been reported.[483-486] There are no other skin, hair, or extracutaneous manifestations.[461,485,487-491]

Mutations in *DSG1* have been found to also result in diffuse and focal hyperkeratosis of the palms and soles with no evidence of striate lesions.[483,486,492]

Etiology and Pathogenesis: SPPK is caused by nonsense and frameshift heterozygous mutations in the *DSG1* or *DSP* genes, demarcating two SPPK subtypes: type I (OMIM #148700) and type II (OMIM #125647), respectively.[489,493,494] The mutations result in haploinsufficiency indicating that decreased expression of these proteins by 50% is sufficient for epidermal function in nonpalmoplantar skin but not at sites subjected to major mechanical trauma such as the palms and soles.[461,493-495]

Of note, SPPK-causing mutations in *DSG1* have recently been shown to be inherited in a semidominant, rather than dominant, fashion. Biallelic mutations in *DSG1* cause skin dermatitis, multiple allergies, and metabolic wasting (SAM) syndrome (OMIM #615508)[496] (Fig. 48-9). Thus, genetic counseling of any patient affected with SPPK should take into consideration these data.

Desmoglein 1 and desmoplakin are important components of the desmosomal plaque. Desmoglein 1, a transmembrane protein that belongs to the family of desmosomal cadherins, is expressed in the upper epidermal layers and plays a critical role in cell–cell adhesion and signal transduction pathways regulating epidermal proliferation and differentiation.[497] Loss of desmoglein 1 results in downregulation of proapoptotic signaling, promotes keratinocytes proliferation, and inhibits epidermal differentiation as a result of unopposed ERK signaling, explaining the hyperkeratotic phenotype seen in SPPK.[498-501] Moreover, it has been suggested that desmoglein 1 deficiency results in SPPK via elevated Ras activity,[502] which is supported by the high rate of PPK in disorders of the Ras–MAPK (mitogen-activated protein kinase) pathway.[501]

Similarly, loss of desmoplakin, a plaque protein that plays a crucial role in anchoring intermediate filaments to desmosomal cadherins, has been shown to result in increased cell proliferation and enhanced G1-to-S-phase entry in the cell cycle associated with elevated phospho-ERK1/2 and phospho-Akt levels.[503]

A heterozygous frameshift mutation affecting the keratin 1 tail domain was found to underlie SPPK type III (OMIM #607654).[79] This mutation leads to the partial loss of the glycine loop motif in the V2 domain and affects the function of the desmosomal plaque during cornification.[78]

Pathology: Histopathology findings in SPPK are orthohyperkeratosis, acanthosis, papillomatosis, widening of the intercellular spaces, and disadhesion of

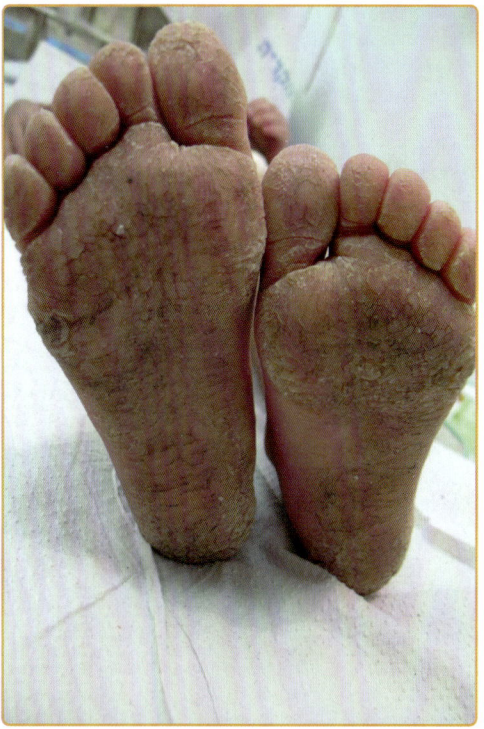

Figure 48-9 Plantar keratoderma in a patient with skin dermatitis, multiple allergies, and metabolic wasting syndrome resulting from biallelic mutations in *DSG1*.

keratinocytes in the upper epidermal layers. Although not entirely specific or sensitive for PPK, the latter two findings serve as a clue for the diagnosis of PPK caused by mutations in genes encoding desmosomal proteins.[484,490,492,504] Immunohistochemical studies demonstrate abnormal perinuclear aggregation of keratin filaments associated with upregulation of KRT16 and abnormal involucrin expression.[493-495] Ultrastructural findings are loosening of intercellular connections and disruption of desmosome–keratin intermediate filament interactions with clumped keratin filaments in a perinuclear distribution. Diminished abnormal-appearing desmosomal structures may be observed.[495]

HEREDITARY KERATOSIS PALMOPLANTARIS VARIANT OF WACHTERS

Clinical Features: Hereditary keratosis palmoplantaris variant of Wachters (PPK varians, Brünauer-Fohs-Siemens syndrome, Siemens syndrome) is a rare autosomal dominant disease with complete penetrance, more common in males, which normally appears in the first or second decade of life. It is characterized by yellowish, nontransgredient, symmetric, nummular, hyperkeratotic plaques localized to pressure points on the soles but that may become more confluent with time. Palmar hyperkeratotic lesions are described as either linear, nummular, membranous, fissured, or periungual. Nummular hyperkeratotic plaques over the elbows, knees, and Achilles tendon were described. Palmoplantar hyperhidrosis, painful transverse fissures, and nail changes (ridging and cuticle hyperkeratosis) may be associated.[505-507] A single case of malignant melanoma arising in the hyperkeratotic lesions on the foot has been described.[508] Varied phenotypic expression with inter- and intrafamilial variability resulted in the description of distinct subtypes and led to the term *keratosis palmoplantaris varians* that was introduced by Wachters in 1963.[509]

Etiology and Pathogenesis: Hereditary keratosis palmoplantaris variant of Wachters is an autosomal dominant disorder, although sporadic cases have been reported. The causative gene is yet to be identified. Immunohistochemical studies show early expression of both filaggrin and involucrin.[505,510]

It is worth mentioning that it is not yet clear whether hereditary keratosis palmoplantaris variant of Wachters and hereditary painful callosities are legitimate distinct entities or are in fact outstanding cases of more common forms of PPK such as PC (KRT16 mutations) or EPPK (KRT1 mutations).

Pathology: Histopathology findings include hyperkeratosis, hypergranulosis, possible focal parakeratosis, and acanthosis with no epidermolytic changes or dermal inflammatory cell infiltrate. Ultrastructural findings are tightly packed tonofibrils and large masses of keratohyaline granules with abnormal configuration.[505,510]

FOCAL INHERITED PALMOPLANTAR KERATODERMA WITH EXTRACUTANEOUS FEATURES, DOMINANT INHERITANCE

PACHYONYCHIA CONGENITA

Clinical Features: PC (OMIM #167200 and 167210) is a group of rare autosomal dominant disorders of keratinization caused by mutations in one of five keratin genes, including *KRT6A, KRT6B, KRT6C, KRT16,* or *KRT17*. PC was first described in the beginning of the 20th century,[511,512] although the causative genes were only identified in the late 1990s.[513-515] PC prevalence in Western countries is 0.9 cases per million with a worldwide PC population estimated to be between 5000 and 10,000.[516-518] The severity of the clinical features varies among and within families as the phenotype may be influenced by modifier genes or environmental factors.[519]

Historically, PC has been divided into two subtypes: PC-1 (Jadassohn-Lewandowski), featuring oral leukokeratosis and caused by mutations in *KRT6A* or *KRT16* and PC-2 (Jackson-Lawler) caused by mutations in *KRT6B* or *KRT17* and featuring cysts and natal teeth. However, phenotypic characterization of more than 1000 mutation-verified PC patients enrolled in the International PC Research Registry showed considerable overlap between these subtypes and lead to a new classification scheme based on the mutant gene. Cases of clinically suspected PC with no identified mutation in the known PC-related genes are termed PC-U (unknown).[518,519]

The three clinical features that are reported in more than 90% of PC patients are thickened toenails, plantar keratoderma, and plantar pain. Thickened toenails, the phenotypic feature that gave its name to the condition, appear during early childhood but may occur also in the first weeks of life (especially with mutations in *KRT6A*). Pachyonychia is characterized by significant subungual hyperkeratosis and very thick nails with a characteristic inverted U or V shape that grow to full length or terminate prematurely (Fig. 48-10A). Paronychia with staphylococcal and candida superinfection may be seen. On average, 9 toenails are involved, and mutations in *KRT6A* carry the highest likelihood of having 10 toenails affected. Nail involvement is variable, even within family members carrying the same mutations. Fingernails, although reported to be involved in many patients (100% of patients with *KRT6A* mutations), may be spared, especially with mutations in *KRT6B*.[518] The most common manifestation of plantar keratoderma is focal PPK (FPPK) with calluses over weight-bearing areas (Fig. 48-10B), although diffuse keratoderma may be observed. Blistering, fissures,

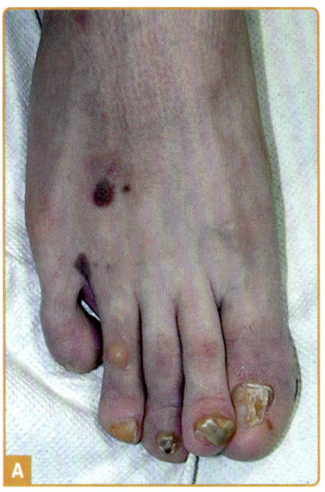 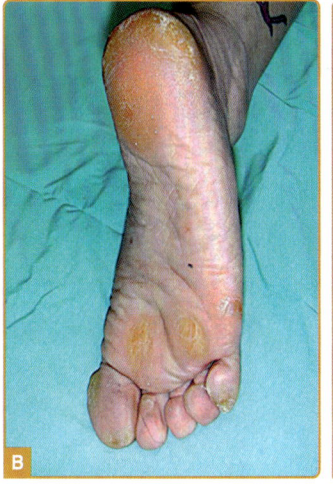 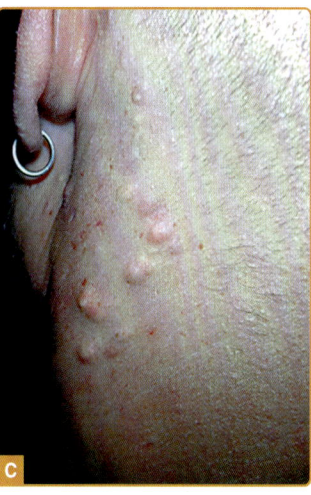

Figure 48-10 Pachyonychia congenita. *KRT6A* mutation with the characteristic nail abnormalities (V-shape thick nails and subungual hyperkeratosis) (**A**) and focal palmoplantar keratoderma with calluses over weight-bearing areas (**B**). Mutations in *KRT17* are typically associated with various types of epidermal inclusion cysts (**C**).

and open sores are common. Palmar lesions are less prominent and usually occur in response to occupational mechanical trauma. The average age of onset of PPK is 4 years, although it may appear at birth or have delayed onset (30 years of age). It is very typical that FPPK starts when children begin to walk. Patients with *KRT16* and *KRT6A* mutations develop keratoderma earlier than patients with *KRT6B* and *KRT17* mutations.[518] Although PC classically causes a nontransgredient FPPK, several cases with transgrediens and involvement of the dorsal feet have been described (mostly with *KRT6A* mutations).[520] Plantar pain occurs in all subtypes, may be more severe in warmer weather, and is considered the most important and debilitating feature that affects patients' quality of life. The severe pain is secondary to blister formation deep underneath the thick callus as demonstrated by high-frequency ultrasound.[521] Approximately 60% of PC patients display neuropathic pain features with the existence of nociceptive pain in the remainder.[517]

Additional features are mucosal involvement, cyst formation, and natal teeth. Oral leukokeratosis was reported in 70% of patients. It tends to appear by 5 years of age, although onset at birth was reported in approximately half of the patients and was most characteristic with mutations in *KRT6A* or *KRT17*. It may be the first manifestation of PC in newborns, is often mistaken for candidiasis, and may alter sucking or feeding, causing failure to thrive. About 40% of patients (mostly with *KRT17* mutations) exhibit various types of epidermal inclusion cysts. Pilosebaceous cysts, such as steatocystomas (Fig. 48-10C), and vellus hair cysts are most common and normally develop during puberty, continue throughout adulthood, and may require surgical removal. The face and trunk are affected. Comedone-like cysts may be found in the axillae, mainly in children.[522] Follicular keratosis on the trunk and extremities, mostly in areas of friction such as the knees and elbows, may be observed in approximately 50% of patients and usually present by early childhood. The phenomenon of natal teeth (erupted teeth present at birth or by 1 month) was reported in 15% of patients with PC, almost exclusively with *KRT17* mutations.[518,519] Primary and secondary dentition is normal.

Less commonly associated features are palmoplantar hyperhidrosis, angular cheilitis, and corneal dystrophy.[523] Alopecia was described in two cases of homozygous, semidominant missense mutations in *KRT17*.[524] Hoarseness with life-threatening respiratory distress secondary to laryngeal leukokeratosis has been seen in infants and children with *KRT6A* mutations. Moreover, infants and children with *KRT6A* mutations may demonstrate severe pain anterior to the ear on first sucking or eating that lasts a few seconds.[525,526]

In PC resulting from mutations in *KRT16*, mild FPPK is a universal finding; however, many mutations in *KRT16* produce a less pronounced phenotype with FPPK restricted to weight-bearing areas of the soles, limited or absent nail involvement, and no evidence of oral leukokeratosis, leading to the diagnosis of focal NEPPK rather than PC.[527-531]

Mutations in *KRT6C* have been reported to be associated with a milder phenotype similar to some of the *KRT16* mutations. These cases are characterized by plantar keratoderma (FPPK over pressure sites or diffuse PPK) and callosities over the palms with absent or minor nail changes, such as hypertrophy of the fifth toenail, and plantar blisters. Leukokeratosis may be seen but with no additional clinical findings.[532,533] Key clinical features of PC with associated mutations are summarized in Table 48-3.

Etiology and Pathogenesis: PC is caused by heterozygous mutations in one of five keratin genes expressed in differentiated epithelial tissues: *KRT6A*, *KRT6B*, *KRT6C*, *KRT16*, and *KRT17*, encoding keratins 6a, 6b, and 6c (type II keratins) and keratins 16 and 17 (type I keratins). The expression of keratins

TABLE 48-3
Pachyonychia Congenita: Key Features

GENE	FREQUENCY (%)	COMMON MUTATION (S)	KEY CLINICAL FEATURES
KRT6A	40	p. Asn172del	Thickened toenails and fingernails since infancy
			Highest likelihood of having 10 toenails affected; Earlier onset of FPPK; transgrediens and involvement of the dorsal feet may occur
			Oral leukokeratosis
			Laryngeal leukokeratosis with hoarseness and life-threatening respiratory distress
KRT16	25–30	p. Arg127Cys (mild)	Mild FPPK with limited or absent nail involvement
		p. Arg127Pro (severe)	Earlier onset FPPK is possible
		p. Leu128Gln (mild)	Coinheritance of *FLG* mutations aggravates the phenotype
		p .Leu128Pro (severe)	
KRT17	20	p. Asn92Ser	Delayed onset of FPPK
			Oral leukokeratosis
			Epidermal inclusion cysts (steatocystomas, vellus hair cysts)
			Natal teeth
			Alopecia[a]
KRT6B	5–9		Fingernails may be spared
			Delayed onset of FPPK
KRT6C	3		Mostly mild FPPK and callosities over the palms with absent or minor nail changes[b]
			Leukokeratosis with no additional clinical features may be seen

[a]In a single case of homozygous semidominant inheritance.
[b]A milder phenotype may be the consequence of more restricted expression of keratin 6c in palmoplantar skin and nails compared with keratins 6a and 6b. *KRT6C* mutation carriers in the general population have been reported.
FPPK, focal palmoplantar keratoderma.

6 and 16 is restricted in normal epidermis to the upper outer hair root sheath and nail bed, palmoplantar skin, and suprabasal orogenital mucosal keratinocytes.[534] In addition, wounding or inflammation induces their expression in interfollicular epidermis, and they are expressed at high levels in cultured keratinocytes from both normal and psoriatic skin.[535]

Autosomal dominant inheritance is observed in more than half of the cases; the remaining cases are caused by spontaneous dominant mutations.[536] There are a few case reports of apparent recessive PC inheritance. However, there are no such cases with confirmed genetic testing, and it is likely that most if not all of these cases represent phenocopies of PC.[537] Semidominant inheritance for *KRT17* mutations has been reported as mentioned earlier.[524] Paternal germ cell mosaicism for a *KRT6A* mutation has also been described.[538] Most mutations are missense mutations, and the remainder are small in-frame deletion, frameshift, nonsense, or splice-site mutations that are likely to exert a dominant-negative effect.[536] The majority of reported mutations to date involve the highly conserved helix boundary domains at either end of the α-helical rod domain, being vital for the elongation phase of filament assembly.[539]

Skin biopsies obtained from PC-involved skin show markedly induced expression of the PC-related genes *KRT6*, *KRT16*, and *KRT17*, which are known to be upregulated in states of stress or injury. Mechanical stress may lead to upregulation of both wild-type and mutant forms of these keratins and perturbed intermediate filament formation caused by mutant keratin incorporation, triggering the PC phenotype. This in turn has been linked to aberrant expression of additional mutant keratin as part of the wound healing response, resulting in a vicious cycle of gradual worsening.[540-542] Moreover, overexpression of genes related to cell adhesion (*DSC2*, *CDSN*, and *GJB2*), cornified cell envelope formation (involucrin and loricrin) and desquamation (kallikrein [KLK]-5; *SPINK6*, and *SERPINs*) and non–PC-related keratins (*KRT75* and *KRT85*) has been observed. Pain-associated genes are also upregulated in PC-involved skin, including *KLK10* (catalyzes the production of bradykinin) and *SPRR1A* (a structural protein in keratinocytes being expressed also by neurons), which may relate to the severe pain featured by PC patients.[542]

Pathology: Skin biopsies obtained from PPK lesions reveal features of NEPPK. Reduced granular layer and cytolysis in the outer root sheath of HFs may be seen.[513,530] Epidermolytic hyperkeratosis has been observed in a case associated with mutation in *KRT16* with striate palmar hyperkeratosis and diffuse PPK of the soles.[101] Ultrastructurally, suprabasal keratinocytes in PC are characterized by densely aggregated keratin filament bundles, predominantly in the perinuclear region and sparing the cell periphery. Reduced desmosome number with widened intercellular spaces and reduced keratohyaline granules are additional findings.[513]

Specific Treatments: Contradictory data regarding the efficacy of retinoids in PC have been published with an improvement in both PPK and nail dystrophy in some reports and no improvement in others. In addition, the treatment had to be withheld in many patients with observed improvement because of increased pain as a result of epidermal thinning and predisposition to infections.[543-546]

In PC, the most effective approach to nail dystrophy consists of mechanical treatments (filing, grinding, cutting, or clipping) and soaking the nails. Surgical avulsion is sometimes ineffective because of regrowth of nails. Oral leukokeratosis may be improved by keeping good oral hygiene, gentle brushing, and oral antibiotics. Follicular hyperkeratosis is treated with oral and topical retinoids, keratolytic agents, and emollients. Steatocystoma multiplex and other pilosebaceous cysts can be treated by incision and drainage, excision, intralesional steroid injection, and oral antibiotics in the case of secondary infections.[544,547-550] Recently, targeted and more specific therapies have been studied in PC. Rapamycin has been shown to result in marked improvement in painful plantar calluses and in quality of life by selectively blocking translation of mRNAs, including *KRT6* mRNA. However, the use of oral rapamycin was limited by side effects, including gastrointestinal symptoms. A clinical trial with topical rapamycin is underway.[526,551] Moreover, a specific siRNA that selectively silences the expression of a specific pathogenic mutation in *KRT6A* has been shown to lead to callus regression and pain control in a phase Ib clinical trial.[552] New approaches for more efficient, safe, and practical ways to deliver siRNA into the epidermis are needed to avoid the painful injections.[548,552-557]

HOWEL-EVANS SYNDROME

Clinical Features: Howel-Evans syndrome (tylosis with esophageal cancer; OMIM #148500) is a rare autosomal dominant disorder with complete penetrance characterized by the association of PPK and mucosal SCCs, particularly of the esophagus. It was first reported by Howel-Evans and coworkers in 1958[558] and has been described in families from a range of countries.[559-565] The estimated prevalence of the disorder in the general population is less than 1 in 1,000,000.[566] The onset of PPK is usually during childhood or adolescence (between 5 and 15 years, although most cases are evident by 7 to 8 years of age). It is characterized by focal, yellowish, thick plaques localized to areas of pressure or friction on the palms and soles (see Fig. 48-7B) that may be associated with painful fissures and secondary infections. Sparing of the palms may be evident.[567] Additional findings are follicular hyperkeratosis, cutaneous horns, and oral leukokeratosis. Cases of SCC of the oropharynx have been recorded.[559-566,568,569]

Esophageal lesions present as few-millimeter, white, polypoid lesions throughout the esophagus. About 95% of patients with Howel-Evans syndrome develop carcinoma by 65 years of age, similar to the onset of sporadic cases.[566]

In patients with Howel-Evans syndrome, screening includes annual gastroscopy. Besides surveillance, diet, and lifestyle modification to reduce risk factors for esophageal carcinoma are recommended.[566]

Etiology and Pathogenesis: Howel-Evans syndrome results from GOF missense mutations in *RHBDF2*, which encodes a catalytically inactive rhomboid intramembrane serine, iRhom2. iRhom2 belongs to a family of seven transmembrane-spanning proteins, which are serine intramembrane proteases associated with EGFR signaling and mitochondrial remodeling.[570,571] RHBDF2 is an iRhom that lost its protease activity during evolution but retained key nonprotease functions (regulation of EGF and TNF-α signaling pathways).[572,753]

Skin biopsies obtained from patients with Howel-Evans syndrome demonstrate cytoplasmic localization of iRhom2 compared with the normal membrane expression seen in normal skin. Similar cytoplasmic localization is observed in biopsies obtained from Howel-Evans syndrome esophageal carcinoma and from sporadic squamous esophageal tumors, suggesting that dysregulation of iRhom2 plays a role in these malignancies.[574,575]

iRhom2 has been shown to regulate the trafficking and activation of ADAM17, a membrane bound sheddase that has been shown to play a pivotal role in the proteolytic cleavage and release of substrates from the cell surface, including TNF-α, members of the EGF family of growth factors, and desmosomes.[573,576] Epidermal keratinocytes from patients with Howel-Evans syndrome show upregulated ADAM17 activity, resulting in increased EGFR activity, increased desmosome processing, immature epidermal desmosomes, upregulated epidermal transglutaminase activity, and resistance to staphylococcal infection.[577] Moreover, these keratinocytes demonstrate features of dysregulated wound repair in vitro.[577,578]

Overexpression of EGFR has been demonstrated in sporadic esophageal SCC and several other carcinomas and correlates with reduced survival. Moreover, expression of ADAM17 has been shown to correlate with progression of esophageal carcinoma.[579-5815] Accordingly, precancerous esophageal lesions seen in Howel-Evans syndrome may be a result of dysregulated EGFR signaling.[574]

Pathology: Affected skin reveals acanthosis, orthohyperkeratosis, and hypergranulosis with no parakeratosis or spongiosis.[566,567]

FOCAL INHERITED PALMOPLANTAR KERATODERMA WITH EXTRACUTANEOUS FEATURES, RECESSIVE INHERITANCE

RICHNER-HANHART SYNDROME

Clinical Features: Richner-Hanhart Syndrome (RHS, tyrosinemia type II, oculocutaneous tyrosinosis, keratosis palmoplantaris with corneal dystrophy;

OMIM #276600) is a rare autosomal recessive disorder named after the original reports of Richner and Hanhart. Its incidence is less than 1 in 250,000, occurring in various ethnic groups, although it seems to be particularly prevalent in Mediterranean countries and in the Arab world.[582-587]

Symptoms typically appear in early childhood and include a triad of painful PPK, bilateral keratitis, and mental retardation that results from intracellular accumulation of tyrosine crystals and a secondary inflammatory response in the involved tissues.

Ocular manifestations include photophobia, pain, tearing, redness, and pseudoherpetiform keratitis with corneal ulcerations. Ocular manifestations occur in 75% of cases, present soon after birth or within the first year of life, and usually antedate the cutaneous manifestations. Skin manifestations usually begin after the first year of life and consist of well-demarcated, focal, palmoplantar, white-yellow, hyperkeratotic plaques surrounded by erythema on the weight-bearing areas of the soles. There is associated pain and often hyperhidrosis. The fingertips, hypothenar, and thenar eminences can also be affected. Sixty percent of cases, particularly untreated ones, present with neurologic manifestations, including mental retardation, nystagmus, tremor, ataxia, and convulsions.[588-591] A case with epileptic seizures, mild mental retardation, and photophobia with no other ophthalmologic or skin manifestations has been reported.[592]

Etiology and Pathogenesis: RHS is an autosomal recessive disorder caused by mutations in the *TAT* gene encoding tyrosine aminotransferase (TAT). As a consequence of TAT deficiency, tyrosine accumulates in tissues. More than 20 mutations have been identified within the *TAT* gene with alteration of the activity and stability of the tyrosine aminotransferase enzyme.[572,587,593-600] It was hypothesized that disease severity, particularly neurologic disabilities, correlates with the presence of a mutant protein but its total absence is associated with more favorable features.[601,602]

Previous reports have suggested that palmoplantar lesions in RHS result from intracellular L-tyrosine crystals that destabilize lysosomal membranes and initiate a cascade of cell injury and inflammation, resulting in the typical skin lesions. This hypothesis is consistent with the presence of crystals in tyrosine-induced lesions in the corneal epithelium of rats and in the spinous layer keratinocytes of patient epidermis.[603-606] However, later studies failed to demonstrate crystals in epidermal keratinocytes and suggested that the palmoplantar hyperkeratosis results from an excessive intracellular concentration of tyrosine that leads to noncovalent cross-links among keratins and the formation of aggregated tonofilaments.[607]

Laboratory Findings: RHS is diagnosed by a high level of serum tyrosine (with normal phenylalanine) and accumulation of tyrosine metabolites in the urine (p-hydroxyphenylpyruvate, p-phenylacetate, p-hydroxyphenylacetate).[601] A static level of urinary succinylacetone distinguishes RHS from type 1 tyrosinemia.

Pathology: Histopathologic findings in RHS include marked acanthosis, hyperkeratosis, and significant hypergranulosis. Parakeratosis, a parakeratotic column in the acrosyringium, and multinucleated keratinocytes in the spinous cell layer are possible findings. Increased mitotic activity in the suprabasal layers and thin, elongated epidermal ridges, may be seen.[586,601,608,609] Intracytoplasmic tyrosine crystals have been reported.[606] Ultrastructural findings include thickening of the granular layer and increased synthesis of tonofibrils and keratohyalin, large numbers of microtubules, and tonofibrillar masses with tubular channels or inclusions of microtubules. Multinucleated keratinocytes in the spinous layer and lipid droplets in the cornified layer may be observed.[586,607,609]

Specific Treatments: The key to the management of RHS is early diagnosis and early initiation of a diet that restricts tyrosine and phenylalanine to reduce the risk and severity of long-term complications of hypertyrosinemia, especially in the eye and skin.[601,609,610] Tandem mass spectrometry newborn screening for inborn errors of metabolism identifies RHS in the asymptomatic neonatal period.[611] Retinoids improve skin and eye lesions, but they do not prevent mental retardation and should be considered discriminately in children.[612] A case in which thigh skin was grafted onto a plantar lesion demonstrated hyperkeratosis that spared the graft area with the formation of a keratotic wall around it.[613]

CARVAJAL SYNDROME

Clinical Features: Carvajal syndrome (CS; OMIM #605676), first reported by Carvajal-Huerta in 1998, is an autosomal recessive disease caused by mutations in the *DSP* gene (encoding desmoplakin) and characterized by a triad of woolly hair, SPPK, and cardiomyopathy. Left ventricular dilated cardiomyopathy develops during childhood; the right ventricle may also be involved.[614-616] Patients may demonstrate only skin or cardiac features or the full phenotype. Woolly hair appears at birth and may be associated with sparse eyebrows and axillary and pubic hair. SPPK develops during childhood, although cases with appearance at birth have been reported. A case featuring alopecia of the scalp, eyebrows, and eyelashes has been described.[617] Additional cutaneous features are linear lichenoid keratotic papules in the flexural folds, follicular hyperkeratosis on the elbows and knees or scattered across the abdomen and lower limbs, nail abnormalities (dystrophy, onychogryphosis, clubbing), transient pruritic vesicles, and psoriasiform plaques.[614-618] CS cases with dominant inheritance are associated with hypo- or oligodontia and leukonychia or brittle nails.[618,619] Co-occurrence with congenital unilateral deafness, recurrent pharyngitis, and diarrhea was reported.[620] The left ventricle is severely affected by the second decade of life in more than 90% of patients, although cardiomyopathy with symptoms of progressive heart failure presenting as early as the first years of life has been reported. Congestive heart failure and ventricular arrhythmia are the most common causes of death during adolescence.[617,621]

Etiology and Pathogenesis: Desmoplakin is a central component of the desmosomes, which are cell-to-cell junctions in simple and stratified squamous epithelia and cardiac muscle that connect intermediate filaments to the desmosomal cadherins in the cytoplasmic membrane. The N-terminal plakin domain of DSP binds PG, plakophilins, and desmosomal cadherins, its C-terminal domain connects the cytoskeleton intermediate filaments, and its central coiled-coil rod domain is responsible for homodimerization.[622] DSP is expressed in all epidermal layers, in the outer root sheath, companion layer, and Henle and Huxley layers of the HF; intercalated discs are important for cardiomyocyte binding in the heart.[623-625]

The first homozygous mutation in *DSP* causing CS was described in an Ecuadorian pedigree and resulted in a truncated protein lacking the C-domain tail region responsible for intermediate filament binding.[614] Another recessive missense mutation that was associated with blisters in early childhood and ARVC during adolescence was described in Arab kindred and affected the C-terminal domain of the protein.[616] Several other homozygous mutations resulting in truncated protein involving the coiled-coil rod domain and the C-terminal domain with impaired intermediate filament binding have been described.[626]

Dominant heterozygous mutations in *DSP* have been reported in cases of tooth agenesis in addition to the common triad of CS (dilated cardiomyopathy with wooly hair, keratoderma, and tooth agenesis; DCWHKTA; OMIM #615821).[618,619,627,628] In these cases, the mutations affect the N-terminal domain of DSP and most involve exon 14, suggesting that this region serves as a hot spot and disrupts desmosome scaffolds in a dominant-negative fashion. The clinical feature of tooth agenesis is in line with studies in mice demonstrating a role of desmosomal proteins in teeth development.[629,630]

Besides DCWHKTA, heterozygous *DSP* mutations are linked to ARVD type 8 (OMIM #607450) and isolated SPPK (see earlier). Homozygous or compound heterozygous *DSP* mutations also result in lethal acantholytic epidermolysis bullosa (OMIM #609638) and skin fragility–wooly hair syndrome (OMIM #607655).[628,631,632]

Pathology: The histopathology findings in CS are hyperkeratosis, papillomatosis, spongiosis, epidermolytic hyperkeratosis, and dyskeratosis. Acantholysis may be seen in the spinous layer.[614]

PUNCTATE INHERITED PALMOPLANTAR KERATODERMA WITHOUT EXTRACUTANEOUS FEATURES, DOMINANT INHERITANCE

PUNCTATE PALMOPLANTAR KERATODERMA TYPE I

Clinical Features: Punctate palmoplantar keratoderma (PPKP) type I (PPKP1; keratosis punctate palmoplantaris type Buschke-Fischer-Brauer; OMIM #148600 [PPKP1A] and 614936 [PPKP1B]) is a rare autosomal dominant disease. The estimated incidence of PPKP1 is approximately 1 to 3 per 100,000 individuals in various populations across Europe, the Middle East, and Asia.[36,588,633-636]

The disease has its onset during the first or second decades of life, although a later onset has also been described.[589,591,633,637-640] It is characterized by multiple hyperkeratotic, centrally indented, yellow to brown papules distributed irregularly over the palmoplantar skin (Fig. 48-11). Lesions may be painful. They increase in size and number with advancing age and coalescence into more confluent plaques, particularly on pressure-bearing areas of plantar skin. A phenotype resembling human papilloma virus–induced papilloma-like lesions has been described.[641,642] Dermoscopic findings of palmoplantar lesions are well-demarcated, structureless, yellow-orange areas

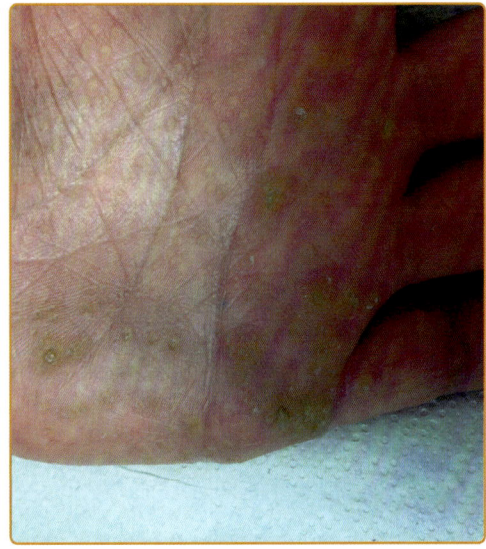

Figure 48-11 Punctate palmoplantar keratoderma type I caused by mutation in *AAGAB*. Multiple hyperkeratotic, centrally indented, yellow to brown papules irregularly distributed over the palmar skin.

surrounded by a whitish halo with no evidence of dotted vessels commonly seen in verruca vulgaris.[37] Lesions reveal white fluorescence with Wood light examination.[643]

Etiology and Pathogenesis: PPKP1 is an autosomal dominant disease that results from heterozygous mutations in two genes, *AAGAB* (PPKP1A) and *COL14A1* (PPKP1B).

AAGAB encodes the α- and γ-adaptin-binding protein p34,[599,634,635,641] which contains an adaptin-binding domain and a Rab-like GTPase domain that might play an important role in clathrin-coated vesicle trafficking as a chaperone and in skin integrity.[635,641,644,645] Inter- and intrafamilial phenotypic variability is common and may be related to the effect of modifier genes or of aging and environmental factors.[36,591] Genetic anticipation (earlier disease onset in later generations) has been reported.[633,639] To date, more than 30 null variants in *AAGAB* have been identified, and haploinsufficiency was suggested as a possible disease-causing mechanism.[635]

A missense mutation in *COL14A1*, encoding collagen type XIV α1 chain, was identified in a large Chinese family with PPKP1 and incomplete penetrance.[646] The protein is mainly expressed in well-differentiated tissues and in late embryonic development, and the reported mutation involves the collagen triple helix repeat region.

Pathology: Histopathologic findings in PPPK include marked hyperkeratosis and acanthosis with epidermal invagination associated with focal parakeratosis, hyper- or hypogranulosis, and overlying orthokeratosis.[634,635,641] Transmission electron microscopy of lesional plantar skin shows an abnormal abundance of small vesicles close to the cell membrane in the basal epidermal layer and prominent dilatation of the Golgi apparatus, consistent with a defect in vesicle transport.[641]

PUNCTATE PALMOPLANTAR KERATODERMA TYPE 2

Clinical Features: PPKP type II (PPKP2; porokeratotic type; OMIM #175860) is an autosomal dominant disease characterized by multiple, firmly attached, tiny, skin-colored to yellow, asymptomatic, keratotic spines arising on the palms and soles around puberty or in the early 20s. Lesions may increase in number over the years with possible extension onto the dorsal and lateral surfaces of the fingers.[646-649] Lesions reveal white fluorescence resembling "stars under the moonlight" with Wood light examination.[650]

Facial sebaceous hypoplasia was reported in male patients.[649] Acquired cases with a similar phenotype have been described in association with internal malignancies.[651]

Etiology and Pathogenesis: The molecular etiology of PPKP2 is unknown. Most described cases are acquired; however, there are also familial cases with autosomal dominant inheritance. The pathogenesis involves enhanced epidermal proliferation of the basal layer under the columnar parakeratoses.[652]

Pathology: Histopathology findings in PPKP2 are compact vertical parakeratotic columns in the stratum corneum overlying hypogranular epidermis resembling cornoid lamellae.[648] Ultrastructural findings are numerous, variable-sized, pyknotic nuclei in the stratum corneum and reduced number of keratohyaline granules in the granular layer.[652]

PUNCTATE PALMOPLANTAR KERATODERMA TYPE 3

Clinical Features: PPKP type III (PPKP3, AKE [of Costa]; OMIM #101850) is a rare autosomal dominant disorder that usually appears during childhood or adolescence, although onset in infancy or adulthood has also been reported. There is no racial or ethnic predilection.[653] AKE is characterized by asymptomatic, round to oval, whitish to yellow and translucent papules, and more rarely nodules and plaques, with a hyperkeratotic surface or umbilication. Changes are located on the palms and soles with predilection for the thenar and hypothenar areas of the hands and pressure sites on the palms and soles. A linear pattern or "paving stones" arrangement over the radial and ulnar margins of the hands may be seen (Fig. 48-12).[654,655] In severe cases, lesions may affect the dorsal aspects of hands and feet (including knuckle pads), wrists, and ankles.[653,656] Aquagenic PPK can be associated,[657] and unilateral involvement has been described.[658,659] Nail dystrophy and hyperhidrosis may be observed.[657,660] Although AKE is usually confined to the skin, a case with reduced elasticity in medium and large arteries and an association with systemic and nodular scleroderma has been reported.[664-663]

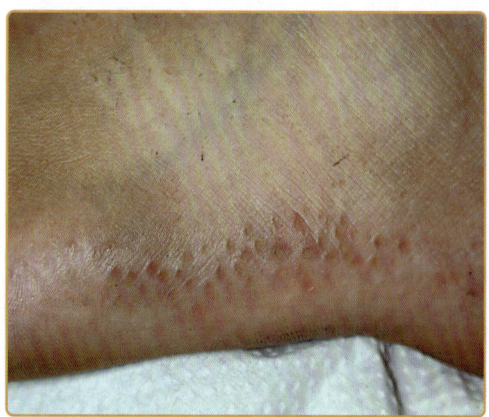

Figure 48-12 Punctate palmoplantar keratoderma type III (acrokeratoelastoidosis). Round to oval yellow papules with central umbilication and a linear pattern of arrangement over the lateral margin of the sole.

TABLE 48-4
Summary for Palmoplantar Keratodermas

	EXTRACUTANEOUS FEATURES	INHERITANCE	FEATURES	GENE	PROTEIN
Diffuse PPK					
Epidermolytic PPK	−	AD	Most common form of diffuse keratoderma, with erythematous sharp margins at the edge of the palms and soles, with thickening and fissuring	*KRT9, KRT1*	Keratin 9, keratin 1
Unna-Thost PPK	−	AD	Diffuse, well-demarcated, yellowish, thick hyperkeratosis with an erythematous rim overlying the palms and soles; smooth and waxy texture	*KRT1*	Keratin 1
Greither syndrome	−	AD	Diffuse, thickened, scaly yellowish PPK, with transgrediens	*KRT1*	Keratin 1
Loricrin keratoderma	−	AD	Honeycomb-like PPK, starfish-like hyperkeratosis, prominent knuckle pads and pseudoainhum	*LOR*	Loricrin
PPK Bothnia type	−	AD	Diffuse, homogenous hyperkeratosis with a yellowish hue; aquagenic wrinkling of palms	*AQP5*	Aquaporin 5
Mal de Meleda	−	AR	Progressive, mutilating PPK with transgrediens; yellowish waxy hyperkeratotic plaques with a red, scaly border over palms and soles; risk for malignancies	*SLURP1*	SLURP1
Nagashima-type PPK	−	AR	Most common type in Asians; transgrediens, nonprogressive, nonmutilating; well-demarcated, erythematous palmoplantar hyperkeratosis	*SERPINB7*	SERPIN7
Olmsted syndrome	+	AD	Mutilating PPK with periorificial keratotic plaques; symmetric, sharply demarcated diffuse PPK with painful fissures and erythematous borders; hair abnormalities are common	*TRPV3* *MBTPS2* (X-linked cases)	TRPV3
Vohwinkel syndrome	+	AD	PPK with hearing impairment; mutilating honeycomb-like PPK, with starfish shaped keratotic plaques, pseudoainhum	*GJB2*	Connexin 26
Keratitis–ichthyosis–deafness syndrome	+	AD	Erythrokeratoderma, grainy PPK with a rough, stippled appearance, chronic cheilitis and perleche, abnormal ectodermal features, progressive keratitis	*GJB2*	Connexin 26
Bart-Pumphrey syndrome	+	AD	Honeycomb-like, diffuse, sharply demarcated PPK, knuckle pads, leukonychia	*GJB2*	Connexin 26
Palmoplantar Keratoderma with deafness	+	AD	Diffuse, transgrediens PPK with underlying erythema, knuckle pads, hearing impairment	*GJB2*	Connexin 26
PPK–congenital alopecia syndrome	+	AD	Well-defined, focal, nonmutilating transgrediens PPK; noncicatricial alopecia; recessive forms may have pseudoainhum and sclerodactyly	*GJB6*	Connexin 30
Hidrotic ectodermal dysplasia (Clouston) syndrome	+	AD	Diffuse, velvety or cobblestone-like PPK with fissures; nail dystrophy and hair loss	*GJB6*	Connexin 30
Huriez syndrome	+	AD	Diffuse, yellowish-grey, nonerythematous PPK, scleroatrophy, sclerodactyly, SCCs	Chromosome 4q23	
Papillon-Lefevre syndrome	+	AR	Diffuse, erythematous, sharply demarcated hyperkeratotic PPK with transgrediens; severe progressive periodontitis and loss of primary and permanent teeth	*CTSC*	Cathepsin C
Naxos disease	+	AR	Diffuse, well-demarcated, nontransgrediens PPK; wooly hair; right ventriculopathy	*JUP*	Plakoglobin

(Continued)

TABLE 48-4
Summary for Palmoplantar Keratodermas (Continued)

	EXTRACUTANEOUS FEATURES	INHERITANCE	FEATURES	GENE	PROTEIN
Palmoplantar hyperkeratosis with SCC of skin and sex reversal syndrome	+	AR	PPK with multiple SCCs and sclerodactyly; chronic periodontal disease leading to loss of teeth; hypogenitalism, altered plasma sex hormone levels, and sex reversal	RSPO1	R-spondin1
PPK with deafness	+	Mitochondrial	Orange-yellow, diffuse, well-demarcated PPK with minimal to no erythema over pressure points; hearing impairment	MTTS1	Decreased serine tRNA levels
Focal PPK					
Striate PPK	−	AD	Linear, thickened hyperkeratotic plaques over palms and volar aspects of digits; circumscribed thickening of soles	DSG1, KRT1	Desmoglein 1, desmoplakin, keratin 1
Hereditary keratosis palmoplantaris variant of Wachters	−	AD	Yellowish, nontransgrediens, symmetric, nummular hyperkeratotic plaques on pressure points of the soles; painful transverse fissures may be present	Unknown	
Pachyonychia congenita	+	AD	Thickened toenails, plantar keratoderma and plantar pain; oral mucosa may be involved, with cyst formation and natal teeth	KRT6A, KRT6B, KRT6C, KRT16, KRT17	Keratin 6a, keratin 6b, keratin 6c, keratin 16, keratin 17
Howel-Evans syndrome	+	AD	Focal yellowish thick plaques over pressure points on the palms and soles, with painful fissures, esophageal SCCs, follicular hyperkeratosis, oral leukokeratosis	RHBDF2	iRohm2
Richner-Hanhart syndrome	+	AR	Well-demarcated, focal, white-yellow painful PPK on pressure points, bilateral keratitis, mental retardation	TAT	Tyrosine aminotransferase
Carvajal syndrome	+	AR	Striate keratoderma; woolly hair, left ventriculopathy; lichenoid keratotic papules in flexural areas, nail abnormalities, unilateral deafness	DSP	desmoplakin
Punctate PPK					
Punctate PPPK type I	−	AD	Painful, hyperkeratotic papules with central indentation irregularly distributed on palms and soles	AAGAB COL14A1	P34 protein Collagen type XIV alpha 1
Punctate PPPK type 2	−	AD	Asymptomatic, firmly attached, yellow keratotic spines on palms and soles	unknown	
Punctate PPPK type 3 (acrokeratoelastoidosis of Costa)	−	AD	Asymptomatic, round-oval, white-yellow translucent hyperkeratotic or umbilicated papules	Chromosome 2p25-p12	
Cole disease	+	AD	Punctate PPK, irregularly shaped, hypopigmented macules over proximal trunk, with internal organ calcification	ENPP1	Endonucleotide pyrophosphatase/phosphodiesterase 1

AD, autosomal dominant; AR, autosomal recessive; PPK, palmoplantar keratoderma; PPPK, punctate palmoplantar keratoderma; SCC, squamous cell carcinoma.

Focal acral hyperkeratosis (FAH) is an autosomal dominant inherited disease with phenotypic resemblance to AKE, including nail abnormalities.[664] However, no elastic tissue abnormalities are observed in these cases. FAH is often considered to be a variant of AKE, although this notion is not accepted by some authors.[654,665-668]

Etiology and Pathogenesis: PPKP3 is an autosomal dominant inherited disorder, although sporadic cases have been described.[669,670] The genetic basis of the disease has yet to be elucidated, although preliminary linkage studies suggest a possible locus on 2p25-p12.[671,672]

Ultrastructural studies support AKE involves a defect in secretion of elastic material and a failure of elastic fiber synthesis rather than degeneration of elastic fibers.[673] In addition, the formation of the keratotic papules are a result of filaggrin overproduction that accumulates over the granular layer before its incorporation into the CCE.[674]

Pathology: AKE lesions show orthokeratotic hyperkeratosis, acanthosis, and hypergranulosis. Both lesional and normal-appearing skin reveal decreased elastic tissue and fragmented, thickened, or thinned elastic fibers (elastorrhexis) in the reticular dermis with sparing of the papillary dermis.[657] Ultrastructural findings are fibroblasts with dense granules at the cytoplasm periphery with reduced extracellular content of elastic fibers.[673]

PUNCTATE INHERITED PALMOPLANTAR KERATODERMA WITH EXTRACUTANEOUS FEATURES, DOMINANT INHERITANCE

COLE DISEASE

Clinical Features: Cole disease (OMIM #615522) is a rare autosomal dominant disorder that presents at birth or during early infancy and is characterized by punctate PPK and irregularly shaped, hypopigmented macules distributed over the proximal extremities or less typically over the trunk.[674-678] Calcifications in several organs (tendons, breast, and spleen) have been described.[678,680]

Etiology and Pathogenesis: Cole disease results from heterozygous mutations in the gene ENPP1, encoding ectonucleotide pyrophosphatase/phosphodiesterase 1, a cell surface protein that generates extracellular inorganic pyrophosphate by catalyzing the hydrolysis of adenosine triphosphate to adenosine monophosphate.[681] ENPP1 is composed of eight domains including phosphodiesterase, nuclease, and somatomedin B–like (SMB) domains.[682] Biallelic mutations affecting the phosphodiesterase domain that mediates ENPP1 catalytic activity or the nuclease domain have been shown to be associated with inherited disorders featuring abnormal calcium homeostasis or ectopic calcifications,[683-685] and mutations associated with Cole disease affect highly conserved cysteine residues clustered within the SMB domains.[678,680] Given the notion that ENPP1 has been shown to inhibit insulin signaling through the interaction between its SMB domain and insulin receptor,[684-687] it is suggested that abnormal insulin signaling plays a role in the pathogenesis of Cole disease.[688-691]

Pathology: Skin biopsies obtained from palmoplantar lesions show hyperkeratosis, orthokeratosis, hypergranulosis, and acanthosis. Calcified deposits in the dermis may be seen.[676] Hypopigmented macules demonstrate hyperkeratosis, reduced melanin content in keratinocytes, and normal or reduced number of melanocytes.[678,680,692] Ultrastructural findings of hypopigmented lesions consist of disproportionately large numbers of melanosomes within the cytoplasm and dendrites of melanocytes with paucity of melanosomes in adjacent keratinocytes, suggesting abnormal melanosome transfer as the primary pathomechanism for hypopigmentation in Cole disease.[678,680]

SUMMARY

See Table 48-4.

REFERENCES

1. Braun-Falco M. Hereditary palmoplantar keratodermas. *J Dtsch Dermatol Ges.* 2009;7(11):971-984; quiz 984-975.
2. Itin PH. Classification of autosomal dominant palmoplantar keratoderma: past-present-future. *Dermatology.* 1992;185(3):163-165.
3. Itin PH, Fistarol SK. Palmoplantar keratodermas. *Clin Dermatol.* 2005;23(1):15-22.
4. Ratnavel RC, Griffiths WA. The inherited palmoplantar keratodermas. *Br J Dermatol.* 1997;137(4):485-490.
5. Kimyai-Asadi A, Kotcher LB, Jih MH. The molecular basis of hereditary palmoplantar keratodermas. *J Am Acad Dermatol.* 2002;47(3):327-343; quiz 344-326.
6. McLean WH, Epithelial Genetics G. Genetic disorders of palm skin and nail. *J Anat.* 2003;202(1):133-141.
7. Paller AS. The molecular bases for the palmoplantar keratodermas. *Pediatr Dermatol.* 1999;16(6):483-486.
8. Has C, Technau-Hafsi K. Palmoplantar keratodermas: clinical and genetic aspects. *J Dtsch Dermatol Ges.* 2016;14(2):123-140.
9. Sakiyama T, Kubo A. Hereditary palmoplantar keratoderma "clinical and genetic differential diagnosis." *J Dermatol.* 2016;43(3):264-274.
10. Schiller S, Seebode C, Hennies HC, et al. Palmoplantar keratoderma (PPK): acquired and genetic causes of a not so rare disease. *J Dtsch Dermatol Ges.* 2014;12(9):781-788.

11. Lind L, Lundstrom A, Hofer PA, et al. The gene for diffuse palmoplantar keratoderma of the type found in northern Sweden is localized to chromosome 12q11-q13. *Hum Mol Genet.* 1994;3(10): 1789-1793.
12. Covello SP, Irvine AD, McKenna KE, et al. Mutations in keratin K9 in kindreds with epidermolytic palmoplantar keratoderma and epidemiology in Northern Ireland. *J Invest Dermatol.* 1998;111(6):1207-1209.
13. Gulati S, Thappa DM, Garg BR. Hereditary palmoplantar keratodermas in South India. *J Dermatol.* 1997;24(12):765-768.
14. Hamm H, Happle R, Butterfass T, et al. Epidermolytic palmoplantar keratoderma of Vorner: is it the most frequent type of hereditary palmoplantar keratoderma? *Dermatologica.* 1988;177(3):138-145.
15. Lopez-Valdez J, Rivera-Vega MR, Gonzalez-Huerta LM, et al. Analysis of the KRT9 gene in a Mexican family with epidermolytic palmoplantar keratoderma. *Pediatr Dermatol.* 2013;30(3):354-358.
16. Patel S, Zirwas M, English JC 3rd. Acquired palmoplantar keratoderma. *Am J Clin Dermatol.* 2007;8(1):1-11.
17. Lucker GP, Van de Kerkhof PC, Steijlen PM. The hereditary palmoplantar keratoses: an updated review and classification. *Br J Dermatol.* 1994;131(1):1-14.
18. Peris K, Salvati EF, Torlone G, et al. Keratoderma hereditarium mutilans (Vohwinkel's syndrome) associated with congenital deaf-mutism. *Br J Dermatol.* 1995;132(4):617-620.
19. Schamroth JM. Mutilating keratoderma. *Int J Dermatol.* 1986;25(4):249-251.
20. Aloi FG, Pippione M. Porokeratotic eccrine ostial and dermal duct nevus. *Arch Dermatol.* 1986;122(8): 892-895.
21. Lederman JS, Sober AJ, Lederman GS. Immunosuppression: a cause of porokeratosis? *J Am Acad Dermatol.* 1985;13(1):75-79.
22. Neumann RA, Knobler RM, Jurecka W, et al. Disseminated superficial actinic porokeratosis: experimental induction and exacerbation of skin lesions. *J Am Acad Dermatol.* 1989;21(6):1182-1188.
23. Wilson NJ, Hansen CD, Azkur D, et al. Recessive mutations in the gene encoding frizzled 6 cause twenty nail dystrophy—expanding the differential diagnosis for pachyonychia congenita. *J Dermatol Sci.* 2013;70(1):58-60.
24. Lucker GP, van de Kerkhof PC, Steijlen PM. Topical calcipotriol in the treatment of epidermolytic palmoplantar keratoderma of Vorner. *Br J Dermatol.* 1994;130(4):543-545.
25. Kanitakis J, Tsoitis G, Kanitakis C. Hereditary epidermolytic palmoplantar keratoderma (Vorner type). Report of a familial case and review of the literature. *J Am Acad Dermatol.* 1987;17(3):414-422.
26. Gruber R, Hennies HC, Romani N, et al. A novel homozygous missense mutation in SLURP1 causing Mal de Meleda with an atypical phenotype. *Arch Dermatol.* 2011;147(6):748-750.
27. Camisa C, Rossana C. Variant of keratoderma hereditaria mutilans (Vohwinkel's syndrome). Treatment with orally administered isotretinoin. *Arch Dermatol.* 1984;120(10):1323-1328.
28. Bondeson ML, Nystrom AM, Gunnarsson U, et al. Connexin 26 (GJB2) mutations in two Swedish patients with atypical Vohwinkel (mutilating keratoderma plus deafness) and KID syndrome both extensively treated with acitretin. *Acta Derm Venereol.* 2006;86(6):503-508.
29. Chang Sing Pang AF, Oranje AP, Vuzveki VD, et al. Successful treatment of keratoderma hereditaria mutilans with an aromatic retinoid. *Arch Dermatol.* 1981;117(4):225-228.
30. O'Driscoll J, Muston GC, McGrath JA, et al. A recurrent mutation in the loricrin gene underlies the ichthyotic variant of Vohwinkel syndrome. *Clin Exp Dermatol.* 2002;27(3):243-246.
31. Hausser I, Frantzmann Y, Anton-Lamprecht I, et al. [Olmsted syndrome. Successful therapy by treatment with etretinate]. *Hautarzt.* 1993;44(6):394-400.
32. Rivers JK, Duke EE, Justus DW. Etretinate: management of keratoma hereditaria mutilans in four family members. *J Am Acad Dermatol.* 1985;13(1):43-49.
33. Tang L, Zhang L, Ding H, et al. Olmsted syndrome: a new case complicated with easily broken hair and treated with oral retinoid. *J Dermatol.* 2012;39(9):816-817.
34. Ueda M, Nakagawa K, Hayashi K, et al. Partial improvement of Olmsted syndrome with etretinate. *Pediatr Dermatol.* 1993;10(4):376-381.
35. Delaporte E, N'Guyen-Mailfer C, Janin A, et al. Keratoderma with scleroatrophy of the extremities or sclerotylosis (Huriez syndrome): a reappraisal. *Br J Dermatol.* 1995;133(3):409-416.
36. Nomura T, Yoneta A, Pohler E, et al. Punctate palmoplantar keratoderma type 1: a novel AAGAB mutation and efficacy of etretinate. *Acta Derm Venereol.* 2015;95(1):110-111.
37. Nomura T, Moriuchi R, Takeda M, et al. Low-dose etretinate shows promise in management of punctate palmoplantar keratoderma type 1: case report and review of the published work. *J Dermatol.* 2015;42(9):889-892.
38. Tekin B, Yucelten D, Beleggia F, et al. Papillon-Lefevre syndrome: report of six patients and identification of a novel mutation. *Int J Dermatol.* 2016;55(8):898-902.
39. Sarma N, Ghosh C, Kar S, et al. Low-dose acitretin in Papillon-Lefevre syndrome: treatment and 1-year follow-up. *Dermatol Ther.* 2015;28(1):28-31.
40. Nazzaro V, Blanchet-Bardon C, Mimoz C, et al. Papillon-Lefevre syndrome. Ultrastructural study and successful treatment with acitretin. *Arch Dermatol.* 1988;124(4):533-539.
41. Grob JJ, Breton A, Bonafe JL, et al. Keratitis, ichthyosis, and deafness (KID) syndrome. Vertical transmission and death from multiple squamous cell carcinomas. *Arch Dermatol.* 1987;123(6):777-782.
42. Langer K, Konrad K, Wolff K. Keratitis, ichthyosis and deafness (KID)-syndrome: report of three cases and a review of the literature. *Br J Dermatol.* 1990;122(5):689-697.
43. Nazzaro V, Blanchet-Bardon C, Lorette G, et al. Familial occurrence of KID (keratitis, ichthyosis, deafness) syndrome. Case reports of a mother and daughter. *J Am Acad Dermatol.* 1990;23(2 Pt 2):385-388.
44. Patel V, Sun G, Dickman M, et al. Treatment of keratitis-ichthyosis- deafness (KID) syndrome in children: a case report and review of the literature. *Dermatol Ther.* 2015;28(2):89-93.
45. Hazen PG, Carney JM, Langston RH, et al. Corneal effect of isotretinoin: possible exacerbation of corneal neovascularization in a patient with the keratitis, ichthyosis, deafness ("KID") syndrome. *J Am Acad Dermatol.* 1986;14(1):141-142.
46. Zhang X, He Y, Zhou H, et al. Severe ichthyosis-related disorders in children: response to acitretin. *J Dermatolog Treat.* 2007;18(2):118-122.
47. Prasad SC, Bygum A. Successful treatment with alitretinoin of dissecting cellulitis of the scalp in

48. Werchau S, Toberer F, Enk A, et al. Keratitis-ichthyosis-deafness syndrome: response to alitretinoin and review of literature. *Arch Dermatol.* 2011;147(8): 993-995.
49. DiGiovanna JJ, Peck GL. Oral synthetic retinoid treatment in children. *Pediatr Dermatol.* 1983;1(1):77-88.
50. Xoagus E, Hudson D, Moodley S. Palmoplantar keratoderma surgical management. *J Plast Reconstr Aesthet Surg.* 2014;67(12):e316-e317.
51. Vorner H. Zur Kenntnis des Keratoma hereditarium palmare et plantare. *Arch Dermatol Syph.* 1901; 56:3-31.
52. Klaus S, Weinstein GD, Frost P. Localized epidermolytic hyperkeratosis. A form of keratoderma of the palms and soles. *Arch Dermatol.* 1970;101(3):272-275.
53. Codispoti A, Colombo E, Zocchi L, et al. Knuckle pads, in an epidermal palmoplantar keratoderma patient with Keratin 9 R163W transgrediens expression. *Eur J Dermatol.* 2009;19(2):114-118.
54. Li M, Yang LJ, Hua HK, et al. Keratin-9 gene mutation in epidermolytic palmoplantar keratoderma combined with knuckle pads in a large Chinese family. *Clin Exp Dermatol.* 2009;34(1):26-28.
55. Chiu HC, Jee SH, Sheen YS, et al. Mutation of keratin 9 (R163W) in a family with epidermolytic palmoplantar keratoderma and knuckle pads. *J Dermatol Sci.* 2007;45(1):63-65.
56. Hamada T, Ishii N, Karashima T, et al. The common KRT9 gene mutation in a Japanese patient with epidermolytic palmoplantar keratoderma and knuckle pad-like keratoses. *J Dermatol.* 2005;32(6):500-502.
57. Kuster W, Reis A, Hennies HC. Epidermolytic palmoplantar keratoderma of Vorner: re-evaluation of Vorner's original family and identification of a novel keratin 9 mutation. *Arch Dermatol Res.* 2002; 294(6):268-272.
58. Lu Y, Guo C, Liu Q, et al. A novel mutation of keratin 9 in epidermolytic palmoplantar keratoderma combined with knuckle pads. *Am J Med Genet A.* 2003;120A(3):345-349.
59. Du ZF, Wei W, Wang YF, et al. A novel mutation within the 2B rod domain of keratin 9 in a Chinese pedigree with epidermolytic palmoplantar keratoderma combined with knuckle pads and camptodactyly. *Eur J Dermatol.* 2011;21(5):675-679.
60. Liang YH, Liu QX, Huang L, et al. A recurrent p.M157R mutation of keratin 9 gene in a Chinese family with epidermolytic palmoplantar keratoderma and literature review. *Int J Dermatol.* 2014;53(8): e375-e379.
61. Funakushi N, Mayuzumi N, Sugimura R, et al. Epidermolytic palmoplantar keratoderma with constriction bands on bilateral fifth toes. *Arch Dermatol.* 2009;145(5):609-610.
62. Umegaki N, Nakano H, Tamai K, et al. Vorner type palmoplantar keratoderma: novel KRT9 mutation associated with knuckle pad-like lesions and recurrent mutation causing digital mutilation. *Br J Dermatol.* 2011;165(1): 199-201.
63. Mofid MZ, Costarangos C, Gruber SB, et al. Hereditary epidermolytic palmoplantar keratoderma (Vorner type) in a family with Ehlers-Danlos syndrome. *J Am Acad Dermatol.* 1998;38(5 Pt 2): 825-830.
64. Sommer G, Vakilzadeh F, Echternacht K, et al. Keratosis palmo-plantaris cum degeneratione granulosa. *Hum Genet.* 1976;33(1):85-87.
65. Chevrant-Breton J, Kerbrat P, Le Marec B, et al. Familial autosomal dominant epidermolytic palmo-plantar keratoderma and adenocarcinoma (study of 4 generations). *Ann Dermatol Venereol.* 1985;112(10):841-844.
66. Reis A, Hennies HC, Langbein L, et al. Keratin 9 gene mutations in epidermolytic palmoplantar keratoderma (EPPK). *Nat Genet.* 1994;6(2):174-179.
67. Hatsell SJ, Eady RA, Wennerstrand L, et al. Novel splice site mutation in keratin 1 underlies mild epidermolytic palmoplantar keratoderma in three kindreds. *J Invest Dermatol.* 2001;116(4):606-609.
68. Terron-Kwiatkowski A, Paller AS, Compton J, et al. Two cases of primarily palmoplantar keratoderma associated with novel mutations in keratin 1. *J Invest Dermatol.* 2002;119(4):966-971.
69. Terron-Kwiatkowski A, Terrinoni A, Didona B, et al. Atypical epidermolytic palmoplantar keratoderma presentation associated with a mutation in the keratin 1 gene. *Br J Dermatol.* 2004;150(6):1096-1103.
70. Terron-Kwiatkowski A, van Steensel MA, van Geel M, et al. Mutation S233L in the 1B domain of keratin 1 causes epidermolytic palmoplantar keratoderma with "tonotubular" keratin. *J Invest Dermatol.* 2006;126(3): 607-613.
71. Uitto J, Richard G, McGrath JA. Diseases of epidermal keratins and their linker proteins. *Exp Cell Res.* 2007;313(10):1995-2009.
72. Langbein L, Heid HW, Moll I, et al. Molecular characterization of the body site-specific human epidermal cytokeratin 9: cDNA cloning, amino acid sequence, and tissue specificity of gene expression. *Differentiation.* 1993;55(1):57-71.
73. Leslie Pedrioli DM, Fu DJ, Gonzalez-Gonzalez E, et al. Generic and personalized RNAi-based therapeutics for a dominant-negative epidermal fragility disorder. *J Invest Dermatol.* 2012;132(6):1627-1635.
74. Liu WT, Ke HP, Zhao Y, et al. The most common mutation of KRT9, c.C487T (p.R163W), in epidermolytic palmoplantar keratoderma in two large Chinese pedigrees. *Anat Rec.* 2012;295(4):604-609.
75. Moll I, Heid H, Franke WW, et al. Distribution of a special subset of keratinocytes characterized by the expression of cytokeratin 9 in adult and fetal human epidermis of various body sites. *Differentiation.* 1987;33(3):254-265.
76. Swensson O, Langbein L, McMillan JR, et al. Specialized keratin expression pattern in human ridged skin as an adaptation to high physical stress. *Br J Dermatol.* 1998;139(5):767-775.
77. Knobel M, O'Toole EA, Smith FJ. Keratins and skin disease. *Cell Tissue Res.* 2015;360(3):583-589.
78. Sprecher E, Ishida-Yamamoto A, Becker OM, et al. Evidence for novel functions of the keratin tail emerging from a mutation causing ichthyosis hystrix. *J Invest Dermatol.* 2001;116(4):511-519.
79. Whittock NV, Smith FJ, Wan H, et al. Frameshift mutation in the V2 domain of human keratin 1 results in striate palmoplantar keratoderma. *J Invest Dermatol.* 2002;118(5):838-844.
80. Bergman R, Khamaysi Z, Sprecher E. A unique pattern of dyskeratosis characterizes epidermolytic hyperkeratosis and epidermolytic palmoplantar keratoderma. *Am J Dermatopathol.* 2008;30(2):101-105.
81. Fuchs-Telem D, Padalon-Brauch G, Sarig O, et al. Epidermolytic palmoplantar keratoderma caused by activation of a cryptic splice site in KRT9. *Clin Exp Dermatol.* 2013;38(2):189-192; quiz 192.
82. Blasik LG, Dimond RL, Baughman RD. Hereditary epidermolytic palmoplantar keratoderma. *Arch Dermatol.* 1981;117(4):229-231.

83. Fritsch P, Honigsmann H, Jaschke E. Epidermolytic hereditary palmoplantar keratoderma. Report of a family and treatment with an oral aromatic retinoid. *Br J Dermatol.* 1978;99(5):561-568.
84. Haneke E. Keratosis palmaris et plantaris with Vorner's granulous degeneration. *Hautarzt.* 1982;33(12):654-656.
85. Laurent R, Prost O, Nicollier M, et al. Composite keratohyaline granules in palmoplantar keratoderma: an ultrastructural study. *Arch Dermatol Res.* 1985;277(5):384-394.
86. Hashimoto K, Mizuguchi R, Tanaka K, et al. Palmoplantar keratoderma (Voerner) with composite keratohyalin granules: studies on keratinization parameters and ultrastructures. *J Dermatol.* 2000;27(1):1-9.
87. Lyu YS, Shi PL, Chen XL, et al. A small indel mutant mouse model of epidermolytic palmoplantar keratoderma and its application to mutant-specific shRNA therapy. *Mol Ther Nucleic Acids.* 2016;5:e299.
88. Devos SA, Delescluse J. An unusual case of palmoplantar keratoderma. *J Eur Acad Dermatol Venereol.* 2003;17(1):68-69.
89. Gamborg Nielsen P, Faergemann J. Dermatophytes and keratin in patients with hereditary palmoplantar keratoderma. A mycological study. *Acta Derm Venereol.* 1993;73(6):416-418.
90. Maruyama R, Katoh T, Nishioka K. A case of Unna-Thost disease accompanied by Epidermophyton floccosum infection. *J Dermatol.* 1999;26(1):63-66.
91. Nielsen PG. Hereditary palmoplantar keratoderma and dermatophytosis in the northernmost county of Sweden (Norrbotten). *Acta Derm Venereol Suppl.* 1994;188:1-60.
92. Kimonis V, DiGiovanna JJ, Yang JM, et al. A mutation in the V1 end domain of keratin 1 in non-epidermolytic palmar-plantar keratoderma. *J Invest Dermatol.* 1994;103(6):764-769.
93. Loh TH, Yosipovitch G, Tay YK. Palmar-plantar keratoderma of Unna Thost associated with atopic dermatitis: an underrecognized entity? *Pediatr Dermatol.* 2003;20(3):195-198.
94. Rogozinski TT, Schwartz RA, Towpik E. Verrucous carcinoma in Unna-Thost hyperkeratosis of the palms and soles. *J Am Acad Dermatol.* 1994;31(6):1061-1062.
95. Sybert VP. *Genetic Skin Disorders.* Oxford: Oxford University Press; 2010.
96. Aguirre-Negrete MG, Hernandez A, Ramirez-Soltero S, et al. Keratosis palmaris et plantaris with clinodactyly. A distinct autosomal dominant genodermatosis. *Dermatologica.* 1981;162(4):300-303.
97. Nielsen PG. Diffuse palmoplantar keratoderma associated with acrocyanosis. A family study. *Acta Derm Venereol.* 1989;69(2):156-161.
98. Kuster W, Becker A. Indication for the identity of palmoplantar keratoderma type Unna-Thost with type Vorner. Thost's family revisited 110 years later. *Acta Derm Venereol.* 1992;72(2):120-122.
99. Candi E, Tarcsa E, Digiovanna JJ, et al. A highly conserved lysine residue on the head domain of type II keratins is essential for the attachment of keratin intermediate filaments to the cornified cell envelope through isopeptide crosslinking by transglutaminases. *Proc Natl Acad Sci U S A.* 1998;95(5):2067-2072.
100. Liu XP, Ling J, Xiong H, et al. Mutation L437P in the 2B domain of keratin 1 causes diffuse palmoplantar keratoderma in a Chinese pedigree. *J Eur Acad Dermatol Venereol.* 2009;23(9):1079-1082.
101. Almutawa F, Thusaringam T, Watters K, et al. Pachyonychia congenita (K16) with unusual features and good response to acitretin. *Case Rep Dermatol.* 2015;7(2):220-226.
102. Akasaka E, Nakano H, Nakano A, et al. Diffuse and focal palmoplantar keratoderma can be caused by a keratin 6c mutation. *Br J Dermatol.* 2011;165(6):1290-1292.
103. Greither A. Keratosis extremitatum hereditaria progrediens mit dominanten Erbgang. *Hautarzt.* 1952;3:198-203.
104. Beylot-Barry M, Taieb A, Surleve-Bazeille JE, et al. Inflammatory familial palmoplantar keratoderma: Greither's disease? *Dermatology.* 1992;185(3):210-214.
105. Fluckiger R, Itin PH. Keratosis extremitatum (Greither's disease): clinical features, histology, ultrastructure. *Dermatology.* 1993;187(4):309-311.
106. Grilli R, Aguilar A, Escalonilla P, et al. Transgrediens et progrediens palmoplantar keratoderma (Greither's disease) with particular histopathologic findings. *Cutis.* 2000;65(3):141-145.
107. Tay YK. What syndrome is this? Greither syndrome. *Pediatr Dermatol.* 2003;20(3):272-275.
108. Gach JE, Munro CS, Lane EB, et al. Two families with Greither's syndrome caused by a keratin 1 mutation. *J Am Acad Dermatol.* 2005;53(5 suppl 1):S225-230.
109. Seike T, Nakanishi H, Urano Y, et al. Malignant melanoma developing in an area of palmoplantar keratoderma (Greither's disease). *J Dermatol.* 1995;22(1):55-61.
110. Sybert VP, Dale BA, Holbrook KA. Palmar-plantar keratoderma. A clinical, ultrastructural, and biochemical study. *J Am Acad Dermatol.* 1988;18(1 Pt 1):75-86.
111. Kansky A, Arzensek J. Is palmoplantar keratoderma of Greither's type a separate nosologic entity? *Dermatologica.* 1979;158(4):244-248.
112. Richard G, Lin JP, Smith L, et al. Linkage studies in erythrokeratodermias: fine mapping, genetic heterogeneity and analysis of candidate genes. *J Invest Dermatol.* 1997;109(5):666-671.
113. Wollina U, Knopf B, Schaaschmidt H, et al. [Familial coexistence of erythrokeratodermia variabilis and keratosis palmoplantaris transgrediens et progrediens]. *Hautarzt.* 1989;40(3):169-172.
114. Porter RM, Lane EB. Phenotypes, genotypes and their contribution to understanding keratin function. *Trends Genet.* 2003;19(5):278-285.
115. Vohwinkel K. Keratoderma hereditaria mutilans. *Arch Dermatol Syphil.* 1929;158:354-364.
116. Maestrini E, Monaco AP, McGrath JA, et al. A molecular defect in loricrin, the major component of the cornified cell envelope, underlies Vohwinkel's syndrome. *Nat Genet.* 1996;13(1):70-77.
117. Hotz A, Bourrat E, Hausser I, et al. Two novel mutations in the LOR gene in three families with loricrin keratoderma. *Br J Dermatol.* 2015;172(4):1158-1162.
118. Pohler E, Cunningham F, Sandilands A, et al. Novel autosomal dominant mutation in loricrin presenting as prominent ichthyosis. *Br J Dermatol.* 2015;173(5):1291-1294.
119. Matsumoto K, Muto M, Seki S, et al. Loricrin keratoderma: a cause of congenital ichthyosiform erythroderma and collodion baby. *Br J Dermatol.* 2001;145(4):657-660.
120. Yeh JM, Yang MH, Chao SC. Collodion baby and loricrin keratoderma: a case report and mutation analysis. *Clin Exp Dermatol.* 2013;38(2):147-150.
121. Gedicke MM, Traupe H, Fischer B, et al. Towards characterization of palmoplantar keratoderma caused by gain-of-function mutation in loricrin: analysis of

a family and review of the literature. *Br J Dermatol.* 2006;154(1):167-171.
122. Armstrong DK, McKenna KE, Hughes AE. A novel insertional mutation in loricrin in Vohwinkel's keratoderma. *J Invest Dermatol.* 1998;111(4):702-704.
123. Kinsler VA, Drury S, Khan A, et al. A novel microdeletion in LOR causing autosomal dominant loricrin keratoderma. *Br J Dermatol.* 2015;172(1):262-264.
124. Song S, Shen C, Song G, et al. A novel c.545-546insG mutation in the loricrin gene correlates with a heterogeneous phenotype of loricrin keratoderma. *Br J Dermatol.* 2008;159(3):714-719.
125. Korge BP, Ishida-Yamamoto A, Punter C, et al. Loricrin mutation in Vohwinkel's keratoderma is unique to the variant with ichthyosis. *J Invest Dermatol.* 1997;109(4):604-610.
126. Ishida-Yamamoto A, Kato H, Kiyama H, et al. Mutant loricrin is not crosslinked into the cornified cell envelope but is translocated into the nucleus in loricrin keratoderma. *J Invest Dermatol.* 2000;115(6):1088-1094.
127. Drera B, Tadini G, Balbo F, et al. De novo occurrence of the 730insG recurrent mutation in an Italian family with the ichthyotic variant of Vohwinkel syndrome, loricrin keratoderma. *Clin Genet.* 2008;73(1):85-88.
128. Takahashi H, Ishida-Yamamoto A, Kishi A, et al. Loricrin gene mutation in a Japanese patient of Vohwinkel's syndrome. *J Dermatol Sci.* 1999;19(1):44-47.
129. Kalinin AE, Kajava AV, Steinert PM. Epithelial barrier function: assembly and structural features of the cornified cell envelope. *BioEssays.* 2002;24(9):789-800.
130. Schmuth M, Fluhr JW, Crumrine DC, et al. Structural and functional consequences of loricrin mutations in human loricrin keratoderma (Vohwinkel syndrome with ichthyosis). *J Invest Dermatol.* 2004;122(4):909-922.
131. Suga Y, Jarnik M, Attar PS, et al. Transgenic mice expressing a mutant form of loricrin reveal the molecular basis of the skin diseases, Vohwinkel syndrome and progressive symmetric erythrokeratoderma. *J Cell Biol.* 2000;151(2):401-412.
132. Ishida-Yamamoto A. Loricrin keratoderma: a novel disease entity characterized by nuclear accumulation of mutant loricrin. *J Dermatol Sci.* 2003;31(1):3-8.
133. Nithya S, Radhika T, Jeddy N. Loricrin—an overview. *J Oral Maxillofac Pathol.* 2015;19(1):64-68.
134. Koch PJ, de Viragh PA, Scharer E, et al. Lessons from loricrin-deficient mice: compensatory mechanisms maintaining skin barrier function in the absence of a major cornified envelope protein. *J Cell Biol.* 2000;151(2):389-400.
135. Elias PM, Schmuth M, Uchida Y, et al. Basis for the permeability barrier abnormality in lamellar ichthyosis. *Exp Dermatol.* 2002;11(3):248-256.
136. Yoneda K, Demitsu T, Nakai K, et al. Activation of vascular endothelial growth factor receptor 2 in a cellular model of loricrin keratoderma. *J Biol Chem.* 2010;285(21):16184-16194.
137. Cao X, Yin J, Wang H, et al. Mutation in AQP5, encoding aquaporin 5, causes palmoplantar keratoderma Bothnia type. *J Invest Dermatol.* 2014;134(1):284-287.
138. Abdul-Wahab A, Takeichi T, Liu L, et al. Autosomal dominant diffuse nonepidermolytic palmoplantar keratoderma due to a recurrent mutation in aquaporin-5. *Br J Dermatol.* 2016;174(2):430-432.
139. Park L, Khani C, Tamburro J. Aquagenic wrinkling of the palms and the potential role for genetic testing. *Pediatr Dermatol.* 2012;29(3):237-242.
140. Rongioletti F, Tomasini C, Crovato F, et al. Aquagenic (pseudo) keratoderma: a clinical series with new pathological insights. *Br J Dermatol.* 2012;167(3):575-582.
141. Blaydon DC, Lind LK, Plagnol V, et al. Mutations in AQP5, encoding a water-channel protein, cause autosomal-dominant diffuse nonepidermolytic palmoplantar keratoderma. *Am J Hum Genet.* 2013;93(2):330-335.
142. Iizuka T, Suzuki T, Nakano K, Sueki H. Immunolocalization of aquaporin-5 in normal human skin and hypohidrotic skin diseases. *J Dermatol.* 2012;39(4):344-349.
143. Kabashima K, Shimauchi T, Kobayashi M, et al. Aberrant aquaporin 5 expression in the sweat gland in aquagenic wrinkling of the palms. *J Am Acad Dermatol.* 2008;59(2 suppl 1):S28-32.
144. Prompt CA, Quinton PM. Functions of calcium in sweat secretion. *Nature.* 1978;272(5649):171-172.
145. Lin Z, Chen Q, Lee M, et al. Exome sequencing reveals mutations in TRPV3 as a cause of Olmsted syndrome. *Am J Hum Genet.* 2012;90(3):558-564.
146. Schnyder UW, Franceschetti AT, Ceszarovic B, et al. [Autochthonous Meleda disease]. *Ann Dermatol Syphiligr (Paris).* 1969;96(5):517-530.
147. Eckl KM, Stevens HP, Lestringant GG, et al. Mal de Meleda (MDM) caused by mutations in the gene for SLURP-1 in patients from Germany, Turkey, Palestine, and the United Arab Emirates. *Hum Genet.* 2003;112(1):50-56.
148. Fischer J, Bouadjar B, Heilig R, et al. Mutations in the gene encoding SLURP-1 in Mal de Meleda. *Hum Mol Genet.* 2001;10(8):875-880.
149. Tjiu JW, Lin PJ, Wu WH, et al. SLURP1 mutation-impaired T-cell activation in a family with mal de Meleda. *Br J Dermatol.* 2011;164(1):47-53.
150. Wajid M, Kurban M, Shimomura Y, et al. Mutations in the SLURP-1 gene underlie Mal de Meleda in three Pakistani families. *J Dermatol Sci.* 2009;56(1):27-32.
151. Sakabe J, Kabashima-Kubo R, Kubo A, et al. A Japanese case of Mal de Meleda with SLURP1 mutation. *J Dermatol.* 2014;41(8):764-765.
152. Taylor JA, Bondavalli D, Monif M, et al. Mal de Meleda in Indonesia: mutations in the SLURP1 gene appear to be ubiquitous. *Australas J Dermatol.* 2016;57(1):e11-13.
153. Nellen RG, Claessens T, Subramaniam R, et al. A novel mutation in SLURP1 in patients with mal de Meleda from the Indian subcontinent. *J Dermatol Sci.* 2015;80(1):76-78.
154. Bchetnia M, Laroussi N, Youssef M, et al. Particular Mal de Meleda phenotypes in Tunisia and mutations founder effect in the Mediterranean region. *BioMed Res Int.* 2013;2013:206803.
155. Nellen RG, Steijlen PM, Hennies HC, et al. Haplotype analysis in western European patients with mal de Meleda: founder effect for the W15R mutation in the SLURP1 gene. *Br J Dermatol.* 2013;168(6):1372-1374.
156. Zhang J, Cheng R, Ni C, et al. First Mal de Meleda report in Chinese Mainland: two families with a recurrent homozygous missense mutation in SLURP-1. *J Eur Acad Dermatol Venereol.* 2016;30(5):871-873.
157. Ward KM, Yerebakan O, Yilmaz E, et al. Identification of recurrent mutations in the ARS (component B) gene encoding SLURP-1 in two families with mal de Meleda. *J Invest Dermatol.* 2003;120(1):96-98.
158. Franceschetti AT, Reinhart V, Schnyder UW. Meleda disease. *J Genet Hum.* 1972;20(4):267-296.
159. Marrakchi S, Audebert S, Bouadjar B, et al. Novel mutations in the gene encoding secreted lymphocyte antigen-6/urokinase-type plasminogen activator receptor-related protein-1 (SLURP-1) and description of five ancestral haplotypes in patients with Mal de Meleda. *J Invest Dermatol.* 2003;120(3):351-355.

160. Bergman R, Bitterman-Deutsch O, Fartasch M, et al. Mal de Meleda keratoderma with pseudoainhum. *Br J Dermatol*. 1993;128(2):207-212.
161. Mokni M, Charfeddine C, Ben Mously R, et al. Heterozygous manifestations in female carriers of Mal de Meleda. *Clin Genet*. 2004;65(3):244-246.
162. Mozzillo N, Nunziata CA, Caraco C, et al. Malignant melanoma developing in an area of hereditary palmoplantar keratoderma (Mal de Meleda). *J Surg Oncol*. 2003;84(4):229-233.
163. Sartore L, Bordignon M, Bassetto F, et al. Melanoma in skin affected with keratoderma palmoplantaris hereditaria (Mal de Meleda): treatment with excision and grafting. *J Am Acad Dermatol*. 2009;61(1):161-163.
164. Baroni A, Piccolo V, Di Maio R, et al. Mal de Meleda with hyperpigmented spots. *Eur J Dermatol*. 2011; 21(3):459-460.
165. Tourlaki A, Bentivogli M, Boneschi V, et al. Genetically proven Mal de Meleda complicated by Bowen's disease of the sole. *Eur J Dermatol*. 2011;21(2):292-294.
166. Nielsen PG. Two different clinical and genetic forms of hereditary palmoplantar keratoderma in the northernmost county of Sweden. *Clin Genet*. 1985; 28:361-366.
167. Kastl I, Anton-Lamprecht I, Gamborg Nielsen P. Hereditary palmoplantar keratosis of the Gamborg Nielsen type. Clinical and ultrastructural characteristics of a new type of autosomal recessive palmoplantar keratosis. *Arch Dermatol Res*. 1990;282(6):363-370.
168. Zhao L, Vahlquist A, Virtanen M, et al. Palmoplantar keratoderma of the Gamborg-Nielsen type is caused by mutations in the SLURP1 gene and represents a variant of Mal de Meleda. *Acta Derm Venereol*. 2014;94(6):707-710.
169. Bickmore WA, Longbottom D, Oghene K, et al. Colocalization of the human CD59 gene to 11p13 with the MIC11 cell surface antigen. *Genomics*. 1993;17(1):129-135.
170. Chimienti F, Hogg RC, Plantard L, et al. Identification of SLURP-1 as an epidermal neuromodulator explains the clinical phenotype of Mal de Meleda. *Hum Mol Genet*. 2003;12(22):3017-3024.
171. van Steensel MA, van Geel MV, Steijlen PM. Mal de Meleda without mutations in the ARS coding sequence. *Eur J Dermatol*. 2002;12(2):129-132.
172. Charfeddine C, Mokni M, Kassar S, et al. Further evidence of the clinical and genetic heterogeneity of recessive transgressive PPK in the Mediterranean region. *J Hum Genet*. 2006;51(10):841-845.
173. Nellen RG, Steijlen PM, van Geel M, et al. Comment on Zhao et al. "Palmoplantar keratoderma of the Gamborg-Nielsen type is caused by mutations in the SLURP1 gene and represents a variant of Mal de Meleda." *Acta Derm Venereol*. 2015;95(8):1034-1035.
174. Arredondo J, Chernyavsky AI, Webber RJ, et al. Biological effects of SLURP-1 on human keratinocytes. *J Invest Dermatol*. 2005;125(6):1236-1241.
175. Fujii T, Horiguchi K, Sunaga H, et al. SLURP-1, an endogenous alpha7 nicotinic acetylcholine receptor allosteric ligand, is expressed in CD205(+) dendritic cells in human tonsils and potentiates lymphocytic cholinergic activity. *J Neuroimmunol*. 2014;267(1-2):43-49.
176. Pham CT, Ivanovich JL, Raptis SZ, et al. Papillon-Lefevre syndrome: correlating the molecular, cellular, and clinical consequences of cathepsin C/dipeptidyl peptidase I deficiency in humans. *J Immunol*. 2004;173(12):7277-7281.
177. Arredondo J, Chernyavsky AI, Grando SA. Overexpression of SLURP-1 and -2 alleviates the tumorigenic action of tobacco-derived nitrosamine on immortalized oral epithelial cells. *Biochem Pharmacol*. 2007;74(8):1315-1319.
178. Pettersson A, Nordlander S, Nylund G, et al. Expression of the endogenous, nicotinic acetylcholine receptor ligand, SLURP-1, in human colon cancer. *Auton Autacoid Pharmacol*. 2008;28(4):109-116.
179. Horiguchi K, Horiguchi S, Yamashita N, et al. Expression of SLURP-1, an endogenous alpha7 nicotinic acetylcholine receptor allosteric ligand, in murine bronchial epithelial cells. *J Neurosci Res*. 2009;87(12):2740-2747.
180. Wang H, Yu M, Ochani M, et al. Nicotinic acetylcholine receptor alpha7 subunit is an essential regulator of inflammation. *Nature*. 2003;421(6921):384-388.
181. Adeyo O, Allan BB, Barnes RH 2nd, et al. Palmoplantar keratoderma along with neuromuscular and metabolic phenotypes in Slurp1-deficient mice. *J Invest Dermatol*. 2014;134(6):1589-1598.
182. Elias PM, Williams ML, Holleran WM, et al. Pathogenesis of permeability barrier abnormalities in the ichthyoses: inherited disorders of lipid metabolism. *J Lipid Res*. 2008;49(4):697-714.
183. Moriwaki Y, Takada K, Nagasaki T, et al. IL-22/STAT3-induced increases in SLURP1 expression within psoriatic lesions exerts antimicrobial effects against Staphylococcus aureus. *PloS One*. 2015;10(10):e0140750.
184. Chernyavsky AI, Kalantari-Dehaghi M, Phillips C, et al. Novel cholinergic peptides SLURP-1 and -2 regulate epithelialization of cutaneous and oral wounds. *Wound Repair Regen*. 2012;20(1):103-113.
185. Frenk E, Guggisberg D, Mevorah B, et al. Meleda disease: report of two cases investigated by electron microscopy. *Dermatology*. 1996;193(4):358-361.
186. Favre B, Plantard L, Aeschbach L, et al. SLURP1 is a late marker of epidermal differentiation and is absent in Mal de Meleda. *J Invest Dermatol*. 2007;127(2):301-308.
187. Nagashima M. Palmoplantar keratoses [in Japanese]. *Jinrui Idengaku Shosho*. 1977;9:23-27.
188. Mitsuhashi Y, Hashimoto I, Takahashi M. Meleda type of keratosis palmoplantaris [in Japanese]. *Hifubyoh Shinryou*. 1989;11:298-299.
189. Kubo A, Shiohama A, Sasaki T, et al. Mutations in SERPINB7, encoding a member of the serine protease inhibitor superfamily, cause Nagashima-type palmoplantar keratosis. *Am J Hum Genet*. 2013;93(5):945-956.
190. Yin J, Xu G, Wang H, et al. New and recurrent SERPINB7 mutations in seven Chinese patients with Nagashima-type palmoplantar keratosis. *J Invest Dermatol*. 2014;134(8):2269-2272.
191. Isoda H, Kabashima K, Tokura Y. "Nagashima-type" keratosis palmoplantaris in two siblings. *J Eur Acad Dermatol Venereol*. 2009;23(6):737-738.
192. Kabashima K, Sakabe J, Yamada Y, et al. "Nagashima-type" keratosis as a novel entity in the palmoplantar keratoderma category. *Arch Dermatol*. 2008;144(3):375-379.
193. Miyauchi T, Nomura T, Suzuki S, et al. Extensive erythema and hyperkeratosis on the extremities and lumbar area as an unusual manifestation of Nagashima-type palmoplantar keratosis. *Acta Derm Venereol*. 2016;96(6):856-858.
194. Nakamizo S, Katoh N, Miyachi Y, et al. Atypical nail dystrophy in a possible case of Nagashima-type palmoplantar keratosis. *J Dermatol*. 2012;39(5):470-471.
195. Nonomura Y, Otsuka A, Miyachi Y, et al. Suspected Nagashima-type palmoplantar keratosis with

195. atypical hyperkeratotic lesions on the ears. *Eur J Dermatol.* 2012;22(3):392-393.
196. Iwata M, Tanizaki H, Endo Y, et al. Malignant melanoma arising in the skin lesions of Nagashima-type palmoplantar keratosis. *Eur J Dermatol.* 2014;24(2):259-260.
197. Kubo A. Nagashima-type palmoplantar keratosis: a common Asian type caused by SERPINB7 protease inhibitor deficiency. *J Invest Dermatol.* 2014;134(8):2076-2079.
198. Shiohama A, Sasaki T, Sato S, et al. Identification and characterization of a recessive missense mutation p.P277L in SERPINB7 in Nagashima-type palmoplantar keratosis. *J Invest Dermatol.* 2016;136(1):325-328.
199. Mizuno O, Nomura T, Suzuki S, et al. Highly prevalent SERPINB7 founder mutation causes pseudodominant inheritance pattern in Nagashima-type palmoplantar keratosis. *Br J Dermatol.* 2014;171(4):847-853.
200. Meyer-Hoffert U. Reddish, scaly, and itchy: how proteases and their inhibitors contribute to inflammatory skin diseases. *Arch Immunol Ther Exp (Warsz).* 2009;57(5):345-354.
201. Ovaere P, Lippens S, Vandenabeele P, et al. The emerging roles of serine protease cascades in the epidermis. *Trends Biochem Sci.* 2009;34(9):453-463.
202. Sakabe JI, Kabashima K, Sugita K, et al. Possible involvement of T lymphocytes in the pathogenesis of Nagashima-type keratosis palmoplantaris. *Clin Exp Dermatol.* 2009;34(7):e282-284.
203. Olmsted HC. Keratodermia palmaris et plantaris congenitalis: report of a case showing associated lesions of unusual location. *Am J Dis Child.* 1927;33:757-764.
204. Wilson NJ, Cole C, Milstone LM, et al. Expanding the phenotypic spectrum of Olmsted syndrome. *J Invest Dermatol.* 2015;135(11):2879-2883.
205. Duchatelet S, Hovnanian A. Olmsted syndrome: clinical, molecular and therapeutic aspects. *Orphanet J Rare Dis.* 2015;10:33.
206. Duchatelet S, Guibbal L, de Veer S, et al. Olmsted syndrome with erythromelalgia caused by recessive transient receptor potential vanilloid 3 mutations. *Br J Dermatol.* 2014;171(3):675-678.
207. Duchatelet S, Pruvost S, de Veer S, et al. A new TRPV3 missense mutation in a patient with Olmsted syndrome and erythromelalgia. *JAMA Dermatol.* 2014;150(3):303-306.
208. Nofal A, Assaf M, Nassar A, et al. Nonmutilating palmoplantar and periorificial kertoderma: a variant of Olmsted syndrome or a distinct entity? *Int J Dermatol.* 2010;49(6):658-665.
209. He Y, Zeng K, Zhang X, et al. A gain-of-function mutation in TRPV3 causes focal palmoplantar keratoderma in a Chinese family. *J Invest Dermatol.* 2015;135(3):907-909.
210. Alotaibi AK, Alotaibi MK, Alsaeed S, et al. Olmsted syndrome with oral involvement, including premature teeth loss. *Odontology.* 2015;103(2):241-245.
211. Poulin Y, Perry HO, Muller SA. Olmsted syndrome—congenital palmoplantar and periorificial keratoderma. *J Am Acad Dermatol.* 1984;10(4):600-610.
212. Attia AM, Bakry OA. Olmsted syndrome. *J Dermatol Case Rep.* 2013;7(2):42-45.
213. Tharini GK, Hema N, Jayakumar S, et al. Olmsted syndrome: report of two cases. *Indian J Dermatol.* 2011;56(5):591-593.
214. Yaghoobi R, Omidian M, Sina N, et al. Olmsted syndrome in an Iranian family: report of two new cases. *Arch Iran Med.* 2007;10(2):246-249.
215. Frias-Iniesta J, Sanchez-Pedreno P, Martinez-Escribano JA, et al A. Olmsted syndrome: report of a new case. *Br J Dermatol.* 1997;136(6):935-938.
216. Judge MR, Misch K, Wright P, et al. Palmoplantar and perioroficial keratoderma with corneal epithelial dysplasia: a new syndrome. *Br J Dermatol.* 1991;125(2):186-188.
217. Dogra D, Ravindraprasad JS, Khanna N, et al. Olmsted syndrome with hypotrichosis. *Indian J Dermatol Venereol Leprol.* 1997;63(2):120-122.
218. Mevorah B, Goldberg I, Sprecher E, et al. Olmsted syndrome: mutilating palmoplantar keratoderma with periorificial keratotic plaques. *J Am Acad Dermatol.* 2005;53(5 suppl 1):S266-272.
219. Tao J, Huang CZ, Yu NW, et al. Olmsted syndrome: a case report and review of literature. *Int J Dermatol.* 2008;47(5):432-437.
220. Requena L, Manzarbeitia F, Moreno C, et al. Olmsted syndrome: report of a case with study of the cellular proliferation in keratoderma. *Am J Dermatopathol.* 2001;23(6):514-520.
221. Cambiaghi S, Tadini G, Barbareschi M, et al. Olmsted syndrome in twins. *Arch Dermatol.* 1995;131(6):738-739.
222. Bergonse FN, Rabello SM, Barreto RL, et al. Olmsted syndrome: the clinical spectrum of mutilating palmoplantar keratoderma. *Pediatr Dermatol.* 2003;20(4):323-326.
223. Larregue M, Callot V, Kanitakis J, et al. Olmsted syndrome: report of two new cases and literature review. *J Dermatol.* 2000;27(9):557-568.
224. Barnett JH, Estes SA. Multiple epitheliomata cuniculata occurring in a mutilating keratoderma. *Cutis.* 1985;35(4):345-347.
225. Dessureault J, Poulin Y, Bourcier M, et al. Olmsted syndrome-palmoplantar and periorificial keratodermas: association with malignant melanoma. *J Cutan Med Surg.* 2003;7(3):236-242.
226. Ogawa F, Udono M, Murota H, et al. Olmsted syndrome with squamous cell carcinoma of extremities and adenocarcinoma of the lung: failure to detect loricrin gene mutation. *Eur J Dermatol.* 2003;13(6):524-528.
227. Yoshizaki Y, Kanki H, Ueda T, et al. A further case of plantar squamous cell carcinoma arising in Olmsted syndrome. *Br J Dermatol.* 2001;145(4):685-686.
228. Ni C, Yan M, Zhang J, et al. A novel mutation in TRPV3 gene causes atypical familial Olmsted syndrome. *Sci Rep.* 2016;6:21815.
229. Georgii A, Przybilla B, Schmoeckel C. Olmstedt syndrome—associated with primary sclerosing cholangitis and immune deficiency of uncertain origin. *Hautarzt.* 1989;40(11):708-712.
230. Atherton DJ, Sutton C, Jones BM. Mutilating palmoplantar keratoderma with periorificial keratotic plaques (Olmsted's syndrome). *Br J Dermatol.* 1990;122(2):245-252.
231. Lai-Cheong JE, Sethuraman G, Ramam M, et al. Recurrent heterozygous missense mutation, p.Gly573Ser, in the TRPV3 gene in an Indian boy with sporadic Olmsted syndrome. *Br J Dermatol.* 2012; 167(2):440-442.
232. Eytan O, Fuchs-Telem D, Mevorach B, et al. Olmsted syndrome caused by a homozygous recessive mutation in TRPV3. *J Invest Dermatol.* 2014;134(6):1752-1754.
233. Cao X, Wang H, Li Y, et al. Semidominant inheritance in Olmsted syndrome. *J Invest Dermatol.* 2016;136(8):1722-1725.
234. Haghighi A, Scott CA, Poon DS, et al. A missense mutation in the MBTPS2 gene underlies the X-linked

form of Olmsted syndrome. *J Invest Dermatol.* 2013;133(2):571-573.
235. Kress DW, Seraly MP, Falo L, et al. Olmsted syndrome. Case report and identification of a keratin abnormality. *Arch Dermatol.* 1996;132(7):797-800.
236. Huang SM, Lee H, Chung MK, et al. Overexpressed transient receptor potential vanilloid 3 ion channels in skin keratinocytes modulate pain sensitivity via prostaglandin E2. *J Neurosci.* 2008;28(51):13727-13737.
237. Yamamoto-Kasai E, Imura K, Yasui K, et al. TRPV3 as a therapeutic target for itch. *J Invest Dermatol.* 2012;132(8):2109-2112.
238. Borbiro I, Lisztes E, Toth BI, et al. Activation of transient receptor potential vanilloid-3 inhibits human hair growth. *J Invest Dermatol.* 2011;131(8):1605-1614.
239. Cheng X, Jin J, Hu L, et al. TRP channel regulates EGFR signaling in hair morphogenesis and skin barrier formation. *Cell.* 16 2010;141(2):331-343.
240. Valdes-Rodriguez R, Kaushik SB, Yosipovitch G. Transient receptor potential channels and dermatological disorders. *Curr Top Med Chem.* 2013;13(3):335-343.
241. Montell C. Preventing a Perm with TRPV3. *Cell.* 2010; 141(2):218-220.
242. Asakawa M, Yoshioka T, Matsutani T, et al. Association of a mutation in TRPV3 with defective hair growth in rodents. *J Invest Dermatol.* 2006;126(12):2664-2672.
243. Megarbane H, Megarbane A. Ichthyosis follicularis, alopecia, and photophobia (IFAP) syndrome. *Orphanet J Rare Dis.* 2011;6:29.
244. Wang HJ, Tang ZL, Lin ZM, et al. Recurrent splice-site mutation in MBTPS2 underlying IFAP syndrome with Olmsted syndrome-like features in a Chinese patient. *Clin Exp Dermatol.* 2014;39(2):158-161.
245. Bedard MS, Powell J, Laberge L, et al. Palmoplantar keratoderma and skin grafting: postsurgical long-term follow-up of two cases with Olmsted syndrome. *Pediatr Dermatol.* 2008;25(2):223-229.
246. Kenner-Bell BM, Paller AS, Lacouture ME. Epidermal growth factor receptor inhibition with erlotinib for palmoplantar keratoderma. *J Am Acad Dermatol.* 2010;63(2):e58-59.
247. Wigley J. A case of hyperkeratosis palmaris et plantaris associated with ainhum-like constriction of the fingers. *Br J Dermatol.* 1929;41:188-191.
248. Bassetto F, Tiengo C, Sferrazza R, et al. Vohwinkel syndrome: treatment of pseudo-ainhum. *Int J Dermatol.* 2010;49(1):79-82.
249. Gibbs RC, Frank SB. Keratoma hereditaria mutilans (Vohwinkel). Differentiating features of conditions with constriction of digits. *Arch Dermatol.* 1966;94(5):619-625.
250. Maestrini E, Korge BP, Ocana-Sierra J, et al. A missense mutation in connexin26, D66H, causes mutilating keratoderma with sensorineural deafness (Vohwinkel's syndrome) in three unrelated families. *Hum Mol Genet.* 1999;8(7):1237-1243.
251. McGibbon DH, Watson RT. Vohwinkel's syndrome and deafness. *J Laryngol Othol.* 1977;91(10):853-857.
252. Wereide K. Mutilating palmoplantar keratoderma successfully treated with etretinate. *Acta Derm Venereol.* 1984;64(6):566-569.
253. Chadhuri A, Haldar B. Keratoderma hereditaria mutilans with acanthosis nigricans (Vohwinkel disease). *Indian J Dermatol Venereol Leprol.* 1980;46:299-304.
254. Gamborg Nielsen P. A curious genetic coincidence found in a study of palmoplantar keratoderma. *Dermatologica.* 1983;167(6):310-313.
255. Sensi A, Bettoli V, Zampino MR, et al. Vohwinkel syndrome (mutilating keratoderma) associated with craniofacial anomalies. *Am J Med Genet.* 1994; 50(2):201-203.
256. Solis RR, Diven DG, Trizna Z. Vohwinkel's syndrome in three generations. *J Am Acad Dermatol.* 2001;44 (2 suppl):376-378.
257. Bhatia KK, Chaudhary S, Pahwa US, et al. Keratoma hereditaria mutilans (Vohwinkel's disease) with congenital alopecia universalis (atrichia congenita). *J Dermatol.* 1989;16(3):231-236.
258. Kikuchi I, Nagata T, Abe S. Keratosis palmoplantaris mutilans. *J Dermatol.* 1976;3:85-88.
259. Serrano Castro PJ, Naranjo Fernandez C, Quiroga Subirana P, et al. Vohwinkel Syndrome secondary to missense mutation D66H in GJB2 gene (connexin 26) can include epileptic manifestations. *Seizure.* 2010;19(2):129-131.
260. Martinez Castrillo JC, Medina S, Gobernado Serrano J. Complex partial seizures in a case of Vohwinkel syndrome (keratoma hereditaria mutilans). *Neurologia.* 1992;7(1):39.
261. Caceres-Rios H, Tamayo-Sanchez L, Duran-Mckinster C, et al. Keratitis, ichthyosis, and deafness (KID syndrome): review of the literature and proposal of a new terminology. *Pediatr Dermatol.* 1996;13(2):105-113.
262. Skinner BA, Greist MC, Norins AL. The keratitis, ichthyosis, and deafness (KID) syndrome. *Arch Dermatol.* 1981;117(5):285-289.
263. Burns FS. A case of generalized congenital erythroderma. *J Cutaneous Dis.* 1915;33.
264. Jan AY, Amin S, Ratajczak P, et al. Genetic heterogeneity of KID syndrome: identification of a Cx30 gene (GJB6) mutation in a patient with KID syndrome and congenital atrichia. *J Invest Dermatol.* 2004;122(5):1108-1113.
265. Wilson FM 2nd, Grayson M, Pieroni D. Corneal changes in ectodermal dysplasia. Case report, histopathology, and differential diagnosis. *Am J Ophthalmol.* 1973;75(1):17-27.
266. Zhang XB, Wei SC, Li CX, et al. Mutation of GJB2 in a Chinese patient with keratitis-ichthyosis-deafness syndrome and brain malformation. *Clin Exp Dermatol.* 2009;34(3):309-313.
267. Derelioglu SS, Yilmaz Y, Keles S. Dental treatments under the general anesthesia in a child with keratitis, ichthyosis, and deafness syndrome. *Case Rep Dent.* 2013;2013:618468.
268. Baden HP, Alper JC. Ichthyosiform dermatosis, keratitis, and deafness. *Arch Dermatol.* 1977;113(12): 1701-1704.
269. Lancaster L Jr, Fournet LF. Carcinoma of the tongue in a child: report of case. *J Oral Surg.* 1969;27(4): 269-270.
270. Tuppurainen K, Fraki J, Karjalainen S, et al. The KID-syndrome in Finland. A report of four cases. *Acta Ophthalmol.* 1988;66(6):692-698.
271. Lazic T, Li Q, Frank M, et al. Extending the phenotypic spectrum of keratitis-ichthyosis-deafness syndrome: report of a patient with GJB2 (G12R) Connexin 26 mutation and unusual clinical findings. *Pediatr Dermatol.* 2012;29(3):349-357.
272. Miteva L. Keratitis, ichthyosis, and deafness (KID) syndrome. *Pediatr Dermatol.* 2002;19(6):513-516.
273. Markova TG, Brazhkina NB, Bliznech EA, et al. Phenotype in a patient with p.D50N mutation in GJB2 gene resemble both KID and Clouston syndromes. *Int J Pediatr Otorhinolaryngol.* 2016;81:10-14.
274. Kutkowska-Kazmierczak A, Niepokoj K, Wertheim-Tysarowska K, et al. Phenotypic variability in gap

junction syndromic skin disorders: experience from KID and Clouston syndromes' clinical diagnostics. *J Appl Genet*. 2015;56(3):329-337.
275. Szymko-Bennett YM, Russell LJ, Bale SJ, et al. Auditory manifestations of keratitis-ichthyosis-deafness (KID) syndrome. *Laryngoscope*. 2002;112(2):272-280.
276. Gilliam A, Williams ML. Fatal septicemia in an infant with keratitis, ichthyosis, and deafness (KID) syndrome. *Pediatr Dermatol*. 2002;19(3):232-236.
277. Haruna K, Suga Y, Oizumi A, et al. Severe form of keratitis-ichthyosis-deafness (KID) syndrome associated with septic complications. *J Dermatol*. 2010;37(7):680-682.
278. Morris MR, Namon A, Shaw GY, et al. The keratitis, ichthyosis, and deafness syndrome. *Otolaryngol Head Neck Surg*. 1991;104(4):526-528.
279. Helm K, Lane AT, Orosz J, et al. Systemic cytomegalovirus in a patient with the keratitis, ichthyosis, and deafness (KID) syndrome. *Pediatr Dermatol*. 1990;7(1):54-56.
280. Coggshall K, Farsani T, Ruben B, et al. Keratitis, ichthyosis, and deafness syndrome: a review of infectious and neoplastic complications. *J Am Acad Dermatol*. 2013;69(1):127-134.
281. Nyquist GG, Mumm C, Grau R, et al. Malignant proliferating pilar tumors arising in KID syndrome: a report of two patients. *Am J Med Genet A*. 2007;143A(7):734-741.
282. Kim KH, Kim JS, Piao YJ, et al. Keratitis, ichthyosis and deafness syndrome with development of multiple hair follicle tumours. *Br J Dermatol*. 2002;147(1):139-143.
283. de Alonso A, Cesarios G, Pecoraro V, et al. Syndrome KID (queratitis, ictiosis sordera) con poromas ecrinos multiples. *Rev Arg Dermatol*. 1993;74:10-14.
284. Bergman R, Mercer A, Indelman M, et al. KID syndrome: histopathological, immunohistochemical and molecular analysis of precancerous and cancerous skin lesions. *Br J Dermatol*. 2012;166(2):455-457.
285. Homeida L, Wiley RT, Fatahzadeh M. Oral squamous cell carcinoma in a patient with keratitis-ichthyosis-deafness syndrome: a rare case. *Oral Surg Oral Med Oral Pathol Oral Radiol*. 2015;119(4):e226-232.
286. Mazereeuw-Hautier J, Bitoun E, Chevrant-Breton J, et al. Keratitis-ichthyosis-deafness syndrome: disease expression and spectrum of connexin 26 (GJB2) mutations in 14 patients. *Br J Dermatol*. 2007;156(5):1015-1019.
287. van Steensel MA, Steijlen PM, Bladergroen RS, et al. A phenotype resembling the Clouston syndrome with deafness is associated with a novel missense GJB2 mutation. *J Invest Dermatol*. 2004;123(2):291-293.
288. Carey AB, Burke WA, Park HM. Malignant fibrous histiocytoma in keratosis, ichthyosis, and deafness syndrome. *J Am Acad Dermatol*. 1988;19(6):1124-1126.
289. Kaku Y, Tanizaki H, Tanioka M, et al. Sebaceous carcinoma arising at a chronic candidiasis skin lesion of a patient with keratitis-ichthyosis-deafness (KID) syndrome. *Br J Dermatol*. 2012;166(1):222-224.
290. Fozza C, Poddie F, Contini S, et al. Keratitis-ichthyosis-deafness syndrome, atypical connexin gjb2 gene mutation, and peripheral T-cell lymphoma: more than a random association? *Case Rep Hematol*. 2011;2011:848461.
291. Maintz L, Betz RC, Allam JP, et al. Keratitis-ichthyosis-deafness syndrome in association with follicular occlusion triad. *Eur J Dermatol*. 2005;15(5):347-352.
292. Montgomery JR, White TW, Martin BL, et al. A novel connexin 26 gene mutation associated with features of the keratitis-ichthyosis-deafness syndrome and the follicular occlusion triad. *J Am Acad Dermatol*. 2004;51(3):377-382.
293. Meigh L, Hussain N, Mulkey DK, et al. Connexin26 hemichannels with a mutation that causes KID syndrome in humans lack sensitivity to CO_2. *eLife*. 2014;3:e04249.
294. Sbidian E, Feldmann D, Bengoa J, et al. Germline mosaicism in keratitis-ichthyosis-deafness syndrome: pre-natal diagnosis in a familial lethal form. *Clin Genet*. 2010;77(6):587-592.
295. Ogawa Y, Takeichi T, Kono M, et al. Revertant mutation releases confined lethal mutation, opening Pandora's box: a novel genetic pathogenesis. *PLoS Genet*. 2014;10(5):e1004276.
296. Bart RS, Pumphrey RE. Knuckle pads, leukonychia and deafness. A dominantly inherited syndrome. *N Engl J Med*. 1967;276(4):202-207.
297. Ramer JC, Vasily DB, Ladda RL. Familial leuconychia, knuckle pads, hearing loss, and palmoplantar hyperkeratosis: an additional family with Bart-Pumphrey syndrome. *J Med Genet*. 1994;31(1):68-71.
298. Richard G. Connexin disorders of the skin. *Clin Dermatol*. 2005;23(1):23-32.
299. Alexandrino F, Sartorato EL, Marques-de-Faria AP, et al. G59S mutation in the GJB2 (connexin 26) gene in a patient with Bart-Pumphrey syndrome. *Am J Med Genet A*. 2005;136(3):282-284.
300. Balighi K, Moeineddin F, Lajevardi V, et al. A family with leukonychia totalis. *Indian J Dermatol*. 2010;55(1):102-104.
301. Gonul M, Gul U, Hizli P, et al. A family of Bart-Pumphrey syndrome. *Indian J Dermatol Venereol Leprol*. 2012;78(2):178-181.
302. Richard G, Brown N, Ishida-Yamamoto A, et al. Expanding the phenotypic spectrum of Cx26 disorders: Bart-Pumphrey syndrome is caused by a novel missense mutation in GJB2. *J Invest Dermatol*. 2004;123(5):856-863.
303. Heathcote K, Syrris P, Carter ND, et al. A connexin 26 mutation causes a syndrome of sensorineural hearing loss and palmoplantar hyperkeratosis (MIM 148350). *J Med Genet*. 2000;37(1):50-51.
304. Richard G, White TW, Smith LE, et al. Functional defects of Cx26 resulting from a heterozygous missense mutation in a family with dominant deafmutism and palmoplantar keratoderma. *Hum Genet*. 1998;103(4):393-399.
305. Uyguner O, Tukel T, Baykal C, et al. The novel R75Q mutation in the GJB2 gene causes autosomal dominant hearing loss and palmoplantar keratoderma in a Turkish family. *Clin Genet*. 2002;62(4):306-309.
306. Kelsell DP, Wilgoss AL, Richard G, et al. Connexin mutations associated with palmoplantar keratoderma and profound deafness in a single family. *Eur J Hum Genet*. 2000;8(2):141-144.
307. Lee JY, In SI, Kim HJ, et al. Hereditary palmoplantar keratoderma and deafness resulting from genetic mutation of Connexin 26. *J Korean Med Sci*. 2010;25(10):1539-1542.
308. Birkenhager R, Lublinghoff N, Prera E, et al. Autosomal dominant prelingual hearing loss with palmoplantar keratoderma syndrome: variability in clinical expression from mutations of R75W and R75Q in the GJB2 gene. *Am J Med Genet A*. 2010;152A(7):1798-1802.

309. de Zwart-Storm EA, van Geel M, van Neer PA, et al. A novel missense mutation in the second extracellular domain of GJB2, p.Ser183Phe, causes a syndrome of focal palmoplantar keratoderma with deafness. *Am J Pathol*. 2008;173(4):1113-1119.
310. Simon AM, Goodenough DA. Diverse functions of vertebrate gap junctions. *Trends Cell Biol*. 1998;8(12):477-483.
311. Oshima A, Doi T, Mitsuoka K, et al. Roles of Met-34, Cys-64, and Arg-75 in the assembly of human connexin 26. Implication for key amino acid residues for channel formation and function. *J Biol Chem*. 2003;278(3):1807-1816.
312. del Castillo FJ, Rodriguez-Ballesteros M, Alvarez A, et al. A novel deletion involving the connexin-30 gene, del(GJB6-d13s1854), found in trans with mutations in the GJB2 gene (connexin-26) in subjects with DFNB1 non-syndromic hearing impairment. *J Med Genet*. 2005;42(7):588-594.
313. Guex N, Peitsch MC. SWISS-MODEL and the Swiss-PdbViewer: an environment for comparative protein modeling. *Electrophoresis*. 1997;18(15):2714-2723.
314. Martinez AD, Acuna R, Figueroa V, et al. Gap-junction channels dysfunction in deafness and hearing loss. *Antioxid Redox Signal*. 2009;11(2):309-322.
315. Scott CA, Tattersall D, O'Toole EA, et al. Connexins in epidermal homeostasis and skin disease. *Biochim Biophys Acta*. 2012;1818(8):1952-1961.
316. Wang CM, Lincoln J, Cook JE, et al. Abnormal connexin expression underlies delayed wound healing in diabetic skin. *Diabetes*. 2007;56(11):2809-2817.
317. Richard G, Rouan F, Willoughby CE, et al. Missense mutations in GJB2 encoding connexin-26 cause the ectodermal dysplasia keratitis-ichthyosis-deafness syndrome. *Am J Hum Genet*. 2002;70(5):1341-1348.
318. Coutinho P, Qiu C, Frank S, et al. Dynamic changes in connexin expression correlate with key events in the wound healing process. *Cell Biol Int*. 2003;27(7):525-541.
319. Lucke T, Choudhry R, Thom R, et al. Upregulation of connexin 26 is a feature of keratinocyte differentiation in hyperproliferative epidermis, vaginal epithelium, and buccal epithelium. *J Invest Dermatol*. 1999;112(3):354-361.
320. Rouan F, White TW, Brown N, et al. trans-dominant inhibition of connexin-43 by mutant connexin-26: implications for dominant connexin disorders affecting epidermal differentiation. *J Cell Sci*. 2001;114(Pt 11):2105-2113.
321. Kelsell DP, Dunlop J, Stevens HP, et al. Connexin 26 mutations in hereditary non-syndromic sensorineural deafness. *Nature*. 1997;387(6628):80-83.
322. Kikuchi T, Kimura RS, Paul DL, et al. Gap junctions in the rat cochlea: immunohistochemical and ultrastructural analysis. *Anat Embryol*. 1995;191(2): 101-118.
323. Rabionet R, Lopez-Bigas N, Arbones ML, et al. Connexin mutations in hearing loss, dermatological and neurological disorders. *Trends Mol Med*. 2002;8(5):205-212.
324. Bergoffen J, Scherer SS, Wang S, et al. Connexin mutations in X-linked Charcot-Marie-Tooth disease. *Science*. 1993;262(5142):2039-2042.
325. Shiels A, Mackay D, Ionides A, et al. A missense mutation in the human connexin50 gene (GJA8) underlies autosomal dominant "zonular pulverulent" cataract, on chromosome 1q. *Am J Hum Genet*. 1998;62(3):526-532.
326. Paznekas WA, Boyadjiev SA, Shapiro RE, et al. Connexin 43 (GJA1) mutations cause the pleiotropic phenotype of oculodentodigital dysplasia. *Am J Hum Genet*. 2003;72(2):408-418.
327. van Steensel MA, van Geel M, Nahuys M, et al. A novel connexin 26 mutation in a patient diagnosed with keratitis-ichthyosis-deafness syndrome. *J Invest Dermatol*. 2002;118(4):724-727.
328. Lamartine J, Munhoz Essenfelder G, Kibar Z, et al. Mutations in GJB6 cause hidrotic ectodermal dysplasia. *Nat Genet*. 2000;26(2):142-144.
329. Richard G, Smith LE, Bailey RA, et al. Mutations in the human connexin gene GJB3 cause erythrokeratodermia variabilis. *Nat Genet*. 1998;20(4):366-369.
330. Yeager M, Nicholson BJ. Structure of gap junction intercellular channels. *Curr Opin Struct Biol*. 1996;6(2):183-192.
331. Marziano NK, Casalotti SO, Portelli AE, et al. Mutations in the gene for connexin 26 (GJB2) that cause hearing loss have a dominant negative effect on connexin 30. *Hum Mol Genet*. 2003;12(8):805-812.
332. Stauffer KA. The gap junction proteins beta 1-connexin (connexin-32) and beta 2-connexin (connexin-26) can form heteromeric hemichannels. *J Biol Chem*. 1995;270(12):6768-6772.
333. Cohen-Salmon M, Ott T, Michel V, et al. Targeted ablation of connexin26 in the inner ear epithelial gap junction network causes hearing impairment and cell death. *Curr Biol*. 2002;12(13):1106-1111.
334. Kudo T, Kure S, Ikeda K, et al. Transgenic expression of a dominant-negative connexin26 causes degeneration of the organ of Corti and non-syndromic deafness. *Hum Mol Genet*. 2003;12(9):995-1004.
335. Bakirtzis G, Choudhry R, Aasen T, et al. Targeted epidermal expression of mutant Connexin 26(D66H) mimics true Vohwinkel syndrome and provides a model for the pathogenesis of dominant connexin disorders. *Hum Mol Genet*. 2003;12(14):1737-1744.
336. Senter TP, Jones KL, Sakati N, et al. Atypical ichthyosiform erythroderma and congenital neurosensory deafness—a distinct syndrome. *J Pediatr*. 1978;92(1):68-72.
337. Rycroft RJ, Moynahan EJ, Wells RS. Atypical ichthyosiform erythrodernam deafness and keratitis. A report of two cases. *Br J Dermatol*. 1976;94(2):211-217.
338. Titeux M, Mendonca V, Decha A, et al. Keratitis-ichthyosis-deafness syndrome caused by GJB2 maternal mosaicism. *J Invest Dermatol*. 2009;129(3):776-779.
339. Neoh CY, Chen H, Ng SK, et al. A rare connexin 26 mutation in a patient with a forme fruste of keratitis-ichthyosis-deafness (KID) syndrome. *Int J Dermatol*. 2009;48(10):1078-1081.
340. Richard G. Connexin disorders of the skin. *Adv Dermatol*. 2001;17:243-277.
341. Sanchez HA, Verselis VK. Aberrant Cx26 hemichannels and keratitis-ichthyosis-deafness syndrome: insights into syndromic hearing loss. *Front Cell Neurosci*. 2014;8:354.
342. Yotsumoto S, Hashiguchi T, Chen X, et al. Novel mutations in GJB2 encoding connexin-26 in Japanese patients with keratitis-ichthyosis-deafness syndrome. *Br J Dermatol*. 2003;148(4):649-653.
343. van Geel M, van Steensel MA, Kuster W, et al. HID and KID syndromes are associated with the same connexin 26 mutation. *Br J Dermatol*. 2002;146(6):938-942.
344. Maeda S, Nakagawa S, Suga M, et al. Structure of the connexin 26 gap junction channel at 3.5 A resolution. *Nature*. 2009;458(7238):597-602.

345. Shurman DL, Glazewski L, Gumpert A, et al. In vivo and in vitro expression of connexins in the human corneal epithelium. *Invest Ophthalmol Visual Sci.* 2005;46(6):1957-1965.

346. Levit NA, Sellitto C, Wang HZ, et al. Aberrant connexin26 hemichannels underlying keratitis-ichthyosis-deafness syndrome are potently inhibited by mefloquine. *J Invest Dermatol.* 2015;135(4):1033-1042.

347. Smith FJ, Morley SM, McLean WH. A novel connexin 30 mutation in Clouston syndrome. *J Invest Dermatol.* 2002;118(3):530-532.

348. Feldmann D, Denoyelle F, Blons H, et al. The GJB2 mutation R75Q can cause nonsyndromic hearing loss DFNA3 or hereditary palmoplantar keratoderma with deafness. *Am J Med Genet A.* 2005;137(2):225-227.

349. Palungwachira P, Iwahara K, Ogawa H. Keratoderma hereditaria mutilans. Etretinate treatment and electron microscope studies. *Australas J Dermatol.* 1992;33(1):19-30.

350. de Berker D, Branford WA, Soucek S, et al. Fatal keratitis ichthyosis and deafness syndrome (KIDS). Aural, ocular, and cutaneous histopathology. *Am J Dermatopathol.* 1993;15(1):64-69.

351. Atabay K, Yavuzer R, Latifoglu O, et al. Keratoderma hereditarium mutilans (Vohwinkel syndrome): an unsolved surgical mystery. *Plast Reconstr Surg.* 2001;108(5):1276-1280.

352. Liebman JJ, Liu Y. Successful surgical management of keratoderma hereditaria mutilans. *Hand.* 2013;8(1):102-104.

353. Zhang M, Song K, Ding N, et al. Using a distant abdominal skin flap to treat digital constriction bands: a case report for Vohwinkel syndrome. *Medicine.* 2016;95(6):e2762.

354. Djalilian AR, Kim JY, Saeed HN, et al. Histopathology and treatment of corneal disease in keratitis, ichthyosis, and deafness (KID) syndrome. *Eye.* 2010;24(4):738-740.

355. Sonoda S, Uchino E, Sonoda KH, et al. Two patients with severe corneal disease in KID syndrome. *Am J Ophthalmol.* 2004;137(1):181-183.

356. Caye L, Scheid K, Pizzol MM, et al. Use of bevacizumab (Avastin) in KID syndrome: case report. *Arq Bras Oftalmol.* 2010;73(3):285-290.

357. Basaran E, Yilmaz E, Alpsoy E, et al. Keratoderma, hypotrichosis and leukonychia totalis: a new syndrome? *Br J Dermatol.* 1995;133(4):636-638.

358. Rai VM, Shenoi SD. Ichthyosis follicularis with congenital atrichia, nail dystrophy and palmoplantar keratoderma. Variant of IFAP syndrome or a new entity? *Dermatol Online J.* 2005;11(3):36.

359. Stevanovic DV. Alopecia congenita: the incomplete dominant form of inheritance with varying expressivity. *Acta Genet Stat Med.* 1959;9:127-132.

360. Stratton RF, Jorgenson RJ, Krause IC. Possible second case of tricho-oculo-dermo-vertebral (Alves) syndrome. *Am J Med Genet.* 1993;46(3):313-315.

361. Wallis C, Ip FS, Beighton P. Cataracts, alopecia, and sclerodactyly: a previously apparently undescribed ectodermal dysplasia syndrome on the island of Rodrigues. *American J Med Genet.* 1989;32(4):500-503.

362. Castori M, Valiante M, Ritelli M, et al. Palmoplantar keratoderma, pseudo-ainhum, and universal atrichia: a new patient and review of the palmoplantar keratoderma-congenital alopecia syndrome. *Am J Med Genet A.* 2010;152A(8):2043-2047.

363. Castori M, Morlino S, Sana ME, et al. Clinical and molecular characterization of two patients with palmoplantar keratoderma-congenital alopecia syndrome type 2. *Clin Exp Dermatol.* 2016;41(6):632-635.

364. Wang H, Cao X, Lin Z, et al. Exome sequencing reveals mutation in GJA1 as a cause of keratoderma-hypotrichosis-leukonychia totalis syndrome. *Hum Mol Genet.* 2015;24(22):6564.

365. Dahl E, Winterhager E, Traub O, et al. Expression of gap junction genes, connexin40 and connexin43, during fetal mouse development. *Anat Embryol.* 1995;191(3):267-278.

366. Tada J, Hashimoto K. Ultrastructural localization of gap junction protein connexin 43 in normal human skin, basal cell carcinoma, and squamous cell carcinoma. *J Cutan Pathol.* 1997;24(10):628-635.

367. Kelly SC, Ratajczak P, Keller M, et al. A novel GJA 1 mutation in oculo-dento-digital dysplasia with curly hair and hyperkeratosis. *Eur J Dermatol.* 2006;16(3):241-245.

368. van Steensel MA, Spruijt L, van der Burgt I, et al. A 2-bp deletion in the GJA1 gene is associated with oculo-dento-digital dysplasia with palmoplantar keratoderma. *Am J Med Genet A.* 2005;132A(2):171-174.

369. Vreeburg M, de Zwart-Storm EA, Schouten MI, et al. Skin changes in oculo-dento-digital dysplasia are correlated with C-terminal truncations of connexin 43. *Am J Med Genet A.* 2007;143(4):360-363.

370. Nicolle G, Hallipre A. Maladie familiale characterisee par des alterations des cheveux et des ongles. *Ann Dermatol Syphilol.* 1895;6(675):804.

371. Clouston HR. A hereditary ectodermal dystrophy. *Can Med Assoc J.* 1929;21(1):18-31.

372. Clouston HR. The major forms of hereditary ectodermal dysplasia (with an autopsy and biopsies on the anhydrotic type). *Can Med Assoc J.* 1939;40(1):1-7.

373. Ando Y, Tanaka T, Horiguchi Y, et al. Hidrotic ectodermal dysplasia: a clinical and ultrastructural observation. *Dermatologica.* 1988;176(4):205-211.

374. Kibar Z, Dube MP, Powell J, et al. Clouston hidrotic ectodermal dysplasia (HED): genetic homogeneity, presence of a founder effect in the French Canadian population and fine genetic mapping. *Eur J Hum Genet.* 2000;8(5):372-380.

375. McNaughton PZ, Pierson DL, Rodman OG. Hidrotic ectodermal dysplasia in a black mother and daughter. *Arch Dermatol.* 1976;112(10):1448-1450.

376. Patel RR, Bixler D, Norins AL. Clouston syndrome: a rare autosomal dominant trait with palmoplantar hyperkeratosis and alopecia. *J Craniofac Genet Dev Biol.* 1991;11(3):176-179.

377. Radhakrishna U, Blouin JL, Mehenni H, et al. The gene for autosomal dominant hidrotic ectodermal dysplasia (Clouston syndrome) in a large Indian family maps to the 13q11-q12.1 pericentromeric region. *Am J Med Genet.* 1997;71(1):80-86.

378. Rajagopalan K, Tay CH. Hidrotic ectodermal dysplasia: study of a large Chinese pedigree. *Arch Dermatol.* 1977;113(4):481-485.

379. Yang R, Hu Z, Kong Q, et al. A known mutation in GJB6 in a large Chinese family with hidrotic ectodermal dysplasia. *J Eur Acad Dermatol Venereol.* 2016;30(8):1362-1365.

380. Marakhonov A, Skoblov M, Galkina V, et al. Clouston syndrome: first case in Russia. *Balkan J Med Genet.* 2012;15(1):51-54.

381. Hassed SJ, Kincannon JM, Arnold GL. Clouston syndrome: an ectodermal dysplasia without significant dental findings. *Am J Med Genet.* 1996;61(3):274-276.

382. Hazen PG, Zamora I, Bruner WE, et al. Premature cataracts in a family with hidrotic ectodermal dysplasia. *Arch Dermatol.* 1980;116(12):1385-1387.
383. Zhang XJ, Chen JJ, Yang S, et al. A mutation in the connexin 30 gene in Chinese Han patients with hidrotic ectodermal dysplasia. *J Dermatol Sci.* 2003;32(1):11-17.
384. Baris HN, Zlotogorski A, Peretz-Amit G, et al. A novel GJB6 missense mutation in hidrotic ectodermal dysplasia 2 (Clouston syndrome) broadens its genotypic basis. *Br J Dermatol.* 2008;159(6):1373-1376.
385. van Steensel MA, Jonkman MF, van Geel M, et al. Clouston syndrome can mimic pachyonychia congenita. *J Invest Dermatol.* 2003;121(5):1035-1038.
386. Hu YH, Lin YC, Hwu WL, et al. Pincer nail deformity as the main manifestation of Clouston syndrome. *Br J Dermatol.* 2015;173(2):581-583.
387. Hale GI, Wilson NJ, Smith FJ, et al. Mutations in GJB6 causing phenotype resembling pachyonychia congenita. *Br J Dermatol.* 2015;172(5):1447-1449.
388. Fraser FC, Der Kaloustian VM. A man, a syndrome, a gene: Clouston's hidrotic ectodermal dysplasia (HED). *Am J Med Genet.* 2001;100(2):164-168.
389. Liu YT, Guo K, Li J, et al. Novel mutations in GJB6 and GJB2 in Clouston syndrome. *Clin Exp Dermatol.* 2015;40(7):770-773.
390. Sugiura K, Teranishi M, Matsumoto Y, et al. Clouston syndrome with heterozygous GJB6 mutation p.Ala88Val and GJB2 variant p.Val27Ile revealing mild sensorineural hearing loss and photophobia. *JAMA Dermatol.* 2013;149(11):1350-1351.
391. Copeland DD, Lamb WA, Klintworth GK. Calcification of basal ganglia and cerebellar roof nuclei in mentally defective patient with hidrotic ectodermal dysplasia. Analysis of intracranial concretions by electron microprobe. *Neurology.* 1977;27(11):1029-1033.
392. Unger VM, Kumar NM, Gilula NB, et al. Three-dimensional structure of a recombinant gap junction membrane channel. *Science.* 1999;283(5405):1176-1180.
393. Sosinsky G. Mixing of connexins in gap junction membrane channels. *Proc Natl Acad Sci U S A.* 1995;92(20):9210-9214.
394. Dahl E, Manthey D, Chen Y, et al. Molecular cloning and functional expression of mouse connexin-30, a gap junction gene highly expressed in adult brain and skin. *J Biol Chem.* 1996;271(30):17903-17910.
395. Lautermann J, Frank HG, Jahnke K, et al. Developmental expression patterns of connexin26 and -30 in the rat cochlea. *Dev Genet.* 1999;25(4):306-311.
396. Nagy JI, Patel D, Ochalski PA, et al. Connexin30 in rodent, cat and human brain: selective expression in gray matter astrocytes, co-localization with connexin43 at gap junctions and late developmental appearance. *Neuroscience.* 1999;88(2):447-468.
397. Essenfelder GM, Bruzzone R, Lamartine J, et al. Connexin30 mutations responsible for hidrotic ectodermal dysplasia cause abnormal hemichannel activity. *Hum Mol Genet.* 2004;13(16):1703-1714.
398. Essenfelder GM, Larderet G, Waksman G, et al. Gene structure and promoter analysis of the human GJB6 gene encoding connexin 30. *Gene.* 2005;350(1):33-40.
399. Fujimoto A, Kurban M, Nakamura M, et al. GJB6, of which mutations underlie Clouston syndrome, is a potential direct target gene of p63. *J Dermatol Sci.* 2013;69(2):159-166.
400. Bosen F, Schutz M, Beinhauer A, et al. The Clouston syndrome mutation connexin30 A88V leads to hyperproliferation of sebaceous glands and hearing impairments in mice. *FEBS Lett.* 2014;588(9):1795-1801.
401. Berger AC, Kelly JJ, Lajoie P, et al. Mutations in Cx30 that are linked to skin disease and non-syndromic hearing loss exhibit several distinct cellular pathologies. *J Cell Sci.* 2014;127(Pt 8):1751-1764.
402. Kellermayer R, Keller M, Ratajczak P, et al. Bigenic connexin mutations in a patient with hidrotic ectodermal dysplasia. *Eur J Dermatol.* 2005;15(2):75-79.
403. Grifa A, Wagner CA, D'Ambrosio L, et al. Mutations in GJB6 cause nonsyndromic autosomal dominant deafness at DFNA3 locus. *Nat Genet.* 1999;23(1):16-18.
404. Huriez C, Deminati M, Agache P, et al. Scleroatrophying and keratodermic genodermatosis of the extremities. *Ann Dermatol Syphiligr (Paris).* 1969;96(2):135-146.
405. Guerriero C, Albanesi C, Girolomoni G, et al. Huriez syndrome: case report with a detailed analysis of skin dendritic cells. *Br J Dermatol.* 2000;143(5):1091-1096.
406. Hamm H, Traupe H, Brocker EB, et al. The scleroatrophic syndrome of Huriez: a cancer-prone genodermatosis. *Br J Dermatol.* 1996;134(3):512-518.
407. Kavanagh GM, Jardine PE, Peachey RD, et al. The scleroatrophic syndrome of Huriez. *Br J Dermatol.* 1997;137(1):114-118.
408. Lambert D, Planche H, Chapuis JL. Sclero-atrophic and keratodermic genodermatosis of the extremities. *Ann Dermatol Venereol.* 1977;104(10):654-657.
409. Watanabe E, Takai T, Ichihashi M, et al. A nonfamilial Japanese case of Huriez syndrome: p53 expression in squamous cell carcinoma. *Dermatology.* 2003;207(1):82-84.
410. Yesudian P, Premalatha S, Thambiah AS. Genetic tylosis with malignancy: a study of a South Indian pedigree. *Br J Dermatol.* 1980;102(5):597-600.
411. Vernole P, Terrinoni A, Didona B, et al. An SRY-negative XX male with Huriez syndrome. *Clin Genet.* 2000;57(1):61-66.
412. Kharge P, Fernendes C, Jairath V, et al. Poikiloderma a varied presentation—Huriez syndrome. *Indian Dermatol Online J.* 2015;6(1):27-30.
413. Patrizi A, Di Lernia V, Patrone P. Palmoplantar keratoderma with sclerodactyly (Huriez syndrome). *J Am Acad Dermatol.* 1992;26(5 Pt 2):855-857.
414. Levi F, Franceschi S, Te VC, et al. Trends of skin cancer in the Canton of Vaud, 1976-92. *Br J Cancer.* 1995;72(4):1047-1053.
415. Deminatti M, Delmas-Marsalet Y, Mennecier M, et al. Study of a probable linkage between a genodermatosis with an autosomal dominant transmission and the MNSs blood group system. *Ann Genet.* 1968;11(4):217-224.
416. Lee YA, Stevens HP, Delaporte E, et al. A gene for an autosomal dominant scleroatrophic syndrome predisposing to skin cancer (Huriez syndrome) maps to chromosome 4q23. *Am J Hum Genet.* 2000;66(1):326-330.
417. Hamon Y, Legowska M, Fergelot P, et al. Analysis of urinary cathepsin C for diagnosing Papillon-Lefevre syndrome. *FEBS J.* 2016;283(3):498-509.
418. Hart TC, Hart PS, Bowden DW, et al. Mutations of the cathepsin C gene are responsible for Papillon-Lefevre syndrome. *J Med Genet.* 1999;36(12):881-887.
419. Papillon M, Lefevre P. 2 Cases of symmetrically, familiarly palmar and plantar hyperkeratosis (Meleda disease) within brother and sister combined with severe dental alterations in both cases. 31, 82-84. *Bull Soc Fr Dermatol Syphiligr.* 1924;31:82-84.

420. Toomes C, James J, Wood AJ, et al. Loss-of-function mutations in the cathepsin C gene result in periodontal disease and palmoplantar keratosis. *Nat Genet.* 1999;23(4):421-424.
421. Wang X, Liu Y, Liu Y, et al. Long-term change of disease behavior in Papillon-Lefevre syndrome: seven years follow-up. *Eur J J Med Genet.* 2015;58(3):184-187.
422. Gorlin RJ, Sedano H, Anderson VE. The syndrome of palmar-plantar hyperkeratosis and premature periodontal destruction of the teeth. A clinical and genetic analysis of the Papillon-Lef'evre syndrome. *J Pediatr.* 1964;65:895-908.
423. Haneke E. The Papillon-Lefevre syndrome: keratosis palmoplantaris with periodontopathy. Report of a case and review of the cases in the literature. *Hum Genet.* 1979;51(1):1-35.
424. Dhanrajani PJ. Papillon-Lefevre syndrome: clinical presentation and a brief review. *Oral Surg Oral Med Oral Pathol Oral Radiol Endod.* 2009;108(1):e1-7.
425. Ullbro C, Crossner CG, Nederfors T, et al. Dermatologic and oral findings in a cohort of 47 patients with Papillon-Lefevre syndrome. *J Am Acad Dermatol.* 2003;48(3):345-351.
426. Pilger U, Hennies HC, Truschnegg A, et al. Late-onset Papillon-Lefevre syndrome without alteration of the cathepsin C gene. *J Am Acad Dermatol.* 2003;49(5 suppl):S240-S243.
427. Ragunatha S, Ramesh M, Anupama P, et al. Papillon-Lefevre syndrome with homozygous nonsense mutation of cathepsin C gene presenting with late-onset periodontitis. *Pediatr Dermatol.* 2015;32(2):292-294.
428. Kobayashi T, Sugiura K, Takeichi T, et al. The novel CTSC homozygous nonsense mutation p.Lys106X in a patient with Papillon-Lefevre syndrome with all permanent teeth remaining at over 40 years of age. *Br J Dermatol.* 2013;169(4):948-950.
429. Shanavas M, Chatra L, Shenai P, et al. Partial expression of the Papillon-Lefevre syndrome. *J Coll Physicians Surg Pak.* 2014;24(suppl 3):S230-S232.
430. Iqtadar S, Mumtaz SU, Abaidullah S. Papillon-Lefevre syndrome with palmoplantar keratoderma and periodontitis, a rare cause of pyrexia of unknown origin: a case report. *medical Med Case Rep.* 2015;9:288.
431. Almuneef M, Al Khenaizan S, Al Ajaji S, et al. Pyogenic liver abscess and Papillon-Lefevre syndrome: not a rare association. *Pediatrics.* 2003;111(1):e85-88.
432. Kanthimathinathan HK, Browne F, Ramirez R, et al. Multiple cerebral abscesses in Papillon-Lefevre syndrome. *Childs Nerv Syst.* 2013;29(8):1227-1229.
433. Wen X, Wang X, Duan X. High immunoglobulin E in a Chinese Papillon-Lefevre syndrome patient with novel compound mutations of cathepsin C. *J Dermatol.* 2012;39(7):664-665.
434. Li Z, Liu J, Fang S, et al. Novel compound heterozygous mutations in CTSC gene cause Papillon-Lefevre syndrome with high serum immunoglobulin E. *J Dermatol Sci.* 2014;76(3):258-260.
435. Nakajima K, Nakano H, Takiyoshi N, et al. Papillon-Lefevre syndrome and malignant melanoma. A high incidence of melanoma development in Japanese palmoplantar keratoderma patients. *Dermatology.* 2008;217(1):58-62.
436. Nagy N, Valyi P, Csoma Z, et al. CTSC and Papillon-Lefevre syndrome: detection of recurrent mutations in Hungarian patients, a review of published variants and database update. *Mol Genet Genom Med.* 2014;2(3):217-228.
437. Sulak A, Toth L, Farkas K, et al. One mutation, two phenotypes: a single nonsense mutation of the CTSC gene causes two clinically distinct phenotypes. *Clin Exp Dermatol.* 2016;41(2):190-195.
438. Hart TC, Hart PS, Michalec MD, et al. Haim-Munk syndrome and Papillon-Lefevre syndrome are allelic mutations in cathepsin C. *J Med Genet.* 2000;37(2):88-94.
439. Hart TC, Hart PS, Michalec MD, et al. Localisation of a gene for prepubertal periodontitis to chromosome 11q14 and identification of a cathepsin C gene mutation. *J Med Genet.* 2000;37(2):95-101.
440. Janjua SA, Iftikhar N, Hussain I, et al. Dermatologic, periodontal, and skeletal manifestations of Haim-Munk syndrome in two siblings. *J Am Acad Dermatol.* 2008;58(2):339-344.
441. Adkison AM, Raptis SZ, Kelley DG, et al. Dipeptidyl peptidase I activates neutrophil-derived serine proteases and regulates the development of acute experimental arthritis. *J Clin Invest.* 2002;109(3):363-371.
442. Dolenc I, Turk B, Pungercic G, et al. Oligomeric structure and substrate induced inhibition of human cathepsin C. *J Biol Chem.* 1995;270(37):21626-21631.
443. Meade JL, de Wynter EA, Brett P, et al. A family with Papillon-Lefevre syndrome reveals a requirement for cathepsin C in granzyme B activation and NK cell cytolytic activity. *Blood.* 2006;107(9):3665-3668.
444. Rawlings ND, Barrett AJ. Evolutionary families of peptidases. *Biochem J.* 1993;290 (Pt 1):205-218.
445. Turk D, Janjic V, Stern I, et al. Structure of human dipeptidyl peptidase I (cathepsin C): exclusion domain added to an endopeptidase framework creates the machine for activation of granular serine proteases. *EMBO J.* 2001;20(23):6570-6582.
446. Wolters PJ, Pham CT, Muilenburg DJ, et al. Dipeptidyl peptidase I is essential for activation of mast cell chymases, but not tryptases, in mice. *J Biol Chem.* 2001;276(21):18551-18556.
447. Rao NV, Rao GV, Hoidal JR. Human dipeptidyl-peptidase I. Gene characterization, localization, and expression. *J Biol Chem.* 1997;272(15):10260-10265.
448. Zhang Y, Hart PS, Moretti AJ, et al. Biochemical and mutational analyses of the cathepsin c gene (CTSC) in three North American families with Papillon Lefevre syndrome. *Hum Mutat.* 2002;20(1):75.
449. Sorensen OE, Clemmensen SN, Dahl SL, et al. Papillon-Lefevre syndrome patient reveals species-dependent requirements for neutrophil defenses. *J Clin Invest.* 2014;124(10):4539-4548.
450. McKoy G, Protonotarios N, Crosby A, et al. Identification of a deletion in plakoglobin in arrhythmogenic right ventricular cardiomyopathy with palmoplantar keratoderma and woolly hair (Naxos disease). *Lancet.* 2000;355(9221):2119-2124.
451. Protonotarios N, Tsatsopoulou A, Patsourakos P, et al. Cardiac abnormalities in familial palmoplantar keratosis. *Br Heart J.* 1986;56(4):321-326.
452. Bukhari I, Juma'a N. Naxos disease in Saudi Arabia. *J Eur Acad Dermatol Venereol.* 2004;18(5):614-616.
453. Meera G, Prabhavathy D, Jayakumar S, et al. Naxos disease in two siblings. *Int J Trichol.* 2010;2(1):53-55.
454. Narin N, Akcakus M, Gunes T, et al. Arrhythmogenic right ventricular cardiomyopathy (Naxos disease): report of a Turkish boy. *Pacing Clin Electrophysiol.* 2003;26(12):2326-2329.
455. Protonotarios N, Tsatsopoulou A, Anastasakis A, et al. Genotype-phenotype assessment in autosomal

455. recessive arrhythmogenic right ventricular cardiomyopathy (Naxos disease) caused by a deletion in plakoglobin. *J Am Coll Cardiol.* 2001;38(5): 1477-1484.
456. Protonotarios N, Tsatsopoulou A, Fontaine G. Naxos disease: keratoderma, scalp modifications, and cardiomyopathy. *J Am Acad Dermatol.* 2001;44(2): 309-311.
457. Coonar AS, Protonotarios N, Tsatsopoulou A, et al. Gene for arrhythmogenic right ventricular cardiomyopathy with diffuse nonepidermolytic palmoplantar keratoderma and woolly hair (Naxos disease) maps to 17q21. *Circulation.* 1998;97(20):2049-2058.
458. Basso C, Tsatsopoulou A, Thiene G, et al. "Petrified" right ventricle in long-standing naxos arrhythmogenic right ventricular cardiomyopathy. *Circulation.* 2001;104(23):E132-E133.
459. Gregoriou S, Kontochristopoulos G, Chatziolou E, et al. Palmoplantar keratoderma, woolly hair and arrhythmogenic right ventricular cardiomyopathy. *Clin Exp Dermatol.* 2006;31(2):315-316.
460. Protonotarios N, Tsatsopoulou A. Naxos disease and Carvajal syndrome: cardiocutaneous disorders that highlight the pathogenesis and broaden the spectrum of arrhythmogenic right ventricular cardiomyopathy. *Cardiovasc Path.* 2004;13(4):185-194.
461. Samuelov L, Sprecher E. Inherited desmosomal disorders. *Cell Tissue Res.* 2015;360(3):457-475.
462. Antoniades L, Tsatsopoulou A, Anastasakis A, et al. Arrhythmogenic right ventricular cardiomyopathy caused by deletions in plakophilin-2 and plakoglobin (Naxos disease) in families from Greece and Cyprus: genotype-phenotype relations, diagnostic features and prognosis. *Eur Heart J.* 2006;27(18): 2208-2216.
463. Cabral RM, Liu L, Hogan C, et al. Homozygous mutations in the 5′ region of the JUP gene result in cutaneous disease but normal heart development in children. *J Invest Dermatol.* 2010;130(6):1543-1550.
464. Asimaki A, Syrris P, Wichter T, et al. A novel dominant mutation in plakoglobin causes arrhythmogenic right ventricular cardiomyopathy. *Am J Hum Genet.* 2007;81(5):964-973.
465. Erken H, Yariz KO, Duman D, et al. Cardiomyopathy with alopecia and palmoplantar keratoderma (CAPK) is caused by a JUP mutation. *Br J Dermatol.* 2011;165(4):917-921.
466. Green KJ, Simpson CL. Desmosomes: new perspectives on a classic. *J Invest Dermatol.* 2007;127(11): 2499-2515.
467. Hobbs RP, Green KJ. Desmoplakin regulates desmosome hyperadhesion. *J Invest Dermatol.* 2012;132(2):482-485.
468. Nie Z, Merritt A, Rouhi-Parkouhi M, et al. Membrane-impermeable cross-linking provides evidence for homophilic, isoform-specific binding of desmosomal cadherins in epithelial cells. *J Biol Chem.* 2011;286(3):2143-2154.
469. Chitaev NA, Troyanovsky SM. Direct Ca2+-dependent heterophilic interaction between desmosomal cadherins, desmoglein and desmocollin, contributes to cell-cell adhesion. *J Cell Biol.* 1997;138(1):193-201.
470. Garrod D, Chidgey M. Desmosome structure, composition and function. *Biochim Biophys Acta.* 2008;1778(3):572-587.
471. Holthofer B, Windoffer R, Troyanovsky S, et al. Structure and function of desmosomes. *Int Rev Cytol.* 2007;264:65-163.
472. Simpson MA, Mansour S, Ahnood D, et al. Homozygous mutation of desmocollin-2 in arrhythmogenic right ventricular cardiomyopathy with mild palmoplantar keratoderma and woolly hair. *Cardiology.* 2009;113(1):28-34.
473. Ramot Y, Molho-Pessach V, Meir T, et al. Mutation in KANK2, encoding a sequestering protein for steroid receptor coactivators, causes keratoderma and woolly hair. *J Med Genet.* 2014;51(6):388-394.
474. Micali G, Nasca MR, Innocenzi D, et al. Association of palmoplantar keratoderma, cutaneous squamous cell carcinoma, dental anomalies, and hypogenitalism in four siblings with 46,XX karyotype: a new syndrome. *J Am Acad Dermatol.* 2005;53(5 suppl 1): S234-S239.
475. Radi O, Parma P, Imbeaud S, et al. XX sex reversal, palmoplantar keratoderma, and predisposition to squamous cell carcinoma: genetic analysis in one family. *Am J Med Genet A.* 2005;138A(3):241-246.
476. Tomaselli S, Megiorni F, De Bernardo C, et al. Syndromic true hermaphroditism due to an R-spondin1 (RSPO1) homozygous mutation. *Hum Mutat.* 2008;29(2):220-226.
477. Kim KA, Zhao J, Andarmani S, et al. R-Spondin proteins: a novel link to beta-catenin activation. *Cell Cycle.* 2006;5(1):23-26.
478. Parma P, Radi O, Vidal V, et al. R-spondin1 is essential in sex determination, skin differentiation and malignancy. *Nat Genet.* 2006;38(11):1304-1309.
479. Martin L, Toutain A, Guillen C, et al. Inherited palmoplantar keratoderma and sensorineural deafness associated with A7445G point mutation in the mitochondrial genome. *Br J Dermatol.* 2000;143(4): 876-883.
480. Sevior KB, Hatamochi A, Stewart IA, et al. Mitochondrial A7445G mutation in two pedigrees with palmoplantar keratoderma and deafness. *Am J Med Genet.* 1998;75(2):179-185.
481. Caria H, Matos T, Oliveira-Soares R, et al. A7445G mtDNA mutation present in a Portuguese family exhibiting hereditary deafness and palmoplantar keratoderma. *J Eur Acad Dermatol Venereol.* 2005;19(4):455-458.
482. Reid FM, Vernham GA, Jacobs HT. A novel mitochondrial point mutation in a maternal pedigree with sensorineural deafness. *Hum Mutat.* 1994;3(3):243-247.
483. Milingou M, Wood P, Masouye I, et al. Focal palmoplantar keratoderma caused by an autosomal dominant inherited mutation in the desmoglein 1 gene. *Dermatology.* 2006;212(2):117-122.
484. Nomura T, Mizuno O, Miyauchi T, et al. Striate palmoplantar keratoderma: report of a novel DSG1 mutation and atypical clinical manifestations. *J Dermatol Sci.* 2015;80(3):223-225.
485. Zamiri M, Smith FJ, Campbell LE, et al. Mutation in DSG1 causing autosomal dominant striate palmoplantar keratoderma. *Br J Dermatol.* 2009;161(3): 692-694.
486. Lovgren ML, McAleer MA, Irvine AD, et al. Mutations in desmoglein-1 cause diverse inherited palmoplantar keratoderma phenotypes: implications for genetic screening. *Br J Dermatol.* 2017;176(5):1345-1350.
487. Barber AG, Wajid M, Columbo M, et al. Striate palmoplantar keratoderma resulting from a frameshift mutation in the desmoglein 1 gene. *J Dermatol Sci.* 2007;45(3):161-166.
488. Dua-Awereh MB, Shimomura Y, Kraemer L, et al. Mutations in the desmoglein 1 gene in five Pakistani

families with striate palmoplantar keratoderma. *J Dermatol Sci.* 2009;53(3):192-197.
489. Hershkovitz D, Lugassy J, Indelman M, et al. Novel mutations in DSG1 causing striate palmoplantar keratoderma. *Clin Exp Dermatol.* 2009;34(2):224-228.
490. Hunt DM, Rickman L, Whittock NV, et al. Spectrum of dominant mutations in the desmosomal cadherin desmoglein 1, causing the skin disease striate palmoplantar keratoderma. *Eur J Hum Genet.* 2001;9(3):197-203.
491. Kljuic A, Gilead L, Martinez-Mir A, et al. A nonsense mutation in the desmoglein 1 gene underlies striate keratoderma. *Exp Dermatol.* 2003;12(4):523-527.
492. Keren H, Bergman R, Mizrachi M, et al. Diffuse nonepidermolytic palmoplantar keratoderma caused by a recurrent nonsense mutation in DSG1. *Arch Dermatol.* 2005;141(5):625-628.
493. Armstrong DK, McKenna KE, Purkis PE, et al. Haploinsufficiency of desmoplakin causes a striate subtype of palmoplantar keratoderma. *Hum Mol Genet.* 1999;8(1):143-148.
494. Rickman L, Simrak D, Stevens HP, et al. N-terminal deletion in a desmosomal cadherin causes the autosomal dominant skin disease striate palmoplantar keratoderma. *Hum Mol Genet.* 1999;8(6):971-976.
495. Whittock NV, Ashton GH, Dopping-Hepenstal PJ, et al. Striate palmoplantar keratoderma resulting from desmoplakin haploinsufficiency. *J Invest Dermatol.* 1999;113(6):940-946.
496. Samuelov L, Sarig O, Harmon RM, et al. Desmoglein 1 deficiency results in severe dermatitis, multiple allergies and metabolic wasting. *Nat Genet.* 2013;45(10):1244-1248.
497. Getsios S, Huen AC, Green KJ. Working out the strength and flexibility of desmosomes. *Nat Rev Mol Cell Biol.* 2004;5(4):271-281.
498. Dusek RL, Getsios S, Chen F, et al. The differentiation-dependent desmosomal cadherin desmoglein 1 is a novel caspase-3 target that regulates apoptosis in keratinocytes. *J Biol Chem.* 2006;281(6):3614-3624.
499. Green KJ, Gaudry CA. Are desmosomes more than tethers for intermediate filaments? *Nat Rev Mol Cell Biol.* 2000;1(3):208-216.
500. Hakimelahi S, Parker HR, Gilchrist AJ, et al. Plakoglobin regulates the expression of the anti-apoptotic protein BCL-2. *J Biol Chem.* 2000;275(15):10905-10911.
501. Harmon RM, Simpson CL, Johnson JL, et al. Desmoglein-1/Erbin interaction suppresses ERK activation to support epidermal differentiation. *J Clin Invest.* 2013;123(4):1556-1570.
502. Hammers CM, Stanley JR. Desmoglein-1, differentiation, and disease. *J Clin Invest.* 2013;123(4):1419-1422.
503. Wan H, South AP, Hart IR. Increased keratinocyte proliferation initiated through downregulation of desmoplakin by RNA interference. *Exp Cell Res.* 2007;313(11):2336-2344.
504. Bergman R, Hershkovitz D, Fuchs D, et al. Disadhesion of epidermal keratinocytes: a histologic clue to palmoplantar keratodermas caused by DSG1 mutations. *J Am Acad Dermatol.* 2010;62(1):107-113.
505. Miteva L, Schwartz RA. Hereditary keratosis palmoplantaris varians of Wachters (keratosis palmoplantaris striata et areata). *Acta Dermatovenerol Alp Pannonica Adriat.* 2010;19(1):33-37.
506. Miteva L, Dourmishev AL. Hereditary palmoplantar keratoderma with nail changes and periodontosis in a father and son. *Cutis.* 1999;63(2):65-68.
507. Paoli S, Mastrolorenzo A. Keratosis palmoplantaris varians of Wachters. *J Eur Acad Dermatol Venereol.* 1999;12(1):33-37.
508. Rubegni P, Poggiali S, Cuccia A, et al. Acral malignant melanoma and striated palmoplantar keratoderma (Brunauer-Fohs-Siemens syndrome): a fortuitous association? *Dermatol Surg.* 2004;30(12 Pt 2):1539-1542.
509. Wachters D. *Over de verschillende morphologische vormen van de keratosis palmoplantaris, in het bijzonder over de "keratosis palmoplantaris varians"* Leiden, The Netherlands: Leiden University; 1963.
510. Fartasch M, Vigneswaran N, Diepgen TL, et al. Abnormalities of keratinocyte maturation and differentiation in keratosis palmoplantaris striata. Immunohistochemical and ultrastructural study before and during etretinate therapy. *Am J Dermatopathol.* 1990;12(3):275-282.
511. Jackson AD, Lawler SD. Pachyonychia congenita; a report of six cases in one family, with a note on linkage data. *Ann Eugen.* 1951;16(2):142-146.
512. Jadassohn J, Lewandowski P. *Pachyonychia congenita: keratosis disseminata circumscripts (follicularis). Tylomata. Leukokeratosis linguae.* Berlin: Urban and Schwarzenberg; 1906.
513. McLean WH, Rugg EL, Lunny DP, et al. Keratin 16 and keratin 17 mutations cause pachyonychia congenita. *Nat Genet.* 1995;9(3):273-278.
514. Munro CS, Carter S, Bryce S, et al. A gene for pachyonychia congenita is closely linked to the keratin gene cluster on 17q12-q21. *J Med Genet.* 1994;31(9):675-678.
515. Smith FJ, Jonkman MF, van Goor H, et al. A mutation in human keratin K6b produces a phenocopy of the K17 disorder pachyonychia congenita type 2. *Hum Mol Genet.* 1998;7(7):1143-1148.
516. Kaspar RL. Challenges in developing therapies for rare diseases including pachyonychia congenita. *J Invest Dermatol Symp Proc.* 2005;10(1):62-66.
517. Wallis T, Poole CD, Hoggart B. Can skin disease cause neuropathic pain? A study in pachyonychia congenita. *Clin Exp Dermatol.* 2016;41(1):26-33.
518. Eliason MJ, Leachman SA, Feng BJ, et al. A review of the clinical phenotype of 254 patients with genetically confirmed pachyonychia congenita. *J Am Acad Dermatol.* 2012;67(4):680-686.
519. McLean WH, Hansen CD, Eliason MJ, et al. The phenotypic and molecular genetic features of pachyonychia congenita. *J Invest Dermatol.* 2011; 131(5):1015-1017.
520. Harris K, Hull PR, Hansen CD, et al. Transgrediens pachyonychia congenita (PC): case series of a nonclassical PC presentation. *Br J Dermatol.* 2012;166(1):124-128.
521. Goldberg I, Sprecher E, Schwartz ME, et al. Comparative study of high-resolution multifrequency ultrasound of the plantar skin in patients with various types of hereditary palmoplantar keratoderma. *Dermatology.* 2013;226(4):365-370.
522. Feng YG, Xiao SX, Ren XR, et al. Keratin 17 mutation in pachyonychia congenita type 2 with early onset sebaceous cysts. *Br J Dermatol.* 2003;148(3):452-455.
523. Guo H, Liu D, Wu J, et al. Pachyonychia congenita with corneal dystrophy. *J Dermatol.* 2013;40(8):681-682.
524. Wilson NJ, Perez ML, Vahlquist A, et al. Homozygous dominant missense mutation in keratin 17 leads to alopecia in addition to severe pachyonychia congenita. *J Invest Dermatol.* 2012;132(7):1921-1924.

525. Haber RM, Drummond D. Pachyonychia congenita with laryngeal obstruction. *Pediatr Dermatol.* 2011;28(4):429-432.
526. O'Toole EA, Kaspar RL, Sprecher E, et al. Pachyonychia congenita cornered: report on the 11th Annual International Pachyonychia Congenita Consortium Meeting. *Br J Dermatol.* 2014;171(5):974-977.
527. Shamsher MK, Navsaria HA, Stevens HP, et al. Novel mutations in keratin 16 gene underly focal non-epidermolytic palmoplantar keratoderma (NEPPK) in two families. *Hum Mol Genet.* 1995;4(10):1875-1881.
528. Liao H, Sayers JM, Wilson NJ, et al. A spectrum of mutations in keratins K6a, K16 and K17 causing pachyonychia congenita. *J Dermatol Sci.* 2007;48(3):199-205.
529. Paris F, Hurtado C, Azon A, et al. A new KRT16 mutation associated with a phenotype of pachyonychia congenita. *Exp Dermatol.* 2013;22(12):838-839.
530. Smith FJ, Fisher MP, Healy E, et al. Novel keratin 16 mutations and protein expression studies in pachyonychia congenita type 1 and focal palmoplantar keratoderma. *Exp Dermatol.* 2000;9(3):170-177.
531. Spaunhurst KM, Hogendorf AM, Smith FJ, et al. Pachyonychia congenita patients with mutations in KRT6A have more extensive disease compared with patients who have mutations in KRT16. *Br J Dermatol.* 2012;166(4):875-878.
532. Wilson NJ, Messenger AG, Leachman SA, et al. Keratin K6c mutations cause focal palmoplantar keratoderma. *J Invest Dermatol.* 2010;130(2):425-429.
533. Wee JS, Smith FJ, Wilson NJ, et al. Focal PPK secondary to a novel KRT6C mutation (Pachyonychia congenita-K6c). *J Eur Acad Dermatol Venereol.* 2016;30(8):1415-1416.
534. Moll R, Franke WW, Schiller DL, et al. The catalog of human cytokeratins: patterns of expression in normal epithelia, tumors and cultured cells. *Cell.* 1982;31(1):11-24.
535. Moll R, Moll I, Wiest W. Changes in the pattern of cytokeratin polypeptides in epidermis and hair follicles during skin development in human fetuses. *Differentiation.* 1982;23(2):170-178.
536. Wilson NJ, O'Toole EA, Milstone LM, et al. The molecular genetic analysis of the expanding pachyonychia congenita case collection. *Br J Dermatol.* 2014;171(2):343-355.
537. Haber RM, Rose TH. Autosomal recessive pachyonychia congenita. *Arch Dermatol.* 1986;122(8):919-923.
538. Pho LN, Smith FJ, Konecki D, et al. Paternal germ cell mosaicism in autosomal dominant pachyonychia congenita. *Arch Dermatol.* 2011;147(9):1077-1080.
539. Steinert PM, Yang JM, Bale SJ, et al. Concurrence between the molecular overlap regions in keratin intermediate filaments and the locations of keratin mutations in genodermatoses. *Biochem Biophys Res Commun.* 1993;197(2):840-848.
540. Godsel LM, Hobbs RP, Green KJ. Intermediate filament assembly: dynamics to disease. *Trends Cell Biol.* 2008;18(1):28-37.
541. Koster MI. Building models for keratin disorders. *J Invest Dermatol.* 2012;132(5):1324-1326.
542. Cao YA, Hickerson RP, Seegmiller BL, et al. Gene expression profiling in pachyonychia congenita skin. *J Dermatol Sci.* 2015;77(3):156-165.
543. Carabott F, Archer CB, Griffiths WA. Etretinate-responsive pachyonychia congenita. *Br J Dermatol.* 1988;119(4):551-553.
544. Gruber R, Edlinger M, Kaspar RL, et al. An appraisal of oral retinoids in the treatment of pachyonychia congenita. *J Am Acad Dermatol.* 2012;66(6):e193-199.
545. Soyuer U, Candan MF. Failure of etretinate therapy in pachyonychia congenita. *Br J Dermatol.* 1987;117(2):264.
546. Thomas DR, Jorizzo JL, Brysk MM, et al. Pachyonychia congenita. Electron microscopic and epidermal glycoprotein assessment before and during isotretinoin treatment. *Arch Dermatol.* 1984;120(11):1475-1479.
547. Gonzalez-Ramos J, Sendagorta-Cudos E, Gonzalez-Lopez G, et al. Efficacy of botulinum toxin in pachyonychia congenita type 1: report of two new cases. *Dermatol Ther.* 2016;29(1):32-36.
548. Goldberg I, Fruchter D, Meilick A, et al. Best treatment practices for pachyonychia congenita. *J Eur Acad Dermatol Venereol.* 2014;28(3):279-285.
549. Swartling C, Karlqvist M, Hymnelius K, et al. Botulinum toxin in the treatment of sweat-worsened foot problems in patients with epidermolysis bullosa simplex and pachyonychia congenita. *Br J Dermatol.* 2010;163(5):1072-1076.
550. Swartling C, Vahlquist A. Treatment of pachyonychia congenita with plantar injections of botulinum toxin. *Br J Dermatol.* 2006;154(4):763-765.
551. Hickerson RP, Leake D, Pho LN, et al. Rapamycin selectively inhibits expression of an inducible keratin (K6a) in human keratinocytes and improves symptoms in pachyonychia congenita patients. *J Dermatol Sci.* 2009;56(2):82-88.
552. Leachman SA, Hickerson RP, Schwartz ME, et al. First-in-human mutation-targeted siRNA phase Ib trial of an inherited skin disorder. *Mol Ther.* 2010;18(2):442-446.
553. Leachman SA, Hickerson RP, Hull PR, et al. Therapeutic siRNAs for dominant genetic skin disorders including pachyonychia congenita. *J Dermatol Sci.* 2008;51(3):151-157.
554. Kaspar RL, Leachman SA, McLean WH, et al. Toward a treatment for pachyonychia congenita: report on the 7th Annual International Pachyonychia Congenita Consortium meeting. *J Invest Dermatol.* 2011;131(5):1011-1014.
555. Smith FJ, Hickerson RP, Sayers JM, et al. Development of therapeutic siRNAs for pachyonychia congenita. *J Invest Dermatol.* 2008;128(1):50-58.
556. Hickerson RP, Smith FJ, McLean WH, et al. SiRNA-mediated selective inhibition of mutant keratin mRNAs responsible for the skin disorder pachyonychia congenita. *Ann N Y Acad Sci.* 2006;1082:56-61.
557. Trochet D, Prudhon B, Vassilopoulos S, et al. Therapy for dominant inherited diseases by allele-specific RNA interference: successes and pitfalls. *Curr Gene Ther.* 2015;15(5):503-510.
558. Howel-Evans W, McConnell RB, Clarke CA, et al. Carcinoma of the oesophagus with keratosis palmaris et plantaris (tylosis): a study of two families. *Q J Med.* 1958;27(107):413-429.
559. de Souza CA, Santos Ada C, Santos Lda C, et al. Hereditary tylosis syndrome and esophagus cancer. *An Bras Dermatol.* 2009;84(5):527-529.
560. Ellis A, Field JK, Field EA, et al. Tylosis associated with carcinoma of the oesophagus and oral leukoplakia in a large Liverpool family—a review of six generations. *Eur J Cancer B Oral Oncol.* 1994;30B(2):102-112.
561. Harper PS, Harper RM, Howel-Evans AW. Carcinoma of the oesophagus with tylosis. *Q J Med.* 1970;39(155):317-333.
562. Hennies HC, Hagedorn M, Reis A. Palmoplantar keratoderma in association with carcinoma of the

esophagus maps to chromosome 17q distal to the keratin gene cluster. *Genomics.* 1995;29(2):537-540.
563. Saarinen S, Vahteristo P, Lehtonen R, et al. Analysis of a Finnish family confirms RHBDF2 mutations as the underlying factor in tylosis with esophageal cancer. *Fam Cancer.* 2012;11(3):525-528.
564. Stevens HP, Kelsell DP, Bryant SP, et al. Linkage of an American pedigree with palmoplantar keratoderma and malignancy (palmoplantar ectodermal dysplasia type III) to 17q24. Literature survey and proposed updated classification of the keratodermas. *Arch Dermatol.* 1996;132(6):640-651.
565. Varela AB, Blanco Rodriguez MM, Boullosa PE, et al. Tylosis A with squamous cell carcinoma of the oesophagus in a Spanish family. *Eur J Gastroenterol Hepatol.* 2011;23(3):286-288.
566. Ellis A, Risk JM, Maruthappu T, et al. Tylosis with oesophageal cancer: diagnosis, management and molecular mechanisms. *Orphanet J Rare Dis.* 2015;10:126.
567. Grundmann JU, Weisshaar E, Franke I, et al. Lung carcinoma with congenital plantar keratoderma as a variant of Clarke-Howel-Evans syndrome. *Int J Dermatol.* 2003;42(6):461-463.
568. Simon M, Hagedorn M. The Clark-Howel-Evans-McConnell syndrome. Observations in one family over 5 generations. *Hautarzt.* 1997;48(11):800-805.
569. Kelsell DP, Risk JM, Leigh IM, et al. Close mapping of the focal non-epidermolytic palmoplantar keratoderma (PPK) locus associated with oesophageal cancer (TOC). *Hum Mol Genet.* 1996;5(6):857-860.
570. McQuibban GA, Saurya S, Freeman M. Mitochondrial membrane remodelling regulated by a conserved rhomboid protease. *Nature.* 2003;423(6939):537-541.
571. Lee MY, Nam KH, Choi KC. iRhoms; its functions and essential roles. *Biomol Ther (Seoul).* 2016;24(2):109-114.
572. Adrain C, Strisovsky K, Zettl M, et al. Mammalian EGF receptor activation by the rhomboid protease RHBDL2. *EMBO Rep.* 2011;12(5):421-427.
573. Adrain C, Zettl M, Christova Y, et al. Tumor necrosis factor signaling requires iRhom2 to promote trafficking and activation of TACE. *Science.* 2012;335(6065):225-228.
574. Blaydon DC, Etheridge SL, Risk JM, et al. RHBDF2 mutations are associated with tylosis, a familial esophageal cancer syndrome. *Am J Hum Genet.* 2012;90(2):340-346.
575. Wojnarowicz PM, Provencher DM, Mes-Masson AM, et al. Chromosome 17q25 genes, RHBDF2 and CYGB, in ovarian cancer. *Int J Oncol.* 2012; 40(6):1865-1880.
576. Zettl M, Adrain C, Strisovsky K, et al. Rhomboid family pseudoproteases use the ER quality control machinery to regulate intercellular signaling. *Cell.* 2011;145(1):79-91.
577. Brooke MA, Etheridge SL, Kaplan N, et al. iRHOM2-dependent regulation of ADAM17 in cutaneous disease and epidermal barrier function. *Hum Mol Genet.* 2014;23(15):4064-4076.
578. Maney SK, McIlwain DR, Polz R, et al. Deletions in the cytoplasmic domain of iRhom1 and iRhom2 promote shedding of the TNF receptor by the protease ADAM17. *Science Signal.* 2015;8(401):ra109.
579. Kitagawa Y, Ueda M, Ando N, et al. Further evidence for prognostic significance of epidermal growth factor receptor gene amplification in patients with esophageal squamous cell carcinoma. *Clin Cancer Res.* 1996;2(5):909-914.
580. Liu HB, Yang QC, Shen Y, et al. [Clinicopathological and prognostic significance of the expression of ADAM17 mRNA and protein in esophageal squamous cell carcinoma]. *Zhonghua Zhong Liu Za Zhi.* 2013;35(5):361-365.
581. Leemans CR, Braakhuis BJ, Brakenhoff RH. The molecular biology of head and neck cancer. *Nat Rev Cancer.* 2011;11(1):9-22.
582. Charfeddine C, Monastiri K, Mokni M, et al. Clinical and mutational investigations of tyrosinemia type II in Northern Tunisia: identification and structural characterization of two novel TAT mutations. *Mol Genet Metab.* 2006;88(2):184-191.
583. Maydan G, Andresen BS, Madsen PP, et al. TAT gene mutation analysis in three Palestinian kindreds with oculocutaneous tyrosinaemia type II; characterization of a silent exonic transversion that causes complete missplicing by exon 11 skipping. *J Inherit Metab Dis.* 2006;29(5):620-626.
584. Hanhart E. Neue Sonderformen von keratosis palmoplantaris, u.a.eine regelmaessigdominante mit systematisierten Lipomen, ferner 2 einfach-rezessive mit Schwachsinn und z.T.mit Hornhautveraenderungen des Auges (Ektodermatosyndrom). *Dermatologica.* 1947(94):286-308.
585. Richner H. Hornhautaffektion bei keratoma palmare et plantare hereditarium. *Klin Mbl Augenheilk.* 1938(100):9.
586. Minami-Hori M, Ishida-Yamamoto A, Katoh N, et al. Richner-Hanhart syndrome: report of a case with a novel mutation of tyrosine aminotransferase. *J Dermatol Sci.* 2006;41(1):82-84.
587. Culic V, Betz RC, Refke M, et al. Tyrosinemia type II (Richner-Hanhart syndrome): a new mutation in the TAT gene. *Eur J Med Genet.* 2011;54(3):205-208.
588. Li M, Yang L, Shi H, et al. Loss-of-function mutation in AAGAB in Chinese families with punctuate palmoplantar keratoderma. *Br J Dermatol.* 2013;169(1):168-171.
589. Brauer A. Uber eine besondere Form des hereditaeren Keratoms (keratoderma disseminatum hereditarium palmare et plantare). *Arch Dermatol Syph.* 1913;114:211-236.
590. Buschke A, Fischer W. Keratodermia mauculosa disseminate symmetrica palmaris and plantaris. *Ikonographia Dermatologica* 1910;51:183-192.
591. Giehl KA, Herzinger T, Wolff H, et al. Eight novel mutations confirm the role of AAGAB in punctate palmoplantar keratoderma type 1 (Buschke-Fischer-Brauer) and show broad phenotypic variability. *Acta Derm Venereol.* 2016;96(4):468-472.
592. Gokay S, Kendirci M, Soylu Ustkoyuncu P, et al. Tyrosinemia type II: novel mutations in the TAT gene in a boy with unusual presentation. *Pediatr Int.* 2016;58(10):1069-1072.
593. Pasternack SM, Betz RC, Brandrup F, et al. Identification of two new mutations in the TAT gene in a Danish family with tyrosinaemia type II. *Br J Dermatol.* 2009;160(3):704-706.
594. Legarda M, Wlodarczyk K, Lage S, et al. A large TAT deletion in a tyrosinaemia type II patient. *Mol Genet Metab.* 2011;104(3):407-409.
595. Natt E, Kida K, Odievre M, et al. Point mutations in the tyrosine aminotransferase gene in tyrosinemia type II. *Proc Natl Acad Sci U S A.* 1992;89(19):9297-9301.
596. Natt E, Westphal EM, Toth-Fejel SE, et al. Inherited and de novo deletion of the tyrosine aminotransferase

596. gene locus at 16q22.1—q22.3 in a patient with tyrosinemia type II. *Hum Genet.* 1987;77(4):352-358.
597. Rettenmeier R, Natt E, Zentgraf H, et al. Isolation and characterization of the human tyrosine aminotransferase gene. *Nucleic Acids Res.* 1990;18(13):3853-3861.
598. Scott CR. The genetic tyrosinemias. *Am J Med Genet C Semin Med Genet.* 2006;142C(2):121-126.
599. Hargrove JL, Scoble HA, Mathews WR, et al. The structure of tyrosine aminotransferase. Evidence for domains involved in catalysis and enzyme turnover. *J Biol Chem.* 1989;264(1):45-53.
600. Huhn R, Stoermer H, Klingele B, et al. Novel and recurrent tyrosine aminotransferase gene mutations in tyrosinemia type II. *Hum Genet.* 1998;102(3):305-313.
601. Bouyacoub Y, Zribi H, Azzouz H, et al. Novel and recurrent mutations in the TAT gene in Tunisian families affected with Richner-Hanhart syndrome. *Gene.* 2013;529(1):45-49.
602. Nouspikel T. DNA repair in mammalian cells: nucleotide excision repair: variations on versatility. *Cell Mol Life Sc.* 2009;66(6):994-1009.
603. Gipson IK, Anderson RA. Response of the lysosomal system of the corneal epithelium to tyrosine-induced cell injury. *J Histochem Cytochem.* 1977;25(12):1351-1362.
604. Gipson IK, Burns RP, Wolfe-Lande JD. Crystals in corneal epithelial lesions of tyrosine-fed rats. *Invest Ophthalmol.* 1975;14(12):937-941.
605. Goldsmith LA. Tyrosine-induced skin disease. *Br J Dermatol.* 1978;98(1):119-123.
606. Shimizu N, Ito M, Ito K, et al. Richner-Hanhart's syndrome. Electron microscopic study of the skin lesion. *Arch Dermatol.* 1990;126(10):1342-1346.
607. Bohnert A, Anton-Lamprecht I. Richner-Hanhart's syndrome: ultrastructural abnormalities of epidermal keratinization indicating a causal relationship to high intracellular tyrosine levels. *J Invest Dermatol.* 1982;79(2):68-74.
608. Viglizzo GM, Occella C, Bleidl D, et al. Richner-Hanhart syndrome (tyrosinemia II): early diagnosis of an incomplete presentation with unusual findings. *Pediatr Dermatol.* 2006;23(3):259-261.
609. Tallab TM. Richner-Hanhart syndrome: importance of early diagnosis and early intervention. *J Am Acad Dermatol.* 1996;35(5 Pt 2):857-859.
610. Farag TI. Dietetic therapy of Richner-Hanhart syndrome. *J R Soc Med.* 1993;86(8):495.
611. Meissner T, Betz RC, Pasternack SM, et al. Richner-Hanhart syndrome detected by expanded newborn screening. *Pediatr Dermatol.* 2008;25(3):378-380.
612. Fraser NG, MacDonald J, Griffiths WA, et al. Tyrosinaemia type II (Richner-Hanhart syndrome)—report of two cases treated with etretinate. *Clin Exp Dermatol.* 1987;12(6):440-443.
613. Crovato F, Desirello G, Gatti R, et al. Richner-Hanhart syndrome spares a plantar autograft. *Arch Dermatol.* 1985;121(4):539-540.
614. Carvajal-Huerta L. Epidermolytic palmoplantar keratoderma with woolly hair and dilated cardiomyopathy. *J Am Acad Dermatol.* 1998;39(3):418-421.
615. Rao BH, Reddy IS, Chandra KS. Familial occurrence of a rare combination of dilated cardiomyopathy with palmoplantar keratoderma and curly hair. *Indian Heart J.* 1996;48(2):161-162.
616. Alcalai R, Metzger S, Rosenheck S, et al. A recessive mutation in desmoplakin causes arrhythmogenic right ventricular dysplasia, skin disorder, and woolly hair. *J Am Coll Cardiol.* 2003;42(2):319-327.
617. Antonov NK, Kingsbery MY, Rohena LO, et al. Early-onset heart failure, alopecia, and cutaneous abnormalities associated with a novel compound heterozygous mutation in desmoplakin. *Pediatr Dermatol.* 2015;32(1):102-108.
618. Bitar F, Najjar T, Hayashi R, et al. A novel heterozygous mutation in desmoplakin gene in a Lebanese patient with Carvajal syndrome and tooth agenesis. *J Eur Acad Dermatol Venereol.* 2016;30(12):e217-e219.
619. Chalabreysse L, Senni F, Bruyere P, et al. A new hypo/oligodontia syndrome: Carvajal/Naxos syndrome secondary to desmoplakin-dominant mutations. *J Dent Res.* 2011;90(1):58-64.
620. Stollberger C, Vujic I, Wollmann E, et al. Carvajal syndrome with oligodontia, hypoacusis, recurrent infections, and noncompaction. *Int J Cardiol.* 2016;203:825-827.
621. Uzumcu A, Norgett EE, Dindar A, et al. Loss of desmoplakin isoform I causes early onset cardiomyopathy and heart failure in a Naxos-like syndrome. *J Med Genet.* 2006;43(2):e5.
622. Huber O. Structure and function of desmosomal proteins and their role in development and disease. *Cell Mol Life Sci.* 2003;60(9):1872-1890.
623. Alibardi L, Bernd N. Immunolocalization of junctional proteins in human hairs indicates that the membrane complex stabilizes the inner root sheath while desmosomes contact the companion layer through specific keratins. *Acta Histochem.* 2013;115(5):519-526.
624. Bierkamp C, Schwarz H, Huber O, et al. Desmosomal localization of beta-catenin in the skin of plakoglobin null-mutant mice. *Development.* 1999;126(2):371-381.
625. Brooke MA, Nitoiu D, Kelsell DP. Cell-cell connectivity: desmosomes and disease. *J Pathol.* 2012;226(2):158-171.
626. Molho-Pessach V, Sheffer S, Siam R, et al. Two novel homozygous desmoplakin mutations in Carvajal syndrome. *Pediatr Dermatol.* 2015;32(5):641-646.
627. Keller DI, Stepowski D, Balmer C, et al. De novo heterozygous desmoplakin mutations leading to Naxos-Carvajal disease. *Swiss medical weekly.* 2012;142:w13670.
628. Norgett EE, Lucke TW, Bowers B, et al. Early death from cardiomyopathy in a family with autosomal dominant striate palmoplantar keratoderma and woolly hair associated with a novel insertion mutation in desmoplakin. *J Invest Dermatol.* 2006;126(7):1651-1654.
629. Lesot H, Kieffer-Combeau S, Fausser JL, et al. Cell-cell and cell-matrix interactions during initial enamel organ histomorphogenesis in the mouse. *Connect tissue Res.* 2002;43(2-3):191-200.
630. Fausser JL, Schlepp O, Aberdam D, et al. Localization of antigens associated with adherens junctions, desmosomes, and hemidesmosomes during murine molar morphogenesis. *Differentiation.* 1998;63(1):1-11.
631. Jonkman MF, Pasmooij AM, Pasmans SG, et al. Loss of desmoplakin tail causes lethal acantholytic epidermolysis bullosa. *Am J Hum Genet.* 2005;77(4):653-660.
632. Rampazzo A, Nava A, Malacrida S, et al. Mutation in human desmoplakin domain binding to plakoglobin causes a dominant form of arrhythmogenic right ventricular cardiomyopathy. *Am J Hum Genet.* 2002;71(5):1200-1206.
633. Charfeddine C, Ktaifi C, Laroussi N, et al. Clinical and molecular investigation of Buschke-Fischer-Brauer

634. Eytan O, Sarig O, Israeli S, et al. A novel splice-site mutation in the AAGAB gene segregates with hereditary punctate palmoplantar keratoderma and congenital dysplasia of the hip in a large family. *Clin Exp Dermatol.* 2014;39(2):182-186.
635. Giehl KA, Eckstein GN, Pasternack SM, et al. Nonsense mutations in AAGAB cause punctate palmoplantar keratoderma type Buschke-Fischer-Brauer. *Am J Hum Genet.* 2012;91(4):754-759.
636. Poonawalla T, Xia L, Patten S, et al. Clouston syndrome and eccrine syringofibroadenomas. *Am J Dermatopathol.* 2009;31(2):157-161.
637. Stanimirovic A, Kansky A, Basta-Juzbasic A, et al. Hereditary palmoplantar keratoderma, type papulosa, in Croatia. *J Am Acad Dermatol.* 1993;29(3):435-437.
638. Kono M, Fukai K, Shimizu N, et al. Punctate palmoplantar keratoderma type 1 with a novel AAGAB frameshift mutation: intrafamilial phenotype variation due to aging. *J Eur Acad Dermatol Venereol.* 2017;31(3):e175-e176.
639. Guo BR, Zhang X, Chen G, et al. Exome sequencing identifies a COL14A1 mutation in a large Chinese pedigree with punctate palmoplantar keratoderma. *J Med Genet.* 2012;49(9):563-568.
640. Miljkovic J, Kansky A. Hereditary palmoplantar keratoderma type papulosa in Slovenia. *Acta Dermatovenerol Alp Pannonica Adriat.* 2009;18(3):114-116.
641. Pohler E, Mamai O, Hirst J, et al. Haploinsufficiency for AAGAB causes clinically heterogeneous forms of punctate palmoplantar keratoderma. *Nat Genet.* 2012;44(11):1272-1276.
642. Emmert S, Kuster W, Hennies HC, et al. 47 patients in 14 families with the rare genodermatosis keratosis punctata palmoplantaris Buschke-Fischer-Brauer. *Eur J Dermatol.* 2003;13(1):16-20.
643. Erkek E, Ayva S. Wood's light excites white fluorescence of type I hereditary punctate keratoderma. *J Eur Acad Dermatol Venereol.* 2007;21(7):993-994.
644. Gorynia S, Lorenz TC, Costaguta G, et al. Yeast Irc6p is a novel type of conserved clathrin coat accessory factor related to small G proteins. *Mol Biol Cell.* 2012;23(22):4416-4429.
645. Page LJ, Sowerby PJ, Lui WW, et al. Gamma-synergin: an EH domain-containing protein that interacts with gamma-adaptin. *J Cell Biol.* 1999;146(5):993-1004.
646. Brown FC. Punctate keratoderma. *Arch Dermatol.* 1971;104(6):682-683.
647. Lestringant GG, Berge T. Porokeratosis punctata palmaris et plantaris. A new entity? *Arch Dermatol.* 1989;125(6):816-819.
648. Sakas EL, Gentry RH. Porokeratosis punctata palmaris et plantaris (punctate porokeratosis). Case report and literature review. *J Am Acad Dermatol.* 1985;13(5 Pt 2):908-912.
649. Schiff BL, Hughes D. Palmoplantar keratosis acuminata with facial sebaceous hyperplasia. *Arch Dermatol.* 1974;109(1):86-87.
650. Erkek E, Atasoy P. Fluorescence of hereditary type II punctate porokeratotic keratoderma (spiny keratoderma) with a Wood's light: stars under the moonlight. *J Am Acad Dermatol.* 2007;57(2 suppl):S63-64.
651. Bianchi L, Orlandi A, Iraci S, et al. Punctate porokeratotic keratoderma—its occurrence with internal neoplasia. *Clin Exp Dermatol.* 1994;19(2):139-141.
652. Kondo S, Shimoura T, Hozumi Y, et al. Punctate porokeratotic keratoderma: some pathogenetic analyses of hyperproliferation and parakeratosis. *Acta Derm Venereol.* 1990;70(6):478-482.
653. Lewis KG, Bercovitch L, Dill SW, et al. Acquired disorders of elastic tissue: part II. decreased elastic tissue. *J Am Acad Dermatol.* 2004;51(2):165-185; quiz 186-168.
654. Costa OG. Akrokerato-elastoidosis; a hitherto undescribed skin disease. *Dermatologica.* 1953;107(3):164-168.
655. Hu W, Cook TF, Vicki GJ, et al. Acrokeratoelastoidosis. *Pediatr Dermatol.* 2002;19(4):320-322.
656. Johansson EA, Kariniemi AL, Niemi KM. Palmoplantar keratoderma of punctate type: acrokeratoelastoidosis Costa. *Acta Derm Venereol.* 1980;60(2):149-153.
657. Poiraud C, Vourc'h-Jourdain M, Cassagnau E, et al. Aquagenic palmoplantar keratoderma associated with acrokeratoelastoidosis. *Clin Exp Dermatol.* 2014;39(5):671-672.
658. Klekowski N, Shwayder T. Unilateral acrokeratoelastoidosis—second reported case. *Pediatr Dermatol.* 2011;28(1):20-22.
659. AlKahtani HS, AlHumidi AA, Al-Hargan AH, et al. A sporadic case of unilateral acrokeratoelastoidosis in Saudi Arabia: a case report. *J Med Case Rep.* 2014;8:143.
660. van Steensel MA, Verstraeten VL, Frank J. Acrokeratoelastoidosis with nail dystrophy: a coincidence or a new entity? *Arch Dermatol.* 2006;142(7):939-941.
661. Scuderi G, Palazzolo A, Massimino SD, et al. Costa's acrokeratoelastoidosis. Apropos of a sporadic case. *G Ital Dermatol Venereol.* 1990;125(10):465-469.
662. Tajima S, Tanaka N, Ishibashi A, et al. A variant of acrokeratoelastoidosis in systemic scleroderma: report of 7 cases. *J Am Acad Dermatol.* 2002; 46(5):767-770.
663. Yoshinaga E, Ohnishi Y, Tajima S. Acrokeratoelastoidosis associated with nodular scleroderma. *Eur J Dermatol.* 2003;13(5):490-492.
664. Khamaysi Z, Bergman R, Sprecher E. Nail dystrophy in focal acral hyperkeratosis: a distinctive feature? *J Eur Acad Dermatol Venereol.* 2008;22(7):891-893.
665. Dowd PM, Harman RR, Black MM. Focal acral hyperkeratosis. *Br J Dermatol.* 1983;109(1):97-103.
666. Rongioletti F, Betti R, Crosti C, et al. Marginal papular acrokeratodermas: a unified nosography for focal acral hyperkeratosis, acrokeratoelastoidosis and related disorders. *Dermatology.* 1994;188(1):28-31.
667. van Steensel MA, Frank J. Focal acral hyperkeratosis and acrokeratoelastoidosis: birds of a feather? *J Eur Acad Dermatol Venereol.* 2009;23(9):1113-1114.
668. Erkek E, Kocak M, Bozdogan O, et al. Focal acral hyperkeratosis: a rare cutaneous disorder within the spectrum of Costa acrokeratoelastoidosis. *Pediatr Dermatol.* 2004;21(2):128-130.
669. Matthews CN, Harman RR. Acrokerato-elastoidosis in a Somerset mother and her two sons. *Br J Dermatol.* 1977;97(suppl 15):42-43.
670. Parker CM. Tender linear lesions of the fingers. Acrokeratoelastoidosis (acquired type) or degenerative collagenous plaques of the hands. *Arch Dermatol.* 1991;127(1):114-115, 117-118.
671. Greiner J, Kruger J, Palden L, et al. A linkage study of acrokeratoelastoidosis. Possible mapping to chromosome 2. *Hum Genet.* 1983;63(3):222-227.
672. Jung EG. Acrokeratoelastoidosis. *Humangenetik.* 1973; 17(4):357-358.
673. Masse R, Quillard A, Hery B, et al. Costa's acrokeratoelastoidosis. Ultrastructural study (author's transl). *Ann Dermatol Venereol.* 1977;104(6-7):441-445.

674. Abulafia J, Vignale RA. Degenerative collagenous plaques of the hands and acrokeratoelastoidosis: pathogenesis and relationship with knuckle pads. *Int J Dermatol.* 2000;39(6):424-432.
675. Cole LA. Hypopigmentation with punctate keratosis of the palms and soles. *Arch Dermatol.* 1976;112(7):998-1000.
676. Moore MM, Orlow SJ, Kamino H, et al. Cole disease: guttate hypopigmentation and punctate palmoplantar keratoderma. *Arch Dermatol.* 2009;145(4):495-497.
677. Schmieder A, Hausser I, Schneider SW, et al. Palmoplantar hyperkeratoses and hypopigmentation. Cole disease. *Acta Derm Venereol.* 2011;91(6):737-738.
678. Vignale R, Yusin A, Panuncio A, et al. Cole disease: hypopigmentation with punctate keratosis of the palms and soles. *Pediatr Dermatol.* 2002;19(4):302-306.
679. Eytan O, Morice-Picard F, Sarig O, et al. Cole disease results from mutations in ENPP1. *Am J Hum Genet.* 2013;93(4):752-757.
680. Schlipf NA, Traupe H, Gilaberte Y, et al. Association of Cole disease with novel heterozygous mutations in the somatomedin-B domains of the ENPP1 gene: necessary, but not always sufficient. *Br J Dermatol.* 2016;174(5):1152-1156.
681. Goding JW, Grobben B, Slegers H. Physiological and pathophysiological functions of the ecto-nucleotide pyrophosphatase/phosphodiesterase family. *Biochim Biophys Acta.* 2003;1638(1):1-19.
682. Jansen S, Perrakis A, Ulens C, et al. Structure of NPP1, an ectonucleotide pyrophosphatase/phosphodiesterase involved in tissue calcification. *Structure.* 2012;20(11):1948-1959.
683. Lorenz-Depiereux B, Schnabel D, Tiosano D, et al. Loss-of-function ENPP1 mutations cause both generalized arterial calcification of infancy and autosomal-recessive hypophosphatemic rickets. *Am J Hum Genet.* 2010;86(2):267-272.
684. Nitschke Y, Baujat G, Botschen U, et al. Generalized arterial calcification of infancy and pseudoxanthoma elasticum can be caused by mutations in either ENPP1 or ABCC6. *Am J Hum Genet.* 2012;90(1):25-39.
685. Rutsch F, Ruf N, Vaingankar S, et al. Mutations in ENPP1 are associated with 'idiopathic' infantile arterial calcification. *Nat Genet.* 2003;34(4):379-381.
686. Kato K, Nishimasu H, Okudaira S, et al. Crystal structure of Enpp1, an extracellular glycoprotein involved in bone mineralization and insulin signaling. *Proc Natl Acad Sci U S A.* 2012;109(42):16876-16881.
687. Maddux BA, Goldfine ID. Membrane glycoprotein PC-1 inhibition of insulin receptor function occurs via direct interaction with the receptor alpha-subunit. *Diabetes.* 2000;49(1):13-19.
688. Boissy RE. Melanosome transfer to and translocation in the keratinocyte. *Exp Dermatol.* 2003;12(suppl 2):5-12.
689. Edmondson SR, Murashita MM, Russo VC, et al. Expression of insulin-like growth factor binding protein-3 (IGFBP-3) in human keratinocytes is regulated by EGF and TGFbeta1. *J Cell Physiol.* 1999;179(2):201-207.
690. Hyun E, Ramachandran R, Cenac N, et al. Insulin modulates protease-activated receptor 2 signaling: implications for the innate immune response. *J Immunol.* 2010;184(5):2702-2709.
691. Stachelscheid H, Ibrahim H, Koch L, et al. Epidermal insulin/IGF-1 signalling control interfollicular morphogenesis and proliferative potential through Rac activation. *EMBO J.* 2008;27(15):2091-2101.
692. Kim JM, Cho HH, Ko HC. Cole disease: a case report and literature review. *J Eur Acad Dermatol Venereol.* 2015;29(12):2492-2493.

Chapter 49 :: Keratosis Pilaris and Other Follicular Keratotic Disorders
:: Anna L. Bruckner

第四十九章
毛周角化病和其他毛囊性角化疾病

中文导读

本章重点介绍了毛周角化病，它是一种常见的良性毛囊角化病，文中详细讲述了其临床表现、病因及发病机制、诊断、鉴别诊断、临床过程、预后及管理。此外，本节还综述了萎缩性毛周角化病、KFSD/IFAP 综合征、小棘毛壅症的特征、病因、诊断及治疗。

〔粟 娟〕

This chapter discusses conditions with the common finding of *follicular keratosis*, defined as orthokeratosis of the follicular ostium and infundibulum. Keratotic plugs protrude from the orifices, producing a rough sensation on palpation of the skin. Keratosis pilaris (KP) is a common, benign form of follicular keratosis; less common variants are associated with follicular inflammation, atrophy, scarring, alopecia, and in rare cases noncutaneous abnormalities. Trichodysplasia spinulosa (TS), a recently described, virally induced follicular dysplasia with similar findings, is also reviewed.

KERATOSIS PILARIS

AT-A-GLANCE

- Common condition of keratotic follicular plugging with variable erythema.
- Mainly involves the cheeks, extensor arms, and thighs.
- Usually improves gradually over years.
- Nonspecific histology of hyperkeratosis distending the follicular orifice.
- Variable response to emollients and keratolytics.
- Variants:
  - Keratosis pilaris rubra: erythema extends beyond perifollicular skin.
  - Erythromelanosis follicularis faciei et colli: erythema and hyperpigmentation.

KP is a common condition characterized by keratotic follicular papules with varying degrees of surrounding erythema. It is common in children and can improve by late adolescence but is often persistent.[1] Studies of healthy school-aged children suggest a prevalence of 1% to 34%.[2-7] The prevalence is higher in populations with associated conditions.

CLINICAL FEATURES

The primary lesions of KP are small (typically 1-mm), keratotic, follicular papules with varying degrees of perifollicular erythema. Expression ranges from a subtle, incidental finding to conspicuous and aesthetically displeasing, often because of striking erythema.

Affected areas include the lateral cheeks, extensor aspects of the upper arms (Fig. 49-1), thighs, and buttocks, and it rarely may be more extensive, extending to the distal limbs and the trunk. Whereas in younger children, the face and arms are mainly involved, the extensor arms and legs are favored in adolescents and adults.

KP is likely accentuated by environmental factors such as ambient humidity. Many with KP experience improvement during the summer as opposed to the winter months or after moving from arid to more humid climates.

Keratosis pilaris rubra (KPR, also called keratosis follicularis rubra) is a variant of KP in which erythema is markedly noticeable, extending beyond the perifollicular skin.[8] Findings are usually limited to the cheeks (Fig. 49-2), forehead, and neck. *Erythromelanosis follicularis faciei et colli* (EFFC) is a similar and likely related condition characterized by hyperpigmentation in addition to erythema and follicular papules.[9] It involves the preauricular and maxillary areas, usually in a symmetric distribution, with spread in some cases to the temples and sides of the neck (the suffix "colli" refers to the neck) and trunk. EFFC is seen primarily in adolescents and young adults, most commonly in males. The hyperpigmentation noted in EFFC may be related to intrinsic skin pigmentation because darker skin types show more evidence of hyperpigmentation (Fig. 49-3). Thus, it is likely that KPR and EFFC are variants of the same clinical spectrum.

ASSOCIATIONS OF KERATOSIS PILARIS

KP is strongly associated with ichthyosis vulgaris (IV) and atopic dermatitis (AD), although the association with AD is not independent of IV.[7,10,11] Other conditions in which KP is more prevalent or more prominent include hypothyroidism, Cushing syndrome, insulin-dependent diabetes, obesity or high body mass index,[12] and Down syndrome. The association of KP with Noonan syndrome (NS) and cardiofaciocutaneous (CFC) syndrome is discussed in the following section. Generalized KP-

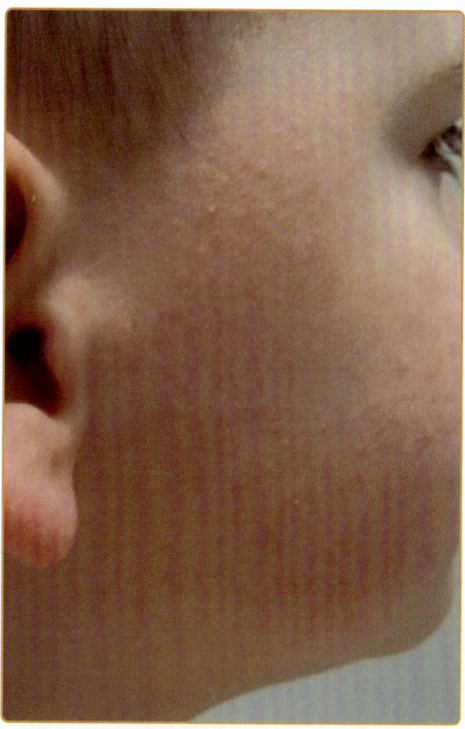

Figure 49-2 Keratosis pilaris rubra with dramatic perifollicular erythema on the cheeks.

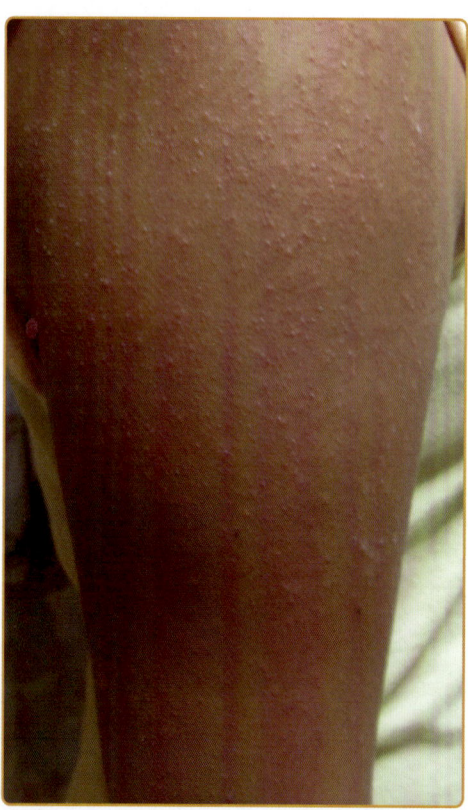

Figure 49-1 Keratosis pilaris in a characteristic distribution on the upper outer arm in a child.

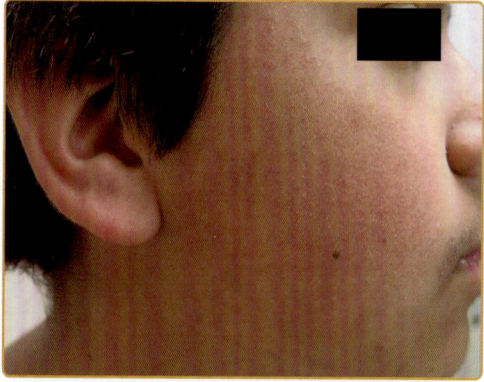

Figure 49-3 Keratosis pilaris rubra with overlapping features of erythromelanosis follicularis faciei et colli in an adolescent with darker skin.

like skin changes have recently been described as a common cutaneous side effect of RAF inhibition.[13]

ETIOLOGY AND PATHOGENESIS

The etiology and pathogenesis of KP are not well understood, and the clinical phenotype may arise by more than one mechanism. KP has been postulated to arise because of defective keratinization of the follicular epithelium. Follicular hyperkeratosis could arise because of mutations in *FLG* (the cause of IV), hyperandrogenism, insulin resistance, or other genetic or metabolic abnormalities. More recent alternative hypotheses include a hair shaft defect or sebaceous etiology. In a study of 25 patients with KP, Thomas and Khopkar identified coiled hair shafts in lesional KP skin, suggesting KP is primarily caused by a hair shaft defect.[14] Gruber and colleagues found atrophic or absent sebaceous glands in KP samples from 20 patients and postulated that this feature could result in follicular plugging and hair shaft defects.[15]

DIAGNOSIS

KP is typically a straightforward clinical diagnosis based on lesional morphology and distribution. Dermoscopic findings of thin, short hair shafts that are coiled or twisted within the follicular ostia are supportive.[14,15]

Biopsy is usually not needed, and the histologic findings are nonspecific. Varying degrees of follicular hyperkeratosis, dilation of the upper dermal vessels, perivascular lymphocytic inflammation, and atrophy or absence of sweat glands are appreciated. In EFFC, hyperpigmentation of the basal layer is also seen.

DIFFERENTIAL DIAGNOSIS

Typical KP should be distinguished from other disorders in the KP spectrum and from other causes of follicular keratosis. Table 49-1 reviews a differential for follicular keratosis.

TABLE 49-1
Differential Diagnosis of Follicular Keratosis

DISORDER	CONSIDERATIONS
Keratosis pilaris	Common; affects lateral cheeks, arms, and legs; associated with xerosis, ichthyosis vulgaris, atopic dermatitis
Ulerythema ophryogenes	Uncommon; loss of eyebrows; strongly associated with Noonan syndrome and cardiofaciocutaneous syndrome
Atrophoderma vermiculatum	Uncommon; honeycomb atrophy affects cheeks
Keratosis follicularis spinulosa decalvans or ichthyosis follicularis, alopecia, and photophobia syndrome	Rare; X-linked; triad of follicular hyperkeratosis, alopecia or atrichia, photophobia
Atrichia with papular lesions	Rare; autosomal recessive; scalp hair fails to regrow after being shed in infancy; follicular plugs or cysts appear later
Hereditary mucoepithelial dysplasia	Rare; autosomal dominant; follicular keratosis, psoriasiform intertrigo, alopecia, fiery-red mucosa, photophobia, pulmonary disease; presumed abnormality of desmosomes or gap junctions
Keratitis, ichthyosis, deafness syndrome	Rare; autosomal dominant; mutations in *GJB2*; characteristic sandpaper-like keratoderma; sensorineural hearing loss
Lichen planopilaris (and Graham Little-Piccardi-Lassueur syndrome)	Adult onset; favors women; keratotic plugs surrounded by violaceous erythema; scarring alopecia
Lichen spinulosus	Round to oval groups of keratotic follicular papules
Monilethrix	Rare; autosomal dominant; characteristic "beaded" pattern of hair on microscopy; perifollicular erythema and follicular keratosis are common; nail changes may occur
Phrynoderma	Caused by vitamin A deficiency; xerosis, keratotic plugs, abnormal hair; ocular disease; poor growth; increased risk of infection-related mortality
Pityriasis rubra pilaris	Erythematous follicular papules; lesions coalesce into plaques with "islands of sparing"; orange-red keratoderma
Trichostasis spinulosa	Comedo-like lesions composed of keratin and vellus hairs; middle to lower central face affected
Trichodysplasia spinulosa	Uncommon; associated with immune suppression; keratotic papules with spiny follicular spicules; most commonly affects central face; variable alopecia (mainly of eyebrows)

CLINICAL COURSE, PROGNOSIS, AND MANAGEMENT

KP tends to improve by adolescence or early adulthood, but it persists into later adult life in at least one third of patients.[1] Patients should be counseled about the benign nature of KP, and expectations should be tempered because treatment may minimize the symptoms but does not eradicate the condition. Most treatments address the rough texture of the skin. Simple steps such as avoiding drying or irritating skin care products and the regular use of bland emollients are reasonable first steps, especially in young children. Keratolytic preparations containing urea, lactic acid, or salicylic acid may soften and smooth KP. Patients should be counseled about the potential burning or stinging sensation of acidic products. Topical retinoids may also be tried if keratolytics are not helpful, but these preparations may aggravate associated erythema, limiting their value. Gentle mechanical exfoliation may also help but has the potential to cause irritation as well.

Short courses of low-potency topical corticosteroids calm irritation and itch that may be seen with KP. Patients should be counseled that corticosteroids do not improve the keratotic plugging, however.

Treatment with vascular- or pigment-specific lasers modestly improves the erythema or hyperpigmentation associated with KP. In a small, randomized clinical trial, Ibrahim and colleagues found a modest reduction in the roughness or bumpiness of KP after three treatments with an 810-nm diode laser. Erythema was unchanged, and long-term outcomes were not evaluated.[16]

KERATOSIS PILARIS ATROPHICANS

AT-A-GLANCE

- Conditions in the keratosis pilaris (KP) spectrum with variable degrees of inflammation and secondary atrophic scarring, alopecia, or both.
- Ulerythema ophryogenes (KP atrophicans faciei) predominantly affects the eyebrow area, causing scarring alopecia.
- Commonly seen in patients with Noonan and cardiofaciocutaneous syndromes
- Atrophoderma vermiculatum predominantly involves the cheeks and leads to a striking honeycomb-like atrophy.

Keratosis pilaris atrophicans (KPA) is a group of rare disorders characterized by follicular keratosis; inflammation; and secondary atrophic scarring, alopecia, or both. The umbrella of KPA has classically covered three clinical entities: ulerythema ophryogenes (UO; also called keratosis pilaris atrophicans faciei [KPAF]), atrophoderma vermiculatum (AV; also called folliculitis ulerythematosa reticulata), and keratosis follicularis spinulosa decalvans (KFSD). Recent work has shown that KFSD is allelic to ichthyosis follicularis, atrichia, and photophobia (IFAP) syndrome, and these two disorders will be discussed in the following section.

KPAF was originally described by Erasmus Wilson in 1878 as folliculitis rubra, and the term *ulerythema ophryogenes*, referring to scarring of the eyebrows, was coined by Taenzer in 1889. AV was originally described by Unna as ulerythema acneiforme in 1894.

CLINICAL FEATURES

UO particularly affects the eyebrows. The onset is in infancy, with erythema and small keratotic follicular papules involving the lateral third of the eyebrows. It may slowly progress through childhood to involve more of the eyebrows, leading to alopecia (Fig. 49-4). Progression usually ceases after puberty, but the sequelae are permanent. Involvement of the cheeks and forehead can occur, but the scalp and eyelash hair are normal. UO is frequently associated with typical KP affecting the arms, legs, or a more generalized distribution. The term *UO* is used interchangeably with *KPAF*, but some prefer the diagnosis of KPAF for patients in whom the initial erythema starts on the cheeks as opposed to the eyebrows.

The characteristic findings of AV are erythema and follicular plugging on the cheeks that progresses to reticular, atrophic scarring (Fig. 49-5). Descriptors such as "worm-eaten" and "honeycomb" aptly capture the

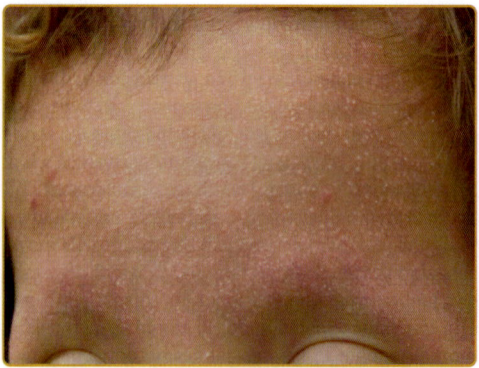

Figure 49-4 Ulerythema ophryogenes involving the forehead and eyebrows in a child with Noonan syndrome. Note the near complete alopecia of the eyebrows.

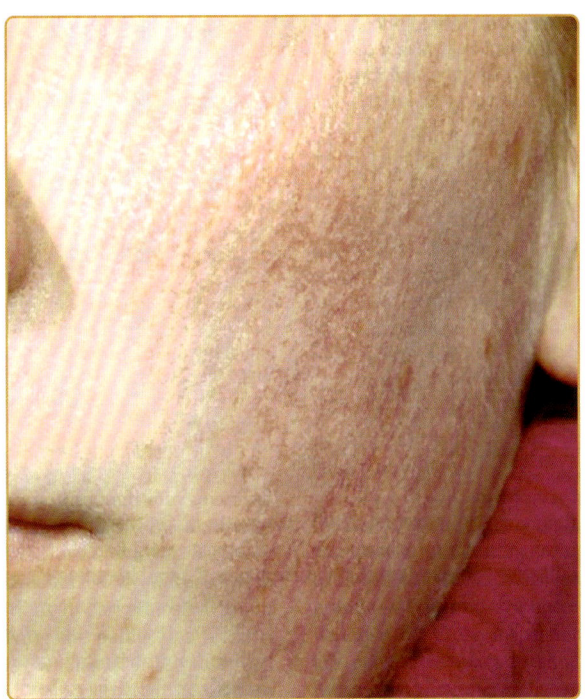

Figure 49-5 Atrophoderma vermiculatum demonstrating honeycomb atrophy on the cheek of an adolescent girl.

morphology. In addition to the cheeks, the forehead, ears, upper lip, and rarely the neck and extremities can be affected as well. Alopecia is not a feature of AV. Sparse open and closed comedones and milia may be found. Typical KP of the extensor aspects of arms and legs is common. AV usually starts in childhood, between 5 and 12 years old, although later onset has also been described.[17] The condition is often sporadic, although an affected father and daughter have been reported, suggesting possible autosomal dominant inheritance.[18] A handful of unilateral, somewhat linear cases have been described, suggesting a mosaic form of the condition (Fig. 49-6).[19] These cases seem to present in infancy, and two have been associated with ipsilateral congenital cataracts.[19,20]

An autosomal recessive form of KPA with overlapping features of AV and KFSD has been described in four children from a large, consanguineous Pakistani family.[21]

SYNDROMES ASSOCIATED WITH ULERYTHEMA OPHRYOGENES AND KERATOSIS PILARIS ATROPHICANS

Although UO may be seen as an isolated finding in otherwise healthy individuals, KP and UO are strongly associated with NS and CFC syndrome. About 80% of patients with genetically confirmed CFC have KP, and 90% have UO.[22] NS affects 1 in 1000 to 2000 newborns, but CFC is quite rare.[23] Both are inherited in an autosomal dominant manner. There is significant overlap in the phenotype of NS and CFC, which includes characteristic craniofacial dysmorphism, congenital cardiac defects, neurocognitive delays, and short stature. Hair anomalies, including sparse, curly, woolly, or brittle hair, are described.

UO has also been reported in association with isolated woolly hair,[24] Rubinstein-Taybi syndrome,[25] Cornelia de Lange syndrome,[26] and 18p monosomy.[27] A family with KP, UO, and koilonychia without evidence of monilethrix has been described.[28]

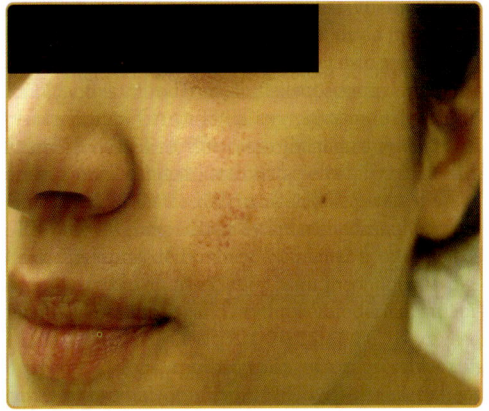

Figure 49-6 Curvilinear follicular atrophy. This finding had been present since early childhood and was stable.

The occurrence of AV in patients with Loeys-Dietz syndrome caused by mutations in *TGFBR2* was recently described.[29] AV-like changes have been reported in adolescents with autosomal dominant hyper-IgE syndrome caused by mutations in *STAT3*.[30]

ETIOLOGY AND PATHOGENESIS

Although the etiology and pathogenesis of UO and AV are not well understood, insights from associated disorders may be informative. NS and CFC are RASopathies, disorders arising because of mutations in genes that encode components or regulators of the Ras–MAPK (mitogen-activated protein kinase) pathway that regulates the cell cycle, cellular growth, differentiation, and senescence.[23] Activating mutations in seven genes have been implicated in NS, the most common being *PTPN11*, *SOS1*, *RAF1*, and *KRAS*. CFC is caused by activating mutations in the *BRAF*, *KRAS*, *MAP2K1*, and *MAP2K2* genes.

A homozygous missense mutation in the *LRP1* gene was identified in the Pakistani family with KPA with features of AV and KFSD. The encoded protein, LRP1, is a multifunctional cell surface receptor that belongs to the low-density lipoprotein receptor family. The pathogenesis of how decreased LRP1 activity produces the phenotype is unclear, and an aberrant inflammatory response or altered follicular adhesion has been hypothesized.[21]

DIAGNOSIS

Like KP, UO and AV are clinical diagnoses. Histologic findings are supportive but not pathognomonic. Follicular hyperkeratosis with atrophy of the pilosebaceous units and varying degrees of perifollicular and perivascular inflammation and perifollicular fibrosis are seen.

DIFFERENTIAL DIAGNOSIS

Follicular atrophy may occur secondary to inflammatory disorders of the pilosebaceous unit such as acne. Table 49-2 reviews other conditions and syndromes in which follicular atrophoderma is a prominent feature.

CLINICAL COURSE, PROGNOSIS, AND MANAGEMENT

Although the progression of UO and AV remit, the resultant changes of alopecia and atrophic scarring are permanent and can negatively impact self-esteem. Unfortunately, the response to therapy is poor for patients with both disorders. Topical options include corticosteroids or calcineurin inhibitors to address inflammation and keratolytics or retinoids for the follicular plugging.[31] Modest improvement with oral

TABLE 49-2
Syndromes Associated with Follicular Atrophoderma

CONDITION	INHERITANCE	MAIN FEATURES	COMMENTS
Bazex syndrome (Bazex-Dupre-Christol syndrome)	X-linked dominant	Hypotrichosis, pili torti, hypohidrosis, milia, development of basal cell carcinomas in adolescence	—
Rombo syndrome	Autosomal dominant	Hypotrichosis, especially of eyelashes; peripheral cyanosis; basal cell carcinomas and trichoepitheliomas	—
Conradi-Hunermann-Happle syndrome (X-linked dominant chondrodysplasia punctate)	X-linked dominant, lethal in males	Congenital onset; blaschkoid erythema with adherent scale; lesions resolve in months, replaced by follicular atrophoderma; cataracts, shortening of limbs, frontal bossing, saddle nose, low-set ears	Mutation in *EBP*, encoding emopamil-binding protein, relevant in cholesterol biosynthesis
Congenital ichthyosis, follicular atrophoderma, hypotrichosis, and hypohidrosis	Autosomal recessive	Congenital, diffuse ichthyosis, hypohidrosis, hypotrichosis; woolly hair in one pedigree	Described in consanguineous families; mutations in *ST14*, encoding matriptase, identified
Nevus comedonicus	Somatic mutation	Blaschkoid distribution of comedo-like plugs in dilated follicular orifices; cribriform atrophy follows extrusion of comedones	Mutations in *FGFR2*, identified in lesional skin (germline mutations in *FGFR2* cause Apert syndrome)

isotretinoin has been reported.[32,33] Pulsed-dye laser may improve the associated erythema, and laser resurfacing can be considered to correct scarring when the condition is quiescent.

KERATOSIS FOLLICULARIS SPINULOSA DECALVANS AND ICHTHYOSIS FOLLICULARIS, ATRICHIA, AND PHOTOPHOBIA SYNDROME

AT-A-GLANCE

- Ultra rare, X-linked disorders characterized by the triad of follicular hyperkeratosis, alopecia or atrichia, and photophobia
- Whereas progressive, scarring alopecia that begins in childhood is seen in KFSD, nonscarring, congenital atrichia is seen in IFAP.
- Females are variably affected with manifestations in a mosaic pattern following the lines of Blaschko.

The term *keratosis follicularis spinulosa decalvans* (KFSD) was first used by Siemens in 1926, who described a scarring follicular condition in a German family and several Dutch cases. IFAP was first reported as a syndrome by McLeod in 1909.

CLINICAL FEATURES

KFSD and IFAP share the features of follicular hyperkeratosis (ichthyosis), alopecia or atrichia, and photophobia. There is significant overlap between the phenotypes, and differentiation on clinical grounds may be difficult. In general, the KFSD phenotype is less severe than IFAP and is distinguished by the hallmark of progressive scarring alopecia. Inheritance of both disorders is X-linked. Males are fully affected, but expression in females varies and follows the lines of Blaschko.

KFSD begins in infancy with spiny lesions affecting hair-bearing areas, especially the scalp (Fig. 49-7), and later the eyebrows, eyelashes, and elsewhere. Varying degrees of inflammation are seen. Progressive, scarring alopecia presents in childhood and continues through adolescence. It is often patchy and is rarely total. Facial lanugo hair is absent, and axillary and pubic hair is often thinned. Associated nail dystrophy and hyperkeratosis of the elbows, knees, palms, and soles occurs.

Ocular findings include photophobia, punctate corneal epithelial defects, corneal dystrophy, and blepharitis.

A variant of KFSD called *folliculitis spinulosa decalvans* is characterized by persistent pustule formation, especially on the scalp.[34] Unlike KFSD, there is more severe inflammation, and alopecia is progressive after puberty. In addition, inheritance appears to be autosomal dominant.

In IFAP syndrome, noninflammatory, spiny, follicular projections occur in a generalized distribution with a predilection for the extensor surfaces and scalp, imparting a rough, "nutmeg-grater" texture to the skin. A lamellar ichthyotic variant has been described, and psoriasiform plaques, keratoderma, angular cheilitis, nail dystrophy, and periungal inflammation may be seen as well.[35] Nonscarring congenital atrichia, often complete, involves the scalp, eyebrows, eyelashes, and body hair. Affected neonates can be born with hair, but their hair does not grow back after being shed in the first few months after birth.

Photophobia can present in infancy or childhood and is thought to arise from abnormal corneal adhesion that leads to superficial corneal erosions, neovascularization, and progressive scarring. Additional noncutaneous findings occur in a subset of patients, including mental retardation, brain anomalies, Hirschsprung disease, corneal opacifications, kidney dysplasia, cryptorchidism, cleft palate, and skeletal malformations, particularly of the vertebrae (the so-called BRESEK or BRESHECK syndrome).[35] A patient with IFAP and additional features of pachyonychia and palmoplantar and periorificial keratoderma reminiscent of Olmsted syndrome has been described.[36]

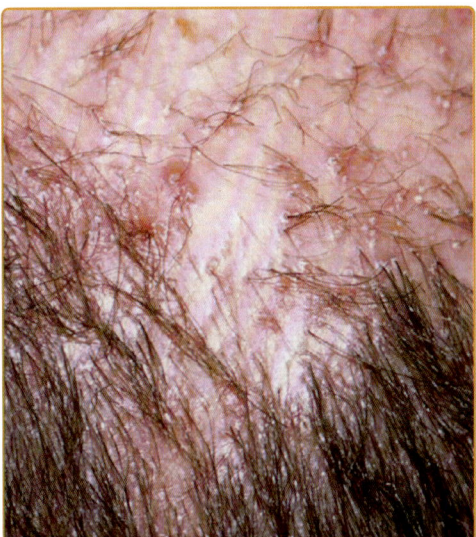

Figure 49-7 Keratosis follicularis spinulosa decalvans with severe scarring alopecia of scalp. (Photograph used with permission from Dr. Peter Hogan.)

ETIOLOGY AND PATHOGENESIS

Oeffner and colleagues identified mutations in *MBTPS2* leading to deficiency in MBTPS2, a metalloprotease essential for cholesterol homeostasis and endoplasmic reticulum stress response, as the cause of IFAP syndrome.[37] Mutations in the *MBTPS2* gene have subsequently been confirmed in both sporadic cases and kindreds with a range of IFAP phenotypes.[35,38-40] Aten and colleagues identified a missense change, c.1523A>G, in *MBTPS2* as the cause of KFSP.[41] This finding was recently verified in a British family as well.[42] The range of genetic variations described thus far includes only missense and intronic mutations, suggesting that changes leading to loss of function in MBTPS2 are nonviable. The range of disease expression in females is due to skewed inactivation of the X chromosome.[35,40]

DIAGNOSIS

The diagnoses of KFSD and IFAP syndrome are suspected in individuals presenting with the triad of follicular keratosis, alopecia or atrichia, and photophobia. A complete ophthalmologic evaluation is recommended. Identification of a pathogenic mutation in the *MBTPS2* gene is confirmatory and should be pursued. Histologic findings are similar to those of KP and KPA, showing follicular hyperkeratosis, perifollicular and dermal inflammation, fibrosis, and distorted follicles at different stages of the condition.

DIFFERENTIAL DIAGNOSIS

See Table 49-1.

CLINICAL COURSE, PROGNOSIS, AND MANAGEMENT

There is a wide range of severity in the KFSP–IFAP spectrum. Aside from patients with IFAP with BRESEK or BRESHECK syndrome, much of the long-term morbidity is associated with ocular disease. The involvement of a skilled ophthalmologist is important. There is no cure or disease-modifying treatment for KFSP or IFAP syndrome at this time, and in general, the results of treatment are unsatisfactory. Improvement of some of the cutaneous changes and regrowth of eyelashes has been reported with oral acitretin.[38,43]

TRICHODYSPLASIA SPINULOSA

AT-A-GLANCE

- Increasingly recognized disorder of viral-induced follicular hyperproliferation that occurs in the setting of immune compromise.
- Characterized by folliculocentric, skin-colored to erythematous papules with spiny spicules, typically affecting the central face
- Histology demonstrates hypertrophic hair bulbs with an expanded inner root sheath containing numerous eosinophilic trichohyaline granules.
- Caused by trichodysplasia spinulosa-associated polyomavirus
- Challenging to manage but tends to resolve when immune function improves

The term *trichodysplasia spinulosa* was proposed in 1999 by Haycox and colleagues,[44] who described an unusual folliculocentric viral infection occurring in the setting of immune suppression. Synonyms include viral-associated trichodysplasia, cyclosporine-induced folliculodystrophy, and pilomatrix dysplasia. TS is rare, although exact epidemiologic data are lacking. Case reports and reviews have increased in the medical literature, and milder forms may be underrecognized. All ages may be affected, and there is no gender predilection.

CLINICAL FEATURES

The distinct skin findings of TS are skin-colored to erythematous, folliculocentric papules with brittle, keratotic spicules (Fig. 49-8A). The central face, including the nose and forehead, is the most common distribution. The entire face, ears, and other parts of the body may be involved. In more severe or long-standing cases, the skin becomes thickened, distorting normal features and sometimes progressing to "leonine" facies. Alopecia is variable, often affecting the eyebrows and eyelashes, and partial loss of scalp and body hair can occur.

TS occurs in the setting of immune compromise because of immune suppression for organ transplantation or treatment of autoimmune disease, chemotherapy for hematopoietic malignancy, or HIV infection. The onset of symptoms varies. Among organ transplant patients, initial lesions appear 8 to 30 months after transplant.[45] There is no consistent pattern of timing with regards to the course of chemotherapy.

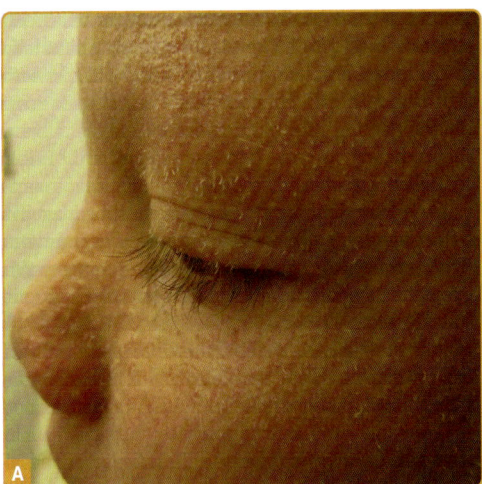
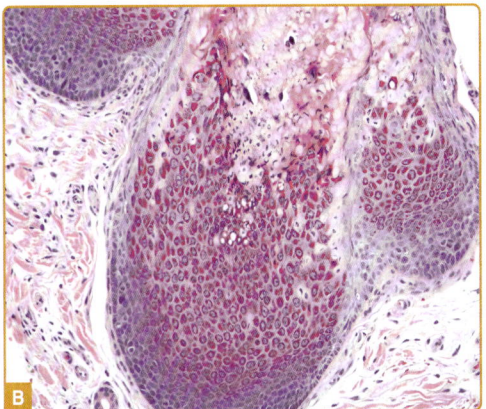

Figure 49-8 Trichodysplasia spinulosa. **A,** Erythematous, folliculocentric papules with keratotic spicules on the face of a child with acute lymphocytic leukemia. Eyebrow alopecia is also seen. **B,** Biopsy from this patient showed an expanded inner root sheath with eosinophilic trichohyaline granules (20× magnification). (Images courtesy of Dr. Lori Prok; used with permission.)

ETIOLOGY AND PATHOGENESIS

Haycox and colleagues were the first to identify intracellular viral particles in affected skin.[44] In 2010, van der Meijden and colleagues characterized this novel polyomavirus, trichodysplasia spinulosa-associated polyomavirus (TSPyV).[46] A precise pathomechanism for TSPyV infection producing clinical symptoms is still being elucidated. The cells of the inner root sheath of the hair follicle are infected in TS. Viral load is high (typically 10^5 copies per cell) in clinically apparent cases, but no or very few asymptomatic control participants have evidence of TSPyV.[47] Seroprevalence studies suggest that asymptomatic infection occurs with increasing prevalence from infancy through adulthood; 70% of adults have IgG antibodies to TSV.[48] A recent publication documenting extensive serologic and viral testing in two adults with TS demonstrates that the disorder is caused by disseminated primary TSPyV infection, not reactivation, in the setting of immune compromise.[49]

DIAGNOSIS

The cutaneous findings of TS are unique, and the diagnosis should be considered in immune compromised patients who develop spiny, folliculocentric papules. Microscopic examination of plucked spicules demonstrates thick concretions of inner root sheath material surrounding a poorly formed hair shaft.[50] The distinct histopathologic finding of TS is a hypertrophic hair bulb with an expanded inner root sheath whose cells contain numerous eosinophilic trichohyaline granules (Fig. 49-8B). In addition, keratotic plugging of the follicular infundibulum and abnormal hair shafts are seen. The presence of the virus can be confirmed by electron microscopy or polymerase chain reaction studies, although the latter may not be widely available.

DIFFERENTIAL DIAGNOSIS

See Table 49-1.

CLINICAL COURSE, PROGNOSIS, AND MANAGEMENT

The clinical findings of TS gradually improve and resolve as immune function is restored. Decreasing immune suppression should be considered when possible. Typical treatments for follicular keratosis, such as emollients, humectants, and retinoids, are not effective for TS. Antiviral therapy with topical cidofovir or systemic valacyclovir is associated with improvement.[47,51]

ACKNOWLEDGMENTS

The author acknowledges the contributions of Paradi Mirmirani and Maureen Rogers, the former authors of this chapter.

REFERENCES

1. Poskitt L, Wilkinson JD. Natural history of keratosis pilaris. *Br J Dermatol.* 1994;130(6):711-713.

2. Fung WK, Lo KK. Prevalence of skin disease among school children and adolescents in a Student Health Service Center in Hong Kong. *Pediatr Dermatol*. 2000; 17(6):440-446.
3. Dogra S, Kumar B. Epidemiology of skin diseases in school children: a study from northern India. *Pediatr Dermatol*. 2003;20(6):470-473.
4. Popescu R, Popescu CM, Williams HC, et al. The prevalence of skin conditions in Romanian school children. *Br J Dermatol*. 1999;140(5):891-896.
5. Inanir I, Sahin MT, Gunduz K, et al. Prevalence of skin conditions in primary school children in Turkey: differences based on socioeconomic factors. *Pediatr Dermatol*. 2002;19(4):307-311.
6. Tay YK, Kong KH, Khoo L, et al. The prevalence and descriptive epidemiology of atopic dermatitis in Singapore school children. *Br J Dermatol*. 2002;146(1):101-106.
7. Brown SJ, Relton CL, Liao H, et al. Filaggrin haploinsufficiency is highly penetrant and is associated with increased severity of eczema: further delineation of the skin phenotype in a prospective epidemiological study of 792 school children. *Br J Dermatol*. 2009;161(4):884-889.
8. Marqueling AL, Gilliam AE, Prendiville J, et al. Keratosis pilaris rubra: a common but underrecognized condition. *Arch Dermatol*. 2006;142(12):1611-1616.
9. Sardana K, Relhan V, Garg V, et al. An observational analysis of erythromelanosis follicularis faciei et colli. *Clin Exp Dermatol*. 2008;33(3):333-336.
10. Mevorah B, Marazzi A, Frenk E. The prevalence of accentuated palmoplantar markings and keratosis pilaris in atopic dermatitis, autosomal dominant ichthyosis and control dermatological patients. *Br J Dermatol*. 1985;112(6):679-685.
11. Bremmer SF, Hanifin JM, Simpson EL. Clinical detection of ichthyosis vulgaris in an atopic dermatitis clinic: implications for allergic respiratory disease and prognosis. *J Am Acad Dermatol*. 2008;59(1):72-78.
12. Yosipovitch G, Mevorah B, Mashiach J, et al. High body mass index, dry scaly leg skin and atopic conditions are highly associated with keratosis pilaris. *Dermatology*. 2000;201(1):34-36.
13. Macdonald JB, Macdonald B, Golitz LE, et al. Cutaneous adverse effects of targeted therapies: part II: inhibitors of intracellular molecular signaling pathways. *J Am Acad Dermatol*. 2015;72(2):221-236; quiz 237-228.
14. Thomas M, Khopkar US. Keratosis pilaris revisited: is it more than just a follicular keratosis? *Int J Trichol*. 2012;4(4):255-258.
15. Gruber R, Sugarman JL, Crumrine D, et al. Sebaceous gland, hair shaft, and epidermal barrier abnormalities in keratosis pilaris with and without filaggrin deficiency. *Am J Pathol*. 2015;185(4):1012-1021.
16. Ibrahim O, Khan M, Bolotin D, et al. Treatment of keratosis pilaris with 810-nm diode laser: a randomized clinical trial. *JAMA Dermatol*. 2015;151(2):187-191.
17. Luria RB, Conologue T. Atrophoderma vermiculatum: a case report and review of the literature on keratosis pilaris atrophicans. *Cutis*. 2009;83(2):83-86.
18. Frosch PJ, Brumage MR, Schuster-Pavlovic C, et al. Atrophoderma vermiculatum. Case reports and review. *J Am Acad Dermatol*. 1988;18(3):538-542.
19. Bhoyrul B, Jones H, Blackford S. Extensive unilateral atrophoderma vermiculatum associated with ipsilateral congenital cataract. *Clin Exp Dermatol*. 2016; 41(2):159-161.
20. Hsu S, Nikko A. Unilateral atrophic skin lesion with features of atrophoderma vermiculatum: a variant of the epidermal nevus syndrome? *J Am Acad Dermatol*. 2000;43(2 Pt 1):310-312.
21. Klar J, Schuster J, Khan TN, et al. Whole exome sequencing identifies LRP1 as a pathogenic gene in autosomal recessive keratosis pilaris atrophicans. *J Med Genet*. 2015;52(9):599-606.
22. Siegel DH, McKenzie J, Frieden IJ, et al. Dermatological findings in 61 mutation-positive individuals with cardio-faciocutaneous syndrome. *Br J Dermatol*. 2011;164(3):521-529.
23. Rauen KA. The RASopathies. *Ann Rev Genom Hum Genet*. 2013;14:355-369.
24. Chien AJ, Valentine MC, Sybert VP. Hereditary woolly hair and keratosis pilaris. *J Am Acad Dermatol*. 2006;54(2 suppl):S35-39.
25. Gomez Centeno P, Roson E, Peteiro C, et al. Rubinstein-Taybi syndrome and ulerythema ophryogenes in a 9-year-old boy. *Pediatr Dermatol*. 1999;16(2):134-136.
26. Florez A, Fernandez-Redondo V, Toribio J. Ulerythema ophryogenes in Cornelia de Lange syndrome. *Pediatr Dermatol*. 2002;19(1):42-45.
27. Liakou AI, Esteves de Carvalho AV, Nazarenko LP. Trias of keratosis pilaris, ulerythema ophryogenes and 18p monosomy: Zouboulis syndrome. *J Dermatol*. 2014; 41(5):371-376.
28. Thai KE, Sinclair RD. Keratosis pilaris and hereditary koilonychia without monilethrix. *J Am Acad Dermatol*. 2001;45(4):627-629.
29. van Dijk FS, Brittain H, Boerma R, et al. Atrophoderma vermiculatum: a cutaneous feature of Loeys-Dietz Syndrome. *JAMA Dermatol*. 2015;151(6):675-677.
30. Olaiwan A, Chandesris MO, Fraitag S, et al. Cutaneous findings in sporadic and familial autosomal dominant hyper-IgE syndrome: a retrospective, single-center study of 21 patients diagnosed using molecular analysis. *J Am Acad Dermatol*. 2011;65(6):1167-1172.
31. Morton CM, Bhate C, Janniger CK, et al. Ulerythema ophryogenes: updates and insights. *Cutis*. 2014;93(2):83-87.
32. Layton AM, Cunliffe WJ. A case of ulerythema ophryogenes responding to isotretinoin. *Br J Dermatol*. 1993; 129(5):645-646.
33. Weightman W. A case of atrophoderma vermiculatum responding to isotretinoin. *Clin Exp Dermatol*. 1998;23(2):89-91.
34. Castori M, Covaciu C, Paradisi M, et al. Clinical and genetic heterogeneity in keratosis follicularis spinulosa decalvans. *Eur J Med Genet*. 2009;52(1):53-58.
35. Bornholdt D, Atkinson TP, Bouadjar B, et al. Genotype-phenotype correlations emerging from the identification of missense mutations in MBTPS2. *Hum Mutat*. 2013;34(4):587-594.
36. Wang HJ, Tang ZL, Lin ZM, et al. Recurrent splice-site mutation in MBTPS2 underlying IFAP syndrome with Olmsted syndrome-like features in a Chinese patient. *Clin Exp Dermatol*. 2014;39(2):158-161.
37. Oeffner F, Fischer G, Happle R, et al. IFAP syndrome is caused by deficiency in MBTPS2, an intramembrane zinc metalloprotease essential for cholesterol homeostasis and ER stress response. *Am J Hum Genet*. 2009;84(4):459-467.
38. Ming A, Happle R, Grzeschik KH, et al. Ichthyosis follicularis, alopecia, and photophobia (IFAP) syndrome due to mutation of the gene MBTPS2 in a large Australian kindred. *Pediatr Dermatol*. 2009;26(4):427-431.

39. Oeffner F, Martinez F, Schaffer J, et al. Intronic mutations affecting splicing of MBTPS2 cause ichthyosis follicularis, alopecia and photophobia (IFAP) syndrome. *Exp Dermatol.* 2011;20(5):447-449.
40. Fong K, Takeichi T, Liu L, et al. Ichthyosis follicularis, atrichia, and photophobia syndrome associated with a new mutation in MBTPS2. *Clin Exp Dermatol.* 2015;40(5):529-532.
41. Aten E, Brasz LC, Bornholdt D, et al. Keratosis follicularis spinulosa decalvans is caused by mutations in MBTPS2. *Hum Mutat.* 2010;31(10):1125-1133.
42. Fong K, Wedgeworth EK, Lai-Cheong JE, et al. MBTPS2 mutation in a British pedigree with keratosis follicularis spinulosa decalvans. *Clin Exp Dermatol.* 2012;37(6):631-634.
43. Khandpur S, Bhat R, Ramam M. Ichthyosis follicularis, alopecia and photophobia (IFAP) syndrome treated with acitretin. *J Eur Acad Dermatol Venereol.* 2005;19(6):759-762.
44. Haycox CL, Kim S, Fleckman P, et al. Trichodysplasia spinulosa—a newly described folliculocentric viral infection in an immunocompromised host. *J Invest Dermatol Symp Proc.* 1999;4(3):268-271.
45. Tan BH, Busam KJ. Virus-associated Trichodysplasia spinulosa. *Adv Anat Pathol.* 2011;18(6):450-453.
46. van der Meijden E, Janssens RW, Lauber C, et al. Discovery of a new human polyomavirus associated with trichodysplasia spinulosa in an immunocompromised patient. *PLoS Pathog.* 2010;6(7):e1001024.
47. Kazem S, van der Meijden E, Feltkamp MC. The trichodysplasia spinulosa-associated polyomavirus: virological background and clinical implications. *APMIS.* 2013;121(8):770-782.
48. Chen T, Mattila PS, Jartti T, et al. Seroepidemiology of the newly found trichodysplasia spinulosa-associated polyomavirus. *J Infect Dis.* 2011;204(10):1523-1526.
49. van der Meijden E, Horvath B, Nijland M, et al. Primary polyomavirus infection, not reactivation, as the cause of Trichodysplasia spinulosa in immunocompromised patients. *J Infect Dis.* 2017;215(7):1080-1084.
50. Lee JS, Frederiksen P, Kossard S. Progressive trichodysplasia spinulosa in a patient with chronic lymphocytic leukaemia in remission. *Australas J Dermatol.* 2008;49(1):57-60.
51. Wu JH, Nguyen HP, Rady PL, et al. Molecular insight into the viral biology and clinical features of trichodysplasia spinulosa. *Br J Dermatol.* 2016;174(3):490-498.

Chapter 50 :: Acantholytic Disorders of the Skin
:: Alain Hovnanian

第五十章

棘层松解性皮肤病

中文导读

棘层松解症是一组具有重叠临床和组织学特征的异质性疾病，其特点为角质形成细胞之间的结合力丧失，导致细胞分离。最常见的棘层松解性疾病有天疱疮、Darier病（DD）、Hailey-Hailey病（HHD）和Grover病（GD）。此外，疣状肢端角化症（AKV）被认为是DD的一种临床变异，丘疹性棘层松解性角化不良（PAD）被认为是DD和HHD的一种可能的临床表现形式。本章主要介绍了DD、AKV、HHD和GD的流行病学、临床特征、病因与发病机制、组织病理学、鉴别诊断、临床病程与预后、疾病管理。

〔粟 娟〕

AT-A-GLANCE

- The acantholytic diseases are a heterogeneous group of diseases with overlapping clinical and histologic features.

- Darier-White disease (DD) and Hailey-Hailey disease (HHD) are uncommon diseases inherited in an autosomal dominant pattern. A defective calcium pump of the sarcoplasmic/endoplasmic reticulum causes DD, and a faulty calcium and manganese pump of the Golgi apparatus underlies HHD.

- Whereas typical DD presents with greasy keratotic papules in a seborrhoeic distribution, HHD is characterized by painful, oozing erosions in flexures and at sites of trauma.

- Nail changes (DD and HHD), flat-topped warty papules on dorsa of hands and feet (DD), and palmar pits (DD and HHD) or palmar keratotic papules (DD) help to confirm the diagnosis.

- Hypertrophic malodorous flexural disease is particularly disabling in DD and HHD.

- Grover disease (GD) is a sporadic papular condition of uncertain etiology that presents most often in sun-damaged skin. Intractable pruritus is common.

- Histopathologicl examination of involved skin in DD, HH, and GD reveals breakdown of intercellular contacts between suprabasal keratinocytes (acantholysis) with variable dyskeratosis.

- Mosaic forms (type 1 and 2) following the lines of Blaschko have been identified in DD and HHD.

- Acrokeratosis verruciformis of Hopf (AKV) mimics acral DD with flat-topped, warty papules on the dorsal hands and feet and nail dystrophy. The histology of AKV is not acantholytic, but several reports have identified a specific *ATP2A2* mutation in patients with AKV, which indicate that some (if not most) cases are allelic variants of DD with limited manifestations.

- Papular acantholytic dyskeratosis (PAD) presents as whitish papules of the genitocrural or anogenital areas (or both). PAD has been associated with a somatic *ATP2A2* mutation and with constitutive *ATP2C1* mutations, indicating that it can be part of the clinical spectrum of DD or HHD.

- Treatment options for these diseases include topical corticosteroids (DD, HHD, GD) and topical or oral retinoids (DD, GD, AKV), but disease-specific therapies are lacking.

INTRODUCTION

Acantholytic diseases are characterized by loss of intercellular cohesion between keratinocytes, resulting in cell separation. Acantholysis can be the major histologic finding but can also be associated with dyskeratosis corresponding to abnormal keratinization with "corps ronds and grains." Acantholysis is caused by rupture of the desmosomal junctions. However, the most frequent acantholytic diseases (pemphigus, Darier disease [DD], Hailey-Hailey disease [HHD], and Grover disease [GD]) are not caused by primary defects in desmosomal components. This chapter describes DD, HHD, and GD; pemphigus is covered in Chap. 52. The relationship between acrokeratosis verruciformis (AKV), also known as Hopf disease, and DD has been debated for decades. AKV can now be considered as a clinical variant of DD since the same Pro602Leu mutation in *ATP2A2* has been identified in five unrelated patients with AKV. Papular acantholytic dyskeratosis (PAD) is presented as a possible clinical form of DD and HHD because PAD has been associated with a somatic *ATP2A2* mutation and germinal *ATP2C1* mutations in distinct patients.

DARIER DISEASE

EPIDEMIOLOGY

DD (Online Mendelian Inheritance in Man [OMIM] #124200) is an autosomal dominant disease affecting both sexes and all ethnic groups. DD was described independently by Darier and by White in 1889 and is also known as Darier-White disease or keratosis follicularis.[1,2] Estimates of prevalence range from 1 in 30,000 (Northeast England, Scotland, Slovenia)[3-5] to 1 in 100,000 (Denmark).[6] Penetrance is complete, but spontaneous mutations are frequent.

CLINICAL FEATURES

CUTANEOUS FINDINGS

The first manifestations usually appear between the ages of 6 and 20 years with a peak between 11 and 15 years, but DD may also develop in infants or older adults.[1,3,7,8] Symptoms include itch, malodor, and pain. Heat, sweating, friction, and sunlight (ultraviolet B [UVB]) exacerbate the signs, which may be noticed for the first time in hot summer months.[2,3]

The discrete, greasy, yellowish-brown keratotic papules (only some are perifollicular) have a predilection for seborrheic areas, including the central chest and upper back, scalp (hair growth is not affected), forehead, neck including the supraclavicular fossae, ears, and skin creases (axillae, groins, and perineum) (Figs. 50-1 and 50-2). Papules tend to coalesce into crusted plaques (Fig. 50-3). Foul-smelling, hypertrophic disease in the groin is particularly disabling (Fig. 50-4). White described the "intolerable stench" that accompanies severe disfiguring disease.[2] DD may affect schooling, work, and relationships.[1,9]

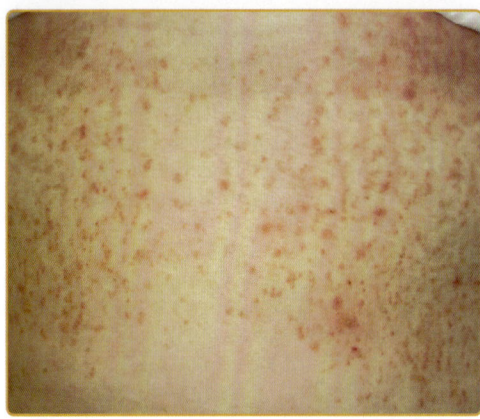

Figure 50-1 Hyperkeratotic, pigmented papules on the trunk of a patient with Darier disease.

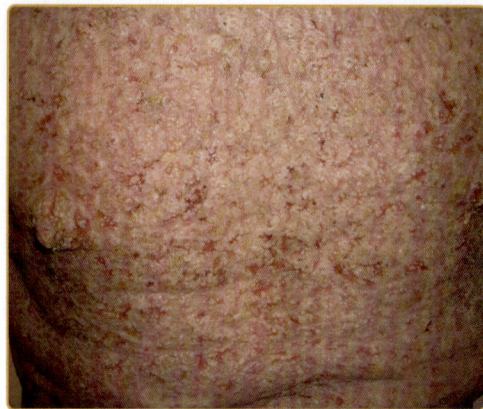

Figure 50-3 Malodorous confluent keratotic papules on the chest with fissuring and hyperkeratosis of the nipples in Darier disease.

The hands, nails, or both are affected in more than 96% of patients and may be the first signs of disease.[1,3] Nail fragility, painful longitudinal splits, or distinctive red and white longitudinal bands terminating in V-shaped nicks are frequent and highly suggestive (Fig. 50-5). Pits or keratotic papules on palms and sometimes soles help to confirm the diagnosis (Fig. 50-6). Many patients (50%–70%) have skin-colored, flat-topped papules on the dorsa of the hands, feet, or both like those of acrokeratosis verruciformis of Hopf (AKV).[10] Hemorrhagic macules with jagged margins, possibly linked to trauma, are the least common acral sign and may blister (Fig. 50-7). Hemorrhagic DD has been reported in some kindreds as well as individuals.[11-14]

Clinical Variants: Variants include painful erosive DD,[15] vesiculobullous DD,[16] grossly hyperkeratotic plaques (cornifying DD),[17-19] nipple hyperkeratosis,[20]

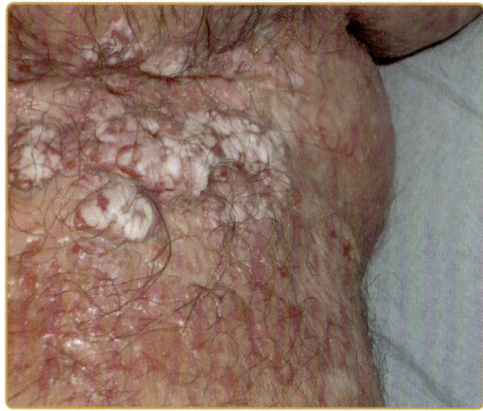

Figure 50-4 Hypertrophic flexural Darier disease may suggest squamous cell carcinoma.

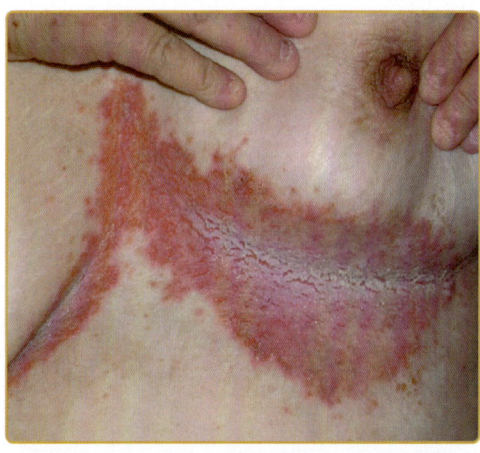

Figure 50-2 Darier disease. Inflammatory plaques with fissures and maceration may simulate Hailey-Hailey disease. Note that the fingernails are dystrophic.

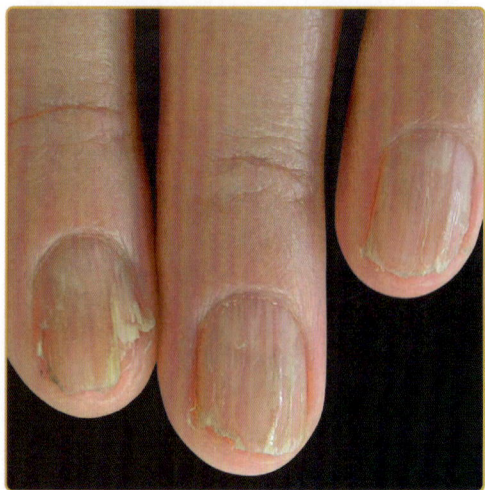

Figure 50-5 Dystrophic fingernails showing fragility, splitting, and red and white longitudinal bands in Darier disease.

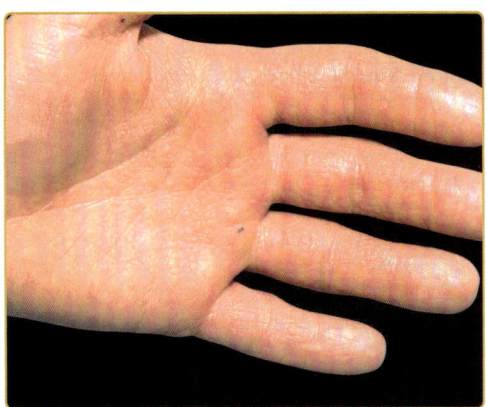

Figure 50-6 Keratotic papules of the palms in Darier disease.

keratoderma (Fig. 50-8), comedonal DD,[21-23] freckled "Groveroid" DD,[24] and guttate leukoderma with confetti-like hypopigmented macules or papules (or both) in pigmented skin.[25,26] AKV is a clinical variant of DD (see later).

Segmental Disease: Type 1 mosaicism presents with one or more unilateral bands of keratotic papules following Blaschko lines. The hands, nails, or both may be affected on the same side.[27,28] This distribution reflects a postzygotic somatic mutation in *ATP2A2* early in embryogenesis.[29-31] Hypopigmented, segmental DD following Blaschko lines has recently been reported on dark skin.[32] Theoretically, patients with segmental Darier and gonadal mosaicism could transmit generalized disease, but no such cases have been reported. Type 2 mosaicism is very rare and was reported only twice. In one case, an excessively pronounced unilateral linear band of DD with a segmental pattern was superimposed on generalized disease.[33] In a second case, a 1-year-old boy born to a mother affected with classic DD developed erosive patches

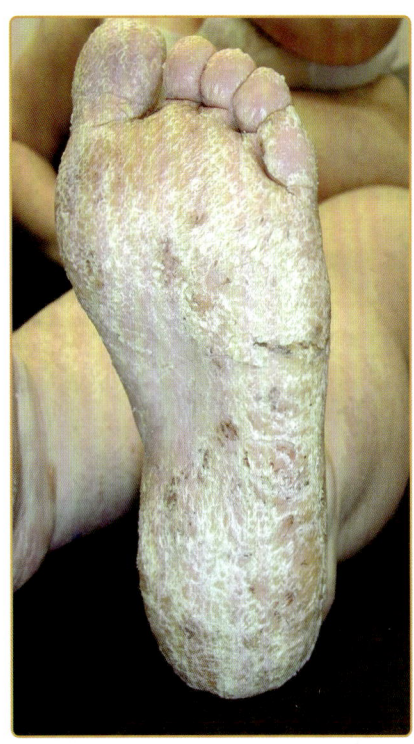

Figure 50-8 Keratoderma in Darier disease.

confined to one side of the abdomen. Molecular analysis of the lesional skin suggested loss of heterozygosity caused by a postzygotic mutation at the *ATP2A2* locus.[34]

NONCUTANEOUS FINDINGS

Oral,[1,35-37] esophageal,[38,39] rectal,[40] and cervical[41] mucosa may be affected in the form of multiple white papules. Corneal abnormalities have been recorded.[42-44] Bone changes, particularly bone cysts, have been reported infrequently.[45-47]

RELATED PHYSICAL FINDINGS

DD has been reported in association with neuropsychiatric disease, including seizures, bipolar disorder, and schizophrenia.[1,48-51] Lithium, which may be prescribed for bipolar disorder, exacerbates DD, possibly by suppressing levels of epidermal SERCA2.[52-55] The lifetime prevalence of major depression (30%), suicide attempts (13%), and suicidal thoughts (31%) appears higher than in the general population, highlighting the need for careful assessment.[51,56] Reports of cosegregation of DD with bipolar disorder in some families support the existence of a bipolar disorder susceptibility gene in the DD region, but *ATP2A2* has been excluded as a common susceptibility gene for bipolar disease.[57-59] Learning difficulties reported in some patients may be, at least in part, secondary to social disability caused by disfigurement.

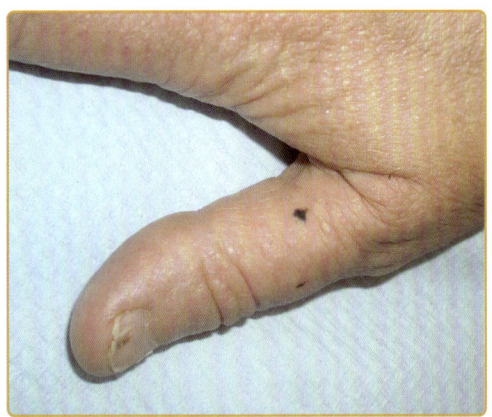

Figure 50-7 Hemorrhagic macule and nail dystrophy in Darier disease.

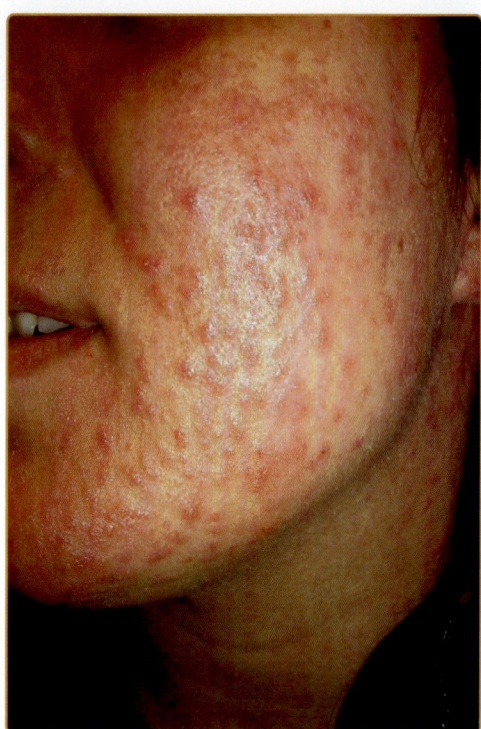

Figure 50-9 Widespread papulovesicular rash caused by infection with herpes simplex virus in Darier disease.

COMPLICATIONS

Impetiginization and eczematization may complicate the picture, and patients have an increased susceptibility to widespread infection with herpes simplex (eczema herpeticum) (Fig. 50-9) and herpes zoster viruses.[60,61] Blockage of salivary glands has been reported.[1,35,62] Squamous cell carcinoma (SCC; scalp, scrotal, vulval, thigh, subungual) has been recorded infrequently, sometimes associated with the presence of human papillomavirus (HPV) 16.[63-66]

ETIOLOGY AND PATHOGENESIS

The gene for DD was mapped by linkage analysis to chromosome region 12q23-24 in 1993,[67] and *ATP2A2* was identified as the defective gene in 1999.[68] *ATP2A2* encodes sarco- and endoplasmic reticulum (ER) Ca^{2+} adenosine triphosphatase (ATPase) isoform 2 (SERCA2), a calcium pump transporting Ca^{2+} from the cytosol to the lumen of the ER.[69-72] DD is caused by mutations inactivating one *ATP2A2* allele.

ATP2A2 spans 76 kilobases (kb), is organized in 21 exons, and encodes a 4.4-kb transcript, which is alternatively spliced into three isoforms: SERCA2a, SERCA2b, and SERCA2c.[73,74] SERCA2a is expressed in slow-twitch skeletal muscles and cardiac muscle, unaffected in DD.[75,76] SERCA2b and SERCA2c are expressed ubiquitously, but SERCA2b is the major isoform detected in the human epidermis.[77] Mutations specific for SERCA2b are sufficient to cause DD (despite the presence of functional SERCA2a from the same allele), confirming that SERCA2b is the predominant functional isoform in epidermis.[78,79] Most tissues may compensate for deficiencies in SERCA2 by mechanisms involving SERCA3, which is not expressed in keratinocytes.[77]

SERCA2 pumps belong to the P-type Ca^{2+} ATPase family. The pumps catalyze the hydrolysis of adenosine triphosphate (ATP) coupled with the translocation of two Ca^{2+} ions from the cytosol to the ER lumen, where Ca^{2+} is stored at high concentrations. SERCA pumps comprise three cytoplasmic domains (the actuator, phosphorylation, and ATP-binding domains) linked to a transmembrane domain with 10 transmembrane helices that contain the two Ca^{2+}-binding sites. After binding of cytosolic Ca^{2+} ions and phosphorylation, the pump undergoes conformational changes and releases Ca^{2+} into the ER lumen.[80]

A recent database of *ATP2A2* mutations created by The Leiden Open Variation Database reported 279 unique *ATP2A2* mutations.[81] A majority (46%) of these mutations are missense mutations, 8% are nonsense mutations, and 10% are splice-site mutations with remaining mutations predicting frameshifts or in-frame deletions or insertions. They are distributed throughout the gene and are mostly family specific. No consistent correlation has been demonstrated between genotype and phenotype, although missense mutations appear to be more often associated with severe forms.[21,48,68,78,79,82-93] The considerable phenotypic variability within and among families suggests that other genetic or environmental factors modify the phenotype.

Although the etiology has been explained, the pathogenesis of DD is only partially understood. High concentrations of Ca^{2+} are required for normal keratinocyte intercellular adhesion and differentiation. Normally, the epidermis displays an increasing epidermal Ca^{2+} gradient from the basal to the superficial layers, but in DD, this gradient is disturbed. The level of Ca^{2+} is reduced in basal cells from both affected and unaffected skin.[94]

The earliest ultrastructural change is breakdown of desmosomes with aggregation of keratin filaments around the cell nucleus.[95] Immunohistologic studies of acantholytic cells reveal internalization of desmosomal components.[96-98] The dyskeratotic cells in the epidermis (grains, corps ronds) are formed through apoptosis, which appears to be triggered by the loss of adhesion.[99] The expression of antiapoptotic proteins in the Bcl-2 gene family is reduced in DD, possibly as a secondary phenomenon, but an alteration in Bcl-2 proteins might also contribute to apoptosis.[100-102] The epidermis is papillomatous and differentiation is abnormal, with the expression of hyperproliferative keratins and premature expression of cornified envelope precursors such as involucrin.[94,103-105] Variations in cellular Ca^{2+} concentrations are likely to have an effect on the expression

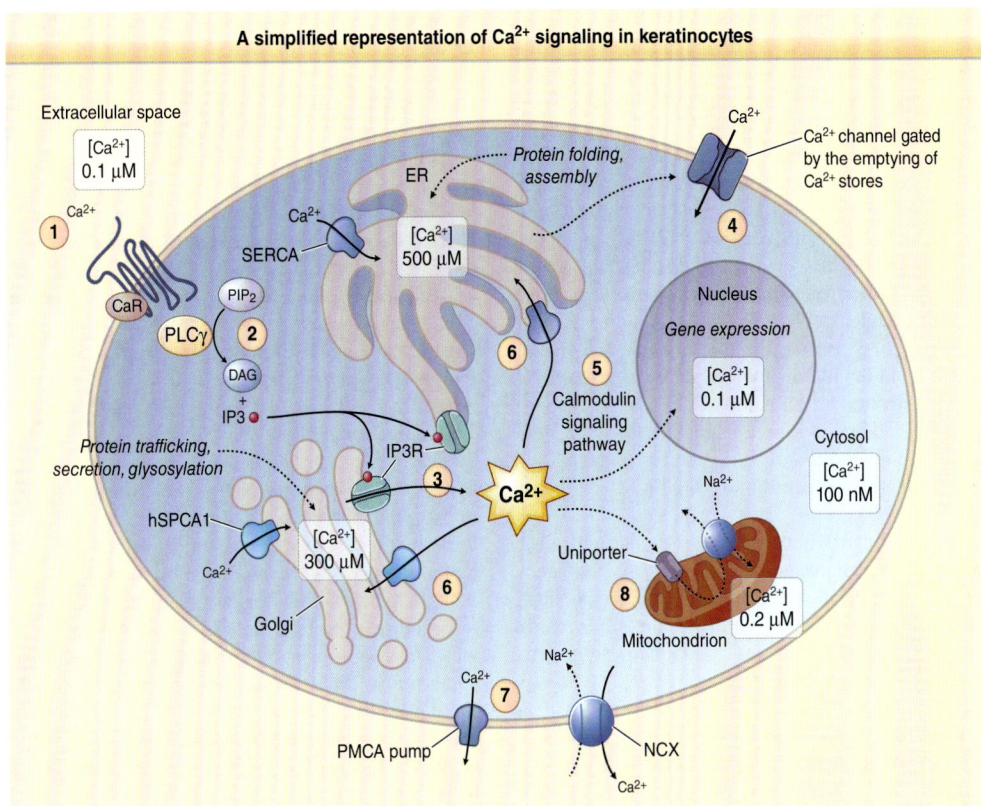

Figure 50-10 A simplified representation of Ca^{2+} signaling in keratinocytes. (1) Ca^{2+} binding to its plasma membrane receptor (CaR) activates phospholipase Cγ (PLCγ). (2) This causes the hydrolysis of phosphatidylinositol 4,5-bisphosphate (PIP2) into inositol 1,4,5-tris-phosphate (IP3) and diacylglycerol.[188] (3) IP3 binds to its receptor (IP3R) at the surface of the endoplasmic reticulum (ER) and Golgi apparatus, which causes the depletion of intracellular stores and induces an increase in intracellular Ca^{2+} levels. (4) This increase triggers the opening of Ca^{2+} release–activated channels in the plasma membrane (store-operated-channels [SOCs]), which leads to a sustained increase in Ca^{2+} intracellular levels. SOCs involve the interaction of stromal interacting molecule (STIM) at the ER membrane with Ora1 at the plasma membrane, which are not shown here. (5) Ca^{2+} binds to calmodulin; this activates calcineurin and calmodulin-dependent protein kinases, which regulate gene transcription through phosphorylation/dephosphorylation of transcription factors. (6) Active Ca^{2+} transport by the different sarcoplasmic reticulum and ER calcium adenosine triphosphatase (ATPase) pumps (SERCA1 to SERCA3) and human secretory pathway Ca^{2+}/Mn^{2+}-ATPase (SPCA1) pump is essential to replenish ER and Golgi Ca^{2+} stores, respectively. SPCA1 is also required for Mn^{2+} influx into the Golgi apparatus (not indicated here). (7) Ca^{2+} efflux to the extracellular space involves plasma membrane Ca^{2+}–ATPases (PMCA) and Na$^+$/Ca^{2+} exchangers (NCX). (8) Mitochondria take up Ca^{2+} released from the internal stores during Ca^{2+} signaling via the Ca^{2+} uniporter and return it to the cytosol through an NCX. Thus, Ca^{2+} homeostasis requires differential Ca^{2+} concentrations in the cytosol, the sarcoplasmic reticulum and ER, the Golgi apparatus, the mitochondria, and the nucleus of the cell. The largest store of cellular Ca^{2+} is located in the ER lumen and in Ca^{2+}-binding proteins. Ca^{2+} signaling is highly regulated and generated by influx through Ca^{2+} receptors, release from internal stores (ER, Golgi apparatus, mitochondrion), and sequestration by Ca^{2+} pumps (SERCAs, SPCA1) and Ca^{2+} exchangers. mNCX, mitochondria Na^{2+}/Ca^{2+} exchanger.

of Ca^{2+}-dependent genes involved in keratinocyte differentiation and adhesion.

SERCA pumps replenish the ER Ca^{2+} pool from cytosolic Ca^{2+}. They play a key role in Ca^{2+} homeostasis of the epidermis, which is described in Fig. 50-10. Because Ca^{2+} signaling plays a major role in keratinocyte growth, differentiation, and cell-to-cell adhesion, SERCA2 dysfunction is expected to have profound consequences in keratinocytes from patients with DD. Mutations disrupting critical functional domains or leading to premature termination codons lead to loss of function of the mutated allele. As a result, global SERCA2 pump activity is reduced, and the ER Ca^{2+} pool is diminished.[69,71] Darier keratinocytes (DK) display abnormal patterns of Ca^{2+} regulation.[106] Several lines of evidence indicate that ER Ca^{2+} store depletion plays a central role in DD pathogenesis. DK and normal keratinocytes treated with the SERCA2-inhibitor thapsigargin (TG) have reduced ER Ca^{2+} stores.[107] Decreased Ca^{2+} stores were shown to impair adherensjunction and desmosome formation and to induce a constitutive ER stress with increased sensitivity to ER stressors in DK and/or TG-treated human keratinocytes (HKs).[108] Specifically, early studies showed that desmoplakin (DP) trafficking was impaired in DK in culture and in HKs treated with thapsigargin.[109,110] This indicated that defective anchorage of desmosomes to the intermediate filament (IF) network is associated with Ca^{2+} store depletion and is likely to contribute to reduced cell-to-cell adhesion in DD. Possible mechanisms for impaired DP localization may involve direct interaction with SERCA2b,[78] impaired membrane translocation of protein kinase Ca (PKCa), a known regulator of DP-IF association and desmosome assembly to the plasma membrane[110] or other mechanisms related to depleted ER Ca^{2+} stores. E-cadherin, desmoglein 3, and desmocollin 2/3 also show reduced expression at the plasma membrane with partial intracellular retention in DK and in TG-treated HKs in culture, providing evidence that immature adherens junctions and desmosomes are associated with Ca^{2+} store depletion and contribute to reduced cell-to-cell adhesion in DD.[108,111,112]

Sphingolipids have recently been implicated in ER Ca^{2+} store depletion and possibly in DD pathogenesis. Among the multiple sphingolipid metabolites, sphingosine can promote cell death, but sphingosine 1-phosphate (S1P) enhances keratinocyte growth and differentiation, inhibits apoptosis,[113,114] and can mobilize Ca^{2+} from the ER stores in HKs.[115] S1P is synthesized from sphingosine by sphingosine kinase (SPHK1) and is degraded by sphingosine phosphatase lyase (SGPL1). Intracellular sphingosine levels were shown to be increased after inactivating SERCA2b with TG (10 nM) or small interfering RNA (siRNA) to SERCA2b in cultured human keratinocytes, but sphingosine kinase levels were reduced.[111] Conversely, inhibiting sphingosine lyase with siRNA rescued the defects in keratinocyte differentiation, E-cadherin and desmoplakin localization, and ER Ca^{2+} stores observed in TG-treated keratinocytes. Extracellular S1P was ineffective to rescue these defects, indicating that intracellular S1P is essential for normalizing the cell phenotype. Although the mechanisms by which sphingosine metabolism interacts with SERCA2 Ca^{2+} signaling are not well understood, these studies suggest that modulating the sphingolipid pathway could have therapeutic implications in DD.

Reduced Ca^{2+} concentration in the ER lumen also predicts dysfunction of Ca^{2+}-dependent proteins involved in posttranslational modifications such as glucosidases involved in glycosylation processes and chaperone molecules implicated in protein folding, which are essential for the proper maturation of transmembrane proteins, such as desmosomal proteins. Exposure of DK or TG-treated HKs to miglustat, a glucosidase inhibitor and pharmacologic chaperone used to treat Gaucher disease, was shown to restore normal E-cadherin and desmosomal localization.[108] Miglustat-treated DK were also less susceptible to mechanical dissociation than untreated DKs. Altogether, these results provided evidence that miglustat restored desmosome and adherens junction formation and improved intercellular strength in DKs. Of note, miglustat treatment did not revert the biochemical markers of ER stress. Possible modes of actions could involve the prevention of interactions between lectins (eg, calnexin) and misfolded E-cadherin or desmosomal proteins during ER quality-control, as described for miglustat and DF508-CFTR mutation.[116] Conversely, miglustat could indirectly impact on sphingosine metabolism and modulate sphingosine and S1P levels. Additional studies are required to test these hypotheses.

Another study has shown that the transport of nascent desmosomal cadherins (DCs) from the ER to the Golgi apparatus is blocked in SERCA2-inhibited keratinocytes.[112] Dsc2/3 and Dsg3 displayed unprocessed high-mannose type N-glycans which were sensitive to EndoH digestion. Dsg3 pro-domain was uncleaved and was sensitive to furin. Dsg3 and Dsc3 colocalized with calnexin and were retained in the ER. These effects were the consequence of a reduction of ER Ca^{2+} below a critical level. However, because neither glycosylation nor prodomain cleavage is required for Dsg trafficking,[117] blockade of DC transport is likely to be due to another consequence of ER Ca^{2+} depletion. A high concentration of Ca^{2+} in the ER is usually thought to be essential for proper folding of the secretory pathway proteins by ER chaperone molecules, which are Ca^{2+}-dependent proteins. Nevertheless, not all secretory pathway proteins are impacted by ER Ca^{2+} depletion. It is therefore possible that Ca^{2+}-binding proteins such as adherens junctions and DC cadherins could be highly sensitive to the reduction of ER Ca^{2+} below a critical level, leading to protein misfolding and subsequent retention by chaperone molecules as described during unfolded protein response.

Overall, these studies have shown that ER Ca^{2+} depletion is crucial for the maturation and trafficking of adherens junction (E-cadherin), DCs (Dsg2-3, Dsc2-3) and the cytolinker molecule desmoplakin. They have pointed to new potential therapeutic directions for DD through modulation of sphingolipids synthesis, the use of miglustat or molecular chaperones to release adhesion molecules trapped in the ER, or the increase of ER Ca^{2+} concentration above the threshold that triggers the disease manifestations.

Other studies have revealed abnormal distribution of purigenic ATP receptors in Darier epidermis.[94] These receptors transmit extracellular calcium and calcium waves into the cytosol. They include direct calcium channels (P2X) and G protein-coupled ATP receptors (P2Y), which result in the production of 1,4,5-triphosphate and calcium signaling (see Fig. 50-10). Impaired expression of these sensors may contribute to dyskeratosis and hyperproliferation.[69,94]

Abnormalities in the regulation of store-operated calcium entry were also reported in DD.[118] This important mechanism allows influx of extracellular Ca^{2+} through plasma membrane Ca^{2+} channels and is triggered by calcium depletion of the ER. It involves stromal interacting molecules (STIMs), calcium release–activated calcium modulator 1 (ORAi1), and transient receptor potential canonical 1 (TRPC1). TRPC1 was shown to be upregulated in keratinocytes from patients with DD or a SERCA2+/− mouse model as a result of depletion of ER Ca^{2+} stores. Increased TRPC1 expression enhanced Ca^{2+} influx, promoted proliferation, restricted apoptosis, and was proposed to contribute to dyskeratosis.[118]

Much of the skin may be able to compensate for the deficiency in SERCA2 by increasing the expression of the normal SERCA2 allele or by upregulating other mechanisms such as the human secretory-pathway Ca^{2+}/Mn^{2+} ATPase isoform 1 (SPCA1) in the Golgi.[107] However, external factors such as UVB irradiation or friction, which are known to exacerbate DD, may disrupt this subtle balance by downregulating ATP2A2 or by increasing the requirement for SERCA2 until the protein reaches a critical level. This hypothesis is supported by the observation that UVB irradiation and proinflammatory cytokines reduce levels of ATP2A2 mRNA in cultured normal keratinocytes, and that retinoids and corticosteroids (used in treatment of DD) prevent this reduction.[119] Lithium, another well-known trigger for DD, reduces epidermal expression of SERCA2 in rats.[52]

Importantly, Serca2 knockout heterozygote mice do not develop signs of DD but papillomas and SCCs.[120] SERCA2 haploinsufficiency in cultured mouse keratinocytes is associated with upregulation of proliferation and downregulation of differentiation markers.[121] SCC has been reported rarely in DD, sometimes in association with HPV16.[63-66,122]

DIFFERENTIAL DIAGNOSIS (SEE TABLE 50-1)

DD may be misdiagnosed as seborrheic dermatitis or acne, particularly in patients without a family history. Signs of DD in the hands or nails are often present. Acneiform facial DD may be confused with familial dyskeratotic comedones[123,124] or comedo-like acantholytic dyskeratosis.[125]

Erosive, bullous, or hypertrophic flexural disease simulates HHD, but HHD tends to present later and patients do not have keratotic papules or nail fragility.[126] Erosive or hypertrophic DD may also resemble pemphigus vulgaris or vegetans (see Chap. 52), but patients do not have mucosal ulcers, and intercellular immunoglobulin and complement are not detected in the epidermis. Localized hypertrophic DD may suggest malignancy (see Fig. 50-4). Freckled or papulovesicular forms may resemble Grover disease (GD, see later),[24] but GD is not familial, or the rare acantholytic variant of Dowling-Degos disease (Galli-Galli disease).[127]

Acral papules resemble flat warts or AKV.[10,128,129] Localized papular vulvocrural acantholytic disease or

HISTOPATHOLOGY

Histologic examination shows downgrowths of narrow cords of keratinocytes, suprabasal acantholysis with suprabasal clefts (lacunae), dyskeratosis (premature and abnormal keratinization), and hyperkeratosis (Fig. 50-11). Apoptosis results in rounded eosinophilic dyskeratotic cells in the epidermis (corps ronds) and flattened parakeratotic cells in the cornified layer (grains).[99] The warty papules on the backs of the hands show the histology of AKV (see later).

TABLE 50-1
Darier Disease: Differential Diagnosis

Seborrheic
- Seborrheic dermatitis (scalp, trunk)
- Grover disease (trunk)
- Acne (forehead)
- Confluent and reticulate papillomatosis (trunk)
- Candida infection (infra-mammary)

Erosive
- Herpes simplex infection
- Bullous impetigo
- Hailey-Hailey disease
- Pemphigus vulgaris

Vegetating Flexural
- Hailey-Hailey disease
- Pemphigus vegetans
- Squamous cell carcinoma

Comedonal
- Acne
- Familial dyskeratotic comedones
- Comedo-like acantholytic dyskeratosis

Acral
- Plane warts
- Acrokeratosis verruciformis of Hopf

Freckled
- Grover disease
- Dowling-Degos disease, acantholytic variant (Galli-Galli disease)

Genital
- Genital warts
- Vulval intraepithelial neoplasia
- Hailey-Hailey disease
- Papular vulvocrural acantholytic disease

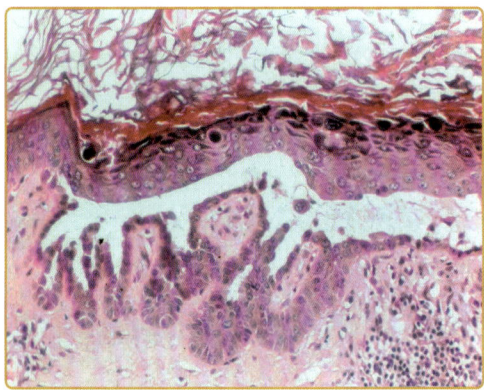

Figure 50-11 Histology of affected skin in Darier disease showing a suprabasal cleft of the epidermis containing acantholytic cells, rounded eosinophilic dyskeratotic cells (corps ronds), hyperkeratosis, and flattened parakeratotic cells in the cornified layer (grains).

papular acantholytic disease[10] may be part of the spectrum of DD or HHD.[130-133]

CLINICAL COURSE AND PROGNOSIS

DD pursues a chronic and relapsing course. The severity is unpredictable and can be influenced by pregnancies. In about 30% of patients, disease becomes less severe in old age, but in others, DD persists or gradually worsens.[1]

MANAGEMENT

Table 50-2 emphasizes several points that are important in the evaluation and ongoing counseling of patients with DD, such as reducing the impact of triggers such as heat and sun. Table 50-3 reviews therapeutic options. These treatments may control, but will not cure, DD.

MEDICATIONS

Emollients containing urea or lactic acid may reduce hyperkeratosis. Topical antiseptics (washes, bath additives), antibiotics, and antifungals help to prevent or treat infection. Herpes simplex causes painful flares that require oral acyclovir or valaciclovir.[60] Topical corticosteroids in combination with antibiotics reduce inflammation. Limited disease may respond to a topical retinoids such as tazarotene[134-136] or (iso)tretinoin[137] prescribed in combination with a topical corticosteroid to reduce irritation. Other topical agents such as adapalene,[138,139] 5-fluorouracil,[140,141] and tacrolimus[142] have been reported to be effective in small numbers of cases.

Oral retinoids such as acitretin 0.25 mg to 0.5 mg/kg, isotretinoin 0.5 mg/kg or alitretinoin (10 or 30 mg/day) reduce hyperkeratosis and malodor but will take 3 to 4 months to achieve maximal effect.[143] The dose needs to be tailored to the response, and adverse effects should be monitored (see Chap. 185). Pregnancy is contraindicated for 2 years after stopping treatment with acitretin and for 1 month after stopping isotretinoin or alitretinoin. Oral antibiotics are useful if lesions are extensive and/or infected. Oral cyclosporin has been advocated for eczematization[144] and in severe vulval disease,[145] but controlled trials are lacking.

Approaches for severe hypertrophic or erosive disease include dermabrasion, laser ablation, and photodynamic therapy, but controlled studies are needed to evaluate these approaches.[15,143,146,147] Botulinum toxin may control flexural exacerbations by reducing sweating. Reduction mammoplasty has been advocated for severe inframammary disease.[148,149]

GENETIC COUNSELING

Genetic counseling should be provided by a medical geneticist, taking into account disease expression and severity within affected members of the family.

ACROKERATOSIS VERRUCIFORMIS OF HOPF OR ACRAL DARIER DISEASE

AKV (OMIM #101900), described by Hopf in 1931,[10] is inherited in an autosomal dominant fashion.[128] Sporadic and familial cases have been reported. Whether AKV is a limited form of DD has been debated for

TABLE 50-3
Darier Disease: Treatment

FIRST LINE	SECOND LINE	THIRD LINE (UNPROVEN EFFICACY)
Discuss how to avoid triggers (heat, sweating, friction) and minimize ultraviolet B–induced exacerbations Antiseptic cleansing products and bath additives Topical antimicrobials (antibacterial, antifungal) Emollients containing urea or lactic acid Moderate or potent topical corticosteroids with topical antibiotics Topical retinoids: isotretinoin, tretinoin, tazarotene, adapalene	Oral acitretin 0.25 mg–0.5 mg/kg/day. Takes 3 months to have a maximal effect. Acitretin should be stopped for 2 years before a woman attempts to conceive. Oral isotretinoin 0.5 mg/kg/day or alitretinoin 10 mg or 30 mg/day. Less effective than acitretin but may be indicated in young women. Isotretinoin and alitretinoin should be stopped for 1 month before a woman attempts to conceive.	Topical 5-fluorouracil Oral ciclosporin for eczematization. Initially 2.5 mg/kg/day Laser surgery, electrosurgery, or dermabrasion Photodynamic therapy Botulinum toxin to reduce sweating in recalcitrant flexural disease Reduction mammoplasty for severe inframammary disease

TABLE 50-2
Darier Disease: What Should I Look for?

- A family history
- Symptoms such as malodor (many patients are relieved to have an opportunity to discuss this distressing problem) or pain (may indicate infection with herpes simplex virus)
- Exacerbating factors: What happens in heat or sun (eg, summer)?
- History of cold sores: Discuss the risk of eczema herpeticum
- Explore the impact of disease, including mood change. Darier disease is associated with depression and suicidal ideation.

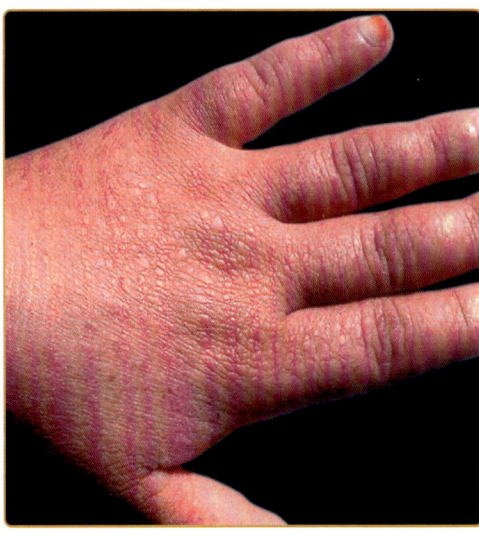

Figure 50-12 Small, skin-colored papules over the dorsum of the hand in acrokeratosis verruciformis of Hopf.

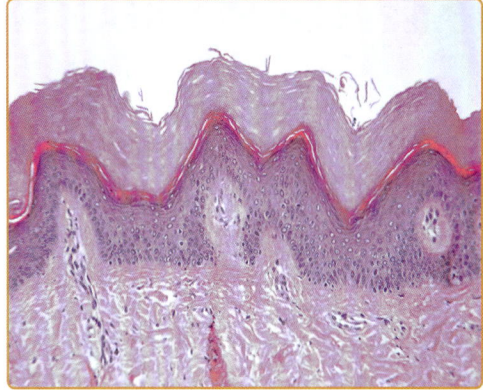

Figure 50-13 Histopathologic features of acrokeratosis verruciformis showing acanthosis and hyperkeratosis with "church spire" elevations of the epidermis but no acantholysis or dyskeratosis. (Used with permission from Dr. Laurence Lamant, Department of Pathology, Purpan Hospital, Toulouse, France.)

decades. The identification of a specific *ATP2A2* mutation in several unrelated patients with familial AKV established that AKV is allelic to DD.[129]

CLINICAL FEATURES

AKV usually presents at birth or in early childhood. The asymptomatic, skin-colored, flat-topped warty papules are distributed symmetrically on the dorsum of the hands and feet (Fig. 50-12). Papules may also develop on knees, elbows, and extensor aspects of the legs and forearms.[10] As in acral DD, punctate keratoses and pits may be present on palms and soles; palmar skin may be thickened; and patients may have subungual hyperkeratosis, longitudinal striations, splits, and V-shaped nicks at the free margin of the nail plates. A linear variant with persistent localized unilateral lesions has been reported in two unrelated Saudi patients.[150]

ETIOLOGY AND PATHOGENESIS

The same heterozygous Pro602Leu missense mutation in *ATP2A2*, the gene that is defective in DD, was identified in five large pedigrees of different geographic origin.[81,129,151,152] The mutation causes complete loss of Ca^{2+} transport activity.[129] Thus, AKV and DD are allelic disorders, and AKV can be considered as a clinical variant of DD, a conclusion that is entirely consistent with the overlapping clinical features. This is further supported by the coexistence (or segregation) of both entities within affected members of the same pedigrees carrying the same Pro602Leu mutation in *ATP2A2*. Nevertheless, mutations in *ATP2A2* were not identified in a Chinese family with AKV in which linkage with the chromosomal region 12q23-12q24 was excluded.[153]

HISTOPATHOLOGY

The classic histopathologic findings are hyperkeratosis, hypergranulosis, and acanthosis with papillomatosis. The spiky elevations of the epidermis are said to resemble "church spires" (Fig. 50-13). The epidermis is neither dyskeratotic nor acantholytic.

DIFFERENTIAL DIAGNOSIS

Acral DD and AKV present similarly, particularly in childhood, when other features of DD may not be apparent. AKV may resemble plane warts, stucco keratoses, or seborrheic warts. However, the family history, symmetrical distribution, and nail changes will suggest the diagnosis.

CLINICAL COURSE AND PROGNOSIS

AKV persists and may worsen slowly with age.

MANAGEMENT

No therapy may be needed. Topical retinoids may flatten lesions. Destruction by cryosurgery, shave, curettage, or laser surgery can be effective. Oral acitretin has been helpful.[154]

HAILEY-HAILEY DISEASE

EPIDEMIOLOGY

HHD (OMIM #169600), also known as familial benign chronic pemphigus, was described by the Hailey brothers in 1939. HHD has an incidence of at least 1 in 50,000, but the prevalence may be higher because misdiagnosis is frequent.[126]

CLINICAL FEATURES (TABLE 50-4)

CUTANEOUS FINDINGS

HHD usually presents between the second and fourth decades of life, predominantly at sites of friction (neck, axillae, inframammary, groin, perineum).[126] The diagnosis is often delayed because HHD simulates common dermatoses such as eczema, tinea, and impetigo. Itch, pain, and malodor are common complaints.

Signs include crusted weeping erosions, vesicopustules, expanding annular plaques with peripheral scaly borders (Figs. 50-14 and 50-15), and vegetating plaques with fissures (rhagades). Postinflammatory hyperpigmentation is frequent. Some patients have longitudinal white lines on the fingernails, and these can help to confirm the diagnosis (Fig. 50-16).[126,155] Disease may be limited to one or two sites, more widespread, or rarely generalized with erythroderma,[156] but even mild disease reduces quality of life.[9,157] Painful malodorous inguinal or perineal disease is particularly disabling. HHD koebnerizes into inflammatory dermatoses and has been exacerbated (or diagnosed) after triggers such as contact dermatitis, removal of adherent patch tests, UV irradiation, cutaneous infections, and scabies infestation.[158-166]

CLINICAL VARIANTS

Segmental Disease: Type 1 mosaicism, in which a postzygotic mutation in *ATP2C1* manifested as localized streaks of HHD along Blaschko lines, was reported in one patient.[167] Type 2 mosaicism has been confirmed in a patient with severe linear involvement superimposed on symmetrical HHD. In the more severely affected skin, a postzygotic mutation caused loss of heterozygosity at the *ATP2C1* locus.[168]

Papular Acantholytic Dyskeratosis: PAD[10] presents as localized, whitish papules that tend to cluster on the genitalia and the inguinal folds. The identification of *ATP2C1* mutations in two unrelated cases[169,170] and occurrence of PAD and HHD in a single

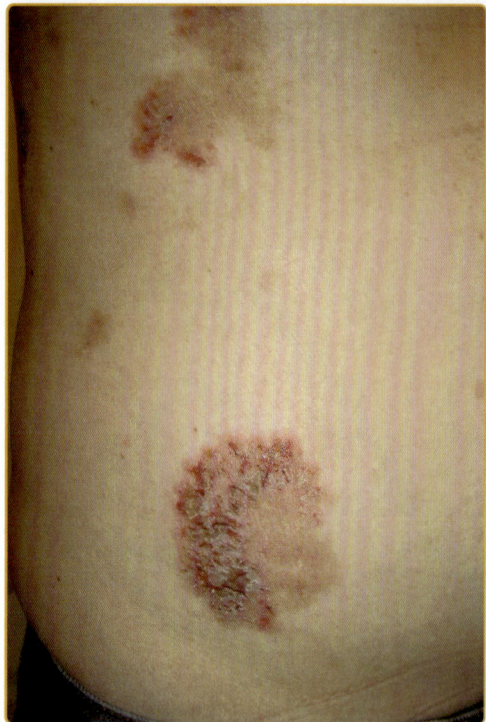

Figure 50-14 Crusted plaques with postinflammatory hyperpigmentation in a patient with Hailey-Hailey disease.

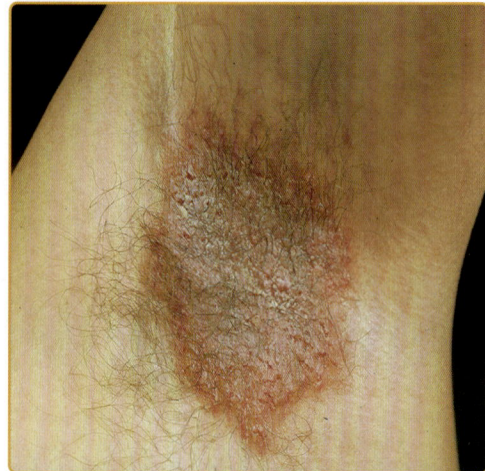

Figure 50-15 Hailey-Hailey disease with a hypertrophic macerated axillary plaque and painful fissures (rhagades).

TABLE 50-4
Hailey-Hailey Disease: What Should I Look for?

Consider the possibility of HHD in any young adult with chronic "eczema" at sites of friction such as the neckline, axilla, or groin. The diagnosis is often missed. Look for:
- Family history
- Exacerbating factors, such as friction, heat, or sweating
- Postinflammatory hyperpigmentation (common)
- Longitudinal white bands in nails (uncommon but very helpful if present)

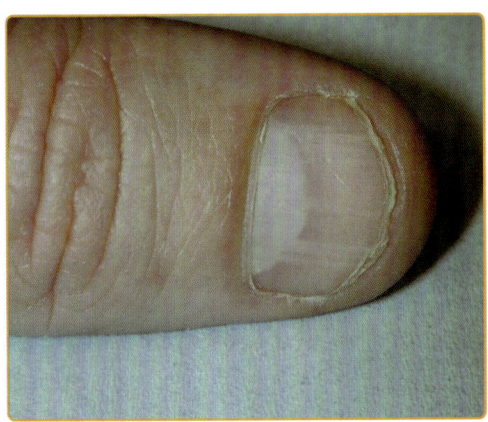

Figure 50-16 White longitudinal lines on the nail of a patient with Hailey-Hailey disease.

family[171] indicate that PAD can be part of the spectrum of HHD.[130,133,172-174]

NONCUTANEOUS FINDINGS

Generally, HHD does not involve mucosa. Rare instances of conjunctival, oral, esophageal, or vaginal involvement may have been initiated by trauma or infection.[175-177]

COMPLICATIONS

Superimposed bacterial or candidal infections are common.[178] Herpes simplex[179,180] causes painful exacerbations, which may disseminate.[181-183] Tinea was a cause of treatment failure in one patient.[184] Allergic contact dermatitis has been described, but the frequency of positive patch tests is probably not increased.[185,186] Skin cancers (SCC more often than basal cell carcinoma) have been reported in association with HHD.[179,180,187,188] SCC may be associated with the presence of HPV.[189-191] SCC of the vulva has been reported in a patient with HHD.[192] Affective disorder cosegregated with HHD in three families.[193-195]

ETIOLOGY AND PATHOGENESIS

The discovery of *ATP2A2* as the causative DD gene raised the possibility that defects in another calcium pump located in chromosomal region 3q21-24 where the HHD locus had been mapped could underlie acantholysis in HHD. Indeed, the defective gene, *ATP2C1*, encodes an ATP-powered calcium and manganese pump on the Golgi membrane, the human secretory-pathway Ca^{2+}/Mn^{2+} ATPase isoform 1 (SPCA1).[196,197] SPCA1 belongs to the family of P-type cation transport ATPases. HHD is dominantly inherited with complete penetrance and is caused by mutations inactivating one *ATP2C1* allele.

The gene spans approximately 30 kb and comprises 28 exons encoding a 4.5-kb transcript. The predicted protein is approximately 115 kDa. Alternative splicing of *ATP2C1* primary transcripts in keratinocytes leads to four splice variants, *ATP2C1a* to *ATP2C1d*, which differ by different splicing of exon 27, 28, or both. *ATP2C1d* is the largest variant, containing exons 27 and 28 in their entirety. The structure of SPCA is similar to that of SERCA, but SPCA only transports a single Ca^{2+} or Mn^{2+} ion into the Golgi lumen.[80,198-200]

The database of *ATP2C1* mutations in the Leiden Open Variation Database reported 177 distinct mutations in HHD scattered across the *ATP2C1* gene.[79,81,196,197,201-212] No correlations have been found between genotype and phenotype, and clinical features show a large range of variability.[201] A majority of these mutations are missense mutations (27%), 16% are nonsense mutations, and 19% are splice-site mutations, with the remaining mutations predicting frameshifts or in-frame deletions or insertions. Mutations predict marked reduction of SPCA1 or cause changes in highly conserved domains that are critical for function.[196,197,205,213,214] Haploinsufficiency appears to be the mechanism for dominant inheritance, but it is not clear how loss of one functional *ATP2C1* allele causes acantholysis.

Ultrastructural studies of acantholytic cells reveal desmosomal breakdown with retraction of keratin filaments from desmosomal plaques to form perinuclear aggregates.[215,216] Desmosomal components, E-cadherin, and connexins are internalized in acantholytic cells, and the expression of keratins is abnormal in lesional skin.[94,96,97,217-221] The abnormality in cell adhesion may be revealed in normal-looking skin in patients with HHD using suction.[222]

Immunohistochemical studies suggest that SPCA1 is localized to the basal layer of normal epidermis.[223] SPCA1 localizes to the Golgi of human keratinocytes and controls Golgi Ca^{2+} stores.[224] Total Ca^{2+} in the epidermal granular layer is reduced, and the normal epidermal Ca^{2+} gradient attenuated in both affected and unaffected skin.[196,224] Golgi Ca^{2+} stores are reduced, Ca^{2+} signaling is abnormal, and the normal upregulation of transcription of *ATP2C1* mRNA by Ca^{2+} stimulation is suppressed in HHD keratinocytes.[196,198,224] Abnormal cytosolic Ca^{2+} levels could influence Ca^{2+}-dependent gene expression or signaling cascades. In addition, low Ca^{2+} or Mn^{2+} concentrations in the Golgi lumen could impair posttranslational modifications, such as Ca^{2+}-dependent proteolytic processing or Mn^{2+}-dependent glycosylation, trafficking, or sorting of proteins important in epidermal cell-to-cell adhesion.

Cultured keratinocytes from involved skin display altered patterns of calcium metabolism and reduced proliferative capacity. Increased oxidative stress in HHD keratinocytes may lead to reduced expression of proteins involved in regulation of the balance between proliferation and differentiation such as Itch and Notch 1.[225] Reorganization of actin is defective, cellular ATP is decreased, and synthesis of involucrin is reduced.[106,226,227] Mice deficient for SPCA1 develop squamous cell papillomas and carcinomas similar to those seen in SERCA2-deficient mice.[228]

Although *ATP2C1* mRNA is expressed ubiquitously, HHD is limited to the skin. Keratinocytes may be more sensitive to levels of SPCA1 than other cells because, unlike most other cells, the Golgi in keratinocytes lack SERCA to compensate for deficient SPCA1.[200] UVB irradiation and proinflammatory cytokines reduce expression of *ATP2C1* mRNA in cultured normal keratinocytes, but suppression is inhibited by retinoids, corticosteroids, cyclosporin, tacrolimus, and vitamin D_3.[119] External factors (UVB, sweating, friction) may reduce the amount of SPCA1 to a critical level, leading to the expression of disease.[200]

In addition to the maintenance of Ca^{2+} and Mn^{2+} concentrations in the Golgi lumen, SPCA1 could also affect cytosolic Ca^{2+} signaling and protein trafficking. For example, Ca^{2+} release from the Golgi results in a localized increase in cytosolic Ca^{2+} levels, which induces vesicle fusion and cargo transport.[229,230] It is therefore conceivable that cell adhesion protein trafficking, such as desmosomal proteins, could be impaired in HHD. In parallel, increased oxidative stress and reduced Notch 1 expression have been reported in cultured keratinocytes derived from skin lesions of patients with HHD.[225,231] Differential gene expression using RNA-sequencing between lesional and nonlesional skin of subjects with HHD showed increased oxidative stress and Notch 1 activation.[232] The DNA damage response, a major target of oxidative stress–induced Notch 1 activation, was downregulated, and the mutation burden was increased in HHD lesions. These results suggested that the *ATP2C1*/NOTCH1 axis may be involved in the pathogenesis of HHD through ROS-induced DNA damage.[232]

HISTOPATHOLOGY

Involved skin displays widespread partial loss of cohesion (keratinocytes may still be linked together by adherens junctions)[233] between suprabasal keratinocytes with an appearance likened to a dilapidated brick wall (Fig. 50-17). Clusters of loosely coherent cells float in suprabasal clefts or bullae. Dyskeratosis,

TABLE 50-5
Hailey-Hailey Disease: Differential Diagnosis

Annular or Crusted Plaques
- Eczema, including allergic contact dermatitis
- Impetigo
- Candidal infection
- Tinea corporis
- Darier disease

Vesicopustules
- Eczema
- Bullous impetigo
- Herpes simplex
- Grover disease
- Pemphigus vulgaris
- Toxic epidermal necrolysis (if widespread)

Vegetating Flexural
- Darier disease
- Pemphigus vegetans
- Squamous cell carcinoma

Localized Genital
- Papular vulvocrural acantholytic disease
- Genital warts
- Darier disease
- Vulval intraepithelial neoplasia

when present, is usually mild, but changes may resemble those in DD.

DIFFERENTIAL DIAGNOSIS (TABLE 50-5)

Eczema or infection (bacterial, fungal or viral) are the most common misdiagnoses. Hypertrophic flexural HHD resembles DD, but acantholysis is more widespread and dyskeratosis less prominent in HHD than in DD. Eroded or vesiculobullous HHD may simulate toxic epidermal necrolysis[234] or pemphigus vulgaris (intercellular immunoglobulin G and complement are not detected in the epidermis). Genital HHD may simulate viral warts[132,235] or vulval intraepithelial neoplasia.[236] PAD[10] limited to the genitalia may be a separate entity, but the identification of *ATP2C1* mutations in two unrelated cases[169,170] and occurrence of PAD and HHD in a single family[171] have shown that PAD can be part of the spectrum of HHD.[133,172-174] A recent report showed that PAD could also be caused by a somatic *ATP2A2* mutation (see section on DD),[134] showing the importance of searching for a familial history of DD and HHD in the presence of PAD.

CLINICAL COURSE AND PROGNOSIS

The course is chronic, punctuated by relapses and remissions, and can be influenced by pregnancies. In some patients, it improves in old age.

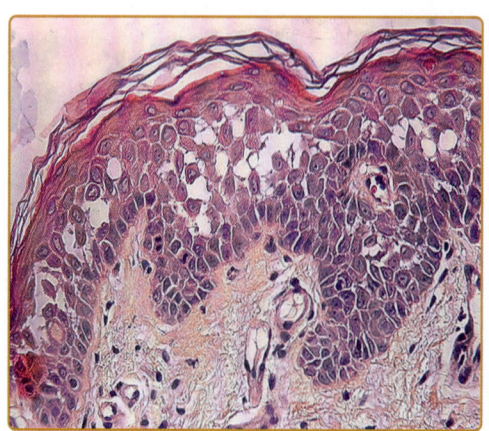

Figure 50-17 Histology of Hailey-Hailey disease. Extensive partial loss of intercellular contacts within the epidermis produces the appearance of a "dilapidated brick wall."

TABLE 50-6
Hailey-Hailey Disease: Treatment

FIRST LINE	SECOND LINE	THIRD LINE (UNPROVEN EFFICACY)
Minimize friction and sweating	Ultrapotent topical corticosteroids in combination with topical or oral antibiotics or antifungal agents to control secondary infection	Antistaphylococcal antibiotics (eg, low-dose tetracycline) for 6 mo or longer
Antiseptic cleansing products and bath additives		Topical tacrolimus
Topical antimicrobials (antibacterial, antifungal)		Topical tacalcitol or calcitriol
Moderately potent or potent topical corticosteroids in combination with topical or oral antibiotics or topical antifungal agents to control secondary infection	Prednisolone 20-30 mg/day; then tapered gradually to control acute exacerbations	Topical 5-fluorouracil
		Oral cyclosporin 2.5 mg/kg
		Oral retinoids: start with a low dose to minimize irritation
		Methotrexate 10–15 mg/wk
Pain relief (topical or oral). Some patients require narcotics		Excision, laser surgery, or dermabrasion
		Botulinum toxin to reduce sweating in recalcitrant flexural disease
		Reduction mammoplasty for severe inframammary disease

MANAGEMENT (TABLE 50-6)

The chronicity of the disease and the multiple recurrence of flares make the management of HHD a challenge for the physicians. Treatment is difficult, and no controlled trials have been performed. Recommendations in the literature are subject to citation bias, and most are based on the response of one or two cases without any long-term follow-up. Suggested recent reviews include Chiaravalotti and coworkers Arora and coworkers, and Farahnik and coworkers.[237-239] Treatment options include nonpharmacologic recommendations, topical and systemic agents, and surgery.

NONPHARMACOLOGIC RECOMMENDATIONS

Triggers such as heat, sweating, and friction should be minimized. Clothing should be soft, loose fitting, and cool. Personal hygiene and frequent cleaning and drying of flexural areas should be recommended to reduce flares. Weight loss may be helpful in case of excess body mass to avoid friction. Physical activity that causes friction should be reduced.

MEDICATIONS

Topical and systemic medications control skin microbial colonization, infection, and inflammation.

Microbial colonization and infections are frequent aggravating factors that can exacerbate lesions or prevent healing. Patients should wash with antimicrobial cleansers during flares, especially when lesions are malodorous or vegetating. Skin swabs should be taken for bacterial and yeast culture to guide local antibacterial and antifungal agents when infection is documented. Testing for herpes simplex virus infection by polymerase chain reaction should be performed with a personal history of herpes or persistence of lesions despite antibiotic or antifungal therapy. Nonadhesive dressings are useful to reduce friction and pain at the site of large erosions and to facilitate reepithelialization. When skin lesions are extensive and infected, oral antibiotics, such as doxycycline, which also has an antiinflammatory effect, can be helpful. Nevertheless, the role of long-term, low-dose systemic antibiotics is unproven. It has been suggested that topical gentamicin may be particularly effective in patients harboring a nonsense mutation in *ATP2C1* through aminoglycoside-induced read-through of nonsense mutations in human cells.[240] Topical application reduces the potential hearing and kidney toxicity of this class of drugs. Considering that 16% of *ATP2C1* mutations are nonsense mutations, patients with HHD carrying such mutations may be eligible for read-through therapy. However, the efficiency by which aminoglycosides induce read-through depends on the nature of the nonsense mutation and its nucleotidic environment. Skin penetration of the molecule may also be limited in the absence of erosions and fissures. Controlled clinical trials are therefore warranted.

Topical corticosteroids are often required to control skin inflammation and to help resolve flares.[126,241] They should be used in combination with topical antimicrobial agents to prevent exacerbation of infection. Pain may limit their application, but potent or ultrapotent topical corticosteroids (aqueous lotions, foams, creams, or ointments) are often efficacious. Their application should be limited to the treatment of acute flares. Prolonged treatment with potent corticosteroids favors superimposed infections, thereby limiting their chronic efficacy. Infection should be prevented or treated with local antiseptics, topical antibiotics, or both. Extensive use of potent topical steroids also increases the risk for cutaneous atrophy, which increases skin fragility. Very early application of topical steroids when only pruritus or limited vesiculopapules are present can significantly reduce the progression of lesions.

Topical calcineurin inhibitors represent a useful alternative to topical steroids for the control of inflammation. Tacrolimus ointment (0.03% or 0.1%) produced lesion resolution in several case reports[241-246] but was ineffective in others.[247,248] Superinfection and irritant contact dermatitis may explain lack of efficacy. Other topical agents that have been recommended include calcitriol,[249,250] tacalcitol,[251] and topical 5-fluorouracil.[252] Analgesia is crucial, and narcotics may be needed in severe disease.

Systemic corticosteroids are a short-term option for widespread disease.[253] Other systemic agents that have been advocated include retinoids,[254,255] methotrexate,[256] cyclosporin,[257,258] dapsone,[259] etanercept,[260] and alefacept.[261] Recently, a phase II open-label pilot study reported the successful use of the α-melanocortin analogue with antioxidant properties, afamelanotide, in two patients.[262] Oral glycopyrrolate (1 mg/day), a systemic anticholinergic drug that reduces hyperhidrosis, was reported to be effective and well tolerated in a patient with a long-standing history of relapsing HHD. Low-dose naltrexone also showed variable efficacy.

PROCEDURES

Alternative approaches have been used in recalcitrant disease. They include excision with or without grafting,[264-266] dermabrasion,[267,268] and laser surgery.[269-271] Other interventions that have been tried include breast reduction surgery for inframammary disease, superficial x-ray therapy (unhelpful),[272] electron-beam therapy,[273] and photodynamic therapy (very painful with variable outcomes).[274,275] Botulinum toxin type A (BTA) may help flexural disease by reducing sweating.[276-279] BTA therapy requires numerous injections at each affected site, which can be painful; has a high cost for a temporary relief; and needs to be regularly repeated every 4 to 6 months.

GENETIC COUNSELING

Genetic counseling should be provided by a medical geneticist, who will take into account the disease severity of the proband and other affected members of the family.

GROVER DISEASE

EPIDEMIOLOGY

GD (also called transient or persistent acantholytic dermatosis) is an acquired condition, first described in 1970, that is most common in fair skinned men older than 40 years old. The male-to-female ratio is 3 to 1.[280-283]

CLINICAL FEATURES

Unlike the other disorders in the chapter, GD is nonfamilial and often self-limited. It typically presents with an itchy rash on sun-damaged skin of the trunk. Itch may be intense and out of proportion to the signs, which comprise scattered pinkish or red-brown papules with variable hyperkeratosis, papulovesicles (rarely bullae), or less often eczematous plaques (Figs. 50-18 and 50-19). The neck, proximal limbs or both can be affected.[283-288] GD has been described in association with widespread sun-induced lentigines.[289,290] Guttate leukoderma, similar to that seen in DD, has been observed in dark skin.[291] Unilateral GD has been reported, but this may have been segmental DD.[292,293]

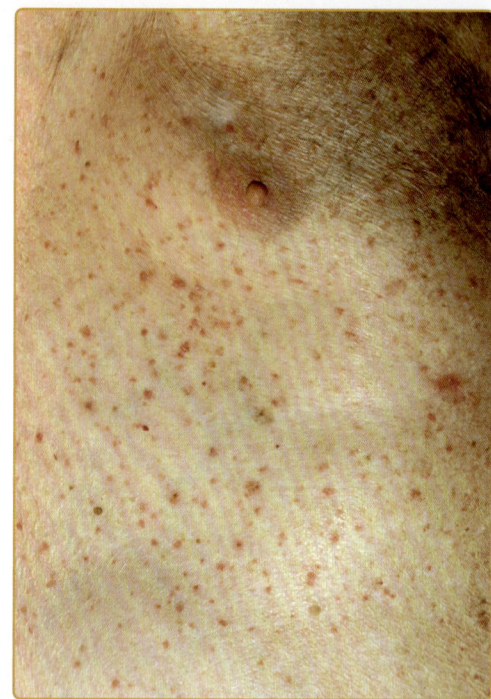

Figure 50-18 Grover disease. Itchy papules on the trunk resembling folliculitis in a 60-year-old man.

ETIOLOGY AND PATHOGENESIS

Although GD shares clinical, histologic, and ultrastructural features with DD, no mutation in *ATP2A2* has been identified in GD[289,294]; the pathogenesis remains unknown.

GD may be triggered by factors that promote sweating, such as febrile illnesses, bed confinement, or

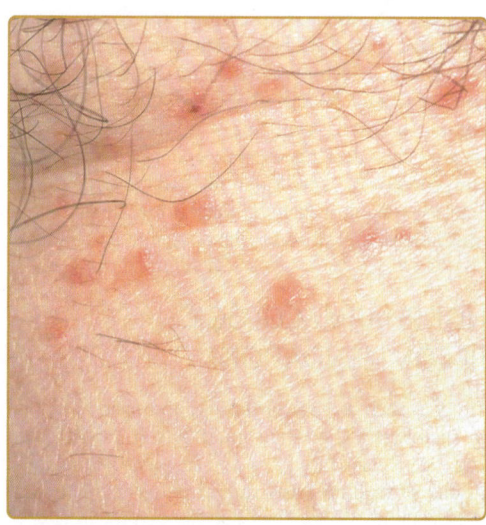

Figure 50-19 Grover disease. Discrete papulovesicular lesions with crusts in a 53-year-old man.

occlusion,[295-298] but is also common in the winter in older men with dry skin.[283,284,299,300] GD has been associated with other factors, including UV or ionizing radiation, inflammatory dermatoses such as atopic eczema, renal failure, HIV infection, malignancies, organ transplant, and some drugs.[282,283,301-305] An observation reported onset of the disease associated with varenicline, a partial agonist of the nicotinic acetylcholine receptor.[306] Electron microscopy shows clumping of keratin filaments with loss of desmosomes, and immunostaining reveals that desmosomal components are internalized.[97] Considering the number of conditions associated with GD, it is possible that multiple causes could result in the clinical and histologic features recognized as GD.[307]

HISTOPATHOLOGY

The histologic picture shows different patterns of acantholysis, which may suggest spongiotic dermatitis, DD, HHD, or pemphigus (although no immunoglobulin or complement are found in the epidermis), the latter being the most frequent pattern. These patterns may occur singly or in combination, which is very suggestive of GD. However, acantholysis can be subtle and focal (Fig. 50-20).[281,284]

DIFFERENTIAL DIAGNOSIS (SEE TABLE 50-7)

Other causes of itching such as scabies, insect bites, and eczema should be excluded. Clinicopathological correlation, including family history and examination of nails and mucous membranes, helps to exclude other causes of acantholysis. Because GD has been associated with many inflammatory and neoplastic conditions, it is essential to search for concomitant disorders, including hematologic malignancies.[307]

TABLE 50-7
Grover Disease: Differential Diagnosis

- Papular eczema or prurigo
- Folliculitis
- Sun damage with solar lentigines and solar keratoses
- Scabies
- Insect bites
- Miliaria rubra
- Darier disease
- Hailey-Hailey disease
- Pemphigus vulgaris

CLINICAL COURSE AND PROGNOSIS

GD may clear within a few months (transient acantholytic dermatosis), or the itch may persist with fluctuating intensity for years (persistent acantholytic dermatosis), especially in older adults.[308,309]

MANAGEMENT

Treatment is symptomatic and difficult, and the therapeutic response (or lack thereof) can be often disappointing.[283,288,310-314] Precipitating factors, including heat, sweating, sunlight, and topical irritants, should be avoided. Emollients and antipruritics may be soothing.

MEDICATIONS

Topical medicaments, such as corticosteroids, retinoids, calcipotriol, or tacalcitol, relieve irritation. Oral retinoids (acitretin), oral corticosteroids, UVB, psoralen and ultraviolet A light (PUVA), and methotrexate

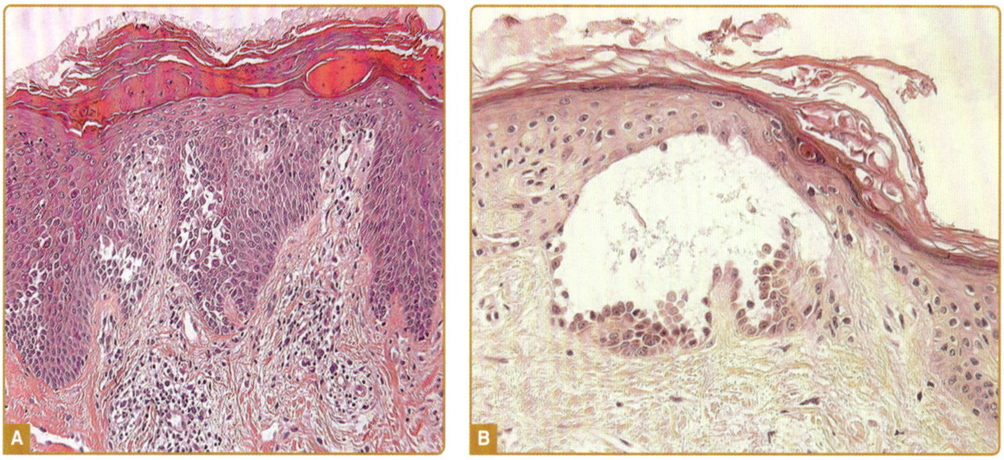

Figure 50-20 **A,** Hailey-Hailey–like histologic pattern in Grover disease with detached keratinocytes (acantholysis), focal spongiosis, and epidermal hyperplasia. **B,** Pemphigus-like pattern in Grover disease with suprabasal acantholytic cleavage.

Differentiating the acantholytic disorders			
	Darier Disease	**Hailey-Hailey Disease**	**Grover Disease**
Distribution	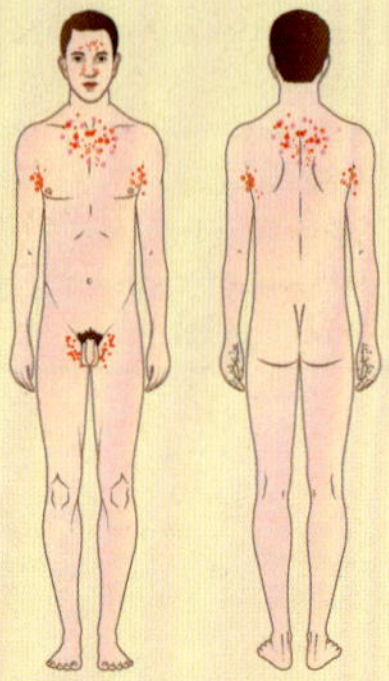	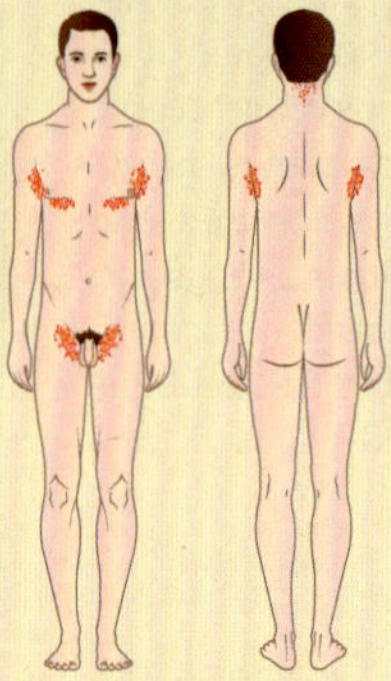	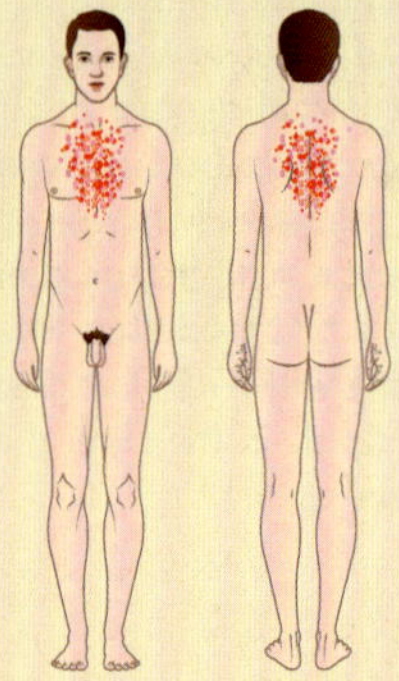
Age at onset	First to second decade	Third to fourth decade	Fifth decade and onward
Gene affected	*ATP2A2*	*ATP2C1*	(Acquired)
Characteristic lesion	Greasy, yellow-brown keratotic papules	Vesicopustules and fissured, vegetating plaques	Papules, crusted or hyperkeratotic
Mucosal involvement	–	–	–
Nail involvement	+	–	–

Figure 50-21 Differentiating the acantholytic disorders.

have been advocated for persistent disease, but controlled trials are lacking at this time. The combination of acitretin and phototherapy has been reported to suppress symptoms.[288]

SUMMARY

See Fig. 50-21.

REFERENCES

1. Burge SM, Wilkinson JD. Darier-White disease: a review of the clinical features in 163 patients. *J Am Acad Dermatol*. 1992;27(1):40-50.
2. Burge S. Darier's disease-the clinical features and pathogenesis. *Clin Exp Dermatol*. 1994;19(3):193-205.
3. Munro CS. The phenotype of Darier's disease: penetrance and expressivity in adults and children. *Br J Dermatol*. 1992;127(2):126-130.
4. Tavadia S, Mortimer E, Munro CS. Genetic epidemiology of Darier's disease: a population study in the west of Scotland. *Br J Dermatol*. 2002;146(1):107-109.
5. Godic A, Miljkovic J, Kansky A, et al. Epidemiology of Darier's disease in Slovenia. *Acta Dermatovenerol Alp Pannonica Adriat*. 2005;14(2):43-48.
6. Svendsen IB, Albrectsen B. The prevalence of dyskeratosis follicularis (Darier's disease) in Denmark: an investigation of the heredity in 22 families. *Acta Derm Venereol*. 1959;39:256-269.
7. Fong G, Capaldi L, Sweeney SM, et al. Congenital Darier disease. *J Am Acad Dermatol*. 2008;59(2 suppl 1):S50-51.
8. Parwanda N, Kumari N, Bhardwaj P. Darier-White disease. *Indian Pediatr*. 2013;50(7):717-718.
9. Harris A, Burge SM, Dykes PJ, et al. Handicap in Darier's disease and Hailey-Hailey disease. *Br J Dermatol*. 1996;135(6):959-963.
10. Rallis E, Economidi A, Papadakis P, et al. Acrokeratosis verruciformis of Hopf (Hopf disease): case report and review of the literature. *Dermatol Online J*. 2005;11(2):10.
11. Jones WN, Nix TE Jr, Clark WH Jr. Hemorrhagic Darier's disease. *Arch Dermatol*. 1964;89:523-527.
12. Coulson IH, Misch KJ. Haemorrhagic Darier's disease. *J R Soc Med*. 1989;82(6):365-366.
13. Foresman PL, Goldsmith LA, Ginn L, et al. Hemorrhagic Darier's disease. *Arch Dermatol*. 1993;129(4):511-512.
14. Regazzini R, Zambruno G, DeFilippi C, et al. Isolated acral Darier's disease with haemorrhagic lesions in a kindred. *Br J Dermatol*. 1996;135(3):495-496.
15. Brown VL, Kelly SE, Burge SM, et al. Extensive recalcitrant Darier disease successfully treated with laser ablation. *Br J Dermatol*. 2010;162(1):227-229.

16. Telfer NR, Burge SM, Ryan TJ. Vesiculo-bullous Darier's disease. *Br J Dermatol*. 1990;122(6):831-834.
17. Rongioletti F, Cestari R, Rebora A. Verrucous and malodorous vegetations on the legs. Darier's disease, cornifying type. *Arch Dermatol*. 1992;128(3):399, 402.
18. Katta R, Reed J, Wolf JE. Cornifying Darier's disease. *Int J Dermatol*. 2000;39(11):844-845.
19. Aliagaoglu C, Atasoy M, Anadolu R, et al. Comedonal, cornifying and hypertrophic Darier's disease in the same patient: a Darier combination. *J Dermatol*. 2006;33(7):477-480.
20. Fitzgerald DA, Lewis-Jones MS. Darier's disease presenting as isolated hyperkeratosis of the breasts. *Br J Dermatol*. 1997;136(2):290.
21. Tsuruta D, Akiyama M, Ishida-Yamamoto A, et al. Three-base deletion mutation c.120_122delGTT in ATP2A2 leads to the unique phenotype of comedonal Darier disease. *Br J Dermatol*. 2010;162(3):687-689.
22. Derrick EK, Darley CR, Burge S. Comedonal Darier's disease. *Br J Dermatol*. 1995;132(3):453-455.
23. Lee MW, Choi JH, Sung KJ, et al. Two cases of comedonal Darier's disease. *Clin Exp Dermatol*. 2002;27(8):714-715.
24. Millard TP, Dhitavat J, Hollowood K, et al. "Groveroid" Darier's disease? *Br J Dermatol*. 2004;150(3):600-602.
25. Ohtake N, Takano R, Saitoh A, et al. Brown papules and leukoderma in Darier's disease: clinical and histological features. *Dermatology*. 1994;188(2):157-159.
26. Goh BK, Ang P, Goh CL. Darier's disease in Singapore. *Br J Dermatol*. 2005;152(2):284-288.
27. Munro CS, Cox NH. An acantholytic dyskeratotic epidermal naevus with other features of Darier's disease on the same side of the body. *Br J Dermatol*. 1992;127(2):168-171.
28. Reese DA, Paul AY, Davis B. Unilateral segmental Darier disease following Blaschko lines: a case report and review of the literature. *Cutis*. 2005;76(3):197-200.
29. Sakuntabhai A, Dhitavat J, Burge S, et al. Mosaicism for ATP2A2 mutations causes segmental Darier's disease. *J Invest Dermatol*. 2000;115(6):1144-1147.
30. Wada T, Shirakata Y, Takahashi H, et al. A Japanese case of segmental Darier's disease caused by mosaicism for the ATP2A2 mutation. *Br J Dermatol*. 2003;149(1):185-188.
31. Gilaberte M, Puig L, Vidal D, et al. Acantholytic dyskeratotic naevi following Blaschko's lines: a mosaic form of Darier's disease. *J Eur Acad Dermatol Venereol*. 2003;17(2):196-199.
32. Morin CB, Netchiporouk E, Billick RC, et al. Hypopigmented segmental Darier disease. *J Cutan Med Surg*. 2015;19(1):69-72.
33. Happle R, Itin PH, Brun AM. Type 2 segmental Darier disease. *Eur J Dermatol*. 1999;9(6):449-451.
34. Folster-Holst R, Nellen RG, Jensen JM, et al. Molecular genetic support for the rule of dichotomy in type 2 segmental Darier disease. *Br J Dermatol*. 2012;166(2):464-466.
35. Macleod RI, Munro CS. The incidence and distribution of oral lesions in patients with Darier's disease. *Br Dent J*. 1991;171(5):133-136.
36. Cardoso CL, Freitas P, Taveira LA, et al. Darier disease: case report with oral manifestations. *Med Oral Patol Oral Circ Bucal*. 2006;11(5):E404-406.
37. Bernabe DG, Kawata LT, Beneti IM, et al. Multiple white papules in the palate: oral manifestation of Darier's disease. *Clin Exp Dermatol*. 2009;34(7):e270-271.
38. Vieites B, Seijo-Rios S, Suarez-Penaranda JM, et al. Darier's disease with esophageal involvement. *Scan J Gastroenterol*. 2008;43(8):1020-1021.
39. Al Robaee A, Hamadah IR, Khuroo S, et al. Extensive Darier's disease with esophageal involvement. *Int J Dermatol*. 2004;43(11):835-839.
40. Klein A, Burns L, Leyden JJ. Rectal mucosa involvement in keratosis follicularis. *Arch Dermatol*. 1974;109(4):560-561.
41. Adam AE. Ectopic Darier's disease of the cervix: an extraordinary cause of an abnormal smear. *Cytopathology*. 1996;7(6):414-421.
42. Blackman HJ, Rodrigues MM, Peck GL. Corneal epithelial lesions in keratosis follicularis (Darier's disease). *Ophthalmology*. 1980;87(9):931-943.
43. Mielke J, Grub M, Besch D, et al. Recurrent corneal ulcerations with perforation in keratosis follicularis (Darier-White disease). *Br J Ophthalmol*. 2002;86(10):1192-1193.
44. Lagali N, Dellby A, Fagerholm P. In vivo confocal microscopy of the cornea in Darier-White disease. *Arch Ophthalmol*. 2009;127(6):816-818.
45. Ramien ML, Prendiville JS, Brown KL, et al. Cystic bone lesions in a boy with Darier disease: a magnetic resonance imaging assessment. *J Am Acad Dermatol*. 2009;60(6):1062-1066.
46. Castori M, Barboni L, Duncan PJ, et al. Darier disease, multiple bone cysts, and aniridia due to double de novo heterozygous mutations in ATP2A2 and PAX6. *Am J Med Genet A*. 2009;149A(8):1768-1772.
47. Crisp AJ, Payne CM, Adams J, et al. The prevalence of bone cysts in Darier's disease: a survey of 31 cases. *Clin Exp Dermatol*. 1984;9(1):78-83.
48. Bchetnia M, Charfeddine C, Kassar S, et al. Clinical and mutational heterogeneity of Darier disease in Tunisian families. *Arch Dermatol*. 2009;145(6):654-656.
49. Ehrt U, Brieger P. Comorbidity of keratosis follicularis (Darier's Disease) and bipolar affective disorder: an indication for valproate instead of lithium. *Gen Hosp Psychiatry*. 2000;22(2):128-129.
50. Wang SL, Yang SF, Chen CC, et al. Darier's disease associated with bipolar affective disorder: a case report. *Kaohsiung J Med Sci*. 2002;18(12):622-626.
51. Gordon-Smith K, Jones LA, Burge SM, et al. The neuropsychiatric phenotype in Darier disease. *Br J Dermatol*. 2010;163(3):515-522.
52. Sule N, Teszas A, Kalman E, et al. Lithium suppresses epidermal SERCA2 and PMR1 levels in the rat. *Pathol Oncol Res*. 2006;12(4):234-236.
53. Clark RD Jr, Hammer CJ, Patterson SD. A cutaneous disorder (Darier's disease) evidently exacerbated by lithium carbonate. *Psychosomatics*. 1986;27(11):800-801.
54. Milton GP, Peck GL, Fu JJ, et al. Exacerbation of Darier's disease by lithium carbonate. *J Am Acad Dermatol*. 1990;23(5 Pt 1):926-928.
55. Rubin MB. Lithium-induced Darier's disease. *J Am Acad Dermatol*. 1995;32(4):674-675.
56. Denicoff KD, Lehman ZA, Rubinow DR, et al. Suicidal ideation in Darier's disease. *J Am Acad Dermatol*. 1990;22(2 Pt 1):196-198.
57. Jones I, Jacobsen N, Green EK, et al. Evidence for familial cosegregation of major affective disorder and genetic markers flanking the gene for Darier's disease. *Mol Psychiatry*. 2002;7(4):424-427.
58. Jacobsen NJ, Franks EK, Elvidge G, et al. Exclusion of the Darier's disease gene, ATP2A2, as a common susceptibility gene for bipolar disorder. *Mol Psychiatry*. 2001;6(1):92-97.

59. Green EK, Grozeva D, Raybould R, et al. P2RX7: a bipolar and unipolar disorder candidate susceptibility gene? *Am J Med Genet B*. 2009;150B(8):1063-1069.
60. Parham DM, Gawkrodger DJ, Vestey JP, Beveridge GW. Disseminated herpes simplex infection complicating Darier's disease: successful treatment with oral acyclovir. *J Infect*. 1985;10(1):77-78.
61. Kandasamy R, Hecker M, Choi M, et al. Darier disease complicated by disseminated zoster. *Dermatol Online J*. 2009;15(2):6.
62. Tegner E, Jonsson N. Darier's disease with involvement of both submandibular glands. *Acta Derm Venereol*. 1990;70(5):451-452.
63. Alexandrescu DT, Dasanu CA, Farzanmehr H, et al. Development of squamous cell carcinomas in Darier disease: a new model for skin carcinogenesis? *Br J Dermatol*. 2008;159(6):1378-1380.
64. Matsui K, Makino T, Nakano H, et al. Squamous cell carcinoma arising from Darier's disease. *Clin Exp Dermatol*. 2009;34(8):e1015-1016.
65. Vazquez J, Morales C, Gonzalez LO, et al. Vulval squamous cell carcinoma arising in localized Darier's disease. *Eur J Obstet Gynecol Reprod Biol*. 2002;102(2):206-208.
66. Orihuela E, Tyring SK, Pow-Sang M, et al. Development of human papillomavirus type 16 associated squamous cell carcinoma of the scrotum in a patient with Darier's disease treated with systemic isotretinoin. *J Urol*. 1995;153(6):1940-1943.
67. Craddock N, Dawson E, Burge S, et al. The gene for Darier's disease maps to chromosome 12q23-q24.1. *Hum Mol Genet*. 1993;2(11):1941-1943.
68. Sakuntabhai A, Ruiz-Perez V, Carter S, et al. Mutations in ATP2A2, encoding a Ca^{2+} pump, cause Darier disease. *Nat Genet*. 1999;21(3):271-277.
69. Pani B, Singh BB. Darier's disease: a calcium-signaling perspective. *Cell Mol Life Sci*. 2008;65(2):205-211.
70. Hovnanian A. Darier's disease: from dyskeratosis to endoplasmic reticulum calcium ATPase deficiency. *Biochem Biophys Res Commun*. 2004;322(4):1237-1244.
71. Hovnanian A. SERCA pumps and human diseases. *Subcell Biochem*. 2007;45:337-363.
72. Dhitavat J, Fairclough RJ, Hovnanian A, et al. Calcium pumps and keratinocytes: lessons from Darier's disease and Hailey-Hailey disease. *Br J Dermatol*. 2004;150(5):821-828.
73. Verboomen H, Wuytack F, De Smedt H, et al. Functional difference between SERCA2a and SERCA2b Ca^{2+} pumps and their modulation by phospholamban. *Biochem J*. 1992;286 (Pt 2):591-595.
74. Verboomen H, Wuytack F, Van den Bosch L, et al. The functional importance of the extreme C-terminal tail in the gene 2 organellar Ca(2+)-transport ATPase (SERCA2a/b). *Biochem J*. 1994;303 (Pt 3):979-984.
75. Tavadia S, Tait RC, McDonagh TA, et al. Platelet and cardiac function in Darier's disease. *Clin Exp Dermatol*. 2001;26(8):696-699.
76. Mayosi BM, Kardos A, Davies CH, et al. Heterozygous disruption of SERCA2a is not associated with impairment of cardiac performance in humans: implications for SERCA2a as a therapeutic target in heart failure. *Heart*. 2006;92(1):105-109.
77. Tavadia S, Authi KS, Hodgins MB, et al. Expression of the sarco/endoplasmic reticulum calcium ATPase type 2 and 3 isoforms in normal skin and Darier's disease. *Br J Dermatol*. 2004;151(2):440-445.
78. Dhitavat J, Dode L, Leslie N, et al. Mutations in the sarcoplasmic/endoplasmic reticulum Ca^{2+} ATPase isoform b cause Darier's disease. *J Invest Dermatol*. 2003;121(3):486-489.
79. Ikeda S, Mayuzumi N, Shigihara T, et al. Mutations in ATP2A2 in patients with Darier's disease. *J Invest Dermatol*. 2003;121(3):475-477.
80. Wuytack F, Raeymaekers L, Missiaen L. Molecular physiology of the SERCA and SPCA pumps. *Cell Calcium*. 2002;32(5-6):279-305.
81. Nellen RG, Steijlen PM, van Steensel MA, et al. Mendelian disorders of cornification caused by defects in intracellular calcium pumps: mutation update and database for variants in atp2a2 and atp2c1 associated with Darier disease and Hailey-Hailey disease. *Hum Mutat*. 2017;38(4):343-356.
82. Sakuntabhai A, Burge S, Monk S, et al. Spectrum of novel ATP2A2 mutations in patients with Darier's disease. *Hum Mol Genet*. 1999;8(9):1611-1619.
83. Jacobsen NJ, Lyons I, Hoogendoorn B, et al. ATP2A2 mutations in Darier's disease and their relationship to neuropsychiatric phenotypes. *Hum Mol Genet*. 1999;8(9):1631-1636.
84. Ruiz-Perez VL, Carter SA, Healy E, et al. ATP2A2 mutations in Darier's disease: variant cutaneous phenotypes are associated with missense mutations, but neuropsychiatric features are independent of mutation class. *Hum Mol Genet*. 1999;8(9):1621-1630.
85. Ringpfeil F, Raus A, DiGiovanna JJ, et al. Darier disease-novel mutations in ATP2A2 and genotype-phenotype correlation. *Exp Dermatol*. 2001;10(1):19-27.
86. Takahashi H, Atsuta Y, Sato K, et al. Novel mutations of ATP2A2 gene in Japanese patients of Darier's disease. *J Dermatol Sci*. 2001;26(3):169-172.
87. Yang Y, Li G, Bu D, et al. Novel point mutations of the ATP2A2 gene in two Chinese families with Darier disease. *J Invest Dermatol*. 2001;116(3):482-483.
88. Pecina-Slaus N, Milavec-Puretic V, Kubat M, et al. Clinical case of acral hemorrhagic Darier's disease is not caused by mutations in exon 15 of the ATP2A2 gene. *Coll Antropol*. 2003;27(1):125-133.
89. Godic A, Glavac D, Korosec B, et al. P160L mutation in the Ca(2+) ATPase 2A domain in a patient with severe Darier disease. *Dermatology*. 2004;209(2):142-144.
90. Onozuka T, Sawamura D, Yokota K, et al. Mutational analysis of the ATP2A2 gene in two Darier disease families with intrafamilial variability. *Br J Dermatol*. 2004;150(4):652-657.
91. Racz E, Csikos M, Kornsee Z, et al. Identification of mutations in the ATP2A2 gene in patients with Darier's disease from Hungary. *Exp Dermatol*. 2004;13(6):396-399.
92. Racz E, Csikos M, Benko R, et al. Three novel mutations in the ATP2A2 gene in Hungarian families with Darier's disease, including a novel splice site generating intronic nucleotide change. *J Dermatol Sci*. 2005;38(3):231-234.
93. Ren YQ, Gao M, Liang YH, et al. Five mutations of ATP2A2 gene in Chinese patients with Darier's disease and a literature review of 86 cases reported in China. *Arch Dermatol Res*. 2006;298(2):58-63.
94. Leinonen PT, Hagg PM, Peltonen S, et al. Reevaluation of the normal epidermal calcium gradient, and analysis of calcium levels and ATP receptors in Hailey-Hailey and Darier epidermis. *J Invest Dermatol*. 2009;129(6):1379-1387.
95. Caulfield JB, Wilgram GF. An electron-microscope study of dyskeratosis and acantholysis in Darier's disease. *J Invest Dermatol*. 1963;41:57-65.

96. Burge SM, Garrod DR. An immunohistological study of desmosomes in Darier's disease and Hailey-Hailey disease. *Br J Dermatol*. 1991;124(3):242-251.
97. Hashimoto K, Fujiwara K, Tada J, et al. Desmosomal dissolution in Grover's disease, Hailey-Hailey's disease and Darier's disease. *J Cutan Pathol*. 1995;22(6):488-501.
98. Hakuno M, Shimizu H, Akiyama M, et al. Dissociation of intra- and extracellular domains of desmosomal cadherins and E-cadherin in Hailey-Hailey disease and Darier's disease. *Br J Dermatol*. 2000;142(4):702-711.
99. Gniadecki R, Jemec GB, Thomsen BM, et al. Relationship between keratinocyte adhesion and death: anoikis in acantholytic diseases. *Arch Dermatol Res*. 1998;290(10):528-532.
100. Dremina ES, Sharov VS, Kumar K, et al. Anti-apoptotic protein Bcl-2 interacts with and destabilizes the sarcoplasmic/endoplasmic reticulum Ca^{2+}-ATPase (SERCA). *Biochem J*. 2004;383(Pt 2):361-370.
101. Bongiorno MR, Arico M. The behaviour of Bcl-2, Bax and Bcl-x in Darier's disease. *Br J Dermatol*. 2002;147(4):696-700.
102. Pasmatzi E, Badavanis G, Monastirli A, et al. Reduced expression of the antiapoptotic proteins of Bcl-2 gene family in the lesional epidermis of patients with Darier's disease. *J Cutan Pathol*. 2007;34(3):234-238.
103. Burge SM, Fenton DA, Dawber RP, et al. Darier's disease: an immunohistochemical study using monoclonal antibodies to human cytokeratins. *Br J Dermatol*. 1988;118(5):629-640.
104. Koizumi H, Kartasova T, Tanaka H, et al. Differentiation-associated localization of small proline-rich protein in normal and diseased human skin. *Br J Dermatol*. 1996;134(4):686-692.
105. Kassar S, Charfeddine C, Zribi H, et al. Immunohistological study of involucrin expression in Darier's disease skin. *J Cutan Pathol*. 2008;35(7):635-640.
106. Leinonen PT, Myllyla RM, Hagg PM, et al. Keratinocytes cultured from patients with Hailey-Hailey disease and Darier disease display distinct patterns of calcium regulation. *Br J Dermatol*. 2005;153(1):113-117.
107. Foggia L, Aronchik I, Aberg K, et al. Activity of the hSPCA1 Golgi Ca^{2+} pump is essential for Ca^{2+}-mediated Ca^{2+} response and cell viability in Darier disease. *J Cell Sci*. 2006;119(Pt 4):671-679.
108. Savignac M, Simon M, Edir A, et al. SERCA2 dysfunction in Darier disease causes endoplasmic reticulum stress and impaired cell-to-cell adhesion strength: rescue by Miglustat. *J Invest Dermatol*. 2014;134(7):1961-1970.
109. Dhitavat J, Cobbold C, Leslie N, et al. Impaired trafficking of the desmoplakins in cultured Darier's disease keratinocytes. *J Invest Dermatol*. 2003;121(6):1349-1355.
110. Hobbs RP, Amargo EV, Somasundaram A, et al. The calcium ATPase SERCA2 regulates desmoplakin dynamics and intercellular adhesive strength through modulation of PKCα signaling. *FASEB J*. 2011;25(3):990-1001.
111. Celli A, Mackenzie DS, Zhai Y, et al. SERCA2-controlled Ca(2)+-dependent keratinocyte adhesion and differentiation is mediated via the sphingolipid pathway: a therapeutic target for Darier's disease. *J Invest Dermatol*. 2012;132(4):1188-1195.
112. Li N, Park M, Xiao S, et al. ER-to-Golgi blockade of nascent desmosomal cadherins in SERCA2-inhibited keratinocytes: implications for Darier's disease. *Traffic*. 2017;18(4):232-241.
113. Hong JH, Youm JK, Kwon MJ, et al. K6PC-5, a direct activator of sphingosine kinase 1, promotes epidermal differentiation through intracellular Ca^{2+} signaling. *J Invest Dermatol*. 2008;128(9):2166-2178.
114. Lichte K, Rossi R, Danneberg K, et al. Lysophospholipid receptor-mediated calcium signaling in human keratinocytes. *J Invest Dermatol*. 2008;128(6):1487-1498.
115. Meyer zu Heringdorf D, Liliom K, Schaefer M, et al. Photolysis of intracellular caged sphingosine-1-phosphate causes Ca^{2+} mobilization independently of G-protein-coupled receptors. *FEBS Lett*. 2003;554(3):443-449.
116. Norez C, Noel S, Wilke M, et al. Rescue of functional delF508-CFTR channels in cystic fibrosis epithelial cells by the alpha-glucosidase inhibitor miglustat. *FEBS Lett*. 2006;580(8):2081-2086.
117. Pasdar M, Nelson WJ. Kinetics of desmosome assembly in Madin-Darby canine kidney epithelial cells: temporal and spatial regulation of desmoplakin organization and stabilization upon cell-cell contact. II. Morphological analysis. *J Cell Biol*. 1988;106(3):687-695.
118. Pani B, Cornatzer E, Cornatzer W, et al. Up-regulation of transient receptor potential canonical 1 (TRPC1) following sarco(endo)plasmic reticulum Ca^{2+} ATPase 2 gene silencing promotes cell survival: a potential role for TRPC1 in Darier's disease. *Mol Biol Cell*. 2006;17(10):4446-4458.
119. Mayuzumi N, Ikeda S, Kawada H, et al. Effects of ultraviolet B irradiation, proinflammatory cytokines and raised extracellular calcium concentration on the expression of ATP2A2 and ATP2C1. *Br J Dermatol*. 2005;152(4):697-701.
120. Liu LH, Boivin GP, Prasad V, et al. Squamous cell tumors in mice heterozygous for a null allele of Atp2a2, encoding the sarco(endo)plasmic reticulum Ca^{2+}-ATPase isoform 2 Ca^{2+} pump. *J Biol Chem*. 2001;276(29):26737-26740.
121. Hong JH, Yang YM, Kim HS, et al. Markers of squamous cell carcinoma in sarco/endoplasmic reticulum Ca^{2+} ATPase 2 heterozygote mice keratinocytes. *Prog Biophys Mol Biol*. 2010;103(1):81-87.
122. Downs AM, Ward KA, Peachey RD. Subungual squamous cell carcinoma in Darier's disease. *Clin Exp Dermatol*. 1997;22(6):277-279.
123. Hall JR, Holder W, Knox JM, et al. Familial dyskeratotic comedones. A report of three cases and review of the literature. *J Am Acad Dermatol*. 1987;17(5 Pt 1):808-814.
124. Hallermann C, Bertsch HP. Two sisters with familial dyskeratotic comedones. *Eur J Dermatol*. 2004;14(4):214-215.
125. Nakagawa T, Masada M, Moriue T, et al. Comedo-like acantholytic dyskeratosis of the face and scalp: a new entity? *Br J Dermatol*. 2000;142(5):1047-1048.
126. Burge SM. Hailey-Hailey disease: the clinical features, response to treatment and prognosis. *Br J Dermatol*. 1992;126(3):275-282.
127. Gilchrist H, Jackson S, Morse L, et al. Galli-Galli disease: a case report with review of the literature. *J Am Acad Dermatol*. 2008;58(2):299-302.
128. Niedleman ML, Mc KV. Acrokeratosis verruciformis (Hopf). A follow-up study. *Arch Dermatol*. 1962;86:779-782.
129. Dhitavat J, Macfarlane S, Dode L, et al. Acrokeratosis verruciformis of Hopf is caused by mutation in

ATP2A2: evidence that it is allelic to Darier's disease. *J Invest Dermatol*. 2003;120(2):229-232.
130. Browne F, Keane H, Walsh M, et al. Papular acantholytic dyskeratosis presenting as genital warts. *Int J STD AIDS*. 2007;18(12):867-868.
131. Salopek TG, Krol A, Jimbow K. Case report of Darier disease localized to the vulva in a 5-year-old girl. *Pediatr Dermatol*. 1993;10(2):146-148.
132. Langenberg A, Berger TG, Cardelli M, et al. Genital benign chronic pemphigus (Hailey-Hailey disease) presenting as condylomas. *J Am Acad Dermatol*. 1992;26(6):951-955.
133. Cooper PH. Acantholytic dermatosis localized to the vulvocrural area. *J Cutan Pathol*. 1989;16(2):81-84.
134. Knopp EA, Saraceni C, Moss J, et al. Somatic ATP2A2 mutation in a case of papular acantholytic dyskeratosis: mosaic Darier disease. *J Cutan Pathol*. 2015;42(11):853-857.
135. Brazzelli V, Prestinari F, Barbagallo T, et al. Linear Darier's disease successfully treated with 0.1% tazarotene gel "short-contact" therapy. *Eur J Dermatol*. 2006;16(1):59-61.
136. Micali G, Nasca MR. Tazarotene gel in childhood Darier disease. *Pediatr Dermatol*. 1999;16(3):243-244.
137. Burge SM, Buxton PK. Topical isotretinoin in Darier's disease. *Br J Dermatol*. 1995;133(6):924-928.
138. Casals M, Campoy A, Aspiolea F, et al. Successful treatment of linear Darier's disease with topical adapalene. *J Eur Acad Dermatol Venereol*. 2009;23(2):237-238.
139. Cianchini G, Colonna L, Camaioni D, et al. Acral Darier's disease successfully treated with adapalene. *Acta Derm Venereol*. 2001;81(1):57-58.
140. Knulst AC, De La Faille HB, Van Vloten WA. Topical 5-fluorouracil in the treatment of Darier's disease. *Br J Dermatol*. 1995;133(3):463-466.
141. Schmidt H, Ochsendorf FR, Wolter M, et al. Topical 5-fluorouracil in Darier disease. *Br J Dermatol*. 2008;158(6):1393-1396.
142. Rubegni P, Poggiali S, Sbano P, et al. A case of Darier's disease successfully treated with topical tacrolimus. *J Eur Acad Dermatol Venereol*. 2006;20(1):84-87.
143. Cooper SM, Burge SM. Darier's disease: epidemiology, pathophysiology, and management. *Am J Clin Dermatol*. 2003;4(2):97-105.
144. Shahidullah H, Humphreys F, Beveridge GW. Darier's disease: severe eczematization successfully treated with cyclosporin. *Br J Dermatol*. 1994;131(5):713-716.
145. Stewart LC, Yell J. Vulval Darier's disease treated successfully with ciclosporin. *J Obstet Gynaecol*. 2008;28(1):108-109.
146. Exadaktylou D, Kurwa HA, Calonje E, et al. Treatment of Darier's disease with photodynamic therapy. *Br J Dermatol*. 2003;149(3):606-610.
147. Minsue Chen T, Wanitphakdeedecha R, Nguyen TH. Carbon dioxide laser ablation and adjunctive destruction for Darier-White disease (keratosis follicularis). *Dermatol Surg*. 2008;34(10):1431-1434.
148. Santiago-et-Sanchez-Mateos JL, Bea S, Fernandez M, et al. Botulinum toxin type A for the preventive treatment of intertrigo in a patient with Darier's disease and inguinal hyperhidrosis. *Dermatol Surg*. 2008;34(12):1733-1737.
149. Cohen PR. Darier disease: sustained improvement following reduction mammaplasty. *Cutis*. 2003;72(2):124-126.
150. Bukhari I. Acrokeratosis verruciformis of Hopf: a localized variant. *J Drugs Dermatol*. 2004;3(6):687-688.
151. Bergman R, Sezin T, Indelman M, et al. Acrokeratosis verruciformis of Hopf showing P602L mutation in ATP2A2 and overlapping histopathological features with Darier disease. *Am J Dermatopathol*. 2012;34(6):597-601.
152. Ronan A, Ingrey A, Murray N, et al. Recurrent ATP2A2 p.(Pro602Leu) mutation differentiates Acrokeratosis verruciformis of Hopf from the allelic condition Darier disease. *Am J Med Genet A*. 2017.
153. Wang PG, Gao M, Lin GS, et al. Genetic heterogeneity in acrokeratosis verruciformis of Hopf. *Clin Exp Dermatol*. 2006;31(4):558-563.
154. Serarslan G, Balci DD, Homan S. Acitretin treatment in acrokeratosis verruciformis of Hopf. *J Dermatolog Treat*. 2007;18(2):123-125.
155. Kirtschig G, Effendy I, Happle R. Leukonychia longitudinalis as the primary symptom of Hailey-Hailey disease. *Hautarzt*. 1992;43(7):451-452.
156. Marsch WC, Stuttgen G. Generalized Hailey-Hailey disease. *Br J Dermatol*. 1978;99(5):553-560.
157. Gisondi P, Sampogna F, Annessi G, et al. Severe impairment of quality of life in Hailey-Hailey disease. *Acta Derm Venereol*. 2005;85(2):132-135.
158. Meffert JJ, Davis BM, Campbell JC. Bullous drug eruption to griseofulvin in a man with Hailey-Hailey disease. *Cutis*. 1995;56(5):279-280.
159. Richard G, Linse R, Harth W. Hailey-Hailey disease. Early detection of heterozygotes by an ultraviolet provocation tests—clinical relevance of the method. *Hautarzt*. 1993;44(6):376-379.
160. Galimberti RL, Kowalczuk AM, Bianchi O, et al. Chronic benign familial pemphigus. *Int J Dermatol*. 1988;27(7):495-500.
161. Marren P, Burge S. Seborrhoeic dermatitis of the scalp—a manifestation of Hailey-Hailey disease in a predisposed individual? *Br J Dermatol*. 1992;126(3):294-296.
162. Ponyai G, Karpati S, Ablonczy E, et al. Benign familial chronic pemphigus (Hailey-Hailey) provoked by contact sensitivity in 2 patients. *Contact Dermatitis*. 1999;40(3):168-169.
163. Peppiatt T, Keefe M, White JE. Hailey-Hailey disease—exacerbation by herpes simplex virus and patch tests. *Clin Exp Dermatol*. 1992;17(3):201-202.
164. Rudolph CM, Kranke B, Turek TD, et al. Contact irritation provoking Hailey-Hailey disease. *Contact Dermatitis*. 2001;44(6):371.
165. Gerdsen R, Hartl C, Christ S, et al. Hailey-Hailey disease: exacerbation by scabies. *Br J Dermatol*. 2001;144(1):211-212.
166. Walker SL, Beck MH. Undiagnosed Hailey-Hailey disease causing painful erosive skin changes during patch testing. *Br J Dermatol*. 2005;153(1):233-234.
167. Hwang LY, Lee JB, Richard G, et al. Type 1 segmental manifestation of Hailey-Hailey disease. *J Am Acad Dermatol*. 2003;49(4):712-714.
168. Poblete-Gutierrez P, Wiederholt T, Konig A, et al. Allelic loss underlies type 2 segmental Hailey-Hailey disease, providing molecular confirmation of a novel genetic concept. *J Clin Invest*. 2004;114(10):1467-1474.
169. Pernet C, Bessis D, Savignac M, et al. Genitoperineal papular acantholytic dyskeratosis is allelic to Hailey-Hailey disease. *Br J Dermatol*. 2012;167(1):210-212.
170. Lipoff JB, Mudgil AV, Young S, et al. Acantholytic dermatosis of the crural folds with ATP2C1 mutation is a possible variant of Hailey-Hailey Disease. *J Cutan Med Surg*. 2009;13(3):151-154.

171. Yu WY, Ng E, Hale C, et al. Papular acantholytic dyskeratosis of the vulva associated with familial Hailey-Hailey disease. *Clin Exp Dermatol*. 2016;41(6):628-631.
172. Wong TY, Mihm MC Jr. Acantholytic dermatosis localized to genitalia and crural areas of male patients: a report of three cases. *J Cutan Pathol*. 1994;21(1):27-32.
173. Dittmer CJ, Hornemann A, Rose C, et al. Successful laser therapy of a papular acantholytic dyskeratosis of the vulva: case report and review of literature. *Arch Gynecol Obstet*. 2010;281(4):723-725.
174. Al-Muriesh M, Abdul-Fattah B, Wang X, et al. Papular acantholytic dyskeratosis of the anogenital and genitocrural area: case series and review of the literature. *J Cutan Pathol*. 2016;43(9):749-758.
175. Kahn D, Hutchinson E. Esophageal involvement in familial benign chronic pemphigus. *Arch Dermatol*. 1974;109(5):718-719.
176. Vaclavinkova V, Neumann E. Vaginal involvement in familial benign chronic pemphigus (Morbus Hailey-Hailey). *Acta Derm Venereol*. 1982;62(1):80-81.
177. Oguz O, Gokler G, Ocakoglu O, et al. Conjunctival involvement in familial chronic benign pemphigus (Hailey-Hailey disease). *Int J Dermatol*. 1997;36(4):282-285.
178. Mashiko M, Akiyama M, Tsuji-Abe Y, et al. Bacterial infection-induced generalized Hailey-Hailey disease successfully treated by etretinate. *Clin Exp Dermatol*. 2006;31(1):57-59.
179. Holst VA, Fair KP, Wilson BB, et al. Squamous cell carcinoma arising in Hailey-Hailey disease. *J Am Acad Dermatol*. 2000;43(2 Pt 2):368-371.
180. Cockayne SE, Rassl DM, Thomas SE. Squamous cell carcinoma arising in Hailey-Hailey disease of the vulva. *Br J Dermatol*. 2000;142(3):540-542.
181. Otsuka F, Niimura M, Harada S, et al. Generalized herpes simplex complicating Hailey-Hailey's disease. *J Dermatol*. 1981;8(1):63-68.
182. Schirren H, Schirren CG, Schlupen EM, et al. Exacerbation of Hailey-Hailey disease by infection with herpes simplex virus. Detection with polymerase chain reaction. *Hautarzt*. 1995;46(7):494-497.
183. Stallmann D, Schmoeckel C. Hailey-Hailey disease with dissemination and eczema herpeticatum in therapy with etretinate. *Hautarzt*. 1988;39(7):454-456.
184. Mak RK, Reynaert SM, Agar N, et al. Hailey-Hailey disease failing to respond to treatment. *Clin Exp Dermatol*. 2005;30(5):598-599.
185. Reitamo S, Remitz A, Lauerma AI, et al. Contact allergies in patients with familial benign chronic pemphigus (Hailey-Hailey disease). *J Am Acad Dermatol*. 1989;21(3 Pt 1):506-510.
186. Remitz A, Lauerma AI, Stubb S, et al. Darier's disease, familial benign chronic pemphigus (Hailey-Hailey disease) and contact hypersensitivity. *J Am Acad Dermatol*. 1990;22(1):134.
187. Furue M, Seki Y, Oohara K, et al. Basal cell epithelioma arising in a patient with Hailey-Hailey's disease. *Int J Dermatol*. 1987;26(7):461-462.
188. Mohr MR, Erdag G, Shada AL, et al. Two patients with Hailey-Hailey disease, multiple primary melanomas, and other cancers. *Arch Dermatol*. 2011;147(2):211-215.
189. Ochiai T, Honda A, Morishima T, et al. Human papillomavirus types 16 and 39 in a vulval carcinoma occurring in a woman with Hailey-Hailey disease. *Br J Dermatol*. 1999;140(3):509-513.
190. Chen MY, Chiu HC, Su LH, et al. Presence of human papillomavirus type 6 DNA in the perineal verrucoid lesions of Hailey-Hailey disease. *J Eur Acad Dermatol Venereol*. 2006;20(10):1356-1357.
191. Chan CC, Thong HY, Chan YC, et al. Human papillomavirus type 5 infection in a patient with Hailey-Hailey disease successfully treated with imiquimod. *Br J Dermatol*. 2007;156(3):579-581.
192. von Felbert V, Hampl M, Talhari C, et al. Squamous cell carcinoma arising from a localized vulval lesion of Hailey-Hailey disease after tacrolimus therapy. *Am J Obstet Gynecol*. 2010;203(3):e5-7.
193. Korner J, Rietschel M, Nothen MM, et al. Familial cosegregation of affective disorder and Hailey-Hailey disease. *Br J Psychiatry*. 1993;163:109-110.
194. Wilk M, Rietschel M, Korner J, et al. Pemphigus chronicus benignus familiaris (Hailey-Hailey disease) and bipolar affective disease in 3 members of a family. *Hautarzt*. 1994;45(5):313-317.
195. Yokota K, Sawamura D. Hailey-Hailey disease with affective disorder: report of a case with novel ATP2C1 gene mutation. *J Dermatol Sci*. 2006;43(2):150-151.
196. Hu Z, Bonifas JM, Beech J, et al. Mutations in ATP2C1, encoding a calcium pump, cause Hailey-Hailey disease. *Nat Genet*. 2000;24(1):61-65.
197. Sudbrak R, Brown J, Dobson-Stone C, et al. Hailey-Hailey disease is caused by mutations in ATP2C1 encoding a novel Ca(2+) pump. *Hum Mol Genet*. 2000;9(7):1131-1140.
198. Missiaen L, Dode L, Vanoevelen J, et al. Calcium in the Golgi apparatus. *Cell Calcium*. 2007;41(5):405-416.
199. Vanoevelen J, Dode L, Raeymaekers L, et al. Diseases involving the Golgi calcium pump. *Subcell Biochem*. 2007;45:385-404.
200. Missiaen L, Raeymaekers L, Dode L, et al. SPCA1 pumps and Hailey-Hailey disease. *Biochem Biophys Res Commun*. 2004;322(4):1204-1213.
201. Dobson-Stone C, Fairclough R, Dunne E, et al. Hailey-Hailey disease: molecular and clinical characterization of novel mutations in the ATP2C1 gene. *J Invest Dermatol*. 2002;118(2):338-343.
202. Chao SC, Tsai YM, Yang MH. Mutation analysis of ATP2C1 gene in Taiwanese patients with Hailey-Hailey disease. *Br J Dermatol*. 2002;146(4):595-600.
203. Yokota K, Yasukawa K, Shimizu H. Analysis of ATP2C1 gene mutation in 10 unrelated Japanese families with Hailey-Hailey disease. *J Invest Dermatol*. 2002;118(3):550-551.
204. Li H, Sun XK, Zhu XJ. Four novel mutations in ATP2C1 found in Chinese patients with Hailey-Hailey disease. *Br J Dermatol*. 2003;149(3):471-474.
205. Fairclough RJ, Lonie L, Van Baelen K, et al. Hailey-Hailey disease: identification of novel mutations in ATP2C1 and effect of missense mutation A528P on protein expression levels. *J Invest Dermatol*. 2004;123(1):67-71.
206. Majore S, Biolcati G, Barboni L, et al. ATP2C1 gene mutation analysis in Italian patients with Hailey-Hailey disease. *J Invest Dermatol*. 2005;125(5):933-935.
207. Ohtsuka T, Okita H, Hama N, et al. Novel mutation in ATP2C1 gene in a Japanese patient with Hailey-Hailey disease. *Dermatology*. 2006;212(2):194-197.
208. Racz E, Csikos M, Karpati S. Novel mutations in the ATP2C1 gene in two patients with Hailey-Hailey disease. *Clin Exp Dermatol*. 2005;30(5):575-577.
209. Zhang XQ, Wu HZ, Li BX, et al. Mutations in the ATP2C1 gene in Chinese patients with Hailey-Hailey disease. *Clin Exp Dermatol*. 2006;31(5):702-705.

210. Li X, Xiao S, Peng Z, et al. Two novel mutations of the ATP2C1 gene in Chinese patients with Hailey-Hailey disease. *Arch Dermatol Res*. 2007;299(4):209-211.
211. Nemoto-Hasebe I, Akiyama M, Osawa R, et al. Diagnosis of Hailey-Hailey disease facilitated by DNA testing: a novel mutation in ATP2C1. *Acta Derm Venereol*. 2008;88(4):399-400.
212. Hamada T, Fukuda S, Sakaguchi S, et al. Molecular and clinical characterization in Japanese and Korean patients with Hailey-Hailey disease: six new mutations in the ATP2C1 gene. *J Dermatol Sci*. 2008;51(1):31-36.
213. Fairclough RJ, Dode L, Vanoevelen J, et al. Effect of Hailey-Hailey disease mutations on the function of a new variant of human secretory pathway Ca^{2+}/Mn^{2+}-ATPase (hSPCA1). *J Biol Chem*. 2003;278(27):24721-24730.
214. Rice WJ, MacLennan DH. Scanning mutagenesis reveals a similar pattern of mutation sensitivity in transmembrane sequences M4, M5, and M6, but not in M8, of the Ca^{2+}-ATPase of sarcoplasmic reticulum (SERCA1a). *J Biol Chem*. 1996;271(49):31412-31419.
215. Wilgram GF, Caulfield JB, Lever WF. An electron-microscopic study of acantholysis and dyskeratosis in Hailey's disease. *J Invest Dermatol*. 1962;39:373-381.
216. Gottlieb SK, Lutzner MA. Hailey-Hailey disease—an electron microscopic study. *J Invest Dermatol*. 1970;54(5):368-376.
217. Inohara S, Tatsumi Y, Tanaka Y, et al. Immunohistochemical localization of desmosomal and cytoskeletal proteins in the epidermis of healthy individuals and patients with Hailey-Hailey's disease. *Acta Derm Venereol*. 1990;70(3):239-241.
218. Bergman R, Levy R, Pam Z, et al. A study of keratin expression in benign familial chronic pemphigus. *Am J Dermatopathol*. 1992;14(1):32-36.
219. Burge SM, Schomberg KH. Adhesion molecules and related proteins in Darier's disease and Hailey-Hailey disease. *Br J Dermatol*. 1992;127(4):335-343.
220. Harada M, Hashimoto K, Fujiwara K. Immunohistochemical distribution of CD44 and desmoplakin I & II in Hailey-Hailey's disease and Darier's disease. *J Dermatol*. 1994;21(6):389-393.
221. Haftek M, Kowalewski C, Mesnil M, et al. Internalization of gap junctions in benign familial pemphigus (Hailey-Hailey disease) and keratosis follicularis (Darier's disease). *Br J Dermatol*. 1999;141(2):224-230.
222. Burge SM, Millard PR, Wojnarowska F. Hailey-Hailey disease: a widespread abnormality of cell adhesion. *Br J Dermatol*. 1991;124(4):329-332.
223. Yoshida M, Yamasaki K, Daiho T, et al. ATP2C1 is specifically localized in the basal layer of normal epidermis and its depletion triggers keratinocyte differentiation. *J Dermatol Sci*. 2006;43(1):21-33.
224. Behne MJ, Tu CL, Aronchik I, et al. Human keratinocyte ATP2C1 localizes to the Golgi and controls Golgi Ca^{2+} stores. *J Invest Dermatol*. 2003;121(4):688-694.
225. Cialfi S, Oliviero C, Ceccarelli S, et al. Complex multipathways alterations and oxidative stress are associated with Hailey-Hailey disease. *Br J Dermatol*. 2010;162(3):518-526.
226. Aberg KM, Racz E, Behne MJ, et al. Involucrin expression is decreased in Hailey-Hailey keratinocytes owing to increased involucrin mRNA degradation. *J Invest Dermatol*. 2007;127(8):1973-1979.
227. Aronchik I, Behne MJ, Leypoldt L, et al. Actin reorganization is abnormal and cellular ATP is decreased in Hailey-Hailey keratinocytes. *J Invest Dermatol*. 2003;121(4):681-687.
228. Okunade GW, Miller ML, Azhar M, et al. Loss of the Atp2c1 secretory pathway Ca(2+)-ATPase (SPCA1) in mice causes Golgi stress, apoptosis, and midgestational death in homozygous embryos and squamous cell tumors in adult heterozygotes. *J Biol Chem*. 2007;282(36):26517-26527.
229. Micaroni M, Perinetti G, Berrie CP, et al. The SPCA1 Ca^{2+} pump and intracellular membrane trafficking. *Traffic*. 2010;11(10):1315-1333.
230. Micaroni M, Giacchetti G, Plebani R, et al. ATP2C1 gene mutations in Hailey-Hailey disease and possible roles of SPCA1 isoforms in membrane trafficking. *Cell Death Dis*. 2016;7(6):e2259.
231. Manca S, Magrelli A, Cialfi S, et al. Oxidative stress activation of miR-125b is part of the molecular switch for Hailey-Hailey disease manifestation. *Exp Dermatol*. 2011;20(11):932-937.
232. Cialfi S, Le Pera L, De Blasio C, et al. The loss of ATP2C1 impairs the DNA damage response and induces altered skin homeostasis: consequences for epidermal biology in Hailey-Hailey disease. *Sci Rep*. 2016;6:31567.
233. Metze D, Hamm H, Schorat A, et al. Involvement of the adherens junction-actin filament system in acantholytic dyskeratosis of Hailey-Hailey disease. A histological, ultrastructural, and histochemical study of lesional and non-lesional skin. *J Cutan Pathol*. 1996;23(3):211-222.
234. Chave TA, Milligan A. Acute generalized Hailey-Hailey disease. *Clin Exp Dermatol*. 2002;27(4):290-292.
235. Ewald K, Gross G. Perianal Hailey-Hailey disease: an unusual differential diagnosis of condylomata acuminata. *Int J STD AIDS*. 2008;19(11):791-792.
236. Evron S, Leviatan A, Okon E. Familial benign chronic pemphigus appearing as leukoplakia of the vulva. *Int J Dermatol*. 1984;23(8):556-557.
237. Chiaravalloti A, Payette M. Hailey-Hailey disease and review of management. *J Drugs Dermatol*. 2014;13(10):1254-1257.
238. Arora H, Bray FN, Cervantes J, et al. Management of familial benign chronic pemphigus. *Clin Cosmet Investig Dermatol*. 2016;9:281-290.
239. Farahnik B, Blattner CM, Mortazie MB, et al. Interventional treatments for Hailey-Hailey disease. *J Am Acad Dermatol*. 2017;76(3):551-558;e553.
240. Kellermayer R, Szigeti R, Keeling KM, et al. Aminoglycosides as potential pharmacogenetic agents in the treatment of Hailey-Hailey disease. *J Invest Dermatol*. 2006;126(1):229-231.
241. Umar SA, Bhattacharjee P, Brodell RT. Treatment of Hailey-Hailey disease with tacrolimus ointment and clobetasol propionate foam. *J Drugs Dermatol*. 2004;3(2):200-203.
242. Rabeni EJ, Cunningham NM. Effective treatment of Hailey-Hailey disease with topical tacrolimus. *J Am Acad Dermatol*. 2002;47(5):797-798.
243. Reuter J, Termeer C, Bruckner-Tuderman L. Tacrolimus-a new therapeutic option for Hailey-Hailey-disease?. *J Dtsch Dermatol Ges*. 2005;3(4):278-279.
244. Sand C, Thomsen HK. Topical tacrolimus ointment is an effective therapy for Hailey-Hailey disease. *Arch Dermatol*. 2003;139(11):1401-1402.
245. Persic-Vojinovic S, Milavec-Puretic V, Dobric I, et al. Disseminated Hailey-Hailey disease treated with

topical tacrolimus and oral erythromycin: case report and review of the literature. *Acta Dermatovenerol Croat.* 2006;14(4):253-257.
246. Rocha Paris F, Fidalgo A, Baptista J, et al. Topical tacrolimus in Hailey-Hailey disease. *Int J Tissue React.* 2005;27(4):151-154.
247. Laffitte E, Panizzon RG. Is topical tacrolimus really an effective therapy for Hailey-Hailey disease? *Arch Dermatol.* 2004;140(10):1282.
248. Pagliarello C, Paradisi A, Dianzani C, et al. Topical tacrolimus and 50% zinc oxide paste for Hailey-Hailey disease: less is more. *Acta Derm Venereol.* 2012;92(4):437-438.
249. Bianchi L, Chimenti MS, Giunta A. Treatment of Hailey-Hailey disease with topical calcitriol. *J Am Acad Dermatol.* 2004;51(3):475-476.
250. Rajpara SM, King CM. Hailey-Hailey disease responsive to topical calcitriol. *Br J Dermatol.* 2005;152(4):816-817.
251. Aoki T, Hashimoto H, Koseki S, et al. 1alpha, 24-dihydroxyvitamin D3 (tacalcitol) is effective against Hailey-Hailey disease both in vivo and in vitro. *Br J Dermatol.* 1998;139(5):897-901.
252. Dammak A, Camus M, Anyfantakis V, et al. Successful treatment of Hailey-Hailey disease with topical 5-fluorouracil. *Br J Dermatol.* 2009;161(4):967-968.
253. Defresne C, Adam C, de Marneffe K. Benign familial chronic pemphigus Hailey-Hailey. *Dermatologica.* 1982;165(6):624-626.
254. Hunt MJ, Salisbury EL, Painter DM, et al. Vesiculobullous Hailey-Hailey disease: successful treatment with oral retinoids. *Australas J Dermatol.* 1996;37(4):196-198.
255. Berger EM, Galadari HI, Gottlieb AB. Successful treatment of Hailey-Hailey disease with acitretin. *J Drugs Dermatol.* 2007;6(7):734-736.
256. Vilarinho C, Ventura F, Brito C. Methotrexate for refractory Hailey-Hailey disease. *J Eur Acad Dermatol Venereol.* 2010;24(1):106.
257. Berth-Jones J, Smith SG, Graham-Brown RA. Benign familial chronic pemphigus (Hailey-Hailey disease) responds to cyclosporin. *Clin Exp Dermatol.* 1995;20(1):70-72.
258. Varada S, Ramirez-Fort MK, Argobi Y, et al. Remission of refractory benign familial chronic pemphigus (Hailey-Hailey disease) with the addition of systemic cyclosporine. *J Cutan Med Surg.* 2015;19(2):163-166.
259. Sire DJ, Johnson BL. Benign familial chronic pemphigus treated with dapsone. *Arch Dermatol.* 1971;103(3):262-265.
260. Norman R, Greenberg RG, Jackson JM. Case reports of etanercept in inflammatory dermatoses. *J Am Acad Dermatol.* 2006;54(3 suppl 2):S139-142.
261. Hurd DS, Johnston C, Bevins A. A case report of Hailey-Hailey disease treated with alefacept (Amevive). *Br J Dermatol.* 2008;158(2):399-401.
262. Biolcati G, Aurizi C, Barbieri L, et al. Efficacy of the melanocortin analogue Nle4-D-Phe7-alpha-melanocyte-stimulating hormone in the treatment of patients with Hailey-Hailey disease. *Clin Exp Dermatol.* 2014;39(2):168-175.
263. Kaniszewska M, Rovner R, Arshanapalli A, et al. Oral glycopyrrolate for the treatment of Hailey-Hailey disease. *JAMA Dermatol.* 2015;151(3):328-329.
264. Shons AR. Wide excision of perineal Hailey-Hailey disease with healing by secondary intention. *Br J Plast Surg.* 1989;42(2):230-232.
265. Menz P, Jackson IT, Connolly S. Surgical control of Hailey-Hailey disease. *Br J Plast Surg.* 1987;40(6):557-561.
266. Guerin-Surville H, Guerin-Surville L, Le Louarn C, et al. Surgical treatment of Hailey-Hailey disease by surgical grafting (2d report): results after a 5-year follow-up. *Ann Dermatol Venereol.* 1989;116(11):904-905.
267. Hamm H, Metze D, Brocker EB. Hailey-Hailey disease. Eradication by dermabrasion. *Arch Dermatol.* 1994;130(9):1143-1149.
268. Kirtschig G, Gieler U, Happle R. Treatment of Hailey-Hailey disease by dermabrasion. *J Am Acad Dermatol.* 1993;28(5 Pt 1):784-786.
269. Kartamaa M, Reitamo S. Familial benign chronic pemphigus (Hailey-Hailey disease). Treatment with carbon dioxide laser vaporization. *Arch Dermatol.* 1992;128(5):646-648.
270. Kruppa A, Korge B, Lasch J, et al. Successful treatment of Hailey-Hailey disease with a scanned carbon dioxide laser. *Acta Derm Venereol.* 2000;80(1):53-54.
271. McElroy JA, Mehregan DA, Roenigk RK. Carbon dioxide laser vaporization of recalcitrant symptomatic plaques of Hailey-Hailey disease and Darier's disease. *J Am Acad Dermatol.* 1990;23(5 Pt 1):893-897.
272. Roos DE, Reid CM. Benign familial pemphigus: little benefit from superficial radiotherapy. *Australas J Dermatol.* 2002;43(4):305-308.
273. Narbutt J, Lesiak A, Arkuszewska C, et al. Effective treatment of recalcitrant Hailey-Hailey disease with electron beam radiotherapy. *J Eur Acad Dermatol Venereol.* 2007;21(4):567-568.
274. Ruiz-Rodriguez R, Alvarez JG, Jaen P, et al. Photodynamic therapy with 5-aminolevulinic acid for recalcitrant familial benign pemphigus (Hailey-Hailey disease). *J Am Acad Dermatol.* 2002;47(5):740-742.
275. Fernandez Guarino M, Ryan AM, Harto A, et al. Experience with photodynamic therapy in Hailey-Hailey disease. *J Dermatolog Treat.* 2008;19(5):288-290.
276. Konrad H, Karamfilov T, Wollina U. Intracutaneous botulinum toxin A versus ablative therapy of Hailey-Hailey disease—a case report. *J Cosmet Laser Ther.* 2001;3(4):181-184.
277. Koeyers WJ, Van Der Geer S, Krekels G. Botulinum toxin type A as an adjuvant treatment modality for extensive Hailey-Hailey disease. *J Dermatolog Treat.* 2008;19(4):251-254.
278. Lapiere JC, Hirsh A, Gordon KB, et al. Botulinum toxin type A for the treatment of axillary Hailey-Hailey disease. *Dermatol Surg.* 2000;26(4):371-374.
279. Ho D, Jagdeo J. Successful botulinum toxin (onabotulinumtoxinA) treatment of Hailey-Hailey disease. *J Drugs Dermatol.* 2015;14(1):68-70.
280. Grover RW. Transient acantholytic dermatosis. *Arch Dermatol.* 1970;101(4):426-434.
281. Chalet M, Grover R, Ackerman AB. Transient acantholytic dermatosis: a reevaluation. *Arch Dermatol.* 1977;113(4):431-435.
282. Heenan PJ, Quirk CJ. Transient acantholytic dermatosis. *Br J Dermatol.* 1980;102(5):515-520.
283. Parsons JM. Transient acantholytic dermatosis (Grover's disease): a global perspective. *J Am Acad Dermatol.* 1996;35(5 Pt 1):653-666; quiz 667-670.
284. Davis MD, Dinneen AM, Landa N, et al. Grover's disease: clinicopathologic review of 72 cases. *Mayo Clinic proceedings.* 1999;74(3):229-234.
285. Maghraoui S, Crickx B, Grossin M, et al. [Transient acantholytic dermatosis (Grover disease)]. *Ann Dermatol Venereol.* 1995;122(11-12):801-806.

286. Streit M, Paredes BE, Braathen LR, et al. Transitory acantholytic dermatosis (Grover disease). An analysis of the clinical spectrum based on 21 histologically assessed cases. *Hautarzt*. 2000;51(4):244-249.
287. Waisman M, Stewart JJ, Walker AE. Bullous transient acantholytic dermatosis. *Arch Dermatol*. 1976;112(10):1440-1441.
288. Quirk CJ, Heenan PJ. Grover's disease: 34 years on. *Australas J Dermatol*. 2004;45(2):83-86; quiz 87-88.
289. Cooper SM, Dhittavat J, Millard P, et al. Extensive Grover's-like eruption with lentiginous "freckling": report of two cases. *Br J Dermatol*. 2004;150(2):350-352.
290. Girard C, Durand L, Guillot B, et al. Persistent acantholytic dermatosis and extensive lentiginous 'freckling': a new entity? *Br J Dermatol*. 2005;153(1):217-218; author reply 218.
291. Rowley MJ, Nesbitt LT Jr, Carrington PR, et al. Hypopigmented macules in acantholytic disorders. *Int J Dermatol*. 1995;34(6):390-392.
292. Fantini F, Kovacs E, Scarabello A. Unilateral transient acantholytic dermatosis (Grover's disease) along Blaschko lines. *J Am Acad Dermatol*. 2002;47(2):319-320.
293. Garcon N, Karam A, Lemasson G, et al. Paraneoplastic transient acantholytic dermatosis (Grover's disease) along Blaschko lines. *Eur J Dermatol*. 2009;19(4):405-406.
294. Powell J, Sakuntabhai A, James M, et al. Grover's disease, despite histological similarity to Darier's disease, does not share an abnormality in the ATP2A2 gene. *Br J Dermatol*. 2000;143(3):658.
295. Hu CH, Michel B, Farber EM. Transient acantholytic dermatosis (Grover's disease). A skin disorder related to heat and sweating. *Arch Dermatol*. 1985;121(11):1439-1441.
296. French LE, Piletta PA, Etienne A, et al. Incidence of transient acantholytic dermatosis (Grover's disease) in a hospital setting. *Dermatology*. 1999;198(4):410-411.
297. Fujita Y, Sato-Matsumura KC, Ohnishi K. Transient acantholytic dermatosis associated with B symptoms of follicular lymphoma. *Clin Exp Dermatol*. 2007;32(6):752-754.
298. Guana AL, Cohen PR. Transient acantholytic dermatosis in oncology patients. *J Clin Oncol*. 1994;12(8):1703-1709.
299. Scheinfeld N, Mones J. Seasonal variation of transient acantholytic dyskeratosis (Grover's disease). *J Am Acad Dermatol*. 2006;55(2):263-268.
300. Grover RW, Rosenbaum R. The association of transient acantholytic dermatosis with other skin diseases. *J Am Acad Dermatol*. 1984;11(2 Pt 1):253-256.
301. Rosina P, Melzani G, Marcelli M, et al. Grover's disease (transient acantholytic dermatosis) associated with atopy. *J Eur Acad Dermatol Venereol*. 2005;19(3):390-391.
302. Ishibashi M, Nagasaka T, Chen KR. Remission of transient acantholytic dermatosis after the treatment with rituximab for follicular lymphoma. *Clin Exp Dermatol*. 2008;33(2):206-207.
303. Held JL, Bank D, Grossman ME. Grover's disease provoked by ionizing radiation. *J Am Acad Dermatol*. 1988;19(1 Pt 1):137-138.
304. Tscharner GG, Buhler S, Borner M, et al. Grover's disease induced by cetuximab. *Dermatology*. 2006;213(1):37-39.
305. Boutli F, Voyatzi M, Lefaki I, et al. Transient acantholytic dermatosis (Grover's disease) in a renal transplant patient. *J Dermatol*. 2006;33(3):178-181.
306. Paslin D. Grover disease may result from the impairment of keratinocytic cholinergic receptors. *J Am Acad Dermatol*. 2012;66(2):332-333.
307. Weaver J, Bergfeld WF. Grover disease (transient acantholytic dermatosis). *Arch Pathol Lab Med*. 2009;133(9):1490-1494.
308. Simon RS, Bloom D, Ackerman AB. Persistent acantholytic dermatosis. A variant of transient acantholytic dermatosis (Grover disease). *Arch Dermatol*. 1976;112(10):1429-1431.
309. Fawcett HA, Miller JA. Persistent acantholytic dermatosis related to actinic damage. *Br J Dermatol*. 1983;109(3):349-354.
310. Eros N, Kovacs A, Karolyi Z. Successful treatment of transient acantholytic dermatosis with systemic steroids. *J Dermatol*. 1998;25(7):469-475.
311. Keohane SG, Cork MJ. Treatment of Grover's disease with calcipotriol (Dovonex). *Br J Dermatol*. 1995;132(5):832-833.
312. Mota AV, Correia TM, Lopes JM, et al. Successful treatment of Grover's disease with calcipotriol. *Eur J Dermatol*. 1998;8(1):33-35.
313. Hayashi H, Yokota K, Koizumi H, et al. Treatment of Grover's disease with tacalcitol. *Clin Exp Dermatol*. 2002;27(2):160-161.
314. Miljkovic J, Marko PB. Grover's disease: successful treatment with acitretin and calcipotriol. *Wien Klin Wochenschr*. 2004;116(suppl 2):81-83.

Chapter 51 :: Porokeratosis
:: Cathal O'Connor, Grainne M. O'Regan, & Alan D. Irvine

第五十一章
汗孔角化症

中文导读

　　汗孔角化症是一种慢性进行性角化疾病，具有遗传异质性，大多数为常染色体显性遗传。目前至少有六种汗孔角化症的临床变异被确认，分别为经典的Mibelli汗孔角化症、播散性浅表光化性汗孔角化症、播散性浅表汗孔角化症、线状汗孔角化症、掌跖播散性汗孔角化症、点状汗孔角化症。一个患者可多种类型并存，受累家庭的多个成员也可表现为不同类型。本章从流行病学、各型临床特征、病因与发病机制、组织病理学、鉴别诊断、治疗、临床病程与预后等方面介绍了汗孔角化症。

〔粟　娟〕

AT-A-GLANCE

- Porokeratosis is a chronic progressive disorders of keratinization characterized clinically by hyperkeratotic papules or plaques surrounded by a threadlike, elevated border that expands centrifugally.
- Porokeratosis is genetically heterogeneous; the majority are inherited as autosomal dominant traits.
- At least six clinical variants of porokeratosis have been described.
- The classic form, porokeratosis of Mibelli, presents in infancy or childhood as asymptomatic, small, brown to skin-colored, annular papules with a characteristic raised border.
- The most common type, disseminated superficial actinic porokeratosis, presents with multiple papules distributed symmetrically on sun-exposed areas.
- Linear porokeratosis presents at birth or in childhood with lesions distributed along Blaschko lines.
- Punctate porokeratosis appears during or after adolescence as 1- to 2-mm papules on the palms or soles.
- In all variants, a thin column of parakeratotic cells (cornoid lamella) corresponds to the hyperkeratotic border and extends throughout the stratum corneum in histologic sections.
- Malignant epithelial neoplasms are reported in all subtypes except the punctate variety.

INTRODUCTION

Porokeratosis is a morphologically distinct disorder of keratinization characterized clinically by hyperkeratotic papules or plaques surrounded by a threadlike elevated border that expands centrifugally. Histologically, a thin column of parakeratotic cells extends throughout the stratum corneum and is seen in all variants. This distinctive histopathologic feature, known as the *cornoid lamella*, corresponds to the raised hyperkeratotic border evident clinically.

At least six clinical variants of porokeratosis are recognized, and recent genetic progress has additionally allowed classification according to the underlying mutation (Table 51-1). Reports of one type of porokeratosis coexisting with other forms and different types developing in multiple members of an affected family suggest more similarities than disparities, particularly in the disseminated forms. Thus, it is important to allow for some flexibility around clinical subcategorization.[1-3]

EPIDEMIOLOGY

The most common variants are disseminated superficial actinic porokeratosis and porokeratosis of Mibelli. The other forms are rare. Porokeratosis usually occurs in fair-skinned individuals and is rare in darker-skinned people. Porokeratosis of Mibelli and porokeratosis palmaris et plantaris disseminata are twice as likely to affect men. Disseminated superficial actinic porokeratosis is twice as likely to occur in women.[4] Linear porokeratosis is seen with equal incidence in men and women. Porokeratosis of Mibelli usually develops in childhood. Disseminated superficial porokeratosis generally develops in the third or fourth decade of life. Porokeratosis palmaris et plantaris disseminata and linear porokeratosis can be seen at any age from birth to adulthood.

CLINICAL FINDINGS

POROKERATOSIS OF MIBELLI

Classic porokeratosis of Mibelli (PM) begins during infancy or childhood as asymptomatic, small, brown

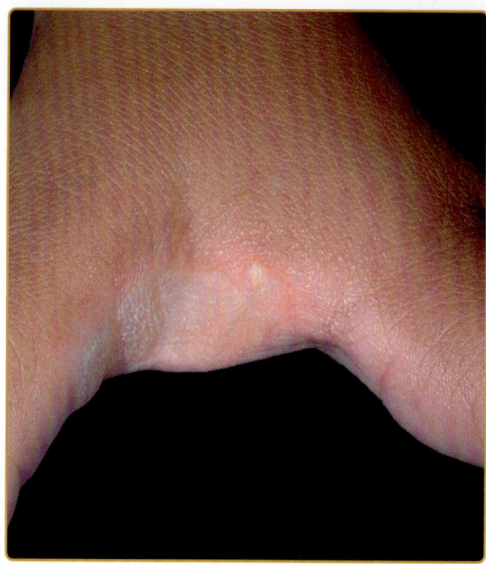

Figure 51-1 Porokeratosis of Mibelli is characterized by a single large lesion with a clearly defined edge. The scaling is not clearly seen at the border because of the interdigital location of this lesion.

to skin-colored, annular papules with a characteristic annular border (Fig. 51-1). The well-demarcated hyperkeratotic border is usually more than 1 mm in height, with a characteristic longitudinal furrow. The center of the lesion may be hyperpigmented, hypopigmented, depressed, atrophic, or anhidrotic. Lesions range in diameter from millimeters to several centimeters, but giant lesions measuring up to 20 cm may occur. Such giant porokeratoses are rare and occur predominantly on the lower leg and foot. Large lesions are associated with a higher malignant potential.[5] Multiple lesions may arise; however, they are usually

TABLE 51-1
Clinical Variants of Porokeratosis and Genes and Genetic Loci Identified to Date

CONDITION	GENE	LOCUS	OMIM	INHERITANCE
Porokeratosis 1 (porokeratosis of Mibelli)	PMVK	1q21.3	175800	AD
Porokeratosis 2 (porokeratosis palmaris et plantaris disseminata)	Not yet identified	12q24.1–q24.2	175850	AD
Porokeratosis 3 (disseminated superficial actinic porokeratosis 1)	MVK	12q24.11	175900	AD
Porokeratosis 4 (disseminated superficial actinic porokeratosis 2)	Not yet identified	15q25.1–15q26.1	607728	AD
Porokeratosis 5 (disseminated superficial actinic porokeratosis 3)	Not yet identified	1p31.3–1p31.1	612293	AD
Porokeratosis 6 (disseminated superficial porokeratosis)	Not yet identified	18p11.3	612353	AD
Porokeratosis 7 (multiple types)	MVD	16q24.2	614714	AD
Porokeratosis 8 (disseminated superficial actinic porokeratosis 4)	SLC17A9	20q13.33	616063	AD
Porokeratosis 9 (multiple types)	FDPS	1q22	616631	
CDAGS syndrome	?RUNX2	22q12–22q13	603116	AR

AD, autosomal dominant; AR, autosomal recessive; CDAGS, craniosynostosis and clavicular hypoplasia, *d*elayed closure of the fontanel, *a*nal anomalies, *g*enitourinary malformations, *s*kin eruption; OMIM, Online Mendelian Inheritance in Man.

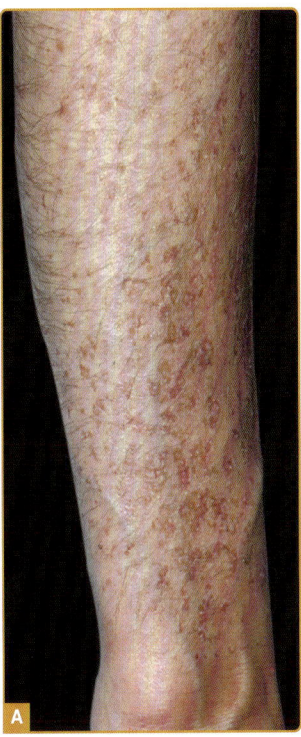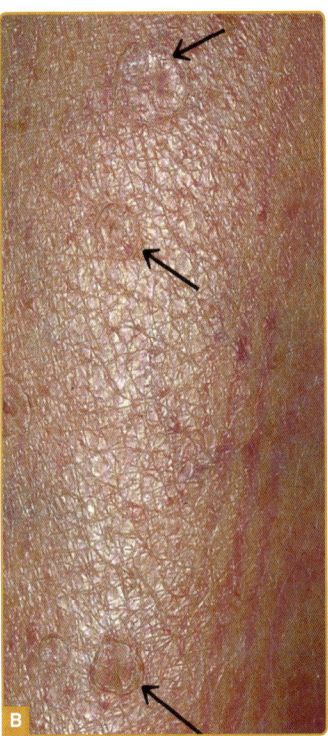

Figure 51-2 **A,** Disseminated superficial actinic porokeratosis with multiple lesions on the forearm in this severely affected individual. **B,** The characteristic furrowing (*arrows*) is clearly demonstrated on the forearm of this patient.

regionally localized and unilateral. The condition is inherited as an autosomal dominant trait. Lesions persist indefinitely.

DISSEMINATED SUPERFICIAL ACTINIC POROKERATOSIS

Disseminated superficial actinic porokeratosis (DSAP) is the most common of the porokeratoses. Lesions are characteristically uniformly small, annular, asymptomatic, or mildly pruritic papules ranging from 2 to 5 mm in diameter, distributed symmetrically on the extremities. Lesions are more generalized than other forms of porokeratosis, with typically more than 50 lesions located predominantly in sun-exposed sites (Fig. 51-2). Although widespread, lesions typically spare the palms, soles, and mucous membranes. Compared with porokeratosis of Mibelli, the hyperkeratotic border is subtler. As the lesions progress, the older, central area becomes atrophic and anhidrotic. DSAP is inherited as an autosomal dominant disorder, with the earliest reported age of onset at 7 years, and is usually fully penetrant by the third or fourth decade of life.[6] Initial reports of induction of lesions by exposure to ultraviolet (UV) light and hypersensitivity of DSAP-derived fibroblasts to x-rays have not been consistently reproduced, and the pathogenesis of DSAP remains unknown.[7-10]

DISSEMINATED SUPERFICIAL POROKERATOSIS

Disseminated superficial porokeratosis (DSP) also shows an autosomal dominant pattern of inheritance and has its onset in the third or fourth decade of life. Lesions primarily are morphologically identical to those of DSAP, occur on the extremities, and are typically distributed symmetrically but do not spare sun-protected areas as in DSAP. Similar to DSAP, more than 100 lesions may be present, with a predilection for the extensor surfaces of the extremities. Notably, involvement of the face is rare in both DSAP and DSP. In both disseminated forms, there is a reported female predominance, with a female-to-male ratio of 2 to 1.

DISSEMINATED SUPERFICIAL POROKERATOSIS OF IMMUNOSUPPRESSION

Disseminated superficial porokeratosis in the context of immunosuppression is recognized after renal, hepatic, and cardiac transplantation; electron-beam irradiation;[11] immunosuppressive chemotherapy;

monoclonal antibodies;[12] systemic corticosteroids with hematopoietic malignancies;[13] and in the setting of HIV infection.[14] It has recently been described in association with type 2 diabetes mellitus as well.[15] Porokeratosis has also been reported after bone marrow transplantation in the absence of ongoing immunosuppressive therapy, which suggests a more complex association than immunosuppression alone.[16] The distribution and morphology of DSP of immunosuppression are similar to those of DSAP, but a history of sun exposure is less evident.

LINEAR POROKERATOSIS

Linear porokeratosis is an uncommon variant, traditionally categorized as a separate entity, but is increasingly recognized as a mosaic manifestation of one of the other types of porokeratosis.[17] Typically, it presents in early childhood, although congenital presentations have been reported.[18] Two distinct clinical variants have been described. The more common presentation consists of a unilateral lesion confined to an extremity following Blaschko lines (Fig. 51-3). In the rare generalized form, multiple lesions affect several extremities and may involve the trunk. Linear variants have the highest potential for malignant degeneration of all the porokeratoses. It has been postulated that this association can be attributed to allelic loss caused by a postzygotic mutation.[19] The proband in Mibelli's original publication most likely had coexistent linear porokeratosis and DSAP, with several subsequent reports confirming this phenomenon.[3,17,20,21] These findings may be explained by the loss of heterozygosity for the DSAP allele and provides an example of the type 2 segmental manifestations of an autosomal dominant disorder.[22,23]

POROKERATOSIS PALMARIS ET PLANTARIS DISSEMINATA

Porokeratosis palmaris et plantaris disseminata (porokeratosis punctata palmaris et plantaris) is a genodermatosis with an autosomal dominant inheritance pattern characterized by small, relatively uniform lesions (Fig. 51-4) that initially appear on the palms and soles. Subsequently, lesions spread to involve other parts of the body, including the mucous membranes and non–sun-exposed sites. The palmar and plantar lesions are generally more hyperkeratotic, and the characteristic longitudinal furrow along this ridge may be quite pronounced (Fig. 51-5). Typically, the lesions appear during adolescence or early adulthood and are bilateral and distributed symmetrically. Porokeratosis palmaris et plantaris disseminata affects males twice as often as females.

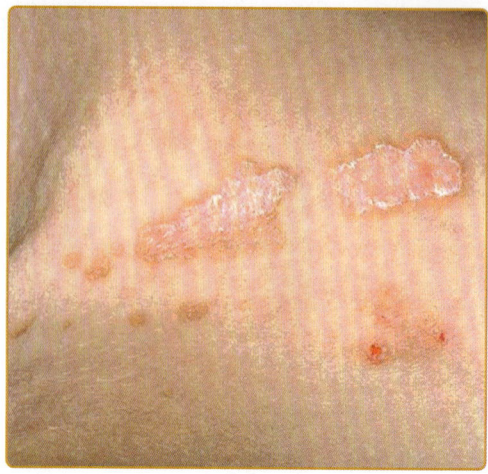

Figure 51-3 Linear porokeratosis showing the characteristic distribution along Blaschko lines.

PUNCTATE POROKERATOSIS

Punctate porokeratosis usually appears during adolescence or adulthood and may be seen concomitantly with other types of porokeratosis. Multiple minute and discrete punctate, hyperkeratotic lesions surrounded by a thin, raised margin are present on the palms and soles. Lesions may occur in a linear arrangement, or

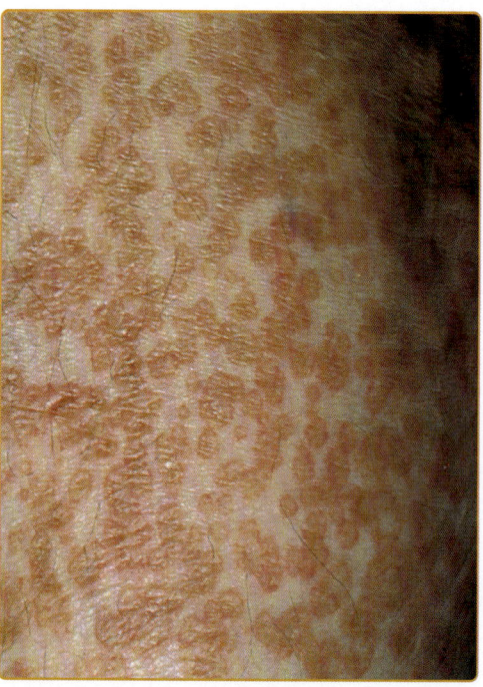

Figure 51-4 Porokeratosis palmaris et plantaris disseminata showing multiple superficial lesions on the calf. Note the similarity to disseminated superficial actinic porokeratosis shown in Fig. 51-2A.

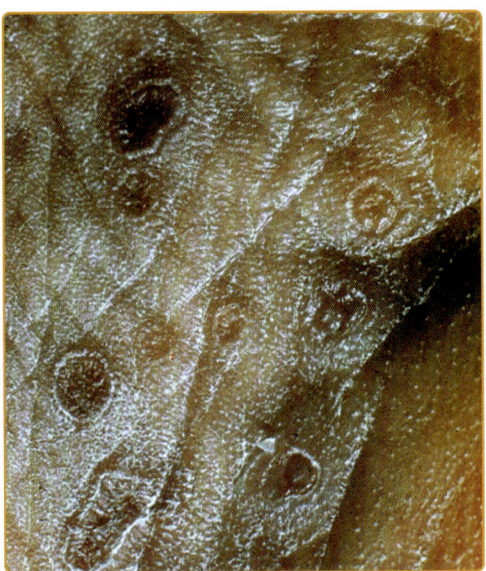

Figure 51-5 Sole of the foot in a patient with porokeratosis palmaris et plantaris disseminata. The ridge and furrow are clearly seen.

they may aggregate to form plaques. Punctate porokeratosis must be differentiated clinically and histologically from punctate keratoderma, also referred to as punctate porokeratotic keratoderma or as porokeratosis punctata palmaris et plantaris (see Chap. 48).

CDAGS SYNDROME

CDAGS syndrome (craniosynostosis and clavicular hypoplasia, delayed closure of the fontanel, anal anomalies, genitourinary malformations, skin eruption), also referred to as CAP syndrome (craniosynostosis, anal anomalies, and porokeratosis), is a rare genodermatosis reported in four ethnically diverse families to date.[24,25] The main phenotypic features consist of craniosynostosis and clavicular hypoplasia, anal anomalies, and porokeratosis. It appears to segregate as an autosomal recessive trait, with possible linkage to chromosome band 22q12–13.[25] The cutaneous manifestations are strikingly consistent, with the development of small, widespread porokeratotic papules from 1 month of age in affected individuals, predominantly affecting the face and extremities, with reported photoaggravation of lesions.

ETIOLOGY AND PATHOGENESIS

Porokeratosis is a genetically heterogeneous disorder with multiple loci identified to date. A splicing mutation in phosphomevalonate kinase (*PMVK*), involved in the cholesterol biosynthetic pathway, has been shown to cause PM.[26] The mevalonate kinase (*MVK*) gene on chromosome 12q24 has recently been identified as a causative gene in DSAP.[27] The product of this gene has a role in regulating calcium-induced keratinocyte differentiation and may confer protection against apoptosis induced by ultraviolet A radiation. Loci at chromosome bands 12q23.2–24.1 and 15q25 (DSAP1 and DSAP2) have been reported in other forms of familial disseminated superficial actinic porokeratoses; a further locus has been identified for disseminated superficial porokeratosis (DSP) at 18p11.3.[28,29] The locus at *DSAP1* includes several candidate genes, including *SART3* (squamous cell antigen recognized by T cells 3), *SSH1* (slingshot 1), and *ARPC3*.[30,31] Porokeratosis punctata palmaris et plantaris maps to a region at chromosome band 12q24.1–24.2, overlapping with the region identified for DSAP1, suggesting that the two forms may be allelic.[32] The centrifugal expansion of lesions is postulated to reflect the migration of a mutant clone of keratinocytes.[33,34] The tumor suppressor proteins p53 and pRb are overexpressed in keratinocytes immediately beneath and adjacent to the cornoid lamella, although to date p53 mutations have not been identified, and there is no significant expression of p53 at the mRNA level.[7,35-38] The increased prevalence of porokeratosis in immunosuppressed patients suggests that impaired immunity may be permissive in genetically predisposed individuals.[39-42] Other reported triggering factors such as exposure to UV light, together with the increased potential for malignant transformation, highlight the dysplastic potential of affected keratinocytes. Malignant degeneration has been described in all variants of porokeratosis, except for the punctate variety.[5,43,44]

HISTOPATHOLOGY

Histopathologic patterns are similar in all forms of porokeratosis, with the characteristic changes evident at the raised and advancing edge of the lesion. The stratum corneum is hyperkeratotic, with a thin column of poorly staining parakeratotic cells, the cornoid lamella, running through the surrounding normal-staining cells (Fig. 51-6). The underlying keratinocytes are edematous with spongiosis and shrunken nuclei, and a striking

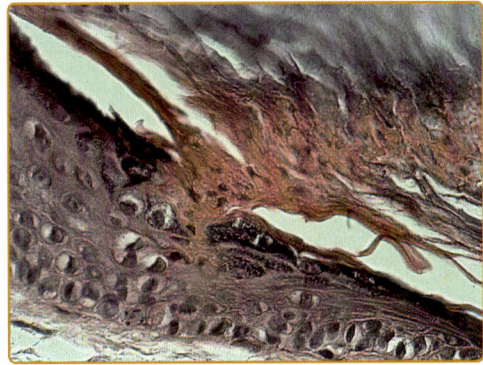

Figure 51-6 The cornoid lamella arises from an indentation of the epidermis and extends as a thin column throughout the stratum corneum. The underlying granular layer is either absent or reduced.

dermal lymphocytic pattern may be evident. Underlying the cornoid lamella, the granular layer is either absent or markedly reduced but is of normal thickness in other areas of the lesion. The epidermis in the central portion of porokeratosis may be normal, hyperplastic, or atrophic. Although characteristic of porokeratosis, the cornoid lamella is not pathognomonic and may also be found in other conditions, such as viral warts, some ichthyoses, and nevoid hyperkeratoses.

DIFFERENTIAL DIAGNOSIS

The classic lesions of porokeratosis are clinically distinctive, and the diagnosis is usually clinically apparent. However, atypical lesions may require differentiation (Table 51-2). Actinic keratoses, for example, may show cornoid lamellae but also show cytologic atypia. Verruca vulgaris often shows mounds of parakeratosis that are sometimes identical to cornoid lamellae, but koilocytosis is usually present. Linear porokeratosis may be clinically confused with other linear lesions (see Table 51-2), none of which has a cornoid lamella.

TREATMENT

Lesions of porokeratosis are chronic, slowly progressive, and relatively asymptomatic, although intense pruritus has been reported.[45] Intervention is usually unnecessary, and disease surveillance is standard. If the lesions are problematic or cosmetically unacceptable, treatment with potent topical steroids, keratolytics, topical retinoids, topical 5-fluorouracil,[46] imiquimod 5%, calcipotriol,[47] anthralin,[48] cryotherapy,[49] carbon dioxide laser,[50] pulsed dye laser,[51] or Nd:YAG (neodymium-doped yttrium aluminum garnet) laser may be considered (Table 51-3). Tacrolimus 0.1% has been shown to be useful in treating patients with linear porokeratosis.[52] Electrochemotherapy with intralesional bleomycin has been successful in treating patients with squamous cell carcinomas (SCCs) associated with linear porokeratosis.[53] To prevent residual lesions or recurrence, ablative measures that reach the middermis are required. Techniques such as curettage, excision, and dermabrasion[54] have been used with variable degrees of success. Oral retinoids have been shown to give the most reproducible results, although the disease typically recurs after their discontinuation. Given the association with malignancy, closer disease surveillance and a lower threshold for biopsy of suspicious lesions may be warranted in cases of giant porokeratoses or linear lesions and in immunosuppressed individuals.

TABLE 51-2
Differential Diagnosis of Porokeratosis

Localized Lesions
Most Likely
- Granuloma annulare
- Tinea corporis
- Actinic keratosis
- Viral warts

Consider
- Elastosis perforans
- Lichen planus
- Focal dermal hypoplasia (Goltz syndrome)

Linear
Consider
- Linear inflammatory verrucous epidermal nevus
- Incontinentia pigmenti (stage II)
- Linear lichen planus
- Ichthyosis linearis circumflexa

TABLE 51-3
Treatment for Porokeratosis

	TOPICAL	SURGICAL	SYSTEMIC
First line	Photoprotection 5-Fluorouracil	Cryotherapy	
Second line	Calcipotriol Imiquimod Topical corticosteroids Topical retinoids	CO_2 laser vaporization	Oral retinoids
Third line	Dermabrasion Nd:YAG laser Grenz ray	Surgical excision	

Nd:YAG, neodymium-doped yttrium aluminum garnet.

COURSE AND PROGNOSIS

The porokeratoses are generally chronic and progressive, with lesions increasing in size and number with time. Typically, this process occurs over decades in PM, but may be rapid in DSAP, particularly after sun exposure. In cases of immune compromise, fluctuations in severity may parallel the state of immune competence, and there are reports of remission after removal of primary malignancy.[42] The disease is generally considered a benign process; however, malignant degeneration may occur. Malignancy is thought to arise in 7% to 11% of individuals, although these figures are likely overestimated. SCC is the most frequently associated tumor and may be invasive. Bowen disease and basal cell carcinoma have also been reported. Spontaneous resolution of lesions has been reported, although it is exceptionally rare.[55]

SUMMARY

A summary of the porokeratosis subtypes can be found in Table 51-4.

TABLE 51-4
Summary of Porokeratosis Subtypes

	INHERITANCE AND RISK FACTORS	EPIDEMIOLOGY	CLINICAL FINDINGS	SPECIAL CONCERNS
Porokeratosis of Mibelli	Autosomal dominant	Onset in infancy or childhood; male predominance	Asymptomatic, small, brown to skin-colored annular papules with an annular border	Large lesions have malignant potential
Disseminated superficial actinic porokeratosis (DSAP)	Autosomal dominant	Most common porokeratosis; as early as childhood; often present by third to fourth decade of life; female predominance	Uniform, small, annular, papules from 2-5 mm, with symmetrical distribution on photoexposed extremities; asymptomatic or mildly pruritic	—
Disseminated superficial porokeratosis	Autosomal dominant	Onset by third to fourth decade of life; female predominance	Similar to above but with distribution to photoprotected sites	—
Disseminated superficial porokeratosis of immunosuppression	Immunosuppression after organ transplantation, drugs, or infections (see text)	Dependent on exposure (see risk factors)	Similar to DSAP	—
Linear porokeratosis	Mosaic manifestation of other porokeratosis variants	Uncommon; presents in early childhood	Primary manifestation dependent on particular variant, however configuration follows lines of Blaschko	Highest potential for malignant degeneration
Porokeratosis palmaris et plantaris disseminata	Autosomal dominant	Appear during adolescence or early adulthood; male predominance	Small, uniform lesions appearing on palms and soles with involvement to other sites; bilateral, symmetric involvement	—
Punctate porokeratosis	Concomitant occurrence with other forms of porokeratosis	Appears during adolescence or adulthood	Multiple discrete punctate hyperkeratotic lesions; may aggregate to form plaques	—

REFERENCES

1. Lin JH, Hsu MM, Sheu HM, et al. Coexistence of three variants of porokeratosis with multiple squamous cell carcinomas arising from lesions of giant hyperkeratotic porokeratosis. *J Eur Acad Dermatol Venereol.* 2006;20:621.
2. Kaur S, Thami GP, Mohan H, et al. Coexistence of variants of porokeratosis: a case report and a review of the literature. *J Dermatol.* 2002;29:305.
3. Mibelli V. Contributo allo studio della ipercheratosi dei canali sudoriferi. *G Ital Mal Venereol Pelle.* 1893;28:313.
4. Sertznig P, von Felbert V, Megahed M. Porokeratosis: present concepts. *J Eur Acad Dermatol Venereol.* 2012; 26(4):404-412.
5. Sasson M, Krain AD. Porokeratosis and cutaneous malignancy. A review. *Dermatol Surg.* 1996;22:339.
6. Zhang SQ, Jiang T, Li M, et al. Exome sequencing identifies MVK mutations in disseminated superficial actinic porokeratosis. *Nat Genet.* 2012;44(10):1156-1160.
7. Arranz-Salas I, Sanz-Trelles A, Ojeda DB. p53 alterations in porokeratosis. *J Cutan Pathol.* 2003;30:455.
8. Chernosky ME, Anderson DE. Disseminated superficial actinic porokeratosis. Clinical studies and experimental production of lesions. *Arch Dermatol.* 1969;99:401.
9. D'Errico M, Teson M, Calcagnile A, et al. Characterization of the ultra-violet B and X-ray response of primary cultured epidermal cells from patients with disseminated superficial actinic porokeratosis. *Br J Dermatol.* 2004;150:47.
10. Schamroth JM, Zlotogorski A, Gilead L. Porokeratosis of Mibelli. Overview and review of the literature. *Acta Derm Venereol.* 1997;77:207.
11. Leibovici V, Zeidenbaum M, Goldenhersh M. Porokeratosis and immunosuppressive treatment for pemphigus foliaceus. *J Am Acad Dermatol.* 1988;19:910.
12. Frew JW, Parsi K. Adalimumab-induced porokeratosis. *Australas J Dermatol.* 2015;56(3):e80-e81.
13. Luelmo-Aguilar J, Gonzalez-Castro U, Mieras-Barcelo C, et al. Disseminated porokeratosis and myelodysplastic syndrome. *Dermatology.* 1992;184:289.
14. Rodriguez EA, Jakubowicz S, Chinchilla DA, et al. Porokeratosis of Mibelli and HIV infection. *Int J Dermatol.* 1996;35:402.
15. Yalcin B, Uysal PI, Kadan E, et al. Eruptive disseminated porokeratosis in a patient with type 2 diabetes mellitus. *Am J Dermatopathol.* 2016;38(8):e125-e127.
16. Alexis AF, Busam K, Myskowski PL. Porokeratosis of Mibelli following bone marrow transplantation. *Int J Dermatol.* 2006;45:361.
17. Happle R. Mibelli revisited: a case of type 2 segmental porokeratosis from 1893. *J Am Acad Dermatol.* 2010; 62(1):136-138.
18. Zhang ZH, Xiang LH, Chen LJ, et al. Congenital facial linear porokeratosis. *Clin Exp Dermatol.* 2005;30:361.
19. Sasaki S, Urano Y, Nakagawa K, et al. Linear porokeratosis with multiple squamous cell carcinomas: study of p53 expression in porokeratosis and squamous cell carcinoma. *Br J Dermatol.* 1996;134:1151.
20. Suh DH, Lee HS, Kim SD, et al. Coexistence of disseminated superficial porokeratosis in childhood with

congenital linear porokeratosis. *Pediatr Dermatol*. 2000;17:466.
21. Welton WA. Linear porokeratosis in a family with DSAP. *Arch Dermatol*. 1972;106:263.
22. Happle R. A rule concerning the segmental manifestation of autosomal dominant skin disorders. Review of clinical examples providing evidence for dichotomous types of severity. *Arch Dermatol*. 1997;133:1505.
23. Happle R. Somatic recombination may explain linear porokeratosis associated with disseminated superficial actinic porokeratosis. *Am J Med Genet*. 1991;39:237.
24. Flanagan N, Boyadjiev SA, Harper J, et al. Familial craniosynostosis, anal anomalies, and porokeratosis: CAP syndrome. *J Med Genet*. 1998;35:763.
25. Mendoza-Londono R, Lammer E, Watson R, et al. Characterization of a new syndrome that associates craniosynostosis, delayed fontanel closure, parietal foramina, imperforate anus, and skin eruption: CDAGS. *Am J Hum Genet*. 2005;77:161.
26. Zeng K, Zhang QG, Li L, et al. Splicing mutation in MVK is a cause of porokeratosis of Mibelli. *Arch Dermatol Res*. 2014;306(8):749-755.
27. Wu LQ, Yang YF, Zheng D, et al. Confirmation and refinement of a genetic locus for disseminated superficial actinic porokeratosis (DSAP1) at 12q23.2-24.1. *Br J Dermatol*. 2004;150:999.
28. Xia K, Deng H, Xia JH, et al. A novel locus (DSAP2) for disseminated superficial actinic porokeratosis maps to chromosome 15q25.1-26.1. *Br J Dermatol*. 2002;147:650.
29. Wei S, Yang S, Lin D, et al. A novel locus for disseminated superficial porokeratosis maps to chromosome 18p11.3. *J Invest Dermatol*. 2004;123:872.
30. Zhang Z, Niu Z, Yuan W, et al. Fine mapping and identification of a candidate gene SSH1 in disseminated superficial actinic porokeratosis. *Hum Mutat*. 2004;24:438.
31. Zhang ZH, Huang W, Niu ZM, et al. Two closely linked variations in actin cytoskeleton pathway in a Chinese pedigree with disseminated superficial actinic porokeratosis. *J Am Acad Dermatol*. 2005;52:972.
32. Wei SC, Yang S, Li M, et al. Identification of a locus for porokeratosis palmaris et plantaris disseminata to a 6.9-cM region at chromosome 12q24.1-24.2. *Br J Dermatol*. 2003;149:261.
33. Reed RJ, Leone P. Porokeratosis—a mutant clonal keratosis of the epidermis. I. Histogenesis. *Arch Dermatol*. 1970;101:340.
34. Otsuka F, Shima A, Ishibashi Y. Porokeratosis has neoplastic clones in the epidermis: microfluorometric analysis of DNA content of epidermal cell nuclei. *J Invest Dermatol*. 1989;92:231S.
35. Chang SE, Lim Y, Lee H, et al. Expression of p53, pRb, p16 and proliferating cell nuclear antigen in squamous cell carcinomas arising on a giant porokeratosis. *Br J Dermatol*. 1999;141:575.
36. Magee JW, McCalmont TH, LeBoit PE. Overexpression of p53 tumor suppressor protein in porokeratosis. *Arch Dermatol*. 1994;130:187.
37. Ninomiya Y, Urano Y, Yoshimoto K, et al. p53 gene mutation analysis in porokeratosis and porokeratosis-associated squamous cell carcinoma. *J Dermatol Sci*. 1997;14:173.
38. Puig L, Alegre M, Costa I, et al. Overexpression of p53 in disseminated superficial actinic porokeratosis with and without malignant degeneration. *Arch Dermatol*. 1995;131:353.
39. Bencini PL, Tarantino A, Grimalt R, et al. Porokeratosis and immunosuppression. *Br J Dermatol*. 1995;132:74.
40. Herranz P, Pizarro A, De Lucas R, et al. High incidence of porokeratosis in renal transplant recipients. *Br J Dermatol*. 1997;136:176.
41. Silver SG, Crawford RI. Fatal squamous cell carcinoma arising from transplant-associated porokeratosis. *J Am Acad Dermatol*. 2003;49:931.
42. Tsambaos D, Spiliopoulos T. Disseminated superficial porokeratosis: complete remission subsequent to discontinuation of immunosuppression. *J Am Acad Dermatol*. 1993;28:651.
43. Maubec E, Duvillard P, Margulis A, et al. Common skin cancers in porokeratosis. *Br J Dermatol*. 2005;152:1389.
44. Otsuka F, Iwata M, Watanabe R, et al. Porokeratosis: clinical and cellular characterization of its cancer-prone nature. *J Dermatol*. 1992;19:702.
45. Kanzaki T, Miwa N, Kobayashi T, et al. Eruptive pruritic papular porokeratosis. *J Dermatol*. 1992;19:109.
46. McDonald SG, Peterka ES. Porokeratosis (Mibelli): treatment with topical 5-fluorouracil. *J Am Acad Dermatol*. 1983;8:107.
47. Harrison PV, Stollery N. Disseminated superficial actinic porokeratosis responding to calcipotriol. *Clin Exp Dermatol*. 1994;19:95.
48. Kosogabe M, Tada J, Arata J. [Punctate porokeratotic keratoderma]. *Nippon Hifuka Gakkai Zasshi*. 1991;101:553.
49. Dereli T, Ozyurt S, Ozturk G. Porokeratosis of Mibelli: successful treatment with cryosurgery. *J Dermatol*. 2004;31:223.
50. Barnett JH. Linear porokeratosis: treatment with the carbon dioxide laser. *J Am Acad Dermatol*. 1986;14:902.
51. Alster TS, Nanni CA. Successful treatment of porokeratosis with 585 nm pulsed dye laser irradiation. *Cutis*. 1999;63:265.
52. Parks AC, Conner KJ, Armstrong CA. Long-term clearance of linear porokeratosis with tacrolimus, 0.1%, ointment. *JAMA Dermatol*. 2014;150(2):194-196.
53. Sommerlad M, Lock A, Moir G, et al. Linear porokeratosis with multiple squamous cell carcinomas successfully treated by electrochemotherapy. *Br J Dermatol*. 2016;175(6):1342-1345.
54. Spencer JM, Katz BE. Successful treatment of porokeratosis of Mibelli with diamond fraise dermabrasion. *Arch Dermatol*. 1992;128:1187.
55. Adriaans B, Salisbury JR. Recurrent porokeratosis. *Br J Dermatol*. 1991;124:383.

Vesiculobullous Disorders

PART 9

第九篇　水疱大疱性疾病

Chapter 52 :: Pemphigus
:: Aimee S. Payne & John R. Stanley

第五十二章

天疱疮

中文导读

天疱疮是指皮肤和黏膜的一组自身免疫性水疱性疾病，其组织学特征是棘层松解所致表皮内水疱，免疫病理显示患者体内有抗角质形成细胞表面物质的自身抗体。

本章从七个方面全面讲述了天疱疮。

1. 流行病学　天疱疮无种族差异，发病率因地区而异，男女比为女:男1.33:1～2.25:1，很少发生在儿童身上。

2. 临床表现　本节介绍了天疱疮主要分为寻常型和落叶型两种类型，但存在几种变异型（表52-2），并介绍了其临床表现。

3. 病因与发病机制　本节介绍了天疱疮抗原及棘层松解的病理生理学、天疱疮免疫应答的遗传特征。其中还提到了B细胞与异种抗原和自身抗原的交叉反应是寻常型天疱疮（PV）和落叶型天疱疮（PF）自身免疫发病的机制。使用B细胞耗竭疗法完全消除这些B细胞克隆，患者可以治愈。

4. 诊断　本节介绍了天疱疮诊断包括皮肤病理和自身抗体检测。

5. 鉴别诊断　天疱疮鉴别诊断见表52-1。

6. 临床病程与预后　系统性糖皮质激素和免疫抑制药的使用极大地改善了天疱疮患者预后，但天疱疮仍然是一种死亡率较高的疾病，感染通常是死亡的原因。用抗CD20单克隆抗体利妥昔单抗治疗可使天疱疮普遍完全缓解。

7. 天疱疮的管理　本节介绍了天疱疮的专家共识或指南，提出PV需尽早治疗，未经治疗者预后很差，死亡率更高。其中糖皮质激素是治疗天疱疮的主要方法。并特别提到了利妥昔单抗能够很好地缓解天疱疮病情，但也有一定风险且可产生抗药性。本章最后展望了天疱疮的未来治疗。

〔陈明亮〕

AT-A-GLANCE

- Two major types: pemphigus vulgaris and pemphigus foliaceus.
- Pemphigus vulgaris: erosions on mucous membranes and skin; flaccid blisters on skin.
- Pemphigus foliaceus: crusted, scaly skin lesions.
- Pemphigus vulgaris histology: suprabasal acantholysis.
- Pemphigus foliaceus histology: subcorneal acantholysis.
- Autoantigens are desmogleins, transmembrane desmosomal adhesion molecules.
- Diagnosis depends on histology showing intraepidermal acantholysis, immunofluorescence studies documenting the presence of cell surface autoantibodies, either bound to patient skin or in the serum, and/or enzyme-linked immunosorbent assay showing anti-desmoglein antibodies
- Therapy includes topical and systemic corticosteroids, oral immunosuppressive agents, intravenous immunoglobulin, and rituximab (anti-CD20 monoclonal antibody).

TABLE 52-1
Nosology and Differential Diagnosis of Pemphigus

Pemphigus Subtypes
- Pemphigus vulgaris
- Pemphigus vegetans
- Pemphigus foliaceus
- Pemphigus erythematosus
- Endemic pemphigus foliaceus (eg, fogo selvagem)
- Immunoglobulin A (IgA) pemphigus
- Subcorneal pustular dermatosis
- Intraepidermal neutrophilic dermatosis
- Paraneoplastic pemphigus

Intraepidermal Blistering Diseases Without Autoantibodies
- Familial benign pemphigus (Hailey-Hailey disease)
- Bullous impetigo, staphylococcal scalded-skin syndrome
- Blisters from herpes simplex and zoster
- Allergic contact dermatitis (eg, rhus dermatitis)
- Epidermolysis bullosa simplex
- Incontinentia pigmenti

Mouth Ulcers/Erosion Without Autoantibodies
- Aphthous ulcers
- Candidiasis
- Lichen planus
- Behçet disease

Subepidermal Blistering Diseases With Autoantibodies
- Bullous pemphigoid
- Herpes gestationis
- Cicatricial pemphigoid
- Epidermolysis bullosa acquisita
- Linear IgA disease and chronic bullous disease of childhood
- Dermatitis herpetiformis
- Bullous lupus erythematosus

Subepidermal Blistering Diseases Without Autoantibodies
- Erythema multiforme
- Toxic epidermal necrolysis
- Porphyria
- Junctional or dystrophic epidermolysis bullosa

INTRODUCTION

DEFINITIONS

The term *pemphigus* refers to a group of autoimmune blistering diseases of skin and mucous membranes that are characterized histologically by intraepidermal blisters due to acantholysis (ie, separation of epidermal cells from each other) and immunopathologically by in vivo bound and circulating immunoglobulin directed against the cell surface of keratinocytes. The nosology of this group of diseases is outlined in Table 52-1. Essentially, pemphigus can be divided into 4 major types: vulgaris, foliaceus (Table 52-2), paraneoplastic (Chap. 53), and IgA pemphigus (Chap. 57). In pemphigus vulgaris (PV), the blister occurs in the deeper part of the epidermis, just above the basal layer, and in pemphigus foliaceus (PF), also called *superficial pemphigus*, the blister is in the granular layer.

HISTORICAL PERSPECTIVE

The history of the discovery of pemphigus, and its various forms, is covered in Walter Lever's classic monograph *Pemphigus* and *Pemphigoid*.[1] Both PV and PF display a spectrum of disease. Various points along these spectra have been given unique names, but because the presentation of these diseases is fluid, patients' disease usually crosses these artificial designations over time. Thus, patients with PV may present with more localized disease, one form of which is called *pemphigus vegetans of Hallopeau*. This may become slightly more extensive and may merge into *pemphigus vegetans of Neumann*. Finally, with more severe disease, full-blown PV may appear. Similarly, patients with PF may present with more localized disease, represented by *pemphigus erythematosus*. However, these patients often go on to more widespread PF.

The discovery by Ernst Beutner and Robert Jordon in 1964 of circulating antibodies against the cell surface of keratinocytes in the sera of patients with PV pioneered our understanding that PV is a tissue-specific autoimmune disease of skin and mucosa.[2] Ultimately, their work led the way to the discoveries of autoantibodies in other autoimmune bullous diseases of the skin.

EPIDEMIOLOGY

INCIDENCE, PREVALENCE, AND SEX RATIO

A few prospective and several retrospective surveys of patients with pemphigus clearly indicate that the epidemiology of pemphigus is dependent on both the area in the world that is studied and the ethnic population in that area.[3-11] PV is more common in Jews and probably in people of Mediterranean descent and from the Middle East. This same ethnic predominance does not exist for PF. Therefore, in areas where the Jewish, Middle Eastern, and Mediterranean population predominates, the ratio of PV to PF cases tends to be higher. For example, in New York, Los Angeles, and Croatia, the ratio of PV to PF cases is approximately 5:1; in Iran the ratio is 12:1; whereas in Singapore it is 2:1 and in Finland, it is only 0.5:1. Similarly, the incidence of pemphigus varies by region. In Jerusalem, the incidence of PV has been estimated to be 1.6 per 100,000 people per year and in Iran approximately 10.0 per 100,000 people per year. In Europe, the incidences are lower, ranging from a high of 0.7 PV cases per 100,000 person years in the United Kingdom to 10-fold less, 0.5 to 1.0 per million person years, in Finland, France, Germany, and Switzerland. In Taiwan, the incidence is 4.7 per million per year.

The prevalence and incidence of PF are also very dependent on its location, as best exemplified by the finding of endemic foci of PF in Brazil, Colombia, and Tunisia. The first recognition of endemic PF was in Brazil and is called *fogo selvagem*, which means "wild fire" in Portuguese. It is a disease that is clinically, histologically, and immunopathologically the same as sporadic PF in any individual patient, but its epidemiology is unique.[12,13] Fogo selvagem is endemic in the rural areas of Brazil, especially along inland riverbeds. The prevalence in some well-studied Indian reservations in rural Brazil can be as high as 3.4%, with the incidence up to 0.8 to 4.0 new cases per 1000 people per year.[13,14] On the reservation in Limao Verde, up to 55% of unaffected individuals have a low-level IgG1 antibody response against desmoglein 1, the PF autoantigen, which becomes an IgG4 response of higher titer against a more pathogenic epitope in disease.[13] Fogo selvagem occurs often in children and young adults, unlike sporadic PF, which is a disease of mostly middle-aged and older patients. Also unlike PF, fogo selvagem occurs not infrequently in genetically related family members, although it is not contagious. There is no known racial or ethnic predominance, and anyone moving into an endemic area may be susceptible to disease. Furthermore, the urban development of rural endemic areas of Brazil decreased the incidence of disease (Fig. 52-1).

These epidemiologic associations suggest that an environmental agent may trigger a low-level autoantibody response that in some genetically susceptible individuals becomes pathogenic against desmoglein 1 by intermolecular epitope spreading. With this theory in mind, it is interesting that 40% to 80% of patients from Brazil with the insect-borne diseases onchocerciasis, leishmaniasis, and Chagas disease have low-level anti-desmoglein 1 antibodies, but patients with other infectious diseases from Brazil rarely have such antibodies.[15] Subsequent studies have shown that IgG4 and IgE antibodies from fogo selvagem patients recognize salivary gland antigens from the sand fly *Lutzomyia longipalpis*, the vector of leishmaniasis.[16] The current theory is that fogo selvagem may initiate with an IgE response against the sand fly salivary antigen LJM11, which cross-reacts with desmoglein 1 and then generalizes to an IgG4 response.[17,18] This fascinating disease holds clues to understanding how this autoimmune response is triggered.

The sex ratio of pemphigus in women versus men ranges from 1.33 to 2.25.[7,9,19-24] Notable outliers to this estimate are the predominance of women (4:1) in an endemic focus of PF in Tunisia,[6] and a predominance of men (19:1) in an endemic focus of PF in Colombia.[25]

AGE OF ONSET

The average age of disease onset also varies by region. In Turkey, Saudi Arabia, Tunisia, and Iran, the mean age of onset is approximately 40 years.[6,19,21,26] Studies in the United States, Europe, and Taiwan demonstrate an average age of onset between 50 and 70 years.[5,6,9-11,20,22,27-29] Pemphigus rarely occurs in children,[30] except in regions of endemic disease.

CLINICAL FEATURES

PEMPHIGUS VULGARIS

CUTANEOUS FINDINGS

The skin lesions in PV can be pruritic or painful. Exposure to ultraviolet radiation may exacerbate disease activity.[31,32] The primary lesion of PV is a flaccid blister, which may occur anywhere on the skin surface, but typically not the palms and soles (Fig. 52-1A, Table 52-2). Usually, the blister arises on normal-appearing skin, but it may develop on erythematous skin. Because PV blisters are fragile, the most common skin lesions observed in patients are erosions resulting from broken blisters. These erosions are often quite large, as they have a tendency to spread at their periphery (Fig. 52-2).

A characteristic finding in pemphigus patients is that erosions can be extended into visibly normal skin by pulling the remnant of the blister wall or rubbing at the periphery of active lesions; additionally, erosions can be induced in normal-appearing skin distant from active lesions by pressure or mechanical shear force. This phenomenon is known as the

TABLE 52-2
Pemphigus Subtypes and Variants

	CUTANEOUS FINDINGS	MUCOUS MEMBRANE INVOLVEMENT	PATHOLOGY	IMMUNOFLUORESCENCE DIRECT (NONQUANTITATIVE)	IMMUNOFLUORESCENCE INDIRECT (SEMIQUANTITATIVE)	ELISA (QUANTITATIVE)
Pemphigus vulgaris	Flaccid blisters, typically sparing palmoplantar surface Large erosions are common presentations (+) Nikolsky sign	Oral and nasal mucous membranes most commonly affected Esophageal Vulvar, cervical, vaginal Ocular	Suprabasal blister with acantholysis "row of tombstones" appearance	IgG bound to surface of keratinocytes (intercellular pattern)	Monkey esophagus substrate ideal IgG in cell surface pattern	Desmogleins 1, 3 (mucosal and skin involvement) Desmoglein 3 (mucosal dominant)
Pemphigus vegetans[a]	Erosions develop excessive papillomatosis tissue and crusting; intertriginous areas, scalp, or face	Oral involvement is common[a]	Suprabasal acantholysis, with papillomatosis of the dermal papillae and downward growth of epidermal strands into the dermis; presence of hyperkeratosis and scale-crust; eosinophilic or neutrophilic intraepidermal abscesses	IgG on cell surface of keratinocytes[a]	IgG in cell surface pattern[a]	Desmoglein 3, sometimes desmoglein 1
Pemphigus foliaceus	Scaly, crusted lesions on erythematous base; seborrheic distribution (face, scalp, upper trunk); small flaccid blisters are transient primary lesions	Very rare	Early lesions show eosinophilic spongiosis; histopathology demonstrates acantholysis below stratum corneum; epidermis beneath the granular layer remains intact; subcorneal pustules containing neutrophils and acantholytic epidermal cells in the blister cavity	IgG bound to surface of keratinocytes (intercellular pattern)	Guinea pig esophagus or human skin substrate ideal IgG in intercellular pattern	Desmoglein 1
Pemphigus erythematosus[b]	Crusted lesions in seborrheic distribution	Rare	Similar to pemphigus foliaceus	IgG and C3 deposition at granular basement membrane zone, IgG with intercellular pattern		Desmoglein 1[†]
Endemic pemphigus foliaceus (fogo selvagem)[c]	Similar to pemphigus foliaceus; characterized by burning sensation, and exacerbation on sun exposure	Rare	Similar to pemphigus foliaceus	Similar to pemphigus foliaceus		Desmoglein 1

[a]Variant of pemphigus vulgaris.
[b]Variant of pemphigus foliaceus.
[c]Similar to pemphigus foliaceus clinically, histologically, and serologically, however with distinct epidemiologic features.[§]

*Ruoco V, Ruoco E, Caccavale S, et al. Pemphigus vegetans of the folds (intertriginous areas). Clin Dermatol. 2015;33(4):471-476.
†Oktarina D, Poot A, Kramer D. The IgG "lupus-band" deposition pattern of pemphigus erythematosus. Association with the desogein 1 ectodomain as revealed by 3 cases. Arch Dermatol. 2012;148(10):1173-1178.
§Rocha-Alvares R, Ortega-Loayza A, Friedman H. Endemic pemphigus vulgaris. Arch Dermatol. 2007;143(7):895-899.

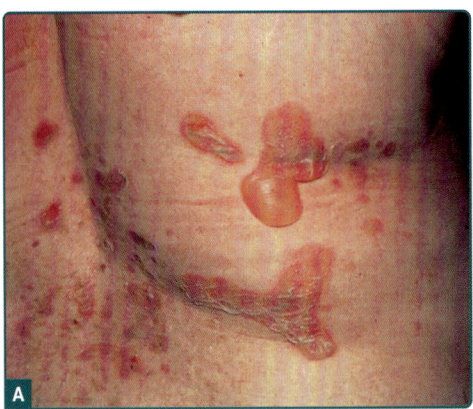 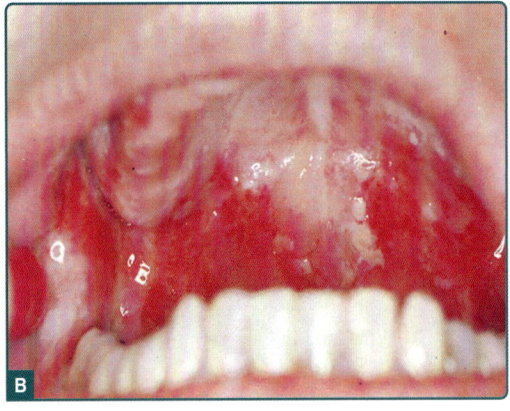

Figure 52-1 Pemphigus vulgaris. **A,** Flaccid blisters. (Used with permission from Lawrence Lieblich, MD.) **B,** Oral erosions.

Nikolsky sign.[33] This sign helps differentiate pemphigus from other blistering diseases of the skin such as pemphigoid (Table 52-1); however, similar findings also can be elicited in staphylococcal scalded skin syndrome, Stevens-Johnson syndrome, and toxic epidermal necrolysis.

In certain patients, erosions have a tendency to develop excessive papillimatosis and crusting, referred to as vegetating lesions (Fig. 52-3). This type of lesion tends to occur more frequently in intertriginous areas, in the scalp, or on the face. Generally, the prognosis for these so-called pemphigus vegetans patients is thought to be better, with milder disease and a higher chance of remission compared to typical PV patients.[34] Some ordinary PV lesions heal with a vegetating morphology and can remain for long periods of time in one place. Thus, vegetating lesions seem to be one reactive pattern of the skin to the autoimmune insult of PV.

Although hair loss is not a usual feature in pemphigus, temporary hair loss can be seen in about 5% of patients and can rarely be a presenting sign of disease.[35]

MUCOUS MEMBRANE LESIONS

The mucous membranes most often affected by PV are those of the oropharyngeal cavity (Fig. 52-1B) and nasal mucosa.[36,37] Endoscopic evaluation revealed that 87% of PV patients had ear, nose, or throat lesions, with involvement of nasal mucosa, pharynx, and larynx being most common at 76%, 66%, and 55%, respectively.[38] Laryngeal involvement was often asymptomatic. As with cutaneous lesions, intact blisters are rare. Oropharyngeal erosions can be so painful that the patient is unable to eat or drink. The inability to eat or drink adequately may require inpatient hospitalization for disease control and intravenous fluid and nutrient repletion.

In the majority of patients, painful mucous membrane erosions are the presenting sign of PV and may be the only sign for an average of 5 months before skin lesions develop.[3] However, the presenting symptoms may vary; in a study from Croatia, painful oral lesions were the presenting symptom in 32% of patients.[23] Most of these patients progressed to a more generalized eruption in 5 months to 1 year; however, some had oral lesions for more than 5 years before generalization. On the other hand, in Tehran, 62% of patients presented with oral lesions only.[7] Skin involvement without mucous membrane involvement in PV is less common, accounting in one study for 11% of PV cases.[39]

GI tract involvement with PV has been described in the esophagus, stomach, duodenum, and anus, although only biopsies of the esophagus have proven the lesions were due to suprabasal acantholysis.[7,40,41] About 27% of PV patients demonstrate such PV histology on blind biopsies of the esophagus.[41] Further-

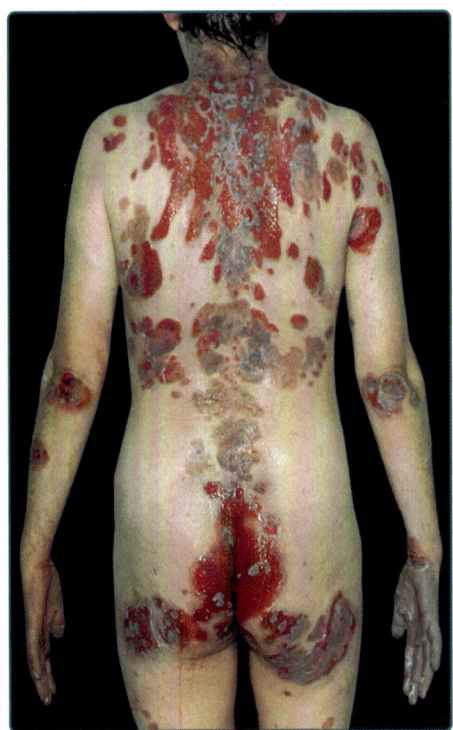

Figure 52-2 Pemphigus vulgaris. Extensive erosions due to blistering. Almost the entire back is denuded. Note intact, flaccid blisters at the lower border of eroded lesions.

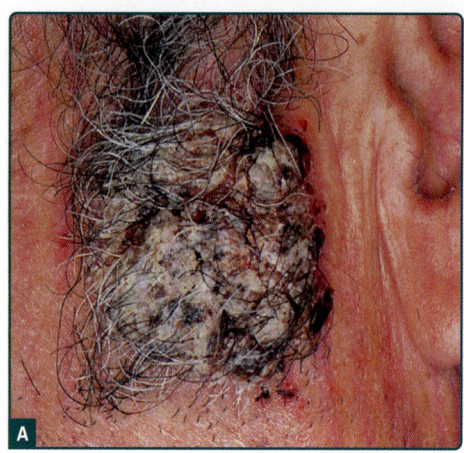
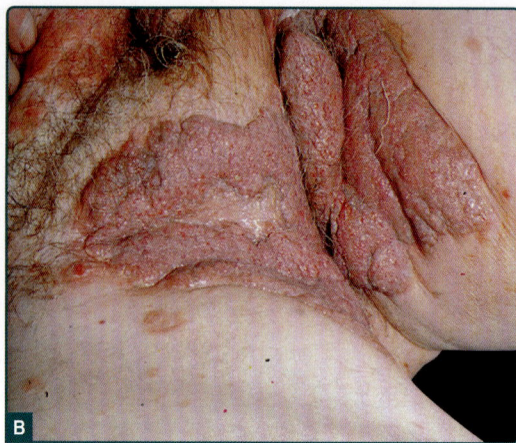

Figure 52-3 **A,** Crusted, vegetating lesions in pemphigus vulgaris. **B,** Extensive, vegetating lesions in intertriginous regions in pemphigus vegetans-type pemphigus vulgaris.

more, esophageal involvement may be asymptomatic but may also lead to esophagitis dissecans, evidenced by sloughing of esophageal casts.[41,42] Involvement of other mucous membranes can also occur, including the vulvovaginal and ocular epithelia.[43-46] Vulvar and cervicovaginal lesions may be found in up to 51% of women with active disease but these lesions may be asymptomatic. Vulvar lesions are most common and may cause severe burning with urination. Even without obvious lesions, Pap smears may be positive in women with pemphigus and the acantholytic cells may be misinterpreted as indicative of cervical dysplasia.[47,48] There is ocular involvement in about 16% of PV patients, some with erosions of the conjunctiva, but findings may be nonspecific.[49] There are rare case reports of corneal erosions in PV patients, but without histologic confirmation of acantholysis.[50]

PEMPHIGUS FOLIACEUS

CUTANEOUS FINDINGS

The characteristic clinical lesions of PF are scaly, crusted erosions, often on an erythematous base. In more localized and early disease, these lesions are usually well demarcated and scattered in a seborrheic distribution, including the face, scalp, and upper trunk (Fig. 52-4A, Table 52-2). The primary lesions of small flaccid blisters are typically not found. Disease may stay localized for years, or it may rapidly progress to generalized involvement, resulting in an exfoliative erythroderma (Fig. 52-4B). Like PV, PF may be exacerbated by ultraviolet radiation.[32,51,52] Patients with PF often complain of pain and burning in the skin lesions. In contrast to patients with PV, those with PF very rarely, if ever, have mucous membrane involvement, even with widespread disease.

The colloquial term for Brazilian endemic pemphigus, fogo selvagem (Portuguese for "wild fire"), takes into account many of the clinical aspects of this disease: the burning feeling of the skin, the exacerbation of disease by the sun, and the crusted lesions that make the patients appear as if they had been burned.

PEMPHIGUS ERYTHEMATOSUS

In 1926, Francis Senear and Barney Usher described 11 patients with features of a pemphigus-lupus erythematosus overlap (*Senear-Usher syndrome*).[53] Over the next several decades, debate over whether these patients had lupus erythematosus, pemphigus, seborrheic dermatitis, or features of all 3 disorders continued, with Senear concluding that the disease is best considered a variant of pemphigus, termed *pemphigus erythematosus*.[54] As these observations were made prior to the development of immunofluorescence testing for both pemphigus and lupus, the diagnosis was primarily based on the clinical presentation: crusted erosions in a seborrheic distribution, at times concurrent with more lupuslike discoid lesions with "carpet-tack" scale. Walter Lever noted that many patients initially categorized as pemphigus erythematosus went on to develop systemic lupus, or more widespread pemphigus foliaceus, or even pemphigus vulgaris, in some cases because of incorrect initial diagnosis. Therefore, rather than perpetuate the use of one term for different diseases, he proposed that pemphigus erythematosus be used to describe a localized form of PF with better prognosis.[1] After the development of immunofluorescence and antinuclear antibody testing for pemphigus and lupus, it was discovered that pemphigus erythematosus patients demonstrate immunologic overlap features; by definition, all demonstrate the cell surface staining pattern classic for pemphigus, approximately 30% have positive antinuclear antibody titers, and 80% have positive lupus band tests, although the latter test is only positive in 20% to 40% of biopsies on non–sun-exposed skin.[55] Subsequent studies have shown that the positive "lupus band" test in pemphigus erythematosus patients is due to granular deposits of IgG

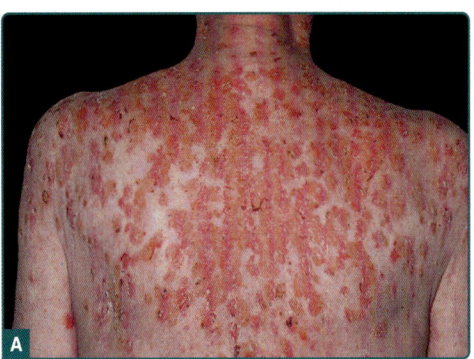 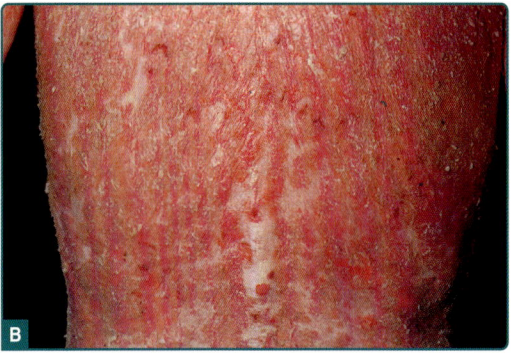

Figure 52-4 Pemphigus foliaceus. **A.** Scaly, crusted lesions on upper back. **B.** Exfoliative erythroderma due to confluent lesions.

and cleaved desmoglein 1 ectodomain deposited at the basement membrane zone, which is thought to occur after ultraviolet light exposure.[56] Thus, because most patients with pemphigus erythematosus do not develop systemic signs or symptoms of lupus, and some may progress from localized disease to generalized PF,[57] the diagnosis of the pemphigus erythematosus variant of PF is largely one of historic, rather than clinical, significance.

NEONATAL PEMPHIGUS

Infants born to mothers with PV may display clinical, histologic, and immunopathologic signs of pemphigus vulgaris.[58,59] The degree of involvement varies from none to severe enough to result in a stillbirth. If the infant survives, disease tends to remit as maternal antibody is catabolized. Mothers with PF may also transmit their autoantibodies to the fetus, but, as discussed in the section "Pathophysiology of Acantholysis", neonatal PF occurs only rarely.[60-62] Neonatal pemphigus should be distinguished from PV and PF that occur in childhood, which are similar to the autoimmune diseases seen in adults.[63]

DRUG-INDUCED PEMPHIGUS

Although there are sporadic case reports of pemphigus associated with the use of several different drugs, the association with penicillamine, and perhaps captopril, is the most significant.[64] The prevalence of pemphigus in penicillamine users is estimated to be approximately 7%. PF (including pemphigus erythematosus) is more common than PV in these penicillamine-treated patients, although either may occur. The findings of direct and indirect immunofluorescence are positive in most of these patients. Three patients with drug-induced PF and one with drug-induced PV have been shown to have autoantibodies to the same molecules involved in sporadic pemphigus, namely, desmoglein 1 and desmoglein 3, respectively.[65] Therefore, by immunofluorescence and immunochemical determinations, these patients with drug-induced pemphigus resemble those with sporadic disease.

Both penicillamine and captopril contain sulfhydryl groups that are postulated to interact with the sulfhydryl groups in desmoglein 1, 3, or both, thereby causing pemphigus either by directly interfering with these adhesion molecules[66] or, alternatively, by modifying them so that they become more antigenic. The use of these drugs may also lead to a more generalized dysregulation of the immune response, as penicillamine has been associated with the onset of several other autoantibody-mediated diseases including myasthenia gravis,[67] Goodpasture syndrome,[68] and antineutrophil cytoplasmic antibody vasculitis.[69] Some, but not all, patients with drug-induced pemphigus go into remission after they stop taking the offending drug.

Additionally, rare anecdotal reports have suggested the association of dietary intake and pemphigus, proposing the hypothesis that thiol-containing foods such as garlic, leeks, and onions may precipitate disease.[70,71] Some patients may note that certain foods aggravate oral lesions, but it is unlikely that dietary intervention alone will remit disease in most patients.

Interestingly, anecdotal case reports have reported improvement of PV with cigarette smoking,[72] as well as with the cholinergic agonists pyridostigmine, carbachol, and pilocarpine.[73,74] Studies suggest that activation of cholinergic receptors may regulate signaling pathways modulated by PV IgG, thereby affecting cell adhesion.[75] These results are intriguing given the clinical benefit of nicotine noted in other inflammatory diseases, such as ulcerative colitis.[76]

ASSOCIATED DISEASES

Myasthenia gravis, thymoma, or both have been associated with pemphigus.[77-79] Approximately one-half of thymoma-associated pemphigus cases are vulgaris; one-half, foliaceus or erythematosus. Most of these data, however, were reported before the recognition of paraneoplastic pemphigus as a distinct entity. Therefore, although thymoma may clearly be associated with PV and PF, it also may be associated with paraneoplastic pemphigus (Chap. 53). Myasthenia gravis is a tissue-specific autoantibody-mediated disease leading to skeletal muscle weakness. Early disease usually affects facial muscles, leading to symptoms of dysarthria, dysphagia, ptosis, or diplopia. Disease may then progress to affect the larger muscles of the trunk and extremities, with potential fatal complications from respiratory muscle involvement. Thymoma, in contrast, is typically asymptomatic in adults. In children, thymomas are more likely to be symptomatic with cough, chest pain, superior vena cava syndrome, dysphagia, and/or hoarseness from localized tumor encroachment. Myasthenia gravis would be best evaluated by a neurologist, who can complete a full neurologic examination and may test for the presence of serum acetylcholine receptor autoantibodies. The course of myasthenia gravis and the course of pemphigus appear to be independent of each other. Likewise, thymic abnormalities may either precede or follow the onset of pemphigus. Posteroanterior and lateral chest radiographs with or without computed tomography follow-up can detect most thymomas. Irradiation of the thymus or thymectomy, although clearly beneficial for myasthenia gravis, may or may not improve the pemphigus disease activity.[80]

Recent epidemiologic studies have identified that pemphigus vulgaris patients have a higher prevalence of autoimmune thyroid disease, rheumatoid arthritis, and Type 1 diabetes compared with the general population.[81] Higher prevalences of these autoimmune diseases are also observed in the family members of PV patients, suggesting a common genetic element that may underlie autoimmune susceptibility.

ETIOLOGY AND PATHOGENESIS

The discovery of pemphigus as an organ-specific, autoantibody-mediated disease of desmosomes highlights the synergy between clinical care and basic science research. The development of light microscopy and electron microscopy allowed dermatologists to identify the morphology and immunopathology of disease. Patient serum IgG served as a key reagent to help identify both the PF and PV antigens.[82-84] The cloning and characterization of the pemphigus antigens have subsequently led to the development of enzyme-linked immunosorbent assays (ELISAs) to improve the sensitivity and specificity of disease diagnosis, and continued studies on pemphigus pathophysiology aim to develop safer and effective therapies for these potentially fatal diseases. A recent in-depth review discusses these issues.[85]

PEMPHIGUS AUTOANTIGENS

Pemphigus antigens are desmogleins, transmembrane glycoproteins of desmosomes (cell-to-cell adhesion structures, reviewed in Chap. 15).[86,87] Desmogleins are part of the cadherin superfamily of calcium-dependent cell-adhesion molecules. The original members of this family (eg, E-cadherin) demonstrate homophilic adhesive interactions (binding between like molecules). Desmogleins similarly demonstrate homophilic binding but likely participate in predominantly heterophilic adhesion by binding desmocollins, the other major transmembrane glycoprotein of desmosomes.[88-90]

The PF antigen (as well as the fogo selvagem antigen) is desmoglein 1, a 160-kDa protein.[82,83,91] The PV antigen is desmoglein 3, a 130-kDa protein that is 64% similar and 46% identical in amino acid sequence to desmoglein 1.[84] All patients with PV have anti–desmoglein 3 antibodies, and some of these patients also have anti–desmoglein 1 antibodies.[92,93] Patients with mucosal-dominant PV tend to have only anti–desmoglein 3 antibodies, whereas those with mucocutaneous disease usually have both anti–desmoglein 3 and anti–desmoglein 1 antibodies.[94-96] PF patients typically have antibodies against only desmoglein 1. However, these rules are not true for every patient.[97,98]

IgG antibodies against another desmosomal cadherin, desmocollin, can be found infrequently in PV, pemphigus vegetans, and atypical pemphigus patients.[99,100] Furthermore, mice with a targeted deletion of desmocollin 3 have PV-like skin lesions,[101] and anti-desmocollin antibodies can cause acantholysis in vitro.[99,102]

Other cell surface molecules such as acetylcholine receptors and E-cadherin also have been identified as immunologic targets of pemphigus serum, although their direct involvement in the pathophysiology of pemphigus has not been well validated.[103-106]

ELECTRON MICROSCOPY

Early ultrastructural studies of the blisters in pemphigus vulgaris and foliaceus focused on the appearance of desmosomes, because these are the most prominent cell-to-cell adhesion junctions in stratified squamous epithelia (Chap. 15). Almost all studies confirm that at various time points during acantholysis, the desmosome is affected and ultimately destroyed, consistent with the cell biologic data discussed in the section below. However, conclusions from electron microscopy studies as to the mechanism of desmosome destruction have varied. Several groups have proposed that the first pathologic event in pemphigus is intercellular widening of interdesmosomal cell membranes, with intact desmosomal junctions.[107-110] Other studies have demonstrated half-split desmosomes without keratin tonofilament retraction, suggesting that pemphigus autoantibodies directly interfere with the trans-adhesive interface of desmosomes, and that keratin retraction is secondary to the loss of intercellular adhesion. Half-desmosomes without tonofilament collapse also have been observed in a mouse model of PV.[111,112] Others have proposed that keratin retraction is a primary pathogenic event in pemphigus, triggered by cellular signaling after PV autoantibody binding.[113] As a potential reconciliation of these findings, one study found that electron microscopic findings may differ depending on the site analyzed: in early blisters, half-desmosomes without keratin retraction are observed; in well-developed lesions, keratin retraction from half-desmosomes occurs; and in spongiotic non-blistered skin, intercellular widening with intact desmosomal junctions can be found, similar to electron microscopy findings in other spongiotic epidermal diseases.[114] Similarly, large-scale electron microscopic maps ("nanotomy") have identified evidence of both half desmosomes and smaller desmosomes in pemphigus patients,[115] and super-resolution microscopy indicates that desmosomes are smaller in PV patients,[116] consistent with a desmoglein nonassembly/desmosome depletion model for pathogenesis as discussed below.

Currently, electron microscopy studies are not part of the clinical diagnostic workup for pemphigus.

PATHOPHYSIOLOGY OF ACANTHOLYSIS

Autoantibodies in pemphigus are pathogenic as suggested by neonatal pemphigus, discussed above, in which mothers with even mild PV can pass IgG autoantibodies to the fetus, causing blistering oral and skin disease that resolves by approximately 6 months, concurrent with the disappearance of maternal IgG from the circulation.[58]

Several lines of evidence indicate that it is the anti-desmoglein 1 and 3 antibodies in pemphigus patients who directly cause blisters and hence are the etiologic agents of disease. Passive transfer of PV or PF IgG to neonatal mice or human skin causes blisters that clinically and histologically mimic the corresponding type of pemphigus in patients.[117-119] The anti-desmoglein antibodies are responsible for blister formation in the passive transfer model, because affinity purified anti-desmoglein 1 and 3 autoantibodies cause PF and PV blisters, respectively, and adsorption of desmoglein-reactive autoantibodies from PF or PV IgG abrogates disease.[120-124] Finally, mice with a targeted deletion of the desmoglein 3 gene have clinical and histologic lesions similar to PV patients,[125] suggesting that inactivation of desmoglein 3 results in a PV-like blister. Similarly, exfoliative toxin, the staphylococcus toxin that causes blisters in bullous impetigo and staphylococcal scalded skin syndrome, cleaves desmoglein 1 and results in a blister with a histology similar or identical to PF.[126]

Unlike many other autoantibody-mediated diseases, such as pemphigoid and epidermolysis bullosa acquisita, in which the constant region of the antibody is required for blister formation to activate complement or bind antibody receptors on inflammatory cells, in pemphigus the variable region of the antibody is sufficient to cause blisters in neonatal mice or human skin.[119,127-129] Furthermore, IgG4, which does not fix complement, has been shown to be both pathogenic and the predominant IgG subclass in both PF and PV.[130-132] For this reason, a significant amount of research on disease pathophysiology has focused on the epitopes bound by pathogenic autoantibodies, as these regions are likely critical for maintaining desmosomal cell adhesion. Epitope mapping studies have shown that pathogenic PV and PF autoantibodies bind calcium-sensitive, conformational epitopes in the amino terminal extracellular domains of desmogleins, whereas nonpathogenic antibodies tend to bind more membrane proximal extracellular domains.[133-136] The amino terminal domains bound by pathogenic autoantibodies are the same domains that are predicted to form the key molecular interactions for desmoglein intercellular adhesion, based on studies of cadherin ultrastructure.[90,137,138] Furthermore, PV IgG have been shown to directly inhibit desmoglein 3–mediated trans-interactions by atomic force microscopy.[139] Collectively, these data form the basis for the "steric hindrance" hypothesis, which proposes that pathogenic antibodies directly interfere with desmoglein adhesive interactions, causing acantholysis.

Studies on cultured keratinocytes have indicated that loss of intercellular adhesion by pathogenic autoantibodies leads to internalization and degradation of desmogleins,[140-143] thereby amplifying the loss of desmoglein function. As discussed above, loss of desmoglein 3 and 1 function results in PV- and PF-like blisters in model systems in which desmogleins are targeted genetically or by enzyme cleavage.

If inactivation of desmoglein isoforms results in blistering, then why do blisters in PV and PF have specific tissue localizations that do not necessarily correlate with the sites at which the antibodies bind by immunofluorescence? In PF, for example, the anti–desmoglein 1 antibodies bind throughout the epidermis and mucous membranes,[144] yet blisters occur only in the superficial epidermis. This apparent paradox can be explained by desmoglein compensation, as outlined in Fig. 52-5. The concept of desmoglein compensation originates in the assumption that autoantibodies against one desmoglein isoform inactivate only that isoform and that another isoform co-expressed in the same area can compensate in adhesion.[145-147] Desmoglein compensation explains why neonatal PF is so unusual, because even though the maternal anti–desmoglein 1 antibodies cross the placenta, in neonatal skin, but not in adult skin, desmoglein 3 is co-expressed with desmoglein 1 in the superficial epidermis, thereby providing protection against the loss of desmoglein 1-based adhesion.[146,148] Desmoglein compensation also offers an explanation for the differing sites of blister formation in PV and PF, both in regard to the histology (ie, suprabasal or superficial), as well as the areas of involvement (mucosa and/or skin).

Further studies have suggested that perturbation of cell signaling pathways can mediate and/or mod-

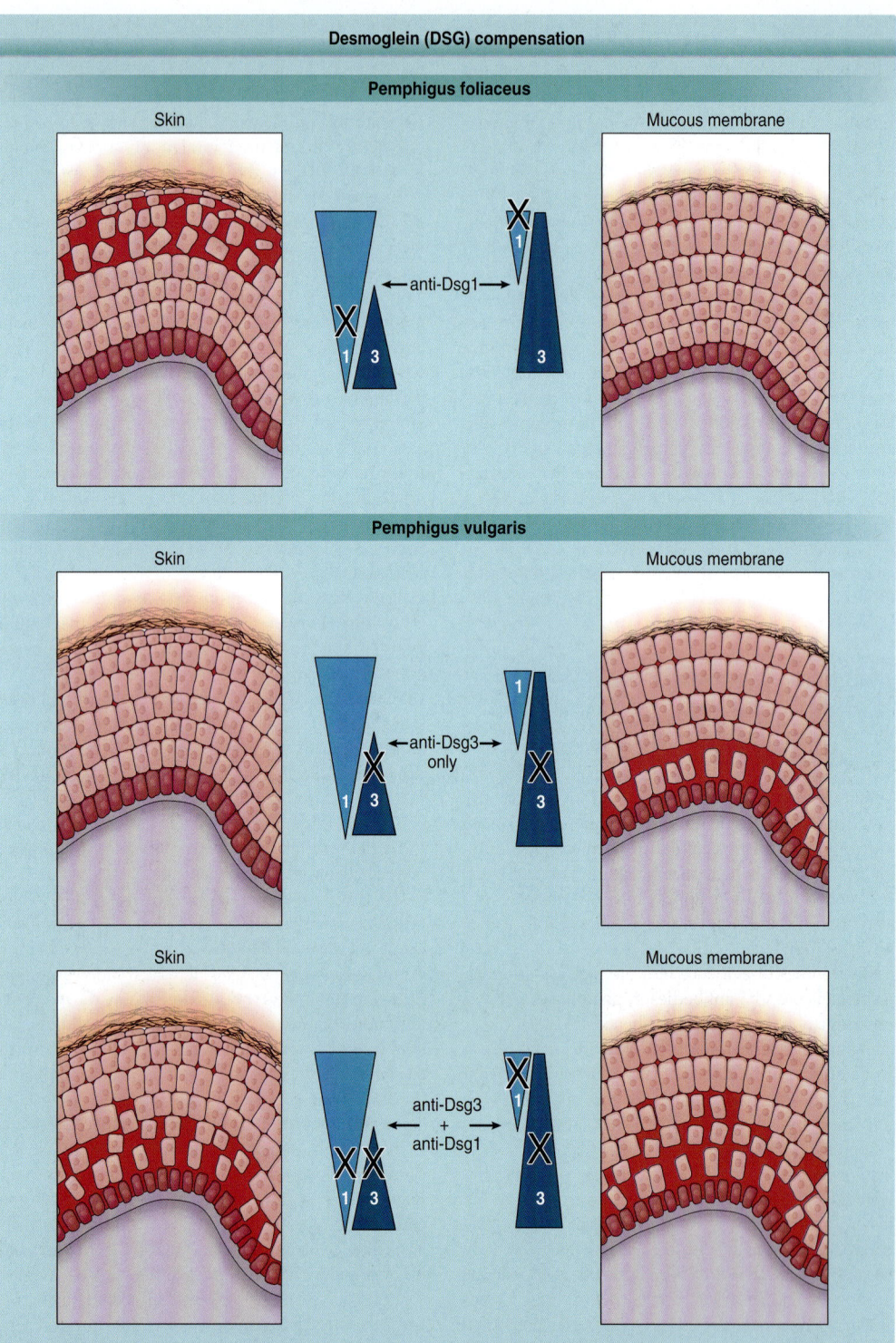

Figure 52-5 Desmoglein (Dsg) compensation. Triangles represent the distribution of Dsg1 and Dsg3 in skin and mucous membranes. Anti-Dsg1 antibodies in pemphigus foliaceus cause acantholysis only in the superficial epidermis of skin. In the deep epidermis and in mucous membranes, Dsg3 compensates for antibody-induced loss of function of Dsg1. In mucosal pemphigus vulgaris, antibodies against Dsg3 are predominant, which cause blisters only in the deep mucous membrane where Dsg3 is present without compensatory Dsg1. However, in mucocutaneous pemphigus, antibodies against both Dsg1 and Dsg3 are present, and blisters form in both mucous membrane and skin. The blister is deep probably because antibodies diffuse from the dermis and interfere first with the function of desmosomes at the base of the epidermis.

ulate blister formation in pemphigus. For example, inhibition of the p38 mitogen activated protein kinase (MAPK) pathway and activation of Rho GTPases, among others, can prevent blister formation after passive transfer of pemphigus IgG in the neonatal mouse model.[149-151] The p38 MAPK pathway has been most studied in this regard. It activates EGF receptor after PV antibody binding, and blocking of this receptor also blocks loss of cell adhesion.[152] Although p38 activation may be secondary to loss of cell adhesion, blocking it does decrease the degree of acantholysis, suggesting that it would be a useful target in pemphigus therapy.[153,154] A more specific target in this pathway, downstream of p38, is MAPK activated protein kinase 2 (MK2), which also can be blocked to modulate pemphigus blister activity, especially spontaneous blistering as opposed to blistering due to trauma (ie, Nikolsky blistering).[155] Finally, in vitro studies with monoclonal anti-desmoglein 3 antibodies and human pemphigus antibodies suggest that acantholysis is a net result of both direct steric hindrance of pathogenic monoclonal antibodies and polyclonal antibodies that may not directly cause steric hindrance but that cause internalization of desmogleins by crosslinking them. This latter effect is dependent on MAPK signaling.[156]

The depletion of desmogleins by pemphigus antibodies may lead to loss of desmogleins in desmosomes resulting in smaller desmosomes and/or their defective function in adhesion, a scenario referred to as the *Dsg nonassembly depletion hypothesis*.[115,140,141,157,158] Consistent with this idea is the observation by direct immunofluorescence of clustering of Dsgs in both PV and PF patients' skin and that forced increased expression of Dsg3 can prevent acantholysis by pemphigus antibodies.[159]

The current general consensus is that desmosomal adhesion is a dynamic process that is perturbed by pemphigus autoantibodies both directly and by signaling pathways.[160] Therefore, therapies that aim to strengthen keratinocyte adhesion by modulation of signaling pathways may have a beneficial effect on pemphigus, regardless of whether cell signaling is a primary pathologic cause of disease.

GENETIC CHARACTERIZATION OF THE PEMPHIGUS IMMUNE RESPONSE

Compared to a matched population, patients with PV have a markedly increased frequency of certain class II major histocompatibility complex (MHC) antigens. Among Ashkenazi Jews with PV, the serologically defined HLA-DR4 haplotype is predominant, whereas in other ethnic groups with PV, the DQ1 allele is more common.[161] However, the association with disease susceptibility becomes even more striking in an analysis of these MHC alleles at a genetic level. Patients with the DR4 serotype almost all have the unusual allele DRB1*0402, and patients with the DQ1 serotype almost all have the rare allele DQB1*0503. Similar, but less restricted, HLA-DR alleles are associated with PF.[162] The protein chains encoded by these PV MHC II alleles vary from those found in HLA-DR4 and DQ1 controls without disease by only a few amino acids. Other studies have confirmed that the immune response in pemphigus is restricted to certain desmoglein peptides and MHC class II alleles.[163-166]

MHC class II alleles encode cell surface molecules that are necessary for antigen presentation to the immune system; therefore, it is hypothesized that PV-associated MHC class II molecules facilitate presentation of desmoglein 3 peptides to T cells.[167] Consistent with this hypothesis, certain peptides from desmoglein 3, predicted to fit into the DRB1*0402 peptide-binding pocket, were found to stimulate T cells from patients.[168] More direct proof of the importance of the DRB1*0402 allele comes from a study of a humanized HLA-transgenic mouse for this allele in which presentation of the immunodominant Dsg3 peptides to human T cells results in production of pemphigus antibodies and the epidermal pathology of PV.[169]

Expression of Dsg3 in the thymus, mediated by the Aire transcription factor, promotes tolerance of CD4 T cells to stimulation by Dsg3.[170] An unexpected observation was that T cells of normal people with the DRB1*0402 or DQB1*0503 respond just as well as those of pemphigus patients to the same desmoglein 3 peptides,[167,171] indicating that T-cell reactivity to desmoglein 3 peptides is not sufficient for disease onset. Dsg-specific CD4+ T cells provide help to simulate anti-Dsg B cells to produce antibodies.[172] In this context, CD4+ T follicular helper cells are thought to be particularly important. Concordantly, there are increased T follicular helper cells with their associated cytokine, IL-27, in PV patients.[173] Another factor that may determine who gets pemphigus and who does not has been proposed to be the presence of regulatory T cells that can suppress the autoimmune response in those who do not.[174] Likely, multiple factors prevent T-cell Dsg responsiveness and subsequent help for B-cell anti-Dsg antibody production.

Cloning of anti-desmoglein B-cell repertoires from PV and PF patients has elucidated the diversity of the antibody variable region genes contributing to the pemphigus immune response.[128,129,175] Shared VH1-46 gene usage has been identified in anti-Dsg3 B cells among PV patients, probably because antibodies using this gene require few or no mutations to bind Dsg3, which may favor the selection of VH1-46 B cells early in the autoimmune response.[176] However, multiple other VH genes have been identified in anti-Dsg3 antibodies among PV patients that are more highly mutated and may not be shared,[128,177-179] although anti-Dsg antibodies from different PV patients have been shown to bind at or near common epitopes on desmoglein 3.[177] Analysis of anti-Dsg1 IgG B-cell repertoires in fogo selvagem patients has identified enrichment for VH3-23 heavy chain gene usage, as well as IGKV1D-39 light chain gene usage, with evidence of shared mutations as well as an increased number of somatic mutations in

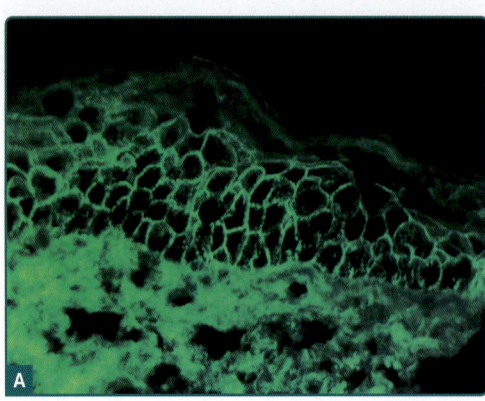 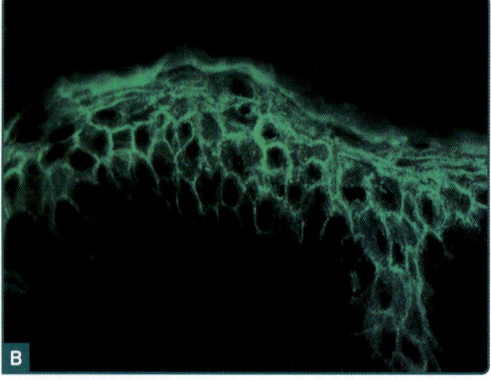

Figure 52-6 Immunofluorescence in pemphigus. **A,** Direct immunofluorescence for immunoglobulin G (IgG) of perilesional skin from a patient with pemphigus vulgaris. Cell surface staining is observed throughout the epidermis with a slight basal predominance. **B,** Indirect immunofluorescence with the serum from a patient with pemphigus foliaceus on normal human skin. IgG is observed on the cell surface throughout the epidermis with a slight superficial predominance.

the antigen-binding regions of Dsg1-reactive antibodies, suggesting antigen-driven selective pressure.[180]

Cross-reactivity in the B-cell repertoire to foreign and self-antigen has been proposed as a mechanism for the onset of autoimmunity in both PV and PF. In addition to the autoantibody cross-reactivity to LJM11 sand fly antigen and Dsg1 discussed previously,[16] Dsg3 autoantibodies in PV have been shown to cross-react with rotavirus VP6 coat protein, and VH1-46 mAbs that both induce suprabasal blisters and inhibit rotavirus infectivity have been identified.[176] Unmutated IgM VH1-46 B cells have a propensity to bind both rotavirus VP6 coat protein,[181] as well as the PV autoantigen Dsg3.[176] However, cross-reactivity to VP6 and Dsg3 in the IgG compartment is rare because of the differing nature of somatic mutations that confer VP6 versus Dsg3 reactivity, thus preventing the onset of pemphigus after rotavirus exposure.

To produce anti-Dsg autoantibodies, B cells must lose tolerance to Dsg, which is a self-antigen. Studies of cloned anti-Dsg B cells have shown that throughout the course of PV, over the years, the same clones of anti-Dsg B cells persist and new ones generally are not produced.[182] These data suggest that some event causes a time-limited loss of tolerance of B cells to Dsg, and if these B-cell clones can be completely eliminated, patients might be cured, thus explaining the rationale for B-cell depletion therapy in pemphigus.

DIAGNOSIS

Diagnosis of pemphigus relies on skin biopsy of a fresh lesion for histology to determine the site of blister formation, as well as a confirmatory immunochemical study to document the presence of skin autoantibodies, either by direct immunofluorescence of perilesional skin, or indirect immunofluorescence or ELISA of patient serum.

LABORATORY TESTING

IMMUNOFLUORESCENCE

The hallmark of pemphigus is the finding of immunoglobulin G (IgG) autoantibodies against the cell surface of keratinocytes. These autoantibodies were first discovered in patients' sera by indirect immunofluorescence techniques and soon thereafter were discovered by direct immunofluorescence of patients' skin.[183]

Direct Immunofluorescence: Essentially all patients with active PV or PF have a positive finding on a direct immunofluorescence study, which tests for IgG bound to the cell surface of keratinocytes in perilesional skin (Fig. 52-6A, Table 52-2).[184] This is a non-quantitative test (either negative or positive). The diagnosis of pemphigus should be seriously questioned if the test result of direct immunofluorescence is negative. It is important that the biopsy for direct immunofluorescence be performed on normal-appearing perilesional skin, as the immune reactants can be difficult to detect in blistered inflamed epidermis (leading to a false negative result). In some cases of pemphigus erythematosus, IgG and C3 are deposited at the basement membrane zone of erythematous facial skin, in addition to the epidermal cell surface IgG, representing a positive lupus band test in addition to the typical pemphigus intercellular pattern.[185] In at least some cases, this band may be the result of UV-induced cleavage of Dsg1 with its accumulation at the basement membrane.[56]

Indirect Immunofluorescence: Indirect immunofluorescence is performed by incubating serial dilutions of patients' sera with epithelial substrates. It is reported as a semiquantitative titer (indicating the last dilution at which the serum demonstrates a positive cell surface staining pattern). The test is offered by most major national laboratories and can remain positive for weeks to months after healing of skin lesions, making it a good diagnostic test if a patient should present with no active skin lesions, for example due to empiric treatment with prednisone by a referring physician. Depending on the substrate used for indirect immunofluorescence, more than 80% of patients with pemphigus have circulating anti–epithelial cell surface IgG (Fig. 52-6B, Table 52-2).[186] The substrate used to detect pemphigus antibody binding in indirect immunofluorescence greatly influences the sensitivity of the test. In general, monkey esophagus is more sensitive for detecting PV antibodies, and guinea pig esophagus or normal human skin is a superior substrate for detecting PF antibodies. Patients with early localized disease and those in remission are most likely to have negative findings on an indirect immunofluorescence test; for these patients, the increased sensitivity of ELISA may help in diagnosis (see below).

Patients with PV and PF usually display similar direct and indirect immunofluorescence findings with IgG on the cell surface of epidermal cells throughout the epidermis, despite the different autoantigen profiles in these 2 diseases. Therefore, it is usually not possible to differentiate the 2 diseases by the pattern of immunofluorescence. There is a positive, but imperfect, correlation between the titer of circulating anti–cell surface antibody and the disease activity in PV and in PF.[187] Although this correlation may hold in general, and although patients in remission often show serologic remission with negative direct and indirect immunofluorescence findings,[188,189] disease activity in individual patients does not necessarily correlate with indirect immunofluorescence titer. Therefore, in the day-to-day management of these patients, following disease activity is more important than following antibody titer.

ENZYME-LINKED IMMUNOSORBENT ASSAY

For diagnosis of disease, antigen-specific ELISAs have been shown to be more sensitive and specific than immunofluorescence, and their titer correlates better than that of indirect immunofluorescence with disease activity.[92,190,191] Additionally, ELISAs are easier to perform and less subjective than immunofluorescence, and have for many physicians replaced the latter as the preferred first diagnostic test for pemphigus (Table 52-2). These assays use desmogleins 1 and 3 bound to plates, which are then incubated with patient sera and developed with anti-human IgG reagents (Fig. 52-7). As an advantage over indirect immunofluorescence, ELISAs can help differentiate between PV and PF because of the different autoantigen profiles in these 2 diseases.[92,190] In most cases, ELISA is positive for desmoglein 3 (but not desmoglein 1) in mucosal PV, is positive for both desmogleins 3 and 1 in PV with both mucosal and significant skin involvement, and is positive for only desmoglein 1 in PF. PV has rarely evolved into PF, and vice versa, as determined by clinical, histologic, and immunochemical criteria.[192-194] A small minority of PF patients may also

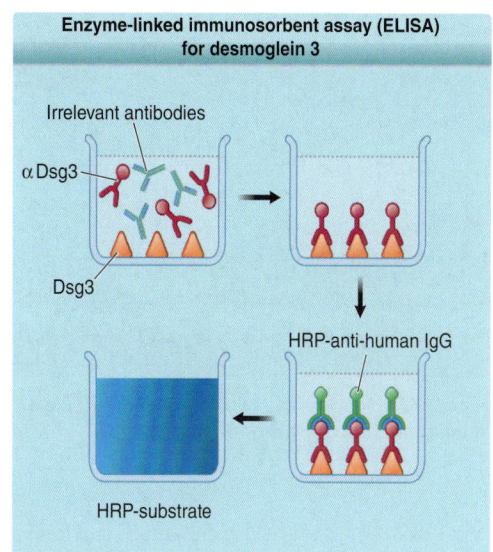

Figure 52-7 Enzyme-linked immunosorbent assay (ELISA) for desmoglein 3. Anti-Dsg3 antibodies (αDsg3) from pemphigus serum binds Dsg3 on the ELISA plate; irrelevant antibodies, that do not bind, are washed off. The plate is then incubated with horseradish peroxidase (HRP) conjugated anti-human IgG, which binds the anti-Dsg3 IgG that is on the plate. HRP is an enzyme that turns a clear substrate blue, and the amount of color, read on spectrophotometer, correlates with the amount of pemphigus (ie, anti-Dsg3) antibody in the patient's serum.

demonstrate autoantibodies to desmoglein 3[195]; therefore, diagnosis should be made based on the clinical-serologic correlation. Additionally, some patients (eg, those with bullous pemphigoid) may demonstrate a low level of anti–desmoglein 3 autoantibodies,[190] which are detectable because of the high sensitivity of the ELISA. Therefore, a result in the indeterminate range should be interpreted carefully, as this may represent a true positive or a false positive, the latter presumably because of formation of nonpathogenic bystander autoantibodies after epidermal damage. As with indirect immunofluorescence, the correlation of ELISA index value with disease activity is not perfect. For example, although ELISA titers correlate with clinical activity, patients in clinical remission (often still on corticosteroid therapy) whose titers have dropped from peak values may still have positive results.[196] In making treatment decisions, a negative result on desmoglein ELISA is more helpful than a positive result, as a patient with the former is more likely to achieve remission off immunosuppressives, whereas a patient with the latter may or may not. In other words, disease activity is the mainstay for determining treatment.

PATHOLOGY

The characteristic histopathologic finding in PV is a suprabasal blister with acantholysis (Fig. 52-8, Table 52-2). Just above the basal cell layer, epidermal

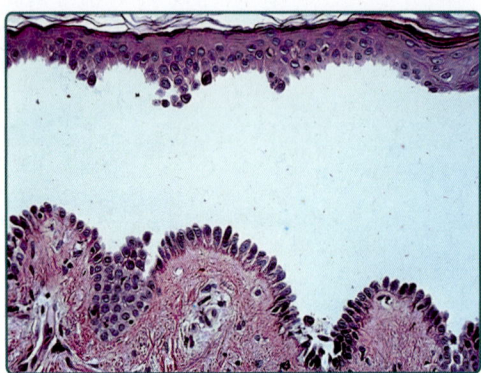

Figure 52-8 Histopathology of pemphigus vulgaris. Suprabasal acantholysis. The row of tombstones.

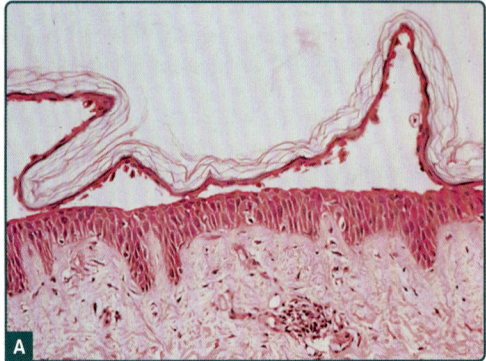
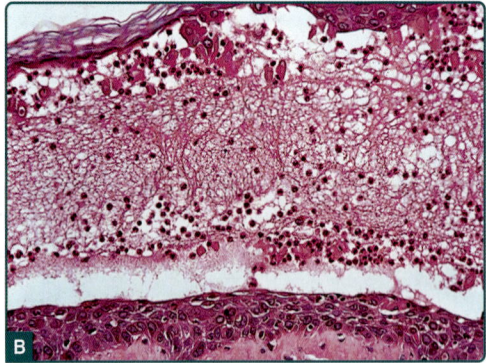

Figure 52-9 Histopathology of pemphigus foliaceus. **A,** Acantholysis in the granular layer. **B,** Subcorneal pustule with acantholysis.

cells lose their normal cell-to-cell contacts and form a blister. Often, a few rounded up (acantholytic) keratinocytes are in the blister cavity. The basal cells stay attached to the basement membrane, but may lose the contact with their neighbors; as a result, they may appear to be a "row of tombstones," symbolic of the potentially fatal prognosis of this disease. Usually, the upper epidermis (from 1 or 2 cell layers above the basal cells) remains intact, as these cells maintain their cell adhesion. Pemphigus vegetans shows not only suprabasal acantholysis but also papillomatosis of the dermal papillae and downward growth of epidermal stands into the dermis, with hyperkeratosis and scale-crust formation. In addition, pemphigus vegetans lesions may show intraepidermal abscesses composed of eosinophils and/or neutrophils.[197] Early PV lesions may show eosinophilic spongiosis.[198]

The histopathology of early blisters in PF patients demonstrates acantholysis (loss of cell-to-cell contact) just below the stratum corneum and in the granular layer (Fig. 52-9A). The stratum corneum is often lost from the surface of these lesions. The deeper epidermis, below the granular layer, remains intact. Another frequent finding is subcorneal pustules, with neutrophils and acantholytic epidermal cells in the blister cavity (Fig. 52-9B). Histologic findings in PF are often indistinguishable from those seen in bullous impetigo/staphylococcal scalded skin syndrome, because blisters in these latter diseases also result from dysfunction of desmoglein 1, in these cases due to proteolytic cleavage by Staphylococcal exfoliative toxins.[87] Therefore, immunochemical studies are essential to confirm a diagnosis of PF, as these would be negative in Staphylococcal-mediated skin blisters. The site of blister formation in pemphigus erythematosus is identical to PF. As in PV lesions, very early PF lesions may show eosinophilic spongiosis.[198]

DIFFERENTIAL DIAGNOSIS

See Table 52-1.

CLINICAL COURSE AND PROGNOSIS

Before the advent of glucocorticoid therapy, PV was almost invariably fatal due to severe blistering of the skin and mucous membranes, leading to malnutrition, dehydration, and sepsis. PF was fatal in approximately 60% of patients. PF was almost always fatal in elderly patients with concurrent medical problems; however, in other patients, its prognosis, without therapy, was much better than PV.[199,200]

The systemic administration of glucocorticoids and the use of immunosuppressive therapy have dramatically improved the prognosis for patients with pemphigus; however, pemphigus is still a disease associated with a significant morbidity and mortality.[201,202] In the United States, the annual mortality rate from pemphigus (age-adjusted to the standard population) is estimated to be 0.023 deaths per 100,000.[203] The inpatient mortality from pemphigus has been estimated at 1.6% to 3.2%, with increased mortality likely due to numerous comorbid health conditions.[79] The risk of death in pemphigus vulgaris patients is 2.36 to 3.3 times greater than for controls in the United Kingdom and Taiwan.[9,11] Infection is often the cause of death, and by causing the immunosuppression necessary in the treatment of active disease, therapy is frequently a contributing factor.[11,204] With glucocorticoid and oral immunosuppressive therapy, the mortality (from disease or therapy) of PV patients followed from 4 to 10 years is approximately 10% or less, whereas that of PF is probably even less. In a study of 40 patients with PV, 2 patients (5%) died of sepsis and 17%, after an average of 18 months of therapy, went into a complete and long-lasting (>4 years, average, thought to be permanent) remission requiring no further therapy.[205] Another 37% of patients achieved remission but relapsed at times after therapy was stopped; most of these also eventually achieved long-lasting remissions. The remainder of patients required continual therapy. In a group of 159 patients with PV from Croatia, only approximately 12% went into long-term remission after therapy with glucocorticoids and immunosuppressives, but most relapsed.[23] In a study from Tehran of 1206 pemphigus patients seen over 20 years, 6.2% of PV and 0.2% of PF patients died, mostly of septicemia; only 9.3% were in complete remission without therapy.[7] Another study showed that; with the use of corticosteroids, about 50% of patients went into at least transient complete remission off therapy after a mean of 3 years.[206] Immunosuppressive adjuvant therapy may reduce the risk of relapse.[207] With the advent of rituximab therapy, complete remission in pemphigus has become more common and is quicker to achieve. Approximately 50-90% of PV patients go into remission off all other immunosuppressive therapy, after 1 or more courses of rituximab.[208] Similar remission rates are found in PF.[209]

MANAGEMENT

Several consensus guidelines for pemphigus disease therapy have been published.[211-214] It is generally agreed that PV, even if initially limited in extent, should be treated at its onset, because it will ultimately generalize and the prognosis without therapy is very poor. In addition, it is probably easier to control early disease than widespread disease, and mortality may be higher if therapy is delayed.[215] Because PF may be localized for many years, and the prognosis without systemic therapy may be good, patients with this type of pemphigus do not necessarily require treatment with systemic therapy; the use of topical corticosteroids may suffice. When the disease is active and widespread, however, the therapy for PF is, in general, similar to that for PV.

A consensus statement on disease definitions and endpoints was proposed by an international committee of pemphigus experts.[216] Additionally, clinical instruments have been developed for tracking disease activity that have been shown to be reliable and valid.[217,218] The standardization of disease definitions and activity scoring will facilitate future clinical trials for pemphigus.

There has been a tremendous advance in the armamentarium of therapies for pemphigus since the time before the development of glucocorticoids when PV was a fatal disease. Thanks to these advances, the "row of tombstones" seen in the pathology of PV no longer alludes to its prognosis for most patients.

CORTICOSTEROIDS

The systemic administration of glucocorticoids, usually prednisone, remains the mainstay of therapy for pemphigus. Before adjuvant immunosuppressive therapy was available, very high initial doses of prednisone (>2.0 mg/kg/d) were used for treatment, although such regimens have retrospectively been associated with significant morbidity and mortality from therapy.[204,219,220] The full systemic dose of glucocorticoids has been defined in the consensus guidelines as 1.5 mg/kg/d of prednisone equivalent for 2 to 3 weeks.[216] However, many patients can be brought under control with a 0.5- to 1.0-mg/kg/d single daily dose, especially if used in combination with adjunctive immunosuppressive therapy, which is thought to result in fewer complications and decreased mortality as compared to higher-dose glucocorticoid regimens.[221,222] For patients who do not initially respond or worsen, splitting the dose using a twice- or 3-times-daily schedule may achieve disease control.

Once disease activity is controlled, tapering prednisone to as low a dose as possible should be the goal. Minimal therapy is defined as 5 to 10 mg daily of prednisone equivalent. Although there are no set guidelines, if disease activity can be fully controlled on minimal-dose prednisone or lower, then glucocorticoid monotherapy may be feasible depending on the patient's other comorbidities and contraindications to alternative immunosuppressive agents. If patients have continued relapses, with daily prednisone doses approaching or exceeding 5 to 10 mg, adjunctive immunosuppressive agents are warranted.

Interestingly, prednisone can control blistering within days, at a time when the autoantibody titer would be unchanged. A possible explanation is that prednisone increases the synthesis of desmogleins or other cell-adhesion molecules or change their posttranscriptional processing to prolong their half-life.[223,224] If pemphigus IgG depletes desmosomes of desmogleins, as discussed above, then prednisone could counteract this effect.

Topical corticosteroids may be used as monotherapy in mild forms of disease, especially PF, or as adjunctive therapy to help heal new lesions. Patients with mucosal disease may benefit from the use of glucocorticoid elixirs as a swish and spit for dental trays to help apply class I corticosteroid gels or ointments to the gingiva. Additionally, class I-IV corticosteroids can be used as topical therapy to help resolve new blisters, even in patients on systemic glucocorticoids.

RITUXIMAB

A very effective therapy for pemphigus, even in cases refractory to standard immunosuppressive therapy, is a monoclonal anti-CD20 antibody, rituximab, which was approved by the FDA for therapy of pemphigus vulgaris in 2018. Rituximab targets B cells, the precursors of antibody-producing plasmablasts. The B cell also acts to process autoantigen and present it to T cells that provide "help" in stimulating the autoantibody response.[225] Rituximab is infused intravenously at a dose of 1000 mg on day 1 and day 15. A maintenance dose of 500 mg can be infused at 12 months and every 6 months thereafter based on clinical evaluation, or a 1000 mg dose if clinical relapse occurs. A pivotal clinical trial comparing first line rituximab therapy plus short-term prednisone (0.5-1.0 mg/kg/day) to high dose (1.5 mg/kg/day) prednisone alone for moderate to severe pemphigus showed superior rates of complete remission off prednisone in the rituximab-treated group (89% versus 34%), although maintenance dosing appears to be required to prevent disease relapse. Although not the FDA-approved dose, a lymphoma dose regimen of 375 mg/m^2 once weekly for four weeks has also been evaluated in a prospective clinical trial.[226] A single cycle of rituximab using the lymphoma dose has been shown to be effective even in relapsed and refractory pemphigus, with 86% of patients experiencing complete healing of skin lesions on or off prednisone.[226] Approximately 80% of patients relapse and require additional therapy to regain disease control,[209] but with repeat cycles of rituximab and/or additional prednisone therapy after clinical relapse, 48% of PV and PF patients, including those with previously refractory disease, are ultimately able to achieve complete remission off prednisone. Disease activity usually begins to remit within 3 months of rituximab infusion; with first-line rituximab therapy, the median time to complete remission off steroids is 9 months. Rituximab has also been shown to be an effective therapy for children with refractory pemphigus.[227-229]

Therapy with rituximab, as with other immunosuppressive treatments, has significant risks.[230] 37% of PV patients treated with rituximab plus prednisone experienced treatment-related infections, similar to the rate (42%) observed in patients treated with high-dose prednisone alone. Grade 3 or higher infectious adverse events requiring hospitalization were observed in 8% of rituximab and prednisone-treated patients, compared to 3% treated with prednisone alone. Fatal infections with rituximab and prednisone therapy have been observed with chronic rituximab therapy, including sepsis, Pneumocystis pneumonia, reactivation of hepatitis B, and JC virus infection reactivation causing progressive multifocal leukoencephalopathy.[209,231-233] In addition, 56% of PV patients treated with rituximab develop anti-drug antibodies. Although the clinical significance of this immunogenicity is currently unclear, one PV patient was reported to develop neutralizing anti-chimeric antibodies to rituximab, associated with infusion reactions and lack of clinical efficacy.[234]

ORAL IMMUNOSUPPRESSIVE AGENTS

As rituximab is not accessible to all pemphigus patients, many experts still use oral immunosuppressive therapy, usually with, but also without, prednisone, from the beginning of therapy. Certainly, when continued doses of glucocorticoids greater than 5 to 10 mg are required for disease control, or if there are contraindications to or intolerable side effects from oral glucocorticoids, adjunctive immunosuppressive agents are used for pemphigus therapy. Prospective randomized studies have shown that immunosuppressive agents such as mycophenolate mofetil and azathioprine have a steroid-sparing effect; retrospective studies suggest decreased mortality with use of adjuvants plus steroids compared to steroids alone.[199,235-238]

Because patients may die from complications of therapy, it is important to monitor all patients closely for potential side effects, such as blood count, liver and kidney laboratory abnormalities, GI ulcer disease, high blood pressure, diabetes, glaucoma, cataracts, osteoporosis, and infection. The decision to use immunosuppressive agents, particularly in young patients, must also take into account the potential incidence of malignancies that might be associated with the long-term use of these drugs, as well as the risks of teratogenicity (for mycophenolate mofetil, azathioprine, and methotrexate). Use of mycophenolate in women of child-bearing potential requires counseling and monitoring regarding pregnancy.

AZATHIOPRINE

Azathioprine is an effective adjunctive immunosuppressive agent for pemphigus, with clinical remission rates of approximately 50% in retrospective studies.[189,229] In a prospective randomized trial of high-dose methylprednisolone (2.0 mg/kg/d) plus azathioprine (2.0 mg/kg/d), 72% of patients achieved clinical remission within a mean of 74 days, although 33% experienced significant adverse effects of therapy, including hyperglycemia, dizziness, abnormal liver enzyme tests, and infection.[235]

Azathioprine is a prodrug, which is converted to active mercaptopurine, thioguanine, and thioinosine metabolites, in part by thiopurine methyltransferase (TPMT), an enzyme whose levels can vary widely in the population. Overall, 89% of whites demonstrate normal to high levels of TPMT, 11% are intermediate, and 0.3% are deficient for TPMT, the latter group representing those who do not tolerate azathioprine therapy.[240] Additionally, 1% to 2% of whites may have "super high" levels of TPMT, which is correlated with both treatment resistance and increased hepatotoxicity from excessive metabolite production.[241] Azathioprine toxicity has also been associated with genetic polymorphisms in nucleotide triphosphate diphosphatase (NUDT15), particularly in Asian populations, and inosine triphosphate pyrophosphatase (ITPA).[242] Altogether, it is estimated that approximately 5% of patients will be azathioprine intolerant.[243]

In patients with normal TPMT levels, the consensus dosing regimen that defines treatment failure is 2.5 mg/kg/d for 12 weeks.[216] From a practical standpoint, however, not all laboratories offer TPMT testing. Additionally, because patients with normal levels of TPMT may also experience azathioprine toxicity, it is reasonable to start all patients at a lower dose (eg, 50 to 100 mg daily) and titrate upward until clinical remission, the target dose of 2.5 mg/kg/d, or unacceptable side effects result. Frequent blood and liver monitoring should continue, particularly over the first 8 to 12 weeks when delayed toxicity from the accumulation of metabolites may emerge.

MYCOPHENOLATE MOFETIL

Mycophenolate mofetil is also an effective steroid-sparing agent for pemphigus. Typical doses range from 30 to 40 mg/kg/d (maximum dose 3 g/d) dosed twice daily (2.0 to 3.0 g/d), although certain patients such as the elderly may achieve disease control with doses as low as 1.0 g/d.

In case series, mycophenolate mofetil has been shown to have a rapid effect in lowering pemphigus antibody titers and decreasing disease activity, even in patients whose disease is unresponsive to azathioprine.[244,245] A prospective randomized trial comparing methylprednisolone (2 mg/kg/d) with azathioprine (2 mg/kg/d) or mycophenolate mofetil (2.0 g/d) in pemphigus patients showed 72% in the azathioprine group and 95% in the mycophenolate mofetil group went in clinical remission in a mean of 74 and 91 days, respectively.[235] Nineteen percent of patients experienced significant side effects of mycophenolate mofetil therapy, compared to 33% in the azathioprine group. None of these differences were statistically significant. Another trial showed that mycophenolate mofetil adjuvant therapy decreased the time to initial response and increased the duration of response to therapy and tended to decrease prednisone dosage, although the latter was not statistically significant.[238] A prospective randomized study indicated that azathioprine was significantly more effective than mycophenolate mofetil as a steroid-sparing agent, although this study compared a full dose of azathioprine (2.5 mg/kg/d) to a partial dose of mycophenolate mofetil (2.0 g/d).[224] Mycophenolate mofetil also has been reported to be an effective therapy for pediatric PV.[246]

Caution with use of mycophenolate mofetil is warranted, as fatal infection and sepsis occurred in 2% to 5% of transplant patients receiving mycophenolate mofetil, and increased risk of infection with or reactivation of cytomegalovirus, herpes zoster, atypical mycobacteria, tuberculosis, and JC virus (in progressive multifocal leukoencephalopathy) have been noted in postmarketing surveillance.[247] Interestingly, mycophenolate mofetil may offer protection against *Pneumocystis carinii* infection.[248]

METHOTREXATE

Once-a-week use of methotrexate is another option for an immunosuppressive therapy in pemphigus, although it is not used as frequently as azathioprine or mycophenolate mofetil.[249]

INTRAVENOUS IMMUNOGLOBULIN

Another method of decreasing serum autoantibodies is the intravenous use of γ-globulin (IVIg) in high doses. IVIg is thought to function by saturating neonatal Fc receptor, thereby increasing catabolism of the patient's serum antibodies, which include the pathogenic autoantibodies.[250-252] It may be useful as adjuvant therapy in those pemphigus patients whose condition does not respond to more conventional therapy.[253,254] A multicenter, randomized, placebo-controlled, double blind study has confirmed its efficacy in pemphigus,[255] but it is expensive and probably requires continued infusions for maintenance of remission. There also can be significant side effects with this therapy, including stroke, deep venous thrombosis, and aseptic meningitis.[256] Some centers will use IVIg to establish initial control of blistering in severely affected patients because it does not increase the risk of infection as do corticosteroids and immunosuppressants. IVIg also has been used in combination with rituximab,[257,258] although it is unclear whether the combination is safer or more effective compared to either alone.

OTHER THERAPIES

There are additional therapies that can be used as adjuncts to standard treatments, or have historically been used for severe or refractory cases of pemphigus.

Cyclophosphamide, although more toxic than azathioprine, mycophenolate mofetil, or rituximab, is thought to be very effective in controlling severe disease, with one report of 19 of 23 patients with pemphigus achieving complete remission in a median time of 8.5 months.[259] A variety of small case series have evaluated different cyclophosphamide regimens for pemphigus, including daily oral therapy (1.1-2.5 mg/kg/d), daily oral therapy (50 mg) with intermittent high-dose intravenous dexamethasone and cyclophosphamide, and immunoablative intravenous cyclophosphamide.[239,260-263] All methods were effective in the short term, although none were curative. Significant side effects, including hematuria, infection, and transitional cell carcinoma of the bladder, were observed with higher dose regimens, although one study using a lower daily dose of cyclophosphamide (1.0-1.5 mg/kg/d) did not report a significantly different safety profile compared with other immunosuppressive agents. Together with the risk of infertility, cyclophosphamide is not considered a first-line steroid-sparing agent in the treatment of PV.

In a case series and randomized double-blind trial, dapsone demonstrated a trend toward efficacy as a steroid-sparing drug in maintenance phase PV, although these results were not statistically significant.[264,265] Dapsone may be used in conjunction with other immunosuppressive agents, particularly rituximab, where it offers the additional benefit of *Pneumocystis* pneumonia prophylaxis.

Plasmapheresis is sometimes used for severe pemphigus, or for pemphigus that is unresponsive to a combination of prednisone and immunosuppressive agents. Although one controlled study found it to be ineffective,[266] other studies have found that it both reduces serum levels of pemphigus autoantibodies and controls disease activity.[267] Plasmapheresis plus intravenous pulse therapy with cyclophosphamide has been reported to result in remissions of PV.[268] For maximum effectiveness, it is necessary to have patients take immunosuppressive agents to prevent the antibody-rebound phenomenon that can follow the removal of IgG. Protein A immunoadsorption, which removes IgG selectively from plasma, also has been used.[269]

Intravenous, pulse administration of methylprednisolone 250 to 1000 mg given over approximately 3 hours daily for 4 to 5 consecutive days, can result in long-term remissions and decrease the total dose of glucocorticoids necessary to control disease.[270] Although the purpose of this therapy is to decrease the incidence of complications of long-term steroid use, it can result in all the usual glucocorticoid complications, as well as cardiac arrhythmias with sudden death, and its use is controversial.[271] Furthermore, a controlled trial found that adjuvant oral dexamethasone pulse therapy in addition to standard therapy with prednisolone and azathioprine for PV is not beneficial.[272] It may be that simply giving divided lower doses of prednisone could accomplish the same result with fewer side effects.

PERSPECTIVES FOR FUTURE THERAPEUTIC STRATEGIES

Given the well-defined nature of disease in pemphigus and unmet need for safe and effective therapies, clinical trials in pemphigus are increasing. As discussed above, inhibitory anti-chimeric antibodies can cause resistance to rituximab. Fc gamma receptor polymorphisms, which can cause decreased antibody-dependent cellular cytotoxic killing of B lymphocytes after rituximab therapy, also have been proposed as a cause of rituximab resistance,[273-276] although these polymorphisms may not always correlate with therapeutic outcome in patients with B-cell cancers.[277,278] Newer, fully humanized or glycoengineered anti-CD20 antibodies may be useful in these situations[279,280], although none are currently in clinical development for pemphigus. PRN1008, an oral covalent inhibitor of the Bruton tyrosine kinase (Btk) required for mature peripheral B cell survival, has entered Phase 2 trials for pemphigus (NCT02704429). The successful clinical development of these B cell–targeted therapies may offer novel strategies for pemphigus treatment in the future.

Agents that block the neonatal Fc receptor (FcRn) have also recently entered clinical trials in pemphigus, including SYNT001 (NCT03075904) and ARGX-113 (NCT03334058). FcRn maintains the serum half-life of IgG and regulates cross-presentation of immune complexes, among other immune functions. Additionally, a phase 1 study (NCT03239470) has been initiated to evaluate the safety and preliminary efficacy of ex vivo expansion and infusion of autologous polyclonal regulatory T cells, which are hypothesized to restore immune tolerance in pemphigus patients. Finally, a novel approach to targeted therapy for pemphigus, called chimeric autoantibody receptor T cell or CAAR-T therapy, has demonstrated preclinical efficacy in experimental PV models.[281] CAAR-T therapy uses the disease autoantigen, Dsg3, as part of a chimeric immunoreceptor to program a patient's own T cells to specifically kill Dsg-specific B cells, and offers the hope of a potentially lasting remission of disease without generalized immune suppression due to the potential for long-term CAART cell engraftment. Efforts are underway to determine the clinical efficacy of CAAR-T technology in pemphigus patients.

REFERENCES

1. Lever WF. *Pemphigus and Pemphigoid*. Springfield, IL: Charles C. Thomas; 1965.
2. Beutner EH, Jordon RE. Demonstration of skin antibodies in sera of pemphigus vulgaris patients by indirect immunofluorescent staining. *Proc Soc Exp Biol Med*. 1964;117:505-510.
3. Krain LS. Pemphigus. Epidemiologic and survival characteristics of 59 patients, 1955-1973. *Arch Dermatol*. 1974;110(6):862-865.
4. Pisanti S, Sharav Y, Kaufman E, et al. Pemphigus vulgaris: incidence in Jews of different ethnic groups, according to age, sex, and initial lesion. *Oral Surg Oral Med Oral Pathol*. 1974;38(3):382-387.
5. Hietanen J, Salo OP. Pemphigus: an epidemiological study of patients treated in Finnish hospitals between 1969 and 1978. *Acta Derm Venereol (Stockh)*. 1982;62(6):491-496.
6. Bastuji-Garin S, Souissi R, Blum L, et al. Comparative epidemiology of pemphigus in Tunisia and France: unusual incidence of pemphigus foliaceus in young Tunisian women. *J Invest Dermatol*. 1995;104(2):302-305.
7. Chams-Davatchi C, Valikhani M, Daneshpazhooh M, et al. Pemphigus: analysis of 1209 cases. *Int J Dermatol*. 2005;44(6):470-476.
8. Goon AT, Tan SH. Comparative study of pemphigus vulgaris and pemphigus foliaceus in Singapore. *Australas J Dermatol*. 2001;42(3):172-175.
9. Langan SM, Smeeth L, Hubbard R, et al. Bullous pemphigoid and pemphigus vulgaris—incidence and mortality in the UK: population based cohort study. *BMJ*. 2008;337:a180.
10. Marazza G, Pham HC, Scharer L, et al. Incidence of bullous pemphigoid and pemphigus in Switzerland: a 2-year prospective study. *Br J Dermatol*. 2009;161(4):861-868.
11. Huang YH, Kuo CF, Chen YH, et al. Incidence, mortality, and causes of death of patients with pemphigus in Taiwan: a nationwide population-based study. *J Invest Dermatol*. 2012;132(1):92-97.
12. Diaz LA, Sampaio SAP, Rivitti EA, et al. Endemic pemphigus foliaceus (fogo selvagem): II. Current and

historical epidemiological aspects. *J Invest Dermatol.* 1989;92(1):4-12.
13. Aoki V, Millikan RC, Rivitti EA, et al. Environmental risk factors in endemic pemphigus foliaceus (fogo selvagem). *J Investig Dermatol Symp Proc.* 2004;9(1):34-40.
14. Warren SJ, Lin MS, Giudice GJ, et al. The prevalence of antibodies against desmoglein 1 in endemic pemphigus foliaceus in Brazil. Cooperative Group on Fogo Selvagem Research. *N Engl J Med.* 2000;343(1):23-30.
15. Diaz LA, Arteaga LA, Hilario-Vargas J, et al. Anti-desmoglein-1 antibodies in onchocerciasis, leishmaniasis and Chagas disease suggest a possible etiological link to fogo selvagem. *J Invest Dermatol.* 2004;123(6):1045-1051.
16. Qian Y, Jeong JS, Maldonado M, et al. Cutting edge: Brazilian pemphigus foliaceus anti-desmoglein 1 autoantibodies cross-react with sand fly salivary LJM11 antigen. *J Immunol.* 2012;189(4):1535-1539.
17. Qian Y, Jeong JS, Abdeladhim M, et al. IgE anti-LJM11 sand fly salivary antigen may herald the onset of fogo selvagem in endemic Brazilian regions. *J Invest Dermatol.* 2015;135(3):913-915.
18. Qian Y, Jeong JS, Ye J, et al. Overlapping IgG4 responses to self- and environmental antigens in endemic pemphigus foliaceus. *J Immunol.* 2016;196(5):2041-2050.
19. Uzun S, Durdu M, Akman A, et al. Pemphigus in the Mediterranean region of Turkey: a study of 148 cases. *Int J Dermatol.* 2006;45(5):523-528.
20. V'lckova-Laskoska MT, Laskoski DS, Kamberova S, et al. Epidemiology of pemphigus in Macedonia: a 15-year retrospective study (1990-2004). *Int J Dermatol.* 2007;46(3):253-258.
21. Salmanpour R, Shahkar H, Namazi MR, et al. Epidemiology of pemphigus in south-western Iran: a 10-year retrospective study (1991-2000). *Int J Dermatol.* 2006;45(2):103-105.
22. Michailidou EZ, Belazi MA, Markopoulos AK, et al. Epidemiologic survey of pemphigus vulgaris with oral manifestations in northern Greece: retrospective study of 129 patients. *Int J Dermatol.* 2007;46(4):356-361.
23. Ljubojevic S, Lipozencic J, Brenner S, et al. Pemphigus vulgaris: a review of treatment over a 19-year period. *J Eur Acad Dermatol Venereol.* 2002;16(6):599-603.
24. Mimouni D, Bar H, Gdalevich M, et al. Pemphigus—analysis of epidemiological factors in 155 patients. *J Eur Acad Dermatol Venereol.* 2008;22(10):1232-1235.
25. Abreu-Velez AM, Hashimoto T, Bollag WB, et al. A unique form of endemic pemphigus in northern Colombia. *J Am Acad Dermatol.* 2003;49(4):599-608.
26. Tallab T, Joharji H, Bahamdan K, et al. The incidence of pemphigus in the southern region of Saudi Arabia. *Int J Dermatol.* 2001;40(9):570-572.
27. Simon DG, Krutchkoff D, Kaslow RA, et al. Pemphigus in Hartford County, Connecticut, from 1972 to 1977. *Arch Dermatol.* 1980;116(9):1035-1037.
28. Tsankov N, Vassileva S, Kamarashev J, et al. Epidemiology of pemphigus in Sofia, Bulgaria. A 16-year retrospective study (1980-1995). *Int J Dermatol.* 2000;39(2):104-108.
29. Micali G, Musumeci ML, Nasca MR. Epidemiologic analysis and clinical course of 84 consecutive cases of pemphigus in eastern Sicily. *Int J Dermatol.* 1998;37(3):197-200.
30. Metry DW, Hebert AA, Jordon RE. Nonendemic pemphigus foliaceus in children. *J Am Acad Dermatol.* 2002;46(3):419-422.
31. Muramatsu T, Iida T, Ko T, et al. Pemphigus vulgaris exacerbated by exposure to sunlight. *J Dermatol.* 1996;23(8):559-563.
32. Reis VM, Toledo RP, Lopez A, et al. UVB-induced acantholysis in endemic pemphigus foliaceus (fogo selvagem) and pemphigus vulgaris. *J Am Acad Dermatol.* 2000;42(4):571-576.
33. Grando SA, Grando AA, Glukhenky BT, et al. History and clinical significance of mechanical symptoms in blistering dermatoses: a reappraisal. *J Am Acad Dermatol.* 2003;48(1):86-92.
34. Ahmed AR, Blose DA. Pemphigus vegetans. Neumann type and Hallopeau type. *Int J Dermatol.* 1984;23(2):135-141.
35. Veraitch O, Ohyama M, Yamagami J, et al. Alopecia as a rare but distinct manifestation of pemphigus vulgaris. *J Eur Acad Dermatol Venereol.* 2013;27(1):86-91.
36. Hale EK, Bystryn JC. Laryngeal and nasal involvement in pemphigus vulgaris. *J Am Acad Dermatol.* 2001;44(4):609-611.
37. Espana A, Fernandez S, del OJ, et al. Ear, nose and throat manifestations in pemphigus vulgaris. *Br J Dermatol.* 2007;156(4):733-737.
38. Kavala M, Altintas S, Kocaturk E, et al. Ear, nose and throat involvement in patients with pemphigus vulgaris: correlation with severity, phenotype and disease activity. *J Eur Acad Dermatol Venereol.* 2011;25(11):1324-1327.
39. Yoshida K, Takae Y, Saito H, et al. Cutaneous type pemphigus vulgaris: a rare clinical phenotype of pemphigus. *J Am Acad Dermatol.* 2005;52(5):839-845.
40. Trattner A, Lurie R, Leiser A, et al. Esophageal involvement in pemphigus vulgaris: a clinical, histologic, and immunopathologic study. *J Am Acad Dermatol.* 1991;24(2, pt 1):223-226.
41. Rao PN, Samarth A, Aurangabadkar SJ, et al. Study of upper gastrointestinal tract involvement in pemphigus by esophago-gastro-duodenoscopy. *Indian J Dermatol Venereol Leprol.* 2006;72(6):421-424.
42. Hokama A, Yamamoto Y, Taira K, et al. Esophagitis dissecans superficialis and autoimmune bullous dermatoses: a review. *World J Gastrointest Endosc.* 2010;2(7):252-256.
43. Malik M, Ahmed AR. Involvement of the female genital tract in pemphigus vulgaris. *Obstet Gynecol.* 2005;106(5, pt 1):1005-1012.
44. Hodak E, Kremer I, David M, et al. Conjunctival involvement in pemphigus vulgaris: a clinical, histopathological and immunofluorescence study. *Br J Dermatol.* 1990;123(5):615-620.
45. Daoud YJ, Cervantes R, Foster CS, et al. Ocular pemphigus. *J Am Acad Dermatol.* 2005;53(4):585-590.
46. Kavala M, Topaloglu Demir F, Zindanci I, et al. Genital involvement in pemphigus vulgaris (PV): correlation with clinical and cervicovaginal Pap smear findings. *J Am Acad Dermatol.* 2015;73(4):655-659.
47. Akhyani M, Chams-Davatchi C, Naraghi Z, et al. Cervicovaginal involvement in pemphigus vulgaris: a clinical study of 77 cases. *Br J Dermatol.* 2008;158(3):478-482.
48. Onuma K, Kanbour-Shakir A, Modery J, et al. Pemphigus vulgaris of the vagina—its cytomorphologic features on liquid-based cytology and pitfalls: case report and cytological differential diagnosis. *Diagn Cytopathol.* 2009;37(11):832-835.

49. Akhyani M, Keshtkar-Jafari A, Chams-Davatchi C, et al. Ocular involvement in pemphigus vulgaris. *J Dermatol.* 2014;41(7):618-621.
50. Suami M, Kato M, Koide K, et al. Keratolysis in a patient with pemphigus vulgaris. *Br J Ophthalmol.* 2001;85(10):1263-1264.
51. Igawa K, Matsunaga T, Nishioka K. Involvement of UV-irradiation in pemphigus foliaceus. *J Eur Acad Dermatol Venereol.* 2004;18(2):216-217.
52. Kano Y, Shimosegawa M, Mizukawa Y, et al. Pemphigus foliaceus induced by exposure to sunlight. Report of a case and analysis of photochallenge-induced lesions. *Dermatology.* 2000;201(2):132-138.
53. Senear FE, Usher B. An unusual type of pemphigus combining features of lupus erythematosus. *Arch Dermatol Syphilol.* 1926;13:761-781.
54. Senear FE, Kingery LB. Pemphigus erythematosus. *Arch Dermatol Syphilol.* 1949;60(2):238-252.
55. Jablonska S, Chorzelski T, Blaszczyk M, et al. Pathogenesis of pemphigus erythematosus. *Arch Dermatol Res.* 1977;258(2):135-140.
56. Oktarina DA, Poot AM, Kramer D, et al. The IgG "lupus-band" deposition pattern of pemphigus erythematosus: association with the desmoglein 1 ectodomain as revealed by 3 cases. *Arch Dermatol.* 2012;148(10):1173-1178.
57. Amerian ML, Ahmed AR. Pemphigus erythematosus. Senear-Usher syndrome. *Int J Dermatol.* 1985;24(1):16-25.
58. Chowdhury MMU, Natarajan S. Neonatal pemphigus vulgaris associated with mild oral pemphigus vulgaris in the mother during pregnancy. *Br J Dermatol.* 1998;139(3):500-503.
59. Fainaru O, Mashiach R, Kupferminc M, et al. Pemphigus vulgaris in pregnancy: a case report and review of literature. *Hum Reprod.* 2000;15(5):1195-1197.
60. Eyre RW, Stanley JR. Maternal pemphigus foliaceus with cell surface antibody bound in neonatal epidermis. *Arch Dermatol.* 1988;124(1):25-27.
61. Avalos-Diaz E, Olague-Marchan M, Lopez-Swiderski A, et al. Transplacental passage of maternal pemphigus foliaceus autoantibodies induces neonatal pemphigus. *J Am Acad Dermatol.* 2000;43(6):1130-1134.
62. Hirsch R, Anderson J, Weinberg JM, et al. Neonatal pemphigus foliaceus. *J Am Acad Dermatol.* 2003;49(2)(Suppl Case Reports):S187-S189.
63. Kanwar AJ, Dhar S, Kaur S. Further experience with pemphigus in children. *Pediatr Dermatol.* 1996;11(2):107-111.
64. Mutasim DF, Pelc NJ, Anhalt GJ. Drug-induced pemphigus. *Dermatol Clin.* 1993;11(3):463-471.
65. Korman NJ, Eyre RW, Zone J, et al. Drug-induced pemphigus: autoantibodies directed against the pemphigus antigen complexes are present in penicillamine and captopril-induced pemphigus. *J Invest Dermatol.* 1991;96(2):273-276.
66. Yokel BK, Hood AF, Anhalt GJ. Induction of acantholysis in organ explant culture by penicillamine and captopril. *Arch Dermatol.* 1989;125(10):1367-1370.
67. Drosos AA, Christou L, Galanopoulou V, et al. D-Penicillamine induced myasthenia gravis: clinical, serological and genetic findings. *Clin Exp Rheumatol.* 1993;11(4):387-391.
68. Sternlieb I, Bennett B, Scheinberg IH. D-Penicillamine induced Goodpasture's syndrome in Wilson's disease. *Ann Intern Med.* 1975;82(5):673-676.
69. Lee Y, Lee ST, Cho H. D-Penicillamine-induced ANA (+) ANCA (+) vasculitis in pediatric patients with Wilson's disease. *Clin Nephrol.* 2016;85(5):296-300.
70. Ruocco V, Brenner S, Lombardi ML. A case of diet-related pemphigus. *Dermatology.* 1996;192(4):373-374.
71. Tur E, Brenner S. Diet and pemphigus. In pursuit of exogenous factors in pemphigus and fogo selvagem. *Arch Dermatol.* 1998;134(11):1406-1410.
72. Mehta JN, Martin AG. A case of pemphigus vulgaris improved by cigarette smoking. *Arch Dermatol.* 2000;136(1):15-17.
73. Nguyen VT, Arredondo J, Chernyavsky AI, et al. Pemphigus vulgaris acantholysis ameliorated by cholinergic agonists. *Arch Dermatol.* 2004;140(3):327-334.
74. Iraji F, Yoosefi A. Healing effect of pilocarpine gel 4% on skin lesions of pemphigus vulgaris. *Int J Dermatol.* 2006;45(6):743-746.
75. Chernyavsky AI, Arredondo J, Piser T, et al. Differential coupling of M1 muscarinic and alpha 7 nicotinic receptors to inhibition of pemphigus acantholysis. *J Biol Chem.* 2008;283(6):3401-3408.
76. Pullan RD, Rhodes J, Ganesh S, et al. Transdermal nicotine for active ulcerative colitis. *N Engl J Med.* 1994;330(12):811-815.
77. Patten SF, Dijkstra JW. Associations of pemphigus and autoimmune disease with malignancy or thymoma. *Int J Dermatol.* 1994;33(12):836-842.
78. Maize JC, Dobson RL, Provost TT. Pemphigus and myasthenia gravis. *Arch Dermatol.* 1975;111(10):1334-1339.
79. Hsu DY, Brieva J, Sinha AA, et al. Comorbidities and inpatient mortality for pemphigus in the U.S.A. *Br J Dermatol.* 2016;174(6):1290-1298.
80. Yoshida M, Miyoshi T, Sakiyama S, et al. Pemphigus with thymoma improved by thymectomy: report of a case. *Surg Today.* 2013;43(7):806-808.
81. Parameswaran A, Attwood K, Sato R, et al. Identification of a new disease cluster of pemphigus vulgaris with autoimmune thyroid disease, rheumatoid arthritis and type I diabetes. *Br J Dermatol.* 2015;172(3):729-738.
82. Koulu L, Kusumi A, Steinberg MS, et al. Human autoantibodies against a desmosomal core protein in pemphigus foliaceus. *J Exp Med.* 1984;160(5):1509-1518.
83. Stanley JR, Koulu L, Klaus Kovtun V, et al. A monoclonal antibody to the desmosomal glycoprotein desmoglein I binds the same polypeptide as human autoantibodies in pemphigus foliaceus. *J Immunol.* 1986;136(4):1227-1230.
84. Amagai M, Klaus-Kovtun V, Stanley JR. Autoantibodies against a novel epithelial cadherin in pemphigus vulgaris, a disease of cell adhesion. *Cell.* 1991;67(5):869-877.
85. Hammers CM, Stanley JR. Mechanisms of disease: pemphigus and bullous pemphigoid. *Annu Rev Pathol.* 2016;11:175-197.
86. Payne AS, Hanakawa Y, Amagai M, et al. Desmosomes and disease: pemphigus and bullous impetigo. *Curr Opin Cell Biol.* 2004;16(5):536-543.
87. Stanley JR, Amagai M. Pemphigus, bullous impetigo, and the staphylococcal scalded-skin syndrome. *N Engl J Med.* 2006;355(17):1800-1810.
88. Amagai M, Karpati S, Klaus-Kovtun V, et al. The extracellular domain of pemphigus vulgaris antigen (desmoglein 3) mediates weak homophilic adhesion. *J Invest Dermatol.* 1994;102(4):402-408.

89. Chitaev NA, Troyanovsky SM. Direct Ca^{2+}-dependent heterophilic interaction between desmosomal cadherins, desmoglein and desmocollin, contributes to cell-cell adhesion. *J Cell Biol.* 1997;138(1):193-201.
90. Harrison OJ, Brasch J, Lasso G, et al. Structural basis of adhesive binding by desmocollins and desmogleins. *Proc Natl Acad Sci U S A.* 2016;113(26):7160-7165.
91. Stanley JR, Klaus Kovtun V, Sampaio SA. Antigenic specificity of fogo selvagem autoantibodies is similar to North American pemphigus foliaceus and distinct from pemphigus vulgaris autoantibodies. *J Invest Dermatol.* 1986;87(2):197-201.
92. Ishii K, Amagai M, Hall RP, et al. Characterization of autoantibodies in pemphigus using antigen-specific enzyme-linked immunosorbent assays with baculovirus-expressed recombinant desmogleins. *J Immunol.* 1997;159(4):2010-2017.
93. Eyre RW, Stanley JR. Identification of pemphigus vulgaris antigen extracted from normal human epidermis and comparison with pemphigus foliaceus antigen. *J Clin Invest.* 1988;81(3):807-812.
94. Ding X, Aoki V, Mascaro JM Jr, et al. Mucosal and mucocutaneous (generalized) pemphigus vulgaris show distinct autoantibody profiles. *J Invest Dermatol.* 1997;109(4):592-596.
95. Amagai M, Tsunoda K, Zillikens D, et al. The clinical phenotype of pemphigus is defined by the anti-desmoglein autoantibody profile. *J Am Acad Dermatol.* 1999;40(167):170.
96. Miyagawa S, Amagai M, Iida T, et al. Late development of antidesmoglein 1 antibodies in pemphigus vulgaris: correlation with disease progression. *Br J Dermatol.* 1999;141(6):1084-1087.
97. Naseer SY, Seiffert-Sinha K, Sinha AA. Detailed profiling of anti-desmoglein autoantibodies identifies anti-Dsg1 reactivity as a key driver of disease activity and clinical expression in pemphigus vulgaris. *Autoimmunity.* 2015;48(4):231-241.
98. Flores G, Culton DA, Prisayanh P, et al. IgG autoantibody response against keratinocyte cadherins in endemic pemphigus foliaceus (fogo selvagem). *J Invest Dermatol.* 2012;132(11):2573-2580.
99. Mao X, Nagler AR, Farber SA, et al. Autoimmunity to desmocollin 3 in pemphigus vulgaris. *Am J Pathol.* 2010;177(6):2724-2730.
100. Ishii N, Teye K, Fukuda S, et al. Anti-desmocollin autoantibodies in nonclassical pemphigus. *Br J Dermatol.* 2015;173(1):59-68.
101. Chen J, Den Z, Koch PJ. Loss of desmocollin 3 in mice leads to epidermal blistering. *J Cell Sci.* 2008;121 (pt 17):2844-2849.
102. Rafei D, Muller R, Ishii N, et al. IgG autoantibodies against desmocollin 3 in pemphigus sera induce loss of keratinocyte adhesion. *Am J Pathol.* 2011;178(2):718-723.
103. Nguyen VT, Ndoye A, Grando SA. Pemphigus vulgaris antibody identifies pemphaxin. *J Biol Chem.* 2000;275(38):29466-29476.
104. Evangelista F, Dasher DA, Diaz LA, et al. E-cadherin is an additional immunological target for pemphigus autoantibodies. *J Invest Dermatol.* 2008;128(7):1710-1718.
105. Oliveira ME, Culton DA, Prisayanh P, et al. E-cadherin autoantibody profile in patients with pemphigus vulgaris. *Br J Dermatol.* 2013;169(4):812-818.
106. Kalantari-Dehaghi M, Anhalt GJ, Camilleri MJ, et al. Pemphigus vulgaris autoantibody profiling by proteomic technique. *PLoS One.* 2013;8(3):e57587.
107. Wilgram GF, Caulfield JB, Madgic EB. An electron microscopic study of acantholysis and dyskeratosis in pemphigus foliaceus. *J Invest Dermatol.* 1964;43:287-299.
108. Guedes AC, Rotta O, Leite HV, et al. Ultrastructural aspects of mucosas in endemic pemphigus foliaceus. *Arch Dermatol.* 2002;138(7):949-954.
109. Hashimoto K, Lever WF. An electron microscopic study on pemphigus vulgaris of the mouth and the skin with special reference to the intercellular cement. *J Invest Dermatol.* 1967;48(6):540-552.
110. Diercks GF, Pas HH, Jonkman MF. The ultrastructure of acantholysis in pemphigus vulgaris. *Br J Dermatol.* 2009;160(2):460-461.
111. Shimizu A, Ishiko A, Ota T, et al. Ultrastructural changes in mice actively producing antibodies to desmoglein 3 parallel those in patients with pemphigus vulgaris. *Arch Dermatol Res.* 2002;294(7):318-323.
112. Shimizu A, Ishiko A, Ota T, et al. IgG binds to desmoglein 3 in desmosomes and causes a desmosomal split without keratin retraction in a pemphigus mouse model. *J Invest Dermatol.* 2004;122(5):1145-1153.
113. Bystryn JC, Grando SA. A novel explanation for acantholysis in pemphigus vulgaris: the basal cell shrinkage hypothesis. *J Am Acad Dermatol.* 2006;54(3):513-516.
114. Wang W, Amagai M, Ishiko A. Desmosome splitting is a primary ultrastructural change in the acantholysis of pemphigus. *J Dermatol Sci.* 2009;54(1):59-61.
115. Sokol E, Kramer D, Diercks GF, et al. Large-scale electron microscopy maps of patient skin and mucosa provide insight into pathogenesis of blistering diseases. *J Invest Dermatol.* 2015;135(7):1763-1770.
116. Stahley SN, Warren MF, Feldman RJ, et al. Super-resolution microscopy reveals altered desmosomal protein organization in tissue from patients with pemphigus vulgaris. *J Invest Dermatol.* 2016;136(1):59-66.
117. Schiltz JR, Michel B. Production of epidermal acantholysis in normal human skin in vitro by the IgG fraction from pemphigus serum. *J Invest Dermatol.* 1976;67(2):254-260.
118. Anhalt GJ, Labib RS, Voorhees JJ, et al. Induction of pemphigus in neonatal mice by passive transfer of IgG from patients with the disease. *N Engl J Med.* 1982;306(20):1189-1196.
119. Rock B, Labib RS, Diaz LA. Monovalent Fab' immunoglobulin fragments from endemic pemphigus foliaceus autoantibodies reproduce the human disease in neonatal Balb/c mice. *J Clin Invest.* 1990;85(1):296-299.
120. Amagai M, Karpati S, Prussick R, et al. Autoantibodies against the amino-terminal cadherin-like binding domain of pemphigus vulgaris antigen are pathogenic. *J Clin Invest.* 1992;90(3):919-926.
121. Amagai M, Hashimoto T, Shimizu N, et al. Absorption of pathogenic autoantibodies by the extracellular domain of pemphigus vulgaris antigen (Dsg3) produced by baculovirus. *J Clin Invest.* 1994;94(1):59-67.
122. Ding X, Diaz LA, Fairley JA, et al. The anti-desmoglein 1 autoantibodies in pemphigus vulgaris sera are pathogenic. *J Invest Dermatol.* 1999;112(5):739-743.
123. Amagai M, Hashimoto T, Green KJ, et al. Antigen-specific immunoabsorption of pathogenic autoantibodies in pemphigus foliaceus. *J Invest Dermatol.* 1995;104(6):895-901.
124. Langenhan J, Dworschak J, Saschenbrecker S, et al. Specific immunoadsorption of pathogenic autoanti-

bodies in pemphigus requires the entire ectodomains of desmogleins. *Exp Dermatol*. 2014;23(4):253-259.
125. Koch PJ, Mahoney MG, Ishikawa H, et al. Targeted disruption of the pemphigus vulgaris antigen (desmoglein 3) gene in mice causes loss of keratinocyte cell adhesion with a phenotype similar to pemphigus vulgaris. *J Cell Biol*. 1997;137(5):1091-1102.
126. Amagai M, Matsuyoshi N, Wang ZH, et al. Toxin in bullous impetigo and staphylococcal scalded-skin syndrome targets desmoglein 1. *Nat Med*. 2000;6(11):1275-1277.
127. Anhalt GJ, Till GO, Diaz LA, et al. Defining the role of complement in experimental pemphigus vulgaris in mice. *J Immunol*. 1986;137(9):2835-2840.
128. Payne AS, Ishii K, Kacir S, et al. Genetic and functional characterization of human pemphigus vulgaris monoclonal autoantibodies isolated by phage display. *J Clin Invest*. 2005;115(4):888-899.
129. Ishii K, Lin CY, Siegel DL, et al. Isolation of pathogenic monoclonal anti-desmoglein 1 human antibodies by phage display of pemphigus foliaceus autoantibodies. *J Invest Dermatol*. 2008;128(4):939-948.
130. Rock B, Martins CR, Theofilopoulos AN, et al. The pathogenic effect of IgG4 autoantibodies in endemic pemphigus foliaceus (fogo selvagem). *N Engl J Med*. 1989;320(22):1463-1469.
131. Futei Y, Amagai M, Ishii K, et al. Predominant IgG4 subclass in autoantibodies of pemphigus vulgaris and foliaceus. *J Dermatol Sci*. 2001;26(1):55-61.
132. Funakoshi T, Lunardon L, Ellebrecht CT, et al. Enrichment of total serum IgG4 in patients with pemphigus. *Br J Dermatol*. 2012;167(6):1245-1253.
133. Futei Y, Amagai M, Sekiguchi M, et al. Use of domain-swapped molecules for conformational epitope mapping of desmoglein 3 in pemphigus vulgaris. *J Invest Dermatol*. 2000;115(5):829-834.
134. Li N, Aoki V, Hans-Filho G, et al. The role of intramolecular epitope spreading in the pathogenesis of endemic pemphigus foliaceus (fogo selvagem). *J Exp Med*. 2003;197(11):1501-1510.
135. Hacker-Foegen MK, Janson M, Amagai M, et al. Pathogenicity and epitope characteristics of anti-desmoglein-1 from pemphigus foliaceus patients expressing only IgG1 autoantibodies. *J Invest Dermatol*. 2003;121(6):1373-1378.
136. Sekiguchi M, Futei Y, Fujii Y, et al. Dominant autoimmune epitopes recognized by pemphigus antibodies map to the N-terminal adhesive region of desmogleins. *J Immunol*. 2001;167(9):5439-5448.
137. Boggon TJ, Murray J, Chappuis-Flament S, et al. C-cadherin ectodomain structure and implications for cell adhesion mechanisms. *Science*. 2002;296(5571):1308-1313.
138. Al-Amoudi A, Diez DC, Betts MJ, et al. The molecular architecture of cadherins in native epidermal desmosomes. *Nature*. 2007;450(7171):832-837.
139. Heupel WM, Zillikens D, Drenckhahn D, et al. Pemphigus vulgaris IgG directly inhibit desmoglein 3-mediated transinteraction. *J Immunol*. 2008;181(3):1825-1834.
140. Aoyama Y, Kitajima Y. Pemphigus vulgaris-IgG causes a rapid depletion of desmoglein 3 (Dsg3) from the Triton X-100 soluble pools, leading to the formation of Dsg3-depleted desmosomes in a human squamous carcinoma cell line, DJM-1 cells. *J Invest Dermatol*. 1999;112(1):67-71.
141. Sato M, Aoyama Y, Kitajima Y. Assembly pathway of desmoglein 3 to desmosomes and its perturbation by pemphigus vulgaris-IgG in cultured keratinocytes, as revealed by time-lapsed labeling immunoelectron microscopy. *Lab Invest*. 2000;80(10):1583-1592.
142. Calkins CC, Setzer SV, Jennings JM, et al. Desmoglein endocytosis and desmosome disassembly are coordinated responses to pemphigus autoantibodies. *J Biol Chem*. 2006;281(11):7623-7634.
143. Mao X, Choi EJ, Payne AS. Disruption of desmosome assembly by monovalent human pemphigus vulgaris monoclonal antibodies. *J Invest Dermatol*. 2009;129(4):908-918.
144. Rivitti EA, Sanches JA, Miyauchi LM, et al. Pemphigus foliaceus autoantibodies bind both epidermis and squamous mucosal epithelium, but tissue injury is detected only in the epidermis. The Cooperative Group on Fogo Selvagem Research. *J Am Acad Dermatol*. 1994;31(6):954-958.
145. Mahoney MG, Wang Z, Rothenberger K, et al. Explanation for the clinical and microscopic localization of lesions in pemphigus foliaceus and vulgaris. *J Clin Invest*. 1999;103(4):461-468.
146. Wu H, Wang ZH, Yan A, et al. Protection of neonates against pemphigus foliaceus by desmoglein 3. *N Engl J Med*. 2000;343(1):31-35.
147. Hanakawa Y, Matsuyoshi N, Stanley JR. Expression of desmoglein 1 compensates for genetic loss of desmoglein 3 in keratinocyte adhesion. *J Invest Dermatol*. 2002;119(1):27-31.
148. Rocha-Alvarez R, Friedman H, et al. Pregnant women with endemic pemphigus foliaceus (Fogo Selvagem) give birth to disease-free babies. *J Invest Dermatol*. 1992;99(1):78-82.
149. Berkowitz P, Hu P, Warren S, et al. p38MAPK inhibition prevents disease in pemphigus vulgaris mice. *Proc Natl Acad Sci U S A*. 2006;103(34):12855-12860.
150. Waschke J, Spindler V, Bruggeman P, et al. Inhibition of Rho A activity causes pemphigus skin blistering. *J Cell Biol*. 2006;175(5):721-727.
151. Sharma P, Mao X, Payne AS. Beyond steric hindrance: the role of adhesion signaling pathways in the pathogenesis of pemphigus. *J Dermatol Sci*. 2007;48(1):1-14.
152. Bektas M, Jolly PS, Berkowitz P, et al. A pathophysiologic role for epidermal growth factor receptor in pemphigus acantholysis. *J Biol Chem*. 2013;288(13):9447-9456.
153. Mao X, Sano Y, Park JM, et al. p38 MAPK activation is downstream of the loss of intercellular adhesion in pemphigus vulgaris. *J Biol Chem*. 2011;286(2):1283-1291.
154. Vielmuth F, Waschke J, Spindler V. Loss of desmoglein binding is not sufficient for keratinocyte dissociation in pemphigus. *J Invest Dermatol*. 2015;135(12):3068-3077.
155. Mao X, Li H, Sano Y, et al. MAPKAP kinase 2 (MK2)-dependent and -independent models of blister formation in pemphigus vulgaris. *J Invest Dermatol*. 2014;134(1):68-76.
156. Saito M, Stahley SN, Caughman CY, et al. Signaling dependent and independent mechanisms in pemphigus vulgaris blister formation. *PLoS One*. 2012;7(12):e50696.
157. Oktarina DA, van der Wier G, Diercks GF, et al. IgG-induced clustering of desmogleins 1 and 3 in skin of patients with pemphigus fits with the desmoglein nonassembly depletion hypothesis. *Br J Dermatol*. 2011;165(3):552-562.

158. van der Wier G, Pas HH, Kramer D, et al. Smaller desmosomes are seen in the skin of pemphigus patients with anti-desmoglein 1 antibodies but not in patients with anti-desmoglein 3 antibodies. *J Invest Dermatol*. 2014;134(8):2287-2290.
159. Jennings JM, Tucker DK, Kottke MD, et al. Desmosome disassembly in response to pemphigus vulgaris IgG occurs in distinct phases and can be reversed by expression of exogenous Dsg3. *J Invest Dermatol*. 2011;131(3):706-718.
160. Kitajima Y. 150(th) anniversary series: Desmosomes and autoimmune disease, perspective of dynamic desmosome remodeling and its impairments in pemphigus. *Cell Commun Adhes*. 2014;21(6):269-280.
161. Wucherpfennig KW, Strominger JL. Selective binding of self peptides to disease-associated major histocompatibility complex (MHC) molecules: a mechanism for MHC- linked susceptibility to human autoimmune diseases [comment]. *J Exp Med*. 1995;181(5):1597-1601.
162. Pavoni DP, Roxo VM, Marquart FA, et al. Dissecting the associations of endemic pemphigus foliaceus (fogo selvagem) with HLA-DRB1 alleles and genotypes. *Genes Immun*. 2003;4(2):110-116.
163. Lin MS, Swartz SJ, Lopez A, et al. Development and characterization of desmoglein-3 specific T cells from patients with pemphigus vulgaris. *J Clin Invest*. 1997;99(1):31-40.
164. Hertl M, Karr RW, Amagai M, et al. Heterogeneous MHC II restriction pattern of autoreactive desmoglein 3 specific T cell responses in pemphigus vulgaris patients and normals. *J Invest Dermatol*. 1998;110(4):388-392.
165. Hertl M, Amagai M, Sundaram H, et al. Recognition of desmoglein 3 by autoreactive T cells in pemphigus vulgaris patients and normals. *J Invest Dermatol*. 1998;110(1):62-66.
166. Yan L, Wang JM, Zeng K. Association between HLA-DRB1 polymorphisms and pemphigus vulgaris: a meta-analysis. *Br J Dermatol*. 2012;167(4):768-777.
167. Hertl M, Eming R, Veldman C. T cell control in autoimmune bullous skin disorders. *J Clin Invest*. 2006;116(5):1159-1166.
168. Wucherpfennig KW, Yu B, Bhol K, et al. Structural basis for major histocompatibility complex (MHC)-linked susceptibility to autoimmunity: charged residues of a single MHC binding pocket confer selective presentation of self-peptides in pemphigus vulgaris. *Proc Natl Acad Sci U S A*. 1995;92(25):11935-11939.
169. Eming R, Hennerici T, Backlund J, et al. Pathogenic IgG antibodies against desmoglein 3 in pemphigus vulgaris are regulated by HLA-DRB1*04:02-restricted T cells. *J Immunol*. 2014;193(9):4391-4399.
170. Wada N, Nishifuji K, Yamada T, et al. Aire-dependent thymic expression of desmoglein 3, the autoantigen in pemphigus vulgaris, and its role in T-cell tolerance. *J Invest Dermatol*. 2011;131(2):410-417.
171. Veldman CM, Gebhard KL, Uter W, et al. T cell recognition of desmoglein 3 peptides in patients with pemphigus vulgaris and healthy individuals. *J Immunol*. 2004;172(6):3883-3892.
172. Zhu H, Chen Y, Zhou Y, et al. Cognate Th2-B cell interaction is essential for the autoantibody production in pemphigus vulgaris. *J Clin Immunol*. 2012;32(1):114-123.
173. Hennerici T, Pollmann R, Schmidt T, et al. Increased frequency of T follicular helper cells and elevated interleukin-27 plasma levels in patients with pemphigus. *PLoS One*. 2016;11(2):e0148919.
174. Veldman C, Höhne A, Dieckmann D, et al. Type I regulatory T cells specific for desmoglein 3 are more frequently detected in healthy individuals than in patients with pemphigus vulgaris. *J Immunol*. 2004;172(10):6468-6475.
175. Yamagami J, Kacir S, Ishii K, et al. Antibodies to the desmoglein 1 precursor proprotein but not to the mature cell surface protein cloned from individuals without pemphigus. *J Immunol*. 2009;183(9):5615-5621.
176. Cho MJ, Lo AS, Mao X, et al. Shared VH1-46 gene usage by pemphigus vulgaris autoantibodies indicates common humoral immune responses among patients. *Nat Commun*. 2014;5:4167.
177. Yamagami J, Payne AS, Kacir S, et al. Homologous regions of autoantibody heavy chain complementarity-determining region 3 (H-CDR3) in patients with pemphigus cause pathogenicity. *J Clin Invest*. 2010;120(11):4111-4117.
178. Di Zenzo G, Di Lullo G, Corti D, et al. Pemphigus autoantibodies generated through somatic mutations target the desmoglein-3 cis-interface. *J Clin Invest*. 2012;122(10):3781-3790.
179. Qian Y, Diaz LA, Ye J, et al. Dissecting the anti-desmoglein autoreactive B cell repertoire in pemphigus vulgaris patients. *J Immunol*. 2007;178(9):5982-5990.
180. Qian Y, Clarke SH, Aoki V, et al. Antigen selection of anti-DSG1 autoantibodies during and before the onset of endemic pemphigus foliaceus. *J Invest Dermatol*. 2009;129(12):2823-2834.
181. Tian C, Luskin GK, Dischert KM, et al. Immunodominance of the VH1-46 antibody gene segment in the primary repertoire of human rotavirus-specific B cells is reduced in the memory compartment through somatic mutation of nondominant clones. *J Immunol*. 2008;180(5):3279-3288.
182. Hammers CM, Chen J, Lin C, et al. Persistence of anti-desmoglein 3 IgG(+) B-cell clones in pemphigus patients over years. *J Invest Dermatol*. 2015;135(3):742-749.
183. Beutner EH, Lever WF, Witebsky E, et al. Autoantibodies in pemphigus vulgaris. *JAMA*. 1965;192:682-688.
184. Judd KP, Lever WF. Correlation of antibodies in skin and serum with disease severity in pemphigus. *Arch Dermatol*. 1979;115(4):428-432.
185. Chorzelski T, Jablonska S, Blaszczyk M. Immunopathological investigations in the Senear-Usher syndrome (coexistence of pemphigus and lupus erythematosus). *Br J Dermatol*. 1968;80(4):211-217.
186. Harman KE, Gratian MJ, Bhogal BS, et al. The use of two substrates to improve the senstivity of indirect immunofluorscence in the diagnosis of pemphigus. *Br J Dermatol*. 2000;142(6):1135-1139.
187. Krasny SA, Beutner EH, Chorzelski TP. Specificity and sensitivity of indirect and direct immunofluorescent findings in the diagnosis of pemphigus. In: Beutner EH, Chorzelski TP, Kumar V, eds. *Immunopathology of the Skin*. New York, NY: John Wiley; 1987:207-247.
188. O'Loughlin S, Goldman GC, Provost TT. Fate of pemphigus antibody following successful therapy. Preliminary evaluation of pemphigus antibody determinations to regulate therapy. *Arch Dermatol*. 1978;114(12):1769-1772.
189. Aberer W, Wolff-Schreiner EC, Stingl G, et al. Azathioprine in the treatment of pemphigus vulgaris. A long-term follow-up. *J Am Acad Dermatol*. 1987;16(3, pt 1):527-533.

190. Amagai M, Komai A, Hashimoto T, et al. Usefulness of enzyme-linked immunosorbent assay using recombinant desmogleins 1 and 3 for serodiagnosis of pemphigus. *Br J Dermatol*. 1999;140(2):351-357.
191. Cheng SW, Kobayashi M, Kinoshita-Kuroda K, et al. Monitoring disease activity in pemphigus with enzyme-linked immunosorbent assay using recombinant desmogleins 1 and 3. *Br J Dermatol*. 2002; 147(2):261-265.
192. Ishii K, Amagai M, Ohata Y, et al. Development of pemphigus vulgaris in a patient with pemphigus foliaceus: antidesmoglein antibody profile confirmed by enzyme-linked immunosorbent assay. *J Am Acad Dermatol*. 2000;42(5, pt 2):859-861.
193. Komai A, Amagai M, Ishii K, et al. The clinical transition between pemphigus foliaceus and pemphigus vulgaris correlates well with the changes in autoantibody profile assessed by an enzyme-linked immunosorbent assay. *Br J Dermatol*. 2001;144(6): 1177-1182.
194. Tsuji Y, Kawashima T, Yokota K, et al. Clinical and serological transition from pemphigus vulgaris to pemphigus foliaceus demonstrated by desmoglein ELISA system. *Arch Dermatol*. 2002;138(1):95-96.
195. Arteaga LA, Prisayanh PS, Warren SJ, et al. CGoFS. A subset of pemphigus foliaceus patients exhibits pathogenic autoantibodies against both desmoglein-1 and desmoglein-3. *J Invest Dermatol*. 2002; 118(5):806-811.
196. Kwon EJ, Yamagami J, Nishikawa T, et al. Antidesmoglein IgG autoantibodies in patients with pemphigus in remission. *J Eur Acad Dermatol Venereol*. 2008;22(9):1070-1075.
197. Udey MC, Stanley JR. Pemphigus: diseases of anti-desmosomal autoimmunity. *JAMA*. 1999;282(6):572-576.
198. Emmerson RW, Wilson-Jones E. Eosinophilic spongiosis in pemphigus. A report of an unusual hitological change in pemphigus *Arch Dermatol*. 1968;97(3):252-257.
199. Carson PJ, Hameed A, Ahmed AR. Influence of treatment on the clinical course of pemphigus vulgaris. *J Am Acad Dermatol*. 1996;34(4):645-652.
200. Bystryn JC, Rudolph JL. Pemphigus. *Lancet*. 2005; 366(9479):61-73.
201. Stanley JR. Therapy of pemphigus vulgaris. *Arch Dermatol*. 1999;135:76-78.
202. Bystryn JC, Steinman NM. The adjuvant therapy of pemphigus. An update. *Arch Dermatol*. 1996; 132(2): 203-212.
203. Risser J, Lewis K, Weinstock MA. Mortality of bullous skin disorders from 1979 through 2002 in the United States. *Arch Dermatol*. 2009;145(9):1005-1008.
204. Ahmed AR, Moy R. Death in pemphigus. *J Am Acad Dermatol*. 1982;7(2):221-228.
205. Herbst A, Bystryn JC. Patterns of remission in pemphigus vulgaris. *J Am Acad Dermatol*. 2000;42(3):422-427.
206. Almugairen N, Hospital V, Bedane C, et al. Assessment of the rate of long-term complete remission off therapy in patients with pemphigus treated with different regimens including medium- and high-dose corticosteroids. *J Am Acad Dermatol*. 2013;69(4):583-588.
207. Atzmony L, Hodak E, Leshem YA, et al. The role of adjuvant therapy in pemphigus: a systematic review and meta-analysis. *J Am Acad Dermatol*. 2015;73(2):264-271.
208. Colliou N, Picard D, Caillot F, et al. Long-term remissions of severe pemphigus after rituximab therapy are associated with prolonged failure of desmoglein B cell response. *Sci Transl Med*. 2013;5(175):175ra30.
209. Joly P, Maho-Vaillant M, Prost-Squarcioni C, et al. First-line rituximab combined with short-term prednisone versus prednisone alone for the treatment of pemphigus (Ritux 3): a prospective, multicentre, parallel-group, open-label randomised trial. *Lancet*. 2017 May 20;389(10083):2031-2040.
210. Mimouni D, Nousari CH, Cummins DL, et al. Differences and similarities among expert opinions on the diagnosis and treatment of pemphigus vulgaris. *J Am Acad Dermatol*. 2003;49(6):1059-1062.
211. Committee for Guidelines for the Management of Pemphigus Disease; Amagai M, Tanikawa A, Shimizu T, et al. Japanese guidelines for the management of pemphigus. *J Dermatol*. 2014;41(6):471-486.
212. Hertl M, Jedlickova H, Karpati S, et al. Pemphigus. S2 Guideline for diagnosis and treatment—guided by the European Dermatology Forum (EDF) in cooperation with the European Academy of Dermatology and Venereology (EADV). *J Eur Acad Dermatol Venereol*. 2015;29(3):405-414.
213. Harman et al, British Association of Dermatologists' guidelines for the management of pemphigus vulgaris 2017, https://doi.org/10.1111/bjd.15930.
214. Murrell et al. Diagnosis and management of pemphigus, *JAAD* 2018, doi: 10.1016/j.JAAD.2018.02.021.
215. Seidenbaum M, David M, Sandbank M. The course and prognosis of pemphigus. A review of 115 patients. *Int J Dermatol*. 1988;27(8):580-584.
216. Murrell DF, Dick S, Amagai M, et al. Consensus statement on definitions of disease endpoints and therapeutic response for pemphigus. *J Am Acad Dermatol*. 2008;58(6):1043-1046.
217. Pfütze M, Niedermeier A, Hertl M, et al. Introducing a novel Autoimmune Bullous Skin Disorder Intensity Score (ABSIS) in pemphigus. *Eur J Dermatol*. 2007;17(1):4-11.
218. Rosenbach M, Murrell DF, Bystryn JC, et al. Reliability and convergent validity of two outcome instruments for pemphigus. *J Invest Dermatol*. 2008; 129(10):2404-2410.
219. Rosenberg FR, Sanders S, Nelson CT. Pemphigus: a 20-year review of 107 patients treated with corticosteroids. *Arch Dermatol*. 1976;112(7):962-970.
220. Hirone T. Pemphigus: a survey of 85 patients between 1970 and 1974. *J Dermatol*. 1978;5(2):43-47.
221. Ratnam KV, Phay KL, Tan CK. Pemphigus therapy with oral prednisolone regimens. A 5-year study. *Int J Dermatol*. 1990;29(5):363-367.
222. Fine JD. Management of acquired bullous skin diseases. *N Engl J Med*. 1995;333(22):1475-1484.
223. Nguyen VT, Arredondo J, Chernyavsky AI, et al. Pemphigus vulgaris IgG and methylprednisolone exhibit reciprocal effects on keratinocytes. *J Biol Chem*. 2004;279(3):2135-2146.
224. Mao et al. *JCI Insight* 2017. doi: 10.1016/j.jaad.2018.02.021.
225. Eming R, Nagel A, Wolff-Franke S, et al. Rituximab exerts a dual effect in pemphigus vulgaris. *J Invest Dermatol*. 2008;128(12):2850-2858.
226. Joly P, Mouquet H, Roujeau JC, et al. A single cycle of rituximab for the treatment of severe pemphigus. *N Engl J Med*. 2007;357(6):545-552.
227. Kincaid L, Weinstein M. Rituximab therapy for childhood pemphigus vulgaris. *Pediatr Dermatol*. 2016;33(2):e61-e64.
228. Vinay K, Kanwar AJ, Sawatkar GU, et al. Successful use of rituximab in the treatment of childhood

and juvenile pemphigus. *J Am Acad Dermatol.* 2014;71(4):669-675.
229. Connelly EA, Aber C, Kleiner G, et al. Generalized erythrodermic pemphigus foliaceus in a child and its successful response to rituximab treatment. *Pediatr Dermatol.* 2007;24(2):172-176.
230. Rituxan [package insert]. South San Francisco: Genentech, 2018.
231. Allen KJ, Wolverton SE. The efficacy and safety of rituximab in refractory pemphigus: a review of case reports. *J Drugs Dermatol.* 2007;6(9):883-889.
232. Cianchini G, Corona R, Frezzolini A, et al. Treatment of severe pemphigus with rituximab: report of 12 cases and a review of the literature. *Arch Dermatol.* 2007;143(8):1033-1038.
233. Kolstad A, Holte H, Fossa A, et al. Pneumocystis jirovecii pneumonia in B-cell lymphoma patients treated with the rituximab-CHOEP-14 regimen. *Haematologica.* 2007;92(1):139-140.
234. Teichmann LL, Woenckhaus M, Vogel C, et al. Fatal Pneumocystis pneumonia following rituximab administration for rheumatoid arthritis. *Rheumatology (Oxford).* 2008;47(8):1256-1257.
235. Beissert S, Werfel T, Frieling U, et al. A comparison of oral methylprednisolone plus azathioprine or mycophenolate mofetil for the treatment of pemphigus. *Arch Dermatol.* 2006;142(11):1447-1454.
236. Chams-Davatchi C, Esmaili N, Daneshpazhooh M, et al. Randomized controlled open-label trial of four treatment regimens for pemphigus vulgaris. *J Am Acad Dermatol.* 2007;57(4):622-628.
237. Chams-Davatchi C, Mortazavizadeh A, Daneshpazhooh M, et al. Randomized double blind trial of prednisolone and azathioprine, vs. prednisolone and placebo, in the treatment of pemphigus vulgaris. *J Eur Acad Dermatol Venereol.* 2013;27(10):1285-1292.
238. Beissert S, Mimouni D, Kanwar AJ, et al. Treating pemphigus vulgaris with prednisone and mycophenolate mofetil: a multicenter, randomized, placebo-controlled trial. *J Invest Dermatol.* 2010;130(8):2041-2048.
239. Olszewska M, Kolacinska-Strasz Z, Sulej J, et al. Efficacy and safety of cyclophosphamide, azathioprine, and cyclosporine (ciclosporin) as adjuvant drugs in pemphigus vulgaris. *Am J Clin Dermatol.* 2007;8(2):85-92.
240. Weinshilboum RM, Sladek SL. Mercaptopurine pharmacogenetics: monogenic inheritance of erythrocyte thiopurine methyltransferase activity. *Am J Hum Genet.* 1980;32(5):651-662.
241. Schaeffeler E, Fischer C, Brockmeier D, et al. Comprehensive analysis of thiopurine S-methyltransferase phenotype-genotype correlation in a large population of German-Caucasians and identification of novel TPMT variants. *Pharmacogenetics.* 2004;14(7):407-417.
242. Yang SK, et al. A common missense variant in NUDT15 confers susceptibility to thiopurine-induced leukopenia. *Nat Genet.* 2014;46:1017-1020.
243. Reuther LO, Vainer B, Sonne J, et al. Thiopurine methyltransferase (TPMT) genotype distribution in azathioprine-tolerant and -intolerant patients with various disorders. The impact of TPMT genotyping in predicting toxicity. *Eur J Clin Pharmacol.* 2004;59(11):797-801.
244. Enk AH, Knop J. Mycophenolate mofetil is effective in the treatment of pemphigus vulgaris. *Arch Dermatol.* 1999;135:54-56.
245. Mimouni D, Anhalt GJ, Cummins DL, et al. Treatment of pemphigus vulgaris and pemphigus foliaceus with mycophenolate mofetil. *Arch Dermatol.* 2003; 139(6):739-742.
246. Baratta A, Camarillo D, Papa C, et al. Pediatric pemphigus vulgaris: durable treatment responses achieved with prednisone and mycophenolate mofetil (MMF). *Pediatr Dermatol.* 2013;30(2):240-244.
247. Cellcept [package insert]. South San Francisco: Genentech, 2015.
248. Oz HS, Hughes WT. Novel anti-*Pneumocystis carinii* effects of the immunosuppressant mycophenolate mofetil in contrast to provocative effects of tacrolimus, sirolimus, and dexamethasone. *J Infect Dis.* 1997;175(4):901-904.
249. Tran KD, Wolverton JE, Soter NA. Methotrexate in the treatment of pemphigus vulgaris: experience in 23 patients. *Br J Dermatol.* 2013;169(4):916-921.
250. Yu Z, Lennon VA. Mechanism of intravenous immune globulin therapy in antibody-mediated autoimmune diseases. *N Engl J Med.* 1999;340(3):227-228.
251. Li N, Zhao M, Hilario-Vargas J, et al. Complete FcRn dependence for intravenous Ig therapy in autoimmune skin blistering diseases. *J Clin Invest.* 2005;115(12):3440-3450.
252. Czernik A, Beutner EH, Bystryn JC. Intravenous immunoglobulin selectively decreases circulating autoantibodies in pemphigus. *J Am Acad Dermatol.* 2008;58(5):796-801.
253. Engineer L, Bhol KC, Ahmed AR. Analysis of current data on the use of intravenous immunoglobulins in management of pemphigus vulgaris. *J Am Acad Dermatol.* 2000;43(6):1049-1057.
254. Ahmed AR, Dahl MV. Consensus statement on the use of intravenous immunoglobulin therapy in the treatment of autoimmune mucocutaneous blistering diseases. *Arch Dermatol.* 2003;139(8):1051-1059.
255. Amagai M, Ikeda S, Shimizu H, et al. A randomized double-blind trial of intravenous immunoglobulin for pemphigus. *J Am Acad Dermatol.* 2009;60(4):595-603.
256. Katz KA, Hivnor CM, Geist DE, et al. Stroke and deep venous thrombosis complicating intravenous immunoglobulin infusions. *Arch Dermatol.* 2003;139(8):991-993.
257. Ahmed AR, Spigelman Z, Cavacini LA, et al. Treatment of pemphigus vulgaris with rituximab and intravenous immune globulin. *N Engl J Med.* 2006;355(17):1772-1779.
258. Ahmed AR, Kaveri S, Spigelman Z. Long-term remissions in Recalcitrant Pemphigus Vulgaris. *N Engl J Med.* 2015;373(27):2693-2694.
259. Cummins DL, Mimouni D, Anhalt GJ, et al. Oral cyclophosphamide for treatment of pemphigus vulgaris and foliaceus. *J Am Acad Dermatol.* 2003;49(2):276-280.
260. Pasricha JS, Das SS. Curative effect of dexamethasone-cyclophosphamide pulse therapy for the treatment of pemphigus vulgaris. *Int J Dermatol.* 1992;31(12):875-877.
261. Kanwar AJ, Kaur S, Thami GP. Long-term efficacy of dexamethasone-cyclophosphamide pulse therapy in pemphigus. *Dermatology.* 2002;204(2):228-231.
262. Hayag MV, Cohen JA, Kerdel FA. Immunoablative high-dose cyclophosphamide without stem cell rescue in a patient with pemphigus vulgaris. *J Am Acad Dermatol.* 2000;43(6):1065-1069.
263. Nousari CH, Brodsky R, Anhalt GJ. Evaluating the role of immunoablative high-dose cyclophosphamide therapy in pemphigus vulgaris. *J Am Acad Dermatol.* 2003;49(1):148-150.
264. Heaphy MR, Albrecht J, Werth VP. Dapsone as a glucocorticoid-sparing agent in maintenance-phase

pemphigus vulgaris. *Arch Dermatol.* 2005; 141(6):699-702.
265. Werth VP, Fivenson D, Pandya AG, et al. Multicenter randomized, double-blind, placebo-controlled, clinical trial of dapsone as a glucocorticoid-sparing agent in maintenance-phase pemphigus vulgaris. *Arch Dermatol.* 2008;144(1):25-32.
266. Guillaume JC, Roujeau JC, Morel P, et al. Controlled study of plasma exchange in pemphigus. *Arch Dermatol.* 1988;124(11):1659-1663.
267. Turner MS, Sutton D, Sauder DN. The use of plasmapheresis and immuosupression in the treatment of pemphigus vulgaris. *J Am Acad Dermatol.* 2000;43(6):1058-1064.
268. Euler HH, Loffler H, Christophers E. Synchronization of plasmapheresis and pulse cyclophosphamide therapy in pemphigus vulgaris. *Arch Dermatol.* 1987;123(9):1205-1210.
269. Shimanovich I, Herzog S, Schmidt E, et al. Improved protocol for treatment of pemphigus vulgaris with protein A immunoadsorption. *Clin Exp Dermatol.* 2006;31(6):768-774.
270. Werth VP. Treatment of pemphigus vulgaris with brief, high-dose intravenous glucocorticoids. *Arch Dermatol.* 1996;132(12):1435-1439.
271. Roujeau JC. Pulse glucocorticoid therapy. The "big shot" revisited. *Arch Dermatol.* 1996;132(12):1499-1502.
272. Mentink LF, Mackenzie MW, Toth GG, et al. Randomized controlled trial of adjuvant oral dexamethasone pulse therapy in pemphigus vulgaris: PEMPULS trial. *Arch Dermatol.* 2006;142(5):570-576.
273. Wu J, Edberg JC, Redecha PB, et al. A novel polymorphism of FcgammaRIIIa (CD16) alters receptor function and predisposes to autoimmune disease. *J Clin Invest.* 1997;100(5):1059-1070.
274. Dall'Ozzo S, Tartas S, Paintaud G, et al. Rituximab-dependent cytotoxicity by natural killer cells: influence of FCGR3A polymorphism on the concentration-effect relationship. *Cancer Res.* 2004;64(13):4664-4669.
275. Weng WK, Levy R. Two immunoglobulin G fragment C receptor polymorphisms independently predict response to rituximab in patients with follicular lymphoma. *J Clin Oncol.* 2003;21(21):3940-3947.
276. Cartron G, Dacheux L, Salles G, et al. Therapeutic activity of humanized anti-CD20 monoclonal antibody and polymorphism in IgG Fc receptor FcgammaRIIIa gene. *Blood.* 2002;99(3):754-758.
277. Farag SS, Flinn IW, Modali R, et al. Fc gamma RIIIa and Fc gamma RIIa polymorphisms do not predict response to rituximab in B-cell chronic lymphocytic leukemia. *Blood.* 2004;103(4):1472-1474.
278. Weng WK, Weng WK, Levy R. Immunoglobulin G Fc receptor polymorphisms do not correlate with response to chemotherapy or clinical course in patients with follicular lymphoma. *Leuk Lymphoma.* 2009;50(9):1494-1500.
279. Ellebrecht CT, Choi EJ, Allman DM, et al. Subcutaneous veltuzumab, a humanized anti-CD20 antibody, in the treatment of refractory pemphigus vulgaris. *JAMA Dermatol.* 2014;150(12):1331-1335.
280. Huang A, Madan RK, Levitt J. Future therapies for pemphigus vulgaris: Rituximab and beyond. *J Am Acad Dermatol.* 2016;74(4):746-753.
281. Ellebrecht CT, Bhoj VG, Nace A, et al. Reengineering chimeric antigen receptor T cells for targeted therapy of autoimmune disease. *Science.* 2016;353(6295);179-184.

Chapter 53 :: Paraneoplastic Pemphigus
:: Grant J. Anhalt & Daniel Mimouni

第五十三章
副肿瘤性天疱疮

中文导读

副肿瘤性天疱疮（PNP）是一种罕见的恶性肿瘤并发症，属于自身免疫疾病，与潜在的淋巴增生性疾病有关。非霍奇金淋巴瘤（NHL）、慢性淋巴细胞白血病（CLL）和Castleman病是最常见的相关肿瘤。皮损特点主要是疼痛、难治性口腔炎和多形性皮损。血清中有抗plakin蛋白自身抗体。本病死亡率高，常因败血症、治疗并发症或闭塞性细支气管炎死亡。没有持续有效的治疗，联合使用利妥昔单抗、糖皮质激素和其他免疫抑制药可取得一定疗效。

本章从八个方面进行了讲述。

1. 流行病学　PNP发病率尚不清楚。有报道在10万例NHL和CLL的患者中，12例患有PNP。

2. 病因和发病机制　PNP的发病可能是肿瘤细胞、免疫系统和特定遗传背景之间复杂的相互作用的结果，本节介绍了HLA Ⅱ类DRB*03和HLA Ⅰ类Cw*14基因具有显著优势。其次PNP患者白细胞介素6（IL-6）明显升高，此外，几乎所有PNP患者都有抗桥粒蛋白自身抗体。

3. 临床表现　本节介绍了PNP的临床表现，最恒定的表现是难治性口腔炎。它是最早出现的症状，且持续存在于整个病程，对治疗极为抵抗。如果缺乏口腔炎，则不能考虑PNP。其皮疹变化不定，不同疾病阶段皮疹形态不同。另外，大约30%～40%患者发生肺损伤，通常致命。少数PNP患者伴有重症肌无力。

4. 实验室检查　本节介绍了PNP最主要的实验室发现是血清中抗plakin蛋白的多克隆IgG自身抗体，主要是桥粒蛋白1和3。其次重点介绍了PNP的组织病理学表现。特殊实验室检查方面，本章提到大约1/3的PNP患者有隐匿的恶性肿瘤。常规生化检查和体格检查往往检测不到肿瘤，最有效的方法是CT扫描或MRI检查。

5. 诊断与鉴别诊断　图53-5列出了诊断方法。表53-4总结了鉴别诊断方法。

6. 预后与临床病程　通常在寻常型天疱疮和其他自身免疫性疾病中有效的免疫抑制，对PNP疗效不好。患者死因包括败血症、胃肠道出血、多器官衰竭和呼吸衰竭等。

7. 治疗　表53-5总结了PNP治疗方案。包括手术完整切除良性或包裹性肿瘤，则疾病通常会明显好转或完全缓解。在恶性肿瘤患者中，始终尚无有效的治疗方案。口服0.5～1.0mg/kg/d泼尼松可部分改善。皮损对治疗反应很快，但口腔炎通常对任何治疗都很难治愈。

8. 预防　没有已知的干预措施可以阻止伴有淋巴样恶性肿瘤PNP患者病情进展。个别病例报告PNP可能是由某些药物、放疗或细胞因子引起，但不清楚这些疗法是否会引发自身免疫疾病，而且肿瘤本身更可能引发自身免疫疾病。

〔陈明亮〕

AT-A-GLANCE

- Rare complication of malignancy, most commonly non-Hodgkin lymphoma, chronic lymphocytic leukemia, or Castleman disease.
- Painful, erosive stomatitis and polymorphous cutaneous lesions that may be blistering and erosive (resembling erythema multiforme), morbilliform, or lichenoid.
- Serum autoantibodies directed against plakin proteins that are detected by indirect immunofluorescence against rodent bladder epithelium.
- High mortality rate, with death from sepsis, complications of treatment, or bronchiolitis obliterans.
- No consistently effective therapy, but some success with the combined use of rituximab, systemic corticosteroids, and other immunosuppressive agents.

Paraneoplastic pemphigus (PNP) is an autoimmune disorder that is almost always linked to an underlying lymphoproliferative disorder. These features define it (Table 53-1): (a) Painful stomatitis and a polymorphous cutaneous eruption with lesions that may be blistering, lichenoid, or resemble erythema multiforme. (b) Histologic findings that reflect the variability of the cutaneous lesions, showing acantholysis, lichenoid, or interface change. (c) Direct immunofluorescence findings of immunoglobulin (Ig) G and complement deposition in the epidermal intercellular spaces, and, often, granular/linear complement deposition along the epidermal basement membrane zone. (d) Serum autoantibodies that bind to the cell surface of skin and mucosae in a pattern typical of pemphigus, which, in addition, also bind to simple, columnar and transitional epithelia. (e) The serum autoantibodies identify desmogleins 1 and 3, in addition to members of the plakin family of epithelial proteins, such as desmoplakins, envoplakins, and periplakins.[1] Non-Hodgkin lymphoma (NHL), chronic lymphocytic leukemia (CLL), and Castleman disease are the neoplasms most commonly associated with PNP. There is no regularly effective treatment. Most patients die from complications of the disease such as pulmonary involvement with respiratory failure.

EPIDEMIOLOGY

The incidence of PNP is unknown, although it is less common than pemphigus vulgaris or foliaceus (see Chap. 52). In an adverse events reporting analysis including 100,000 patients with known NHL and CLL, 12 were found to have PNP.[2] Only 3 of the 12 patients were identified by the reporting physician, and the remainder were identified only by retrospective data analysis, suggesting that the majority of cases of PNP are not being properly diagnosed. In this series, the most common misdiagnoses were erythema multiforme, Stevens-Johnson syndrome, toxic epidermal necrolysis (TEN), and drug reaction.

ETIOLOGY AND PATHOGENESIS

In almost all cases, PNP is associated with a limited number of lymphoproliferative neoplasms. On the basis of 140 cases of PNP confirmed by immunoprecipitation findings of the characteristic autoantibody profile, the estimated frequencies of specific neoplasms are 44% NHL, 19% CLL, 16% Castleman disease (giant follicular hyperplasia), 8% thymoma (malignant and benign), 7% sarcomas that are retroperitoneal and often poorly differentiated, 4% Waldenström macroglobulinemia, and in 2% the neoplasms were too poorly differentiated to categorize (Fig. 53-1). The disproportionate representation of Castleman disease is notable, given its overall rarity. In children with PNP, Castleman disease is almost always the underlying neoplasm.[3] Before the description of PNP, many cases of Castleman disease associated with atypical forms of pemphigus had been reported, and we suspect that most were PNP. Furthermore, this association was emphasized in a retrospective study of 114 patients with Castleman disease identified 37 cases of PNP confirmed by the specific autoantibodies.[4]

With very rare exceptions, more common cancers, such as adenocarcinomas of breast, bowel, and lung, or basal cell and squamous cell carcinoma of skin, have not been associated with PNP. There are a few reports of PNP and squamous cell carcinoma, but in most of them, the diagnosis was made with immunofluorescent techniques only, which have significant false-positive and false-negative rates, and were not confirmed immunochemically, so the association remains unproven.

The mechanisms by which these tumors induce autoimmunity against epithelial proteins remain speculative. One hypothesis states that the tumors constitutively or anomalously express epithelial proteins. These proteins are targeted by the antitumor immune response that cross-reacts with normal constitutive epithelial proteins of the host. This mechanism occurs in several neurologic paraneoplastic syndromes.[5] This antitumor immune response may be initiated by

TABLE 53-1
Defining Features of Paraneoplastic Pemphigus

a. Painful stomatitis and a polymorphous cutaneous eruption
b. Histologic findings that reflect cutaneous lesions (acantholysis, lichenoid or interface changes)
c. IgG complement deposition in the epidermal intercellular spaces and/or along basement membrane zone with granular/linear component (Direct Immunofluorescence)
d. Serum IgG autoantibodies that bind of cell surface of skin and mucosae, but also to simple, columnar and transitional epithelia
e. Serum IgG autoantibodies to desmogleins 1 and 3, desmoplakins, envoplakin and periplakin

reactivity against plakin proteins, and the antitumor immune response may cross-react with normal constitutive proteins of epithelia. However, to date, there are no data to support this hypothesis.

It is more likely that this autoimmune disease is a result of more complex interactions between the tumor cells, the immune system, and specific genetic background. In many autoimmune diseases, specific genetic predispositions have been found, and human leukocyte antigen (HLA) studies performed on 2 different series of PNP patients revealed a significant predominance of HLA-class II DRB*03 and HLA-class I Cw*14 genes. It is interesting to note that these 2 HLA molecules are not those associated with development of pemphigus vulgaris, providing another argument to consider PNP as a distinct entity.[6,7]

There is evidence that dysregulated cytokine production by tumor cells drives the development of autoimmunity. Patients with PNP have evidence of markedly elevated levels of interleukin (IL)-6.[8] It has been observed that in a subset of cases of NHLs,[9] CLL, and Castleman tumors, the tumor cells secrete massive amounts of IL-6 in vitro. IL-6 is known to promote B-cell differentiation and to drive Ig production, and dysregulated IL-6 production has been implicated in certain autoimmune diseases. Castleman tumors are known to be associated with other autoimmune phenomena such as myasthenia gravis and autoimmune cytopenias, and these patients also have high serum levels of IL-6. Symptoms attributable to Castleman tumors are routinely reversed by complete excision of the affected node(s), and, coincidentally, serum IL-6 levels revert to normal. Administration of anti–IL-6 receptor monoclonal antibodies also effectively reverses systemic manifestations of Castleman disease and is currently being studied in clinical trials.[10]

It had also been proposed that the autoantibody may derive from the lymphoid tumor itself. Cultures of Castleman tumors have been shown to contain B cells that produce specific autoantibody.[11] However, Castleman tumors are unique in that they are not clonal neoplasms, and these studies showed the expansion of several immunologically active B-cell clones within the tumors. In Waldenström macroglobulinemia, the autoantibody is polyclonal and IgG class, not IgM, and therefore, cannot be produced by the tumor cells.

Almost all patients with PNP have autoantibodies against desmogleins, demonstrable by enzyme-linked immunosorbent assay (ELISA), and when the desmoglein autoantibodies from these patients are affinity purified and injected into neonatal mice, acantholytic skin lesions are induced.[12] It also has been demonstrated that pathogenic autoantibodies from PNP patients bind to the middle portion of desmoglein 3—extracellular domains 2 and 3—in contrast to pemphigus vulgaris patients where the pathogenic autoantibodies bind to extracellular domain 1.[13] However, none of features of the disease that appear to be induced by cell-mediated autoimmunity are recreated by the Ig injections. No internal organs, like the lungs are involved, and there are no findings of lymphocyte-mediated lichenoid or interface epithelial injury. This is another indication that humoral immunity alone reproduces features of acantholysis, but passive transfer of autoimmune cells from these patients may be necessary to induce the complete spectrum of the disease in animals.

It has been demonstrated in a mouse model that the cellular autoimmune response, which is represented by interface dermatitis, is caused by desmoglein 3–specific CD4+ T cells. This specific response is mediated by interferon-γ and is the dominant response in the lichenoid variant of PNP.[14]

There is evidence that ectopic desmoglein 3 expression is present in the lungs in the PNP mouse model. This squamous metaplasia of the lungs is probably the cause for the fatal bronchiolitis obliterans involvement in PNP.[15]

CLINICAL FINDINGS

HISTORY

CUTANEOUS LESIONS

The most constant clinical feature of the disease is the presence of intractable stomatitis (Fig. 53-2A,B). It is

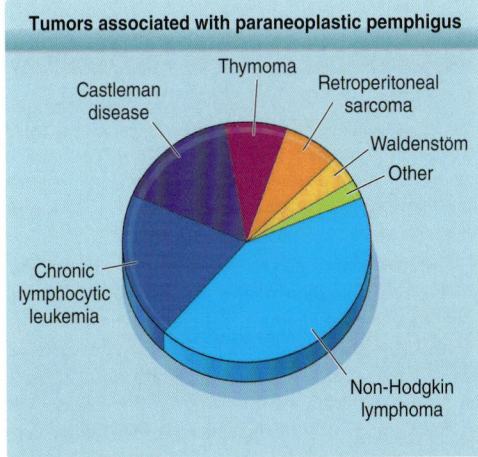

Figure 53-1 Tumors associated with paraneoplastic pemphigus.

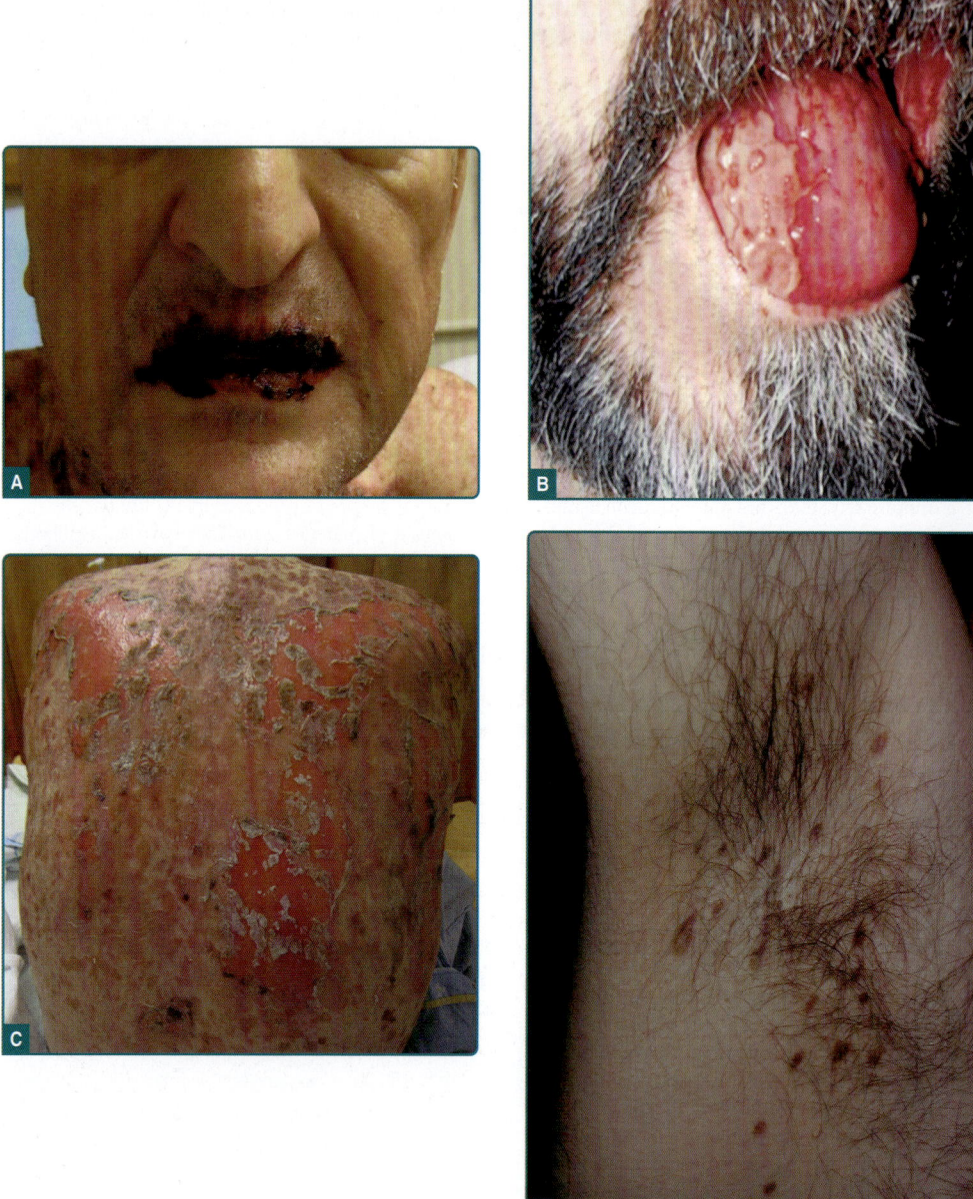

Figure 53-2 **A,** Extensive erosions involving the vermilion of the lips in a patient presenting with paraneoplastic pemphigus and lymphoma. The characteristic severe stomatitis, accompanied by polymorphous cutaneous lesions, is the most consistent feature of the disease. **B,** Painful ulcerations tend to localize to the lateral border of the tongue. **C,** Widespread erosions and sloughing involving the majority of the back from the same patient pictured in **A**. **D,** Lesions from the axilla of a patient with paraneoplastic pemphigus. These lesions clinically resemble lichen planus.

the earliest presenting sign and the one feature that persists throughout the course of the disease, even after treatment and is extremely resistant to therapy. This finding is so consistent that in its absence, PNP should not be considered in the differential diagnosis.

This stomatitis consists of erosions and ulcerations that can affect all surfaces of the oropharynx. The lesions differ from those seen in pemphigus vulgaris in that they show more necrosis and lichenoid change. They also preferentially localize to the lateral borders of the tongue, and characteristically extend onto and involve the vermilion of the lips. Occasionally, oral lesions are the only manifestation of the disease.

The cutaneous lesions of PNP are quite variable, and different morphologies may occur in an individual patient according to the stage of the disease (see Fig. 53-2C,D). The initial patients reported with the syndrome had episodes of waves of blistering affecting the upper trunk, head and neck, and proximal extremities. These lesions consisted of blisters that ruptured easily, leaving erosions. The blisters on the extremities were sometimes quite tense, resembling those seen in bullous pemphigoid, or they had surrounding erythema, clinically resembling erythema multiforme (see Fig. 53-2D). On the upper chest and back, confluent erosive lesions can develop, producing a picture resembling TEN. The similarity of the mucocutaneous features to erythema multiforme and TEN explains why this is the most common differential diagnosis for PNP. However, it is important to note that erythema multiforme and TEN are self-limited events that evolve and resolve over several weeks, whereas PNP is a relentlessly progressive and evolves continuously over months.

Cutaneous lichenoid eruptions are very common, and they may be the only cutaneous signs of the disease, or may develop in lesions that had previously been blistered. When cutaneous lichenoid lesions are present, severe stomatitis is also invariably present. In the chronic form of the disease and after treatment, this lichenoid eruption may predominate over blistering on the cutaneous surface. The common presence of both blisters and lichenoid lesions affecting the palms and the soles as well as the paronychial tissues helps distinguish PNP from pemphigus vulgaris, in which acral and paronychial lesions are uncommon.

There are a small number of patients who appear to have PNP but who do not have demonstrable circulating autoantibodies.[16] These patients tend to have predominantly lichenoid skin and mucosal lesions, but behave in every other way like antibody-positive patients. They have the same underlying neoplasms, and frequently develop bronchiolitis obliterans. Because the definition of the disease relies so heavily on demonstration of the specific autoantibody markers, further study is required to determine the exact classification of what is presently termed the *lichenoid variant of paraneoplastic pemphigus*.

The disease also has been identified in a horse and 2 dogs. In animal species, the disease is associated with the same neoplasms and has the same clinical outcomes.[17]

RELATED CLINICAL FINDINGS

PNP is the only form of pemphigus that involves nonstratified squamous epithelium. Approximately 30% to 40% of cases develop pulmonary injury, often with a fatal outcome.[18] The earliest symptoms are progressive dyspnea associated initially with an absence of findings on chest radiography. Pulmonary functions studies show airflow obstruction in large and small airways. Inflammation of the large airways evolves and is evidenced by endoscopic biopsy showing acantholysis of bronchial respiratory epithelium. Pulmonary function deteriorates in most cases despite immunosuppressive therapy, and radiologic, histologic, and functional changes characteristic of bronchiolitis obliterans develop. Another interesting clinical association of PNP is with myasthenia gravis, diagnosed in 20 (35%) of patients in a recent cohort of 59 patients with PNP.[19]

LABORATORY TESTS

The key finding is the serologic identification of polyclonal IgG autoantibodies against plakin proteins and, in most cases, desmogleins 1 and 3. The plakins are a group of sequence-related proteins that form the intracellular plaque of desmosomes and hemidesmosomes, and mediate attachment of cytoskeletal intermediate filaments to transmembrane adhesion molecules such as the desmogleins (see Chap. 48). Autoantibodies against these proteins are the most characteristic surrogate markers for the disease. The pattern of antigens recognized by individual patients shows considerable variability, but the most characteristic and consistently recognized plakin antigens are envoplakin[20] and periplakin[21] (210 and 190 kDa, respectively; Fig. 53-3). The next most frequently detected are antibodies against desmoplakin I and desmoplakin II (250 and 210 kDa, respectively). Autoantibodies against α_2-macroglobulin-like-1 a 170-kDa protein, was identified in the sera of 70% of PNP patients. This recently reported autoantibody may be pathogenic by decreasing the normal keratinocyte adhesion.[22] Less commonly, patients recognize bullous pemphigoid Ag 1 (230 kDa), plectin (400 kDa), and plakoglobin (82 kDa) (Table 53-2). PNP patients may also have clinical and serologic evidence of other autoimmune phenomena such as myasthenia gravis and autoimmune cytopenias (Fig. 53-3).

To screen for PNP autoantibodies, one can test for IgG autoantibodies by indirect immunofluorescence reactive with rodent urinary bladder epithelium. A positive result implies the presence of plakin autoantibodies; however, the sensitivity and specificity of this serologic test are only approximately 75% and 83%, respectively.[23] ELISA kits using recombinant proteins containing subdomains of envoplakin and periplakin have been developed and demonstrate high sensitivity and specificity for the diagnosis of PNP.[24,25] More specific and sensitive tests, which are more time-consuming, technically demanding, and of limited availability, include immunoblotting against epidermal cell extracts that can effectively detect antibodies against envoplakin, periplakin, and desmoplakin, and immunoprecipitation, using radiolabeled keratinocyte extracts, which can detect antibodies against any of the plakin proteins. The combination of rodent urinary bladder and immunoblotting has equal specificity and sensitivity to the detection of autoantibodies against the plakin proteins and the α_2-macroglobulin-like-1 protein.[26]

The PNP autoantibody profile is more complex than that observed in pemphigus vulgaris or foliaceus, where there are autoantibodies produced only against the desmogleins. The humoral immunity in PNP may represent an example of epitope spreading in which patients develop autoantibodies against structurally related plakin proteins and structurally unrelated transmembrane cell-surface proteins (the desmogleins) that are physically linked to the plakin proteins in the desmosome and hemidesmosome.

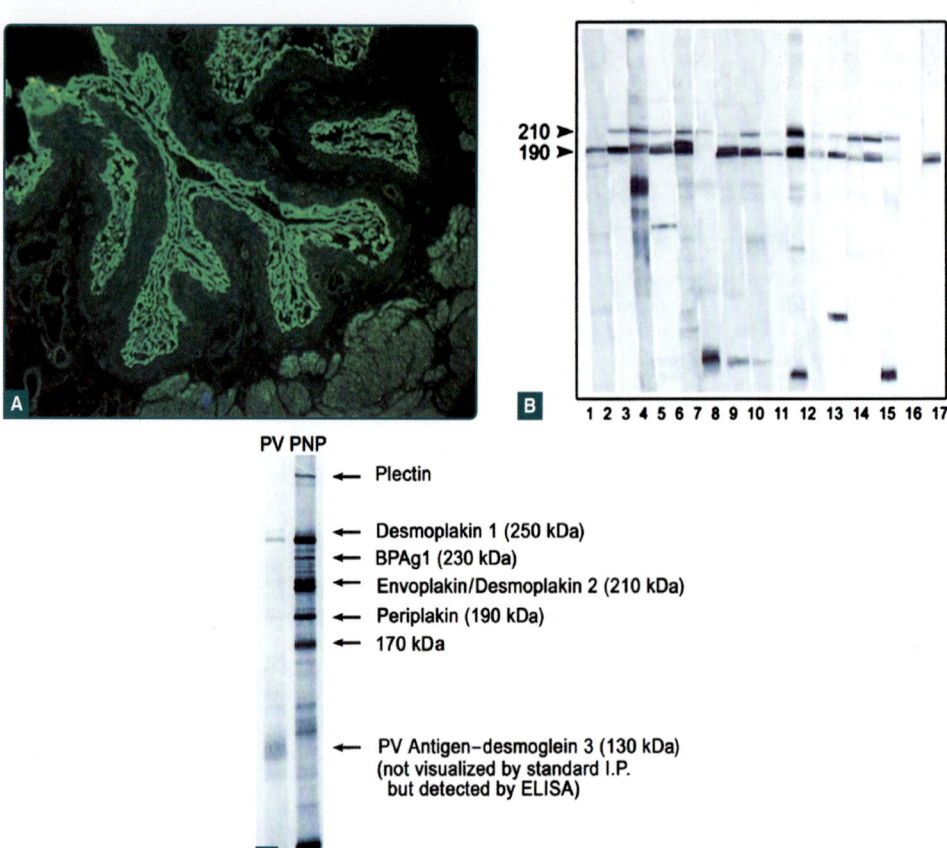

Figure 53-3 Diagnosis of paraneoplastic pemphigus (PNP) depends on the demonstration of antiplakin antibodies. **A,** This can be accomplished by indirect immunofluorescence of patient serum on rodent urinary bladder demonstrating binding of immunoglobulin G to the cell surface of transitional epithelial cells. A positive result implies the presence of antiplakin antibodies. This technique, although easily performed, has the lowest sensitivity and specificity. **B,** Immunoblotting against epidermal cell extracts is much more sensitive and specific. This shows detection of envoplakin (210 kDa) and/or periplakin (190 kDa) in 15 patients with PNP. Lane 16 is a normal control, and lane 17 shows a monoclonal antibody against periplakin. This technique uses denatured antigen extracts, so it does not reliably detect some of the PNP antigens, but antibodies against the most characteristic plakin antigens, envoplakin and periplakin, are easily detected. **C,** Immunoprecipitation using radiolabeled, nondenatured epidermal extracts and serum from a patient with PNP and pemphigus vulgaris (PV). In this case, the PNP patient's serum identifies all the plakin antigens. Envoplakin and desmoplakin II migrate as a doublet at 210 kDa. This technique is the most sensitive and specific test for demonstration of antiplakin antibodies in PNP, but has limited availability. Although this technique readily detects the antiplakin antibodies, desmoglein 3 is not always efficiently identified, and this is best shown by using enzyme-linked immunosorbent assay (ELISA).

TABLE 53-2
Target Antigens in Paraneoplastic Pemphigus

AUTOANTIGEN	MOLECULAR WEIGHT (KDA)
Desmoglein 1	160
Desmoglein 3	130
Desmoplakin 1	250
Desmoplakin 2	210
Bullous pemphigoid antigen 1	230
Envoplakin	210
Periplakin	190
Plectin	500
α_2-Macroglobulin-like-1 protease inhibitor	170

HISTOPATHOLOGY

The histopathology of PNP is distinctive from that of pemphigus vulgaris and foliaceus for 2 reasons. First, because the lesions can be clinically very polymorphous, there is substantial variability in the histologic findings.[27] Second, findings resulting from cell-mediated cytotoxicity are frequently observed.

Owing to the severe mucositis, many biopsies of oral lesions yield nonspecific changes of inflammation and ulceration. If one can biopsy perilesional epithelium, a lichenoid mucositis with variable degrees of individual cell necrosis and suprabasilar acantholysis can be observed.

TABLE 53-3
Typical Histologic Findings

RESULTING FROM HUMORAL IMMUNE RESPONSE	RESULTING FROM CELLULAR IMMUNE RESPONSE
Suprabasilar acantholysis	Individual keratinocyte necrosis
	Thick lichenoid band along the dermal–epidermal junction
	Basal cell vacuolar changes

When evaluating biopsies from skin lesions, one must recognize that lesions with different clinical morphologies yield differing histologic findings (Table 53-3). In noninflammatory cutaneous blisters, suprabasilar acantholysis is expected to be more prominent than the interface/lichenoid change (Fig. 53-4A). When erythematous macules and papules are sampled, interface and lichenoid dermatitis is predominant (Fig. 53-4B,C). Lesions with a mixed clinical pattern also show mixed histologic features of concomitant suprabasilar acantholysis and interface/lichenoid dermatitis.

There is also observed variability of the interface and lichenoid dermatitis. The spectrum of changes can include: (a) individual keratinocyte necrosis with lymphocytic infiltration into the epidermis, reminiscent of that seen in erythema multiforme or graft-versus-host disease; (b) vacuolar interface change with sparse lymphocytic infiltrate of the basilar epithelium, resembling cutaneous lupus erythematosus or dermatomyositis; and (c) a thick lichenoid band along the dermal–epidermal junction similar to that seen in lichen planus. Although most of the specimens show a complex overlap of histologic patterns, there is a relatively good correlation between the clinical and the predominant histologic pattern.

The histopathologic variability of this disease may be related to the fact that it is a presumed antitumor immune response. If this speculation is correct, one would expect to observe a combination of both humoral and cell-mediated immunity that is aberrantly directed against normal epithelium. In such a setting, one would expect to see changes of the sort described in the previous paragraph. This degree of cell-mediated immunity is not seen in pemphigus vulgaris or foliaceus (see Chap. 52); hence the unique histopathologic features, and, presumably, the unique clinical features as well. the presence of T-cell–mediated epithelial cytotoxicity has been demonstrated in histologic studies.[2]

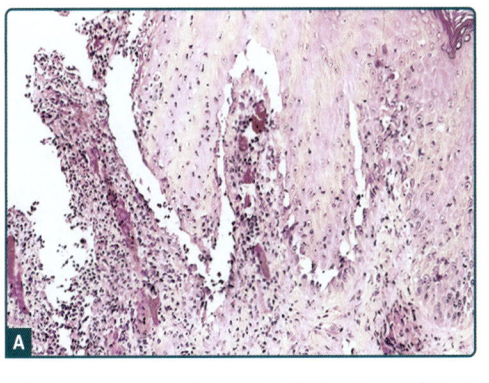
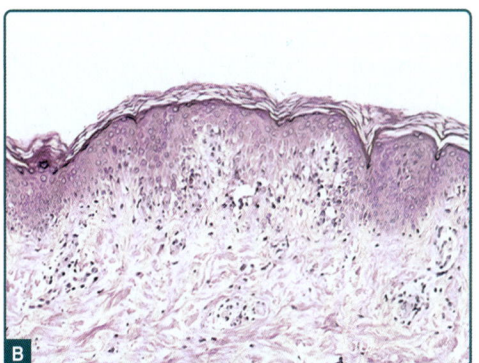
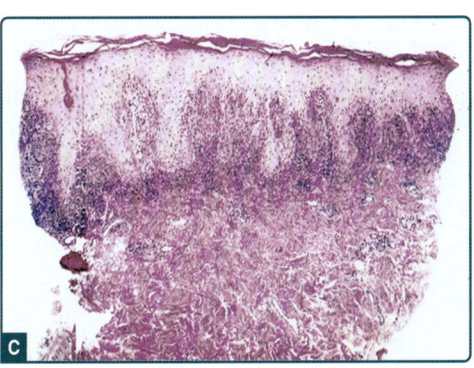
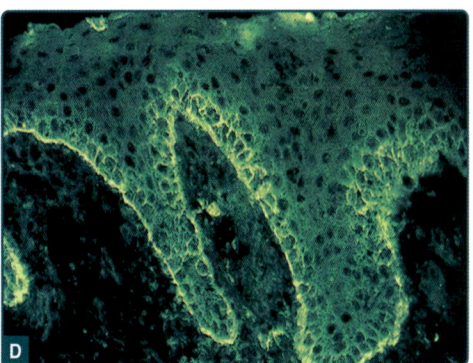

Figure 53-4 **A,** Histopathology of a blistering cutaneous lesion in paraneoplastic pemphigus. This demonstrates the characteristic presence of vacuolar interface change and suprabasilar acantholysis (Hematoxylin and eosin [H&E], ×200). **B,** Macular and papular lesions may show just vacuolar interface change (H&E, ×100). **C,** Lichenoid lesions demonstrate lichenoid infiltrates on histologic examination (H&E, ×40). The presence of these varied histologic findings help differentiate paraneoplastic pemphigus from pemphigus vulgaris. **D,** Direct immunofluorescence can be negative in a significant number of cases, but when positive, the most characteristic changes are those of deposition of immunoglobulin G and complement components on both the surface of basilar and suprabasilar keratinocytes and along the epidermal basement membrane zone (immunofluorescence with fluoresceinated anti–immunoglobulin G, ×200).

IMMUNOPATHOLOGY

Patients with PNP should have evidence of IgG autoantibodies bound to the cell surface of affected epithelium by direct immunofluorescence. However, false negatives are more common in PNP than in pemphigus vulgaris, and repeated biopsies may be necessary, as well as careful investigation of the adnexal structures, which may be the only positive site.[28] In a minority of cases, one might also see a combination of both cell-surface and basement membrane zone deposition of IgG and complement components, but the absence of this combined cell-surface/basement membrane zone staining does not negate the diagnosis (see Fig. 53-4D).

SPECIAL TESTS

Approximately one-third of patients have an occult malignancy at the time they develop PNP. Neoplasms that would not be detected by routine complete blood count, serum chemistries, and physical examination are most likely to be intraabdominal lymphoma, intrathoracic or retroperitoneal Castleman tumors, or retroperitoneal sarcomas. The most effective and efficient method for screening for these tumors is either computer-aided tomography or MRI of the body from the neck to the base of the bladder. If available, positron emission tomography/CT using fluorodeoxyglucose as a biologically active molecule, can be a more specific technique for identifying an occult lymphoma. Other studies, such as endoscopy, are not required.

DIAGNOSIS AND DIFFERENTIAL DIAGNOSIS

The diagnosis can best be made if the algorithm shown in Figure 53-5 is followed. Table 53-4 summarizes the clinical differential diagnosis.

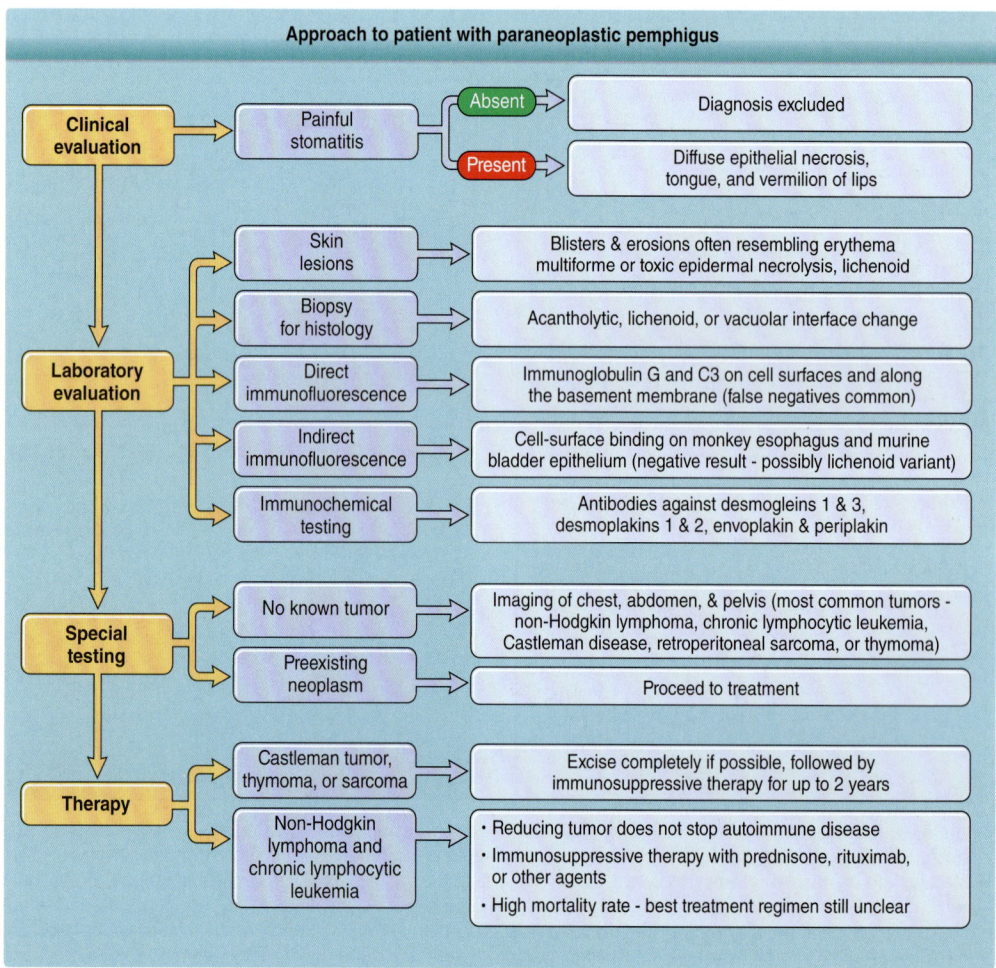

Figure 53-5 Approach to a patient with paraneoplastic pemphigus.

TABLE 53-4
Differential Diagnosis of Paraneoplastic Pemphigus

- Oral lesions
  - Pemphigus vulgaris
  - Stevens-Johnson syndrome
  - Mucous membrane pemphigoid
  - Oral lichen planus
  - Chemotherapy-induced stomatitis
  - Major aphthous stomatitis
- Cutaneous lesions
  - Erythema multiforme/Stevens-Johnson syndrome/toxic epidermal necrolysis
  - Pemphigus vulgaris
  - Drug eruption
  - Lichen planus
  - Subepidermal blistering disorders

PROGNOSIS AND CLINICAL COURSE

It is not known why PNP is so refractory to the type of immunosuppressive treatments that are usually effective in pemphigus vulgaris and other autoimmune diseases.

In those patients who do succumb, death has been attributed in individual cases to multiple factors, including sepsis, GI bleeding, "multiorgan failure," and respiratory failure. Patients with autoimmune disease associated with B-cell neoplasms are known to have a high frequency of autoimmune cytopenias, and some fatal episodes of sepsis are suspected to have occurred because of sudden and unexplained neutropenia, possibly caused by this mechanism. Respiratory failure is a common terminal event. The development of shortness of breath with obstructive disease progressing to bronchiolitis obliterans is a terminal complication in most cases. Because these patients have autoantibodies that react with desmoplakins, and because desmoplakins are present in respiratory epithelium, respiratory failure may be a result of autoantibody-mediated injury to bronchial epithelium, with plugging of terminal bronchioles, resulting in airflow obstruction and ventilation–perfusion abnormalities. Additionally, direct damage to alveolar epithelium could cause a diffusion barrier and subsequent intractable hypoxia. One autopsy study showed an absence of autoantibodies and a marked infiltration of bronchioles with cytotoxic T cells in a patient who died from PNP and bronchiolitis obliterans. This shows that there may be similar complex humoral and cell-mediated autoimmune injury to the lung, similar to what is seen in the skin. The pulmonary injury does not respond well to medical treatment, and the development of shortness of breath and hypoxia in a patient with this syndrome is an ominous prognostic sign. A recent long-term multicenter retrospective cohort study with 18 years of followup performed in France found that presentation with erythema multiforme–like lesions and keratinocyte necrosis in skin histology examination with were significant negative prognostic factors[29]

There is no definite correlation between tumor burden and the activity of the autoimmune syndrome in patients with malignant neoplasms. Treatment of the primary malignancy does not affect the activity of the autoimmune disease. It seems that once the process is initiated by the malignancy, the autoimmunity progresses independently. An example of the disconnect between tumor burden and autoimmunity is found in the case reported by Fullerton et al,[30] in which PNP occurred after successful autologous bone marrow transplantation for NHL. This patient was free of detectable tumor burden at the time of his death, but died from pulmonary injury secondary to PNP. It is notable that the patient underwent autologous bone marrow transplantation, and therefore received his own memory T cells, or possibly individual malignant lymphoid cells that were not detectable by routine autopsy methods.

TREATMENT

Table 53-5 summarizes PNP treatment options.

Individuals with benign or encapsulated tumors such as Castleman tumors or thymoma should have

TABLE 53-5
Treatments for Paraneoplastic Pemphigus

	DRUG	USUAL DOSE	OTHER DOSING
First line	Prednisone	0.5-1.0 mg/kg	Methylprednisolone, 1000 mg IV daily × 3 days
	Rituximab	375 mg/m² IV weekly × 4 wk, repeat every 6 months	1000 mg IV weekly × 2 wk
	Daclizumab	2 mg/kg IV weekly × 4 wk, then every other week indefinitely	
	Basiliximab	20 mg IV on day 0 and day 4, repeat every 3-4 months	
Second line	Cyclosporine	5 mg/kg daily	
	Cyclophosphamide	2.5 mg/kg daily	
	Mycophenolate mofetil	1000 mg by mouth twice daily	
	High-dose IV immunoglobulin	2 g/kg IV, repeat every 3-4 wk	
	Plasmapheresis	Every other day for 6 total treatments	

them surgically excised. If the entire lesion is removed, the disease generally improves substantially or goes into complete remission. The remission of the autoimmune disease may take 1 to 2 years after surgery, so continued immunosuppression during this period is required. The usual treatment involves combined use of prednisone and rituximab.[31] In pediatric cases with respiratory disease, the persistent autoimmunity immediately after surgery can cause ongoing pulmonary injury, and lung transplantation might be required for long-term survival.[32]

In patients with malignant neoplasms, there is no consensus regarding a therapeutic regimen that is consistently effective. Despite scattered individual reports of long-term survivors, almost all patients with NHL or CLL succumb in a period of 1 month to 2 years after diagnosis. Oral corticosteroids in a dose of 0.5 to 1.0 mg/kg produce partial improvement, but not complete resolution of lesions. Cutaneous lesions respond quickly to therapy, but the stomatitis is generally quite refractory to any treatment. Systemic corticosteroids and many other agents have been tried in individual cases, but none has proven to be particularly effective. Methods that have been tried and often failed include immunosuppression with cyclophosphamide, mycophenolate mofetil or azathioprine, gold, dapsone, plasmapheresis, and photopheresis. A small number of patients have shown a good response to combination treatment directed at both humoral and cell-mediated autoimmunity. These patients received oral prednisone, rituximab, and daclizumab or basiliximab (both are nondepleting monoclonal antibody against CD25, the high-affinity IL-2 receptor of T cells). This appears to be a less toxic way of downregulating both humoral and cell-mediated autoimmunity, with promising early results.

PREVENTION

There is no known intervention that may prevent the development of PNP in a patient with a known lymphoid malignancy. Although there have been individual case reports of PNP perhaps being triggered by certain drugs, radiation therapy, or cytokine administration, it is still not clear that any of these treatments triggered the autoimmune disease, and it appears more likely that the neoplasm itself triggers the autoimmunity.

REFERENCES

1. Anhalt GJ, Kim SC, Stanley JR, et al. Paraneoplastic pemphigus: an autoimmune mucocutaneous disease associated with neoplasia. *N Engl J Med*. 1990;323:1729.
2. Nguyen VT, Ndoye A, Bassler KD, et al. Classification, clinical manifestations, and immunopathological mechanisms of the epithelial variant of paraneoplastic autoimmune multiorgan syndrome: a reappraisal of paraneoplastic pemphigus. *Arch Dermatol*. 2001;137:193.
3. Mimouni D, Anhalt GJ, Lazarova Z, et al. Paraneoplastic pemphigus in children and adolescents. *Br J Dermatol*. 2002;147:725.
4. Dong Y, Wang M, Nong L, et al. Clinical and laboratory characterization of 114 cases of Castleman disease patients from a single centre: paraneoplastic pemphigus is an unfavourable prognostic factor. *Br J Haematol*. 2015;169:834.
5. Posner JB. Immunology of paraneoplastic syndromes: Overview. *Ann N Y Acad Sci*. 2003;998:178.
6. Martel P, Loiseau P, Joly P, et al. Paraneoplastic pemphigus is associated with the DRB1*03 allele. *J Autoimmun*. 2003;20:91.
7. Liu Q, Bu DF, Li D, et al. Genotyping of HLA-I and HLA-II alleles in Chinese patients with paraneoplastic pemphigus. *Br J Dermatol*. 2008;158:587.
8. Nousari HC, Kimyai-Asadi A, Anhalt GJ. Elevated levels of interleukin-6 in paraneoplastic pemphigus. *J Invest Dermatol*. 1999;112:396.
9. Nishimoto N, Kanakura Y, Aozasa K, et al. Humanized anti-interleukin-6 receptor antibody treatment of multicentric Castleman disease. *Blood*. 2005;06:2627.
10. Nishimoto N, Terao K, Mima T, et al. Mechanisms and pathological significances in increase in serum interleukin-6 (IL-6) and soluble IL-6 receptor after administration of an anti-IL-6 receptor antibody, tocilizumab, in patients with rheumatoid arthritis and Castleman disease. *Blood*. 2008;112:3959.
11. Wang L, Bu D, Yang Y, et al. Castleman's tumors and production of auto antibody in paraneoplastic pemphigus. *Lancet*. 2004;363:525.
12. Amagai M, Nishikawa T, Nousari HC, et al. Antibodies against desmoglein 3 (pemphigus vulgaris antigen) are present in sera from patients with paraneoplastic pemphigus and cause acantholysis in vivo in neonatal mice. *J Clin Invest*. 1998;102:775.
13. Sugiura K, Koga H, Ishikawa R, et al. Paraneoplastic pemphigus with anti-laminin-332 autoantibodies in a patient with follicular dendritic cell sarcoma. *JAMA Dermatol*. 2013;149:111.
14. Hata T, Nishimoto S, Nagao K, et al. Ectopic expression of epidermal antigens renders the lung a target organ in paraneoplastic pemphigus. *J Immunol*. 2013;191:89.
15. Takahashi H, Kouno M, Nagao K, et al. Desmoglein 3-specific CD4+ T cells induce pemphigus vulgaris and interface dermatitis in mice. *J Clin Invest*. 2011;121:3677.
16. Cummins DL, Mimouni D, Tzu J, et al. Lichenoid paraneoplastic pemphigus in the absence of detectable antibodies. *J Am Acad Dermatol*. 2007;56:153.
17. de Bruin A, Müller E, Wyder M, et al. Periplakin and envoplakin are target antigens in canine and human paraneoplastic pemphigus. *J Am Acad Dermatol*. 1999;40:682.
18. Nousari HC, Deterding R, Wojtczack H, et al: The mechanism of respiratory failure in paraneoplastic pemphigus. *N Engl J Med*. 1999;340:1406.
19. Wang R, Li J, Wang M, et al. Prevalence of myasthenia gravis and associated autoantibodies in paraneoplastic pemphigus and their correlations with symptoms and prognosis. *Br J Dermatol*. 2015;172:968.
20. Kim SC, Kwon YD, Lee IJ, et al. cDNA cloning of the 210-kDa paraneoplastic pemphigus antigen reveals that envoplakin is a component of the antigen complex. *J Invest Dermatol*. 1997;109:365.
21. Mahoney MG, Aho S, Uitto J, et al. The members of the plakin family of proteins recognized by paraneoplastic pemphigus antibodies include periplakin. *J Invest Dermatol*. 1998;111:308.

22. Numata S, Teye K, Tsuruta D, et al. Anti-α-2-macroglobulin-like-1 autoantibodies are detected frequently and may be pathogenic in paraneoplastic pemphigus. *J Invest Dermatol*. 2013;133:1785.
23. Huang Y, Li J, Zhu X. Detection of anti-envoplakin and anti-periplakin autoantibodies by ELISA in patients with paraneoplastic pemphigus. *Arch Dermatol Res*. 2009;301:703.
24. Probst C, Schlumberger W, Stöcker W, et al. Development of ELISA for the specific determination of autoantibodies against envoplakin and periplakin in paraneoplastic pemphigus. *Clin Chim Acta*. 2009;410:13.
25. Helou J, Allbritton J, Anhalt GJ. Accuracy of indirect immunofluorescent testing in the diagnosis of paraneoplastic pemphigus. *J Am Acad Dermatol*. 1995;32:441.
26. Poot AM, Diercks GF, Kramer D, et al. Laboratory diagnosis of paraneoplastic pemphigus. *Br J Dermatol*. 2013;169:1016.
27. Horn TD, Anhalt GJ. Histologic features of paraneoplastic pemphigus. *Arch Dermatol*. 1991;128:1091.
28. Barnadas MA, Curell R, Alomar A, et al. Paraneoplastic pemphigus with negative direct immunofluorescence in epidermis or mucosa but positive findings in adnexal structures. *J Cutan Pathol*. 2009;36:34.
29. Leger S, Picard D, Ingen-Housz-Oro S, et al. Prognostic factors of paraneoplastic pemphigus. *Arch Dermatol*. 2012;148:1165.
30. Fullerton SH, Woodley DT, Smoller BR, et al. Paraneoplastic pemphigus with immune deposits in bronchial epithelium. *JAMA*. 1992;267:1550.
31. Borradori L, Lombardi T, Samson J, et al. Anti-CD20 monoclonal antibody (rituximab) for refractory erosive stomatitis secondary to CD20(+) follicular lymphoma-associated paraneoplastic pemphigus. *Arch Dermatol*. 2001;137:269.
32. Chin AC, Stich D, White FV, et al. Paraneoplastic pemphigus and bronchiolitis obliterans associated with a mediastinal mass: a rare case of Castleman's disease with respiratory failure requiring lung transplantation. *J Pediatr Surg*. 2001;36:E22.

Chapter 54 :: Bullous Pemphigoid
:: Donna A. Culton, Zhi Liu, & Luis A. Diaz

第五十四章
大疱性类天疱疮

中文导读

大疱性类天疱疮好发于老年人，表现为瘙痒性荨麻疹样斑块和张力性大疱。少数人有口腔黏膜糜烂。皮肤病理显示表皮下水疱伴嗜酸性粒细胞浸润。直接免疫荧光（DIF）显示皮损周围基底膜区C3和IgG沉积。间接免疫荧光（IIF）显示血清中有IgG抗基底膜自身抗体。自身抗原BP180和BP230是角质形成细胞半桥粒蛋白质。治疗包括局部和全身糖皮质激素和免疫抑制药。

本章内容包括以下七个方面。

1. 流行病学　大疱性类天疱疮通常发生在60岁以上者，没有种族和性别差异，其发病率逐渐增加。

2. 临床表现　本节介绍了大疱性类天疱疮的典型表现及其他特异性表现。同时提到了大疱性类天疱疮可与其他皮肤病共存，尤其是扁平苔藓，具有两种疾病典型临床、病理学和免疫病理学特征。

3. 病因与发病机制　本节介绍了大疱性类天疱疮多为偶发性，无明显诱因。有报道大疱性类天疱疮可与紫外线、某些药物等相关。大疱性类天疱疮患者有两种半桥粒抗原。

4. 诊断　本节介绍了是根据临床表现、组织学和免疫荧光特征来诊断的。

5. 鉴别诊断　本节介绍了大疱性类天疱疮的鉴别诊断包括自身免疫性水疱性疾病（表54-1）和非自身免疫性水疱性疾病。组织病理学、直接和间接IF检查很容易将大疱性类天疱疮与这些疾病区分开来（表54-2）。

6. 临床病程与预后　大疱性类天疱疮的特征是在不治疗时偶尔自行缓解，局限性病变更可能自行缓解。老年人、一般健康状况差者、有神经系统疾病者、有多系统疾病者、血清中有抗BP180抗体者预后不良，治疗后第1年内复发。

7. 类天疱疮的管理　本节介绍了局限性大疱性类天疱疮患者仅外用糖皮质激素有效（表54-3），广泛皮损者需要口服泼尼松治疗，局部糖皮质激素治疗对中度和重度大疱性天疱疮也有效。

〔陈明亮〕

AT-A-GLANCE

- Bullous pemphigoid usually occurs in older adults.
- The yearly mortality rate varies from 6% to 40%.
- Bullous pemphigoid consists of pruritic urticarial plaques and tense, large blisters. Oral mucous membrane erosions occur in a minority of patients.
- Skin pathology shows subepidermal blisters with eosinophils and other inflammatory cells.
- Direct immunofluorescence (IF) shows C3 and immunoglobulin (Ig) G at epidermal basement membrane zone of perilesional skin. Indirect IF shows IgG anti–basement membrane autoantibodies in the serum.
- The autoantigens BP180 and BP230 are proteins of the keratinocyte hemidesmosome, a basal cell–basement membrane adhesion structure.
- Therapy includes topical and systemic corticosteroids and immunosuppressives.

INTRODUCTION

Bullous pemphigoid is the most common autoimmune blistering disorder in the adult population. The disease typically presents as pruritic, tense blisters often on a background of urticarial plaques. It occurs most frequently in older adults. It is mediated by autoantibodies directed against hemidesmosomal proteins BP180 and BP230, which trigger an inflammatory cascade that ultimately leads to blister formation. This chapter addresses the epidemiology, clinical features, pathogenesis, diagnosis, and treatment of bullous pemphigoid.

HISTORICAL PERSPECTIVE

Bullous pemphigoid was originally described as a subepidermal blistering disease with distinctive clinical and histologic features by Walter Lever in 1953.[1] Antibodies against the dermal–epidermal junction were first described in perilesional skin and in the serum of patients by Jordon and Beutner 14 years later, confirming the separation of bullous pemphigoid from pemphigus.[2] Over the following years, the antigenic targets were fully characterized as hemidesmosomal proteins BP180 and BP230.[3-5]

EPIDEMIOLOGY

Bullous pemphigoid typically occurs in patients older than 60 years of age, with a peak incidence in the 70s.[6] There are exceptions in which classic bullous pemphigoid occurs in middle-aged adults and even infants and children, which is especially rare.[7-10] There is no known ethnic, racial, or sexual predilection for developing bullous pemphigoid.

The incidence of bullous pemphigoid is estimated to be 7 per 1 million per year in Germany and 14 per 1 million per year in Scotland.[6,11] Recent studies suggest that the incidence of bullous pemphigoid is increasing and may be as high as 22 to 24 per 1 million per year in the United States and France and 43 per 1 million per year in the United Kingdom.[12-14]

CLINICAL FEATURES

CUTANEOUS FINDINGS

The classic form of bullous pemphigoid is characterized by large, tense blisters arising on normal skin or on an erythematous or urticarial base (Fig. 54-1A).[15,16] These lesions are most commonly found on flexural surfaces, the lower abdomen, and the thighs, although they may occur anywhere. The bullae are typically filled with serous fluid but may be hemorrhagic. The Nikolsky and Asboe-Hansen signs are negative. Eroded skin from ruptured blisters usually heals spontaneously without scarring, although milia can occur, and postinflammatory pigmentation is common. Pruritus is usually intense but may be minimal in some patients.

Although the more classic presentation of bullous pemphigoid consists of tense bullae on an erythematous or urticarial base, a noninflammatory form of bullous pemphigoid may also be seen presenting as tense bullae on normal-appearing skin (Fig. 54-1B). The noninflammatory form of bullous pemphigoid may be associated with a sparser inflammatory infiltrate histologically (see Diagnosis: Pathology).

Nonbullous lesions are the first manifestation of bullous pemphigoid in almost half of patients.[17] Often, urticarial type lesions precede the more classic tense bullae early in the course of disease. Other early nonbullous findings include eczematous, serpiginous, or targetoid erythema multiforme-like lesions (Fig. 54-1C). Atypical clinical presentations can also be seen in more established disease and include erythroderma and prurigo nodularis–like or vegetative lesions.[18-24]

Although bullous pemphigoid is typically widespread, localized forms of disease have been reported and are becoming increasingly recognized.[14] Localized disease often presents as tense bullae restricted to localized areas of involvement, most commonly the lower legs.[18,25] Dyshidrotic dermatitis–like lesions have also been reported localized to the hands and feet.[26-30] Changes induced by radiation, trauma, or surgery (colostomy, urostomy, or skin graft donor site) may precipitate localized disease in these areas.[31-39] Childhood bullous pemphigoid, although rare, most often presents as localized disease with acral and vulvar or perivulvar distribution being common.[7-10,40-42] In these cases, the diagnosis is confirmed by routine histology, direct immunofluorescence (IF), and indirect IF or enzyme-linked immunosorbent assay (ELISA)

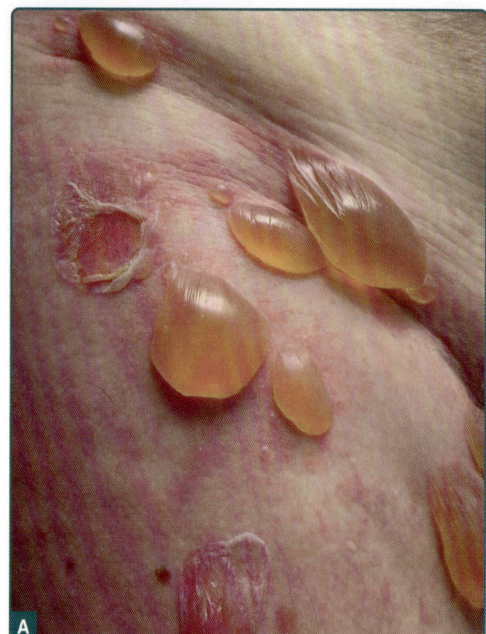
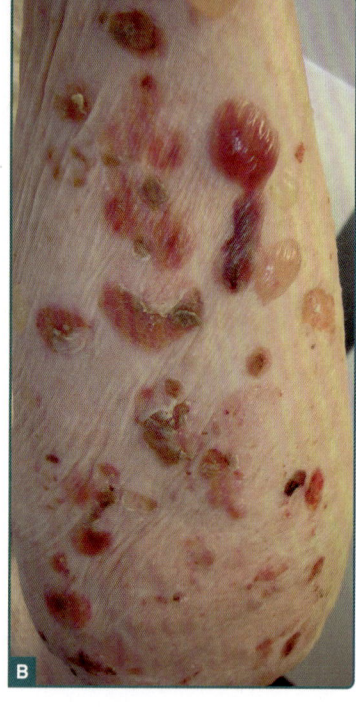
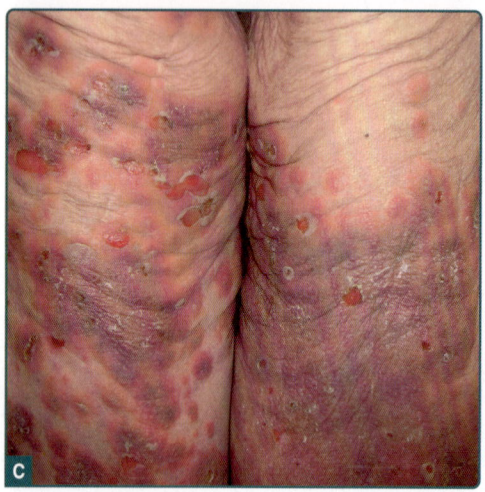

Figure 54-1 Bullous pemphigoid. **A,** Large, tense bullae, some of which are denuded on the upper leg. **B,** An example of the noninflammatory form of bullous pemphigoid. **C,** Urticarial and erythema multiforme–like lesions of bullous pemphigoid on the thighs.

studies. Autoantibodies from these patients show typical IF localization and bind classic pemphigoid antigens, although resuls of indirect IF and ELISA may be negative because of low levels of circulating autoantibodies.[19-24,28-30,43]

Mucous membrane lesions occur in approximately 10% of patients and are almost always limited to the oral mucosa.[15,44-46] Intact blisters are rare, with erosions more commonly seen. The lesions heal without scarring. The presence of scarring or mucosal predominant disease in the absence of classic cutaneous findings is more suggestive of mucous membrane pemphigoid as discussed in Chap. 55.

Bullous pemphigoid may also coexist with other cutaneous diseases, notably lichen planus. Lichen planus pemphigoides describes the coexistence of bullous pemphigoid and lichen planus with typical clinical, histologic, and immunopathologic features of both diseases.[47-50] Lichen planus pemphigoides more often presents in middle-aged patients (mean age of onset, 35 to 45 years of age) and is more localized to the extremities with a less severe clinical course compared with classic bullous pemphigoid.

The Bullous Pemphigoid Disease Area Index (or BPDAI) is a recently developed and validated tool that may be used to objectively measure of clinical disease activity in patients with bullous pemphigoid.[51,52] Although originally designed for use in clinical trials, it can be useful in the clinical setting as well to objectively document the level of disease activity.

NONCUTANEOUS FINDINGS

Approximately 75% of patients have elevated total serum immunoglobulin (Ig) E levels, which often correlates with titers of bullous pemphigoid IgG autoantibodies by IF.[53-55] More than half of patients have peripheral blood eosinophilia as well.[55-58]

COMPLICATIONS

Complications in untreated patients include skin infection developing within denuded bullae, dehydration, electrolyte imbalance, and possibly death from sepsis. Most often complications are related to treatment with systemic corticosteroids or other immunosuppressive medications. Complications caused by bacterial (pneumonia, urinary tract infection, soft tissue infection) and viral (disseminated or localized herpes) mediated infections are common, especially among patients with low functional status and dementia, and contribute to morbidity and mortality.[59-61]

ETIOLOGY AND PATHOGENESIS

Most cases of bullous pemphigoid occur sporadically without any obvious precipitating factors. However, there are reports in which bullous pemphigoid appears to be triggered by ultraviolet (UV) light, either UVB or after psoralen and ultraviolet A light (PUVA) therapy, and radiation therapy.[62-64] Certain medications have also been associated with the development of bullous pemphigoid, including penicillamine, efalizumab, etanercept, and furosemide, among others.[65-71] Recent reports suggest that bullous pemphigoid may also develop after immune checkpoint blockade with anti–programmed cell death receptor 1 (anti–PD-1) treatment.[72-74]

IMMUNOPATHOLOGY

Remarkable advances have been made characterizing the pathophysiology of bullous pemphigoid as a multistep process involving autoantibody binding to hemidesmosomal antigens, which triggers an inflammatory cascade that ultimately results in blister formation. The development of animal models has been instrumental in demonstrating the pathogenicity of bullous pemphigoid autoantibodies and dissecting the factors that contribute to blister formation.

BULLOUS PEMPHIGOID ANTIGENS

IF techniques demonstrate that patients with bullous pemphigoid exhibit circulating and tissue-bound autoantibodies directed against antigens of the cutaneous basement membrane zone (BMZ).[2] Immunoelectron microscopy studies localize bullous pemphigoid antigens to the hemidesmosome, an organelle that is important in anchoring the basal cell to the underlying basement membrane.[75] These autoantibodies bind to both the intracellular plaque of the hemidesmosome and the extracellular face of the hemidesmosome. Bullous pemphigoid autoantibodies recognize two distinct antigens with molecular weights of 230 kDa and 180 kDa by immunoblot analysis of human skin extracts.[76]

The 230-kDa molecule is termed BP230, BPAG1, or BPAG1e (indicating epidermal expression).[4,76-78] BP230 belongs to the plakin family of proteins.[79,80] By immunoelectron microscopy, BP230 is located in the intracellular plaque of the hemidesmosome, where keratin intermediate filaments insert.[81] Analysis of BP230-deficient mouse strain generated by transgenic knockout technology further demonstrates that the function of BP230 is to anchor keratin intermediate filaments to the hemidesmosome.[82] Mice lacking BP230 show fragility of basal cells caused by collapse of the keratin filament network but no epidermal-dermal adhesion defect. Interestingly, an alternatively spliced form of BP230 is expressed in neural tissue, termed BPAG1n. BPAG1n stabilizes the cytoskeleton of sensory neurons[83,84] just as BP230 stabilizes the cytoskeleton of epidermal cells. The lack of dermal–epidermal separation in the BP230-null mice indicates that pathogenic autoantibodies in bullous pemphigoid do not act simply by inhibiting the function of BP230.

The 180-kDa bullous pemphigoid autoantigen is termed BP180, BPAG2, or type XVII collagen.[3,85,86] BP180 is a transmembrane protein of the collagen family with an intracellular amino-terminal domain and an extracellular carboxy-terminal domain that spans the lamina lucida and projects into the lamina densa of the basement membrane.[87-91] Its intracellular or cytoplasmic domain is located in the plaque of the hemidesmosome, and its extracellular domain is linked to anchoring filaments.[92-94] The extracellular domain of BP180 contains a series of 15 collagen regions interrupted by 16 noncollagen sequences.[89] The noncollagen region 16A, also known as the NC16A domain, is adjacent to the membrane-spanning region and harbors the major autoantibody-reactive epitopes.[95,96] ELISA to measure antibodies against the BP180 NC16A domain is both sensitive and specific for a diagnosis of bullous pemphigoid,[97-99] and its titers correlate with disease activity.[98,100] Further evidence that BP180 mediates dermal–epidermal adhesion comes from analysis of the gene defect in patients with the inherited junctional subepidermal blistering disease, non-Herlitz junctional epidermolysis bullosa (JEB-nH), previously known as generalized atrophic benign epidermolysis bullosa. These patients have recessively inherited mutations in the *BP180* gene that result in a missing or dysfunctional protein.[101-103]

PATHOPHYSIOLOGY OF SUBEPIDERMAL BLISTERING

The distinctive feature of bullous pemphigoid is the presence of circulating and tissue-bound autoantibodies against BP180 and BP230. Autoantibodies of various Ig isotypes and IgG subclasses are present in bullous pemphigoid sera with IgG being predominant followed by IgE.[104-106] Serum levels of anti-BP180-NC16A IgG correlate well with disease activity in bullous pemphigoid patients.[85,86,100]

Inflammatory cells are present in the upper dermis and bullous cavity, including eosinophils (the predominant cell type), neutrophils, lymphocytes, and monocytes and macrophages. Both intact and degranulating eosinophils, neutrophils, and mast cells (MCs) are found in the dermis.[107-110] Local activation of these cells may occur via the multiple inflammatory mediators present in the lesional skin or blister fluid.[54,111-118] Several proteinases are found in bullous pemphigoid blister fluid, including plasmin, collagenase, neutrophil elastase, and matrix metalloproteinase (MMP)-9,[119-126] which may play a crucial role in subepidermal blister formation by their ability to degrade extracellular matrix (ECM) proteins.

Both in vitro and in vivo data demonstrate that autoantibodies, particularly those against BP180, are pathogenic suggesting that the autoantibodies trigger the entire inflammatory cascade that ultimately leads to tissue injury and blister formation. In vitro studies using normal human skin sections indicate that bullous pemphigoid IgG is capable of generating dermal-epidermal separation in the presence of complement and leukocytes.[127,128] Early attempts to demonstrate the pathogenicity of patient autoantibodies by a passive transfer mouse model were unsuccessful because bullous pemphigoid anti-BP180-NC16A autoantibodies fail to cross-react with the murine BP180.[129] To overcome this difficulty, rabbit antibodies were raised against the epitope on mouse BP180. Passive transfer of these rabbit antibodies to neonatal mice induces blisters that show some of the key features of human bullous pemphigoid, including in situ deposition of rabbit IgG and mouse C3 at the BMZ, dermal-epidermal separation, and an inflammatory cell infiltrate.[129] These and other studies demonstrate that experimental blistering in animals requires activation of the classical pathway of complement system, MC degranulation, and neutrophil infiltration.[130-134] A well-orchestrated proteolytic event occurs during the disease progression. Plasmin activates proenzyme MMP-9 and activated MMP-9 then degrades α1-proteinase inhibitor, the physiological inhibitor of neutrophil elastase. Unchecked neutrophil elastase degrades BP180 and other ECM components, resulting dermal-epidermal junction separation[135-138] (Fig. 54-2). To directly test the pathogenicity of anti-BP180 IgG autoantibodies from bullous pemphigoid patients, humanized BP180 mouse strains were generated, in which the human BP180 or NC16A domain replaces the murine BP180 or corresponding domain.[139,140] These humanized mice, upon injection with anti-BP180 IgG from bullous pemphigoid patients, develop subepidermal blisters.[139,140] Like the rabbit antimurine BP180 IgG-induced model, the humanized NC16A mouse model of bullous pemphigoid also requires complement, MCs, and neutrophils (Fig. 54-3).[139]

IgE anti-BP180 autoantibodies may also play a role in blister formation. Human skin grafts onto immune-deficient mice injected with an IgE hybridoma to the extracellular portion of BP180 or total IgE from bullous pemphigoid patients' sera exhibit histologic dermal-epidermal separation,[141,142] suggesting that anti-BP180 IgE antibodies may also participate in pathogenesis of bullous pemphigoid through activating MCs and recruitment of eosinophils.

Although most animal model studies clearly show that complement deposition and the subsequent inflammatory cascade triggered by BP180-specific antibodies is essential for blister formation, direct interference of hemidesmosome-mediated cell-cell matrix adhesion by anti-BP180 autoantibodies and BP180 depletion via the ubiquitin/proteasome pathway may represent complement-independent mechanisms of anti-BP180 autoantibody pathogenicity.[143,144] Interestingly, recent studies have shown that deletion of the dominant BP180 epitope domain results in the development of anti-BP180 antibodies, blistering and itching in mice, suggesting a more complex and expanding role for this region.[145] Involvement of anti-BP230 autoantibodies in bullous pemphigoid blistering is also implicated in some animal model studies[146,147]; however, direct evidence in humans is lacking.

Autoreactive T lymphocytes that recognize BP180 are present in addition to autoreactive B lymphocytes,[148-151] supporting the concept that bullous pemphigoid is a T cell-dependent antibody-mediated skin autoimmune disease. As in most autoimmune diseases, the initial trigger for induction of autoreactive lymphocytes and autoantibody production in bullous pemphigoid remains unknown.

Several other subepidermal blistering diseases also show autoimmune responses to BP180. These include pemphigoid gestationis (or herpes gestationis), cicatricial pemphigoid (or mucous membrane pemphigoid), linear IgA bullous dermatosis, and lichen planus pemphigoid.[152-162] It is possible they may share some common immunopathological mechanisms with bullous pemphigoid.

RISK FACTORS

No specific environmental risk factors have been identified for bullous pemphigoid. In terms of genetic risk factors, certain human leukocyte antigens (HLA) alleles have been associated with bullous pemphigoid. HLA-DQB1*0301 has been associated with classic bullous pemphigoid, as well as cicatricial pemphigoid in whites.[163,164] HLA-DRB1*04, DRB1*1101, and

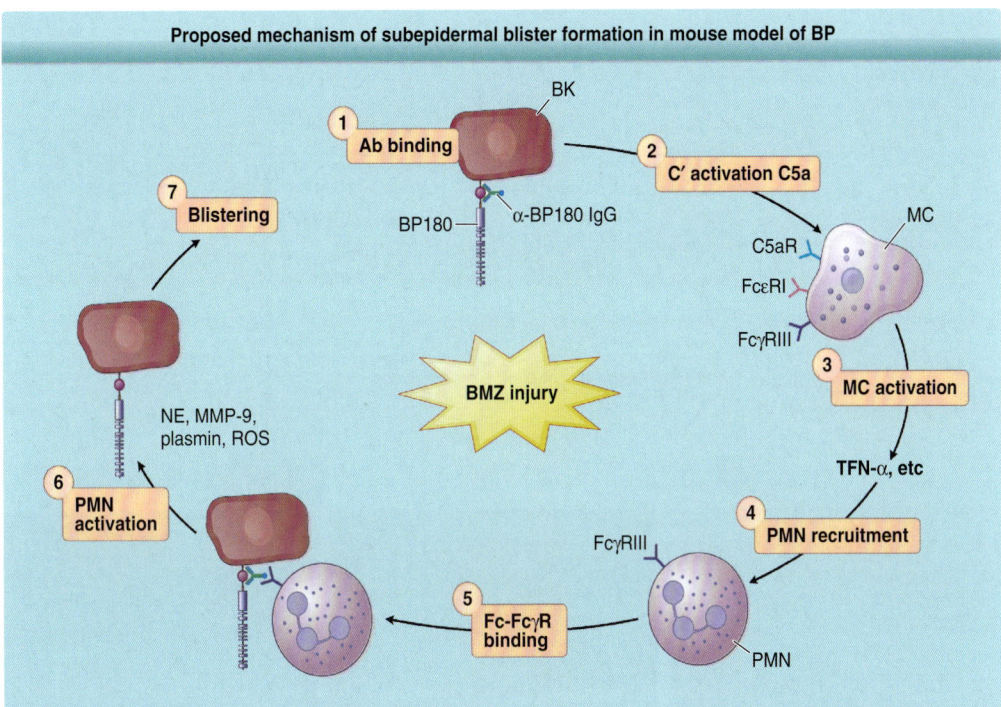

Figure 54-2 Proposed mechanism of subepidermal blister formation in mouse model of bullous pemphigoid (BP). Subepidermal blistering is an inflammatory process that involves the following steps: (1) anti-BP180 IgG binds to the pathogenic epitope of BP180 antigen on the surface of basal keratinocytes (BK). (2) The molecular interaction between BP180 antigen and anti-BP180 IgG activates the classical pathway of the complement system (C') (3) C' activation products C3a and C5a cause mast cells (MCs) to degranulate. (4) Tumor necrosis factor-α and other proinflammatory mediators released by MCs recruit neutrophils (PMNs). (5) Infiltrating PMNs bind to the BP180-anti-BP180 immune complex via the molecular interaction between Fcγ receptor III (FcγRIII) on neutrophils and the Fc domain of anti-BP180 IgG. (6) The interaction between Fc and FcγRIII activates PMNs to release neutrophil elastase (NE), gelatinase B (MMP-9), plasminogen activators (PAs), and reactive oxygen species (ROS). (7) Proteolytic enzymes and ROS work together to degrade BP180 and other extracellular matrix proteins, leading to subepidermal blistering.

DQB1*0302 alleles are associated with an increased risk of bullous pemphigoid among patients of Japanese descent.[165]

Neurologic disease is seen frequently in bullous pemphigoid patients. Recent studies have shown that patients with neurologic disease, including dementia, stroke, and Parkinson disease, have a significantly higher risk of developing bullous pemphigoid than those without neurological disease.[166,167]

Although there have been many case reports of bullous pemphigoid associated with malignancy, case-control studies have revealed conflicting data regarding the frequency of malignancy in bullous pemphigoid patients compared with age-matched control participants.[168-171] Most studies have shown no increased risk of malignancy in bullous pemphigoid patients.[172,173] However, recent evidence suggests that hematologic malignancies may be increased in patients with bullous pemphigoid.[174] Although a thorough review of systems and symptom guided workup is indicated in patients with a new diagnosis of bullous pemphigoid, extensive screening for an asymptomatic malignancy is not necessary.

DIAGNOSIS

The diagnosis of bullous pemphigoid is made based on clinical, histologic, and IF features.

PATHOLOGY

Biopsy of an early small vesicle is diagnostic with histology revealing a subepidermal blister with a superficial dermal infiltrate consisting of eosinophils, neutrophils, lymphocytes, and monocytes and macrophages (Fig. 54-4).[15] The infiltrate ranges from intense (classic) to sparse (cell poor) but characteristically contains eosinophils and neutrophils, which may also be seen in the blister cavity. The blister roof is usually viable without evidence of necrosis. Histology of urticarial lesions may only show a superficial dermal infiltrate of lymphocytes, monocytes and macrophages, and eosinophils with papillary dermal edema or eosinophilic spongiosis.[175]

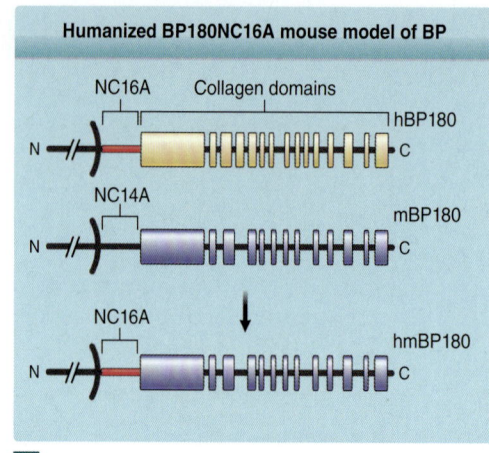
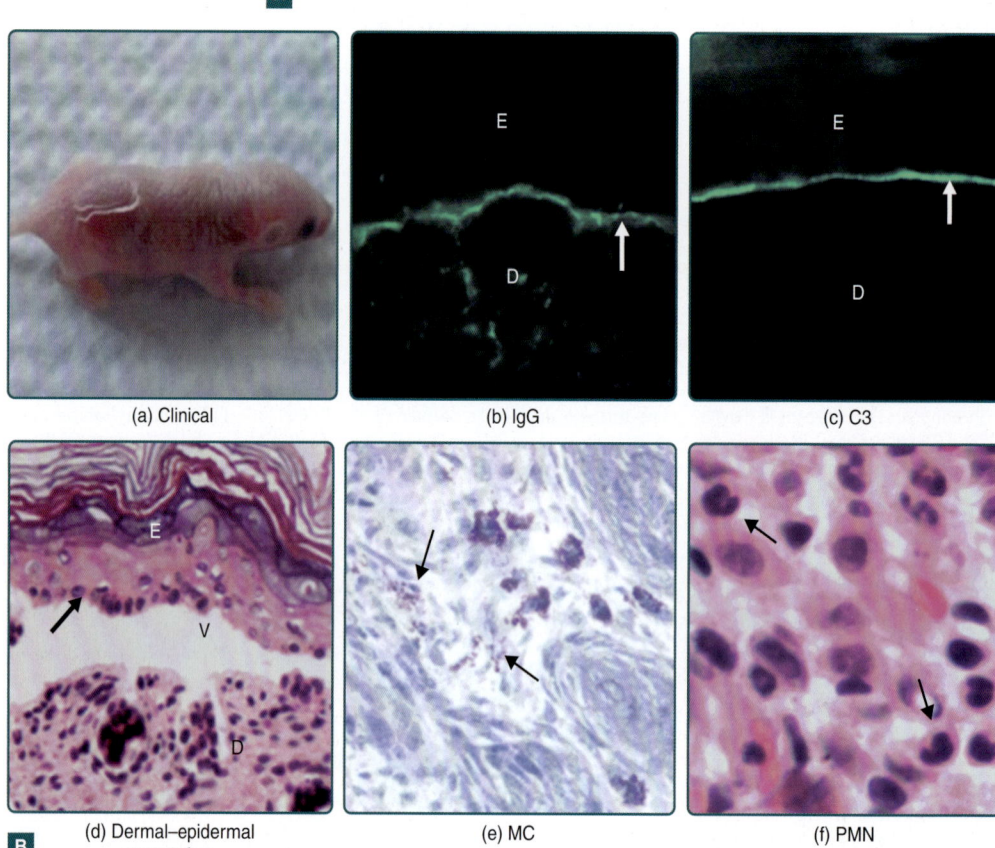

Figure 54-3 Humanized BP180NC16A mouse model of bullous pemphigoid (BP). **A,** Human BP180 (*top panel*) is a transmembrane protein of basal keratinocytes. It contains a single transmembrane domain. The extracellular region is consisted of 15 interrupted collagen domains (yellow bars) and 16 noncollagen domains (black lines). The NC16A domain (red line) harbors immunodominant epitopes recognized by BP autoantibodies. The extracellular region of mouse BP180 (*middle panel*) contains 13 collagen domains (blue bars) and 14 noncollagen domain (black lines). In humanized BP180NC16A mice, the mouse BP180NC14A domain was replaced by the human NC16A domain (*lower panel*). **B,** Neonatal NC16A mice injected intradermally (i.d.) with BP180NC16A-specific immunoglobulin (Ig) G autoantibodies developed clinical blistering (*a*). Direct immunofluorescence showed basement membrane zone (BMZ)deposition of human IgG (*b*) and murine C3 (*c*). Histologic sections of lesional skin showed dermal–epidermal separation (*d*). Examination of toluidine blue–stained skin sections revealed degranulating mast cells (MCs) (*e*). Hematoxylin and eosin staining showed infiltrating neutrophils (PMNs) in the upper dermis (400× magnification). (*f*).Arrows in *b* to *d* indicate basal keratinocytes. D, dermis; E, epidermis; V, vesicle.

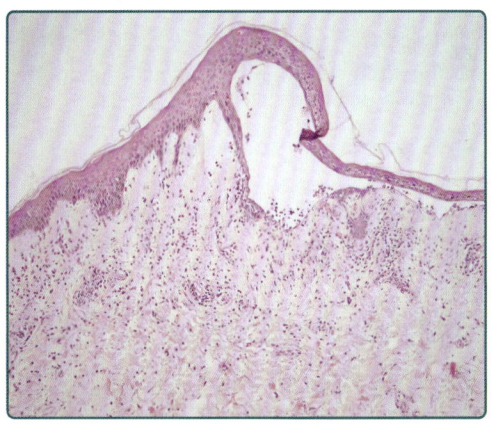

Figure 54-4 Histopathology of bullous pemphigoid. Subepidermal blister with an inflammatory cell infiltrate containing eosinophils in the superficial dermis (100× magnification).

IMMUNOFLUORESCENCE

Direct IF of perilesional skin shows linear IgG (usually IgG1 and IgG4, although all IgG subclasses and IgE have been reported) and C3 along the basement membrane[2,44,55,176,177] (Fig. 54-5). In approximately 70% of patients, there are circulating IgG autoantibodies that bind the BMZ on normal human skin or monkey esophagus by indirect IF.[44,55,57,105,176,178-180] The use of 1-M NaCl split skin, which separates the epidermis from the dermis at the lamina lucida, as the substrate for indirect IF testing is more sensitive for the detection of circulating anti-BMZ autoantibodies.[181,182] In addition to being more sensitive, the other advantage of the 1-M NaCl-split skin substrate is that it allows for the differentiation between bullous pemphigoid and epidermolysis bullosa acquisita (EBA) antibodies. Whereas bullous pemphigoid antibodies bind the epidermal side of the artificially induced blister (ie, the bottom of the basal cells), antibodies from EBA bind the dermal side of split skin (Fig. 54-6). In contrast to pemphigus, indirect IF antibody titers do not usually correlate with disease extent or activity in bullous pemphigoid.[183]

ELISA testing has also proven to be useful in both clinical and research settings for the detection of circulating antigen-specific autoantibodies. Commercial kits are available for detection of both BP-180 (NC16A and total) and BP-230 IgG antibodies. A sensitivity of 89% and specificity of 98% when used with appropriate cutoff values are reported with these assays.[97]

As many as 75% of patients also have antigen specific IgE with anti-BP180 and anti-BP230 IgE antibodies detectable by IF and ELISA.[104,106,179,184-187] Antigen-specific IgE antibodies may correlate with

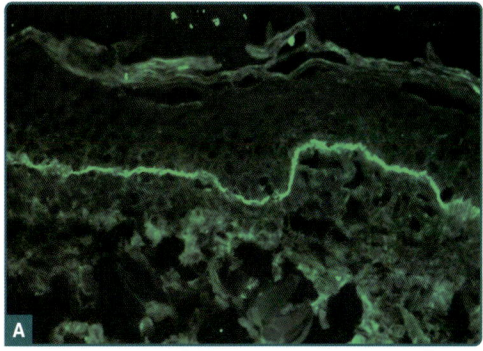

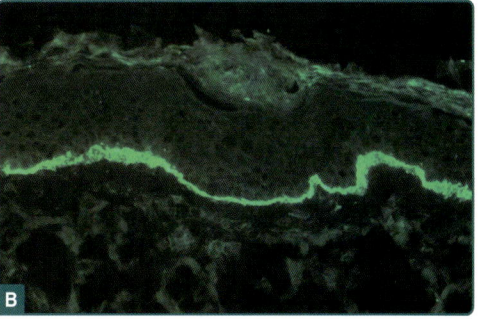

Figure 54-5 Direct immunofluorescence of bullous pemphigoid perilesional tissue shows a linear pattern of immunoglobulin G (**A**) and C3 (**B**) deposition along the epidermal–dermal junction.

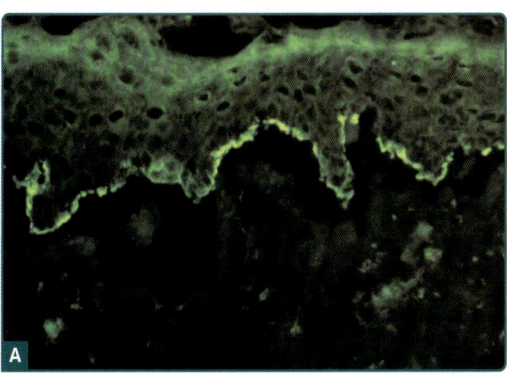

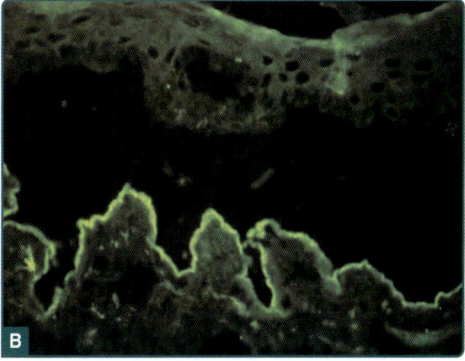

Figure 54-6 Indirect immunofluorescence on normal skin previously incubated in 1-M NaCl to induce a split through the lamina lucida of the dermal epidermal junction. **A,** Immunoglobulin (Ig) G antibodies from bullous pemphigoid serum binds to the epidermal side (roof) of the artificial blister (BP180 and BP230 of hemidesmosomes). **B,** IgG antibodies from epidermolysis bullosa acquisita (EBA) serum binds to the dermal side (floor) of the split (collagen VII of anchoring fibers).

disease severity and could play a role in recruiting eosinophils to skin lesions.[141,184,188]

Approximately 7% of the normal population has anti-BP180 antibodies detectable by ELISA in the absence of clinical and histologic features of disease without age or gender predilection. The relevance of this positivity is not known because long-term follow-up data are not available. However, this finding underscores the importance of using ELISA in appropriate clinical settings and not as a screening tool in patients who lack other features of disease.[189,190]

DIFFERENTIAL DIAGNOSIS

The differential diagnosis for bullous pemphigoid includes other autoimmune-mediated blistering diseases, such as linear IgA disease, dermatitis herpetiformis, EBA and pemphigus (Table 54-1) but also non–autoimmune-mediated disorders that can result in blistering, including contact dermatitis, dyshidrosis, bullous bite reactions, and stasis dermatitis with bullae formation. Histology, direct IF, and indirect IF studies can easily distinguish bullous pemphigoid from these diseases (Table 54-2). Distinguishing bullous pemphigoid from EBA and cicatricial pemphigoid may be difficult because histology and direct IF may be identical.[46,191] EBA can usually be distinguished from bullous pemphigoid by indirect or direct IF on salt split skin as stated earlier.[192]

As opposed to bullous pemphigoid, cicatricial pemphigoid usually presents with mucosal lesions predominantly, if not exclusively (see Chap. 55). Cicatricial pemphigoid is characterized by desquamative gingivitis as well as inflammation and scarring of conjunctiva. If there is blistering of the skin, it may be localized to the head and neck and may also result in scarring. Large, tense blisters, which are characteristic of bullous pemphigoid, are usually not seen in cicatricial pemphigoid.

CLINICAL COURSE AND PROGNOSIS

Bullous pemphigoid is characterized by a waxing and waning course with occasional spontaneous remission in the absence of treatment. Localized disease is more likely to resolve spontaneously, but spontaneous remission can even occur in patients with more generalized disease. For example, before the availability of systemic corticosteroids, Lever reported that 8 of 30 adults with bullous pemphigoid went into remission after approximately 15 months (range, 3 to 38 months) of active disease.[15] In treated patients, the length of disease ranges from 9 weeks to 17 years with a median treatment period of 2 years and 50% remission rates in patients followed for at least 3 years.[193] Clinical remission with reversion of direct and indirect IF to negative has been noted in patients, even those with severe generalized disease treated with oral corticosteroids alone or with azathioprine.[55,194] High ELISA

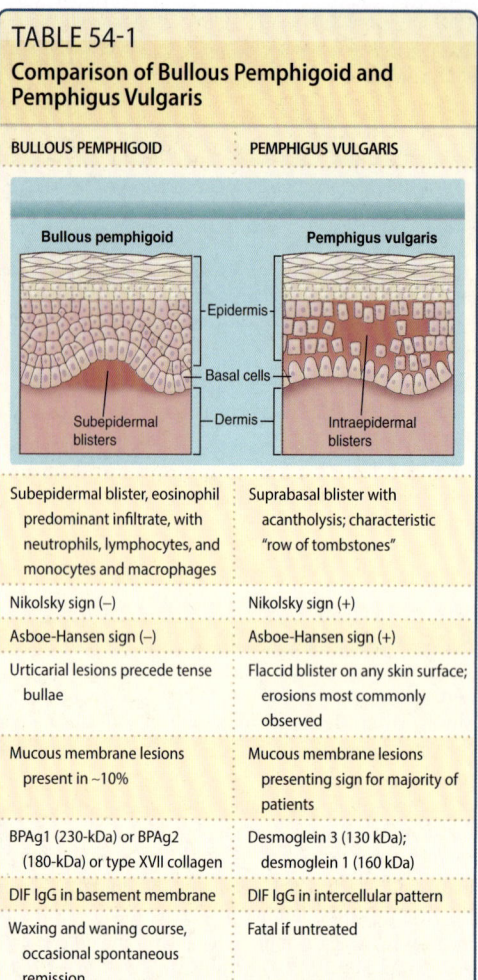

TABLE 54-1
Comparison of Bullous Pemphigoid and Pemphigus Vulgaris

BULLOUS PEMPHIGOID	PEMPHIGUS VULGARIS
Subepidermal blister, eosinophil predominant infiltrate, with neutrophils, lymphocytes, and monocytes and macrophages	Suprabasal blister with acantholysis; characteristic "row of tombstones"
Nikolsky sign (−)	Nikolsky sign (+)
Asboe-Hansen sign (−)	Asboe-Hansen sign (+)
Urticarial lesions precede tense bullae	Flaccid blister on any skin surface; erosions most commonly observed
Mucous membrane lesions present in ~10%	Mucous membrane lesions presenting sign for majority of patients
BPAg1 (230-kDa) or BPAg2 (180-kDa) or type XVII collagen	Desmoglein 3 (130 kDa); desmoglein 1 (160 kDa)
DIF IgG in basement membrane	DIF IgG in intercellular pattern
Waxing and waning course, occasional spontaneous remission	Fatal if untreated

DIF, direct immunofluorescence; IgG, immunoglobulin G.

TABLE 54-2
Differential Diagnosis of Bullous Pemphigoid

Subepidermal Blistering Diseases with Autoantibodies
- Pemphigoid gestationis
- Cicatricial pemphigoid
- Epidermolysis bullosa acquisita (EBA)
- Linear immunoglobulin A disease
- Dermatitis herpetiformis
- Bullous lupus erythematosus, described as an EBA phenotype

Subepidermal Blistering Diseases without Autoantibodies
- Erythema multiforme and toxic epidermal necrolysis
- Porphyria
- Epidermolysis bullosa (genodermatoses)

Intraepidermal Blistering Diseases with Autoantibodies
- Pemphigus

Intraepidermal Blistering Diseases without Autoantibodies
- Allergic contact dermatitis
- Bullous impetigo, staphylococcal scalded-skin syndrome
- Friction blisters
- Hailey-Hailey disease
- Incontinentia pigmenti

titers and positive direct IF at the time of therapy cessation has been associated with a high risk of relapse within the first year after cessation of therapy.[194,195] At least one of these tests should be considered before therapy is discontinued. Old age, poor general health, neurologic disease, extensive disease, and the presence of anti-BP180 antibodies have been associated with a poor prognosis and relapse within the first year of treatment.[196-200]

Early mortality rates in untreated patients were reported to be 25%.[15] Newer studies have shown the 1-year mortality rate of patients with bullous pemphigoid to be between 19% and 40% in Europe but possibly lower (6% to 19%) in the United States.[13,14,196-198,201-204] The factors underlying this discrepancy in mortality rates between Europe and the United States are not clear; in fact, recent studies have suggested a slow, steady increase in mortality rate over the past 24 years in the United States.[205] Extent of disease does not contribute to differences in overall survival.[14]

TABLE 54-3
Treatments for Bullous Pemphigoid

Corticosteroids
- High-potency topical steroids
- Prednisone

Other Immunosuppressive Agents
- Azathioprine
- Mycophenolate mofetil
- Methotrexate

Modulators of Antibody Levels
- Intravenous gammaglobulin
- Plasmapheresis

Other
- Tetracycline or erythromycin and nicotinamide
- Dapsone
- Omalizumab

B-Cell Depletion
- Rituximab

MANAGEMENT

MEDICATIONS

Treatment depends on multiple factors, including extent of disease and patient comorbidities.[206] Patients with localized bullous pemphigoid often can be treated successfully with topical corticosteroids alone (Table 54-3).[55,176,207]

Patients with more extensive disease are usually treated with oral prednisone.[207-209] Despite the lack of randomized controlled trials, oral prednisone remains the mainstay of therapy. Studies also suggest that potent topical steroids, such as clobetasol proprionate cream 0.05% applied twice daily, are also effective in both moderate and severe bullous pemphigoid and may be safer than oral prednisone.[203] High-potency topical treatment does result in significant systemic absorption and therefore may act via local and systemic effects.[210] Such topical therapy can be expensive and difficult to apply, which may prove prohibitive in many patients.

In older adult patients, the complications of systemic glucocorticoid therapy (eg, osteoporosis, diabetes, and immunosuppression) may be especially severe.[211] Therefore, it is important to try to minimize the total dose and duration of therapy with oral glucocorticoids. Starting doses of prednisone of 0.75 to 1.0 mg/kg/day or even less may be adequate for disease control.[212] In addition, immunosuppressive agents such as methotrexate, azathioprine, and mycophenolate mofetil are often used in conjunction with prednisone for their potential steroid-sparing effects,[207,209,213-222] although very few controlled trials have addressed this common approach to therapy. After the development of blisters has been arrested (consolidation phase), a careful tapering of the prednisone is recommended.[51] A weekly lowering of 5 mg to reach 30 mg is recommended, after which an alternating-day tapering regimen is typically initiated. Prednisone tapering must be done according to the clinical response and side effects of the patient. The majority of disease may be controlled with small amounts of prednisone and immunosuppressive drugs.

Sulfones may be effective in a minority of patients. Dapsone and sulfapyridine have been reported to control disease activity in 15% to 44% of patients with bullous pemphigoid.[209,223-225] Reports have described successful treatment of some bullous pemphigoid patients with tetracycline and nicotinamide or variations on this theme, such as erythromycin and nicotinamide or tetracycline alone.[226-228] Other effective therapies include plasmapheresis,[229] intravenous immunoglobulins,[230-232] omalizumab,[233,234] and rituximab.[235,236]

REFERENCES

1. Lever WF. Pemphigus. *Medicine (Baltimore)*. 1953; 32(1):1-123.
2. Jordon RE, Beutner EH, Witebsky E, et al. Basement zone antibodies in bullous pemphigoid. *JAMA*. 1967;200(9):751-756.
3. Labib RS, Anhalt GJ, Patel HP, et al. Molecular heterogeneity of the bullous pemphigoid antigens as detected by immunoblotting. *J Immunol*. 1986;136(4):1231-1235.
4. Stanley JR, Hawley-Nelson P, Yuspa SH, et al. Characterization of bullous pemphigoid antigen: a unique basement membrane protein of stratified squamous epithelia. *Cell*. 1981;24(3):897-903.
5. Mutasim DF, Takahashi Y, Labib RS, et al. A pool of bullous pemphigoid antigen(s) is intracellular and associated with the basal cell cytoskeleton-hemidesmosome complex. *J Invest Dermatol*. 1985; 84(1):47-53.
6. Gudi VS, White MI, Cruickshank N, et al. Annual incidence and mortality of bullous pemphigoid in the Grampian Region of North-east Scotland. *Br J Dermatol*. 2005;153(2):424-427.
7. Amos B, Deng JS, Flynn K, et al. Bullous pemphigoid in infancy: case report and literature review. *Pediatr Dermatol*. 1998;15(2):108-111.

8. Fisler RE, Saeb M, Liang MG, et al. Childhood bullous pemphigoid: a clinicopathologic study and review of the literature. *Am J Dermatopathol*. 2003; 25(3):183-189.
9. Gajic-Veljic M, Nikolic M, Medenica L. Juvenile bullous pemphigoid: the presentation and follow-up of six cases. *J Eur Acad Dermatol Venereol*. 2010;24(1):69-72.
10. Trueb RM, Didierjean L, Fellas A, et al. Childhood bullous pemphigoid: report of a case with characterization of the targeted antigens. *J Am Acad Dermatol*. 1999;40(2 Pt 2):338-344.
11. Zillikens D, Wever S, Roth A, et al. Incidence of autoimmune subepidermal blistering dermatoses in a region of central Germany. *Arch Dermatol*. 1995;131(8):957-958.
12. Joly P, Baricault S, Sparsa A, et al. Incidence and mortality of bullous pemphigoid in France. *J Invest Dermatol*. 2012;132(8):1998-2004.
13. Langan SM, Smeeth L, Hubbard R, et al. Bullous pemphigoid and pemphigus vulgaris—incidence and mortality in the UK: population based cohort study. *BMJ*. 2008;337:a180.
14. Brick KE, Weaver CH, Lohse CM, et al. Incidence of bullous pemphigoid and mortality of patients with bullous pemphigoid in Olmsted County, Minnesota, 1960 through 2009. *J Am Acad Dermatol*. 2014;71(1): 92-99.
15. Lever WF. *Pemphigus and Pemphigoid*. Springfield, IL: Charles C Thomas;1965.
16. Yancey KB, Egan CA. Pemphigoid: clinical, histologic, immunopathologic, and therapeutic considerations. *JAMA*. 2000;284(3):350-356.
17. Sun C, Chang B, Gu H. Non-bullous lesions as the first manifestation of bullous pemphigoid: a retrospective analysis of 24 cases. *J Dermatolog Treat*. 2009;20(4):233-237.
18. Borradori L, Prost C, Wolkenstein P, et al. Localized pretibial pemphigoid and pemphigoid nodularis. *J Am Acad Dermatol*. Nov 1992;27(5 Pt 2):863-867.
19. Amato L, Gallerani I, Mei S, et al. Erythrodermic bullous pemphigoid. *Int J Dermatol*. 2001;40(5):343-346.
20. Chan LS, Dorman MA, Agha A, et al. Pemphigoid vegetans represents a bullous pemphigoid variant. Patient's IgG autoantibodies identify the major bullous pemphigoid antigen. *J Am Acad Dermatol*. 1993;28(2 Pt 2):331-335.
21. Kim J, Chavel S, Girardi M, et al. Pemphigoid vegetans: a case report and review of the literature. *J Cutan Pathol*. 2008;35(12):1144-1147.
22. Korman NJ, Woods SG. Erythrodermic bullous pemphigoid is a clinical variant of bullous pemphigoid. *Br J Dermatol*. 1995;133(6):967-971.
23. Scrivener Y, Heid E, Grosshans E, et al. Erythrodermic bullous pemphigoid. *J Am Acad Dermatol*. 1999; 41(4):658-659.
24. Tashiro H, Arai H, Hashimoto T, et al. Pemphigoid nodularis: two case studies and analysis of autoantibodies before and after the development of generalized blistering. *J Nippon Med Sch*. 2005;72(1):60-65.
25. Person JR, Rogers RS 3rd, Perry HO. Localized pemphigoid. *Br J Dermatol*. 1976;95(5):531-534.
26. Provost TT, Maize JC, Ahmed AR, et al. Unusual subepidermal bullous diseases with immunologic features of bullous pemphigoid. *Arch Dermatol*. 1979;115(2):156-160.
27. Ogbechie OA, Eastham AB, Vleugels RA. Tense bullae on the palms and soles. *JAMA Dermatol*. 2015; 151(1):99-100.
28. Kim YJ, Kim MY, Kim HO, et al. Dyshidrosiform bullous pemphigoid. *Acta Derm Venereol*. 2004;84(3): 253-254.
29. Sugimura C, Katsuura J, Moriue T, et al. Dyshidrosiform pemphigoid: report of a case. *J Dermatol*. 2003;30(7): 525-529.
30. Yasuda M, Miyachi Y, Utani A. Two cases of dyshidrosiform pemphigoid with different presentations. *Clin Exp Dermatol*. 2009;34(5):e151-153.
31. Calikoglu E, Anadolu R, Erdem C, et al. Localized bullous pemphigoid as an unusual complication of radiation therapy. *J Eur Acad Dermatol Venereol*. 2002;16(6):646-647.
32. Hafejee A, Coulson IH. Localized bullous pemphigoid 20 years after split skin grafting. *Clin Exp Dermatol*. 2005;30(2):187-188.
33. Macfarlane AW, Verbov JL. Trauma-induced bullous pemphigoid. *Clin Exp Dermatol*. 1989;14(3):245-249.
34. Massa MC, Freeark RJ, Kang JS. Localized bullous pemphigoid occurring in a surgical wound. *Dermatol Nurs*. 1996;8(2):101-103.
35. Melani L, Giomi B, Antiga E, et al. Radiation therapy as a trigger factor for initially localized bullous pemphigoid. *Breast J*. 2005;11(6):485-486.
36. Ohata C, Shirabe H, Takagi K, et al. Localized bullous pemphigoid after radiation therapy: two cases. *Acta Derm Venereol*. 1997;77(2):157.
37. Pardo J, Rodrguez-Serna M, Mercader P, et al. Localized bullous pemphigoid overlying a fistula for hemodialysis. *J Am Acad Dermatol*. 2004;51(2 suppl):S131-132.
38. Torchia D, Caproni M, Ketabchi S, et al. Bullous pemphigoid initially localized around a urostomy. *Int J Dermatol*. 2006;45(11):1387-1389.
39. Vande Maele DM, Reilly JC. Bullous pemphigoid at colostomy site: report of a case. *Dis Colon Rectum*. 1997;40(3):370-371.
40. Nemeth AJ, Klein AD, Gould EW, et al. Childhood bullous pemphigoid. Clinical and immunologic features, treatment, and prognosis. *Arch Dermatol*. 1991; 127(3):378-386.
41. Farrell AM, Kirtschig G, Dalziel KL, et al. Childhood vulval pemphigoid: a clinical and immunopathological study of five patients. *Br J Dermatol*. 1999;140(2):308-312.
42. Schumann H, Amann U, Tasanen K, et al. A child with localized vulval pemphigoid and IgG autoantibodies targeting the C-terminus of collagen XVII/BP180. *Br J Dermatol*. 1999;140(6):1133-1138.
43. Domloge-Hultsch N, Utecht L, James W, et al. Autoantibodies from patients with localized and generalized bullous pemphigoid immunoprecipitate the same 230-kd keratinocyte antigen. *Arch Dermatol*. 1990;126(10):1337-1341.
44. Person JR, Rogers RS 3rd. Bullous and cicatricial pemphigoid. Clinical, histopathologic, and immunopathologic correlations. *Mayo Clin Proc*. 1977;52(1):54-66.
45. Sollecito TP, Parisi E. Mucous membrane pemphigoid. *Dent Clin North Am*. 2005;49(1):91-106, viii.
46. Venning VA, Frith PA, Bron AJ, et al. Mucosal involvement in bullous and cicatricial pemphigoid. A clinical and immunopathological study. *Br J Dermatol*. 1988;118(1):7-15.
47. Demircay Z, Baykal C, Demirkesen C. Lichen planus pemphigoides: report of two cases. *Int J Dermatol*. 1;40(12):757-759.
48. Hsu S, Ghohestani RF, Uitto J. Lichen planus pemphigoides with IgG autoantibodies to the 180 kd bullous

48. ...pemphigoid antigen (type XVII collagen). *J Am Acad Dermatol*. 000;42(1 Pt 1):136-141.
49. Maceyko RF, Camisa C, Bergfeld WF, et al. Oral and cutaneous lichen planus pemphigoides. *J Am Acad Dermatol*. 1992;27(5 Pt 2):889-892.
50. Stingl G, Holubar K. Coexistence of lichen planus and bullous pemphigoid. A immunopathological study. *Br J Dermatol*. 1975;93(3):313-320.
51. Murrell DF, Daniel BS, Joly P, et al. Definitions and outcome measures for bullous pemphigoid: recommendations by an international panel of experts. *J Am Acad Dermatol*. 2012;66(3):479-485.
52. Wijayanti A, Zhao CY, Boettiger D, et al. The reliability, validity and responsiveness of two disease scores (BPDAI and ABSIS) for bullous pemphigoid: which one to use? *Acta Derm Venereol*. 2017, 4; 97(1):24-31.
53. Arbesman CE, Wypych JI, Reisman RE, et al. IgE levels in sera of patients with pemphigus or bullous pemphigoid. *Arch Dermatol*. 1974;110(3): 378-381.
54. Baba T, Sonozaki H, Seki K, et al. An eosinophil chemotactic factor present in blister fluids of bullous pemphigoid patients. *J Immunol*. 1976;116(1):112-116.
55. Hadi SM, Barnetson RS, Gawkrodger DJ, et al. Clinical, histological and immunological studies in 50 patients with bullous pemphigoid. *Dermatologica*. 1988;176(1):6-17.
56. Bernard P, Venot J, Constant F, et al. Blood eosinophilia as a severity marker for bullous pemphigoid. *J Am Acad Dermatol*. 1987;16(4):879-881.
57. Bushkell LL, Jordon RE. Bullous pemphigoid: a cause of peripheral blood eosinophilia. *J Am Acad Dermatol*. 1983;8(5):648-651.
58. van Beek N, Schulze FS, Zillikens D, et al. IgE-mediated mechanisms in bullous pemphigoid and other autoimmune bullous diseases. *Expert Rev Clin Immunol*. 2016;12(3):267-277.
59. Phoon YW, Fook-Chong SM, Koh HY, et al. Infectious complications in bullous pemphigoid: an analysis of risk factors. *J Am Acad Dermatol*. 2015;72(5):834-839.
60. Lehman JS, el-Azhary RA. Kaposi varicelliform eruption in patients with autoimmune bullous dermatoses. *Int J Dermatol*. 2016;55(3):e136-140.
61. Barrick BJ, Barrick JD, Weaver CH, et al. Herpes zoster in patients with bullous pemphigoid: a population-based case-control and cohort study. *Br J Dermatol*. 2016;174(5):1112-1114.
62. Cram DL, Fukuyama K. Immunohistochemistry of ultraviolet-induced pemphigus and pemphigoid lesions. *Arch Dermatol*. 1972;106(6):819-824.
63. Mul VE, van Geest AJ, Pijls-Johannesma MC, et al. Radiation-induced bullous pemphigoid: a systematic review of an unusual radiation side effect. *Radiother Oncol*. 2007;82(1):5-9.
64. Thomsen K, Schmidt H. PUVA-induced bullous pemphigoid. *Br J Dermatol*. 1976;95(5):568-569.
65. Bastuji-Garin S, Joly P, Picard-Dahan C, et al. Drugs associated with bullous pemphigoid. A case-control study. *Arch Dermatol*. 1996;132(3):272-276.
66. Bordignon M, Belloni-Fortina A, Pigozzi B, et al. Bullous pemphigoid during long-term TNF-alpha blocker therapy. *Dermatology*. 2009;219(4):357-358.
67. Duong TA, Buffard V, Andre C, et al. Efalizumab-induced bullous pemphigoid. *J Am Acad Dermatol*. 2010;62(1):161-162.
68. Lee JJ, Downham TF 2nd. Furosemide-induced bullous pemphigoid: case report and review of literature. *J Drugs Dermatol*. 2006;5(6):562-564.
69. Monnier-Murina K, Du Thanh A, Merlet-Albran S, et al. Bullous pemphigoid occurring during efalizumab treatment for psoriasis: a paradoxical auto-immune reaction? *Dermatology*. 2009;219(1):89-90.
70. Popadic S, Skiljevic D, Medenica L. Bullous pemphigoid induced by penicillamine in a patient with Wilson disease. *Am J Clin Dermatol*. 2009;10(1):36-38.
71. Stavropoulos PG, Soura E, Antoniou C. Drug-induced pemphigoid: a review of the literature. *J Eur Acad Dermatol Venereol*. 2014;28(9):1133-1140.
72. Jour G, Glitza IC, Ellis RM, et al. Autoimmune dermatologic toxicities from immune checkpoint blockade with anti-PD-1 antibody therapy: a report on bullous skin eruptions. *J Cutan Pathol*. 2016;43(8):688-696.
73. Naidoo J, Schindler K, Querfeld C, et al. Autoimmune bullous skin disorders with immune checkpoint inhibitors targeting PD-1 and PD-L1. *Cancer Immunol Res*. 2016;4(5):383-389.
74. Hwang SJ, Carlos G, Chou S, et al. Bullous pemphigoid, an autoantibody-mediated disease, is a novel immune-related adverse event in patients treated with anti-programmed cell death 1 antibodies. *Melanoma Res*. 2016;26(4):413-416.
75. Mutasim DF, Morrison LH, Takahashi Y, et al. Definition of bullous pemphigoid antibody binding to intracellular and extracellular antigen associated with hemidesmosomes. *J Invest Dermatol*. 1989;92(2):225-230.
76. Stanley JR. Cell adhesion molecules as targets of autoantibodies in pemphigus and pemphigoid, bullous diseases due to defective epidermal cell adhesion. *Adv Immunol*. 1993;53:291-325.
77. Thoma-Uszynski S, Uter W, Schwietzke S, et al. BP230- and BP180-specific auto-antibodies in bullous pemphigoid. *J Invest Dermatol*. 2004;122(6):1413-1422.
78. Yoshida M, Hamada T, Amagai M, et al. Enzyme-linked immunosorbent assay using bacterial recombinant proteins of human BP230 as a diagnostic tool for bullous pemphigoid. *J Dermatol Sci*. 2006; 41(1):21-30.
79. Green KJ, Virata ML, Elgart GW, et al. Comparative structural analysis of desmoplakin, bullous pemphigoid antigen and plectin: members of a new gene family involved in organization of intermediate filaments. *Int J Biol Macromol*. 1992;14(3):145-153.
80. Stanley JR, Tanaka T, Mueller S, et al. Isolation of complementary DNA for bullous pemphigoid antigen by use of patients' autoantibodies. *J Clin Invest*. 1988;82(6):1864-1870.
81. Tanaka T, Korman NJ, Shimizu H, et al. Production of rabbit antibodies against carboxy-terminal epitopes encoded by bullous pemphigoid cDNA. *J Invest Dermatol*. 1990;94(5):617-623.
82. Guo L, Degenstein L, Dowling J, et al. Gene targeting of BPAG1: abnormalities in mechanical strength and cell migration in stratified epithelia and neurologic degeneration. *Cell*. 1995;81(2):233-243.
83. Brown A, Bernier G, Mathieu M, et al. The mouse dystonia musculorum gene is a neural isoform of bullous pemphigoid antigen 1. *Nat Genet*. 1995; 10(3):301-306.
84. Yang Y, Dowling J, Yu QC, et al. An essential cytoskeletal linker protein connecting actin microfilaments to intermediate filaments. *Cell*. 1996;86(4):655-665.
85. Haase C, Budinger L, Borradori L, et al. Detection of IgG autoantibodies in the sera of patients with bullous and gestational pemphigoid: ELISA studies utilizing

a baculovirus-encoded form of bullous pemphigoid antigen 2. *J Invest Dermatol.* 1998;110(3):282-286.
86. Zillikens D, Mascaro JM, Rose PA, et al. A highly sensitive enzyme-linked immunosorbent assay for the detection of circulating anti-BP180 autoantibodies in patients with bullous pemphigoid. *J Invest Dermatol.* 1997;109(5):679-683.
87. Bedane C, McMillan JR, Balding SD, et al. Bullous pemphigoid and cicatricial pemphigoid autoantibodies react with ultrastructurally separable epitopes on the BP180 ectodomain: evidence that BP180 spans the lamina lucida. *J Invest Dermatol.* 1997;108(6):901-907.
88. Diaz LA, Ratrie H 3rd, Saunders WS, et al. Isolation of a human epidermal cDNA corresponding to the 180-kD autoantigen recognized by bullous pemphigoid and herpes gestationis sera. Immunolocalization of this protein to the hemidesmosome. *J Clin Invest.* 1990;86(4):1088-1094.
89. Giudice GJ, Emery DJ, Diaz LA. Cloning and primary structural analysis of the bullous pemphigoid autoantigen BP180. *J Invest Dermatol.* 1992;99(3):243-250.
90. Giudice GJ, Squiquera HL, Elias PM, et al. Identification of two collagen domains within the bullous pemphigoid autoantigen, BP180. *J Clin Invest.* 1991;87(2):734-738.
91. Hopkinson SB, Riddelle KS, Jones JC. Cytoplasmic domain of the 180-kD bullous pemphigoid antigen, a hemidesmosomal component: molecular and cell biologic characterization. *J Invest Dermatol.* 1992;99(3):264-270.
92. Borradori L, Koch PJ, Niessen CM, et al. The localization of bullous pemphigoid antigen 180 (BP180) in hemidesmosomes is mediated by its cytoplasmic domain and seems to be regulated by the beta4 integrin subunit. *J Cell Biol.* 1997;136(6):1333-1347.
93. Ishiko A, Shimizu H, Kikuchi A, et al. Human autoantibodies against the 230-kD bullous pemphigoid antigen (BPAG1) bind only to the intracellular domain of the hemidesmosome, whereas those against the 180-kD bullous pemphigoid antigen (BPAG2) bind along the plasma membrane of the hemidesmosome in normal human and swine skin. *J Clin Invest.* 1993;91(4):1608-1615.
94. Masunaga T, Shimizu H, Yee C, et al. The extracellular domain of BPAG2 localizes to anchoring filaments and its carboxyl terminus extends to the lamina densa of normal human epidermal basement membrane. *J Invest Dermatol.* 1997;109(2):200-206.
95. Giudice GJ, Emery DJ, Zelickson BD, et al. Bullous pemphigoid and herpes gestationis autoantibodies recognize a common non-collagenous site on the BP180 ectodomain. *J Immunol.* 1993;151(10):5742-5750.
96. Zillikens D, Rose PA, Balding SD, et al. Tight clustering of extracellular BP180 epitopes recognized by bullous pemphigoid autoantibodies. *J Invest Dermatol.* 1997;109(4):573-579.
97. Sakuma-Oyama Y, Powell AM, Oyama N, et al. Evaluation of a BP180-NC16a enzyme-linked immunosorbent assay in the initial diagnosis of bullous pemphigoid. *Br J Dermatol.* 2004;151(1):126-131.
98. Schmidt E, Obe K, Brocker EB, et al. Serum levels of autoantibodies to BP180 correlate with disease activity in patients with bullous pemphigoid. *Arch Dermatol.* 2000;136(2):174-178.
99. Tsuji-Abe Y, Akiyama M, Yamanaka Y, et al. Correlation of clinical severity and ELISA indices for the NC16A domain of BP180 measured using BP180 ELISA kit in bullous pemphigoid. *J Dermatol Sci.* 2005;37(3):145-149.
100. Hofmann S, Thoma-Uszynski S, Hunziker T, et al. Severity and phenotype of bullous pemphigoid relate to autoantibody profile against the NH2- and COOH-terminal regions of the BP180 ectodomain. *J Invest Dermatol.* 2002;119(5):1065-1073.
101. Jonkman MF, de Jong MC, Heeres K, et al. 180-kD bullous pemphigoid antigen (BP180) is deficient in generalized atrophic benign epidermolysis bullosa. *J Clin Invest.* 1995;95(3):1345-1352.
102. McGrath JA, Darling T, Gatalica B, et al. A homozygous deletion mutation in the gene encoding the 180-kDa bullous pemphigoid antigen (BPAG2) in a family with generalized atrophic benign epidermolysis bullosa. *J Invest Dermatol.* 1996;106(4):771-774.
103. McGrath JA, Gatalica B, Christiano AM, et al. Mutations in the 180-kD bullous pemphigoid antigen (BPAG2), a hemidesmosomal transmembrane collagen (COL17A1), in generalized atrophic benign epidermolysis bullosa. *Nat Genet.* 1995;11(1):83-86.
104. Christophoridis S, Budinger L, Borradori L, et al. IgG, IgA and IgE autoantibodies against the ectodomain of BP180 in patients with bullous and cicatricial pemphigoid and linear IgA bullous dermatosis. *Br J Dermatol.* 2000;143(2):349-355.
105. Dimson OG, Giudice GJ, Fu CL, et al. Identification of a potential effector function for IgE autoantibodies in the organ-specific autoimmune disease bullous pemphigoid. *J Invest Dermatol.* 2003;120(5):784-788.
106. Dopp R, Schmidt E, Chimanovitch I, et al. IgG4 and IgE are the major immunoglobulins targeting the NC16A domain of BP180 in Bullous pemphigoid: serum levels of these immunoglobulins reflect disease activity. *J Am Acad Dermatol.* 2000;42(4):577-583.
107. Borrego L, Maynard B, Peterson EA, et al. Deposition of eosinophil granule proteins precedes blister formation in bullous pemphigoid. Comparison with neutrophil and mast cell granule proteins. *Am J Pathol.* 1996;148(3):897-909.
108. Czech W, Schaller J, Schopf E, et al. Granulocyte activation in bullous diseases: release of granular proteins in bullous pemphigoid and pemphigus vulgaris. *J Am Acad Dermatol.* 1993;29(2 Pt 1):210-215.
109. Dvorak AM, Mihm MC Jr, Osage JE, et al. Bullous pemphigoid, an ultrastructural study of the inflammatory response: eosinophil, basophil and mast cell granule changes in multiple biopsies from one patient. *J Invest Dermatol.* 1982;78(2):91-101.
110. Wintroub BU, Mihm MC Jr, Goetzl EJ, et al. Morphologic and functional evidence for release of mast-cell products in bullous pemphigoid. *N Engl J Med.* 1978;298(8):417-421.
111. D'Auria L, Cordiali Fei P, Ameglio F. Cytokines and bullous pemphigoid. *Eur Cytokine Netw.* 1999;10(2):123-134.
112. Diaz-Perez JL, Jordon RE. The complement system in bullous pemphigoid. IV. Chemotactic activity in blister fluid. *Clin Immunol Immunopathol.* 1976;5(3):360-370.
113. Katayama I, Doi T, Nishioka K. High histamine level in the blister fluid of bullous pemphigoid. *Arch Dermatol Res.* 1984;276(2):126-127.
114. Kawana S, Ueno A, Nishiyama S. Increased levels of immunoreactive leukotriene B4 in blister fluids of bullous pemphigoid patients and

effects of a selective 5-lipoxygenase inhibitor on experimental skin lesions. *Acta Derm Venereol*. 1990;70(4):281-285.

115. Schmidt E, Ambach A, Bastian B, et al. Elevated levels of interleukin-8 in blister fluid of bullous pemphigoid compared with suction blisters of healthy control subjects. *J Am Acad Dermatol*. 1996;34(2 Pt 1):310-312.

116. Schmidt E, Bastian B, Dummer R, et al. Detection of elevated levels of IL-4, IL-6, and IL-10 in blister fluid of bullous pemphigoid. *Arch Dermatol Res* 1996;288(7):353-357.

117. Schmidt E, Mittnacht A, Schomig H, et al. Detection of IL-1 alpha, IL-1 beta and IL-1 receptor antagonist in blister fluid of bullous pemphigoid. *J Dermatol Sci*. 1996;11(2):142-147.

118. Wakugawa M, Nakamura K, Hino H, et al. Elevated levels of eotaxin and interleukin-5 in blister fluid of bullous pemphigoid: correlation with tissue eosinophilia. *Br J Dermatol*. 2000;143(1):112-116.

119. Baird J, Lazarus GS, Belin D, et al. mRNA for tissue-type plasminogen activator is present in lesional epidermis from patients with psoriasis, pemphigus, or bullous pemphigoid, but is not detected in normal epidermis. *J Invest Dermatol*. 1990;95(5):548-552.

120. Gissler HM, Simon MM, Kramer MD. Enhanced association of plasminogen/plasmin with lesional epidermis of bullous pemphigoid. *Br J Dermatol*. 1992;127(3):272-277.

121. Kramer MD, Reinartz J. The autoimmune blistering skin disease bullous pemphigoid. The presence of plasmin/alpha 2-antiplasmin complexes in skin blister fluid indicates plasmin generation in lesional skin. *J Clin Invest*. 1993;92(2):978-983.

122. Lauharanta J, Salonen EM, Vaheri A. Plasmin-like proteinase associated with high molecular weight complexes in blister fluid of bullous pemphigoid. *Acta Derm Venereol*. 1989;69(6):527-529.

123. Oikarinen AI, Zone JJ, Ahmed AR, et al. Demonstration of collagenase and elastase activities in the blister fluids from bullous skin diseases. Comparison between dermatitis herpetiformis and bullous pemphigoid. *J Invest Dermatol*. 1983;81(3):261-266.

124. Schaefer BM, Jaeger C, Drepper E, et al. Plasminogen activation in bullous pemphigoid immunohistology reveals urokinase type plasminogen activator, its receptor and plasminogen activator inhibitor type-2 in lesional epidermis. *Autoimmunity*. 1996;23(3):155-164.

125. Stahle-Backdahl M, Inoue M, Guidice GJ, et al. 92-kD gelatinase is produced by eosinophils at the site of blister formation in bullous pemphigoid and cleaves the extracellular domain of recombinant 180-kD bullous pemphigoid autoantigen. *J Clin Invest*. 1994;93(5):2022-2030.

126. Verraes S, Hornebeck W, Polette M, et al. Respective contribution of neutrophil elastase and matrix metalloproteinase 9 in the degradation of BP180 (type XVII collagen) in human bullous pemphigoid. *J Invest Dermatol*. 2001;117(5):1091-1096.

127. Gammon WR, Merritt CC, Lewis DM, et al. An in vitro model of immune complex-mediated basement membrane zone separation caused by pemphigoid antibodies, leukocytes, and complement. *J Invest Dermatol*. 1982;78(4):285-290.

128. Sitaru C, Schmidt E, Petermann S, et al. Autoantibodies to bullous pemphigoid antigen 180 induce dermal-epidermal separation in cryosections of human skin. *J Invest Dermatol*. 2002;118(4):664-671.

129. Liu Z, Diaz LA, Troy JL, et al. A passive transfer model of the organ-specific autoimmune disease, bullous pemphigoid, using antibodies generated against the hemidesmosomal antigen, BP180. *J Clin Invest*. 1993;92(5):2480-2488.

130. Chen R, Ning G, Zhao ML, et al. Mast cells play a key role in neutrophil recruitment in experimental bullous pemphigoid. *J Clin Invest*. 2001;108(8):1151-1158.

131. Liu Z, Giudice GJ, Swartz SJ, et al. The role of complement in experimental bullous pemphigoid. *J Clin Invest*. 1995;95(4):1539-1544.

132. Liu Z, Giudice GJ, Zhou X, et al. A major role for neutrophils in experimental bullous pemphigoid. *J Clin Invest*. 1997;100(5):1256-1263.

133. Nelson KC, Zhao M, Schroeder PR, et al. Role of different pathways of the complement cascade in experimental bullous pemphigoid. *J Clin Invest*. 2006;116(11):2892-2900.

134. Liu Z. Bullous pemphigoid: using animal models to study the immunopathology. *J Investig Dermatol Symp Proc*. 2004;9(1):41-46.

135. Liu Z, Li N, Diaz LA, et al. Synergy between a plasminogen cascade and MMP-9 in autoimmune disease. *J Clin Invest*. 2005;115(4):879-887.

136. Liu Z, Shapiro SD, Zhou X, et al. A critical role for neutrophil elastase in experimental bullous pemphigoid. *J Clin Invest*. 2000;105(1):113-123.

137. Liu Z, Shipley JM, Vu TH, et al. Gelatinase B-deficient mice are resistant to experimental bullous pemphigoid. *J Exp Med*. 1998;188(3):475-482.

138. Liu Z, Zhou X, Shapiro SD, et al. The serpin alpha1-proteinase inhibitor is a critical substrate for gelatinase B/MMP-9 in vivo. *Cell*. 2000;102(5):647-655.

139. Liu Z, Sui W, Zhao M, et al. Subepidermal blistering induced by human autoantibodies to BP180 requires innate immune players in a humanized bullous pemphigoid mouse model. *J Autoimmun*. 2008;31(4):331-338.

140. Nishie W, Sawamura D, Goto M, et al. Humanization of autoantigen. *Nat Med*. 2007;13(3):378-383.

141. Fairley JA, Burnett CT, Fu CL, et al. A pathogenic role for IgE in autoimmunity: bullous pemphigoid IgE reproduces the early phase of lesion development in human skin grafted to nu/nu mice. *J Invest Dermatol*. 2007;127(11):2605-2611.

142. Zone JJ, Taylor T, Hull C, et al. IgE basement membrane zone antibodies induce eosinophil infiltration and histological blisters in engrafted human skin on SCID mice. *J Invest Dermatol*. 2007;127(5):1167-1174.

143. Kitajima Y, Nojiri M, Yamada T, et al. Internalization of the 180 kDa bullous pemphigoid antigen as immune complexes in basal keratinocytes: an important early event in blister formation in bullous pemphigoid. *Br J Dermatol*. 1998;138(1):71-76.

144. Ujiie H, Sasaoka T, Izumi K, et al. Bullous pemphigoid autoantibodies directly induce blister formation without complement activation. *J Immunol*. 2014;193(9):4415-4428.

145. Hurskainen T, Kokkonen N, Sormunen R, et al. Deletion of the major bullous pemphigoid epitope region of collagen XVII induces blistering, autoimmunization, and itching in mice. *J Invest Dermatol*. 2015;135(5):1303-1310.

146. Hall R 3rd, Murray JC, McCord MM, et al. Rabbits immunized with a peptide encoded for by the 230-kD bullous pemphigoid antigen cDNA develop an enhanced inflammatory response to UVB irradiation: a potential animal model for bullous pemphigoid. *J Invest Dermatol*. 1993;101(1):9-14.

147. Kiss M, Husz S, Janossy T, et al. Experimental bullous pemphigoid generated in mice with an antigenic epitope of the human hemidesmosomal protein BP230. *J Autoimmun*. 2005;24(1):1-10.
148. Budinger L, Borradori L, Yee C, et al. Identification and characterization of autoreactive T cell responses to bullous pemphigoid antigen 2 in patients and healthy controls. *J Clin Invest*. 1998;102(12):2082-2089.
149. Leyendeckers H, Tasanen K, Bruckner-Tuderman L, et al. Memory B cells specific for the NC16A domain of the 180 kDa bullous pemphigoid autoantigen can be detected in peripheral blood of bullous pemphigoid patients and induced in vitro to synthesize autoantibodies. *J Invest Dermatol*. 2003;120(3):372-378.
150. Warren SJ, Lin MS, Giudice GJ, et al. The prevalence of antibodies against desmoglein 1 in endemic pemphigus foliaceus in Brazil. Cooperative Group on Fogo Selvagem Research. *N Engl J Med*. 2000;343(1):23-30.
151. Pickford WJ, Gudi V, Haggart AM, et al. T cell participation in autoreactivity to NC16a epitopes in bullous pemphigoid. *Clin Exp Immunol*. 2015;180(2):189-200.
152. Balding SD, Prost C, Diaz LA, et al. Cicatricial pemphigoid autoantibodies react with multiple sites on the BP180 extracellular domain. *J Invest Dermatol*. 1996;106(1):141-146.
153. Bernard P, Prost C, Durepaire N, et al. The major cicatricial pemphigoid antigen is a 180-kD protein that shows immunologic cross-reactivities with the bullous pemphigoid antigen. *J Invest Dermatol*. 1992;99(2):174-179.
154. Jordon RE, Heine KG, Tappeiner G, et al. The immunopathology of herpes gestationis. Immunofluorescence studies and characterization of "HG factor." *J Clin Invest*. 1976;57(6):1426-1431.
155. Katz SI, Hertz KC, Yaoita H. Herpes gestationis. Immunopathology and characterization of the HG factor. *J Clin Invest*. 1976;57(6):1434-1441.
156. Lin MS, Gharia MA, Swartz SJ, et al. Identification and characterization of epitopes recognized by T lymphocytes and autoantibodies from patients with herpes gestationis. *J Immunol*. 1999;162(8):4991-4997.
157. Murakami H, Nishioka S, Setterfield J, et al. Analysis of antigens targeted by circulating IgG and IgA autoantibodies in 50 patients with cicatricial pemphigoid. *J Dermatol Sci*. 1998;17(1):39-44.
158. Provost TT, Tomasi TB Jr. Evidence for complement activation via the alternate pathway in skin diseases, I. Herpes gestationis, systemic lupus erythematosus, and bullous pemphigoid. *J Clin Invest*. 1973;52(7):1779-1787.
159. Shornick JK, Bangert JL, Freeman RG, et al. Herpes gestationis: clinical and histologic features of twenty-eight cases. *J Am Acad Dermatol*. 1983;8(2):214-224.
160. Tamada Y, Yokochi K, Nitta Y, et al. Lichen planus pemphigoides: identification of 180 kd hemidesmosome antigen. *J Am Acad Dermatol*. 1995;32(5 Pt 2):883-887.
161. Zone JJ, Taylor TB, Kadunce DP, et al. Identification of the cutaneous basement membrane zone antigen and isolation of antibody in linear immunoglobulin A bullous dermatosis. *J Clin Invest*. 1990;85(3):812-820.
162. Zone JJ, Taylor TB, Meyer LJ, et al. The 97 kDa linear IgA bullous disease antigen is identical to a portion of the extracellular domain of the 180 kDa bullous pemphigoid antigen, BPAg2. *J Invest Dermatol*. 1998;110(3):207-210.
163. Delgado JC, Turbay D, Yunis EJ, et al. A common major histocompatibility complex class II allele HLA-DQB1*0301 is present in clinical variants of pemphigoid. *Proc Natl Acad Sci U S A*. 1996;93(16):8569-8571.
164. Oyama N, Setterfield JF, Powell AM, et al. Bullous pemphigoid antigen II (BP180) and its soluble extracellular domains are major autoantigens in mucous membrane pemphigoid: the pathogenic relevance to HLA class II alleles and disease severity. *Br J Dermatol*. 2006;154(1):90-98.
165. Okazaki A, Miyagawa S, Yamashina Y, et al. Polymorphisms of HLA-DR and -DQ genes in Japanese patients with bullous pemphigoid. *J Dermatol*. 2000;27(3):149-156.
166. Langan SM, Groves RW, West J. The relationship between neurological disease and bullous pemphigoid: a population-based case-control study. *J Invest Dermatol*. 2011;131(3):631-636.
167. Bastuji-Garin S, Joly P, Lemordant P, et al. Risk factors for bullous pemphigoid in the elderly: a prospective case-control study. *J Invest Dermatol*. 2011;131(3):637-643.
168. Jedlickova H, Hlubinka M, Pavlik T, et al. Bullous pemphigoid and internal diseases—a case-control study. *Eur J Dermatol*. 2010;20(1):96-101.
169. Lindelof B, Islam N, Eklund G, et al. Pemphigoid and cancer. *Arch Dermatol*. 1990;126(1):66-68.
170. Stone SP, Schroeter AL. Bullous pemphigoid and associated malignant neoplasms. *Arch Dermatol*. 1975;111(8):991-994.
171. Venning VA, Wojnarowska F. The association of bullous pemphigoid and malignant disease: a case control study. *Br J Dermatol*. 1990;123(4):439-445.
172. Cai SC, Allen JC, Lim YL, et al. Association of bullous pemphigoid and malignant neoplasms. *JAMA Dermatol*. 2015;151(6):665-667.
173. Ong E, Goldacre R, Hoang U, et al. Associations between bullous pemphigoid and primary malignant cancers: an English national record linkage study, 1999-2011. *Arch Dermatol Res*. 2014;306(1):75-80.
174. Schulze F, Neumann K, Recke A, et al. Malignancies in pemphigus and pemphigoid diseases. *J Invest Dermatol*. 2015;135(5):1445-1447.
175. Crotty C, Pittelkow M, Muller SA. Eosinophilic spongiosis: a clinicopathologic review of seventy-one cases. *J Am Acad Dermatol*. 1983;8(3):337-343.
176. Ahmed AR, Maize JC, Provost TT. Bullous pemphigoid. Clinical and immunologic follow-up after successful therapy. *Arch Dermatol*. 1977;113(8):1043-1046.
177. Beutner EH, Lever WF, Witebsky E, et al. Autoantibodies in pemphigus vulgaris: response to an intercellular substance of epidermis. *JAMA*. 1965;192:682-688.
178. Beutner EH, Jordon RE, Chorzelski TP. The immunopathology of pemphigus and bullous pemphigoid. *J Invest Dermatol*. 1968;51(2):63-80.
179. Fairley JA, Fu CL, Giudice GJ. Mapping the binding sites of anti-BP180 immunoglobulin E autoantibodies in bullous pemphigoid. *J Invest Dermatol*. 2005;125(3):467-472.
180. Parodi A, Rebora A. Serum IgE antibodies bind to the epidermal side of the basement membrane zone splits in bullous pemphigoid. *Br J Dermatol*. 1992;126(5):526-527.
181. Gammon WR, Briggaman RA, Inman AO 3rd, et al. Differentiating anti-lamina lucida and anti-sublamina densa anti-BMZ antibodies by indirect immunofluorescence on 1.0 M sodium chloride-separated skin. *J Invest Dermatol*. 1984;82(2):139-144.
182. Kelly SE, Wojnarowska F. The use of chemically split tissue in the detection of circulating anti-basement membrane zone antibodies in bullous

182. pemphigoid and cicatricial pemphigoid. *Br J Dermatol*. 1988;118(1):31-40.
183. Sams WM Jr, Jordon RE. Correlation of pemphigoid and pemphigus antibody titres with activity of disease. *Br J Dermatol*. 1971;84(1):7-13.
184. Ishiura N, Fujimoto M, Watanabe R, et al. Serum levels of IgE anti-BP180 and anti-BP230 autoantibodies in patients with bullous pemphigoid. *J Dermatol Sci*. 2008;49(2):153-161.
185. Iwata Y, Komura K, Kodera M, et al. Correlation of IgE autoantibody to BP180 with a severe form of bullous pemphigoid. *Arch Dermatol*. 2008;144(1):41-48.
186. Messingham KA, Noe MH, Chapman MA, et al. A novel ELISA reveals high frequencies of BP180-specific IgE production in bullous pemphigoid. *J Immunol Methods*. 2009;346(1-2):18-25.
187. Woodley DT. The role of IgE anti-basement membrane zone autoantibodies in bullous pemphigoid. *Arch Dermatol*. 2007;143(2):249-250.
188. Kalowska M, Ciepiela O, Kowalewski C, et al. Enzyme-linked Immunoassay Index for anti-NC16a IgG and IgE auto-antibodies correlates with severity and activity of bullous pemphigoid. *Acta Derm Venereol*. 2016;96(2):191-196.
189. Wieland CN, Comfere NI, Gibson LE, et al. Anti-bullous pemphigoid 180 and 230 antibodies in a sample of unaffected subjects. *Arch Dermatol*. 2010;146(1):21-25.
190. Keller JJ, Kittridge AL, Debanne SM, et al. Evaluation of ELISA testing for BP180 and BP230 as a diagnostic modality for bullous pemphigoid: a clinical experience. *Arch Dermatol Res*. 2016;308(4): 269-272.
191. Gammon WR, Inman AO 3rd, Wheeler C, Jr. Differences in complement-dependent chemotactic activity generated by bullous pemphigoid and epidermolysis bullosa acquisita immune complexes: demonstration by leukocytic attachment and organ culture methods. *J Invest Dermatol*. 1984;83(1): 57-61.
192. Gammon WR, Kowalewski C, Chorzelski TP, et al. Direct immunofluorescence studies of sodium chloride-separated skin in the differential diagnosis of bullous pemphigoid and epidermolysis bullosa acquisita. *J Am Acad Dermatol* 1990;22(4):664-670.
193. Venning VA, Wojnarowska F. Lack of predictive factors for the clinical course of bullous pemphigoid. *J Am Acad Dermatol*. 1992;26(4):585-589.
194. Bernard P, Reguiai Z, Tancrede-Bohin E, et al. Risk factors for relapse in patients with bullous pemphigoid in clinical remission: a multicenter, prospective, cohort study. *Arch Dermatol*. 2009;145(5):537-542.
195. Ingen-Housz-Oro S, Plee J, Belmondo T, et al. Positive direct immunofluorescence is of better value than ELISA-BP180 and ELISA-BP230 values for the prediction of relapse after treatment cessation in bullous pemphigoid: a retrospective study of 97 patients. *Dermatology*. 2015;231(1):50-55.
196. Joly P, Benichou J, Lok C, et al. Prediction of survival for patients with bullous pemphigoid: a prospective study. *Arch Dermatol*. 2005;141(6):691-698.
197. Roujeau JC, Lok C, Bastuji-Garin S, et al. High risk of death in elderly patients with extensive bullous pemphigoid. *Arch Dermatol*. 1998;134(4):465-469.
198. Rzany B, Partscht K, Jung M, et al. Risk factors for lethal outcome in patients with bullous pemphigoid: low serum albumin level, high dosage of glucocorticosteroids, and old age. *Arch Dermatol*. 2002;138(7):903-908.
199. Tanaka M, Hashimoto T, Dykes PJ, et al. Clinical manifestations in 100 Japanese bullous pemphigoid cases in relation to autoantigen profiles. *Clin Exp Dermatol*. 1996;21(1):23-27.
200. Fichel F, Barbe C, Joly P, et al. Clinical and immunologic factors associated with bullous pemphigoid relapse during the first year of treatment: a multicenter, prospective study. *JAMA Dermatol*. 2014;150(1):25-33.
201. Bystryn JC, Rudolph JL. Why is the mortality of bullous pemphigoid greater in Europe than in the US? *J Invest Dermatol*. 2005;124(3):xx-xxi.
202. Colbert RL, Allen DM, Eastwood D, et al. Mortality rate of bullous pemphigoid in a US medical center. *J Invest Dermatol*. 2004;122(5):1091-1095.
203. Joly P, Roujeau JC, Benichou J, et al. A comparison of oral and topical corticosteroids in patients with bullous pemphigoid. *N Engl J Med*. 2002;346(5): 321-327.
204. Parker SR, Dyson S, Brisman S, et al. Mortality of bullous pemphigoid: an evaluation of 223 patients and comparison with the mortality in the general population in the United States. *J Am Acad Dermatol*. 2008;59(4):582-588.
205. Risser J, Lewis K, Weinstock MA. Mortality of bullous skin disorders from 1979 through 2002 in the United States. *Arch Dermatol*. 2009;145(9):1005-1008.
206. Feliciani C, Joly P, Jonkman MF, et al. Management of bullous pemphigoid: the European Dermatology Forum consensus in collaboration with the European Academy of Dermatology and Venereology. *Br J Dermatol*. 2015;172(4):867-877.
207. Fine JD. Management of acquired bullous skin diseases. *N Engl J Med*. 1995;333(22):1475-1484.
208. Patton T, Korman NJ. Bullous pemphigoid treatment review. *Expert Opin Pharmacother*. 2006;7(17): 2403-2411.
209. Wojnarowska F, Kirtschig G, Highet AS, et al. Guidelines for the management of bullous pemphigoid. *Br J Dermatol*. 2002;147(2):214-221.
210. Bystryn JC, Wainwright BD, Shupack JL. Oral and topical corticosteroids in bullous pemphigoid. *N Engl J Med*. 2002;347(2):143-145; author reply 143-145.
211. Savin JA. The events leading to the death of patients with pemphigus and pemphigoid. *Br J Dermatol*. 1979;101(5):521-534.
212. Khumalo NP, Murrell DF, Wojnarowska F, et al. A systematic review of treatments for bullous pemphigoid. *Arch Dermatol*. Mar 2002;138(3):385-389.
213. Bara C, Maillard H, Briand N, et al. Methotrexate for bullous pemphigoid: preliminary study. *Arch Dermatol*. Nov 2003;139(11):1506-1507.
214. Gurcan HM, Ahmed AR. Analysis of current data on the use of methotrexate in the treatment of pemphigus and pemphigoid. *Br J Dermatol*. 2009;161(4):723-731.
215. Kjellman P, Eriksson H, Berg P. A retrospective analysis of patients with bullous pemphigoid treated with methotrexate. *Arch Dermatol*. 2008;144(5):612-616.
216. Bohm M, Beissert S, Schwarz T, et al. Bullous pemphigoid treated with mycophenolate mofetil. *Lancet*. 1997;349(9051):541.
217. Burton JL, Harman RR, Peachey RD, et al. Azathioprine plus prednisone in treatment of pemphigoid. *Br Med J*. 1978;2(6146):1190-1191.
218. Guillaume JC, Vaillant L, Bernard P, et al. Controlled trial of azathioprine and plasma exchange in addition to prednisolone in the treatment of bullous pemphigoid. *Arch Dermatol*. 1993;129(1):49-53.
219. Heilborn JD, Stahle-Backdahl M, Albertioni F, et al. Low-dose oral pulse methotrexate as monotherapy

in elderly patients with bullous pemphigoid. *J Am Acad Dermatol*. 1999;40(5 Pt 1):741-749.
220. Nousari HC, Griffin WA, Anhalt GJ. Successful therapy for bullous pemphigoid with mycophenolate mofetil. *J Am Acad Dermatol*. 1998;39(3):497-498.
221. Paul MA, Jorizzo JL, Fleischer AB Jr, et al. Low-dose methotrexate treatment in elderly patients with bullous pemphigoid. *J Am Acad Dermatol*. 1994;31(4):620-625.
222. Beissert S, Werfel T, Frieling U, et al. A comparison of oral methylprednisolone plus azathioprine or mycophenolate mofetil for the treatment of bullous pemphigoid. *Arch Dermatol*. 2007;143(12):1536-1542.
223. Bouscarat F, Chosidow O, Picard-Dahan C, et al. Treatment of bullous pemphigoid with dapsone: retrospective study of thirty-six cases. *J Am Acad Dermatol*. 1996;34(4):683-684.
224. Person JR, Rogers RS 3rd. Bullous pemphigoid responding to sulfapyridine and the sulfones. *Arch Dermatol*. 1977;113(5):610-615.
225. Venning VA, Millard PR, Wojnarowska F. Dapsone as first line therapy for bullous pemphigoid. *Br J Dermatol*. 1989;120(1):83-92.
226. Berk MA, Lorincz AL. The treatment of bullous pemphigoid with tetracycline and niacinamide. A preliminary report. *Arch Dermatol*. 1986;122(6):670-674.
227. Fivenson DP, Breneman DL, Rosen GB, et al. Nicotinamide and tetracycline therapy of bullous pemphigoid. *Arch Dermatol*. 1994;130(6):753-758.
228. Kolbach DN, Remme JJ, Bos WH, et al. Bullous pemphigoid successfully controlled by tetracycline and nicotinamide. *Br J Dermatol*. 1995;133(1):88-90.
229. Roujeau JC, Guillaume JC, Morel P, et al. Plasma exchange in bullous pemphigoid. *Lancet*. 1984;2(8401):486-488.
230. Ahmed AR. Intravenous immunoglobulin therapy for patients with bullous pemphigoid unresponsive to conventional immunosuppressive treatment. *J Am Acad Dermatol*. 2001;45(6):825-835.
231. Ahmed AR, Dahl MV. Consensus statement on the use of intravenous immunoglobulin therapy in the treatment of autoimmune mucocutaneous blistering diseases. *Arch Dermatol*. 2003;139(8):1051-1059.
232. Engineer L, Ahmed AR. Role of intravenous immunoglobulin in the treatment of bullous pemphigoid: analysis of current data. *J Am Acad Dermatol*. 2001;44(1):83-88.
233. Fairley JA, Baum CL, Brandt DS, et al. Pathogenicity of IgE in autoimmunity: successful treatment of bullous pemphigoid with omalizumab. *J Allergy Clin Immunol*. 2009;123(3):704-705.
234. Yu KK, Crew AB, Messingham KA, et al. Omalizumab therapy for bullous pemphigoid. *J Am Acad Dermatol*. 2014;71(3):468-474.
235. Cho YT, Chu CY, Wang LF. First-line combination therapy with rituximab and corticosteroids provides a high complete remission rate in moderate-to-severe bullous pemphigoid. *Br J Dermatol*. 2015;173(1):302-304.
236. Shetty S, Ahmed AR. Treatment of bullous pemphigoid with rituximab: critical analysis of the current literature. *J Drugs Dermatol*. 2013;12(6):672-677.

Chapter 55 :: Mucous Membrane Pemphigoid :: Kim B. Yancey

第五十五章　黏膜类天疱疮

中文导读

黏膜类天疱疮（MMP）是一种罕见的慢性自身免疫性表皮下水疱性疾病，其特征是黏膜和皮肤糜烂，引起受累部位瘢痕形成。

本章内容包括以下七个方面。

1. 流行病学　MMP发病率为（1~2）/100万/年；女性发病率为男性的1.5~2.0倍。MMP平均发病年龄为60岁左右，没有种族或地域差异。

2. 临床表现　本节介绍了MMP的临床表现，口腔是MMP患者最常见的第一个也可能是唯一受累部位。口腔内病变可导致白色网状瘢痕。此外，还有眼部、鼻咽、喉部、食管和肛门生殖器黏膜等受累。25%~35%MMP患者皮肤受累，其并发症详见表55-1。

3. 病因与发病机制　本病的危险因素包括高龄、女性和拥有HLADQB1*0301等位基因。极少数情况下可由药物、外伤（如眼科手术）或过敏反应引起。MMP自身抗体识别不同的自身抗原，被认为是一种疾病表型，而不是独立的一种疾病。表55-2总结了MMP患者自身抗体识别的自身抗原。

4. 诊断　本节介绍了MMP的组织病理学改变、直接免疫荧光等特征。

5. 鉴别诊断　本节介绍了若出现黏膜糜烂性病变、表皮下大疱和皮损周围基底膜免疫反应物沉积时，提示MMP的诊断。鉴别诊断包括其他免疫性大疱性疾病、多形红斑、Stevens-Johnson综合征、中毒性表皮坏死松解症、药物反应性黏膜炎、扁平苔藓和红斑狼疮等。

6. 临床病程与预后　本节概述了MMP病程慢性，可局限于某一部位（如口、眼）数年，也可进行性累及其他黏膜。MMP很少自行缓解，治疗效果取决于其严重程度和受累部位。瘢痕只能预防，不能逆转。

7. 黏膜类天疱疮的管理　本节介绍了治疗MMP的主要目的是阻止疾病进展，防止组织炎症、被破坏和瘢痕形成。所有MMP患者都需要长期随访，因为这种慢性病复发的可能性大。表55-4总结了MMP的治疗方法。

〔陈明亮〕

AT-A-GLANCE

- A chronic autoimmune subepithelial blistering disease characterized by erosive lesions of mucous membranes and skin that typically results in scarring in at least some sites of involvement.

- Lesions commonly involve the oral and ocular mucosae; other sites that may be involved include the nasopharyngeal, laryngeal, esophageal, and anogenital mucosae.

- A rare disorder with a predominance in the elderly and an estimated incidence of 1 to 2 cases per million annually; females are affected 1.5 to 2 times as often as males.

- A progressive disorder that may result in serious complications (eg, blindness, loss of the airway, esophageal stricture formation).

- Severity of involvement in one organ does not necessarily correlate with the presence or severity of disease at other sites.

- Immunopathologic studies of perilesional mucosa and skin demonstrate in situ deposits of immunoreactants in epithelial basement membranes; circulating anti–basement membrane autoantibodies are detected in the sera of some but not all patients.

- A variety of different autoantigens are recognized by autoantibodies from patients, suggesting that mucous membrane pemphigoid is not a single nosologic entity but a disease phenotype.

DEFINITION

Mucous membrane pemphigoid (MMP) is a rare chronic autoimmune subepithelial blistering disease characterized by erosive lesions of mucous membranes and skin that typically results in scarring of at least some sites of involvement.[1-4]

HISTORICAL PERSPECTIVE

In 1794, Wichmann described a chronic blistering disorder characterized by ocular involvement.[5] What are thought to be related cases were reported by Thost in 1911.[6] In 1949, Civatte separated this disorder from pemphigus on the basis of histopathologic findings.[5] Lever affirmed this distinction and suggested that this disorder be named "benign mucous membrane pemphigoid," a designation now regarded a misnomer given the potential devastating consequences of MMP.[4] Over the years, a variety of alternate designations, such as cicatricial pemphigoid, oral pemphigoid, desquamative gingivitis, ocular pemphigoid, ocular cicatricial pemphigoid, essential shrinkage of the conjunctivae, ocular pemphigus, have been applied to MMP.

In 2002, an international consensus conference agreed upon the designation of this disorder as MMP in that this nomenclature is inclusive of patients with disease affecting any mucosal surface and that it emphasizes the mucosal predominant character of this disorder.[1] In 2015, an international panel of experts issued a consensus statement providing accurate and reproducible definitions for disease extent, activity, outcome measures, end points, and therapeutic response.[7]

EPIDEMIOLOGY

MMP has been estimated to have an incidence of 1 to 2 cases per million annually; females are affected 1.5 to 2.0 times as often as males.[8-10] MMP has a mean age of onset in the early to middle 60s.[10] Although there is no known racial or geographic predilection, the *HLADQB1*0301* allele is significantly increased in frequency in patients with oral, ocular, and generalized bullous pemphigoid; amino acid residues at positions 57 and 71 to 77 of the DQB1 protein may represent a disease-susceptibility marker.[11-15]

CLINICAL FEATURES

CUTANEOUS FINDINGS

Patients typically describe the onset of painful, erosive, and/or blistering lesions on 1 or more mucosal surfaces.[16] A few skin lesions on the upper body are also sometimes noted. Associated symptoms are typically site specific. The mouth is the most frequent site of involvement in patients with MMP; it is often the first (and only) site affected.[1,5,16] In the mouth, lesions often involve the gingiva, buccal mucosa, and palate (Fig. 55-1); other sites, such as the alveolar ridge, tongue, and lips, are also susceptible. Erosive lesions of the gingiva resulting in tissue retraction and loss are

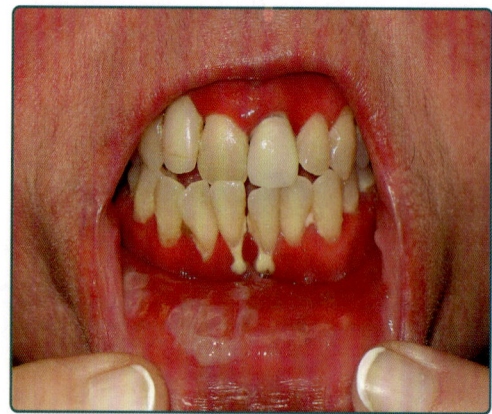

Figure 55-1 Denuded and inflamed sites on the oral mucosa are seen in association with sites of gingiva recession and loss.

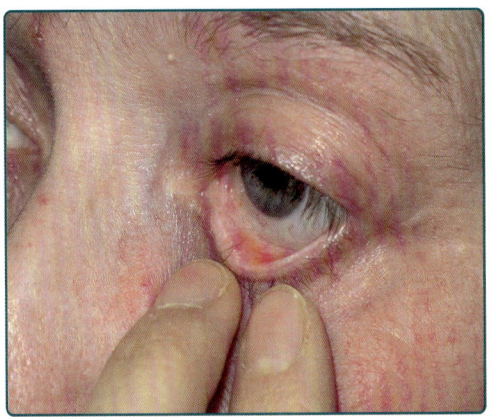

Figure 55-2 The medial aspects of the lower conjunctival fornix and eyelid show shortening, fibrosis, and malaligned eyelashes.

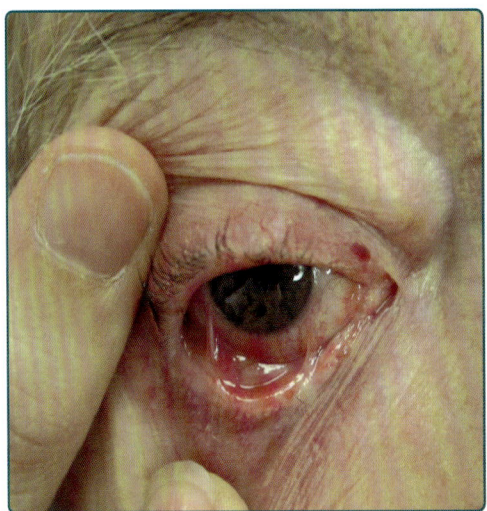

Figure 55-3 Ocular involvement has resulted in conjunctivitis, a shortened conjunctival fornix, and symblepharon formation.

a frequent manifestation of MMP. Other sites of intraoral involvement may show tense blisters that rupture easily or mucosal erosions that form as a consequence of epithelial fragility. Lesions in the mouth may result in a delicate white pattern of reticulated scarring; oral lesions can heal without scarring in some instances. In severe disease, adhesions may develop between the buccal mucosa and the alveolar process, around the uvula and tonsillar fossae, and between the tongue and the floor of the mouth. Gingival involvement can result in tissue loss and dental complications (eg, caries, periodontal ligament damage, and loss of bone mass and teeth).

Ocular involvement in patients with MMP is common and may become sight threatening (Figs. 55-2 and 55-3).[17,18] Ocular lesions typically manifest as conjunctivitis that progresses insidiously to scarring. Early ocular disease can be quite subtle and nonspecific. Although disease is usually bilateral, it often begins unilaterally and progresses to both eyes within several years. Patients may complain of burning, dryness, or a foreign-body sensation in one or both eyes; frank blisters on conjunctival surfaces are rarely seen. Early disease is best appreciated by slitlamp examination. Because disease may be localized to the upper tarsal conjunctiva, it may escape detection without eversion of the eyelids. Chronic ocular involvement can result in scarring characterized by shortened fornices, symblepharons (ie, fibrous tracts between bulbar and palpebral conjunctival surfaces), and, in severe disease, ankyloblepharons (ie, fibrous tracts fusing the superior and inferior palpebral conjunctivae with obliteration of the conjunctival sac). Conjunctival scarring also can cause entropion and trichiasis (ie, in-turning of the eyelashes) that result in corneal irritation, superficial punctate keratopathy, corneal neovascularization, corneal ulceration, and/or blindness. Additional ocular complications include scarring of the lacrimal ducts, decreased tear secretion, and loss of mucosal goblet cells leading to decreased tear mucus content and unstable tear films. It is very important for patients with suspected ocular involvement to be examined by an ophthalmologist because early disease may be subtle, only identified by slitlamp examination, and hold potential for severe complications. MMP may be limited to the eyes.

Other sites that may be affected by MMP include the nasopharyngeal, laryngeal, esophageal, and anogenital mucosae. Nasopharyngeal lesions can result in discharge, epistaxis, excessive crust formation, impaired airflow, chronic sinusitis, scarring, and tissue loss. Laryngeal involvement may present as hoarseness, sore throat, and/or loss of phonation. Chronic laryngeal erosions, edema, and scarring may result in supraglottic stenosis and airway compromise that eventually necessitates tracheostomy. Esophageal involvement may result in stricture formation, dysphagia, odynophagia, weight loss, and/or aspiration. It has been suggested that esophageal dysfunction and gastroesophageal reflux may elicit or exacerbate laryngeal disease and/or bronchospasm in such patients. Although involvement of the genital and/or rectal mucosae in patients with MMP is relatively rare, it can be a source of substantial pain and morbidity (Fig. 55-4). Cases of urethral stricture, vaginal stenosis, and anal narrowing have developed as a consequence of this disease.

The skin is involved in 25% to 35% of patients with MMP. The most frequently affected areas are the scalp, head, neck, and upper trunk (Fig. 55-5). Lesions typically consist of small vesicles or bullae situated on erythematous and/or urticarial bases. Lesions rupture easily and are often seen as small, crusted papules or plaques. The extent and number of cutaneous lesions are generally small; lesions sometimes recur in the same areas.

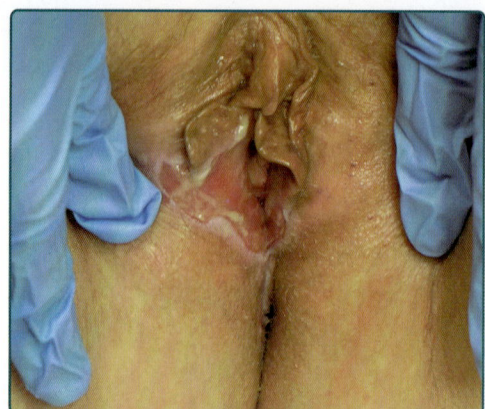

Figure 55-4 Scalloped erosions and sites of denuded vulvar and vaginal mucosae represent painful sites of disease in a patient with mucous membrane pemphigoid.

In 1957, Brunsting and Perry described 7 patients with recurrent scarring subepidermal blistering lesions on the head or neck that for many years was considered a variant form of MMP.[19] Similar patients were subsequently identified by others.[20-25] Although such patients are typically elderly and demonstrate deposits of immunoreactants in epidermal basement membranes like other patients with MMP, Brunsting-Perry pemphigoid predominates in men, lacks mucous membrane involvement, and only in selected cases is associated with immunoglobulin (Ig) G autoantibodies against BP230 (also termed bullous pemphigoid antigen 1 [BPAG1] or dystonin) or BP180 (also termed bullous pemphigoid antigen 2 [BPAG2] or type XVII collagen).[21-24] Because some patients with the same clinical, histologic, and immunopathologic features have been reported to have autoantibodies directed against type VII collagen and blister planes beneath the lamina densa, it has been suggested that a subset of such patients may have a localized forms of epidermolysis bullosa acquisita.[21,22] Rare patients with this phenotype and autoantibodies directed against laminin-332 and/or other skin autoantigens also have been described.[24,25]

NONCUTANEOUS FINDINGS

In 2001, a cohort of 35 patients with MMP and IgG autoantibodies directed against laminin-332 (ie, anti–laminin 332 MMP [formerly called antiepiligrin cicatricial pemphigoid]) was shown to have an increased relative risk for cancer.[26] Ten patients in this cohort had solitary solid cancers (3 lung, 3 gastric, 2 colon, 2 endometrial); 8 patients developed cancer after the onset of MMP (6 within a year, 7 within 14 months). The time between blister onset and cancer diagnosis was approximately 14 months in 9 of the 10 patients. Eight patients in this cohort died as a consequence of their cancer; all deaths occurred within 21 months. This study showed that this form of MMP has an increased relative risk for malignancy that approximates that for adults with dermatomyositis; as is true for dermatomyositis, the risk for cancer appears to be particularly high in the first year of disease. Other patients with this form of MMP and cancer have been described by numerous sources.[26-36] Interestingly, subsequent studies suggest that the relative risk for cancer among patients with ocular or oral MMP and autoantibodies versus integrin subunit β_4 or integrin subunit α_6, respectively, may be reduced.[37,38]

COMPLICATIONS

Site-specific complications of MMP were outlined earlier and are summarized in Table 55-1.

ETIOLOGY AND PATHOGENESIS

RISK FACTORS FOR DISEASE

Risk factors for disease include advanced age, female gender, and possession of the *HLADQB1*0301* allele.[1,5,16,39] In rare cases, disease may be provoked by prescription drugs, trauma (eg, eye surgery), or hypersensitivity reactions.

Autoantibodies directed against autoantigens in epidermal basement membrane are held responsible for the pathogenesis of MMP (Fig. 55-6).[1,5,16,39] Because different autoantigens are recognized by circulating autoantibodies from different patients with MMP, this disorder is considered a disease phenotype rather than a single nosologic entity. Table 55-2 summarizes the autoantigens recognized by autoantibodies from patients with MMP. Even though autoantibodies

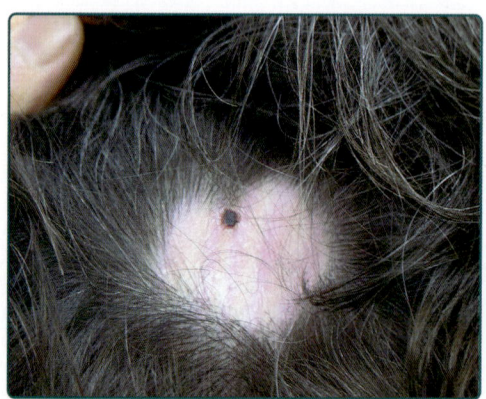

Figure 55-5 The scalp displays scarring alopecia and a focal hemorrhagic crust as a consequence of involvement with mucous membrane pemphigoid.

TABLE 55-1
Potential Complications of Mucous Membrane Pemphigoid

SITE	POTENTIAL COMPLICATIONS
Mouth	
Mucosa	Painful, erosive scarring lesions; adhesions between the buccal mucosa and the alveolar process, the uvula and the tonsillar fossae, and the tongue and the floor of the mouth
Gingiva	Painful, erosive scarring lesions; loss of gingival tissue; caries; periodontal ligament damage; loss of alveolar bone; loss of teeth
Eyes	
Conjunctivae	Painful, erosive conjunctivitis; foreign-body sensations; photophobia; scarring; shortened fornices; loss of goblet cells; decrease in tear mucus content and unstable tear films; symblepharons; ankyloblepharons
Eyelids	Ectropion; trichiasis; ankyloblepharons
Cornea	Corneal irritation; superficial punctate keratopathy; corneal neovascularization; corneal ulcers; blindness
Tear ducts	Scarring; occlusion; secondary infection
Nose	Discharge; epistaxis; excessive crust formation; impaired airflow; recurrent and chronic sinusitis; scarring and tissue loss
Larynx	Hoarseness; impaired phonation; loss of voice; scarring, supraglottic stenosis, airway compromise and loss
Esophagus	Dysphagia, odynophagia, impaired swallowing; stricture formation; weight loss; aspiration
Anogenital region	Painful erosions; stenosis and strictures; secondary infections

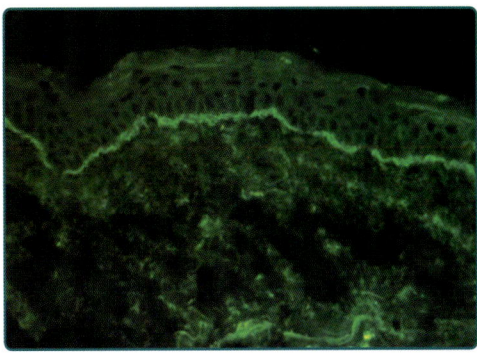

Figure 55-6 Direct immunofluorescence microscopy of normal-appearing perilesional skin from a patient with mucous membrane pemphigoid shows continuous linear deposits of C3 in the epidermal basement membrane.

directed against some of these autoantigens are pathogenic in vivo (Table 55-2), it is conceivable that other mechanisms may contribute to disease pathogenesis. As scarring is a major pathologic manifestation of MMP, profibrotic processes have been studied in biopsy samples and cultured fibroblasts from lesional tissue. Examples of profibrotic factors that have been identified in such studies include serpin h1; transforming growth factor beta; interleukins 4, 5, and 13; and connective tissue growth factor.[40,41] What accounts for the loss of immunologic tolerance to skin in patients with MMP is unknown.

BP180 appears to represent a major MMP autoantigen[16,42-44]; other autoantigens of particular interest include laminin 332, integrin subunit β_4, integrin subunit α_6, type VII collagen, and BP230.[16] Most patients with MMP have IgG anti–basement membrane autoantibodies; some patients have IgA anti–basement membrane autoantibodies alone or in conjunction with IgG anti–basement membrane autoantibodies.

TABLE 55-2
Major Mucous Membrane Pemphigoid Autoantigens

AUTOANTIGEN	MW (KDA)	LOCATION SSS/ULTRA	PASSIVE TRANSFER STUDIES
BP230	230	Epid/HD	
BP180	180	Epid/HD-af	IgG vs. the NC16A domain of BP180 creates subepidermal blisters in newborn mice that resemble those seen in patients with BP[94,95]
Integrin β_4	~205	Epid/HD-af	
Integrin α_6	~120	Epid/HD-af	
Laminin 332	400–440	Derm/LL-LD interface	Experimental IgG (intact IgG and Fab fragments alone) vs. laminin 332 create subepidermal blisters in newborn and adult mice that resemble those seen in patients with AECP[96]
			Patient IgG creates subepidermal blisters in human skin grafts on immunodeficient adult mice that resemble those seen in patients with AECP[97]
Type VII collagen	290	Derm/AF	Experimental and patient IgG vs. the NC1 domain of type VII collagen create subepidermal blisters in adult mice that resemble those seen in patients with EBA[98-100]

AECP, antiepiligrin cicatricial pemphigoid; AF, anchoring fibril; BP, bullous pemphigoid; BP230, bullous pemphigoid antigen 1; BP180, bullous pemphigoid antigen 2; Derm, dermal; EBA, epidermolysis bullosa acquisita; Epid, epidermal; HD, hemidesmosome; HD-af, hemidesmosome–anchoring filament complexes; IgG, immunoglobulin G; LL-LD interface, lamina lucida–lamina densa interface; Location SSS/Ultra, localization in 1 M NaCl–split-skin/ultrastructural localization in epidermal basement membrane; MW (kDa), molecular weight in kilodaltons.

The most common IgA autoantigen linked to the MMP phenotype is BP180.[45-47]

DIAGNOSIS

LIGHT MICROSCOPY

Although the findings of light microscopy studies of lesional skin or mucosa from patients with MMP are often nonspecific, they characteristically show a subepidermal blister and a dermal leukocytic infiltrate composed of lymphocytes and histiocytes as well as variable numbers of neutrophils and eosinophils.[1,20,48,49] Plasma cells can be seen in mucosal lesions, whereas eosinophils and neutrophils are more commonly seen in skin lesions. Biopsy specimens of older lesions may be relatively "cell poor" and show features that correlate with the noninflammatory character of such sites clinically. Light microscopy studies of older lesions often show fibroblast proliferation and lamellar fibrosis (ie, fibrosis characterized by collagen bundles ordered parallel to the surface epithelium). It is not always possible (or in the case of ocular disease, appropriate) to biopsy blistered mucosa for light microscopy studies.

ELECTRON MICROSCOPY

Ultrastructural studies of lesional skin or mucosa from patients with MMP show that blisters typically develop within the lamina lucida and eventuate in partial or complete destruction of the basal lamina in older lesions.[48-52] A generally held idea is that blisters form below those of bullous pemphigoid, because scarring is more common in patients with this disease. Reports of patients with blisters in the sublamina densa region are thought to represent mucosa-predominant forms of epidermolysis bullosa acquisita.

IMMUNOFLUORESCENCE MICROSCOPY

Direct immunofluorescence microscopy of normal-appearing perilesional tissue from patients with MMP shows continuous deposits of immunoreactants in epithelial basement membranes.[1,3,5,16,52] The most commonly detected immunoreactants are IgG and C3 (see Fig. 55-6); the predominant subclass of these autoantibodies is IgG_4.[53] In situ deposits of IgA, IgM, and/or fibrin are found in some patients.[54] Multiple biopsies may be required to demonstrate in situ deposits of immunoreactants in some patients. One study comparing direct immunofluorescence microscopy findings on skin and mucosal samples from 10 patients found immunoreactants more commonly in perilesional mucosal biopsy specimens, suggesting that mucous membranes are the preferred biopsy site for direct immunofluorescence microscopy studies in these patients.[52] Subsequent studies showed that splitting tissue samples with 1 M NaCl increases the sensitivity of direct immunofluorescence microscopy and facilitates identification of immunoreactants as well as their relative distribution within epithelial basement membranes.[55,56]

Indirect immunofluorescence microscopy studies using intact skin or mucosa often find low-titer IgG (and/or IgA) anti–basement membrane autoantibodies in the blood of patients with MMP.[1,5,16,52,57] The use of 1 M NaCl split-skin as a test substrate in these studies substantially increases the detection of such autoantibodies.[58-61] In such studies, IgG (and/or IgA) binding is usually directed against the epidermal side of 1 M NaCl split-skin, although combined epidermal and dermal or exclusively dermal binding can occur. In fact, this heterogeneity in autoantibody binding patterns was one of the first clues that MMP is a disease phenotype that is associated with different autoantigens (see Table 55-2). Although some studies suggest that the use of human mucosal tissue substrates increases the likelihood of detecting autoantibodies in patients with MMP by indirect immunofluorescence microscopy, other studies have not obtained such results.[4,52] Patients with both IgG and IgA anti–basement membrane autoantibodies appear to have a worse prognosis as defined by requirements for medications to control disease as well as overall clinical severity score.[45,47]

OTHER IMMUNOPATHOLOGY STUDIES

Selected cases may require specialized immunochemical studies (eg, immunoblot studies of keratinocyte or skin extracts, immunoprecipitation studies of biosynthetically radiolabeled keratinocytes) to identify the autoantigen targeted by circulating anti–basement membrane autoantibodies from patients with MMP. Perilesional tissue from seronegative patients may be further characterized by immunoelectron microscopy to determine if in situ deposits of immunoreactants reside above or below the lamina densa of epidermal basement membrane.

DIAGNOSTIC ALGORITHM

The diagnosis of MMP should be based on alignment of all clinical, histopathologic, and/or immunopathologic findings.

DIFFERENTIAL DIAGNOSIS

The diagnosis of MMP is suggested when patients present with erosive lesions of mucous membranes, subepidermal bullae, and continuous deposits of immunoreactants in epithelial basement membranes of perilesional tissue. Participants in a 2002 international consensus conference concluded that clinical features and direct immunofluorescence microscopy features are essential findings that should be demonstrated before the diagnosis of MMP is assigned.[1] Distinguishing MMP from other autoimmune bullous diseases can be difficult and may require specialized immunopathologic studies. The differential diagnosis of MMP includes other immunobullous diseases (eg, pemphigus vulgaris, paraneoplastic pemphigus, bullous pemphigoid, linear IgA dermatosis, epidermolysis bullosa acquisita), erythema multiforme, Stevens-Johnson syndrome, toxic epidermal necrolysis, drug reactions (ie, hypersensitivity reactions or chemotherapy-induced mucositis), lichen planus, and lupus erythematosus (Table 55-3). In respect to early disease in the mouth, MMP may resemble pemphigus vulgaris, paraneoplastic pemphigus, erosive lichen planus, erythema multiforme, Stevens-Johnson syndrome, or early toxic epidermal necrolysis; in respect to early disease in the genital region, MMP may resemble pemphigus vulgaris, bullous pemphigoid, erosive lichen planus, or lichen sclerosus. In the case of ocular disease, cicatrizing or inflammatory conjunctivitis resembling MMP can result from long-term use of certain ophthalmologic preparations (eg, pilocarpine, guanethidine, or ephedrine used in the treatment of glaucoma or idoxuridine used as an antiviral) or exposure to selected biologics (eg, epidermal growth factor receptor tyrosine kinase inhibitors).[5,18,39] It has also been demonstrated that some cases of ocular MMP can develop after severe ocular inflammatory injury caused by Stevens-Johnson syndrome or toxic epidermal necrolysis.[5,62] Interestingly, the time between the development of Stevens-Johnson syndrome and the onset of ocular MMP in these patients ranges from a few months to more than 30 years. Finally, rare patients with cicatrizing conjunctivitis who lack in situ deposits of immunoreactants in conjunctival or epidermal basement membranes are sometimes encountered. Although immunopathology studies in such patients are negative, because their disease is inflammatory and sight-threatening, they are often treated with immunosuppressive agents as if they have MMP.

CLINICAL COURSE AND PROGNOSIS

MMP is typically a chronic disease. Involvement may be limited to a given anatomic site (eg, the mouth, the eyes) for years; some cases show progressive involvement of other mucosae. Even localized involvement can have a major negative impact on quality of life. In many ways, sites of involvement significantly influence the prognosis of MMP. Uncontrolled or aggressive disease in the eyes, hypopharynx, esophagus, or genital regions can compromise vision, respiration, swallowing, and genitourinary function. MMP rarely goes into spontaneous remission; its treatment is largely determined by its severity and sites of involvement. Scarring can only be prevented in these patients; it cannot be reversed. As noted above, some reports have suggested that patients with high titers and/or dual isotypes of anti–basement membrane autoantibodies (ie, both IgG and IgA anti–basement membrane autoantibodies) tend to have more severe and/or persistent disease.

MANAGEMENT

The primary goal of treatment of MMP is to halt progression of disease and prevent tissue inflammation, destruction, and scarring. Treatment of MMP is largely determined by its site(s) of involvement, its relative severity, and its rate of progression. Treatment regimens are largely derived from clinical experience rather than clinical trials; virtually all treatment interventions are "off-label."[63-65] All patients with MMP require long-term followup because of the possibility for this chronic disease to relapse.

LOCAL CARE MEASURES

Table 55-4 summarizes the treatment options for MMP. Mild lesions of the oral mucosa and skin can often be

---

TABLE 55-3
Differential Diagnosis of Mucous Membrane Pemphigoid

Most Likely
- Pemphigus
  - Pemphigus vulgaris
  - Paraneoplastic pemphigus
- Other subepidermal immunobullous diseases
  - Epidermolysis bullosa acquisita
  - Bullous pemphigoid
  - Linear immunoglobulin A dermatosis
- Erythema multiforme
- Lupus erythematosus
- Lichen planus

Consider
- Drug-induced hypersensitivity reactions
- Lichen sclerosus (especially in the anogenital area)

Always Rule Out
- Pemphigus (specifically, pemphigus vulgaris, paraneoplastic pemphigus)
- Other subepidermal immunobullous diseases
- Erythema multiforme
- Lupus erythematosus
- Lichen planus

treated effectively with moderate- to high-potency topical glucocorticoids (or calcineurin inhibitors such as tacrolimus) in a gel or ointment base applied 2 to 4 times each day.[64-67] Blotting lesional sites dry with a soft disposable tissue can enhance the adherence and effectiveness of topical agents applied to lesional sites in the mouth. These agents are particularly effective before bed, because oral secretions tend to diminish during sleep. These agents are easily applied, can be used widely on mucosal surfaces, and lack the grittiness encountered with agents formulated in dental pastes. Because it is difficult to maintain contact of topical corticosteroids with mucous membranes (and because lesions often are localized to the gingiva), customized delivery trays to occlude topical glucocorticoids over lesional sites in the mouth are also useful.[64,65,68,69] Such delivery trays should be fashioned in soft vinyl and fitted to cover the patient's gingiva (ie, not the patient's teeth). Topical agents can be applied under occlusion in such trays for 10 to 20 minutes 1 to 4 times daily for 1 to 2 weeks then tapered (or interrupted for a break in therapy). Patients with intraoral involvement should follow a strict regimen of oral hygiene that includes brushing of the teeth 2 to 3 times each day along with daily flossing and regular dental cleanings 2 to 3 times each year. These interventions are essential to avert the accumulation of plaque, the loss of gingiva, and acceleration of tooth decay. Use of a pediatric toothbrush with soft bristles, toothpaste that lacks sodium lauryl sulfate, and mouthwashes free of alcohol facilitate patient compliance with oral hygiene measures. Some sources recommend use of topical anesthetics for painful intraoral lesions in patients with MMP. Such agents should be applied carefully and locally (ie, not as a "rinse") before meals, brushing teeth, dental procedures, or other occasions when pain control is required. Care should be taken to avoid introduction of topical anesthetics into pharyngeal, hypopharyngeal, or laryngeal areas to diminish the likelihood of aspiration. Medicated mouthwashes (eg, dexamethasone 100 mcg/mL, 5 mL per rinse) used in a "swish-and-spit" regimen for 5 minutes 2 to 3 times each day represents another approach for topical therapy. For oral disease resistant to topical glucocorticoids, these agents can (in some instances) be administered intralesionally. Comanagement of such patients with a dentist familiar with MMP is key.

Because of potentially severe complications, ocular, laryngeal, esophageal, and/or anogenital involvement requires aggressive management by teams of physicians familiar with specialized care of these organ systems.[1,5,16,64,65] Early and regular evaluation by an ophthalmologist experienced in the management of patients with MMP is also important. Local eye care measures include prompt identification of ocular inflammation and management of eyelid hygiene, ocular lubrication, and secondary ocular infections (infections are more common in patients undergoing treatment with immunosuppressive drugs than in other patients). Patients whose ocular disease is complicated by trichiasis (ie, misdirected eyelashes that grow inward toward the eye and damage the cornea, conjunctivae, or under surface of the eyelid) may benefit from epilation, although this decision is best made by an ophthalmologist. Patients with nasal involvement benefit from irrigations, humidified environments, emollients, and topical corticosteroids (sprays or drops). Twice daily irrigation of nasal passages with saline or tap water delivered via bulb syringe, piston syringe, or other nasal irrigation devices removes

TABLE 55-4
Treatments for Mucous Membrane Pemphigoid

Mild Involvement	
SITES	LOCAL CARE MEASURES
Mouth	Topical corticosteroid (gels or ointments) twice daily/4 times daily; topical corticosteroids under occlusion (eg, dental trays); topical calcineurin inhibitors; intralesional corticosteroids
Nose	Irrigation with isotonic saline twice daily/thrice daily; nasal lubricants; topical corticosteroids (eg, via sprays, inhalers)
Anogenital region	Topical corticosteroids; topical calcineurin inhibitors
Skin	Topical corticosteroids; topical calcineurin inhibitors
Moderate Involvement	
SITES	THERAPEUTIC OPTIONS
Mouth, eyes, nose, larynx, esophagus, anogenital region	Local care measures outlined above plus dapsone 50-200 mg daily, prednisone 20-60 mg each morning, or both of these agents simultaneously
Severe Involvement	
SITES	THERAPEUTIC OPTIONS
Mouth, eyes, nose, larynx, esophagus, anogenital region	Local care measures outlined above plus prednisone (1 mg/kg each morning), intravenous immunoglobulin (2 g/kg body weight over 2-3 days every 2-6 weeks for 4-6 months), or both of these agents simultaneously in conjunction with azathioprine (2-2.5 mg/kg/day), mycophenolate mofetil (1-2.5 g/day), cyclophosphamide (1-2 mg/kg/day), or rituximab (375 mg/m^2 weekly × 4 then every 4-6 months as needed, or 1000 mg on days 1 and 15 and then 500 mg at month 6)

crusts over mucosal erosions and diminishes the likelihood of secondary complications such as infection and/or bleeding. Irrigations also increase the relative efficacy of topical corticosteroids delivered to nasal passages by spray or drops. Use of intranasal emollients after irrigation of nasal passages limits reaccumulation of crusts. Esophageal involvement requires early diagnosis and aggressive medical management to avert esophageal dysfunction, gastroesophageal reflux, stricture formation, aspiration, laryngeal irritation, and/or bronchospastic pulmonary disease. Soft diets, agents to diminish gastroesophageal reflux and/or gastric acidity, and/or esophageal dilation may be required. Urologists and colorectal surgeons provide important care for the rare patients who develop anogenital lesions. Such patients may require local topical therapy, dilations, stool softeners, and/or evaluation of adjacent internal mucosal surfaces.

SYSTEMIC THERAPIES

For patients with disease resistant to local therapy or of greater severity, treatment with systemic agents in combination with local care measures is indicated. A number of reports suggest that dapsone (50 to 200 mg by mouth daily) may be effective.[70-73] Others have found that patients with MMP do not respond to this agent. Other systemic agents reported to be of benefit in patients with mild disease include sulfapyridine, minocycline, or a combination of tetracycline and niacinamide. For mild or moderate ocular involvement, systemic glucocorticoids (eg, 20 to 60 mg of prednisone by mouth each morning) alone or in conjunction with daily dapsone may be effective. For nonresponsive or severe disease affecting the ocular, pharyngeal, or urogenital epithelia, a combination of systemic glucocorticoids and an additional immunosuppressive is indicated.[74-79] In such cases, azathioprine (2.0 to 2.5 mg/kg/day), mycophenolate mofetil (1.0 to 2.5 g/day), or cyclophosphamide (1 to 2 mg/kg/day) are often used in conjunction with daily prednisone (1 mg/kg/day). In this regimen, daily prednisone is tapered gradually over approximately 6 months, and the patient is maintained on the alternate agent alone for an additional 6 to 12 months before further reductions in therapy are pursued. Such combined regimens have had success in halting the progression of severe disease, limiting scarring, and producing long-term remissions. In an effort to avoid adverse effects and complications produced by prolonged treatment with immunosuppressive agents, some groups treat patients with intravenous Ig (ie, intravenous Ig 2 g/kg of body weight administered over 2 to 3 days every 2 to 6 weeks for 4 to 6 months).[80-85] Biologic agents that antagonize tumor necrosis factor-α (eg, etanercept, infliximab) have shown efficacy in selected patients with MMP.[86] Increasing numbers of patients with MMP are being treated with daily corticosteroids (alone or in combination with the other immunosuppressive agents listed above) plus rituximab (1000 mg on days 1 and 15, 500 mg at month 6; or 375 mg/m^2 weekly × 4 then every 4-6 months as needed).[87-93]

When MMP is stabilized, treatment should be tapered slowly (eg, over 6 to 12 months). Flares of disease justify reinstitution of systemic therapies. Some patients require long-term maintenance therapy. In selected cases, immunopathology studies (eg, indirect immunofluorescence microscopy studies of 1 M NaCl split-skin, autoantibody-specific enzyme-linked immunosorbent assays) can be used to determine if seropositive patients convert to a seronegative status following treatment—a laboratory observation that may identify patients who are better candidates for a reduction (or cessation) of therapy.

REFERENCES

1. Chan LS, Ahmed AR, Anhalt GJ, et al. The first international consensus on mucous membrane pemphigoid: definition, diagnostic criteria, pathogenic factors, medical treatment, and prognostic indicators. *Arch Dermatol*. 2002;138(3):370.
2. Yancey KB, Egan CA. Pemphigoid: clinical, histologic, immunopathologic, and therapeutic considerations. *JAMA*. 2000;284(3):350.
3. Bean SF, Waisman M, Michel B, et al. Cicatricial pemphigoid. Immunofluorescent studies. *Arch Dermatol*. 1972;106(2):195.
4. Lever WF. *Pemphigus and Pemphigoid*. Springfield, IL: Charles C Thomas; 1965.
5. Bernard P, Borradori L. Pemphigoid group. In: Bolognia J, Jorizzo J, Schaffer J, eds. *Dermatology*. 3rd ed. Oxford, UK: Elsevier; 2012:475-490.
6. Thost A. Der chronische Schleimhautpemphigus der oberen Luftwege. *Arch Laryng Rhinol*. 1911;25:459.
7. Murrell DF, Marinovic B, Caux F, et al. Definitions and outcome measures for mucous membrane pemphigoid: recommendations of an international panel of experts. *J Am Acad Dermatol*. 2015;72(1):168.
8. Bernard P, Vaillant L, Labeille B, et al. Incidence and distribution of subepidermal autoimmune bullous skin diseases in three French regions. Bullous Diseases French Study Group. *Arch Dermatol*. 1995;131(1):48.
9. Zillikens D, Wever S, Roth A, et al. Incidence of autoimmune subepidermal blistering dermatoses in a region of central Germany. *Arch Dermatol*. 1995;131(8):957.
10. Laskaris G, Sklavounou A, Stratigos J. Bullous pemphigoid, cicatricial pemphigoid, and pemphigus vulgaris. A comparative clinical survey of 278 cases. *Oral Surg Oral Med Oral Pathol*. 1982;54(6):656.
11. Ahmed AR, Foster S, Zaltas M, et al. Association of DQw7 (DQB1*0301) with ocular cicatricial pemphigoid. *Proc Natl Acad Sci U S A*. 1991;88(24):11579.
12. Yunis JJ, Mobini N, Yunis EJ, et al. Common major histocompatibility complex class II markers in clinical variants of cicatricial pemphigoid. *Proc Natl Acad Sci U S A*. 1994;91(16):7747.
13. Delgado JC, Turbay D, Yunis EJ, et al. A common major histocompatibility complex class II allele HLA-DQB1*0301 is present in clinical variants of pemphigoid. *Proc Natl Acad Sci U S A*. 1996;93(16):8569.
14. Chan LS, Hammerberg C, Cooper KD. Significantly increased occurrence of HLA-DQB1*0301 allele in

patients with ocular cicatricial pemphigoid. *J Invest Dermatol*. 1997;108(2):129.
15. Setterfield J, Theron J, Vaughan RW, et al. Mucous membrane pemphigoid: HLA-DQB1*0301 is associated with all clinical sites of involvement and may be linked to antibasement membrane IgG production. *Br J Dermatol*. 2001;145(3):406.
16. Schmidt E, Zillikens D. Pemphigoid diseases. *Lancet*. 2013;381(9863):320.
17. Foster CS. Cicatricial pemphigoid. *Trans Am Ophthalmol Soc*. 1986;84:527.
18. Thorne JE, Anhalt GJ, Jabs DA. Mucous membrane pemphigoid and pseudopemphigoid. *Ophthalmology*. 2004;111(1):45.
19. Brunsting LA, Perry HO. Benign pemphigoid; a report of seven cases with chronic, scarring, herpetiform plaques about the head and neck. *AMA Arch Derm*. 1957;75(4):489.
20. Fleming TE, Korman NJ. Cicatricial pemphigoid. *J Am Acad Dermatol*. 2000;43(4):571.
21. Kurzhals G, Stolz W, Meurer M, et al. Acquired epidermolysis bullosa with the clinical feature of Brunsting-Perry cicatricial bullous pemphigoid. *Arch Dermatol*. 1991;127(3):391.
22. Joly P, Ruto F, Thomine E, et al. Brunsting-Perry cicatricial bullous pemphigoid: a clinical variant of localized acquired epidermolysis bullosa? *J Am Acad Dermatol*. 1993;28(1):89.
23. Daito J, Katoh N, Asai J, et al. Brunsting-Perry cicatricial pemphigoid associated with autoantibodies to the C-terminal domain of BP180. *Br J Dermatol*. 2008;159(4):984.
24. Jedlickova H, Niedermeier A, Zgazarova S, et al. Brunsting-Perry pemphigoid of the scalp with antibodies against laminin 332. *Dermatology*. 2011;222(3):193.
25. Fukuda S, Tsuruta D, Uchiyama M, et al. Brunsting-Perry type pemphigoid with IgG autoantibodies to laminin-332, BP230 and desmoplakins I/II. *Br J Dermatol*. 2011;165(2):433.
26. Egan CA, Lazarova Z, Darling TN, et al. Anti-epiligrin cicatricial pemphigoid and relative risk for cancer. *Lancet*. 2001;357(9271):1850.
27. Egan CA, Lazarova Z, Darling TN, et al. Anti-epiligrin cicatricial pemphigoid: clinical findings, immunopathogenesis, and significant associations. *Medicine (Baltimore)*. 2003;82(3):177.
28. Matsushima S, Horiguchi Y, Honda T, et al. A case of anti-epiligrin cicatricial pemphigoid associated with lung carcinoma and severe laryngeal stenosis: review of Japanese cases and evaluation of risk for internal malignancy. *J Dermatol*. 2004;31(1):10.
29. Chamberlain AJ, Cooper SM, Allen J, et al. Paraneoplastic immunobullous disease with an epidermolysis bullosa acquisita phenotype: two cases demonstrating remission with treatment of gynaecological malignancy. *Australas J Dermatol*. 2004;45(2):136.
30. Shannon JF, Mackenzie-Wood A, Wood G, et al. Cicatricial pemphigoid in non-Hodgkin's lymphoma. *Intern Med J*. 2003;33(8):396.
31. Parisi E, Raghavendra S, Werth VP, et al. Modification to the approach of the diagnosis of mucous membrane pemphigoid: A case report and literature review. *Oral Surg Oral Med Oral Pathol Oral Radiol Endod*. 2003;95(2):182.
32. Sadler E, Lazarova Z, Sarasombath P, et al. A widening perspective regarding the relationship between anti-epiligrin cicatricial pemphigoid and cancer. *J Dermatol Sci*. 2007;47(1):1.
33. Fukushima S, Egawa K, Nishi H, et al. Two cases of anti-epiligrin cicatricial pemphigoid with and without associated malignancy. *Acta Derm Venereol*. 2008;88(5):484.
34. Mitsuya J, Hara H, Ito K, et al. Metastatic ovarian carcinoma-associated subepidermal blistering disease with autoantibodies to both the p200 dermal antigen and the gamma 2 subunit of laminin 5 showing unusual clinical features. *Br J Dermatol*. 2008;158(6):1354.
35. Demitsu T, Yoneda K, Iida E, et al. A case of mucous membrane pemphigoid with IgG antibodies against all the alpha3, beta3 and gamma2 subunits of laminin-332 and BP180 C-terminal domain, associated with pancreatic cancer. *Clin Exp Dermatol*. 2009;34(8):e992.
36. Takahara M, Tsuji G, Ishii N, et al. Mucous membrane pemphigoid with antibodies to the beta(3) subunit of Laminin 332 in a patient with acute myeloblastic leukemia and graft-versus-host disease. *Dermatology*. 2009;219(4):361.
37. Malik M, Gurcan HM, Christen W, et al. Relationship between cancer and oral pemphigoid patients with antibodies to alpha6-integrin. *J Oral Pathol Med*. 2007;36(1):1.
38. Letko E, Gurcan HM, Papaliodis GN, et al. Relative risk for cancer in mucous membrane pemphigoid associated with antibodies to the beta4 integrin subunit. *Clin Exp Dermatol*. 2007;32(6):637.
39. Xu HH, Werth VP, Parisi E, et al. Mucous membrane pemphigoid. *Dent Clin North Am*. 2013;57(4):611.
40. Foster CS, Sainz De La Maza M. Ocular cicatricial pemphigoid review. *Curr Opin Allergy Clin Immunol*. 2004;4(5):435.
41. Saw VP, Offiah I, Dart RJ, et al. Conjunctival interleukin-13 expression in mucous membrane pemphigoid and functional effects of interleukin-13 on conjunctival fibroblasts in vitro. *Am J Pathol*. 2009;175(6):2406.
42. Bernard P, Prost C, Durepaire N, et al. The major cicatricial pemphigoid antigen is a 180-kD protein that shows immunologic cross-reactivities with the bullous pemphigoid antigen. *J Invest Dermatol*. 1992;99(2):174.
43. Balding SD, Prost C, Diaz LA, et al. Cicatricial pemphigoid autoantibodies react with multiple sites on the BP180 extracellular domain. *J Invest Dermatol*. 1996;106(1):141.
44. Bedane C, McMillan JR, Balding SD, et al. Bullous pemphigoid and cicatricial pemphigoid autoantibodies react with ultrastructurally separable epitopes on the BP180 ectodomain: evidence that BP180 spans the lamina lucida. *J Invest Dermatol*. 1997;108(6):901.
45. Setterfield J, Shirlaw PJ, Bhogal BS, et al. Cicatricial pemphigoid: serial titres of circulating IgG and IgA antibasement membrane antibodies correlate with disease activity. *Br J Dermatol*. 1999;140(4):645.
46. Egan CA, Taylor TB, Meyer LJ, et al. The immunoglobulin A antibody response in clinical subsets of mucous membrane pemphigoid. *Dermatology*. 1999;198(4):330.
47. Setterfield J, Shirlaw PJ, Kerr-Muir M, et al. Mucous membrane pemphigoid: a dual circulating antibody response with IgG and IgA signifies a more severe and persistent disease. *Br J Dermatol*. 1998;138(4):602.
48. Mutasim DF, Pelc NJ, Anhalt GJ. Cicatricial pemphigoid. *Dermatol Clin*. 1993;11(3):499.

49. Rose C, Schmidt E, Kerstan A, et al. Histopathology of anti-laminin 5 mucous membrane pemphigoid. *J Am Acad Dermatol*. 2009;61(3):433.
50. Bernard P, Prost C, Lecerf V, et al. Studies of cicatricial pemphigoid autoantibodies using direct immunoelectron microscopy and immunoblot analysis. *J Invest Dermatol*. 1990;94(5):630.
51. Meyer JR, Migliorati CA, Daniels TE, et al. Localization of basement membrane components in mucous membrane pemphigoid. *J Invest Dermatol*. 1985;84(2):105.
52. Fine JD, Neises GR, Katz SI. Immunofluorescence and immunoelectron microscopic studies in cicatricial pemphigoid. *J Invest Dermatol*. 1984;82(1):39.
53. Hsu R, Lazarova Z, Yee C, et al. Noncomplement fixing, IgG4 autoantibodies predominate in patients with anti-epiligrin cicatricial pemphigoid. *J Invest Dermatol*. 1997;109(4):557.
54. Leonard JN, Wright P, Williams DM, et al. The relationship between linear IgA disease and benign mucous membrane pemphigoid. *Br J Dermatol*. 1984;110(3):307.
55. Gammon WR, Kowalewski C, Chorzelski TP, et al. Direct immunofluorescence studies of sodium chloride-separated skin in the differential diagnosis of bullous pemphigoid and epidermolysis bullosa acquisita. *J Am Acad Dermatol*. 1990;22(4):664.
56. Domloge-Hultsch N, Bisalbutra P, Gammon WR, et al. Direct immunofluorescence microscopy of 1 mol/L sodium chloride-treated patient skin. *J Am Acad Dermatol*. 1991;24:946.
57. Oyama N, Setterfield JF, Powell AM, et al. Bullous pemphigoid antigen II (BP180) and its soluble extracellular domains are major autoantigens in mucous membrane pemphigoid: the pathogenic relevance to HLA class II alleles and disease severity. *Br J Dermatol*. 2006;154(1):90.
58. Domloge-Hultsch N, Anhalt GJ, Gammon WR, et al. Antiepiligrin cicatricial pemphigoid. A subepithelial bullous disorder. *Arch Dermatol*. 1994;130(12):1521.
59. Lazarova Z, Yancey KB. Reactivity of autoantibodies from patients with defined subepidermal bullous diseases against 1 mol/L salt-split skin. Specificity, sensitivity, and practical considerations. *J Am Acad Dermatol*. 1996;35(3, pt 1):398.
60. Kelly SE, Wojnarowska F. The use of chemically split tissue in the detection of circulating anti-basement membrane zone antibodies in bullous pemphigoid and cicatricial pemphigoid. *Br J Dermatol*. 1988;118(1):31.
61. Lazarova Z, Sitaru C, Zillikens D, et al. Comparative analysis of methods for detection of anti-laminin 5 autoantibodies in patients with anti-epiligrin cicatricial pemphigoid. *J Am Acad Dermatol*. 2004;51(6):886.
62. Chan LS, Soong HK, Foster CS, et al. Ocular cicatricial pemphigoid occurring as a sequela of Stevens-Johnson syndrome. *JAMA*. 1991;266(11):1543.
63. Kirtschig G, Murrell D, Wojnarowska F, et al. Interventions for mucous membrane pemphigoid/cicatricial pemphigoid and epidermolysis bullosa acquisita: a systematic literature review. *Arch Dermatol*. 2002;138(3):380.
64. Kourosh AS, Yancey KB. Therapeutic approaches to patients with mucous membrane pemphigoid. *Dermatol Clin*. 2011;29(4):637.
65. Yancey KB. Management of mucous membrane pemphigoid. *UpToDate*. 2016. https://www.uptodate.com/contents/management-of-mucous-membrane-pemphigoid?search=Yancey%20KB.%20Management%20of%20mucous%20membrane%20pemphigoid&source=search_result&selectedTitle=1~150&usage_type=default&display_rank=1
66. Assmann T, Becker J, Ruzicka T, et al. Topical tacrolimus for oral cicatricial pemphigoid. *Clin Exp Dermatol*. 2004;29(6):674.
67. Lee HY, Blazek C, Beltraminelli H, et al. Oral mucous membrane pemphigoid: complete response to topical tacrolimus. *Acta Derm Venereol*. 2011;91(5):604.
68. Lee MS, Wakefield PE, Konzelman JL Jr, et al. Oral insertable prosthetic device as an aid in treating oral ulcers. *Arch Dermatol*. 1991;127(4):479.
69. Gonzalez-Moles MA, Ruiz-Avila I, Rodriguez-Archilla A, et al. Treatment of severe erosive gingival lesions by topical application of clobetasol propionate in custom trays. *Oral Surg Oral Med Oral Pathol Oral Radiol Endod*. 2003;95(6):688.
70. Rogers RS 3rd, Seehafer JR, Perry HO. Treatment of cicatricial (benign mucous membrane) pemphigoid with dapsone. *J Am Acad Dermatol*. 1982;6(2):215.
71. Ciarrocca KN, Greenberg MS. A retrospective study of the management of oral mucous membrane pemphigoid with dapsone. *Oral Surg Oral Med Oral Pathol Oral Radiol Endod*. 1999;88(2):159.
72. Arash A, Shirin L. The management of oral mucous membrane pemphigoid with dapsone and topical corticosteroid. *J Oral Pathol Med*. 2008;37(6):341.
73. Hegarty AM, Ormond M, Sweeney M, et al. Dapsone efficacy and adverse events in the management of mucous membrane pemphigoid. *Eur J Dermatol*. 2010;20(2):223.
74. Korman NJ. Update on the use of azathioprine in the management of pemphigus and bullous pemphigoid. *Med Surg Dermatol*. 1996;3:209.
75. Korman NJ. Update on the use of cyclophosphamide in the management of pemphigus, bullous pemphigoid, and cicatricial pemphigoid. *Med Surg Dermatol*. 1998;5.
76. Megahed M, Schmiedeberg S, Becker J, et al. Treatment of cicatricial pemphigoid with mycophenolate mofetil as a steroid-sparing agent. *J Am Acad Dermatol*. 2001;45(2):256.
77. Saw VP, Dart JK, Rauz S, et al. Immunosuppressive therapy for ocular mucous membrane pemphigoid strategies and outcomes. *Ophthalmology*. 2008;115(2):253.
78. Doycheva D, Deuter C, Blumenstock G, et al. Long-term results of therapy with mycophenolate mofetil in ocular mucous membrane pemphigoid. *Ocul Immunol Inflamm*. 2011;19(6):431.
79. Staines K, Hampton PJ. Treatment of mucous membrane pemphigoid with the combination of mycophenolate mofetil, dapsone, and prednisolone: a case series. *Oral Surg Oral Med Oral Pathol Oral Radiol*. 2012;114(1):e49.
80. Ahmed AR, Dahl MV. Consensus statement on the use of intravenous immunoglobulin therapy in the treatment of autoimmune mucocutaneous blistering diseases. *Arch Dermatol*. 2003;139(8):1051.
81. Foster CS, Ahmed AR. Intravenous immunoglobulin therapy for ocular cicatricial pemphigoid: a preliminary study. *Ophthalmology*. 1999;106(11):2136.
82. Sami N, Letko E, Androudi S, et al. Intravenous immunoglobulin therapy in patients with ocular-cicatricial pemphigoid: a long-term follow-up. *Ophthalmology*. 2004;111(7):1380.
83. Wetter DA, Davis MD, Yiannias JA, et al. Effectiveness of intravenous immunoglobulin therapy for skin

disease other than toxic epidermal necrolysis: a retrospective review of Mayo Clinic experience. *Mayo Clin Proc*. 2005;80(1):41.
84. Letko E, Miserocchi E, Daoud YJ, et al. A nonrandomized comparison of the clinical outcome of ocular involvement in patients with mucous membrane (cicatricial) pemphigoid between conventional immunosuppressive and intravenous immunoglobulin therapies. *Clin Immunol*. 2004;111(3):303.
85. Ahmed AR, Colon JE. Comparison between intravenous immunoglobulin and conventional immunosuppressive therapy regimens in patients with severe oral pemphigoid: effects on disease progression in patients nonresponsive to dapsone therapy. *Arch Dermatol*. 2001;137(9):1181.
86. Sacher C, Rubbert A, Konig C, et al. Treatment of recalcitrant cicatricial pemphigoid with the tumor necrosis factor alpha antagonist etanercept. *J Am Acad Dermatol*. 2002;46(1):113.
87. Ross AH, Jaycock P, Cook SD, et al. The use of rituximab in refractory mucous membrane pemphigoid with severe ocular involvement. *Br J Ophthalmol*. 2009;93(4):421.
88. Foster CS, Chang PY, Ahmed AR. Combination of rituximab and intravenous immunoglobulin for recalcitrant ocular cicatricial pemphigoid: a preliminary report. *Ophthalmology*. 2010;117(5):861.
89. Le Roux-Villet C, Prost-Squarcioni C, Alexandre M, et al. Rituximab for patients with refractory mucous membrane pemphigoid. *Arch Dermatol*. 2011;147(7):843.
90. Kasperkiewicz M, Shimanovich I, Ludwig RJ, et al. Rituximab for treatment-refractory pemphigus and pemphigoid: a case series of 17 patients. *J Am Acad Dermatol*. 2011;65(3):552.
91. Shetty S, Ahmed AR. Critical analysis of the use of rituximab in mucous membrane pemphigoid: a review of the literature. *J Am Acad Dermatol*. 2013;68(3):499.
92. Heelan K, Walsh S, Shear NH. Treatment of mucous membrane pemphigoid with rituximab. *J Am Acad Dermatol*. 2013;69(2):310.
93. Maley A, Warren M, Haberman I, et al. Rituximab combined with conventional therapy versus conventional therapy alone for the treatment of mucous membrane pemphigoid (MMP). *J Am Acad Dermatol*. 2016;74(5):835.
94. Liu Z, Diaz LA, Troy JL, et al. A passive transfer model of the organ-specific autoimmune disease, bullous pemphigoid, using antibodies generated against the hemidesmosomal antigen, BP180. *J Clin Invest*. 1993;92(5):2480.
95. Nishie W, Sawamura D, Goto M, et al. Humanization of autoantigen. *Nat Med*. 2007;13(3):378.
96. Lazarova Z, Yee C, Darling T, et al. Passive transfer of anti-laminin 5 antibodies induces subepidermal blisters in neonatal mice. *J Clin Invest*. 1996;98(7):1509.
97. Lazarova Z, Hsu R, Yee C, et al. Human anti-laminin 5 autoantibodies induce subepidermal blisters in an experimental human skin graft model. *J Invest Dermatol*. 2000;114(1):178.
98. Woodley DT, Ram R, Doostan A, et al. Induction of epidermolysis bullosa acquisita in mice by passive transfer of autoantibodies from patients. *J Invest Dermatol*. 2006;126(6):1323.
99. Sitaru C, Mihai S, Otto C, et al. Induction of dermal-epidermal separation in mice by passive transfer of antibodies specific to type VII collagen. *J Clin Invest*. 2005;115(4):870.
100. Woodley DT, Chang C, Saadat P, et al. Evidence that anti-type VII collagen antibodies are pathogenic and responsible for the clinical, histological, and immunological features of epidermolysis bullosa acquisita. *J Invest Dermatol*. 2005;124(5):958.

Chapter 56 :: Epidermolysis Bullosa Acquisita
:: David T. Woodley & Mei Chen

第五十六章
获得性大疱性表皮松解症

中文导读

获得性大疱性表皮松解症（EBA）是一种罕见的病因不明的自身免疫性表皮下大疱性疾病，由抗Ⅶ型胶原IgG抗体引起，表现为皮肤脆弱、表皮下水疱、愈合后瘢痕和粟丘疹。好发于易受创伤部位，如手、足、肘、膝、骶部、甲和口，潜在系统性疾病如炎症性肠病，可有黏膜糜烂和食管狭窄。病理为表皮下大疱、纤维化和粟丘疹，直接免疫荧光显示表皮-真皮交界处IgG沉积。治疗方案有限且难有效。

本章内容包括以下几个方面。

1. 流行病学　本病无性别、种族或地域差别。EBA和大疱性SLE具有免疫遗传相关性，HLADR2基因与锚定纤维的自身免疫有关，也可能是与之存在连锁不平衡的其他基因标记。

2. 病因与发病机制　EBA是一种慢性表皮下水疱性疾病，与位于真皮-表皮交界处（DEJ）的锚定纤维结构内的Ⅶ型胶原自身免疫有关，EBA抗体与锚定纤维内的Ⅶ型胶原结合。EBA患者皮肤直接免疫荧光显示DEJ处IgG沉积。

3. 临床表现　本节介绍了EBA的皮损多种多样，可以模拟其他获得性自身免疫大疱性疾病，目前至少有5种临床表现，并且可能与各种系统性疾病有关。

4. 实验室检查　本节介绍了EBA的组织病理学、直接免疫荧光、免疫电镜等特征。尚可利用Western blot和ELISA检查EBA患者血清中Ⅶ型胶原抗体。

5. 鉴别诊断　见表56-1。怀疑遗传性营养不良型EB者可能是罕见的EBA儿童患者，检测抗体可以排除。

6. 诊断　本节介绍了Yaoita等制定的EBA诊断标准仍然适用，并列出了这些标准，对其稍加修改。

7. 并发症　EBA引起的并发症包括通常由葡萄球菌或链球菌引起的继发皮肤感染，有明显黏膜受累，导致食管狭窄，甚至喉瘢痕。

8. 治疗　EBA通常治疗反应差。所有EBA患者都需要支持治疗，包括开放式伤口护理和避免创伤。患者不应过度清洗或过度使用热水或刺激性肥皂，避免毛巾长期或剧烈摩擦皮肤。长时间日晒可加重或促进手背和指关节新的损伤，应避免日晒并使用防晒霜。局部皮肤感染时应立即就医和使用抗生素。

〔陈明亮〕

AT-A-GLANCE

- Rare, autoimmune subepidermal bullous disease due to immunoglobulin G autoantibodies to Type VII collagen.
- Etiology is unknown.
- Skin fragility, subepidermal blisters, residual scarring, and milia formation. Common sites are trauma-prone areas such as hands, feet, elbows, knees, sacrum, nails, and mouth.
- Related features may include an underlying systemic disease such as inflammatory bowel disease. May have erosions of the mucosa and esophageal stenosis.
- Pathology shows subepidermal bulla, fibrosis, milia formation, and positive direct immunofluorescence for immunoglobulin G deposits at the epidermal–dermal junction.
- Treatment options are limited and often difficult.

EPIDEMIOLOGY

Epidermolysis bullosa acquisita (EBA) is a sporadic autoimmune bullous disease of unknown etiology. The disease has no gender, racial, ethnic, or geographical predisposition. There may be some genetic predisposition to EBA and autoimmunity in African Americans who live in the southeastern part of the United States.[1] African American patients in the southeastern part of the United States who have either EBA or bullous systemic lupus erythematosus (SLE) have a high incidence of the HLA-DR2 phenotype. The calculated relative risk for EBA in HLA-DR2+ individuals is 13.1 in these patients. These results also suggest that EBA and bullous SLE are immunogenetically related and that the *HLADR2* gene either is involved with autoimmunity to anchoring fibril collagen or is some sort of a marker for some other gene that exists in linkage disequilibrium with it.[1]

In another study examining HLA genotypes in EBA patients, it was found that HLA-DRB1*15:03 was overrepresented.[2]

In concordance with the genetic permissiveness towards EBA in humans, an active murine model of EBA in which mice are immunized with murine Type VII collagen, the development of EBA depends on the strain of mouse used.[3,4]

EBA is an exceedingly rare disease and considerably less frequent than other autoimmune bullous diseases (bullous pemphigoid, pemphigus vulgaris, dermatitis herpetiformis, etc.), which themselves are quite rare. In unselected bullous disease patients who exhibited an anti–basement membrane zone autoantibody in their blood, approximately 5% had the diagnosis of EBA or bullous SLE.[5] This incidence is similar to those reported by other investigators.[6] A prospective French study using electron and immune-electron microscopy to confirm the diagnosis of EBA, found an incidence rate as 0.17 to 0.26 per million people and accounted for only 2% to 3% of all patients with a subepidermal autoimmune bullous disease.[7] The incidence of EBA in a region of Germany was 0.17, again confirming the rarity of EBA.[8]

ETIOLOGY AND PATHOGENESIS

EBA is a chronic, subepidermal blistering disease associated with autoimmunity to the collagen (Type VII collagen) within anchoring fibril structures that are located at the dermal–epidermal junction (DEJ). Although the precise etiology of EBA is unknown, most of the evidence suggests an autoimmune etiology. The immunoglobulin G (IgG) autoantibodies to Type VII collagen are associated with a paucity of normal anchoring fibrils at the basement membrane zone (BMZ) separating the epidermis from the dermis and poor epidermal–dermal adherence. Although it is an acquired disease that usually begins in adulthood, it was placed in the category epidermolysis bullosa (EB) more than 100 years ago because physicians were struck by how similar the clinical lesions of EBA were to those seen in children with hereditary dystrophic forms of EB. Direct immunofluorescence (DIF) of perilesional skin biopsies from EBA patients reveals IgG deposits at the DEJ.[9] EBA antibodies bind to Type VII collagen within anchoring fibrils.[10,11]

Anchoring fibrils anchor the epidermis and its underlying BMZ to the papillary dermis. Patients with hereditary forms of dystrophic EB (Chap. 60) and EBA have decreased numbers of anchoring fibrils in their DEJ. This paucity of anchoring fibrils is associated with 2 similar clinical phenotypes, EBA and dystrophic forms of hereditary EB, because both diseases are characterized by skin fragility, subepidermal blisters, milia formation, and scarring. Although both EBA and hereditary forms of dystrophic EB are etiologically unrelated in terms of their underlying pathogenesis, they share the common feature of decreased anchoring fibrils. In the case of dystrophic forms of hereditary EB, the cause of decreased or absent anchoring fibrils is a genetic defect in the *COL7A1* gene, which encodes for Type VII collagen α chains, that ultimately results in small, nonfunctional, or decreased anchoring fibrils.[12,13] The gene coding for Type VII collagen is located on the short arm of chromosome 3.[14] The gene defects involved in hereditary forms of dystrophic EB have been identified at variable locations, but the severity of the disease appears to correlate with the degree of Type VII collagen and anchoring fibril perturbations.[13] In EBA, the IgG autoantibodies binding to the Type VII collagen α chains result in decreased anchoring fibrils, but the pathway leading to this reduction is unknown. It may be that Type VII collagen α chains that are newly synthesized but decorated with EBA autoantibodies cannot form triple-helical structures and stable anchoring fibrils. Healed burn wounds that have been covered with cultured keratinocyte sheets also have decreased numbers of anchoring fibrils within the first year after transplantation, and this is associated with spontaneous blister formation, shortened suction blistering times, and skin fragility.[15] These observations provide indirect evidence that anchoring fibrils play a role in maintaining adherence between the epidermis and dermis.

The Type VII collagen α chain has a molecular mass of 290 kDa and the collagen consists of a homotrimer of 3 identical α chains (Chap. 15). Each α chain consists of a large globular noncollagenous amino terminus called the *noncollagenous 1* (NC-1) *domain* that is approximately one-half the entire mass of the α chain. Next, there is a helical domain with typical glycine-X-Y repeats. At the carboxyl terminus is a second globular noncollagenous domain, NC-2, that is much smaller than NC-1.[16] Most EBA autoantibodies recognize 4 predominant antigenic epitopes within the NC-1 domain and do not recognize the helical or NC-2 domains.[17,18] There may be something intrinsically "antigenic" about the NC-1 domain because the available monoclonal antibodies that have been generated against Type VII collagen (anti–C-VII antibodies) specifically recognize only NC-1 subdomains.

A reduction in the number of anchoring fibrils is seen in the lesional and perilesional skin of EBA patients, but the pathway leading to this reduction is unknown.

Several independent lines of evidence have implicated autoimmune responses as a key element in the pathogenesis of EBA. First, the pathogenic role of EBA antibodies is suggested by the observation that when patients with SLE develop autoantibodies to the Type VII collagen, they develop widespread skin blisters and fall into a rare subset of SLE called *bullous SLE*.[19] This "experiment of nature" suggests that EBA autoantibodies are pathogenic and capable of inducing disadherence between the epidermis and dermis. Second, direct proof that EBA autoantibodies are pathogenic comes from recent passive transfer studies. We immunized rabbits and raised a high-titer antiserum to the NC-1 domain of human Type VII collagen. We injected this antibody into hairless immune-competent mice, and the mice developed bullous skin disease with many of the features of EBA in humans.[20] The mice developed subepidermal blisters and lost nails on their feet. They also had circulating NC-1 antibodies in their blood and anti–NC-1 IgG antibody deposits at their DEJ. In addition, the mice had murine complement deposits at the DEJ induced by the autoantibody–antigen complex.[20] Another study by Sitaru and colleagues[21] showed that the injection of rabbit polyclonal antibodies to the NC-1 domain of mouse Type VII collagen into mice also induced subepidermal skin blisters that were reminiscent of human EBA.[21] Further, we have also affinity-purified human EBA autoantibodies against an NC-1 column and injected them into mice. The mice then developed clinical, histologic, immunologic, and ultrastructural features akin to human EBA.[22] Taken together, these successful passive transfer experiments and the observations with bullous SLE strongly suggest that EBA autoantibodies are "pathogenic" and capable of causing epidermal–dermal separation in skin.

Using clinical patient studies, *in vitro* assays and murine models of EBA, much has been learned about the details of the immune responses of EBA patients harboring anti–Type VII collagen autoantibodies. EBA IgG autoantibodies in both the patients' blood and tissue bound in the patients' DEJ represent all 4 subclasses of IgG, particulary IgG1 and IgG4.[23] Circulating EBA autoantibodies consist of both complement binding and non–complement binding populations.[24] Nevertheless, when compared with BP, EBA patients had a higher presence of C3b and C5 (90% vs 33%, 90% vs 58%, respectively). These studies provided evidence[3] for complement activation at the DEJ in the majority of EBA patients and that EBA antibodies were more potent activators of C5 than BP antibodies.[25] Gammon and co-workers developed an *in vitro* assay to look at the functions of bullous pemphigoid and EBA immune complexes in skin. A slide chamber was made consisting of a cryostat section of human skin (normal skin or skin from patients with BP or EBA) with and without the additions of leukocytes and the additions of complement. The readout was the migration and attraction of the leukocytes to the DEJ of the human skin cryosections.[26] When cryostat sections of bullous pemphigoid skin and EBA skin were compared, the EBA immune complexes again generated more complement activation than bullous pemphigoid immune complexes.

In addition to murine models of EBA created by the passive transfer of anti–Type VII collagen antibodies, as noted in the sections "Epidemiology" above, an active murine model of EBA has been established by immunizing certain strains of mice with murine Type VII collagen. This active murine EBA model invokes complement fixing anti-Type VII collagen antibodies and requires T cells for disease induction.

CLINICAL FINDINGS

See Fig. 56-1. If a patient presents with bullae on the skin with no reasonable explanation despite a thorough history and physical examination, 3 tests should be done: a skin biopsy for routine hematoxylin and eosin histology, a second biopsy juxtaposed to a lesion but on normal-appearing skin for DIF and a blood draw to test for antibodies against the BMZ and/or Type VII collagen by indirect immunofluorescence (IIF) or enzyme-linked immunosorbent assay (ELISA).

The cutaneous lesions of EBA can be quite varied and can mimic other types of acquired autoimmune bullous diseases. The common denominator for patients with EBA is autoimmunity to Type VII (anchoring fibril) collagen. There are at least 5 clinical presentations: (1) a classic presentation, (2) a bullous pemphigoid (BP)-like presentation, (3) a mucous membrane pemphigoid (MMP)-like presentation, (4) a presentation reminiscent of Brunsting–Perry pemphigoid with scarring lesions and a predominant head and neck distribution, and (5) a presentation reminiscent of linear IgA bullous dermatosis or chronic bullous disease of childhood. The classical presentation and the BP-like presentation are the most commonly reported presentations of this very rare disease.

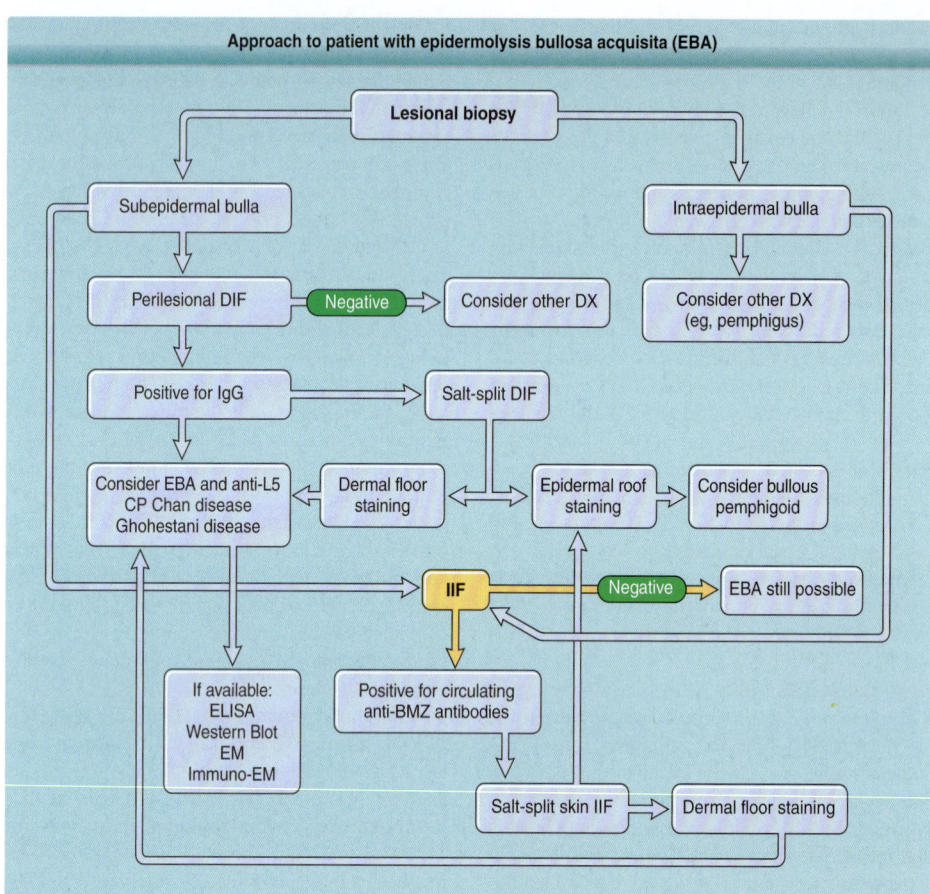

Figure 56-1 Approach to the patient with epidermolysis bullosa acquisita (EBA). BMZ, basement membrane zone; DIF, direct immunofluorescence; DX, diagnosis; ELISA, enzyme-linked immunosorbent assay; IgG, immunoglobulin G; IIF, indirect immunofluorescence.

CLASSIC PRESENTATION

The classic presentation (Figs. 56-2 and 56-3A) is of a noninflammatory bullous disease with an acral distribution that heals with scarring and milia formation. This presentation is reminiscent of porphyria cutanea tarda (PCT; Chap. 124) when it is mild and of the hereditary form of recessive dystrophic EB when it is severe (Chap. 60). The classic form of EBA is thus a mechanobullous disease marked by skin fragility. These patients have erosions, tense blisters within noninflamed skin, and scars over trauma-prone surfaces such as the backs of the hands, knuckles, elbows, knees, sacral area, and toes (Figs. 56-2, 56-3A, and 56-4). Some blisters may be hemorrhagic or develop scales, crusts, or erosions. The lesions heal with scarring and frequently with the formation of pearl-like milia cysts within the scarred areas (Fig. 56-3A). Although this presentation may be reminiscent of PCT, these patients do not have other hallmarks of PCT, such as hirsutism, a photodistribution of the eruption, or scleroderma-like changes, and their urinary porphyrins are within normal limits. A scarring alopecia and some degree of nail dystrophy may be seen.

Although the disease is usually not as severe as that of patients with hereditary forms of recessive dystrophic EB, EBA patients with the classic form of the disease may have many of the same sequelae, such as

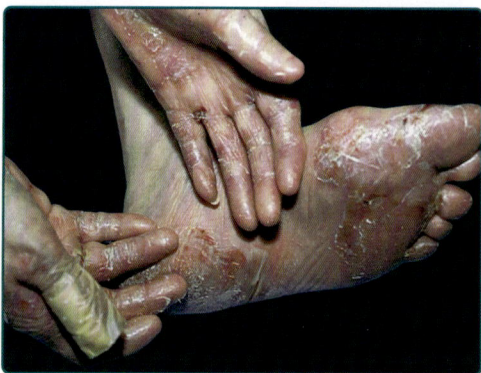

Figure 56-2 Patient with epidermolysis bullosa acquisita who has severe blistering, erosions, scarring, and milia formation on trauma-prone areas of her skin. This is the classic presentation.

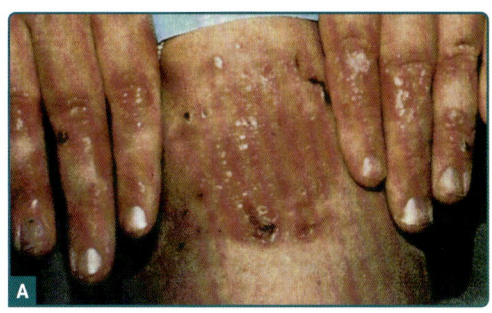
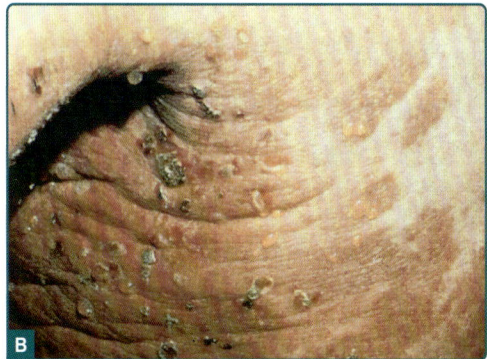
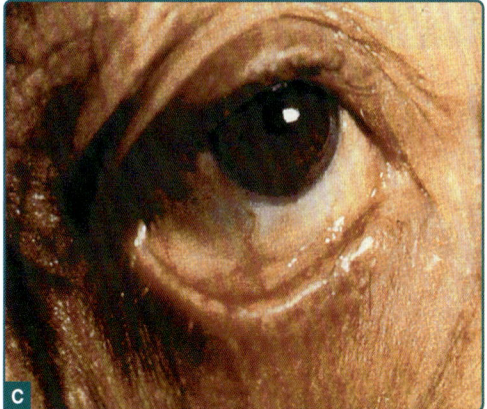
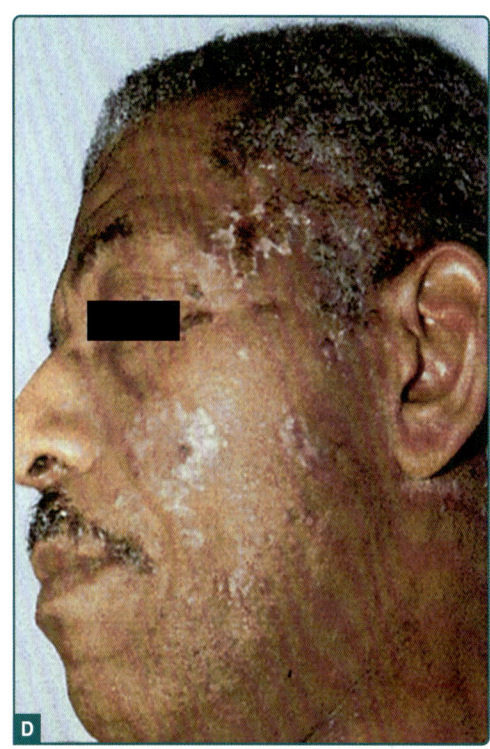

Figure 56-3 A, Classic presentation of epidermolysis bullosa acquisita with scarring and milia over trauma-prone areas of skin. **B,** Bullous pemphigoid–like presentation of epidermolysis bullosa acquisita with a widespread inflammatory vesiculobullous dermatosis. **C,** Cicatricial pemphigoid–like presentation of epidermolysis bullosa acquisita with a mucosal-centered bullous scarring eruption. **D,** Brunsting–Perry pemphigoid–like presentation of epidermolysis bullosa acquisita with bullous and scarring lesions predominantly on the head and neck.

scarring, loss of scalp hair, loss of nails, fibrosis of the hands and fingers, and esophageal stenosis.[27]

BULLOUS PEMPHIGOID–LIKE PRESENTATION

A second clinical presentation of EBA is of a widespread, inflammatory vesiculobullous eruption involving the trunk, central body, and skin folds in addition to the extremities.[6] The bullous lesions are tense and surrounded by inflamed or even urticarial skin. Large areas of inflamed skin may be seen without any blisters and only erythema or urticarial plaques. These patients often complain of pruritus and do not demonstrate prominent skin fragility, scarring, or milia formation. This clinical constellation is more reminiscent of BP (Figs. 56-3B and 56-4) than a mechanobullous disorder. Similar to BP, the distribution of the lesions may show an accentuation within flexural areas and skin folds.

MUCOUS MEMBRANE PEMPHIGOID-LIKE PRESENTATION

Both the classic and BP-like forms of EBA may have involvement of mucosal surfaces. However, EBA also may present with such predominant mucosal involvement that the clinical appearance is reminiscent of MMP (Fig. 56-3C).[28] These patients usually have erosions and scars on the mucosal surfaces of the mouth, upper esophagus, conjunctiva, anus, or vagina with or without similar lesions on the glabrous skin.

BRUNSTING–PERRY PEMPHIGOID-LIKE PRESENTATION

Brunsting–Perry cicatricial BP is a chronic, recurrent vesiculobullous eruption localized to the head and neck and characterized by residual scars, subepidermal bullae, IgG deposits at the DEJ, and minimal or no mucosal involvement. The antigenic target for the IgG autoantibodies, however, has not been defined. Nevertheless, a patient reported with this constellation of findings had IgG autoantibodies directed to anchoring fibrils below the lamina densa.[29] We have seen 3 additional patients with the features of Brunsting–Perry pemphigoid and autoantibodies directed to Type VII collagen (unpublished observations). Therefore, it appears that EBA patients may present with a clinical phenotype of Brunsting–Perry pemphigoid (Fig. 56-3D).

IMMUNOGLOBULIN A BULLOUS DERMATOSIS–LIKE PRESENTATION

IgA bullous dermatosis–like presentation of EBA is manifested by a subepidermal bullous eruption, a neutrophilic infiltrate, and linear IgA deposits at the BMZ when viewed by DIF. It may resemble linear IgA bullous dermatosis (LABD), dermatitis herpetiformis, or chronic bullous disease of childhood and may feature tense vesicles arranged in an annular fashion and involvement of mucous membranes.[30] The autoantibodies are usually IgA, IgG, or both.

The diagnosis of these subepidermal blistering cases with IgA anti–Type VII collagen antibodies showing linear IgA deposition at the BMZ is disputable. Some clinicians regard the patients as having purely LABD, whereas others regard them as having a subset of EBA. Further, the majority of EBA patients have low-titer IgA antibodies in their blood directed against Type VII collagen.

Childhood EBA is a rare disease. It has a variable presentation, including an LABD-like disease, a BP-like disease, and the classic mechanobullous EBA presentation. Although mucosal involvement is frequent and severe in childhood EBA, the overall prognosis is more favorable than in adult EBA.

INCIDENCE OF THE CLINICAL PRESENTATIONS OF EPIDERMOLYSIS BULLOSA ACQUISITA

According to the authors' experience, approximately 25% of patients with EBA may present with a BP-like clinical appearance. The disease of some of these patients eventually smolders into a more non-inflammatory mechanobullous form. However, both the classic and BP-like forms of the disease may coexist in the same patient (Fig. 56-5). The clinical phenotype of EBA that is reminiscent of pure CP occurs in fewer than 10% of all EBA cases.

RELATED PHYSICAL FINDINGS

EBA patients may have many physical findings similar to patients with hereditary dystrophic EB due to gene defects in the Type VII collagen gene. These include oral erosions, esophageal strictures, hypo- and hyperpigmentation skin mottling, nail loss, milia formation, scarring, and a degree of fibrosis of the hands.

A number of published reports suggest that EBA may be associated with various systemic diseases[18] such as inflammatory bowel disease, SLE, amyloidosis, thyroiditis, multiple endocrinopathy syndrome, rheumatoid arthritis, pulmonary fibrosis, chronic lymphocytic leukemia, thymoma, diabetes, multiple myeloma and other diseases in which an autoimmune pathogenesis has been implicated. At the University of North Carolina, Stanford, Northwestern, and University of Southern California, with a combined experience of following more than 62 EBA

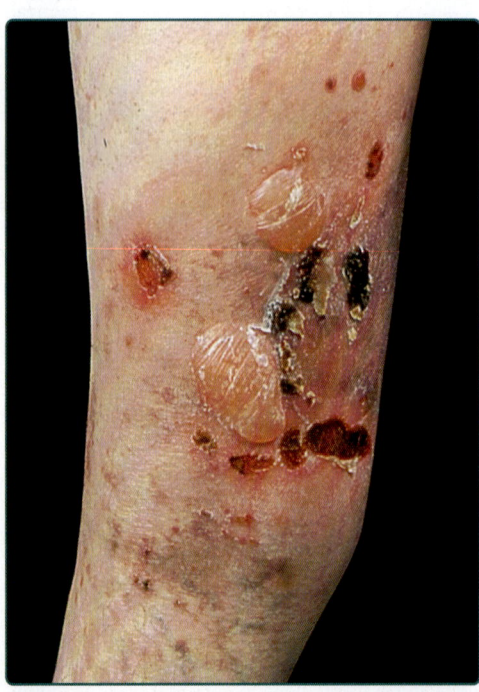

Figure 56-4 An epidermolysis bullosa acquisita patient with involvement of the leg. Note bullae, erosions, and crusts.

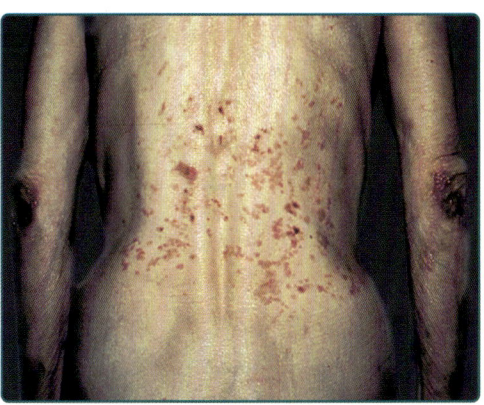

Figure 56-5 An epidermolysis bullosa acquisita patient demonstrating 2 presentations of the disease: The classic mechanobullous presentation with erosions, scarring, and milia over the elbows and the more inflammatory bullous pemphigoid-like lesions on her trunk.

patients, it appears that inflammatory bowel disease is the systemic disease most frequently associated with EBA.

LABORATORY TESTS

HISTOPATHOLOGY

Routine histologic examination of lesional skin obtained from EBA patients shows a subepidermal blister and a clean separation between the epidermis and dermis. The degree of inflammatory infiltrate within the dermis usually reflects the degree of inflammation of the lesion observed by the clinician. Lesions that are reminiscent of recessive dystrophic EB or PCT usually have a notable scarcity of inflammatory cells within the dermis. Lesions that are clinically reminiscent of BP usually have significantly more inflammatory cells within the dermis, and these cells may be a mixture of lymphocytes, monocytes, neutrophils, and eosinophils. The histology of EBA skin specimens obtained from BP-like lesions may be difficult to distinguish from BP itself.

DIRECT IMMUNOFLUORESCENCE

Patients with EBA have IgG deposits within the DEJ of their skin.[10,27] This is best detected by DIF of a biopsy specimen obtained from a perilesional site (Fig. 56-6). IgG is the predominant immunoglobulin class, but deposits of complement, IgA, IgM, factor B, and properdin also may be detected. The DIF staining demonstrates an intense linear fluorescent band at the DEJ. Yaoita et al.[9] have suggested that a positive DIF and IgG deposits within the sublamina densa zone are necessary criteria for the diagnosis of EBA.

Patients with PCT, which may mimic EBA clinically, frequently have IgG and complement deposits at the DEJ similar to those of EBA patients (Chap. 124). However, the DIF feature that distinguishes PCT from EBA is that PCT skin also demonstrates immune deposits around the dermal blood vessels.

Patients with EBA may have autoantibodies in their blood directed against the DEJ.[10] These antibodies can be detected by IIF of the patient's serum on a substrate of monkey or rabbit esophagus or human skin and stain the DEJ in a linear fashion that may be indistinguishable from BP sera.[22]

IMMUNOELECTRON MICROSCOPY

The localization of the immune deposits within the DEJ of the skin of EBA patients by immunoelectron microscopy is the "gold standard" for the diagnosis. As demonstrated by Nieboer et al.[31] and Yaoita et al.,[9] patients with EBA have immune deposits within the sublamina densa zone of the cutaneous BMZ. This localization is clearly distinct from the deposits in BP, which are higher up in the hemidesmosome area or lamina lucida area of the basement membrane. It is also distinct from CP, which has antigenic targets confined to the lamina lucida.

INDIRECT SALT-SPLIT SKIN IMMUNOFLUORESCENCE

When human skin is incubated in 1 molar sodium chloride, the DEJ fractures cleanly through the lamina lucida zone. This fracture places the BP antigen on the epidermal side of the split and all other basement membrane structures on the dermal side of the separa-

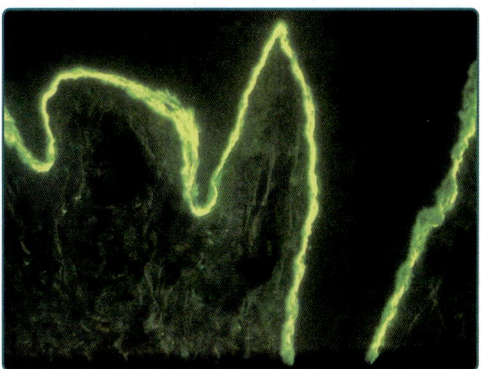

Figure 56-6 Direct immunofluorescence staining for immunoglobulin G deposits in perilesional skin of an epidermolysis bullosa acquisita patient. Note the dense deposits within the dermal–epidermal junction (the epidermis is on top in this section).

tion. Salt-split skin substrate can be used to distinguish EBA and BP sera.[10]

If the serum antibody is IgG and labels the epidermal roof, the patient does not have EBA, and BP should be considered. If, on the other hand, the antibody labels the dermal side of the separation, the patient usually has either EBA or bullous SLE. The latter can be ruled out by other serology and by clinical criteria.

DIRECT SALT-SPLIT SKIN IMMUNOFLUORESCENCE

Perilesional skin incubated in cold 1 molar sodium chloride is fractured through the DEJ, which effectively places the BP antigen (and any associated immune deposits) on the epidermal roof and the EBA antigen (and any associated immune deposits) on the dermal floor of the separation (Fig. 56-7).[27] If the patient has EBA, IgG immune deposits are detected on the dermal side of the separation by a routine DIF method using fluorescein-conjugated anti-human IgG.

WESTERN IMMUNOBLOTTING

Antibodies in EBA sera bind to a 290-kDa band in Western blots of human skin basement membrane proteins containing Type VII collagen, whereas sera from all other primary blistering diseases do not.[10] This band is the α chain of Type VII collagen. Often, a second band of 145 kDa is labeled with EBA antibodies. This band is the amino-terminal globular NC-1 domain of the Type VII collagen α chain, which is rich in carbohydrate and contains the antigenic epitopes of EBA autoantibodies, bullous SLE autoantibodies, and monoclonal antibodies against Type VII collagen.[17]

ENZYME-LINKED IMMUNOSORBENT ASSAY

Chen et al.[30] have produced milligram quantities of recombinant, purified, posttranslationally modified NC-1 in stably transfected human cells and have used this NC-1 to develop an ELISA for autoantibody detection in EBA patients and in patients with bullous SLE. This ELISA is more sensitive than immunofluorescence and Western blotting, and yet it is very specific for antibodies to Type VII collagen. There is now a commercially available ELISA for the detection of anti–Type VII collagen in the sera of patients.

DIFFERENTIAL DIAGNOSIS

See Table 56-1. Because EBA has been described in infants and children, it is worth considering that a

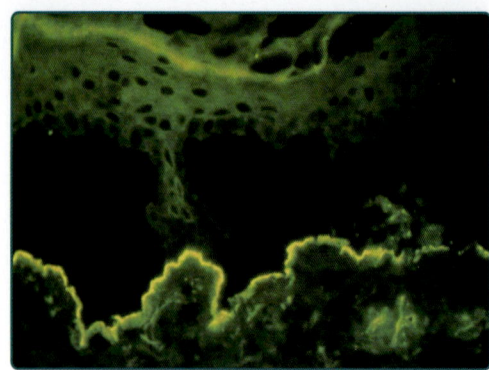

Figure 56-7 Direct immunofluorescence (DIF) staining of a patient's perilesional skin biopsy after incubation in 1 molar cold saline for 72 hours and probed with anti-human IgG antibodies. The cold salt incubation fractures the dermal–epidermal junction of the skin specimen. In EBA patients, the IgG deposits remain with the dermal floor of the fractured skin. In contrast, in patients with bullous pemphigoid, the deposits would remain with the epidermal roof of the fractured skin (not shown). Likewise, if the serum of an EBA patient has a circulating IgG antibody to Type VII (anchoring fibril) collagen and indirect immunofluorescence (IIF) is performed, the serum will label the dermal floor of salt-split human skin substrate and leave the epidermal roof unlabeled. These results are because incubating human skin in cold 1 molar salt fractures the dermal–epidermal junction such that the hemidesmosomes of the epidermis and the bullous pemphigoid autoantigens associated with hemidesmosomes remain with the epidermal roof, whereas anchoring fibrils and Type VII collagen, the autoantigen in EBA, remain with the dermal floor.

patient thought to have genetic dystrophic EB just might be a rare childhood patient with EBA. This can be ruled out by the antibody tests outlined in the section "Laboratory Tests." PCT can look clinically very much like classic EBA and can be ruled out by a urine or plasma test for uroporphyrins. Pseudo-PCT, usually caused by drugs such as nonsteroidal anti-inflammatory agents, can look similar to EBA with skin fragility, erosions, and blisters over trauma-prone areas, scarring, and milia formation. Nevertheless, the DIF appears different in that pseudo-PCT,

TABLE 56-1
Differential Diagnosis of Epidermolysis Bullosa Acquisita

Most Likely
- Porphyria cutanea tarda
- Pseudo-porphyria cutanea tarda
- Bullous pemphigoid
- Cicatricial pemphigoid

Consider
- Linear immunoglobulin A bullous disease
- Brunsting–Perry pemphigoid
- Bullous systemic lupus erythematosus

like PCT, shows IgG deposits at both the BMZ at the DEJ and around dermal blood vessels (which are not stained in EBA).

The BP-like EBA can be eliminated by several methods listed above, but the first-line test would be indirect and direct salt-split immunofluorescence.

DIAGNOSIS

The diagnostic criteria developed by Yaoita et al.[9] for the diagnosis of EBA still stand. These criteria, with slightly updated modifications, are shown in Table 56-2. Alternatives for the last item in the table are indirect or direct salt-split skin immunofluorescence, Western blotting, and ELISA.

COMPLICATIONS

The complications caused by EBA include secondary skin infections, usually due to *Staphylococcus* or *Streptococcus*, because the blisters and erosions compromise the skin's barrier. Scarring and milia formation are naturally occurring complications or sequelae of the deep blistering process. Severe EBA patients may develop significant fibrosis of the hands with decreased range of motion of the palm and digits. Because of wounds and fibrosis of the soles of the feet and toes, some EBA patients have difficulty walking. Many patients with EBA lose their fingernails. EBA patients with significant mucosal involvement may develop esophageal strictures and even laryngeal scarring.

TREATMENT

EBA usually responds poorly to treatment. Supportive therapy is warranted in all patients with EBA. This includes instruction in open wound care and strategies for avoiding trauma. Patients should be warned not to over wash or overuse hot water or harsh soaps and to avoid prolonged or vigorous rubbing of their skin with a washcloth or towel. In some patients, it appears that prolonged sun exposure may aggravate or promote new lesions on the dorsal hands and knuckles. Thus, avoidance of prolonged sun exposure and the use of sunscreens are helpful. The patient should be educated to recognize localized skin infections and to seek medical care and antibiotic therapy promptly when they occur.

EBA patients are often refractory to high doses of systemic glucocorticoids, azathioprine, methotrexate, and cyclophosphamide, especially when they have the classic mechanobullous form of the disease. These agents may be somewhat helpful in controlling EBA when it appears as an inflammatory BP-like disease. Some EBA patients improve on dapsone, especially when neutrophils are present in their dermal infiltrate.

Cyclosporine has been shown to be beneficial in EBA.[32] However, the long-term toxicity of this drug limits its use.

There are also independent reports of EBA patients responding to high doses of colchicine.[33] This is often used as a first-line drug because its side effects are relatively benign compared with other therapeutic choices. Diarrhea is a common side effect of colchicine, however, which makes it difficult for many patients to achieve a high enough dose to control the disease. Moreover, because of this side effect, we are hesitant to use colchicine in EBA patients who also have inflammatory bowel disease. In addition, there are patients who do not respond to colchicine. Colchicine is a well-known microtubule inhibitor, but it also appears to have properties that have the potential to inhibit antigen presentation to T cells, which could downregulate autoimmunity.

Photopheresis improves the clinical features of EBA and remarkably lengthens the suction blistering times

TABLE 56-2
Diagnostic Criteria for Epidermolysis Bullosa Acquisita

- A bullous disorder within the clinical spectrum outlined earlier (see "Clinical Findings").
- No family history of a bullous disorder.
- Histology showing a subepidermal blister.
- Deposition of immunoglobulin G deposits within the dermal–epidermal junction (ie, a positive direct immunofluorescence of perilesional skin).
- Immunoglobulin G deposits localized to the lower lamina densa and/or sublamina densa zone of the dermal–epidermal junction when perilesional skin is examined by direct immunoelectron microscopy.

TABLE 56-3
Treatments for Epidermolysis Bullosa Acquisita (EBA)

MEDICATION	DOSE RANGE
Colchicine[a]	0.6-3.0 mg/d
Cyclosporine A	6 mg/kg/d
Dapsone[b]	100-300 mg/d
Cytoxan	50-200 mg/d
Prednisone[c]	1.0-1.5 mg/kg
Intravenous immunoglobulin[d]	3 g/kg divided over 5 d
Infliximab	5 mg/kg at 0, 2, 4, and 6 wk
Rituximab	375 mg/m² of BSA, IV weekly × 4 wk Or 1000 mg IV on week 1 and week 3

[a]Must start with 0.4 to 0.6 mg/d and each 1 to 2 weeks double this dose as tolerated. When patient develops diarrhea, back off 1 tablet (0.4-0.6 mg).
[b]Begin at 25 mg/d and double each week after the complete blood count and liver function tests. Most patients need between 100 and 250 mg/d. Increasing the dose slowly helps the patient tolerate the anemia that develops (ie, less orthostatic light-headedness, etc.). Expect a 1- to 2-g drop in the patient's hemoglobin on therapeutic doses.
[c]Usually does not help the classic, mechanobullous type of EBA with minimal inflammation. However, it may be somewhat helpful in the bullous pemphigoid–like type of EBA.
[d]Intravenous immunoglobulin is given over 4 to 5 days every month for 5 or 6 months to give it an adequate trial.

of the patients, suggesting an improvement in their dermal–epidermal adherence.[34]

In addition to photophoresis, plasmapheresis and removal of the antibodies to Type VII collagen in an EBA patient's plasma is useful for gaining control of EBA patients similar to pemphigus patients. Given that the autoantibodies are pathogenic, this is not surprising, but when plasmapheresis is performed it is necessary to have the patient also treated with a chemotherapy agent (such as azathioprine, cyclophosphamide, mycotile mofelate, methotrexate).

Intravenous immunoglobulin (IVIG) has been reported to be effective in patients with EBA.[35] The mechanism by which γ-globulin may invoke a positive response in EBA is unknown.

The anti–TNF-α biologics (such as infliximab) have been tried in EBA with some success in uncontrolled open trials. Rituximab, a monoclonal antibody against the CD20 protein on the surface of B lymphocytes induces markedly decreased B-cell lymphocytes in the patients and has shown efficacy in recalcitrant EBA patients.[36,37] Table 56-3 outlines treatment options in EBA that have some support in the medical literature.

REFERENCES

1. Gammon WR, Heise ER, Burke WA, et al. Increased frequency of HLA DR2 in patients with autoantibodies to EBA antigen: evidence that the expression of autoimmunity to type VII collagen is HLA class II allele associated. *J Invest Dermatol*. 1988;91:228-232.
2. Zumelzu C, Le Roux-Villet C, Loiseau P, et al. Black patients of African Descent and HLA-DRB1*15:03 frequency overrepresented in epidermolysis bullosa acquisita. *J Invest Dermatol*. 2011;131(12):2366-2393.
3. Sitaru C, Chiriac MT, Mihai S, et al. Induction of complement fixing autoantibodies against type VII collagen results in subepidermal blistering in mice. *J Immunol*. 2006;177(5):3461-3468.
4. Ludwig RJ, Recke A, Bieber K, et al. Generation of antibodies of distinct subclasses and specificity is linked to H2s in an active mouse model of epidermolysis bullosa acquisita. *J Invest Dermatol*. 2011;131(1):167-176.
5. Zhu X-J, Niimi Y, Bystryn J-C. Epidermolysis bullosa acquisita. Incidence in patients with basement membrane zone antibodies. *Arch Dermatol*. 1990; 126(2):171-174.
6. Gammon WR, Briggaman RA, Woodley DT, et al. Epidermolysis bullosa acquisita: a pemphigoid-like disease. *J Am Acad Dermatol*. 1984;11(5, pt 1):820-832.
7. Bernard P, Vaillant L, Labeille B, et al. Incidence and distribution of subepidermal autoimmune bullous skin diseases in three French regions. Bullous Diseases French Study Group. *Arch Dermatol*. 1995;131(1):48-52.
8. Zillikens D, Wever S, Roth A, et al. Incidence of autoimmune subepidermal blistering dermatoses in a region of central Germany. *Arch Dermatol*. 1995;131(8):957-958.
9. Yaoita H, Briggaman RA, Lawley TJ, et al. Epidermolysis bullosa acquisita: ultrastructural and immunological studies. *J Invest Dermatol*. 1981;76(4):288-292.
10. Woodley DT, Briggaman RA, O'Keefe EJ, et al. Identification of the skin basement membrane autoantigen in epidermolysis bullosa acquisita. *N Engl J Med*. 1984;310(16):1007-1013.
11. Woodley DT, Burgeson RE, Lunstrum G, et al. The epidermolysis bullosa acquisita antigen is the globular carboxyl terminus of type VII procollagen. *J Clin Invest*. 1988;81(3):683-687.
12. Christiano AM, D'Alessio M, Paradisi M, et al. A common insertion mutation in COL7A1 in two Italian families with recessive dystrophic epidermolysis bullosa. *J Invest Dermatol*. 1996;106(4):679-684.
13. Shimizu H. Molecular basis of recessive dystrophic epidermolysis bullosa: genotype/phenotype correlation in a case of moderate clinical severity. *J Invest Dermatol*. 1996;106(1):119-124.
14. Parente MG, Chung LC, Ryynänen J, et al. Human type VII collagen: cDNA cloning and chromosomal mapping of the gene. *Proc Natl Acad Sci U S A*. 1991;88(16):6931-6935.
15. Woodley DT, Peterson HD, Herzog SR, et al. Burn wounds resurfaced by cultured epidermal autografts show abnormal reconstitution of anchoring fibrils. *JAMA*. 1988;259(17):2566-2571.
16. Christiano AM, Greenspan DS, Lee S, et al. Cloning of human type VII collagen: complete primary sequence of the alpha 1(VII) chain and identification of intragenic polymorphisms. *J Biol Chem*. 1994;269(32):20256.
17. Lapiere J-C, Woodley DT, Parente MG, et al. Epitope mapping of type VII collagen: identification of discrete peptide sequences recognized by sera from patients with acquired epidermolysis bullosa. *J Clin Invest*. 1993;92(4):1831-1839.
18. Jones DA, Hunt SW 3rd, Prisayanh PS, et al. Immunodominant autoepitopes of type VII collagen are short, paired peptide sequences within the fibronectin type III homology region of the non-collagenous (NC1) domain. *J Invest Dermatol*. 1995;104(2):231-235.
19. Gammon WR, Woodley DT, Dole KC, et al. Evidence that antibasement membrane zone antibodies in bullous eruption of systemic lupus erythematosus recognize epidermolysis bullosa acquisita autoantigens. *J Invest Dermatol*. 1985;84(6):472-476.
20. Woodley DT, Chang C, Saadat P, et al. Evidence that anti-type VII collagen antibodies are pathogenic and responsible for the clinical, histological, and immunological features of epidermolysis bullosa acquisita. *J Invest Dermatol*. 2005;124(5):958-964.
21. Sitaru C, Mihai S, Otto C, et al. Induction of dermal-epidermal separation in mice by passive transfer of antibodies specific to type VII collagen. *J Clin Invest*. 2005;115(4):870-878.
22. Woodley DT, Ram R, Doostan A, et al. Induction of epidermolysis bullosa acquisita in mice by passive transfer of autoantibodies from patients. *J Invest Dermatol*. 2006;126(6):1323-1330.
23. Mooney E, Gammon WR. Heavy and light chain isotypes of immunoglobulin in epidermolysis bullosa acquisita. *J Invest Dermatol*. 1990;95(3):317-319.
24. Briggaman RA, Gammon WR, Woodley DT. Epidermolysis bullosa acquisita of the immunopathological type (dermolytic pemphigoid). *J Invest Dermatol*. 1985;85(1)(suppl):79s–84s.
25. Mooney E, Falk RJ, Gammon WR. Studies on complement deposits in epidermolysis bullosa and bullous pemphigoid. *Arch Dermatol*. 1992;128(1):58-60.
26. Gammon WR, Lewis DM, Carlo JR, et al. Pemphigoid antibody mediated attachment of peripheral blood

leukocytes at the dermal-epidermal junction of human skin. *J Invest Dermatol*. 1980;75(4):334-339.
27. Woodley DT. Epidermolysis bullosa acquisita. *Prog Dermatol*. 1988;22:1-13.
28. Roenigk HH Jr, Ryan JG, Bergfeld WF. Epidermolysis bullosa acquisita: report of three cases and review of all published cases. *Arch Dermatol*. 1971;103(1):1-10.
29. Kurzhals G, Stolz W, Meurer M, et al. Acquired epidermolysis bullosa with the clinical features of Brunsting-Perry cicatricial bullous pemphigoid. *Arch Dermatol*. 1991;127(3):391-395.
30. Chen M, Chan LS, Cai X, et al. Development of an ELISA for rapid detection of anti-type VII collagen autoantibodies in epidermolysis bullosa acquisita. *J Invest Dermatol*. 1997;108(1):68-72.
31. Nieboer C, Boorsma DM, Woerdeman MJ, et al. Epidermolysis bullosa acquisita: immunofluorescence, electron microscopic and immunoelectron microscopic studies in four patients. *Br J Dermatol*. 1980;102(4):383-392.
32. Crow LL, Finkle JP, Gammon WR, et al. Clearing of epidermolysis bullosa acquisita on cyclosporin A. *J Am Acad Dermatol*. 1988;19(5, pt 2):937-942.
33. Cunningham BB, Kirchmann TT, Woodley D. Colchicine for epidermolysis bullosa (EBA). *J Am Acad Dermatol*. 1996;34(5, pt 1):781-784.
34. Gordon KB, Chan LS, Woodley DT. Treatment of refractory epidermolysis bullosa acquisita with extracorporeal photochemotherapy. *Br J Dermatol*. 1997;136(3):415-420.
35. Meier F, Sönnichsen K, Schaumburg-Lever G, et al. Epidermolysis bullosa acquisita: efficacy of high dose intravenous immunoglobulins. *J Am Acad Dermatol*. 1993;29(2, pt 2):334-337.
36. Schmidt E, Benoit S, Brocker EB, et al. Successful adjuvant treatment of recalcitrant epidermolysis bullosa acquisita with anti-CD20 antibody rituximab. *Arch Dermatol*. 2006;142(2):147-150.
37. Sadler E, Schafleitner B, Lanschueter C, et al. Treatment-resistant classical epidermolysis bullosa acquisita responding to rituximab. *Br J Dermatol*. 2007;157(2):417-419.

Chapter 57 :: Intercellular Immunoglobulin (Ig) A Dermatosis (IgA Pemphigus)
:: Takashi Hashimoto

第五十七章
细胞间IgA皮病（IgA天疱疮）

中文导读

　　细胞间IgA皮病（IAD）是一种由IgA抗体引起的慢性水疱性和/或脓疱性自身免疫性皮肤病。

　　本章从以下七个方面对本病进行了详细介绍。

　　1．流行病学　尚无明确的IAD流行病学资料。世界各地均有个案报道，IAD发病与种族、人种、性别无关。IAD平均发病年龄为45.9岁，偶见儿童IAD。

　　2．病因与发病机制　获得性免疫性大疱性皮病（AIBDs）患者有IgG或IgA自身抗体，它们与角质形成细胞表面或表皮基底膜区成分发生反应。IAD是AIBDs的一种，各种类型IAD具有针对不同桥粒糖蛋白和桥粒胶体蛋白的自身抗体，表明IgA自身抗体与皮肤病变的发生有关。

　　3．临床表现　本节分别介绍了角层下脓疱性皮病型细胞间IgA皮病、表皮内中性粒细胞IgA皮病型细胞间IgA皮病、增殖性天疱疮型细胞间IgA皮病、落叶型天疱疮和寻常型天疱疮型细胞间IgA皮病、未定型细胞间IgA皮病的临床表现。

　　4．诊断　本节介绍了IAD的组织病理学、免疫荧光检查的特征。

　　5．鉴别诊断　本节在表57-3中总结了IAD的鉴别诊断，提到了IAD除了需要区别于其他AIBDs，还需要与脓疱型银屑病、多形红斑、干燥综合征、SCLE相鉴别。

　　6．临床病程与预后　一般而言，IAD可用氨苯砜控制，合并使用或不使用低剂量糖皮质激素。IAD虽然不是致命性的，但极其难治。

　　7．治疗　由于IAD罕见，目前尚无IAD治疗性临床研究，无令人满意的IAD治疗指南，本节介绍了氨苯砜和其他磺胺类药物、糖皮质激素和免疫抑制剂等治疗药物。

〔陈明亮〕

AT-A-GLANCE

- Intercellular immunoglobulin (Ig) A dermatosis (IAD) is a chronic vesicular and/or pustular autoimmune skin disease caused by IgA, not by IgG, antibodies.
- Two major types: subcorneal pustular dermatosis (SPD)-type IAD and intraepidermal neutrophilic IgA dermatosis (IEN)-type IAD.
- SPD-type IAD clinically shows superficial pustules on the intertriginous areas.
- IEN-type IAD clinically shows atypical pustular skin lesions with a sunflower-like configuration.
- Diagnosis is made by histopathology showing intraepidermal pustules, immunofluorescence detecting in vivo bound and/or circulating IgA antikeratinocyte cell-surface autoantibodies, and various biochemical and molecular biologic methods demonstrating reactivity with various autoantigens.
- SPD-type IAD shows histopathologically subcorneal neutrophilic pustules.
- IEN-type IAD shows histopathologically neutrophilic pustules in the middle epidermis.
- Major autoantigens are desmogleins (Dsg) and desmocollins (Dsc), cadherin-type cell-to-cell adhesion molecules found in desmosomes.
- Patients are treated mainly with dapsone and systemic corticosteroids; other treatment options include immunosuppressive agents, tetracycline, colchicine, plasmapheresis, retinoids, adalimumab, and psoralen and ultraviolet A.

This chapter discusses findings, pathogenesis, diagnosis, and treatments for intercellular immunoglobulin (Ig) A dermatosis (also called IgA pemphigus): Other synonyms are intraepidermal neutrophilic IgA dermatosis, intercellular IgA vesiculopustular dermatosis and IgA pemphigus foliaceus.

In addition to clinical and histopathologic assessments, detection of autoantibodies to the skin by immunofluorescence is still a hallmark for the diagnoses of various autoimmune bullous diseases (AIBDs), which are organ-specific autoimmune diseases of the skin and mucous membranes.[1-4] In addition, according to the progress in recent biochemical and molecular biologic techniques, various methods detecting autoantigen, including immunoblotting and enzyme-linked immunosorbent assays (ELISAs), are performed to make precise diagnoses of various AIBDs.[1-8] Based on the results of these antigen detection analyses, AIBDs are currently classified into a large number of different diseases with distinct autoantibodies and autoantigens.[1,2]

The term *intercellular IgA dermatosis* (IAD) (also frequently called *IgA pemphigus*) refers to a group of AIBDs of skin and mucous membranes. IAD is characterized clinically by pustular skin lesions, histopathologically by intraepidermal neutrophilic pustules, and immunopathologically by in vivo bound and circulating IgA antibodies directed against the keratinocytes cell surfaces.[9-14]

This disease entity was first reported by Daniel Wallach.[15] IAD/IgA pemphigus shows variable clinical, histopathologic, and immunologic features. As a result, this condition has been reported under a variety of names, including IAD,[14] intraepidermal neutrophilic IgA dermatosis (IEN),[16] intercellular IgA vesiculopustular dermatosis,[17] and IgA pemphigus foliaceus.[18]

However, clinical, histopathologic, and immunologic features of this disease are considerably different from those in classical IgG types of pemphigus. Therefore, the term IAD was proposed as the name most suitable for this disorder.[9-11,14]

In the current classification of IAD,[9-13] 2 major subtypes of IAD are subcorneal pustular dermatosis (SPD)-type IAD and IEN-type IAD. There also are minor subtypes, including IgA pemphigus vegetans (PVeg), IgA pemphigus foliaceus (PF), IgA pemphigus vulgaris (PV), and undetermined-type IAD. Table 57-1 outlines the classification of the IAD subtypes with their autoantigens.

SPD-type IAD develops the pustules in the uppermost epidermis, just below the cornified layer, whereas IEN-type IAD develops the pustule in the middle or entire epidermis. IgA PVeg clinically shows PVeg-like vegetating skin lesions, whereas IgA PF and IgA PV show IgA autoantibodies against desmoglein (Dsg) 1 and Dsg3, respectively.

EPIDEMIOLOGY

PV, the representative disease of classical IgG-type pemphigus, is known to have human leukocyte antigen–related genetic background and to be more prevalent in Jewish, Middle Eastern, and Japanese populations. In contrast, the epidemiology of IAD has not been studied because of IAD's rarity. However, because sporadic cases have been reported through the world evenly,[9-13] incidence and prevalence of IAD seem to be indepen-

TABLE 57-1
Classification of Subtypes of Intercellular IgA Dermatosis and Their Autoantigens

DISEASES	AUTOANTIGENS
Subcorneal pustular dermatosis (SPD)-type intercellular IgA dermatosis (IAD)	Desmocollin 1 (Dsc1)
Intraepidermal neutrophilic IgA dermatosis (IEN)-type IAD	Unknown
IgA pemphigus vegetans (PVeg)	Desmogleins or desmocollins
IgA pemphigus foliaceus (PF)	Desmoglein 1 (Dsg1)
IgA pemphigus vulgaris (PV)	Desmoglein 3 (Dsg3)
Undetermined-type IAD	Undetermined, desmogleins or desmocollins

dent of the ethnic population. There is no gender prevalence.[9] The average age of disease onset is around 45.9 years.[9] This age of onset is younger than those in other AIBDs. There are also a few cases of IAD occurring in a child.[9]

ETIOLOGY AND PATHOGENESIS

AIBDs show autoantibodies of either IgG or IgA classes, which react with various cutaneous structural components at either keratinocyte cell surfaces or epidermal basement membrane zone. IAD is one of AIBDs, and shows anti–cell-surface autoantibodies exclusively of IgA class. Basic research revealed that various types of IAD have IgA autoantibodies against different autoantigens, mainly desmogleins and desmocollins, and suggested that the IgA autoantibodies are related to development of the skin lesions.

Although a passive transfer of IgG from patients to neonatal mice induced blisters with typical histology for PV or PF, no animal disease models were able to reproduce the human phenotype of IAD. Thus, the pathogenic role of IgA autoantibodies is still unclear.

AUTOANTIGENS

Earlier studies using immunoblotting techniques suggested that IAD sera contained IgA autoantibodies reactive most frequently with desmocollins,[17] and less frequently desmogleins.[19] However, sensitivity of immunoblotting to detect antigens for IgA autoantibodies in IAD sera was very low, probably because the IgA autoantibodies react with conformation dependent epitopes on the autoantigens, which are destroyed during the immunoblotting procedure.[17]

Desmogleins[6] and desmocollins[8] are transmembrane glycoproteins, and consist of the desmosomal cadherin superfamily of calcium-dependent cell-adhesion molecules. Each desmocollin (ie, Dsc1, Dsc2, and Dsc3) is composed of the 110-kDa a form (ie, Dsc1a, Dsc2a, Dsc3a) and the 100-kDa b form (ie, Dsc1b , Dsc2b , Dsc3b), which are produced by alternative splicing.[8] Dsc1 is expressed in the keratinocyte cell surfaces in the uppermost epidermis,[8] where subcorneal pustules and IgA deposition are found in the skin lesions of SPD-type IAD, strongly suggesting that IgA anti-Dsc1 autoantibodies play a pathogenic role in SPD-type IAD. In contrast, Dsc2 is expressed in the entire epidermis and Dsc3 is expressed more strongly in the low epidermis.

Then, the sophisticated technique of transfection of complementary DNAs (cDNAs) of human Dsc1, Dsc2, and Dsc3 into cultured COS-7 cells was developed.[20] In the cDNA transfection method, IgA autoantibodies in the SPD-type IAD sera react with Dsc1, while IgA antibodies in IEN-type IAD sera react with none of Dsc1, Dsc2, or Dsc3.[20]

Subsequently, IgA ELISAs using baculovirus-producing recombinant proteins of Dsg1 and Dsg3 were developed.[21] In this ELISA, IgA antibodies in IgA PF and IgA PV sera react with Dsg1 and Dsg3, respectively.[21]

To detect autoantibodies to Dsc1, Dsc2, and Dsc3 for both IgG and IgA antibodies, ELISAs using baculovirus-producing recombinant proteins of human Dsc1, Dsc2, and Dsc3 were developed.[22] However, sensitivity of this method was proved to be very low, and even IgA antibodies in SPD-type IAD sera rarely reacted with Dsc1. The reason for this low sensitivity was thought to be because antidesmocollin autoantibodies cannot react with baculovirus-producing desmocollin-recombinant proteins, whereas antidesmoglein autoantibodies can react with baculovirus-producing desmoglein-recombinant proteins.

Consequently, novel ELISAs were developed using mammalian recombinant proteins of human Dsc1, Dsc2, and Dsc3, in which IgG antibodies in sera from patients with paraneoplastic pemphigus and atypical pemphigus, but not classical IgG-types of pemphigus, frequently reacted with desmocollins.[8] Subsequently, using the IgG ELISAs of mammalian recombinant proteins of Dsc1, Dsc2, and Dsc3, IgA ELISAs were developed.[23] In the IgA ELISAs, IgA antibodies in sera from most patients with SPD-type IAD react with Dsc1, whereas Dsc2 and Dsc3 react with sera from particular IAD sera.[23]

The autoantigen for IEN-type IAD are still unidentified. Immunoelectron-microscopy study indicated that IgA antibodies in IEN-type IAD sera react with cell surfaces at the interdesmosomal area in keratinocytes, suggesting that an autoantigen for IEN-type IAD is nondesmosomal protein.[24] Previous biochemical studies using either immunoblotting[17] or proteomics techniques[25] have not identified autoantigen in IEN-type IAD.

CLINICAL FINDINGS

Table 57-2 provides a summary of IAD subtypes.

SUBCORNEAL PUSTULAR DERMATOSIS–TYPE INTERCELLULAR IgA DERMATOSIS

The typical skin lesions of SPD-type IAD are superficial flaccid pustules developed in the periphery of annular or herpetiform erythemas on the entire body, most prevalently intertriginous regions, such as axillae and groins (Figs. 57-1 and 57-2).[9,10,13,14,26,27] Because pustules in SPD-type IAD are extremely superficial, the most pustular skin lesions turn into erosions and crusts, resulting in postinflammatory pigmentation. The Nikolsky sign is usually absent.

These clinical features are indistinguishable from those seen in patients with classical SPD without IgA autoantibodies.

INTRAEPIDERMAL NEUTROPHILIC IgA DERMATOSIS–TYPE INTERCELLULAR IgA DERMATOSIS

The characteristic skin lesions of IEN-type IAD are demarcated atypical pustular lesions scattered on the entire body, in which relatively deep pustules develop on the slightly elevated periphery of annular erythemas of 10 mm to 30 mm and generate a so-called sunflower-like configuration (Figs. 57-3 and 57-4).[9,10,13,16,27] Whereas SPD-type IAD never develops mucous membrane lesions, particular cases of IEN-type IAD show oral mucosal lesions.

PEMPHIGUS VEGETANS–TYPE INTERCELLULAR IgA DERMATOSIS

PVeg-type IAD patients develop PVeg-like vegetating skin lesions with erosions, prevalently in the intertriginous areas and the scalp (Fig. 57-5).[9,10,13,28]

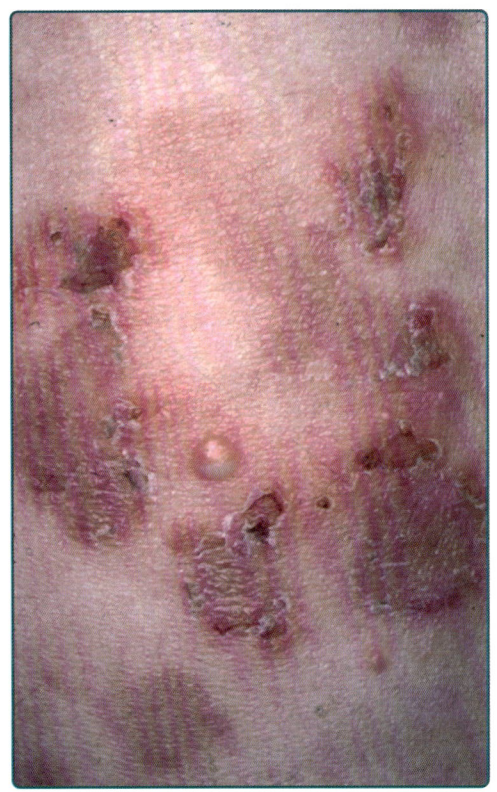

Figure 57-1 Clinical feature of subcorneal pustular dermatosis–type intercellular IgA dermatosis showing superficial pustules on herpetiform erythemas and hypopyon. (From Hashimoto T, Inamoto N, Nakamura K, et al. Intercellular IgA dermatosis with clinical features of subcorneal pustular dermatosis. *Arch Dermatol*. 1987; 123(8):1062-1065, with permission. Copyright © 1987 American Medical Association. All rights reserved.)

TABLE 57-2
Summary of Intercellular IgA Dermatosis Subtypes

IAD SUBTYPE	CLINICAL FEATURES
SPD-type IAD	Superficial flaccid pustules in the periphery of annular of herpetiform erythemas, most prominent in axillae and groin; (−) Nikolsky; no mucosal involvement
IEN-type IAD	Demarcated atypical pustular lesions scattered on entire body; "sunflower like" configuration; may have mucosal involvement
PVeg-type IAD	Vegetating skin lesions with erosions; scalp and intertriginous areas most affected
PF and PV-type IAD	Clinical and histopathologic similarity to PF and PV, but with IgA reactivity mainly with Dsg1 and Dsg3
Undetermined-type IAD	IAD patients that do not meet any of the above-mentioned subtypes.

Dsg, desmoglein; IAD, intercellular IgA dermatosis; IEN, intraepidermal neutrophilic IgA dermatosis; PF, pemphigus foliaceus; PV, pemphigus vulgaris; PVeg, pemphigus vegetans; SPD, subcorneal pustular dermatosis.

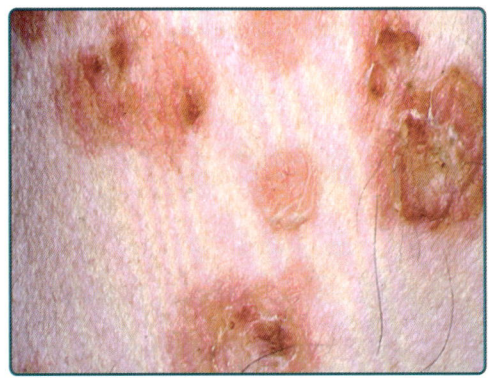

Figure 57-2 Clinical feature of subcorneal pustular dermatosis–type intercellular IgA dermatosis showing superficial pustules and flaccid bullae on the herpetiform erythemas. (From Hashimoto T, Teye K, Ishii N. Clinical and immunological studies of 49 cases of various types of intercellular IgA dermatosis and 13 cases of classical subcorneal pustular dermatosis examined at Kurume University. *Br J Dermatol*. 2017;176(1):168-75, with permission. Copyright © 2017, John Wiley & Sons.)

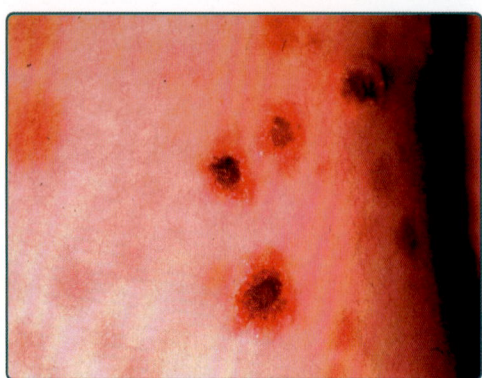

Figure 57-3 Clinical feature of intraepidermal neutrophilic IgA dermatosis–type intercellular IgA dermatosis showing elevated annular erythema with pustules on the periphery and crusts in the center.

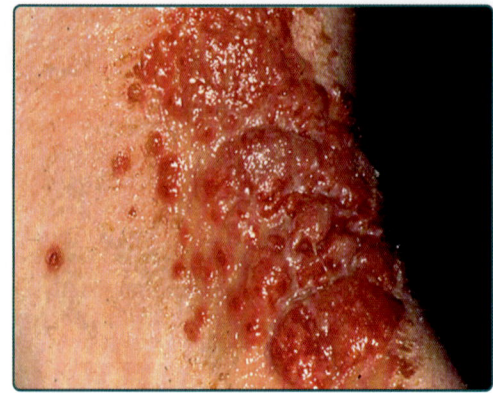

Figure 57-5 Clinical feature of IgA pemphigus vegetans showing vegetating erosive skin lesions. (From Weston WL, Friednash M, Hashimoto T, et al. A novel childhood pemphigus vegetans variant of intraepidermal neutrophilic IgA dermatosis. *J Am Acad Dermatol.* 1998;38(4): 635-38, with permission. Copyright © American Academy of Dermatology.)

PEMPHIGUS FOLIACEUS AND PEMPHIGUS VULGARIS–TYPE INTERCELLULAR IgA DERMATOSIS

While SPD-type IAD, IEN-type IAD, and PVeg-type IAD are diagnosed based on the clinical and histopathologic features, the diagnoses of PF-type IAD and PV-type IAD are made for the patients who show IgA reactivity mainly or exclusively with Dsg1 and Dsg3, respectively, in ELISAs or immunoblotting.[9,10,13,21] PF-type IAD shows clinical and histopathologic features that mimic either PF or IEN-type IAD.[9,10,13,19] PV-type IAD shows mainly clinical and histopathologic features of either PV or IEN-type IAD.[9,10,13,29] Some patients with PV-type IAD show PV-like oral mucosal erosive lesions (Fig. 57-6).[29]

UNDETERMINED-TYPE INTERCELLULAR IgA DERMATOSIS

Some IAD patients show clinical and histopathologic features that do not meet the criteria of SPD-type IAD, IEN-type IAD, or PVeg-type IAD, and do not show exclusive IgA reactivity with either Dsg1 or Dsg3. These cases are tentatively classified as undetermined-type IAD.[9] One patient with undetermined-type IAD showed paraneoplastic pemphigus–like clinical features with severe oral mucosal lesions.[30] However, these cases may progress to show

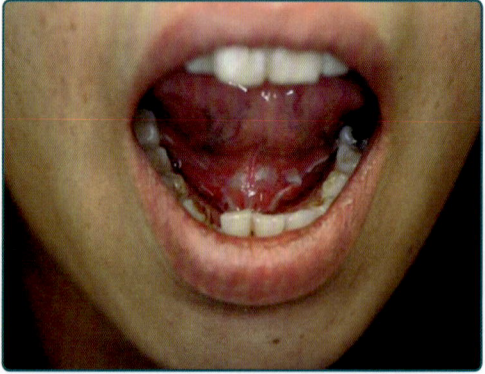

Figure 57-6 Clinical feature of IgA pemphigus vulgaris showing blisters and erosions on the oral mucosa. (From Hashimoto T, Teye K, Ishii N. Clinical and immunological studies of 49 cases of various types of intercellular IgA dermatosis and 13 cases of classical subcorneal pustular dermatosis examined at Kurume University. *Br J Dermatol.* 2017;176(1):168-75, and used with permission from Professor Hiroyuki Matsue, Department of Dermatology, Chiba University School of Medicine, Chiba, Japan.)

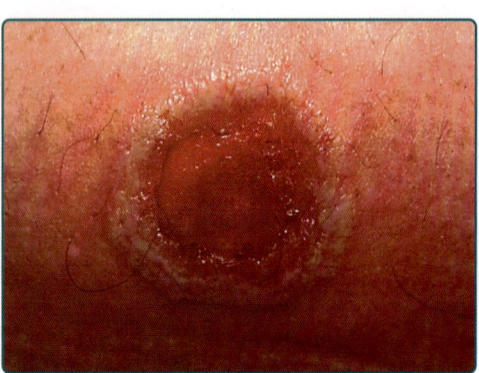

Figure 57-4 Clinical feature of intraepidermal neutrophilic IgA dermatosis–type intercellular IgA dermatosis showing atypical pustular skin lesion with so-called sunflower-like configuration.

characteristics of other types of IAD. Alternatively, futures studies may suggest additional types of IAD for these patients.

ASSOCIATED DISEASES

Underlying disease most frequently found in IAD is ulcerative colitis.[9] Interestingly, ulcerative colitis is associated with either IEN-type IAD or PV-type IAD, but never with SPD-type IAD.[9] IAD is also associated with either multiple myeloma[9,31] or B-cell lymphoma.[32] Considering that elevation of total serum level of IgA is also found in IAD patients,[9] B-cell or plasma cell proliferative disorders may trigger development of IAD. There is no particular association with nonhematologic malignant tumors.

DIAGNOSIS

For the diagnosis of IAD, in addition to inspection of skin lesions, various laboratory tests are necessary.[9-13] Histopathologic examination and direct immunofluorescence of biopsies taken from lesional skin and perilesional skin, respectively, are first performed. In serologic tests, circulating IgA autoantibodies and their autoantigens are determined by indirect immunofluorescence, immunoblotting mainly using normal human epidermal extracts, and ELISAs using recombinant proteins of desmogleins and desmocollins, as well as cDNA transfection methods for Dsc1, Dsc2, and Dsc3.[9-13]

HISTOPATHOLOGY

Histopathologically, SPD-type IAD shows subcorneal neutrophilic pustule in the uppermost epidermis (Fig. 57-7), which is identical to histopathologic findings seen in classical SPD without IgA antibodies. In contrast, IEN-type IAD develops intraepidermal neutrophilic pustules in the middle or entire epidermis (Fig. 57-8). In both SPD-type and IEN-type IAD, eosinophils and acantholytic cells are also occasionally seen in the pustules. PVeg-type IAD shows PVeg-like acanthosis with intraepidermal neutrophilic/eosinophilic pustules. PF-type IAD usually shows either IEN-type IAD-like intraepidermal neutrophilic pustules in the entire epidermis or PF-like acantholytic blister in the upper epidermis. PV-type IAD usually shows IEN-type IAD-like pustules containing either neutrophils or eosinophils in the entire epidermis, or PV-like suprabasilar acantholytic blisters (Fig. 57-9).

IMMUNOFLUORESCENCE

DIRECT IMMUNOFLUORESCENCE

For the diagnosis of IAD, direct immunofluorescence using perilesional skin biopsy, which detects in vivo bound IgA autoantibodies, is essential. When a negative result is obtained for direct immunofluorescence, the diagnosis of IAD should be seriously doubted. SPD-type IAD shows IgA deposition to keratinocyte cell surfaces in the uppermost epidermis (Fig. 57-10). In contrast, IEN-type IAD shows IgA deposition to the cell surfaces in the entire epidermis (Fig. 57-11). PVeg-type IAD shows IgA deposition to various levels in the epidermis, which depends on the autoantigens in each patient. PF-type IAD shows IgA deposition to the cell surfaces in the entire epidermis, being stronger in the upper epidermis. PV-type IAD shows IgA deposition to the cell surfaces in the lower epidermis (Fig. 57-12). Undermined-type IAD shows IgA reactivity with various epidermal layers, depending on the autoantigens in each patient.

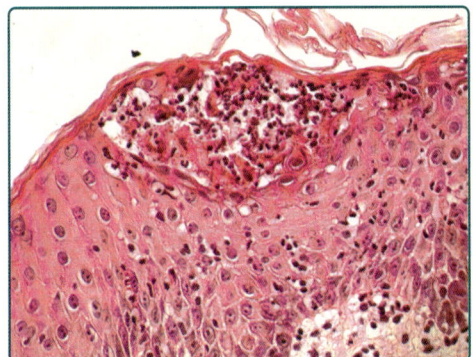

Figure 57-7 Histopathologic feature of subcorneal pustular dermatosis–type intercellular IgA dermatosis showing subcorneal pustules in the upper epidermis. (From Robinson ND, Hashimoto T, Amagai M, et al. The new pemphigus variants. *J Am Acad Dermatol*. 1999;40(5, pt 1): 649-71, Table II, 5th picture, with permission. Copyright © American Academy of Dermatology.)

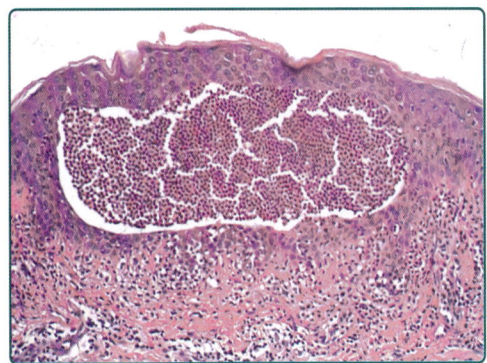

Figure 57-8 Histopathologic feature of intraepidermal neutrophilic IgA dermatosis–type intercellular IgA dermatosis showing neutrophilic pustule formation in the middle epidermis. (From Hashimoto T, Yasumoto S, Nagata Y, et al. Clinical, histopathological and immunological distinction in two cases of IgA pemphigus. *Clin Exp Dermatol*. 2002; 27(8):636-40, Fig. 2. Copyright © 2002, John Wiley & Sons.)

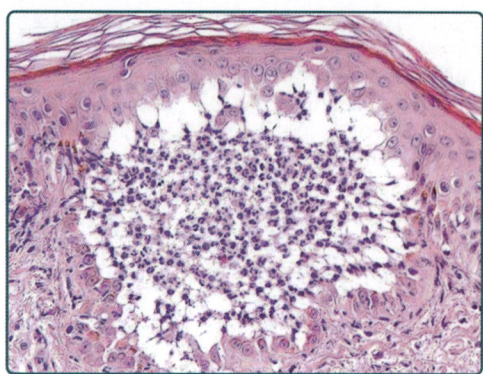

Figure 57-9 Histopathologic feature of IgA pemphigus vulgaris showing suprabasal blister containing neutrophils. (From Hashimoto T, Teye K, Ishii N. Clinical and immunological studies of 49 cases of various types of intercellular IgA dermatosis and 13 cases of classical subcorneal pustular dermatosis examined at Kurume University. Br J Dermatol. 2017;176(1):168-75, and used with permission from Professor Hiroyuki Matsue, Department of Dermatology, Chiba University School of Medicine, Chiba, Japan.)

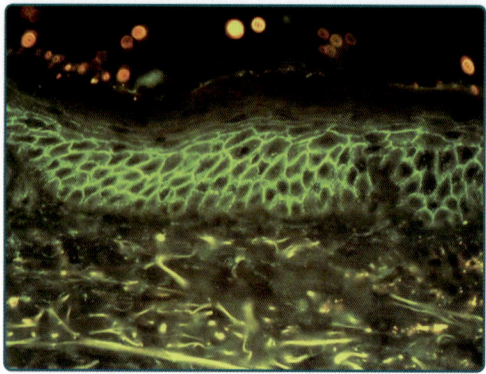

Figure 57-11 Direct immunofluorescence result of intraepidermal neutrophilic IgA dermatosis–type intercellular IgA dermatosis showing IgA reactivity with keratinocyte cell surfaces in the entire epidermis. (From Hashimoto T, Teye K, Ishii N. Clinical and immunological studies of 49 cases of various types of intercellular IgA dermatosis and 13 cases of classical subcorneal pustular dermatosis examined at Kurume University. Br J Dermatol. 2017;176(1):168-75, with permission. Copyright © 2017, John Wiley & Sons.)

INDIRECT IMMUNOFLUORESCENCE

Because titers of IgA antikeratinocyte cell-surface autoantibodies in the sera of various types of IAD are in general very low, IAD patient sera occasionally shows negative results in indirect immunofluorescence with sections of normal human skin or monkey esophagus as substrates. Thus, sensitivity of indirect immunofluorescence for the diagnosis of IAD is lower than that of direct immunofluorescence.

In indirect immunofluorescence using normal human skin, circulating IgA antibodies in various types of IAD show IgA reactivity to keratinocyte cell surfaces at the same levels in the epidermis as those of IgA deposition detected by direct immunofluorescence. Thus, the sera of SPD-type IAD show exclusive IgA binding to cell surfaces in the uppermost epidermis (Fig. 57-13), whereas IEN-type IAD shows IgA reactivity with the cell surfaces in the entire epidermis (Fig. 57-14). PVeg-type IAD shows IgA binding to various levels in the epidermis. IgA PF shows IgA reactivity with the cell surfaces in the entire epidermis, being stronger in the upper epidermis (Fig. 57-15), whereas PV-type IAD shows IgA reactivity with the cell surfaces in the lower epidermis (Fig. 57-16). Undetermined-type IAD shows IgA reactivity with various epidermal layers.

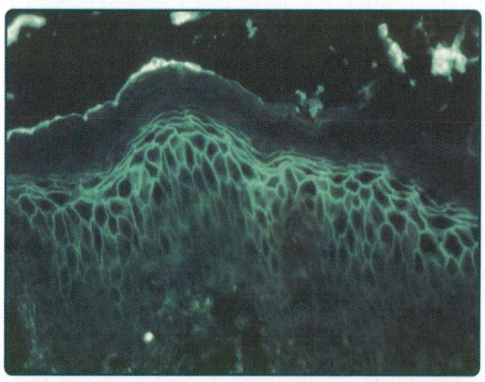

Figure 57-10 Direct immunofluorescence result of subcorneal pustular dermatosis–type intercellular IgA dermatosis showing IgA reactivity with keratinocyte cell surfaces in the uppermost epidermis. (From Hashimoto T, Teye K, Ishii N. Clinical and immunological studies of 49 cases of various types of intercellular IgA dermatosis and 13 cases of classical subcorneal pustular dermatosis examined at Kurume University. Br J Dermatol. 2017;176(1):168-75, with permission. Copyright © 2017, John Wiley & Sons.)

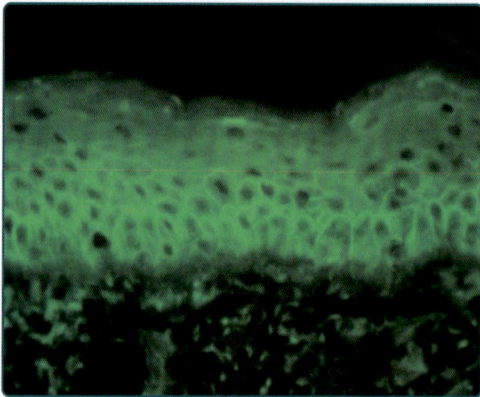

Figure 57-12 Direct immunofluorescence result of pemphigus vulgaris–type intercellular IgA dermatosis showing IgA reactivity with keratinocyte cell surfaces in the lower epidermis. (From Hashimoto T, Teye K, Ishii N. Clinical and immunological studies of 49 cases of various types of intercellular IgA dermatosis and 13 cases of classical subcorneal pustular dermatosis examined at Kurume University. Br J Dermatol. 2017;176(1):168-75, and used with permission from Professor Hiroyuki Matsue, Department of Dermatology, Chiba University School of Medicine, Chiba, Japan.)

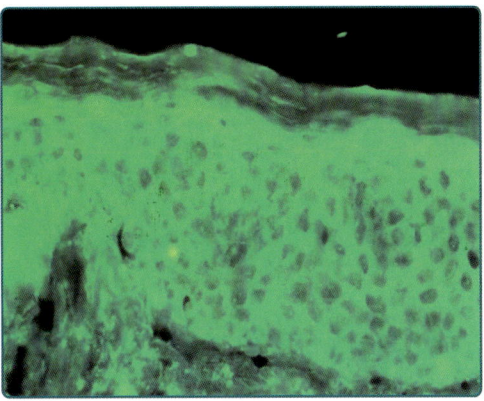

Figure 57-13 Indirect immunofluorescence result of subcorneal pustular dermatosis–type intercellular IgA dermatosis showing IgA reactivity with keratinocyte cell surfaces in the uppermost epidermis.

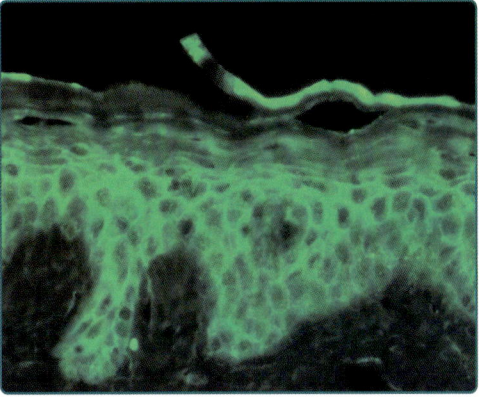

Figure 57-15 Indirect immunofluorescence result of pemphigus foliaceus–type intercellular IgA dermatosis showing IgA reactivity with keratinocyte cell surfaces in the entire epidermis, being stronger in the upper epidermis.

Although direct immunofluorescence is nonquantitative test, indirect immunofluorescence is performed for serially diluted patient sera and thus is a semiquantitative method. In some reported cases, titers of IgA anti–cell-surface antibodies in IAD sera decreased or disappeared after the resolution of the skin lesions. Thus, the titers in indirect immunofluorescence may be a good parameter to determine disease activity in IAD patients, and may be useful for choosing treatment options and determining doses of drugs during disease course. However, the correlation of IgA antibody titers with disease activity is, in general, less apparent than that in classical IgG-types of pemphigus.

IMMUNOBLOTTING

In original studies to determine autoantigens for classical IgG-types of pemphigus, immunoprecipitation using extracts of radiolabeled cultured keratinocytes was performed. However, because the procedures of immunoprecipitation are time-consuming and hazardous, this method is not widely used today.

Following immunoprecipitation, immunoblotting using various substrates are used to determine the autoantigens for patients in various AIBDs.[1,2] Immunoblotting of normal human epidermal extracts is currently most frequently performed for detection of autoantigen in various types of pemphigus.[1,2]

Immunoblotting was also applied to determine the autoantigens in various types of IAD. In earlier immunoblotting studies using either purified bovine desmosome or normal human epidermal extract, sera of a few IAD patients showed IgA reactivity with 2 protein bands corresponding to the a and b forms of the desmocollins.[17] However, because the sensitivity of immunoblotting for diagnosis of IAD is very low, this technique is infrequently used to determine the autoantigens in IAD today.

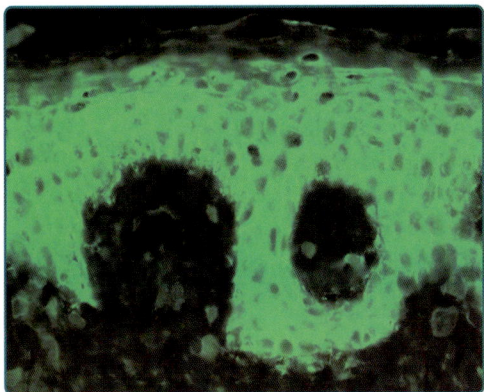

Figure 57-14 Indirect immunofluorescence result of intraepidermal neutrophilic IgA dermatosis–type intercellular IgA dermatosis showing IgA reactivity with keratinocyte cell surfaces in the entire epidermis.

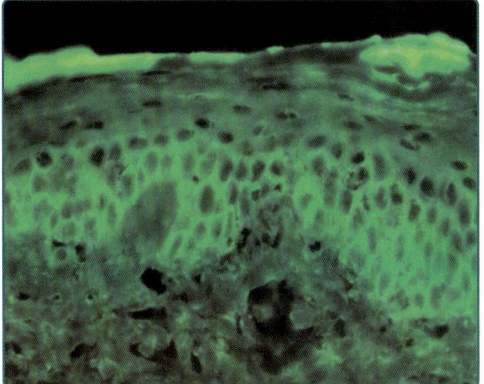

Figure 57-16 Indirect immunofluorescence result of pemphigus vulgaris–type intercellular IgA dermatosis showing IgA reactivity with keratinocyte cell surfaces in the lower epidermis.

COMPLEMENTARY DNA TRANSFECTION METHOD

The cDNA transfection method is a more sensitive method for detecting IgA autoantibodies to Dsc1, Dsc2, and Dsc3 in the sera from patients with various types of IAD because this method can detect IgA reactivity with the epitopes on the native desmocollin proteins.[20] In this method, full-length cDNAs of human desmocollins are transfected into COS-7 cells, and reactivity of IgA autoantibodies in IAD sera with each desmocollin molecule expressed on the cell surface of the transfected COS-7 is detected by immunofluorescence without fixation.[20] In this method, almost all patients with SPD-type IAD show IgA reactivity with Dsc1 (Figs. 57-17 and 57-18), while the IEN-type of IAD does not react with Dsc1, Dsc2, or Dsc3.[20] However, this method needs a special molecular biologic facility and is time-consuming. In addition, high background staining may interfere with detection of positive reactivity.

ENZYME-LINKED IMMUNOSORBENT ASSAYS

Currently, ELISAs using recombinant proteins of Dsg1, Dsg3, BP180, BP230, and Type VII collagen are commercially available, and are useful for the diagnosing various types of pemphigus, bullous pemphigoid, and epidermolysis bullosa acquisita. In general, ELISA is more sensitive than either indirect immunofluorescence, immunoblotting, or cDNA transfection. In addition, ELISA is a quantitative method and can manipulate many samples simultaneously; as a result, ELISA is the preferred diagnostic method for various AIBDs.

To detect IgA autoantibodies to Dsg1 and Dsg3, IgA ELISAs of Dsg1 and Dsg3 were developed by modification of IgG ELISAs using baculovirus-producing recombinant proteins.[21] These ELISAs detect IgA antibodies to Dsg1 and Dsg3 in the sera from minor subsets of IAD, which are diagnosed as PF-type IAD and PV-type IAD, respectively.

IgA ELISA using mammalian recombinant proteins of Dsc1, Dsc2, and Dsc3 can detect IgA anti-Dsc1 antibodies in most cases of SPD-type IAD.[8] In addition, this method also detects IgA antibodies to Dsc1, Dsc2, and Dsc3 in various combinations in some cases of other types of IAD. Thus, the IgA ELISA using mammalian recombinant proteins is the preferred test for detecting IgA reactivity with Dsc1, Dsc2, and Dsc3 in various types of IAD.

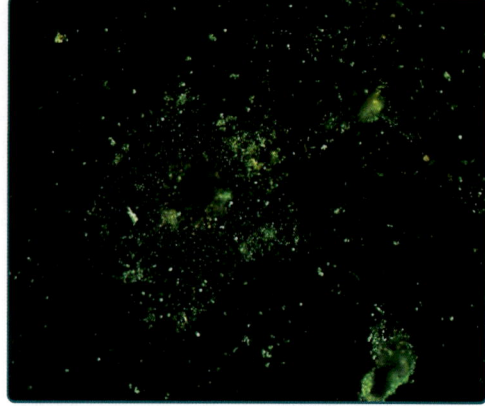

Figure 57-18 Result of complementary DNA transfection method for negative reactivity with Dsc1 by IgA antibodies in healthy normal serum.

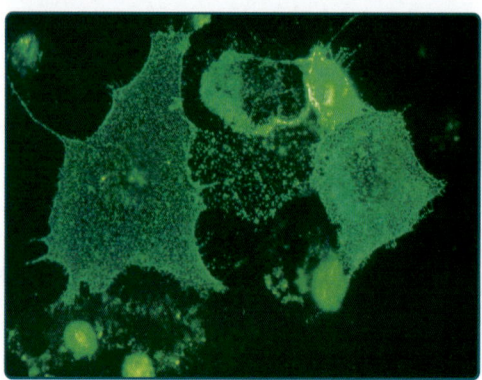

Figure 57-17 Result of complementary DNA transfection method for positive reactivity with Dsc1 by IgA antibodies in the serum of the subcorneal pustular dermatosis–type intercellular IgA dermatosis patient.

DIFFERENTIAL DIAGNOSIS

Table 57-3 summarizes the differential diagnoses for IAD.

Because SPD-type IAD and classical SPD without IgA antibodies show exactly the same clinical and histopathologic features,[9] these 2 diseases should be differentiated by detection IgA anti–cell-surface antibodies by direct immunofluorescence.

IAD also needs to be differentiated from other AIBDs. IAD shows clinically and histopathologically

TABLE 57-3

Differential Diagnoses for Intercellular IgA Dermatosis

- Classical subcorneal pustular dermatosis
- Pemphigus foliaceus
- Pemphigus vulgaris
- Pemphigus vegetans
- Paraneoplastic pemphigus
- Dermatitis herpetiformis
- Linear IgA bullous dermatosis
- Pustular psoriasis
- Erythema multiforme
- Sjögren syndrome
- Subacute cutaneous lupus erythematosus

bullous and pustular skin lesions, which are similar to those seen in PF, PV, PVeg, and paraneoplastic pemphigus. Therefore, these IgG types of pemphigus should also be differentiated. Because IAD frequently shows annular and herpetiform erythematous lesions, dermatitis herpetiformis Duhring and linear IgA bullous dermatosis are also considered to be differential diagnoses.

Pustular psoriasis, particularly recurrent annular-type pustular psoriasis, also shows clinical and histopathologic features indistinguishable from IAD. Erythema multiforme, Sjögren syndrome and subacute cutaneous lupus erythematosus may show annular erythematous skin lesions, which are similar to those seen in IAD. These diseases should also be differentiated.

To exclude the possibility of the patient having one of the diseases mentioned above, both direct and indirect immunofluorescence tests, as well as other immunologic and biochemical examination, are necessary.

PROGNOSIS AND CLINICAL COURSE

In contrast to various classical IgG types of pemphigus, IAD has a much better prognosis and is rarely fatal. Although the systemic administration of high doses of corticosteroids and immunosuppressive agents are inevitable therapy in classical IgG types of pemphigus, except for PF and pemphigus erythematosus, these aggressive therapies are unnecessary in most IAD patients. In general, IAD patients can be controlled with dapsone with or without low doses of systemic corticosteroids.

The disease course of IAD is usually refractory, and skin lesions frequently recur upon withdrawal of the drugs. Some patients, who could be followed for a long time, continued to show recurrence after more than 30 years.[9,14] Thus, IAD is considered to be not fatal disease but extremely intractable disease condition. Various types of treatments are tried, but show inconsistent effectiveness among individual IAD patients.

TREATMENTS

Because of the rarity of IAD, systematic clinical trial studies have never been performed for any treatments for IAD.[33] Therefore, no satisfactory guidelines of treatment of IAD are currently available.

DAPSONE AND OTHER SULFONES

Oral dapsone 50 to 200 mg/day is the most common therapy in IAD.[9,10,13] Other sulfones, including salazosulfapyridine, sulfamethoxypyridazine, and sulfamethoxazole-trimethoprim, were also occasionally used in patients, who showed less response to dapsone. A considerable number of IAD patients can be controlled sufficiently or even completely by sole treatment of dapsone or other sulfones.[9,10,13] However, in IAD cases with insufficient response to dapsone or sulfones, a variety of other types of treatments are used.

CORTICOSTEROIDS AND IMMUNOSUPPRESSIVE AGENTS

The systemic corticosteroids, most commonly prednisolone, are the second choice of therapy for IAD.[9,10,13] In contrast to classical IgG types of pemphigus, which are treated with high doses of glucocorticoids (0.5 to 1.0 mg/kg/day, equivalent to prednisolone), relatively low doses of corticosteroids (0.2 to 0.5 mg/kg/day, equivalent to prednisolone) are given in IAD. A combination of dapsone and low-dose systemic corticosteroids is also frequently used. Either pulsed corticosteroid (intravenous administration of a high dose of methylprednisolone) or various types of immunosuppressive agents are rarely used in IAD. However, very refractory IAD patients have been treated with aggressive immunosuppressive therapy with either high-dose systemic corticosteroids or various immunosuppressive agents, including azathioprine, mycophenolate mofetil, cyclosporine, cyclophosphamide, and methotrexate.[34]

OTHER THERAPIES

A number of other types of therapy are used in IAD patients in whom systemic dapsone and corticosteroids are not effective.

Like treatments for bullous pemphigoid, antibiotics, including tetracycline, minocycline, doxycycline, and macrolides, are used in IAD, mainly for their antiinflammatory effects. To suppress activity of neutrophils, colchicine is also used. However, the effectiveness of these drugs in IAD is inconsistent.

Although experimental disease models have not been established, IgA autoantibodies in IAD are considered to be pathogenic. Therefore, plasmapheresis is sometimes used for patients with severe IAD to remove IgA autoantibodies. Intravenous Ig therapy is another therapy used to reduce activity of autoantibodies, but its use in IAD has not been reported.

Because of the clinical and histopathologic similarity of IAD to pustular psoriasis, IAD patients are also treated with therapies for psoriasis and pustular psoriasis; that is, systemic retinoids, including etretinate, isotretinoin,[35] and acitretin,[36] adalimumab infusion, and psoralen and ultraviolet A.[14] These treatments show some effectiveness in particular IAD patients, but not in all IAD patients. A combination of dapsone and acitretin also has been successfully used.[37]

Because IAD usually shows very refractory disease course, treatment with anti-CD20 monoclonal antibodies, most commonly rituximab, may be a therapeutic option for IAD in the future, particularly for patients with extremely intractable IAD and frequent recurrences.

PERSPECTIVES

Because IAD is a very rare disease, a number of questions about its pathophysiology remain unsolved and should be the subject of study. Among the questions to resolved are these: The pathogenic activity of IgA autoantibodies in the sera of IAD patients should be examined by specific disease models in the future. As mentioned above, the autoantigen for IEN-type IAD is considered to be a nondesmosomal protein (Fig. 57-19),[24] and therefore may be a unique protein as an autoantigen in pemphigus. Finally, the mechanism for production of IgA autoantibodies in IAD, including class-switch from IgM to IgA, should also be examined.

REFERENCES

1. Hashimoto T, Tsuruta D, Koga H, et al. Summary of results of serological tests and diagnoses for 4774 cases of various autoimmune bullous diseases consulted to Kurume University. *Br J Dermatol.* 2016;175(5):953-965.
2. Otten JV, Hashimoto T, Hertl M, et al. Molecular diagnosis in autoimmune skin blistering conditions. *Curr Mol Med.* 2014;14(1):69-95.
3. Hashimoto T, Ishii N, Ohata C, et al. Pathogenesis of epidermolysis bullosa acquisita, an autoimmune subepidermal bullous disease. *J Pathol.* 2012;228(1):1-7.
4. Tsuruta D, Ishii N, Hashimoto T. Diagnosis and treatment of pemphigus. *Immunotherapy.* 2012;4(7):735-745.
5. Hashimoto T, Ogawa MM, Konohana A, et al. Detection of pemphigus vulgaris and pemphigus foliaceus antigens by immunoblot analysis using different antigen sources. *J Invest Dermatol.* 1990;94(3):327-331.
6. Ishii K, Amagai M, Hall RP, et al. Characterization of autoantibodies in pemphigus using antigen-specific enzyme-linked immunosorbent assays with baculovirus-expressed recombinant desmogleins. *J Immunol.* 1997;159(4):2010-2017.
7. Ohzono A, Sogame R, Li X, et al. Clinical and immunological findings in 104 cases of paraneoplastic pemphigus. *Br J Dermatol.* 2015;173(6):1447-1452.
8. Ishii N, Teye K, Fukuda S, et al. Anti-desmocollin autoantibodies in nonclassical pemphigus. *Br J Dermatol.* 2015;173(1):59-68.
9. Hashimoto T, Teye K, Ishii N. Clinical and immunological studies of 49 cases of various types of intercellular IgA dermatosis and 13 cases of classical subcorneal pustular dermatosis examined at Kurume University. *Br J Dermatol.* 2017;176(1):168-175.
10. Hashimoto T, Nishikawa T. Nomenclature for diseases with IgA antikeratinocyte cell surface autoantibodies. *Br J Dermatol.* 2015;173(3):868-869.
11. Nishikawa T, Hashimoto T, Teraki Y, et al. The clinical and histopathological spectrum of IgA pemphigus. *Clin Exp Dermatol.* 1991;16(5):401-402.
12. Hashimoto T. Immunopathology of IgA pemphigus. *Clin Dermatol.* 2001;19(6):683-689.
13. Tsuruta D, Ishii N, Hamada T, et al. IgA pemphigus. *Clin Dermatol.* 2011;29(4):437-442.
14. Hashimoto T, Inamoto N, Nakamura K, et al. Intercellular IgA dermatosis with clinical features of subcorneal pustular dermatosis. *Arch Dermatol.* 1987;123(8):1062-1065.
15. Wallach D, Cottenot F, Pelbois G, et al. Subcorneal pustular dermatosis and monoclonal IgA. *Br J Dermatol.* 1982;107(2):229-234.
16. Huff JC, Golitz LE, Kunke KS. Intraepidermal neutrophilic IgA dermatosis. *N Engl J Med.* 1985;313(26):1643-1645.
17. Ebihara T, Hashimoto T, Iwatsuki K, et al. Autoantigens for IgA anti-intercellular antibodies of intercellular IgA vesiculopustular dermatosis. *J Invest Dermatol.* 1991;97(4):742-745.
18. Beutner EH, Chorzelski TP, Wilson RM, et al. IgA pemphigus foliaceus. Report of two cases and a review of the literature. *J Am Acad Dermatol.* 1989;20(1):89-97.
19. Karpati S, Amagai M, Liu WL, et al. Identification of desmoglein 1 as autoantigen in a patient with

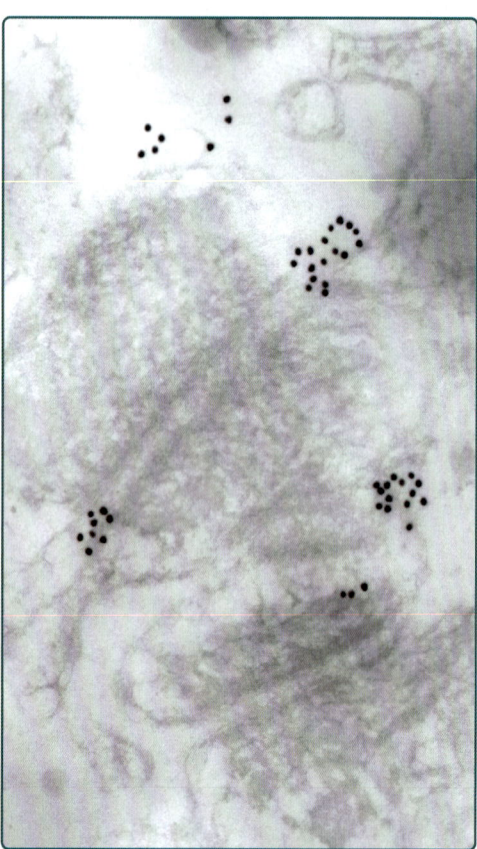

Figure 57-19 Immunogold electron microscopy with sera from intraepidermal neutrophilic dermatosis–type intercellular IgA dermatosis showing binding of gold particles to cell surfaces in the interdesmosomal region, but not in desmosomes, in cultured normal human keratinocyte. (From Ishii N, Ishida-Yamamoto A, Hashimoto T. Immunolocalization of target autoantigens in IgA pemphigus. *Clin Exp Dermatol.* 2004;29(1):62-66, Fig. 3D, with permission. Copyright © 2004, John Wiley & Sons.)

19. intraepidermal neutrophilic IgA dermatosis type of IgA pemphigus. *Exp Dermatol*. 2000;9(3):224-228.
20. Hashimoto T, Kiyokawa C, Mori O, et al. Human desmocollin 1 (Dsc1) is an autoantigen for the subcorneal pustular dermatosis type of IgA pemphigus. *J Invest Dermatol*. 1997;109(2):127-131.
21. Hashimoto T, Komai A, Futei Y, et al. Detection of IgA autoantibodies to desmogleins by an enzyme-linked immunosorbent assay: the presence of new minor subtypes of IgA pemphigus. *Arch Dermatol*. 2001;137(6):735-738.
22. Hisamatsu Y, Amagai M, Garrod DR, et al. The detection of IgG and IgA autoantibodies to desmocollins 1-3 by enzyme-linked immunosorbent assays using baculovirus-expressed proteins, in atypical pemphigus but not in typical pemphigus. *Br J Dermatol*. 2004;151(1):73-83.
23. Teye K, Numata S, Ohzono A, et al. Establishment of IgA ELISAs of mammalian recombinant proteins of human desmocollins 1-3. *J Dermatol Sci*. 2016;83(1):75-77.
24. Ishii N, Ishida-Yamamoto A, Hashimoto T. Immunolocalization of target autoantigens in IgA pemphigus. *Clin Exp Dermatol*. 2004;29(1):62-66.
25. Tsuchisaka A, Ishii N, Hamada T, et al. Epidermal polymeric immunoglobulin receptors: leads from intraepidermal neutrophilic IgA dermatosis-type IgA pemphigus. *Exp Dermatol*. 2015;24(3):217-219.
26. Yasuda H, Kobayashi H, Hashimoto T, et al. Subcorneal pustular dermatosis type of IgA pemphigus: demonstration of autoantibodies to desmocollin-1 and clinical review. *Br J Dermatol*. 2000;143(1):144-148.
27. Hashimoto T, Yasumoto S, Nagata Y, et al. Clinical, histopathological and immunological distinction in two cases of IgA pemphigus. *Clin Exp Dermatol*. 2002;27(8):636-640.
28. Weston WL, Friednash M, Hashimoto T, et al. A novel childhood pemphigus vegetans variant of intraepidermal neutrophilic IgA dermatosis. *J Am Acad Dermatol*. 1998;38(4):635-638.
29. Tajima M, Mitsuhashi Y, Irisawa R, et al. IgA pemphigus reacting exclusively to desmoglein 3. *Eur J Dermatol*. 2010;20(5):626-629.
30. Ueda A, Ishii N, Temporin K, et al. IgA pemphigus with paraneoplastic pemphigus-like clinical features showing IgA antibodies to desmoglein 1/3 and desmocollin 3, and IgG and IgA antibodies to the basement membrane zone. *Clin Exp Dermatol*. 2013;38(4):370-373.
31. Espana A, Gimenez-Azcarate A, Ishii N, et al. Antidesmocollin 1 autoantibody negative subcorneal pustular dermatosis-type IgA pemphigus associated with multiple myeloma. *Br J Dermatol*. 2015;172(1):296-298.
32. Asahina A, Koga H, Suzuki Y, et al. IgA pemphigus associated with diffuse large B-cell lymphoma showing unique reactivity with desmocollins: unusual clinical and histopathological features. *Br J Dermatol*. 2013;168(1):224-226.
33. Moreno AC, Santi CG, Gabbi TV, et al. IgA pemphigus: case series with emphasis on therapeutic response. *J Am Acad Dermatol*. 2014;70(1):200-201.
34. Sibley Hash K, Rencic A, Hernandez MI, et al. Aggressive immunosuppressive therapy for a refractory case of IgA pemphigus. *Arch Dermatol*. 2002;138(6):744-746.
35. Gruss C, Zillikens D, Hashimoto T, et al. Rapid response of IgA pemphigus of subcorneal pustular dermatosis type to treatment with isotretinoin. *J Am Acad Dermatol*. 2000;43(5, pt 2):923-926.
36. Ruiz-Genao DP, Hernandez-Nunez A, Hashimoto T, et al. A case of IgA pemphigus successfully treated with acitretin. *Br J Dermatol*. 2002;147(5):1040-1042.
37. Monshi B, Richter L, Hashimoto T, et al. IgA pemphigus of the subcorneal pustular dermatosis type. Successful therapy with a combination of dapsone and acitretin [in German]. *Hautarzt*. 2012;63(6):482-486.

Chapter 58 :: Linear Immunoglobulin A Dermatosis and Chronic Bullous Disease of Childhood
:: Matilda W. Nicholas, Caroline L. Rao, & Russell P. Hall III

第五十八章
线状IgA皮病和儿童慢性大疱性皮病

中文导读

线状IgA皮病是一种罕见的免疫介导的水疱性皮病，其特征是在表皮基底膜均匀一致的线状IgA沉积（图58-1）。线状IgA皮病可表现为获得性大疱性表皮松解症（EBA）、疱疹样皮炎（DH）、大疱性类天疱疮（BP）、扁平苔藓、结节性痒疹或瘢痕性类天疱疮样症状。

儿童慢性大疱性皮病（CBDC）是一种罕见的水疱性皮病，主要发生在5岁以下儿童，特征为表皮基底膜均匀线状IgA沉积。

1. 流行病学　线状IgA皮病最常发生在青春期后，大多数出现在40岁后。而CBDC最常出现在5岁之前。与线状IgA皮病一样，CBDC患者中女性占主导地位。高达76%CBDC患者表达HLA-B8。成人和儿童线状IgA皮病中，TNF2等位基因频率都有所增加。

2. 病因与发病机制：免疫病理学　线状IgA皮病和CBDC是指真皮-表皮交界处基底膜区均匀线状IgA荧光沉积。少数人有其他免疫反应物沉积，最常见的是IgG，偶尔见补体C3。目前尚不清楚患者皮肤中IgA沉积的真正来源。

3. 临床表现　本节介绍了线状IgA皮病的临床表现是异质性的，通常与DH患者没有区别。患者可能出现环形或成群的丘疹、水疱和大疱。

4. 组织病理学　本节介绍了线状IgA皮病和CBDC的组织病理学表现、电镜下表现。

5. 鉴别诊断　线状IgA皮病常与DH临床表现相似。有些与BP、瘢痕性类天疱疮、EBA相似，很少有中毒性表皮坏死松解症样表现。CBDC患者要与儿童DH和儿童BP相鉴别。

6. 治疗和预后　本节介绍了线状IgA皮病、药物诱导IgA皮病和CBDC的临床特征，并且提出线状IgA皮病患者常对氨苯砜或磺胺吡啶反应敏感。CBDC有自限性，大多数在起病后两年内缓解。

〔陈明亮〕

AT-A-GLANCE

Linear Immunoglobulin A Dermatosis

- Rare blistering disease with onset typically after fourth decade of life.
- Linear band of immunoglobulin (Ig) A at the dermal–epidermal basement membrane.
- Clinical presentations may mimic dermatitis herpetiformis, bullous pemphigoid, and cicatricial pemphigoid.
- May occur in association with many drugs, including vancomycin.
- May occur in association with inflammatory bowel diseases, but is only rarely associated with gluten-sensitive enteropathy.
- Rarely seen in association with malignancy, specifically lymphoid malignancy.
- Histology shows subepidermal collection of neutrophils at the basement membrane, often collecting in papillary tips with subepidermal blisters.
- Patients have relatively low titers of circulating IgA autoantibodies, most frequently against portions of BPAG2 (type XVII collagen), or rarely against BPAG1, LAD 285, type VII collagen, and others.
- Most patients respond dramatically to treatment with dapsone; some require adjunctive systemic corticosteroids.
- Prognosis is variable with both spontaneous remissions and longstanding disease.

Chronic Bullous Disease of Childhood

- Rare blistering disorder of childhood presenting predominantly in children younger than 5 years of age.
- Linear IgA at the dermal–epidermal basement membrane.
- Clinical presentation of tense bullae, often in perineum and perioral regions, giving a "cluster-of-jewels" appearance. New lesions sometimes appear around the periphery of previous lesions with a collarette of blisters.
- Histology shows subepidermal collection of neutrophils at the basement membrane, similar to linear IgA bullous dermatosis.
- Most patients respond dramatically to treatment with dapsone.
- Spontaneous remissions, often within 2 years, are frequent.

Linear immunoglobulin (Ig) A dermatosis is a rare, immune-mediated, blistering skin disease that is defined by the presence of homogeneous linear deposits of IgA at the cutaneous basement membrane (Fig. 58-1). Although in the original description of patients with linear IgA dermatosis it was considered to be a manifestation of dermatitis herpetiformis (DH), it has now been clearly separated from DH on the basis of its immunopathology, immunogenetics, and lack of consistent association with a gluten-sensitive enteropathy.[1-4] Patients with linear IgA dermatosis can present with lesions suggestive of epidermolysis bullosa acquisita (EBA), DH, bullous pemphigoid (BP), lichen planus, prurigo nodularis, or cicatricial pemphigoid.[1-6]

Drug-induced linear IgA was initially described in association with vancomycin and is now associated with a wide variety of drugs.[7-15] Drug-induced linear IgA differs somewhat from classic linear IgA in clinical presentation with a wider variety of clinical presentations, including morbilliform, erythema multiforme–like, and toxic epidermal necrolysis–like.[7-11,16-18]

Chronic bullous disease of childhood (CBDC) is a rare blistering disease that occurs predominantly in children younger than 5 years of age and has an identical pattern of homogeneous linear IgA deposits at the epidermal basement membrane.[19,20] Studies demonstrate that in some patients CBDC and linear IgA dermatosis represent different presentations of the same disease process.[21,22]

EPIDEMIOLOGY

Linear IgA dermatosis occurs most often after puberty, with most patients presenting after the fourth decade of life.[2,4,23] A slight predominance of females has been noted in several studies,[2,4,23] although others have noted the opposite.[24,25] In contrast, CBDC presents most often before the age of 5 years.[26] As in patients with linear IgA dermatosis, there is a slight female predominance in patients with CBDC in several,[20,26] but not all, studies.[24,27]

Evaluation of the human leukocyte antigen (HLA) association in patients with linear IgA dermatosis and CBDC has yielded conflicting results. Some investigators have found an increased frequency of the human histocompatibility antigen HLA-B8 in patients with linear IgA dermatosis, whereas others have found no increased frequency.[28-30] In CBDC, an increased frequency of HLA-B8 has been noted, with up to 76% of patients expressing HLA-B8.[26] Collier et al demonstrated an increased frequency of HLA-B8, HLA-DR3, and HLA-DQ2 in CBDC that was not seen in adults with linear IgA dermatosis.[28] These authors suggested that these haplotypes may have a role in earlier disease presentation. In addition, the *TNF2* allele was found with increased frequency in both adults and children with linear IgA disease when compared with unaffected subjects. There was, however, no increase seen in either adults or children when compared with HLA-DR3+ controls.

ETIOLOGY AND PATHOGENESIS: IMMUNOPATHOLOGY

Linear IgA dermatosis and CBDC are defined by the presence of a homogeneous linear band of IgA at the dermal–epidermal basement membrane zone (Table 58-1). A minority of patients in both groups have additional deposits of other immunoreactants, most often IgG and occasionally the third component of complement (C3).[26] A recent retrospective study noted that 40% of cases of idiopathic linear IgA disease had C3 deposits on direct immunofluorescence, but no cases of drug-induced linear IgA dermatosis in adults had C3 deposits.[24] Because IgA is the predominant Ig of the secretory immune system, numerous investigators have attempted to determine if the IgA present in the skin of these patients is of mucosal origin. Characterization of the IgA subclass in the skin has revealed almost exclusively IgA1 and not the subclass most often associated with mucosa, IgA2.[23,31,32] In addition, neither secretory piece nor J chain, both of which are present in secretory IgA, has been found in the IgA present in the skin of patients with linear IgA deposits.[33] Although these data have led to suggestions that the IgA is not of mucosal origin, the true origin of the IgA deposits in the skin of these patients is not known.

Initially it was thought that patients with linear IgA dermatosis and CBDC rarely had circulating IgA antibodies against the epidermal basement membrane (see Table 58-2). Indirect immunofluorescence, using 1 M NaCl-split normal human skin as a substrate, demonstrates that the majority of patients with CBDC have low-titer circulating antibodies against the epidermal side of the split skin.[10,23] Circulating low-titer IgA antibodies directed against the epidermal basement membrane also have been found in adults with linear IgA dermatosis.[26,34] Others have reported binding of IgA antibodies from some patients to the dermal side of normal human split skin, suggesting that more than 1 antigen may be the target for the IgA anti–basement membrane antibodies.[34-36] Immunoelectron

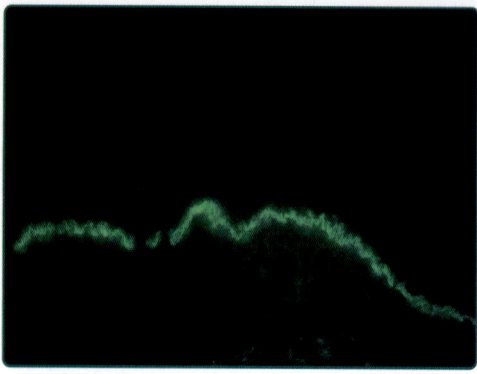

Figure 58-1 Direct immunofluorescence of normal-appearing perilesional skin from a patient with linear immunoglobulin A dermatosis. A homogeneous band of immunoglobulin A is present at the dermal–epidermal junction.

microscopy studies have been performed to determine the exact location of the IgA in the skin of patients with both linear IgA dermatosis and CBDC. Immunoelectron microscopy of the skin of patients with linear IgA deposits has revealed 3 distinct patterns of immunoreactants. In some patients with linear IgA dermatosis, the IgA deposits are found in the lamina lucida region of the basement membrane zone, similar to the location of immunoreactants present in the skin of patients with BP.[35,37] A second pattern of IgA deposition has been detected in which the IgA deposits are present at and below the lamina densa in a pattern similar to that seen in EBA.[35,37,38] Prost et al have described a third pattern of immunoreactants in some patients with linear IgA dermatosis in which the IgA deposits are found both above and below the lamina densa.[35] In a similar manner, immunoelectron microscopy studies of skin of patients with CBDC have shown the IgA immunoreactants to be in either the lamina lucida or a sublamina densa location.[21,38] These findings further support the probability that multiple antigens may be involved as the targets in both adults and children with linear IgA deposits in the skin. Horiguchi et al reviewed 213 cases of linear IgA in Japan and found a strong association between older

TABLE 58-1
Immunoreactants and Circulating Antibodies

TYPE	COMPOSITION OF CUTANEOUS IMMUNOREACTANTS	LOCATION OF IMMUNOREACTANTS	CIRCULATING IgA AUTOANTIBODIES
Linear IgA	40% have C3 24% have IgG Almost all IgA1	1. Lamina lucida (BP-like) 2. At and below lamina lucida (EBA-like) 3. Above and below lamina lucida	May have low titer against epidermal basement membrane antigens
Drug-induced IgA	None reported with C3 Almost all have IgA1		
CBDC	9% have IgG May have C3 Almost all have IgA1	Lamina lucida or sublamina densa	Most have low titer against epidermal side of sodium split-skin

BP, bullous pemphigoid; CBDC, chronic bullous disease of childhood; EBA, epidermolysis bullosa acquisita; Ig, immunoglobulin.

TABLE 58-2
Pharmacological Treatments

First-line	Dapsone
	Sulfapyridine
First-line adjuvant	Low-dose prednisone
Second-line	Mycophenolate mofetil
	Intravenous immunoglobulin
Second-line adjuvant	Antibiotics (including trimethoprim-sulfamethoxazole, dicloxacillin, erythromycin, flucloxacillin)
	Topical tacrolimus

age of onset and both IgG/IgA type and dermal binding. IgG was found in approximately 9% of patients with the infantile (CBDC) type whereas in adults (older than age 16 years), IgG was found in 24% of patients. Interestingly, when comparing the different groups based on patterns of antigen binding (eg, dermal vs epidermal and IgA vs IgG/IgA) no significant clinical differences were found.[39]

Although the relatively low titer of IgA antibodies against the basement membrane present in the sera of patients with both linear IgA dermatosis and CBDC has complicated the search for specific antigenic targets for the IgA, several investigators have made significant observations regarding the antigenic targets in these diseases (see Table 58-2). Zone et al studied sera from patients who had circulating IgA antibodies that bound to the epidermal side of 1 M NaCl-split normal human skin, as shown by indirect immunofluorescence.[40] They found that serum IgA from patients with either CBDC or linear IgA dermatosis bound to a 97-kDa protein. Immunoelectron microscopy revealed that the 97-kDa antigen is present in the lamina lucida, below the hemidesmosome of normal human skin, in a location similar to where the IgA is localized in patients with CBDC and linear IgA dermatosis.[41] Subsequently, Zone et al determined that the 97-kDa linear IgA bullous disease antigen is identical to a portion of the extracellular domain of the 180-kDa BP antigen (BPAG2 or collagen XVII), which is essential in anchoring basal keratinocytes to the epidermal basement membrane.[42] The BP antigen (BPAG2) consists of a 180-kDa transmembrane protein and 120-kDa portion that corresponds to the collagenous ectodomain. Roh et al and Schumann et al reported that autoantibodies in patients with linear IgA dermatosis recognize the soluble 120-kDa ectodomain of type XVII collagen.[43,44] The 120-kDa antigen target is not unique to linear IgA dermatosis because it is also the antigen targeted by autoantibodies in some patients with cicatricial pemphigoid and BP.[43,44] Furthermore, IgA antibodies and T cells from patients with linear IgA bullous dermatosis have been found to be directed against the NC-16A region of collagen type XVII, which is the same region against which the IgG and T cells from patients with BP are directed.[45,46] This may explain in part the overlap in clinical and histologic features of these conditions. Wojnarowska et al identified another possible target antigen in patients with linear IgA dermatosis and CBDC. Using sera from patients in whom the IgA bound to the epidermal side of 1 M NaCl split-skin on routine indirect immunofluorescence, they found that IgA in the sera of some patients with these diseases bound to a 285-kDa protein (LAD 285) that was not the 230-kDa BP antigen or type VII collagen, the EBA antigen.[47] Allen and Wojnarowska have analyzed the sera of more than 70 patients with both linear IgA dermatosis and CBDC and found that the predominant antigenic target in these patients is the BP180 antigen (collagen XVII), but that some patients react with multiple antigens including the BP230, LAD 285, and other yet-to-be-identified proteins.[48] Ishii et al described a patient with Linear IgA who had antibodies directed at the NC16a domain of BP180 without evidence of antibody formation to 120-kDa LAD-1.[49] Izaki et al reported a case of linear IgA/IgG bullous dermatosis with anti–laminin-332 autoantibodies.[50] Tsuchisaka et al showed that in 8 of 12 patients with sublamina densa pattern direct immunofluorescence, type VII collagen appeared to be the antibody target.[51] In many patients, IgA appears to bind to several different antigenic targets, suggesting the possibility that there is epitope spreading. The clinical significance of these findings however, has not been established.[48]

CLINICAL FINDINGS

CUTANEOUS MANIFESTATIONS

The clinical manifestations of linear IgA dermatosis are heterogeneous and often indistinguishable from those seen in patients with DH.[2,4,26,52] Patients may present with combinations of annular or grouped papules, vesicles, and bullae (Figs. 58-2 and 58-3). Typically, these lesions are distributed symmetrically on extensor surfaces, including elbows, knees, and buttocks. Lesions most often are very pruritic,

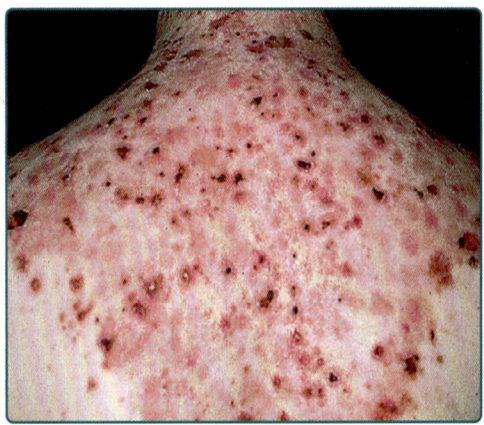

Figure 58-2 Patient with linear immunoglobulin A dermatosis with crusted erosions, papules, and vesicles on the back and neck.

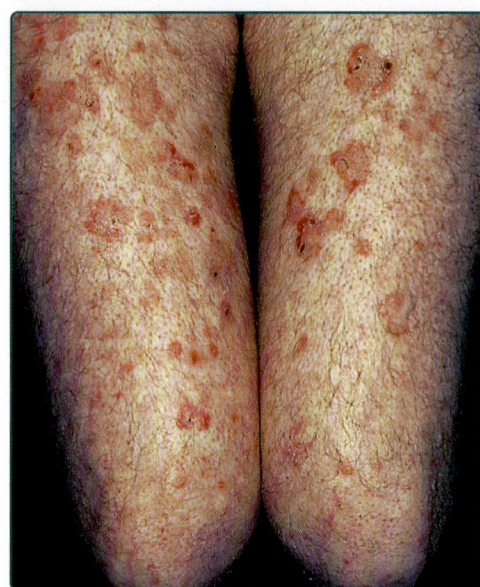

Figure 58-3 Patient with linear immunoglobulin A dermatosis with annular erythematous plaques on the thighs.

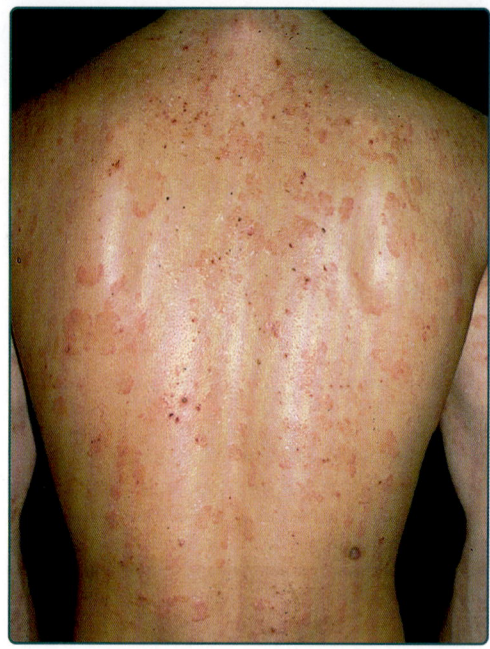

Figure 58-4 Patient with linear immunoglobulin A dermatosis with grouped urticarial papules on the back with scattered crusted erosions.

resulting in numerous crusted papules (Fig. 58-4). The clinical presentation can be difficult to distinguish from that seen in patients with DH. However, the degree of pruritus seen in patients with linear IgA dermatosis is variable and, in general, less severe than that seen in patients with DH. Some patients with linear IgA dermatosis present with larger bullae, in a pattern more consistent with that seen in patients with BP, or occasionally with cutaneous findings similar to those seen in patients with EBA.

Patients with drug-induced linear IgA bullous dermatosis have been reported with erythema multiforme–like findings and a toxic epidermal necrolysis–like presentation, with widespread bullae.[7,11,17] Localized palmar and morbilliform variants also have been described.[16,18,53] The Koebner phenomenon has also been reported in drug-induced linear IgA dermatosis.[54] While vancomycin is most closely associated with the drug-induced linear IgA, a number of other medications also have been implicated, including lithium, phenytoin, sulfamethoxazole-trimethoprim, furosemide, atorvastatin, captopril, diclofenac, ketoprofen, and infliximab.[13,14,17] In addition, a localized linear IgA in the setting of an acute contact dermatitis has been reported.[55] Recovery has been reported with discontinuation of the offending agent alone, but these patients may benefit from dapsone therapy (see "Treatment and Prognosis" below).[7,11,56]

The clinical presentation of CBDC is characterized most often by the development of tense bullae, often on an inflammatory base.[19] These lesions occur most frequently in the perineum and perioral region, and often may occur in clusters, giving a "cluster of jewels" appearance (Figs. 58-5, 58-6, and 58-7). New lesions sometimes appear around the periphery of previous lesions, with a resulting "collarette" of blisters. Patients often report significant pruritus and/or a burning of the skin with the development of skin lesions. Patients with CBDC often present with the acute development of large numbers of tense blisters, which may rupture and become secondarily infected. CBDC differs from linear IgA bullous dermatosis of adults in its typical clinical appearance, relative paucity of serious mucosal involvement, and good prognosis.[39]

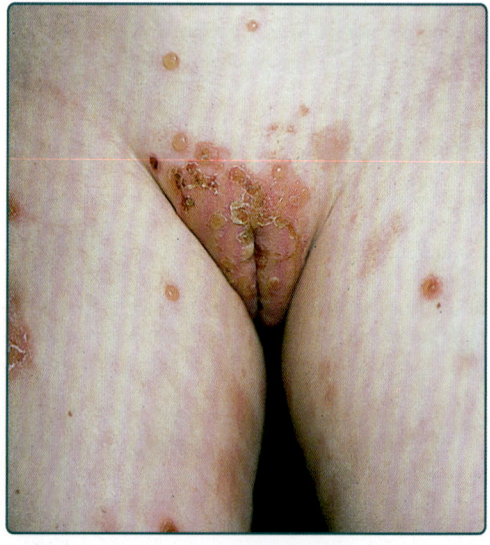

Figure 58-5 Patient with chronic bullous disease of childhood. Tense bullae and crusted papules are present on the abdomen, with a clustering of bullae noted in the perineal region.

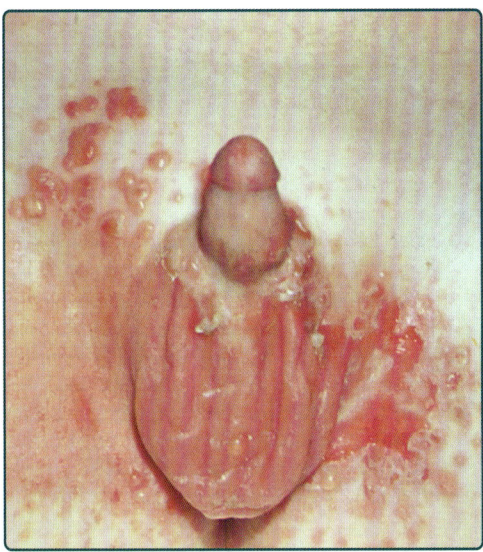

Figure 58-6 Chronic bullous disease of childhood. Tense blisters on erythematous bases in the pubic and inguinal areas.

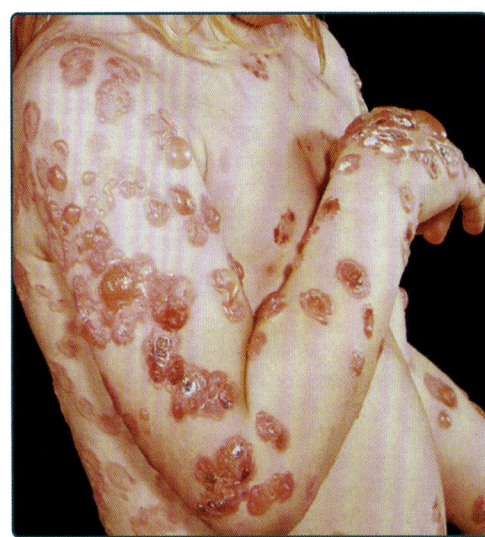

Figure 58-7 Extensive chronic bullous disease of childhood. Note tense and flaccid blisters without notable inflammation.

Rarely, patients with linear IgA dermatosis may present with an acute febrile illness with arthritis, arthralgias, and generalized malaise.[57,58] The presence of multiple papules and vesicles in a patient with systemic signs and symptoms has led to the evaluation of these patients for systemic infections, including viral infections. Routine direct immunofluorescence, however, has revealed linear deposits of IgA, and these patients have responded to conventional therapy.

MUCOSAL INVOLVEMENT

Mucosal involvement is an important clinical manifestation seen in patients with linear IgA dermatosis and CBDC. This involvement can range from largely asymptomatic oral ulcerations and erosions to severe oral disease alone, as well as to severe conjunctival and oral disease typical of that seen in cicatricial pemphigoid.[26,59,60] Oral lesions may occur in up to 70% of patients with linear IgA disease.[26] Mucosal invasion with complication is less often seen in CBDC.[39,61] Although most patients with linear IgA dermatosis and mucosal involvement have significant cutaneous disease, cases have been reported in the literature in which the presenting and predominant clinical manifestations are lesions of the mucous membranes.[60,62] These patients may present with desquamative gingivitis and oral lesions consistent with those seen in patients with cicatricial pemphigoid (see Chap. 55). Patients also may present with conjunctival disease and scar formation typical of that seen in patients with cicatricial pemphigoid (see Chap. 55). Mucosal involvement also appears to be less prominent in patients with drug-induced linear IgA.[17] Patients with linear IgA bullous dermatosis also have been reported to present with severe laryngeal and pharyngeal involvement before the development of more typical cutaneous manifestitations.[63,64]

DISEASE ASSOCIATIONS

The similar clinical presentation of many patients with linear IgA disease to that seen in patients with DH led to the investigation of patients with linear IgA disease for an associated gluten-sensitive enteropathy. Although some investigators have found evidence of minimal inflammatory changes in the small bowel of patients with linear IgA disease, numerous investigators have been unable to show that the majority of patients with linear IgA disease have significant evidence of the villous atrophy characteristically seen in patients with DH.[3,65] In addition, the clinical manifestations of linear IgA disease have not been controlled by the use of a gluten-free diet.[66] Circulating autoantibodies against tissue transglutaminase, which occur with high frequency in patients with untreated gluten-sensitive enteropathy and DH, have not been found in most patients with linear IgA diseases.[67]

Other conditions have been reported in association with linear IgA disease. One example is ulcerative colitis and Crohn disease, which can result in a clinical syndrome where the activity of both diseases is linked (ie, as one disease flares, so does the other).[68,69] Paige and coworkers reviewed 70 patients with linear IgA bullous dermatosis and found 5 (7.1%) had associated ulcerative colitis. The extent and reason for this association has yet to be established. Perhaps, the abnormal mucosal IgA1 production seen in patients with ulcerative colitis may play a role.[69] In 1 case, an ulcerative colitis patient developed linear IgA disease only after treatment with infliximab.[14] In patients with CBDC, Horiguchi reported associated systemic disease in only 13 of 213 cases reviewed.[39] CBDC also has been reported in association with acute mononucleosis and *Paecilomyces* lung infection in the setting of chronic granulomatous disease.[70] The relationship between these conditions and CBDC has yet to be established.

The relatively acute onset of clinical, histologic, and immunopathologic findings consistent with linear IgA disease has been seen in patients who have been taking a variety of drugs, including vancomycin, lithium phenytoin, sulfamethoxazole-trimethoprim, furosemide, atorvastatin, captopril, diclofenac, ketoprofen, and infliximab.[7-9,13,14,17,56] Vancomycin is the most common drug that is associated with the development of linear IgA bullous dermatosis, and linear IgA bullous dermatosis is the most common nonimmediate hypersensitivity reaction to vancomycin.[71] Linear IgA dermatosis has similarly been described with interferon-α2a and was temporally related to the influenza vaccine. While these may reflect an induction of a previously unrecognized autoimmune process, in both cases the eruption was self-limited, in contrast to classic linear IgA, which follows a chronic, waxing-and-waning course.[72,73] The mechanism of this interaction is not known; however, a small number of patients with vancomycin-induced linear IgA disease have been reported to have circulating IgA antibodies directed against the BP180, BP230, and LAD 285 antigens.[74,75] In 1 case of vancomycin-induced linear IgA bullous dermatosis, rechallenge with vancomycin in a gradual manner did not result in a recurrence of the eruption.[76] Identifying the causative agent in a patient receiving multiple potential triggers may be difficult, although recently, a drug-induced lymphocyte stimulation test was successfully employed to identify the triggering agent in 1 patient.[77] This has yet to be studied more broadly.

Rarely, physical exposures can also trigger linear IgA bullous dermatosis, chief among them ultraviolet light.[78] Development in association with varicella zoster has also been reported.[79]

Linear IgA disease also has been associated rarely with a variety of malignancies. Patients with linear IgA disease have been reported with both lymphoid and nonlymphoid malignancies.[80-82] An unusual urticarial form of linear IgA with oral lesions was reported as a presenting sign of chronic lymphocytic leukemia.[83] Godfrey et al reported 3 cases of lymphoid malignancies in 70 patients with linear IgA disease followed for a mean of 8.5 years. This represented an increase over the predicted number of 0.2 cases in an age- and sex-matched population.[80] No increase in the rate of nonlymphoid malignancies was seen. These findings suggest a small risk of lymphoid malignancy in these patients. However, larger population-based studies need to be done to confirm these findings.

Although limitation of manifestations to the skin and mucous membranes is the rule, a few cases of IgA nephropathy in association with linear IgA dermatosis have been reported.[12]

HISTOPATHOLOGY

Routine histopathology of an early lesion in patients with linear IgA dermatosis and CBDC reveals a subepidermal bulla with collections of neutrophils along the basement membrane, often accumulating at the papillary tips (Fig. 58-8). A mild lymphocytic infiltrate may be present around the superficial dermal blood vessels without any evidence of neutrophilic vasculitis. Occasionally, the inflammatory infiltrate is composed of eosinophils, but most frequently neutrophils are the major component of the subepidermal inflammation.[26,84,85] Electron microscopic examination of the blisters found in patients with both linear IgA dermatosis and CBDC revealed that the blister forms either within the lamina lucida or in a sublamina densa location.[21,37] Usually the histopathology seen in linear IgA disease is difficult to distinguish from that seen in patients with DH. Smith et al[85] reported that patients with linear IgA disease tended to have fewer papillary microabscesses and a more diffuse infiltrate of neutrophils at the basement membrane zone. However, Blenkinsopp et al found no significant difference between the histopathology found in patients with linear IgA disease and those with DH.[84] In general, the histopathology of blisters in linear IgA disease, CBDC, and DH is virtually indistinguishable.

DIFFERENTIAL DIAGNOSIS

Linear IgA dermatosis often closely mimics the clinical pattern seen in patients with DH. Some patients may have findings that resemble those seen in patients with BP, cicatricial pemphigoid, EBA, and, rarely, toxic epidermal necrolysis. In a similar manner, patients with CBDC must be differentiated from those with DH of childhood and childhood BP. The findings of linear IgA deposits at the basement membrane by direct immunofluorescence, most often in the absence of IgG and C3, can distinguish this disease from BP, cicatricial pemphigoid, and EBA, whereas granular IgA deposits are found at the basement membrane in patients with DH (Table 58-3).

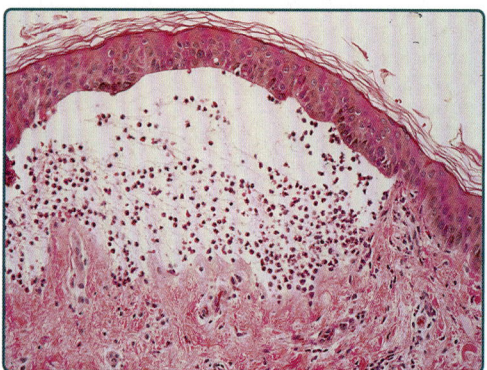

Figure 58-8 Histopathology of lesional skin from a patient with linear immunoglobulin A dermatosis showing a subepidermal blister filled with neutrophils. (Used with permission from Kim B. Yancey, MD.)

TABLE 58-3
Linear Immunoglobulin A Bullous Dermatosis Differential Diagnosis

- Dermatitis herpetiformis
- Bullous pemphigoid
- Epidermolysis bullosa acquisita
- Bullous eruption of systemic lupus erythematosus
- Cicatricial pemphigoid
- Lichen planus
- Toxic epidermal necrolysis

TREATMENT AND PROGNOSIS

Table 58-4 provides a clinical comparison between linear IgA, drug-induced IgA, and CBDC. Adults with linear IgA dermatosis have an unpredictable course.[4,26]

Many patients have disease that continues for years, with few, if any, episodes of remission. Occasionally, patients may have a spontaneous remission with loss of clinical features of the disease and disappearance of the linear IgA deposits in the skin. Patients with severe mucosal disease, especially of the eyes, may have persistent problems with symblepharon formation and resulting structural problems with the eyelids and cornea, even after active blistering has remitted. Untreated ocular involvement can lead to cicatrix and loss of vision.[86]

Patients with linear IgA disease most often respond dramatically to dapsone or sulfapyridine (see Table 58-2). This response usually occurs within 24 to 48 hours, in a manner similar to that seen with DH; as such, it is not a helpful diagnostic sign for linear IgA disease.[2,4,26] Although most patients are well controlled with dapsone or sulfapyridine alone, some patients require low-dose prednisone therapy to suppress blister formation.[26] In patients who are unresponsive or intolerant of these medications, mycophenolate mofetil

TABLE 58-4
Clinical Comparison between Linear IgA, Drug-Induced IgA, and Chronic Bullous Disease of Childhood

	EPIDEMIOLOGY	CLINICAL PRESENTATION	MUCOSAL INVOLVEMENT	DISEASE ASSOCIATIONS AND TRIGGERS	COURSE	TREATMENT
Linear IgA dermatosis	Often adults at the 4th decade of life; slight female predominance	Similar to Dermatitis herpetiformis (DH; see Chap. 59); annular or grouped papules, vesicles, and bullae on extensors, including elbows, knees, and buttocks; pruritus is less severe than in DH	Oral involvement in up to 70% of patients with linear IgA disease	Possible association with ulcerative colitis; ultraviolet light is the chief physical trigger	Unpredictable course; varies from spontaneous remission to longstanding disease	Dapsone, sulfapyridine; response within 24-48 h; low-dose prednisone may suppress blister formation
Drug-induced linear IgA	Adults[a]	Vary from erythema multiforme–like, to toxic epidermal necrolysis–like with widespread bullae; Koebner phenomenon may be present	Mucosal involvement less prominent than with linear IgA dermatosis	Vancomycin most commonly implicated; interferon-α, influenza vaccine, lithium, phenytoin, sulfamethoxazole-trimethoprim, furosemide, atorvastatin, captopril, diclofenac, ketoprofen, and infliximab	Rechallenge of drug may not result in recurrence	Discontinuation of causative drug; sometimes initiation of dapsone is helpful
Chronic bullous disease of childhood	Occurs before 5 years of age; slight female predominance	Tense bullae in a "cluster-of-jewels" appearance; collarette of blisters may be present	Mucosal involvement noted, but less commonly than in linear IgA dermatosis	Possible association with infectious mononucleosis and *Paecilomyces* lung infection in the setting of chronic granulomatous disease	Self-limited; remission within 2 years of onset	Dapsone, sulfapyridine; small doses of prednisone may be of use. mycophenolate mofetil as a steroid-sparing agent; topical tacrolimus

[a]In a single-center cohort study of 28 patients comparing drug-induced linear IgA bullous dermatosis and linear IgA bullous dermatosis, the median age of occurrence in drug-induced cases was 75 years, whereas the median age of occurrence in spontaneous linear IgA bullous dermatosis was 44.5 years. (Data from Chanal J, Ingen-Housz-Oro S, Ortonne N, et al. Linear IgA bullous dermatosis: comparison between the drug-induced and spontaneous forms. *Br J Dermatol*. 2013;169(5):1041-1048.)

is useful as a steroid-sparing agent.[87] Trimethoprim-sulfamethoxazole is reported to be helpful when used in conjunction with other immunosuppressives.[88] The majority of patients with linear IgA disease cannot control their skin disease with a gluten-free diet.[66]

CBDC is most often a self-limited disease, with most children going into remission within 2 years of the onset of the disease.[19,20,26] Occasionally, the disease persists well into puberty, but often is less severe than the initial eruption. Patients with CBDC respond in a similar dramatic fashion to dapsone or sulfapyridine.[19,20,26] Many children, however, require the addition of relatively small doses of prednisone to bring the disease under control.[19,20] Mycophenolate mofetil is used as a steroid-sparing agent in isolated cases.[89] Intravenous immunoglobulins also have been proposed in the rare patient who is not responding to, or is intolerant of, dapsone therapy.[90,91] Topical tacrolimus also may be a useful tool in minimizing systemic therapy.[92] Several case reports suggest that some patients with CBDC may respond to antibiotics, including sulfonamides, dicloxacillin, and erythromycin.[93,94] In one case series, 7 children with linear IgA disease were treated with flucloxacillin and demonstrated improvement, with 4 children achieving remission within 3 months.[95] However, spontaneous remission in these patients cannot be ruled out.

REFERENCES

1. Chorzelski TP, Beutner EH, Jablonska S, et al. Immunofluorescence studies in the diagnosis of dermatitis herpetiformis and its differentiation from bullous pemphigoid. *J Invest Dermatol*. 1971;56:373-380.
2. Chorzelski TP, Jablonska S, Maciejowska E. Linear IgA bullous dermatosis of adults. *Clin Dermatol*. 1991;9:383-392.
3. Lawley TJ, Strober W, Yaoita H, et al. Small intestinal biopsies and HLA types in dermatitis herpetiformis patients with granular and linear IgA skin deposits. *J Invest Dermatol*. 1980;74:9-12.
4. Leonard JN, Haffenden GP, Ring NP, et al. Linear IgA disease in adults. *Br J Dermatol*. 1982;107:301-316.
5. Cohen DM, Bhattacharyya I, Zunt SL, et al. Linear IgA disease histopathologically and clinically masquerading as lichen planus. *Oral Surg Oral Med Oral Pathol Oral Radiol Endod*. 1999;88:196-201.
6. Torchia D, Caproni M, Del Bianco E, et al. Linear IgA disease presenting as prurigo nodularis. *Br J Dermatol*. 2006;155(2):479-480.
7. Armstrong AW, Fazeli A, Yeh SW, et al. Vancomycin-induced linear IgA disease manifesting as bullous erythema multiforme. *J Cutan Pathol*. 2004;31:393-397.
8. Baden LA, Apovian C, Imber MJ, et al. Vancomycin-induced linear IgA bullous disease. *Arch Dermatol*. 1988;124:1186-1188.
9. Carpenter S, Berg D, Sidhu-Malik N, et al. Vancomycin-associated linear IgA dermatosis. *J Am Acad Dermatol*. 1992;26:45-48.
10. McWhirter JD, Hashimoto K, Fayne S, et al. Linear IgA bullous dermatosis related to lithium carbonate. *Arch Dermatol*. 1987;123:1120-1122.
11. Waldman MA, Black DR, Callen JP. Vancomycin-induced linear IgA bullous disease presenting as toxic epidermal necrolysis. *Clin Exp Dermatol*. 2004;29:633-636.
12. Kim JS, Choi M, Nam CH, et al. Concurrent drug-induced linear immunoglobulin A dermatosis and immunoglobulin A nephropathy. *Ann Dermatol*. 2015;27(3):315-318.
13. Concha-Garzón MJ, Pérez-Gala S, Solano-López G, et al. Ketoprofen-induced lamina lucida-type linear IgA bullous dermatosis. *J Eur Acad Dermatol Venereol*. 2016;30(2):350-352.
14. Hoffmann J, Hadaschik E, Enk A, et al. Linear IgA bullous dermatosis secondary to infliximab therapy in a patient with ulcerative colitis. *Dermatology*. 2015;231(2):112-115.
15. Akasaka E, Kayo SJ, Nakano H, et al. Diaminodiphenyl sulfone-induced hemolytic anemia and alopecia in a case of linear IgA bullous dermatosis. *Case Rep Dermatol*. 2015;7(2):183-186.
16. Billet SE, Kortuem KR, Gibson LE, et al. A morbilliform variant of vancomycin-induced linear IgA bullous dermatosis. *Arch Dermatol*. 2008;144(6):774-778.
17. Khan I, Hughes R, Curran S, et al. Drug-associated linear IgA disease mimicking toxic epidermal necrolysis. *Clin Exp Dermatol*. 2009;34(6):715-717.
18. Walsh SN, Kerchner K, Sangueza OP. Localized palmar vancomycin-induced linear IgA bullous dermatosis occurring at supratherapeutic levels. *Arch Dermatol*. 2009;145(5):603-604.
19. Chorzelski TP, Jablonska S. IgA linear dermatosis of childhood (chronic bullous disease of childhood). *Br J Dermatol*. 1979;101:535-542.
20. Jabłońska S, Chorzelski TP, Rosinska D, et al. Linear IgA bullous dermatosis of childhood (chronic bullous dermatosis of childhood). *Clin Dermatol*. 1992;9:393-401.
21. Dabrowski J, Chorzelski TP, Jablońska S, et al. The ultrastructural localization of IgA deposits in chronic bullous disease of childhood (CBDC). *J Invest Dermatol*. 1979;72:291-295.
22. Zone JJ, Pazderka Smith E, Powell D, et al. Antigenic specificity of antibodies from patients with linear basement membrane deposition of IgA. *Dermatology*. 1994;189(suppl 1):64-66.
23. Wojnarowska F, Bhogal BS, Black MM. Chronic bullous disease of childhood and linear IgA disease of adults are IgA1-mediated diseases. *Br J Dermatol*. 1994;131:201-204.
24. Ling, K, Bygum A. Linear IgA bullous dermatosis: a retrospective study of 23 patients in Denmark. *Acta Derm Venereol*. 2015;95(4):466-471.
25. Sobjanek M, Sokolowska-Wojdylo M, Sztaba-Kania M, et al. Clinical and immunopathological heterogeneity of 22 cases of linear IgA bullous dermatosis. *J Eur Acad Dermatol Venereol*. 2008;22(9):1131.
26. Wojnarowska F, Marsden RA, Bhogal B, et al. Chronic bullous disease of childhood, childhood cicatricial pemphigoid and linear IgA disease of adults. A comparative study demonstrating clinical and immunopathologic overlap. *J Am Acad Dermatol*. 1988;19(5, pt 1):792-805.
27. Kanwar AJ, Sandhu K, Handa S. Chronic bullous dermatosis of childhood in north India. *Pediatr Dermatol*. 2004;21(5):610-612.
28. Collier PM, Wojnarowska F, Welsh K, et al. Adult linear IgA disease and chronic bullous disease of childhood: the association with human lymphocyte antigens Cw7, B8, DR3 and tumour necrosis factor influences disease expression. *Br J Dermatol*. 1999;141:867-875.

29. Sachs JA, Leonard J, Awad J, et al. A comparative serological and molecular study of linear IgA disease and dermatitis herpetiformis. *Br J Dermatol*. 1988;118: 759-764.
30. Venning VA, Taylor CJ, Ting A, et al. HLA type in bullous pemphigoid, cicatricial pemphigoid and linear IgA disease. *Clin Exp Dermatol*. 1989;14:283-285.
31. Flotte TJ, Olbricht SM, Collins AB, et al. Immunopathologic studies of adult linear IgA bullous dermatosis. *Arch Pathol Lab Med*. 1985;109:457-459.
32. Hall RP, Lawley TJ. Characterization of circulating and cutaneous IgA immune complexes in patients with dermatitis herpetiformis. *J Immunol*. 1985;135:1760-1765.
33. Leonard JN, Haffenden GP, Unsworth DJ, et al. Evidence that the IgA in patients with linear IgA disease is qualitatively different from that of patients with dermatitis herpetiformis. *Br J Dermatol*. 1983;110:315-321.
34. Wojnarowska F, Collier PM, Allen J, et al. The localization of the target antigens and antibodies in linear IgA disease is heterogeneous and dependent on the methods used. *Br J Dermatol*. 1995;132:750-757.
35. Prost C, De Leca AC, Combemale P, et al. Diagnosis of adult linear IgA dermatosis by immunoelectronmicroscopy in 16 patients with linear IgA deposits. *J Invest Dermatol*. 1989;92:39-45.
36. Kárpáti S, Meurer M, Stolz W, et al. Ultrastructural binding sites of endomysium antibodies from sera of patients with dermatitis herpetiformis and coeliac disease. *Gut*. 1992;33(2):191-193.
37. Kárpáti S, Stolz W, Meurer M, et al. Ultrastructural immunogold studies in two cases of linear IgA dermatosis. Are there two distinct types of this disease? *Br J Dermatol*. 1992;127:112-118.
38. Bhogal B, Wojnarowska F, Marsden RA, et al. Linear IgA bullous dermatosis of adults and children: an immunoelectron microscopic study. *Br J Dermatol*. 1987;117:289-296.
39. Horiguchi Y, Ikoma A, Sakai R, et al. Linear IgA dermatosis: report of an infantile case and analysis of 213 cases in Japan. *J Dermatol*. 2008;35(11):737-743.
40. Zone JJ, Taylor TB, Kadunce DP, et al. Identification of the cutaneous basement membrane zone antigen and isolation of antibody in linear immunoglobulin A bullous dermatosis. *J Clin Invest*. 1990;85:812-820.
41. Ishiko A, Shimizu H, Masunaga T, et al. 97-kDa linear IgA bullous dermatosis (LAD) antigen localizes to the lamina lucida of the epidermal basement membrane. *J Invest Dermatol*. 1996;106:739-743.
42. Zone JJ, Taylor TB, Meyer LJ, et al. The 97 kDa linear IgA bullous disease antigen is identical to a portion of the extracellular domain of the 180 kDa bullous pemphigoid antigen, BPAg2. *J Invest Dermatol*. 1998;110:207-210.
43. Roh JY, Yee C, Lazarova Z, et al. The 120-kDa soluble ectodomain of type XVII collagen is recognized by autoantibodies in patients with pemphigoid and linear IgA dermatosis. *Br J Dermatol*. 2000;143:104-111.
44. Schumann H, Baetge J, Tasanen K, et al. The shed ectodomain of collagen XVII/BP 180 is targeted by autoantibodies in different blistering skin diseases. *Am J Pathol*. 2000;156:685-695.
45. Lin MS, Fu CL, Olague-Marchan M, et al. Autoimmune responses in patients with linear IgA bullous dermatosis: both autoantibodies and T lymphocytes recognize the NC16A domain of the BP180 molecule. *Clin Immunol*. 2002;102:310-319.
46. Zillikens D, Herzele K, Georgi M, et al. Autoantibodies in a subgroup of patients with linear IgA disease react with the NC16A domain of BP1801. *J Invest Dermatol*. 1999;113:947-953.
47. Wojnarowska F, Whitehead P, Leigh IM, et al. Identification of the target antigen in chronic bullous disease of childhood and linear IgA disease of adults. *Br J Dermatol*. 1991;124:157-162.
48. Allen J, Wojnarowska F. Linear IgA disease: the IgA and IgG response to the epidermal antigens demonstrates that intermolecular epitope spreading is associated with IgA rather than IgG antibodies, and is more common in adults. *Br J Dermatol*. 2003;149:977-985.
49. Ishii N, Ohyama B, Yamaguchi Z, et al. IgA autoantibodies against the NC16a domain of BP180 but not 120-kDa LAD-1 detected in a patient with linear IgA disease. *Br J Dermatol*. 2008;158(5):1151-1153.
50. Izaki S, Mitsuya J, Okada T, et al. A case of linear IgA/IgG bullous dermatosis with anti-laminin-332 autoantibodies. *Acta Derm Venereol*. 2015;95(3):359-360.
51. Tsuchisaka A, Ohara K, Ishii N, et al. Type VII collagen is the major autoantigen for sublamina densa-type linear IgA bullous dermatosis. *J Invest Dermatol*. 2015;135(2):626-629.
52. Peters MS, Rogers RS III. Clinical correlations of linear IgA deposition at the cutaneous basement membrane zone. *J Am Acad Dermatol*. 1989;20:761-770.
53. Norris IN, Haeberle MT, Callen JP, et al. Generalized linear IgA dermatosis with palmar involvement. *Dermatol Online J*. 2015;21(9).
54. Choudhry SZ, Kashat M, Lim HW. Vancomycin-induced linear IgA bullous dermatosis demonstrating the isomorphic phenomenon. *Int J Dermatol*. 2015;54(11):1211-1213.
55. Perrett CM, Evans AV, Russell-Jones R. Tea tree oil dermatitis associated with linear IgA disease. *Clin Exp Dermatol*. 2003;28(2):167-170.
56. Tran D, Kossard S, Shumack S. Phenytoin-induced linear IgA dermatosis mimicking toxic epidermal necrolysis. *Australas J Dermatol*. 2003;44:284-286.
57. Blockmans D, Bossuyt L, Degreef H, et al. Linear IgA dermatosis: a new cause of fever of unknown origin. *Neth J Med*. 1995;47:214-218.
58. Leigh G, Marsden RA, Wojnarowska F. Linear IgA dermatosis with severe arthralgia. *Br J Dermatol*. 1988; 119:789-792.
59. Kelly SE, Frith PA, Millard PR, et al. A clinicopathological study of mucosal involvement in linear IgA disease. *Br J Dermatol*. 1988;119:161-170.
60. Leonard JN, Wright P, Williams DM, et al. The relationship between linear IgA disease and benign mucous membrane pemphigoid. *Br J Dermatol*. 1984;110:307-314.
61. Romani L, Diociaiuti A, D'Argenio P, et al. A case of neonatal linear IgA bullous dermatosis with severe eye involvement. *Acta Derm Venereol*. 2015;95(8):1015-1017.
62. Porter SR, Bain SE, Scully CM. Linear IgA disease manifesting as recalcitrant desquamative gingivitis. *Oral Surg*. 1992;74:179-182.
63. Sato K, Hanazawa H, Sato Y, et al. Initial presentation and fatal complications of linear IgA bullous dermatosis in the larynx and pharynx. *J Laryngol Otol*. 2005;119:314-318.
64. Joseph TI, Sathyan P, Goma Kumar KU. Linear IgA dermatosis adult variant with oral manifestation: a rare case report. *J Oral Maxillofac Pathol*. 2015;19(1):83-87.
65. deFranchis R, Primignani M, Cipolla M, et al. Small-bowel involvement in dermatitis herpetiformis and in linear IgA bullous dermatosis. *J Clin Gastroenterol*. 1983;5:429-436.

66. Leonard JN, Griffiths CE, Powles AV, et al. Experience with a gluten free diet in the treatment of linear IgA disease. *Acta Derm Venereol*. 1987;67:145-148.
67. Rose C, Dieterich W, Bröcker EB, et al. Circulating autoantibodies to tissue transglutaminase differentiate patients with dermatitis herpetiformis from those with linear IgA disease. *J Am Acad Dermatol*. 1999;41:957-961.
68. Birnie AJ, Perkins W. A case of linear IgA disease occurring in a patient with colonic Crohn's disease. *Br J Dermatol*. 2005;153(5):1050-1052.
69. Paige DG, Leonard JN, Wojnarowska F, et al. Linear IgA disease and ulcerative colitis. *Br J Dermatol*. 1997;136:779-782.
70. Sillevis Smitt JH, Leusen JH, Stas HG, et al. Chronic bullous disease of childhood and a paecilomyces lung infection in chronic granulomatous disease. *Arch Dis Child*. 1997;77:150-152.
71. Minhas JS, Wickner PG, Long AA, et al. Immune-mediated reactions to vancomycin: a systematic case review and analysis. *Ann Allergy Asthma Immunol*. 2016;116(6):544-553.
72. Alberta-Wszolek L, Mousette AM, Mahalingam M, et al. Linear IgA bullous dermatosis following influenza vaccination. *Dermatol Online J*. 2009;15(11):3.
73. Kocyigit P, Akay BN, Karaosmanoglu N. Linear IgA bullous dermatosis induced by interferon-alpha 2a. *Clin Exp Dermatol*. 2009;34(5):e123-124.
74. Palmer RA, Ogg G, Allen J, et al. Vancomycin-induced linear IgA disease with autoantibodies to BP180 and LAD 285. *Br J Dermatol*. 2001;145:816-820.
75. Paul C, Wolkenstein P, Prost C, et al. Drug-induced linear IgA disease: target antigens are heterogeneous. *Br J Dermatol*. 1997;136(3):406-411.
76. Joshi S, Scott G, Looney RJ. A successful challenge in a patient with vancomycin-induced linear IgA dermatosis. *Ann Allergy Asthma Immunol*. 2004;93:101-103.
77. Tomida E, Kato Y, Ozawa H, et al. Causative drug detection by drug-induced lymphocyte stimulation test in drug-induced linear IgA bullous dermatosis. *Br J Dermatol*. 2016;175(5):1106-1108.
78. Wozniak K, Kalinska-Bienias A, Hashimoto T, et al. Ultraviolet-induced linear IgA bullous dermatosis: a case report and literature survey. *Br J Dermatol*. 2014;171(6):1578-1581.
79. Blickenstaff RD, Perry HO, Peters MS. Linear IgA deposition associated with cutaneous varicella-zoster infection: a case report. *J Cutan Pathol*. 1988;15(1):49-52.
80. Godfrey K, Wojnarowska F, Leonard J. Linear IgA disease of adults: association with lymphoproliferative malignancy and possible roel of other triggering factors. *Br J Dermatol*. 1990;123:447-452.
81. McEvoy MT, Connolly SM. Linear IgA dermatosis: Association with malignancy. *J Am Acad Dermatol*. 1990;22:59-63.
82. Yang CS, Robinson-Bostom L, Landow S. Linear IgA bullous dermatosis associated with metastatic renal cell carcinoma. *JAAD Case Rep*. 2015;1(2):91-92.
83. Tiger JB, Rush JT, Barton DT, et al. Urticarial linear IgA bullous dermatosis (LABD) as a presenting sign of chronic lymphocytic leukemia (CLL). *JAAD Case Rep*. 2015;1(6):412-414.
84. Blenkinsopp WK, Haffenden GP, Fry L, et al. Histology of linear IgA disease, dermatitis herpetiformis and bullous pemphigoid. *Am J Dermatopathol*. 1983;5:547-554.
85. Smith SB, Harrist TJ, Murphy GF, et al. Linear IgA bullous dermatosis v dermatitis herpetiformis: quantitative measurements of dermoepidermal alterations. *Arch Dermatol*. 1984;120:324-328.
86. Talhari C, Althaus C, Megahed M. Ocular linear IgA disease resulting in blindness. *Arch Dermatol*. 2006;142(6):786-787.
87. Talhari C, Mahnke N, Ruzicka T, et al. Successful treatment of linear IgA disease with mycophenolate mofetil as a corticosteroid sparing agent. *Clin Exp Dermatol*. 2005;30(3):297-298.
88. Peterson JD, Chan LS. Linear IgA bullous dermatosis responsive to trimethoprim-sulfamethoxazole. *Clin Exp Dermatol*. 2007;32(6):756-758.
89. Farley-Li J, Mancini AJ. Treatment of linear IgA bullous dermatosis of childhood with mycophenolate mofetil. *Arch Dermatol*. 2003;139:1121-1124.
90. Goebeler M, Seitz C, Rose C, et al. Successful treatment of linear IgA disease with salazosulphapyridine and intravenous immunoglobulins. *Br J Dermatol*. 2003;149:912-914.
91. Kroiss MM, Vogt M, Landthaler WS. High-dose intravenous immune globulin is also effective in linear IgA disease. *Br J Dermatol*. 2000;142:582-582.
92. Dauendorffer JN, Mahe E, Saiag P. Tacrolimus ointment, an interesting adjunctive therapy for childhood linear IgA bullous dermatosis. *J Eur Acad Dermatol Venereol*. 2008;22(3):364-365.
93. Cooper SM, Powell J, Wojnarowska F. Linear IgA disease: successful treatment with erythromycin. *Clin Exp Dermatol*. 2002;27(8):677-679.
94. Siegfried EC, Sirawan S. Chronic bullous disease of childhood: successful treatment with dicloxacillin. *J Am Acad Dermatol*. 1998;39:797-800.
95. Alajlan A, Al-Khawajah M, Al-Sheikh O, et al. Treatment of linear IgA bullous dermatosis of childhood with flucloxacillin. *J Am Acad Dermatol*. 2006;54:652-656.

Chapter 59 :: Dermatitis Herpetiformis
:: Stephen I. Katz

第五十九章
疱疹样皮炎

中文导读

疱疹样皮炎（DH）是一种慢性、剧烈瘙痒性、丘疹水疱性皮肤病，皮疹对称分布于肢体伸侧。组织病理以真皮乳头中性粒细胞聚集为特征，正常皮肤免疫荧光检测发现颗粒状IgA沉积可以确诊。表皮谷氨酰胺转化酶（eTG）是其主要的自身抗原。大多数DH患者有谷胶敏感性肠病。氨苯砜起效迅速，许多患者须严格禁止谷胶饮食。

本章从七个方面介绍。

1. 流行病学 不同白种人群DH发病率在10/10万~75/10万。男女比例为1.1:1~1.5:1。本病可发生在任何年龄，20岁、30岁和40岁年龄段最常见。

2. 临床表现 本节介绍了DH的临床表现，包括其原发病变表现，但黏膜损伤罕见。其次提出了DH常与恶性肿瘤、胃肠道疾病、某些自身免疫性疾病相关。

3. 病因与发病机制 本节介绍了谷蛋白在DH发病中起至关重要作用，可能与干扰素、IL-2和IL-8、内皮细胞E-选择素等相关。

4. 诊断 本节介绍了DH的直接免疫荧光及组织病理学特点。

5. 鉴别诊断 本节介绍了DH皮疹多形、缺乏诊断性皮损，易与许多其他疾病混淆，在临床和病理学上可能较难与线状IgA皮病区分，但有独特的免疫学特征。

6. 临床病程与预后 大多数DH患者病程无限期存在，但病情严重程度不一。大约10%~12% DH患者可以最终缓解。

7. 疾病管理 本节介绍了氨苯砜、重氮酮和磺胺吡啶可迅速改善病情，停止谷胶饮食后患者病情可好转。同时介绍了由坚持高蛋白、无限制脂肪、低糖饮食组成的"阿特金斯饮食"。

〔陈明亮〕

AT-A-GLANCE

- Intensely itchy, chronic papulovesicular eruption distributed symmetrically on extensor surfaces.
- Characterized histologically by dermal papillary collections of neutrophils.
- Granular immunoglobulin A deposits in normal-appearing skin are diagnostic.
- Epidermal transglutaminases appear to be the dominant autoantigens.
- Most, if not all, dermatitis herpetiformis patients have an associated gluten-sensitive enteropathy.
- The rash responds rapidly to dapsone therapy and, in many patients, to strict adherence to a gluten-free diet.

HISTORICAL PERSPECTIVE

In 1884, Louis Duhring first described the clinical features and natural history of a polymorphous pruritic disorder that he called *dermatitis herpetiformis* (DH); however, the critical elements in the pathogenesis of DH remained unknown until the 1960s.[1] In 1888, Brocq described patients with a very similar disorder and called it *dermatite polymorphe prurigineuse*.[2] In addition, he analyzed Duhring's report and excluded several types of patients from the diagnosis. Since 1888, several important discoveries have been made. In 1940, Costello[3] demonstrated the efficacy of sulfapyridine in the treatment of DH. In early 1960s, Pierard and Whimster[4] and MacVicar et al[5] found that early lesions of DH are characterized by neutrophilic microabscesses in the dermal papillae. In 1967, Cormane[6] found that the skin of DH patients contained granular immunoglobulin deposits in dermal papillary tips, and in 1969, van der Meer[7] extended these studies and found that the most regularly detected immunoglobulin (Ig) deposited in DH is IgA. The association between DH and intestinal abnormalities was first observed by Marks et al[8] in 1966. Fry et al[9] and Shuster et al[10] identified the intestinal findings as a gluten-sensitive enteropathy. In 1973, Fry et al[11] demonstrated that strict adherence to a gluten-free diet would improve the skin disease as well as reverse the intestinal abnormality, as occurs in celiac disease. Katz et al[12] identified a strong association between DH and certain histocompatibility antigens in 1972. In 1979, Jablonska and Chorzelski[13] distinguished those patients with linear IgA deposits from those with granular IgA deposits and defined a distinct entity. In 1999, Dieterich et al[14] identified antibodies to tissue transglutaminases in the sera from DH patients. Distinguishing between various types of transglutaminases enabled Sárdy et al,[15] in 2002, to demonstrate that epidermal transglutaminase (eTG) is the dominant autoantigen in DH. In 2016, Görög et al[16] demonstrated circulating transglutaminase 3–IgA immune complexes in DH patients.

EPIDEMIOLOGY

The prevalence of DH in various white populations varies between 10 in 100,000 persons and 75 in 100,000 persons.[17-19] The male-to-female ratio ranges from 1.1 to 1 to 1.5 to 1. It may start at any age, including in childhood; however, the second, third, and fourth decades of life are the most common ages. After presentation, DH persists indefinitely in most patients, although with varying severity.

Patients with DH have an associated gluten-sensitive enteropathy (celiac disease) that is usually asymptomatic.

CLINICAL FEATURES

CUTANEOUS FINDINGS

The primary lesion of DH is an erythematous papule, an urticaria-like plaque, or, most commonly, a vesicle (Figs. 59-1, 59-2, and 59-3). Large bullae occur infrequently. Vesicles, especially if they occur on the palms, may be hemorrhagic. The continual appearance and disappearance of lesions may result in hyperpigmentation and/or hypopigmentation. Patients may present with only crusted lesions, and

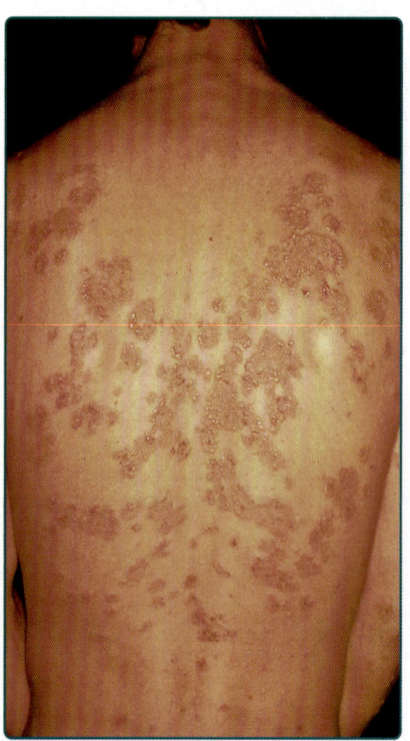

Figure 59-1 Extensive eruption with grouped papules, vesicles, and crusts on the back.

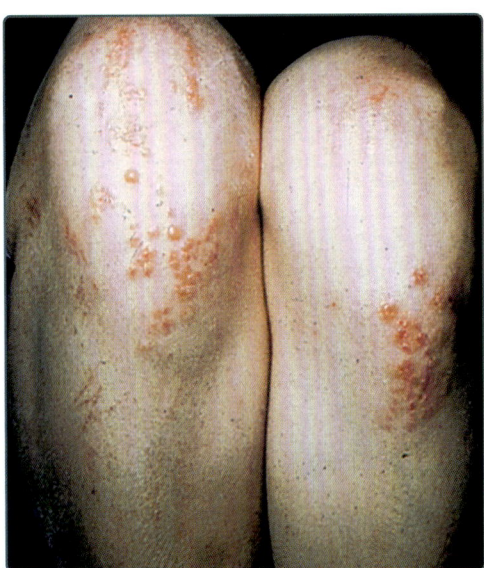

Figure 59-2 Papules, vesicles, and crusts on knees.

a thorough search may not reveal a primary lesion. The herpetiform (herpes-like) grouping of lesions is often present in some areas (Figs. 59-1 and 59-3), but patients also may have many individual nongrouped lesions. Symptoms vary considerably from the usually severe burning and itching in most patients to the almost complete lack of symptoms in a rare patient. Most patients usually can predict the eruption of a lesion as much as 8 to 12 hours before its appearance because of localized stinging, burning, or itching. The usual symmetric distribution of lesions on elbows, knees, buttocks, shoulders, and sacral areas is seen in most patients at one time or another (Figs. 59-1 to 59-4). Although these regions are affected most commonly, most patients have scalp lesions and/or lesions in the posterior nuchal area. Another commonly affected area is the face, especially along the mandible, on the upper eyelid, and facial hairline. Mucous membrane lesions are rare.

NONCUTANEOUS FINDINGS

GASTROINTESTINAL FINDINGS

Most, if not all, DH patients have an associated GI abnormality that is caused by gluten sensitivity.[8-10,20] The pathology of the gluten-sensitive enteropathy (gluten-sensitive enteropathy) is described below.

MALIGNANCY

Most large studies have reported a significant increase in non-Hodgkin lymphomas in patients with DH and an occasional GI lymphoma, but no other increased risk of malignancy.[21-23] Retrospective studies suggest a protective role for a gluten-free diet against GI lymphomas.[24] Hervonen and coworkers reported that 11 (1%) of 1104 patients with DH developed a lymphoma from 2 to 31 years after the diagnosis of DH.[25] Of interest, only 2 lymphomas were of the enteropathy-associated type, whereas 8 were B-cell type lymphomas and 1 was unclassified. The patients with DH who developed lymphoma had adhered to a gluten-free diet less strictly than did patients without lymphoma.[25] Of interest, the mortality rate for patients with DH was equal to or lower than in the general population.[23,26] Lewis et al used the General Practice

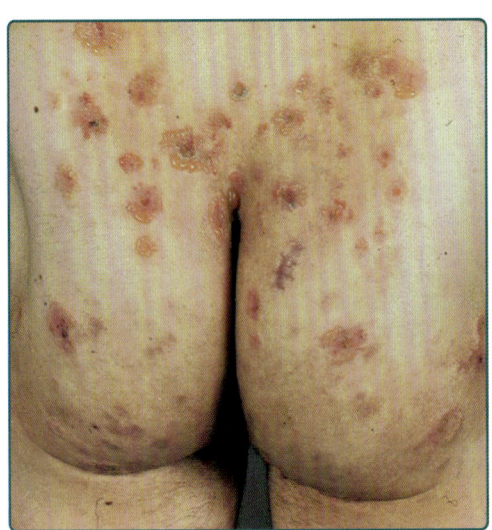

Figure 59-3 This patient has many firm-topped vesicles and bullae, some erosions, and residual hyperpigmentation. Some of the vesicles are arranged in an annular pattern.

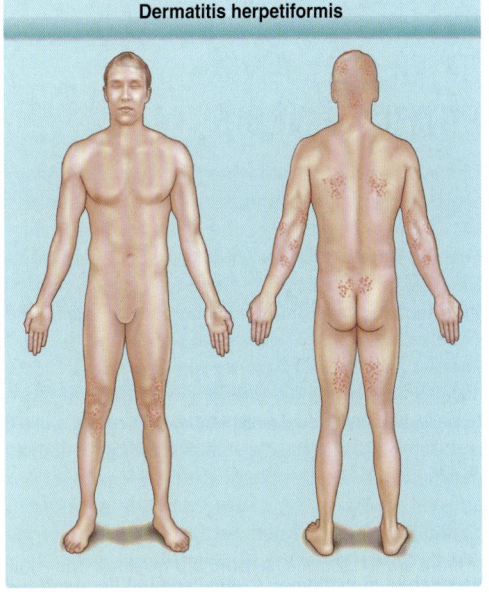

Figure 59-4 Pattern of distribution.

Research Database in the United Kingdom to study a cohort of 846 DH patients and 4225 matched controls. They report no increased risk of malignancy in the DH patients. They suggest a population bias of hospitalized patients in smaller studies resulted in either differences in the degree of intestinal inflammation or unrelated illnesses increasing frequencies of malignancy in the DH patients.[26] These studies suggest that patients with DH may not have an increased risk of malignancy.

OTHER DISEASES

In addition to celiac disease, atrophic gastritis, and pernicious anemia, DH patients have a higher incidence of other autoimmune diseases, such as thyroid disease, insulin-dependent diabetes, lupus erythematosus, Sjögren syndrome, and vitiligo.[27-29] This predilection for associated autoimmune diseases may be a result of the high frequency of the 8.1 ancestral haplotype in these DH patients.[30] Neurologic disease has been reported in patients with isolated celiac disease, including epilepsy, ataxia, opsoclonus-myoclonus, and dementia; however, confirmation of these findings awaits confirmation with large epidemiologic studies.[31,32] Some authors have proposed that patients with DH may be at higher risk for these neurologic complications as a consequence of longstanding ingestion of gluten; however, Wills and coworkers found no evidence of immune-mediated neurologic disease in their evaluation of patients with DH.[33]

Patients with untreated celiac disease also have been found to have an increased frequency of bone loss.[34] Patients with DH frequently continue on gluten-containing diets with a longstanding, albeit low grade, malabsorption. Di Stefano et al demonstrated a significantly reduced bone mineral density in patients with DH on gluten-containing diets.[35] Other studies have refuted this and still others have found no increase in fracture rate in patients with DH.[27,36]

ETIOLOGY AND PATHOGENESIS

Gluten, a protein found in wheat, barley, and rye, plays a critical role in the pathogenesis of DH. Oats, long thought to contain gluten and play a role in inducing DH lesions, are devoid of toxicity in patients with DH.[37,38] As in celiac disease, there is an increased density of small bowel intraepithelial T cells with a γ/δ T-cell receptor in the jejunum of patients with DH.[39] The finding that T-cell lines from patients with DH produce significantly more interleukin (IL) 4 than those from patients with celiac disease and that gut biopsies from symptomatic patients with isolated celiac disease show increased expression of interferon-γ suggests that different cytokine patterns may play a role in the varied clinical manifestations of these 2 diseases.[40,41] Systemic evidence of the gut mucosal immune response has also been found in the serum and the skin of patients with DH. Patients with DH on regular gluten-containing diets have increased serum IL-2 receptor levels and serum IL-8 levels, increased endothelial cell E-selectin expression in skin, and an increased expression of CD11b on circulating neutrophils.[42-44] These systemic manifestations of the gut mucosal immune response may play a role in creating the proinflammatory environment in the skin necessary for the development of skin lesions. The enteropathy seen in DH patients probably relates to the IgA deposits that are found in the skin of these patients, although a direct relationship has not been demonstrated. Patients with a clinical picture consistent with DH and partial IgA deficiency have been reported.[45]

eTGs appear to be the dominant autoantigens in DH.[14,15] Dermal deposits of eTG have been shown to colocalize with cutaneous deposits of IgA, in the papillary tips and because eTGs are strongly expressed in the upper epidermis, it has been suggested that in regions of trauma they may diffuse through the basement membrane after release from epidermal keratinocytes.[46] eTGs were also found in uninvolved skin at least 5 cm away from the lesion suggesting additional factors involved in the production of DH lesions.[46] It is also known that patients with both gluten-sensitive enteropathy and DH have circulating IgA antibodies directed against eTGs.[14,47] There appears to be a predilection for these circulating IgA autoantibodies to bind to eTG in DH, whereas the predilection is for autoantibodies to bind tissue transglutaminases in patients with celiac disease.[15] The precise role of the circulating IgA anti-eTG in the development of skin lesions in patients with DH is not known but circulating IgA anti-eTG does decrease after the institution of a gluten-free diet.[48] However, children with celiac disease have lower levels of circulating IgA anti-eTG when compared to adults with celiac disease, whereas levels of circulating IgA antibodies against tissue transglutaminase are not significantly different between children and adults with celiac disease.[49] This observation has led to the hypothesis that epitope spread over time results in the development of IgA anti-eTG and that this late onset of IgA anti-eTG antibodies may play a role in the typical development of DH in the second to third decade of life.[49] The mechanism whereby the IgA anti-eTG binds to skin in patients with DH is not fully understood. One longstanding hypothesis is that IgA-containing circulating immune complexes are responsible for the IgA deposits in DH skin. The discovery of IgA anti-eTG antibodies has led to the suggestion that IgA–eTG immune complexes may be depositing in the skin of DH patients. This concept has recently received considerable traction in that circulating IgA–TG immune complexes have been identified in DH patients at higher levels before instituting a gluten-free diet.[16] It is possible that the IgA anti-eTG binds initially via antigen–antibody circulating immune complexes and that ability of transglutaminase to crosslink proteins results in the IgA crosslinking to dermal proteins, perhaps fibrin or fibrinogen, resulting in the stable, long-lasting IgA deposits seen in the skin of patients with DH.[50] This hypothesis awaits confirmation. Whether the IgA skin deposits play a role in the pathophysiology of blister formation is not known. The finding of IgA and complement in almost all skin sites, not only in lesional skin, makes one postulate that if IgA (either alone or as a part of an immune complex) does play a role, additional factors are still needed to explain the initiation of lesions. Takeuchi et al demonstrated that minor trauma to skin results in increased expression of IL-8 and E-selectin, both of which may predispose to a neutrophilic inflammatory infiltrate.[51] These findings, coupled with the typical appearance of DH lesions on extensor surfaces at sites of trauma, suggest that local cytokine/chemokine production after trauma may be one of the inciting factors of DH skin lesions. It may be that after the initial neutrophilic infiltrate binds to the cutaneous IgA, factors such as cytokines, chemokines, and proteases are released that both directly result in blister formation and induce basal keratinocytes to produce collagenases or stromelysin-1 that further contributes to the formation of blisters.[52,53] Other studies suggest that T cells may play a role in the pathogenesis of the skin lesions; however, no specific T-cell responses to gluten have been detected.[54,55]

It has been known for some time that iodides, administered orally, can exacerbate or elicit eruptions of DH, and this has, in former times, been used for diagnostic purposes. The availability of immunopathologic techniques for the detection of IgA deposits in skin has made such provocation tests obsolete.

There is a marked increase in the incidence of certain major histocompatibility complex antigens in patients with DH. Worldwide studies have found that 77% to 87% of DH patients have human leukocyte antigen (HLA)-B8 (compared with 20% to 30% of unaffected individuals).[12,55,56,57] In addition, the class II major histocompatibility complex antigens HLA-DR and HLA-DQ are associated with DH even more frequently than is HLA-B8.[58,59] Park et al[60] reported that more than 90% of patients expressed Te24, which was later shown to be similar to HLA-DQw2; this finding has been confirmed by others. Molecular studies indicate that susceptibility to DH is not associated with a unique HLA-DQw2 molecule.[61,62] Virtually all patients with DH have genes that encode the HLA-DQ ($\alpha1*0501$, $\beta1*02$) or the HLA-DQ ($\alpha1*03$, $\beta1*0302$) heterodimers, a pattern identical to that seen in celiac disease.[61,63] This strong association between susceptibility genes and DH and celiac disease is important clinically and pathophysiologically in that there is a strong concordance of these 2 diseases in monozygotic twins.[62] Furthermore, first-degree relatives of both DH and celiac disease patients are often (4% to 5%) affected with one or the other of these diseases.[64] Non–major histocompatibility complex susceptibility genes are also associated with DH.

DNase-hypersensitivity regions 1 and 2, which function as enhancers for the Ig heavy-chain regulatory region, are found with higher frequencies in DH patients.[65]

Marietta et al have reported an HLA-DQ8 transgenic nonobese diabetic mouse that when immunized with gluten developed neutrophilic skin lesions along with cutaneous deposits of IgA; withdrawal of dietary gluten resulted in resolution of the skin lesions.[66] Although differences between the animal model and DH in patients exist, further investigation of this mouse model may provide important information regarding the pathogenesis of DH.

DIAGNOSIS

LABORATORY TESTING

DIRECT IMMUNOFLUORESCENCE

After Cormane demonstrated that both perilesional and uninvolved skin of patients with DH contained granular Ig deposits located in dermal papillary tips, van der Meer found that the most regularly detected Ig class in DH skin was IgA (Fig. 59-5).[6,7] Although most patients have granular IgA deposits in their skin, some deposits have a more distinct fibrillary pattern of IgA deposits.[67] For the most part, IgA deposits have not been seen in the skin of patients with celiac disease except for the study of Cannistraci et al.[68,69] The significance of the latter findings in the pathogenesis of DH is not known.[69]

Finding granular IgA deposits in normal-appearing skin is the most reliable criterion for the diagnosis of DH.[70,71] These IgA deposits are unaffected by treatment with drugs, but may decrease in intensity or disappear after long-term adherence to a gluten-free diet.[72,73] The IgA deposits are not uniformly intense throughout

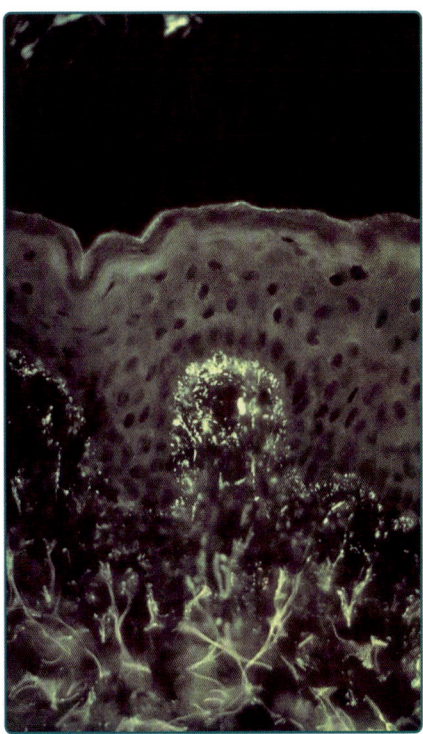

Figure 59-5 Direct immunofluorescence showing granular dermal papillary deposits of immunoglobulin A.

the skin and may be detected more easily in normal-appearing skin near active lesions.[74] In DH, other immunoglobulins are sometimes bound to the skin in the same areas as the IgA.[71] IgA deposits also may be seen in the skin of patients with bullous pemphigoid, scarring pemphigoid, Henoch-Schönlein purpura, and alcoholic liver disease, although in different patterns of distribution than those seen in DH.

Because of the IgA skin deposits and the association between DH and celiac disease, several groups have studied the IgA subclasses in DH. IgA1 is the predominant (or exclusive) subclass that has been identified in the skin of DH patients.[75,76] Most IgA1 is produced in the bone marrow, whereas most IgA2 is produced at mucosal sites. This does not negate the possibility that the IgA1 in skin may still be of mucosal origin because IgA1 is the predominant IgA subclass of IgA antibodies directed against dietary proteins produced in gut secretions in patients with DH.[77,78]

Kantele et al reported a DH association with an increase in circulating IgA1-plasmoblasts with skin-homing receptors (CLA) as compared to those with IgA2.[78] The third component of complement (C3) is frequently found in the same location as IgA. The presence of C3 in both perilesional and normal-appearing skin is not affected by treatment with dapsone (diaminodiphenyl sulfone), but C3 may not be detectable after treatment with a gluten-free diet.[73,80] C5 and components of the alternative complement pathway also may be seen in areas corresponding to the IgA deposits. The C5–C9 membrane attack complex, which is formed as the terminal event in complement activation, is also seen in normal-appearing and perilesional skin of patients.[81] The exact site of the IgA deposits in DH skin has been studied by immunoelectron microscopy. Early studies indicated that IgA is preferentially associated with bundles of microfibrils and with anchoring fibrils of the papillary dermis immediately below the basal lamina.[82,83] Other studies, however, indicate that some or almost all of the IgA deposits are related to nonfibrillar components of skin and other connective tissues.[83-85] There is also no agreement as to whether the IgA deposits in DH colocalize to fibrillin, a major component of the elastic microfibrillar bundles.[85,86]

SERUM STUDIES

Chorzelski et al described an IgA antibody that binds to an intermyofibril substance (endomysium) of smooth muscle.[87] Sárdy et al showed that these IgA autoantibodies have specificity for transglutaminase, particularly for eTG.[15] Although a majority of DH patients on gluten-containing diets have circulating anti eTG antibodies, and this serum assay is thought to be quite sensitive, a significant number of patients do not have circulating anti-eTG antibodies.[49,88,89]

PATHOLOGY

The histology of an early skin lesion (clinically nonvesicular) is characterized by dermal papillary collections of neutrophils (microabscesses), neutrophilic fragments, varying numbers of eosinophils, fibrin, and, at times, separation of the papillary tips from the overlying epidermis (Fig. 59-6). In addition, in such early lesions, the upper and middle dermal blood vessels are surrounded by a lymphohistiocytic infiltrate, as well as some neutrophils and an occasional eosinophil.[4,5] At times, early lesions may be difficult or impossible to differentiate from those of linear IgA disease (see Chap. 58), the bullous eruption of lupus erythematosus (see Chap. 61), bullous pemphigoid (see Chap. 54), or the neutrophil-rich form of epidermolysis bullosa acquisita (see Chap. 56). The histology of older lesions shows subepidermal vesicles that may be impossible to differentiate from other subepidermal bullous eruptions, such as bullous pemphigoid, erythema multiforme, bullous drug eruption, and pemphigoid gestationis. Immunofluorescent localization and ultrastructural studies of the site of blister formation in DH demonstrate that the blister forms above the lamina densa, within the lamina lucida. This is thought to occur because the lamina lucida is the most vulnerable component of the dermal–epidermal junction.[90]

The pathology of the DH-associated enteropathy is essentially the same as seen in celiac disease that is unassociated with DH, although the lesion in the latter is usually much more severe; this applies to the epithelial cell derangement as well as to the character of the

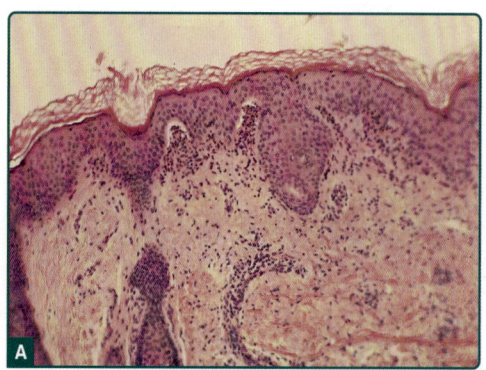
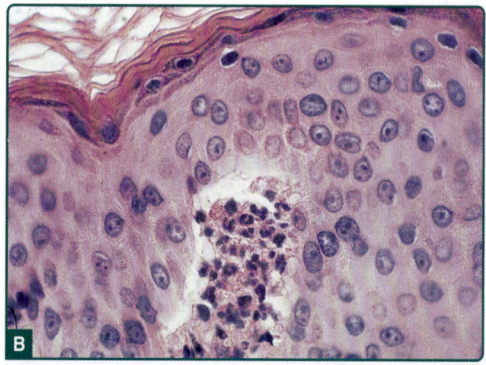

Figure 59-6 Biopsy of an early lesion showing dermal papillary collections of neutrophils and eosinophils and subepidermal vesiculation at low (**A**) and high (**B**) magnification.

lymphoplasmacytic infiltrate. Over the past 45 years the prevalence of severe villous atrophy in DH patients has decreased in Finland.[91] The distribution of the GI lesion in the small intestine is, as a general rule, more widespread in celiac disease. The functional changes in the bowel and clinical sequelae encountered in the enteropathy associated with DH and those seen in celiac disease are similar but again differ in degree, those in the latter being more severe. Thus, in DH one observes steatorrhea (20% to 30% of patients), abnormal D-xylose absorption (10% to 33% of patients), and occasional anemia secondary to iron or folate deficiency. In patients not taking dapsone or related drugs, the anemia is usually caused by malabsorption. In addition to the small intestinal lesion, patients with DH have an increased incidence of achlorhydria and atrophic gastritis.[92,93] Reports of pernicious anemia and antibodies to gastric parietal cells are thus likely to be more than the result of chance.

DIFFERENTIAL DIAGNOSIS

DH may be confused with numerous other conditions because of its pleomorphic manifestations and the occasional lack of diagnostic lesions (Table 59-1). Neurotic excoriations, eczema, papular urticaria, transient acantholytic dermatosis, pemphigoid, pemphigoid gestationis, erythema multiforme, and various other dermatoses can be differentiated easily on the basis of histologic and immunologic criteria. Linear IgA disease may be more difficult to differentiate clinically and histologically, but it is distinctive immunologically. A high index of suspicion is very helpful in that even in the absence of primary lesions, DH can be diagnosed based on the typical in vivo–bound granular IgA deposits in normal-appearing skin.

CLINICAL COURSE AND PROGNOSIS

After presentation, DH persists indefinitely in most patients, although with varying severity. A rare patient will have extreme waxing and waning of disease whereby they may be free of disease for up to a year at a time even without treatment. Two long-term studies of immunologically verified patients have suggested that the disease in approximately 10% to 12% of DH patients eventually remits.[94,95] Nonsteroidal antiinflammatory drugs may cause an exacerbation of the DH even in those who disease is well controlled with either dapsone or gluten-free diet.[96]

MANAGEMENT

SULFONES

Diaminodiphenyl sulfone (dapsone), sulfoxone (diazone—not available in the United States), and sulfapyridine (not generally available in the United States) provide prompt improvement in symptoms and signs of the disease. Symptoms may abate in as few as 3 hours or as long as a few days after the first pill is taken, and new lesions no longer erupt after 1 to 2 days of treatment. Exacerbations occur from hours to days after cessation of treatment. This response to therapy was, for a long time, the most important element in making a diagnosis. The preferred treatment for an adult is dapsone at an initial dosage of 100 to 150 mg/day (this usually can be taken once a day). A rare patient may require 300 to 400 mg of dapsone for initial improvement. Patients should be instructed to take the minimal dose required to suppress signs and symptoms. Not all patients require daily treatment; in rare cases, 25 mg weekly is sufficient. Sulfapyridine, in a dosage of 1.0 to 1.5 g daily, is particularly useful in patients intolerant of dapsone, in elderly patients, and in those with cardiopulmonary problems. The pharmacology, mechanism(s) of action, adverse effects, and monitoring of dapsone are discussed in Chap. 187.

GLUTEN-FREE DIET

EFFECT ON THE SMALL INTESTINE

The intestinal lesion in DH responds to dietary gluten withdrawal. The time course of the response in adults with DH is the same as that in adults with celiac disease.

EFFECT ON THE SKIN DISEASE

Strict adherence to a gluten-free diet will, after variable periods of time (from 4 months to 1 year), reduce or completely eliminate the requirement for medication in most, but not all, patients. The most extensive early study by Fry et al has been confirmed by several groups.[97] However, it is only the very highly motivated patient who can adhere to the diet, which requires counseling by a dietitian who is very familiar with its use. The general availability of gluten-free foods (and

---

TABLE 59-1
Differential Diagnosis of Dermatitis Herpetiformis

Consider
- Eczema
- Atopic dermatitis
- Papular urticaria
- Neurotic excoriations
- Bullous pemphigoid
- Pemphigoid gestationis
- Linear immunoglobulin A dermatosis
- Atopic dermatitis

Rule Out
- Scabies

standardized labelling in the United States) in most food markets has made adherence to this diet much easier than in previous times. Despite this, there are still patients who remain refractory to gluten-free diet treatment.[97]

ELEMENTAL AND OTHER DIET THERAPY

Studies in small numbers of DH patients have indicated that elemental diets (composed of free amino acids, short-chain polysaccharides, and small amounts of triglycerides) can be very beneficial in alleviating the skin disease within a few weeks.[98,99] The beneficial effect on the skin disease may be achieved even if the patient ingests large amounts of gluten.[100] Unfortunately, elemental diets are difficult to tolerate for long periods. Interestingly, complete resolution of the skin lesions of DH has also been reported by adherence to the high-protein, unlimited fat, low-carbohydrate diet popularized as the "Atkins Diet."[100] Further studies are needed to confirm this report.

REFERENCES

1. Duhring LA. Dermatitis herpetiformis. *J Am Med Assoc*. 1884;3:225.
2. Brocq L. De la dermatite herpetiforme de Duhring. *Ann Dermatol Syphiligr (Paris)*. 1888:152.
3. Costello M. Dermatitis herpetiformis treated with sulfapyridine. *Arch Dermatol Syph*. 1974;41:134.
4. Pierard J, Whimster I. The histological diagnosis of dermatitis herpetiformis, bullous pemphigoid and erythema multiforme. *Br J Dermatol*. 1961;73:253-266.
5. MacVicar DN, Graham JH, Burgoon CF. Dermatitis herpetiformis, erythema multiforme and bullous pemphigoid: a comparative histopathological and histochemical study. *J Invest Dermatol*. 1963;41:289-300.
6. Cormane RH. Immunofluorescent studies of the skin in lupus erythematosus and other diseases. *Pathol Eur*. 1967;2:170-187.
7. van der Meer JB. Granular deposits of immunoglobulins in the skin of patients with dermatitis herpetiformis: an immunofluorescent study. *Br J Dermatol*. 1969;81:493-503.
8. Marks J, Shuster S, Watson AJ. Small bowel changes in dermatitis herpetiformis. *Lancet*. 1966;2(7476):1280-1282.
9. Fry L, McMinn RM, Cowan JD, et al. Effect of gluten free-diet on dermatological, intestinal and haematological manifestations of dermatitis herpetiformis. *Lancet*. 1968;1:557-561.
10. Shuster S, Watson AJ, Marks J. Coeliac syndrome in dermatitis herpetiformis. *Lancet*. 1968;1(7552):1101-1106.
11. Fry L, Seah PP, Riches DJ, et al. Clearance of skin lesions in dermatitis herpetiformis after gluten withdrawal. *Lancet*. 1973;1(7798):288-291.
12. Katz SI, Falchuk ZM, Dahl MV, et al. HL-A8: a genetic link between dermatitis herpetiformis and gluten-sensitive enteropathy. *J Clin Invest*. 1972;51(11):2977-2980.
13. Jablonska S, Chorzelski T. IgA linear dermatosis. *Ann Dermatol Venereol*. 1979;106 (8-9):651-655.
14. Dieterich W, Ehnis T, Bauer M, et al. Identification of tissue transglutaminase as the autoantigen of celiac disease. *Nat Med*. 1997;3:797-801.
15. Sárdy M, Kárpáti S, Merkl B, et al: Epidermal transglutaminase (TGase 3) is the autoantigen of dermatitis herpetiformis. *J Exp Med*. 2002;195:747-757.
16. Görög A, Németh K, Kolev K, et al. Circulating transglutaminase 3-immunoglobulin A immune complexes in dermatitis herpetiformis. *J Invest Dermatol*. 2016;136(8):1729-1731.
17. Salmi TT, Hervonen K, Kautiainen H, et al. Prevalence and incidence of dermatitis herpetiformis: a 40-year prospective study from Finland. *Br J Dermatol*. 2011;165(2):354-359.
18. Bolotin D, Petronic-Rosic V. Dermatitis herpetiformis. Part I. Epidemiology, pathogenesis, and clinical presentation. *J Am Acad Dermatol*. 2011;64(6):1017-1024.
19. Smith JB, Tulloch JE, Meyer LJ, et al. The incidence and prevalence of dermatitis herpetiformis in Utah. *Arch Dermatol*. 1992;128(12):1608-1610.
20. Reunala T, Lokki J. Dermatitis herpetiformis in Finland. *Acta Derm Venereol*. 1978;58:505-510.
21. Leonard JN, Tucker WF, Fry JS, et al. Increased incidence of malignancy in dermatitis herpetiformis. *Br Med J (Clin Res Ed)*. 1983;286(6358):16-18.
22. Collin P, Pukkala E, Reunala T. Malignancy and survival in dermatitis herpetiformis: a comparison with coeliac disease. *Gut*. 1996;38:528-530.
23. Grainge MJ, West J, Solaymani-Dodaran M, et al. The long-term risk of malignancy following a diagnosis of coeliac disease or dermatitis herpetiformis: a cohort study. *Aliment Pharmacol Ther*. 2012;35(6):730-739.
24. Lewis HM, Renaula TL, Garioch JJ, et al. Protective effect of gluten-free diet against development of lymphoma in dermatitis herpetiformis. *Br J Dermatol*. 1996;135(3):363-367.
25. Hervonen K, Vornanen M, Kautiainen H, et al. Lymphoma in patients with dermatitis herpetiformis and their first-degree relatives. *Br J Dermatol*. 2005;152(1):82-86.
26. Viljamaa M, Kaukinen K, Pukkala E, et al. Malignancy and mortality in patients with coeliac disease and dermatitis herpetiformis: 30-year population based study. *Dig Liver Dis*. 2006;38:374-380.
27. Lewis NR, Logan RF, Hubbard RB, et al. No increase in risk of fracture, malignancy or mortality in dermatitis herpetiformis: a cohort study. *Aliment Pharmacol Ther*. 2008;27(11):1140-1147.
28. Fry L. Dermatitis herpetiformis. *Bailliers Clin Gastroenterol*. 1995;9:371-393.
29. Reunala T, Collin P. Diseases associated with dermatitis herpetiformis. *Br J Dermatol*. 1997;136:315-318.
30. Price P, Witt C, Allcock R, et al. The genetic basis for the association of the 8.1 ancestral haplotype (A1, B8, DR3) with multiple immunopathological diseases. *Immunol Rev*. 1999;167:257-274.
31. Bushara KO. Neurologic presentation of celiac disease. *Gastroenterology*. 2005;128:S92-S97.
32. Helsing P, Froen H. Dermatitis herpetiformis presenting as ataxia in a child. *Acta Derm Venereol*. 2007;87:163-165.
33. Wills AJ, Turner B, Lock RJ, et al. Dermatitis herpetiformis and neurological dysfunction. *J Neurol Neurosurg Psychiatry*. 2002;72(2):259-261.
34. Corazza GR, Di Stefano M, Mauriño E, et al. Bones in coeliac disease: diagnosis and treatment. *Best Pract Res Clin Gastroenterol*. 2005;19(3):453-465.

35. Di Stefano M, Jorizzo RA, Veneto G, et al. Bone mass and metabolism in dermatitis herpetiformis. *Dig Dis Sci*. 1999;44(10):2139-2143.
36. Abuzakouk M, Barnes L, O'Gorman N, et al. Dermatitis herpetiformis: no evidence of bone disease despite evidence of enteropathy. *Dig Dis Sci*. 2007;52(3):659-664.
37. Reunala T, Collin P, Holm K, et al. Tolerance to oats in dermatitis herpetiformis. *Gut*. 1998;43(4):490-493.
38. Hardman CM, Garioch JJ, Leonard JN, et al. Absence of toxicity of oats in patients with dermatitis herpetiformis. *N Engl J Med*. 1997;337(26):1884-1887.
39. Savilahti E, Ormälä T, Arato A, et al. Density of gamma/delta+ T cells in the jejunal epithelium of patients with coeliac disease and dermatitis herpetiformis is increased with age. *Clin Exp Immunol*. 1997;109(3):464-467.
40. Smith AD, Bagheri B, Streilein RD, et al. Expression of interleukin-4 and interferon-gamma in the small bowel of patients with dermatitis herpetiformis and isolated gluten-sensitive enteropathy. *Dig Dis Sci*. 1999;44(10):2124-2132.
41. Hall RP, Smith AD, Streilein RD. Increased production of IL-4 by T cell lines from patients with dermatitis herpetiformis compared to patients with isolated gluten sensitive enteropathy. *Dig Dis Sci*. 2000;45:2036-2043.
42. Hall RP 3rd, Takeuchi F, Benbenisty KM, et al. Cutaneous endothelial cell activation in normal skin of patients with dermatitis herpetiformis associated with increased serum levels of IL-8, sE-Selectin and TNF-alpha. *J Invest Dermatol*. 2006;126(6):1331-1337.
43. Ward MM, Pisetsky DS, Hall RP. Soluble interleukin-2 receptor levels in patients with dermatitis herpetiformis. *J Invest Dermatol*. 1991;97:568-572.
44. Smith AD, Streilein RD, Hall RP. Neutrophil CD11b, L-selectin and Fc IgA receptors in patients with dermatitis herpetiformis. *Br J Dermatol*. 2002;147:1109-1117.
45. Samolitis NJ, Hull CM, Leiferman KM, et al. Dermatitis herpetiformis and partial IgA deficiency. *J Am Acad Dermatol*. 2006;54(5 suppl):S206-S209.
46. Dieterich W, Laag E, Bruckner-Tuderman L, et al. Antibodies to tissue transglutaminase as serologic markers in patients with dermatitis herpetiformis. *J Invest Dermatol*. 1999;113(1):133-136.
47. Donaldson MR, Zone JJ, Schmidt LA, et al. Epidermal transglutaminase deposits in perilesional and uninvolved skin in patients with dermatitis herpetiformis. *J Invest Dermatol*. 2007;127(5):1268-1271.
48. Reunala T, Salmi TT, Hervonen K, et al. IgA antiepidermal transglutaminase antibodies in dermatitis herpetiformis: a significant but not complete response to a gluten-free diet treatment. *Br J Dermatol*. 2015;172:1139-1141.
49. Hull CM, Liddle M, Hansen N, et al. Elevation of IgA anti-epidermal transglutaminase antibodies in dermatitis herpetiformis. *Br J Dermatol*. 2008;159(1):120-124.
50. Taylor TB, Schmidt LA, Meyer LJ, et al. Transglutaminase 3 present in the IgA aggregates in dermatitis herpetiformis skin is enzymatically active and binds soluble fibrinogen. *J Invest Dermatol*. 2015;135(2):623-625.
51. Takeuchi F, Streilein RD, Hall RP. Increased E-selectin, IL-8 and IL-10 gene expression in human skin after minimal trauma: a potential explanation of regional distribution of skin lesions. *Exp Dermatol*. 2003;12:777-783.
52. Airola K, Vaalamo M, Reunala T, et al. Enhanced expression of interstitial collagenase, stromelysin-1, and urokinase plasminogen activator in lesions of dermatitis herpetiformis. *J Invest Dermatol*. 1995;105(2):184-189.
53. Salmela MT, Pender SL, Reunala T, et al. Parallel expression of macrophage metalloelastase (MMP-12) in duodenal and skin lesions of patients with dermatitis herpetiformis. *Gut*. 2001;48(4):496-502.
54. Baker BS, Garioch JJ, Bokth S, et al. Lack of proliferative response by gluten specific T cells in the blood and gut of patients with dermatitis herpetiformis. *J Autoimmun*. 1995;8(4):561-574.
55. Garioch JJ, Baker BS, Leonard JN, et al. T lymphocytes in lesional skin of patients with dermatitis herpetiformis. *Br J Dermatol*. 1994;131(6):822-826.
56. Katz SI, Hertz KC, Rogentine N, et al. HLA-B8 and dermatitis herpetiformis in patients with IgA deposits in skin. *Arch Dermatol*. 1977;113(2):155-156.
57. Reunala T, Salo OP, Tiilikainen A, et al. Histocompatibility antigens and dermatitis herpetiformis with special reference to jejunal abnormalities and acetylator phenotype. *Br J Dermatol*. 1976;94(2):139-143.
58. Thomsen M, Platz P, Marks J, et al. Association of LD-8a and LD-12a with dermatitis herpetiformis. *Tissue Antigens*. 1976;7(1):60-62.
59. Keuning, JJ, Peña AS, van Leeuwen A, et al. HLA-DW3 associated with coeliac disease. *Lancet*. 1976;1(7958):506-508.
60. Park MS, Terasaki PI, Ahmed AR, et al. The 90% incidence of HLA antigen (Te24) in dermatitis herpetiformis. *Tissue Antigens*. 1983;22(4):263-266.
61. Otley CC, Wenstrup RJ, Hall RP. DNA sequence analysis and restriction fragment length polymorphism (RFLP) typing of the HLA-DQw2 alleles associated with dermatitis herpetiformis. *J Invest Dermatol*. 1991;97:318-322.
62. Hervonen K, Karell K, Holopainen P, et al. Concordance of dermatitis herpetiformis and celiac disease in monozygous twins. *J Invest Dermatol*. 2000;115(6):990-993.
63. Spurkland A, Ingvarsson G, Falk ES, et al. Dermatitis herpetiformis and celiac disease are both primarily associated with the HLA-DQ (alpha 1*0501, beta 1*02) or the HLA- DQ (alpha 1*03, beta 1*0302) heterodimers. *Tissue Antigens*. 1997;49(1):29-34.
64. Hervonen K, Hakanen M, Kaukinen K, et al. First-degree relatives are frequently affected in coeliac disease and dermatitis herpetiformis. *Scand J Gastroenterol*. 2002;37(1):51-55.
65. Cianci R, Giambra V, Mattioli C, et al. Increased frequency of Ig heavy-chain HS1,2-A enhancer *2 allele in dermatitis herpetiformis, plaque psoriasis, and psoriatic arthritis. *J Invest Dermatol*. 2008;128(8):1920-1924.
66. Marietta EV, Rashtak S, Pittelkow MR. Experiences with animal models of dermatitis herpetiformis: a review. *Autoimmunity*. 2012;45(1):81-90.
67. Ko CJ, Colegio OR, Moss JE, et al. Fibrillar IgA deposition in dermatitis herpetiformis–an underreported pattern with potential clinical significance. *J Cutan Pathol*. 2010;37(4):475-477.

68. Seah PP, Fry L, Stewart JS, et al. Immunoglobulins in the skin in dermatitis herpetiformis and coeliac disease. *Lancet*. 1972;1(7751):611-614.
69. Cannistraci C, Lesnoni La Parola I, Cardinali G, et al. Co-localization of IgA and TG3 on healthy skin of coeliac patients. *J Eur Acad Dermatol Venereol*. 2007;21(4):509-514.
70. Seah PP, Fry L. Immunoglobulins in the skin in dermatitis herpetiformis and their irrelevance in the diagnosis. *Br J Dermatol*. 1975;92:157-166.
71. Leonard J, Haffenden G, Tucker W, et al. Gluten challenge in dermatitis herpetiformis. *N Engl J Med*. 1983;308(14):816-819.
72. Reunala T. Gluten-free diet in dermatitis herpetiformis II. Morphological and immunological findings in the skin and small intestine of 12 patients and matched controls. *Br J Dermatol*. 1978;98:69-78.
73. Zone JJ, Meyer LJ, Petersen MJ. Deposition of granular IgA relative to clinical lesions in dermatitis herpetiformis. *Arch Dermatol*. 1996;132:912-918.
74. Hall RP, Lawley TJ. Characterization of circulating and cutaneous IgA immune complexes in patients with dermatitis herpetiformis. *J Immunol*. 1985;135:1760-1765.
75. Barghuthy FS, Kumar V, Valeski E, et al. Identification of IgA subclasses in skin of dermatitis herpetiformis patients. *Int Arch Allergy Appl Immunol*. 1988;85(3):268-271.
76. Hall RP, Waldbauer GV. Characterization of the mucosal immune response to dietary antigens in patients with dermatitis herpetiformis. *J Invest Dermatol*. 1988;90:658-663.
77. Hall RP, McKenzie KD. Comparison of the intestinal and serum antibody response in patients with dermatitis herpetiformis. *Clin Immunol Immunopathol*. 1992;62(1, pt 1):33-41.
78. Kantele JM, Savilahti E, Westerholm-Ormio M, et al. Decreased numbers of circulating plasmablast and differences in IgA1-plasmablast homing to skin in coeliac disease and dermatitis herpetiformis. *Clin Exp Immunol*. 2009;156(3):535-541.
79. Katz SI, Hertz KC, Crawford PS, et al. Effect of sulfones on complement deposition in dermatitis herpetiformis and on complement-mediated guinea-pig reactions. *J Invest Dermatol*. 1976;67(6):688-690.
80. Ljunghall K, Tjernlund U. Dermatitis herpetiformis: effect of gluten-restricted and gluten-free diet on dapsone requirement and on IgA and C3 deposits in uninvolved skin. *Acta Derm Venereol*. 1983;63:129-136.
81. Dahlback K, Lofberg H, Dahlback B. Vitronectin colocalizes with Ig deposits and C9 neoantigen in discoid lupus erythematosus and dermatitis herpetiformis, but not in bullous pemphigoid. *Br J Dermatol*. 1989;120:725-733.
82. Stingl G, Hönigsmann H, Holubar K, et al: Ultrastructural localization of immunoglobulins in skin of patients with dermatitis herpetiformis. *J Invest Dermatol*. 1976;67(4):507-512.
83. Yaoita H. Identification of IgA binding structures in skin of patients with dermatitis herpetiformis. *J Invest Dermatol*. 1978;71:213-216.
84. Kárpáti S, Meurer M, Stolz W, et al. Dermatitis herpetiformis bodies. Ultrastructural study on the skin of patients using direct preembedding immunogold labeling. *Arch Dermatol*. 1990;126(11):1469-1474.
85. Lightner VA, Sakai LY, Hall RP. IgA-binding structures in dermatitis herpetiformis skin are independent of elastic-microfibrillar bundles. *J Invest Dermatol*. 1991;96:88-92.
86. Dahlback K, Sakai L. IgA immunoreactive deposits colocal with fibrillin immunoreactive fibers in dermatitis herpetiformis skin. *Acta Derm Venereol*. 1990;70:194-198.
87. Chorzelski TP, Sulej J, Tchorzewska H, et al. IgA class endomysium antibodies in dermatitis herpetiformis and coeliac disease. *Ann N Y Acad Sci*. 1983;420:325-334.
88. Rose C, Armbruster FP, Ruppert J, et al. Autoantibodies against epidermal transglutaminase are a sensitive diagnostic marker in patients with dermatitis herpetiformis on a normal or gluten-free diet. *J Am Acad Dermatol*. 2009;61(1):39-43.
89. Borroni G, Biagi F, Ciocca O, et al. IgA anti-epidermal transglutaminase autoantibodies: a sensible and sensitive marker for diagnosis of dermatitis herpetiformis in adult patients. *J Eur Acad Dermatol Venereol*. 2013;27(7):836-841.
90. Smith JB, Taylor TB, Zone JJ. The site of blister formation in dermatitis herpetiformis is within the lamina lucida. *J Am Acad Dermatol*. 1992;27:209-213.
91. Mansikka E, Hervonen K, Salmi TT, et al. The decreasing prevalence of severe villous atrophy in dermatitis herpetiformis: a 45-year experience in 393 patients. *J Clin Gastroenterol*. 2017;51(3):235-239.
92. Stockbrugger R, Andersson H, Gillberg R, et al: Auto-immune atrophic gastritis in patient with dermatitis herpetiformis. *Acta Derm Venereol*. 1997;56(2):111-113.
93. O'Donoghue DP, Lancaster-Smith M, Johnson GD, et al. Gastric lesion in dermatitis herpetiformis. *Gut*. 1976;17(3):185-188.
94. Paek SY, Steinberg SM, Katz SI. Remission in dermatitis herpetiformis: a cohort study. *Arch Dermatol*. 2011;147(3):301-305.
95. Garioch JJ, Lewis HM, Sargent SA, et al. 25 years' experience of a gluten-free diet in the treatment of dermatitis herpetiformis. *Br J Dermatol*. 1994;131(4):541-545.
96. Griffiths CE, Leonard JN, Fry L. Dermatitis herpetiformis exacerbated by indomethacin. *Br J Dermatol*. 1985;112:443-445.
97. Hervonen K, Salmi TT, Ilus T, et al. Dermatitis herpetiformis refractory to gluten-free dietary treatment. *Acta Derm Venereol*. 2016;96(1):82-86.
98. Kadunce DP, McMurry MP, Avots-Avotins A, et al. The effect of an elemental diet with and without gluten on disease activity in dermatitis herpetiformis. *J Invest Dermatol*. 1991;97(2):175-182.
99. Zeedijk N, van der Meer JB, Poen H, et al. Dermatitis herpetiformis: consequences of elemental diet. *Acta Derm Venereol*. 1986;66(4):316-320.
100. Sladden MJ, Johnston GA. Complete resolution of dermatitis herpetiformis with the Atkins' diet. *Br J Dermatol*. 2006;154:565-566.

Chapter 60 :: Inherited Epidermolysis Bullosa :: M. Peter Marinkovich

第六十章
遗传性大疱性表皮松解症

中文导读

遗传性大疱性表皮松解症（EB）是一种家族遗传性皮肤病，其特征是轻微创伤后出现水疱。按水疱发生位置分为单纯型、半桥粒型、交界型和营养不良型。借助免疫荧光和电镜诊断EB，尚需进行DNA分析。

本章内容从以下六个方面简述。

1. 引言　EB是一个家族性疾病，共同特点是轻度创伤后起水疱，严重者累及黏膜。病情严重程度因EB亚型而异，取决于潜在的遗传性分子缺陷。根据临床特征、免疫学、电镜、分子生物学、遗传和蛋白质缺陷等确定EB的主要亚型。

2. 病因与发病机制　EB源于基底细胞与下方真皮之间连接结构的缺陷。这些缺陷可能来自角质形成细胞浆膜内或真皮-表皮基底膜区（BMZ）的细胞外。本章详细介绍了组成BMZ结构的成分、生理作用和引起EB的机制，这些成分包括角蛋白细丝、半桥粒、锚定细丝、锚定纤维。

3. 临床表现　EB分为单纯型、交界型和营养不良型。电镜是EB分型"金标准"，间接免疫荧光检测基底膜抗原对区分EB亚型非常有用。根据临床、遗传、组织学和生化评估，每型又分为几种不同亚型，表60-1总结了这些临床亚型。

4. 诊断　本节介绍了诊断EB的第一步是详询病史和体查，皮肤活检是另一个重要的诊断步骤，尽可能取新鲜水疱。需要通过透射电镜（TEM）或间接免疫荧光显微镜（IDDF）来确定水疱发生在BMZ的具体层次，基因突变分析也很重要，全外显子测序可能使EB突变检测更方便易行。

5. 治疗　本节介绍了大多数EB治疗实质是支持治疗。根据皮肤和器官受累严重程度制订具体方案，包括伤口护理、控制感染、手术管理和营养支持。局部治疗的目的是避免外伤。

6. 总结　本节最后概述和总结了EB的类型和临床表现。

〔陈明亮〕

AT-A-GLANCE

- Epidermolysis bullosa is a family of inherited genodermatoses characterized by blistering in response to minor trauma.
- Blistering level categories are the simplex, hemidesmosomal, junctional, and dystrophic subtypes.
- Cutaneous involvement varies from localized to widespread blistering depending on subtype.
- Extracutaneous involvement varies from none to severely debilitating or lethal.
- The oropharynx, trachea, esophagus, eyes, teeth, nails, hair can be involved depending on subtype.
- Diagnosis is made by immunofluorescent or electron microscopy followed by DNA analysis.

INTRODUCTION

Inherited epidermolysis bullosa (EB, is a family of diseases with the common feature of blistering in response to mild trauma. Patients with EB can show blistering in the form of small vesicles or larger bullae, occurring on cutaneous surfaces and, in the severe forms, on mucosal tissues as well. Although skin and mucosa fragility and trauma-induced painful blisters are hallmarks across the EB spectrum, the distribution of the involvement, the depth of blister formation, any associated extracutaneous involvement, and the severity of the blistering process vary with the different EB subtypes and depend on the underlying heritable molecular defect. EB diseases vary also in the way in which blistered areas heal. The wound repair responses are often abnormal and can eventuate into chronic erosions, hypertrophic granulation tissue, scarring, or even invasive carcinoma. Although the milder EB subtypes are associated with a normal lifespan and little or no internal involvement, the most severe recessively inherited forms are mutilating, multiorgan disorders that threaten both the quality and length of life.

A number of early studies identified the major subtypes of EB. Studies of von Hebra[1-3] were the first to distinguish pemphigus from inherited blistering, and the term *epidermolysis bullosa hereditaria* was first suggested by Koebner.[4] Hallopeau was the first to distinguish between simplex (nonscarring) and dystrophic (scarring) forms of the disease,[5] and Weber,[6] and Cockayne,[7] Dowling and Meara,[8] and Koebner[4] each described unique forms of epidermolysis bullosa simplex. Hoffman,[9] Cockayne,[10] Touraine,[11] Pasini,[12] and Bart[13] provided much of the information about subtypes of DEB. Herlitz described epidermolysis bullosas letalis,[14] which was later found to be a part of the third major category of EB: the junctional form. The use of electron microscopy in EB diagnosis led to the studies of Pearson and collaborators,[15] who classified the patients not only on the basis of clinical findings but also on the existence of ultrastructural changes. A comprehensive classification of EB based on a combination of ultrastructural and clinical findings was completed in an early landmark treatise by Gedde-Dahl.[16] Recent major advances have led to the identification of protein and genetic abnormalities in most types of EB patients. These studies have led to an improved understanding of the biological basis of EB and culminating in the current EB classification based on genetic and protein defects,[17] which provides a rational approach to specific molecular therapy.

ETIOLOGY AND PATHOGENESIS

OVERVIEW

EB arises from defects of attachment of basal keratinocytes to the underlying dermis. These defects can arise from inside the keratinocyte plasma membrane or extracellularly in the dermal-epidermal basement membrane zone (BMZ). Many tissues such as the skin and cornea, which are subjected to external disruptive forces, contain a complex BMZ composed of a group of specialized components that assemble into anchoring complexes (Fig. 60-1). At the most superior aspect of the BMZ, keratin-containing intermediate filaments of the basal cell cytoskeleton insert upon electron-dense condensations of the basal cell plasma membrane termed *hemidesmosomes*. Anchoring filaments span the lamina lucida, connecting hemidesmosomes with the lamina densa and anchoring filaments. At the most inferior aspect of the BMZ, collagen VII–containing anchoring fibrils extend from the lamina densa into the papillary dermis and combine with the lamina densa and anchoring plaques, trapping interstitial collagen fibrils. Thus, the cutaneous BMZ connects the extensive basal cell cytoskeletal network with the abundant network of interstitial collagen fibrils in the dermis.[18,19]

KERATIN FILAMENTS

Keratins are obligate heteropolymers that are composed of pairs of acidic and basic monomers. The keratin pair 5 and 14 assemble to form the extensive intermediate filament network of the basal cell cytoskeleton.[20] Keratins contain a central α-helical rod with several nonhelical interruptions as well as nonhelical carboxy and amino terminal regions. The regions of highest conservation between the keratins are located on the ends of the keratin rod in the helix boundary motifs. Whereas extensive mutagenesis studies suggest that helical regions near the ends of the central rod are important in keratin filament elongation, the nonhelical domains may be important in forming lateral associations.[21] Keratin intermediate filaments insert upon electron-dense structures known as hemidesmosomes.

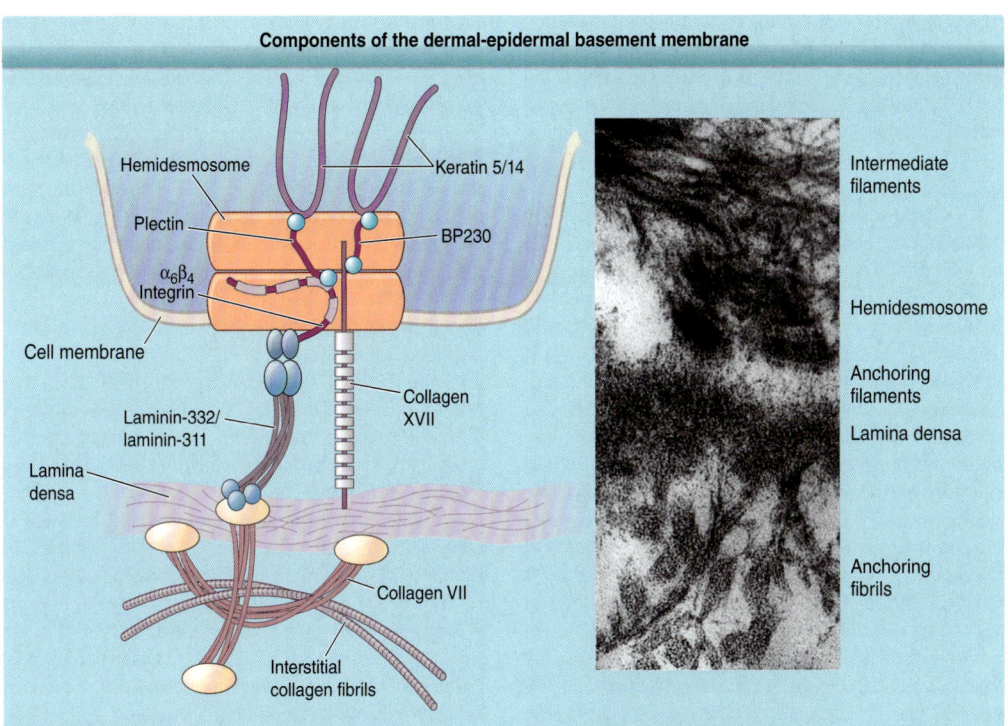

Figure 60-1 Schematic of the components of the dermal–epidermal basement membrane on the left compared with ultrastructural appearance of basement membrane morphological entities on the right.

HEMIDESMOSOMES

Hemidesmosomes contain intracellular proteins including plectin and BP230. Plectin is a 500-kD protein that acts as an intermediate filament binding protein. It is possible that plectin also interacts with microfilaments because plectin contains a domain with similarity to the actin binding domain of spectrin.[22,23] BP230, also known as BPAG1, is a 230-kD protein that has homology both to desmoplakin[24] and to plectin. Several splicing variants of BP230 are of vital importance in the nervous system.[25-27] BP230 localizes to a region referred to as the inner plate on the cytoplasmic surface of the hemidesmosome and like plectin functions in the connection between hemidesmosomes and intermediate filaments. BP230 negative transgenic mice lack a hemidesmosomal inner plate and the connection between hemidesmosomes and intermediate filaments is severed, creating a cytoplasmic zone of mechanical fragility just above the hemidesmosomes.

ANCHORING FILAMENTS

Hemidesmosomes also contain the transmembrane proteins collagen XVII (also termed BPAG2 and BP180)[28] and α6β4 integrin.[29] The cytoplasmic portions of these molecules make up part of the hemidesmosome-dense plaque, and the extracellular portions of these molecules make up portions of the anchoring filament and probably contribute to the structure known as the subbasal dense plate that underlies hemidesmosomes in the lamina lucida region. β4 Integrin only pairs with the α6 subunit, but the α6 subunit can combine either with the β4 integrin or with the β1 integrin. Both the α6β1 or α6β4 integrin combinations have been shown to act as receptors for laminins, and α6β4 integrin acts as a specific receptor for laminin-332. α6β4 Integrin plays a central role in organization of the hemidesmosome. The β4 integrin contains an especially large cytoplasmic domain, which functions in the interaction with other proteins of the hemidesmosomal plaque including collagen XVII and plectin.[30] Skin from transgenic mice lacking β4 integrin is devoid of hemidesmosomes and shows severe deficits in cell adhesion.[31] Interactions between plectin and α6β4 integrin appear to be critical both in the assembly as well as the disassembly of hemidesmosomes.[32]

Collagen XVII (BPAG2, BP180) is a collagenous protein with a type II transmembrane orientation. Based on electron microscopy and crosslinking studies, collagen XVII assembles into a triple-helical homotrimer and contains three main regions: an intracellular amino-terminal globular head, a central rod, and an extracellular flexible tail.[33] Collagen XVII associates with laminin-332 and α6β4 integrin in adhesion structures termed *stable anchoring contacts* formed by keratinocytes in vivo, which are thought to represent prehemidesmosomes.[34] The autoantigen in linear immunoglobulin (Ig) A bullous dermatosis, LAD-1,[35,36] is a 120-kD protein that has been shown by peptide sequencing to be the cleaved exodomain of collagen XVII.[37] Collagen XVII undergoes processing in keratinocyte cultures and in skin through the action of sheddases, membrane-associated proteases that solubilize cell surface receptors.[38,39]

In addition to α6β4 integrin and collagen XVII, anchoring filaments contain the molecules laminin-332 and laminin-311. Like all members of the family of laminin proteins,[40-42] laminin-332 is a large heterotrimeric molecule and contains α3, β3, and γ2 chains.[43,44] The first laminins to be described contained 3 short arms and 1 long arm, forming a cross shape as shown by rotary shadowing analysis. In contrast, laminin-332 contains truncations of each short arm.[45-47] Because of these short arm truncations, laminin-332 cannot self-polymerize with other laminins or bind to nidogen. Instead, laminin-332 forms a disulfide bonded attachment to laminin-311,[48] the other known anchoring filament laminin[43] that contains α3, β1, and γ1 chains. Laminin-332 also undergoes processing of its γ2 and α3 chains.[49] Although rat laminin γ2 chain has been previously been shown to be processed by metalloproteinase-2[50] and membrane-type metalloproteinase type 1,[51] the predominant site of cleavage by these enzymes is not conserved in human laminin-332.[52] Other studies have shown that processing of laminin γ2 chain takes place through a special class of proteins termed C-proteinases, which also process C-terminal domains of procollagen molecules.[53] Although one member of this class of proteins, bone morphogenic protein 1,[54] is capable of performing this action, a splice variant of this protein termed *mammalian tolloid* is the enzyme that is predominantly expressed in keratinocytes and fibroblasts, and mammalian tolloid is the thus the enzyme that likely performs this function in the skin.[52] Mammalian tolloid also processes the laminin α3 chain,[52] although other enzymes such as plasmin,[55] matrix metalloproteinase (MMP)-2[50] and membrane type MMP-1[51] are also capable of this function. The γ2 chain short arm appears important in the assembly of laminin-332 into basement membrane.[56] The antigen recognized by monoclonal antibody (mAb) 19-DEJ-1[57] also localizes to anchoring filaments, but its molecular identity remains unknown.

ANCHORING FIBRILS

Collagen VII is the major constituent of anchoring fibrils. Analysis of the deduced amino acid sequence of collagen VII[58] reveals the presence of a long central collagenous region characterized by repeating Gly-X-Y sequences that contains a number of noncollagenous interruptions, including a 39–amino acid noncollagenous segment in the center of the helix that corresponds to the "hinge region" predicted by biochemical studies.[59,60] These interruptions account for the flexibility of the collagen VII molecule and explain its ability to loop around and entrap dermal matrix molecules to provide its function of stabilizing the basement membrane to the underlying papillary dermis.[61] A 50-kD component of anchoring fibrils has also been identified that appears to localize to the insertion sites of anchoring fibrils to the lamina densa.[62]

The 145-kD N-terminal end of collagen VII contains the largest noncollagenous domain that inserts onto the lamina densa and anchoring plaques. Collagen IV, the most abundant component of these structures, binds to the collagen VII NC1 domain. A direct interaction between anchoring filaments and anchoring fibrils exists from a specific interaction between the anchoring filament component laminin-332 and collagen VII NC1 domain.[63,64] Collagen VII binds the β3 chain on laminin-332.[63,65-67] This appears to be a critical factor in the maintenance of dermal–epidermal cohesion. Like all collagens, collagen VII assembles into a triple helix. Only one chain of collagen VII, the α1 chain, has been identified; one gene codes for an entire molecule, and thus collagen VII is a homotrimer. Collagen VII triple helices are joined together at their processed NC-2 globular domains to form antiparallel dimers.[61,68] Processing of the NC-2 domains takes place via the same family of C-proteinases (bone morphogenic protein 1 and/or mammalian tolloid) that are known to process laminin-332, a closely associated molecule. Anchoring fibrils may derive from lateral associations of collagen VII antiparallel dimers.

CLINICAL FINDINGS

A classification of EB is made based on the ultrastructural level within which the cleavage plane of the blister occurs. EB has been traditionally classified according to the level of BMZ separation on transmission electron microscopy into simplex, junctional, and dystrophic subtypes[69] (Fig. 60-2). Although traditionally the diagnostic "gold standard" for grouping EB has been electron microscopy, immunomapping of basement membrane antigens as viewed by indirect immunofluorescence can also be quite useful in distinguishing subtypes of EB. Within each of these groups, there are several distinct types of EB based on clinical, genetic, histologic, and biochemical evaluation.[17] When possible, molecular characterization at the protein or DNA levels should be appended to the clinical subtype (termed the "onion skin approach") to better delineate the diagnosis and to aid in delivery of emerging molecular therapies. These clinical subtypes are summarized in Table 60-1.

EPIDERMOLYSIS BULLOSA SIMPLEX

Epidermolysis bullosa simplex (EBS) is a disease group characterized by intraepidermal blistering and most often is associated with keratin gene mutations. The range of disease phenotypes range from mild to severe among different subgroups.[70] The common EBS types are dominantly inherited and include generalized severe (Dowling-Meara), generalized intermediate

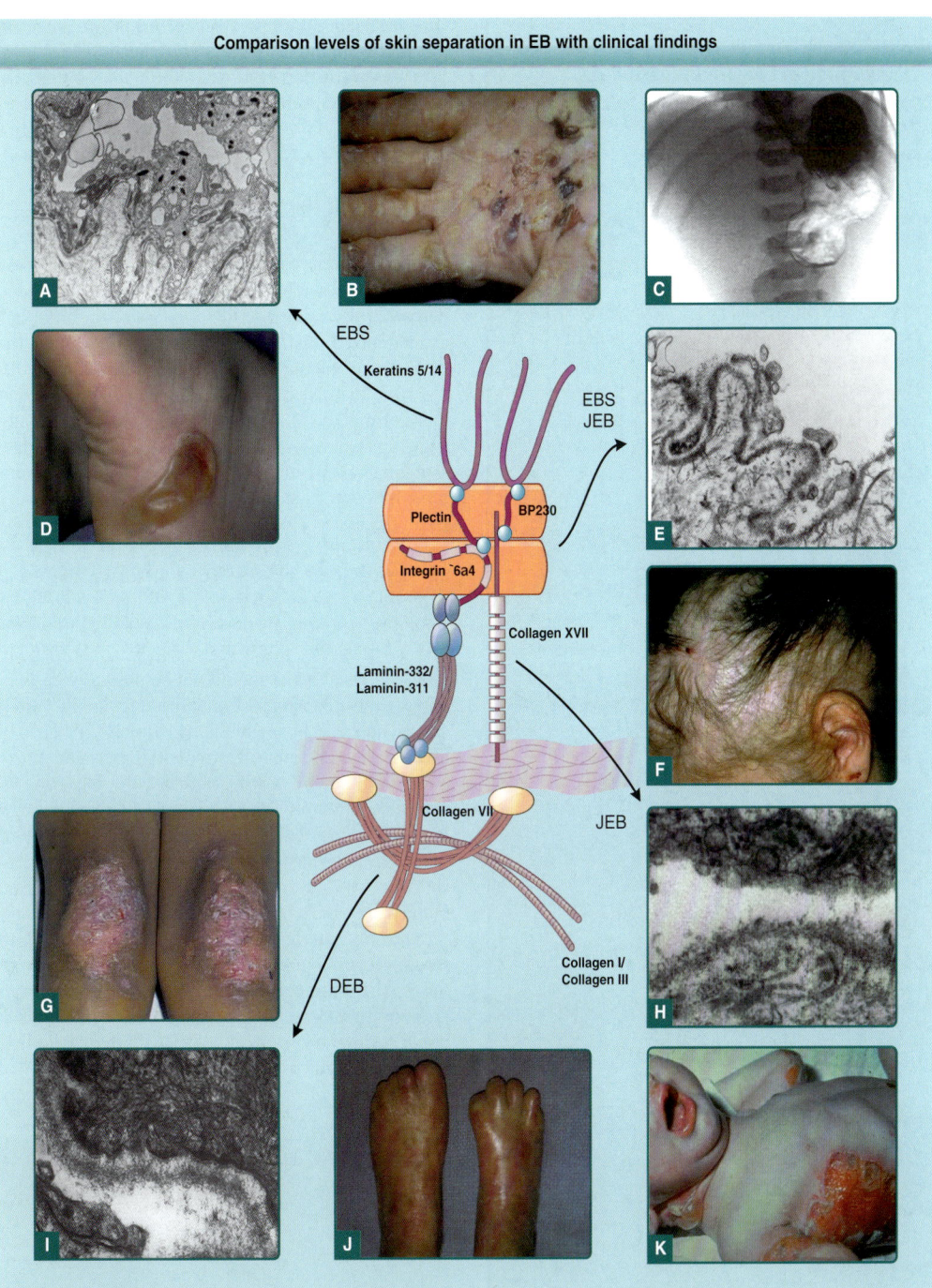

Figure 60-2 Comparison of levels of skin separation in epidermolysis bullosa (EB) with clinical findings. **A,** Transmission electron micrograph showing typical intraepidermal separation in epidermolysis bullosa simplex (EBS). **B,** Palmar hyperkeratosis and erosions in EB herpetiformis. **C,** Radiograph showing pyloric atresia associated with EB. **D,** Localized blister on heel in EBS Weber-Cockayne. **E,** Transmission electron micrograph showing typical separation at level of hemidesmosome in EB with pyloric atresia, alternatively classified as EBS or junctional epidermolysis bullosa (JEB). **F,** Nonscarring diffuse alopecia and scalp erosions in generalized atrophic benign epidermolysis bullosa. **G,** Localized dystrophic changes with milia in dominant dystrophic epidermolysis bullosa (DEB). **H,** Transmission electron microscopy showing typical intralamina lucida separation in JEB. **I,** Transmission electron microscopy showing typical sublamina densa separation in DEB. **J,** Pseudosyndactly in recessive DEB. **K,** Generalized blistering in Herlitz JEB.

TABLE 60-1
Classification of Epidermolysis Bullosa

DISEASE	AFFECTED GENE	AFFECTED PROTEIN
Simplex		
Generalized severe	KRT5/KRT14	Keratin 5/keratin 14
Generalized intermediate	RT5/KRT14	Keratin 5/keratin 14
Localized	RT5/KRT14	Keratin 5/keratin 14
Mottled pigmentation	KRT5	Keratin 5
EB with muscular dystrophy	PLEC1	Plectin
Superficialis	Unknown	Unknown
Acantholytic	DSP, JUP	Desmoplakin, plakoglobin
Plakophillin deficiency	PKP1	Plakophillin 1
Plakoglobin deficiency	JUP	Plakoglobin
Ogna	PLEC1	Plectin
BP230 deficiency	DST-e	BP230/BPAG1
Exophillin-5 deficiency	EXPH5	Exophillin 5
Acral peeling skin syndrome	TGM5	Transglutaminase 5
Junctional		
EB with pyloric atresia[a]	ITGB4/ITGA6/PLEC1	Integrin α6, integrin β4, plectin
Generalized severe	LAMB3/LAMA3/LAMC2	Laminin-332
Generalized intermediate	LAMB3/LAMA3/LAMC2/COL17A1	Laminin-332, collagen XVII
Localized	LAMB3/LAMA3/LAMC2/COL17A1	Laminin-332, collagen XVII
Inversa	LAMB3/LAMA3/LAMC2	Laminin-332
Laryngo-onycho-cutaneous	LAMA3A	Laminin α3
Respiratory and Renal	ITGA3	Integrin α3
Dystrophic		
Generalized dominant	COL7A1	Collagen VII
Localized dominant	COL7A1	Collagen VII
Generalized severe recessive	COL7A1	Collagen VII
Generalized intermediate recessive	COL7A1	Collagen VII
Localized recessive	COL7A1	Collagen VII
Inversa recessive	COL7A1	Collagen VII
Bullous dermolysis of the newborn	COL7A1	Collagen VII
Kindler syndrome	KIND1	Kindlin

[a]Alternatively classified as simplex.
EB, epidermolysis bullosa.

(Koebner), and localized (Weber-Cockayne). There are several uncommon varieties, which include EBS Ogna, EBS with muscular dystrophy, EBS with mottled pigmentation, and a group of suprabasal EBS subtypes.

GENERALIZED SEVERE EPIDERMOLYSIS BULLOSA SIMPLEX

This subtype is also known as the Dowling Meara, herpetiformis variant of EBS. It presents at birth, has a generalized distribution, and is regarded as the most severe of the EBS subtypes (Fig. 60-3). It differs from the generalized intermediate variant in that the oral mucosa is more often involved, occasionally showing extensive erosions. Milium formation may sometimes occur in infancy in patients with this subtype; however, this postwound phenomenon usually resolves later in childhood. The disease can often be associated with spontaneous appearance of grouped or "herpetiform" blisters. These occur on the trunk and proximal extremities and heal without scarring. It should be noted that often when patients show a generalized blistering, this herpetiform pattern is not seen; therefore, its absence should not be used as a basis to exclude this EB subtype. Generalized severe EBS often shows nail involvement. In this disease, nails may become shed and may regrow with dystrophy. Interestingly, although heat exacerbates the blistering in other EBS subtypes, it does not appear to have a major impact in generalized severe EBS. Hyperkeratosis of the palms and soles often develops beginning in early childhood and can progress to confluent keratoderma of the palms and soles. These can be quite painful, and occasionally interference with ambulation has led to flexural contractures. Occasionally, involvement of the esophagus in generalized severe EBS ranging from erosions to pyloric atresia[71] has been reported. The upper respiratory tract can also be affected, including the laryngeal mucosa.[72]

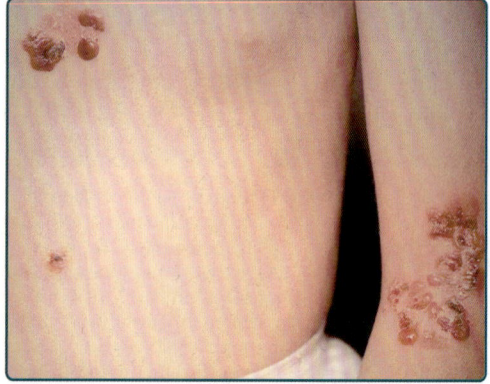

Figure 60-3 Characteristic blister formation on trunk and arm in patient with Dowling-Meara epidermolysis bullosa simplex.

GENERALIZED INTERMEDIATE EPIDERMOLYSIS BULLOSA SIMPLEX

The other common form of generalized EBS is the intermediate form, also known as the Koebner EBS. This subtype shows an onset of generalized blistering at birth or at latest during early infancy. The hands, feet, and extremities usually show the most involvement. Lesions often heal with postinflammatory hyper or hypopigmentation, and although occasional atrophy and milia can occur, they are rare and much less frequent than in generalized severe EBS. Palmar-plantar hyperkeratosis and erosions may be present (Fig. 60-4). Thickening of the soles is common but often does not present until later childhood. The oral mucosa sometimes shows mild erosive activity, but these usually improve with increasing age. Usually there is not a severe growth retardation in this EB subtype.

LOCALIZED EPIDERMOLYSIS BULLOSA SIMPLEX

This is a mild form of EB, previously referred to as the Weber-Cockayne subtype of EBS (Fig. 60-5). This disease is the most common form of EB and often presents during infancy or childhood. Occasionally, it presents in early adulthood, such as when blisters are noted after marching during military service. It is speculated that there are a number of undiagnosed cases of this form of EB because it can be mild enough to escape reporting or detection during clinical visits. Hyperhidrosis of the palms and soles is a common association. Blisters can occasionally become secondarily infected. Postinflammatory pigmentary abnormalities occur with this variant, but milia and scarring as a rule are absent. Blistering activity usually follows areas of trauma, with the hands and feet being the most common and the scalp being the least common. Mild oral erosions are present only rarely and usually resolve with increasing age. Nail involvement is rare with this EB subtype.

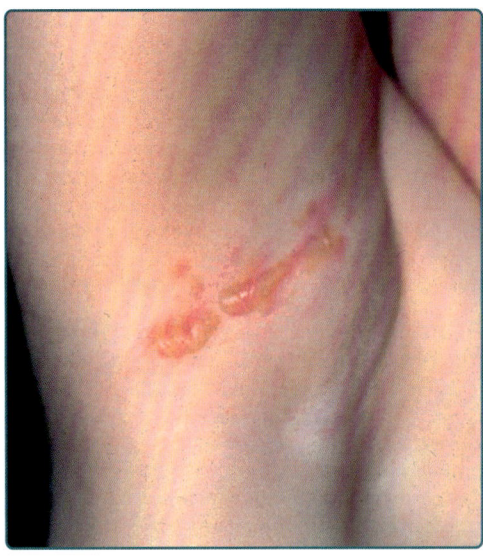

Figure 60-5 Trauma-induced blistering from clothing in patient with localized epidermolysis bullosa simplex.

ADDITIONAL VARIANTS OF EPIDERMOLYSIS BULLOSA SIMPLEX

Epidermolysis Bullosa Simplex of Ogna: Onset in infancy is common with seasonal blistering (summer) on the acral areas. Small hemorrhagic and serous blisters occur primarily on the extremities. Healing occurs without scarring. This disease was originally reported in patients from Norway. These patients also show a characteristic onychogryphosis of the great toenails.

Epidermolysis Bullosa Simplex with Muscular Dystrophy: This rare clinical entity is an autosomal recessive disorder that consists of generalized blistering of the skin at birth or shortly thereafter. This is accompanied by a progressive muscular dystrophy.[73] It presents with generalized blistering similar to generalized intermediate EBS. These patients have been shown to harbor mutations in the gene coding for HD1/plectin.[74-76]

Epidermolysis Bullosa Simplex with Mottled Pigmentation: This form of EB, as its name implies, is characterized by mottled hyperpigmentation of the trunk and proximal extremities. There is blistering in a generalized distribution beginning at birth or early infancy. Pigmentary alterations and blistering may improve with increasing age. Mild oral mucosal involvement may be present in infancy.

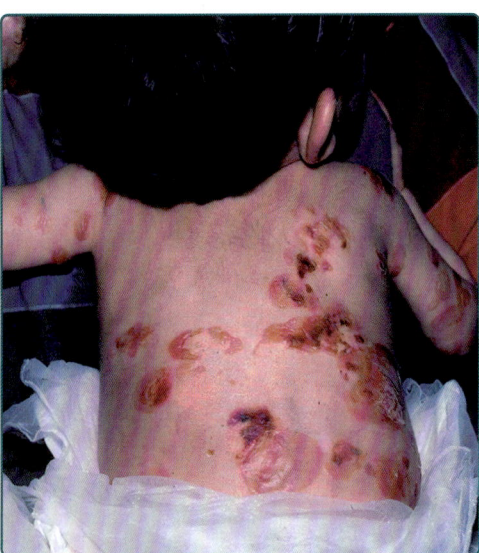

Figure 60-4 Widespread blistering in an infant with generalized epidermolysis bullosa simplex.

This condition is distinct from the large melanocytic nevi, which can be seen in all three EB types.[77]

Epidermolysis Bullosa Simplex Superficialis: This is an uncommon form of EBS is named after the subcorneal separation that produces the blisters in this disease.[78] Erosions and crusts, rather than intact bullae, are usually seen in these patients, and heal with postinflammatory pigmentary changes. Despite the superficial cleavage plane, nail involvement, atrophic scarring, and milia have been observed in this disease.

Acantholytic Epidermolysis Bullosa Simplex: This subtype[79] is a rare recessively inherited and lethal disorder characterized by generalized erosions at birth. As in the superficialis subtype, blisters are not normally seen because of the very superficial level of epidermal separation, which has been described as sheetlike. Nails are dystrophic. Alopecia, neonatal teeth, oral erosions, and respiratory involvement distinguish this disorder from other superficial EBS subtypes.

Plakophilin Deficiency: This subtype, also known as ectodermal dysplasia skin fragility syndrome, is another inherited disorder of suprabasilar epidermal separation characterized by generalized erosions and sometimes superficial blisters at birth.[80] Alopecia is also very common, as are palmoplantar keratoderma, painful fissures, and nail dystrophy. Patients may sometimes demonstrate failure to thrive, cheilitis, hypohidrosis, and pruitis. Like the other superficial EBS subtypes, this disorder is associated with dystrophic nails.

BP230 Deficiency: This is an extremely rare variant of EB caused by mutations of the *DST-e* gene, which has been described in a small collection of Kuwaiti and Iranian families. Blistering onset is usually at birth, and the phenotype is localized, often affecting the feet, without significant mucosal or other extracutaneous involvement. Like other forms of EBS, blisters may heal with postinflammatory pigment changes but no scarring. Inheritance appears autosomal recessive, but some heterozygous carriers have also reported self-limiting mild blistering in the first and second decades of life.

Exophillin-5 Deficiency: This is a very rare autosomal recessive EBS variant caused by mutations of the *EXPH5* gene. Blistering is high in the epidermis, resulting in trauma-induced crusting or fragile blisters and vesicles. The disease is overall mild and has no extracutaneous involvement, and remission or improvement during childhood is characteristic of this disease.[81]

Acral Peeling Skin Syndrome: This EB variant[82] is characterized by superficial and painless skin peeling occurring most commonly on the hands and feet. Humidity, heat, and water exposure can exacerbate this condition. The level of separation histologically is between the stratum granulosum and stratum corneum.

MOLECULAR PATHOLOGY OF EPIDERMOLYSIS BULLOSA SIMPLEX

Most of the patients with EB simplex analyzed at the genetic level have been found to be associated with mutations of the genes coding for keratins 5 and 14.[21,70] The level of separation of the skin in these patients is at the midbasal cell, shown in Fig. 60-4, associated with variable intermediate filament clumping. Hemidesmosomes and other BMZ structures are normal by electron microscopy. The majority of keratin gene mutations associated with EBS are dominantly inherited because of abnormalities in the multimeric assembly of keratin filaments. There is a smaller subset of patients with recessively inherited disease of varying severity.[83,84]

Mutations coding for the most conserved regions of keratins 5 and 14, the helix boundary domains,[85] correlate with the most severe forms of EBS, such as the Dowling-Meara subtype, which exhibits intermediate filament clumping seen by transmission electron microscopy. On the other hand, milder types of disease, such as the Weber-Cockayne subtype, are associated with mutations coding for regions of keratins 5 and 14, which are less conserved. Mutations that code for a specific region of the amino terminus of keratin 5 are present in patients having EBS with mottled pigmentation.[86] Although significance of this type of mutation and its association with pigmentary abnormalities remains unclear,[87,88] it has been suggested that the keratin 5 globular head domain is responsible for keratin filament insertion onto melanosomes. Recent studies have shown that some mutations of the keratin 5 gene may produce protein that is unstable under increased temperatures.[89] This could help to explain the well observed exacerbation of some subtypes of EBS to warm temperatures.

The mutations associated with EBS with muscular dystrophy produce premature termination codons, splice-site, or other mutations that result in lack of expression or defective expression of plectin.[90] Although the form of EB associated with plectin abnormalities is classified as simplex, it has an identical level of skin separation to that seen in junctional epidermolysis bullosa (JEB) with pyloric atresia.[69] Specifically, the separation is present just above the level of the hemidesmosome in the intracellular part of the BMZ. This separation of EBS with muscular dystrophy and JEB with pyloric atresia, diseases with identical levels of separation, into two distinct EB categories illustrates the limitations of the current EB classification system. Plectin defects, like α6β4 integrin defects, can also be associated with pyloric atresia.[90]

Plectin is normally expressed in a wide range of tissues, including muscle.[22] Although the mechanism of muscular dystrophy in plectin-deficient patients is unknown, it has been observed that disorganization of muscle sarcomeres occurs in the absence of plectin. It is possible that absence of plectin's spectrin-like domain, which may normally interact with actin filaments in muscle, may be a key factor in the muscle pathology.[91]

The underlying molecular defect of ectodermal dysplasia skin fragility syndrome has been shown to be loss of function of the desmosomal protein plakophilin 1.[80] Plakophilin is expressed mainly in suprabasilar keratinocytes and outer root sheath cells. Microscopic findings in this disease usually show intraepidermal acantholysis located in the areas where plakophilin 1 is normally expressed. The molecular defect involves loss-of-function mutations in the PKP1 gene coding for plakophilin 1.[92-97]

Deficiency of BP230 (an alternatively spliced dystrophic variant sometimes termed DST-e) is characterized by decreased or absent expression of BP230 by immunofluorescence microscopy and loss of the inner hemidesmosomal plate as seen by transmission electron microscopy. Homozygous premature termination codon mutations as well as point mutations of the *DST*-e gene in the area coding for the coiled-coil domain of BP230 have been associated with this disorder.[81] Exophillin-5 deficiency is associated with loss-of-function mutations of the *EXPH5* gene. This disease can show a complete absence of expression of this protein in the skin by immunofluorescence microscopy, and electron microscopy may show abnormal collections of basal keratinocyte perinuclear vesicles.[98,99] Mutations of TGM5, which encodes a member of the multigene transglutaminase family, produces alterations of transglutaminase expression associated with the underlying cause of acral peeling skin syndrome.[82]

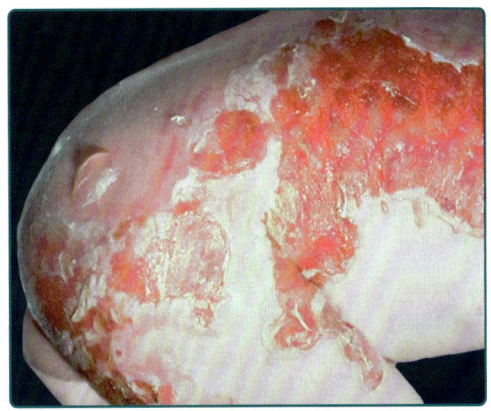

Figure 60-6 Widespread blistering at birth in an infant with Herlitz junctional epidermolysis bullosa.

JUNCTIONAL EPIDERMOLYSIS BULLOSA

All patients with JEB share the common histopathologic feature of blister formation within the lamina lucida of the BMZ caused by either a defect of anchoring filaments located in the lamina lucida and superior lamina densa. This group of diseases is inherited in an autosomal recessive manner, and there is considerable variation of the individual clinical phenotypes depending on the molecular defect. Three principal forms of JEB are most common. Patients with severe generalized JEB (previously termed Herlitz disease, JEB gravis, or lethal JEB) present with the most severe disease phenotype.[14,100] It is unfortunate that this most severe subtype of JEB is also the most common.

GENERALIZED SEVERE JUNCTIONAL EPIDERMOLYSIS BULLOSA

Generalized severe JEB is one of the most severe EB subtypes, resulting in lethality during infancy or early childhood.[101] This disease is characterized by generalized and often extensive blistering at birth (Fig. 60-6). Later during infancy, a distinctive periorificial granulation tissue manifests. This can occur around the mouth, eyes, and nares most commonly but also can be present in the scalp; around the ears; and less frequently, in other locations besides the head and neck. This hypertrophic granulation tissue can also occur in nonlethal subtypes. Nails are usually severely affected and often are lost during infancy. When nails are still present, they are usually dystrophic and often associated with hypertrophic granulation tissue. Dental defects are present in this disease characterized by pitting of the tooth enamel. Oropharyngeal mucosal erosions are usually present and may be widespread. Erosions of all stratified squamous epithelial tissues, including nasal, conjunctival, esophageal, tracheal, laryngeal, rectal, and urethral mucosa can be affected. Associated systemic findings in severe cases are important factors in the lethality of this disease. Involvement of the large airways including tracheolaryngeal stenosis or obstruction are commonly associated with Herlitz JEB disease and hoarseness in early infancy is an ominous sign. There is a characteristic failure to thrive and growth retardation in this disease, often with a mixed anemia. Sepsis is a common and often lethal complication.

GENERALIZED INTERMEDIATE JUNCTIONAL EPIDERMOLYSIS BULLOSA

Sometimes patients initially presenting with a generalized severe phenotype survive infancy. These patients eventually prove to have a severity of blistering and oral erosions less than the lethal form. In particular, a lack of significant hoarseness is regarded as a favorable prognostic sign, indicative of less severe internal disease manifestations. Scalp and nail lesions and periorificial nonhealing erosions are among the most common findings in these patients during childhood. Despite the lack of lethality in infancy, these patients nonetheless can have severe epithelial adhesion abnormalities, and tracheostomies or gastrostomy tubes may help in patient survival (Fig. 60-7). The nonlethal status of these patients distinguishes them from the Herlitz group and the terms *nonlethal JEB* or *JEB mitis* have been used in the past to describe these patients. They are much less common than severe generalized JEB patients. There are other rare variants of nonlethal JEB that present with localized junctional blistering of the extremities or with blistering in an inversa distribution on the trunk and intertriginous areas.

A distinct subset of generalized intermediate JEB (previously termed *generalized atrophic benign EB*) presents at birth with generalized cutaneous involvement.[102] However, despite the widespread cutaneous blistering, there is a relative paucity of oral erosions or other mucosal disease. Although enamel pitting is present, resulting in extensive dental caries, and nail dystrophy can often be severe, there is little other extracutaneous involvement noted in these patients. The blisters in these patients, which heal with a characteristic atrophic scarring, are debilitating and can be widespread, but nonetheless these patients generally have a normal lifespan. Blistering improves with age, growth is normal, and anemia is rarely seen. Some patients with this disease subtype have undergone normal uncomplicated pregnancies and deliveries. One peculiar characteristic of these patients is a progressive alopecia of the scalp and terminal hairs elsewhere in the body. The hair loss starts to become severe after the onset of puberty, and although patchy hair loss associated with atrophic scarring has been described, often the alopecia is quite diffuse, and scarring is subtle or nonexistent.

LOCALIZED JUNCTIONAL EPIDERMOLYSIS BULLOSA

A rare subtype of JEB is the localized variant, previously known as minimus JEB. These patients generally show mild disease, which can be accentuated in localized areas, most often the hands, feet, and pretibial regions. Nails can sometimes be shed or become dystrophic, and enamel pitting can occur. Oral or nasal erosions can also occur, but there is an absence of any internal involvement. These patients generally have a favorable prognosis and a normal lifespan.

JUNCTIONAL EPIDERMOLYSIS BULLOSA WITH PYLORIC ATRESIA

These patients exhibit extreme mucosal and cutaneous fragility and may also have various urologic abnormalities, including hydronephrosis and nephritis. Mutations of the genes coding for the β4 and α6 integrin have been associated with EB,[103] and in this group of diseases, pyloric atresia is present. Although pyloric stenosis is relatively more common, the distinct association of pyloric atresia, a rare condition,

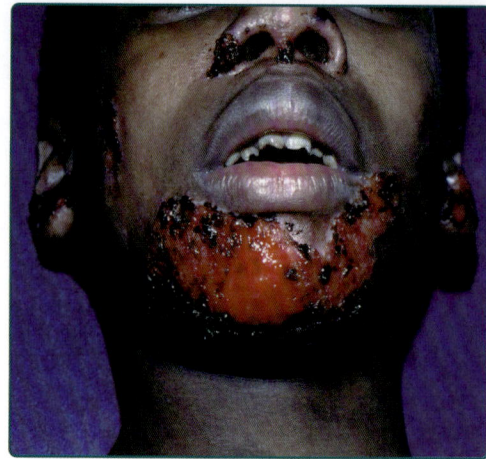

Figure 60-7 Periorificial erosions and hypertrohic granulation tissue in a patient with non-Herlitz junctional epidermolysis bullosa.

with EB makes this disease particularly unique. In these patients, hemidesmosomes are usually absent or rudimentary, and the level of separation is a low intrabasal epidermal at the level of the hemidesmosome as seen in EBS with muscular dystrophy described earlier. Most cases of this disease are quite severe and lethal in infancy caused by extensive extracutaneous epithelial sloughing in addition to widespread blistering of the skin and mucosa. Rare nonlethal cases of this disease have been characterized that appear to result from a partial loss of function of β4 integrin.[104] Interestingly, nonlethal JEB can sometimes ameliorate itself through alterations in mRNA splicing.[105,106]

JUNCTIONAL EPIDERMOLYSIS BULLOSA WITH RESPIRATORY AND RENAL INVOLVEMENT

Blistering of the skin starts early in life, is generally mild or even absent, and may be associated with a diffuse alopecia and nail dystrophy. Extracutaneous involvement, however, presents at birth and is quite severe, consisting of interstitial lung disease, resulting in respiratory distress and lung infections. Kidney manifestations of this disease include renal failure, nephrotic syndrome, renal hypoplasia, and hydronephrosis. Despite aggressive neonatal supportive care, patients die in infancy because of these severe respiratory or renal complications.

LARYNGO-ONYCHO-CUTANEOUS SYNDROME

This rare autosomal recessive condition[107] is characterized by nail dystrophy, cutaneous erosions, and extensive granulation tissue, especially localizing to the conjunctiva and larynx. Sites of cutaneous involvement include areas of repeated trauma or pressure such as the elbows, knees, fingers, and toes.

MOLECULAR PATHOLOGY OF JUNCTIONAL EPIDERMOLYSIS BULLOSA

JEB can be associated with mutations of the genes coding for the α3, β3, or γ2 subunits of laminin-332.[108,109] Absence of any of the three chains results in a lack of trimeric laminin-332 assembly and secretion, which results in a similar blistering phenotype. Patients with mutations of genes coding for the α3 or γ2 laminin subunits still show normal expression of laminin-311, which contains α3, β1, and γ1 chains.[44] Therefore, positive linear BMZ staining of JEB skin for α3 chain on indirect immunofluorescence microscopy (IDIF) with absent expression of the other chains is an indication of either a α3 or γ2 chain defect. Conversely, absence of α3 staining on IDIF can be indicative of a mutation of the α3 gene. About 80% of laminin-332 mutations can be traced to one of two recurrent nonsense mutations in the *LAMB3* gene, making prenatal testing for laminin-332 lesions easier than other EB candidate genes.[110] In patients with Herlitz disease, all of the mutations so far detected have been those producing premature termination codons, resulting in absence of expression of laminin-332. Although patients with Herlitz disease generally show a complete lack of expression of laminin-332, patients without Herlitz disease who have abnormal granulation tissue and significant mucosal involvement often show reduced expression of laminin-332. This is due to expression of a molecule with deletions or missense mutations resulting in partial loss of laminin-332 function. This can lead to cases clinically classified as non-Herlitz JEB, especially cases with significant mucosal involvement.[76,111,112] In some cases, spontaneous amelioration of blistering in severe JEB cases has taken place, which has been associated with genetic mechanisms that result in the reexpression of laminin-332.[106]

In the non-Herlitz JEB variant, generalized atrophic benign junctional EB (GABEB), blistering occurs in the lamina lucida region and abnormalities of hemidesmosomes or anchoring filaments are usually present (Fig. 60-8). Although laminin-332 mutations underlie a subset of GABEB patients, the majority of these patients have abnormalities of the hemidesmosomal protein collagen XVII (also known as BP180 or BPAG2). A number of mutations of the gene coding for collagen XVII have been described in patients with GABEB, including premature termination codon mutations, missense mutations, splice-site mutations, truncations, and a glycine substitution mutation.[113,114] Although intralamina lucida or junctional skin separation has been shown in all patients with this disease, one patient was described with a cytoplasmic deletion of collagen XVII who showed intrabasal epidermal skin separation.[115] Localized JEB has been shown to be associated with COL17A1 mutations.[116] Laryngo-onycho-cutaneous syndrome is characterized by N-terminal mutations of the *LAMA3* gene leading to deletion of the laminin α3 LE domain.[107]

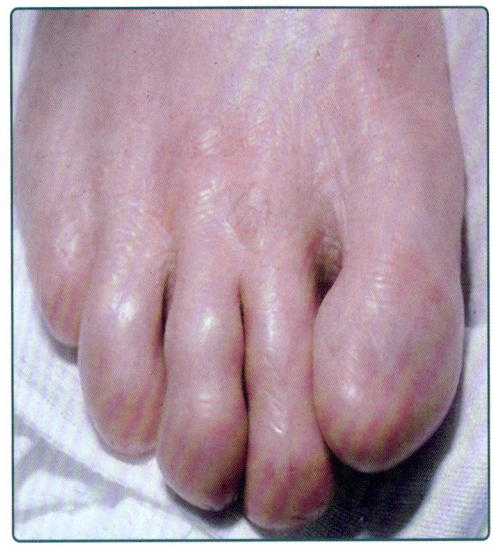

Figure 60-8 Loss of nails and skin atrophy a patient with non-Herlitz junctional epidermolysis bullosa or generalized atrophic benign epidermolysis bullosa.

Of interest, mosaic GABEB patients have been identified who demonstrate well defined areas of blistering associated with absence of collagen XVII expression as well as areas of nonblistering skin associated with normal collagen XVII expression. Careful analysis of these patients' keratinocytes revealed reversion of one of the two alleles of the mutation, most likely caused by a mitotic gene conversion involving nonreciprocal exchange of parental allele DNA.[117,118] Understanding how EB can undergo spontaneous molecular correction in these cases could help in the design of future molecular therapeutic strategies.

JEB with respiratory and renal involvement is caused by mutations of the *ITGA3* gene.[119,120] These patients can show an absence of expression of integrin α3 in skin biopsies by immunofluorescence microscopy. Electron microscopy shows intralamina lucida separation, like other JEB subtypes.[119]

DYSTROPHIC EPIDERMOLYSIS BULLOSA

Dystrophic EB (DEB) is characterized by blisters that heal with scarring and milium formation. DEB can be inherited either in an autosomal recessive (RDEB) or dominant fashion (DDEB). One of the most important reasons to distinguish between these two subtypes is the increased prevalence of invasive squamous cell carcinoma (SCC) associated with the recessive but not the dominant form. Regardless of the mode of

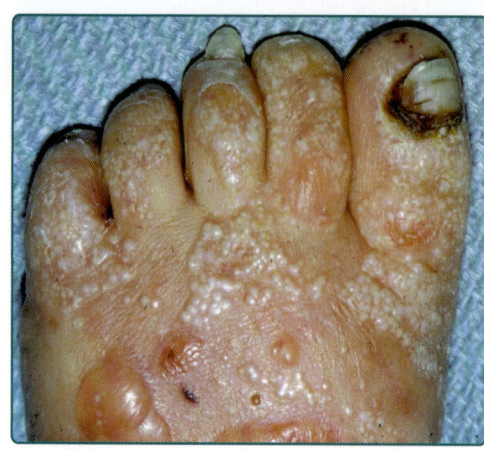

Figure 60-9 Localized trauma-induced blistering with secondary milia in a patient with dominant dystrophic epidermolysis bullosa.

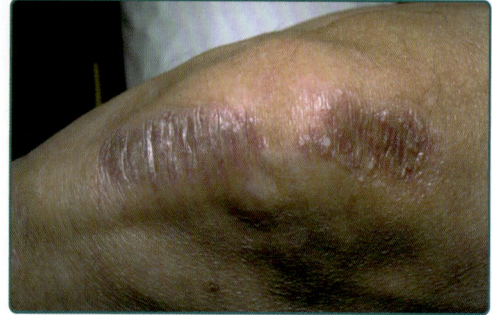

Figure 60-11 Milia in a patient with dominant dystrophic epidermolysis bullosa.

inheritance, DEB is derived from defects of the ultrastructural entity known as the anchoring fibril, which results in sublamina densa separation.

LOCALIZED AUTOSOMAL DOMINANT DYSTROPHIC EPIDERMOLYSIS BULLOSA

The localized subtype of dominant DDEB (sometimes called the Cockayne-Touraine of DDEB) can present at birth, but occasionally it is not appreciated until childhood. Although generalized blistering can sometimes take place, especially early in life, the blistering usually becomes localized to repetitively traumatized areas such as the knees, sacrum, and acral surfaces (Figs. 60-9 and 60-10). These areas show a characteristic scarred, dystrophic appearance. Often the scarring is hypertrophic. Milia are common accompanying features of the healing process in these patients (Fig. 60-11). Nail dystrophy and nail loss with atrophic scarring of the distal digits are common. Occasionally, nail abnormalities can be the only presenting abnormality in DDEB. Oral lesions are not common, and teeth are usually unaffected. These patients have a good prognosis and a normal lifespan.

GENERALIZED AUTOSOMAL DOMINANT DYSTROPHIC EPIDERMOLYSIS BULLOSA

The generalized form of DDEB (sometimes referred to as the Pasini subtype of DDEB) presents at birth with a generally more severe and widespread blistering phenotype compared with the localized subtype. Blisters in generalized DDEB heal with scarring plaques and milia in a fashion similar to other DEB subtypes. In addition, this disease is sometimes distinguished by the spontaneous appearance of distinctive scarlike, flesh-colored papules on the truck. These albopapuloid lesions are not pathognomonic because these lesions can also be seen in other EB subtypes. As patients get older, the generalized blistering may eventually localize to the extremities. Patients often show dystrophic or absent nails. Oral erosions can often be present but usually are not extensive, and enamel defects can be seen in some patients. A rare variant of self-remitting generalized DDEB, termed *bullous dermolysis of the newborn*, consists of generalized blistering that gradually recedes after infancy.[121] Skin biopsies from these patients often show basal epidermal intracytoplasmic accumulations of collagen VII when examined by immunofluorescence microscopy.[122]

RECESSIVE DYSTROPHIC EPIDERMOLYSIS BULLOSA

Recessive DEB (RDEB) can be quite variable in its severity. Although the severe subtype is the most common, a localized form can occasionally be seen that has been previously termed *RDEB mitis*. Similar to localized DDEB, localized RDEB is usually confined to repetitively traumatized skin surfaces, most often in an acral distribution. Scarring and milium formation accompany the healing of blisters. Mucosal involvement in localized RDEB, if present, is mild.

Severe RDEB, previously known by the eponym the Hallopeau-Siemens, is a devastating disease

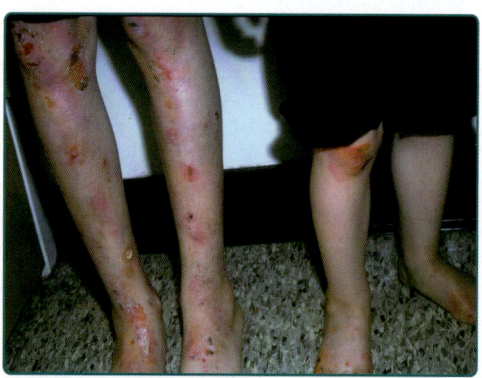

Figure 60-10 Cutaneous lesions in siblings with dominant dystrophic epidermolysis bullosa.

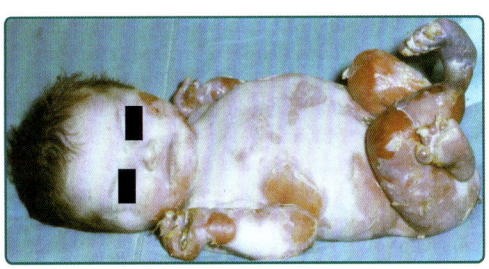

Figure 60-12 Widespread blistering with localized absence of skin at birth in a patient with recessive dystrophic epidermolysis bullosa.

(Fig. 60-12). This disease presents with generalized blistering at birth. Occasionally, there is extensive denudation of an entire region of skin at birth, often involving one of the limbs. This congenital absence of skin is sometimes termed Bart syndrome. Healing and blistering cycles occurring during infancy can lead to a progressive scarring, which can become quite extensive. Pseudosyndactyly resulting from a closure of the digits in a "mitten" of skin is an extremely common feature of this disease (Fig. 60-13). Scarring can lead to flexion contracture of the hands (Fig. 60-14), as well as the limbs. In contrast to the patients with severe JEB, these patients do not show significant periorificial involvement. Instead, the scalp is the most commonly affected area on the head and neck of these patients.

The oropharynx can be extensively involved in both dominant and recessive DEB (Fig. 60-15) with generalized erosions evolving into a scarring that limits the movement of the tongue and narrows the opening of the oral cavity. The teeth can show significant enamel pitting, and caries can be extensive, leading to loss of teeth. Involvement of the trachea or larynx can lead to a narrowing of the airway, which could require intervention with a tracheostomy. Mucosal erosions of the esophagus can lead to stricture formation and

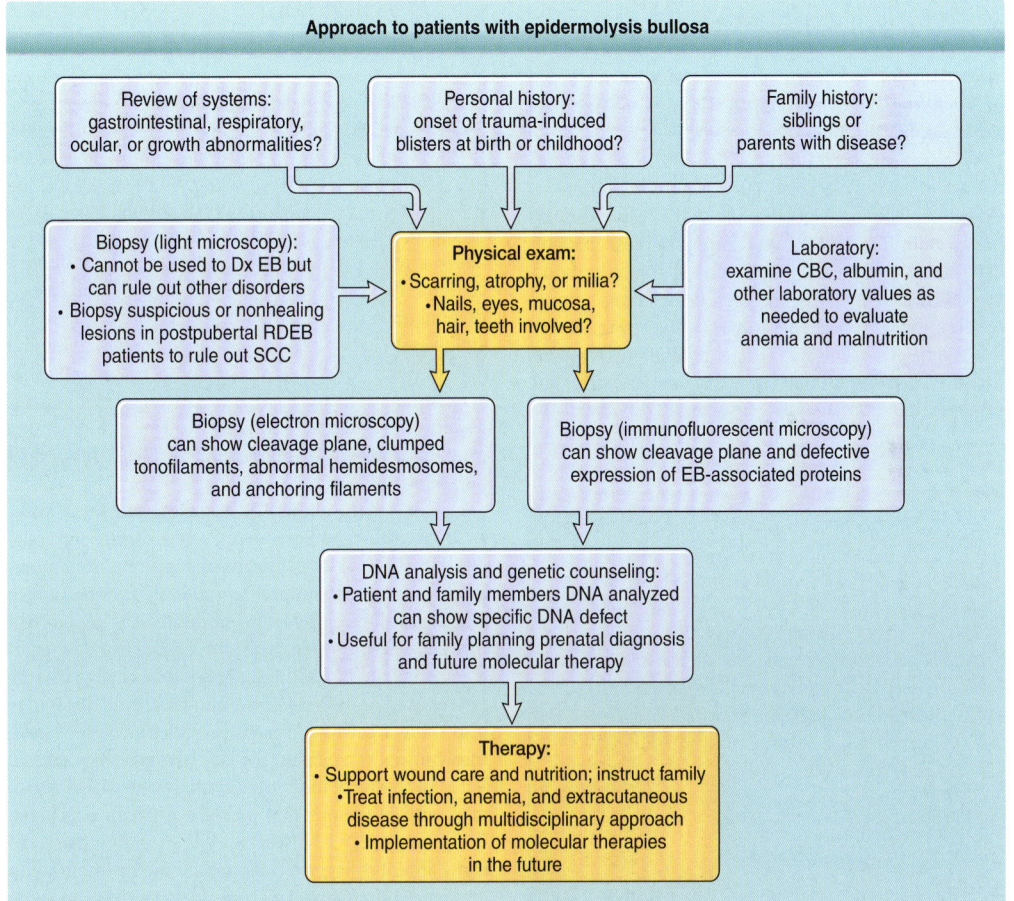

Figure 60-13 Approach to patients with epidermolysis bullosa (EB). A complete history, including family history and review of systems, is essential. Physical examination can provide important clues, and laboratory values can help identify associated anemia and malnutrition. Electron microscopy or indirect immunofluorescent microscopy is required for diagnosis. DNA analysis is helpful for determining prognosis and family planning. Therapy is mainly supportive. Teaching and working with nursing staff and especially families is critical, as are interdisciplinary interactions with other specialists in the treatment of extracutaneous complications. CBC, complete blood count; Dx, diagnosis; RDEB, autosomal recessive epidermolysis bullosa; SCC, squamous cell carcinoma.

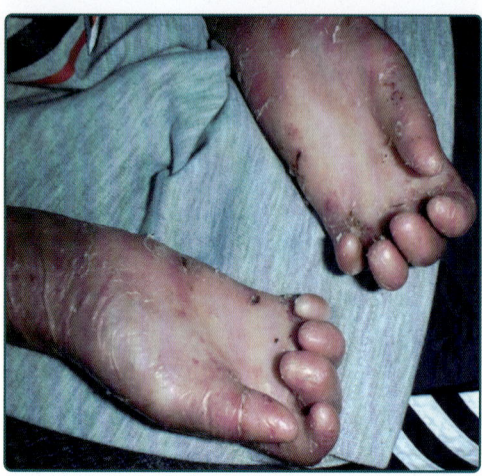

Figure 60-14 Scarring of the hands in patient with recessive dystrophic epidermolysis bullosa.

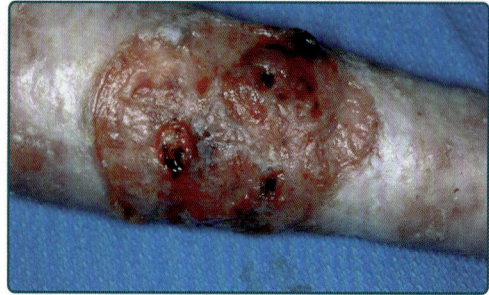

Figure 60-16 Squamous cell carcinoma in patient with recessive dystrophic epidermolysis bullosa.

webbing. The combination of oral lesions, dental caries, esophageal strictures, and increased caloric needs from extensive wound healing can lead these patients toward malnutrition and growth retardation. These patients usually have problems with anemia and may show a deficiency of iron absorption.

In the more distant past, most severe RDEB patients died in infancy of sepsis and other complications of extensive blistering. More recently, with improved nutritional, infection, and wound support, these patients usually can survive into their teens or into adulthood. However, after puberty, another devastating complication, SCC, can and often does appear (Fig. 60-16). It is estimated that 50% to 80% of patients with severe-RDEB eventually develop these carcinomas, and many of these die of metastatic disease. RDEB-associated carcinomas are distinct from most other cutaneous SCCs in that they are extremely aggressive with strong tendencies for invasion and metastasis.

MOLECULAR PATHOLOGY OF DYSTROPHIC EPIDERMOLYSIS BULLOSA

Abnormalities of anchoring fibrils are present in DEB patients, which range from subtle changes in some patients with dominant disease to absence of anchoring fibrils in patients with the severe recessive form of this disease, are present, and a sublamina densa plane of blister cleavage is present (see Fig. 60-4). These observations correlate with indirect immunofluorescent microscopic analysis of patients with DEB, which demonstrates varying degrees of linear collagen VII staining at the dermal–epidermal junction in dominant patients and totally absent staining in severe recessive patients. In some patients, there is a cytoplasmic retention of collagen VII, which can be demonstrated in patient biopsy sections and analysis of patient keratinocytes.[123]

DEB has been shown to be associated in all cases thus far with mutations of the gene coding for collagen VII (COL7A1). In the recessive forms, mutations usually cause premature termination codons, which result in lack of collagen VII in tissue. It is known that mRNAs bearing premature stop codons show accelerated turnover.[124] In addition, truncated proteins that are not secreted or not assembled into anchoring fibrils may also show accelerated turnover. Either or both of these mechanisms can explain the lack of detectable collagen VII in the tissue of individuals with severe RDEB associated with mutations that produce premature termination codons.[61,125,126] However, even in individuals who show absent collagen VII tissue staining by immunofluorescence microscopy, analysis of patient keratinocytes can in many cases still demonstrate low levels of mutant collagen VII expression.[127,128] Recently, in addition to cases reported in JEB patients, a revertant mosaicism phenotype has also been reported in RDEB.[129]

Generally, COL7A1 mutations that do not cause premature termination codons produce less severe

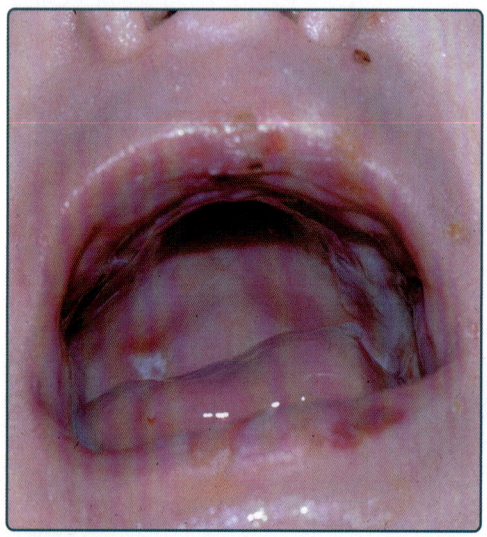

Figure 60-15 Oral erosions in a patient with dominant dystrophic epidermolysis bullosa.

disease.[108,114] For example, mutations that produce glycine substitutions of the triple helical region interfere with triple helical assembly of the collagen VII molecule. These types of mutations are present in many patients with milder dominant forms of this disease. In these patients, collagen VII molecules may not be able to assume the proper conformation needed to polymerize into anchoring fibrils. One subtype of DEB associated with increased pruritus, EB pruriginosa, has also been described to be associated with glycine mutations.[130] Other COL7A1 mutations have been shown to be associated with impaired secretion of collagen VII, resulting in intracellular accumulation of this molecule. In one study, DEB patient mutations that involve the area of the gene coding for the collagen VII NC2 domain were shown to interfere with NC2 processing and the assembly of anchoring fibrils.[131]

KINDLER SYNDROME

New advances in our understanding of the molecular pathology of the skin have brought to light the underlying pathophysiology of a disease related to EB, Kindler syndrome. Kindler syndrome was first described by Theresa Kindler in 1954.[132] It is characterized by EB-like trauma-induced blistering at birth and during infancy, with atrophic changes during healing reminiscent or JEB or DEB.[133-139] However, in late childhood, the blistering usually subsides and gives way to a progressive poikiloderma, which distributes to sun-exposed areas. The poikiloderma may show areas of atrophy and hyperkeratosis, as well as hypopigmentation, hyperpigmentation, and telangiectasias. These patients often show photosensitivity. Nail changes and webbing of the toes and fingers are also sometimes present. Internal complications include oral inflammation, esophageal or ureteral strictures, and ectropion. Ultrastructurally, these patients show reduplication of the basement membrane, which is the most consistent feature seen. Although there is often a sublamina densa split with anchoring fibril abnormalities, sometimes lamina lucida or intraepidermal separation can be seen associated with the blistering phenotype. Molecular investigation of this disease led to the discovery of a new epidermal protein, kindlin-1, which shows decreased expression by immunofluorescent microscopy in this disease. Kindlin-1 appears to have some homology to signaling proteins such as talin, which suggests a signaling function, but its role in Kindler syndrome remains unclear.[140] A number of mutations of the gene coding for kindlin-1, KIND1, have been described.[141-143] These include nonsense, frameshift, and splice-site mutations that underlie the observed decreased kindlin-1 expression in affected skin. Why the disease evolves from a blistering to a poikilodermatous phenotype and the exact function of kindlin-1 in epidermal homeostasis remains to be fully elucidated.

DIAGNOSIS

The first step toward making the diagnosis of EB begins with a thorough history and physical examination (see Fig. 60-13). Useful historical information includes the age of onset of blistering and the presence of blistering in other family members. A review of gastrointestinal (GI), respiratory, ocular, dental, and genitourinary systems is important as is evaluation of general growth and development. Physical examination requires not only a complete skin examination but also a thorough evaluation of mucosal tissues, hair, nails, and teeth. Laboratory measurements of importance in the initial visit include evaluation for anemia and for measures of nutrition, such as serum albumin.

Skin biopsy is another important diagnostic step. Routine histologic analysis cannot be used to diagnose EB but can be useful for excluding other causes of blistering. The dermal–epidermal BMZ is simply too small to be visualized by light microscopy. To differentiate levels of BMZ separation in skin biopsies, transmission electron microscopy (TEM) or indirect immunofluorescent microscopy (IDDF) must be used. The interior of blisters rapidly reepithelialize, which can obscure correct determination of blister levels. For this reason, it is critical to biopsy a blister that is as fresh as possible. One way to ensure a fresh blister is for the clinician to induce it in the office. This can be accomplished by gently rotating a pencil eraser over an intact area of patient's skin until separation of the epidermis from the dermis can be observed. This is more easily performed with patients who have more severe disease variants compared with patients with milder disease. When actually doing the biopsy, its best to place the circular biopsy punch so that only 10% of the punch covers the visible blister with 90% covering intact skin. This is because it is helpful to have both intact and blistered skin on the same biopsy specimen, and extension of the blister is likely to occur either during the biopsy process or during shipping.

TEM has been regarded for many years as the gold standard for determining the level of blistering in EB subtypes. In addition to determining the level of blistering, ultrastructural entities can also be analyzed by TEM for characteristic alterations. For example, clumping of keratin intermediate filaments in basal keratinocyte cytoplasm is a pathognomonic finding for severe generalized (Dowling-Meara) EBS. Rudimentary hemidesmosomes can be an important clue to the diagnosis of JEB. Absent or altered anchoring fibrils often occur in DEB subtypes, especially the recessive forms.

IDDF microscopy can provide additional information on the level of blistering, as well as important clues to the underlying molecular defects. In this technique, an antibody panel against known BMZ antigens is applied to frozen sections of blistered patient skin. The localization of the antigens to the epidermal or dermal portion of the blister indicates the level of skin separation in the BMZ. In EBS samples, for example, intracellular hemidesmosomal components such as BP230 and a lamina densa protein such as type IV collagen would each localize to the floor of the blister. In JEB cases, BP230 would localize to the roof of the blister, and type IV collagen would localize to the floor. In DEB, collagen VII and BP230 would localize to the roof of the blister. The specific absence or presence of staining with a particular antibody in frozen sections of intact portions of patient skin give important clues to the specific molecular defect. Whereas samples that lack staining with antibodies specific to laminin-332 would further support a JEB diagnosis, a lack of staining for collagen VII would support a DEB diagnosis. Absence of staining for collagen XVII would support a generalized intermediate JEB diagnosis.

A complete panel of antibodies to support IDDF-based diagnosis of EB would include antibodies against laminin-332 (Herlitz and non-Herlitz JEB), as well as antibodies against BP180/collagen XVII (non-Herlitz JEB or generalized atrophic benign EB), collagen VII (RDEB), α6 and β4 integrins (JEB with pyloric atresia), plectin (EBS with muscular dystrophy), and keratins 5 and 14 (recessive EBS). Antibodies against the individual chains α3, γ2, and β3 chains of laminin-332 are especially helpful.

Its known that laminin-311 (which shares the same laminin α3 chain as laminin-332) is expressed in Herlitz JEB associated with null mutations of genes coding for β3 chain (LAMB3) and γ2 chain (LAMC2) but not in Herlitz JEB associated with null mutations of the α3 chain gene (LAMA3).[44] Therefore, if laminin β3 and γ2 antibodies are negative and α3 antibody is positive, this could point the genetic analysis to examine the LAMB3 and LAMC2. Conversely, if all three laminin-332 chains are absent by IDIF, this could point the genetic investigation toward LAMA3, saving time and effort in arriving at the final molecular diagnosis.

Gene mutation analysis has revolutionized our understanding of the EB family of diseases and is considered the ultimate final step in arriving at the molecular diagnosis in EB. Concurrent advances in our knowledge of the biochemical structure and supramolecular assembly of BMZ proteins have both facilitated and complemented the molecular biology studies. Thus, EB patient diagnosis requires both clinical and molecular information. Blood samples or buccal swabs are taken from the patient as well as the parents and siblings for genetic analysis. Whole-exome sequencing will likely make EB mutation detection easier, faster and less expensive as this practice becomes more widespread.[144]

DIFFERENTIAL DIAGNOSIS

See Table 60-2.

TABLE 60-2
Differential Diagnosis of Epidermolysis Bullosa

Most Likely
- Pompholyx
- Insect bites
- Friction blisters
- Thermal burns
- Bullous impetigo

Consider
- Chronic bullous dermatosis of childhood (linear immunoglobulin A disease)
- Bullous pemphigoid
- Epidermolysis bullosa acquisita
- Bullous systemic lupus erythematosus
- Cicatritial pemphigoic
- Pemphigus vulgaris

Always Rule Out
- Stevens-Johnson syndrome
- Toxic epidermal necrolysis

GENETIC COUNSELING

DNA mutation analyses can be extremely helpful to EB patients. The prognostic benefit to the patient can often be highly significant. For example, recessive DEB cases may have equivalent blistering activity compared with the more severe dominant cases, but their risk of invasive SCC is much greater. Through DNA diagnosis, these two groups can be distinguished, thereby identifying patients potentially at risk for invasive SCC.

Prenatal diagnosis of EB in affected families can be an extremely accurate technique, especially if the original proband has previously had mutational analysis or identification of the defective gene. Fetal skin biopsies and fetoscopy with their increased risk of pregnancy loss can now be avoided by analysis of either chorionic villus sampling as early as 8 to 10 weeks[145] or gestation or amniocentesis in the second trimester.[146] The development of highly informative intragenic and flanking polymorphic DNA markers in EB candidate genes together with rapid screening of genetic "hotspots" makes genetic screening of at-risk pregnancies a viable option.[110,147] Coupling of the technique of in vitro fertilization with EB prenatal diagnosis, preimplantation diagnosis has now been successfully performed for EB cases.[148] Another promising area of prenatal diagnosis with potential future applications to EB is the detection and analysis of fetal cells in the maternal circulation.[149]

TREATMENT

Most therapy for EB is supportive in nature. The regimen is tailored to the severity and extent of skin and systemic involvement and usually entails a combination of wound management, infection control, surgical management as needed, and nutritional support. Skin care and supportive care for other organ systems in certain EB subtypes are most optimally coordinated through a multidisciplinary approach. Comprehensive topical therapy is a mainstay of treatment in EB, with avoidance of trauma as a primary goal. Wound healing is impaired by endogenous factors, including foreign bodies, bacteria, nutritional deficiencies, anemia, and repeated trauma. Therefore, optimizing wound healing in patients with EB involves control of all of these factors.[150]

SUPPORTIVE SKIN CARE

Extensive areas of denuded skin can result in the loss of the barrier provided by the stratum corneum. Subsequent microbial penetration can result in the accumulation of serum and moisture that further enhances bacterial propagation. The above factors combined with immunosuppressive therapy facilitate development of infections. Prevention of infection is obviously the preferred strategy.

A modified Dakin solution (0.025% w/v sodium hypochlorite) can be helpful in reducing the bacterial load in patient skin. Soaking wounds in this solution for 20 minutes before dressing changes also helps to free adherent bandages that have dried onto the wound bed. After soaking, wounds can be dressed with mupirocin or other topical antibiotics and covered with semiocclusive nonadhesive dressings. Tape causes further blistering and peeling of the skin, so it is essential to use self-adhering (clinging) gauze or self-adherent paper to hold nonadherent dressings in place.

For patients with generalized or localized subtypes of EBS, controlling exposure to heat may prove helpful in controlling blister formation. Advising patients to use soft, well-ventilated shoes is also recommended. Patients with Herlitz JEB, lacking functional laminin-332, an extracellular matrix protein shown to be involved in keratinocyte adhesion and migration, may have especially difficult problems with wound healing. For patients with DEB, use of finger splinting or diligent hand wrapping and appropriate hand protection against trauma are helpful, especially after hand surgery (see later).

INFECTION

Management of skin infections is a critical part of EB patient care. Large areas of denuded skin, a common finding in patients with EB, provides an inadequate barrier to microbial penetration and can lead to both skin infections as well as the more devastating complication of sepsis. *Staphylococcus aureus* and *Streptococcus pyogenes* are common infectious agents. Gram-negative infections with *Pseudomonas aeruginosa* can also occur. Skin cultures and the use of the appropriate systemic antibiotics are indicated for wound infection. Gentle whirlpool therapy, frequent (daily) dressing changes, dilute chlorine baths, rotation of topical antibiotics, and use of topical disinfectants such as iodine–povidone are all helpful ways to reduce resistant bacteria.

SURGICAL TREATMENT

Among the EB patient population, those with the severe recessive DEB (Hallopeau-Siemens) variant are generally the most in need of surgical intervention.[151] Mitten pseudosyndactyly in these patients can be surgically released; however, this procedure may have to be repeated periodically because of the strong tendency of this condition to recur.[151-154] Splinting after surgery is essential to reducing recurrence of hand deformities. Surgery may also be used to correct limb, perioral, and perineal contracture deformities, but unfortunately, a high rate of recurrence is common. Extra care must be taken to minimize trauma to oral mucosa in EB patients during intubation.

TUMORS

SCC often arises after puberty in patients with recessive DEB. SCC may arise in multiple primary sites, especially in nonhealing areas. Careful surveillance of nonhealing areas is of utmost importance because patients often die from metastatic disease.[155] Surgical excision using either Mohs or non-Mohs approaches is an important first-line modality with radiation therapy as a useful adjunct in some cases.[156] Isotretinoin has been used for patients with RDEB for chemoprevention of SCC. Although it appears well tolerated, it is not clear whether in can increase the overall survival rate of these patients.[157] Cetuximab therapy has been demonstrated to offer some benefit,[155,158] but the cutaneous side effects can sometimes be problematic.

CARE FOR EXTRACUTANEOUS INVOLVEMENT

GASTROINTESTINAL MANAGEMENT

Esophageal lesions are often the most disabling complication found in recessive DEB and JEB of both the severe and intermediate generalized variants. Esophageal strictures usually respond to dilation; however, recurrence of strictures after dilation is common.[159] Colonic interposition has proven effective in advanced cases but is rarely used. Gastrostomy tube insertion has been effective in providing nutrition to individuals with esophageal strictures.[160]

Increased fluid and fiber intake and stool softeners may also be of value in EB patients with constipation and colitis.[161]

EYE LESIONS

Patients with EBS, particularly those with the Dowling-Meara subtype, can experience recurrent inflammation of the eyelid, with bullous lesions in the conjunctivae. Patients with JEB and patients with recessive DEB can experience corneal ulcerations with scarring, obliteration of tear ducts, and eyelid lesions.[162] Cicatricial conjunctivitis can also occur in patients with recessive DEB. Corneal erosions are treated supportively with application of antibiotic ointments and use of cycloplegic agents to reduce ciliary spasms and provide comfort. Moisture chambers and ocular lubricants are also commonly used. Severely affected upper eyelids may be surgically managed with full-thickness skin grafting. Complete correction of any eye disorder in EB patients is difficult to achieve. Proper management of eye lesions in EB patients must include the assistance of an ophthalmologist to prevent serious visual compromise.[163] Surgical and ocular surface reconstruction can help reduce granulation tissue in laryngo-onycho-cutaneous syndrome.[164]

OROPHARYNGEAL LESIONS

Good dental hygiene is essential for EB patients, and regular visits to the dentist are especially important. Enamel defects in JEB patients and pain on brushing and flossing in patients with severe JEB and DEB often lead to dental carries.[165,166] The softest brush available should be used for regular cleansing. Oral mucosal blistering may also accompany forms of JEB and DEB, especially in severe DEB subtypes such as the severe generalized recessive form, narrowing of the mouth opening (microstomia), and scarring induced limitation of movement of the tongue (ankyloglossia) and be particularly debilitating. Normal saline rinses are effective for gentle cleaning of the mucosal surfaces. Mouthwashes containing alcohol or other harsh agents should be avoided. Erosions and scarring involving the trachea and larynx with resultant narrowing of the airway. In patients with airway involvement, there is danger of pulmonary aspiration.[167] Surgical intubation should be performed gently with small bore airways by anesthesiologists experienced in the care of EB patients.[168]

NUTRITION, ANEMIA, AND CARDIOVASCULAR DISEASE

Nutritional assessment and support can be critical in patients with EB[169] for several reasons. Extensive cutaneous injury is associated with marked alterations in hemodynamic and metabolic responses, with increased caloric and protein requirements. Oropharyngeal and GI lesions provide the greatest overall threat to nutritional well-being. These include oral blistering, abnormal esophageal motility, strictures, dysphagia, diarrhea, malabsorption, and dental problems. Nutritional assessment must take into account these factors to develop a supplemental regimen to replenish nutritional deficiencies.[170] Patients are often unable to increase their food intake to balance this increased caloric need. For example, hypoplastic enamel formation in JEB may lead to tooth decay, mucosal blistering, and oral candidiasis. All of these potential complications may compromise patients' ability to eat. Extensive internal mucosal disadhesion in the GI tract may cause abnormal GI motility, strictures, and diarrhea are complications that may lead to malabsorption of iron and other nutrients. Anemia of chronic disease can certainly affect all severe EB subtypes. Recessive DEB patients often show a particularly severe iron deficiency that may not responsive to oral iron supplementation. For these patients, parenteral iron can be helpful. Furthermore, if a lack of a reticulocyte response to iron supplementation is seen in iron-deficient patients, it is helpful to assess the erythropoietin level and to treat with recombinant erythropoietin if necessary.[171] Transfusion is also useful in the treatment of anemia in EB, especially when symptoms require a rapid correction. Dilated cardiomyopathy is a devastating and potentially fatal complication of severe DEB and JEB patients that is highly associated with chronic anemia.[172]

PSYCHOLOGICAL ASPECTS OF EPIDERMOLYSIS BULLOSA

Patients with EB, especially the severe subtypes, can be plagued with chronic pain.[173-175] Although many, despite extremely adverse conditions, seem to find a way to maintain a surprisingly positive outlook on life, others lapse into depression.[176,177] Patients with severe EB can also create stress for their families and loved ones.[178,179] Thus, it is important to identify the warning signs of depression when they arise and to work in a multidisciplinary approach with psychiatrists and clinical psychologists as needed. Supportive psychotherapy and patient support group meetings can help patients and their families in this regard. An additional source of support for patients and families include several important patient-based organizations that assist with education and support, including the Dystrophic Epidermolysis Bullosa Research Association and Epidermolysis Bullosa Medical Research Foundation.

ANTIINFLAMMATORY THERAPIES

A number of new therapies are emerging for EB, which are listed in Fig. 60-17 and described later.

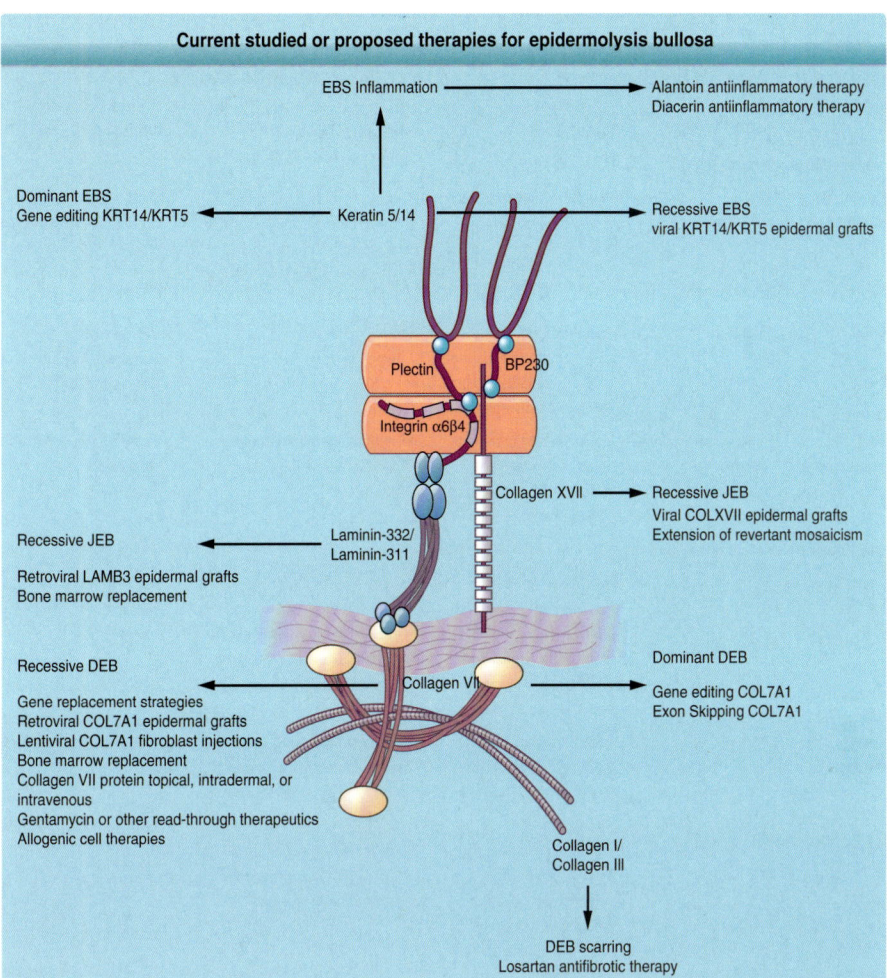

Figure 60-17 Current studied or proposed therapies for epidermolysis bullosa. DEB, dystrophic epidermolysis bullosa; EBS, epidermolysis bullosa simplex; JBS, junctional epidermolysis bullosa.

Repetitive scratching–induced trauma and an exuberant inflammatory wound each contribute to wound chronicity, especially in patients with inflammatory subtypes of EBS or EB pruriginosa. Although topical corticosteroids can produce short-term relief from itching and reduce inflammation, in the long term, these agents induce skin atrophy, which exacerbates the intrinsic fragility of EB skin and worsens blistering/healing. Tetracycline and phenytoin have been used in the past for EB but are not currently indicated treatment.[180] The naturally occurring component of rhubarb root, and interleukin-β blocker diacerein[181] was found to be well tolerated and to reduce blister formation in patients with severe EBS with inflammatory skin phenotypes.[182] Losartan, a small-molecule angiotensin II type I receptor antagonist used to treat hypertension, has shown promise in preclinical studies in reducing the fibrosis accompanying DEB wounding. Losartan achieves this effect by reducing transforming growth factor-β expression in the skin.[183]

ALLOGENEIC CELL THERAPIES

Allogeneic cell therapies including, allogeneic keratinocyte skin equivalents,[184] allogeneic fibroblast injections,[185,186] and mesenchymal stem cell infusions,[187] have shown positive short-term effects on EB wound healing. However, they fail to show any long-term benefits. Allogeneic bone marrow transplantation performed on a group of seven children with recessive DEB. Some patients demonstrated noticeable clinical benefit, as well as collagen VII staining at the dermal–epidermal junction for 1 year or longer; however, restoration of anchoring fibrils was incomplete.[188] Of note, this procedure demonstrated a mortality rate of approximately 30%. Contributing to the mortality rate observed may have been the combination of widespread cutaneous erosions and the immunomyeloablative-induced immunosuppression required for successful bone marrow transplant take.

TABLE 60-3
Summary of the Types of Epidermolysis Bullosa and their Clinical Manifestations

	AGE OF ONSET	DISTRIBUTION	CLINICAL MANIFESTATIONS	SEQUELAE AND COMPLICATIONS
Epidermolysis Bullosa Simplex (EBS)				
Generalized severe (Dowling-Meara)	Birth	Generalized; oral mucosal involvement; nail involvement	Sudden onset of grouped or herpetiform blisters, extensive erosions; nail shedding and dystrophy palmoplantar hyperkeratosis in older children	Milia formation, contractures, esophageal erosions, pyloric atresia
Generalized intermediate (Koebner)	Birth	Generalized but most prominent on hands, feet, and extremities; mild oral mucosal involvement	Erosions, palmoplantar hyperkeratosis	Postinflammatory hyperpigmentation or hypopigmentation, milia formation
Localized (Weber-Cockayne)	Infancy, childhood, occasionally adulthood	Areas of friction or trauma, most commonly the hands and feet; mild oral involvement	Blistering after trauma; palmoplantar hyperhidrosis	No milia formation; no scarring sequelae
Junctional Epidermolysis Bullosa (JEB)				
Generalized severe JEB (Herlitz)	Birth	Generalized; mucosal involvement (nasal, conjunctival, esophageal, tracheal, laryngeal, rectal, urethral); nail involvement; dental involvement	Extensive blistering; periorificial granulation tissue (mouth, eyes, nares); loss of nails or dystrophic nails with granulation tissue; pitted tooth enamel	Tracheolaryngeal stenosis or obstruction, failure to thrive, sepsis
Generalized intermediate JEB	Birth	Generalized; minimal oral or other mucosal involvement; dental involvement	Widespread blistering; extensive dental caries; nail dystrophy; may have progressive alopecia of scalp	Atrophic scars, normal growth
Localized JEB		Localized (most often hands, feet, pretibial regions); oral mucosal involvement (minimal); nail involvement; dental involvement	Localized erosions; nail shedding and dystrophy; enamel pitting; oral and nasal erosions	
JEB with pyloric atresia	Birth	Generalized; mucosal involvement; systemic involvement	Extensive cutaneous sloughing, with widespread blistering	Pyloric stenosis, hydronephrosis, nephritis
Dystrophic Epidermolysis Bullosa (DEB)				
Localized DDEB (Cockayne-Touraine)	Birth or childhood	Generalized early in life but localizes to sites of trauma (knees, sacrum, acral areas); nail involvement	Blisters; nail dystrophy or nail loss may be presenting symptoms	Milia, hypertrophic scarring
Generalized DDEB (Pasini)	Birth	Generalized early in life but may localize to extremities; nail involvement	Widespread severe blistering; albopauloid lesions; oral erosions; dystrophic or absent nails; enamel defects	Milia, scarring plaques
Localized RDEB	Birth	Acral distribution	Blisters; mild oral mucosal erosions	Milia, scarring
Severe RDEB (Hallopeau-Siemens)	Birth	Generalized; mucosal involvement; dental involvement	Extensively denuded skin; enamel pitting with caries and loss of teeth	Pseudosyndactyly, flexion contractures of hands and limbs, tracheal and laryngeal involvement, esophageal structures, malnutrition, growth retardation, anemia, iron deficiency, SCC

DDEB, dominant dystrophic epidermolysis bullosa; RDEB, recessive dystrophic epidermolysis bullosa; SSC, squamous cell carcinoma.

AUTOLOGOUS GENETIC THERAPIES

Retroviral ex vivo gene therapy using autologous keratinocytes was performed for one patient with JEB.[189] In this study, a patient with a missense mutation of laminin-332 was grafted with genetically corrected keratinocyte monolayers expressing wild-type laminin-332. After 6.5 years of postgrafting follow-up, grafts still showed positive expression of laminin-332 and resistance to blistering.[190] More recently, this therapy was extended in a widespread and remarkable manner to another JEB patient with genetically corrected epidermal grafts covering more than 80% of skin surfaces.[191] A similar approach was more recently performed on a clinical trial of four patients with recessive DEB.[127] In this study, full-length *COL7A1* gene, coding for collagen VII was transferred ex vivo to primary recessive DEB patient keratinocytes. Collagen VII engineered patient cells were expanded then grafted as monolayers to patient wounds (six grafts per patient). Results showed clinical improvement as well as restoration of collagen VII expression and anchoring fibril formation as long as 1 year. Gene editing via CRISPER/Cas9 combined with the use of induced pluripotent stem cells[192-194] is another promising future therapy for Exon skipping has shown promise in as a potential future therapy in both JEB[195] as well as DEB skin.[196,197] The potential to extend skin in patients with COL17A1 and COL7A1 self-correcting mutations by autologous grafting has also been proposed as a novel therapy.[198]

SUMMARY

A summary of the types of EB and their clinical manifestations is shown in Table 60-3.

REFERENCES

1. Hebra FV. *Arztlicher Bericht des K.K allegemeinen Krankenhauses zu Wien vom Jare 1870*. Pemphigus. Vienna; 1870:362.
2. Fox T. Notes on unusual or rare forms of skin disease. *Lancet*. 1879;1:766.
3. Goldscheider A. Hereditare Neigung zer Blasenbildung. *Monatsschr Prakt Dermatol*. 1882;1:163.
4. Koebner H. Hereditare Anlage zur Blasenbildung. *Dtsch Med Wochenschr*. 1886;12:21.
5. Hallopeau MH. Nouvelle etude sur la dermatite bulleuse congenitale avec kysts epidermiques. *Ann Dermatol Syphiligr (Paris)*. 1896;7:453.
6. Weber FP. Recurrent bullous eruption on the feet in a child. *Proc R Soc Med*. 1926;19:72.
7. Cockayne EA. Recurrent bullous eruption of feet. *Br J Dermatol*. 1938;50:358.
8. Dowling GB. Epidermolysis bullosa resembling juvenile dermatitis herpetiformis. *Br J Dermatol*. 1954; 66:139.
9. Hoffman E. Uber den Erbgang bei Epidermolysis bullosa hereditaria. *Arch Rassen Gesellsch Biol*. 1926; 18:353.
10. Cockayne EA. *Inherited Abnormalities of the Skin and Its Appendages*. London: Oxford University Press; 1933.
11. Touraine MA. Classification des epidermolyses bulleuses. *Ann Dermatol Syphiligr (Paris)*. 1942;2:141.
12. Pasini A. Dystrophie cutanee bulleuse atrophiante et albopapuloide. *Ann Dermatol Syphiligr (Paris)*. 1928;9:1044.
13. Bart BJ, Gorlin RJ, Anderson VE, et al. Congenital localized absence of skin and associated abnormalities resembling epidermolysis bullosa. *Arch Dermatol*. 1966;93:293.
14. Herlitz G. Kongenitaler, nicht syphilitischer Pemphigus: Eine Ubersicht nebst Beschreibung einer neuen Krankheitsform. *Acta Paediatr*. 1935;7:315.
15. Pearson RW. Studies on the pathogenesis of epidermolysis bullosa. *J Invest Dermatol*. 1962;39:551-575.
16. Gedde-Dahl T. *Epidermolysis Bullosa: A Clinical, Genetic and Epidemiologic Study*. Baltimore: The John Hopkins Press; 1971:1-180.
17. Fine JD, Bruckner-Tuderman L, Eady RA, et al. Inherited epidermolysis bullosa: updated recommendations on diagnosis and classification. *J Am Acad Dermatol*. 2014;70(6):1103-1126.
18. Kanasaki K, Kanda Y, Palmsten K, et al. Integrin beta1-mediated matrix assembly and signaling are critical for the normal development and function of the kidney glomerulus. *Dev Biol*. 2008;313(2):584-593.
19. Yoshida-Moriguchi T, Yu L, Stalnaker SH, et al. O-mannosyl phosphorylation of alpha-dystroglycan is required for laminin binding. *Science*. 2010;327(5961):88-92.
20. Arin MJ. The molecular basis of human keratin disorders. *Hum Genet*. 2009;125(4):355-373.
21. Coulombe PA, Kerns ML, Fuchs E. Epidermolysis bullosa simplex: a paradigm for disorders of tissue fragility. *J Clin Invest*. 2009;119(7):1784-1793.
22. Rezniczek GA, Janda L, Wiche G. Plectin. *Methods Cell Biol*. 2004;78:721-755.
23. Andreu P, Johansson M, Affara NI, et al. FcRγ activation regulates inflammation-associated squamous carcinogenesis. *Cancer Cell*. 2010;17(2):121-134.
24. Jefferson JJ, Ciatto C, Shapiro L, et al. Structural analysis of the plakin domain of bullous pemphigoid antigen1 (BPAG1) suggests that plakins are members of the spectrin superfamily. *J Mol Biol*. 2007; 366(1):244-257.
25. Young KG, Kothary R. Dystonin/Bpag1 is a necessary endoplasmic reticulum/nuclear envelope protein in sensory neurons. *Exp Cell Res*. 2008;314(15): 2750-2761.
26. Young KG, Kothary R. Dystonin/Bpag1—a link to what? *Cell Motil Cytoskeleton*. 2007;64(12):897-905.
27. Leung CL, Zheng M, Prater SM, et al. The BPAG1 locus: Alternative splicing produces multiple isoforms with distinct cytoskeletal linker domains, including predominant isoforms in neurons and muscles. *J Cell Biol*. 2001;154(4):691-697.
28. Has C, Kern JS. Collagen XVII. *Dermatol Clin*. 2010;28(1): 61-66.
29. Litjens S, de Pereda J, Sonnenberg A. Current insights into the formation and breakdown of hemidesmosomes. *Trends Cell Biol*. 2006;16:376-383.
30. de Pereda JM, Lillo MP, Sonnenberg A. Structural basis of the interaction between integrin alpha6beta4 and plectin at the hemidesmosomes. *EMBO J*. 2009;28: 1180-1190.

31. Dowling J, Yu QC, Fuchs E. Beta4 integrin is required for hemidesmosome formation, cell adhesion and cell survival. *J Cell Biol*. 1996;134(2):559-572.
32. Margadant C, Frijns E, Wilhelmsen K, Sonnenberg A. Regulation of hemidesmosome disassembly by growth factor receptors. *Curr Opin Cell Biol*. 2008;20(5): 589-596.
33. Hirako Y, Usukura J, Nishizawa Y, et al. Demonstration of the molecular shape of BP180, a 180-kDa bullous pemphigoid antigen and its potential for trimer formation. *J Biol Chem*. 1996;271(23):13739-13745.
34. Carter WG, Kaur P, Gil SG, et al. Distinct functions for integrins alpha 3 beta 1 in focal adhesions and alpha 6 beta 4/bullous pemphigoid antigen in a new stable anchoring contact (SAC) of keratinocytes: relation to hemidesmosomes. *J Cell Biol*. 1990;111(6 Pt 2): 3141-3154.
35. Zone JJ, Taylor TB, Kadunce DP, et al. Identification of the cutaneous basement membrane antigen in linear IgA bullous dermatosis. *J Clin Invest*. 1990;85: 812-820.
36. Marinkovich MP, Taylor TB, Keene DR, et al. LAD-1, the linear IgA bullous dermatosis autoantigen, is a novel 120- kDa anchoring filament protein synthesized by epidermal cells. *J Invest Dermatol*. 1996;106(4): 734-738.
37. Zone JJ, Taylor TB, Meyer LJ, et al. The 97 kDa linear IgA bullous disease antigen is identical to a portion of the extracellular domain of the 180 kDa bullous pemphigoid antigen, BPAg2. *J Invest Dermatol*. 1998;110(3):207-210.
38. Franzke CW, Bruckner P, Bruckner-Tuderman L. Collagenous transmembrane proteins: recent insights into biology and pathology. *J Biol Chem*. 2005; 280(6):4005-4008.
39. Franzke CW, Tasanen K, Borradori L, et al. Shedding of collagen XVII/BP180: structural motifs influence cleavage from cell surface. *J Biol Chem*. 2004;279(23): 24521-24529.
40. Durbeej M. Laminins. *Cell Tissue Res*. 2010;339(1): 259-268.
41. Miner JH. Laminins and their roles in mammals. *Microsc Res Tech*. 2008;71(5):349-356.
42. Schéele S, Nyström A, Durbeej M, et al. Laminin isoforms in development and disease. *J Mol Med*. 2007;85:825-836.
43. Marinkovich MP, Lunstrum GP, Keene DR, et al. The dermal-epidermal junction of human skin contains a novel laminin variant. *J Cell Biol*. 1992;119(3): 695-703.
44. Meneguzzi G, Marinkovich MP, Aberdam D, et al. Kalinin is abnormally expressed in epithelial basement membranes of Herlitz's junctional epidermolysis bullosa patients. *Exp Dermatol*. 1992;1(5):221-229.
45. Gerecke DR, Cordon MK, Wagman WW. Hemidesmosomes, anchoring fibrils. In: Mecham RP, Birk DE, Yurchenko PD, eds. *Extracellular Matrix Assembly and Structure*. San Diego: Academic Press; 1994:417-439.
46. Ryan MC, Tizard R, VanDevanter DR, et al. Cloning of the LamA3 gene encoding the alpha 3 chain of the adhesive ligand epiligrin. Expression in wound repair. *J Biol Chem*. 1994;269(36):22779-22787.
47. Kallunki P, Sainio K, Eddy R, et al. A truncated laminin chain homologous to the B2 chain: structure, spatial expression, and chromosomal assignment. *J Cell Biol*. 1992;119(3):679-693.
48. Champliaud MF, Lunstrum GP, Rousselle P, et al. Human amnion contains a novel laminin variant, laminin 7, which like laminin 6, covalently associates with laminin 5 to promote stable epithelial-stromal attachment. *J Cell Biol*. 1996;132(6):1189-1198.
49. Marinkovich M, Lunstrum G, Burgeson R. The anchoring filament protein kalinin is synthesized and secreted as a high molecular weight precursor. *J Biol Chem*. 1992;267(25):17900-17906.
50. Giannelli G, Falk-Marzillier J, Schiraldi O, et al. Induction of cell migration by matrix metalloprotease-2 cleavage of laminin-5. *Science*. 1997;277(5323): 225-228.
51. Koshikawa N, Giannelli G, Cirulli V, et al. Role of cell surface metalloprotease MT1-MMP in epithelial cell migration over laminin-5. *J Cell Biol*. 2000;148(3): 615-624.
52. Veitch DP, Nokelainen P, McGowan KA, et al. Mammalian tolloid metalloproteinase, and not matrix metalloprotease 2 or membrane type 1 metalloprotease, processes laminin-5 in keratinocytes and skin. *J Biol Chem*. 2003;278(18):15661-15668.
53. Ge G, Greenspan D. Developmental roles of the BMP1/TLD metalloproteinases. *Birth Defects Res C Embryo Today*. 2006;78(1):47-68.
54. Amano S, Scott IC, Takahara K, et al. Bone morphogenetic protein 1 is an extracellular processing enzyme of the laminin 5 gamma 2 chain. *J Biol Chem*. 2000;275(30):22728-22735.
55. Goldfinger LE, Hopkinson SB, deHart GW, et al. The alpha3 laminin subunit, alpha6beta4 and alpha-3beta1 integrin coordinately regulate wound healing in cultured epithelial cells and in the skin. *J Cell Sci*. 1999;112:2615-2629.
56. Gagnoux-Palacios L, Allegra M, Spirito F, et al. The short arm of the laminin gamma2 chain plays a pivotal role in the incorporation of laminin 5 into the extracellular matrix and in cell adhesion. *J Cell Biol*. 2001;153(4):835-850.
57. Fine JD, Horiguchi Y, Couchman JR. 19-DEJ-1, a hemidesmosome-anchoring filament complex associated monoclonal antibody. Definition of a new skin basement membrane antigenic defect in junctional and dystrophic epidermolysis bullosa. *Arch Dermatol*. 1989;125:520-523.
58. Parente MG, Chung LC, Ryynänen J, et al. Human type VII collagen: cDNA cloning and chromosomal mapping of the gene (COL7A1) on chromosome 3 to dominant dystrophic epidermolysis bullosa. *Am J Hum Genet*. 1991;24:119-135.
59. Burgeson RE, Lundstrum GP, Rokosova B. The structure and function of type VII collagen. *Ann N Y Acad Sci*. 1990;580:32-43.
60. Bachinger HP, Morris NP, Lundstrum GP. The relationship of the biophysical and biochemical characteristics of type VII collagen to the function of anchoring fibrils. *J Biol Chem*. 1990;265:10095-10101.
61. Bruckner-Tuderman L, Hopfner B, Hammami-Hauasli N. Biology of anchoring fibrils: lessons from dystrophic epidermolysis bullosa. *Matrix Biol*. 1999; 18(1):43-54.
62. Gayraud B, Höpfner B, Jassim A, et al. Characterization of a 50-kDa component of epithelial basement membranes using GDA-J/F3 monoclonal antibody. *J Biol Chem*. 1997;272(14):9531-9538.
63. Chen M, Marinkovich MP, Jones JC, et al. NC1 domain of type VII collagen binds to the beta3 chain of laminin 5 via a unique subdomain within the fibronectin-like repeats. *J Invest Dermatol*. 1999; 112(2):177-183.

64. Rousselle P, Keene DR, Ruggiero F, et al. Laminin 5 binds the NC-1 domain of type VII collagen. *J Cell Biol*. 1997;138(3):719-728.
65. Nakashima Y, Kariya Y, Yasuda C, et al. Regulation of cell adhesion and type VII collagen binding by the beta3 chain short arm of laminin-5: effect of its proteolytic cleavage. *J Biochem (Tokyo)*. 2005;138(5):539-552.
66. Waterman EA, Sakai N, Nguyen NT, et al. A laminin-collagen complex drives human epidermal carcinogenesis through phosphoinositol-3-kinase activation. *Cancer Res*. 2007;67(9):4264-4270.
67. Ortiz-Urda S, Garcia J, Green CL, et al. Type VII collagen is required for Ras-driven human epidermal tumorigenesis. *Science*. 2005;307(5716):1773-1776.
68. Chen M, Keene DR, Costa FK, et al. The carboxyl terminus of type VII collagen mediates antiparallel-dimer formation and constitutes a new antigenic epitope for EBA autoantibodies. *J Biol Chem*. 2001;27:27.
69. Smith LT. Ultrastructural findings in epidermolysis bullosa. *Arch Dermatol*. 1993;129(12):1578-1584.
70. Sprecher E. Epidermolysis bullosa simplex. *Dermatol Clin*. 2010;28(1):23-32.
71. Morrell DS, Rubenstein DS, Briggaman RA, et al. Congenital pyloric atresia in a newborn with extensive aplasia cutis congenita and epidermolysis bullosa simplex. *Br J Dermatol*. 2000;143(6):1342-1343.
72. Shemanko CS, Horn HM, Keohane SG, et al. Laryngeal involvement in the Dowling-Meara variant of epidermolysis bullosa simplex with keratin mutations of severely disruptive potential. *Br J Dermatol*. 2000;142(2):315-320.
73. Chavanas S, Pulkkinen L, Gache Y, et al. A homozygous nonsense mutation in the PLEC1 gene in patients with epidermolysis bullosa simplex with muscular dystrophy. *J Clin Invest*. 1996;98(10):2196-2200.
74. Gache Y, Chavanas S, Lacour JP, et al. Defective expression of plectin/HD1 in epidermolysis bullosa simplex with muscular dystrophy. *J Clin Invest*. 1996;97(10):2289-2298.
75. McLean WH, Pulkkinen L, Smith FJ, et al. Loss of plectin causes epidermolysis bullosa with muscular dystrophy: cDNA cloning and genomic organization. *Genes Dev*. 1996;10(14):1724-1735.
76. Dang M, Pulkkinen L, Smith FJ, et al. Novel compound heterozygous mutations in the plectin gene in epidermolysis bullosa with muscular dystrophy and the use of protein truncation test for detection of premature termination codon mutations. *Lab Invest*. 1998;78(2):195-204.
77. Bauer JW, Schaeppi H, Kaserer C, et al. Large melanocytic nevi in hereditary epidermolysis bullosa. *J Am Acad Dermatol*. 2001;44(4):577-584.
78. Fine JD, Johnson L, Wright T. Epidermolysis bullosa simplex superficialis. *Arch Dermatol*. 1989;125:633-638.
79. McGrath JA, Bolling MC, Jonkman MF. Lethal acantholytic epidermolysis bullosa. *Dermatol Clin*. 2010;28(1):131-135.
80. McGrath J. A novel genodermatosis caused by mutations in plakophilin 1, a structural component of desmosomes. *J Dermatol*. 1999;26(11):764-769.
81. McGrath JA. Recently identified forms of epidermolysis bullosa. *Ann Dermatol*. 2015;27(6):658-666.
82. Kiritsi D, Cosgarea I, Franzke CW, et al. Acral peeling skin syndrome with TGM5 gene mutations may resemble epidermolysis bullosa simplex in young individuals. *J Invest Dermatol*. 2010;130(6):1741-1746.
83. Hovnanian A, Duquesnoy P, Amselem S. Genetic linkage of recessive epidermolysis bullosa to the type VII collagen gene. *J Clin Invest*. 1992;90:1033-1037.
84. Jonkman MF, Heeres K, Pas HH, et al. Effects of keratin 14 ablation on the clinical and cellular phenotype in a kindred with recessive epidermolysis bullosa simplex. *J Invest Dermatol*. 1996;107(5):764-769.
85. Coulombe PA. The cellular and molecular biology of keratins: beginning a new era. *Curr Opin Cell Biol*. 1993;5(1):17-29.
86. Uttam J, Hutton E, Coulombe PA, et al. The genetic basis of epidermolysis bullosa simplex with mottled pigmentation. *Proc Natl Acad Sci U S A*. 1996;93(17):9079-9084.
87. Irvine AD, Rugg EL, Lane EB, et al. Molecular confirmation of the unique phenotype of epidermolysis bullosa simplex with mottled pigmentation. *Br J Dermatol*. 2001;144(1):40-45.
88. Moog U, de Die-Smulders CE, Scheffer H, et al. Epidermolysis bullosa simplex with mottled pigmentation: clinical aspects and confirmation of the P24L mutation in the KRT5 gene in further patients. *Am J Med Genet*. 1999;86(4):376-379.
89. Chamcheu JC, Virtanen M, Navsaria H, et al. Epidermolysis bullosa simplex due to KRT5 mutations: mutation-related differences in cellular fragility and the protective effects of trimethylamine N-oxide in cultured primary keratinocytes. *Br J Dermatol*. 2010;162(5):980-989.
90. Rezniczek GA, Walko G, Wiche G. Plectin gene defects lead to various forms of epidermolysis bullosa simplex. *Dermatol Clin*. 2010;28(1):33-41.
91. Konieczny P, Wiche G. Muscular integrity—a matter of interlinking distinct structures via plectin. *Adv Exp Med Biol*. 2008;642:165-175.
92. Fassihi H, Grace J, Lashwood A, et al. Preimplantation genetic diagnosis of skin fragility-ectodermal dysplasia syndrome. *Br J Dermatol*. 2006;154(3):546-550.
93. Ersoy-Evans S, Erkin G, Fassihi H, et al. Ectodermal dysplasia-skin fragility syndrome resulting from a new homozygous mutation, 888delC, in the desmosomal protein plakophilin 1. *J Am Acad Dermatol*. 2006;55(1):157-161.
94. Fassihi H, Wessagowit V, Ashton GH, et al. Complete paternal uniparental isodisomy of chromosome 1 resulting in Herlitz junctional epidermolysis bullosa. *Clin Exp Dermatol*. 2005;30(1):71-74.
95. Hamada T, South AP, Mitsuhashi Y, et al. Genotype-phenotype correlation in skin fragility-ectodermal dysplasia syndrome resulting from mutations in plakophilin 1. *Exp Dermatol*. 2002;11(2):107-114.
96. Whittock N, Haftek M, Angoulvant N, et al. Genomic amplification of the human plakophilin 1 gene and detection of a new mutation in ectodermal dysplasia/skin fragility syndrome. *J Invest Dermatol*. 2000;115(3):368-374.
97. McGrath J, Hoeger PH, Christiano AM, et al. Skin fragility and hypohidrotic ectodermal dysplasia resulting from ablation of plakophilin 1. *Br J Dermatol*. 1999;140(2):297-307.
98. Bruckner Tuderman L, McGrath JA, Robinson EC, et al. Progress in epidermolysis bullosa research: summary of DEBRA International Research Conference 2012. *J Invest Dermatol*. 2013;133(9):2121-2126.
99. Rashidghamat E, Ozoemena L, Liu L, et al. Mutations in EXPH5 underlie a rare subtype of autosomal recessive epidermolysis bullosa simplex. *Br J Dermatol*. 2016;174(2):452-453.

100. Fattah A. Epidermolysis bullosa hereditaria letalis (Herlitz). *Dermatologica*. 196;133(6):475-481.
101. Laimer M, Lanschuetzer CM, Diem A, et al. Herlitz junctional epidermolysis bullosa. *Dermatol Clin*. 2010;28(1):55-60.
102. Hintner H, Wolff K. Generalized atrophic benign epidermolysis bullosa. *Arch Dermatol*. 1982;118(6):375-384.
103. Vidal F, Aberdam D, Miquel C, et al. Integrin beta 4 mutations associated with junctional epidermolysis bullosa with pyloric atresia. *Nat Genet*. 1995;10(2):229-234.
104. Inoue M, Tamai K, Shimizu H, et al. A homozygous missense mutation in the cytoplasmic tail of beta4 integrin, G931D, that disrupts hemidesmosome assembly and underlies non-Herlitz junctional epidermolysis bullosa without pyloric atresia? *J Invest Dermatol*. 2000;114(5):1061-1064.
105. Chavanas S, Gache Y, Vailly J, et al. Splicing modulation of integrin beta4 pre-mRNA carrying a branch point mutation underlies epidermolysis bullosa with pyloric atresia undergoing spontaneous amelioration with ageing. *Hum Mol Genet*. 1999;8(11):2097-2105.
106. Gache Y, Allegra M, Bodemer C, et al. Genetic bases of severe junctional epidermolysis bullosa presenting spontaneous amelioration with aging. *Hum Mol Genet*. 2001;10(21):2453-2461.
107. McLean WH, Irvine AD, Hamill KJ, et al. An unusual N-terminal deletion of the laminin alpha3a isoform leads to the chronic granulation tissue disorder laryngo-onycho-cutaneous syndrome. *Hum Mol Genet*. 2003;12(18):2395-2409.
108. Pfendner EG, Bruckner A, Conget P, et al. Basic science of epidermolysis bullosa and diagnostic and molecular characterization: proceedings of the IInd International Symposium on Epidermolysis Bullosa, Santiago, Chile, 2005. *Int J Dermatol*. 2007;46(8):781-794.
109. Varki R, Sadowski S, Pfendner E, et al. Epidermolysis bullosa. I. Molecular genetics of the junctional and hemidesmosomal variants. *J Med Genet*. 2006;43(8):641-652.
110. Kivirikko S, McGrath JA, Pulkkinen L, et al. Mutational hotspots in the LAMB3 gene in the lethal (Herlitz) type of junctional epidermolysis bullosa. *Hum Mol Genet*. 1996;5:231-237.
111. McGrath JA, Pulkkinen L, Christiano AM, et al. Altered laminin 5 expression due to mutations in the gene encoding the B3 chain in generalized atrophic benign epidermolysis bullosa. *J Invest Dermatol*. 1995;104:467-474.
112. Cserhalmi-Friedman PB, Baden H, Burgeson RE, et al. Molecular basis of non-lethal junctional epidermolysis bullosa: identification of a 38 basepair insertion and a splice site mutation in exon 14 of the LAMB3 gene. *Exp Dermatol*. 1998;7(2-3):105-111.
113. Varki R, Sadowski S, Uitto J, et al. Epidermolysis bullosa. II. Type VII collagen mutations and phenotype-genotype correlations in the dystrophic subtypes. *J Med Genet*. 2007;44(3):181-192.
114. Vaisanen L, Has C, Franzke C, et al. Molecular mechanisms of junctional epidermolysis bullosa: Col 15 domain mutations decrease the thermal stability of collagen XVII. *J Invest Dermatol*. 2005;125(6):1112-1118.
115. Fontao L, Tasanen K, Huber M, et al. Molecular consequences of deletion of the cytoplasmic domain of bullous pemphigoid 180 in a patient with predominant features of epidermolysis bullosa simplex. *J Invest Dermatol*. 2004;122(1):65-72.
116. Floeth M, Fiedorowicz J, Schäcke H, et al. Novel homozygous and compound heterozygous COL17A1 mutations associated with junctional epidermolysis bullosa. *J Invest Dermatol*. 1998;111(3):528-533.
117. Jonkman MF, Scheffer H, Stulp R, et al. Revertant mosaicism in epidermolysis bullosa caused by mitotic gene conversion. *Cell*. 1997;88(4):543-551.
118. Pasmooij A, Pas HH, Deviaene FC, et al. Multiple correcting COL17A1 mutations in patients with revertant mosaicism of epidermolysis bullosa. *Am J Hum Genet*. 2005;77(5):727-740.
119. Has C, Spartà G, Kiritsi D, et al. Integrin alpha3 mutations with kidney, lung, and skin disease. *N Engl J Med*. 2012;366(16):1508-1514.
120. He Y, Balasubramanian M, Humphreys N, et al. Intronic ITGA3 mutation impacts splicing regulation and causes interstitial lung disease, nephrotic syndrome, and epidermolysis bullosa. *J Invest Dermatol*. 2016;136(5):1056-1059.
121. Hashimoto K, Matsumoto M, Iacobelli D. Transient bullous dermolysis of the newborn. *Arch Dermatol*. 1985;121:1429-1438.
122. Heinecke G, Marinkovich MP, Rieger KE. Intraepidermal type VII collagen by immunofluorescence mapping: a specific finding for bullous dermolysis of the newborn. *Pediatr Dermatol*. 2017;34(3):308-314.
123. Smith LT, Sybert VP. Intra-epidermal retention of type VII collagen in a patient with recessive dystrophic epidermolysis bullosa. *J Invest Dermatol*., 1990;94:261.
124. Cui Y, Hagan KW, Zhang S, et al. Identification and characterization of genes that are required for the accelerated degradation of mRNAs containing a premature translational termination codon. *Genes Dev*. 1995;9:423-436.
125. Uitto J, Pulkkinen L, Christiano AM. Molecular basis of the dystrophic and junctional form of epidermolysis bullosa: mutations in the type VII collagen and kalinin (laminin-5) genes. *J Invest Dermatol*. 1994;103:39S-45S.
126. Christiano AM, Anhalt G, Gibbons S, et al. Premature termination codons in the type VII collagen gene (COL7A1) underlie severe, mutilating recessive dystrophic epidermolysis bullosa. *Genomics*. 1994;21(1):160-168.
127. Siprashvili Z, Nguyen NT, Gorell ES, et al. Safety and wound outcomes following genetically corrected autologous epidermal grafts in patients with recessive dystrophic epidermolysis bullosa. *JAMA*. 2016;316(17):1808-1817.
128. Gorell ES, Nguyen N, Siprashvili Z, et al. Characterization of patients with dystrophic epidermolysis bullosa for collagen VII therapy. *Br J Dermatol*. 2015;173(3):821-823.
129. Almaani N, Liu L, Perez A, et al. Epidermolysis bullosa pruriginosa in association with lichen planopilaris. *Clin Exp Dermatol*. 2009;34(8):e825-e828.
130. Mellerio JE, Ashton GH, Mohammedi R, et al. Allelic heterogeneity of dominant and recessive COL7A1 mutations underlying epidermolysis bullosa pruriginosa. *J Invest Dermatol*. 1999;112(6):984-987.
131. Bruckner-Tuderman L, Nilssen O, Zimmermann DR, et al. Immunohistochemical and mutation analyses demonstrate that procollagen VII is processed to collagen VII through removal of the NC-2 domain. *J Cell Biol*. 1995;131(2):551-559.
132. Kindler T. Congenital poikiloderma with traumatic bulla formation and progressive cutaneous atrophy. *Br J Dermatol*. 1954;66(3):104-111.

133. Ashton G, McLean WH, South AP, et al. Recurrent mutations in kindlin-1, a novel keratinocyte focal contact protein, in the autosomal recessive skin fragility and photosensitivity disorder, Kindler syndrome. *J Invest Dermatol*. 2004;122(1):78-83.
134. Patrizi A, Pauluzzi P, Neri I, et al. Kindler syndrome: report of a case with ultrastructural study and review of the literature. *Pediatr Dermatol*. 1996;13(5):397-402.
135. Haber R, Hanna W. Kindler syndrome. Clinical and ultrastructural findings. *Arch Dermatol*. 1996;132(12):1487-1490.
136. Forman A, Prendiville JS, Esterly NB, et al. Kindler syndrome: report of two cases and review of the literature. *Pediatr Dermatol*. 1989;6(2):91-101.
137. Hovnanian A, Blanchet-Bardon C, de Prost Y. Poikiloderma of Theresa Kindler: report of a case with ultrastructural study, and review of the literature. *Pediatr Dermatol*. 1989;6(2):82-90.
138. Hacham-Zadeh S, Garfunkel A. Kindler syndrome in two related Kurdish families. *Am J Med Genet*. 1985;20(1):43-48.
139. Verret J, Avenel M, Larrègue M, et al. Kindler syndrome. Case report with ultrastructure study. *Ann Dermatol Venereol*. 1984;111(3):259-269.
140. Lai-Cheong JE, Tanaka A, Hawche G, et al. Kindler syndrome: a focal adhesion genodermatosis. *Br J Dermatol*. 2009;160(2):233-242.
141. Has C, Wessagowit V, Pascucci M, et al. Molecular basis of Kindler syndrome in Italy: novel and recurrent Alu/Alu recombination, splice site, nonsense, and frameshift mutations in the KIND1 gene. *J Invest Dermatol*. 2006;126(8):1776-1783.
142. Lanschuetzer C, Muss WH, Emberger M, et al. Gene symbol: Kind1. Disease: Kindler syndrome. *Hum Genet*. 2004;115(2):175.
143. Ashton G. Kindler syndrome. *Clin Exp Dermatol*. 2004;29(2):116-121.
144. Takeichi T, Liu L, Fong K, et al. Whole-exome sequencing improves mutation detection in a diagnostic epidermolysis bullosa laboratory. *Br J Dermatol*. 2015;172(1):94-100.
145. Fassihi H, Eady RA, Mellerio JE, et al. Prenatal diagnosis for severe inherited skin disorders: 25 years' experience. *Br J Dermatol*. 2006;154(1):106-113.
146. Marinkovich MP, Meneguzzi G, Burgeson RE, et al. Prenatal diagnosis of Herlitz junctional epidermolysis bullosa by amniocentesis. *Prenat Diagn*. 1995;15(11):1027-1034.
147. Ashton GH, Mellerio JE, Dunnill MG, et al. A recurrent laminin 5 mutation in British patients with lethal (Herlitz) junctional epidermolysis bullosa: evidence for a mutational hotspot rather than propagation of an ancestral allele. *Br J Dermatol*. 1997;136(5):674-677.
148. Cserhalmi-Friedman PB, Tang Y, Adler A, et al. Preimplantation genetic diagnosis in two families at risk for recurrence of Herlitz junctional epidermolysis bullosa. *Exp Dermatol*. 2000;9(4):290-297.
149. Kaiser J. Prenatal diagnosis. An earlier look at baby's genes. *Science*. 2005;309(5740):1476-1478.
150. Lin AN, Carter DM. Medical and surgical treatment of the skin in epidermolysis bullosa. In: Lin AN, Carter DM, eds. *Epidermolysis Bullosa—Basic and Clinical Aspects*. New York: Springer-Verlag; 1992.
151. Terrill PJ, Mayou BJ, Pemberton J. Experience in the surgical management of the hand in dystrophic epidermolysis bullosa. *Br J Plast Surg*. 1992;45(6):435-442.
152. Ladd AL, Kibele A, Gibbons S. Surgical treatment and postoperative splinting of recessive dystrophic epidermolysis bullosa. *J Hand Surg*. 1996;21(5):888-897.
153. Greider JL, Flatt AE. Surgical restoration of the hand in epidermolysis bullosa. *Arch Dermatol*. 1988;124:765-767.
154. Glicenstein J, Mariani D, Haddad R. The hand in recessive dystrophic epidermolysis bullosa. *Hand Clin*. 2000;16(4):637-645.
155. Mellerio JE, Robertson SJ, Bernardis C, et al. Management of cutaneous squamous cell carcinoma in patients with epidermolysis bullosa: best clinical practice guidelines. *Br J Dermatol*. 2016;174(1):56-67.
156. Bastin KT, Steeves RA, Richards MJ. Radiation therapy for squamous cell carcinoma in dystrophic epidermolysis bullosa: case reports and literature review. *Am J Clin Oncol*. 1997;20(1):55-58.
157. Fine J, Johnson LB, Weiner M, et al. Chemoprevention of squamous cell carcinoma in recessive dystrophic epidermolysis bullosa: results of a phase 1 trial of systemic isotretinoin. *J Am Acad Dermatol*. 2004;50(4):563-571.
158. Arnold AW, Bruckner-Tuderman L, Zuger C, et al. Cetuximab therapy of metastasizing cutaneous squamous cell carcinoma in a patient with severe recessive dystrophic epidermolysis bullosa. *Dermatology*. 2009;219(1):80-83.
159. Ergun G, Schaefer RA. Gastrointestinal aspects of epidermolysis bullosa. In: Lin AN, Carter DM, eds. *Epidermolysis Bullosa—Basic and Clinical Aspects*. New York: Springer-Verlag; 1992.
160. Haynes L, Atherton DJ, Ade-Ajayi N, et al. Gastrostomy and growth in dystrophic epidermolysis bullosa. *Br J Dermatol*. 1996;134(5):872-879.
161. Freeman EB, Köglmeier J, Martinez AE, et al. Gastrointestinal complications of epidermolysis bullosa in children. *Br J Dermatol*. 2008;158(6):1308-1314.
162. McDonnell PJ, Schofield OMV, Spalton DJ. Eye involvement in junctional epidermolysis bullosa. *Arch Ophthalmol*. 1989;107:1635-1637.
163. Tong L, Hodgkins PR, Denyer J, et al. The eye in epidermolysis bullosa. *Br J Ophthalmol*. 1999;83(3):323-326.
164. Kadyan A, Aralikatti A, Shah S, et al. Laryngo-onycho-cutaneous syndrome. *Ophthalmology*. 2010;117(5):1056-1056; e2.
165. Kirkham J, Robinson C, Strafford SM, et al. The chemical composition of tooth enamel in junctional epidermolysis bullosa. *Arch Oral Biol*. 2000;45(5):377-386.
166. Serrano Martinez C, Silvestre Donat FJ, et al. Hereditary epidermolysis bullosa. Dental management of three cases. *Med Oral*. 2001;6(1):48-56.
167. Travis SP, McGrath JA, Turnbull AJ, et al. Oral and gastrointestinal manifestation s of epidermolysis bullosa. *Lancet*. 1992;340:1505-1506.
168. Lin AN, Lateef F, Kelly R, et al. Anesthetic management in epidermolysis bullosa: review of 129 anesthetic episodes in 32 patients. *J Am Acad Dermatol*. 1994;30(3):412-416.
169. Tesi D, Lin AN. Nutritional management of the epidermolysis bullosa patient. In: Lin AN, Carter DM, eds. *Epidermolysis Bullosa—Basic and Clinical Aspects*. New York: Springer-Verlag; 1992.
170. Hubbard L, Haynes L, Sklar M, et al. The challenges of meeting nutritional requirements in children and adults with epidermolysis bullosa: proceedings of a multidisciplinary team study day. *Clin Exp Dermatol*. 2011;36(6):579-583; quiz 583-584.

171. Fridge JL, Vichinsky EP. Correction of the anemia of epidermolysis bullosa with intravenous iron and erythropoietin. *J Pediatr*. 1998;132(5):871-873.
172. Lara-Corrales I, Mellerio JE, Martinez AE, et al. Dilated cardiomyopathy in epidermolysis bullosa: a retrospective, multicenter study. *Pediatr Dermatol*. 2010;27(3):238-243.
173. Dietz M. A day in the life of a patient with DDEB. *J Am Acad Dermatol*. 2004;51(1 suppl):S58-S59.
174. Goldschneider KR, Lucky AW. Pain management in epidermolysis bullosa. *Dermatol Clin*. 2010;28(2):273-282, ix.
175. Tabolli S, Sampogna F, Di Pietro C, et al. Quality of life in patients with epidermolysis bullosa. *Br J Dermatol*. 2009;161(4):869-877.
176. Schomer H, Vergunst R. Psychological factors in epidermolysis bullosa. *S Afr Med J*. 1992;81(11):580.
177. Moss K. Contact at the borderline: psychoanalytic psychotherapy with EB patients. *Br J Nurs*. 2008;17(7):449-455.
178. Lansdown R, Atherton D, Dale A, et al. Practical and psychological problems for parents of children with epidermolysis bullosa. *Child Care Health Dev*. 1986;12(4):251-256.
179. Fine JD, Johnson LB, Weiner M, et al. Impact of inherited epidermolysis bullosa on parental interpersonal relationships, marital status and family size. *Br J Dermatol*. 2005;152(5):1009-1014.
180. Caldwell-Brown D, Stern RS, Lin AN, et al. Lack of efficacy of phenytoin in recessive dystrophic epidermolysis bullosa. Epidermolysis Bullosa Study Group. *N Engl J Med*. 1992;327(3):163-167.
181. Wally V, Lettner T, Peking P, et al. The pathogenetic role of IL-1beta in severe epidermolysis bullosa simplex. *J Invest Dermatol*. 2013;133(7):1901-1903.
182. Wally V, Kitzmueller S, Lagler F, et al. Topical diacerein for epidermolysis bullosa: a randomized controlled pilot study. *Orphanet J Rare Dis*. 2013;8:69.
183. Nystrom A, Thriene K, Mittapalli V, et al. Losartan ameliorates dystrophic epidermolysis bullosa and uncovers new disease mechanisms. *EMBO Mol Med*. 2015;7(9):1211-1228.
184. Falabella AF, Valencia IC, Eaglstein WH, et al. Tissue-engineered skin (Apligraf) in the healing of patients with epidermolysis bullosa wounds. *Arch Dermatol*. 2000;136(10):1225-1230.
185. Petrof G, Martinez-Queipo M, Mellerio JE, et al. Fibroblast cell therapy enhances initial healing in recessive dystrophic epidermolysis bullosa wounds: results of a randomized, vehicle-controlled trial. *Br J Dermatol*. 2013;169(5):1025-1033.
186. Venugopal SS, Yan W, Frew JW, et al. A phase II randomized vehicle-controlled trial of intradermal allogeneic fibroblasts for recessive dystrophic epidermolysis bullosa. *J Am Acad Dermatol*. 2013;69(6):898-908; e7.
187. Petrof G, Lwin SM, Martinez-Queipo M, et al. Potential of systemic allogeneic mesenchymal stromal cell therapy for children with recessive dystrophic epidermolysis bullosa. *J Invest Dermatol*. 2015;135(9):2319-2321.
188. Wagner JE, Ishida-Yamamoto A, McGrath JA, et al. Bone marrow transplantation for recessive dystrophic epidermolysis bullosa. *N Engl J Med*. 2010;363(7):629-639.
189. Mavilio F, Pellegrini G, Ferrari S, et al. Correction of junctional epidermolysis bullosa by transplantation of genetically modified epidermal stem cells. *Nat Med*. 2006;12(12):1397-1402.
190. De Rosa L, Carulli S, Cocchiarella F, et al. Long-term stability and safety of transgenic cultured epidermal stem cells in gene therapy of junctional epidermolysis bullosa. *Stem Cell Reports*. 2014;2(1):1-8.
191. Hirsch T, Rothoeft T, Teig N, et al. Regeneration of the entire human epidermis using transgenic stem cells. *Nature*. 2017;551(7680):327-332.
192. Hainzl S, Peking P, Kocher T, et al. COL7A1 Editing via CRISPR/Cas9 in recessive dystrophic epidermolysis bullosa. *Mol Ther*. 2017;25(11):2573-2584.
193. Webber BR, Osborn M, McElroy AN, et al. CRISPR/Cas9-based genetic correction for recessive dystrophic epidermolysis bullosa. *NPJ Regen Med*. 2016;1.
194. Sebastiano V, Zhen HH, Haddad B, et al. Human COL7A1-corrected induced pluripotent stem cells for the treatment of recessive dystrophic epidermolysis bullosa. *Sci Transl Med*. 2014;6(264):264ra163.
195. Kowalewski C, Bremer J, Gostynski A, et al. Amelioration of junctional epidermolysis bullosa due to exon skipping. *Br J Dermatol*. 2016;174(6):1375-1379.
196. Bornert O, Kühl T, Bremer J, et al. Analysis of the functional consequences of targeted exon deletion in COL7A1 reveals prospects for dystrophic epidermolysis bullosa therapy. *Mol Ther*. 2016;24(7):1302-1311.
197. Schwieger-Briel A, Weibel L, Chmel N, et al. A COL7A1 variant leading to in-frame skipping of exon 15 attenuates disease severity in recessive dystrophic epidermolysis bullosa. *Br J Dermatol*. 2015;173(5):1308-1311.
198. Kiritsi D, Garcia M, Brander R, et al. Mechanisms of natural gene therapy in dystrophic epidermolysis bullosa. *J Invest Dermatol*. 2014;134(8):2097-2104.

Autoimmune Connective Tissue and Rheumatologic Disorders

PART 10

第十篇 自身免疫结缔组织病和风湿病

Chapter 61 :: Lupus Erythematosus
:: Clayton J. Sontheimer, Melissa I. Costner, & Richard D. Sontheimer

第六十一章
红斑狼疮

中文导读

红斑狼疮（LE）是一组对自身核酸及相关蛋白发生免疫反应的异质性疾病，病谱的一端只累及皮肤，而另一端可以引起严重的内脏损害。本章从流行病学、病因学和发病机制、临床症状、诊断标准、鉴别诊断、疾病进程及预后、疾病治疗及管理等七个方面全面阐述了红斑狼疮各型的特点。LE特异性皮肤病的发病机制与SLE的发病机制密不可分。强调了识别LE特异性皮损的重要性，LE的皮损特点可以反应SLE潜在的活动性。急性、亚急性和慢性皮肤型红斑狼疮与发病时间无关而与疾病的病程和严重程度及与是否发展为SLE相关。分别对于ACLE，SCLE，CCLE包括经典型DLE，肥厚型DLE，黏膜DLE，深在性LE/狼疮性脂膜炎，冻疮样狼疮，肿胀型红斑狼疮等的临床特点、好发年龄、好发部位等进行了详细的描述；提及了罕见变体如肥厚性红斑狼疮、苔藓样红斑狼疮、毛细血管扩张性红斑狼疮、线状红斑狼疮和水肿性红斑狼疮及非特异性皮损；并从实验室检查、组织病理、免疫组织病理等方面就各型红斑狼疮对应的特点进行了详细的阐述。列举了需要与皮肤红斑狼疮相鉴别的皮肤疾病，包括临床表现非常相似，需要考虑及通常需要排除的皮肤病。并综述了各型CLE的疾病进程与预后，最后从健康教育、局部治疗用药、全身治疗、外科及美容治疗等多维度阐述了CLE治疗用药的阶梯选择。

〔施 为〕

AT-A-GLANCE

- A group of heterogeneous illnesses that have in common the development of immunity to self-nucleic acids and their associated proteins, with skin-only disease at one end of the spectrum and severe visceral involvement at the other.

- Skin lesions may be specific to lupus or nonspecific, being seen in other conditions as well.

- Acute cutaneous lupus erythematosus (malar rash) is almost always associated with underlying visceral involvement. Subacute cutaneous lupus patients meet American College of Rheumatology systemic lupus erythematosus criteria approximately 50% of the time (but typically express only mild systemic clinical manifestations). Chronic cutaneous lupus (classic discoid lupus erythematosus, lupus panniculitis, chilblain lupus, and tumid lupus erythematosus) patients most often have skin-only or skin-predominant disease.

- Classical discoid lupus erythematosus causes scarring and can be permanently disfiguring.

- Subacute cutaneous lupus and acute cutaneous lupus erythematosus are highly photosensitive and are characteristically nonscarring.

- Lupus erythematosus–nonspecific skin lesions include nonscarring alopecia, mouth ulcers, photosensitivity, Raynaud phenomenon, vasculitis/vasculopathy, and bullous systemic lupus erythematosus, among others. They often herald a systemic lupus erythematosus flare.

- Treatment consists of physical sun protection, topical sunscreens, local and short-term systemic glucocorticoids, antimalarials, retinoids, thalidomide/lenalidomide, conventional immunosuppressives, and biologic therapies.

- Lupus erythematosus occurs much more commonly in women (9:1 female-to-male ratio).

- Both systemic lupus erythematosus and cutaneous lupus erythematosus are associated with upregulation of type 1 interferon signaling.

Lupus erythematosus (LE) is the root designation for a diverse array of clinical illnesses that are linked together by the development of autoimmunity directed predominantly at the molecular constituents of nucleosomes and ribonucleoproteins. Some patients present with life-threatening manifestations of systemic LE (SLE), whereas others, who are affected with what represents the same basic underlying disease process, express little more than isolated discoid LE (DLE) skin lesions throughout their illness. It is convenient to conceptualize LE as a clinical spectrum (Fig. 61-1) ranging from mildly affected patients with only localized DLE skin lesions to those at risk of dying from the systemic manifestations of LE such as nephritis, CNS disease, or vasculitis. The pattern of skin involvement expressed by an individual patient with LE can provide insight about the position on the spectrum where the patient's illness might best be placed.

The nomenclature and classification system originally devised by James N. Gilliam divides the cutaneous manifestations of LE into those lesions that show characteristic histologic changes of LE (LE-specific skin disease; ie, an interface dermatitis) and those that are not histopathologically distinct for LE and/or may be seen as a feature of another disease processes (LE-nonspecific skin disease).[1] Within this context, the term *LE-specific* relates to those lesions displaying an interface dermatitis. The term *cutaneous LE* (CLE) is often used synonymously with "LE-specific skin disease" as an umbrella designation for the 3 major categories of LE-specific skin disease: acute cutaneous LE (ACLE), subacute cutaneous LE (SCLE), and chronic cutaneous LE (CCLE). This will be the framework used in our discussion of the extraordinarily diverse set of cutaneous lesions that occur in patients with LE (Table 61-1).

The essence of LE is in its heterogeneity, and the challenge for those who treat it is to recognize clinically useful patterns within the mosaic of features that constitute this protean illness. An overview of the systemic manifestations of LE can be seen in the American College of Rheumatology's (ACR) classification criteria for SLE,[2] which are presented in Table 61-2,

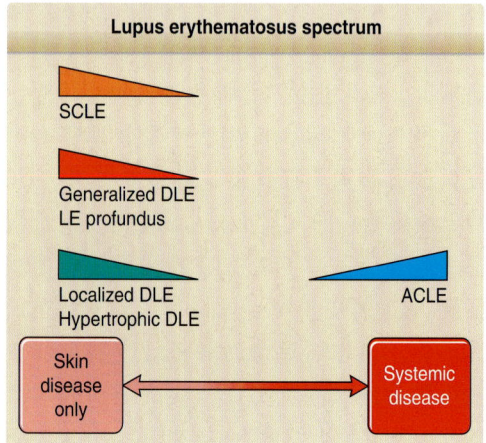

Figure 61-1 Spectrum of disease: local involvement to systemic disease. ACLE, acute cutaneous lupus erythematosus; DLE, discoid lupus erythematosus; LE, lupus erythematosus; SLE, systemic lupus erythematosus.

and from the outline of the systemic manifestations of SLE presented in Table 61-3.

EPIDEMIOLOGY

The epidemiology and socioeconomic impact of LE in general,[3] and CLE specifically,[4] have been reviewed.

TABLE 61-1
The Gilliam Classification of Skin Lesions Associated with Lupus Erythematosus

LE-SPECIFIC SKIN DISEASE (CUTANEOUS LE/CLE)	LE-NONSPECIFIC SKIN DISEASE

A. ACLE
  1. Localized ACLE (malar rash, butterfly rash)
  2. Generalized ACLE (lupus maculopapular lupus rash, SLE rash, rash, photosensitive lupus dermatitis)
    a. TEN-like ACLE
B. SCLE
  1. Annular SCLE (syn. Lupus marginatus, symmetric erythema centrifugum, autoimmune annular erythema, lupus erythematosus gyrates repens)
  2. Papulosquamous SCLE (syn. Disseminated DLE, subacute disseminated LE, superficial disseminated LE, psoriasiform LE, pityriasiform LE, maculopapular photosensitive LE)
C. CCLE
  1. Classic DLE
    a. Localized DLE
    b. Generalized DLE
  2. Hypertrophic/verrucous DLE
  3. Lupus profundus/lupus panniculitis
  4. Mucosal DLE
  5. Oral DLE
  6. Conjunctival DLE
  7. Lupus tumidus (urticarial plaque phase of LE)
  8. Chilblain LE (chilblain lupus, perniotic lupus)
  9. Lichenoid DLE (LE/lichen planus overlap, lupus planus)
	A. Cutaneous vascular disease
	  1. Vasculitis
	    a. Leukocytoclastic
	      i. Palpable purpura
	      ii. Urticarial vasculitis
	    b. Polyarteritis nodosa-like cutaneous lesions
	  2. Vasculopathy
	    a. Degos disease-like lesions
	    b. Secondary atrophie blanche (syn. livedoid vasculitis, livedo vasculitis)
	  3. Periungual telangiectasia
	  4. Livedo reticularis
	  5. Thrombophlebitis
	  6. Raynaud phenomenon
	  7. Erythromelalgia
	B. Nonscarring alopecia
	  1. "Lupus hair"
	  2. Telogen effluvium
	  3. Alopecia areata
	C. Sclerodactyly
	D. Rheumatoid nodules
	E. Calcinosis cutis
	F. LE-nonspecific bullous lesions
	G. Urticaria
	H. Papulonodular mucinosis
	I. Cutis laxa/anetoderma
	J. Acanthosis nigricans
	K. Erythema multiforme (syn. Rowell syndrome)
	L. Leg ulcers
	M. Lichen planus

ACLE, acute cutaneous lupus erythematosus; CCLE, chronic cutaneous lupus erythematosus; DLE, discoid lupus erythematosus; LE, lupus erythematosus; SCLE, subacute cutaneous lupus erythematosus; SLE, systemic lupus erythematosus; TEN, toxic epidermal necrolysis.

Adapted from Sontheimer RD. The lexicon of cutaneous lupus erythematosus—a review and personal perspective on the nomenclature and classification of the cutaneous manifestations of lupus erythematosus. *Lupus*. 1997;6(2):84-95. Copyright © Stockton Press. Reprinted with permission of SAGE Publications.

Skin disease is the second most frequent clinical manifestation of LE after joint inflammation. As many as 45% of patients with CLE experience some degree of vocational handicap. Recent quality-of-life studies suggested that the impact of skin manifestations in patients with SLE was preceded only by pain and fatigue related to their disease.[5] The Dermatology Life Quality Index and SF-36 have been used to measure quality of life in patients with CLE. Both questionnaires showed that patients with active skin lesions had lower quality of life and that patients with associated alopecia were particularly impacted.[6]

Malar, or butterfly rash (localized ACLE), has been reported in 20% to 60% of large cohorts of patients with LE. Limited data suggest that the maculopapular or SLE rash of generalized ACLE is present in approximately 35% to 60% of patients with SLE. ACLE, like SLE in general, is 8 times more common in women than men. All races are affected; however, the early clinical manifestations of ACLE can be overlooked in a dark-skinned individual.

Patients presenting with SCLE lesions constitute 7% to 27% of LE patient populations. SCLE is primarily a disease of white females, with the mean age of onset being in the fifth decade. Drug-induced SCLE patients are somewhat older at disease onset, perhaps reflecting greater exposure to drugs for age-related medical problems (hypertension, cardiovascular disease).

The most common form of CCLE, a classic DLE skin lesion, is present in 15% to 30% of SLE populations selected in various ways. Approximately 5% of patients presenting with isolated localized DLE subsequently develop SLE. Published population-based data have argued strongly that the incidence and prevalence of isolated forms of CLE are equivalent to those of SLE.[7] Although DLE can occur in infants and the elderly, it is most common in individuals between 20 and 40 years of age. DLE has a female-to-male ratio of 3:2 to 3:1, which is much lower than that of SLE. All races are affected, but investigations suggest that DLE might be more prevalent in blacks.

ETIOLOGY AND PATHOGENESIS

The cause(s) of and pathogenic mechanisms responsible for LE-specific skin disease are not fully understood, although recent work has provided many new insights. The pathogenesis of LE-specific skin disease is inextricably intertwined with SLE pathogenesis. Simply put, SLE is a disorder in which the interplay between host factors (susceptibility genes, hormonal milieu, etc) and environmental factors (ultraviolet [UV] radiation, viruses, and drugs) leads to loss of self-tolerance, and induction of autoimmunity. This is followed by activation and expansion of the immune system, and eventuates in immunologic injury to end organs and clinical expression of disease.[8] Recent work highlights the important role of interferon-α signaling in the pathogenesis of both SLE and LE-specific skin disease.

TABLE 61-2
The 1982 Revised Criteria for Classification of Systemic Lupus Erythematosus[a]

CRITERION	DEFINITION
1. Malar rash	Fixed erythema, flat or raised, over the malar eminences, tending to spare the nasolabial folds
2. Discoid rash	Erythematous raised patches with adherent keratotic scaling and follicular plugging; atrophic scarring may occur in older lesions
3. Photosensitivity	Skin rash as a result of unusual reaction to sunlight, by patient history or physician observation
4. Oral ulcers	Oral or nasopharyngeal ulceration, usually painless, observed by a physician
5. Arthritis	Nonerosive arthritis involving 2 or more peripheral joints, characterized by tenderness, swelling, or effusion
6. Serositis	a. Pleuritis—convincing history of pleuritic pain or rub heard by a physician or evidence of pleural effusion
	or
	b. Pericarditis—documented by electrocardiogram or rub or evidence of pericardial effusion
7. Renal disorder	a. Persistent proteinuria— >0.5 g/day or greater than 3+ if quantitation not performed
	or
	b. Cellular casts—may be red cell, hemoglobin, granular, tubular, or mixed
8. Neurologic disorder	a. Seizures—in the absence of offending drugs or known metabolic derangements (eg, uremia, ketoacidosis, or electrolyte imbalance)
	or
	b. Psychosis—in the absence of offending drugs or known metabolic derangements (eg, uremia, ketoacidosis, or electrolyte imbalance)
9. Hematologic disorder	a. Hemolytic anemia—with reticulocytosis
	or
	b. Leukopenia— <4000 µL total on 2 or more occasions
	or
	c. Lymphopenia— <1500/µL on 2 or more occasions
	or
	d. Thrombocytopenia— <100,000 µL in the absence of offending drugs
10. Immunologic disorder	a. Anti-DNA—antibody to native DNA in abnormal titer
	or
	b. Anti–Smith antigen—presence of antibody to Smith nuclear antigen
	or
	c. Positive finding of antiphospholipid antibodies based on (1) an abnormal serum level of immunoglobulin G or immunoglobulin M anticardiolipin antibodies, (2) a positive test result for lupus anticoagulant using a standard method, or (3) a false-positive serologic test for syphilis known to be positive for at least 6 months and confirmed by *Treponema pallidum* immobilization or fluorescent treponemal antibody absorption test
11. Antinuclear antibody	An abnormal titer of antinuclear antibody by immunofluorescence of an equivalent assay at any point in time and in the absence of drugs known to be associated with "drug-induced lupus" syndrome

[a]The proposed classification is based on 11 criteria. For the purpose of identifying patients in clinical studies, a person shall be said to have systemic lupus erythematosus if any 4 or more of the 11 criteria are present, serially or simultaneously, during any interval or observation.

From Tan EM, Cohen AS, Fries JF, et al. The 1982 revised criteria for the classification of systemic lupus erythematosus. *Arthritis Rheum*. 1982;25(11): 1271-1277, copyright 1982, with permission of the American College of Rheumatology.

IMMUNOLOGIC FACTORS

Multiple studies highlight the important role of plasmacytoid dendritic cells (PDCs) and type 1 interferon (IFN) signaling, comprised of interferon-α and interferon-β, in the pathogenesis of both SLE and LE-specific skin disease. type 1 IFN is the most upregulated gene pathway identified in microarray studies in SLE patients, and increased type 1 IFN has been seen in the blood and skin of patients with CLE.[9,10]

Large numbers of PDCs are present in skin lesions of patients with CLE.[11] PDCs produce large amounts of type 1 IFN in response to DNA and RNA stimulation through toll-like receptors 7 and 9. In healthy state conditions, PDCs recognize viral DNA and RNA and not self-DNA; however, immune complexes generated by autoantibody binding of DNA and RNA from apoptotic cells are recognized by PDCs and lead to activation and production of type 1 IFN. Chronic type 1 IFN, in turn, promotes loss of tolerance in SLE through its actions of B and T cells.[12,13]

TABLE 61-3
Overview of the Extracutaneous Manifestations of Systemic Lupus Erythematosus

- General
  - Fever, fatigue, malaise, weight loss
  - Alopecia
- Musculoskeletal
  - Arthralgia, arthritis, morning stiffness
  - Myalgia, myositis
  - Avascular necrosis
- Hematologic
  - Anemia
    - Anemia of chronic disease (normocytic)
    - Autoimmune hemolytic anemia (Coombs positive)
  - Leukopenia, lymphopenia, neutropenia
  - Thrombocytopenia
  - Antiphospholipid syndrome, thrombosis (thrombophlebitis, deep vein thrombosis)
- Cardiopulmonary
  - Pleurisy, pleural effusion, aseptic pneumonitis, pulmonary hemorrhage, Interstitial lung disease, pulmonary embolism, coronary artery disease
  - Chest pain, pericarditis, myocarditis Libman-Sacks endocarditis
- Renal
  - Membranoproliferative glomerulonephritis (World Health Organization [WHO] classes II-IV)
    - Proteinuria, hematuria, red blood cell casts
  - Membranous glomerulonephritis (WHO class V)
    - Severe proteinuria, nephrotic syndrome
- Neuropsychiatric
  - Peripheral neuropathy, transverse myelitis, Guillain-Barré syndrome
  - Chorea, choreoathetosis
  - Seizures
  - Headaches
  - Acute confusional state, psychosis
  - Cognitive dysfunction
  - Aseptic meningitis
- GI
  - Anorexia, nausea, vomiting, abdominal pain
  - Hepatitis, hepatomegaly
  - Pancreatitis
  - Mesenteric vasculitis
  - Protein-losing enteropathy
- Ocular
  - Retinal vascular disease, optic neuropathy
  - Conjunctivitis, episcleritis
  - Dry eyes, keratitis
- Nasooral
  - Palatal ulceration
  - Sicca syndrome, secondary Sjögren Syndrome
- Lymphatic system
  - Lymphadenopathy
  - Splenomegaly

Recent work has identified a separate DNA-sensing and RNA-sensing pathway, termed the *immunostimulatory DNA pathway*, that is active within the cytoplasm in contrast to endosomal toll-like receptors. Monogenetic syndrome caused by mutations in immunostimulatory DNA pathway genes, as seen in Aicardi-Goutières syndrome and SAVI, result in upregulated immunostimulatory DNA pathway activity and chronic IFN-β production, and share many features with spontaneous LE.[14] Single-nucleotide polymorphisms in immunostimulatory DNA pathway genes are associated with CLE and SLE.[15] Insights from these diseases, termed *interferonopathies*, further support the role for inappropriate type 1 IFN activity, whether IFN-α or IFN-β, as a proximal and driving event in lupus pathogenesis.

ENVIRONMENTAL FACTORS

Genetic predisposition for a lupus diathesis does not, in itself, produce disease. Rather, it appears that induction of autoimmunity in such patients is triggered by some inciting event, likely an environmental exposure. Drugs, viruses, UV light, and, possibly, tobacco induce development of SLE.

UV radiation is probably the most important environmental factor in the induction phase of SLE, especially of LE-specific skin disease. UV light likely leads to self-immunity and loss of tolerance because it causes apoptosis of keratinocytes, which in turn, makes previously cryptic peptides available for immunosurveillance. UVB radiation displaces autoantigens such as Ro/SS-A and related autoantigens, La/SS-B, and calreticulin, from their normal locations inside epidermal keratinocytes to the cell surface.[16] UVB irradiation induces the release of CCL27 (cutaneous T cell-attracting chemokine), which upregulates the expression of chemokines that activate autoreactive T cells and type 1 IFN, producing dendritic cells, which likely play a central role in lupus pathogenesis.[17,18]

A recent, large, case-control study reported that smokers are at a greater risk of developing SLE than are nonsmokers and former smokers. A cross-sectional analysis of a collaborative Web-based database established by Werth and colleagues documented that patients with treatment-resistant CLE were much more likely to smoke.[19] Several authors have shown that patients with LE-specific skin disease who smoke are less responsive to antimalarial treatment.[20-22]

Numerous drugs are implicated in inducing various features of SLE (Table 61-4). The drugs that induce CLE can be linked by their photosensitizing properties. It is suggested that these drugs cause an increase in keratinocyte apoptosis, exposure of previously intracellular peptides on epidermal cell surfaces, and enhance proinflammatory cytokines such as tumor necrosis factor (TNF)-α and type 1 IFN.[23,24]

There is much speculation about the role of infectious agents, particularly viruses, in the induction of SLE and CLE. Seroconversion to Epstein-Barr virus among patients with SLE is nearly universal, and recent data demonstrate that patients with SLE have defective control of latent Epstein-Barr virus infection that probably stems from altered T-cell responses against Epstein-Barr virus.

TABLE 61-4
Causes of Drug-Induced Lupus

Drug-Induced Subacute Cutaneous Lupus Erythematosus

Antacids[a]
  Protein pump inhibitors (esomeprazole, lansoprazole, omeprazole, pantoprazole)

Antibiotics (Amoxicillin/clavulanic acid, doxycycline, minocycline, nitrofurantoin, norfloxacin)

Anticonvulsants/antiepileptics (carbamazepine, phenytoin, lamotrigine)

Antifungals[a] (griseofulvin, terbinafine)

Antihistamines (brompheniramine, ranitidine)

Antiinflammatory
  Nonsteroidal antiinflammatories (naproxen, piroxicam)

Immunomodulators (hydroxychloroquine, imiquimod, interferon-α, interferon-β, leflunomide)

Biologics[a] (adalimumab, bevacizumab, efalizumab, etanercept, golimumab, infliximab, ranibizumab, rituximab)

Cardiovascular
  Antihypertensives
    Angiotensin-converting enzyme (ACE) inhibitors (captopril, cilazapril, enalapril, lisinopril, ramipril)
    ACEII receptor antagonists (losartan)
    Beta blockers (acebutolol, oxypurinol)
    Calcium channel blockers (amlodipine, diltiazem, nifedipine, nitrendipine, verapamil)
    Diuretics (chlorothiazide, hydrochlorothiazide, hydrochlorothiazide/triamterene)
  Statins (pravastatin, simvastatin)

Chemotherapeutic[a] (capecitabine, docetaxel, doxorubicin, doxorubicin/cyclophosphamide, fluorouracil, gemcitabine, mitotane, paclitaxel, pazopanib, pemetrexed/carboplatin, tamoxifen)

Hormone-altering (anastrozole, leuprorelin)

Ultraviolet therapy (psoralen and ultraviolet A [PUVA])

Others (allopurinol, amiodarone, bupropion, citalopram, iodine-131, torsemide, tiotropium, ticlopidine)

Drug-Induced Systemic Lupus Erythematosus (Typically without Skin Involvement)

Antihyperlipidemic agents
Anti–tumor necrosis factor biologics
Hydralazine
Isoniazid
Minocycline
Procainamide

[a]Indicates most commonly imputed drug classes. Imputed drugs are listed alphabetically by class.
Data summarized from Michaelis TC, Sontheimer RD, Lowe GC. An update in drug-induced subacute cutaneous lupus erythematosus. *Dermatol Online J.* 2017;23(3).

CLINICAL FINDINGS

It is important to distinguish among the subtypes of LE-specific skin disease, because the type of skin involvement in LE can reflect the underlying pattern of SLE activity. In fact, the designations acute, subacute, and chronic, in regard to CLE, refer to the pace and severity of any associated SLE and are not necessarily related to how long individual lesions have been present. For example, ACLE almost always occurs in the setting of acutely flaring SLE, whereas CCLE often occurs in the absence of SLE or in the presence of mild, smoldering SLE. SCLE occupies an intermediate position in this clinical spectrum. Subclassification, although important for assigning risk, is sometimes difficult, as it is not uncommon to see more than 1 subtype of LE-specific skin disease in the same patient, especially in patients with SLE.

ACUTE CUTANEOUS LUPUS ERYTHEMATOSUS

Although ACLE localized to the face is the usual pattern of presentation, ACLE can assume a generalized distribution. Localized ACLE has commonly been referred to as the *classic butterfly rash* or *malar rash of SLE* (Fig. 61-2). In localized ACLE, confluent symmetric erythema and edema are centered over the malar eminences and bridges over the nose (unilateral involvement with ACLE has been described). The nasolabial folds are characteristically spared. The forehead, chin, and V area of the neck can be involved, and severe facial swelling may occur. Occasionally, ACLE begins as small macules and/or papules on the face that later may become confluent and hyperkeratotic. Generalized ACLE presents as a widespread morbilliform or exanthematous eruption often focused over the extensor aspects of the arms and hands and characteristically sparing the knuckles (Fig. 61-3A). Although perivascular nail fold erythema and telangiectasia can occur (Fig. 61-3B), they are considerably more common and occur in more exaggerated forms in dermatomyositis and systemic sclerosis. Generalized ACLE has been indiscriminately referred to as

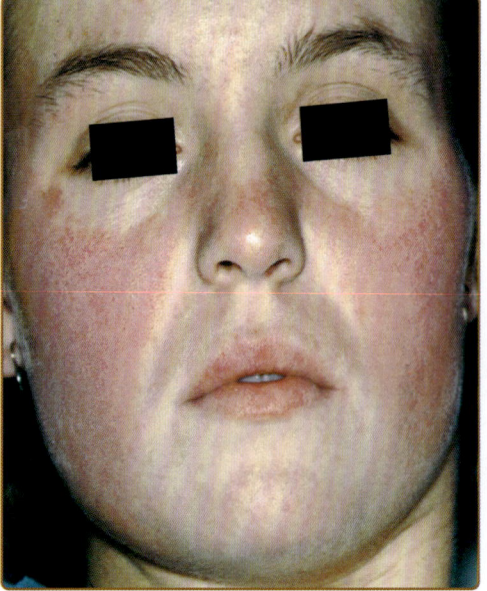

Figure 61-2 Localized acute cutaneous lupus erythematosus. Erythematous, slightly edematous, sharply demarcated erythema is seen on the malar areas in a "butterfly" distribution.

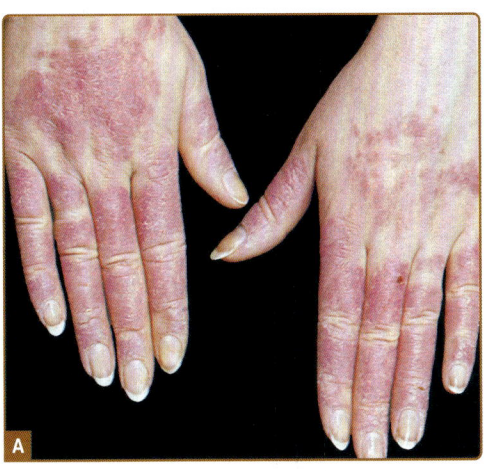
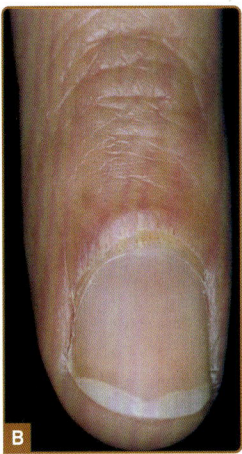

Figure 61-3 Generalized acute cutaneous lupus erythematosus. **A,** Well-demarcated patches of erythema with fine overlying scale on the dorsal aspect of the hands, fingers, and periungual areas. Note the characteristic sparing of the knuckles, which are preferentially involved in dermatomyositis. **B,** Closeup view of periungual erythema and grossly visible telangiectasia. Although these lesions can be seen in lupus erythematosus, they are much more typical of dermatomyositis.

the *maculopapular rash of SLE*, *photosensitive lupus dermatitis*, and *SLE rash*. An extremely acute form of ACLE is rarely seen that can simulate toxic epidermal necrolysis (TEN; Fig. 61-4). This form of LE-specific vesiculobullous disease results from widespread apoptosis of epidermal keratinocytes, and eventuates in areas of full-thickness epidermal skin necrosis, which is subsequently denuded. ACLE can be differentiated from true TEN because it occurs on predominantly sun-exposed skin and has a more insidious onset. The mucosa may or may not be involved, as in TEN.

ACLE is typically precipitated or exacerbated by exposure to UV light. This form of CLE can be quite ephemeral, lasting only hours, days, or weeks; however, some patients experience more prolonged periods of activity. Postinflammatory pigmentary change is most prominent in patients with heavily pigmented skin. Atrophic scarring does not occur in ACLE unless the process is complicated by secondary bacterial infection.

SUBACUTE CUTANEOUS LUPUS ERYTHEMATOSUS

The presence of SCLE skin lesions was first characterized as a distinctive immunogenetic subset of LE in 1979.[25] A disease presentation dominated by SCLE lesions marks the presence of a distinct subset of LE having characteristic clinical, serologic, and genetic features. Although a finding of circulating autoantibodies to the Ro/SS-A ribonucleoprotein particle strongly supports a diagnosis of SCLE, the presence of this autoantibody specificity is not required to make a diagnosis of SCLE.

SCLE initially presents as erythematous macules and/or papules that evolve into hyperkeratotic papulosquamous or annular/polycyclic plaques (Fig. 61-5). Whereas most patients have either annular or papulosquamous SCLE, a few develop elements of both morphologic varieties. SCLE lesions are characteristically photosensitive and occur in predominantly sun-exposed areas (ie, upper back, shoulders, extensor aspects of the arms, V area of the neck, and, less commonly, the face). SCLE lesions typically heal without scarring but can resolve with long-lasting, if not permanent, vitiligo-like leukoderma, and telangiectasias.

Several variants of SCLE have been described. On occasion, SCLE lesions present initially with an appearance of erythema multiforme. Such cases are similar to Rowell syndrome (erythema multiforme–like lesions occurring in patients with SLE in the presence of La/SS-B autoantibodies). As a result of intense injury to epidermal basal cells, the active edge of an annular SCLE lesion occasionally undergoes a vesiculobullous change that can subsequently produce a strikingly crusted appearance. Such lesions can mimic Stevens-Johnson syndrome/TEN. Pathogenesis is similar to that described above for TEN-like ACLE. Rarely, SCLE presents with exfoliative erythroderma or displays a curious acral distribution of annular lesions. Pityriasiform and exanthematous variants of SCLE have been reported. The skin lesions of neonatal LE (transient, photosensitive, nonscarring LE-specific skin lesions in neonates who have received immunoglobulin (Ig) G anti-Ro/SS-A, and, occasionally, other autoantibody specificities transplacentally) share many features with SCLE.

Unlike ACLE skin lesions, SCLE lesions tend to be less transient than ACLE lesions and heal with more pigmentary change. They are also less edematous and more hyperkeratotic than ACLE lesions. SCLE more commonly involves the neck, shoulders, upper extremities, and trunk, whereas ACLE more commonly affects the malar areas of the face. When the face is involved with SCLE, it is most often the lateral face, with sparing of the central, malar regions. In comparison to SCLE lesions, DLE lesions are generally associ-

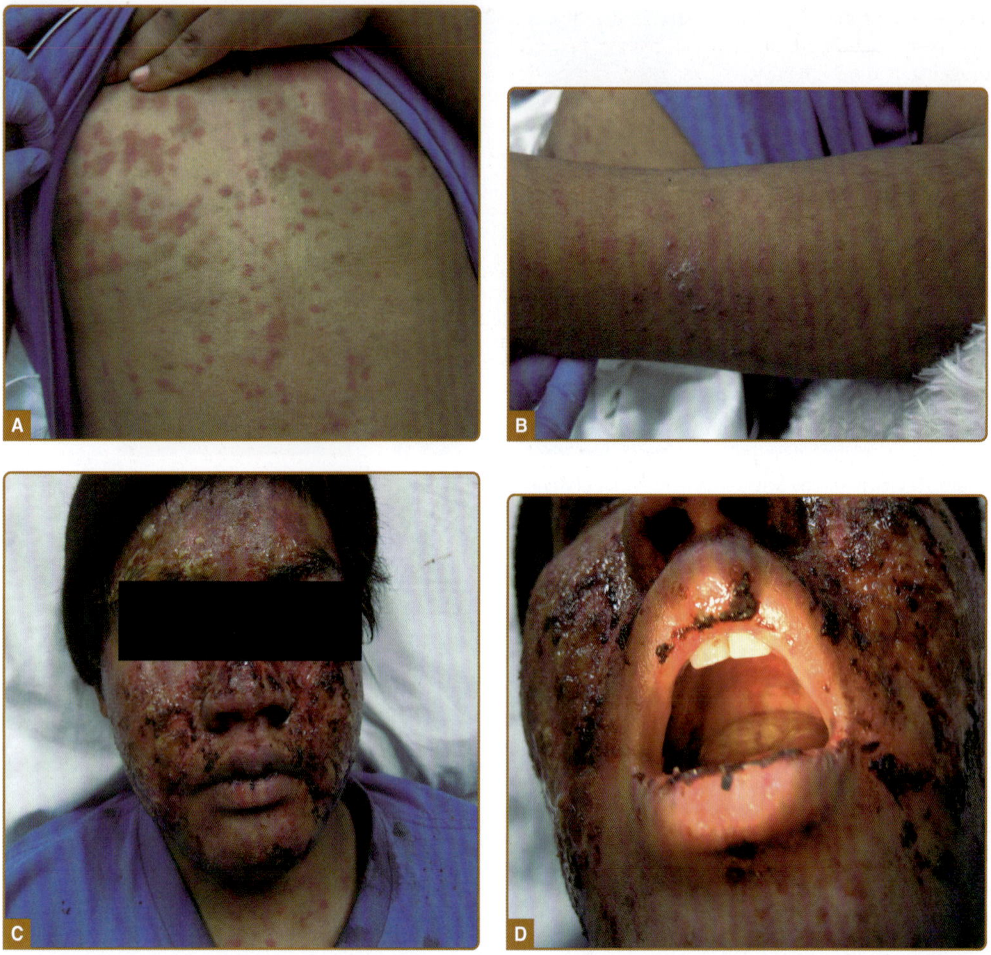

Figure 61-4 Toxic epidermal necrolysis (TEN)-like acute cutaneous lupus in a 16-year-old boy. **A,** Widespread erythematous papules with vesiculobullous changes over the trunk. **B,** Similar changes over the arm. **C,** Severe epidermal loss and denuding over the face in a 16-year-old boy. **D,** Painless palatal ulceration characteristic of systemic lupus erythematosus was present as opposed to severe mucosal involvement of TEN.

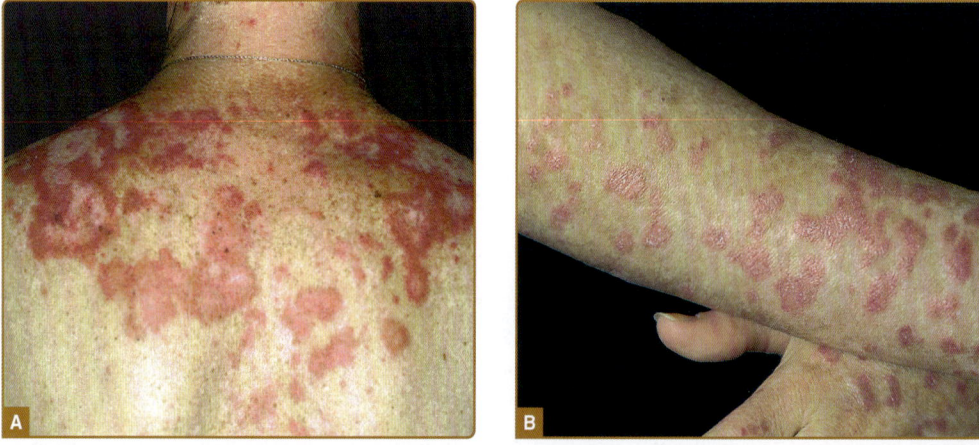

Figure 61-5 Subacute cutaneous lupus erythematosus (SCLE). **A,** Annular SCLE on the upper back of a 38-year-old woman. Note the central areas of hypopigmentation in which no dermal atrophy is present. **B,** Papulosquamous SCLE over the extensor aspect of the forearm of a 26-year-old woman.

ated with a greater degree of hyperpigmentation and hypopigmentation, atrophic dermal scarring, follicular plugging, and adherent scale. A consistent clinical difference is that DLE lesions are characteristically indurated, whereas SCLE lesions are not; this difference reflects the greater depth of inflammation seen histopathologically in DLE lesions.

Approximately one-half of patients with SCLE meet the ACR's revised criteria for the classification of SLE. However, manifestations of severe SLE, such as nephritis, CNS disease, and systemic vasculitis, develop in only 10% to 15% of patients with SCLE. It has been suggested that the papulosquamous type of SCLE, leukopenia, high titer of antinuclear antibody (ANA) (>1:640), and anti–double-stranded DNA (dsDNA) antibodies are risk factors for the development of SLE in a patient presenting with SCLE lesions.

SCLE can overlap with other autoimmune diseases that share the 8.1 ancestral haplotype (human leukocyte antigen A1-B8-DR3-DQ2), including Sjögren's syndrome, dermatitis herpetiformis, sarcoidosis, and Hashimoto thyroiditis. Other disorders that have been anecdotally related to SCLE are rheumatoid arthritis, Sweet syndrome, porphyria cutanea tarda, gluten-sensitive enteropathy, and Crohn disease. There has also been the suggestion anecdotally that SCLE may be associated with internal malignancy (breast, lung, gastric, uterine, hepatocellular, and laryngeal carcinomas, as well as with Hodgkin lymphoma).[26] Several different types of chemotherapeutic agents are known to be capable of triggering drug-induced SCLE. This could perhaps confound the possibility that SCLE has a significant association with internal malignancy.

of life. Follicular involvement in DLE is a prominent feature. Keratotic plugs accumulate in dilated follicles that soon become devoid of hair. When the adherent scale is lifted from more advanced lesions, keratotic spikes similar in appearance to carpet tacks can be seen to project from the undersurface of the scale (ie, the "carpet tack" sign). DLE lesions can be difficult to diagnose in white patients because the characteristic peripheral hyperpigmentation is often absent. Hypertrophic DLE lesions can be confused with hypertrophic actinic keratosis, keratoacanthoma, and squamous cell carcinoma.

DLE lesions are most frequently encountered on the face, scalp, ears, V area of the neck, and extensor aspects of the arms. Any area of the face, including the eyebrows, eyelids, nose, and lips, can be affected. A symmetric, hyperkeratotic, butterfly-shaped DLE plaque is occasionally found over the malar areas of the face and bridge of the nose. Such lesions should not be confused with the more transient, edematous, minimally scaling ACLE erythema reactions that occur in the same areas. Facial DLE, like ACLE and SCLE, usually spares the nasolabial folds. It may be difficult to distinguish early lesions of malar DLE from ACLE, but induration and recalcitrance to topical steroids/calcineurin inhibitors favor the former diagnosis. When DLE lesions occur perioorally, they can resolve with a striking acneiform pattern of pitted scarring. DLE characteristically affects the external ear, including the conchal bowl and outer portion of the external auditory canal (Fig. 61-8A). Such lesions often present initially as dilated, hyperpigmented follicles. The scalp is involved in 60% of patients with DLE; irreversible, scarring alopecia resulting from

CHRONIC CUTANEOUS LUPUS ERYTHEMATOSUS

CLASSIC DISCOID LUPUS ERYTHEMATOSUS

Classic DLE lesions, the most common form of CCLE, begin as red-purple macules, papules, or small plaques and rapidly develop a hyperkeratotic surface. Early classic DLE lesions typically evolve into sharply demarcated, coin-shaped (ie, discoid) erythematous plaques covered by a prominent, adherent scale that extends into the orifices of dilated hair follicles (Fig. 61-6).

DLE lesions typically expand with erythema and hyperpigmentation at the periphery, leaving hallmark atrophic central scarring, telangiectasia, and hypopigmentation (Fig. 61-7). DLE lesions at this stage can merge to form large, confluent, disfiguring plaques. DLE in persons of certain ethnic backgrounds, such as Asian Indians, can present clinically as isolated areas of macular hyperpigmentation. When present on hair-bearing skin (scalp, eyelid margins, and eyebrows), DLE causes scarring alopecia, which can lead to disfigurement and markedly impact quality

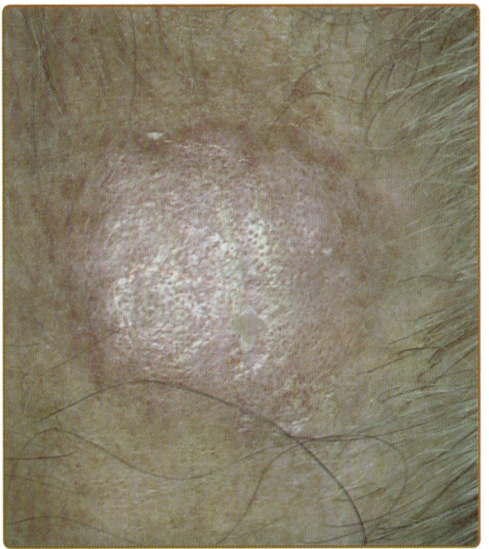

Figure 61-6 Classic discoid lupus erythematosus. Typical early erythematous plaque on the forehead demonstrating hyperkeratosis and accentuation of follicle orifices in a 60-year-old man with a 25-year history of cutaneous lupus erythematosus. The lesion had been present for 3 months; no dermal atrophy was present at this stage.

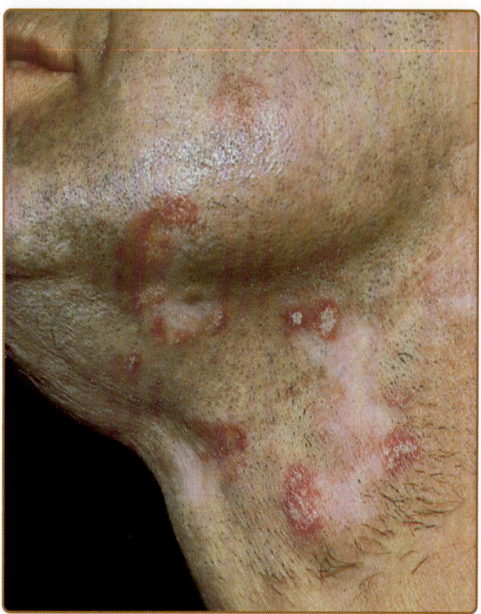

Figure 61-7 Classic discoid lupus erythematosus. Sharply demarcated, round-to-ovoid slightly indurated, erythematous plaques on the neck and face. Most plaques show a mild degree of hyperkeratosis, and some show dermal atrophy. Noninflamed areas of hypopigmentation and scarring mark the sites of prior lesions that have resolved.

such involvement has been reported in one-third of patients (Fig. 61-8B). The irreversible, scarring alopecia resulting from DLE differs from the reversible, nonscarring alopecia that patients with SLE often develop during periods of systemic disease activity. This type of hair loss, so-called *lupus hair*, may represent telogen effluvium occurring as the result of flaring systemic disease.

Localized DLE lesions occur only on the head or neck, whereas generalized DLE lesions occur both above and below the neck. Generalized DLE is more commonly associated with underlying SLE and is often more recalcitrant to standard therapy, frequently requiring layering of antimalarial and immunosuppressive medications. DLE lesions below the neck most commonly occur on the extensor aspects of the arms, forearms, and hands, although they can occur at virtually any site on the body. The palms and soles can be the sites of painful, and at times disabling, erosive DLE lesions. On occasion, small DLE lesions occurring only around follicular orifices appear at the elbow and elsewhere (follicular DLE). We have observed that elbow/extensor arm lesions seem to occur with acral finger lesions of DLE, and that patients with this combination of findings more frequently have active systemic disease. DLE activity can localize to the nail unit. The nail can be impacted by other forms of CLE as well as SLE, producing nail fold erythema and telangiectasia, red lunulae, clubbing, paronychia, pitting, leukonychia striata, and onycholysis.

DLE lesions can be potentiated by sunlight exposure but to a lesser extent than ACLE and SCLE lesions. DLE, as well as other forms of LE skin disease activity, can be precipitated by any form of cutaneous trauma (ie, the Koebner phenomenon or isomorphic effect).

The relationship between classic DLE and SLE has been the subject of much debate.[27] The following summary points can be made: (a) 5% of patients presenting with classic DLE lesions subsequently develop unequivocal evidence of SLE and (b) patients with generalized DLE (ie, lesions both above and below the neck) have somewhat higher rates of immunologic abnormalities, a higher risk for progressing to SLE, and a higher risk for developing more severe manifestations of SLE than patients with localized DLE.

Roughly one-fourth of patients with SLE develop DLE lesions at some point in the course of their disease, and such patients tend to have less-severe forms of SLE.

Aside from classic DLE, there are several other less-common variants of CCLE, which are subclassified as such because of their overlapping histologies and tendency to occur in a low frequency in association with underlying SLE.

HYPERTROPHIC DISCOID LUPUS ERYTHEMATOSUS

Hypertrophic DLE, also referred to as *hyperkeratotic* or *verrucous DLE*, is a rare variant of CCLE in which the hyperkeratosis normally found in classic DLE lesions is greatly exaggerated. The extensor aspects of the arms, the upper back, and the face are the areas most frequently affected. Overlapping features of hypertrophic LE and lichen planus have been described under the rubric *lupus planus*. The entity *lupus erythematosus hypertrophicus et profundus* appears to represent a rare form of hypertrophic DLE. Patients with hypertrophic DLE probably do not have a greater risk for developing SLE than do patients with classic DLE lesions.

MUCOSAL DISCOID LUPUS ERYTHEMATOSUS

Mucosal DLE occurs in approximately 25% of patients with CCLE. The oral mucosa is most frequently affected; however, nasal, conjunctival, and genital mucosal surfaces can be targeted. In the mouth, the buccal mucosal surfaces are most commonly involved, with the palate, alveolar processes, and tongue being sites of less frequent involvement. Lesions begin as painless, erythematous patches that evolve to chronic plaques that can be confused with lichen planus. Chronic buccal mucosal plaques are sharply marginated and have irregularly scalloped, white borders with radiating white striae and telangiectasia. The surfaces of these plaques overlying the

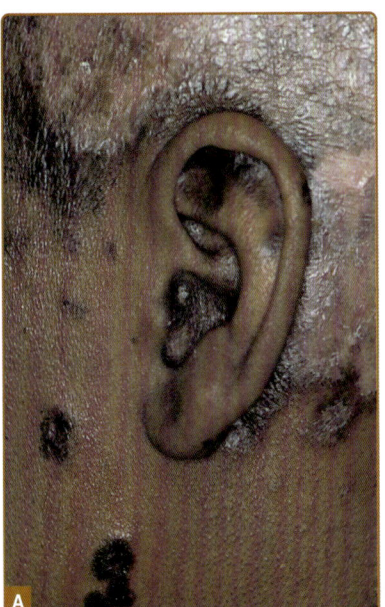
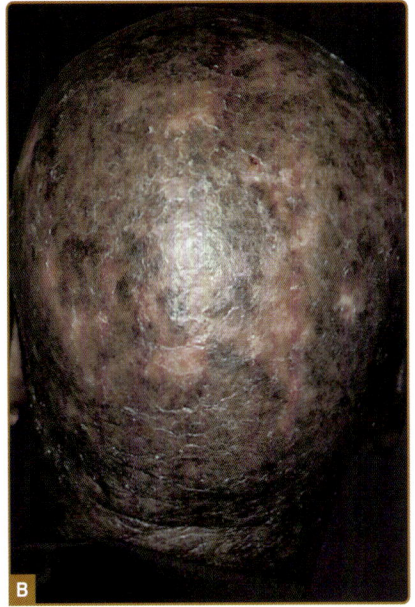
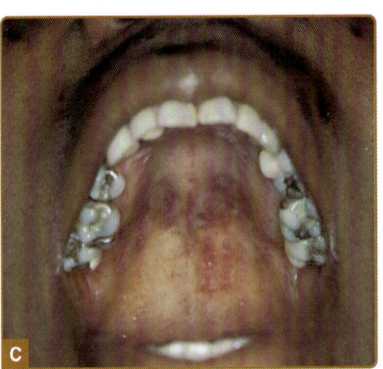

Figure 61-8 Classic discoid lupus erythematosus (DLE) and mucosal DLE in a 45-year-old African American woman with a 20-year history of untreated cutaneous lupus erythematosus. **A,** Characteristic involvement of the ear shows lesions with atrophy and postinflammatory hyperpigmentation as well as inflammatory red plaques on the scalp with postinflammatory hypopigmentation. **B,** Confluent lesions on the scalp have resulted in extensive scarring alopecia. **C,** Plaques of DLE on the palatal mucosa showing morphologic features similar to those of cutaneous lesions.

palatal mucosa often have a honeycomb appearance. Central depression often occurs in older lesions, and painful ulceration can develop. Rarely, oral mucosal DLE lesions can degenerate into squamous cell carcinoma, similar to longstanding cutaneous DLE lesions. Any degree of nodular asymmetry within a mucosal DLE lesion should be evaluated for the possibility of malignant degeneration. Chronic DLE plaques also appear on the vermilion border of the lips. At times, DLE involvement of the lips can present as a diffuse cheilitis, especially on the more sun-exposed lower lip.

DLE lesions may present on the nasal, conjunctival, and anogenital mucosa. Perforation of the nasal septum is more often associated with SLE than DLE. Conjunctival DLE lesions affect the lower lid more often than the upper lid. Lesions begin as focal areas of nondescript inflammation most commonly affecting the palpebral conjunctivae or the lid margin. Scarring becomes evident as lesions mature, and the permanent loss of eyelashes and ectropion can develop, producing considerable disability.

LUPUS ERYTHEMATOSUS PROFUNDUS/LUPUS ERYTHEMATOSUS PANNICULITIS

LE profundus/LE panniculitis (Kaposi-Irrgang disease) is a rare form of CCLE typified by inflammatory lesions in the lower dermis and subcutaneous tissue. Approximately 70% of patients with this type of CCLE also have typical DLE lesions, often overlying the panniculitis lesions. Some have used the term *LE profundus* to designate those patients who have both LE panniculitis and DLE lesions, and *LE panniculitis* to refer to those having only subcutaneous involvement. Typical subcutaneous lesions present as firm nodules, 1 to 3 cm in diameter. The overlying skin often becomes attached to the subcutaneous nodules and is drawn inward to produce deep, saucerized depressions (Fig. 61-9). The head, proximal upper arms, chest, back, breasts, buttocks, and thighs are the sites frequently affected. LE panniculitis, in the absence of overlying DLE, may produce breast nodules that can

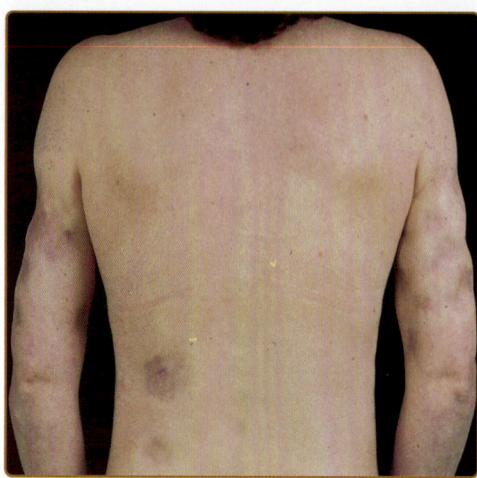

Figure 61-9 Lupus erythematosus panniculitis. Lupus panniculitis has resulted in large, sunken areas of overlying skin; erythema and atrophy of the skin are present.

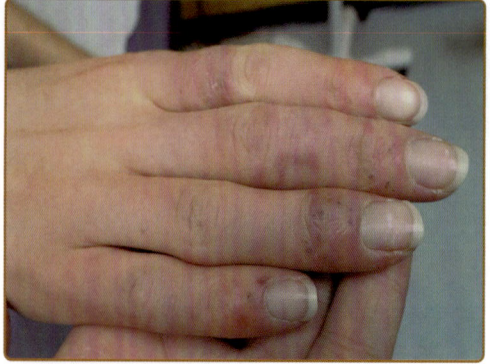

Figure 61-10 Chilblain lupus. Chilblain lesions affecting the fingers in a patient with longstanding lupus and lupus nephritis. The skin lesions were chronic and occurred without cold exposure.

mimic carcinoma clinically and radiologically (lupus mastitis). Medically unresponsive extensive breast involvement can be so severe as to require radical mastectomy. Confluent facial involvement can simulate the appearance of lipoatrophy. Dystrophic calcification frequently occurs in older lesions of LE profundus/LE panniculitis, and pain associated with such calcification can, at times, be the dominant clinical problem. Roughly 50% of patients with LE profundus/panniculitis have evidence of SLE. However, the systemic features of patients with LE panniculitis/profundus tend to be less severe, similar to those of patients with SLE who have DLE skin lesions.

CHILBLAIN LUPUS ERYTHEMATOSUS

Chilblain LE lesions initially develop as purple-red patches, papules, and plaques on the toes, fingers, and face, which are precipitated by cold, damp climates and are clinically and histologically similar to idiopathic chilblains (pernio) (Fig. 61-10). As they evolve, these lesions usually assume the appearance of scarred atrophic plaques with associated telangiectases. They may resemble old lesions of DLE or may mimic acral lesions of small vessel vasculitis. Histologic findings include a superficial and deep lymphocytic vascular reaction in addition to fibrin deposition in reticular, dermal-based blood vessels. Patients with chilblain LE often have typical DLE lesions on the face and head. It is possible that chilblain LE begins as a classic acral, cold-induced lesion that then Koebnerizes DLE lesions, thus explaining the spectrum of clinicohistologic findings, which seem to vary based on when, in the course of the lesion, the biopsy sample is taken.

Chilblain LE appears to be associated with anti-Ro/SS-A antibodies,[28] and is linked to Raynaud phenomenon in many cases.[29] Persistence of lesions beyond the cold months, a positive ANA, or presence of one of the other ACR criteria for SLE at the time of diagnosis of chilblain lesions helps to distinguish chilblain LE from idiopathic chilblains.[30] Approximately 20% of patients presenting with chilblain LE later develop SLE. Chilblain LE is an underrecognized entity, yet it is likely that it is one of the most common causes of digital lesions in patients with LE. It is sometimes misdiagnosed as vasculitis and may overlap with acral DLE as mentioned above. An autosomal dominant, familial form of Chilblain LE has been described, and is caused by a missense mutation in the *TREX 1* (endonuclease repair) gene.[31]

LUPUS ERYTHEMATOSUS TUMIDUS

Lupus erythematosus tumidus (LET; tumid LE) is a variant of CCLE in which the dermal findings of DLE, namely, excessive mucin deposition and superficial perivascular and periadnexal inflammation, are found on histologic evaluation. The characteristic epidermal histologic changes of LE-specific skin disease are only minimally expressed, if at all. This results in succulent, edematous, urticaria-like plaques with little surface change (Fig. 61-11). Annular urticaria-like plaques can also be seen. The paucity of epidermal change often produces confusion concerning the diagnosis of LET as a form of CCLE.[32,33]

Several recent reports support this subclassification and further characterize this subtype of CCLE.[34-39] Although described to occur in some patients with SLE, most patients with LET have a negative ANA and a benign disease course. LET appears to be the most photosensitive subtype of cutaneous lupus, and typically demonstrates a good response to antimalarials. Additionally, LET lesions tend to resolve completely without either scarring or atrophy.

There continues to be debate about the validity of LET as an authentic form of LE-skin disease. Some argue that LET lesions may in fact not be a form of CLE[32] while others feel that LET deserves to be recognized as a distinct type of CLE (intermittent CLE) equivalent in importance to ACLE, SCLE, and CCLE.[35] Evidence of type I interferon upregulation in skin lesions of UV light-induced LE tumidus support the latter argument.[40]

OTHER VARIANTS

Other rare forms of CCLE CLE have been described. These include, LE hypertrophicus et profundus, lichenoid DLE, LE vermiculatus, LE telangiectaticus, linear CLE, and LE edematous (probably a historical designation for urticaria-like plaque variant of DLE and/or tumid LE). Further information on these clinical entities is available.[41]

LUPUS ERYTHEMATOSUS NONSPECIFIC SKIN DISEASE

Many other cutaneous findings have been found in patients with lupus patients, particularly SLE; they are listed in Table 61-1. Of note, the presence of LE-nonspecific skin changes, especially when seen in conjunction with LE-specific rashes, corresponds with higher systemic disease activity.[42] Specific findings such as livedo reticularis, thrombophlebitis, or cutaneous infarct may suggest the presence of secondary antiphospholipid syndrome. Space constraints do not allow specific discussions of these entities here.

NONCUTANEOUS FINDINGS

Systemic lupus can cause a myriad of extracutaneous manifestations, which manifestations are outlined in Table 61-3.

DIAGNOSIS

Figure 61-12 outlines approaches to the patient with skin lesions suspicious for CLE.

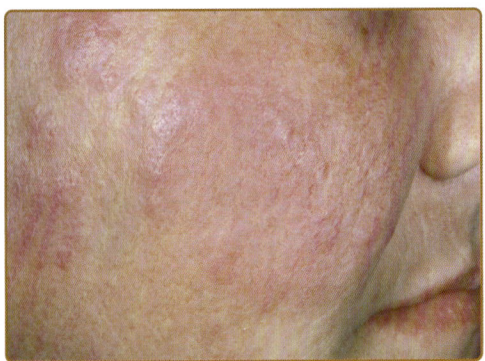

Figure 61-11 Lupus erythematosus tumidus. Note succulent, indurated plaques.

LABORATORY TESTING

Because of the strong association between ACLE and SLE, the immunologic laboratory features of ACLE are those associated with SLE (high-titer ANA, anti-dsDNA, anti-Smith antigen, hypocomplementemia, hypergammaglobinemia, etc). Other laboratory findings, such as cytopenias, decreased kidney function, and urine changes (hematuria, proteinuria), reflect disease activity and can vary from patient to patient depending on the extent of end-organ involvement.

The laboratory markers for SCLE are the presence of anti-Ro/SS-A (70% to 90%) and, less commonly, anti-La/SS-B (30% to 50%) autoantibodies. ANA are present in 60% to 80% of patients with SCLE, and rheumatoid factor is present in approximately 33%. Other autoantibodies in patients with SCLE include false-positive serologic tests for syphilis (Venereal Disease Research Laboratory [VDRL] rapid plasma reagin; 7% to 33%), anticardiolipin (10% to 16%), antithyroid (18% to 44%), anti-Smith antigen (10%), anti-dsDNA (10%), and anti-U1 ribonucleoprotein (10%). Patients with SCLE, particularly those with systemic involvement, may have a number of laboratory abnormalities, including anemia, leukopenia, thrombocytopenia, elevated erythrocyte sedimentation rate, hypergammaglobulinemia, proteinuria, hematuria, urine casts, elevated serum creatine and blood urea nitrogen, and depressed complement levels (resulting from genetic deficiency or increased complement consumption).

ANA are present in low titer in 30% to 40% of patients with DLE; however, fewer than 5% have the higher ANA levels that are characteristic of patients with overt SLE (>1:320 titer by indirect immunofluorescence assay). Antibodies to single-stranded DNA are not uncommon in DLE, but antibodies to dsDNA are distinctly uncommon. Precipitating antibodies to U1 ribonucleoprotein are sometimes found in patients whose disease course is dominated by DLE lesions; however, such patients usually have only mild manifestations of SLE or overlapping connective tissue disorders such as mixed connective tissue disease. Precipitating Ro/SS-A and La/SS-B autoantibodies are rare in patients with DLE; low levels of anti-Ro/SS-A antibody detected by enzyme-linked immunoassay are more common. A small percentage of patients with DLE have low-grade anemia, biologic false-positive serologic tests for syphilis (VDRL rapid plasma reagent), positive rheumatoid factor tests, slight depressions in serum complement levels, modest elevations in γ-globulin, and modest leukopenia. It has been suggested that such findings are risk factors for the development of SLE. ANA are present in 70% to 75% of patients with LE profundus/panniculitis, but anti-dsDNA antibodies are rare.

The laboratory findings associated with SLE, as well as with CLE, in both adults and children, are reviewed elsewhere.[43,44] It should be noted that the assay methodologies for the detection of the autoantibodies discussed above continue to evolve over time. Commercial reference laboratories at the time of this publication have largely moved to the use of solid-phase immunoassay

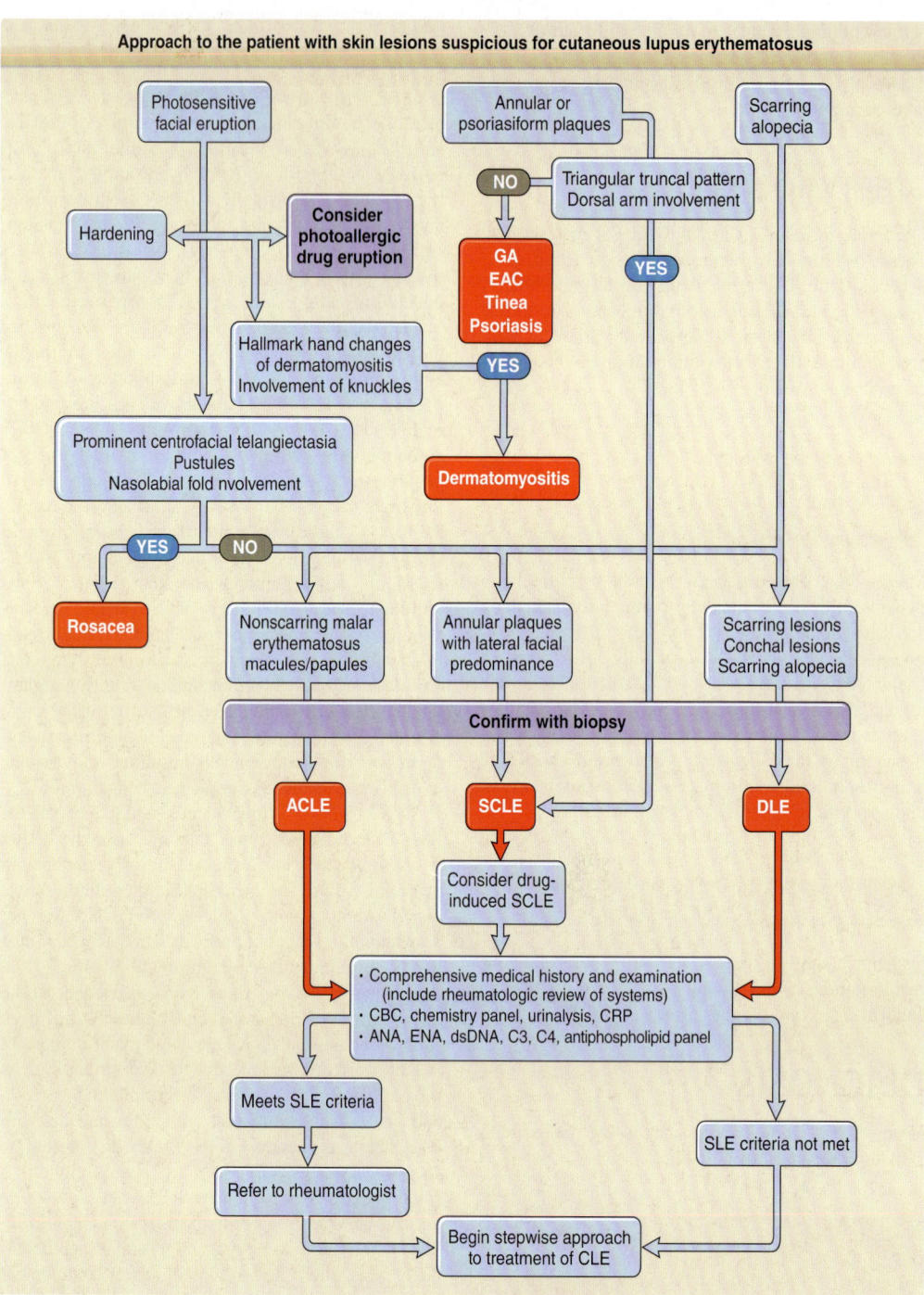

Figure 61-12 Approach to the patient with skin lesions suspicious for cutaneous lupus erythematosus. ACLE, acute cutaneous lupus erythematosus; ANA, antinuclear antibody; CBC, complete blood cell count; CLE, cutaneous lupus erythematosus; CRP, C-reactive protein; DLE, discoid lupus erythematosus; dsDNA, doubled-stranded DNA; EAC, erythema annulare centrifugum; ENA, extractable nuclear antibody; GA, granuloma annulare; SCLE, subacute cutaneous lupus erythematosus; SLE, systemic lupus erythematosus.

techniques, especially multiplex flow immunoassay. The disease incidence/prevalence of the autoantibodies discussed in the section above might vary somewhat from the results of the autoantibody assays that one might receive from commercial laboratories today.

HISTOPATHOLOGY

The LE-specific skin disease histopathology is a distinctive constellation of hyperkeratosis, epidermal atrophy, vacuolar basal cell degeneration, dermal–epidermal junction basement membrane thickening, dermal edema, dermal mucin deposition, and mononuclear cell infiltration of the dermal–epidermal junction and dermis, focused in a perivascular and periappendageal distribution. Variable degrees of these features are encountered in the different forms of LE-specific skin disease. Differences of opinion exist as to whether ACLE, SCLE, and DLE lesions can be distinguished reliably on the basis of their histopathologic appearances alone.[44-46]

ACUTE CUTANEOUS LUPUS ERYTHEMATOSUS

The histopathologic changes in ACLE lesions are generally less impressive than those in SCLE and DLE lesions, and are mainly those of a cell-poor interface dermatitis (Fig. 61-13A). The lymphohistiocytic cellular infiltrate is relatively sparse. Some authors have noted an increase in the number of neutrophils in the infiltrate, especially when recent-onset lesions are biopsied. A mild degree of focal vacuolar alteration of basal keratinocytes can be seen, in addition to telangiectases and extravasation of erythrocytes. One may see individually necrotic keratinocytes, and in its most severe form, ACLE can display extensive epidermal necrosis similar to TEN. The upper dermis usually shows pronounced mucinosis and may be very helpful in distinguishing ACLE from other causes of a cell-poor interface dermatitis. It is uncommon to see basement membrane zone thickening, follicular plugging, or alteration of epidermal thickness in ACLE, although epidermal atrophy is sometimes present.[45,46]

SUBACUTE CUTANEOUS LUPUS ERYTHEMATOSUS

SCLE also typically presents as an interface dermatitis, with foci of vacuolar alteration of basal keratinocytes alternating with areas of lichenoid dermatitis (see Fig. 61-13B). Pronounced epidermal atrophy is often present. SCLE is in the differential diagnosis of atrophic lichenoid dermatitis, along with atrophic lichen planus and lichenoid drug eruptions. Dermal changes include edema, prominent mucin deposition, and sparse mononuclear cell infiltration usually limited to areas around blood vessels and periadnexal structures in the upper one-third of the dermis. Lesser degrees of hyperkeratosis, follicular plugging, mononuclear cell

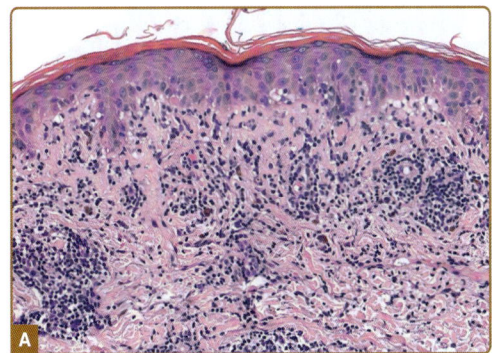
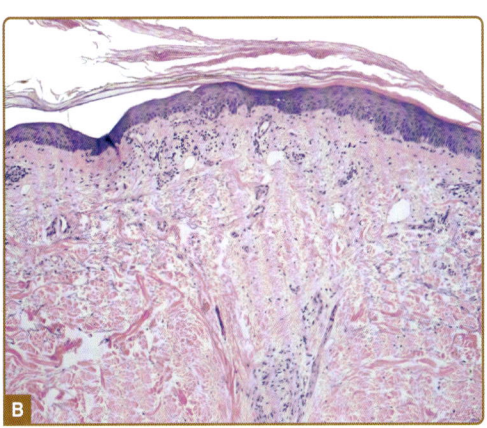
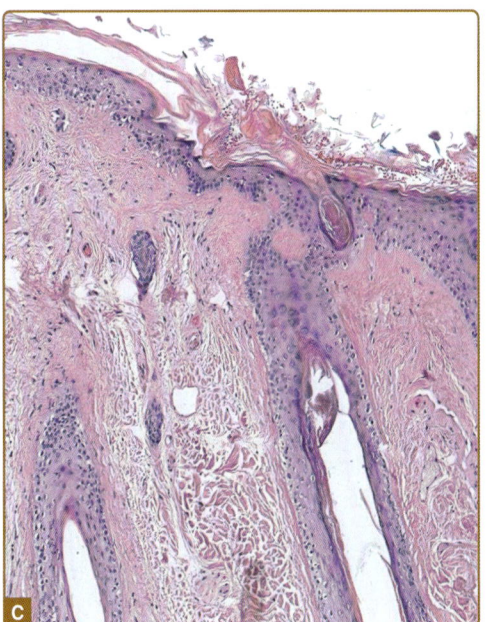

Figure 61-13 Histopathology of lupus erythematosus-specific skin disease. **A,** Acute cutaneous lupus lesion (hematoxylin and eosin [H&E] stain) showing interface dermatitis and vacuolar changes as well as perivascular inflammatory cell infiltrate (×128). **B,** Subacute cutaneous lupus lesion (H&E stain) with mild interface dermatitis, vacuolar changes, and mild hyperkeratosis. Mild epidermal atrophy and prominent mucinosis in upper dermis are also seen (×100). **C,** Discoid lupus lesion showing typical interface changes as well as hyperkeratosis, follicular plugging. Mild dermal fibroplasia is also seen (×84).

infiltration of adnexal structures, and dermal melanophages might help distinguish SCLE lesions from DLE lesions. It has not been possible to reliably differentiate papulosquamous from annular SCLE by histopathologic criteria alone.[43]

CHRONIC CUTANEOUS LUPUS ERYTHEMATOSUS

In classic DLE lesions, epidermal changes include hyperkeratosis, variable atrophy, and interface changes similar to those described for SCLE (see Fig. 61-13C). The epidermal basement membrane is markedly thickened. Dermal changes include a dense mononuclear cell infiltrate composed primarily of CD4 T lymphocytes and macrophages predominantly in the periappendageal and perivascular areas, melanophages, and dermal mucin deposition. The infiltrate is often quite dense and typically extends well into the deeper reticular dermis and/or subcutis, which may help to distinguish it from ACLE or SCLE. In chronic scarring DLE lesions, the dense inflammatory cell infiltrate subsides and is replaced by dermal fibroplasia. A folliculotropic variant of DLE, in which the inflammatory infiltrate is predominantly around hair follicles, has been described, as have lymphomatoid variants, in which there are extremely dense infiltrates that may contain atypical lymphoid cells.[45]

IMMUNOHISTOLOGY

Immunohistology is often helpful in confirming a diagnosis of LE-specific skin disease and has been shown to boost the sensitivity and specificity of diagnosis.[45] Because it is not uncommon to see negative immunofluorescence studies in patients with acute, subacute, and chronic LE, and false-positive studies in healthy individuals, immunohistology must be interpreted in the context of clinical and histologic findings in a given patient.

IgG, IgA, IgM, and complement components (C3, C4, C1q, properdin, factor B, and the membrane attack complex C5b-C9) deposited in a continuous granular or linear band-like array at the dermal–epidermal junction have been observed in the lesional and nonlesional skin of patients with LE since the early 1960s (Fig. 61-14). However, debate about terminology in this area continues to cloud the field. Some restrict the use of the term *lupus band test* to refer to the examination of nonlesional skin biopsies for the presence of this band-like array of immunoreactants at the dermal-epidermal junction. Others qualify the lupus band test as being either "lesional" or "nonlesional." Less confusion might exist if the terms *lesional lupus band test* and *nonlesional lupus band test* were uniformly adopted.

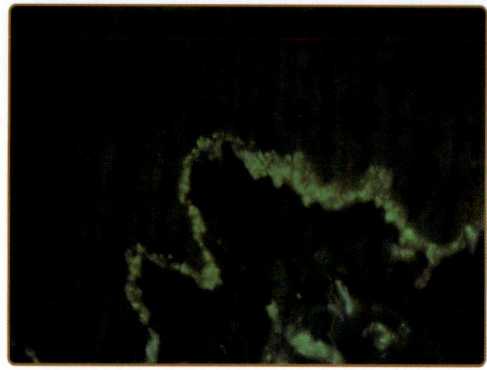

Figure 61-14 Immunopathology of lupus erythematosus–specific skin disease. Direct immunofluorescence examination of a discoid lupus erythematosus lesional skin biopsy showing a continuous band of granular fluorescence at the dermal–epidermal junction as a result of staining with fluorescein isothiocyanate–conjugated goat anti–immunoglobulin G.

ACUTE CUTANEOUS LUPUS ERYTHEMATOSUS

The sparse data that exist suggest that 60% to 100% of ACLE lesions display a lesional lupus band. However, the realization that sun-damaged skin from otherwise healthy individuals can display similar immunopathology has diluted the clinical value of this finding.

SUBACUTE CUTANEOUS LUPUS ERYTHEMATOSUS

Initial studies indicated that approximately 60% of patients with SCLE had lesional lupus bands. A "dust-like particle" pattern of IgG deposition focused around epidermal basal keratinocytes has been suggested to be more specific for SCLE by reflecting the presence of in vivo bound Ro/SS-A autoantibody.

CHRONIC CUTANEOUS LUPUS ERYTHEMATOSUS

Early reports suggested that more than 90% of classic DLE lesions had lesional immunoreactants at the dermal–epidermal junction, often extending along the basement membrane of the hair follicle, but subsequent studies report somewhat lower rates. Lesions on the head, neck, and arms are positive more frequently (80%) than those on the trunk (20%). The lesional lupus band also appears to be a function of the age of the lesion being examined, with older lesions (>3 months) being positive more often than younger ones. Ultrastructural localization of immunoglobulin at the dermal–epidermal junction confirms that these proteins are deposited on the upper dermal collagen fibers and along the lamina densa of the epidermal basement membrane zone.

In LE profundus, immunoglobulin and complement deposits are usually found in blood vessel walls of the deep dermis and subcutis. Immunoglobulin deposits at the dermal–epidermal junction may or may not be present, depending on the site biopsied, the presence or absence of accompanying SLE, and the presence or absence of overlying changes of DLE at the dermal–epidermal junction.

NONLESIONAL LUPUS BAND TEST

There has been much debate over the past 3 decades regarding the diagnostic and prognostic significance of an immunoglobulin/complement band at the dermal–epidermal junction of nonlesional skin taken from patients with LE.[44] When totally sun-protected nonlesional skin (eg, buttocks) is sampled, the diagnostic specificity for SLE appears to be very high when 3 or more immunoreactants are present at the dermal–epidermal junction. Prospectively ascertained followup data also suggest that the presence of a nonlesional lupus band test correlates positively with risk for developing LE nephritis. However, the nonlesional lupus band test has fallen out of favor as a clinical tool largely because the information gained has not been proven to be of significantly greater value than the results of more readily available serologic assays such as antibody to dsDNA.

DIFFERENTIAL DIAGNOSIS

Table 61-5 outlines the differential diagnosis of CLE. In addition, reticulated erythematosus mucinosis has been suggested by some to be a form of photosensitive CLE perhaps related to LE tumidus. Reticulated erythematosus mucinosis presents as a reticulated array of macules and/or papules on the upper chest and back.

CLINICAL COURSE AND PROGNOSIS

ACUTE CUTANEOUS LUPUS ERYTHEMATOSUS

Both localized and generalized forms of ACLE lesions flare and abate in parallel with underlying SLE disease

TABLE 61-5
Differential Diagnosis of Lupus Erythematosus

MOST LIKELY	CONSIDER	ALWAYS RULE OUT
■ ACLE	■ ACLE	■ ACLE
■ Localized	■ Localized	■ Generalized
■ Acne rosacea	■ Seborrheic dermatitis	■ Toxic epidermal necrolysis
■ Dermatomyositis	■ Polymorphous light eruption	■ CCLE
■ Generalized	■ Photoallergic contact dermatitis	■ DLE
■ Drug hypersensitivity reaction	■ Generalized	■ Tinea incognito
■ Photoallergic/phototoxic drug reactions	■ Dermatomyositis	■ Cutaneous T-cell lymphoma
■ Viral exanthems	■ SCLE	■ Lupus panniculitis
■ SCLE	■ Papulosquamous	■ Infectious panniculitis (deep fungal/atypical mycobacterial organisms)
■ Papulosquamous	■ Photoallergic/photo lichenoid drug reaction	■ Calciphylaxis
■ Photosensitive psoriasis	■ Annular	
■ Annular	■ Erythema gyratum repens	
■ Erythema annulare centrifugum	■ DLE	
■ Granuloma annulare	■ Early DLE/LET	
■ CCLE	■ Granuloma faciale	
■ Early DLE/LET	■ Sarcoidosis	
■ Polymorphous light eruption	■ Jessner benign lymphocytic infiltration of the skin	
■ Fully evolved DLE/hypertrophic DLE	■ Pseudolymphoma	
■ Squamous cell carcinoma	■ Lymphoma cutis	
■ Hypertrophic actinic keratosis	■ Lupus vulgaris/cutaneous tuberculosis	
■ Keratoacanthoma	■ Urticaria	
■ Lupus panniculitis	■ Urticarial vasculitis	
■ Morphea profundus	■ Fully evolved DLE/hypertrophic DLE	
	■ Prurigo nodularis	
	■ Hypertrophic lichen planus	
	■ Lupus panniculitis	
	■ Subcutaneous sarcoidosis	
	■ Traumatic panniculitis	
	■ Eosinophilic fasciitis	

ACLE, acute cutaneous lupus erythematosus; CCLE, chronic cutaneous lupus erythematosus; DLE, discoid lupus erythematosus; LET, lupus erythematosus tumidus; SCLE, subacute cutaneous lupus erythematosus.

activity. Therefore, the prognosis for any given patient with ACLE is dictated by the pattern of the underlying SLE. Both 5-year (80% to 95%) and 10-year (70% to 90%) survival rates for SLE have progressively improved over the past 4 decades as a result of earlier diagnosis made possible by more sensitive laboratory testing and improved immunosuppressive treatment regimens. Ominous prognostic signs in SLE are hypertension, nephritis, systemic vasculitis, and CNS disease.

SUBACUTE CUTANEOUS LUPUS ERYTHEMATOSUS

Because SCLE has been recognized as a separate disease entity for only 2 decades, the long-term outcome associated with SCLE lesions has yet to be determined. It is the authors' experience that most patients with SCLE have intermittent recurrences of skin disease activity over long periods of time without significant progression of systemic involvement (we are aware of only 1 death directly attributable to SLE in approximately 150 patients with SCLE). Other patients enjoy long-term if not permanent remissions of their skin disease activity. A few patients have experienced unremitting cutaneous disease.

It has also been the authors' experience that approximately 10% of the patients with SCLE develop active SLE, including lupus nephritis. This subgroup of patients is marked by the presence of papulosquamous SCLE, localized ACLE, high-titer ANA, leukopenia, and/or antibodies to dsDNA. Long-term followup studies of SCLE are required to determine the true risk of severe systemic disease progression in patients presenting with SCLE skin lesions. CCLE lesions, typically classic DLE, have also arisen in patients initially presenting with SCLE.

Evidence suggests that overlap occurs between SCLE and Sjögren syndrome. Patients with SCLE who develop Sjögren syndrome are at risk for developing the extraglandular systemic complications associated with Sjögren syndrome, including vasculitis, peripheral neuropathy, autoimmune thyroiditis, renal tubular acidosis, myositis, chronic hepatitis, primary biliary cirrhosis, psychosis, lymphadenopathy, splenomegaly, and B-cell lymphoma.

CHRONIC CUTANEOUS LUPUS ERYTHEMATOSUS

Most patients with untreated classic DLE lesions suffer indolent progression to large areas of cutaneous dystrophy and scarring alopecia that can be psychosocially devastating and occupationally disabling. However, with treatment, skin disease can be largely controlled. Spontaneous remission occurs occasionally, and the disease activity can recrudesce at the sites of older, inactive lesions. Rebound after discontinuation of treatment is typical, and slower taper of medications during periods of inactivity is recommended. Squamous cell carcinoma occasionally develops in chronic smoldering DLE lesions.

Death from SLE is distinctly uncommon in patients who present initially with localized DLE. As discussed in "Epidemiology" above, patients presenting with localized DLE have only a 5% chance of subsequently developing clinically significant SLE disease activity. Generalized DLE and persistent, low-grade laboratory abnormalities appear to be risk factors for such disease progression. Unrecognized squamous cell carcinoma developing within a longstanding DLE skin lesion could be a cause of morbidity and mortality.

OUTCOME MEASURES

The recent development of a validated instrument to measure activity of CLE, the Cutaneous Lupus Erythematosus Disease Area and Severity Index (CLASI), has made it possible to objectively follow patients' disease course and response to therapy. The instrument has separate scores for damage (scarring) and activity which is important, because one would not expect a "burned-out" scarred area to normalize with drugs that were meant to abate LE activity.[47] It has been validated as a useful tool to measure clinical response.[48]

MANAGEMENT

The initial management of patients with any form of CLE should include an evaluation to rule out underlying SLE disease activity at the time of diagnosis. All patients with CLE should receive instruction about protection from sunlight and artificial sources of UV radiation, and should be advised to avoid the use of potentially photosensitizing drugs such as hydrochlorothiazide, tetracycline, griseofulvin, and piroxicam. With regard to specific medical therapy, local measures should be maximized and systemic agents used if significant local disease activity persists or systemic activity is superimposed.

ACLE lesions usually respond to the systemic immunosuppressive measures required to treat the underlying SLE disease activity that so frequently accompanies this form of CLE (eg, systemic glucocorticoids, azathioprine, and cyclophosphamide). Increasing evidence suggests that aminoquinoline antimalarial agents such as hydroxychloroquine can have a steroid-sparing effect on SLE, and these drugs can be of value in ACLE. The local measures discussed in "Local Therapy" below can also be of value in treating ACLE. Because the lesions of SCLE and CCLE are often found in patients who have little or no evidence of underlying systemic disease activity, unlike the lesions of ACLE, nonimmunosuppressive treatment modalities are preferred for SCLE and CCLE (Table 61-6). For the most part, SCLE and CCLE lesions respond equally to such agents.

Accurate diagnosis is always the key to optimal medical management. In genetically complex clinical

TABLE 61-6
Therapeutic Options for Lupus Erythematosus–Specific Skin Disease

	DRUG	DOSE
First line	Topical glucocorticoids, topical calcineurin inhibitor	Class I topical steroid daily to twice daily for 2 weeks alternating with pimecrolimus 1% or tacrolimus 0.1% twice daily for 2 weeks
	Intralesional triamcinolone acetonide	2.5-10 mg/cc
Second line	Hydroxychloroquine	6.5 mg/kg/day based on ideal body weight
	Chloroquine	3-3.5 mg/kg/day based on ideal body weight
	Quinacrine	100 mg/day (available at compounding pharmacies
	If monotherapy fails, add quinacrine to either hydroxychloroquine or chloroquine	
Short course only (2-16 weeks)	Prednisone	5-60 mg/day
	Thalidomide	50-200 mg/day; taper to 50 mg every other day on response
Third line (safer immunosuppressives)	Azathioprine	1.5-2.5 mg/kg/day
	Mycophenolate mofetil	1-1.5 g/dose, twice daily
	Methotrexate	7.5-25 mg by mouth or subcutaneously, once weekly
Worth considering	Dapsone	50-200 mg/day
	Accutane	0.5-2 mg/kg/day
	Acitretin	10-50 mg/day
	Gold	Titrate to 50 mg intramuscularly weekly, taper after 1 g
Investigational (some currently available for other indications)	Leflunomide	
	Anti–tumor necrosis factor biologics	
	Rituximab	
	Belimumab	
	Abatacept	
	Janus kinase (JAK) inhibitors (tofacitinib, ruxolitinib)	
	Antiinterferon antibodies	
	CXCR3 receptor inhibitors	

disorders that are variably expressed clinically from one person to another, such as LE, there is a tendency to over ascribe new clinical findings to LE once a diagnosis of LE has been established. To call attention to this important clinical axiom, Robert Greenwald, a rheumatologist, formulated his "Law of Lupus." It states that "SLE is often falsely accused of causing *anything and everything* that might happen to a patient subsequent to the diagnosis of SLE."[49] Failure to recognize this principle in an acute medical setting can result in misdiagnosis and potentially serious mismanagement. Common inflammatory skin lesions, such as psoriasis and eczematous dermatitis, can occur in individuals with LE. These skin lesions are completely independent of LE and its treatment. Likewise, confusion can arise as a result of skin changes that occur as a result of systemic immunosuppressive therapy that might be needed to treat LE patients (eg, herpes zoster, steroid-induced acne, drug eruptions, opportunistic infections).

LOCAL THERAPY

SUN PROTECTION

Advise patients to avoid direct sun exposure, wear tightly woven clothing and broad-brimmed hats, and regularly use broad-spectrum, water-resistant sunscreens (SPF [sun protection factor] ≥30 with an efficient ultraviolet A blocking agent such as a photostabilized form of avobenzone [Parsol 1789], micronized titanium dioxide, micronized zinc oxide, or ecamsule [Mexoryl SX]). UV-blocking films should be applied to home and automobile windows, and acrylic diffusion shields should be placed over fluorescent lighting. Corrective camouflage cosmetics such as Dermablend and Covermark offer the dual benefit of being highly effective physical sunscreens as well as aesthetically pleasing cosmetic masking agents. Ting and Sontheimer provide an in-depth discussion of practical and theoretical photoprotection and local therapy for autoimmune connective tissue skin disease.[50]

As a result of the need for sun avoidance, and perhaps of other factors as well, both CLE and SLE patients are often found to be vitamin D insufficient or deficient.[51,52] There are clear human health benefits to normalizing vitamin D metabolism. Whether correcting vitamin D insufficiency/deficiency has a therapeutic impact on the cutaneous and SLE disease activity is under study.

TOPICAL GLUCOCORTICOIDS

Although some prefer intermediate-strength preparations, such as triamcinolone acetonide 0.1%, for sensitive areas such as the face, superpotent topical class I agents, such as clobetasol propionate 0.05% or betamethasone dipropionate 0.05%, produce the greatest benefit in CLE. Twice-daily application of the superpotent preparations to lesional skin for 2 weeks followed by a 2-week rest period can minimize the risk of local complications such as steroid atrophy and telangiectasia. Alternatively, a topical calcineurin inhibitor can be used daily during the 2-week rest period from topical corticosteroids. Ointments are more effective than creams for more hyperkeratotic lesions such as hypertrophic DLE. Occlusive therapy with glucocorticoid-impregnated tape (eg, flurandrenolide) or glucocorticoids with plastic food wrap (eg, Saran or Glad Press-N-Seal) can potentiate the beneficial effects of topical glucocorticoids but also carries a higher risk of local side effects. Class I or class II topical glucocorticoid solutions and gels are best for treating the scalp. Unfortunately, even the most aggressive regimen of topical glucocorticoids by itself does not provide adequate improvement for most patients with SCLE and CCLE.

TOPICAL CALCINEURIN INHIBITORS

Pimecrolimus 1% cream and tacrolimus 0.1% ointment have demonstrated efficacy in the treatment of ACLE, DLE, and SCLE.[53-55] A double-blind, placebo-controlled pilot study showed that pimecrolimus 1% cream had equal efficacy with betamethasone valerate 0.1% cream in treating facial DLE,[56] and a different study demonstrated the efficacy of topical tacrolimus 0.3% compound in clobetasol propionate 0.05% for recalcitrant CLE.[57]

It remains to be demonstrated whether topical delivery of newer classes of targeted nonsteroidal antiinflammatory agents that are being developed for other clinical indications might be of benefit for CLE (eg, topical apremilast, topical tofacitinib).

INTRALESIONAL GLUCOCORTICOIDS

Intralesional glucocorticoids (eg, triamcinolone acetonide suspension, 2.5 to 5 mg/mL for the face with higher concentrations allowable in less-sensitive sites) are more useful in the management of DLE than SCLE. Intralesional glucocorticoids themselves can produce cutaneous and subcutaneous atrophy (deep injections into the subcutaneous tissue enhances this risk). A 30-gauge needle is preferred because it produces only mild discomfort on penetration, especially when injected perpendicularly to the skin. The active borders of lesions should be thoroughly infiltrated. Intralesional therapy is indicated for particularly hyperkeratotic lesions or lesions that are unresponsive to topical glucocorticoids, but most patients with CLE have too many lesions to be managed exclusively by intralesional glucocorticoid injections.

SYSTEMIC THERAPY

ANTIMALARIALS

One or a combination of the aminoquinoline antimalarials can be effective for approximately 75% of patients with CLE who have failed to benefit adequately from the local measures described in "Local Therapy" above. The risks of retinal toxicity should be discussed with the patient, and a pretreatment ophthalmologic examination should be performed. However, the risk of antimalarial retinopathy is extremely rare, particularly in the first 10 years of therapy, if the recommended daily dose maximum levels of these agents are not exceeded (hydroxychloroquine, 6.5 mg/kg/day based on ideal body weight; chloroquine, 3 to 4 mg/kg/day). Patients should have followup ophthalmologic evaluations every 6 to 12 months while on therapy.

Hydroxychloroquine sulfate (Plaquenil), 6 to 6.5 mg/kg of lean body mass, should be given daily, either once daily or in 2 divided doses to prevent GI side effects. Approximately 6 weeks are required to reach equilibrium blood levels of hydroxychloroquine. Patients should be informed about a 2- to 3-month delayed onset of therapeutic benefit. If no response is seen after 8 to 12 weeks, quinacrine hydrochloride, 100 mg/day (currently available in the United States only through compounding pharmacies), can be added to the hydroxychloroquine without enhancing the risk of retinopathy (quinacrine does not cause retinopathy). If, after 4 to 6 weeks of this combined regimen adequate clinical control has not been achieved, consideration should be given to replacing the hydroxychloroquine in this combined regimen with chloroquine diphosphate (Aralen), 3 to 4 mg/kg/day. Doses may need to be adjusted for patients with decreased renal or hepatic function. In Europe, chloroquine is generally felt to be more efficacious than hydroxychloroquine in treating CLE, perhaps because of the earlier therapeutic responses that might occur as a result of the shorter time period required to reach steady-state blood levels with chloroquine as compared to hydroxychloroquine. Hydroxychloroquine and chloroquine should not be used simultaneously because of enhanced risk for retinal toxicity. There is some evidence that chloroquine may be more retinotoxic than hydroxychloroquine.

It is now possible to assay serum levels of hydroxychloroquine. However, this assay has not yet been made available widely by commercial testing laboratories in the United States. Recent studies examining this end point have found that up to 10% of CLE and SLE patients are not compliant in taking their hydroxychloroquine therapy as prescribed.[58,59] In addition, these and other studies have suggested that hydroxychloroquine serum levels and disease activity measures are inversely correlated in both cutaneous and SLE patients undergoing hydroxychloroquine therapy.[60]

It is now generally agreed that the modern hydroxychloroquine regimen can be used safely in children (with the appropriate dose adjustment based on lean body mass) and in women who are pregnant. However, the therapeutic index in children is quite narrow. Therefore, extra caution should be taken to prevent accidental overdosing of children.

Multiple side effects other than retinal toxicity are associated with the use of antimalarials. Quinacrine is associated with a higher incidence of side effects, such as headache, GI intolerance, hematologic toxicity, pruritus, lichenoid drug eruptions, and mucosal or cutaneous pigmentary deposition, than is either hydroxychloroquine or chloroquine. However, at the currently recommended dose of no more than 100 mg/day, such adverse effects are extremely rare. Quinacrine commonly produces a yellow discoloration of the entire skin and sclera in fair-skinned individuals, which is completely reversible when the dose of the drug is reduced or discontinued altogether. Quinacrine can produce significant hemolysis in patients with glucose-6-phosphate dehydrogenase (G6PD) deficiency (this adverse effect has also been reported to occur rarely with hydroxychloroquine and chloroquine). Each of the aminoquinoline antimalarials can produce bone marrow suppression, including aplastic anemia, although this effect is exceedingly rare with the current dosage regimens. Toxic psychosis, grand mal seizures, neuromyopathy, and cardiac arrhythmias occurred with the use of high doses of these drugs in the past; these reactions are uncommon with the lower daily dose regimens used today.

Before therapy with hydroxychloroquine and chloroquine is begun, complete blood cell counts, as well as liver and renal function tests, should be performed; these tests should be repeated 4 to 6 weeks after therapy is initiated, and every 4 to 6 months thereafter. A screen for hematologic toxicity when quinacrine is used is recommended more often. Patients with overt or subclinical porphyria cutanea tarda are at particularly high risk for developing acute hepatotoxicity, which often simulates an acute surgical abdomen, when treated with therapeutic doses of antimalarials for CLE.

NONIMMUNOSUPPRESSIVE OPTIONS FOR ANTIMALARIAL-REFRACTORY DISEASE

Some patients with refractory CLE (SCLE more than DLE) respond to diaminodiphenylsulfone (dapsone).[61] An initial dose of 25 mg by mouth twice daily can be increased up to 200 to 400 mg/day, if necessary. Significant dose-related hemolysis and/or methemoglobinemia can result from the use of dapsone, especially in individuals deficient in G6PD activity. Consequently, complete blood counts and liver function tests should be performed regularly, and testing for G6PD status should be considered prior to starting treatment, especially in high-risk populations. Isotretinoin, 0.5 to 2.0 mg/kg/day, and acitretin, 10 to 50 mg/day, also have been used in this setting, but their efficacy is limited by their side effects (teratogenicity, mucocutaneous dryness, and hyperlipidemia). In addition, breakthrough of CLE activity has been a problem with the long-term use of retinoids.

Thalidomide (50 to 200 mg/day) is strikingly effective for CLE that is refractory to other medications. Numerous studies cite response rates between 85% and 100%, with many patients experiencing complete remission.[62] However, strict prescribing regulations put in place in the United States in 1998 because of severe teratogenicity, make thalidomide challenging to dispense to women of childbearing potential. Sensory neuropathy is another toxicity associated with thalidomide, and 25% to 75% of patients with CLE develop peripheral neuropathy while taking the drug. Most cases are reversible when therapy is stopped. Neuropathy seems to correlate with total treatment times so that short courses are preferred. Relapses after the drug is stopped are common. Excess somnolence as well as constipation and other minor side effects sometimes limit its use, although these effects usually abate with lower daily doses.[63] Thromboembolism is a serious adverse event that may occur in patients with a preexisting hypercoagulable state (eg, presence of antiphospholipid antibodies). Oncologists who use thalidomide for multiple myeloma frequently initiate concomitant anticoagulation therapy to prevent this side effect. Lenalidomide (Revlimid, Celgene), a thalidomide analog, is U.S. Food and Drug Administration (FDA) approved for the treatment of multiple myeloma. In preliminary studies, its efficacy rate in CLE appears to be similar to that of thalidomide. Safety data to date indicates a much lower rate of peripheral neuropathy compared to thalidomide; however, it has a similar rate of thromboembolism (especially when combined with glucocorticoids) and leukopenia compared to thalidomide. Its potential teratogenicity in humans has yet to be determined.

Other drugs reported to be of value in the treatment of refractory CLE are gold and clofazimine; however, the benefit varies from case to case and both of these agents are associated with the risk of significant side effects. Vitamin E, phenytoin, sulfasalazine, danazol, DHEA, and phototherapy (UVA1 phototherapy, photopheresis) also have been reported clinical trials to be of potential value in CLE.

IMMUNOSUPPRESSIVE OPTIONS FOR ANTIMALARIAL-REFRACTORY DISEASE

Systemic Glucocorticoids: Every effort should be made to avoid the use of systemic glucocorticoids in patients with LE limited to the skin. However, in occasional patients who have especially severe and symptomatic skin disease, intravenous pulse methylprednisolone has been used. In less-acute cases, moderate daily doses of oral glucocorticoids (prednisone, 20 to 40 mg/day, given as a single morning dose) can be used as supplemental therapy during the loading phase of therapy with an antimalarial agent. The dose should be reduced at the earliest possible time because of the complications of long-term glucocorticoid therapy, especially avascular (aseptic) bone necrosis, a side effect to which patients with LE are particularly susceptible.

Because steroid-induced bone loss occurs most rapidly in the first 6 months of use, all patients who do not have contraindications should begin agents to prevent osteoporosis with the initiation of steroid therapy. An excellent review describing current recommendations for prevention of bone loss and other side effects of systemic glucocorticoids has been published.[64] When the disease activity is controlled, the daily dosage should be reduced by 5- to 10-mg decrements until activity flares again or until a daily dosage of 20 mg/day is achieved. The daily dose should then be lowered by 2.5-mg decrements (some physicians prefer to use 1-mg dose decrements below 10 mg/day). Alternate-day glucocorticoid therapy has not been successful in suppressing disease activity in most patients with CLE or SLE. Prednisolone rather than prednisone should be used in patients who have significant underlying liver disease, because prednisone requires hydroxylation in the liver to become biologically active. Any amount of prednisone given as a single oral dose in the morning has less adrenal-suppressing activity than the same amount given in divided doses throughout the day. However, any given amount of this drug, taken in divided doses, has a greater LE-suppressing activity than does the same amount of drug given as a single morning dose. Daily doses of prednisone less than or equal to 7.5 mg/day eliminate glucocorticoid-induced damage accrual in SLE patients.[65]

Traditional Immunosuppressives: Azathioprine (Imuran) (1.5 to 2 mg/kg per day orally) can play a glucocorticoid-sparing role in the severely affected patient with CLE. Mycophenolate mofetil (CellCept) (2.5 to 3 g divided twice daily orally) is a purine analog similar to azathioprine, but with more specific inhibition of the de novo pathway in lymphocytes. This characteristic may allow for more efficacy and less toxicity in treating severe, recalcitrant CLE, and such results have been reported in several studies.[66,67] Methotrexate (7.5 to 25 mg orally 1 day per week) is effective for severe refractory CLE. A double-blind, randomized, placebo-controlled trial in patients with SLE showed that moderate doses of methotrexate (15 to 20 mg weekly) effectively controlled cutaneous and articular activity and permitted a reduction in prednisone dose.[68] Other immunosuppressives that have been used anecdotally include cytosine arabinoside (Cytarabine) and cyclosporine. Immunotherapy with high-dose IV gammaglobulin has also been used.

Biologic Therapies: There have been reports documenting efficacy of anti-TNF medications (etanercept, adalimumab, infliximab) in the treatment of recalcitrant CLE, particularly SCLE.[69-71] However, these agents are also well-known to induce both SLE and CLE, highlighting the importance of TNF homeostasis in patients predisposed to LE.[72,73]

B-lymphocyte stimulator (BLyS [synonym: B-cell activating factor (BAFF)]), is a recently discovered member of the TNF cytokine family. BLyS is made by monocytes and macrophages with subsequent release when these cells are activated. BLyS binds to a receptor found only on B cells which stimulates maturation into antibody-secreting plasma cells. A fully human monoclonal antibody directed against BLyS (belimumab [Benlysta]) inhibits the biologic activity of BLyS. Belimumab is now FDA approved for SLE. In the clinical trials of belimumab in SLE, the cutaneous end points in SLE patients were met in addition to the systemic end points. However, little has been reported to date concerning the clinical efficacy of belimumab in isolated CLE.

As previously discussed abnormal regulation of interferon-α appears to play a central role in the pathogenesis of both cutaneous and systemic manifestations of LE by upregulating proinflammatory cytokines and chemokines. Three biologics that target type 1 IFN are currently being tested for their efficacy and safety in active SLE patients (2 anti–interferon-α monoclonal antibodies [rontalizumab and sifalimumab] and one monoclonal antibody that binds to a type 1 IFN receptor [anifrolumab]).[74] Recombinant humanized antibodies to type 1 IFN and to the interferon receptor are under development. If these new biologics prove to be of benefit in SLE disease activity, one could extrapolate that they might be helpful in CLE disease activity.

Class I interferon actions are transduced through the Janus kinase (JAK)-signal transducer and activator of transcription (STAT) intracellular signaling pathway. Disrupting this intracellular signaling pathway might provide another approach to downregulating SLE and CLE disease activity and damage. Two orally administered JAK isoenzyme inhibitors have been approved by the FDA for other clinical disorders: tofacitinib (JAK 1/3) for rheumatoid arthritis and ruxolitinib (JAK 1/2) for myelodysplastic disorders. There are case reports in which these 2 drugs appeared to have clinical benefit in both CLE and cutaneous dermatomyositis.[75,76] More specific JAK1 isoenzyme inhibitors are currently under development (eg, filgotinib) which promise to lessen the side effects of this new class of targeted, small-molecule therapy.

SURGICAL AND COSMETIC THERAPY

DLE lesions can produce permanent scarring alopecia, cosmetically disturbing dermal atrophy, and long-lasting pigmentary changes. Patients so affected often ask about the possibility of cosmetic correction of these changes. Surgical interventions such as hair transplantation and dermabrasion carry finite risks because CLE is characterized by a tendency for nonspecific mechanical trauma, including surgical incision or laser ablation, to exacerbate disease activity (ie, Koebner phenomenon/isomorphic phenomenon). Some patients tolerate scar revision techniques, including dermabrasion, if they are on maintenance systemic therapy (eg, antimalarials). There are anecdotal reports of the successful management of active CLE with argon and pulsed-dye laser therapy.[77] Resurfacing of atrophic scars with the Erbium:YAG or Fraxel carbon dioxide resurfacing laser is reported to be beneficial.[78,79] Autologous fat transplantation can be of clinical value in patients with atrophic scarring from burned out lupus panniculitis/profundus. The injection of atrophic lesions with collagen or other similar foreign cosmetic materials should be avoided.

TREATMENT ALGORITHM

Treatment of CLE with the aforementioned agents is typically done in a stepwise manner to minimize the risk of side effects and is outlined in Table 61-6.

PREVENTION

Predicting and preventing the initial clinical manifestation of LE, whether it is skin disease or systemic, is not feasible at this time. However, as many LE patients exhibit worsening of their skin disease activity with UV light exposure, physical protection from sunlight and artificial sources of UV light as well as the regular use of broad-spectrum sunscreens having a SPF of 30 or greater should be encouraged.

CLE patients should be encouraged to discontinue cigarette smoking. CLE patients who smoke cigarettes are not as responsive to antimalarial therapy compared to those who do not smoke. CLE patients who smoke and are not responding to antimalarial therapy have been observed to experience complete remission in their CLE activity after they discontinue smoking with no other change in their therapy. Cigarette smoking does not alter antimalarial metabolism. It has been suggested that cigarette smoking, irrespective of antimalarial therapy, is strongly associated with CLE and somewhat less so with SLE.[80,81]

REFERENCES

1. Gilliam JN, Sontheimer RD. Distinctive cutaneous subsets in the spectrum of lupus erythematosus. *J Am Acad Dermatol*. 1981;4(4):471-475.
2. Tan EM, Cohen AS, Fries JF, et al. The 1982 revised criteria for the classification of systemic lupus erythematosus. *Arthritis Rheum*. 1982;25(11):1271-1277.
3. Watanabe T, Tsuchida T. Classification of lupus erythematosus based upon cutaneous manifestations. Dermatological, systemic and laboratory findings in 191 patients. *Dermatology*. 1995;190(4):277-283.
4. Tebbe B, Orfanos CE. Epidemiology and socioeconomic impact of skin disease in lupus erythematosus. *Lupus*. 1997;6(2):96-104.
5. Robinson D Jr, Aguilar D, Schoenwetter M, et al. Impact of systemic lupus erythematosus on health, family, and work: the patient perspective. *Arthritis Care Res (Hoboken)*. 2010;62(2):266-273.
6. Ferraz LB, Almeida FA, Vasconcellos MR, et al. The impact of lupus erythematosus cutaneous on the quality of life: the Brazilian-Portuguese version of DLQI. *Qual Life Res*. 2006;15(3):565-570.
7. Durosaro O, Davis MD, Reed KB, et al. Incidence of cutaneous lupus erythematosus, 1965-2005: a population-based study. *Arch Dermatol*. 2009;145(3):249-253.
8. Lin JH, Dutz JP, Sontheimer RD, et al. Pathophysiology of cutaneous lupus erythematosus. *Clin Rev Allergy Immunol*. 2007;33(1-2):85-106.
9. Braunstein I, Klein R, Okawa J, Werth VP. The interferon-regulated gene signature is elevated in subacute cutaneous lupus erythematosus and discoid lupus erythematosus and correlates with the cutaneous lupus area and severity index score. *Br J Dermatol*. 2012;166(5):971-975.
10. Bennett L, Palucka AK, Arce E, et al. Interferon and granulopoiesis signatures in systemic lupus erythematosus blood. *J Exp Med*. 2003;197(6):711-723.
11. Farkas L, Beiske K, Lund-Johansen F, et al. Plasmacytoid dendritic cells (natural interferon-alpha/beta-producing cells) accumulate in cutaneous lupus erythematosus lesions. *Am J Pathol*. 2001;159(1):237-243.
12. Jego G, Palucka AK, Blanck JP, et al. Plasmacytoid dendritic cells induce plasma cell differentiation through type I interferon and interleukin 6. *Immunity*. 2003;19(2):225-234.
13. Kiefer K, Oropallo MA, Cancro MP, et al. Role of type I interferons in the activation of autoreactive B cells. *Immunol Cell Biol*. 2012;90(5):498-504.
14. Crow YJ, Chase DS, Lowenstein Schmidt J, et al. Characterization of human disease phenotypes associated with mutations in TREX1, RNASEH2A, RNASEH2B, RNASEH2C, SAMHD1, ADAR, and IFIH1. *Am J Med Genet A*. 2015;167A(2):296-312.
15. Namjou B, Kothari PH, Kelly JA, et al. Evaluation of the TREX1 gene in a large multi-ancestral lupus cohort. *Genes Immun*. 2011;12(4):270-279.
16. Casciola-Rosen L, Rosen A. Ultraviolet light-induced keratinocyte apoptosis: a potential mechanism for the induction of skin lesions and autoantibody production in LE. *Lupus*. 1997;6(2):175-180.
17. Meller S, Winterberg F, Gilliet M, et al. Ultraviolet radiation-induced injury, chemokines, and leukocyte recruitment: an amplification cycle triggering cutaneous lupus erythematosus. *Arthritis Rheum*. 2005;52(5):1504-1516.
18. Lehmann P, Homey B. Clinic and pathophysiology of photosensitivity in lupus erythematosus. *Autoimmun Rev*. 2009;8(6):456-461.
19. Moghadam-Kia S, Chilek K, Gaines E, et al. Cross-sectional analysis of a collaborative Web-based data-

20. Rahman P, Gladman DD, Urowitz MB. Smoking interferes with efficacy of antimalarial therapy in cutaneous lupus. *J Rheumatol*. 1998;25(9):1716-1719.
21. Hardy CJ, Palmer BP, Muir KR, et al. Smoking history, alcohol consumption, and systemic lupus erythematosus: a case-control study. *Ann Rheum Dis*. 1998;57(8):451-455.
22. Jewell ML, McCauliffe DP. Patients with cutaneous lupus erythematosus who smoke are less responsive to antimalarial treatment. *J Am Acad Dermatol*. 2000;42(6):983-987.
23. Kang I, Park SH. Infectious complications in SLE after immunosuppressive therapies. *Curr Opin Rheumatol*. 2003;15(5):528-534.
24. Yung RL, Quddus J, Chrisp CE, et al. Mechanism of drug-induced lupus. I. Cloned Th2 cells modified with DNA methylation inhibitors in vitro cause autoimmunity in vivo. *J Immunol*. 1995;154(6):3025-3035.
25. Sontheimer RD, Thomas JR, Gilliam JN. Subacute cutaneous lupus erythematosus: a cutaneous marker for a distinct lupus erythematosus subset. *Arch Dermatol*. 1979;115(12):1409-1415.
26. Chaudhry SI, Murphy LA, White IR. Subacute cutaneous lupus erythematosus: a paraneoplastic dermatosis? *Clin Exp Dermatol*. 2005;30(6):655-658.
27. Jou IM, Liu MF, Chao SC. Widespread cutaneous necrosis associated with antiphospholipid syndrome. *Clin Rheumatol*. 1996;15(4):394-398.
28. Franceschini F, Calzavara-Pinton P, Quinzanini M, et al. Chilblain lupus erythematosus is associated with antibodies to SSA/Ro. *Lupus*. 1999;8(3):215-219.
29. Hedrich CM, Fiebig B, Hauck FH, et al. Chilblain lupus erythematosus—a review of literature. *Clin Rheumatol*. 2008;27(8):949-954.
30. Viguier M, Pinquier L, Cavelier-Balloy B, et al. Clinical and histopathologic features and immunologic variables in patients with severe chilblains. A study of the relationship to lupus erythematosus. *Medicine (Baltimore)*. 2001;80(3):180-188.
31. Lee-Kirsch MA, Chowdhury D, Harvey S, et al. A mutation in TREX1 that impairs susceptibility to granzyme A-mediated cell death underlies familial chilblain lupus. *J Mol Med (Berl)*. 2007;85(5):531-537.
32. Callen JP. Clinically relevant information about cutaneous lupus erythematosus. *Arch Dermatol*. 2009;145(3):316-319.
33. Maize JC Jr, Costner M. Tumid lupus erythematosus: a form of lupus erythematosus. *Arch Dermatol*. 2010;146(4):451; author reply 450-451.
34. Ruiz H, Sanchez JL. Tumid lupus erythematosus. *Am J Dermatopathol*. 1999;21(4):356-360.
35. Kuhn A, Sonntag M, Richter-Hintz D, et al. Phototesting in lupus erythematosus: a 15-year experience. *J Am Acad Dermatol*. 2001;45(1):86-95.
36. Dekle CL, Mannes KD, Davis LS, et al. Lupus tumidus. *J Am Acad Dermatol*. 1999;41(2, pt 1):250-253.
37. Vieira V, Del Pozo J, Yebra-Pimentel MT, et al. Lupus erythematosus tumidus: a series of 26 cases. *Int J Dermatol*. 2006;45(5):512-517.
38. Stead J, Headley C, Ioffreda M, et al. Coexistence of tumid lupus erythematosus with systemic lupus erythematosus and discoid lupus erythematosus: a report of two cases of tumid lupus. *J Clin Rheumatol*. 2008;14(6):338-341.
39. Tomasini D, Mentzel T, Hantschke M, et al. Plasmacytoid dendritic cells: an overview of their presence and distribution in different inflammatory skin diseases, with special emphasis on Jessner's lymphocytic infiltrate of the skin and cutaneous lupus erythematosus. *J Cutan Pathol*. 2010;37(11):1132-1139.
40. Obermoser G, Schwingshackl P, Weber F, et al. Recruitment of plasmacytoid dendritic cells in ultraviolet irradiation-induced lupus erythematosus tumidus. *Br J Dermatol*. 2009;160(1):197-200.
41. Obermoser G, Sontheimer RD, Zelger B. Overview of common, rare and atypical manifestations of cutaneous lupus erythematosus and histopathological correlates. *Lupus*. 2010;19(9):1050-1070.
42. Zecevic RD, Vojvodic D, Ristic B, et al. Skin lesions—an indicator of disease activity in systemic lupus erythematosus? *Lupus*. 2001;10(5):364-367.
43. Lee LA, Weston WL. Cutaneous lupus erythematosus during the neonatal and childhood periods. *Lupus*. 1997;6(2):132-138.
44. David-Bajar KM, Davis BM. Pathology, immunopathology, and immunohistochemistry in cutaneous lupus erythematosus. *Lupus*. 1997;6(2):145-157.
45. Crowson AN, Magro C. The cutaneous pathology of lupus erythematosus: a review. *J Cutan Pathol*. 2001;28(1):1-23.
46. Baltaci M, Fritsch P. Histologic features of cutaneous lupus erythematosus. *Autoimmun Rev*. 2009;8(6):467-473.
47. Albrecht J, Taylor L, Berlin JA, et al. The CLASI (Cutaneous Lupus Erythematosus Disease Area and Severity Index): an outcome instrument for cutaneous lupus erythematosus. *J Invest Dermatol*. 2005;125(5):889-894.
48. Bonilla-Martinez ZL, Albrecht J, Troxel AB, et al. The cutaneous lupus erythematosus disease area and severity index: a responsive instrument to measure activity and damage in patients with cutaneous lupus erythematosus. *Arch Dermatol*. 2008;144(2):173-180.
49. Greenwald RA. Greenwald's law of lupus. *J Rheumatol*. 1992;19(9):1490.
50. Ting WW, Sontheimer RD. Local therapy for cutaneous and systemic lupus erythematosus: practical and theoretical considerations. *Lupus*. 2001;10(3):171-184.
51. Cusack C, Danby C, Fallon JC, et al. Photoprotective behaviour and sunscreen use: impact on vitamin D levels in cutaneous lupus erythematosus. *Photodermatol Photoimmunol Photomed*. 2008;24(5):260-267.
52. Watad A, Neumann SG, Soriano A, et al. Vitamin D and systemic lupus erythematosus: myth or reality? *Isr Med Assoc J*. 2016;18(3-4):177-182.
53. Kreuter A, Gambichler T, Breuckmann F, et al. Pimecrolimus 1% cream for cutaneous lupus erythematosus. *J Am Acad Dermatol*. 2004;51(3):407-410.
54. Lampropoulos CE, Sangle S, Harrison P, et al. Topical tacrolimus therapy of resistant cutaneous lesions in lupus erythematosus: a possible alternative. *Rheumatology (Oxford)*. 2004;43(11):1383-1385.
55. von Pelchrzim R, Schmook T, Friedrich M, et al. Efficacy of topical tacrolimus in the treatment of various cutaneous manifestations of lupus erythematosus. *Int J Dermatol*. 2006;45(1):84-85.
56. Barikbin B, Givrad S, Yousefi M, et al. Pimecrolimus 1% cream versus betamethasone 17-valerate 0.1% cream in the treatment of facial discoid lupus erythematosus: a double-blind, randomized pilot study. *Clin Exp Dermatol*. 2009;34(7):776-780.

57. Madan V, August PJ, Chalmers RJ. Efficacy of topical tacrolimus 0.3% in clobetasol propionate 0.05% ointment in therapy-resistant cutaneous lupus erythematosus: a cohort study. *Clin Exp Dermatol*. 2010;35(1):27-30.
58. Frances C, Cosnes A, Duhaut P, et al. Low blood concentration of hydroxychloroquine in patients with refractory cutaneous lupus erythematosus: a French multicenter prospective study. *Arch Dermatol*. 2012;148(4):479-484.
59. Mok CC, Penn HJ, Chan KL, et al. Hydroxychloroquine serum concentrations and flares of systemic lupus erythematosus: a longitudinal cohort analysis. *Arthritis Care Res (Hoboken)*. 2016;68(9):1295-1302.
60. Durcan L, Clarke WA, Magder LS, et al. hydroxychloroquine blood levels in systemic lupus erythematosus: clarifying dosing controversies and improving adherence. *J Rheumatol*. 2015;42(11):2092-2097.
61. Neri R, Mosca M, Bernacchi E, et al. A case of SLE with acute, subacute and chronic cutaneous lesions successfully treated with dapsone. *Lupus*. 1999;8(3):240-243.
62. Briani C, Zara G, Rondinone R, et al. Positive and negative effects of thalidomide on refractory cutaneous lupus erythematosus. *Autoimmunity*. 2005;38(7):549-555.
63. Wu JJ, Huang DB, Pang KR, et al. Thalidomide: dermatological indications, mechanisms of action and side-effects. *Br J Dermatol*. 2005;153(2):254-273.
64. Dooley MA, Ginzler EM. Newer therapeutic approaches for systemic lupus erythematosus: immunosuppressive agents. *Rheum Dis Clin North Am*. 2006;32(1):91-102, ix.
65. Ruiz-Arruza I, Ugarte A, Cabezas-Rodriguez I, et al. Glucocorticoids and irreversible damage in patients with systemic lupus erythematosus. *Rheumatology (Oxford)*. 2014;53(8):1470-1476.
66. Hanjani NM, Nousari CH. Mycophenolate mofetil for the treatment of cutaneous lupus erythematosus with smoldering systemic involvement. *Arch Dermatol*. 2002;138(12):1616-1618.
67. Kreuter A, Tomi NS, Weiner SM, et al. Mycophenolate sodium for subacute cutaneous lupus erythematosus resistant to standard therapy. *Br J Dermatol*. 2007;156(6):1321-1327.
68. Carneiro JR, Sato EI. Double blind, randomized, placebo controlled clinical trial of methotrexate in systemic lupus erythematosus. *J Rheumatol*. 1999;26(6):1275-1279.
69. Norman R, Greenberg RG, Jackson JM. Case reports of etanercept in inflammatory dermatoses. *J Am Acad Dermatol*. 2006;54(3)(suppl 2):S139-S142.
70. Fautrel B, Foltz V, Frances C, et al. Regression of subacute cutaneous lupus erythematosus in a patient with rheumatoid arthritis treated with a biologic tumor necrosis factor alpha-blocking agent: comment on the article by Pisetsky and the letter from Aringer et al. *Arthritis Rheum*. 2002;46(5):1408-1409; author reply 1409.
71. Aringer M, Graninger WB, Steiner G, et al. Safety and efficacy of tumor necrosis factor alpha blockade in systemic lupus erythematosus: an open-label study. *Arthritis Rheum*. 2004;50(10):3161-3169.
72. Ramos-Casals M, Brito-Zeron P, Munoz S, et al. Autoimmune diseases induced by TNF-targeted therapies: analysis of 233 cases. *Medicine (Baltimore)*. 2007;86(4):242-251.
73. Wetter DA, Davis MD. Lupus-like syndrome attributable to anti-tumor necrosis factor alpha therapy in 14 patients during an 8-year period at Mayo Clinic. *Mayo Clin Proc*. 2009;84(11):979-984.
74. Kalunian KC. Interferon-targeted therapy in systemic lupus erythematosus: Is this an alternative to targeting B and T cells? *Lupus*. 2016;25(10):1097-1101.
75. Wenzel J, van Holt N, Maier J, et al. JAK1/2 inhibitor ruxolitinib controls a case of chilblain lupus erythematosus. *J Invest Dermatol*. 2016;136(6):1281-1283.
76. Kurtzman DJ, Wright NA, Lin J, et al. Tofacitinib citrate for refractory cutaneous dermatomyositis: an alternative treatment. *JAMA Dermatol*. 2016;152(8):944-945.
77. Erceg A, Bovenschen HJ, van de Kerkhof PC, et al. Efficacy and safety of pulsed dye laser treatment for cutaneous discoid lupus erythematosus. *J Am Acad Dermatol*. 2009;60(4):626-632.
78. Tremblay JF, Carey W. Atrophic facial scars secondary to discoid lupus erythematous: treatment using the erbium:YAG laser. *Dermatol Surg*. 2001;27(7):675-677.
79. Walker SL, Harland CC. Carbon dioxide laser resurfacing of facial scarring secondary to chronic discoid lupus erythematosus. *Br J Dermatol*. 2000;143(5):1101-1102.
80. Chasset F, Frances C, Barete S, et al. Influence of smoking on the efficacy of antimalarials in cutaneous lupus: a meta-analysis of the literature. *J Am Acad Dermatol*. 2015;72(4):634-639.
81. Jiang F, Li S, Jia C. Smoking and the risk of systemic lupus erythematosus: an updated systematic review and cumulative meta-analysis. *Clin Rheumatol*. 2015;34(11):1885-1892.

Chapter 62 :: Dermatomyositis
:: Matthew Lewis & David Fiorentino

第六十二章
皮肌炎

中文导读

皮肌炎（DM）是一种全身性自身免疫性疾病，具有影响儿童和成人的双峰分布，其特征是皮肤和肌肉的炎症和损伤，10%～20%的成人皮肌炎可合并内脏恶性肿瘤。本章从概述、流行病学、临床特征、皮肤外表现、病因学和发病机理、诊断、病理、鉴别诊断、临床进程和预后、管理、干预等方面详细地全方位阐述了皮肌炎的特征；也阐述了无肌病性皮肌炎的概念；详细描述了皮肌炎典型皮损的常见、少见皮疹及罕见表现。临床医生应该区分皮疹是疾病活跃时的表现还是疾病导致的皮肤损伤，因为前者是可逆的而后者不会因为免疫抑制治疗而得到改善。对于皮疹进行活动性评估有益于临床治疗决策的制定。疾病活跃的皮疹特征是红斑、瘙痒、硬结（丘疹或斑块）、皮屑及溃疡，但是也需要注意到红斑虽然大多数情况下是活跃的标志，但是也可能是后期皮肤损伤的特点（如弥漫性毛细血管扩张性红斑），因而注意避免仅仅因为红斑而没有其他疾病活跃表现时升级治疗。文中讨论了几种皮肤损害而非皮疹活跃的皮肤临床特征。皮外表现分别阐述了肺部、肌肉、关节、消化道、心血管、内脏恶性肿瘤等各器官受累的临床特征。皮肌炎主要是一种免疫介导的疾病，分子和组织学证据支持先天性和适应性免疫的作用。激活先天免疫系统是疾病发病和发展的关键点。诊断仍然依赖于临床医生基于病史和体检实验室结果的综合分析。皮肌炎的皮肤组织病理经典表现为少细胞的界面皮炎。文中列举了与皮肌炎皮疹相似的皮肤病变的临床特点及鉴别要点。疾病管理的基本原则是评估潜在影响的器官，即皮肤、肌肉和肺。筛查恶性肿瘤是至关重要的。由于皮肌炎多器官受累，包括皮肤科、风湿科、呼吸科及神经科医生的多科合作是必要的。并分别就局部治疗、全身治疗、物理治疗及康复、特殊情况下如手术切除钙质沉着等多方面阐述了疾病的治疗及干预。

〔施 为〕

AT-A-GLANCE

- Dermatomyositis (DM) is a systemic autoimmune disease with a bimodal distribution affecting children and adults, characterized by inflammation and damage to the skin and muscle.
- Interstitial lung disease (ILD) affects 20% of patients and is a major source of morbidity and mortality in these patients.
- In adults, DM heralds the diagnosis of a coexisting internal malignancy in 10% to 20% of cases. A thorough review of systems and malignancy workup, including computed tomography scans of the chest, abdomen, and pelvis, may be prudent to detect occult cancers that are missed on routine age-appropriate screening.
- The diagnosis is established with a combination of the hallmark cutaneous findings and supportive skin histopathology, with or without evidence of a proximal myopathy. The diagnosis may be challenging because 20% of patients never manifest clinically significant muscle weakness.
- The cutaneous manifestations are typified by violaceous erythema in many sites, most notably the eyelids, upper chest, back, elbows, knees, and lateral hips in addition to proximal nailfold capillary dilation and pericapillary hemorrhage.
- Characteristic autoantibodies (antisynthetase, anti–Mi-2, anti–transcriptional intermediary factor [TIF1]-γ, anti–melanoma differentiation–associated gene 5 [*MDA5*], anti–nuclear matrix protein 2 [NXP2], and anti–small ubiquitin-like modifier activating enzyme [SAE] autoantibodies) may be useful in identifying clinical subsets and establishing the diagnosis in cases without the classic clinical or histopathologic features.
- The presence or absence of certain autoantibodies assists with risk stratification for organ involvement as well as for associated malignancy. Notably, the presence of anti-MDA5 and antisynthetase autoantibodies is associated with an increased risk of ILD, and the presence of anti–TIF1-γ and anti-NXP2 autoantibodies is associated with an increased risk of having an associated cancer.
- Treatment of cutaneous DM can be challenging, and most patients with significant skin disease require systemic therapy. Multiple agents may be necessary to achieve complete remission; the risks and benefits each agent should be considered carefully given the potentially prolonged treatment course.

INTRODUCTION

DEFINITIONS

Dermatomyositis (DM) continues to be classified as a form of myositis and, in fact, is traditionally considered one of the idiopathic inflammatory myopathies. Implicit in this classification is that myositis is required to make this diagnosis, as well as the characteristic rash—the often used criteria of Bohan and Peter exemplify this.[1,2] This is problematic because it is widely accepted now that a proportion of patients, perhaps 20%,[3] have the characteristic rash but no clinical signs or symptoms of myositis. These patients make up a population now defined as clinically amyopathic dermatomyositis (CADM), a term coined by Sontheimer in 1991.[4] Patients with CADM have the characteristic DM rash (with a consistent skin biopsy) for at least 6 months' duration but no evidence of weakness by history or clinical examination; earlier concepts also require demonstration of normal muscle enzyme levels,[5-7] but this definition was later refined that a patient with normal strength and abnormal muscle enzyme levels could still be included under the CADM definition.[8] If not CADM, then the rest of patients with DM have what is often termed "classic dermatomyositis," referring to the traditionally recognized disease with symptomatic myositis. CADM is a useful term for physicians because it is defined clinically and makes no attempt to deny the presence of subclinical muscle inflammation. The CADM umbrella can further be subclassified into exactly two groups depending on the results of further imaging (eg, magnetic resonance imaging [MRI]), electromyographic, muscle biopsy, or (now) laboratory studies of muscle enzymes: hypomyopathic DM, in which at least one of these test results is abnormal, and amyopathic DM, in which all the test results are normal.

It should be noted that several other groups have proposed classification criteria for DM that focus on muscle histology,[9] clinical findings,[10,11] or combinations of these.[12] It has become clear that muscle histology and clinical findings cannot be defined that are specific to DM, although it remains possible that novel serotypes may have sufficient sensitivity and specificity to play a major role in defining DM.

The definition of exactly what constitutes a "DM rash" has been elusive. Sontheimer has proposed formal cutaneous criteria for making a diagnosis of CADM in 2002.[5] Three major criteria include the pathognomonic heliotrope sign (violaceous erythema on the upper eyelids), Gottron papules (papules overlying the metacarpophalangeal [MCP] and interphalangeal [IP] joints), and Gottron sign (erythema overlying the knees, elbows, or IP joints) and 14 additional minor criteria (Fig. 62-1). Sontheimer suggested that a diagnosis of CADM could be made if two major criteria were present or one major criterion and two minor criteria were present in addition to biopsy of at least one region showing histopathologic changes consistent with DM.[5] Although these criteria seem comprehensive and reasonable, they have not yet been validated in any way.

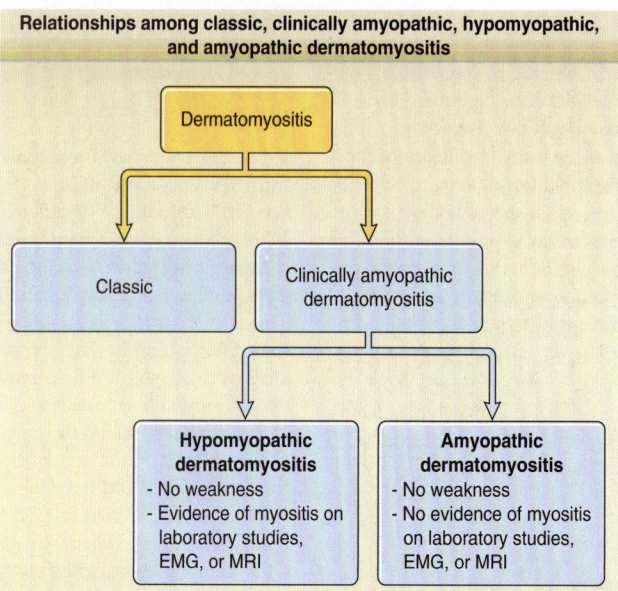

Figure 62-1 Display of the relationships among classic, clinically amyopathic, hypomyopathic, and amyopathic dermatomyositis. EMG, electromyography; MRI, magnetic resonance imaging.

It will continue to be important to recognize patients with CADM even though there is no evidence that this group of patients is pathogenically, histologically, or serologically different from the classic group except with regards to absence of clinical weakness. Even if these patients were managed the same as patients with myositis regarding aggressive immunotherapy (which is not necessarily the case), they are an important group to recognize because these patients appear to harbor the same risks for systemic disease (eg, interstitial lung disease [ILD]) and malignancy as their classic counterparts.[8] Thus, for now, recognizing the prototypical and also atypical or subtle cutaneous presentations of CADM is especially important for dermatologists because these clues may provide the only data upon which the diagnosis is based.

EPIDEMIOLOGY

DM has a bimodal distribution in the age of disease onset, occurring at two peaks, at 5 to 14 years and 45 to 64 years of life. The disease affects women two to three times more than often than men. As discussed earlier, DM is typically classified as an idiopathic inflammatory myopathy, a group of disorders that includes polymyositis, inclusion body myositis, nonspecific myositis, and immune-mediated necrotizing myopathy. Estimating the incidence and prevalence of pure DM is challenging because of a lack of precision and standardization regarding diagnostic criteria (with many studies even grouping DM and polymyositis into one disease), differing methods of case ascertainment, differing study design, and possible geographic influences.[13,14] Despite this, using data from the few population-based studies or largest databases available, estimates of incidence and prevalence are remarkably similar, with incidence rates ranging from 5 to 10 per 1 million per year and prevalence estimates of 10 to 20 per 100,000. Data from the largest population-based study in southeast Norway (>2.6 million people) estimated a point prevalence of total polymyositis or DM of 8.7 (95% confidence interval [CI], 4.5–11.2) per 100,000, of which about half of cases were DM. This study estimated an incidence of 6 to 10 cases per 1 million each year.[15] Bendewald and coworkers provided population estimates for adult-onset DM from Olmstead County, Minnesota. The age- and sex-adjusted incidence was 9.63 (95% CI, 6.09–13.17) per 1 million per decade, and the prevalence was 21.42 per 100,000 persons (95% CI, 13.07–29.77).[3] In their small cohort, 20% (6 of 29 cases) were clinically amyopathic. Analysis of data from large insurance claims databases in Japan and Taiwan estimated an annual incidence of 10 to 13 and 6 to 10 per million annually, respectively.[16,17] Based on registry data, the annual incidence of juvenile-onset DM in the United States among children ages 2 to 17 was estimated between 2.5 and 4.1 per million.[18]

CLINICAL FEATURES

CUTANEOUS FINDINGS

Elements of the patient history may be useful in distinguishing DM from mimicking eruptions. Triggers may be present such as substantial ultraviolet exposure, strenuous activity (for the patient with concurrent myositis), or recent malignancy. There is often significant pruritus associated with affected skin, particularly on the scalp, which may also be described as a "tightness" or burning or with other dysesthetic qualities such as crawling or tingling. This severe pruritus on the scalp may be caused by structural damage to epidermal small-fiber nerves.[19] The natural history of the eruption is chronic and often progressive, ultimately resulting in a background of dyspigmentation, atrophy, and telangiectasias. An evanescent or wholly intermittent eruption is unlikely to represent DM. With treatment, however, many patients can ultimately enter remission in which no further activity is present but residual damage features (eg, poikiloderma) may remain.

The characteristic cutaneous feature of affected skin in DM is violaceous patches and plaques, varying from a bright pink to a deep violet color. In darker skin types, the erythema is often subtle, and careful examination is important to detect skin involvement. To heighten the sensitivity of the exam and appreciate these, at times, subtle color changes, patient positioning, and proper lighting in the examination room are critical. Many types of overhead direct lighting tend to obscure the subtle color changes seen in DM skin, and thus natural lighting is recommended for the clinical examination. Evaluating the patient in a reclined or supine position helps minimize shadows, particularly on the face, and overexposure with direct lighting.

The scalp is one of the most commonly involved sites, often only with pink to red erythema (Fig. 62-2), but there may be associated fine white scale. The pruritus and dysesthesia are often severe and out of proportion to the erythema on examination. The scalp can be affected in any location but often involves a linear band just above and below the frontal hairline. Examination findings alone are not always specific enough to differentiate it from seborrheic dermatitis, psoriasis, and contact dermatitis. Subtle erythema is often perceptible on the vertex scalp or along the hair part or borders of the hairline even when the remainder of the cutaneous disease is quiescent.

The heliotrope sign (Fig. 62-3) may exemplify the pink to purple violet hue of the eruption, resembling the color of the flower petals after which the sign is named. The eyelid eruption can be associated with periorbital edema, and patients are often initially misdiagnosed with allergic contact dermatitis or angioedema. In addition, erythema of the lateral canthi, medial canthi, and adjacent nasal sidewalls can be seen (Fig. 62-4). The forehead, cheeks, ears, and chin may vary from uninvolved to focal patches or plaques to diffuse erythema.

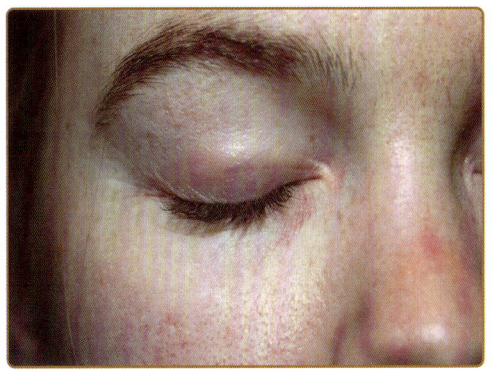

Figure 62-3 Heliotrope sign. Violaceous to pink erythema and edema on the upper eyelid.

The skin changes in DM are often distributed to prototypical regions on the body Table 62-1). Trunk involvement is often seen on the posterior neck, upper back, and shoulders, known as the shawl sign (Fig. 62-5), which may extend to the posterior upper arms. Patients can display symmetric violaceous erythema, often with a livedo character, symmetrically on the lateral lower back. Confluent violaceous erythema on the sun-exposed areas of the lower anterior neck and anterior chest is termed the V-neck sign (Fig. 62-6). The violaceous to pink papules over the IP and MCP joints are termed Gottron papules (Fig. 62-7). They may display the same range of features seen elsewhere such as poikiloderma, atrophy, hypopigmentation, hyperkeratosis, or ulceration (Fig. 62-8). They may take the form of larger, ill-defined, round circular plaques (often with scale) or of 2- to 4-mm, smooth, well-demarcated, often umbilicated papules. Gottron sign is symmetric macular violaceous erythema over the IP joints, olecranon processes (Fig. 62-9), patellae, and medial malleoli. Generally, juvenile DM more characteristically displays atrophy and poikiloderma in classic areas of Gottron sign.

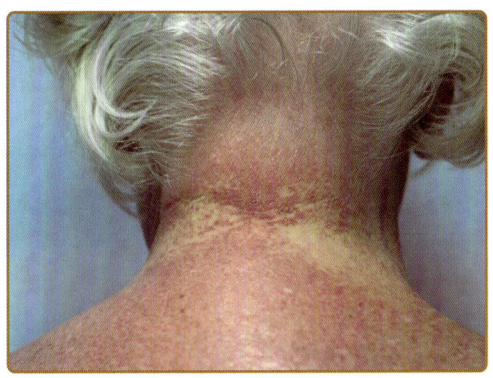

Figure 62-2 Diffuse pink psoriasiform plaques on the posterior neck and nuchal scalp.

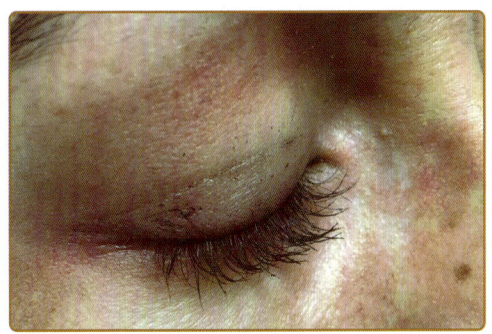

Figure 62-4 Red ill-defined macules on the medial and lateral canthi, often seen in conjunction with the heliotrope sign.

TABLE-62-1
Sontheimer's Proposed Diagnostic Criteria for Cutaneous Dermatomyositis[1]

Diagnosis of cutaneous dermatomyositis requires:
1. Presence of two major criteria or one major criterion and two minor criteria *and*
2. Skin biopsy changes consistent with cutaneous dermatomyositis

Major Criteria
Heliotrope sign
Gottron papules
Gottron sign

Minor Criteria
Macular violaceous erythema involving (each area counts as one minor criterion)
- Scalp or anterior hairline
- Malar eminences of face, forehead, or chin
- V-area of neck or upper chest (V-neck sign)
- Posterior neck or posterior shoulders (shawl sign)
- Extensor surfaces of arms or forearms
- Linear streaking overlying extensor tendons of dorsal hands
- Periungal skin
- Lateral thighs or hips (holster sign)
- Medial malleoli

Nailfold capillary telangiectasia, hemorrhage-infarct
Poikiloderma
Mechanic's hands
Cutaneous calcinosis
Cutaneous ulcers
Pruritus

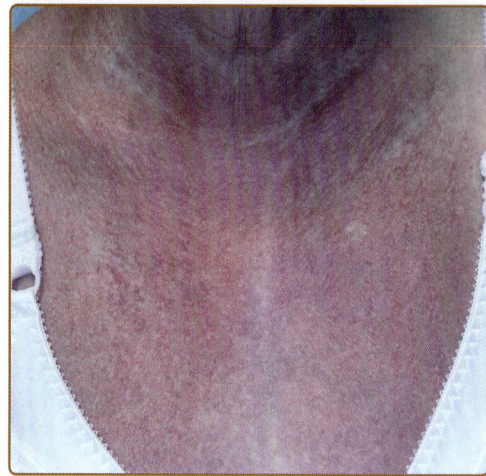

Figure 62-6 V-neck sign. Red, ill-defined telangiectatic patches on the upper chest.

this is patterned as violaceous, folliculocentric macules or subtle papules and can be confused with keratosis pilaris. The violaceous and typically macular nature of the eruption, usually in the absence of involvement of other areas typical for keratosis pilaris (eg, upper outer arms) helps to characterize this finding of DM. In addition, flagellate erythema may be found as widespread linear patches or urticarial plaques, typically on the middle and lower back, and flanks, possibly caused by excoriation or imprinting from clothing or bed sheets.

Of note, many of sites of cutaneous DM skin involvement areas are *not* necessarily in areas of ultraviolet (UV) exposure (so-called "photodistributed"), including the scalp, lower back, and lateral thighs. Some patients can present with a classic photodistributed eruption, but more often the erythema is patchy even in sites with high risk of UV exposure. The violaceous erythema and poikiloderma on the lateral hips and lateral thighs is termed the Holster sign (Fig. 62-10). Often

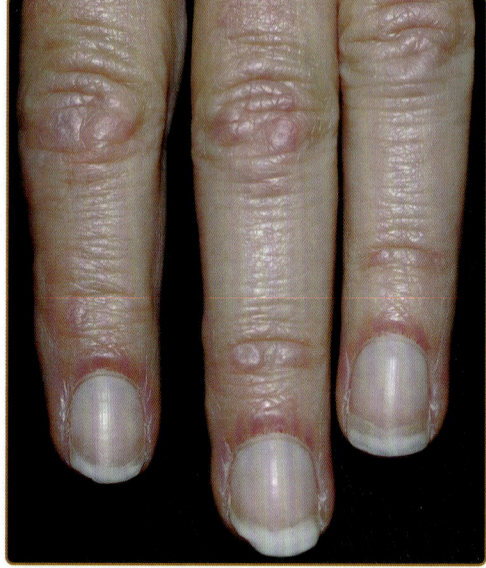

Figure 62-7 Gottron papules. Light pink, ill-defined papules over the proximal and distal interphalangeal joints, few with central umbilication. Deep red erythema, edema of the proximal nailfolds, and dilated nailfold capillaries are evident.

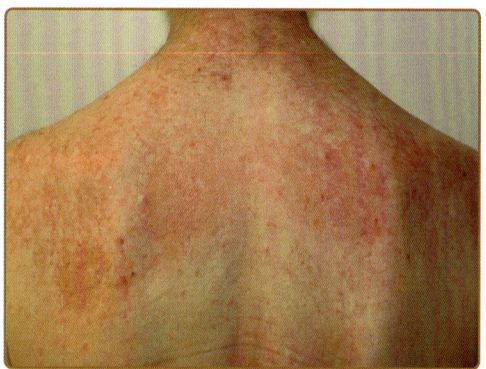

Figure 62-5 Shawl sign. Pink to red thin patches and plaques, often with thin white scale, on the upper posterior back characteristic of the shawl sign.

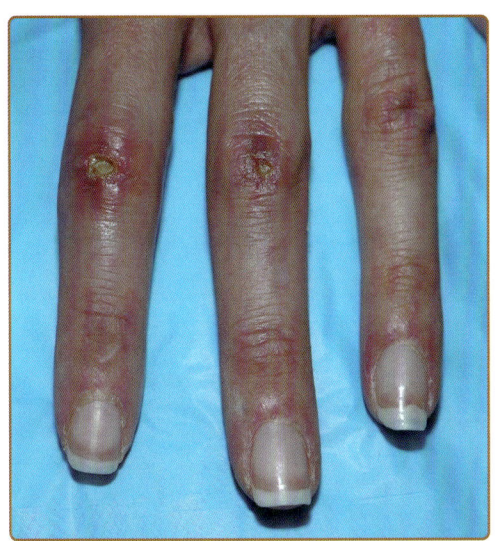

Figure 62-8 Ulcerated Gottron papules. Well-demarcated 3- to 4-mm ulcers with surrounding erythema and edema on the second and third proximal interphalangeal joints exemplify the vasculopathy seen in dermatomyositis.

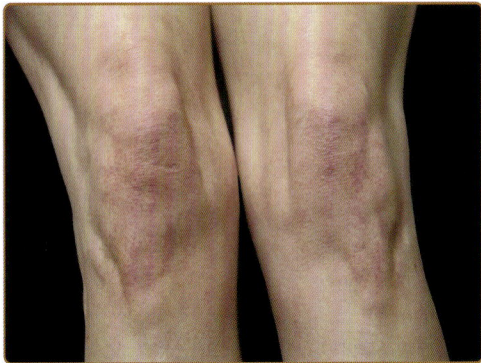

Figure 62-9 Gottron sign. Ill-defined violaceous erythema on the knees is seen, which has follicular accentuation in this patient.

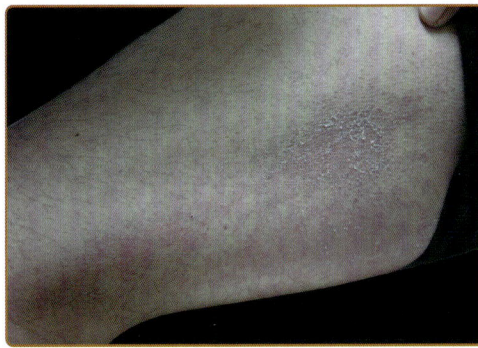

Figure 62-10 Holster sign. On the lateral thigh are ill-defined pink papules coalescing into plaques are seen with scale and follicular accentuation.

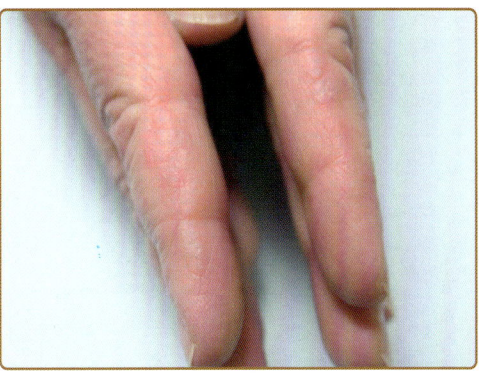

Figure 62-11 Mechanic's hands. On the lateral second digits are hyperkeratotic pink ill-defined papules with scale.

Other characteristic hand findings include the, so-called "mechanic's" hands. This finding was initially described as hyperkeratosis and fissuring along the medial thumb and lateral second and third digits in 1979.[20] This finding may be subtle and often requires palpating the fingers to appreciate the rough texture (Fig. 62-11). This lateral second digit hyperkeratosis seems to differ in quality and severity with the findings in patients with antisynthetase antibodies, the latter associated with fissuring and scaling that tends to also involve the distal fingertips.

In 2012, Sato and coworkers found an increased prevalence of ILD among their patients with DM with mechanic's hands (78%, 7 of 9) compared with without mechanic's hands (40%, 12 of 30),[21] supporting that mechanic's hands is a cutaneous clue to the possible presence of ILD. A recent study by Werth and coworkers found that in 101 patients with DM, mechanic's hands was associated with an odds ratio of 3.28 (95% CI, 1.36–7.88; $P = 0.01$) of having ILD.

Evidence of vasculopathy is manifested in many ways on the skin. Proximal nailfold involvement can present as subtle edema or erythema as well as microscopic or clinically obvious capillary dilation. When pronounced and easily visualized with the naked eye, these nailfold capillary changes can be highly suggestive of DM over other connective tissue disorders. The classic findings include red, edematous, often tender proximal nailfolds with ramified and dilated capillary loops with intervening pale to white avascular areas with capillary drop-out, cuticular hemorrhages, and elongated, ragged cuticles (Fig. 62-12). Although these changes are a sign of ongoing cutaneous disease activity,[22] in longstanding DM, damage may be evident as persistently dilated and arborizing capillaries.[23] Sensitive nailfolds can be a helpful diagnostic symptom for DM. In addition, gingival telangiectasias have been described in DM.[24] In addition, livedo reticularis can be seen in a minority of patients.

Cutaneous ulceration can be an exemplary sign of vasculopathy, although it can also be the result of robust, liquefactive interface dermatitis, or excoriation. Ulceration may be present in 30% of patients and

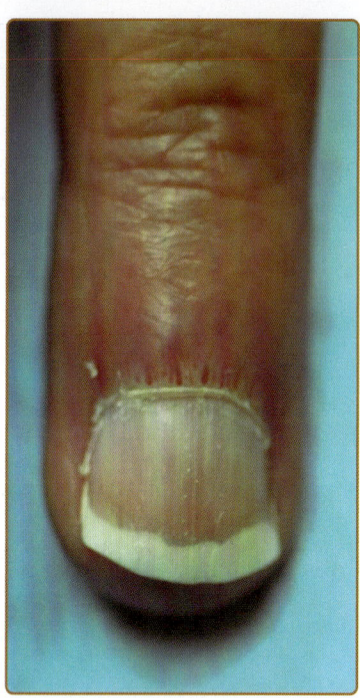

Figure 62-12 Dilated proximal nailfold capillary loops with intervening avascular areas.

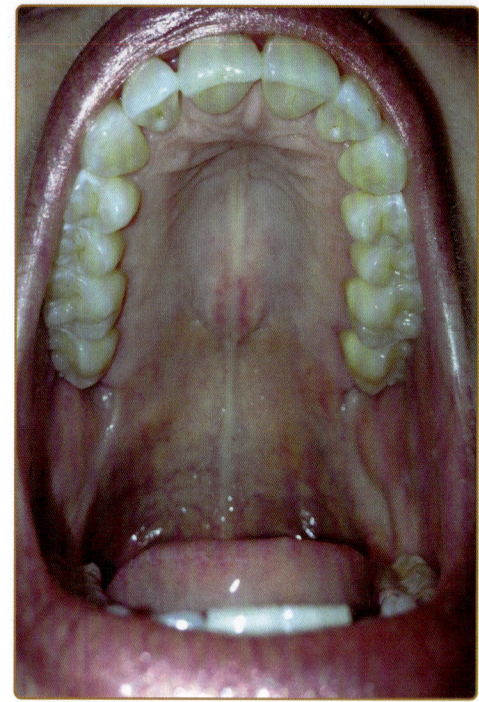

Figure 62-13 Ovoid palatal patch. This symmetric violaceous patch is seen symmetrically across the posterior hard palate and may aid in distinguishing dermatomyositis from other cutaneous eruptions, namely lupus.

often affects the skin over the extensor joint surfaces, although it can be found anywhere.[25] Cutaneous ulceration in DM warrants concern for the presence of anti-MDA5 antibodies or malignancy (especially if necrosis is seen). In the setting of anti-MDA5 antibodies, cutaneous ulceration commonly occurs over Gottron papules (see Fig. 62-8) or in areas of Gottron sign (eg, extensor surfaces).[25,26] Ulcers have been correlated with the presence of ILD, but this is likely through their association with anti-MDA5 antibodies.[25,27] As such, worsening cutaneous ulceration in a patient with anti-MDA5 antibodies may be a cutaneous sign of worsening ILD.

Visualization of the oral mucosa, particularly the hard palate, may provide a valuable sign to aid in the diagnosis of DM. One can observe a symmetric violaceous patch across the midline of the hard palate, termed the *ovoid palatal patch* (Fig. 62-13), most frequently in the subset of patients with DM with anti–transcriptional intermediary factor 1γ (TIF1-γ) antibodies.[28] Biopsies from these lesions appear to demonstrate interface mucositis, consistent with typical findings of DM. Like nailfold capillary changes described later, these hard palate changes appear to fade with control of disease activity. These lesions could be confused with oral findings of discoid lupus or lichen planus, but their consistent localization to the center of the hard palate may aid in the diagnosis of DM when other cutaneous features are nondiagnostic. In addition, other oral mucosal findings include gingival telangiectasias (noted earlier) as well as more classic lichen planus–like lesions around the gingiva or buccal mucosa. Whether or not these latter lesions represent coexisting lichen planus or are part of the DM disease spectrum is not clear.

In general, the clinician should be always differentiating signs of skin activity, which may be reversible with therapy, versus damage. The distinction between activity and damage in DM skin is critical for clinical decision making so immunosuppressive treatments are not escalated for signs of skin damage. Cutaneous disease activity is characterized by erythema, itch, induration (papules or plaques), scale, or ulceration. Although erythema is often an important sign of activity, it can often be a sign of damage as well (eg, diffuse telangiectatic erythema), and thus care must be taken not to inadvertently escalate therapy solely caused by erythema that has no other qualities of disease activity. This phenomenon can be especially true on the face and chest, and faint erythema in the absence of symptoms or other skin changes is often mild damage and may not respond to traditional immunosuppressive therapies. Also, a reticular pattern of pink to red erythema on the palms and volar surfaces (more commonly seen in the anti-MDA5 group, Fig. 62-14), in addition to more classic livedo reticularis (including that found on the lateral flanks) represents vascular changes that have unclear association with disease activity.

When substantial inflammation has been present, a distinctive and pathognomonic pattern may be seen composed of reticulated, sometimes atrophic white macules adjacent to erythema or telangiectasias, which

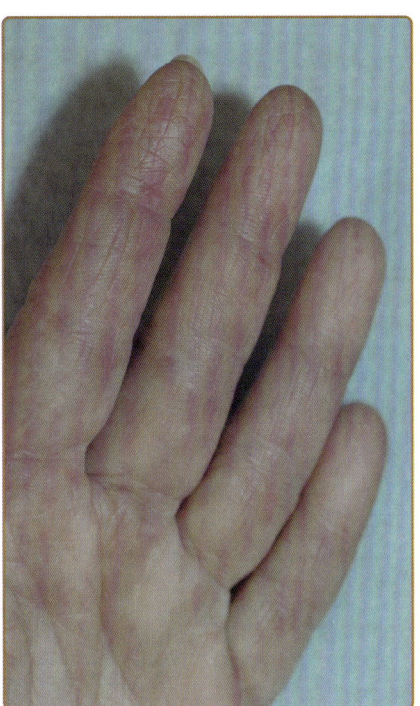

Figure 62-14 A reticular pattern of deep red erythema on the palmar fingers is more commonly seen in the anti–melanoma differentiation–associated gene 5 (*MDA5*) dermatomyositis group.

the authors have termed "red on white" (Fig. 62-15).[29] The thin skin along the bitemporal hairline is a frequent place to visualize the "red-on-white" pattern, but notably, this pattern does not necessarily follow patterns of sun exposure and may be found on the hair-bearing scalp. It is becoming increasingly clear that many of these areas do not represent permanent damage per se because these lesions may slowly resolve with time, even in areas with atrophy. However, this morphology is a very useful diagnostic tool because it does not seem to be associated with other connective tissue diseases, such as cutaneous lupus.

Skin damage from DM is reflected by brown, often reticulated, postinflammatory hyperpigmented patches in areas of prior disease activity. Longstanding disease activity, typically in sun-exposed areas, results in more significant damage, characterized by atrophy, hypopigmentation, hyperpigmentation, and telangiectasias, termed *poikiloderma* (Fig. 62-16). Poikiloderma (as opposed to the "red-on-white" manifestation discussed earlier) is a late manifestation and is not diagnostically specific because many other acquired and congenital diseases result in poikiloderma such as cutaneous lupus, chronic actinic damage (poikiloderma of Civatte), poikilodermatous mycosis fungoides (poikiloderma vasculare atrophicans), *Borrelia* infection (acrodermatitis chronica atrophicans), chronic radiation dermatitis, graft-versus-host disease, hydroxyurea, and dyskeratosis congenita. Therefore, ancillary cutaneous findings are necessary to discern the cause of poikiloderma.

Calcinosis is typically a late manifestation in the skin, subcutaneous tissue, fascia, or muscle and typically affects the trunk, proximal extremities, or areas of previous disease activity. The prevalences of calcinosis are 20% in adult DM[30] and up to 40% in juvenile DM.[31] Calcinosis also occurs more rapidly after disease onset in juvenile versus adult DM (2.9 years vs 7.9 years, respectively).[32] In juvenile DM, risk factors for development of calcinosis include longer disease duration, younger age of disease onset, sustained disease activity, and internal organ involvement.[33,34] Calcinosis is most frequent on the extremities in DM, in contrast to systemic sclerosis in which digital calcinosis is most frequent.[32] In both juvenile and adult DM, the presence of anti–nuclear matrix protein 2 (NXP-2) antibodies is associated with an increased risk of calcinosis.[35,36] In adults, fingertip ulceration has been associated with calcinosis,[36] suggesting that vascular insufficiency or damage may be involved in the pathogenesis of calcinosis. Calcinosis is also commonly seen in the anti-MDA5 subset (especially in patients with longstanding disease),[36] which is associated with known vasculopathy.

Figure 62-15 "Red on white." Reticulated white macules surrounded by telangiectatic red macules are seen on the distal thigh and knee. This cutaneous finding is specific to dermatomyositis and is valuable in differentiating dermatomyositis from cutaneous lupus.

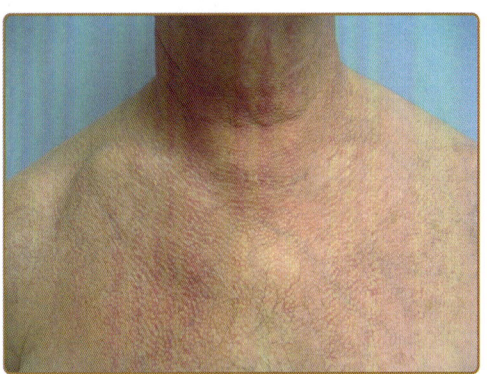

Figure 62-16 Poikiloderma. This triad of hyperpigmentation, hypopigmentation, and telangiectasias is a sign of damage, as shown on the chest.

Panniculitis reflects active disease in DM, typically affecting the buttocks, trunk, and proximal extremities; it may progress to calcinosis or lipoatrophy.[37] Histopathology shows a lobular panniculitis but may have features of lupus panniculitis with lipomembranous changes or with septal thickening as in deep morphea.

Alopecia in DM is most commonly nonscarring and diffuse, although patchy involvement, rarely with scarring, can also be seen. Alopecia can be caused by DM disease, coexisting disorders, medications, or telogen effluvium. Patients with anti-MDA5 antibodies have a higher risk of alopecia, which commonly is severe and occurs early in the disease.

RARE PRESENTATIONS OF CUTANEOUS DERMATOMYOSITIS

Subcutaneous edema that is either generalized or located in the limbs has been recognized as a rare manifestation of DM.[38] Interestingly, edema in the distal extremities has recently been found to be associated with anti-NXP2 antibodies and may predict more severe muscle disease.[38,39] It is unclear what the relationship is between anti-NXP2 antibodies and the more severe, generalized presentations described in the literature. Rarely, DM may present erythroderma in which 90% or more of the body surface shows confluent erythema. Generalized ichthyosis can also be a presenting sign of DM.

There is a subset of patients with DM with clinical manifestations with overlapping features of both psoriasis and DM.[40,41] Their skin disease may show psoriasiform, well-demarcated thick plaques over the MCPs and proximal interphalangeal (PIP) joints, elbows, and knees in addition to dilated and abnormal nailfold capillaries. Skin biopsies tend to reveal both epidermal hyperplasia and interface dermatitis. Some of these patients have a history of psoriasis, and it is unclear if these lesions represent concomitant psoriasis or a psoriasiform manifestation of DM.

EXTRACUTANEOUS FINDINGS

PULMONARY INVOLVEMENT

ILD is the most common pulmonary manifestation in DM and is a leading cause of morbidity and mortality in these patients.[42] Other pulmonary manifestations in DM include aspiration pneumonia; drug-induced pneumonitis; and, rarely, pulmonary hypertension. ILD affects between 15% and 50% of patients with DM, depending on the population and autoantibody distribution.[43-46]

There are three clinically described patterns of lung involvement, which may precede or proceed muscle involvement[47,48]: it may be asymptomatic with only radiologic evidence of ILD; it may have an insidious onset with gradual development of decreased exercise capacity, dyspnea on exertion, or a dry cough; finally, it may be acute onset with hypoxia and possibly respiratory failure, necessitating hospitalization.

In a recent study from a large US cohort of 438 patients with polymyositis or DM ($n = 393$), the presence of ILD in patients with DM was associated with an increased risk of death with a hazard ratio of 2.13 (95% CI, 1.06–4.25; $P = 0.03$).[49] Large case series have suggested that more than 75% to 86% of patients who have an antisynthetase antibody will develop ILD.[47,50] Similarly, patients with DM with anti-MDA5 antibodies have a marked increased risk of developing ILD with estimates between 50% and 100%[25,51] Table 62-2). Rapidly progressive ILD is an aggressive form that responds poorly to immunosuppressive therapies, having a 6-month survival rate of approximately 40%.[52] Rapidly progressive ILD may affect 40% to 60% of patients with anti-MDA5 antibodies.[53-56]

Pulmonary function tests (PFTs) show a restrictive disease pattern with a decreased forced vital capacity (FVC)[57] or a decreased diffusion capacity of carbon monoxide. Exertional oxygenation desaturation on the 6-minute walk test provides a global assessment of cardiopulmonary function and exercise performance. However, confounding factors such as deconditioning, myopathy, arthritis, respiratory muscle weakness, and pulmonary hypertension may also produce reduced FVC and diffusion capacity of carbon monoxide.[58] Therefore, high-resolution computed tomography (CT) of the chest is a necessary step in establishing the diagnosis of ILD.

High-resolution CT scan of the chest is a valuable diagnostic test and may show subclinical fibrosis before symptom onset. Up to 65% of patients with polymyositis and DM will have subclinical CT evidence of ILD.[59] The most common radiographic and histologic pattern in DM is nonspecific interstitial pneumonia, reported in 81.8% (18 of 22 cases).[60] Radiographically, basilar and peripheral ground-glass opacities and subpleural sparing characterize nonspecific interstitial pneumonia. Other patterns of involvement include usual interstitial pneumonia, cryptogenic organizing pneumonia, and diffuse alveolar damage, the latter with a poor prognosis.

Pulmonary arterial hypertension is a rare manifestation in DM. Symptoms may include increased fatigue, shortness of breath, dyspnea on exertion, palpitations, chest pain, edema, lightheadedness, and rarely presyncopal or syncopal episodes. PFT revealing a disproportionately low diffusion capacity of carbon monoxide compared with a relatively normal FVC should prompt further screening for pulmonary artery hypertension. If a high-resolution CT scan is checked for worsening shortness of breath and abnormal PFT results, it may show an enlarged pulmonary artery but no evidence of ILD. Echocardiographic findings suggestive of pulmonary hypertension include a right ventricular systolic pressure greater than 40 mm Hg, right ventricular

TABLE 62-2
Clinical Associations with Autoantibodies Associated with Dermatomyositis[1,2]

AUTOANTIBODY	AUTOANTIGEN	CLINICAL PHENOTYPE IN ADULT DERMATOMYOSITIS	FREQUENCY IN ADULT DERMATOMYOSITIS	FREQUENCY AND PHENOTYPE IN JUVENILE DERMATOMYOSITIS
Anti-tRNA synthetase	Jo-1: histidyl PL-7: threonyl PL-12: alanyl EJ: glycyl OJ: isoleucyl KS: asparaginyl Ha: tyrosinyl Zo: phenylalanyl	Increased risk of ILD PL-7: mild skin or muscle disease[3] PL-12, KS, OJ: isolated ILD[4-6] Variable spectrum of findings of the antisynthetase syndrome: ILD, fever, arthritis, myositis, mechanic's hands, Raynaud phenomenon	Jo-1 is the most frequent, up to 20% Non–Jo-1 anti-tRNA synthetase antibodies between 1% and 5%[7]	4%–5%[8] Older onset Antisynthetase syndrome with ILD, fever, nonerosive polyarthritis, Raynaud phenomenon, mechanic's hands
Anti–Mi-2	Mi-2; regulates transcription as a component of nucleosome remodeling and deacetylase (NuRD) complex	Hallmark cutaneous disease, good prognosis and response to therapy; relapses common; high CK values (>5000 U/L); rare ILD, cancer; not amyopathic	Ethnogeographic variation: 20% in US[9] and Japan[10] 6.7% in Glasgow 60% in Guatemala[11]	3%[8,12] Classic skin disease Myositis Good therapeutic response; more likely to be in remission at 2 yr
Anti–transcriptional intermediary factor (TIF1)-γ	p155; TIF; role in apoptosis, ubiquitination, and innate immunity	Increased cancer risk in adults Severe cutaneous disease Red-on-white skin lesions Ovoid palatal patch Low ILD risk Low CK values (200–2000 U/L)	21%–38%[13,14]	23%–35%[8] Severe skin disease Lipodystrophy
Anti–melanoma differentiation–associated gene 5 (MDA5)	Melanoma differentiation-associated protein 5; cytosolic receptor for viral dsRNA; mediates type I IFN innate immune response	High ILD risk, RP-ILD, especially in Asians Skin ulceration, red palmar papules, alopecia, gingival pain Arthritis Often isolated high aldolase	7%–10% in US[15,16] 20%–35% in Asia[17,18]	7%–14%[19,20] ILD in Japanese cohort Skin ulceration, arthritis, milder myositis
Anti–nuclear matrix protein 2 (NXP2)	Nuclear matrix protein; transcription	Increased cancer risk in adults Increased risk of calcinosis Peripheral edema, myalgia, severe dysphagia Distal weakness	1.6%–30%[14,21-23]	20%–25%[8,12] Calcinosis, more severe myositis, poorer functional status
Anti–small ubiquitin-like modifier activating enzyme (SAE)	Small ubiquitin-like modifier activating enzyme; posttranslational modification	Skin disease onset before myositis May have severe skin disease Dysphagia	1.5%–10%[24-27]	1%[12]

CK, creatine kinase; IFN, interferon; ILD, interstitial lung disease; RP-ILD, rapidly progressive interstitial lung disease.

enlargement, maximum tricuspid regurgitant velocity greater than 3.0 m/s, and presence of a pericardial effusion.[61] Transthoracic echocardiography only has a sensitivity of 82% and specificity of 69% to detect pulmonary hypertension[61] and cannot differentiate patients with pulmonary arterial hypertension from those with left heart disease or ILD associated pulmonary hypertension. The gold standard for the diagnosis of pulmonary arterial hypertension is right heart catheterization showing a mean pulmonary artery pressure of 25 mm Hg or greater at rest and an end-expiratory pulmonary artery wedge pressure of 15 mm Hg or less.[62]

MUSCLE INVOLVEMENT

Myositis in DM typically presents as symmetrical proximal muscle weakness. About 20% of patients with DM, those with CADM, do not have clinical evidence or symptoms of weakness, although it is unclear what proportion of those patients might actually have subclinical myositis. If patients with DM do develop weakness, then about 80% of patients develop weakness within the first year of symptom onset.[63] The temporal course of myositis may be acute, subacute, or chronic and progressive.

Patients often report weakness in the extensor muscles surrounding the shoulder and pelvic girdles and proximal limbs. Quadriceps and gluteal muscle weakness may manifest as difficulty rising from a chair or toilet, climbing stairs, or stepping onto curbs. Patients may report shoulder and upper extremity weakness as difficulty washing their hair or reaching for items in overhead cupboards. Neck flexor muscle involvement is also common with difficulty raising the head off the bed while laying supine.

Patients may also complain of myalgias, which can occur even in the absence of frank clinical weakness. Approximately 30% of patients complain of muscle pain with or without muscle weakness.[9] Myalgias are described as soreness or muscle tightness or burning, but muscles are not tender to palpation. Care should be taken to distinguish this pain from other causes of pain, such as joint pain or fibromyalgia,[64] and care must be taken to not escalate immunosuppression for what may be symptoms of a pain disorder.

Involvement of respiratory muscles of the chest wall or diaphragm may also lead to respiratory insufficiency and occasionally respiratory failure. Patients may note a hoarse or raspy voice (dysphonia) from cricoarytenoid muscle involvement, which occurs in up to 40% of patients with DM.[65] Also, dysphagia may occur in 20% to 50% of cases because of weak pharyngeal musculature and thus an inability to propel food in the pharyngeal phase of swallowing.[66] Interestingly, there is a high correlation between dysphagia and weakness of the anterior neck muscles (eg, sternocleidomastoids).[67] Distal muscle weakness in the hands, manifesting as difficulty opening jars or holding onto objects, more typically occurs late in disease or in patients with anti-NXP2 antibodies.

JOINT INVOLVEMENT

Arthralgias are common in DM, reported in 30% to 40% of patients.[68-70] In general, the arthralgias in DM are mild to moderate in severity and involve the small joints of the hands, including the wrists, MCP and PIP joints, and the shoulders, elbows, and ankles.[71] More rarely, patients can have a true arthritis, often presenting as a symmetric polyarthropathy affecting the distal joints and often clinically indistinguishable from rheumatoid arthritis. Thus, patients with DM with arthritis as the presenting symptom may be diagnosed as having rheumatoid arthritis or a rheumatoid arthritis overlap disease before evolution of the skin, muscle, or pulmonary manifestations.[72,73] Illustrative historical questions eliciting symptoms of an inflammatory arthritis include joint swelling, morning stiffness for 30 minutes or longer, or joint pain that improves with activity. Evaluation for synovitis, indicative of active joint inflammation, can be determined by palpation for warmth; range of motion; swelling or palpable fluid; and tenderness of each small joint of the hand, elbows, shoulders, knees, and other symptomatic joints.

Arthritis and arthralgias are more common among patients with DM with anti-MDA5 and anti-synthetase antibodies. However, erosive changes have been reported, more commonly in the anti–synthetase antibody subset.[74-77] Hall and coworkers found that 9 of 11 (81.8%) anti-MDA5 patients versus 40 of 149 (26.7%) non-MDA5 patients with DM exhibited an inflammatory arthritis ($P <0.001$).[78] Patients with DM with antisynthetase antibodies, the most common of which is Jo-1, may also manifest a nonerosive arthritis in up to 93% of cases.[71] In these patients with antisynthetase antibodies, the nonerosive arthritis may occur in the setting of "antisynthetase syndrome" consisting of fever, arthritis, myositis, ILD, mechanic's hands, or Raynaud phenomenon. The arthritis may flare in 50% of patients during disease relapse.[71]

GASTROINTESTINAL INVOLVEMENT

Gastrointestinal (GI) involvement is an uncommon manifestation in juvenile DM, reported in 4% of juvenile patients with DM.[79] It is associated with more severe disease[80] and is thought to result from a vasculopathy affecting the bowel wall.[81] The sequelae include ulceration and perforation, which may be life threatening. The presenting symptoms include persistent and worsening abdominal pain. They also may have nonspecific accompanying symptoms such as diarrhea, vomiting, constipation, and more rarely frank hematemesis or hematochezia; juvenile patients may not initially have evidence of hemorrhage such as melena, occult blood in the stool, or radiographic evidence of perforation.[82] Therefore, judicious monitoring of juvenile patients with DM with abdominal pain is warranted to recognize and intervene early in cases with GI involvement.

CARDIOVASCULAR INVOLVEMENT

Cardiac involvement in DM is increasingly being recognized as an important clinical feature. Cardiac involvement is usually subclinical. The most common electrocardiographic abnormalities are ST-T segment changes in 12.5% to 56.7% and conduction abnormalities in 25% to 38.5% of patients with DM.[83] Echocardiographic findings have shown left ventricular hypertrophy in 8% to 15% and left ventricular diastolic dysfunction in 42% of patients.[84] Myocarditis may lead to myocardial fibrosis and ventricular dysfunction and thus cardiomyopathy. Rosenbohm and coworkers screened 11 patients with DM with cardiac MRI and found that 54% (6 of 11) displayed evidence of late gadolinium enhancement, consistent with myocardial inflammation.[85] Cardiac troponin I may be a useful biomarker in detecting subclinical cardiac muscle involvement.[86] Patients with the anti-MDA5 antibody subtype may be at higher risk for cardiac involvement.[87,88]

INTERNAL MALIGNANCY

DM is associated with an internal malignancy in 10% to 20% of cases.[89] Malignancies tend to occur within the first 1 to 2 years of disease onset and can be many types. Multiple population-based studies have estimated a standardized incidence ratio of 4 to 6 for malignancy compared with the normal population.[90] The cancer types that are overrepresented may vary depending on the population studied but appear to involve both solid tumors as well as hematopoietic malignancies. Common types of solid tumors include breast, lung, ovarian, prostate, colorectal, gastric, and pancreatic,[91-93] with nasopharyngeal cancer being more common in Southeast Asians.[94] The mechanism of the relationship between DM and malignancy is unknown but may include increased risk of cancer in the setting of immunosuppressive therapy, increased detection in the setting of heightened surveillance, and DM occurring in the setting of an immunologic response to internal malignancy.

There are several clinical risk factors associated with risk of malignancy, which include increasing age, male gender, cutaneous necrosis, dysphagia, and rapid onset of myositis.[95] Factors protective of malignancy include ILD, arthritis, and Raynaud phenomenon. Recently, malignancies have also been found to be more associated with particular DM-specific autoantibodies. The major antibody associated with malignancy is anti–TIF1-γ, although the precise elevation in risk appears to vary among studies and populations studied.[96,97] More recent data suggest that anti-NXP2 antibodies may also be associated with cancer, although this association is not as strong.[97,98]

Cancer screening is a source of controversy because no guidelines currently exist to direct screening in newly diagnosed patients with DM. Most authorities would agree with age-appropriate, routine cancer screening at a very minimum. However, in a small study, Sparsa and coworkers reported that initial routine cancer screening failed to discover 4 of 13 malignancies in their cohort.[99] A recent study of 400 patients showed that a substantial number of occult cancers (17 of 29) were only discovered using tests, usually CT scans, beyond what would be considered "age appropriate." Identifying which tests to order and in what patient population is of high priority.

ETIOLOGY AND PATHOGENESIS

DM is primarily an immune-mediated disorder with molecular and histologic evidence supporting a role for both innate and adaptive immunity. Muscle and skin biopsies show infiltration of CD3+ T cells, plasmacytoid dendritic cells, and macrophages as well as B cells (especially in muscle).[100,101] Parenchymal cell injury is manifested in the skin by interface dermatitis with keratinocyte injury and in muscle by atrophy, degeneration, and regeneration of muscle fibers, typically in a perifascicular distribution.

There is strong evidence for activation of the innate immune system as a critical step in disease pathogenesis and propagation. High levels of interferon (IFN)-induced genes and proteins found in blood, muscle, and skin and have been shown to correlate with disease activity.[102] There is some evidence that this response may be driven by IFN-β, although this is not yet clear. There are multiple pathways that could lead to activation of IFNs, most arising from so-called pattern recognition receptors in the cytoplasm. Many of these receptors are activated by aberrant quantity or structure of nucleic acids, which could come from viruses or the host, the latter in the form of damaged DNA or improperly processed RNA. High levels of IFN can induce DM autoantigens (eg, MDA5), activate immature dendritic cells to become effective antigen-presenting cells, and upregulate major histocompatibility (MHC) class I expression, and activate lymphocytes. In both skin and muscle, the cells expressing these IFN-induced gene products appear most concentrated in the areas of tissue damage and may play a role in recruiting and activating cytotoxic effector cells.

There is also abundant evidence for activation of the adaptive immune system in DM. Genetic studies have shown that polymorphisms in the human leukocyte antigen (HLA) region are highly associated with risk of DM, implicating activation of T cells. In addition, DM is associated with the presence of several, highly specific, circulating autoantibodies that are evidence of T- and B-cell activation. As mentioned, CD3+ T cells are found in tissue biopsies. The exact role of these antigen-specific responses is at present unclear, but the correlation between clinical phenotypes and specific autoantibodies suggests that these immune responses lie at the heart of disease pathogenesis. In addition, an animal model of myositis can be created by inducing anti–Jo1 immune responses in mice. Although some of these antigens have now been discovered, it remains unclear what cell type(s) or structures are the targets of such an immune response. Of interest, expression of several DM autoantigens is increased in damaged and regenerating muscle cells, suggesting that muscle fibers themselves might be direct targets of antigen-specific CD3+ cells.

The immune response may not be the entire story because histologic data support that a vasculopathy is a primary event in DM. Biopsies of both skin and muscle show endothelial degeneration and capillary dropout as some of the earliest findings. Deposition of the membrane attack complex of complement, consisting of C5b-9, is seen on the capillaries at the dermal–epidermal junction (DEJ) in skin and in the perifascicular blood vessels of the muscle.[103] However, there is no other evidence that membrane attack complex deposition is the result of an immune attack on the vessels. Greenberg and coworkers have hypothesized that increased production of IFN-α/β–inducible proteins by plasmacytoid dendritic cells and myocytes can also result in endothelial damage.[104]

Genetics likely play a large role in the risk for developing DM. Certain HLA alleles are clearly some of the greatest risk factors for the development of DM. The HLA-B8 allele was the first allele found in increased prevalence in 12 of 17 (75%) juvenile patients with DM compared to 21% of control participants.[105] Subsequently, multiple other HLA alleles, largely consisting of the HLA 8.1 ancestral haplotype (HLA-A*0101, -C*0701, -B*0801, -DRB1*0301, -DQA1*0501, and -DQB1*0201) have been enriched in patients with DM.[106,107] Genome-wide studies have confirmed a role for MHC class I and II genes but have also uncovered other loci conferring risk; these include the *BLK* gene involved in B-cell activation and the *TYK2* gene, which plays a role in signaling from IFN receptors.

In addition, other nonimmune events may play a role in features of the disease. Currently, one area of investigation centers around the endoplasmic reticulum stress response that may be partially responsible for some of the weakness symptoms seen in DM. Endoplasmic stress could be the result of upregulation of MHC class I or other proteins and induces an unfolded protein response that results in activation of inflammatory nuclear factor kappa B (NF-κB) signaling pathways, mitochondrial dysfunction, and elevated reactive oxygen species, all of which can contribute to weakness.

Current models suggest that DM is initiated in a genetically predisposed individual who is then subjected to an environmental trigger. The nature of that trigger could vary and could include UV exposure, infection, and malignancy. On the cellular level, these triggers could result in antigen modification or upregulation, cellular death, and activation of nucleic acid response with increased production of IFN, endoplasmic stress, and activation of the innate immune system. There is likely redundant interplay between the innate and adaptive immune system that allows not only initiation but also disease propagation.

DIAGNOSIS

Unfortunately, there are no adequate, validated diagnostic criteria for DM. Like most rheumatic diseases, DM variably affects different organ systems and with varying degrees of severity. Because of this, it is difficult to define this disease on either clinical or histologic criteria. We have already discussed that using clinical, histologic, electromyographic, or histologic criteria of muscle involvement for diagnosis will not diagnose the population of patients with amyopathic disease. However, the same may hold true for skin disease; although some would argue that the characteristic rash is the key to diagnosis, it is not clear that the skin needs to be involved in the DM disease process any more than does the muscle. A practical approach is not to require specific muscle or skin involvement but to have organ-specific criteria that must be met if indeed an organ is involved. Unfortunately, there are no validated clinical skin criteria that can serve to diagnose DM skin disease. It has been suggested that vascular membrane attack complex deposition may serve to distinguish this disease from cutaneous lupus, but unfortunately, there are no data regarding membrane attack complex deposition in other skin diseases. It is thought that certain features on muscle biopsy characterize DM, namely perifascicular atrophy, but recent studies challenge this notion.[108] The recent characterization of several DM-specific autoantibodies gives the hope of making this diagnosis with a blood test, but sensitivity and specificity data of these assays across multiple mimicking skin and muscle diseases are still lacking. It is likely that optimization of future diagnostic criteria will require a combination of clinical, histologic, and serologic data.

Thus, at present, establishing a diagnosis of DM continues to rely on the clinician's impression based on history and physical examination findings.

HELPFUL SKIN FINDINGS

Features of the skin examination that we find particularly sensitive are microscopic periungual telangiectasias, lateral digit hyperkeratosis, and scalp erythema and dysesthesia. Some elements that are more specific are the "red-on-white" patches, the ovoid palatal patch, grossly visible periungual telangiectasias, and Gottron papules.

MUSCLE DISEASE

As discussed, myositis is not a requirement for the diagnosis. However, tests supporting the presence of an inflammatory myopathy are helpful when a patient presents with a suspicious rash. In this way, a clinical suspicion of DM is a necessary but not always sufficient for diagnosing DM. Muscle involvement by history (including dysphagia, dysphonia, and myalgia) and weakness on examination will serve to increase suspicion for myositis but are not confirmatory. Elevation of muscle enzymes, however, should be the next step in nailing down the diagnosis (see later). Electromyography or MRI can be used in situations when the clinical suspicion is still high for myopathy but muscle enzymes are normal. Finally, a muscle biopsy can be performed in cases in which a cause for muscle symptoms is still not clear.

SYNDROMIC PRESENTATIONS

Certain combinations of symptoms, although not necessarily common, have reasonably high specificity to be helpful in making a diagnosis of DM, regardless of the presence of the more "typical" cutaneous features of DM. A patient presenting with alopecia, cutaneous or mucosal ulceration, palmar erythematous papules, severe arthralgia or arthritis, and shortness of breath, even with a few of these symptoms, should trigger the clinician to consider anti-MDA5 DM. Patients with mechanic hands, arthritis, Raynaud phenomenon, and lung symptoms are at high risk of having antisynthetase disease, which some consider to fall under the umbrella of DM if there are particular DM-like signs present on the skin. Patients with extreme myalgia, peripheral edema, and distal weakness should be ruled out for DM specifically with anti-NXP2 antibodies even if the rash is subtle. Knowledge of these phenotypes will increase the clinician's sensitivity for making the DM diagnosis.

DIAGNOSTIC LABORATORY EVALUATION

AUTOANTIBODIES

Myositis-specific autoantibodies associated with DM are evolving as key tools in assisting in establishing the diagnosis. These MSAs include TIF1-γ, NXP2, MDA5, small ubiquitin-like modifier activating enzyme (SAE), Mi-2, Jo-1, and the other antisynthetase antibodies (PL-7, PL-12, EJ, OJ, SRP). In our US cohort, these antibody tests have an 80% to 85% sensitivity for diagnosing DM. Thus, these MSAs may provide pivotal information to establish the diagnosis of DM in subtle or complex cases.

Importantly, MSAs are becoming increasingly relevant to identify clinical subsets and disease associations (see Table 62-2). As clinical phenotyping improves with respect to disease features and clinical course and increasing availability of testing for MSAs, this classification method will likely add value to current definitions by allowing improved prognostication, targeted screening, and potentially tailored therapy.

ANA testing, if performed, should be done using method of direct immunofluorescence. ANA test results can be negative in DM 50% of the time but are usually positive in systemic lupus erythematosus, and thus a negative test result can help point away from systemic lupus if that is in the differential diagnosis.

MUSCLE ENZYMES

Early in the course of myositis, serum muscle enzymes (ie, creatine kinase, aldolase, lactate dehydrogenase [LDH], aspartate aminotransferase [AST]), alanine aminotransferase [ALT]) are reasonably sensitive biomarkers of muscle inflammation. However, mid to late in the course of myositis, their sensitivity decreases. It is unclear why the sensitivity of muscle enzyme drops as myositis continues, but it may be a result of perifascicular muscle atrophy and fibrosis, resulting in less dramatic changes in these tests even while inflammation persists. Additionally, often only the creatine kinase or only the aldolase will be elevated in a single patient. To increase the sensitivity of detecting myositis on laboratory testing, the clinician should evaluate creatine kinase, aldolase, and LDH as a group when testing muscle enzymes.

There are a few practical issues to be aware of when evaluating muscle enzymes. First, all muscle enzymes can be elevated after strenuous activity; in questionable cases, the enzyme levels can be rechecked after 10-14 days following the activity. Second, aldolase (and AST and ALT) can be elevated with liver disease or hemolysis of the blood sample. Very high levels should be rechecked. γ-Glutamyl transferase will be elevated with hepatic injury but will not be elevated in myositis and is a helpful addition to laboratory testing for myositis if hepatic sources are suspected.

ELECTROMYOGRAPHIC STUDIES

Similar to muscle enzyme abnormalities, early in the disease course, myositis may be detectable on electromyographic studies in 70% to 90% of patients with DM with active muscle disease and the sensitivity to detect myositis decreases over time. The classic triad electromyographic findings of myositis is small amplitude, short duration, polyphasic motor unit potentials; fibrillations and positive sharp waves; and complex repetitive discharges.[109] These findings reflect active muscle inflammation and may be seen in other inflammatory myopathies such as polymyositis.[110] Late in the course of the disease, the sensitivity decreases.

OTHER DIAGNOSTIC LABORATORY TESTS

Most other laboratory tests performed at disease onset would be to evaluate for target organ involvement and not necessarily be used in making the diagnosis. However, serum ferritin is often highly elevated (>500 mg/dL) in anti-MDA5 patients with DM[111] and may be helpful in diagnosis anti-MDA5 disease when serologic testing is unavailable or of inadequate sensitivity. In addition, it may be a useful biomarker to assess the severity and follow the clinical response of ILD in anti-MDA5 patients with DM.[112,113]

IMAGING

MRI provides a detailed view of the muscle anatomy, allowing for localization and discrimination of the type of pathologic process (eg, edema, inflammation, fibrosis, calcifications, or atrophy). MRI can be useful to differentiate weakness caused by damage or steroid-myopathy versus active myositis when muscle enzymes and electromyographic studies are inconclusive. MRI can also be used in directing the site of a diagnostic biopsy, if needed,[114] or may be used to assess clinical response to treatment.[115] Muscle edema is a sensitive indicator of myositis and correlates with creatine kinase levels.[116] On short tau inversion recovery, in which normal muscle is dark and inflamed muscle is bright, an increased signal intensity within muscle tissue suggests muscle inflammation, necrosis, or degeneration.[117] Yoshida and coworkers also identified fasciitis on MRI in 12 of 14 patients with DM, suggesting that the fascial microvasculature may be a primary site of involvement.[118] Muscle damage may be identified on T1-weighted images, in which there is fatty replacement of skeletal muscle.[73]

PATHOLOGY

SKIN HISTOPATHOLOGY

Skin biopsies from affected skin in DM classically show a cell-poor interface dermatitis, increased dermal mucin, a perivascular lymphocytic infiltrate, and vascular ectasia (Fig. 62-17). Other inconstant findings include epidermal atrophy and basement membrane thickening. However, frequently many of these findings are subtle or absent. Smith and coworkers reviewed 40 DM skin biopsies and noted that when interface dermatitis was absent (20% of cases), increased dermal mucin was always present.[119] It has been suggested that whereas DM is characterized by increased presence of plasmacytoid dendritic cells in mostly an epidermal location, in cutaneous lupus, they are situated primarily in the dermis.[120]

The role of direct immunofluorescence testing in DM diagnosis is still unclear. It has been reported that DM biopsies do not demonstrate immunoreactants along the DEJ, the so-called "lupus band," but this finding is not uniformly defined in terms of its intensity and antibody composition. Magro and coworkers found that if the definition of a lupus band is made stringent, only 1 of 24 patients with DM has a positive lupus band test result. However, in addition to most patients with DM, more than 35% of cutaneous lupus biopsies were also negative for the lupus band test. So, if a stringently defined lupus band (eg, interrupted deposition of immunoglobulin [Ig] G or continuous deposition of IgM) is present on biopsy, these data suggest that a diagnosis of DM is unlikely. In addition, Mascaró and coworkers found that deposition of the membrane attack complex or C5b-9, at either the DEJ or around vessels of DM occurs in 77% to 86% of patients.[103] Magro and coworkers repeated this testing in 24 patients with DM and found that membrane attack complex deposition at both the DEJ and around vessels along with a negative lupus band test result was 78% sensitive and 93% specific for making a diagnosis of DM over cutaneous lupus.[121]

MUSCLE HISTOPATHOLOGY

In patients referred to a dermatology clinic with a rash and weakness, muscle biopsy is seldom necessary to establish the diagnosis of DM. Evidence of myositis on laboratory testing, electromyography, or MRI is often sufficient in the setting of a cutaneous eruption supporting DM. Muscle biopsy can yield false-negative results, both because of immunosuppressive medications and the patchy nature of the inflammation. MRI can be used to as a guide to selecting a biopsy site. If a muscle biopsy is necessary to confirm the diagnosis of DM, it has the highest yield if performed within 2 weeks of beginning any immunomodulatory therapy.

Typical muscle histopathology findings in DM include perifascicular atrophy, degenerating and regenerating myofibers, membrane attack complex deposition in the endomysial capillary walls,[122] endothelial cell swelling, and capillary necrosis. The inflammatory cell infiltrate consists of CD4+ T cells,[123] plasmacytoid dendritic cells secreting IFN-α,[101] B lymphocytes, macrophages, and plasma cells. However, there is a range of histologic findings even in clear DM cases, and histologic findings of inflammatory myopathies often cluster according to other criteria and do not necessarily respect the clinical boundaries of idiopathic inflammatory myopathy categories that have been defined.

DIFFERNTIAL DIAGNOSIS OF DERMATOMYOSITIS

See Table 62-3.

CLINICAL COURSE AND PROGNOSIS

The long-term survival rate for adults with DM is approximately 65% to 75%, but there are relatively little data regarding specific organ outcomes such as muscle

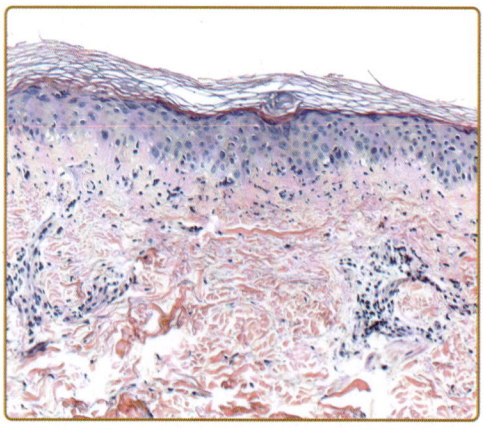

Figure 62-17 Histopathology of cutaneous dermatomyositis. Skin biopsy shows vacuolar interface dermatitis, basement membrane thickening, perivascular lymphocytic infiltrate, and increased dermal mucin.

TABLE 62-3
Patients with Skin Findings That Are Similar to Dermatomyositis

CONDITION	DESCRIPTION
Acute cutaneous lupus	Characterized by malar pink patches and plaques; may generalize to rest of face and body; generally spares PIP and DIP joints; spares nasolabial folds; usually does not have significant pruritus; 5%–15% of patients with SLE may have myositis; patients have systemic lupus and positive lupus serologies
Photoallergic or airborne contact dermatitis	Patients have new exposure before onset of eruption; distribution is to skin that was exposed to allergen or sun exposure, not in DM distribution; patients often have itching or burning; patients do not have nailfold capillary changes or systemic symptoms
Acne rosacea (erythematotelangiectatic or neurogenic)	May have itching, burning quality but erythema is limited to face; absence of damage (hyperpigmentation, atrophy); no systemic symptoms
Polymorphous light eruption	Sun-exposed sites are affected, typically immediately after sun exposure (delayed 1–2 days in DM); rash not in classic DM extensor distribution; eruption may resolve completely in 1–2 wk with sun avoidance; no systemic symptoms
	Characterized by annular or psoriasiform plaques on sun-exposed skin; 30%–60% have SLE; 80% have positive anti-Ro antibody; may be medication associated; lacks pathognomonic DM skin findings (eg, Gottron papules, Gottron sign, heliotrope)
Seborrheic dermatitis	Scalp disease may be challenging to separate from DM; has greasy scale and orange-red quality instead of violaceous; may affect central chest, upper back, and neck but spares extremities; patients do not have systemic symptoms
Psoriasis	Tends to spare the face; lacks characteristic damage of DM; lacks nailfold capillary changes; rarely, patients may have both DM and psoriasis
Phototoxic or photoallergic drug eruption	Patients have a recently added medication; distribution is to sun-exposed areas, not extensor; eruption often has sharp borders and substantial edema; no nailfold capillary changes; patients are without systemic symptoms
Lichenoid drug eruption	Patients are taking medication associated with lichenoid dermatitis; eruption is often widespread and papular; not in DM distribution
Pityriasis rubra pilaris	Typically involves palms and soles; may have islands of sparing; has an orange-red quality as opposed to violaceous; lacks nailfold capillary changes
Atopic dermatitis	Distribution is usually flexural in adults; lichenification present in chronic cases; may have history of seasonal allergies or asthma; generally improves with sun exposure; lacks atrophy; nailfold capillary changes
Patients with Weakness and other Skin or Systemic Findings	
Mixed connective tissue disease	Patients may have facial, chest, or scalp rash with poikiloderma, nailfold capillary changes, calcinosis, and myositis; patients do not have Gottron papules; arthritis, Raynaud phenomenon, cutaneous sclerosis, GERD, and cytopenias are prominent symptoms; patients have anti-U1RNP antibodies
Systemic sclerosis	May have myositis, depigmented and hyperpigmented patches, nailfold capillary changes, pruritus, and calcinosis but not the erythema of DM; telangiectasias aree matted; patients have Raynaud phenomenon, GERD, and often cutaneous sclerosis
Polymyositis	May have periungual capillary changes but not the cutaneous eruption of DM
Immune-mediated necrotizing myopathy	History of statin use; patients do not have cutaneous eruption of DM

anti-U1RNP, anti-U1 ribonucleoprotein; DM, dermatomyositis; GERD, gastroesophageal reflux disease; PIP, proximal interphalangeal; SLE, systemic lupus erythematosus.

or skin disease.[124] Remission rates of 25% to 70% have been reported, but most studies suggest that number is probably closer to 20% to 40% at 5 years. Major causes of death include malignancy, pulmonary or cardiac disease, and infection, but other predictors have variably been reported, including older age, male gender, nonwhite race, and longer duration of symptoms. Outcomes may also relate to autoantibody status; studies in both Japan and the United States have shown that presence of anti-MDA5 antibodies is a risk factor for death.[125,126]

For children, long-term registries have provided clearer data regarding remission rates, including that for skin disease. Most studies suggest that approximately 60% of patients have chronic disease (eg, past 5 years), with major risk factors for chronicity being a delay in therapy and early persistent (eg, 3 months) skin disease or decline in nailfold capillary density. Most reports suggest that the most common source of persistent disease activity is in the skin over muscles or other organs.[127-129]

MANAGEMENT

PRINCIPLES OF MANAGEMENT

Treatment of DM first requires assessing the potentially affected organs, namely the skin, muscle, and lungs. It should be emphasized that ILD and associated cancers are leading causes of disease-related death and are prioritized during treatment selection. Screening for malignancy is critical because the treatment of a cancer associated with DM may result in a reduced disease severity or, at times, disease remission. Cutaneous DM often has discordant treatment response with the muscle disease,[130] with recalcitrant skin disease continuing years after the muscle disease is in remission. Given the chronicity of the skin disease, it is worthwhile to weigh the long-term toxicity of the prescribed therapy against the achieved or potential cutaneous benefit. With that in mind, one should first select the appropriate agents to target the affected organs, consider patient comorbidities and preferences, and discuss the risks and benefits of each with the patient before deciding upon a regimen. Establishing collaborative relationships with the co-managing providers (rheumatologist, dermatologist, neurologist, and pulmonologist) is critical for the treatment of patients in whom multiple organs are involved.

CANCER SCREENING

Given that 10% to 20% of patients with DM have an associated malignancy, a thorough investigation is justified upon initial diagnosis. In addition to a complete history and physical exam, routine age-appropriate cancer screening studies (colonoscopy, mammogram, prostate examination) and relevant screening blood work (complete blood count, renal and liver function tests) as well as a urinalysis are indicated. The role of other blood work (eg, erythrocyte sedimentation rate, C-reactive protein, cancer markers, serum and urine protein immunofixation electrophoresis) in identifying cancer in a patient with DM is currently not established. The role of testing for anti–TIF1-γ and anti–NXP-2 antibodies in risk stratification is not yet known given the fact that, at least in the US population, most patients with these antibodies still do not harbor a malignancy. The role for more aggressive screening (eg, CT scans, positron emission tomography) is unclear, although as discussed earlier, this imaging may detect occult malignancies not found on routine age-appropriate screening in the higher risk period (2–3 years from diagnosis). The role for rescreening is even less clear. It would be prudent to consider blind rescreening be considered in patients with disease that is difficult to control or who have experienced an unexplained disease flare after a sustained quiescent period, especially in patients with a history of malignancy.

MONITORING OF EXTRACUTANEOUS DISEASE

MUSCLE DISEASE

Manual muscle testing is helpful to gauge changes in strength between visits. Even a busy dermatologist can check a few muscle groups such as the neck flexors, deltoids, and quadriceps at each visit to assess gross changes in muscle strength. If more time is available, then the manual muscle testing for a subset of eight muscle groups (MMT8) may be performed, which is a validated muscle test in which eight major muscle group (neck flexors, deltoids, biceps, wrist extensors, gluteus maximus, gluteus medius, quadriceps, ankles dorsiflexors) that are highest yield in idiopathic inflammatory myopathies.[131] Other factors such as pain, joint contracture, and fatigue may impact this measurement. Serum muscle enzymes (creatine kinase, aldolase, and LDH) are checked at each visit as biomarkers of myositis. However, as the duration of myositis increases, they become insensitive markers of myositis. Electromyography and MRI remain as more sensitive tests for active myositis in the setting of increasing weakness and normal muscle enzymes. The clinician must consider other causes of weakness, including muscle damage from prior myositis versus deconditioning, steroid myopathy, hydroxychloroquine-induced myopathy, or thyroid myopathy, for example. In this way, it is important not to reflexively treat weakness with increased immunosuppression until active myositis is identified as the cause.

PULMONARY DISEASE

Although there are no formalized guidelines for screening for ILD, it is valuable to obtain baseline PFTs with diffusion capacity in case there is future development of pulmonary symptoms and then annual screening as long as other symptoms of DM continue. Screening PFTs with diffusion capacity of carbon monoxide can be performed up to every 3 to 6 months if new pulmonary symptoms develop. PFT results are effort dependent and therefore influenced by following instructions during the test, muscle strength, and energy level. If PFTs show concerning changes for new or worsening ILD, then a high-resolution CT scan of the chest is the next step to evaluate the lung parenchyma.

CARDIOVASCULAR INVOLVEMENT

Consideration should be given to evaluating for cardiac muscle disease. The creatine kinase-MB isoform is found in both cardiac as well as regenerating skeletal muscle, so it is not a specific test, although it could be used as a screening test for cardiac involvement. We prefer to use cardiac troponin I testing because it is specific for myocardial damage. There are no standard recommendations for screening for cardiac involvement, but some authorities suggest using cardiac troponin I as a screening test for subclinical myocardial involvement followed by echocardiography or electrocardiography if the result is positive.[86] Patients with DM with anti-MDA5 antibodies may be at higher risk for clinically evident and, at times, fatal cardiac involvement.[87,88]

INTERVENTIONS

Evidence for medical therapies and treatment ladders in DM arise largely from single-center, retrospective case reports, case series, and expert opinion[132-136] (Table 62-4).

TOPICAL THERAPY

Although photoprotection is a key first step in management, up to 60% of patients with DM are actually minimally photosensitive, and as few as 20% may report disease exacerbation after UV exposure.[130,137] Despite this finding, it is helpful to carefully review the basic concepts of UV protection.

Topical corticosteroids may have a palliative effect on DM skin disease by reducing erythema, scale, and pruritus and play an adjunctive role to systemic agents. However, they are unlikely to fully control skin symptoms except in the mildest cases. Class I or II topical steroid creams or ointments are used on the thick skin of the elbows, knees, and hyperkeratosis on the hands and can be tried to mitigate the common complaint of nailfold sensitivity, and occlusion with plastic wrap can be added at night to increase the potency further.

Scalp pruritus may improve with topical steroid solutions or oils, although systemic agents are often needed in severe cases.

Topical calcineurin inhibitors such as tacrolimus 0.1% ointment or pimecrolimus 1% cream may have modest efficacy in some cases of cutaneous DM.[138-142] In practice, these agents have comparable efficacy to low- to midpotency topical corticosteroids (class IV to class VI). They do offer the benefit of being used safely on the face without concern for atrophy or hypopigmentation.

SYSTEMIC THERAPY

Systemic corticosteroids are undesirable agents as monotherapy for cutaneous DM because they usually elicit only partial responses and are associated with long-term side effects. However, systemic corticosteroids are first-line therapy in the treatment of myositis.[143] Complete clinical responses in muscle inflammation with prednisone monotherapy at doses greater than 0.5 mg/kg/day have been achieved in 27%[144] to 87%[11] of patients with DM.[145] They can also be used for joint disease and ILD, although often a corticosteroid-sparing agent is required.

The addition of corticosteroid-sparing agents may improve control of myositis and extracutaneous manifestations, but their critical role is to minimize toxicities of oral corticosteroids, including the risk for corticosteroid-induced myopathy.[146]

Antimalarials are typically regarded as first-line agents for skin disease. These agents have modest benefit for skin disease in DM with retrospective studies suggesting that improvement is seen in approximately 30% to 50% of patients.[147] In addition, up to 30% of patients with DM may experience a drug eruption on initiation of hydroxychloroquine.[148] The addition of quinacrine to hydroxychloroquine or chloroquine may be more effective than a single agent.[149] Hydroxychloroquine may also be useful for mild symptoms of inflammatory arthritis, and chloroquine has been reported to ameliorate arthritis in DM in one case report.[150]

Methotrexate is effective in significantly reducing cutaneous disease severity in 50% to 100% of patients with DM.[151-154] Similarly, methotrexate is a first-line treatment for myositis in combination with prednisone, and often dosages of 20 to 25 mg/wk are typically necessary to control muscle inflammation.[68,155] Methotrexate is also an effective treatment choice when concomitant arthritis is present.[156] In patients with DM with suspected or diagnosed ILD, it is prudent to select a different agent than methotrexate because of its potential to induce acute pneumonitis and pulmonary fibrosis,[157,158] thereby complicating the evaluation and management of ILD.

Mycophenolate mofetil has been shown to be effective at dosages of 2 to 3 g/day in reducing cutaneous disease severity[159,160] and myositis.[161-163] It is considered a first-line oral agent when ILD is present.[164-168] About 20% of patients experience nausea or diarrhea

TABLE 62-4
Treatment Ladder in Dermatomyositis

	SKIN DISEASE	MUSCLE DISEASE
First Line	Photoprotection Topical steroids Hydroxychloroquine or Chloroquine Quinacrine	Systemic corticosteroids
Second Line	Methotrexate Mycophenolate mofetil Intravenous immune globulin Azathioprine	
Third Line	Tofacitinib Leflunomide Dapsone Thalidomide Cyclosporine Cyclophosphamide	Rituximab Leflunomide Cyclosporine Cyclophosphamide

at 2 g/day.[169] If GI side effects are dose limiting, then switching to enteric-coated mycophenolate sodium is an option for maintaining a patient on therapy.[170]

Intravenous immunoglobulin (IVIG) is most likely the single most effective agent for cutaneous DM, with consistently 70% to 80% of patients achieving an almost complete or complete response.[171,172] IVIG is also effective for myositis.[173,174] A randomized placebo-controlled crossover trial of 15 patients with DM by Dakalas and coworkers in 1993[175] showed a significant improvement in muscle strength in 9 of 12 patients (75%) and a dramatic improvement in skin disease based on clinical photographs in 8 of 12 patients (67%) who received IVIG. The standard dosing regimen is 2 g/kg/mo divided over 3 to 5 days. The therapeutic effect may be perceived as early as 1 week, but it may not be apparent until the second or third month. Because IVIG works relatively quickly, it can be used in patients who are rapidly declining or are acutely ill with dysphagia or respiratory muscle involvement. Headaches may occur in up to 56% of patients and may be severe and debilitating. The rate of infusion, the total dose,[176] the formulation of IVIG,[177] and the volume status of the patient may influence the occurrence of headache. Aseptic meningitis is a rare adverse event manifesting as fever, headache, photophobia, meningismus, neutrophilic pleocytosis, or eosinophilia in the cerebrospinal fluid.[178,179] Anaphylaxis is also rare but may occur in primary IgA deficiency; therefore, checking serum IgA levels before infusion is recommended. However, there is no evidence that having low but detectable immunoglobulin levels confers any increased risk for anaphylaxis.[176] Also, venous thrombosis and renal injury[179] are risks of IVIG, particularly among patients with preexisting thrombophilias or chronic kidney disease, respectively.

Azathioprine has not been assessed specifically for cutaneous DM. In combined studies of DM and polymyositis, azathioprine has shown efficacy in improving myositis in up to 75% of cases[180-182] and improving survival.[183] The first randomized controlled trial of 28 patients with polymyositis or DM compared prednisolone with azathioprine 2.5 mg/kg/day versus prednisolone with methotrexate 15 mg/wk and found no difference in efficacy for myositis.[187] The second randomized controlled crossover trial of 30 patients with polymyositis or DM showed improved response in the group receiving combination oral methotrexate and azathioprine (8 of 15; 53%) compared with methotrexate alone (3 of 15; 20%).[185] The authors occasionally combine low dose azathioprine with methotrexate when myositis is persistent with methotrexate alone. Azathioprine is commonly used as maintenance therapy in the treatment of ILD associated with idiopathic inflammatory myopathies,[47,60] typically after induction with cyclophosphamide.[186,187]

Rituximab has mixed results in cutaneous DM with a clinical trial reporting no benefit[188] one report of moderate improvement in cutaneous DM.[189] Rituximab can be of benefit for myositis, especially those with anti–Jo-1 and anti–Mi-2 autoantibodies.[190] A large randomized clinical trial did not show benefit with rituximab, although this may center around difficult issues with trial design.[191] Rituximab has been reported to be successful in retrospective studies for the treatment of ILD.[192] Dosing in DM typically follows the rheumatoid arthritis protocol of 1000 mg intravenously on days 0 and 14.[188] Infectious complications are the most frequent[193] serious adverse effects in patients with DM, with rare reports of progressive multifocal leukoencephalopathy.[193-195]

Calcineurin inhibitors (eg, cyclosporine and tacrolimus) are not commonly used to treat muscle or skin inflammation, although a randomized clinical trial of 36 patients with DM ($n = 20$) or polymyositis ($n = 16$) comparing cyclosporine (3–3.5 mg/kg/day) with methotrexate (7.5–15 mg/wk) in addition to oral corticosteroids found decreases in creatine kinase, and improvements in strength were comparable between the groups at 6 months.[196] Its primary use is in the setting of ILD, especially severe ILD in the setting of anti-MDA5 or antisynthetase antibodies.[197,198] Nephrotoxicity risk is highest above 3 mg/kg/day and requires careful monitoring of renal function and blood pressure.[199,200]

Other treatments reported for use in DM skin disease include dapsone and thalidomide, but evidence of their efficacy is scant.

PHYSICAL MEDICINE AND REHABILITATION

Strength training has been shown to improve muscle strength and function,[201-203] and aerobic exercise has been shown to improve endurance[204,205] in patients with chronic DM. In active DM and polymyositis, a home strength training program has been shown to be safe[206] but did not show benefit in strength or disease control over the control group that performed range of motion exercises in a randomized clinical trial.[207] We advise all patients to enroll in a physical therapy program early after diagnosis so as to prevent injury and to maintain as much mobility and muscle strength as possible.

SPECIAL CIRCUMSTANCES

Calcinosis remains one of the most formidable therapeutic challenging in DM. Surgical excision for localized lesions remains the most effective and definitive therapy.[208] Multiple medical therapies have been proposed, including anti-inflammatory medications and calcium and phosphate modulators, but no single agent is reliably effective.[31] IVIG has been reported to work well in some cases[209-211] but not in others.[212] Bisphosphonates have been cited as effective for calcinosis in juvenile DM, although controlled studies are needed.[213-215]

REFERENCES

1. Bohan A, Peter JB. Polymyositis and dermatomyositis (second of two parts). *N Engl J Med*. 1975;292:403-407.
2. Bohan A, Peter JB. Polymyositis and dermatomyositis (first of two parts). *N Engl J Med*. 1975;292:344-347.
3. Bendewald MJ, Wetter DA, Li X, et al. Incidence of dermatomyositis and clinically amyopathic dermatomyositis: a population-based study in Olmsted County, Minnesota. *Arch Dermatol*. 2010;146:26-30.
4. Euwer RL, Sontheimer RD. Amyopathic dermatomyositis (dermatomyositis sine myositis). Presentation of six new cases and review of the literature. *J Am Acad Dermatol*. 1991;24:959-966.
5. Sontheimer RD. Dermatomyositis: an overview of recent progress with emphasis on dermatologic aspects. *Dermatol Clin*. 2002;20:387-408.
6. Sontheimer RD. Cutaneous features of classic dermatomyositis and amyopathic dermatomyositis. *Curr Opin Rheumatol*. 1999;11:475-482.
7. Sontheimer RD. Skin disease in dermatomyositis—what patients and their families often want to know. *Dermatol Online J*. 2002;8:6.
8. Gerami P, Schope JM, McDonald L, et al. A systematic review of adult-onset clinically amyopathic dermatomyositis (dermatomyositis sine myositis): a missing link within the spectrum of the idiopathic inflammatory myopathies. *J Am Acad Dermatol*. 2006;54:597-613.
9. Dalakas MC, Hohlfeld R. Polymyositis and dermatomyositis. *Lancet*. 2003;362:971-982.
10. Hoogendijk JE, Amato AA, Lecky BR, et al. 119th ENMC international workshop: trial design in adult idiopathic inflammatory myopathies, with the exception of inclusion body myositis, 10-12 October 2003, Naarden, The Netherlands. *Neuromuscul Disord*. 2004;14:337-345.
11. Troyanov Y, Targoff IN, Tremblay JL, et al. Novel classification of idiopathic inflammatory myopathies based on overlap syndrome features and autoantibodies: analysis of 100 French Canadian patients. *Medicine (Baltimore)*. 2005;84:231-249.
12. Fernandez C, Bardin N, De Paula AM, et al. Correlation of clinicoserologic and pathologic classifications of inflammatory myopathies: study of 178 cases and guidelines for diagnosis. *Medicine (Baltimore)*. 2013;92:15-24.
13. Meyer A, Meyer N, Schaeffer M, et al. Incidence and prevalence of inflammatory myopathies: a systematic review. *Rheumatology (Oxford)*. 2015;54:50-63.
14. Bernatsky S, Joseph L, Pineau CA, et al. Estimating the prevalence of polymyositis and dermatomyositis from administrative data: age, sex and regional differences. *Ann Rheum Dis*. 2009;68:1192-1196.
15. Dobloug C, Garen T, Bitter H, et al. Prevalence and clinical characteristics of adult polymyositis and dermatomyositis; data from a large and unselected Norwegian cohort. *Ann Rheum Dis*. 2015;74:1551-1556.
16. Ohta A, Nagai M, Nishina M, et al. Prevalence and incidence of polymyositis and dermatomyositis in Japan. *Mod Rheumatol*. 2014;24:477-480.
17. Kuo CF, See LC, Yu KH, et al. Incidence, cancer risk and mortality of dermatomyositis and polymyositis in Taiwan: a nationwide population study. *Br J Dermatol*. 2011;165:1273-1279.
18. Mendez EP, Lipton R, Ramsey-Goldman R, et al. US incidence of juvenile dermatomyositis, 1995-1998: results from the National Institute of Arthritis and Musculoskeletal and Skin Diseases Registry. *Arthritis Rheum*. 2003;49:300-305.
19. Hurliman E, Groth D, Wendelschafer-Crabb G, et al. Small fiber neuropathy in a patient with dermatomyositis and severe scalp pruritus. *Br J Dermatol*. 2016.
20. Taggart AJ, Finch MB, Courtney PA, et al. Anti Jo-1 myositis. "Mechanic's hands" and interstitial lung disease. *Ulster Med J*. 2002;71:68-71.
21. Sato Y, Teraki Y, Izaki S, et al. Clinical characterization of dermatomyositis associated with mechanic's hands. *J Dermatol*. 2012;39:1093-1095.
22. Smith RL, Sundberg J, Shamiyah E, et al. Skin involvement in juvenile dermatomyositis is associated with loss of end row nailfold capillary loops. *J Rheumatol*. 2004;31:1644-1649.
23. Manfredi A, Sebastiani M, Cassone G, et al. Nailfold capillaroscopic changes in dermatomyositis and polymyositis. *Clin Rheumatol*. 2015;34:279-284.
24. Ghali FE, Stein LD, Fine JD, et al. Gingival telangiectases: an underappreciated physical sign of juvenile dermatomyositis. *Arch Dermatol*. 1999;135:1370-1374.
25. Narang NS, Casciola-Rosen L, Li S, et al. Cutaneous ulceration in dermatomyositis: association with anti-melanoma differentiation-associated gene 5 antibodies and interstitial lung disease. *Arthritis Care Res (Hoboken)*. 2014;67(5):667-672.
26. Cao H, Xia Q, Pan M, et al. Gottron papules and Gottron sign with ulceration: a distinctive cutaneous feature in a subset of patients with classic dermatomyositis and clinically amyopathic dermatomyositis. *J Rheumatol*. 2016;43(9):1735-1742.
27. Xu Y, Yang CS, Li YJ, et al. Predictive factors of rapidly progressive-interstitial lung disease in patients with clinically amyopathic dermatomyositis. *Clin Rheumatol*. 2016;35:113-116.
28. Bernet LL, Lewis MA, Rieger KE, et al. Ovoid palatal patch in dermatomyositis: a novel finding associated with anti-TIF1gamma (p155) antibodies. *JAMA Dermatol*. 2016;152(9):1049-1051.
29. Fiorentino DF, Kuo K, Chung L, et al. Distinctive cutaneous and systemic features associated with antitranscriptional intermediary factor-1gamma antibodies in adults with dermatomyositis. *J Am Acad Dermatol*. 2015;72:449-455.
30. Walsh JS, Fairley JA. Calcifying disorders of the skin. *J Am Acad Dermatol*. 1995;33:693-706; quiz 707-710.
31. Hoeltzel MF, Oberle EJ, Robinson AB, et al. The presentation, assessment, pathogenesis, and treatment of calcinosis in juvenile dermatomyositis. *Curr Rheumatol Rep*. 2014;16:467-014-0467-y.
32. Balin SJ, Wetter DA, Andersen LK, et al. Calcinosis cutis occurring in association with autoimmune connective tissue disease: the Mayo Clinic experience with 78 patients, 1996-2009. *Arch Dermatol*. 2012;148:455-462.
33. Sallum AM, Pivato FC, Doria-Filho U, et al. Risk factors associated with calcinosis of juvenile dermatomyositis. *J Pediatr (Rio J)*. 2008;84:68-74.
34. Sanner H, Gran JT, Sjaastad I, et al. Cumulative organ damage and prognostic factors in juvenile dermatomyositis: a cross-sectional study median 16.8 years after symptom onset. *Rheumatology (Oxford)*. 2009;48:1541-1547.
35. Gunawardena H, Wedderburn LR, Chinoy H, et al. Autoantibodies to a 140-kd protein in juvenile dermatomyositis are associated with calcinosis. *Arthritis Rheum*. 2009;60:1807-1814.

36. Valenzuela A, Chung L, Casciola-Rosen L, et al. Identification of clinical features and autoantibodies associated with calcinosis in dermatomyositis. *JAMA Dermatol*. 2014;150:724-729.
37. Hansen CB, Callen JP. Connective tissue panniculitis: lupus panniculitis, dermatomyositis, morphea/scleroderma. *Dermatol Ther*. 2010;23:341-349.
38. Milisenda JC, Doti PI, Prieto-Gonzalez S, et al. Dermatomyositis presenting with severe subcutaneous edema: five additional cases and review of the literature. *Semin Arthritis Rheum*. 2014;44:228-233.
39. Tu J, McLean-Tooke A, Junckerstorff R. Increasing recognition of dermatomyositis with subcutaneous edema—is this a poorer prognostic marker? *Dermatol Online J*. 2014;20:21244.
40. Kim NN, Lio PA, Morgan GA, et al. Double trouble: therapeutic challenges in patients with both juvenile dermatomyositis and psoriasis. *Arch Dermatol*. 2011;147:831-835.
41. Sarin KY, Chung L, Kim J, et al. Molecular profiling to diagnose a case of atypical dermatomyositis. *J Invest Dermatol*. 2013;133:2796-2799.
42. Marie I, Hatron PY, Dominique S, et al. Short-term and long-term outcomes of interstitial lung disease in polymyositis and dermatomyositis: a series of 107 patients. *Arthritis Rheum*. 2011;63:3439-3447.
43. Kang EH, Lee EB, Shin KC, et al. Interstitial lung disease in patients with polymyositis, dermatomyositis and amyopathic dermatomyositis. *Rheumatology (Oxford)*. 2005;44:1282-1286.
44. Fiorentino D, Chung L, Zwerner J, et al. The mucocutaneous and systemic phenotype of dermatomyositis patients with antibodies to MDA5 (CADM-140):a retrospective study. *J Am Acad Dermatol*. 2011;65:25-34.
45. Sun Y, Liu Y, Yan B, et al. Interstitial lung disease in clinically amyopathic dermatomyositis (CADM) patients: a retrospective study of 41 Chinese Han patients. *Rheumatol Int*. 2013;33:1295-1302.
46. Mukae H, Ishimoto H, Sakamoto N, et al. Clinical differences between interstitial lung disease associated with clinically amyopathic dermatomyositis and classic dermatomyositis. *Chest*. 2009;136:1341-1347.
47. Connors GR, Christopher-Stine L, Oddis CV, et al. Interstitial lung disease associated with the idiopathic inflammatory myopathies: what progress has been made in the past 35 years? *Chest*. 2010;138:1464-1474.
48. Fathi M, Lundberg IE. Interstitial lung disease in polymyositis and dermatomyositis. *Curr Opin Rheumatol*. 2005;17:701-706.
49. Johnson C, Pinal-Fernandez I, Parikh R, et al. Assessment of mortality in autoimmune myositis with and without associated interstitial lung disease. *Lung*. 2016;194(5):733-737.
50. Richards TJ, Eggebeen A, Gibson K, et al. Characterization and peripheral blood biomarker assessment of anti-Jo-1 antibody-positive interstitial lung disease. *Arthritis Rheum*. 2009;60:2183-2192.
51. Cao H, Pan M, Kang Y, et al. Clinical manifestations of dermatomyositis and clinically amyopathic dermatomyositis patients with positive expression of anti-melanoma differentiation-associated gene 5 antibody. *Arthritis Care Res (Hoboken)*. 2012;64:1602-1610.
52. Chen Z, Cao M, Plana MN, et al. Utility of anti-melanoma differentiation-associated gene 5 antibody measurement in identifying patients with dermatomyositis and a high risk for developing rapidly progressive interstitial lung disease: a review of the literature and a meta-analysis. *Arthritis Care Res (Hoboken)*. 2013;65:1316-1324.
53. Hamaguchi Y, Kuwana M, Hoshino K, et al. Clinical correlations with dermatomyositis-specific autoantibodies in adult Japanese patients with dermatomyositis: a multicenter cross-sectional study. *Arch Dermatol*. 2011;147:391-398.
54. Cao H, Pan M, Kang Y, et al. Clinical manifestations of dermatomyositis and clinically amyopathic dermatomyositis patients with positive expression of anti-melanoma differentiation-associated gene 5 antibody. *Arthritis Care Res (Hoboken)*. 2012;64:1602-1610.
55. Gono T, Kawaguchi Y, Satoh T, et al. Clinical manifestation and prognostic factor in anti-melanoma differentiation-associated gene 5 antibody-associated interstitial lung disease as a complication of dermatomyositis. *Rheumatology (Oxford)*. 2010;49:1713-1719.
56. Labrador-Horrillo M, Martinez MA, Selva-O'Callaghan A, et al. Anti-MDA5 antibodies in a large Mediterranean population of adults with dermatomyositis. *J Immunol Res*. 2014;2014:290797.
57. Martinez FJ, Flaherty K. Pulmonary function testing in idiopathic interstitial pneumonias. *Proc Am Thorac Soc*. 2006;3:315-321.
58. Da Silva JA, Jacobs JW, Kirwan JR, et al. Safety of low dose glucocorticoid treatment in rheumatoid arthritis: published evidence and prospective trial data. *Ann Rheum Dis*. 2006;65:285-293.
59. Fathi M, Dastmalchi M, Rasmussen E, et al. Interstitial lung disease, a common manifestation of newly diagnosed polymyositis and dermatomyositis. *Ann Rheum Dis*. 2004;63:297-301.
60. Douglas WW, Tazelaar HD, Hartman TE, et al. Polymyositis-dermatomyositis-associated interstitial lung disease. *Am J Respir Crit Care Med*. 2001;164:1182-1185.
61. Zhang RF, Zhou L, Ma GF, et al. Diagnostic value of transthoracic Doppler echocardiography in pulmonary hypertension: a meta-analysis. *Am J Hypertens*. 2010;23:1261-1264.
62. Hoeper MM, Bogaard HJ, Condliffe R, et al. Definitions and diagnosis of pulmonary hypertension. *J Am Coll Cardiol*. 2013;62:D42-50.
63. Cosnes A, Amaudric F, Gherardi R, et al. Dermatomyositis without muscle weakness. Long-term follow-up of 12 patients without systemic corticosteroids. *Arch Dermatol*. 1995;131:1381-1385.
64. Smith BW, McCarthy JC, Dawley CA. Suspect myopathy? Take this approach to the work-up. *J Fam Pract*. 2014;63:631-638.
65. Pachman LM, Hayford JR, Chung A, et al. Juvenile dermatomyositis at diagnosis: clinical characteristics of 79 children. *J Rheumatol*. 1998;25:1198-1204.
66. Parodi A, Caproni M, Marzano AV, et al. Dermatomyositis in 132 patients with different clinical subtypes: cutaneous signs, constitutional symptoms and circulating antibodies. *Acta Derm Venereol*. 2002;82:48-51.
67. Mugii N, Hasegawa M, Matsushita T, et al. Oropharyngeal dysphagia in dermatomyositis: associations with clinical and laboratory features including autoantibodies. *PLoS One*. 2016;11:e0154746.
68. Koh ET, Seow A, Ong B, et al. Adult onset polymyositis/dermatomyositis: clinical and laboratory features and treatment response in 75 patients. *Ann Rheum Dis*. 1993;52:857-861.

69. Citera G, Goni MA, Maldonado, et al. Joint involvement in polymyositis/dermatomyositis. *Clin Rheumatol*. 1994;13:70-74.
70. Porkodi R, Shanmuganandan K, Parthiban M, et al. Clinical spectrum of inflammatory myositis in South India—a ten year study. *J Assoc Physicians India*. 2002;50:1255-1258.
71. Klein M, Mann H, Plestilova L, et al. Arthritis in idiopathic inflammatory myopathy: clinical features and autoantibody associations. *J Rheumatol*. 2014;41:1133-1139.
72. Mumm GE, McKown KM, Bell CL. Antisynthetase syndrome presenting as rheumatoid-like polyarthritis. *J Clin Rheumatol*. 2010;16:307-312.
73. Mammen AL. Autoimmune myopathies: autoantibodies, phenotypes and pathogenesis. *Nat Rev Neurol*. 2011;7:343-354.
74. Wasko MC, Carlson GW, Tomaino MM, et al. Dermatomyositis with erosive arthropathy: association with the anti-PL-7 antibody. *J Rheumatol*. 1999;26:2693-2694.
75. Oddis CV, Medsger TA Jr, Cooperstein LA. A subluxing arthropathy associated with the anti-Jo-1 antibody in polymyositis/dermatomyositis. *Arthritis Rheum*. 1990;33:1640-1645.
76. Schumacher HR, Schimmer B, Gordon GV, et al. Articular manifestations of polymyositis and dermatomyositis. *Am J Med*. 1979;67:287-292.
77. Levin J, Werth VP. Skin disorders with arthritis. *Best Pract Res Clin Rheumatol*. 2006;20:809-826.
78. Hall JC, Casciola-Rosen L, Samedy LA, et al. Anti-melanoma differentiation-associated protein 5-associated dermatomyositis: expanding the clinical spectrum. *Arthritis Care Res (Hoboken)*. 2013;65:1307-1315.
79. Robinson AB, Hoeltzel MF, Wahezi DM, et al. Clinical characteristics of children with juvenile dermatomyositis: the Childhood Arthritis and Rheumatology Research Alliance Registry. *Arthritis Care Res (Hoboken)*. 2014;66:404-410.
80. Gitiaux C, De Antonio M, Aouizerate J, et al. Vasculopathy-related clinical and pathological features are associated with severe juvenile dermatomyositis. *Rheumatology (Oxford)*. 2016;55:470-479.
81. Tweezer-Zaks N, Ben-Horin S, Schiby G, et al. Severe gastrointestinal inflammation in adult dermatomyositis: characterization of a novel clinical association. *Am J Med Sci*. 2006;332:308-313.
82. Mamyrova G, Kleiner DE, James-Newton L, et al. Late-onset gastrointestinal pain in juvenile dermatomyositis as a manifestation of ischemic ulceration from chronic endarteropathy. *Arthritis Rheum*. 2007;57:881-884.
83. Zhang L, Wang GC, Ma L, et al. Cardiac involvement in adult polymyositis or dermatomyositis: a systematic review. *Clin Cardiol*. 2012;35:686-691.
84. Gonzalez-Lopez L, Gamez-Nava JI, Sanchez L, et al. Cardiac manifestations in dermato-polymyositis. *Clin Exp Rheumatol*. 1996;14:373-379.
85. Rosenbohm A, Buckert D, Gerischer N, et al. Early diagnosis of cardiac involvement in idiopathic inflammatory myopathy by cardiac magnetic resonance tomography. *J Neurol*. 2015;262:949-956.
86. Hughes M, Lilleker JB, Herrick AL, et al. Cardiac troponin testing in idiopathic inflammatory myopathies and systemic sclerosis-spectrum disorders: biomarkers to distinguish between primary cardiac involvement and low-grade skeletal muscle disease activity. *Ann Rheum Dis*. 2015;74:795-798.
87. Pau-Charles I, Moreno PJ, Ortiz-Ibanez K, et al. Anti-MDA5 positive clinically amyopathic dermatomyositis presenting with severe cardiomyopathy. *J Eur Acad DermatolJ Eur Acad Dermatol Venereol*. 2014;28:1097-1102.
88. Sakurai N, Nagai K, Tsutsumi H, et al. Anti-CADM-140 antibody-positive juvenile dermatomyositis with rapidly progressive interstitial lung disease and cardiac involvement. *J Rheumatol*. 2011;38:963-964.
89. Madan V, Chinoy H, Griffiths CE, et al. Defining cancer risk in dermatomyositis. Part I. *Clin Exp Dermatol*. 2009;34:451-455.
90. Olazagasti JM, Baez PJ, Wetter DA, et al. Cancer risk in dermatomyositis: a meta-analysis of cohort studies. *Am J Clin Dermatol*. 2015;16:89-98.
91. Hill CL, Zhang Y, Sigurgeirsson B, et al. Frequency of specific cancer types in dermatomyositis and polymyositis: a population-based study. *Lancet*. 2001;357:96-100.
92. Chow WH, Gridley G, Mellemkjaer L, et al. Cancer risk following polymyositis and dermatomyositis: a nationwide cohort study in Denmark. *Cancer Causes Control*. 1995;6:9-13.
93. Sigurgeirsson B, Lindelof B, Edhag O, et al. Risk of cancer in patients with dermatomyositis or polymyositis. A population-based study. *N Engl J Med*. 1992;326:363-367.
94. Huang YL, Chen YJ, Lin MW, et al. Malignancies associated with dermatomyositis and polymyositis in Taiwan: a nationwide population-based study. *Br J Dermatol*. 2009;161:854-860.
95. Lu X, Yang H, Shu X, et al. Factors predicting malignancy in patients with polymyositis and dermatomyositis: a systematic review and meta-analysis. *PLoS One*. 2014;9:e94128.
96. Trallero-Araguas E, Rodrigo-Pendas JA, Selva-O'Callaghan A, et al. Usefulness of anti-p155 autoantibody for diagnosing cancer-associated dermatomyositis: a systematic review and meta-analysis. *Arthritis Rheum*. 2012;64:523-532.
97. Fiorentino DF, Chung LS, Christopher-Stine L, et al. Most patients with cancer-associated dermatomyositis have antibodies to nuclear matrix protein NXP-2 or transcription intermediary factor 1gamma. *Arthritis Rheum*. 2013;65:2954-2962.
98. Ichimura Y, Matsushita T, Hamaguchi Y, et al. Anti-NXP2 autoantibodies in adult patients with idiopathic inflammatory myopathies: possible association with malignancy. *Ann Rheum Dis*. 2012;71:710-713.
99. Sparsa A, Liozon E, Herrmann F, et al. Routine vs extensive malignancy search for adult dermatomyositis and polymyositis: a study of 40 patients. *Arch Dermatol*. 2002;138:885-890.
100. Caproni M, Torchia D, Cardinali C, et al. Infiltrating cells, related cytokines and chemokine receptors in lesional skin of patients with dermatomyositis. *Br J Dermatol*. 2004;151:784-791.
101. Greenberg SA, Pinkus JL, Pinkus GS, et al. Interferon-alpha/beta-mediated innate immune mechanisms in dermatomyositis. *Ann Neurol*. 2005;57:664-678.
102. Baechler EC, Bauer JW, Slattery CA, et al. An interferon signature in the peripheral blood of dermatomyositis patients is associated with disease activity. *Mol Med*. 2007;13:59-68.
103. Mascaro JM Jr, Hausmann G, Herrero C, et al. Membrane attack complex deposits in cutaneous lesions of dermatomyositis. *Arch Dermatol*. 1995;131:1386-1392.

104. Greenberg SA. Dermatomyositis and type 1 interferons. *Curr Rheumatol Rep*. 2010;12:198-203.
105. Reed AM, Pachman LM, Hayford J, et al. Immunogenetic studies in families of children with juvenile dermatomyositis. *J Rheumatol*. 1998;25:1000-1002.
106. Mallen SR, Essex MN, Zhang R. Gastrointestinal tolerability of NSAIDs in elderly patients: a pooled analysis of 21 randomized clinical trials with celecoxib and nonselective NSAIDs. *Curr Med Res Opin*. 2011;27:1359-1366.
107. Reed AM, Pachman L, Ober C. Molecular genetic studies of major histocompatibility complex genes in children with juvenile dermatomyositis: increased risk associated with HLA-DQA1 *0501. *Hum Immunol*. 1991;32:235-240.
108. Pinal-Fernandez I, Casciola-Rosen LA, Christopher-Stine L, et al. The prevalence of individual histopathologic features varies according to autoantibody status in muscle biopsies from patients with dermatomyositis. *J Rheumatol*. 2015;42:1448-1454.
109. Bohan A, Peter JB, Bowman RL, et al. Computer-assisted analysis of 153 patients with polymyositis and dermatomyositis. *Medicine (Baltimore)*. 1977;56:255-286.
110. Briani C, Doria A, Sarzi-Puttini P, et al. Update on idiopathic inflammatory myopathies. *Autoimmunity*. 2006;39:161-170.
111. Horai Y, Koga T, Fujikawa K, et al. Serum interferon-alpha is a useful biomarker in patients with anti-melanoma differentiation-associated gene 5 (MDA5) antibody-positive dermatomyositis. *Mod Rheumatol*. 2015;25:85-89.
112. Gono T, Sato S, Kawaguchi Y, et al. Anti-MDA5 antibody, ferritin and IL-18 are useful for the evaluation of response to treatment in interstitial lung disease with anti-MDA5 antibody-positive dermatomyositis. *Rheumatology (Oxford)*. 2012;51:1563-1570.
113. Mimori T, Nakashima R, Hosono Y. Interstitial lung disease in myositis: clinical subsets, biomarkers, and treatment. *Curr Rheumatol Rep*. 2012;14:264-274.
114. Del Grande F, Carrino JA, Del Grande M, et al. Magnetic resonance imaging of inflammatory myopathies. *Top Magn Reson Imaging*. 2011;22:39-43.
115. Curiel RV, Jones R, Brindle K. Magnetic resonance imaging of the idiopathic inflammatory myopathies: structural and clinical aspects. *Ann N Y Acad Sci*. 2009;1154:101-114.
116. Barsotti S, Zampa V, Talarico R, et al. Thigh magnetic resonance imaging for the evaluation of disease activity in patients with idiopathic inflammatory myopathies followed in a single center. *Muscle Nerve*. 2016;54(4):666-672.
117. Adams EM, Chow CK, Premkumar A, et al. The idiopathic inflammatory myopathies: spectrum of MR imaging findings. *Radiographics*. 1995;15:563-574.
118. Yoshida K, Kurosaka D, Joh K, et al. Fasciitis as a common lesion of dermatomyositis, demonstrated early after disease onset by en bloc biopsy combined with magnetic resonance imaging. *Arthritis Rheum*. 2010;62:3751-3759.
119. Smith ES, Hallman JR, DeLuca AM, et al. Dermatomyositis: a clinicopathological study of 40 patients. *Am J Dermatopathol*. 2009;31:61-67.
120. McNiff JM, Kaplan DH. Plasmacytoid dendritic cells are present in cutaneous dermatomyositis lesions in a pattern distinct from lupus erythematosus. *J Cutan Pathol*. 2008;35:452-456.
121. Magro CM, Crowson AN. The immunofluorescent profile of dermatomyositis: a comparative study with lupus erythematosus. *J Cutan Pathol*. 1997;24:543-552.
122. Kissel JT, Mendell JR, Rammohan KW. Microvascular deposition of complement membrane attack complex in dermatomyositis. *N Engl J Med*. 1986;314:329-334.
123. Arahata K, Engel AG. Monoclonal antibody analysis of mononuclear cells in myopathies. I: quantitation of subsets according to diagnosis and sites of accumulation and demonstration and counts of muscle fibers invaded by T cells. *Ann Neurol*. 1984;16:193-208.
124. Marie I. Morbidity and mortality in adult polymyositis and dermatomyositis. *Curr Rheumatol Rep*. 2012;14:275-285.
125. Moghadam-Kia S, Oddis CV, Sato S, et al. Anti-melanoma differentiation-associated gene 5 is associated with rapidly progressive lung disease and poor survival in US patients with amyopathic and myopathic dermatomyositis. *Arthritis Care Res (Hoboken)*. 2016;68:689-694.
126. Koga T, Fujikawa K, Horai Y, et al. The diagnostic utility of anti-melanoma differentiation-associated gene 5 antibody testing for predicting the prognosis of Japanese patients with DM. *Rheumatology (Oxford)*. 2012;51:1278-1284.
127. Christen-Zaech S, Seshadri R, Sundberg J, et al. Persistent association of nailfold capillaroscopy changes and skin involvement over thirty-six months with duration of untreated disease in patients with juvenile dermatomyositis. *Arthritis Rheum*. 2008;58:571-576.
128. Stringer E, Singh-Grewal D, Feldman BM. Predicting the course of juvenile dermatomyositis: significance of early clinical and laboratory features. *Arthritis Rheum*. 2008;58:3585-3592.
129. Sanner H, Sjaastad I, Flato B. Disease activity and prognostic factors in juvenile dermatomyositis: a long-term follow-up study applying the Paediatric Rheumatology International Trials Organization criteria for inactive disease and the myositis disease activity assessment tool. *Rheumatology (Oxford)*. 2014;53:1578-1585.
130. Dourmishev L, Meffert H, Piazena H. Dermatomyositis: comparative studies of cutaneous photosensitivity in lupus erythematosus and normal subjects. *Photodermatol Photoimmunol Photomed*. 2004;20:230-234.
131. Rider LG, Koziol D, Giannini EH, et al. Validation of manual muscle testing and a subset of eight muscles for adult and juvenile idiopathic inflammatory myopathies. *Arthritis Care Res (Hoboken)*. 2010;62:465-472.
132. Femia AN, Vleugels RA, Callen JP. Cutaneous dermatomyositis: an updated review of treatment options and internal associations. *Am J Clin Dermatol*. 2013;14:291-313.
133. Lam C, Vleugels RA. Management of cutaneous dermatomyositis. *Dermatol Ther*. 2012;25:112-134.
134. Strowd LC, Jorizzo JL. Review of dermatomyositis: establishing the diagnosis and treatment algorithm. *J Dermatolog Treat*. 2013;24:418-421.
135. Jorizzo J, Vleugels RA. Dermatomyositis. In: Bolognia J, Jorizzo J, Schaffer J, eds. *Dermatology*. Vol 1. 3rd ed. St. Louis: Saunders; 2012:639.
136. Mathai SC, Danoff SK. Management of interstitial lung disease associated with connective tissue disease. *BMJ*. 2016;352:h6819.
137. Cheong WK, Hughes GR, Norris PG, et al. Cutaneous photosensitivity in dermatomyositis. *Br J Dermatol*. 1994;131:205-208.

138. Peyrot I, Sparsa A, Loustaud-Ratti V, et al. Topical tacrolimus and resistant skin lesions of dermatomyositis. *Rev Med Interne*. 2006;27:730-735.
139. Lampropoulos CE, D'Cruz DP. Topical tacrolimus treatment in a patient with dermatomyositis. *Ann Rheum Dis*. 2005;64:1376-1377.
140. Hollar CB, Jorizzo JL. Topical tacrolimus 0.1% ointment for refractory skin disease in dermatomyositis: a pilot study. *J Dermatolog Treat*. 2004;15:35-39.
141. Yoshimasu T, Ohtani T, Sakamoto T, et al. Topical FK506 (tacrolimus) therapy for facial erythematous lesions of cutaneous lupus erythematosus and dermatomyositis. *Eur J Dermatol*. 2002;12:50-52.
142. Kim JE, Jeong MG, Lee HE, et al. Successful treatment of cutaneous lesions of dermatomyositis with topical pimecrolimus. *Ann Dermatol*. 2011;23:348-351.
143. Iorizzo LJ 3rd, Jorizzo JL. The treatment and prognosis of dermatomyositis: an updated review. *J Am Acad Dermatol*. 2008;59:99-112.
144. Chwalinska-Sadowska H, Maldykowa H. Polymyositis-dermatomyositis:25 years of follow-up of 50 patients disease course, treatment, prognostic factors. *Mater Med Pol*. 1990;22:213-218.
145. Marie I, Hachulla E, Hatron PY, et al. Polymyositis and dermatomyositis: short term and long term outcome, and predictive factors of prognosis. *J Rheumatol*. 2001;28:2230-2237.
146. Dalakas MC. Inflammatory myopathies: management of steroid resistance. *Curr Opin Neurol*. 2011; 24:457-462.
147. Woo TY, Callen JP, Voorhees JJ, et al. Cutaneous lesions of dermatomyositis are improved by hydroxychloroquine. *J Am Acad Dermatol*. 1984;10:592-600.
148. Pelle MT, Callen JP. Adverse cutaneous reactions to hydroxychloroquine are more common in patients with dermatomyositis than in patients with cutaneous lupus erythematosus. *Arch Dermatol*. 2002;138: 1231-1233; discussion 1233.
149. Ang GC, Werth VP. Combination antimalarials in the treatment of cutaneous dermatomyositis: a retrospective study. *Arch Dermatol*. 2005;141:855-859.
150. Climent-Albaladejo A, Saiz-Cuenca E, Rosique-Roman J, et al. Dermatomyositis sine myositis and antisynthetase syndrome. *Joint Bone Spine*. 2002;69:72-75.
151. Zieglschmid-Adams ME, Pandya AG, Cohen SB, et al. Treatment of dermatomyositis with methotrexate. *J Am Acad Dermatol*. 1995;32:754-757.
152. Kasteler JS, Callen JP. Low-dose methotrexate administered weekly is an effective corticosteroid-sparing agent for the treatment of the cutaneous manifestations of dermatomyositis. *J Am Acad Dermatol*. 1997;36:67-71.
153. Hornung T, Ko A, Tuting T, et al. Efficacy of low-dose methotrexate in the treatment of dermatomyositis skin lesions. *Clin Exp Dermatol*. 2012;37:139-142.
154. Click JW, Qureshi AA, Vleugels RA. Methotrexate for the treatment of cutaneous dermatomyositis. *J Am Acad Dermatol*. 2013;68:1043-1045.
155. Metzger AL, Bohan A, Goldberg LS, et al. Polymyositis and dermatomyositis: combined methotrexate and corticosteroid therapy. *Ann Intern Med*. 1974;81:182-189.
156. Tse S, Lubelsky S, Gordon M, et al. The arthritis of inflammatory childhood myositis syndromes. *J Rheumatol*. 2001;28:192-197.
157. Camus P, Fanton A, Bonniaud P, et al. Interstitial lung disease induced by drugs and radiation. *Respiration*. 2004;71:301-326.
158. Kim YJ, Song M, Ryu JC. Mechanisms underlying methotrexate-induced pulmonary toxicity. *Expert Opin Drug Saf*. 2009;8:451-458.
159. Edge JC, Outland JD, Dempsey JR, et al. Mycophenolate mofetil as an effective corticosteroid-sparing therapy for recalcitrant dermatomyositis. *Arch Dermatol*. 2006;142:65-69.
160. Gelber AC, Nousari HC, Wigley FM. Mycophenolate mofetil in the treatment of severe skin manifestations of dermatomyositis: a series of 4 cases. *J Rheumatol*. 2000;27:1542-1545.
161. Majithia V, Harisdangkul V. Mycophenolate mofetil (CellCept): an alternative therapy for autoimmune inflammatory myopathy. *Rheumatology (Oxford)*. 2005;44:386-389.
162. Pisoni CN, Cuadrado MJ, Khamashta MA, et al. Mycophenolate mofetil treatment in resistant myositis. *Rheumatology (Oxford)*. 2007;46:516-518.
163. Rowin J, Amato AA, Deisher N, et al. Mycophenolate mofetil in dermatomyositis: is it safe? *Neurology*. 2006;66:1245-1247.
164. Tsuchiya H, Tsuno H, Inoue M, et al. Mycophenolate mofetil therapy for rapidly progressive interstitial lung disease in a patient with clinically amyopathic dermatomyositis. *Mod Rheumatol*. 2014;24:694-696.
165. Cozzani E, Cinotti E, Felletti R, et al. Amyopathic dermatomyositis with lung involvement responsive to mycophenolate mofetil. *Immunopharmacol Immunotoxicol*. 2013;35:687-692.
166. Morganroth PA, Kreider ME, Werth VP. Mycophenolate mofetil for interstitial lung disease in dermatomyositis. *Arthritis Care Res (Hoboken)*. 2010;62:1496-1501.
167. Mira-Avendano IC, Parambil JG, Yadav R, et al. A retrospective review of clinical features and treatment outcomes in steroid-resistant interstitial lung disease from polymyositis/dermatomyositis. *Respir Med*. 2013;107:890-896.
168. Saketkoo LA, Espinoza LR. Experience of mycophenolate mofetil in 10 patients with autoimmune-related interstitial lung disease demonstrates promising effects. *Am J Med Sci*. 2009;337:329-335.
169. Kitchin JE, Pomeranz MK, Pak G, et al. Rediscovering mycophenolic acid: a review of its mechanism, side effects, and potential uses. *J Am Acad Dermatol*. 1997;37:445-449.
170. Sterneck M, Settmacher U, Ganten T, et al. Improvement in gastrointestinal and health-related quality of life outcomes after conversion from mycophenolate mofetil to enteric-coated mycophenolate sodium in liver transplant recipients. *Transplant Proc*. 2014;46:234-240.
171. Femia AN, Eastham AB, Lam C, et al. Intravenous immunoglobulin for refractory cutaneous dermatomyositis: a retrospective analysis from an academic medical center. *J Am Acad Dermatol*. 2013;69:654-657.
172. Bounfour T, Bouaziz JD, Bezier M, et al. Clinical efficacy of intravenous immunoglobulins for the treatment of dermatomyositis skin lesions without muscle disease. *J Eur Acad Dermatol Venereol*. 2014;28:1150-1157.
173. Cherin P, Herson S, Wechsler B, et al. Efficacy of intravenous gammaglobulin therapy in chronic refractory polymyositis and dermatomyositis: an open study with 20 adult patients. *Am J Med*. 1991;91:162-168.
174. Cherin P, Herson S, Wechsler B, et al. Intravenous immunoglobulin for polymyositis and dermatomyositis. *Lancet*. 1990;336:116.

175. Dalakas MC, Illa I, Dambrosia JM, et al. A controlled trial of high-dose intravenous immune globulin infusions as treatment for dermatomyositis. *N Engl J Med.* 1993;329:1993-2000.
176. Caress JB, Kennedy BL, Eickman KD. Safety of intravenous immunoglobulin treatment. *Expert Opin Drug Saf.* 2010;9:971-979.
177. Feldmeyer L, Benden C, Haile SR, et al. Not all intravenous immunoglobulin preparations are equally well tolerated. *Acta Derm Venereol.* 2010;90:494-497.
178. Sekul EA, Cupler EJ, Dalakas MC. Aseptic meningitis associated with high-dose intravenous immunoglobulin therapy: frequency and risk factors. *Ann Intern Med.* 1994;121:259-262.
179. Obando I, Duran I, Martin-Rosa L, et al. Aseptic meningitis due to administration of intravenous immunoglobulin with an unusually high number of leukocytes in cerebrospinal fluid. *Pediatr Emerg Care.* 2002;18:429-432.
180. Ramirez G, Asherson RA, Khamashta MA, et al. Adult-onset polymyositis-dermatomyositis: description of 25 patients with emphasis on treatment. *Semin Arthritis Rheum.* 1990;20:114-120.
181. Hollingworth P, de Vere Tyndall A, Ansell BM, et al. Intensive immunosuppression versus prednisolone in the treatment of connective tissue diseases. *Ann Rheum Dis.* 1982;41:557-562.
182. Joffe MM, Love LA, Leff RL, et al. Drug therapy of the idiopathic inflammatory myopathies: predictors of response to prednisone, azathioprine, and methotrexate and a comparison of their efficacy. *Am J Med.* 1993;94:379-387.
183. Yu KH, Wu YJ, Kuo CF, et al. Survival analysis of patients with dermatomyositis and polymyositis: analysis of 192 Chinese cases. *Clin Rheumatol.* 2011;30:1595-1601.
184. Miller J, Walsh Y, Saminaden S, et al. Randomised double blind controlled trial of methotrexate and steroids compared with azathioprine and steroids in the treatment of idiopathic inflammatory myopathy *J Neurol Sci.* 2002;199:S53.
185. Villalba L, Hicks JE, Adams EM, et al. Treatment of refractory myositis: a randomized crossover study of two new cytotoxic regimens. *Arthritis Rheum.* 1998;41:392-399.
186. Hoyles RK, Ellis RW, Wellsbury J, et al. A multicenter, prospective, randomized, double-blind, placebo-controlled trial of corticosteroids and intravenous cyclophosphamide followed by oral azathioprine for the treatment of pulmonary fibrosis in scleroderma. *Arthritis Rheum.* 2006;54:3962-3970.
187. Mok CC, To CH, Szeto ML. Successful treatment of dermatomyositis-related rapidly progressive interstitial pneumonitis with sequential oral cyclophosphamide and azathioprine. *Scand J Rheumatol.* 2003;32:181-183.
188. Chung L, Genovese MC, Fiorentino DF. A pilot trial of rituximab in the treatment of patients with dermatomyositis. *Arch Dermatol.* 2007;143:763-767.
189. Dinh HV, McCormack C, Hall S, et al. Rituximab for the treatment of the skin manifestations of dermatomyositis: a report of 3 cases. *J Am Acad Dermatol.* 2007;56:148-153.
190. Aggarwal R, Bandos A, Reed AM, et al. Predictors of clinical improvement in rituximab-treated refractory adult and juvenile dermatomyositis and adult polymyositis. *Arthritis Rheumat.* 2014;66:740-749.
191. Oddis CV, Reed AM, Aggarwal R, et al. Rituximab in the treatment of refractory adult and juvenile dermatomyositis and adult polymyositis: a randomized, placebo-phase trial. *Arthritis Rheum.* 2013;65:314-324.
192. Andersson H, Sem M, Lund MB, et al. Long-term experience with rituximab in anti-synthetase syndrome-related interstitial lung disease. *Rheumatology (Oxford).* 2015;54(8):1420-1428.
193. Marie I, Menard JF, Hachulla E, et al. Infectious complications in polymyositis and dermatomyositis: a series of 279 patients. *Semin Arthritis Rheum.* 2011;41:48-60.
194. Belhassen-Garcia M, Rabano-Gutierrez A, Velasco-Tirado V, et al. Atypical progressive multifocal leukoencephalopathy in a patient with antisynthetase syndrome. *Intern Med.* 2015;54:519-524.
195. Vulliemoz S, Lurati-Ruiz F, Borruat FX, et al. Favourable outcome of progressive multifocal leucoencephalopathy in two patients with dermatomyositis. *J Neurol Neurosurg Psychiatry.* 2006;77:1079-1082.
196. Vencovsky J, Jarosova K, Machacek S, et al. Cyclosporine A versus methotrexate in the treatment of polymyositis and dermatomyositis. *Scand J Rheumatol.* 2000;29:95-102.
197. Takada K, Nagasaka K, Miyasaka N. Polymyositis/dermatomyositis and interstitial lung disease: a new therapeutic approach with T-cell-specific immunosuppressants. *Autoimmunity.* 2005;38:383-392.
198. Kameda H, Nagasawa H, Ogawa H, et al. Combination therapy with corticosteroids, cyclosporin A, and intravenous pulse cyclophosphamide for acute/subacute interstitial pneumonia in patients with dermatomyositis. *J Rheumatol.* 2005;32:1719-1726.
199. Ryan C, Amor KT, Menter A. The use of cyclosporine in dermatology: part II. *J Am Acad Dermatol.* 2010;63:949-972; quiz 973-974.
200. Amor KT, Ryan C, Menter A. The use of cyclosporine in dermatology: part I. *J Am Acad Dermatol.* 2010;63:925-946; quiz 947-948.
201. Mattar MA, Gualano B, Perandini LA, et al. Safety and possible effects of low-intensity resistance training associated with partial blood flow restriction in polymyositis and dermatomyositis. *Arthritis Res Ther.* 2014;16:473-014-0473-5.
202. Alexanderson H, Dastmalchi M, Esbjornsson-Liljedahl M, et al. Benefits of intensive resistance training in patients with chronic polymyositis or dermatomyositis. *Arthritis Rheum.* 2007;57:768-777.
203. Wiesinger GF, Quittan M, Aringer M, et al. Improvement of physical fitness and muscle strength in polymyositis/dermatomyositis patients by a training programme. *Br J Rheumatol.* 1998;37:196-200.
204. Riisager M, Mathiesen PR, Vissing J, et al. Aerobic training in persons who have recovered from juvenile dermatomyositis. *Neuromuscul Disord.* 2013;23: 962-968.
205. Omori CH, Silva CA, Sallum AM, et al. Exercise training in juvenile dermatomyositis. *Arthritis Care Res (Hoboken).* 2012;64:1186-1194.
206. Alexanderson H, Stenstrom CH, Jenner G, Lundberg I. The safety of a resistive home exercise program in patients with recent onset active polymyositis or dermatomyositis. *Scand J Rheumatol.* 2000;29:295-301.
207. Alexanderson H, Munters LA, Dastmalchi M, et al. Resistive home exercise in patients with recent-onset polymyositis and dermatomyositis—a randomized controlled single-blinded study with a 2-year followup. *J Rheumatol.* 2014;41:1124-1132.
208. Welborn MC, Gottschalk H, Bindra R. Juvenile dermatomyositis: a case of calcinosis cutis of the elbow

and review of the literature. *J Pediatr Orthop*. 2014 35(5):e43-e46.
209. Shahani L. Refractory calcinosis in a patient with dermatomyositis: response to intravenous immune globulin. *BMJ Case Rep*. 2012;pii: bcr2012006629.
210. Penate Y, Guillermo N, Melwani P, et al. Calcinosis cutis associated with amyopathic dermatomyositis: response to intravenous immunoglobulin. *J Am Acad Dermatol*. 2009;60:1076-1077.
211. Schanz S, Ulmer A, Fierlbeck G. Response of dystrophic calcification to intravenous immunoglobulin. *Arch Dermatol*. 2008;144:585-587.
212. Kalajian AH, Perryman JH, Callen JP. Intravenous immunoglobulin therapy for dystrophic calcinosis cutis: unreliable in our hands. *Arch Dermatol*. 2009;145:334; author reply 335.
213. Palaniappan P, Lionel AP, Kumar S. Successful treatment of calcinosis cutis in juvenile dermatomyositis with pamidronate. *J Clin Rheumatol*. 2014;20:454-455.
214. Tayfur AC, Topaloglu R, Gulhan B, et al. Bisphosphonates in juvenile dermatomyositis with dystrophic calcinosis. *Mod Rheumatol*. 2015:1-6.
215. Saini I, Kalaivani M, Kabra SK. Calcinosis in juvenile dermatomyositis: frequency, risk factors and outcome. *Rheumatol Int*. 2016;36:961-965.

Chapter 63 :: Systemic Sclerosis
:: Pia Moinzadeh, Christopher P. Denton, Carol M. Black, & Thomas Krieg

第六十三章
系统性硬皮病

中文导读

硬皮病（系统性硬皮病，SSc）是一种多系统自身免疫性疾病，其特点是血管病、炎症、皮肤和许多其他器官的纤维化。鉴别诊断包括严重的局限性硬皮病，以及许多其他类似硬皮病的情况。本章从定义、流行病学、系统性硬皮病的临床特征、病因学及发病机制、诊断、鉴别诊断、临床进程及预后、疾病管理等各方面全面阐述了系统性硬皮病。本病皮肤和器官受累的程度以及疾病进展和预后都有很大的个体差异。SSc的异质性来源于患者器官受累程度和严重程度不同。皮肤、食道、肺、心脏和肾脏是最常见的受累器官。临床表现很大程度上依赖于确诊时疾病的阶段和亚类。文中从临床分类及不同亚类的定义，器官受累的特点如雷诺现象、皮肤损害、心肺系统、胃肠道受累、肾脏受累等各方面详细描述了与SSc相关的临床特点。遗传因素决定了疾病的严重程度和易感性，但也有强有力的论据支持环境和化学因素是疾病的诱因。SSc发病机制的关键是自身免疫、血管病变和纤维化之间的密切联系。本章总结了系统性硬皮病的临床诊断思路及需要与SSc相鉴别的疾病类型。疾病的发展在很大程度上取决于特定的亚类。另外，提倡对患者进行多学科管理，及早发现和治疗并发症，可能会大大改善患者生命中的预后。本章基于疾病调整的治疗方法讨论SSc的治疗，也总结了肢端血管病及并发症，皮肤受累，心肺表现，胃肠道受累及硬皮病肾脏危象的处理以及其他支持治疗措施。

〔施　为〕

AT-A-GLANCE

- Scleroderma (systemic sclerosis [SSc]) is a multisystemic autoimmune disease characterized by vasculopathy, inflammation, and fibrosis of the skin and many other organs.

- Differential diagnosis of SSc includes severe forms of localized scleroderma, as well as many other scleroderma-like conditions.

- Raynaud phenomenon, circulating autoantibodies, and skin sclerosis are almost always present and are important for the early diagnosis.

- Patients with SSc are classified into 2 major subtypes depending on the extent of skin sclerosis (diffuse cutaneous systemic sclerosis and limited cutaneous systemic sclerosis).

- Patients with an overlap syndrome, including mixed connective tissue disease, are characterized by additional clinical features of other rheumatic diseases.

- Involvement of internal organs (digestive tract, lung, kidney, and heart) can lead to severe dysfunction and determines the prognosis.

- The heterogeneity and clinical course of SSc and SSc overlap syndromes require the urgent need of interdisciplinary collaborations and regular followup visits.

- Although the disease is still not curable, there have been substantial advances in developing new therapeutic approaches and treating organ-based complications based on a better understanding of the pathophysiology.

DEFINITIONS

Scleroderma (systemic sclerosis [SSc]) is a multisystem disease, characterized by autoimmunologic processes, vascular endothelial cell injury, inflammation, and an extensive activation of fibroblasts. There is a large individual variability in the extent of skin and organ involvement, as well as in disease progression and prognosis. Skin, esophagus, lung, heart, and kidneys are the most frequently affected organs.

EPIDEMIOLOGY

Women are more frequently affected by SSc, with a female-to-male ratio between 3:1 and 14:1.[1-4] The age of disease onset ranges between 30 and 50 years.[1] However, male patients have earlier onset than female patients. Blacks with SSc are frequently younger than whites.

SSc is a rare disease; however, incidence rates increased from 0.6 to 16 patients per million inhabitants and prevalence rates rose from 2 to 233 patients per million inhabitants per year,[2-5] depending on methodologic differences in case definition and ascertainment as well as the investigated time period. It can be assumed that these numbers represent an underestimation as patients with mild disease remain often undiagnosed.

SSc has the highest case-specific mortality of any of the autoimmune rheumatic diseases, but it varies individually, depending on racial or ethnic differences, presence and severity of organ involvement, SSc subsets, age at diagnosis, and gender differences. Although not curable, there have been substantial advances in treatment options for organ-based complications of SSc.

CLINICAL FEATURES OF SYSTEMIC SCLEROSIS

SSc usually starts with a Raynaud phenomenon, which can precede the disease for many years. The clinical manifestations depend to a large extent on the subset and stage of disease. The clinical features of established SSc are diverse with severe fibrosis of the skin and all additional cutaneous manifestations. These include hardening of the skin, development of contractures, digital ulcerations and calcifications. They also reflect the multiple patterns of internal organ involvement and the consequences of progression of the underlying pathologic processes of vasculopathy, inflammation, and fibrosis. Particular consideration must be given to the hallmark complications of hypertensive scleroderma renal crisis (SRC), pulmonary arterial hypertension (PAH), pulmonary fibrosis (PF), and GI dysmotility.

CLASSIFICATION AND DEFINITION OF DIFFERENT SSc SUBSETS

The heterogeneity of SSc arises from the range of disease manifestations that vary in extent and severity of organ involvement between patients. However, some clinical features that are almost always present are Raynaud phenomenon (RP) and skin sclerosis. The extent of skin sclerosis defines each major disease subset, each of which has particular clinical characteristics, although there are also common features to each.

In 1980, the American College of Rheumatology (ACR) published preliminary classification criteria for SSc for patients with established disease,[6] which criteria showed 97% sensitivity and 98% specificity for SSc. According to the criteria, the diagnosis is proven, if either 1 major criterion or at least 2 minor criteria are found. The major criterion are scleroderma proximal to the metacarpophalangeal or metatarsophalangeal joints; the minor criteria include sclerodactyly, digital ulcerations and/or pitting digital scars, and bibasilar PF. Although these criteria have been used for many years they do not allow the inclusion of patients with early SSc and some patients with limited cutaneous systemic sclerosis. As a result, new ACR/European League Against Rheumatism criteria were developed, which are based on a score system and consider several additional criteria such as abnormal nailfold capillaries, fingertip lesions, and autoantibodies. These new criteria now allow early diagnosis of patients and include those patients in clinical trials before extensive fibrosis develops.[7]

In 1988, a descriptive subclassification of limited versus diffuse SSc was introduced by LeRoy,[8] which was primarily associated with the extent of cutaneous involvement. This classification has been widely accepted and used in clinical practice. In 2001, LeRoy and Medsger[9] published amended criteria, with the additional presence of autoantibodies and nailfold capillaroscopic alterations. Furthermore, these criteria include a separate group of patients with early onset of SSc, with minimal skin thickening. It was mandatory that patients with early (limited) SSc have evidence of RP plus scleroderma-specific autoantibodies and/or nailfold capillaroscopic manifestations.[10,11] Although there are several other classifications published, for example, by Nadashkevich and colleagues and by Maricq and Valter,[10,12] the initial LeRoy classification is still widely used in daily clinical practice.

Diffuse cutaneous SSc is defined as a progressive form of SSc with an early onset of RP, usually within 1 year of onset of skin thickening. This subset is characterized by rapid skin involvement of trunk, face, upper arms, and thighs, showing very frequently, anti–scleroderma 70 (antitopoisomerase-I) or anti-RNA polymerase III antibodies.[8] Furthermore, there is a higher propensity to develop PF, cardiac involvement, and SRC (Fig. 63-1).

Limited cutaneous SSc is characterized by a long preexisting history of RP and skin changes of the extremities distal to the knee and elbow joints, including facial skin.[8] This SSc-subset variant often (50% to 70% of cases) presents with anticentromere antibodies and is frequently associated with isolated PAH. The traditional acronym CREST (calcinosis, RP, esophageal dysmotility, sclerodactyly, and telangiectasias) is assigned to the limited form of SSc (Fig. 63-2).

Patients suffering from early SSc, also known as undifferentiated SSc, are defined by positive RP and at least 1 additional feature of SSc (positive nailfold capillary alterations, puffy fingers, pulmonary hypertension) and/or detectable scleroderma-associated autoantibodies without fulfilling the ACR criteria.[1,13,14]

A very small proportion of cases (1.5%) develop vascular (RP and/or PAH), immunologic (most commonly anticentromere antibodies), and organ-based fibrotic features of SSc, but do not show skin sclerosis.[15] Patients suffering from this subset are classified as *SSc sine scleroderma*.

Patients with features of scleroderma together with those of another autoimmune rheumatic disease are designated *SSc overlap syndrome* (Fig. 63-3 and Table 63-1). SSc overlap syndrome is defined as a disease occurring with clinical aspects of SSc (according to the ACR criteria) or main symptoms of SSc simultaneously with those of other connective tissue diseases or other autoimmune diseases, such as dermatomyositis, Sjögren syndrome, systemic lupus erythematosus, vasculitis, and polyarthritis. These patients present mostly high titers of anti-U1RNP, anti-nRNP, antifibrillarin, or anti-PmScl antibodies.[16]

This group of patients includes well-defined patients suffering from mixed connective tissue disease (MCTD), characterized by high titers of circulating anti-U1RNP antibodies (Table 63-2). There is still an ongoing discussion, whether MCTD represents a distinct disease entity or may be an early form of another connective tissue disease. These MCTD patients have varying clinical features with symptoms of systemic lupus erythematosus or rheumatoid arthritis with Raynaud syndrome, and later developing sclerodermatous lesions. They have swollen fingers and puffy hands. Non-Raynaud symptoms are skin sclerosis at acral regions and internal manifestations that occur later. There are often intense inflammatory symptoms with heavy arthralgia. MCTD patients can develop pericarditis, pleuritis, and pulmonary hypertension. However, there is a good response to antiinflammatory/anti-immune therapy and the prognosis is clearly better than in patients with classic scleroderma.[17,18]

Another already well-defined subset within the overlap syndromes are patients with sclerodermatous lesions, who also suffer from an intense myositis. These patients are usually characterized by specific Pm-Scl autoantibodies, have typical mechanic hands, and develop early intense subcutaneous calcifications. Similar to MCTD patients, they respond well to an early antiinflammatory treatment (eg, methotrexate/glucocorticosteroids).[19]

Other overlap syndromes include patients with Raynaud and lupus erythematosus or rheumatoid arthritis symptoms, who later develop sclerodermatous lesions. Many of these patients have specific circulating autoantibodies that probably represent distinct disease entities. However further studies using molecular markers are still required to clarify their disease identity within the spectrum of scleroderma-related diseases.[19]

In addition, the frequency and timing of different visceral manifestations of SSc differs between major subsets. However, there is some overlap between subsets in terms of organ-based disease and the extent and severity of skin sclerosis.

In all patients, the extent and severity of skin sclerosis can be assessed by the modified Rodnan skin score. Skin score at baseline correlates with disease severity and outcome in diffuse cutaneous SSc. Thickening and fibrosis of the skin as one of the first recognized phenomenon in SSc still forms the basis of most classification criteria and proposed subsets of this disease spectrum.

It also has to be mentioned that another classification of SSc-related diseases, which is completely based on autoantibodies, has been proposed. There is evidence from association studies that this may be clinically

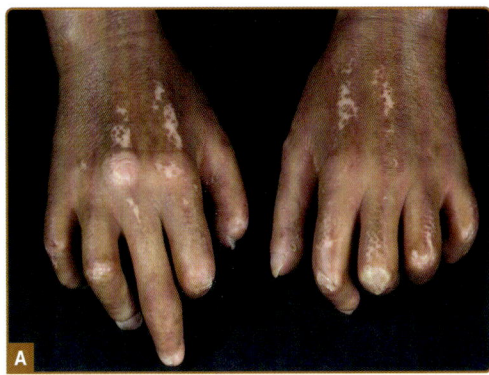
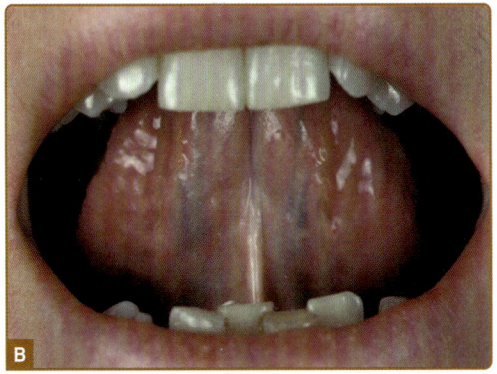
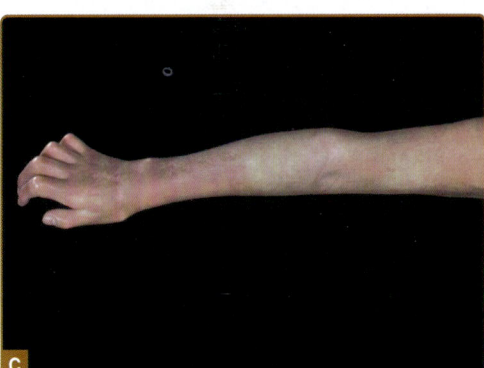
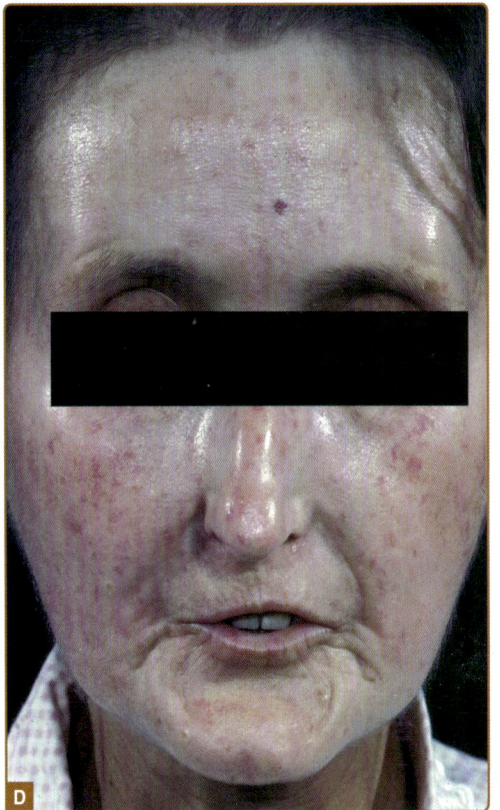

Figure 63-1 Extensive skin involvement in patients with diffuse cutaneous systemic sclerosis. **A,** Sclerodactyly with dermatogenous contractures (restricted mobility of digital joints) and salt-and-pepper hyperpigmentations and hypopigmentations. **B,** Microstomia (radial furrowing around the mouth) with frenulum sclerosis. **C,** Skin thickening proximal of the metacarpophalangeal joints. **D,** Typical scleroderma facial physiognomy with hypermimia, microstomia, telangiectasias, and a beaked nose.

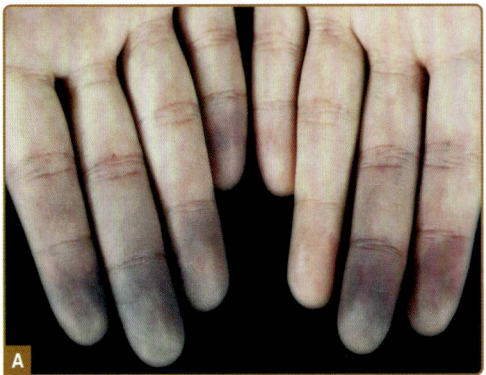
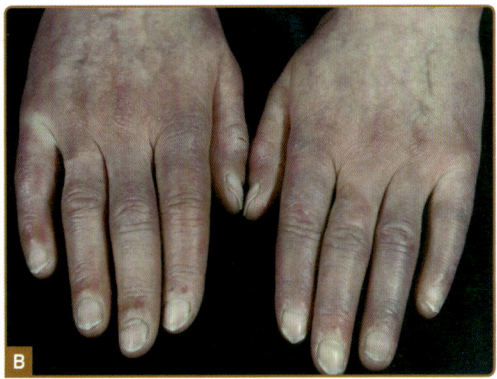

Figure 63-2 Clinical feature of patients with early disease. **A,** Raynaud phenomenon with typical discoloration (blue-white pallor), localized mostly at fingers and/or toes as the result of vasospasm. Coldness and emotional stress are the most frequent triggers for these attacks. **B,** Limited disease with puffy fingers.

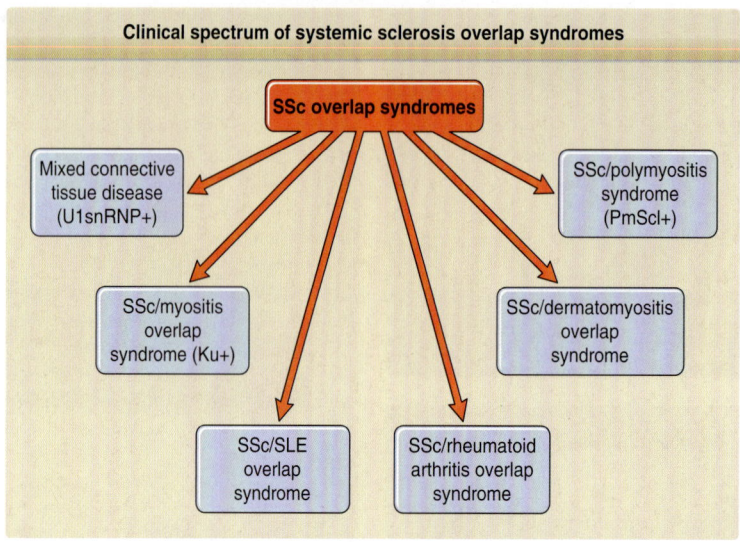

Figure 63-3 Clinical spectrum of systemic sclerosis (SSc) overlap syndromes. Patients with clinical features of scleroderma together with features of at least 1 additional autoimmune rheumatic disease are designated SSc overlap syndromes. SLE, systemic lupus erythematosus.

meaningful, as indicated in Table 63-3. Moreover, genetic association analysis using a candidate gene approach has demonstrated an association between serologically based subsets of SSc that are stronger than with SSc overall. The significance of this is uncertain, and it should be noted that a genetic basis for autoantibody reactivity has been well described, leading to the suggestion that the serologic subsets may be more genetically homogeneous than unselected SSc cases or clinically defined subsets of SSc. Large-scale studies in multinational patient cohorts using molecular and clinical markers are probably required to revise the current classification system of this heterogeneous spectrum of diseases.

ORGAN MANIFESTATION

RAYNAUD PHENOMENON

Distinctive for this disease is the initial onset of RP, which appears in more than 90% of SSc patients (see Fig. 63-2).[1] It is defined by recurrent attacks of vasospasm of small digital arterioles/arteries at fingers and toes, usually caused by cold and/or other stimuli, for example, emotional stress. RP clinically appears suddenly and is clearly restricted and is accompanied by painful pallor/ischemia of single or several digits/toes, followed by reactive hyperemia after reheating at the end of a RP attack, in some cases cyanosis (triphasic RP) also ensues (see Fig. 63-2).

SKIN INVOLVEMENT

Skin involvement is a cardinal feature of SSc and usually appears first in the fingers and hands. Within time, patients develop nonpitting edema of the fingers (puffy fingers), hands, and extremities, followed by an increasing induration and skin thickening (sclerodactyly) (see Figs. 63-1 and 63-2). Depending on the localization of skin thickening, restricted mobility of joints (dermatogenous contractures), and/or restricted breath excursion may be present. Typical facial features include telangiectasias, a beak-shaped nose, and reduced mouth aperture (microstomia). The typical

TABLE 63-1
Clinical Features of Systemic Sclerosis/Myositis Overlap Syndrome

- Raynaud phenomenon
- Sclerodactyly
- Mechanic hands
- Myositis
- Pulmonary involvement
- Calcinosis cutis
- Serositis
- PmScl autoantibodies

TABLE 63-2
Clinical Features of Mixed Connective Tissue Disease[17,18]

- Raynaud phenomenon
- Puffy fingers/hands
- Sclerodactyly
- Oesophageal involvement
- Pulmonary hypertension/interstitial lung disease
- Myositis
- Arthritis and arthralgia
- Serositis
- Anemia/lymphopenia
- High titers of U1RNP antibodies

TABLE 63-3
Clinical Association of Hallmark Autoantibodies in Systemic Sclerosis[47]

REACTIVITY	TARGET ANTIGEN	FREQUENCY IN SSc (%)	HLA ASSOCIATION	CLINICAL ASSOCIATION
Centromere	CENP proteins speckled pattern	20 to 30	HLA-DRB1 HLA-DQB1	Limited skin sclerosis, severe gut disease, isolated PAH, calcinosis
Scl-70	Topoisomerase-1 speckled pattern	15 to 20	HLA-DRB1 HLA-DQB1 HLA-DPB1	Diffuse skin sclerosis, pulmonary fibrosis and secondary PAH, increased SSc-related mortality rate
RNAP III	RNA polymerase III speckled pattern	20	HLA-DQB1	Diffuse skin sclerosis, hypertensive renal crisis, correlated with a higher mortality rate
nRNP	U1RNP speckled pattern	15	HLA-DR2, HLA-DR4 HLA-DQw5, DQw8	Overlap features of SLE, arthritis
Pm-Scl	Polymyositis/Scl nuclear staining pattern	3	HLA-DQA1 HLA-DRB1	Limited skin sclerosis, myositis–sclerosis overlap, calcinosis
Fibrillarin	U3RNP nuclear staining pattern	4	HLA-DQB1	Diffuse skin sclerosis, myositis, PAH, renal disease
Th/To	7-2RNP nuclear staining pattern	2–5	HLA-DRB1	Limited skin sclerosis, pulmonary fibrosis

PAH, pulmonary arterial hypertension; SLE, systemic lupus erythematosus; SSc, systemic sclerosis.

facial appearance of SSc patients is characterized by a radial furrowing around the mouth, no expression, a stiff and mask-like facial appearance, and sclerosis of the frenulum. Besides cosmetic/aesthetic problems, this causes considerable difficulties regarding eating and oral hygiene (see Fig. 63-1).

The abnormal deposition of cutaneous and/or subcutaneous calcium (calcinosis cutis), usually occurs over pressure points (acral, joints) (Fig. 63-4). Calcinosis cutis next to joints is Thibierge-Weissenbach syndrome. Further skin manifestations include hypopigmented and hyperpigmented (salt-and-pepper) skin (see Fig. 63-1), and loss of hair follicles and sweat glands (hypohidrosis/anhydrosis).[20]

Approximately 50% of patients with SSc are affected by digital ulceration associated with vasculopathy at some point in their disease. This is the major external feature of structural vessel disease, probably attributable to thickened intima and lumen-occluded vessels. Tender and painful pitting scars are very frequent and, on occasion, progress to ulcers. These occur on the finger- or toe-tips, over the extensor surfaces of the joints as a result of microtrauma or in association with the abovementioned calcinosis cutis. Digital ulcers are associated with strong, local pain and a major impact on quality of life regarding all-day functions (eg, dressing, eating). Other complications include critical digital ischemia, paronychia, infections, gangrene, osteomyelitis, and finger pulp loss or amputation.

CARDIOPULMONARY MANIFESTATIONS

There are different ways that the cardiopulmonary system may be involved, most often appearing as fibrosis and PAH. The differentiation between these manifestations is often clinically difficult because of similar overlapping clinical features, such as dyspnea, nonproductive cough, disturbed diffusion capacity, and cyanoses. PAH is currently the most common cause of disease-related death in SSc.[21] It occurs in both limited and diffuse cutaneous subsets, although the most typical cases are those of limited SSc associated with isolated PAH. This condition has substantial similarities to idiopathic PAH. Thus, 2 patterns of disease occur in SSc. Most cases have PAH, but there are some patients with late-stage extensive interstitial lung fibrosis in SSc that develop a true secondary pulmonary hypertension.[22] Besides the right-heart worsening caused by PAH, the heart could also be involved by diffuse or focal fibrosis or from inflammatory myocarditis. This may lead to diastolic or systolic dysfunction, as well as a restricted contractibility of the myocardium. These patients clinically present cardiac arrhythmia, paroxysmal tachycardia, incomplete or complete right-heart blocks, and heart insufficiency.[23]

GI INVOLVEMENT

GI involvement is the most common internal organ involvement in patients suffering from both limited and diffuse SSc (>60%).[1] Many parts of the GI tract may be impaired, affecting motility, digestion, absorption, and excretion.[24]

Esophageal involvement includes symptoms like dysphagia, heartburn resulting from reflux, nausea, and/or vomiting. A weakened lower esophageal sphincter and impaired peristalsis increase the risk for esophagitis. If untreated, this could lead to peptic esophagitis, gastric/esophageal ulcerations, peptic stricture formations, and fistulae. Chronic gastroesophageal reflux can be complicated after a time

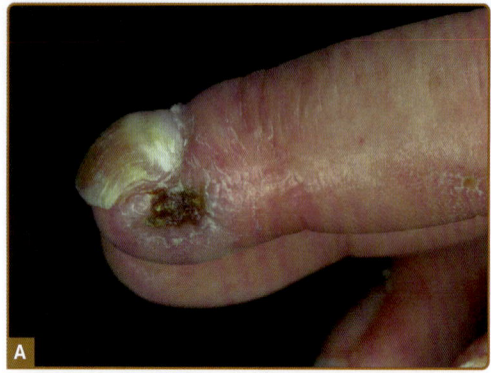 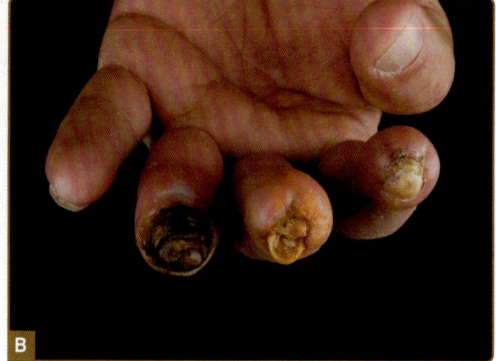
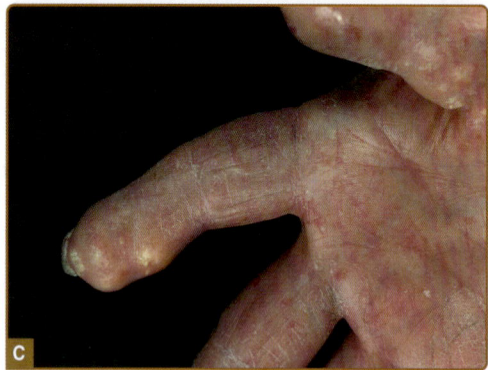 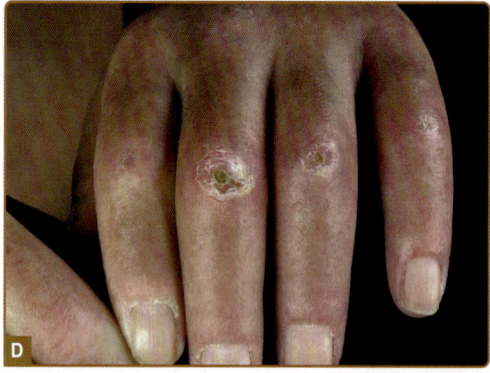

Figure 63-4 Digital alterations with complications. **A,** Digital ulcerations at the fingertips. **B,** Digital ulcerations and necrosis of the fingertips. **C,** Severe calcifications with deposition of subcutaneous masses. **D,** Multiple ulcerations at bone protuberants with inflammation in the surrounding sclerotic skin.

by a higher risk for Barrett esophagus, which may progress into an adenocarcinoma.

Possible gastric manifestations include atrophy of mucous membrane–associated ulcerations and delayed gastric emptying. Gastric antral vascular ectasia is also an important complication in some SSc patients and needs to be detected by endoscopy because it can lead to severe, often not recognized, bleeding.[25]

SSc can also affect the intestine, and includes atonic dilation, constrictions, malabsorption, pseudoobstruction, diarrhea, constipation, fecal incontinence, and severe malnutrition.

KIDNEY INVOLVEMENT

SRC appears in 5% to 10% of SSc patients, and may cause an abrupt onset of significant systemic hypertension (>140/90 mm Hg, or a rise in systolic/diastolic blood pressure ≥30/≥20 mm Hg), together with an increase in serum creatinine, proteinuria, hematuria, thrombocytopenia, or hemolysis followed by an acute renal failure.[26] Studies suggest that a chronic vasculopathy with reduced glomerular filtration rate is frequent. In addition, there is evidence of an increase in fibrillar collagen deposition within the renal interstitium in SSc. Many cases occur within the first 12 months of disease, and in up to 25% of patients with SRC, the diagnosis of SSc is made at the time of the renal presentation. End-organ damage can result in encephalopathy with generalized seizures or flash pulmonary edema. Microangiopathic anemia is common, and sometimes disseminated, intravascular coagulation develops. Nephrotoxic drugs and high-dose prednisolone (>7.5 mg/day) should be avoided in patients suffering from SSc.[27]

ETIOLOGY AND PATHOGENESIS

The pathogenesis of this complex autoimmune disease involves multiple cell types (endothelial cells, epithelial cells, fibroblasts, and lymphocytic cells) interacting through a variety of mechanisms that are dependent on their microenvironment and several key mediators.

Major facets of the disease include inflammation, vasculature, and the activation of connective tissue-producing cells (Fig. 63-5). The clinical heterogeneity of SSc makes it likely that distinct pathogenetic mechanisms predominate in particular patients or subsets of disease. Similarly, the key pathways are not necessarily the same at different stages of SSc. Although a genetic component to etiopathogenesis is likely and evidence supports genetic factors determining severity and susceptibility, there are also strong arguments, supporting environmental and chemical factors as triggers for the disease.[28]

GENETIC FACTORS

The best evidence for a genetic contribution to SSc and related diseases comes from studies that report familial clustering and from the limited twin studies that have been undertaken. Although the absolute risk for familial-occurring SSc is relative low, the relative risk for first-degree relatives is 13-fold higher compared to the normal population.[29] Several studies suggest that a positive family history for SSc is the strongest risk factor, but ethnicity also contributes.[29] Assassi and colleagues suggest that members of SSc-affected families tend to show concordant scleroderma-specific autoantibodies.[30] Further support is provided from genetic association studies with candidate gene approaches. Most success has been observed in genetic analysis of individual components of the disease such

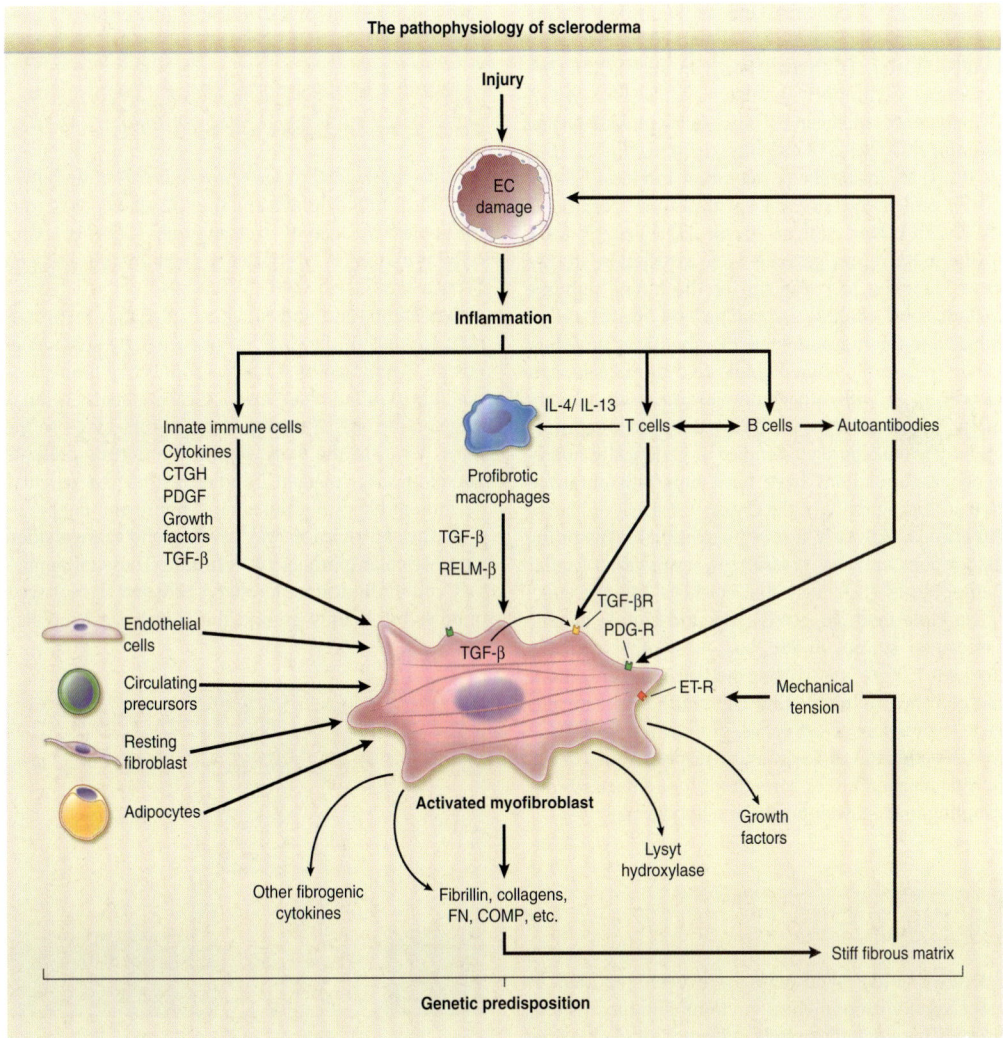

Figure 63-5 Pathogenesis of systemic sclerosis. The schematic shows how the development of systemic sclerosis results from a complex interplay between cells within the immune system, including adaptive and innate compartments, the vasculature, and the connective tissue. Cell–matrix interactions are important regulators of cellular functions. Early vascular events lead to later development of an autonomous population of activated fibroblasts and myofibroblasts that contract soft tissue and deposit excessive extracellular matrix proteins. These cells may develop from resident connective tissue fibroblasts; transdifferentiation from other cell types, including activated microvascular pericytes; and recruitment of circulating progenitor cells (fibrocytes). The contribution of each lineage to the fibrotic lesion is still unclear. Many growth factors and cytokines are implicated as mediators of this process, and complex reciprocal networks may lead to a profibrotic microenvironment. Potential disease-modifying therapies could target individual mediators alone or in combination (eg, tumor growth factor-β [TGF-β], endothelin [ET-1], connective tissue growth factor [CTGF], platelet-derived growth factor [PDGF]) or modulate immune cells (eg, cyclophosphamide) or the endothelial cell (eg, prostacyclin analogs). The extracellular matrix is an important repository for mediators that are later released and play a key role in pathogenesis. CCL, CC chemokine ligand; COMP, cartilage oligomeric matrix protein; EC, extracellular; ET-R, endothelin receptor; FN, fibronectin; Ig, immunoglobulin; IL, interleukin; RELM-β, resistin like molecule-β.

as autoantibody profiles. These appear to have a strong genetic determinant, and this may underlie the apparent mutual exclusivity of the SSc hallmark reactivities. It has been demonstrated that the ability to mount an immune response to a particular SSc-associated antigen is restricted by major histocompatibility complex haplotype. Several studies suggest an association of HLA-DRB1*1302 and HLA-DQB1*0604/0605 haplotypes with antifibrillarin-positive patients,[31] while HLA-SRB1*0301 occurs in patients with anti–Pm-Scl antibodies.[32] Observation from a large number of studies examining genetic markers has identified a number of candidate genes (eg, anemia-inducing factor [AIF]-1, cluster of differentiation [CD] 19, CD22, CD86, cytotoxic T-lymphocyte antigen [CTLA]-4, CCL-2, CCL-5, chemokine ligand [CXCL]-8, chemokine-related receptor [CXCR]-2, interleukin [IL]-1α, IL-1β, IL-2, IL-10, IL-13, macrophage migration inhibitory factor (MIF), protein tyrosine phosphatase non-receptor 22 (PTPN22) tumor necrosis factor [TNF]-α).[29,33] Most of the more recent genome-wide association studies have identified loci relevant for the innate immune system; some of these associations are already rather robust and might lead to new therapeutic approaches. Others reflect the altered connective tissue response. However, as with other complex diseases, in very many instances, it has not always possible to replicate initially promising data. Studies of genetically homogeneous populations have been especially informative, including those of the Choctaw Nation of Native Americans. However, it is of interest that some of the associations are very plausible in terms of molecular pathogenesis. It is likely that epistasis and the effect of multiple modifier genes confound simple genetic association studies in SSc, just as in other complex diseases.[34] There is increasing evidence that epigenetic mechanisms by modulating chromatin structure and gene expression of cytokines/growth factors critical for the activation of the immune response and/or the fibrotic reaction are important additional factors contributing to the development of scleroderma.

ENVIRONMENTAL FACTORS

Scleroderma-like syndromes have been reported in association with numerous environmental toxins and drugs. These agents include solvents (vinyl chloride, benzene, toluene, epoxy resins), drugs (bleomycin, carbidopa, pentazocine, cocaine, docetaxel, metaphenylenediamine), and miscellaneous substances.[35]

SSc was reported to occur in underground coal and gold miners. In male patients with silicosis who were older than 40 years of age, the likelihood of developing SSc was approximately 190 times greater than in males not exposed to silica, and 50 times greater than in males without silicosis but exposed to silica dust.[36] The role of silicone gel implants and other silicone products in the development of scleroderma has been questioned.[37] However, most epidemiologic studies have failed to show a significant association. An unusual form of scleroderma characterized by RP, morphea-like skin changes, capillary abnormalities of the nailfold (similar to those in SSc), osteolysis of the distal phalanges, and hepatic and PF may occur in workers exposed to polyvinyl chloride. Bleomycin also produces PF, RP, and cutaneous changes indistinguishable from those of SSc.[37] The development of these changes appears to be dose-dependent and is reversible on discontinuation of the drug. Collectively, chemical exposures account for a small fraction of scleroderma-like diseases. Large epidemiologic studies have not yet revealed a significant role for toxins and drugs in scleroderma.

HISTOPATHOLOGY

The histopathology of SSc shows fibrosis of the lower two-thirds of the dermis and the subcutaneous fibrous trabeculae, because of excessive deposition of extracellular matrix (ECM) proteins, most notably collagen Types I and III (Fig. 63-6).[28]

Panniculitis and mucoid edema also may be prominent features in the early stages, whereby subcutaneous fat is replaced by a fibrous connective tissue. It is possible to differentiate histologically an early cellular stage on the one hand and a later fibrotic stage on the other hand. In the early stages, the dermis presents pathologically collagen bundles within the reticular dermis, and appear pale, homogenous, running parallel to the skin surface, and swollen, and there is often a perivascular lymphocytic infiltrate. These inflammatory cell infiltrates are localized between the collagen bundles but mainly around the vessels, and can also

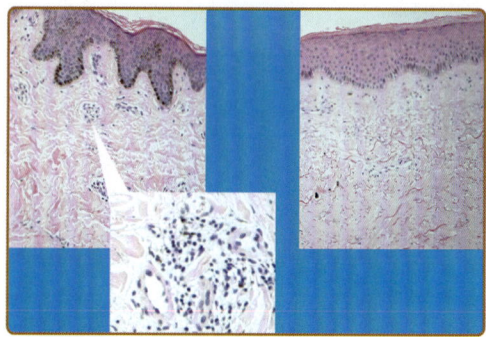

Figure 63-6 Histologic appearance of skin in early and late-stage diffuse cutaneous systemic sclerosis (SSc). In SSc, there is perivascular mononuclear cell infiltrate at the early stages of disease. This precedes the development of skin sclerosis. Perivascular changes are shown at high power in the *left panel*. Later stage disease is accompanied by skin sclerosis, a low density of blood vessels, and absence of inflammatory cells. At this stage, there may be associated epidermal changes with thickening and loss of secondary skin structures, including hair follicles and sweat glands. Absence of the rete ridges is also characteristic at the later stages of diffuse cutaneous SSc. Similar changes are predicted in localized cutaneous SSc, but this is rarely biopsied because of limited skin sclerosis and concerns about healing.

spread into subcutaneous fat tissue. The infiltrate can also entrap sweat glands. The epidermis often becomes atrophic in the overlying areas. Vessels of all sizes may be involved in SSc. In the early stages, there may only be dilation of capillaries, then endothelial proliferation and complete occlusion of vessels occur. With the progression of scleroderma, the involved skin becomes more avascular and inflammation decreases. In later stages, pilosebaceous units and eccrine glands disappear, collagen bundles appear to be packed closely, and there may be an effacement of the rete ridges.[20]

VASCULOPATHY

Vasculopathy in SSc is an early event and is based on inappropriate vascular remodeling and repair processes. It involves the microcirculation and arterioles and is very likely a primary event in the pathogenetic processes of the disease. Vascular abnormalities are characterized by vasoconstriction, adventitial and intimal proliferation, inflammation, and thrombosis.[28] The earliest signs of vascular dysfunction are represented by enhanced vascular permeability with an imbalance between vasodilatory (nitric oxide, prostacyclin, calcitonin gene-related peptide) and vasoconstrictive mediators (endothelin-1, angiotensin II, α_2-adrenoreceptors). Consequently, the impaired blood flow leads to tissue hypoxia, which induces strong expression of vascular endothelial growth factor and its receptors, associated with a defect of vasculogenesis. However, inflammatory cytokines like TNF-α may stimulate or inhibit angiogenesis depending on the duration of the stimulus.[38]

In addition to these functional abnormalities, intravascular and structural changes contribute to overt RP, and in the course of time to progressive reduction of vessels and blood flow. This pattern of obliterative vasculopathy may clinically manifest in all vessels of virtually all organs. Early lesions in the microcirculation because of structural damage are initially seen in the nailfold capillaries and as vasospastic responses in RP. Furthermore, vascular changes, that is, overgrowth of the endothelium and deposition of scar tissue, produce some of the major complications of SSc, including PAH, SRC, and digital vasculopathy.

IMMUNE EVENTS

There are early inflammatory changes in the skin and lung of patients with SSc. The first inflammatory infiltrates in lesional skin are predominantly cells of the monocyte lineage (T cells, macrophages, B cells, and mast cells).[39] There are several lines of evidence for the crucial role of the innate immune system in SSc. This is underlined by the association of interferon regulatory factor-5 variants with scleroderma.[40,41] Several studies also demonstrate the role of macrophages as important contributors of cytokines, which influence the fibrotic response.[42]

Later, T lymphocytes predominate and are detectable in both the circulation and affected organs. These T cells are predominantly CD4+, bear markers of activation, exhibit oligoclonal expansion, which suggests an antigen-driven proliferation, and show a predominant T-helper 2 phenotype.[43,44] Consequently, increased serum levels of T-helper 2 cell–derived cytokines (IL-2, IL-4, IL-10, IL-13, and IL-17) have been observed in scleroderma patients.[45,46]

In addition to T cells, B cells are also found in involved skin. Several studies suggest that B cells are able to induce ECM production through secretion of IL-6 and transforming growth factor-β (TGF-β) and are involved in the production of autoantibodies.

Several of these autoantibodies are associated with defined subsets of the disease and are important diagnostic markers (see Table 63-3).[47] The potential role of autoantibodies in pathogenesis is a fascinating and exciting area. The majority of SSc cases have circulating antibodies. These include a number of hallmark reactivities, as well as autoantibodies, that occur in other autoimmune rheumatic diseases (eg, anticyclic citrullinated peptide, rheumatoid factor) but also antibodies that may have functional significance, as they are directed against cell-surface antigens (eg, antiendothelial cell antibodies, antifibrillin antibodies, anti–platelet-derived growth factor [PDGF] receptor antibodies) (Table 63-4).[48-50] However, functional impact of these antibodies remains an area of investigation. There is growing evidence of functional significance for antiendothelial cell autoantibodies and for antifibroblast-reacting antibodies. Reports also suggest the presence of antifibrillin autoantibodies and stimulatory autoantibodies reacting with PDGF receptors.[48-50] Microchimerism and graft-versus-host disease mechanisms have been suggested in some cases, although the relatively high frequency of microchimerism in healthy individuals or other disease states suggests that this may be contributory rather than causal if it has a role in SSc.

Careful clinical studies have identified a subset of SSc patients (characterized by RNA polymerase antibodies), who develop the disease in association with the occurrence of malignancies.[51-53] This led to the hypothesis that fibrosis may represent an immune response against tumor antigens and initiated a discussion on the relationship of autoimmunity and malignancy in general. Further studies are required to clarify this issue.

FIBROSIS

SSc is a multisystem fibrotic disease. The initial inflammation and hypoxia induces in fibroblasts the production of several proteins that are involved in ECM remodeling as, for example, thrombospondin-1, fibronectin-1, lysylhydroxylase-2, and TGF-β–induced proteins.[54] At the same time there is a disturbed balance

TABLE 63-4
Functional Autoantibodies in Systemic Sclerosis and Their Association to Pathophysiology[48-50]

FUNCTIONAL ANTIBODY	FREQUENCY IN SYSTEMIC SCLEROSIS	CLINICAL ASSOCIATION
Anti–platelet-derived growth factor receptor	33% to 100%	• Seem to induce skin fibrosis as a result of activation of fibroblasts into myofibroblasts and fibroblast-like cells • First functional antibodies discovered in systemic sclerosis (SSc)
Antiendothelial cell antibodies	44% to 84%	• Mediates endothelial cell damage and activation of fibroblasts resulting from stimulation of proinflammatory and fibrotic cytokines • Associated with severe organ manifestation • Associated with perivascular, vascular (digital ulcers [DUs]) and lung involvement (pulmonary arterial hypertension [PAH]) • Also found in other rheumatic diseases
Antifibroblast antibodies	26% to 58%	• Associated with Scl-70 antibodies and the prevalence of interstitial lung disease and PAH • Increased prevalence in diffuse cutaneous SSc compared to limited cutaneous SSc
Antifibrillin-1	>50%	• Activates fibroblasts by stimulation of the release of transforming growth factor-ββ
Anti–matrix metalloproteinase (MMP) 1, anti-MMP3	49% to 52%	• Inhibits the degradation of extracellular matrix proteins, because of an inhibition of MMP collagenase activity • Correlates with the extent of fibrosis (skin, lung, kidney)
Angiotensin II Type 1 receptor and endothelin Type A receptor	82% to 83%	• Simultaneous presence has been described in SSc patients (cross-reactivity) • Associated with early and severe disease, PAH, DUs, renal crisis, diffuse cutaneous SSc, and lung fibrosis

between synthesis and degradation mechanisms leading to the excess of ECM in specialized organs, which is then responsible for much of the morbidity and mortality of the disease. The key event in the development of fibrosis is the induction of fibroblasts into activated myofibroblasts. Alternatively, also other cell types (eg, circulating precursor cells, endothelial cells, and epithelial cells) can be converted into myofibroblasts. The initiation of this process includes a number of key cytokines and growth factors that may represent logical therapeutic targets. These include fibrogenic cytokines such as TGF-β, connective tissue growth factor, PDGF, and endothelin-1.[28,55-57] Especially TGF-β has been shown to play a central role,[58] which is also underscored by extensive expression profiling studies using skin biopsies from scleroderma patients in different stages of the diseases.[59] This has already led to therapeutic approaches using antibodies against TGF-β in early clinical studies.[60]

Myofibroblasts are characterized by a high contractility, ECM production, and cytokine release. This function together with altered biophysical properties of the resulting connective tissue lead to persistent activation of fibroblasts with an excessive deposition of ECM components. However, crucial for understanding the mechanisms of this disease is the close connection between autoimmunity, vasculopathy, and fibrosis. This was recently demonstrated in a mouse model characterized by downregulation of the transcription factors Friend leukemia integration 1 (Fli1) and Kruppel-like factor 5 (KLF5), which develop a scleroderma like disease with the production of autoantibodies.[61]

Figure 63-5 is a schematic that summarizes the pathogenetic mechanisms.

DIAGNOSIS

RAYNAUD PHENOMENON

Patients presenting only with RP should be studied for capillary alterations as well as autoantibody status. All these are predictors for the development of SSc, which together make the diagnosis of SSc rather likely. To identify and visualize vascular cutaneous alterations caused by SSc, nailfold capillaroscopy is a noninvasive, simple, and one of the most useful diagnostic and prognostic methods (Table 63-5). Furthermore, it is a useful tool to categorize capillary changes into early, active, and late patterns. Laser Doppler perfusion imaging is also a noninvasive microvascular imaging technique able to provide maps of the cutaneous blood flow.[62]

SKIN SCLEROSIS

Skin involvement should be evaluated using the modified Rodnan Skin Score. Usually, 17 sites are assessed and skin thickness is categorized to grade 1, 2, or 3, corresponding to mild, medium, and severe, according to palpation of the skin by a trained examiner (Fig. 63-7). Newer techniques for calculating skin thickening also have been evaluated. In addition to the modified Rodnan skin score,[63] the 20-MHz ultrasonography,[64] MRI,[65] and plicometer[66] methods are useful for assessing skin thickening (recommended diagnostic procedures are listed in Table 63-5). Further physical procedures to monitor skin fibrosis are the

TABLE 63-5
Recommended Diagnostic Procedures in Systemic Sclerosis[71]

ORGAN INVOLVEMENT	CLINICAL FEATURE	DIAGNOSTIC PROCEDURES
Vascular system	Raynaud phenomenon	- Coldness provocation - Nailfold capillaroscopy - Antinuclear antibody levels
Skin	Scleroderma Calcinosis cutis	- Clinical assessment regarding puffy fingers, telangiectasias, mechanic hands, hypopigmentations/hyperpigmentations, digital ulcerations, dermatogenous contractures - Modified Rodnan skin score - 20-MHz ultrasonography - Radiography (X-ray, MRI, CT)
Musculoskeletal system	Arthralgia Synovitis Muscle weakness	- Clinical assessment regarding fist closure deficiency, joint contractures, tendon friction rub, muscle weakness - Laboratory parameters: erythrocyte sedimentation rate, rheumatoid factor, antinuclear autoantibodies - Creatine kinase (greater than threefold?) - MRI, electromyography - Muscle biopsy
GI tract	Reflux Dysphagia Gastric antral vascular ectasia Diarrhea, obstipation	- Gastro-/esophageal endoscopy - Esophageal scintigraphy, esophagus manometry - Gastro-/esophageal endoscopy with laser coagulation, if necessary - Colonoscopy
Respiratory system	Dyspnea	- Lung function test (carbon monoxide transfer factor corrected for hemoglobin [TLCOc] single breath (SB), total lung capacity [TLC], forced vital capacity [FVC]) - Radiography (X-ray or high resolution CT) - Bronchoalveolar lavage (BAL) (optional)
Cardiac system	Dyspnea, arrhythmia	- Electrocardiography (conduction blocks?) - Echocardiography (mean pulmonary artery pressure, diastolic dysfunction?, ventricular ejection fraction) - (Spiro-)Ergometry - 24-Hour blood pressure controls - Right-heart catheterization - Cardio MRI
Kidney	Renal function failure	- Regular blood pressure controls (>140/90 mm Hg) - Ultrasonography - Serum levels of creatinine, urine analyses (protein, albuminuria, microelectrophoresis)

durometer,[67] cutometer,[68] and elastometer.[69] In addition to these noninvasive methods, skin biopsy with histologic evaluation of the dermal skin thickness is an appropriate but invasive method. This method enables the characterization of the inflammatory infiltrates.

CARDIOPULMONARY INVOLVEMENT

Individuals with SSc and cardiopulmonary symptoms should be followed up at least annually using pulmonary function tests, echocardiography, a 6-minute walk test, and high-resolution CT (HRCT).[70] Pulmonary function tests are the most important techniques to determine possible cardiopulmonary involvement, because of impaired diffusion capacity of the lung for carbon monoxide (DLCO ≤75%) being an early marker of both lung fibrosis and PAH.[71]

To determine the presence of interstitial lung involvement, that is, subpleural localized line opacities, ground-glass opacities, and subpleural cysts with honeycomb formations, HRCT and/or thoracic radiography should be used.

Followup should also include transthoracic Doppler echocardiography, a noninvasive procedure, that can indicate a hypertrophy with or without enlargement of the right ventricle, paradoxical motion of the interventricular septum, tricuspid valve insufficiency, and pericardial effusion. Right-heart catheterization is indeed the gold standard, but is an invasive diagnostic procedure to determine PAH. PAH is defined as a mean pulmonary artery pressure of ≥25 mm Hg at rest together with a pulmonary capillary wedge pressure of ≤15 mm Hg as determined by right-heart catheterization.[70,72,73]

Cardiac MRI is also a potential strategy for assessing myocardiac involvement in SSc. Besides imaging procedures, there is also some promise for the use of N-terminal brain natriuretic peptide to detect right ventricular impairment (see Table 63-5). Early detec-

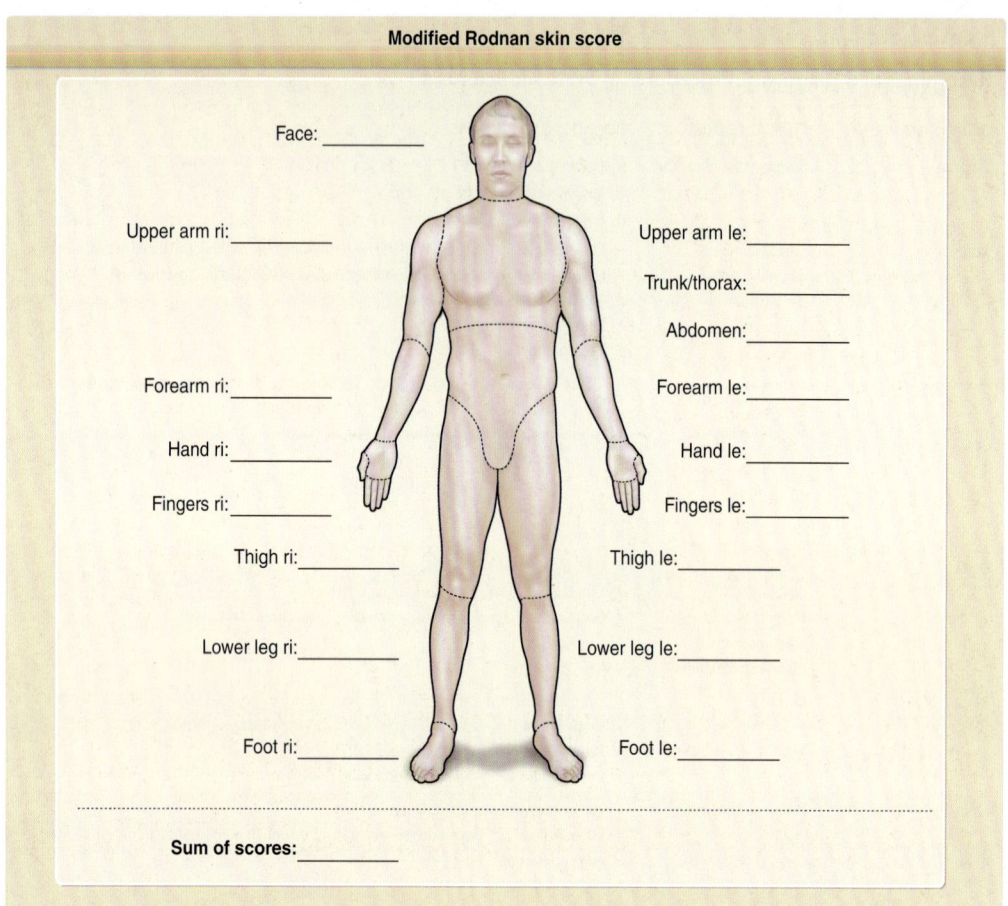

Figure 63-7 Modified Rodnan skin score (mRSS). Skin hardening evaluation using the modified mRSS is usually performed by assessing the skin thickness at 17 different areas. The skin sclerosis is categorized by palpation to grade 1, corresponding to mild, grade 2, corresponding to moderate, and grade 3, corresponding to severe. le, Left; ri, right.

tion of cardiac involvement is crucial to prevent and to allow early treatment of cardiomyopathy and severe cardiac arrhythmias.[70]

GI INVOLVEMENT

The presence of esophagitis can be determined by upper GI endoscopy with histologic evaluations. Impaired motility of the esophagus can usually be diagnosed by scintigraphic evaluation following a radiolabeled meal or 24-hour pH manometry (see Table 63-5).[71]

KIDNEY INVOLVEMENT

Early diagnosis is the key role in improving the outcome of SRC using regular blood pressure monitoring, urine analysis microelectrophoresis, and determination of creatinine clearance (see Table 63-5).[26]

DIFFERENTIAL DIAGNOSIS

The diagnosis of SSc is clinical. Although there are criteria that were developed to facilitate the distinction of SSc from other connective tissue diseases, no formal diagnostic criteria have been developed. However, determination of the correct subset of the disease, including the SSc overlap syndromes, is required to enable judging of prognosis and involvement of certain organs and for determining the therapeutic approach. There are several differential diagnoses that imitate scleroderma: circumscript (localized) scleroderma; eosinophilic fasciitis; sclerodermiform genodermatoses; acrodermatitis chronica atrophicans; scleroderma-like syndromes induced by environmental factors; scleroderma adultorum Buschke; scleroderma diabeticorum; scleromyxedema; nephrogenic fibrosing dermopathy; porphyria cutanea tarda; graft-versus-host disease; and scleroderma-like lesions in malignancies. These certainly have to be excluded. Table 63-6 outlines the differential diagnosis of SSc.

CLINICAL COURSE AND PROGNOSIS

The development of the disease depends very much on the specific subset. Patients with the limited form develop RP already many years prior to the onset of other organ manifestations. Skin fibrosis remains localized to the acral areas and the main complications are the development of digital ulcerations and pulmonary hypertension. In the diffuse form, however, fibrosis occurs early and together with inflammation, joint pain and shows a rapid spreading to almost all parts of the integument. In these patients, manifestations of the lung (lung fibrosis), heart, and kidney occur early in the disease course and often determine the prognosis. There is still a high number of deaths associated with this disease subset. Several studies indicate that the diffuse cutaneous SSc patients show a rapid worsening of the disease in the initial years. In later years, the activity of the disease is reduced and symptoms can improve. Surprisingly, the sclerotic skin also can become softer and contractures can be diminished.

Although SSc is still a life-threatening disease, a multidisciplinary management of the patients with early detection and treatment of complications may lead to a much-improved prognosis during the patient's life.

MANAGEMENT

DISEASE-MODIFYING TREATMENT

Three facets of SSc are potentially amenable to therapeutic modulation, which raises the possibility of true disease-modifying treatment. At present, vascular therapies and immunomodulation have the widest range of candidate therapies. Tables 63-7 and 63-8 summarize these approaches. General immunosuppression can be of benefit by improving skin involvement and interstitial lung disease. The best evidence is available for cyclophosphamide but more recently mycophenolate mofetil (MMF) has been shown to be as effective as oral cyclophosphamide and is used by many centers.[74,75] There is also evidence that rituximab can lead to improvement of the disease course in a select group of patients, if standard immunosuppression has failed.[76] Efficiency of immunosuppression in general is demonstrated by trials from the United States and Europe using high-intensity immunosuppression with autologous hemopoietic stem cell transplantation in some selected patients.[77-80] However, side effects always have to be considered (Table 63-9).

Antifibrotic treatment remains still a challenge, although during the last few years a number of new approaches have been generated mainly based on the better understanding of the underlying mechanisms. A newer study using a new antibody against TGF-β led to an improvement of the severity of skin involvement and a reduction of the expression of several TGF-β–dependent genes.[60] Some encouragement is also provided by newer clinical trials of idiopathic PF. However, at present there is no proven antifibrotic agent. Figure 63-8 is a simplified schematic for integrating putative disease-modifying therapy with programs of screening and surveillance that permit timely intervention in SSc with organ-based strategies that currently form the basis of the majority of SSc therapeutics. Possibilities for targeted disease modifying therapy depend on the availability of therapeutic agents and a clear understanding of their role in pathogenesis.

There has been much more success in the field of organ-based therapeutics in SSc, which already had a high impact especially on the quality of life of many patients. Early detection of these organ-specific complications is required to enable early intervention.

DIGITAL VASCULOPATHY AND ITS COMPLICATIONS

Simple but important recommendations for reducing the frequency of Raynaud attacks include reducing vasoconstriction by avoiding precipitating factors like nicotine, sympathomimetics, emotional stress and coldness, and instead to have good home heating, thick and airtight clothes, thermochemical or microwaveable hand warmers, electrically heated gloves, soles, or infrared hyperthermy, regular paraffin wax bath treatments, and minimizing finger trauma.

Therapy requires a close interaction between several medical disciplines applying topical and systemic therapies. Current local management of digital ulcers includes a combination of nonphar-

TABLE 63-6
Differential Diagnosis of Systemic Sclerosis

Differential Diagnosis
- Circumscript (localized) scleroderma (morphea)
- Eosinophilic fasciitis
- Lichen sclerosus et atrophicans
- Sclerodermiform genodermatoses (eg, progeria, acrogeria)
- Sclerodermiform acrodermatitis chronica atrophicans
- Scleroderma adultorum Buschke
- Scleroderma diabeticorum
- Scleroderma amyloidosus
- Scleromyxedema
- Mixed connective tissue disease (MCTD)
- Nephrogenic fibrosing dermopathy
- Sclerodermiform porphyria cutanea tarda
- Sclerodermiform chronic graft-versus-host disease
- Eosinophilia-myalgia syndrome

TABLE 63-7
Recommended Therapeutic Strategies for Internal Organ Involvement in Systemic Sclerosis[105]

ORGAN INVOLVEMENT	CLINICAL FEATURE	THERAPEUTIC OPTIONS
Vasculopathy	Raynaud phenomenon	Consistent warm keeping, paraffin-bath, patient education
		Calcium channel blockers (eg, nifedipine) by mouth
		Angiotensin receptor antagonists
		Alternatives: selective serotonin reuptake inhibitors (SSRIs), α-blockers, sympathectomy with or without botulinum toxin injection
	Digital ulcers	Prostacyclin (eg, iloprost) IV[87,88]
		Endothelin receptor blockade (eg, bosentan by mouth)[81,106]
		Phosphodiesterase Type 5 inhibitors (off-label)[90]
		Wound dressing (hydrocolloid membrane, Mepilex)
Musculoskeletal system	Synovitis/myositis	Methotrexate (by mouth, IM), rituximab (off-label)
GI tract	Reflux	Proton pump inhibitors, prokinetics
	Dysphagia	H_2-receptor antagonists
	Diarrhea, obstipation	Change habit of eating, parenteral nutrition
		Antibiotics (eg, ciprofloxacin)
		Symptomatic management with antidiarrheal agents or laxatives
Respiratory system	Dyspnea	Oxygen, if necessary
	Alveolitis/lung fibrosis	Cyclophosphamide IV
		Mycophenolate mofetil by mouth (used as an alternative or after cyclophosphamide)
		Glucocorticoids (short dated, if necessary)
Cardiac system	Pulmonary arterial hypertension	Oxygen, if necessary
		Diuretics
		Endothelin receptor blockade (eg, bosentan by mouth, macitentan)[107]
		Inhaled iloprost[107]
		Phosphodiesterase Type 5 inhibitors (eg, sildenafil by mouth, tadalafil)[107,108]
		Epoprostenol by mouth[107]
		Combination of different agents
	Systolic heart failures	Immunosuppression with or without pacemaker
		Cardioverter defibrillator
		Angiotensin-converting enzyme inhibitors and carvedilol (selective β-blockers may be considered, but consider worsening of Raynaud phenomenon)
	Diastolic heart failure	Diuretics
		Calcium channel inhibitors
Kidney	Scleroderma renal crisis	Angiotensin-converting enzyme–Hemmer (high-dosed)

macologic care, antibiotics (in case of infection), analgesia, and individually applied wound dressings, if necessary.

Potential pharmacologic treatment requires optimal therapy for RP, including agents that have the potential for vascular remodeling and/or dilation, such as calcium channel blockers and angiotensin II receptor antagonists,[81,82] which should be considered first-line therapy. The results have been contradictory with other pharmacologic treatment options, such as diltiazem and angiotensin-converting enzyme inhibitors.[83-86]

Parenteral prostacyclin derivatives, in particular iloprost, are widely used, and help to heal digital ulcers and may prevent recurrent lesions. Prostacyclin derivatives by IV infusion are the mainstay of therapy for critical digital ischemia.[87,88] Antiplatelet agents, such as aspirin and clopidogrel, are also used, especially in critical digital ischemia.

There has been enthusiasm about therapies that are effective for PAH in digital vasculopathy. Thus, in 2 large, controlled trials, bosentan, an oral dual-specificity endothelin receptor antagonist, was shown to significantly reduce the number of new digital ulcers, compared with placebo.[89] However, no positive effect on healing of established ulcers was demonstrated. Other agents, such as phosphodiesterase Type 5 inhibitors sildenafil and tadalafil, also have been used for treatment of RP and digital ulcers,

TABLE 63-8
Therapeutic Options for Skin Involvement in Systemic Sclerosis[20,105]

CLINICAL FEATURE	THERAPEUTIC OPTIONS
Skin hardening	- Lymphatic drainage - Physiotherapy - Topical treatment with steroids or calcineurin inhibitors - Systemic treatment with steroids (short dated) and/or immunosuppressants - Phototherapy (psoralen and ultraviolet A, ultraviolet A1, extracorporeal photochemotherapy)
Dryness and itching	- Topical treatment with steroids, capsaicin - Cannabinoid agonists - Emollients - Phototherapy (psoralen and ultraviolet A, ultraviolet A1) - Systemic treatment with antihistamines or gabapentin
Digital ulcerations	- IV iloprost - Bosentan by mouth - Hydrocolloid dressings - Skin substitutes - Physical therapy
Calcifications	- Bisphosphonate by mouth - Local corticosteroid injection - Laser therapy - Surgery
Telangiectases	- Laser therapy - Camouflage
Hyperpigmentation and hypopigmentation	- Bleaching agents, camouflage, sunscreens - Salicylic acid and chemical peelings - Hydroquinone, retinoids, corticosteroids

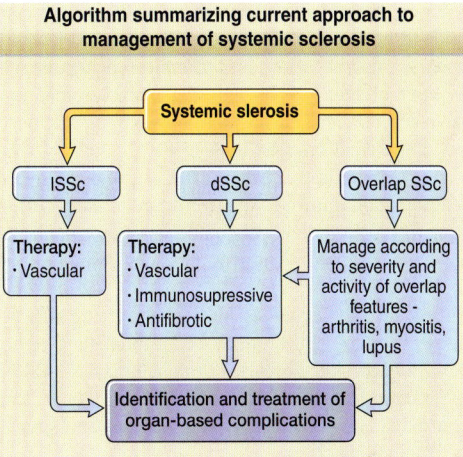

Figure 63-8 Algorithm summarizing the current approach to management of systemic sclerosis (SSc). The principles of therapy for SSc include accurate diagnosis and treatment according to the disease subset, the presence of overlap features, and the likely predominant pathologic process according to the stage of disease. In all cases, screening for and treatment of organ-based complications has a major role in successful management. Education of patients and a multidisciplinary team, including specialist nurses, physiotherapists, occupational therapists and many subspecialty physicians, and surgeons, are central to providing appropriate care for severe cases of SSc. dSSc, Diffuse cutaneous systemic sclerosis; lSSc, limited cutaneous systemic sclerosis.

but prospective clinical trial data are not available.[90] Surgical treatments include digital microarteriolysis, which can benefit single fingers with refractory ulcers. Whenever possible, surgical amputation of digits is avoided, and prolonged treatment with parenteral prostacyclin in combination with phosphodiesterase Type 5 inhibitors and potent analgesia may help with this. Lumbar sympathectomy may be helpful for lower-limb RP or ulceration. Generally, a temporary procedure is performed initially to determine the likely benefit from a definitive sympathectomy. In cases of critical digital ischemia, antiplatelet therapies are often given, with anecdotal reports of the benefit of clopidogrel in preventing digital infarction (see Table 63-7).

SKIN INVOLVEMENT

Key elements in the management of skin manifestations of SSc are physical therapy and regular exercise to maintain circulation, joint mobility, and muscle strength, all aimed at improving the quality of life of SSc patients. Skin affected by scleroderma tends to be very dry, taut, and susceptible to trauma.

Skin hardening can be improved by physical therapy and exercise, lymphatic drainage, topical treatment with steroids, calcineurin inhibitors, and moisturizing crèmes. Systemic therapies include immunosuppressive drugs, systemic steroids (for just a short time), and phototherapy (ultraviolet A1 or psoralen and ultraviolet A). Ultraviolet A1 phototherpay appears to inhibit fibrotic and inflammatory processes and reduce the amount of sclerotic skin.[91]

Dry and itching skin should be treated topically with corticosteroids, cannabinoid agonists, capsaicin, emollients, and phototherapy (see above). Local steroid injections and laser or surgical therapies could also be tried for the treatment of calcinosis cutis.

TABLE 63-9
Stem Cell Transplantation (ASCT) for Early Diffuse Cutaneous Systemic Sclerosis[78-80]

- Recommended in poor-prognosis diffuse cutaneous systemic sclerosis (SSc)
- Patients should not have severe organ manifestations, which render this option highly toxic

Pro	Contra
- Improved long-term survival - Improved event-free survival	- 10% Transplant-related mortality - Patients with cardiopulmonary disease have to be excluded

Laser therapies or noninvasive methods like camouflage have been used for telangiectases. Bleaching agents, salicylic acids, and chemical peels, as well as camouflage, retinoids, and corticosteroids, may have the potential to improve hyperpigmentation or hypopigmentations (see Table 63-8).

Two randomized clinical trials have shown that methotrexate improves the skin score in early diffuse SSc, while positive effects on other organ manifestations have not been established.[92,93] On the other hand, in two randomized clinical trials, cyclophosphamide improved skin sclerosis.[94,95] For balancing efficacy and side effects, MMF might be an interesting option to influence skin fibrosis.[74] Protein kinase inhibitors (eg, imatinib) have been used, but as of this writing, controlled clinical trials have been mixed and suggest poor tolerability.[96,97]

CARDIOPULMONARY MANIFESTATIONS

It is increasingly appreciated that a group of patients with some lung fibrosis have predominantly PAH and that this group may respond to standard PAH therapies. There have been substantial advances in the treatment of PAH over the past decade. Most cases are treated with oral agents, either an endothelin receptor antagonist (eg, bosentan, ambrisentan) or a phosphodiesterase 5 inhibitor (eg, sildenafil, tadalafil), once the PAH is significantly functionally limited (New York Heart Association class III). Later, if progression takes place, a combination of oral treatment or introduction of parenteral prostacyclin is used, by either the IV or subcutaneous route. Inhaled delivery systems for iloprost are available.

Although PAH is probably responsible for more deaths than lung fibrosis in SSc, lung fibrosis remains an important complication. Treatment of SSc-PF remains challenging.[98] Adding to a substantial body of uncontrolled or retrospective data suggesting benefit for cyclophosphamide in SSc-PF, the results of 2 randomized, double-blind, placebo-controlled trials have been reported. Both show a modest placebo-subtracted benefit for cyclophosphamide.[99-101] For change in forced vital capacity (percent predicted), this was statistically significant for the Scleroderma Lung Study comparing oral cyclophosphamide with placebo, showing a strong trend ($p = 0.06$) in the trial of IV cyclophosphamide followed by oral azathioprine. At present, most centers use cyclophosphamide as treatment for severe or progressive SSc-PF, defining the extent and severity by pulmonary function tests and HRCT. The extent of disease by HRCT and a history of progressive restrictive abnormality on pulmonary function tests is the best predictor of future decline in lung function and is generally used to make decisions about therapy. Newer clinical trials have shown equal efficacy in the treatment of both MMF and cyclophosphamide for stabilizing lung function of patients with scleroderma and ILD.[74] MMF therapy is associated with a stability of lung function for up to 36 months, with a better side-effect profile than in patients treated with azathioprine.[102] Other therapies that are in use include carbocysteine and low-dose corticosteroids. The place of other immunosuppressive strategies remains uncertain and requires evaluation in prospective multicenter clinical trials. It is noteworthy that despite there being a strong theoretic rationale for using the endothelin receptor antagonist bosentan as a therapy for lung fibrosis, bosentan was not superior to placebo in a recent large multicenter study of SSc-PF cases.

Cardiac involvement from SSc is also an important contributor to mortality but remains one of the least-well understood and poorly recognized of the internal organ complications of SSc. A large number of studies confirm that radionuclide imaging, electrophysiologic, and functional abnormalities are frequent in SSc, but the significance of these findings is uncertain. Hemodynamically significant cardiac involvement occurs in up to 10% of cases of diffuse cutaneous SSc. An inflammatory component of myocarditis may respond to immunosuppressive treatment, and so an operational approach to management of cardiac scleroderma. Although this is not yet based on sufficient reliable data, it could form a basis for prospective evaluation of the significance of impaired left ventricular ejection fraction and elevated circulating troponin levels in SSc.

There have been many advances in SSc, including a better appreciation of the diversity of the condition, improved understanding of the underlying pathologic mechanisms, and major progress in treating organ-based complications. This includes the accumulation of robust clinical trial data that demonstrate effectiveness or lack of benefit of individual therapies and in validation of measures of disease assessment.[103]

GI INVOLVEMENT

Involvement of the GI tract occurs frequently in SSc. Esophageal symptoms can respond very well to proton pump inhibitors and agents that increase lower esophageal sphincter tone such as domperidone, although high-dose treatment may be associated with an increased risk of cardiac arrhythmia. Midgut involvement takes many forms. Pseudoobstruction requires conservative management initially, but subsequently may require parenteral nutritional supplementation. Small intestinal bacterial overgrowth can be treated using broad-spectrum antibiotics, and pancreatic insufficiency may require enzyme supplements. Large bowel involvement is a major challenge. Anorectal incontinence sometimes responds well to an implanted sacral nerve stimulator or to less-elaborate approaches, such as bioplastic injection to increase the internal anal sphincter bulk. Associated rectal prolapse may require additional surgical intervention. Chronic constipation, sometimes with overflow diarrhea, is a common problem. An adjustment to diet and judicious use of stimulating, softening, or bulking aperients is recommended, but an individualized approach with substantial patient involvement is generally the most successful approach. On occasion, defunctioning colostomy is needed, but this is only appropriate in a very limited number of cases.

SCLERODERMA RENAL CRISIS

Overall, approximately two-thirds of the cases of SRC that present to a specialist center require renal replacement therapy. Of these, approximately one-half of cases eventually recover sufficiently to discontinue dialysis. This can occur over 24 months after the renal crisis, and so decisions about renal transplantation should be postponed depending on the outcome. The possibility of late recovery distinguishes SRC from other causes of end-stage renal failure. These outcomes are possible through the use of angiotensin-converting enzyme inhibitors as routine therapy for SRC. Before their availability, the mortality from established SRC was greater than 90% at 12 months. The most critical aspect of management of SRC is prompt identification and treatment of significant hypertension in the context of scleroderma, with initiation of angiotensin-converting enzyme inhibitors. This is a medical emergency and any features of renal impairment or end-organ damage should prompt hospitalization.[104]

Table 63-10 illustrates the frequency of organ involvement in 2 networks for SSc (Germany and United Kingdom).

TABLE 63-10

Frequency of Organ Involvement in Two Networks for Systemic Sclerosis (Germany and United Kingdom)

CLINICAL FEATURES	DIFFUSE CUTANEOUS SYSTEMIC SCLEROSIS		LIMITED CUTANEOUS SYSTEMIC SCLEROSIS	
	GERMANY (n = 780)	UNITED KINGDOM (n = 741)	GERMANY (n = 1190)	UNITED KINGDOM (n = 1505)
Raynaud phenomenon	95.3%	97%	96.3%	99%
Skin Hardening	95.9%	100%	90%	90%
Digital ulcerations	36%	28%	24.3%	13%
PAH	20.2%	12%	14%	15%
Lung fibrosis	62.9%	38%	26.7%	16%
GI tract involvement	65.2%	90%	60.7%	90%
Heart involvement	20%	3%	9.9%	1%
Kidney involvement	15.9%	19%	9.7%	3%
Musculoskeletal involvement	48.8%	45%	38.8%	35%

OTHER SUPPORTIVE PROCEDURES

All these organ-specific therapeutic approaches have to be supported by several general measures to help the patients. These general measures include recommendations for keeping the home and the body warm, and for optimizing nutritional status. Paraffin waxing and physical therapy has to be provided. Patients need to be taught to deal with the complications of daily life and to recognize early those symptoms that indicate disease progression and new organ involvement.

REFERENCES

1. Hunzelmann N, Genth E, Krieg T, et al. The registry of the German Network for Systemic Scleroderma: frequency of disease subsets and patterns of organ involvement. *Rheumatology (Oxford)*. 2008;47(8):1185-1192.
2. Mayes MD, Lacey JV Jr, Beebe-Dimmer J, et al. Prevalence, incidence, survival, and disease characteristics of systemic sclerosis in a large US population. *Arthritis Rheum*. 2003;48(8):2246-2255.
3. Silman AJ. Epidemiology of scleroderma. *Curr Opin Rheumatol*. 1991;3(6):967-972.
4. Tamaki T, Mori S, Takehara K. Epidemiological study of patients with systemic sclerosis in Tokyo. *Arch Dermatol Res*. 1991;283(6):366-371.
5. Medsger TA Jr, Masi AT. Epidemiology of systemic sclerosis (scleroderma). *Ann Intern Med*. 1971;74(5):714-721.
6. Preliminary criteria for the classification of systemic sclerosis (scleroderma). Subcommittee for scleroderma criteria of the American Rheumatism Association Diagnostic and Therapeutic Criteria Committee. *Arthritis Rheum*. 1980;23(5):581-590.
7. van den Hoogen F, Khanna D, Fransen J, et al. 2013 Classification criteria for systemic sclerosis: an American College of Rheumatology/European League Against Rheumatism collaborative initiative. *Arthritis Rheum*. 2013;65(11):2737-2747.
8. LeRoy EC, Black C, Fleischmajer R, et al. Scleroderma (systemic sclerosis): classification, subsets and pathogenesis. *J Rheumatol*. 1988;15(2):202-205.
9. LeRoy EC, Medsger TA Jr. Criteria for the classification of early systemic sclerosis. *J Rheumatol*. 2001;28(7):1573-1576.
10. Nadashkevich O, Davis P, Fritzler MJ. Revising the classification criteria for systemic sclerosis. *Arthritis Rheum*. 2006;55(6):992-993.
11. Walker JG, Pope J, Baron M, et al. The development of systemic sclerosis classification criteria. *Clin Rheumatol*. 2007;26(9):1401-1409.
12. Maricq HR, Valter I. A working classification of scleroderma spectrum disorders: a proposal and the results of testing on a sample of patients. *Clin Exp Rheumatol*. 2004;22(3)(suppl 33):S5-S13.
13. LeRoy EC, Maricq HR, Kahaleh MB. Undifferentiated connective tissue syndromes. *Arthritis Rheum*. 1980;23(3):341-343.
14. Alarcon GS. Unclassified or undifferentiated connective tissue disease. *Baillieres Best Pract Res Clin Rheumatol*. 2000;14(1):125-137.

15. Poormoghim H, Lucas M, Fertig N, et al. Systemic sclerosis sine scleroderma: demographic, clinical, and serologic features and survival in forty-eight patients. *Arthritis Rheum*. 2000;43(2):444-451.
16. Bennett RM. Scleroderma overlap syndromes. *Rheum Dis Clin North Am*. 1990;16(1):185-198.
17. Ciang NC, Pereira N, Isenberg DA. Mixed connective tissue disease-enigma variations? *Rheumatology (Oxford)*. 2017;56(3):326-333.
18. Gunnarsson R, Hetlevik SO, Lilleby V, et al. Mixed connective tissue disease. *Best Pract Res Clin Rheumatol*. 2016;30(1):95-111.
19. Iaccarino L, Gatto M, Bettio S, et al. Overlap connective tissue disease syndromes. *Autoimmun Rev*. 2013;12(3):363-373.
20. Krieg T, Takehara K. Skin disease: a cardinal feature of systemic sclerosis. *Rheumatology (Oxford)*. 2009;48(suppl 3):iii14-iii18.
21. Chaisson NF, Hassoun PM. Systemic sclerosis-associated pulmonary arterial hypertension. *Chest*. 2013;144(4):1346-1356.
22. Thakkar V, Nikpour M, Stevens WM, et al. Prospects for improving outcomes in systemic sclerosis-related pulmonary hypertension. *Intern Med J*. 2015;45(3):248-254.
23. Allanore Y, Meune C, Kahan A. Outcome measures for heart involvement in systemic sclerosis. *Rheumatology (Oxford)*. 2008;47(suppl 5):v51-v53.
24. Forbes A, Marie I. Gastrointestinal complications: the most frequent internal complications of systemic sclerosis. *Rheumatology (Oxford)*. 2009;48(suppl 3):iii36-iii39.
25. Parrado RH, Lemus HN, Coral-Alvarado PX, et al. Gastric antral vascular ectasia in systemic sclerosis: current concepts. *Int J Rheumatol*. 2015;2015:762546.
26. Hudson M. Scleroderma renal crisis. *Curr Opin Rheumatol*. 2015;27(6):549-554.
27. Hunzelmann N, Moinzadeh P, Genth E, et al. High frequency of corticosteroid and immunosuppressive therapy in patients with systemic sclerosis despite limited evidence for efficacy. *Arthritis Res Ther*. 2009;11(2):R30.
28. Gabrielli A, Avvedimento EV, Krieg T. Scleroderma. *N Engl J Med*. 2009;360(19):1989-2003.
29. Agarwal SK, Tan FK, Arnett FC. Genetics and genomic studies in scleroderma (systemic sclerosis). *Rheum Dis Clin North Am*. 2008;34(1):17-40; v.
30. Assassi S, Arnett FC, Reveille JD, et al. Clinical, immunologic, and genetic features of familial systemic sclerosis. *Arthritis Rheum*. 2007;56(6):2031-2037.
31. Arnett FC, Reveille JD, Goldstein R, et al. Autoantibodies to fibrillarin in systemic sclerosis (scleroderma). An immunogenetic, serologic, and clinical analysis. *Arthritis Rheum*. 1996;39(7):1151-1160.
32. Marguerie C, Bunn CC, Copier J, et al. The clinical and immunogenetic features of patients with autoantibodies to the nucleolar antigen PM-Scl. *Medicine (Baltimore)*. 1992;71(6):327-336.
33. Assassi S, Tan FK. Genetics of scleroderma: update on single nucleotide polymorphism analysis and microarrays. *Curr Opin Rheumatol*. 2005;17(6):761-767.
34. Herrick AL, Worthington J. Genetic epidemiology: systemic sclerosis. *Arthritis Res*. 2002;4(3):165-168.
35. Nietert PJ, Silver RM. Systemic sclerosis: environmental and occupational risk factors. *Curr Opin Rheumatol*. 2000;12(6):520-526.
36. Mayes MD. Epidemiologic studies of environmental agents and systemic autoimmune diseases. *Environ Health Perspect*. 1999;107(suppl 5):743-748.
37. Jablonska S, Blaszczyk M. Scleroderma-like disorders. *Semin Cutan Med Surg*. 1998;17(1):65-76.
38. Sainson RC, Johnston DA, Chu HC, et al. TNF primes endothelial cells for angiogenic sprouting by inducing a tip cell phenotype. *Blood*. 2008;111(10):4997-5007.
39. Kraling BM, Maul GG, Jimenez SA. Mononuclear cellular infiltrates in clinically involved skin from patients with systemic sclerosis of recent onset predominantly consist of monocytes/macrophages. *Pathobiology*. 1995;63(1):48-56.
40. Saigusa R, Asano Y, Taniguchi T, et al. Multifaceted contribution of the TLR4-activated IRF5 transcription factor in systemic sclerosis. *Proc Natl Acad Sci U S A*. 2015;112(49):15136-15141.
41. Xu Y, Wang W, Tian Y, et al. Polymorphisms in STAT4 and IRF5 increase the risk of systemic sclerosis: a meta-analysis. *Int J Dermatol*. 2016;55(4):408-416.
42. Stifano G, Christmann RB. Macrophage involvement in systemic sclerosis: do we need more evidence? *Curr Rheumatol Rep*. 2016;18(1):2.
43. Mavalia C, Scaletti C, Romagnani P, et al. Type 2 helper T-cell predominance and high CD30 expression in systemic sclerosis. *Am J Pathol*. 1997;151(6):1751-1758.
44. Roumm AD, Whiteside TL, Medsger TA Jr, et al. Lymphocytes in the skin of patients with progressive systemic sclerosis. Quantification, subtyping, and clinical correlations. *Arthritis Rheum*. 1984;27(6):645-653.
45. Hasegawa M, Fujimoto M, Kikuchi K, et al. Elevated serum levels of interleukin 4 (IL-4), IL-10, and IL-13 in patients with systemic sclerosis. *J Rheumatol*. 1997;24(2):328-332.
46. Kurasawa K, Hirose K, Sano H, et al. Increased interleukin-17 production in patients with systemic sclerosis. *Arthritis Rheum*. 2000;43(11):2455-2463.
47. Ho KT, Reveille JD. The clinical relevance of autoantibodies in scleroderma. *Arthritis Res Ther*. 2003;5(2):80-93.
48. Choi MY, Fritzler MJ. Progress in understanding the diagnostic and pathogenic role of autoantibodies associated with systemic sclerosis. *Curr Opin Rheumatol*. 2016;28(6):586-594.
49. Gunther J, Rademacher J, van Laar JM, et al. Functional autoantibodies in systemic sclerosis. *Semin Immunopathol*. 2015;37(5):529-542.
50. Kill A, Riemekasten G. Functional autoantibodies in systemic sclerosis pathogenesis. *Curr Rheumatol Rep*. 2015;17(5):34.
51. Moinzadeh P, Fonseca C, Hellmich M, et al. Association of anti-RNA polymerase III autoantibodies and cancer in scleroderma. *Arthritis Res Ther*. 2014;16(1):R53.
52. Shah AA, Casciola-Rosen L. Cancer and scleroderma: a paraneoplastic disease with implications for malignancy screening. *Curr Opin Rheumatol*. 2015;27(6):563-570.
53. Shah AA, Hummers LK, Casciola-Rosen L, et al. Examination of autoantibody status and clinical features associated with cancer risk and cancer-associated scleroderma. *Arthritis Rheumatol*. 2015;67(4):1053-1061.
54. Brinckmann J, Kim S, Wu J, et al. Interleukin 4 and prolonged hypoxia induce a higher gene expression of lysyl hydroxylase 2 and an altered cross-link pattern: important pathogenetic steps in early and

late stage of systemic scleroderma? *Matrix Biol.* 2005;24(7):459-468.
55. Abraham DJ, Krieg T, Distler J, et al. Overview of pathogenesis of systemic sclerosis. *Rheumatology (Oxford).* 2009;48(suppl 3):iii3-iii7.
56. Baroni SS, Santillo M, Bevilacqua F, et al. Stimulatory autoantibodies to the PDGF receptor in systemic sclerosis. *N Engl J Med.* 2006;354(25):2667-2676.
57. Kawakami T, Ihn H, Xu W, et al. Increased expression of TGF-beta receptors by scleroderma fibroblasts: evidence for contribution of autocrine TGF-beta signaling to scleroderma phenotype. *J Invest Dermatol.* 1998;110(1):47-51.
58. Lafyatis R. Transforming growth factor beta—at the centre of systemic sclerosis. *Nat Rev Rheumatol.* 2014;10(12):706-719.
59. Pendergrass SA, Lemaire R, Francis IP, et al. Intrinsic gene expression subsets of diffuse cutaneous systemic sclerosis are stable in serial skin biopsies. *J Invest Dermatol.* 2012;132(5):1363-1373.
60. Rice LM, Padilla CM, McLaughlin SR, et al. Fresolimumab treatment decreases biomarkers and improves clinical symptoms in systemic sclerosis patients. *J Clin Invest.* 2015;125(7):2795-2807.
61. Noda S, Asano Y, Nishimura S, et al. Simultaneous downregulation of KLF5 and Fli1 is a key feature underlying systemic sclerosis. *Nat Commun.* 2014;5:5797.
62. Rosato E, Roumpedaki E, Pisarri S, et al. Digital ischemic necrosis in a patient with systemic sclerosis: the role of laser Doppler perfusion imaging. *Vasa.* 2009;38(4):390-393.
63. Clements PJ, Hurwitz EL, Wong WK, et al. Skin thickness score as a predictor and correlate of outcome in systemic sclerosis: high-dose versus low-dose penicillamine trial. *Arthritis Rheum.* 2000;43(11):2445-2454.
64. Moore TL, Lunt M, McManus B, et al. Seventeen-point dermal ultrasound scoring system—a reliable measure of skin thickness in patients with systemic sclerosis. *Rheumatology (Oxford).* 2003;42(12):1559-1563.
65. Akesson A, Fiori G, Krieg T, et al. Assessment of skin, joint, tendon and muscle involvement. *Clin Exp Rheumatol.* 2003;21(3)(suppl 29):S5-S8.
66. Nives Parodi M, Castagneto C, Filaci G, et al. Plicometer skin test: a new technique for the evaluation of cutaneous involvement in systemic sclerosis. *Br J Rheumatol.* 1997;36(2):244-250.
67. Kissin EY, Schiller AM, Gelbard RB, et al. Durometry for the assessment of skin disease in systemic sclerosis. *Arthritis Rheum.* 2006;55(4):603-609.
68. Balbir-Gurman A, Denton CP, Nichols B, et al. Noninvasive measurement of biomechanical skin properties in systemic sclerosis. *Ann Rheum Dis.* 2002;61(3):237-241.
69. Enomoto DN, Mekkes JR, Bossuyt PM, et al. Quantification of cutaneous sclerosis with a skin elasticity meter in patients with generalized scleroderma. *J Am Acad Dermatol.* 1996;35(3, pt 1):381-387.
70. Vandecasteele EH, De Pauw M, Brusselle G, et al. The heart and pulmonary arterial hypertension in systemic sclerosis. *Acta Clin Belg.* 2016;71(1):1-18.
71. Hunzelmann N, Genth E, Krieg T, et al. Organ-specific diagnosis in patients with systemic sclerosis: Recommendations of the German Network for Systemic Sclerosis (DNSS) [in German]. *Z Rheumatol.* 2008;67(4):334-336, 337-340.
72. Badesch DB, Abman SH, Simonneau G, et al. Medical therapy for pulmonary arterial hypertension: updated ACCP evidence-based clinical practice guidelines. *Chest.* 2007;131(6):1917-1928.
73. Wells AU, Steen V, Valentini G. Pulmonary complications: one of the most challenging complications of systemic sclerosis. *Rheumatology (Oxford).* 2009;48(suppl 3):iii40-iii44.
74. Shenoy PD, Bavaliya M, Sashidharan S, et al. Cyclophosphamide versus mycophenolate mofetil in scleroderma interstitial lung disease (SSc-ILD) as induction therapy: a single-centre, retrospective analysis. *Arthritis Res Ther.* 2016;18(1):123.
75. Tashkin DP, Roth MD, Clements PJ, et al. Mycophenolate mofetil versus oral cyclophosphamide in scleroderma-related interstitial lung disease (SLS II): a randomised controlled, double-blind, parallel group trial. *Lancet Respir Med.* 2016;4(9):708-719.
76. Giuggioli D, Lumetti F, Colaci M, et al. Rituximab in the treatment of patients with systemic sclerosis. Our experience and review of the literature. *Autoimmun Rev.* 2015;14(11):1072-1078.
77. Burt RK, Shah SJ, Dill K, et al. Autologous non-myeloablative haemopoietic stem-cell transplantation compared with pulse cyclophosphamide once per month for systemic sclerosis (ASSIST): an open-label, randomised phase 2 trial. *Lancet.* 2011;378(9790):498-506.
78. Tyndall A, Furst DE. Adult stem cell treatment of scleroderma. *Curr Opin Rheumatol.* 2007;19(6):604-610.
79. van Laar JM, Farge D, Sont JK, et al. Autologous hematopoietic stem cell transplantation vs intravenous pulse cyclophosphamide in diffuse cutaneous systemic sclerosis: a randomized clinical trial. *JAMA.* 2014;311(24):2490-2498.
80. van Laar JM, Farge D, Tyndall A. Stem cell transplantation: a treatment option for severe systemic sclerosis? *Ann Rheum Dis.* 2008;67(suppl 3):iii35-iii38.
81. Denton CP, Howell K, Stratton RJ, et al. Long-term low molecular weight heparin therapy for severe Raynaud's phenomenon: a pilot study. *Clin Exp Rheumatol.* 2000;18(4):499-502.
82. Dziadzio M, Denton CP, Smith R, et al. Losartan therapy for Raynaud's phenomenon and scleroderma: clinical and biochemical findings in a fifteen-week, randomized, parallel-group, controlled trial. *Arthritis Rheum.* 1999;42(12):2646-2655.
83. Challenor VF. Angiotensin converting enzyme inhibitors in Raynaud's phenomenon. *Drugs.* 1994;48(6):864-867.
84. Kahan A, Foult JM, Weber S, et al. Nifedipine and alpha 1-adrenergic blockade in Raynaud's phenomenon. *Eur Heart J.* 1985;6(8):702-705.
85. Meyrick Thomas RH, Rademaker M, Grimes SM, et al. Nifedipine in the treatment of Raynaud's phenomenon in patients with systemic sclerosis. *Br J Dermatol.* 1987;117(2):237-241.
86. Rhedda A, McCans J, Willan AR, et al. A double blind placebo controlled crossover randomized trial of diltiazem in Raynaud's phenomenon. *J Rheumatol.* 1985;12(4):724-727.
87. Wigley FM, Korn JH, Csuka ME, et al. Oral iloprost treatment in patients with Raynaud's phenomenon secondary to systemic sclerosis: a multicenter, placebo-controlled, double-blind study. *Arthritis Rheum.* 1998;41(4):670-677.
88. Wigley FM, Seibold JR, Wise RA, et al. Intravenous iloprost treatment of Raynaud's phenomenon and

88. ischemic ulcers secondary to systemic sclerosis. *J Rheumatol.* 1992;19(9):1407-1414.
89. Korn JH, Mayes M, Matucci Cerinic M, et al. Digital ulcers in systemic sclerosis: prevention by treatment with bosentan, an oral endothelin receptor antagonist. *Arthritis Rheum.* 2004;50(12):3985-3993.
90. Fries R, Shariat K, von Wilmowsky H, et al. Sildenafil in the treatment of Raynaud's phenomenon resistant to vasodilatory therapy. *Circulation.* 2005;112(19):2980-2985.
91. Rose RF, Turner D, Goodfield MJ, et al. Low-dose UVA1 phototherapy for proximal and acral scleroderma in systemic sclerosis. *Photodermatol Photoimmunol Photomed.* 2009;25(3):153-155.
92. Das SN, Alam MR, Islam N, et al. Placebo controlled trial of methotrexate in systemic sclerosis. *Mymensingh Med J.* 2005;14(1):71-74.
93. van den Hoogen FH, Boerbooms AM, Swaak AJ, et al. Comparison of methotrexate with placebo in the treatment of systemic sclerosis: a 24 week randomized double-blind trial, followed by a 24 week observational trial. *Br J Rheumatol.* 1996;35(4):364-372.
94. Nadashkevich O, Davis P, Fritzler M, et al. A randomized unblinded trial of cyclophosphamide versus azathioprine in the treatment of systemic sclerosis. *Clin Rheumatol.* 2006;25(2):205-212.
95. Tashkin DP, Elashoff R, Clements PJ, et al. Cyclophosphamide versus placebo in scleroderma lung disease. *N Engl J Med.* 2006;354(25):2655-2666.
96. Gordon J, Udeh U, Doobay K, et al. Imatinib mesylate (Gleevec) in the treatment of diffuse cutaneous systemic sclerosis: results of a 24-month open label, extension phase, single-centre trial. *Clin Exp Rheumatol.* 2014;32(6)(suppl 86):S189-S193.
97. Prey S, Ezzedine K, Doussau A, et al. Imatinib mesylate in scleroderma-associated diffuse skin fibrosis: a phase II multicentre randomized double-blinded controlled trial. *Br J Dermatol.* 2012;167(5):1138-1144.
98. Hachulla E, Coghlan JG. A new era in the management of pulmonary arterial hypertension related to scleroderma: endothelin receptor antagonism. *Ann Rheum Dis.* 2004;63(9):1009-1014.
99. Merkel PA, Clements PJ, Reveille JD, et al. Current status of outcome measure development for clinical trials in systemic sclerosis. Report from OMERACT 6. *J Rheumatol.* 2003;30(7):1630-1647.
100. Steen VD. The lung in systemic sclerosis. *J Clin Rheumatol.* 2005;11(1):40-46.
101. Khanna D, Yan X, Tashkin DP, et al. Impact of oral cyclophosphamide on health-related quality of life in patients with active scleroderma lung disease: results from the scleroderma lung study. *Arthritis Rheum.* 2007;56(5):1676-1684.
102. Owen C, Ngian GS, Elford K, et al. Mycophenolate mofetil is an effective and safe option for the management of systemic sclerosis-associated interstitial lung disease: results from the Australian Scleroderma Cohort Study. *Clin Exp Rheumatol.* 2016;34(5)(suppl 100):170-176.
103. Denton CP, Black CM. Targeted therapy comes of age in scleroderma. *Trends Immunol.* 2005;26(11):596-602.
104. Ghossein C, Varga J, Fenves AZ. Recent developments in the classification, evaluation, pathophysiology, and management of scleroderma renal crisis. *Curr Rheumatol Rep.* 2016;18(1):5.
105. Denton CP, Hughes M, Gak N, et al. BSR and BHPR guideline for the treatment of systemic sclerosis. *Rheumatology (Oxford).* 2016;55(10):1906-1910.
106. Wise RA, Wigley FM, White B, et al. Efficacy and tolerability of a selective alpha(2C)-adrenergic receptor blocker in recovery from cold-induced vasospasm in scleroderma patients: a single-center, double-blind, placebo-controlled, randomized crossover study. *Arthritis Rheum.* 2004;50(12):3994-4001.
107. Murdaca G, Spano F, Puppo F. Current therapies for the treatment of systemic sclerosis-related pulmonary arterial hypertension: efficacy and safety. *Expert Opin Drug Saf.* 2014;13(3):295-305.
108. Kumar U, Sankalp G, Sreenivas V, et al. Prospective, open-label, uncontrolled pilot study to study safety and efficacy of sildenafil in systemic sclerosis-related pulmonary artery hypertension and cutaneous vascular complications. *Rheumatol Int.* 2013;33(4):1047-1052.

Chapter 64 :: Morphea and Lichen Sclerosus
:: Nika Cyrus & Heidi T. Jacobe

第六十四章

硬斑病和硬化性萎缩性苔藓

中文导读

　　硬斑病是针对皮肤的自限性和慢性复发性自身免疫性疾病，主要特征为炎症、硬化、萎缩、皮肤增厚硬化，少数人有系统受累包括关节炎和神经系统。与硬皮病的区别在于缺乏肢端硬化。本章从流行病学、临床特征、病因学及发病机制、诊断、鉴别诊断、临床进程及预后、管理等方面阐述该病的特点。硬斑病目前分为5个公认的亚型，任何亚型都可以累及浅表或深部皮肤（累及皮下、筋膜或者以下），也可以与硬化性萎缩性苔藓重叠，文中概述了硬斑病不同时期的皮肤表现。介绍了局限型、泛发型及线状硬斑病、深在性硬斑病、混合型硬斑病、嗜酸性筋膜炎的临床特点以及组织病理学特点，实验室检查及影像学特点，列举了需要鉴别的疾病特点。该病会导致功能障碍及美感受损。自限性和慢性、复发的疾病进程会产生重大的疾病负担。本章全面综述了从疾病活动性评估及器官损害评估、受累深度评估、疾病进展评估、系统受累评估、疾病亚型评估至各个阶段需要采取的干预措施及治疗选择。

　　硬化性苔藓（LS）是一种慢性炎症性皮肤病，由于严重的瘙痒、疤痕和解剖/功能损伤而影响生活质量。LS也可能出现在生殖器外。外阴疾病增加了患鳞状细胞癌的风险。本章也从流行病学、临床特征、病因学及发病机制、诊断、鉴别诊断、临床进程及预后、管理及预防各方面阐述了该疾病的特征。

〔施　为〕

MORPHEA

AT-A-GLANCE

- Occurs in children and adults.
- Linear subtype predominates in children.
- Circumscribed and generalized predominate in adults.
- A self-limited or chronically relapsing autoimmune disorder targeting the skin with the following major features:
  - Inflammatory, sclerotic, atrophic phases.
  - Thickened sclerotic skin.
  - Systemic disease, including arthritis and neurologic disorders, in a minority.
  - Differentiated from scleroderma by lack of acrosclerosis/sclerodactyly.
- Complications may cause significant irreversible cosmetic and functional impairment including the following:
  - Atrophy of dermis, fat, and subcutaneous structures.
  - Contracture.
  - Limb-length discrepancy.
  - Bony abnormalities.
- Effective treatment reduces signs of disease activity and does not produce complete resolution of lesions. Treatment based on the following:
  - Disease subtype.
  - Depth of involvement.
  - Stage (inflammatory, sclerotic, atrophic).
  - Potential for complications.

Morphea is a chronic inflammatory disease characterized by sclerosis of the skin. The term *localized scleroderma* is also used in some texts. This causes confusion with systemic sclerosis (scleroderma), often resulting in unnecessary evaluation and anxiety. It is the opinion of the authors that the term *localized scleroderma* should be avoided. Morphea itself has a spectrum of manifestations ranging from skin only to multiple organ involvement. Of note, organ involvement in morphea is distinctly different from systemic sclerosis (Table 64-1).

EPIDEMIOLOGY

Morphea has an estimated incidence of 2.7 per 100,000 with a female-to-male ratio of 2 to 3:1.[1] Morphea is more common in whites, although population-based studies have not verified this observation.[2-5] The relative frequency of the different subtypes varies between studies. This is likely due to use of different classification systems. Twenty to thirty percent of morphea begins in childhood, but it can occur at any age.[2-5] Linear morphea is the most common pediatric subtype (although all subtypes occur at any age).[1,2,6] Twenty-five percent to 87% of pediatric cases are linear morphea, with limb or trunk involvement in approximately 70% to 80% and en coup de sabre or progressive hemifacial atrophy (formerly described as Parry-Romberg syndrome) in 22% to 30%.[1,2,4,5,7,8] In adults, circumscribed and generalized subtypes predominate.[5] Deep morphea/morphea profunda is uncommon in both adults and children, with a frequency of 2% to 4%.[1,2,4,7,8] Periods of disease activity vary from 3 to 6 years.[2,8] Newer studies demonstrate morphea has a relapsing remitting course in some patients. Although longitudinal studies are needed to better determine the frequency and associated clinical factors of recurrence, the frequency of recurrence maybe 20% of cases or more. Others have a chronic course persisting for decades. The prognostic markers for recurrent or chronic disease have yet to be determined.[9,10]

CLINICAL FEATURES

Morphea is currently divided into 5 putative subtypes (Table 64-2).[11] Superficial or deep disease (involving subcutis, fascia, or below) may occur with any subtype. Morphea lesions may also occur with overlying lichen sclerosus change (Fig. 64-1).

CUTANEOUS FINDINGS

Stages of Cutaneous Lesions: Figure 64-2 outlines the stages of morphea lesions.

TABLE 64-1 Differential Diagnosis of Morphea
Most Likely
- Scleroderma (systemic sclerosis)
- Lipodermatosclerosis
- Eosinophilic fasciitis
- Morpheaform injection-site reactions
- Nephrogenic systemic fibrosis
- Chronic graft-versus-host disease
Consider
- Lichen sclerosus
- Pretibial myxedema
- Connective tissue nevi
- Morpheaform basal cell carcinoma
- Chemical-mediated sclerosing skin conditions (toxic oil syndrome, rapeseed oil, etc)
- Lyme disease (acrodermatitis atrophicans)
- Phenylketonuria
- Scleromyxedema, scleredema, pretibial myxedema
- Polyneuropathy, organomegaly, endocrinopathy, M protein, and skin changes (POEMS) syndrome
Always Rule Out
- Carcinoma of the breast metastatic to skin (carcinoma en cuirasse)
- Porphyria cutanea tarda

TABLE 64-2
Proposed Classification of Morphea Subtypes

MORPHEA SUBTYPE	MODIFIERS	CLINICAL
Circumscribed	Superficial	Single or multiple oval/round lesions limited to epidermis and dermis
	Deep	Single or multiple oval/round lesions involving subcutaneous tissue, fascia, or muscle
Linear	Trunk/limbs	Linear lesions involving dermis subcutaneous tissue with/without involvement of skin, dermis, subcutaneous tissue, muscle, or bone
	Head	En coup de sabre, progressive facial hemiatrophy, linear lesions of the face (may involve underlying soft tissue, bone, or brain/gingiva/etc.)
Generalized		
1. Coalescent plaque		More than or equal to 4 plaques in at least 2 of 7 anatomic sites (head–neck, right/left upper extremity, right/left lower extremity, anterior/posterior trunk); isomorphic pattern: coalescent plaques inframammary fold, waistline, lower abdomen, proximal thighs; symmetric pattern: symmetric plaques circumferential around breasts, umbilicus, arms, and legs
2. Pansclerotic		Circumferential involvement of majority of body surface area (sparing fingertips and toes), affecting skin, subcutaneous tissue, muscle or bone; no internal organ involvement
3. Mixed		Combination of any above subtype: eg, linear-circumscribed

Adapted from Laxer RM, Zulian F. Localized scleroderma. *Curr Opin Rheumatol*. 2006;18:606-613, with permission. https://journals.lww.com/co-rheumatology.

Morphea begins as erythematous plaques or patches, sometimes with a reticulated appearance. Later, hypopigmented sclerotic plaques develop at the center of the lesion, surrounded by an erythematous or violaceous border (inflammatory stage) (Fig. 64-3A). Pain and/or itching can occur with active lesions. Sclerosis develops centrally, has a shiny white color with surrounding hyperpigmentation (sclerotic stage). There may be loss of hair follicles, producing alopecia. Over months to years, the sclerotic plaque softens and becomes atrophic with hypopigmentation or hyperpigmentation (atrophic stage) (Fig. 64-3B). The atrophic stage is associated with cigarette paper wrinkling (papillary dermis), cliff drop (dermal), or deep indentions altering the contour of the affected body part (subcutis or deeper atrophy).

Circumscribed Morphea: Circumscribed morphea presents as oval to round lesions that are of limited cutaneous distribution so do not meet criteria for generalized disease (see Table 64-2). Patients with circumscribed morphea should be closely followed, as both linear and generalized morphea may begin with circumscribed lesions.

Atrophoderma of Pasini and Pierini is thought to be the residua of plaque-type morphea. The borders of the atrophoderma lesions have a "cliff-drop" appearance resembling "burnt-out" morphea lesions.

Generalized Morphea: Generalized morphea is characterized by more than or equal to 4 lesions on at least 2 of 7 different anatomic sites. There are likely 3 variants of generalized morphea: (a) isomorphic, (b) symmetric, and (c) pansclerotic (see Table 64-2 and

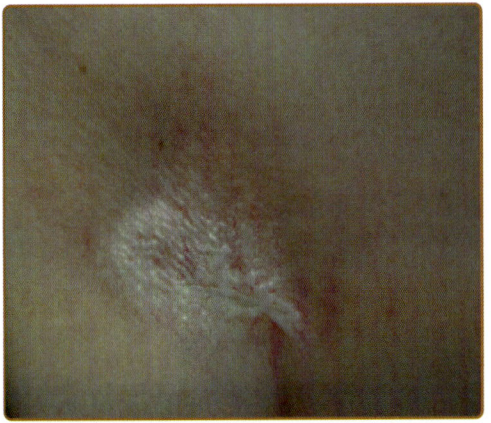

Figure 64-1 Lichen sclerosis can overlie morphea lesions.

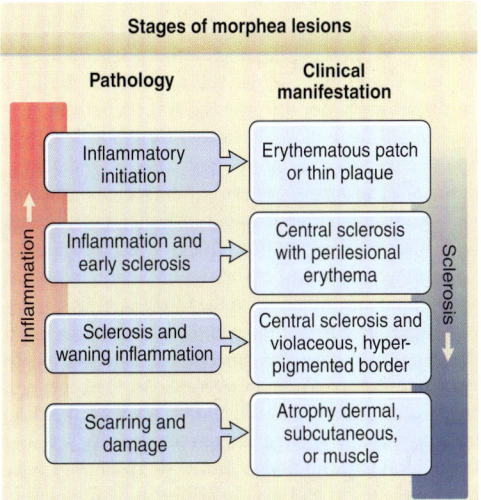

Figure 64-2 Stages of morphea lesions. (Reproduced with permission from Jacobe H. Pathogenesis, clinical manifestations, and diagnosis of morphea [localized scleroderma] in adults. In: Post TW, ed. *UpToDate*. Waltham, MA: UpToDate, Inc. Copyright © 2017. For more information visit www.uptodate.com.)

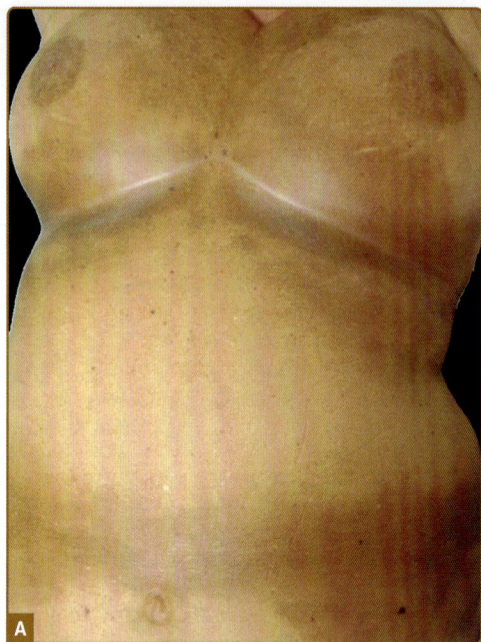
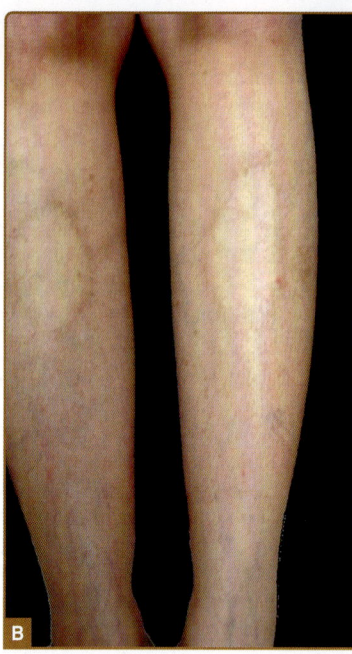

Figure 64-3 Generalized morphea. **A.** Isomorphic plaques involving bra and waistband areas. **B.** Symmetric plaques on a patient with generalized morphea. (Reproduced with permission from Jacobe H. Pathogenesis, clinical manifestations, and diagnosis of morphea [localized scleroderma] in adults. In: Post TW, ed. *UpToDate*. Waltham, MA: UpToDate, Inc. Copyright © 2017. For more information visit www.uptodate.com.)

Figs. 64-3 and 64-4).[12-14] In direct contrast to systemic sclerosis, generalized morphea does not present with acrosclerosis or sclerodactyly. Instead, lesions frequently begin on the trunk and spread acrally, sparing the fingers and toes (Fig. 64-4).

Linear Morphea: Linear morphea usually affects the extremities and face, but it can occur on the trunk (where it is often misclassified as circumscribed) (see Table 64-2 and Fig. 64-5A). The presence of multiple linear lesions is not uncommon. A recent study suggests that linear morphea may follow the Blaschko lines.[15] Linear morphea may involve the dermis, subcutaneous tissue, muscle, or even underlying bone, causing significant cosmetic and functional impairment. Bone marrow inflammation has also been reported.[16,17] En coup de sabre ("cut of the sword") may present as an atrophic linear plaque on the forehead (Fig. 64-5B), extending to the scalp (where cicatricial alopecia occurs), brow, nose, and lip. These lesions start with an inflammatory phase, but because of their location on the scalp, they do not illicit the patients' attention until pigmentary change and atrophy develops. Other linear lesions on the head and neck present on any part of the face, and are generally hyperpigmented atrophic plaques (Fig. 64-5C). Progressive hemifacial atrophy is characterized by a slowly progressive, unilateral atrophy of skin, soft tissues, muscles, and/or bony structures. The atrophy may be accompanied by classic linear morphea lesions on the face or elsewhere. Examination of the face from multiple perspectives and with facial expressions can elicit subtle anatomic asymmetry in early progressive hemifacial atrophy.

Deep Morphea: Deep morphea, or morphea profunda, involves the deep dermis, subcutaneous tissue, fascia, and muscle. Plaques are poorly circumscribed and symmetrical (Fig. 64-6). The skin feels thickened and bound down to the underlying fascia and muscle. A "groove sign" (depression) may be present at the site of tendons and ligaments. Deep morphea lesions may underlie any clinical subtype of morphea, particularly linear and generalized, or occur alone. Progressive hemifacial atrophy is simply deep morphea affecting the face.

Mixed Morphea: Mixed morphea is a combination of any of the above subtypes, although most commonly it denotes linear and circumscribed lesions in combination.[11]

Eosinophilic Fasciitis: Eosinophilic fasciitis, or Shulman syndrome, is a related disorder presenting with rapid onset of symmetric areas of pain and poorly circumscribed indurated, plaques, usually on the extremities. Eosinophilic fasciitis may occur with cutaneous lesions similar to morphea in 30% of cases, or remain without skin involvement. Deep subcutaneous and fascial involvement and peripheral eosinophilia are common.[18]

NONCUTANEOUS FINDINGS

Extracutaneous manifestations develop in 22% to 56% of morphea patients.[1,4,5,7,8,19] Musculoskeletal involve-

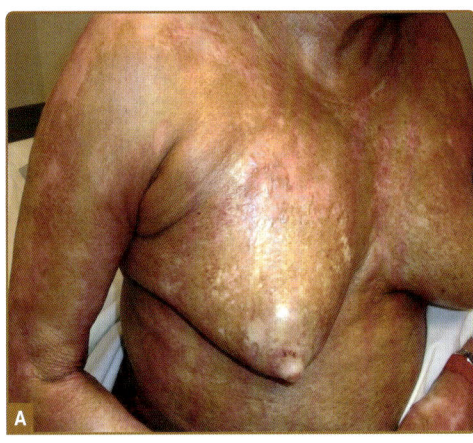
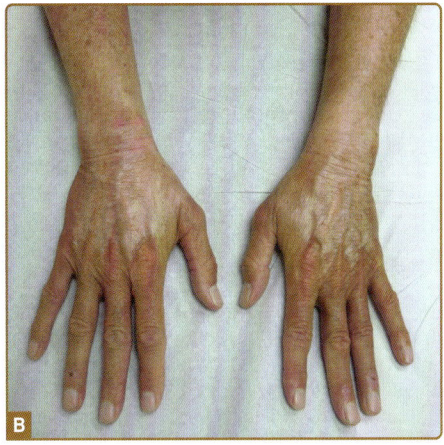

Figure 64-4 Pansclerotic morphea: sclerosis encompassing majority of body surface area (**A**), characteristically sparing the fingertips (**B**). (Reproduced with permission from Jacobe H. Pathogenesis, clinical manifestations, and diagnosis of morphea [localized scleroderma] in adults. In: Post TW, ed. *UpToDate*. Waltham, MA: UpToDate, Inc. Copyright © 2017. For more information visit www.uptodate.com.)

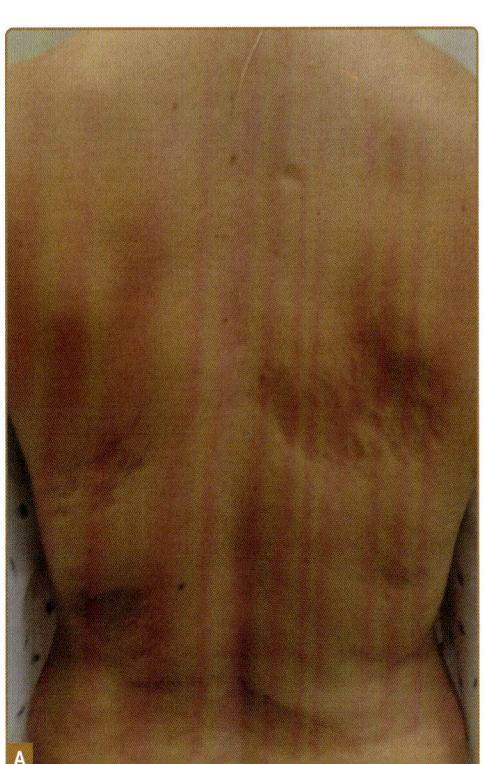
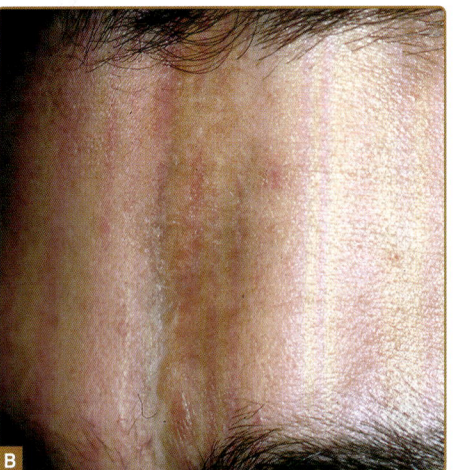
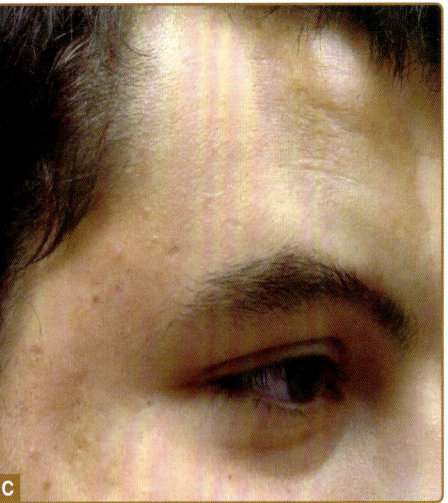

Figure 64-5 **A,** Multiple linear lesions involving trunk. **B,** En coup de sabre. **C,** Multiple hyperpigmented linear morphea lesions on the face. (Reproduced with permission from Jacobe H. Pathogenesis, clinical manifestations, and diagnosis of morphea [localized scleroderma] in adults. In: Post TW, ed. *UpToDate*. Waltham, MA: UpToDate, Inc. Copyright © 2017. For more information visit www.uptodate.com.)

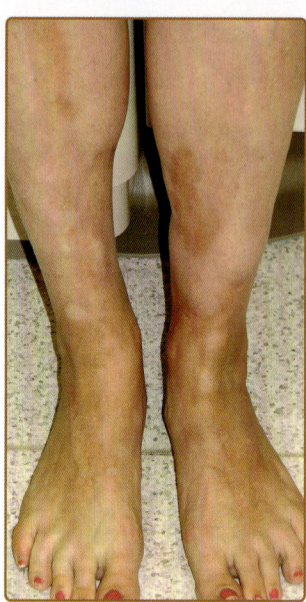

Figure 64-6 Morphea profunda: involved areas have "cobblestone" appearance with subcutaneous atrophy. (Reproduced with permission from Jacobe H. Pathogenesis, clinical manifestations, and diagnosis of morphea [localized scleroderma] in adults. In: Post TW, ed. *UpToDate*. Waltham, MA: UpToDate, Inc. Copyright © 2017. For more information visit www.uptodate.com.)

ment is the most common finding (12%) and can occur unrelated to skin lesions.[20,21] Musculoskeletal involvement can include arthritis, myalgias, neuropathies, and carpal tunnel syndrome. En coup de sabre is associated with neurologic and ocular complications (3.6%) including seizures, headaches, adnexal abnormalities (eyelids, eyelashes), uveitis, and episcleritis.[20-24] Rarely, serious complications, such as CNS vasculitis, can develop, which is an emergency. Facial morphea may produce dental malocclusion, altered dentition, gingivitis, deviation of the uvula, and atrophy of the tongue and salivary glands. Morphea can also rarely involve the genitals typically in postmenopausal women with generalized subtype[25] or coexist with genital lichen sclerosus.

COMPLICATIONS

Cutaneous disease itself produces limited range of motion, limb-length discrepancy, joint deformity, and contracture (45% to 56% linear morphea). Patients with lesions crossing joint lines are most at risk.[8,19,20]

Children with morphea can have significant morphea-related morbidity, including effects on growth, function, and quality of life (fewer studies exist in adults).[26,27] Muscle weakness may occur in affected extremities or face. Behavioral changes, learning disabilities, and seizure (sometimes preceding cutaneous lesions)[23,24] have been reported in children with (and without) facial involvement. In addition, disfigurement and physical symptoms (fatigue, pain, itch) associated with morphea affect psychosocial development and play a substantial role in the quality of life for patients with morphea.

Pansclerotic morphea is associated with an increased risk of squamous cell carcinoma caused by chronic ulcers. The resulting sclerosis of the skin can cause significant contracture, and produces restrictive pulmonary defects and dysphagia. Circumferential sclerosis of the arms or legs may also produce compartment syndrome, bullae, and ulcers.[13]

Morphea can coexist with other autoimmune diseases such as lichen sclerosus, systemic lupus erythematosus, vitiligo, primary biliary sclerosis, autoimmune hepatitis, Hashimoto thyroiditis, and myasthenia gravis.[22,28-33] In particular, generalized morphea is associated with an increased rate of autoimmune disease.[5] Despite this association, screening in the absence of symptoms is not indicated.

ETIOLOGY AND PATHOGENESIS

The etiology and pathogenesis of morphea is poorly understood. Most pathologic events ascribed to morphea are extrapolated from studies in systemic sclerosis (assuming the 2 disorders arise from the same etiology). Morphea likely arises from a genetic background that increases disease susceptibility, combined with other causative factors (eg, infectious, environmental exposures) that modulate disease expression. HLA-DRB1*04:04 and HLA-B37 confer an increased risk for morphea.[34] The presence of a human leukocyte antigen association along with familial clustering and higher-than-expected rates of familial autoimmune disorders implicate a genetic predisposition.[9,35,36] Although there are no definitive associations, development of morphea lesions is linked to local tissue trauma, including radiation, surgery, insect bites, and intramuscular injections.[12] Sixteen percent of patients develop initial lesions of morphea at sites of trauma resulting from chronic friction or surgery.[12]

Increasing amounts of evidence support autoimmune-mediated inflammation early in the course of morphea.[37] Early morphea lesions are characterized by the influx of large amounts of mononuclear lymphocytes (usually activated T lymphocytes), plasma cells, and eosinophils. This is likely the result of autoimmunity, as there is widespread autoimmune reactivity in morphea patients (elevated antinuclear antibodies [ANAs], cytokines, and adhesion molecules). Morphea patients also have concomitant autoimmune disease at a higher-than-expected frequency than occurs in a healthy population.[31] Vessel damage and upregulation of adhesion molecules (intercellular adhesion molecule-1, vascular cell adhesion molecule-1, and E-selectin) occur related to the inflammatory cell infiltrate that facilitates local monocyte recruitment.[38]

T-helper (Th) 1-associated cytokines and chemokines including interleukin (IL)-12, IL-2 interferon (IFN)-γ, IFN-α2, and CXCL-10 are increased in the serum of morphea patients compared to controls.[39,40] Macrophage cytokines and growth factors including granulocyte-macrophage colony-stimulating factor and monocyte chemoattractant protein-1 are also increased in morphea serum.[39] In addition, CXCL-9, a key Th1 chemokine, is significantly elevated in the sera of patients with active morphea compared to controls (unpublished data). CXCL-9 and CXCL-10 are produced by macrophages after stimulation by IFN-γ. CXCL-9 subsequently binds to CXCR3 on T cells, leading to migration of Th1 and cytotoxic T cells from peripheral blood into target tissues. Interestingly, there is a positive correlation between CXCL-9 levels and disease severity scores in morphea, suggesting that CXCL-9 may potentially serve as a useful biomarker in morphea (unpublished data). CXCL-10 levels in serum also correlate with disease activity in morphea patients.[39] Gene expression analysis of inflammatory border of morphea also shows upregulation of Th1 and IFN-regulated pathways compared to unaffected skin, which is consistent with the findings in serum (unpublished data).

On the other hand, there is also evidence of elevation of Th2-related cytokines in morphea including IL-4 and IL-13.[40,41] These cytokines (especially IL-4) upregulate transforming growth factor-β, initiating a cascade of events resulting in increased production of collagen and other extracellular matrix components via induction of connective tissue growth factor, platelet-derived growth factor, and matrix metalloproteinases. These cytokines and growth factors inhibit IFN-γ (a suppressor of collagen synthesis and Th1-related cytokine). Taken together, the pathogenesis of morphea appears to involve a transition from a predominantly Th1 profile in the early inflammatory stage of morphea to a Th2 profile in the later sclerotic stage. The factors mediating the transition of Th1 to Th2 remain unknown. Some reports indicate that chimerism or nonself cells may play a role in the pathogenesis of morphea by initiating a local inflammatory reaction.[42]

DIAGNOSIS

The diagnosis of morphea is usually made by the characteristic clinical appearance of the lesions. Histologic examination should be used to exclude other disorders on the differential, particularly in the case of lesions on the breast, in which carcinoma of the breast should be excluded. Histologic examination may aid therapeutic decision making because it is sometimes difficult to determine the degree of activity or depth of involvement by clinical examination alone. Biopsy of the advancing edge of a lesion may provide insight into both (Fig. 64-7).

LABORATORY TESTING

Although a large number of laboratory-based assessments are reported to reflect disease activity and prognosis in morphea, promising new biomarkers need further validation. Consequently, laboratory-based tests are not recommended for evaluation morphea in the absence of specific signs and symptoms indicating the need for further assessment.

Serum Autoantibodies: Autoantibodies reported in patients with morphea include ANA, anti–single-stranded DNA, anti–double-stranded DNA, anti-histone, antitopoisomerase IIα, antiphospholipid, anticentromere, anti-Scl-70, rheumatoid factor, and matrix metalloproteinase-1.[5,19,43-48] ANAs occur in 34% to 80% of patients and are more common in patients with linear or generalized disease.[58,19,43,49] A case-control study of 187 adults and children showed positive ANA and antihistone antibodies in 34% and 12% of morphea patients compared to 11% and 2% of controls respectively ($P < 0.001$).[49] The majority (81%) had a speckled pattern of ANA. In terms of prognostic significance, only in the subset of linear morphea, antihistone antibodies were associated with functional limitation, and ANA was associated with extensive body surface area involvement.[49] Overall, the clinical and prognostic significance of autoantibodies in morphea remains unclear and testing for them is not indicated.

Other Serum Abnormalities: Peripheral eosinophilia, hypergammaglobulinemia, and increased erythrocyte sedimentation rate or C-reactive protein may occur with active disease of any type, but particularly deep morphea. Additionally, patients with muscle involvement may have elevation of creatine kinase and aldolase.

PATHOLOGY

Biopsies should be taken from the inflammatory or indurated border when present (indicate on pathology requisition) or sclerotic center and include subcutaneous fat. For lesions with minimal clinical change, biopsy of site-matched unaffected skin is helpful. Findings depend on where the biopsy was taken, stage of the lesion, and depth of involvement (see Fig. 64-7). The inflammatory phase demonstrates an interstitial

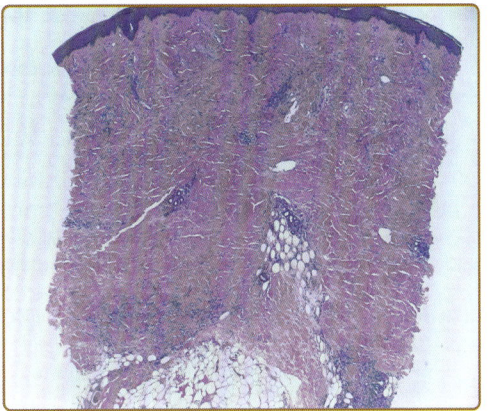

Figure 64-7 Morphea histology demonstrates perivascular, interstitial, and subcutaneous inflammatory cell infiltrate with marked dermal fibrosis.

and perivascular inflammatory cell infiltrate in the dermis and sometimes subcutaneous tissue, composed mostly of lymphocytes and plasma cells, but eosinophils, mast cells, and macrophages also may be present. There is also tissue edema, enlarged tortuous vessels, and thickened collagen bundles. In sclerotic lesions there is homogenization of the papillary dermis and sclerosis extending to the reticular dermis (or beyond depending on depth of involvement) with thickened collagen bundles. With severe sclerosis there is compression and loss of appendageal structures. In deep morphea, the deep reticular dermis, subcutis, and fascia show similar changes. The atrophic phase is characterized by loss of inflammatory cell infiltrate, lessening of sclerosis, and absence of appendageal structures. Telangiectasia may occur.

IMAGING

Assessment via MRI and ultrasonography is becoming increasingly useful for determination of lesion activity and depth and should be considered when deep morphea is present or suspected. MRI provides a complete assessment of the extent of disease, including depth of involvement and disease activity.[50] MRI findings include fascial thickening and enhancement, subcutaneous septal thickening, articular synovitis, tenosynovitis, perifascial enhancement, myositis, enthesitis, and, rarely, bone marrow involvement.[50] Musculoskeletal involvement was seen with MRI in 38% of patients in whom it was not clinically suspected.[50] It is also possible to evaluate the response to treatment, although not currently routine practice.

Ultrasonography is a sensitive tool usable for evaluating or monitoring tissue thickness, loss of subcutaneous fat and muscle, or other architectural alterations. Disease activity can be correlated with the detection of hyperemia and echogenicity.[51] Discussion with the radiologist performing the MRI or ultrasonography studies is crucial to adequately detect and evaluate change related to the morphea.

DIFFERENTIAL DIAGNOSIS

The differential diagnosis of morphea includes systemic sclerosis and other sclerodermoid conditions, including graft-versus-host disease, sclerodermoid porphyria cutanea tarda (especially with photodistributed sclerodermoid eruptions), lipodermatosclerosis, lichen sclerosus, and others (see Table 64-1). It is important to note that morphea and systemic sclerosis are distinct entities. Systemic sclerosis is characterized by acral sclerosis/sclerodactyly, nail-fold capillary changes, Raynaud phenomenon, characteristic internal organ involvement (eg, pulmonary, renal, and GI), and hallmark autoantibodies. These features are absent in morphea. For a morpheaform plaque on the breast, carcinoma en cuirasse resulting from metastatic breast cancer is an important diagnosis to rule out. Morpheaform reactions can also develop secondary to vitamin K_1 injections, taxanes, IFN-β1a, and balicatib.[52-55]

CLINICAL COURSE AND PROGNOSIS

Although morphea causes functional and aesthetic impairment, it is rarely life-threatening. Morphea may be self-limited, but frequently has a remitting relapsing or chronic course that produces significant disease burden over time.[9] Recurrences occur in approximately 25% of patients.[56] A higher risk of recurrence (31% of patients) has been reported for linear morphea of the extremities as compared to other subtypes.[56]

MANAGEMENT

OVERVIEW

The natural history of morphea is poorly understood. At least some cases undergo spontaneous remission after a few years of activity. However, even when spontaneous remission occurs, residual damage created by active disease remains. In addition, new evidence suggests at least a subset of morphea patients has continued disease activity over many years, ultimately leading to extensive disease burden and related morbidity.[9] Despite the large number of reported treatments, no consistent recommendations exist for therapy. This section provides an evidence-based algorithm for the rational evaluation and management of morphea patients (Fig. 64-8). It is important to understand what constitutes therapeutic success in morphea when treating patients. Therapeutic success is defined by resolution of erythema, typically over 2 to 3 months, lesion softening, which can take 12 months or more, cessation of lesion growth, and no new lesion development. In general, active lesions are most amenable to treatment. A morphea-specific outcome measure known as localized scleroderma cutaneous assessment tool (LoSCAT) has been validated and consists of 2 scores: LoSSI (localized scleroderma severity index) and LoSDI (localized scleroderma damage index), which are useful for monitoring disease activity and damage, respectively, especially in clinical trials and research. Serial photography is helpful in clinical practice.

PATIENT EVALUATION

In determining which therapy is appropriate, the following must be considered:

- *Disease activity and damage*: Existing studies indicate that early, active disease is most responsive to therapy.[57] Indicators of active disease include development of new lesions or extension of existing lesions (photographs are critical), erythema and/or induration of the advancing edge of the lesion, and patient-reported symptoms, such as itch or tingling. Disease damage (reversible or irreversible) includes pigmentary change, sclerosis of the lesion center, atrophy (dermal, subcutaneous, muscle), contracture, limb-length discrepancy, and scarring alopecia. Disease damage is much more difficult to treat and therapy should be aimed at preventing disease damage. Furthermore, patients with active disease at risk for significant damage (facial lesions, progressive hemifacial atrophy, lesions crossing joint lines, large body surface area involvement, rapid progression) likely need aggressive therapy (phototherapy and/or systemic immunosuppressives).

- *Depth of involvement*: Morphea involving the superficial to mid-dermis would logically be amenable to topical therapy or phototherapy; however, involvement of the deep dermis and beyond should be treated systemically. Deep involvement can occur in all subtypes of morphea, but is especially prominent among linear and some generalized patients, and is associated with functional impairment and pain.
- *Disease progression*: Many generalized and linear morphea patients are initially diagnosed with circumscribed morphea, but progress to have much more extensive disease.[9] Therefore, patients who initially present with 1 to 3 plaques (which may be amenable to localized therapy) should be closely followed. If these patients progress, therapy should then be aimed at preventing further progression (ie, phototherapy or systemic therapy).
- *Systemic involvement*: Systemic involvement is an indication for systemic immunosuppressive therapy.
- *Disease subtype*: Patients with linear and generalized (particularly those with rapid onset of confluent plaques) are likely at risk for severe,

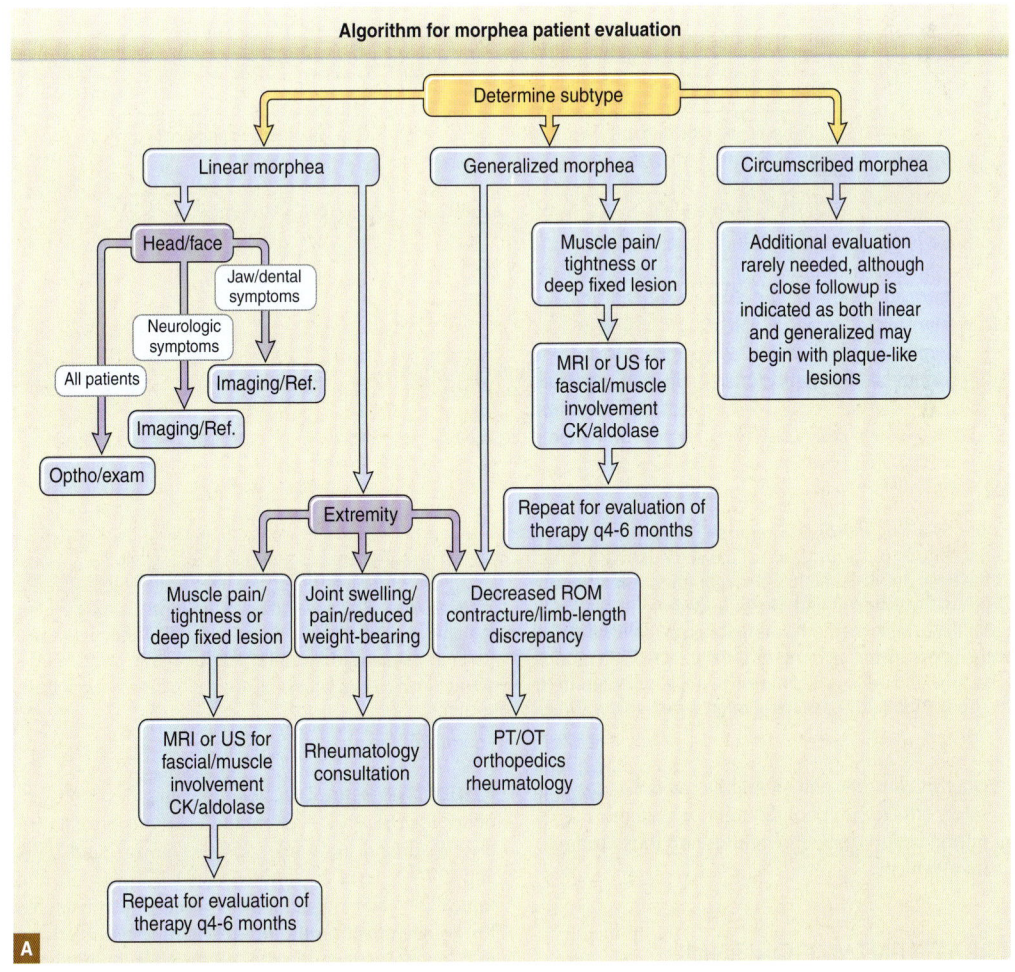

Figure 64-8 **A,** Algorithm for the evaluation of patients with morphea. Optho, ophthalmologic; OT, occupational therapy; PT, physical therapy; ROM, range of motion; US, ultrasonography.

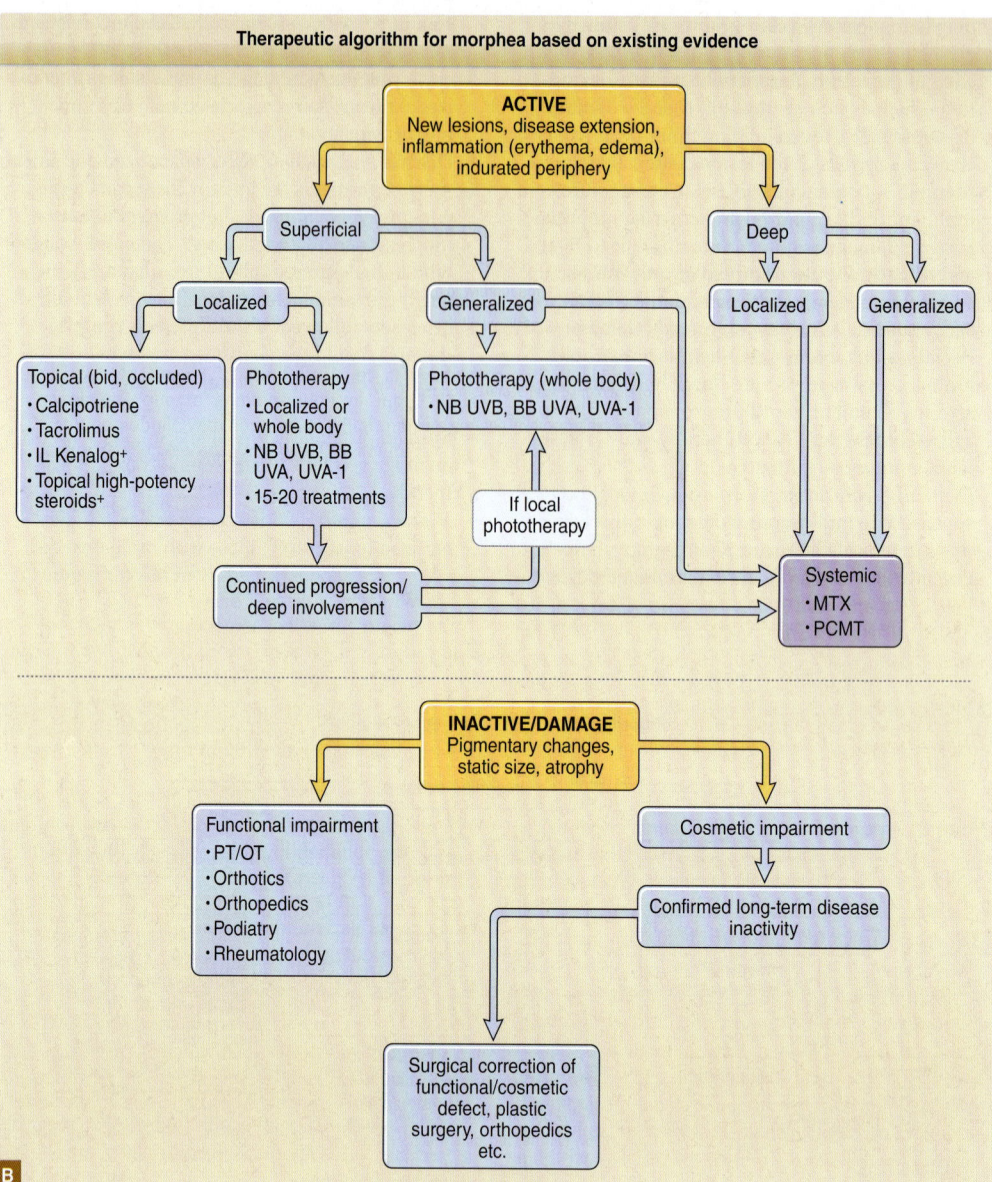

Figure 64-8 (*continued*) **B,** Therapeutic algorithm for morphea based on existing evidence. Superficial involvement is defined by histologic evidence of papillary dermal involvement. Deep involvement is defined as sclerosis or inflammation of the deep dermis, subcutis, fascia, or muscle. Histologic examination and/or MRI are encouraged to evaluate lesions for depth of involvement and, likewise, determine appropriate treatment as well as evaluation of therapeutic efficacy. BB, broadband; MTX, methotrexate; NB, narrowband; OT, occupational therapy; PCMT, pulsed corticosteroids and methatrexate; PT, physical therapy; UVA/B, ultraviolet A/B. (Reproduced with permission from Jacobe H. Pathogenesis, clinical manifestations, and diagnosis of morphea (localized scleroderma) in adults. In: Post TW, ed. *UpToDate*. Waltham, MA: UpToDate, Inc. Copyright © 2017. For more information visit www.uptodate.com.)

extensive disease and should be treated aggressively either with phototherapy or systemic immunosuppressives depending on the depth of involvement.

TREATMENT ALGORITHM

Table 64-3 outlines morphea therapy.

Phototherapy: Phototherapy has level 1 evidence for efficacy (level 1, randomized controlled trials: broadband ultraviolet (UV) A, narrowband UVB, and UVA-1; level 2: psoralen and UVA systemic and topical).[58-63] Narrowband UVB should be considered for lesions affecting the superficial dermis (relatively thin on palpation or with sclerosis and inflammation in the papillary and superficial reticular dermis). UVA-based therapies are more appropriate for deeper dermal lesions because of a greater depth of penetration. UVA-1 in particular has evidence for normalization of dermal collagen and effect on inflammation in morphea so is appropriate for both inflammatory and sclerotic disease.[63] In the absence of access to UVA-1 phototherapy, use of broadband UVA is also supported by the literature.[58] Disease is expected to improve (progression halted and erythema improved) after 10 to 20 treatments and most trials stopped after 20 to 30 treatments. Evidence suggests that patients continue to improve after cessation of therapy, and some authors recommend using a greater number of treatments[9,12,29,30,34-36,48-51,54,60-67] for further therapeutic benefit. Uncontrolled trials demonstrated increased benefit with a medium to high dose of UVA-1 versus a low dose, but controlled trials were less convincing.[59] Typically, UVA-1 is administered 3 to 5 times a week for 30 to 40 treatments. Optimum dose and regimen for UVA-1 phototherapy has yet to be determined. Recurrence can develop in approximately half of patients within 3 years of stopping UVA-1 phototherapy, emphasizing the need for close follow up.[65] A second course of UVA-1 phototherapy or systemic treatments can be considered in these cases of recurrence. Phototherapy is likely ineffective for deep involvement (subcutis, fascia, muscle), and therefore should not be considered as primary therapy.

Vitamin D Derivative: Only 1 study provides level 1 evidence on the effect of vitamin D derivatives in morphea, and it showed no difference between oral calcitriol and placebo.[66] In fact, placebo and treatment groups improved equally. The authors also point out that the study was underpowered by their own calculations, making definitive conclusions regarding the efficacy of oral calcitriol difficult. The efficacy of topical vitamin D derivatives has been explored via uncontrolled trials and case reports[67] (level 2 evidence) and showed improvement in most or all patients, albeit over several months of therapy (an interval in which lesions might improve independent of therapy). Importantly, calcipotriene was applied under occlusion in these studies.

IMMUNOMODULATORS

Methotrexate with or without Corticosteroids: The use of methotrexate (monotherapy) and methotrexate combined with systemic corticosteroids is effective based on level 1 evidence.[22,57,68-71] Methotrexate is considered a first-line systemic treatment for morphea, especially for deep morphea and rapidly progressive or disabling morphea. In most studies with combined therapy, corticosteroids are used for induction therapy either orally or via intravenous pulse (intravenous methylprednisolone 30 mg/kg/day for 3 days per month or 1 mg/kg/day prednisone) over the first 3 to 4 months. Methotrexate is used as steroid-sparing agent and started simultaneously (0.6 mg/kg/week in children or 15 to 25 mg/week in adults administered orally or with subcutaneous injection). Most study participants responded in a mean of 2 to 5 months defined by no new lesions and resolution of inflammation, not resolution of sclerosis. The best responders were all early in their disease course. In a randomized, double-blind, controlled trial, methotrexate plus prednisone was compared to prednisone alone in pediatric morphea.[71] Prednisone was administered for 4 months, while methotrexate or placebo were continued for 12 months. Responders met 3 criteria: absence of new lesions, computerized skin score rate ≤1, and decreased percentage temperature change of at least 10% compared to baseline. Methotrexate was significantly more effective than prednisone alone at 12 months (67.4% vs 29.2%). In addition, the chance of recurrence in the prednisone-only group was 3 times higher than in the methotrexate group. Optimum dose, route, and indications for addition of corticosteroids, and duration of therapy have not been determined. The authors taper methotrexate after 6 months of inactivity by 2.5 to 5 mg every 4 weeks. The average duration of methotrexate use ranges from 21 to 27 months. Approximately 15% of patients relapse at 2-year followup after starting methotrexate, which suggests the need for close followup.[72]

TABLE 64-3
Morphea Therapy

TREATMENT	LEVEL OF EVIDENCE[a]
BB UVA	1,2
UVA-1	1,2
Calcitriol, oral (inefficacy 1)	1,2
IFN-γ (inefficacy 1)	1
PUVA bath	2
PUVA cream	2
ECP	2
Calcipotriene, topical	2
MTX monotherapy, MTX plus steroids	1,2
PCMT	2
Tacrolimus, topical	2
Steroids, oral	2
Hydroxychloroquine, MMF, cyclosporine, Bosentan, infliximab, imiquimod, antimicrobials, D-penicillamine, 585-nm long-pulse laser, wide surgical resection, orthopedic surgery, Apligraf	Minimal evidence (≥level 3)

[a]Level of Evidence: 1, indicates randomized controlled trial; 2, uncontrolled trial; and 3, case report, case series.
BB, broadband; ECP, eosinophil cationic protein; IFN, IF; MMF, mycophenolate mofetil; MTX, methotrexate; PUVA, psoralen and ultraviolet A; UVA/B, ultraviolet A/B.
Reproduced with permission from Jacobe H. Pathogenesis, clinical manifestations, and diagnosis of morphea (localized scleroderma) in adults. In: Post TW, ed. *UpToDate*. Waltham, MA: UpToDate, Inc. Copyright © 2017. For more information visit www.uptodate.com.

Mycophenolate Mofetil: Case series using oral mycophenolate mofetil indicate potential utility in patients refractory to methotrexate or sensitive to side effects.[57,73-75] In the experience of the authors, mycophenolate mofetil can be used as a second-line systemic treatment, and is effective for morphea refractory to methotrexate or patients with contraindications or intolerance of methotrexate. In a case series of 10 patients with morphea refractory to methotrexate and prednisone, all patients treated with mycophenolate mofetil experienced clinical improvement on average 3.5 months after starting treatment.[74] Further controlled trials are needed to clarify the role of mycophenolate mofetil in treatment of morphea.

Other Immunomodulators: Level 2 evidence suggests the use of occluded topical tacrolimus 0.1% ointment might be effective for active, inflammatory superficial plaque-type morphea.[76,77] Case reports on the use of oral cyclosporine, imatinib, bosentan, abatacept, infliximab, and topical imiquimod also have reported some efficacy, but more definitive studies are lacking.

Antimicrobials: Despite the widespread use of antimicrobials in morphea (antibiotics and hydroxychloroquine), no published clinical trials exist.[78] Literature supporting the use of antimalarials is limited to a case series in which 2 patients improved with hydroxychloroquine (while simultaneously receiving oral steroids and methotrexate).[79] In a retrospective review, 7 (64%) of 11 patients continued to have active disease 3 to 15 months after starting hydroxychloroquine.[4] At this time, the use of these agents in severe morphea is not indicated pending more definitive evidence of efficacy.

Lack of Evidence: The most commonly used treatment for morphea, topical steroids, has not been investigated in a clinical trial. There are also no studies investigating the use of intralesional steroids. In the hands of the authors, intralesional steroids have been extremely effective in treating circumscribed plaques or as an adjuvant for recalcitrant areas in patients receiving phototherapy or systemic treatment. Current evidence does not support the use of penicillamine or IFN-γ.[80]

Adjunctive Therapy: A significant number of morphea patients suffer irreversible sequelae. When these patients come to medical attention, they may no longer have disease activity, but rather damage from the past or a mixture of active disease and damage. Consequently, every morphea patient should be examined for the presence of limitation in range of motion, contracture, limb-length discrepancy, or other functional impairment. In these cases, consultation with rheumatology, physical/occupational therapy, physical medicine and rehabilitation, plastic surgery, orthopedics, and oral maxillofacial surgery is highly recommended to maximize cosmesis, function, and minimize further damage.

LICHEN SCLEROSUS

AT-A-GLANCE

- Infrequent chronic inflammatory dermatosis with anogenital and extragenital manifestations.
- Preferentially affects women in the fifth or sixth decade of life and children younger than age 10 years; the female-to-male ratio is 5:1.
- Antibodies to extracellular matrix protein-1 and predominance of Th1 pathway point to an autoimmune pathogenesis.
- Anogenital manifestations cause severe discomfort (pruritus, dyspareunia, dysuria, and painful defecation) and present with polygonal papules and porcelain-white plaques, erosions, and various degrees of sclerosis. If left untreated, scarring and resultant functional impairment can occur.
- Vulvar lichen sclerosus is associated with an increased risk of squamous cell carcinoma.
- Potent topical corticosteroids and skin care are the most successful therapeutics; calcineurin inhibitors have also demonstrated benefit.
- Interdisciplinary management is essential for long-term control.

Lichen sclerosus (LS) is a chronic inflammatory dermatosis of the anogenital area that affects quality of life because of severe itching, scarring, and anatomic/functional impairment. LS may also present with extragenital manifestations. Of note, vulvar disease has an increased risk of squamous cell carcinoma, particularly if untreated.

EPIDEMIOLOGY

The incidence of LS has not been precisely determined. It has been estimated to be in the order of 14 per 100,000 persons per year.[81] LS is more frequent in females, accounting for a 5:1 female-to-male ratio. It preferentially affects women in the fifth or sixth decade of life and children younger than age 10 years.[81,82] Up to 15% of LS cases occur in children, particularly in girls, and one study reported a prevalence of 1 in 900 premenarchal girls.[83] A 0.07% incidence in males was determined in a study of 153,432 male soldiers.[84] Among blacks and Hispanics, the incidence was 1.06%, whereas the incidence was only 0.051% in white soldiers.[84] LS seems to be a prominent cause of phimosis; in one study, 14% of adolescent boys with phimosis had LS, whereas 40% of phimosis cases in adult men were associated with LS.[84] Similarly, a study of foreskins examined after therapeutic circumcision for phimosis confirmed many cases of unrecognized

LS.[85] As genital LS in males is almost exclusively seen in uncircumcised men, the rate of circumcision in a given population has a strong impact on the occurrence of the disease.

CLINICAL FEATURES

CUTANEOUS FINDINGS

Vulvar LS presents with porcelain-white atrophic papules coalescing into plaques on the labia minora and majora.[86] Follicular plugging may be seen in early LS.[86] Fissures, erosions, telangiectasias, purpura, erythema, hyperkeratosis, and different degrees of sclerosis can be present in the anogenital area (Fig. 64-9); often the classical figure-8 pattern of the vulva and anus may be observed (Fig. 64-9E). Bullae (occasionally hemorrhagic) may develop when the lichenoid infiltrate separates epidermis from the sclerotic dermis. Anogenital LS frequently causes intractable itching, soreness, dyspareunia, dysuria, discomfort with defecation, or genital bleeding, and, with time, may lead to destructive scarring (Fig. 64-9F). Gradual obliteration or synechiae of the labia minora and clitoris, burying of the clitoris, as well as stenosis of the introitus, may also result. Male genital LS (also known as balanitis xerotica obliterans) is usually confined to the

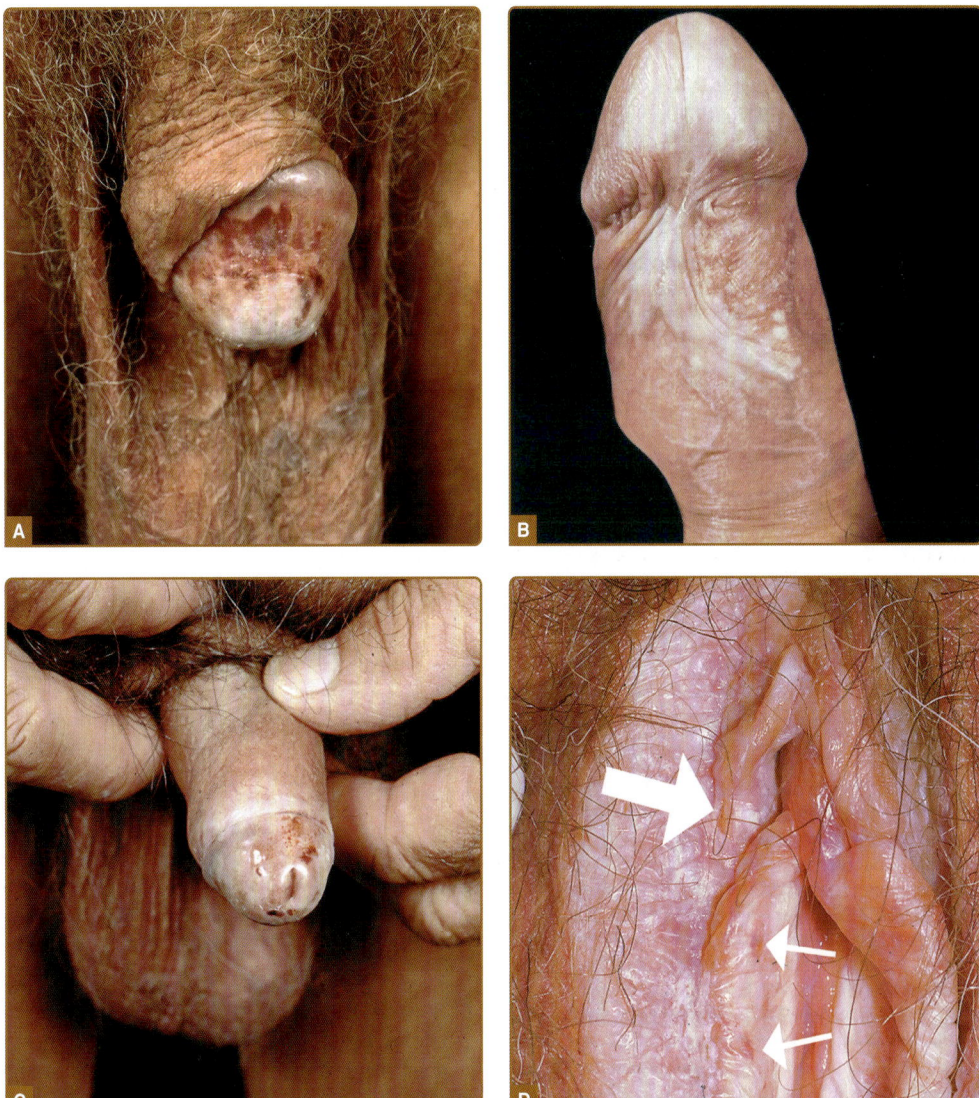

Figure 64-9 **A,** Early sclerosis and significant hemorrhage on the glans in early lichen sclerosus. **B,** Sclerosis of the frenulum and increased vulnerability with bleeding upon sexual intercourse. **C,** Significant sclerosis of the glans and conglutination with the preputium in advanced lichen sclerosus. Note narrowing of the urethral orifice and hemorrhage. **D,** In addition to the well-demarcated white vulvar plaque that is classic for lichen sclerosus, the waxy and crinkled texture, purpura (*small arrows*), and erosions (*large arrow*) are diagnostic.

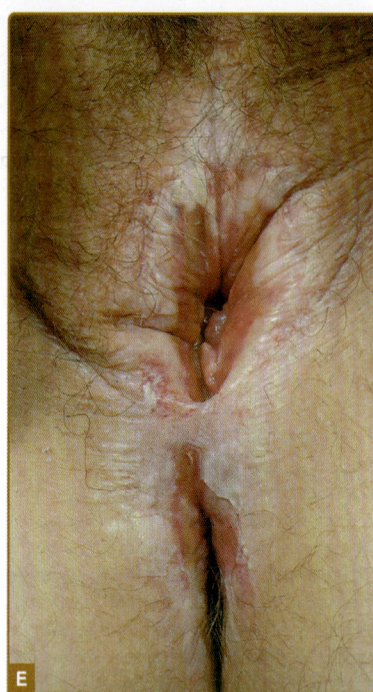
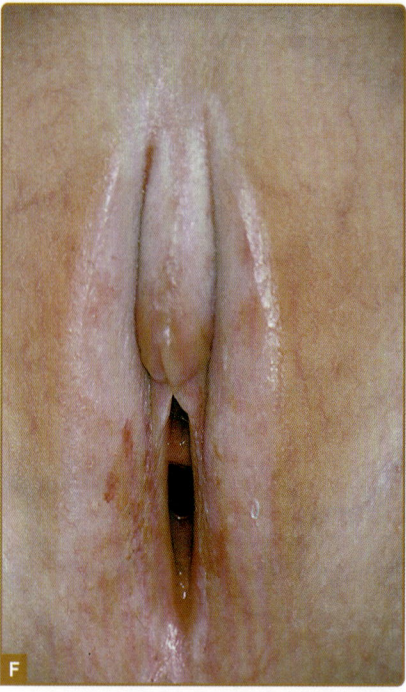

Figure 64-9 (*continued*) **E,** Sclerotic vulva with disappearance of the smaller labia and shrinkage of the introitus. Significant erythema and erosions are seen on the vulva and the anus in a figure-8 configuration. The patient complained of severe pruritus and dyspareunia. **F,** Erosive, sclerotic vulva in an 8-year-old girl.

glans penis, prepuce, or foreskin remnants (Fig. 64-9A–C). Penile shaft involvement is less common, whereas scrotal involvement is rare. Many male genital LS cases are simply diagnosed as phimosis. In severe cases, erections may become painful. Urethral strictures with decreased urinary stream and difficulty voiding can result.

Extragenital LS typically affects the thighs, neck, trunk, and lips; lesions are associated with pruritus, burning, or maybe asymptomatic (Fig. 64-10). The size of LS lesions may vary from a few millimeters to large portions of the trunk. A clinical histopathologic study has revealed 27 adult cases with lip involvement.[87] Clinical presentation consisted of asymptomatic vitiligo-like lesions in 70% with a variable degree of dermal sclerosis confined to the papillary layer. Consequently, vitiligo-like LS needs to be added to this spectrum of oral lichenoid lesions.

NONCUTANEOUS FINDINGS

Except for the association with autoimmune thyroid disease, alopecia areata, pernicious anemia, morphea, and vitiligo, no additional related findings have been reported. Except in cases where a thorough history and examination indicate the presence of concomitant autoimmune diseases, laboratory testing is not recommended.

COMPLICATIONS

Dyspareunia, urinary obstruction, constipation, secondary infection related to ulceration, steroid use, and squamous cell carcinoma represent the main complications in females (Fig. 64-11). The lifetime risk of developing squamous cell carcinoma as a complication of longstanding LS has been estimated in the order of 4% to 6%.[81,88] In a study of 2875 women with LS, incidence of vulvar squamous cell carcinoma was 2.1% after

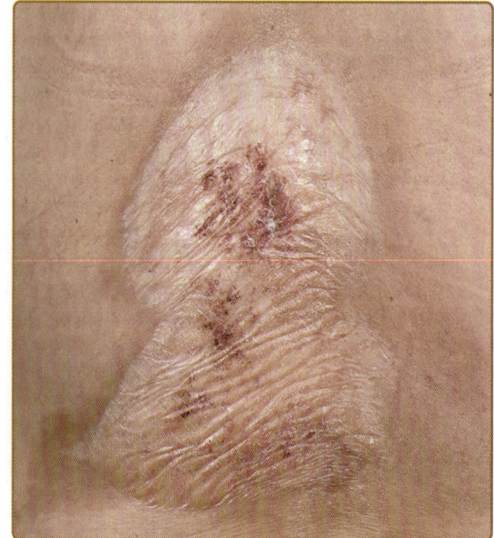

Figure 64-10 Extragenital lichen sclerosus with confluent whitish papules and plaques on the skin over the thoracic and lumbar spine.

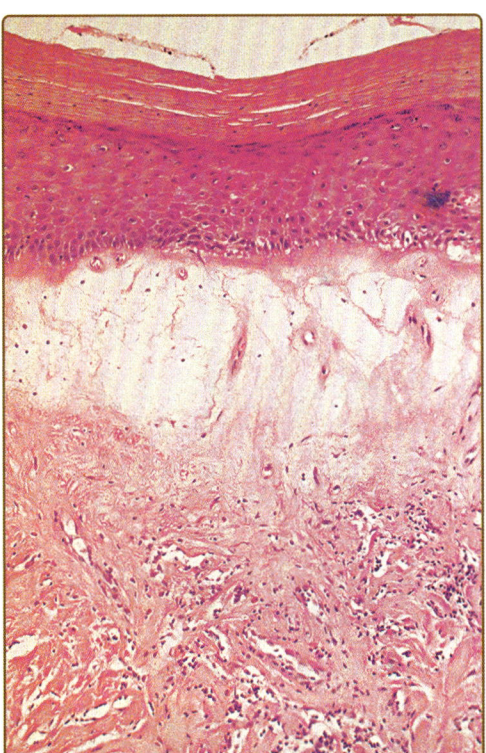

Figure 64-11 Hyperkeratotic epithelium without rete ledges and basal degeneration of keratinocytes. Collagen fibers are homogenized in the papillary dermis, and a lichenoid lymphocytic infiltrate is present. The dermal vessels are dilated.

5 years, 3.3% after 10 years, and 6.7% after 20 years, highlighting the need for long-term followup.[89] Age, long duration of LS, human papillomavirus infection, and evidence of hyperplastic changes represent significant risk factors.[90,91] *IRF6*, a tumor-suppressor gene, is downregulated in vulvar squamous cell carcinoma associated with LS, and maybe involved in early carcinogenesis of squamous cell carcinoma in LS.[92] In males, painful erections and urinary obstruction represent the most frequent complications.

ETIOLOGY AND PATHOGENESIS

The cause of LS is unknown. A recent cohort study reported a high rate of familial LS cases.[93] Of 1052 females with LS, 126 (12%) had a positive family history of LS. Vulvar cancer was significantly increased in those patients with a family history of LS compared with those without (4.1% vs. 1.2%).[93] This report proposes a likely genetic component in the etiology of LS. Local irritation and trauma (Koebner phenomenon) also seem to play a role in some cases. The disturbed function of fibroblasts with increased production of collagen has been demonstrated in LS.[94,95] Evidence for a presumed infectious cause, such as acid-fast rods, spirochetes, or *Borrelia*, has not been found.[96]

Autoimmune diseases are found at increased frequency in LS patients, which suggests that LS may result from a common genetic predisposition to this group of disorders. A study of 350 patients with LS revealed that 21.5% had 1 or more autoimmune diseases.[96] Serologic and clinical evidence of thyroid disease, alopecia areata, pernicious anemia, and vitiligo suggested an association with LS. Low-titer autoantibodies against the extracellular matrix protein-1 (ECM-1) and collagen XVII have been identified in 67% of LS cases.[97,98] ECM-1 may be involved in basement membrane and interstitial collagenous fiber assembly and growth-factor binding,[99] and may also regulate blood vessel function.[100]

The immune infiltrate in LS contains abundant T cells, B cells, and antigen-presenting dendritic cells.[101,102] Further characterization of the infiltrate has shown a predominance of CD8 cytotoxic T cells over CD4 T cells, and presence of regulatory T cells.[103,104] A monoclonal T-cell receptor γ-chain rearrangement has alluded to the existence of an LS antigen, potentially the ECM-1 protein, which is also recognized by anti–ECM-1 autoantibodies.[93,105] Gene expression profiling of LS has shown significant upregulation of Th1 and Type I IFN-regulated cytokines and chemokines, including IFN-γ, CXCL-9, CXCL-10, CXCL-11, CXCR3, CCR5, CCL4, and CCL5.[104] No upregulation of Th2 or Th17 pathways was seen. Plasmacytoid dendritic cells, present in LS lesions, may be the source of Type I IFN production.[103] The IFN-regulated chemokines, CXCL-9, CXCL-10, and CXCL-11, are involved in migration of Th1 cells into tissues through binding to CXCR3. Notably, these findings are similar to pathogenesis of active inflammatory morphea as described earlier. Extragenital and genital LS is commonly seen in association with plaque-type morphea, and some authors have suggested a common pathomechanism. Pathogenesis of LS is likely a multifactorial process involving the interaction of genetic predisposition, autoimmunity (with predominance of Th1 cells), and local factors, such as trauma and chronic irritation. Further studies are needed to elucidate the pathogenesis of LS.

DIAGNOSIS

A skin punch biopsy of a mature lesion will confirm the diagnosis if the diagnosis is not obvious by clinical examination. Despite the described association with autoimmune diseases, an autoimmune workup (eg, antinuclear antibody, parietal cell antibody, vitamin B_{12} levels, thyroid function tests) is not generally recommended because of their relatively low occurrence, but should be considered if review of systems raises the possibility of a concomitant autoimmune disease.[106] *Borrelia* antibody titers should not be analyzed, as they are not associated with LS.[107] To exclude squamous cell carcinoma, serial biopsies may be indicated or involvement of gynecology oncology.

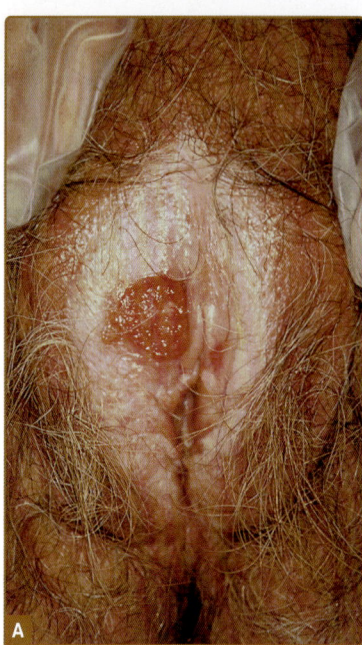
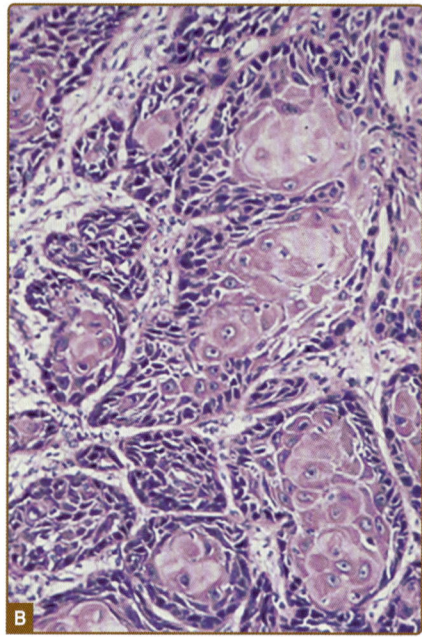

Figure 64-12 **A.** A 1.5-cm, sharply demarcated ulcer of longstanding lichen sclerosus on the right labia majora. **B.** Histology reveals squamous cell carcinoma.

PATHOLOGY

Classical LS shows an atrophic epidermis and a lichenoid infiltrate at the dermal–epidermal junction.[108] Papillary edema is usually seen in early LS, but is gradually replaced by fibrosis with homogenization of collagen and acid mucopolysaccharides as the lesion matures (Fig. 64-12). Epidermal hyperplasia and/or dysplasia associated with LS on vulvar specimens are associated with an increased risk of malignant transformation, especially in conjunction with infection by high-risk human papillomaviruses.

IMAGING

Imaging studies are only needed in special situations (eg, urinary obstruction secondary to stenosing genital LS). High-resolution ultrasonography is occasionally used to document the depth of sclerosis.

DIFFERENTIAL DIAGNOSIS

The differential diagnosis of LS includes a variety of other conditions including lichen simplex chronicus, lichen planus, contact dermatitis, morphea, vitiligo, and other conditions (Table 64-4). Vulvar lichen planus more commonly involves the vagina, whereas LS spares the vagina. Clinically, extragenital LS maybe confused with morphea or lichen planus (see Fig. 64-12). Typical early plaque-type morphea lesions show an erythematous ring with progressive central induration and whitening. Patients have been described with lesions typical of both plaque-type morphea and the chalky white, atrophic plaques of LS.[109]

Constipation is a common complication in children with anogenital LS.[110] The associated purpura and discoloration often raise a concern about child abuse, especially if LS is not recognized. It should be noted, however, that LS and child abuse may coexist[111] and that some cases of LS have been linked with trauma of the anogenital region. LS in children has occasionally been associated with a perineal pyramidal protrusion, a common lesion that can be confused with condyloma and is also associated with constipation. Table 64-5 outlines the pitfalls in diagnosing LS.

CLINICAL COURSE AND PROGNOSIS

LS is a chronic, relapsing condition with possibility of long-term functional and anatomic impairment if left untreated. The prognosis of LS is generally favorable in patients who are diagnosed and treated in the early nonscarring stages, and in patients compliant with initial and maintenance therapy with topical corticosteroids. Importantly, childhood-onset vulvar LS does not always resolve at puberty and may remain persistent.[112] A prospective study of 12 cases of childhood LS showed that 9 patients, still had active LS at puberty, and continued to require maintenance therapy after menarche. Six of the 12 experienced significant disturbance of the vulvar architecture. A further case series reported the efficacy of topical clobetasol propionate

TABLE 64-4
Differential Diagnosis of Lichen Sclerosus

Genital Manifestations

Consider
- Zoon balanitis
- Child abuse (sexual)
- Radiation dermatitis (for vulvar cancer)
- Contact dermatitis, including excessive genital hygiene
- Lichen planus
- Lichen simplex chronicus
- Vitiligo

Rule Out
- Cicatricial pemphigoid
- Erythroplasia of Queyrat (Bowen disease)
- Leukoplakia
- Squamous cell carcinoma
- Paget disease

Extragenital Manifestations

Consider
- Anetoderma
- Atrophoderma of Pasini and Pierini
- Idiopathic guttate hypomelanosis
- Lipoid proteinosis (mild forms; see Chap. 133)
- Lichen planus
- Morphea
- Pinta
- Tinea versicolor

Rule Out
- Discoid lupus erythematosus
- Graft-versus-host disease (scleroderma-like)
- Extramammary Paget disease
- Squamous cell carcinoma

0.05% in childhood LS.[113] Nine of 15 young girls suffered from a relapse approximately 1 year following the first clearing of the lesions. The authors also concluded that early aggressive treatment with ultrapotent corticosteroids enables the best clinical course of childhood LS.[113] Recalcitrant chronic LS that causes erosions and progressive scarring may result in severe dysfunction of urination, sexual function, and defecation. Furthermore, the scarring nature of advanced LS produces resorption of the labia, alopecia, and altered anatomic structure of the vulva.

TABLE 64-5
Pitfalls in the Diagnosis of Lichen Sclerosus

- Wrong/incomplete diagnosis in the case of squamous cell carcinoma.
- Lichen sclerosus, especially when bullous, hemorrhagic, or erosive; may be confused with child abuse.
- Inappropriate surveillance for steroid adverse effects.
- Irritant dermatitis caused by overwashing of the anogenital area may imitate lichen sclerosus and facilitate the occurrence of contact dermatitis.

MANAGEMENT

TOPICAL TREATMENTS

Treatment should be initiated in all patients with LS, not only to improve symptoms, but also to prevent long-term complications such as anatomic distortion, scarring, and impaired function. Ultrapotent topical corticosteroids, most commonly clobetasol propionate 0.05%, are the first-line treatment for genital LS based on randomized controlled trials (RCTs).[114-116] A metaanalysis including 7 RCTs supported efficacy of clobetasol, mometasone, and calcineurin inhibitors in the treatment of genital LS, but showed no evidence for topical androgens or progesterone.[117] Consequently, the use of topical androgens and progesterone as monotherapy is not supported by current evidence. Head-to-head RCTs comparing clobetasol versus pimecrolimus, and clobetasol versus tacrolimus, have demonstrated superior efficacy of clobetasol compared to calcineurin inhibitors.[115,116] Clobetasol should also be used for treatment of vulvar LS in children. A study of 72 children demonstrated efficacy and safety of clobetasol for vulvar LS.[118] Mometasone furoate 0.1% is also effective in the treatment of vulvar LS.[119] Mometasone furoate 0.1% and clobetasol propionate 0.05% had comparable efficacy for treatment of vulvar LS in a head-to-head RCT.[119]

We typically initiate therapy with clobetasol propionate 0.05% ointment once to twice daily until remission is achieved, typically after 2 to 3 months. Alternatively, a tapering regimen with clobetasol once daily for 4 weeks, every other day for 4 weeks, and then twice a week for 4 weeks can be used.[120] Approximately 50% to 60% of patients experience complete remission. Ointments tend to be less irritating and better tolerated than creams. A lower-potency corticosteroid or calcineurin inhibitors can be considered if there is cutaneous atrophy from use of ultrapotent topical steroids. It is important for patients to receive exact instructions on where to apply ointment.

PHOTOTHERAPY AND SYSTEMIC TREATMENTS

Evidence for phototherapy and systemic treatments is limited to small clinical trials and case series. A small RCT comparing clobetasol versus UVA-1 phototherapy in 30 female patients with vulvar LS showed clinical improvement with both treatments.[121] However, clobetasol was more effective than UVA-1 in relief of pruritus and quality of life. In the authors' experience, phototherapy should be used as an adjunct to topical steroids, not in place of them as severe flares may occur. Preliminary studies with photodynamic therapy with 5-aminolevulinic acid have shown efficacy in treatment of vulvar LS.[122] UVA-1 or photodynamic therapy can be considered as a second-line treatment if topical corticosteroids are ineffective or not tolerated. Systemic therapy with acitretin has been effective in small RCTs for penile and severe vulvar LS.[123,124]

ADJUNCTIVE TREATMENTS

It is thought that irritation from urinary and fecal incontinence exacerbates vulvar LS. Therefore, referral for treatment of these conditions is important. Furthermore, addition of barrier creams containing zinc oxide is important to protect the vulvar and perianal skin. The functional impairment from advanced LS is a significant problem and needs to be discussed with the patient. This can include difficulty with urination, sexual intercourse, and defecation/constipation. Referral to urogynecology and gastroenterology should be considered. In addition, pelvic floor therapists can teach patients gentle stretching exercises and counselors can help address the emotional toll of the disease. These interventions can have a positive impact on the quality of life of patients with LS.

MAINTENANCE THERAPY

The importance of maintenance therapy in treatment of genital LS has been recognized. In a prospective longitudinal cohort of 507 women with vulvar LS, clinical outcomes were compared between compliant patients, who used topical corticosteroids consistently as maintenance therapy, versus partially compliant patients over the period of 2 to 7 years.[125] Compliant patients had improved symptom control and function compared to partially compliant patients. In addition, vulvar carcinoma developed in 0% of compliant patients versus 4.7% of partially compliant patients ($P <0.001$).[125] The risk of relapse of LS is also reduced with maintenance therapy. For instance, use of mometasone furoate twice a week reduces the risk of relapse of vulvar LS compared to placebo over a 52-week period (0% in mometasone vs. 62% in placebo).[119] Taken together, current evidence supports continuation of maintenance therapy with topical corticosteroids twice to 3 times a week, even with asymptomatic genital LS. Both clobetasol and mometasone are effective for maintenance treatment.[126] Potency of topical corticosteroids should be adjusted based on level of hyperkeratosis or presence of corticosteroid-induced atrophy.[125] Further studies are needed to elucidate the duration of maintenance therapy in LS.

TREATMENT OF MALE GENITAL LICHEN SCLEROSUS

In general, much less is known about the treatment and course of male genital LS. Circumcision will generally resolve male genital LS and the associated phimosis, although potent topical steroids may obviate the need for surgery.

TREATMENT OF EXTRAGENITAL LICHEN SCLEROSUS

Current evidence for treatment of extragenital LS is limited to case series and uncontrolled trials. Overall, the treatment modalities utilized for treatment of extragenital LS are similar to morphea. Active lesions may present with peripheral erythema like morphea. Extragenital LS lesions may respond to treatment with topical corticosteroids, topical calcineurin inhibitors, UVA-1 phototherapy, or methotrexate in combination with prednisone.[127,128] Extragenital LS, with a limited surface area of involvement, can be treated with superpotent topical steroids such as clobetasol propionate. For generalized extragenital LS or for cases resistance to topical steroids, UVA-1 phototherapy can be beneficial. In a case series of patients with extragenital LS, 10 patients were treated with low-dose UVA-1 phototherapy (20 J/cm^2) 4 times a week for 10 weeks.[127] All patients experienced decreased number of sclerotic skin lesions, softening of lesions, and repigmentation after completing therapy. Systemic therapy is rarely used for treatment of extragenital LS. Use of pulsed glucocorticoids plus methotrexate, is supported by a small retrospective study of 7 patients.[128] Further controlled trials are warranted to elucidate the treatment of extragenital LS.

PREVENTION

No truly preventive measures of LS have been reported. An interdisciplinary management team is essential for the long-term control of LS. Specialists from gynecology, urology, pediatrics, and pain medicine should be involved in patient care and collaborate to prevent significant complications, including the monitoring for squamous cell carcinoma and corticosteroid adverse events. It has also been helpful to circulate information via patient organizations for LS.

ACKNOWLEDGMENTS

We acknowledge the contribution of previous authors Stephanie Saxton-Daniels and Ulrich R. Hengge.

REFERENCES

1. Peterson LS, Nelson AM, Su WP, et al. The epidemiology of morphea (localized scleroderma) in Olmsted County 1960-1993. *J Rheumatol.* 1997;24:73-80.
2. Greenberg A, Falanga V. Localized cutaneous sclerosis. In: *Cutaneous Manifestations of Rheumatic Diseases.* Baltimore, MD: Williams & Wilkins; 1996.

3. Sehgal VN, Srivastava G, Aggarwal AK, et al. Localized scleroderma/morphea. *Int J Dermatol*. 2002;41:467-475.
4. Christen-Zaech S, Hakim MD, Afsar FS, et al. Pediatric morphea (localized scleroderma): review of 136 patients. *J Am Acad Dermatol*. 2008;59:385-396.
5. Leitenberger JJ, Cayce RL, Haley RW, et al. Distinct autoimmune syndromes in morphea: a review of 245 adult and pediatric cases. *Arch Dermatol*. 2009;145:545-550.
6. Vierra E, Cunningham BB. Morphea and localized scleroderma in children. *Semin Cutan Med Surg*. 1999;18:210-225.
7. Zulian F, Athreya BH, Laxer R, et al. Juvenile localized scleroderma: clinical and epidemiological features in 750 children. An international study. *Rheumatology (Oxford)*. 2006;45:614-620.
8. Marzano AV, Menni S, Parodi A, et al. Localized scleroderma in adults and children. Clinical and laboratory investigations on 239 cases. *Eur J Dermatol*. 2003;13:171-176.
9. Saxton-Daniels S, Jacobe HT. An evaluation of long-term outcomes in adults with pediatric-onset morphea. *Arch Dermatol*. 2010;146:1044-1045.
10. Condie D, Grabell D, Jacobe H. Comparison of outcomes in adults with pediatric-onset morphea and those with adult-onset morphea: a cross-sectional study from the morphea in adults and children cohort. *Arthritis Rheumatol*. 2014;66:3496-3504.
11. Laxer RM, Zulian F. Localized scleroderma. *Curr Opin Rheumatol*. 2006;18:606-613.
12. Grabell D, Hsieh C, Andrew R, et al. The role of skin trauma in the distribution of morphea lesions: a cross-sectional survey of the Morphea in Adults and Children cohort IV. *J Am Acad Dermatol*. 2014;71:493-498.
13. Kim A, Marinkovich N, Vasquez R, et al. Clinical features of patients with morphea and the pansclerotic subtype: a cross-sectional study from the Morphea in Adults and Children cohort. *J Rheumatol*. 2014;41:106-112.
14. Teske N, Welser J, Jacobe H. Skin mapping for the classification of generalized morphea. *J Am Acad Dermatol*. 2016;78:351-357.
15. Weibel L, Harper JI. Linear morphoea follows Blaschko's lines. *Br J Dermatol*. 2008;159:175-181.
16. Muroi E, Ogawa F, Yamaoka T, et al. Case of localized scleroderma associated with osteomyelitis. *J Dermatol*. 2010;37:81-84.
17. Horger M, Fierlbeck G, Kuemmerle-Deschner J, et al. MRI findings in deep and generalized morphea (localized scleroderma). *AJR Am J Roentgenol*. 2008;190:32-39.
18. Lakhanpal S, Ginsburg WW, Michet CJ, et al. Eosinophilic fasciitis: clinical spectrum and therapeutic response in 52 cases. *Semin Arthritis Rheum*. 1988;17:221-231.
19. Falanga V, Medsger TA Jr, Reichlin M. Antinuclear and anti-single-stranded DNA antibodies in morphea and generalized morphea. *Arch Dermatol*. 1987;123:350-353.
20. Zulian F, Vallongo C, Woo P, et al. Localized scleroderma in childhood is not just a skin disease. *Arthritis Rheum*. 2005;52:2873-2881.
21. Zulian F. New developments in localized scleroderma. *Curr Opin Rheumatol*. 2008;20:601-607.
22. Tollefson MM, Witman PM. En coup de sabre morphea and Parry-Romberg syndrome: a retrospective review of 54 patients. *J Am Acad Dermatol*. 2007;56:257-263.
23. Sartori S, Martini G, Calderone M, et al. Severe epilepsy preceding by four months the onset of scleroderma en coup de sabre. *Clin Exp Rheumatol*. 2009;27:64-67.
24. Chiang KL, Chang KP, Wong TT, et al. Linear scleroderma "en coup de sabre": initial presentation as intractable partial seizures in a child. *Pediatr Neonatol*. 2009;50:294-298.
25. Schlosser BJ. Practice gaps. Missing genital lichen sclerosus in patients with morphea: don't ask? Don't tell?: comment on "high frequency of genital lichen sclerosus in a prospective series of 76 patients with morphea." *Arch Dermatol*. 2012;148:28-29.
26. Klimas NK, Shedd AD, Bernstein IH, et al. Health-related quality of life in morphea. *Br J Dermatol*. 2015;172:1329-1337.
27. Das S, Bernstein I, Jacobe H. Correlates of self-reported quality of life in adults and children with morphea. *J Am Acad Dermatol*. 2014;70:904-910.
28. Gonzalez-Lopez MA, Drake M, Gonzalez-Vela MC, et al. Generalized morphea and primary biliary cirrhosis coexisting in a male patient. *J Dermatol*. 2006;33:709-713.
29. Khalifa M, Ben Jazia E, Hachfi W, et al. Autoimmune hepatitis and morphea: a rare association [in French]. *Gastroenterol Clin Biol*. 2006;30:917-918.
30. Dervis E, Acbay O, Barut G, et al. Association of vitiligo, morphea, and Hashimoto's thyroiditis. *Int J Dermatol*. 2004;43:236-237.
31. Harrington CI, Dunsmore IR. An investigation into the incidence of auto-immune disorders in patients with localized morphoea. *Br J Dermatol*. 1989;120:645-648.
32. Bonifati C, Impara G, Morrone A, et al. Simultaneous occurrence of linear scleroderma and homolateral segmental vitiligo. *J Eur Acad Dermatol Venereol*. 2006;20:63-65.
33. Majeed M, Al-Mayouf SM, Al-Sabban E, et al. Coexistent linear scleroderma and juvenile systemic lupus erythematosus. *Pediatr Dermatol*. 2000;17:456-459.
34. Jacobe H, Ahn C, Arnett F, et al. Major histocompatibility complex (MHC) class I and II alleles which confer susceptibility or protection in the Morphea in Adults and Children (MAC) cohort. *Arthritis Rheumatol*. 2014;66:3170-3177.
35. Wadud MA, Bose BK, Al Nasir T. Familial localised scleroderma from Bangladesh: two case reports. *Bangladesh Med Res Counc Bull*. 1989;15:15-19.
36. Rees RB, Bennett J. Localized scleroderma in father and daughter. *AMA Arch Derm Syphilol*. 1953;68:360.
37. Gabrielli A, Avvedimento EV, Krieg T. Scleroderma. *N Engl J Med*. 2009;360:1989-2003.
38. Gruschwitz MS, Hornstein OP, von Den Driesch P. Correlation of soluble adhesion molecules in the peripheral blood of scleroderma patients with their in situ expression and with disease activity. *Arthritis Rheum*. 1995;38:184-189.
39. Torok KS, Kurzinski K, Kelsey C, et al. Peripheral blood cytokine and chemokine profiles in juvenile localized scleroderma: T-helper cell-associated cytokine profiles. *Semin Arthritis Rheum*. 2015;45:284-293.
40. Ihn H, Sato S, Fujimoto M, et al. Demonstration of interleukin-2, interleukin-4 and interleukin-6 in sera

from patients with localized scleroderma. *Arch Dermatol Res.* 1995;287:193-197.
41. Hasegawa M, Sato S, Nagaoka T, et al. Serum levels of tumor necrosis factor and interleukin-13 are elevated in patients with localized scleroderma. *Dermatology.* 2003;207:141-147.
42. McNallan KT, Aponte C, el-Azhary R, et al. Immunophenotyping of chimeric cells in localized scleroderma. *Rheumatology (Oxford).* 2007;46:398-402.
43. Takehara K, Moroi Y, Nakabayashi Y, et al. Antinuclear antibodies in localized scleroderma. *Arthritis Rheum.* 1983;26:612-616.
44. Rosenberg AM, Uziel Y, Krafchik BR, et al. Antinuclear antibodies in children with localized scleroderma. *J Rheumatol.* 1995;22:2337-2343.
45. Sato S, Kodera M, Hasegawa M, et al. Antinucleosome antibody is a major autoantibody in localized scleroderma. *Br J Dermatol.* 2004;151:1182-1188.
46. Sato S, Ihn H, Soma Y, et al. Antihistone antibodies in patients with localized scleroderma. *Arthritis Rheum.* 1993;36:1137-1141.
47. Tomimura S, Ogawa F, Iwata Y, et al. Autoantibodies against matrix metalloproteinase-1 in patients with localized scleroderma. *J Dermatol Sci.* 2008; 52:47-54.
48. Kroft EB, de Jong EM, Evers AW. Psychological distress in patients with morphea and eosinophilic fasciitis. *Arch Dermatol.* 2009;145:1017-1022.
49. Dharamsi JW, Victor S, Aguwa N, et al. Morphea in Adults and Children cohort III: nested case-control study: the clinical significance of autoantibodies in morphea. *JAMA Dermatol.* 2013;149:1159-1165.
50. Schanz S, Fierlbeck G, Ulmer A, et al. Localized scleroderma: MR findings and clinical features. *Radiology.* 2011;260:817-824.
51. Li SC, Liebling MS, Haines KA. Ultrasonography is a sensitive tool for monitoring localized scleroderma. *Rheumatology (Oxford).* 2007;46:1316-1319.
52. Alonso-Llamazares J, Ahmed I. Vitamin K1-induced localized scleroderma (morphea) with linear deposition of IgA in the basement membrane zone. *J Am Acad Dermatol.* 1998;38:322-324.
53. Bouchard SM, Mohr MR, Pariser RJ. Texane-induced morphea in a patient with CREST syndrome. *Dermatol Reports.* 2010;2:23-24.
54. Bezalel SA, Strober BE, Ferenczi K. Interferon beta-1a-induced morphea. *JAAD Case Rep.* 2015;1:15-17.
55. Runger TM, Adami S, Benhamou CL, et al. Morphea-like skin reactions in patients treated with the cathepsin K inhibitor balicatib. *J Am Acad Dermatol.* 2012;66:e89-e96.
56. Mertens JS, Seyger MM, Kievit W, et al. Disease recurrence in localized scleroderma: a retrospective analysis of 344 patients with paediatric- or adult-onset disease. *Br J Dermatol.* 2015;172:722-728.
57. Uziel Y, Feldman BM, Krafchik BR, et al. Methotrexate and corticosteroid therapy for pediatric localized scleroderma. *J Pediatr.* 2000;136:91-95.
58. El-Mofty M, Zaher H, Bosseila M, et al. Low-dose broad-band UVA in morphea using a new method for evaluation. *Photodermatol Photoimmunol Photomed.* 2000;16:43-49.
59. Kreuter A, Hyun J, Stucker M, et al. A randomized controlled study of low-dose UVA1, medium-dose UVA1, and narrowband UVB phototherapy in the treatment of localized scleroderma. *J Am Acad Dermatol.* 2006;54:440-447.
60. de Rie MA, Enomoto DN, de Vries HJ, et al. Evaluation of medium-dose UVA1 phototherapy in localized scleroderma with the cutometer and fast Fourier transform method. *Dermatology.* 2003;207:298-301.
61. Kerscher M, Meurer M, Sander C, et al. PUVA bath photochemotherapy for localized scleroderma. Evaluation of 17 consecutive patients. *Arch Dermatol.* 1996;132:1280-1282.
62. Grundmann-Kollmann M, Behrens S, Gruss C, et al. Chronic sclerodermic graft-versus-host disease refractory to immunosuppressive treatment responds to UVA1 phototherapy. *J Am Acad Dermatol.* 2000;42:134-136.
63. El-Mofty M, Mostafa W, Esmat S, et al. Suggested mechanisms of action of UVA phototherapy in morphea: a molecular study. *Photodermatol Photoimmunol Photomed.* 2004;20:93-100.
64. Torrelo A, Suarez J, Colmenero I, et al. Deep morphea after vaccination in two young children. *Pediatr Dermatol.* 2006;23:484-487.
65. Vasquez R, Jabbar A, Khan F, et al. Recurrence of morphea after successful ultraviolet A1 phototherapy: a cohort study. *J Am Acad Dermatol.* 2014;70:481-488.
66. Hulshof MM, Bouwes Bavinck JN, Bergman W, et al. Double-blind, placebo-controlled study of oral calcitriol for the treatment of localized and systemic scleroderma. *J Am Acad Dermatol.* 2000;43:1017-1023.
67. Cunningham BB, Landells ID, Langman C, et al. Topical calcipotriene for morphea/linear scleroderma. *J Am Acad Dermatol.* 1998;39:211-215.
68. Seyger MM, van den Hoogen FH, de Boo T, et al. Low-dose methotrexate in the treatment of widespread morphea. *J Am Acad Dermatol.* 1998;39:220-225.
69. Kreuter A, Gambichler T, Breuckmann F, et al. Pulsed high-dose corticosteroids combined with low-dose methotrexate in severe localized scleroderma. *Arch Dermatol.* 2005;141:847-852.
70. Weibel L, Sampaio MC, Visentin MT, et al. Evaluation of methotrexate and corticosteroids for the treatment of localized scleroderma (morphoea) in children. *Br J Dermatol.* 2006;155:1013-1020.
71. Zulian F, Martini G, Vallongo C, et al. Methotrexate treatment in juvenile localized scleroderma: a randomized, double-blind, placebo-controlled trial. *Arthritis Rheum.* 2011;63:1998-2006.
72. Zulian F, Vallongo C, Patrizi A, et al. A long-term follow-up study of methotrexate in juvenile localized scleroderma (morphea). *J Am Acad Dermatol.* 2012;67:1151-1156.
73. Schlaak M, Friedlein H, Kauer F, et al. Successful therapy of a patient with therapy recalcitrant generalized bullous scleroderma by extracorporeal photopheresis and mycophenolate mofetil. *J Eur Acad Dermatol Venereol.* 2008;22:631-633.
74. Martini G, Ramanan AV, Falcini F, et al. Successful treatment of severe or methotrexate-resistant juvenile localized scleroderma with mycophenolate mofetil. *Rheumatology (Oxford).* 2009;48:1410-1413.
75. Mertens JS, Marsman D, van de Kerkhof PC, et al. Use of mycophenolate mofetil in patients with severe localized scleroderma resistant or intolerant to methotrexate. *Acta Derm Venereol.* 2016;96:510-513.
76. Mancuso G, Berdondini RM. Localized scleroderma: response to occlusive treatment with tacrolimus ointment. *Br J Dermatol.* 2005;152:180-182.
77. Kroft EB, Groeneveld TJ, Seyger MM, et al. Efficacy of topical tacrolimus 0.1% in active plaque morphea:

77. (cont.) randomized, double-blind, emollient-controlled pilot study. *Am J Clin Dermatol*. 2009;10:181-187.
78. Mohrenschlager M, Jung C, Ring J, Abeck D. Effect of penicillin G on corium thickness in linear morphea of childhood: an analysis using ultrasound technique. *Pediatr Dermatol*. 1999;16:314-316.
79. Maragh SH, Davis MD, Bruce AJ, et al. Disabling pansclerotic morphea: clinical presentation in two adults. *J Am Acad Dermatol*. 2005;53:S115-S119.
80. Hunzelmann N, Anders S, Fierlbeck G, et al. Double-blind, placebo-controlled study of intralesional interferon gamma for the treatment of localized scleroderma. *J Am Acad Dermatol*. 1997;36:433-435.
81. Powell JJ, Wojnarowska F. Lichen sclerosus. *Lancet*. 1999;353:1777-1783.
82. Marini A, Blecken S, Ruzicka T, et al. Lichen sclerosus. New aspects of pathogenesis and treatment [in German]. *Hautarzt*. 2005;56:550-555.
83. Powell J, Wojnarowska F. Childhood vulvar lichen sclerosus: an increasingly common problem. *J Am Acad Dermatol*. 2001;44:803-806.
84. Kizer WS, Prarie T, Morey AF. Balanitis xerotica obliterans: epidemiologic distribution in an equal access health care system. *South Med J*. 2003;96:9-11.
85. Tokgoz H, Polat F, Tan MO, et al. Histopathological evaluation of the preputium in preschool and primary school boys. *Int Urol Nephrol*. 2004;36:573-576.
86. Funaro D. Lichen sclerosus: a review and practical approach. *Dermatol Ther*. 2004;17:28-37.
87. Attili VR, Attili SK. Lichen sclerosus of lips: a clinical and histopathologic study of 27 cases. *Int J Dermatol*. 2010;49:520-525.
88. Hagedorn M, Buxmeyer B, Schmitt Y, et al. Survey of genital lichen sclerosus in women and men. *Arch Gynecol Obstet*. 2002;266:86-91.
89. Bleeker MC, Visser PJ, Overbeek LI, et al. Lichen sclerosus: incidence and risk of vulvar squamous cell carcinoma. *Cancer Epidemiol Biomarkers Prev*. 2016;25:1224-1230.
90. von Krogh G, Dahlman-Ghozlan K, Syrjanen S. Potential human papilloma-virus reactivation following topical corticosteroid therapy of genital lichen sclerosus and erosive lichen planus. *J Eur Acad Dermatol Venereol*. 2002;16:130.
91. Jones RW, Sadler L, Grant S, et al. Clinically identifying women with vulvar lichen sclerosus at increased risk of squamous cell carcinoma: a case-control study. *J Reprod Med*. 2004;49:808-811.
92. Rotondo JC, Borghi A, Selvatici R, et al. Hypermethylation-induced inactivation of the *IRF6* gene as a possible early event in progression of vulvar squamous cell carcinoma associated with lichen sclerosus. *JAMA Dermatol*. 2016;152:928-933.
93. Sherman V, McPherson T, Baldo M, et al. The high rate of familial lichen sclerosus suggests a genetic contribution: an observational cohort study. *J Eur Acad Dermatol Venereol*. 2010;24:1031-1034.
94. Carli P, Moretti S, Spallanzani A, et al. Fibrogenic cytokines in vulvar lichen sclerosus. An immunohistochemical study. *J Reprod Med*. 1997;42:161-165.
95. Scrimin F, Rustja S, Radillo O, et al. Vulvar lichen sclerosus: an immunologic study. *Obstet Gynecol*. 2000;95:147-150.
96. Meyrick Thomas RH, Ridley CM, McGibbon DH, et al. Lichen sclerosus et atrophicus and autoimmunity—a study of 350 women. *Br J Dermatol*. 1988;118:41-46.
97. Oyama N, Chan I, Neill SM, et al. Autoantibodies to extracellular matrix protein 1 in lichen sclerosus. *Lancet*. 2003;362:118-123.
98. Howard A, Dean D, Cooper S, et al. Circulating basement membrane zone antibodies are found in lichen sclerosus of the vulva. *Australas J Dermatol*. 2004;45:12-15.
99. Chan I. The role of extracellular matrix protein 1 in human skin. *Clin Exp Dermatol*. 2004;29:52-56.
100. Kowalewski C, Kozlowska A, Chan I, et al. Three-dimensional imaging reveals major changes in skin microvasculature in lipoid proteinosis and lichen sclerosus. *J Dermatol Sci*. 2005;38:215-224.
101. Farrell AM, Marren P, Dean D, et al. Lichen sclerosus: evidence that immunological changes occur at all levels of the skin. *Br J Dermatol*. 1999;140:1087-1092.
102. Carlson JA, Grabowski R, Chichester P, et al. Comparative immunophenotypic study of lichen sclerosus: epidermotropic CD57+ lymphocytes are numerous—implications for pathogenesis. *Am J Dermatopathol*. 2000;22:7-16.
103. Wenzel J, Wiechert A, Merkel C, et al. IP10/CXCL10-CXCR3 interaction: a potential self-recruiting mechanism for cytotoxic lymphocytes in lichen sclerosus et atrophicus. *Acta Derm Venereol*. 2007;87:112-117.
104. Terlou A, Santegoets LA, van der Meijden WI, et al. An autoimmune phenotype in vulvar lichen sclerosus and lichen planus: a Th1 response and high levels of microRNA-155. *J Invest Dermatol*. 2012;132:658-666.
105. Regauer S, Reich O, Beham-Schmid C. Monoclonal gamma-T-cell receptor rearrangement in vulvar lichen sclerosus and squamous cell carcinomas. *Am J Pathol*. 2002;160:1035-1045.
106. Foldes-Papp Z, Reich O, Demel U, et al. Lack of specific immunological disease pattern in vulvar lichen sclerosus. *Exp Mol Pathol*. 2005;79:176-185.
107. De Vito JR, Merogi AJ, Vo T, et al. Role of *Borrelia burgdorferi* in the pathogenesis of morphea/scleroderma and lichen sclerosus et atrophicus: a PCR study of thirty-five cases. *J Cutan Pathol*. 1996;23:350-358.
108. Fung M, LeBoit P. Light microscopic criteria for the diagnosis of early vulvar lichen sclerosus: a comparison with lichen planus. *Am J Surg Pathol*. 1998;22:473-478.
109. Khachemoune A, Guldbakke KK, Ehrsam E. Infantile perineal protrusion. *J Am Acad Dermatol*. 2006;54:1046-1049.
110. Maronn ML, Esterly NB. Constipation as a feature of anogenital lichen sclerosus in children. *Pediatrics*. 2005;115:e230-e232.
111. Powell J, Wojnarowska F. Childhood vulval lichen sclerosus and sexual abuse are not mutually exclusive diagnoses. *BMJ*. 2000;320:311.
112. Smith SD, Fischer G. Childhood onset vulvar lichen sclerosus does not resolve at puberty: a prospective case series. *Pediatr Dermatol*. 2009;26:725-729.
113. Patrizi A, Gurioli C, Medri M, et al. Childhood lichen sclerosus: a long-term follow-up. *Pediatr Dermatol*. 2010;27:101-103.
114. Bracco GL, Carli P, Sonni L, et al. Clinical and histologic effects of topical treatments of vulval lichen sclerosus. A critical evaluation. *J Reprod Med*. 1993;38:37-40.
115. Goldstein AT, Creasey A, Pfau R, et al. A double-blind, randomized controlled trial of clobetasol versus pimecrolimus in patients with vulvar lichen sclerosus. *J Am Acad Dermatol*. 2011;64:e99-e104.
116. Funaro D, Lovett A, Leroux N, et al. A double-blind, randomized prospective study evaluating topical clobetasol propionate 0.05% versus topical tacrolimus 0.1% in patients with vulvar lichen sclerosus. *J Am Acad Dermatol*. 2014;71:84-91.

117. Chi CC, Kirtschig G, Baldo M, et al. Systematic review and meta-analysis of randomized controlled trials on topical interventions for genital lichen sclerosus. *J Am Acad Dermatol.* 2012;67:305-312.
118. Casey GA, Cooper SM, Powell JJ. Treatment of vulvar lichen sclerosus with topical corticosteroids in children: a study of 72 children. *Clin Exp Dermatol.* 2015;40:289-292.
119. Virgili A, Borghi A, Minghetti S, et al. Mometasone fuoroate 0.1% ointment in the treatment of vulvar lichen sclerosus: a study of efficacy and safety on a large cohort of patients. *J Eur Acad Dermatol Venereol.* 2014;28:943-948.
120. Neill SM, Lewis FM, Tatnall FM, et al; British Association of Dermatologists. British Association of Dermatologists' guidelines for the management of lichen sclerosus 2010. *Br J Dermatol.* 2010;163: 672-682.
121. Terras S, Gambichler T, Moritz RK, et al. UV-A1 phototherapy vs clobetasol propionate, 0.05%, in the treatment of vulvar lichen sclerosus: a randomized clinical trial. *JAMA Dermatol.* 2014;150:621-627.
122. Shi L, Miao F, Zhang LL, et al. Comparison of 5-aminolevulinic acid photodynamic therapy and clobetasol propionate in treatment of vulvar lichen sclerosus. *Acta Derm Venereol.* 2016;96:684-688.
123. Ioannides D, Lazaridou E, Apalla Z, et al. Acitretin for severe lichen sclerosus of male genitalia: a randomized, placebo controlled study. *J Urol.* 2010; 183:1395-1399.
124. Bousema MT, Romppanen U, Geiger JM, et al. Acitretin in the treatment of severe lichen sclerosus et atrophicus of the vulva: a double-blind, placebo-controlled study. *J Am Acad Dermatol.* 1994;30:225-231.
125. Lee A, Bradford J, Fischer G. Long-term management of adult vulvar lichen sclerosus: a prospective cohort study of 507 women. *JAMA Dermatol.* 2015;151:1061-1067.
126. Corazza M, Borghi A, Minghetti S, et al. Clobetasol propionate vs. mometasone furoate in 1-year proactive maintenance therapy of vulvar lichen sclerosus: results from a comparative trial. *J Eur Acad Dermatol Venereol.* 2016;30:956-961.
127. Kreuter A, Gambichler T, Avermaete A, et al. Low-dose ultraviolet A1 phototherapy for extragenital lichen sclerosus: results of a preliminary study. *J Am Acad Dermatol.* 2002;46:251-255.
128. Kreuter A, Gambichler T. Narrowband UV-B phototherapy for extragenital lichen sclerosus. *Arch Dermatol.* 2007;143:1213.

Chapter 65 :: Psoriatic Arthritis and Reactive Arthritis
:: Ana-Maria Orbai & John A. Flynn

第六十五章
银屑病性关节炎和反应性关节炎

中文导读

银屑病性关节炎（Psoriatic Arthritis，PsA）是一种进行性炎症性肌肉骨骼疾病。本章从流行病学、临床特征、病因学及发病机制、诊断、鉴别诊断、临床进程及预后、管理及预防等各方面阐述了疾病的特征。PsA在全球银屑病患者中均存在诊断不足的问题。本章从伴有PsA的银屑病皮疹特点、关节表现、非皮肤非关节的表现、医疗风险和PsA合并症等角度描述PsA的临床特点。头皮、间擦部位、指甲部位银屑病与PsA相关，皮肤银屑病的严重程度也与PsA的高风险有关。PsA的临床表现是异质性的，不仅包括炎症性关节炎，还包括附着炎、手指炎和脊椎炎。文章描述了各类型关节炎的临床特点及影像学检查特点。PsA的延迟诊断常见，需要皮肤科医生提高警惕性。皮肤科医生的高怀疑指数仍然是检测PsA的关键。早期诊断和治疗可以减低残疾发生，本章列出了根据疾病症状及受累程度选择相关药物及副作用，以及欧洲风湿病联盟（EULAR）和银屑病研究和评估小组（GRAPPA）制定的PsA治疗指南。达标治疗不仅需要关注疾病还需要患者参与日常管理。

反应性关节炎以前被称为Reiter或Fiessinger-Leroy综合征，典型的三种临床表现包括尿道炎症、眼部症状和关节炎，是典型的少关节炎，通常发生在肠道或尿道感染后1~4周。本章从流行病学、临床特征、遗传特点、危险因素、诊断、鉴别诊断、治疗、预后及总结等各方面阐述了该疾病的特征。

〔施　为〕

PSORIATIC ARTHRITIS

AT-A-GLANCE

- Psoriatic arthritis is a progressive inflammatory musculoskeletal disease occurring in about a third of people with psoriasis.
- Psoriatic arthritis is underdiagnosed.
- Clinical presentation is heterogeneous and variably includes the following manifestations: peripheral arthritis, spondyloarthritis (inflammatory arthritis of the spine), enthesitis (inflammation at the insertion sites of ligaments and tendons onto bone), and dactylitis (full-thickness inflammation of digits and toes).
- Associated extramusculoskeletal manifestations in addition to skin and nail psoriasis are inflammatory eye disease and inflammatory bowel disease.
- Several genetic risk factors have been identified for psoriatic arthritis.
- Serology for the rheumatoid factor is usually negative and inflammatory markers may be normal.
- Prompt recognition, pharmacologic treatment, and disease monitoring are necessary to prevent damage and improve long-term outcomes for psoriatic arthritis.

Psoriatic arthritis (PsA) was first linked to psoriasis in 1818 by French dermatologist Jean L. M. Alibert while caring for patients with chronic diseases at Hopital Saint-Louis in Paris. He noticed the association of psoriasis with inflammatory joint disease flares. The first case series was described by French dermatologist Charles Bourdillon in his doctoral thesis in 1888 and included descriptions of the PsA characteristic involvement of the distal interphalangeal joints as well as the disability potentially associated with PsA.[1,2]

Almost a century later, in 1973 John H. M. Moll and Verna Wright characterized PsA in great clinical detail and developed the first classification rule for PsA[3] consisting of inflammatory arthritis compatible with a PsA phenotype, psoriasis, and seronegative status for the rheumatoid factor. Several other classification schemes were developed. The Classification criteria for PsA (CASPAR)[4] are now the most widely accepted and define inclusion of participants in PsA clinical trials (Table 65-1).

Much progress has been made in recent years in understanding PsA pathophysiology through the discovery of specific molecular pathways involved in disease initiation and progression. A number of new targeted pharmacologic treatments have become available in addition to traditional medications.

Early diagnosis and treatment of PsA have been recognized as key to preventing damage and improving function and long-term outcomes. In addition, PsA has a significant association with multiple health risk factors and comorbidities that need to be identified and concomitantly managed.

EPIDEMIOLOGY

PsA prevalence is highly variable depending on the study and the case definition used, and it is estimated to be 0.02% to 0.25% in the general population. PsA occurs most frequently in people with psoriasis, and prevalence estimates in this population range from 3.2% to 41%.[5] PsA is underdiagnosed in people with psoriasis worldwide based on studies from Australia,[6] China,[7] North America, and Europe,[8,9] as well as a systematic literature review and meta-analysis.[10] Prevalence is equal in men and women and unlike psoriasis which has a bimodal incidence, PsA onset is most commonly seen in adulthood with a mean age of onset at 39.2 years.[7]

The annual incidence rate of PsA was 2.7 cases per 100 psoriasis patients (95% confidence interval [CI] 2.1-3.6) in the Toronto cohort.[11] The incidence of PsA mirrors incidence of psoriasis without evidence of change in PsA risk over time for people with psoriasis.[11,12]

Clinical predictors of PsA are nail psoriasis,[7,11,12] severe psoriasis,[7,11] scalp, intergluteal, or perianal psoriasis,[7,12] and the presence of uveitis.[11]

CLINICAL FEATURES

CUTANEOUS FINDINGS

Scalp and intergluteal psoriasis are more likely to be associated with PsA. Severity of skin psoriasis also has been linked to higher PsA risk.[13] Clinical nail disease with a prevalence of 40% in psoriasis is a known risk factor for PsA. In PsA, nail disease prevalence is 80%. Both the nail plate and nail matrix are affected, with nail pitting being the most common.[14] Association of nail psoriasis with distal interphalangeal joint arthritis has been noted since the initial descriptions of PsA. Association of onycholysis with axial PsA has recently been described.[15] Severe psoriasis, nail, scalp, and intergluteal psoriasis should prompt dermatologists to consider PsA when caring for patients with psoriasis (Fig. 65-1).

NONCUTANEOUS FINDINGS

It has recently been recognized that PsA is preceded by nonspecific musculoskeletal and systemic symptoms consisting of joint pain, fatigue, and stiffness in the year prior to diagnosis.[16] This is relevant to dermatologists and primary care physicians caring for patients with psoriasis and should prompt referral to a rheumatologist. The clinical spectrum of PsA musculoskeletal

TABLE 65-1
The Classification Criteria for PsA (CASPAR)

ENTRY CRITERIA: INFLAMMATORY ARTICULAR DISEASE OF THE JOINTS, SPINE, OR ENTHESES

Classification Criteria	Points
1. Psoriasis (mutually exclusive categories for scoring)	
• Current	2 points
• Personal history	1 point
• Family history (first- or second-degree relative)	1 point
2. Nail dystrophy typical of psoriasis (onycholysis, pitting, hyperkeratosis), must be current	1 point
3. Negative rheumatoid factor (any method except latex)	1 point
4. Dactylitis (current, or historical if recorded by a rheumatologist)	1 point
5. Juxtaarticular new bone formation (ill-defined ossification near joint margins excluding osteophytes) on plain hand/feet radiographs	1 point
A classification of PsA is met if the final score is equal to or more than 3 points. Specificity is 98.7% and sensitivity is 91.4% against the criterion standard, which is a diagnosis established by the rheumatologist.	

Adapted from Taylor W, et al. Classification criteria for PsA. *Arthritis Rheum.* 2006;54(8):2665-2673, Table 6, p. 2671.

TABLE 65-2
Psoriatic Arthritis Phenotypes

Oligoarthritis	>70%
Polyarthritis/symmetric	15%
Distal interphalangeal joint predominant	5%
Spondyloarthritis	5%
Arthritis mutilans	5%

ously thought in association with peripheral PsA. Correct quantification of joints affected is important for treating and monitoring PsA. Joint inflammation in PsA is more vascular and less tender than in rheumatoid arthritis, and joint tenderness and swelling each predict subsequent joint damage (Fig. 65-2).[18]

Dactylitis: Dactylitis is full-thickness inflammation of a digit (finger or toe). Acute dactylitis is tender. It has a prevalence of 20% to 59%[19-23] in PsA and is a sign of disease severity associated with radiographic damage.[24,25] Inflammation affects the joints, entheses, and subcutaneous tissues of the digits. Dactylitis assessed with high-resolution MRI is characterized by multiple lesions spanning multiple musculoskeletal structures: diffuse extracapsular soft tissue edema (92%), diffuse or focal increased bone marrow edema (83%), enthesitis at the collateral ligament (75%) and extensor tendon (50%) insertions, flexor tenosynovitis (75%), synovitis (68%), signal intensity changes in the tendon pulleys (fingers), and fibrous sheaths (toes). Dactylitis is one of the criteria scored in the CASPAR classification as a result of its specificity for PsA. In the CASPAR sample, acute dactylitis increased the odds of PsA by 20 (95% CI 5.9-67) whereas historical dactylitis increased the odds for PsA by 5.5 (95% CI 1.8-17) (Fig. 65-3).[4]

Enthesitis: Entheses are anatomical structures formed by tendon, ligament, and joint capsule insertions on bone. They function together with bone and synovium as the synovio-entheseal complex (SEC) to distribute biomechanical stress in musculoskeletal

manifestations is heterogeneous (Table 65-2), encompassing not only inflammatory arthritis but also enthesitis, dactylitis, and spondylitis, all described below.

Arthritis: PsA clinical presentations have been described by Moll and Wright[3] as 5 distinct phenotypes (percentage of patients): oligoarticular (>70%), polyarticular/symmetrical (15%), distal interphalangeal joint predominant (5%), spondyloarthritis (5%), and arthritis mutilans (5%).[3] These phenotypes tend to overlap with cumulative disease duration. For example, the oligoarticular presentation tends to become symmetric over time as more joints become involved.[17] Spondyloarthritis occurs more frequently than previ-

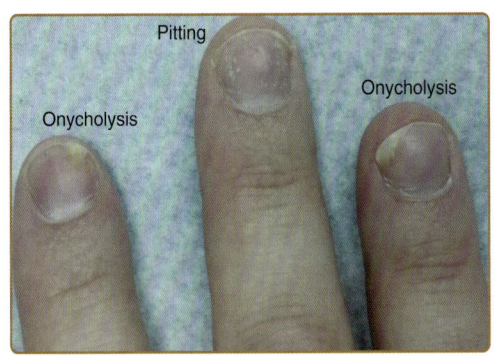

Figure 65-1 Psoriatic nail pitting at the third finger and onycholysis at the index and fourth fingers. Small splinter hemorrhages also can be observed at the index nail.

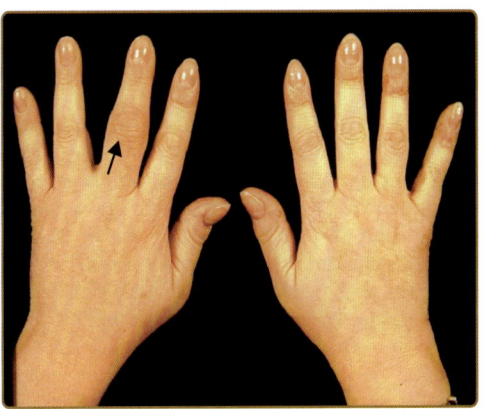

Figure 65-2 Swelling and erythema of the left third metacarpophalangeal joint (*arrow*) indicating inflammatory arthritis in a patient with psoriatic arthritis.

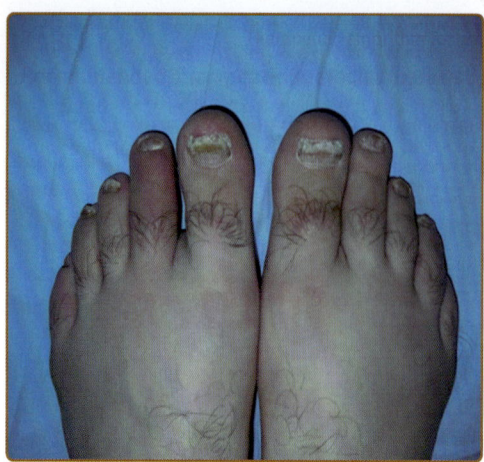

Figure 65-3 Psoriatic nail dystrophy and arthritis of the fifth distal interphalangeal joint in a patient with psoriatic arthritis. (Image used with permission from Dr. Umut Kalyoncu, Division of Rheumatology, Hacettepe University School of Medicine, Ankara, Turkey.)

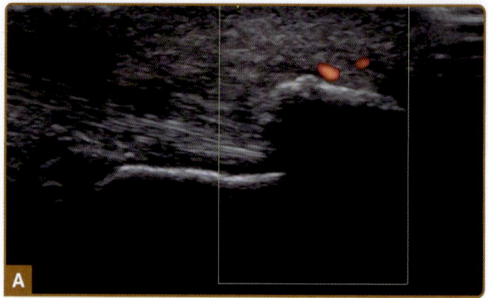

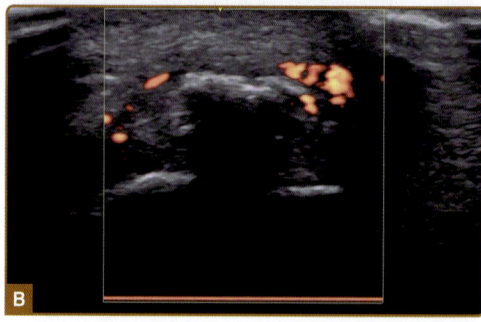

Figure 65-4 **A,** Enthesitis of the Achilles tendon is illustrated on ultrasonograph. Longitudinal tendon microfibers are disrupted. Image inset shows red Doppler signal corresponding to abnormal vascularity secondary to inflammation. **B,** Enthesitis of the Achilles tendon illustrated on ultrasonograph. Inset pictures enthesophyte (light gray with dark shadow) and red Doppler signal corresponding to abnormal vascularity at the entheseal insertion site. (Images used with permission from Dr. Jemima Albayda, Division of Rheumatology, Johns Hopkins University School of Medicine.)

structures.[26,27] Enthesitis is inflammation at entheseal sites and has an important role in PsA pathophysiology, with studies supporting a link between biomechanical damage as the initiating event of autoimmunity in PsA. Clinically, enthesitis is diagnosed as tenderness to pressure at entheseal insertion sites. There are multiple enthesitis indices that differ by the location and number of entheseal sites included in the count. Clinical enthesitis occurs in 35% of people with PsA, with an annual incidence of 0.9%. The most common sites of involvement are the Achilles tendons, plantar fascia, and lateral epicondyles at the elbows (Figs. 65-4, 65-5 and 65-15).[28] Subclinical enthesitis demonstrated with ultrasonography has been shown to exist in a significant proportion of patients (7% to 11%) with psoriasis.[29] In addition, the nail–entheseal complex has been invoked as a mediator of nail psoriasis based on evidence from nail ultrasonographic studies.[30]

Spondyloarthritis: Spondyloarthritis is defined as inflammatory arthritis affecting the axial skeleton leading to spondylitis and/or sacroiliitis. An isolated spondyloarthritis/axial phenotype is rare in PsA and occurs in 2% to 4% of cases. More commonly, axial PsA overlaps with peripheral PsA, and 30% to 40% or people with PsA are affected.[15,21] Risk factors for axial PsA are the presence of onycholysis, inflammatory back pain symptoms, PsA duration/young age at onset, positive HLA-B27, and inflammatory bowel disease. There are significant differences between axial PsA and ankylosing spondylitis (AS), which were explored in several studies. AS is significantly more likely to present with bilateral sacroiliitis, complete ankylosis of the sacroiliac joints, bridging syndesmophytes formed in a caudal to cranial progression, and more severe osteoproliferation than axial PsA.[15,31,32] Axial PsA is more likely to present as isolated spondylitis, manifest with random syndesmophyte formation, isolated involvement of the cervical spine,[32] and although sacroiliitis is also most commonly symmetric it is less likely so than in AS.[15] Axial PsA with isolated spondylitis is about 4 times more likely to be asymptomatic than axial PsA with sacroiliitis (OR 0.26, 95% CI 0.11-0.61, P = .002) (Fig. 65-6).[15]

Noncutaneous Extraarticular Manifestations:

Eye Disease: Eye involvement manifests in a third of people with PsA[33] and about 10% in people with psoriasis.[34] Complications from psoriatic skin inflammation can cause blepharitis and dry eye. In addition, people with PsA may also develop conjunctivitis, uveitis, episcleritis, scleritis, keratoconjunctivitis sicca, and keratitis.[33] Uveitis is defined as inflammation of the iris, ciliary body, or choroid, and prevalence is variably estimated at 7% to 25% in people with PsA.[33,35] This is much less than in AS, where uveitis occurs in about 40%.[34] Uveitis risk is higher in PsA than in psoriasis.[35,36] There are differences in ocular manifestations of uveitis between people with axial versus peripheral PsA. In axial PsA, uveitis is diagnosed at a younger age (mean [standard deviation] 37.9 [9.6] years) than in psoriasis (43.3 [16.5]) and peripheral PsA (48.3 [22.4]), more likely to present in males who are HLA-B27 posi-

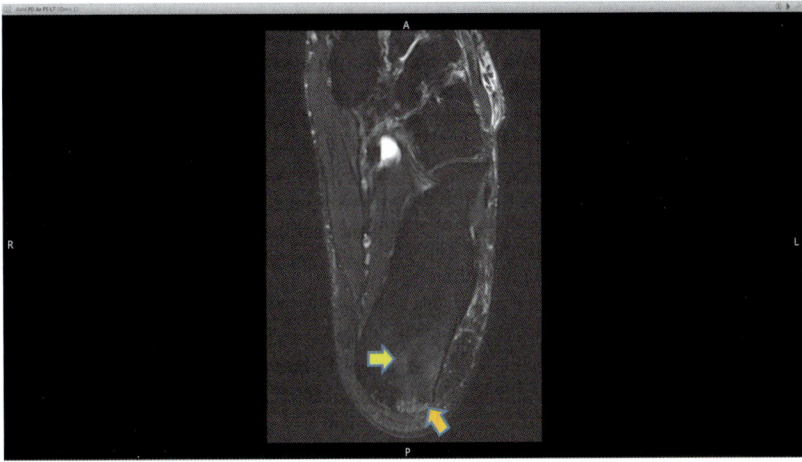

Figure 65-5 Enthesitis of the Achilles tendon demonstrated on MRI.

tive and more likely to involve the anterior segment. In contrast, uveitis in peripheral PsA is more likely to be insidious, bilateral, and to involve the posterior segment.[37] Perhaps because of later diagnosis or increased severity, uveitis in patients with PsA is more likely to lead to ocular complications than in psoriasis (Figs. 65-7 and 65-8).[35]

Inflammatory Bowel Disease: Psoriasis, PsA, and inflammatory bowel disease partially overlap in their genetic determinants, immune effectors, and therapeutics. Risk of inflammatory bowel disease was increased in a Danish nationwide study in psoriasis and PsA versus the general population without psoriatic disease.[38] In the US Nurses' Health Study II (NHS II), women with psoriasis and especially with PsA had an increased risk of incident Crohn disease: relative risk (RR) for Crohn disease in psoriasis 3.86 (95% CI 2.23-6.67) and RR for Crohn disease in PsA 6.43 (95% CI 2.04-20.32).[39] In a case–control study of 15 patients with active psoriasis and PsA but without any GI symptoms versus normal controls, all PsA patients had microscopic colitis with increased lamina propria cellularity and lymphoid aggregates. Additionally, the majority had active inflammation, with polymorphonuclear leukocyte infiltration.[40]

MEDICAL RISK FACTORS AND COMORBIDITIES ASSOCIATED WITH PsA

Cardiovascular risk is increased in people with PsA versus the general population as recently shown in a systematic review and meta-analysis of observational studies. Pooled relative risk for myocardial infarction was 1.57 (95% CI 1.19-2.06), and there was also evidence of increased risk for cerebrovascular events and congestive heart failure.[41] In the Toronto longitudinal cohort study, 1091 PsA patients followed over 35 years had the following independent predictors of cardio-

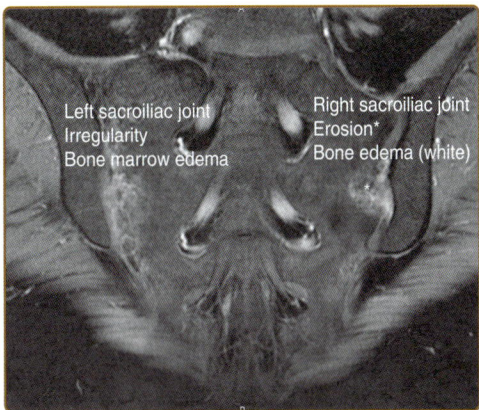

Figure 65-6 Sacroiliitis illustrated on MRI: at the left sacroiliac joint, there is joint space narrowing and irregularity with adjacent subchondral bone marrow edema in the ilium and the sacrum. At the right sacroiliac joint, there is joint space narrowing and an erosion with adjacent subchondral bone marrow edema in the sacrum.

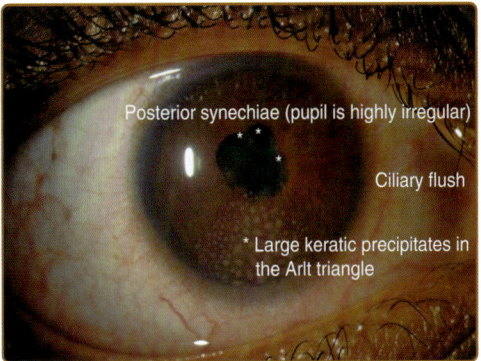

Figure 65-7 Large keratic precipitates in the Arlt's triangle region, mild ciliary flush (conjunctival injection at the limbus), and posterior synechiae (adhesions of the iris to the lens). (Image used with permission from Dr. Bryn Melissa Burkholder, Wilmer Eye Institute, Johns Hopkins University School of Medicine.)

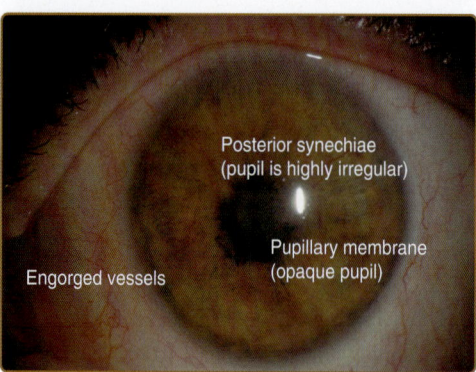

Figure 65-8 HLA-B27-associated uveitis demonstrates extensive posterior synechiae, a pupillary membrane, and engorged iris vessels. (Image used with permission from Dr. Bryn Melissa Burkholder, Wilmer Eye Institute, Johns Hopkins University School of Medicine.)

vascular events in the multivariate analysis: hypertension, diabetes, the number of dactylitis digits, and elevated erythrocyte sedimentation rate—the latter a predictor only in women.[42] The implications of these studies are that cardiovascular risk may be underestimated by taking into account traditional cardiovascular risk factors only, and that PsA activity may need to be considered as an independent predictor. Current recommendations state to control disease activity to lower cardiovascular risk in rheumatoid arthritis as well as PsA and AS.[43] However, evidence for psoriasis and PsA treatment specific effects on cardiovascular risk is inconclusive as of this writing.

In addition to cardiovascular disease, obesity, type 2 diabetes mellitus, nonalcoholic fatty liver disease, and the metabolic syndrome are all increased in people with PsA versus the general population. These potential comorbidities are relevant for PsA disease activity and treatment and should be taken into account for a comprehensive management of patients with PsA.[44] An important link between obesity and PsA disease activity has been identified in several studies. Overweight and obese patients are less likely to achieve minimal disease activity compared to PsA patients with normal weight in 2 independent cohort studies.[45,46] Furthermore, overweight and obese patients who lost 5% or more of their body weight were more likely to achieve minimal disease activity on tumor necrosis factor (TNF) inhibitor therapy compared to controls that did not lose weight.[47]

ETIOLOGY AND PATHOGENESIS

GENETICS

Moll and Wright were the first to study PsA heritability in families with PsA (including 253 first-degree relatives of 88 PsA probands) and concluded that prevalence of PsA in first-degree relatives is 5.5%.[48] This translates to a PsA risk around 100 times higher in first-degree relatives than the general population, suggesting a strong genetic component for the disease. As of this writing, HLA-B27 has the strongest evidence for being a genetic risk factor for PsA in people with psoriasis.[49,50] HLA-B27 haplotypes also hold prognostic value through association with disease characteristics: PsA onset within 1 year from psoriasis diagnosis, axial PsA, enthesitis, dactylitis, and uveitis.[33,49,50] However, HLA-B27 prevalence in PsA is 19% to 35%, supporting the notion that PsA heritability is multifactorial.

Additional HLA-independent genetic risk factors specific for PsA (vs psoriasis) have been discovered and confirmed in the past few years using genomewide association studies. These additional PsA-specific susceptibility genes are located as follows: upstream of *IL23R* gene on chromosome 1,[51,52] in the *PTPN22* gene on chromosome 1,[53] the 5q31 locus,[54] and upstream of *TNFAIP3* on chromosome 6.[51] Interestingly, susceptibility loci for both psoriasis and PsA have been confirmed within the *IL23R* and *TNFAIP3* genes, whereas the signals upstream of these genes represent PsA-specific variants.[51] PTPN22 encodes a lymphoid-specific intracellular phosphatase involved in T-cell signaling pathways and has been associated with rheumatoid arthritis, type 1 diabetes, systemic lupus erythematosus, and Grave disease, whereas the 5q31 locus is common to inflammatory bowel disease, juvenile idiopathic arthritis, and asthma.

We are now beginning to discern genetic susceptibilities specific to PsA versus psoriasis that support the existence of differences in pathophysiology inferred from clinical experience, tissue studies, and differential response to targeted therapeutics. PsA susceptibility genes encode multiple immune functions from antigen presentation and processing to innate and adaptive immunity pathways. In addition to genetic susceptibility and possibly other host factors, environmental factors must also play a role in determining the significant heterogeneity observed in PsA expression among individuals.

RISK FACTORS

Implicit to the PsA case definition, people with psoriasis represent the population at greatest risk for developing PsA. Several risk factors associated with developing PsA have been identified in people with psoriasis: psoriasis type/location such as scalp and intergluteal, psoriasis severity, psoriatic nail disease, positive HLA-B27,[13] and uveitis.[11] In addition to these clinical factors, the following environmental and individual factors increase the risk of PsA: physical trauma, smoking, overweight, and obese physique.[55] Increased weight has been recognized as a risk factor for incident PsA in several population studies. In the U.S. NHS II, incident PsA relative risk in overweight and obese versus ideal BMI range was RR 1.83 (95% CI 1.15-2.89) for BMI 25 to 29.9, RR 3.12 (95% CI 1.9-5.11) for BMI 30 to 34.9, and RR 6.46 (95% CI 4.11-10.16) for BMI greater than 35.[56] In the UK Health Improvement Network study, PsA risk in people with psoriasis who were obese versus normal weight was RR 1.22 (95% CI 1.02-1.47) for BMI 30 to 34.9 and RR 1.48 (95% CI 1.2-1.81) for BMI greater than 35.[57] Smoking was a factor increasing the relative risk of incident PsA versus nonsmokers in U.S. women NHS II participants with an RR 3.13 (95% CI 2.08-4.71), a dose–response relationship for smoking duration and pack-years, as well as an association between smoking and higher disease severity.[58] Congruently, smoking has been shown to be associated with poor PsA functional outcome in the Bath longitudinal cohort.[59] However, in the Toronto cohort, findings were divergent and current smoking status versus lifetime nonsmoker status was associated with lower odds of incident PsA.[60]

PATHOGENESIS

PsA is associated with genetic risk factors encoding immune system functions that include antigen presentation (MHC class I alleles, especially HLA-B27 for PsA), antigen processing, and innate and adaptive immune responses. Central to innate immunity in both psoriasis and PsA is TNF-induced NF-kB signaling with transcription of inflammatory mediators.[61] Adaptive immune system responses are characterized by selective transcription of mediators favoring Th1 and Th17 cells: IL12/Tbet signaling leading to Th1 cell differentiation and proliferation; and RORγt signaling in the presence of IL23 leading to Th17 cell differentiation and proliferation.[62,63] The agent precipitating the cascade of immune events leading to PsA phenotypes is currently unknown, and therefore alternate hypothesis have been sought. The biomechanical stress/synovio-entheseal complex (SEC) hypothesis connects damage at entheseal insertion sites in the presence of a genetically susceptible background with erroneous tissue repair responses and self-propagating inflammation leading to PsA.[26,27] This model posits that micro-damaged entheses release local tissue factors that in turn couple with pattern recognition molecules and activate the innate immune system. These events are followed by aberrant adaptive immune responses central to the pathophysiology of the disease. In mouse models of PsA, innate IL23 responsive cells localized at the entheseal bone interface were inducible (with IL23 stimulation) to express IL22, which promoted entheseal inflammation and periosteal new bone formation through STAT3 phosphorylation and signaling.[63,64] The SEC hypothesis corresponds with the fact that as of this writing no specific autoantigens have been identified in PsA.

Comparatively, in psoriasis there are protein targets that have been hypothesized to catalyze initiation of immune system responses in the skin. Cathelicidin LL37 complexed with damaged keratinocyte DNA has long been postulated as the initiator of psoriatic inflammation via toll-like receptor 9 in the presence of damaged skin. This leads to interferon-α, which together with TNF-α, IL-1β, and IL-6 stimulate dermal dendritic cells to migrate to lymphoid organs and stimulate Th1 and Th17 cell differentiation.[65] Just recently, an autoantigen was discovered and shown to trigger psoriasis-specific cytokines in the skin supporting the exciting hypothesis that psoriasis is an autoimmune disease. The melanocyte-derived protein ADAMTSL5 was shown to mediate MHC class I–dependent CD8+ T-cell activation in the skin, leading to overproduction of IL-17—the signature cytokine of psoriatic lesions.[66]

DIAGNOSIS

EARLY PsA

It is increasingly recognized that delaying rheumatologic care in PsA is linked not only to suffering but also to long-term joint damage and disability. Current estimates from research studies have shown that delay in diagnosis of 6 months or more versus less than 6 months are linked to significantly more disability in people with PsA.[59,67] Furthermore, associated manifestations (lower extremity arthritis, uveitis, sacroiliitis, enthesitis, inflammatory bowel disease, etc.), and health risk factors (cardiovascular disease, hypertension, metabolic syndrome, liver disease) in individuals with PsA are underrecognized and undertreated without a specialist's care, compromising chances of improved patient outcomes.[44] There is increased interest in screening for early PsA, with dermatology clinics representing the ideal setting. Several PsA screening questionnaires have been validated in patients with psoriasis, and a positive score should prompt referral to a rheumatologist (Table 65-3).

Unfortunately, screening questionnaires may miss a significant proportion of PsA patients, close to 30%, because of best performance of these questionnaires in the polyarticular PsA pattern and therefore dermatologists' high index of suspicion remains key for detecting PsA.[9] Recent findings that a diagnosis of PsA is preceded by stiffness, fatigue and joint pain support implementation of screening procedures and keeping a high index of suspicion for PsA in the psoriasis patient population.[16]

PsA CLASSIFICATION

The CASPAR criteria (Table 65-1) are used for classification of PsA and participant inclusion in PsA clinical trials. Even after meeting CASPAR criteria patients with PsA represent a highly heterogeneous clinical population. The involvement of a rheumatologist early in the PsA course is essential. To diagnose PsA, several clinical indicators in people with psoriasis are helpful, as outlined in the discussion above on risk factors for PsA. Laboratory tests for rheumatoid factor and anticyclic citrullinated peptides (anti-CCP) are important to exclude rheumatoid arthritis. Genotyping for HLA-B27 has clinical and prognostic value because

TABLE 65-3
PsA Screening Tools for People with Psoriasis

QUESTIONNAIRES	PASE[a]	TOPAS[b]	TOPAS2	PEST[c]	EARP[d]
Target population	Psoriasis	Psoriasis and general population	Psoriasis and general population	Psoriasis	Psoriasis
Domains	Symptom and function subscales	Skin, joint, nail	Skin, joint, nail, spine	Joint, nail, enthesitis, dactylitis	Joint, antiinflammatories, low back pain, stiffness, dactylitis, enthesitis
Number of items	15	12	13	5	10
Feasibility completion, min, mean (SD)	4-6	NR	NR	NR	2 (1.5)
Feasibility scoring, min	1 	NR Weighted sum	NR Weighted sum	NR Simple sum	NR Simple sum
Reliability, (ICC)	0.9	NR	NR	NR	NR
Internal consistency Cronbach's alpha	NR	NR	NR	NR	0.83
Sensitivity % (95% CI)	82 (57-96)	86.8	87.2 92	92	85.2
Specificity, % (95% CI)	73 (59-84)	93.1	82.7 77.2	78	91.6
Score range	15-75	0-12	0-12	0-5	0-10
Value of cut-off score suggestive of PsA	≥47 ≥44	≥8	≥7 ≥8	≥3	≥3

[a]PsA Screening and Evaluation.[68,69]
[b]Toronto PsA Screen.[70]
[c]Psoriasis Epidemiology Screening Tool.
[d]The Early PsA Screening Questionnaire.[71]
NR, not reported.

HLA-B27-positive individuals are at higher risk for early PsA, axial PsA, severe enthesitis, and uveitis. Radiographs are recommended to evaluate PsA characteristic joint damage such as juxta-articular bone erosions and new bone formation. These may also show enthesophytes at sites of prior entheseal trauma or inflammation. For capturing disease activity, imaging techniques that can distinguish tissue edema and vascularization are needed. These are musculoskeletal ultrasonography and MRI. Images of power Doppler signal for enthesitis are presented in Figs. 65-5, and MRI showing enthesitis, enthesophyte, and bone marrow edema are represented in Fig. 65-6.

DIFFERENTIAL DIAGNOSIS

Other types of inflammatory arthritis that can co-occur with psoriasis should be considered (please see diagnostic algorithm in Fig. 65-9). Rheumatoid arthritis is usually positive for the rheumatoid factor or anti-CCP. Reactive arthritis is more likely to occur after a GI or sexually transmitted infection (see section "Reactive Arthritis"). Gout is more common in people with psoriasis than in the general population likely due to increased skin turnover and increased association with cardiovascular comorbidities and medications used to treat them. The most common differential diagnosis may be osteoarthritis (OA) because of its high prevalence and overlapping predilection for a similar patient population in terms of comorbidities. OA is usually less inflammatory than PsA, worsening with activities and at the end of the day, and lacking PsA-specific manifestations like dactylitis, enthesitis, and/or spondylitis. In the subset of patients with erosive OA, differentiation may be difficult and needs to be determined by the treating rheumatologist while considering additional clinical, laboratory, and imaging characteristics. Techniques such as musculoskeletal ultrasonography and MRI may be useful to make the distinction.

CLINICAL COURSE AND PROGNOSIS

Delayed PsA diagnosis and effective treatment are associated with disability and radiographic damage. There is a window of opportunity of about 6 months to initiate therapy to maximize chances of minimal disease damage.

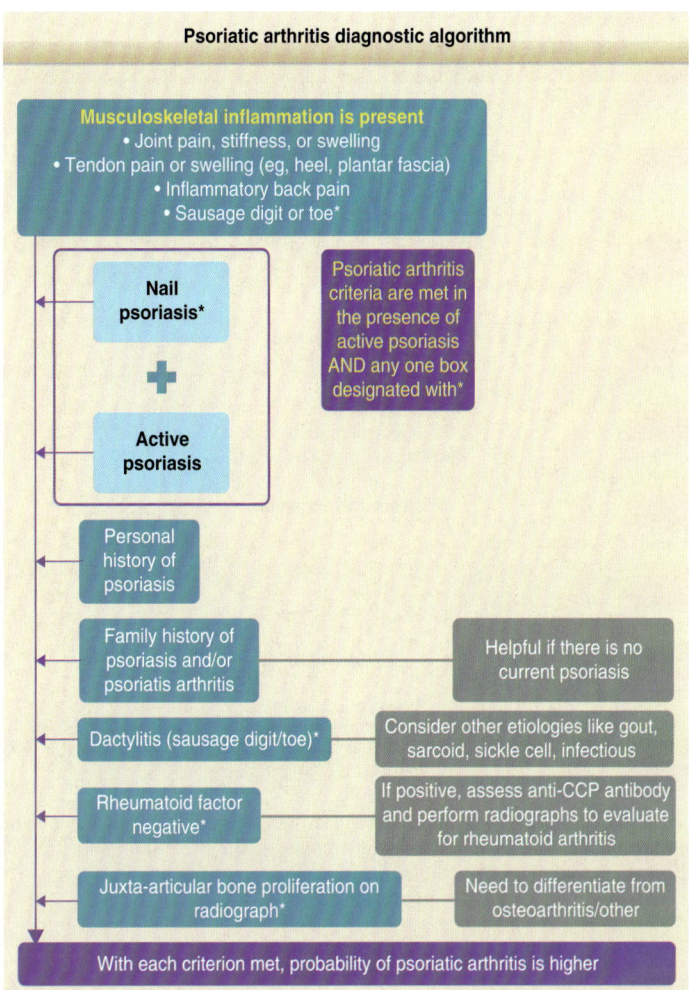

Figure 65-9 Psoriatic arthritis (PsA) diagnostic algorithm.

Multiple new therapeutic agents have been approved in PsA in the past 5 years. These therapeutics showed efficacy in decreasing PsA disease activity, slowing damage progression and improving fatigue and additional patient health outcomes.[72] There is now evidence that disease-modifying treatment for PsA is effective for controlling disease activity and decreasing work disability in PsA.[73]

MANAGEMENT

The highest quality evidence underlying PsA management is extrapolated based on the efficacy of therapeutic interventions in PsA randomized controlled trials. However, PsA is a complex disease with multiple pathophysiologic manifestations and broad life impact, as well as significant heterogeneity among individuals. Although as of this writing is has been difficult to capture individual heterogeneity in clinical trials, advances in the science of outcome measurement are making this increasingly possible. To this end, the core set of PsA outcomes to be measured in upcoming PsA clinical trials has recently been updated to reflect PsA manifestations and both patients' and physicians' priorities (Fig. 65-10).[74] In addition to comprehensive assessment of pathophysiologic manifestations like musculoskeletal and skin disease activity, fatigue is now included as a mandatory outcome, whereas additional patient relevant aspects such as participation in daily life activities (according the International Classification of Functioning definition, participation is the ability to be involved in life, to perform societal tasks and responsibilities, to work, and to take part in social events, leisure and family life) and emotional well-being are strongly recommended to be measured in clinical trials. As these outcomes begin to be systematically measured and reported, information on treatment efficacy for multiple aspects of PsA will become more complete and helpful for decision making in clinical care.

Current treatment recommendations for PsA mandate beginning treatment according to the clinical phenotype and assessing disease activity every 3 months

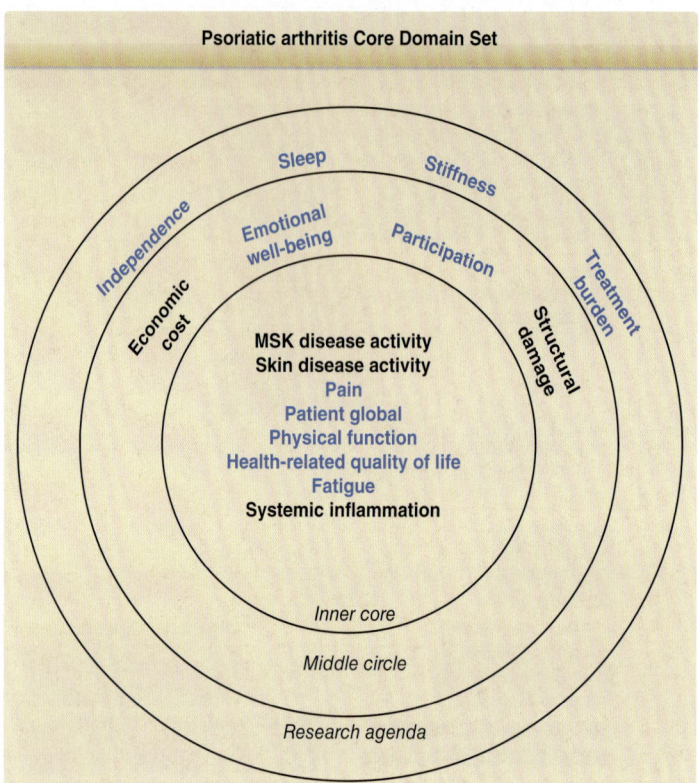

Figure 65-10 Psoriatic arthritis (PsA) Core Domain Set to be measured in PsA clinical trials and longitudinal observational studies. Blue font represents patient reported outcomes. (Reproduced with permission from BMJ Publishing Group Ltd: Orbai AM, et al. *Ann Rheum Dis*. 2017;76(4):673-680, Fig. 3.)

at least in the beginning or until the treatment target is achieved. The goal of therapy is to achieve minimal or low disease activity and escalating therapy until this goal is achieved as standard of care.[72] However, in a recent U.S. national survey of psoriasis and PsA, among patients reporting high disease burden, only 10% with psoriasis and only 25% with PsA reported treatment with biologics.[75]

PsA treatment guideline sets have been updated in 2015-2016.[76] The disease-modifying antirheumatic drugs (DMARDs) methotrexate, sulfasalazine, and leflunomide (Table 65-4) are generally recommended as first-line agents. Antimalarials (hydroxychloroquine) are not used in PsA because of the potential for worsening or precipitating development of psoriasis. Methotrexate is approved for treating psoriasis and is being used off-label in the United States to treat PsA based on data extrapolated from rheumatoid arthritis and clinical practice. The MIPA randomized controlled trial (RCT) of methotrexate versus placebo for PsA[77] showed numerical benefit but no significant treatment effect difference between methotrexate and placebo groups; however, the RCT used a low target methotrexate dose (15 mg/wk) and had a high dropout rate (30%). In the Toronto longitudinal cohort methotrexate >15 mg/wk versus 15 mg/wk or lower improved disease activity and slowed damage progression, suggesting a benefit for methotrexate doses above 15 mg/wk.[78] However, experts still question the utility of methotrexate as a disease-modifying drug in PsA as it has not been consistently linked to comprehensive long-term patient outcomes such as PsA-specific manifestations or slowing damage progression, improving quality of life for patients, and reducing comorbidities. As an adjunct to biologic therapy, infliximab methotrexate in particular, not only prevented the formation of antiinfliximab antibodies but also increased efficacy.[79] Methotrexate can cause mucosal ulcerations and an oral exam should be part of any routine rheumatologic examination. Kidney function is an important consideration with methotrexate dosing. Daily folic acid supplementation is recommended with both sulfasalazine and methotrexate.

Sulfasalazine has been shown to improve psoriatic joint swelling with no effect on psoriasis or enthesitis. Sulfasalazine is the preferred DMARD in peripheral spondyloarthritis considering risk and benefits in individual patients.

Leflunomide is effective for both psoriasis and PsA with mild to moderate improvements.[80] Hepatic toxicity and the risk of anemia need to be considered during

TABLE 65-4
Medications

	PSORIATIC DISEASE SPECIFIC INDICATIONS							
	CUTANEOUS		MUSCULOSKELETAL					
DRUG	SKIN	NAIL	ARTHRITIS	DACTYLITIS	ENTHESITIS	AXIAL SPONDYLOARTHRITIS	OTHER	SIDE EFFECTS AND SPECIAL CONSIDERATIONS
methotrexate	+		+					Risk of mucosal ulcerations, hepatotoxicity, teratogenic. Liver function tests, blood counts and renal function need to be monitored. Folic acid 1 mg daily mandatory for the duration of methotrexate therapy
Sulfasalazine			+					Monitor liver function, blood counts. Reversible azoorspermia. Folic acid supplementation indicated
Leflunomide	+		+					Risk of hepatotoxicity, teratogenic. Monitor liver function, blood counts. Long half-life, stores in adipose tissue.
Etanercept	+	+	+			+		Drug induced SLE, Demyelinating disease, CHF, cancer
Infliximab	+	+	+	+	+	+	+uveitis +IBD	
Adalimumab	+	+	+	+[d]	+[d]	+	+uveitis +IBD	
Certolizumab	+	+	+	+	+	+	+IBD [Crohn disease]	
Golimumab	+	+	+	+	+	+	+IBD [Ulcerative colitis]	
Apremilast	+	+	+	+[d]	+[d]			Weight loss (10%). Depression (1%)
Ustekinumab	+	+	+	+[d]	+[d]		+IBD [Crohn disease]	Increased risk of eosinophilic pneumonia, cancer
Secukinumab	+	+	+	+	+	+		Increased risk of candidiasis, exacerbation of IBD
Ixekizumab	+	+	+		+[d]			Increased risk of candidiasis, exacerbation of IBD, neutropenia
Tofacitinib	+	+	+	+[d]	+[d]		+IBD [Ulcerative colitis]	Increased risk of elevated LDL and HDL (10-19%), pulmonary embolism, herpes zoster, neutropenia, lymphopenia, GI perforation, cancer
Abatacept			+					Chronic obstructive pulmonary disease exacerbation, cancer

[a]Eye disease, Inflammatory bowel disease.
[b]First line agents in the treatment of PsA.
[c]First line biologic agents; first line treatments for enthesitis, spondyloarthritis PsA.
[d]Efficacy not reproduced in some trials.
PsA, psoriatic arthritis; IBD, inflammatory bowel disease.

use of traditional synthetic disease-modifying drugs and therapy monitored with serial liver function tests and complete blood counts, particularly in the beginning of therapy and regularly thereafter.

Apremilast, a selective inhibitor of the enzyme phosphodiesterase 4 (PDE4), is a targeted synthetic disease-modifying medication with moderate effects for PsA for skin, nails, arthritis, enthesitis, dactylitis, as well as patient-reported outcomes including physical function. Long-term structural damage data are currently lacking for this medication. Side-effect profile is favorable; however, a 1% risk of depression has been observed and needs to be considered in this patient population.

In some patients, it is difficult to achieve current treatment targets with classical synthetic DMARDs even in combination, and side effects can be severe for patients.[81] However, in the era of multiple targeted therapies for PsA and psoriasis, disease remission is possible more than ever before. TNF inhibitors (adalimumab, certolizumab, golimumab, etanercept, infliximab) are generally the first-line biologic agents and have been used for PsA for almost 2 decades. They have excellent efficacy for all PsA pathophysiologic manifestations including skin disease, arthritis, dactylitis, enthesitis, spondylitis, and nail disease. Adalimumab and infliximab are also effective for PsA-associated manifestations of uveitis and inflammatory bowel disease (it should be noted that certolizumab is also effective for Crohn disease, whereas golimumab is effective for ulcerative colitis). These agents are first-line treatment for enthesitis and axial PsA, where classical synthetic disease-modifying drugs will not help. There are no head-to-head trials of TNF inhibitors in PsA, and these are prescribed taking into account the patient's context and potential additional indications or risks.

Ustekinumab, an inhibitor of the common p40 subunit of both IL12 and IL23, is approved for the treatment of psoriasis and PsA. In psoriasis, it is labeled for people who are candidates for phototherapy or systemic therapy. Ustekinumab is also approved for Crohn disease in people who failed TNF inhibitors.

IL17 inhibitors are the most efficacious medication class approved as of this writing for psoriasis. Secukinumab and ixekizumab are both IL17 inhibitors. Secukinumab is labeled for PsA and AS, in addition to psoriasis. Ixekizumab is approved for psoriasis and psoriatic arthritis and is being evaluated in phase III clinical trials for AS. Tofacitinib, a jak/stat inhibitor was recently labeled for psoriatic arthritis and ulcerative colitis. Abatacept, an anti-T cell therapy/CTLA4 inhibitor was labeled for psoriatic arthritis. For both these therapies, efficacy for psoriasis has not met primary endpoints in clinical trials.

NEW MOLECULES

Additional molecules are under study with 3 IL23 inhibitors currently in various clinical trial stages. Guselkumab is an IgG1 antibody binding the p19 subunit specific to IL23. This is being evaluated in 3 Phase III studies for psoriasis, and results are awaited. Tildrakizumab is another IL23 monoclonal antibody currently in Phase III psoriasis studies. Risankizumab is a third compound in the IL23/p19 inhibitor family and also currently in Phase III psoriasis clinical trials.

Additional JAK pathway inhibitors are being developed. Upadacitinib is a JAK inhibitor in phase III clinical trials in psoriatic arthritis.

There are also additional IL17 inhibitors being developed with one of them, bimekizumab, currently in phase III clinical trials.

An additional immunologic target being evaluated in psoriasis/PsA is RORγt, a transcription factor on which IL17 production is dependent.

TREATMENT ALGORITHM

The European League against Rheumatism (EULAR) and the Group for Research and Assessment of Psoriasis and PsA (GRAPPA) have both designed treatment guidelines for PsA (Fig. 65-11).[76] The underlying principles of these guidelines are tight control of PsA inflammation until a status of PsA minimal disease activity or PsA remission is reached. Regular assessment is required ideally every 3 months and at least every 6 months to assess PsA disease activity and tailor therapy to target.

The treatment algorithm starts with initiation of DMARDs followed by biologic medications with TNF inhibitors as first-line biologics. It should be noted that in the case of enthesitis or spondylitis, the first-line medication becomes a TNF inhibitor as DMARDs are not effective for these manifestations. Second-line biologics are interleukin 12/23 inhibitors (IL12/23i, ustekinumab), which are highly effective for skin disease, followed by arthritis, enthesitis, dactylitis, and inflammatory back pain symptoms. Ustekinumab is also U.S. FDA–approved for Crohn inflammatory bowel disease. Interleukin 17 (IL17) inhibitors have the highest efficacy of any approved PsA medication as of this writing for psoriasis, and one is approved for AS. IL17i are also effective for arthritis, dactylitis, enthesitis, and psoriatic nail disease. There is a concern for worsening inflammatory bowel disease with IL17 inhibitors and that aspect is currently under study. There are no data on efficacy of IL12/23 and IL17 inhibitors for uveitis.

The GRAPPA treatment guideline requires systematic PsA assessments for all pathophysiologic domains potentially affected, including arthritis, dactylitis, enthesitis, spondylitis, skin psoriasis, and nail psoriasis. Treatment is adjusted at every assessment to cover most efficiently all disease manifestations, considering each patient's individual health context.[72]

PREVENTION/SCREENING

Prevention of PsA is an area worthy of further exploration. The population at risk, people with psoriasis, is well defined, and there is considerable overlap

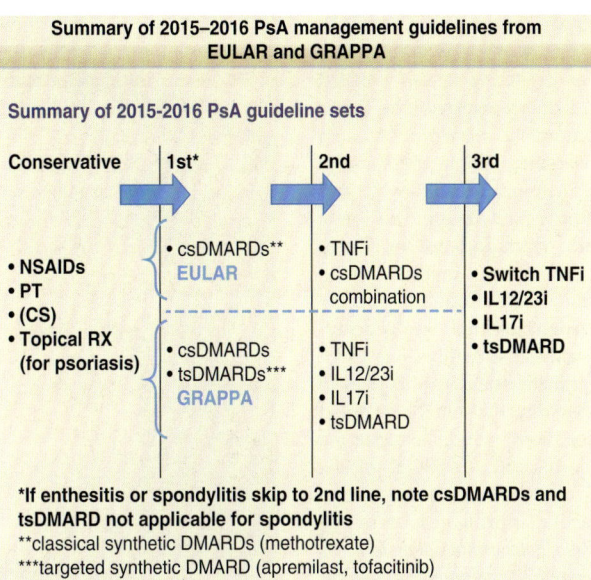

Figure 65-11 Summary of 2015-2016 PsA management guidelines from EULAR and GRAPPA. NSAIDs, Nonsteroidal anti-inflammatory drugs; PT, physical therapy; CS, corticosteroid injections recommended with caution; DMARD, disease-modifying antirheumatic drug; TNFi, tumor necrosis factor inhibitor; IL12/23i, interleukin 12/23 inhibitor; IL17i, interleukin 17 inhibitor. [a]If enthesitis or spondylitis skip to second line, note csDMARDs not applicable for enthesitis and tsDMARD not applicable for spondylitis. [b]Classical synthetic DMARDs (methotrexate, sulfasalazine, or leflunomide). [c]Targeted synthetic DMARD (apremilast). Dashed arrows designate less stringent concept of first- and second-line agents, with the algorithm being tailored to as many affected pathophysiologic domains as possible with the simplest regimen and the patients' individual health context.

between psoriasis and PsA treatment. However, it is unknown if biologic treatments in psoriasis prevent PsA onset. This seems unlikely given the need for chronic treatment and high rate of PsA relapse with discontinuation of therapy even for people in remission. Because both skin and joint disease require monitoring to ensure achievement of treatment targets, it is highly recommended that musculoskeletal symptoms be assessed and monitored on therapy by a rheumatologist for best patient outcomes. Prevention and modification of known personal and environmental risk factors for PsA (smoking, obesity, and physical trauma) have a plausible role in preventing or delaying PsA onset.

There is increased focus on the importance of early diagnosis of PsA.[13] It was recently described in a PsA inception cohort that musculoskeletal pain, fatigue, and stiffness preceded PsA onset by several months. It is therefore important that high-risk psoriasis patients be quickly referred to rheumatologists for diagnostic evaluation for PsA[16] so they can commence treatment and monitoring. PsA screening questionnaires attempt to capture people with psoriasis and those with a high probability of inflammatory musculoskeletal disease. These are easy to administer in the waiting room (Table 65-3). Probing for musculoskeletal symptoms during the dermatology visit could help close the gap of undiagnosed PsA in people with psoriasis.

REACTIVE ARTHRITIS

AT-A-GLANCE

- Reactive arthritis is typically an oligoarthritis that develops 1 to 4 weeks following an enteric or urethral infection.
- Inciting infections agents include *Chlamydia trachomatis*, *Yersinia*, *Shigella*, *Salmonella*, *Campylobacter*, *Clostridium difficile*, and *Escherichia coli*.
- It is classified as a spondyloarthritis, with common clinical features including arthritis of the spine and sacroiliac joints, enthesitis, dactylitis, and the absence of serologies associated with rheumatoid arthritis.
- Cutaneous manifestations include keratoderma blenorrhagicum, circinate balanitis, aphthous ulcers, and nail changes.
- Associated extramusculoskeletal manifestations in addition to cutaneous findings include inflammatory eye and cardiac disease.
- The HLA-B27 haplotype appears to be a risk factor and is associated with a more chronic prognosis.
- Although reactive arthritis often is self-limited in weeks to months, as much as a third of patients may develop chronic disease.

INTRODUCTION

Reactive arthritis (ReA), formerly referred to as Reiter or Fiessinger–Leroy syndrome, along with PsA, is an inflammatory arthritis classified within the spondyloarthritis (SpA) family.[82,83] SpA also includes AS and the arthritis of inflammatory bowel disease. The classic triad of symptoms in ReA, which does not develop in the majority of patients, encompasses urethral, ocular, and articular inflammation. This inflammation occurs as a reaction to an antecedent infection and is generally self-limited. Within articular structures, it is a separate entity from septic arthritis due to the inability to recover any infectious agent directly from the inflamed joints. Cutaneous manifestations include keratoderma blenorrhagicum, circinate balanitis, aphthous ulcers, and nail changes. The infectious agents most commonly implicated in reactive arthritis include the GI pathogens (*Yersinia*, *Shigella*, *Salmonella*, *Campylobacter*, and *Clostridium difficile*) as well as venereal urogenital infection (*Chlamydia trachomatis*).

EPIDEMIOLOGY

The lack of consensus and standardization of the diagnostic criteria for reactive arthritis makes epidemiologic studies challenging. The post-venereal urogenital type typically presents in younger adults in their third to fifth decade of life where there is a male predominance. Studies have suggested that up to 8% of patients with chlamydial infections may develop a subsequent reactive arthritis.[84] Unlike enteric infections that are nearly always symptomatic, urogenital infections may be asymptomatic in the majority of patients. Most epidemiologic studies of reactive arthritis are in the setting of infection by enteric pathogens. In outbreaks of enteric infection due to food contamination, up to 20% of patients have developed articular symptoms. The overall prevalence is estimated at 20 to 40 per 100,000, with a yearly incidence of 25 per 100,000.[85]

CLINICAL FEATURES

One to 4 weeks following the triggering infection, the patent will develop an oligoarthritis (2 to 4 joints) that is asymmetric.[86] The predominant symptom in patients with enteric infection is diarrhea, which can be bloody. With urogenital infections, the patient may describe dysuria with a purulent urethral discharge or may be without symptoms. The classic triad of urethral, ocular, and articular inflammation is rarely present together. Although it is felt that the majority of patients with reactive arthritis have a self-limited course, a significant portion can have symptoms extending beyond 6 months at which point they are considered as having chronic ReA.

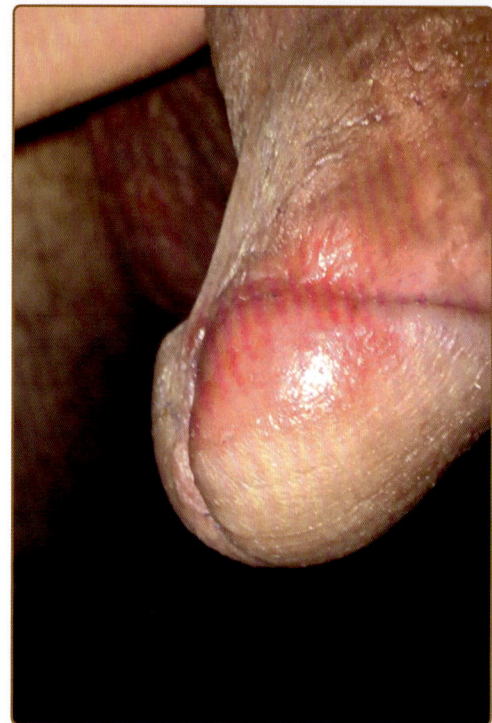

Figure 65-12 Circinate balanitis.

CUTANEOUS

Several cutaneous manifestations are seen in ReA. Circinate balanitis is the inflammatory skin lesion that develops on the shaft or glans of the penis and more rarely on the scrotum (Figs. 65-12 and 65-13). This erythematous lesion can be both papular and pustular and develop raised borders around the meatus. In an uncircumcised patient, identification of the lesion will require retraction of the foreskin where the lesions are moist and generally painless. In a circumcised patient, the lesions may harden to a hyperkeratotic dry crust resembling a psoriatic plaque that can be painful

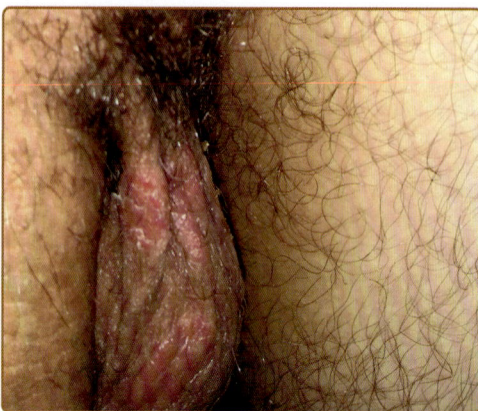

Figure 65-13 Scrotal involvement.

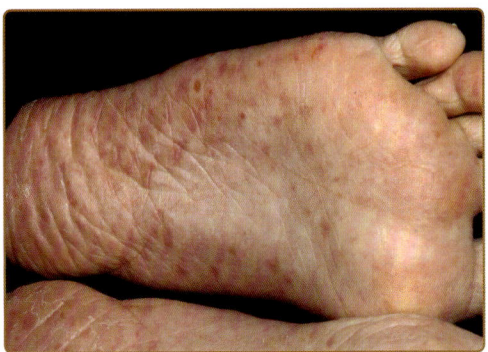

Figure 65-14 Keratoderma blenorrhagicum.

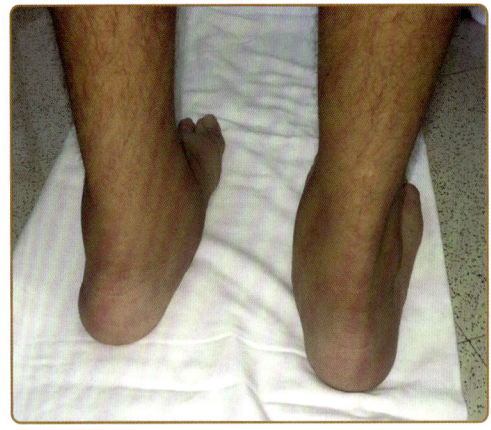

Figure 65-15 Enthesitis of left Achilles tendon ("Lover's heel").

with subsequent scarring. Rarely, female patients can develop erythematous vulvar ulcerative lesions.

Keratoderma blenorrhagicum resembles a pustular psoriasis and is generally found on the palms and soles. Initially it is an erythematous vesicular lesion that develops into pustular keratotic lesions before coalescing into psoriatic-like plaques. These skin lesions occur in 10% to 30% of cases and sometimes be seen in other parts of the body (Fig. 65-14).

A typically self-limited stomatitis may rarely develop. This is characterized by superficial ulcerations or erythematous grayish plaques involving the buccal mucosa, palate, and tongue. These are painless, though they may bleed.

Psoriatic-like nail lesions may develop with subungual accumulation of debris and potential abscess formation. Onycholysis, nail pitting, transverse ridging, or periungual scaling can be seen in the minority of patients.

MUSCULOSKELETAL

The typical pattern of joint involvement is an asymmetric peripheral oligoarthritis that may also involve the axial skeleton with the symptoms of inflammatory back and buttock pain.[87] These axial symptoms manifest with spinal stiffness and pain early in the morning and after periods of prolonged rest, as a result of inflammation involving the spine and sacroiliac joints. The lumbar spine is more frequently involved than the cervical and thoracic spine. Although an oligoarthritis in the lower extremities is the most common pattern of peripheral joint involvement, there also may be a monoarticular or polyarticular presentation.

ENTHESITIS

As described in PsA, enthesitis includes inflammation of tendons, fascia, and ligaments with a predilection for where these structures insert onto bone. This is a common finding in all forms of spondyloarthritis. In ReA, swelling and discomfort of the heel ("Lover's heel") results from Achilles tendon involvement (Fig. 65-15). With inflammation of the plantar fascial insertion site, patients will describe the early morning posterior foot when first getting out of bed.

DACTYLITIS

As described above, this is the result of enthesitis involving the toes and fingers leading to a diffuse swelling of the entire digit, sometimes referred to as a "sausage digit." Seen predominately in SpA, this also has been described in sarcoidosis and polyarticular gout.[88]

OCULAR

Although the original description of ReA included conjunctivitis, other forms of inflammatory eye disease can develop, including keratitis, scleritis, episcleritis, and iritis. Presenting symptoms typically include photophobia and visual clouding from inflammatory cells in the anterior chamber. This can be a relapsing condition leading to a chronic uveitis with visual loss.

CARDIAC

Cardiac involvement with aortic valvular inflammation is rare. This can lead to aortic insufficiency and has been described in both the acute and chronic settings.[89] Heart block may also develop if there is involvement of the atrioventricular node or conducting pathway.

GENETICS

Genetic susceptibility appears to play a role in ReA.[90] Similar to the other forms of spondyloarthritis, HLA-B27 is seen as a risk factor with studies suggesting, depending in part on the background genetic prevalence of HLA-B27, that up to 30% to 40% of patients with ReA are positive for this antigen. Given that this haplotype is seen in 7% to 9% of the white population, there is a greater prevalence of ReA in this group compared with other ethnic populations such as Asians with a lower prevalence of HLA-B27. Multiple studies demonstrate that HLA-B27-positive patients have more severe symptoms and are more likely to develop chronic disease.

RISK FACTORS

In addition to the genetic susceptibility, the infectious agents most commonly implicated in ReA are the GI pathogens (*Yersinia*, *Shigella*, *Salmonella*, *Campylobacter*, and *C. difficile*) as well as venereal urogenital infection with *C. trachomatis*.[91,92] It also has been described with *Chlamydia pneumoniae*, *Ureaplasma urealyticum*, and intravesicular Bacille Calmette-Guérin.

DIAGNOSIS

There are no standardized criteria for ReA that have been validated. In 1995, the Third International Workshop on Reactive Arthritis established criteria for diagnosing ReA.[93] These criteria are:

- The arthritis should predominantly involve the lower limb, involve one or only a few joints, and not equally involve both sides of the body (asymmetric).
- There should be evidence or a history of preceding infection. Although it is ideal to have a culture that is positive for an infectious agent that is recognized to be associated with this condition, if the patient has documented diarrhea or urethritis in the prior 4 weeks, laboratory confirmation is not required.
- The patient should not have evidence that the joint itself is infected (ie, septic arthritis). Also, other causes of monoarthritis (such as gout) or oligoarthritis (such as rheumatoid arthritis) should be ruled out.

LABORATORY FINDINGS

There are no definitive laboratory tests available to diagnosis ReA. Although nonspecific acute-phase reactants (eg, erythrocyte sedimentation rate, C-reactive protein, platelet count) may be elevated, there is no association with known autoantibodies such as rheumatoid factor or antinuclear antibody. The presence of the HLA-B27 haplotype can be seen in up to half of the patients who develop sacroiliitis. Its presence is more helpful in suggesting a prognosis of greater chronicity than in establishing the diagnosis, given the background prevalence of up to 8% HLA-B27 positivity in asymptomatic individuals.

Synovial fluid analysis of an involved joint typically show evidence of sterile inflammation with 4,000 to 50,000 white blood cells per microliter with a polymorphonuclear cell predominance. Crystal analysis is negative as is Gram stain and microbial culture.

Given the association with precedent GI and urogenital infections, it is important to determine if there is ongoing infection. With symptoms of urethritis, appropriate cultures should be obtained for *C. trachomatis*.[94] For gastroenteritis, cultures for active disease or serologic testing can be obtained for *Shigella*, *Salmonella*, *Yersinia*, *Campylobacter*, and *C. difficile*. Serologic testing for antibodies to these causative organisms is not reliable.

IMAGING

Plain radiographic findings develop in the minority of patients with ReA, typically only after months of ongoing inflammation. Axial imaging can demonstrate sacroiliac erosions that are frequently unilateral.[95] Similar to other forms of spondyloarthritis, there also can be formation of syndesmophytes where the longitudinal spinal ligaments calcify, leading to ankyloses and the development of a "bamboo spine." Periosteal inflammation may develop in the involved peripheral joints, leading to a "whiskering" appearance along with bone erosions.

DIFFERENTIAL DIAGNOSIS

Other infectious etiologies must be considered. These include disseminated gonococcal infection, Lyme disease, and subacute bacterial endocarditis. These present frequently with an oligoarthritis and different skin manifestations. Viral infections such as HIV and parvovirus B19 will present as a polyarthritis. Septic arthritis is generally a monoarthritis in which the infectious agent can be cultured directly from the joint. Arthrocentesis demonstrates highly inflamed synovial fluid, typically greater than 50,000 leukocytes/μL with neutrophilic predominance. A Gram stain may visualize the organism, and the culture will be positive. With ReA, the synovial fluid has a lower leukocyte count with a sterile culture.

Microcrystalline disease in the form of gout or pseudogout generally presents with a severe monoarthritis or more rarely as an oligoarthritis. Arthrocentesis demonstrates highly inflammatory synovial fluid with the diagnostic findings of monosodium urate crystals in gout and calcium pyrophosphate dehydrate crystals in pseudogout.

The articular manifestation of systemic lupus erythematosus and rheumatoid arthritis is generally quite distinct from ReA in that these conditions usually present with a symmetric and progressive small joint polyarthritis. The characteristic serologies, rheumatoid factor and anticyclic citrullinated peptide in rheumatoid arthritis and antinuclear antibody in lupus, are typically not seen in ReA. Other forms of SpA (PsA, arthritis of inflammatory bowel disease and AS) may mimic ReA with the presence of oligoarthritis, enthesitis, dactylitis, and the presence of HLA-B27.

TREATMENT

ANTIBIOTICS

Given the correlation of specific infections with the subsequent development of ReA, it is understandable that treating any underlying infection is often attempted. In most cases the underlying infection is self-limited and can no longer be identified. If the inciting infectious agent can be determined, it must be treated aggressively with antibiotics. In the case of infection with *C. trachomatis*, the appropriate partners should be treated as well. There is no convincing evidence to support the long-term use of antibiotics in patients with ongoing synovitis.[96]

NONSTEROIDAL ANTIINFLAMMATORY DRUGS

In the acute setting, a symptomatic approach with nonsteroidal antiinflammatory drugs (NSAIDs) is appropriate initial therapy for both antiinflammatory and analgesic effects, especially given that the natural history of many of the symptoms of acute ReA is self-limiting. Various preparations have been studied at prescription strength.[90] Appropriate caution should be used in patients with underlying renal or hepatic insufficiency and in those with GI side effects.

CORTICOSTEROIDS

When ReA involves only a few joints, intraarticular injection of corticosteroids can be administered to provide short-term relief of joint inflammation. For more involved articular inflammation, systemic steroid administration can be considered, though this rarely provides sufficient benefit to the symptoms of axial inflammation.

Topical corticosteroids are also used as initial treatment of many of the extraarticular features of ReA, including inflammatory eye disease along with the cutaneous manifestations of keratoderma blenorrhagicum and circinate balanitis. Other treatments for these cutaneous manifestations are similar to what has been used for cutaneous psoriasis including keratolytics, coal tar, and phototherapy, with etretinate and oral methotrexate being reserved for more severe cases.

DISEASE-MODIFYING ANTIRHEUMATIC DRUGS

In patients who do not respond to NSAIDs and corticosteroids, several DMARDs have been used in the treatments of ReA. These include sulfasalazine, methotrexate, azathioprine, and cyclosporine. In chronic ReA, sulfasalazine also has been shown in clinical trials to provide marginal benefit in overall response.[97] There have been no such trials conducted for methotrexate, azathioprine, and cyclosporine though there are numerous case reports suggesting benefit with peripheral arthritis.

With the remarkable success of biologic therapies, especially TNF inhibitors, in other forms of spondyloarthritis (namely AS and PsA) their use has been reported. Several case reports along with an open-label study indicate there may be clinical benefit with these drugs in the treatment of ReA, though no randomized controlled studies have been conducted.[98,99]

PROGNOSIS

Although the majority of patients with ReA have a self-limited course within a few months of onset of the condition, relapses can develop leading to a chronic course manifested by recurrent uveitis, urethritis or erosive arthritis.

CONCLUSION

Unlike the other forms of SpA, the etiologic triggers of ReA are well described. While the association with specific infectious agents is undeniable, it is also clear that the involved articular and extraarticular tissues remain culture-free. The diagnosis, in the absence of any available definitive testing, remains to be established on clinical grounds. Fortunately, the natural history in the majority of cases is self-limited. The cornerstone of therapy remains suppression of inflammation in a supportive fashion.

REFERENCES

1. Moll JM. Psoriatic arthritis. *Br J Rheumatol*. 1984; 23(4): 241-244.
2. Pasero G, Marson P. The antiquity of psoriatic arthritis. *Clin Exp Rheumatol*. 2006;24(4):351-353.
3. Moll JM, Wright V. Psoriatic arthritis. *Semin Arthritis Rheum*. 1973;3(1):55-78.
4. Taylor W, Gladman D, Helliwell P, et al. Classification criteria for psoriatic arthritis: development of new criteria from a large international study. *Arthritis Rheum*. 2006;54(8):2665-2673.
5. Ogdie A, Weiss P. The epidemiology of psoriatic arthritis. *Rheum Dis Clin North Am*. 2015;41(4):545-568.
6. Spelman L, Su JC, Fernandez-Penas P, et al. Frequency of undiagnosed psoriatic arthritis among psoriasis patients in Australian dermatology practice. *J Eur Acad Dermatol Venereol*. 2015;29(11):2184-2191.
7. Yang Q, Qu L, Tian H, et al. Prevalence and characteristics of psoriatic arthritis in Chinese patients with psoriasis. *J Eur Acad Dermatol Venereol*. 2011;25(12):1409-1414.
8. Mease PJ, Gladman DD, Papp KA, et al. Prevalence of rheumatologist-diagnosed psoriatic arthritis in patients with psoriasis in European/North American dermatology clinics. *J Am Acad Dermatol*. 2013;69(5):729-735.

9. Haroon M, Kirby B, FitzGerald O. High prevalence of psoriatic arthritis in patients with severe psoriasis with suboptimal performance of screening questionnaires. *Ann Rheum Dis.* 2013;72(5):736-740.
10. Villani AP, Rouzaud M, Sevrain M, et al. Prevalence of undiagnosed psoriatic arthritis among psoriasis patients: systematic review and meta-analysis. *J Am Acad Dermatol.* 2015;73(2):242-248.
11. Eder L, Haddad A, Rosen CF, et al. The incidence and risk factors for psoriatic arthritis in patients with psoriasis: a prospective cohort study. *Arthritis Rheumatol.* 2016;68(4):915-923.
12. Wilson FC, Icen M, Crowson CS, et al. Incidence and clinical predictors of psoriatic arthritis in patients with psoriasis: a population-based study. *Arthritis Rheum.* 2009;61(2):233-239.
13. McHugh NJ. Early psoriatic arthritis. *Rheum Dis Clin North Am.* 2015;41(4):615-622.
14. Choi JW, Kim BR, Seo E, et al. Identification of nail features associated with psoriasis severity. *J Dermatol.* 2017;44(2):147-153.
15. Jadon DR, Sengupta R, Nightingale A, et al. Axial disease in psoriatic arthritis study: defining the clinical and radiographic phenotype of psoriatic spondyloarthritis. *Ann Rheum Dis.* 2017;76(4):701-707.
16. Eder L, Polachek A, Rosen CF, et al. The development of PsA in patients with psoriasis is preceded by a period of non-specific musculoskeletal symptoms: a prospective cohort study. *Arthritis Rheumatol.* 2017;69(3):622-629.
17. Helliwell PS, Hetthen J, Sokoll K, et al. Joint symmetry in early and late rheumatoid and psoriatic arthritis: comparison with a mathematical model. *Arthritis Rheum.* 2000;43(4):865-871.
18. Cresswell L, Chandran V, Farewell VT, et al. Inflammation in an individual joint predicts damage to that joint in psoriatic arthritis. *Ann Rheum Dis.* 2011;70(2):305-308.
19. Ranza R, Carneiro S, Qureshi AA, et al. Prevalence of psoriatic arthritis in a large cohort of Brazilian patients with psoriasis. *J Rheumatol.* 2015;42(5):829-834.
20. Gladman DD, Ziouzina O, Thavaneswaran A, et al. Dactylitis in psoriatic arthritis: prevalence and response to therapy in the biologic era. *J Rheumatol.* 2013;40(8):1357-1359.
21. Gladman DD. Clinical features and diagnostic considerations in psoriatic arthritis. *Rheum Dis Clin North Am.* 2015;41(4):569-579.
22. Helliwell PS, Porter G, Taylor WJ. Polyarticular psoriatic arthritis is more like oligoarticular psoriatic arthritis, than rheumatoid arthritis. *Ann Rheum Dis.* 2007;66(1):113-117.
23. Yamamoto T, Ohtsuki M, Sano S, et al. Epidemiological analysis of psoriatic arthritis patients in Japan. *J Dermatol.* 2016;43(10):1193-1196.
24. Brockbank JE, Stein M, Schentag CT, et al. Dactylitis in psoriatic arthritis: a marker for disease severity? *Ann Rheum Dis.* 2005;64(2):188-190.
25. Geijer M, Lindqvist U, Husmark T, et al. The Swedish Early Psoriatic Arthritis Registry 5-year followup: substantial radiographic progression mainly in men with high disease activity and development of dactylitis. *J Rheumatol.* 2015;42(11):2110-2117.
26. McGonagle D, Lories RJ, Tan AL, et al. The concept of a "synovio-entheseal complex" and its implications for understanding joint inflammation and damage in psoriatic arthritis and beyond. *Arthritis Rheum.* 2007;56(8):2482-2491.
27. Benjamin M, McGonagle D. Histopathologic changes at "synovio-entheseal complexes" suggesting a novel mechanism for synovitis in osteoarthritis and spondylarthritis. *Arthritis Rheum.* 2007;56(11):3601-3609.
28. Polachek A, Li S, Chandran V, et al. Clinical enthesitis in a prospective longitudinal psoriatic arthritis cohort: incidence, prevalence, characteristics and outcome. *Arthritis Care Res (Hoboken).* 2017;69(11):1685-1691.
29. Naredo E, Moller I, de Miguel E, et al. High prevalence of ultrasonographic synovitis and enthesopathy in patients with psoriasis without psoriatic arthritis: a prospective case-control study. *Rheumatology (Oxford).* 2011;50(10):1838-1848.
30. Aydin SZ, Castillo-Gallego C, Ash ZR, et al. Ultrasonographic assessment of nail in psoriatic disease shows a link between onychopathy and distal interphalangeal joint extensor tendon enthesopathy. *Dermatology.* 2012;225(3):231-235.
31. Gladman DD, Brubacher B, Buskila D, et al. Differences in the expression of spondyloarthropathy: a comparison between ankylosing spondylitis and psoriatic arthritis. *Clin Invest Med.* 1993;16(1):1-7.
32. Helliwell PS, Hickling P, Wright V. Do the radiological changes of classic ankylosing spondylitis differ from the changes found in the spondylitis associated with inflammatory bowel disease, psoriasis, and reactive arthritis? *Ann Rheum Dis.* 1998;57(3):135-140.
33. Lambert JR, Wright V. Eye inflammation in psoriatic arthritis. *Ann Rheum Dis.* 1976;35(4):354-356.
34. Murray PI, Rauz S. The eye and inflammatory rheumatic diseases: the eye and rheumatoid arthritis, ankylosing spondylitis, psoriatic arthritis. *Best Pract Res Clin Rheumatol.* 2016;30(5):802-825.
35. Abbouda A, Abicca I, Fabiani C, et al. Psoriasis and psoriatic arthritis-related uveitis: different ophthalmological manifestations and ocular inflammation features. *Semin Ophthalmol.* 2017;32(6):715-720.
36. Egeberg A, Khalid U, Gislason GH, et al. Association of psoriatic disease with uveitis: a Danish nationwide cohort study. *JAMA Dermatol.* 2015;151(11):1200-1205.
37. Paiva ES, Macaluso DC, Edwards A, et al. Characterisation of uveitis in patients with psoriatic arthritis. *Ann Rheum Dis.* 2000;59(1):67-70.
38. Egeberg A, Mallbris L, Warren RB, et al. Association between psoriasis and inflammatory bowel disease: a Danish nationwide cohort study. *Br J Dermatol.* 2016;175(3):487-492.
39. Li WQ, Han JL, Chan AT, et al. Psoriasis, psoriatic arthritis and increased risk of incident Crohn's disease in US women. *Ann Rheum Dis.* 2013;72(7):1200-1205.
40. Scarpa R, Manguso F, D'Arienzo A, et al. Microscopic inflammatory changes in colon of patients with both active psoriasis and psoriatic arthritis without bowel symptoms. *J Rheumatol.* 2000;27(5):1241-1246.
41. Polachek A, Touma Z, Anderson M, et al. Risk of cardiovascular morbidity in patients with psoriatic arthritis: a meta-analysis of observational studies. *Arthritis Care Res (Hoboken).* 2017;69(1):67-74.
42. Eder L, Wu Y, Chandran V, et al. Incidence and predictors for cardiovascular events in patients with psoriatic arthritis. *Ann Rheum Dis.* 2016;75(9):1680-1686.
43. Agca R, Heslinga SC, Rollefstad S, et al. EULAR recommendations for cardiovascular disease risk management in patients with rheumatoid arthritis and other forms of inflammatory joint disorders: 2015/2016 update. *Ann Rheum Dis.* 2017;76(1):17-28.
44. Husni ME. Comorbidities in psoriatic arthritis. *Rheum Dis Clin North Am.* 2015;41(4):677-698.

45. Eder L, Thavaneswaran A, Chandran V, et al. Obesity is associated with a lower probability of achieving sustained minimal disease activity state among patients with psoriatic arthritis. *Ann Rheum Dis.* 2015;74(5):813-817.
46. Hojgaard P, Glintborg B, Kristensen LE, et al. The influence of obesity on response to tumour necrosis factor-alpha inhibitors in psoriatic arthritis: results from the DANBIO and ICEBIO registries. *Rheumatology (Oxford).* 2016;55(12):2191-2199.
47. Di Minno MN, Peluso R, Iervolino S, et al. Weight loss and achievement of minimal disease activity in patients with psoriatic arthritis starting treatment with tumour necrosis factor alpha blockers. *Ann Rheum Dis.* 2014;73(6):1157-1162.
48. Moll JM, Wright V. Familial occurrence of psoriatic arthritis. *Ann Rheum Dis.* 1973;32(3):181-201.
49. Eder L, Chandran V, Pellet F, et al. Human leucocyte antigen risk alleles for psoriatic arthritis among patients with psoriasis. *Ann Rheum Dis.* 2012;71(1):50-55.
50. Winchester R, Minevich G, Steshenko V, et al. HLA associations reveal genetic heterogeneity in psoriatic arthritis and in the psoriasis phenotype. *Arthritis Rheum.* 2012;64(4):1134-1144.
51. Stuart PE, Nair RP, Tsoi LC, et al. Genome-wide association analysis of psoriatic arthritis and cutaneous psoriasis reveals differences in their genetic architecture. *Am J Hum Genet.* 2015;97(6):816-836.
52. Budu-Aggrey A, Bowes J, Loehr S, et al. Replication of a distinct psoriatic arthritis risk variant at the IL23R locus. *Ann Rheum Dis.* 2016;75(7):1417-1418.
53. Bowes J, Loehr S, Budu-Aggrey A, et al. PTPN22 is associated with susceptibility to psoriatic arthritis but not psoriasis: evidence for a further PsA-specific risk locus. *Ann Rheum Dis.* 2015;74(10):1882-1885.
54. Bowes J, Budu-Aggrey A, Huffmeier U, et al. Dense genotyping of immune-related susceptibility loci reveals new insights into the genetics of psoriatic arthritis. *Nat Commun.* 2015;6:6046.
55. Thorarensen SM, Lu N, Ogdie A, et al. Physical trauma recorded in primary care is associated with the onset of psoriatic arthritis among patients with psoriasis. *Ann Rheum Dis.* 2017;76(3):521-525.
56. Li W, Han J, Qureshi AA. Obesity and risk of incident psoriatic arthritis in US women. *Ann Rheum Dis.* 2012;71(8):1267-1272.
57. Love TJ, Zhu Y, Zhang Y, et al. Obesity and the risk of psoriatic arthritis: a population-based study. *Ann Rheum Dis.* 2012;71(8):1273-1277.
58. Li W, Han J, Qureshi AA. Smoking and risk of incident psoriatic arthritis in US women. *Ann Rheum Dis.* 2012;71(6):804-808.
59. Tillett W, Jadon D, Shaddick G, et al. Smoking and delay to diagnosis are associated with poorer functional outcome in psoriatic arthritis. *Ann Rheum Dis.* 2013;72(8):1358-1361.
60. Eder L, Shanmugarajah S, Thavaneswaran A, et al. The association between smoking and the development of psoriatic arthritis among psoriasis patients. *Ann Rheum Dis.* 2012;71(2):219-224.
61. De Wilde K, Martens A, Lambrecht S, et al. A20 inhibition of STAT1 expression in myeloid cells: a novel endogenous regulatory mechanism preventing development of enthesitis. *Ann Rheum Dis.* 2017;76(3):585-592.
62. Manel N, Unutmaz D, Littman DR. The differentiation of human T(H)-17 cells requires transforming growth factor-beta and induction of the nuclear receptor RORgammat. *Nat Immunol.* 2008;9(6):641-649.
63. Sherlock JP, Joyce-Shaikh B, Turner SP, et al. IL-23 induces spondyloarthropathy by acting on ROR-gammat+ CD3+CD4-CD8- entheseal resident T cells. *Nat Med.* 2012;18(7):1069-1076.
64. Barnas JL, Ritchlin CT. Etiology and pathogenesis of psoriatic arthritis. *Rheum Dis Clin North Am.* 2015;41(4):643-663.
65. Nestle FO, Kaplan DH, Barker J. Psoriasis. *N Engl J Med.* 2009;361(5):496-509.
66. Arakawa A, Siewert K, Stohr J, et al. Melanocyte antigen triggers autoimmunity in human psoriasis. *J Exp Med.* 2015;212(13):2203-2212.
67. Haroon M, Gallagher P, FitzGerald O. Diagnostic delay of more than 6 months contributes to poor radiographic and functional outcome in psoriatic arthritis. *Ann Rheum Dis.* 2015;74(6):1045-1050.
68. Husni ME, Meyer KH, Cohen DS, et al. The PASE questionnaire: pilot-testing a psoriatic arthritis screening and evaluation tool. *J Am Acad Dermatol.* 2007;57(4):581-587.
69. Dominguez PL, Husni ME, Holt EW, et al. Validity, reliability, and sensitivity-to-change properties of the psoriatic arthritis screening and evaluation questionnaire. *Arch Dermatol Res.* 2009;301(8):573-579.
70. Gladman DD, Schentag CT, Tom BD, et al. Development and initial validation of a screening questionnaire for psoriatic arthritis: the Toronto Psoriatic Arthritis Screen (ToPAS). *Ann Rheum Dis.* 2009;68(4):497-501.
71. Tinazzi I, Adami S, Zanolin EM, et al. The early psoriatic arthritis screening questionnaire: a simple and fast method for the identification of arthritis in patients with psoriasis. *Rheumatology (Oxford).* 2012;51(11):2058-2063.
72. Coates LC, Kavanaugh A, Mease PJ, et al. Group for research and assessment of psoriasis and psoriatic arthritis 2015 treatment recommendations for psoriatic arthritis. *Arthritis Rheumatol.* 2016;68(5):1060-1071.
73. Tillett W, Shaddick G, Jobling A, et al. Effect of anti-TNF and conventional synthetic disease-modifying anti-rheumatic drug treatment on work disability and clinical outcome in a multicentre observational cohort study of psoriatic arthritis. *Rheumatology (Oxford).* 2017;56(4):603-612.
74. Orbai AM, de Wit M, Mease P, et al. International patient and physician consensus on a psoriatic arthritis core outcome set for clinical trials. *Ann Rheum Dis.* 2017;76(4):673-680.
75. Lebwohl MG, Kavanaugh A, Armstrong AW, et al. US Perspectives in the management of psoriasis and psoriatic arthritis: patient and physician results from the population-based Multinational Assessment of Psoriasis and Psoriatic Arthritis (MAPP) Survey. *Am J Clin Dermatol.* 2016;17(1):87-97.
76. Gossec L, Coates LC, de Wit M, et al. Management of psoriatic arthritis in 2016: a comparison of EULAR and GRAPPA recommendations. *Nat Rev Rheumatol.* 2016;12(12):743-750.
77. Kingsley GH, Kowalczyk A, Taylor H, et al. A randomized placebo-controlled trial of methotrexate in psoriatic arthritis. *Rheumatology (Oxford).* 2012;51(8):1368-1377.
78. Chandran V, Schentag CT, Gladman DD. Reappraisal of the effectiveness of methotrexate in psoriatic arthritis: results from a longitudinal observational cohort. *J Rheumatol.* 2008;35(3):469-471.
79. Baranauskaite A, Raffayova H, Kungurov NV, et al. Infliximab plus methotrexate is superior to methotrexate alone in the treatment of psoriatic arthritis in methotrexate-naive patients: the RESPOND study. *Ann Rheum Dis.* 2012;71(4):541-548.

80. Behrens F, Finkenwirth C, Pavelka K, et al. Leflunomide in psoriatic arthritis: results from a large European prospective observational study. *Arthritis Care Res (Hoboken)*. 2013;65(3):464-470.
81. Coates LC, Moverley AR, McParland L, et al. Effect of tight control of inflammation in early psoriatic arthritis (TICOPA): a UK multicentre, open-label, randomised controlled trial. *Lancet*. 2015;386(10012):2489-2498.
82. Reiter H. Uber eine bisher unerkannte Spirochateninfektion (Spirochetosis arthritica). *Dtsch Med Wochensohr*. 1916;42:1535.
83. Fiessinger M, Leroy E. Contribution a l'etude d'une epidemie de dysenterie dans le somme. *Bull Mem Soc Med Hop Paris*. 1916;40:2030.
84. Rich E, Hook EW 3rd, Alarcón GS, et al. Reactive arthritis in patients attending and urban sexually transmitted disease clinic. *Arthritis Rheum*. 1996;39:1172.
85. Townes JM, Deodhar AA, Laine ES, et al. Reactive arthritis following culture-confirmed infections with bacterial enteric pathogens in Minnesota and Oregon: a population-based study. *Ann Rheum Dis*. 2008;67(12):1689.
86. Carter JD, Hudson AP. Reactive arthritis: clinical aspects and medical management. *Rheum Dis Clin North Am*. 2009;35:21.
87. Leirisalo-Repo M. Reactive arthritis. *Scand J Rheumatol*. 2005;34:251.
88. Rothschild BM, Pingitore C, Eaton M. Dactylitis: implications for clinical practice. *Semin Arthritis Rheum*. 1998;28:41.
89. Brown LE, Forfia P, Flynn JA. Aortic insufficiency in a patient with reactive arthritis: case report and review of the literature. *HSS J*. 2011;7(2):187.
90. Hannu T. Reactive arthritis. *Best Pract Res Clin Rheumatol*. 2011;25(3):347.
91. Carter JD, Inman RD. Chlamydia-induced reactive arthritis: hidden in plain sight? *Best Pract Res Clin Rheumatol*. 2011;25(3):359.
92. Kvien TK, Glennås A, Melby K, et al. Reactive arthritis: incidence, triggering agents and clinical presentation. *J Rheumatol*. 1994;21(1):115-122.
93. Kingsley G, Sieper J. Third international workshop on reactive arthritis. 23-26 September 1995, Berlin, Germany. Report and abstracts. *Ann Rheum Dis*. 1996;55: 564-584.
94. Fendler C, Laitko S, Sörensen H, et al. Frequency of triggering bacteria in patients with reactive arthritis and undifferentiated oligoarthritis and the relative importance of the tests used for diagnosis. *Ann Rheum Dis*. 2001;60(4):337-343.
95. Ozgül A, Dede I, Taskaynatan MA, et al. Clinical presentations of chlamydial and non-chlamydial reactive arthritis. *Rheumatol Int*. 2006;26(10):879-885.
96. Kvien TK, Gaston JS, Bardin T, et al. Three month treatment of reactive arthritis with azithromycin: a EULAR double blind, placebo controlled study. *Ann Rheum Dis*. 2004;63(9):1113-1119.
97. Clegg DO, Reda DJ, Weisman MH, et al. Comparison of sulfasalazine and placebo in the treatment of reactive arthritis. *Arthritis Rheum*. 1996;39(12):2021-2027.
98. Meyer A, Chatelus E, Wendling D, et al. Safety and efficacy of anti-tumor necrosis factorαtherapy in ten patients with recent-onset refractory reactive arthritis. *Arthritis Rheum*. 2011;63(5):1274-1280.
99. Flagg SD, Meador R, Hsia E, et al. Decreased pain and synovial inflammation after etanercept therapy in patients with reactive and undifferentiated arthritis: an open-label trial. *Arthritis Rheum*. 2005;53(4):613-617.

Chapter 66 :: Rheumatoid Arthritis, Juvenile Idiopathic Arthritis, Adult-Onset Still Disease, and Rheumatic Fever
:: Warren W. Piette

第六十六章
类风湿性关节炎、幼年特发性关节炎、成人Still病和风湿热

中文导读

　　本章讨论的疾病主要累及肌肉骨骼系统，是常见的风湿性疾病，这些疾病均有皮肤受累。类风湿性关节炎（RA）以近端指间关节和掌指关节对称关节炎中最常见。皮肤表现相当多，包括多种组织病理表现的丘疹、斑块和结节、血管炎、坏疽性脓皮病/溃疡。疾病的进展最终导致关节功能受限，限制关节功能状态，可能导致过早死亡。通常基于疾病严重程度选择相应的治疗。本节从定义、临床特征、病因及发病学、诊断、临床进程、预后及管理等方面详细阐述该病。临床表现分别从一般特征、皮肤表现、血管病变、非皮肤发现讨论了RA的临床特征。重点放在皮肤表现上，并阐述了皮疹相应的组织病理特点。列出了修正的诊断标准，概述了RA的健康管理及治疗用药、干预措施。

　　幼年特发性关节炎是一组包括各种病因不明的关节炎的疾病，既往命名为幼年性类风湿关节炎、幼年性Still病。包含了七种类型。通常在16岁前发病，持续至少6周。本章从临床特征、病因及发病机制、诊断、鉴别诊断、临床进程及预后、管理等方面对于该病进行了阐述。成人Still病（AOSD）是一个累及多系统的综合征，特征性的表现为血清阴性多关节炎和发热；其经典皮疹表现为三文鱼色红斑和一过性消失，血沉升高，中性粒细胞增高。目前识别了几个非典型的新的皮疹；与恶性肿瘤有关，尤其是伴有非典型持久性皮疹的患者中。本章从流行病学、临床特征、诊断、鉴别诊断、临床进程及预后方面就该病进行了阐述。急性风湿热是一种对A组链球菌感染的炎症反应，通常发生在咽喉感染后2～3周；是aβ-溶血性链球菌口咽感染的迟发性后遗症。它是一种可影响心脏、关节、中枢神经系统、皮肤和皮下组织的炎性疾病。治疗潜在的感染可以预防风湿热。本章从流行病学、临床特征、诊断、治疗等方面阐述了该病的特点。

〔施　为〕

This chapter discusses common rheumatologic diseases that have predominantly musculoskeletal presentations; however, all of these conditions have cutaneous manifestations.

RHEUMATOID ARTHRITIS

AT-A-GLANCE

- Affects roughly 1% of the world population.
- Chronic, disfiguring, inflammatory condition.
- Genetics and environment play a role in etiology.
- Symmetric arthritis of the proximal interphalangeal and metacarpophalangeal joints most common.
- Skin findings quite varied, including papules, plaques, and nodules with multiple histologic types, vasculitis/Bywaters lesions, pyoderma gangrenosum/Felty ulcers.
- Treatment based on severity of disease.

Rheumatoid arthritis (RA) is a systemic inflammatory autoimmune disease that is characterized by debilitating chronic, symmetric polyarthritis. Important extraarticular manifestations are many, including, in part, rheumatoid nodules, pyoderma gangrenosum, granulomatous and other skin lesions, vasculitis, and internal organ involvement. The disease process is often progressive, resulting in limitation of joint function, decline in functional status, and possibly premature death. Permanent remission is unusual.

DEFINITIONS

The revised diagnostic criteria approved in 2010 by the board of directors of the American College of Rheumatology and the executive directors of the European League Against Rheumatism focuses on identifying patients earlier in the course of their disease than was allowed by previous criteria.[1] Table 66-1 outlines these

TABLE 66-1

2010 American College of Rheumatology/European League Against Rheumatism Classification Criteria for Arthritis[a]

Target population: patients who (a) have at least 1 joint with definite clinical synovitis (swelling), (b) with the synovitis not better explained by another disease.[a]

CLASSIFICATION CRITERIA FOR RHEUMATOID ARTHRITIS (RA) (ADD SCORE OF CATEGORIES A TO D; SCORE ≥6/10 IS NEEDED FOR DEFINITE RA CLASSIFICATION)	SCORE
A. Joint Involvement: tender or swollen joint on examination, *excluding* distal IP joints, first MCP joints, and first MTP joints	
1 large joint (shoulder, elbow, hip, knee, or ankle)	0
2 to 10 large joints	1
1 to 3 small joints (MCP, proximal IP, 2nd to 5th MTP, thumb IP, wrists) with or without large joints	2
4-10 small joints with or without large joints	3
>10 joints (must have at least 1 small joint; other joints can include joints not specifically listed elsewhere, eg, TM, AC, SC)	5
B. Serology (at least 1 test result is needed for classification)	
Negative RF and negative ACPA	0
Low-positive RF or low-positive ACPA[b]	2
High-positive RF or high-positive ACPA[b]	3
C. Acute-phase reactants (at least 1 result needed for classification)	
Normal CRP *and* normal ESR	0
Abnormal CRP *or* abnormal ESR	1
D. Duration of symptoms[c]	
<6 weeks	0
≥6 weeks	1

[a]Differential diagnosis to exclude other diseases varies by presentation, but may include, for example, systemic lupus erythematosus, psoriatic arthritis, and gout.
[b]Negative = less than upper limits normal (ULN); low-positive = greater than ULN but <3 times ULN; high-positive = >3 times ULN.
[c]Patient self-report of the duration of signs or symptoms of synovitis (eg, pain, swelling, tenderness) of joints that are clinically involved at the time of assessment, regardless of treatment status.

AC, acromioclavicular; ACPA, anticitrullinated protein antibody; CRP, C-reactive protein; ESR, erythrocyte sedimentation rate; IP, interphalangeal; MCP, metacarpophalangeal; MTP, metatarsophalangeal; RF, rheumatoid factor; SC, sternoclavicular; TM, temporomandibular.

Criteria aimed at newly presenting patients. Patients with erosive disease or with longstanding but now inactive disease meeting prior 2010 requirements are considered to have RA.

Modified from Aletaha D, Neogi T, Silman AJ, et al. 2010 Rheumatoid arthritis classification criteria. An American College Rheumatology/European League Against Rheumatism collaborative initiative. *Arthritis Rheum*. 2010;62(9):2569-2581. With permission of John Wiley & Sons. Copyright © 2010, American College of Rheumatology.

revised criteria. Even though cutaneous findings may be a key to diagnosis, none are considered diagnostic as no extraarticular physical findings are included in the criteria.

EPIDEMIOLOGY

RA has an annual incidence of approximately 0.4 per 1000 in females and 0.2 per 1000 in males, with a prevalence of approximately 0.4% to 1% of the adult population in diverse populations worldwide.[2-4] RA has a peak onset of approximately 50 years of age.[2,3]

CLINICAL FEATURES

RA often begins with general constitutional symptoms such as fatigue, anorexia, vague musculoskeletal complaints, and generalized weakness. It may be weeks or months before the characteristic synovitis presents. It is in these early stages that diagnosis is most difficult, but early diagnosis and treatment are essential because most joint damage occurs early in the disease process. The American College of Rheumatology guidelines proposed in 1987 were thought to be too insensitive to recognize RA during this critical early phase, leading to the revised criteria in 2010 (see Table 66-1).[1]

CUTANEOUS FINDINGS

Rheumatoid Nodules and Nodulosis: The most common dermatologic finding in RA has been the rheumatoid nodule, although as patients are treated earlier and more aggressively, this cutaneous finding may become less common. Classically a subcutaneous nodule, the rheumatoid nodule occurs in approximately 25% of patients with RA (Fig. 66-1A).[5-8] More than 90% of patients with rheumatoid nodules have seropositive RA. The usual location is over pressure points such as the olecranon, the extensor surface of the forearms, and the Achilles tendon, but they have been described in almost every location, including viscera.[7,8] The main histologic findings (Fig. 66-1B) are palisaded granulomas in the deep dermis or subcutaneous tissues with fibrinoid degeneration of collagen, a multitude of neutrophils and neutrophilic dust, with surrounding fibrosis and proliferation of vessels. The main differential diagnoses histopathologically include subcutaneous granuloma annulare, necrobiosis lipoidica, foreign-body or infectious granulomatous reaction, and epithelioid sarcoid. Although rheumatoid nodules are benign, they can lead to complications, including ulceration, infection, joint effusion (rheumatoid chyliform bursitis), and fistulas (fistulous rheumatism). All conditions may lead to the need for surgical excision, although excision of asymptomatic nodules can itself lead to complications.[5,8]

Rheumatoid nodulosis is the development of rheumatoid nodules in patients without chronic synovitis or radiographic findings, and mild or no systemic manifestations. This involves men predominantly, and many develop frank RA. In children, similar lesions are termed *pseudorheumatoid nodulosis*. Their distribution differs by localizing over the tibia, the dorsal foot, or scalp. They may be large but there is no systemic disease nor positive serology. Most regress within 2 years; progression to RA is extremely rare.[8] Table 66-2 outlines the differential diagnosis of rheumatoid nodules.

Methotrexate-Related Cutaneous Reactions: Low-dose methotrexate, often used for the treatment of RA, may precipitate erythema in and enlargement of preexisting rheumatoid nodules, known as *accelerated nodulosis*.[5-8] Regression of these changes is expected when the methotrexate dose is decreased or discontinued.

A papular reaction to methotrexate has been reported as a syndrome of clustered, erythematous, indurated papules arising most commonly on the proximal extremities and buttocks.[6] This has been reported not only in patients with RA, but also in association with

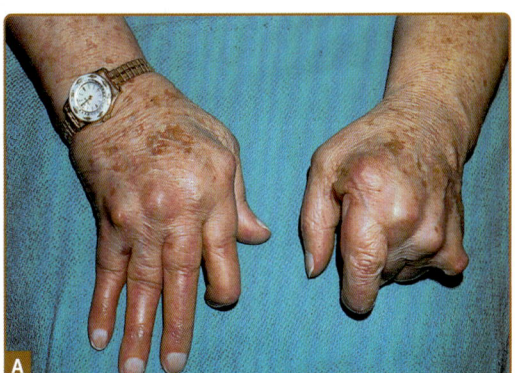 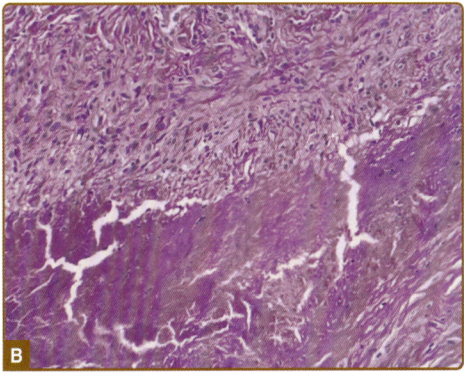

Figure 66-1 Rheumatoid nodules. **A,** Severely affected joints of a patient with rheumatoid arthritis with overlying rheumatoid nodules. **B,** Histopathologically, rheumatoid nodules are palisaded granulomas in the deep reticular dermis surrounding degenerated collagen.

> **TABLE 66-2**
> **Differential Diagnosis of Rheumatoid Nodules**
>
> **Consider**
> - Subcutaneous granuloma annulare
> - Pseudorheumatoid nodulosis (children)
> - Foreign-body granuloma
> - Infectious granuloma
> - Sarcoid granuloma
> - Myxoid cyst
> - Traumatic epidermal cyst
> - Xanthoma
>
> **Rule Out**
> - Epithelioid sarcoma
> - Fibromatous nodules in Lyme borreliosis

other diseases, especially collagen vascular diseases. In rare instances, some lesions may develop erosions or surrounding livedo. The histologic pattern seen is mostly a histiocytic infiltrate arranged interstitially between collagen bundles in the dermis, intermixed with a few neutrophils. Small rosettes of histiocytes may surround thick collagen bundles in the reticular dermis.

Yet another possible cutaneous complication of methotrexate therapy (occasionally other immunosuppressive drugs) in RA is the development of Epstein-Barr virus-associated multifocal cutaneous lymphoproliferative disease, which may regress on discontinuation of therapy.[9,10]

Granulomatous Dermatoses (Reactive Granulomatous Dermatitis): Reactive granulomatous dermatitis has been proposed as an inclusive term for the following 3 syndromes: interstitial granulomatous dermatitis (IGD), palisaded neutrophilic and granulomatous dermatitis (PNGD), and interstitial granulomatous drug reaction (IGDR). IGD and PNGD are associated with autoimmune diseases, including RA; IGDR is a drug-associated syndrome that may be included in IGD and PNGD.[11]

PNGD has been reported as Churg-Strauss granuloma, cutaneous extravascular necrotizing granuloma, rheumatoid papules, Winkelmann granuloma, and, by some authors, IGD.[11] It presents as symmetric skin-colored to erythematous smooth, umbilicated, or crusted papules, primarily on elbows and extremities: 51% involve upper extremities, 27% lower extremities, 21% trunk, head, and neck. Less common are urticarial plaques; erythematous nodules with scale; papulonodules; pink-to-red papules and plaques; erythematous edematous plaques; violaceous patches and plaques; annular papules and plaques; annular gyrate plaques; and linear bands.[6,11]

Histopathologically, early features include intense neutrophilic inflammation, karyorrhectic debris, and leukocytoclastic vasculitis. Later findings are piecemeal areas of collagen degeneration and palisades of histiocytes and small granulomas, eventually accompanied by areas of fibrosis.

Spontaneous resolution occurs in 20%, sometimes as quickly as 1 week. Most treatment is directed at underlying disease. Tumor necrosis factor (TNF) inhibitors and allopurinol have been implicated as causes, so stopping them may induce remission. Treatments include intralesional corticosteroid, nonsteroidal anti-inflammatory drugs (NSAIDs), dapsone, colchicine, systemic corticosteroids, oral tacrolimus, and TNF inhibitors. Topical therapy is generally not effective.[6,11]

IGD has been previously reported as IGD with arthritis, IGD with cords and arthritis, linear subcutaneous bands of RA, linear rheumatoid nodules, linear granuloma annulare, railway track dermatitis, and Ackerman syndrome. IGD also has been described in association with a number of disorders, including RA. Usually asymptomatic, this syndrome presents symmetrically on the lateral upper trunk and proximal inner arms and thighs, and occasionally on the buttocks, abdomen, breast, and umbilicus.[6,11] Initially, IGD was reported in patients with inflammatory arthritis and pathognomonic linear bands or cords on the upper trunk. It is now recognized that less than 10% of IGD cases present this way. Other morphologic presentations include erythematous to violaceous patches or plaques; diffuse macular erythema; annular plaques; polycyclic indurated plaques; cockades of color with violaceous centers surrounded by erythema; annular scaly plaques; subcutaneous nodules; large atrophic hyperpigmented plaques; disseminated indurated violaceous papules and plaques; periungual and mucosal erythema; and elbow papules and nodules similar to those of PNGD.[6,11]

Histopathologic findings include a dense, diffuse infiltrate of histiocytes arranged in a band-like configuration in middle or deep reticular dermis. There may be foci of basophilic collagen surrounded by palisaded histiocytes. These cells may also exhibit large and pleomorphic nuclei; scattered mitotic figures are readily seen. Neutrophils and eosinophils may be present, most notably in areas of degenerated collagen. Variably dense interstitial CD68+ epithelioid histiocytes often surround foci of abnormal collagen, which leads to clefting away of the altered collagen and histiocyte section (the "floating sign," reported in 67% of cases). Vasculitis is usually absent. Lymphocytes abutting epidermis with basal vacuolization is rarely seen, but may distinguish IGDR from pure IGD. Mucin deposition is minimal or absent. Most medications are actually associated with IGDR; previous IGD associations with TNF inhibitors, soy, angiotensin-converting enzyme inhibitors, and furosemide may actually be IGDR. Treatment includes stopping any causative drug and treating underlying disease.

Probably often used interchangeably with IGD, IGDR was reported to present as erythematous to violaceous plaques, often annular, concentrated on inner arms, proximal medial thighs, proximal trunk, and intertriginous sites.[11] Subsequent reports added isolated plaque, erythroderma, subcutaneous nodules on palms and soles, erythema nodosum-like lesions, and scalp, cheeks, and extensor forearms involvement.

Histologic findings are similar to IGD and include diffuse interstitial histiocytes with granulomas, and rare giant cells surrounding piecemeal fragmentation of collagen. Mucin is scant; vasculitis absent. IGDR should include interface dermatitis with basal vacuolar degeneration, areas of dyskeratosis, and prominent tissue eosinophilia. Lymphoid atypia is frequent, with large cells, hyperchromatic nuclei, and occasional convoluted nuclei. Commonly implicated drugs include calcium channel blockers, beta-blockers, lipid-lowering agents, and angiotensin-converting enzyme inhibitors. Treatment involves stopping the drug.

Neutrophilic Dermatoses: Rheumatoid neutrophilic dermatosis is a very rare cutaneous manifestation in patients with severe RA; it was first described by Ackerman in 1978. Lesions are usually chronic, erythematous, and urticaria-like plaques and papules that are sharply marginated (Fig. 66-2A). Histopathologically, these lesions have a dense infiltrate of neutrophils without leukocytoclasia, in the setting of a mixed infiltrate and papillary edema (Fig. 66-2B).[12,13] It may be difficult to differentiate from acute febrile neutrophilic dermatosis (Sweet syndrome) (see Chap. 36). Some authors accept PNGD as a histologic finding consistent with rheumatoid neutrophilic dermatitis.[13] However, in the absence of granuloma formation, it seems reasonable to separate rheumatoid neutrophilic dermatitis from multiple named entities that seem to be now included under the term *IGD*. Five patents have been reported with tense blister formation, typically on the lower extremities in older females.[14]

Autoimmune neutrophilic dermatoses syndrome produces urticarial lesions in association with systemic lupus erythematosus, RA, and secondary Sjögren syndrome, which lesions regress within 24 hours, but unlike urticaria they are typically nonpruritic. Histopathologically, lesions show interstitial and perivascular neutrophilic infiltrate with leukocytoclasia without vasculitis, vacuolar alteration at the dermal–epidermal junction. Remission follows administration of immunomodulating drugs.[15,16] A figurate erythema, consisting of annular lesions, often with vesicles or purpura, with a histology resembling mild Sweet syndrome has been reported as a mostly idiopathic condition, but association with systemic lupus erythematosus (not yet with RA) has been reported.[17]

Patients treated with TNFα inhibitors may develop an eruption that is clinically and histologically indistinguishable from psoriasis. This can occur in those receiving these agents for any condition, but those with RA appear to be at greatest risk. The eruption typically clears with drug cessation, and may or may not reoccur during treatment with other drugs of this class.[6]

VASCULAR MANIFESTATIONS

Rheumatoid Vasculitis: With an estimated annual incidence of less than 1%, this syndrome most often affects men and smokers with longstanding disease, who are seropositive to rheumatoid factor and to citrullinated peptides.[6,18-22] Previously, rheumatoid vasculitis affected 1 in 8 males with RA versus 1 in 38 females; male sex is now associated with an odds ratio of 1.98.[17,19] Smoking remains the most consistently demonstrated environmental risk factor for rheumatoid vasculitis, particularly in male seropositive patients. A declining trend in the incidence of rheumatoid vasculitis was noted beginning in the 1990s and reconfirmed in newer studies. Population-based data from the Norwich cohort in the United Kingdom noted a drop in the average incidence of rheumatoid vasculitis from 9.1 per million between 1988 and 2002 to 3.9 per million between 2001 and 2010. These declines are largely attributed to improved treatment of RA, roughly coinciding with the advent of biologic response modifiers, but another explanation may be the decline in rates of cigarette smoking.[19,20] There also appears to be a higher risk of rheumatoid vasculitis among RA patients with peripheral vascular disease (odds ratio: 3.98) and cerebrovascular disease (odds ratio: 6.48).[19]

In a large study of rheumatoid vasculitis, the median age of participants at presentation was 63 years and the median duration of RA was 10.8 years. One-third of participants were current smokers. The majority

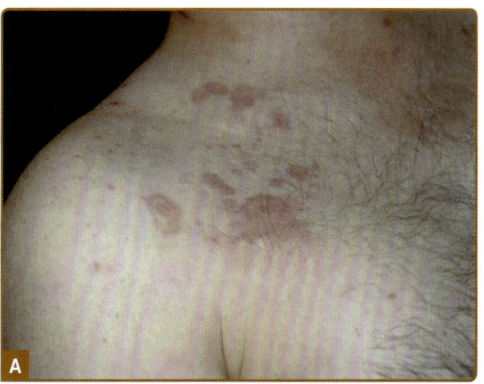
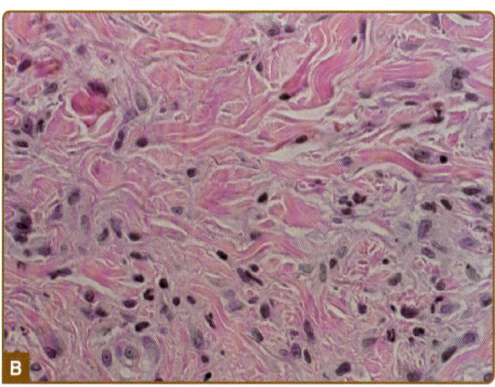

Figure 66-2 Rheumatoid neutrophilic dermatosis. **A,** Lesions are erythematous urticarial papules that often coalesce into plaques in a patient with rheumatoid arthritis. **B,** Histopathologically, there is an interstitial mixed dermal infiltrate that is predominated by neutrophils without leukocytoclasis. This infiltrate is often accompanied by papillary edema.

were seropositive and had elevated inflammatory markers.[19] In rheumatoid vasculitis patients, the mean duration between the diagnosis of RA and the onset of vasculitic symptoms was 10 to 14 years, and presentation within the first 5 years of the RA diagnosis is unusual.[19,20] Cutaneous vasculitis was the most common presentation, followed by vasculitic neuropathy. Patients often have rheumatoid nodules, although newer studies find a lower percentage than was previously reported (44% of patients compared with 86%).[19] These observations may be the result of improved control of RA in recent years.

Although severe RA increases the odds of rheumatoid vasculitis, the vasculitis often develops at a time when the inflammatory arthritis has burned out. Despite this, the onset of rheumatoid vasculitis is often heralded by constitutional symptoms (fever, weight loss), an escalation of the acute-phase markers (erythrocyte sedimentation rate and/or C-reactive protein), thrombocytosis, and anemia of chronic disease. Although complement levels are normal or elevated in RA, hypocomplementemia is often seen in patients with rheumatoid vasculitis.

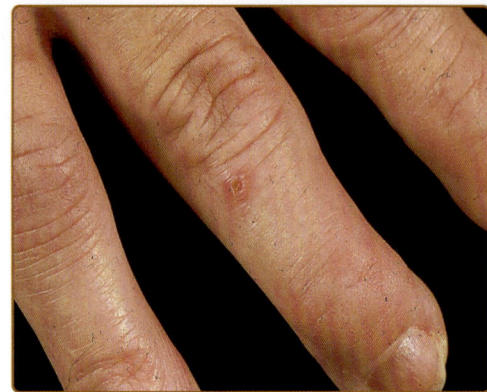

Figure 66-3 Bywaters lesions. Note the purpuric papule on the dorsal finger.

Vasculitis Pathology: Rheumatoid vasculitis primarily affects small- to medium-sized vessels systemically and shares many features with polyarteritis nodosa, albeit without the development of microaneurysms.[20] Histopathologic examination reveals mononuclear or neutrophilic infiltration of the vessel walls and elements of vessel wall destruction (necrosis, leukocytoclasis, and disruption of the elastic laminae).[20] Isolated capillaritis or perivascular infiltrates without vessel wall involvement can be seen in RA, but are not adequate for a histopathologic diagnosis of rheumatoid vasculitis.

Cutaneous Rheumatoid Vasculitis: The skin is involved in 75% to 89% of patients with rheumatoid vasculitis, often as the presenting sign of the condition.[6] Somewhat confusing the interpretation of vasculitis incidence in many studies is the inclusion of purpura, livedo reticularis, atrophie blanche, and ulcers as cutaneous signs of rheumatoid vasculitis, despite the often nonvasculitic histology.[6] Exclusion of nailfold involvement in a recent study found rheumatoid vasculitis involved skin in 65% of patients. Some patients may have nailfold telangiectasias, with minute digital ulcerations or petechiae and digital pulp papules (Bywaters lesions; Fig. 66-3). These papules are a manifestation of mild vasculitis and typically occur without systemic signs of vasculitis.

Pyoderma Gangrenosum and Felty Syndrome Ulcers: Vasculitis, along with certain other extraarticular manifestations of RA (pericarditis, pleuritis, amyloidosis sacculitis) can present as lower-extremity ulcers. However, pyoderma gangrenosum (see Chap. 37) should be suspected if deep liquefying ulcers with a characteristic purple, undermined border occur in patients with RA. The ulcers may occur at any site, but are most common on the lower extremities and abdomen. Pyoderma gangrenosum occurs more frequently and more severely in females and may take years to heal. Leg ulcers may also appear in patients with Felty syndrome, a combination of chronic RA, hypersplenism, and leukopenia (Fig. 66-4).[12] In some instances, the ulcers of Felty syndrome exhibit the same morphologic characteristics and behavior of pyoderma gangrenosum ulcers, suggesting that these ulcers are not necessarily a manifestation of rheumatoid vasculitis.

TNF-inhibitor therapy is associated with both onset and improvement of rheumatoid vasculitis. Other vasculitis syndromes, such as cryoglobulinemic vasculitis (see Chap. 144), erythema elevatum diutinum (see Chap. 140), benign cutaneous polyarteritis nodosa, and livedo vasculitis (segmental hyalinizing vasculitis/atrophie blanche; see Chap. 148), and reactive angioendotheliomatosis,[12] also have been described in patients with RA. Treatment with argatroban, an antithrombin agent, in a patient with antiphosphatidylserine prothrombin complex antibodies led to resolution

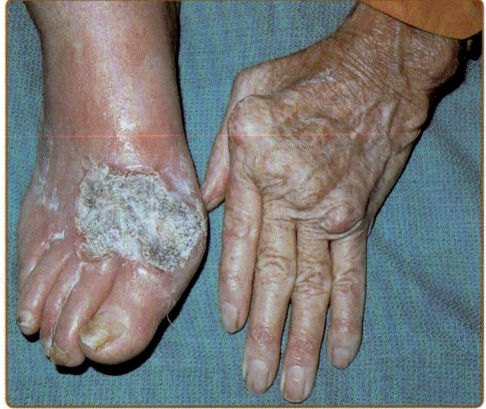

Figure 66-4 Felty syndrome ulcer. A refractory ulcer on the foot of a patient with rheumatoid arthritis and hypersplenism.

of ulcers refractory to immunosuppressive therapy, consistent with occlusive, rather than vasculitic, mechanisms in some patients. Raynaud phenomenon affects 5% to 17% of RA patients.[7]

Intravascular or Intralymphatic Histiocytosis: Indurated erythema, livedo-like erythema, and papules over the elbows have been reported as clinical findings of intravascular or intralymphatic histiocytosis in RA.[23,24]

OTHER SKIN MANIFESTATIONS

Palmar erythema, erythromelalgia, autoimmune bullous diseases such as epidermolysis bullosa acquisita (see Chap. 56), yellow nail syndrome (see Chap. 91), erythema multiforme (see Chap. 43), erythema nodosum (see Chap. 73), and urticaria (see Chap. 41) also have been reported in patients with RA.[25]

NONCUTANEOUS FINDINGS

In addition to systemic vasculitis, which can affect numerous organ systems, there are multiple nondermatologic extraarticular manifestations of RA. Table 66-3 lists the more common ones.

Articular Manifestations: The articular manifestations of RA relate to an inflammatory synovitis that can affect joints, tendons, and bursae. Synovial inflammation usually results in warmth, but not erythema of the affected area. Significant pain is associated with stretching of the joint capsule. Hand and foot involvement is predominant in most patients. Although the initial manifestations in the hand may be asymmetric, the clinical course subsequently takes on a symmetric and diffuse pattern. The pattern of joint involvement is highly suggestive of the diagnosis with characteristic involvement of the proximal interphalangeal and metacarpophalangeal joints with sparing of the distal interphalangeal joints.

Chronic inflammation may result in irreversible structural damage of the joint, including cartilage destruction and bony erosion. Late structural deformities may result from soft-tissue contractures or from bony ankylosis. Characteristic deformities include radial deviation of the hand with ulnar deviation of the digits, the "swan neck" deformity from hyperextension of the proximal interphalangeal joint and compensatory flexion of the distal interphalangeal joint, and the boutonnière deformity from flexion contracture of the proximal interphalangeal joint and extension of the distal interphalangeal joint. Similar structural deformities can occur in the feet, and all can be debilitating. Involvement of the thoracic and lumbar spine in RA is exceptional. Although the shoulder joint is often affected, it is soft-tissue structures, which include the rotator cuff tendons and muscles and the subacromial bursa, that are usually symptomatic.[26]

ETIOLOGY AND PATHOGENESIS

An important posttranslational modification of protein is the conversion of arginine to its polar analog, citrulline. This greatly enhances immune recognition of joint-associated proteins, which are selectively targeted by autoreactive T and B cells in patients with RA.[21,22] The selective recognition of citrullinated synovial proteins is important in pathogenesis.[21,22] Anticitrullinated protein antibodies (ACPAs) are of particular interest, as these autoantibodies are highly specific for RA and can be found in approximately 50% of early RA patients. In addition, the presence of anticyclic citrullinated peptide antibodies predicts disease severity and radiologic damage. Therefore, ACPA could also be used as a biomarker for patients with a more-severe disease phenotype to target those patients for more aggressive treatment. In addition, the number of citrullinated antigens identified by ACPA increases exponentially through epitope spreading leading up to disease onset.

It is now known that breaking tolerance to posttranslationally modified proteins in arthritis is not exclusively confined to citrullination. Proteins that have undergone a different type of posttranslational modification are also recognized by autoantibodies. One of these posttranslational processes is carbamylation, where the amino acid lysine is changed to become homocitrulline. Smoking can enhance carbamylation and extensive carbamylation is especially likely during chronic inflammation. Antibodies to carbamylated proteins were found to be present not only in ACPA+ patients but also in ACPA– RA patients.[21,22]

The progression toward RA almost certainly begins long before the disease manifests as arthritis, and this progression depends on both important genetic factors

TABLE 66-3
Nondermatologic Manifestations of Rheumatoid Arthritis

TYPE	MANIFESTATIONS
Ocular	Keratoconjunctivitis sicca, scleritis, episcleritis, scleromalacia
Renal	Amyloidosis, vasculitis
Hematologic	Anemia, thrombocytosis, lymphadenopathy, Felty syndrome
Neurologic	Entrapment neuropathy, cervical myelopathy, mononeuritis multiplex (from vasculitis), peripheral neuropathy
Lung	Pleural effusions, pulmonary fibrosis, bronchiolitis obliterans, rheumatoid nodules, vasculitis
Cardiac	Pericarditis, premature atherosclerosis, vasculitis, nodules, aortic root dilation

and less-well-defined environmental factors.[22] Twin studies have shown heritability of RA to be 60%, with the remaining risk presumably a result of environmental factors. More than 100 genetic loci are associated with RA, the most important being within the human leukocyte antigen (HLA) class II region, encoding the HLA-DRB1 molecule. Recent evidence suggests that this locus is associated not with a risk of becoming ACPA+, but rather with the risk of progressing from ACPA+ to ACPA+ RA.

DIAGNOSIS

Several conditions can mimic RA, and must be considered in the differential diagnosis of early disease, such as viral syndromes (especially parvovirus B19, rubella, hepatitides B and C); psoriatic arthritis; polymyalgia rheumatica; remitting seronegative symmetric synovitis with pitting edema; palindromic rheumatism; adult Still disease; systemic lupus erythematosus; gout; multicentric reticulohistiocytosis; and leprosy.[26-28] Table 66-1 lists the diagnostic criteria.

SUPPORTIVE STUDIES AND LABORATORY TESTING

There is no one specific histologic, radiographic, or laboratory test that conclusively permits the diagnosis of RA. Rheumatoid factor, an autoantibody that reacts with the Fc portion of immunoglobulin G, is found in sera of 85% of patients with RA. Rheumatoid factor positivity is not definitive because it can be found in other disease processes, for example, lupus erythematosus, Sjögren/sicca syndrome, myositis, sarcoidosis, liver diseases, pulmonary fibrotic processes, and cryoglobulinemia. It is also found in 3% to 5% of the unaffected population.[29] A false-positive rheumatoid factor can be caused by many factors, including chronic bacterial infections such as infective endocarditis, hepatitis C, tuberculosis, and Lyme disease, as well as by viral diseases such as rubella and infectious mononucleosis.[30,31]

ACPAs are a more specific marker than rheumatoid factor, particularly in early disease where specificity ranges from 94% to 100%, compared to 23% to 94% for rheumatoid factor, with roughly equivalent sensitivities.[32]

Several studies confirm the increased sensitivity of ultrasonography compared with the standard clinical examination to define typical joint or tissue pathologies. Ultrasonography provides detailed information about the status of the synovial membrane, tendons, cartilage, bursae, and cortical bones. Ultrasonography allows the detection and characterization of intraarticular and periarticular inflammatory processes, such as effusion versus synovial hypertrophy, fundamental to the correct interpretation of the pathologic process.[33]

CLINICAL COURSE, PROGNOSIS, AND MANAGEMENT

Because the exact cause of RA is unknown, treatment has been directed against various components of the inflammatory process.[22] In the past, most patients with early disease were started on NSAIDs until joint erosions were evident. Although useful to alleviate symptoms, these medications do not alter disease progression. The genetic susceptibility variants identified as of this writing strongly implicate several immune pathways in the development of RA.[22] In addition, there is already significant overlap between the targets of several approved RA therapies and identified susceptibility genes for RA (cytotoxic T-lymphocyte antigen [CTLA]-4: abatacept; tyrosine kinase [TYK]-2: tofacitinib; interleukin [IL]-6: tocilizumab) demonstrating the potential of genetics not only to identify biologic pathways that lead to RA, but also that these pathways can be targeted and lead to the successful treatment of disease symptoms.

European League Against Rheumatism recommendations for management of RA were updated in 2016.[34] In part, they maintain that rheumatologists are the specialists who should primarily care for patients with RA, that treatment decisions should be shared with the patient, and that treatment decisions should be based on disease activity, progression of structural damage, comorbidities, and safety issues. This new recommendation means that therapy with disease-modifying antirheumatic drugs (DMARDs) should be started as soon as the diagnosis is made, with the aim of sustained remission or low disease activity.[34] Methotrexate should be part of the first treatment strategy unless contraindicated, when leflunomide or sulfasalazine are suggested. Short-term glucocorticoids should be considered when initiating or changing conventional DMARDs. Failure of response or poor prognostic factors should prompt consideration for use of biologic DMARDs, including TNF inhibitors (adalimumab, certolizumab, etanercept, golimumab, and infliximab), a costimulation inhibitor (abatacept), an IL-6 receptor blocker (tocilizumab, possibly sarilumab in the future), IL-6 inhibitors (possibly clazakizumab or sirukumab in the future), an anti–B-cell agent (rituximab), as well as synthetic targeted DMARDs, primarily Janus kinase (JAK) inhibitors, tofacitinib, and perhaps baricitinab.[34-36] Anakinra competitively inhibits IL-1 effects, but is currently thought to be a less-effective biologic DMARD for RA.[37]

Treatment of rheumatoid vasculitis is difficult. Use of hydroxychloroquine and low-dose aspirin is associated with lower odds of developing rheumatoid vasculitis among RA patients, thus conferring a possible protective effect.[20] Despite aggressive use of cyclophosphamide and biologics, rheumatoid vasculitis remains difficult to treat, with high relapse and mortality rates that have not changed in more than 40 years, with 5-year mortality rates ranging from 26% to 60%.[20]

JUVENILE IDIOPATHIC ARTHRITIS

AT-A-GLANCE

- There are multiple forms of juvenile idiopathic arthritis (JIA) (formerly juvenile rheumatoid arthritis).
- The multisystemic form of JIA is often referred to as juvenile Still syndrome (sJIA).
- The eruption, along with fever and arthralgia/arthritis can trigger consideration of this systemic form, and is limited to this form.
- There are more recently recognized variants of the eruption.

Juvenile idiopathic arthritis (JIA) is a group of conditions encompassing all forms of arthritis of unknown etiology lasting for at least 6 weeks and with an onset before 16 years of age.[38] It replaces the previous terms juvenile RA and Still disease, and currently encompasses 7 entities: systemic onset arthritis, oligoarthritis (persistent or extended), rheumatoid factor–negative polyarthritis, rheumatoid factor–positive polyarthritis, psoriatic arthritis, enthesitis-related arthritis, and undifferentiated.[38,39] Of these, only the systemic-onset form (sJIA) and the psoriatic arthritis form have skin findings. The diagnosis of juvenile psoriatic arthritis requires the coexistence of arthritis and a typical psoriatic rash or, when the rash is missing, the presence of arthritis and any 2 of the following: family history of psoriasis in a first-degree relative, dactylitis (sausage-like swelling of individual digits that extends beyond the joint margins), and nail pitting or onycholysis.[38] There is increasing evidence that juvenile psoriatic arthritis is not a homogeneous disease entity, but includes at least 2 distinct subgroups: one shares the same characteristics as early-onset antinuclear antibody–positive JIA (antinuclear antibody positivity bridges several subsets); the other belongs to the spectrum of spondyloarthropathies.[38] As psoriatic skin disease is well characterized elsewhere, this chapter focuses predominantly on sJIA.

EPIDEMIOLOGY

The reported incidence and prevalence of JIA in European and North American populations range from 2 to 20 and from 16 to 150 per 100,000, respectively.[38,40] sJIA accounts for 5% to 15% of children with JIA in North America and Europe.[38] One study of JIA patients over a 53-year period (1960-2013) found no significant change in overall incidence; however, the incidence decreased among females ($P = 0.003$).[40] A cyclic pattern of incidence was observed, with peaks approximately every 10 years.

CLINICAL FEATURES

sJIA accounts for 5% to 15% of children with JIA in North America and Europe.[38] The Internation League of Associations for Rheumatology criteria for sJIA require the presence of arthritis accompanied or preceded by a documented quotidian fever of at least 2 weeks duration, plus at least 1 of the following: characteristic rash, generalized symmetrical lymphadenopathy, enlargement of liver or spleen, or serositis (pericarditis, pleural or pericardial effusion, [rarely] peritonitis).[38] The fever has a typical intermittent pattern, with 1 or 2 daily spikes, up to 39°C (102.2°F) or higher, followed by rapid return to baseline. The erythematous, salmon pink, evanescent macular rash usually appears with the fever. Arthritis is often symmetrical and polyarticular, but may be absent at onset and develop much later. Diagnosis cannot be considered definite until arthritis is present. Signs of systemic inflammation are invariably present, but there are no specific laboratory abnormalities.[38,39]

CUTANEOUS FINDINGS

The classic sJIA eruption has been a very transient salmon pink mostly macular eruption (Fig. 66-5) coincident with febrile episodes. It may at times be indistinguishable from urticaria but is typically not pruritic. The eruption is identical to that often seen in adult-onset Still disease.[38] However, very different cutaneous presentations have been newly recognized in adult-onset Still disease. Of these variants, one also has been described (rarely) in sJIA—persistent pruritic papules and plaques (see section "Adult-onset Still Disease"). Perhaps the others will subsequently be reported in JIA.

NONCUTANEOUS FINDINGS

Enthesitis: Because enthesitis is common to both the psoriatic arthritis and the enthesitis-related arthritis category of JIA, it is important to be aware of enthesi-

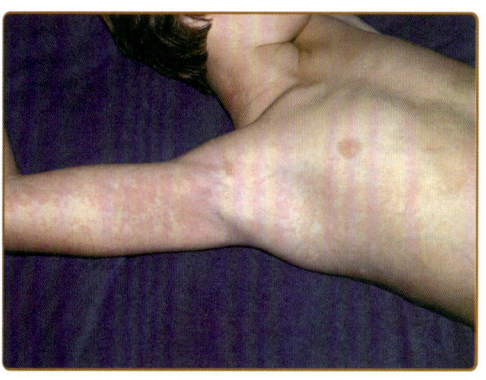

Figure 66-5 Juvenile idiopathic arthritis. (Used with permission from the William Weston, MD Collection.)

tis-related arthritis. It usually affects boys older than age 6 years and presents with lower-limb asymmetrical arthritis associated with enthesitis. Later, these children can develop inflammatory lumbosacral pain and are at risk of developing acute anterior uveitis. Almost two-third of patients with enthesitis-related arthritis have persistent disease. The presence of hip or ankle arthritis and a family history of spondyloarthropathy or polyarticular joint involvement at onset are associated with poorer prognosis. Psoriatic arthritis can also present as enthesitis, with evolution of cutaneous findings later.[41,42]

Macrophage Activation Syndrome: A secondary or acquired form of hemophagocytic lymphohistiocytosis (HLH), macrophage activation syndrome (MAS) is a potentially life-threatening complication of rheumatic disorders, most commonly with sJIA and adult-onset Still disease.[38,43] The full syndrome is thought to occur in roughly 10% of children with sJIA, but may be partially expressed in as high as 30% to 40%. A change in the fever pattern from the intermittent spikes of sJIA to a continuous high level is often the heralding clinical manifestation. Hepatosplenomegaly, generalized lymphadenopathy may worsen acutely. CNS dysfunction develops in one-third of children, typically as lethargy, irritability, disorientation, headache, seizures, or coma. These may be explained by the association of MAS with thrombotic thrombocytopenic purpura. Skin or mucosal hemorrhage may be seen in 20% of all MAS. Heart, lung, and kidney failure may eventuate in the sickest patients. Typically, cytopenia, abnormal liver function tests, a prolonged prothrombin time and partial thromboplastin time, and serum ferritin 5000 to 10,000 ng/mL are present.[39]

In 2016, collaborative guidelines were proposed for the classification of MAS in sJIA. MAS is considered present if a *febrile* patient with *known* or *suspected sJIA* who has a *ferritin* value >684 ng/mL also exhibits any 2 of the following: *platelet count* ≤181 × 10^9/L, *aspartate aminotransferase* >48 units/L, *triglycerides* >156 mg/dL, or *fibrinogen* ≤360 mg/dL.[43] It was also noted that treatments for sJIA such as IL-1 blocker canakinumab and IL-6 blocker tocilizumab might inhibit the full expression of MAS, thereby clouding the diagnosis.

ETIOLOGY AND PATHOGENESIS

The factors leading to JIA are poorly understood. The concordance rates for JIA among monozygotic twins ranges from 25% to 40%, and disease phenotypes are very similar in both twin and sibling pairs for onset and disease course.[44] There appears to be a familial link between RA and JIA, as well a familial risk of autoimmunity, such as thyroid disease. Gene associations vary between the subsets of JIA. sJIA seems to be strongly associated with HLA DRB1:11,[44] while HLA-B27, the microbiome, γ/δ-T cells and the IL-23/IL-17 axis all likely contribute to enthesitis-related arthritis pathogenesis.[45]

DIAGNOSIS

Dermatologic expertise can be crucial to recognizing the expanding spectrum of cutaneous findings in sJIA and adult-onset Still disease, especially with the newly recognized cutaneous variants of these syndromes (see "Adult-Onset Still Disease" below). In addition, dermatologists can offer insight into the differential diagnosis of the variable morphologic patterns seen in sJIA and their associations with other conditions, especially with autoimmune and autoinflammatory syndromes.

SUPPORTIVE STUDIES AND LABORATORY TESTING

Conventional radiographs are poor at assessing joint inflammation in JIA.[38] An MRI is more sensitive but difficult to use routinely, especially in children. Ultrasonography may be very sensitive in detecting early inflammation and minimal effusions, but is also very operator dependent and not routinely available in clinic or at bedside.

DIFFERENTIAL DIAGNOSIS

The differential diagnosis of JIA, in the absence of helpful skin findings, is extensive and is essentially a diagnosis of exclusion. The systemic onset form can be mimicked or confused with many different syndromes in pediatric patients, such as: (a) infections (septicemia, bacterial endocarditis, brucellosis, typhoid fever, leishmaniasis, viral); (b) malignancy/lymphoproliferative (leukemia, lymphoma, neuroblastoma, Castleman syndrome); (c) acute rheumatic fever; (d) connective tissue diseases (especially systemic lupus, Kawasaki syndrome, systemic vasculitides); (e) inflammatory bowel disease; (f) sarcoidosis; and (g) autoinflammatory syndromes.[38] Other than sJIA and the psoriatic subset of JIA, dermatologists will probably not be involved in the diagnosis of JIA.

CLINICAL COURSE, PROGNOSIS, AND MANAGEMENT

Because JIA affects individuals who are rapidly developing physically, mentally, and socially, treatment must be multifaceted and include counseling and encouragement to negotiate the challenges of participating in daily activities, along with physical therapy and occupational therapy. NSAIDs have been used as short-term monotherapy for JIA, but are not disease modifying. Intraarticular corticosteroid injections are frequently used, particularly in oligoarthritis.[38] Methotrexate remains the most widely used conventional DMARD in management of JIA; leflunomide may have similar effectiveness but there is little experience in children. Systemic glucocorticoids are mainly used to manage more-severe extraarticular manifestations such as high fever unresponsive to NSAIDs, severe anemia, myocarditis, pericarditis, and MAS.[38] TNF inhibitors are increasingly used to treat JIA.[38,46,47] Other biologics have been reported successful in treating JIA, including anakinra (anti–IL-1) abatacept (inhibits T-cell activation), tocilizumab (inhibits IL-6), and rituximab (anti–B-cell), but none are yet approved for treating JIA. Unfortunately, TNF blockers, and anti–IL-1 and anti–IL-6 agents, while improving some patients with JIA, also have been implicated in triggering MAS.[47] Whether this is a causal association is not known.

Treatment of MAS is less certain. High-dose corticosteroids are typically given, but cyclosporine and IL-1 inhibitors have shown some efficacy in resistant cases, as has etoposide, which is used for hemophagocytic lymphohistiocytosis.[48]

ADULT-ONSET STILL DISEASE

AT-A-GLANCE

- Multisystem syndrome that can mimic infection.
- Classic eruption is well described, but several new atypical variants are now recognized.
- Appears to have an association with malignancy, perhaps more so in those with atypical cutaneous presentations.

The expression *adult-onset Still disease* (AOSD) was introduced by Bywaters in 1971 to characterize a syndrome of seronegative polyarthritis, salmon-colored mostly macular and evanescent eruption, fever, and raised erythrocyte sedimentation rate, which, along with neutrophilic leukocytosis, mirrors the presentation of sJIA.[49,50]

EPIDEMIOLOGY

This syndrome most often affects younger adults, and females more often in Eastern than in Western countries.[49] Its incidence has been estimated at 0.16 per 100,000 in France, and 0.22 and 0.34 per 100,000 for men and women in Japan. Its prevalence was calculated at 0.73 and 1.74 for men and women in Japan.[49,50]

CLINICAL FEATURES

High fever of unknown origin exceeding 39°C is the presenting sign of AOSD in most patients.[49-51] Classically, patients present with 1 to 2 daily fever spikes above 39°C (102.2°F) occurring in the afternoon or evening and receding within hours. A retrospective review of 245 Italian patients combined with other recent series of AOSD patients resulted in a total of 731 patients.[51] Findings in the cumulative group included 61% were female, the average age at onset was 42.4 years, and there was an average delay in diagnosis of 2.33 months. The frequency of symptoms and signs in descending order was fever 93%, arthralgia 90%, rash 70% (Fig. 66-6), sore throat 64%, lymphadenopathy/splenomegaly 53%, hepatomegaly 39%, and pericarditis 13%.[51] Myalgia was not reported but other reviews find that myalgia occurred in 35% to 44% of patients.[49,50] The course of the disease was monocyclic in 24% to 30%, polycyclic in 41% to 44% (intermittent episodes with remission in between), and chronic articular in 26% to 36% of patients.[49,51]

CUTANEOUS FINDINGS

Table 66-4 outlines the cutaneous manifestations of AOSD.

Classical Cutaneous Presentation: The skin is involved in 60% to 70% of cases.[49,51] It is seen more often in the febrile presentation than in the solely arthritic form of disease. It most characteristically occurs on the chest, abdomen, and extensor surfaces

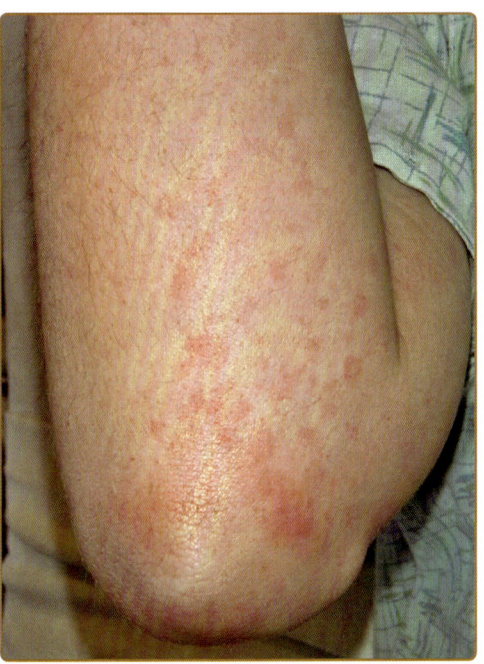

Figure 66-6 Adult-onset Still disease. Lesions are discrete pink to red macules and slightly edematous papules. (Used with permission from James E. Fitzpatrick, MD.)

of the arms, and tends to peak with the fever in the late afternoon, and then disappears, only to recur with fever the following day.[52] The rash consists of discrete pink to red macules or slightly edematous papules ranging in size from 5 to 10 mm (see Fig. 66-6). The lesions tend to be relatively fixed in shape and site during their daily eruption and seldom itch. Koebner phenomena may be seen. This is also the typical eruption of sJIA.

Atypical Cutaneous Presentations: In one series of 81 patients with atypical cutaneous AOSD, 87% were female, ages ranged from 8 to 83 years (median: 36 ± 16 years), and 64% were from East Asia.[53] Atypical cutaneous features were often present in addition to the typical evanescent rash,[54] but in 30% to 43% of the cases the only skin manifestations were atypical.[53,54] The most often reported atypical presentation is that of persistent, pruritic papules and plaques,[54,55] which are present in 75% of patients, and pruritic 87% of the time.[53] Rarely, this presentation also is seen in sJIA.[55] These lesions may develop fine scale, and are most commonly located on trunk, extremities, head, and/or neck. In some cases, plaques are linear suggesting triggering by local trauma (Koebner phenomenon). The color of the atypical eruption was either erythematous or brown, and less commonly violaceous.[54] Table 66-4 lists other less-common atypical variants. More than one morphology or distribution pattern was observed in several patients. The most commonly involved areas were the back, followed by chest, abdomen, and extensor surface of extremities.[53]

NONCUTANEOUS FINDINGS

In 731 patients with arthritis, 23.7% had monoarthritis, 44.3% had oligoarthritis, and 32% had polyarthritis.[51] Fever >39.5°C (103.1°F) seemed predictive of monocyclic AOSD, whereas arthritis and thrombocytopenia were associated with chronic and complicated AOSD, respectively.[49]

COMPLICATIONS

Two serious complications associated with AOSD are reactive hemophagocytic syndrome (2.85% to 6%) and thrombotic thrombocytopenic purpura.[49,51,53,56,57] Reactive hemophagocytic syndrome is similar if not identical to MAS, and both are essentially part of the hemophagocytic lymphohistiocytosis spectrum. Both are rare, and the reasons for these associations are unknown.

An important newly recognized complication of AOSD is its association with malignancy.[54,58] Initially, this association was thought to be more common with the classical skin eruption,[54] but there is conflicting data suggesting atypical skin disease may increase the risk.[58] Malignancy may precede, appear concurrently, or present months or years after symptoms and signs of AOSD.[54] The diagnosis of malignancy did not precede or immediately follow a clinical presentation otherwise consistent with AOSD in a considerable subset of patients (42%).[54] Median time between diagnosis of AOSD and detection of malignancy was 9 months.[58] The malignancies were 50% hematopoietic (mostly lymphomas), 50% solid tumors (breast, lung, esophagus, and liver angiosarcoma).[58] Others were myeloproliferative, myelodysplastic, papillary thyroid, laryngeal squamous cell, melanoma, ovarian, kidney.[54,58] In some patients, AOSD resolved after successful therapy for tumor.[58] With regard to hematologic malignancies, lactate dehydrogenase, atypical cells in the blood count, and possibly also elevated soluble IL-2 receptor levels are red flags. A bone marrow biopsy should be of considered in the initial workup and any accessible enlarged lymph node should be biopsied.[58]

Myocarditis is a rare but potentially life-threatening complication that responds positively to corticosteroids and other immunomodulatory drugs.[59]

TABLE 66-4
Cutaneous Manifestations of Adult-Onset Still Disease

Classical Presentations
- Salmon-colored, macular or slightly papular evanescent eruption usually concurrent with fever spikes; may show Koebner phenomenon[52]
- Urticarial eruption morphologically, but typically nonpruritic

Atypical Variants
- Up to 81% had concurrent classical eruption with adult-onset Still disease[54]

Most Common
- Persistent, pruritic papules and plaques[54,55]
- Pigmented >50% cases[53]

Rare
- Urticarial erythema and papules
- Dermatographism-like
- Generalized or widespread persistent nonpruritic erythema[53]
- Flagellate erythema
- Lichenoid papules
- Dermatomyositis-like
- Dermatomyositis-like edema of lids without other findings[53]
- Lichen amyloidosis-like
- Prurigo pigmentosa-like
- Vesiculopustular eruption hands and feet or trunk and limbs[53]
- Widespread peau d'orange skin change (cutaneous mucinosa)[53]
- Photoaccentuation noted occasionally
- More than one morphology or distribution pattern observed in several patients
- Most commonly involved

DIAGNOSIS

AOSD remains difficult to diagnose. Exclusion of causes of fever of unknown origin is essential, and use of published criteria for AOSD is important. The standard criteria set for AOSD has been the Yamaguchi criteria. Alternative criteria have been proposed; one (Fautrel) has a recent supportive large comparison study, includes glycosylated ferritin as a specific criteria, and does not require exclusion criteria. Table 66-5 includes both sets of criteria.[60,61]

SUPPORTIVE STUDIES AND LABORATORY TESTING

In the largest review of AOSD, leukocytosis occurred in 85% of patients and was composed of ≥80% polymorphonuclear neutrophils in 69% of patients.[51] In decreasing order of frequency, the following values were noted: increased C-reactive protein 93%, elevated erythrocyte sedimentation rate (≥20 mm/h) 85%, elevated hepatic enzymes 62%, and thrombocytosis (>400 × 10^9/L) 46%. Antinuclear antibody, rheumatoid factor, and cyclic citrullinated peptide antibodies were rarely positive.[51] Anemia <10 g/dL has been reported in 50% to 75% of patients.[61]

Serum ferritin above normal levels was observed in 56.4% of patients with elevations of more than 3 times normal in 60%.[51] A very elevated serum ferritin with a lowered concentration of glycosylated ferritin, is strongly suggestive of, but not specific for, this diagnosis. Perhaps more specific is the fraction of glycosylated ferritin. In healthy individuals, 50% to 80% of serum ferritin is glycosylated, but this drops to 20% to 50% in patients with inflammatory diseases.[61] The assessment of glycosylated ferritin was correlated with early diagnosis in one study.[49]

PATHOLOGY

Classical Cutaneous: The histopathology of the classical eruption of AOSD is characterized by a mild inflammatory cell infiltration (lymphocytic, lymphohistiocytic, mixed, or predominantly neutrophilic, occasionally eosinophilic) in the upper dermis, basal vacuolization, keratinocyte necrosis, presence of karyorrhexis, and mucin in the dermis. Some of the histologic findings from lesions submitted to pathology as acute (such as acanthosis, parakeratosis, and rarely reported neutrophilic eccrine hidradenitis and neutrophilic urticarial dermatosis) seem to be more chronic changes.[62-64] Whether the specimens were actually from some of the more chronic lesions of atypical skin in AOSD patients who had both classical and atypical lesions will no doubt be sorted out in future studies.

Atypical Cutaneous: The histopathology of lesions in the persistent pruritic papule and plaque variant includes dyskeratosis present mainly in the superficial epidermis without accompanying basilar dyskeratosis, and a sparse superficial dermal infiltrate often with neutrophils but without vasculitis.[54,55] Occasionally dermal mucin deposition, subcorneal or intracorneal pustules, acanthosis or spongiosis were noted.[55]

Extracutaneous: Aside from the skin, pathologic findings have shown lymph node findings of paracortical or diffuse hyperplasia pattern with immunoblastic and vascular proliferation, which can mimic angioimmunoblastic T-cell lymphoma in nodes.[64] Liver biopsies showed sparse portal and sinusoidal inflammatory cell infiltration, with various degrees of Kupffer cell hyperplasia. The cellularity of bone marrow varied from 20% to 80%. Myeloid cell hyperplasia was frequent. On immunohistochemistry, the number of CD8+ lymphocytes was greater than that of CD4+ lymphocytes in the skin, liver, and bone marrow, but the number of CD4+ lymphocytes was greater than that of CD8+ lymphocytes in the lymph nodes.[64]

TABLE 66-5
Adult-Onset Still Disease Criteria

Yamaguchi et al	Fautrel et al
■ At least 5 criteria, 2 of which must be major, *and* ■ No exclusion criteria	■ Four major criteria *or* ■ Three major criteria and 2 minor criteria
Major Criteria	**Major Criteria**
■ Fever ≥39°C (102.2°F) lasting 1 week or more ■ Arthralgia lasting 2 weeks or more ■ Typical skin rash: maculopapular, nonpruritic, salmon-pink rash with concomitant fever spikes ■ Leucocytosis ≥10,000/mm³ with neutrophil polymorphonuclear count ≥80%	■ Spiking fever 39°C (102.2°F) ■ Arthralgia ■ Transient erythema ■ Pharyngitis ■ Neutrophil polymorphonuclear count ≥80% ■ Glycosylated ferritin fraction ≤20%
Minor	**Minor**
■ Pharyngitis or sore throat ■ Lymphadenopathy and/or splenomegaly ■ Liver enzyme abnormalities (aminotransferases) ■ Negative for rheumatoid factor or antinuclear antibodies	■ Typical rash ■ Leucocytosis >10,000/mm³
Exclusion Criteria	**Exclusion Criteria**
■ Absence of infection, especially sepsis and Epstein-Barr viral infection ■ Absence of malignant diseases, especially lymphomas ■ Absence of inflammatory disease, especially polyarteritis nodosa	■ None

DIFFERENTIAL DIAGNOSIS

The differential diagnosis of the cutaneous manifestations is extensive, based on the cutaneous manifestations present, as listed in Table 66-4. The differential diagnosis of AOSD in general often falls into the category of fever of unknown origin, and is quite extensive, focusing particularly on acute or subacute infections autoinflammatory diseases, and systemic autoimmune diseases.

CLINICAL COURSE AND PROGNOSIS

Acute disease is often treated with NSAIDs, particularly enteric-coated aspirin, although this is often ineffective, with response rates of 20% to 25%.[51] Corticosteroids are often used acutely. Steroid-sparing medications are often required, and include IM gold, D-penicillamine, sulfasalazine, hydroxychloroquine, methotrexate, thalidomide, azathioprine, cyclosporine, cyclophosphamide, and IV immunoglobulin. Biologic agents are increasingly reported for resistant or chronic cases, and are sometimes used as first-line therapy. These include anti-TNF agents, anakinra (anti–IL-1), rituximab, tocilizumab, and canakinumab (an IL-6 receptor inhibitor).[41,42,47,49,51,53]

The treatment guidelines for reactive hemophagocytic syndrome in AOSD have not been established. For JIA-associated reactive hemophagocytic syndrome, the main treatment is the administration of high-dose steroids.[65] However, refractory cases of reactive hemophagocytic syndrome require additional therapy. In adults, medications which may be effective include methotrexate, azathioprine, high-dose IV immunoglobulins, cyclosporine, cyclophosphamide, plasma exchange, etoposide, and anti-TNF agents.[65]

RHEUMATIC FEVER

AT-A-GLANCE

- Incidence has rapidly declined in more-developed nations.
- Rare complication of oropharyngeal group A streptococcal infection.
- Distinctive but uncommon cutaneous manifestation of erythema marginatum.
- Erythema marginatum has been used to describe different skin manifestations in other clinical settings, which can be confusing.

Acute rheumatic fever is an inflammatory response to group A streptococcal infection, which typically occurs 2 to 3 weeks after a throat infection.[66] It is a delayed sequel to group A β-hemolytic streptococcal infection of the oropharynx. It is an inflammatory disease that can affect the heart, joints, CNS, skin, and subcutaneous tissues. It is a clinical diagnosis made on the basis of criteria, the latest from 2015.[67] Treatment of the underlying infection, if recognized, prevents rheumatic fever,

EPIDEMIOLOGY

The incidence of acute rheumatic fever (ARF) and the prevalence of rheumatic heart disease substantially declined in the last century in Europe, North America, and other developed nations.[67] This decline is attributed to improved hygiene, improved access to antibiotic drugs and medical care, reduced household crowding, and possibly changes in the epidemiology of specific group A streptococcal strains, as well as other social and economic changes. The major burden is currently found in low- and middle-income countries and in selected indigenous populations elsewhere, especially among Pacific people, New Zealand Maori, and indigenous Australians.[66,67] A resurgence of ARF in the intermountain areas of the United States, occurred in the 1980s.[66]

The pattern of disease in the high-prevalence regions is often hyperendemic, with cases occurring throughout the year and near absence of outbreaks. In contrast, high-income settings experience a low background incidence of ARF with periodic outbreaks.[67] Currently, the average incidence in most developed communities is less than 5 per 100,000 population.[68] Most cases of ARF occur in children ages 5 to 15 years, but it may occasionally occur in young adults.[66]

Streptococcal pharyngitis is a common infection in childhood. Pharyngitis caused by rheumatogenic strains of group A *Streptococcus* in a susceptible host triggers an abnormal immune inflammatory response.[66] This response most probably involves cross reactivity of streptococcal antibodies against myocardium, synovial tissue, and, in chorea, the basal ganglia. In carditis, activated monoclonal autoantibodies produce T-cell infiltration in the valve endothelium.[66] Oddly, however, the morbidity and mortality of rheumatic fever results from valvular disease rather than acute carditis.[68]

CLINICAL FEATURES

ARF is characterized by a clinical syndrome, typically presenting as migratory polyarthritis, especially knees, ankles, elbows, and wrists.[66,67] Carditis occurs in approximately 80% of people with rheumatic fever and commonly affects the mitral and aortic valves, resulting in regurgitation. Other less-common clinical features include abnormal involuntary movements (chorea), and the skin findings of erythema marginatum and subcutaneous nodules.[66,67] A history of rapid improvement with salicylates or NSAIDs is also characteristic. Generally, the arthritis in ARF runs a self-limited course, even without therapy, lasting approximately 4 weeks.[67] In practice, the joint manifestations can be difficult to assess because of good response to NSAIDs, which can mask the symptoms. Monoarthritis, particularly involving the hip, also has been described as a presenting feature in populations

TABLE 66-6

Diagnosis of Acute Rheumatic Fever in Patient Populations with Evidence of Preceding Group A Streptococcal Infection Using the 2015 Revised Jones Criteria[a]

- Diagnosis of initial acute rheumatic fever: 2 major criteria *or* 1 major plus 2 minor criteria
- Diagnosis of recurrent acute rheumatic fever: 2 major criteria *or* 1 major plus 2 minor *or* 3 minor criteria

MAJOR CRITERIA	MINOR CRITERIA
Carditis: clinical and/or subclinical	*ECG abnormality*[b]: prolonged PR interval, after accounting for age variability
Chorea	*Laboratory values*: ■ CRP ≥3.0 mg/dL and/or ESR ≥60 mm/h in LR population ■ CRP ≥3.0 mg/dL and/or ESR ≥30 mm/h in MR and HR populations
Erythema marginatum	*Fever*: ■ ≥38.5°C (101.3°F) in LR population ■ ≥38°C (100.4°F) in MR and HR populations
Subcutaneous nodules	
Arthritis: ■ Polyarthritis only in LR population ■ Monoarthritis or polyarthritis or polyarthralgia in MR and HR populations	*Arthritis*[c]: ■ Polyarthralgia in LR population ■ Monoarthralgia in MR and HR populations

[a]LR population defined as acute rheumatic fever incidence ≤2/100,000 school-aged children *or* rheumatic heart disease prevalence of ≤1 per 1,000 all-age population per year.
[b]Unless carditis is a major criterion.
[c]Unless joint manifestation is a major criterion.
CRP, C-reactive protein; ECG, electrocardiogram; ESR, erythrocyte sedimentation rate; HR, high risk; LR, low risk; MR, moderate risk.
Data from Gewitz MH, Baltimore RS, Tani LY, et al. Revision in the Jones Criteria for the diagnosis of acute rheumatic fever in the era of Doppler echocardiography. A scientific statement from the American Heart Association. *Circulation*. 2015;131:1806-1818.

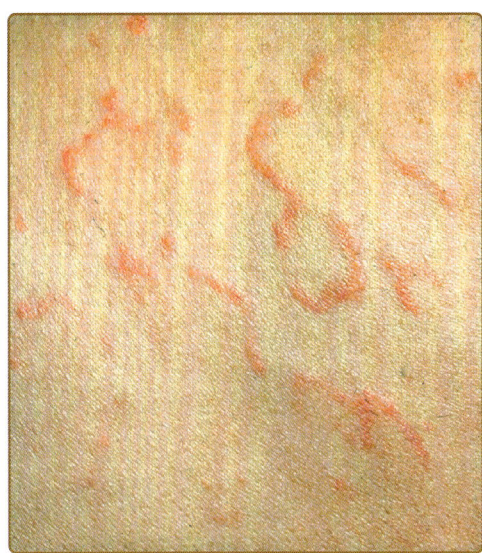

Figure 66-7 Erythema marginatum of rheumatic fever. Enlarging and shifting transient annular and polycyclic lesions.

with a high incidence of rheumatic fever, and is included in diagnostic guidelines (Table 66-6).[66]

CUTANEOUS FINDINGS

Both erythema marginatum and subcutaneous nodules are rare in ARF, each occurring in less than 5% of cases.[66,67] Erythema marginatum, much like the eruption in sJIA and Still disease, is evanescent, but differs by its tendency to develop annular or serpiginous erythema (Fig. 66-7). It typically occurs on the torso, upper arms, and legs, and spares the face. Erythema marginatum can fluctuate over many weeks, may be exacerbated by heat, and blanches with pressure. It is not itchy or painful. Histopathologically, there is a sparse superficial perivascular infiltrate of lymphocytes and neutrophils.

In dermatologic literature erythema marginatum is usually considered unique to ARF. However, other literature does contain very different cutaneous syndromes given the same name, both as part of hereditary angioedema and as an unusual drug eruption. Skin findings may be the presenting sign of hereditary angioedema attacks, and a prodrome of erythema marginatum had been reported in up to 25% of patients.[69] Recently, 49 (56%) of 87 patients with hereditary angioedema were reported with erythema marginatum. It had frequently been confused with urticaria, leading to a delay in the correct diagnosis in half the patients with the rash. It often preceded angioedema attacks, but could develop concurrently or even recur independently of the angioedema attacks.[70] The term "chicken wire erythema" also has been applied to this eruption. The second non-ARF syndrome involving a marginatum-type eruption is as a side effect of the oral multikinase inhibitor sorafenib, reported as erythema marginatum hemorrhagicum. This was distinguished by a purpuric margin and presumably was less labile than the erythema marginatum of ARF.[71]

Subcutaneous nodules are typically less than 2 cm in diameter, firm, painless, and mobile nodules that usually appear during the first weeks of the inflammatory phase. They tend to localize over extensor surfaces—elbows, wrists, knees, and ankles, and sometimes Achilles tendon, occiput, or thoracic or lumbar spine.[66,67] Nodules may last for up 2 weeks, and often occur in association with carditis. The histopathology generally consists of a central zone of fibrinoid necrotic material surrounded by histiocytes and fibroblasts and around small vessels are collection of lymphocytes and polymorphs.[72] Small focal lesions similar or identical to the myocardial Aschoff nodule are frequently seen. Surprisingly, the nodules heal without residual damage.

NONCUTANEOUS FINDINGS

Globally, approximately 50% to 65% of people with rheumatic fever have clinically detectable carditis (inflammation of the heart valve leaflets leading to valvular regurgitation). The mitral valve is most often affected, followed by the aortic valve. Pericarditis and myocarditis also occasionally occur, though isolated pericarditis or myocarditis should never be considered rheumatic in origin.[66,67] Severe carditis can occur and can lead to congestive heart failure.[66] Milder rheumatic carditis may be subclinical in approximately 30% of all individuals with rheumatic fever—that is, detected by echocardiography but not audible by stethoscope.[66,67] Rheumatic carditis can evolve over weeks to months, underscoring the importance of repeating echocardiography in 2 to 4 weeks if the first echocardiogram is normal. Chorea affects up to 15% of people with ARF, is more common in females and adolescents, and consists of purposeless, involuntary, jerky movements which may be asymmetrical (hemichorea), facial grimacing, fidgeting, clumsiness, and emotional lability. Patients may experience deterioration in handwriting, inability to feed themselves, and unsteady gait leading to falls.[66,67] Chorea typically occurs after a longer latent period (up to 6 months) after a streptococcal infection, by which time the other inflammatory features of rheumatic fever have resolved. It can follow a fluctuating course over many months or years, before eventually resolving.[67]

DIAGNOSIS

The diagnosis of ARF depends exclusion of other syndromes that may mimic ARF, similar to those diseases to be excluded in the differential of sJIA and Still disease, and on the constellation of clinical findings as detailed by current criteria, which now also support the use of echocardiographic findings to confirm subclinical carditis. Table 66-6 details these criteria.

TREATMENT

Treatment is first directed at eradication of group A β-hemolytic streptococci from the oropharynx using phenoxymethylpenicillin (penicillin VK) (250 mg twice daily in children; 500 mg twice daily in adolescents) or a single dose of IM benzathine penicillin, followed by institution of long-term prophylaxis. Erythromycin is the recommended alternative in instances of penicillin allergy.[66] Neither salicylates nor corticosteroids have shown sustained effects on outcome, but both are sometimes still used. Chorea treatment is supportive, and even though the course may last for months, it generally enters remission. Naproxen 10 to 20 mg/kg/day is given divided into 2 daily doses for treatment of acute joint manifestations. Patients require long-term followup, primarily for complications of valvulitis.

SUMMARY

Table 66-7 summarizes the common dermatologic findings and associations for RA, JIA, AOSD, and rheumatic fever.

TABLE 66-7
Summary of Common Dermatologic Findings and Associations

DERMATOLOGIC FINDING	CLINICAL APPEARANCE
Rheumatoid Arthritis	
Rheumatoid nodule	Subcutaneous nodule over pressure points (olecranon, extensor forearm, Achilles tendon)
Rheumatoid vasculitis	Purpura, livedo reticularis, atrophie blanche, ulcers
Pyoderma gangrenosum	Deep, liquefying ulcers with a purple, undermined border, commonly affecting the lower extremities and abdomen
Juvenile Idiopathic Arthritis	
Classic cutaneous presentation	Transient, salmon pink macular eruption coincident with febrile episodes
Adult-Onset Still Disease	
Classic cutaneous presentation	Transient, discrete, pink to red macules or edematous papules distributed over the chest, abdomen, and extensor arms, peaking with febrile episodes
Atypical cutaneous presentation	Persistent pruritic papules and plaques with or without a fine scale, distributed over trunk, extremities, head, or neck; Koebner phenomenon may occur
Rheumatic Fever	
Erythema marginatum	Evanescent, erythematous patches in annular or serpiginous configuration distributed over the torso, upper arms, and legs with facial sparing
Subcutaneous nodules	Firm, painless, and mobile nodules localizing over extensor surfaces (elbows, wrists, knees), and often associated with carditis

REFERENCES

1. Aletaha D, Neogi T, Silman AJ, et al. 2010 Rheumatoid arthritis classification criteria. An American College Rheumatology/European League Against Rheumatism collaborative initiative. *Arthritis Rheum.* 2010;62(9):2569-2581.
2. Alamanos Y, Drosos AA. Epidemiology of adult rheumatoid arthritis. *Autoimmun Rev.* 2005;4:130-136.
3. Scott D, Wolfe F, Huizinga TW. Rheumatoid arthritis. *Lancet.* 2010;376(9746):1094-1108.
4. Liao KP, Karlson EW. Classification and epidemiology of rheumatoid arthritis. In: Hochberg MC, Silman AJ, Smolen JS, et al, eds. *Rheumatology.* 5th ed. Philadelphia, PA: Mosby; 2010.
5. Sayah A, English JC 3rd. Rheumatoid arthritis: a review of the cutaneous manifestations. *J Am Acad Dermatol.* 2005;53:191-2009.
6. Clarke JT, Werth VP. Rheumatic manifestations of skin disease. *Curr Opin Rheumatol.* 2010;22:78-84.
7. Prete M, Racanelli V, Digiglio L, et al. Extra-articular manifestations of rheumatoid arthritis: an update. *Autoimmun Rev.* 2011;11:123-131.
8. Tilstra JS, Lienesch DW. Rheumatoid nodules. *Dermatol Clin.* 2015;33:361-371.
9. Maruani A, Wierzbicka E, Machet MC, et al. Reversal of multifocal cutaneous lymphoproliferative disease associated with Epstein-Barr virus after withdrawal of methotrexate therapy for rheumatoid arthritis. *J Am Acad Dermatol.* 2007;57(5)(suppl):S69-S71.
10. Kameda T, Dobashi H, Miyatake N, et al. Association of higher methotrexate dose with lymphoproliferative disease onset in rheumatoid arthritis patients. *Arthritis Care Res (Hoboken).* 2014;56:1302-1309.
11. Rosenbach M, English JC 3rd. Reactive granulomatous dermatitis. A review of palisaded granulomatous dermatitis, interstitial granulomatous dermatitis, interstitial granulomatous drug reaction, and a proposed reclassification. *Dermatol Clin.* 2015;33(3):373-387.
12. Magro CM, Crowson AN. The spectrum of cutaneous lesions in rheumatoid arthritis: a clinical and pathological study of 43 patients. *J Cutan Pathol.* 2003;30:1-10.
13. Sangueza OP, Caudell MD, Mengesha YM, et al. Palisaded neutrophilic granulomatous dermatitis in rheumatoid arthritis. *J Am Acad Dermatol.* 2002;47:251-257.
14. Fujio Y, Funakoshi T, Nakayama K, et al. Rheumatoid neutrophilic dermatosis with tense blister formation: a case report and review of the literature. *Australas J Dermatol.* 2014;5:e12-e14.
15. Saeb-Lima M, Charli-Joseph Y, Rodriguez-Acosta ED, et al. Autoimmunity-related neutrophilic dermatosis: a newly described entity that is not exclusive of systemic lupus erythematosus. *Am J Dermatopathol.* 2013;35:655-660.
16. Gasdorf L, Bessis D, Lipsker D. Lupus erythematosus and neutrophilic urticarial dermatosis. A retrospective study of 7 patients. *Medicine (Baltimore).* 2014;93:e351.
17. Wu YH, Hsiao PF. Neutrophilic figurate erythema. *Am J Dermatopathol.* 2017;39:344-350.
18. Watts RA, Carruthers DM, Symmons DP, et al. The incidence of rheumatoid vasculitis in the Norwich Health Authority. *Br J Rheumatol.* 1994;33(9):832-833.
19. Makol A, Crowson CS, Wetter DA, et al. Vasculitis associated with rheumatoid arthritis: a case control study. *Rheumatology (Oxford).* 2014;53:890-899.
20. Makol A, Matteson EL, Warrington KJ. Rheumatoid vasculitis: an update. *Curr Opin Rheumatol.* 2015;27:63-70.
21. Nguyen H, James EA. Immune recognition of citrullinated epitopes. *Immunology.* 2016;149:131-1388.
22. Yarwood A, Huizinga TW, Worthington J. The genetics of rheumatoid arthritis: risk and protection in different stages of the evolution of RA. *Rheumatology (Oxford).* 2016;55(2):199-209.
23. Requena L, El-Shabrawi-Caelen L, Walsh S, et al. Intralymphatic histiocytosis. A clinicopathologic study of 16 cases. *Am J Dermatopathol.* 2009;31:140-151.
24. Huang HY, Liang CW, Hu SL, et al. Cutaneous intravascular histiocytosis associated with rheumatoid arthritis: a case report and review of the literature. *Clin Exp Dermatol.* 2009;34:e302-e303.
25. Jorizzo JL, Daniels JC. Dermatologic conditions reported in patients with rheumatoid arthritis. *J Am Acad Dermatol.* 1983;8:439.
26. Brasington RD Jr. Clinical features of rheumatoid arthritis. In: Hochberg MC, Silman AJ, Smolen JS, et al, eds. *Rheumatology.* 5th ed. Philadelphia, PA: Mosby; 2010.
27. Kerr JR. Role of parvovirus B19 in the pathogenesis of autoimmunity and autoimmune disease. *J Clin Pathol.* 2016;69:279-291.
28. El-Gendy HJ, El-Gohary RM, Shohdy KS, et al. Leprosy masquerading as systemic rheumatic diseases. *Clin Rheumatol.* 2016;22:264-271.
29. Meyer PW, Ally MM, Anderson R. Reliable and cost-effective serodiagnosis of rheumatoid arthritis. *Rheumatol Int.* 2016;36:751-758.
30. Harris E, Budd R, Firestein G, et al, eds. *Kelley's Textbook of Rheumatology.* 7th ed. Philadelphia, PA: Elsevier Saunders; 2004.
31. Gardner GC, Kadel NJ. Ordering and interpreting rheumatologic laboratory tests. *J Am Acad Orthop Surg.* 2003;11:60-67.
32. Liao KP, Karlson EW. Classification and epidemiology of rheumatoid arthritis. In: Hochberg MC, Silman AJ, Smolen JS, et al, eds. *Rheumatology.* 5th ed. Philadelphia, PA: Mosby; 2010.
33. Ruta S, Reginato AM, Pineda C, et al. General applications of ultrasound in rheumatology. Why we need it in our daily practice. *J Clin Rheumatol.* 2015;21(3):133-143.
34. Smolen JS, Landewe R, Bijlsma J, et al. EULAR recommendations for the management of rheumatoid arthritis with synthetic and biological disease-modifying antirheumatic drugs: a 2016 update. *Ann Rheum Dis.* 2017;76:960-977.
35. Lee YH, Bae SC. Comparative efficacy and safety of tocilizumab, rituximab, abatacept and tofacitinib in patients with active rheumatoid arthritis that inadequately responds to tumor necrosis factor inhibitors: a Bayesian network meta-analysis of randomized controlled trials. *Int J Rheum Dis.* 2016;19:1103-1111.
36. Alfons-Cristancho R, Armstrong N, Arjunji R, et al. Comparative effectiveness of biologics for the management of rheumatoid arthritis: a systematic review and network meta-analysis. *Clin Rheumatol.* 2017;36:25-34.
37. Singh JA, Christensen R, Wells GA, et al. Biologics for rheumatoid arthritis: an overview of Cochrane reviews. *Cochrane Database Syst Rev.* 2009;(4):CD007848.
38. Giancane G, Consolaro A, Lanni S, et al. Juvenile idiopathic arthritis: diagnosis and treatment. *Rheumatol Ther.* 2016;3:187-207.
39. Eisenstein EM, Berkun Y. Diagnosis and classification of juvenile idiopathic arthritis. *J Autoimmun.* 2014;48-49:31-33.

40. Krause ML, Crowson CS, Michet CJ, et al. Juvenile idiopathic arthritis in Olmsted County, Minnesota, 1960-2013. *Arthritis Rheum.* 2016;68:247-254.
41. Aggarwal A, Misra DP. Enthesitis-related arthritis. *Clin Rheumatol.* 2015;34(11):1839-1846.
42. Weiss PF. Update on enthesitis-related arthritis. *Curr Opin Rheumatol.* 2016;28:530-536.
43. Ravelli A, Minoia F, Davi S, et al. Classification criteria for macrophage activation syndrome complicating systemic juvenile idiopathic arthritis: a European League Against Rheumatism/American College of Rheumatology/Paediatric Rheumatology International Trials Organization collaborative initiative. *Arthritis Rheumatol.* 2016;68:566-576.
44. Hersh AO, Prahalad S. Genetics of juvenile idiopathic arthritis. *Rheum Dis Clin North Am.* 2017;43:435-448.
45. Weiss PF. Update on enthesitis-related arthritis. *Curr Opin Rheumatol.* 2016;28:530-536.
46. Cimaz R, Marino A, Martini A. How I treat juvenile idiopathic arthritis: a state of the art review. *Autoimmun Rev.* 2017;16:1008-1015.
47. Vanoni F, Minoia F, Malattia C. Biologics in juvenile idiopathic arthritis: a narrative review. *Eur J Pediatr.* 2017;176:1147-1153.
48. Ravelli A, Davi S, Minoia F, et al. Macrophage activation syndrome. *Hematol Oncol Clin North Am.* 2015;29:927-941.
49. Gerfaud-Valentin M, Maucort-Boulch D, Hot A, et al. Adult-onset Still disease: Manifestations, treatment, outcome, and prognostic factors. *Medicine (Baltimore).* 2014;93(2):91-99.
50. Lebrun D, Mestrallet S, Dehoux M, et al. Validation of the Fautrel classification criteria for adult-onset Still's disease. *Semin Arthritis Rheum.* 2018;47(4):578-585.
51. Sfriso P, Priori R, Valesini G, et al. Adult-onset Still's disease: an Italian multicenter retrospective observational study of manifestations and treatments in 245 patients. *Clin Rheumatol.* 2016;35:1683-1689.
52. Braverman IM. Hypersensitivity syndromes. In: *Skin Signs of Systemic Disease*. 3rd ed. Philadelphia, PA: Saunders; 1998.
53. Narvaez Garcia FJ, Pascual M, Lopez de Recalde M, et al. Adult-onset Still's disease with atypical cutaneous manifestations. *Medicine (Baltimore).* 2017;96(11):e6318.
54. Sun N, Brezinski EA, Berliner J, et al. Updates in adult-onset Still disease: atypical cutaneous manifestations and associations with delayed malignancy. *J Am Acad Dermatol.* 2015;73(2):294-303.
55. Fortna RR, Gudjonsson JE, Seidel G, et al. Persistent pruritic papules and plaques: a characteristic histopathologic presentation seen in a subset of patients with adult-onset and juvenile Still's disease. *J Cutan Pathol.* 2010;37(9):932-937.
56. Gopal M, Cohn CD, McEntire MR, et al. Thrombotic thrombocytopenic purpura and adult onset Still's disease. *Am J Med Sci.* 2009; 337(5):373-376.
57. Hot A, Toh ML, Coppéré B, et al. Reactive hemophagocytic syndrome in adult-onset Still disease: clinical features and long-term outcome: a case-control study of 8 patients. *Medicine (Baltimore).* 2010;89(1):37-46.
58. Hofheinz K, Schett G, Manger B. Adult onset Still's disease associated with malignancy—cause or coincidence? *Semin Arthritis Rheum.* 2016;45:621-626.
59. Gerfaud-Valentin M, Seve P, Iwaz J, et al. Myocarditis in adult-onset Still disease. *Medicine (Baltimore).* 2014;93:280-289.
60. Yamaguchi M, Ohta A, Tsunematsu T, et al. Preliminary criteria for classification of adult Still's disease. *J Rheumatol.* 1992;19:424-430.
61. Fautrel B, Zing E, Golmard JL, et al. Proposal for a new set of classification criteria for adult-onset still disease. *Medicine (Baltimore).* 2002;81:194-200.
62. Kiefer C, Bernard C, Dan L. Neutrophilic urticaria dermatosis: a variant of neutrophilic urticaria strongly associated with systemic disease. Report of 9 cases and review of the literature. *Medicine (Baltimore).* 2009;88:23-31.
63. Larson AR, Laga AC, Granter SR. The spectrum of histopathologic findings in cutaneous lesions in patients with Still disease. *Am J Clin Pathol.* 2015;144:945-951.
64. Kim HA, Kwon JE, Yim H, et al. The pathologic findings of skin, lymph node, liver, and bone marrow in patients with adult-onset Still disease. A comprehensive analysis of 40 cases. *Medicine (Baltimore).* 2015;94:1-9.
65. Bae CB, Jung JY, Kim HA, et al. Reactive hemophagocytic syndrome in adult-onset Still disease: clinical features, predictive factors, and prognosis in 21 patients. *Medicine (Baltimore).* 2015;94(4):e451.
66. Webb RH, Grant C, Hamden A. Acute rheumatic fever. *BMJ.* 2015;351:h3443.
67. Gewitz MH, Baltimore RS, Tani LY, et al. Revision of the Jones Criteria for the diagnosis of acute rheumatic fever in the era of Doppler echocardiography: a scientific statement from the American Heart Association. *Circulation.* 2015;131(20):1806-1818.
68. Carapetis JR, McDonald M, Wilson NJ. Acute rheumatic fever. *Lancet.* 2005;366:155-168.
69. Parish LC. Hereditary angioedema: diagnosis and management—a perspective for the dermatologist. *J Am Acad Dermatol.* 2011;65:843-850.
70. Rasmussen ER, Valente de Freitas P, Bygum A. Urticaria and prodromal symptoms including erythema marginatum in Danish patients with hereditary angioedema. *Acta Derm Venereol.* 2001;81:376-377.
71. Rubsam K, Flaig MJ, Ruzicka T, et al. Erythema marginatum hemorrhagicum: a unique cutaneous side effect of sorafenib. *J Am Acad Dermatol.* 2011;64:1194-1196.
72. Tandon R. Rheumatic fever pathogenesis: approach in research needs change. *Ann Pediatr Cardiol.* 2012;5:169-178.

Chapter 67 :: Scleredema and Scleromyxedema
:: Roger H. Weenig & Mark R. Pittelkow

第六十七章
硬肿症和硬化性黏液水肿

中文导读

硬化性黏液水肿顾名思义即具有硬化和黏蛋白沉积的特点，感染、炎症、糖尿病、药物、重金属、基因突变和毒素及某些特殊的介质如细胞因子、趋化因子、球蛋白-副球蛋白及循环因子都可以刺激细微细胞过度产生黏蛋白或者胶原。本章聚焦于硬肿症和硬化性黏液水肿两种疾病。硬肿症是一种以真皮黏蛋白沉积和轻度硬化为特征的急性皮肤硬结为表现的疾病。年轻发病与感染、成人发病与糖尿病，以及副蛋白血症相关，其各具临床特点。罕见的相关性疾病还包括甲状旁腺功能亢进、结缔组织疾病、艾滋病毒感染。组织病理学表现为真皮全层增厚伴胶原束增宽被黏蛋白沉积物分割，主要为透明质酸。本章从历史发展、流行病学、发病机制、临床表现、病理特点、预后及临床进程、治疗等各方面阐述了硬肿症的疾病特点。硬化性黏液水肿是慢性进展性的疾病，特征性表现为真皮纤维化、黏蛋白沉积和甲状腺功能正常。通常与副蛋白血症（通常为免疫球蛋白G-Kappa）有关。临床变异型包括泛发性融合性苔藓样疹（硬化黏液水肿）、婴儿丘疹性黏蛋白沉积症、成年丘疹性黏蛋白沉积症、自愈性丘疹黏蛋白沉积症、肢端持续性丘疹性黏蛋白沉积症、结节性黏蛋白病、局限性或泛发性苔藓样斑块。本章从流行病学、发病机制、临床特征、组织病理、预后及临床进程、治疗等各方面对该病进行了阐述。伴随着慢性的、进行性的临床进程的硬化性黏液水肿，常有更多的全身器官和组织受累，预后很差。治疗上列举了美法仑、糖皮质激素、静脉注射免疫球蛋白、沙利度胺、体外光化学治疗、干扰素-α、联合化疗、补骨脂素和UVA等方法。自体外周血干细胞移植在伴有严重疾病的硬化性黏液水肿患者中取得显著疗效。

〔施　为〕

Skin disorders that are characterized by increased mucin content, excessive collagen deposition, or fibrocyte hyperplasia are designated as mucinoses, sclerosing disorders, or fibrosing disorders, respectively. As the fibrocyte (fibroblast) is the cellular component of their pathogenesis, these conditions are aptly viewed as various forms of "fibropathy." In some conditions, one fibrocyte product predominates, such as excessive mucin production in pretibial myxedema or collagen deposition in scleroderma. In others conditions there is a combination of excessive mucin and collagen deposition (scleredema) or excessive mucin deposition and fibrocyte hyperplasia (scleromyxedema and nephrogenic systemic fibrosis). Hence, the nosology of some of these conditions does not accurately describe what is observed histopathologically. For example, "fibromyxedema" more accurately depicts the histopathogenesis of scleromyxedema, as scleromyxedema implies a combination of sclerosis and mucinosis, which more accurately describes scleredema.

Fibroblasts are derived from CD34-positive hematopoietic precursors that originate in the bone marrow and populate the skin during development and wound repair. The chief role of the skin fibroblast is to deposit collagen, elastin, and ground substance, the major constituents of the dermis and pannicular septae and the substrate to which the epidermis and skin appendages attach.

Stimuli that cause fibrocytes to overproduce mucin or collagen, or to proliferate are protean and broad ranging. Infectious triggers, inflammatory states, diabetes mellitus, drugs, heavy metals (eg, gadolinium), genetic mutations, and toxins (eg, tainted rapeseed oil and L-tryptophan in eosinophilia myalgia syndrome), as well as specific mediators, such as eicosenoids, growth factors, cytokines, chemokines, immunoglobulins-paraproteins, and other circulating factors, have been implicated, but the precise mechanisms that result in the varied forms of fibrocyte pathology (fibropathy) are poorly characterized. Some of these stimuli may recruit bone-marrow derived fibrocyte precursors to the skin; others may act directly on fibrocytes already residing in the skin.

This chapter focuses on the distinctive conditions of scleredema and scleromyxedema (Table 67-1.). Other diseases relevant to cutaneous fibrocytes are discussed separately in other chapters and are listed in Table 67-2.

SCLEREDEMA

AT-A-GLANCE

- Acute skin induration characterized by dermal mucinosis and mild sclerosis.
- Disease associations:
  - Postinfectious scleredema of youth.
  - Diabetes mellitus–associated scleredema of adulthood.
  - Paraproteinemia-associated scleredema.
  - Rare associations: hyperparathyroidism, connective tissue disease, HIV infection.
- Histopathology: pandermal thickening with broad collagen bundles separated by mucin deposits, chiefly hyaluronate.

- Clinical course:
  - Postinfectious: usually resolves in 1 to 2 years.
  - Diabetes mellitus–associated: may improve with better control of diabetes, but a prolonged course is expected.
  - Paraprotein associated: often more chronic although remissions observed with specific treatments.
- Treatment: treat underlying disease; UVA-1; psoralen plus ultraviolet A light.

HISTORICAL ASPECTS

Scleredema was described by Buschke in 1902[1] and is also designated as scleredema of Buschke and scleredema adultorum, although the latter is a misleading term because children or adolescents can develop the condition.

EPIDEMIOLOGY

Scleredema is rare, although the precise incidence and prevalence are unknown. Men and women are affected with equal frequency. More than half of cases of scleredema occur in childhood or adolescence, most commonly after an upper respiratory tract infection.[2] Streptococcal infection is most commonly identified, but other infectious agents also have been implicated. Disease development in adulthood in association with adult-onset diabetes mellitus is the second most common presentation of scleredema. Uncommonly, scleredema occurs in association with paraproteinemia or multiple myeloma, and this association possibly is becoming more common as other causes diminish in frequency with better treatment and management of underlying disease.

PATHOGENESIS

Type 1 collagen and hyaluronate appear to be the major fibroblast products that are increased in scleredema-affected skin.[3-5] The precise mechanism(s) for increased collagen and glycosaminoglycan production in scleredema is not known. Stimulation of

TABLE 67-1
Scleredema and Scleromyxedema

CONDITION	EPIDEMIOLOGY	ASSOCIATED CONDITIONS	CLINICAL MANIFESTATIONS	HISTOLOGIC FINDINGS	COURSE/ PROGNOSIS	TREATMENT OPTIONS
Scleredema	Childhood or adolescence Adulthood Adulthood	Postinfectious Diabetes mellitus Paraproteinemia Also hyperparathyroidism, connective tissue disease, HIV	Acute onset, nonpitting neck induration; shoulders, upper back, face, and arms may be affected. Affected skin feels smooth and waxy.	"Squared" appearance on low-power microscopy; more dermis in affected skin compared to adjacent unaffected skin; decreased number/higher placement of eccrine glands; mucin stains (Alcian blue, colloidal iron) can identify mucin deposits	Abates in 1-2 years Protracted course Chronic, resistant to therapies	Treatment of underlying condition (except for postinfectious scleredema); UVA-1 phototherapy may be effective
Scleromyxedema (also, lichen myxedematosus)	Mid to late adulthood, males and females equally affected	Paraproteinemia	Generalized lichenoid eruption has minute papules on extremities and trunk Confluent, lichenoid plaques	Superficial to mid-dermal fibroplasia and mucin deposition	Chronic, progressive course	Treatment of underlying cause

fibroblasts by serum factors or immunoglobulin may be related to the pathogenesis of scleredema, particularly cases associated with infectious agents or a paraproteinemia. Serum from a patient with scleredema associated with paraproteinemia was able to increase collagen production by cultured fibroblasts in vitro.[6] However, the factor(s) involved has not been elucidated. Other soluble circulating cytokines and small molecule mediators likely also play critical roles.

CLINICAL FINDINGS

The clinical findings of scleredema are distinctive. An acute onset of nonpitting induration of neck, shoulders, and upper back skin may be followed by involvement of the face and arms. Characteristically, the affected skin appears smooth and waxy, with tense dermal induration and prominent follicular ostia, at times imparting a "peau d'orange" appearance (Fig. 67-1). In general, however, skin changes are better felt on palpation than seen. The skin of the upper trunk (especially the back) is a favored site for scleredema, but more widespread involvement may be observed. The affected and unaffected skin blend imperceptibly. Scleredema involving the esophagus, bone marrow, nerve, liver, or salivary glands has been described rarely.[7,8] However, investigations to identify internal organ involvement by scleredema are infrequently pursued. Patients may report symptoms of restricted motion of joints, the tongue, or eyes, as well as weak or tender muscles.

HISTOPATHOLOGY

Punch biopsies of affected skin reveal a nontapered (square) appearance on low power. The proportion of dermis in dramatically increased in comparison to adjacent nonaffected skin (Fig. 67-2A). A decreased number or higher placement of eccrine units may be appreciated. Fibroblasts are normal in number and morphology. The collagen bundles are slightly thickened and separated from each other by subtle deposits of mucin. Stains for mucin (Alcian blue, colloidal iron) are often used to identify the mucin deposits (Fig. 67-2B).

PROGNOSIS AND CLINICAL COURSE

Postinfectious scleredema usually abates in 1 to 2 years. Scleredema associated with adult-onset diabetes tends to be protracted, although some patients appear to improve with better glucose control. Gammopathy-associated scleredema is more chronic and can be resistant to many therapies.

TREATMENT

Antibiotics do not appear to affect the course of postinfectious scleredema. Treatment of the associated

TABLE 67-2
Selected Fibroblast Disorders

	CHAPTER
Excessive Collagen Production by Fibroblasts—*Sclerosing Disorders*	
• Scleroderma	63
• Morphea	64
• Sclerodermoid graft-versus-host disease	129
• Sclerodermoid porphyria cutanea tarda	124
• Eosinophilic fasciitis	40, 63
• Sclerodermoid drug reactions (bleomycin, epoxy resin, pentazocine)	63
• Lipodermatosclerosis (sclerosing panniculitis)	73, 148
• Collagenoma	136
Fibroblast Hyperplasia—*Fibrosing Disorders*	
• Fibromatosis (Dupuytren contracture, Peyronie disease)	72
Excessive Collagen and Mucin Production by Fibroblasts—*Scleromucinoses*	
• Scleredema	67
Fibroblast Hyperplasia and Excessive Mucin Production by Fibroblasts—*Fibromucinoses*	
• Lichen myxedematosus and scleromyxedema	67
• Nephrogenic systemic fibrosis/ nephrogenic fibrosing dermopathy	133
• Toxic oil syndrome	64
• Eosinophilia-myalgia syndrome	40
Fibroblast Hyperplasia and Excessive Collagen Production by Fibroblasts—*Fibrosclerosing Disorders*	
• Juvenile hyaline fibromatosis	72
• Gingival fibromatosis	72
Excessive Mucin Production by Fibroblasts—*Mucinoses*	
• Pretibial myxedema	137
• Generalized myxedema	137
• Localized myxedema	137
• Reticular erythematous mucinosis and plaque-like mucinosis	62
• Connective tissue disease	61, 62, 63, 66, 68, 69
• Degos disease	146

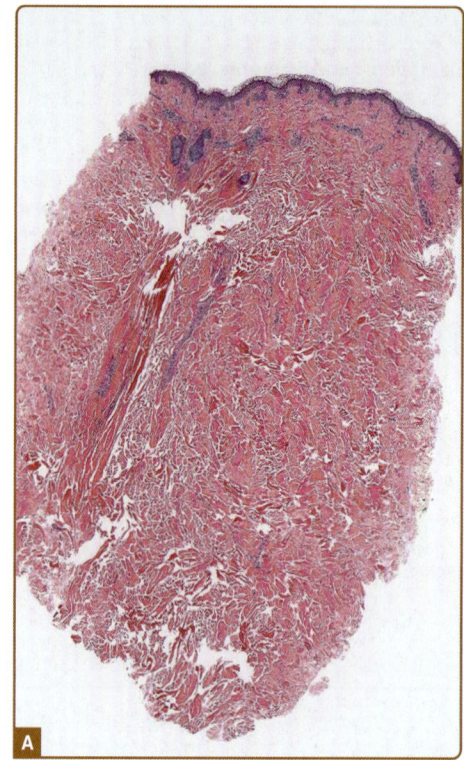

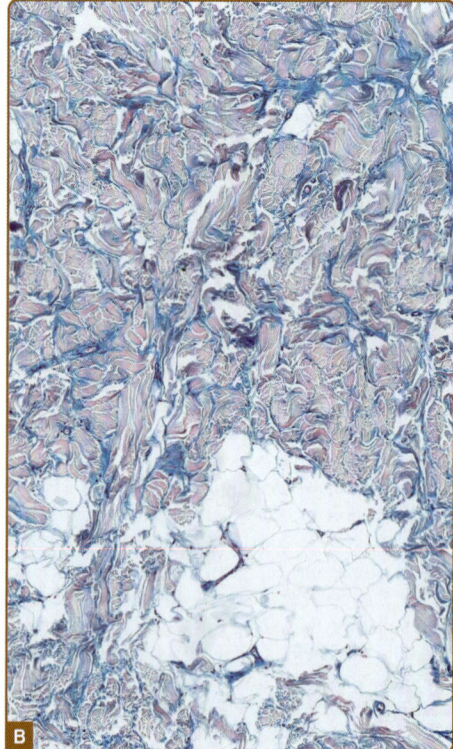

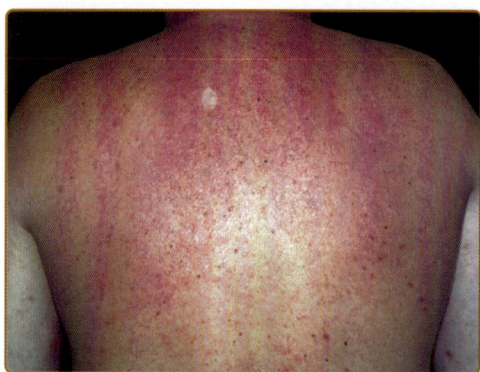

Figure 67-1 Scleredema. Waxy, nonpitting induration of back skin.

Figure 67-2 **A,** Scleredema. Thickened dermis characterized by enlarged collagen bundles separated by clear spaces (×15 original magnification). **B,** Scleredema. Mucin deposition identified in clear spaces by acid mucopolysaccharide stain (×80 original magnification).

disease (eg, improved glucose control or treatment of paraproteinemia) may lead to improvement. Ultraviolet A1 phototherapy has been variably effective in some patients,[9-11] as has psoralen plus ultraviolet A phototherapy.[11,12] Treatment with methotrexate did not provide benefit in a series of cases of scleredema. Scleredema has responded to local radiotherapy or electron-beam irradiation. Scleredema associated with monoclonal gammopathy has responded to extracorporeal photopheresis and intravenous immunoglobulin.[13]

SCLEROMYXEDEMA

AT-A-GLANCE

- Chronic, progressive condition characterized by dermal fibrosis and mucinosis and normal thyroid function.
- Usually associated with paraproteinemia (typically immunoglobulin G-kappa).
- Clinical variants
  - Generalized, confluent lichenoid eruption (scleromyxedema).
  - Discrete papular (rarely nodular) eruption on the trunk or extremities (lichen myxedematosus).
    - Papular mucinosis of infancy.
    - Papular mucinosis of adulthood.
    - Self-healing papular mucinosis.
    - Acral persistent papular mucinosis.
    - Nodular variant.
  - Localized or generalized lichenoid plaques (but distinct from plaque-like mucinosis/reticulated erythematous mucinosis).
  - Urticarial plaques
- Histopathology: superficial to mid-dermal fibroplasia and mucin deposition.
- Clinical course: chronic progressive course and poor outcome in generalized, systemic cases; localized and self-healing forms have a better prognosis.
- Treatment: correct paraproteinemia: through clonal plasma cell targeted therapies, intravenous immune globulin, autologous stem-cell transplant.

EPIDEMIOLOGY

Lichen myxedematosus/scleromyxedema is a rare disease afflicting men and women with equal frequency and symptom onset in mid to later life.[14-16]

PATHOGENESIS

The pathogenesis of scleromyxedema is unknown. Most patients with scleromyxedema have a monoclonal paraproteinemia, typically designated as monoclonal gammopathy of undetermined significance. Rare patients meet criteria for multiple myeloma. Excessive hyaluronate production and fibroblast proliferation are observed, but support for a direct effect of the monoclonal protein on fibroblasts is lacking.[17,18] Indirect mechanisms appear to include circulating cytokines, inflammatory mediators, and fibroblast precursor cell lineages that migrate from the blood, take up residence in the dermis and, in more extensive cases, in other tissues, and synthesize mucin.

CLINICAL FINDINGS

Several distinct clinical presentations, and hence nosologic designations have been recognized. Although there is considerable clinical overlap and patients may show progression from limited to widespread involvement, it is useful to distinguish localized from generalized disease as well as patients that present with discrete papules from those with confluent plaques. The generalized lichenoid eruption consists of numerous minute (1 to 3 mm) papules scattered on the extremities and the trunk. Scleromyxedema presents with confluent lichenoid plaques. Individual lesions and plaques may exhibit marked erythema or hyperpigmentation. The face is involved in most cases, resulting in significant deformity, "bovine facies" (Fig. 67-3). The trunk and extremities are usually affected (Fig. 67-4A) and often results in decreased

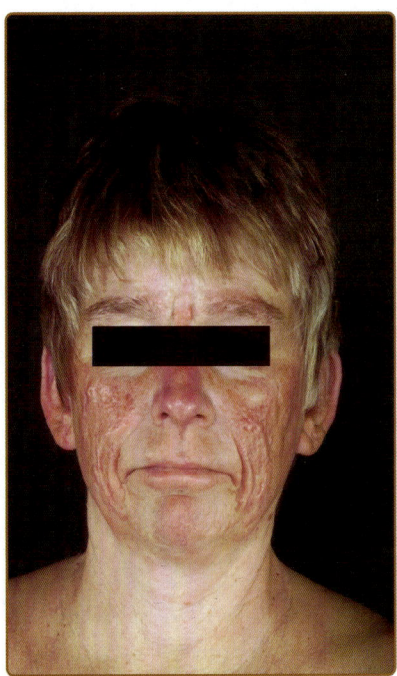

Figure 67-3 Scleromyxedema. Marked, nodular induration of facial skin with accentuation of skin folds.

flexibility and range of motion in the involved areas (Fig. 67-4B).

A monoclonal paraproteinemia of undetermined significance, usually immunoglobulin G λ (IgG-λ) type is identified in most patients. Paraproteinemia is less common in localized variants. Progression to multiple myeloma occurs rarely.

Muscle weakness, contractures, restrictive lung disease, upper airway involvement, pulmonary hypertension, esophageal dysmotility, and neurologic disorders (seizures, motor impairment, carpal tunnel syndrome, depression, memory loss, aphasia, peripheral neuropathy, and psychosis) have been reported in association with scleromyxedema. Thyroid function is normal by definition.

HISTOPATHOLOGY

The classical histopathologic findings in scleromyxedema consist of superficial to mid-dermal mucin deposition with admixed fibroblast proliferation (Fig. 67-5). Recently, Rongioletti et al reported an interstitial proliferation of epithelioid histiocytes imparting a granuloma annulare-like pattern in 10 of 44 patients studied.[19] A mild perivascular and interstitial T-cell infiltrate is also seen, but inflammation is rarely a prominent feature. Occasional multinucleated histiocytes with or without elastophagocytosis may be identified in biopsies of scleromyxedema. A highly unusual histologic presentation with a marked dermal granulomatous infiltrate was observed in association with fibromucinous deposition in a 56-year-old male with scleromyxedema.[20]

Moreover, scleromyxedema is histologically distinct from other mucinoses as well as sclerosing and fibrosing conditions. Nephrogenic systemic fibrosis (previously designated nephrogenic fibrosing dermopathy) shows close histologic resemblance to scleromyxedema. However, the pannicular septae are the focus for histologic distinction: they are consistently involved in nephrogenic systemic fibrosis and never involved in scleromyxedema. Moreover, scleromyxedema tends to be restricted to the upper half of the dermis and nephrogenic systemic fibrosis becomes more prominent in the lower dermis and then extends to pannicular septae.

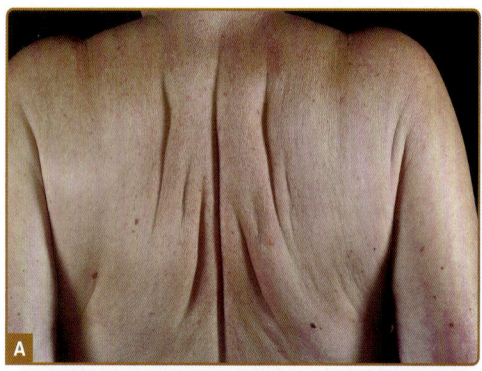

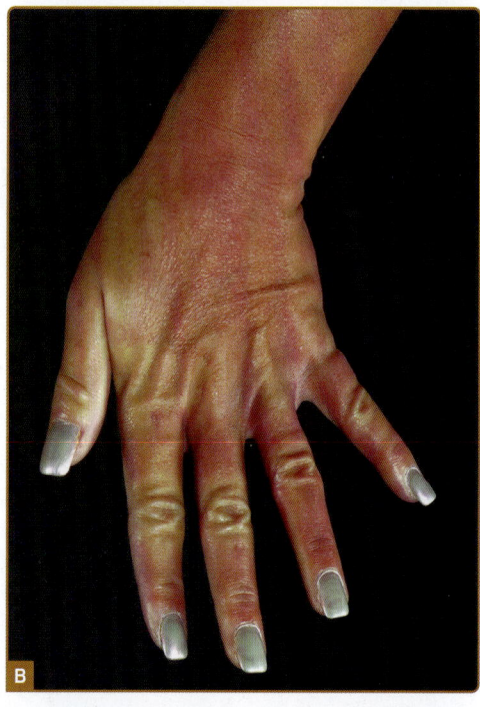

Figure 67-4 **A,** Scleromyxedema. Thickened bound-down skin of the back. **B,** Scleromyxedema. Confluent lichenoid papules and indurated skin of the hand and wrist.

PROGNOSIS AND CLINICAL COURSE

Localized, "self-healing" variants are usually confined to the skin and are self-limiting. However, prospective followup and caution is advised as some cases fitting criteria for localized disease have been associated with internal organ involvement or progression to more

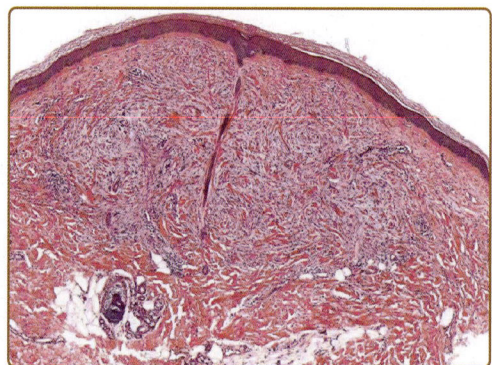

Figure 67-5 Scleromyxedema. Superficial to mid-dermal fibroplasia and increased mucin (×40 original magnification).

generalized disease (so-called atypical papular mucinosis). Scleromyxedema usually follows a chronic and progressive clinical course with more systemic organ and tissue involvement, and a poor outcome is expected. Respiratory failure, cerebral disease, and infection usually lead to a gradual decline and death.

TREATMENT

Melphalan had been used for decades to treat scleromyxedema with variable efficacy.[21-23] Other therapies directed toward quantitatively reducing or ameliorating the effects of the paraproteinemia have shown variable results. Agents or therapies with reported efficacy include: glucocorticoids,[24] intravenous immunoglobulin,[25] thalidomide,[26] extracorporeal photophoresis,[27] interferon-α,[28] combination chemotherapy,[29] and psoralen and ultraviolet A.[30] Partial to complete remission was achieved in 8 of 10 patients treated with intravenous immunoglobulin.[31] Autologous peripheral blood stem cell transplantation has resulted in dramatic remission of scleromyxedema in patients with severe disease.[32]

REFERENCES

1. Buschke A. Ueber Sclerodermie. *Berl Klin Wochenschr*. 1902;39:955.
2. Greenberg LM, Geppert C, Worthen HG, et al. Scleredema adultorum in children. *Pediatrics*. 1963;32:1044.
3. Oikarinen A, Ala-Kokko L, Palatsi R, et al. Scleredema and paraproteinemia. Enhanced collagen production and elevated type I procollagen messenger RNA level in fibroblasts grown from cultures from the fibrotic skin of a patient. *Arch Dermatol*. 1987;123:226.
4. Haapasaari KM, Kallioinen M, Tasanen K, et al. Increased collagen propeptides in the skin of a scleredema patient but no change in re-epithelialisation rate. *Acta Derm Venereol*. 1996;76:305.
5. Kobayashi T, Yamasaki Y, Watanabe T. Diabetic scleredema: a case report and biochemical analysis for glycosaminoglycans. *J Dermatol*. 1997;24:100.
6. Ohta A, Uitto J, Oikarinen AI, et al. Paraproteinemia in patients with scleredema: clinical findings and serum effects on skin fibroblasts in vitro. *J Am Acad Dermatol*. 1987;16:96.
7. Wright RA, Bernie H. Scleredema adultorum of Buschke with upper esophageal involvement. *Am J Gastroenterol*. 1982;77:9.
8. Basarab T, Burrows NP, Munn SE, et al. Systemic involvement in scleredema of Buschke associated with IgG-kappa paraproteinaemia. *Br J Dermatol*. 1997;136:939.
9. Janiga JJ, Ward DH, Lim HW. UVA-1 as a treatment for scleredema. *Photodermatol Photoimmunol Photomed*. 2004;20:210.
10. Eberlein-König B, Vogel M, Katzer K, et al. Successful UVA1 phototherapy in a patient with scleredema adultorum. *J Eur Acad Dermatol Venereol*. 2005;19:203.
11. Rongioletti F, Kaiser F, Cinotti E, et al. Scleredema. A multicentre study of characteristics, comorbidities, course and therapy in 44 patients. *J Eur Acad Dermatol Venereol*. 2015;29:2399.
12. Hager CM, Sobhi HA, Hunzelmann N, et al. Bath-PUVA therapy in three patients with scleredema adultorum. *J Am Acad Dermatol*. 1998;38:240.
13. Eastham AB, Femia AN, Velez NF, et al. Paraproteinemia-associated scleredema treated successfully with intravenous immunoglobulin. *JAMA Dermatol*. 2014;150:788.
14. Montgomery H, Underwood LJ. Lichen myxedematosus; differentiation from cutaneous myxedemas or mucoid states. *J Invest Dermatol*. 1953;20:213.
15. Gottron HA. Skleromyxodem (eine eigenartige euscheinungs-form von myxothesaurodermie). *Arch Dermatol Syph*. 1954;199:71.
16. Montgomery H. Diseases of metabolism. In: *Dermatopathology*. New York, NY: Harper & Row; 1967:830.
17. Harper RA, Rispler J. Lichen myxedematosus serum stimulates skin fibroblast proliferation. *Science*. 1978;199:545.
18. Yaron M, Yaron I, Yust I, et al. Lichen myxedematosus (scleromyxedema) serum stimulates hyaluronic acid and prostaglandin E production by human fibroblasts. *J Rheumatol*. 1985;12:171.
19. Rongioletti F, Merlo G, Carli C, et al. Histopathologic characteristics of scleromyxedema: a study of a series of 34 cases. *J Am Acad Dermatol*. 2016;74:1194.
20. Stetsenko GY, Vary JC Jr, Olerud JE, et al. Unusual granulomatous variant of scleromyxedema. *J Am Acad Dermatol*. 2008;59:346.
21. Feldman P, Shapiro L, Pick AI, et al. Scleromyxedema. A dramatic response to melphalan. *Arch Dermatol*. 1969;99:51.
22. Harris RB, Perry HO, Kyle RA, et al. Treatment of scleromyxedema with melphalan. *Arch Dermatol*. 1979;115:295.
23. Dinneen AM, Dicken CH. Scleromyxedema. *J Am Acad Dermatol*. 1995;33:37-43.
24. Rayson D, Lust JA, Duncan A, et al. Scleromyxedema: a complete response to prednisone. *Mayo Clin Proc*. 1999;74:481.
25. Lister RK, Jolles S, Whittaker S, et al. Scleromyxedema: response to high-dose intravenous immunoglobulin (hdIVIg). *J Am Acad Dermatol*. 2000;43:403.
26. Caradonna S, Jacobe H. Thalidomide as a potential treatment for scleromyxedema. *Arch Dermatol*. 2004;140:277.
27. Berkson M, Lazarus GS, Uberti-Benz M, et al. Extracorporeal photochemotherapy: a potentially useful treatment for scleromyxedema. *J Am Acad Dermatol*. 1991;25:724.
28. Tschen JA, Chang JR. Scleromyxedema: treatment with interferon alfa. *J Am Acad Dermatol*. 1999;40:303.
29. Farr PM, Ive FA. PUVA treatment of scleromyxoedema. *Br J Dermatol*. 1984;110:347.
30. Laimer M, Namberger K, Massone C, et al. Vincristine, idarubicin, dexamethasone and thalidomide in scleromyxedema. *Acta Derm Venereol*. 2009;89:631.
31. Blum M, Wigley FM, Hummers LK. Scleromyxedema: a case series highlighting long-term outcomes of treatment with intravenous immunoglobulin (IVIG). *Medicine (Baltimore)*. 2008;87:10.
32. Lacy MQ, Hogan WJ, Gertz MA, et al. Successful treatment of scleromyxedema with autologous peripheral blood stem cell transplantation. *Arch Dermatol*. 2005;141:1277.

Chapter 68 :: Sjögren Syndrome
:: Akiko Tanikawa

第六十八章
干燥综合征

中文导读

Sjögren综合征（SS）是一种慢性系统性自身免疫性疾病，其特征是淋巴细胞浸润，外分泌腺和上皮破坏，导致口干、眼干和B淋巴细胞高反应性。本章从流行病学、病因及发病机制、临床特征、诊断和诊断试验、临床进程及预后、治疗等方面阐述了该病的特点。诊断SS最好的自身抗体是抗Ro/SSA和抗La/SSB抗体。临床表现非常广泛，从干眼症、口干、全身乏力、低热、肌痛和关节痛，到多器官功能障碍。外泌腺外受累的临床症状重点描述了皮肤受累的各种皮损表现，还介绍了非皮肤非外泌腺的组织器官受累可以出现的临床症状和体征；并讨论了对怀孕的影响。与原发性干燥综合征相关的环状红斑，与SCLE难以鉴别。SS患者的淋巴瘤发病率增加，淋巴结病、腮腺肿大、可触及的紫癜、低C4血清水平和冷球蛋白是非霍奇金淋巴瘤/淋巴增殖性疾病预测因子。口腔干燥和眼干燥患者的SS诊断需要牙医或唾液腺专家（如耳鼻喉科医生和眼科医生）的评估，本章列出了Sjögren综合征国际分类标准的修订。并总结了高危类型和低风险类型的特点，列举了SS综合征口干、眼干症状的治疗。同时对于腺外临床表现的治疗也进行了阐述。讨论了生物制剂分子靶向治疗在SS中的应用经验。

〔施 为〕

AT-A-GLANCE

- A chronic, multisystem autoimmune disease, characterized by chronic inflammation involving the exocrine glands.
- Salivary and lachrymal glands are affected predominantly, leading to dry mouth and dry eyes.
- May occur alone (primary Sjögren syndrome, pSS), or may coexist with other systemic connective tissue disorders (secondary Sjögren syndrome).
- Extraglandular manifestations of primary Sjögren syndrome include fatigue, Raynaud phenomenon, purpura, arthritis, vasculitis, interstitial pulmonary disease, peripheral or central neuropathy, and autonomic nervous dysfunction.
- Patients with systemic manifestations are at higher risk of developing lymphoma.
- Treatment of sicca symptoms is mainly symptomatic, whereas management of extraglandular manifestations is similar to that of other autoimmune diseases.
- Both innate and adaptive immunity contribute to pSS pathogenesis and pSS is associated with upregulation of the Type 1 interferon signaling pathway.

INTRODUCTION

Sjögren syndrome (SS) is a chronic systemic autoimmune disorder characterized by lymphocytic infiltration and destruction of exocrine glands and epithelia leading to dry mouth, dry eyes, and B lymphocyte hyperreactivity. SS can occur as an isolated disorder; primary Sjögren syndrome (pSS); it also may occur in association with other autoimmune condition such as rheumatoid arthritis, systemic lupus erythematosus (SLE) and other collagen disease; secondary SS. Disease may be localized to the salivary and lachrymal glands, but more than one-third of patients develop systemic manifestations. The clinical presentation can vary from mild sicca symptoms, fatigue, and arthralgias to severe systemic symptoms involving multiple organ systems. A small but definitely number of patients of the pSS develop lymphoma with higher incidence than that of the general population or patients with other autoimmune diseases (Fig. 68-1).

EPIDEMIOLOGY

SS is one of the most common rheumatic autoimmune diseases. SS predominantly affects women, with a female to male ratio of 9:1. Patients are most commonly diagnosed in their fourth and fifth decades of life, but it can affect any age, including the elderly and children. SS has a worldwide distribution. The estimated annual incidence rate of pSS ranged from 3.9 to 5.3 per 100,000 in several studies.[1] The prevalence rates can vary considerably, depending on the classification criteria used. The estimated prevalence rate in the adult general population from previous studies, mainly in whites, was between 0.2% and 2.7%, whereas the estimated prevalence rate from Asian studies was 0.03% to 0.77%.[2,3]

ETIOLOGY AND PATHOGENESIS

Although the precise pathogenesis of SS remains largely unknown, genetic and epigenetic disposition, various environmental factors, including viral and other pathogenic infections, and hormones have been implicated in the pathogenesis of the disease. Recent studies have shown that both innate and adaptive immunity contribute to the development of pSS; the Type 1 interferon (IFN) signaling pathway plays a central role in the pathogenesis of the disease. Increasing apoptosis in epithelial cells of damaged salivary glands, plasmacytoid dendritic cells (pDCs), autoreactive lymphocytes, and autoantibodies are considered to play significant roles in perpetuating the chronic auto-feedback inflammatory process.[4]

IMMUNOGENETIC FACTORS

The role of genetic factors in SS was recognized in family studies where first-degree relatives of patients had an increased prevalence of SS.[5,6] Such family clustering was further observed among first-degree relatives of individuals with anti-Ro/SSA antibodies, regardless of their clinical diagnoses (SS, systemic lupus erythematosus, or even healthy controls).[7]

There is a well-established association between SS or anti-Ro/SSA and anti-La/SSB antibodies with HLA class genes.[8] The genetic loci significantly associated with pSS are HLA DQA1*0501 and HLA DQB1*0201 in white patients, but the pattern differs among ethnic groups, studies, and populations.[9,10] In 2013, the first genomewide association study (GWAS) identified several susceptibility genes, such as IRF5 (interferon regulatory factor), STAT4 (signal transducer and activator of transcription 4), IL12A (gene regulating innate and adaptive immunity), BLK (B lymphoid tyrosine kinase), and CXCR5 (encoding a protein related to B-cell activation and localization), as risk variant genes related to SLE and SS.[11] IRF5 is an important transcription factor involved in upregulating the Type I IFN pathway, which is activated by toll-like receptor (TLR) signals or viral infection and the production of inflammatory cytokines, whereas STAT 4 is a protein involved in the Type II IFN pathway and activating the adaptive immune system.[11-13] TNFAIP3 and TNIP genes were also identified in GWAS, which regulate nuclear factor kappa-light-chain enhancer of activated B-cell (NF-κB) signaling. A TNFAIP3 mutation found in the coding region of TNFAIP3 has been correlated with an increased risk of lymphoma.[14]

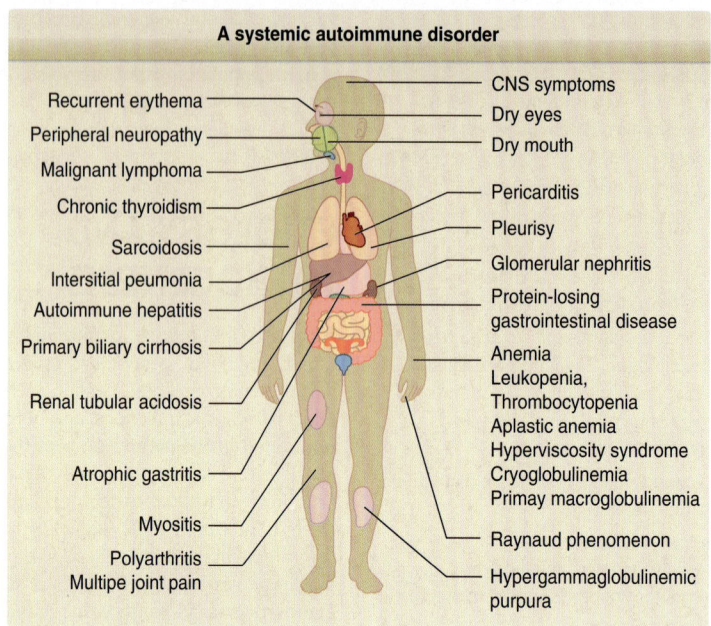

Figure 68-1 Sjögren syndrome. A systemic autoimmune disorder.

A recent epigenome-wide DNA methylation association study (EWAS) highlighted new links between epigenetic changes and disease-related inflammatory processes in the salivary glands, which is a major target organ in pSS. It also suggests the possibility that epigenetic factors contribute to the pathogenesis of pSS. MicroRNA expression patterns in the salivary glands have been demonstrated linked with the disease.[15] Recent studies have shown that the Ro60 autoantigen binds endogenous retroelements and regulates inflammatory gene expression,[16] but knowledge in this area is still limited.[4]

INNATE AND ADAPTIVE IMMUNITY

Type I IFN (IFN) is a key cytokine in the innate immune system, activating antigen-presenting cells and influencing autoimmune responses. Increased Type I IFN activity has been shown in the sera of pSS patients, and IFN-α also has been detected in the minor salivary glands of patients. Many IFN-stimulated genes and proteins are overexpressed, which has been called the "IFN signature." This has been found in about 50% of pSS patients and confirmed in the peripheral blood and/or salivary glands of patients.[17] Previous studies have shown that when the Type I IFN receptor or IFN itself is eliminated, many features of the disease are also eliminated. This supports the theory, based on previous SS research, that Type I IFN has a central role in the pathogenesis of SS.[18-22] Discovery of risk variants in IRF5, STAT4, and other susceptibility loci suggests that genetic polymorphism is a major factor in the onset of SS, activating the IFN pathway that regulates T-cell and B-cell immune responses.

BAFF (B-cell activating factor), a member of the TNF family and a cytokine produced by the activated IFN signaling pathway, is related to the adaptive immune system. BAFF promotes B-cell maturation, proliferation, and survival. BAFF has been shown to contribute to the pathogenesis of SS. First, levels of BAFF are increased in the salivary glands of SS patients and upregulated by IFN-α.[23] Second, transgenic mice that overexpress BAFF develop clinical manifestations of SS and SLE and have an increased risk of developing lymphoma versus wild-type mice.[24] Third, BAFF is usually produced in innate immune responses, but after damage to salivary gland cells by RNA viruses or TLR3 ligands, large amounts of BAFF can be produced by epithelial cells. Furthermore, the serum level of BAFF is known to correlate with the levels of anti-Ro/SSA antibodies, anti-La/SSB antibodies, and rheumatoid factor.[25] BAFF is also related to follicular structure (also called germinal center [GC]-like structure) formation. GC-like structures are known to be associated with an increased risk of lymphoma and may occur in one-fifth of patients with pSS.[26]

ENVIRONMENTAL FACTORS

Several factors are considered major environmental triggers that interact with genetic and epigenetic factors to cause disease onset. The strong predominance of females with the disease suggests gender-specific predisposing factors. Although sex hormones are obvious targets, there is no proof that the difference in the pathogenesis between males and females is due to sex hormones alone.[27,28]

Viruses, especially Epstein–Barr virus (EBV), are known to replicate in oropharyngeal and lachrymal glands, resulting in the hypothesis that these viruses may be involved in the pathogenesis of SS. In fact, genetic material from EBV was detected by DNA hybridization in SS salivary tissue, but it was also found in normal individuals, so the result is controversial.[29,30] In a Japanese cohort, defective human T-lymphotropic virus-I genome was isolated from salivary gland tissue.[31] Hepatitis C virus[32-34] and HIV are also thought of as initiators of the disease, with the presence of chronic inflammation in salivary glands, and presenting clinical symptoms similar to SS.[35] Other viruses, such as cytomegalovirus,[36] coxsackie A virus,[37] and endogenous retroviruses, also have been proposed as causative agents.[38] Recent studies further showed that EBV infections promoted the release of Ro/SSA and La/SSB ribonucleoprotein complexes through epithelial apoptosis.[39] The EBV-encoded small RNA and La/SSB complex is known to activate Type I IFN expression through activating TLR 3.[40] However, no single virus has been clearly implicated in the pathogenesis of SS. Animal model studies support the hypothesis that there can be a delay, for years, between viral infections (such as cytomegalovirus) and the development of SS.[36] Stress,[41] occupational exposure,[42] and personality features also have been proposed as triggers of the disease.[43,44]

GLANDULAR EPITHELIUM

In histopathology, sections of salivary and lachrymal glands in pSS are characterized by periductal mononuclear infiltrate. Most of the infiltrating cells are CD4+ T lymphocytes, although CD8+ cytotoxic T cells and plasmacytoid dendritic cells (pDCs) are also detected. Activated B lymphocytes, including immunoglobulin-secreting cells, are also present.

The salivary glands are thought to be the first and main target in pSS. The role of the salivary gland epithelial cells in pSS has been established. Studies have indicated that epithelial cells play an active role in disease pathogenesis and this is referred to as "autoimmune epithelitis."[45] First, glandular cells, including duct and acinar epithelial cells, express HLA class II major histocompatibility complex (MHC) molecules and costimulator CD86; these interact with CD28 on T cells and contribute to recruiting inflammatory cells.[46] Second, damage to the salivary gland by environmental factors, such as viruses, causes dysfunction in the gland, leading to activation of epithelial cells, increasing apoptosis, and elevated Type I IFN production by pDCs. Apoptotic keratinocytes are known to relocalize Ro/SSA and La/SSB from the nucleus to the cell surfaces in a complex, presenting autoantigens to autoantibodies. Thus, epithelial cells may not only be the target of the disease but may also function as antigen-presenting cells, inducing further autoimmune responses through activating TLR and IFN signaling pathways.[47-49] Previous studies have shown that epithelial cells express TLR 3, 7, and 9 when in an activated condition.[39,50] They can also produce Type I IFN by themselves, inappropriately, through activated TLR 3 within the gland[50] and become involved in perpetuating this chronic autofeedback inflammation. Third, such epithelial cells also produce large amounts of BAFF.[17] Finally, some epithelial cells express Fas and Fas ligand[51] and, as a consequence, undergo apoptosis; others may be destroyed by perforin, granzymes, and other cytotoxins produced by lymphocytes.[52] Extraglandular manifestations occur as a result of similar lymphocytic infiltration in other organs. "Autoimmune epithelitis" well describes the systemic nature of SS.

AUTOANTIBODIES

Autoantibodies are hallmarks of systemic autoimmune diseases, including SS. The best-defined autoantibodies in SS are the anti-Ro/SSA and anti-La/SSB antibodies.[53] Although the pathogenic role of any particular autoantibody remains undefined, both are targeted against ribonucleoprotein antigens. Anti-Ro/SSA recognizes 2 RNA-binding proteins (the 52-kDa or the 60-kDa protein), whereas anti-La/SSB antibodies recognize RNA polymerase III. Anti-Ro/SSA antibodies are found in more than 70% of patients with SS but are not specific for SS and are frequently found in SLE and other autoimmune diseases, even when there is no symptom or sign of oral or ocular dryness. Anti-La/SSB antibodies are more specific; it is present in 50% of patients with pSS or SS/SLE but is rarely seen in other diseases.[54] Although the pathogenic role of these antibodies is undefined, previous studies showed that Ro and La are expressed on the surface of apoptotic epithelial cells[48]; it is possible that an immune response against these antigens contributes to inflammation in the gland and further immunoreactive pathways. The most compelling in vivo evidence for a pathogenic role for these autoantibodies comes from newborns with fetal heart block, born to women with anti-Ro/SSA and/or anti-La/SSB antibodies. These antibodies can cross the placenta and bind to Ro and La antigens located on the cell surface of fetal myocardial tissue, leading to fetal heart block.[55] Other autoantibodies, such as antinuclear antibodies (ANA) and rheumatoid factor (RF), are frequently present in patients with both primary and secondary SS. Although they lack specificity, they are markers of a systemic autoimmune response and thus can help distinguish SS from other causes of salivary or lachrymal gland dysfunction. A large clinical study performed in Spain suggested the group of patients with anti-Ro/La antibodies had the highest prevalence among most systemic, hematologic, and immunologic alternations (higher frequency of Raynaud phenomenon, altered parotid scintigraphy, positive salivary gland biopsies, peripheral neuropathy, thrombocytopenia, and rheumatoid factor). Hypocomplementemia was associated with a higher frequency of vasculitis, lymphoma, and cryoglobulins, and higher frequencies of parotid enlargement, vasculitis, and leucopenia.[56] SSA positivity could also be related to extraglandular manifestations, vasculitis, hematologic abnormalities, and serological hyperreactivity.[57,58]

Further research has focused on identifying antibodies more specific for SS, such as anti-α-fodrin and anti-muscarinic acetylcholine receptor antibodies,[59] but the results have been controversial. The major stimulus for saliva production is the binding of acetylcholine to muscarinic acetylcholine receptors. The hypothesis that oral and ocular dryness could result from antibodies antagonizing the muscarinic acetylcholine receptor-3 is intriguing.[59] These antibodies have been demonstrated to play an essential role in glandular dysfunction in the non-obese diabetic (NOD) mouse model of SS, possibly through an inhibitory effect on the receptor.[60] In humans, however, results are still contradictory because multiple attempts to detect these antibodies with conventional immunologic methods have failed.[61,62]

A small group of patients positive for anticentromere autoantibody (ACA) present a clinical picture similar to that of limited scleroderma. About 1% to 17% of SS patients have been reported to be positive for ACA.[55,63] There is no difference between ACA-positive and ACA-negative patients in terms of female dominance or salivary gland damage and dysfunction. The ACA-positive group usually has a higher prevalence of Raynaud phenomenon and thyroid dysfunction than ACA-negative patients. This group also shows a higher frequency of vasculitis, peripheral neuropathy, and primary biliary cirrhosis, but lymphoma is the same as in the ACA-negative group.[64-68] Positivity for antimitochondrial antibody (AMA) also has been demonstrated to be related to primary biliary cirrhosis.[69]

CLINICAL FINDINGS

Sjögren syndrome (SS) is a multifocal autoimmune disease, with systemic involvement in one-third of patients. The clinical presentation is very wide-ranging, from dry eyes, dry mouth, general fatigue, subfever, myalgia, and arthralgia, to multiple organ dysfunction.[70]

EXOCRINE GLAND INVOLVEMENT

The characteristic feature of SS is exocrine gland dysfunction, leading to the classic sicca symptoms of xerostomia (dry mouth) and xerophthalmia or keratoconjunctivitis sicca (dry eyes).

XEROSTOMIA

Oral dryness is a principal symptom of SS, caused by decreased saliva secretion, which is persistent and continuous throughout the day and night and can significantly compromise quality of life. Reduced salivation causes difficulty in chewing and swallowing dry foods. Dryness of the tongue and oral mucosa leads to an altered sense of taste and, at times, produces burning discomfort, especially when eating acidic or spicy foods. Physical examination may reveal a red and fissured tongue with characteristic atrophy of the filiform papillae (Fig. 68-2) or angular cheilitis. Ulcerations may be found, particularly in SS patients with dentures, usually in proximity to the mucosal surface that makes contact with the denture.

Normal saliva has antimicrobial properties, so a lack of saliva can predispose to infections. Oral thrush is common and can be manifested as pseudomembranous or erythematous mucosal lesions. Furthermore, patients with SS have an increased incidence of caries. A characteristic feature of caries in SS is its primary location, at the cervical and incisal regions of the teeth.

Bilateral salivary gland enlargement typically occurs in the parotid glands of SS patients. It is frequently nontender, and it can be recurrent or chronic. Painful, unilateral parotid enlargement should raise the suspicion of an infection or a salivary gland stone. In cases of persistent unilateral parotid gland enlargement, the presence of lymphoma should be excluded (Table 68-1). Medical causes of oral dryness, such as dehydration, diabetes, viral infections, and drug treatment, should be considered when evaluating a patient for Sjögren syndrome.

KERATOCONJUNCTIVITIS SICCA

Ocular dryness is the other dominant feature of SS. A burning and itching sensation in the eyes, commonly exacerbated by smoke, is caused by lack of tear production. Patients frequently complain of intolerance to contact lenses. Paradoxically, the quantity of tears produced during crying may not be affected. Physical evaluation shows corneal injection and mucous dis-

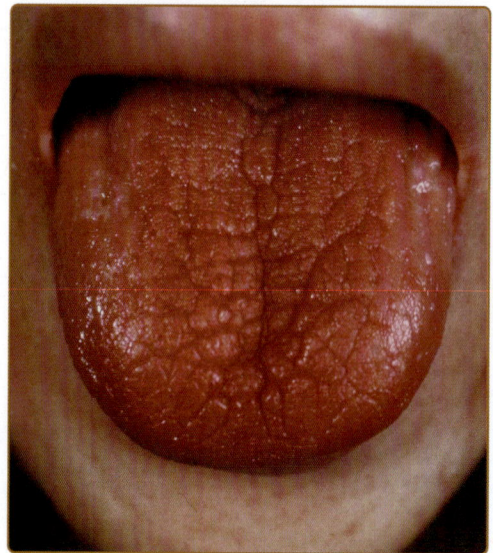

Figure 68-2 The characteristic tongue of patients with Sjögren syndrome. A red and fissured tongue with characteristic atrophy of the filiform papillae.

TABLE 68-1
Differential Diagnosis of Parotid Gland Swelling[a]

Bilateral	Viral infections	Mumps
		Epstein–Barr, cytomegalovirus, coxsackie, influenza
		HIV, Human T-lymphotropic virus-I (HTLV-I)
		Hepatitis C
	Immune mediated	Sjögren syndrome
		Sarcoidosis
		IgG4-related disease
		Amyloidosis
	Metabolic	Diabetes mellitus
		Hyperlipoproteinemia
		Hepatic cirrhosis
		Chronic pancreatitis
	Endocrine	Acromegaly
		Gonadal hypofunction
Unilateral	Other	Alcohol
		Recurrent parotitis of the childhood
	Bacterial infections	
	Neoplasms	Mainly lymphomas, salivary gland tumor
	Sialolithiasis	

[a]Medical causes of oral dryness, such as dehydration, diabetes, viral infections, or drug treatment, should be considered when evaluating a patient for Sjögren syndrome.

charge in the lower fornix. Enlarged lachrymal glands have been described in Sjögren patients, but occur less commonly than enlarged salivary glands. The constellation of symptoms and signs indicating dry eyes constitutes keratoconjunctivitis sicca.

OTHER SICCA MANIFESTATIONS

Cutaneous xerosis, a term used to describe dryness of the skin, is very common in SS, with a frequency varying between 23% and 68%. The most common symptoms of xerosis are nonspecific pruritus, burning sensations, and a pin prick–like feeling. Physical examination reveals roughness, fine scaling, and loss of elasticity in the skin. The pathogenesis of xerosis is unknown. Impairment of the sweat glands is considered an important factor because decreased sweating has been reported in SS patients. A recent study indicated that xerosis may be related to increased epidermal proliferation with disturbed epidermal differentiation.[71]

Xerostomia predisposes to angular cheilitis, which presents as recurrent, symmetric, itching fissures.

Eyelid dermatitis is defined by the presence of erythematous, infiltrated, and lichenified lesions of the eyelids associated with itching and foreign body sensations.

Anhidrosis/hypohidrosis also has been reported as an exocrine manifestation, but is rare.[72,73]

Dryness of the upper respiratory tract can cause epistaxis, hoarseness, and bronchial hyperresponsiveness. Another common complaint in women with the disease is vaginal dryness, which may lead to an increased incidence of vaginal infections and dyspareunia.

EXTRAGLANDULAR INVOLVEMENT

SKIN INVOLVEMENT

Cutaneous manifestations are common extraglandular features of SS (Table 68-2).[74]

Hypergammaglobulinemic Purpura: Purpuric macules are very common in SS (Fig. 68-3). Flat, nonpalpable, blanching purpura has been associated with an entity called benign hyperglobulinemic purpura, characterized by polyclonal hypergammaglobulinemia and rheumatoid factor positivity. Skin biopsies reveal ruptured blood vessels with complement deposition.[75]

Cutaneous Vasculitis: Cutaneous vasculitis (CV) can present as palpable purpura or urticarial vasculitis and occurs in about 9% of patients.[76]

Palpable purpura, which does not blanch when pressure is applied to the skin, is due to dermal vasculitis with extravasation of red blood cells, and typically involves the lower extremities and buttocks (Chap. 138). It represents an important marker of more severe disease and is associated with an increased risk of lymphoma development and mortality.[55] Histopathologically, palpable purpura can be divided into 2 groups. Neutrophilic inflammatory vascular disease is characterized by a predominantly neutrophilic infiltrate, fibrinoid

TABLE 68-2
Cutaneous Manifestations of Sjögren Syndrome

- Hypergammaglobulinemic purpura
- Cutaneous vasculitis
  - Nonpalpable purpura
  - Palpable purpura
  - Urticarial vasculitis
  - Necrotizing vasculitis
- Annular erythema associated with primary Sjögren syndrome
- Erythema multiforme
- Erythema perstans
- Erythema nodosum
- Oral
  - Dry mucous membranes
  - Papillary atrophy of the tongue
  - Candidiasis
  - Angular cheilosis
- Eyelid dermatitis
- Alopecia
- Vitiligo

with perinuclear fluorescence can be found, but are uncommon in SS.

Annular Erythema Associated with Primary Sjögren Syndrome:
Annular erythema associated with pSS is found primarily among Asian pSS patients who have anti-Ro/SSA (> 90%) and anti-La/SSB (~70%) antibodies. The characteristic and typical rash is an erythematous lesion with a wide elevated border and central clearing; fine scale, erosion, or a crust can be seen in some cases.[78,79] The lesion usually starts from a small indurate erythema that expands to an annular form; it can sometimes be polycyclic, and may heal without atrophy, scar, or pigmentation (Fig. 68-4). They are localized mainly on the faces of Asian patients (81%), but can also occur on the arms, trunk, and proximal thighs. Sunlight and cold exposure, mental stress, and pregnancy may be triggers of the lesions. Annular erythema associated with pSS occur in Asian patients with an occurrence of up to 47%, but is less common in whites, with an occurrence of 9%.[80] Because annular erythema associated with pSS shares a clinical presentation with subacute cutaneous lupus (SCLE), it is still debatable whether annular erythema associated with pSS is a variant of SCLE (annular SCLE), as proposed by Sontheimer in 1979,[81] but it seems to represent a distinct clinical and histopathologic entity.

The 2 conditions can hardly be distinguished from clinical presentations or laboratory investigations, such as positivity for anti-SSA/Ro and anti-SSB/La

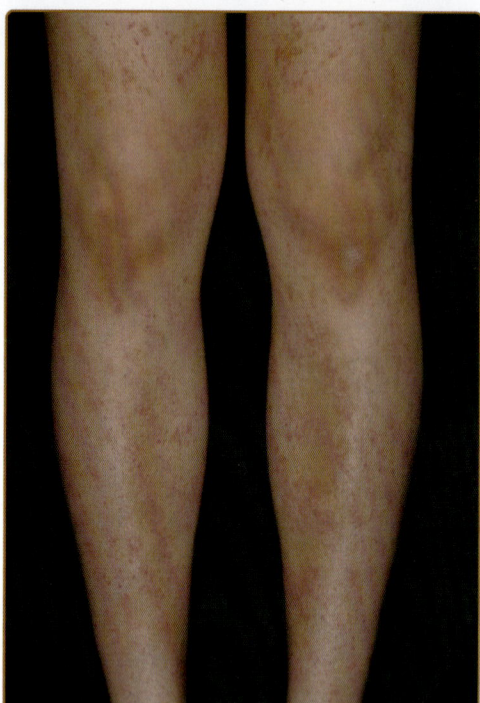

Figure 68-3 Non-palpable purpura with pigmentation in a patient with primary Sjögren syndrome.

necrosis, occlusion of the lumen, and extravasation of red blood cells, and is indistinguishable from classical leukocytoclastic vasculitis (Chap. 138). However, mononuclear inflammatory vascular disease is characterized by a mononuclear inflammatory infiltrate, with invasion of the blood vessel walls. Fibrinoid necrosis is present but less prominent. The clinical presentation of these 2 forms are indistinguishable, but neutrophilic inflammatory vascular disease is associated more strongly with markers of systemic autoimmunity, such as antinuclear antibodies and anti-Ro/SSA and anti-La/SSB antibodies, hypergammaglobulinemia, rheumatoid factor, and hypocomplementemia. Cryoglobulinemic vasculitis also can be seen in Sjögren patients and has the same cutaneous manifestations (Chap. 138).

Urticarial vasculitis is the second most frequent form of CV in SS and presents as pruritic wheals with erythema (Chap. 138). In contrast to true urticaria, individual lesions last for more than 24 hours and often resolve with hyperpigmentation. Biopsy of the skin lesions demonstrates a perivascular neutrophilic infiltrate, accompanied by leukocytoclasia.

Necrotizing vasculitis is not commonly seen in Sjögren syndrome.[77] It can present as palpable purpuric lesions of the lower extremities, which may ulcerate, finally resolving within 1 to 4 weeks. They heal with atrophy or scar tissue formation. This form of vasculitis has been observed more frequently in patients with more active disease; it has been associated with arthritis, Raynaud phenomenon, peripheral neuropathy, fever, and pulmonary or glomerular involvement. Antineutrophil cytoplasmic antibodies

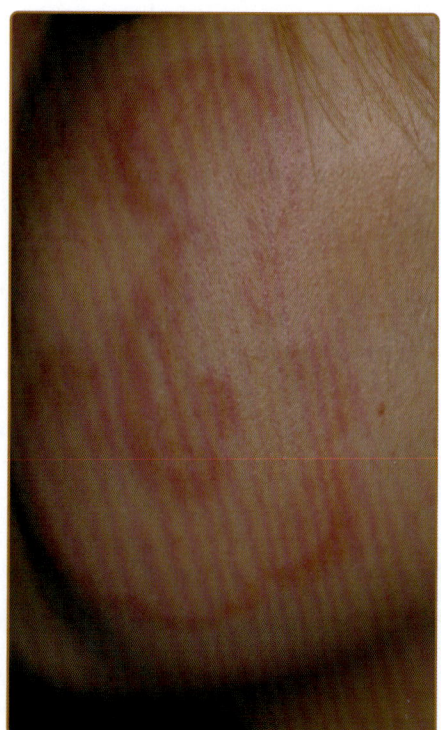

Figure 68-4 Annular erythema associated with primary Sjögren syndrome in a young female patient presented with figurate annular erythema with raised border.

antibodies; they even show similar Ro/SS-A autoantibody epitopes and titer responses, but there are some distinct differences between the 2 conditions. First, annular erythema associated with pSS are located mainly on the face (>80%) in Oriental patients, but mainly on the trunk in white patients; second, the percentage of anti-SSA/Ro antibody–positive patients is different between annular erythema associated with pSS in Asians and SCLE in non-Asian patients; third, in histopathologic findings and finally, in HLA DR3 and 8 expression.[80,82,83] In histopathology, SCLE presents with liquefaction degeneration in the basal membrane zone, positivity for IgM/IgG in the dermal–epidermal junction with direct immunofluorescence (DIF), and cell infiltration being, basically, in the upper dermis, whereas in annular erythema associated with pSS, the dense cell infiltration is localized mainly around sweat glands, and nuclear dust also can be seen when they have vasculitis. Usually, no vacuolar changes are found in the dermal–epidermal junction, and no other findings suggest lupus erythematosus, such as epidermal atrophy or follicular plugging, and are usually negative for DIF.

SS and SLE share common genetic polymorphisms, such as IRF5, STAT4, and BLK[11]; thus, it is possible patients present similar manifestations in both conditions.[84] However, other studies have demonstrated notable differences in populations with risk haplotypes and risk alleles, including HLA.[85] Previous studies have also shown that Oriental patients have higher anti-SSA/Ro antibody titers and are more commonly negative for HLA DR3 and DR8, which show a high incidence in American patients.[82] It is well known that annular erythema associated with pSS are common in Asians but rare in whites, whereas SCLE are more common in whites but rare in Asians. The similarity between annular erythema associated with pSS and SCLE may be explained as a phenotype variation, from sharing the same genetic polymorphisms but having different risk haplotypes/alleles in different ethnic groups. At present, annular erythema associated with pSS is included in the EULAR-SS Disease Activity Index (ESSDAI), cutaneous domain, and classified as a moderate activity level manifestation in SS.[86]

Erythema Nodosum: Erythema nodosum, a painful nodular eruption of the anterior surface of the lower extremities, may occur but is rare in SS patients. Its presence should raise suspicion for sarcoidosis. Erythema multiforme–like lesions and superficial ill-defined patches (erythema perstans) also have been described in SS.

Other Skin Manifestations Related to Peripheral Circulation and Temperature:
Raynaud phenomenon is probably the most common abnormality. It can be seen in 15% to 35% of patients and can precede sicca symptoms by many years. Raynaud phenomenon in SS is not accompanied by telangiectasias, as seen in systemic sclerosis. Calcifications have been described, but are uncommon. Although Raynaud phenomenon is usually mild in pSS, it is a marker of a subgroup with increased risk of extraglandular manifestations.[87] Acrocyanosis, pernio-like eruptions (Fig. 68-5), livedo, and periungual hemorrhage also may be observed.

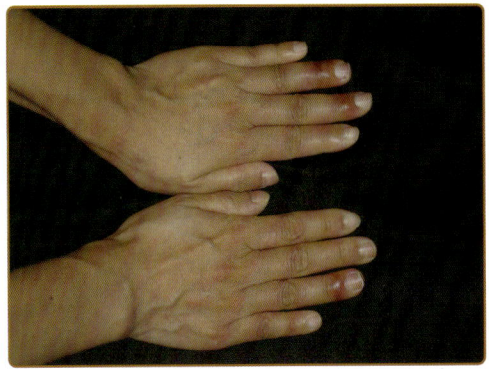

Figure 68-5 Pernio-like eruption in a patient with primary Sjögren syndrome.

Other Cutaneous Manifestations: Other cutaneous manifestations including photosensitivity, indurated erythema, alopecia, vitiligo vulgaris, lichen planus, sarcoidosis, granuloma annulare, and psoriasis also may be seen in SS, albeit infrequently.

NONCUTANEOUS EXTRAGLANDULAR MANIFESTATIONS

Musculoskeletal Manifestations: A symmetric nonerosive polyarthritis is frequently seen in pSS. The distinction between pSS and rheumatoid arthritis may be difficult in this regard; the absence of rheumatoid factor and anti-CCP antibodies, and the absence of erosions on radiographs would favor SS over rheumatoid arthritis. Arthralgias and myalgias are common complaints but true myositis is rare in pSS.

Fatigue and Fibromyalgia: Fatigue is a common complaint in SS, but the pathogenesis remains unknown. Fibromyalgia is a distinct condition, rather similar to SS, and should always be considered in the differential diagnosis.

Thyroid Dysfunction: Thyroid dysfunction is a very common symptom, occurring in 10% to 70% of SS patients. It often presents as fatigue and patients easily become tired.

Visceral Manifestations: *Lungs.* Dry cough due to dryness of the tracheal mucosa is common (tracheobronchitis sicca). Rarely, patients may develop interstitial pneumonitis. Patients may also develop mucosa-associated lymphoid tissue (MALT) lymphoma in the lungs.

Renal and genitourinary manifestations include interstitial cystitis (50%), renal tubular acidosis, interstitial nephritis and, rarely, glomerulonephritis.

Gastrointestinal. Dysphagia due to xerostomia and esophageal dysmotility is common. *Helicobacter pylori* is associated with an increased risk of MALT lymphomas; thus, patients with gastritis should be checked for *H. pylori* and treated if found positive. An asymptomatic, chemical pancreatitis with high-serum amylase concentrations has been reported in 25% of patients.

Other conditions, such as celiac disease, primary biliary cirrhosis, and hypothyroidism may also occur with pSS. Because of these associations, a high index of diagnostic suspicion is warranted to identify and treat these conditions.

Neurologic manifestations can be divided into those that involve the CNS, and those that involve the peripheral nervous system and autonomic dysfunction.

The peripheral nervous system is involved in ~20% of patients with pSS.[88] However, this can increase to 70% when the patient has cutaneous vasculitis. The most common manifestations are peripheral axonal polyneuropathies, which are typically sensory. Another entity that has been described is a ganglionopathy involving the sensory ganglia of the posterior column. This starts with unilateral peripheral paresthesias, evolving over months to years to deep sensory impairment, positive Romberg sign, generalized areflexia, and ataxia.[89] Cranial neuropathies are also frequent. The most common form is unilateral trigeminal neuropathy; it usually spares the ophthalmic division, preserving the corneal reflex. Other cranial neuropathies may lead to Bell palsy (facial nerve), neural deafness, vestibular dysfunction (vestibule-cochlear), and diplopia (oculomotor, trochlear, abducent nerve).

The CNS also may be involved, although the prevalence and the spectrum of manifestations remain controversial. Manifestations similar to multiple sclerosis as well as transverse myelitis have been described. The latter is frequently associated with antiaquaporin-4 autoantibodies.

Lymphoma/Lymphoproliferative Disease:
The incidence of lymphoma in SS patients is increased 15- to 44-fold, according to various studies[90]; 4% of patients during the first 5 years, 10% at 15 years, and 18% after 20 years, postdiagnosis, develop lymphomas.[91] Most of these are indolent, extranodal, marginal-zone B-cell lymphomas of MALT, but higher-grade lymphomas are also seen.[90] It has been proposed that at least a proportion of DLBCLs arise from MALT transformation, and lifelong follow-up of patients with pSS and MALT lymphoma is recommended.[92]

Various clinical and laboratory features have been correlated with an increased risk of lymphoma development. Lymphadenopathy, parotid enlargement, palpable purpura, low C4 serum levels, and cryoglobulins are the most consistent non-Hodgkin lymphoma/lymphoproliferative disease predictors. Some studies have also identified splenomegaly, low C3 serum levels, lymphopenia, and neutropenia as significant prognostic factors. Histopathologically, the presence of germinal center–like (GC-like) lesions in salivary biopsies of pSS are associated with an enhanced possibility of developing lymphoma. *TNFAIP3* and *TNIP1* gene variants were identified together with the *IRF5*, *STAT4*, and *CXCR5* genes in GWAS; polymorphisms in these genes also have been suggested to contribute to GC-like structure formation, and further studies have demonstrated associations between the gene variants and pSS and non-Hodgkin lymphoma.[93-95] In contrast, anti-Ro, anti-La, and antinuclear antibodies, rheumatoid factor, male gender, hypergammaglobulinemia, and anemia were not associated with lymphoma/lymphoproliferative diseases.[91,96-98]

Pregnancy: Recent studies have suggested that women with pSS may experience more complications in pregnancy than healthy controls. Significant increases in the rates of spontaneous abortions, preterm deliveries, and low-body-weight infants were reported. The mechanism of the lower body weight was suggested to be due to underlying placental insufficiency, related to the autoimmune background.[99] Moreover, carriers of the Ro/SSA and La/SSB antibody can transmit it through the placental circulation to the fetus. These antibodies (anti-Ro/SSA, anti-La/SSB) can cause congenital heart block (CHB) or neonatal lupus (NLE), characterized by an annular rash with central regression or mild atrophy in the scalp and around the eyes, as well as hepatic and hematologic abnormalities. The skin lesions can be variable and appears in infants at a few weeks of age. Although the rash typically resolves spontaneously at 6-8 months of age, the heart block is permanent and requires the placement of a pacemaker in ~60% of patients. Expectant mothers with Ro/SSA and La/SSB antibodies should be counseled about this risk, and their fetuses should be followed closely for the development of fetal heart block.

DIAGNOSIS AND DIAGNOSIS TESTS

The diagnosis of SS in a patient with complaints of oral and ocular dryness requires evaluation by a dentist or salivary gland specialist, such as an otorhinolaryngologist, and an ophthalmologist, for specialized tests to quantify mucosal dryness, as well as laboratory evidence of autoantibodies and a salivary gland biopsy for evidence of inflammation within the gland itself. Unlike other autoimmune disorders, SS still lacks universally accepted classification criteria. Several sets of diagnostic criteria have been developed and used by various groups over time, creating some confusion with regard to how to define SS. Recently, an international consensus group agreed on a set of criteria, and this revised American–European classification system has been widely accepted (Table 68-3).[100] Six features are taken into consideration: subjective complaints and objective evidence of dry eyes or dry mouth, objective evidence of salivary gland inflammation, and the presence of specific autoantibodies in the serum. For the diagnosis of pSS, at least 4 criteria should be present, and at least one of them should be evidence of lymphocytic infiltration or the presence of autoantibodies. Patients with a coexisting connective tissue disease are

TABLE 68-3
Revised International Classification Criteria for Sjögren Syndrome

I. Ocular Symptoms: A positive response to at least one of the following questions:
1. Have you had daily, persistent, troublesome dry eyes for more than 3 mo?
2. Do you have a recurrent sensation of sand or gravel in the eyes?
3. Do you use tear substitutes more than 3 times a day?

II. Oral symptoms: A positive response to at least one of the following questions:
1. Have you had a daily feeling of dry mouth for more than 3 mo?
2. Have you had recurrently or persistently swollen salivary glands as an adult?
3. Do you frequently drink liquids to aid in swallowing dry food?

III. Ocular signs: Objective evidence of ocular involvement defined as a positive result for at least one of the following 2 tests:
1. Schirmer test, performed without anesthesia (≤5 mm in 5 min)
2. Rose Bengal score or other ocular dye score (≥4 according to the van Bijsterveld scoring system)

IV. Histopathology: In minor salivary glands (obtained through normal-appearing mucosa) focal lymphocytic sialoadenitis, evaluated by an expert histopathologist, with a focus score ≥1, defined as a number of lymphocytic foci (which are adjacent to normal-appearing mucous acini and contain more than 50 lymphocytes) per 4 mm^3 per glandular tissue

V. Salivary gland involvement: Objective evidence of salivary gland involvement defined as a positive result for at least one of the following diagnostic tests:
1. Unstimulated whole salivary flow (<1.5 mL/15 min)
2. Parotid sialography showing the presence of diffuse sialectasias (punctuate, cavitary, or destructive pattern), without evidence of obstruction in the major ducts
3. Salivary scintigraphy showing delayed uptake, reduced concentration, and/or reduced excretion of tracer

VI. Autoantibodies: Presence in the serum of the following autoantibodies: antibodies to Ro/SSA, La/SSB or both

Reproduced with permission from BMJ Publishing Group Ltd: Vitali C et al. Classification criteria for Sjögren's syndrome: A revised version of the European criteria proposed by the American-European Consensus Group. *Ann Rheum Dis*. 2002;61:554.

TABLE 68-4
Proposed Classification Criteria for Sjögren Syndrome

The classification of SS, which applies to individuals with signs/symptoms that may be suggestive of SS, will be met in patients who have at least 2 of the following 3 objective features:
1. Positive serum anti-SSA/Ro and/or anti-SSB/La or (positive rheumatoid factor and ANA titer ≥1:320)
2. Keratoconjunctivitis sicca with ocular staining score ≥3 (assuming that individual is not currently using daily eye drops for glaucoma and has not had corneal surgery or cosmetic eyelid surgery in the last 5 y)
3. Labial salivary gland biopsy exhibiting focal lymphocytic sialadenitis with a focus score of ≥1 focus/4 mm^2

Exclusion Criteria
History of head and neck radiation treatment
Acquired immunodeficiency syndrome
Hepatitis C infection
Sarcoidosis
Amyloidosis
Graft-vs-host disease
IgG4-related disease

Modified from Shiboski SC, et al. American College of Rheumatology classification criteria for Sjögren's syndrome: A data-driven, expert consensus approach in the Sjögren's International Collaborative Clinical Alliance cohort. *Arthritis Care Res (Hoboken)*. 2012;64(4):475-87, with permission.

labeled secondary SS. Exclusions include other diseases and medications that may cause sicca symptoms.

In 2012, the American College of Rheumatology provided new criteria (Table 68-4).[101] The new criteria require at least 2 of the following 3:

- Positive serum anti-SSA/anti-SSB antibodies or positive rheumatoid factor (RF) and antinuclear antibody titer ≥1:320,
- Keratoconjunctivitis sicca with ocular staining score ≥3,
- Labial salivary gland biopsy showing focal lymphocytic sialadenitis with a focus score ≥1 focus/4 mm^2.

These criteria are thought to be stricter than those previously applied, and so the prevalence may decline.[102]

ORAL DRYNESS

SIALOMETRY

Sialometry involves measurement of the total saliva produced from all salivary glands in a time period of 15 min. The whole unstimulated salivary flow is considered suggestive of SS if it is <1.5 mL in 15 minutes. A "stimulated" salivary flow can be measured after administration of lemon juice or citric acid, and low values are also suggestive of SS.

SALIVARY GLAND SCINTIGRAPHY

Salivary gland scintigraphy (SGS) is a functional study to assess saliva production by measuring the secretion of a radioisotope (^{99m}technetium sodium pertechnetate) into the oral cavity. SGS provides functional information about individual salivary glands and can potentially distinguish between decreased production and/or decreased excretion of saliva. The past decade has seen a shift toward the quantitative evaluation of SGS based on various parameters generated from time-activity curves.[103] Given the high cost and the exposure to radiation, routine use may not yet be justified but it is a useful diagnostic tool in selected cases. Sialography is an imaging method based on retrograde injection of contrast media into the parotid duct. Dilation of salivary ducts and sialolithiases are the most common findings.

OCULAR DRYNESS

The diagnosis of keratoconjuctivitis sicca is based on the demonstration of decreased tear production, corneal damage, or both. Tear production is usually measured using Schirmer test. This is performed by placing a standardized paper strip in the inferior fornix of each eye and measuring the length of filter paper that becomes wet after 5 minutes. The American–European classification system uses a cut-off value of 5 mm in 5 minutes, below which a diagnosis of dry eye is made. An alternative method is staining with a dye (rose Bengal or lissamine green) that preferentially stains the devitalized cornea and conjunctiva. This staining is evaluated through the van Bijsterveld scoring system; a score of 4 or more indicates keratoconjunctivitis sicca. These tests have high sensitivity but low specificity; they identify ocular dryness, but cannot attribute abnormal findings to SS.

LABORATORY TESTING

High levels of inflammatory markers, such as high sedimentation rates and signs of chronic inflammation (anemia, hypoalbuminemia), are common in SS patients. Serologic tests may demonstrate hyperglobulinemia in as many as 80% of pSS patients. Autoantibodies commonly include Ro/SSA and La/SSB antibodies, as well as rheumatoid factor and ANA. Hypocomplement has been associated with a higher frequency of vasculitis and lymphoma, and cryoglobulins with higher frequencies of parotid enlargement, vasculitis, and leukoplakia.

HISTOPATHOLOGY

None of the above diagnostic procedures is specific for SS. The most reliable objective diagnostic feature is seen on a biopsy of the minor salivary gland. A small incision is made on the inner surface of the lip, and a minor salivary gland tissue sample is collected. Evidence of a focal, periductal infiltrate, composed of T and B lymphocytes and few plasma cells, is the histologic hallmark of SS (Fig. 68-6). The degree of lymphocytic infiltration is evaluated semiquantitatively by means of a focus scoring system. Evidence of one or more foci is considered indicative of SS, and a focus is considered a conglomeration of at least 50 lymphocytes per 4 mm^2 of glandular tissue. GC-like structures are thought to be a risk factor for developing lymphoma.[104] Atrophy and fat tissue are other findings that may be present in SS patients, but also can be present in healthy, elderly individuals. Although a salivary gland biopsy provides important clues that may lead to a definitive diagnosis, some controversy still exists regarding its sensitivity and specificity. Some patients with pSS, diagnosed on the basis of reduced salivary flow and evidence of anti-SSA and anti-SSB antibodies, have no lymphocytic infiltration in biopsy specimens from the minor salivary glands. Additionally, some healthy individuals may demonstrate lymphocytic foci in their salivary glands.

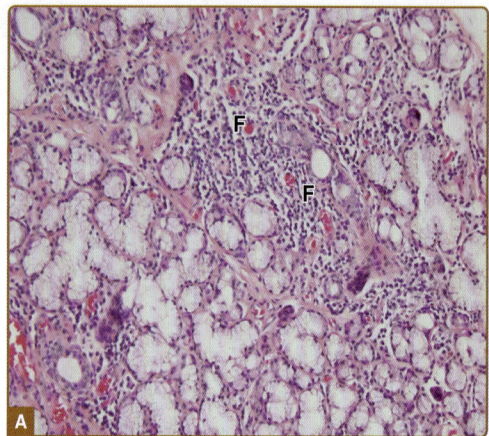
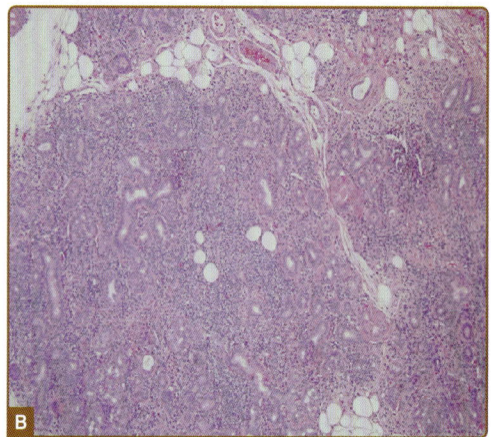
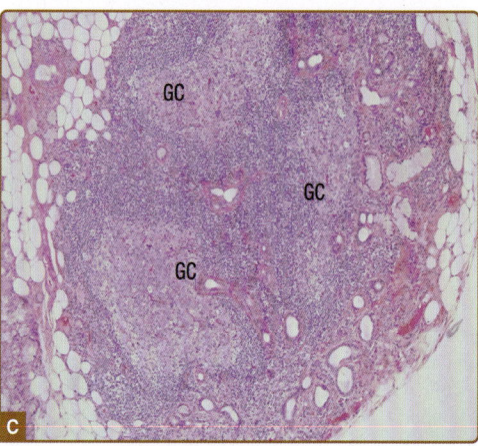

Figure 68-6 Histopathology of the minor salivary gland in Sjögren's syndrome. The degree of lymphocytic infiltration varies from moderate (**A**) to diffuse (**B**). In the most severe forms, germinal center formation can be observed (**C**). F = lymphocytic focus; GC = germinal center.

CLINICAL COURSE AND PROGNOSIS

There are 2 patterns of pSS that define 2 distinct disease categories with very different clinical risks. Patients with low complement C4 levels and/or palpable purpura early in their disease course may be classified as a high-risk disease syndrome (Type I). This group comprises ~20% of pSS diagnoses and carries a significantly increased risk of lymphoproliferative disease; it also has an increased mortality rate. Most severe extraglandular manifestations also occur in this group. Patients without these 2 predictors (80% of all pSS diagnoses) may be reassured that they have a low-risk (Type II) form of pSS that carries no increased risk of death and, in general, has a more benign course, dominated by sicca symptom.[97,105,106]

TREATMENT

TREATMENT OF DRY MOUTH (TABLE 68-5)

The treatment of oral dryness is largely symptomatic.[107] Nonpharmacologic strategies remain the mainstay of treatment. Adequate hydration, and reducing irritants like coffee, alcohol, and nicotine, as well as the substitution of drugs that can lead to dry mouth (diuretics, tricyclics, antihistamines, β-blockers) when possible are important. Frequent sips of water are recommended initially to maintain moisture. Patients should also be encouraged to use sugar-free candies and chewing gum to increase saliva production. Saliva substitutes are available in the form of gels, oils, and sprays, but the need for frequent application is inconvenient for many patients.

Sugar-containing foods should be avoided because they contribute to an increased risk of dental caries and oral candidiasis. Meticulous dental hygiene is essential for SS patients to prevent or treat dental caries. Caries prevention with fluoride application, including prescription-strength toothpaste, fluoride gels, and oral rinses, is further recommended.

Oral candidiasis is treated with oral and systemic antifungal therapy. To prevent candidiasis, patients should not wear dentures at night and dentures should be soaked in 2% chlorhexidine. Nystatin or clotrimazole cream can be used to treat angular cheilitis.

If dry mouth is not adequately controlled with replacement methods, pharmacologic therapy with secretagogue drugs is an option. Two drugs are approved for this indication: (1) pilocarpine (5 mg 4 times/d)[108] and (2) cevimeline (30 mg 3 times/d).[109] Both act on muscarinic receptors and increase exocrine gland secretion. They are contraindicated in narrow-angle glaucoma and uncontrolled asthma. Cholinergic side effects, such as excessive sweating, urinary frequency, flushing, and headaches, are common with both. Tolerability may be increased if treatment is started at a lower dose, which is then increased gradually (Table 68-5).

TREATMENT OF DRY EYES (TABLE 68-5)

Nonpharmacologic measures are important therapeutic interventions; avoidance of dry, smoky, and windy environments; avoiding contact lenses or opting for those higher in water content; and minimizing medications that inhibit tear production (diuretics, β-blockers, tricyclic antidepressants, antihistamines) are first-line measures.

Many tear substitutes are available and are commonly used by patients to alleviate ocular dryness. Preservative-free preparations are preferred, especially if used more than 4 times per day. Methylcellulose-containing ointments may provide longer relief, but their use is limited to nighttime use because of the risk of blurred vision.

A frequently used surgical option is occlusion of the puncta to block tear drainage and, consequently, increase moisture. The occlusion can be transient, with the insertion of collagen or silicone plugs, or permanent, with electrocautery.

Cyclosporine 0.05% ophthalmic solution has been approved by the FDA for the treatment of keratoconjunctivitis sicca.[110] Topical corticosteroids are rarely needed and should probably only be prescribed after an ophthalmic examination. Infections may present with aggravation of symptoms or increased mucus secretion and should be promptly treated with topical antibiotics. Pilocarpine and cevimeline can be effective for dry eyes, too, especially in patients with the most severe dryness.[109]

TABLE 68-5

Management of Sicca Symptoms in Sjögren Syndrome

Dry mouth	- Frequent water - Mechanical stimulation of saliva secretion (sugar-free gum and candies) - Artificial saliva - Meticulous oral hygiene - Caries prevention with fluoride-containing toothpaste and rinses - Aggressive treatment of candidiasis with topical and systemic antifungals - Sialogogues: pilocarpine (5 mg orally 3 times/d) or cevimeline (30 mg orally 3 times/d)
Dry eyes	- Frequent use of preservative-free artificial tears - Nighttime use of moisturizing ointments - Topical cyclosporine ophthalmic solution (0.05%, one drop every 12 h) - Surgical: punctal plug placement - Sialogogues

TREATMENT OF EXTRAGLANDULAR MANIFESTATIONS

The treatment of the musculoskeletal manifestations of SS is similar to that of other systemic rheumatologic diseases.[111] Because of reduced saliva production and esophageal dysmotility, these patients have reduced tolerance to nonsteroidal antiinflammatory drugs. Antimalarial drugs, such as hydroxychloroquine, are effective for arthralgia/arthritis, myalgia, fatigue, and annular erythema.[112] Dryness of the eyes and mouth may also improve slightly in some cases.[113] Visceral manifestations, such as vasculitis, pneumonitis, and glomerulonephritis, and neurologic manifestations are treated with corticosteroids and immunosuppressive drugs, it doses similar to those used in systemic lupus erythematosus.[114] Recently, a large-scale cohort study of pSS patients from Spain focused on the adequacy of therapies for the level of systemic activity, measured by the ESSDAI score.[115]

Treatment of lymphoma in SS is the same as in the population generally. Most SS-associated lymphomas are low-grade B-cell lymphomas, localized to the exocrine glands. For these cases, watchful waiting may be the most appropriate approach. Higher-grade lymphomas require more aggressive treatment with a rituximab, cytotoxic regimen, and/or radiation therapy.

MOLECULAR TARGET THERAPY

Several randomized case–control studies have focused on therapy for SS using biologic agents, such as the TNF-blocking agents, infliximab[116] and etanercept,[117] but none of the studies showed clinical benefit. There is increasing interest in therapies targeting B cells, such as monoclonal antibodies against CD20 (rituximab) or CD22 (epratuzumab). A recent randomized placebo-controlled study demonstrated the efficacy of rituximab over placebo in patients with active pSS.[118] Rituximab improved stimulated salivary flows, laboratory parameters of inflammation, and subjective symptoms. This clinical efficacy was supported by reduced glandular infiltration and morphologic improvements in epithelial cells on salivary gland biopsies.[119,120] Other potential targets for biologic therapy include cytokines, such as IL-6 and BlyS (BAFF), interferons, adhesion molecules, and chemokines. However, even if effective, systemic immunomodulatory therapy may be associated with unwanted side effects and may not be justified in patients with pSS whose disease is limited to exocrine glands. An alternative approach is to develop a localized form of immunotherapy by using gene therapy restricted to the salivary and lachrymal glands. This approach would most likely alter the abnormal immune response locally, but possibly avoid the systemic side effects.[114,121,122]

REFERENCES

1. Patel R, Shahane A. The epidemiology of Sjögren's syndrome. *Clin Epidemiol.* 2014;6:247-255.
2. Qin B, Wang J, Yang Z, et al. Epidemiology of primary Sjögren's syndrome: a systematic review and meta-analysis. *Ann Rheum Dis.* 2015;74(11):1983-1989.
3. Miyasaka N. Epidemiology and pathogenesis of Sjögren's syndrome. *Nihon Rinsho.* 1995;53(10):2367-2370.
4. Nocturne G, Marette X. Advances in understanding the pathogenesis of primary Sjögren's syndrome. *Nat Rev Rheumatol.* 2013;9(9):544-556.
5. Foster H, Walker D, Charles P, et al. Association of DR3 with susceptibility to and severity of primary Sjögren's syndrome in a family study. *Br J Rheumatol.* 1992;31(5):309-314.
6. Kuo CF, Grainge MJ, Valdes AM, et al. Familial risk of Sjögren's syndrome and co-aggregation of autoimmune disease in affected families. A nation wide study. *Arthritis Rheum.* 2015;67(7):1904-1912.
7. Arnett FC, Hamilton RG, Reveille JD, et al. Genetic studies of Ro (SS-A) and La (SS-B) autoantibodies in families with systemic lupus erythematosus and primary Sjögren's syndrome. *Arthritis Rheum.* 1989;32(4):413-419.
8. Cobb BL, Lessard CJ, Harley JB, et al. Genes and Sjogren's syndrome. *Rheum Dis Clin North Am.* 2008;34(4):847-868.
9. Li YZ, Zhabg KL, Chen H, et al. A genome-wide association study in Han Chinese identifies a susceptibility locus for primary Sjögren's syndrome at 7q11.23. *Nat Genet.* 2013;45(11):1361-1365.
10. Hernandez-Molina G, Vargas-Alarcon G, Rodriguez-Perez JM, et al. High-resolution HLA analysis of primary and secondary Sjögren's syndrome: a common immunogenetic background in Mexican patients. *Rheumatol Int.* 2015;35(4):643-649.
11. Lessard CJ, Li H, Adrianto I, et al. Variants at multiple loci implicated in both innate and adaptive immune responses are associated with Sjögren's syndrome. *Nat Genet.* 2013;45(11):1284-1292.
12. Nordmark G, Kristjansdottir G, Theander E, et al. Additive effects of the major risk alleles of IRF5 and STAT4 in primary Sjögren's syndrome. *Genes Immun.* 2009;10(1):68-76.
13. Gestermann N, Mekinian A, Comets E, et al. STAT4 is a confirmed genetic risk factor for Sjögren's syndrome and could be involved in type 1 interferon pathway signaling. *Genes Immun.* 2010;11(5):432-438.
14. Noctume G, Tam J, boudaoud S, et al. Germline variation of INFAIP3 in primary Sjögren's syndrome-associated lymphoma. *Ann Rheum Dis.* 2016;75(4):780-783.
15. Alevizos I, Alexander S, Turner RJ, et al. MicroRNA expression profiles as biomarkers of minor salivary gland inflammation and dysfunction in Sjögren's syndrome. *Arthritis Rheum.* 2011;63(2):535-544.
16. Hung T, Pratt GA, Sundaraman B, et al. The Ro60 autoantigen binds endogenous retroelements and regulates inflammatory gene expression. *Science.* 2015;350(6259):455-459.

17. Brkic Z, Maria NI, van Helden-Meeuwsen CG. Prevalence of interferon type I signature in CD14 monocytes of patients with Sjögren's syndrome and association with disease activity and BAFF gene expression. *Ann Rheum Dis.* 2013;72(5):728-735.
18. Ambrus JL, Suresh L, Peck A. Multiple roles for B-lymphocytes in Sjogren's syndrome. *J Clin Med.* 2016;5(10):87.
19. Szczerba BM, Rybakowska PD, Dey P, et al. Type I interferon receptor deficiency prevents murine Sjögren's syndrome. *J Dent Res.* 2013;92(5):444-449.
20. Banchereau J, Pascual V. Type I interferon in systemic lupus erythematosus and other autoimmune diseases. *Immunity.* 2006;25(3):383-392.
21. Bave U, Nordmark G, Lovgren T, et al. Activation of the type I interferon system in primary Sjögren's syndrome—a possible etiopathogenic mechanism. *Arthritis Rheum.* 2005;52(4):1185-1195.
22. Brkic Z, Versnel MA. Type I IFN signature in primary Sjögren's syndrome patients. *Expert Rev Clin Immunol.* 2014;10(4):457-467.
23. Groom J, Kalled SL, Cutler AH, et al. Association of BAFF/BLyS overexpression and altered B cell differentiation with Sjögren's syndrome. *J Clin Invest.* 2002;109(1):59-68.
24. Mackay F, Woodcock SA, Lawton P, et al. Mice transgenic for Baff develop lymphocytic disorders along with autoimmune manifestations. *J Exp Med.* 1999;190(11):1697-1710.
25. Mariette X, Roux S, Zhang J, et al. The level of BLyS (BAFF) correlates with the titer of autoantibodies in human Sjögren's syndrome. *Ann Rheum Dis.* 2003;62(2):168-171.
26. Theander E, Vasaitis L, Baecklund E, et al. Lymphoid organization in labial salivary gland biopsies is a possible predictor for the development of malignant lymphoma in primary Sjögren's syndrome. *Ann Rheum Dis.* 2011;70(8):1363-1368.
27. Porola P, Virkki L, Przybyla BD, et al. Androgen deficiency and defective intracrine processing of dehydroepiandrosterone in salivary glands in Sjögren's syndrome. *J Rheumatol.* 2008;35(11):2229-2235.
28. Liu K, Kurien BT, Zimmerman SL, et al. X chromosome dose and sex bias in autoimmune diseases: increased 47,XXX in systemic lupus erythematosus and Sjögren's syndrome. *Arthritis Rheumatol.* 2016;68(5):1290-1300.
29. Xavier M, Joel G, Didier C, et al. Detection of Epstein-Barr virus DNA by in situ hybridization and polymerase chain reaction in salivary gland biopsy specimens from patients with Sjögren's syndrome. *Am J Med.* 1991;90(1):286-294.
30. Karameris A, Gorgoulis V, Lliopoulos A, et al. Detection of Epstein Barr viral genome by an in situ hybridization method in salivary gland biopsies from patients with secondary Sjögren's syndrome. *Clin Exp Rheumatol.* 1992;10(4):327-332.
31. Sumida T, Yonaha F, Maeda T, et al. Expression of sequences homologous to HTLV-I tax gene in the labial salivary glands of Japanese patients with Sjögren's syndrome. *Arthritis Rheum.* 1994;37(4):545-550.
32. Mariette X, Zerbib M, Jaccar A, et al. Hepatitis C virus and Sjögren's syndrome. *Arthritis Rheum.* 1993;36(2):280-281.
33. Manuel RC, Sandra M, Pilar BZ. Hepatitis C virus and Sjögren's syndrome: trigger or mimic? *Rheum Dis Clin North Am.* 2008;34(4):869-884.
34. Wang Y, Dou H, Liu G, et al. Hepatitis C virus infection and the risk of Sjögren's or sicca syndrome: a meta-analysis. *Microbiol Immunol.* 2014;58(12):675-687.
35. Kordossis T, Paikos S, Aroni K, et al. Prevalence of Sjögren's-like syndrome in a cohort of HIV-1-positive patients: descriptive pathology and immunopathology. *Br J Rheumatol.* 1998;37(6):691-695.
36. Fleck M, Kern ER, Zhou T, et al. Murine cytomegalovirus induces a Sjögren's syndrome-like disease in C57Bl/6-lpr/lpr mice. *Arthritis Rheum.* 1998;41(12):2175-2184.
37. Triantafyllopoulou A, Tapinos N, Moutsopoulos HM. Evidence for coxsackievirus infection in primary Sjögren's syndrome. *Arthritis Rheum.* 2004;50(9):2897-2902.
38. Moyes DL, Martin A, Sawcer S, et al. The distribution of the endogenous retroviruses HERV-K113 and HERV-K115 in health and disease. *Genomics.* 2005;86(3):337-341.
39. Nocturne G, Mriette X. Advances in understanding the pathogenesis of primary Sjögren's syndrome. *Nat Rev Rheumatol.* 2013;9(9):544-556.
40. Iwakiri D, Zhou L, Samanta M, et al. Epstein-Barr virus (EBV)-encoded small RNA is released from EBV-infected cells and activates signaling from Toll-like receptor 3. *J Exp Med.* 2009;206(10):2091-2099.
41. Karaiskos D, Mavragani CP, Makaroni S, et al. Stress, coping strategies and social support in patients with primary Sjögren's syndrome prior to disease onset: a retrospective case-control study. *Ann Rheum Dis.* 2009;68(1):40-46.
42. Chaigne B, Lasfargues G, Marie I, et al. Primary Sjögren's syndrome and occupational risk factors: a case-control study. *J Autoimmun.* 2015;60:80-85.
43. Karaiskos D, Mavragani CP, Sinno MF, et al. Psychopathological and personality features in primary Sjögren's syndrome—associations with autoantibodies to neuropeptides. *Rheumatology (Oxford).* 2010;49(9):1762-1769.
44. Nezos A, Mavragani CP. Contribution of genetic factors to Sjögren's syndrome and related lymphogenesis. *J Immunol Res.* 2015;2015:754825.
45. Mitsias DI, Kapsogeorgou EK, Moutsopoulos HM. The role of epithelial cells in the initiation and perpetuation of autoimmune lesions: lessons from Sjögren's syndrome (autoimmune epithelitis). *Lupus.* 2006;15(5):255-261.
46. Jonsson R, Klareskog L, Backman K, et al. Expression of HLA-D-locus (DP, DQ, DR)-coded antigens, beta 2-microglobulin, and the interleukin 2 receptor in Sjögren's syndrome. *Clin Immunol Immunopathol.* 1987;45(2):235-243.
47. Mavragani CP, Moutsopoulos HM. The geoepidemiology of Sjögren's syndrome. *Autoimmun Rev.* 2010;9(5):A305-A310.
48. Ohlsson M, Jonsson R, Brokstad KA. Subcellular redistribution and surface exposure of the Ro52, Ro60 and La48 autoantigens during apoptosis in human ductal epithelial cells: a possible mechanism in the pathogenesis of Sjögren's syndrome. *Scand J Immunol.* 2002;56(5):456-469.
49. Bolstad AI, Jonsson R. The role of apoptosis in Sjögren's syndrome. *Ann Med Onterne (Paris).* 1998;149(1):25-29.
50. Spachidou MP, Bourazopoulou E, Maratheftis CI, et al. Expression of functional Toll-like receptors by salivary gland epithelial cells: increased mRNA expression in cells derived from patients with primary Sjögren's syndrome. *Clin Exp Immunol.* 2007;147(3):497-503.
51. Bolstad AI, Eiken HG, Rosenlund B, et al. Increased salivary gland tissue expression of Fas, Fas ligand, cytotoxic T lymphocyte-associated antigen 4, and programmed cell death 1 in primary Sjögren's syndrome. *Arthritis Rheum.* 2003;48(1):174-185.

52. Alperr S, kang HI, Weissman I, et al. Expression of granzyme A in salivary gland biopsies from patients with primary Sjögren's syndrome. *Arthritis Rheum.* 1994;37(7):1046-1054.
53. Mavragani CP, Tzioufas AG, Moutsopoulos HM. Sjögren's syndrome: autoantibodies to cellular antigens. Clinical and molecular aspects. *Int Arch Allergy Immunol.* 2000;123(1): 46-57.
54. Tzioufas AG, Tatouli IP, Moutsopoulos HM. Autoantibodies in Sjögren's syndrome: clinical presentation and regulatory mechanisms. *Presse Med.* 2012; 41(9, pt 2):e451-e460.
55. Kyriakidis NC, Kapsogeorgou EK, Tzioufas AG. A comprehensive review of autoantibodies in primary Sjögren's syndrome: clinical phenotypes and regulatory mechanisms. *J Autoimmun.* 2014;51:67-74.
56. Manuel RC, Roser S, Jose R, et al. Primary Sjögren's syndrome in Spain: clinical and immunologic expression in 1010 patients. *Medicine (Baltimore).* 2008; 87(4):210-219.
57. Mario GC, Claudia MP, Cesar JH, et al. Serologic features of primary Sjögren's syndrome: clinical and prognostic correlation. *Int J Clin Rheumatol.* 2012;7(6):651-659.
58. Alexander EL, Arnett FC, Provost TT, et al. Sjögren's syndrome: association of anti-Ro (SS-A) antibodies with vasculitis, hematologic abnormalities, and serologic hyperreactivity. *Ann Intern Med.* 1983;98(2):155-159.
59. Zuo J, Willicams AEG, Park YJ, et al. Muscarinic type 3 receptor autoantibodies are associated with anti-SSA/Ro autoantibodies in Sjögren's syndrome. *J Immunol Methods.* 2016;437:28-36.
60. Robinson CP, Brayer J, Yamachika S, et al. Transfer of human serum IgG to non-obese diabetic Igmu null mice reveals a role for autoantibodies in the loss of secretory function of exocrine tissues in Sjögren's syndrome. *Proc Natl Acad Sci U S A.* 1998;95(13): 7538-7543.
61. Dawson L, Tobin A, Smith P, et al. Antimuscarinic antibodies in Sjögren's syndrome: where are we, and where are we going? *Arthritis Rheum.* 2005;52(10): 2984-2995.
62. Roescher N, Kingman A, Shirota Y, et al. Peptide-based ELISAs are not sensitive and specific enough to detect muscarinic receptor type 3 autoantibodies in serum from patients with Sjögren's syndrome. *Ann Rheum Dis.* 2011;70(1):235-236.
63. Baer AN, Medrano L, DeMacro MM, et al. Association of anticentromere antibodies with more severe exocrine glandular dysfunction in Sjögren's Syndrome: analysis of the Sjögren's international collaborative clinical alliance cohort. *Arthritis Care Res (Hoboken).* 2016;68(10): 1554-1559.
64. Lee KE, Kang JH, Lee JW, et al. Anti-centromere antibody-positive Sjögren's syndrome: a distinct clinical subgroup? *Int J Rheum Dis.* 2015;18(7):776-782.
65. Katano K, Kawano M, Koni I, et al. Clinical and laboratory features of anticentromere antibody positive primary Sjögren's syndrome. *J Rheumatol.* 2001;28(10): 2238-2244.
66. Kitagawa T, Shibasaki K, Toya S. Clinical significance and diagnostic usefulness of anti-centromere antibody in Sjögren's syndrome. *Clin Rheumatol.* 2012;31(1):105-112.
67. Nakamura H, Kawakami A, Hayashi T, et al. Anti-centromere antibody-seropositive Sjögren's syndrome differs from conventional subgroup in clinical and pathological study. *BMC Musculoskelet Disord.* 2010;11:140.
68. Bournia VK, Diamanti KD, Vlachoyiannopoulos PG, et al. Anticentromere antibody positive Sjögren's syndrome: a retrospective descriptive analysis. *Arthritis Res Ther.* 2010;12(2):R47.
69. Selmi C, Meroni PL, Gershwin ME. Primary biliary cirrhosis and Sjögren's syndrome: Autoimmune epithelitis. *J Autoimmun.* 2012;39(1-2):34-42.
70. Malladi AS, Sack KE, Shiboski SC, et al. Primary Sjögren's syndrome as a systemic disease: a study of participants enrolled in an international Sjögren's syndrome registry. *Arthritis Care Res (Hoboken).* 2012;64(6):911-918.
71. Bernacchi E, Bianchi B, Amato L, et al. Xerosis in primary Sjögren's syndrome: immunohistochemical and functional investigations. *J Dermatol Sci.* 2005;39(1):53-55.
72. Mitchell J, Greenspan J, Daniels T, et al. Anhidrosis (hypohidrosis) in Sjögren's syndrome. *J Am Acad Dermatol.* 1987;16(1, pt 2):233-235.
73. Katayama I, Yokozeki H, Nishioka K. Impaired sweating as an exocrine manifestation in Sjögren's syndrome. *Br J Dermatol.* 1995;133(5):716-720.
74. Roguedas AM, Misery L, Sassolas B, et al. Cutaneous manifestations of primary Sjögren's syndrome are underestimated. *Clin Exp Rheumatol.* 2004;22(5):632-636.
75. Fox RI, Liu AY. Sjögren's syndrome in dermatology. *Clin Dermatol.* 2006;24(5):393-413.
76. Ramos-Casals M, Anaya JM, García-Carrasco M, et al. Cutaneous vasculitis in primary Sjögren syndrome: classification and clinical significance of 52 patients. *Medicine (Baltimore).* 2004;83(2):96-106.
77. Scofield RH. Vasculitis in Sjögren's syndrome. *Curr Rheumatol Rep.* 2011;13(6):482-488.
78. Teramoto N, Katayama I, Arai H, et al. Annular erythema: a possible association with primary Sjögren's syndrome. *J Am Acad Dermatol.* 1989;20(4):596-601.
79. Katayama I, Teramoto N, Arai H, et al. Annular erythema. A comparative study of Sjögren syndrome with subacute cutaneous lupus erythematosus. *Int J Dermatol.* 1991;30(9):635-639.
80. Brito-Zerón P, Retamozo S, Akasbi M, et al. Annular erythema in primary Sjögren's syndrome: description of 43 non-Asian cases. *Lupus.* 2014;23(2):166-175.
81. Sontheimer RD, Thomas JR, Gilliam JN. Subacute cutaneous lupus erythematosus: a cutaneous marker for a distinct lupus erythematosus subset. *Arch Dermatol.* 1979;115(12):1409-1415.
82. Provost TT. Anti-Ro (SSA) and andi-La(SSB) antibodies in lupus erythematosus and Sjögren's syndrome. *Keio J Med.* 1991;40(2):72-77.
83. McCauliffe DP, Faircloth E, Wang L, et al. Similar Ro/SS-A autoantibody epitope and titer responses in annular erythema of Sjögren's syndrome and subacute cutaneous lupus erythematosus. *Arch Dermatol.* 1996;132(5):528-531.
84. Ramos-Casals M, Brito-Zeron P, Font J. The overlap of Sjögren's syndrome with other systemic autoimmune diseases. *Semin Arthritis Rheum.* 2007;36(4):246-255.
85. Tushiya N, Ito I, Kawasaki A. Association of IRF5, STAT4, and BLK with systemic erythematosus and other rheumatic disease. *Nihon Rinsho Meneki Gakkai Kaishi.* 2010;33(2):57-65.
86. Ramos-Casals M, Brito-Zeron P, Seror R, et al. Characterization of systemic disease in primary Sjögren's syndrome: EULAR-SS Task Force recommendations for articular, cutaneous, pulmonary and renal involvements. *Rheumatology (Oxford).* 2015;54(12):2230-2238.
87. Mario GC, Antoni S, Manuel RC, et al. Raynaud's phenomenon in primary Sjögren's syndrome. Prevalence and clinical characteristics in a series of 320 patients. *J Rheumatol.* 2002;29(4):726-730.

88. Mellgren SI, Goransson LG, Omdal R. Primary Sjögren's syndrome associated neuropathy. *Can J Neurol Sci.* 2007;34(3):280-287.
89. Mori K, Iijima M, Koike H, et al. The wide spectrum of clinical manifestations in Sjögren's syndrome-associated neuropathy. *Brain.* 2005;128(pt 11):2518-2534.
90. Kassan SS, Moutsopoulos HM. Clinical manifestations and early diagnosis of Sjögren's syndrome. *Arch Intern Med.* 2004;164(12):1275-1284.
91. Nishishinya MB, Pereda CA, Muñoz-Fernández S, et al. Identification of lymphoma predictors in patients with primary Sjögren's syndrome: a systematic literature review and meta-analysis. *Rheumatology (Oxford).* 2015;35(1):17-26.
92. Solans LR, Lopez HA, Bosch GJA, et al. Risk, predictors, and clinical characteristics of lymphoma development in primary Sjögren's syndrome. *Semin Arthritis Rheum.* 2011;41(3):415-423.
93. Song H, Tong D, Cha Z, et al. C-X-C chemokine receptor type 5 gene polymorphisms are associated with non-Hodgkin lymphoma. *Mol Biol.* 2012;39(9):8629-8635.
94. Urban N, Andrea R, Ivo K, et al. The NF-κB negative regulator TNFAIP3 (A20) is inactivated by somatic mutations and genomic deletions in marginal zone lymphomas. *Blood.* 2009;113(20):4918-4921.
95. Charbonneau B, Wang AH, Maurer MJ, et al. CXCR5 polymorphisms in non-Hodgkin lymphoma risk and prognosis. *Cancer Immunol Immunother.* 2013;62(9):1475-1484.
96. Baimpa E, Dahabreh IJ, Voulgarelis M, et al. Hematologic manifestations and predictors of lymphoma development in primary Sjögren's syndrome: clinical and pathophysiologic aspects. *Medicine (Baltimore).* 2009;88(5):284-293.
97. Ioannidis JP, Vassiliou VA, Moutsopoulos HM. Long-term risk of mortality and lymphoproliferative disease and predictive classification of primary Sjögren's syndrome. *Arthritis Rheum.* 2002;46(3):741-747.
98. Giannouli S, Voulgarelis M. Predicting progression to lymphoma in Sjögren's syndrome patients. *Expert Rev Clin Immunol.* 2014;10(4):501-512.
99. Carolis SD, Salvi S, Botta A, et al. The impact of primary Sjögren's syndrome on pregnancy outcome: our series and review of the literature. *Autoimmun Rev.* 2013;13(2):103-107.
100. Vitali C, Bombardieri S, Jonsson R. Classification criteria for Sjögren's syndrome: a revised version of the European criteria proposed by the American-European Consensus Group. *Ann Rheum Dis.* 2002;61(6):554-558.
101. Shiboski SC, Shibioski CH, Criswell LA, et al. American College of Rheumatology classification criteria for Sjogren syndrome: a data-driven, expert consensus approach in the Sjögren's international collaborative clinical alliance cohort. *Arthritis Care Res.* 2012;64(4):475-487.
102. Mario GC, Claidoa MP, Cesar JH, at al. Serologic features of primary Sjögren's syndrome: clinical and prognostic correlation. *Int J Clin Rheumatol.* 2012;7(6):651-659.
103. Roescher N, Illei GG. Can quantified salivary gland scintigraphy results aid diagnosis of patients with sicca symptoms? *Nat Clin Pract Rheumatol.* 2008;4(4):178-179.
104. Theander E, Vasaitis L, Baecklind E, et al. Lymphoid organization in labral salivary gland biopsies is a possible predictor for the development of malignant lymphoma in primary Sjögren's syndrome. *Ann Rheum Dis.* 2011;70(8):1363-1368.
105. Horvath IF, Szanto A, Papp G, et al. Clinical course, prognosis, and cause of death in primary Sjögren's syndrome. *J Immunol Res.* 2014;2014:647507.
106. Moutsopoulos HM. Sjögren's syndrome: a forty-year scientific journey. *J Autoimmun.* 2014;51:1-9.
107. Mavragani CP, Moutsopoulos NM, Moutsopoulos HM. The management of Sjögren's syndrome. *Nat Clin Pract Rheumatol.* 2006;2(5):252-261.
108. Vivino FB, Al-Hashimi I, Khan Z, et al. Pilocarpine tablets for the treatment of dry mouth and dry eye symptoms in patients with Sjögren Syndrome: a randomized, placebo-controlled, fixed-dose, multicenter trial. *Arch Intern Med.* 1999;159(2):174-181.
109. Petrone D, Condemi JJ, Fife R, et al. A double-blind, randomized, placebo-controlled study of cevimeline in Sjögren's syndrome patients with xerostomia and keratoconjunctivitis sicca. *Arthritis Rheum.* 2002;46(3):748-754.
110. Sall K, Stevenson OD, Mundorf TK, et al. Two multicenter, randomized studies of the efficacy and safety of cyclosporine ophthalmic emulsion in moderate to severe dry eye disease. CsA Phase 3 Study Group. *Ophthalmology.* 2000;107(4):631-639.
111. Mavragani CP, Moutsopoulos HM. Conventional therapy of Sjögren's syndrome. *Clin Rev Allergy Immunol.* 2007;32(3):284-291.
112. Fos RI, Chan E, Benton L, et al. Treatment of primary Sjögren's syndrome with hydroxychloroquine. *Am J Med.* 1988;85(4A):62-67.
113. Tishler M, Yaron I, Shirazi I, et al. Hydroxychloroquine treatment for primary Sjögren's syndrome: its effect on salivary and serum inflammatory markers. *Ann Rheum Dis.* 1999;58(4):253-256.
114. Saraux A, Pers JO, Devauchelle-Pensec V. Treatment of primary Sjögren syndrome. *Nat Rev Rheumatol.* 2016;12(8):456-471.
115. Gheitasi H, Kostov B, Solans R, et al. How are we treating our systemic patients with primary Sjögren syndrome? Analysis of 1120 patients. *Int Immunopharmacol.* 2015;27(2):194-199.
116. Mariette X, Ravaud P, Steinfeld S, et al. Inefficacy of infliximab in primary Sjögren's syndrome: Results of the randomized, controlled Trial of Remicade in Primary Sjogren's Syndrome (TRIPSS). *Arthritis Rheum.* 2004;50(4):1270-1276.
117. Sankar V, Brennan MT, Kok MR, et al. Etanercept in Sjögren's syndrome: a twelve-week randomized; double-blind, placebo-controlled pilot clinical trial. *Arthritis Rheum.* 2004;50(7):2240-2245.
118. Meijer JM, Meiners PM, Vissink A, et al. Effectiveness of rituximab treatment in primary Sjögren's syndrome: a randomized, double-blind, placebo-controlled trial. *Arthritis Rheum.* 2010;62(4):960-968.
119. Carubbi F, Alunno A, Cipriani P, et al. Rituximab in primary Sjögren's syndrome: a ten-year journey. *Lupus.* 2014;23(13):1337-1349.
120. Pijpe J, Meijer JM, Bootsma H, et al. Clinical and histologic evidence of salivary gland restoration supports the efficacy of rituximab treatment in Sjögren's syndrome. *Arthritis Rheum.* 2009;60(11):3251-3256.
121. Lodde BM, Baum BJ, Tak PP, et al. Experience with experimental biological treatment and local gene

therapy in Sjögren's syndrome: implications for exocrine pathogenesis and treatment. *Ann Rheum Dis.* 2006;65(11):1406-1413.

122. Ramos-Casals M, Tzioufas AG, Stone JH, et al. Treatment of primary Sjögren's syndrome: a systematic review. *JAMA.* 2010;304(4):452-460.

Chapter 69 :: Relapsing Polychondritis
:: Camille Francès

第六十九章

复发性多软骨炎

中文导读

复发性多软骨炎（RP）是一种罕见的多系统自身免疫性疾病，软骨炎的反复发作导致软骨结构的逐渐破坏，其他富含蛋白聚糖的结构，如眼睛、血管或内耳也受到影响。皮肤表现常见，尤其与骨髓增生异常有关。本章从流行病学、临床特征、病因及发病机制、诊断、临床进程及预后、管理等方面对本病进行了阐述。耳廓软骨炎最常见，引起耳廓软骨部分的疼痛、红肿和肿胀，最后软骨破坏，非软骨处不受累。鼻软骨受累可以出现鞍鼻。皮肤损害大多为非特异性的，如结节性红斑、固定环形荨麻疹丘疹、紫癜、口腔复杂性口疮、浅静脉炎、网状青斑、四肢溃疡、远端坏死，以及无菌性脓疱、Sweet综合征及其组织细胞样亚型、持久性隆起性红斑和坏疽性脓皮病等中性粒细胞皮病。非皮肤的临床表现描述了呼吸道软骨炎、关节症状、眼部炎症、听力障碍、心血管症状等。临床可以分为三个亚型：血液学受累为主、呼吸受累为主及轻度患者。个体化治疗是优化管理的关键。本章介绍了非甾体抗炎药、秋水仙碱、氨苯砜、糖皮质激素、免疫抑制药及生物制剂的应用。少数难治性重症RP患者可进行自体干细胞移植。

〔施　为〕

AT-A-GLANCE

- Relapsing polychondritis is a rare multisystem autoimmune disease.
- Different factors are implicated in the pathogenesis, including a genetic susceptibility, immunization against cartilaginous structures, and modification of cytokine and chemokine signatures.
- More than 30% of patients have an associated disease, mainly of autoimmune or hematologic origin.
- Recurrent episodes of chondritis lead to progressive destruction of cartilaginous structures.
- Other proteoglycan-rich structures, such as eyes, blood vessels, or inner ear, are also affected.
- Dermatologic manifestations occur frequently, especially in association with myelodysplasia. They are nonspecific and resemble those observed in Behçet disease and inflammatory bowel diseases.

EPIDEMIOLOGY

Relapsing polychondritis (RP) is a rare inflammatory disease with an estimated prevalence of 4.5 per million people.[1] The incidence of RP has been estimated to be 0.71/million/year in the United Kingdom, being slightly higher in women than men (0.76 vs 0.66). The mean age (range) at diagnosis in men was 55 years (range: 17-81 years) and in women 51 years (range: 11-79 years).[2] Development of the disease may occur in young children and in the elderly. Although most cases have been reported in whites, there is no evidence supporting the role of ethnic or geographical factors.

CLINICAL FEATURES

Disease onset is usually sudden with characteristic chondritis, and/or, less frequently, arthritis or ocular inflammation. Nonspecific initial symptoms, such as fever or weight loss, are rare.

CUTANEOUS FINDINGS

Attacks of chondritis usually occur in a relapsing–remitting pattern. Inflammatory episodes generally last a few days or weeks and may subside spontaneously or upon treatment; recurrences after weeks or months occur and subsequently result in cartilage destruction.[3] Auricular chondritis is the most frequent occurrence (85% of cases), causing pain, redness, and swelling of the cartilaginous portion of the pinna, sparing the noncartilaginous lobe (Fig. 69-1). Biopsy of the auricular cartilage is unnecessary for diagnosis. After several attacks, the pinna may become soft and sloppy with a cauliflower aspect (Fig. 69-2); sometimes it is stiff from calcifications. Nasal chondritis (65% of cases) is less inflammatory, presenting with nasal pain, stuffiness, rhinorrhea, and sometimes epistaxis. The characteristic saddle-nose deformity (Fig. 69-3) may appear secondly or without previous inflammatory episodes.

Other dermatologic manifestations are sometimes the presenting feature of RP (12% of cases), noticed subsequently in more than one-third of patients of a large series.[4] The other dermatologic manifestations are nonspecific and include nodules on the limbs (Fig. 69-4) with an aspect of erythema nodosum, fixed annular urticarial papules on the trunk,[5] purpura (Fig. 69-5), oral or complex aphthosis (Fig. 69-6), super-

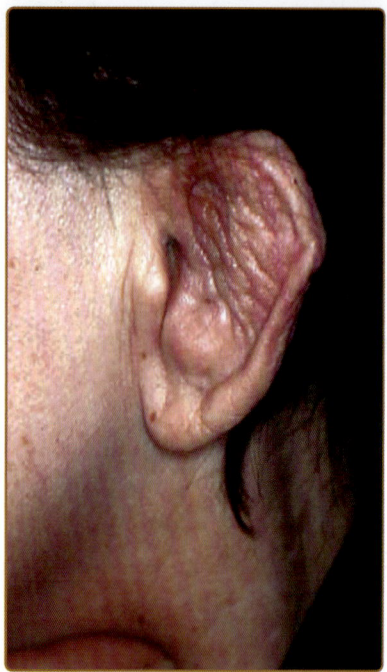

Figure 69-2 Relapsing polychondritis. Soft and sloppy ear with a "cauliflower" aspect.

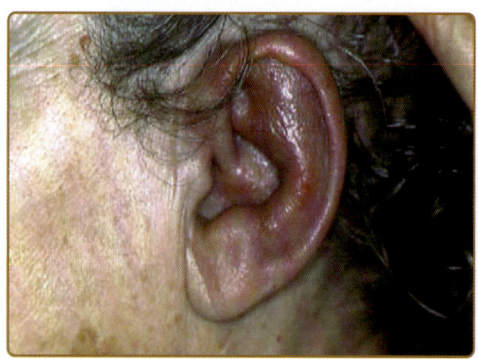

Figure 69-1 Relapsing polychondritis. Painful inflammation of the cartilaginous portion of ear.

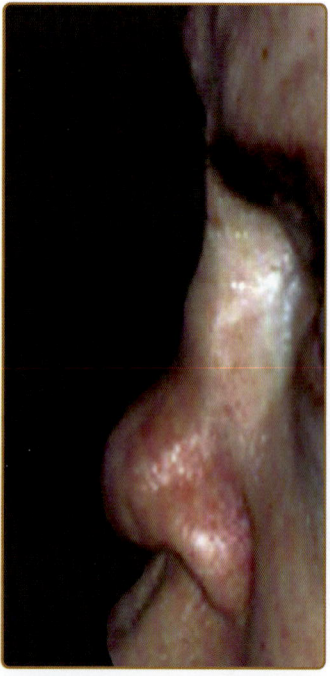

Figure 69-3 Relapsing polychondritis. Saddle-nose deformity.

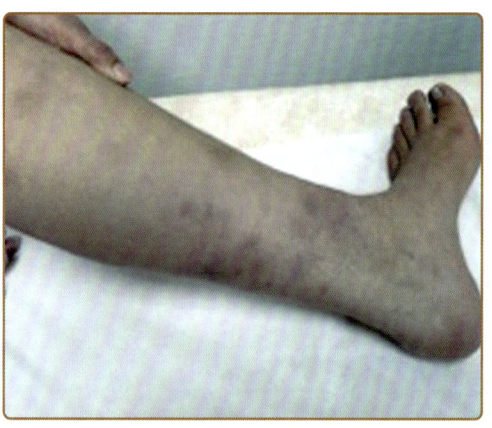

Figure 69-4 Relapsing polychondritis. Nodules of the limbs that may be secondary to septal panniculitis, vasculitis, thrombosis, or deep neutrophils infiltrate.

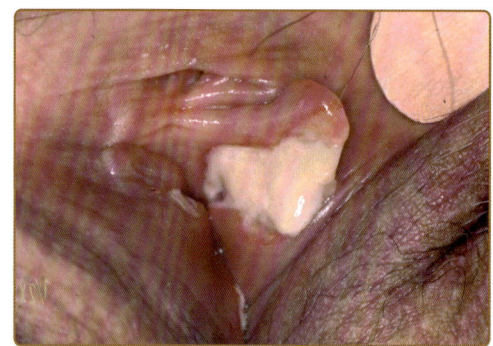

Figure 69-6 Relapsing polychondritis. Giant vulvar aphtha contemporary to acute auricular chondritis.

ficial phlebitis, livedo reticularis (Fig. 69-7), ulcerations on the limbs, distal necrosis. Neutrophilic dermatoses are mainly observed in association with hematologic abnormalities: sterile pustules (Fig. 69-8), Sweet syndrome and its histiocytoid subtype, erythema elevatum diutinum, and pyoderma gangrenosum. Skin lesions appear either concomitantly or not with attacks of chondritis. Pathologic features include neutrophilic or lymphocytic vasculitis, thrombotic vascular lesions, neutrophil infiltrates, and nonspecific inflammation of the dermis or subcutis. Patients with and without dermatologic manifestations have similar clinical manifestations of RP. However, the frequency of dermatologic manifestations (>90%), age at first chondritis, and male-to-female ratio seems higher when RP is associated with myelodysplasia[4]; so, their presence in an old person warrants repeated blood cell counts to detect a smouldering myelodysplasia.

NONCUTANEOUS FINDINGS

Respiratory tract chondritis, although uncommon at presentation, occurs in up to 50% of RP patients, and may be lethal. Respiratory involvement is manifested by hoarseness, nonproductive persistent cough, dyspnea, and/or wheezing. Complications of respiratory tract chondritis include upper airway collapse,

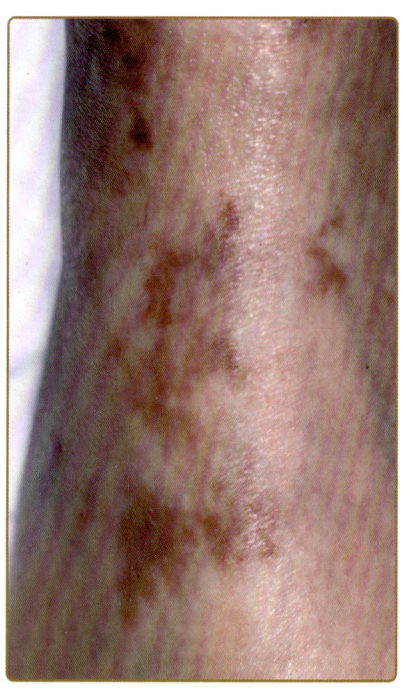

Figure 69-5 Relapsing polychondritis. Purpura secondary to leukocytoclastic vasculitis.

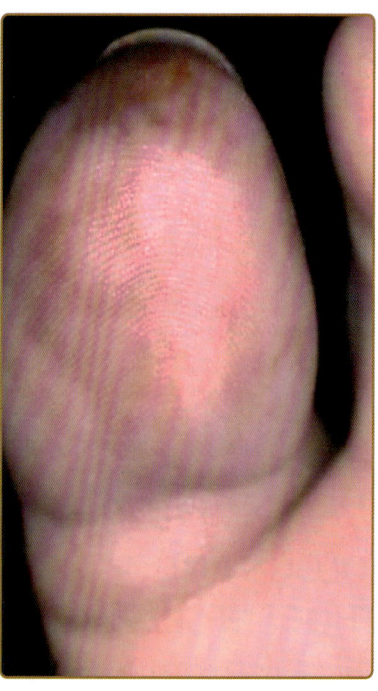

Figure 69-7 Relapsing polychondritis. Necrotic livedo secondary to leukocytoclastic vasculitis.

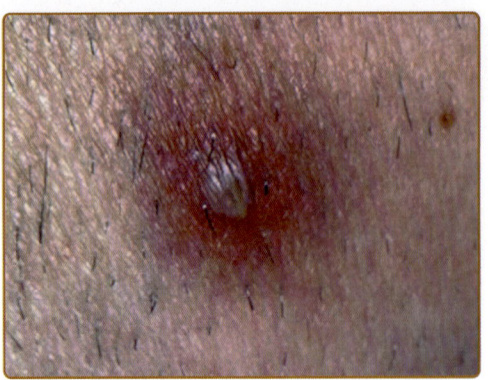

Figure 69-8 Relapsing polychondritis. Sterile pustule as observed in Behçet disease.

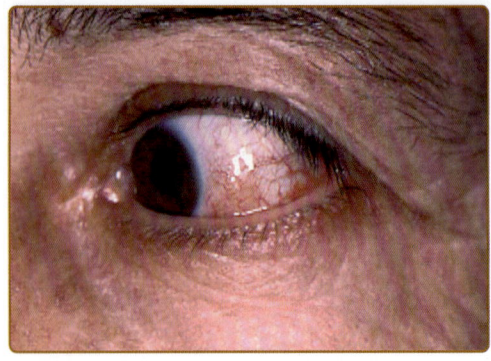

Figure 69-9 Relapsing polychondritis. Red eye suggestive of scleritis, which must be confirmed by an ophthalmologist.

obstructive respiratory insufficiency, and secondary infections. Costochondritis (35% of RP patients) induces parietal pains, which may also compromise respiration.

Joint pain is a common presenting feature (30% of RP patients). Large and small joints of the peripheral or axial skeleton may all be affected. Arthritis is intermittent, migratory, asymmetric, seronegative, and usually nonerosive.

Nearly 60% of RP patients developed ocular inflammation. Episcleritis and scleritis (Fig. 69-9) are the most common manifestations, followed by keratoconjunctivitis sicca, iritis, retinopathy, and keratitis. Rarely, corneal perforation, retinal vasculitis, and optic neuritis will lead to blindness.

Conductive hearing loss is secondary to stenosis of the external auditory canal, eustachian tube chondritis, or serous otitis media, whereas perception hearing loss may occur as a consequence of sensorineural involvement. Symptoms of vestibular dysfunction such as dizziness, ataxia, nausea, and vomiting are usually acute and improve with time.

The spectrum of cardiovascular manifestations is wide and includes different heart tissues (aortic and/or mitral regurgitation, impairment of the conduction system, pericarditis) and all types of vessels (thoracic and abdominal aortitis leading to aneurysms, Takayasu-like aortic arch syndrome, medium-vessel and large-vessel vasculitis, leukocytoclastic vasculitis, and thrombophlebitis). Lesions are inflammatory and/or thrombotic. Some, but not all, thrombotic manifestations have been linked to antiphospholipid syndrome. Large-vessel vasculitis tends to occur after several years of smoldering and, often, occult disease, despite immunosuppressive therapy.

ETIOLOGY AND PATHOGENESIS

To date, the etiology of RP is still poorly known.

The inflammation is initially perichondrial, characterized by an inflammatory polymorphic infiltrate with lymphocytes, neutrophils, macrophages, and plasma cells. The T cells are primarily CD4; the antigen-presenting cells are activated with expression of human leukocyte antigen-D related (HLA-DR). Direct immunofluorescence inconsistently shows immunoglobulins and C3 deposits at the junction perichondrium-cartilage. With the progression of the disease, the cartilage is invaded by inflammatory cells with release of proteolytic enzymes such as matrix proteinase (MMP)-3 and cathepsins K and L. MMP-8, MMP-9, and elastase are localized at the periphery of the cartilage that gradually deteriorated with loss of basophilia, release of glycosaminoglycans, fragmentation of collagen and elastic tissue. At a late stage, it is replaced by fibrous connective tissue that may contain gelatinous cysts and calcifications.

The role of the humoral immune response was based on the presence of antibodies to collagen type II in a third of patients with RP, especially in the acute phase of RP. Antibody titers seemed to correlate with the severity of symptoms. Other antibodies also detected in patients with RP include antibodies to collagen type IX and type XI; minor collagens that represent 5% to 10% of cartilage collagens; antibodies to matrilin-1, an extracellular matrix protein, predominantly expressed in upper respiratory tract cartilage; and antibodies to cartilage oligomeric matrix protein, additional cartilage protein, expressed in auricular, tracheal, and nasal cartilage. Several animal models have been published in which immunization with these various cartilage proteins induced a variety of chondritis manifestations that mimic those seen in patients.[6] Although human studies and murine models strongly support a prominent role for collagen type II, matrilin-1, and cartilage oligomeric matrix protein, as potential target antigens, the detection of antibodies toward these proteins has low sensitivity and specificity, and therefore not used in clinical practice. Triggering events of RP include mechanical stimuli such as traumas and piercing, which may expose cryptic antigens of the cartilaginous matrix and induce an autoimmune process.

Influence of T cells in RP pathogenesis, although less investigated, also has been demonstrated in patients and in animal models with specificity against the same cartilage proteins. T-cell clones isolated from an RP patient were found to be specific for a peptide corresponding to residues 261 to 273 of the type II collagen and were restricted to either the DRBI*0101 or the DRBI*0401 allele.[7] RP is likely a T-helper-1–mediated disease as serum levels of interferon-γ, interleukin (IL)-12, and IL-2 parallel changes in disease activity, while the levels of T-helper-2 cytokines do not. Other mediators are involved in the pathogenesis such as sTREM-1, MCP-1, MIP-1β, and IL-8. A complex cytokine network orchestrates the recruitment of infiltrating cells in RP lesions.

The genetic background of RP seems to be different according to the different populations. HLA-DR4 was found to be associated with RP in the German but not in the Japanese population. In the Japanese population RP was associated with HLA-DRB*16:02, HLA-DQB1*05:02, and HLA-B*67:01, and differs genetically from other rheumatic diseases.[8]

DIAGNOSIS

The different diagnostic criteria for RP are based on characteristic clinical manifestations.[9] A positive histologic confirmation is rarely required (Table 69-1). Table 69-2 shows the main differential diagnoses and diseases that may be associated with RP.

Laboratory findings in RP are nonspecific, but consistent with an acute or chronic inflammation. Urinalysis may be abnormal in case of renal involvement (mesangial expansion, immunoglobulin A nephropathy, tubulointerstitial nephritis, or necrotizing glomerulonephritis).

Pulmonary function tests, including inspiratory and expiratory flow volume curves, should be performed systematically to detect occult involvement. Imaging diagnosis delivers information about the degree of disease activity that correlates better with clinical features than unspecific inflammatory laboratory markers. Additionally, clinically unapparent cartilage involvement can be detected. Indeed, most disease manifestations can be objectified by means of cross-sectional imaging (computed tomography or MRI). The complementary use of functional data like those obtained with aid of diffusion-weighted imaging and glucose metabolism analysis (eg, fluorodeoxyglucose-positron emission tomography [FDG-PET]), allow a correct evaluation of the disease activity.[13]

TABLE 69-1
Different Diagnostic Criteria[9]

1. McAdam et al.[10]
   (1) Bilateral auricular chondritis
   (2) Nonerosive seronegative inflammatory polyarthritis
   (3) Nasal chondritis
   (4) Ocular inflammation
   (5) Respiratory chondritis
   (6) Cochlear and/or vestibular damage

   For the diagnosis of RP, patients must have 3 of 6 of the above criteria.

2. Damiani and Levine[11]
   For the diagnosis of RP, patients must have
   (1) At least 3 of the McAdam clinical criteria
   (2) One or more of the McAdam clinical criteria + biopsy confirmation of cartilage inflammation
   (3) Chondritis at 2 or more separate anatomic locations with response to steroids and/or dapsone

3. Michet et al.[12]
   (1) Major criteria
      – Auricular chondritis
      – Nasal chondritis
      – Laryngotracheal chondritis
   (2) Minor criteria
      – Conjunctivitis, episcleritis, scleritis, or uveitis
      – Hearing loss
      – Vestibular dysfunction
      – Seronegative polyarthritis

   For the diagnosis of RP, patients must have 2 major criteria or 1 major criteria + 2 minor criteria.

TABLE 69-2
Differential Diagnosis

AURICULAR CHONDRITIS	NASAL CHONDRITIS
Bacterial cellulitis	Sinusitis
Leishmaniasis	Infectious perichondritis
Leprosy	Granulomatosis with polyangiitis
Traumatisms (rugbyman, boxer)	Congenital syphilis

Main Diseases Associated with Relapsing Polychondritis and/or with Clinical Similar Manifestations

Autoimmune Diseases	Vascular Diseases
Rheumatoid arthritis	Leukocytoclastic vasculitis
Systemic lupus erythematosus	Granulomatosis with polyangiitis
Sjögren syndrome	Polyarteritis nodosa
Mixed connective tissue disease	Microscopic polyangiitis
Thyroid autoimmune disease	Eosinophilic granulomatosis with polyangiitis
Diabetes mellitus	Behçet disease
	MAGIC (mouth and genital ulcers with inflamed cartilage) syndrome
	Takayasu arteritis
	Antiphospholipid syndrome
Hematologic Disorders	
Myelodysplastic syndromes	
Immunoglobulin A myeloma	
Immunoglobulin A deficiency	
Others	
Skin Diseases	**Intestinal Diseases**
Vitiligo	Crohn disease
Psoriasis	Ulcerative colitis
Alopecia areata	**Others**
Lichen planus	Ankylosing spondylitis
	Reiter syndrome

CLINICAL COURSE AND PROGNOSIS

The clinical course of RP is progressive with intermittent flares. The number of different organ manifestations, their severity, and the response to treatment are unpredictable.[3] The Relapsing Polychondritis Disease Activity Index (RPDAI) was developed to assess disease activity thanks to an international cooperation.[14] Cluster analysis of a large series of patients permitted to separate patients into 3 clinical phenotypes: hematologic, respiratory, and mild. The first group of patients with myelodysplasia was associated with death; the second group of patients with tracheobronchial involvement was associated with infections. By contrast, patients included in the mild phenotype had no severe complication and the possible occurrence of clinical remission. Factors associated with death on multivariable analysis were male sex, cardiac abnormalities, and concomitant myelodysplasia.[15] The United Kingdom population-based cohort study suggested that the relative mortality in RP may be 2 to 3 times higher than in the general population.[2]

MANAGEMENT

Because of the highly variable course of RP, individualized therapy is the key to optimum management without standardized guidelines. An algorithm for treatment cannot be established. General therapeutic guidelines are based on retrospective analyses of series of patients or isolated case reports. Nonsteroidal antiinflammatory drugs, colchicine, or dapsone may be useful for patients with mild auricular or nasal chondritis, arthralgia, or mild arthritis. More serious manifestations required oral corticosteroids in dose of 0.3 to 1 mg/kg of body weight according to their severity. Pulse intravenous steroids are prescribed for acute airway obstruction, sudden hearing loss, and/or before surgical intervention (tracheostomy, aortic aneurysm repair, cardiac valve replacement). Long-term corticosteroids decrease the frequency and severity of recurrences, although they do not prevent vital organ involvement. Whether steroid therapy should be continued during clinical remission periods remains unclear. Many kinds of immunosuppressants have been used with some success as disease-modifying and steroid-sparing agents. Methotrexate (0.3 mg/kg/week) is often effective. Cyclophosphamide is used in severe forms of RP. Azathioprine, mycophenolate mofetil, cyclosporine, leflunomide, and chlorambucil have produced inconsistent effects.

Although serum levels of IL-6 and tumor necrosis factor-α are usually not elevated in patients with active RP, infliximab has been the most frequently used biologic agent with variable results—frequently partial or complete efficacy, sometimes secondary to loss of efficacy or severe infection. Rituximab usually has no treatment effect. Other biologic agents tried in RP include tocilizumab, anakinra, etanercept, adalimumab, and certolizumab. The number of treated patients is too low to allow definitive conclusions.[3] In a few patients with refractory severe RP, treatment intensification followed by autologous stem cell transplantation has been performed.

REFERENCES

1. Mathew SD, Battafarano DF, Morris MJ. Relapsing polychondritis in the Department of Defense population and review of the literature. *Semin Arthritis Rheum*. 2012;42(1):70.
2. Hazra N, Dregan A, Charlton J, et al. Incidence and mortality of relapsing polychondritis in the UK: a population-based cohort study. *Rheumatology (Oxford)*. 2015;54(12):2181.
3. Vitale A, Sota J, Rigante D, et al. Relapsing polychondritis: an update on pathogenesis, clinical features, diagnostic tools and therapeutic perspectives. *Curr Rheumatol Rep*. 2016;18(1):3.
4. Frances C, El Rassi R, Laporte JL, et al. Dermatologic manifestations of relapsing polychondritis. *Medicine (Baltimore)*. 2001;80(3):173.
5. Tronquoy AF, de Quatrebarbes J, Picard D, et al. Papular and annular fixed urticarial eruption: a characteristic skin manifestation in patients with relapsing polychondritis. *J Am Acad Dermatol*. 2011;65(6):1161.
6. Arnaud L, Mathian A, Haroche J, et al. Pathogenesis of relapsing polychondritis: a 2013 update. *Autoimmun Rev*. 2014;13(2):90.
7. Buckner JH, Van Landeghen M, Kwok WW, et al. Identification of type II collagen peptide 261-273-specific T-cell clones in a patient with relapsing polychondritis. *Arthritis Rheum*. 2002;46(1):238.
8. Terao C, Yoshifuji H, Yamano Y, et al. Genotyping of relapsing polychondritis identified novel susceptibility HLA alleles and distinct genetic characteristics from other rheumatic diseases. *Rheumatology (Oxford)*. 2016;55(9):1686-1692.
9. Longo L, Greco A, Rea A, et al. Relapsing polychondritis: a clinical update. *Autoimmun Rev*. 2016;15(6):539.
10. McAdam LP, O'Hanlan MA, Bluestone R, Pearson CM. Relapsing polychondritis: prospective study of 23 patients and a review of the literature. *Medicine (Baltimore)*. 1976;55(3):193-215.
11. Damiani JM, Levine HL. Relapsing polychondritis–report of ten cases. *Laryngoscope*. 1979;89(6 Pt 1):929-946.
12. Michet CJ Jr, McKenna CH, Luthra HS, O'Fallon WM. Relapsing polychondritis. Survival and predictive role of early disease manifestations. *Ann Intern Med*. 1986;104(1):74-78.
13. Thaiss WM, Nikolaou K, Spengler W, et al. Imaging diagnosis in relapsing polychondritis and correlation with clinical and serological data. *Skeletal Radiol*. 2016;45(3):339.
14. Arnaud L, Devilliers H, Peng SL, et al. The relapsing polychondritis activity index: development of a disease activity score for relapsing polychondritis. *Autoimmun Rev*. 2012;12(2):204.
15. Dion J, Costedoat-Chalumeau N, Sène D, et al. Relapsing polychondritis can be characterized by 3 different clinical phenotypes: analysis of a recent series of 142 patients. *Arthritis Rheumatol*. 2016;68(12):2992-3001.

Dermal Connective Tissue Disorders PART 11

第十一篇　真皮结缔组织异常

Chapter 70 :: Anetoderma and Other Atrophic Disorders of the Skin
:: Catherine Maari & Julie Powell

第七十章　斑状萎缩和其他萎缩性皮病

中文导读

　　斑状萎缩表现为局限性 1～2 厘米左右隆起或者凹陷的斑片，局部常有囊样凸起，可以是原发性疾病，也可以继发。与抗磷脂综合征相关。病理学表现为真皮弹性组织的丢失。本节从流行病学、发病机制、临床特征、病理表现、鉴别诊断、治疗等方面对于该病进行了阐述。所有类型的斑状萎缩的特征都是正常皮肤弹性的局限性丧失。特征性病变是松弛区域真皮物质消失，形成凹陷、皱纹或囊样突起。文章提到了可以产生继发斑状萎缩的相关皮肤疾病。不论是原发还是继发都需要关注潜在的疾病，主要是抗凝脂抗体综合征、自身免疫性甲状腺炎和HIV。斑状萎缩必须区别于其他弹性组织疾病和结缔组织萎缩，文中进行了较为详细的描述。并对于该病目前的治疗药物及治疗方法进行了介绍。其他萎缩性皮肤病包括从发病机制、临床特征、组织病理、鉴别诊断、治疗等方面阐述了真皮中层弹性组织溶解，从发病机制、临床特征、组织病理、鉴别诊断、治疗等方面探讨了膨胀纹的特征，从病因学及发病机制、临床特征、组织病理、鉴别诊断、治疗等方面阐述了特发性Pasini 和 Pierini皮肤萎缩症。简单介绍了网状红斑萎缩性毛囊炎和萎缩性毛周角化病。包括一组密切相关的疾病，如小棘状毛囊角化症和眉部瘢痕性红斑。这些疾病的特征是毛周角化性丘疹、不同程度的炎症和继发性萎缩性瘢痕。该节还简要介绍了Bazex-Dupré-Christol综合征和Conradi-Hünermann-Happle 综合征。

〔施　为〕

ANETODERMA

> **AT-A-GLANCE**
> - Circumscribed 1- to 2-cm areas of flaccid skin that may be elevated, macular, or depressed.
> - Often circumscribed sac-like protrusions.
> - Primary or secondary to a preceding dermatosis in the same location.
> - Association with antiphospholipid syndrome.
> - Pathology consists of loss of elastic tissue in the dermis.

EPIDEMIOLOGY

The lesions in anetoderma usually occur in young adults between the ages of 15 and 30 years and more often in women than men. Anetoderma is rare, and the incidence is unknown. Several hundred cases have been reported.[1-4]

PATHOGENESIS

The pathogenesis of anetoderma is unknown. The key defect is damage to the dermal elastic fibers. Anetoderma may be considered to be unusual scars, because scars also have decreased elastic tissue. The loss of dermal elastin could be the result of an impaired turnover of elastin caused by either increased destruction or decreased synthesis of elastic fibers.[4,5] Recently, a decrease in fibulin protein expression was described, suggesting that not only elastolytic overactivity, but also defective elastic fiber reassembly, may be involved.[6] Immunologic mechanisms may also play a role, as it can be associated with various systemic conditions, primarily antiphospholipid antibodies.

CLINICAL FEATURES

All types of anetoderma are characterized by a circumscribed loss of normal skin elasticity. The characteristic lesions are flaccid circumscribed areas of slack skin with the impression of loss of dermal substance forming depressions, wrinkling, or sac-like protrusions (Fig. 70-1). These atrophic, skin-colored, or blue-white lesions are 5 to 30 mm in diameter. The number varies from a few to hundreds. The skin surface can be wrinkled, thinned, and often depigmented, and a central depression may be seen. Coalescence of smaller lesions can give rise to larger herniations. The examining finger sinks without resistance into a distinct pit with sharp borders as if into a hernia ring (buttonhole

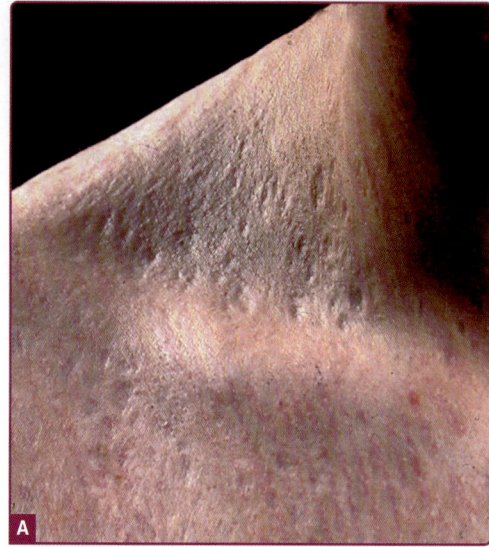

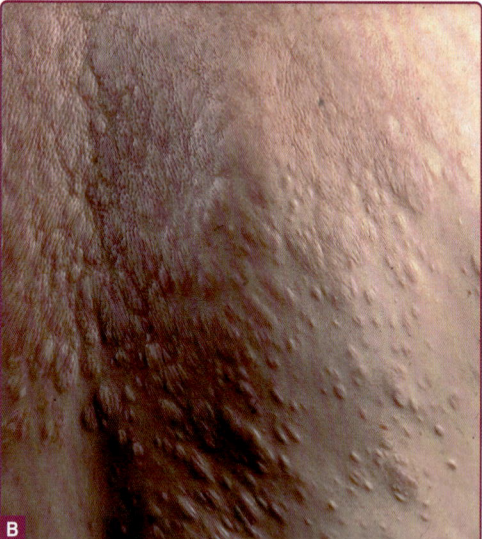

Figure 70-1 Anetoderma. Primary anetoderma. **A,** Multiple, sharply defined, depressed lesions that look punched out in the supraclavicular region. **B,** Soft, sac-like protrusions on the back. When depressed, there is the buttonhole phenomenon. This is the same patient as in **A**.

sign). The protrusion reappears as soon as the pressure from the finger is removed.[4]

The most common sites for these asymptomatic lesions are the chest, back, neck, and upper extremities. They usually develop in young adults, and new lesions often continue to form for many years as the older lesions fail to resolve.

Primary anetoderma occurs when there is no underlying associated skin disease (ie, it arises on clinically normal skin). It is historically subdivided into 2 types: (a) those with preceding inflammatory lesions, mainly erythema (the Jadassohn-Pellizzari type), and (b) those without preceding inflammatory lesions (the Schweninger-Buzzi type). This classification is only of historical interest, because the 2 types of lesions can coexist in the same patient; the prognosis and the histopathology are also the same.[4]

True secondary anetoderma implies that the characteristic atrophic lesion has appeared in the exact same site as a previous specific pathology; the most common causes are probably acne and varicella. Numerous and heterogeneous dermatoses have been associated with secondary anetoderma (Table 70-1), namely infectious (syphilis, Lyme disease, leprosy, molluscum contagiosum), inflammatory (granuloma annulare, discoid lupus, sarcoidosis, lichen planus) and tumoral (pilomatricomas, juvenile xanthogranuloma, xanthomas, involuted infantile hemangiomas, cutaneous B-cell lymphoma) to mention only a few. Anetoderma also has been described in premature infants, possibly related to the use of cutaneous monitoring leads or adhesives as well as extreme prematurity.[7] Both primary and secondary types of anetoderma may be associated with an underlying disease, mainly antiphospholipid syndrome[8] autoimmune thyroiditis and HIV, in which cases the atrophic lesions do not necessarily develop in areas of skin inflammation. Although most cases are sporadic, rare cases of familial anetoderma have been recently described and are usually not associated with preexisting lesions.[9]

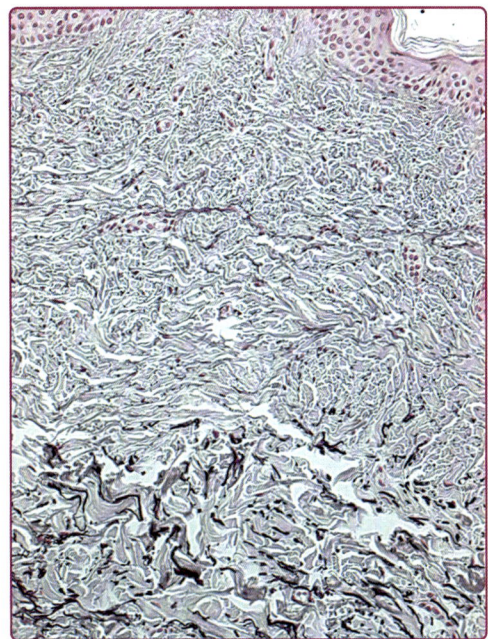

Figure 70-2 Anetoderma. Pathology shows decrease of elastic fibers in the papillary and reticular dermis (Weigert stain). (Used with permission from Victor Kokta, MD.)

PATHOLOGY

In routinely stained sections, the collagen fibers within the dermis of affected skin appear normal. Perivascular lymphocytes, in majority T-helper cells, are often present in all types of anetoderma and do not correlate with clinical inflammatory findings.[10]

The predominant defect as revealed by elastic tissue stains is a focal partial or complete loss of elastic tissue in the papillary and/or midreticular dermis. There are usually some residual abnormal, irregular, and fragmented elastic fibers (Fig. 70-2). Presumably, the weakening of the elastic network leads to flaccidity and herniation. Direct immunofluorescence sometimes shows linear or granular deposits of immunoglobulins and complement along the dermal–epidermal junction or around the dermal blood vessels in affected skin.[11] Electron microscopy demonstrates that the elastic fibers are fragmented and irregular in shape, occasionally engulfed within macrophages.

DIFFERENTIAL DIAGNOSIS

Anetoderma must be differentiated from other disorders of elastic tissue as well as atrophies of the connective tissue (Table 70-2).

Keloids form nodules that are much firmer on palpation. A history of trauma is often elicited, and the pathology is very distinct.

Glucocorticoid-induced atrophy occurs most commonly over the triceps or buttocks at sites where injections are usually given. Clinically, the lesions resemble atrophoderma. History is obviously most helpful in making the diagnosis. On histopathology, polarization may show the steroid crystals in the dermis.

Nevus lipomatosus superficialis of Hoffman and Zurhelle presents as a clustered group of soft, skin-

TABLE 70-1
Conditions Associated with Secondary Anetoderma

Infectious
- Syphilis
- Lyme disease
- Leprosy
- Molluscum contagiosum

Inflammatory
- Granuloma annulare
- Discoid lupus erythematosus
- Sarcoidosis
- Lichen planus

Tumoral
- Pilomatricomas
- Juvenile xanthogranuloma
- Xanthomas
- Involuted infantile hemangiomas
- Cutaneous B-cell lymphoma

Other Conditions[a]
- Antiphospholipid syndrome
- Autoimmune thyroiditis
- HIV

[a]Also associated with primary anetoderma.

TABLE 70-2
Differential Diagnosis of Primary Anetoderma

ELEVATED	DEPRESSED
Secondary anetoderma	Secondary anetoderma
Acne scars	Glucocorticoid-induced atrophy
Keloids	Acne scars
Nevus lipomatosus superficialis	
Papular elastorrhexis	
Connective tissue nevi	

colored to yellow nodules usually on the lower trunk and buttocks and present since birth. Histology shows ectopic mature lipocytes located in the dermis.

Papular elastorrhexis is an acquired disorder characterized by white, firm nonfollicular papules measuring 1 to 3 mm, evenly scattered on the chest, abdomen, and back. It usually appears in adolescence or early adulthood. The pathology demonstrates focal degeneration of elastic fibers and normal collagen. There are no associated extracutaneous abnormalities. This is believed by some authors to be a variant of connective tissue nevi[12] or an abortive form of the Buschke-Ollendorff syndrome,[13] whereas others think that these represent papular acne scars.[14] They are differentiated from anetoderma by being firm noncompressible lesions.

Middermal elastolysis (MDE) usually consists of larger areas with diffuse wrinkling without herniation and with elastolysis limited to the middermis (see "Middermal Elastolysis" section).

TREATMENT

There is no regularly effective treatment. In secondary anetoderma, appropriate treatment of the inflammatory underlying condition might prevent new lesions. Various therapeutic modalities have been tried but with no improvement of existing atrophic lesions, including intralesional injections of triamcinolone, and systemic administration of aspirin, dapsone, phenytoin, penicillin G (benzylpenicillin), and vitamin E. Some authors have reported improvement with hydroxychloroquine. In patients with limited lesions that are cosmetically objectionable, surgical excision may be useful. Ablative and nonablative fractionated lasers have shown some improvement in limited cases.[15,16] The use of soft-tissue fillers is inconclusive.

OTHER ATROPHIC DISORDERS OF THE SKIN

MIDDERMAL ELASTOLYSIS

MDE is a rare acquired disorder of elastic tissue. It is characterized by patches and plaques of diffuse, fine, wrinkled skin, most often located on the trunk, neck, and arms. In 1977, Shelley and Wood reported the first case of "wrinkles due to idiopathic loss of middermal elastic tissue."[17] Since then, approximately 100 cases have been reported. The vast majority of patients are white women between the ages of 30 and 50 years.[17-19]

PATHOGENESIS

The pathogenesis of this acquired elastic tissue degeneration is still unknown. Ultraviolet exposure has been postulated to be a major contributing factor in the degeneration of elastic fibers,[20] including natural sunlight and narrowband ultraviolet B phototherapy.[21] Other possible mechanisms include defects in the synthesis of elastic fibers, autoimmunity against elastic fibers, and damage to elastic fibers through the release of elastase by inflammatory cells or fibroblasts. Of interest, MDE has been reported in a case of immune reconstitution inflammatory syndrome.[22] Some data suggest that inflammatory processes and an imbalance between matrix metalloproteinases and tissue inhibitor of metalloproteinases are probably involved in the pathogenesis of MDE, in addition to CD34+ dendritic fibroblasts.[23] A decrease of lysyl oxidase-like 2 expression potentially has an effect on elastin renewal.[24] A recent study has shown that dermal fibulin-4 and fibulin-5 are significantly diminished in MDE compared with controls. This data indicates that the pathogenesis is not only secondary to an elastolytic overactivity, but also altered reassembly of elastic fibers.[6]

CLINICAL FEATURES

MDE is characterized by asymptomatic, well-demarcated, or diffuse areas of fine wrinkling (type I), usually in a symmetric distribution (Fig. 70-3A). Discrete perifollicular papules can be seen in some cases (type II), leaving the hair follicle itself as an indented center. More rarely, a reticular pattern (type III) with erythematous patches and telangiectasia can be seen. Lesions are typically found on the trunk, neck, and upper extremities. They are chronic and give the skin a prematurely aged appearance. There is usually no history of a preceding inflammatory dermatosis, but some patients report mild-to-moderate erythema and more rarely urticarial lesions or granuloma annulare. There is usually no associated systemic involvement.

Although the diagnosis of MDE is mainly based on clinical and histopathologic features, noninvasive diagnostic techniques (optical coherence microscopy or high-frequency ultrasound) may be helpful.[25]

PATHOLOGY

Histopathology shows a normal epidermis and, occasionally, a mild perivascular infiltrate in the dermis. The characteristic features are seen on elastic tissue stains (such as Verhoeff-van Gieson or Weigert) and reveal a selective band-like loss of elastic fibers in the

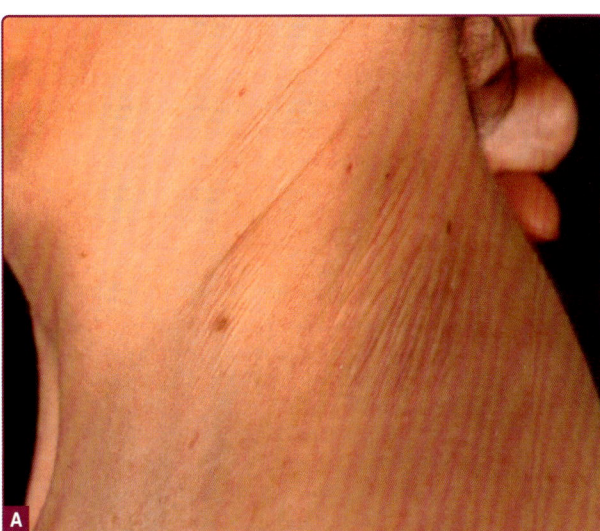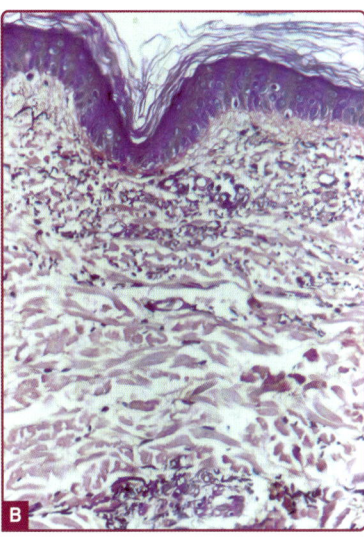

Figure 70-3 Middermal elastolysis. **A,** Well-circumscribed area of fine wrinkling on the neck of a middle-aged woman. (Used with permission from Richard Dubuc, MD.) **B,** Histology of middermal elastolysis. Note selective loss of elastic fibers in the middermis. Normal elastic tissue is preserved in the superficial papillary dermis and in the reticular dermis (Weigert stain). (Used with permission from Danielle Bouffard, MD.)

middermis (see Fig. 70-3B). Macrophagic elastophagocytosis can occasionally be seen. There is preservation of normal elastic tissue in the superficial papillary dermis above, in the reticular dermis below, and along adjacent hair follicles. Electron microscopy studies have shown phagocytosis by macrophages of both normal and degenerated elastic fiber tissue.[26]

DIFFERENTIAL DIAGNOSIS

MDE must be differentiated from the other common disorders of elastic tissue.

Solar elastosis differs by its onset in an older age group, location in only sun-exposed areas, yellowish color, and coarser wrinkling, as well as by hyperplasia and abnormalities of elastic fibers and basophilic degeneration of the collagen in the papillary dermis.

Anetoderma is characterized clinically by smaller soft macules and papules instead of diffuse wrinkling, and histologically by elastolysis that can occur in any layer of the dermis.

Perifollicular elastolysis[27] differs by a selective and almost complete loss of elastic fibers surrounding hair follicles compared with preservation of elastic fibers around follicles in MDE. Elastase-producing *Staphylococcus epidermidis* was found in the hair follicles and is the presumed etiology of this condition.

Postinflammatory elastolysis and cutis laxa were originally described in young girls of African descent. An inflammatory phase, consisting of indurated plaques or urticaria, malaise, and fever, preceded the diffuse wrinkling, atrophy, and severe disfigurement. Insect bites may be the trigger for the initial inflammatory lesions.[28]

TREATMENT

There is no known effective treatment for MDE. Sunscreens, colchicine, chloroquine, vitamin E, and topical retinoic acid have been tried without good success.[17-19] Topical soybean extract and eicosapentaenoic acid may prove to be interesting options.[18]

STRIAE

Chapters 105 and 137 provide additional discussion of striae.

Striae are very common and usually develop between the ages of 5 and 50 years.[29] They occur about twice as frequently in women as in men. They commonly develop during puberty, with an overall incidence of 25% to 35%,[30] or during pregnancy, with an incidence of up to 90%.[31]

PATHOGENESIS

The factors leading to the development of striae have not been fully elucidated. Striae distensae are the results of breaks in the connective tissue, resulting in dermal atrophy. Many factors, including hormones (particularly corticosteroids), mechanical stress, and genetic predisposition, appear to play a role.

CLINICAL FEATURES

Striae are usually multiple, symmetric, well-defined linear atrophic lesions that follow the lines of cleavage.

Initially, striae appear as red-to-violaceous elevated lines (striae rubra). Over time, the color gradually fades, and the lesions become atrophic, with the skin surface exhibiting a fine, white, wrinkled appearance (striae alba). The striae can measure several centimeters in length and a few millimeters to a few centimeters in width.

During puberty, striae appear in areas where there is a rapid increase in size. In girls, the most common sites are the breasts, thighs, hips, and buttocks, whereas in boys, they are seen on the shoulders, lumbosacral region, and thighs. Other less-common sites include the abdomen, upper arms, neck, and axillae.

Striae distensae are a common finding on the abdomen, and less so on the breasts and thighs, of pregnant women, especially during the last trimester. They are more common in younger primigravidas than in older pregnant women, and are associated with larger weight gain and/or with babies of higher birth weight. Striae gravidarum can be associated with a higher risk of lacerations during vaginal delivery,[32] as well as the development of pelvic relaxation and clinical prolapse.[33]

The striae associated with systemic corticosteroid therapy and Cushing syndrome can be larger and more widely distributed.

PATHOLOGY

Histologic findings show a decrease in dermal thickness and in collagen in the upper dermis. The collagen bundles are thinned and lie parallel to the epidermis, but they are also arranged transversely to the direction of the striae. Alterations in elastic fibers are variable, but dermal elastin can be fragmented, and specific elastin staining can demonstrate a marked reduction in visible elastin content compared with adjacent normal dermis.[34] There is absence of both hair follicles and other appendages.

DIFFERENTIAL DIAGNOSIS

The diagnosis of striae distensae is usually straightforward, but the differential diagnosis does include linear focal elastosis (elastotic striae) that was first described by Burket and colleagues in 1989.[35] Linear focal elastosis is characterized by rows of yellow palpable striae-like bands on the lower back. Unlike striae, the lesions are raised and yellow rather than depressed and white. Elderly men are most commonly affected, although cases in teenagers have been described. Linear focal elastosis is probably not an uncommon condition. Histologically, there is a focal increase in the number of elongated or fragmented elastic fibers and a thickened dermis. It is postulated that linear focal elastosis may represent an excessive regenerative process of elastic fibers and could be thought of as a keloidal repair of striae distensae.[36]

TREATMENT[37]

Striae distensae have no medical consequences, but they are frequently distressing to those affected. As stretch marks tend to regress spontaneously to some degree over time, the usefulness of treatments that have been tried without case controls is difficult to assess. Topical treatments that have shown some improvement of early stage striae are tretinoin 0.1% cream,[38] a combination of 0.05% tretinoin/20% glycolic acid, or 10% L-ascorbic acid/20% glycolic acid.[39] Several lasers[40] have been used in treating striae: the 585-nm pulsed-dye laser has been demonstrated to be of some efficacy in improving the appearance of striae rubra but has no effect on striae alba. Preliminary data have shown improvement of striae alba with fractionated microneedle radiofrequency in combination with fractional carbon dioxide laser.[41] Microneedling and combination treatment with radiofrequency and pulsed magnetic fields also appear promising.[42,43] The long-term future of treatment strategies is encouraging with the advance in laser technologies.

IDIOPATHIC ATROPHODERMA OF PASINI AND PIERINI

Idiopathic atrophoderma of Pasini and Pierini is a form of dermal atrophy that presents as 1 or several sharply demarcated depressed patches with no outpouching, usually on the back of adolescents or young adults.[44] Whether atrophoderma is a nonsclerotic, primarily atrophic variant of morphea or a separate distinct entity is still debated.[45]

EPIDEMIOLOGY AND PATHOGENESIS

This disorder is more frequently encountered in women than in men, with a ratio of 6:1. It usually starts insidiously in young individuals in the second or third decades of life. Congenital cases have been reported.[46]

Its relationship to morphea is favored by its striking clinical and histologic similarities to the atrophy seen at sites of regressing plaques of morphea. Antibodies to *Borrelia burgdorferi* have been reported.[47] Typical lesions of morphea, lichen sclerosus, and atrophoderma have been observed to occur simultaneously in the same patient, but in different areas, supporting the view that these conditions are related.[48] In a series of 139 patients, 24 (17%) had white induration in the central portions of their atrophic lesions, and 30 (22%) had superficial plaques of morphea coexisting in areas outside of their atrophic foci.[49] However, to some, the different course and outcome of atrophoderma of Pierini and Pasini as compared with morphea justifies preservation of a distinct name.

CLINICAL FEATURES

The lesions are well-demarcated depressed patches, usually occurring on the trunk, especially on the back and lumbosacral region, followed in frequency by the chest, arms, and abdomen.[47,49] The distribution is often symmetric and bilateral.

The lesions are single or multiple and usually round or ovoid, ranging in size from a few centimeters to patches covering large areas of the trunk (Fig. 70-4). They are usually asymptomatic and lack inflammation. When lesions coalesce, they can form large, irregular, brown patches but can be hypopigmented.[49] The surface of the skin is normal in appearance, and there is no skin induration or sclerosis.

The borders or edges of these lesions are sharply defined, and they are usually described as abrupt, "cliff-drop" borders ranging from 1 to 8 mm in depth, although they can have a gradual slant.[46] These depressed patches are characteristic and give the impression of inverted plateaus, or, if multiple lesions are present, they can have the appearance of Swiss cheese. They are even more apparent when present on the back because the dermis is thicker in this area. The skin surrounding the patches is normal in appearance, and there is no erythema or lilac ring as in morphea.

The course of this benign disease is progressive, and lesions can continue to appear for decades before reaching a standstill. Transformation to generalized morphea has not been observed.

PATHOLOGY

The histologic picture is generally not diagnostic.[47,49] The epidermis is usually normal. Collagen bundles in the middermis and reticular dermis show varying degrees of homogenization and clumping. Dermal thickness is eventually reduced when compared with adjacent normal skin. Some irregular clumping and loss of elastic fibers were described in earlier case reports, but in most series, no abnormality was seen with elastic tissue stains; consequently, this is not of diagnostic value. The appendages are usually preserved. If sclerodermatous changes appear in preexisting patches, the histology reveals varying degrees of collagen sclerosis resembling morphea. A recent study using multiphoton microscopy suggests that the atrophic appearance of atrophoderma lesions reflect changes in the organization of collagen and elastic fibers and not variation in their content.[50]

DIFFERENTIAL DIAGNOSIS

The differential diagnosis is to be made with active lesions of morphea that usually present as indurated, often hyperpigmented plaques with a characteristic peripheral lilac rim.

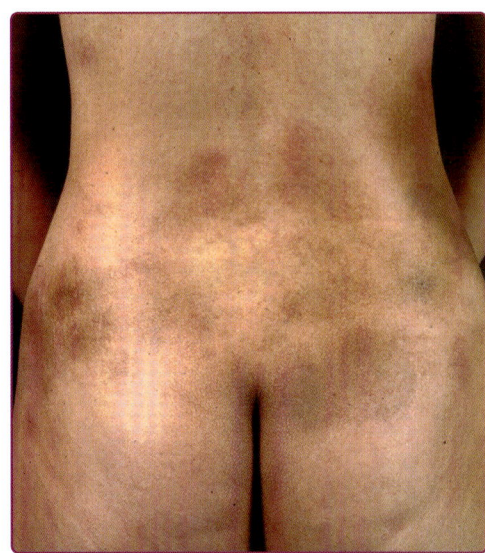

Figure 70-4 Atrophoderma of Pasini and Pierini. Brownish depressed lesions on the lower back.

TREATMENT

No treatment has proven effective. Penicillin and doxycycline have been used with poor results. Dramatic response to oral hydroxychloroquine was reported in 1 patient.[51] Q-switched alexandrite laser can maybe help decrease hyperpigmentation.[52]

FOLLICULAR ATROPHODERMA

Follicular atrophoderma refers to dimple-like depressions at the follicular orifices. It can occur as an isolated defect of limited extent, in association with a variety of disorders in which hair follicles are plugged with keratin, or with rare genodermatoses.[53,54]

Distinctive ice-pick depressions around hair follicles can be seen most commonly on the cheeks and on the back of the hands or feet. These pitted scars can present at birth or early in life. A family history may be present. Follicular atrophoderma occurs in the conditions described in the following sections.

ATROPHODERMA VERMICULATUM

Atrophoderma vermiculatum is a term that applies when the lesions are found exclusively on the cheeks.[55] It is a condition that can either occur sporadically, be inherited as an autosomal dominant disorder, be part of a group of related diseases including keratosis pilaris atrophicans, or be associated with various syndromes.

Multiple inflammatory symmetric papules on the cheeks, presumably centered around hair follicles, may precede the atrophic lesions. These papules then go on to develop pitted, atrophic, and depressed scars in a reticulated or honeycomb pattern (Fig. 70-5). These lesions can extend to the forehead and preauricular regions. This condition usually has its onset in childhood or, less often, around puberty. Men and women seem to be affected equally. It usually has a slow progressive course.

KERATOSIS PILARIS ATROPHICANS

Keratosis pilaris atrophicans[55,56] can include atrophoderma vermiculatum but also a group of closely related disorders that includes keratosis follicularis spinulosa decalvans and ulerythema ophryogenes. These conditions are characterized by keratotic follicular papules, variable degrees of inflammation, and secondary atrophic scarring. Keratosis follicularis spinulosa decalvans begins in infancy with keratotic follicular papules over the malar area and progresses to involve the eyebrows, scalp, and extremities, with scarring alopecia. This condition is inherited in an X-linked recessive fashion in some patients. Ulerythema ophryogenes (or keratosis pilaris atrophicans faciei) differs from atrophoderma vermiculatum by affecting primarily the lateral portion of the eyebrows (ophryogenes) with erythema, follicular papules, and alopecia (Fig. 70-6).

The underlying pathologic defect in these disorders appears to be abnormal follicular hyperkeratinization of the upper third of the hair shaft leading to obstruction of the growing hair and production of chronic inflammation. The end result of this process is scarring below that level. Histopathology is usually not very helpful and shows dilated follicles, sometimes associated with plugging, inflammation, and sclerosis of dermal collagen.

ASSOCIATED SYNDROMES

The various syndromes that include atrophoderma vermiculatum are Rombo syndrome (milia, telangiectasias, basal cell carcinomas, hypotrichosis, acral cyanosis, and, rarely, trichoepitheliomas), Nicolau-Balus syndrome (syringomas and milia), Tuzun syndrome (scrotal tongue), Loeys-Dietz syndrome,[57] and finally the Braun-Falco-Marghescu syndrome (palmoplantar hyperkeratosis and keratosis pilaris).

THERAPY

These disorders are mainly a cosmetic but vexing problem. Various topical treatments, including emollients, corticosteroids, tretinoin, and keratolytics, have shown no consistent benefit. Systemic isotretinoin has been shown to stop progression and to induce remission in some cases.[55] Dermabrasion as well as carbon dioxide and 585-nm pulsed-dye lasers are other options to improve the appearance of the atrophic scars.[58]

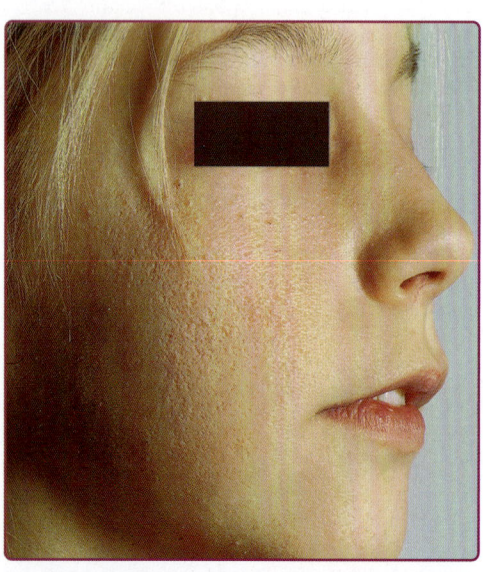

Figure 70-5 Atrophoderma vermiculatum. Multiple, small, pitted scars on the cheek of a young girl.

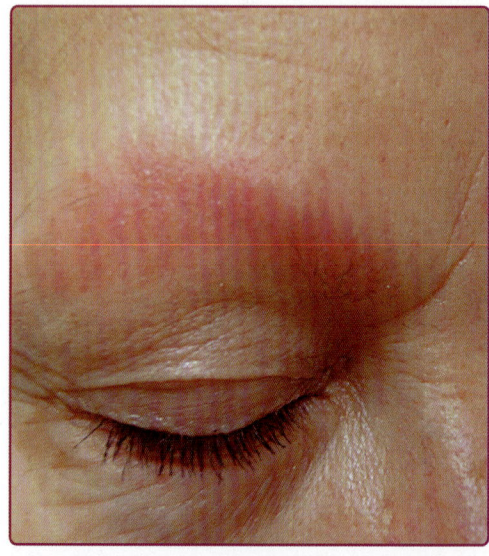

Figure 70-6 Ulerythema ophryogenes. Erythematous follicular papules and scarring alopecia of the eyebrow.

BAZEX-DUPRÉ-CHRISTOL SYNDROME (OMIM 301845)

Bazex-Dupré-Christol syndrome is characterized by follicular atrophoderma, milia, multiple basal cell carcinomas, hypotrichosis, and localized hypohidrosis.[59] The follicular atrophoderma described as multiple ice-pick marks or patulous follicles can be found most commonly on the dorsa of the hands. It is inherited in an X-linked dominant fashion, and the gene has been linked to Xq24-q27.[60] Additional reported findings include facial hyperpigmentation, hair shaft dystrophy, and multiple trichoepitheliomas. This syndrome might be better considered as an ectodermal dysplasia.[61]

CONRADI-HÜNERMANN-HAPPLE SYNDROME (X-LINKED DOMINANT CHONDRODYSPLASIA PUNCTATA, CDPX2, OMIM 302960)

Conradi-Hünermann-Happle syndrome is an X-linked dominant disorder that occurs only in girls because it is usually lethal in hemizygous males. The underlying molecular defect consists of mutations in the emopamil-binding protein gene at Xp11.23-p11.22.[62] The clinical manifestations include an ichthyosiform scaling erythroderma patterned along the lines of Blaschko that usually resolves during the first year of life and is replaced by bands of follicular atrophoderma. Hyperpigmentation, cataracts, scarring alopecia, saddle-nose deformity, asymmetric limb reduction defects, and stippled calcifications of the epiphyses can be seen. Ichthyosis with keratotic follicular plugs containing dystrophic calcification in newborns are distinctive histopathologic features.[63]

OTHER ATROPHIES OF THE CONNECTIVE TISSUE

Many systemic conditions (scleroderma [see Chap. 63], lupus erythematosus [see Chap. 61], dermatomyositis [see Chap. 62]), and genodermatoses (poikiloderma congenitale, dyskeratosis congenita, Cockayne syndrome, Hallermann-Streiff syndrome) have skin atrophy as an associated finding and are described in other chapters.

REFERENCES

1. Jadassohn J. Uber eine eigenartige form von "atrophica maculosa cutis". *Arch Derm Syphilol.* 1892;24:342-358.
2. Schweninger E, Buzzi F. Multiple benign tumor-like new growths of the skin. In: Internationaler Atlas Sellltener Hautkrankheiten, plate 15. Leipzig, Germany: L Voss; 1891.
3. Venencie PY, Winkelmann RK, Moore BA. Anetoderma: clinical findings, associations, and long-term follow-up evaluations. *Arch Dermatol.* 1984;120:1032-1039.
4. Kineston DP, Xia Y, Turiansky GW. Anetoderma: a case report and review of the literature. *Cutis.* 2008; 81:501-506.
5. Venencie PY, Bonnefoy A, Gogly B, et al. Increased expression of gelatinases A and B by skin explants from patients with anetoderma. *Br J Dermatol.* 1997;137:517-525.
6. Gambichler T, Reininghaus L, Skrygan M, et al. Fibulin protein expression in mid-dermal elastolysis and anetoderma: a study of 23 cases. *Acta Derm Venereol.* 2016;96:708-710.
7. Gougeon E, Beer F, Gay S, et al. Anetoderma of prematurity: an iatrogenic consequence of neonatal intensive care. *Arch Dermatol.* 2010;146:565-567.
8. Hodak E, David M. Primary anetoderma and antiphospholipid antibodies—review of the literature. *Clin Rev Allergy Immunol.* 2007;32:162-166.
9. Patrizi A, Neri I, Virdi A, et al. Familial anetoderma: a report of two families. *Eur J Dermatol.* 2011;21:680-685.
10. Venecie PY, Wilkelmann RK. Histopathologic findings in anetoderma. *Arch Dermatol.* 1984;120:1040-1044.
11. Bergman R, Friedman-Birnbaum R, Hazaz B, et al. An immunofluorescence study of primary anetoderma. *Clin Exp Dermatol.* 1990;15:124-130.
12. Sears J, Stone M, Argenyi Z. Papular elastorrhexis: a variant of connective tissue nevus: case reports and review of the literature. *J Am Acad Dermatol.* 1988;19:409-414.
13. Schirren H, Schirren C, Stolz W, et al. Papular elastorrhexis: a variant of dermatofibrosis lenticularis disseminata (Buschke-Ollendorff syndrome). *Dermatology.* 1994;189:368-372.
14. Wilson B, Dent C, Cooper P. Papular acne scars; a common cutaneous finding. *Arch Dermatol.* 1990;126: 797-800.
15. Wang K, Ross NA, Saedi N. Anetoderma treated with combined 595-nm pulsed-dye laser and 1550-nm non-ablative fractionated laser. *J Cosmet Laser Ther.* 2016;18:38-40.
16. Cho S, Jung JY, Lee JH. Treatment of anetoderma occurring after resolution of Stevens-Johnson syndrome using an ablative 10,600-nm carbon dioxide fractional laser. *Dermatol Surg.* 2012;38:677-679.
17. Shelley WB, Wood MG. Wrinkles due to idiopathic loss of mid-dermal elastic tissue. *Br J Dermatol.* 1977; 97:441-445.
18. Hardin J, Dupuis E, Haber RM. Mid-dermal elastolysis: a female-centric disease; case report and updated review of the literature. *Int J Women's Dermatol.* 2015;1:126-130.
19. Gambichler T. Mid-dermal elastolysis revisited. *Arch Dermatol Res.* 2010;302:85-93.
20. Snider RL, Lang PG, Maize JC. The clinical spectrum of mid-dermal elastolysis and the role of UV light in its pathogenesis. *J Am Acad Dermatol.* 1993;28: 938-942.
21. Vatve M, Morton R, Bilsland D. A case of mid-dermal elastolysis after narrowband ultraviolet B phototherapy. *Clin Exp Dermatol.* 2009;34:263-264.
22. Cota C, Latini A, Lora V, et al. Mid-dermal elastolysis as a manifestation of immune reconstitution inflammatory

syndrome in an HIV-infected patient. *J Am Acad Dermatol.* 2014;71:e134-e135.
23. Gambichler T, Breuckmann F, Kreuter A, et al. Immunohistochemical investigation of mid-dermal elastolysis. *Clin Exp Dermatol.* 2004;29:192-195.
24. Gambichler T, Skyrgan M. Decreased lysyl oxidase-like 2 expression in mid-dermal elastolysis. *Arch Dermatol Res.* 2013;305:359-363.
25. Scola N, Goulimus A, Gambichler T. Non-invasive imaging of mid-dermal elastolysis. *Clin Exp Dermatol.* 2011;36:155-160.
26. Harmon CB, Su WP, Gagne EJ, et al. Ultrastructural evaluation of mid-dermal elastolysis. *J Cutan Pathol.* 1994;21:233-238.
27. Varadi DP, Saqueton AC. Perifollicular elastolysis. *Br J Dermatol.* 1970;83:143.
28. Verhagen AR, Woederman MJ. Post-inflammatory elastolysis and cutis laxa. *Br J Dermatol.* 1975;92:183-190.
29. Garcia-Hidalgo L, Orozco-Topete R, Gonzalez-Barranco J, et al. Dermatoses in 156 obese adults. *Obes Res.* 1999;7:299-302.
30. Ammar NM, Rao B, Schwartz RA, et al. Adolescent striae. *Cutis.* 2000;65:69-70.
31. Farahnik B, Park K, Kroumpouzos G, et al. Striae gravidarum: risk factors, prevention and management. *Int J Womens Dermatol.* 2017;3:77-85.
32. Wahman AJ, Finan MA, Emerson SC. Striae gravidarum as a predictor of vaginal lacerations at delivery. *South Med J.* 2000;93:873-876.
33. Salter SA, Batra RS, Rohrer TE, et al. Striae and pelvic relaxation: two disorders of connective tissue with a strong association. *J Invest Dermatol.* 2006;126:1745-1748.
34. Arem A, Ward Kisher C. Analysis of striae. *Plast Reconstr Surg.* 1980;65:22-29.
35. Burket JM, Zelickson AS, Padilla RS. Linear focal elastosis (elastotic striae). *J Am Acad Dermatol.* 1989;20:633-636.
36. Hashimoto K. Linear focal elastosis: keloidal repair of striae distensae. *J Am Acad Dermatol.* 1998;39:309-313.
37. Al-Himdani S, Ud-Din S, Gilmore S, et al. Striae distensae: a comprehensive review and evidence-based evaluation of prophylaxis and treatment. *Br J Dermatol.* 2014;170:527-547.
38. Kang S. Topical tretinoin therapy for management of early striae. *J Am Acad Dermatol.* 1998;39:S90-S92.
39. Ash K, Lord J, Zukowski M, et al. Comparison of topical therapy for striae alba (20% glycolic acid/0.05% tretinoin versus 20% glycolic acid/10% L-ascorbic acid). *Dermatol Surg.* 1998;24:849-856.
40. Aldahan AS, Shah VV, Mlacker S, et al. Laser and light treatments for striae distensae: a comprehensive review of the literature. *Am J Clin Dermatol.* 2016;17:239-256.
41. Fatemi Naeini F, Behfar S, Abtahi-Naeini B, et al. Promising option for treatment of striae alba: fractionated microneedle radiofrequency in combination with fractional carbon dioxide laser. *Dermatol Res Pract.* 2016;2016:2896345.
42. Ramaut L, Hoeksema H, Pirayesh A, et al. Microneedling: where do we stand now? A systematic review of the literature. *J Plast Reconstr Aesthet Surg.* 2018;71:1-14.
43. Dover JS, Rothaus K, Gold MH. Evaluation of safety and patient subjective efficacy of using radiofrequency and pulsed magnetic fields for the treatment of striae (stretch marks). *J Clin Aesthet Dermatol.* 2014;7:30-33.
44. Canizares O, Sachs PM, Jaimovich L, et al. Idiopathic atrophoderma of Pasini and Pierini. *Arch Dermatol.* 1958;77:42-60.
45. Jablonska S, Blaszczyk M. Is superficial morphea synonymous with atrophoderma Pierini-Pasini? *J Am Acad Dermatol.* 2004;50:979-980.
46. Kang CY, Lam J. Congenital idiopathic atrophoderma of Pierini and Pasini. *Int J Dermatol.* 2015;54:e44-e46.
47. Buechner SA, Rufli T. Atrophoderma of Pasini and Pierini: clinical and histopathologic findings and antibodies to *Borrelia burgdorferi* in thirty-four patients. *J Am Acad Dermatol.* 1994;30:441-446.
48. Amano H, Nagai Y, Ishikawa O. Multiple morphea coexistent with atrophoderma of Pierini-Pasini (APP): APP could be abortive morphea. *J Eur Acad Dermatol Venereol.* 2007;21:1254-1256.
49. Saleh Z, Abbas O, Dahdah MJ, et al. Atrophoderma of Pierini and Pasini: a clinical and histopathological study. *J Cutan Pathol.* 2008;35:1108-1114.
50. Vieira-Damiani G, Lage D, Christofoletti Daldon PÉ, et al. Idiopathic atrophoderma of Pasini and Pierini: a case study of collagen and elastin texture by multiphoton microscopy. *J Am Acad Dermatol.* 2017;77:930-937.
51. Carter JD, Valeriano J, Vasey FB. Hydroxychloroquine as treatment for atrophoderma of Pierini and Pasini. *Int J Dermatol.* 2006;45:1255-1256.
52. Arpey CJ, Patel DS, Stone MS, et al. Treatment of atrophoderma of Pierini and Pasini-associated hyperpigmentation with the Q-switched alexandrite laser: a clinical, histologic, and ultrastructural appraisal. *Lasers Surg Med.* 2000;27:206-212.
53. Miescher G. Atypische Chondrodystrophie, Typus morquino kombiniert mit follikularer atrophodermie. *Dermatologica.* 1944;89:38-51.
54. Curth HO. The genetics of follicular atrophoderma. *Arch Dermatol.* 1978;114:1479-1483.
55. Luria RB, Conologue T. Atrophoderma vermiculatum: a case report and review of the literature on keratosis pilaris atrophicans. *Cutis.* 2009;83:83-86.
56. Callaway SR, Lesher JL. Keratosis pilaris atrophicans: case series and review. *Pediatr Dermatol.* 2004;21:14-17.
57. van Dijk FS, Brittain H, Boerma R, et al. Atrophoderma vermiculatum: a cutaneous feature of Loeys-Dietz syndrome. *JAMA Dermatol.* 2015;151:675-677.
58. Handrick C, Alster T. Laser treatment of atrophoderma vermiculata. *J Am Acad Dermatol.* 2001;44:693-695.
59. Torrelo A, Sprecher E, Medeiro IG, et al. What syndrome is this? Basex-Dupré-Christol syndrome. *Pediatr Dermatol.* 2006;23:286-290.
60. Parren LJ, Abuzahra F, Wagenvoort T, et al. Linkage refinement of Bazex-Dupré-Christol syndrome to an 11·4-Mb interval on chromosome Xq25-27.1. *Br J Dermatol.* 2011;165:201-203.
61. Castori M, Castiglia D, Passarelli F, et al. Bazex-Dupré-Christol syndrome: an ectodermal dysplasia with skin appendage neoplasms. *Eur J Med Genet.* 2009:52:250-255.
62. Canueto J, Giros M, Ciria S, et al. Clinical, molecular and biochemical characterization of nine Spanish families with Conradi-Hünermann-Happle syndrome: new insights into X-linked dominant chondrodysplasia punctata with a comprehensive review of the literature. *Br J Dermatol.* 2012;166:830-838.
63. Hoang MP, Carder KR, Pandya AG, et al. Ichthyosis and keratotic follicular plugs containing dystrophic calcification in newborns: distinctive histopathologic features of X-linked dominant chondrodysplasia punctata (Conradi-Hünermann-Happle syndrome). *Am J Dermatopathol.* 2004;26:53-58.

Chapter 71 :: Acquired Perforating Disorders
:: Garrett T. Desman & Raymond L. Barnhill

第七十一章
获得性穿通性皮病

中文导读

获得性穿通性皮病（APD）是一组独立确诊的疾病，通常继发于糖尿病和慢性肾脏疾病。这组疾病揽括了此前认识的Kyrle病、获得性匍行性穿通性弹性组织变性、获得性穿通性胶原病和穿通性毛囊炎。本章从临床特征、相关疾病、病因及发病机制、诊断、鉴别诊断、临床进程、预后及管理几个方面描述了本病。获得性穿通性皮病是一组成人发病的获得性穿通性皮病的总称。这一组疾病具有共同的临床特征及好发部位。皮损表现为脐状丘疹和/或结节，中央有角化的栓子或结痂，好发于四肢伸侧。组织病理显示真皮内物质（胶原、弹性蛋白和/或纤维蛋白）通过杯状表皮凹陷处排出。目前无特效治疗，病程慢性。尽管这组疾病可能是家族性原发或获得性全身疾病（如慢性肾功能衰竭、糖尿病）的主要表现，但穿出的真皮成分也可能是其他原发性皮肤病（如穿通性环状肉芽肿、痛风、穿通性弹性假黄瘤）的继发成分。本节也描述了其他关联的疾病和综合征及相关药物。这组疾病由于穿通排出的物质不同而诊断各异，APC在角质栓中是胶原束，AEPS是弹力纤维，KD是无定型包括纤维素和角质成分的物质，穿通性毛囊炎是特征性的退行性胶原和细胞外基质从毛囊上皮穿通排出。有时可以同时发现胶原和弹力纤维排出。进一步强调了APD的重叠。由于该病与系统疾病相关，需要完善血糖、糖耐量实验、肝肾功能及甲状腺功能等检查。鉴别诊断非常广泛包括感染性、炎症性、肿瘤性皮病。本章详细说明了文献中描述的治疗方案。

〔施 为〕

AT-A-GLANCE

- Acquired perforating disorders represent a group of separately identified cutaneous disorders that occur most often in the setting of chronic renal disease or diabetes mellitus.

- The previously recognized Kyrle disease (KD), acquired elastosis perforans serpiginosa (AEPS), acquired perforating collagenosis (APC), and perforating folliculitis (PF) are now classified under the umbrella term of acquired perforating dermatosis.

- Lesions present as umbilicated papules and/or nodules with a central keratotic plug or crust distributed preferentially on extensor surfaces of the extremities.

- Histopathologic examination of lesional skin demonstrates invagination of the epidermis with extrusion of dermal material (collagen, elastin, and/or fibrin) through the cup-shaped epidermal depression.

- Treatment is challenging with no universally effective therapy, and patients often exhibit a chronic course.

The perforating disorders are a group of conditions characterized by the transepidermal elimination of connective tissue elements. Although this finding may be the primary manifestation of familial or acquired systemic conditions (ie, chronic renal failure, diabetes mellitus), the perforation of dermal elements also may be seen as a secondary component to other primary dermatoses (eg, perforating granuloma annulare, gout, perforating pseudoxanthoma elasticum) (Table 71-1). Rare familial primary perforating disorders typically present in childhood and are characterized histopathologically by the transepidermal elimination of collagen (reactive perforating collagenosis) or elastic fibers (elastosis perforans serpiginosa). Similar adult-onset nonfamilial/acquired lesions are most commonly associated with chronic kidney disease and diabetes mellitus. These cases were originally given various appellations within the medical literature, complicating the subject matter (Table 71-2). Eventually, comprehensive review of the literature concluded that 4 separate clinicopathologic entities characterized the adult-onset acquired primary perforating disorders: Kyrle disease (KD), acquired perforating collagenosis (APC), perforating folliculitis, and acquired elastosis perforans serpiginosa (AEPS).[1-4] Further studies, however, have reported more clinicopathologic similarities than differences among these acquired conditions, in particular, a varied composition of extruded contents (ie, collagen, elastin fibers, fibrin) from lesion to lesion in the same patient. This has resulted in some authors advocating for a combined designation of acquired perforating dermatosis (APD).[5,6] Although the use of this unified designation is encouraged, an acknowledgment of the clinical and histopathologic manifestations of these 4 described conditions is important for understanding the spectrum of findings as well as possible correlations with systemic disease (Table 71-3).

TABLE 71-1
Secondary Perforating Disorders

Hematomas
Perforating calcinosis cutis
Gout (urate crystals)
Papular mucinosis (mucin)
Perforating pseudoxanthoma elasticum
Granuloma annulare
Necrobiosis lipoidica
Rheumatoid nodule
Sarcoidosis
Foreign body (silica, wood splinter, glass, metal)
Infection (chromomycosis, leprosy)
Tumor cells (melanoma, pilomatrixoma, epithelioid sarcoma)

TABLE 71-2
Synonyms for Acquired Perforating Dermatosis

Acquired reactive perforating collagenosis[38]
Hyperkeratosis follicularis et parafollicularis in cutem penetrans[4]
Hyperkeratosis penetrans[39]
Keratosis follicularis serpiginosa[40]
Kyrle disease[41]
Kyrle-like lesions[42]
Perforating disorder[23]
Perforating folliculitis[43]
Perforating folliculitis of hemodialysis[35]
Reactive perforating collagenosis of diabetes mellitus and renal failure[44]
Uremic follicular hyperkeratosis[45]

CLINICAL FEATURES

APD is an umbrella designation for adult-onset acquired perforating disease encompassing KD, APC, perforating folliculitis, and AEPS, with AEPS exhibiting distinctive clinical findings and disease associations. No geographic or clear racial predilection has been established. APD is characterized clinically by round, umbilicated, skin-colored, erythematous or hyperpigmented papules and nodules with a central crust or keratotic plug, predominantly involving the extensor surfaces of the extremities and the trunk (APC, KD) (Fig. 71-1). Lesions less commonly involve the face or scalp. Although the central keratotic core is the most specific clinical finding, it is occasionally removed by the patient, leaving behind only a shallow crater. Mucous membranes are spared. In rare cases, purple annular plaques or pustules mixed with papules have been observed. Scratching of APD lesions can lead to koebnerization with linear umbilicated papules arising in excoriated skin. Some lesions may exhibit a follicular-based distribution with minimal

TABLE 71-3
Presentations of Acquired Perforating Dermatosis

	KYRLE DISEASE/ACQUIRED PERFORATING COLLAGENOSIS	PERFORATING FOLLICULITIS	ACQUIRED ELASTOSIS PERFORANS SERPIGINOSA
Age of onset	4th decade (average)	3rd decade (average)	2nd decade (average)
Site	Extensor lower and upper extremities; head, neck, and trunk	Hair-bearing portions of extremities	Nape of neck; upper extremities; face; lower extremities
Cutaneous findings	Round, umbilicated, skin-colored, erythematous or hyperpigmented papules and nodules with a central crust or keratotic plug	Similar to Kyrle disease/acquired perforating collagenosis, but with follicular distribution and variable central crusting	Papules in serpiginous configuration with central atrophy
Disease associations	Renal failure, hemodialysis, diabetes mellitus, hepatic insufficiency	Idiopathic, minor association with renal failure, hemodialysis, diabetes mellitus	Down syndrome; Ehlers-Danlos syndrome; osteogenesis imperfecta; pseudoxanthoma elasticum; minor association with renal failure
Koebner phenomenon	Positive	Negative	Occasionally

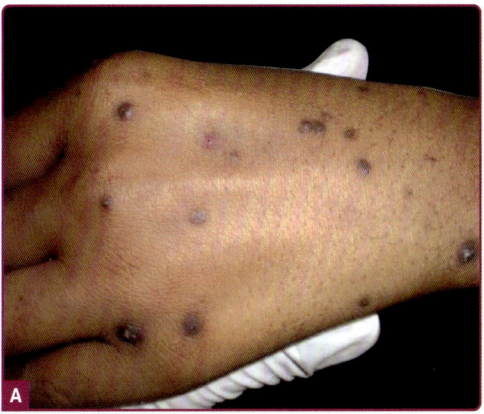
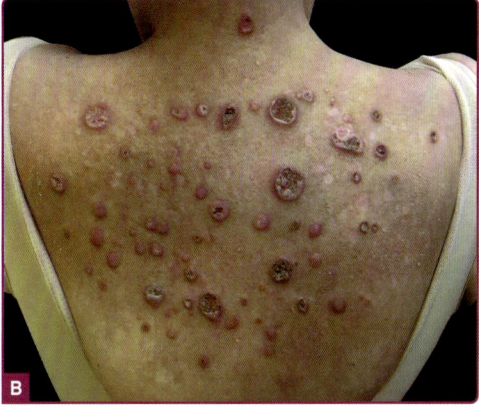

Figure 71-1 Acquired perforating dermatosis. **A,** Acquired perforating collagenosis type. Multiple, round, hyperpigmented papules, each with a central keratotic plug, distributed on the extensor aspects of the hand and wrist in a patient with chronic kidney disease. **B,** Kyrle disease type. Multiple large crateriform nodules with central keratinous contents on the back of a patient with hypothyroidism. (Image **B**, used with permission from Drs. Megan Rogge and Tamara Lazic-Strugar, Icahn School of Medicine at The Mount Sinai Hospital, New York, NY.)

Koebner response (perforating folliculitis; Fig. 71-2). Lesional pain and pruritus, ranging from mild-to-severe and intractable, have been reported.[6]

Elastosis perforans serpiginosa, whether familial or acquired, exhibits papules in a serpiginous configuration, often with central atrophy, and typically is localized to 1 region of the body, such as the neck, trunk, or the extremities (Fig. 71-3). These lesions are frequently asymptomatic and only occasionally manifest a koebnerization response. Elastosis perforans serpiginosa affects nearly 4 times more males than females. The familial form of the disease has a reported autosomal dominant mode of inheritance.[7]

The term *reactive perforating collagenosis* refers to an extremely rare familial disorder that most commonly presents in early childhood with an equal sex distribution. Both autosomal dominant and recessive modes of inheritance have been reported. Similar to KD and

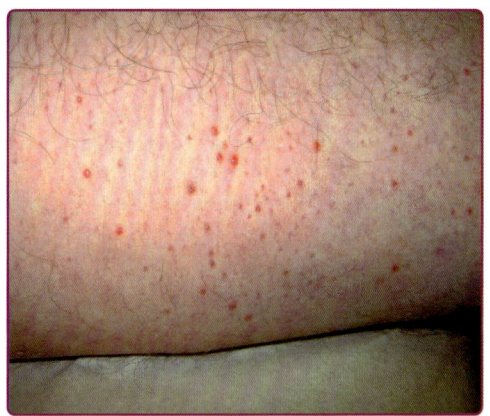

Figure 71-2 Acquired perforating dermatosis, perforating folliculitis type. Multiple follicular, erythematous, firm papules with variable central crusting.

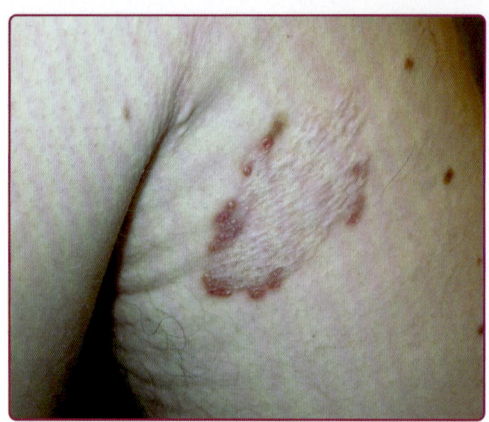

Figure 71-3 Acquired perforating dermatosis, acquired elastosis perforans serpiginosa type. Annular plaque with variably crusted erythematous papules at the periphery and central cribriform scarring in a patient taking penicillamine for Wilson disease.

APC, following superficial trauma, small keratotic papules develop on the upper and lower extremities, and occasionally on the face. This form of disease has the strongest koebnerization response.[8]

ASSOCIATIONS OF ACQUIRED PERFORATING DISORDERS

The most common systemic conditions associated with adult-onset APD are chronic kidney disease (CKD) and diabetes mellitus (DM). APD has been documented in 4.5% to 10% of hemodialysis patients in North America and in 11% of a dialysis population (both hemodialysis and peritoneal dialysis) in Great Britain.[9,10] Not surprisingly, the most common cause of CKD among APD patients is diabetic nephropathy.[10] APD also has occurred in patients with chronic renal dysfunction who are not undergoing dialysis, as well as in those patients who have received renal transplants. Interestingly, in a series of 22 patients with APD, 3 were healthy with no known associated illnesses.[6] Some advocate that the phenomenon of APD simply represents a form of prurigo nodularis owing to its association with other pruritic conditions, such as insect bites and scabies, lymphoma, and hepatobiliary diseases.[11-18] Lesions associated with CKD and DM typically follow a chronic course that parallels systemic disease (KD, acquired reactive perforating collagenosis). Follicular-based lesions unassociated with CKD or DM typically lack a Koebner response and may follow a waxing-and-waning course. APD has rarely been associated with the use of certain therapeutics, including tumor necrosis factor-α inhibitors, indinavir, and sorafenib.[19-22] AEPS is well recognized as a potential adverse effect of prolonged D-penicillamine therapy.[22] As mentioned earlier in this section, some elastosis perforans serpiginosa cases are familial and associated with an autosomal dominant mode of inheritance. Other associations include Down syndrome and various inborn disorders of connective tissue metabolism, such as Ehlers-Danlos syndrome, Marfan syndrome, osteogenesis imperfecta, scleroderma, and pseudoxanthoma elasticum. However, rare cases of AEPS have been reported in patients with CKD in the absence of penicillamine exposure or other known associations.[1] Table 71-3 lists less-commonly reported associations with APD.

ETIOLOGY AND PATHOGENESIS

Although the precise etiology and pathogenesis of APD are unknown, a complex interaction between epithelium, connective tissue, and inflammatory mediators is most likely involved. According to the current trend for unification, perforating folliculitis and APC may be phenotypic variants of a disease spectrum or merely different stages in lesional development. KD most likely represents an extreme phenotype or end-stage manifestation of the 2 former conditions. Controversy still exists regarding whether perforating folliculitis represents a true primary perforating disease as ruptured follicles with extruded stromal elements are a feature of many infectious conditions, such as *Pityrosporum* folliculitis.

Regardless, as APD is most strongly associated with pruritic conditions, superficial trauma to the epidermis most likely represents the primary inciting factor in susceptible patients. This is highlighted by the fact that many patients have common prurigo nodules in addition to classic perforating lesions. Additionally, resolution of APD lesions with discontinuation of manipulation/trauma supports this mechanism.[6] Predisposing conditions include vasculopathy/angiopathy (related to DM), microdeposition of exogenous materials within the dermis (including calcium salts and silicon, pertinent to the increased frequency of APD in dialysis patients), and epidermal or dermal change related to metabolic derangements including vitamin A deficiency.[10,23-26]

A recent study indicates a role of advanced glycation end product–modified collagens I and III, where traumatized keratinocytes bind to these extracellular matrix proteins via advanced glycation end product receptor CD36, inducing keratinocyte terminal differentiation and upward movement of keratinocytes along with glycated collagen.[27] Fibronectin also has been implicated because it links keratinocytes with Type IV collagen within the basement membrane and plays a vital role in epithelial cell signaling, migration, and differentiation. Increased fibronectin levels have been documented in the serum of patients with DM and uremia, as well as within the skin at sites of transepidermal elimination.[28] Imbalances in transforming growth factor-β3, matrix metalloproteinase-1, and tissue inhibitor of metalloproteinase-1 also have been demonstrated in APD lesions; whether these alterations are pathogenic or reflective of normal wound healing is currently unknown.[26,29]

Whether the pathogenesis of the familial primary perforating dermatoses is different from the acquired forms is also unknown. Transepidermal elimination of Type IV collagen has been documented in both familial reactive perforating collagenosis and APC.[30] In elastosis perforans serpiginosa, enhanced expression of elastin receptors has been detected in the epidermis surrounding the elastic material in both familial and acquired conditions.[31] However, in penicillamine-associated AEPS, it is hypothesized that penicillamine alters dermal elastic fibers in affected patients.[32] Elastic fiber abnormalities, including "bramble bush–appearing" fibers of variable thickness and increased numbers of fibers in the papillary and reticular dermis, have been described in patients with penicillamine-induced AEPS.[33]

DIAGNOSIS

HISTOPATHOLOGY

The diagnosis of APD is based on clinical and histopathologic findings. Folliculitis and prurigo nodularis may occur concomitantly, especially in patients with CKD, therefore multiple biopsies should be taken if lesions show different clinical morphologies. APD is characterized histologically by transepidermal elimination of dermal material through an epidermal invagination, which may be follicular or perifollicular. Lesions typically demonstrate a central keratotic plug with crusting or hyperkeratosis; parakeratosis is variable. Within the dermis surrounding the perforation, there is often a focal inflammatory infiltrate with neutrophils predominating in early lesions and lymphocytes, macrophages, or multinucleated giant cells present in older lesions.

The 4 initially identified acquired perforating disorders (APC, AEPS, KD, and perforating folliculitis) were classically differentiated histopathologically on the basis of the nature of the eliminated dermal material. In APC, collagen bundles are detected within the plug (Fig. 71-4); in AEPS, elastic fibers are instead noted (Fig. 71-5). In KD, amorphous dermal material with fibrin and/or keratin comprises the extruded contents. Perforating folliculitis is characterized by perforation of the follicular epithelium by degenerating collagen and extracellular matrix (Fig. 71-6). Clear identification of the eliminated material may be impossible and, in addition, multiple substances (ie, collagen and elastic fibers) may be simultaneously detected, reinforcing the clinical and histopathologic overlap within APD.[5,6]

Lesions of familial reactive perforating collagenosis and elastosis perforans serpiginosa characteristically contain extruded collagen and elastin, respectively.[7,8]

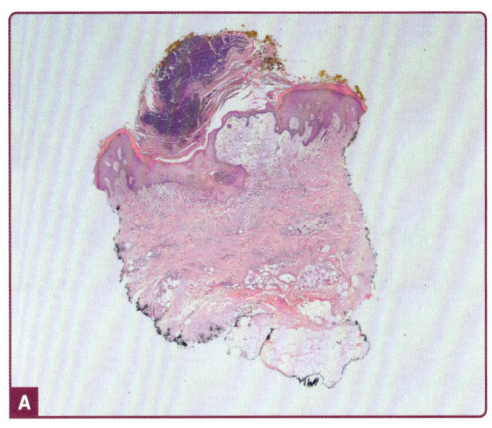

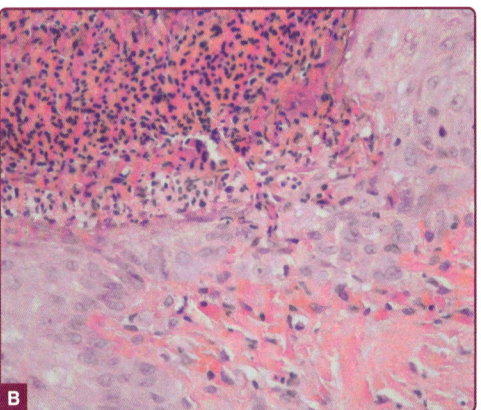

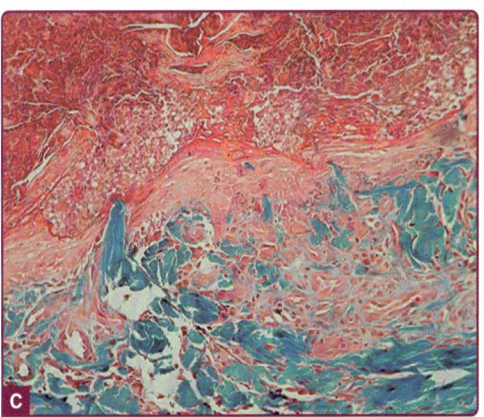

Figure 71-4 Acquired perforating dermatosis, acquired perforating collagenosis type. **A,** There is a crateriform epidermal invagination filled with necrotic material and inflammatory cells. **B,** Individual collagen bundles penetrate through the epidermis and into the core of necrotic material. **C,** Trichrome stain highlights the collagen bundles *(blue)* from the reticular dermis penetrating through the epidermis.

LABORATORY TESTS

Laboratory evaluation for comorbidities should include fasting blood glucose; glucose tolerance test; serum creatinine; glomerular filtration rate or creati-

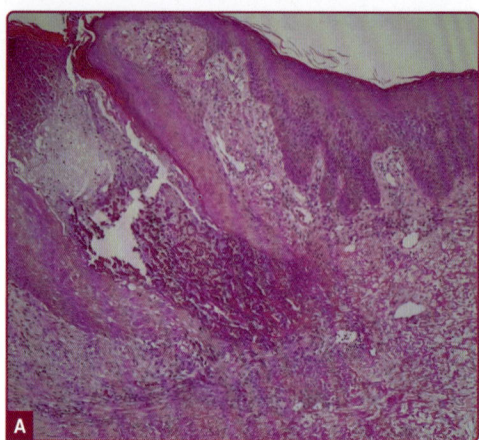

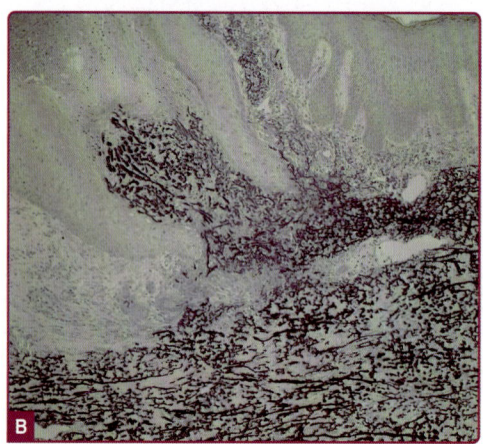

Figure 71-5 Acquired perforating dermatosis, acquired elastosis perforans serpiginosa type. **A,** Dilated follicular structure with transepidermal elimination of densely eosinophilic elongated bundles (hematoxylin and eosin stain). **B,** Transepidermally eliminated elongated bundles are elastin fibers (elastin stain).

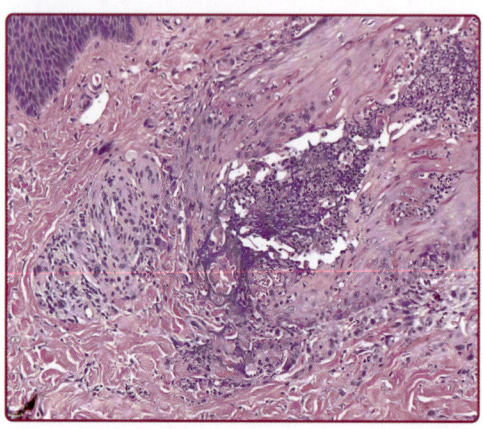

Figure 71-6 Acquired perforating dermatosis, perforating folliculitis type. A dilated follicular unit exhibits disruption of the outer root sheath epithelium by perforating dermal collagen. The follicular ostium is filled with necrotic debris and acute inflammatory cells. (Used with permission from Garrett Desman, MD. From Desman GT, Barnhill RL: *Barnhill's Dermatopathology Challenge*. New York, NY: McGraw-Hill Education; 2016:346.)

TABLE 71-4
Conditions Associated with Acquired Perforating Dermatosis

Common Associations
Chronic kidney disease
Diabetes mellitus (insulin-dependent and noninsulin-dependent)
Scabies[12,13]

Rare Associations
AIDS[46,47]
Arthropod bites[14,48]
Atopic dermatitis[34]
Cutaneous cytomegalovirus infection[49]
Hyperparathyroidism[38]
Liver diseases (hepatitis C, hepatitis B, steatohepatitis, primary biliary cirrhosis)[6,15]
Lupus vulgaris[50]
Myelodysplastic syndrome[49]
Malignancy (Hodgkin lymphoma, mixed histiocytic–lymphocytic lymphoma, hepatocellular carcinoma, pancreatic carcinoma, prostate carcinoma, papillary thyroid carcinoma)[17,18,51-56]
Mikulicz disease[57]
Neurodermatitis[38]
Poland syndrome[58]
Primary sclerosing cholangitis[59]
Pulmonary aspergillosis[60]
Pulmonary fibrosis[34]
Salt water application[23]
Thyroid disease (hypothyroidism, sick euthyroid syndrome, Hashimoto thyroiditis)[15,38,61]
Vitamin A deficiency[24]

nine clearance; serum uric acid; liver function tests; and thyroid function tests. A comprehensive family and past medical history, as well as review of systems, should be obtained. Additional diagnostic testing for associated conditions (Table 71-4) should be performed as indicated.

DIFFERENTIAL DIAGNOSIS

The differential diagnosis of APD is broad and includes infectious, inflammatory, and neoplastic disorders, including those that koebnerize (Table 71-5). APD can be especially difficult to differentiate from prurigo nodularis. Perforating pseudoxanthoma elasticum should be distinguished from AEPS.

CLINICAL COURSE, PROGNOSIS, AND MANAGEMENT

COMPLICATIONS

Most complications that occur in patients with APD arise from underlying systemic illnesses. However, patients should be monitored for secondary infection (bacterial, fungal, and viral) as well as parasitic infestation. In an

TABLE 71-5
Differential Diagnosis of Acquired Perforating Dermatosis

- Actinic granuloma (annular elastolytic giant cell granuloma)
- Arthropod bites
- Discoid lupus erythematous
- Flegel disease (hyperkeratosis follicularis perstans)
- Folliculitis (bacterial, yeast)
- Keratosis follicularis (Darier disease)
- Keratosis pilaris
- Lichen planus
- Multiple keratoacanthomas (Ferguson-Smith familial keratoacanthomas, Grzybowski eruptive keratoacanthomas)
- Perforating granuloma annulare
- Perforating periumbilical calcific elastosis
- Perforating pseudoxanthoma elasticum
- Porokeratosis
- Prurigo nodularis
- Psoriasis
- Sarcoidosis
- Scabies

TABLE 71-6
Treatment of Acquired Perforating Dermatosis

TREATMENT	ACTION	DOSING
Topical Therapies		
Retinoic acid[a]	Retinoid	0.025% gel[62]
Tretinoin[a]	Retinoid	0.1% cream one to three times daily[63,64]
Tazarotene[a]	Retinoid	0.1% gel daily[65]
Beclomethasone[a]	Corticosteroid	0.1% cream[9]
Triamcinolone acetonide[a]	Corticosteroid	10 mg/mL intralesional injection[9]
Imiquimod	Immune response modifier	Daily for 6 weeks then 3 times per week for 4 weeks[32]
Phenol	Antipruritic	0.5% phenol with 10% glycerin in Sorbolene cream[66]
Capsaicin	Capsaicinoid	0.025%-0.075% ointment
Systemic Therapies		
Isotretinoin[b]	Retinoid	Isotretinoin 0.5 mg/kg/day[67,68]
Acitretin[b]	Retinoid	25-30 mg daily[66,69]
Prednisolone	Corticosteroid	30 mg daily[70]
Allopurinol[b]	Xanthine oxidase inhibitor	100 mg daily[71,72]
Doxycycline	Antibiotic	100 mg daily[13,73,74]
Metronidazole	Antibiotic	500 mg twice daily[75]
Clindamycin	Antibiotic	300 mg three times daily[76]
Hydroxychloroquine	Antimalarial	200 mg daily[77]
Physical Modalities		
UVB[a]	Phototherapy	MED for 2 minutes every other day with increments of 30 seconds for 2–4 weeks[78]
NUVB[a]	Phototherapy	Three times a week for 2-3 months[33] 400 mJ/cm², increased to 1,500 mJ/cm², two to three times per week, 10–15 exposures[37]
PUVA[b,74]	Phototherapy	Four times per week for total of 326 J/cm²[79]
Liquid nitrogen	Cryotherapy	10 seconds, on five occasions over 4 months, one occasion 3 months later[80]
Carbon dioxide laser	Laser	Five lesional passes at 300 J (pattern 5, size 7, density 7), followed by 3 resurfacing passes at 300 J (pattern 2, size 8, density 5), power of 80 W[81]
TENS	Other	1 hour daily for 3 weeks[82]
Surgical debridement[76,83]		

[a]First-line therapy.
[b]Second-line therapy.
NUVB, narrowband ultraviolet B; PUVA, psoralen and ultraviolet A; TENS, transcutaneous electrical nerve stimulation; UVB, ultraviolet B.

attempt to relieve the associated pruritus, patients may apply products to their skin that may result in irritant or allergic contact dermatitis. In darker-skinned patients with more excoriations, postinflammatory pigmentary alteration and scarring can be significant.

PROGNOSIS

The prognosis of APD is heavily linked to the presence of underlying diseases. Some studies have shown that APD may improve with successful treatment of the underlying illness.[34] Most cases of APD continue for years unless treated.

MANAGEMENT

Treatment of APD is difficult. Table 71-6 details the therapeutic options that are described in the literature to date. There have not been any well-designed clinical trials of treatment for APD, and current treatment strategies are based largely on anecdotal reports. In patients with CKD, improvement in APD lesions has been reported after changing the type of dialysis tubing or modification of the dialysis procedure.[10] In a few cases, APD has resolved following renal transplantation.[9,35,36] The most commonly employed treatments for APD include topical and oral retinoids, topical and intradermal corticosteroids, and ultraviolet B phototherapy. Phototherapy is effective for uremic pruritus and therefore may be particularly beneficial for patients with CKD by reducing koebnerization.[37] Several authors have reported improvement in APD following treatment with allopurinol in cases of elevated or normal uric acid levels.[37] Currently available therapeutic options may not provide complete resolution of APD lesions or associated symptoms.

REFERENCES

1. Schamroth JM, Kellen P, Grieve TP. Elastosis perforans serpiginosa in a patient with renal disease. *Arch Dermatol*. 1986;122(1):82-84.
2. Poliak SC, Lebwohl MG, Parris A, et al. Reactive perforating collagenosis associated with diabetes mellitus. *N Engl J Med*. 1982;306(2):81-84.
3. Mehregan AH, Coskey RJ. Perforating folliculitis. *Arch Dermatol*. 1968;97(4):394-399.
4. Kyrle J. Uber einen ungewohnlichen fall von universeller follicularer und parafollikularer hyperkeratose (hyperkeratosis follicularis et parafollicularis in cutem penetrans). *Arch Dermatol Syph*. 1916;123.
5. Rapini RP, Herbert AA, Drucker CR. Acquired perforating dermatosis. Evidence for combined transepidermal elimination of both collagen and elastic fibers. *Arch Dermatol*. 1989;125(8):1074-1078.
6. Saray Y, Seckin D, Bilezikci B. Acquired perforating dermatosis: clinicopathological features in twenty-two cases. *J Eur Acad Dermatol Venereol*. 2006;20(6):679-688.
7. Langeveld-Wildschut EG, Toonstra J, van Vloten WA, et al. Familial elastosis perforans serpiginosa. *Arch Dermatol*. 1993;129(2):205-207.
8. Pai VV, Naveen KN, Athanikar SB, et al. Familial reactive perforating collagenosis: a report of two cases. *Indian J Dermatol*. 2014;59(3):287-289.
9. Morton CA, Henderson IS, Jones MC, et al. Acquired perforating dermatosis in a British dialysis population. *Br J Dermatol*. 1996;135(5):671-677.
10. Kurban MS, Boueiz A, Kibbi AG. Cutaneous manifestations of chronic kidney disease. *Clin Dermatol*. 2008;26(3):255-264.
11. Kestner RI, Stander S, Osada N, et al. Acquired reactive perforating dermatosis is a variant of prurigo nodularis. *Acta Derm Venereol*. 20178;97(2):249-254.
12. Hinrichs W, Breuckmann F, Altmeyer P, et al. Acquired perforating dermatosis: a report on 4 cases associated with scabies infection. *J Am Acad Dermatol*. 2004;51(4):665-667.
13. Brinkmeier T, Herbst RA, Frosch PJ. Reactive perforating collagenosis associated with scabies in a diabetic. *J Eur Acad Dermatol Venereol*. 2004;18(5):588-590.
14. Kim EJ, Kim MY, Kim HO, et al. Acquired reactive perforating collagenosis triggered by insect bite. *J Dermatol*. 2007;34(9):677-679.
15. Chiu MW, Haley JC. Acquired perforating dermatosis associated with primary biliary cirrhosis and Hashimoto thyroiditis. *Cutis*. 2007;79(6):451-455.
16. Karpouzis A, Tsatalas C, Sividris E, et al. Acquired reactive perforating collagenosis associated with myelodysplastic syndrome evolving to acute myelogenous leukaemia. *Australas J Dermatol*. 2004;45(1):78-79.
17. Eigentler TK, Metzler G, Brossart P, et al. Acquired perforating collagenosis in Hodgkin's disease. *J Am Acad Dermatol*. 2005;52(5):922.
18. Henry JC, Jorizzo JL, Apisarnthanarax P. Reactive perforating collagenosis in the setting of prurigo nodularis. *Int J Dermatol*. 1983;22(6):386-387.
19. Gilaberte Y, Coscojuela C, Vázquez C, et al. Perforating folliculitis associated with tumour necrosis factor-alpha inhibitors administered for rheumatoid arthritis. *Br J Dermatol*. 2007;156(2):368-371.
20. Calista D, Morri M. Acquired reactive perforating collagenosis induced by indinavir in 2 patients with HIV disease. *Eur J Dermatol*. 2008;18(1):84-85.
21. Wolber C, Udvardi A, Tatzreiter G, et al. Perforating folliculitis, angioedema, hand-foot syndrome—multiple cutaneous side effects in a patient treated with sorafenib. *J Dtsch Dermatol Ges*. 2009;7(5):449-452.
22. Pass F, Goldfischer S, Sternlieb I, et al. Elastosis perforans serpiginosa during penicillamine therapy for Wilson disease. *Arch Dermatol*. 1973;108(5):713-715.
23. Lee SJ, Jang JW, Lee WC, et al. Perforating disorder caused by salt-water application and its experimental induction. *Int J Dermatol*. 2005;44(3):210-214.
24. Barr DJ, Riley RJ, Greco DJ. Bypass phrynoderma. Vitamin A deficiency associated with bowel-bypass surgery. *Arch Dermatol*. 1984;120(7):919-921.
25. Kawakami T, Saito R. Acquired reactive perforating collagenosis associated with diabetes mellitus: eight cases that meet Faver's criteria. *Br J Dermatol*. 1999;140(3):521-524.
26. Patterson JW. Progress in the perforating dermatoses. *Arch Dermatol*. 1989;125(8):1121-1123.
27. Fujimoto E, Kobayashi T, Fujimoto N, et al. AGE-modified collagens I and III induce keratinocyte terminal differentiation through AGE receptor CD36: epidermal-dermal interaction in acquired perforating dermatosis. *J Invest Dermatol*. 2010;130(2):405-414.
28. Bilezikci B, Seckin D, Demirhan B. Acquired perforating dermatosis in patients with chronic renal failure: a possible pathogenetic role for fibronectin. *J Eur Acad Dermatol Venereol*. 2003;17(2):230-232.
29. Gambichler T, Birkner L, Stücker M, et al. Up-regulation of transforming growth factor-beta3 and extracellular matrix proteins in acquired reactive perforating collagenosis. *J Am Acad Dermatol*. 2009;60(3):463-469.
30. Herzinger T, Schirren CG, Sander CA, et al. Reactive perforating collagenosis-transepidermal elimination of type IV collagen. *Clin Exp Dermatol*. 1996;21(4):279-282.
31. Fujimoto N, Akagi A, Tajima S, et al. Expression of 67-kDa elastin receptor in perforating skin disorders. *Br J Dermatol*. 2002;146(1):74-79.
32. Kelly SC, Purcell SM. Imiquimod therapy for elastosis perforans serpiginosa. *Arch Dermatol*. 2006;142(7):829-830.
33. Hashimoto K, McEvoy B, Belcher R. Ultrastructure of penicillamine-induced skin lesions. *J Am Acad Dermatol*. 1981;4(3):300-315.
34. Tsuboi H, Katsuoka K. Characteristics of acquired reactive perforating collagenosis. *J Dermatol*. 2007;34(9):640-644.
35. White CR Jr, Heskel NS, Pokorny DJ. Perforating folliculitis of hemodialysis. *Am J Dermatopathol*. 1982;4(2):109-116.
36. Saldanha LF, Gonick HC, Rodriguez HJ, et al. Silicon-related syndrome in dialysis patients. *Nephron*. 1997;77(1):48-56.
37. Ohe S, Danno K, Sasaki H, et al. Treatment of acquired perforating dermatosis with narrowband ultraviolet B. *J Am Acad Dermatol*. 2004;50(6):892-894.
38. Faver IR, Daoud MS, Su WP. Acquired reactive perforating collagenosis. Report of six cases and review of the literature. *J Am Acad Dermatol*. 1994;30(4):575-580.

39. Abele DC, Dobson RL. Hyperkeratosis penetrans (Kyrle's disease). Report of a case in a Negro with autopsy findings. *Arch Dermatol*. 1961;83:277-283.
40. Lutz W. Keratosis follicularis serpiginosa [in undetermined language]. *Dermatologica*. 1953;106(3-5):318-319.
41. Hood AF, Hardegen GL, Zarate AR, et al. Kyrle's disease in patients with chronic renal failure. *Arch Dermatol*. 1982;118(2):85-88.
42. Stone RA. Kyrle-like lesions in two patients with renal failure undergoing dialysis. *J Am Acad Dermatol*. 1981;5(6):707-709.
43. Mehregan AH, Schwartz OD, Livingood CS. Reactive perforating collagenosis. *Arch Dermatol*. 1967;96(3):277-282.
44. Cochran RJ, Tucker SB, Wilkin JK. Reactive perforating collagenosis of diabetes mellitus and renal failure. *Cutis*. 1983;31(1):55-58.
45. Garcia-Bravo B, Rodriguez-Pichardo A, Camacho F. Uraemic follicular hyperkeratosis. *Clin Exp Dermatol*. 1985;10(5):448-454.
46. Bank DE, Cohen PR, Kohn SR. Reactive perforating collagenosis in a setting of double disaster: acquired immunodeficiency syndrome and end-stage renal disease. *J Am Acad Dermatol*. 1989;21(2, pt 2):371-374.
47. Rubio FA, Herranz P, Robayna G, et al. Perforating folliculitis: report of a case in an HIV-infected man. *J Am Acad Dermatol*. 1999;40(2, pt 2):300-302.
48. Ghosh SK, Bandyopadhyay D, Chatterjee G. Acquired reactive perforating collagenosis following insect bite. *Indian J Dermatol Venereol Leprol*. 2009;75(3):306-307.
49. Yamashita N, Watanabe D, Ozawa H, et al. Reactive perforating collagenosis with cutaneous cytomegalovirus infection. *Eur J Dermatol*. 2006;16(6):696-697.
50. Zelger B, Hintner H, Auböck J, et al. Acquired perforating dermatosis. Transepidermal elimination of DNA material and possible role of leukocytes in pathogenesis. *Arch Dermatol*. 1991;127(5):695-700.
51. Pedragosa R, Knobel HJ, Huguet P, et al. Reactive perforating collagenosis in Hodgkin's disease. *Am J Dermatopathol*. 1987;9(1):41-44.
52. Bong JL, Fleming CJ, Kemmett D. Reactive perforating collagenosis associated with underlying malignancy. *Br J Dermatol*. 2000;142(2):390-391.
53. Chae KS, Park YM, Cho SH, et al. Reactive perforating collagenosis associated with periampullary carcinoma. *Br J Dermatol*. 1998;139(3):548-550.
54. Boeck K, Mempel M, Hein R, et al. Acquired perforating collagenosis in a patient with carcinoma of the prostate. *Acta Derm Venereol*. 1997;77(6):486-487.
55. Kilic A, Gönül M, Cakmak SK, et al. Acquired reactive perforating collagenosis as a presenting sign of hepatocellular carcinoma. *Eur J Dermatol*. 2006;16(4):447.
56. Yazdi S, Saadat P, Young S, et al. Acquired reactive perforating collagenosis associated with papillary thyroid carcinoma: a paraneoplastic phenomenon? *Clin Exp Dermatol*. 2010;35(2):152-155.
57. Shiomi T, Yoshida Y, Horie Y, et al. Acquired reactive perforating collagenosis with the histological features of IgG4-related sclerosing disease in a patient with Mikulicz's disease. *Pathol Int*. 2009;59(5):326-331.
58. Fistarol SK, Itin PH. Acquired perforating dermatosis in a patient with Poland syndrome. *Dermatology*. 2003;207(4):390-394.
59. Skiba G, Milkiewicz P, Mutimer D, et al. Successful treatment of acquired perforating dermatosis with rifampicin in an Asian patient with sclerosing cholangitis. *Liver*. 1999;19(2):160-163.
60. Kim JH, Kang WH. Acquired reactive perforating collagenosis in a diabetic patient with pulmonary aspergillosis. *Cutis*. 2000;66(6):425-430.
61. Fatani MI, Al-Ghamdi YM, Al-Afif KA, et al. Acquired reactive perforating collagenosis associated with sick euthyroid syndrome. *Saudi Med J*. 2002;23(11):1408-1410.
62. Berger RS. Reactive perforating collagenosis of renal failure/diabetes responsive to topical retinoic acid. *Cutis*. 1989;43(6):540-542.
63. Petrozzi JW, Warthan TL. Kyrle disease. Treatment with topically applied tretinoin. *Arch Dermatol*. 1974;110(5):762-765.
64. Cullen SI. Successful treatment of reactive perforating collagenosis with tretinoin. *Cutis*. 1979;23(2):187-191, 193.
65. Outland JD, Brown TS, Callen JP. Tazarotene is an effective therapy for elastosis perforans serpiginosa. *Arch Dermatol*. 2002;138(2):169-171.
66. Satchell AC, Crotty K, Lee S. Reactive perforating collagenosis: a condition that may be underdiagnosed. *Australas J Dermatol*. 2001;42(4):284-287.
67. Ratnavel RC, Norris PG. Penicillamine-induced elastosis perforans serpiginosa treated successfully with isotretinoin. *Dermatology*. 1994;189(1):81-83.
68. Jan V, Saugier J, Arbeille B, et al. Elastosis perforans serpiginosa with vitamin A deficiency in a child with trisomy 21 [in French]. *Ann Dermatol Venereol*. 1996;123(3):188-190.
69. Baumer FE, Wolter M, Marsch WC. The Kyrle disease entity and its therapeutic modification by acitretin (etretin) [in German]. *Z Hautkr*. 1989;64(4):286, 289-291.
70. Iwamoto I, Baba S, Suzuki H. Acquired reactive perforating collagenosis with IgA nephropathy. *J Dermatol*. 1998;25(9):597-600.
71. Hoque SR, Ameen M, Holden CA. Acquired reactive perforating collagenosis: four patients with a giant variant treated with allopurinol. *Br J Dermatol*. 2006;154(4):759-762.
72. Gnanaraj P, Venugopal V, Sangitha C, et al. A giant variant of acquired reactive perforating collagenosis associated with hydronephrosis: successful treatment with allopurinol. *Int J Dermatol*. 2009;48(2):204-206.
73. Gönül M, Cakmak SK, Gül U, et al. Two cases of acquired perforating dermatosis treated with doxycycline therapy. *Int J Dermatol*. 2006;45(12):1461-1463.
74. Brinkmeier T, Schaller J, Herbst RA, et al. Successful treatment of acquired reactive perforating collagenosis with doxycycline. *Acta Derm Venereol*. 2002;82(5):393-395.
75. Khalifa M, Slim I, Kaabia N, et al. Regression of skin lesions of Kyrle's disease with metronidazole in a diabetic patient. *J Infect*. 2007;55(6):e139-e140.
76. Kasiakou SK, Peppas G, Kapaskelis AM, et al. Regression of skin lesions of Kyrle's disease with clindamycin: implications for an infectious component in the etiology of the disease. *J Infect*. 2005;50(5):412-416.
77. Lubbe J, Sorg O, Malé PJ, et al. Sirolimus-induced inflammatory papules with acquired reactive perforating collagenosis. *Dermatology*. 2008;216(3):239-242.

78. Hurwitz RM. The evolution of perforating folliculitis in patients with chronic renal failure. *Am J Dermatopathol*. 1985;7(3):231-239.
79. Serrano G, Aliaga A, Lorente M. Reactive perforating collagenosis responsive to PUVA. *Int J Dermatol*. 1988;27(2):118-119.
80. Tuyp EJ, McLeod WA. Elastosis perforans serpiginosa: treatment with liquid nitrogen. *Int J Dermatol*. 1990;29(9):655-656.
81. Abdullah A, Colloby PS, Foulds IS, et al. Localized idiopathic elastosis perforans serpiginosa effectively treated by the Coherent Ultrapulse 5000C aesthetic laser. *Int J Dermatol*. 2000;39(9):719-720.
82. Chan LY, Tang WY, Lo KK. Treatment of pruritus of reactive perforating collagenosis using transcutaneous electrical nerve stimulation. *Eur J Dermatol*. 2000;10(1):59-61.
83. Oziemski MA, Billson VR, Crosthwaite GL, et al. A new treatment for acquired reactive perforating collagenosis. *Australas J Dermatol*. 1991;32(2):71-74.

Chapter 72 :: Genetic Disorders Affecting Dermal Connective Tissue
:: Jonathan A. Dyer

第七十二章

影响真皮结缔组织的遗传性疾病

中文导读

遗传性结缔组织疾病的临床和基因背景各不相同，影响皮肤、关节，及各种其他的皮肤外组织器官，包括心血管系统。皮肤表型的性质和严重程度取决于突变类型以及受影响蛋白质对皮肤结构和功能的作用。本章从流行病学、临床特征、病因学及发病学、实验室检验、鉴别诊断及预防和治疗等方面描述了Ehlers-Danlos综合征（EDS）疾病。这是一组以不同程度的皮肤脆弱性和过度伸展性增加以及关节过度活动为特征的遗传和临床异质性疾病。EDS的严重程度范围从只有轻微的临床症状到严重衰弱均可见到。皮肤特征包括不同程度的皮肤脆弱性和过度伸展性。经典型表现为柔软、光滑的皮肤，容易擦伤，伤口愈合为薄、萎缩、裂开的疤痕。皮肤外表现包括关节活动过度伴经常脱位，妊娠和分娩并发症，以及较少见的心血管表现，特别是主动脉根部扩张。几种罕见的EDS临床特征在文中也有描述；特别列出了经典样EDS、血管亚型、超活动型的临床特点。并详细描述了导致该病的基因突变问题，对于怀疑有EDS变异的患者，目前的指导原则建议尽可能使用二代序列对多个已知EDS基因进行并行测序。对于那些未发现突变或仅有一个AR突变的患者，进一步进行拷贝数变异分析或全外显子组测序/全基因组测序，重点是EDS基因以及它们的调控序列。要意识到不确定意义的变异（VUS），使一些患者的遗传评估复杂化。多学科预防策略是管理EDS患者最有效的方法。早期识别受影响的患者并进行适当的干预（疼痛管理、物理治疗、手术）和教育是很重要的。马凡氏综合征是一种主要影响骨骼、眼部和心血管（CV）系统的常染色体显性遗传疾病。本节从流行病学、临床特征、病因及发病机制、实验室检查、鉴别诊断及治疗方面对本病进行了阐述。本病表现为3个主要器官系统的异常：眼（典型的晶状体脱位）、骨骼（四肢过长、关节松动、前胸畸形和后凸畸形），最重要的是心血管（典型的动脉瘤和二尖瓣赘）。马凡氏综合征的诊断是基于一系列临床发现。实验室检查或组织学检查无诊断性帮助。基因检测有助于诊断。本节从流行病学、临床特征、病因及发病机制、实验室检查、鉴别诊断、预防及治疗方面阐述了弹性纤维假黄瘤。PXE中的皮肤在颈部两侧和脖颈（图72-8）、会阴、腋窝、脐部和弯曲褶皱处显示出淡黄色、平顶、离散和融合的丘疹，皮肤松弛程度随年龄增长而增加。皮肤外表现包括血管样条纹、视力损害、视网膜色素沉着、心血管疾病和出血。乳腺和睾丸发生微钙化，可能被误认为恶性肿瘤。PXE患者皮损活检的组织学改变是诊断性的，表现为明显的嗜碱性弹性纤维断裂卷曲，von-Kossa染色能很容易地检测到弹性纤维上的钙沉积。PXE没有治愈方法，需要多学科合作来解决该疾病的各种表现。本节从流行病学、临床特征、病因及发病机制、实验室检查、鉴别诊断、获得性皮肤松弛症、治疗等方面阐述了皮肤松弛症（泛发性弹性组织溶解），该病以AD、AR和X连锁形式存在，其中隐性形式最为常见。本章描述了各型的临床特点及受累器官相关症状。列出了与继发性CL相关的药物及疾病以及临床表现和组织学特点。应尽可能进行遗传检测，以确定潜在的遗传缺陷。本节从流行病学、临床特征、病因及发病机制、诊断、鉴别诊断、临床进程及预后、管理等方面描述了BUSCHKE-OLLEN-DORFF综合征，皮肤特征包括弹性瘤和胶原瘤（播散性豆状皮肤纤维化）。皮肤外表现包括可能被误认为恶性肿瘤的骨斑点症。无严重全身后遗症。诊断主要基于临床怀疑或影像学特征性骨异常的检测。鉴别诊断包括无骨病变的结缔组织痣、硬斑病和PXE。诊断后一般不需要进行任何干预。本节从流行病学、临床特征、病因及发病机制、实验室检查、特殊检查、鉴别诊断、预后及临床进程、治疗、预防等方面全面介绍了类脂蛋白沉积的特点。诊断LP最可靠的临床征象是声音嘶哑，舌下系带增厚阻碍患者舌头伸出，次要特征包括眼睑珠状丘疹、肘部和前臂伸侧周围皮肤疣状丘疹浸润和轻度脱发。

〔施　为〕

Inherited connective tissue disorders are clinically and genetically diverse conditions affecting the skin, joints, and a variety of extracutaneous tissues, including the cardiovascular (CV) system. The nature and severity of the skin phenotype is dependent on the type of mutation as well as the role of the affected protein on dermal structure and function (see Chaps. 15 and 18). The diagnosis of many inherited connective tissue disorders is clinical, although Clinical Laboratory Improvement Amendments (1988) (CLIA)-approved genetic testing is increasingly available. A listing of research laboratories that might offer testing can be found at http://www.genetests.org.

EHLERS-DANLOS SYNDROMES

AT-A-GLANCE

- Combined incidence of almost 1 in 5000 persons.
- Thirteen subtypes.
- Most commonly autosomal dominant (classical and hypermobile types).
- Defects in the Type V collagen gene most commonly cause the classical subtype.
- Cutaneous features include varying degrees of skin fragility and hyperextensibility. The classical subtype exhibits soft, velvety skin that bruises easily and wounds that heal as thin, atrophic, gaping scars.
- Extracutaneous manifestations include hypermobile joints with frequent dislocations, complications with pregnancy and delivery, and, less commonly, cardiovascular manifestations, particularly aortic root dilation.
- Information for patients and professionals at http://www.ehlers-danlos.org and https://www.ehlers-danlos.com/.

A variety of genetically and clinically heterogeneous inherited conditions characterized by varying degrees of skin fragility and hyperextensibility, and joint hypermobility have been collected under the rubric of the Ehlers-Danlos syndromes (EDS). A new classification system published in 2017[1] attempted to consolidate and simplify existing subgroups (Table 72-1) as well as reconcile new genetic discoveries with existing clinical phenotypes. Major and minor diagnostic criteria were developed for each major subtype of EDS. Despite these revisions, many patients defy clear-cut classification. The spectrum of EDS severity ranges from subtle clinical findings to severe, debilitating disease.

TABLE 72-1
The Ehlers-Danlos Syndromes: Clinical Subtypes and Associated Defects

CLINICAL EDS SUBTYPE (ABBREVIATION: OMIM #)	CLINICAL FEATURES	INHERITANCE	PROTEIN/(GENE DEFECT)
Classical (cEDS:130000 and 130010)	Hyperextensible skin; easy bruising; wide, atrophic scars; hypermobile joints	AD	Collagen Type V/(COL5A1, COL5A2)
Classical-like EDS (clEDS: 606408)	Similar to cEDS but without atrophic scarring; foot deformities; muscle weakness; acrogeria; axonal polyneuropathy	AR	Tenascin XB/(TNXB)
Cardiac-valvular EDS (cvEDS:225320)	Similar to cEDS but with severe, progressive, cardiac valvular disease	AR	Type I collagen/(COL1A2—biallelic mutations leading to nonsense-mediated messenger RNA decay and loss of pro a2(I) collagen chains
Vascular EDS (vEDS:130050)	Thin, translucent skin with easy bruising; arterial and visceral rupture; typical facies	AD	Major: collagen Type III/(COL3A1) Rare: Type I collagen/(COL1A1: c.934C>T, p.[Arg312 Cys]; c.1720C>T, p.[Arg574Cys]; c.3227C>T, p.[Arg1093Cys])
Hypermobile EDS (hEDS: 130020)	Smooth, velvety skin; joint hypermobility	AD/AR	Unclear for most; collagen Type III; tenascin XB/(COL3A1; TNXB)[a]
Arthrochalasia EDS (aEDS: 130060)	Hyperextensible and fragile skin; severe joint hypermobility; congenital hip dislocation	AD	Collagen Type I/(COL1A1; COL1A2)
Dermatosparaxis EDS (dEDS: 225410)	Severely fragile, sagging, redundant skin; hernias and premature rupture of fetal membranes	AR	Procollagen I N-peptidase/(ADAMTS2)
Kyphoscoliotic EDS (kEDS: 225400 and 229200)	Atrophic scars, easy bruising; neonatal hypotonia; scoliosis; ocular rupture; marfanoid habitus	AR	Lysyl hydroxylase/(PLOD1) FKBP22/(FKBP14)
Brittle cornea syndrome (BCS: 229200/614170)	Thin cornea; early-onset progressive keratoconus/keratoglobus; blue sclerae; corneal scarring; retinal detachment; deafness; developmental hip dysplasia; scoliosis; arachnodactyly; distal joint hypermobility; soft, velvety, thin skin	AR	ZNF469/(ZNF469) PRDM5/(PRDM5)
Spondylodysplastic EDS (spEDS: 612350/130070/271640)	Progressive short stature; variable muscle hypotonia; limb bowing; hyperextensible skin; delayed motor and cognitive development; osteopenia; characteristic radiographic findings	AR	B4GalT7/(B4GALT7) B3GalT6/(B3GALT6) ZIP13/(SLC39A13)
Musculocontractural EDS (mcEDS: 601776)	Congenital multiple contractures; characteristic craniofacial features; skin hyperextensibility; easy bruising; skin fragility with atrophic scars; increased palmar wrinkling; recurrent/chronic dislocations; chronic constipation and colonic diverticula; pneumothorax/pneumohemothorax	AR	D4ST1/(CHST14) DSE/(DSE)
Myopathic EDS (mEDS: 616470)	Congenital muscle hypotonia and/or atrophy improving with age; proximal joint contractures; distal joint hypermobility; soft, doughy skin with atrophic scarring; motor developmental delay with myopathy on biopsy	AD/AR	Type XII collagen/(COL12A1)
Periodontal EDS (pEDS: 130080/617174)	Severe, intractable, early-onset periodontitis; gingival detachment; pretibial plaques; family history; easy bruising; distal joint hypermobility; skin hyperextensibility, fragility, abnormal scarring (wide/atrophic); increased rate of infections; marfanoid facial features; acrogeria; prominent vasculature	AD	C1r/(C1R) C1s/(C1S)

[a]Few reported cases.
AD, autosomal dominant; AR, autosomal recessive; EDS, Ehlers-Danlos syndrome; OMIM, Online Mendelian Inheritance in Man.
Table adapted from Malfait F, Francomano C, Byers P, et al. The 2017 international classification of the Ehlers-Danlos syndromes. Am J Med Genet C Semin Med Genet. 2017;175(1):8-26.

TABLE 72-2
Revised Diagnostic Criteria for Ehlers-Danlos Syndrome Subtypes

EHLERS-DANLOS SYNDROME (EDS) SUBTYPE	MAJOR CRITERIA	MINOR CRITERIA	MINIMAL DIAGNOSTIC CRITERIA
Classical EDS (cEDS)	1. Skin hyperextensibility (Remvig; see Table 72-3) and atrophic scarring 2. Generalized joint hypermobility (GJH) (Beighton; see Table 72-4)	1. Easy bruising 2. Soft, doughy skin 3. Skin fragility (or traumatic splitting) 4. Molluscoid pseudotumors 5. Subcutaneous spheroids 6. Hernia (or history thereof) 7. Epicanthal folds 8. Complications of joint hypermobility (eg, sprains, luxation/subluxation, pain, flexible flatfoot) 9. Family history of a first-degree relative who meets clinical criteria	– Major criterion (1): skin hyperextensibility and atrophic scarring *plus* – Either major criterion (2): GJH – And/or: at least 3 minor criteria Confirmatory molecular testing obligatory to reach a final diagnosis
Classical-like EDS (clEDS)	1. Skin hyperextensibility, velvety skin texture, but *no* atrophic scarring 2. GJH with or without dislocations (shoulder/ankle) 3. Easy or spontaneous bruising	1. Foot deformities including brachydactyly with excessive skin; piezogenic papules; hallux valgus; pes planus; a "broad/plump forefoot" 2. Leg edema—without cardiac failure 3. Mild proximal and distal muscle weakness 4. Axonal polyneuropathy 5. Muscle atrophy of hands/feet 6. Acrogeria (hands) 7. Prolapse of the vagina/uterus/rectum	3 Major *and* family history consistent with autosomal recessive (AR) transmission Confirmatory molecular testing is necessary for diagnosis
Cardiac-valvular EDS (cvEDS)	1. Severe progressive cardiac-valvular problems (aortic valve, mitral valve) 2. Skin involvement: skin hyperextensibility, atrophic scars, thin skin, easy bruising 3. Joint hypermobility (generalized or restricted to small joints)	1. Inguinal hernia 2. Pectus deformity (especially excavatum) 3. Joint dislocations 4. Foot deformities: pes planus, pes planovalgus, hallux valgus	Major criterion (1): severe progressive cardiac-valvular problems *and* a family history compatible with AR inheritance *plus* – Either: 1 other major criterion – And/or: at least 2 minor criteria Confirmatory molecular testing is obligatory to reach a final diagnosis
Vascular EDS (vEDS)	1. Family history of vEDS with documented causative variant in *COL3A1* 2. Arterial rupture at a young age 3. Spontaneous sigmoid colon perforation in the absence of known diverticular disease or other bowel pathology 4. Uterine rupture during the third trimester in the absence of previous C-section and/or severe peripartum perineum tears 5. Carotid-cavernous sinus fistula (CCSF) formation in the absence of trauma	1. Bruising unrelated to identified trauma and/or in unusual sites such as cheeks and back 2. Thin, translucent skin with increased venous visibility 3. Characteristic facial appearance 4. Spontaneous pneumothorax 5. Acrogeria 6. Talipes equinovarus 7. Congenital hip dislocation 8. Hypermobility of small joints 9. Tendon and muscle rupture 10. Keratoconus 11. Gingival recession and gingival fragility 12. Early-onset varicose veins (younger than age 30 years and nulliparous if female)	1. A family history consistent with or suggestive of vEDS *or*: 2. Arterial rupture/dissection in individual younger than age 40 years 3. Unexplained sigmoid colon rupture 4. Spontaneous pneumothorax + other suggestive features 5. Any of the above should lead to testing to rule out vEDS; if multiple other "minor" features listed above are present then testing should also be considered; because of the difficulty in making a clinical diagnosis of vEDS, there is a very low threshold for genetic testing of *COL3A1* in patients with suspicious findings

(Continued)

TABLE 72-2
Revised Diagnostic Criteria for Ehlers-Danlos Syndrome Subtypes (*Continued*)

EHLERS-DANLOS SYNDROME (EDS) SUBTYPE	MAJOR CRITERIA	MINOR CRITERIA	MINIMAL DIAGNOSTIC CRITERIA

Hypermobile EDS (hEDS)	1. GJH (varies with gender/age)
	  a. Beighton score: ≥6 (prepubertal children/adolescents); ≥5 (puberty to 50 years old); ≥4 (>50 years old)
	  b. If acquired joint limitations affecting score calculation then include 5-point questionnaire (5PQ)
	2. Two or more of the following
	  a. Systemic manifestations of a more generalized connective tissue disorder (total of 5 of the following)
	    i. Unusually soft/velvety skin
	    ii. Mild skin hyperextensibility
	    iii. Unexplained striae
	    iv. Bilateral piezogenic papules of the heel
	    v. Recurrent/multiple abdominal hernia (umbilical/inguinal crural)
	    vi. Atrophic scarring of at least 2 sites (but not as severe as cEDS)
	    vii. Pelvic floor, rectal, and/or uterine prolapse in children, men, nulliparous women without predisposing conditions
	    viii. Dental crowding/high/narrow palate
	    ix. Arachnodactyly + Wrist (Steinberg) sign bilaterally + Thumb (Walker) sign bilaterally
	    x. Arm span-to-height ratio ≥1.05
	    xi. Mitral valve prolapse: mild or greater
	    xii. Aortic root dilation with Z-score greater than +2
	  b. Positive family history (using current diagnostic criteria)
	  c. Musculoskeletal complications (at least 1)
	    i. Musculoskeletal pain in 2 or more limbs; daily for at least 3 months
	    ii. Chronic, widespread pain for ≥3 months
	    iii. Recurrent joint dislocations/joint instability without trauma
	      Three or more atraumatic dislocations of same joint or 2 or more atraumatic dislocations in 2 different joints at different times
	      Medical confirmation of joint instability at 2 or more sites not related to trauma
	3. All of the following:
	  a. No unusual skin fragility
	  b. Exclusion of other inherited/acquired connective tissue disorders
	  c. Exclusion of alternative diagnoses causing joint hypermobility
		—	All 3 of the major criteria must be met

(*Continued*)

TABLE 72-2
Revised Diagnostic Criteria for Ehlers-Danlos Syndrome Subtypes (*Continued*)

EHLERS-DANLOS SYNDROME (EDS) SUBTYPE	MAJOR CRITERIA	MINOR CRITERIA	MINIMAL DIAGNOSTIC CRITERIA
Arthrochalasia EDS (aEDS)	1. Congenital bilateral hip dislocation (1 unilateral case) 2. Severe GJH—multiple dislocations/subluxations 3. Skin hyperextensibility	1. Muscle hypotonia 2. Kyphoscoliosis 3. Radiologically mild osteopenia 4. Tissue fragility; atrophic scars 5. Easy bruising	Major criterion 1 plus either major criterion 2 and at least 2 minor criteria or major criterion 3 Confirmatory molecular testing is necessary Heterozygous mutations in *COL1A1* or *COL1A2* causing partial/entire loss of exon 6

Dermatosparaxis EDS (dEDS)	1. Extreme skin fragility: congenital or postnatal skin tearing
	2. Typical craniofacial features: may present at birth or develop in childhood
	  a. Prominent/protuberant eyes—puffy eyelids with edema
	  b. Excess periorbital skin
	  c. Epicanthal folds
	  d. Downslanting palpebral fissures
	  e. Blue sclerae
	  f. Large fontanels/wide cranial sutures; delayed closure of fontanels
	  g. Hypoplastic chin
	3. Redundant skin, excess folds at wrists/ankles—almost lax
	4. Increased palmar wrinkling
	5. Severe bruising: subcutaneous hematoma/hemorrhage
	6. Umbilical hernia
	7. Postnatal growth retardation
	8. Short limbs, hands, feet
	9. Perinatal complications from connective tissue fragility: congenital skull fractures, intracerebral hemorrhage, friable umbilical cord, congenital skin tearing, neonatal pneumothorax
		1. Soft, doughy skin
		2. Skin hyperextensibility
		3. Atrophic scars
		4. GJH
		5. Complications of visceral fragility
		  a. Bladder rupture
		  b. Diaphragm rupture
		  c. Rectal prolapse
		6. Delayed motor development
		7. Osteopenia
		8. Hirsutism
		9. Abnormal teeth
		10. Refractive errors
		11. Strabismus
			Major criteria 1 and 2 plus 1 other major and/or 3 minor criteria
			Confirmatory testing is necessary: *ADAMTS2* # encodes ADAMTS-2, the main procollagen I *N*-proteinase

Kyphoscoliotic (kEDS)	1. Congenital muscle hypotonia—often striking
	2. Congenital/early-onset kyphoscoliosis (progressive or nonprogressive)
	3. GJH with dislocations/subluxation (especially shoulders/hips/knees)
		1. Skin hyperextensibility
		2. Easy bruising
		3. Rupture/aneurysms of medium sized arteries
		4. Osteopenia/osteoporosis
		5. Blue sclerae
		6. Hernia (umbilical/inguinal)
		7. Pectus
		8. Marfanoid habitus
		9. Talipes equinovarus
		10. Refractive errors
		Gene-specific minor criteria:
		1. *PLOD1* (Majority of kEDS patients)
		  a. Skin fragility (easy bruising; friable skin; poor healing; widened atrophic scars)
		  b. Scleral/ocular fragility/rupture
		  c. Microcornea
		  d. Facial dysmorphology:
		    i. Low-set ears
		    ii. Epicanthal folds
		    iii. Down-slanting palpebral fissures
		    iv. Synophrys
		    v. High palate
		2. *FKBP14*
		  a. Congenital hearing impairment
		  b. Follicular hyperkeratosis
		  c. Muscle atrophy
		  d. Bladder diverticula
			Major criteria 1 and 2 plus major criterion 3 and/or 3 minor criteria (general or gene-specific)
			Confirmatory molecular testing is necessary
			Laboratory confirmation of kEDS: quantification of deoxypyridinoline and pyridinoline crosslinks in urine by high-performance liquid chromatography; an increased deoxypyridinoline-to-pyridinoline ratio (often 2-9 [10 to 40 times the reference range of 0.2]) is a highly sensitive and specific test for kEDS caused by biallelic PLOD1 mutations (kEDS-PLOD1), but is normal for biallelic *FKBP14* mutations (kEDS-FKBP14); this rapid and cost-effective test can also determine the importance of variants of uncertain significance detected in PLOD1

(*Continued*)

TABLE 72-2
Revised Diagnostic Criteria for Ehlers-Danlos Syndrome Subtypes (*Continued*)

EHLERS–DANLOS SYNDROME (EDS) SUBTYPE	MAJOR CRITERIA	MINOR CRITERIA	MINIMAL DIAGNOSTIC CRITERIA
Brittle cornea syndrome (BCS)	1. Thin cornea—with or without rupture 2. Early-onset progressive keratoconus 3. Early-onset progressive keratoglobus 4. Blue sclerae	1. Enucleation/corneal scarring from previous rupture 2. Progressive loss of corneal stromal depth 3. High myopia 4. Retinal detachment 5. Deafness 6. Hypercompliant tympanic membranes 7. Developmental dysplasia of the hip 8. Infantile hypotonia (mild) 9. Scoliosis 10. Arachnodactyly 11. Distal joint hypermobility 12. Pes planes; hallux valgus 13. Mild fifth finger contracture 14. Soft, velvety skin; translucent skin	Major criterion 1 plus 1 other major criterion and/or 3 minor criteria Confirmatory molecular testing is necessary AR mutations in *ANF469* (encodes ZNF469, a zinc finger protein) or *PRDM5* (encodes a DNA binding transcription factor of the PR-SET protein family and lacks intrinsic histone methyltransferase activity)

Spondylodysplastic EDS (spEDS)	1. Short stature (progressive during childhood)
	2. Muscle hypotonia (variable severity)
	3. Limb bowing
		1. Skin hyperextensibility, soft, doughy skin, thin translucent skin
		2. Pes planus
		3. Delayed motor development
		4. Osteopenia
		5. Delayed cognitive development
		Gene-specific minor criteria:
		B3GALT6
		  1. Kyphoscoliosis
		  2. Joint hypermobility: either GJH or distal joints
		  3. Joint contractures (especially hands)
		  4. Abnormal fingers (slender; tapered; arachnodactyly; spatulate, broad distal phalanges)
		  5. Talipes
		  6. Characteristic Craniofacial features
		  7. Tooth discoloration, dysplasia
		  8. Characteristic radiologic findings
		  9. Osteoporosis with multiple spontaneous fractures
		  10. Ascending aortic aneurysm
		  11. Lung hypoplasia; restrictive lung disease
		B4GALT7
		  1. Radioulnar synostosis
		  2. Bilateral elbow contracture/limited movement
		  3. GJH
		  4. Single transverse palmar crease
		  5. Characteristic facial features
		  6. Characteristic radiographic findings
		  7. Severe hypermetropia
		  8. Clouded cornea
		SLC39A13
		  1. Protuberant eyes/bluish sclerae
		  2. Fine palmar wrinkles
		  3. Thenar muscle atrophy; tapered fingers
		  4. Distal joint hypermobility
		  5. Characteristic radiologic findings
			Major criteria 1 and 2 plus characteristic radiographic findings and at least 3 minor criteria (general or type specific)

(*Continued*)

TABLE 72-2
Revised Diagnostic Criteria for Ehlers-Danlos Syndrome Subtypes (Continued)

EHLERS-DANLOS SYNDROME (EDS) SUBTYPE	MAJOR CRITERIA	MINOR CRITERIA	MINIMAL DIAGNOSTIC CRITERIA
Musculocontractural EDS (mcEDS)	1. Congenital multiple contractures 2. Characteristic craniofacial features (birth/early infancy) 3. Skin hyperextensibility; easy bruising; skin fragility with atrophic scars; increased palmar wrinkling	1. Recurrent/chronic dislocations 2. Pectus 3. Spinal deformities 4. Abnormal fingers 5. Progressive talipes deformities 6. Large subcutaneous hematomas 7. Chronic constipation 8. Colonic diverticulae 9. Pneumothorax/pneumohemothorax 10. Nephrolithiasis/cystolithiasis 11. Hydronephrosis 12. Cryptorchidism 13. Strabismus 14. Refractive errors 15. Glaucoma	*Birth thru early childhood:* Major criteria 1 and 2 *Adolescence thru Adulthood:* Major criteria 1 and 3 Confirmatory molecular testing is necessary to confirm
Myopathic EDS (mEDS)	1. Congenital muscle hypotonia and/or atrophy a. Improves with age 2. Proximal joint contractures 3. Distal joint hypermobility	1. Soft, doughy skin 2. Atrophic scarring 3. Motor developmental delay 4. Muscle biopsy shows myopathy	Major criterion 1 plus 1 other major criterion and/or 3 minor criteria Confirmatory molecular testing is necessary to confirm mEDS caused by heterozygous or biallelic mutations in *COL12A1*—encodes Type XII collagen; high overlap with Type VI related myopathies such as Bethlem myopathy and Ulrich congenital muscular dystrophy
Periodontal EDS (pEDS)	1. Severe, intractable periodontitis—early onset 2. Lack of attached gingiva 3. Pretibial plaques 4. Family history: first-degree relative meeting diagnostic criteria	1. Easy bruising 2. Joint hypermobility—mostly distal 3. Skin hyperextensibility, fragility, abnormal scarring (wide/atrophic) 4. Increase rate of infections 5. Hernia 6. Marfanoid facial features 7. Acrogeria 8. Prominent vasculature	Major criterion 1 or 2 plus at least 2 other major criteria and 1 minor criteria Confirmatory molecular testing is necessary to confirm pEDS caused by heterozygous gain-of-function mutations in *C1R* or *C1S*—first components (subunits C1r and C1s) of classical complement pathway

Adapted from Malfait F, Francomano C, Byers P, et al. The 2017 international classification of the Ehlers-Danlos syndromes. *Am J Med Genet C Semin Med Genet.* 2017;175(1):8-26.

EPIDEMIOLOGY

EDS prevalence may be as high as 1:5000 individuals. Classical EDS (cEDS) occurs in 1 in 10,000 to 20,000 newborns. The vascular subtype is the most clinically significant EDS subtype because of the risk of arterial or major organ rupture. Inherited in an autosomal dominant (AD) fashion, the incidence is approximately 1 in 50,000 to 200,000 individuals.[2] The kyphoscoliosis, arthrochalasia, and dermatosparaxis subtypes are considerably less common than the classical, hypermobility, and vascular types. Confusion over the diagnosis of the hypermobility type and its overlap with joint hypermobility syndrome interferes with prevalence estimates, but if inclusive definitions are used, it may be the most common subtype.

CLINICAL FEATURES

Table 72-2 summarizes the clinical diagnostic criteria for EDS subtypes.

CLASSICAL EHLERS-DANLOS SYNDROME

Patients with cEDS (Online Mendelian Inheritance in Man [OMIM]: 130000) typically exhibit skin hyperextensibility and fragility along with atrophic scarring, and generalized joint hypermobility. In the past, patients exhibiting very mild features were termed "mitis." The skin in cEDS patients is hyperextensible (Fig. 72-1) but recoils easily to its normal

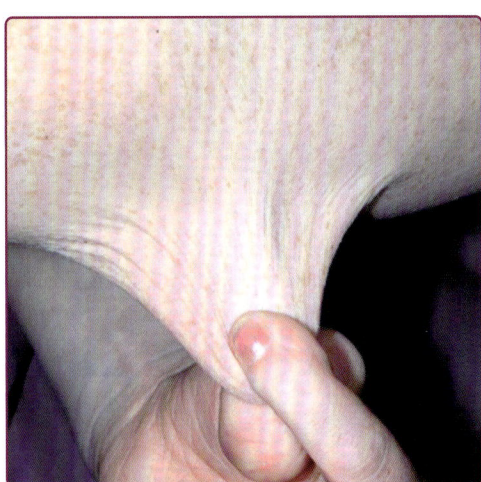

Figure 72-1 Classical Ehlers-Danlos syndrome. Dermal elasticity is demonstrated. Unlike cutis laxa, the skin returns to original shape after stretching.

position after stretching, in contrast to the skin in cutis laxa (CL).

Skin hyperextensibility should be assessed using the Remvig et al[3] criteria (Table 72-3) by pinching and lifting the skin, pulling until resistance is met, at a site not subjected to mechanical forces or scarring, such as the volar surface of the nondominant forearm. Hyperextensibility is present if the skin can be stretched beyond 1.5 cm on the distal forearms and/or dorsal hands and beyond 3 cm at the neck, elbow, and/or knees.

The skin is velvety, thin, and bruises easily. Fetuses with cEDS may exhibit growth retardation, hernias, and joint dislocations. Bruising manifests early in childhood and is often persistent in areas prone to trauma, especially the shins (Fig. 72-2). Tissue fragility can be striking, with innocuous trauma resulting in disproportionately large skin tears that are relatively painless without excessive bleeding. Wounds often gape.

Even with surgical repair, wounds in EDS often exhibit slow healing and frequent infection. Postoperative wound dehiscence is common, especially if wounds are inadequately secured, often necessitating repeated repairs or secondary intention healing (Fig. 72-3). Even with surgical repair, dehiscence upon suture removal can occur. Healed wounds result in atrophic, often widened cigarette paper-like (or "fish mouth") scars, especially on pressure points (knees,

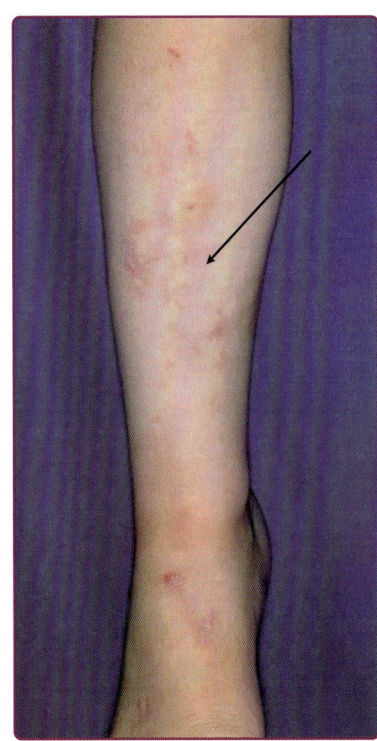

Figure 72-2 Classical Ehlers-Danlos syndrome. Chronic discolored scars on the shin and ankle after repeated trauma. This is often associated with firm subcutaneous nodules that can be confused with subcutaneous granuloma annulare. Note the widened scars along the anterior shin (arrow).

elbows, forehead, chin) (see Figs. 72-2 and 72-3). Hematoma formation and/or recurrent ecchymoses often results in persistent hyperpigmentation. Calcification and fibrosis of hematomas produce subcu-

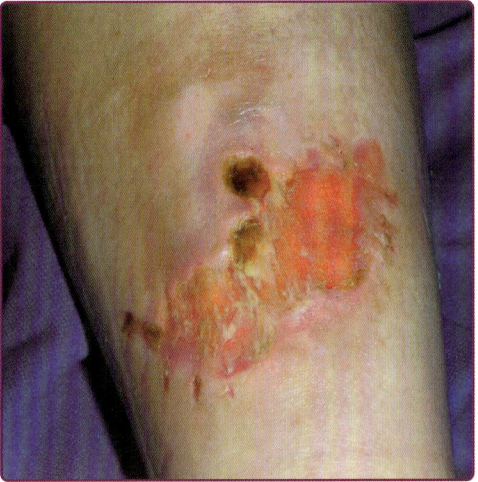

Figure 72-3 Classical Ehlers-Danlos syndrome. After suturing for a laceration, the wound dehisced with secondary infection and marked widening. Note the evidence of former sutures at the lower border, now 3 weeks after the injury and treatment with antibiotics. Scars tend to stretch further in the 6 months after closure.

TABLE 72-3
Criteria for Skin Hyperextensibility[3]

1. Pinch and lift the skin,[a] pulling until resistance is met. Hyperextensibility is present if the skin can be stretched beyond:
2. 1.5 cm on distal forearms and/or dorsal hands
3. 3 cm at neck, elbow, and/or knees.

[a]Best assessed at a site not subjected to mechanical forces or scarring, such as the volar surface of the nondominant forearm.

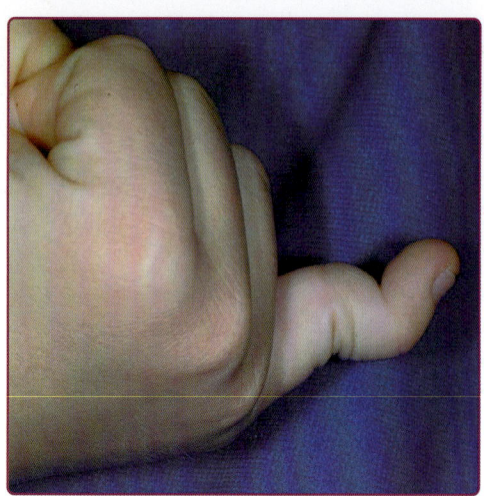

Figure 72-4 Classical Ehlers-Danlos syndrome. Hyperextensibility of digits is demonstrated.

TABLE 72-5
5-Point Questionnaire

An answer in the affirmative to 2 or more of the questions has 85% sensitivity and specificity (tested internationally and in different languages):

1. Can you now (or could you ever) place your hands flat on the floor without bending your knees?
2. Can you now (or could you ever) bend your thumb to touch your forearm?
3. As a child did you amuse your friends by contorting your body into strange shapes or could you do the splits?
4. As a child or teenager did your shoulder or kneecap dislocate on more than 1 occasion?
5. Do you consider yourself double-jointed?

taneous, nodular molluscoid pseudotumors, most frequently around the elbows, fingers, and knee. These are often associated with scars. Spheroids are small subcutaneous spherical hard nodules, usually on the forearms and shins that may become calcified and thus detectable radiographically. Additionally, subcutaneous fat herniation on the medial or lateral aspects of the heels or wrists with pressure (piezogenic pedal papules) may be seen. Epicanthal folds are often present in childhood, although they may not persist in adulthood. Acrocyanosis and chilblains also have been described in affected individuals.

Joint hypermobility is frequent (Fig. 72-4), and often greatest at the fingers and/or wrists. In suspected patients, including older children and adolescents, it is assessed using the Beighton scale (Table 72-4) with a score of 5 or greater out of 9 confirming joint hypermobility. Sprains, dislocations or subluxations, scoliosis, and pes planus are common complications and patients frequently describe chronic joint and limb pain, although skeletal radiographs may be normal. Patients are typically "double-jointed" and often able to perform various "tricks" with their joints as a result. It is important to recognize that chronic and excessive joint hypermobility frequently leads to early-onset osteoarthritis. Joint laxity decreases with age and criteria have been developed (5-point questionnaire; Table 72-5) to address this when evaluating adult patients. Osteoporosis is more common when compared to age-matched controls. Muscle hypotonia and delayed gross motor development are also described. EDS patients are often diagnosed with chronic fatigue syndrome or fibromyalgia because of persistent fatigue and chronic pain. Temporomandibular joint dysfunction is common and a frequent cause of secondary headache in cEDS.

Most patients with cEDS or hypermobile EDS (hEDS) are able to extend the tongue to touch the tip of the nose (Gorlin sign; Fig. 72-5), although this sign can be displayed by approximately 10% of individuals without inherited disorders of connective tissue. Lack of lingual and labial frenula has been described as a minor feature of EDS, and is particularly common in patients with the vascular type.[4] Hypermobility and absence of the frenula allow some EDS patients to "swallow" their own tongue. Hiatal and postoperative hernias, as well as

TABLE 72-4
Beighton Criteria for Joint Hypermobility

1. Passive dorsiflexion of the fifth finger >90 degrees.
2. Passive apposition of the thumbs to the flexor aspect of the forearm (Beighton sign).
3. Hyperextension of the elbow >10 degrees.
4. Hyperextension of the knees >10 degrees.
5. Ability of the palms to completely touch the floor during forward flexion of the trunk with knees fully extended.

Numbers 1 to 4 are scored for each side, so that a maximal score of 2 is possible if both left and right sides meet criterion; number 5 is scored as 1. A person who scores 5 or greater out of 9 is hypermobile.

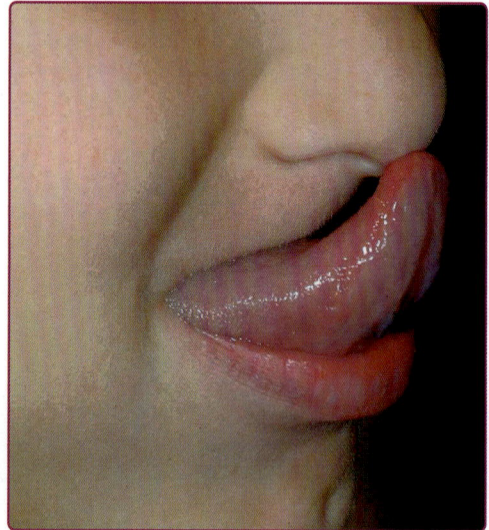

Figure 72-5 Classical Ehlers-Danlos syndrome (EDS). Gorlin sign is the ability to touch the tip of the nose with the tongue and is described in approximately 50% of patients with Ehlers-Danlos, in contrast to 10% of individuals who do not have EDS.

anal prolapse, have been noted as manifestations of the tissue hyperextensibility and fragility. Sexual dysfunction, including dyspareunia is reported, and functional bowel disorders occur in up to half of patients.

Approximately 40% to 50% of affected individuals (in addition to approximately 20% of infants born to affected mothers) are born prematurely (32 to 37 weeks), either as a result of premature rupture of fetal membranes or chorioamnionitis.[5] Monitoring during pregnancy and the postpartum period is recommended, because of the risk of premature labor during the third trimester, the increased risk for skin tears, postpartum hemorrhage, and uterine/bladder prolapse. The fragility of the already abnormal connective tissue may be worsened by the effect of pregnancy-related hormones that soften connective tissue, such as relaxin.

Patients with cEDS occasionally exhibit structural heart malformations. Mitral valve prolapse (MVP), and less often tricuspid valve prolapse, has been noted in approximately 6% of cEDS patients; recent reports suggest that aortic root dilation (typically nonprogressive) may occur more frequently than previously thought.[6] Arterial rupture, intracranial aneurysms, and arteriovenous fistulas have been described in classic EDS, typically in patients exhibiting severe clinical phenotypes, but are much less common than in Marfan syndrome. Baseline echocardiography with measurement of aortic diameter is recommended with CT or MRI examinations if needed. The current recommendation is yearly echocardiogram if cardiac abnormalities (aortic dilation, MVP) are present. If no abnormalities are noted, subsequent studies are only recommended as dictated by symptoms. Blood pressure control, including β-blocker therapy, has been anecdotally successful and should be considered if patients have a glycine substitution near the C-terminus of the triple helix as a result of increased vascular fragility concerns.

Several rare forms of EDS present with skin and joint findings similar to cEDS but with additional important clinical features.

Classical-like EDS with propensity for arterial rupture/vascular-like cEDS is caused by heterozygous COL1A1 c.934C>T, p.(Arg312Cys) substitutions. The substitution of arginine for cysteine in COL1A1 increases the risk for vascular rupture mimicking COL3A1-vascular Ehlers-Danlos syndrome (vEDS). The clinical similarity between this rare variant and cEDS because of COL5A mutations reinforces the value of genetic testing even in "typical" cEDS patients, and the importance of investigating the family history for vascular rupture.[7,8]

An autosomal recessive (AR) *cardiac valvular subtype of EDS* exhibits clinical findings of cEDS as well as the onset of severe cardiac valve problems later in life and results from total loss of the proa2(I) chains of Type I collagen as a result of homozygous or compound heterozygous mutations in COL1A2.[7]

Osteogenesis imperfecta EDS overlap syndrome occurs as a result of mutations at the N-terminal end of both COL1A1 and COL1A2, which affect processing of the N-propeptide; such patients phenotypically present as EDS rather than osteogenesis imperfecta. Mutations

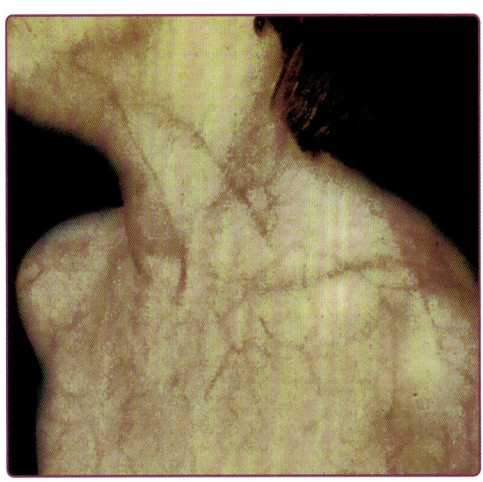

Figure 72-6 Vascular Ehlers-Danlos syndrome. The venous pattern is apparent in a fair-skinned individual. (To enhance visibility of the venous network, the image was colorized.)

in the same area that do not result in delays in Type I procollagen N-propeptide processing present as osteogenesis imperfecta.

CLASSICAL-LIKE EHLERS-DANLOS SYNDROME

An AR form of EDS resembling a mild version of cEDS can result from homozygous tenascin-XB (TNXB) deficiency. Heterozygotes (especially females) for these mutations may exhibit hypermobility EDS.[9,10]

VASCULAR TYPE

The classic quadrad of vEDS includes a characteristic facial appearance (which may be subtle), thin, translucent skin with a prominent venous pattern (Fig. 72-6), extensive bruising or hematomas, and vascular or visceral rupture (or both).[2] Excessive bleeding with circumcision may occur. Joint hypermobility is usually minimal and limited to the digits. The facial features include a thin nose and upper lip, small earlobes, and sunken, pigmented periocular regions. Subcutaneous fat is decreased, especially of the face and limbs. Acrogeria is described, but rare, and often associated with mutations near the carboxyl-terminal end of the COL3A1 triple helical domain. Alopecia is a variable finding but has been significant in some female patients. Widened, thin (papyraceous) scars may be noted on bony prominences. Hematomas, which may be frequent and/or quite large, may develop after minimal to no trauma, such as sphygmomanometer inflation. Ecchymoses during childhood may raise concerns for abuse, similar to cEDS. The development of superficial venous insufficiency before the age of 20 years can be a clinical indicator of vEDS. Superficial venous insufficiency is more common in vEDS, and an unusually complicated response to a vein stripping procedure in a relatively young patient should raise concern for vEDS. Endovenous laser and radiofrequency ablations have been successfully reported in vEDS patients. Gum fragility has been noted in some vEDS patients with loss of gingival tissue and tooth loss that mimics periodontal EDS.

Spontaneous rupture of arteries, particularly mid-sized arteries, may occur during childhood, although the peak age of incidence is the third or fourth decade of life. There may be an increased risk of sudden death from spontaneous vascular rupture in males younger than 20 years old. Mesenchymal abdominal, splenic, and renal arteries are often involved, as is the descending aorta. Aortic rupture/dissection is typically not preceded by detectable aortic dilation,[6] occurs distal to the midaortic arch, and exhibits distal extension. Arterial or intestinal rupture often presents as acute abdominal or flank pain; arterial rupture is the most common cause of death. Stroke is also reported in vEDS. A carotid-cavernous sinus fistula may occur in these patients and represents a medical emergency. Patients note the sudden onset of a temporal swishing sound, with injection of the affected eye, pain, and protrusion of the globe. Pregnancies may be complicated by prepartum and postpartum arterial bleeding, and by intrapartum uterine rupture. Pregnancies carry a 12% to 25% fatality rate. Vaginal and perineal tears from delivery heal poorly and caesarean wounds often dehisce.[2]

Bowel rupture occurs in approximately 25% to 30% of vEDS patients and usually occurs in the sigmoid colon. Spontaneous pneumothorax occurs in approximately 12% of vEDS patients, often later in childhood, and there is a high risk of recurrence. The median life span for vEDS patients is approximately 51 years.[2]

HYPERMOBILITY TYPE

The diagnosis of hEDS is difficult and new diagnostic criteria (see Table 72-2) were developed in an attempt to clarify this complicated category of EDS. Current criteria are clinical and based on appropriate examination and family history. Phenotypic findings are quite variable and many patients who seek medical care are female. Patients with hEDS have abnormal skin, with changes similar to, yet more subtle than cEDS or vEDS. Patients with hEDS have soft, velvety skin with occasional mild hyperextensibility but no fragility. Because hyperextensibility in hEDS can be subtle, the so-called rubber glove skin test is used to distinguish hEDS skin from normal. In this clinical test, the skin of the patient's dorsal hand is pulled upwards and is noted to stretch over a much wider area than typical, often extending to the wrist and beyond. The stretching of the skin mimics that seen when pulling on the back of a rubber glove while wearing it on the hand.

Patients often note easy bruising and piezogenic papules may be seen. The skin may be slightly transparent with more visible veins and tendons, yet it is not nearly as striking as vEDS. In occasional patients, mild prolongation of bleeding can mimic von Willebrand disease. Scarring is variable, and even though some atrophic changes may be noted, these changes are milder and less striking than the changes seen in cEDS. Striae may occur during adolescence in the absence of sudden weight gain. Molluscoid pseudotumors are not seen.[11]

Joint hypermobility is generalized and dislocations of the shoulder, patella, and temporomandibular joints are particularly common. The hips and digits also may be involved and scoliosis and pes planus are also seen. Musculoskeletal pain often has an early onset, is chronic, and often debilitating. Fatigue and sleep disturbances are typical and hEDS patients are often diagnosed with a variety of psychiatric conditions or fibromyalgia. Headaches are common. Temporomandibular joint disorder is more frequent and a pain syndrome (regional) is associated with hEDS that may result from chronic stretch injury to the nerves passing over hypermobile joints as well as the fragility of the neural connective tissue. Depression is common in these patients, often related to their chronic pain. Early onset of osteoarthritis may occur and osteoporosis is more common than in age-matched controls. Functional bowel disorders may occur in up to 50% of patients. Pelvic prolapse and dyspareunia also have been noted.

One-third to one-half of hEDS patients will note some type of atypical chest pain, heart palpitations, and/or orthostatic intolerance. Aortic root dilation can occur in 25% to 33% of hEDS patients; however, it is usually mild and in the absence of significant dilation its long-term risk is unclear. Increased elastic fiber degeneration relative to unaffected controls has been demonstrated on electron microscopy and dilation and/or rupture of the ascending aorta has been described in these patients.

Three discreet phases of clinical progression are recognized in hEDS, although the timing of individual phases is highly variable and not all patients exhibit all 3 phases. Infants first exhibit the "hypermobility" phase, which by the second decade evolves to a "pain" phase, during which joint hypermobility decreases (although still hypermobile by the Beighton scale), but worsening pain progressively impacts quality of life and function. During childhood pain is often described in the lower limbs, often termed *growing pains*, and pain with repetitive tasks also may be noted. The third phase, *stiffness*, is characterized by progressive limitation of joint mobility and a dramatic impact on the quality of life. Depression and anxiety are common during this phase. Additional findings in these patients are dysphonia, headache, and dolichocolon.[11]

ETIOLOGY AND PATHOGENESIS

CLASSICAL EHLERS-DANLOS SYNDROME

More than 90% of cEDS cases are caused by AD mutations in the α_1 or α_2 chain of Type V collagen (COL5A1 and COL5A2) with the majority occurring in COL5A1. Approximately 50% are de novo mutations. Type V collagen is a minor fibrillar collagen that regulates collagen fibril diameter. These mutations may result in dominant negative or haploinsufficient states and approximately one-third of cases are caused by haploinsufficiency of the COL5A1 gene.[9] Mutations in the signal peptide region of COL5A1, which disrupt Type V collagen secretion, also have been identified in patients with cEDS.[12] COL5A2 mutations may result in more-severe phenotypes overall. An additional locus may exist, as several families do not exhibit linkage to COL5A1 or COL5A2.

Patients with features of cEDS exhibiting defective Type I collagen caused by AD COL1A1 mutations also have been described. In particular, patients with the heterozygous COL1A1 c.934C>T, p.(Arg312Cys) substitution are at high risk for vascular rupture,[8] similar to the complications of the vEDS subtype. The Classical-like and cardiac-valvular subtypes, which may exhibit skin and joint findings similar to cEDS are described above.

Electron microscopy of the skin in EDS reveals thickened collagen fibrils, highlighting the role of Type V collagen in regulating their size. It is proposed that the amino terminus of $\alpha_1(V)$ carries a negative charge, conferred by abundant tyrosine residues, and appears to limit fibril growth. Less than 5% of fibrils may exhibit "collagen flowers," which are rare composite fibrils.[13]

VASCULAR EHLERS-DANLOS SYNDROME

vEDS is associated with dominant negative mutations in the Type III collagen gene (COL3A1), resulting in reduced amounts of Type III collagen in the dermis, vessels, and viscera, as well as decreased production and secretion of Type III collagen by cultured fibroblasts. More than 320 different mutations (exon-skipping or missense) have been reported; these mutations typically lead to disruption of the triple-helical structure of Type III collagen. As Type III collagen is a homotrimer, mutant proα1(III) chains affect most fibrils, interfering with secretion and leading to intracellular accumulation. Type III collagen plays an important role in the integrity of the walls of both blood vessels and hollow organs, in addition to the upper dermis. Analysis of Type III procollagen and collagen chains and direct genetic testing of COL3A1 have been used to test for vEDS.

The inheritance of hEDS is typically AD. The molecular basis for hEDS is largely unclear. One family was found to have haploinsufficiency of COL3A1. Approximately 5% of patients with the hypermobility form show diminished levels of tenascin X from heterozygous mutations in the TNXB gene, which encodes tenascin-X (TNX). The phenotype in these patients is intermediate between cEDS and hEDS; approximately 40% of patients exhibit abnormal skin findings similar to cEDS but milder and without atrophic scarring. TNXB is located near the CYP21A2 gene, which is associated with congenital adrenal hyperplasia, and microdeletions in the region affecting both genes have been described in patients with congenital adrenal hyperplasia who also exhibit clinical features of hEDS.

LABORATORY INVESTIGATION

Routine histopathologic examination of the skin from EDS patients is typically normal. Electron microscopy demonstrates abnormalities in the appearance of collagen fibrils as noted above. Despite the bruising and increased bleeding, tests of platelet function and coagulation are usually normal, further highlighting the underlying defects in skin and blood vessel structural integrity. As noted above for specific subtypes, while genetic diagnosis is possible, especially as a research tool, a variety of biochemical tests are available as well.

MOLECULAR TESTING IN EHLERS-DANLOS SYNDROME SUBTYPES

Advances in next-generation sequencing have allowed more frequent genetic evaluation of patients suspected of having EDS and broadened the spectrum of genetic etiologies recognized to cause EDS subtypes. For patients suspected of having a variant of EDS, current guidelines recommend, where possible, using next-generation sequencing strategies for parallel sequencing of multiple known EDS genes. For those patients where no mutation or only a single AR mutation is identified, further investigations, such as copy number variant analysis or whole-exome sequencing/whole-genome sequencing, with focus on EDS genes of interest and their regulatory regions, should be undertaken.

Even though more frequent employment of these testing strategies enables the identification of new mutations and new genes of interest in the pathogenesis of EDS, it also generates variants of uncertain significance (VUS), which complicate the genetic evaluation of these patients. Appropriate interpretation of VUS, especially missense variants, must be correlated with the clinical phenotype. American College of Medical Genetics and Genomics (ACMG) guidelines suggest that VUS supported by other data regarding pathogenicity, such as strong in silico predictive scoring or mutations occurring in known functionally active areas of a protein, can be considered "likely pathogenic." Further workups, including familial studies and more detailed protein assays, are necessary in such cases to better clarify the relationship of the VUS with the individual patient's clinical condition. While further evaluations are being done, patients with "likely pathogenic" mutations should be followed as clinically appropriate. The rapid expansion of the availability of genetic testing highlights the critical role of medical genetics in evaluating and managing these patients. Where possible, genetic testing and interpretation should include a medical geneticist or genetic counselors.

For patients who meet minimum clinical criteria for a specific EDS subtype but either lack genetic confirmation, or have a VUS, or have no known causative genetic variants detected, a "provisional clinical diagnosis" of EDS may be made. Clinical followup in such patients is warranted.

Additionally, a pathogenetic classification of EDS subtypes has been proposed with subtypes grouped by known or suspected shared molecular pathways.[1]

DIFFERENTIAL DIAGNOSIS

EDS must be distinguished clinically and histologically from CL. In CL, the hyperelastic skin does not return to its normal position after stretching. The kyphoscoliotic and hypermobility forms of EDS must be distinguished from Marfan syndrome, which additionally is characterized by ectopia lentis and characteristic skeletal abnormalities. Molluscoid pseudotumors of the lower legs may mimic subcutaneous granuloma annulare. The easy bruisability and poor wound healing of EDS patients has led to concerns of child abuse.[2]

vEDS exhibits significant clinical similarities to Loeys-Dietz syndrome Type 2, an aortic aneurysm syndrome caused by mutations in transforming growth factor (TGF)-β receptors 1 and 2 (*TGFBR1* and *TGFBR2*) genes. These patients also exhibit skin findings, including velvety translucent skin, easy bruising, and widened, atrophic scars.[14] Prior to detection of arterial anomalies Loeys-Dietz syndrome patients may be misdiagnosed as cEDS or hEDS.

PREVENTION AND TREATMENT

A multidisciplinary preventive strategy is the most productive approach to the management of EDS patients. Early identification of affected patients with appropriate intervention (pain management, physical therapy, surgery) and education is important. Non–weight-bearing exercise (eg, swimming) can promote muscle development. Exercise regimens are typically designed to strengthen muscles to stabilize joints and relieve stress. Physical therapy focused on shoulder girdle strengthening has decreased the frequency of shoulder dislocations in patients with a history of chronic or recurrent dislocation. Some patients use orthopedic devices, such as orthotics and braces, with benefit.

Avoiding and preventing injuries is of great importance. Assessment of the home environment with modifications to make homes "EDS safe," such as avoiding hard, sharp edges on furniture and arrangement to prevent or minimize falls, can be helpful. Patients with significant skin fragility or bruising may require protective padding or bandaging and should avoid contact sports and heavy exercise.

When cutaneous wounds do occur, they should be sutured using both subcuticular and cuticular sutures, which are tightly spaced and left in place for a prolonged duration (at least twice as long as standard). Adhesive tapes, bolsters, or pressure bandages are necessary to aid healing, diminish scarring, and lower the risk of hematoma and pseudotumor formation. Close monitoring for postoperative infection is critical and preventive antibiotic therapy is often employed. Pseudotumors of the elbows or knees are typically more easily surgically removed than those on the heels.[9]

Ongoing rheumatologic and orthopedic care may be required to prevent progressive joint disease in certain patients. Low-impact sports are preferable to contact sports and weight training for patients with hEDS. Ascorbate therapy (approximately 2 g/day in adults with proportional decreases in pediatric patients) may improve bruising (but not other findings) in cEDS. Antiinflammatory drugs may improve the musculoskeletal pain associated with EDS, but those interfering with platelet function (especially aspirin) should be avoided in patients with significant bruising. Patients with valvular heart disease should be followed by cardiologists, and a baseline echocardiogram with measurement of aortic diameter is recommended before 10 years of age.[9]

Joint dislocation (with the exception of congenital dislocation of the hip) in EDS typically spontaneously resolves or can be remedied with closed reduction. Patients with EDS (especially hEDS) may benefit from a variety of physical therapy interventions, such as myofascial release therapies and low-resistance exercises for muscle toning. Exercise progression should involve increasing the number of repetitions, frequency, or duration of exercise, rather than increasing resistance and should progress slowly. Isometric exercises and swimming are often beneficial in cEDS and hEDS. Pain from writing utensils can be lessened by altering the grip to rest the shaft of writing utensils on the thenar web and holding the tip between the index and ring fingers. Transvaginal pelvic physical therapy has been successfully used for abdominal and back pain, as well as for radicular pain of the lower extremities and dyspareunia. Braces are commonly used to stabilize joints. Intervention is typically multidisciplinary and should involve rheumatology, orthopedic surgery, physical and occupational therapy, and pain management specialists, as appropriate. Pain in hEDS is often undertreated. Even though reparative or corrective surgical procedures are often delayed as long as possible, the perioperative complication rate in patients with hEDS is not increased. GI symptoms may be quite troublesome and require aggressive therapy with proton pump inhibitors, H_2-blockers, and other agents. Calcium and vitamin D supplementation is typically encouraged.

Ideally, patients with vEDS are cared for by a team of physicians with expertise or awareness of the condition at a center with the capabilities to handle the medical complications that can arise. A protocol for managing suspected complications should be devised between the medical team and the vEDS patient. Patients with vEDS should have an emergency care card or medical alert document (a "vEDS passport") describing the condition so that emergency department physicians caring for the patient in an emergency situation can be made aware of the disease. vEDS patients who are or are planning to become pregnant should be cared for by high-risk obstetrics teams. No consensus exists for surveillance recommendations in patients with vEDS; however, a recent review suggested annual review of the vascular tree by Doppler ultrasonography, CT angiography, or magnetic resonance angiography when feasible.[2]

Patients with vEDS should refrain from contact sports and avoid medications that impair platelet function. Invasive vascular procedures should be avoided, unless absolutely necessary (such as with arterial rupture), because of the extremely high risk of vascular rupture. Many symptomatic vascular events in vEDS patients are dissections that resolve on their own. However, arterial ruptures must be repaired. When necessary, tissues must be handled with extreme caution because of pronounced intraoperative tissue fragility. One published series suggested early intervention by skilled surgeons could be more safely performed than previously thought and provided suggestions for management.[15] Maintaining blood pressure in the normal to low-normal reference range and preventing blood pressure surges is often a goal of therapy. Studies examining the use of β blockers in vEDS are in progress.

Fatigue is present in more than 75% of EDS patients of most types. It appears most often in hEDS, but is seen in other forms of EDS as well. Contributing factors include disruptions of sleep, impaired self-efficacy, and pain.[11] A variety of neuromuscular findings, including reduction in vibration sense and mild-to-moderate muscle weakness, were commonly found in a small group of multiple types of EDS. These symptomatic findings correlated with myopathic features on needle electromyography (a mixed neurogenic–myopathic pattern in 60%), as well as with muscle ultrasonography, showing increased echo intensity and atrophy. The subset of patients with hEDS resulting from TNXB haploinsufficiency seem to have fewer neuromuscular issues, although TNXB levels correlate inversely with neuromuscular symptoms.[16]

Pregnancy in the EDS patient should be considered high risk. The effects of hormonally mediated connective tissue softening on the abnormal connective tissue of EDS have not been studied, but may account for the increased skin fragility and other EDS sequelae that occur during pregnancy and the immediate postpartum period. Prenatal diagnosis is possible by genetic and biochemical analyses. Unless children are severely affected by their disorder, they generally adjust well to the skin findings and joint hypermobility.

The Ehlers-Danlos Society is a national support group that can be contacted through its website (https://www.ehlers-danlos.com).

MARFAN SYNDROME

AT-A-GLANCE

- Incidence: ~1 in 5000 (OMIM: 154700).
- Autosomal dominant; caused by mutations in fibrillin 1 (*FBN1*; chromosome 15q21.1).
- Cutaneous features include striae distensae (two-thirds of patients), inguinal or incisional hernias, and, rarely, elastosis perforans serpiginosa.
- Extracutaneous manifestations include hyperextensible joints, upward lens displacement, skeletal abnormalities, and cardiac aberrations, such as aortic aneurysm and rupture.
- Information for patients and professionals is available at The Marfan Foundation website (http://www.marfan.org).

Marfan syndrome is an AD disorder that primarily affects the skeletal, ocular, and cardiovascular (CV) systems.[17] The prognosis for patients with Marfan syndrome has improved over the past three decades as a result of better medical and surgical treatments.[18]

EPIDEMIOLOGY

Approximately 25% of Marfan syndrome cases occur sporadically, particularly in patients born of older fathers. Parental germline mosaicism has been described.[19] Marfan syndrome is a very common connective tissue disorder, with the overall prevalence estimated at approximately 1:3000 to 5000 persons with no racial, gender, or geographic predilection.[14]

CLINICAL FEATURES

Marfan syndrome is a generalized connective tissue disorder exhibiting abnormalities of 3 primary organ systems: ocular (typically lens dislocation), skeletal (excessive extremity length, loose joints, anterior chest deformities, and kyphoscoliosis), and most importantly, CV (classically aortic aneurysm and mitral valve redundancy). Many of the typical physical features of Marfan syndrome are age-dependent, making diagnosis in childhood more difficult. No single clinical sign is pathognomonic.[14,20]

Marfan syndrome patients may present to the dermatologist for evaluation of striae or for other skin disorders unrelated to the condition. Recognition of the other clinical findings of Marfan syndrome may trigger the detection of unrecognized patients.

The "marfanoid habitus" is characteristically dolichostenomelic (tall and thin), with a lower-body segment (pubic symphysis to floor) that is longer than the upper segment (height minus lower segment) (Fig. 72-7). Characteristically, the arm span exceeds the person's height by several centimeters. The distal bones are excessively long (arachnodactyly). Skeletal features of Marfan syndrome are characterized by bone overgrowth and joint laxity. Kyphoscoliosis may be severe and increases with the adolescent growth spurt. Thoracic cage abnormalities, such as pectus excavatum (sternal depression) and carinatum (sternal projection), result from excessive rib overgrowth and are common. The combination of kyphoscoliosis and pectus excavatum rarely compromises cardiopulmonary function. Joint laxity from capsular, ligamentous, and tendinous involvement may cause flat feet, knee or elbow hyperextensibility (genu recurvatum), and occasional joint dislocation. Patellar dislocation is not uncommon; dislocation of the hip, often detected during the newborn period, may be the first sign of Marfan syndrome. Screening tests for joint hypermobility are the thumb (or Steinberg) sign, in which the thumb extends well beyond the ulnar border of the hand when overlapped by the fingers, and the wrist (or Walker-Murdoch) sign, in which the thumb overlaps the fifth finger as they grasp the opposite wrist. The underlying joint hyperextensibility and long extremities of Marfan patients often enable them to reach around their back and touch their umbilicus from the opposite side (Fig. 72-7).

Most patients with Marfan syndrome exhibit myopia caused by flattening of the corneas and an abnormally long anterior–posterior orbital axis. An estimated 50% to 70% of patients have ectopia lentis, typically with upward lens displacement. Subluxation and complete dislocation of the lens often lead to secondary ocular abnormalities, including ametropia, myopia, acute glaucoma, and increased risk of retinal detachment. As mild displacements may be missed with standard ocular exams, referral to an ophthalmologist for a dilated slitlamp examination is necessary if a diagnosis of Marfan syndrome is suspected.

CV abnormalities are responsible for the majority of the morbidity and mortality in Marfan patients. CV abnormalities are detected in approximately 40% of patients with Marfan syndrome by cardiac examination and almost 100% of patients by autopsy examination. Medial necrosis of the aorta is the most common defect and diffuse dilation of the proximal segment of the ascending aorta with aortic regurgitation often occurs. Such dilation is progressive, and may even be detected in utero. The progression of dilation is not always continuous and this unpredictability mandates frequent monitoring. Death in Marfan patients usually occurs in adulthood as a result of CV sequelae, most commonly secondary to dilation of the aortic root, leading to aortic dissection or rupture and pericardial tamponade. MVP results from dilation of the mitral valve annulus, with stretching of the chordae and mitral valve leaflet redundancy. It occurs in approximately 25% of affected children and adolescents, and in 86% of those with associated pectus excavatum.[21] MVP increases with age, and eventually occurs in approximately 75% of patients. MVP may lead to abnormal findings on electrocardiogram, mitral valvular regurgitation, and even cardiac arrhythmias leading to sudden death.[20]

Lack of subcutaneous fat and the presence of striae, most prominent on the upper chest, arms, thighs, and abdomen, are the most common cutaneous manifestations of Marfan syndrome. These cutaneous features are found in up to two-third of patients. Elastosis perforans serpiginosa (see Chap. 71) is more common in individuals with Marfan syndrome, and inguinal or incisional hernias may occur. Skin findings are considered minor diagnostic features in the revised diagnostic criteria.[14,20]

Dural ectasia (stretching of the dural sac in the lumbosacral region) often develops in patients with Marfan syndrome. Emphysema has been described, and lung bullae increase the risk of pneumothorax, particularly involving the upper lobes. Oral findings may include a high-arched palate and crowding of anterior teeth.

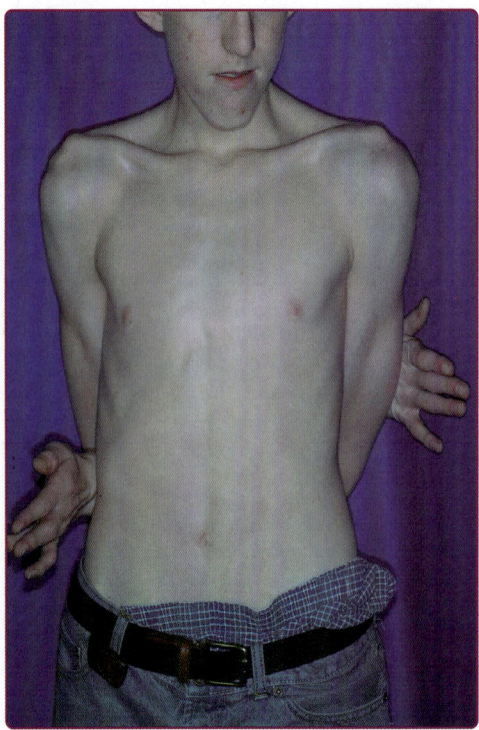

Figure 72-7 Marfan syndrome. Frontal view of teenage boy with Marfan syndrome. Note the tall stature, arachnodactyly, long arms, and ability to cross them behind the back and nearly reach around to the umbilicus.

NEONATAL MARFAN SYNDROME

Infants with the neonatal form of Marfan syndrome have the body disproportion of Marfan syndrome in addition to lax skin, emphysema, ocular abnormalities, joint contractures, kyphoscoliosis, adducted thumbs, crumpled ears, micrognathia, muscle hypoplasia, and deficient subcutaneous fat over joints. Severe cardiac valve insufficiency and aortic dilation result in death during the first 2 years of life.[20,22]

MARFAN SYNDROME IN PEDIATRIC PATIENTS

The clinical features necessary for diagnosing Marfan syndrome develop with age. Pediatric patients often do not meet international criteria for the diagnosis of Marfan syndrome at the time of first examination. Followup examination is critical in suspected pediatric cases to identify affected patients.[23]

ETIOLOGY AND PATHOGENESIS

Even though standard histopathology of affected skin appears normal, with electron microscopy dermal collagen in Marfan syndrome exhibits abnormal thickness, array, and shape, including fibrils of variable thickness, disarray, twisted fibrils, and fibrils with a flower-like appearance and ragged margins, similar to those found in EDS. The content ratio of collagen Type I to collagen Type III is also decreased.[24] Defects occur in the architecture of the collagen microfibrils of large vessels, rather than collagen content or crosslinking.[25] These defects are similar to those seen in abdominal aortic aneurysms and are proposed to explain the weakened aneurysmal vessels in Marfan syndrome.

Marfan syndrome results from heterozygous mutations in the profibrillin 1 gene on chromosome 15q21.1. The spectrum of clinical phenotypes resulting from *FBN1* defects extends beyond classical Marfan syndrome, and these disparate conditions have been termed *fibrillopathies* or *fibrillinopathies*.[26] These range from the severe neonatal Marfan phenotype to isolated aortic root dilation or marfanoid skeletal features without typical CV pathology or ectopia lentis.

Fibrillin is a 350-kDa glycoprotein that is a major component of extracellular matrix (ECM) microfibrils, which are structural components of the zonular fibers of the suspensory ligament of the lens and associated with elastic fibers in the aorta and skin. Virtually every family's mutation is different and more than 500 mutations have been reported occurring in any of the 65 exons of the gene. No hot spots have been identified, except in cases of neonatal Marfan syndrome. Mutations creating premature termination codons appear to lead to milder disease, whereas those in exons 24 to 31 are associated with neonatal Marfan syndrome and more-severe disease. Marfan syndrome Type II is caused by mutations at the *TGFBR2* gene locus. Recently, mutations in *FBN1* were found in 4% of patients with sporadic nonsyndromic aortic dissection.[27]

Fibrillin also modulates the activities of adjacent cells via interactions with mechanosensors as well as syndecan and integrin receptors. Fibrillin also interacts with latent TGF-β binding protein, sequestering it, and controlling TGF-β availability. Deficiency of fibrillin increases TGF-β availability and fibrillin-1 mutation leads to constitutive activation of latent TGF-β signaling through both "classic" and noncanonical TGF-β pathways. How this results in the phenotypic changes seen in Marfan patients is unclear but under investigation.[28] In addition to the action of activated TGF-β, macroaggregates of fibrillin monomers form the basic scaffold on which mature elastin fibers are assembled; as a result, abnormal fibrillin creates a disordered microfibril matrix that may further lead to disordered and weak elastic fiber formation and disruption of the microfibril network that connects elastic lamellae to neighboring interstitial cells.[29]

Research into the impact of these pathways and their potential therapeutic implications for Marfan syndrome is ongoing.

LABORATORY INVESTIGATION

The diagnosis of Marfan syndrome is based on a constellation of clinical findings. There is no diagnostic laboratory test or histologic abnormality. Referral to medical genetics with genetic testing in suspected cases is typical. Diagnosis of Marfan syndrome in a new patient (without a known family history of Marfan syndrome) is made with detection of a FBN1 pathogenic variant of known association with Marfan syndrome along with 1 of the following features: (a) aortic root enlargement (Z-score ≥2) or (b) ectopia lentis. Alternatively, a positive Z-score along with enough additional clinical features to yield a systemic score of 7 or higher is diagnostic. A systemic score calculator is available on the website of the Marfan Foundation (http://www.marfan.org/dx/score). For patients with a known family history of Marfan syndrome, the presence of any of these features is adequate to make the diagnosis: (a) ectopia lentis; (b) a systemic score of 7 or higher; or (c) significant aortic root dilation (Z-score ≥2 if older than 20 years and ≥3 if younger than 20 years).[14]

TABLE 72-6
Differential Diagnoses for Marfan Syndrome

DISORDER	CLINICAL SIMILARITIES TO MARFAN	CLINICAL DIFFERENCES FROM MARFAN	DEFECT
Homocystinuria	Dolichostenomelia Orthopedic abnormalities Ectopia lentis (downward displacement)	Elevated fasting homocysteine levels Autosomal recessive	Cystathionine β synthetase deficiency causes abnormal methionine metabolism and increased levels of urinary homocysteine
MASS (mitral valve prolapse, aortic root diameter, stretch marks, skeletal features) syndrome	Mitral valve prolapse Myopia Skin—striae Skeletal findings Autosomal dominant (AD)	Borderline aortic enlargement is not progressive	Heterozygous fibrillin-1 mutations
Mitral valve prolapse (MVP) syndrome	MVP Skeletal findings AD	Lack of other features	Fibrillin-1
Familial ectopia lentis	Ectopia lentis Skeletal changes	Questionable risk of eventual aortic enlargement; current recommendations are for periodic imaging	Heterozygous fibrillin-1 mutations
Shprintzen-Goldberg syndrome	Dolichostenomelia Arachnodactyly Scoliosis Pectus Highly arched palate Occasional aortic root enlargement	Craniosynostosis Developmental delay Hypertelorism Proptosis Rib anomalies Chiari malformation Equinovarus deformity	Fibrillin mutations not present in most cases
Loeys-Dietz syndrome (LDS)	Generalized arterial tortuosity with aneurysms and dissection occurring throughout Aneurysms more labile than Marfan syndrome Early dissections and ruptures even in childhood AD	No ectopia lentis Dolichostenomelia less frequent/obvious Hypertelorism Cleft palate with broad/bifid uvula Learning disabilities Chiari I malformation Hydrocephalus Blue sclerae Craniosynostosis Talipes Exotropia Soft, velvety, translucent, easily bruised skin	Mutations in *TGFBR1* and *TGFBR2*
Hemizygous X-linked biglycan deficiency syndrome	Early-onset thoracic aortic aneurysms Dissection occurs	Pectus Hypertelorism Joint hypermobility Contractures Mild skeletal dysplasia	*BGN*—hemizygous mutations; loss of function; X-linked gene
Familial thoracic aortic aneurysms and aortic dissection (FTAAD) syndrome	Vascular disease AD	No other typical clinical features	*TGFBR2* mutations and other loci
Ehlers-Danlos syndrome (EDS)	Kyphoscoliotic form EDS may exhibit increased risk for rupture of medium-sized arteries Vascular EDS has joint laxity (often only small joints), translucent skin, characteristic facies, organ rupture, and tendency for aneurysm or dissection of medium to large muscular arteries AD	Vascular pathology not limited to the aortic root, although this may be involved	

(Continued)

TABLE 72-6
Differential Diagnoses for Marfan Syndrome (*Continued*)

DISORDER	CLINICAL SIMILARITIES TO MARFAN	CLINICAL DIFFERENCES FROM MARFAN	DEFECT
Weil-Marchesani syndrome	Ectopia lentis	Orthopedic features differ Short stature Brachydactyly Spherophakia Stiff joints	
Congenital contractural arachnodactyly (CCA; Beals syndrome)	Congenital contractures (elbows, knees, hips, and fingers)—improve with time Ocular (keratoconus) and/or cardiovascular (aortic root dilation, MVP, and septal defects) findings rare Arachnodactyly, progressive severe Kyphoscoliosis High-arched palate Muscular hypoplasia/weakness	Characteristic folded upper helix—"crumpled" appearance of ear—improves with time	Defects in second fibrillin gene (*FBN2*- typically in the "neonatal region" of exons 23 to 34) Likely locus heterogeneity

DIFFERENTIAL DIAGNOSIS

Although Marfan syndrome in its most typical form is rarely confused with other conditions, milder cases share great phenotypic overlap with other hereditary aneurysmal and connective tissue disorders, such as homocystinuria. A number of different conditions exhibit partial phenotypic overlap with Marfan syndrome, including some also caused by fibrillin-1 mutations. Table 72-6 summarizes these conditions.

TREATMENT

Management of Marfan syndrome has focused on prevention of the disabling and life-threatening potential complications. Medical genetics coordination with a multidisciplinary team composed of cardiology, ophthalmology, orthopaedics, and cardiothoracic surgery is typical where available. With appropriate management the life expectancy of patients with Marfan syndrome is similar to the general population.[20]

Early and regular ophthalmologic examinations are required to detect correctable amblyopia and retinal detachment. Ectopia lentis and even complete subluxation may be tolerated for decades. Lens extraction may be required to treat diplopia, glaucoma, cataracts, or retinal detachment. LASIK (laser-assisted in situ keratomileusis) surgery is contraindicated.

Repair of pectus excavatum is appropriate if cardiopulmonary compromise develops, but is delayed until skeletal maturation is nearly complete to prevent recurrence and should use internal stabilization. Scoliosis may be lessened in adolescent girls by estrogen therapy, but this may produce an overall decrease in height. Bracing, physical therapy, and vertebral fusion may all be required to prevent severe scoliosis.

A family history of early aortic dissection mandates aggressive monitoring. At a minimum, patients with Marfan syndrome should undergo yearly monitoring. Aortic complications have not been reported in patients with an aortic diameter normal for age or less than 40 mm in diameter (in adults). Long-term propranolol therapy has been administered to prevent aortic dilation by decreasing myocardial contractility, but may not affect survival. An early small trial in children with Marfan syndrome who were recalcitrant to β blockers using angiotensin II Type 1 receptor blockers (losartan and irbesartan) led to a significant decrease in aortic root diameter and dilation of the sinotubular junction. Larger randomized trials, however, did not show any greater benefit of these therapies over β-adrenergic blockers. Aneurysmal and valvular heart defects may require prosthetic replacement, but this should be delayed for as long as possible to avoid recurrent prosthesis replacement, particularly in growing children. Replacement of the aortic root has led to increased life expectancy and is indicated once the maximal measurement is greater than 5 cm in adults and older children, the rate of size increase is approximately 1 cm/year, or progressive aortic regurgitation develops. Patients with pulmonary involvement should avoid situations with rapid changes in air pressure, such as scuba diving or flying, and, of course, should not smoke. Doxycycline inhibits matrix metalloproteinase, and in mouse models has been shown to improve aortic wall architecture and delay aortic dissection. Prophylaxis is recommended for dental work in Marfan syndrome patients with mitral or aortic valve regurgitation. Historically, patients with known aortic dilation were instructed to avoid caffeine, stressful circumstances, and vigorous exercise. Newer studies, however, in mouse models of Marfan syndrome have shown a benefit from regular moderate exercise with reduced aneurysm progression. Further studies are needed to assess whether these findings are applicable to human Marfan syndrome patients.[30,31]

Children should be excused from participation in physical education so as to avoid potentially harmful exertion, contact sports, and isometric exercises, which might lead to aortic rupture or congenital heart failure. Unfortunately, this can add to the isolation of a child who may already be concerned about an unusual body image or is socially ostracized because of looking "different" or being excessively tall. Importantly, not all patients with Marfan syndrome exhibit striking "classic" phenotypes. When the diagnosis in a patient with an atypical presentation is suspected, one must make certain that appropriate studies are performed, so that potentially lethal internal manifestations are not neglected. The website for the National Marfan Foundation is www.marfan.org.

PSEUDOXANTHOMA ELASTICUM

AT-A-GLANCE (Continued)

- Incidence: 1 in 25,000 to 100,000 live births (OMIM: 177850 and 264800).
- Autosomal recessive inheritance, occasionally pseudodominant.
- Mutations in *ABCC6* gene on chromosome 16q13.1.
- Cutaneous features include yellow, flat papules in the neck, flexures, and periumbilical areas. Less-frequent skin lesions include acneiform lesions, elastosis perforans serpiginosa, reticulate pigmentation, and granulomatous nodules.
- Extracutaneous manifestations include angioid streaks, visual impairment, peau d'orange retinal hyperpigmentation, cardiovascular disease, and bleeding. Breast and testicular microcalcifications occur and may be mistaken for malignancy.
- Histopathology shows swollen, clumped, fragmented elastic fibers and calcium deposits in the mid and deep reticular dermis. Alterations are easily visualized with calcium (ie, von Kossa) and elastic (ie, Verhoeff-van Gieson or orcein) stains.
- Information for patients and professionals is available at the PXE International (http://www.pxe.org) and the National Association for Pseudoxanthoma Elasticum (http://www.napeusa.com) websites.

EPIDEMIOLOGY

Also known as *Grönblad-Strandberg syndrome*, this rare entity is a heritable ectopic mineralization disorder exhibiting progressive deposition of calcium hydroxyapatite on elastic tissue. It occurs in approximately 1 in 25,000 to 100,000 individuals, but is likely underdiagnosed. Now classified as an AR disorder, occasional pseudodominance is reported and heterozygous carriers may exhibit a phenotype closely resembling pseudoxanthoma elasticum (PXE).[32] PXE appears to be more severe in female patients.[33] The average age of diagnosis in patients with a positive family history is 8 to 12 years.[34]

CLINICAL FEATURES

Patients with PXE show marked clinical heterogeneity, with some patients displaying lesions of the skin, eye, and systemic vasculature (eg, GI and coronary vessels), while others in the same family (presumably with the same gene mutations) show only involvement of 1 system. Typically, the skin in PXE demonstrates yellowish, flat-topped, discrete, and confluent papules in the skin creases of the sides and nape of the neck (Fig. 72-8), perineum, axillae, umbilicus, and flexural folds with skin redundancy that increases with advancing age. These changes are often termed *plucked chicken skin*. Calcification of affected skin is common. Multiple comedones have been described in association with the typical skin changes, likely related to elastic fiber degeneration similar to solar elastosis.[34] Perforating periumbilical PXE also has been described.[35] Infiltrative oral, anal, and vaginal mucosal lesions may also occur.[36] The dermatologic features generally begin in the second

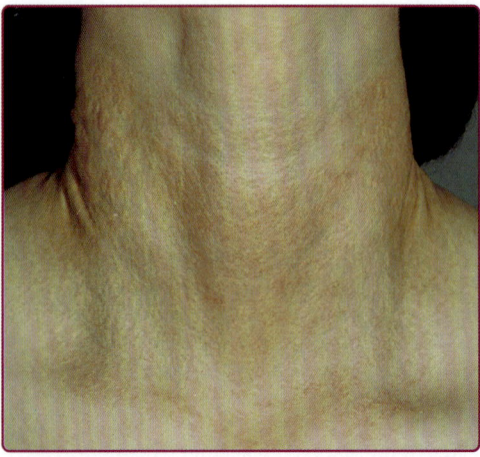

Figure 72-8 Pseudoxanthoma elasticum papules on the neck. There is a distinct yellowish hue. Loose, thickened skin with a pebbled appearance on the neck.

TABLE 72-7
Differential Diagnosis of the Skin Lesions of Pseudoxanthoma Elasticum

DISORDER	MORPHOLOGY	DISTRIBUTION	ASSOCIATIONS	DIFFERENTIATION
Dermatofibroma lenticularis	Asymptomatic, flat-topped yellowish papules and nodules, which, when grouped, form large plaques several centimeters in diameter	Often proximal extremities, truncal; symmetric; may be more widespread	Osteopoikilosis, fractures in Buschke-Ollendorff syndrome—caused by *LEMD3* (*MAN1*) mutations	Clinical; biopsy shows increased elastic tissue
Localized acquired cutaneous pseudoxanthoma elasticum (PXE)	Asymptomatic, coalescing yellow macules and papules, occasional reticulate or checkered pattern; lax, redundant areas	Neck, axillae, groin, flexural surfaces, areas exposed to saltpeter fertilizer (calcium-ammonium-nitrate)	Older age, exposure to saltpeter fertilizer in Norwegian farmers, uremia	Histology shows fragmented, thickened, mineralized elastic fibers in mid- and deep-reticular dermis
Perforating periumbilical PXE[35]	Asymptomatic or pruritic, erythematous lesions that progress to hyperpigmented plaques, with central atrophy, a red, scaly border, and peripheral hyperkeratotic papules, sometimes expressing elastotic debris	Periumbilical or breast area	Multiparity, ascites, abdominal surgery; uremia, and hyperphosphatemia in chronic renal failure	Histopathology shows elimination of basophilic, elastotic debris through channels in addition to thickened and mineralized elastic fibers in mid- and deep-reticular dermis
Long-term penicillamine therapy[44,46]	Varied presentations; may resemble PXE, elastosis perforans serpiginosa, cutis laxa, and anetoderma	Similar to those seen in idiopathic forms of disease (ie, neck and flexures for PXE, flexures in elastosis perforans serpiginosa)	Use of D-penicillamine	Histopathology shows thickened elastic bundles with prominent lateral protrusions ("bramble-bush"), granulomatous dermal inflammation, infrequent calcification, and transepidermal elimination of elastic fibers
Actinic damage to neck	Numerous small, asymptomatic, discrete, white papules	Neck	Middle-aged to elderly individuals	Histology shows elastolysis and fibrosis in papillary and midreticular dermis
Papular elastorrhexis	Asymptomatic, firm, nonfollicular 1- to 5-mm whitish papules on trunk and upper extremities	Chest, abdomen, shoulders, back, proximal extremities	Sporadic occurrence; rarely familial	Loss of elastic tissue in reticular dermis (relative increase in fibrillar component) and fragmentation, with occasional perivascular mixed infiltrate

decade, but are often subtle and overlooked. Rarely, progression may lead to diffuse skin involvement and/or CL-like laxity in the flexures. Some authors suggest that prominence of the horizontal and oblique mental creases (which separate the lower lip from the chin) prior to 30 years of age is highly specific for PXE. Skin biopsy can be quite helpful, as the typical histologic findings may be found even with minimal or absent skin lesions.[37] Table 72-7 outlines a differential diagnosis for the characteristic skin lesions of PXE.

Elastosis perforans serpiginosa is reported in patients with PXE (see Chap. 71). Hyperpigmented, reticulated macules, lip telangiectasias, and acneiform and granulomatous lesions also have been described.[38] Although cosmetic concerns over cutaneous lesions may prompt some patients to seek medical input, it is more commonly a visual or vascular complication, such as a GI tract hemorrhage, which prompts patients to seek medical attention.

The most common ophthalmologic finding are angioid streaks (87% of patients). These are radial curvilinear extensions of gray, brown, or reddish coloration from the optic disc, caused by visualization of the choroid through tears in the elastic-rich Bruch membrane. Calcification of its outer layer, the lamina elastica, leads to fragility and fissuring. Angioid streaks often develop during the third or fourth decade of life, although the youngest patient described was 10 years of age.[39] Angioid streaks rarely interfere with visual acuity and may progress or remain stationary. Trauma is likely a precipitating factor in the development of neovascularization and hemorrhagic complications. Characteristic irregular retinal epithelial mottling ("peau d'orange") is commonly seen resulting from degenerated elastic tissue. Peau d'orange retinal changes precede angioid streaks and are the more common ocular finding in children with PXE. Drusen of the optic nerve also have been described, and drusen-like lesions of the posterior pole have been reported in a 12-year-old boy with PXE. Additional ocular changes reported in PXE include healing subretinal hemorrhages ("salmon patches"); small scars or white foci that represent residua of past hemorrhage ("pearls"); and pigmented foci from previous hemorrhage ("black dots").

Loss of vision in PXE tends to occur later in life and is a result of scarring and fibrosis from choroidal neovascularization and retinal hemorrhage. It can lead to a disc-shaped degeneration of the central visual area causing central visual loss, although peripheral vision often remains intact.

Calcification of degenerated elastic tissue of the internal lamina of blood vessels with subsequent hemorrhage and/or intimal proliferation is a common and potentially serious complication of PXE. The GI tract and renal vasculature are sites of early manifestations of this degenerative damage, which often presents as acute-onset hemorrhage in the second to fourth decade. It is estimated that 10% to 15% of PXE patients will have at least 1 GI hemorrhagic event. Both hypertension from renal artery stenosis and GI bleeding (especially gastric) may occur as early as adolescence. Late vascular sequelae in PXE include cerebrovascular accidents (subarachnoid hemorrhage has been a significant cause of mortality in PXE), intermittent claudication (most common), and myocardial infarction. Severe coronary artery disease has been noted, even in adolescents with PXE; coronary artery bypass surgery may be ameliorative.[40] Physical signs may include diminished peripheral pulses, hypertension (3 times more common in persons with PXE than in the general population), murmurs related to MVP and/or congestive heart failure, and peripheral gangrene. Rectovesical prolapse may also occur.[36] Pulmonary and pulmonary vascular involvement is described, but not common.

Breast and testicular microcalcifications occur and may be mistaken for malignancy. There is not an increased risk for breast or testicular cancer in PXE.[34]

Pregnancy is not contraindicated, but miscarriage rates may be higher in the first trimester, and multiple pregnancies may accelerate the pace of the disease.[36]

ETIOLOGY AND PATHOGENESIS

The mutated gene in typical PXE is *ABCC6*, a member of the adenosine triphosphate-binding cassette transmembrane transporter family (subfamily C member 6; OMIM: 603234) located on chromosome 16p13.1. Most mutations are unique, although 2 occur more frequently: *R1141X*, found predominantly in Europe (28.4% of European patients and 18.8% overall), and *ABCC6del23-29*, which occurs at an overall frequency of 12.9% and is most prevalent in U.S. patients (28.4%).[41] The ABCC6 protein is a putative efflux transporter expressed primarily in the basolateral plasma membrane of liver hepatocytes and proximal tubules of the kidney, 2 sites not affected by PXE. Little to no ABCC6 is expressed in tissues affected by PXE. Evidence supports the concept that PXE is a "metabolic" disease, with deficiency of hepatic ABCC6 leading to the deficiency of adenosine triphosphate excretion into the intracellular space, where it is typically hydrolyzed to produce the potent mineralization inhibitor inorganic pyrophosphate. The ratio of inorganic pyrophosphate to inorganic phosphate is tightly controlled to prevent tissue mineralization, and when disturbed, triggers ectopic mineralization as seen in PXE, generalized arterial calcification of infancy (GACI), and arterial calcification caused by deficiency of CD73.[42]

The great phenotypic heterogeneity exhibited by PXE patients suggests that additional genes or environmental factors contribute to and modify the development of clinical findings. Certain polymorphisms in the promoter of the *SPP1* gene (osteopontin) are more frequent in PXE patients than controls, and 1 is associated with a significantly reduced PXE risk.

Mutations in *GGCX*, which encodes an enzyme necessary for γ-glutamyl carboxylation of gla proteins, have been described in patients with PXE associated with multiple coagulation factor deficiency.

GACI (OMIM: 208000) is an AR disorder characterized by onset of widespread arterial calcification in infancy. A variety of extracardiac findings are reported, including skin and retinal findings identical to PXE. Mutations in ectonucleotide pyrophosphatase/phosphodiesterase 1 (OMIM: 173335) or, less commonly, ABCC6 have been reported in these patients.

Arterial calcification caused by CD73 (OMIM: 129190) deficiency (OMIM: 211800) is a late-onset AR mineralization disorder with vascular calcification similar to PXE and GACI.[34]

LABORATORY INVESTIGATION

The histologic changes on biopsy of lesional skin from patients with PXE are diagnostic, showing distinctive broken curls of basophilic elastic fibers with routine hematoxylin and eosin or Verhoeff-van Gieson staining (Fig. 72-9). Calcium deposition on elastic fibers can be easily detected with von Kossa stain. Similar dystrophic fibers have been noted histologically as an incidental finding in inflammatory skin diseases in patients who do not have PXE.[43] Electron microscopy shows calcification in a centripetal pattern within elastic fibers.[44] Soft-tissue radiographs of the upper and lower extremities may reveal vessel wall calcification. Dental radiographs may demonstrate early vascular calcification. Ultrasonography shows a characteristic pattern of dotted increased echogenicity of renal arteries.[45] Similar patterns have been described on ultrasonography of affected pancreas and spleen. Table 72-8 summarizes the recommended testing for patients with PXE.

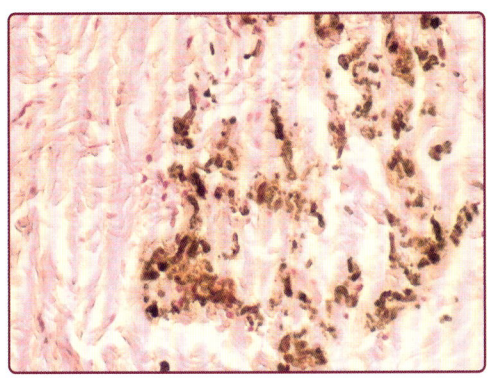

Figure 72-9 Pseudoxanthoma elasticum, elastic tissue stain. The elastic fibers show marked degeneration: They are swollen, tortuous, and irregularly clumped.

DIFFERENTIAL DIAGNOSIS

Table 72-7 outlines the differential diagnosis of PXE.

The pebbly pattern and yellow discoloration of flexural skin of classical PXE is quite distinctive. The later development of redundancy may be confused with the sagging skin of CL. Ten percent of patients with β-thalassemia have both angioid streaks and the skin manifestations of PXE, while 16% have only the skin lesions that are clinically and histopathologically typical of PXE.[43] D-Penicillamine may induce an acquired form of PXE, but elastic fibers do not become calcified.[44,46] PXE-like changes also have been noted both clinically and histologically in longstanding nephrogenic systemic fibrosis.[47]

TABLE 72-8
Monitoring Studies for Patients with Pseudoxanthoma Elasticum

STUDY	REASON
Complete blood cell count	Occult blood loss; iron-deficiency anemia
Calcium, phosphate	Rare reports of hypercalcemia and hyperphosphatemia
Fasting lipids	Hyperlipidemia aggravates risk of cardiovascular disease
Urinalysis	Hemorrhage from urinary tract
Fecal test for blood	Occult blood loss from GI hemorrhage
Eye examination	To detect angioid streaks, retinal hemorrhage, early retinopathy
Endoscopy	If evidence of GI bleeding
Echocardiography	If murmur, angina, or personal or family history of coronary artery disease
Doppler blood pressure (ankle, brachial)	To investigate claudication or if decreases peripheral pulses
CT of head	If focal neurologic problems or evidence of cerebral hemorrhage
Radiographs	If seeking calcifications

Angioid streaks have been described in a variety of disorders, among them EDS, Marfan syndrome, lead poisoning, sickle cell anemia, thalassemia, Paget disease of bone, acromegaly and other pituitary disorders, and familial hyperphosphatemia.[39]

PREVENTION AND TREATMENT

There is no cure for PXE and a multidisciplinary approach is required to address the myriad manifestations of the disease. Plastic surgery may improve the appearance of sagging skin, although extrusion of calcium particles through the surgical wound may result in delayed healing and unsightly scars.[48] Fillers or autologous fat injections have been used to soften the prominent facial creases. GI bleeding can usually be managed conservatively with iced saline lavage and transfusion and rarely requires balloon embolization or surgery for control.[49] Anticoagulants (nonsteroidal antiinflammatory drugs/aspirin) are typically avoided in PXE patients. All patients should be followed by a retina specialist and instructed in the use of an Amsler grid to detect early symptoms of retinal hemorrhage. Laser photocoagulation (such as verteporfin photodynamic therapy every 3 months) has been used to treat the choroidal neovascularization.[50] Recently, intravitreal injections of the vascular endothelial growth factor inhibitor bevacizumab have been rapidly adopted to stop the choroidal neovascularization of PXE.[34]

With recent progress in elucidating the pathogenesis of PXE, a variety of treatments are under investigation. Bisphosphonates, such as etidronate, are stable inorganic pyrophosphate analogs that have been tested in mouse models of PXE with promising results. Additionally, etidronate has been used as prenatal therapy for pregnant mothers with a history of GACI or when fetal GACI is detected on ultrasonography with apparent decrease in maternal mortality. A variety of additional approaches have been considered, including the use of amlexanox to promote read through of premature termination codons.[34]

Although low calcium (60 to 1200 mg/day) and low-lipid diets have been advocated, their value has not been clinically tested and following the recommended daily allowance for these nutrients is recommended. A report describing the use of aluminum hydroxide as an oral phosphate binder noted improvement in PXE skin lesions in 3 of 6 patients treated.[51] Oral ascorbic acid and tocopherol were administered to a single patient with apparent positive response after several years.[52] A diet with fivefold the standard of magnesium to ABCC6 null mice prevented the development of connective tissue mineralization.[53]

Dietary supplementation with magnesium carbonate, which is used as an antacid and commonly added to table salt to prevent caking, is a simple and attractive therapeutic intervention and studies have been completed assessing magnesium supplementation as a treatment for PXE.[34]

Regular evaluation and followup with a cardiologist should be encouraged. Patients should be advised to protect their eyes from even mild trauma, and about the potential for future visual loss. Because of the potential risk to eyes and calcified vessels when traumatized, contact sports and high-intensity CV exercise should be prohibited for persons with PXE. This can be quite life altering for the child or adolescent who may not fully understand the consequences of the seemingly minor skin changes. Avoidance of high-cholesterol foods and smoking, control of blood pressure, and safe aerobic exercises may be recommended by the physician. Patient support groups include the National Association for Pseudoxanthoma Elasticum (www.napeusa.com) and PXE International (www.pxe.org).

CUTIS LAXA (GENERALIZED ELASTOLYSIS)

> ### AT-A-GLANCE
>
> - Inheritance may be autosomal dominant (AD; OMIM: 123700), autosomal recessive (AR; OMIM: 219100 or 219200), or X-linked recessive (XLR; also known as *occipital horn syndrome* [OMIM: 304150]).
> - Mutations in elastin (*ELN*) or fibulin-5 (*FBLN5*) in AD; in fibulin-5 (*FBLN5, EVEC, DANCE*) or fibulin-4 (*FBLN4*), or variety of additional genes (see Table 72-9) in AR; in copper transport adenosine triphosphatase (*ATP7A*) in XLR.
> - Cutaneous features include pendulous, inelastic skin, with an aged facies.
> - Extracutaneous manifestations may include pulmonary emphysema, aortic aneurysm, pulmonary artery and valve stenosis, hernias, GI diverticula, joint laxity, low serum ceruloplasmin, and bilateral exostoses of the occiput (or occipital horn syndrome).
> - Histopathology shows sparse and fragmented elastic fibers, better visualized with stains (ie, Verhoeff-van Gieson or orcein).
> - Information for patients and professionals is available at the Cutis Laxa International website (http://www.cutislaxa.org).

CL is a heterogeneous group of disorders (Table 72-9) that result from abnormalities in elastic tissue. It is characterized by widespread laxity of skin and, in some cases, involvement of other organs.

EPIDEMIOLOGY

AD, AR, and X-linked forms exist, with recessive forms the most common. Estimated incidence is 1 in 1,000,000 live births. Review of the world literature suggests only a few hundreds of cases reported in approximately 400 families. Importantly, historically only a minority of CL patients have had identified molecular causes, although this is changing because of next-generation sequencing. It is estimated that the success for detecting mutations in patients with the AR form of CL (ARCL) Type I is only approximately 10%.[54]

CLINICAL FEATURES

The skin in CL is inelastic and appears pendulous. At birth infants appear to have unusually soft and loose skin. The skin is hyperextensible, but does not resume or slowly resumes its normal shape after stretching. Persons with CL are often described as having a bloodhound-like facial appearance (Fig. 72-10) and loose skin of the face, neck, shoulders, and thighs often first attracts attention. Young, affected children appear aged. Signs of skin fragility, easy bruising, or abnormal scarring are typically absent in contrast to EDS. The viscoelastic modulus of the skin in patients with CL is significantly altered compared to normal patients and CL appears to result in similar changes in skin mechanics as aging.[55] Both AR and X-linked forms of CL can exhibit congenital onset. Joint hypermobility can occur. Internal organ involvement may be seen with both inherited and acquired CL. Table 72-9 summarizes the clinical features of the described CL subtypes.

Autosomal dominant cutis laxa (ADCL) (OMIM: 123700) primarily affects the skin. It may present at any age, from infancy to adulthood and all ages in between, and tends to be relatively benign with a normal/near-normal life expectancy. Patients may exhibit distinctive facial features, including a beaked nose, long philtrum, high forehead, and large ears. Internal involvement is less common but may occur.

X-linked CL (OMIM: 304150) typically affects males and includes patients with the *occipital horn syndrome* and Menkes disease. Clinical findings in X-linked CL often begin around 2 to 3 months of age. Patients exhibit hypotonia, skin laxity (often distal), a thin face with long philtrum and short columella, inverted lower eyelids, a high forehead, and a hooked/beaked nose, as well as large fontanels and brittle hair. Without treatment there is progressive failure to thrive and developmental delay. In severe forms, seizures may develop with progressive neurologic decline, and respiratory and feeding difficulties. Patients may die within the first decade. In less-severe cases, mild mental retardation is common and progressive development of the characteristic occipital exostoses occurs. These exostosis are often first detectable by 5 to 10 years of age.

TABLE 72-9
Cutis Laxa Syndromes: Clinical Subtypes and Associated Defects

SUBTYPE (OMIM #)	CLINICAL FEATURES	INHERITANCE	PROTEIN (GENE DEFECT/OMIM #)	CELLULAR DEFECT
ADCL (123700)	Congenital Primarily cutaneous (hyperextensible loose hanging skin folds) Hernias Rare vascular complications Acute respiratory disease, 55%; emphysema, approximately 35% (Near-)normal life expectancy Some clinical variability	AD	Elastin (*ELN*/130160) Fibulin 5 (*FBLN5*/604580)	Abnormal elastic fibers
XLR (304150)	Mild mental retardation Exostoses Congenital wrinkling of the skin (mainly distal) and skin hyperextensibility Pili torti Distal joint laxity Progressive exostoses including "occipital horns" Skeletal abnormalities Failure to thrive Genitourinary (GU) diverticula Retinal artery tortuosity	XLR	α Polypeptide of Cu^{2+} transporting adenosine triphosphatase (ATPase) (*ATP7A*/300011)	Defective copper metabolism Reduced functionality of Cu^{2+}-dependent enzymes including lysyl oxidases
ARCL Type 1 (219100) (including Urban-Rifkin-Davis syndrome [URDS])	Emphysema Congenital Severe Loose hanging redundant skin Early lethality Supravalvular and aortic and Pulmonary artery stenosis Hernias (various including diaphragmatic) Mucosal prolapse (Congenital or early onset) No hip dislocation GI and GU diverticula with secondary infections Arterial tortuosity Aneurysm formation (more common in FBLN4-related CL) Marfanoid habitus Osteoporosis (*FBLN4*) Diaphragmatic hernia; corneal thinning (*SLC2A10*)	AR	Fibulin 5 (ARCL1a) (*FBLN5*/604580) LTBP4 (URDS) Fibulin 4 (ARCL1b) (*FBLN4*/EFEMP2/604633) *SLC2A10*; facilitative glucose transporter GLUT10	Defective elastic fiber assembly Severely underdeveloped elastic fibers
Metabolic CL Type 2 (ARCL)	No ocular involvement + abnormal glycosylation = ATP6V subunit mutations			
ARCL2A ranges from Debre type (severe) to wrinkly skin (mild) (219200)	Clinical variability Downslanting palpebral fissures Long philtrum Microcephaly Developmental delay Hypotonia Congenital hip dislocation Mental retardation Delayed fontanel closure Cobblestone brain malformation Congenital CL improves over time, especially after puberty Dental caries common Cardiopulmonary involvement is very rare Apolipoprotein C-III isoelectric focusing is diagnostic	AR	$α_2$ Subunit of V-type H^+-ATPase (*ATP6V0A2*/611716)	Congenital disorder of glycosylation (CDG-II) Abnormal pH regulation of Golgi compartments Leads to impaired retrograde Golgi trafficking Increased cellular apoptosis ?Impaired transport of tropoelastin from cell Increased vascularization of dermis; reduced collagen

(Continued)

TABLE 72-9
Cutis Laxa Syndromes: Clinical Subtypes and Associated Defects (Continued)

SUBTYPE (OMIM #)	CLINICAL FEATURES	INHERITANCE	PROTEIN (GENE DEFECT/OMIM #)	CELLULAR DEFECT
ARCL2 (ATP6V1E1, ATP6V1A)	Generalized CL Dysmorphic facies Hypotonia Joint contractures Congenital hip dysplasia Cardiac abnormalities[a] Pneumothorax Aortic root dilation Marfanoid habitus ATP6V1E1 – generalized skin wrinkling ATP6V1A – larger skin folds/abnormal fat distribution	AR	V-ATPase: E1 subunit of V1 domain/(ATP6V1E1: 108746) Subunit A of V1 domain/(ATP6V1A: 607027)	Also CDG-II
ARCL2 – conserved oligomeric Golgi (COG) 7	Severe phenotype Neurologic symptoms Microcephaly Intrauterine growth retardation (IUGR) Cholestatic liver disease: elevated transaminases; creatine kinase; bilirubin Skeletal dysplasia Cardiac anomalies Recurrent infections Hyperthermia Early fatality	AR	Conserved oligomeric Golgi complex sub-unit 7/(COG7)	Combined N- and O-glycosylation defects present
ARCL2B (progeroid forms) (612940)	Progeroid appearance Osteopenia Wormian bones Variable connective tissue weakness Wrinkly, lax skin—especially over hands Finger contractures Triangular facies with mandibular hypoplasia causing prognathism Adulthood: long facies with prominent chin Lipodystrophy Variable Intellectual disability is common Agenesis of corpus callosum Cataracts/corneal clouding Athetoid movements	AR	Pyrroline-5-carboxylate reductase 1(PYCR1/179035)	Abnormal mitochondrial proline metabolism PYCR1 catalyzes reduction of Δ^1-pyrroline-5-carboxylate (P5C) to proline; final step in proline synthesis from glutamate Increased cellular apoptosis Mitochondrial defects Elastic fiber abnormalities similar to other ARCL Highly variable severity
ARCL Type 3a (ARCL3A) (219150)	CL Joint laxity/hypotonia Microcephaly Intrauterine and postnatal growth retardation Congenital hip dislocation Bilateral subcapsular cataract Severe mental retardation Structural brain abnormalities Progressive neurodegeneration Seizures Dystonia (hands/feet) Peripheral neuropathy Paradoxical hyperammonemia with hyperprolinemia and urea cycle deficiency in some patients	AR	Δ^1-Pyrroline-5-carboxylate synthase (P5CS) deficiency/ALDH18A1	Catalyzes reduction of glutamate to P5C, a precursor of proline and ornithine Proline may play role in neurotransmission Ornithine is urea cycle intermediate Dietary arginine temporarily restores urea cycle, leading to paradoxical hyperammonemia
ARCL Type 3b (ARCL3B) (614438) - De Barsy syndrome (DBS)	CL Significant mental retardation Eye anomalies (cataract) Dystonia Progeroid features Progressive No glycosylation defects	AR	PYCR1	Frayed elastic fibers

(Continued)

TABLE 72-9
Cutis Laxa Syndromes: Clinical Subtypes and Associated Defects (Continued)

SUBTYPE (OMIM #)	CLINICAL FEATURES	INHERITANCE	PROTEIN (GENE DEFECT/OMIM #)	CELLULAR DEFECT
Gerodermia osteodysplastica (GO) (231070)	Progeroid features Malar/maxillary hypoplasia "Droopy" face: oblique furrows from lateral edge of supraorbital ridge to outer canthus Sagging cheeks Joint laxity Short-stature dwarfism but may be normal weight/length at birth Normal mental development Osteoporosis/osteopenia Frequent fractures, especially vertebral Improvement in progeroid features and joint laxity over time No glycosylation defects	AR	SCYL1-binding protein 1 (GORAB /607983)	Soluble protein present in both skin and osteoblasts Interacts with Rab6, which interacts with COG complex Disrupted Golgi trafficking
MACS/RIN2 syndrome (macrocephaly; alopecia; CL; scoliosis) (613075)	Characteristic facial features: puffy eyelids; soft, redundant facial skin; sagged cheeks; lower lip eversion; micrognathia; gingival hypertrophy; abnormal dentition; sparse scalp hair Macrocephaly Severe joint laxity Scoliosis Normal psychomotor development	AR	Ras and Rab interactor 2 protein (RIN2/610222)	RIN2 interacts with Rab5 protein, which is important for endosomal and likely other intracellular trafficking RIN proteins can act as regulators of Ras pathway, which suggests weak pathomechanistic overlap with Costello syndrome
Additional Syndromes				
Transaldolase deficiency	Congenital CL in some patients Cutaneous telangiectasia Hydrops fetalis Aortic coarctation Bleeding tendency Dysmorphic features Hypertrichosis Variable multiorgan involvement Hepatosplenomegaly Clitoral enlargement Cirrhosis Liver failure Hemolytic anemia GU malformation Renal Thrombocytopenia Erythronic acid is novel biomarker of disease Many exhibit gradual improvement including skin—except for liver and renal	AR	Transaldolase/*TALDO1* gene/(602063)	Inborn error in pentose phosphate metabolic pathway
Costello syndrome (218040); Noonan syndrome (163950); Cardiofaciocutaneous syndrome (115150)	Loose, soft doughy skin Inguinal, axillary, hands/feet Feeding problems Pulmonary artery stenosis Bleeding tendency Dry skin Characteristic facies	AD	Ras-MAPK pathway defects	

*a*Patients with mutations in these genes have been reported as wrinkly skin syndrome prior to identification of their underlying mutation.
AD, autosomal dominant; AR, autosomal recessive; CL, cutis laxa; OMIM, Online Mendelian Inheritance in Man; XLR, X-linked recessive.
Data from Mohamed M, Voet M, Gardeitchik T, et al. Cutis laxa. *Adv Exp Med Biol*. 2014;802:161-184; and Morava E, Lefeber DJ, Urban Z, et al. Defining the phenotype in an autosomal recessive cutis laxa syndrome with a combined congenital defect of glycosylation. *Eur J Hum Genet*. 2008;16(1):28-35.

Early intervention with copper replacement therapy can be helpful in some patients.

Clinical findings in the ARCL syndromes are heterogeneous in both severity and organ involvement. ARCL Type 1 (ARCL1; OMIM: 219100) can exhibit great variability. ARCL1A often presents with a severe phenotype that includes emphysema, hernias, pulmonary artery stenosis, and visceral involvement such as GI and genitourinary (GU) diverticula, as well as early lethality resulting from profound elastic tissue defects in several organs. Cardiopulmonary insufficiency may develop with time. The cutaneous findings in such patients are often pronounced, with loose, hanging, pendulous skin. Some patients with ARCL Type 1 have milder involvement.

ARCL1B (OMIM: 614437) is also highly variable. Some patients exhibit severe complications such as CV or pulmonary failure early in life. Arterial tortuosity is often a prominent feature. Other patients with milder presentations exhibit craniofacial abnormalities and additional vascular issues such as aneurysms and pulmonary artery hypoplasia. Cardiac hypertrophy can occur. Emphysema of the lungs can develop in some patients and may lead to pulmonary failure. Patients with hypotonia and bone fragility, as well as diaphragmatic hernias, are described. Characteristic facial features include hypertelorism, abnormal ears, high-arched palate, and retrognathia. Patients often exhibit lax joints and arachnodactyly.

ARCL1C (OMIM: 613177) is also known as Urban-Rifkin-Davis syndrome. Patients exhibit CL of the skin and severe pulmonary, GU, and GI complications; CV complications, however, are often quite mild. Pulmonary emphysema, cystic degeneration, and atelectasis can occur. Tracheomalacia, as well as diaphragmatic hernias and pulmonary artery stenosis, develop in some patients. Hydronephrosis and GI diverticula are reported. Characteristic facial features such as macrognathia, wide anterior fontanels, hypertelorism, and (occasionally) a flattened midface or prominent ears may be noted. Some patients have had growth deficiencies.

Children with ARCL Type 2 have distinct clinical findings and can be divided into 2 groups based on the presence or absence of *N*- and *O*-linked glycosylation defects (congenital disorder of glycosylation [CDG] Type II). While these subtypes share many common features such as CL, hyperextensible joints (including flat feet), and progeroid features, other clinical differences between these subtypes are becoming evident.[56]

ARCL2A (OMIM: 219200) is caused by ATP6V0A2 (OMIM: 611716) mutations (a subunit of the V-adenosine triphosphatase [ATPase] pump). The clinical findings in these patients range from mild wrinkly skin to severe ("Debre-type") CL. Often patients with more pronounced wrinkly skin phenotypes (OMIM: 278250) exhibit milder developmental delays and neurodegeneration, while the more severe "Debre-type" individuals exhibit milder skin involvement but more pronounced neurologic and developmental abnormalities. Improvement in the skin symptoms with time may be noted. CNS malformations are common leading to developmental delay and intellectual disability. Microcephaly may occur. Neurologic regression may begin near the end of the first decade of life and may present with slurring of speech, ataxia, and progressive spasticity. Seizures may develop, often between 8 and 12 years of age. Affected infants may exhibit hypotonia, feeding problems, and failure to thrive. Enlarged fontanels with delayed closure are described. Characteristic facial features include downslanting palpebral fissures; a long philtrum; a broadened and flattened nasal bridge; large, anteverted nares; enlarged ears; and microstomia. Full, sagging cheeks are common. Joint laxity, including congenital hip dislocation, may occur, as well as inguinal hernias, and ocular abnormalities such as strabismus and myopia. Of note, these patients very rarely exhibit cardiopulmonary involvement.

ARCL2 caused by ATP6V1E1 (ARCL Type IIC; OMIM: 617402; OMIM: 108746) and ATP6V1A (ARCL Type IID; OMIM: 617403; OMIM: 607027) mutations exhibit generalized CL, dysmorphic facies, hypotonia, joint contractures, congenital hip dysplasia, and cardiac abnormalities. ATP6V1E1 mutations led to generalized skin wrinkling whereas ATP6V1A mutations led to larger skin folds and abnormal fat distribution that improved over time. CNS abnormalities were noted with nearly 80% of reported ARCL2A patients exhibiting intellectual disabilities. Both ATP6V1E1 and ATP6V1A mutations led to increased risk for life-threatening complications such as pneumothorax, aortic root dilation, cardiomyopathy, and congenital heart defects. These features also distinguish these forms of ARCL from the more common forms.[57]

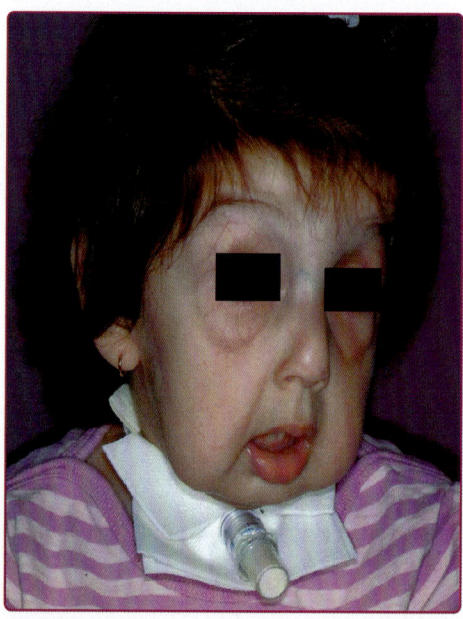

Figure 72-10 Cutis laxa caused by fibulin-4 mutation. The facial skin hangs in loose folds, giving the appearance of premature aging. Note the prominent periorbital vessels. The tracheostomy was placed for diaphragmatic eventration and respiratory difficulty.

ARCL2B (OMIM: 612940) includes so called "progeroid" forms of CL and is caused by pyrroline-5-carboxylate reductase (PYCR; OMIM: 179035) mutations. CL is most notable in the arms and legs. Affected infants often exhibit failure to thrive and growth and developmental delays. Agenesis or hypoplasia of the corpus callosum is common. Distinctive facial features noted in this subtype of ARCL include a thin, pinched nose, large ears and forehead, blue sclera, triangular facies with a wizened appearance, and thin skin. The sagging cheeks noted in ARCL1A are not typically present. Severe wrinkling of the dorsal hands and feet, wormian bones, lipodystrophy, cataracts/corneal clouding, and athetoid movements may occur, and when present, strongly suggest the diagnosis of ARCL2B. As patients age the triangular facies disappear and by adulthood these patients exhibit elongated facies with a prominent chin. Lipodystrophy is commonly noted in adults with ARCL2B. Scoliosis, bowing of the long bones of the upper and lower extremities, arachnodactyly, osteopenia, osteoporosis, and congenital hip dislocation are described.

ARCL Type 3a (ARCL3A; OMIM: 219150) results from mutations in *ALDH18A1* (OMIM: 138250), which encodes Δ¹-pyrroline-5-carboxylate synthase (P5CS). Affected infants exhibit CL, loose joints, growth impairment, intellectual delay that is moderate to severe, cataracts, and corneal anomalies. Some patients develop dystonia and posturing. CV or pulmonary involvement is rare. This ARCL subgroup includes many infants previously diagnosed with de Barsy syndrome. ARCL Type 3b (ARCL3B; OMIM: 614438) results from PYCR1 (OMIM: 179035) defects leading to a more-severe phenotype.

Gerodermia osteodysplastica (GO; OMIM: 231070) also has been termed *Walt Disney dwarfism*. Affected infants/children exhibit loose skin acrally, as well as on the face and stomach. Oblique furrows from the lateral border of the supraorbital ridge to the outer canthus are a recently reported distinguishing finding.[56] Malar/maxillary hypoplasia, prognathism, sagging cheeks, and a prematurely aged appearance are noted. Even though GO patients may exhibit growth deficiency and short stature, they often have normal weights and lengths at birth. Lax joints, hip dislocations and hernias occur. Osteopenia/osteoporosis is common and pathologic fractures (particularly of vertebral column) occur, but CV or pulmonary involvement is rare. Patients have normal cognition. Improvement of progeroid features and joint laxity over time occurs in most patients with these ARCL subtypes.[56,57]

Table 72-9 summarizes additional syndromes considered to be subtypes of CL.

ETIOLOGY AND PATHOGENESIS

Skin elasticity (reversible deformability), as well as elasticity of other tissues such as lung or larger arterial vessels, results from a network composed of elastin fibers. Abnormalities in elastic fiber synthesis, stabilization, or degradation may all lead to the clinical phenotype of CL.

Elastic fibers are composed of an amorphous elastin component (90% of fibril) surrounded by a microfibrillar sheath based on fibrillin. Elastic fibers do not spontaneously assemble; their construction requires a carefully orchestrated sequence of reactions.[58] Elastin is synthesized from individual tropoelastin molecules aligned on a network of elastic fibers and the alignment is stabilized via the formation of intermolecular crosslinks mediated by copper-dependent lysyl oxidase. Mutations in the elastin gene (45 kb in length and mapped to 7q11.2.) typically shift the reading frame at the 3' end, causing read through of the 3' untranslated region. The resulting abnormal protein is deposited in the ECM and the tropoelastin monomers prematurely activate, disrupting deposition on microfibrils and preventing maturation to insoluble elastin. These abnormal elastic fibers are responsible for many cases of ADCL (OMIM: 123700).

Interestingly some patients with acquired CL have an underlying p.(G773D) variant at the C-terminus of the elastin gene, which increases the protein's sensitivity to inflammation-mediated destruction.[59]

The structure of the elastic fiber network is diverse and varies based on location within the dermis. Superficial oxytalan fibers extend from the dermoepidermal junction and are composed primarily of microfibril bundles. These extend through elaunin fibers, which run perpendicularly in the papillary dermis and contain a small amount of elastin. Deeper, in the reticular dermis, thick horizontal elastic fibers contain higher amounts of elastin.[60] Mutations in genes whose protein products form part of the elastic fiber interface such as fibulin 4 (*FBLN4*; OMIM: 604633) and fibulin 5 (*FBLN5, EVEC*, or *DANCE*; OMIM: 604580) are associated with the frequently fatal ARCL Type I (OMIM: 219100) in humans. Fibulin 5 binds cell surface integrin receptors and key components of elastic fibers, suggesting a role in cell-directed elastic fiber assembly. ARCL Type I fibulin 5 mutations lead to abnormal protein folding, decreased secretion, and decreased interaction with elastin and fibrillin-1. One patient with ADCL and a duplication in the fibulin 5 gene has been reported.[61] Missense mutations in fibulin 4 (epidermal growth factor–containing fibulin-like ECM protein 2 [EFEMP2]; OMIM: 604633) have been noted in several patients with unusually severe ARCL Type I with a primary CV phenotype. These patients have severe arterial tortuosity, arterial stenosis, along with aneurysms. Elastic fibers in these patients are severely underdeveloped.

ARCL Type 1c (Urban-Rifkin-Davis syndrome; OMIM: 604710) also exhibits lung, GI, and GU abnormalities and is caused by mutations in LTBP4 (latent TGF-β binding protein 4), which binds the latent TGF-β complex resulting in TGF-β sequestration. LTBP4 may function to guide FBLN5-coated elastin globules toward microfibrils, explaining the phenotypic similarities between patients deficient in either FBLN5 or LTBP4.

DEFECTS IN INTRACELLULAR TRAFFICKING

ARCL2A (Debre type; OMIM: 219200) patients exhibit loss-of-function mutations in *ATP6V0A2*, which encodes the a2 subunit of the V-type H+ ATPase, which is mainly located in the Golgi apparatus. Defects in *ATP6V0A2* result in CDG-II, as a consequence of defective serum protein *N*- and *O*-linked glycosylation. Increased intravesicular pH in dermal fibroblasts likely leads to impaired crosslinking and maturation of elastin as well as affect function of glycosylation enzymes. Fibroblasts from affected patients demonstrate impaired Golgi trafficking, likely because of abnormal pH regulation in the Golgi compartments. Increased cellular apoptosis also occurs. Analysis of apolipoprotein C-III isoelectric focusing is diagnostic in all cases.

Recently, biallelic mutations in *ATP6V1E1* (OMIM: 108746) and *ATP6V1A* (OMIM: 607027) encoding the E1 and A subunits of the V1 domain of V-ATPase were reported in patients with ARCL2 (see Table 72-9). The causative mutations affected assembly and structure of the V-ATPase, glycosylation of proteins, and trafficking in the Golgi, as well as lysosomal function, which caused defects in ECM architecture and homeostasis.[57]

Mutations in COG7 (component of oligomeric Golgi complex subunit 7; OMIM: 606978) exhibit a severe phenotype, with pronounced neurologic symptoms, intrauterine growth retardation and cholestatic liver disease causing early fatality. Glycosylation defects are also present, likely because of defective localization of glycosylation enzymes caused by impaired retrograde Golgi transport.[62]

The MACS/RIN2 syndrome (macrocephaly, alopecia, CL, and scoliosis [OMIM: 613075]/Ras and Rab interactor 2 [OMIM: 610222]) exhibits hyperextensible/lax skin, macrocephaly, distinct facies, slow/thin hair growth, and scoliosis. It is considered part of the ARCL2 spectrum and mild protein hypoglycosylation can be observed. The protein encoded by the RIN2 gene is a guanine nucleotide exchange factor which interacts with R-RAS and Rab5 in early endocytosis.

GO (OMIM: 231070) results from mutations in *SCYL1BP1* whose protein product, termed GORAB (OMIM: 607983), is a soluble protein highly expressed both in skin and osteoblasts. It interacts with RAB6 and ARF5, which interact with the conserved oligomeric Golgi complex and is important in Golgi trafficking.[63] In contrast to ARCL of the Debre type, no glycosylation defects are present in GO.

DEFECTS IN METABOLISM

Mutations in PYCR1 (OMIM: 179035), a mitochondrial enzyme involved in proline synthesis from pyrroline-5-carboxylate (P5C), were initially reported in a group of patients who had previously been diagnosed with a variety of disorders, including wrinkly skin syndrome, De Barsy syndrome, and GO. The resulting abnormal proline metabolism leads to mitochondrial defects and increased cellular apoptosis. ARCL2B (OMIM: 612940) also has been termed *PYCR1-related CL*.

ARCL Type 3 (ARCL3A [OMIM: 219150] and ARCL3B [OMIM: 614438]) include patients historically termed *De Barsy syndrome*. These patients represent an extreme form of the ARCL2B spectrum with more striking progeroid appearance, cataracts/corneal clouding, and significant intellectual disability. Most ARCL3 patients have PYCR1 mutations. PYCR2 (OMIM: 616406) mutations result in a phenotype devoid of cutaneous findings, although affected patients exhibit microcephaly and hypomyelination.[64]

Patients with defects in *ALDH18A1* (ARCL3B; OMIM: 138250), which encodes the mitochondrial enzyme Δ^1-P5C synthase, responsible for converting glutamic acid to P5C, often manifest a similar, yet strikingly severe, phenotype of ARCL Type 3a, including thin translucent skin and occasional arterial malformations. Increased sensitivity to oxidative stress may play a role in the clinical findings.

Mutations in the *ATP7A* gene (OMIM: 300011), which encodes a protein member of the *P*-type ATPase family responsible for copper transport into the Golgi apparatus, cause X-linked CL, which is allelic to Menkes disease (OMIM: 309400) and occipital horn syndrome (OMIM: 304150). *ATP7A* mediates copper transport from the GI tract, efflux of excess copper from cells, and delivery of intracellular stores of copper to cuproenzymes such as lysyl oxidase.

Acquired forms of CL present after skin inflammation and structural damage of elastic fibers. Increased neutrophil elastase present in affected skin is presumed to disrupt elastic fiber integrity. Abnormalities in the genes in which mutations lead to hereditary CL may also play a role in acquired forms of CL. For example, a patient with compound heterozygous elastin mutations showed partial rescue of elastic fiber synthesis by a heterozygous missense mutation in fibulin 5. The resultant elastic fiber system functioned normally, until challenged by *Toxocara canis* parasite infestation during adolescence, leading to acquired CL.[59]

LABORATORY INVESTIGATION

Special stains for elastic tissue (Verhoeff-van Gieson stain) of skin biopsy specimens demonstrate significantly decreased or absent dermal elastic fibers (in both AD and AR forms of CL). Remaining fibers are often clumped, short, granular, and fragmented. Increased elastin-associated microfibrils are noted on electron microscopy. Calcification is not typically seen. Electron microscopy is considered diagnostic for most cases of ARCL, revealing moth-eaten elastic fibers, with abnormal elastin fiber branching and reduced elastin synthesis creating loose microfibrils. Importantly, in both ADCL and ARCL some patients exhibit relatively normal electron microscopy and thus the presence or absence of histologic or electron microscopic findings is not necessary for the diagnosis of CL in the clinical setting of loose, hanging skin with decreased elasticity.[54] In acquired cases, a mononuclear or mixed inflammatory infiltrate containing neutrophils may be present.

Transferrin isoelectric focusing studies and apolipoprotein C-III immunoelectric focusing should be considered in all patients with AR or sporadic CL (especially those with typical facies, late fontanel closure, and developmental delay or CNS involvement). It is important to note that CDG may be missed by the transferrin immunoelectric focusing method in young children. However, the apolipoprotein C-III immunoelectric focusing pattern is typically abnormal, even in very young patients. In cases where suspicion is high but these studies are normal early in infancy, they should likely both be repeated after 6 months of age.[54]

DIFFERENTIAL DIAGNOSIS

Patients with EDS have skin that regains a normal appearance when released after stretching. Other features of EDS, including joint laxity, increased bruising, and poor wound healing, are not seen with CL. Older patients with PXE may have laxity of skin, especially in flexural areas, but the skin shows a pebbly, yellow appearance. Histologic examination of lesional skin further distinguishes these entities. A disorder with features of both PXE and CL, as well as deficiency in multiple coagulation factors, results from mutations in the γ-glutamyl carboxylase (*GGCX*) gene. These patients exhibit mineralized elastic fibers with positive dermal von Kossa staining, and mild retinopathy similar to PXE, but with the pronounced skin folds more typical of CL. Patients also exhibit an abnormal bleeding tendency from deficiency of vitamin K–dependent clotting factors (factors II, VII, IX, and X), atherosclerosis, and possibly cerebral aneurysms.[65] As in PXE, CL-like changes are also reported in longstanding nephrogenic systemic fibrosis.[66]

ACQUIRED CUTIS LAXA

Acquired forms of generalized and localized CL occasionally occur. In Type I-acquired CL, ill-defined areas of loose skin appear insidiously but progressively with elastolysis occurring beyond inflammatory areas in many cases. Type I skin lesions involve the head and neck and progress in a cephalocaudal direction. The development of CL is preceded by an inflammatory eruption (urticaria, erythema multiforme, eczematous eruption) in approximately 50% of cases. Although Type I acquired CL usually begins in adulthood, children have been described with this condition. Pulmonary involvement presents as emphysema and is the most frequent cause of death in acquired cases.[67] Severe tracheobronchomegaly is described. Aortic aneurysms with subsequent rupture, and GI and GU diverticula have also lead to mortality in these patients. Most affected children have not had evidence of systemic elastolysis.

Type II-acquired CL (Marshall syndrome) is a postinflammatory elastolysis characterized by more localized, well-demarcated, nonpruritic erythematous plaques that extend peripherally and have a hypopigmented center. These appear in crops over a period of days to weeks, often in association with fever, malaise, and peripheral eosinophilia. Localized, or less commonly generalized, areas of CL gradually occur at sites of previous inflammation.[68] Although systemic involvement is rare, fatal aortitis has been reported.[69]

Acquired CL may develop after drug exposure to penicillin, D-penicillamine,[70] or isoniazid. It has been associated with $α_1$-antitrypsin deficiency, complement deficiency (C3, C4), sarcoidosis, syphilis, systemic lupus erythematosus, systemic amyloidosis, cutaneous mastocytosis,[71] and multiple myeloma.

Acquired CL is one of the primary presenting features of hereditary gelsolin amyloidosis (AGel amyloidosis), an AD condition resulting from mutations in gelsolin, an actin-modulating protein. Cleavage of the mutant protein creates amyloidogenic protein fragments, which accumulate into amyloid fibrils and are deposited in most tissues. While normal at birth, CL develops with age, initially involving eyelid and scalp skin, but eventually becoming more widespread. Patients also note dry skin, pruritus, and fissuring, as well as loss of hair. Petechiae and ecchymoses are also common. Noncutaneous findings includes corneal lattice dystrophy, as well as cranial and peripheral polyneuropathy. Skin biopsy reveals elastic fiber diminution and fragmentation, as well as widespread deposition of AGel amyloid, including around elastic fibers. How this leads to destruction of the elastic fibers over time is unknown.[72]

A transient form of neonatal CL with generalized skin laxity and inguinal hernias has been described in infants born to mothers who were administered D-penicillamine during pregnancy.[73,74] In these cases, the loose skin resolved during the first year of life.

TREATMENT

Although some forms of CL improve with time, others worsen with age. The physical sequelae of the more-severe forms of CL require a multidisciplinary approach to address complications. In addition to the physical complications associated with CL, it is important for the clinician to recognize that patients with CL often sustain significant psychological trauma because of their appearance. Intervention as appropriate or desired by the patient, addressing not only the physical aspects of the disease, but the psychological and emotional aspects as well, is critical.

Genetic testing should be undertaken to determine the underlying genetic defect where possible. Identification of a specific genetic defect can guide further testing and monitoring. Avoiding environmental exposures known to exacerbate CL-related changes (ultraviolet light for the skin or smoking for the lungs) is important. When appropriate, ongoing regular cardiac and pulmonary evaluations and monitoring are typical. In cases where cardiopulmonary failure occurs, appropriate drug and ventilatory support is managed by the appropriate specialties.

Plastic surgery has been somewhat successful in improving the physical appearance of some patients temporarily and is a reasonable consideration as vasculature and wound healing capability are normal.[75] Numerous procedures may be necessary. Herniations are typically repaired when clinically indicated.

Acquired CL is often recalcitrant to treatment. Dapsone is reported to control acute swelling, which may support a role for neutrophil elastase.[76] Botulinum toxin has been used to improve facial cosmesis.[77] Recently, rescue of elastin insufficiency in mice via introduction of the human elastin gene was described, suggesting a potential avenue for future molecular therapies.[34]

Lastly, a variety of resources exist to support CL patients and their families, including Cutis Laxa Internationale (www.cutislaxa.org).

BUSCHKE-OLLENDORFF SYNDROME

AT-A-GLANCE

- Autosomal dominant syndrome with an incidence of 1:20,000 people (OMIM: 166700).
- Mutations in *LEMD3* gene (OMIM: 607844).
- Cutaneous features include elastomas and collagenomas (dermatofibrosis lenticularis disseminata).
- Extracutaneous manifestations include osteopoikilosis, which may be mistaken for malignancy.
- No serious systemic sequelae.

Buschke and Ollendorff originally reported the association of connective tissue nevi and osteopoikilosis.[78]

EPIDEMIOLOGY

The disorder is inherited in an AD manner with variable expressivity, but usually complete penetrance. The estimated incidence is 1:20,000 people.[79]

CLINICAL FEATURES

CUTANEOUS FINDINGS

Characteristic connective tissue nevi appear as collections of skin-colored to yellow papules or plaques (dermatofibrosis lenticularis disseminata) most commonly located on the buttocks, proximal trunk, and limbs. Many patients begin to develop lesions in early childhood, although later onset and emergence of new lesions while others disappear also have been reported. Histopathologic examination of lesional skin may show increased amounts of elastic tissue (elastoma) or collagen, although decreased or normal amounts of elastic tissue and abnormalities of collagen also have been described.

NONCUTANEOUS FINDINGS

The bony lesions most frequently appear after 15 years of age. They are discrete spherical areas of increased radiodensity, most frequently noted in the epiphyses and metaphyses of long bone, pelvis, scapulae, carpal, and tarsal bones. The radiographic appearance of the lesions may raise concerns for neoplasia. Although the osteopoikilosis is typically asymptomatic, functional limitation as a consequence of decreased mobility of an affected cutaneous area has been reported. Other skeletal abnormalities, including short stature, otosclerosis, and supernumerary vertebrae and ribs have been described. Cataracts and peptic ulcer disease have rarely been reported in patients with Buschke-Ollendorff syndrome.

COMPLICATIONS

No complications from Buschke-Ollendorff syndrome have been reported.

ETIOLOGY AND PATHOGENESIS

Buschke-Ollendorff syndrome results from loss-of-function mutations in the *LEMD3* gene (also called *MAN1*). *LEMD3* appears to antagonize both bone morphogenetic protein and TGF-β signaling pathways in human cell lines; consequently, loss of *LEMD3* leads to enhanced TGF-β signaling. Defects in *LEMD3* also have been detected in cases of both isolated osteopoikilosis and osteopoikilosis with melorheostosis ("flowing" hyperostosis over the cortex of tubular bones), but not in cases of sporadic isolated melorheostosis.[80]

DIAGNOSIS

The diagnosis of Buschke-Ollendorff syndrome is primarily based on clinical suspicion or the detection of characteristic bony abnormalities on radiography.

DIFFERENTIAL DIAGNOSIS

Connective tissue nevi without associated bony changes, morphea, and PXE are the most frequent disorders considered in the differential diagnosis.

CLINICAL COURSE AND PROGNOSIS

No interventions are typically necessary apart from informing the patient of the suspected diagnosis and the associated bony findings.

MANAGEMENT

No therapy is available or necessary.

LIPOID PROTEINOSIS

AT-A-GLANCE

- Rare worldwide, with the greatest incidence (1 in 300 population) in the Namaqualand region of South Africa.
- Autosomal recessive disorder with variable phenotype, even within families.
- Caused by defects in extracellular matrix protein-1 (ECM-1; OMIM: 602201).
- Hoarseness is the most frequent finding, occurring from infancy.
- Skin fragility and blistering occur in some affected children; blisters heal as infiltrated lesions with scar-like appearance.
- Progressive development of infiltrated papules and plaques is seen, as well as verrucous hyperkeratotic lesions, especially on the elbows and extensor aspects of the arms and lower legs.
- Beaded papules on the eyelid margin (moniliform blepharosis) are a classic finding in adolescents and adults, but are not always present.
- Calcification of the temporal lobes and amygdala may lead to neurologic and/or psychiatric symptoms such as epilepsy, neuropsychiatric disorders, and spontaneous CNS hemorrhage.
- Upper airway infiltration can lead to airway compromise.
- Periodic acid–Schiff–positive, diastase-resistant thickening is seen at the dermal–epidermal junction, perivascularly, and along adnexal epithelia with hyaline material in the dermis.
- Electron microscopy reveals deposited dermal material and excess basement membrane material around blood vessels with irregular duplication of the lamina densa at the dermal–epidermal junction.
- No effective treatment exists. Laser ablation/dermabrasion of papules is helpful in some cases.

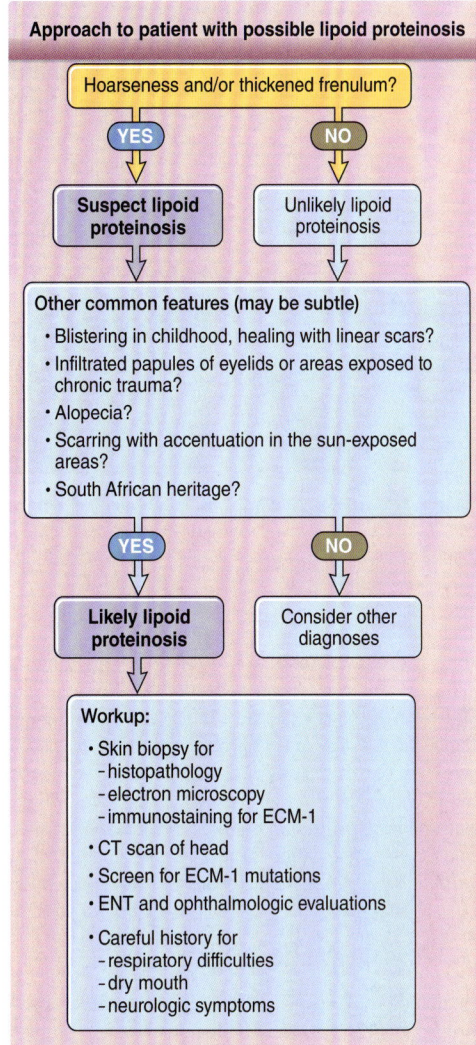

Figure 72-11 Approach to the patient with possible lipoid proteinosis. ECM-1, extracellular matrix protein-1; ENT, ear, nose, and throat.

EPIDEMIOLOGY

Lipoid proteinosis (LP) is also known as *hyalinosis cutis et mucosae* or Urbach-Wiethe disease (OMIM: 247100). Fewer than 500 cases have been reported worldwide. However, it is relatively common in the Namaqualand area of Northern Cape Province in South Africa (frequency of 1 in 300 population). As of this writing, all South African LP patients studied have carried the same mutation (*Q276X*), likely contributed by a German settler who arrived in 1652 (founder effect).[81]

CLINICAL FEATURES

The most reliable clinical signs for diagnosing LP are a hoarse voice and thickened sublingual frenulum,

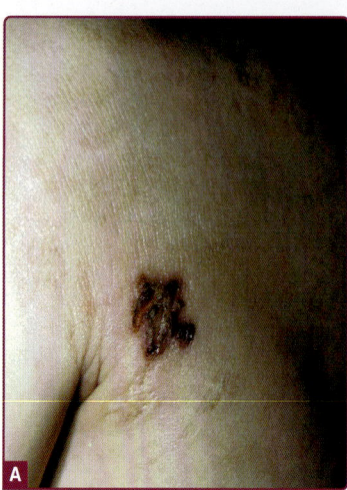
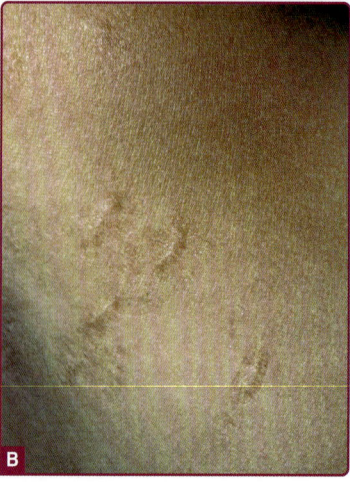

Figure 72-12 Lipoid proteinosis. **A,** Early bullous lesion with typical hemorrhagic crust. **B,** Healing with scarring. (From Dyer JA, Yu QC, Paller AS. "Free-floating" desmosomes in lipoid proteinosis: an inherent defect in keratinocyte adhesion? *Pediatr Dermatol.* 2006;23:1, with permission. Copyright © 2006 John Wiley & Sons.)

which prevents patients from protruding the tongue. Secondary features include beaded eyelid papules, infiltration of warty papules of the skin around the elbows and extensor forearms, and mild alopecia. Increased scarring and photoaging of sun-exposed skin may be seen. Scars or scar-like lesions are present in areas of minor trauma but are not increased at sites of surgery or vaccination. Figure 72-11 is an algorithm outlining an approach to the patient with suspected LP.

CUTANEOUS LESIONS

The phenotypic features of LP are quite variable, even within families. This is well demonstrated in studies of South African patients, all of whom share the same mutation yet exhibit highly variable phenotypes. The variable expressivity can lead to difficulty in diagnosis of affected patients. The earliest finding in LP is hoarseness from vocal cord infiltration, which occurs at birth or in the first few years of life. Initially, this may be noted as a faint or weak cry and is one of the most striking and consistent features. Hoarseness may progress during the lifetime of a patient. Dysphagia may occur from involvement of the upper aerodigestive tract and esophagus.[82] Skin lesions usually develop in the first years of life, although the timing of their onset is variable.

Importantly, 2 stages of skin lesions may be noted. An underappreciated clinical feature of LP is erosions that can develop during childhood in up to 50% of patients. Blistering can be extensive enough to mimic epidermolysis bullosa. The associated vesicles (and rarely bullae) are typically noninflammatory and heal slowly with hemorrhagic crusting and resultant scarring (Fig. 72-12). Scars may be linear and resemble pseudoporphyria on the face. In some patients, blistering is worse during warmer weather. Skin fragility and easy wounding with minor trauma or friction are noted. Spontaneous development of extrafacial pustular lesions also has been noted. Shedding of sheets of skin, which leaves red oozing areas, also has been described.

The skin lesions of the second stage are better recognized. Although beaded papules along the eyelid margins (moniliform blepharosis; Fig. 72-13) are considered a pathognomonic clinical finding, they are variable and may be subtle. Other cutaneous stigmata include generalized skin thickening with a waxy, yellow appearance and areas of distinct papules and nodules. Areas subject to repeated friction or trauma, such as the elbows, hallunces, and extensor aspects of the arms and lower legs, may develop overlying hyperkeratosis, which may be quite striking and verrucous. The scarring usually begins during childhood and is often worst on the face. It may follow trauma or occur

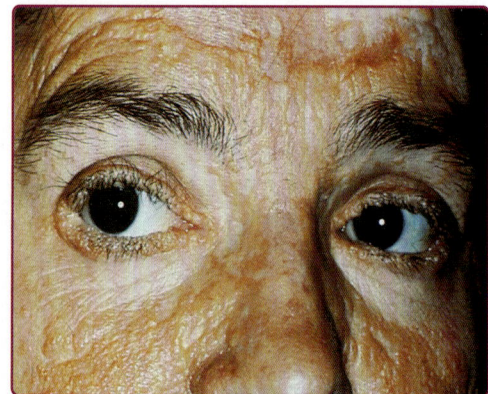

Figure 72-13 Lipoid proteinosis. Beaded papules along margin of the eyelids (moniliform blepharosis). Note increased severity of yellowish, waxy lesions in sun-exposed areas. (Used with permission from O. Braun-Falco, Munich.)

spontaneously, yet no tendency to excessive scarring is noted after surgery or vaccination. Pock-like and acneiform scarring are well described in LP, especially on the face and extremities. Some areas may resemble solar elastosis. Flexural lichenification also may be seen, and patients with LP have been misdiagnosed as having atopic dermatitis. Some patients report increased photosensitivity, and, in some patients, sun-exposed areas exhibit the greatest amount of scarring. Significant pruritus, alterations in the ability to sweat, and abnormal pain sensation have been noted. Alopecia may occur, although it is variable in severity. Nails are normal.

RELATED PHYSICAL FINDINGS

The mucosa of patients with LP exhibit infiltration and thickening. Early in life, oral erosions may be noted and these may persist.[83] Thickening of the lingual frenulum leads to inability to protrude the tongue (Fig. 72-14). The pharynx, tongue, soft palate, tonsils, and lips are typically involved and loss of the tongue papillae resulting in a smooth surface may occur. Laryngeal and pharyngeal involvement may be severe enough to trigger respiratory difficulty, and tracheostomy has been required in rare cases. Shortness of breath or worsening of respiratory difficulties, as well as swelling of the salivary glands (submandibular and parotid), may be triggered by upper respiratory tract infections. Xerostomia and dental caries may be seen.[84] Dental abnormalities (absent permanent upper lateral incisors) also have been described. Parotitis from infiltration of the Stenson duct and subsequent blockage can occur.

CNS involvement is a well-recognized, but variable, feature of LP. Amygdala dysfunction has been described, which leads to abnormal perception and appraisal of fear. More recent studies have demonstrated subtle differences between LP patients and normal controls in the judgment of facial expression and emotion, in memory for negative and positive pictures, and in odor-figure association tests. Because of the frequent bilateral amygdala damage, LP has been used as a model disorder for investigation of the function of the amygdala. Neurologic and psychiatric findings include seizures (often temporal lobe), memory deficits, social and behavioral changes, paranoid symptoms, mental retardation, and aggressiveness. Severe generalized dystonia also has been reported.[85] Calcification of the temporal lobes in the region of the amygdala or hippocampi may be detected on brain imaging. Spontaneous hemorrhage in the CNS may also occur.[82]

The ocular examination may reveal drusen-like fundal lesions. Eyelid infiltration may induce corneal ulcers caused by abnormal eyelash positioning, and alopecia of the eyebrows and eyelashes can occur. The abnormal deposition of hyaline material has been detected histopathologically in many internal organs, although this is typically asymptomatic.

ETIOLOGY AND PATHOGENESIS

LP is inherited in an AR fashion and is caused by mutations in the gene encoding ECM-1 (OMIM: 602201). Although given this name because of its discovery among various connective tissue proteins in a murine stromal cell line, ECM-1 likely has broader functions. ECM-1 is known to inhibit bone mineralization, contribute to epidermal differentiation, and stimulate angiogenesis.[86]

The *ECM1* gene is located next to the epidermal differentiation complex on chromosome band 1q21. ECM-1 is present both in the epidermis and as a secreted protein in the dermis. There are 4 splice variants: ECM-1a is encoded by the full gene, ECM-1b lacks exon 7, ECM-1c contains an additional exon 5a, and a fourth form shows truncation of 57 amino acids.[86] ECM-1a is widely expressed, whereas ECM-1b is expressed only in tonsils, keratinocytes, and the upper respiratory tract. ECM-1c is also expressed in the skin.

ECM-1 appears to have several functions. In the skin, it interacts with several ECM proteins, including perlecan (a heparin sulfate proteoglycan present in basement membranes), fibulin 1C, fibulin 1D, fibulin 3, matrix metalloproteinase 9, fibronectin, the β_3 chain of laminin 332, and collagen Type IV. ECM-1 may well serve as a "binding core" for cutaneous extracellular and basement membrane proteins.[87] The second tandem repeat of ECM-1, encoded by exon 7, binds fibulin-1, an extracellular component of most basement membranes. Thus, ECM-1a binds to fibulin, whereas ECM-1b, lacking exon 7, does not.[87] Whereas ECM-1a is expressed in basal keratinocytes, ECM-1b is only expressed in terminally differentiated keratinocytes. Given the differential expression of ECM-1 isoforms in skin, the ability to bind fibulin-1 may be important in keratinocyte differentiation. A report describing ultrastructural evidence of desmosomal detachment in cultured keratinocytes from a pediatric patient with the vesicular lesions of LP suggests a role in normal

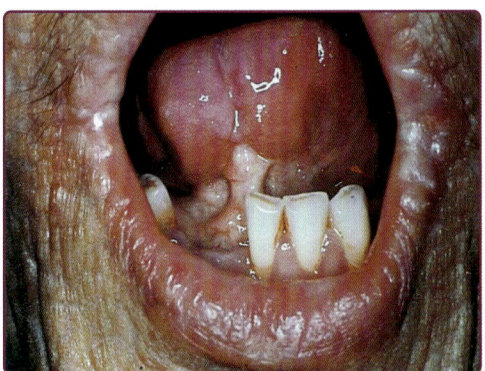

Figure 72-14 Restricted mobility of the tongue as a result of infiltration of the frenulum is seen in most patients with lipoid proteinosis. Note discoloration of the lips as well. (Used with permission from O. Braun-Falco, Munich.)

differentiation as well.[88] A recent report in mice found no epidermal alteration in association with overexpression or underexpression of ECM-1, arguing against a role in epidermal differentiation in murine systems, but the relevance for human skin is unclear. Both ECM-1a and ECM-1b may stimulate blood vessel endothelial cell proliferation and promote angiogenesis in chicken embryo. Abnormalities of the cutaneous vasculature are described in LP.[89]

Mutations in *ECM1* in LP lead to loss-of-function of ECM-1. The majority of mutations occur in exon 7, with frameshift mutations leading to ablation of the ECM-1a transcript but not that of ECM-1b, which typically lacks exon 7. Mutations outside of exon 7 typically occur in exon 6 and are nonsense or frameshift mutations. Patients with exon 7 mutations may have a slightly milder phenotype than those with non–exon 7 mutations with regard to respiratory and skin (but not neurologic) manifestations.

Antibodies to ECM-1 have been detected in adult patients with lichen sclerosus (see Chap. 64).[90]

LABORATORY INVESTIGATION

Light microscopic evaluation of lesional sections reveals deposition of amorphous eosinophilic material at the dermal–epidermal junction, perivascularly, and along adnexal epithelia. There is deposition of hyaline material in the dermis, often perpendicular to the basement membrane (Fig. 72-15). The hyaline material is periodic acid–Schiff positive and diastase resistant, with a composition similar to that of basement membrane. Often arranged in concentric, "onion-skin" layers around vessels, these layers include Type III and Type IV collagen, as well as laminin. Electron microscopy reveals irregular duplication of the lamina densa at the dermal–epidermal junction. Cytoplasmic vacuoles are noted in dermal fibroblasts.[91] The presence of lipids varies and is considered a secondary phenomenon that results from lipid adherence to glycoproteins present in the hyaline material rather than a primary defect of LP.

The histologic features of the early bullous lesions of LP have only recently been described. Acantholysis of keratinocytes apparently is the cause.[92] Electron microscopy suggests an abnormality of desmosomal attachment, with "free-floating" desmosomes noted in bullous lesions. These preliminary findings require confirmation; but are intriguing given the pattern of expression of ECM-1 in the epidermis.[88]

Three-dimensional analysis of the cutaneous vasculature in LP shows enlarged vessels in the mid- and deep dermis with an orientation parallel to the dermal–epidermal junction. The dermal papillary plexus also lacks capillary loops. As in lichen sclerosus, the subcutaneous plexus and transverse connecting vessels are atretic or poorly formed.[89] Such vascular abnormalities may reflect a disturbance of ECM-1 function during angiogenesis.

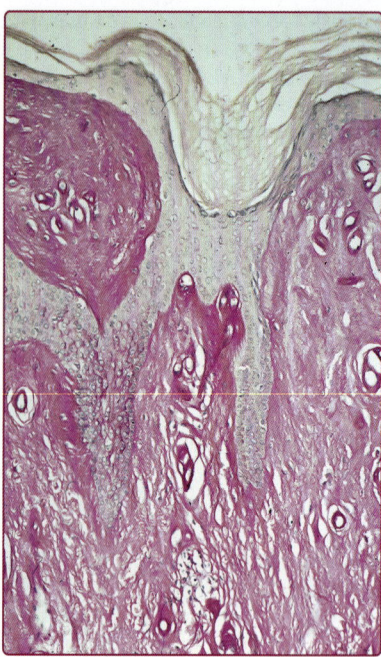

Figure 72-15 Extensive deposition of periodic acid–Schiff–positive, diastase-resistant hyaline material in the dermis of a scar-like lesion of lipoid proteinosis.

SPECIAL TESTS

CT scans of the brain reveal bilateral anterior medial temporal lobe calcifications, often bean-shaped, and especially within the amygdala, in 50-75% of LP patients.[82,93]

Histopathologic evaluation of these lesions shows amorphous masses of calcium and bone along with multiple haphazardly arranged small blood vessels with wall calcification and gliotic adjacent tissue. The cortex and white matter show isolated blood vessels occluded by fibrin, parietal calcification, small perivascular infarctions, and demyelination.[93] Immunohistochemical staining of skin biopsy specimens may show absence or attenuation of ECM-1. This may prove to be a valid diagnostic test, not only to aid in diagnosis in mild cases but also potentially to direct molecular investigations.[94]

DIFFERENTIAL DIAGNOSIS

Table 72-10 outlines the differential diagnosis of LP.

PROGNOSIS AND CLINICAL COURSE

The prognosis of LP is variable. Often, there is progressive worsening of cutaneous features, with clearance

TABLE 72-10
Differential Diagnosis of Lipoid Proteinosis

Clinical

Most Likely
- Erythropoietic protoporphyria (EPP) or pseudoporphyria (clinically and histologically)—in EPP most changes are in sun-exposed areas, whereas in lipoid proteinosis they are present in non–sun-exposed sites as well; EPP has no beading of the eyelids
- Variegate porphyria—especially in South Africa
- Epidermolysis bullosa—hoarseness with blistering (infancy)
- Impetigo—childhood blisters and erosions

Consider
- Scarring from acne
- Scleromyxedema
- Amyloidosis
- Residual lichenification from atopic dermatitis

Histopathologic
- Erythropoietic protoporphyria
- Diabetic microangiopathy
- Amyloidosis
- Lichen sclerosus

---

during childhood of blistering lesions and progressive development of infiltrative lesions. The hoarseness and mucosal lesions also may progress with time. Although some patients have experienced respiratory complications from upper respiratory tract infiltration that have, in rare cases, led to early mortality, most patients have a normal life span. It is important to recognize the impact of LP on the quality of life of affected patients. The disfiguring nature of the skin lesions, along with the abnormal voice, significantly impacts the interactions of LP patients with others. Patients have increased difficulty in holding jobs.[81]

TREATMENT

Many agents, including topical and systemic corticosteroids, oral dimethyl sulfoxide,[95] and intralesional heparin, have been investigated and used in the treatment of LP. None of these agents has demonstrated any sustained benefits. Improvement of various aspects of LP following treatment with acitretin is described in individual case reports.[96,97] Given the apparent photoexacerbation of lesions in a subset of LP patients, photoprotection is reasonable, although there are no data confirming benefit. Additionally, avoidance of friction or trauma may be helpful given the prominence of lesions on frequently traumatized sites. Early intervention for developmental problems is important, and management of other stigmata by the appropriate specialists is warranted. Various surgical modalities, such as dermabrasion and CO_2 laser procedures, have been used to treat cutaneous lesions. CO_2 laser surgery for vocal cord lesions and eyelid papules has been helpful. Microlaryngoscopic excision of laryngeal lesions has improved voice quality and airway access in some patients. Seizures and other neurologic complications should be managed by a neurologist.[82]

PREVENTION

Prenatal genetic testing in families at risk is theoretically possible using DNA-based analysis.

REFERENCES

1. Malfait F, Francomano C, Byers P, et al. The 2017 international classification of the Ehlers-Danlos syndromes. *Am J Med Genet C Semin Med Genet.* 2017;175(1):8-26.
2. Byers PH, Belmont J, Black J, et al. Diagnosis, natural history, and management in vascular Ehlers-Danlos syndrome. *Am J Med Genet C Semin Med Genet.* 2017;175(1):40-47.
3. Remvig L, Duhn PH, Ullman S, et al. Skin extensibility and consistency in patients with Ehlers-Danlos syndrome and benign joint hypermobility syndrome. *Scand J Rheumatol.* 2009;38(3):227-230.
4. Machet L, Huttenberger B, Georgesco G, et al. Absence of inferior labial and lingual frenula in Ehlers-Danlos syndrome: a minor diagnostic criterion in French patients. *Am J Clin Dermatol.* 2010;11(4):269-273.
5. Ramos-E-Silva M, Libia Cardozo Pereira A, Bastos Oliveira G, et al. Connective tissue diseases: pseudoxanthoma elasticum, anetoderma, and Ehlers-Danlos syndrome in pregnancy. *Clin Dermatol.* 2006;24(2):91-96.
6. Wenstrup RJ, Meyer RA, Lyle JS, et al. Prevalence of aortic root dilation in the Ehlers-Danlos syndrome. *Genet Med.* 2002;4(3):112-117.
7. Brady AF, Demirdas S, Fournel-Gigleux S, et al. The Ehlers-Danlos syndromes, rare types. *Am J Med Genet C Semin Med Genet.* 2017;175(1):70-115.
8. Malfait F, Symoens S, De Backer J, et al. Three arginine to cysteine substitutions in the pro-alpha (I)-collagen chain cause Ehlers-Danlos syndrome with a propensity to arterial rupture in early adulthood. *Hum Mutat.* 2007;28(4):387-395.
9. Bowen JM, Sobey GJ, Burrows NP, et al. Ehlers-Danlos syndrome, classical type. *Am J Med Genet C Semin Med Genet.* 2017;175(1):27-39.
10. Burch GH, Gong Y, Liu W, et al. Tenascin-X deficiency is associated with Ehlers-Danlos syndrome. *Nat Genet.* 1997;17(1):104-108.
11. Tinkle B, Castori M, Berglund B, et al. Hypermobile Ehlers-Danlos syndrome (a.k.a. Ehlers-Danlos syndrome type III and Ehlers-Danlos syndrome hypermobility type): clinical description and natural history. *Am J Med Genet C Semin Med Genet.* 2017;175(1):48-69.
12. Symoens S, Malfait F, Renard M, et al. COL5A1 signal peptide mutations interfere with protein secretion and cause classic Ehlers-Danlos syndrome. *Hum Mutat.* 2009;30(2):E395-E403.
13. Mao JR, Bristow J. The Ehlers-Danlos syndrome: on beyond collagens. *J Clin Invest.* 2001;107(9):1063-1069.
14. Bradley TJ, Bowdin SC, Morel CF, et al. The expanding clinical spectrum of extracardiovascular and cardiovascular manifestations of heritable thoracic aortic aneurysm and dissection. *Can J Cardiol.* 2016;32(1):86-99.
15. Brooke BS, Arnaoutakis G, McDonnell NB, et al. Contemporary management of vascular complications associated with Ehlers-Danlos syndrome. *J Vasc Surg.* 2010;51(1):131-138; discussion 138-139.

16. Voermans NC, van Alfen N, Pillen S, et al. Neuromuscular involvement in various types of Ehlers-Danlos syndrome. *Ann Neurol.* 2009;65(6):687-697.
17. Pyeritz RE. The Marfan syndrome. *Annu Rev Med.* 2000;51:481-510.
18. Pearson GD, Devereux R, Loeys B, et al. Report of the National Heart, Lung, and Blood Institute and National Marfan Foundation Working Group on research in Marfan syndrome and related disorders. *Circulation.* 2008;118(7):785-791.
19. Rantamaki T, Kaitila I, Syvanen AC, et al. Recurrence of Marfan syndrome as a result of parental germ-line mosaicism for an FBN1 mutation. *Am J Hum Genet.* 1999;64(4):993-1001.
20. Dietz H. Marfan syndrome. In: Adam MP, Ardinger HH, Pagon RA, et al, eds. GeneReviews(R) [Internet]. Seattle (WA): University of Washington; 1993-2018. Last update: October 12, 2017. Available at https://www.ncbi.nlm.nih.gov/books/NBK1335/
21. Seliem MA, Duffy CE, Gidding SS, et al. Echocardiographic evaluation of the aortic root and mitral valve in children and adolescents with isolated pectus excavatum: comparison with Marfan patients. *Pediatr Cardiol.* 1992;13(1):20-23.
22. Liu LH, Lin SM, Lin DS, et al. Losartan in combination with propranolol slows the aortic root dilatation in neonatal Marfan syndrome. *Pediatr Neonatol.* 2018;59(2):211-213.
23. Faivre L, Masurel-Paulet A, Collod-Beroud G, et al. Clinical and molecular study of 320 children with Marfan syndrome and related type I fibrillinopathies in a series of 1009 probands with pathogenic FBN1 mutations. *Pediatrics.* 2009;123(1):391-398.
24. Kobayasi T. Dermal elastic fibres in the inherited hypermobile disorders. *J Dermatol Sci.* 2006;41(3):175-185.
25. Lindeman JH, Ashcroft BA, Beenakker JW, et al. Distinct defects in collagen microarchitecture underlie vessel-wall failure in advanced abdominal aneurysms and aneurysms in Marfan syndrome. *Proc Natl Acad Sci U S A.* 2010;107(2):862-865.
26. Robinson PN, Arteaga-Solis E, Baldock C, et al. The molecular genetics of Marfan syndrome and related disorders. *J Med Genet.* 2006;43(10):769-787.
27. Tan L, Li Z, Zhou C, et al. FBN1 mutations largely contribute to sporadic non-syndromic aortic dissection. *Hum Mol Genet.* 2017;26(24):4814-4822.
28. Ramirez F, Caescu C, Wondimu E, et al. Marfan syndrome; a connective tissue disease at the crossroads of mechanotransduction, TGFβ signaling and cell stemness. *Matrix Biol.* 2017 [Epub ahead of print].
29. Goumans MJ, Liu Z, ten Dijke P. TGF-beta signaling in vascular biology and dysfunction. *Cell Res.* 2009;19(1):116-127.
30. Mas-Stachurska A, Siegert AM, Batlle M, et al. Cardiovascular benefits of moderate exercise training in Marfan syndrome: insights from an animal model. *J Am Heart Assoc.* 2017;6(9).
31. de Waard V. Marfan on the move. *J Am Heart Assoc.* 2017;6(9).
32. Martin L, Maitre F, Bonicel P, et al. Heterozygosity for a single mutation in the ABCC6 gene may closely mimic PXE: consequences of this phenotype overlap for the definition of PXE. *Arch Dermatol.* 2008;144(3):301-306.
33. Uitto J, Jiang Q. Pseudoxanthoma elasticum-like phenotypes: more diseases than one. *J Invest Dermatol.* 2007;127(3):507-510.
34. Uitto J, Li Q, van de Wetering K, et al. Insights into pathomechanisms and treatment development in heritable ectopic mineralization disorders: summary of the PXE International Biennial Research Symposium-2016. *J Invest Dermatol.* 2017;137(4):790-795.
35. Kazakis AM, Parish WR. Periumbilical perforating pseudoxanthoma elasticum. *J Am Acad Dermatol.* 1988;19(2, pt 2):384-388.
36. Viljoen DL, Beatty S, Beighton P. The obstetric and gynaecological implications of pseudoxanthoma elasticum. *Br J Obstet Gynaecol.* 1987;94(9):884-888.
37. Lebwohl M, Phelps RG, Yannuzzi L, et al. Diagnosis of pseudoxanthoma elasticum by scar biopsy in patients without characteristic skin lesions. *N Engl J Med.* 1987;317(6):347-350.
38. Li TH, Tseng CR, Hsiao GH, et al. An unusual cutaneous manifestation of pseudoxanthoma elasticum mimicking reticulate pigmentary disorders. *Br J Dermatol.* 1996;134(6):1157-1159.
39. Georgalas I, Papaconstantinou D, Koutsandrea C, et al. Angioid streaks, clinical course, complications, and current therapeutic management. *Ther Clin Risk Manag.* 2009;5(1):81-89.
40. Nishida H, Endo M, Koyanagi H, et al. Coronary artery bypass in a 15-year-old girl with pseudoxanthoma elasticum. *Ann Thorac Surg.* 1990;49(3):483-485.
41. Le Saux O, Beck K, Sachsinger C, et al. Evidence for a founder effect for pseudoxanthoma elasticum in the Afrikaner population of South Africa. *Hum Genet.* 2002;111(4-5):331-338.
42. Zhao J, Kingman J, Sundberg JP, et al. Plasma PPi deficiency is the major, but not the exclusive, cause of ectopic mineralization in an abcc6–/– mouse model of PXE. *J Invest Dermatol.* 2017;137(11):2336-2343.
43. Aessopos A, Farmakis D, Loukopoulos D. Elastic tissue abnormalities resembling pseudoxanthoma elasticum in beta thalassemia and the sickling syndromes. *Blood.* 2002;99(1):30-35.
44. Becuwe C, Dalle S, Ronger-Savle S, et al. Elastosis perforans serpiginosa associated with pseudo-pseudoxanthoma elasticum during treatment of Wilson's disease with penicillamine. *Dermatology.* 2005;210(1):60-63.
45. Suarez MJ, Garcia JB, Orense M, et al. Sonographic aspects of pseudoxanthoma elasticum. *Pediatr Radiol.* 1991;21(7):538-539.
46. Coatesworth AP, Darnton SJ, Green RM, et al. A case of systemic pseudo-pseudoxanthoma elasticum with diverse symptomatology caused by long-term penicillamine use. *J Clin Pathol.* 1998;51(2):169-171.
47. Lewis KG, Lester BW, Pan TD, et al. Nephrogenic fibrosing dermopathy and calciphylaxis with pseudoxanthoma elasticum-like changes. *J Cutan Pathol.* 2006;33(10):695-700.
48. Viljoen DL, Bloch C, Beighton P. Plastic surgery in pseudoxanthoma elasticum: experience in nine patients. *Plast Reconstr Surg.* 1990;85(2):233-238.
49. Cunningham JR, Lippman SM, Renie WA, et al. Pseudoxanthoma elasticum: treatment of gastrointestinal hemorrhage by arterial embolization and observations on autosomal dominant inheritance. *Johns Hopkins Med J.* 1980;147(4):168-173.
50. Browning AC, Chung AK, Ghanchi F, et al. Verteporfin photodynamic therapy of choroidal neovascularization in angioid streaks: one-year results of a prospective case series. *Ophthalmology.* 2005;112(7):1227-1231.
51. Sherer DW, Singer G, Uribarri J, et al. Oral phosphate binders in the treatment of pseudoxanthoma elasticum. *J Am Acad Dermatol.* 2005;53(4):610-615.
52. Takata T, Ikeda M, Kodama H, et al. Treatment of pseudoxanthoma elasticum with tocopherol acetate and ascorbic acid. *Pediatr Dermatol.* 2007;24(4):424-425.

53. LaRusso J, Li Q, Jiang Q, et al. Elevated dietary magnesium prevents connective tissue mineralization in a mouse model of pseudoxanthoma elasticum (Abcc6(−/−)). *J Invest Dermatol*. 2009;129(6):1388-1394.
54. Morava E, Lefeber DJ, Urban Z, et al. Defining the phenotype in an autosomal recessive cutis laxa syndrome with a combined congenital defect of glycosylation. *Eur J Hum Genet*. 2008;16(1):28-35.
55. Kozel BA, Su CT, Danback JR, et al. Biomechanical properties of the skin in cutis laxa. *J Invest Dermatol*. 2014;134(11):2836-2838.
56. Kariminejad A, Afroozan F, Bozorgmehr B, et al. Discriminative features in three autosomal recessive cutis laxa syndromes: cutis laxa IIa, cutis laxa IIb, and geroderma osteoplastica. *Int J Mol Sci*. 2017;18(3). pii: E635.
57. Van Damme T, Gardeitchik T, Mohamed M, et al. Mutations in ATP6V1E1 or ATP6V1A cause autosomal-recessive cutis laxa. *Am J Hum Genet*. 2017;100(2):216-227.
58. Vanakker O, Callewaert B, Malfait F, et al. The genetics of soft connective tissue disorders. *Annu Rev Genomics Hum Genet*. 2015;16:229-255.
59. Hu Q, Reymond JL, Pinel N, et al. Inflammatory destruction of elastic fibers in acquired cutis laxa is associated with missense alleles in the elastin and fibulin-5 genes. *J Invest Dermatol*. 2006;126(2):283-290.
60. Baldwin AK, Simpson A, Steer R, et al. Elastic fibres in health and disease. *Expert Rev Mol Med*. 2013;15:e8.
61. Markova D, Zou Y, Ringpfeil F, et al. Genetic heterogeneity of cutis laxa: a heterozygous tandem duplication within the fibulin-5 (*FBLN5*) gene. *Am J Hum Genet*. 2003;72(4):998-1004.
62. Wu X, Steet RA, Bohorov O, et al. Mutation of the COG complex subunit gene COG7 causes a lethal congenital disorder. *Nat Med*. 2004;10(5):518-523.
63. Hennies HC, Kornak U, Zhang H, et al. Gerodermia osteodysplastica is caused by mutations in SCYL1BP1, a Rab-6 interacting golgin. *Nat Genet*. 2008;40(12):1410-1412.
64. Fischer-Zirnsak B, Escande-Beillard N, Ganesh J, et al. Recurrent de novo mutations affecting residue Arg138 of pyrroline-5-carboxylate synthase cause a progeroid form of autosomal-dominant cutis laxa. *Am J Hum Genet*. 2015;97(3):483-492.
65. De Vilder EY, Debacker J, Vanakker OM. GGCX-associated phenotypes: an overview in search of genotype-phenotype correlations. *Int J Mol Sci*. 2017;18(2).
66. Bangsgaard N, Marckmann P, Rossen K, et al. Nephrogenic systemic fibrosis: late skin manifestations. *Arch Dermatol*. 2009;145(2):183-187.
67. Lewis KG, Bercovitch L, Dill SW, et al. Acquired disorders of elastic tissue: part II. Decreased elastic tissue. *J Am Acad Dermatol*. 2004;51(2):165-185; quiz 186-188.
68. Haider M, Alfadley A, Kadry R, et al. Acquired cutis laxa type II (Marshall syndrome) in an 18-month-old child: a case report. *Pediatr Dermatol*. 2010;27(1):89-91.
69. Muster AJ, Bharati S, Herman JJ, et al. Fatal cardiovascular disease and cutis laxa following acute febrile neutrophilic dermatosis. *J Pediatr*. 1983;102(2):243-248.
70. Hill VA, Seymour CA, Mortimer PS. Penicillamine-induced elastosis perforans serpiginosa and cutis laxa in Wilson's disease. *Br J Dermatol*. 2000;142(3):560-561.
71. Mahajan VK, Sharma NL, Garg G. Cutis laxa acquisita associated with cutaneous mastocytosis. *Int J Dermatol*. 2006;45(8):949-951.
72. Kiuru-Enari S, Keski-Oja J, Haltia M. Cutis laxa in hereditary gelsolin amyloidosis. *Br J Dermatol*. 2005;152(2):250-257.
73. Linares A, Zarranz JJ, Rodriguez-Alarcon J, et al. Reversible cutis laxa due to maternal D-penicillamine treatment. *Lancet*. 1979;2(8132):43.
74. Solomon L, Abrams G, Dinner M, et al. Neonatal abnormalities associated with D-penicillamine treatment during pregnancy. *N Engl J Med*. 1977;296(1):54-55.
75. Nahas FX, Sterman S, Gemperli R, et al. The role of plastic surgery in congenital cutis laxa: a 10-year follow-up. *Plast Reconstr Surg*. 1999;104(4):1174-1178; discussion 1179.
76. Fisher BK, Page E, Hanna W. Acral localized acquired cutis laxa. *J Am Acad Dermatol*. 1989;21(1):33-40.
77. Tamura BM, Lourenco LM, Platt A, et al. Cutis laxa: Improvement of facial aesthetics by using botulinum toxin. *Dermatol Surg*. 2004;30(12, pt 2):1518-1520.
78. Gass JK, Hellemans J, Mortier G, et al. Buschke-Ollendorff syndrome: a manifestation of a heterozygous nonsense mutation in the LEMD3 gene. *J Am Acad Dermatol*. 2008;58(5)(suppl 1):S103-S104.
79. Schena D, Germi L, Zamperetti MR, et al. Buschke-Ollendorff syndrome. *Int J Dermatol*. 2008;47(11):1159-1161.
80. Hellemans J, Preobrazhenska O, Willaert A, et al. Loss-of-function mutations in LEMD3 result in osteopoikilosis, Buschke-Ollendorff syndrome and melorheostosis. *Nat Genet*. 2004;36(11):1213-1218.
81. Van Hougenhouck-Tulleken W, Chan I, Hamada T, et al. Clinical and molecular characterization of lipoid proteinosis in Namaqualand, South Africa. *Br J Dermatol*. 2004;151(2):413-423.
82. Vahidnezhad H, Youssefian L, Uitto J. Lipoid proteinosis. In: Adam MP, Ardinger HH, Pagon RA, et al, eds. GeneReviews(R). Seattle (WA): University of Washington.; 1993-2018. Initially posted: January 21, 2016. Available at https://www.ncbi.nlm.nih.gov/books/NBK338540/
83. Sargenti Neto S, Batista JD, Durighetto AF Jr. A case of oral recurrent ulcerative lesions in a patient with lipoid proteinosis (Urbach-Wiethe disease). *Br J Oral Maxillofac Surg*. 2010;48(8):654-655.
84. Cote DN. Head and neck manifestations of lipoid proteinosis. *Otolaryngol Head Neck Surg*. 1998;119(1):144-145.
85. Siebert M, Markowitsch HJ, Bartel P. Amygdala, affect and cognition: evidence from 10 patients with Urbach-Wiethe disease. *Brain*. 2003;126(pt 12):2627-2637.
86. Hamada T, Wessagowit V, South AP, et al. Extracellular matrix protein 1 gene (ECM1) mutations in lipoid proteinosis and genotype-phenotype correlation. *J Invest Dermatol*. 2003;120(3):345-350.
87. Sercu S, Lambeir AM, Steenackers E, et al. ECM1 interacts with fibulin-3 and the beta 3 chain of laminin 332 through its serum albumin subdomain-like 2 domain. *Matrix Biol*. 2009;28(3):160-169.
88. Dyer JA, Yu QC, Paller AS. "Free-floating" desmosomes in lipoid proteinosis: an inherent defect in keratinocyte adhesion? *Pediatr Dermatol*. 2006;23(1):1-6.
89. Kowalewski C, Kozlowska A, Chan I, et al. Three-dimensional imaging reveals major changes in skin microvasculature in lipoid proteinosis and lichen sclerosus. *J Dermatol Sci*. 2005;38(3):215-224.
90. Oyama N, Chan I, Neill SM, et al. Autoantibodies to extracellular matrix protein 1 in lichen sclerosus. *Lancet*. 2003;362(9378):118-123.
91. Paller AS. Histology of lipoid proteinosis. *JAMA*. 1994;272(7):564-565.
92. Ko C, Barr RJ. Vesicular lesions in a patient with lipoid proteinosis: a probable acantholytic dermatosis. *Am J Dermatopathol*. 2003;25(4):335-337.

93. Teive HA, Pereira ER, Zavala JA, et al. Generalized dystonia and striatal calcifications with lipoid proteinosis. *Neurology*. 2004;63(11):2168-2169.
94. Chan I, South AP, McGrath JA, et al. Rapid diagnosis of lipoid proteinosis using an anti-extracellular matrix protein 1 (ECM1) antibody. *J Dermatol Sci*. 2004;35(2):151-153.
95. Ozkaya-Bayazit E, Ozarmagan G, Baykal C, et al. Oral DMSO therapy in 3 patients with lipoidproteinosis. Results of long-term therapy [in German]. *Hautarzt*. 1997;48(7):477-481.
96. Carnevale C, Castiglia D, Diociaiuti A, et al. Lipoid proteinosis: a previously unrecognized mutation and therapeutic response to acitretin. *Acta Derm Venereol*. 2017;97(10):1249-1251.
97. Toosi S, Ehsani AH. Treatment of lipoid proteinosis with acitretin: a case report. *J Eur Acad Dermatol Venereol*. 2009;23(4):482-483.
98. Banne E, Meiner V, Shaag A, et al. Transaldolase deficiency: a new case expands the phenotypic spectrum. *JIMD Rep*. 2016;26:31-36.

Subcutaneous Tissue Disorders PART 12

第十二篇　皮下脂肪疾病

Chapter 73 :: Panniculitis
:: Eden Pappo Lake, Sophie M. Worobec, & Iris K. Aronson

第七十三章

脂膜炎

中文导读

皮下脂肪的炎症（脂膜炎）的诊断常存在困难，目前使用较多的分类方法通过组织学特征常将脂膜炎分为"间隔型"和"小叶型"（表73-2），在这个基础上再进一步参照是否存在血管炎及所浸润炎症细胞的成分进行分类（表73-1）。本章首先对脂肪组织的功能特别是其通过TLRs介导免疫包括先天性免疫和适应性应答的功能进行了介绍，同时对脂肪细胞如何参与炎症反应保护宿主免受感染性疾病和环境危害作了详细阐述。接下来将脂膜炎按病种进行介绍，共分为十四节：①结节性红斑；②硬红斑和结节性血管炎；③硬化性脂膜炎；④感染诱发的脂膜炎；⑤α1-抗胰蛋白酶脂膜炎；⑥胰腺性脂膜炎；⑦狼疮性脂膜炎；⑧组织细胞吞噬性脂膜炎；⑨新生儿皮下脂肪坏死；⑩寒冷性脂膜炎；⑪人工性和外伤性脂膜炎；⑫结缔组织病相关性脂膜炎；⑬痛风脂膜炎；⑭激素后脂膜炎。分别对这些疾病的流行病学、临床特征、病因和病理学机制、诊断、鉴别诊断及治疗进行了介绍，重点阐述了前十种疾病。

1．结节性红斑　结节性红斑（EN）是间隔性脂膜炎的代表，它的发生与多种病因有关，其临床过程往往具有自限性。本节从该病的流行病学、临床特征、病因和发病机制、诊断和鉴别诊断、临床过程和预后及治疗等方面进行了详细阐述。

2．硬红斑和结节性血管炎　硬红斑（EI）和结节性血管炎（NV）由于临床上表现非常相似，经常被放在一起描述视作同一个疾病，是最常见的伴有血管炎的脂膜炎，与结核分枝杆菌感染相关。本节从该病的流行病学、临床特征、病因和发病机制、诊断和鉴别诊断、临床过程和预后及治疗等方面进行了详细阐述。

3.硬化性脂膜炎 硬化性脂膜炎有多个同义词，包括硬皮病样皮下脂膜炎、具有膜性坏死的慢性脂膜炎、硬化性萎缩性蜂窝织炎和静脉淤积性脂膜炎等。它是一种发生在小腿的硬化性脂膜炎，通常与血管功能障碍有关。本节从该病的流行病学、临床特征、病因和发病机制、诊断和鉴别诊断、临床过程、预后及治疗等方面进行了详细阐述。

4.感染诱发的脂膜炎 感染诱发的脂膜炎（IIP）是由病原体直接引起的脂膜炎，可以由细菌、分枝杆菌、真菌、原生动物或病毒引起，可分为原发性感染和由败血症或血源性播散引起的继发性感染。本节从流行病学、临床特征、病因和发病机制、诊断和鉴别诊断、临床过程和预后及治疗等方面对该病进行了详细阐述。

5.α1-抗胰蛋白酶脂膜炎 α1-抗胰蛋白酶（α1AT）是在肝脏中产生的一种糖蛋白。它是一种功能广泛的丝氨酸蛋白酶抑制剂，并可作为急性期反应物在应激时分泌增加。α1AT缺乏症被认为是一种共显性遗传疾病，可出现脂膜炎表现。本节从该病的流行病学、临床特征、病因和发病机制、诊断和鉴别诊断、临床过程和预后及治疗等方面进行了详细阐述。

6.胰腺性脂膜炎 胰腺的各种病理改变都可诱发胰腺炎，包括急性胰腺炎，甚至可发生在内镜下胰胆管逆行造影术后。本节从该病的流行病学、临床特征、病因和发病机制、诊断和鉴别诊断、临床过程和预后及治疗等方面对该病进行了详细阐述。

7.狼疮性脂膜炎 红斑狼疮性脂膜炎（LEP），也称为深在性狼疮、皮下红斑狼疮和Irrgang-Kaposi综合征，由Kaposi于1883年首次描述。本节从流行病学、临床特征、病因和发病机制、诊断和鉴别诊断、临床过程和预后及治疗等方面对该病进行了详细阐述。

8.组织细胞吞噬性脂膜炎 吞噬性组织细胞性脂膜炎（CHP）是一种罕见的可能致命的脂膜炎。如果与嗜血细胞型淋巴细胞组织细胞增生症（HLH）或巨噬细胞活化综合征相关，则可能需要化疗。CHP本身可能代表"缓慢进展"的淋巴瘤而不是单纯的炎症性疾病。本节从流行病学、临床特征、病因和发病机制、诊断和鉴别诊断、临床过程和预后及治疗等方面对该病进行了详细阐述。

9.新生儿皮下脂肪坏死 新生儿的皮下脂肪坏死（SCFN）是一种罕见的脂膜炎，通常发生在生命的最初几天至几周，可自发缓解。本节从流行病学、临床特征、病因和发病机制、诊断和鉴别诊断、临床过程和预后及治疗等方面对该病进行了详细阐述。

10.寒冷性脂膜炎 寒冷的脂膜炎，也称为Haxthausen病，是一种皮肤暴露于寒冷的天气或冰块应用后（如在室上性心动过速的冷敷应用中）发生在皮下脂肪的炎症反应，也可在黏膜上发生（冰棒性脂膜炎）。本节从流行病学、临床特征、病因和发病机制、诊断和鉴别诊断、临床过程和预后及治疗等方面对该病进行了详细阐述。

在接下来的四个小节中，分别对人工性和外伤性脂膜炎、结缔组织病相关性脂膜炎、痛风脂膜炎、激素后脂膜炎的临床和组织学特征以及治疗要点进行了简单介绍。

〔黄莹雪〕

Inflammation in subcutaneous fat (panniculitis) often poses a diagnostic problem as the clinical and histopathologic findings in the various inflammatory disorders of adipose tissue (AT) have overlapping features (Table 73-1).[1],[2] A useful histopathologic classification divides the panniculitides into "septal" and "lobular" (Table 73-2), although several diagnoses exhibit overlapping features.[1] This classification is expanded by noting the presence or absence of vasculitis,[2] and the composition of the inflammatory infiltrate (Table 73-1).

AT functions in energy storage and expenditure, appetite modulation, insulin sensitivity, endocrine and reproductive systems, bone metabolism, inflammation, and immunity.[3] Its origin is traced back to the invertebrate fat body, which has innate immune system, metabolic, and lipid, glycogen and protein storage functions. In the evolution of vertebrates these functions were divided up between the liver and AT with both retaining innate immune system functions.[4,5] The human adipocyte is equipped to protect the organism from pathogenic microbes by recognition of pathogen-associated molecular patterns via receptors called pattern recognition receptors (PRRs).[6] Toll-like receptors (TLRs) are a type of transmembrane PRR, expressed either on the plasma membrane where they detect cell-surface microbial patterns such as lipopolysaccharides of Gram-negative bacteria, or in endosomal/lysosomal organelles, where they recognize mainly microbial nucleic acids.[4,7] Secreted PRRs bind to the surface of microbes, activate the complement system, and opsonize microbes for phagocytosis.[7] Once activated, the PRRs activate proinflammatory signaling pathways, especially activation of transcription factors nuclear factor κB, interferon regulatory factor 3, or nuclear factor of activated T cells, that promote expression of genes involved in the immune response.[7,8] TLRs also trigger activation of adaptive immunity responses that include antibody responses, T-helper type 1, T-helper type 17 CD4+ T cell, CD8+ T-cell responses, and T-helper type 2 (via TLR4) and immunoglobulin E response.[7]

Adipocytes are the most abundant cells in white AT, but other cell types include pericytes, fibroblasts, endothelial cells, vascular smooth muscle cells and inflammatory cells, especially macrophages.[3,9] Macrophage-derived cytokines and chemokines, including tumor necrosis factor (TNF)-α, induce adipocyte lipolysis, which leads to release of free fatty acids from the adipocyte, which induces proinflammatory signaling.[10] This paracrine loop involving inflammatory cytokines and free fatty acids propagates inflammation.[11] AT also contains lymphocytes that contribute to AT inflammation.[5] Adipocytes interact with blood vessels, and bidirectional crosstalk between perivascular AT and blood vessels exists.[12] Perivascular AT secretes high levels of proinflammatory cytokines such as interleukin (IL)-6, IL-8, and monocyte chemotactic protein-1 compared to antiinflammatory adiponectin, when compared to other AT depots.[13] Adipocyte transmembrane PRRs and TLRs, and receptors for interaction with macrophages and lymphocytes, as well as production and secretion of multiple cytokines and adipokines reflect the role of the adipocyte in protecting the host from infectious disease and other environmental dangers.

ERYTHEMA NODOSUM

AT-A-GLANCE

Clinical

- Symmetric, tender, erythematous, nodules, and plaques on the anterior aspects of the lower extremities.
- Acute onset; no ulceration or scarring.
- Fever, fatigue, arthralgias, arthritis, headache are common.
- More common in women.
- Lasts from 3 to 6 weeks, with new lesions appearing for up to 6 weeks.

Histopathology

- Mostly septal panniculitis without vasculitis.
- Thickened, fibrotic septae with inflammatory cells.
- Neutrophils in early lesions.
- Histiocytes and Miescher granulomas in late-stage lesions.

Treatment

- Treatment of any associated disorder.
- Bed rest, aspirin, nonsteroidal antiinflammatory drugs.

Erythema nodosum (EN) is the prototypic septal panniculitis. It is a common panniculitis and multiple etiologies are associated with EN, although many cases are idiopathic. The frequency of EN caused by a single agent has changed greatly over the past century, and is influenced by geography and endemic disease.[14,15] Although the diagnosis is often clinical, the histopathology can be helpful, demonstrating septal inflammation and thickened and fibrotic septae. The clinical findings are usually self-limiting, but an underlying etiology must be investigated as associated diseases have significance for the patient.

EPIDEMIOLOGY

EN occurs in person of all ages, and most cases affect young women in the second to fourth decades of life.[15] Larger studies show more than 80% of EN patients are female, or a female-to-male ratio of 5:1.[16] However, in pediatric cases there is no gender difference.[17] Prevalence in England and Spain varies from 0.38% to 0.5% of patients seen in clinics.[18,19]

TABLE 73-1
Summary of Different Types of Panniculitis

PANNICULITIS	AGE GROUPS	ASSOCIATED FACTORS	CLINICAL COURSE AND MANIFESTATIONS	HISTOPATHOLOGY	TREATMENT
Erythema nodosum	Young women, 2nd to 4th decades	Infections (commonly streptococcal), medications, malignancies (leukemias, lymphomas)	Acute onset; symmetric, tender, nodules & plaques Affecting anterior lower extremities Fever, fatigue, arthralgias, arthritis, headache, no ulceration, no atrophy, no scarring	Septal Panniculitis No vasculitis Neutrophils (early), Meischer granulomas (late)	Bed rest, aspirin, NSAIDs SSKI, 2-10 drops thrice daily Colchicine Corticosteroids (rarely indicated)
Erythema induratum	Young/middle-aged women	Venous insufficiency, obesity Infectious etiology: MTB, hepatitides B, C	Erythematous SQ nodules on lower extremities May affect calves, anterolateral leg Tenderness, ulceration, scarring Protracted course, with recurrent episodes 3-6 weeks duration	Lobular, often with vasculitis (90%). Early central necrosis of adipocytes; neutrophilic infiltrate In older lesions, epithelioid histiocytes, multinucleated giant cells	If MTB testing is positive, full course of multidrug therapy Treat underlying cause SSKI, NSAIDs, colchicine, antimalarials, corticosteroids, gold Bed rest Pentoxifylline, compression
Lipodermatosclerosis (sclerosing panniculitis, hypodermitis sclerodermiformis, chronic panniculitis with lipomembranous changes, sclerotic atrophic cellulitis, venous stasis panniculitis)	Overweight women older than 40 years	Venous insufficiency Obesity Systemic sclerosis Pulmonary Infarction Hypertension	Indurated, woody plaques on lower extremities, with acute & chronic changes (most commonly, anteromedial calf area) Intense pain is the most frequent symptom Stage: acute inflammatory Chronic fibrosis Inverted champagne bottle	Stasis changes Lobular panniculitis No vasculitis Ischemic necrosis at center Thickened, fibrotic septa, atrophy of subcutaneous fat Membranocystic changes	Compression therapy is the major recommended treatment (30-40 mm Hg) Stanozolol: to decrease pain, erythema, induration Pentoxifylline, horse chestnut seed extract, oxerutins, flavonoid fraction Weight loss
Infectious panniculitis	—	Wide variety of bacteria, fungi, parasites, viruses Either primarily inoculated, or hematogenous Staphylococcus aureus panniculitis with juvenile diabetes Panniculitis of mycetoma, chromoblastomycosis, sporotrichosis	Erythematous plaques, nodules, abscess with purulent discharge (fluctuant/abscess-type lesions) Most commonly on legs and feet Upper extremities, trunk, face may be involved	Mostly lobular panniculitis, but with a mixed pattern Pattern dependent on whether infection was inoculation related or hematogenous Neutrophilic infiltrate	Depends on the known organisms

α_1-Antitrypsin panniculitis	Most common in 30-60 years of age groups MM: most common phenotype (normal AAT) ZZ: 10%-15% of N levels; associated with >60% of cases	Pulmonary and hepatic disease (emphysema in COPD, cirrhosis, hepatocellular CA), highest risk ZZ phenotype Panniculitis uncommon in AAT deficiency	Painful erythematous nodules and plaques Cellulitis, fluctuant abscess type Most common site: lower trunk, also buttocks, proximal extremities May be life-threatening	Early necrosis of SQ fat Splaying of neutrophils between collagen bundles is characteristic Liquefactive necrosis	MILD-MODERATE: dapsone, doxycycline SEVERE: protein replacement therapy
Pancreatic panniculitis	Occurs in 2%-3% of patients with pancreatic disorders	Pancreatitis, pancreatic CA	Erythematous nodules with spontaneous ulceration Lower extremities, especially periarticular areas (knee, ankle) Crops of lesions; red-brown Atrophic, hyperpigmented scarring Oily abscesses	Lobular panniculitis No vasculitis Intense necrosis at center of lobule Ghost adipocytes Saponification and calcification	Octreotide Plasmapheresis
Lupus panniculitis	Females more frequently affected than males (4:1) 30-60 years old, also in childhood May occur before or after diagnosis of lupus erythematosus or discoid lupus erythematosus	Systemic lupus erythematosus Sjogren's Syndrome Rheumatoid arthritis	UPPER ARMS (lateral), shoulders, face, scalp, hips, buttocks, breasts Rare on lower extremities Deep, tender SQ nodules; no surface changes Resolves with depressed lipoatrophic areas Chronic, with yearly/periodic flares Duration: average of 6 years	Vacuolar alteration of basal cell layer, thickened basement membrane, mucin deposition, superficial and deep perivascular infiltrate Mostly lobular panniculitis, with lymphoid follicles, variable hyaline fat necrosis, sclerotic collagen bundles, lymphocytic and plasma cell infiltrate	Hydroxychloroquine is first-line treatment Quinacrine
Panniculitis with dermatomyositis	Very rare	Dermatomyositis	Erythematous nodules and plaques, affecting arms, buttocks, thighs, abdomen	Mixed septal and lobular panniculitis, lymphocytic and plasma cell infiltrate, hyaline sclerosis of septal collagen; calcification, membranocystic changes in late stages	Corticosteroids alone, or corticosteroids with methotrexate
Cytophagic histiocytic panniculitis	Rare; seen in adults, adolescents, and children	HLH MAS	SQ erythematous to violaceous plaques on extremities, trunk Fulminant cases may have: ulceration, fever, hepatosplenomegaly, hemocytophagocytosis in BM, LN, liver, CNS May be acute and intermittent, or have a rapidly fatal course	Lobular panniculitis No vasculitis Bean bag cells: macrophages with intact or fragmented erythrocytes, leukocytes, or platelets Necrosis	Corticosteroids Cyclosporine Multidisciplinary care in a hospital setting

(Continued)

TABLE 73-1
Summary of Different Types of Panniculitis (Continued)

PANNICULITIS	AGE GROUPS	ASSOCIATED FACTORS	CLINICAL COURSE AND MANIFESTATIONS	HISTOPATHOLOGY	TREATMENT
Subcutaneous fat necrosis of the newborn	Rare, first few weeks of life	History of perinatal complications (meconium aspiration, hypothermia, hypoxemia, gestational diabetes)	Erythematous to violaceous, firm nodules or plaques affecting buttocks, back, shoulders, cheeks, thighs Anterior trunk spared Oily/chalky white material Late hypercalcemia (monitor for 6 months)	Lobular panniculitis No vasculitis Needle-shaped clefts in radial array Nodules and plaques, resolving spontaneously	Spontaneous resolution Monitor serum calcium for hypercalcemia Systemic glucocorticoids may be considered; nephrocalcinosis
Cold panniculitis (Haxthausen disease)	Scrotal cold panniculitis in 9–14-year-old males	Exposure to cold weather, popsicles, ice packs, swimming	Indurate, erythematous plaques or nodules at sites of cold exposure; affects face, thighs, scrotal fat of prepubertal boys Resolution within 3 months	Lobular panniculitis No vasculitis Perivascular lymphohistiocytic infiltrate	Spontaneous resolution
Factitial panniculitis	—	Associated with personality aberrations	SQ implantation (medications, cosmetic fillers, oils, human waste)	Lobular panniculitis No vasculitis Suppurative granuloma involving fat lobule Refractile foreign material	Psychiatric treatment; Intralesional steroids, surgical excision

AAT, α_1-antitrypsin; BM, bone marrow; CA, cancer; COPD, chronic obstructive pulmonary disease; HLH, hemophagocytic lymphohistiocytosis; MAS, macrophage activation syndrome; MTB, *Mycobacterium tuberculosis*; NSAID, nonsteroidal antiinflammatory drug; SQ, subcutaneous; SSKI, saturated solution of potassium iodide.

TABLE 73-2
Differentiating Septal vs Lobular Panniculitis

	SEPTAL PANNICULITIS	LOBULAR PANNICULITIS
Origin of inflammation	Interlobular septa	Primarily the lobule or blood vessel
Appearance of lobule	Lobule appears intact, individual adipocytes well defined	Lobule is necrotic, lipophages common; free liquid may accumulate in pools of varying shapes
Necrosis	Absent	Common
Inflammatory cell	Neutrophils (acute) Mononuclear cells, multinucleated giant cells (chronic)	Lymphoid infiltrates Plasma cells are common
Vasculitis	Absent	May be present
Characteristic findings	Miescher granuloma	
Associated conditions	Erythema nodosum	Erythema induratum Lupus panniculitis Pancreatic panniculitis Lipodermatosclerosis α_1-Antitrypsin deficiency

CLINICAL FEATURES

EN presents with tender, erythematous, warm nodules and plaques on the lower legs (see Fig. 73-1). The anterior lower legs and ankles are most commonly involved, but the forearms, upper legs, trunk, and even the face can be involved; with more atypical locations seen in children.[17,18] The nodules may become confluent and violaceous and bruise-like, termed *erythema contusiformis* when hemorrhage is present.[15] Ulceration and scarring are not seen.[15] EN may be associated with systemic symptoms of fever, malaise, fatigue, arthralgia, arthritis, headache, and, more rarely, abdominal pain, vomiting, diarrhea, or cough.[15,16] Upper respiratory tract infection precedes the onset of EN in 20% to 30% of cases.[16,18,19] Laboratory abnormalities frequently indicate the etiology; that is, a positive throat culture and leukocytosis in streptococcal infections.[20,21] A positive purified protein derivative suggests tuberculosis infection in endemic areas and high-risk individuals. An abnormal chest radiograph may be seen with either sarcoidosis or pulmonary infections.

ETIOLOGY AND PATHOGENESIS

ETIOLOGY

EN is associated with numerous etiologies (Table 73-3). The abundance of idiopathic cases of EN (37% to 60%) reported in large reviews,[17,22] reflects the difficulty of defining a specific causation of EN. Infections, medications, malignancies, autoimmune disease, and inflammatory disorders have all been documented to provoke the clinical findings of EN. Infectious causes include bacterial, viral, fungal, and protozoan, with streptococcal respiratory tract infections being the most common etiology in pediatric cases of EN.[16,17] Viral etiologies are difficult to diagnose and may confound idiopathic EN.[16] EN secondary to tuberculosis varies with higher rates seen in endemic areas but is rare in the United States and Europe.[16]

Common causative medications include antibiotics, oral contraceptives and other hormonal therapies, and nonsteroidal antiinflammatories.[16,23] More recent cases have suggested an association between EN and omeprazole use,[24] leukotriene inhibitors,[20] and vemurafenib.[25] The prevalence of oral contraceptive-induced EN has decreased since the introduction of low-dose estrogen therapy.[23] Malignancies related to EN most often include leukemias or lymphomas.[15] Sarcoidosis and inflammatory bowel disease are also known etiologies. Sarcoidosis-induced EN prevalence varies by geography and patient population

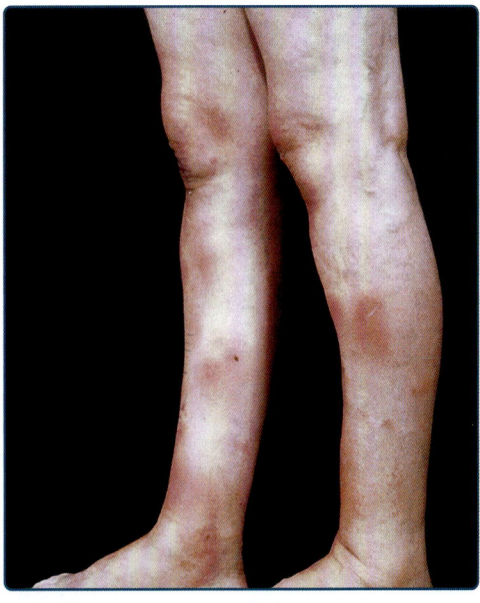

Figure 73-1 Erythema nodosum. Erythematous nodules located mainly on the anterior lower legs.

but can be a cause of up to one-third of EN cases.[26] Temporal arteritis also has been noted to cause EN.[22]

PATHOGENESIS

The cutaneous findings of EN are considered to be a hypersensitivity reaction to the above etiologies. Other theories suggest immune complex deposition[27] and neutrophilic involvement.[28] Overall, the pathophysiologic mechanism is not understood. Early studies showed the presence of interferon-γ and IL-2, activation of leukocytes,[29] upregulation of various adhesion molecules,[30] and genetic polymorphisms in TNF-α promoter, macrophage migration inhibitory factor, or RANTES (regulated upon activation, normal T-cell expressed and secreted).[31-33]

AT can activate innate and adaptive immune responses to destroy pathogens.[34] Excessive adipocyte production and secretion of proinflammatory adipokines and adipocytokines is associated with obesity, cardiovascular disease, hypertension, and diabetes.[34] In contrast, EN is associated with a more limited coccidiomycosis infection[35] and with a less severe and shorter duration of sarcoidosis,[35,36] especially in those carrying the HLA-DRB1*03-positive leukocyte antigen.[37] Therefore, certain genetic mutations associated with enhanced inflammatory reactions may confer resistance to certain pathogens.[35,37] Further evidence of the innate immune system's function is the neutrophilic involvement seen in EN cytokine profiles, with high expression of TNF-α, IL-8, IL-6, monocyte chemoattractant protein-1, and granulocyte colony-stimulating factor.[28]

DIAGNOSIS

All of the above etiologies present with similar histopathologic features, and the spectrum of histopathologic features in EN and other panniculitides may be variable.[38] This necessitates correlation with clinical features, including location of lesions, systemic symptoms, and laboratory findings. Examination of AT requires large excisional biopsies, as the inflammatory infiltrate can be missed. Inflammation in AT is not a static process, and more than 1 biopsy may be necessary to come to a conclusive diagnosis. EN is generally a "septal" pattern with inflammation confined predominantly to the septa. Of note the "lobular" form implies inflammation predominantly involving the fat lobule itself.

Early EN shows edema of the adipose septae with neutrophils and extravasated red blood cells. As EN develops, the septae widen and become fibrosed, and a mixed infiltrate that includes lymphocytes, histiocytes, neutrophils, and some eosinophils is seen.[15] Fibrotic, wide septae characterize late EN lesions, often with granulomas, and fat lobules may be encroached upon and partially effaced (Fig. 73-2A). An overlying superficial and deep dermal perivascular infiltrate is frequently present in EN.[39]

EN has characteristic, but not sensitive or specific, groupings of histiocytes surrounding a central stellate cleft called Miescher granuloma (see Fig. 73-2B).[15] It is considered characteristic of early EN, but is not universally found in EN,[39] and has been described in other types of panniculitis.[39] Some authors believe the Miescher granulomas are consistently found in EN.[15] Late EN lesions may demonstrate lipomembranous change.[15,40] Although by definition, vasculitis is characteristically absent in EN, thrombophlebitis has been emphasized by some as a feature in early EN,[41] and medium-vessel arteritis may (rarely) occur.[38]

DIFFERENTIAL DIAGNOSIS

Table 73-4 outlines the differential diagnosis of EN.

CLINICAL COURSE AND PROGNOSIS

EN is a benign, self-limiting subcutaneous disease that resolves a few weeks after initial presentation;

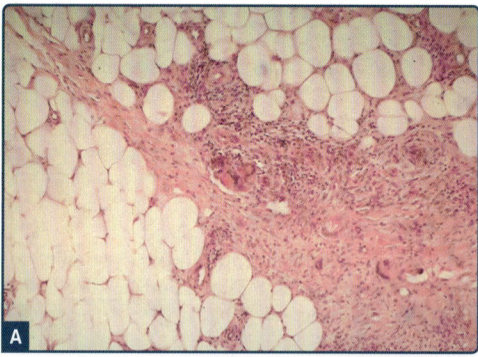
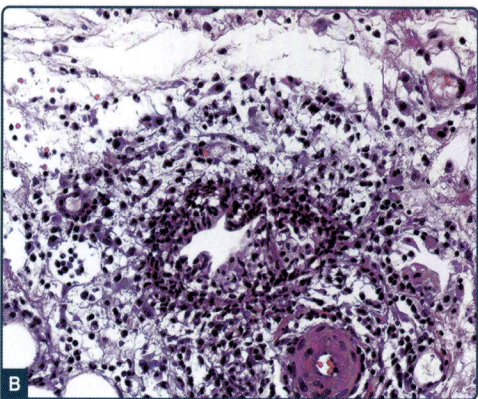

Figure 73-2 **A,** Widened septa with inflammatory infiltrate including multinucleated giant cells. **B,** High-power magnification of a Miescher granuloma shows a discrete micronodular aggregate of small histiocytes around a central stellate cleft.

TABLE 73-3
Reported Etiologies of Erythema Nodosum

Bacterial Infections
- **Streptococcal infections**
- **Tuberculosis**
- ***Yersinia* infections**
- ***Salmonella* infections**
- ***Campylobacter* infections**
- Brucellosis
- Tularemia
- Atypical mycobacterial infections
- Chancroid
- Meningococcemia
- *Corynebacterium diphtheriae* infections
- Cat-scratch disease
- *Propionibacterium acnes*
- *Shigella* infections
- Gonorrhea
- Syphilis
- Leptospirosis
- Q fever
- Lymphogranuloma venereum
- *Chlamydophila psittaci* infections
- *Mycoplasma pneumoniae* infections
- *Helicobacter pylori* infection

Viral Infections
- Infectious mononucleosis
- Hepatitis B
- Milker nodules
- Orf (contagious ecthyma)
- Herpes simplex
- Measles
- Cytomegalovirus infections

Fungal Infections
- Dermatophytes
- Blastomycosis
- Histoplasmosis
- Coccidioidomycosis
- Sporotrichosis
- Aspergillosis

Protozoal Infections
- Toxoplasmosis
- Ancylostomiasis
- Amebiasis
- Giardiasis
- Ascariasis

Drugs
- **Sulfonamides**
- **Bromides**
- **Iodides**
- **Oral contraceptives, progesterone**
- Minocycline
- Gold salts
- **Penicillin**
- Salicylates
- Chlorothiazides
- Phenytoin
- Aminopyrine
- Arsphenamine
- Hepatitis B vaccine
- Nitrofurantoin
- Pyritinol
- D-Penicillamine
- Thalidomide
- Isotretinoin
- Interleukin-2
- Omeprazole
- Valproate
- Tdap (tetanus, diphtheria, and pertussis) vaccine
- Leukotriene-modifying agents
- Vemurafenib

Miscellaneous Conditions
- **Sarcoidosis**
- Ulcerative colitis
- Colon diverticulosis
- **Crohn disease**
- Behçet disease
- Reactive arthritis
- Sweet syndrome
- Pregnancy
- Takayasu arteritis
- Immunoglobulin A nephropathy
- Chronic active hepatitis
- Granulomatous mastitis
- Vogt-Koyanagi disease
- Sjögren syndrome
- Temporal arteritis
- Systemic lupus erythematosus
- Dental infection

Malignant Diseases
- Hodgkin disease
- Non-Hodgkin lymphoma, including mucosa-associated lymphoid tissue (MALT) lymphoma
- Leukemia
- Sarcoma
- Renal carcinoma
- Postradiotherapy for pelvic carcinoma

the course, however, varies based on the etiology. Medication-induced EN may improve after discontinuation of the drug with reappearance of clinical findings when the drug is reintroduced. New lesions of EN are uncommon after 6 weeks, with persistent and recurrent cases reported.[18] After avoidance of causative factors, recurrence is more common if no etiology is identified.[21] EN secondary to a malignancy, a severe systemic disease, or infection may have a more complicated course as a result of the prognosis of the primary disease. Patients with EN secondary to sarcoidosis have an improved prognosis.[36] Patients with Crohn disease and EN are more likely to have colonic involvement of inflammatory bowel disease.[42] While recurrence of EN is rare, it is more frequent when associated with sarcoidosis, hormonal therapy and pregnancy, and streptococcal infection.[26] Most cases of EN heal well with no recurrence, but relapses occur in 6% to 34% of reported cases.[20]

TABLE 73-4
Differential Diagnosis of Erythema Nodosum

DIAGNOSIS	CHARACTERISTIC FEATURES
Erythema induratum/nodular vasculitis	Most common on posterior calves with ulceration.
Simple bruising	History of trauma or anticoagulation, with no history of ongoing lesions. Lack of inflammatory features such as warmth. Tender only to palpation and heal spontaneously.
Cutaneous polyarteritis nodosa	Nodules in association with livedo reticularis and arterial inflammation on histology, possibly with neuropathy.
Sarcoidosis	Can occur as nodules or plaques or patches on extremities. Sarcoidal granulomas in dermis or subcutis of cutaneous nodules on skin biopsy. Often with systemic sarcoidosis.
Cellulitis	Larger plaques that are erythematous and lack the violaceous bruising. More tender and warm.
Lipodermatosclerosis	Firm plaques nearly circumferential around lower leg.
Pancreatic panniculitis	Occurs anywhere on the legs; ulceration and drainage. Serum lipase and amylase often elevated.
Behçet syndrome occurring in the fat	Vasculitis occurring in the fat tissue, either lymphocytic or neutrophilic, small arterial involvement with either lobular or mixed lobular and septal pattern.
Sweet syndrome	Erythematous nodules may be present on the face, neck, upper trunk, as well as extremities. Nodules may have vesicles, pustules, or bullae. Histology with intense dermal edema; diffuse, deep neutrophilic infiltrate with karyorrhexis.
Subcutaneous tuberculosis or other atypical mycobacterial infection	Nodules or plaques occurring in endemic areas. Habitation or travel to endemic areas; possible history of trauma. Characteristic features on microbiology and positive acid-fast bacilli on histopathology.

nonsteroidal antiinflammatory agents are recommended. Supersaturated potassium iodide solution (SSKI) can be used, but thyroid disorder and pregnancy screening must be done prior to administration, and there are risks of hypothyroidism, goiter, and heart and lung toxicity.[43] Dosing SSKI is via drops in water or juice, using 2-10 drops (1 drop = 0.03 mL = 30 mg) 3 times per day.[43] Colchicine is effective in Behçet-related EN specifically.[44] Etanercept[45] and infliximab[46] are options for inflammatory bowel disease–associated EN. Other potential treatment options include oxyphenbutazone[47] and hydroxychloroquine,[48] with limited, randomized, controlled trials. Corticosteroids are not first-line therapy as there is a risk of infectious etiology in idiopathic EN.

ERYTHEMA INDURATUM AND NODULAR VASCULITIS

AT-A-GLANCE

Clinical
- Erythematous subcutaneous nodules and plaques of lower legs; common on calves, but also on anterolateral legs, feet, and thighs; rarely also on arms, forearms, and face.
- Associated with venous insufficiency; more frequent in middle-aged women.
- Often, ulceration and scarring present.
- Chronic, relapsing course.
- Infectious etiologies include bacterial (especially *Mycobacterium tuberculosis*), fungal, viral, and protozoal.

Histopathology
- Mostly lobular or mixed lobular and septal panniculitis with vasculitis in 90%.
- Extensive necrosis of the adipocytes in the center of the adipose lobule.
- Variable inflammatory infiltrate: neutrophils in early lesions and epithelioid histiocytes and multinucleated giant cells in fully developed lesions.
- Vasculitis of the small veins and venules of the fat lobule.

Treatment
- With positive *Mycobacterium tuberculosis* studies: a full course of antituberculosis triple-agent therapy.
- Complete treatment of infectious etiologies.
- In other cases: potassium iodide, other antiinflammatory drugs, supporting bandages and hose, leg elevation, bed rest.

MANAGEMENT

If there is an identifiable etiologic factor, management of EN focuses on eliminating the exposure, or treating the underlying diseases. Potential infection must be sought and treated and suspected medications should be discontinued. An extensive review of all medications (including nonprescription and supplemental products), medical supplements and a thorough medical history, including symptoms several weeks prior to the EN onset, travel history, and family history of infections are critical to the workup.[18]

Supportive care is the mainstay of treatment after removing or treating the provoking factors: bed rest if severe, with lower-extremity elevation, and

Erythema induratum (EI) and nodular vasculitis (NV) also present as nodular lesions on the legs. They were first described as early as 1945, with a relationship with *Mycobacterium tuberculosis* (MTB).[49] The clinical presentation and histopathology differentiate EI/NV from EN, cutaneous polyarteritis nodosa, or other nodules seen on the legs. EI most commonly presents with ulcerated nodules on the calves, and is associated with MTB infection. A similar disorder, appearing in calves and other lower-extremity sites was subsequently described without MTB association and was called NV. However, clinically the 2 nodular leg syndromes are so similar that it is impossible to separate them.[50-52] Consequently, the terms are most often used interchangeably.

EPIDEMIOLOGY

The EI/NV grouping is the most common diagnosis of a panniculitis with vasculitis.[53] EI/NV is seen most commonly in young to middle-aged women,[51,54] as dominant as a 9:1 ratio.[55] Ages range from 8 months to 66 years with a mean age of 36.6 years.[56,57] In a review of 165 patients with cutaneous tuberculosis (TB), only 2 presented with EI.[58] This varies by time of study and location, as a study in Hong Kong showed 79.5% of cutaneous TB cases to be EI.[59] Pediatric cutaneous TB accounts for 1% to 2% of cases. The highest rates of pediatric cutaneous TB are seen in Pakistan.[60] EI lesions develop more frequently during winter, and are associated with obesity and venous insufficiency.[51]

CLINICAL FEATURES

EI/NV is known for affecting the calves as recurrent, erythematous to violaceous nodules and deep plaques that may be tender[51] (Fig. 73-3) but often are not painful.[50] Ulceration often leads to scarring.[51] Surface changes include crusting of the ulcers and a surrounding collarette of scale (Fig. 73-4).[50] Although the posterior calf is the most frequent location, lesions may also appear in the anterolateral areas of the feet,[61] thighs, and, rarely, the arms and face.[50] A consistent systemic finding in patients with MTB-associated EI is a positive tuberculoid skin test, including the Mantoux test or tuberculin-purified protein derivative. Systemic findings related to the etiology, TB or otherwise, vary greatly.

ETIOLOGY AND PATHOGENESIS

Although EI was frequently associated with MTB, the etiology was controversial because organisms are not always identified in the biopsies and tissue cultures. With the advent of polymerase chain reaction (PCR) techniques, multiple culture-negative cases were shown to contain MTB DNA.[62]

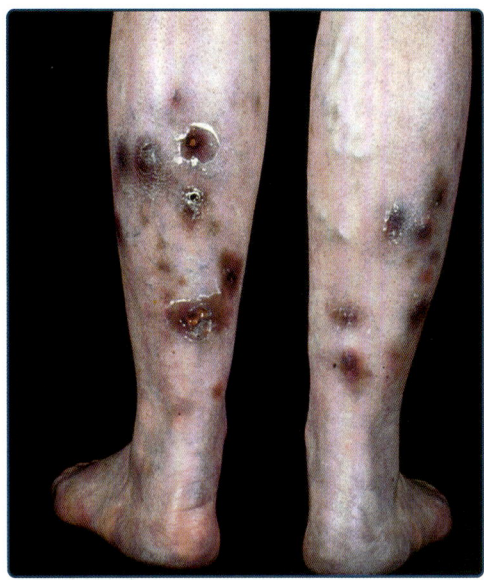

Figure 73-3 Erythema induratum. Erythematous to brown and bluish nodules with ulceration on calves.

In vitro studies show that MTB can bind to scavenger receptors, enter adipocytes, and, via the nearly 20 lipases of MTB, can appropriate the host lipids, accumulate intracytoplasmic lipid inclusions, and survive in a nonreplicating state that is insensitive to the major antimycobacterial medication isoniazid.[63] However, rifampin and ethambutol can reduce MTB bacterial load in adipocytes by 80% to 90%.[63] Other organisms that can infect adipocytes and serve as a reservoir of reactivation include cytomegalovirus, *Chlamydophila pneumoniae*, adenovirus, influenza virus, respiratory syncytial virus, *Rickettsia prowazekii*, and *Trypanosoma cruzi*.[64-67] Infection of adipocytes leads to activation of cytokines and adipokines that bring other innate immune cells (macrophages, neutrophils, mast cells, natural killer cells) as well as adaptive immune cells (sensitized T cells) to the infection site to help contain the infection.[57]

EI is considered to be a hypersensitivity disorder mediated by immune complexes or cell-mediated hypersensitivity, manifested by the presence of tuberculin skin tests and highly positive interferon-γ release assay tests to MTB.[68,69] The T cells, monocytes, and macrophages as well as Langerhans cells may suggest a type IV hypersensitivity reaction.[70]

Extracutaneous MTB is found in many EI patients, and may be present in the lung, lymph nodes, kidney, bowel,[51] or adrenal glands, presenting as Addison disease.[55] Rare species, including *Mycobacterium monacense*, can also cause the EI/NV clinical and histopathologic presentation.[71] Other infections and disorders also have been associated with NV, including hepatitis B, hepatitis C (red finger syndrome and panniculitis), ulcerative colitis, leukemia, rheumatoid arthritis, hypothyroidism, and *Nocardia* infection.[51,72-74] Crohn disease is also a rare cause of NV, and when present it may be metastatic disese.[75] *Chlamydophila pneumoniae* has been reported to induce NV.[76] Medications,

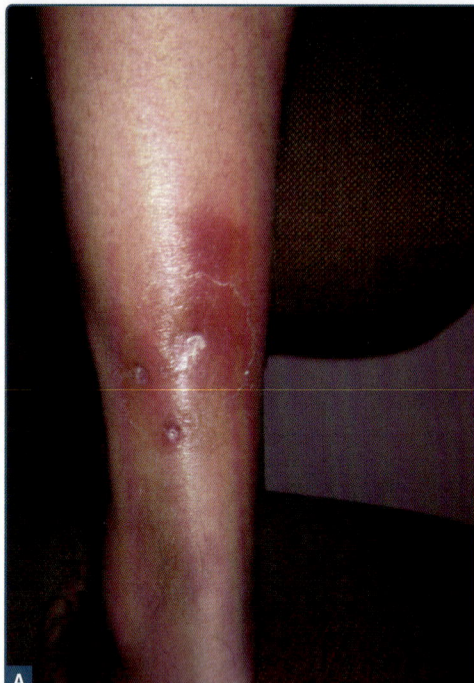

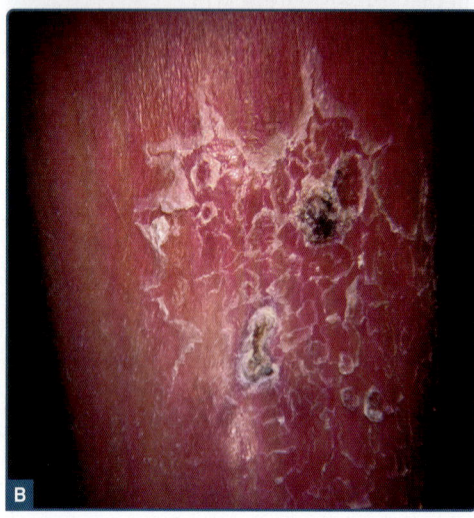

Figure 73-4 A and **B,** Erythema induratum with surrounding collarette of scale.

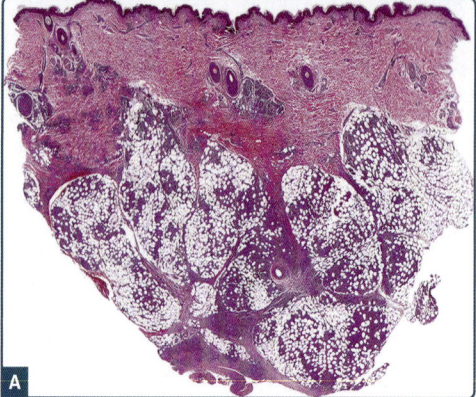

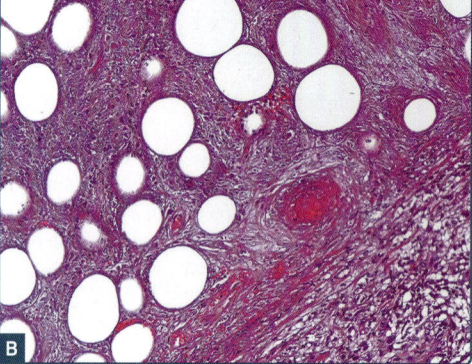

Figure 73-5 Erythema induratum nodular vasculitis. **A,** Low-power magnification shows a mostly lobular panniculitis. **B,** Higher-power magnification shows extensive adipocyte necrosis and vascular damage—necrotizing vasculitis of small venules in the fat lobule.

including propylthiouracil[77] and etanercept,[78] also are associated with NV. Bacillus Calmette-Guérin vaccination is reported to cause EI, 2 and 3 months after injection.[56,57]

DIAGNOSIS

Histopathologic findings correlate with lesion duration, but the common denominator is a mostly lobular or mixed septal and lobular panniculitis (Fig. 73-5A). In early lesions, fat lobules contain discrete aggregates of inflammatory cells, with neutrophils predominating without leukocytoclasia.[53] Adipocyte necrosis is present, which leads to foamy histiocytes. In established lesions of EI/NV, collections of epithelioid histiocytes, multinucleated giant cells, and lymphocytes produce a granulomatous appearance.[52,53] Intense vascular damage, when present, is accompanied by extensive areas of caseous necrosis (Fig. 73-5B), eventuating in tuberculoid granuloma formation.[52] The caseous necrosis may involve the overlying dermis to such an extent that ulceration occurs.[52] Eosinophils may be present and do not conflict the diagnosis.[79]

In a review of 101 cases consistent with EI, vasculitis (of lobular venules, septal veins, and septal arteries) was present in 90% of cases.[51] Lack of vasculitis has been seen on the histopathology in severely immunocompromised patients.[80] Importantly, MTB can cause both EN and EI, and thus in a patient with appropriate travel and exposures, clinical and pathologic characteristics may not rule out a diagnosis of TB.[81]

DIFFERENTIAL DIAGNOSIS

Table 73-5 outlines the differential diagnosis of erythema induratum/nodular vasculitis.

TABLE 73-5
Differential Diagnosis of Erythema Induratum/Nodular Vasculitis

DIAGNOSIS	CHARACTERISTIC FEATURES
Erythema nodosum	Most common on anterior legs with no ulceration and no scarring.
Cutaneous polyarteritis nodosa	Nodules in association with livedo reticularis and arterial inflammation on histology, possibly with neuropathy.
Sarcoidosis	Can occur as nodules or plaques or patches on extremities. Sarcoidal granulomas in dermis or subcutis of cutaneous nodules on ski biopsy. Often occurs with systemic sarcoidosis.
Lipodermatosclerosis	Firm plaques that can become nearly circumferential around lower leg. In morbid obesity, can occur on breasts and abdomen.
Pancreatic panniculitis	Occurs anywhere on the legs, with ulceration and drainage. Serum lipase and amylase are often elevated.
Behçet syndrome occurring in the fat	Vasculitis occurring in the fat tissue, either lymphocytic or neutrophilic; small arterial involvement with either lobular or mixed lobular and septal pattern.
Subcutaneous Sweet syndrome	Erythematous nodules may be present on the face, neck, and upper trunk, as well as extremities. Nodules may have vesicles, pustules, or bullae. Histology with intense dermal edema; diffuse, deep neutrophilic infiltrate with karyorrhexis.

Antiinflammatory treatments that have been used in NV not associated with MTB include SSKI, nonsteroidal antiinflammatory agents, corticosteroids, and gold, as well as bed rest with leg elevation, and treatment of venous insufficiency with compression and pentoxifylline, and even mycophenolate mofetil.[54,83,84] If immunosuppressive agents are used, monitoring for possible infectious etiology is recommended.

LIPODERMATOSCLEROSIS

AT-A-GLANCE

Clinical
- Indurated, firm plaques of wood-like consistency on the lower legs.
- Associations: chronic venous insufficiency, elevated body mass index, female gender, arterial hypertension, arterial ischemia, and thrombophlebitis.

Histopathology
- Background of stasis changes; mostly lobular panniculitis without vasculitis.
- Ischemic necrosis at the center of fat lobule.
- Thickened and fibrotic septae and atrophy of the subcutaneous fat, with marked fibrosis and sclerosis in late-stage severe cases.

Treatment
- Compression stockings, ultrasound therapy, pentoxifylline.
- Successful response to anabolic steroids, platelet-rich plasma, in cases.

CLINICAL COURSE AND PROGNOSIS

EI/NV can have a protracted course with recurrent episodes over months[50] to years.[51,52] Patients with EI/NV are generally healthy, except for the associated disease. The course of EI is also often more chronic than EN, and the ulceration and scarring of EI leads to a worse cosmetic and potentially debilitating outcome than EN.[70]

MANAGEMENT

In patients with positive MTB cultures, positive tuberculoid skin test or positive interferon-γ release assay such as the QuantiFERON-TB Gold in-tube assay, treatment with multiple agent anti-TB therapy is indicated.[70] If an interferon-γ release assay is negative but clinical suspicion in a high-risk TB area persists, lesional PCR is recommended.[82] Patients with hepatitis B or hepatitis C should receive appropriate antiviral intervention. Other infectious etiologies should be sought and treated if present. Potentially causative medications should be discontinued.

Lipodermatosclerosis (LDS) has multiple synonyms, including sclerosing panniculitis, hypodermitis sclerodermiformis, chronic panniculitis with lipomembranous changes, sclerotic atrophic cellulitis, and venous stasis panniculitis. It is a form of sclerosing panniculitis involving the lower legs, often related to vascular malfunction. The first name used was *hypodermitis sclerodermiformis*, which was used as early as the 1950s.[85]

EPIDEMIOLOGY

LDS is the most common form of panniculitis, seen by clinicians far more frequently than EN. LDS occurs with venous insufficiency, mostly in overweight women older than 40 years,[86,87] with age ranges varying from 31 to 74 years and older.[88] The female-to-male ratio is 4:1,[88] and in some studies it is as high as 12:1.[89] White race has been associated more often with LDS.[89] Obesity is common, with 85% of affected patients having a body mass index greater than 30.[90] Comorbidities include hypertension, thyroid disease, diabetes mellitus, prior history of lower-extremity cellulitis, and deep vein thrombosis.[90] Obstructive sleep apnea and arthritis (both osteoarthritic and rheumatoid) also are associated with LDS.[88]

CLINICAL FEATURES

LDS has an acute inflammatory stage and a chronic fibrotic stage. In patients presenting with the acute form, very painful, poorly demarcated, cellulitis-like erythematous plaques persist and evolve to violaceous, edematous, or indurated plaques or nodules, which are seen on the lower legs, most commonly on the lower anteromedial calf (Fig. 73-6).[87,91] Unilateral

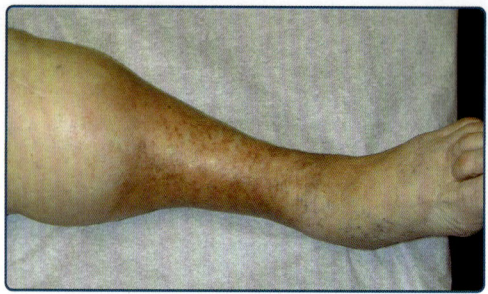

Figure 73-7 Chronic lipodermatosclerosis with champagne bottle/bowling pin deformity.

involvement is seen in 55%, a localized plaque in 51%, and ulceration in 13% of cases.[90] Lesions can be very painful, leading to misdiagnoses of EN, cellulitis, or thrombophlebitis.[87,91] Although patients in this acute phase may lack obvious venous disease,[87] vascular studies show venous insufficiency in the majority.[91] In those patients with normal venous studies, most have a high body mass index.[90]

The chronic form of LDS does not always follow an obvious acute phase.[87] Chronic LDS presents as indurated[92] to sclerotic, depressed and hyperpigmented skin. These findings occur on the lower portion of the lower leg, predominantly on the medial aspect, or in a stocking distribution. This is described as an "inverted champagne bottle" or a "bowling pin" appearance (Fig. 73-7).[86,87,91]

ETIOLOGY AND PATHOGENESIS

A few medications are reported to induce LDS, including gemcitabine[93] and pemetrexed.[94] Additional pathogenic features may include elevated hydrostatic pressure-induced vascular permeability secondary to downregulation of tight junctions[95] with extravascular diffusion of fibrin[90]; microthrombi[96]; abnormalities in protein S and protein C[97]; hypoxia[98]; damage to endothelial cells by inflammatory cells[99]; upregulation of intercellular adhesion molecules and platelet-derived and endothelial-derived factors[100]; and inflammation with wound healing and local collagen stimulation leading to fibrosis and further vascular and lymphatic damage.[90] The fibrosis is accompanied by increased transforming growth factor-β1 gene and protein expression,[101] as well as an increase in procollagen type 1 gene expression.[102]

Hypoxia in AT induces chronic inflammation with macrophage infiltration and inflammatory cytokine expression.[103] The adipocyte produces multiple matrix metalloproteinases as well as tissue inhibitors of metalloproteinases,[104] which may contribute to tissue remodeling seen in LDS. Studies have linked expansion of AT (as in obesity) to hypoxia, causing an increase in hypoxia-inducible factor 1α expression.[105] This stimulates extracellular factors, including collagen I and collagen III, leading to fibrosis.[106]

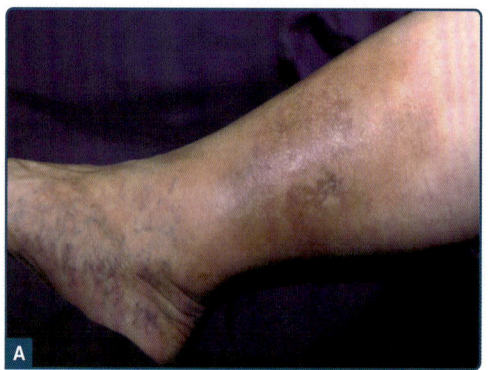

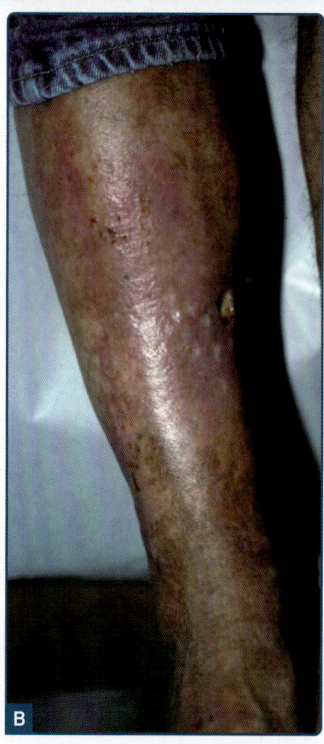

Figure 73-6 **A,** Chronic lipodermatosclerosis (LDS) with mild erythema of the medial lower leg, indicating presence of active inflammation. Cellulitis-like plaques on the medial lower leg. **B,** Severe acute inflammation with ulcerations superimposed on chronic LDS.

DIAGNOSIS

The diagnosis is often clinical, and biopsy of LDS skin can have a difficult course of healing.[92] Of note, concern for poor healing and delay of biopsy would have failed to identify 2 cases of malignancy in case reports of cutaneous T-cell lymphoma[107] and angiosarcoma.[108] Biopsies are best taken from the proximal edge of involvement for highest rates of healing. Less-invasive options, such as MRI, have been used to view the extent of disease.[109]

Histopathologic findings reflect the evolution of disease. Dermal stasis changes are present at any stage, including a proliferation of capillaries and venules, small thick-walled blood vessels, extravasated erythrocytes, hemosiderin-laden macrophages, lymphohistiocytic inflammation, and fibrosis.[52,110] In the subcutis, early lesions of LDS show a sparse infiltrate of lymphocytes in the septa, with central lobular ischemic fat necrosis. Capillary congestion is observed within fat lobules, often with endothelial cell necrosis, thrombosis, red cell extravasation, and hemosiderin deposition.[52,110]

Lipomembranous or membranocystic changes may be present with small pseudocystic spaces within necrotic fat. The spaces are lined by a membranous lining of hyaline eosinophilic material, which is highlighted by periodic acid-Schiff staining. Lipomembranous changes are not exclusive to LDS.[52,111]

With progression of LDS, the spectrum of histopathologic changes encompasses increasing degrees of fat necrosis, septal fibrosis, and thickening; an inflammatory infiltrate of lymphocytes, histiocytes, and foamy macrophages; and partial to extensive atrophy of fat lobules.[52,87,110] Advanced lesions show septal sclerosis with marked atrophy of fat lobules secondary to lipophagic fat necrosis, accompanied by lipomembranous change and a marked reduction in inflammation.[52,110]

DIFFERENTIAL DIAGNOSIS

Table 73-6 outlines the differential diagnosis of LDS.

TABLE 73-6
Differential Diagnosis of Lipodermatosclerosis

DIAGNOSIS	CHARACTERISTICS
Erythema nodosum (EN)	Warm, tender, erythematous subcutaneous nodules on pretibial areas; a lack of preceding venous insufficiency is common. Sarcoidosis or other high-risk medication exposure.
Erythema induratum (EI)/nodular vasculitis	Tender nodules and plaques on calf areas; living in an area endemic for tuberculosis (EI). Vasculitis on histopathology.
Cellulitis	Can occur with chronic edema, venous insufficiency. More likely unilateral and after injury or animal bite.
Infection-induced panniculitis	EN-like nodules, deep inflamed nodules or abscesses; older lesions may show fibrosis. Commonly on legs. Often seen in severely immunosuppressed patients with malignancies.
Scleroderma/morphea	Scleroderma or morphea involvement elsewhere. May have associated venous insufficiency of legs.
Deep vein thrombosis	Pain and edema of posterior calf with positive Doppler examination.
Nephrogenic systemic fibrosis	Subsequent to MRI with gadolinium exposure in patients with renal dysfunction. Can occur on areas other than legs.
Malignancies	Persistent, worsening disease, often with systemic symptoms. Presence of cutaneous T-cell lymphoma, angiosarcoma, or other sarcomas on leg. More likely in patients who underwent transplantation and in immunosuppressed patients.
Necrobiosis lipoidica	Clinically, the lesions consist of yellow-brown, indurated plaques with an atrophic, depressed area.
Eosinophilic fasciitis/Shulman syndrome	Coarse, thickened skin with peau d'orange appearance. A "groove sign" or "dry riverbed sign" can be seen along lines of vessels when arms are lifted or extended laterally. Peripheral blood eosinophilia and hyperglobulinemia are common.

CLINICAL COURSE AND PROGNOSIS

The course of LDS is variable and depends on the patient's comorbidities and compliance with the treatment regimen, particularly compression, which can be difficult to adhere to daily. The acute form may last months or even a year.[91] The chronic form can last years and can be refractory to standard treatment regimens. The ulcerations and resulting scarring are permanent and can be cosmetically distressful. Secondary infection of ulcers must be avoided. Dermatosclerosis in patients with systemic sclerosis has been associated with pulmonary infarction and hypertension secondary to leg thrombi.[112] Additionally, untreated LDS can result in venolymphedema.[92]

MANAGEMENT

Diagnostic tests to evaluate peripheral vascular disease include the ankle brachial index for arterial evaluation, as well as venous Doppler examinations to detect thrombi and duplex sonography to detect direction of flow and severity of venous reflux.[91] A patient with arterial compromise should not undergo compression therapy, which is a first-line treatment for LDS.[87,90] Higher compression gradient (30 to 40 mm Hg) may be more effective, but lower pressure (15 to 20 mm Hg or 20 to 30 mm Hg) encourages compliance, especially in the elderly, and effectively decreases edema.[113] Compression tightens vascular tight junctions, inhibiting permeability of fluid into the perivascular tissue.[95,114] Stockings must be worn all day; a few days without compression may lead to recurrence of edema and inflammation.[113] Because of the difficulty of wearing stockings, adaptive compression modalities have been developed, which use sustained or intermittent pneumatic compression.

Stanozolol is effective in LDS; it decreases pain, erythema, and induration.[115] Patients tolerate the treatment well, and the risk of hepatotoxicity has been evaluated as an asymptomatic increase in liver transaminases that resolves with medication cessation.[116] This drug is not available in the United States. Other anabolic steroids, such as oxandrolone and danazol, also have been used.[117,118]

Pentoxifylline has been successfully used in LDS cases with and without associated ulceration and is a useful adjunct to compression for treating venous ulcers and may be effective as monotherapy.[119] In fact, in one study, hydroxychloroquine and pentoxifylline combined therapy, without compression, led to a 50% reduction in pain from baseline.[120]

Ultrasound therapy can reduce and even resolve induration, tenderness, and erythema.[121,122] Available through physical therapy departments, it is a simple and safe treatment and may be used as adjunctive therapy.[121,122] Because obesity is a common condition among affected patients, weight loss is critical. Capsaicin may alleviate pain associated with LDS.[123] Finally, refractory disease has responded to intralesional, autologous, platelet-rich plasma, injected in a grid-like pattern, and repeated every 2 weeks.[124]

One author (IKA) has noted improvement in patients treated with rutin and vitamin C, particularly adjunctive to compression therapy.

INFECTION-INDUCED PANNICULITIS

AT-A-GLANCE

Clinical
- Caused by multiple infectious agents: bacteria, fungi, parasites, and viruses.
- AT may serve as reservoir for various infections.
- Patients may be immunosuppressed with primary inoculation or hematogenous spread.
- Erythematous plaques, nodules, abscesses, ulcers with purulent discharge.

Histopathology
- Suppurative granulomas within fat lobule.
- In primary cutaneous infections, epicenter of inflammation is superficial dermis; in secondary infections, epicenter is deep reticular dermis and subcutaneous fat.
- Special stains, cultures, and serologic studies for detection of microorganisms.

Treatment
- Appropriate antimicrobial therapy selected according to susceptibility tests.

Infection-induced panniculitis (IIP), also termed *infectious panniculitis* and *infective panniculitis*, is panniculitis directly caused by an infectious agent.[74] AT infection can be caused by bacteria, mycobacteria, fungi, protozoa, or viruses.[52,74,125] Primary infections produced by direct inoculation at a wound site (injury, surgical procedure, catheter, injection, acupuncture) usually result in a single lesion which may spread locally.[52,74,125] Secondary infections caused by sepsis and hematogenous spread may manifest as single or multiple lesions.[52,74,125] In immunosuppressed patients, microorganisms may be numerous and identified on routine histopathology, or with special stains. In immunocompetent patients, microorganisms may be sparse, requiring positive cultures, lesional PCR, or serologic studies for identification.[52,74,125]

EPIDEMIOLOGY

IIP is most frequently seen in immunocompromised hosts, including those with diabetes mellitus.[126] The epidemiology depends on the infectious etiology with geographic and host susceptibility. Recent reports of infectious etiologies in association with various autoimmune disorders include *Staphylococcus aureus* panniculitis with juvenile dermatomyositis,[127] mucormycosis in systemic lupus erythematosus (SLE),[126] *Mycobacterium*-associated and *Histoplasma*-associated panniculitis with rheumatoid arthritis,[128,129] as well as *Histoplasma* causing panniculitis in 2 patients with polymyositis.[130] Complicating these associations is the fact that autoimmune disorders are often treated with immunosuppressive therapies.

CLINICAL FEATURES

The clinical appearance of IIP varies from fluctuant or abscess-like lesions with purulence and ulcerations to nonspecific erythematous, firm subcutaneous plaques, purpuric plaques, and EN-like lesions.[74,125,131] Deep nodules or plaques may not always appear fluctuant, and pustules, fluctuant papules, and ulcers can be superimposed on top of firm, deep nodules.[125] The most common sites of infection are the legs and feet, but upper extremities, trunk, and face also may be involved.[74,125] Immunosuppression of varying etiology is the most frequent association.[52,74,125] Immunosuppression is associated with more widespread and abscess-type lesions. In immunocompetent patients, granulomas are common.[125,132] Clinical features vary with the setting, the infective organism and patient's immunocompetence.[125,131]

ETIOLOGY AND PATHOGENESIS

Innumerable infectious agents can cause IIP via direct inoculation or hematologic spread. Diffuse fusariosis has presented with panniculitis in a patient with acute lymphoblastic leukemia.[133] One case reported cutaneous aspergillosis panniculitis in a patient with acute lymphoblastic leukemia, and gouty panniculitis was suspected with the presence of urate crystals. This patient also had the characteristic "ghost cell" changes of pancreatic panniculitis, which along with the urate crystals may be secondary to fungal enzymatic changes.[134] These findings have been appreciated in mucormycoses as well.[126] Transplantation patients are at risk for disseminated infections, as seen in a review of 15 solid-organ transplantation patients (mainly renal transplantations) with cryptococcal panniculitis. Duration between transplantation and infection ranged from 3 months to 31 years.[135] Cryptococcal infection in the transplantation group is highest in heart transplant recipients.[136] *Pseudomonas aeruginosa* may cause panniculitis, most often as a disseminated infection, but it has presented without septicemia.[137] Epstein-Barr virus also has been reported to cause IIP localized to the trunk in a patient with methotrexate-associated lymphoproliferative disorder, with resolution after discontinuation of methotrexate.[138]

Immunocompetent patients with IIP also have been reported. Panniculitis caused by syphilis has presented with cutaneous findings of secondary syphilis, with an infiltrate containing many plasma cells and positive *Treponema pallidum* immunohistochemical staining.[139] Cutaneous leishmaniasis has also presented as inflammation of the AT, noted in 2 Iraqi cases with both septal and lobular histopathology, improving with local treatment standard for cutaneous leishmaniasis.[140] *Borrelia burgdorferi* is also associated with panniculitis, in an immunocompetent host, mimicking a subcutaneous panniculitis-like T-cell lymphoma (SPTCL), which responded promptly to doxycycline.[141]

The adipocyte is an innate immune cell that tailors specific and distinct receptor-mediated transcriptional responses to the various microbial infections.[142] Adipocytes can be infected in vitro with infectious agents, including *Chlamydophila pneumoniae*, cytomegalovirus, adenovirus, respiratory syncytial virus, influenza,[64] MTB,[63] *R. prowazekii*,[65] *T. cruzi*,[143] *Coxiella burnetii*,[65] and HIV.[144]

In vitro infection of adipocytes with *T. cruzi* (the cause of Chagas disease) results in increased expression of multiple proinflammatory cytokines and chemokines, increased expression of TLR2 and TLR9 and acute-phase reactants, but decreased expression of adiponectin and peroxisome-proliferator-activated receptor γ, the negative regulators of inflammation.[9,66] In mice, real-time PCR has shown that at 300 days postinfection with *T. cruzi*, a comparable number of parasites are present in both AT and heart tissue, indicating that AT is a reservoir for the parasites.[9] Interestingly, the *T. cruzi* amastigotes are more numerous in brown AT than in white α_1-antitrypsin.[9]

In another murine study, *Mycobacterium leprae* had very limited growth potential in AT, as preadipocytes and adipocytes were not permissive for *M. leprae* multiplication and logarithmic growth.[145] Because adipocytes have high expression of TLR4, adipocytes are responsive to endotoxin, producing proinflammatory cytokines at comparable or higher levels than macrophages.[9] TLR2 induction in adipocytes confers a high degree of sensitivity to fungal cell-wall components.[9]

Mutations coding TLRs or downstream signaling proteins can increase the risk of infections.[146] The genetic variants in TLRs, and other innate immune signaling components and their effect on adipocyte function and development of panniculitis are not yet known.

DIAGNOSIS

Evaluation includes histopathologic studies with stains for organisms as well as tissue culture, with sensitivities. Immunosuppression may lead to the presence of numerous microorganisms but diagnosis is more difficult in immunocompetent patients.[52,74,125] Molecular PCR techniques have increased detection of mycobacterium infections.[62,79] Histopathologic features vary with the organism and its virulence, the host immune status, and the duration of the lesion.[74] A mostly lobular panniculitis,[52] IIP often reveals a mixed septal and lobular pattern.[74] The superficial dermis has more inflammation in infections acquired by direct inoculation, while infections secondary to hematogenous spread involve the deep reticular dermis and subcutaneous fat.[52]

Additional features of IIP include hemorrhage, vascular proliferation, foci of basophilic necrosis, and sweat gland necrosis.[74] Overlying epidermal changes, such as parakeratosis, acanthosis, and spongiosis are seen in nonulcerated specimens. Dermal findings include edema, a diffuse perivascular inflammatory infiltrate, proliferation of thick-walled vessels, and focal or diffuse hemorrhage.[74] Observation of these features warrants stains for bacteria, mycobacteria, and fungi, and additional immunohistochemistry or PCR amplification techniques may be necessary. Occasionally histopathologic changes suggest a particular etiology. Suppurative granulomas formed by epithelioid histiocytes surrounding aggregated neutrophils are common with atypical mycobacteria.[52] Viral inclusions within endothelial cells may be seen in cytomegalovirus-associated panniculitis.[147]

DIFFERENTIAL DIAGNOSIS

Table 73-7 outlines the differential diagnosis of IIP.

CLINICAL COURSE AND PROGNOSIS

The clinical course and prognosis of IIP are affected by the infective organism and whether the organism was introduced locally or hematologically. Organisms treated with antibiotics, and a prompt diagnosis, portend a good prognosis. Immunocompromised patients are at risk for a more complicated course.

TABLE 73-7
Differential Diagnosis of Infection-Induced Panniculitis

DIAGNOSIS	CHARACTERISTICS
α_1-Antitrypsin panniculitis	Nodules, plaques, and cellulitis-like lesions to fluctuant abscess-like lesions that tend to ulcerate and drain, and appear on lower trunk and proximal extremities.
Pancreatic panniculitis	Occurs anywhere on the legs, with ulceration and drainage. Serum lipase and amylase often elevated. Fungal strains should be used to rule out mucormycosis or aspergillosis which can cause "ghost cell" adipocytes, especially in immunocompromised patients.
Traumatic/factitial panniculitis	Variable nodules, plaques, ulceration. Need high index of suspicion by caring physicians. Trauma can predispose to infection-induced panniculitis.
Erythema induratum/nodular vasculitis	Crops of tender nodules and plaques on posterior lower legs, often develop ulceration and drainage.
Pyoderma gangrenosum	Can present at any location. Highly inflammatory with characteristic rolled, elevated edges. Related to trauma. Not classically confined to the lower legs.
Cutaneous/subcutaneous lymphomas	Nodules and plaques, some with ulceration, predominantly on legs. Can be mimicked by *Borrelia burgdorferi*–induced panniculitis in an immunocompetent host.[141]
Lymphoproliferative disorders	Immunocompromised or posttransplantation patient (but not restricted to such). Must be differentiated into benign and malignant behavior/characteristics both clinically and with histopathology.

MANAGEMENT

Treatment varies depending on the suspected or known organisms and their cultures and sensitivities. In cases involving bacteria such as MTB and parasites such as *T. cruzi*, the capability to remain dormant in AT necessitates the use of appropriate antibiotics, often for extended treatment courses.[9,63]

α_1-ANTITRYPSIN PANNICULITIS

AT-A-GLANCE

Clinical
- ZZ-, MZ-, MS-, and SS-phenotype-associated panniculitis. Rare, with >60% occurring in ZZ cases.
- Low levels of α_1-antitrypsin are associated with emphysema, hepatitis, cirrhosis, vasculitis, and angioedema.

(Continued)

AT-A-GLANCE (Continued)

- Subcutaneous nodules mostly located on the lower abdomen, buttocks, and proximal extremities.
- Frequent ulceration, draining lesions, poor healing after surgery, and isomorphic phenomenon.

Histopathology
- Mostly lobular panniculitis without vasculitis.
- Dense inflammatory infiltrate of neutrophils and neutrophils between collagen bundles of deep reticular dermis.
- Normal fat adjacent to necrotic adipocytes.

Treatment
- Dapsone, doxycycline.
- Supplemental intravenous infusion of α_1-antitrypsin or liver transplantation for severe forms of homozygous ZZ disease.

α_1-Antitrypsin (α_1AT) is a glycoprotein made in the liver. It is a serine protease inhibitor that has widespread function as well as an acute phase reactant, increased in times of stress. α_1AT deficiency is inherited as a codominant disorder, and more than 100 alleles have been identified.[148,149] The α_1AT phenotypes are classified according to gel electrophoresis migration as F (fast), M (medium), S (slow), and Z (very slow), and null variants that do not produce any α_1AT and patients may have dysfunctional α_1AT with normal levels.[150] Deficiency in α_1AT was first seen in the 1960s with protein electrophoresis isolation.[151] The first description of panniculitis secondary to glycoprotein deficiency was in 1972.[152]

EPIDEMIOLOGY

Panniculitis uncommonly occurs in α_1AT deficiency, fewer than 50 cases having been reported[153] in ZZ, MZ, MS, and SS phenotypes. More than 60% involve ZZ phenotypes and 65% affect women.[153] Homozygous MM represents 90% to 97% of the population.[154] Presenting in all ages, panniculitis is most often seen between ages 30 and 60 years.[153,155] The estimated prevalence of α_1AT deficiency in whites is 1 per 3000 to 5000 in the United States, with incidence in white newborns similar to that of cystic fibrosis.[150] Cases also have been noted to initially present after pregnancy as acute-phase reactants (including α_1AT) rise and fall.[156] Up to 35% of cases have preceding trauma.[154]

CLINICAL FEATURES

Patients present with painful erythematous nodules and plaques, but early lesions may have a cellulitic or fluctuant abscess-type appearance (Fig. 73-8A).

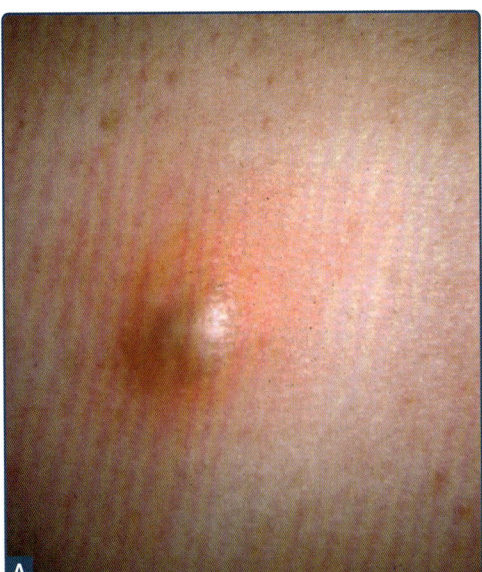

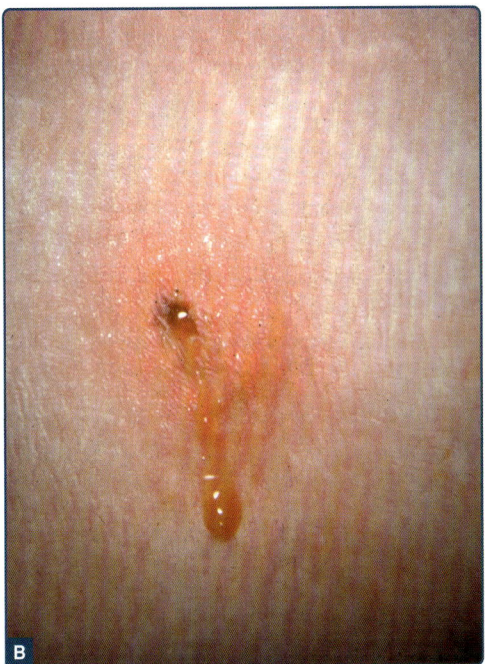

Figure 73-8 α₁-Antitrypsin deficiency–associated panniculitis. **A,** Fluctuant abscess appearance. **B,** Discharge of oily material from lesion.

Lesions may ulcerate with oily or serosanguinous discharge (Fig. 73-8B) and resolve with atrophic scars.[52] The lesions appear most commonly on the lower trunk (buttocks) (Fig. 73-9) and proximal extremities, but the lower legs and other sites may be affected.[52,153,157] α_1AT panniculitis may coexist with autoimmune disease, cancer, or infection,[158,159] thus the presence of α_1AT deficiency in association with panniculitis should not preclude a search for infection or other underlying medical problems such as autoimmune disorders or malignancies.

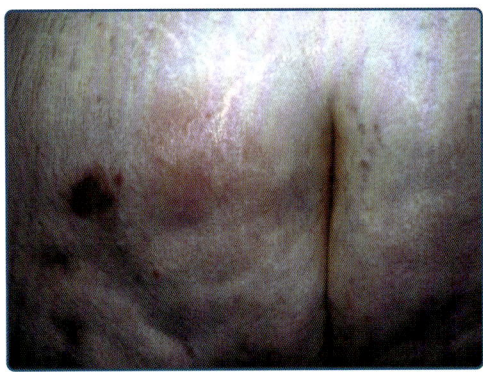

Figure 73-9 α_1-Antitrypsin deficiency–associated panniculitis. Nodular lesion on the buttock.

α_1AT deficiency is associated with pulmonary and hepatic disease, leading to chronic obstructive pulmonary disease, hepatic cirrhosis, or hepatocellular carcinoma[150]; the ZZ phenotype is at highest risk. There is no association of the null variant with hepatic disease, as it is the accumulation of polymerized α_1AT in the liver that induces damage, and accumulation does not occur in this variant.[150]

ETIOLOGY AND PATHOGENESIS

α_1AT is a glycoprotein that is produced and secreted mainly by hepatocytes, but also in small amounts by monocytes/macrophages and neutrophils,[160] and is known to inhibit numerous proteases. α_1AT may also help regulate complement activation.[161,162]

Homozygous MM is associated with normal levels of α_1AT (90 to 220 mg/dL),[163] whereas those homozygous for ZZ have low levels at 10% to 15% of normal, and those heterozygous for S or Z allele have levels in between.[150] ZZ is the most common phenotype to induce panniculitis. MS heterozygous individuals may have low-normal serum levels causing panniculitis clinically[164,165] and the F variant may increase lung disease[166] and is associated with panniculitis only as the FZ phenotype.[154,167]

Possible mechanisms leading to the development of α_1AT panniculitis include lack of interference with the various proteases that lead to activation of lymphocytes, macrophages, complement, activation of the autoinflammatory cascade mediated by activation of IL-1 and IL-1β,[168] and lysis and destruction of connective tissue at sites of inflammation. Trauma to adipocytes may result in release of adipokines and cytokines that are chemotactic to inflammatory cells, whose released proteases are unopposed because of the absence of the α_1AT, leading to severe damage in involved tissue.[154,169,170] Animal models of soft-tissue injury show elevated levels of IL-6 and monocyte chemotactic protein-1, and increased systemic inflammatory mediators.[169] Interestingly, a case has been reported of a patient with MM phenotype acquiring a ZZ phenotype from a donor liver; after the transplantation patient developed panniculitis.[171]

DIAGNOSIS

Histopathologic findings vary with the age and type of lesion biopsied. Early in development, nodular lesions reveal edema and degeneration of adipocytes, with ruptured and collapsed cell membranes and a perivascular mononuclear infiltrate.[172] Also reported at this stage is a mild infiltrate of neutrophils and macrophages in septa and lobules, with foci of early necrosis of subcutaneous fat. This may be accompanied by splaying of neutrophils between collagen bundles throughout the overlying reticular dermis, considered an early and distinctive diagnostic clue.[173] More advanced lesions have masses of neutrophils and histiocytes associated with necrosis and replacement of fat lobules (Fig. 73-10). Involvement also may be focal, manifested by large areas of normal fat in immediate proximity to necrotic septa and fat lobules.[174] Liquefactive necrosis and dissolution of dermal collagen may be accompanied by ulceration, and degeneration of elastic tissue may lead to septal destruction and the appearance of "floating" necrotic fat lobules.[159,175] Neutrophils and necrotic adipocytes are less prevalent in late-stage lesions, with replacement by lymphocytes, foamy histiocytes, and variable amount of fibrosis within fat lobules.[159,176]

At times the histopathology fails to demonstrate the characteristic features.[177] These rare cases suggest that this disease should be considered in a patient with ulcerative lesions if pathology is not suggestive of a diagnosis with serum protein levels and phenotype testing in the correct clinical setting. Because of the complex nature of these proteins, it is best to obtain serum protein levels as well as phenotyping.[150]

DIFFERENTIAL DIAGNOSIS

Table 73-8 outlines the differential diagnosis of α_1AT. Neutrophilic panniculitis can be seen as part of the histopathology in numerous diseases:

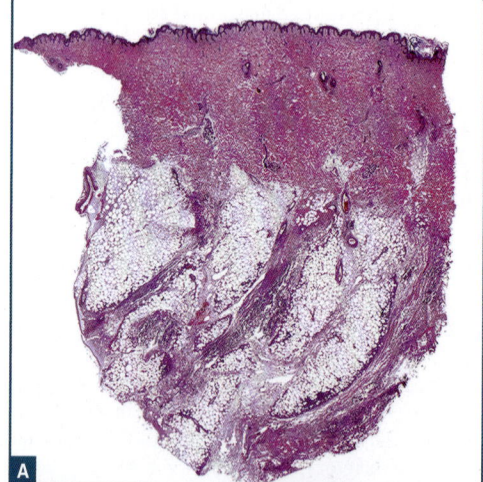
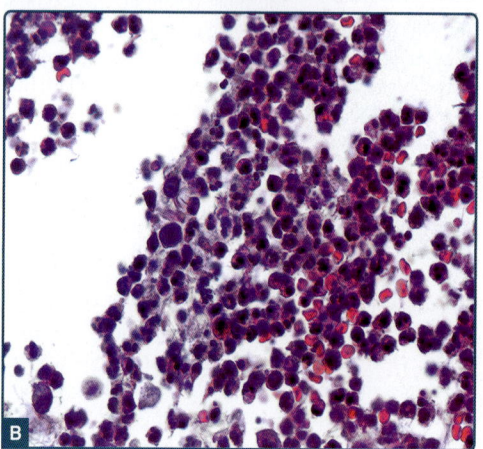

Figure 73-10 α_1-Antitrypsin deficiency–associated panniculitis. **A,** Low-power magnification shows a mostly lobular panniculitis. **B,** High-power magnification shows dense inflammatory infiltrate of neutrophils in the fat lobule.

TABLE 73-8
Differential Diagnosis of α_1-Antitrypsin Deficiency Panniculitis

DIAGNOSIS	CHARACTERISTICS
Infection-induced panniculitis	Erythema nodosum–like nodules, deep inflamed nodules or abscesses; older lesions may show fibrosis. Commonly on legs. Often seen in severely immunosuppressed patients with malignancies.
Factitial panniculitis	Geometric morphology. Patient often has an underlying psychiatric disturbance. Identifying foreign material is helpful. Histopathology varies based on mechanism.
Erythema induratum/ nodular vasculitis	Tender nodules and plaques on calf areas, living in an area endemic for tuberculosis (erythema induratum). Vasculitis on histopathology.
Pancreatic panniculitis	Occurs anywhere on the legs, ulceration and drainage. Serum lipase and amylase often elevated.
Subcutaneous Sweet syndrome	Erythematous nodules may be present on the face, neck, upper trunk, as well as extremities. Nodules may have vesicles, pustules or bullae. Histology with intense dermal edema; diffuse, deep neutrophilic infiltrate with karyorrhexis.
Pyoderma gangrenosum	Violaceous, undermined borders with isomorphic response.

α_1AT-deficiency panniculitis, IIP, factitial or traumatic panniculitis, pancreatic panniculitis, medication-associated panniculitis (vemurafenib, ponatinib); subcutaneous sweets syndrome or neutrophilic panniculitis associated with myelodysplasia. Additionally cutaneous Crohn disease, familial Mediterranean fever, rheumatoid arthritis and cases of idiopathic neutrophilic panniculitis can cause a neutrophilic panniculitis.

CLINICAL COURSE AND PROGNOSIS

Cutaneous and subcutaneous necrosis can develop rapidly. Fatal cases have been reported, mainly the ZZ variant.[178,179] A rare fatal case with MZ phenotype that mimicked pyoderma gangrenosum also has been reported.[180] Prompt diagnosis and treatment of severe disease with α_1AT augmentation may significantly improve the panniculitis and may induce clinical remission, requiring augmentation therapy infusions only with recurrence. Although the panniculitis may lead to significant morbidity, the lung and liver disease associated with α_1AT deficiency are a much higher priority and comanagement with pulmonologists and hepatologists is ideal.

MANAGEMENT

Many medications have been used in the treatment of α_1AT-deficiency panniculitis including colchicine, antimalarials, dapsone, doxycycline, plasma infusion and plasma exchange, intravenous augmentation therapy of α_1AT protein, and liver transplantation.[157,181,182] Steroids, immunosuppressives, and cytotoxic agents are less effective. Doxycycline, and especially dapsone, may be useful in mild to moderate disease, especially in heterozygous cases such as MZ. Severe panniculitis unresponsive to standard treatment requires protein-replacement therapy (augmentation therapy).[183] For severe panniculitis, α_1AT infusions are recommended at 60 mg/kg, often with a few weekly infusions, with repeat infusions for recurrence.[183] Long-term supplementation may be required in severe cases.[149]

Panniculitis has also resolved with liver transplantation,[184] and panniculitis acquired after liver transplantation has successfully been treated with retransplantation.[171] It is critical to note the tendency of α_1AT-deficiency panniculitis for poor wound healing, as a case of an untreated α_1AT patient resulted in poor healing after intraabdominal surgery.[185] Not initiating augmentation therapy in a timely fashion may cause significant complications and must be considered in the appropriate clinical setting.[185] As trauma may induce lesions in one-third of patients, debridement is discouraged.[52]

PANCREATIC PANNICULITIS

AT-A-GLANCE

Clinical
- Erythematous subcutaneous nodules that often ulcerate spontaneously.
- Lower extremities (around ankles and knees) are the most frequent sites of involvement.
- Regression of pancreatitis-associated cutaneous lesions occurs as pancreas improves, but those associated with pancreatic carcinoma tend to persist; may be fatal.

Histopathology
- Mostly lobular panniculitis without vasculitis.
- Intense necrosis of adipocytes at center of fat lobule.
- "Ghost cell" adipocytes with finely granular and basophilic intracytoplasmic material.

Treatment
- Treatment of the underlying pancreatic disease.
- Additional treatment options: octreotide, plasmapheresis.
- Stop precipitating medications.

Panniculitis associated with and secondary to underlying pancreatic disease was first noted in 1883.[186] Variable pathologies of the pancreas can induce panniculitis, including acute pancreatitis, even following endoscopic retrograde cholangiopancreatography procedures.[187] The panniculitis resolves as the pancreatic disease improves, which may be difficult or impossible in cases of malignancy.

EPIDEMIOLOGY

Panniculitis in association with pancreatic disease is an uncommon occurrence, developing in 0.3% to 3% of patients with pancreatic disorders such as acute or chronic pancreatitis, pancreatic carcinoma, or pancreatic pseudocysts.[188-190] Pancreatic disease of any kind may be associated with pancreatic panniculitis. Although pancreatitis is most commonly a result of alcohol abuse, cholelithiasis, medications, trauma, and viral infections are also known etiologic factors.[190,191] Congenital pancreatic abnormalities may also cause panniculitis.[190]

CLINICAL FEATURES

The cutaneous lesions appear as crops on the lower legs, especially the periarticular areas, but are also on the arms, wrists,[192] thighs, and trunk.[188] The lesions are ill-defined erythematous to red-brown edematous and tender nodules, which may involute and resolve with atrophic hyperpigmented scars.[188] They may have central "softer" areas or may become fluctuant, abscess-like, and drain an oily material similar to lesions of α_1AT-deficiency panniculitis (Fig. 73-11).[188] The cutaneous panniculitis may precede the diagnosis of the associated pancreatic disease by weeks to months in up to 45% of patients.[188,191]

Extracutaneous manifestations include periarticular fat necrosis with concomitant arthritis,[188,193] and painful medullary fat necrosis in bone.[194,195] Monoarticular or oligoarticular arthritis secondary to periarticular fat necrosis may be present in more than half of patients.[188] This triad of pancreatic disease, panniculitis, and polyarthritis (PPP syndrome) is very rare and is associated with both pancreatitis and pancreatic carcinoma.[194,196] Osteonecrosis may also develop as enzymes extend to the joint capsules and cause purulent joints.[195]

Pleural effusions and serositis also may be seen with pancreatic panniculitis,[194,197] and pleural effusions are associated with a high mortality rate.[197] Eosinophilia may be seen in pancreatic panniculitis resulting from either pancreatitis or pancreatic malignancies.[190,197] A pancreatic tumor (or pancreatitis) in association with panniculitis, polyarthritis, and eosinophilia (the Schmid triad) imparts a poor prognosis.[198,199] An important complication of pancreatic panniculitis is secondary infection.[200]

ETIOLOGY AND PATHOGENESIS

Pancreatic panniculitis has generally been attributed to release of pancreatic enzymes such as lipase, amylase, and trypsin into the circulation, promoting vascular permeability and damage, leading to release of fatty acids from adipocytes and subsequent fat necrosis.[194,201] However, there are reports of pancreatic panniculitis in the setting of normal serum levels of pancreatic enzymes.[188] Additionally, incubation of normal AT with amylase, lipase and a pancreatitis patient's serum failed to induce fat necrosis in vitro.[202] Resistin and leptin are potential markers of extrapancreatic fat necrosis.[203]

Other than the more common causes of pancreatitis, pancreatic panniculitis may be seen in association with pancreatitis following renal or combined renal and pancreatic transplantation,[204,205] liver transplantation,[206] with SLE with hemophagocytic syndrome,[207] as well as HIV with hemophagocytic syndrome.[208] Pancreatic cancer and metastatic disease can cause a panniculitis that improves with resection of the malignant tissue.[209] Panniculitis also may be associated with acute fatty liver of pregnancy and HELLP syndrome (hemolysis, elevated liver enzymes, low platelet count).[210] Rare drug-induced cases have been reported, including to L-asparaginase in the setting of treating acute lymphoblastic leukemia,[211] and treatment of hepatitis C.[212] Identical histopathology has been seen at the site of subcutaneous interferon β injections.[213]

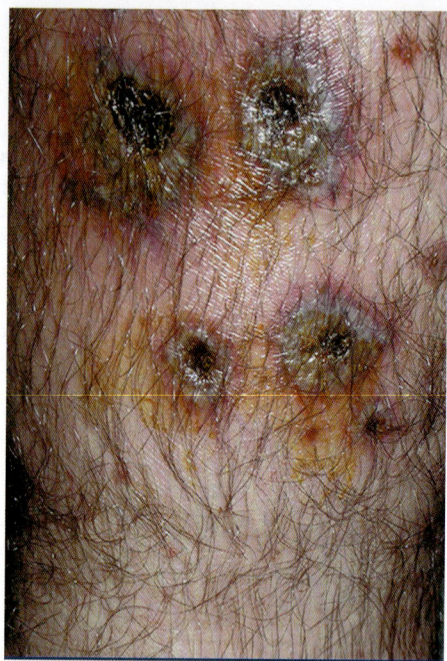

Figure 73-11 Pancreatic panniculitis. Erythematous subcutaneous nodules that ulcerate and exude an oily material.

TABLE 73-9
Differential Diagnosis of Pancreatic Panniculitis

DIAGNOSIS	CHARACTERISTICS
α_1-Antitrypsin deficiency	Tender, erythematous nodules, often with a suppurative exudate. Located on the abdomen, buttocks, and proximal extremities.
Erythema induratum/nodular vasculitis	Tender nodules and plaques on calf areas, living in an area endemic for tuberculosis (erythema induratum). Vasculitis present on histopathology.
Cutaneous polyarteritis nodosa	Nodules in association with livedo reticularis and arterial inflammation on histology, possibly with neuropathy.
Infection-induced panniculitis	Erythema nodosum–like nodules, deep inflamed nodules or abscesses; older lesions may show fibrosis. Most commonly on legs. Often seen in severely immunosuppressed patients. "Ghost cell" changes and urate crystals secondary to fungal enzymatic changes can be seen in mucormycosis and aspergillosis associated pancreatitis.[126,134]
Pyoderma gangrenosum	Violaceous, undermined borders with isomorphic response.
Malignancies	Persistent, worsening disease, often with systemic symptoms. Presence of cutaneous T-cell lymphoma, angiosarcoma, or other sarcomas on leg with/without venous hypertension. More likely in patients with solid-organ transplants or other immunosuppressed states.
Behçet syndrome occurring in the fat	Vasculitis occurring in the fat tissue, either lymphocytic or neutrophilic, small arterial involvement with either lobular or mixed lobular and septal pattern.

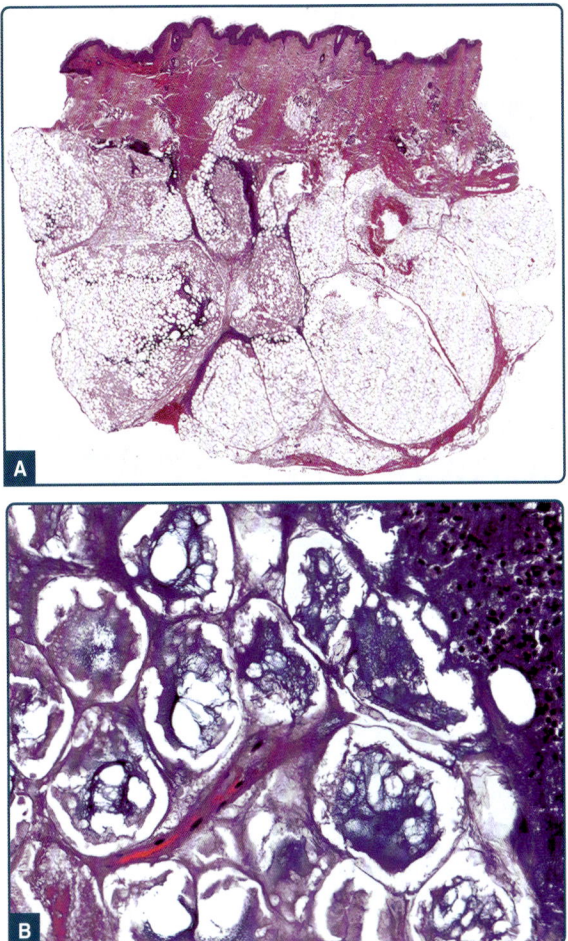

Figure 73-12 Pancreatic panniculitis. **A,** Low-power magnification shows a mostly lobular panniculitis with adipocyte necrosis at the center of the fat lobule. **B,** Higher-power magnification shows ghost adipocytes, necrotic adipocytes without nuclei and with cytoplasmic fine, granular basophilic material resulting from calcification.

DIAGNOSIS

Developed lesions of pancreatic panniculitis demonstrate lobular fat necrosis (Fig. 73-12A). Adipocytes lose their nuclei but maintain peripheral outlines, forming characteristic "ghost cells" (Fig. 73-12B). Saponification causes calcification, producing fine, granular basophilic deposits within and around necrotic adipocytes. The ghost cells are frequently aggregated in small clusters at the center of fat lobules, with a peripheral inflammatory infiltrate of neutrophils.[52] In older lesions, necrosis and ghost cells are replaced by foamy histiocytes, multinucleated giant cells, lymphocytes, and, eventually, fibrosis.[52,214]

DIFFERENTIAL DIAGNOSIS

Table 73-9 outlines the differential diagnosis of pancreatic panniculitis.

CLINICAL COURSE AND PROGNOSIS

Overall, when the pancreatic pathology resolves, the cutaneous symptoms subsequently improve. Panniculitis associated with pancreatic disease may be fatal, with a mortality rate of 24%[196] to 42%,[197] and mortality rates near 100% in those with pancreatic carcinoma. Acute pancreatitis may be treated and may resolve promptly with supportive care, however pancreatic carcinoma and associated panniculitis is far more difficult to treat.

MANAGEMENT

The focus of treatment of pancreatic panniculitis is on the underlying pancreatic disease. Care is often supportive. Because patients may lack abdominal symptoms at presentation, pancreatic panniculitis should be considered in any patient with panniculitis. Octreotide,[215] a somatostatin analog, and plasmapheresis are associated with resolution of pancreatic panniculitis.[216] Treating pancreatic cancer with surgical resection and combination chemotherapy may ameliorate the cutaneous findings.[192]

LUPUS PANNICULITIS

AT-A-GLANCE

Clinical
- Erythematous nodules on face, shoulders, upper arms, scalp, chest, buttocks; rarely on lower extremities.
- Persistent areas of lipoatrophy in regressed lesions.

Histopathology
- Mostly lobular panniculitis (with or without lymphocytic vasculitis).
- Lobular lymphocytic infiltrate; may include plasma cells and eosinophils.
- Lymphoid follicles and sclerotic collagen bundles within septae.
- Hyaline necrosis and atrophy of entire fat lobule in late-stage lesions.
- Interface changes of discoid lupus erythematosus in 20% to 30% of cases.

Treatment
- Antimalarials, thalidomide, topical steroids.
- If active and severely inflamed, short oral courses of corticosteroids.
- Dapsone, cyclosporine, methotrexate, intravenous immunoglobulin, rituximab, azathioprine, tacrolimus.

Lupus erythematosus panniculitis (LEP), also termed *lupus profundus, subcutaneous lupus erythematosus,* and *Irrgang-Kaposi syndrome,* was first described in 1883 by Kaposi and named lupus erythematous profundus by Irrgang in 1940.[217] Overall, it is very rare, even among the lupus erythematosus cohort.

EPIDEMIOLOGY

LEP is a rare variant of lupus erythematosus, presenting as inflammation in the AT. LEP may appear as the sole manifestation of lupus erythematosus or may occur prior to or after the onset of discoid lupus erythematosus (DLE) or SLE.[218,219] The incidence of SLE in patients with LEP is reported to range from 10% to 41%.[220] DLE in patients with LEP has a higher incidence, ranging from 21% to 60%.[218] Among those who have SLE, only 2% to 5% will have LEP.[218] Although rare, LEP occurs worldwide, more frequently among women than men, with a female-to-male ratio of approximately 4:1.[221] LEP is most common between the ages of 30 and 60 years, but may rarely be seen in childhood or even as neonatal lupus.[222,223] When present in association with SLE, LEP tends to occur with less-severe SLE.[221,224] Patients with LEP may have other autoimmune disorders such as Sjögren syndrome and rheumatoid arthritis.[218] Raynaud phenomenon is present in 10% of LEP patients.[221]

Other associations with LEP include TNF inhibitors, which caused SLE-like reactions as well as LEP in a patient with rheumatoid arthritis.[225] Treatment of a female patient with hairy cell leukemia with interferon has been associated with emergence of disseminated ulcerating lupus panniculitis.[226]

CLINICAL FEATURES

LEP lesions may be tender and painful and usually appear on the lateral upper arms, shoulders, face, scalp, hips, buttocks, breasts, and, rarely, on the lower extremities (Fig. 73-13).[218,224] Orbital involvement may present with periorbital edema,[227] and Blaschko linear patterns have been reported.[228] The lesions are deep subcutaneous nodules either with or without surface changes, including erythema and DLE features such as atrophy, hyperkeratosis, hyperpigmentation or hypopigmentation, telangiectasia, follicular plugging, and focal necrosis.[218] Ulceration can be seen in up to 28% of cases.[221] Areas of ongoing indurated panniculitis may coexist with DLE and lead to subcutaneous atrophy and scar formation on the cutaneous surface. Atrophy of facial lesions leads to severe cosmetic alterations. Lesions may be induced by trauma, including injections and surgical procedures.[218,224]

Serology may be normal or abnormal.[218,224] Patients with associated SLE tend to have higher positive antinuclear antibody (ANA) titers[224] and C4 deficiency may be found.[218,229] Other laboratory findings may include rheumatoid factor, false-positive Venereal Disease Research Laboratory, ANA, leukopenia, anemia, or thrombocytopenia.[230] Antiphospholipid antibodies may be positive, and if thrombi are noted on histopathology, testing for antiphospholipid antibodies should be performed.[231]

Lupus mastitis is a rare form of lupus panniculitis involving the breast. It may clinically mimic Paget disease. On mammography there is calcification paralleling the course of fat necrosis, and early deposition is concerning for malignancy. MRI shows the extent of lupus mastitis and nonspecific fat necrosis; adding contrast may significantly aid in diagnosis.[232]

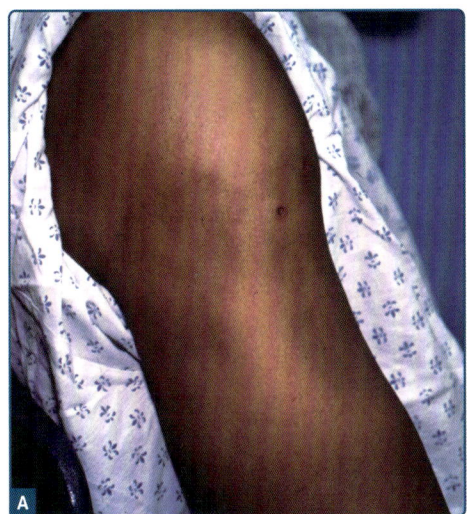

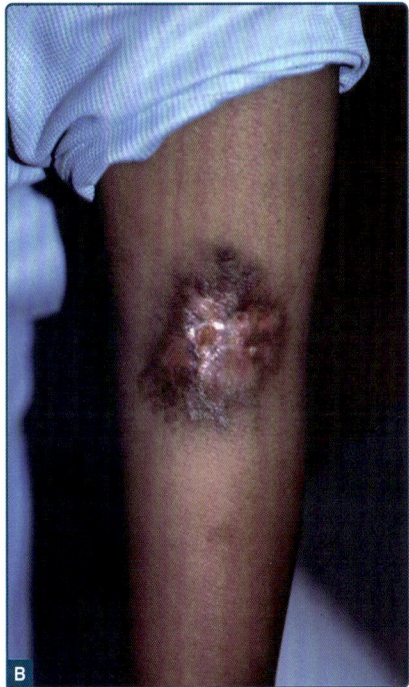

Figure 73-13 Lupus panniculitis. **A,** Atrophic upper arm lesion with superficial hyperpigmentation. **B,** With superimposed discoid lupus erythematosus and ulceration.

ETIOLOGY AND PATHOGENESIS

The innate immune system plays a significant role in the development of LEP. Adipocytes are important cells of the innate immune system expressing TLR1, TLR2, TLR3, TLR4, and TLR6.[233] The stromovascular fraction of AT expresses TLR5, TLR7, TLR8, TLR9, and TLR10.[233] In SLE, TLR7 and TLR9 recognize RNA and DNA patterns, respectively, and appear to provide a mechanism for recognition of self-DNA or self-RNA, with subsequent activation of the adaptive immune system and production of autoantibodies to nucleic acids and proteins bound to nucleic acids.[234,235] Inhibitors of TLR7 and TLR9 can prevent disease in mouse models of autoimmunity.[234] Genetic variations in TLR9 receptor predispose to SLE[236] and regression of SLE was seen in a patient who acquired TLR7 and TLR9 defects and antibody deficiency.[237] Both receptors have been suggested as therapeutic targets.[234,235] Interestingly, hydroxychloroquine blocks intracellular TLRs in vitro.[238]

DIAGNOSIS

Histopathologic features of DLE are seen in approximately 20% to 30% of LEP cases. These features include vacuolization of the basal cell layer, thickened basement membrane, mucin deposition between dermal collagen bundles, and a superficial and deep perivascular inflammatory infiltrate of lymphocytes.[52,224] The AT shows a lobular or mixed lobular and septal panniculitis, with lymphocytes, formation of lymphoid follicles (20% germinal centers),[218] variable hyaline fat necrosis,[52,224] and hyalinized and sclerotic septal collagen bundles associated with an interstitial infiltrate of lymphocytes and plasma cells.[52] Karyorrhexis, lymphocytic vasculitis, and membranocystic changes may be seen.[218] Calcification and/or fibrin thrombi also may be noted in 10% of cases.[224] Eosinophils may be seen in 22% to 41% of cases.[218]

Direct immunofluorescence of blood vessels and basement membrane demonstrates positive findings in almost all SLE-associated LEP, and a high percentage of positive findings in LEP without SLE.[224] Immunohistochemical studies of LEP show a predominance of lymphocytes, with both αβ T-helper (CD4+) and cytotoxic (CD8+) lymphocytes mixed with (CD20+) B cells and plasma cells.[220]

In cases with only AT involvement and without other features specific for DLE or SLE, differentiation from subcutaneous T-cell lymphoma is essential and difficult.[239] Anaplastic large-cell lymphoma may also have overlapping features with LEP.[240] There are reports of a spectrum of subcutaneous lymphoid dyscrasias, with lesions originally diagnosed as LEP, progressing to indeterminate lymphocytic lobular panniculitis and eventuating in a diagnosis of SPTCL.[241] Lymphocytic atypia and lymphocytic rimming is seen in SPTCL.[242] SPTCL may coexist with LEP, and must be distinguished from atypical lymphocytic panniculitis in which clonal T-cell infiltrates are associated with indolent behavior.[243-245] There may be epidermal involvement in SPTCL,[246-248] making the distinction more difficult from LEP. Lack of adipocyte membrane disruption suggests LEP.[242] Hyaline lipomembranous change is common in LEP, but seen infrequently in SPTCL.[242]

In 1 study, high levels of the interferon-α protein marker human myxovirus resistance protein 1 (MxA) were found in the infiltrate of LEP lesions.[249] Minimal, less than 20% staining, with MxA suggests a lymphoma.[249] CCL5 (the ligand of the receptor often expressed in adipocytes CCR5) expression is much higher in lymphomas compared to LEP.[250] Ki-67 staining of greater than 20% and focal areas of increased uptake are more suggestive of SPTCL.[242,251] Presence of CD123-positive staining also suggests LEP[242] and is an important prognostic indicator.

Even though serology is not specific it should be added to the workup, because SLE will require further treatment. ANA serology has a high false-positive rate, and may be positive in patients with SPTCL.[242]

DIFFERENTIAL DIAGNOSIS

Table 73-10 outlines the differential diagnosis of LEP.

TABLE 73-10

Differential Diagnosis of Lupus Erythematosus Panniculitis

DIAGNOSIS	CHARACTERISTICS
Tumid lupus	Erythematous, edematous plaques mainly in photoexposed areas with extensive mucin deposition on histopathology without epidermal change.
Cutaneous lymphoma (including subcutaneous panniculitis-like T-cell lymphoma [SPTCL])	Persistent, worsening disease, often with systemic symptoms. Histopathology is critical if no surface changes or additional signs or symptoms suggest lupus erythematosus panniculitis (LEP). LEP more often involves the face, whereas SPTCL more often involves the scalp, lower extremities, and buttocks.[242] Lymphocytic atypia and lymphocytic rimming is seen in SPTCL. Up to 19% of SPTCL cases with an αβ phenotype can have an associated autoimmune disorder with lupus erythematosus being the most common.[247]
Erythema induratum/nodular vasculitis	Tender nodules and plaques on calf areas, living in an area endemic for tuberculosis (erythema induratum). Vasculitis on histopathology.
Morphea/systemic sclerosis	Early lymphocytic panniculitis with subsequent subcutaneous septal and dermal sclerosis. In association with clinical features of morphea and systemic sclerosis.
Pancreatic panniculitis	Occurs most commonly on the legs with ulceration and drainage. Serum lipase and amylase often elevated.

CLINICAL COURSE AND PROGNOSIS

LEP is a chronic inflammatory disorder with periodic flares or long remissions. Average disease duration is 6 years, with a range of less than 1 year to 38 years.[221] CD123 immunohistochemical staining can be a helpful prognostic indicator, as a higher percentage of CD123 positive cells has a greater response to steroid therapy.[252] Prompt treatment aids in reducing permanent and potentially disfiguring scarring.

MANAGEMENT

Treatment is challenging, as is assessment of response to therapy, other than clinical assessment of erythema, induration, and tenderness. Just as in other forms of cutaneous lupus, sun protection and avoidance are often recommended.[253] Antimalarials are the first-line treatment of LEP[218,254] and may be the only medications needed.[254] When monotherapy with hydroxychloroquine is ineffective, combination with quinacrine has been used successfully but is difficult to obtain.[218,255] Antimalarials interfere with both inflammatory cytokines[256] and TLRs.[238] Antimalarials have a diminished effect in smokers.[257,258]

Topical steroids also may be successful, particularly under occlusion.[253] Systemic corticosteroids are effective and useful if the disease is active and severe,[224] and used as short courses or during antimalarial initiation. Long-term use of corticosteroids is avoided because of the chronic nature of LEP. Intralesional steroids are not recommended as the trauma may induce further activation as well as atrophy. Other treatments include dapsone,[259] thalidomide,[260] cyclosporine,[261] methotrexate,[262] azathioprine,[253] intravenous immunoglobulin (IVIG),[262] and tacrolimus.[263] Severe, recalcitrant cases may require rituximab[264] or infliximab, although caution must be advised with this modality because of its association with known activation of lupus erythematosus in some instances.[265] Considering the common calcification seen in LEP histopathology, calcium-channel blockers such as diltiazem are effective adjuncts, improving the calcinosis.[266]

CYTOPHAGIC HISTIOCYTIC PANNICULITIS

AT-A-GLANCE

Clinical

- Subcutaneous erythematous to violaceous plaques and nodules on extremities, trunk, and less frequently elsewhere; lesions may ulcerate.
- Fever, hepatosplenomegaly, 2 or more cytopenias; hemocytophagocytosis in bone marrow, lymph nodes, liver, or CNS.
- Hypertriglyceridemia, ferritin >500 mg/L; increased soluble CD25, CD163 levels.
- Low or absent natural killer cell activity, fibrinogen levels.
- Potentially rapidly fatal disease course if associated with hemophagocytic lymphohistiocytosis and macrophage activation syndrome; intermittent

remissions and exacerbations prior to death; or nonfatal acute or intermittent course.

Histopathologic
- Mostly lobular panniculitis without vasculitis.
- Histiocytes and mature lymphocytes within fat lobules with necrosis of adipocytes.
- "Bean-bag" cells: macrophages that contain intact or fragmented erythrocytes, leukocytes or platelets within their cytoplasm; may be focal.

Treatment
- First-line treatment is immunosuppression with cyclosporine and corticosteroids. Other options include tacrolimus, azathioprine, anakinra, cyclophosphamide with IVIG.
- Cytophagic histiocytic panniculitis with hemophagocytic lymphohistiocytosis or macrophage activation syndrome requires combined chemotherapy and aggressive supportive care.
- Diagnose and treat associated malignancies or infections.

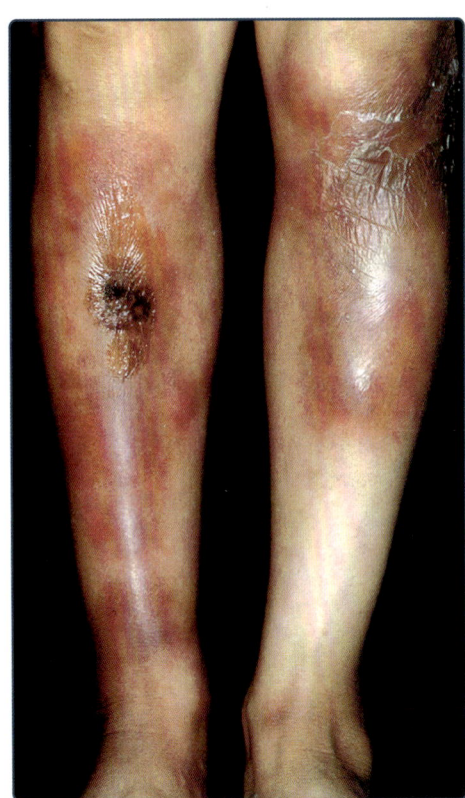

Figure 73-14 Cytophagic histiocytic panniculitis. Multiple erythematous plaques and nodules on the lower extremity.

Cytophagic histiocytic panniculitis (CHP) is a rare panniculitis that varies in duration from 3 months to 27 years and may be fatal.[267-269] It may be an aggressive disease requiring chemotherapy if related to hemophagocytic lymphohistiocytosis (HLH) or macrophage activation syndrome, but a more indolent course requiring immunosuppressant therapy with an excellent remission rate is also reported. Of note, HLH may be primary (genetic) or secondary (to infections, autoimmune disease), but CHP is only secondary in etiology. CHP itself may represent a "smoldering" lymphoma rather than a purely inflammatory disease.[270]

EPIDEMIOLOGY

CHP is rare, but is seen in adults, adolescents, and children. The oldest patient reported was 80[271] years old at time of diagnosis. Children affected include one with a perforin gene mutation (likely suffering from familial HLH).[272] One adult with familial multiple lipomatosis syndrome developed CHP at age 43 years.[273] As a consequence of the variable etiologies, epidemiology is largely based on the cause of CHP.

CLINICAL FEATURES

Lesions are subcutaneous plaques and nodules of variable sizes that may coalesce on the extremities and trunk and less frequently on the head and neck (Fig. 73-14).[267,274,275] Mucosal involvement is rare.[275] Features vary from skin colored to erythematous, purpuric, ecchymotic, or hyperpigmented; flat or raised; well circumscribed or diffuse; and indurated to fluctuant or ulcerated.[269,274] Individual lesions can reach 20 cm in diameter.[276]

Fulminant forms of the disease may be associated with fever, hepatosplenomegaly, lymphadenopathy, serosal effusions, pancytopenia, intravascular coagulation, liver failure, hemorrhagic diatheses, and death.[268,269,274,277] Laboratory tests should include a complete blood count with differential, liver function, ferritin, erythrocyte sedimentation rate, and lipid profile. Interestingly, erythrocyte sedimentation rate is often normal or low.[275] Soluble hemoglobin-haptoglobin scavenger receptor CD163 serum levels are associated with hemophagocytic disease activity and correlate with serum ferritin levels.[278] Serum CD163 level in CHP is much higher than levels seen in sepsis and in normal controls.[278] Other tests are determined by history and physical findings and the clinical course. A positive ANA may be detected and does not alone prove LEP.[279,280]

As CHP may cause hypertriglyceridemia, highly elevated serum lipid levels cause pancreatitis, which may improve with plasmapheresis.[281] Elevated cholesterol levels may persist for years after improvement of the panniculitis.[279] The elevated triglycerides during the hemophagocytic disease are secondary to inhibition of lipoprotein lipase, leading to IL-6, IL-1, and TNF secretion from macrophages.[281,282]

ETIOLOGY AND PATHOGENESIS

CHP may belong to a spectrum of panniculitides with benign lymphocytic infiltrate that develop reactive HLH/macrophage activation syndrome.[269,271,275] Secondary HLH is associated with infections, connective tissue diseases, and malignancies, or precipitated by medication.[283-285] Infections associated with HLH/macrophage activation syndrome include Epstein-Barr virus, cytomegalovirus, parvovirus, varicella, human herpesviruses 6 and 8, avian influenza, rubella, adenovirus, hepatitis B, HIV, bacterial, acid-fast bacterial, parasitic, and fungal infections.[285,286] CHP has presented after H1N1 influenza vaccine[287] and visceral leishmaniasis.[288] Trauma-induced CHP also has been reported.[280]

HLH is considered an autoinflammatory disease, with impairment of cytolytic T-cell and natural killer cell functions leading to a compensatory cascade of potentially fatal reactions.[289] Underlying gene mutations affect vesicular transport, granule shedding, and pore-forming cytolytic proteins involved in granule-mediated cytotoxicity.[251,286,289,290] Inability of the cytotoxic cells to eliminate infected cells leads to increased activation and proliferation of T cells, which produce high levels of cytokines that stimulate and activate macrophages without the ability to terminate the reaction via apoptosis.[251,289]

Both LEP and CHP may, in some cases, fit into a spectrum of subcuticular lymphoid dyscrasia, ranging from benign reactive changes to SPTCL, including atypical indeterminate lobular panniculitis.[241-244,270] Immunophenotyping and genotyping studies are important for differentiating malignant SPTCL, which may have αβ or γδ rearranged T cells, from CHP with benign T cells. Monitoring biopsies is prudent as transformation has been reported.[277] Both SPTCL types can be associated with hemophagocytic syndrome/HLH and present with CHP; the incidence of HLH is much higher among γδ cases than among αβ cases.[247]

DIAGNOSIS

Multiple biopsies may be needed to establish the diagnosis of CHP as cytophagocytosis on histopathology may be focal. The histopathology is principally a lobular panniculitis (Fig. 73-15A) with fat lobules containing an infiltrate of histiocytes and mature lymphocytes with variable plasma cells, neutrophils, and eosinophils.[52] Phagocytic histiocytes contain intact or fragmented cells and nuclear debris within their cytoplasm; this represents the characteristic "beanbag cell" (Fig. 73-15B).[52] This is unlike emperipolesis (the presence of an intact cell within the cytoplasm of another cell) in which inflammatory cells pass through a histiocyte and no nuclear debris is seen.[291]

Immunohistochemical studies demonstrate that cytophagic histiocytes express histiocytic markers such as CD68, whereas most lymphocytes show a

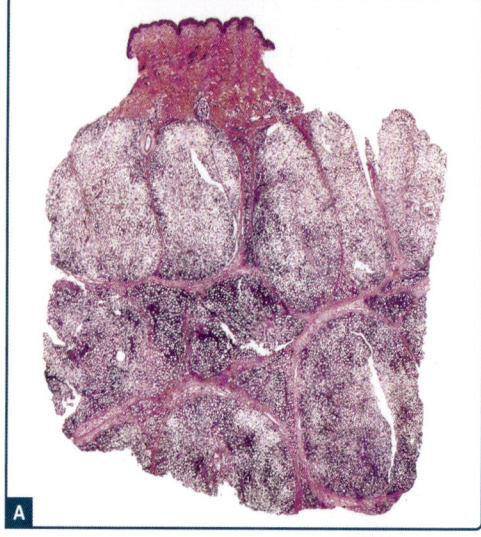
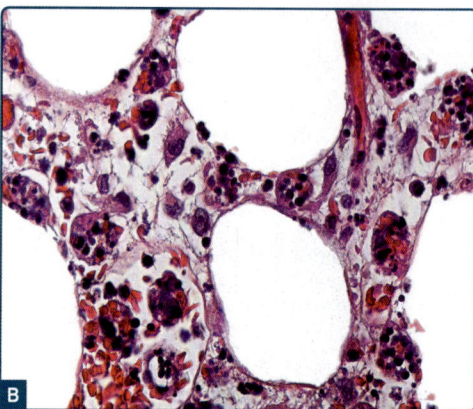

Figure 73-15 Cytophagic histiocytic panniculitis. **A,** Low-power magnification histologic image shows lobular panniculitis. **B.** Cytophagocytic "bean bag" cells in the adipose tissue.

T-cell immunophenotype. The presence of atypical lymphocytes, lymphocytic rimming of adipocytes, and clonality are concerning for lymphoma.[242,247] In rapidly progressive cases of CHP with HLH, cytophagic features can also be seen in internal organs including lymph nodes, spleen, liver, and bone marrow, and in cerebrospinal fluid fluid.[267-269,274,277]

DIFFERENTIAL DIAGNOSIS

Table 73-11 outlines the differential diagnosis of CHP.

CLINICAL COURSE AND PROGNOSIS

Patients may have a rapidly fatal disease course, a longer disease course with intermittent remissions and exacerbations for many years prior to death, or

TABLE 73-11
Differential Diagnosis of Cytophagic Histiocytic Panniculitis

DIAGNOSIS	CHARACTERISTICS
α_1-Antitrypsin deficiency	Tender, erythematous nodules that often have a suppurative exudate. Located on the lower abdomen, buttocks, and proximal extremities. Serology for enzymatic levels and phenotype helpful.
Erythema induratum/ nodular vasculitis	Tender nodules and plaques on calf areas, living in an area endemic for tuberculosis (erythema induratum). Vasculitis present on histopathology.
Cutaneous polyarteritis nodosa	Nodules in association with livedo reticularis and arterial inflammation on histology, possibly with neuropathy.
Infection-induced panniculitis	Erythema nodosum–like nodules, deep and inflamed nodules, or abscesses; older lesions may show fibrosis. Most commonly on legs. Systemic symptoms possible with fever. Often seen in severely immunosuppressed patients with malignancies. "Ghost cell" changes and urate crystals secondary to fungal enzymatic changes can be seen in mucormycosis and aspergillosis associated pancreatitis.[126,134]
Pyoderma gangrenosum	Violaceous, undermined borders with isomorphic response. Rare to mild systemic symptoms.
Malignancies	Persistent, worsening disease, often with systemic symptoms. Subcutaneous panniculitis-like T-cell lymphoma must be distinguished from atypical lymphocytic panniculitis. Presence of cutaneous T-cell lymphoma, angiosarcoma, or other sarcomas on leg with or without venous hypertension. More likely, but not exclusively, in patients with solid-organ transplants or other immunosuppressed states. Systemic symptoms possible.

a nonfatal acute or intermittent course responsive to treatment.[268,274,277,292] Patients with the benign, nonfatal course were found to have less-severe laboratory abnormalities.[292] Prompt treatment with corticosteroids and cyclosporine in the appropriate patient may reduce a 70% mortality rate to near 0%.[267,279] The panniculitis by itself is not always a marker of disease severity as 1 patient with CHP had resolution of cutaneous lesions with high-dose corticosteroid and cyclosporine therapy followed by recurrence 5 months later, progression, and death with generalized HLH.[293] This 1998 case was the first report of the failure of cyclosporine, and highlights the need for careful followup for systemic involvement even after an apparent therapeutic response.[293]

MANAGEMENT

Multidisciplinary care is critical in CHP management owing to its potentially rapidly fatal course. Hospitalization may be required for a rapid workup and institution of treatment. In HLH associated with an infection, treating the pathogen may result in recovery, but this is unpredictable.[294]

Treatment of CHP includes immunosuppressive, immunomodulating, or cytotoxic agents that target activated macrophages/histiocytes (steroids, etoposide, high-dose IVIG) and T cells (steroids, cyclosporine, antithymocyte globulin).[275] Among the published cases, cyclosporine and corticosteroids are often used and are often successful. In patients with both SLE and CHP, the combination of corticosteroids with cyclosporine may induce remission of both diseases.[276]

Cyclosporine-resistant disease also has been reported to respond to tacrolimus.[295] Tacrolimus may be an option for patients who have adverse effects with cyclosporine, and it may be a more realistic long-term treatment option for cases of CHP that are not able to taper off therapy.[296] Resistant cases may warrant a trial with cyclophosphamide and IVIG.[297] Addition of combined chemotherapy may be helpful.[275,298] Multiple rounds of combination chemotherapy or autologous stem cell transplantation may be required to induce remission.[299]

Cyclosporine, and cyclosporine with etoposide,[280] are effective regimens for CHP in both children and adults. In 2 pediatric patients, who developed CHP after viral infections, focal areas within the histopathology suggested SPTCL versus a reactive T-cell proliferation with in situ T-cell clonality; however, cyclosporine with corticosteroids induced remission for 69 and 29 months, respectively.[300] This report highlights the need to discriminate between CHP associated with a nonmalignant condition or with SPTCL. This report also suggests that when the diagnosis suggests a reactive T-cell proliferation rather than true lymphoma, cyclosporine may be used because nonmalignant CHP often improves with cyclosporine and prednisone whereas CHP with SPTCL is best treated aggressively.[300] One adolescent with lifelong CHP and severe HLH experienced improvement signs with anakinra, an IL-1 receptor antagonist, in addition to prednisone and cyclosporine.[301]

SUBCUTANEOUS FAT NECROSIS OF THE NEWBORN

AT-A-GLANCE

Clinical

- Circumscribed, red to violaceous, subcutaneous nodules, or plaques with predilection for buttocks, shoulders, cheeks, and thighs.
- Hypercalcemia in some cases, even presenting after the acute episode. Rarely, hypertriglyceridemia, hypoglycemia, thrombocytopenia, anemia.

Histopathology

- Mostly lobular panniculitis without vasculitis.
- Dense inflammatory infiltrate of lymphocytes, histiocytes, lipophages, and multinucleated giant cells.
- Needle-shaped clefts, often in radial array, within cytoplasm of histiocytes and multinucleated giant cells.

Treatment

- Nodules and plaques usually resolve spontaneously.
- Monitor for hypercalcemia for 6 months following onset, treat if hypercalcemia develops.

Subcutaneous fat necrosis of the newborn (SCFN) is a rare panniculitis that occurs in the first few days to weeks of life. Nearly all cases resolve spontaneously. The most common complication is hypercalcemia. Additional secondary effects include hypertriglyceridemia, hypoglycemia, thrombocytopenia, and anemia.[302-304]

EPIDEMIOLOGY

SCFN presents in full-term or postterm newborns (preterm cases also have been noted[305]) with a preceding history of perinatal complications, including meconium aspiration, asphyxia, hypothermia (eg, for cardiac surgery or ice pack application for supraventricular tachycardia, or for hypoxic ischemic encephalopathy complicating lack of respiratory effort[306]), hypoxemia, seizures, sepsis, gestational diabetes, preeclampsia, factors requiring cesarean section, forceps delivery, severe neonatal anemia, maternal cocaine use, and/or failure to thrive.[302-304,307,308] Within the population requiring hypothermic treatment of asphyxia, macrosomia and hemodynamic instability represent additional risk factors.[309]

CLINICAL FEATURES

Lesions are sharply demarcated, erythematous to violaceous, firm, indurated nodules or plaques located on the back, shoulders, arms, buttocks, thighs, or face, but rarely on the anterior trunk or the anterolateral shins (Fig. 73-16A).[303,306,307] Visceral involvement has been reported with MRI findings in one case consistent with abdominal wall, perihepatic, perisplenic, and perirenal fat necrosis.[310] The subcutaneous nodules range in size from several millimeters to up to 11 cm in diameter,[311,312] may be single or multiple, and are usually well defined.[311] Rarely, fluctuant nodules may drain an oily or chalky white material.[312] Larger blisters may form and may need drainage.[306] Lesions are not warm to touch[311] and are commonly painless; rarely, morphine is needed for pain control.[311] While often asymptomatic, the location and the size of the lesions can have local mass effect, such as in a case of radial nerve palsy secondary to SCFN that improved spontaneously within 10 weeks.[313]

There are several metabolic complications that may occur during and even after resolution of the panniculitis.[303] These include hypercalcemia (which affects 36% to 56% of patients with SCFN),[314] thrombocytopenia,[302,303] hypertriglyceridemia (likely related to the fat necrosis), hypoglycemia,[303,304] and anemia.[303] It is unclear if the glucose and hematologic abnormalities are secondary to the SCFN or to the initial insult that provokes the SCFN, as they may precede onset of cutaneous findings.[305,315] Hypercalcemia may be asymptomatic,[304] or may progress to symptomatic failure to thrive, irritability, fever, vomiting, hypotonia, seizures, polyuria and polydipsia, and even death.[311,312] Soft tissue and organ calcification may occur with variable outcomes.[302,311]

ETIOLOGY AND PATHOGENESIS

The ultimate cause of SCFN is not known, but hypothermia and hypoxia are presumed to be involved. Therapeutic hypothermia is used in pediatric intensive care in cases of asphyxia. It is unclear whether the hypothermia assists with the process or is a direct cause of the SCFN.[316] Cold exposure during surgical procedures may also induce SCFN.[317] Possible explanations have included a biochemical defect in the composition or metabolism of neonatal fat, leading to crystallization, fat necrosis, and subsequent inflammation after cold stress.[303,318] The hypercalcemia may be related to increased 25-hydroxyvitamin D_3–1α hydroxylase within the granulomatous infiltrates.[319]

Brown adipose tissue (BAT) in neonates rapidly converts fat stores to heat under conditions of cold stress.[320] SCFN affecting BAT has been confirmed with immunohistochemical staining, as well as uncoupling protein isoform 1, found specifically in BAT.[321] The BAT cells generate heat. The mechanism is complex, and uses uncoupling protein isoform 1, cytosolic fatty acids, and Ca^{2+} ions.[322]

DIAGNOSIS

Characteristically, SCFN is a mostly lobular panniculitis (see Fig. 73-16B), with focal necrosis of the fat lobule and a dense inflammatory infiltrate of lymphocytes, histiocytes, and foreign-body giant cells; a few eosinophils are possible.[52,303,323]

A primarily neutrophilic infiltrate may mimic an infection, especially if lesions are biopsied when 1 day old.[324] Many adipocytes retain their cellular outlines, but contain fine eosinophilic strands and granules, as well as needle-shaped clefts in radial array (see

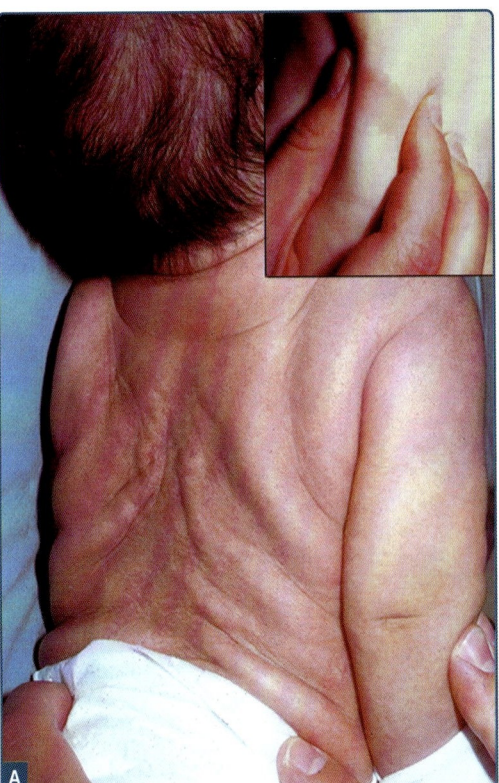
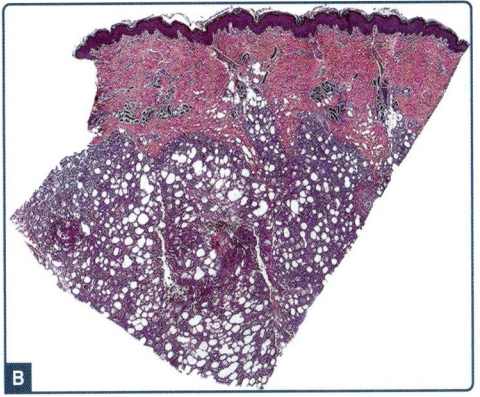
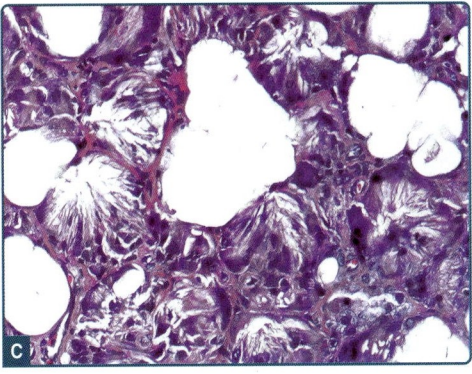

Figure 73-16 Subcutaneous fat necrosis of the newborn. **A,** Circumscribed, indurated subcutaneous nodules on the back. **B,** Low-power magnification histology shows mostly lobular panniculitis. **C,** Higher-power magnification shows needle-shaped clefts of adipocytes, histiocytes, and multinucleated giant cells.

Fig. 73-16C).[52,303,323] On frozen section, these clefts are occupied by doubly refractile crystals, representing triglycerides. Similar clefts and crystals also may be seen within the cytoplasm of the multinucleated giant cells.[52,303,323] Late-stage lesions may demonstrate fibrosis and calcified areas within fat lobules.[52,311] Fine-needle aspiration may be less painful, more cost-effective, and a more rapid diagnosis.[325,326] Ultrasonography also may be an adjunctive noninvasive diagnostic tool. AT is hyperechoic with high blood flow on Doppler and calcifications are seen.[327]

DIFFERENTIAL DIAGNOSIS

Table 73-12 outlines the differential diagnosis of SCFN.

CLINICAL COURSE AND PROGNOSIS

SCFN is a benign process with an excellent prognosis. Lesions regress in a few weeks to 6 months, with some eventuating in atrophy.[303,304,310] Hypercalcemia is the most severe potential adverse outcome and may cause nephrocalcinosis.[329] Even severe hypercalcemia may be asymptomatic.[314] The hypercalcemia may have a delayed onset up to 6 months after appearance of the skin lesions; therefore, serial monitoring of serum calcium levels is necessary.[303,304]

MANAGEMENT

SCFN nodules resolve spontaneously, and treatment should be conservative in most cases, except for lesions that may benefit from aspiration to prevent rupture, infections, necrosis, and scarring.[302,303] Surgical management has been used in severe cases that persist for months with incision and curettage of small calcifications.[330]

Serum calcium should be monitored serially, for several months after presentation in case of delayed elevations. If hypercalcemia is present, management includes hydration, use of the calcium-wasting diuretic furosemide, and a low calcium formula.[303,314] Systemic glucocorticoids may be used to inhibit vitamin D production by the macrophages in the inflamed AT.[303,307,312] Bisphosphonates, including alendronate,[331] etidronate,[332] and pamidronate,[333] treat hypercalcemia in SCFN.

Importantly, nephrocalcinosis may still develop in spite of cutaneous response.[301] The degree and duration of hypercalcemia and hypercalciuria may

TABLE 73-12

Differential Diagnosis of Subcutaneous Fat Necrosis of the Newborn

DIAGNOSIS	CHARACTERISTICS
Cellulitis	Larger plaques that are erythematous, usually lacking the violaceous bruising. Tender and warm.
Cold panniculitis	With any exposure to cold in both children and adults, not specific to the setting of hypoxia. Histopathology lacks needle-shaped clefts within the subcutaneous adipose tissue. Resolves with rewarming.
Sclerema neonatorum	Diffuse skin hardening, particularly on buttocks and thighs, in stressed infants in the first week of life, who are often low weight and premature.[52,328] Histopathology also shows needle-shaped clefts, with minimal inflammation. Poor prognosis with systemic illness.[52]
Poststeroid panniculitis	Occurs in children, usually 10 days after rapid cessation of high-dose systemic corticosteroid therapy. Similar histopathology to subcutaneous fat necrosis of the newborn.

be critical in development of nephrocalcinosis, encouraging early monitoring and recognition of hypercalcemia, as rapid therapeutic intervention may prevent dystrophic calcification.[334] Renal ultrasound detects nephrocalcinosis.[314] Persistent nephrocalcinosis does not result consistently in renal dysfunction.[314]

For prevention of SCFN, a specific nursing protocol has reduced the risk of SCFN while cooling. It includes rotation of the neonate every 3 hours and a gentler cooling surface–cooling device.[335]

COLD PANNICULITIS

AT-A-GLANCE

Clinical
- Circumscribed, red to violaceous, subcutaneous plaques or nodules on the face and thighs, and rarely of the scrotal fat in prepubertal boys.
- Follows exposure to cold weather, water, popsicles, and ice packs.

Histopathology
- Mostly lobular panniculitis with a lymphohistiocytic or mixed infiltrate, without vasculitis.
- Perivascular lymphohistiocytic infiltrate involving blood vessels at the dermal–subcutaneous junction and within overlying dermis.
- Findings may be similar to those seen in perniosis.

Treatment
- Avoid direct ice placement on skin and cold exposure.
- Spontaneous resolution within 3 months.

Cold panniculitis, also known as Haxthausen disease,[336] was first described in 1902 with hardening of a child's chin after cold weather exposure.[337] When occurring in equestrians, the terms *horse rider's pernio* and *equestrian panniculitis* are also used.[338] Cold panniculitis is an inflammatory reaction of AT that occurs after skin is exposed to cold weather and ice application (as in cold pack application for supraventricular tachycardia),[336] and can occur on mucosae as well (popsicle panniculitis).[337,339]

EPIDEMIOLOGY

Cold panniculitis occurs in children and in young female horseback riders as well as other adults with appropriate exposures. Symptoms may be secondary to intraoral frozen teething rings,[340] or after ice packs are applied to treat febrile episodes.[341] Scrotal cold panniculitis presents in 9- to 14-year-old overweight boys after cold exposure (including swimming in cold ocean water).[342] Symptoms of cold panniculitis in horseback riders have been reported in both males and females. A survey in Finland suggested 25% of riders have symptoms in the winter months.[338] Moderate smoking is statistically significant for an increased risk of cold panniculitis in equestrians, as is wearing tight riding clothes throughout the day, riding for long periods, and being younger than 35 years old.[338] Other risk factors for equestrian-like panniculitis include motorbike or open vehicle riding, wading through cold rivers, and young women wearing tight jeans.[343,344]

CLINICAL FEATURES

Clinical findings of indurated, erythematous plaques or nodules occur at sites of cold exposure and may include mucosa. The onset ranges from 6 to 72 hours after exposure,[345] appearing directly at sites that have contact with cold.[336] In equestrians with cold panniculitis, the presentation is on the lateral thighs.[338]

Scrotal cold panniculitis, also known as scrotal fat necrosis, manifests as unilateral or bilateral tender masses below the testes. Recognizing these changes is important to avoid unnecessary biopsy or intervention, as spontaneous resolution over days to several weeks will occur.[342] Equestrian panniculitis appears hours after long outdoor cold exposure while wearing tight-fitting, noninsulated pants. The lesions are pruritic, erythematous nodules and plaques that may focally ulcerate, crust, and drain.[337,338]

ETIOLOGY AND PATHOGENESIS

In affected infants, the mechanism of inflammation has been attributed to a higher proportion of saturated fat to unsaturated fat in infants, with the composition becoming more unsaturated with age.[337,346] Other mechanisms include the effects of cold on BAT, which is more prevalent in infants than adults, and its activation to generate heat.[347] Cold exposure leads to changes in BAT including increased vascular endothelial growth factor, enhanced free fatty acid degradation, and metabolic changes.[348,349] Scrotal cold panniculitis may be related to the greater concentration of scrotal fat and the increased cold sensitivity of the scrotal AT of younger males.[350]

Equestrian panniculitis may represent perniosis/chilblains, rather than a true panniculitis.[343,344,351] Although high levels of cold agglutinins were detected in 2 Scottish women with equestrian panniculitis,[351] other series do not show this abnormality[338,346] and cryoglobulins and cold agglutinins are not thought to play a role.[352]

DIAGNOSIS

The diagnosis is often clinical given the history of the cold exposure to the affected areas. In general, the histopathologic picture of cold panniculitis is a mostly lobular panniculitis, with a lymphohistiocytic or mixed inflammatory infiltrate present within fat lobules.[52,337] There is a superficial and deep perivascular, as well as periadnexal, lymphocytic infiltrate with prominent inflammation of veins most notable at the dermal–subcutaneous fat junction; these histopathologic findings closely resemble those seen in perniosis.[343,346] The title "cold-associated perniosis of the thighs" has been suggested.[343] In scrotal cases, ultrasound findings may help confirm the diagnosis.[342]

DIFFERENTIAL DIAGNOSIS

Table 73-13 outlines the differential diagnosis of cold panniculitis.

CLINICAL COURSE AND PROGNOSIS

Cold panniculitis is self-limiting and resolves upon rewarming without continued exposure to cold. Full improvement may be seen over days[341] to 3 months.[340] Postinflammatory hyperpigmentation may remain.[352]

MANAGEMENT

There is no additional treatment needed of cold panniculitis other than avoidance of further cold exposure; the best prevention is avoidance of cold exposure.[340] Equestrians with cold panniculitis may benefit from warm clothing and local topical corticosteroid application. Prevention in this population includes warm and loose-fitting clothing both while riding and during the day, as well as smoking cessation.[338] Nifedipine is not an effective treatment.[338,345]

TABLE 73-13
Differential Diagnosis of Cold Panniculitis

DIAGNOSIS	CHARACTERISTICS
Cellulitis	Large plaques that are often unilateral, erythematous, tender and warm. Systemic findings may include fever and leukocytosis.
Subcutaneous fat necrosis of the newborn	Cold exposure in infants in the setting of hypoxia. Histopathology with needle-shaped clefts within the adipose tissue. Complications such as hypercalcemia are possible.
Sclerema neonatorum	Diffuse skin hardening, particularly on buttocks and thighs, in stressed infants in the first week of life, who are often low weight and premature.[52,328] Histopathology also shows needle-shaped clefts with minimal inflammation.[52] Poor prognosis with systemic illness.[52]
Poststeroid panniculitis	Occurs in children, usually within 10 days after rapid cessation of high-dose systemic corticosteroid therapy. Similar histopathology to subcutaneous fat necrosis of the newborn.
Erythema nodosum	Violaceous or red plaques on the anterior legs with no ulceration.

FACTITIAL AND TRAUMATIC PANNICULITIS

AT-A-GLANCE

Clinical

- In factitial panniculitis (a variant of Munchausen syndrome),[353] self-induced trauma (mechanical, physical, or chemical) causes subcutaneous inflammation. In trauma-induced panniculitis the injury is not induced by the patient, such as in a postsurgical panniculitis or panniculitis following a sport injury.[354,355]
- Erythematous geometric papules and nodules with erosions or ulcerations (Fig. 73-17),[356] with disparate location or appearance.
- Factitial panniculitis is often seen in patients with personality aberrations and subcutaneous implantation may include medications, cosmetic fillers, oils, and food or human waste.[356]
- Traumatic panniculitis may be secondary to cupping, acupuncture, and electropuncture,[357,358] or may be iatrogenic from immunizations or therapeutic injections.[356]
- Secondary hypertrichosis at affected sites is rare.[359,360]

Histopathology

- Mostly a nonspecific lobular panniculitis without vasculitis, varying with the cause.
- Suppurative granuloma involving the fat lobule; requires cultures for various organisms. Necrosis is often present.[361]
- Polarization of the slide may identify refractile foreign material within macrophages.[356]
- Late stages may show foamy histocytes with fibrotic changes and dystrophic calcific deposits.[356,362] Foamy lipophagic histiocytes, adipocyte anisocytosis with pseudocystic degeneration, single adipocyte necrosis, erythrocyte extravasation, and foreign-body granuloma with multinucleated giant cells are all potential features. Frank scarring, deep phlebitis, and traumatic neuromas may be present in postsurgical panniculitis.[354]

Treatment

- Psychiatric treatment for self-inflicted factitial panniculitis.[52]
- Supportive care and interference with injection of responsible agents.
- Often the implanted material must be surgically excised.[356,357]
- Prevention of ongoing trauma and supportive care is needed for traumatic panniculitis as it is self-limiting without further trauma.[361]

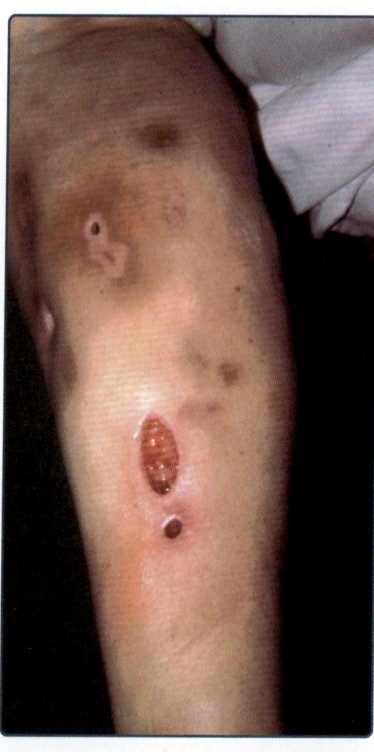

Figure 73-17 Factitial panniculitis. Self-induced round and angulated ulceration on the leg at sites of injections and trauma.

CONNECTIVE TISSUE DISEASE-ASSOCIATED PANNICULITIS

AT-A-GLANCE

Clinical

- Most often associated with dermatomyositis, and may precede, occur with, or appear late in the disease course, with severity correlating with disease flares.[363]
- Erythematous, tender to painful nodules and plaques on the arms, buttocks, thighs, and abdomen. Complications include ulceration and lipoatrophy.[364,365]
- Rarely, panniculitis is the primary presentation of dermatomyositis,[52,366] and juvenile dermatomyositis-associated panniculitis is uncommon but has been reported.[367] Panniculitis in a child should prompt workup for connective tissue disease.[368]
- Infection may occur concurrently and must be treated prior to immunosuppression.[367]
- Panniculitis is also associated with morphea and systemic sclerosis, but the association is rare.
- SPTCL must be considered in the differential diagnosis of a connective tissue disease panniculitis. Up to 19% of SPTCL with an αβ phenotype in one series had an associated autoimmune disorder.[247] SPTCL with a γδ phenotype was reported as developing in a patient with rheumatoid arthritis after 3 years of anti-TNF therapy.[247] One patient with SPTCL presented with clinical features of dermatomyositis.[369]

Histopathology

- Mostly lobular panniculitis with a lymphocytic and plasma cell infiltrate, with dermal mucin and vacuolar interface change, similar to lupus panniculitis.[52,370]
- Calcification may be present.[363]
- Membranocystic change may be present in late-stage lesions,[52,230] and indicate a worse prognosis.[371]

Treatment

- Same as for dermatomyositis: corticosteroids, immunosuppressants (including azathioprine, mycophenolate mofetil, and methotrexate[370]) and IVIG.[364,366,371,372]
- Calcification within lesions may benefit from IVIG.[373]
- Antimalarials are not effective in dermatomyositis-associated panniculitis.[370]

GOUTY PANNICULITIS

AT-A-GLANCE

Clinical

- Subcutaneous urate crystals are a rare manifestation of gout.[374]
- Most commonly firm, indurated nodules or plaques, with variable tenderness on the lower extremities,[375] with possible urate crystal deposition in bone marrow[375] and otherwise diffuse involvement.[376]
- A chalky substance may overly ulceration.[376,377]
- Massive AT hypertrophy may be seen, requiring surgical resection.[378]
- Hyperuricemia is associated,[379] as well as arthralgias (gouty arthritis).[380]
- The lesions may precede a diagnosis of gout,[376] but they are often a late consequence of chronic gout.[377]
- Differential diagnosis includes foreign-body panniculitis, calcium, and other crystal deposition diseases.[375]

Histopathology

- Fine, radially oriented, needle-shaped urate crystals within AT are surrounded by granulomatous inflammation. The monosodium urate crystals are refractile and negatively birefringent.[375,378,379]
- Alcohol fixation allows for enhanced crystal visualization.[375]
- There is no evidence of vasculitis.[379]

Treatment

- Standard treatments for gout include allopurinol (high doses),[380] probenecid, and antiinflammatory medications, including colchicine, which can be used to reduce uric acid levels.[375]
- Acute panniculitis may benefit from corticosteroids.[379]
- Surgery may be necessary for ulcerated lesions that do not heal.[377]

POSTSTEROID PANNICULITIS

AT-A-GLANCE

Clinical

- Poststeroid panniculitis is rare, most often seen in children after high doses of systemic corticosteroid treatment, days to weeks after abrupt corticosteroid withdrawal.[303,381] Cases in adults are very rare.[382,383]
- Erythematous, tender nodules and plaques on the cheeks, trunk, arms,[382] and legs.[381]

(Continued)

AT-A-GLANCE (Continued)

- Resolves in weeks or months without scarring; can leave residual hyperpigmentation. Most common complication is ulceration; systemic symptoms are rare.[382]

Histopathology

- Lobular panniculitis with a lymphocytic and granulomatous infiltrate, without vasculitis. Lipophages and crystals can be present.[382]
- Needle-shaped clefts in a radial orientation are seen, similar to those seen in SCFN and sclerema neonatorum; sclerema neonatorum lacks or has sparse inflammation.[382]
- Multinucleated giant cells may contain the needle-shaped clefts with foamy histiocytes.[382,383]

Treatment

- Lesions resolve within weeks or months without scarring even without treatment, leaving residual hyperpigmentation.[382,383]
- It has been postulated that gradual tapering of steroids can eliminate the risk of poststeroid panniculitis.[381]

ACKNOWLEDGMENTS

The authors wish to acknowledge Dr. Patricia Fishman for her work on the prior edition of this chapter.

REFERENCES

1. Patterson JW. Panniculitis. New findings in the "third compartment." *Arch Dermatol*. 1987;123:1615-1618.
2. Requena L. Normal subcutaneous fat, necrosis of adipocytes and classification of the panniculitides. *Semin Cutan Med Surg*. 2007;26:66-70.
3. Fantuzzi G. Adipose tissue, adipokines, and inflammation. *J Allergy Clin Immunol*. 2005;115:911-919; quiz 920.
4. Ferrandon D, Imler JL, Hetru C, et al. The Drosophila systemic immune response: sensing and signalling during bacterial and fungal infections. *Nat Rev Immunol*. 2007;7:862-874.
5. Caspar-Bauguil S, Cousin B, Galinier A, et al. Adipose tissues as an ancestral immune organ: site-specific change in obesity. *FEBS Lett*. 2005;579:3487-3492.
6. Janeway CA Jr, Medzhitov R. Innate immune recognition. *Annu Rev Immunol*. 2002;20:197-216.
7. Iwasaki A, Medzhitov R. Regulation of adaptive immunity by the innate immune system. *Science*. 2010;327:291-295.
8. Miller LS. Toll-like receptors in skin. *Adv Dermatol*. 2008;24:71-87.
9. Desruisseaux MS, Nagajyothi, Trujillo ME, et al. Adipocyte, adipose tissue, and infectious disease. *Infect Immun*. 2007;75:1066-1078.
10. Schaffler A, Scholmerich J, Salzberger B. Adipose tissue as an immunological organ: Toll-like

receptors, C1q/TNFs and CTRPs. *Trends Immunol.* 2007;28:393-399.
11. Nishimura S, Manabe I, Nagai R. Adipose tissue inflammation in obesity and metabolic syndrome. *Discov Med.* 2009;8:55-60.
12. Rajsheker S, Manka D, Blomkalns AL, et al. Crosstalk between perivascular adipose tissue and blood vessels. *Curr Opin Pharmacol.* 2010;10:191-196.
13. Chatterjee TK, Stoll LL, Denning GM, et al. Proinflammatory phenotype of perivascular adipocytes: influence of high-fat feeding. *Circ Res.* 2009;104:541-549.
14. Crawley FE. Erythema nodosum as initial manifestation of Boeck's sarcoidosis. *Br Med J.* 1950;2:1362-1364.
15. Requena L, Yus ES. Panniculitis. Part I. Mostly septal panniculitis. *J Am Acad Dermatol.* 2001;45:163-183; quiz 184-186.
16. Cribier B, Caille A, Heid E, et al. Erythema nodosum and associated diseases. A study of 129 cases. *Int J Dermatol.* 1998;37:667-672.
17. Aydin-Teke T, Tanir G, Bayhan GI, et al. Erythema nodosum in children: evaluation of 39 patients. *Turk J Pediatr.* 2014;56:144-149.
18. Requena L, Requena C. Erythema nodosum. *Dermatol Online J.* 2002;8:4.
19. Garcia-Porrua C, Gonzalez-Gay MA, Vazquez-Caruncho M, et al. Erythema nodosum: etiologic and predictive factors in a defined population. *Arthritis Rheum.* 2000;43:584-592.
20. Papagrigoraki A, Gisondi P, Rosina P, et al. Erythema nodosum: etiological factors and relapses in a retrospective cohort study. *Eur J Dermatol.* 2010;20:773-777.
21. Mert A, Kumbasar H, Ozaras R, et al. Erythema nodosum: an evaluation of 100 cases. *Clin Exp Rheumatol.* 2007;25:563-570.
22. Kisacik B, Onat AM, Pehlivan Y. Multiclinical experiences in erythema nodosum: rheumatology clinics versus dermatology and infection diseases clinics. *Rheumatol Int.* 2013;33:315-318.
23. Bartelsmeyer JA, Petrie RH. Erythema nodosum, estrogens, and pregnancy. *Clin Obstet Gynecol.* 1990;33:777-781.
24. Ricci RM, Deering KC. Erythema nodosum caused by omeprazole. *Cutis.* 1996;57:434.
25. Degen A, Volker B, Kapp A, et al. Erythema nodosum in a patient undergoing vemurafenib therapy for metastatic melanoma. *Eur J Dermatol.* 2013;23:118.
26. Hannuksela M. Erythema nodosum. *Clin Dermatol.* 1986;4:88-95.
27. Jones JV, Cumming RH, Asplin CM. Evidence for circulating immune complexes in erythema nodosum and early sarcoidosis. *Ann N Y Acad Sci.* 1976;278:212-219.
28. De Simone C, Caldarola G, Scaldaferri F, et al. Clinical, histopathological, and immunological evaluation of a series of patients with erythema nodosum. *Int J Dermatol.* 2016;55(5):e289-e294.
29. Kunz M, Beutel S, Brocker E. Leucocyte activation in erythema nodosum. *Clin Exp Dermatol.* 1999;24:396-401.
30. Senturk T, Aydintug O, Kuzu I, et al. Adhesion molecule expression in erythema nodosum-like lesions in Behçet's disease. A histopathological and immunohistochemical study. *Rheumatol Int.* 1998;18:51-57.
31. Labunski S, Posern G, Ludwig S, et al. Tumour necrosis factor-alpha promoter polymorphism in erythema nodosum. *Acta Derm Venereol.* 2001;81:18-21.
32. Amoli MM, Donn RP, Thomson W, et al. Macrophage migration inhibitory factor gene polymorphism is associated with sarcoidosis in biopsy proven erythema nodosum. *J Rheumatol.* 2002;29:1671-1673.
33. Amoli MM, Miranda-Filloy JA, Vazquez-Rodriguez TR, et al. Regulated upon activation normal T-cell expressed and secreted (RANTES) and epithelial cell-derived neutrophil-activating peptide (ENA-78) gene polymorphisms in patients with biopsy-proven erythema nodosum. *Clin Exp Rheumatol.* 2009;27:S142-S143.
34. Schaffler A, Muller-Ladner U, Scholmerich J, et al. Role of adipose tissue as an inflammatory organ in human diseases. *Endocr Rev.* 2006;27:449-467.
35. Braverman IM. Protective effects of erythema nodosum in coccidioidomycosis. *Lancet.* 1999;353:168.
36. Marcoval J, Mana J, Rubio M. Specific cutaneous lesions in patients with systemic sarcoidosis: relationship to severity and chronicity of disease. *Clin Exp Dermatol.* 2011;36:739-744.
37. Grunewald J, Eklund A. Löfgren's syndrome: human leukocyte antigen strongly influences the disease course. *Am J Respir Crit Care Med.* 2009;179:307-312.
38. Thurber S, Kohler S. Histopathologic spectrum of erythema nodosum. *J Cutan Pathol.* 2006;33:18-26.
39. White WL, Hitchcock MG. Diagnosis: erythema nodosum or not? *Semin Cutan Med Surg.* 1999;18:47-55.
40. Requena L, Sanchez Yus E. Erythema nodosum. *Semin Cutan Med Surg.* 2007;26:114-125.
41. Winkelmann RK, Forstrom L. New observations in the histopathology of erythema nodosum. *J Invest Dermatol.* 1975;65:441-446.
42. Weizman A, Huang B, Berel D, et al. Clinical, serologic, and genetic factors associated with pyoderma gangrenosum and erythema nodosum in inflammatory bowel disease patients. *Inflamm Bowel Dis.* 2014;20:525-533.
43. Sterling JB, Heymann WR. Potassium iodide in dermatology: a 19th century drug for the 21st century—uses, pharmacology, adverse effects, and contraindications. *J Am Acad Dermatol.* 2000;43:691-697.
44. Davatchi F, Sadeghi Abdollahi B, Tehrani Banihashemi A, et al. Colchicine versus placebo in Behçet's disease: randomized, double-blind, controlled crossover trial. *Mod Rheumatol.* 2009;19:542-549.
45. Boyd AS. Etanercept treatment of erythema nodosum. *Skinmed.* 2007;6:197-199.
46. Hanauer SB. How do I treat erythema nodosum, aphthous ulcerations, and pyoderma gangrenosum? *Inflamm Bowel Dis.* 1998;4:70; discussion 73.
47. Golding D. Treating erythema nodosum. *Br Med J.* 1969;4:560-561.
48. Alloway JA, Franks LK. Hydroxychloroquine in the treatment of chronic erythema nodosum. *Br J Dermatol.* 1995;132:661-662.
49. Montgomery H, O'Leary PA, Parker NW. Nodular vascular diseases of the legs: erythema induratum and allied conditions. *JAMA.* 1945;128:335-345.
50. Mascaro JM Jr, Baselga E. Erythema induratum of bazin. *Dermatol Clin.* 2008;26:439-445, v.
51. Segura S, Pujol RM, Trindade F, et al. Vasculitis in erythema induratum of Bazin: a histopathologic study of 101 biopsy specimens from 86 patients. *J Am Acad Dermatol.* 2008;59:839-851.
52. Requena L, Sanchez Yus E. Panniculitis. Part II. Mostly lobular panniculitis. *J Am Acad Dermatol.* 2001;45:325-361; quiz 362-364.
53. Ferrara G, Stefanato CM, Gianotti R, et al. Panniculitis with vasculitis. *G Ital Dermatol Venereol.* 2013;148:387-394.

54. Gilchrist H, Patterson JW. Erythema nodosum and erythema induratum (nodular vasculitis): diagnosis and management. *Dermatol Ther*. 2010;23:320-327.
55. Brandao Neto RA, Carvalho JF. Erythema induratum of Bazin associated with Addison's disease: first description. *Sao Paulo Med J*. 2012;130:405-408.
56. Inoue T, Fukumoto T, Ansai S, et al. Erythema induratum of Bazin in an infant after Bacille Calmette-Guerin vaccination. *J Dermatol*. 2006;33:268-272.
57. Sekiguchi A, Motegi S, Ishikawa O. Erythema induratum of Bazin associated with bacillus Calmette-Guerin vaccination: implication of M1 macrophage infiltration and monocyte chemotactic protein-1 expression. *J Dermatol*. 2016;43:111-113.
58. Sharma S, Sehgal VN, Bhattacharya SN, et al. Clinicopathologic spectrum of cutaneous tuberculosis: a retrospective analysis of 165 Indians. *Am J Dermatopathol*. 2015;37:444-450.
59. Chong LY, Lo KK. Cutaneous tuberculosis in Hong Kong: a 10-year retrospective study. *Int J Dermatol*. 1995;34:26-29.
60. Sethuraman G, Ramesh V. Cutaneous tuberculosis in children. *Pediatr Dermatol*. 2013;30:7-16.
61. Oshio A, Yoshii Y, Ono K, et al. Erythema induratum of Bazin with anti-phospholipid antibodies. *J Dtsch Dermatol Ges*. 2015;13:810-811.
62. Baselga E, Margall N, Barnadas MA, et al. Detection of *Mycobacterium tuberculosis* DNA in lobular granulomatous panniculitis (erythema induratum-nodular vasculitis). *Arch Dermatol*. 1997;133:457-462.
63. Neyrolles O, Hernandez-Pando R, Pietri-Rouxel F, et al. Is adipose tissue a place for *Mycobacterium tuberculosis* persistence? *PLoS One*. 2006;1:e43.
64. Bouwman JJ, Visseren FL, Bouter KP, et al. Infection-induced inflammatory response of adipocytes in vitro. *Int J Obes (Lond)*. 2008;32:892-901.
65. Bechah Y, Paddock CD, Capo C, et al. Adipose tissue serves as a reservoir for recrudescent *Rickettsia prowazekii* infection in a mouse model. *PLoS One*. 2010;5:e8547.
66. Nagajyothi F, Desruisseaux MS, Thiruvur N, et al. *Trypanosoma cruzi* infection of cultured adipocytes results in an inflammatory phenotype. *Obesity (Silver Spring)*. 2008;16:1992-1997.
67. Nagajyothi F, Desruisseaux MS, Weiss LM, et al. Chagas disease, adipose tissue and the metabolic syndrome. *Mem Inst Oswaldo Cruz*. 2009;104(suppl 1):219-225.
68. Angus J, Roberts C, Kulkarni K, et al. Usefulness of the QuantiFERON test in the confirmation of latent tuberculosis in association with erythema induratum. *Br J Dermatol*. 2007;157:1293-1294.
69. Lighter J, Tse DB, Li Y, et al. Erythema induratum of Bazin in a child: evidence for a cell-mediated hyper-response to *Mycobacterium tuberculosis*. *Pediatr Infect Dis J*. 2009;28:326-328.
70. Cho KH, Lee DY, Kim CW. Erythema induratum of Bazin. *Int J Dermatol*. 1996;35:802-808.
71. Romero JJ, Herrera P, Cartelle M, et al. Panniculitis caused by *Mycobacterium monacense* mimicking erythema induratum: a case in Ecuador. *New Microbes New Infect*. 2016;10:112-115.
72. Gimenez-Garcia R, Sanchez-Ramon S, Sanchez-Antolin G, et al. Red fingers syndrome and recurrent panniculitis in a patient with chronic hepatitis C. *J Eur Acad Dermatol Venereol*. 2003;17:692-694.
73. Pozdnyakova O, Garg A, Mahalingam M. Nodular vasculitis—a novel cutaneous manifestation of autoimmune colitis. *J Cutan Pathol*. 2008;35:315-319.
74. Patterson JW, Brown PC, Broecker AH. Infection-induced panniculitis. *J Cutan Pathol*. 1989;16:183-193.
75. Misago N, Narisawa Y. Erythema induratum (nodular vasculitis) associated with Crohn's disease: a rare type of metastatic Crohn's disease. *Am J Dermatopathol*. 2012;34:325-329.
76. Sakuma H, Niiyama S, Amoh Y, et al. Chlamydophila pneumoniae Infection Induced Nodular Vasculitis. *Case Rep Dermatol*. 2011;3:263-267.
77. Wolf D, Ben-Yehuda A, Okon E, et al. Nodular vasculitis associated with propylthiouracil therapy. *Cutis*. 1992;49:253-255.
78. Park SB, Chang IK, Im M, et al. Nodular vasculitis that developed during etanercept (Enbrel) treatment in a patient with psoriasis. *Ann Dermatol*. 2015;27:605-607.
79. Schneider JW, Jordaan HF, Geiger DH, et al. Erythema induratum of Bazin. A clinicopathological study of 20 cases and detection of *Mycobacterium tuberculosis* DNA in skin lesions by polymerase chain reaction. *Am J Dermatopathol*. 1995;17:350-356.
80. Tehrany YA, Toutous-Trellu L, Trombert V, et al. A case of tuberculous granulomatous panniculitis without vasculitis. *Case Rep Dermatol*. 2015;7:141-145.
81. Chen S, Chen J, Chen L, et al. *Mycobacterium tuberculosis* infection is associated with the development of erythema nodosum and nodular vasculitis. *PLoS One*. 2013;8:e62653.
82. Teramura K, Fujimoto N, Nakanishi G, et al. Disseminated erythema induratum of Bazin. *Eur J Dermatol*. 2014;24:697-698.
83. Shaffer N, Kerdel FA. Nodular vasculitis (erythema induratum): treatment with auranofin. *J Am Acad Dermatol*. 1991;25:426-429.
84. Taverna JA, Radfar A, Pentland A, et al. Case reports: nodular vasculitis responsive to mycophenolate mofetil. *J Drugs Dermatol*. 2006;5:992-993.
85. Huriez C, Desmons F, Agache P, et al. Patchy and diffuse hypodermitis and dermo-hypodermitis [in French]. *Presse Med*. 1962;70:2743-2746.
86. Jorizzo JL, White WL, Zanolli MD, et al. Sclerosing panniculitis. A clinicopathologic assessment. *Arch Dermatol*. 1991;127:554-558.
87. Kirsner RS, Pardes JB, Eaglstein WH, et al. The clinical spectrum of lipodermatosclerosis. *J Am Acad Dermatol*. 1993;28:623-627.
88. Choonhakarn C, Chaowattanapanit S, Julanon N. Lipodermatosclerosis: a clinicopathologic correlation. *Int J Dermatol*. 2016;55:303-308.
89. Walsh SN, Santa Cruz DJ. Lipodermatosclerosis: a clinicopathological study of 25 cases. *J Am Acad Dermatol*. 2010;62:1005-1012.
90. Bruce AJ, Bennett DD, Lohse CM, et al. Lipodermatosclerosis: review of cases evaluated at Mayo Clinic. *J Am Acad Dermatol*. 2002;46:187-192.
91. Greenberg AS, Hasan A, Montalvo BM, et al. Acute lipodermatosclerosis is associated with venous insufficiency. *J Am Acad Dermatol*. 1996;35:566-568.
92. Alavi A, Sibbald RG, Phillips TJ, et al. What's new: management of venous leg ulcers: approach to venous leg ulcers. *J Am Acad Dermatol*. 2016;74:627-640.
93. Chu CY, Yang CH, Chiu HC. Gemcitabine-induced acute lipodermatosclerosis-like reaction. *Acta Derm Venereol*. 2001;81:426-428.
94. Shuster M, Morley K, Logan J, et al. Lipodermatosclerosis secondary to pemetrexed use. *J Thorac Oncol*. 2015;10:e11-e12.

95. Herouy Y, Kahle B, Idzko M, et al. Tight junctions and compression therapy in chronic venous insufficiency. *Int J Mol Med*. 2006;18:215-219.
96. Leu HJ. Morphology of chronic venous insufficiency—light and electron microscopic examinations. *Vasa*. 1991;20:330-342.
97. Falanga V, Bontempo FA, Eaglstein WH. Protein C and protein S plasma levels in patients with lipodermatosclerosis and venous ulceration. *Arch Dermatol*. 1990;126:1195-1197.
98. Schmeller W, Roszinski S, Huesmann M. Tissue oxygenation and microcirculation in dermatoliposclerosis with different degrees of erythema at the margins of venous ulcers. A contribution to hypodermitis symptoms [in German]. *Vasa*. 1997;26:18-24.
99. Saharay M, Shields DA, Porter JB, et al. Leukocyte activity in the microcirculation of the leg in patients with chronic venous disease. *J Vasc Surg*. 1997;26:265-273.
100. Peschen M, Grenz H, Brand-Saberi B, et al. Increased expression of platelet-derived growth factor receptor alpha and beta and vascular endothelial growth factor in the skin of patients with chronic venous insufficiency. *Arch Dermatol Res*. 1998;290:291-297.
101. Pappas PJ, You R, Rameshwar P, et al. Dermal tissue fibrosis in patients with chronic venous insufficiency is associated with increased transforming growth factor-beta1 gene expression and protein production. *J Vasc Surg*. 1999;30:1129-1145.
102. Degiorgio-Miller AM, Treharne LJ, McAnulty RJ, et al. Procollagen type I gene expression and cell proliferation are increased in lipodermatosclerosis. *Br J Dermatol*. 2005;152:242-249.
103. Ye J, Gao Z, Yin J, et al. Hypoxia is a potential risk factor for chronic inflammation and adiponectin reduction in adipose tissue of ob/ob and dietary obese mice. *Am J Physiol Endocrinol Metab*. 2007;293:E1118-E1128.
104. Halberg N, Wernstedt-Asterholm I, Scherer PE. The adipocyte as an endocrine cell. *Endocrinol Metab Clin North Am*. 2008;37:753-768, x-xi.
105. Halberg N, Khan T, Trujillo ME, et al. Hypoxia-inducible factor 1alpha induces fibrosis and insulin resistance in white adipose tissue. *Mol Cell Biol*. 2009;29:4467-4483.
106. Khan T, Muise ES, Iyengar P, et al. Metabolic dysregulation and adipose tissue fibrosis: role of collagen VI. *Mol Cell Biol*. 2009;29:1575-1591.
107. Tidwell WJ, Malone J, Callen JP. Cutaneous T-cell lymphoma misdiagnosed as lipodermatosclerosis. *JAMA Dermatol*. 2016;152:487-488.
108. Jowett AJ, Parvin SD. Angiosarcoma in an area of lipodermatosclerosis. *Ann R Coll Surg Engl*. 2008;90:W15-W16.
109. Chan CC, Yang CY, Chu CY. Magnetic resonance imaging as a diagnostic tool for extensive lipodermatosclerosis. *J Am Acad Dermatol*. 2008;58:525-527.
110. Huang TM, Lee JY. Lipodermatosclerosis: a clinicopathologic study of 17 cases and differential diagnosis from erythema nodosum. *J Cutan Pathol*. 2009;36:453-460.
111. Alegre VA, Winkelmann RK, Aliaga A. Lipomembranous changes in chronic panniculitis. *J Am Acad Dermatol*. 1988;19:39-46.
112. Jinnin M, Ihn H, Asano Y, et al. Sclerosing panniculitis is associated with pulmonary hypertension in systemic sclerosis. *Br J Dermatol*. 2005;153:579-583.
113. Gniadecka M, Karlsmark T, Bertram A. Removal of dermal edema with class I and II compression stockings in patients with lipodermatosclerosis. *J Am Acad Dermatol*. 1998;39:966-970.
114. Kahle B, Idzko M, Norgauer J, et al. Tightening tight junctions with compression therapy. *J Invest Dermatol*. 2003;121:1228-1229.
115. Vesic S, Vukovic J, Medenica LJ, et al. Acute lipodermatosclerosis: an open clinical trial of stanozolol in patients unable to sustain compression therapy. *Dermatol Online J*. 2008;14:1.
116. Carson P, Hong CJ, Otero-Vinas M, et al. Liver enzymes and lipid levels in patients with lipodermatosclerosis and venous ulcers treated with a prototypic anabolic steroid (stanozolol): a prospective, randomized, double-blinded, placebo-controlled trial. *Int J Low Extrem Wounds*. 2015;14:11-18.
117. Segal S, Cooper J, Bolognia J. Treatment of lipodermatosclerosis with oxandrolone in a patient with stanozolol-induced hepatotoxicity. *J Am Acad Dermatol*. 2000;43:558-559.
118. Hafner C, Wimmershoff M, Landthaler M, et al. Lipodermatosclerosis: successful treatment with danazol. *Acta Derm Venereol*. 2005;85:365-366.
119. Jull A, Arroll B, Parag V, et al. Pentoxifylline for treating venous leg ulcers. *Cochrane Database Syst Rev*. 2007:CD001733.
120. Choonhakarn C, Chaowattanapanit S. Lipodermatosclerosis: improvement noted with hydroxychloroquine and pentoxifylline. *J Am Acad Dermatol*. 2012;66:1013-1014.
121. Rowe L, Cantwell A Jr. Hypodermitis sclerodermiformis. Successful treatment with ultrasound. *Arch Dermatol*. 1982;118:312-314.
122. Damian DL, Yiasemides E, Gupta S, et al. Ultrasound therapy for lipodermatosclerosis. *Arch Dermatol*. 2009;145:330-332.
123. Boyd K, Shea SM, Patterson JW. The role of capsaicin in dermatology. *Prog Drug Res*. 2014;68:293-306.
124. Jeong KH, Shin MK, Kim NI. Refractory lipodermatosclerosis treated with intralesional platelet-rich plasma. *J Am Acad Dermatol*. 2011;65:e157-e158.
125. Delgado-Jimenez Y, Fraga J, Garcia-Diez A. Infective panniculitis. *Dermatol Clin*. 2008;26:471-480, vi.
126. Requena L, Sitthinamsuwan P, Santonja C, et al. Cutaneous and mucosal mucormycosis mimicking pancreatic panniculitis and gouty panniculitis. *J Am Acad Dermatol*. 2012;66:975-984.
127. Spalding SJ, Meza MP, Ranganathan S, et al. *Staphylococcus aureus* panniculitis complicating juvenile dermatomyositis. *Pediatrics*. 2007;119:e528-e530.
128. Chen WS, Lee YF, Wang HP, et al. *Mycobacterium*-associated lobular panniculitis, mimicking a rheumatoid nodule in a patient with rheumatoid arthritis. *J Formos Med Assoc*. 2009;108:673-676.
129. Bourre-Tessier J, Fortin C, Belisle A, et al. Disseminated *Histoplasma capsulatum* infection presenting with panniculitis and focal myositis in rheumatoid arthritis treated with etanercept. *Scand J Rheumatol*. 2009;38:311-316.
130. Quinter S, Cheng CL, Prakash N, et al. Disseminated histoplasmosis presenting as panniculitis in two immunosuppressed patients. *Dermatol Online J*. 2012;18:3.
131. Morrison LK, Rapini R, Willison CB, et al. Infection and panniculitis. *Dermatol Ther*. 2010;23:328-340.
132. Bartralot R, Garcia-Patos V, Sitjas D, et al. Clinical patterns of cutaneous nontuberculous mycobacterial infections. *Br J Dermatol*. 2005;152:727-734.
133. Zhang CZ, Fung MA, Eisen DB. Disseminated fusariosis presenting as panniculitis-like lesions on the legs

of a neutropenic girl with acute lymphoblastic leukemia. *Dermatol Online J.* 2009;15:5.
134. Colmenero I, Alonso-Sanz M, Casco F, et al. Cutaneous aspergillosis mimicking pancreatic and gouty panniculitis. *J Am Acad Dermatol.* 2012;67:789-791.
135. Kothiwala SK, Prajapat M, Kuldeep CM, et al. Cryptococcal panniculitis in a renal transplant recipient: case report and review of literature. *J Dermatol Case Rep.* 2015;9:76-80.
136. Abuav R, McGirt LY, Kazin RA. Cryptococcal panniculitis in an immunocompromised patient: a case report and review of the literature. *Cutis.* 2010;85:303-306.
137. Roriz M, Maruani A, Le Bidre E, et al. Locoregional multiple nodular panniculitis induced by Pseudomonas aeruginosa without septicemia: three cases and focus on predisposing factors. *JAMA Dermatol.* 2014;150:628-632.
138. Nemoto Y, Taniguchi A, Kamioka M, et al. Epstein-Barr virus-infected subcutaneous panniculitis-like T-cell lymphoma associated with methotrexate treatment. *Int J Hematol.* 2010;92:364-368.
139. Plotner AN, Mutasim DF. A case of "syphilis panniculitis" caused by direct fat inoculation by treponema pallidum. *Arch Dermatol.* 2012;148:269-270.
140. Sharquie KE, Hameed AF. Panniculitis is an important feature of cutaneous leishmaniasis pathology. *Case Rep Dermatol Med.* 2012;2012:612434.
141. Kempf W, Kazakov DV, Kutzner H. Lobular panniculitis due to *Borrelia burgdorferi* infection mimicking subcutaneous panniculitis-like T-cell lymphoma. *Am J Dermatopathol.* 2013;35:e30-e33.
142. Leber JH, Crimmins GT, Raghavan S, et al. Distinct TLR- and NLR-mediated transcriptional responses to an intracellular pathogen. *PLoS Pathog.* 2008;4:e6.
143. Combs TP, Nagajyothi, Mukherjee S, et al. The adipocyte as an important target cell for *Trypanosoma cruzi* infection. *J Biol Chem.* 2005;280:24085-24094.
144. Maurin T, Saillan-Barreau C, Cousin B, et al. Tumor necrosis factor-alpha stimulates HIV-1 production in primary culture of human adipocytes. *Exp Cell Res.* 2005;304:544-551.
145. Godard CM. Attempts to cultivate *Mycobacterium leprae* in fat tissue. *Acta Leprol.* 1993;8:133-135.
146. Pamer EG. TLR polymorphisms and the risk of invasive fungal infections. *N Engl J Med.* 2008;359:1836-1838.
147. Ballestero-Diez M, Alvarez-Ruiz SB, Aragues Montanes M, et al. Septal panniculitis associated with cytomegalovirus infection. *Histopathology.* 2005;46:720-722.
148. Stoller JK, Aboussouan LS. Alpha1-antitrypsin deficiency. *Lancet.* 2005;365:2225-2236.
149. Gross B, Grebe M, Wencker M, et al. New Findings in PiZZ alpha1-antitrypsin deficiency-related panniculitis. Demonstration of skin polymers and high dosing requirements of intravenous augmentation therapy. *Dermatology.* 2009;218:370-375.
150. Silverman EK, Sandhaus RA. Clinical practice. Alpha1-antitrypsin deficiency. *N Engl J Med.* 2009;360:2749-2757.
151. Erikkson S. Alpha1-antitrypsin deficiency: lessons learned from the bedside to the gene and back again. *Chest.* 1989;95:181-189.
152. Warter J, Storck D, Grosshans E, et al. Weber-Christian syndrome associated with an alpha-1 antitrypsin deficiency. Familial investigation [in French]. *Ann Med Interne (Paris).* 1972;123:877-882.
153. Geraminejad P, DeBloom JR 2nd, Walling HW, et al. Alpha-1-antitrypsin associated panniculitis: the MS variant. *J Am Acad Dermatol.* 2004;51:645-655.
154. Blanco I, Lipsker D, Lara B, et al. Neutrophilic panniculitis associated with alpha-1 antitrypsin deficiency: an update. *Br J Dermatol.* 2016;174(4):753-762.
155. Pittelkow MR, Smith KC, Su WP. Alpha-1-antitrypsin deficiency and panniculitis. Perspectives on disease relationship and replacement therapy. *Am J Med.* 1988;84:80-86.
156. Yesudian PD, Dobson CM, Wilson NJ. Alpha1-antitrypsin deficiency panniculitis (phenotype PiZZ) precipitated postpartum and successfully treated with dapsone. *Br J Dermatol.* 2004;150:1222-1223.
157. Chng WJ, Henderson CA. Suppurative panniculitis associated with alpha 1-antitrypsin deficiency (PiSZ phenotype) treated with doxycycline. *Br J Dermatol.* 2001;144:1282-1283.
158. Pottage JC Jr, Trenholme GM, Aronson IK, et al. Panniculitis associated with histoplasmosis and alpha 1-antitrypsin deficiency. *Am J Med.* 1983;75:150-153.
159. Smith KC, Su WP, Pittelkow MR, et al. Clinical and pathologic correlations in 96 patients with panniculitis, including 15 patients with deficient levels of alpha 1-antitrypsin. *J Am Acad Dermatol.* 1989;21:1192-1196.
160. Andersen MM. Leucocyte-associated plasma proteins. Association of prealbumin, albumin, orosomucoid, alpha 1-antitrypsin, transferrin and haptoglobin with human lymphocytes, monocytes, granulocytes and a promyelocytic leukaemic cell line (HL-60). *Scand J Clin Lab Invest.* 1983;43:49-59.
161. Breit SN, Wakefield D, Robinson JP, et al. The role of alpha 1-antitrypsin deficiency in the pathogenesis of immune disorders. *Clin Immunol Immunopathol.* 1985;35:363-380.
162. Ades EW, Hinson A, Chapuis-Cellier C, et al. Modulation of the immune response by plasma protease inhibitors. I. Alpha 2-macroglobulin and alpha 1-antitrypsin inhibit natural killing and antibody-dependent cell-mediated cytotoxicity. *Scand J Immunol.* 1982;15:109-113.
163. Olson JM, Moore EC, Valasek MA, et al. Panniculitis in alpha-1 antitrypsin deficiency treated with enzyme replacement. *J Am Acad Dermatol.* 2012;66: e139-e141.
164. Loche F, Tremeau-Martinage C, Laplanche G, et al. Panniculitis revealing qualitative alpha 1 antitrypsine deficiency (MS variant). *Eur J Dermatol.* 1999;9:565-567.
165. Laureano A, Carvalho R, Chaveiro A, et al. Alpha-1-antitrypsin deficiency-associated panniculitis: a case report. *Dermatol Online J.* 2014;20:21245.
166. Sinden NJ, Koura F, Stockley RA. The significance of the F variant of alpha-1-antitrypsin and unique case report of a PiFF homozygote. *BMC Pulm Med.* 2014;14:132.
167. Elsensohn AN, Liaqat M, Powell G, et al. Alpha-1-antitrypsin associated panniculitis and corneal ulcer with a rare allelic variant (PiFZ): a case report. *Int J Dermatol.* 2016;55(6):698-699.
168. Marzano AV, Damiani G. Neutrophilic panniculitis and autoinflammation: what's the link? *Br J Dermatol.* 2016;175(3):646-647.
169. Kobbe P, Vodovotz Y, Kaczorowski DJ, et al. The role of fracture-associated soft tissue injury in the induction of systemic inflammation and remote organ dysfunction after bilateral femur fracture. *J Orthop Trauma.* 2008;22:385-390.
170. Boden G, Silviera M, Smith B, et al. Acute tissue injury caused by subcutaneous fat biopsies produces

endoplasmic reticulum stress. *J Clin Endocrinol Metab.* 2010;95:349-352.
171. Fernandez-Torres R, Garcia-Silva J, Robles O, et al. Alfa-1-antitrypsin deficiency panniculitis acquired after liver transplant and successfully treated with retransplant. *J Am Acad Dermatol.* 2009;60:715-716.
172. Eng A, Aronson IK. Dermatopathology of panniculitis. *Semin Dermatol.* 1984;3:1-13.
173. Geller JD, Su WP. A subtle clue to the histopathologic diagnosis of early alpha 1-antitrypsin deficiency panniculitis. *J Am Acad Dermatol.* 1994;31:241-245.
174. Su WP, Smith KC, Pittelkow MR, et al. Alpha 1-antitrypsin deficiency panniculitis: a histopathologic and immunopathologic study of four cases. *Am J Dermatopathol.* 1987;9:483-490.
175. Hendrick SJ, Silverman AK, Solomon AR, et al. Alpha 1-antitrypsin deficiency associated with panniculitis. *J Am Acad Dermatol.* 1988;18:684-692.
176. Smith KC, Pittelkow MR, Su WP. Panniculitis associated with severe alpha 1-antitrypsin deficiency. Treatment and review of the literature. *Arch Dermatol.* 1987;123:1655-1661.
177. Streicher JL, Sheehan MP, Armstrong AB, et al. Cutaneous manifestation of alpha(1)-antitrypsin deficiency: panniculitis absent on biopsy. *Cutis.* 2014;93:303-306.
178. Rubinstein HM, Jaffer AM, Kudrna JC, et al. Alpha1-antitrypsin deficiency with severe panniculitis. Report of two cases. *Ann Intern Med.* 1977;86:742-744.
179. Balk E, Bronsveld W, Van der Deyl JA, et al. Alpha 1-antitrypsin deficiency with vascular leakage syndrome and panniculitis. *Neth J Med.* 1982;25:138-141.
180. Vigl K, Monshi B, Vujic I, et al. Pyoderma gangrenosum-like necrotizing panniculitis associated with alpha-1 antitrypsin deficiency: a lethal course. *J Dtsch Dermatol Ges.* 2015;13:1180-1184.
181. Ortiz PG, Skov BG, Benfeldt E. Alpha1-antitrypsin deficiency-associated panniculitis: case report and review of treatment options. *J Eur Acad Dermatol Venereol.* 2005;19:487-490.
182. Furey NL, Golden RS, Potts SR. Treatment of alpha-1-antitrypsin deficiency, massive edema, and panniculitis with alpha-1 protease inhibitor. *Ann Intern Med.* 1996;125:699.
183. Blanco I, Lara B, de Serres F. Efficacy of alpha1-antitrypsin augmentation therapy in conditions other than pulmonary emphysema. *Orphanet J Rare Dis.* 2011;6:14.
184. O'Riordan K, Blei A, Rao MS, et al. alpha 1-antitrypsin deficiency-associated panniculitis: resolution with intravenous alpha 1-antitrypsin administration and liver transplantation. *Transplantation.* 1997;63:480-482.
185. Cathomas M, Schuller A, Candinas D, et al. Severe postoperative wound healing disturbance in a patient with alpha-1-antitrypsin deficiency: the impact of augmentation therapy. *Int Wound J.* 2015;12:601-604.
186. Zheng ZJ, Gong J, Xiang GM, et al. Pancreatic panniculitis associated with acinar cell carcinoma of the pancreas: a case report. *Ann Dermatol.* 2011;23:225-228.
187. Hu JC, Gutierrez MA. Pancreatic panniculitis after endoscopic retrograde cholangiopancreatography. *J Am Acad Dermatol.* 2011;64:e72-e74.
188. Dahl PR, Su WP, Cullimore KC, et al. Pancreatic panniculitis. *J Am Acad Dermatol.* 1995;33:413-417.
189. Lopez A, Garcia-Estan J, Marras C, et al. Pancreatitis associated with pleural-mediastinal pseudocyst, panniculitis and polyarthritis. *Clin Rheumatol.* 1998;17:335-339.
190. Rongioletti F, Caputo V. Pancreatic panniculitis. *G Ital Dermatol Venereol.* 2013;148:419-425.
191. Hughes SH, Apisarnthanarax P, Mullins F. Subcutaneous fat necrosis associated with pancreatic disease. *Arch Dermatol.* 1975;111:506-510.
192. Callata-Carhuapoma HR, Pato Cour E, Garcia-Paredes B, et al. Pancreatic acinar cell carcinoma with bilateral ovarian metastases, panniculitis and polyarthritis treated with FOLFIRINOX chemotherapy regimen. A case report and review of the literature. *Pancreatology.* 2015;15:440-444.
193. Kalwaniya S, Choudhary P, Aswani Y, et al. Pancreatic panniculitis. *Indian J Dermatol Venereol Leprol.* 2015;81:282-283.
194. Cutlan RT, Wesche WA, Jenkins JJ 3rd, et al. A fatal case of pancreatic panniculitis presenting in a young patient with systemic lupus. *J Cutan Pathol.* 2000;27:466-471.
195. Langenhan R, Reimers N, Probst A. Osteomyelitis: a rare complication of pancreatitis and PPP-syndrome. *Joint Bone Spine.* 2016;83:221-224.
196. Narvaez J, Bianchi MM, Santo P, et al. Pancreatitis, panniculitis, and polyarthritis. *Semin Arthritis Rheum.* 2010;39:417-423.
197. Potts DE, Mass MF, Iseman MD. Syndrome and pancreatic disease, subcutaneous fat necrosis and polyserositis. Case report and review of literature. *Am J Med.* 1975;58:417-423.
198. Beltraminelli HS, Buechner SA, Hausermann P. Pancreatic panniculitis in a patient with an acinar cell cystadenocarcinoma of the pancreas. *Dermatology.* 2004;208:265-267.
199. Arbelaez-Cortes A, Vanegas-Garcia AL, Restrepo-Escobar M, et al. Polyarthritis and pancreatic panniculitis associated with pancreatic carcinoma: review of the literature. *J Clin Rheumatol.* 2014;20:433-436.
200. Omland SH, Ekenberg C, Henrik-Nielsen R, et al. Pancreatic panniculitis complicated by infection with *Corynebacterium tuberculostearicum*: a case report. *IDCases.* 2014;1:45-46.
201. Wilson HA, Askari AD, Neiderhiser DH, et al. Pancreatitis with arthropathy and subcutaneous fat necrosis. Evidence for the pathogenicity of lipolytic enzymes. *Arthritis Rheum.* 1983;26:121-126.
202. Berman B, Conteas C, Smith B, et al. Fatal pancreatitis presenting with subcutaneous fat necrosis. Evidence that lipase and amylase alone do not induce lipocyte necrosis. *J Am Acad Dermatol.* 1987;17:359-364.
203. Schaffler A, Landfried K, Volk M, et al. Potential of adipocytokines in predicting peripancreatic necrosis and severity in acute pancreatitis: pilot study. *J Gastroenterol Hepatol.* 2007;22:326-334.
204. Echeverria CM, Fortunato LP, Stengel FM, et al. Pancreatic panniculitis in a kidney transplant recipient. *Int J Dermatol.* 2001;40:751-753.
205. Pike JL, Rice JC, Sanchez RL, et al. Pancreatic panniculitis associated with allograft pancreatitis and rejection in a simultaneous pancreas-kidney transplant recipient. *Am J Transplant.* 2006;6:2502-2505.
206. Anders M, Gonzalez VM, Ruiz J, et al. An unreported case of pancreatic panniculitis in a liver transplant patient. *Acta Gastroenterol Latinoam.* 2014;44:239-242.
207. Abdallah M, B'Chir Hamzaoui S, Bouslama K, et al. Acute pancreatitis associated with hemophagocytic syndrome in systemic lupus erythematous: a case report [in French]. *Gastroenterol Clin Biol.* 2005;29:1054-1056.

208. Martinez-Escribano JA, Pedro F, Sabater V, et al. Acute exanthem and pancreatic panniculitis in a patient with primary HIV infection and haemophagocytic syndrome. *Br J Dermatol*. 1996;134:804-807.
209. Banfill KE, Oliphant TJ, Prasad KR. Resolution of pancreatic panniculitis following metastasectomy. *Clin Exp Dermatol*. 2012;37:440-441.
210. Kirkland EB, Sachdev R, Kim J, et al. Early pancreatic panniculitis associated with HELLP syndrome and acute fatty liver of pregnancy. *J Cutan Pathol*. 2011;38:814-817.
211. Chiewchengchol D, Wananukul S, Noppakun N. Pancreatic panniculitis caused by L-asparaginase induced acute pancreatitis in a child with acute lymphoblastic leukemia. *Pediatr Dermatol*. 2009;26:47-49.
212. Pfaundler N, Kessebohm K, Blum R, et al. Adding pancreatic panniculitis to the panel of skin lesions associated with triple therapy of chronic hepatitis C. *Liver Int*. 2013;33:648-649.
213. Ball NJ, Cowan BJ, Hashimoto SA. Lobular panniculitis at the site of subcutaneous interferon beta injections for the treatment of multiple sclerosis can histologically mimic pancreatic panniculitis. A study of 12 cases. *J Cutan Pathol*. 2009;36:331-337.
214. Weedon D. Panniculitis. In: *Weedon's Skin Pathology*. 3rd ed. London, UK: Churchill Livingstone Elsevier; 2010,460-480.
215. Hudson-Peacock MJ, Regnard CF, Farr PM. Liquefying panniculitis associated with acinous carcinoma of the pancreas responding to octreotide. *J R Soc Med*. 1994;87:361-362.
216. Francombe J, Kingsnorth AN, Tunn E. Panniculitis, arthritis and pancreatitis. *Br J Rheumatol*. 1995;34:680-683.
217. Irgang SS. Lupus erythematosus profundus: Report of an example with clinical resemblance to Darier-Roussy sarcoid. *Arch Derm Syphilol*. 1940;42:97-108.
218. Fraga J, Garcia-Diez A. Lupus erythematosus panniculitis. *Dermatol Clin*. 2008;26:453-463, vi.
219. Zhao YK, Wang F, Chen WN, et al. Lupus panniculitis as an initial manifestation of systemic lupus erythematosus: a case report. *Medicine (Baltimore)*. 2016;95:e3429.
220. Massone C, Kodama K, Salmhofer W, et al. Lupus erythematosus panniculitis (lupus profundus): clinical, histopathological, and molecular analysis of nine cases. *J Cutan Pathol*. 2005;32:396-404.
221. Martens PB, Moder KG, Ahmed I. Lupus panniculitis: clinical perspectives from a case series. *J Rheumatol*. 1999;26:68-72.
222. Nitta Y. Lupus erythematosus profundus associated with neonatal lupus erythematosus. *Br J Dermatol*. 1997;136:112-114.
223. Fernandes S, Santos S, Freitas I, et al. Linear lupus erythematosus profundus as an initial manifestation of systemic lupus erythematosus in a child. *Pediatr Dermatol*. 2014;31:378-380.
224. Arai S, Katsuoka K. Clinical entity of lupus erythematosus panniculitis/lupus erythematosus profundus. *Autoimmun Rev*. 2009;8:449-452.
225. Lee H, Kim DS, Chung KY. Adalimumab-induced lupus panniculitis. *Lupus*. 2014;23:1443-1444.
226. Urosevic-Maiwald M, Nobbe S, Kerl K, et al. Disseminated ulcerating lupus panniculitis emerging under interferon therapy of hairy cell leukemia: treatment- or disease-related? *J Dermatol*. 2014;41:329-333.
227. Magee KL, Hymes SR, Rapini RP, et al. Lupus erythematosus profundus with periorbital swelling and proptosis. *J Am Acad Dermatol*. 1991;24:288-290.
228. Tsuzaka S, Ishiguro N, Akashi R, et al. A case of lupus erythematosus profundus with multiple arc-shaped erythematous plaques on the scalp and a review of the literature. *Lupus*. 2012;21:662-665.
229. Nousari HC, Kimyai-Asadi A, Provost TT. Generalized lupus erythematosus profundus in a patient with genetic partial deficiency of C4. *J Am Acad Dermatol*. 1999;41:362-364.
230. Winkelmann RK. Panniculitis in connective tissue disease. *Arch Dermatol*. 1983;119:336-344.
231. Arai S, Katsuoka K, Eto H. An unusual form of lupus erythematosus profundus associated with antiphospholipid syndrome: report of two cases. *Acta Derm Venereol*. 2013;93:581-582.
232. Mosier AD, Boldt B, Keylock J, et al. Serial MR findings and comprehensive review of bilateral lupus mastitis with an additional case report. *J Radiol Case Rep*. 2013;7:48-58.
233. Kopp A, Buechler C, Neumeier M, et al. Innate immunity and adipocyte function: ligand-specific activation of multiple Toll-like receptors modulates cytokine, adipokine, and chemokine secretion in adipocytes. *Obesity (Silver Spring)*. 2009;17:648-656.
234. Barrat FJ, Coffman RL. Development of TLR inhibitors for the treatment of autoimmune diseases. *Immunol Rev*. 2008;223:271-283.
235. Kono DH, Haraldsson MK, Lawson BR, et al. Endosomal TLR signaling is required for anti-nucleic acid and rheumatoid factor autoantibodies in lupus. *Proc Natl Acad Sci U S A*. 2009;106:12061-12066.
236. Tao K, Fujii M, Tsukumo S, et al. Genetic variations of Toll-like receptor 9 predispose to systemic lupus erythematosus in Japanese population. *Ann Rheum Dis*. 2007;66:905-909.
237. Visentini M, Conti V, Cagliuso M, et al. Regression of systemic lupus erythematosus after development of an acquired Toll-like receptor signaling defect and antibody deficiency. *Arthritis Rheum*. 2009;60:2767-2771.
238. Lafyatis R, York M, Marshak-Rothstein A. Antimalarial agents: closing the gate on Toll-like receptors? *Arthritis Rheum*. 2006;54:3068-3070.
239. Arps DP, Patel RM. Lupus profundus (panniculitis): a potential mimic of subcutaneous panniculitis-like T-cell lymphoma. *Arch Pathol Lab Med*. 2013;137:1211-1215.
240. Papalas JA, Wang E. Clinical and histopathologic overlap between subcutaneous panniculitis-like T-cell lymphoma with systemic features and small cell CD8+ ALK+ systemic anaplastic large cell lymphoma with cutaneous involvement. *J Cutan Pathol*. 2016;43:480-481.
241. Magro CM, Crowson AN, Kovatich AJ, et al. Lupus profundus, indeterminate lymphocytic lobular panniculitis and subcutaneous T-cell lymphoma: a spectrum of subcuticular T-cell lymphoid dyscrasia. *J Cutan Pathol*. 2001;28:235-247.
242. LeBlanc RE, Tavallaee M, Kim YH, et al. Useful parameters for distinguishing subcutaneous panniculitis-like T-cell lymphoma from lupus erythematosus panniculitis. *Am J Surg Pathol*. 2016;40(6):745-754.
243. Magro CM, Crowson AN, Byrd JC, et al. Atypical lymphocytic lobular panniculitis. *J Cutan Pathol*. 2004;31:300-306.

244. Magro CM, Schaefer JT, Morrison C, et al. Atypical lymphocytic lobular panniculitis: a clonal subcutaneous T-cell dyscrasia. *J Cutan Pathol*. 2008;35:947-954.
245. Pincus LB, LeBoit PE, McCalmont TH, et al. Subcutaneous panniculitis-like T-cell lymphoma with overlapping clinicopathologic features of lupus erythematosus: coexistence of 2 entities? *Am J Dermatopathol*. 2009;31:520-526.
246. Wang CY, Su WP, Kurtin PJ. Subcutaneous panniculitic T-cell lymphoma. *Int J Dermatol*. 1996;35:1-8.
247. Willemze R, Jansen PM, Cerroni L, et al. Subcutaneous panniculitis-like T-cell lymphoma: definition, classification, and prognostic factors: an EORTC Cutaneous Lymphoma Group Study of 83 cases. *Blood*. 2008;111:838-845.
248. Aguilera P, Mascaro JM Jr, Martinez A, et al. Cutaneous gamma/delta T-cell lymphoma: a histopathologic mimicker of lupus erythematosus profundus (lupus panniculitis). *J Am Acad Dermatol*. 2007;56:643-647.
249. Wang X, Magro CM. Human myxovirus resistance protein 1 (MxA) as a useful marker in the differential diagnosis of subcutaneous lymphoma vs. lupus erythematosus profundus. *Eur J Dermatol*. 2012;22:629-633.
250. Magro CM, Wang X. CCL5 expression in panniculitic T-cell dyscrasias and its potential role in adipocyte tropism. *Am J Dermatopathol*. 2013;35:332-337.
251. Vastert SJ, Kuis W, Grom AA. Systemic JIA: new developments in the understanding of the pathophysiology and therapy. *Best Pract Res Clin Rheumatol*. 2009;23:655-664.
252. Miyashita A, Fukushima S, Makino T, et al. The proportion of lymphocytic inflammation with CD123-positive cells in lupus erythematous profundus predict a clinical response to treatment. *Acta Derm Venereol*. 2014;94:563-567.
253. Braunstein I, Werth VP. Update on management of connective tissue panniculitides. *Dermatol Ther*. 2012;25:173-182.
254. Callen JP. Management of skin disease in patients with lupus erythematosus. *Best Pract Res Clin Rheumatol*. 2002;16:245-264.
255. Chung HS, Hann SK. Lupus panniculitis treated by a combination therapy of hydroxychloroquine and quinacrine. *J Dermatol*. 1997;24:569-572.
256. Wozniacka A, Lesiak A, Boncela J, et al. The influence of antimalarial treatment on IL-1beta, IL-6 and TNF-alpha mRNA expression on UVB-irradiated skin in systemic lupus erythematosus. *Br J Dermatol*. 2008;159:1124-1130.
257. Jewell ML, McCauliffe DP. Patients with cutaneous lupus erythematosus who smoke are less responsive to antimalarial treatment. *J Am Acad Dermatol*. 2000;42:983-987.
258. Kreuter A, Gaifullina R, Tigges C, et al. Lupus erythematosus tumidus: response to antimalarial treatment in 36 patients with emphasis on smoking. *Arch Dermatol*. 2009;145:244-248.
259. Ujiie H, Shimizu T, Ito M, et al. Lupus erythematosus profundus successfully treated with dapsone: review of the literature. *Arch Dermatol*. 2006;142:399-401.
260. Hansen CB, Callen JP. Connective tissue panniculitis: lupus panniculitis, dermatomyositis, morphea/scleroderma. *Dermatol Ther*. 2010;23:341-349.
261. Ishiguro N, Iwasaki T, Kawashima M, et al. Intractable ulceration in a patient with lupus erythematosus profundus successfully treated with cyclosporine. *Int J Dermatol*. 2012;51:1131-1133.
262. Espirito Santo J, Gomes MF, Gomes MJ, et al. Intravenous immunoglobulin in lupus panniculitis. *Clin Rev Allergy Immunol*. 2010;38:307-318.
263. Ueda T, Eto H, Katsuoka K, et al. Lupus erythematosus panniculitis treated with tacrolimus. *Eur J Dermatol*. 2012;22:260-261.
264. Moreno-Suarez F, Pulpillo-Ruiz A. Rituximab for the treatment of lupus erythematosus panniculitis. *Dermatol Ther*. 2013;26:415-418.
265. Gunther C, Aringer M, Lochno M, et al. TNF-alpha blockade with infliximab in a patient with lupus erythematosus profundus. *Acta Derm Venereol*. 2012;92:401-403.
266. Morgan KW, Callen JP. Calcifying lupus panniculitis in a patient with subacute cutaneous lupus erythematosus: response to diltiazem and chloroquine. *J Rheumatol*. 2001;28:2129-2132.
267. Alegre VA, Winkelmann RK. Histiocytic cytophagic panniculitis. *J Am Acad Dermatol*. 1989;20:177-185.
268. Craig AJ, Cualing H, Thomas G, et al. Cytophagic histiocytic panniculitis—a syndrome associated with benign and malignant panniculitis: case comparison and review of the literature. *J Am Acad Dermatol*. 1998;39:721-736.
269. Crotty CP, Winkelmann RK. Cytophagic histiocytic panniculitis with fever, cytopenia, liver failure, and terminal hemorrhagic diathesis. *J Am Acad Dermatol*. 1981;4:181-194.
270. Wick MR, Patterson JW. Cytophagic histiocytic panniculitis—a critical reappraisal. *Arch Dermatol*. 2000;136:922-924.
271. Winkelmann RK, Bowie EJ. Hemorrhagic diathesis associated with benign histiocytic, cytophagic panniculitis and systemic histiocytosis. *Arch Intern Med*. 1980;140:1460-1463.
272. Chen RL, Hsu YH, Ueda I, et al. Cytophagic histiocytic panniculitis with fatal haemophagocytic lymphohistiocytosis in a paediatric patient with perforin gene mutation. *J Clin Pathol*. 2007;60:1168-1169.
273. Krilis M, Miyakis S. Cytophagic histiocytic panniculitis with haemophagocytosis in a patient with familial multiple lipomatosis and review of the literature. *Mod Rheumatol*. 2012;22:158-162.
274. Aronson IK, West DP, Variakojis D, et al. Fatal panniculitis. *J Am Acad Dermatol*. 1985;12:535-551.
275. Aronson IK, Worobec SM. Cytophagic histiocytic panniculitis and hemophagocytic lymphohistiocytosis: an overview. *Dermatol Ther*. 2010;23:389-402.
276. Hasegawa H, Mizoguchi F, Kohsaka H, et al. Systemic lupus erythematosus with cytophagic histiocytic panniculitis successfully treated with high-dose glucocorticoids and cyclosporine A. *Lupus*. 2013;22:316-319.
277. Marzano AV, Berti E, Paulli M, et al. Cytophagic histiocytic panniculitis and subcutaneous panniculitis-like T-cell lymphoma: report of 7 cases. *Arch Dermatol*. 2000;136:889-896.
278. Schaer DJ, Schleiffenbaum B, Kurrer M, et al. Soluble hemoglobin-haptoglobin scavenger receptor CD163 as a lineage-specific marker in the reactive hemophagocytic syndrome. *Eur J Haematol*. 2005;74:6-10.
279. Ostrov BE, Athreya BH, Eichenfield AH, et al. Successful treatment of severe cytophagic histiocytic panniculitis with cyclosporine A. *Semin Arthritis Rheum*. 1996;25:404-413.
280. Pasqualini C, Jorini M, Carloni I, et al. Cytophagic histiocytic panniculitis, hemophagocytic

lymphohistiocytosis and undetermined autoimmune disorder: reconciling the puzzle. *Ital J Pediatr*. 2014;40:17.
281. Coman T, Dalloz MA, Coolen N, et al. Plasmapheresis for the treatment of acute pancreatitis induced by hemophagocytic syndrome related to hypertriglyceridemia. *J Clin Apher*. 2003;18:129-131.
282. Tengku-Muhammad TS, Hughes TR, Cryer A, et al. Differential regulation of lipoprotein lipase in the macrophage J774.2 cell line by cytokines. *Cytokine*. 1996;8:525-533.
283. Risdall RJ, McKenna RW, Nesbit ME, et al. Virus-associated hemophagocytic syndrome: a benign histiocytic proliferation distinct from malignant histiocytosis. *Cancer*. 1979;44:993-1002.
284. Janka G, Imashuku S, Elinder G, et al. Infection- and malignancy-associated hemophagocytic syndromes. Secondary hemophagocytic lymphohistiocytosis. *Hematol Oncol Clin North Am*. 1998;12:435-444.
285. Tristano AG. Macrophage activation syndrome: a frequent but under-diagnosed complication associated with rheumatic diseases. *Med Sci Monit*. 2008;14:Ra27-Ra36.
286. Filipovich AH. Hemophagocytic lymphohistiocytosis and other hemophagocytic disorders. *Immunol Allergy Clin North Am*. 2008;28:293-313, viii.
287. Pauwels C, Livideanu CB, Maza A, et al. Cytophagic histiocytic panniculitis after H1N1 vaccination: a case report and review of the cutaneous side effects of influenza vaccines. *Dermatology*. 2011;222:217-220.
288. Merelli M, Quartuccio L, Bassetti M, et al. Efficacy of intravenous cyclosporine in a case of cytophagic histiocytic panniculitis complicated by haemophagocytic syndrome after visceral leishmania infection. *Clin Exp Rheumatol*. 2015;33:906-909.
289. Masters SL, Simon A, Aksentijevich I, et al. Horror autoinflammaticus: the molecular pathophysiology of autoinflammatory disease (*). *Annu Rev Immunol*. 2009;27:621-668.
290. Badolato R, Parolini S. Novel insights from adaptor protein 3 complex deficiency. *J Allergy Clin Immunol*. 2007;120:735-741; quiz 742-743.
291. Rastogi V, Sharma A, Misra SR, et al. Emperipolesis—a review. *J Clin Diagn Res*. 2014;8:Zm01-Zm02.
292. White JW Jr, Winkelmann RK. Cytophagic histiocytic panniculitis is not always fatal. *J Cutan Pathol*. 1989;16:137-144.
293. Guitart J, Sethi R, Gordon K. Fatal cytophagic histiocytic panniculitis after a short response to cyclosporine. *J Eur Acad Dermatol Venereol*. 1998;10:267-268.
294. Rouphael NG, Talati NJ, Vaughan C, et al. Infections associated with haemophagocytic syndrome. *Lancet Infect Dis*. 2007;7:814-822.
295. Miyabe Y, Murata Y, Baba Y, et al. Successful treatment of cyclosporine-A-resistant cytophagic histiocytic panniculitis with tacrolimus. *Mod Rheumatol*. 2011;21:553-556.
296. Rios Fernandez R, Callejas Rubio JL, Sanchez Cano D, et al. Long-term evolution of cytophagic histiocytic panniculitis. *J Cutan Med Surg*. 2010;14:136-140.
297. Mori Y, Sugiyama T, Chiba R, et al. A case of systemic lupus erythematosus with hemophagocytic syndrome and cytophagic histiocytic panniculitis [in Japanese]. *Ryumachi*. 2001;41:31-36.
298. Matsue K, Itoh M, Tsukuda K, et al. Successful treatment of cytophagic histiocytic panniculitis with modified CHOP-E. Cyclophosphamide, adriamycin, vincristine, predonisone, and etoposide. *Am J Clin Oncol*. 1994;17:470-474.
299. Koizumi K, Sawada K, Nishio M, et al. Effective high-dose chemotherapy followed by autologous peripheral blood stem cell transplantation in a patient with the aggressive form of cytophagic histiocytic panniculitis. *Bone Marrow Transplant*. 1997;20:171-173.
300. Bader-Meunier B, Fraitag S, Janssen C, et al. Clonal cytophagic histiocytic panniculitis in children may be cured by cyclosporine A. *Pediatrics*. 2013;132:e545-e549.
301. Behrens EM, Kreiger PA, Cherian S, et al. Interleukin 1 receptor antagonist to treat cytophagic histiocytic panniculitis with secondary hemophagocytic lymphohistiocytosis. *J Rheumatol*. 2006;33:2081-2084.
302. Tran JT, Sheth AP. Complications of subcutaneous fat necrosis of the newborn: a case report and review of the literature. *Pediatr Dermatol*. 2003;20:257-261.
303. Torrelo A, Hernandez A. Panniculitis in children. *Dermatol Clin*. 2008;26:491-500, vii.
304. Mahe E, Girszyn N, Hadj-Rabia S, et al. Subcutaneous fat necrosis of the newborn: a systematic evaluation of risk factors, clinical manifestations, complications and outcome of 16 children. *Br J Dermatol*. 2007;156:709-715.
305. Mitra S, Dove J, Somisetty SK. Subcutaneous fat necrosis in newborn—an unusual case and review of literature. *Eur J Pediatr*. 2011;170:1107-1110.
306. Thomas JM, Bhandari J, Rytina E, et al. Subcutaneous fat necrosis of the neonate with a delayed second eruption. *Pediatr Dermatol*. 2016;33:e134-e136.
307. Burden AD, Krafchik BR. Subcutaneous fat necrosis of the newborn: a review of 11 cases. *Pediatr Dermatol*. 1999;16:384-387.
308. Carraccio C, Papadimitriou J, Feinberg P. Subcutaneous fat necrosis of the newborn: link to maternal use of cocaine during pregnancy. *Clin Pediatr (Phila)*. 1994;33:317-318.
309. Courteau C, Samman K, Ali N, et al. Macrosomia and hemodynamic instability may represent risk factors for subcutaneous fat necrosis in asphyxiated newborns treated with hypothermia. *Acta Paediatr*. 2016;105(9):e396-e405.
310. Vasireddy S, Long SD, Sacheti B, et al. MRI and US findings of subcutaneous fat necrosis of the newborn. *Pediatr Radiol*. 2009;39:73-76.
311. Norwood-Galloway A, Lebwohl M, Phelps RG, et al. Subcutaneous fat necrosis of the newborn with hypercalcemia. *J Am Acad Dermatol*. 1987;16:435-439.
312. Balfour E, Antaya RJ, Lazova R. Subcutaneous fat necrosis of the newborn presenting as a large plaque with lobulated cystic areas. *Cutis*. 2002;70:169-173.
313. Haider S. Images in paediatrics: subcutaneous fat necrosis causing radial nerve palsy. *BMJ Case Rep*. 2012;2012.
314. Shumer DE, Thaker V, Taylor GA, et al. Severe hypercalcaemia due to subcutaneous fat necrosis: presentation, management and complications. *Arch Dis Child Fetal Neonatal Ed*. 2014;99:F419-F421.
315. Varan B, Gurakan B, Ozbek N, et al. Subcutaneous fat necrosis of the newborn associated with anemia. *Pediatr Dermatol*. 1999;16:381-383.
316. Hakan N, Aydin M, Zenciroglu A, et al. Is therapeutic hypothermia real cause of subcutaneous fat necrosis in newborns? *Indian J Pediatr*. 2013;80:355.
317. Akin MA, Akin L, Coban D, et al. Post-operative subcutaneous fat necrosis in a newborn: a case report. *Fetal Pediatr Pathol*. 2011;30:363-369.

318. Silverman AK, Michels EH, Rasmussen JE. Subcutaneous fat necrosis in an infant, occurring after hypothermic cardiac surgery. Case report and analysis of etiologic factors. *J Am Acad Dermatol*. 1986;15:331-336.
319. Farooque A, Moss C, Zehnder D, et al. Expression of 25-hydroxyvitamin D3-1alpha-hydroxylase in subcutaneous fat necrosis. *Br J Dermatol*. 2009;160:423-425.
320. Heaton JM. The distribution of brown adipose tissue in the human. *J Anat*. 1972;112:35-39.
321. Ichimiya H, Arakawa S, Sato T, et al. Involvement of brown adipose tissue in subcutaneous fat necrosis of the newborn. *Dermatology*. 2011;223:207-210.
322. de Meis L, Ketzer LA, da Costa RM, et al. Fusion of the endoplasmic reticulum and mitochondrial outer membrane in rats brown adipose tissue: activation of thermogenesis by Ca2+. *PLoS One*. 2010;5:e9439.
323. Tajirian A, Ross R, Zeikus P, et al. Subcutaneous fat necrosis of the newborn with eosinophilic granules. *J Cutan Pathol*. 2007;34:588-590.
324. Ricardo-Gonzalez RR, Lin JR, Mathes EF, et al. Neutrophil-rich subcutaneous fat necrosis of the newborn: A potential mimic of infection. *J Am Acad Dermatol*. 2016;75(1):177-185.e17.
325. Schubert PT, Razack R, Vermaak A, et al. Fine-needle aspiration cytology of subcutaneous fat necrosis of the newborn: the cytology spectrum with review of the literature. *Diagn Cytopathol*. 2012;40:245-247.
326. Schubert PT, Razak R, Jordaan HF. Fine-needle aspiration as a method of diagnosis of subcutaneous fat necrosis of the newborn. *Pediatr Dermatol*. 2016;33:e220-e221.
327. Tognetti L, Filippou G, Bertrando S, et al. Subcutaneous fat necrosis in a newborn after brief therapeutic hypothermia: ultrasonographic examination. *Pediatr Dermatol*. 2015;32:427-429.
328. Fretzin DF, Arias AM. Sclerema neonatorum and subcutaneous fat necrosis of the newborn. *Pediatr Dermatol*. 1987;4:112-122.
329. Gomes C, Lobo L, Azevedo AS, et al. Nephrocalcinosis and subcutaneous fat necrosis [in Portuguese]. *Acta Med Port*. 2015;28:119-122.
330. Beuzeboc Gerard M, Aillet S, Bertheuil N, et al. Surgical management of subcutaneous fat necrosis of the newborn required due to a lack of improvement: a very rare case. *Br J Dermatol*. 2014;171:183-185.
331. Hakan N, Aydin M, Zenciroglu A, et al. Alendronate for the treatment of hypercalcaemia due to neonatal subcutaneous fat necrosis. *Eur J Pediatr*. 2011;170:1085-1086; author reply 1087.
332. Perez Martinez E, Camprubi Camprubi M, Ramos Cebrian M, et al. Treatment with bisphosphonates in severe hypercalcemia due to subcutaneous fat necrosis in an infant with hypoxic-ischemic encephalopathy. *J Perinatol*. 2014;34:492-493.
333. Samedi VM, Yusuf K, Yee W, et al. Neonatal hypercalcemia secondary to subcutaneous fat necrosis successfully treated with pamidronate: a case series and literature review. *AJP Rep*. 2014;4:e93-e96.
334. Lombet J. Commentary on "Pamidronate: treatment for severe hypercalcemia in neonatal subcutaneous fat necrosis" by Alos N, et al. *Hormone Research* 2006;65:289-294. *Horm Res*. 2008;70:254-255; author reply 256.
335. Filippi L, Catarzi S, Padrini L, et al. Strategies for reducing the incidence of skin complications in newborns treated with whole-body hypothermia. *J Matern Fetal Neonatal Med*. 2012;25:2115-2121.
336. Bolotin D, Duffy KL, Petronic-Rosic V, et al. Cold panniculitis following ice therapy for cardiac arrhythmia. *Pediatr Dermatol*. 2011;28:192-194.
337. Quesada-Cortes A, Campos-Munoz L, Diaz-Diaz RM, et al. Cold panniculitis. *Dermatol Clin*. 2008;26: 485-489, vii.
338. Pekki A, Sauni R, Vaalasti A, et al. Cold panniculitis in Finnish horse riders. *Acta Derm Venereol*. 2011;91:463-464.
339. Epstein EH Jr, Oren ME. Popsicle panniculitis. *N Engl J Med*. 1970;282:966-967.
340. Bournas VG, Eilbert W. Infant with facial lesions. Cold panniculitis. *Ann Emerg Med*. 2011;58:216-221.
341. Patel AR, Husain S, Lauren CT, et al. Circular erythematous patch in a febrile infant. Cold panniculitis. *Pediatr Dermatol*. 2012;29:659-660.
342. Harkness G, Meikle G, Craw S, et al. Ultrasound appearance of scrotal fat necrosis in prepubertal boys. *Pediatr Radiol*. 2007;37:370-373.
343. Ferrara G, Cerroni L. Cold-associated perniosis of the thighs ("equestrian-type") chilblain): a reappraisal based on a clinicopathologic and immunohistochemical study of 6 cases. *Am J Dermatopathol*. 2016;38(10):726-731.
344. Price RD, Murdoch DR. Perniosis (chilblains) of the thigh: report of five cases, including four following river crossings. *High Alt Med Biol*. 2001;2:535-538.
345. Tlougan BE, Mancini AJ, Mandell JA, et al. Skin conditions in figure skaters, ice-hockey players and speed skaters: part II-cold-induced, infectious and inflammatory dermatoses. *Sports Med*. 2011;41:967-984.
346. West SE, McCalmont TH, North JP. Ice-pack dermatosis: a cold-induced dermatitis with similarities to cold panniculitis and perniosis that histopathologically resembles lupus. *JAMA Dermatol*. 2013;149:1314-1318.
347. Gesta S, Tseng YH, Kahn CR. Developmental origin of fat: tracking obesity to its source. *Cell*. 2007;131:242-256.
348. Fredriksson JM, Nikami H, Nedergaard J. Cold-induced expression of the VEGF gene in brown adipose tissue is independent of thermogenic oxygen consumption. *FEBS Lett*. 2005;579:5680-5684.
349. Gasparetti AL, de Souza CT, Pereira-da-Silva M, et al. Cold exposure induces tissue-specific modulation of the insulin-signalling pathway in Rattus norvegicus. *J Physiol*. 2003;552:149-162.
350. Justrabo E, Martin L, Athias A, et al. Bilateral scrotal panniculitis in a prepubescent child [in French]. *Arch Anat Cytol Pathol*. 1998;46:208-212.
351. De Silva BD, McLaren K, Doherty VR. Equestrian perniosis associated with cold agglutinins: a novel finding. *Clin Exp Dermatol*. 2000;25:285-288.
352. Ter Poorten JC, Hebert AA, Ilkiw R. Cold panniculitis in a neonate. *J Am Acad Dermatol*. 1995;33:383-385.
353. Boyd AS. Revision: cutaneous Munchausen syndrome: clinical and histopathologic features. *J Cutan Pathol*. 2014;41:333-336.
354. Grassi S, Rosso R, Tomasini C, et al. Post-surgical lipophagic panniculitis: a specific model of traumatic panniculitis and new histopathological findings. *G Ital Dermatol Venereol*. 2013;148:435-441.
355. Shellagi N, Rodrigues G. Traumatic panniculitis of the right thigh: a case report. *Oman Med J*. 2011;26:436-437.
356. Sanmartin O, Requena C, Requena L. Factitial panniculitis. *Dermatol Clin*. 2008;26:519-527, viii.
357. Lee JS, Ahn SK, Lee SH. Factitial panniculitis induced by cupping and acupuncture. *Cutis*. 1995;55:217-218.

358. Jeong KH, Lee MH. Two cases of factitial panniculitis induced by electroacupuncture. *Clin Exp Dermatol.* 2009;34:e170-e173.
359. Lee JH, Jung KE, Kim HS, et al. Traumatic panniculitis with localized hypertrichosis: two new cases and considerations. *J Dermatol.* 2013;40:139-141.
360. Oh CC, Tan KB, Thirumoorthy T, et al. Traumatic panniculitis in a Chinese woman. *Skinmed.* 2014;12:127-128.
361. Moreno A, Marcoval J, Peyri J. Traumatic panniculitis. *Dermatol Clin.* 2008;26:481-483, vii.
362. Weedon D. Traumatic fat necrosis. In: *Skin Pathology.* 2nd ed. London, UK: Churchill Livingstone; 2002, 349-368.
363. Chairatchaneeboon M, Kulthanan K, Manapajon A. Calcific panniculitis and nasopharyngeal cancer-associated adult-onset dermatomyositis: a case report and literature review. *Springerplus.* 2015;4:201.
364. Solans R, Cortes J, Selva A, et al. Panniculitis: a cutaneous manifestation of dermatomyositis. *J Am Acad Dermatol.* 2002;46:S148-S150.
365. Hemmi S, Kushida R, Nishimura H, et al. Magnetic resonance imaging diagnosis of panniculitis in dermatomyositis. *Muscle Nerve.* 2010;41:151-153.
366. Neidenbach PJ, Sahn EE, Helton J. Panniculitis in juvenile dermatomyositis. *J Am Acad Dermatol.* 1995;33:305-307.
367. Salman A, Kasapcopur O, Ergun T, et al. Panniculitis in juvenile dermatomyositis: Report of a case and review of the published work. *J Dermatol.* 2016;43(8):951-953.
368. Otero Rivas MM, Vicente Villa A, Gonzalez Lara L, et al. Panniculitis in juvenile dermatomyositis. *Clin Exp Dermatol.* 2015;40:574-575.
369. Chiu HY, He GY, Chen JS, et al. Subcutaneous panniculitis-like T-cell lymphoma presenting with clinicopathologic features of dermatomyositis. *J Am Acad Dermatol.* 2011;64:e121-e123.
370. Girouard SD, Velez NF, Penson RT, et al. Panniculitis associated with dermatomyositis and recurrent ovarian cancer. *Arch Dermatol.* 2012;148:740-744.
371. Douvoyiannis M, Litman N, Dulau A, et al. Panniculitis, infection, and dermatomyositis: case and literature review. *Clin Rheumatol.* 2009;28(suppl 1):S57-S63.
372. Winkelman WJ, Billick RC, Srolovitz H. Dermatomyositis presenting as panniculitis. *J Am Acad Dermatol.* 1990;23:127-128.
373. Penate Y, Guillermo N, Melwani P, et al. Calcinosis cutis associated with amyopathic dermatomyositis: response to intravenous immunoglobulin. *J Am Acad Dermatol.* 2009;60:1076-1077.
374. Snider AA, Barsky S. Gouty panniculitis: a case report and review of the literature. *Cutis.* 2005;76:54-56.
375. Choi CM, Lew BL, Lee SH, et al. Gouty panniculitis also involving the bone marrow. *Acta Derm Venereol.* 2013;93:189-190.
376. Pattanaprichakul P, Bunyaratavej S, McLain PM, et al. Disseminated gouty panniculitis: an unusual presentation of extensive cutaneous tophi. *Dermatol Pract Concept.* 2014;4:33-35.
377. Wang L, Rose C, Mellen P, et al. Gouty panniculitis with ulcerations in a patient with multiple organ dysfunctions. *Case Rep Rheumatol.* 2014;2014:320940.
378. Gaviria JL, Ortega VG, Gaona J, et al. Unusual dermatological manifestations of gout: review of literature and a case report. *Plast Reconstr Surg Glob Open.* 2015;3:e445.
379. Ochoa CD, Valderrama V, Mejia J, et al. Panniculitis: another clinical expression of gout. *Rheumatol Int.* 2011;31:831-835.
380. Penaranda-Parada E, Bejarano NS, Mejia J, et al. Gouty arthritis and panniculitis: extensive involvement of the dermis and severe joint damage. *J Clin Rheumatol.* 2012;18:142-143.
381. Sacchidanand SA, Kanathur S, Somaiah S, et al. Poststeroid panniculitis: a rare case report. *Indian Dermatol Online J.* 2013;4:318-320.
382. de-Andres-del-Rosario A, Verea-Hernando MM, Yebra-Pimentel MT, et al. Poststeroid panniculitis in an adult. *Am J Dermatopathol.* 2011;33:e77-e80.
383. Kim ST, Kim TK, Lee JW, et al. Post-steroid panniculitis in an adult. *J Dermatol.* 2008;35:786-788.

Chapter 74 :: Lipodystrophy
:: Abhimanyu Garg

第七十四章
脂肪营养不良

中文导读

脂肪营养不良是一组以脂肪组织的选择性缺失为特征的异质性疾病，可分为遗传性和获得性。本章从流行病学、不同类型脂肪营养不良的临床特征和发病机制、诊断和鉴别诊断、临床过程和预后及治疗等方面对该组疾病进行了详细介绍。

1. 流行病学　脂肪营养不良是罕见病，本章对不同类型的脂肪营养不良的发病情况进行了介绍。

2. 遗传性脂肪营养不良　近十年来，在遗传性脂肪营养不良的分子基础方面取得了相当大的进展。

（1）先天性全身脂肪营养不良（BERARDINELLI-SEIP综合症）临床特征：在出生时或出生后不久出现身体脂肪几乎完全缺乏。患者还伴有明显的肌肉丰富、皮下静脉突出、肢端肥大症、黑棘皮病、肝肿大和脐突出(图74-1A，表74-2)。本章还介绍了该病可能合并的疾病，以及男女性患者性腺和生殖有关的异常。病因和发病机制：利用定位克隆策略和候选基因方法进行全基因组连锁分析，已确定常染色体隐性先天性全身脂肪营养不良（CGL）的四个基因位点即AGPAT2，BSCL2，CAV1和CAVIN1。详细介绍了这几个基因的功能及突变后的功能变化。

（2）家族性部分脂肪营养不良临床特征：四肢脂肪缺失程度与躯干不同，非脂肪营养不良区域皮下脂肪沉积增加(见图74-1B)。大多数FPL患者为lamin A/C (LMNA)基因的杂合突变的Dunnigan变异型。这些患者在儿童早期有正常的体脂分布，但在青春期前后，四肢和躯干的皮下脂肪逐渐丢失(见图74-1B)。PPARG基因杂合突变导致的FPL患者，也有来自四肢特别是四肢远端的脂肪损失，但面部、颈部和躯干区域的脂肪无影响。同时对FPL存在的其他突变也作了简单描述。病因和发病机制：常染色体显性家族性部分脂肪营养不良（FPL）的五个基因位点即LMNA，PPARG，AKT2，PLIN1和ADRA2A。详细介绍了这几个基因的功能及突变后的功能变化。

（3）下颌末端发育不良相关的脂肪营养不良临床特征：MAD患者具有典型的骨骼异常，包括下颌骨和锁骨发育不全、牙髓溶解、皮肤萎缩、类早衰特征如尖嘴鼻/脱发/皮肤薄伴浅表血管显露和点状色素沉着、出牙延迟，以及颅骨闭合、关节僵硬和脂肪营养不良。病因和发病机制：染色体1p34上的LMNA和锌金属蛋白酶(ZMP-STE24)突变可引起常染色体隐性MAD相关的脂肪营养不良。

（4）其他类型临床特征：本章介绍了一种新的综合征，表现为下颌发育不全、耳聋及早衰特征相关的脂肪营养不良，并介绍了CANDLE综合症(伴有脂肪营养不良和体温升高的慢性非典型中性粒细胞性皮肤病）、JMP综合征及其他罕见的脂肪营养不良综合征如常染色体隐性FPL和SHORT（身材矮小、过度伸展或腹股沟疝、眼部凹陷、Rieger异常和出牙延迟）综合征及新生儿早老综合征（Wiedemann-Rautenstrauch）。病因和发病机制：本章对上述疾病的基因突变位点进行了详细介绍，但也指出还有许多其他遗传性脂肪营养不良综合征的分子遗传学机制仍不清楚(见表74-1)

3. 获得性脂肪营养不良

（1）获得性部分脂肪营养不良（BARRAQUER-SIMONS综合症）临床特征：大多数获得性部分脂肪营养不良在患者15岁之前就开始出现，表现为面部、颈部、上肢和躯干脂肪减少，腹部和下肢保留SQ脂肪（见图74-1C）。接着作者对该病可能出现的肾病并发症进行了介绍。病因和发病机制：SQ脂肪丢失的确切发病机制仍不清楚，但由自身免疫所介导的证据较充分。

（2）获得性全身脂肪营养不良(LAWRENCE综合征)临床特征：获得性全身脂肪营养不良通常在儿童时期表现为不同程度的SQ脂肪减少，往往会发展为严重的难治性肝脂肪变性和纤维化、糖尿病和高甘油三酯血症。病因和发病机制：确切机制尚不清楚，作者指出可能与脂膜炎或自身免疫介导有关，部分为特发性。

（3）HIV感染患者高活性抗逆转录病毒治疗诱发的脂肪营养不良临床特征：艾滋病毒感染者在接受含有蛋白酶抑制剂的高活性抗逆转录病毒治疗2年或更长时间后，面部、躯干和四肢的SQ脂肪减少(见图74-1E、74-3A和74-3B)。有些人还伴有水牛背、双下巴及腹部脂肪增加。病因和发病机制：蛋白酶抑制药引起HIV感染患者的脂肪营养不良可能通过抑制ZMPSTE24，导致prelamin A的聚集有关。

（4）局限性脂肪营养不良临床特征：局部的脂肪营养不良表现为局部区域的SQ脂肪减少导致组织凹陷。病因和发病机制：可能与各种药物的SQ注射、脂膜炎、压力及其他机制有关。

4. 诊断　患有糖尿病、高甘油三酯血症、肝脂肪变性、黑棘皮病和多囊卵巢综合征的"苗条或不胖"的患者应高度怀疑脂肪营养不良。对于童年时期出现全身性脂肪营养不良的人，根据出生时脂肪减少的证据来判断遗传性或获得性。本章从患者的病史、皮肤表现、合并疾病、实验室检查和特殊检查详细阐述了该病的诊断要点。

5. 鉴别诊断　全身性脂肪营养不良最重要的鉴别诊断是严重的体重下降。本章列出了部分脂肪营养不良及综合征相关脂肪营养不良的鉴别诊断。

6. 临床过程和预后　预后不好主要与合并症相关，本章对导致不同类型脂肪营养预后不良的合并症及致死原因进行了详细阐述。

7. 治疗　目前尚无逆转体内脂肪丢失的治疗方法。治疗的主要手段包括美容手术和面部整容。一般治疗建议包括低脂饮食，除心肌病患者，应鼓励运动以减轻胰岛素抵抗及其并发症。对脂肪营养不良所合并的代谢并发症，本章也提出了治疗建议并介绍了治疗进展。

〔黄莹雪〕

AT-A-GLANCE

- Lipodystrophies are genetic or acquired disorders characterized by selective loss of body fat. The extent of fat loss determines the severity of associated metabolic complications such as diabetes mellitus, hypertriglyceridemia, hepatic steatosis, and acanthosis nigricans.

- Four loci have been identified for the autosomal recessive congenital generalized lipodystrophy (CGL), namely, *AGPAT2*, *BSCL2*, *CAV1*, and *CAVIN1*.

- Five loci have been identified for autosomal dominant familial partial lipodystrophy (FPL), namely, *LMNA*, *PPARG*, *AKT2*, *PLIN1*, and *ADRA2A*.

- *LIPE*, *CIDEC*, *PCYT1A*, and *RECQL2* are loci for autosomal recessive FPL, and *LMNA* and *ZMPSTE24* are loci for mandibuloacral dysplasia-associated lipodystrophy.

- Molecular basis of many extremely rare forms of genetic lipodystrophies remains to be elucidated.

- The most prevalent variety of lipodystrophy develops after prolonged duration of protease inhibitor containing highly active antiretroviral therapy in HIV-infected patients.

- The acquired generalized lipodystrophy and acquired partial lipodystrophy are mainly autoimmune in origin.

- Localized lipodystrophies occur as a result of drug or vaccine injections, pressure, and panniculitis, as well as other unknown reasons.

- Current management includes cosmetic surgery and early identification and treatment of metabolic and other complications.

- Metreleptin replacement therapy is beneficial for treating metabolic complications in hypoleptinemic patients with generalized lipodystrophies.

Lipodystrophies are a heterogeneous group of disorders characterized by selective loss of adipose tissue.[1,2] The extent of fat loss varies, with some patients losing fat from small areas (localized lipodystrophy), and others having more extensive fat loss, for example, involving the extremities (partial lipodystrophy) or the entire body (generalized lipodystrophy). Depending upon the extent of fat loss, patients may be predisposed to develop complications associated with insulin resistance such as diabetes mellitus, dyslipidemia, hepatic steatosis, acanthosis nigricans, polycystic ovarian disease, and coronary heart disease.[3-5] There are 2 main types of lipodystrophies: genetic and acquired. Table 74-1 provides a detailed classification of various types of lipodystrophies.

EPIDEMIOLOGY

Although the genetic lipodystrophies are rare, recent advances, such as improved definition of the phenotypes and elucidation of the molecular defects, have led to increased recognition of these syndromes. Overall, based on literature reports of approximately 1200 patients, the estimated prevalence of genetic lipodystrophies may be less than 1 in a million. Affected females are recognized easily and thus are reported more often than males.

The autosomal-recessive congenital generalized lipodystrophy (CGL) has been reported in approximately 500 patients, with clustering of patients reported in Lebanon and Brazil, where there is increased prevalence of consanguinity. Recently, prevalence of CGL was reported to be approximately 1 in 2 million general population in Turkey.[6] The autosomal-dominant familial partial lipodystrophy (FPL) of the Dunnigan variety is the most common with approximately 500 patients being reported; and FPL caused by *PPARG* mutations has been reported in approximately 40 patients. As a result of founder mutations, FPL Dunnigan type prevalence has been estimated to be as high as 1:200,000 general population from the Canadian province of Ontario[7] and approximately 1:20,000 of the general population of the Reunion Island located in the Indian Ocean.[8] The autosomal-recessive mandibuloacral dysplasia (MAD) that is caused by *LMNA* mutations has been reported in approximately 30 patients; MAD caused by *ZMPSTE24* mutations has been reported in 15 patients.

Acquired partial lipodystrophy was recognized approximately 125 years ago and only approximately 250 to 300 cases of various ethnicities with a male-to-female ratio of 1:4 have been reported.[9] Acquired generalized lipodystrophy has been reported in fewer than 100 cases, mostly in whites with a male-to-female ratio of 1:3.[10] The most common type at present is highly active antiretroviral therapy (containing protease inhibitors [PIs])-induced lipodystrophy in HIV-infected patients, which is estimated to be affecting more than 100,000 patients in the United States and many more in other countries.[1,11,12]

GENETIC LIPODYSTROPHIES

In the last decade or so, considerable progress has been made in elucidation of the molecular basis of many types of genetic lipodystrophies. In general, mutations

TABLE 74-1
Classification of Lipodystrophies

Genetic Lipodystrophies
1. Autosomal recessive, congenital generalized lipodystrophy (CGL)
   a. Type 1: *AGPAT2* mutations
   b. Type 2: *BSCL2* mutations
   c. Type 3: *CAV1* mutation
   d. Type 4: *CAVIN1* mutations
   e. Others
2. Autosomal dominant, familial partial lipodystrophy (FPL)
   a. Dunnigan variety: *LMNA* mutations
   b. *PPARG* mutations
   c. *AKT2* mutation
   d. *PLIN1* mutations
   e. *ADRA2A* (adrenoceptor α_{2A}) mutation
   f. Others
3. Autosomal recessive, familial partial lipodystrophy (FPL)
   a. *CIDEC* mutation
   b. *LIPE* mutations
   c. *PCYT1A* mutations
   d. *RECQL2* mutations
4. Autosomal recessive, mandibuloacral dysplasia (MAD)–associated lipodystrophy
   a. *LMNA* mutations
   b. *ZMPSTE24* mutations
   c. Others
5. Other lipodystrophies associated with *LMNA* mutations
   a. Atypical progeroid syndrome
   b. Hutchinson-Gilford progeria syndrome
6. SHORT (short stature, hyperextensibility of joints or hernia, ocular depression, Rieger anomaly, teething) syndrome
   a. *PIK3R1* mutations
7. Neonatal progeroid (Weidemann-Rautenstrauch) syndrome
   a. *FBN1* mutations
   b. *CAV1* mutations
   c. *POLR3A* mutation
8. Mandibular hypoplasia, deafness, progeroid (MDP) syndrome
   a. *POLD1* mutations
9. Autoinflammatory lipodystrophy (joint contractures, microcytic anemia, panniculitis-associated [JMP] lipodystrophy syndrome spectrum including chronic atypical neutrophilic dermatosis with lipodystrophy and elevated temperature [CANDLE] syndrome)
   a. *PSMB8* mutations

Acquired Lipodystrophies
1. Highly active antiretroviral therapy–induced lipodystrophy in HIV-infected patients
2. Acquired generalized lipodystrophy
   a. Panniculitis induced
   b. Autoimmune diseases associated
   c. Idiopathic
3. Acquired partial (Barraquer-Simons) lipodystrophy
   a. Autoimmune diseases associated
   b. Membranoproliferative glomerulonephritis associated
   c. Idiopathic
4. Localized lipodystrophies
   a. Panniculitis induced
   b. Pressure induced
   c. Drug induced
   d. Centrifugal
   e. Idiopathic

in genes involved in adipocyte differentiation, triglyceride synthesis, lipid droplet formation, and adipocyte survival have been reported to cause lipodystrophies.

CONGENITAL GENERALIZED LIPODYSTROPHY (BERARDINELLI-SEIP SYNDROME)

CLINICAL FEATURES

This autosomal recessive disorder has 4 subtypes and can be recognized at birth or soon thereafter from the near total lack of body fat.[13] Patients also have marked muscularity, prominent subcutaneous veins, acromegaloid features, acanthosis nigricans, hepatomegaly, and umbilical prominence (Fig. 74-1A, Table 74-2). During childhood, they have a voracious appetite, and accelerated linear growth. Females usually have hirsutism, clitoromegaly, oligomenorrhea, and polycystic ovaries. Only a few women have had successful pregnancies. Fertility may be affected in some men with CGL because of teratozoospermia. Some CGL patients develop hypertrophic cardiomyopathy, mild mental retardation, and focal lytic lesions in the appendicular bones after puberty.[13] Metabolic abnormalities related to insulin resistance, such as diabetes mellitus, hyperlipidemia, and hepatic steatosis, may manifest at a young age and are often difficult to control.

ETIOLOGY AND PATHOGENESIS

Genome-wide linkage analysis with positional cloning strategy and candidate gene approach have led to the identification of 4 genetic loci for CGL: 1-acylglycerol-3-phosphate-*O*-acyltransferase 2 (*AGPAT2*) gene on chromosome 9q34[14,15]; Berardinelli-Seip congenital lipodystrophy 2 (*BSCL2*) gene on chromosome 11q13[16]; caveolin 1 (*CAV1*) gene on chromosome 7q31[17]; and caveolae associated protein 1 (*CAVIN1*), also known as polymerase I and transcript release factor (*PTRF*) gene on chromosome 17q21.[18] AGPAT2 is a critical enzyme involved in the biosynthesis of triglycerides and phospholipids from glycerol-3-phosphate and is expressed highly in the adipose tissue.[19] The *BSCL2*-encoded protein, seipin, plays a role in lipid droplet fusion and also may be involved in adipocyte differentiation.[20-22] Caveolin 1 is an integral component of caveolae, specialized microdomains seen in abundance on adipocyte membranes. Caveolin 1 binds fatty acids and translocates them to lipid droplets. *CAVIN1* is involved in biogenesis of caveolae and regulates expression of caveolins 1 and 3.[18] Patients with *BSCL2* mutations lack mechanical fat located in the orbital region, palm, sole, and in periarticular regions, as well as metabolically active adipose tissue located in the subcutaneous (SQ), intraabdominal, intrathoracic, and other areas as compared to those with *AGPAT2*, *CAV1*, and *PTRF* mutations where mechanical fat is preserved.[17,23] The only reported patient with *CAV1* mutation also had short stature and presumed vitamin D resistance.[17] Only approximately 15 patients with *CAVIN1* mutations have been reported

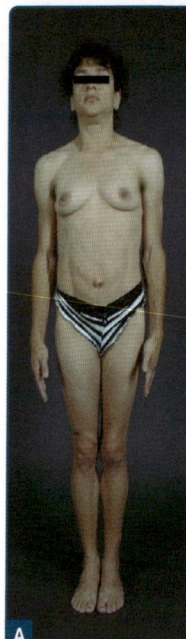 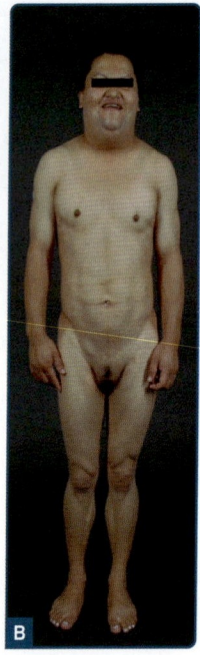 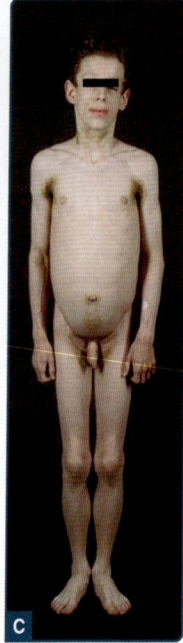 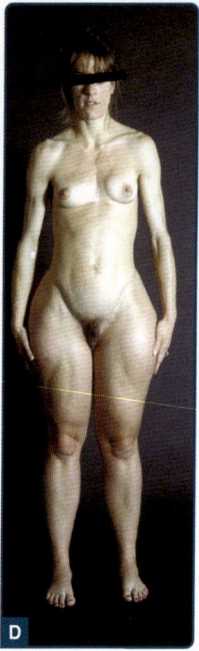 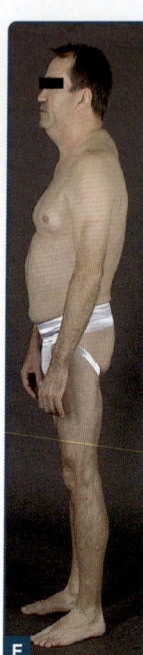

Figure 74-1 Clinical features of patients with various types of lipodystrophies. **A,** Anterior view of a 33-year-old Hispanic female with congenital generalized lipodystrophy (also known as Berardinelli-Seip congenital lipodystrophy), Type 1 caused by homozygous c.589–2A>G; p.(Val197Glufs*32) mutation in the *AGPAT2* gene. The patient had generalized loss of subcutaneous fat with acanthosis nigricans in the axillae and neck. She has umbilical prominence and acromegaloid features (enlarged mandible, hands, and feet). **B,** Anterior view of a 27-year-old Native American Hispanic female with familial partial lipodystrophy of the Dunnigan variety caused by heterozygous p.Arg482Trp mutation in *LMNA* gene. She had marked loss of subcutaneous fat from the limbs and anterior truncal region. The breasts were atrophic. She had increased subcutaneous fat deposits in the face, anterior neck, and vulvar regions. **C,** Anterior view of an 8-year-old German boy with acquired generalized lipodystrophy. He had severe generalized loss of subcutaneous fat with marked acanthosis nigricans in the neck, axillae, and groin. **D,** Anterior view of a 39-year-old white female with acquired partial lipodystrophy (Barraquer-Simons syndrome). She had marked loss of subcutaneous fat from the face, neck, upper extremities, and chest, but had lipodystrophy on localized regions on anterior thighs. She had increased subcutaneous fat deposition in the lower extremities. **E,** Lateral view of a 53-year-old white male infected with HIV with highly active antiretroviral therapy–induced lipodystrophy. He had marked loss of subcutaneous fat from the face and limbs, but had increased subcutaneous fat deposition in the neck region anteriorly and posteriorly showing buffalo hump. Abdomen was protuberant because of excess intraabdominal fat. He had been on protease inhibitor–containing antiretroviral therapy for more than 8 years.

and they have congenital myopathy, increased creatine kinase levels, percussion-induced myoedema, pyloric stenosis, atlantoaxial instability, and cardiac rhythm disturbances including prolonged QT interval and exercise-induced ventricular tachycardia, which can result in sudden death.[18,24,25] Patients of Lebanese origin harbor homozygous c.315_319delGTATC; p.(Tyr106Cysfs*6) mutation in *BSCL2*, whereas those of African origin nearly always have either homozygous or compound heterozygous c.589–2A>G; p.(Val197Glufs*32) mutation in *AGPAT2* gene.[15,16,26]

FAMILIAL PARTIAL LIPODYSTROPHY

CLINICAL FEATURES

FPL in most patients is transmitted in an autosomal dominant fashion and is characterized by fat loss from the limbs with variable fat loss from the trunk and increased SQ fat deposition in nonlipodystrophic regions (see Fig. 74-1B). Most FPL patients have the Dunnigan variety as a result of heterozygous mutations in lamin A/C (*LMNA*) gene. These patients have normal body fat distribution during early childhood, but around the time of puberty, SQ fat from the extremities and trunk is progressively lost (see Fig. 74-1B). The face, neck, and intraabdominal region are spared, and often excess fat accumulates there.[27,28] Affected men are often more difficult to diagnose clinically, as many normal men are also quite muscular. Women are more severely affected metabolically.[29]

Patients with FPL caused by heterozygous mutations in *PPARG* gene also have fat loss from the extremities, especially from distal regions, but the fat from the face, neck, and truncal areas is spared.[30] There is increased prevalence of hypertension among the affected subjects. Four subjects from a single family with diabetes and insulin resistance were reported to harbor a heterozygous mutation in *AKT2* gene.[31] The female proband had lipodystrophy of the

TABLE 74-2
Clinical Features of Various Types of Congenital Generalized Lipodystrophy

CHARACTERISTIC	SUBTYPE OF CONGENITAL GENERALIZED LIPODYSTROPHY (CGL)			
	CGL1	CGL2	CGL3	CGL4
Gene	AGPAT2	BSCL2	CAV1	CAVIN1
Loss of metabolically active adipose tissue	+++	+++	++	++
Loss of mechanical adipose tissue	−	+	−	−
Bone marrow fat	−	−	+	+
Lytic bone lesions	++	+	−	−
Mild mental retardation	−	+	−	−
Cardiomyopathy	−	+	−	+
Echocardiogram	Normal	Abnormal	Normal	Normal
Catecholaminergic polymorphic ventricular tachycardia	−	−	−	+
Prolonged QT interval	−	−	−	+
Sudden death	−	−	−	+
Congenital pyloric stenosis	−	−	−	+
Atlantoaxial instability	−	−	−	+
Acanthosis nigricans	+++	+++	++	+/−
Hepatomegaly	+	+	+	+
Congenital myopathy	−	−	−	+
Diabetes mellitus	+	+	+	−
Hypertriglyceridemia	+	+	+	+
Hypocalcemia	−	−	+	−
Hyperinsulinemia	+	+	+	+/−
Cirrhosis	+	++	−	−

−, absent; +/−, absent/present; +, mild; ++, moderate; +++, severe.

limbs, although detailed studies of body fat distribution were not performed. Recently, 12 FPL patients were reported to harbor *PLIN1* mutations.[32,33] Three patients from a single family with atypical FPL and marked buffalo hump had a heterozygous *ADRA2A* mutation.[34]

ETIOLOGY AND PATHOGENESIS

FPL results from heterozygous missense mutations in 1 of the 5 genes: lamin A/C (*LMNA*) on chromosome 1q21–22,[35-38] an integral component of nuclear lamina; peroxisome proliferator-activated receptor γ (*PPARG*) on chromosome 3p25,[30,39,40] a key transcription factor involved in adipocyte differentiation; v-AKT murine thymoma oncogene homolog 2 (*AKT2*) on chromosome 19q13,[31] which is involved in downstream insulin signaling; perilipin 1 (*PLIN1*) on chromosome 15q26, a key component of lipid droplets[32]; and adrenoreceptor α$_{2A}$ (*ADRA2A*), the main presynaptic inhibitory feedback G-protein–coupled receptor regulating norepinephrine release.[34] Adipocyte loss in patients with *LMNA* mutations may be a result of disruption of nuclear envelope function and integrity resulting in premature cell death. Some patients with mutations in the aminoterminal region of lamin A/C also develop myopathy, cardiomyopathy, and conduction system abnormalities indicative of a multisystem dystrophy.[41] On the other hand, others with mutations in the extreme C-terminal region of lamin A may have mild lipodystrophy.[42]

MANDIBULOACRAL DYSPLASIA–ASSOCIATED LIPODYSTROPHY

CLINICAL FEATURES

Patients with MAD have characteristic skeletal abnormalities including hypoplasia of the mandible and clavicles, acroosteolysis, cutaneous atrophy, progeroid features such as thin beaked nose, hair loss, thin skin with prominent superficial vasculature and mottled hyperpigmentation, delayed dentition and closure of cranial sutures, joint stiffness, and lipodystrophy.[43,44]

ETIOLOGY AND PATHOGENESIS

Mutations in *LMNA* and zinc metalloproteinase (*ZMPSTE24*) on chromosome 1p34 cause autosomal-recessive MAD-associated lipodystrophies.[45,46] *ZMPSTE24* is involved in posttranslational proteolytic processing of prelamin A to mature lamin A and its deficiency can result in accumulation of prelamin A in cells which is supposed to cause toxicity. Those persons with *ZMPSTE24* mutations develop clinical manifestations earlier in life, are premature at birth, and can develop focal segmental glomerulosclerosis, calcified skin nodules, and thin shiny skin.[47,48]

OTHER TYPES

CLINICAL FEATURES

My colleagues and I reported a novel syndrome with mandibular hypoplasia, deafness, progeroid features–associated lipodystrophy.[49] All males with mandibular hypoplasia, deafness, progeroid features had undescended testes and were hypogonadal. One adult female showed lack of breast development. Patients with autoinflammatory lipodystrophy present as a spectrum of clinical manifestations, with onset ranging from during the first months of life[50] to later during childhood.[51] Early features are recurrent fevers, annular violaceous plaques, poor weight and height gain, persistent violaceous eyelid swelling, hepatomegaly, arthralgias, variable muscle atrophy, and progressive lipodystrophy.[52-54] Histopathologic examination of lesional skin shows atypical mononuclear infiltrates of myeloid lineage and mature neutrophils, and laboratory abnormalities include chronic anemia, elevated acute-phase reactants, and raised liver enzymes with a cytokine profile showing high levels of interferon-inducible protein–1, monocyte chemotactic protein–1, interleukin-6, and interleukin-1 receptor antagonist, consistent with an interferon signaling signature.[52,53] This presentation has been called CANDLE syndrome (chronic atypical neutrophilic dermatosis with lipodystrophy and elevated temperature).[50] Older individuals with *PSMB8* mutations show joint contractures, muscle atrophy, microcytic anemia, and panniculitis-induced (JMP) childhood-onset lipodystrophy (Fig. 74-2).[51] Other features of JMP syndrome include hypergammaglobulinemia, elevated erythrocyte sedimentation rate, hepatosplenomegaly, and calcification of basal ganglia.[51] Other rare syndromes of lipodystrophy include autosomal-recessive FPL and SHORT (short stature, hyperextensibility or inguinal hernia, ocular depression, Rieger anomaly, and teething delay) syndrome.[55,56] The fat loss is usually confined to the face, upper extremities, and trunk, and sometimes the buttocks.[55,56] Patients with neonatal progeroid (Wiedemann-Rautenstrauch) syndrome present with generalized loss of body fat and muscle mass and progeroid appearance at birth.[57] There is a marked heterogeneity in the phenotype of patients with Wiedemann-Rautenstrauch syndrome.

ETIOLOGY AND PATHOGENESIS

De novo recurrent heterozygous mutation in polymerase (DNA) delta 1, catalytic subunit (*POLD1*) gene has been reported in patients with mandibular hypoplasia, deafness, progeroid features syndrome.[58] Most patients with SHORT syndrome have a de novo recurrent heterozygous missense mutation in phosphoinositide-3-kinase regulatory subunit 1 (PIK3R1) gene.[59] De novo heterozygous mutations in fibrillin 1 (*FBN1*)[60] and caveolin 1 (*CAV1*)[61] and biallelic mutations in RNA polymerase III subunit A (*POLR3A*)[62] have been reported in Wiedemann-Rautenstrauch syndrome patients. Recently, a single patient with autosomal recessive, FPL phenotype was found to harbor a homozygous missense mutation in cell death-inducing DNA fragmentation factor a-like effector c (*CIDEC*) gene on chromosome 3p25, involved in lipid droplet formation.[63] The histopathology of the SQ adipose tissue of the patient revealed multilocular, small lipid droplets in adipocytes. Two additional patients with autosomal recessive partial and generalized lipodystrophy phenotype had mutations in phosphate cytidylyltransferase 1α (*PCYT1A*) gene that encodes the rate-limiting enzyme in phosphatidyl choline biosynthetic pathway.[64] Loss-of-function mutations in hormone sensitive lipase (*LIPE*) gene have been reported to cause an autosomal recessive FPL phenotype with multiple symmetric lipomatosis and myopathy.[65-67] Two women with FPL and features of Werner syndrome have been reported to harbor null mutations in Werner syndrome RecQ like helicase (*WRN*) gene.[68]

Heterozygous *LMNA* mutations can also cause partial or generalized lipodystrophy in patients with atypical progeroid syndrome[69] and generalized loss of SQ fat in Hutchinson-Gilford progeria syndrome.[70] Autoinflammatory lipodystrophy syndrome results from mutations in proteasome subunit, beta-type, 8 (*PSMB8*).[52,53] *PSMB8* encodes the β5i subunit of the immunoproteasome involved in proteolytic cleavage of immunogenic epitopes presented by major histocompatibility complex Class I molecules.[52] The molecular genetic basis of many other genetic lipodystrophy syndromes remains unclear (see Table 74-1).

ACQUIRED LIPODYSTROPHIES

Despite recognition of acquired lipodystrophies for more than a century, progress in understanding underlying pathogenic mechanisms has been slow.

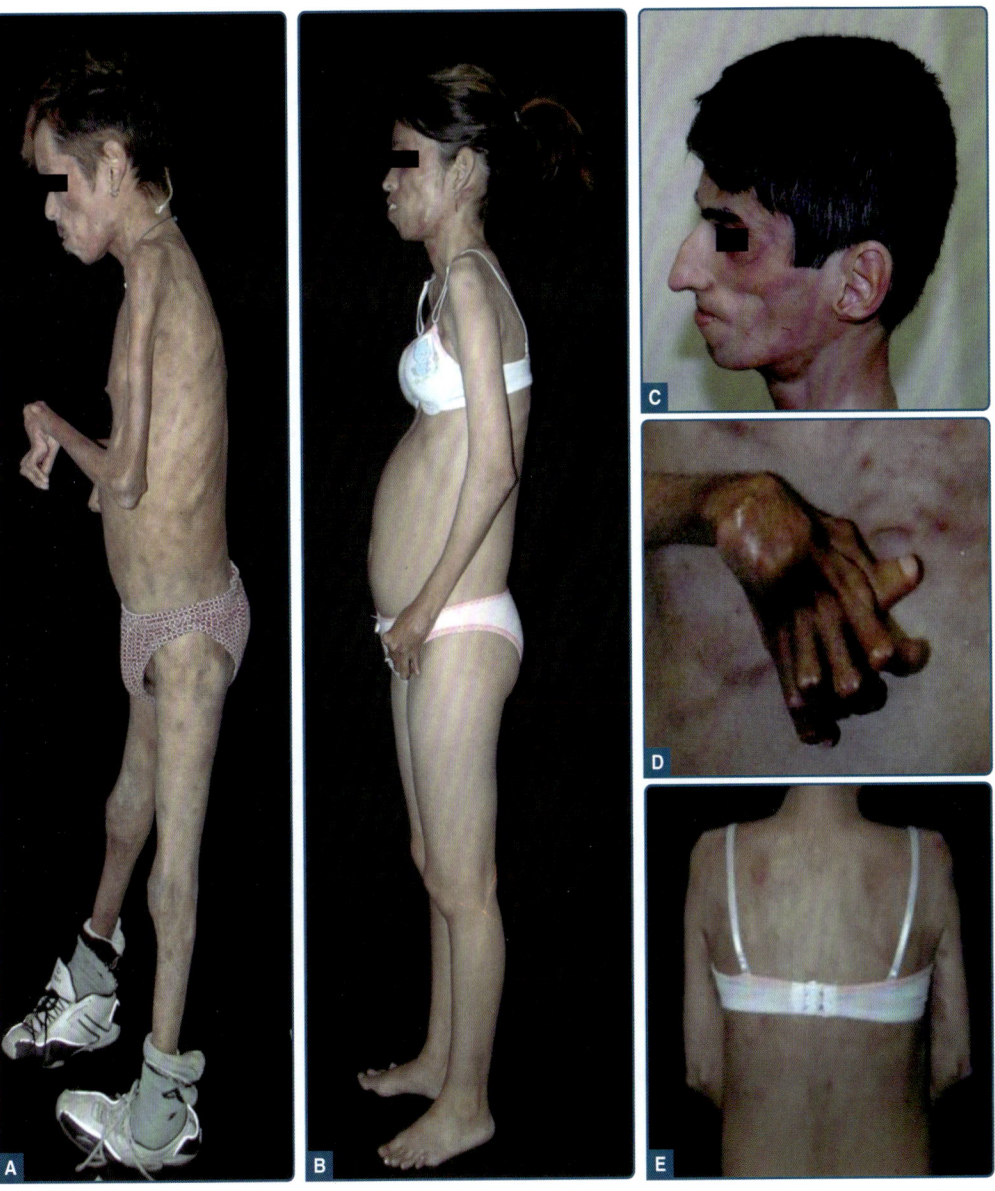

Figure 74-2 Phenotype of patients with joint contractures, muscle atrophy, microcytic anemia, and panniculitis-induced lipodystrophy (JMP) syndrome. **A,** Left lateral view of a 30-year-old Mexican male with JMP syndrome showing marked generalized loss of subcutaneous fat and muscle mass from the face, neck, chest, and extremities. Flexion contracture at the elbow, wrist, and hand are seen. **B,** Left lateral view of a 26-year-old Mexican female with JMP syndrome showing lipodystrophy affecting mostly the upper body, that is, the face, neck, thorax, and upper extremities. **C,** Left lateral view of the face of a 35-year-old Portuguese male with JMP syndrome showing marked loss of subcutaneous fat. **D,** Dorsal view of the hand from a 35-year-old Portuguese male showing flexion contractures of the wrist, proximal and distal interphalangeal joints and hyperextension of the metacarpophalangeal joints. **E,** Posterior view of the chest of a 26-year-old Mexican female with JMP syndrome showing many discrete, small, erythematous maculopapular and nodular skin lesions on the chest and medial side of right arm. (Reproduced with permission from Agarwal AK, Xing C, DeMartino GN, et al. PSMB8 encoding the β5i proteasome subunit is mutated in joint contractures, muscle atrophy, microcytic anemia, and panniculitis-induced lipodystrophy syndrome. *Am J Hum Genet.* 2010;87:866-872. Copyright © Elsevier.)

ACQUIRED PARTIAL LIPODYSTROPHY (BARRAQUER-SIMONS SYNDROME)

CLINICAL FEATURES

Acquired partial lipodystrophy develops in most patients before age 15 years. Patients lose SQ fat gradually in a symmetric fashion starting with the face and then spreading downward. Most patients present with fat loss from the face, neck, upper extremities, and trunk, with sparing of SQ abdominal fat and lower extremities (see Fig. 74-1C). Approximately, 20% of the patients develop mesangiocapillary (membranoproliferative) glomerulonephritis, and some develop drusen.[9] Usually, patients do not develop metabolic complications.

ETIOLOGY AND PATHOGENESIS

The exact pathogenesis of SQ fat loss remains unclear but there is strong evidence of autoimmune-mediated adipocyte loss as more than 80% of the patients have low levels of complement 3 (C3) and presence of a circulating immunoglobulin G, a C3-nephritic factor that blocks degradation of the enzyme C3 convertase.[9] Loss of fat could be the result of C3-nephritic factor–induced lysis of adipocytes expressing factor D.

ACQUIRED GENERALIZED LIPODYSTROPHY (LAWRENCE SYNDROME)

CLINICAL FEATURES

Acquired generalized lipodystrophies present with variable amount of SQ fat loss usually during childhood. Although many patients have generalized loss of fat, some areas are spared (see Fig. 74-1D). Usually, intraabdominal or bone marrow fat is spared.[10] However, patients develop extremely severe hepatic steatosis and fibrosis, diabetes, and hypertriglyceridemia, which are difficult to manage.

ETIOLOGY AND PATHOGENESIS

The exact mechanisms of fat loss are not known. In approximately 25% of patients, SQ fat loss occurs following development of SQ inflammatory nodules that on biopsy reveal panniculitis.[10] These lesions initially result in localized fat loss followed by generalized loss of fat. Another 25% of the patients have associated autoimmune diseases, especially juvenile dermatomyositis.[10,71] In the remaining patients with the idiopathic variety, multiple unknown mechanisms are likely involved.[10] Patients with the panniculitis-associated variety have less-severe fat loss and metabolic complications than seen in other types. Some patients have been reported to have low serum levels of complement 4.[72]

HIGHLY ACTIVE ANTIRETROVIRAL THERAPY–INDUCED LIPODYSTROPHY IN HIV-INFECTED PATIENTS

CLINICAL FEATURES

Patients infected with HIV who are receiving PI-containing highly active antiretroviral therapy usually lose SQ fat from the face, trunk, and extremities 2 years or more after initiation of therapy (see Figs. 74-1E, 74-3A, and 74-3B). Fat loss from the face can be so severe as to result in an emaciated appearance. Some of them develop buffalo hump, double chin, and also gain intraabdominal fat. The fat loss progressively gets worse with ongoing highly active antiretroviral therapy and does not reverse on discontinuation of PIs. Some cases develop diabetes mellitus and many develop combined hyperlipidemia that can predispose the patients to coronary heart disease.[12]

ETIOLOGY AND PATHOGENESIS

Drugs such as HIV-1 PIs and nucleoside analogs are implicated in causing lipodystrophy in HIV-infected patients. Many, but not all, PIs may induce lipodystrophy by inhibiting ZMPSTE24, resulting in accumulation of prelamin A.[73] Other mechanisms may include PI-induced alteration of expression of key transcription factors involved in lipogenesis and adipocyte differentiation, such as sterol regulatory element-binding protein 1c and PPARG.[74] PIs also reduce glucose transporter 4 expression, which may be a mechanism for inducing insulin resistance.[75] Nucleoside analogs, especially zidovudine and stavudine, may induce fat loss by inhibiting polymerase-γ, a mitochondrial enzyme involved in replication of mitochondrial DNA.[76] As most patients receive multiple antiretroviral drugs together, the individual effects of PIs or nucleoside reverse transcriptase inhibitors on the phenotype are not clear.

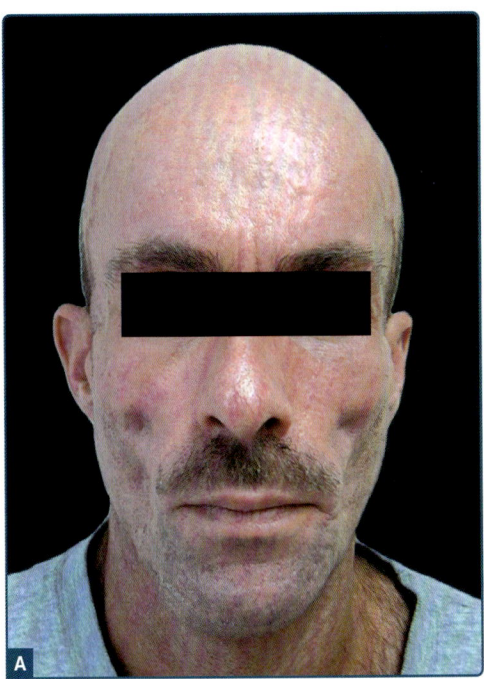
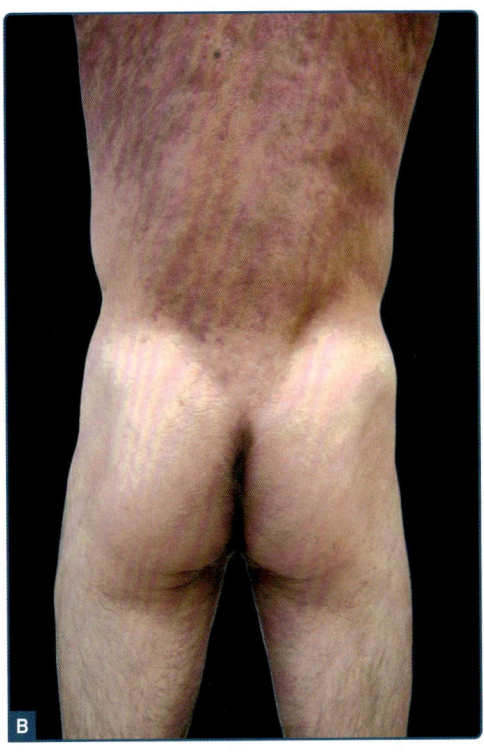

Figure 74-3 **A,** Highly active antiretroviral therapy–induced lipodystrophy in a patient with HIV infection–associated lipodystrophy. Loss of buccal fat results in prominence of the zygomatic arch **B,** Highly active antiretroviral therapy-induced lipodystrophy with loss of subcutaneous fat from the lateral buttock and deposit in the trunk, causing an increased waist-to-hip ratio.

LOCALIZED LIPODYSTROPHY

CLINICAL FEATURES

Localized lipodystrophies present with SQ fat loss from a focal region resulting in a dimple or a crater with overlying skin usually unaffected. In some patients, large contiguous or anatomically distinct areas on any region of the body may be involved.[3]

ETIOLOGY AND PATHOGENESIS

This can occur from SQ injection of various drugs, panniculitis, pressure, and other mechanisms.[3]

DIAGNOSIS

Lipodystrophies should be strongly suspected in "lean or nonobese" patients who present with premature onset of diabetes, hypertriglyceridemia, hepatic steatosis, acanthosis nigricans, and polycystic ovarian syndrome. These patients should be examined carefully for evidence of loss of SQ fat especially from the hips and thighs, as well as excess SQ fat deposition in various anatomic regions. For those presenting with generalized lipodystrophy during childhood, pictures at birth should be evaluated for evidence of fat loss. If lipodystrophy phenotype is discovered at or shortly after birth, CGL should be considered; otherwise, the patient may have acquired lipodystrophy.

HISTORY

Patients should be asked about their age at time of onset and the progression of the lipodystrophy and other associated manifestations. Taking a detailed family history, including the history of consanguinity, is very important to understand the mode of inheritance of genetic lipodystrophies. Associated autoimmune diseases, especially juvenile dermatomyositis, should be considered in patients with acquired lipodystrophies. Those with localized lipodystrophies should be asked about local injections, trauma, pressure, or other insults. A detailed history of duration and type of antiretroviral therapy should be obtained from HIV-infected patients with lipodystrophy.

CUTANEOUS LESIONS

The most common cutaneous lesion seen in patients with lipodystrophies is acanthosis nigricans in the axillae,

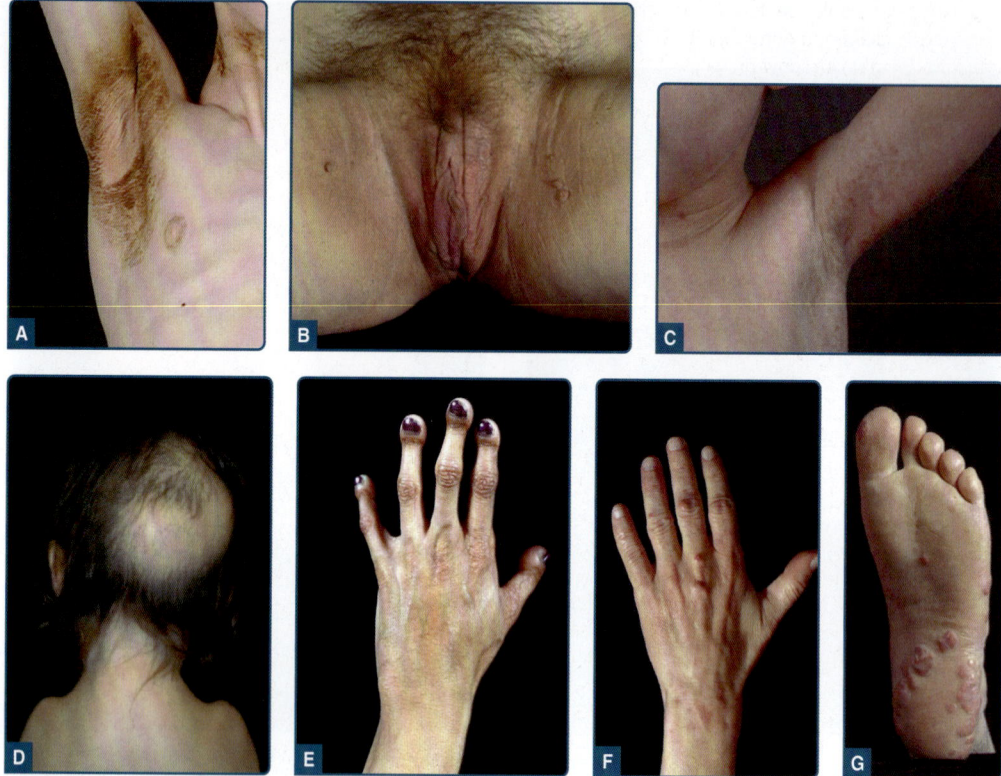

Figure 74-4 Dermatologic manifestations seen in patients with lipodystrophies. **A,** Acanthosis nigricans (brownish discoloration with thickening of the skin) in the axilla and anterior neck in an 8-year-old white boy with acquired generalized lipodystrophy. **B,** Acanthosis nigricans in the perineum and medial parts of the proximal thighs in a 37-year-old female with familial partial lipodystrophy (FPL). Multiple, small skin tags accompany increased pigmentation and thick skin. **C,** Multiple, slightly hyperpigmented flat plaques (freckles) in a 7-year-old boy with atypical progeroid syndrome caused by a heterozygous p.(Cys588Arg) mutation in the *LMNA* gene. **D,** Loss of hair from the posterior scalp region in a 5-year-old girl with severe mandibuloacral dysplasia (MAD) caused by a homozygous p.(Arg527Cys) mutation in the *LMNA* gene. She had narrow shoulders as a result of clavicular hypoplasia. **E,** Acroosteolysis in a 20-year-old Hispanic woman with MAD caused by a homozygous p.(Arg527His) mutation in the *LMNA* gene. The terminal digits appear short and bulbous because of resorption of the terminal phalanges. The skin on the dorsum of the hand is atrophic, especially over the proximal interphalangeal and metacarpophalangeal joints. **F,** Tuberous xanthomas over the middle finger of a 45-year-old white patient with severe hyperlipidemia associated with FPL of the Dunnigan variety caused by a heterozygous p.(Arg482Gln) mutation in the *LMNA* gene. **G,** Planar xanthomas on the sole of the patient described in **F**. (Panel C reproduced with permission from Garg A, Subramanyam L, Agarwal AK, et al. Atypical progeroid syndrome due to heterozygous missense *LMNA* mutations. *J Clin Endocrinol Metab*. 2009;94:4971-4983. Copyright 2009, The Endocrine Society. Panel G reproduced with permission from Simha V, Garg A. Lipodystrophy: lessons in lipid and energy metabolism. *Curr Opin Lipidol*. 2006;17: 162-169. Wolters Kluwer/Lippincott Williams & Wilkins.)

groins, neck, and sometimes even on the knuckles, Achilles tendons, and trunk (Figs. 74-4A and B). Many patients develop clitoromegaly and hirsutism as a result of associated polycystic ovarian syndrome. Freckles were noted in a patient with atypical progeroid syndrome (Fig. 74-4C). A thin, beaked nose with loss of scalp, eyebrow, and axillary hair with cutaneous atrophy and mottled hyperpigmentation can be seen in patients with progeroid syndromes and MAD (Fig. 74-4D), along with acroosteolysis (Fig. 74-4E).[43,69,70] Rare patients with MAD develop shiny, taut, atrophic skin with a tendency to breakdown. Eruptive, tuberous, and planar xanthomas are also commonly seen in patients with extreme hypertriglyceridemia (Figs. 74-4F and G). Loss of SQ fat from the soles can result in plantar calluses. SQ nodules with overlying erythema may be seen in patients with panniculitis.

LABORATORY TESTING

Laboratory testing depends upon the type of lipodystrophy. Except for patients with localized lipodystrophies, a serum chemistry profile for glucose, lipids, liver enzymes, and uric acid should be obtained. Measurement of fasting and postprandial serum glucose and insulin during an oral glucose tolerance test can provide some estimate of insulin resistance. Serum leptin measurements are not diagnostic, but can help guide treatment decisions as far as investigational human recombinant leptin (metreleptin) replacement therapy is concerned. Serum leptin and adiponectin levels are very low in patients with generalized lipodystrophies.[77] Patients with acquired partial lipodystrophy should be tested for serum C3 and C3-nephritic factor and annually checked for proteinuria. Radiographs can show presence of lytic lesions in appendicular bones in patients with CGL and skeletal defects in those with MAD. Skin biopsy is useful for patients with localized lipodystrophy or panniculitis-associated varieties.

SPECIAL TESTS (INCLUDING IMAGING STUDIES)

Distinction between various types of lipodystrophies can be made by physical examination and supported by anthropometry, including measurement of skinfold thickness with calipers at various sites. For in-depth phenotyping of body fat distribution, whole-body dual-energy X-ray absorptiometry, and T1-weighted MRI can be conducted. For those genetic lipodystrophies whose molecular basis is known, various commercial and research laboratories offer genetic testing. Prenatal genetic testing is also feasible. FPL patients, atypical progeroid syndrome patients and CGL, Type 4 patients who are predisposed to cardiomyopathy should undergo electrocardiography and Holter monitoring to detect arrhythmias and echocardiography to assess cardiac function.

DIFFERENTIAL DIAGNOSIS

The most important differential diagnosis of generalized lipodystrophies is with conditions presenting with severe weight loss, such as malnutrition, famine, starvation, anorexia nervosa, uncontrolled diabetes mellitus, thyrotoxicosis, adrenocortical insufficiency, cancer cachexia, HIV-associated wasting, diencephalic syndrome, and chronic infections. For partial lipodystrophies, distinction should be made with Cushing syndrome, generalized and truncal obesity, and multiple symmetric lipomatosis (Madelung disease). Patients with MAD and progeroid syndromes-associated lipodystrophies should be differentiated from those with Werner syndrome and leprechaunism (Donahue syndrome).

CLINICAL COURSE AND PROGNOSIS

Some patients develop extreme hypertriglyceridemia and chylomicronemia, which result in acute pancreatitis and even death. Long-term complications of diabetes such as nephropathy, neuropathy, and retinopathy are frequently seen. Many patients develop coronary heart disease and other atherosclerotic vascular complications.[29,78] Hepatic steatosis can lead to cirrhosis, necessitating liver transplantation. Sudden death has been reported during childhood in CGL, Type 4, likely from arrhythmias.[24] Some patients with acquired partial lipodystrophy and membranoproliferative glomerulonephritis may require kidney transplantation.[9] Patients with Hutchinson-Gilford progeria syndrome die of acute myocardial infarction or cerebrovascular accidents during their teenage years.[79] Some patients with atypical progeroid syndrome and FPL-Dunnigan develop cardiomyopathy with valvular dysfunction, congestive heart failure, and arrhythmias requiring pacemaker implantation.[41,69] Two adult patients with MAD caused by ZMPSTE24 mutations died of renal failure resulting from focal segmental glomerulosclerosis.[47] Some patients with acquired generalized lipodystrophy have been reported to develop peripheral T-cell lymphomas.[80]

The prognosis is dependent upon the type of lipodystrophy. In most of the published cases of CGL the patients have been children, resulting in a lack of data about their prognosis. In my experience, some patients have died of complications of acute pancreatitis or cirrhosis, or developed end-stage renal disease, requiring renal transplantation, and blindness as a consequence of diabetic retinopathy. Patients with FPL are also predisposed to metabolic complications and die of atherosclerotic vascular and coronary heart disease or cardiomyopathy and rhythm disturbances. Some patients with MAD have reportedly died during childhood and some died later in their third and fourth decades from complications of renal failure.[47,81] Patients with acquired generalized lipodystrophy suffer severe metabolic complications. Patients with acquired partial lipodystrophy and membranoproliferative glomerulonephritis develop renal failure, but others have a normal life span as do those with localized lipodystrophy. HIV-infected patients with lipodystrophy are predisposed to developing coronary heart disease.

MANAGEMENT

Treatment of various types of lipodystrophies is quite challenging. There is no specific treatment available to reverse the loss of body fat. The mainstay of treatment includes cosmetic surgery and management of complications. Patients with partial lipodystrophies can undergo autologous adipose tissue transplantation or implantation of dermal fillers such as hyaluronic acid, calcium hydroxylapatite, silicone, polyacrylamide gels, or poly-L-lactic acid.[82] Unwanted excess adipose tissue can be surgically excised or removed by liposuction. Those with CGL can undergo reconstructive facial surgery, including facial grafts from thighs, free flaps from anterolateral thigh, anterior abdomen, or temporalis muscle.[1] Support of the parents is critical for preventing unwanted stress and psychological sequelae in children affected with lipodystrophies.

All patients are advised to consume low-fat diets. These diets can improve chylomicronemia in patients with extreme hypertriglyceridemia. However, high carbohydrate intake may also raise very low-density lipoprotein triglyceride concentrations. Increased physical activity should be encouraged to mitigate insulin resistance and its complications except in those who have cardiomyopathy. Lytic bone lesions in appendicular bones in patients with CGL usually do not pose an increased risk of fractures.

There are no well-controlled trials available to guide treatment decisions about how to manage metabolic complications. For severe hypertriglyceridemia, an extremely low-fat diet along with fibrates and n-3 polyunsaturated fatty acids from fish oils should be used.[5] Statins can be added if required. Any form of estrogen therapy should be avoided, as it can pose the risk of severe hypertriglyceridemia-induced acute pancreatitis. Diabetes should be managed initially with metformin. Thiazolidinediones should be used with caution in patients with partial lipodystrophies as they can potentially increase unwanted fat deposition in nonlipodystrophic regions.[83] Although thiazolidinediones can be useful in FPL patients with *PPARG* mutations, the data on their efficacy are equivocal.[84] If hyperglycemia persists despite using various combinations of oral antidiabetic drugs, insulin therapy should be initiated. For those with extreme insulin resistance, highly concentrated U-200 or U-500 insulin should be used. Although SQ metreleptin replacement therapy improves diabetes control, hepatic steatosis, and hypertriglyceridemia in markedly hypoleptinemic patients with generalized lipodystrophies,[85,86] its effects in patients with FPL so far have been equivocal.[87,88] Metreleptin may be effective in selected FPL patients with severe metabolic derangements or low serum leptin levels.[89] Metreleptin therapy is approved by the U.S. Food and Drug Administration for patients with generalized lipodystrophies to treat metabolic complications and in Japan for both generalized and partial lipodystrophies. Frequent side effects of metreleptin include injection-site reactions and hypoglycemia (in patients on concomitant insulin therapy). The significance of reported neutralizing antibodies to leptin remains unclear. There is also a risk of developing T-cell lymphoma in acquired generalized lipodystrophy patients. Switching from PIs and nucleoside reverse transcriptase inhibitors strongly associated with lipodystrophy to other regimens may improve dyslipidemia and insulin resistance in HIV-infected patients with lipodystrophy; however, loss of SQ fat may not improve.[90]

With the discovery of the molecular genetic basis of many types of inherited lipodystrophies, prenatal diagnosis can be offered for those families with an affected child. Premarital genetic counseling can be provided to those with a high prevalence of consanguinity and CGL, such as those from Lebanon and certain regions of Brazil. If the newer highly active antiretroviral therapy regimens (not including PIs) are proven not to be associated with lipodystrophy and are deemed to be efficacious and safe, we may be able to prevent development of lipodystrophy in HIV-infected patients.

REFERENCES

1. Garg A. Acquired and inherited lipodystrophies. *N Engl J Med*. 2004;350:1220-1234.
2. Garg A. Clinical review#: Lipodystrophies: genetic and acquired body fat disorders. *J Clin Endocrinol Metab*. 2011;96:3313-3325.
3. Garg A. Lipodystrophies. *Am J Med*. 2000;108:143-152.
4. Hussain I, Garg A. Lipodystrophy syndromes. *Endocrinol Metab Clin North Am*. 2016;45:783-797.
5. Brown RJ, Araujo-Vilar D, Cheung PT, et al. The diagnosis and management of lipodystrophy syndromes: a multi-society practice guideline. *J Clin Endocrinol Metab*. 2016;101(12):4500-4511.
6. Akinci B, Onay H, Demir T, et al. Natural history of congenital generalized lipodystrophy: a nationwide study from Turkey. *J Clin Endocrinol Metab*. 2016;101:2759-2767.
7. Al-Shali KZ, Hegele RA. Laminopathies and atherosclerosis. *Arterioscler Thromb Vasc Biol*. 2004;24:1591-1595.
8. Andre P, Schneebeli S, Vigouroux C, et al. Metabolic and cardiac phenotype characterization in 37 atypical Dunnigan patients with nonfarnesylated mutated prelamin A. *Am Heart J*. 2015;169:587-593.
9. Misra A, Peethambaram A, Garg A. Clinical features and metabolic and autoimmune derangements in acquired partial lipodystrophy: report of 35 cases and review of the literature. *Medicine (Baltimore)*. 2004;83:18-34.
10. Misra A, Garg A. Clinical features and metabolic derangements in acquired generalized lipodystrophy: case reports and review of the literature. *Medicine (Baltimore)*. 2003;82:129-146.
11. Chen D, Misra A, Garg A. Lipodystrophy in human immunodeficiency virus-infected patients. *J Clin Endocrinol Metab*. 2002;87:4845-4856.
12. Grinspoon S, Carr A. Cardiovascular risk and body-fat abnormalities in HIV-infected adults. *N Engl J Med*. 2005;352:48-62.
13. Patni N, Garg A. Congenital generalized lipodystrophies—new insights into metabolic dysfunction. *Nat Rev Endocrinol*. 2015;11:522-534.
14. Garg A, Wilson R, Barnes R, et al. A gene for congenital generalized lipodystrophy maps to human chromosome 9q34. *J Clin Endocrinol Metab*. 1999;84:3390-3394.
15. Agarwal AK, Arioglu E, De Almeida S, et al. AGPAT2 is mutated in congenital generalized lipodystrophy linked to chromosome 9q34. *Nat Genet*. 2002;31:21-23.
16. Magre J, Delepine M, Khallouf E, et al. Identification of the gene altered in Berardinelli-Seip congenital lipodystrophy on chromosome 11q13. *Nat Genet*. 2001;28:365-370.
17. Kim CA, Delepine M, Boutet E, et al. Association of a homozygous nonsense caveolin-1 mutation with Berardinelli-Seip congenital lipodystrophy. *J Clin Endocrinol Metab*. 2008;93:1129-1134.
18. Hayashi YK, Matsuda C, Ogawa M, et al. Human PTRF mutations cause secondary deficiency of caveolins resulting in muscular dystrophy with generalized lipodystrophy. *J Clin Invest*. 2009;119:2623-2633.
19. Agarwal AK, Garg A. Congenital generalized lipodystrophy: significance of triglyceride biosynthetic pathways. *Trends Endocrinol Metab*. 2003;14:214-221.
20. Szymanski KM, Binns D, Bartz R, et al. The lipodystrophy protein seipin is found at endoplasmic reticulum lipid droplet junctions and is important for droplet morphology. *Proc Natl Acad Sci U S A*. 2007;104:20890-20895.
21. Fei W, Shui G, Gaeta B, et al. Fld1p, a functional homologue of human seipin, regulates the size of lipid droplets in yeast. *J Cell Biol*. 2008;180:473-482.
22. Payne VA, Grimsey N, Tuthill A, et al. The human lipodystrophy gene BSCL2/seipin may be essential for normal adipocyte differentiation. *Diabetes*. 2008;57:2055-2060.

23. Simha V, Garg A. Phenotypic heterogeneity in body fat distribution in patients with congenital generalized lipodystrophy due to mutations in the *AGPAT2* or *Seipin* genes. *J Clin Endocrinol Metab*. 2003;88:5433-5437.
24. Rajab A, Straub V, McCann LJ, et al. Fatal cardiac arrhythmia and long-QT syndrome in a new form of congenital generalized lipodystrophy with muscle rippling (CGL4) due to PTRF-CAVIN mutations. *PLoS Genet*. 2010;6:e1000874.
25. Shastry S, Delgado MR, Dirik E, et al. Congenital generalized lipodystrophy, type 4 (CGL4) associated with myopathy due to novel PTRF mutations. *Am J Med Genet A*. 2010;152A:2245-2253.
26. Agarwal AK, Simha V, Oral EA, et al. Phenotypic and genetic heterogeneity in congenital generalized lipodystrophy. *J Clin Endocrinol Metab*. 2003;88:4840-4847.
27. Dunnigan MG, Cochrane MA, Kelly A, et al. Familial lipoatrophic diabetes with dominant transmission. A new syndrome. *Q J Med*. 1974;43:33-48.
28. Garg A, Peshock RM, Fleckenstein JL. Adipose tissue distribution in patients with familial partial lipodystrophy (Dunnigan variety). *J Clin Endocrinol Metab*. 1999;84:170-174.
29. Garg A. Gender differences in the prevalence of metabolic complications in familial partial lipodystrophy (Dunnigan variety). *J Clin Endocrinol Metab*. 2000;85:1776-1782.
30. Agarwal AK, Garg A. A novel heterozygous mutation in peroxisome proliferator-activated receptor-g gene in a patient with familial partial lipodystrophy. *J Clin Endocrinol Metab*. 2002;87:408-411.
31. George S, Rochford JJ, Wolfrum C, et al. A family with severe insulin resistance and diabetes due to a mutation in AKT2. *Science*. 2004;304:1325-1328.
32. Gandotra S, Le Dour C, Bottomley W, et al. Perilipin deficiency and autosomal dominant partial lipodystrophy. *N Engl J Med*. 2011;364:740-748.
33. Kozusko K, Tsang VH, Bottomley W, et al. Clinical and molecular characterization of a novel PLIN1 frameshift mutation identified in patients with familial partial lipodystrophy. *Diabetes*. 2015;64:299-310.
34. Garg A, Sankella S, Xing C, et al. Whole-exome sequencing identifies ADRA2A mutation in atypical familial partial lipodystrophy. *JCI Insight*. 2016;16;1(9).
35. Peters JM, Barnes R, Bennett L, et al. Localization of the gene for familial partial lipodystrophy (Dunnigan variety) to chromosome 1q21-22. *Nat Genet*. 1998;18:292-295.
36. Cao H, Hegele RA. Nuclear lamin A/C R482Q mutation in Canadian kindreds with Dunnigan-type familial partial lipodystrophy. *Hum Mol Genet*. 2000;9:109-112.
37. Shackleton S, Lloyd DJ, Jackson SN, et al. *LMNA*, encoding lamin A/C, is mutated in partial lipodystrophy. *Nat Genet*. 2000;24:153-156.
38. Speckman RA, Garg A, Du F, et al. Mutational and haplotype analyses of families with familial partial lipodystrophy (Dunnigan variety) reveal recurrent missense mutations in the globular C-terminal domain of lamin A/C. *Am J Hum Genet*. 2000;66:1192-1198.
39. Hegele RA, Cao H, Frankowski C, et al. PPARG F388L, a transactivation-deficient mutant, in familial partial lipodystrophy. *Diabetes*. 2002;51:3586-3590.
40. Semple RK, Chatterjee VK, O'Rahilly S. PPAR gamma and human metabolic disease. *J Clin Invest*. 2006;116:581-589.
41. Garg A, Speckman RA, Bowcock AM. Multisystem dystrophy syndrome due to novel missense mutations in the amino-terminal head and alpha-helical rod domains of the lamin A/C gene. *Am J Med*. 2002;112:549-555.
42. Garg A, Vinaitheerthan M, Weatherall P, et al. Phenotypic heterogeneity in patients with familial partial lipodystrophy (Dunnigan variety) related to the site of missense mutations in Lamin A/C (*LMNA*) gene. *J Clin Endocrinol Metab*. 2001;86:59-65.
43. Simha V, Garg A. Body fat distribution and metabolic derangements in patients with familial partial lipodystrophy associated with mandibuloacral dysplasia. *J Clin Endocrinol Metab*. 2002;87:776-785.
44. Simha V, Agarwal AK, Oral EA, et al. Genetic and phenotypic heterogeneity in patients with mandibuloacral dysplasia-associated lipodystrophy. *J Clin Endocrinol Metab*. 2003;88:2821-2824.
45. Novelli G, Muchir A, Sangiuolo F, et al. Mandibuloacral dysplasia is caused by a mutation in LMNA-encoding lamin A/C. *Am J Hum Genet*. 2002;71:426-431.
46. Agarwal AK, Fryns JP, Auchus RJ, et al. Zinc metalloproteinase, ZMPSTE24, is mutated in mandibuloacral dysplasia. *Hum Mol Genet*. 2003;12:1995-2001.
47. Agarwal AK, Zhou XJ, Hall RK, et al. Focal segmental glomerulosclerosis in patients with mandibuloacral dysplasia due to zinc metalloproteinase deficiency. *J Investig Med*. 2006;54:208-213.
48. Ahmad Z, Zackai E, Medne L, et al. Early onset mandibuloacral dysplasia due to compound heterozygous mutations in ZMPSTE24. *Am J Med Genet A*. 2010;152A:2703-2710.
49. Shastry S, Simha V, Godbole K, et al. A novel syndrome of mandibular hypoplasia, deafness, and progeroid features associated with lipodystrophy, undescended testes, and male hypogonadism. *J Clin Endocrinol Metab*. 2010;95:E192-E197.
50. Torrelo A, Patel S, Colmenero I, et al. Chronic atypical neutrophilic dermatosis with lipodystrophy and elevated temperature (CANDLE) syndrome. *J Am Acad Dermatol*. 2010;62:489-495.
51. Garg A, Hernandez MD, Sousa AB, et al. An autosomal recessive syndrome of joint contractures, muscular atrophy, microcytic anemia, and panniculitis-associated lipodystrophy. *J Clin Endocrinol Metab*. 2010;95:E58-E63.
52. Agarwal AK, Xing C, DeMartino GN, et al. PSMB8 encoding the beta5i proteasome subunit is mutated in joint contractures, muscle atrophy, microcytic anemia, and panniculitis-induced lipodystrophy syndrome. *Am J Hum Genet*. 2010;87:866-872.
53. Liu Y, Ramot Y, Torrelo A, et al. Mutations in proteasome subunit beta type 8 cause chronic atypical neutrophilic dermatosis with lipodystrophy and elevated temperature with evidence of genetic and phenotypic heterogeneity. *Arthritis Rheum*. 2012;64:895-907.
54. Torrelo A, Colmenero I, Requena L, et al. Histologic and immunohistochemical features of the skin lesions in CANDLE syndrome. *Am J Dermatopathol*. 2015;37:517-522.
55. Sensenbrenner JA, Hussels IE, Levin LS. CC-A low birthweight syndrome, Rieger syndrome. *Birth Defects Orig Artic Ser*. 1975;11:423-426.
56. Gorlin RJ, Cervenka J, Moller K, et al. Rieger anomaly and growth retardation (the S-H-O-R-T syndrome). *Birth Defects Orig Artic Ser*. 1975;11:46-48.
57. O'Neill B, Simha V, Kotha V, et al. Body fat distribution and metabolic variables in patients with neonatal progeroid syndrome. *Am J Med Genet A*. 2007;143:1421-1430.

58. Weedon MN, Ellard S, Prindle MJ, et al. An in-frame deletion at the polymerase active site of POLD1 causes a multisystem disorder with lipodystrophy. *Nat Genet.* 2013;45:947-950.
59. Avila M, Dyment DA, Sagen JV, et al. Clinical reappraisal of SHORT syndrome with PIK3R1 mutations: towards recommendation for molecular testing and management. *Clin Genet.* 2015. [Epub ahead of print]
60. Garg A, Xing C. De novo heterozygous FBN1 mutations in the extreme C-terminal region cause progeroid fibrillinopathy. *Am J Med Genet A.* 2014;164A:1341-1345.
61. Garg A, Kircher M, Del Campo M, et al; University of Washington Center for Mendelian Genomics. Whole exome sequencing identifies de novo heterozygous CAV1 mutations associated with a novel neonatal onset lipodystrophy syndrome. *Am J Med Genet A.* 2015;167A:1796-1806.
62. Jay AM, Conway RL, Thiffault I, et al. Neonatal progeroid syndrome associated with biallelic truncating variants in POLR3A. *Am J Med Genet A.* 2016;170:3343-3346.
63. Rubio-Cabezas O, Puri V, Murano I, et al. Partial lipodystrophy and insulin resistant diabetes in a patient with a homozygous nonsense mutation in CIDEC. *EMBO Mol Med.* 2009;1:280-287.
64. Payne F, Lim K, Girousse A, et al. Mutations disrupting the Kennedy phosphatidylcholine pathway in humans with congenital lipodystrophy and fatty liver disease. *Proc Natl Acad Sci U S A.* 2014;111:8901-8906.
65. Farhan SM, Robinson JF, McIntyre AD, et al. A novel LIPE nonsense mutation found using exome sequencing in siblings with late-onset familial partial lipodystrophy. *Can J Cardiol.* 2014;30:1649-1654.
66. Albert JS, Yerges-Armstrong LM, Horenstein RB, et al. Null mutation in hormone-sensitive lipase gene and risk of type 2 diabetes. *N Engl J Med.* 2014;370:2307-2315.
67. Zolotov S, Xing C, Mahamid R, et al. Homozygous LIPE mutation in siblings with multiple symmetric lipomatosis, partial lipodystrophy, and myopathy. *Am J Med Genet A.* 2017;173(1):190-194.
68. Donadille B, D'Anella P, Auclair M, et al. Partial lipodystrophy with severe insulin resistance and adult progeria Werner syndrome. *Orphanet J Rare Dis.* 2013;8:106.
69. Garg A, Subramanyam L, Agarwal AK, et al. Atypical progeroid syndrome due to heterozygous missense LMNA mutations. *J Clin Endocrinol Metab.* 2009;94:4971-4983.
70. Merideth MA, Gordon LB, Clauss S, et al. Phenotype and course of Hutchinson-Gilford progeria syndrome. *N Engl J Med.* 2008;358:592-604.
71. Bingham A, Mamyrova G, Rother KI, et al. Predictors of acquired lipodystrophy in juvenile-onset dermatomyositis and a gradient of severity. *Medicine (Baltimore).* 2008;87:70-86.
72. Savage DB, Semple RK, Clatworthy MR, et al. Complement abnormalities in acquired lipodystrophy revisited. *J Clin Endocrinol Metab.* 2009;94:10-16.
73. Hudon SE, Coffinier C, Michaelis S, et al. HIV-protease inhibitors block the enzymatic activity of purified Ste24p. *Biochem Biophys Res Commun.* 2008;374:365-368.
74. Bastard JP, Caron M, Vidal H, et al. Association between altered expression of adipogenic factor SREBP1 in lipoatrophic adipose tissue from HIV-1-infected patients and abnormal adipocyte differentiation and insulin resistance. *Lancet.* 2002;359:1026-1031.
75. Murata H, Hruz PW, Mueckler M. The mechanism of insulin resistance caused by HIV protease inhibitor therapy. *J Biol Chem.* 2000;275:20251-20254.
76. Carr A, Miller J, Law M, et al. A syndrome of lipoatrophy, lactic acidaemia and liver dysfunction associated with HIV nucleoside analogue therapy: contribution to protease inhibitor-related lipodystrophy syndrome. *AIDS.* 2000;14:F25-F32.
77. Haque WA, Shimomura I, Matsuzawa Y, et al. Serum adiponectin and leptin levels in patients with lipodystrophies. *J Clin Endocrinol Metab.* 2002;87:2395-2398.
78. Hegele RA. Premature atherosclerosis associated with monogenic insulin resistance. *Circulation.* 2001;103:2225-2229.
79. Hennekam RC. Hutchinson-Gilford progeria syndrome: review of the phenotype. *Am J Med Genet A.* 2006;140:2603-2624.
80. Brown RJ, Chan JL, Jaffe ES, et al. Lymphoma in acquired generalized lipodystrophy. *Leuk Lymphoma.* 2016;57:45-50.
81. Agarwal AK, Kazachkova I, Ten S, et al. Severe mandibuloacral dysplasia-associated lipodystrophy and progeria in a young girl with a novel homozygous Arg527Cys LMNA mutation. *J Clin Endocrinol Metab.* 2008;93:4617-4623.
82. Sturm LP, Cooter RD, Mutimer KL, et al. A systematic review of permanent and semipermanent dermal fillers for HIV-associated facial lipoatrophy. *AIDS Patient Care STDS.* 2009;23:699-714.
83. Arioglu E, Duncan-Morin J, Sebring N, et al. Efficacy and safety of troglitazone in the treatment of lipodystrophy syndromes. *Ann Intern Med.* 2000;133:263-274.
84. Savage DB, Tan GD, Acerini CL, et al. Human metabolic syndrome resulting from dominant-negative mutations in the nuclear receptor peroxisome proliferator-activated receptor-gamma. *Diabetes.* 2003;52:910-917.
85. Oral EA, Simha V, Ruiz E, et al. Leptin-replacement therapy for lipodystrophy. *N Engl J Med.* 2002;346:570-578.
86. Simha V, Szczepaniak LS, Wagner AJ, et al. Effect of leptin replacement on intrahepatic and intramyocellular lipid content in patients with generalized lipodystrophy. *Diabetes Care.* 2003;26:30-35.
87. Simha V, Subramanyam L, Szczepaniak L, et al. Comparison of efficacy and safety of leptin replacement therapy in moderately and severely hypoleptinemic patients with familial partial lipodystrophy of the Dunnigan variety. *J Clin Endocrinol Metab.* 2012;97:785-792.
88. Park JY, Javor ED, Cochran EK, et al. Long-term efficacy of leptin replacement in patients with Dunnigan-type familial partial lipodystrophy. *Metabolism.* 2007;56:508-516.
89. Diker-Cohen T, Cochran E, Gorden P, et al. Partial and generalized lipodystrophy: comparison of baseline characteristics and response to metreleptin. *J Clin Endocrinol Metab.* 2015;100:1802-1810.
90. Carr A, Hudson J, Chuah J, et al. HIV protease inhibitor substitution in patients with lipodystrophy: a randomized, controlled, open-label, multicentre study. *AIDS.* 2001;15:1811-1822.